SAUNDERS

2005
ICD-9-CM
Volumes 1, 2, & 3
AND
HCPCS Level II

SAUNDERS

2005
ICD-9-CM
Volumes 1, 2, & 3
AND
HCPCS Level II

Includes Official Coding Guidelines!

Carol J. Buck, MS, CPC

Program Director (Ret.), Medical Secretary Programs
Northwest Technical College
East Grand Forks, Minnesota

Technical Collaborator:
Karla R. Lovaasen, RHIA, CCS, CCS-P
Coding and Consulting Services
Whapeton, North Dakota

An Imprint of Elsevier

SAUNDERS
An Imprint of Elsevier

11830 Westline Industrial Drive
St. Louis, Missouri 63146

DISCLAIMER

Every effort has been made to make this text complete and accurate, but no guarantee, warranty, or representation is made for its accuracy or completeness.

Elsevier and Carol J. Buck are not providing any legal or professional service/advice in presenting these codes and bear no liability for how the codes are used.

THE PUBLISHER

Publishing Director: Andrew Allen
Senior Acquisitions Editor: Susan Cole
Developmental Editor: Beth LoGiudice
Publishing Services Manager: Linda McKinley
Project Manager: Ellen Kunkelmann
Designer: Kathi Gosche

Saunders 2005 ICD-9-CM, Volumes 1, 2, and 3, and HCPCS Level II   ISBN 1-416-00138-7

Printed in the United States of America.

Last digit is the print number: 9   8   7   6   5   4   3   2   1

GUIDE TO USING THE SAUNDERS 2005 ICD-9-CM, Volumes 1, 2, and 3, AND HCPCS Level II

Medical coding has long been a part of the health care profession. Through the years medical coding systems have become more complex and extensive. Today, medical coding is an intricate and immense process that is present in every health care setting. The increased use of electronic submissions for health care services only increases the need for coders who understand the coding process.

Saunders 2005 ICD-9-CM Volumes 1, 2, & 3 and HCPCS Level II was developed to help meet the needs of students preparing for a career in medical coding by offering a comprehensive coding text at a reasonable price. This text combines the official coding guidelines, all three volumes of the ICD-9-CM, and HCPCS in one book—three books in one.

All material strictly adheres to the latest government versions available at the time of printing.

ILLUSTRATIONS AND ITEMS

The ICD-9-CM, Volume 1, Tabular List contains illustrations, pictures, and items to assist you in understanding difficult terminology, diseases/conditions, or coding in a specific category. Items are always printed in ▆▆▆ ink so the added material is not mistaken for official notations or instructions. Your ideas on what other descriptions or illustrations should be in future editions of this text are always appreciated.

Annotated

Throughout this text revisions and additions are indicated by the following symbols:

◀▥▥▶ **Revised:** Revisions within the line or code from the previous edition are indicated by the black arrow.

◀▶ **New:** Additions to the previous edition are indicated by the color triangle.

The revision and addition symbols are the only symbols that appear in the ICD-9-CM indexes.

ICD-9-CM, Volume 1, Tabular List Symbols

● **Not a principal diagnosis:** These codes have a black dot before them. These codes give additional information or describe the circumstances affecting the health care encounter but are unacceptable as principal diagnosis for inpatient admission.

● **Use additional digit(s):** The color dot cautions you that the code requires additional digit(s) to insure the greatest specificity.

❑ **Nonspecific code:** These have a square before the code. Although these codes are valid as a principal diagnosis, they are usually too general to be used as a principal diagnosis for Medicare, and you should continue to seek a code that is more specific.

ICD-9-CM, Volume 3, Tabular List Symbols

● **Use additional digit(s):** The color dot cautions you that the code requires additional digit(s) to insure the greatest specificity.

✖ **Valid O.R. procedure:** The color "x" is placed before a code that is a valid operating room (O.R.) procedure according to the DRG grouper.

In addition to the symbols, the official ICD-9-CM conventions appear throughout the text. Refer to the illustrations of conventions on the following pages and to the Introduction for further information on conventions.

HCPCS Symbols

☉ **Special coverage instructions** apply to these codes. Usually these special coverage instructions are included in the Medicare Carrier Manual (MCM) select references in Appendix A or in the Coverage Issues Manual (CIM) in Appendix B of this text.

◆ **Not covered by or valid for Medicare** is indicated by the diamond. Usually the reason for the exclusion is included in the Medicare Carrier Manual (MCM) select references in Appendix A or in the Coverage Issues Manual (CIM) in Appendix B of this text.

✳ **Carrier discretion** is an indication that you must contact the individual third-party payors to find out the coverage available for codes identified by this symbol.

SAUNDERS
2005 ICD-9-CM, Volumes 1, 2, and 3, and HCPCS LEVEL II

Symbols Used in All Volumes of ICD-9-CM to Identify New or Revised Material

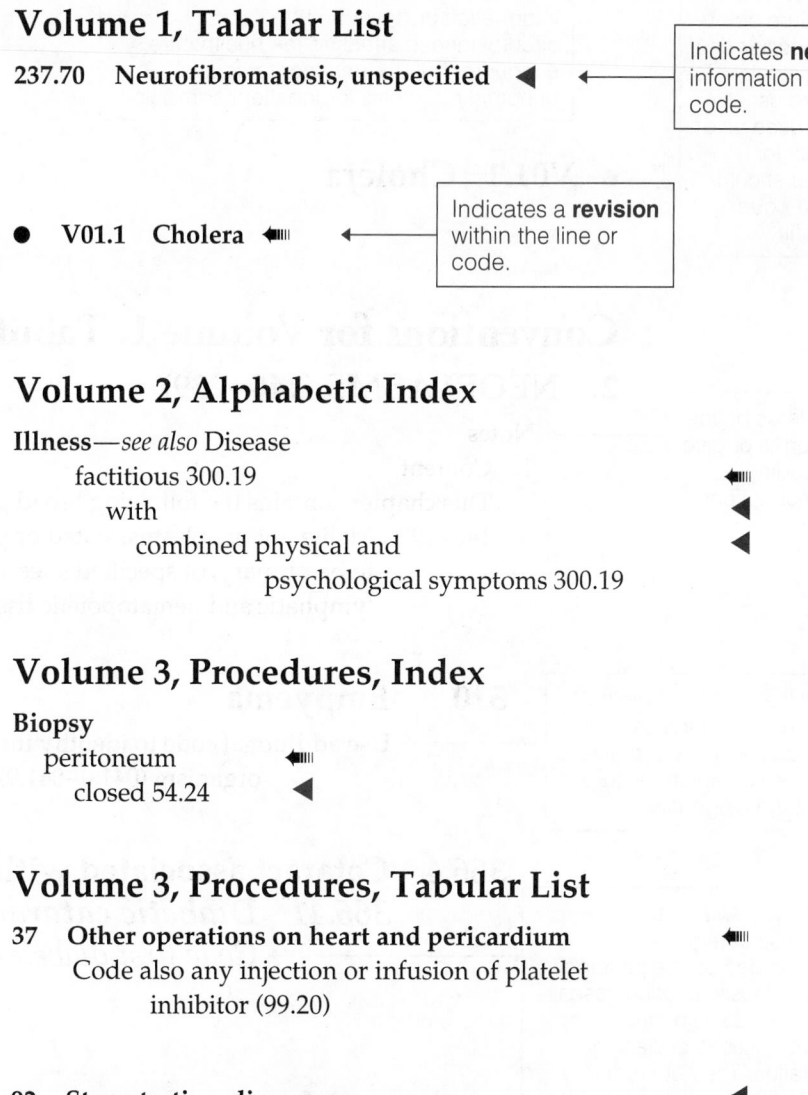

Volume 1, Tabular List

237.70   **Neurofibromatosis, unspecified** ◄ ← Indicates **new** information or a new code.

● **V01.1   Cholera** ◄ ← Indicates a **revision** within the line or code.

Volume 2, Alphabetic Index

Illness—*see also* Disease
    factitious 300.19 ◄
       with ◄
          combined physical and ◄
             psychological symptoms 300.19

Volume 3, Procedures, Index

Biopsy
    peritoneum ◄
       closed 54.24 ◄

Volume 3, Procedures, Tabular List

37   **Other operations on heart and pericardium** ◄
    Code also any injection or infusion of platelet
       inhibitor (99.20)

92   **Stereotactic radiosurgery** ◄

Symbols for Volume 1, Tabular List

Use Additional Digit(s): The color dot cautions you that the code requires additional digit(s) to ensure the greatest specificity.

● **237.7   Neurofibromatosis**
      von Recklinghausen's disease
  □ **237.70   Neurofibromatosis,**
                unspecified

Not a Principal Diagnosis: These codes have a black dot before them. These codes give additional information or describe the circumstances affecting the health care encounter but are unacceptable as principal diagnosis for inpatient admission.

Nonspecific code: These codes have a square before them. Although these codes are valid as a principal diagnosis, they are usually too general to be used as a principal diagnosis for Medicare, and you should continue to seek a code that is more specific.

● **V01.1   Cholera**

Conventions for Volume 1, Tabular List

2.   NEOPLASMS (140–239)

Notes define terms or give coding instructions.

Notes
1. Content
    This chapter contains the following broad groups:
    140–195   Malignant neoplasms, stated or presumed
              to be primary, of specified sites, except of
              lymphatic and hematopoietic tissue.

"Use additional digit(s)" directs you to use an additional code to give a more complete picture of the diagnosis.

510   Empyema
    Use additional code to identify infectious
            organism (041.0–041.9)

366.4   Cataract associated with other disorders
  366.41   Diabetic cataract
       Code first diabetes (250.5)

"*Code first*" is used in those categories not intended as the principal diagnosis. In such cases, the code, title, and instructions appear in italics. The note requires that the underlying disease (etiology) be sequenced first.

428   Heart failure
    Code, if applicable, heart failure due to
    hypertension first (402.0-402.9, with fifth-digit
    1 or 404.0-404.9 with fifth-digit 1 or 3)

A code with this note may be principal if no causal condition is applicable or known

474   Chronic disease of tonsils and adenoids

"and" indicates a code that can be assigned if either of the conditions is present or if both of the conditions are present.

366.4   Cataract associated with other disorders

"with" indicates a code that can only be used if both conditions are present.

The "Includes" note appears immediately under a code to further define, or give example of, the contents of the code.

087   Relapsing fever
Includes: recurrent fever

420.0   *Acute pericarditis in disease classified elsewhere*

Italicized type is used for all exclusion notes and to identify those codes that are not usually sequenced as the principal diagnosis.

Terms following the word "Excludes" are to be coded elsewhere. The term "Excludes" means "Do Not Code Here."

150.2   Abdominal esophagus
Excludes: *recurrent fever*

244.8   Other specified acquired hypothyroidism
        Secondary hypothyroidism NEC

NEC means Not Elsewhere Classifiable and is to be used only when the information at hand specifies a condition but there is no more specific code for that condition.

Bold type is used for all codes and titles.

159.0   Intestinal tract, part unspecified
        Intestine NOS

NOS means Not Otherwise Specified and is the equivalent of "unspecified."

426.89   Other
        Dissociation:
            atrioventricular [AV]

Brackets are used to enclose synonyms, alternative wording, or explanatory phrases.

158.8   Specified parts of peritoneum
        Cul-de-sac (of Douglas)
        Mesentery

Parentheses are used to enclose supplementary words that may be present or absent in the statement of a disease without affecting the code.

628.4   Of cervical or vaginal origin
        Infertility associated with:
            anomaly of cervical mucus
            congenital structural anomaly

A colon is used after an incomplete term that needs one or more of the modifiers that follow in order to make it assignable to a given category.

Conventions for Volume 2, Alphabetic Index

Nonessential modifiers are enclosed in parentheses and are words that may be used to clarify the diagnosis but do not affect the code.

Ileus (adynamic) (bowel) (colon) (inhibitory) (intestine) (neurogenic) (paralytic)

Essential modifiers are NOT enclosed in parentheses and are subterms that DO affect the selection of the appropriate code.

Incoordination
esophageal-pharyngeal (newborn) 787.2

Hereditary—*see* condition

"see" is a cross reference directing you to look elsewhere.

Paralysis
embolic (current episode) (*see also* Embolism, brain) 434.1

"*see also*" is a cross reference directing you to look under another main term if all the information being searched for cannot be located under the first main term entry.

Delivery
completely normal case—*see* category 650

"*see* category" is a cross reference directing you to Volume 1, Tabular List for important information governing the use of the specific code.

Amputation
traumatic (complete) (partial)

"Notes" are used to define terms and give coding instructions

Note "Complicated" includes traumatic amputation with delayed healing, delayed treatment, foreign body, or major infection.

Adolescence NEC V21.2

NEC means Not Elsewhere Classifiable.

Conventions for Volume 3, Procedures Index

Arthrotomy 80.10

     as operative approach—*omit code*

> "*omit code*" identifies procedures or services that are included in another larger procedure or service. For example, an incision that is part of the main surgical procedure is not coded separately.

Ileal

     bladder

         closed 57.87 [45.51]

> For some operative procedures it is necessary to record the individual components of the procedure.
> These procedures are termed **"synchronous procedures"** and are listed together in the Index. The codes are sequenced in the same order as displayed in the Index.

Operation

     Thompson

         cleft lip repair 27.54

         correction of lymphedema 40.9

         quadricepsplasty 83.86

> Eponyms are operations named for people and are listed in the Index both under the eponym and under the term "Operation."

Thompson operation

     cleft lip repair 27.54

     correction of lymphedema 40.9

     quadricepsplasty 83.86

Volume 3, Index to Procedures, also contains "*see*," "*see also*," "*see* category," "essential modifiers," "nonessential modifiers," "notes," NEC, and NOS as in Volume 2, Alphabetic Index.

Symbols for Volume 3, Procedures, Tabular List

Use additional digit(s):
The color dot cautions you that the code requires additional digit(s) to ensure the greatest specificity.

● 31.9   **Other operations on larynx and trachea**
✖ 31.91   **Division of laryngeal nerve**

Valid O.R. procedure:
The red X is placed before a code that is a valid operating room (O.R.) procedure according to the DRG grouper.

Conventions for Volume 3, Procedures, Tabular List

The "Includes" note appears to further define, or give example of, the contents of the code.

88.4   **Arteriography using contrast material**

Bold type is used for all codes and titles.

Includes: angiography of arteries
arterial puncture for injection of contrast material
radiography of arteries (by fluoroscopy)
retrograde arteriography

The fifth-digit subclassification identifies the site to be viewed, not the site of injection

Terms following the word "Excludes" are to be coded elsewhere. The term means "Do Not Code Here."

Excludes: *arteriography using:*

radioisotopes or radionuclides (92.01–92.19)

For some operative procedures it is necessary to record the individual components of the procedure. These procedures are termed "synchronous procedures."

45.5   **Isolation of intestinal segment**

Code also any synchronous:

anastomosis other than end-to-end (45.90–45.94)

enterostomy (46.10–46.39)

Symbols for HCPCS

Special coverage instructions apply to these codes. Usually these instructions are included in the Medicare Carrier Manual (MCM) select references in Appendix A or in the Coverage Issues Manual (CIM) in Appendix B of this text.

→ ✲

L3540 Miscellaneous shoe additions, sole, full
MCM 2079, CIM 70-3

Medicare Carrier Manual (MCM) and Coverage Issues Manual (CIM) give instructions regarding use of the code. MCM and CIM select references are located in the appendices of this text.

Not covered by or valid for Medicare is indicated by the diamond. Usually the reason for the exclusion is included in the Medicare Carrier Manual (MCM) references in Appendix A or in the Coverage Issues Manual (CIM) in Appendix B of this text.

→ ◆

A5074 Pouch, urinary; with faceplate attached; plastic or rubber
MCM 2130

Carrier discretion is an indication that you must contact the individual third-party payors to find out the coverage available for these codes.

→ ✱

A6154 Wound pouch, each

Indicates **new** information or a new code.

→ ▶

A4614 Peak expiratory flow rate meter, hand held

Indicates a **revision** within the line or code.

→ ⏩

J0270 Injection alprostadil, per 1.25 mcg

GUIDE TO THE 2005 ICD-9-CM UPDATES and 2004 HCPCS Updates

VOLUME 1 CHANGES EFFECTIVE OCTOBER 1, 2004 AND CLASSIFICATION OF DISEASES AND E CODES

Special note: The Glossary of Mental Disorders, one of the appendices, will be removed from the official ICD-9-CM CD-ROM effective with this update.

1. **INFECTIOUS AND PARASITIC DISEASES (001–139)**
   008 Intestinal infections due to other organisms
   008.4 Other specified bacteria
   008.46 Other anaerobes
   Anaerobic enteritis NOS

   Delete — ~~Gram-negative anaerobes~~
   Bacteroides (fragilis)

   Add — Gram-negative anaerobes

   041 Bacterial infection in conditions classified elsewhere and of unspecified site

   Revise — **041.82** ~~Bacillus~~ Bacteroides fragilis
   041.84 Other anaerobes

   Delete — ~~Bacteroides (fragilis)~~

   042 Human immunodeficiency virus [HIV] disease

   Revise — **Excludes** *exposure to HIV virus (V01.79)*

   062 Mosquito-borne viral encephalitis
   062.8 Other specified mosquito-borne viral encephalitis

   Revise — **Excludes** *West Nile virus (066.40–066.49)*

   066 Other arthropod-borne viral diseases
   066.4 West Nile fever

   Delete — ~~West Nile encephalitis~~
   ~~West Nile encephalomyelitis~~
   ~~West Nile virus~~

   New code — **066.40 West Nile fever, unspecified**
   West Nile fever NOS
   West Nile fever without complications
   West Nile virus NOS

   New code — **066.41 West Nile fever with encephalitis**
   West Nile encephalitis
   West Nile encephalomyelitis

   New code — **066.42 West Nile fever with other neurologic manifestation**
   Use additional code to specify the neurologic manifestation

   New code — **066.49 West Nile fever with other complications**
   Use additional code to specify the other conditions

   070 Viral hepatitis
   070.4 Other specified viral hepatitis with hepatic coma

   Revise — **070.41 Acute** ~~or unspecified~~ **hepatitis C with hepatic coma**

   070.5 Other specified viral hepatitis without mention of hepatic coma

   Revise — **070.51 Acute** ~~or unspecified~~ **hepatitis C without mention of hepatic coma**

   070.6 Unspecified viral hepatitis with hepatic coma

   Add — **Excludes** *unspecified viral hepatitis C with hepatic coma (070.71)*

   New subcategory — **070.7 Unspecified viral hepatitis C**
   New code — **070.70 Unspecified viral hepatitis C without hepatic coma**
   Unspecified viral hepatitis C NOS

   New code — **070.71 Unspecified viral hepatitis C with hepatic coma**

   070.9 Unspecified viral hepatitis without mention of hepatic coma

   Add — **Excludes** *unspecified viral hepatitis C without hepatic coma (070.70)*

2. **NEOPLASMS (140–239)**
   176 Kaposi's sarcoma
   176.1 Soft tissue
   Revise — Includes: Blood vessel
   Revise — Connective tissue
   Revise — Fascia
   Revise — Ligament
   Revise — Lymphatic(s) NEC
   Revise — Muscle

   176.8 Other specified sites
   Revise — Includes: Oral cavity NEC

   233 Carcinoma in situ of breast and genitourinary system
   233.1 Cervix uteri
   Add — Cervical intraepithelial neoplasia III [CIN III]
   Add — Severe dysplasia of cervix

   Add — **Excludes** *cervical intraepithelial neoplasia II [CIN II] (622.12)*
   cytologic evidence of malignancy without histologic confirmation (795.04)
   high grade squamous intraepithelial lesion (HGSIL) (795.04)
   moderate dysplasia of cervix (622.12)

3. **ENDOCRINE, NUTRITIONAL AND METABOLIC DISEASES, AND IMMUNITY DISORDERS (240–279)**
   250 Diabetes mellitus
   The following fifth-digit subclassification is for use with category 250:

   Revise — 0 type II ~~[non-insulin dependent type] [NIDDM type] [adult-onset type]~~ or unspecified type, not stated as uncontrolled
   Fifth-digit 0 is for use for type II, ~~adult-onset diabetic~~ patients, even if the patient requires insulin

   Add — Use additional code, if applicable, for associated long-term (current) insulin use V58.67

   Revise — 1 type I ~~[insulin dependent type] [IDDM]~~ [juvenile type], not stated as uncontrolled

   Revise — 2 type II ~~[non-insulin dependent type] [NIDDM type] [adult-onset type]~~ or unspecified type, uncontrolled
   Fifth-digit 2 is for use for type II, ~~adult-onset diabetic~~ patients, even if the patient requires insulin

   Add — Use additional code, if applicable, for associated long-term (current) insulin use V58.67

   250.6 Diabetes with neurological manifestations
   Use additional code to identify manifestation, as:
   diabetic:
   Add — gastroparalysis (536.3)
   Add — gastroparesis (536.3)

   252 Disorders of parathyroid gland

	252.0 Hyperparathyroidism
Delete	~~Hyperplasia of parathyroid~~
	~~Osteitis fibrosa cystica generalisata~~
	~~von Recklinghausen's disease of bone~~
Delete	**Excludes** ~~secondary hyperparathyroidism (of renal origin) (588.8)~~
New code	252.00 Hyperparathyroidism, unspecified
New code	252.01 Primary hyperparathyroidism
	Hyperplasia of parathyroid
New code	252.02 Secondary hyperparathyroidism, non-renal
	Excludes secondary hyperparathyroidism (of renal origin) (588.81)
New code	252.08 Other hyperparathyroidism
	Tertiary hyperparathyroidism

255 Disorders of adrenal glands
255.1 Hyperaldosteronism
255.10 Primary aldosteronism

Add	**Excludes** Conn's syndrome (255.12)
	255.11 Glucocorticoid-remediable aldosteronism
Add	**Excludes** Conn's syndrome (255.12)

273 Disorders of plasma protein metabolism

New code	273.4 Alpha-1-antitrypsin deficiency
	AAT deficiency

275 Disorders of mineral metabolism
275.4 Disorders of calcium metabolism

Revise	**Excludes** parathyroid disorders (252.00–252.9)

277 Other and unspecified disorders of metabolism
277.6 Other deficiencies of circulating enzymes

Delete	~~Alpha-1-antitrypsin deficiency~~

277.8 Other specified disorders of metabolism

New code	277.85 Disorders of fatty acid oxidation
	Carnitine palmitoyltransferase deficiencies (CPT1, CPT2)
	Glutaric aciduria type II (type IIA, IIB, IIC)
	Long chain 3-hydroxyacyl CoA dehydrogenase deficiency (LCHAD)
	Long chain/very long chain acyl CoA dehydrogenase deficiency (LCAD, VLCAD)
	Medium chain acyl CoA dehydrogenase deficiency (MCAD)
	Short chain acyl CoA dehydrogenase deficiency (SCAD)
	Excludes primary carnitine deficiency (277.81)
New code	277.86 Peroxisomal disorders
	Adrenomyeloneuropathy
	Neonatal adrenoleukodystrophy
	Rhizomelic chrondrodysplasia punctata
	X-linked adrenoleukodystrophy
	Zellweger syndrome
Add	**Excludes** infantile Refsum disease (356.3)
New code	277.87 Disorders of mitochondrial metabolism
	Kearns-Sayre syndrome
	Mitochondrial Encephalopathy, Lactic Acidosis and Stroke-like episodes (MELAS syndrome)
	Mitochondrial Neurogastrointestinal Encephalopathy syndrome (MNGIE)
	Myoclonus with Epilepsy and with Ragged Red Fibers (MERRF syndrome)
	Neuropathy, Ataxia and Retinitis Pigmentosa (NARP syndrome)
Add	Use additional code for associated conditions
Add	**Excludes** disorders of pyruvate metabolism (271.8)

Add	Leber's optic atrophy (377.16)
Add	Leigh's subacute necrotizing encephalopathy (330.8)
Add	Reye's syndrome (331.81)

4. DISEASES OF THE BLOOD AND BLOOD-FORMING ORGANS (280–289)

286 Coagulation defects

Revise	286.5 Hemorrhagic disorder due to intrinsic circulating anticoagulants
Add	Secondary hemophilia
Delete	~~Use additional E code to identify cause, if drug induced~~

5. MENTAL DISORDERS (290–319)

Revise	290 ~~Senile and presenile organic psychotic conditions~~ Dementias
Add	**Excludes** dementia due to alcohol (291.0–291.2)
Add	dementia due to drugs (292.82)
Revise	290.4 ~~Arteriosclerotic~~ Vascular dementia
Revise	290.40 ~~Arteriosclerotic~~ Vascular dementia, uncomplicated
Revise	290.41 ~~Arteriosclerotic~~ Vascular dementia, with delirium
Revise	290.42 ~~Arteriosclerotic~~ Vascular dementia, with ~~delusional features~~ delusions
Revise	290.43 ~~Arteriosclerotic~~ Vascular dementia, with ~~depressive features~~ depressed mood
Revise	291 ~~Alcoholic psychoses~~ Alcohol-induced mental disorders
Revise	291.1 Alcohol-induced persisting amnestic ~~syndrome~~ disorder
Revise	291.2 ~~Other alcoholic~~ Alcohol-induced persisting dementia
Revise	291.3 Alcohol ~~withdrawal hallucinosis~~-induced psychotic disorder with hallucinations
Revise	291.5 Alcohol~~ic jealousy~~-induced psychotic disorder with delusions
Revise	291.8 Other specified ~~alcoholic psychosis~~ alcohol-induced mental disorders
	291.89 Other
Add	Alcohol-induced anxiety disorder
Add	Alcohol-induced mood disorder
Add	Alcohol-induced sexual dysfunction
Add	Alcohol-induced sleep disorder
Revise	291.9 Unspecified ~~alcoholic psychosis~~ alcohol-induced mental disorders
Add	Alcohol-related disorder NOS
Revise	292 ~~Drug psychoses~~ Drug-induced mental disorders
Delete	Includes: ~~drug-induced mental disorders~~
Revise	292.0 Drug withdrawal ~~syndrome~~
Revise	292.1 ~~Paranoid and/or hallucinatory states induced by drugs~~ Drug-induced psychotic disorders
Revise	292.11 Drug-induced ~~organic delusional syndrome~~ psychotic disorder with delusions
Revise	292.12 Drug-induced ~~hallucinosis~~ psychotic disorder with hallucinations
	292.8 Other specified drug-induced mental disorders
Revise	292.82 Drug-induced persisting dementia
Revise	292.83 Drug-induced persisting amnestic ~~syndrome~~ disorder
Revise	292.84 Drug-induced ~~organic affective syndrome~~ mood disorder
	292.89 Other
Add	Drug-induced anxiety disorder
Add	Drug-induced sexual dysfunction
Add	Drug-induced sleep disorder
Add	Drug intoxication
	292.9 Unspecified drug-induced mental disorder
Add	Drug-related disorder NOS

Revise	293	Transient ~~organic psychotic conditions~~ <u>mental disorders</u> due to conditions classified elsewhere
Revise	293.0	~~Acute delirium~~ <u>Delirium</u> due to conditions classified elsewhere
Revise	293.8	Other specified transient ~~organic~~ mental disorders <u>due to conditions classified elsewhere</u>
Revise	293.81	~~Organic delusional syndrome~~ <u>Psychotic disorder with delusions in conditions classified elsewhere</u>
Revise	293.82	~~Organic hallucinosis syndrome~~ <u>Psychotic disorder with hallucinations in conditions classified elsewhere</u>
Revise	293.83	~~Organic affective syndrome~~ <u>Mood disorder in conditions classified elsewhere</u>
Revise	293.84	~~Organic anxiety syndrome~~ <u>Anxiety disorder in conditions classified elsewhere</u>
	293.89	Other
Add		Catatonic disorder in conditions classified elsewhere
Revise	293.9	Unspecified transient ~~organic~~ mental disorder in conditions classified elsewhere
Revise	294	~~Other organic psychotic conditions (chronic)~~ <u>Persistent mental disorders due to conditions classified elsewhere</u>
Revise	294.0	Amnestic ~~syndrome~~ <u>disorder in conditions classified elsewhere</u>
Add		Code first underlying condition
	294.1	Dementia in conditions classified elsewhere
Add		Dementia of the Alzheimer's type
Revise	294.8	Other ~~specified organic brain syndromes (chronic)~~ <u>persistent mental disorders due to conditions classified elsewhere</u>
Add		Amnestic disorder NOS
Add		Dementia NOS
Revise	294.9	Unspecified ~~organic brain syndrome (chronic)~~ <u>persistent mental disorders due to conditions classified elsewhere</u>
Add		Cognitive disorder NOS
	295	Schizophrenic disorders
Revise	295.4	~~Acute schizophrenic episode~~ <u>Schizophreniform disorder</u>
Delete		~~Schizophreniform disorder~~
Revise	295.6	Residual type ~~schizophrenia~~
Revise	295.7	~~Schizo-affective type~~ <u>Schizoaffective disorder</u>
	295.9	Unspecified schizophrenia
Add		Schizophrenia, undifferentiated type
Revise	296	~~Affective psychoses~~ <u>Episodic mood disorders</u>
Revise	296.0	Bipolar I disorder, single manic ~~disorder, single~~ episode
Revise	296.4	Bipolar ~~affective~~ <u>I</u> disorder, <u>most recent episode (or current)</u> manic
Revise	296.5	Bipolar ~~affective~~ <u>I</u> disorder, <u>most recent episode (or current)</u> depressed
Revise	296.6	Bipolar ~~affective~~ <u>I</u> disorder, <u>most recent episode (or current)</u> mixed
Revise	296.7	Bipolar ~~affective~~ <u>I</u> disorder, <u>most recent episode (or current)</u> unspecified
Revise	296.8	~~Manic-depressive psychosis,~~ <u>Other and unspecified bipolar disorders</u>
Revise	296.80	~~Manic-depressive psychosis,~~ <u>Bipolar disorder, unspecified</u>
Add		Bipolar disorder NOS
	296.89	Other
Add		Bipolar II disorder
Revise	296.9	Other and unspecified ~~affective psychoses~~ <u>episodic mood disorder</u>
Revise	296.90	Unspecified ~~affective psychosis~~ <u>episodic mood disorder</u>
Add		Mood disorder NOS
Revise	296.99	Other specified ~~affective psychoses~~ <u>episodic mood disorder</u>
Revise	297	~~Paranoid states [Delusional disorders]~~
Revise	297.1	~~Paranoia~~ <u>Delusional disorder</u>
Revise	297.3	Shared ~~paranoid~~ <u>psychotic</u> disorder
	298	Other nonorganic psychoses
	298.8	Other and unspecified reactive psychosis
Add		Brief psychotic disorder
	298.9	Unspecified psychosis
Add		Psychotic disorder NOS
Revise	299	~~Psychoses with origin specific to childhood~~ <u>Pervasive developmental disorders</u>
Delete		Includes: ~~pervasive developmental disorders~~
Revise	299.0	~~Infantile autism~~ <u>Autistic disorder</u>
Revise	299.1	~~Disintegrative psychosis~~ <u>Childhood disintegrative disorder</u>
Revise	299.8	Other specified ~~early childhood psychoses~~ <u>Pervasive developmental disorders</u>
Add		Asperger's disorder
Revise	299.9	Unspecified <u>pervasive developmental disorder</u>
Add		Pervasive developmental disorder NOS
Revise	300	~~Neurotic disorders~~ <u>Anxiety, dissociative and somatoform disorders</u>
	300.0	Anxiety states
Revise	300.01	Panic disorder <u>without agoraphobia</u>
Add		**Excludes** *panic disorder with agoraphobia (300.21)*
Revise	300.1	~~Hysteria~~ <u>Dissociative, conversion and factitious disorders</u>
Revise	300.12	~~Psychogenic~~ <u>Dissociative</u> amnesia
Revise	300.13	~~Psychogenic~~ <u>Dissociative</u> fugue
Revise	300.14	~~Multiple personality~~ <u>Dissociative identity disorder</u>
Delete		~~Dissociative identity disorder~~
Revise	300.16	Factitious ~~illness~~ <u>disorder</u> with predominantly psychological <u>signs and symptoms</u>
	300.19	Other and unspecified factitious illness
Revise		Factitious ~~illness~~ <u>disorder (with combined psychological and physical signs and symptoms) (with predominantly physical signs and symptoms)</u> NOS
	300.2	Phobic disorders
Revise	300.21	Agoraphobia with panic ~~attacks~~ <u>disorder</u>
Add		Panic disorder with agoraphobia
Add		**Excludes** *agoraphobia without panic disorder (300.22)*
Add		*panic disorder without agoraphobia (300.01)*
Revise	300.29	Other isolated or ~~simple~~ <u>specific</u> phobias
Revise	300.4	~~Neurotic depression~~ <u>Dysthymic disorder</u>
Delete		~~Dysthymic disorder~~
Revise	300.6	Depersonalization ~~syndrome~~ <u>disorder</u>
Delete		~~Depersonalization disorder~~
Revise	300.8	~~Other neurotic disorders~~ <u>Somatoform disorders</u>
Revise	300.89	Other somatoform disorders
Revise	300.9	~~Unspecified neurotic disorder~~ <u>Unspecified nonpsychotic mental disorder</u>
Delete		~~Neurosis NOS~~
	301	Personality disorders
	301.2	Schizoid personality disorder
Revise	301.22	Schizotypal personality <u>disorder</u>
Revise	301.4	Obsessive-compulsive personality disorder
	301.8	Other personality disorders
Revise	301.81	Narcissistic personality <u>disorder</u>
Revise	301.82	Avoidant personality <u>disorder</u>
Revise	301.83	Borderline personality <u>disorder</u>
Revise	302	Sexual ~~deviations~~ and gender identity disorders
Revise	302.0	Ego-dystonic ~~homosexuality~~ <u>sexual orientation</u>

Revise   Sexual orientation ~~Homosexual~~ conflict disorder

Revise   302.3 ~~Transvestism~~ Transvestic fetishism

Revise   302.6 ~~Disorders of psychosexual identify~~ Gender identity disorder in children

Delete   ~~Gender identity disorder of childhood~~

Add   Gender identity disorder NOS

Delete   **Excludes** ~~homosexuality (302.0)~~

302.7 Psychosexual dysfunction

302.70 Psychosexual dysfunction, unspecified

Add   Sexual dysfunction NOS

Revise   302.71 ~~With inhibited~~ Hypoactive sexual desire disorder

302.72 With inhibited sexual excitement

Add   Female sexual arousal disorder

Add   Male erectile disorder

Revise   302.73 ~~With inhibited~~ female orgasmic disorder

Revise   302.74 ~~With inhibited~~ male orgasmic disorder

Revise   302.75 ~~With~~ Premature ejaculation

Revise   302.76 ~~With functional~~ Dyspareunia, psychogenic

Delete   ~~Dyspareunia, psychogenic~~

302.79 With other specified psychosexual dysfunctions

Add   Sexual aversion disorder

302.8 Other specified psychosexual disorders

Revise   302.85 Gender identity disorder ~~of adolescent or adult life~~ in adolescents or adults

Add   **Excludes** gender identity disorder NOS (302.6)

Add   gender identity disorder in children (302.6)

302.89 Other

Add   Frotteurism

302.9 Unspecified psychosexual disorder

Add   Paraphilia NOS

Add   Sexual disorder NOS

304 Drug dependence

Revise   304.1 ~~Barbiturate and similarly acting~~ Sedative, or hypnotic or anxiolytic dependence

304.6 Other specified drug dependence

Add   Inhalant dependence

Add   Phencyclidine dependence

305 Nondependent abuse of drugs

Revise   305.4 ~~Barbiturate and similarly acting~~ Sedative, or hypnotic or anxiolytic abuse

305.9 Other, mixed, or unspecified drug abuse

Add   Caffeine intoxication

Add   Inhalant abuse

Add   Phencyclidine abuse

307 Special symptoms or syndromes, not elsewhere classified

Revise   307.0 ~~Stammering and~~ Stuttering

307.2 Tics

307.20 Tic disorder, unspecified

Add   Tic disorder NOS

Revise   307.21 Transient tic disorder ~~of childhood~~

Revise   307.22 Chronic motor or vocal tic disorder

Revise   307.23 ~~Gilles de la~~ Tourette's disorder

Revise   307.3 ~~Stereotyped repetitive movements~~ Stereotypic movement disorder

307.4 Specific disorders of sleep of nonorganic origin

Revise   **Excludes** narcolepsy (347.00–347.11)

Revise   307.45 ~~Phase-shift disruption of 24-hour sleep-wake cycle~~ Circadian rhythm sleep disorder

Revise   307.46 ~~Somnambulism or night terrors~~ Sleep arousal disorder

Add   Night terror disorder

Add   Night terrors

Add   Sleep terror disorder

Add   Sleepwalking

Add   Somnambulism

307.47 Other dysfunctions of sleep stages or arousal from sleep

Add   Dyssomnia NOS

Add   Nightmare disorder

Add   Parasomnia NOS

307.5 Other and unspecified disorders of eating

307.50 Eating disorder, unspecified

Add   Eating disorder NOS

Revise   307.51 Bulimia nervosa

Revise   307.53 ~~Psychogenic~~ Rumination disorder

307.59 Other

Add   Feeding disorder of infancy or early childhood

Revise   307.8 ~~Psychalgia~~ Pain disorders related to psychological factors

307.89 Other

Delete   ~~Psychogenic backache~~

Add   Code first to site of pain

Add   **Excludes** pain disorder exclusively attributed to psychological factors (307.80)

Add   psychogenic pain (307.80)

Delete   **Excludes** ~~pain not specifically attributed to a psychological cause (in):~~
~~back (724.5)~~
~~joint (719.4)~~
~~limb (729.5)~~
~~lumbago (724.2)~~
~~rheumatic (729.0)~~

307.9 Other and unspecified special symptoms or syndromes, not elsewhere classified

Add   Communication disorder NOS

308 Acute reaction to stress

308.3 Other acute reactions to stress

Delete   ~~Brief or acute posttraumatic stress disorder~~

Add   Acute stress disorder

309 Adjustment reaction

Revise   309.0 ~~Brief depressive reaction~~ Adjustment disorder with depressed mood

Delete   ~~Adjustment disorder with depressed mood~~

309.2 With predominant disturbance of other emotions

Revise   309.24 Adjustment ~~reaction~~ disorder with ~~anxious mood~~ anxiety

Revise   309.28 Adjustment ~~reaction~~ disorder with mixed ~~emotional features~~ anxiety and depressed mood

Revise   309.3 Adjustment disorder with ~~predominant~~ disturbance of conduct

Revise   309.4 Adjustment disorder with mixed disturbance of emotions and conduct

309.8 Other specified adjustment reactions

Revise   309.81 ~~Prolonged~~ Posttraumatic stress disorder

Add   Posttraumatic stress disorder NOS

Add   **Excludes** acute stress disorder (308.3)

Revise   310 Specific nonpsychotic mental disorders due to organic brain damage

Revise   310.1 ~~Organic~~ Personality change ~~syndrome~~ due to conditions classified elsewhere

Delete   Mild memory disturbance

310.8 Other specified nonpsychotic mental disorders following organic brain damage

Add   Mild memory disturbance

312 Disturbance of conduct, not elsewhere classified

312.3 Disorders of impulse control, not elsewhere classified

312.39 Other

Add   Trichotillomania

312.8 Other specified disturbances of conduct, not elsewhere classified

	312.89 Other conduct disorder
Add	Conduct disorder of unspecified onset
	312.9 Unspecified disturbance of conduct
Add	Disruptive behavior disorder NOS
	313 Disturbance of emotions specific to childhood and adolescence
	313.2 Sensitivity, shyness, and social withdrawal disorder
Revise	313.23 ~~Elective~~ Selective mutism
	313.8 Other or mixed emotional disturbances of childhood or adolescence
Revise	313.81 Oppositional <u>defiant</u> disorder
	313.82 Identity disorder
Add	Identity problem
	313.89 Other
Add	Reactive attachment disorder of infancy or early childhood
Revise	313.9 Unspecified emotional disturbance of child<u>hood or adolescence</u>
Add	Mental disorder of infancy, childhood or adolescence NOS
	315 Specific delays in development
Revise	315.1 ~~Specific arithmetical~~ Mathematics disorder
	315.2 Other specific learning difficulties
Add	Disorder of written expression
	315.3 Developmental speech or language disorder
Revise	315.31 ~~Developmental~~ Expressive language disorder
Delete	~~Expressive language disorder~~
Revise	315.32 Mixed receptive-expressive language disorder ~~(mixed)~~
Delete	~~Receptive expressive language disorder~~
	315.39 Other
Add	Phonological disorder
Revise	315.4 Developmental coordination disorder
	315.9 Unspecified delay in development
Add	Learning disorder NOS

6. DISEASES OF THE NERVOUS SYSTEM AND SENSE ORGANS (320–389)

	337 Disorders of the autonomic nervous system
	337.3 Autonomic dysreflexia
	Use additional code to identify the cause, such as:
Revise	decubitus ulcer (707.00–707.09)
	347 Cataplexy and narcolepsy
New subcategory	347.0 Narcolepsy
New code	347.00 Without cataplexy
	Narcolepsy NOS
New code	347.01 With cataplexy
New subcategory	347.1 Narcolepsy in conditions classified elsewhere
	Code first underlying condition
New code	347.10 Without cataplexy
New code	347.11 With cataplexy
	380 Disorders of external ear
Revise	380.0 Perichondritis <u>and chondritis</u> of pinna
Add	Chondritis of auricle
New Code	380.03 Chondritis of pinna

7. DISEASES OF THE CIRCULATORY SYSTEM (390–459)

	402 Hypertensive heart disease
Revise	Includes: any condition classifiable to ~~428~~, 429.0–429.3, 429.8, 429.9 due to hypertension
Add	436 Acute, but ill-defined cerebrovascular disease
Delete	~~Cerebrovascular accident [CVA] NOS~~
Delete	~~Stroke~~
Add	**Excludes** *cerebrovascular accident (434.91)*
	CVA (ischemic) (434.91)
	embolic (434.11)
	hemorrhagic (430, 431, 432.0–432.9)
	thrombotic (434.01)

	stroke (ischemic) (434.91)
	embolic (434.11)
	hemorrhagic (430, 431, 432.0–432.9)
	thrombotic (434.01)
	453 Other venous embolism and thrombosis
New subcategory	453.4 Venous embolism and thrombosis of deep vessels of lower extremity
New code	453.40 Venous embolism and thrombosis of unspecified deep vessels of lower extremity
	Deep vein thrombosis NOS
	DVT NOS
New code	453.41 Venous embolism and thrombosis of deep vessels of proximal lower extremity
	Femoral
	Iliac
	Popliteal
	Thigh
	Upper leg NOS
New code	453.42 Venous embolism and thrombosis of deep vessels of distal lower extremity
	Calf
	Lower leg NOS
	Peroneal
	Tibial

8. DISEASES OF THE RESPIRATORY SYSTEM (460–519)

	466 Acute bronchitis and bronchiolitis
	466.0 Acute bronchitis
Add	**Excludes** *acute bronchitis with chronic obstructive pulmonary disease (491.22)*
	477 Allergic rhinitis
New code	477.2 Due to animal (cat) (dog) hair and dander
	491 Chronic bronchitis
	491.2 Obstructive chronic bronchitis
	491.21 With (acute) exacerbation
Delete	~~Acute and chronic obstructive bronchitis~~
Delete	~~Emphysema with acute and chronic bronchitis~~
New code	491.22 With acute bronchitis
	492 Emphysema
	492.8 Other emphysema
	Excludes *emphysema:*
Revise	*with chronic bronchitis (491.20–491.22)*
	493 Asthma
	493.2 Chronic obstructive asthma
Revise	**Excludes** *chronic obstructive bronchitis (491.20–491.22)*
	496 Chronic airway obstruction, not elsewhere classified
	Excludes *chronic obstructive lung disease [COPD] specified (as) (with):*
Revise	*bronchitis (491.20–491.22)*
Revise	*with emphysema (491.20–491.22)*

9. DISEASES OF THE DIGESTIVE SYSTEM (520–579)

	520 Disorders of tooth development and eruption
	520.6 Disturbances in tooth eruption
Delete	**Excludes** ~~impacted or embedded teeth with abnormal position of such teeth or adjacent teeth (524.3)~~
	521 Diseases of hard tissues of teeth
	521.0 Dental caries
	521.05 Odontoclasia
Revise	**Excludes** *internal and external resorption of teeth (521.40–521.49)*
New code	521.06 Dental caries pit and fissure
New code	521.07 Dental caries of smooth surface
New code	521.08 Dental caries of root surface
Revise	521.1 Excessive attrition <u>(approximal wear) (occlusal wear)</u>

Delete	~~Approximal wear~~
Delete	~~Occlusal wear~~
New code	521.10 Excessive attrition, unspecified
New code	521.11 Excessive attrition, limited to enamel
New code	521.12 Excessive attrition, extending into dentine
New code	521.13 Excessive attrition, extending into pulp
New code	521.14 Excessive attrition, localized
New code	521.15 Excessive attrition, generalized
	521.2 Abrasion
New code	521.20 Abrasion, unspecified
New code	521.21 Abrasion, limited to enamel
New code	521.22 Abrasion, extending into dentine
New code	521.23 Abrasion, extending into pulp
New code	521.24 Abrasion, localized
New code	521.25 Abrasion, generalized
	521.3 Erosion
New code	521.30 Erosion, unspecified
New code	521.31 Erosion, limited to enamel
New code	521.32 Erosion, extending into dentine
New code	521.33 Erosion, extending into pulp
New code	521.34 Erosion, localized
New code	521.35 Erosion, generalized
	521.4 Pathological resorption
Delete	~~Internal granuloma of pulp~~
Delete	~~Resorption of tooth or root (external) (internal)~~
New code	521.40 Pathological resorption, unspecified
New code	521.41 Pathological resorption, internal
New code	521.42 Pathological resorption, external
New code	521.49 Other pathological resorption
	Internal granuloma of pulp
Revise	521.7 **Intrinsic posteruptive color changes**
Add	**Excludes** extrinsic color changes (523.6)
	523 Gingival and periodontal diseases
	523.2 Gingival recession
Revise	Gingival recession ~~(generalized) (localized)~~ (postinfective) (postoperative)
New code	523.20 Gingival recession, unspecified
New code	523.21 Gingival recession, minimal
New code	523.22 Gingival recession, moderate
New code	523.23 Gingival recession, severe
New code	523.24 Gingival recession, localized
New code	523.25 Gingival recession, generalized
	523.6 Accretions on teeth
Add	Extrinsic discoloration of teeth
Add	**Excludes** intrinsic discoloration of teeth (521.7)
	524 Dentofacial anomalies, including malocclusion
	524.0 Major anomalies of jaw size
New code	524.07 Excessive tuberosity of jaw
	524.2 Anomalies of dental arch relationship
Delete	~~Crossbite (anterior) (posterior)~~
	~~Disto-occlusion~~
	~~Mesio-occlusion~~
	~~Midline deviation~~
	~~Open bite (anterior) (posterior)~~
	~~Overbite (excessive):~~
	~~deep~~
	~~horizontal~~
	~~vertical~~
	~~Overjet~~
	~~Posterior lingual occlusion of mandibular teeth~~
	~~Soft tissue impingement~~
Add	**Excludes** soft tissue impingement (524.81–524.82)
New code	524.20 Unspecified anomaly of dental arch relationship
New code	524.21 Angle's class I
	Neutro-occlusion
New code	524.22 Angle's class II
	Disto-occlusion Division I
	Disto-occlusion Division II

New code	524.23 Angle's class III
	Mesio-occlusion
New code	524.24 Open anterior occlusal relationship
New code	524.25 Open posterior occlusal relationship
New code	524.26 Excessive horizontal overlap
New code	524.27 Reverse articulation
	Anterior articulation
	Posterior articulation
New code	524.28 Anomalies of interarch distance
	Excessive interarch distance
	Inadequate interarch distance
New code	524.29 Other anomalies of dental arch relationship
Revise	524.3 Anomalies of tooth position of fully erupted teeth
Delete	~~Crowding of tooth, teeth~~
	~~Diastema of tooth, teeth~~
	~~Displacement of tooth, teeth~~
	~~Rotation of tooth, teeth~~
	~~Spacing, abnormal, of tooth, teeth~~
	~~Transposition of tooth, teeth~~
	~~Impacted or embedded teeth with abnormal position of such teeth or adjacent teeth~~
Add	**Excludes** impacted or embedded teeth with abnormal position of such teeth or adjacent teeth (520.6)
New code	524.30 Unspecified anomaly of tooth position
	Diastema of teeth NOS
	Displacement of teeth NOS
	Transposition of teeth NOS
New code	524.31 Crowding of teeth
New code	524.32 Excessive spacing of teeth
New code	524.33 Horizontal displacement of teeth
	Tipping of teeth
New code	524.34 Vertical displacement of teeth
	Infraeruption of teeth
	Supraeruption of teeth
New code	524.35 Rotation of teeth
New code	524.36 Insufficient interocclusal distance of teeth (ridge)
New code	524.37 Excessive interocclusal distance of teeth
	Loss of occlusal vertical dimension
New code	524.39 Other anomalies of tooth position
	524.5 Dentofacial functional abnormalities
Delete	~~Abnormal jaw closure~~
Delete	~~Malocclusion due to:~~
Delete	~~abnormal swallowing~~
Delete	~~mouth breathing~~
Delete	~~tongue, lip, or finger habits~~
New code	524.50 Dentofacial functional abnormality, unspecified
New code	524.51 Abnormal jaw closure
	Dyskinesia
New code	524.52 Limited mandibular range of motion
New code	524.53 Deviation in opening and closing of the mandible
New code	524.54 Insufficient anterior guidance
New code	524.55 Centric occlusion maximum intercuspation discrepancy
New code	524.56 Non-working side interference
New code	524.57 Lack of posterior occlusal support
New code	524.59 Other dentofacial functional abnormalities
	Abnormal swallowing
	Mouth breathing
	Sleep postures
	Tongue, lip, or finger habits
	524.6 Temporomandibular joint disorders
New code	524.64 Temporomandibular joint sounds on opening and/or closing the jaw
	524.7 Dental alveolar anomalies

New code   **524.75 Vertical displacement of alveolus and teeth**
            Extrusion of alveolus and teeth
New code   **524.76 Occlusal plane deviation**
            524.8 Other specified dentofacial anomalies
New code   **524.81 Anterior soft tissue impingement**
New code   **524.82 Posterior soft tissue impingement**
New code   **524.89 Other specified dentofacial anomalies**
        525 Other diseases and conditions of the teeth and supporting structures
            525.2 Atrophy of edentulous alveolar ridge
New code   **525.20 Unspecified atrophy of edentulous alveolar ridge**
            Atrophy of the mandible NOS
            Atrophy of the maxilla NOS
New code   **525.21 Minimal atrophy of the mandible**
New code   **525.22 Moderate atrophy of the mandible**
New code   **525.23 Severe atrophy of the mandible**
New code   **525.24 Minimal atrophy of the maxilla**
New code   **525.25 Moderate atrophy of the maxilla**
New code   **525.26 Severe atrophy of the maxilla**
        528 Diseases of the oral soft tissues, excluding lesions specific for gingiva and tongue
            528.6 Leukoplakia of oral mucosa, including tongue
Revise   **Excludes** *leukokeratosis nicotina palati (528.79)*
            528.7 Other disturbances of oral epithelium, including tongue
Delete   ~~Erythroplakia of mouth or tongue~~
                ~~Focal epithelial hyperplasia of mouth or tongue~~
                ~~Leukoedema of mouth or tongue~~
                ~~Leukokeratosis nicotina palati~~
New code   **528.71 Minimal keratinized residual ridge mucosa**
New code   **528.72 Excessive keratinized residual ridge mucosa**
New code   **528.79 Other disturbances of oral epithelium, including tongue**
                Erythroplakia of mouth or tongue
                Focal epithelial hyperplasia of mouth or tongue
                Leukoedema of mouth or tongue
                Leukokeratosis nicotina palate
        529 Diseases and other conditions of the tongue
            529.8 Other specified conditions of the tongue
Revise   **Excludes** *erythroplasia of tongue (528.79)*
        530 Diseases of esophagus
            530.8 Other specified disorders of esophagus
New code   **530.86 Infection of esophagostomy**
                Use additional code to specify infection
New code   **530.87 Mechanical complication of esophagostomy**
                Malfunction of esophagostomy
        536 Disorders of function of stomach
            536.3 Gastroparesis
Add   Gastroparalysis
        560 Intestinal obstruction without mention of hernia
            560.8 Other specified intestinal obstruction
                560.89 Other
Add   Acute pseudo-obstruction of intestine

10.   DISEASES OF THE GENITOURINARY SYSTEM (580–629)
        588 Disorders resulting from impaired renal function
            588.8 Other specified disorders resulting from impaired renal function
Delete   ~~Hypokalemic nephropathy~~
                ~~Secondary hyperparathyroidism (of renal origin)~~
New code   **588.81 Secondary hyperparathyroidism (of renal origin)**
                Secondary hyperparathyroidism NOS

New code   **588.89 Other specified disorders resulting from impaired renal function**
                Hypokalemic nephropathy
        596 Other disorders of bladder
            596.8 Other specified disorders of bladder
Revise   **Excludes** *cystocele, female (618.01–618.02, 618.09, 618.2–618.4)*
Revise   *hernia or prolapse of bladder, female (618.01–618.02, 618.09, 618.2–618.4)*
        599 Other disorders of urethra and urinary tract
            599.5 Prolapsed urethral mucosa
Revise   **Excludes** *urethrocele, female (618.03, 618.09, 618.2–618.4)*
        615 Inflammatory diseases of uterus, except cervix
Revise   **Excludes** *hyperplastic endometritis (621.30–621.33)*
        618 Genital prolapse
            618.0 Prolapse of vaginal walls without mention of uterine prolapse
Delete   ~~Cystocele~~
                ~~Cystourethrocele~~
                ~~Proctocele, female, without mention of uterine prolapse~~
                ~~Rectocele, without mention of uterine prolapse~~
                ~~Urethrocele, female, without mention of uterine prolapse~~
                ~~Vaginal prolapse, without mention of uterine prolapse~~
New code   **618.00 Unspecified prolapse of vaginal walls**
                Vaginal prolapse NOS
New code   **618.01 Cystocele, midline**
                Cystocele NOS
New code   **618.02 Cystocele, lateral**
                Paravaginal
New code   **618.03 Urethrocele**
New code   **618.04 Rectocele**
                Proctocele
New code   **618.05 Perineocele**
New code   **618.09 Other prolapse of vaginal walls without mention of uterine prolapse**
                Cystourethrocele
            618.8 Other specified genital prolapse
Delete   ~~Incompetence or weakening of pelvic fundus~~
                ~~Relaxation of vaginal outlet or pelvis~~
New code   **618.81 Incompetence or weakening of pubocervical tissue**
New code   **618.82 Incompetence or weakening of rectovaginal tissue**
New code   **618.83 Pelvic muscle wasting**
                Disuse atrophy of pelvic muscles and anal sphincter
New code   **618.89 Other specified genital prolapse**
        621 Disorders of uterus, not elsewhere classified
Revise   **621.3 Endometrial cystic hyperplasia**
New code   **621.30 Endometrial hyperplasia, unspecified**
                Endometrial hyperplasia NOS
New code   **621.31 Simple endometrial hyperplasia without atypia**
New code   **621.32 Complex endometrial hyperplasia without atypia**
New code   **621.33 Endometrial hyperplasia with atypia**
        622 Noninflammatory disorders of cervix
            622.1 Dysplasia of cervix (uteri)
Delete   ~~Anaplasia of cervix~~
Delete   ~~Cervical atypism~~
Delete   ~~Cervical intraepithelial neoplasia I (CIN I)~~
Delete   ~~Cervical intraepithelial neoplasia II (CIN II)~~
Delete   ~~High grade squamous intraepithelial dysplasia (HGSIL)~~
Delete   ~~Low grade squamous intraepithelial dysplasia (LGSIL)~~

Add	Excludes	*abnormal results from cervical cytologic examination without histologic confirmation (795.00–795.09)*

New code	**622.10**	**Dysplasia of cervix, unspecified**
		Anaplasia of cervix
		Cervical atypism
		Cervical dysplasia NOS
New code	**622.11**	**Mild dysplasia of cervix**
		Cervical intraepithelial neoplasia I [CIN I]
New code	**622.12**	**Moderate dysplasia of cervix**
		Cervical intraepithelial neoplasia II [CIN II]

Add	Excludes	*carcinoma in situ of cervix (233.1)*
		cervical intraepithelial neoplasia III [CIN III] (233.1)
		severe dysplasia (233.1)

629 Other disorders of female genital organs

New subcategory	**629.2**	**Female genital mutilation status**
		Female circumcision status
New code	**629.20**	**Female genital mutilation status, unspecified**
		Female genital mutilation status NOS
New code	**629.21**	**Female genital mutilation Type I status**
		Clitorectomy status
New code	**629.22**	**Female genital mutilation Type II status**
		Clitorectomy with excision of labia minora status
New code	**629.23**	**Female genital mutilation Type III status**
		Infibulation status

11. COMPLICATIONS OF PREGNANCY, CHILDBIRTH, AND THE PUERPERIUM (630–677)

648 Other current conditions in the mother classifiable elsewhere, but complicating pregnancy, childbirth or the puerperium

  648.6 Other cardiovascular diseases

Add	Excludes	*peripartum cardiomyopathy (674.5)*

692 Contact dermatitis and other eczema

  692.8 Due to other specified agents

New code	**692.84**	**Due to animal (cat) (dog) dander**
		Due to animal (cat) (dog) hair
	692.89	**Other**
		Dermatitis due to:
Delete		~~furs~~

Delete	Excludes	~~*allergy NOS, due to animal hair, dander (animal), or dust (477.8)*~~
Add		*allergy (NOS) (rhinitis) due to animal hair or dander (477.2)*
Add		*allergy to dust (477.8)*

12. DISEASES OF THE SKIN AND SUBCUTANEOUS TISSUE (680–709)

705 Disorders of sweat glands

New subcategory	**705.2**	**Focal hyperhidrosis**

Add	Excludes	*generalized (secondary) hyperhidrosis (780.8)*

New code	**705.21**	**Primary focal hyperhidrosis**
		Focal hyperhidrosis NOS
		Hyperhidrosis NOS
		Hyperhidrosis of:
		axilla
		face
		palms
		soles
New code	**705.22**	**Secondary focal hyperhidrosis**
		Frey's syndrome

  705.8 Other specified disorders of sweat glands

    705.89 Other

Revise	Excludes	*generalized hyperhidrosis (780.8)*

707 Chronic ulcer of skin

  707.0 Decubitus ulcer

New code	**707.00**	**Unspecified site**
New code	**707.01**	**Elbow**
New code	**707.02**	**Upper back**
Add		Shoulder blades
New code	**707.03**	**Lower back**
Add		Sacrum
New code	**707.04**	**Hip**
New code	**707.05**	**Buttock**
New code	**707.06**	**Ankle**
New code	**707.07**	**Heel**
New code	**707.09**	**Other site**
		Head

13. DISEASES OF THE MUSCULOSKELETAL SYSTEM AND CONNECTIVE TISSUE (710–739)

713 Arthropathy associated with other disorders classified elsewhere

  713.0 Arthropathy associated with other endocrine and metabolic disorders

    Code first underlying disease, as:

Revise	hyperparathyroidism (252.00–252.08)

718 Other derangement of joint

Revise	Excludes	*jaw (524.60–524.69)*

719 Other and unspecified disorders of joint

Revise	Excludes	*jaw (524.60–524.69)*

  719.8 Other specified disorders of joint

Revise	Excludes	*temporomandibular joint-pain-dysfunction syndrome [Costen's syndrome] (524.60)*

728 Disorders of muscle, ligament, and fascia

  728.2 Muscular wasting and disuse atrophy, not elsewhere classified

Add	Excludes	*pelvic muscle wasting and disuse atrophy (618.83)*

733 Other disorders of bone and cartilage

Revise	Excludes	*osteitis fibrosa cystica generalisata (252.01)*

  733.2 Cyst of bone

    733.29 Other

Revise	Excludes	*osteitis fibrosa cystica (252.01)*

737 Curvature of spine

  737.4 Curvature of spine associated with other conditions

    Code first associated condition, as:

Revise	osteitis fibrosa cystica (252.01)

14. CONGENITAL ANOMALIES (740–759)

758 Chromosomal anomalies

Add	Use additional codes for conditions associated with the chromosomal anomalies

  758.3 Autosomal deletion syndromes

Delete		~~Antimongolism syndrome~~
Delete		~~Cri-du-chat syndrome~~
New code	**758.31**	**Cri-du-chat syndrome**
		Deletion 5p
New code	**758.32**	**Velo-cardio-facial syndrome**
		Deletion 22q11.2
New code	**758.33**	**Other microdeletions**
		Miller-Dieker syndrome
		Smith-Magenis syndrome
New code	**758.39**	**Other autosomal deletions**

15. CERTAIN CONDITIONS ORIGINATING IN THE PERINATAL PERIOD (760–779)

760 Fetus or newborn affected by maternal conditions which may be unrelated to present pregnancy

Revise	**760.7**	**Noxious influences affecting fetus or newborn via placenta or breast milk**

771 Infections specific to the perinatal period

  771.8 Other infections specific to the perinatal period

Revise	Use additional code to identify organism (041.0–041.9)

16. SYMPTOMS, SIGNS, AND ILL-DEFINED CONDITIONS (780–799)

780 General symptoms
780.5 Sleep disturbances
New code   **780.58 Sleep related movement disorder**
     Periodic limb movement disorder
Add   **Excludes** *restless leg syndrome (333.99)*
Revise   **780.8 Generalized hyperhidrosis**
Add   Secondary hyperhidrosis
Add   **Excludes** *focal (localized) (primary) (secondary) hyperhidrosis (705.21–705.22)*
Add   Frey's syndrome (705.22)
785 Symptoms involving the cardiovascular system
785.52 Septic shock
Add   endotoxic
Add   gram-negative
Revise   **Code first:**
     systemic inflammatory response syndrome due to infectious process with organ dysfunction (995.92)
Add   systemic inflammatory response syndrome due to non-infectious process with organ dysfunction (995.94)
785.59 Other
Delete   ~~endotoxic~~
Delete   ~~gram-negative~~
788 Symptoms involving urinary system
Revise   **788.3 Urinary incontinence**
     Code, if applicable, any causal condition first, such as:
Revise   genital prolapse (618.00–618.9)
New code   **788.38 Overflow incontinence**
790 Nonspecific findings on examination of blood
790.9 Other nonspecific findings on examination of blood
New code   **790.95 Elevated C-reactive protein (CRP)**
Revise   **795 Other and nonspecific abnormal cytological, histological, ~~and~~ immunological and DNA test findings**
Revise   **795.0 ~~Nonspecific~~ Abnormal Papanicolaou smear of cervix and cervical HPV**
Add   Abnormal thin preparation smear of cervix
Add   Abnormal cervical cytology
Revise   **Excludes** *cervical intraepithelial neoplasia I [CIN I] (622.11)*
Revise   cervical intraepithelial neoplasia II [CIN II] (622.12)
Revise   dysplasia (histologically confirmed) of cervix (uteri) NOS (622.10)
Delete   ~~high grade squamous intraepithelial dysplasia (HGSIL) (622.1)~~
Delete   ~~low grade squamous intraepithelial dysplasia (LGSIL) (622.1)~~
Add   mild dysplasia (histologically confirmed) (622.11)
Add   moderate dysplasia (histologically confirmed) (622.12)
Add   severe dysplasia (histologically confirmed) (233.1)
Revise   **795.00 ~~Nonspecific a~~Abnormal glandular Papanicolaou smear of cervix, ~~unspecified~~**
Add   Atypical endocervical cells NOS
Add   Atypical endometrial cells NOS
Add   Atypical glandular cells NOS
Revise   **795.01 ~~Atypical squamous cell changes of undetermined significance favor benign (ASCUS favor benign)~~**
     Papanicolaou smear of cervix with atypical squamous cells of undetermined significance (ASC-US)
Delete   ~~Atypical glandular cell changes of undetermined significance favor benign (AGCUS favor benign)~~

Revise   **795.02 ~~Atypical squamous cell changes of undetermined significance favor dysplasia (ASCUS favor dysplasia)~~**
     Papanicolaou smear of cervix with atypical squamous cells cannot exclude high grade squamous intraepithelial lesion (ASC-H)
Delete   ~~Atypical glandular cell changes of undetermined significance favor dysplasia (AGCUS favor dysplasia)~~
New code   **795.03 Papanicolaou smear of cervix with low grade squamous intraepithelial lesion (LGSIL)**
New code   **795.04 Papanicolaou smear of cervix with high grade squamous intraepithelial lesion (HGSIL)**
     Cytologic evidence of carcinoma
New code   **795.05 Cervical high risk human papillomavirus (HPV) DNA test positive**
New code   **795.08 Unsatisfactory smear**
     Inadequate sample
Revise   **795.09 Other ~~nonspecific~~ abnormal Papanicolaou smear of cervix and cervical HPV**
Delete   ~~Benign cellular changes~~
Delete   ~~Unsatisfactory smear~~
Add   Papanicolaou smear of cervix with low risk human papillomavirus (HPV) DNA test positive
Add   Use additional code for associated human papillomavirus (079.4)
Add   **Excludes** *encounter for Papanicolaou cervical smear to confirm findings of recent normal smear following initial abnormal smear (V72.32)*
796 Other nonspecific abnormal findings
New code   **796.6 Abnormal findings on neonatal screening**
Add   **Excludes** *nonspecific serologic evidence of human immunodeficiency virus [HIV] (795.71)*

17. INJURY AND POISONING (800–999)

995 Certain adverse effects not elsewhere classified
995.9 Systemic inflammatory response syndrome (SIRS)
Revise   Code first underlying condition systemic infection
     995.92 Systemic inflammatory response syndrome due to infectious process with organ dysfunction
     Use additional code to specify organ dysfunction, such as:
Delete   ~~kidney failure (584.5–584.9, 585, 586)~~
     995.94 Systemic inflammatory response syndrome due to noninfectious process with organ dysfunction
     Use additional code to specify organ dysfunction, such as:
Delete   ~~kidney failure (584.5–584.9, 585, 586)~~
996 Complications peculiar to certain specified procedures
996.4 Mechanical complication of internal orthopedic device, implant, and graft
Revise   **Excludes** *pressure ulcer due to cast (707.00–707.09)*
997 Complications affecting specified body systems, not elsewhere classified
997.4 Digestive system complications
     Excludes *specified gastrointestinal complications classified elsewhere, such as:*
Add   *infection of esophagostomy (530.86)*
Add   *mechanical complication of esophagostomy (530.87)*

Revise **SUPPLEMENTARY CLASSIFICATION OF FACTORS IN-FLUENCING HEALTH STATUS AND CONTACT WITH HEALTH SERVICES (V01–V84)**

V01 Contact with or exposure to communicable diseases

V01.7 Other viral diseases

New code   **V01.71 Varicella**

New code   **V01.79 Other viral diseases**

V01.8 Other communicable diseases

New code   **V01.83 Escherichia coli (E. coli)**

New code   **V01.84 Meningococcus**

V07 Need for isolation and other prophylactic measures

Revise   **V07.4** ~~Postmenopausal h~~Hormone replacement therapy (postmenopausal)

V08 Asymptomatic human immunodeficiency virus [HIV] infection status

Revise   **Excludes** *exposure to HIV (V01.79)*

V09 Infection with drug-resistant microorganisms

V09.0 Infection with microorganisms resistant to penicillins

Add   Methicillin-resistant staphylococcus aureus (MRSA)

V09.8 Infection with microorganisms resistant to other specified drugs

Add   Vancomycin (glycopeptide) intermediate staphylococcus aureus (VISA/GISA)

Add   Vancomycin (glycopeptide) resistant enterococcus (VRE)

Add   Vancomycin (glycopeptide) resistant staphylococcus aureus (VRSA/GRSA)

V22 Normal pregnancy

Revise   **Excludes** *pregnancy examination or test, pregnancy unconfirmed (V72.40)*

V45 Other postprocedural states

V45.7 Acquired absence of organ

V45.77 Genital organs

Add   **Excludes** *female genital mutilation status (629.20–629.23)*

V46 Other dependence on machines

V46.1 Respirator

New code   **V46.11 Dependence on respirator, status**

New code   **V46.12 Encounter for respirator dependence during power failure**

V49 Other conditions influencing health status

V49.8 Other specified conditions influencing health status

New code   **V49.83 Awaiting organ transplant status**

V58 Encounter for other and unspecified procedures and aftercare

V58.4 Other aftercare following surgery

New code   **V58.44 Aftercare following organ transplant**

Use additional code to identify the organ transplanted (V42.0–V42.9)

V58.6 Long-term (current) drug use

Add   **Excludes** *hormone replacement therapy (postmenopausal) (V07.4)*

V58.61 Long-term (current) use of anticoagulants

Add   **Excludes** *long-term (current) use of aspirin (V58.66)*

V58.63 Long-term (current) use of antiplatelets/antithrombotics

Add   **Excludes** *long-term (current) use of aspirin (V58.66)*

V58.64 Long-term (current) use of non-steroidal antiinflammatories (NSAID)

Add   **Excludes** *long-term (current) use of aspirin (V58.66)*

New code   **V58.66 Long-term (current) use of aspirin**

New code   **V58.67 Long-term (current) use of insulin**

V58.7 Aftercare following surgery to specified body systems, not elsewhere classified

Add   **Excludes** *aftercare following organ transplant (V58.44)*

Add   *aftercare following surgery for neoplasm (V58.42)*

V69 Problems related to lifestyle

New code   **V69.4 Lack of adequate sleep**

Sleep deprivation

Add   **Excludes** *insomnia (780.52)*

Revise **PERSONS WITHOUT REPORTED DIAGNOSIS ENCOUNTERED DURING EXAMINATION AND INVESTIGATION OF INDIVIDUALS AND POPULATIONS (V70–V84)**

V72 Special investigations and examinations

V72.3 Gynecological examination

Delete   ~~Papanicolaou cervical smear as part of general gynecological examination~~

Delete   ~~Pelvic examination (annual) (periodic)~~

Delete   ~~Use additional code to identify routine vaginal Papanicolaou smear (V76.47)~~

New code   **V72.31 Routine gynecological examination**

General gynecological examination with or without Papanicolaou cervical smear

Pelvic examination (annual) (periodic)

Use additional code to identify routine vaginal Papanicolaou smear (V76.47)

New code   **V72.32 Encounter for Papanicolaou cervical smear to confirm findings of recent normal smear following initial abnormal smear**

Revise   **V72.4 Pregnancy examination or test, pregnancy unconfirmed**

Delete   ~~Possible pregnancy, not (yet) confirmed~~

New code   **V72.40 Pregnancy examination or test, pregnancy unconfirmed**

Possible pregnancy, not (yet) confirmed

New code   **V72.41 Pregnancy examination or test, negative result**

V76 Special screening for malignant neoplasms

V76.2 Cervix

Revise   **Excludes** *that as part of a general gynecological examination (V72.31)*

V82 Special screening for other conditions

V82.8 Other specified conditions

V82.81 Osteoporosis

Use additional code to identify:

Revise   hormone replacement therapy (postmenopausal) status (V07.4)

New category **V84 Genetic susceptibility to disease**

Add   **Includes:** Confirmed abnormal gene

Add   Use additional code, if applicable, for any associated family history of the disease (V16–V19)

New subcategory **V84.0 Genetic susceptibility to malignant neoplasm**

Add   Code first, if applicable, any current malignant neoplasms (140.0–195.8, 200.0–208.9, 230.0–234.9)

Add   Use additional code, if applicable, for any personal history of malignant neoplasm (V10.0–V10.9)

New code   **V84.01 Genetic susceptibility to malignant neoplasm of breast**

New code   **V84.02 Genetic susceptibility to malignant neoplasm of ovary**

New code   **V84.03 Genetic susceptibility to malignant neoplasm of prostate**

New code   **V84.04 Genetic susceptibility to malignant neoplasm of endometrium**

New code   **V84.09 Genetic susceptibility to other malignant neoplasm**

New code   **V84.8 Genetic susceptibility to other disease**

VOLUME 3 CHANGES EFFECTIVE OCTOBER 1, 2004

00.0 Therapeutic ultrasound

Add exclusion term   **Excludes** *diagnostic ultrasound (non-invasive) (88.71–88.79)*

     intracardiac echocardiography [ICE] (heart chamber(s)) (37.28)

     intravascular imaging (adjunctive) (00.21–00.29)

New code   **00.16 Pressurized treatment of venous bypass graft [conduit] withpharmaceutical substance**

     Ex-vivo treatment of vessel

     Hyperbaric pressurized graft [conduit]

New code   **00.17 Infusion of vasopressor agent**

New subcategory **00.2 Intravascular imaging of blood vessels**

     Endovascular ultrasonography

     Intravascular ultrasound (IVUS)

     Code also any synchronous diagnostic or therapeutic procedures

     Excludes *therapeutic ultrasound (00.01–00.09)*

New code   **00.21 Intravascular imaging of extracranial cerebral vessels**

     Common carotid vessels and branches

     Intravascular ultrasound (IVUS), extracranial cerebral vessels

     Excludes *diagnostic ultrasound (non-invasive) of head and neck (88.71)*

New code   **00.22 Intravascular imaging of intrathoracic vessels**

     Aorta and aortic arch

     Intravascular ultrasound (IVUS), intrathoracic vessels

     Vena cava (superior) (inferior)

     Excludes *diagnostic ultrasound (non-invasive) of other sites of thorax (88.73)*

New code   **00.23 Intravascular imaging of peripheral vessels**

     Imaging of:

       vessels of arm(s)

       vessels of leg(s)

     Intravascular ultrasound (IVUS), peripheral vessels

     Excludes *diagnostic ultrasound (non-invasive) of peripheral vascular system (88.77)*

New code   **00.24 Intravascular imaging of coronary vessels**

     Intravascular ultrasound (IVUS), coronary vessels

     Excludes *diagnostic ultrasound (non-invasive) of heart (88.72)*

     intracardiac echocardiography [ICE] (ultrasound of heart chamber(s)) (37.28)

New code   **00.25 Intravascular imaging of renal vessels**

     Intravascular ultrasound (IVUS), renal vessels

     Renal artery

     Excludes *diagnostic ultrasound (non-invasive) of urinary system (88.75)*

New code   **00.28 Intravascular imaging, other specified vessel(s)**

New code   **00.29 Intravascular imaging, unspecified vessel(s)**

New subcategory **00.3 Computer assisted surgery [CAS]**

     CT-free navigation

     Image guided navigation (IGN)

     Image guided surgery (IGS)

     Imageless navigation

     Code also diagnostic or therapeutic procedure

     Excludes *stereotactic frame application only (93.59)*

New code   **00.31 Computer assisted surgery with CT/CTA**

New code   **00.32 Computer assisted surgery with MR/MRA**

New code   **00.33 Computer assisted surgery with fluoroscopy**

New code   **00.34 Imageless computer assisted surgery**

New code   **00.35 Computer assisted surgery with multiple datasets**

New code   **00.39 Other computer assisted surgery**

     Computer assisted surgery NOS

Revise code title   **00.55 Insertion of drug-eluting ~~non-coronary artery~~ peripheral vessel stent(s)**

Revise code also note   Code also any ~~non-coronary~~ angioplasty or atherectomy of other non-coronary vessel(s) (39.50)

Revise exclusion term   **Excludes** *drug-coated peripheral stents, e.g. heparin coated (39.90)*

Add exclusion term   *insertion of cerebrovascular stent(s) (00.63–00.65)*

Revise exclusion term   *insertion of non-drug-eluting stent(s): ~~non-coronary artery~~ peripheral vessel (39.90)*

New subcategory **00.6 Procedures on blood vessels**

     Excludes *angioplasty or atherectomy of other non-coronary vessel(s) (39.50)*

     insertion of coronary artery stent(s) (36.06–36.07)

     insertion of drug-eluting peripheral vessel stent(s) (00.55)

     insertion of non-drug-eluting peripheral vessel stent(s) (39.90)

New code   **00.61 Percutaneous angioplasty or atherectomy of precerebral (extracranial) vessel(s)**

     Basilar

     Carotid

     Vertebral

     Code also any:

     injection or infusion of thrombolytic agent (99.10)

     percutaneous insertion of carotid artery stent(s) (00.63)

     percutaneous insertion of other precerebral artery stent(s) (00.64)

     Excludes *angioplasty or atherectomy of other non-coronary vessel(s) (39.50)*

     removal of cerebrovascular obstruction of vessel(s) by open approach (38.01–38.02, 38.11–38.12, 38.31–38.32, 38.41–38.42)

New code   **00.62 Percutaneous angioplasty or atherectomy of intracranial vessel(s)**

     Code also any:

     injection or infusion of thrombolytic agent (99.10)

     percutaneous insertion of intracranial stent(s) (00.65)

     Excludes *angioplasty or atherectomy of other non-coronary vessel(s)(39.50)*

     removal of cerebrovascular obstruction of vessel(s) by open approach (38.01–38.02, 38.11–38.12, 38.31–38.32, 38.41–38.42)

New code   **00.63 Percutaneous insertion of carotid artery stent(s)**

     Includes the use of any embolic protection device, distal protection device, filter device, or stent delivery system

     Non-drug-eluting stent

	Code also percutaneous angioplasty or atherectomy of precerebral vessel(s) (00.61)
New code	**00.64 Percutaneous insertion of other precerebral (extracranial) artery stent(s)**
	Includes the use of any embolic protection device, distal protection device, filter device, or stent delivery system
	Basilar stent
	Vertebral stent
	Code also percutaneous angioplasty or atherectomy of precerebral vessel(s) (00.61)
New code	**00.65 Percutaneous insertion of intracranial vascular stent(s)**
	Includes the use of any embolic protection device, distal protection device, filter device, or stent delivery system
	Code also percutaneous angioplasty or atherectomy of intracranial vessel(s) (00.62)
New subcategory	**00.9 Other procedures and interventions**
New code	**00.91 Transplant from live related donor**
	Code also organ transplant procedure
New code	**00.92 Transplant from live non-related donor**
	Code also organ transplant procedure
New code	**00.93 Transplant from cadaver**
	Code also organ transplant procedure
Revise code title	**01.22 Removal of intracranial neurostimulator lead(s)**
Add code also note	Code also any removal of neurostimulator pulse generator (86.05)
Revise code title	**02.93 Implantation or replacement of intracranial neurostimulator lead(s)**
Add code also note	Code also any insertion of neurostimulator pulse generator (86.94–86.96)
Revise code title	**03.93 ~~Insertion~~ Implantation or replacement of spinal neurostimulator lead(s)**
Add code also note	Code also any insertion of neurostimulator pulse generator (86.94–86.96)
Revise code title	**03.94 Removal of spinal neurostimulator lead(s)**
Add code also note	Code also any removal of neurostimulator pulse generator (86.05)
Revise code title	**04.92 Implantation or replacement of peripheral neurostimulator lead(s)**
Add code also note	Code also any insertion of neurostimulator pulse generator (86.94–86.96)
Revise code title	**04.93 Removal of peripheral neurostimulator lead(s)**
Add code also note	Code also any removal of neurostimulator pulse generator (86.05)
	11.60 Corneal transplant, not otherwise specified
Add note	Note: To report donor source—*see* codes 00.91–00.93
New code	**27.64 Insertion of palatal implant**
	27.69 Other plastic repair of palate
Add code also note	Code also any insertion of palatal implant (27.64)
	33.5 Lung transplant
Add note	Note: To report donor source—*see* codes 00.91–00.93
	33.6 Combined heart-lung transplantation
Add note	Note: To report donor source—*see* codes 00.91–00.93
	36.1 Bypass anastomosis for heart revascularization
Add code also note	Code also:
	pressurized treatment of venous bypass graft [conduit] with pharmaceutical substance, if performed (00.16)
Revise code title	**36.11 (Aorto)coronary bypass of one coronary artery**

Revise code title	**36.12 (Aorto)coronary bypass of two coronary arteries**
Revise code title	**36.13 (Aorto)coronary bypass of three coronary arteries**
Revise code title	**36.14 (Aorto)coronary bypass of four or more coronary arteries**
	37.26 Cardiac electrophysiologic stimulation and recording studies
Add exclusion term	**Excludes** *device interrogation only without arrhythmia induction (bedside check) (89.45–89.49)*
	37.28 Intracardiac echocardiography
Add inclusion term	Echocardiography of heart chambers
Add exclusion term	**Excludes** *intravascular imaging of coronary vessels (intravascular ultrasound) (IVUS) (00.24)*
	37.52 Implantation of total replacement heart system
Revise exclusion term	**Excludes** *implantation of heart assist system [VAD] (37.62, 37.65, 37.66)*
	37.53 Replacement or repair of thoracic unit of total replacement heart system
Revise exclusion term	**Excludes** *replacement and repair of heart assist system [VAD] (37.63)*
	37.54 Replacement or repair of other implantable component of total replacement heart system
Revise exclusion term	**Excludes** *replacement and repair of heart assist system [VAD] (37.63)*
Revise subcategory title	**37.6 Implantation of heart and circulatory assist system**
Revise code title	**37.62 ~~Implant~~ Insertion of ~~other~~ non-implantable heart assist system**
Delete inclusion term	~~Insertion of centrifugal pump~~
Delete inclusion term	~~Insertion of heart assist system, not specified as pulsatile~~
Add exclusion term	**Excludes** *insertion of percutaneous external heart assist device (37.68)*
Revise code title	**37.63 ~~Replacement and r~~ Repair of heart assist system**
Add inclusion term	Replacement of parts of an existing ventricular assist device (VAD)
Revise exclusion term	**Excludes** *replacement or repair of other implantable component of total replacement heart system [artificial heart] (37.54)*
Revise exclusion term	*replacement or repair of thoracic unit of total replacement heart system [artificial heart] (37.53)*
	37.64 Removal of heart assist system
Add exclusion term	**Excludes** *explantation [removal] of percutaneous external heart assist device (97.44)*
Revise code title	**37.65 Implant of ~~an~~ external, ~~pulsatile~~ heart assist system**
Revise note	Note: Device ~~not implantable~~ (outside the body but connected to heart) with external circulation and pump. Includes open chest (sternotomy) procedure for cannulae attachments
Add exclusion term	**Excludes** *insertion of percutaneous external heart assist device (37.68)*
Revise code title	**37.66 ~~Implant~~ Insertion of ~~an~~ implantable, ~~pulsatile~~ heart assist system**
Add inclusion term	Axial flow heart assist system
Add inclusion term	Diagonal pump heart assist system
Add inclusion term	Left ventricular assist device (LVAD)
Add inclusion term	Pulsatile heart assist system
Add inclusion term	Right ventricular assist device (RVAD)
Add inclusion term	Rotary pump heart assist system
Add inclusion term	Ventricular assist device (VAD) not otherwise specified

Revise exclusion term | **Excludes** | *implantation of total replacement heart system [artificial heart] (37.52)*

Add exclusion term   *insertion of percutaneous external heart assist device (37.68)*

New code   **37.68 Insertion of percutaneous external heart assist device**
Includes percutaneous [femoral] insertion of cannulae attachments
Circulatory assist device
Extrinsic heart assist device
pVAD
Percutaneous heart assist device

New code   **37.90 Insertion of left atrial appendage device**
Left atrial filter
Left atrial occluder
Transseptal catheter technique

37.99 Other

Add exclusion term | **Excludes** | *insertion of left atrial appendage device (37.90)*

39.2 Other shunt or vascular bypass

Add code also note   Code also pressurized treatment of venous bypass graft [conduit] with pharmaceutical substance, if performed (00.16)

Revise code title   **39.50 Angioplasty or atherectomy of other non-coronary vessel(s)**
Percutaneous transluminal angioplasty (PTA) of non-coronary vessel:

Delete inclusion term   ~~head and neck arteries:~~
Delete inclusion term   ~~basilar~~
Delete inclusion term   ~~carotid~~
Delete inclusion term   ~~vertebral~~

Add code also note   Code also any:
percutaneous insertion of carotid artery stent(s) (00.63)

Add exclusion term | **Excludes** | *percutaneous angioplasty or atherectomy of precerebral or cerebral vessel(s) (00.61–00.62)*

39.7 Endovascular repair of vessel

Revise exclusion term | **Excludes** | *angioplasty or atherectomy of other non-coronary vessel(s) (39.50)*

Revise exclusion term   *insertion of non-drug-eluting ~~non-coronary~~ peripheral vessel stent(s) ~~or stents~~ (39.90)*

Add exclusion term   *percutaneous insertion of carotid artery stent(s) (00.63)*

Add exclusion term   *percutaneous insertion of intracranial stent(s) (00.65)*

Add exclusion term   *percutaneous insertion of other precerebral artery stent(s) (00.64)*

39.79 Other endovascular repair (of aneurysm) of other vessels

Revise exclusion term | **Excludes** | *insertion of drug-eluting ~~non-coronary artery~~ peripheral vessel stent(s) (00.55)*

Revise exclusion term | **Excludes** | *insertion of non-drug-eluting ~~non-coronary artery~~ peripheral vessel stent(s) (for other than aneurysm repair) (39.90)*

Revise code title   **39.90 Insertion of non-drug-eluting, ~~non-coronary artery~~ peripheral vessel stent(s)**

Revise exclusion term | **Excludes** | *insertion of drug-eluting, ~~non-coronary artery~~ peripheral vessel stent(s) (00.55)*

Add exclusion term   *percutaneous insertion of carotid artery stent(s) (00.63)*

Add exclusion term   *percutaneous insertion of intracranial stent(s) (00.65)*

Add exclusion term   *percutaneous insertion of other precerebral artery stent(s) (00.64)*

41.0 Bone marrow or hematopoietic stem cell transplant

Add note   Note: To report donor source—*see* codes 00.91–00.93

New code   **44.38 Laparoscopic gastroenterostomy**
Bypass: gastroduodenostomy
gastroenterostomy
gastrogastrostomy
Laparoscopic gastrojejunostomy without gastrectomy NEC

| **Excludes** | *gastroenterostomy, open approach (44.39)*

44.66 Other procedures for creation of esophagogastric sphincteric competence

Add exclusion term | **Excludes** | *that by laparoscopy (44.67)*

New code   **44.67 Laparoscopic procedures for creation of esophagogastric sphincteric competence**
Fundoplication
Gastric cardioplasty
Nissen's fundoplication
Restoration of cardio-esophageal angle

New code   **44.68 Laparoscopic gastroplasty**
Banding
Silastic vertical banding
Vertical banded gastroplasty (VBG)
Code also any synchronous laparoscopic gastroenterostomy (44.38)

| **Excludes** | *insertion, laparoscopic adjustable gastric band (restrictive procedure) (44.95)*
other repair of stomach, open approach (44.61–44.65, 44.69)

New code   **44.95 Laparoscopic gastric restrictive procedure**
Adjustable gastric band and port insertion

| **Excludes** | *laparoscopic gastroplasty (44.68)*
other repair of stomach (44.69)

New code   **44.96 Laparoscopic revision of gastric restrictive procedure**
Revision or replacement of:
adjustable gastric band
subcutaneous gastric port device

New code   **44.97 Laparoscopic removal of gastric restrictive device(s)**
Removal of either or both:
adjustable gastric and
subcutaneous port device

| **Excludes** | *nonoperative removal of gastric restrictive device(s) (97.86)*
open removal of gastric restrictive device(s) (44.99)

New code   **44.98 (Laparoscopic) adjustment of size of adjustable gastric restrictive device**
Infusion of saline for device tightening
Withdrawal of saline for device loosening
Code also any:
abdominal ultrasound (88.76)
abdominal wall fluoroscopy (88.09)
barium swallow (87.61)

46.97 Transplant of intestine

Add note   Note: To report donor source—*see* codes 00.91–00.93

50.19 Other diagnostic procedures on liver

Add inclusion term   Laparoscopic liver biopsy

50.5 Liver transplant

Add note   Note: To report donor source—*see* codes 00.91–00.93

52.8 Transplant of pancreas

Add note   Note: To report donor source—*see* codes 00.91–00.93

55.5 Complete nephrectomy
Code also any synchronous excision of:

Add code also note   adrenal gland (07.21–07.3)

55.6 Transplant of kidney

Add note   Note: To report donor source—*see* codes 00.91–00.93

65.99 Other
Add inclusion term — Ovarian drilling
75.34 Other fetal monitoring
Add inclusion term — Antepartum fetal nonstress test
78.6 Removal of implanted devices from bone
Add inclusion term — Removal of internal limb lengthening device
80.51 Excision of intervertebral disc
Add exclusion term — **Excludes** *that for insertion of (non-fusion) spinal disc replacement device (84.60–84.69)*
New code — **81.65 Vertebroplasty**
Injection of bone void filler (cement) (polymethylmethacrylate) (PMMA) into the diseased or fractured vertebral body
Excludes *kyphoplasty (81.66)*
New code — **81.66 Kyphoplasty**
Insertion of inflatable balloon, bone tamp, or other device to create a cavity for partial restoration of height of diseased or fractured vertebral body prior to injection of bone void filler (cement) (polymethylmethacrylate) (PMMA)
Excludes *vertebroplasty (81.65)*
84.5 Implantation of other musculoskeletal devices and substances
Add exclusion term — **Excludes** *insertion of (non-fusion) spinal disc replacement device (84.60–84.69)*
New code — **84.53 Implantation of internal limb lengthening device with kinetic distraction**
Code also limb lengthening procedure (78.30–78.39)
New code — **84.54 Implantation of other internal limb lengthening device**
Implantation of internal limb lengthening device, Not Otherwise Specified (NOS)
Code also limb lengthening procedure (78.30–78.39)
New code — **84.55 Insertion of bone void filler**
Insertion of:
acrylic cement (PMMA)
bone void cement
calcium based bone void filler
polymethylmethacrylate (PMMA)
Excludes *that with kyphoplasty (81.66)*
that with vertebroplasty (81.65)
New code — **84.59 Insertion of other spinal devices**
New subcategory **84.6 Replacement of spinal disc**
Includes: non-fusion arthroplasty of the spine with insertion of artificial disc prosthesis
New code — **84.60 Insertion of spinal disc prosthesis, not otherwise specified**
Replacement of spinal disc, NOS
Includes: diskectomy (discectomy)
New code — **84.61 Insertion of partial spinal disc prosthesis, cervical**
Nuclear replacement device, cervical
Partial artificial disc prosthesis (flexible), cervical
Replacement of nuclear disc (nucleus pulposus), cervical
Includes: diskectomy (discectomy)
New code — **84.62 Insertion of total spinal disc prosthesis, cervical**
Replacement of cervical spinal disc, NOS
Replacement of total spinal disc, cervical
Total artificial disc prosthesis (flexible), cervical
Includes: diskectomy (discectomy)

New code — **84.63 Insertion of spinal disc prosthesis, thoracic**
Artificial disc prosthesis (flexible), thoracic
Replacement of thoracic spinal disc, partial or total
Includes: diskectomy (discectomy)
New code — **84.64 Insertion of partial spinal disc prosthesis, lumbosacral**
Nuclear replacement device, lumbar
Partial artificial disc prosthesis (flexible), lumbar
Replacement of nuclear disc (nucleus pulposus), lumbar
Includes: diskectomy (discectomy)
New code — **84.65 Insertion of total spinal disc prosthesis, lumbosacral**
Replacement of lumbar spinal disc, NOS
Replacement of total spinal disc, lumbar
Total artificial disc prosthesis (flexible), lumbar
Includes: diskectomy (discectomy)
New code — **84.66 Revision or replacement of artificial spinal disc prosthesis, cervical**
Removal of (partial) (total) spinal disc prosthesis with synchronous insertion of new (partial) (total) spinal disc prosthesis, cervical
Repair of previously inserted spinal disc prosthesis, cervical
New code — **84.67 Revision or replacement of artificial spinal disc prosthesis, thoracic**
Removal of (partial) (total) spinal disc prosthesis with synchronous insertion of new (partial) (total) spinal disc prosthesis, thoracic
Repair of previously inserted spinal disc prosthesis, thoracic
New code — **84.68 Revision or replacement of artificial spinal disc prosthesis, lumbosacral**
Removal of (partial) (total) spinal disc prosthesis with synchronous insertion of new (partial) (total) spinal disc prosthesis, lumbosacral
Repair of previously inserted spinal disc prosthesis, lumbosacral
New code — **84.69 Revision or replacement of artificial spinal disc prosthesis, not otherwise specified**
Removal of (partial) (total) spinal disc prosthesis with synchronous insertion of new (partial) (total) spinal disc prosthesis
Repair of previously inserted spinal disc prosthesis
Revise code title — **86.05 Incision with removal of foreign body or device from skin and subcutaneous tissue**
Add inclusion term — Removal of neurostimulator pulse generator (single array, dual array)
86.09 Other incision of skin and subcutaneous tissue
Add inclusion term — Relocation of subcutaneous device pocket NEC
Add inclusion term — Reopening subcutaneous pocket for device revision without replacement
New code — **86.94 Insertion or replacement of single array neurostimulator pulse generator**
Pulse generator (single array, single channel) for intracranial, spinal, and peripheral neurostimulator
Code also any associated lead implantation (02.93, 03.93, 04.92)

New code   **86.95 Insertion or replacement of dual array neurostimulatorpulse generator**

Pulse generator (dual array, dual channel) for intracranial, spinal, and peripheral neurostimulator

Code also any associated lead implantation (02.93, 03.93, 04.92)

New code   **86.96 Insertion or replacement of other neurostimulator pulse generator**

Code also any associated lead implantation (02.93, 03.93, 04.92)

Excludes *insertion of dual array neurostimulator pulse generator (86.95)*

insertion of single array neurostimulator pulse generator (86.94)

88.7 Diagnostic ultrasound

Add inclusion term   Non-invasive ultrasound

Add exclusion term   **Excludes** *intravascular imaging (adjunctive) (IVUS) (00.21–00.29)*

88.72 Diagnostic ultrasound of heart

Delete exclusion term   ~~Intravascular ultrasound of heart~~

Add inclusion term   Transesophageal echocardiography

Add exclusion term   **Excludes** *echocardiography of heart chambers (37.28)*

intracardiac echocardiography (ICE) (37.28)

intravascular (IVUS) imaging of coronary vessels (00.24)

Revise subcategory title   **89.4 Cardiac stress tests, pacemaker and defibrillator checks**

89.45 Artificial pacemaker rate check

Add inclusion term   Bedside device check of pacemaker or cardiac resynchronization pacemaker [CRT-P]

Add inclusion term   Interrogation only without arrhythmia induction

Add exclusion term   **Excludes** *electrophysiologic studies [EPS] (37.26)*

Add exclusion term   *non-invasive programmed electrical stimulation [NIPS] (arrhythmia induction) (37.26)*

New code   **89.49 Automatic implantable cardioverter/defibrillator (AICD) check**

Bedside check of an AICD or cardiac resynchronization defibrillator [CRT-D]

Checking pacing thresholds of device

Interrogation only without arrhythmia induction

Excludes *electrophysiologic studies [EPS] (37.26)*

non-invasive programmed electrical stimulation [NIPS] (arrhythmia induction) (37.26)

93.90 Continuous positive airway pressure [CPAP]

Add inclusion term   Bi-level airway pressure

Add inclusion term   Non-invasive positive pressure (NIPPV)

96.7 Other continuous mechanical ventilation

Add exclusion term   **Excludes** *non-invasive positive pressure (NIPPV) (93.90)*

97.44 Nonoperative removal of heart assist system

Add inclusion term   Explantation [removal] of circulatory assist device

Add inclusion term   Explantation [removal] of percutaneous external heart assist device

Add inclusion term   Removal of extrinsic heart assist device

Add inclusion term   Removal of pVAD

Add inclusion term   Removal of percutaneous heart assist device

New code   **99.78 Aquapheresis**

Plasma water removal

Ultrafiltration [for water removal]

Excludes *hemodiafiltration (39.95)*

hemodialysis (39.95)

therapeutic plasmapheresis (99.71)

HCPCS 2004 New/Revised/Deleted Codes and Modifiers

2005 HCPCS Updates and quarterly updates will be posted on the companion website (http://evolve.elsevier.com/Buck/icd) when available

NEW CODES/MODIFIERS

CD	A6447	C1757	C2617	E1004	E2599	H2031	K0642	Q3031
CE	A6448	C1758	C2619	E1005	G0296	H2032	K0643	Q4054
CF	A6449	C1759	C2620	E1006	G0297	H2033	K0644	Q4055
KD	A6450	C1760	C2621	E1007	G0298	H2034	K0645	Q4075
KF	A6451	C1762	C2622	E1008	G0299	H2035	K0646	Q4076
KZ	A6452	C1763	C2625	E1009	G0300	H2036	K0647	Q4077
SM	A6453	C1764	C2626	E1010	G0302	H2037	K0648	S0104
SN	A6454	C1766	C2627	E1019	G0303	J0152	K0649	S0107
SQ	A6455	C1767	C2628	E1021	G0304	J0215	K0650	S0115
SW	A6456	C1768	C2629	E1028	G0305	J0583	K0651	S0136
UF	A6550	C1769	C2630	E1029	G0306	J0595	K0652	S0137
UG	A6551	C1770	C2631	E1030	G0307	J1335	K0653	S0138
UH	A7046	C1771	C2633	E1391	G0308	J1595	K0654	S0139
UJ	A7520	C1772	C8918	E1634	G0309	J2001	K0655	S0140
UK	A7521	C1773	C8919	E2120	G0310	J2185	K0656	S0141
UN	A7522	C1776	C8920	E2201	G0311	J2280	K0657	S0158
UP	A7523	C1777	C9123	E2202	G0312	J2353	K0658	S0159
UQ	A7524	C1778	C9202	E2203	G0313	J2354	K0659	S0160
UR	A7525	C1779	C9203	E2204	G0314	J2505	K0660	S0161
US	A7526	C1780	C9205	E2300	G0315	J2783	K0661	S0162
A0800	A9280	C1781	C9207	E2301	G0316	J3411	K0662	S0163
A4216	A9525	C1782	C9208	E2310	G0317	J3415	K0663	S0164
A4217	A9526	C1784	C9209	E2311	G0318	J3465	K0664	S0165
A4248	A9528	C1785	C9210	E2320	G0319	J3486	K0665	S0194
A4366	A9529	C1786	C9211	E2321	G0320	J7303	K0666	S0201
A4416	A9530	C1787	C9212	E2322	G0321	J7621	K0667	S0207
A4417	A9531	C1788	C9704	E2323	G0322	J9098	K0668	S0115
A4418	A9532	C1789	E0118	E2324	G0323	J9178	K0669	S0136
A4419	A9533	C1813	E0140	E2325	G0324	J9263	L0112	S0137
A4420	A9534	C1814	E0190	E2326	G0325	J9395	L0861	S0138
A4423	A9999	C1815	E0240	E2327	G0326	K0552	L1831	S0139
A4424	C1080	C1816	E0247	E2328	G0327	K0601	L1907	S0140
A4425	C1081	C1817	E0248	E2329	G0328	K0602	L1951	S0141
A4426	C1082	C1818	E0300	E2330	G0338	K0603	L1971	S0158
A4427	C1083	C1819	E0301	E2331	G0339	K0604	L3031	S0159
A4428	C1713	C1874	E0302	E2340	G0340	K0605	L3917	S0160
A4429	C1714	C1875	E0303	E2341	G3001	K0606	L5673	S0161
A4430	C1715	C1876	E0304	E2342	H2010	K0607	L5679	S0162
A4431	C1717	C1877	E0470	E2343	H2011	K0608	L5681	S0163
A4432	C1721	C1878	E0471	E2351	H2012	K0609	L5683	S0164
A4433	C1722	C1879	E0472	E2360	H2013	K0618	L8511	S0165
A4434	C1724	C1880	E0561	E2361	H2014	K0619	L8512	S0194
A4638	C1725	C1881	E0562	E2362	H2015	K0620	L8513	S0315
A4644	C1726	C1882	E0637	E2363	H2016	K0627	L8514	S0316
A4645	C1727	C1883	E0638	E2364	H2017	K0628	L8631	S0317
A4646	C1728	C1884	E0675	E2365	H2018	K0629	L8659	S0320
A4671	C1729	C1885	E0955	E2366	H2019	K0630	P9051	S0618
A4672	C1730	C1887	E0956	E2367	H2020	K0631	P9052	S1040
A4673	C1731	C1891	E0957	E2399	H2021	K0632	P9053	S2070
A4674	C1732	C1892	E0960	E2402	H2022	K0633	P9054	S2082
A4728	C1733	C1893	E0981	E2500	H2023	K0634	P9055	S2083
A6407	C1750	C1894	E0982	E2502	H2024	K0635	P9056	S2085
A6441	C1751	C1895	E0983	E2504	H2025	K0636	P9057	S2090
A6442	C1752	C1896	E0984	E2506	H2026	K0637	P9058	S2091
A6443	C1753	C1897	E0985	E2508	H2027	K0638	P9059	S2095
A6444	C1754	C1898	E0986	E2510	H2028	K0639	P9060	S2113
A6445	C1755	C1899	E1002	E2511	H2029	K0640	Q0137	S2131
A6446	C1756	C2615	E1003	E2512	H2030	K0641	Q0182	S2135

xxix

NEW CODES/MODIFIERS — *Continued*

S2152	S3828	S3890	S5136	S5550	S9335	T2019	T2037	V2756
S2213	S3829	S5100	S5140	S5551	S9434	T2020	T2038	V2761
S2225	S3833	S5101	S5141	S5552	S9476	T2021	T2039	V2762
S2230	S3834	S5102	S5145	S5553	S9484	T2022	T2040	V2782
S2235	S3840	S5105	S5146	S5560	S9490	T2023	T2041	V2783
S2255	S3841	S5108	S5150	S5561	S9900	T2024	T2042	V2784
S2262	S3842	S5109	S5151	S5565	S9976	T2025	T2043	V2786
S2265	S3843	S5110	S5160	S5566	S9977	T2026	T2044	V2797
S2266	S3844	S5111	S5161	S5570	S9988	T2027	T2045	
S2267	S3845	S5115	S5162	S5571	T2010	T2028	T2046	
S2362	S3846	S5116	S5165	S8004	T2011	T2029	T2048	
S2363	S3847	S5120	S5170	S8075	T2012	T2030	T2101	
S3000	S3848	S5121	S5175	S8120	T2013	T2031	T5001	
S3625	S3849	S5125	S5180	S8121	T2014	T2032	T5999	
S3655	S3850	S5126	S5181	S8460	T2015	T2033	V2121	
S3820	S3851	S5130	S5185	S8948	T2016	T2034	V2221	
S3822	S3852	S5131	S5190	S8990	T2017	T2035	V2321	
S3823	S3853	S5135	S5199	S9150	T2018	T2036	V2745	

REVISED CODES/MODIFIERS

CB	C1718	E0149	E0967	E1225	L1844	L5648	L8658	V5363
A4232	C1719	E0950	E0972	E1226	L1950	L5848	M0100	V5364
A4326	C1720	E0951	E0973	E1390	L2405	L5984	M0301	
A4421	C2616	E0952	E0974	G0247	L3902	L6620	P9017	
A4538	E0141	E0958	E0978	J0880	L4350	L6675	S0199	
A4623	E0143	E0959	E0990	J7308	L4360	L6676	S2150	
A6025	E0144	E0961	E0992	K0455	L4386	L8110	S9123	
C1716	E0147	E0966	E0995	L1843	L5646	L8120	V5362	

DELETED CODES/MODIFIERS

A4214	C1018	E1065	K0025	K0087	K0550	K0613	Q9925	S8945
A4319	C1020	E1066	K0026	K0088	K0556	K0614	Q9926	S9524
A4323	C1021	E1069	K0027	K0089	K0557	K0615	Q9927	S9546
A4621	C1022	G0111	K0028	K0100	K0558	K0616	Q9928	S9802
A4622	C1166	G0112	K0029	K0103	K0559	K0617	Q9929	S9803
A4631	C1167	G0113	K0030	K0107	K0560	K0621	Q9930	S9806
A4712	C1207	G0114	K0031	K0112	K0581	K0622	Q9931	T1008
A6421	C1774	G0115	K0032	K0113	K0582	K0623	Q9932	T1011
A6422	C9010	G0116	K0033	K0268	K0583	K0624	Q9933	V2116
A6424	C9111	G0025	K0035	K0460	K0584	K0625	Q9934	V2117
A6426	C9116	G0167	K0036	K0461	K0585	K0626	Q9935	V2216
A6428	C9119	G0236	K0048	K0531	K0586	L1885	Q9936	V2217
A6430	C9120	G0256	K0049	K0532	K0587	L2102	Q9937	V2316
A6432	C9204	G0261	K0054	K0533	K0588	L2104	Q9938	V2317
A6434	C9503	G0262	K0055	K0534	K0589	L2122	Q9939	V2740
A6436	C9711	G0272	K0057	K0538	K0590	L2124	Q9940	V2741
A6438	E0142	G0273	K0058	K0539	K0591	Q0086	S0009	V2742
A6440	E0145	G0274	K0062	K0540	K0592	Q2010	S0079	V2743
A7019	E0146	J0151	K0063	K0541	K0593	Q4052	S0124	
A7020	E0165	J1910	K0079	K0542	K0594	Q4053	S0130	
A9518	E0943	J2000	K0080	K0543	K0595	Q4078	S0135	
C1010	E0975	J2352	K0082	K0544	K0596	Q9920	S0193	
C1011	E0976	J7508	K0083	K0545	K0597	Q9921	S0830	
C1015	E0979	J9180	K0084	K0546	K0610	Q9922	S8180	
C1016	E0991	K0016	K0085	K0547	K0611	Q9923	S8181	
C1017	E0993	K0022	K0086	K0549	K0612	Q9924	S8470	

CONTENTS

UNIT ONE

ICD-9-CM

UNIT ONE

ICD-9-CM

PART I

Introduction

ICD-9-CM BACKGROUND

The International Classification of Diseases, 9th Revision, Clinical Modification (ICD-9-CM) is based on the official version of the World Health Organization's 9th Revision, International Classification of Diseases (ICD-9). ICD-9 is designed for the classification of morbidity and mortality information for statistical purposes, and for the indexing of hospital records by disease and operations, for data storage and retrieval. The historical background of the International Classification of Diseases may be found in the Introduction to ICD-9 (Manual of the International Classification of Diseases, Injuries, and Causes of Death, World Health Organization, Geneva, Switzerland, 1977).

ICD-9-CM is a clinical modification of the World Health Organization's International Classification of Diseases, 9th Revision (ICD-9). The term "clinical" is used to emphasize the modification's intent: to serve as a useful tool in the area of classification of morbidity data for indexing of medical records, medical care review, and ambulatory and other medical care programs, as well as for basic health statistics. To describe the clinical picture of the patient, the codes must be more precise than those needed only for statistical groupings and trend analysis.

COORDINATION AND MAINTENANCE COMMITTEE

Annual modifications are made to the ICD-9-CM through the ICD-9-CM Coordination and Maintenance Committee (C&M). The Committee is made up of representatives from two Federal Government agencies, the National Center for Health Statistics and the Health Care Financing Administration. The Committee holds meetings twice a year which are open to the public. Modification proposals submitted to the Committee for consideration are presented at the meetings for public discussion. Those modification proposals which are approved are incorporated into the official government version of the ICD-9-CM and become effective for use October 1 of the year following their presentation. This CD-ROM contains the modifications approved from the 1995 C&M cycle.

This CD-ROM is the only official federal government version of the ICD-9-CM. It may be purchased through the Government Printing Office.

CHARACTERISTICS OF ICD-9-CM

ICD-9-CM far exceeds its predecessors in the number of codes provided. The disease classification has been expanded to include health-related conditions and to provide greater specificity at the fifth-digit level of detail. These fifth digits are not optional; they are intended for use in recording the information substantiated in the clinical record.

Volume I of ICD-9-CM contains five appendices:

Appendix A   Morphology of Neoplasms
Appendix B   Glossary of Mental Disorders
Appendix C   Classification of Drugs by American Hospital Formulary Service List Number and Their ICD-9-CM Equivalents
Appendix D   Classification of Industrial Accidents According to Agency
Appendix E   List of Three-Digit Categories

3

These appendices are included as a reference to the user in order to provide further information about the patient's clinical picture, to further define a diagnostic statement, to aid in classifying new drugs, or to reference three-digit categories.

Volume 2 of ICD-9-CM contains many diagnostic terms which do not appear in Volume 1 since the index includes most diagnostic terms currently in use.

The Disease Classification

ICD-9-CM is totally compatible with its parent system, ICD-9, thus meeting the need for comparability of morbidity and mortality statistics at the international level. A few fourth-digit codes were created in existing three-digit rubrics only when the necessary detail could not be accommodated by the use of a fifth-digit subclassification. To ensure that each rubric of ICD-9-CM collapses back to its ICD-9 counterpart the following specifications governed the ICD-9-CM disease classification:

Specifications for the Tabular List

1. Three-digit rubrics and their contents are unchanged from ICD-9.
2. The sequence of three-digit rubrics is unchanged from ICD-9.
3. Unsubdivided three-digit rubrics are subdivided where necessary to:
   a) Add clinical detail
   b) Isolate terms for clinical accuracy
4. The modification in ICD-9-CM is accomplished by the addition of a fifth digit to existing ICD-9 rubrics.
5. The optional dual classification in ICD-9 is modified.
   a) Duplicate rubrics are deleted:
      1) Four-digit manifestation categories duplicating etiology entries.
      2) Manifestation inclusion terms duplicating etiology entries.
   b) Manifestations of diseases are identified, to the extent possible, by creating five-digit codes in the etiology rubrics.
   c) When the manifestation of a disease cannot be included in the etiology rubrics, provision for its identification is made by retaining the ICD-9 rubrics used for classifying manifestations of disease.
6. The format of ICD-9-CM is revised from that used in ICD-9.
   a) American spelling of medical terms is used.
   b) Inclusion terms are indented beneath the titles of codes.
   c) Codes not to be used for principal tabulation of disease are printed with the notation, "Code first underlying disease."

Specifications for the Alphabetic Index

1. Format of the Alphabetic Index follows the format of ICD-9.
2. When two codes are required to indicate etiology and manifestation, the manifestation code appears in brackets, e.g., diabetic cataract 250.5X [366.41]. The etiology code is always sequenced first followed by the manifestation code.

ICD-9-CM Official Guidelines For Coding and Reporting

NOTE: Effective 10/1/03

The Centers for Medicare and Medicaid Services (CMS) formerly the Health Care Financing Administration (HCFA) and the National Center for Health Statistics (NCHS), two departments within the Department of Health and Human Services (DHHS) present the following guidelines for coding and reporting using the International Classification of Diseases, 9th Revision, Clinical Modification (ICD-9-CM). These guidelines should be used as a companion document to the official versions of the ICD-9-CM as published on CD-ROM.

These guidelines for coding and reporting have been developed and approved by the Cooperating Parties for ICD-9-CM: the American Hospital Association, the American Health Information Management Association, CMS, and the NCHS. These guidelines, published by the Department of Health and Human Services have also appeared in the Coding Clinic for ICD-9-CM, published by the American Hospital Association.

These guidelines have been developed to assist the user in coding and reporting in situations where the ICD-9-CM does not provide direction. Coding and sequencing instructions in volumes I, II, and III of ICD-9-CM take precedence over any guidelines. The conventions, general guidelines and chapter-specific guidelines apply to the proper use of ICD-9-CM, regardless of the health care setting. A joint effort between the attending physician and coder is essential to achieve complete and accurate documentation, code assignment, and reporting of diagnoses and procedures. These guidelines have been developed and approved by the Cooperating Parties to assist both the physician and the coder in identifying those diagnoses that are to be reported. The importance of consistent, complete documentation in the medical record cannot be overemphasized. Without such documentation the application of all coding guidelines is a difficult, if not impossible, task.

These guidelines are not exhaustive. The cooperating parties are continuing to conduct reviews of these guidelines and develop new guidelines as needed. Users of the ICD-9-CM should be aware that only guidelines approved by the cooperating parties are official. Revision of these guidelines and new guidelines will be published by the U.S. Department of Health and Human Services when they are approved by the cooperating parties. The term "admitted" is used generally to mean a health care encounter in any setting.

The guidelines have been reorganized into several new sections including an enhanced introduction that provides more detail about the structure and conventions of the classification usually found in the classification itself. The other new section, General Guidelines, brings together overarching guidelines that were previously found throughout the various sections of the guidelines. The new format of the guidelines also includes a resequencing of the disease-specific guidelines. They are sequenced in the same order as they appear in the tabular list chapters (Infectious and Parasitic Diseases, Neoplasms, etc.)

These changes will make it easier for coders, experienced and beginners, to more easily find the specific portion of the coding guideline information they seek.

Table of Contents

Section I Conventions, General Coding Guidelines and Chapter-Specific Guidelines

The conventions, general guidelines and chapter-specific guidelines are applicable to all health care settings unless otherwise indicated.

A. Conventions for the ICD-9-CM

The conventions for the ICD-9-CM are the general rules for use of the classification independent of the guidelines. These conventions are incorporated within the index and tabular of the ICD-9-CM as instructional notes. The conventions are as follows:

1. Format: The ICD-9-CM uses an indented format for ease in reference

2. Abbreviations
   a. Index Abbreviations
      NEC "Not elsewhere classifiable"

      This abbreviation in the index represents "other specified" When a specific code is not available for a condition the index directs the coder to the "other specified" code in the tabular.

   b. Tabular Abbreviations
      NEC "Not elsewhere classifiable"

      This abbreviation in the tabular represents "other specified" When a specific code is not available for a condition the tabular includes an NEC entry under a code to identify the code as the "other specified" code. (see "Other" codes)

      NOS "Not otherwise specified" This abbreviation is the equivalent of unspecified. (see "Unspecified" codes)

3. Punctuation

   [ ] Brackets are used in the tabular list to enclose synonyms, alternative wording or explanatory phrases. Brackets are used in the index to identify manifestation codes. (see etiology/manifestations)

   ( ) Parentheses are used in both the index and tabular to enclose supplementary words which may be present or absent in the statement of a disease or procedure without affecting the code number to which it is assigned. The terms within the parentheses are referred to as nonessential modifiers.

   : Colons are used in the Tabular list after an incomplete term which needs one or more of the modifiers following the colon to make it assignable to a given category.

4. Includes and Excludes Notes and Inclusion terms

   Includes: This note appears immediately under a three-digit code title to further define, or give examples of, the content of the category.

   Excludes: An excludes note under a code indicate that the terms excluded from the code are to be coded elsewhere. In some cases the codes for the excluded terms should not be used in conjunction with the code from which it is excluded. An example of this is a congenital condition excluded from an acquired form of the same condition. The congenital and acquired codes should not be used together. In other cases, the excluded terms may be used together with an excluded code. An example of this is when fractures of different bones are coded to different codes. Both codes may be used together if both types of fractures are present.

   Inclusion terms: List of terms are included under certain four and five digit codes. These terms are the conditions for which that code number is to be used. The terms may be synonyms of the code title, or, in the case of "other specified" codes, the terms are a list of the various conditions assigned to that code. The inclusion terms are not necessarily exhaustive. Additional terms found only in the index may also be assigned to a code.

5. Other and Unspecified codes

   a. "Other" codes

      Codes titled "other" or "other specified" (usually a code with a 4th digit 8 or fifth-digit 9 for diagnosis codes) are for use when the information in the medical record provides detail for which a specific code does not exist. Index entries with NEC in the line designate "other" codes in the tabular. These index entries represent specific disease entities for which no specific code exists so the term is included within an "other" code.

   b. "Unspecified" codes

      Codes (usually a code with a 4th digit 9 or 5th digit 0 for diagnosis codes) titled "unspecified" are for use when the information in the medical record is insufficient to assign a more specific code.

6. Etiology/manifestation convention ("code first", "use additional code" and "in diseases classified elsewhere" notes)

   Certain conditions have both an underlying etiology and multiple body system manifestations due to the underlying etiology. For such conditions the ICD-9-CM has a coding convention that requires the underlying condition be sequenced first followed by the manifestation. Wherever such a combination exists there is a "use additional code" note at the etiology code, and a "code first" note at the manifestation code. These instructional notes indicate the proper sequencing order of the codes, etiology followed by manifestation.

In most cases the manifestation codes will have in the code title, "in diseases classified elsewhere." Codes with this title are a component of the etiology/ manifestation convention. The code title indicates that it is a manifestation code. "In diseases classified elsewhere" codes are never permitted to be used as first listed or principle diagnosis codes. They must be used in conjunction with an underlying condition code and they must be listed following the underlying condition.

There are manifestation codes that do not have "in diseases classified elsewhere" in the title. For such codes a "use additional code" note will still be present and the rules for sequencing apply.

In addition to the notes in the tabular, these conditions also have a specific index entry structure. In the index both conditions are listed together with the etiology code first followed by the manifestation codes in brackets. The code in brackets is always to be sequenced second.

The most commonly used etiology/manifestation combinations are the codes for Diabetes mellitus, category 250. For each code under category 250 there is a use additional code note for the manifestation that is specific for that particular diabetic manifestation. Should a patient have more than one manifestation of diabetes more than one code from category 250 may be used with as many manifestation codes as are needed to fully describe the patient's complete diabetic condition. The 250 diabetes codes should be sequenced first, followed by the manifestation codes.

"Code first" and "Use additional code" notes are also used as sequencing rules in the classification for certain codes that are not part of an etiology/ manifestation combination. See - Other multiple coding for a single condition in the General Guidelines section.

B. General Coding Guidelines

1. Use of Both Alphabetic Index and Tabular List

   Use both the Alphabetic Index and the Tabular List when locating and assigning a code. Reliance on only the Alphabetic Index or the Tabular List leads to errors in code assignments and less specificity in code selection.

2. Locate each term in the Alphabetic Index and verify the code selected in the Tabular List. Read

and be guided by instructional notations that appear in both the Alphabetic Index and the Tabular List.

3. Level of Detail in Coding

   Diagnosis and procedure codes are to be used at their highest number of digits available.

   ICD-9-CM diagnosis codes are composed of codes with either 3, 4, or 5 digits. Codes with three digits are included in ICD-9-CM as the heading of a category of codes that may be further subdivided by the use of fourth and/or fifth digits, which provide greater detail.

   A three-digit code is to be used only if it is not further subdivided. Where fourth-digit subcategories and/or fifth-digit subclassifications are provided, they must be assigned. A code is invalid if it has not been coded to the full number of digits required for that code. For example, Acute myocardial infarction, code 410, has fourth digits that describe the location of the infarction (e.g., 410.2, Of inferolateral wall), and fifth digits that identify the episode of care. It would be incorrect to report a code in category 410 without a fourth and fifth digit.

   ICD-9-CM Volume 3 procedure codes are composed of codes with either 3 or 4 digits. Codes with two digits are included in ICD-9-CM as the heading of a category of codes that may be further subdivided by the use of third and/or fourth digits, which provide greater detail.

4. The appropriate code or codes from 001.0 through V83.89 must be used to identify diagnoses, symptoms, conditions, problems, complaints or other reason(s) for the encounter/ visit.

5. The selection of codes 001.0 through 999.9 will frequently be used to describe the reason for the admission/encounter. These codes are from the section of ICD-9-CM for the classification of diseases and injuries (e.g., infectious and parasitic diseases; neoplasms; symptoms, signs, and ill-defined conditions, etc.).

6. Codes that describe symptoms and signs, as opposed to diagnoses, are acceptable for reporting purposes when a related definitive diagnosis has not been established (confirmed) by the physician. Chapter 16 of ICD-9-CM, Symptoms, Signs, and Ill-defined conditions (codes 780.0 - 799.9) contain many, but not all codes for symptoms.

7. Conditions that are an integral part of a disease process

   Signs and symptoms that are integral to the disease process should not be assigned as additional codes.

8. Conditions that are not an integral part of a disease process

   Additional signs and symptoms that may not be

associated routinely with a disease process should be coded when present.

9. Multiple coding for a single condition

In addition to the etiology/manifestation convention that requires two codes to fully describe a single condition that affects multiple body systems, there are other single conditions that also require more than one code. "Use additional code" notes are found in the tabular at codes that are not part of an etiology/manifestation pair where a secondary code is useful to fully describe a condition. The sequencing rule is the same, "use additional code" indicates that a secondary code should be added.

For example, for infections that are not included in chapter 1, a secondary code from category 041, Bacterial infection in conditions classified elsewhere and of unspecified site, may be required to identify the bacterial organism causing the infection. A "use additional code" note will normally be found at the infection code indicates a need for the organism code to be added as a secondary code.

"Code first" notes are also under certain codes that are not specifically manifestation codes but may be due to an underlying cause. When a "code first" note is present and an underlying condition is present the underlying condition should be sequenced first. "Code, if applicable, any causal condition first", notes indicate that this code may be assigned as a principal diagnosis when the causal condition is unknown or not applicable. If a causal condition is known, then the code for that condition should be sequenced as the principal or first-listed diagnosis.

Multiple codes may be needed for late effects, complication codes and obstetric codes to more fully describe a condition. See the specific guidelines for these conditions for further instruction.

10. Acute and Chronic Conditions

If the same condition is described as both acute (subacute) and chronic, and separate subentries exist in the Alphabetic Index at the same indentation level, code both and sequence the acute (subacute) code first.

11. Combination Code

A combination code is a single code used to classify:

two diagnoses, or

A diagnosis with an associated secondary process (manifestation)

A diagnosis with an associated complication

Combination codes are identified by referring to subterm entries in the Alphabetic Index and by reading the inclusion and exclusion notes in the Tabular List.

Assign only the combination code when that code fully identifies the diagnostic conditions involved or when the Alphabetic Index so directs. Multiple coding should not be used when the classification provides a combination code that clearly identifies all of the elements documented in the diagnosis. When the combination code lacks necessary specificity in describing the manifestation or complication, an additional code may be used as a secondary code.

12. Late Effects

A late effect is the residual effect (condition produced) after the acute phase of an illness or injury has terminated. There is no time limit on when a late effect code can be used. The residual may be apparent early, such as in cerebrovascular accident cases, or it may occur months or years later, such as that due to a previous injury. Coding of late effects generally requires two codes sequenced in the following order: The condition or nature of the late effect is sequenced first. The late effect code is sequenced second.

An exception to the above guidelines are those instances where the code for late effect is followed by a manifestation code identified in the Tabular List and title, or the late effect code has been expanded (at the fourth and fifth-digit levels) to include the manifestation(s). The code for the acute phase of an illness or injury that led to the late effect is never used with a code for the late effect.

13. Impending or Threatened Condition

Code any condition described at the time of discharge as "impending" or "threatened" as follows:

If it did occur, code as confirmed diagnosis.

If it did not occur, reference the Alphabetic Index to determine if the condition has a subentry term for "impending" or "threatened" and also reference main term entries for "Impending" and for "Threatened."

If the subterms are listed, assign the given code.

If the subterms are not listed, code the existing underlying condition(s) and not the condition described as impending or threatened.

C. Chapter-Specific Coding Guidelines

In addition to general coding guidelines, there are guidelines for specific diagnoses and/or conditions in the classification. Unless otherwise indicated, these guidelines apply to all health care settings.

C1. Infectious and Parasitic Diseases

A. Human Immunodeficiency Virus (HIV) Infections

1. Code only confirmed cases of HIV infection/illness. This is an exception to the hospital inpatient guideline Section II, H.

In this context, "confirmation" does not require documentation of positive serology or culture for HIV; the physician's diagnostic statement that the patient is HIV positive, or has an HIV-related illness is sufficient.

2. Selection and sequencing

   a. If a patient is admitted for an HIV-related condition, the principal diagnosis should be 042, followed by additional diagnosis codes for all reported HIV-related conditions.

   b. If a patient with HIV disease is admitted for an unrelated condition (such as a traumatic injury), the code for the unrelated condition (e.g., the nature of injury code) should be the principal diagnosis. Other diagnoses would be 042 followed by additional diagnosis codes for all reported HIV-related conditions.

   c. Whether the patient is newly diagnosed or has had previous admissions/encounters for HIV conditions (or has expired) is irrelevant to the sequencing decision.

   d. V08 Asymptomatic human immunodeficiency virus [HIV] infection, is to be applied when the patient without any documentation of symptoms is listed as being "HIV positive," "known HIV," "HIV test positive," or similar terminology. Do not use this code if the term "AIDS" is used or if the patient is treated for any HIV-related illness or is described as having any condition(s) resulting from his/her HIV positive status; use 042 in these cases.

   e. Patients with inconclusive HIV serology, but no definitive diagnosis or manifestations of the illness, may be assigned code 795.71, Inconclusive serologic test for Human Immunodeficiency Virus [HIV]

   f. Previously diagnosed HIV-related illness

      Patients with any known prior diagnosis of an HIV-related illness should be coded to 042. Once a patient had developed an HIV-related illness, the patient should always be assigned code 042 on every subsequent admission/encounter. Patients previously diagnosed with any HIV illness (042) should never be assigned to 795.71 or V08.

   g. HIV Infection in Pregnancy, Childbirth and the Puerperium

      During pregnancy, childbirth or the puerperium, a patient admitted (or presenting for a health care encounter) because of an HIV-related illness should receive a principal diagnosis of 647.6X, Other specified infectious and parasitic diseases in the mother classifiable elsewhere, but complicating the pregnancy, childbirth or the puerperium, followed by 042 and the code(s) for the HIV-related illness(es). Codes from Chapter 15 always take sequencing priority.

      Patients with asymptomatic HIV infection status admitted (or presenting for a health care encounter) during pregnancy, childbirth, or the puerperium should receive codes of 647.6X and V08.

   h. Encounters for Testing for HIV

      If a patient is being seen to determine his/her HIV status, use code V73.89, Screening for other specified viral disease. Use code V69.8, Other problems related to lifestyle, as a secondary code if an asymptomatic patient is in a known high risk group for HIV. Should a patient with signs or symptoms or illness, or a confirmed HIV related diagnosis be tested for HIV, code the signs and symptoms or the diagnosis. An additional counseling code V65.44 may be used if counseling is provided during the encounter for the test.

      When a patient returns to be informed of his/her HIV test results use code V65.44, HIV counseling, if the results of the test are negative.

      If the results are positive but the patient is asymptomatic use code V08, Asymptomatic HIV infection. If the results are positive and the patient is symptomatic use code 042, HIV infection, with codes for the HIV related symptoms or diagnosis. The HIV counseling code may also be used if counseling is provided for patients with positive test results.

B. Septicemia, Systemic Inflammatory Response Syndrome (SIRS), Sepsis, Severe Sepsis, and Septic Shock

   1. In most cases, it will be a code from category 038, Septicemia, that will be used

in conjunction with a code from subcategory 995.9

   a. If the documentation in the record states streptococcal sepsis, codes 038.0 and code 995.91 should be used, in that sequence.

   b. If the documentation states streptococcal septicemia, only code 038.0 should be assigned, however, the physician should be queried whether the patient has sepsis, an infection with SIRS.

   c. Either the term sepsis or SIRS must be documented, to assign a code from subcategory 995.9.

2. If the terms sepsis, severe sepsis, or SIRS are used with an underlying infection other than septicemia, such as pneumonia, cellulitis or a nonspecified urinary tract infection, code 038.9 should be assigned first, then code 995.91, followed by the code for the initial infection. The use of the terms sepsis or SIRS indicates that the patient's infection has advanced to the point of a systemic infection so the systemic infection should be sequenced before the localized infection. The instructional note under subcategory 995.9 instructs to assign the underlying condition first.

Note: The term urosepsis is a nonspecific term. If that is the only term documented then only code 599.0 should be assigned based on the default for the term in the ICD-9-CM index, in addition to the code for the causal organism if known.

3. For patients with severe sepsis, the code for the systemic infection (038.x) or trauma should be sequenced first, followed by either code 995.92, Systemic inflammatory response syndrome due to infectious process with organ dysfunction, or code 995.94, Systemic inflammatory response syndrome due to noninfectious process with organ dysfunction. Codes for the specific organ dysfunctions should also be assigned.

4. If septic shock is documented, it is necessary to code first the initiating system infection or trauma, then either code 995.92 or 995.94, followed by code 785.52, Septic shock.

5. Sepsis and septic shock associated with abortion, ectopic pregnancy, and molar pregnancy are classified to category codes in Chapter 11 (630-639).

6. Negative or inconclusive blood cultures do not preclude a diagnosis of septicemia or sepsis in patients with clinical evidence of the condition, however, the physician should be queried.

  C2. Neoplasms

Chapter 2 of the ICD-9-CM contains the code for most benign and all malignant neoplasms. Certain benign neoplasms, such as prostatic adenomas, may be found in the specific body system chapters. To properly code a neoplasm it is necessary to determine from the record if the neoplasm is benign, in-situ, malignant, or of uncertain histologic behavior. If malignant, any secondary (metastatic) sites should also be determined.

The neoplasm table in the Alphabetic Index should be referenced first. If the histological term is documented, that term should be referenced first, rather than going immediately to the Neoplasm Table, in order to determine which column in the Neoplasm Table is appropriate. For example, if the documentation indicates "adenoma," refer to the term in the Alphabetic Index to review the entries under this term and the instructional note to "see also neoplasm, by site, benign." The table provides the proper code based on the type of neoplasm and the site. It is important to select the proper column in the table that corresponds to the type of neoplasm. The tabular should then be referenced to verify that the correct code has been selected from the table and that a more specific site code does not exist.

A. If the treatment is directed at the malignancy, designate the malignancy as the principal diagnosis.

B. When a patient is admitted because of a primary neoplasm with metastasis and treatment is directed toward the secondary site only, the secondary neoplasm is designated as the principal diagnosis even though the primary malignancy is still present.

C. Coding and sequencing of complications associated with the malignant neoplasm or with the therapy thereof are subject to the following guidelines:

1. When admission/encounter is for management of an anemia associated with the malignancy, and the treatment is only for anemia, the anemia is designated at the principal diagnosis and is followed by the appropriate code(s) for the malignancy.

2. When the admission/encounter is for management of an anemia associated with chemotherapy or radiotherapy and the only treatment is for the anemia, the anemia is sequenced first followed by the appropriate code(s) for the malignancy.

3. When the admission/encounter is for management of dehydration due to the malignancy or the therapy, or a combination of both, and only the dehydration is being treated (intravenous rehydration), the dehydration is sequenced first, followed by the code(s) for the malignancy.

11

4. When the admission/encounter is for treatment of a complication resulting from a surgical procedure performed for the treatment of an intestinal malignancy, designate the complication as the principal or first-listed diagnosis if treatment is directed at resolving the complication.

D. When a primary malignancy has been previously excised or eradicated from its site and there is no further treatment directed to that site and there is no evidence of any existing primary malignancy, a code from category V10, Personal history of malignant neoplasm, should be used to indicate the former site of the malignancy. Any mention of extension, invasion, or metastasis to another site is coded as a secondary malignant neoplasm to that site. The secondary site may be the principal or first-listed with the V10 code used as a secondary code.

E. Admissions/Encounters involving chemotherapy and radiation therapy

1. When an episode of care involves the surgical removal of a neoplasm, primary or secondary site, followed by chemotherapy or radiation treatment, the neoplasm code should be assigned as principal or first-listed diagnosis. When an episode of inpatient care involves surgical removal of a primary site or secondary site malignancy followed by adjunct chemotherapy or radiotherapy, code the malignancy as the principal or first-listed diagnosis, using codes in the 140-198 series or where appropriate in the 200-203 series.

2. If a patient admission/encounter is solely for the administration of chemotherapy or radiation therapy code V58.0, Encounter for radiation therapy, or V58.1, Encounter for chemotherapy, should be the first-listed or principal diagnosis. If a patient receives both chemotherapy and radiation therapy both codes should be listed, in either order of sequence.

3. When a patient is admitted for the purpose of radiotherapy or chemotherapy and develops complications such as uncontrolled nausea and vomiting or dehydration, the principal or first-listed diagnosis is V58.0, Encounter for radiotherapy, or V58.1, Encounter for chemotherapy.

F. When the reason for admission/encounter is to determine the extent of the malignancy, or for a procedure such as paracen-

tesis or thoracentesis, the primary malignancy or appropriate metastatic site is designated as the principal or first-listed diagnosis, even though chemotherapy or radiotherapy is administered.

G. Symptoms, signs, and ill-defined conditions listed in Chapter 16 characteristic of, or associated with, an existing primary or secondary site malignancy cannot be used to replace the malignancy as principal or first-listed diagnosis, regardless of the number of admissions or encounters for treatment and care of the neoplasm.

C3. Endocrine, Nutritional, and Metabolic Diseases and Immunity Disorders

Reserved for future guideline expansion

C4. Diseases of Blood and Blood Forming Organs

Reserved for future guideline expansion

C5. Mental Disorders

Reserved for future guideline expansion

C6. Diseases of Nervous System and Sense Organs

Reserved for future guideline expansion

C7. Diseases of Circulatory System

A. Hypertension

The Hypertension Table, found under the main term, "Hypertension", in the Alphabetic Index, contains a complete listing of all conditions due to or associated with hypertension and classifies them according to malignant, benign, and unspecified.

1. Hypertension, Essential, or NOS Assign hypertension (arterial) (essential) (primary) (systemic) (NOS) to category code 401 with the appropriate fourth digit to indicate malignant (.0), benign (.1), or unspecified (.9). Do not use either .0 malignant or .1 benign unless medical record documentation supports such a designation.

2. Hypertension with Heart Disease

Heart conditions (425.8, 429.0-429.3, 429.8, 429.9) are assigned to a code from category 402 when a causal relationship is stated (due to hypertension) or implied (hypertensive). Use an additional code from category 428 to identify the type of heart failure in those patients with heart failure. More than one code from category 428 may be assigned if the patient has systolic or diastolic failure and congestive heart failure.

The same heart conditions (425.8, 428, 429.0-429.3, 429.8, 429.9) with hypertension, but without a stated casual relationship, are coded separately. Sequence according to the circumstances of the admission/encounter.

3. Hypertensive Renal Disease with Chronic Renal Failure

   Assign codes from category 403, Hypertensive renal disease, when conditions classified to categories 585-587 are present. Unlike hypertension with heart disease, ICD-9-CM presumes a cause-and-effect relationship and classifies renal failure with hypertension as hypertensive renal disease.

4. Hypertensive Heart and Renal Disease

   Assign codes from combination category 404, Hypertensive heart and renal disease, when both hypertensive renal disease and hypertensive heart disease are stated in the diagnosis. Assume a relationship between the hypertension and the renal disease, whether or not the condition is so designated. Assign an additional code from category 428, to identify the type of heart failure. More than one code from category 428 may be assigned if the patient has systolic or diastolic failure and congestive heart failure.

5. Hypertensive Cerebrovascular Disease

   First assign codes from 430-438, Cerebrovascular disease, then the appropriate hypertension code from categories 401-405.

6. Hypertensive Retinopathy

   Two codes are necessary to identify the condition. First assign the code from subcategory 362.11, Hypertensive retinopathy, then the appropriate code from categories 401-405 to indicate the type of hypertension.

7. Hypertension, Secondary

   Two codes are required: one to identify the underlying etiology and one from category 405 to identify the hypertension. Sequencing of codes is determined by the reason for admission/encounter.

8. Hypertension, Transient

   Assign code 796.2, Elevated blood pressure reading without diagnosis of hypertension, unless patient has an established diagnosis of hypertension. Assign code 642.3x for transient hypertension of pregnancy.

9. Hypertension, Controlled

   Assign appropriate code from categories 401-405. This diagnostic statement usually refers to an existing state of hypertension under control by therapy.

10. Hypertension, Uncontrolled

    Uncontrolled hypertension may refer to untreated hypertension or hypertension not responding to current therapeutic regimen. In either case, assign the appropriate code from categories 401-405 to designate the stage and type of hypertension. Code to the type of hypertension.

11. Elevated Blood Pressure

    For a statement of elevated blood pressure without further specificity, assign code 796.2, Elevated blood pressure reading without diagnosis of hypertension, rather than a code from category 401.

Late Effects of Cerebrovascular Disease Category 438 is used to indicate conditions classifiable to categories 430-437 as the causes of late effects (neurologic deficits), themselves classified elsewhere. These "late effects" include neurologic deficits that persist after initial onset of conditions classifiable to 430-437. The neurologic deficits caused by cerebrovascular disease may be present from the onset or may arise at any time after the onset of the condition classifiable to 430-437. Codes from category 438 may be assigned on a health care record with codes from 430-437, if the patient has a current cerebrovascular accident (CVA) and deficits from an old CVA. Assign code V12.59 (and not a code from category 438) as an additional code for history of cerebrovascular disease when no neurologic deficits are present.

C8. Diseases of Respiratory System

   Reserved for future guideline expansion

C9. Diseases of Digestive System

   Reserved for future guideline expansion

C10. Diseases of Genitourinary System

   Reserved for future guideline expansion

C11. Complications of Pregnancy, Childbirth, and the Puerperium

   A. General Rules for Obstetric Cases

      1. Obstetric cases require codes from chapter 11, codes in the range 630-677, Complications of Pregnancy, Childbirth, and the Puerperium. Should the physician document that the pregnancy is incidental to the encounter, then code V22.2 should be used in place of any chapter 11 codes. It is the physician's responsibility to state that the condition being treated is not affecting the pregnancy.

      2. Chapter 11 codes have sequencing pri-

ority over codes from other chapters. Additional codes from other chapters may be used in conjunction with chapter 11 codes to further specify conditions. For example, sepsis and septic shock associated with abortion, ectopic pregnancy, and molar pregnancy are classified to category codes in Chapter 11 (630-639).

3. Chapter 11 codes are to be used only on the maternal record, never on the record of the newborn.

4. Categories 640-648, 651-676 have required fifth-digits, which indicate whether the encounter is antepartum, postpartum and whether a delivery has also occurred.

5. The fifth-digits, which are appropriate for each code number, are listed in brackets under each code. The fifth-digits on each code should all be consistent with each other. That is, should a delivery occur all of the fifth-digits should indicate the delivery.

6. For prenatal outpatient visits for patients with high-risk pregnancies, a code from category V23, Supervision of high-risk pregnancy, should be used as the principal or first-listed diagnosis. Secondary chapter 11 codes may be used in conjunction with these codes if appropriate. A thorough review of any pertinent excludes note is necessary to be certain that these V codes are being used properly.

7. An outcome of delivery code, V27.0-V27.9, should be included on every maternal record when a delivery has occurred. These codes are not to be used on subsequent records or on the newborn record.

8. For routine outpatient prenatal visits when no complications are present codes V22.0, Supervision of normal first pregnancy, and V22.1, Supervision of other normal pregnancy, should be used as the first-listed diagnoses. These codes should not be used in conjunction with chapter 11 codes.

B. Selection of OB Principal or First-listed Diagnosis

1. In episodes when no delivery occurs, the principal diagnosis should correspond to the principal complication of the pregnancy, which necessitated the encounter. Should more than one complication exist, all of which are treated or monitored, any of the complications codes may be sequenced first.

2. When a delivery occurs, the principal diagnosis should correspond to the main circumstances or complication of the delivery.

In cases of cesarean delivery, the selection of the principal diagnosis should correspond to the reason the cesarean delivery was performed unless the reason for admission/encounter was unrelated to the condition resulting in the cesarean delivery.

C. Fetal Conditions Affecting the Management of the Mother

Codes from category 655, Known or suspected fetal abnormality affecting management of the mother, and category 656, Other fetal and placental problems affecting the management of the mother, are assigned only when the fetal condition is actually responsible for modifying the management of the mother, i.e., by requiring diagnostic studies, additional observation, special care, or termination of pregnancy. The fact that the fetal condition exists does not justify assigning a code from this series to the mother's record.

D. HIV Infection in Pregnancy, Childbirth and the Puerperium

During pregnancy, childbirth or the puerperium, a patient admitted because of an HIV-related illness should receive a principal diagnosis of 647.6X, Other specified infectious and parasitic diseases in the mother classifiable elsewhere, but complicating the pregnancy, childbirth or the puerperium, followed by 042 and the code(s) for the HIV-related illness(es). This is an exception to the sequencing rule found in above.

Patients with asymptomatic HIV infection status admitted during pregnancy, childbirth, or the puerperium should receive codes of 647.6X and V08.

E. Normal Delivery, 650

1. Code 650 is for use in cases when a woman is admitted for a full-term normal delivery and delivers a single, healthy infant without any complications antepartum, during the delivery, or postpartum during the delivery episode.

2. Code 650 may be used if the patient had a complication at some point during her pregnancy but the complication is not present at the time of the admission for delivery.

3. Code 650 is always a principal diagnosis. It is not to be used if any other code

from chapter 11 is needed to describe a current complication of the antenatal, delivery, or perinatal period. Additional codes from other chapters may be used with code 650 if they are not related to or are in any way complicating the pregnancy.

4. V27.0, Single liveborn, is the only outcome of delivery code appropriate for use with 650.

F. The Postpartum Period

1. The postpartum period begins immediately after delivery and continues for six weeks following delivery.

2. A postpartum complication is any complication occurring within the six-week period.

3. Chapter 11 codes may also be used to describe pregnancy-related complications after the six-week period should the physician document that a condition is pregnancy related.

4. Postpartum complications that occur during the same admission as the delivery are identified with a fifth digit of "2." Subsequent admissions/encounters for postpartum complications should identified with a fifth digit of "4."

5. When the mother delivers outside the hospital prior to admission and is admitted for routine postpartum care and no complications are noted, code V24.0, Postpartum care and examination immediately after delivery, should be assigned as the principal diagnosis.

6. A delivery diagnosis code should not be used for a woman who has delivered prior to admission to the hospital. Any postpartum procedures should be coded.

G. Code 677, Late effect of complication of pregnancy, childbirth, and the puerperium

1. Code 677, Late effect of complication of pregnancy, childbirth, and the puerperium is for use in those cases when an initial complication of a pregnancy develops a sequelae requiring care or treatment at a future date.

2. This code may be used at any time after the initial postpartum period.

3. This code, like all late effect codes, is to be sequenced following the code describing the sequelae of the complication.

H. Abortions

1. Fifth-digits are required for abortion categories 634-637. Fifth-digit 1, incom-

plete, indicates that all of the products of conception have not been expelled from the uterus. Fifth-digit 2, complete, indicates that all products of conception have been expelled from the uterus prior to the episode of care.

2. A code from categories 640-648 and 651-657 may be used as additional codes with an abortion code to indicate the complication leading to the abortion.

Fifth digit 3 is assigned with codes from these categories when used with an abortion code because the other fifth digits will not apply. Codes from the 660-669 series are not to be used for complications of abortion.

3. Code 639 is to be used for all complications following abortion. Code 639 cannot be assigned with codes from categories 634-638.

4. Abortion with Liveborn Fetus.

When an attempted termination of pregnancy results in a liveborn fetus assign code 644.21, Early onset of delivery, with an appropriate code from category V27, Outcome of Delivery. The procedure code for the attempted termination of pregnancy should also be assigned.

5. Retained Products of Conception following an abortion.

Subsequent admissions for retained products of conception following a spontaneous or legally induced abortion are assigned the appropriate code from category 634, Spontaneous abortion, or legally induced abortion, with a fifth digit of "1" (incomplete). This advice is appropriate even when the patient was discharged previously with a discharge diagnosis of complete abortion.

C12. Diseases Skin and Subcutaneous Tissue

Reserved for future guideline expansion

C13. Diseases of Musculoskeletal and Connective Tissue

Reserved for future guideline expansion

C14. Congenital Anomalies

Reserved for future guideline expansion

C15. Newborn (Perinatal) Guidelines

For coding and reporting purposes the perinatal period is defined as birth through the 28th day following birth. The following guidelines are provided for reporting purposes. Hospitals may record other diagnoses as needed for internal data use.

A. General Perinatal Rule

All clinically significant conditions noted

on routine newborn examination should be coded. A condition is clinically significant if it requires:

clinical evaluation; or

therapeutic treatment; or

diagnostic procedures; or

extended length of hospital stay; or

increased nursing care and/or monitoring; or

has implications for future health care needs.

Note: The perinatal guidelines listed above are the same as the general coding guidelines for "additional diagnoses," except for the final point regarding implications for future health care needs. Whether or not a condition is clinically significant can only be determined by the physician.

B. Use of Codes V30-V39

When coding the birth of an infant, assign a code from categories V30-V39, according to the type of birth. A code from this series is assigned as a principal diagnosis, and assigned only once to a newborn at the time of birth.

C. Newborn Transfers

If the newborn is transferred to another institution, the V30 series is not used at the receiving hospital.

D. Use of Category V29

1. Assign a code from category V29, Observation and evaluation of newborns and infants for suspected conditions not found, to identify those instances when a healthy newborn is evaluated for a suspected condition that is determined after study not to be present. Do not use a code from category V29 when the patient has identified signs or symptoms of a suspected problem; in such cases, code the sign or symptom.

2. A V29 code is to be used as a secondary code after the V30, Outcome of delivery, code. It may also be assigned as a principal code for readmissions or encounters when the V30 code no longer applies. It is for use only for healthy newborns and infants for which no condition after study is found to be present.

E. Maternal Causes of Perinatal Morbidity

Codes from categories 760-763, Maternal causes of perinatal morbidity and mortality, are assigned only when the maternal condition has actually affected the fetus or newborn. The fact that the mother has an associated medical condition or experiences some complication of pregnancy, labor or delivery does not justify the routine assignment of codes from these categories to the newborn record.

F. Congenital Anomalies

Assign an appropriate code from categories 740-759, Congenital Anomalies, as an additional diagnosis when a specific abnormality is diagnosed for an infant. Congenital anomalies may also be the principal or first listed diagnosis for admissions/encounters subsequent to the newborn admission. Such abnormalities may occur as a set of symptoms or multiple malformations. A code should be assigned for each presenting manifestation of the syndrome if the syndrome is not specifically indexed in ICD-9-CM.

G. Coding of Additional Perinatal Diagnoses

1. Assign codes for conditions that require treatment or further investigation, prolong the length of stay, or require resource utilization.

2. Assign codes for conditions that have been specified by the physician as having implications for future health care needs.

Note: This guideline should not be used for adult patients.

3. Assign a code for Newborn conditions originating in the perinatal period (categories 760-779), as well as complications arising during the current episode of care classified in other chapters, only if the diagnoses have been documented by the responsible physician at the time of transfer or discharge as having affected the fetus or newborn.

H. Prematurity and Fetal Growth Retardation

Codes from category 764 and subcategories 765.0 and 765.1 should not be assigned based solely on recorded birthweight or estimated gestational age, but on the attending physician's clinical assessment of maturity of the infant. NOTE: Since physicians may utilize different criteria in determining prematurity, do not code the diagnosis of prematurity unless the physician documents this condition.

A code from subcategory 765.2, Weeks of gestation, should be assigned as an additional code with category 764 and codes from 765.0 and 765.1 to specify weeks of gestation as documented by the physician.

C16. Signs, Symptoms and Ill-Defined Conditions

Reserved for future guideline expansion

C17. Injury and Poisoning

A. Coding of Injuries

When coding injuries, assign separate codes for each injury unless a combination code is provided, in which case the combination code is assigned. Multiple injury codes are provided in ICD-9-CM, but should not be assigned unless information for a more specific code is not available. These codes are not to be used for normal, healing surgical wounds or to identify complications of surgical wounds.

The code for the most serious injury, as determined by the physician, is sequenced first.

1. Superficial injuries such as abrasions or contusions are not coded when associated with more severe injuries of the same site.

2. When a primary injury results in minor damage to peripheral nerves or blood vessels, the primary injury is sequenced first with additional code(s) from categories 950-957, Injury to nerves and spinal cord, and/or 900-904, Injury to blood vessels. When the primary injury is to the blood vessels or nerves, that injury should be sequenced first.

B. Coding of Fractures

The principles of multiple coding of injuries should be followed in coding fractures. Fractures of specified sites are coded individually by site in accordance with both the provisions within categories 800-829 and the level of detail furnished by medical record content. Combination categories for multiple fractures are provided for use when there is insufficient detail in the medical record (such as trauma cases transferred to another hospital), when the reporting form limits the number of codes that can be used in reporting pertinent clinical data, or when there is insufficient specificity at the fourth-digit or fifth-digit level. More specific guidelines are as follows:

1. Multiple fractures of same limb classifiable to the same three-digit or four-digit category are coded to that category.

2. Multiple unilateral or bilateral fractures of same bone(s) but classified to different fourth-digit subdivisions (bone part) within the same three-digit category are coded individually by site.

3. Multiple fracture categories 819 and 828 classify bilateral fractures of both upper limbs (819) and both lower limbs (828), but without any detail at the fourth-digit level other than open and closed type of fractures.

4. Multiple fractures are sequenced in accordance with the severity of the fracture and the physician should be asked to list the fracture diagnoses in the order of severity.

C. Coding of Burns

Current burns (940-948) are classified by depth, extent and by agent (E code). Burns are classified by depth as first degree (erythema), second degree (blistering), and third degree (full-thickness involvement).

1. Sequence first the code that reflects the highest degree of burn when more than one burn is present.

2. Classify burns of the same local site (three-digit category level, (940-947) but of different degrees to the subcategory identifying the highest degree recorded in the diagnosis.

3. Non-healing burns are coded as acute burns.

   Necrosis of burned skin should be coded as a non-healed burn.

4. Assign code 958.3, Posttraumatic wound infection, not elsewhere classified, as an additional code for any documented infected burn site.

5. When coding burns, assign separate codes for each burn site. Category 946 Burns of Multiple specified sites, should only be used if the location of the burns are not documented.

   Category 949, Burn, unspecified, is extremely vague and should rarely be used.

6. Assign codes from category 948, Burns classified according to extent of body surface involved, when the site of the burn is not specified or when there is a need for additional data. It is advisable to use category 948 as additional coding when needed to provide data for evaluating burn mortality, such as that needed by burn units. It is also advisable to use category 948 as an additional code for reporting purposes when there is mention of a third-degree burn involving 20 percent or more of the body surface.

   In assigning a code from category 948:
   Fourth-digit codes are used to identify the percentage of total body surface involved in a burn (all degree).

   Fifth-digits are assigned to identify the percentage of body surface involved in third-degree burn.

   Fifth-digit zero (0) is assigned when less

than 10 percent or when no body surface is involved in a third-degree burn.

Category 948 is based on the classic "rule of nines" in estimating body surface involved: head and neck are assigned nine percent, each arm nine percent, each leg 18 percent, the anterior trunk 18 percent, posterior trunk 18 percent, and genitalia one percent. Physicians may change these percentage assignments where necessary to accommodate infants and children who have proportionately larger heads than adults and patients who have large buttocks, thighs, or abdomen that involve burns.

7. Encounters for the treatment of the late effects of burns (i.e., scars or joint contractures) should be coded to the residual condition (sequelae) followed by the appropriate late effect code (906.5-906.9). A late effect E code may also be used, if desired.

8. When appropriate, both a sequelae with a late effect code, and a current burn code may be assigned on the same record.

D. Coding of Debridement of Wound, Infection, or Burn

Excisional debridement may be performed by a physician and/or other health care provider and involves an excisional, as opposed to a mechanical (brushing, scrubbing, washing) debridement.

For coding purposes, excisional debridement, 86.22.

Nonexcisional debridement is assigned to 86.28.

Modified based on Coding Clinic, 2nd Quarter 2000, p. 9.

E. Adverse Effects, Poisoning and Toxic Effects

The properties of certain drugs, medicinal and biological substances or combinations of such substances, may cause toxic reactions. The occurrence of drug toxicity is classified in ICD-9-CM as follows:

1. Adverse Effect

When the drug was correctly prescribed and properly administered, code the reaction plus the appropriate code from the E930-E949 series. Codes from the E930-E949 series must be used to identify the causative substance for an adverse effect of drug, medicinal and biological substances, correctly prescribed and properly administered. The effect,

such as tachycardia, delirium, gastrointestinal hemorrhaging, vomiting, hypokalemia, hepatitis, renal failure, or respiratory failure, is coded and followed by the appropriate code from the E930-E949 series.

Adverse effects of therapeutic substances correctly prescribed and properly administered (toxicity, synergistic reaction, side effect, and idiosyncratic reaction) may be due to (1) differences among patients, such as age, sex, disease, and genetic factors, and (2) drug-related factors, such as type of drug, route of administration, duration of therapy, dosage, and bioavailability.

2. Poisoning

a. When an error was made in drug prescription or in the administration of the drug by physician, nurse, patient, or other person, use the appropriate poisoning code from the 960-979 series.

b. If an overdose of a drug was intentionally taken or administered and resulted in drug toxicity, it would be coded as a poisoning (960-979 series).

c. If a nonprescribed drug or medicinal agent was taken in combination with a correctly prescribed and properly administered drug, any drug toxicity or other reaction resulting from the interaction of the two drugs would be classified as a poisoning.

d. When coding a poisoning or reaction to the improper use of a medication (e.g., wrong dose, wrong substance, wrong route of administration) the poisoning code is sequenced first, followed by a code for the manifestation. If there is also a diagnosis of drug abuse or dependence to the substance, the abuse or dependence is coded as an additional code.

C18. Classification of Factors Influencing Health Status and Contact with Health Service

A. ICD-9-CM provides codes to deal with encounters for circumstances other than a disease or injury. The Supplementary Classification of Factors Influencing Health Status and Contact with Health Services (V01.0-V83.89) is provided to deal with occasions when circumstances other than a disease or injury (codes 001-999) are recorded as a diagnosis or problem.

There are four primary circumstances for the use of V codes:

1. When a person who is not currently sick encounters the health services for some specific reason, such as to act as an organ donor, to receive prophylactic care, such as inoculations or health screenings, or to receive counseling on health related issue.

2. When a person with a resolving disease or injury, or a chronic, long-term condition requiring continuous care, encounters the health care system for specific aftercare of that disease or injury (e.g., dialysis for renal disease; chemotherapy for malignancy; cast change). A diagnosis/symptom code should be used whenever a current, acute, diagnosis is being treated or a sign or symptom is being studied.

3. When circumstances or problems influence a person's health status but are not in themselves a current illness or injury.

4. For newborns, to indicate birth status.

B. V codes are for use in both the inpatient and outpatient setting but are generally more applicable to the outpatient setting. V codes may be used as either a first listed (principal diagnosis code in the inpatient setting) or secondary code depending on the circumstances of the encounter. Certain V codes may only be used as first listed, others only as secondary codes.

C. V Codes indicate a reason for an encounter. They are not procedure codes. A corresponding procedure code must accompany a V code to describe the procedure performed.

D. Categories of V Codes

1. Contact/Exposure

Category V01 indicates contact with or exposure to communicable diseases. These codes are for patients who do not show any sign or symptom of a disease but have been exposed to it by close personal contact with an infected individual or are in an area where a disease is epidemic. These codes may be used as a first listed code to explain an encounter for testing, or, more commonly, as a secondary code to identify a potential risk.

2. Inoculations and vaccinations

Categories V03-V06 are for encounters for inoculations and vaccinations. They indicate that a patient is being seen to receive a prophylactic inoculation against a disease. The injection itself must be represented by the appropriate procedure code. A code from V03-V06 may be used as a secondary code if the inoculation is given as a routine part of preventive health care, such as a well-baby visit.

3. Status

Status codes indicate that a patient is either a carrier of a disease or has the sequelae or residual of a past disease or condition. This includes such things as the presence of prosthetic or mechanical devices resulting from past treatment. A status code is informative because the status may affect the course of treatment and its outcome. A status code is distinct from a history code. The history code indicates that the patient no longer has the condition.

The status V codes/categories are:

V02 Carrier or suspected carrier of infectious diseases

Carrier status, indicates that a person harbors the specific organisms of a disease without manifest symptoms and is capable of transmitting the infection.

V08 Asymptomatic HIV infection status

This code indicates that a patient has tested positive for HIV but has manifested no signs or symptoms of the disease.

V09 Infection with drug-resistant microorganisms

This category indicates that a patient has an infection which is resistant to drug treatment. Sequence the infection code first.

V21 Constitutional states in development

V22.2 Pregnant state, incidental

This code is a secondary code only for use when the pregnancy is in no way complicating the reason for visit. Otherwise, a code from the obstetric chapter is required.

V26.5x Sterilization status

V42 Organ or tissue replaced by transplant

V43 Organ or tissue replaced by other means

V44 Artificial opening status

V45 Other postsurgical states

V46 Other dependence on machines

V49.6 Upper limb amputation status

V49.7 Lower limb amputation status

V48.81 Postmenopausal status

V49.82 Dental sealant status

V58.6 Long-term (current) drug use

This subcategory indicates a patient's continuous use of a prescribed drug (including such things as aspirin therapy) for the long-term treatment of a condition or for prophylactic use. It is not for use for patients who have addictions to drugs.

V83 Genetic carrier status

Categories V42-V46, and subcategories V49.6, V49.7 are for use only if there are no complications or malfunctions of the organ or tissue replaced, the amputation site or the equipment on which the patient is dependent. These are always secondary codes.

4. History (of)

There are two types of history V codes, personal and family. Personal history codes explain a patient's past medical condition that no longer exists and is not receiving any treatment but that has the potential for recurrence, and, therefore, may require continued monitoring. The exceptions to this general rule are category V14, Personal history of allergy to medicinal agents and subcategory V15.0, Allergy, other than to medicinal agents. A person who has had an allergic episode to a substance or food in the past should always be considered allergic to the substance.

Family history codes are for use when a patient has a family member(s) who has had a particular disease that causes the patient to be at higher risk of also contracting the disease.

Personal history codes may be used in conjunction with follow-up codes and family history codes may be use in conjunction with screening codes to explain the need for a test or procedure. History codes are also acceptable on any medical record regardless of the reason for visit. A history of an illness, even if no longer present, is important information that may alter the type of treatment ordered.

The history V code categories are:

V10 Personal history of malignant neoplasm

V12 Personal history of certain other diseases

V13 Personal history of other diseases

Except: V13.4, Personal history of arthritis, and V13.6, Personal history of congenital malformations. These conditions are lifelong so are not true history codes.

V14 Personal history of allergy to medicinal agents

V15 Other personal history presenting hazards to health

Except: V15.7, Personal history of contraception.

V16 Family history of malignant neoplasm

V17 Family history of certain chronic disabling diseases

V18 Family history of certain other specific diseases

V19 Family history of other conditions

5. Screening

Screening is the testing for disease or disease precursors in seemingly well individuals so that early detection and treatment can be provided for those who test positive for the disease. Screenings that are recommended for many subgroups in a population include: routine mammograms for women over 40, a fecal occult blood test for everyone over 50, an amniocentesis to rule out a fetal anomaly for pregnant women over 35, because the incidence of breast cancer and colon cancer in these subgroups is higher than in the general population, as is the incidence of Down's syndrome in older mothers.

The testing of a person to rule out or confirm a suspected diagnosis because the patient has some sign or symptom is a diagnostic examination, not a screening. In these cases, the sign or symptom is used to explain the reason for the test.

A screening code may be a first listed code if the reason for the visit is specifically the screening exam. It may also be used as an additional code if the screening is done during an office visit for other health problems. A screening code is not necessary if the screening is inherent to a routine examination, such as a pap smear done during a routine pelvic examination.

Should a condition be discovered during the screening then the code for the condition may be assigned as an additional diagnosis.

The V code indicates that a screening exam is planned. A procedure code is required to confirm that the screening was performed.

The screening V code categories:

V28 Antenatal screening

V73-V82 Special screening examinations

6. Observation

There are two observation V code categories. They are for use in very limited circumstances when a person is being observed for a suspected condition that is ruled out. The observation codes are not for use if an injury or illness or any signs or symptoms related to the suspected condition are present. In such cases the diagnosis/symptom code is used with the corresponding E code to identify any external cause.

The observation codes are to be used as principal diagnosis only. The only exception to this is when the principal diagnosis is required to be a code from the V30, Live born infant, category. Then the V29 observation code is sequenced after the V30 code. Additional codes may be used in addition to the observation code but only if they are unrelated to the suspected condition being observed.

The observation V code categories:

V29 Observation and evaluation of newborns for suspected condition not found

A code from category V30 should be sequenced before the V29 code.

V71 Observation and evaluation for suspected condition not found

7. Aftercare

Aftercare visit codes cover situations when the initial treatment of a disease or injury has been performed and the patient requires continued care during the healing or recovery phase, or for the long-term consequences of the disease. The aftercare V code should not be used if treatment is directed at a current, acute disease or injury, the diagnosis code is to be used in these cases. Exceptions to this rule are codes V58.0, Radiotherapy, and V58.1, Chemotherapy. These codes are to be first listed, followed by the diagnosis code when a patient's encounter is solely to receive radiation therapy or chemotherapy for the treatment of a neoplasm. Should a patient receive both chemotherapy and radiation therapy during the same encounter code V58.0 and V58.1 may be used together on a record with either one being sequenced first.

The aftercare codes are generally first listed to explain the specific reason for the encounter. An aftercare code may be used as an additional code when some type of aftercare is provided in addition to the reason for admission and no diagnosis code is applicable. An example of this would be the closure of a colostomy during an encounter for treatment of another condition.

Certain aftercare V code categories need a secondary diagnosis code to describe the resolving condition or sequelae, for others, the condition is inherent in the code title.

Additional V code aftercare category terms include, fitting and adjustment, and attention to artificial openings.

The aftercare V category/codes:

V52 Fitting and adjustment of prosthetic device and implant

V53 Fitting and adjustment of other device

V54 Other orthopedic aftercare

V55 Attention to artificial openings

V56 Encounter for dialysis and dialysis catheter care

V57 Care involving the use of rehabilitation procedures

V58.0 Radiotherapy

V58.1 Chemotherapy

V58.3 Attention to surgical dressings and sutures

V58.41 Encounter for planned post-operative wound closure

V53.42 Aftercare, surgery, neoplasm

V53.43 Aftercare, surgery, trauma

V58.49 Other specified aftercare following surgery

V53.71-V53.78 Aftercare following surgery

V58.81 Fitting and adjustment of vascular catheter

V58.82 Fitting and adjustment of non-vascular catheter

V53.83 Monitoring therapeutic drug

V58.89 Other specified aftercare

8. Follow-up

The follow-up codes are for use to explain continuing surveillance following completed treatment of a disease, condition, or injury. They infer that the condition has been fully treated and no longer exists. They should not be confused with aftercare codes which explain current treatment for a healing condition or its sequelae. Follow-up codes may be used in conjunction with history codes to provide the full picture of the healed condition and its treatment. The follow-up code is sequenced first, followed by the history code.

A follow-up code may be used to explain repeated visits. Should a condition be found to have recurred on the follow-up visit, then the diagnosis code should be used in place of the follow-up code.

The follow-up V code categories:

V24 Postpartum care and evaluation

V67 Follow-up examination

9. Donor

Category V59 is the donor codes. They are for use for living individuals who are donating blood or other body tissue. These codes are only for individuals donating for others, not for self donations. They are not for use to identify cadaveric donations.

10. Counseling

Counseling V codes are for use for when a patient or family member receives assistance in the aftermath of an illness or injury, or when support is required in coping with family or social problems. They are not necessary for use in conjunction with a diagnosis code when the counseling component of care is considered integral to standard treatment.

The counseling V categories/codes:

V25.0 General counseling and advice for contraceptive management

V26.3 Genetic counseling

V26.4 General counseling and advice for procreative management

V61 Other family circumstances

V65.1 Person consulted on behalf of another person

V65.3 Dietary surveillance and counseling

V65.4 Other counseling, not elsewhere classified

11. Obstetrics and related conditions

See the Obstetrics guidelines for further instruction on the use of these codes.

V codes for pregnancy are for use in those circumstances when none of the problems or complications included in the codes from the Obstetrics chapter exist (a routine prenatal visit or post-partum care) V22.0, Supervision of normal first pregnancy, and V22.1, Supervision of other normal pregnancy, are always first listed and are not to be used with any other code from the OB chapter.

The outcome of delivery, category V27, should be included on all maternal delivery records. It is always a secondary code.

V codes for family planning (contraceptive) or procreative management and counseling should be included on an obstetric record either during the pregnancy or the postpartum stage, if applicable.

Obstetrics and related conditions V code categories:

V22 Normal pregnancy

V23 Supervision of high-risk pregnancy

Except: V23.2, Pregnancy with history of abortion. Code 646.3, Habitual aborter, from the OB chapter is required to indicate a history of abortion during a pregnancy.

V24 Postpartum care and evaluation

V25 Encounter for contraceptive management

Except V25.0x (See counseling above)

V26 Procreative management

Except V26.5x, Sterilization status, V26.3 and V26.4 (Counseling)

V27 Outcome of delivery

V28 Antenatal screening

See Screening—see section 5 of this article

12. Newborn, infant and child

See the newborn guidelines for further instruction on the use of these codes.

Newborn V code categories:

V20 Health supervision of infant or child

V29 Observation and evaluation of newborns for suspected condition not found—see Observation, section 6 of this article.

V30-V39 Liveborn infant according to type of birth

13. Routine and administrative examinations

The V codes allow for the description of encounters for routine examinations, such as, a general check-up, or, examinations for administrative purposes, such as, a pre-employment physical. The codes are for use as first listed codes only and are not to be used if the examination is for diagnosis of a suspected condition or for treatment purposes. In such cases the diagnosis code is used. During a routine exam, should a diagnosis or condition be discovered, it should be coded as an additional code. Pre-existing and chronic conditions, and history codes may also be included as additional codes as long as the examination is for administrative purposes and not focused on any particular condition.

Pre-operative examination V codes are for use only in those situations when a patient is being cleared for surgery and no treatment is given.

The V codes categories/code for routine and administrative examinations:

V20.2 Routine infant or child health check

> Any injections given should have a corresponding procedure code.

V70 General medical examination

V72 Special investigations and examinations

> Except V72.5 and V72.6

14. Miscellaneous V codes

The miscellaneous V codes capture a number of other health care encounters that do not fall into one of the other categories. Certain of these codes identify the reason for the encounter, others are for use as additional codes which provide useful information on circumstances which may affect a patient's care and treatment.

Miscellaneous V code categories/codes:

V07 Need for isolation and other prophylactic measures

V50 Elective surgery for purposes other than remedying health states

V58.5 Orthodontics

V60 Housing, household, and economic circumstances

V62 Other psychosocial circumstances

V63 Unavailability of other medical facilities for care

V64 Persons encountering health services for specific procedures, not carried out

V66 Convalescence and Palliative Care

V68 Encounters for administrative purposes

V69 Problems related to lifestyle

15. Nonspecific V codes

Certain V codes are so non-specific, or potentially redundant with other codes in the classification that there can be little justification for their use in the inpatient setting. Their use in the outpatient setting should be limited to those instances when there is no further documentation to permit more precise coding. Otherwise, any sign or symptom or any other reason for visit which is captured in another code should be used.

Nonspecific V code categories/codes:

V29 Personal history of mental disorder

> A code from the mental disorders chapter, with an in remission fifth-digit, should be used.

V13.4 Personal history of arthritis

V13.6 Personal history of congenital malformations

V15.7 Personal history of contraception

V23.2 Pregnancy with history of abortion

V40 Mental and behavioral problems

V41 Problems with special senses and other special functions

V47 Other problems with internal organs

V48 Problems with head, neck, and trunk

V49 Problems with limbs and other problems

> Exceptions:
>
> > V49.6 Upper limb amputation status
> >
> > V49.7 Lower limb amputation status

V49.81 Postmenopausal status

V49.82 Dental sealant status

V51 Aftercare involving the use of plastic surgery

V58.2 Blood transfusion, without reported diagnosis

V58.9 Unspecified aftercare

V72.5 Radiological examination, NEC

V72.6 Laboratory examination

Codes V72.5 and V72.6 are not to be used if any sign or symptoms, or reason for a test is documented. See section K and L of the outpatient guidelines.

C19. Supplemental Classification of External Causes of Injury and Poisoning (E codes)

Introduction: These guidelines are provided for those who are currently collecting E codes in order that there will be standardization in the process. If your institution plans to begin collecting E codes, these guidelines are to be applied. The use of E codes is supplemental to the application of ICD-9-CM diagnosis codes. E codes are never to be recorded as principal diagnosis (first-listed in noninpatient setting) and are not required for reporting to CMS.

External causes of injury and poisoning codes (E codes) are intended to provide data for injury research and evaluation of injury prevention strategies. E codes capture how the injury or poisoning happened (cause), the intent (unintentional or accidental; or intentional, such as suicide or assault), and the place where the event occurred. Some major categories of E codes include:

transport accidents

poisoning and adverse effects of drugs, medicinal substances and biologicals

accidental falls

accidents caused by fire and flames

accidents due to natural and environmental factors

late effects of accidents, assaults or self injury

assaults or purposely inflicted injury

suicide or self inflicted injury

These guidelines apply for the coding and collection of E codes from records in hospitals, outpatient clinics, emergency departments, other ambulatory care settings and physician offices, and nonacute care settings, except when other specific guidelines apply. (See Section III, Reporting Diagnostic Guidelines for Hospital-based Outpatient Services/Reporting Requirements for Physician Billing.)

A. General E Code Coding Guidelines

1. An E code may be used with any code in the range of 001-V83.02, which indicates an injury, poisoning, or adverse effect due to an external cause.

2. Assign the appropriate E code for all initial treatments of an injury, poisoning, or adverse effect of drugs.

3. Use a late effect E code for subsequent visits when a late effect of the initial injury or poisoning is being treated. There is no late effect E code for adverse effects of drugs.

4. Use the full range of E codes to completely describe the cause, the intent and the place of occurrence, if applicable, for all injuries, poisonings, and adverse effects of drugs.

5. Assign as many E codes as necessary to fully explain each cause. If only one E code can be recorded, assign the E code most related to the principal diagnosis.

6. The selection of the appropriate E code is guided by the Index to External Causes, which is located after the alphabetical index to diseases and by Inclusion and Exclusion notes in the Tabular List.

7. An E code can never be a principal (first listed) diagnosis.

B. Place of Occurrence Guideline

Use an additional code from category E849 to indicate the Place of Occurrence for injuries and poisonings. The Place of Occurrence describes the place where the event occurred and not the patient's activity at the time of the event.

Do not use E849.9 if the place of occurrence is not stated.

C. Adverse Effects of Drugs, Medicinal and Biological Substances Guidelines

1. Do not code directly from the Table of Drugs and Chemicals. Always refer back to the Tabular List.

2. Use as many codes as necessary to describe completely all drugs, medicinal or biological substances.

3. If the same E code would describe the causative agent for more than one adverse reaction, assign the code only once.

4. If two or more drugs, medicinal or bio-

logical substances are reported, code each individually unless the combination code is listed in the Table of Drugs and Chemicals. In that case, assign the E code for the combination.

5. When a reaction results from the interaction of a drug(s) and alcohol, use poisoning codes and E codes for both.

6. If the reporting format limits the number of E codes that can be used in reporting clinical data, code the one most related to the principal diagnosis. Include at least one from each category (cause, intent, place) if possible.

   If there are different fourth digit codes in the same three digit category, use the code for "Other specified" of that category. If there is no "Other specified" code in that category, use the appropriate "Unspecified" code in that category.

   If the codes are in different three digit categories, assign the appropriate E code for other multiple drugs and medicinal substances.

7. Codes from the E930-E949 series must be used to identify the causative substance for an adverse effect of drug, medicinal and biological substances, correctly prescribed and properly administered. The effect, such as tachycardia, delirium, gastrointestinal hemorrhaging, vomiting, hypokalemia, hepatitis, renal failure, or respiratory failure, is coded and followed by the appropriate code from the E930-E949 series.

D. Multiple Cause E Code Coding Guidelines

If two or more events cause separate injuries, an E code should be assigned for each cause. The first listed E code will be selected in the following order:

E codes for child and adult abuse take priority over all other E codes—see Child and Adult abuse guidelines

E codes for terrorism events take priority over all other E codes except child and adult abuse

E codes for cataclysmic events take priority over all other E codes except child and adult abuse and terrorism

E codes for transport accidents take priority over all other E codes except cataclysmic events and child and adult abuse and terrorism

The first-listed E code should correspond to the cause of the most serious diagnosis due to an assault, accident, or self-harm, following the order of hierarchy listed above.

E. Child and Adult Abuse Guideline

1. When the cause of an injury or neglect is intentional child or adult abuse, the first listed E code should be assigned from categories E960-E968, Homicide and injury purposely inflicted by other persons, (except category E967). An E code from category E967, Child and adult battering and other maltreatment, should be added as an additional code to identify the perpetrator, if known.

2. In cases of neglect when the intent is determined to be accidental E code E904.0, Abandonment or neglect of infant and helpless person, should be the first listed E code.

F. Unknown or Suspected Intent Guideline

1. If the intent (accident, self-harm, assault) of the cause of an injury or poisoning is unknown or unspecified, code the intent as undetermined E980-E989.

2. If the intent (accident, self-harm, assault) of the cause of an injury or poisoning is questionable, probable or suspected, code the intent as undetermined E980-E989.

G. Undetermined Cause

When the intent of an injury or poisoning is known, but the cause is unknown, use codes: E928.9, Unspecified accident, E958.9, Suicide and self-inflicted injury by unspecified means, and E968.9, Assault by unspecified means.

These E codes should rarely be used, as the documentation in the medical record, in both the inpatient outpatient and other settings, should normally provide sufficient detail to determine the cause of the injury.

H. Late Effects of External Cause Guidelines

1. Late effect E codes exist for injuries and poisonings but not for adverse effects of drugs, misadventures and surgical complications.

2. A late effect E code (E929, E959, E969, E977, E989, or E999.1) should be used with any report of a late effect or sequela resulting from a previous injury or poisoning (905-909).

3. A late effect E code should never be used with a related current nature of injury code.

I. Misadventures and Complications of Care Guidelines

1. Assign a code in the range of E870-E876 if misadventures are stated by the physician.

2. Assign a code in the range of E878-E879

if the physician attributes an abnormal reaction or later complication to a surgical or medical procedure, but does not mention misadventure at the time of the procedure as the cause of the reaction.

J. Terrorism Guidelines

1. When the cause of an injury is identified by the Federal Government (FBI) as terrorism, the first-listed E-code should be a code from category E979, Terrorism. The definition of terrorism employed by the FBI is found at the inclusion note at E979. The terrorism E-code is the only E-code that should be assigned. Additional E codes from the assault categories should not be assigned.

2. When the cause of an injury is suspected to be the result of terrorism a code from category E979 should not be assigned. Assign a code in the range of E codes based circumstances on the documentation of intent and mechanism.

3. Assign code E979.9, Terrorism, secondary effects, for conditions occurring subsequent to the terrorist event. This code should not be assigned for conditions that are due to the initial terrorist act.

4. For statistical purposes these codes will be tabulated within the category for assault, expanding the current category from E960-E969 to include E979 and E999.1.

Section II Selection of Principal Diagnos(es) for Inpatient, Short-term, Acute Care, and Long Term Care Hospital Records

The circumstances of inpatient admission always govern the selection of principal diagnosis. The principal diagnosis is defined in the Uniform Hospital Discharge Data Set (UHDDS) as "that condition established after study to be chiefly responsible for occasioning the admission of the patient to the hospital for care."

The UHDDS definitions are used by acute care short-term hospitals to report inpatient data elements in a standardized manner. These data elements and their definitions can be found in the July 31, 1985, Federal Register (Vol. 50, No, 147), pp. 31038-40.

In determining principal diagnosis the coding conventions in the ICD-9-CM, Volumes I and II take precedence over these official coding guidelines. (See Section IA).

The importance of consistent, complete documentation in the medical record cannot be overemphasized. Without such documentation the application of all coding guidelines is a difficult, if not impossible, task.

A. Codes for symptoms, signs, and ill-defined conditions

Codes for symptoms, signs, and ill-defined conditions from Chapter 16 are not to be used as principal diagnosis when a related definitive diagnosis has been established.

B. Two or more interrelated conditions, each potentially meeting the definition for principal diagnosis.

When there are two or more interrelated conditions (such as diseases in the same ICD-9-CM chapter or manifestations characteristically associated with a certain disease) potentially meeting the definition of principal diagnosis, either condition may be sequenced first, unless the circumstances of the admission, the therapy provided, the Tabular List, or the Alphabetic Index indicate otherwise.

C. Two or more diagnoses that equally meet the definition for principal diagnosis.

In the unusual instance when two or more diagnoses equally meet the criteria for principal diagnosis as determined by the circumstances of admission, diagnostic workup and/or therapy provided, and the Alphabetic Index, Tabular List, or another coding guidelines does not provide sequencing direction, any one of the diagnoses may be sequenced first.

D. Two or more comparative or contrasting conditions.

In those rare instances when two or more contrasting or comparative diagnoses are documented as "either/or" (or similar terminology), they are coded as if the diagnoses were confirmed and the diagnoses are sequenced according to the circumstances of the admission. If no further determination can be made as to which diagnosis should be principal, either diagnosis may be sequenced first.

E. A symptom(s) followed by contrasting/comparative diagnoses.

When a symptom(s) is followed by contrasting/comparative diagnoses, the symptom code is sequenced first. All the contrasting/comparative diagnoses should be coded as additional diagnoses.

F. Original treatment plan not carried out.

Sequence as the principal diagnosis the condition, which after study occasioned the admission to the hospital, even though treatment may not have been carried out due to unforeseen circumstances.

G. Complications of surgery and other medical care.

When the admission is for treatment of a complication resulting from surgery or other medical care, the complication code is sequenced as the principal diagnosis. If the complication is classified to the 996-999 series, an additional code for the specific complication may be assigned.

H. Uncertain Diagnosis.

If the diagnosis documented at the time of discharge is qualified as "probable", "suspected", "likely", "questionable", "possible", or "still to be ruled out", code the condition as if it existed or was established. The bases for these guidelines are the diagnostic workup, arrangements for further workup or observation, and initial therapeutic approach that correspond most closely with the established diagnosis.

Section III Reporting Additional Diagnoses for Inpatient, Short-term, Acute Care, and Long Term Care Hospital Records

GENERAL RULES FOR OTHER (ADDITIONAL) DIAGNOSES

For reporting purposes the definition for—other diagnoses" is interpreted as additional conditions that affect patient care in terms of requiring:

clinical evaluation; or

therapeutic treatment; or

diagnostic procedures; or

extended length of hospital stay; or

increased nursing care and/or monitoring.

The UHDDS item #11-b defines Other Diagnoses as "all conditions that coexist at the time of admission, that develop subsequently, or that affect the treatment received and/or the length of stay. Diagnoses that relate to an earlier episode which have no bearing on the current hospital stay are to be excluded." UHDDS definitions apply to inpatients in acute care, short-term, hospital setting. THe UHDDS definitions are used by acute care short-term hospitals to report inpatient data elements in a standardized manner. These data elements and their definitions can be found in the July 31, 1985, Federal Register (Vol. 50, No, 147), pp. 31038–40.

The following guidelines are to be applied in designating "other diagnoses" when neither the Alphabetic Index nor the Tabular List in ICD-9-CM provide direction. The listing of the diagnoses in the patient record is the responsibility of the attending physician.

A. Previous conditions

If the physician has included a diagnosis in the final diagnostic statement, such as the discharge summary or the face sheet, it should ordinarily be coded. Some physicians include in the diagnostic statement resolved conditions or diagnoses and status-post procedures from previous admission that have no bearing on the current stay. Such conditions are not to be reported and are coded only if required by hospital policy.

However, history codes (V10-V19) may be used as secondary codes if the historical condition or family history has an impact on current care or influences treatment.

B. Abnormal findings

Abnormal findings (laboratory, x-ray, pathologic, and other diagnostic results) are not coded and reported unless the physician indicates their clinical significance. If the findings are outside the normal range and the attending physician has ordered other tests to evaluate the condition or prescribed treatment, it is appropriate to ask the physician whether the abnormal finding should be added.

Please note: This differs from the coding practices in the outpatient setting for coding encounters for diagnostic tests that have been interpreted by a physician.

C. Uncertain Diagnosis

If the diagnosis documented at the time of discharge is qualified as "probable", "suspected", "likely", "questionable", "possible", or "still to be ruled out", code the condition as if it existed or was established. The bases for these guidelines are the diagnostic workup, arrangements for further workup or observation, and initial therapeutic approach that correspond most closely with the established diagnosis.

Section IV Diagnostic Coding and Reporting Guidelines for Outpatient Services

These coding guidelines for outpatient diagnoses have been approved for use by hospitals/physicians in coding and reporting hospital-based outpatient services and physician office visits.

Information about the use of certain abbreviations, punctuation, symbols, and other conventions used in the ICD-9-CM Tabular List (code numbers and titles), can be found in Section IA of these guidelines, under "Conventions Used in the Tabular List." Information about the correct sequence to use in finding a code is also described in Section I.

The terms encounter and visit are often used interchangeably in describing outpatient service contacts and, therefore, appear together in these guidelines without distinguishing one from the other.

Though the conventions and general guidelines apply to all settings, coding guidelines for outpatient and physician reporting of diagnoses will vary in a number of instances from those for inpatient diagnoses, recognizing that:

The Uniform Hospital Discharge Data Set (UHDDS) definition of principal diagnosis applies only to inpatients in acute, short-term, and Long Term Care hospitals.

Coding guidelines for inconclusive diagnoses (probable, suspected, rule out, etc.) were developed for inpatient reporting and do not apply to outpatients.

A. Selection of first-listed condition

In the outpatient setting, the term first-listed diagnosis is used in lieu of principal diagnosis.

In determining the first-listed diagnosis the coding conventions of ICD-9-CM, as well as the general and disease specific guidelines take precedence over the outpatient guidelines.

Diagnoses often are not established at the time of the initial encounter/visit. It may take two or more visits before the diagnosis is confirmed.

The most critical rule involves beginning the search for the correct code assignment through the Alphabetic Index. Never begin searching initially in the Tabular List as this will lead to coding errors.

B. The appropriate code or codes from 001.0 through V83.89 must be used to identify diagnoses, symptoms, conditions, problems, complaints, or other reason(s) for the encounter/visit.

C. For accurate reporting of ICD-9-CM diagnosis codes, the documentation should describe the patient's condition, using terminology which includes specific diagnoses as well as symptoms, problems, or reasons for the encounter. There are ICD-9-CM codes to describe all of these.

D. The selection of codes 001.0 through 999.9 will frequently be used to describe the reason for the encounter. These codes are from the section of ICD-9-CM for the classification of diseases and injuries (e.g. infectious and parasitic diseases; neoplasms; symptoms, signs, and ill-defined conditions, etc.).

E. Codes that describe symptoms and signs, as opposed to diagnoses, are acceptable for reporting purposes when a diagnosis has not been established (confirmed) by the physician. Chapter 16 of ICD-9-CM, Symptoms, Signs, and Ill-defined conditions (codes 780.0 - 799.9) contain many, but not all codes for symptoms.

F. ICD-9-CM provides codes to deal with encounters for circumstances other than a disease or injury. The Supplementary Classification of factors Influencing Health Status and Contact with Health Services (V01.0- V83.89) is provided to deal with occasions when circumstances other than a disease or injury are recorded as diagnosis or problems.

G. Level of Detail in Coding

1. ICD-9-CM is composed of codes with either 3, 4, or 5 digits. Codes with three digits are included in ICD-9-CM as the heading of a category of codes that may be further subdivided by the use of fourth and/or fifth digits, which provide greater specificity.

2. A three-digit code is to be used only if it is not further subdivided. Where fourth-digit subcategories and/or fifth-digit subclassifications are provided, they must be assigned. A code is invalid if it has not been coded to the full number of digits required for that code. See also discussion under Section I, General Coding Guidelines, Level of Detail.

H. List first the ICD-9-CM code for the diagnosis, condition, problem, or other reason for encounter/visit shown in the medical record to be chiefly responsible for the services provided. List additional codes that describe any coexisting conditions.

I. Do not code diagnoses documented as "probable", "suspected," "questionable," "rule out," or "working diagnosis". Rather, code the condition(s) to the highest degree of certainty for that encounter/visit, such as symptoms, signs, abnormal test results, or other reason for the visit.

Please note: This differs from the coding practices used by hospital medical record departments for coding the diagnosis of acute care, short-term hospital inpatients.

J. Chronic diseases treated on an ongoing basis may be coded and reported as many times as the patient receives treatment and care for the condition(s).

K. Code all documented conditions that coexist at the time of the encounter/visit, and require or affect patient care treatment or management. Do not code conditions that were previously treated and no longer exist. However, history codes (V10-V19) may be used as secondary codes if the historical condition or family history has an impact on current care or influences treatment.

L. For patients receiving diagnostic services only during an encounter/visit, sequence first the diagnosis, condition, problem, or other reason for encounter/visit shown in the medical record to be chiefly responsible for the outpatient services provided during the encounter/visit. Codes for other diagnoses (e.g., chronic conditions) may be sequenced as additional diagnoses.

For outpatient encounters for diagnostic tests that have been interpreted by a physician, and the final report is available at the time of coding, code any confirmed or definitive diagnosis(es) documented in the interpretation. Do not code related signs and symptoms as additional diagnoses.

Please note: This differs from the coding practice in the hospital inpatient setting regarding abnormal findings on test results.

M. For patients receiving therapeutic services only during an encounter/visit, sequence first the diagnosis, condition, problem, or other reason for encounter/visit shown in the medical record to be chiefly responsible for the outpatient services provided during the encounter/visit. Codes for other diagnoses (e.g., chronic conditions) may be sequenced as additional diagnoses.

The only exception to this rule is that when the primary reason for the admission/encounter is chemotherapy, radiation therapy, or rehabilitation, the appropriate V code for the service is listed first, and the diagnosis or problem for which the service is being performed listed second.

N. For patients receiving preoperative evaluations only, sequence a code from category V72.8, Other specified examinations, to describe the pre-op consultations. Assign a code for the condition to describe the reason for the surgery as an additional diagnosis. Code also any findings related to the pre-op evaluation.

O. For ambulatory surgery, code the diagnosis for which the surgery was performed. If the postop-erative diagnosis is known to be different from the preoperative diagnosis at the time the diagnosis is confirmed, select the postoperative diagnosis for coding, since it is the most definitive.

P. For routine outpatient prenatal visits when no complications are present codes V22.0, Supervision of normal first pregnancy, and V22.1, Supervision of other normal pregnancy, should be used as principal diagnoses. These codes should not be used in conjunction with chapter 11 codes.

PART II

Alphabetic Index, Volume 2

SECTION I INDEX TO DISEASES

A

AAT (alpha-1 antitrypsin) deficiency 273.4 ◄

AAV (disease) (illness) (infection) - *see* Human immunodeficiency virus (disease) (illness) (infection)

Abactio - *see* Abortion, induced

Abactus venter - *see* Abortion, induced

Abarognosis 781.99

Abasia (-astasia) 307.9
  atactica 781.3
  choreic 781.3
  hysterical 300.11
  paroxysmal trepidant 781.3
  spastic 781.3
  trembling 781.3
  trepidans 781.3

Abderhalden-Kaufmann-Lignac syndrome (cystinosis) 270.0

Abdomen, abdominal - *see also* condition
  accordion 306.4
  acute 789.0
  angina 557.1
  burst 868.00
  convulsive equivalent (*see also* Epilepsy) 345.5
  heart 746.87
  muscle deficiency syndrome 756.79
  obstipum 756.79

Abdominalgia 789.0
  periodic 277.3

Abduction contracture, hip or other joint - *see* Contraction, joint

Abercrombie's syndrome (amyloid degeneration) 277.3

Aberrant (congenital) - *see also* Malposition, congenital
  adrenal gland 759.1
  blood vessel NEC 747.60
    arteriovenous NEC 747.60
    cerebrovascular 747.81
    gastrointestinal 747.61
    lower limb 747.64
    renal 747.62
    spinal 747.82
    upper limb 747.63
  breast 757.6
  endocrine gland NEC 759.2
  gastrointestinal vessel (peripheral) 747.61
  hepatic duct 751.69
  lower limb vessel (peripheral) 747.64
  pancreas 751.7
  parathyroid gland 759.2
  peripheral vascular vessel NEC 747.60
  pituitary gland (pharyngeal) 759.2
  renal blood vessel 747.62
  sebaceous glands, mucous membrane, mouth 750.26
  spinal vessel 747.82
  spleen 759.0
  testis (descent) 752.51
  thymus gland 759.2
  thyroid gland 759.2
  upper limb vessel (peripheral) 747.63

Aberratio
  lactis 757.6
  testis 752.51

Aberration - *see also* Anomaly
  chromosome - *see* Anomaly, chromosome(s)
  distalial 368.9

Aberration *(Continued)*
  mental (*see also* Disorder, mental, nonpsychotic) 300.9

Abetalipoproteinemia 272.5

Abionarce 780.79

Abiotrophy 799.89

Ablatio
  placentae - *see* Placenta, ablatio
  retinae (*see also* Detachment, retina) 361.9

Ablation
  pituitary (gland) (with hypofunction) 253.7
  placenta - *see* Placenta, ablatio
  uterus 621.8

Ablepharia, ablepharon, ablephary 743.62

Ablepsia - *see* Blindness

Ablepsy - *see* Blindness

Ablutomania 300.3

Abnormal, abnormality, abnormalities - *see also* Anomaly
  acid-base balance 276.4
    fetus or newborn - *see* Distress, fetal
  adaptation curve, dark 368.63
  alveolar ridge 525.9
  amnion 658.9
    affecting fetus or newborn 762.9
  anatomical relationship NEC 759.9
  apertures, congenital, diaphragm 756.6
  auditory perception NEC 388.40
  autosomes NEC 758.5
    13 758.1
    18 758.2
    21 or 22 758.0
    D_1 758.1
    E_3 758.2
    G 758.0
  ballistocardiogram 794.39
  basal metabolic rate (BMR) 794.7
  biosynthesis, testicular androgen 257.2
  blood level (of)
    cobalt 790.6
    copper 790.6
    iron 790.6
    lithium 790.6
    magnesium 790.6
    mineral 790.6
    zinc 790.6
  blood pressure
    elevated (without diagnosis of hypertension) 796.2
    low (*see also* Hypotension) 458.9
      reading (incidental) (isolated) (nonspecific) 796.3
  bowel sounds 787.5
  breathing behavior - *see* Respiration
  caloric test 794.19
  cervix (acquired) NEC 622.9
    congenital 752.40
    in pregnancy or childbirth 654.6
      causing obstructed labor 660.2
        affecting fetus or newborn 763.1
  chemistry, blood NEC 790.6
  chest sounds 786.7
  chorion 658.9
    affecting fetus or newborn 762.9
  chromosomal NEC 758.89
    analysis, nonspecific result 795.2
    autosomes (*see also* Abnormal, autosomes NEC) 758.5
    fetal (suspected), affecting management of pregnancy 655.1
    sex 758.81

Abnormal, abnormality, abnormalities *(Continued)*
  clinical findings NEC 796.4
  communication - *see* Fistula
  configuration of pupils 379.49
  coronary
    artery 746.85
    vein 746.9
  cortisol-binding globulin 255.8
  course, Eustachian tube 744.24
  dentofacial NEC 524.9
    functional 524.50 ◄▦
    specified type NEC 524.89 ◄▦
  development, developmental NEC 759.9
    bone 756.9
    central nervous system 742.9
  direction, teeth 524.30 ◄▦
  dynia (*see also* Defect, coagulation) 286.9
  Ebstein 746.2
  echocardiogram 793.2
  echoencephalogram 794.01
  echogram NEC - *see* Findings, abnormal, structure
  electrocardiogram (ECG) (EKG) 794.31
  electroencephalogram (EEG) 794.02
  electromyogram (EMG) 794.17
    ocular 794.14
  electro-oculogram (EOG) 794.12
  electroretinogram (ERG) 794.11
  erythrocytes 289.9
    congenital, with perinatal jaundice 282.9 [774.0]
  eustachian valve 746.9
  excitability under minor stress 301.9
  fat distribution 782.9
  feces 787.7
  fetal heart rate - *see* Distress, fetal
  fetus NEC
    affecting management of pregnancy - *see* Pregnancy, management affected by, fetal
    causing disproportion 653.7
      affecting fetus or newborn 763.1
      causing obstructed labor 660.1
        affecting fetus or newborn 763.1
  findings without manifest disease - *see* Findings, abnormal
  fluid
    amniotic 792.3
    cerebrospinal 792.0
    peritoneal 792.9
    pleural 792.9
    synovial 792.9
    vaginal 792.9
  forces of labor NEC 661.9
    affecting fetus or newborn 763.7
  form, teeth 520.2
  function studies
    auditory 794.15
    bladder 794.9
    brain 794.00
    cardiovascular 794.30
    endocrine NEC 794.6
    kidney 794.4
    liver 794.8
    nervous system
      central 794.00
      peripheral 794.19
    oculomotor 794.14
    pancreas 794.9

ICD-9-CM

A

Vol. 2

Abnormal, abnormality, abnormalities
(*Continued*)
function studies (*Continued*)
placenta 794.9
pulmonary 794.2
retina 794.11
special senses 794.19
spleen 794.9
thyroid 794.5
vestibular 794.16
gait 781.2
hysterical 300.11
gastrin secretion 251.5
globulin
cortisol-binding 255.8
thyroid-binding 246.8
glucagon secretion 251.4
glucose 790.29
in pregnancy, childbirth, or puerperium 648.8
fetus or newborn 775.0
non-fasting 790.29
gravitational (G) forces or states 994.9
hair NEC 704.2
hard tissue formation in pulp 522.3
head movement 781.0
heart
rate
fetus affecting livreborninfant
before the onset of labor 763.81
during labor 763.82
unspecified as to time of onset 763.83
intrauterine
before the onset of labor 763.81
during labor 763.82
unspecified as to time of onset 763.83
newborn
before the onset of labor 763.81
during labor 763.82
unspecified as to time of onset 763.83
shadow 793.2
sounds NEC 785.3
hemoglobin (*see also* Disease, hemoglobin) 282.7
trait - *see* Trait, hemoglobin, abnormal
hemorrhage, uterus - *see* Hemorrhage, uterus
histology NEC 795.4
increase
in
appetite 783.6
development 783.9
involuntary movement 781.0
jaw closure 524.51　　　　◀▥▥
karyotype 795.2
knee jerk 796.1
labor NEC 661.9
affecting fetus or newborn 763.7
laboratory findings - *see* Findings, abnormal
length, organ or site, congenital - *see* Distortion
loss of height 781.91
loss of weight 783.21
lung shadow 793.1
mammogram 793.80
microcalcification 793.81
Mantoux test 795.5

Abnormal, abnormality, abnormalities
(*Continued*)
membranes (fetal)
affecting fetus or newborn 762.9
complicating pregnancy 658.8
menstruation - *see* Menstruation
metabolism (*see also* condition) 783.9
movement 781.0
disorder NEC 333.90
sleep related 780.58　　　◀
specified NEC 333.99
head 781.0
involuntary 781.0
specified type NEC 333.99
muscle contraction, localized 728.85
myoglobin (Aberdeen) (Annapolis) 289.9
narrowness, eyelid 743.62
optokinetic response 379.57
organs or tissues of pelvis NEC
in pregnancy or childbirth 654.9
affecting fetus or newborn 763.89
causing obstructed labor 660.2
affecting fetus or newborn 763.1
origin - *see* Malposition, congenital
palmar creases 757.2
Papanicolaou (smear)
cervix 795.00
with　　　　　　　　　　◀
atypical squamous cells　　◀▥▥
cannot exclude high grade squamous intraepithelial lesion (ASC-H) 795.01　　　◀▥▥
of undetermined significance (ASC-US) 795.02　　◀▥▥
high grade squamous intraepithelial lesion (HGSIL) 795.04　　　　　　◀
low grade squamous intraepithelial lesion (LGSIL) 795.03　　　　　　◀
nonspecific findings NEC 795.09
other site 795.1
parturition
affecting fetus or newborn 763.9
mother - *see* Delivery, complicated
pelvis (bony) - *see* Deformity, pelvis
percussion, chest 786.7
periods (grossly) (*see also* Menstruation) 626.9
phonocardiogram 794.39
placenta - *see* Placenta, abnormal
plantar reflex 796.1
plasma protein - *see* Deficiency, plasma, protein
pleural folds 748.8
position - *see also* Malposition
gravid uterus 654.4
causing obstructed labor 660.2
affecting fetus or newborn 763.1
posture NEC 781.92
presentation (fetus) - *see* Presentation, fetus, abnormal
product of conception NEC 631
puberty - *see* Puberty
pulmonary
artery 747.3
function, newborn 770.89
test results 794.2
ventilation, newborn 770.89
hyperventilation 786.01
pulsations in neck 785.1
pupil reflexes 379.40
quality of milk 676.8

Abnormal, abnormality, abnormalities
(*Continued*)
radiological examination 793.9
abdomen NEC 793.6
biliary tract 793.3
breast 793.89
mammogram NOS 793.80
mammographic microcalcification 793.81
gastrointestinal tract 793.4
genitourinary organs 793.5
head 793.0
intrathoracic organ NEC 793.2
lung (field) 793.1
musculoskeletal system 793.7
retroperitoneum 793.6
skin and subcutaneous tissue 793.9
skull 793.0
red blood cells 790.09
morphology 790.09
volume 790.09
reflex NEC 796.1
renal function test 794.4
respiration signs - *see* Respiration
response to nerve stimulation 794.10
retinal correspondence 368.34
rhythm, heart - *see also* Arrhythmia
fetus - *see* Distress, fetal
saliva 792.4
scan
brain 794.09
kidney 794.4
liver 794.8
lung 794.2
thyroid 794.5
secretion
gastrin 251.5
glucagon 251.4
semen 792.2
serum level (of)
acid phosphatase 790.5
alkaline phosphatase 790.5
amylase 790.5
enzymes NEC 790.5
lipase 790.5
shape
cornea 743.41
gallbladder 751.69
gravid uterus 654.4
affecting fetus or newborn 763.89
causing obstructed labor 660.2
affecting fetus or newborn 763.1
head (*see also* Anomaly, skull) 756.0
organ or site, congenital NEC - *see* Distortion
sinus venosus 747.40
size
fetus, complicating delivery 653.5
causing obstructed labor 660.1
gallbladder 751.69
head (*see also* Anomaly, skull) 756.0
organ or site, congenital NEC - *see* Distortion
teeth 520.2
skin and appendages, congenital NEC 757.9
soft parts of pelvis - *see* Abnormal, organs or tissues of pelvis
spermatozoa 792.2
sputum (amount) (color) (excessive) (odor) (purulent) 786.4
stool NEC 787.7
bloody 578.1
occult 792.1

Abnormal, abnormality, abnormalities
  (Continued)
  stool NEC *(Continued)*
    bulky 787.7
    color (dark) (light) 792.1
    content (fat) (mucus) (pus) 792.1
    occult blood 792.1
  synchondrosis 756.9
  test results without manifest disease -
    see Findings, abnormal
  thebesian valve 746.9
  thermography - *see* Findings, abnor-
    mal, structure
  threshold, cones or rods (eye) 368.63
  thyroid-binding globulin 246.8
  thyroid product 246.8
  toxicology (findings) NEC 796.0
  tracheal cartilage (congenital) 748.3
  transport protein 273.8
  ultrasound results - *see* Findings, ab-
    normal, structure
  umbilical cord
    affecting fetus or newborn 762.6
    complicating delivery 663.9
    specified NEC 663.8
  union
    cricoid cartilage and thyroid carti-
      lage 748.3
    larynx and trachea 748.3
    thyroid cartilage and hyoid bone
      748.3
  urination NEC 788.69
    psychogenic 306.53
    stream
      intermittent 788.61
      slowing 788.62
      splitting 788.61
      weak 788.62
    urgency 788.63
  urine (constituents) NEC 791.9
  uterine hemorrhage (*see also* Hemor-
    rhage, uterus) 626.9
    climacteric 627.0
    postmenopausal 627.1
  vagina (acquired) (congenital)
    in pregnancy or childbirth 654.7
      affecting fetus or newborn 763.89
      causing obstructed labor 660.2
        affecting fetus or newborn 763.1
  vascular sounds 785.9
  vectorcardiogram 794.39
  visually evoked potential (VEP) 794.13
  vulva (acquired) (congenital)
    in pregnancy or childbirth 654.8
      affecting fetus or newborn 763.89
      causing obstructed labor 660.2
        affecting fetus or newborn 763.1
  weight
    gain 783.1
      of pregnancy 646.1
        with hypertension - *see* Tox-
          emia, of pregnancy
    loss 783.21
  x-ray examination - *see* Abnormal, ra-
    diological examination
Abnormally formed uterus - *see* Anomaly, uterus
Abnormity (any organ or part) - *see*
  Anomaly
ABO
  hemolytic disease 773.1
  incompatibility reaction 999.6
Abocclusion 524.20 ◄▥
Abolition, language 784.69

Aborter, habitual or recurrent NEC
  without current pregnancy 629.9
  current abortion (*see also* Abortion,
    spontaneous) 634.9
    affecting fetus or newborn 761.8
  observation in current pregnancy 646.3
Abortion (complete) (incomplete) (inevi-
  table) (with retained products of
  conception) 637.9

Note	Use the following fifth-digit sub-classification with categories 634-637:
0	unspecified
1	incomplete
2	complete

  with
    complication(s) (any) following pre-
      vious abortion - *see* category 639
    damage to pelvic organ (laceration)
      (rupture) (tear) 637.2
    embolism (air) (amniotic fluid)
      (blood clot) (pulmonary) (pye-
      mic) (septic) (soap) 637.6
    genital tract and pelvic infection 637.0
    hemorrhage, delayed or excessive
      637.1
    metabolic disorder 637.4
    renal failure (acute) 637.3
    sepsis (genital tract) (pelvic organ)
      637.0
      urinary tract 637.7
    shock (postoperative) (septic) 637.5
    specified complication NEC 637.7
    toxemia 637.3
    unspecified complication(s) 637.8
    urinary tract infection 637.7
  accidental - *see* Abortion, spontaneous
  artificial - *see* Abortion, induced
  attempted (failed) - *see* Abortion, failed
  criminal - *see* Abortion, illegal
  early - *see* Abortion, spontaneous
  elective - *see* Abortion, legal
  failed (legal) 638.9
    with
      damage to pelvic organ (lacera-
        tion) (rupture) (tear) 638.2
      embolism (air) (amniotic fluid)
        (blood clot) (pulmonary) (pye-
        mic) (septic) (soap) 638.6
      genital tract and pelvic infection
        638.0
      hemorrhage, delayed or excessive
        638.1
      metabolic disorder 638.4
      renal failure (acute) 638.3
      sepsis (genital tract) (pelvic organ)
        638.0
        urinary tract 638.7
      shock (postoperative) (septic) 638.5
      specified complication NEC 638.7
      toxemia 638.3
      unspecified complication(s) 638.8
      urinary tract infection 638.7
  fetal indication - *see* Abortion, legal
  fetus 779.6
  following threatened abortion - *see*
    Abortion, by type
  habitual or recurrent (care during
    pregnancy) 646.3
    with current abortion (*see also* Abor-
      tion, spontaneous) 634.9
      affecting fetus or newborn 761.8
    without current pregnancy 629.9

Abortion *(Continued)*
  homicidal - *see* Abortion, illegal
  illegal 636.9
    with
      damage to pelvic organ (lacera-
        tion) (rupture) (tear) 636.2
      embolism (air) (amniotic fluid)
        (blood clot) (pulmonary)
        (pyemic) (septic) (soap) 636.6
      genital tract and pelvic infection
        636.0
      hemorrhage, delayed or excessive
        636.1
      metabolic disorder 636.4
      renal failure 636.3
      sepsis (genital tract) (pelvic organ)
        636.0
        urinary tract 636.7
      shock (postoperative) (septic)
        636.5
      specified complication NEC 636.7
      toxemia 636.3
      unspecified complication(s) 636.8
      urinary tract infection 636.7
    fetus 779.6
  induced 637.9
    illegal - *see* Abortion, illegal
    legal indications - *see* Abortion, legal
    medical indications - *see* Abortion,
      legal
    therapeutic - *see* Abortion, legal
  late - *see* Abortion, spontaneous
  legal (legal indication) (medical indica-
    tion) (under medical supervision)
    635.9
    with
      damage to pelvic organ (lacera-
        tion) (rupture) (tear) 635.2
      embolism (air) (amniotic fluid)
        (blood clot) (pulmonary) (pye-
        mic) (septic) (soap) 635.6
      genital tract and pelvic infection
        635.0
      hemorrhage, delayed or excessive
        635.1
      metabolic disorder 635.4
      renal failure (acute) 635.3
      sepsis (genital tract) (pelvic organ)
        635.0
        urinary tract 635.7
      shock (postoperative) (septic) 635.5
      specified complication NEC 635.7
      toxemia 635.3
      unspecified complication(s) 635.8
      urinary tract infection 635.7
    fetus 779.6
  medical indication - *see* Abortion, legal
  mental hygiene problem - *see* Abor-
    tion, legal
  missed 632
  operative - *see* Abortion, legal
  psychiatric indication - *see* Abortion,
    legal
  recurrent - *see* Abortion, spontaneous
  self-induced - *see* Abortion, illegal
  septic - *see* Abortion, by type, with
    sepsis
  spontaneous 634.9
    with
      damage to pelvic organ (lacera-
        tion) (rupture) (tear) 634.2
      embolism (air) (amniotic fluid)
        (blood clot) (pulmonary) (pye-
        mic) (septic) (soap) 634.6

ICD-9-CM

◄

Vol. 2

Abortion (*Continued*)
  spontaneous (*Continued*)
    with (*Continued*)
      genital tract and pelvic infection 634.0
      hemorrhage, delayed or excessive 634.1
      metabolic disorder 634.4
      renal failure 634.3
      sepsis (genital tract) (pelvic organ) 634.0
        urinary tract 634.7
      shock (postoperative) (septic) 634.5
      specified complication NEC 634.7
      toxemia 634.3
      unspecified complication(s) 634.8
      urinary tract infection 634.7
    fetus 761.8
    threatened 640.0
      affecting fetus or newborn 762.1
  surgical - *see* Abortion, legal
  therapeutic - *see* Abortion, legal
  threatened 640.0
    affecting fetus or newborn 762.1
  tubal - *see* Pregnancy, tubal
  voluntary - *see* Abortion, legal
Abortus fever 023.9
Aboulomania 301.6
Abrachia 755.20
Abrachiatism 755.20
Abrachiocephalia 759.89
Abrachiocephalus 759.89
Abrami's disease (acquired hemolytic jaundice) 283.9
Abramov-Fiedler myocarditis (acute isolated myocarditis) 422.91
Abrasion - *see also* Injury, superficial, by site
  cornea 918.1
  dental 521.20 ◄▥
    extending into ◄
      dentine 521.22 ◄
      pulp 521.23 ◄
    generalized 521.25 ◄
    limited to enamel 521.21 ◄
    localized 521.24 ◄
  teeth, tooth (dentifrice) (habitual) (hard tissues) (occupational) (ritual) (traditional) (wedge defect) (*see also* Abrasion, dental) 521.20 ◄▥
Abrikossov's tumor (M9580/0) - *see also* Neoplasm, connective tissue, benign
  malignant (M9580/3) - *see* Neoplasm, connective tissue, malignant
Abrism 988.8
Abruption, placenta - *see* Placenta, abruptio
Abruptio placentae - *see* Placenta, abruptio
Abscess (acute) (chronic) (infectional) (lymphangitic) (metastatic) (multiple) (pyogenic) (septic) (with lymphangitis) (*see also* Cellulitis) 682.9
  abdomen, abdominal
    cavity - *see* Abscess, peritoneum
    wall 682.2
  abdominopelvic - *see* Abscess, peritoneum
  accessory sinus (chronic) (*see also* Sinusitis) 473.9
  adrenal (capsule) (gland) 255.8
  alveolar 522.5
    with sinus 522.7
  amebic 006.3
    bladder 006.8

Abcess (*Continued*)
  amebic (*Continued*)
    brain (with liver or lung abscess) 006.5
    liver (without mention of brain or lung abscess) 006.3
      with
        brain abscess (and lung abscess) 006.5
        lung abscess 006.4
    lung (with liver abscess) 006.4
      with brain abscess 006.5
    seminal vesicle 006.8
    specified site NEC 006.8
    spleen 006.8
  anaerobic 040.0
  ankle 682.6
  anorectal 566
  antecubital space 682.3
  antrum (chronic) (Highmore) (*see also* Sinusitis, maxillary) 473.0
  anus 566
  apical (tooth) 522.5
    with sinus (alveolar) 522.7
  appendix 540.1
  areola (acute) (chronic) (nonpuerperal) 611.0
    puerperal, postpartum 675.1
  arm (any part, above wrist) 682.3
  artery (wall) 447.2
  atheromatous 447.2
  auditory canal (external) 380.10
  auricle (ear) (staphylococcal) (streptococcal) 380.10
  axilla, axillary (region) 682.3
    lymph gland or node 683
  back (any part) 682.2
  Bartholin's gland 616.3
    with
      abortion - *see* Abortion, by type, with sepsis
      ectopic pregnancy (*see also* categories 633.0-633.9) 639.0
      molar pregnancy (*see also* categories 630-632) 639.0
    complicating pregnancy or puerperium 646.6
    following
      abortion 639.0
      ectopic or molar pregnancy 639.0
  bartholinian 616.3
  Bezold's 383.01
  bile, biliary, duct or tract (*see also* Cholecystitis) 576.8
  bilharziasis 120.1
  bladder (wall) 595.89
    amebic 006.8
  bone (subperiosteal) (*see also* Osteomyelitis) 730.0
    accessory sinus (chronic) (*see also* Sinusitis) 473.9
    acute 730.0
    chronic or old 730.1
    jaw (lower) (upper) 526.4
    mastoid - *see* Mastoiditis, acute
    petrous (*see also* Petrositis) 383.20
    spinal (tuberculous) (*see also* Tuberculosis) 015.0 [730.88]
      nontuberculous 730.08
  bowel 569.5
  brain (any part) 324.0
    amebic (with liver or lung abscess) 006.5

Abscess (*Continued*)
  brain (*Continued*)
    cystic 324.0
    late effect - *see* category 326
    otogenic 324.0
    tuberculous (*see also* Tuberculosis) 013.3
  breast (acute) (chronic) (nonpuerperal) 611.0
    newborn 771.5
    puerperal, postpartum 675.1
    tuberculous (*see also* Tuberculosis) 017.9
  broad ligament (chronic) (*see also* Disease, pelvis, inflammatory) 614.4
    acute 614.3
  Brodie's (chronic) (localized) (*see also* Osteomyelitis) 730.1
  bronchus 519.1
  buccal cavity 528.3
  bulbourethral gland 597.0
  bursa 727.89
    pharyngeal 478.29
  buttock 682.5
  canaliculus, breast 611.0
  canthus 372.20
  cartilage 733.99
  cecum 569.5
    with appendicitis 540.1
  cerebellum, cerebellar 324.0
    late effect - *see* category 326
  cerebral (embolic) 324.0
    late effect - *see* category 326
  cervical (neck region) 682.1
    lymph gland or node 683
    stump (*see also* Cervicitis) 616.0
  cervix (stump) (uteri) (*see also* Cervicitis) 616.0
  cheek, external 682.0
    inner 528.3
  chest 510.9
    with fistula 510.0
    wall 682.2
  chin 682.0
  choroid 363.00
  ciliary body 364.3
  circumtonsillar 475
  cold (tuberculous) - *see also* Tuberculosis, abscess
    articular - *see* Tuberculosis, joint
  colon (wall) 569.5
  colostomy or enterostomy 569.61
  conjunctiva 372.00
  connective tissue NEC 682.9
  cornea 370.55
    with ulcer 370.00
  corpus
    cavernosum 607.2
    luteum (*see also* Salpingo-oophoritis) 614.2
  Cowper's gland 597.0
  cranium 324.0
  cul-de-sac (Douglas') (posterior) (*see also* Disease, pelvis, inflammatory) 614.4
    acute 614.3
  dental 522.5
    with sinus (alveolar) 522.7
  dentoalveolar 522.5
    with sinus (alveolar) 522.7
  diaphragm, diaphragmatic - *see* Abscess, peritoneum
  digit NEC 681.9

Abscess *(Continued)*
  Douglas' cul-de-sac or pouch *(see also Disease, pelvis, inflammatory)* 614.4
    acute 614.3
  Dubois' 090.5
  ductless gland 259.8
  ear
    acute 382.00
    external 380.10
    inner 386.30
    middle - *see* Otitis media
  elbow 682.6
  endamebic - *see* Abscess, amebic
  entamebic - *see* Abscess, amebic
  enterostomy 569.61
  epididymis 604.0
  epidural 324.9
    brain 324.0
    late effect - *see* category 326
    spinal cord 324.1
  epiglottis 478.79
  epiploon, epiploic - *see* Abscess, peritoneum
  erysipelatous *(see also* Erysipelas) 035 ◄
  esophagostomy 530.86
  esophagus 530.19
  ethmoid (bone) (chronic) (sinus) *(see also* Sinusitis, ethmoidal) 473.2
  external auditory canal 380.10
  extradural 324.9
    brain 324.0
    late effect - *see* category 326
    spinal cord 324.1
  extraperitoneal - *see* Abscess, peritoneum
  eye 360.00
  eyelid 373.13
  face (any part, except eye) 682.0
  fallopian tube *(see also* Salpingo-oophoritis) 614.2
  fascia 728.89
  fauces 478.29
  fecal 569.5
  femoral (region) 682.6
  filaria, filarial *(see also* Infestation, filarial) 125.9
  finger (any) (intrathecal) (periosteal) (subcutaneous) (subcuticular) 681.00
  fistulous NEC 682.9
  flank 682.2
  foot (except toe) 682.7
  forearm 682.3
  forehead 682.0
  frontal (sinus) (chronic) *(see also* Sinusitis, frontal) 473.1
  gallbladder *(see also* Cholecystitis, acute) 575.0
  gastric 535.0
  genital organ or tract NEC
    female 616.9
      with
        abortion - *see* Abortion, by type, with sepsis
        ectopic pregnancy *(see also* categories 633.0-633.9) 639.0
        molar pregnancy *(see also* categories 630-632) 639.0
      following
        abortion 639.0
        ectopic or molar pregnancy 639.0
      puerperal, postpartum, childbirth 670
    male 608.4

Abscess *(Continued)*
  genitourinary system, tuberculous *(see also* Tuberculosis) 016.9
  gingival 523.3
  gland, glandular (lymph) (acute) NEC 683
  glottis 478.79
  gluteal (region) 682.5
  gonorrheal NEC *(see also* Gonococcus) 098.0
  groin 682.2
  gum 523.3
  hand (except finger or thumb) 682.4
  head (except face) 682.8
  heart 429.89
  heel 682.7
  helminthic *(see also* Infestation, by specific parasite) 128.9
  hepatic 572.0
    amebic *(see also* Abscess, liver, amebic) 006.3
    duct 576.8
  hip 682.6
    tuberculous (active) *(see also* Tuberculosis) 015.1
  ileocecal 540.1
  ileostomy (bud) 569.61
  iliac (region) 682.2
    fossa 540.1
  iliopsoas (tuberculous) *(see also* Tuberculosis) 015.0 *[730.88]*
    nontuberculous 728.89
  infraclavicular (fossa) 682.3
  inguinal (region) 682.2
    lymph gland or node 683
  intersphincteric (anus) 566
  intestine, intestinal 569.5
    rectal 566
  intra-abdominal *(see also* Abscess, peritoneum) 567.2
    postoperative 998.59
  intracranial 324.0
    late effect - *see* category 326
  intramammary - *see* Abscess, breast
  intramastoid *(see also* Mastoiditis, acute) 383.00
  intraorbital 376.01
  intraperitoneal - *see* Abscess, peritoneum
  intraspinal 324.1
    late effect - *see* category 326
  intratonsillar 475
  iris 364.3
  ischiorectal 566
  jaw (bone) (lower) (upper) 526.4
    skin 682.0
  joint *(see also* Arthritis, pyogenic) 711.0
    vertebral (tuberculous) *(see also* Tuberculosis) 015.0 *[730.88]*
      nontuberculous 724.8
  kidney 590.2
    with
      abortion - *see* Abortion, by type, with urinary tract infection
      calculus 592.0
      ectopic pregnancy *(see also* categories 633.0-633.9) 639.8
      molar pregnancy *(see also* categories 630-632) 639.8
      complicating pregnancy or puerperium 646.6
        affecting fetus or newborn 760.1
      following
        abortion 639.8
        ectopic or molar pregnancy 639.8

Abscess *(Continued)*
  knee 682.6
    joint 711.06
    tuberculous (active) *(see also* Tuberculosis) 015.2
  labium (majus) (minus) 616.4
    complicating pregnancy, childbirth, or puerperium 646.6
  lacrimal (passages) (sac) *(see also* Dacryocystitis) 375.30
    caruncle 375.30
    gland *(see also* Dacryoadenitis) 375.00
  lacunar 597.0
  larynx 478.79
  lateral (alveolar) 522.5
    with sinus 522.7
  leg, except foot 682.6
  lens 360.00
  lid 373.13
  lingual 529.0
    tonsil 475
  lip 528.5
  Littre's gland 597.0
  liver 572.0
    amebic 006.3
      with
        brain abscess (and lung abscess) 006.5
        lung abscess 006.4
      due to Entamoeba histolytica 006.3
    dysenteric *(see also* Abscess, liver, amebic) 006.3
    pyogenic 572.0
    tropical *(see also* Abscess, liver, amebic) 006.3
  loin (region) 682.2
  lumbar (tuberculous) *(see also* Tuberculosis) 015.0 *[730.88]*
    nontuberculous 682.2
  lung (miliary) (putrid) 513.0
    amebic (with liver abscess) 006.4
      with brain abscess 006.5
  lymph, lymphatic, gland or node (acute) 683
    any site, except mesenteric 683
    mesentery 289.2
  lymphangitic, acute - *see* Cellulitis
  malar 526.4
  mammary gland - *see* Abscess, breast
  marginal (anus) 566
  mastoid (process) *(see also* Mastoiditis, acute) 383.00
    subperiosteal 383.01
  maxilla, maxillary 526.4
    molar (tooth) 522.5
      with sinus 522.7
    premolar 522.5
    sinus (chronic) *(see also* Sinusitis, maxillary) 473.0
  mediastinum 513.1
  meibomian gland 373.12
  meninges *(see also* Meningitis) 320.9
  mesentery, mesenteric - *see* Abscess, peritoneum
  mesosalpinx *(see also* Salpingo-oophoritis) 614.2
  milk 675.1
  Monro's (psoriasis) 696.1
  mons pubis 682.2
  mouth (floor) 528.3
  multiple sites NEC 682.9
  mural 682.2
  muscle 728.89

◄ **New**   ◄▥▥ **Revised**

Abscess *(Continued)*
  myocardium 422.92
  nabothian (follicle) *(see also* Cervicitis)
      616.0
  nail (chronic) (with lymphangitis) 681.9
      finger 681.02
      toe 681.11
  nasal (fossa) (septum) 478.1
      sinus (chronic) *(see also* Sinusitis) 473.9
  nasopharyngeal 478.29
  nates 682.5
  navel 682.2
      newborn NEC 771.4
  neck (region) 682.1
      lymph gland or node 683
  nephritic *(see also* Abscess, kidney) 590.2
  nipple 611.0
      puerperal, postpartum 675.0
  nose (septum) 478.1
      external 682.0
  omentum - *see* Abscess, peritoneum
  operative wound 998.59
  orbit, orbital 376.01
  ossifluent - *see* Abscess, bone
  ovary, ovarian (corpus luteum) *(see
      also* Salpingo-oophoritis) 614.2
  oviduct *(see also* Salpingo-oophoritis)
      614.2
  palate (soft) 528.3
      hard 526.4
  palmar (space) 682.4
  pancreas (duct) 577.0
  paradontal 523.3
  parafrenal 607.2
  parametric, parametrium (chronic) *(see
      also* Disease, pelvis, inflammatory)
      614.4
      acute 614.3
  paranephric 590.2
  parapancreatic 577.0
  parapharyngeal 478.22
  pararectal 566
  parasinus *(see also* Sinusitis) 473.9
  parauterine *(see also* Disease, pelvis, in-
      flammatory) 614.4
      acute 614.3
  paravaginal *(see also* Vaginitis) 616.10
  parietal region 682.8
  parodontal 523.3
  parotid (duct) (gland) 527.3
      region 528.3
  parumbilical 682.2
      newborn 771.4
  pectoral (region) 682.2
  pelvirectal - *see* Abscess, peritoneum
  pelvis, pelvic
      female (chronic) *(see also* Disease,
          pelvis, inflammatory) 614.4
          acute 614.3
      male, peritoneal (cellular tissue) - *see*
          Abscess, peritoneum
      tuberculous *(see also* Tuberculosis)
          016.9
  penis 607.2
      gonococcal (acute) 098.0
          chronic or duration of 2 months
              or over 098.2
  perianal 566
  periapical 522.5
      with sinus (alveolar) 522.7
  periappendiceal 540.1
  pericardial 420.99
  pericecal 540.1
  pericemental 523.3

Abscess *(Continued)*
  pericholecystic *(see also* Cholecystitis,
      acute) 575.0
  pericoronal 523.3
  peridental 523.3
  perigastric 535.0
  perimetric *(see also* Disease, pelvis, in-
      flammatory) 614.4
      acute 614.3
  perinephric, perinephritic *(see also* Ab-
      scess, kidney) 590.2
  perineum, perineal (superficial) 682.2
      deep (with urethral involvement) 597.0
      urethra 597.0
  periodontal (parietal) 523.3
      apical 522.5
  periosteum, periosteal *(see also* Periosti-
      tis) 730.3
      with osteomyelitis *(see also* Osteomy-
          elitis) 730.2
          acute or subacute 730.0
          chronic or old 730.1
  peripleuritic 510.9
      with fistula 510.0
  periproctic 566
  periprostatic 601.2
  perirectal (staphylococcal) 566
  perirenal (tissue) *(see also* Abscess, kid-
      ney) 590.2
  perisinuous (nose) *(see also* Sinusitis)
      473.9
  peritoneum, peritoneal (perforated)
      (ruptured) 567.2
      with
          abortion - *see* Abortion, by type,
              with sepsis
          appendicitis 540.1
          ectopic pregnancy *(see also* catego-
              ries 633.0-633.9) 639.0
          molar pregnancy *(see also* catego-
              ries 630-632) 639.0
      following
          abortion 639.0
          ectopic or molar pregnancy 639.0
      pelvic, female *(see also* Disease, pel-
          vis, inflammatory) 614.4
          acute 614.3
      postoperative 998.59
      puerperal, postpartum, childbirth
          670
      tuberculous *(see also* Tuberculosis)
          014.0
  peritonsillar 475
  perityphlic 540.1
  periureteral 593.89
  periurethral 597.0
      gonococcal (acute) 098.0
          chronic or duration of 2 months
              or over 098.2
  periuterine *(see also* Disease, pelvis, in-
      flammatory) 614.4
      acute 614.3
  perivesical 595.89
  pernicious NEC 682.9
  petrous bone - *see* Petrositis
  phagedenic NEC 682.9
      chancroid 099.0
  pharynx, pharyngeal (lateral) 478.29
  phlegmonous NEC 682.9
  pilonidal 685.0
  pituitary (gland) 253.8
  pleura 510.9
      with fistula 510.0
  popliteal 682.6

Abscess *(Continued)*
  postanal 566
  postcecal 540.1
  postlaryngeal 478.79
  postnasal 478.1
  postpharyngeal 478.24
  posttonsillar 475
  posttyphoid 002.0
  Pott's *(see also* Tuberculosis) 015.0
      [730.88]
  pouch of Douglas (chronic) *(see also* Dis-
      ease, pelvis, inflammatory) 614.4
  premammary - *see* Abscess, breast
  prepatellar 682.6
  prostate *(see also* Prostatitis) 601.2
      gonococcal (acute) 098.12
          chronic or duration of 2 months
              or over 098.32
  psoas (tuberculous) *(see also* Tuberculo-
      sis) 015.0 *[730.88]*
      nontuberculous 728.89
  pterygopalatine fossa 682.8
  pubis 682.2
  puerperal - *see* Puerperal, abscess, by site
  pulmonary - *see* Abscess, lung
  pulp, pulpal (dental) 522.0
      finger 681.01
      toe 681.10
  pyemic - *see* Septicemia
  pyloric valve 535.0
  rectovaginal septum 569.5
  rectovesical 595.89
  rectum 566
  regional NEC 682.9
  renal *(see also* Abscess, kidney) 590.2
  retina 363.00
  retrobulbar 376.01
  retrocecal - *see* Abscess, peritoneum
  retrolaryngeal 478.79
  retromammary - *see* Abscess, breast
  retroperineal 682.2
  retroperitoneal - *see* Abscess, peritoneum
  retropharyngeal 478.24
      tuberculous *(see also* Tuberculosis)
          012.8
  retrorectal 566
  retrouterine *(see also* Disease, pelvis, in-
      flammatory) 614.4
      acute 614.3
  retrovesical 595.89
  root, tooth 522.5
      with sinus (alveolar) 522.7
  round ligament *(see also* Disease, pel-
      vis, inflammatory) 614.4
      acute 614.3
  rupture (spontaneous) NEC 682.9
  sacrum (tuberculous) *(see also* Tubercu-
      losis) 015.0 *[730.88]*
      nontuberculous 730.08
  salivary duct or gland 527.3
  scalp (any part) 682.8
  scapular 730.01
  sclera 379.09
  scrofulous *(see also* Tuberculosis) 017.2
  scrotum 608.4
  seminal vesicle 608.0
      amebic 006.8
  septal, dental 522.5
      with sinus (alveolar) 522.7
  septum (nasal) 478.1
  serous *(see also* Periostitis) 730.3
  shoulder 682.3
  side 682.2
  sigmoid 569.5

ICD-9-CM

A

Vol. 2

Abscess *(Continued)*
   sinus (accessory) (chronic) (nasal) *(see also* Sinusitis) 473.9
      intracranial venous (any) 324.0
         late effect - *see* category 326
   Skene's duct or gland 597.0
   skin NEC 682.9
      tuberculous (primary) *(see also* Tuberculosis) 017.0
   sloughing NEC 682.9
   specified site NEC 682.8
      amebic 006.8
   spermatic cord 608.4
   sphenoidal (sinus) *(see also* Sinusitis, sphenoidal) 473.3
   spinal
      cord (any part) (staphylococcal) 324.1
         tuberculous *(see also* Tuberculosis) 013.5
      epidural 324.1
   spine (column) (tuberculous) *(see also* Tuberculosis) 015.0 *[730.88]*
      nontuberculous 730.08
   spleen 289.59
      amebic 006.8
   staphylococcal NEC 682.9
   stitch 998.59
   stomach (wall) 535.0
   strumous (tuberculous) *(see also* Tuberculosis) 017.2
   subarachnoid 324.9
      brain 324.0
      cerebral 324.0
      late effect - *see* category 326
      spinal cord 324.1
   subareolar - *see also* Abscess, breast
      puerperal, postpartum 675.1
   subcecal 540.1
   subcutaneous NEC 682.9
   subdiaphragmatic - *see* Abscess, peritoneum
   subdorsal 682.2
   subdural 324.9
      brain 324.0
      late effect - *see* category 326
      spinal cord 324.1
   subgaleal 682.8
   subhepatic - *see* Abscess, peritoneum
   sublingual 528.3
      gland 527.3
   submammary - *see* Abscess, breast
   submandibular (region) (space) (triangle) 682.0
      gland 527.3
   submaxillary (region) 682.0
      gland 527.3
   submental (pyogenic) 682.0
      gland 527.3
   subpectoral 682.2
   subperiosteal - *see* Abscess, bone
   subperitoneal - *see* Abscess, peritoneum
   subphrenic - *see also* Abscess, peritoneum
      postoperative 998.59
   subscapular 682.2
   subungual 681.9
   suburethral 597.0
   sudoriparous 705.89
   suppurative NEC 682.9
   supraclavicular (fossa) 682.3
   suprahepatic - *see* Abscess, peritoneum
   suprapelvic *(see also* Disease, pelvis, inflammatory) 614.4
      acute 614.3
   suprapubic 682.2

Abscess *(Continued)*
   suprarenal (capsule) (gland) 255.8
   sweat gland 705.89
   syphilitic 095.8
   teeth, tooth (root) 522.5
      with sinus (alveolar) 522.7
      supporting structures NEC 523.3
   temple 682.0
   temporal region 682.0
   temporosphenoidal 324.0
      late effect - *see* category 326
   tendon (sheath) 727.89
   testicle - *see* Orchitis
   thecal 728.89
   thigh (acquired) 682.6
   thorax 510.9
      with fistula 510.0
   throat 478.29
   thumb (intrathecal) (periosteal) (subcutaneous) (subcuticular) 681.00
   thymus (gland) 254.1
   thyroid (gland) 245.0
   toe (any) (intrathecal) (periosteal) (subcutaneous) (subcuticular) 681.10
   tongue (staphylococcal) 529.0
   tonsil(s) (lingual) 475
   tonsillopharyngeal 475
   tooth, teeth (root) 522.5
      with sinus (alveolar) 522.7
      supporting structure NEC 523.3
   trachea 478.9
   trunk 682.2
   tubal *(see also* Salpingo-oophoritis) 614.2
   tuberculous - *see* Tuberculosis, abscess
   tubo-ovarian *(see also* Salpingo-oophoritis) 614.2
   tunica vaginalis 608.4
   umbilicus NEC 682.2
      newborn 771.4
   upper arm 682.3
   upper respiratory 478.9
   urachus 682.2
   urethra (gland) 597.0
   urinary 597.0
   uterus, uterine (wall) *(see also* Endometritis) 615.9
      ligament *(see also* Disease, pelvis, inflammatory) 614.4
         acute 614.3
      neck *(see also* Cervicitis) 616.0
   uvula 528.3
   vagina (wall) *(see also* Vaginitis) 616.10
   vaginorectal *(see also* Vaginitis) 616.10
   vas deferens 608.4
   vermiform appendix 540.1
   vertebra (column) (tuberculous) *(see also* Tuberculosis) 015.0 *[730.88]*
      nontuberculous 730.0
   vesical 595.89
   vesicouterine pouch *(see also* Disease, pelvis, inflammatory) 614.4
   vitreous (humor) (pneumococcal) 360.04
   vocal cord 478.5
   von Bezold's 383.01
   vulva 616.4
      complicating pregnancy, childbirth, or puerperium 646.6
   vulvovaginal gland *(see also* Vaginitis) 616.3
   web-space 682.4
   wrist 682.4

Absence (organ or part) (complete or partial)
   acoustic nerve 742.8
   adrenal (gland) (congenital) 759.1
      acquired V45.79
   albumin (blood) 273.8
   alimentary tract (complete) (congenital) (partial) 751.8
      lower 751.5
      upper 750.8
   alpha-fucosidase 271.8
   alveolar process (acquired) 525.8
      congenital 750.26
   anus, anal (canal) (congenital) 751.2
   aorta (congenital) 747.22
   aortic valve (congenital) 746.89
   appendix, congenital 751.2
   arm (acquired) V49.60
      above elbow V49.66
      below elbow V49.65
      congenital *(see also* Deformity, reduction, upper limb) 755.20
         lower - *see* Absence, forearm, congenital
         upper (complete) (partial) (with absence of distal elements, incomplete) 755.24
         with
            complete absence of distal elements 755.21
            forearm (incomplete) 755.23
   artery (congenital) (peripheral) NEC *(see also* Anomaly, peripheral vascular system) 747.60
      brain 747.81
      cerebral 747.81
      coronary 746.85
      pulmonary 747.3
      umbilical 747.5
   atrial septum 745.69
   auditory canal (congenital) (external) 744.01
   auricle (ear) (with stenosis or atresia of auditory canal), congenital 744.01
   bile, biliary duct (common) or passage (congenital) 751.61
   bladder (acquired) V45.74
      congenital 753.8
   bone (congenital) NEC 756.9
      marrow 284.9
         acquired (secondary) 284.8
         congenital 284.0
         hereditary 284.0
         idiopathic 284.9
      skull 756.0
   bowel sounds 787.5
   brain 740.0
      specified part 742.2
   breast(s) (acquired) V45.71
      congenital 757.6
   broad ligament (congenital) 752.19
   bronchus (congenital) 748.3
   calvarium, calvaria (skull) 756.0
   canaliculus lacrimalis, congenital 743.65
   carpal(s) (congenital) (complete) (partial) (with absence of distal elements, incomplete) *(see also* Deformity, reduction, upper limb) 755.28
      with complete absence of distal elements 755.21
   cartilage 756.9

◀ **New**   ◀|||| **Revised**

Absence *(Continued)*
  caudal spine 756.13
  cecum (acquired) (postoperative) (post-
      traumatic) V45.72
    congenital 751.2
  cementum 520.4
  cerebellum (congenital) (vermis)
      742.2
  cervix (acquired) (uteri) V45.77
    congenital 752.49
  chin, congenital 744.89
  cilia (congenital) 743.63
    acquired 374.89
  circulatory system, part NEC 747.89
  clavicle 755.51
  clitoris (congenital) 752.49
  coccyx, congenital 756.13
  cold sense (*see also* Disturbance, sensa-
      tion) 782.0
  colon (acquired) (postoperative)
      V45.72
    congenital 751.2
  congenital
    lumen - *see* Atresia
    organ or site NEC - *see* Agenesis
    septum - *see* Imperfect, closure
  corpus callosum (congenital) 742.2
  cricoid cartilage 748.3
  diaphragm (congenital) (with hernia)
      756.6
    with obstruction 756.6
  digestive organ(s) or tract, congenital
      (complete) (partial) 751.8
    acquired V45.79
    lower 751.5
    upper 750.8
  ductus arteriosus 747.89
  duodenum (acquired) (postoper-
      ative) V45.72
    congenital 751.1
  ear, congenital 744.09
    acquired V45.79
    auricle 744.01
    external 744.01
    inner 744.05
    lobe, lobule 744.21
    middle, except ossicles 744.03
      ossicles 744.04
    ossicles 744.04
  ejaculatory duct (congenital) 752.89
  endocrine gland NEC (congenital)
      759.2
  epididymis (congenital) 752.89
    acquired V45.77
  epiglottis, congenital 748.3
  epileptic (atonic) (typical) (*see also* Epi-
      lepsy) 345.0
  erythrocyte 284.9
  erythropoiesis 284.9
    congenital 284.0
  esophagus (congenital) 750.3
  eustachian tube (congenital) 744.24
  extremity (acquired)
    congenital (*see also* Deformity, reduc-
      tion) 755.4
    lower V49.70
    upper V49.60
  extrinsic muscle, eye 743.69
  eye (acquired) V45.78
    adnexa (congenital) 743.69
    congenital 743.00
    muscle (congenital) 743.69
  eyelid (fold), congenital 743.62
    acquired 374.89

Absence *(Continued)*
  face
    bones NEC 756.0
    specified part NEC 744.89
  fallopian tube(s) (acquired) V45.77
    congenital 752.19
  femur, congenital (complete) (partial)
      (with absence of distal elements,
      incomplete) (*see also* Deformity, re-
      duction, lower limb) 755.34
    with
      complete absence of distal ele-
        ments 755.31
      tibia and fibula (incomplete) 755.33
  fibrin 790.92
  fibrinogen (congenital) 286.3
    acquired 286.6
  fibula, congenital (complete) (partial)
      (with absence of distal elements,
      incomplete) (*see also* Deformity, re-
      duction, lower limb) 755.37
    with
      complete absence of distal ele-
        ments 755.31
      tibia 755.35
        with
          complete absence of distal ele-
            ments 755.31
          femur (incomplete) 755.33
            with complete absence of
              distal elements 755.31
  finger (acquired) V49.62
    congenital (complete) (partial) (*see
      also* Deformity, reduction, upper
      limb) 755.29
    meaning all fingers (complete)
      (partial) 755.21
    transverse 755.21
  fissures of lungs (congenital) 748.5
  foot (acquired) V49.73
    congenital (complete) 755.31
  forearm (acquired) V49.65
    congenital (complete) (partial) (with
      absence of distal elements, in-
      complete) (*see also* Deformity,
      reduction, upper limb) 755.25
    with
      complete absence of distal ele-
        ments (hand and fingers)
        755.21
      humerus (incomplete) 755.23
  fovea centralis 743.55
  fucosidase 271.8
  gallbladder (acquired) V45.79
    congenital 751.69
  gamma globulin (blood) 279.00
  genital organs
    acquired V45.77
    congenital
      female 752.89
        external 752.49
        internal NEC 752.89
      male 752.89
        penis 752.69
  genitourinary organs, congenital NEC
      752.89
  glottis 748.3
  gonadal, congenital NEC 758.6
  hair (congenital) 757.4
    acquired - *see* Alopecia
  hand (acquired) V49.63
    congenital (complete) (*see also* Defor-
      mity, reduction, upper limb)
      755.21

Absence *(Continued)*
  heart (congenital) 759.89
    acquired - *see* Status, organ replacement
  heat sense (*see also* Disturbance, sensa-
      tion) 782.0
  humerus, congenital (complete) (partial)
      (with absence of distal elements, in-
      complete) (*see also* Deformity, reduc-
      tion, upper limb) 755.24
    with
      complete absence of distal ele-
        ments 755.21
      radius and ulna (incomplete) 755.23
  hymen (congenital) 752.49
  ileum (acquired) (postoperative) (post-
      traumatic) V45.72
    congenital 751.1
  immunoglobulin, isolated NEC 279.03
    IgA 279.01
    IgG 279.03
    IgM 279.02
  incus (acquired) 385.24
    congenital 744.04
  internal ear (congenital) 744.05
  intestine (acquired) (small) V45.72
    congenital 751.1
      large 751.2
    large V45.72
      congenital 751.2
  iris (congenital) 743.45
  jaw - *see* Absence, mandible
  jejunum (acquired) V45.72
    congenital 751.1
  joint, congenital NEC 755.8
  kidney(s) (acquired) V45.73
    congenital 753.0
  labium (congenital) (majus) (minus)
      752.49
  labyrinth, membranous 744.05
  lacrimal apparatus (congenital) 743.65
  larynx (congenital) 748.3
  leg (acquired) V49.70
    above knee V49.76
    below knee V49.75
    congenital (partial) (unilateral) (*see
      also* Deformity, reduction, lower
      limb) 755.31
      lower (complete) (partial) (with
        absence of distal elements, in-
        complete) 755.35
        with
          complete absence of distal ele-
            ments (foot and toes)
            755.31
          thigh (incomplete) 755.33
            with complete absence of
              distal elements 755.31
    upper - *see* Absence, femur
  lens (congenital) 743.35
    acquired 379.31
  ligament, broad (congenital) 752.19
  limb (acquired)
    congenital (complete) (partial) (*see
      also* Deformity, reduction)
      755.4
    lower 755.30
      complete 755.31
      incomplete 755.32
      longitudinal - *see* Deficiency,
        lower limb, longitudinal
      transverse 755.31
    upper 755.20
      complete 755.21
      incomplete 755.22

ICD-9-CM

A

Vol. 2

Absence *(Continued)*
  limb *(Continued)*
    congenital *(Continued)*
      upper *(Continued)*
        longitudinal - *see* Deficiency, upper limb, longitudinal
        transverse 755.21
    lower NEC V49.70
    upper NEC V49.60
  lip 750.26
  liver (congenital) (lobe) 751.69
  lumbar (congenital) (vertebra) 756.13
    isthmus 756.11
    pars articularis 756.11
  lumen - *see* Atresia
  lung (bilateral) (congenital) (fissure) (lobe) (unilateral) 748.5
    acquired (any part) V45.76
  mandible (congenital) 524.09
  maxilla (congenital) 524.09
  menstruation 626.0
  metacarpal(s), congenital (complete) (partial) (with absence of distal elements, incomplete) (*see also* Deformity, reduction, upper limb) 755.28
    with all fingers, complete 755.21
  metatarsal(s), congenital (complete) (partial) (with absence of distal elements, incomplete) (*see also* Deformity, reduction, lower limb) 755.38
    with complete absence of distal elements 755.31
  muscle (congenital) (pectoral) 756.81
    ocular 743.69
  musculoskeletal system (congenital) NEC 756.9
  nail(s) (congenital) 757.5
  neck, part 744.89
  nerve 742.8
  nervous system, part NEC 742.8
  neutrophil 288.0
  nipple (congenital) 757.6
  nose (congenital) 748.1
    acquired 738.0
  nuclear 742.8
  ocular muscle (congenital) 743.69
  organ
    of Corti (congenital) 744.05
    or site
      acquired V45.79
      congenital NEC 759.89
  osseous meatus (ear) 744.03
  ovary (acquired) V45.77
    congenital 752.0
  oviduct (acquired) V45.77
    congenital 752.19
  pancreas (congenital) 751.7
    acquired (postoperative) (posttraumatic) V45.79
  parathyroid gland (congenital) 759.2
  parotid gland(s) (congenital) 750.21
  patella, congenital 755.64
  pelvic girdle (congenital) 755.69
  penis (congenital) 752.69
    acquired V45.77
  pericardium (congenital) 746.89
  perineal body (congenital) 756.81
  phalange(s), congenital 755.4
    lower limb (complete) (intercalary) (partial) (terminal) (*see also* Deformity, reduction, lower limb) 755.39

Absence *(Continued)*
  phalange(s) *(Continued)*
    lower limb *(Continued)*
      meaning all toes (complete) (partial) 755.31
      transverse 755.31
    upper limb (complete) (intercalary) (partial) (terminal) (*see also* Deformity, reduction, upper limb) 755.29
      meaning all digits (complete) (partial) 755.21
      transverse 755.21
  pituitary gland (congenital) 759.2
  postoperative - *see* Absence, by site, acquired
  prostate (congenital) 752.89
    acquired V45.77
  pulmonary
    artery 747.3
    trunk 747.3
    valve (congenital) 746.01
    vein 747.49
  punctum lacrimale (congenital) 743.65
  radius, congenital (complete) (partial) (with absence of distal elements, incomplete) 755.26
    with
      complete absence of distal elements 755.21
      ulna 755.25
        with
          complete absence of distal elements 755.21
          humerus (incomplete) 755.23
  ray, congenital 755.4
    lower limb (complete) (partial) (*see also* Deformity, reduction, lower limb) 755.38
      meaning all rays 755.31
      transverse 755.31
    upper limb (complete) (partial) (*see also* Deformity, reduction, upper limb) 755.28
      meaning all rays 755.21
      transverse 755.21
  rectum (congenital) 751.2
    acquired V45.79
  red cell 284.9
    acquired (secondary) 284.8
    congenital 284.0
    hereditary 284.0
    idiopathic 284.9
  respiratory organ (congenital) NEC 748.9
  rib (acquired) 738.3
    congenital 756.3
  roof of orbit (congenital) 742.0
  round ligament (congenital) 752.89
  sacrum, congenital 756.13
  salivary gland(s) (congenital) 750.21
  scapula 755.59
  scrotum, congenital 752.89
  seminal tract or duct (congenital) 752.89
    acquired V45.77
  septum (congenital) - *see also* Imperfect, closure, septum
    atrial 745.69
      and ventricular 745.7
    between aorta and pulmonary artery 745.0
    ventricular 745.3
      and atrial 745.7

Absence *(Continued)*
  sex chromosomes 758.81
  shoulder girdle, congenital (complete) (partial) 755.59
  skin (congenital) 757.39
  skull bone 756.0
    with
      anencephalus 740.0
      encephalocele 742.0
      hydrocephalus 742.3
        with spina bifida (*see also* Spina bifida) 741.0
      microcephalus 742.1
  spermatic cord (congenital) 752.89
  spinal cord 742.59
  spine, congenital 756.13
  spleen (congenital) 759.0
    acquired V45.79
  sternum, congenital 756.3
  stomach (acquired) (partial) (postoperative) V45.75
    with postgastric surgery syndrome 564.2
    congenital 750.7
  submaxillary gland(s) (congenital) 750.21
  superior vena cava (congenital) 747.49
  tarsal(s), congenital (complete) (partial) (with absence of distal elements, incomplete) (*see also* Deformity, reduction, lower limb) 755.38
  teeth, tooth (congenital) 520.0
    with abnormal spacing 524.30 ◄▥
    acquired 525.10
      with malocclusion 524.30 ◄▥
      due to
        caries 525.13
        extraction 525.10
        periodontal disease 525.12
        trauma 525.11
  tendon (congenital) 756.81
  testis (congenital) 752.89
    acquired V45.77
  thigh (acquired) 736.89
  thumb (acquired) V49.61
    congenital 755.29
  thymus gland (congenital) 759.2
  thyroid (gland) (surgical) 246.8
    with hypothyroidism 244.0
    cartilage, congenital 748.3
    congenital 243
  tibia, congenital (complete) (partial) (with absence of distal elements, incomplete) (*see also* Deformity, reduction, lower limb) 755.36
    with
      complete absence of distal elements 755.31
      fibula 755.35
        with
          complete absence of distal elements 755.31
          femur (incomplete) 755.33
            with complete absence of distal elements 755.31
  toe (acquired) V49.72
    congenital (complete) (partial) 755.39
      meaning all toes 755.31
      transverse 755.31
    great V49.71
  tongue (congenital) 750.11

ICD-9-CM

Vol. 2

Absence *(Continued)*
tooth, teeth (congenital) 520.0
  with abnormal spacing 524.30 ◀▥
  acquired 525.10
    with malocclusion 524.30 ◀▥
    due to
      caries 525.13
      extraction 525.10
      periodontal disease 525.12
      trauma 525.11
trachea (cartilage) (congenital) (rings) 748.3
transverse aortic arch (congenital) 747.21
tricuspid valve 746.1
ulna, congenital (complete) (partial) (with absence of distal elements, incomplete) *(see also* Deformity, reduction, upper limb) 755.27
  with
    complete absence of distal elements 755.21
    radius 755.25
      with
        complete absence of distal elements 755.21
        humerus (incomplete) 755.23
umbilical artery (congenital) 747.5
ureter (congenital) 753.4
  acquired V45.74
urethra, congenital 753.8
  acquired V45.74
urinary system, part NEC, congenital 753.8
  acquired V45.74
uterus (acquired) V45.77
  congenital 752.3
uvula (congenital) 750.26
vagina, congenital 752.49
  acquired V45.77
vas deferens (congenital) 752.89
  acquired V45.77
vein (congenital) (peripheral) NEC *(see also* Anomaly, peripheral vascular system) 747.60
  brain 747.81
  great 747.49
  portal 747.49
  pulmonary 747.49
vena cava (congenital) (inferior) (superior) 747.49
ventral horn cell 742.59
ventricular septum 745.3
vermis of cerebellum 742.2
vertebra, congenital 756.13
vulva, congenital 752.49
Absentia epileptica *(see also* Epilepsy) 345.0
Absinthemia *(see also* Dependence) 304.6
Absinthism *(see also* Dependence) 304.6
Absorbent system disease 459.89
Absorption
alcohol, through placenta or breast milk 760.71
antibiotics, through placenta or breast milk 760.74
anti-infective, through placenta or breast milk 760.74
chemical NEC 989.9
  specified chemical or substance - *see* Table of Drugs and Chemicals
  through placenta or breast milk (fetus or newborn) 760.70
    alcohol 760.71
    anti-infective agents 760.74

Absorption *(Continued)*
chemical NEC *(Continued)*
  through placenta or breast milk *(Continued)*
    cocaine 760.75
    "crack" 760.75
    diethylstilbestrol [DES] 760.76
    hallucinogenic agents 760.73
    medicinal agents NEC 760.79
    narcotics 760.72
    obstetric anesthetic or analgesic drug 763.5
    specified agent NEC 760.79
    suspected, affecting management of pregnancy 655.5
cocaine, through placenta or breast milk 760.75
drug NEC *(see also* Reaction, drug)
  through placenta or breast milk (fetus or newborn) 760.70
    alcohol 760.71
    anti-infective agents 760.74
    cocaine 760.75
    "crack" 760.75
    diethylstilbestrol (DES) 760.76
    hallucinogenic agents 760.73
    medicinal agents NEC 760.79
    narcotics 760.72
    obstetric anesthetic or analgesic drug 763.5
    specified agent NEC 760.79
    suspected, affecting management of pregnancy 655.5
fat, disturbance 579.8
hallucinogenic agents, through placenta or breast milk 760.73
immune sera, through placenta or breast milk 760.79
lactose defect 271.3
medicinal agents NEC, through placenta or breast milk 760.79
narcotics, through placenta or breast milk 760.72
noxious substance - *see* Absorption, chemical
protein, disturbance 579.8
pus or septic, general - *see* Septicemia
quinine, through placenta or breast milk 760.74
toxic substance - *see* Absorption, chemical
uremic - *see* Uremia
Abstinence symptoms or syndrome
alcohol 291.81
drug 292.0
Abt-Letterer-Siwe syndrome (acute histiocytosis X) (M9722/3) 202.5
Abulia 799.89
Abulomania 301.6
Abuse
adult 995.80
  emotional 995.82
  multiple forms 995.85
  neglect (nutritional) 995.84
  physical 995.81
  psychological 995.82
  sexual 995.83
alcohol *(see also* Alcoholism) 305.0
  dependent 303.9
  nondependent 305.0
child 995.50
  counseling
    perpetrator
      non-parent V62.83
      parent V61.22
    victim V61.21

Abuse *(Continued)*
child *(Continued)*
  emotional 995.51
  multiple forms 995.59
  neglect (nutritional) 995.52
  physical 995.54
    shaken infant syndrome 995.55
  psychological 995.51
  sexual 995.53
drugs, nondependent 305.9

> Note   Use the following fifth-digit subclassification with the following codes: 305.0, 305.2-305.9:
>
> 0   unspecified
> 1   continuous
> 2   episodic
> 3   in remission

amphetamine type 305.7
antidepressants 305.8
anxiolytic 305.4 ◀
barbiturates 305.4
caffeine 305.9
cannabis 305.2
cocaine type 305.6
hallucinogens 305.3
hashish 305.2
hypnotic 305.4 ◀
inhalant 305.9 ◀
LSD 305.3
marijuana 305.2
mixed 305.9
morphine type 305.5
opioid type 305.5
phencyclidine (PCP) 305.9
sedative 305.4 ◀
specified NEC 305.9
tranquilizers 305.4
spouse 995.80
tobacco 305.1
Acalcerosis 275.40
Acalcicosis 275.40
Acalculia 784.69
developmental 315.1
Acanthocheilonemiasis 125.4
Acanthocytosis 272.5
Acanthokeratodermia 701.1
Acantholysis 701.8
bullosa 757.39
Acanthoma (benign) (M8070/0) - *see also* Neoplasm, by site, benign
malignant (M8070/3) - *see* Neoplasm, by site, malignant
Acanthosis (acquired) (nigricans) 701.2
adult 701.2
benign (congenital) 757.39
congenital 757.39
glycogenic
  esophagus 530.89
juvenile 701.2
tongue 529.8
Acanthrocytosis 272.5
Acapnia 276.3
Acarbia 276.2
Acardia 759.89
Acardiacus amorphus 759.89
Acardiotrophia 429.1
Acardius 759.89
Acariasis 133.9
sarcoptic 133.0
Acaridiasis 133.9
Acarinosis 133.9

Acariosis 133.9
Acarodermatitis 133.9
  urticarioides 133.9
Acarophobia 300.29
Acatalasemia 277.89
Acatalasia 277.89
Acatamathesia 784.69
Acataphasia 784.5
Acathisia 781.0
  due to drugs 333.99
Acceleration, accelerated
  atrioventricular conduction 426.7
  idioventricular rhythm 427.89
Accessory (congenital)
  adrenal gland 759.1
  anus 751.5
  appendix 751.5
  atrioventricular conduction 426.7
  auditory ossicles 744.04
  auricle (ear) 744.1
  autosome(s) NEC 758.5
    21 or 22 758.0
  biliary duct or passage 751.69
  bladder 753.8
  blood vessels (peripheral) (congenital)
    NEC (*see also* Anomaly, peripheral
    vascular system) 747.60
    cerebral 747.81
    coronary 746.85
  bone NEC 756.9
    foot 755.67
  breast tissue, axilla 757.6
  carpal bones 755.56
  cecum 751.5
  cervix 752.49
  chromosome(s) NEC 758.5
    13-15 758.1
    16-18 758.2
    21 or 22 758.0
    autosome(s) NEC 758.5
    D_1 758.1
    E_3 758.2
    G 758.0
    sex 758.81
  coronary artery 746.85
  cusp(s), heart valve NEC 746.89
    pulmonary 746.09
  cystic duct 751.69
  digits 755.00
  ear (auricle) (lobe) 744.1
  endocrine gland NEC 759.2
  external os 752.49
  eyelid 743.62
  eye muscle 743.69
  face bone(s) 756.0
  fallopian tube (fimbria) (ostium)
    752.19
  fingers 755.01
  foreskin 605
  frontonasal process 756.0
  gallbladder 751.69
  genital organ(s)
    female 752.89
      external 752.49
      internal NEC 752.89
    male NEC 752.89
      penis 752.69
  genitourinary organs NEC 752.89
  heart 746.89
    valve NEC 746.89
      pulmonary 746.09
  hepatic ducts 751.69
  hymen 752.49
  intestine (large) (small) 751.5
  kidney 753.3

Accessory (*Continued*)
  lacrimal canal 743.65
  leaflet, heart valve NEC 746.89
    pulmonary 746.09
  ligament, broad 752.19
  liver (duct) 751.69
  lobule (ear) 744.1
  lung (lobe) 748.69
  muscle 756.82
  navicular of carpus 755.56
  nervous system, part NEC 742.8
  nipple 757.6
  nose 748.1
  organ or site NEC - *see* Anomaly, spec-
    ified type NEC
  ovary 752.0
  oviduct 752.19
  pancreas 751.7
  parathyroid gland 759.2
  parotid gland (and duct) 750.22
  pituitary gland 759.2
  placental lobe - *see* Placenta, abnormal
  preauricular appendage 744.1
  prepuce 605
  renal arteries (multiple) 747.62
  rib 756.3
    cervical 756.2
  roots (teeth) 520.2
  salivary gland 750.22
  sesamoids 755.8
  sinus - *see* Condition
  skin tags 757.39
  spleen 759.0
  sternum 756.3
  submaxillary gland 750.22
  tarsal bones 755.67
  teeth, tooth 520.1
    causing crowding 524.31   ◀▥
  tendon 756.89
  thumb 755.01
  thymus gland 759.2
  thyroid gland 759.2
  toes 755.02
  tongue 750.13
  tragus 744.1
  ureter 753.4
  urethra 753.8
  urinary organ or tract NEC 753.8
  uterus 752.2
  vagina 752.49
  valve, heart NEC 746.89
    pulmonary 746.09
  vertebra 756.19
  vocal cords 748.3
  vulva 752.49
Accident, accidental - *see also* Condition
  birth NEC 767.9
  cardiovascular (*see also* Disease, cardio-
    vascular) 429.2
  cerebral (*see also* Disease, cerebrovascu-
    lar, acute) 434.91   ◀▥
  cerebrovascular (current) (CVA) (*see*
    also Disease, cerebrovascular,
    acute) 434.91   ◀▥
    embolic 434.11   ◀
    healed or old V12.59
    impending 435.9
    ischemic 434.91   ◀
    late effect - *see* Late effect(s) (of)
      cerebrovascular disease
    postoperative 997.02
    thrombotic 434.01   ◀
  coronary (*see also* Infarct, myocardium)
    410.9

Accident, accidental (*Continued*)
  craniovascular (*see also* Disease, cere-
    brovascular, acute) 436
  during pregnancy, to mother, affecting
    fetus or newborn 760.5
  heart, cardiac (*see also* Infarct, myocar-
    dium) 410.9
  intrauterine 779.89
  vascular - *see* Disease, cerebrovascular,
    acute
Accommodation
  disorder of 367.51
    drug-induced 367.89
    toxic 367.89
  insufficiency of 367.4
  paralysis of 367.51
    hysterical 300.11
  spasm of 367.53
Accouchement - *see* Delivery
Accreta placenta (without hemorrhage)
  667.0
  with hemorrhage 666.0
Accretio cordis (nonrheumatic) 423.1
Accretions on teeth 523.6
Accumulation secretion, prostate 602.8
Acephalia, acephalism, acephaly 740.0
Acephalic 740.0
Acephalobrachia 759.89
Acephalocardia 759.89
Acephalocardius 759.89
Acephalochiria 759.89
Acephalochirus 759.89
Acephalogaster 759.89
Acephalostomus 759.89
Acephalothorax 759.89
Acephalus 740.0
Acetonemia 790.6
  diabetic 250.1
Acetonglycosuria 982.8
Acetonuria 791.6
Achalasia 530.0
  cardia 530.0
  digestive organs, congenital NEC
    751.8
  esophagus 530.0
  pelvirectal 751.3
  psychogenic 306.4
  pylorus 750.5
  sphincteral NEC 564.89
Achard-Thiers syndrome (adrenogenital)
  255.2
Ache(s) - *see* Pain
Acheilia 750.26
Acheiria 755.21
Achillobursitis 726.71
Achillodynia 726.71
Achlorhydria, achlorhydric 536.0
  anemia 280.9
  diarrhea 536.0
  neurogenic 536.0
  postvagotomy 564.2
  psychogenic 306.4
  secondary to vagotomy 564.2
Achloroblepsia 368.52
Achloropsia 368.52
Acholia 575.8
Acholuric jaundice (familial) (splenome-
  galic) (*see also* Spherocytosis) 282.0
  acquired 283.9
Achondroplasia 756.4
Achrestic anemia 281.8
Achroacytosis, lacrimal gland 375.00
  tuberculous (*see also* Tuberculosis) 017.3
Achroma, cutis 709.00

◀   **New**   ◀▥   **Revised**

Achromate (congenital) 368.54
Achromatopia 368.54
Achromatopsia (congenital) 368.54
Achromia
  congenital 270.2
  parasitica 111.0
  unguium 703.8
Achylia
  gastrica 536.8
    neurogenic 536.3
    psychogenic 306.4
  pancreatica 577.1
Achylosis 536.8
Acid
  burn - *see also* Burn, by site
    from swallowing acid - *see* Burn, in-
      ternal organs
  deficiency
    amide nicotinic 265.2
    amino 270.9
    ascorbic 267
    folic 266.2
    nicotinic (amide) 265.2
    pantothenic 266.2
  intoxication 276.2
  peptic disease 536.8
  stomach 536.8
    psychogenic 306.4
Acidemia 276.2
  arginosuccinic 270.6
  fetal
    affecting management of pregnancy
      656.3
    before onset of labor, in
      liveborn infant 768.2
    during labor, in liveborn infant
      768.3
    intrauterine—*see* Distress fetal
      656.3
    unspecified as to time of onset,
      in liveborn infant 768.4
  pipecolic 270.7
Acidity, gastric (high) (low) 536.8
  psychogenic 306.4
Acidocytopenia 288.0
Acidocytosis 288.3
Acidopenia 288.0
Acidosis 276.2
  diabetic 250.1
  fetal
    affecting management of
      pregnancy 656.8
    affecting newborn 768.9
  kidney tubular 588.89 ◄▥
  lactic 276.2
  metabolic NEC 276.2
    with respiratory acidosis 276.4
    late, of newborn 775.7
  renal
    hyperchloremic 588.89 ◄▥
    tubular (distal) (proximal) 588.89 ◄▥
  respiratory 276.2
    complicated by
      metabolic acidosis 276.4
      metabolic alkalosis 276.4
Aciduria 791.9
  arginosuccinic 270.6
  beta-aminoisobutyric (BAIB) 277.2
  glutaric ◄
    type I 270.7 ◄
    type II (type IIA, IIB, IIC) 277.85 ◄
    type III 277.86 ◄
  glycolic 271.8
  methylmalonic 270.3
    with glycinemia 270.7

Aciduria (*Continued*)
  organic 270.9
  orotic (congenital) (hereditary) (pyrimi-
    dine deficiency) 281.4
Acladiosis 111.8
  skin 111.8
Aclasis
  diaphyseal 756.4
  tarsoepiphyseal 756.59
Acleistocardia 745.5
Aclusion 524.4
Acmesthesia 782.0
Acne (pustular) (vulgaris) 706.1
  agminata (*see also* Tuberculosis) 017.0
  artificialis 706.1
  atrophica 706.0
  cachecticorum (Hebra) 706.1
  conglobata 706.1
  conjunctiva 706.1
  cystic 706.1
  decalvans 704.09
  erythematosa 695.3
  eyelid 706.1
  frontalis 706.0
  indurata 706.1
  keloid 706.1
  lupoid 706.0
  necrotic, necrotica 706.0
    miliaris 704.8
  nodular 706.1
  occupational 706.1
  papulosa 706.1
  rodens 706.0
  rosacea 695.3
  scorbutica 267
  scrofulosorum (Bazin) (*see also* Tuber-
    culosis) 017.0
  summer 692.72
  tropical 706.1
  varioliformis 706.0
Acneiform drug eruptions 692.3
Acnitis (primary) (*see also* Tuberculosis)
  017.0
Acomia 704.00
Acontractile bladder 344.61
Aconuresis (*see also* Incontinence) 788.30
Acosta's disease 993.2
Acousma 780.1
Acoustic - *see* Condition
Acousticophobia 300.29
Acquired - *see* Condition
Acquired immune deficiency syndrome
  - *see* Human immunodeficiency vi-
  rus (disease) (illness) (infection)
Acquired immunodeficiency syndrome -
  see Human immunodeficiency virus
  (disease) (illness) (infection)
Acragnosis 781.99
Acrania 740.0
Acroagnosis 781.99
Acroasphyxia, chronic 443.89
Acrobrachycephaly 756.0
Acrobystiolith 608.89
Acrobystitis 607.2
Acrocephalopolysyndactyly 755.55
Acrocephalosyndactyly 755.55
Acrocephaly 756.0
Acrochondrohyperplasia 759.82
Acrocyanosis 443.89
  newborn 770.83
Acrodermatitis 686.8
  atrophicans (chronica) 701.8
  continua (Hallopeau) 696.1
  enteropathica 686.8

Acrodermatitis (*Continued*)
  Hallopeau's 696.1
  perstans 696.1
  pustulosa continua 696.1
  recalcitrant pustular 696.1
Acrodynia 985.0
Acrodysplasia 755.55
Acrohyperhidrosis (*see also* Hyperhidro-
  sis) 780.8 ◄▥
Acrokeratosis verruciformis 757.39
Acromastitis 611.0
Acromegaly, acromegalia (skin) 253.0
Acromelalgia 443.89
Acromicria, acromikria 756.59
Acronyx 703.0
Acropachy, thyroid (*see also* Thyrotoxico-
  sis) 242.9
Acropachyderma 757.39
Acroparesthesia 443.89
  simple (Schultz's type) 443.89
  vasomotor (Nothnagel's type) 443.89
Acropathy thyroid (*see also* Thyrotoxico-
  sis) 242.9
Acrophobia 300.29
Acroposthitis 607.2
Acroscleriasis (*see also* Scleroderma)
  710.1
Acroscleroderma (*see also* Scleroderma)
  710.1
Acrosclerosis (*see also* Scleroderma) 710.1
Acrosphacelus 785.4
Acrosphenosyndactylia 755.55
Acrospiroma, eccrine (M8402/0) - *see*
  Neoplasm, skin, benign
Acrostealgia 732.9
Acrosyndactyly (*see also* Syndactylism)
  755.10
Acrotrophodynia 991.4
Actinic - *see also* Condition
  cheilitis (due to sun) 692.72
    chronic NEC 692.74
    due to radiation, except from sun
      692.82
  conjunctivitis 370.24
  dermatitis (due to sun) (*see also* Der-
    matitis, actinic) 692.70
    due to
      roentgen rays or radioactive sub-
        stance 692.82
      ultraviolet radiation, except from
        sun 692.82
      sun NEC 692.70
  elastosis solare 692.74
  granuloma 692.73
  keratitis 370.24
  ophthalmia 370.24
  reticuloid 692.73
Actinobacillosis, general 027.8
Actinobacillus
  lignieresii 027.8
  mallei 024
  muris 026.1
Actinocutitis NEC (*see also* Dermatitis,
  actinic) 692.70
Actinodermatitis NEC (*see also* Dermatitis, actinic) 692.70
Actinomyces
  israelii (infection) - *see* Actinomycosis
  muris-ratti (infection) 026.1
Actinomycosis, actinomycotic 039.9
  with
    pneumonia 039.1
  abdominal 039.2
  cervicofacial 039.3

Actinomycosis, actinomycotic
  (Continued)
  cutaneous 039.0
  pulmonary 039.1
  specified site NEC 039.8
  thoracic 039.1
Actinoneuritis 357.89
Action, heart
  disorder 427.9
    postoperative 997.1
  irregular 427.9
    postoperative 997.1
    psychogenic 306.2
Active - *see* Condition
Activity decrease, functional 780.99
Acute - *see also* Condition
  abdomen NEC 789.0
  gallbladder (*see also* Cholecystitis, acute) 575.0
Acyanoblepsia 368.53
Acyanopsia 368.53
Acystia 753.8
Acystinervia - *see* Neurogenic, bladder
Acystineuria - *see* Neurogenic, bladder
Adactylia, adactyly (congenital) 755.4
  lower limb (complete) (intercalary) (partial) (terminal) (*see also* Deformity, reduction, lower limb) 755.39
    meaning all digits (complete) (partial) 755.31
    transverse (complete) (partial) 755.31
  upper limb (complete) (intercalary) (partial) (terminal) (*see also* Deformity, reduction, upper limb) 755.29
    meaning all digits (complete) (partial) 755.21
    transverse (complete) (partial) 755.21
Adair-Dighton syndrome (brittle bones and blue sclera, deafness) 756.51
Adamantinoblastoma (M9310/0) - *see* Ameloblastoma
Adamantinoma (M9310/0) - *see* Ameloblastoma
Adamantoblastoma (M9310/0) - *see* Ameloblastoma
Adams-Stokes (-Morgagni) disease or syndrome (syncope with heart block) 426.9
Adaptation reaction (*see also* Reaction, adjustment) 309.9
Addiction - *see also* Dependence
  absinthe 304.6
  alcoholic (ethyl) (methyl) (wood) 303.9
    complicating pregnancy, childbirth, or puerperium 648.4
      affecting fetus or newborn 760.71
      suspected damage to fetus affecting management of pregnancy 655.4
  drug (*see also* Dependence) 304.9
  ethyl alcohol 303.9
  heroin 304.0
  hospital 301.51
  methyl alcohol 303.9
  methylated spirit 303.9
  morphine (-like substances) 304.0
  nicotine 305.1
  opium 304.0
  tobacco 305.1
  wine 303.9

Addison's
  anemia (pernicious) 281.0
  disease (bronze) (primary adrenal insufficiency) 255.4
    tuberculous (*see also* Tuberculosis) 017.6
  keloid (morphea) 701.0
  melanoderma (adrenal cortical hypofunction) 255.4
Addison-Biermer anemia (pernicious) 281.0
Addison-Gull disease - *see* Xanthoma
Addisonian crisis or melanosis (acute adrenocortical insufficiency) 255.4
Additional - *see also* Accessory
  chromosome(s) 758.5
    13-15 758.1
    16-18 758.2
    21 758.0
    autosome(s) NEC 758.5
    sex 758.81
Adduction contracture, hip or other joint - *see* Contraction, joint
Adenasthenia gastrica 536.0
Aden fever 061
Adenitis (*see also* Lymphadenitis) 289.3
  acute, unspecified site 683
    epidemic infectious 075
  axillary 289.3
    acute 683
    chronic or subacute 289.1
  Bartholin's gland 616.8
  bulbourethral gland (*see also* Urethritis) 597.89
  cervical 289.3
    acute 683
    chronic or subacute 289.1
  chancroid (Ducrey's bacillus) 099.0
  chronic (any lymph node, except mesenteric) 289.1
    mesenteric 289.2
  Cowper's gland (*see also* Urethritis) 597.89
  epidemic, acute 075
  gangrenous 683
  gonorrheal NEC 098.89
  groin 289.3
    acute 683
    chronic or subacute 289.1
  infectious 075
  inguinal (region) 289.3
    acute 683
    chronic or subacute 289.1
  lymph gland or node, except mesenteric 289.3
    acute 683
    chronic or subacute 289.1
    mesenteric (acute) (chronic) (nonspecific) (subacute) 289.2
  mesenteric (acute) (chronic) (nonspecific) (subacute) 289.2
    due to Pasteurella multocida (P. septica) 027.2
  parotid gland (suppurative) 527.2
  phlegmonous 683
  salivary duct or gland (any) (recurring) (suppurative) 527.2
  scrofulous (*see also* Tuberculosis) 017.2
  septic 289.3
  Skene's duct or gland (*see also* Urethritis) 597.89
  strumous, tuberculous (*see also* Tuberculosis) 017.2
  subacute, unspecified site 289.1

Adenitis *(Continued)*
  sublingual gland (suppurative) 527.2
  submandibular gland (suppurative) 527.2
  submaxillary gland (suppurative) 527.2
  suppurative 683
  tuberculous - *see* Tuberculosis, lymph gland
  urethral gland (*see also* Urethritis) 597.89
  venereal NEC 099.8
  Wharton's duct (suppurative) 527.2
Adenoacanthoma (M8570/3) - *see* Neoplasm, by site, malignant
Adenoameloblastoma (M9300/0) 213.1
  upper jaw (bone) 213.0
Adenocarcinoma (M8140/3) - *see also* Neoplasm, by site, malignant

---

Note The list of adjectival modifiers below is not exhaustive. A description of adenocarcinoma that does not appear in this list should be coded in the same manner as carcinoma with that description. Thus, "mixed acidophil-basophil adenocarcinoma" should be coded in the same manner as "mixed acidophil-basophil carcinoma," which appears in the list under "Carcinoma."

Except where otherwise indicated, the morphological varieties of adenocarcinoma in the list below should be coded by site as for "Neoplasm, malignant."

---

  with
    apocrine metaplasia (M8573/3)
    cartilaginous (and osseous) metaplasia (M8571/3)
    osseous (and cartilaginous) metaplasia (M8571/3)
    spindle cell metaplasia (M8572/3)
    squamous metaplasia (M8570/3)
  acidophil (M8280/3)
    specified site - *see* Neoplasm, by site, malignant
    unspecified site 194.3
  acinar (M8550/3)
  acinic cell (M8550/3)
  adrenal cortical (M8370/3) 194.0
  alveolar (M8251/3)
  and
    epidermoid carcinoma, mixed (M8560/3)
    squamous cell carcinoma, mixed (M8560/3)
  apocrine (M8401/3)
    breast - *see* Neoplasm, breast, malignant
    specified site NEC - *see* Neoplasm, skin, malignant
    unspecified site 173.9
  basophil (M8300/3)
    specified site - *see* Neoplasm, by site, malignant
    unspecified site 194.3
  bile duct type (M8160/3)
    liver 155.1
    specified site NEC - *see* Neoplasm, by site, malignant
    unspecified site 155.1

ICD-9-CM

A

Vol. 2

Adenocarcinoma (Continued)
bronchiolar (M8250/3) - see Neoplasm, lung, malignant
ceruminous (M8420/3) 173.2
chromophobe (M8270/3)
specified site - see Neoplasm, by site, malignant
unspecified site 194.3
clear cell (mesonephroid type) (M8310/3)
colloid (M8480/3)
cylindroid type (M8200/3)
diffuse type (M8145/3)
specified site - see Neoplasm, by site, malignant
unspecified site 151.9
duct (infiltrating) (M8500/3)
with Paget's disease (M8541/3) - see Neoplasm, breast, malignant
specified site - see Neoplasm, by site, malignant
unspecified site 174.9
embryonal (M9070/3)
endometrioid (M8380/3) - see Neoplasm, by site, malignant
eosinophil (M8280/3)
specified site - see Neoplasm, by site, malignant
unspecified site 194.3
follicular (M8330/3)
and papillary (M8340/3) 193
moderately differentiated type (M8332/3) 193
pure follicle type (M8331/3) 193
specified site - see Neoplasm, by site, malignant
trabecular type (M8332/3) 193
unspecified type 193
well differentiated type (M8331/3) 193
gelatinous (M8480/3)
granular cell (M8320/3)
Hürthle cell (M8290/3) 193
in
adenomatous
polyp (M8210/3)
polyposis coli (M8220/3) 153.9
polypoid adenoma (M8210/3)
tubular adenoma (M8210/3)
villous adenoma (M8261/3)
infiltrating duct (M8500/3)
with Paget's disease (M8541/3) - see Neoplasm, breast, malignant
specified site - see Neoplasm, by site, malignant
unspecified site 174.9
inflammatory (M8530/3)
specified site - see Neoplasm, by site, malignant
unspecified site 174.9
in situ (M8140/2) - see Neoplasm, by site, in situ
intestinal type (M8144/3)
specified site - see Neoplasm, by site, malignant
unspecified site 151.9
intraductal (noninfiltrating) (M8500/2)
papillary (M8503/2)
specified site - see Neoplasm, by site, in situ
unspecified site 233.0
specified site - see Neoplasm, by site, in situ
unspecified site 233.0

Adenocarcinoma (Continued)
islet cell (M8150/3)
and exocrine, mixed (M8154/3)
specified site - see Neoplasm, by site, malignant
unspecified site 157.9
pancreas 157.4
specified site NEC - see Neoplasm, by site, malignant
unspecified site 157.4
lobular (M8520/3)
specified site - see Neoplasm, by site, malignant
unspecified site 174.9
medullary (M8510/3)
mesonephric (M9110/3)
mixed cell (M8323/3)
mucinous (M8480/3)
mucin-producing (M8481/3)
mucoid (M8480/3) - see also Neoplasm, by site, malignant
cell (M8300/3)
specified site - see Neoplasm, by site, malignant
unspecified site 194.3
nonencapsulated sclerosing (M8350/3) 193
oncocytic (M8290/3)
oxyphilic (M8290/3)
papillary (M8260/3)
and follicular (M8340/3) 193
intraductal (noninfiltrating) (M8503/2)
specified site - see Neoplasm, by site, in situ
unspecified site 233.0
serous (M8460/3)
specified site - see Neoplasm, by site, malignant
unspecified site 183.0
papillocystic (M8450/3)
specified site - see Neoplasm, by site, malignant
unspecified site 183.0
pseudomucinous (M8470/3)
specified site - see Neoplasm, by site, malignant
unspecified site 183.0
renal cell (M8312/3) 189.0
sebaceous (M8410/3)
serous (M8441/3) - see also Neoplasm, by site, malignant
papillary
specified site - see Neoplasm, by site, malignant
unspecified site 183.0
signet ring cell (M8490/3)
superficial spreading (M8143/3)
sweat gland (M8400/3) - see Neoplasm, skin, malignant
trabecular (M8190/3)
tubular (M8211/3)
villous (M8262/3)
water-clear cell (M8322/3) 194.1
Adenofibroma (M9013/0)
clear cell (M8313/0) - see Neoplasm, by site, benign
endometrioid (M8381/0) 220
borderline malignancy (M8381/1) 236.2
malignant (M8381/3) 183.0
mucinous (M9015/0)
specified site - see Neoplasm, by site, benign
unspecified site 220

Adenofibroma (Continued)
prostate 600.20
with urinary retention 600.21
serous (M9014/0)
specified site - see Neoplasm, by site, benign
unspecified site 220
specified site - see Neoplasm, by site, benign
unspecified site 220
Adenofibrosis
breast 610.2
endometrioid 617.0
Adenoiditis 474.01
acute 463
chronic 474.01
with chronic tonsillitis 474.02
Adenoids (congenital) (of nasal fossa) 474.9
hypertrophy 474.12
vegetations 474.2
Adenolipomatosis (symmetrical) 272.8
Adenolymphoma (M8561/0)
specified site - see Neoplasm, by site, benign
unspecified 210.2
Adenoma (sessile) (M8140/0) - see also Neoplasm, by site, benign

> Note   Except where otherwise indicated, the morphological varieties of adenoma in the list below should be coded by site as for "Neoplasm, benign."

acidophil (M8280/0)
specified site - see Neoplasm, by site, benign
unspecified site 227.3
acinar (cell) (M8550/0)
acinic cell (M8550/0)
adrenal (cortex) (cortical) (functioning) (M8370/0) 227.0
clear cell type (M8373/0) 227.0
compact cell type (M8371/0) 227.0
glomerulosa cell type (M8374/0) 227.0
heavily pigmented variant (M8372/0) 227.0
mixed cell type (M8375/0) 227.0
alpha cell (M8152/0)
pancreas 211.7
specified site NEC - see Neoplasm, by site, benign
unspecified site 211.7
alveolar (M8251/0)
apocrine (M8401/0)
breast 217
specified site NEC - see Neoplasm, skin, benign
unspecified site 216.9
basal cell (M8147/0)
basophil (M8300/0)
specified site - see Neoplasm, by site, benign
unspecified site 227.3
beta cell (M8151/0)
pancreas 211.7
specified site NEC - see Neoplasm, by site, benign
unspecified site 211.7
bile duct (M8160/0) 211.5
black (M8372/0) 227.0

Adenoma (Continued)
bronchial (M8140/1) 235.7
carcinoid type (M8240/3) - see Neoplasm, lung, malignant
cylindroid type (M8200/3) - see
Neoplasm, lung, malignant
ceruminous (M8420/0) 216.2
chief cell (M8321/0) 227.1
chromophobe (M8270/0)
specified site - see Neoplasm, by site,
benign
unspecified site 227.3
clear cell (M8310/0)
colloid (M8334/0)
specified site - see Neoplasm, by site,
benign
unspecified site 226
cylindroid type, bronchus (M8200/3) -
see Neoplasm, lung, malignant
duct (M8503/0)
embryonal (M8191/0)
endocrine, multiple (M8360/1)
single specified site - see Neoplasm,
by site, uncertain behavior
two or more specified sites 237.4
unspecified site 237.4
endometrioid (M8380/0) - see also
Neoplasm, by site, benign
borderline malignancy (M8380/1) -
see Neoplasm, by site, uncertain
behavior
eosinophil (M8280/0)
specified site - see Neoplasm, by site,
benign
unspecified site 227.3
fetal (M8333/0)
specified site - see Neoplasm, by site,
benign
unspecified site 226
follicular (M8330/0)
specified site - see Neoplasm, by site,
benign
unspecified site 226
hepatocellular (M8170/0) 211.5
Hürthle cell (M8290/0) 226
intracystic papillary (M8504/0)
islet cell (functioning) (M8150/0)
pancreas 211.7
specified site NEC - see Neoplasm,
by site, benign
unspecified site 211.7
liver cell (M8170/0) 211.5
macrofollicular (M8334/0)
specified site NEC - see Neoplasm,
by site, benign
unspecified site 226
malignant, malignum (M8140/3) - see
Neoplasm, by site,
malignant
mesonephric (M9110/0)
microfollicular (M8333/0)
specified site - see Neoplasm, by site,
benign
unspecified site 226
mixed cell (M8323/0)
monomorphic (M8146/0)
mucinous (M8480/0)
mucoid cell (M8300/0)
specified site - see Neoplasm, by site,
benign
unspecified site 227.3
multiple endocrine (M8360/1)
single specified site - see Neoplasm,
by site, uncertain behavior

Adenoma (Continued)
multiple endocrine (Continued)
two or more specified sites 237.4
unspecified site 237.4
nipple (M8506/0) 217
oncocytic (M8290/0)
oxyphilic (M8290/0)
papillary (M8260/0) - see also Neoplasm, by site, benign
intracystic (M8504/0)
papillotubular (M8263/0)
Pick's tubular (M8640/0)
specified site - see Neoplasm, by site,
benign
unspecified site
female 220
male 222.0
pleomorphic (M8940/0)
polypoid (M8210/0)
prostate (benign) 600.20
with urinary retention 600.21
rete cell 222.0
sebaceous, sebaceum (gland) (senile)
(M8410/0) - see also Neoplasm,
skin, benign
disseminata 759.5
Sertoli cell (M8640/0)
specified site - see Neoplasm, by site,
benign
unspecified site
female 220
male 222.0
skin appendage (M8390/0) - see Neoplasm, skin, benign
sudoriferous gland (M8400/0) - see Neoplasm, skin, benign
sweat gland or duct (M8400/0) - see
Neoplasm, skin, benign
testicular (M8640/0)
specified site - see Neoplasm, by site,
benign
unspecified site
female 220
male 222.0
thyroid 226
trabecular (M8190/0)
tubular (M8211/0) - see also Neoplasm,
by site, benign
papillary (M8460/3)
Pick's (M8640/0)
specified site - see Neoplasm, by
site, benign
unspecified site
female 220
male 222.0
tubulovillous (M8263/0)
villoglandular (M8263/0)
villous (M8261/1) - see Neoplasm, by
site, uncertain behavior
water-clear cell (M8322/0) 227.1
wolffian duct (M9110/0)
Adenomatosis (M8220/0)
endocrine (multiple) (M8360/1)
single specified site - see Neoplasm,
by site, uncertain behavior
two or more specified sites
237.4
unspecified site 237.4
erosive of nipple (M8506/0) 217
pluriendocrine - see Adenomatosis, endocrine
pulmonary (M8250/1) 235.7
malignant (M8250/3) - see Neoplasm, lung, malignant

Adenomatosis (Continued)
specified site - see Neoplasm, by site,
benign
unspecified site 211.3
Adenomatous
cyst, thyroid (gland) - see Goiter, nodular
goiter (nontoxic) (see also Goiter, nodular) 241.9
toxic or with hyperthyroidism 242.3
Adenomyoma (M8932/0) - see also Neoplasm, by site, benign
prostate 600.20
with urinary retention 600.21
Adenomyometritis 617.0
Adenomyosis (uterus) (internal) 617.0
Adenopathy (lymph gland) 785.6
inguinal 785.6
mediastinal 785.6
mesentery 785.6
syphilitic (secondary) 091.4
tracheobronchial 785.6
tuberculous (see also Tuberculosis)
012.1
primary, progressive 010.8
tuberculous (see also Tuberculosis,
lymph gland) 017.2
tracheobronchial 012.1
primary, progressive 010.8
Adenopharyngitis 462
Adenophlegmon 683
Adenosalpingitis 614.1
Adenosarcoma (M8960/3) 189.0
Adenosclerosis 289.3
Adenosis
breast (sclerosing) 610.2
vagina, congenital 752.49
Adentia (complete) (partial) (see also Absence, teeth) 520.0
Adherent
labium (minus) 624.4
pericardium (nonrheumatic) 423.1
rheumatic 393
placenta 667.0
with hemorrhage 666.0
prepuce 605
scar (skin) NEC 709.2
tendon in scar 709.2
Adhesion(s), adhesive (postinfectional)
(postoperative)
abdominal (wall) (see also Adhesions,
peritoneum) 568.0
amnion to fetus 658.8
affecting fetus or newborn
762.8
appendix 543.9
arachnoiditis - see Meningitis
auditory tube (Eustachian) 381.89
bands - see also Adhesions, peritoneum
cervix 622.3
uterus 621.5
bile duct (any) 576.8
bladder (sphincter) 596.8
bowel (see also Adhesions, peritoneum)
568.0
cardiac 423.1
rheumatic 398.99
cecum (see also Adhesions, peritoneum)
568.0
cervicovaginal 622.3
congenital 752.49
postpartal 674.8
old 622.3

◀ **New**   ◀▥ **Revised**

ICD-9-CM

Vol. 2

Adhesion(s) (*Continued*)
cervix 622.3
clitoris 624.4
colon (*see also* Adhesions, peritoneum) 568.0
common duct 576.8
congenital - *see also* Anomaly, specified type NEC
    fingers (*see also* Syndactylism, fingers) 755.11
    labium (majus) (minus) 752.49
    omental, anomalous 751.4
    ovary 752.0
    peritoneal 751.4
    toes (*see also* Syndactylism, toes) 755.13
    tongue (to gum or roof of mouth) 750.12
conjunctiva (acquired) (localized) 372.62
    congenital 743.63
    extensive 372.63
cornea - *see* Opacity, cornea
cystic duct 575.8
diaphragm (*see also* Adhesions, peritoneum) 568.0
due to foreign body - *see* Foreign body
duodenum (*see also* Adhesions, peritoneum) 568.0
    with obstruction 537.3
ear, middle - *see* Adhesions, middle ear
epididymis 608.89
epidural - *see* Adhesions, meninges
epiglottis 478.79
Eustachian tube 381.89
eyelid 374.46
    postoperative 997.99
        surgically created V45.69
gallbladder (*see also* Disease, gallbladder) 575.8
globe 360.89
heart 423.1
    rheumatic 398.99
ileocecal (coil) (*see also* Adhesions, peritoneum) 568.0
ileum (*see also* Adhesions, peritoneum) 568.0
intestine (postoperative) (*see also* Adhesions, peritoneum) 568.0
    with obstruction 560.81
        with hernia - *see also* Hernia, by site, with obstruction
            gangrenous - *see* Hernia, by site, with gangrene
intra-abdominal (*see also* Adhesions, peritoneum) 568.0
iris 364.70
    to corneal graft 996.79
joint (*see also* Ankylosis) 718.5
kidney 593.89
labium (majus) (minus), congenital 752.49
liver 572.8
lung 511.0
mediastinum 519.3
meninges 349.2
    cerebral (any) 349.2
        congenital 742.4
    congenital 742.8
    spinal (any) 349.2
        congenital 742.59
    tuberculous (cerebral) (spinal) (*see also* Tuberculosis, meninges) 013.0

Adhesion(s) (*Continued*)
mesenteric (*see also* Adhesions, peritoneum) 568.0
middle ear (fibrous) 385.10
    drum head 385.19
        to
            incus 385.11
            promontorium 385.13
            stapes 385.12
        specified NEC 385.19
nasal (septum) (to turbinates) 478.1
nerve NEC 355.9
    spinal 355.9
        root 724.9
            cervical NEC 723.4
            lumbar NEC 724.4
            lumbosacral 724.4
            thoracic 724.4
ocular muscle 378.60
omentum (*see also* Adhesions, peritoneum) 568.0
organ or site, congenital NEC - *see* Anomaly, specified type NEC
ovary 614.6
    congenital (to cecum, kidney, or omentum) 752.0
parauterine 614.6
parovarian 614.6
pelvic (peritoneal)
    female (postoperative) (postinfection) 614.6
    male (postoperative) (postinfection) (*see also* Adhesions, peritoneum) 568.0
    postpartal (old) 614.6
    tuberculous (*see also* Tuberculosis) 016.9
penis to scrotum (congenital) 752.69
periappendiceal (*see also* Adhesions, peritoneum) 568.0
pericardium (nonrheumatic) 423.1
    rheumatic 393
    tuberculous (*see also* Tuberculosis) 017.9 [420.0]
pericholecystic 575.8
perigastric (*see also* Adhesions, peritoneum) 568.0
periovarian 614.6
periprostatic 602.8
perirectal (*see also* Adhesions, peritoneum) 568.0
perirenal 593.89
peritoneum, peritoneal (fibrous) (postoperative) 568.0
    with obstruction (intestinal) 560.81
        with hernia - *see also* Hernia, by site, with obstruction
            gangrenous - *see* Hernia, by site, with gangrene
        duodenum 537.3
    congenital 751.4
    female (postoperative) (postinfective) 614.6
    pelvic, female 614.6
    pelvic, male 568.0
    postpartal, pelvic 614.6
    to uterus 614.6
peritubal 614.6
periureteral 593.89
periuterine 621.5
perivesical 596.8
perivesicular (seminal vesicle) 608.89

Adhesion(s) (*Continued*)
pleura, pleuritic 511.0
    tuberculous (*see also* Tuberculosis, pleura) 012.0
pleuropericardial 511.0
postoperative (gastrointestinal tract) (*see also* Adhesions, peritoneum)
    eyelid 997.99
        surgically created V45.69
    pelvic female 614.9
    pelvic, male 568.0
    urethra 598.2
postpartal, old 624.4
preputial, prepuce 605
pulmonary 511.0
pylorus (*see also* Adhesions, peritoneum) 568.0
Rosenmüller's fossa 478.29
sciatic nerve 355.0
seminal vesicle 608.89
shoulder (joint) 726.0
sigmoid flexure (*see also* Adhesions, peritoneum) 568.0
spermatic cord (acquired) 608.89
    congenital 752.89
spinal canal 349.2
    nerve 355.9
        root 724.9
            cervical NEC 723.4
            lumbar NEC 724.4
            lumbosacral 724.4
            thoracic 724.4
stomach (*see also* Adhesions, peritoneum) 568.0
subscapular 726.2
tendonitis 726.90
    shoulder 726.0
testicle 608.89
tongue (congenital) (to gum or roof of mouth) 750.12
    acquired 529.8
trachea 519.1
tubo-ovarian 614.6
tunica vaginalis 608.89
ureter 593.89
uterus 621.5
    to abdominal wall 614.6
        in pregnancy or childbirth 654.4
            affecting fetus or newborn 763.89
vagina (chronic) (postoperative) (postradiation) 623.2
vaginitis (congenital) 752.49
vesical 596.8
vitreous 379.29
Adie (-Holmes) syndrome (tonic pupillary reaction) 379.46
Adiponecrosis neonatorum 778.1
Adiposa dolorosa 272.8
Adiposalgia 272.8
Adiposis
    cerebralis 253.8
    dolorosa 272.8
    tuberosa simplex 272.8
Adiposity 278.00
    heart (*see also* Degeneration, myocardial) 429.1
    localized 278.1
Adiposogenital dystrophy 253.8
Adjustment
    prosthesis or other device - *see* Fitting of
    reaction - *see* Reaction, adjustment

Administration, prophylactic
  antibiotics V07.39
  antitoxin, any V07.2
  antivenin V07.2
  chemotherapeutic agent NEC V07.39
  chemotherapy NEC V07.39
  diphtheria antitoxin V07.2
  fluoride V07.31
  gamma globulin V07.2
  immune sera (gamma globulin) V07.2
  passive immunization agent V07.2
  RhoGAM V07.2
Admission (encounter)
  as organ donor - *see* Donor
  by mistake V68.9
  for
    adequacy testing (for)
      hemodialysis V56.31
      peritoneal dialysis V56.32
    adjustment (of)
      artificial
        arm (complete) (partial) V52.0
        eye V52.2
        leg (complete) (partial) V52.1
      brain neuropacemaker V53.02
      breast
        implant V52.4
        prosthesis V52.4
      cardiac device V53.39
        defibrillator, automatic implant-
          able V53.32
        pacemaker V53.31
          carotid sinus V53.39
      catheter
        non-vascular V58.82
        vascular V58.81
      cerebral ventricle (communicating)
        shunt V53.01
      colostomy belt V55.3
      contact lenses V53.1
      cystostomy device V53.6
      dental prosthesis V52.3
      device, unspecified type V53.90
        abdominal V53.5
        cardiac V53.39
          defibrillator, automatic im-
            plantable V53.32
          pacemaker V53.31
        carotid sinus V53.39
        cerebral ventricle (communicat-
          ing) shunt V53.01
        insulin pump V53.91
        intrauterine contraceptive V25.1
        nervous system V53.09
        orthodontic V53.4
        other device V53.99
        prosthetic V52.9
          breast V52.4
          dental V52.3
          eye V52.2
          specified type NEC V52.8
        special senses V53.09
        substitution
          auditory V53.09
          nervous system V53.09
          visual V53.09
        urinary V53.6
      dialysis catheter
        extracorporeal V56.1
        peritoneal V56.2
      diaphragm (contraceptive) V25.02
      growth rod V54.02
      hearing aid V53.2
      ileostomy device V55.2

Admission *(Continued)*
  for *(Continued)*
    adjustment (of) *(Continued)*
      intestinal appliance or device NEC
        V53.5
      intrauterine contraceptive device
        V25.1
      neuropacemaker (brain) (peripheral
        nerve) (spinal cord) V53.02
      orthodontic device V53.4
      orthopedic (device) V53.7
        brace V53.7
        cast V53.7
        shoes V53.7
      pacemaker
        brain V53.02
        cardiac V53.31
        carotid sinus V53.39
        peripheral nerve V53.02
        spinal cord V53.02
      prosthesis V52.9
        arm (complete) (partial) V52.0
        breast V52.4
        dental V52.3
        eye V52.2
        leg (complete) (partial) V52.1
        specified type NEC V52.8
      spectacles V53.1
      wheelchair V53.8
    adoption referral or proceedings
      V68.89
    aftercare (*see also* Aftercare) V58.9
      cardiac pacemaker V53.31
      chemotherapy V58.1
      dialysis
        extracorporeal (renal) V56.0
        peritoneal V56.8
        renal V56.0
      fracture (*see also* Aftercare, frac-
        ture) V54.9
      medical NEC V58.89
      organ transplant V58.44   ◄
      orthopedic V54.9
        specified type NEC V54.89
      pacemaker device
        brain V53.02
        cardiac V53.31
        carotid sinus V53.39
        nervous system V53.02
        spinal cord V53.02
      postoperative NEC V58.49
        wound closure, planned V58.41
      postpartum
        immediately after delivery V24.0
        routine follow-up V24.2
      postradiation V58.0
      radiation therapy V58.0
      removal of
        non-vascular catheter V58.82
        vascular catheter V58.81
      specified NEC V58.89
      surgical NEC V58.49
        wound closure, planned V58.41
    artificial insemination V26.1
    attention to artificial opening (of)
      V55.9
      artificial vagina V55.7
      colostomy V55.3
      cystostomy V55.5
      enterostomy V55.4
      gastrostomy V55.1
      ileostomy V55.2
      jejunostomy V55.4
      nephrostomy V55.6

Admission *(Continued)*
  for *(Continued)*
    attention to artificial opening
      (Continued)
      specified site NEC V55.8
        intestinal tract V55.4
        urinary tract V55.6
      tracheostomy V55.0
      ureterostomy V55.6
      urethrostomy V55.6
    battery replacement
      cardiac pacemaker V53.31
    boarding V65.0
    breast
      augmentation or reduction V50.1
      removal, prophylactic V50.41
    change of
      cardiac pacemaker (battery) V53.31
      carotid sinus pacemaker V53.39
      catheter in artificial opening - *see*
        Attention to, artificial, opening
      dressing V58.3
      fixation device
        external V54.89
        internal V54.01
      Kirschner wire V54.89
      neuropacemaker device (brain) (pe-
        ripheral nerve) (spinal cord)
        V53.02
      pacemaker device
        brain V53.02
        cardiac V53.31
        carotid sinus V53.39
        nervous system V53.02
      plaster cast V54.89
      splint, external V54.89
      Steinmann pin V54.89
      surgical dressing V58.3
      traction device V54.89
    checkup only V70.0
    chemotherapy V58.1
    circumcision, ritual or routine (in ab-
      sence of medical indication)
      V50.2
    clinical research investigation
      (control) (normal comparison)
      (participant) V70.7
    closure of artificial opening - *see*
      Attention to, artificial, opening
    contraceptive
      counseling V25.09
        emergency V25.03
        postcoital V25.03
      management V25.9
        specified type NEC V25.8
    convalescence following V66.9
      chemotherapy V66.2
      psychotherapy V66.3
      radiotherapy V66.1
      surgery V66.0
      treatment (for) V66.5
        combined V66.6
        fracture V66.4
        mental disorder NEC V66.3
        specified condition NEC V66.5
    cosmetic surgery NEC V50.1
      following healed injury or opera-
        tion V51
    counseling (*see also* Counseling)
      V65.40
      without complaint or sickness
        V65.49
    contraceptive management V25.09
      emergency V25.03
      postcoital V25.03

Admission (*Continued*)
for (*Continued*)
counseling (*Continued*)
dietary V65.3
exercise V65.41
for nonattending third party
V65.19
for pediatric pre-birth visit for expectant mother V65.11
genetic V26.3
gonorrhea V65.45
HIV V65.44
human immunodeficiency virus
V65.44
injury prevention V65.43
insulin pump training V65.46
procreative management V26.4
sexually transmitted disease NEC
V65.45
HIV V65.44
specified reason NEC V65.49
substance use and abuse V65.42
syphilis V65.45
victim of abuse
child V61.21
partner or spouse V61.11
desensitization to allergens V07.1
dialysis V56.0
catheter
fitting and adjustment
extracorporeal V56.1
peritoneal V56.2
removal or replacement
extracorporeal V56.1
peritoneal V56.2
extracorporeal (renal) V56.0
peritoneal V56.8
renal V56.0
dietary surveillance and counseling
V65.3
drug monitoring, therapeutic V58.83
ear piercing V50.3
elective surgery
breast
augmentation or reduction V50.1
removal, prophylactic V50.41
circumcision, ritual or routine (in
absence of medical indication)
V50.2
cosmetic NEC V50.1
following healed injury or operation V51
ear piercing V50.3
face-lift V50.1
hair transplant V50.0
plastic
cosmetic NEC V50.1
following healed injury or operation V51
prophylactic organ removal V50.49
breast V50.41
ovary V50.42
repair of scarred tissue (following
healed injury or operation)
V51
specified type NEC V50.8
end-of-life care V66.7
examination (*see also* Examination)
V70.9
administrative purpose NEC V70.3
adoption V70.3
allergy V72.7
at health care facility V70.0
athletic team V70.3

Admission (*Continued*)
for (*Continued*)
examination (*Continued*)
camp V70.3
cardiovascular, preoperative V72.81
clinical research investigation (control) (participant) V70.7
dental V72.2
developmental testing (child) (infant) V20.2
donor (potential) V70.8
driver's license V70.3
ear V72.1
employment V70.5
eye V72.0
follow-up (routine) - *see* Examination, follow-up
for admission to
old age home V70.3
school V70.3
general V70.9
specified reason NEC V70.8
gynecological V72.31 ◀▥
health supervision (child) (infant)
V20.2
hearing V72.1
immigration V70.3
insurance certification V70.3
laboratory V72.6
marriage license V70.3
medical (general) (*see also* Examination, medical) V70.9
medicolegal reasons V70.4
naturalization V70.3
pelvic (annual) (periodic) V72.31◀▥
postpartum checkup V24.2
pregnancy (possible) (unconfirmed) V72.40 ◀▥
negative result V72.41 ◀
preoperative V72.84
cardiovascular V72.81
respiratory V72.82
specified NEC V72.83
prison V70.3
psychiatric (general) V70.2
requested by authority V70.1
radiological NEC V72.5
respiratory, preoperative V72.82
school V70.3
screening - *see* Screening
skin hypersensitivity V72.7
specified type NEC V72.85
sport competition V70.3
vision V72.0
well baby and child care V20.2
exercise therapy V57.1
face-lift, cosmetic reason V50.1
fitting (of)
artificial
arm (complete) (partial) V52.0
eye V52.2
leg (complete) (partial) V52.1
biliary drainage tube V58.82
brain neuropacemaker V53.02
breast V52.4
implant V50.1
prosthesis V52.4
cardiac pacemaker V53.31
catheter
non-vascular V58.82
vascular V58.81
cerebral ventricle (communicating)
shunt V53.01
chest tube V58.82

Admission (*Continued*)
for (*Continued*)
fitting (*Continued*)
colostomy belt V55.2
contact lenses V53.1
cystostomy device V53.6
dental prosthesis V52.3
device, unspecified type V53.90
abdominal V53.5
cerebral ventricle (communicating) shunt V53.01
insulin pump V53.91
intrauterine contraceptive
V25.1
nervous system V53.09
orthodontic V53.4
other device V53.99
prosthetic V52.9
breast V52.4
dental V52.3
eye V52.2
special senses V53.09
substitution
auditory V53.09
nervous system V53.09
visual V53.09
diaphragm (contraceptive)
V25.02
fistula (sinus tract) drainage tube
V58.82
growth rod V54.02
hearing aid V53.2
ileostomy device V55.2
intestinal appliance or device NEC
V53.5
intrauterine contraceptive device
V25.1
neuropacemaker (brain) (peripheral
nerve) (spinal cord) V53.02
orthodontic device V53.4
orthopedic (device) V53.7
brace V53.7
cast V53.7
shoes V53.7
pacemaker
brain V53.02
cardiac V53.31
carotid sinus V53.39
spinal cord V53.02
pleural drainage tube V58.82
prosthesis V52.9
arm (complete) (partial) V52.0
breast V52.4
dental V52.3
eye V52.2
leg (complete) (partial) V52.1
specified type NEC V52.8
spectacles V53.1
wheelchair V53.8
follow-up examination (routine) (following) V67.9
cancer chemotherapy V67.2
chemotherapy V67.2
high-risk medication NEC V67.51
injury NEC V67.59
psychiatric V67.3
psychotherapy V67.3
radiotherapy V67.1
specified surgery NEC V67.09
surgery V67.00
vaginal pap smear V67.01
treatment (for) V67.9
combined V67.6
fracture V67.4

Admission (*Continued*)
for (*Continued*)
follow-up examination (*Continued*)
treatment (*Continued*)
involving high-risk medication NEC V67.51
mental disorder V67.3
specified NEC V67.59
hair transplant, for cosmetic reason V50.0
health advice, education, or instruction V65.4
hormone replacement therapy (postmenopausal) V07.4 ◄
hospice care V66.7
insertion (of)
subdermal implantable contraceptive V25.5
insulin pump titration V53.91
insulin pump training V65.46
intrauterine device
insertion V25.1
management V25.42
investigation to determine further disposition V63.8
isolation V07.0
issue of
medical certificate NEC V68.0
repeat prescription NEC V68.1
contraceptive device NEC V25.49
kidney dialysis V56.0
lenghtening of growth rod V54.02
mental health evaluation V70.2
requested by authority V70.1
nonmedical reason NEC V68.89
nursing care evaluation V63.8
observation (without need for further medical care) (*see also* Observation) V71.9
accident V71.4
alleged rape or seduction V71.5
criminal assault V71.6
following accident V71.4
at work V71.3
foreign body ingestion V71.89
growth and development variations, childhood V21.0
inflicted injury NEC V71.6
ingestion of deleterious agent or foreign body V71.89
injury V71.6
malignant neoplasm V71.1
mental disorder V71.09
newborn - *see* Observation, suspected, condition, newborn
rape V71.5
specified NEC V71.89
suspected disorder V71.9
abuse V71.81
accident V71.4
at work V71.3
benign neoplasm V71.89
cardiovascular V71.7
exposure
anthrax V71.82
biological agent NEC V71.83
heart V71.7
inflicted injury NEC V71.6
malignant neoplasm V71.1
mental NEC V71.09
neglect V71.81
SARS V71.83
specified condition NEC V71.89
tuberculosis V71.2
tuberculosis V71.2

Admission (*Continued*)
for (*Continued*)
occupational therapy V57.21
organ transplant, donor - *see* Donor
ovary, ovarian removal, prophylactic V50.42
palliative care V66.7
Papanicolaou smear
cervix V76.2
vaginal V76.47
following hysterectomy for malignant condition V67.01
for suspected malignant neoplasm V76.2
no disease found V71.1
routine, as part of gynecological examination V72.31 ◄▦
to confirm findings of recent normal smear following initial abnormal smear V72.32 ◄
passage of sounds or bougie in artificial opening - *see* Attention to, artificial, opening
paternity testing V70.4
peritoneal dialysis V56.8
physical therapy NEC V57.1
plastic surgery
cosmetic NEC V50.1
following healed injury or operation V51
postmenopausal hormone replacement therapy V07.4
postpartum observation
immediately after delivery V24.0
routine follow-up V24.2
poststerilization (for restoration) V26.0
procreative management V26.9
specified type NEC V26.8
prophylactic
administration of
antibiotics V07.39
antitoxin, any V07.2
antivenin V07.2
chemotherapeutic agent NEC V07.39
chemotherapy NEC V07.39
diphtheria antitoxin V07.2
fluoride V07.31
gamma globulin V07.2
immune sera (gamma globulin) V07.2
RhoGAM V07.2
tetanus antitoxin V07.2
breathing exercises V57.0
chemotherapy NEC V07.39
fluoride V07.31
measure V07.9
specified type NEC V07.8
organ removal V50.49
breast V50.41
ovary V50.42
psychiatric examination (general) V70.2
requested by authority V70.1
radiation management V58.0
radiotherapy V58.0
reforming of artificial opening - *see* Attention to, artificial, opening
rehabilitation V57.9
multiple types V57.89
occupational V57.21
orthoptic V57.4
orthotic V57.81
physical NEC V57.1
specified type NEC V57.89
speech V57.3
vocational V57.22

Admission (*Continued*)
for (*Continued*)
removal of
cardiac pacemaker V53.31
cast (plaster) V54.89
catheter from artificial opening - *see* Attention to, artificial, opening
cerebral ventricle (communicating) shunt V53.01
cystostomy catheter V55.5
device
cerebral ventricle (communicating) shunt V53.01
fixation
external V54.89
internal V54.01
intrauterine contraceptive V25.42
traction, external V54.89
dressing V58.3
fixation device
external V54.89
internal V54.01
intrauterine contraceptive device V25.42
Kirschner wire V54.89
neuropacemaker (brain) (peripheral nerve) (spinal cord) V53.02
orthopedic fixation device
external V54.89
internal V54.01
pacemaker device
brain V53.02
cardiac V53.31
carotid sinus V53.39
nervous system V53.02
plaster cast V54.89
plate (fracture) V54.01
rod V54.01
screw (fracture) V54.01
splint, traction V54.89
Steinmann pin V54.89
subdermal implantable contraceptive V25.43
surgical dressing V58.3
sutures V58.3
traction device, external V54.89
ureteral stent V53.6
repair of scarred tissue (following healed injury or operation) V51
reprogramming of cardiac pacemaker V53.31
respirator dependence, during power failure V46.12 ◄
restoration of organ continuity (poststerilization) (tuboplasty) (vasoplasty) V26.0
sensitivity test - *see also* Test, skin
allergy NEC V72.7
bacterial disease NEC V74.9
Dick V74.8
Kveim V82.89
Mantoux V74.1
mycotic infection NEC V75.4
parasitic disease NEC V75.8
Schick V74.3
Schultz-Charlton V74.8
social service (agency) referral or evaluation V63.8
speech therapy V57.3
sterilization V25.2
suspected disorder (ruled out) (without need for further care) - *see* Observation
terminal care V66.7

◄ **New**   ◄▦ **Revised**

Admission (Continued)
for (Continued)
  tests only - see Test
  therapeutic drug monitoring V58.83
  therapy
    blood transfusion, without reported diagnosis V58.2
    breathing exercises V57.0
    chemotherapy V58.1
      prophylactic NEC V07.39
        fluoride V07.31
    dialysis (intermittent) (treatment)
      extracorporeal V56.0
      peritoneal V56.8
      renal V56.0
      specified type NEC V56.8
    exercise (remedial) NEC V57.1
      breathing V57.0
    long-term (current) drug use NEC V58.69
      antibiotics V58.62
      anticoagulants V58.61
      anti-inflammatories, non-steroidal (NSAID) V58.64
      antiplatelets V58.63
      antithrombotics V58.63
      aspirin V58.66
      insulin V58.67
      steroids V58.65
    occupational V57.21
    orthoptic V57.4
    physical NEC V57.1
    radiation V58.0
    speech V57.3
    vocational V57.22
  toilet or cleaning
    of artificial opening - see Attention to, artificial, opening
    of non-vascular catheter V58.82
    of vascular catheter V58.81
  tubal ligation V25.2
  tuboplasty for previous sterilization V26.0
  vaccination, prophylactic (against)
    arthropod-borne virus, viral NEC V05.1
      disease NEC V05.1
      encephalitis V05.0
    Bacille Calmette-Guérin (BCG) V03.2
    BCG V03.2
    chickenpox V05.4
    cholera alone V03.0
      with typhoid-paratyphoid (cholera + TAB) V06.0
    common cold V04.7
    dengue V05.1
    diphtheria alone V03.5
    diphtheria-tetanus-pertussis (DTP) (DTaP) V06.1
      with
        poliomyelitis (DTP + polio) V06.3
        typhoid-paratyphoid (DTP + TAB) V06.2
    diphtheria-tetanus [Td] [DT] without pertussis V06.5
    disease (single) NEC V05.9
      bacterial NEC V03.9
        specified type NEC V03.89
      combinations NEC V06.9
        specified type NEC V06.8
      specified type NEC V05.8
      viral NEC V04.89
    encephalitis, viral, arthropod-borne V05.0

Admission (Continued)
for (Continued)
  vaccination (Continued)
    Hemophilus influenzae, type B [Hib] V03.81
    hepatitis, viral V05.3
    immune sera (gamma globulin) V07.2
    influenza V04.81
      with
        Streptococcus pneumoniae [pneumococcus] V06.6
    Leishmaniasis V05.2
    measles alone V04.2
    measles-mumps-rubella (MMR) V06.4
    mumps alone V04.6
      with measles and rubella (MMR) V06.4
    not done because of contraindication V64.0
    pertussis alone V03.6
    plague V03.3
    pneumonia V03.82
    poliomyelitis V04.0
      with diphtheria-tetanuspertussis (DTP + polio) V06.3
    rabies V04.5
    respiratory syncytial virus (RSV) V04.82
    rubella alone V04.3
      with measles and mumps (MMR) V06.4
    smallpox V04.1
    specified type NEC V05.8
    Streptococcus pneumoniae [pneumococcus] V03.82
      with
        influenza V06.6
    tetanus toxoid alone V03.7
      with diphtheria [Td] [DT] V06.5
        and pertussis (DTP) (DTaP) V06.1
    tuberculosis (BCG) V03.2
    tularemia V03.4
    typhoid alone V03.1
      with diphtheria-tetanus-pertussis (TAB + DTP) V06.2
    typhoid-paratyphoid alone (TAB) V03.1
    typhus V05.8
    varicella V05.4
    viral encephalitis, arthropod-borne V05.0
    viral hepatitis V05.3
    yellow fever V04.4
  vasectomy V25.2
  vasoplasty for previous sterilization V26.0
  vision examination V72.0
  vocational therapy V57.22
  waiting period for admission to other facility V63.2
    undergoing social agency investigation V63.8
  well baby and child care V20.2
  x-ray of chest
    for suspected tuberculosis V71.2
    routine V72.5
Adnexitis (suppurative) (see also Salpingo-oophoritis) 614.2
Adolescence NEC V21.2
Adoption
  agency referral V68.89
  examination V70.3
  held for V68.89

Adrenal gland - see condition
Adrenalism 255.9
  tuberculous (see also Tuberculosis) 017.6
Adrenalitis, adrenitis 255.8
  meningococcal hemorrhagic 036.3
Adrenarche, precocious 259.1
Adrenocortical syndrome 255.2
Adrenogenital syndrome (acquired) (congenital) 255.2
  iatrogenic, fetus or newborn 760.79
Adrenoleukodystropy 277.86 ◄
  neonatal 277.86 ◄
  x-linked 277.86 ◄
Adrenomyeloneuropathy 277.86 ◄
Adventitious bursa - see Bursitis
Adynamia (episodica) (hereditary) (periodic) 359.3
Adynamic
  ileus or intestine (see also Ileus) 560.1
  ureter 753.22
Aeration lung, imperfect, newborn 770.5
Aerobullosis 993.3
Aerocele - see Embolism, air
Aerodermectasia
  subcutaneous (traumatic) 958.7
    surgical 998.81
  surgical 998.81
Aerodontalgia 993.2
Aeroembolism 993.3
Aerogenes capsulatus infection (see also Gangrene, gas) 040.0
Aero-otitis media 993.0
Aerophagy, aerophagia 306.4
  psychogenic 306.4
Aerosinusitis 993.1
Aerotitis 993.0
Affection, affections - see also Disease
  sacroiliac (joint), old 724.6
  shoulder region NEC 726.2
Afibrinogenemia 286.3
  acquired 286.6
  congenital 286.3
  postpartum 666.3
African
  sleeping sickness 086.5
  tick fever 087.1
  trypanosomiasis 086.5
    Gambian 086.3
    Rhodesian 086.4
Aftercare V58.9
  artificial openings - see Attention to, artificial, opening
  blood transfusion without reported diagnosis V58.2
  breathing exercise V57.0
  cardiac device V53.39
    defibrillator, automatic implantable V53.32
    pacemaker V53.31
      carotid sinus V53.39
  carotid sinus pacemaker V53.39
  cerebral ventricle (communicating) shunt V53.01
  chemotherapy session (adjunctive) (maintenance) V58.1
  defibrillator, automatic implantable cardiac V53.32
  exercise (remedial) (therapeutic) V57.1
    breathing V57.0
  extracorporeal dialysis (intermittent) (treatment) V56.0
  following surgery NEC V58.49
    for
      injury V58.43
      neoplasm V58.42

ICD-9-CM

A

Vol. 2

Aftercare (*Continued*)
following surgery NEC (*Continued*)
for (*Continued*)
organ transplant V58.44 ◄
trauma V58.43
joint replacement V54.81
of
circulatory system V58.73
digestive system V58.75
genital system V58.76
genitourinary system V58.76
musculoskeletal system V58.78
nervous system V58.72
oral cavity V58.75
respiratory system V58.74
sense organs V58.71
skin V58.77
subcutaneous tissue V58.77
teeth V58.75
urinary system V58.76
wound closure, planned V58.41
fracture V54.9
healing V54.89
pathologic
ankle V54.29
arm V54.20
lower V54.22
upper V54.21
finger V54.29
foot V54.29
hand V54.29
hip V54.23
leg V54.24
lower V54.26
upper V54.25
pelvis V54.29
specified site NEC V54.29
toe(s) V54.29
vertebrae V54.27
wrist V54.29
traumatic
ankle V54.19
arm V54.10
lower V54.12
upper V54.11
finger V54.19
foot V54.19
hand V54.29
hip V54.13
leg V54.14
lower V54.16
upper V54.15
pelvis V54.19
specified site NEC V54.19
toe(s) V54.19
vertebrae V54.17
wrist V54.19
removal of
external fixation device V54.89
internal fixation device V54.01
specified care NEC V54.89
gait training V57.1
for use of artificial limb(s) V57.81
internal fixation device V54.09
involving
dialysis (intermittent) (treatment)
extracorporeal V56.0
peritoneal V56.8
renal V56.0
gait training V57.1
for use of artificial limb(s) V57.81
growth rod
adjustment V54.02
lengthening V54.02

Aftercare (*Continued*)
involving (*Continued*)
internal fixation device V54.09
orthoptic training V57.4
orthotic training V57.81
radiotherapy session V58.0
removal of
dressings V58.3
fixation device
external V54.89
internal V54.01
fracture plate V54.01
pins V54.01
plaster cast V54.89
rods V54.01
screws V54.01
surgical dressings V58.3
sutures V58.3
traction device, external V54.89
neuropacemaker (brain) (peripheral
nerve) (spinal cord) V53.02
occupational therapy V57.21
orthodontic V58.5
orthopedic V54.9
change of external fixation or traction device V54.89
following joint replacement V54.81
internal fixation device V54.09
removal of fixation device
external V54.89
internal V54.01
specified care NEC V54.89
orthoptic training V57.4
orthotic training V57.81
pacemaker
brain V53.02
cardiac V53.31
carotid sinus V53.39
peripheral nerve V53.02
spinal cord V53.02
peritoneal dialysis (intermittent) (treatment) V56.8
physical therapy NEC V57.1
breathing exercises V57.0
radiotherapy session V58.0
rehabilitation procedure V57.9
breathing exercises V57.0
multiple types V57.89
occupational V57.21
orthoptic V57.4
orthotic V57.81
physical therapy NEC V57.1
remedial exercises V57.1
specified type NEC V57.89
speech V57.3
therapeutic exercises V57.1
vocational V57.22
renal dialysis (intermittent) (treatment)
V56.0
specified type NEC V58.89
removal of non-vascular cathether
V58.82
removal of vascular catheter V58.81
speech therapy V57.3
vocational rehabilitation V57.22
After-cataract 366.50
obscuring vision 366.53
specified type, not obscuring vision
366.52
Agalactia 676.4
Agammaglobulinemia 279.00
with lymphopenia 279.2
acquired (primary) (secondary) 279.06
Bruton's X-linked 279.04

Agammaglobulinemia (*Continued*)
infantile sex-linked (Bruton's) (congenital) 279.04
Swiss-type 279.2
Aganglionosis (bowel) (colon) 751.3
Age (old) (*see also* Senile) 797
Agenesis - *see also* Absence, by site, congenital
acoustic nerve 742.8
adrenal (gland) 759.1
alimentary tract (complete) (partial)
NEC 751.8
lower 751.2
upper 750.8
anus, anal (canal) 751.2
aorta 747.22
appendix 751.2
arm (complete) (partial) (*see also* Deformity, reduction, upper limb) 755.20
artery (peripheral) NEC (*see also*
Anomaly, peripheral vascular system) 747.60
brain 747.81
coronary 746.85
pulmonary 747.3
umbilical 747.5
auditory (canal) (external) 744.01
auricle (ear) 744.01
bile, biliary duct or passage 751.61
bone NEC 756.9
brain 740.0
specified part 742.2
breast 757.6
bronchus 748.3
canaliculus lacrimalis 743.65
carpus NEC (*see also* Deformity, reduction, upper limb) 755.28
cartilage 756.9
cecum 751.2
cerebellum 742.2
cervix 752.49
chin 744.89
cilia 743.63
circulatory system, part NEC 747.89
clavicle 755.51
clitoris 752.49
coccyx 756.13
colon 751.2
corpus callosum 742.2
cricoid cartilage 748.3
diaphragm (with hernia) 756.6
digestive organ(s) or tract (complete)
(partial) NEC 751.8
lower 751.2
upper 750.8
ductus arteriosus 747.89
duodenum 751.1
ear NEC 744.09
auricle 744.01
lobe 744.21
ejaculatory duct 752.89
endocrine (gland) NEC 759.2
epiglottis 748.3
esophagus 750.3
Eustachian tube 744.24
extrinsic muscle, eye 743.69
eye 743.00
adnexa 743.69
eyelid (fold) 743.62
face
bones NEC 756.0
specified part NEC 744.89
fallopian tube 752.19
femur NEC (*see also* Absence, femur,
congenital) 755.34

◄ **New** ◄▦ **Revised**

Agenesis (*Continued*)
fibula NEC (*see also* Absence, fibula, congenital) 755.37
finger NEC (*see also* Absence, finger, congenital) 755.29
foot (complete) (*see also* Deformity, reduction, lower limb) 755.31
gallbladder 751.69
gastric 750.8
genitalia, genital (organ)
  female 752.89
    external 752.49
    internal NEC 752.89
  male 752.89
    penis 752.69
glottis 748.3
gonadal 758.6
hair 757.4
hand (complete) (*see also* Deformity, reduction, upper limb) 755.21
heart 746.89
  valve NEC 746.89
    aortic 746.89
    mitral 746.89
    pulmonary 746.01
hepatic 751.69
humerus NEC (*see also* Absence, humerus, congenital) 755.24
hymen 752.49
ileum 751.1
incus 744.04
intestine (small) 751.1
  large 751.2
iris (dilator fibers) 743.45
jaw 524.09
jejunum 751.1
kidney(s) (partial) (unilateral) 753.0
labium (majus) (minus) 752.49
labyrinth, membranous 744.05
lacrimal apparatus (congenital) 743.65
larynx 748.3
leg NEC (*see also* Deformity, reduction, lower limb) 755.30
lens 743.35
limb (complete) (partial) (*see also* Deformity, reduction) 755.4
  lower NEC 755.30
  upper 755.20
lip 750.26
liver 751.69
lung (bilateral) (fissures) (lobe) (unilateral) 748.5
mandible 524.09
maxilla 524.09
metacarpus NEC 755.28
metatarsus NEC 755.38
muscle (any) 756.81
musculoskeletal system NEC 756.9
nail(s) 757.5
neck, part 744.89
nerve 742.8
nervous system, part NEC 742.8
nipple 757.6
nose 748.1
nuclear 742.8
organ
  of Corti 744.05
  or site not listed - *see* Anomaly, specified type NEC
osseous meatus (ear) 744.03
ovary 752.0
oviduct 752.19
pancreas 751.7
parathyroid (gland) 759.2

Agenesis (*Continued*)
patella 755.64
pelvic girdle (complete) (partial) 755.69
penis 752.69
pericardium 746.89
perineal body 756.81
pituitary (gland) 759.2
prostate 752.89
pulmonary
  artery 747.3
  trunk 747.3
  vein 747.49
punctum lacrimale 743.65
radioulnar NEC (*see also* Absence, forearm, congenital) 755.25
radius NEC (*see also* Absence, radius, congenital) 755.26
rectum 751.2
renal 753.0
respiratory organ NEC 748.9
rib 756.3
roof of orbit 742.0
round ligament 752.89
sacrum 756.13
salivary gland 750.21
scapula 755.59
scrotum 752.89
seminal duct or tract 752.89
septum
  atrial 745.69
  between aorta and pulmonary artery 745.0
  ventricular 745.3
shoulder girdle (complete) (partial) 755.59
skull (bone) 756.0
  with
    anencephalus 740.0
    encephalocele 742.0
    hydrocephalus 742.3
      with spina bifida (*see also* Spina bifida) 741.0
    microcephalus 742.1
spermatic cord 752.89
spinal cord 742.59
spine 756.13
  lumbar 756.13
    isthmus 756.11
    pars articularis 756.11
spleen 759.0
sternum 756.3
stomach 750.7
tarsus NEC 755.38
tendon 756.81
testicular 752.89
testis 752.89
thymus (gland) 759.2
thyroid (gland) 243
  cartilage 748.3
tibia NEC (*see also* Absence, tibia, congenital) 755.36
tibiofibular NEC 755.35
toe (complete) (partial) (*see also* Absence, toe, congenital) 755.39
tongue 750.11
trachea (cartilage) 748.3
ulna NEC (*see also* Absence, ulna, congenital) 755.27
ureter 753.4
urethra 753.8
urinary tract NEC 753.8
uterus 752.3
uvula 750.26
vagina 752.49

Agenesis (*Continued*)
vas deferens 752.89
vein(s) (peripheral) NEC (*see also* Anomaly, peripheral vascular system) 747.60
  brain 747.81
  great 747.49
  portal 747.49
  pulmonary 747.49
vena cava (inferior) (superior) 747.49
vermis of cerebellum 742.2
vertebra 756.13
  lumbar 756.13
    isthmus 756.11
    pars articularis 756.11
vulva 752.49
Ageusia (*see also* Disturbance, sensation) 781.1
Aggressiveness 301.3
Aggressive outburst (*see also* Disturbance, conduct) 312.0
in children or adolescents 313.9 ◀▥
Aging skin 701.8
Agitated - *see* condition
Agitation 307.9
catatonic (*see also* Schizophrenia) 295.2
Aglossia (congenital) 750.11
Aglycogenosis 271.0
Agnail (finger) (with lymphangitis) 681.02
Agnosia (body image) (tactile) 784.69
verbal 784.69
  auditory 784.69
    secondary to organic lesion 784.69
  developmental 315.8
  secondary to organic lesion 784.69
  visual 784.69
    developmental 315.8
    secondary to organic lesion 784.69
visual 368.16
  developmental 315.31
Agoraphobia 300.22
with panic disorder 300.21 ◀▥
Agrammatism 784.69
Agranulocytopenia 288.0
Agranulocytosis (angina) (chronic) (cyclical) (genetic) (infantile) (periodic) (pernicious) 288.0
Agraphia (absolute) 784.69
with alexia 784.61
developmental 315.39
Agrypnia (*see also* Insomnia) 780.52
Ague (*see also* Malaria) 084.6
brass-founders' 985.8
dumb 084.6
tertian 084.1
Agyria 742.2
Ahumada-del Castillo syndrome (nonpuerperal galactorrhea and amenorrhea) 253.1
AIDS 042
AIDS-associated retrovirus (disease) (illness) 042
infection - *see* Human immunodeficiency virus, infection
AIDS-associated virus (disease) (illness) 042
infection - *see* Human immunodeficiency virus, infection
AIDS-like disease (illness) (syndrome) 042
AIDS-related complex 042
AIDS-related conditions 042

ICD-9-CM

◀

Vol. 2

AIDS-related virus (disease) (illness) 042
  infection - *see* Human immunodeficiency virus, infection
AIDS virus (disease) (illness) 042
  infection - *see* Human immunodeficiency virus, infection
Ailment, heart - *see* Disease, heart
Ailurophobia 300.29
Ainhum (disease) 136.0
Air
  anterior mediastinum 518.1
  compressed, disease 993.3
  embolism (any site) (artery) (cerebral) 958.0
    with
      abortion - *see* Abortion, by type, with embolism
      ectopic pregnancy (*see also* categories 633.0-633.9) 639.6
      molar pregnancy (*see also* categories 630-632) 639.6
      due to implanted device - *see* Complications, due to (presence of) any device, implant, or graft classified to 996.0-996.5 NEC
    following
      abortion 639.6
      ectopic or molar pregnancy 639.6
      infusion, perfusion, or transfusion 999.1
    in pregnancy, childbirth, or puerperium 673.0
    traumatic 958.0
  hunger 786.09
    psychogenic 306.1
  leak (lung) (pulmonary) (thorax) 512.8
    iatrogenic 512.1
    postoperative 512.1
  rarefied, effects of - *see* Effect, adverse, high altitude
  sickness 994.6
Airplane sickness 994.6
Akathisia, acathisia 781.0
  due to drugs 333.99
Akinesia algeria 352.6
Akiyami 100.89
Akureyri disease (epidemic neuromyasthenia) 049.8
Alacrima (congenital) 743.65
Alactasia (hereditary) 271.3
Alalia 784.3
  developmental 315.31
    receptive-expressive 315.32
  secondary to organic lesion 784.3
Alaninemia 270.8
Alastrim 050.1
Albarrán's disease (colibacilluria) 791.9
Albers-Schönberg's disease (marble bones) 756.52
Albert's disease 726.71
Albinism, albino (choroid) (cutaneous) (eye) (generalized) (isolated) (ocular) (oculocutaneous) (partial) 270.2
Albinismus 270.2
Albright (-Martin) (-Bantam) disease (pseudohypoparathyroidism) 275.49
Albright (-McCune) (-Sternberg) syndrome (osteitis fibrosa disseminata) 756.59
Albuminous - *see* condition

Albuminuria, albuminuric (acute) (chronic) (subacute) 791.0
  Bence-Jones 791.0
  cardiac 785.9
  complicating pregnancy, childbirth, or puerperium 646.2
    with hypertension - *see* Toxemia, of pregnancy
    affecting fetus or newborn 760.1
  cyclic 593.6
  gestational 646.2
  gravidarum 646.2
    with hypertension - *see* Toxemia, of pregnancy
    affecting fetus or newborn 760.1
  heart 785.9
  idiopathic 593.6
  orthostatic 593.6
  postural 593.6
  pre-eclamptic (mild) 642.4
    affecting fetus or newborn 760.0
    severe 642.5
      affecting fetus or newborn 760.0
  recurrent physiologic 593.6
  scarlatinal 034.1
Albumosuria 791.0
  Bence-Jones 791.0
  myelopathic (M9730/3) 203.0
Alcaptonuria 270.2
Alcohol, alcoholic
  abstinence 291.81
  acute intoxication 305.0
    with dependence 303.0
  addiction (*see also* Alcoholism) 303.9
    maternal
      with suspected fetal damage affecting management of pregnancy 655.4
      affecting fetus or newborn 760.71
  amnestic disorder, persisting 291.1
  anxiety 291.89
  brain syndrome, chronic 291.2
  cardiopathy 425.5
  chronic (*see also* Alcoholism) 303.9
  cirrhosis (liver) 571.2
  delirium 291.0
    acute 291.0
    chronic 291.1
    tremens 291.0
    withdrawal 291.0
  dementia NEC 291.2
  deterioration 291.2
  drunkenness (simple) 305.0
  hallucinosis (acute) 291.3
  induced   ◄
    mental disorder 291.9   ◄
      anxiety 291.89   ◄
      mood 291.89   ◄
      sexual 291.89   ◄
      sleep 291.89   ◄
      specified type 291.89   ◄
    persisting   ◄
      amnestic disorder 291.1   ◄
      dementia 291.2   ◄
    psychotic disorder   ◄
      with   ◄
        delusions 291.5   ◄
        hallucinations 291.3   ◄
  insanity 291.9
  intoxication (acute) 305.0
    with dependence 303.0
    pathological 291.4

Alcohol, alcoholic (*Continued*)
  jealousy 291.5
  Korsakoff's, Korsakov's, Korsakow's 291.1
  liver NEC 571.3
    acute 571.1
    chronic 571.2
  mania (acute) (chronic) 291.9
  mood 291.89
  paranoia 291.5
  paranoid (type) psychosis 291.5
  pellagra 265.2
  poisoning, accidental (acute) NEC 980.9
    specified type of alcohol - *see* Table of Drugs and Chemicals
  psychosis (*see also* Psychosis, alcoholic) 291.9
    Korsakoff's, Korsakov's, Korsakow's 291.1
    polyneuritic 291.1
      with
        delusions 291.5
        hallucinations 291.3
  related disorder 291.9   ◄
  withdrawal symptoms, syndrome NEC 291.81
    delirium 291.0
    hallucinosis 291.3
Alcoholism 303.9

> Note   Use the following fifth-digit subclassification with category 303:
>
> | 0 | unspecified |
> | 1 | continuous |
> | 2 | episodic |
> | 3 | in remission |

  with psychosis (*see also* Psychosis, alcoholic) 291.9
  acute 303.0
  chronic 303.9
    with psychosis 291.9
  complicating pregnancy, childbirth, or puerperium 648.4
    affecting fetus or newborn 760.71
  history V11.3
  Korsakoff's, Korsakov's, Korsakow's 291.1
  suspected damage to fetus affecting management of pregnancy 655.4
Alder's anomaly or syndrome (leukocyte granulation anomaly) 288.2
Alder-Reilly anomaly (leukocyte granulation) 288.2
Aldosteronism (primary) 255.11
  congenital 255.10
  familial type I 255.11
  glucocorticoid-remediable 255.11
  secondary 255.14
Aldosteronoma (M8370/1) 237.2
Aldrich (-Wiskott) syndrome (eczema-thrombocytopenia) 279.12
Aleppo boil 085.1
Aleukemic - *see* condition
Aleukia
  congenital 288.0
  hemorrhagica 284.9
    acquired (secondary) 284.8
    congenital 284.0
    idiopathic 284.9
  splenica 289.4
Alexia (congenital) (developmental) 315.01
  secondary to organic lesion 784.61

ICD-9-CM

A

Vol. 2

Algoneurodystrophy 733.7
Algophobia 300.29
Alibert's disease (mycosis fungoides)
(M9700/3) 202.1
Alibert-Bazin disease (M9700/3) 202.1
Alice in Wonderland syndrome 293.89
Alienation, mental (see also Psychosis)
298.9
Alkalemia 276.3
Alkalosis 276.3
metabolic 276.3
with respiratory acidosis 276.4
respiratory 276.3
Alkaptonuria 270.2
Allen-Masters syndrome 620.6
Allergic bronchopulmonary aspergillo-
sis 518.6
Allergy, allergic (reaction) 995.3
air-borne substance (see also Fever,
hay) 477.9
specified allergen NEC 477.8
alveolitis (extrinsic) 495.9
due to
Aspergillus clavatus 495.4
cryptostroma corticale 495.6
organisms (fungal, thermophilic
actinomycete, other) growing
in ventilation (air conditioning systems) 495.7
specified type NEC 495.8
anaphylactic shock 999.4
due to food - see Anaphylactic
shock, due to, food
angioneurotic edema 995.1
animal (cat) (dog) (epidermal) 477.8 ◀▥
dander 477.2 ◀
hair 477.2 ◀
arthritis (see also Arthritis, allergic)
716.2
asthma - see Asthma
bee sting (anaphylactic shock) 989.5
biological - see Allergy, drug
bronchial asthma - see Asthma
conjunctivitis (eczematous) 372.14
dander, animal (cat) (dog) 477.2 ◀▥
dandruff 477.8
dermatitis (venenata) - see Dermatitis
diathesis V15.09
drug, medicinal substance, and biological (any) (correct medicinal substance properly administered) (external) (internal) 995.2
wrong substance given or taken
NEC 977.9
specified drug or substance - see
Table of Drugs and Chemicals
dust (house) (stock) 477.8
eczema - see Eczema
endophthalmitis 360.19
epidermal (animal) 477.8
feathers 477.8
food (any) (ingested) 693.1
atopic 691.8
in contact with skin 692.5
gastritis 535.4
gastroenteritis 558.3
gastrointestinal 558.3
grain 477.0
grass (pollen) 477.0
asthma (see also Asthma) 493.0
hay fever 477.0
hair, animal (cat) (dog) 477.2 ◀▥
hay fever (grass) (pollen) (ragweed)
(tree) (see also Fever, hay)
477.9

Allergy, allergic (Continued)
history (of) V15.09
to
eggs V15.03
food additives V15.05
insect bite V15.06
latex V15.07
milk products V15.02
nuts V15.05
peanuts V15.01
radiographic dye V15.08
seafood V15.04
specified food NEC V15.05
spider bite V15.06
horse serum - see Allergy, serum
inhalant 477.9
dust 477.8
pollen 477.0
specified allergen other than pollen
477.8
kapok 477.8
medicine - see Allergy, drug
migraine 346.2
milk protein 558.3
pannus 370.62
pneumonia 518.3
pollen (any) (hay fever) 477.0
asthma (see also Asthma) 493.0
primrose 477.0
primula 477.0
purpura 287.0
ragweed (pollen) (Senecio jacobae)
477.0
asthma (see also Asthma) 493.0
hay fever 477.0
respiratory (see also Allergy, inhalant)
477.9
due to
drug - see Allergy, drug
food - see Allergy, food
rhinitis (see also Fever, hay) 477.9
due to food 477.1
rose 477.0
Senecio jacobae 477.0
serum (prophylactic) (therapeutic)
999.5
anaphylactic shock 999.4
shock (anaphylactic) (due to adverse effect of correct medicinal substance
properly administered) 995.0
food - see Anaphylactic shock, due
to, food
from serum or immunization
999.5
anaphylactic 999.4
sinusitis (see also Fever, hay) 477.9
skin reaction 692.9
specified substance - see Dermatitis,
due to
tree (any) (hay fever) (pollen) 477.0
asthma (see also Asthma) 493.0
upper respiratory (see also Fever, hay)
477.9
urethritis 597.89
urticaria 708.0
vaccine - see Allergy, serum
Allescheriosis 117.6
Alligator skin disease (ichthyosis congenita) 757.1
acquired 701.1
Allocheiria, allochiria (see also Disturbance, sensation) 782.0
Almeida's disease (Brazilian blastomycosis) 116.1

Alopecia (atrophicans) (pregnancy) (premature) (senile) 704.00
adnata 757.4
areata 704.01
celsi 704.01
cicatrisata 704.09
circumscripta 704.01
congenital, congenitalis 757.4
disseminata 704.01
effluvium (telogen) 704.02
febrile 704.09
generalisata 704.09
hereditaria 704.09
marginalis 704.01
mucinosa 704.09
postinfectional 704.09
seborrheica 704.09
specific 091.82
syphilitic (secondary) 091.82
telogen effluvium 704.02
totalis 704.09
toxica 704.09
universalis 704.09
x-ray 704.09
Alpers' disease 330.8
Alpha-lipoproteinemia 272.4
Alpha thalassemia 282.49
Alphos 696.1
Alpine sickness 993.2
Alport's syndrome (hereditary hematuria-nephropathy-deafness) 759.89
Alteration (of), altered
awareness 780.09
transient 780.02
consciousness 780.09
persistent vegetative state 780.03
transient 780.02
mental status 780.99
amnesia (retrograde) 780.93
memory loss 780.93
Alternaria (infection) 118
Alternating - see condition
Altitude, high (effects) - see Effect, adverse, high altitude
Aluminosis (of lung) 503
Alvarez syndrome (transient cerebral ischemia) 435.9
Alveolar capillary block syndrome
516.3
Alveolitis
allergic (extrinsic) 495.9
due to organisms (fungal, thermophilic actinomycete, other)
growing in ventilation (air conditioning systems) 495.7
specified type NEC 495.8
due to
Aspergillus clavatus 495.4
Cryptostroma corticale 495.6
fibrosing (chronic) (cryptogenic) (lung)
516.3
idiopathic 516.3
rheumatoid 714.81
jaw 526.5
sicca dolorosa 526.5
Alveolus, alveolar - see condition
Alymphocytosis (pure) 279.2
Alymphoplasia, thymic 279.2
Alzheimer's
dementia (senile)
with behavioral disturbance 331.0
[294.11]
without behavioral disturbance
331.0 [294.10]

Alzheimer's *(Continued)*
  disease or sclerosis 331.0
    with dementia - *see* Alzheimer's, dementia
Amastia *(see also* Absence, breast)
  611.8
Amaurosis (acquired) (congenital) *(see also* Blindness) 369.00
  fugax 362.34
  hysterical 300.11
  Leber's (congenital) 362.76
  tobacco 377.34
  uremic - *see* Uremia
Amaurotic familial idiocy (infantile) (juvenile) (late) 330.1
Ambisexual 752.7
Amblyopia (acquired) (congenital) (partial) 368.00
  color 368.59
    acquired 368.55
  deprivation 368.02
  ex anopsia 368.00
  hysterical 300.11
  nocturnal 368.60
    vitamin A deficiency 264.5
  refractive 368.03
  strabismic 368.01
  suppression 368.01
  tobacco 377.34
  toxic NEC 377.34
  uremic - *see* Uremia
Ameba, amebic (histolytica) - *see also* Amebiasis
  abscess 006.3
    bladder 006.8
    brain (with liver and lung abscess) 006.5
    liver 006.3
      with
        brain abscess (and lung abscess) 006.5
        lung abscess 006.4
    lung (with liver abscess) 006.4
      with brain abscess 006.5
    seminal vesicle 006.8
    spleen 006.8
  carrier (suspected of) V02.2
  meningoencephalitis
    due to Naegleria (gruberi) 136.2
    primary 136.2
Amebiasis NEC 006.9
  with
    brain abscess (with liver or lung abscess) 006.5
    liver abscess (without mention of brain or lung abscess) 006.3
    lung abscess (with liver abscess) 006.4
      with brain abscess 006.5
  acute 006.0
  bladder 006.8
  chronic 006.1
  cutaneous 006.6
  cutis 006.6
  due to organism other than Entamoeba histolytica 007.8
  hepatic *(see also* Abscess, liver, amebic) 006.3
  nondysenteric 006.2
  seminal vesicle 006.8
  specified
    organism NEC 007.8
    site NEC 006.8
Ameboma 006.8

Amelia 755.4
  lower limb 755.31
  upper limb 755.21
Ameloblastoma (M9310/0) 213.1
  jaw (bone) (lower) 213.1
    upper 213.0
  long bones (M9261/3) - *see* Neoplasm, bone, malignant
  malignant (M9310/3) 170.1
    jaw (bone) (lower) 170.1
      upper 170.0
  mandible 213.1
  tibial (M9261/3) 170.7
Amelogenesis imperfecta 520.5
  nonhereditaria (segmentalis) 520.4
Amenorrhea (primary) (secondary) 626.0
  due to ovarian dysfunction 256.8
  hyperhormonal 256.8
Amentia *(see also* Retardation, mental) 319
  Meynert's (nonalcoholic) 294.0
    alcoholic 291.1
  nevoid 759.6
American
  leishmaniasis 085.5
  mountain tick fever 066.1
  trypanosomiasis - *see* Trypanosomiasis, American
Ametropia *(see also* Disorder, accommodation) 367.9
Amianthosis 501
Amimia 784.69
Amino acid
  deficiency 270.9
    anemia 281.4
  metabolic disorder *(see also* Disorder, amino acid) 270.9
Aminoaciduria 270.9
  imidazole 270.5
Amnesia (retrograde) 780.93
  auditory 784.69
    developmental 315.31
    secondary to organic lesion 784.69
  dissociative 300.12   ◄
  hysterical or dissociative type 300.12
  psychogenic 300.12
  transient global 437.7
Amnestic (confabulatory) syndrome 294.0
  alcohol-induced persisting 291.1   ◄⫶
  drug-induced persisting 292.83   ◄⫶
  posttraumatic 294.0
Amniocentesis screening (for) V28.2
  alpharetoprotein level, raised V28.1
  chromosomal anomalies V28.0
Amnion, amniotic - *see also* condition
  nodosum 658.8
Amnionitis (complicating pregnancy) 658.4
  affecting fetus or newborn 762.7
Amoral trends 301.7
Amotio retinae *(see also* Detachment, retina) 361.9
Ampulla
  lower esophagus 530.89
  phrenic 530.89
Amputation
  any part of fetus, to facilitate delivery 763.89
  cervix (supravaginal) (uteri) 622.8
    in pregnancy or childbirth 654.6
      affecting fetus or newborn 763.89

Amputation *(Continued)*
  clitoris - *see* Wound, open, clitoris
  congenital
    lower limb 755.31
    upper limb 755.21
  neuroma (traumatic) - *see also* Injury, nerve, by site
    surgical complication (late) 997.61
  penis - *see* Amputation, traumatic, penis
  status (without complication) - *see* Absence, by site, acquired
  stump (surgical) (posttraumatic)
    abnormal, painful, or with complication (late) 997.60
    healed or old NEC - *see also* Absence, by site, acquired
      lower V49.70
      upper V49.60
  traumatic (complete) (partial)

> Note "Complicated" includes traumatic amputation with delayed healing, delayed treatment, foreign body, or infection.

  arm 887.4
    at or above elbow 887.2
      complicated 887.3
    below elbow 887.0
      complicated 887.1
    both (bilateral) (any level(s)) 887.6
      complicated 887.7
    complicated 887.5
  finger(s) (one or both hands) 886.0
    with thumb(s) 885.0
      complicated 885.1
    complicated 886.1
  foot (except toe(s) only) 896.0
    and other leg 897.6
      complicated 897.7
    both (bilateral) 896.2
      complicated 896.3
    complicated 896.1
  toe(s) only (one or both feet) 895.0
    complicated 895.1
  genital organ(s) (external) NEC 878.8
    complicated 878.9
  hand (except finger(s) only) 887.0
    and other arm 887.6
      complicated 887.7
    both (bilateral) 887.6
      complicated 887.7
    complicated 887.1
  finger(s) (one or both hands) 886.0
    with thumb(s) 885.0
      complicated 885.1
    complicated 886.1
    thumb(s) (with fingers of either hand) 885.0
      complicated 885.1
  head 874.9
  late effect - *see* Late, effects (of), amputation
  leg 897.4
    and other foot 897.6
      complicated 897.7
    at or above knee 897.2
      complicated 897.3
    below knee 897.0
      complicated 897.1
    both (bilateral) 897.6
      complicated 897.7
    complicated 897.5

Amputation (*Continued*)
lower limb(s) except toe(s) - *see* Amputation, traumatic, leg
nose - *see* Wound, open, nose
penis 878.0
complicated 878.1
sites other than limbs - *see* Wound, open, by site
thumb(s) (with finger(s) of either hand) 885.0
complicated 885.1
toe(s) (one or both feet) 895.0
complicated 895.1
upper limb(s) - *see* Amputation, traumatic, arm
Amputee (bilateral) (old) - *see* Absence, by site, acquired V49.70
Amusia 784.69
developmental 315.39
secondary to organic lesion 784.69
Amyelencephalus 740.0
Amyelia 742.59
Amygdalitis - *see* Tonsillitis
Amygdalolith 474.8
Amyloid disease or degeneration 277.3
heart 277.3 [*425.7*]
Amyloidosis (familial) (general) (generalized) (genetic) (primary) (secondary) 277.3
with lung involvement 277.3 [*517.8*]
heart 277.3 [*425.7*]
nephropathic 277.3 [*583.81*]
neuropathic (Portuguese) (Swiss) 277.3 [*357.4*]
pulmonary 277.3 [*517.8*]
systemic, inherited 277.3
Amylopectinosis (brancher enzyme deficiency) 271.0
Amylophagia 307.52
Amyoplasia congenita 756.89
Amyotonia 728.2
congenita 358.8
Amyotrophia, amyotrophy, amyotrophic 728.2
congenita 756.89
diabetic 250.6 [*358.1*]
lateral sclerosis (syndrome) 335.20
neuralgic 353.5
sclerosis (lateral) 335.20
spinal progressive 335.21
Anacidity, gastric 536.0
psychogenic 306.4
Anaerosis of newborn 768.9
Analbuminemia 273.8
Analgesia (*see also* Anesthesia) 782.0
Analphalipoproteinemia 272.5
Anaphylactic shock or reaction (correct substance properly administered) 995.0
due to
food 995.60
additives 995.66
crustaceans 995.62
eggs 995.68
fish 995.65
fruits 995.63
milk products 995.67
nuts (tree) 995.64
peanuts 995.61
seeds 995.64,
specified NEC 995.69
tree nuts 995.64
vegetables 995.63
immunization 999.4

Anaphylactic shock or reaction
(*Continued*
due to (*Continued*)
overdose or wrong substance given or taken 977.9
specified drug - *see* Table of Drugs and Chemicals
serum 999.4
following sting(s) 989.5
purpura 287.0
serum 999.4
Anaphylactoid shock or reaction - *see* Anaphylactic shock
Anaphylaxis - *see* Anaphylactic shock
Anaplasia, cervix 622.10 ◀▥
Anarthria 784.5
Anarthritic rheumatoid disease 446.5
Anasarca 782.3
cardiac (*see also* Failure, heart 428.0
fetus or newborn 778.0
lung 514
nutritional 262
pulmonary 514
renal (*see also* Nephrosis) 581.9
Anaspadias 752.62
Anastomosis
aneurysmal - *see* Aneurysm
arteriovenous, congenital NEC (*see also* Anomaly, arteriovenous) 747.60
ruptured, of brain (*see also* Hemorrhage, subarachnoid) 430
intestinal 569.89
complicated NEC 997.4
involving urinary tract 997.5
retinal and choroidal vessels 743.58
acquired 362.17
Anatomical narrow angle (glaucoma) 365.02
Ancylostoma (infection) (infestation) 126.9
americanus 126.1
braziliense 126.2
caninum 126.8
ceylanicum 126.3
duodenale 126.0
Necator americanus 126.1
Ancylostomiasis (intestinal) 126.9
Ancylostoma
americanus 126.1
caninum 126.8
ceylanicum 126.3
duodenale 126.0
braziliense 126.2
Necator americanus 126.1
Anders' disease or syndrome (adiposis tuberosa simplex) 272.8
Andersen's glycogen storage disease 271.0
Anderson's disease 272.7
Andes disease 993.2
Andrews' disease (bacterid) 686.8
Androblastoma (M8630/1)
benign (M8630/0)
specified site - *see* Neoplasm, by site, benign
unspecified site
female 220
male 222.0
malignant (M8630/3)
specified site - *see* Neoplasm, by site, malignant
unspecified site
female 183.0
male 186.9

Androblastoma (*Continued*)
specified site - *see* Neoplasm, by site, uncertain behavior
tubular (M8640/0)
with lipid storage (M8641/0)
specified site - *see* Neoplasm, by site, benign
unspecified site
female 220
male 222.0
specified site - *see* Neoplasm, by site, benign
unspecified site
female 220
male 222.0
unspecified site
female 236.2
male 236.4
Android pelvis 755.69
with disproportion (fetopelvic) 653.3
affecting fetus or newborn 763.1
causing obstructed labor 660.1
affecting fetus or newborn 763.1
Anectasis, pulmonary (newborn or fetus) 770.5
Anemia 285.9
with
disorder of
anaerobic glycolysis 282.3
pentose phosphate pathway 282.2
koilonychia 280.9
6-phosphogluconic dehydrogenase deficiency 282.2
achlorhydric 280.9
achrestic 281.8
Addison's (pernicious) 281.0
Addison-Biermer (pernicious) 281.0
agranulocytic 288.0
amino acid deficiency 281.4
aplastic 284.9
acquired (secondary) 284.8
congenital 284.0
constitutional 284.0
due to
chronic systemic disease 284.8
drugs 284.8
infection 284.8
radiation 284.8
idiopathic 284.9
myxedema 244.9
of or complicating pregnancy 648.2
red cell (acquired) (pure) (with thymoma) 284.8
congenital 284.0
specified type NEC 284.8
toxic (paralytic) 284.8
aregenerative 284.9
congenital 284.0
asiderotic 280.9
atypical (primary) 285.9
autohemolysis of Selwyn and Dacie (type I) 282.2
autoimmune hemolytic 283.0
Baghdad Spring 282.2
Balantidium coli 007.0
Biermer's (pernicious) 281.0
blood loss (chronic) 280.0
acute 285.1
bothriocephalus 123.4
brickmakers' (*see also* Ancylostomiasis) 126.9
cerebral 437.8
childhood 282.9 ◀▥

ICD-9-CM

◀

Vol. 2

Anemia (*Continued*)
  chlorotic 280.9
  chronica congenita aregenerativa 284.0
  chronic simple 281.9
  combined system disease NEC 281.0
    [336.2]
    due to dietary deficiency 281.1
      [336.2]
  complicating pregnancy or childbirth
    648.2
  congenital (following fetal blood loss)
    776.5
    aplastic 284.0
    due to isoimmunization NEC 773.2
    Heinz-body 282.7
    hereditary hemolytic NEC 282.9
    nonspherocytic
      type I 282.2
      type II 282.3
    pernicious 281.0
    spherocytic (*see also* Spherocytosis)
      282.0
  Cooley's (erythroblastic) 282.49
  crescent - *see* Disease, sickle-cell
  cytogenic 281.0
  Dacie's (nonspherocytic)
    type I 282.2
    type II 282.3
  Davidson's (refractory) 284.9
  deficiency 281.9
    2,3 diphosphoglycurate mutase
      282.3
    2,3 PG 282.3
    6-PGD 282.2
    6-phosphogluronic dehydrogenase
      282.2
    amino acid 281.4
    combined B_{12} and folate 281.3
    enzyme, drug-induced (hemolytic)
      282.2
    erythrocytic glutathione 282.2
    folate 281.2
      dietary 281.2
      drug-induced 281.2
    folic acid 281.2
      dietary 281.2
      drug-induced 281.2
    G-6-PD 282.2
    GGS-R 282.2
    glucose-6-phosphate dehydrogenase
      (G-6-PD) 282.2
    glucose-phosphate isomerase 282.3
    glutathione peroxidase 282.2
    glutathione reductase 282.2
    glyceraldehyde phosphate dehydro-
      genase 282.3
    GPI 282.3
    G SH 282.2
    hexokinase 282.3
    iron (Fe) 280.9
      specified NEC 280.8
    nutritional 281.9
      with
        poor iron absorption 280.9
        specified deficiency NEC 281.8
        due to inadequate dietary iron in-
          take 280.1
      specified type NEC 281.8
    of or complicating pregnancy
      648.2
    pentose phosphate pathway 282.2
    PFK 282.3
    phosphofructo-aldolase 282.3
    phosphofructokinase 282.3

Anemia (*Continued*)
  deficiency (*Continued*)
    phosphoglycerate kinase 282.3
    PK 282.3
    protein 281.4
    pyruvate kinase (PK) 282.3
    TPI 282.3
    triosephosphate isomerase 282.3
    vitamin B_{12} NEC 281.1
      dietary 281.1
      pernicious 281.0
  Diamond-Blackfan (congenital hypo-
    plastic) 284.0
  dibothriocephalus 123.4
  dimorphic 281.9
  diphasic 281.8
  diphtheritic 032.89
  Diphyllobothrium 123.4
  drepanocytic (*see also* Disease, sickle-
    cell) 282.60
  due to
    blood loss (chronic) 280.0
      acute 285.1
    defect of Embden-Meyerhof path-
      way glycolysis 282.3
    disorder of glutathione metabolism
      282.2
    fetal blood loss 776.5
    fish tapeworm (D. latum) infestation
      123.4
    glutathione metabolism disorder
      282.2
    hemorrhage (chronic) 280.0
      acute 285.1
    hexose monophosphate (HMP)
      shunt deficiency 282.2
    impaired absorption 280.9
    loss of blood (chronic) 280.0
      acute 285.1
    myxedema 244.9
    Necator americanus 126.1
    prematurity 776.6
    selective vitamin B_{12} malabsorption
      with proteinuria 281.1
  Dyke-Young type (secondary)
    (symptomatic) 283.9
  dyserythropoietic (congenital) (types I,
    II, III) 285.8
  dyshemopoietic (congenital) 285.8
  Egypt (*see also* Ancylostomiasis) 126.9
  elliptocytosis (*see also* Elliptocytosis)
    282.1
  enzyme deficiency, drug-induced 282.2
  epidemic (*see also* Ancylostomiasis) 126.9
  EPO resistant 285.21
  erythroblastic
    familial 282.49
    fetus or newborn (*see also* Disease,
      hemolytic) 773.2
    late 773.5
  erythrocytic glutathione deficiency
    282.2
  erythropoietin-resistant (EPO resistant
    anemia) 285.21
  essential 285.9
  Faber's (achlorhydric anemia) 280.9
  factitious (self-induced bloodletting)
    280.0
  familial erythroblastic (microcytic)
    282.49
  Fanconi's (congenital pancytopenia)
    284.0
  favism 282.2
  fetal, following blood loss 776.5

Anemia (*Continued*)
  fetus or newborn
    due to
      ABO
        antibodies 773.1
        incompatibility, maternal/fetal
          773.1
        isoimmunization 773.1
      Rh
        antibodies 773.0
        incompatibility, maternal/fetal
          773.0
        isoimmunization 773.0
    following fetal blood loss 776.5
  fish tapeworm (D. latum) infestation
    123.4
  folate (folic acid) deficiency 281.2
    dietary 281.2
    drug-induced 281.2
  folate malabsorption, congenital 281.2
  folic acid deficiency 281.2
    dietary 281.2
    drug-induced 281.2
  G-6-PD 282.2
  general 285.9
  glucose-6-phosphate dehydrogenase
    deficiency 282.2
  glutathione-reductase deficiency 282.2
  goat's milk 281.2
  granulocytic 288.0
  Heinz-body, congenital 282.7
  hemoglobin deficiency 285.9
  hemolytic 283.9
    acquired 283.9
      with hemoglobinuria NEC 283.2
      autoimmune (cold type) (idiopathic)
        (primary) (secondary) (sympto-
        matic) (warm type) 283.0
      due to
        cold reactive antibodies 283.0
        drug exposure 283.0
        warm reactive antibodies 283.0
      fragmentation 283.19
      idiopathic (chronic) 283.9
      infectious 283.19
        autoimmune 283.0
      non-autoimmune 283.10
      toxic 283.19
      traumatic cardiac 283.19
    acute 283.9
      due to enzyme deficiency NEC
        282.3
      fetus or newborn (*see also* Disease,
        hemolytic) 773.2
      late 773.5
      Lederer's (acquired infectious he-
        molytic anemia) 283.19
    autoimmune (acquired) 283.0
    chronic 282.9
      idiopathic 283.9
    cold type (secondary) (symptomatic)
      283.0
    congenital (spherocytic) (*see also*
      Spherocytosis) 282.0
      nonspherocytic - *see* Anemia, he-
        molytic, nonspherocytic, con-
        genital
    drug-induced 283.0
      enzyme deficiency 282.2
    due to
      cardiac conditions 283.19
      drugs 283.0
      enzyme deficiency NEC 282.3
        drug-induced 282.2

◀ **New**   ◀▥ **Revised**

Anemia *(Continued)*
hemolytic *(Continued)*
due to *(Continued)*
presence of shunt or other internal prosthetic device 283.19
thrombotic thrombocytopenic purpura 446.6
elliptocytotic *(see also* Elliptocytosis) 282.1
familial 282.9
hereditary 282.9
due to enzyme deficiency NEC 282.3
specified NEC 282.8
idiopathic (chronic) 283.9
infectious (acquired) 283.19
mechanical 283.19
microangiopathic 283.19
nonautoimmune 283.10
nonspherocytic
congenital or hereditary NEC 282.3
glucose-6-phosphate dehydrogenase deficiency 282.2
pyruvate kinase (PK) deficiency 282.3
type I 282.2
type II 282.3
type I 282.2
type II 282.3
of or complicating pregnancy 648.2
resulting from presence of shunt or other internal prosthetic device 283.19
secondary 283.19
autoimmune 283.0
sickle-cell - *see* Disease, Hb-E, sickle-cell
Stransky-Regala type (Hb-E) *(see also* Disease, hemoglobin) 282.7
symptomatic 283.19
autoimmune 283.0
toxic (acquired) 283.19
uremic (adult) (child) 283.11
warm type (secondary) (symptomatic) 283.0
hemorrhagic (chronic) 280.0
acute 285.1
HEMPAS 285.8
hereditary erythroblast multinuclearity-positive acidified serum test 285.8
Herrick's (hemoglobin S disease) 282.61
hexokinase deficiency 282.3
high A$_2$ 282.49
hookworm *(see also* Ancylostomiasis) 126.9
hypochromic (idiopathic) (microcytic) (normoblastic) 280.9
with iron loading 285.0
due to blood loss (chronic) 280.0
acute 285.1
familial sex linked 285.0
pyridoxine-responsive 285.0
hypoplasia, red blood cells 284.8
congenital or familial 284.0
hypoplastic (idiopathic) 284.9
congenital 284.0
familial 284.0
of childhood 284.0
idiopathic 285.9
hemolytic, chronic 283.9
in
chronic illness NEC 285.29
end-stage renal disease 285.21
neoplastic disease 285.22
infantile 285.9

Anemia *(Continued)*
infective, infectional 285.9
intertropical *(see also* Ancylostomiasis) 126.9
iron (Fe) deficiency 280.9
due to blood loss (chronic) 280.0
acute 285.1
of or complicating pregnancy 648.2
specified NEC 280.8
Jaksch's (pseudoleukemia infantum) 285.8
Joseph-Diamond-Blackfan (congenital hypoplastic) 284.0
labyrinth 386.50
Lederer's (acquired infectious hemolytic anemia) 283.19
leptocytosis (hereditary) 282.49
leukoerythroblastic 285.8
macrocytic 281.9
nutritional 281.2
of or complicating pregnancy 648.2
tropical 281.2
malabsorption (familial), selective B$_{12}$ with proteinuria 281.1
malarial *(see also* Malaria) 084.6
malignant (progressive) 281.0
malnutrition 281.9
marsh *(see also* Malaria) 084.6
Mediterranean (with hemoglobinopathy) 282.49
megaloblastic 281.9
combined B$_{12}$ and folate deficiency 281.3
nutritional (of infancy) 281.2
of infancy 281.2
of or complicating pregnancy 648.2
refractory 281.3
specified NEC 281.3
megalocytic 281.9
microangiopathic hemolytic 283.19
microcytic (hypochromic) 280.9
due to blood loss (chronic) 280.0
acute 285.1
familial 282.49
hypochromic 280.9
microdrepanocytosis 282.49
miners' *(see also* Ancylostomiasis) 126.9
myelopathic 285.8
myelophthisic (normocytic) 285.8
newborn *(see also* Disease, hemolytic) 773.2
due to isoimmunization *(see also* Disease, hemolytic) 773.2
late, due to isoimmunization 773.5
posthemorrhagic 776.5
nonregenerative 284.9
nonspherocytic hemolytic - *see* Anemia, hemolytic, nonspherocytic
normocytic (infectional) (not due to blood loss) 285.9
due to blood loss (chronic) 280.0
acute 285.1
myelophthisic 284.8
nutritional (deficiency) 281.9
with
poor iron absorption 280.9
specified deficiency NEC 281.8
due to inadequate dietary iron intake 280.1
megaloblastic (of infancy) 281.2 ◀▥
of childhood 282.9
of chronic illness NEC 285.29
of or complicating pregnancy 648.2
affecting fetus or newborn 760.8

Anemia *(Continued)*
of prematurity 776.6
orotic aciduric (congenital) (hereditary) 281.4
osteosclerotic 289.89
ovalocytosis (hereditary) *(see also* Elliptocytosis) 282.1
paludal *(see also* Malaria) 084.6
pentose phosphate pathway deficiency 282.2
pernicious (combined system disease) (congenital) (dorsolateral spinal degeneration) (juvenile) (myelopathy) (neuropathy) (posterior sclerosis) (primary) (progressive) (spleen) 281.0
of or complicating pregnancy 648.2
pleochromic 285.9
of sprue 281.8
portal 285.8
posthemorrhagic (chronic) 280.0
acute 285.1
newborn 776.5
postoperative ◀
due to blood loss 285.1 ◀
other 285.9 ◀
postpartum 648.2
pressure 285.9
primary 285.9
profound 285.9
progressive 285.9
malignant 281.0
pernicious 281.0
protein-deficiency 281.4
pseudoleukemia infantum 285.8
puerperal 648.2
pure red cell 284.8
congenital 284.0
pyridoxine-responsive (hypochromic) 285.0
pyruvate kinase (PK) deficiency 282.3
refractoria sideroblastica 285.0
refractory (primary) 284.9
with hemochromatosis 285.0
megaloblastic 281.3
sideroblastic 285.0
sideropenic 280.9
Rietti-Greppi-Micheli (thalassemia minor) 282.49
scorbutic 281.8
secondary (to) 285.9
blood loss (chronic) 280.0
acute 285.1
hemorrhage 280.0
acute 285.1
inadequate dietary iron intake 280.1
semiplastic 284.9
septic 285.9
sickle-cell *(see also* Disease, sickle-cell) 282.60
sideroachrestic 285.0
sideroblastic (acquired) (any type) (congenital) (drug-induced) (due to disease) (hereditary) (primary) (refractory) (secondary) (sex-linked hypochromic) (vitamin B$_6$ responsive) 285.0
sideropenic (refractory) 280.9
due to blood loss (chronic) 280.0
acute 285.1
simple chronic 281.9
specified type NEC 285.8
spherocytic (hereditary) *(see also* Spherocytosis) 282.0

Anemia (Continued)
  splenic 285.8
    familial (Gaucher's) 272.7
  splenomegalic 285.8
  stomatocytosis 282.8
  syphilitic 095.8
  target cell (oval) 282.49
  thalassemia 282.49
  thrombocytopenic (see also Thrombocy-
    topenia) 287.5
  toxic 284.8
  triosephosphate isomerase deficiency
    282.3
  tropical, macrocytic 281.2
  tuberculous (see also Tuberculosis) 017.9
  vegan's 281.1
  vitamin
    B₆-responsive 285.0
    B₁₂ deficiency (dietary) 281.1
      pernicious 281.0
  von Jaksch's (pseudoleukemia infan-
    tum) 285.8
  Witts' (achlorhydric anemia) 280.9
  Zuelzer (-Ogden) (nutritional megalo-
    blastic anemia) 281.2
Anencephalus, anencephaly 740.0
  fetal, affecting management of preg-
    nancy 655.0
Anergasia (see also Psychosis, organic)
  294.9
  senile 290.0
Anesthesia, anesthetic 782.0
  complication or reaction NEC 995.2
    due to
      correct substance properly admin-
        istered 995.2
      overdose or wrong substance
        given 968.4
      specified anesthetic - see Table
        of Drugs and Chemicals
  cornea 371.81
  death from
    correct substance properly adminis-
      tered 995.4
    during delivery 668.9
    overdose or wrong substance given
      968.4
    specified anesthetic - see Table of
      Drugs and Chemicals
  eye 371.81
  functional 300.11
  hyperesthetic, thalamic 348.8
  hysterical 300.11
  local skin lesion 782.0
  olfactory 781.1
  sexual (psychogenic) 302.72
  shock
    due to
      correct substance properly admin-
        istered 995.4
      overdose or wrong substance
        given 968.4
      specified anesthetic - see Table
        of Drugs and Chemicals
  skin 782.0
  tactile 782.0
  testicular 608.9
  thermal 782.0
Anetoderma (maculosum) 701.3
Aneuploidy NEC 758.5
Aneurin deficiency 265.1
Aneurysm (anastomotic) (artery) (cirsoid)
  (diffuse) (false) (fusiform) (multiple)
  (ruptured) (saccular) (varicose) 442.9

Aneurysm (Continued)
  abdominal (aorta) 441.4
    ruptured 441.3
    syphilitic 093.0
  aorta, aortic (nonsyphilitic) 441.9
    abdominal 441.4
      dissecting 441.02
      ruptured 441.3
      syphilitic 093.0
    arch 441.2
      ruptured 441.1
    arteriosclerotic NEC 441.9
      ruptured 441.5
    ascending 441.2
      ruptured 441.1
    congenital 747.29
    descending 441.9
      abdominal 441.4
        ruptured 441.3
      ruptured 441.5
      thoracic 441.2
        ruptured 441.1
    dissecting 441.00
      abdominal 441.02
      thoracic 441.01
      thoracoabdominal 441.03
    due to coarctation (aorta) 747.10
    ruptured 441.5
    sinus, right 747.29
    syphilitic 093.0
    thoracoabdominal 441.7
      ruptured 441.6
    thorax, thoracic (arch) (nonsyphilitic)
      441.2
      dissecting 441.01
      ruptured 441.1
      syphilitic 093.0
    transverse 441.2
      ruptured 441.1
    valve (heart) (see also Endocarditis,
      aortic) 424.1
  arteriosclerotic NEC 442.9
    cerebral 437.3
      ruptured (see also Hemorrhage,
        subarachnoid) 430
  arteriovenous (congenital) (peripheral)
    NEC (see also Anomaly, arteriove-
    nous) 747.60
    acquired NEC 447.0
      brain 437.3
        ruptured (see also Hemorrhage,
          subarachnoid) 430
      coronary 414.11
      pulmonary 417.0
    brain (cerebral) 747.81
      ruptured (see also Hemorrhage,
        subarachnoid) 430
    coronary 746.85
    pulmonary 747.3
    retina 743.58
    specified site NEC 747.89
      acquired 447.0
    traumatic (see also Injury, blood ves-
      sel, by site) 904.9
  basal - see Aneurysm, brain
  berry (congenital) (ruptured) (see also
    Hemorrhage, subarachnoid) 430
  brain 437.3
    arteriosclerotic 437.3
      ruptured (see also Hemorrhage,
        subarachnoid) 430
    arteriovenous 747.81
      acquired 437.3
        ruptured (see also Hemorrhage,
          subarachnoid) 430

Aneurysm (Continued)
  brain (Continued)
    arteriovenous (Continued)
      ruptured (see also Hemorrhage,
        subarachnoid) 430
    berry (congenital) (ruptured) (see
      also Hemorrhage, subarachnoid)
      430
    congenital 747.81
      ruptured (see also Hemorrhage,
        subarachnoid) 430
    meninges 437.3
      ruptured (see also Hemorrhage,
        subarachnoid) 430
    miliary (congenital) (ruptured) (see
      also Hemorrhage, subarachnoid)
      430
    mycotic 421.0
      ruptured (see also Hemorrhage,
        subarachnoid) 430
    nonruptured 437.3
    ruptured (see also Hemorrhage, sub-
      arachnoid) 430
    syphilitic 094.87
    syphilitic (hemorrhage) 094.87
    traumatic - see Injury, intracranial
  cardiac (false) (see also Aneurysm,
    heart) 414.10
  carotid artery (common) (external)
    442.81
    internal (intracranial portion) 437.3
      extracranial portion 442.81
      ruptured into brain (see also Hem-
        orrhage, subarachnoid) 430
    syphilitic 093.89
      intracranial 094.87
  cavernous sinus (see also Aneurysm,
    brain) 437.3
    arteriovenous 747.81
      ruptured (see also Hemorrhage,
        subarachnoid) 430
    congenital 747.81
      ruptured (see also Hemorrhage,
        subarachnoid) 430
  celiac 442.84
  central nervous system, syphilitic 094.89
  cerebral - see Aneurysm, brain
  chest - see Aneurysm, thorax
  circle of Willis (see also Aneurysm,
    brain) 437.3
    congenital 747.81
      ruptured (see also Hemorrhage,
        subarachnoid) 430
    ruptured (see also Hemorrhage, sub-
      arachnoid) 430
  common iliac artery 442.2
  congenital (peripheral) NEC 747.60
    brain 747.81
      ruptured (see also Hemorrhage,
        subarachnoid) 430
    cerebral - see Aneurysm, brain, con-
      genital
    coronary 746.85
    gastrointestinal 747.61
    lower limb 747.64
    pulmonary 747.3
    renal 747.62
    retina 743.58
    specified site NEC 747.89
    spinal 747.82
    upper limb 747.63
  conjunctiva 372.74
  conus arteriosus (see also Aneurysm,
    heart) 414.10

◀ **New**   ◀▥▥ **Revised**

Aneurysm (Continued)
coronary (arteriosclerotic) (artery) (vein) (see also Aneurysm, heart) 414.11
  arteriovenous 746.85
  congenital 746.85
  syphilitic 093.89
cylindrical 441.9
  ruptured 441.5
  syphilitic 093.9
dissecting 442.9
  aorta 441.00
    abdominal 441.02
    thoracic 441.01
    thoracoabdominal 441.03
    syphilitic 093.9
ductus arteriosus 747.0
embolic - see Embolism, artery
endocardial, infective (any valve) 421.0
femoral 442.3
gastroduodenal 442.84
gastroepiploic 442.84
heart (chronic or with a stated duration of over 8 weeks) (infectional) (wall) 414.10
  acute or with a stated duration of 8 weeks or less (see also Infarct, myocardium) 410.9
  congenital 746.89
  valve - see Endocarditis
hepatic 442.84
iliac (common) 442.2
infective (any valve) 421.0
innominate (nonsyphilitic) 442.89
  syphilitic 093.89
interauricular septum (see also Aneurysm, heart) 414.10
interventricular septum (see also Aneurysm, heart) 414.10
intracranial - see Aneurysm, brain
intrathoracic (nonsyphilitic) 441.2
  ruptured 441.1
  syphilitic 093.0
jugular vein 453.8
lower extremity 442.3
lung (pulmonary artery) 417.1
malignant 093.9
mediastinal (nonsyphilitic) 442.89
  syphilitic 093.89
miliary (congenital) (ruptured) (see also Hemorrhage, subarachnoid) 430
mitral (heart) (valve) 424.0
mural (arteriovenous) (heart) (see also Aneurysm, heart) 414.10
mycotic, any site 421.0
  ruptured, brain (see also Hemorrhage, subarachnoid) 430
myocardium (see also Aneurysm, heart) 414.10
neck 442.81
pancreaticoduodenal 442.84
patent ductus arteriosus 747.0
peripheral NEC 442.89
  congenital NEC (see also Aneurysm, congenital) 747.60
popliteal 442.3
pulmonary 417.1
  arteriovenous 747.3
    acquired 417.0
  syphilitic 093.89
  valve (heart) (see also Endocarditis, pulmonary) 424.3
racemose 442.9
  congenital (peripheral) NEC 747.60
radial 442.0

Aneurysm (Continued)
Rasmussen's (see also Tuberculosis) 011.2
renal 442.1
retinal (acquired) 362.17
  congenital 743.58
  diabetic 250.5 [362.01]
sinus, aortic (of Valsalva) 747.29
specified site NEC 442.89
spinal (cord) 442.89
  congenital 747.82
  syphilitic (hemorrhage) 094.89
spleen, splenic 442.83
subclavian 442.82
  syphilitic 093.89
superior mesenteric 442.84
syphilitic 093.9
  aorta 093.0
  central nervous system 094.89
  congenital 090.5
  spine, spinal 094.89
thoracoabdominal 441.7
  ruptured 441.6
thorax, thoracic (arch) (nonsyphilitic) 441.2
  dissecting 441.01
  ruptured 441.1
  syphilitic 093.0
traumatic (complication) (early) - see Injury, blood vessel, by site
tricuspid (heart) (valve) - see Endocarditis, tricuspid
ulnar 442.0
upper extremity 442.0
valve, valvular - see Endocarditis
venous 456.8
  congenital NEC (see also Aneurysm, congenital) 747.60
ventricle (arteriovenous) (see also Aneurysm, heart) 414.10
visceral artery NEC 442.84
Angiectasis 459.89
Angiectopia 459.9
Angiitis 447.6
allergic granulomatous 446.4
hypersensitivity 446.20
  Goodpasture's syndrome 446.21
  specified NEC 446.29
necrotizing 446.0
Wegener's (necrotizing respiratory granulomatosis) 446.4
Angina (attack) (cardiac) (chest) (effort) (heart) (pectoris) (syndrome) (vasomotor) 413.9
abdominal 557.1
accelerated 411.1
agranulocytic 288.0
aphthous 074.0
catarrhal 462
crescendo 411.1
croupous 464.4
cruris 443.9
  due to atherosclerosis NEC (see also Arteriosclerosis, extremities) 440.20
decubitus 413.0
diphtheritic (membranous) 032.0
erysipelatous 034.0
erythematous 462
exudative, chronic 476.0
faucium 478.29
gangrenous 462
  diphtheritic 032.0
infectious 462

Angina (Continued)
initial 411.1
intestinal 557.1
ludovici 528.3
Ludwig's 528.3
malignant 462
  diphtheritic 032.0
membranous 464.4
  diphtheritic 032.0
mesenteric 557.1
monocytic 075
nocturnal 413.0
phlegmonous 475
  diphtheritic 032.0
preinfarctional 411.1
Prinzmetal's 413.1
progressive 411.1
pseudomembranous 101
psychogenic 306.2
pultaceous, diphtheritic 032.0
scarlatinal 034.1
septic 034.0
simple 462
stable NEC 413.9
staphylococcal 462
streptococcal 034.0
stridulous, diphtheritic 032.3
syphilitic 093.9
  congenital 090.5
tonsil 475
trachealis 464.4
unstable 411.1
variant 413.1
Vincent's 101
Angioblastoma (M9161/1) - see Neoplasm, connective tissue, uncertain behavior
Angiocholecystitis (see also Cholecystitis, acute) 575.0
Angiocholitis (see also Cholecystitis, acute) 576.1
Angiodysgensis spinalis 336.1
Angiodysplasia (intestinalis) (intestine) 569.84
with hemorrhage 569.85
duodenum 537.82
  with hemorrhage 537.83
stomach 537.82
  with hemorrhage 537.83
Angioedema (allergic) (any site) (with urticaria) 995.1
hereditary 277.6
Angioendothelioma (M9130/1) - see also Neoplasm, by site, uncertain behavior
benign (M9130/0) (see also Hemangioma, by site) 228.00
bone (M9260/3) - see Neoplasm, bone, malignant
Ewing's (M9260/3) - see Neoplasm, bone, malignant
nervous system (M9130/0) 228.09
Angiofibroma (M9160/0) - see also Neoplasm, by site, benign
juvenile (M9160/0) 210.7
  specified site - see Neoplasm, by site, benign
  unspecified site 210.7
Angiohemophilia (A) (B) 286.4
Angioid streaks (choroid) (retina) 363.43
Angiokeratoma (M9141/0) - see also Neoplasm, skin, benign
corporis diffusum 272.7
Angiokeratosis
diffuse 272.7

Angioleiomyoma (M8894/0) - *see* Neoplasm, connective tissue, benign
Angioleucitis 683
Angiolipoma (M8861/0) (*see also* Lipoma, by site) 214.9
  infiltrating (M8861/1) - *see* Neoplasm, connective tissue, uncertain behavior
Angioma (M9120/0) (*see also* Hemangioma, by site) 228.00
  capillary 448.1
  hemorrhagicum hereditaria 448.0
  malignant (M9120/3) - *see* Neoplasm, connective tissue, malignant
  pigmentosum et atrophicum 757.33
  placenta - *see* Placenta, abnormal
  plexiform (M9131/0) - *see* Hemangioma, by site
  senile 448.1
  serpiginosum 709.1
  spider 448.1
  stellate 448.1
Angiomatosis 757.32
  bacillary 083.8
  corporis diffusum universale 272.7
  cutaneocerebral 759.6
  encephalocutaneous 759.6
  encephalofacial 759.6
  encephalotrigeminal 759.6
  hemorrhagic familial 448.0
  hereditary familial 448.0
  heredofamilial 448.0
  meningo-oculofacial 759.6
  multiple sites 228.09
  neuro-oculocutaneous 759.6
  retina (Hippel's disease) 759.6
  retinocerebellosa 759.6
  retinocerebral 759.6
  systemic 228.09
Angiomyolipoma (M8860/0)
  specified site - *see* Neoplasm, connective tissue, benign
  unspecified site 223.0
Angiomyoliposarcoma (M8860/3) - *see* Neoplasm, connective tissue, malignant
Angiomyoma (M8894/0) - *see* Neoplasm, connective tissue, benign
Angiomyosarcoma (M8894/3) - *see* Neoplasm, connective tissue, malignant
Angioneurosis 306.2
Angioneurotic edema (allergic) (any site) (with urticaria) 995.1
  hereditary 277.6
Angiopathia, angiopathy 459.9
  diabetic (peripheral) 250.7 [443.81]
  peripheral 443.9
    diabetic 250.7 [443.81]
    specified type NEC 443.89
  retinae syphilitica 093.89
  retinalis (juvenilis) 362.18
    background 362.10
    diabetic 250.5 [362.01]
    proliferative 362.29
    tuberculous (*see also* Tuberculosis) 017.3 [362.18]
Angiosarcoma (M9120/3) - *see* Neoplasm, connective tissue, malignant
Angiosclerosis - *see* Arteriosclerosis
Angioscotoma, enlarged 368.42
Angiospasm 443.9
  brachial plexus 353.0
  cerebral 435.9
  cervical plexus 353.2

Angiospasm (*Continued*)
  nerve
    arm 354.9
      axillary 353.0
      median 354.1
      ulnar 354.2
    autonomic (*see also* Neuropathy, peripheral, autonomic) 337.9
    axillary 353.0
    leg 355.8
      plantar 355.6
    lower extremity - *see* Angiospasm, nerve, leg
    median 354.1
    peripheral NEC 355.9
    spinal NEC 355.9
    sympathetic (*see also* Neuropathy, peripheral, autonomic) 337.9
    ulnar 354.2
    upper extremity - *see* Angiospasm, nerve, arm
  peripheral NEC 443.9
  traumatic 443.9
    foot 443.9
    leg 443.9
  vessel 443.9
Angiospastic disease or edema 443.9
Angle's ◄
    class I 524.21 ◄
    class II 524.22 ◄
    class III 524.23 ◄
Anguillulosis 127.2
Angulation
  cecum (*see also* Obstruction, intestine) 560.9
  coccyx (acquired) 738.6
    congenital 756.19
  femur (acquired) 736.39
    congenital 755.69
  intestine (large) (small) (*see also* Obstruction, intestine) 560.9
  sacrum (acquired) 738.5
    congenital 756.19
  sigmoid (flexure) (*see also* Obstruction, intestine) 560.9
  spine (*see also* Curvature, spine) 737.9
  tibia (acquired) 736.89
    congenital 755.69
  ureter 593.3
  wrist (acquired) 736.09
    congenital 755.59
Angulus infectiosus 686.8
Anhedonia 302.72
Anhidrosis (lid) (neurogenic) (thermogenic) 705.0
Anhydration 276.5
  with
    hypernatremia 276.0
    hyponatremia 276.1
Anhydremia 276.5
  with
    hypernatremia 276.0
    hyponatremia 276.1
Anidrosis 705.0
Aniridia (congenital) 743.45
Anisakiasis (infection) (infestation) 127.1
Anisakis larva infestation 127.1
Aniseikonia 367.32
Anisocoria (pupil) 379.41
  congenital 743.46
Anisocytosis 790.09
Anisometropia (congenital) 367.31
Ankle - *see* condition

Ankyloblepharon (acquired) (eyelid) 374.46
  filiforme (adnatum) (congenital) 743.62
  total 743.62
Ankylodactly (*see also* Syndactylism) 755.10
Ankyloglossia 750.0
Ankylosis (fibrous) (osseous) 718.50
  ankle 718.57
  any joint, produced by surgical fusion V45.4
  cricoarytenoid (cartilage) (joint) (larynx) 478.79
  dental 521.6
  ear ossicle NEC 385.22
    malleus 385.21
  elbow 718.52
  finger 718.54
  hip 718.55
  incostapedial joint (infectional) 385.22
  joint, produced by surgical fusion NEC V45.4
  knee 718.56
  lumbosacral (joint) 724.6
  malleus 385.21
  multiple sites 718.59
  postoperative (status) V45.4
  sacroiliac (joint) 724.6
  shoulder 718.51
  specified site NEC 718.58
  spine NEC 724.9
  surgical V45.4
  teeth, tooth (hard tissues) 521.6
  temporomandibular joint 524.61
  wrist 718.53
Ankylostoma - *see* Ancylostoma
Ankylostomiasis (intestinal) - *see* Ancylostomiasis
Ankylurethria (*see also* Stricture, urethra) 598.9
Annular - *see also* condition
  detachment, cervix 622.8
  organ or site, congenital NEC - *see* Distortion
  pancreas (congenital) 751.7
Anodontia (complete) (partial) (vera) 520.0
  with abnormal spacing 524.30 ◄▥
  acquired 525.10
    causing malocclusion 524.30 ◄▥
    due to
      caries 525.13
      extraction 525.10
      periodontal disease 525.12
      trauma 525.11
Anomaly, anomalous (congenital) (unspecified type) 759.9
  abdomen 759.9
  abdominal wall 756.70
  acoustic nerve 742.9
  adrenal (gland) 759.1
  Alder (-Reilly) (leukocyte granulation) 288.2
  alimentary tract 751.9
    lower 751.5
    specified type NEC 751.8
    upper (any part, except tongue) 750.9
      tongue 750.10
        specified type NEC 750.19
  alveolar 524.70 ◄▥
    ridge (process) 525.8 ◄
    specified NEC 524.79 ◄
  ankle (joint) 755.69
  anus, anal (canal) 751.5

◄ **New** ◄▥ **Revised**

Anomaly, anomalous (Continued)
    aorta, aortic 747.20
        arch 747.21
        coarctation (postductal) (preductal)
            747.10
        cusp or valve NEC 746.9
        septum 745.0
        specified type NEC 747.29
    aorticopulmonary septum 745.0
    apertures, diaphragm 756.6
    appendix 751.5
    aqueduct of Sylvius 742.3
        with spina bifida (see also Spina bi-
            fida) 741.0
    arm 755.50
        reduction (see also Deformity, reduc-
            tion, upper limb) 755.20
    arteriovenous (congenital) (peripheral)
        NEC 747.60
        brain 747.81
        cerebral 747.81
        coronary 746.85
        gastrointestinal 747.61
        lower limb 747.64
        renal 747.62
        specified site NEC 747.69
        spinal 747.82
        upper limb 747.63
    artery (see also Anomaly, peripheral
        vascular system) NEC 747.60
        brain 747.81
        cerebral 747.81
        coronary 746.85
        eye 743.9
        pulmonary 747.3
        renal 747.62
        retina 743.9
        umbilical 747.5
    arytenoepiglottic folds 748.3
    atrial
        bands 746.9
        folds 746.9
        septa 745.5
    atrioventricular
        canal 745.69
        common 745.69
        conduction 426.7
        excitation 426.7
        septum 745.4
    atrium - see Anomaly, atrial
    auditory canal 744.3
        specified type NEC 744.29
            with hearing impairment 744.02
    auricle
        ear 744.3
            causing impairment of hearing
                744.02
        heart 746.9
            septum 745.5
    autosomes, autosomal NEC 758.5
    Axenfeld's 743.44
    back 759.9
    band
        atrial 746.9
        heart 746.9
        ventricular 746.9
    Bartholin's duct 750.9
    biliary duct or passage 751.60
        atresia 751.61
    bladder (neck) (sphincter) (trigone)
        753.9
        specified type NEC 753.8
    blood vessel 747.9
        artery - see Anomaly, artery

Anomaly, anomalous (Continued)
    blood vessel (Continued)
        peripheral vascular - see Anomaly,
            peripheral vascular system
        vein - see Anomaly, vein
    bone NEC 756.9
        ankle 755.69
        arm 755.50
        chest 756.3
        cranium 756.0
        face 756.0
        finger 755.50
        foot 755.67
        forearm 755.50
        frontal 756.0
        head 756.0
        hip 755.63
        leg 755.60
        lumbosacral 756.10
        nose 748.1
        pelvic girdle 755.60
        rachitic 756.4
        rib 756.3
        shoulder girdle 755.50
        skull 756.0
            with
                anencephalus 740.0
                encephalocele 742.0
                hydrocephalus 742.3
                    with spina bifida (see also
                        Spina bifida) 741.0
                microcephalus 742.1
        toe 755.66
    brain 742.9
        multiple 742.4
        reduction 742.2
        specified type NEC 742.4
        vessel 747.81
    branchial cleft NEC 744.49
        cyst 744.42
        fistula 744.41
        persistent 744.41
        sinus (external) (internal) 744.41
    breast 757.9
    broad ligament 752.10
        specified type NEC 752.19
    bronchus 748.3
    bulbar septum 745.0
    bulbus cordis 745.9
        persistent (in left ventricle) 745.8
    bursa 756.9
    canal of Nuck 752.9
    canthus 743.9
    capillary NEC (see also Anomaly, pe-
        ripheral vascular system) 747.60
    cardiac 746.9
        septal closure 745.9
            acquired 429.71
        valve NEC 746.9
            pulmonary 746.00
            specified type NEC 746.89
    cardiovascular system 746.9
        complicating pregnancy, childbirth,
            or puerperium 648.5
    carpus 755.50
    cartilage, trachea 748.3
    cartilaginous 756.9
    caruncle, lacrimal, lachrymal 743.9
    cascade stomach 750.7
    cauda equina 742.59
    cecum 751.5
    cerebral - see also Anomaly, brain ves-
        sels 747.81
    cerebrovascular system 747.81

Anomaly, anomalous (Continued)
    cervix (uterus) 752.40
        with doubling of vagina and uterus
            752.2
        in pregnancy or childbirth 654.6
            affecting fetus or newborn 763.89
            causing obstructed labor 660.2
                affecting fetus or newborn 763.1
    Chédiak-Higashi (-Steinbrinck) (con-
        genital gigantism of peroxidase
        granules) 288.2
    cheek 744.9
    chest (wall) 756.3
    chin 744.9
        specified type NEC 744.89
    chordae tendineae 746.9
    choroid 743.9
        plexus 742.9
    chromosomes, chromosomal 758.9
        13 (13-15) 758.1
        18 (16-18) 758.2
        21 or 22 758.0
        autosomes NEC (see also Abnormal,
            autosomes) 758.5
            deletion 758.39   ◄▥
        Christchurch 758.39   ◄▥
        D₁ 758.1
        E₃ 758.2
        G 758.0
        mitochondrial 758.9
        mosaics 758.89
        sex 758.81
            complement, XO 758.6
            complement, XXX 758.81
            complement, XXY 758.7
            complement, XYY 758.81
            gonadal dysgenesis 758.6
            Klinefelter's 758.7
            Turner's 758.6
        trisomy 21 758.0
    cilia 743.9
    circulatory system 747.9
        specified type NEC 747.89
    clavicle 755.51
    clitoris 752.40
    coccyx 756.10
    colon 751.5
    common duct 751.60
    communication
        coronary artery 746.85
        left ventricle with right atrium
            745.4
    concha (ear) 744.3
    connection
        renal vessels with kidney 747.62
        total pulmonary venous 747.41
    connective tissue 756.9
        specified type NEC 756.89
    cornea 743.9
        shape 743.41
        size 743.41
        specified type NEC 743.49
    coronary
        artery 746.85
        vein 746.89
    cranium - see Anomaly, skull
    cricoid cartilage 748.3
    cushion, endocardial 745.60
        specified type NEC 745.69
    cystic duct 751.60
    dental arch relationship 524.20   ◄▥
        angle's class I 524.21   ◄
        angle's class II 524.22   ◄
        angle's class III 524.23   ◄

Anomaly, anomalous *(Continued)*
  dental arch relationship *(Continued)*
    articulation ◄
      anterior 524.27 ◄
      posterior 524.27 ◄
      reverse 524.27 ◄
    disto-occlusion 524.22 ◄
      division I 524.22 ◄
      division II 524.22 ◄
    excessive horizontal overlap 524.26◄
    interarch distance (excessive)
        (inadequate) 524.28 ◄
    mesio-occlusion 524.23 ◄
    neutro-occlusion 524.21 ◄
    open ◄
      anterior occlusal relationship
          524.24 ◄
      posterior occlusal relationship
          524.25 ◄
    specified NEC 524.29 ◄
  dentition 520.6
  dentofacial NEC 524.9
    functional 524.50 ◄▥
    specified type NEC 524.89 ◄▥
  dermatoglyphic 757.2
  Descemet's membrane 743.9
    specified type NEC 743.49
  development
    cervix 752.40
    vagina 752.40
    vulva 752.40
  diaphragm, diaphragmatic (apertures)
      NEC 756.6
  digestive organ(s) or system 751.9
    lower 751.5
    specified type NEC 751.8
    upper 750.9
  distribution, coronary artery 746.85
  ductus
    arteriosus 747.0
    Botalli 747.0
  duodenum 751.5
  dura 742.9
    brain 742.4
    spinal cord 742.59
  ear 744.3
    causing impairment of hearing
        744.00
      specified type NEC 744.09
    external 744.3
      causing impairment of hearing
          744.02
      specified type NEC 744.29
    inner (causing impairment of hear-
        ing) 744.05
    middle, except ossicles (causing im-
        pairment of hearing) 744.03
      ossicles 744.04
    ossicles 744.04
    prominent auricle 744.29
    specified type NEC 744.29
    with hearing impairment 744.09
  Ebstein's (heart) 746.2
    tricuspid valve 746.2
  ectodermal 757.9
  Eisenmenger's (ventricular septal de-
      fect) 745.4
  ejaculatory duct 752.9
    specified type NEC 752.89
  elbow (joint) 755.50
  endocardial cushion 745.60
    specified type NEC 745.69
  endocrine gland NEC 759.2
  epididymis 752.9

Anomaly, anomalous *(Continued)*
  epiglottis 748.3
  esophagus 750.9
    specified type NEC 750.4
  Eustachian tube 744.3
    specified type NEC 744.24
  eye (any part) 743.9
    adnexa 743.9
      specified type NEC 743.69
    anophthalmos 743.00
    anterior
      chamber and related structures
          743.9
        angle 743.9
          specified type NEC 743.44
        specified type NEC 743.44
      segment 743.9
        combined 743.48
        multiple 743.48
        specified type NEC 743.49
    cataract (*see also* Cataract) 743.30
    glaucoma (*see also* Buphthalmia) 743.20
    lid 743.9
      specified type NEC 743.63
    microphthalmos (*see also* Micro-
        phthalmos) 743.10
    posterior segment 743.9
      specified type NEC 743.59
      vascular 743.58
      vitreous 743.9
        specified type NEC 743.51
    ptosis (eyelid) 743.61
    retina 743.9
      specified type NEC 743.59
    sclera 743.9
      specified type NEC 743.47
    specified type NEC 743.8
  eyebrow 744.89
  eyelid 743.9
    specified type NEC 743.63
  face (any part) 744.9
    bone(s) 756.0
    specified type NEC 744.89
  fallopian tube 752.10
    specified type NEC 752.19
  fascia 756.9
    specified type NEC 756.89
  femur 755.60
  fibula 755.60
  finger 755.50
    supernumerary 755.01
    webbed (*see also* Syndactylism, fin-
        gers) 755.11
  fixation, intestine 751.4
  flexion (joint) 755.9
    hip or thigh (*see also* Dislocation,
        hip, congenital) 754.30
  folds, heart 746.9
  foot 755.67
  foramen
    Botalli 745.5
    ovale 745.5
  forearm 755.50
  forehead (*see also* Anomaly, skull)
      756.0
  form, teeth 520.2
  fovea centralis 743.9
  frontal bone (*see also* Anomaly, skull)
      756.0
  gallbladder 751.60
  Gartner's duct 752.11
  gastrointestinal tract 751.9
    specified type NEC 751.8
    vessel 747.61

Anomaly, anomalous *(Continued)*
  genitalia, genital organ(s) or system
    female 752.9
      external 752.40
        specified type NEC 752.49
      internal NEC 752.9
    male (external and internal)
        752.9
      epispadias 752.62
      hidden penis 752.65
      hydrocele, congenital 778.6
      hypospadias 752.61
      micropenis 752.64
      testis, undescended 752.51
        retractile 752.52
      specified type NEC 752.89
    genitourinary NEC 752.9
  Gerbode 745.4
  globe (eye) 743.9
  glottis 748.3
  granulation or granulocyte, genetic
      288.2
    constitutional 288.2
    leukocyte 288.2
  gum 750.9
  gyri 742.9
  hair 757.9
    specified type NEC 757.4
  hand 755.50
  hard tissue formation in pulp 522.3
  head (*see also* Anomaly, skull) 756.0
  heart 746.9
    auricle 746.9
    bands 746.9
    fibroelastosis cordis 425.3
    folds 746.9
    malposition 746.87
    maternal, affecting fetus or newborn
        760.3
    obstructive NEC 746.84
    patent ductus arteriosus (Botalli)
        747.0
    septum 745.9
      acquired 429.71
      aortic 745.0
      aorticopulmonary 745.0
      atrial 745.5
      auricular 745.5
      between aorta and pulmonary ar-
          tery 745.0
      endocardial cushion type 745.60
        specified type NEC 745.69
      interatrial 745.5
      interventricular 745.4
        with pulmonary stenosis or
            atresia, dextraposition of
            aorta, and hypertrophy of
            right ventricle 745.2
        acquired 429.71
      specified type NEC 745.8
      ventricular 745.4
        with pulmonary stenosis or
            atresia, dextraposition of
            aorta, and hypertrophy of
            right ventricle 745.2
        acquired 429.71
    specified type NEC 746.89
    tetralogy of Fallot 745.2
    valve NEC 746.9
      aortic 746.9
        atresia 746.89
        bicuspid valve 746.4
        insufficiency 746.4

ICD-9-CM

A

Vol. 2

Anomaly, anomalous (*Continued*)
  heart (*Continued*)
    valve NEC (*Continued*)
      aortic (*Continued*)
        specified type NEC 746.89
        stenosis 746.3
          subaortic 746.81
          supravalvular 747.22
      mitral 746.9
        atresia 746.89
        insufficiency 746.6
        specified type NEC 746.89
        stenosis 746.5
      pulmonary 746.00
        atresia 746.01
        insufficiency 746.09
        stenosis 746.02
          infundibular 746.83
          subvalvular 746.83
      tricuspid 746.9
        atresia 746.1
        stenosis 746.1
    ventricle 746.9
  heel 755.67
  Hegglin's 288.2
  hemianencephaly 740.0
  hemicephaly 740.0
  hemicrania 740.0
  hepatic duct 751.60
  hip (joint) 755.63
  hourglass
    bladder 753.8
    gallbladder 751.69
    stomach 750.7
  humerus 755.50
  hymen 752.40
  hypersegmentation of neutrophils, hereditary 288.2
  hypophyseal 759.2
  ileocecal (coil) (valve) 751.5
  ileum (intestine) 751.5
  ilium 755.60
  integument 757.9
    specified type NEC 757.8
  interarch distance (excessive) (inadequate) 524.28 ◄
  intervertebral cartilage or disc 756.10
  intestine (large) (small) 751.5
    fixational type 751.4
  iris 743.9
    specified type NEC 743.46
  ischium 755.60
  jaw NEC 524.9
    closure 524.51 ◄▥
    size (major) NEC 524.00
    specified type NEC 524.89 ◄▥
  jaw-cranial base relationship 524.10
    specified NEC 524.19
  jejunum 751.5
  joint 755.9
    hip
      dislocation (*see also* Dislocation, hip, congenital) 754.30
      predislocation (*see also* Subluxation, congenital, hip) 754.32
      preluxation (*see also* Subluxation, congenital, hip) 754.32
      subluxation (*see also* Subluxation, congenital, hip) 754.32
    lumbosacral 756.10
      spondylolisthesis 756.12
      spondylosis 756.11
    multiple arthrogryposis 754.89
    sacroiliac 755.69

Anomaly, anomalous (*Continued*)
  Jordan's 288.2
  kidney(s) (calyx) (pelvis) 753.9
    vessel 747.62
  Klippel-Feil (brevicollis) 756.16
  knee (joint) 755.64
  labium (majus) (minus) 752.40
  labyrinth, membranous (causing impairment of hearing) 744.05
  lacrimal
    apparatus, duct or passage 743.9
      specified type NEC 743.65
    gland 743.9
      specified type NEC 743.64
  Langdon Down (mongolism) 758.0
  larynx, laryngeal (muscle) 748.3
    web, webbed 748.2
  leg (lower) (upper) 755.60
    reduction NEC (*see also* Deformity, reduction, lower limb) 755.30
  lens 743.9
    shape 743.36
    specified type NEC 743.39
  leukocytes, genetic 288.2
    granulation (constitutional) 288.2
  lid (fold) 743.9
  ligament 756.9
    broad 752.10
    round 752.9
  limb, except reduction deformity 755.9
    lower 755.60
      reduction deformity (*see also* Deformity, reduction, lower limb) 755.30
      specified type NEC 755.69
    upper 755.50
      reduction deformity (*see also* Deformity, reduction, upper limb) 755.20
      specified type NEC 755.59
  lip 750.9
    harelip (*see also* Cleft, lip) 749.10
    specified type NEC 750.26
  liver (duct) 751.60
    atresia 751.69
  lower extremity 755.60
    vessel 747.64
  lumbosacral (joint) (region) 756.10
  lung (fissure) (lobe) NEC 748.60
    agenesis 748.5
    specified type NEC 748.69
  lymphatic system 759.9
  Madelung's (radius) 755.54
  mandible 524.9
    size NEC 524.00
  maxilla 524.90
    size NEC 524.00
  May (-Hegglin) 288.2
  meatus urinarius 753.9
    specified type NEC 753.8
  meningeal bands or folds, constriction of 742.8
  meninges 742.9
    brain 742.4
    spinal 742.59
  meningocele (*see also* Spina bifida) 741.9
  mesentery 751.9
  metacarpus 755.50
  metatarsus 755.67
  middle ear, except ossicles (causing impairment of hearing) 744.03
    ossicles 744.04

Anomaly, anomalous (*Continued*)
  mitral (leaflets) (valve) 746.9
    atresia 746.89
    insufficiency 746.6
    specified type NEC 746.89
    stenosis 746.5
  mouth 750.9
    specified type NEC 750.26
  multiple NEC 759.7
    specified type NEC 759.89
  muscle 756.9
    eye 743.9
      specified type NEC 743.69
    specified type NEC 756.89
  musculoskeletal system, except limbs 756.9
    specified type NEC 756.9
  nail 757.9
    specified type NEC 757.5
  narrowness, eyelid 743.62
  nasal sinus or septum 748.1
  neck (any part) 744.9
    specified type NEC 744.89
  nerve 742.9
    acoustic 742.9
      specified type NEC 742.8
    optic 742.9
      specified type NEC 742.8
    specified type NEC 742.8
  nervous system NEC 742.9
    brain 742.9
      specified type NEC 742.4
    specified type NEC 742.8
  neurological 742.9
  nipple 757.6 ◄▥
  nonteratogenic NEC 754.89
  nose, nasal (bone) (cartilage) (septum) (sinus) 748.1
  ocular muscle 743.9
  omphalomesenteric duct 751.0
  opening, pulmonary veins 747.49
  optic
    disc 743.9
      specified type NEC 743.57
    nerve 742.9
  opticociliary vessels 743.9
  orbit (eye) 743.9
    specified type NEC 743.66
  organ
    of Corti (causing impairment of hearing) 744.05
    or site 759.9
      specified type NEC 759.89
  origin
    both great arteries from same ventricle 745.11
    coronary artery 746.85
    innominate artery 747.69
    left coronary artery from pulmonary artery 746.85
    pulmonary artery 747.3
    renal vessels 747.62
    subclavian artery (left) (right) 747.21
  osseous meatus (ear) 744.03
  ovary 752.0
  oviduct 752.10
  palate (hard) (soft) 750.9
    cleft (*see also* Cleft, palate) 749.00
  pancreas (duct) 751.7
  papillary muscles 746.9
  parathyroid gland 759.2
  paraurethral ducts 753.9
  parotid (gland) 750.9
  patella 755.64

Anomaly, anomalous *(Continued)*
    Pelger-Huët (hereditary hyposegmentation) 288.2
    pelvic girdle 755.60
        specified type NEC 755.69
    pelvis (bony) 755.60
        complicating delivery 653.0
        rachitic 268.1
            fetal 756.4
    penis (glans) 752.69
    pericardium 746.89
    peripheral vascular system NEC 747.60
        gastrointestinal 747.61
        lower limb 747.64
        renal 747.62
        specified site NEC 747.69
        spinal 747.82
        upper limb 747.63
    Peter's 743.44
    pharynx 750.9
        branchial cleft 744.41
        specified type NEC 750.29
    Pierre Robin 756.0
    pigmentation 709.00
        congenital 757.33
        specified NEC 709.09
    pituitary (gland) 759.2
    pleural folds 748.8
    portal vein 747.40
    position tooth, teeth 524.30 ◀▥
        crowding 524.31 ◀
        displacement 524.30 ◀
            horizontal 524.33 ◀
            vertical 524.34 ◀
        distance ◀
            interocclusal ◀
                excessive 524.37 ◀
                insufficient 524.36 ◀
        excessive spacing 524.32 ◀
        rotation 524.35 ◀
        specified NEC 524.39 ◀
    preauricular sinus 744.46
    prepuce 752.9
    prostate 752.9
    pulmonary 748.60
        artery 747.3
        circulation 747.3
        specified type NEC 748.69
        valve 746.00
            atresia 746.01
            insufficiency 746.09
            specified type NEC 746.09
            stenosis 746.02
                infundibular 746.83
                subvalvular 746.83
        vein 747.40
        venous
            connection 747.49
                partial 747.42
                total 747.41
            return 747.49
                partial 747.42
                total (TAPVR) (complete) (subdiaphragmatic) (supradiaphragmatic) 747.41
    pupil 743.9
    pylorus 750.9
        hypertrophy 750.5
        stenosis 750.5
    rachitic, fetal 756.4
    radius 755.50
    rectovaginal (septum) 752.40
    rectum 751.5
    refraction 367.9

Anomaly, anomalous *(Continued)*
    renal 753.9
        vessel 747.62
    respiratory system 748.9
        specified type NEC 748.8
    rib 756.3
        cervical 756.2
    Rieger's 743.44
    rings, trachea 748.3
    rotation - *see also* Malrotation
        hip or thigh (*see also* Subluxation, congenital, hip) 754.32
    round ligament 752.9
    sacroiliac (joint) 755.69
    sacrum 756.10
    saddle
        back 754.2
        nose 754.0
            syphilitic 090.5
    salivary gland or duct 750.9
        specified type NEC 750.26
    scapula 755.50
    sclera 743.9
        specified type NEC 743.47
    scrotum 752.9
    sebaceous gland 757.9
    seminal duct or tract 752.9
    sense organs 742.9
        specified type NEC 742.8
    septum
        heart - *see* Anomaly, heart, septum
        nasal 748.1
    sex chromosomes NEC (*see also* Anomaly, chromosomes) 758.81
    shoulder (girdle) (joint) 755.50
        specified type NEC 755.59
    sigmoid (flexure) 751.5
    sinus of Valsalva 747.29
    site NEC 759.9
    skeleton generalized NEC 756.50
    skin (appendage) 757.9
        specified type NEC 757.39
    skull (bone) 756.0
        with
            anencephalus 740.0
            encephalocele 742.0
            hydrocephalus 742.3
                with spina bifida (*see also* Spina bifida) 741.0
            microcephalus 742.1
    specified type NEC
        adrenal (gland) 759.1
        alimentary tract (complete) (partial) 751.8
            lower 751.5
            upper 750.8
        ankle 755.69
        anus, anal (canal) 751.5
        aorta, aortic 747.29
            arch 747.21
        appendix 751.5
        arm 755.59
        artery (peripheral) NEC (*see also* Anomaly, peripheral vascular system) 747.60
            brain 747.81
            coronary 746.85
            eye 743.58
            pulmonary 747.3
            retinal 743.58
            umbilical 747.5
        auditory canal 744.29
            causing impairment of hearing 744.02

Anomaly, anomalous *(Continued)*
    specified type NEC *(Continued)*
        bile duct or passage 751.69
        bladder 753.8
            neck 753.8
        bone(s) 756.9
            arm 755.59
            face 756.0
            leg 755.69
            pelvic girdle 755.69
            shoulder girdle 755.59
            skull 756.0
                with
                    anencephalus 740.0
                    encephalocele 742.0
                    hydrocephalus 742.3
                        with spina bifida (*see also* Spina bifida) 741.0
                    microcephalus 742.1
        brain 742.4
        breast 757.6
        broad ligament 752.19
        bronchus 748.3
        canal of Nuck 752.89
        cardiac septal closure 745.8
        carpus 755.59
        cartilaginous 756.9
        cecum 751.5
        cervix 752.49
        chest (wall) 756.3
        chin 744.89
        ciliary body 743.46
        circulatory system 747.89
        clavicle 755.51
        clitoris 752.49
        coccyx 756.19
        colon 751.5
        common duct 751.69
        connective tissue 756.89
        cricoid cartilage 748.3
        cystic duct 751.69
        diaphragm 756.6
        digestive organ(s) or tract 751.8
            lower 751.5
            upper 750.8
        duodenum 751.5
        ear 744.29
            auricle 744.29
                causing impairment of hearing 744.02
            causing impairment of hearing 744.09
            inner (causing impairment of hearing) 744.05
            middle, except ossicles 744.03
                ossicles 744.04
        ejaculatory duct 752.89
        endocrine 759.2
        epiglottis 748.3
        esophagus 750.4
        eustachian tube 744.24
        eye 743.8
            lid 743.63
            muscle 743.69
        face 744.89
            bone(s) 756.0
        fallopian tube 752.19
        fascia 756.89
        femur 755.69
        fibula 755.69
        finger 755.59
        foot 755.67
        fovea centralis 743.55
        gallbladder 751.69

Anomaly, anomalous *(Continued)*
  specified type NEC *(Continued)*
    Gartner's duct 752.89
    gastrointestinal tract 751.8
    genitalia, genital organ(s)
      female 752.89
        external 752.49
        internal NEC 752.89
      male 752.89
        penis 752.69
        scrotal transposition 752.81
    genitourinary tract NEC 752.89
    glottis 748.3
    hair 757.4
    hand 755.59
    heart 746.89
      valve NEC 746.89
        pulmonary 746.09
    hepatic duct 751.69
    hydatid of Morgagni 752.89
    hymen 752.49
    integument 757.8
    intestine (large) (small) 751.5
      fixational type 751.4
    iris 743.46
    jejunum 751.5
    joint 755.8
    kidney 753.3
    knee 755.64
    labium (majus) (minus) 752.49
    labyrinth, membranous 744.05
    larynx 748.3
    leg 755.69
    lens 743.39
    limb, except reduction deformity
        755.8
      lower 755.69
        reduction deformity *(see also* De-
            formity, reduction, lower
            limb) 755.30
      upper 755.59
        reduction deformity *(see also* De-
            formity, reduction, upper
            limb) 755.20
    lip 750.26
    liver 751.69
    lung (fissure) (lobe) 748.69
    meatus urinarius 753.8
    metacarpus 755.59
    mouth 750.26
    muscle 756.89
      eye 743.69
    musculoskeletal system, except limbs
        756.9
    nail 757.5
    neck 744.89
    nerve 742.8
      acoustic 742.8
      optic 742.8
    nervous system 742.8
    nipple 757.6
    nose 748.1
    organ NEC 759.89
      of Corti 744.05
    osseous meatus (ear) 744.03
    ovary 752.0
    oviduct 752.19
    pancreas 751.7
    parathyroid 759.2
    patella 755.64
    pelvic girdle 755.69
    penis 752.69
    pericardium 746.89

Anomaly, anomalous *(Continued)*
  specified type NEC *(Continued)*
    peripheral vascular system NEC *(see
        also* Anomaly, peripheral vascu-
        lar system) 747.60
    pharynx 750.29
    pituitary 759.2
    prostate 752.89
    radius 755.59
    rectum 751.5
    respiratory system 748.8
    rib 756.3
    round ligament 752.89
    sacrum 756.19
    salivary duct or gland 750.26
    scapula 755.59
    sclera 743.47
    scrotum 752.89
      transposition 752.81
    seminal duct or tract 752.89
    shoulder girdle 755.59
    site NEC 759.89
    skin 757.39
    skull (bone(s)) 756.0
      with
        anencephalus 740.0
        encephalocele 742.0
        hydrocephalus 742.3
          with spina bifida *(see also*
              Spina bifida) 741.0
        microcephalus 742.1
    specified organ or site NEC 759.89
    spermatic cord 752.89
    spinal cord 742.59
    spine 756.19
    spleen 759.0
    sternum 756.3
    stomach 750.7
    tarsus 755.67
    tendon 756.89
    testis 752.89
    thorax (wall) 756.3
    thymus 759.2
    thyroid (gland) 759.2
      cartilage 748.3
    tibia 755.69
    toe 755.66
    tongue 750.19
    trachea (cartilage) 748.3
    ulna 755.59
    urachus 753.7
    ureter 753.4
      obstructive 753.29
    urethra 753.8
      obstructive 753.6
    urinary tract 753.8
    uterus 752.3
    uvula 750.26
    vagina 752.49
    vascular NEC *(see also* Anomaly, pe-
        ripheral vascular system) 747.60
      brain 747.81
    vas deferens 752.89
    vein(s) (peripheral) NEC *(see also*
        Anomaly, peripheral vascular
        system) 747.60
      brain 747.81
      great 747.49
      portal 747.49
      pulmonary 747.49
    vena cava (inferior) (superior) 747.49
    vertebra 756.19
    vulva 752.49
  spermatic cord 752.9

Anomaly, anomalous *(Continued)*
  spine, spinal 756.10
    column 756.10
    cord 742.9
      meningocele *(see also* Spina bifida)
          741.9
      specified type NEC 742.59
      spina bifida *(see also* Spina bifida)
          741.9
      vessel 747.82
    meninges 742.59
    nerve root 742.9
  spleen 759.0
  Sprengel's 755.52
  sternum 756.3
  stomach 750.9
    specified type NEC 750.7
  submaxillary gland 750.9
  superior vena cava 747.40
  talipes - *see* Talipes
  tarsus 755.67
    with complete absence of distal ele-
        ments 755.31
  teeth, tooth NEC 520.9
    position 524.30 ◀▥
      crowding 524.31 ◀
      displacement 524.30 ◀
        horizontal 524.33 ◀
        vertical 524.34 ◀
      distance ◀
        interocclusal ◀
          excessive 524.37 ◀
          insufficient 524.36 ◀
      excessive spacing 524.32 ◀
      rotation 524.35 ◀
      specified NEC 524.39 ◀
    spacing 524.30 ◀▥
  tendon 756.9
    specified type NEC 756.89
  termination
    coronary artery 746.85
  testis 752.9
  thebesian valve 746.9
  thigh 755.60
    flexion *(see also* Subluxation, congen-
        ital, hip) 754.32
  thorax (wall) 756.3
  throat 750.9
  thumb 755.50
    supernumerary 755.01
  thymus gland 759.2
  thyroid (gland) 759.2
    cartilage 748.3
  tibia 755.60
    saber 090.5
  toe 755.66
    supernumerary 755.02
    webbed *(see also* Syndactylism, toes)
        755.13
  tongue 750.10
    specified type NEC 750.19
  trachea, tracheal 748.3
    cartilage 748.3
    rings 748.3
  tragus 744.3
  transverse aortic arch 747.21
  trichromata 368.59
  trichromatopsia 368.59
  tricuspid (leaflet) (valve) 746.9
    atresia 746.1
    Ebstein's 746.2
    specified type NEC 746.89
    stenosis 746.1
  trunk 759.9

ICD-9-CM

◢

Vol. 2

Anomaly, anomalous *(Continued)*
Uhl's (hypoplasia of myocardium, right ventricle) 746.84
ulna 755.50
umbilicus 759.9
artery 747.5
union, trachea with larynx 748.3
unspecified site 759.9
upper extremity 755.50
vessel 747.63
urachus 753.7
specified type NEC 753.7
ureter 753.9
obstructive 753.20
specified type NEC 753.4
obstructive 753.29
urethra (valve) 753.9
obstructive 753.6
specified type NEC 753.8
urinary tract or system (any part, except urachus) 753.9
specified type NEC 753.8
urachus 753.7
uterus 752.3
with only one functioning horn 752.3
in pregnancy or childbirth 654.0
affecting fetus or newborn 763.89
causing obstructed labor 660.2
affecting fetus or newborn 763.1
uvula 750.9
vagina 752.40
valleculae 748.3
valve (heart) NEC 746.9
formation, ureter 753.29
pulmonary 746.00
specified type NEC 746.89
vascular NEC (*see also* Anomaly, peripheral vascular system) 747.60
ring 747.21
vas deferens 752.9
vein(s) (peripheral) NEC (*see also* Anomaly, peripheral vascular system) 747.60
brain 747.81
cerebral 747.81
coronary 746.89
great 747.40
specified type NEC 747.49
portal 747.40
pulmonary 747.40
retina 743.9
vena cava (inferior) (superior) 747.40
venous return (pulmonary) 747.49
partial 747.42
total 747.41
ventricle, ventricular (heart) 746.9
bands 746.9
folds 746.9
septa 745.4
vertebra 756.10
vesicourethral orifice 753.9
vessels NEC (*see also* Anomaly, peripheral vascular system) 747.60
optic papilla 743.9
vitelline duct 751.0
vitreous humor 743.9
specified type NEC 743.51
vulva 752.40
wrist (joint) 755.50
Anomia 784.69
Anonychia 757.5
acquired 703.8

Anophthalmos, anophthalmus (clinical) (congenital) (globe) 743.00
acquired V45.78
Anopsia (altitudinal) (quadrant) 368.46
Anorchia 752.89
Anorchism, anorchidism 752.89
Anorexia 783.0
hysterical 300.11
nervosa 307.1
Anosmia (*see also* Disturbance, sensation) 781.1
hysterical 300.11
postinfectional 478.9
psychogenic 306.7
traumatic 951.8
Anosognosia 780.99
Anosphrasia 781.1
Anosteoplasia 756.50
Anotia 744.09
Anovulatory cycle 628.0
Anoxemia 799.0
newborn 768.9
Anoxia 799.0
altitude 993.2
cerebral 348.1
with
abortion - *see* Abortion, by type, with specified complication NEC
ectopic pregnancy (*see also* categories 633.0-633.9) 639.8
molar pregnancy (*see also* categories 630-632) 639.8
complicating
delivery (cesarean) (instrumental) 669.4
ectopic or molar pregnancy 639.8
obstetric anesthesia or sedation 668.2
during or resulting from a procedure 997.01
following
abortion 639.8
ectopic or molar pregnancy 639.8
newborn (*see also* Distress, fetal, liveborn infant) 768.9
due to drowning 994.1
fetal, affecting newborn 768.9
heart - *see* Insufficiency, coronary
high altitude 993.2
intrauterine
fetal death (before onset of labor) 768.0
during labor 768.1
liveborn infant - *see* Distress, fetal, liveborn infant
myocardial - *see* Insufficiency, coronary
newborn 768.9
mild or moderate 768.6
severe 768.5
pathological 799.0
Anteflexion - *see* Anteversion
Antenatal
care, normal pregnancy V22.1
first V22.0
screening (for) V28.9
based on amniocentesis NEC V28.2
chromosomal anomalies V28.0
raised alphafetoprotein levels V28.1
chromosomal anomalies V28.0
fetal growth retardation using ultrasonics V28.4
isoimmunization V28.5

Antenatal *(Continued)*
screening *(Continued)*
malformations using ultrasonics V28.3
raised alphafetoprotein levels in amniotic fluid V28.1
specified condition NEC V28.8
Streptococcus B V28.6
Antepartum - *see* condition
Anterior - *see also* condition
spinal artery compression syndrome 721.1
Antero-occlusion 524.24 ◀▦
Anteversion
cervix (*see also* Anteversion, uterus) 621.6
femur (neck), congenital 755.63
uterus, uterine (cervix) (postinfectional) (postpartal, old) 621.6
congenital 752.3
in pregnancy or childbirth 654.4
affecting fetus or newborn 763.89
causing obstructed labor 660.2
affecting fetus or newborn 763.1
Anthracosilicosis (occupational) 500
Anthracosis (lung) (occupational) 500
lingua 529.3
Anthrax 022.9
with pneumonia 022.1 *[484.5]*
colitis 022.2
cutaneous 022.0
gastrointestinal 022.2
intestinal 022.2
pulmonary 022.1
respiratory 022.1
septicemia 022.3
specified manifestation NEC 022.8
Anthropoid pelvis 755.69
with disproportion (fetopelvic) 653.2
affecting fetus or newborn 763.1
causing obstructed labor 660.1
affecting fetus or newborn 763.1
Anthropophobia 300.29
Antibioma, breast 611.0
Antibodies
maternal (blood group) (*see also* Incompatibility) 656.2
anti-D, cord blood 656.1
fetus or newborn 773.0
Antibody deficiency syndrome
agammaglobulinemic 279.00
congenital 279.04
hypogammaglobulinemic 279.00
Anticoagulant, circulating (*see also* Circulating anticoagulants) 286.5
Antimongolism syndrome 758.39 ◀▦
Antimonial cholera 985.4
Antisocial personality 301.7
Antithrombinemia (*see also* Circulating anticoagulants) 286.5
Antithromboplastinemia (*see also* Circulating anticoagulants) 286.5
Antithromboplastinogenemia (*see also* Circulating anticoagulants) 286.5
Antitoxin complication or reaction - *see* Complications, vaccination
Anton (-Babinski) syndrome (hemiasomatognosia) 307.9
Antritis (chronic) 473.0
acute 461.0
Antrum, antral - *see* condition
Anuria 788.5
with
abortion - *see* Abortion, by type, with renal failure

Anuria *(Continued)*
with *(Continued)*
ectopic pregnancy *(see also* categories
633.0-633.9) 639.3
molar pregnancy *(see also* categories
630-632) 639.3
calculus (impacted) (recurrent) 592.9
kidney 592.0
ureter 592.1
congenital 753.3
due to a procedure 997.5
following
abortion 639.3
ectopic or molar pregnancy 639.3
newborn 753.3
postrenal 593.4
puerperal, postpartum, childbirth 669.3
specified as due to a procedure 997.5
sulfonamide
correct substance properly administered 788.5
overdose or wrong substance given
or taken 961.0
traumatic (following crushing) 958.5
Anus, anal - *see* condition
Anusitis 569.49
Anxiety (neurosis) (reaction) (state) 300.00
alcohol-induced 291.89
depression 300.4
drug-induced 292.89
due to or associated with physical condition 293.84
generalized 300.02
hysteria 300.20
in
acute stress reaction 308.0
transient adjustment reaction 309.24
panic type 300.01
separation, abnormal 309.21
syndrome (organic) (transient) 293.84
Aorta, aortic - *see* condition
Aortectasia 441.9
Aortitis (nonsyphilitic) 447.6
arteriosclerotic 440.0
calcific 447.6
Döhle-Heller 093.1
luetic 093.1
rheumatic *(see also* Endocarditis, acute,
rheumatic) 391.1
rheumatoid - *see* Arthritis, rheumatoid
specific 093.1
syphilitic 093.1
congenital 090.5
Apathetic thyroid storm *(see also* Thyrotoxicosis) 242.9
Apepsia 536.8
achlorhydric 536.0
psychogenic 306.4
Aperistalsis, esophagus 530.0
Apert's syndrome (acrocephalosyndactyly) 755.55
Apert-Gallais syndrome (adrenogenital)
255.2
Apertognathia 524.20
Aphagia 787.2
psychogenic 307.1
Aphakia (acquired) (bilateral) (postoperative) (unilateral) 379.31
congenital 743.35
Aphalangia (congenital) 755.4
lower limb (complete) (intercalary)
(partial) (terminal) 755.39
meaning all digits (complete) (partial) 755.31
transverse 755.31

Aphalangia *(Continued)*
upper limb (complete) (intercalary)
(partial) (terminal) 755.29
meaning all digits (complete) (partial) 755.21
transverse 755.21
Aphasia (amnestic) (ataxic) (auditory)
(Broca's) (choreatic) (classic) (expressive) (global) (ideational) (ideokinetic) (ideomotor) (jargon) (motor)
(nominal) (receptive) (semantic)
(sensory) (syntactic) (verbal) (visual)
(Wernicke's) 784.3
developmental 315.31
syphilis, tertiary 094.89
uremic - *see* Uremia
Aphemia 784.3
uremic - *see* Uremia
Aphonia 784.41
clericorum 784.49
hysterical 300.11
organic 784.41
psychogenic 306.1
Aphthae, aphthous - *see also* condition
Bednar's 528.2
cachectic 529.0
epizootic 078.4
fever 078.4
oral 528.2
stomatitis 528.2
thrush 112.0
ulcer (oral) (recurrent) 528.2
genital organ(s) NEC
female 629.8
male 608.89
larynx 478.79
Apical - *see* condition
Aplasia - *see also* Agenesis
alveolar process (acquired) 525.8
congenital 750.26
aorta (congenital) 747.22
aortic valve (congenital) 746.89
axialis extracorticalis (congenital)
330.0
bone marrow (myeloid) 284.9
acquired (secondary) 284.8
congenital 284.0
idiopathic 284.9
brain 740.0
specified part 742.2
breast 757.6
bronchus 748.3
cementum 520.4
cerebellar 742.2
congenital pure red cell 284.0
corpus callosum 742.2
erythrocyte 284.8
congenital 284.0
extracortical axial 330.0
eye (congenital) 743.00
fovea centralis (congenital) 743.55
germinal (cell) 606.0
iris 743.45
labyrinth, membranous 744.05
limb (congenital) 755.4
lower NEC 755.30
upper NEC 755.20
lung (bilateral) (congenital) (unilateral)
748.5
nervous system NEC 742.8
nuclear 742.8
ovary 752.0
Pelizaeus-Merzbacher 330.0
prostate (congenital) 752.89

Aplasia *(Continued)*
red cell (pure) (with thymoma) 284.8
acquired (secondary) 284.8
congenital 284.0
hereditary 284.0
of infants 284.0
primary 284.0
round ligament (congenital) 752.89
salivary gland 750.21
skin (congenital) 757.39
spinal cord 742.59
spleen 759.0
testis (congenital) 752.89
thymic, with immunodeficiency
279.2
thyroid 243
uterus 752.3
ventral horn cell 742.59
Apleuria 756.3
Apnea, apneic (spells) 786.03
newborn, neonatorum 770.81
essential 770.81
obstructive 770.82
primary 770.81
sleep 770.81
specified NEC 770.82
psychogenic 306.1
sleep NEC 780.57
with
hypersomnia 780.53
hyposomnia 780.51
insomnia 780.51
sleep disturbance NEC 780.57
Apneumatosis newborn 770.4
Apodia 755.31
Apophysitis (bone) *(see also* Osteochondrosis) 732.9
calcaneus 732.5
juvenile 732.6
Apoplectiform convulsions *(see also* Disease, cerebrovascular, acute) 436
Apoplexia, apoplexy, apoplectic *(see also*
Disease, cerebrovascular, acute)
436
abdominal 569.89
adrenal 036.3
attack 436
basilar *(see also* Disease, cerebrovascular, acute) 436
brain *(see also* Disease, cerebrovascular,
acute) 436
bulbar *(see also* Disease, cerebrovascular, acute) 436
capillary *(see also* Disease, cerebrovascular, acute) 436
cardiac *(see also* Infarct, myocardium)
410.9
cerebral *(see also* Disease, cerebrovascular, acute) 436
chorea *(see also* Disease, cerebrovascular, acute) 436
congestive *(see also* Disease, cerebrovascular, acute) 436
newborn 767.4
embolic *(see also* Embolism, brain) 434.1
fetus 767.0
fit *(see also* Disease, cerebrovascular,
acute) 436
healed or old V12.59
heart (auricle) (ventricle) *(see also* Infarct, myocardium) 410.9
heat 992.0
hemiplegia *(see also* Disease, cerebrovascular, acute) 436

ICD-9-CM
Vol. 2

Apoplexia, apoplexy, apoplectic
  (Continued)
  hemorrhagic (stroke) (*see also* Hemorrhage, brain) 432.9
  ingravescent (*see also* Disease, cerebrovascular, acute) 436
  late effect - *see* Late effect(s) (of) cerebrovascular disease
  lung - *see* Embolism, pulmonary
  meninges, hemorrhagic (*see also* Hemorrhage, subarachnoid) 430
  neonatorum 767.0
  newborn 767.0
  pancreatitis 577.0
  placenta 641.2
  progressive (*see also* Disease, cerebrovascular, acute) 436
  pulmonary (artery) (vein) - *see* Embolism, pulmonary
  sanguineous (*see also* Disease, cerebrovascular, acute) 436
  seizure (*see also* Disease, cerebrovascular, acute) 436
  serous (*see also* Disease, cerebrovascular, acute) 436
  spleen 289.59
  stroke (*see also* Disease, cerebrovascular, acute) 436
  thrombotic (*see also* Thrombosis, brain) 434.0
  uremic - *see* Uremia
  uteroplacental 641.2
Appendage
  fallopian tube (cyst of Morgagni) 752.11
  intestine (epiploic) 751.5
  preauricular 744.1
  testicular (organ of Morgagni) 752.89
Appendicitis 541
  with
    perforation, peritonitis (generalized), or rupture 540.0
     with peritoneal abscess 540.1
    peritoneal abscess 540.1
  acute (catarrhal) (fulminating) (gangrenous) (inflammatory) (obstructive) (retrocecal) (suppurative) 540.9
    with
     perforation, peritonitis, or rupture 540.0
      with peritoneal abscess 540.1
     peritoneal abscess 540.1
  amebic 006.8
  chronic (recurrent) 542
  exacerbation - *see* Appendicitis, acute
  fulminating - *see* Appendicitis, acute
  gangrenous - *see* Appendicitis, acute
  healed (obliterative) 542
  interval 542
  neurogenic 542
  obstructive 542
  pneumococcal 541
  recurrent 542
  relapsing 542
  retrocecal 541
  subacute (adhesive) 542
  subsiding 542
  suppurative - *see* Appendicitis, acute
  tuberculous (*see also* Tuberculosis) 014.8
Appendiclausis 543.9
Appendicolithiasis 543.9

Appendicopathia oxyurica 127.4
Appendix, appendicular - *see also* condition
  Morgagni (male) 752.89
    fallopian tube 752.11
Appetite
  depraved 307.52
  excessive 783.6
    psychogenic 307.51
  lack or loss (*see also* Anorexia) 783.0
    nonorganic origin 307.59
  perverted 307.52
    hysterical 300.11
Apprehension, apprehensiveness (abnormal) (state) 300.00
  specified type NEC 300.09
Approximal wear 521.10 ◀▥
Apraxia (classic) (ideational) (ideokinetic) (ideomotor) (motor) 784.69
  oculomotor, congenital 379.51
  verbal 784.69
Aptyalism 527.7
Aqueous misdirection 365.83
Arabicum elephantiasis (*see also* Infestation, filarial) 125.9
Arachnidism 989.5
Arachnitis - *see* Meningitis
Arachnodactyly 759.82
Arachnoidism 989.5
Arachnoiditis (acute) (adhesive) (basic) (brain) (cerebrospinal) (chiasmal) (chronic) (spinal) (*see also* Meningitis) 322.9
  meningococcal (chronic) 036.0
  syphilitic 094.2
  tuberculous (*see also* Tuberculosis, meninges) 013.0
Araneism 989.5
Arboencephalitis, Australian 062.4
Arborization block (heart) 426.6
Arbor virus, arbovirus (infection) NEC 066.9
ARC 042
Arches - *see* condition
Arcuatus uterus 752.3
Arcus (cornea)
  juvenilis 743.43
    interfering with vision 743.42
  senilis 371.41
Arc-welders' lung 503
Arc-welders' syndrome (photokeratitis) 370.24
Areflexia 796.1
Areola - *see* condition
Argentaffinoma (M8241/1) - *see also* Neoplasm, by site, uncertain behavior
  benign (M8241/0) - *see* Neoplasm, by site, benign
  malignant (M8241/3) - *see* Neoplasm, by site, malignant
  syndrome 259.2
Argentinian hemorrhagic fever 078.7
Arginosuccinicaciduria 270.6
Argonz-del Castillo syndrome (nonpuerperal galactorrhea and amenorrhea) 253.1
Argyll-Robertson phenomenon, pupil, or syndrome (syphilitic) 094.89
  atypical 379.45
  nonluetic 379.45
  nonsyphilitic 379.45
  reversed 379.45

Argyria, argyriasis NEC 985.8
  conjunctiva 372.55
  cornea 371.16
  from drug or medicinal agent
    correct substance properly administered 709.09
    overdose or wrong substance given or taken 961.2
Arhinencephaly 742.2
Arias-Stella phenomenon 621.30 ◀▥
Ariboflavinosis 266.0
Arizona enteritis 008.1
Arm - *see* condition
Armenian disease 277.3
Arnold-Chiari obstruction or syndrome (*see also* Spina bifida) 741.0
  type I 348.4
  type II (*see also* Spina bifida) 741.0
  type III 742.0
  type IV 742.2
Arrest, arrested
  active phase of labor 661.1
    affecting fetus or newborn 763.7
  any plane in pelvis
    complicating delivery 660.1
     affecting fetus or newborn 763.1
  bone marrow (*see also* Anemia, aplastic) 284.9
  cardiac 427.5
    with
     abortion - *see* Abortion, by type, with specified complication NEC
     ectopic pregnancy (*see also* categories 633.0-633.9) 639.8
     molar pregnancy (*see also* categories 630-632) 639.8
    complicating
     anesthesia
      correct substance properly administered 427.5
      obstetric 668.1
      overdose or wrong substance given 968.4
      specified anesthetic - *see* Table of Drugs and Chemicals
     delivery (cesarean) (instrumental) 669.4
    ectopic or molar pregnancy 639.8
    surgery (nontherapeutic) (therapeutic) 997.1
    fetus or newborn 779.89
    following
     abortion 639.8
     ectopic or molar pregnancy 639.8
    postoperative (immediate) 997.1
     long-term effect of cardiac surgery 429.4
  cardiorespiratory (*see also* Arrest, cardiac) 427.5
  deep transverse 660.3
    affecting fetus or newborn 763.1
  development or growth
    bone 733.91
    child 783.40
    fetus 764.9
     affecting management of pregnancy 656.5
    tracheal rings 748.3
  epiphyseal 733.91
  granulopoiesis 288.0
  heart - *see* Arrest, cardiac

◀ **New**　　◀▥ **Revised**

Arrest, arrested (*Continued*)
 respiratory 799.1
  newborn 770.89
 sinus 426.6
 transverse (deep) 660.3
  affecting fetus or newborn
   763.1
Arrhenoblastoma (M8630/1)
 benign (M8630/0)
  specified site - *see* Neoplasm, by site,
   benign
  unspecified site
   female 220
   male 222.0
 malignant (M8630/3)
  specified site - *see* Neoplasm, by site,
   malignant
  unspecified site
   female 183.0
   male 186.9
 specified site - *see* Neoplasm, by site,
  uncertain behavior
 unspecified site
  female 236.2
  male 236.4
Arrhinencephaly 742.2
 due to
  trisomy 13 (13-15) 758.1
  trisomy 18 (16-18) 758.2
Arrhythmia (auricle) (cardiac) (cordis)
  (gallop rhythm) (juvenile) (nodal)
  (reflex) (sinus) (supraventricular)
  (transitory) (ventricle) 427.9
 bigeminal rhythm 427.89
 block 426.9
 bradycardia 427.89
 contractions, premature 427.60
 coronary sinus 427.89
 ectopic 427.89
 extrasystolic 427.60
 postoperative 997.1
 psychogenic 306.2
 vagal 780.2
Arrillaga-Ayerza syndrome (pulmonary
  artery sclerosis with pulmonary hypertension) 416.0
Arsenical
 dermatitis 692.4
 keratosis 692.4
 pigmentation 985.1
  from drug or medicinal agent
   correct substance properly admin-
    istered 709.09
   overdose or wrong substance
    given or taken 961.1
Arsenism 985.1
 from drug or medicinal agent
  correct substance properly administered 692.4
  overdose or wrong substance given
   or taken 961.1
Arterial - *see* condition
Arteriectasis 447.8
Arteriofibrosis - *see* Arteriosclerosis
Arteriolar sclerosis - *see* Arteriosclerosis
Arteriolith - *see* Arteriosclerosis
Arteriolitis 447.6
 necrotizing, kidney 447.5
 renal - *see* Hypertension, kidney
Arteriolosclerosis - *see* Arteriosclerosis
Arterionephrosclerosis (*see also* Hyper-
  tension, kidney) 403.90
Arteriopathy 447.9

Arteriosclerosis, arteriosclerotic (artery)
  (deformans) (diffuse) (disease) (endarteritis) (general) (obliterans) (obliterative) (occlusive) (senile) (with calcification) 440.9
 with
  gangrene 440.24
  psychosis (*see also* Psychosis, arteriosclerotic) 290.40
  ulceration 440.23
 aorta 440.0
 arteries of extremities - *see* Arteriosclerosis, extremities
 basilar (artery) (*see also* Occlusion, artery, basilar) 433.0
 brain 437.0
 bypass graft
  coronary artery 414.05
   autologous artery (gastroepiploic)
    (internal mammary) 414.04
   autologous vein 414.02
   of transplanted heart 414.07
   nonautologous biological 414.03
  extremity 440.30
   autologous vein 440.31
   nonautologous biological 440.32
 cardiac - *see* Arteriosclerosis, coronary
 cardiopathy - *see* Arteriosclerosis, coronary
 cardiorenal (*see also* Hypertension, cardiorenal) 404.90
 cardiovascular (*see also* Disease, cardiovascular) 429.2
 carotid (artery) (common) (internal)
  (*see also* Occlusion, artery, carotid)
  433.1
 central nervous system 437.0
 cerebral 437.0
  late effect - *see* Late effect(s) (of)
   cerebrovascular disease
 cerebrospinal 437.0
 cerebrovascular 437.0
 coronary (artery) 414.00
  graft - *see* Arteriosclerosis, bypass
   graft
  native artery 414.01
  of transplanted heart 414.06
 extremities (native artery) NEC
  440.20
  bypass graft 440.30
   autologous vein 440.31
   nonautologous biological 440.32
  claudication (intermittent) 440.21
   and
    gangrene 440.24
    rest pain 440.22
     and
      gangrene 440.24
      ulceration 440.23
       and gangrene 440.24
    ulceration 440.23
     and gangrene 440.24
  gangrene 440.24
  rest pain 440.22
   and
    gangrene 440.24
    ulceration 440.23
     and gangrene 440.24
  specified site NEC 440.29
  ulceration 440.23
   and gangrene 440.24
 heart (disease) - *see also* Arteriosclerosis, coronary

Arteriosclerosis, arteriosclerotic
  (*Continued*)
 heart (*Continued*)
  valve 424.99
   aortic 424.1
   mitral 424.0
   pulmonary 424.3
   tricuspid 424.2
 kidney (*see also* Hypertension, kidney)
  403.90
 labyrinth, labyrinthine 388.00
 medial NEC (*see also* Arteriosclerosis,
  extremities) 440.20
 mesentery (artery) 557.1
 Mönckeberg's (*see also* Arteriosclerosis,
  extremities) 440.20
 myocarditis 429.0
 nephrosclerosis (*see also* Hypertension,
  kidney) 403.90
 peripheral (of extremities) - *see* Arteriosclerosis, extremities
 precerebral 433.9
  specified artery NEC 433.8
 pulmonary (idiopathic) 416.0
 renal (*see also* Hypertension, kidney)
  403.90
  arterioles (*see also* Hypertension, kidney) 403.90
  artery 440.1
 retinal (vascular) 440.8 [362.13]
 specified artery NEC 440.8
  with gangrene 440.8 [785.4]
 spinal (cord) 437.0
 vertebral (artery) (*see also* Occlusion,
  artery, vertebral) 433.2
Arteriospasm 443.9
Arteriovenous - *see* condition
Arteritis 447.6
 allergic (*see also* Angiitis, hypersensitivity) 446.20
 aorta (nonsyphilitic) 447.6
  syphilitic 093.1
 aortic arch 446.7
 brachiocephalica 446.7
 brain 437.4
  syphilitic 094.89
 branchial 446.7
 cerebral 437.4
  late effect - *see* Late effect(s) (of)
   cerebrovascular disease
  syphilitic 094.89
 coronary (artery) - *see also* Arteriosclerosis, coronary
  rheumatic 391.9
   chronic 398.99
  syphilitic 093.89
 cranial (left) (right) 446.5
 deformans - *see* Arteriosclerosis
 giant cell 446.5
 necrosing or necrotizing 446.0
 nodosa 446.0
 obliterans - *see also* Arteriosclerosis
  subclavicocarotica 446.7
 pulmonary 417.8
 retina 362.18
 rheumatic - *see* Fever, rheumatic
 senile - *see* Arteriosclerosis
 suppurative 447.2
 syphilitic (general) 093.89
  brain 094.89
  coronary 093.89
  spinal 094.89
 temporal 446.5
 young female, syndrome 446.7

ICD-9-CM

A

Vol. 2

Artery, arterial - *see* condition
Arthralgia (*see also* Pain, joint) 719.4
  allergic (*see also* Pain, joint) 719.4
  in caisson disease 993.3
  psychogenic 307.89
  rubella 056.71
  Salmonella 003.23
  temporomandibular joint 524.62
Arthritis, arthritic (acute) (chronic) (sub-
    acute) 716.9
  meaning Osteoarthritis - *see* Osteoar-
    throsis

Note   Use the following fifth-digit
subclassification with categories 711-
712, 715-716:

  0   site unspecified
  1   shoulder region
  2   upper arm
  3   forearm
  4   hand
  5   pelvic region and thigh
  6   lower leg
  7   ankle and foot
  8   other specified sites
  9   multiple sites

---

  allergic 716.2
  ankylosing (crippling) (spine) 720.0
    [713.2]
    sites other than spine 716.9
  atrophic 714.0
    spine 720.9
  back (*see also* Arthritis, spine) 721.90
  Bechterew's (ankylosing spondylitis)
    720.0
  blennorrhagic 098.50 [711.6]
  cervical, cervicodorsal (*see also* Spondy-
    losis, cervical) 721.0
  Charcôt's 094.0 [713.5]
    diabetic 250.6 [713.5]
    syringomyelic 336.0 [713.5]
    tabetic 094.0 [713.5]
  chylous (*see also* Filariasis) 125.9 [711.7]
  climacteric NEC 716.3
  coccyx 721.8
  cricoarytenoid 478.79
  crystal (-induced) - *see* Arthritis, due to
    crystals
  deformans (*see also* Osteoarthrosis)
    715.9
    spine 721.90
      with myelopathy 721.91
  degenerative (*see also* Osteoarthrosis)
    715.9
    idiopathic 715.09
    polyarticular 715.09
    spine 721.90
      with myelopathy 721.91
  dermatoarthritis, lipoid 272.8 [713.0]
  due to or associated with
    acromegaly 253.0 [713.0]
    actinomycosis 039.8 [711.4]
    amyloidosis 277.3 [713.7]
    bacterial disease NEC 040.89 [711.4]
    Behçet's syndrome 136.1 [711.2]
    blastomycosis 116.0 [711.6]
    brucellosis (*see also* Brucellosis) 023.9
      [711.4]
    caisson disease 993.3
    coccidioidomycosis 114.3 [711.6]
    coliform (Escherichia coli) 711.0
    colitis, ulcerative - (*see also* Colitis,
      ulcerative) 556.9 [713.1]

Arthritis, arthritic (*Continued*)
  due to or associated with (*Continued*)
    cowpox 051.0 [711.5]
    crystals -(*see also* Gout)
      dicalcium phosphate 275.49 [712.1]
      pyrophosphate 275.49 [712.2]
      specified NEC 275.49 [712.8]
    dermatoarthritis, lipoid 272.8 [713.0]
    dermatological disorder NEC 709.9
      [713.3]
    diabetes 250.6 [713.5]
    diphtheria 032.89 [711.4]
    dracontiasis 125.7 [711.7]
    dysentery 009.0 [711.3]
    endocrine disorder NEC 259.9
      [713.0]
    enteritis NEC 009.1 [711.3]
      infectious (*see also* Enteritis, infec-
        tious) 009.0 [711.3]
        specified organism NEC 008.8
          [711.3]
      regional (*see also* Enteritis, re-
        gional) 555.9 [713.1]
        specified organism NEC 008.8
          [711.3]
    epiphyseal slip, nontraumatic (old)
      716.8
    erysipelas 035 [711.4]
    erythema
      epidemic 026.1
      multiforme 695.1 [713.3]
      nodosum 695.2 [713.3]
    Escherichia coli 711.0
    filariasis NEC 125.9 [711.7]
    gastrointestinal condition NEC 569.9
      [713.1]
    glanders 024 [711.4]
    Gonococcus 098.50
    gout 274.0
    H. influenzae 711.0
    helminthiasis NEC 128.9 [711.7]
    hematological disorder NEC 289.9
      [713.2]
    hemochromatosis 275.0 [713.0]
    hemoglobinopathy NEC (*see also*
      Disease, hemoglobin) 282.7
      [713.2]
    hemophilia (*see also* Hemophilia)
      286.0 [713.2]
    Hemophilus influenzae (H. influen-
      zae) 711.0
    Henoch (-Schönlein) purpura 287.0
      [713.6]
    histoplasmosis NEC (*see also* Histo-
      plasmosis) 115.99 [711.6]
    hyperparathyroidism 252.00
      [713.0]   ◀▥
    hypersensitivity reaction NEC 995.3
      [713.6]
    hypogammaglobulinemia (*see also*
      Hypogammaglobulinemia)
      279.00 [713.0]
    hypothyroidism NEC 244.9 [713.0]
    infection (*see also* Arthritis, infec-
      tious) 711.9
    infectious disease NEC 136.9 [711.8]
    leprosy (*see also* Leprosy) 030.9
      [711.4]
    leukemia NEC (M9800/3) 208.9
      [713.2]
    lipoid dermatoarthritis 272.8 [713.0]
    Lyme disease 088.81 [711.8]
    Mediterranean fever, familial 277.3
      [713.7]
    meningococcal infection 036.82

Arthritis, arthritic (*Continued*)
  due to or associated with (*Continued*)
    metabolic disorder NEC 277.9 [713.0]
    multiple myelomatosis (M9730/3)
      203.0 [713.2]
    mumps 072.79 [711.5]
    mycobacteria 031.8 [711.4]
    mycosis NEC 117.9 [711.6]
    neurological disorder NEC 349.9
      [713.5]
    ochronosis 270.2 [713.0]
    O'Nyong Nyong 066.3 [711.5]
    parasitic disease NEC 136.9 [711.8]
    paratyphoid fever (*see also* Fever,
      paratyphoid) 002.9 [711.3]
    Pneumococcus 711.0
    poliomyelitis (*see also* Poliomyelitis)
      045.9 [711.5]
    Pseudomonas 711.0
    psoriasis 696.0
    pyogenic organism (E. coli) (H. in-
      fluenzae) (Pseudomonas) (Strep-
      tococcus) 711.0
    rat-bite fever 026.1 [711.4]
    regional enteritis (*see also* Enteritis,
      regional) 555.9 [713.1]
    Reiter's disease 099.3 [711.1]
    respiratory disorder NEC 519.9
      [713.4]
    reticulosis, malignant (M9720/3)
      202.3 [713.2]
    rubella 056.71
    salmonellosis 003.23
    sarcoidosis 135 [713.7]
    serum sickness 999.5 [713.6]
    Staphylococcus 711.0
    Streptococcus 711.0
    syphilis (*see also* Syphilis) 094.0
      [711.4]
    syringomyelia 336.0 [713.5]
    thalassemia 282.49 [713.2]
    tuberculosis (*see also* Tuberculosis,
      arthritis) 015.9 [711.4]
    typhoid fever 002.0 [711.3]
    ulcerative colitis - (*see also* Colitis, ul-
      cerative) 556.9 [713.1]
    urethritis
      nongonococcal (*see also* Urethritis,
        nongonococcal) 099.40 [711.1]
      nonspecific (*see also* Urethritis,
        nongonococcal) 099.40 [711.1]
      Reiter's 099.3 [711.1]
    viral disease NEC 079.99 [711.5]
  erythema epidemic 026.1
  gonococcal 098.50
  gouty (acute) 274.0
  hypertrophic (*see also* Osteoarthrosis)
    715.9
    spine 721.90
      with myelopathy 721.91
  idiopathic, blennorrheal 099.3
  in caisson disease 993.3 [713.8]
  infectious or infective (acute) (chronic)
    (subacute) NEC 711.9
    nonpyogenic 711.9
    spine 720.9
  inflammatory NEC 714.9
  juvenile rheumatoid (chronic) (polyar-
    ticular) 714.30
    acute 714.31
    monoarticular 714.33
    pauciarticular 714.32
  lumbar (*see also* Spondylosis, lumbar)
    721.3

Arthritis, arthritic *(Continued)*
  meningococcal 036.82
  menopausal NEC 716.3
  migratory - *see* Fever, rheumatic
  neuropathic (Charcôt's) 094.0 *[713.5]*
    diabetic 250.6 *[713.5]*
    nonsyphilitic NEC 349.9 *[713.5]*
    syringomyelic 336.0 *[713.5]*
    tabetic 094.0 *[713.5]*
  nodosa (*see also* Osteoarthrosis) 715.9
    spine 721.90
      with myelopathy 721.91
  nonpyogenic NEC 716.9
    spine 721.90
      with myelopathy 721.91
  ochronotic 270.2 *[713.0]*
  palindromic (*see also* Rheumatism, pal-
      indromic) 719.3
  pneumococcal 711.0
  postdysenteric 009.0 *[711.3]*
  postrheumatic, chronic (Jaccoud's)
      714.4
  primary progressive 714.0
    spine 720.9
  proliferative 714.0
    spine 720.0
  psoriatic 696.0
  purulent 711.0
  pyogenic or pyemic 711.0
  rheumatic 714.0
    acute or subacute - *see* Fever, rheu-
        matic
    chronic 714.0
    spine 720.9
  rheumatoid (nodular) 714.0
    with
      splenoadenomegaly and leuko-
          penia 714.1
      visceral or systemic involvement
          714.2
    aortitis 714.89
    carditis 714.2
    heart disease 714.2
    juvenile (chronic) (polyarticular)
        714.30
      acute 714.31
      monoarticular 714.33
      pauciarticular 714.32
    spine 720.0
  rubella 056.71
  sacral, sacroiliac, sacrococcygeal (*see
      also* Spondylosis, sacral) 721.3
  scorbutic 267
  senile or senescent (*see also* Osteoar-
      throsis) 715.9
    spine 721.90
      with myelopathy 721.91
  septic 711.0
  serum (nontherapeutic) (therapeutic)
      999.5 *[713.6]*
  specified form NEC 716.8
  spine 721.90
    with myelopathy 721.91
    atrophic 720.9
    degenerative 721.90
      with myelopathy 721.91
    hypertrophic (with deformity) 721.90
      with myelopathy 721.91
    infectious or infective NEC 720.9
    Marie-Strümpell 720.0
    nonpyogenic 721.90
      with myelopathy 721.91
    pyogenic 720.9
    rheumatoid 720.0

Arthritis, arthritic *(Continued)*
  spine *(Continued)*
    traumatic (old) 721.7
    tuberculous (*see also* Tuberculosis)
        015.0 *[720.81]*
  staphylococcal 711.0
  streptococcal 711.0
  suppurative 711.0
  syphilitic 094.0 *[713.5]*
    congenital 090.49 *[713.5]*
  syphilitica deformans (Charcôt) 094.0
      [713.5]
  temporomandibular joint 524.69
  thoracic (*see also* Spondylosis, thoracic)
      721.2
  toxic of menopause 716.3
  transient 716.4
  traumatic (chronic) (old) (post) 716.1
    current injury - *see* Nature of injury
  tuberculous (*see also* Tuberculosis, ar-
      thritis) 015.9 *[711.4]*
  urethritica 099.3 *[711.1]*
  urica, uratic 274.0
  venereal 099.3 *[711.1]*
  vertebral (*see also* Arthritis, spine)
      721.90
  villous 716.8
  von Bechterew's 720.0
Arthrocele (*see also* Effusion, joint) 719.0
Arthrochondritis - *see* Arthritis
Arthrodesis status V45.4
Arthrodynia (*see also* Pain, joint) 719.4
  psychogenic 307.89
Arthrodysplasia 755.9
Arthrofibrosis, joint (*see also* Ankylosis)
    718.5
Arthrogryposis 728.3
  multiplex, congenita 754.89
Arthrokatadysis 715.35
Arthrolithiasis 274.0
Arthro-onychodysplasia 756.89
Arthro-osteo-onychodysplasia 756.89
Arthropathy (*see also* Arthritis) 716.9

Note   Use the following fifth-digit
subclassification with categories 711-
712, 716:

  0   site unspecified
  1   shoulder region
  2   upper arm
  3   forearm
  4   hand
  5   pelvic region and thigh
  6   lower leg
  7   ankle and foot
  8   other specified sites
  9   multiple sites

  Behçet's 136.1 *[711.2]*
  Charcôt's 094.0 *[713.5]*
    diabetic 250.6 *[713.5]*
    syringomyelic 336.0 *[713.5]*
    tabetic 094.0 *[713.5]*
  crystal (-induced) - *see* Arthritis, due to
      crystals
  gouty 274.0
  neurogenic, neuropathic (Charcôt's)
      (tabetic) 094.0 *[713.5]*
    diabetic 250.6 *[713.5]*
    nonsyphilitic NEC 349.9 *[713.5]*
    syringomyelic 336.0 *[713.5]*
  postdysenteric NEC 009.0 *[711.3]*
  postrheumatic, chronic (Jaccoud's)
      714.4

Arthropathy *(Continued)*
  psoriatic 696.0
  pulmonary 731.2
  specified NEC 716.8
  syringomyelia 336.0 *[713.5]*
  tabes dorsalis 094.0 *[713.5]*
  tabetic 094.0 *[713.5]*
  transient 716.4
  traumatic 716.1
  uric acid 274.0
Arthrophyte (*see also* Loose, body, joint)
    718.1
Arthrophytis 719.80
  ankle 719.87
  elbow 719.82
  foot 719.87
  hand 719.84
  hip 719.85
  knee 719.86
  multiple sites 719.89
  pelvic region 719.85
  shoulder (region) 719.81
  specified site NEC 719.88
  wrist 719.83
Arthropyosis (*see also* Arthritis, pyo-
    genic) 711.0
**Arthroscopic surgical procedure con-
    verted to open procedure** V64.43
Arthrosis (deformans) (degenerative) (*see
    also* Osteoarthrosis) 715.9
  Charcôt's 094.0 *[713.5]*
  polyarticular 715.09
  spine (*see also* Spondylosis) 721.90
Arthus' phenomenon 995.2
  due to
    correct substance properly adminis-
        tered 995.2
    overdose or wrong substance given
        or taken 977.9
      specified drug - *see* Table of Drugs
          and Chemicals
    serum 999.5
Articular - *see also* condition
Articulation   ◀
  anterior 524.27   ◀
  posterior 524.27   ◀
  reverse 524.27   ◀
  disc disorder (reducing or non-reduc-
      ing) 524.63
  spondylolisthesis 756.12
Artificial
  device (prosthetic) - *see* Fitting, device
  insemination V26.1
  menopause (states) (symptoms) (syn-
      drome) 627.4
  opening status (functioning) (without
      complication) V44.9
    anus (colostomy) V44.3
    colostomy V44.3
    cystostomy V44.50
      appendico-vesicostomy V44.52
      cutaneous-vesicostomy V44.51
      specified type NEC V44.59
    enterostomy V44.4
    gastrostomy V44.1
    ileostomy V44.2
    intestinal tract NEC V44.4
    jejunostomy V44.4
    nephrostomy V44.6
    specified site NEC V44.8
    tracheostomy V44.0
    ureterostomy V44.6
    urethrostomy V44.6
    urinary tract NEC V44.6

ICD-9-CM

◀

Vol. 2

Artificial (*Continued*)
vagina V44.7
vagina status V44.7
ARV (disease) (illness) (infection) - *see*
Human immunodeficiency virus
(disease) (illness) (infection)
Arytenoid - *see* condition
Asbestosis (occupational) 501
Asboe-Hansen's disease (incontinentia
pigmenti) 757.33
Ascariasis (intestinal) (lung) 127.0
Ascaridiasis 127.0
Ascaridosis 127.0
Ascaris 127.0
lumbricoides (infestation) 127.0
pneumonia 127.0
Ascending - *see* condition
Aschoff's bodies (*see also* Myocarditis,
rheumatic) 398.0
Ascites 789.5
abdominal NEC 789.5
cancerous (M8000/6) 197.6
cardiac 428.0
chylous (nonfilarial) 457.8
filarial (*see also* Infestation, filarial)
125.9
congenital 778.0
due to S. japonicum 120.2
fetal, causing fetopelvic disproportion
653.7
heart 428.0
joint (*see also* Effusion, joint) 719.0
malignant (M8000/6) 197.6
pseudochylous 789.5
syphilitic 095.2
tuberculous (*see also* Tuberculosis)
014.0
Ascorbic acid (vitamin C) deficiency
(scurvy) 267
**ASC-H (atypical squamous cells cannot
exclude high grade squamous intraepithelial lesion)** 795.02 ◀
**ASC-US (atypical squamous cells of un-
determined significance** 795.01 ◀◖◖◖
ASCVD (arteriosclerotic cardiovascular
disease) 429.2
Aseptic - *see* condition
Asherman's syndrome 621.5
Asialia 527.7
Asiatic cholera (*see also* Cholera) 001.9
Asocial personality or trends 301.7
Asomatognosia 781.8
Aspergillosis 117.3
with pneumonia 117.3 [484.6]
allergic bronchopulmonary 518.6
nonsyphilitic NEC 117.3
Aspergillus (flavus) (fumigatus) (infection) (terreus) 117.3
Aspermatogenesis 606.0
Aspermia (testis) 606.0
Asphyxia, asphyxiation (by) 799.0
antenatal - *see* Distress, fetal
bedclothes 994.7
birth (*see also* Asphyxia, newborn)
768.9
bunny bag 994.7
carbon monoxide 986
caul (*see also* Asphyxia, newborn) 768.9
cave-in 994.7
crushing - *see* Injury, internal, intrathoracic organs
constriction 994.7
crushing - *see* Injury, internal, intrathoracic organs

Asphyxia, asphyxiation (*Continued*)
drowning 994.1
fetal, affecting newborn 768.9
food or foreign body (in larynx)
933.1
bronchioles 934.8
bronchus (main) 934.1
lung 934.8
nasopharynx 933.0
nose, nasal passages 932
pharynx 933.0
respiratory tract 934.9
specified part NEC 934.8
throat 933.0
trachea 934.0
gas, fumes, or vapor NEC 987.9
specified - *see* Table of Drugs and
Chemicals
gravitational changes 994.7
hanging 994.7
inhalation - *see* Inhalation
intrauterine
fetal death (before onset of labor)
768.0
during labor 768.1
liveborn infant - *see* Distress, fetal,
liveborn infant
local 443.0
mechanical 994.7
during birth (*see also* Distress, fetal)
768.9
mucus 933.1
bronchus (main) 934.1
larynx 933.1
lung 934.8
nasal passages 932
newborn 770.1
pharynx 933.0
respiratory tract 934.9
specified part NEC 934.8
throat 933.0
trachea 934.0
vaginal (fetus or newborn) 770.1
newborn 768.9
with neurologic involvement 768.5
blue 768.6
livida 768.6
mild or moderate 768.6
pallida 768.5
severe 768.5
white 768.5
pathological 799.0
plastic bag 994.7
postnatal (*see also* Asphyxia, newborn)
768.9
mechanical 994.7
pressure 994.7
reticularis 782.61
strangulation 994.7
submersion 994.1
traumatic NEC - *see* Injury, internal,
intrathoracic organs
vomiting, vomitus - *see* Asphyxia, food
or foreign body
Aspiration
acid pulmonary (syndrome) 997.3
obstetric 668.0
amniotic fluid 770.1
bronchitis 507.0
contents of birth canal 770.1
fetal pneumonitis 770.1
food, foreign body, or gasoline (with
asphyxiation) - *see* Asphyxia, food
or foreign body

Aspiration (*Continued*)
meconium 770.1
mucus 933.1
into
bronchus (main) 934.1
lung 934.8
respiratory tract 934.9
specified part NEC 934.8
trachea 934.0
newborn 770.1
vaginal (fetus or newborn) 770.1
newborn 770.1
pneumonia 507.0
pneumonitis 507.0
fetus or newborn 770.1
obstetric 668.0
syndrome of newborn (massive) (meconium) 770.1
vernix caseosa 770.1
Asplenia 759.0
with mesocardia 746.87
Assam fever 085.0
Assimilation, pelvis
with disproportion 653.2
affecting fetus or newborn 763.1
causing obstructed labor 660.1
affecting fetus or newborn 763.1
Assmann's focus (*see also* Tuberculosis)
011.0
Astasia (-abasia) 307.9
hysterical 300.11
Asteatosis 706.8
cutis 706.8
Astereognosis 780.99
Asterixis 781.3
in liver disease 572.8
Asteroid hyalitis 379.22
Asthenia, asthenic 780.79
cardiac (*see also* Failure, heart) 428.9
psychogenic 306.2
cardiovascular (*see also* Failure, heart)
428.9
psychogenic 306.2
heart (*see also* Failure, heart) 428.9
psychogenic 306.2
hysterical 300.11
myocardial (*see also* Failure, heart)
428.9
psychogenic 306.2
nervous 300.5
neurocirculatory 306.2
neurotic 300.5
psychogenic 300.5
psychoneurotic 300.5
psychophysiologic 300.5
reaction, psychoneurotic 300.5
senile 797
Stiller's 780.79
tropical anhidrotic 705.1
Asthenopia 368.13
accommodative 367.4
hysterical (muscular) 300.11
psychogenic 306.7
Asthenospermia 792.2
Asthma, asthmatic (bronchial) (catarrh)
(spasmodic) 493.9

Note   The following fifth digit subclassification is for use with codes
493.0-493.2 493.9:

0	unspecified
1	with status asthmaticus
2	with (acute) exacerbation

Asthma, asthmatic *(Continued)*
with
chronic obstructive pulmonary disease (COPD) 493.2
hay fever 493.0
rhinitis, allergic 493.0
allergic 493.9
stated cause (external allergen) 493.0
atopic 493.0
cardiac *(see also* Failure, ventricular,
left) 428.1
cardiobronchial *(see also* Failure, ventricular, left) 428.1
cardiorenal *(see also* Hypertension, cardiorenal) 404.90
childhood 493.0
Colliers' 500
cough variant 493.82
croup 493.9
detergent 507.8
due to
detergent 507.8
inhalation of fumes 506.3
internal immunological process 493.0
endogenous (intrinsic) 493.1
eosinophilic 518.3
exercise induced bronchospasm
493.81
exogenous (cosmetics) (dander or dust)
(drugs) (dust) (feathers) (food)
(hay) (platinum) (pollen) 493.0
extrinsic 493.0
grinders' 502
hay 493.0
heart *(see also* Failure, ventricular, left)
428.1
IgE 493.0
infective 493.1
intrinsic 493.1
Kopp's 254.8
late-onset 493.1
meat-wrappers' 506.9
Millar's (laryngismus stridulus) 478.75
millstone makers' 502
miners' 500
Monday morning 504
New Orleans (epidemic) 493.0
platinum 493.0
pneumoconiotic (occupational) NEC
505
potters' 502
psychogenic 316 *[493.9]*
pulmonary eosinophilic 518.3
red cedar 495.8
Rostan's *(see also* Failure, ventricular,
left) 428.1
sandblasters' 502
sequoiosis 495.8
stonemasons' 502
thymic 254.8
tuberculous *(see also* Tuberculosis, pulmonary) 011.9
Wichmann's (laryngismus stridulus)
478.75
wood 495.8
Astigmatism (compound) (congenital)
367.20
irregular 367.22
regular 367.21
Astroblastoma (M9430/3)
nose 748.1
specified site - *see* Neoplasm, by site,
malignant
unspecified site 191.9

Astrocytoma (cystic) (M9400/3)
anaplastic type (M9401/3)
specified site - *see* Neoplasm, by site,
malignant
unspecified site 191.9
fibrillary (M9420/3)
specified site - *see* Neoplasm, by site,
malignant
unspecified site 191.9
fibrous (M9420/3)
specified site - *see* Neoplasm, by site,
malignant
unspecified site 191.9
gemistocytic (M9411/3)
specified site - *see* Neoplasm, by site,
malignant
unspecified site 191.9
juvenile (M9421/3)
specified site - *see* Neoplasm, by site,
malignant
unspecified site 191.9
nose 748.1
pilocytic (M9421/3)
specified site - *see* Neoplasm, by site,
malignant
unspecified site 191.9
piloid (M9421/3)
specified site - *see* Neoplasm, by site,
malignant
unspecified site 191.9
protoplasmic (M9410/3)
specified site - *see* Neoplasm, by site,
malignant
unspecified site 191.9
specified site - *see* Neoplasm, by site,
malignant
subependymal (M9383/1) 237.5
giant cell (M9384/1) 237.5
unspecified site 191.9
Astroglioma (M9400/3)
nose 748.1
specified site - *see* Neoplasm, by site,
malignant
unspecified site 191.9
Asymbolia 784.60
Asymmetrical breathing 786.09
Asymmetry - *see also* Distortion
chest 786.9
face 754.0
jaw NEC 524.12
maxillary 524.11
pelvis with disproportion 653.0
affecting fetus or newborn 763.1
causing obstructed labor 660.1
affecting fetus or newborn 763.1
Asynergia 781.3
Asynergy 781.3
ventricular 429.89
Asystole (heart) *(see also* Arrest, cardiac)
427.5
Ataxia, ataxy, ataxic 781.3
acute 781.3
brain 331.89
cerebellar 334.3
hereditary (Marie's) 334.2
in
alcoholism 303.9 *[334.4]*
myxedema *(see also* Myxedema)
244.9 *[334.4]*
neoplastic disease NEC 239.9 *[334.4]*
cerebral 331.89
family, familial 334.2
cerebral (Marie's) 334.2
spinal (Friedreich's) 334.0

Ataxia, ataxy, ataxic *(Continued)*
Friedreich's (heredofamilial) (spinal)
334.0
frontal lobe 781.3
gait 781.2
hysterical 300.11
general 781.3
hereditary NEC 334.2
cerebellar 334.2
spastic 334.1
spinal 334.0
heredofamilial (Marie's) 334.2
hysterical 300.11
locomotor (progressive) 094.0
diabetic 250.6 *[337.1]*
Marie's (cerebellar) (heredofamilial)
334.2
nonorganic origin 307.9
partial 094.0
postchickenpox 052.7
progressive locomotor 094.0
psychogenic 307.9
Sanger-Brown's 334.2
spastic 094.0
hereditary 334.1
syphilitic 094.0
spinal
hereditary 334.0
progressive locomotor 094.0
telangiectasia 334.8
Ataxia-telangiectasia 334.8
Atelectasis (absorption collapse) (complete)
(compression) (massive) (partial)
(postinfective) (pressure collapse)
(pulmonary) (relaxation) 518.0
newborn (congenital) (partial) 770.5
primary 770.4
primary 770.4
tuberculous *(see also* Tuberculosis, pulmonary) 011.9
Ateleiosis, ateliosis 253.3
Atelia - *see* Distortion
Ateliosis 253.3
Atelocardia 746.9
Atelomyelia 742.59
Athelia 757.6
Atheroembolism
extremity
lower 445.02
upper 445.01
kidney 445.81
specified site NEC 445.89
Atheroma, atheromatous *(see also* Arteriosclerosis) 440.9
aorta, aortic 440.0
valve *(see also* Endocarditis, aortic)
424.1
artery - *see* Arteriosclerosis
basilar (artery) *(see also* Occlusion, artery, basilar) 433.0
carotid (artery) (common) (internal)
(see also Occlusion, artery, carotid)
433.1
cerebral (arteries) 437.0
coronary (artery) - *see* Arteriosclerosis,
coronary
degeneration - *see* Arteriosclerosis
heart, cardiac - *see* Arteriosclerosis,
coronary
mitral (valve) 424.0
myocardium, myocardial - *see* Arteriosclerosis, coronary
pulmonary valve (heart) *(see also* Endocarditis, pulmonary) 424.3

ICD-9-CM

Vol. 2

Atheroma, atheromatous (Continued)
  skin 706.2
  tricuspid (heart) (valve) 424.2
  valve, valvular - see Endocarditis
  vertebral (artery) (see also Occlusion,
    artery, vertebral) 433.2
Atheromatosis - see also Arteriosclerosis
  arterial, congenital 272.8
Atherosclerosis - see Arteriosclerosis
Athetosis (acquired) 781.0
  bilateral 333.7
  congenital (bilateral) 333.7
  double 333.7
  unilateral 781.0
Athlete's
  foot 110.4
  heart 429.3
Athletic team examination V70.3
Athrepsia 261
Athyrea (acquired) (see also Hypothyroidism) 244.9
  congenital 243
Athyreosis (congenital) 243
  acquired - see Hypothyroidism
Athyroidism (acquired) (see also Hypothyroidism) 244.9
  congenital 243
Atmospheric pyrexia 992.0
Atonia, atony, atonic
  abdominal wall 728.2
  bladder (sphincter) 596.4
    neurogenic NEC 596.54
      with cauda equina syndrome
        344.61
  capillary 448.9
  cecum 564.89
    psychogenic 306.4
  colon 564.89
    psychogenic 306.4
  congenital 779.89
  dyspepsia 536.3
    psychogenic 306.4
  intestine 564.89
    psychogenic 306.4
  stomach 536.3
    neurotic or psychogenic 306.4
    psychogenic 306.4
  uterus 666.1
    affecting fetus or newborn 763.7
  vesical 596.4
Atopy NEC V15.09
Atransferrinemia, congenital 273.8
Atresia, atretic (congenital) 759.89
  alimentary organ or tract NEC
    751.8
    lower 751.2
    upper 750.8
  ani, anus, anal (canal) 751.2
  aorta 747.22
    with hypoplasia of ascending aorta
      and defective development of
      left ventricle (with mitral valve
      atresia) 746.7
    arch 747.11
    ring 747.21
  aortic (orifice) (valve) 746.89
    arch 747.11
  aqueduct of Sylvius 742.3
    with spina bifida (see also Spina bi-
      fida) 741.0
  artery NEC (see also Atresia, blood ves-
    sel) 747.60
    cerebral 747.81

Atresia, atretic (Continued)
  artery NEC (Continued)
    coronary 746.85
    eye 743.58
    pulmonary 747.3
    umbilical 747.5
  auditory canal (external) 744.02
  bile, biliary duct (common) or passage
    751.61
    acquired (see also Obstruction, bili-
      ary) 576.2
  bladder (neck) 753.6
  blood vessel (peripheral) NEC
    747.60
    cerebral 747.81
    gastrointestinal 747.61
    lower limb 747.64
    pulmonary artery 747.3
    renal 747.62
    spinal 747.82
    upper limb 747.63
  bronchus 748.3
  canal, ear 744.02
  cardiac
    valve 746.89
      aortic 746.89
      mitral 746.89
      pulmonary 746.01
      tricuspid 746.1
  cecum 751.2
  cervix (acquired) 622.4
    congenital 752.49
    in pregnancy or childbirth 654.6
      affecting fetus or newborn
        763.89
      causing obstructed labor
        660.2
        affecting fetus or newborn
          763.1
  choana 748.0
  colon 751.2
  cystic duct 751.61
    acquired 575.8
      with obstruction (see also Obstruc-
        tion, gallbladder) 575.2
  digestive organs NEC 751.8
  duodenum 751.1
  ear canal 744.02
  ejaculatory duct 752.89
  epiglottis 748.3
  esophagus 750.3
  Eustachian tube 744.24
  fallopian tube (acquired) 628.2
    congenital 752.19
  follicular cyst 620.0
  foramen of
    Luschka 742.3
      with spina bifida (see also Spina
        bifida) 741.0
    Magendie 742.3
      with spina bifida (see also Spina
        bifida) 741.0
  gallbladder 751.69
  genital organ
    external
      female 752.49
      male NEC 752.89
        penis 752.69
    internal
      female 752.89
      male 752.89
  glottis 748.3
  gullet 750.3

Atresia, atretic (Continued)
  heart
    valve NEC 746.89
      aortic 746.89
      mitral 746.89
      pulmonary 746.01
      tricuspid 746.1
  hymen 752.42
    acquired 623.3
    postinfective 623.3
  ileum 751.1
  intestine (small) 751.1
    large 751.2
  iris, filtration angle (see also Buphthal-
    mia) 743.20
  jejunum 751.1
  kidney 753.3
  lacrimal, apparatus 743.65
    acquired - see Stenosis, lacrimal
  larynx 748.3
  ligament, broad 752.19
  lung 748.5
  meatus urinarius 753.6
  mitral valve 746.89
    with atresia or hypoplasia of aortic
      orifice or valve, with hypoplasia
      of ascending aorta and defective
      development of left ventricle
      746.7
  nares (anterior) (posterior)
    748.0
  nasolacrimal duct 743.65
  nasopharynx 748.8
  nose, nostril 748.0
    acquired 738.0
  organ or site NEC - see Anomaly, spec-
    ified type NEC
  osseous meatus (ear) 744.03
  oviduct (acquired) 628.2
    congenital 752.19
  parotid duct 750.23
    acquired 527.8
  pulmonary (artery) 747.3
    valve 746.01
    vein 747.49
  pulmonic 746.01
  pupil 743.46
  rectum 751.2
  salivary duct or gland 750.23
    acquired 527.8
  sublingual duct 750.23
    acquired 527.8
  submaxillary duct or gland
    750.23
    acquired 527.8
  trachea 748.3
  tricuspid valve 746.1
  ureter 753.29
  ureteropelvic junction 753.21
  ureterovesical orifice 753.22
  urethra (valvular) 753.6
  urinary tract NEC 753.29
  uterus 752.3
    acquired 621.8
  vagina (acquired) 623.2
    congenital 752.49
    postgonococcal (old) 098.2
    postinfectional 623.2
    senile 623.2
  vascular NEC (see also Atresia, blood
    vessel) 747.60
    cerebral 747.81
  vas deferens 752.89

◀ New   ◀▥ Revised

ICD-9-CM

Vol. 2

Atresia, atretic *(Continued)*
vein NEC (*see also* Atresia, blood vessel) 747.60
cardiac 746.89
great 747.49
portal 747.49
pulmonary 747.49
vena cava (inferior) (superior) 747.49
vesicourethral orifice 753.6
vulva 752.49
acquired 624.8
Atrichia, atrichosis 704.00
congenital (universal) 757.4
Atrioventricularis commune 745.69
Atrophia - *see also* Atrophy
alba 709.09
cutis 701.8
idiopathica progressiva 701.8
senilis 701.8
dermatological, diffuse (idiopathic) 701.8
flava hepatis (acuta) (subacuta) (*see also* Necrosis, liver) 570
gyrata of choroid and retina (central) 363.54
generalized 363.57
senilis 797
dermatological 701.8
unguium 703.8
congenita 757.5
Atrophoderma, atrophodermia 701.9
diffusum (idiopathic) 701.8
maculatum 701.3
et striatum 701.3
due to syphilis 095.8
syphilitic 091.3
neuriticum 701.8
pigmentosum 757.33
reticulatum symmetricum faciei 701.8
senile 701.8
symmetrical 701.8
vermiculata 701.8
Atrophy, atrophic
adrenal (autoimmune) (capsule) (cortex) (gland) 255.4
with hypofunction 255.4
alveolar process or ridge (edentulous) 525.20
mandible 525.20
minimal 525.21
moderate 525.22
severe 525.23
maxilla 525.20
minimal 525.24
moderate 525.25
severe 525.26
appendix 543.9
Aran-Duchenne muscular 335.21
arm 728.2
arteriosclerotic - *see* Arteriosclerosis
arthritis 714.0
spine 720.9
bile duct (any) 576.8
bladder 596.8
blanche (of Milian) 701.3
bone (senile) 733.99
due to
disuse 733.7
infection 733.99
tabes dorsalis (neurogenic) 094.0

Atrophy, atrophic *(Continued)*
bone *(Continued)*
posttraumatic 733.99
brain (cortex) (progressive) 331.9
with dementia 290.10
Alzheimer's 331.0
with dementia - *see* Alzheimer's, dementia
circumscribed (Pick's) 331.11
with dementia
with behavioral disturbance 331.11 [294.11]
without behavioral disturbance 331.11 [294.10]
congenital 742.4
hereditary 331.9
senile 331.2
breast 611.4
puerperal, postpartum 676.3
buccal cavity 528.9
cardiac (brown) (senile) (*see also* Degeneration, myocardial) 429.1
cartilage (infectional) (joint) 733.99
cast, plaster of Paris 728.2
cerebellar - *see* Atrophy, brain
cerebral - *see* Atrophy, brain
cervix (endometrium) (mucosa) (myometrium) (senile) (uteri) 622.8
menopausal 627.8
Charcôt-Marie-Tooth 356.1
choroid 363.40
diffuse secondary 363.42
hereditary (*see also* Dystrophy, choroid) 363.50
gyrate
central 363.54
diffuse 363.57
generalized 363.57
senile 363.41
ciliary body 364.57
colloid, degenerative 701.3
conjunctiva (senile) 372.89
corpus cavernosum 607.89
cortical (*see also* Atrophy, brain) 331.9
Cruveilhier's 335.21
cystic duct 576.8
dacryosialadenopathy 710.2
degenerative
colloid 701.3
senile 701.3
Déjérine-Thomas 333.0
diffuse idiopathic, dermatological 701.8
disuse
bone 733.7
muscle 728.2
pelvic muscles and anal sphincter 618.83
Duchenne-Aran 335.21
ear 388.9
edentulous alveolar ridge 525.20
mandible 525.20
minimal 525.21
moderate 525.22
severe 525.23
maxilla 525.20
minimal 525.24
moderate 525.25
severe 525.26
emphysema, lung 492.8

Atrophy, atrophic *(Continued)*
endometrium (senile) 621.8
cervix 622.8
enteric 569.89
epididymis 608.3
eyeball, cause unknown 360.41
eyelid (senile) 374.50
facial (skin) 701.9
facioscapulohumeral (Landouzy-Déjérine) 359.1
fallopian tube (senile), acquired 620.3
fatty, thymus (gland) 254.8
gallbladder 575.8
gastric 537.89
gastritis (chronic) 535.1
gastrointestinal 569.89
genital organ, male 608.89
glandular 289.3
globe (phthisis bulbi) 360.41
gum (*see also* Recession, gingival) 523.20
hair 704.2
heart (brown) (senile) (*see also* Degeneration, myocardial) 429.1
hemifacial 754.0
Romberg 349.89
hydronephrosis 591
infantile 261
paralysis, acute (*see also* Poliomyelitis, with paralysis) 045.1
intestine 569.89
iris (generalized) (postinfectional) (sector shaped) 364.59
essential 364.51
progressive 364.51
sphincter 364.54
kidney (senile) (*see also* Sclerosis, renal) 587
with hypertension (*see also* Hypertension, kidney) 403.90
congenital 753.0
hydronephrotic 591
infantile 753.0
lacrimal apparatus (primary) 375.13
secondary 375.14
Landouzy-Déjérine 359.1
laryngitis, infection 476.0
larynx 478.79
Leber's optic 377.16
lip 528.5
liver (acute) (subacute) (*see also* Necrosis, liver) 570
chronic (yellow) 571.8
yellow (congenital) 570
with
abortion - *see* Abortion, by type, with specified complication NEC
ectopic pregnancy (*see also* categories 633.0-633.9) 639.8
molar pregnancy (*see also* categories 630-632) 639.8
chronic 571.8
complicating pregnancy 646.7
following
abortion 639.8
ectopic or molar pregnancy 639.8
from injection, inoculation or transfusion (onset within 8

Atrophy, atrophic (Continued)
liver (Continued)
  yellow (Continued)
    months after administration) -
      see Hepatitis, viral
    healed 571.5
    obstetric 646.7
    postabortal 639.8
    postimmunization - see Hepatitis,
      viral
    posttransfusion - see Hepatitis,
      viral
    puerperal, postpartum 674.8
lung (senile) 518.89
  congenital 748.69
macular (dermatological) 701.3
  syphilitic, skin 091.3
    striated 095.8
muscle, muscular 728.2
  disuse 728.2
  Duchenne-Aran 335.21
  extremity (lower) (upper) 728.2
  familial spinal 335.11
  general 728.2
  idiopathic 728.2
  infantile spinal 335.0
  myelopathic (progressive) 335.10
  myotonic 359.2
  neuritic 356.1
  neuropathic (peroneal) (progressive)
    356.1
  peroneal 356.1
  primary (idiopathic) 728.2
  progressive (familial) (hereditary)
    (pure) 335.21
    adult (spinal) 335.19
    infantile (spinal) 335.0
    juvenile (spinal) 335.11
    spinal 335.10
      adult 335.19
      hereditary or familial 335.11
      infantile 335.0
  pseudohypertrophic 359.1
  spinal (progressive) 335.10
    adult 335.19
    Aran-Duchenne 335.21
    familial 335.11
    hereditary 335.11
    infantile 335.0
    juvenile 335.11
  syphilitic 095.6
myocardium (see also Degeneration,
  myocardial) 429.1
myometrium (senile) 621.8
  cervix 622.8
myotatic 728.2
myotonia 359.2
nail 703.8
  congenital 757.5
nasopharynx 472.2
nerve - see also Disorder, nerve
  abducens 378.54
  accessory 352.4
  acoustic or auditory 388.5
  cranial 352.9
    first (olfactory) 352.0
    second (optic) (see also Atrophy,
      optic nerve) 377.10
    third (oculomotor) (partial)
      378.51
      total 378.52
    fourth (trochlear) 378.53
    fifth (trigeminal) 350.8

Atrophy, atrophic (Continued)
nerve (Continued)
  cranial (Continued)
    sixth (abducens) 378.54
    seventh (facial) 351.8
    eighth (auditory) 388.5
    ninth (glossopharyngeal) 352.2
    tenth (pneumogastric) (vagus)
      352.3
    eleventh (accessory) 352.4
    twelfth (hypoglossal) 352.5
  facial 351.8
  glossopharyngeal 352.2
  hypoglossal 352.5
  oculomotor (partial) 378.51
    total 378.52
  olfactory 352.0
  peripheral 355.9
  pneumogastric 352.3
  trigeminal 350.8
  trochlear 378.53
  vagus (pneumogastric) 352.3
nervous system, congenital 742.8
neuritic (see also Disorder, nerve)
  355.9
neurogenic NEC 355.9
  bone
    tabetic 094.0
nutritional 261
old age 797
olivopontocerebellar 333.0
optic nerve (ascending) (descending)
  (infectional) (nonfamilial) (papillo-
  macular bundle) (postretinal) (secondary NEC) (simple) 377.10
  associated with retinal dystrophy
    377.13
  dominant hereditary 377.16
  glaucomatous 377.14
  hereditary (dominant) (Leber's)
    377.16
  Leber's (hereditary) 377.16
  partial 377.15
  postinflammatory 377.12
  primary 377.11
  syphilitic 094.84
    congenital 090.49
    tabes dorsalis 094.0
orbit 376.45
ovary (senile), acquired 620.3
oviduct (senile), acquired 620.3
palsy, diffuse 335.20
pancreas (duct) (senile) 577.8
papillary muscle 429.81
paralysis 355.9
parotid gland 527.0
patches skin 701.3
  senile 701.8
penis 607.89
pharyngitis 472.1
pharynx 478.29
pluriglandular 258.8
polyarthritis 714.0
prostate 602.2
pseudohypertrophic 359.1
renal (see also Sclerosis, renal) 587
reticulata 701.8
retina (see also Degeneration, retina)
  362.60
  hereditary (see also Dystrophy, ret-
    ina) 362.70
rhinitis 472.0
salivary duct or gland 527.0

Atrophy, atrophic (Continued)
scar NEC 709.2
sclerosis, lobar (of brain) 331.0
  with dementia
    with behavioral disturbance 331.0
      [294.11]
    without behavioral disturbance
      331.0 [294.10]
scrotum 608.89
seminal vesicle 608.89
senile 797
  degenerative, of skin 701.3
skin (patches) (senile) 701.8
spermatic cord 608.89
spinal (cord) 336.8
  acute 336.8
  muscular (chronic) 335.10
    adult 335.19
    familial 335.11
    juvenile 335.10
  paralysis 335.10
    acute (see also Poliomyelitis, with
      paralysis) 045.1
spine (column) 733.99
spleen (senile) 289.59
spots (skin) 701.3
  senile 701.8
stomach 537.89
striate and macular 701.3
  syphilitic 095.8
subcutaneous 701.9
  due to injection 999.9
sublingual gland 527.0
submaxillary gland 527.0
Sudeck's 733.7
suprarenal (autoimmune) (capsule)
  (gland) 255.4
  with hypofunction 255.4
tarso-orbital fascia, congenital
  743.66
testis 608.3
thenar, partial 354.0
throat 478.29
thymus (fat) 254.8
thyroid (gland) 246.8
  with
    cretinism 243
    myxedema 244.9
  congenital 243
tongue (senile) 529.8
  papillae 529.4
  smooth 529.4
trachea 519.1
tunica vaginalis 608.89
turbinate 733.99
tympanic membrane (nonflaccid)
  384.82
  flaccid 384.81
ulcer (see also Ulcer, skin) 707.9
upper respiratory tract 478.9
uterus, uterine (acquired) (senile)
  621.8
  cervix 622.8
  due to radiation (intended effect)
    621.8
vagina (senile) 627.3
vascular 459.89
vas deferens 608.89
vertebra (senile) 733.99
vulva (primary) (senile) 624.1
Werdnig-Hoffmann 335.0
yellow (acute) (congenital) (liver) (subacute) (see also Necrosis, liver) 570

◀ **New**   ◀⃛ **Revised**

Atrophy, atrophic (Continued)
  yellow (Continued)
    chronic 571.8
    resulting from administration of blood, plasma, serum, or other biological substance (within 8 months of administration) - see Hepatitis, viral

Attack
  akinetic (see also Epilepsy) 345.0
  angina - see Angina
  apoplectic (see also Disease, cerebrovascular, acute) 436
  benign shuddering 333.93
  bilious - see Vomiting
  cataleptic 300.11
  cerebral (see also Disease, cerebrovascular, acute) 436
  coronary (see also Infarct, myocardium) 410.9
  cyanotic, newborn 770.83
  epileptic (see also Epilepsy) 345.9
  epileptiform 780.39
  heart (see also Infarct, myocardium) 410.9
  hemiplegia (see also Disease, cerebrovascular, acute) 436
  hysterical 300.11
  jacksonian (see also Epilepsy) 345.5
  myocardium, myocardial (see also Infarct, myocardium) 410.9
  myoclonic (see also Epilepsy) 345.1
  panic 300.01
  paralysis (see also Disease, cerebrovascular, acute) 436
  paroxysmal 780.39
  psychomotor (see also Epilepsy) 345.4
  salaam (see also Epilepsy) 345.6
  schizophreniform (see also Schizophrenia) 295.4
  sensory and motor 780.39
  syncope 780.2
  toxic, cerebral 780.39
  transient ischemic (TIA) 435.9
  unconsciousness 780.2
    hysterical 300.11
  vasomotor 780.2
  vasovagal (idiopathic) (paroxysmal) 780.2

Attention to
  artificial
    opening (of) V55.9
      digestive tract NEC V55.4
      specified site NEC V55.8
      urinary tract NEC V55.6
      vagina V55.7
  colostomy V55.3
  cystostomy V55.5
  gastrostomy V55.1
  ileostomy V55.2
  jejunostomy V55.4
  nephrostomy V55.6
  surgical dressings V58.3
  sutures V58.3
  tracheostomy V55.0
  ureterostomy V55.6
  urethrostomy V55.6

Attrition
  gum (see also Recession, gingival) 523.20 ◄‖

Attrition (Continued)
  teeth (hard tissues) 521.10 ◄‖
    excessive 521.10 ◄
      extending into
        dentine 521.12 ◄
        pulp 521.13 ◄
      generalized 521.15 ◄
      limited to enamel 521.11 ◄
      localized 521.14 ◄

Atypical - see also condition
  cells
    endocervical 795.00 ◄
    endometrial 795.00 ◄
    glandular 795.00 ◄
  distribution, vessel (congenital) (peripheral) NEC 747.60
  endometrium 621.9
  kidney 593.89

Atypism, cervix 622.10 ◄‖

Audible tinnitus (see also Tinnitus) 388.30

Auditory - see condition

Audry's syndrome (acropachyderma) 757.39

Aujeszky's disease 078.89

Aura, jacksonian (see also Epilepsy) 345.5

Aurantiasis, cutis 278.3

Auricle, auricular - see condition

Auriculotemporal syndrome 350.8

Australian
  Q fever 083.0
  X disease 062.4

Autism, autistic (child) (infantile) 299.0

Autodigestion 799.89

Autoerythrocyte sensitization 287.2

Autographism 708.3

Autoimmune
  cold sensitivity 283.0
  disease NEC 279.4
  hemolytic anemia 283.0
  thyroiditis 245.2

Autoinfection, septic - see Septicemia

Autointoxication 799.89

Automatism 348.8
  epileptic (see also Epilepsy) 345.4
  paroxysmal, idiopathic (see also Epilepsy) 345.4

Autonomic, autonomous
  bladder 596.54
    neurogenic 596.54
      with cauda equina 344.61
  dysreflexia 337.3
  faciocephalalgia (see also Neuropathy, peripheral, autonomic) 337.9
  hysterical seizure 300.11
  imbalance (see also Neuropathy, peripheral, autonomic 337.9

Autophony 388.40

Autosensitivity, erythrocyte 287.2

Autotopagnosia 780.99

Autotoxemia 799.89

Autumn - see condition

Avellis' syndrome 344.89

Aviators'
  disease or sickness (see also Effect, adverse, high altitude) 993.2
  ear 993.0
  effort syndrome 306.2

Avitaminosis (multiple NEC) (see also Deficiency, vitamin) 269.2
  A 264.9
  B 266.9
    with
      beriberi 265.0
      pellagra 265.2
  B_1 265.1
  B_2 266.0
  B_6 266.1
  B_{12} 266.2
  C (with scurvy) 267
  D 268.9
    with
      osteomalacia 268.2
      rickets 268.0
  E 269.1
  G 266.0
  H 269.1
  K 269.0
  multiple 269.2
  nicotinic acid 265.2
  P 269.1

Avulsion (traumatic) 879.8
  blood vessel - see Injury, blood vessel, by site
  cartilage - see also Dislocation, by site
    knee, current (see also Tear, meniscus) 836.2
    symphyseal (inner), complicating delivery 665.6
  complicated 879.9
  diaphragm - see Injury, internal, diaphragm
  ear - see Wound, open, ear
  epiphysis of bone - see Fracture, by site
  external site other than limb - see Wound, open, by site
  eye 871.3
  fingernail - see Wound, open, finger
  fracture - see Fracture, by site
  genital organs, external - see Wound, open, genital organs
  head (intracranial) NEC - see also Injury, intracranial, with open intracranial wound
    complete 874.9
    external site NEC 873.8
      complicated 873.9
  internal organ or site - see Injury, internal, by site
  joint - see also Dislocation, by site
    capsule - see Sprain, by site
  ligament - see Sprain, by site
  limb - see also Amputation, traumatic, by site
    skin and subcutaneous tissue - see Wound, open, by site
  muscle - see Sprain, by site
  nerve (root) - see Injury, nerve, by site
  scalp - see Wound, open, scalp
  skin and subcutaneous tissue - see Wound, open, by site
  symphyseal cartilage (inner), complicating delivery 665.6
  tendon - see also Sprain, by site
    with open wound - see Wound, open, by site
  toenail - see Wound, open, toe(s)
  tooth 873.63
    complicated 873.73

◄ **New**   ◄‖ **Revised**

Awaiting organ transplant status
 V49.83 ◀
Awareness of heart beat 785.1
Axe grinders' disease 502
Axenfeld's anomaly or syndrome 743.44
Axilla, axillary - *see also* condition
 breast 757.6

Axonotmesis - *see* Injury, nerve, by site
Ayala's disease 756.89
Ayerza's disease or syndrome (pulmo-
nary artery sclerosis with pulmonary
hypertension) 416.0
Azoospermia 606.0

Azorean disease (of the nervous system)
 334.8
Azotemia 790.6
 meaning uremia (*see also* Uremia) 586
Aztec ear 744.29
Azygos lobe, lung (fissure) 748.69

B

Baader's syndrome (erythema multiforme exucatiuum) 695.1
Baastrup's syndrome 721.5
Babesiasis 088.82
Babesiosis 088.82
Babington's disease (familial hemorrhagic telangiectasia) 448.0
Babinski's syndrome (cardiovascular syphilis) 093.89
Babinski-Fröhlich syndrome (adiposogenital dystrophy) 253.8
Babinski-Nageotte syndrome 344.89
Bacillary - *see* condition
Bacilluria 791.9
  asymptomatic, in pregnancy or puerperium 646.5
  tuberculous (*see also* Tuberculosis) 016.9
Bacillus - *see also* Infection, bacillus
  abortus infection 023.1
  anthracis infection 022.9
  coli
    infection 041.4
      generalized 038.42
      intestinal 008.00
      pyemia 038.42
      septicemia 038.42
  Flexner's 004.1
  fusiformis infestation 101
  mallei infection 024
  Shiga's 004.0
  suipestifer infection (*see also* Infection, Salmonella) 003.9
Back - *see* condition
Backache (postural) 724.5
  psychogenic 307.89
  sacroiliac 724.6
Backflow (pyelovenous) (*see also* Disease, renal) 593.9
Backknee (*see also* Genu, recurvatum) 736.5
Bacteremia 790.7
Bacteria
  in blood (*see also* Bacteremia) 790.7
  in urine (*see also* Bacteriuria) 791.9
Bacterial - *see* condition
Bactericholia (*see also* Cholecystitis, acute) 575.0
Bacterid, bacteride (Andrews' pustular) 686.8
Bacteriuria, bacteruria 791.9
  with
    urinary tract infection 599.0
  asymptomatic 791.9
    in pregnancy or puerperium 646.5
      affecting fetus or newborn 760.1
Bad
  breath 784.9
  heart - *see* Disease, heart
  trip (*see also* Abuse, drugs, nondependent) 305.3
Baehr-Schiffrin disease (thrombotic thrombocytopenic purpura) 446.6
Baelz's disease (cheilitis glandularis apostematosa) 528.5
Baerensprung's disease (eczema marginatum) 110.3
Bagassosis (occupational) 495.1
Baghdad boil 085.1

Bagratuni's syndrome (temporal arteritis) 446.5
Baker's
  cyst (knee) 727.51
    tuberculous (*see also* Tuberculosis) 015.2
  itch 692.89
Bakwin-Krida syndrome (craniometaphyseal dysplasia) 756.89
Balanitis (circinata) (gangraenosa) (infectious) (vulgaris) 607.1
  amebic 006.8
  candidal 112.2
  chlamydial 099.53
  due to Ducrey's bacillus 099.0
  erosiva circinata et gangraenosa 607.1
  gangrenous 607.1
  gonococcal (acute) 098.0
    chronic or duration of 2 months or over 098.2
  nongonococcal 607.1
  phagedenic 607.1
  venereal NEC 099.8
  xerotica obliterans 607.81
Balanoposthitis 607.1
  chlamydial 099.53
  gonococcal (acute) 098.0
    chronic or duration of 2 months or over 098.2
  ulcerative NEC 099.8
Balanorrhagia - *see* Balanitis
Balantidiasis 007.0
Balantidiosis 007.0
Balbuties, balbutio 307.0
Bald
  patches on scalp 704.00
  tongue 529.4
Baldness (*see also* Alopecia) 704.00
Balfour's disease (chloroma) 205.3
Balint's syndrome (psychic paralysis of visual fixation) 368.16
Balkan grippe 083.0
Ball
  food 938
  hair 938
Ballantyne (-Runge) syndrome (postmaturity) 766.22
Balloon disease (*see also* Effect, adverse, high altitude) 993.2
Ballooning posterior leaflet syndrome 424.0
Baló's disease or concentric sclerosis 341.1
Bamberger's disease (hypertrophic pulmonary osteoarthropathy) 731.2
Bamberger-Marie disease (hypertrophic pulmonary osteoarthropathy) 731.2
Bamboo spine 720.0
Bancroft's filariasis 125.0
Band(s)
  adhesive (*see also* Adhesions, peritoneum) 568.0
  amniotic 658.8
    affecting fetus or newborn 762.8
  anomalous or congenital - *see also* Anomaly, specified type NEC
    atrial 746.9
    heart 746.9
    intestine 751.4
    omentum 751.4
    ventricular 746.9

Band(s) *(Continued)*
  cervix 622.3
  gallbladder (congenital) 751.69
  intestinal (adhesive) (*see also* Adhesions, peritoneum) 568.0
    congenital 751.4
    obstructive (*see also* Obstruction, intestine) 560.81
  periappendiceal (congenital) 751.4
  peritoneal (adhesive) (*see also* Adhesions, peritoneum) 568.0
    with intestinal obstruction 560.81
    congenital 751.4
  uterus 621.5
  vagina 623.2
Bandl's ring (contraction)
  complicating delivery 661.4
    affecting fetus or newborn 763.7
Bang's disease (Brucella abortus) 023.1
Bangkok hemorrhagic fever 065.4
Bannister's disease 995.1
Bantam-Albright-Martin disease (pseudohypoparathyroidism) 275.49
Banti's disease or syndrome (with cirrhosis) (with portal hypertension) - *see* Cirrhosis, liver
Bar
  calcaneocuboid 755.67
  calcaneonavicular 755.67
  cubonavicular 755.67
  prostate 600.90
    with urinary retention 600.91
  talocalcaneal 755.67
Baragnosis 780.99
Barasheh, barashek 266.2
Barcoo disease or rot (*see also* Ulcer, skin) 707.9
Bard-Pic syndrome (carcinoma, head of pancreas) 157.0
Bärensprung's disease (eczema marginatum) 110.3
Baritosis 503
Barium lung disease 503
Barlow's syndrome (meaning mitral valve prolapse) 424.0
Barlow (-Möller) disease or syndrome (meaning infantile scurvy) 267
Barodontalgia 993.2
Baron Münchausen syndrome 301.51
Barosinusitis 993.1
Barotitis 993.0
Barotrauma 993.2
  odontalgia 993.2
  otitic 993.0
  sinus 993.1
Barraquer's disease or syndrome (progressive lipodystrophy) 272.6
Barré-Guillain syndrome 357.0
Barré-Liéou syndrome (posterior cervical sympathetic) 723.2
Barrel chest 738.3
Barrett's esophagus 530.85 ◀
Barrett's syndrome or ulcer (chronic peptic ulcer of esophagus) 530.85
Bársony-Polgár syndrome (corkscrew esophagus) 530.5
Bársony-Teschendorf syndrome (corkscrew esophagus) 530.5
Bartholin's
  adenitis (*see also* Bartholinitis) 616.8
  gland - *see* condition

ICD-9-CM

B

Vol. 2

Bartholinitis (suppurating) 616.8
    gonococcal (acute) 098.0
        chronic or duration of 2 months or over 098.2
Bartonellosis 088.0
Bartter's syndrome (secondary hyperaldosteronism with juxtaglomerular hyperplasia) 255.13
Basal - *see* condition
Basan's (hidrotic) ectodermal dysplasia 757.31
Baseball finger 842.13
Basedow's disease or syndrome (exophthalmic goiter) 242.0
Basic - *see* condition
Basilar - *see* condition
Bason's (hidrotic) ectodermal dysplasia 757.31
Basopenia 288.0
Basophilia 288.8
Basophilism (corticoadrenal) (Cushing's) (pituitary) (thymic) 255.0
Bassen-Kornzweig syndrome (abetalipoproteinemia) 272.5
Bat ear 744.29
Bateman's
    disease 078.0
    purpura (senile) 287.2
Bathing cramp 994.1
Bathophobia 300.23
Batten's disease, retina 330.1 *[362.71]*
Batten-Mayou disease 330.1 *[362.71]*
Batten-Steinert syndrome 359.2
Battered
    adult (syndrome) 995.81
    baby or child (syndrome) 995.54
    spouse (syndrome) 995.81
Battey mycobacterium infection 031.0
Battledore placenta - *see* Placenta, abnormal
Battle exhaustion (*see also* Reaction, stress, acute) 308.9
Baumgarten-Cruveilhier (cirrhosis) disease, or syndrome 571.5
Bauxite
    fibrosis (of lung) 503
    workers' disease 503
Bayle's disease (dementia paralytica) 094.1
Bazin's disease (primary) (*see also* Tuberculosis) 017.1
Beach ear 380.12
Beaded hair (congenital) 757.4
Beals syndrome 759.82 ◄
Beard's disease (neurasthenia) 300.5
Bearn-Kunkel (-Slater) syndrome (lupoid hepatitis) 571.49
Beat
    elbow 727.2
    hand 727.2
    knee 727.2
Beats
    ectopic 427.60
    escaped, heart 427.60
        postoperative 997.1
    premature (nodal) 427.60
        atrial 427.61
        auricular 427.61
        postoperative 997.1
        specified type NEC 427.69
        supraventricular 427.61
        ventricular 427.69
Beau's
    disease or syndrome (*see also* Degeneration, myocardial) 429.1

Beau's (*Continued*)
    lines (transverse furrows on fingernails) 703.8
Bechterew's disease (ankylosing spondylitis) 720.0
Bechterew-Strümpell-Marie syndrome (ankylosing spondylitis) 720.0
Beck's syndrome (anterior spinal artery occlusion) 433.8
Becker's
    disease (idiopathic mural endomyocardial disease) 425.2
    dystrophy 359.1
Beckwith (-Wiedemann) syndrome 759.89
Bedclothes, asphyxiation or suffocation by 994.7
Bednar's aphthae 528.2
Bedsore 707.00 ◄▥
    with gangrene 707.00 *[785.4]* ◄▥
Bedwetting (*see also* Enuresis) 788.36
Beer-drinkers' heart (disease) 425.5
Bee sting (with allergic or anaphylactic shock) 989.5
Begbie's disease (exophthalmic goiter) 242.0
Behavior disorder, disturbance - *see also* Disturbance, conduct
    antisocial, without manifest psychiatric disorder
        adolescent V71.02
        adult V71.01
        child V71.02
    dyssocial, without manifest psychiatric disorder
        adolescent V71.02
        adult V71.01
        child V71.02
    high-risk- see problem
Behçet's syndrome 136.1
Behr's disease 362.50
Beigel's disease or morbus (white piedra) 111.2
Bejel 104.0
Bekhterev's (Bechterew's) **disease** (ankylosing spondylitis) 720.0
Bekhterev-Strümpell-Marie syndrome (ankylosing spondylitis) 720.0
Belching (*see also* Eructation) 787.3
Bell's
    disease (*see also* Psychosis, affective) 296.0
    mania (*see also* Psychosis, affective) 296.0
    palsy, paralysis 351.0
        infant 767.5
        newborn 767.5
        syphilitic 094.89
    spasm 351.0
Bence-Jones albuminuria, albuminosuria, or proteinuria 791.0
Bends 993.3
Benedikt's syndrome (paralysis) 344.89
Benign - *see also* condition
    cellular changes, cervix 795.09
    prostate
        hyperplasia 600.20 ◄▥
            with urinary retention 600.21 ◄▥
        neoplasm 222.2
Bennett's
    disease (leukemia) 208.9
    fracture (closed) 815.01
        open 815.11

Benson's disease 379.22
Bent
    back (hysterical) 300.11
    nose 738.0
        congenital 754.0
Bereavement V62.82
    as adjustment reaction 309.0
Berger's paresthesia (lower limb) 782.0
Bergeron's disease (hysteroepilepsy) 300.11
Beriberi (acute) (atrophic) (chronic) (dry) (subacute) (wet) 265.0
    with polyneuropathy 265.0 *[357.4]*
    heart (disease) 265.0 *[425.7]*
    leprosy 030.1
    neuritis 265.0 *[357.4]*
Berlin's disease or edema (traumatic) 921.3
Berloque dermatitis 692.72
Bernard-Horner syndrome (*see also* Neuropathy, peripheral, autonomic) 337.9
Bernard-Sergent syndrome (acute adrenocortical insufficiency) 255.4
Bernard-Soulier disease or thrombopathy 287.1
Bernhardt's disease or paresthesia 355.1
Bernhardt-Roth disease or syndrome (paresthesia) 355.1
Bernheim's syndrome (*see also* Failure, heart) 428.0
Bertielliasis 123.8
Bertolotti's syndrome (sacralization of fifth lumbar vertebra) 756.15
Berylliosis (acute) (chronic) (lung) (occupational) 503
Besnier's
    lupus pernio 135
    prurigo (atopic dermatitis) (infantile eczema) 691.8
Besnier-Boeck disease or sarcoid 135
Besnier-Boeck-Schaumann disease (sarcoidosis) 135
Best's disease 362.76
Bestiality 302.1
Beta-adrenergic hyperdynamic circulatory state 429.82
Beta-aminoisobutyric aciduria 277.2
Beta-mercaptolactate-cysteine disulfiduria 270.0
Beta thalassemia (major) (minor) (mixed) 282.49
Beurmann's disease (sporotrichosis) 117.1
Bezoar 938
    intestine 936
    stomach 935.2
Bezold's abscess (*see also* Mastoiditis) 383.01
Bianchi's syndrome (aphasia-apraxia-alexia) 784.69
Bicornuate or bicornis uterus 752.3
    in pregnancy or childbirth 654.0
        with obstructed labor 660.2
            affecting fetus or newborn 763.1
        affecting fetus or newborn 763.89
Bicuspid aortic valve 746.4
Biedl-Bardet syndrome 759.89
Bielschowsky's disease 330.1
Bielschowsky-Jansky
    amaurotic familial idiocy 330.1
    disease 330.1

Biemond's syndrome (obesity, polydactyly, and mental retardation) 759.89
Biermer's anemia or disease (pernicious anemia) 281.0
Biett's disease 695.4
Bifid (congenital) - *see also* Imperfect, closure
  apex, heart 746.89
  clitoris 752.49
  epiglottis 748.3
  kidney 753.3
  nose 748.1
  patella 755.64
  scrotum 752.89
  toe 755.66
  tongue 750.13
  ureter 753.4
  uterus 752.3
  uvula 749.02
    with cleft lip (*see also* Cleft, palate, with cleft lip) 749.20
Biforis uterus (suprasimplex) 752.3
Bifurcation (congenital) - *see also* Imperfect, closure
  gallbladder 751.69
  kidney pelvis 753.3
  renal pelvis 753.3
  rib 756.3
  tongue 750.13
  trachea 748.3
  ureter 753.4
  urethra 753.8
  uvula 749.02
    with cleft lip (*see also* Cleft, palate, with cleft lip) 749.20
  vertebra 756.19
Bigeminal pulse 427.89
Bigeminy 427.89
Big spleen syndrome 289.4
Bilateral - *see* condition
Bile duct - *see* condition
Bile pigments in urine 791.4
Bilharziasis (*see also* Schistosomiasis) 120.9
  chyluria 120.0
  cutaneous 120.3
  galacturia 120.0
  hematochyluria 120.0
  intestinal 120.1
  lipemia 120.9
  lipuria 120.0
  Oriental 120.2
  piarhemia 120.9
  pulmonary 120.2
  tropical hematuria 120.0
  vesical 120.0
Biliary - *see* condition
Bilious (attack) - *see also* Vomiting
  fever, hemoglobinuric 084.8
Bilirubinuria 791.4
Biliuria 791.4
Billroth's disease
  meningocele (*see also* Spina bifida) 741.9
Bilobate placenta - *see* Placenta, abnormal
Bilocular
  heart 745.7
  stomach 536.8
Bing-Horton syndrome (histamine cephalgia) 346.2
Binswanger's disease or dementia 290.12

Biörck (-Thorson) syndrome (malignant carcinoid) 259.2
Biparta, bipartite - *see also* Imperfect, closure
  carpal scaphoid 755.59
  patella 755.64
  placenta - *see* Placenta, abnormal
  vagina 752.49
Bird
  face 756.0
  fanciers' lung or disease 495.2
Bird's disease (oxaluria) 271.8
Birth
  abnormal fetus or newborn 763.9
  accident, fetus or newborn - *see* Birth, injury
  complications in mother - *see* Delivery, complicated
  compression during NEC 767.9
  defect - *see* Anomaly
  delayed, fetus 763.9
  difficult NEC, affecting fetus or newborn 763.9
  dry, affecting fetus or newborn 761.1
  forced, NEC, affecting fetus or newborn 763.89
  forceps, affecting fetus or newborn 763.2
  hematoma of sternomastoid 767.8
  immature 765.1
    extremely 765.0
  inattention, after or at 995.52
  induced, affecting fetus or newborn 763.89
  infant - *see* Newborn
  injury NEC 767.9
    adrenal gland 767.8
    basal ganglia 767.0
    brachial plexus (paralysis) 767.6
    brain (compression) (pressure) 767.0
    cerebellum 767.0
    cerebral hemorrhage 767.0
    conjunctiva 767.8
    eye 767.8
    fracture
      bone, any except clavicle or spine 767.3
      clavicle 767.2
      femur 767.3
      humerus 767.3
      long bone 767.3
      radius and ulna 767.3
      skeleton NEC 767.3
      skull 767.3
      spine 767.4
      tibia and fibula 767.3
    hematoma 767.8
      liver (subcapsular) 767.8
      mastoid 767.8
      skull 767.19
      sternomastoid 767.8
      testes 767.8
      vulva 767.8
    intracranial (edema) 767.0
    laceration
      brain 767.0
      by scalpel 767.8
      peripheral nerve 767.7
    liver 767.8
    meninges
      brain 767.0
      spinal cord 767.4

Birth (*Continued*)
  injury NEC (*Continued*)
    nerves (cranial, peripheral) 767.7
      brachial plexus 767.6
      facial 767.5
    paralysis 767.7
      brachial plexus 767.6
      Erb (-Duchenne) 767.6
      facial nerve 767.5
      Klumpke (-Déjérine) 767.6
      radial nerve 767.6
      spinal (cord) (hemorrhage) (laceration) (rupture) 767.4
    rupture
      intracranial 767.0
      liver 767.8
      spinal cord 767.4
      spleen 767.8
      viscera 767.8
    scalp 767.19
    scalpel wound 767.8
    skeleton NEC 767.3
    specified NEC 767.8
    spinal cord 767.4
    spleen 767.8
    subdural hemorrhage 767.0
    tentorial, tear 767.0
    testes 767.8
    vulva 767.8
  instrumental, NEC, affecting fetus or newborn 763.2
  lack of care, after or at 995.52
  multiple
    affected by maternal complications of pregnancy 761.5
    healthy liveborn - *see* Newborn, multiple
  neglect, after or at 995.52
  newborn - *see* Newborn
  palsy or paralysis NEC 767.7
  precipitate, fetus or newborn 763.6
  premature (infant) 765.1
  prolonged, affecting fetus or newborn 763.9
  retarded, fetus or newborn 763.9
  shock, newborn 779.89
  strangulation or suffocation
    due to aspiration of amniotic fluid 770.1
    mechanical 767.8
  trauma NEC 767.9
  triplet
    affected by maternal complications of pregnancy 761.5
    healthy liveborn - *see* Newborn, multiple
  twin
    affected by maternal complications of pregnancy 761.5
    healthy liveborn - *see* Newborn, twin
  ventouse, affecting fetus or newborn 763.3
Birthmark 757.32
Bisalbuminemia 273.8
Biskra button 085.1
Bite(s)
  with intact skin surface - *see* Contusion
  animal - *see* Wound, open, by site
    intact skin surface - *see* Contusion
  centipede 989.5
  chigger 133.8
  fire ant 989.5

ICD-9-CM

B

Vol. 2

Bite(s) (*Continued*)
flea - *see* Injury, superficial, by site
human (open wound) - *see also*
    Wound, open, by site
    intact skin surface - *see* Contusion
insect
    nonvenomous - *see* Injury, superfi-
        cial, by site
    venomous 989.5
mad dog (death from) 071
poisonous 989.5
red bug 133.8
reptile 989.5
    nonvenomous - *see* Wound, open, by
        site
snake 989.5
    nonvenomous - *see* Wound, open, by
        site
spider (venomous) 989.5
    nonvenomous - *see* Injury, superfi-
        cial, by site
venomous 989.5
Biting
cheek or lip 528.9
nail 307.9
Black
death 020.9
eye NEC 921.0
hairy tongue 529.3
lung disease 500
Blackfan-Diamond anemia or syndrome
    (congenital hypoplastic anemia)
    284.0
Blackhead 706.1
Blackout 780.2
Blackwater fever 084.8
Bladder - *see* condition
Blast
blindness 921.3
concussion - *see* Blast, injury
injury 869.0
    with open wound into cavity
        869.1
    abdomen or thorax - *see* Injury, in-
        ternal, by site
    brain (*see also* Concussion, brain)
        850.9
        with skull fracture - *see* Fracture,
            skull
    ear (acoustic nerve trauma) 951.5
        with perforation, tympanic mem-
            brane - *see* Wound, open, ear,
            drum
    lung (*see also* Injury, internal, lung)
        861.20
    otitic (explosive) 388.11
Blastomycosis, blastomycotic (chronic)
    (cutaneous) (disseminated) (lung)
    (pulmonary) (systemic) 116.0
Brazilian 116.1
European 117.5
keloidal 116.2
North American 116.0
primary pulmonary 116.0
South American 116.1
Bleb(s) 709.8
emphysematous (bullous) (diffuse)
    (lung) (ruptured) (solitary)
    492.0
filtering, eye (postglaucoma) (status)
    V45.69
    with complication 997.99
    postcataract extraction (complica-
        tion) 997.99

Bleb(s) (*Continued*)
lung (ruptured) 492.0
    congenital 770.5
subpleural (emphysematous) 492.0
Bleeder (familial) (hereditary) (*see also*
    Defect, coagulation) 286.9
nonfamilial 286.9
Bleeding (*see also* Hemorrhage) 459.0
anal 569.3
anovulatory 628.0
atonic, following delivery 666.1
capillary 448.9
due to subinvolution 621.1
    puerperal 666.2
ear 388.69
excessive, associated with menopausal
    onset 627.0
familial (*see also* Defect, coagulation)
    286.9
following intercourse 626.7
gastrointestinal 578.9
gums 523.8
hemorrhoids - *see* Hemorrhoids, bleed-
    ing
intermenstrual
    irregular 626.6
    regular 626.5
intraoperative 998.11
irregular NEC 626.4
menopausal 627.0
mouth 528.9
nipple 611.79
nose 784.7
ovulation 626.5
postclimacteric 627.1
postcoital 626.7
postmenopausal 627.1
    following induced menopause 627.4
postoperative 998.11
preclimacteric 627.0
puberty 626.3
    excessive, with onset of menstrual
        periods 626.3
rectum, rectal 569.3
tendencies (*see also* Defect, coagulation)
    286.9
throat 784.8
umbilical stump 772.3
umbilicus 789.9
unrelated to menstrual cycle 626.6
uterus, uterine 626.9
    climacteric 627.0
    dysfunctional 626.8
    functional 626.8
    unrelated to menstrual cycle 626.6
vagina, vaginal 623.8
    functional 626.8
vicarious 625.8
Blennorrhagia, blennorrhagic - *see* Blen-
    norrhea
Blennorrhea (acute) 098.0
adultorum 098.40
alveolaris 523.4
chronic or duration of 2 months or
    over 098.2
gonococcal (neonatorum) 098.40
inclusion (neonatal) (newborn) 771.6
neonatorum 098.40
Blepharelosis (*see also* Entropion)
    374.00
Blepharitis (eyelid) 373.00
angularis 373.01
ciliaris 373.00
    with ulcer 373.01

Blepharitis (*Continued*)
marginal 373.00
    with ulcer 373.01
scrofulous (*see also* Tuberculosis)
    017.3 [373.00]
squamous 373.02
ulcerative 373.01
Blepharochalasis 374.34
congenital 743.62
Blepharoclonus 333.81
Blepharoconjunctivitis (*see also* Conjunc-
    tivitis) 372.20
angular 372.21
contact 372.22
Blepharophimosis (eyelid) 374.46
congenital 743.62
Blepharoplegia 374.89
Blepharoptosis 374.30
congenital 743.61
Blepharopyorrhea 098.49
Blepharospasm 333.81
Blessig's cyst 362.62
Blighted ovum 631
Blind
bronchus (congenital) 748.3
eye - *see also* Blindness
    hypertensive 360.42
    hypotensive 360.41
loop syndrome (postoperative) 579.2
sac, fallopian tube (congenital)
    752.19
spot, enlarged 368.42
tract or tube (congenital) NEC - *see*
    Atresia
Blindness (acquired) (congenital) (both
    eyes) 369.00
blast 921.3
    with nerve injury - *see* Injury, nerve,
        optic
Bright's - *see* Uremia
color (congenital) 368.59
    acquired 368.55
    blue 368.53
    green 368.52
    red 368.51
    total 368.54
concussion 950.9
cortical 377.75
day 368.10
    acquired 368.10
    congenital 368.10
    hereditary 368.10
    specified type NEC 368.10
due to
    injury NEC 950.9
    refractive error - *see* Error, refractive
eclipse (total) 363.31
emotional 300.11
hysterical 300.11
legal (both eyes) (USA definition)
    369.4
    with impairment of better (less im-
        paired) eye
    near-total 369.02
        with
            lesser eye impairment 369.02
                near-total 369.04
                total 369.03
    profound 369.05
        with
            lesser eye impairment 369.05
                near-total 369.07
                profound 369.08
                total 369.06

◀ **New**   ◀▥ **Revised**

Blindness (Continued)
legal (Continued)
with impairment of better (less impaired) eye (Continued)
severe 369.21
with
lesser eye impairment 369.21
blind 369.11
near-total 369.13
profound 369.14
severe 369.22
total 369.12
total
with lesser eye impairment
total 369.01
mind 784.69
moderate
both eyes 369.25
with impairment of lesser eye (specified as)
blind, not further specified 369.15
low vision, not further specified 369.23
near-total 369.17
profound 369.18
severe 369.24
total 369.16
one eye 369.74
with vision of other eye (specified as)
near-normal 369.75
normal 369.76
near-total
both eyes 369.04
with impairment of lesser eye (specified as)
blind, not further specified 369.02
total 369.03
one eye 369.64
with vision of other eye (specified as)
near-normal 369.65
normal 369.66
night 368.60
acquired 368.62
congenital (Japanese) 368.61
hereditary 368.61
specified type NEC 368.69
vitamin A deficiency 264.5
nocturnal - see Blindness, night
one eye 369.60
with low vision of other eye 369.10
profound
both eyes 369.08
with impairment of lesser eye (specified as)
blind, not further specified 369.05
near-total 369.07
total 369.06
one eye 369.67
with vision of other eye (specified as)
near-normal 369.68
normal 369.69
psychic 784.69
severe
both eyes 369.22
with impairment of lesser eye (specified as)
blind, not further specified 369.11

Blindness (Continued)
severe (Continued)
both eyes (Continued)
with impairment of lesser eye (specified as) (Continued)
low vision, not further specified 369.21
near-total 369.13
profound 369.14
total 369.12
one eye 369.71
with vision of other eye (specified as)
near-normal 369.72
normal 369.73
snow 370.24
sun 363.31
temporary 368.12
total
both eyes 369.01
one eye 369.61
with vision of other eye (specified as)
near-normal 369.62
normal 369.63
transient 368.12
traumatic NEC 950.9
word (developmental) 315.01
acquired 784.61
secondary to organic lesion 784.61
Blister - see also Injury, superficial, by site
beetle dermatitis 692.89
due to burn - see Burn, by site, second degree
fever 054.9
multiple, skin, nontraumatic 709.8
Bloating 787.3
Bloch-Siemens syndrome (incontinentia pigmenti) 757.33
Bloch-Stauffer dyshormonal dermatosis 757.33
Bloch-Sulzberger disease or syndrome (incontinentia pigmenti) (melanoblastosis) 757.33
Block
alveolar capillary 516.3
arborization (heart) 426.6
arrhythmic 426.9
atrioventricular (AV) (incomplete) (partial) 426.10
with
2:1 atrioventricular response block 426.13
atrioventricular dissociation 426.0
first degree (incomplete) 426.11
second degree (Mobitz type I) 426.13
Mobitz (type II) 426.12
third degree 426.0
complete 426.0
congenital 746.86
congenital 746.86
Mobitz (incomplete)
type I (Wenckebach's) 426.13
type II 426.12
partial 426.13
auriculoventricular (see also Block, atrioventricular) 426.10
complete 426.0
congenital 746.86
congenital 746.86
bifascicular (cardiac) 426.53

Block (Continued)
bundle branch (complete) (false) (incomplete) 426.50
bilateral 426.53
left (complete) (main stem) 426.3
with right bundle branch block 426.53
anterior fascicular 426.2
with
posterior fascicular block 426.3
right bundle branch block 426.52
hemiblock 426.2
incomplete 426.2
with right bundle branch block 426.53
posterior fascicular 426.2
with
anterior fascicular block 426.3
right bundle branch block 426.51
right 426.4
with
left bundle branch block (incomplete) (main stem) 426.53
left fascicular block 426.53
anterior 426.52
posterior 426.51
Wilson's type 426.4
cardiac 426.9
conduction 426.9
complete 426.0
eustachian tube (see also Obstruction, Eustachian tube) 381.60
fascicular (left anterior) (left posterior) 426.2
foramen Magendie (acquired) 331.3
congenital 742.3
with spina bifida (see also Spina bifida) 741.0
heart 426.9
first degree (atrioventricular) 426.11
second degree (atrioventricular) 426.13
third degree (atrioventricular) 426.0
bundle branch (complete) (false) (incomplete) 426.50
bilateral 426.53
left (see also Block, bundle branch, left) 426.3
right (see also Block, bundle branch, right) 426.4
complete (atrioventricular) 426.0
congenital 746.86
incomplete 426.13
intra-atrial 426.6
intraventricular NEC 426.6
sinoatrial 426.6
specified type NEC 426.6
hepatic vein 453.0
intraventricular (diffuse) (myofibrillar) 426.6
bundle branch (complete) (false) (incomplete) 426.50
bilateral 426.53
left (see also Block, bundle branch, left) 426.3
right (see also Block, bundle branch, right) 426.4
kidney (see also Disease, renal) 593.9
postcystoscopic 997.5

ICD-9-CM

B

Vol. 2

Block (*Continued*)
  myocardial (*see also* Block, heart)
    426.9
  nodal 426.10
  optic nerve 377.49
  organ or site (congenital) NEC - *see*
    Atresia
  parietal 426.6
  peri-infarction 426.6
  portal (vein) 452
  sinoatrial 426.6
  sinoauricular 426.6
  spinal cord 336.9
  trifascicular 426.54
  tubal 628.2
  vein NEC 453.9
Blocq's disease or syndrome (astasia-
  abasia) 307.9
Blood
  constituents, abnormal NEC 790.6
  disease 289.9
    specified NEC 289.89
  donor V59.01
    other blood components V59.09
    stem cells V59.02
    whole blood V59.01
  dyscrasia 289.9
    with
      abortion - *see* Abortion, by type,
        with hemorrhage, delayed or
        excessive
      ectopic pregnancy (*see also* catego-
        ries 633.0-633.9) 639.1
      molar pregnancy (*see also* catego-
        ries 630-632) 639.1
    fetus or newborn NEC 776.9
    following
      abortion 639.1
      ectopic or molar pregnancy
        639.1
    puerperal, postpartum 666.3
  flukes NEC (*see also* Infestation, Schis-
    tosoma) 120.9
  in
    feces (*see also* Melena) 578.1
      occult 792.1
    urine (*see also* Hematuria) 599.7
  mole 631
  occult 792.1
  poisoning (*see also* Septicemia) 038.9
  pressure
    decreased, due to shock following
      injury 958.4
    fluctuating 796.4
    high (*see also* Hypertension) 401.9
      incidental reading (isolated) (non-
        specific), without diagnosis of
        hypertension 796.2
    low (*see also* Hypotension) 458.9
      incidental reading (isolated) (non-
        specific), without diagnosis of
        hypotension 796.3
  spitting (*see also* Hemoptysis) 786.3
  staining cornea 371.12
  transfusion
    without reported diagnosis V58.2
    donor V59.01
      stem cells V59.02
    reaction or complication - *see* Com-
      plications, transfusion
  tumor - *see* Hematoma
  vessel rupture - *see* Hemorrhage
  vomiting (*see also* Hematemesis)
    578.0

Blood-forming organ disease 289.9
Bloodgood's disease 610.1
Bloodshot eye 379.93
Bloom (-Machacek) (-Torre) syndrome
  757.39
Blotch, palpebral 372.55
Blount's disease (tibia vara) 732.4
Blount-Barber syndrome (tibia vara)
  732.4
Blue
  baby 746.9
  bloater 491.20
    with   ◀▥
      acute bronchitis 491.22   ◀
      exacerbation (acute) 491.21   ◀
  diaper syndrome 270.0
  disease 746.9
  dome cyst 610.0
  drum syndrome 381.02
  sclera 743.47
    with fragility of bone and deafness
      756.51
  toe syndrome 445.02
Blueness (*see also* Cyanosis) 782.5
Blurring, visual 368.8
Blushing (abnormal) (excessive) 782.62
Boarder, hospital V65.0
  infant V65.0
Bockhart's impetigo (superficial folliculitis) 704.8
Bodechtel-Guttmann disease (subacute sclerosing panencephalitis)
  046.2
Boder-Sedgwick syndrome (ataxia-telangiectasia) 334.8
Body, bodies
  Aschoff (*see also* Myocarditis, rheu-
    matic) 398.0
  asteroid, vitreous 379.22
  choroid, colloid (degenerative)
    362.57
    hereditary 362.77
  cytoid (retina) 362.82
  drusen (retina) (*see also* Drusen) 362.57
    optic disc 377.21
  fibrin, pleura 511.0
  foreign - *see* Foreign body
  Hassall-Henle 371.41
  loose
    joint (*see also* Loose, body, joint)
      718.1
      knee 717.6
    knee 717.6
    sheath, tendon 727.82
  Mallory's 034.1
  Mooser 081.0
  Negri 071
  rice (joint) (*see also* Loose, body, joint)
    718.1
    knee 717.6
  rocking 307.3
Boeck's
  disease (sarcoidosis) 135
  lupoid (miliary) 135
  sarcoid 135
Boerhaave's syndrome (spontaneous
  esophageal rupture) 530.4
Boggy
  cervix 622.8
  uterus 621.8
Boil (*see also* Carbuncle) 680.9
  abdominal wall 680.2
  Aleppo 085.1
  ankle 680.6

Boil (*Continued*)
  anus 680.5
  arm (any part, above wrist) 680.3
  auditory canal, external 680.0
  axilla 680.3
  back (any part) 680.2
  Baghdad 085.1
  breast 680.2
  buttock 680.5
  chest wall 680.2
  corpus cavernosum 607.2
  Delhi 085.1
  ear (any part) 680.0
  eyelid 373.13
  face (any part, except eye) 680.0
  finger (any) 680.4
  flank 680.2
  foot (any part) 680.7
  forearm 680.3
  Gafsa 085.1
  genital organ, male 608.4
  gluteal (region) 680.5
  groin 680.2
  hand (any part) 680.4
  head (any part, except face) 680.8
  heel 680.7
  hip 680.6
  knee 680.6
  labia 616.4
  lacrimal (*see also* Dacryocystitis)
    375.30
    gland (*see also* Dacryoadenitis)
      375.00
    passages (duct) (sac) (*see also* Dac-
      ryocystitis) 375.30
  leg, any part, except foot 680.6
  multiple sites 680.9
  Natal 085.1
  neck 680.1
  nose (external) (septum) 680.0
  orbit, orbital 376.01
  partes posteriores 680.5
  pectoral region 680.2
  penis 607.2
  perineum 680.2
  pinna 680.0
  scalp (any part) 680.8
  scrotum 608.4
  seminal vesicle 608.0
  shoulder 680.3
  skin NEC 680.9
  specified site NEC 680.8
  spermatic cord 608.4
  temple (region) 680.0
  testis 608.4
  thigh 680.6
  thumb 680.4
  toe (any) 680.7
  tropical 085.1
  trunk 680.2
  tunica vaginalis 608.4
  umbilicus 680.2
  upper arm 680.3
  vas deferens 608.4
  vulva 616.4
  wrist 680.4
Bold hives (*see also* Urticaria) 708.9
Bolivian hemorrhagic fever 078.7
Bombé, iris 364.74
Bomford-Rhoads anemia (refractory)
  284.9
Bone - *see* condition
Bonnevie-Ullrich syndrome 758.6
Bonnier's syndrome 386.19

Bonvale Dam fever 780.79
Bony block of joint 718.80
  ankle 718.87
  elbow 718.82
  foot 718.87
  hand 718.84
  hip 718.85
  knee 718.86
  multiple sites 718.89
  pelvic region 718.85
  shoulder (region) 718.81
  specified site NEC 718.88
  wrist 718.83
Borderline
  intellectual functioning V62.89
  pelvis 653.1
    with obstruction during labor
      660.1
      affecting fetus or newborn 763.1
  psychosis (*see also* Schizophrenia)
    295.5
    of childhood (*see also* Psychosis,
      childhood) 299.8
  schizophrenia (*see also* Schizophrenia)
    295.5
Borna disease 062.9
Bornholm disease (epidemic pleurodynia) 074.1
Borrelia vincentii (mouth) (pharynx)
  (tonsils) 101
Bostock's catarrh (*see also* Fever, hay)
  477.9
Boston exanthem 048
Botalli, ductus (patent) (persistent)
  747.0
Bothriocephalus latus infestation 123.4
Botulism 005.1
Bouba (*see also* Yaws) 102.9
Bouffée délirante 298.3
Bouillaud's disease or syndrome (rheu-
  matic heart disease) 391.9
Bourneville's disease (tuberous sclerosis)
  759.5
Boutonneuse fever 082.1
Boutonniere
  deformity (finger) 736.21
  hand (intrinsic) 736.21
Bouveret (-Hoffmann) **disease or syn-
  drome** (paroxysmal tachycardia)
  427.2
Bovine heart - *see* Hypertrophy, cardiac
Bowel - *see* condition
Bowen's
  dermatosis (precancerous) (M8081/2) -
    see Neoplasm, skin, in situ
  disease (M8081/2) - *see* Neoplasm,
    skin, in situ
  epithelioma (M8081/2) - *see* Neoplasm,
    skin, in situ
  type
    epidermoid carcinoma in situ
      (M8081/2) - *see* Neoplasm, skin,
      in situ
    intraepidermal squamous cell carci-
      noma (M8081/2) - *see* Neo-
      plasm, skin, in situ
Bowing
  femur 736.89
    congenital 754.42
  fibula 736.89
    congenital 754.43
  forearm 736.09
    away from midline (cubitus valgus)
      736.01

Bowing (*Continued*)
  forearm (*Continued*)
    toward midline (cubitus varus)
      736.02
  leg(s), long bones, congenital 754.44
  radius 736.09
    away from midline (cubitus valgus)
      736.01
    toward midline (cubitus varus)
      736.02
  tibia 736.89
    congenital 754.43
Bowleg(s) 736.42
  congenital 754.44
  rachitic 268.1
Boyd's dysentery 004.2
Brachial - *see* condition
Brachman-de Lange syndrome (Amsterdam dwarf, mental retardation, and
  brachycephaly) 759.89
Brachycardia 427.89
Brachycephaly 756.0
Brachymorphism and ectopia lentis
  759.89
Bradley's disease (epidemic vomiting)
  078.82
Bradycardia 427.89
  chronic (sinus) 427.81
  newborn 779.81
  nodal 427.89
  postoperative 997.1
  reflex 337.0
  sinoatrial 427.89
    with paroxysmal tachyarrhythmia or
      tachycardia 427.81
    chronic 427.81
  sinus 427.89
    with paroxysmal tachyarrhythmia or
      tachycardia 427.81
    chronic 427.81
    persistent 427.81
    severe 427.81
  tachycardia syndrome 427.81
  vagal 427.89
Bradypnea 786.09
Brailsford's disease 732.3
  radial head 732.3
  tarsal scaphoid 732.5
**Brailsford-Morquio disease or syn-
  drome** (mucopolysaccharidosis IV)
  277.5
Brain - *see also* condition
  death 348.8
  syndrome (acute) (chronic) (nonpsy-
    chotic) (organic) (with neurotic
    reaction) (with behavioral reac-
    tion) (*see also* Syndrome, brain)
    310.9
    with
      presenile brain disease 290.10
      psychosis, psychotic reaction (*see
        also* Psychosis, organic) 294.9
    congenital (*see also* Retardation, men-
      tal) 319
Branched-chain amino-acid disease 270.3
Branchial - *see* condition
Brandt's syndrome (acrodermatitis en-
  teropathica) 686.8
Brash (water) 787.1
Brass-founders' ague 985.8
Bravais-Jacksonian epilepsy (*see also* Ep-
  ilepsy) 345.5
Braxton Hicks contractions 644.1
Braziers' disease 985.8

Brazilian
  blastomycosis 116.1
  leishmaniasis 085.5
BRBPR (bright red blood per rectum)
  569.3 ◀
Break
  cardiorenal - *see* Hypertension, cardio-
    renal
  retina (*see also* Defect, retina) 361.30
Breakbone fever 061
Breakdown
  device, implant, or graft - *see* Compli-
    cations, mechanical
  nervous (*see also* Disorder, mental,
    nonpsychotic) 300.9
  perineum 674.2
Breast - *see* condition
Breast feeding difficulties 676.8
Breath
  foul 784.9
  holder, child 312.81
  holding spells 786.9
  shortness 786.05
Breathing
  asymmetrical 786.09
  bronchial 786.09
  exercises V57.0
  labored 786.09
  mouth 784.9
  periodic 786.09
  tic 307.20
Breathlessness 786.09
Breda's disease (*see also* Yaws) 102.9
Breech
  delivery, affecting fetus or newborn
    763.0
  extraction, affecting fetus or newborn
    763.0
  presentation (buttocks) (complete)
    (frank) 652.2
    with successful version 652.1
    before labor, affecting fetus or new-
      born 761.7
    during labor, affecting fetus or new-
      born 763.0
Breisky's disease (kraurosis vulvae) 624.0
Brennemann's syndrome (acute mesen-
  teric lymphadenitis) 289.2
Brenner's
  tumor (benign) (M9000/0) 220
    borderline malignancy (M9000/1)
      236.2
    malignant (M9000/3) 183.0
    proliferating (M9000/1) 236.2
Bretonneau's disease (diphtheritic malig-
  nant angina) 032.0
Breus' mole 631
Brevicollis 756.16
Bricklayers' itch 692.89
Brickmakers' anemia 126.9
Bridge
  myocardial 746.85
Bright red blood per rectum (BRBPR)
  569.3 ◀
Bright's
  blindness - *see* Uremia
  disease (*see also* Nephritis) 583.9
    arteriosclerotic (*see also* Hyperten-
      sion, kidney) 403.90
Brill's disease (recrudescent typhus) 081.1
  flea-borne 081.0
  louse-borne 081.1
Brill-Symmers disease (follicular lym-
  phoma) (M9690/3) 202.0

ICD-9-CM

B

Vol.

Brill-Zinsser disease (recrudescent typhus) 081.1
Brinton's disease (linitis plastica) (M8142/3) 151.9
Brion-Kayser disease (*see also* Fever, paratyphoid) 002.9
Briquet's disorder or syndrome 300.81
Brissaud's
  infantilism (infantile myxedema) 244.9
  motor-verbal tic 307.23
Brissaud-Meige syndrome (infantile myxedema) 244.9
Brittle
  bones (congenital) 756.51
  nails 703.8
    congenital 757.5
Broad - *see also* condition
  beta disease 272.2
  ligament laceration syndrome 620.6
Brock's syndrome (atelectasis due to enlarged lymph nodes) 518.0
Brocq's disease 691.8
  atopic (diffuse) neurodermatitis 691.8
  lichen simplex chronicus 698.3
  parakeratosis psoriasiformis 696.2
  parapsoriasis 696.2
Brocq-Duhring disease (dermatitis herpetiformis) 694.0
Brodie's
  abscess (localized) (chronic) (*see also* Osteomyelitis) 730.1
  disease (joint) (*see also* Osteomyelitis) 730.1
Broken
  arches 734
    congenital 755.67
  back - *see* Fracture, vertebra, by site
  bone - *see* Fracture, by site
  compensation - *see* Disease, heart
  implant or internal device - *see* listing under Complications, mechanical
  neck - *see* Fracture, vertebra, cervical
  nose 802.0
    open 802.1
  tooth, teeth 873.63
    complicated 873.73
Bromhidrosis 705.89
Bromidism, bromism
  acute 967.3
    correct substance properly administered 349.82
    overdose or wrong substance given or taken 967.3
  chronic (*see also* Dependence) 304.1
Bromidrosiphobia 300.23
Bromidrosis 705.89
Bronchi, bronchial - *see* Condition
Bronchiectasis (cylindrical) (diffuse) (fusiform) (localized) (moniliform) (postinfectious) (recurrent) (saccular) 494.0
  with acute exacerbation 494.1
  congenital 748.61
  tuberculosis (*see also* Tuberculosis) 011.5
Bronchiolectasis - *see* Bronchiectasis
Bronchiolitis (acute) (infectious) (subacute) 466.19
  with
    bronchospasm or obstruction 466.19
    influenza, flu, or grippe 487.1

Bronchiolitis (*Continued*)
  catarrhal (acute) (subacute) 466.19
  chemical 506.0
    chronic 506.4
  chronic (obliterative) 491.8
  due to external agent - *see* Bronchitis, acute, due to
  fibrosa obliterans 491.8
  influenzal 487.1
  obliterans 491.8
    with organizing pneumonia (B.O.O.P.) 516.8
    status post lung transplant 996.84
  obliterative (chronic) (diffuse) (subacute) 491.8
    due to fumes or vapors 506.4
  respiratory syncytial virus 466.11
  vesicular - *see* Pneumonia, broncho-
Bronchitis (diffuse) (hypostatic) (infectious) (inflammatory) (simple) 490
  with
    emphysema - *see* Emphysema
    influenza, flue, or grippe 487.1
    obstruction airway, chronic 491.20
      with ◀▥
        acute bronchitis 491.22 ◀
        exacerbation (acute) 491.21 ◀
    tracheitis 490
      acute or subacute 466.0
        with bronchospasm or obstruction 466.0
      chronic 491.8
  acute or subacute 466.0
    with
      bronchospasm 466.0
      obstruction 466.0
      tracheitis 466.0
    chemical (due to fumes or vapors) 506.0
    due to
      fumes or vapors 506.0
      radiation 508.8
  allergic (acute) (*see also* Asthma) 493.9
  arachidic 934.1
  aspiration 507.0
    due to fumes or vapors 506.0
  asthmatic (acute) 493.90
    with
      acute exacerbation 493.92
      status asthmaticus 493.91
    chronic 493.2
  capillary 466.19
    with bronchospasm or obstruction 466.19
    chronic 491.8
  caseous (*see also* Tuberculosis) 011.3
  Castellani's 104.8
  catarrhal 490
    acute - *see* Bronchitis, acute
    chronic 491.0
  chemical (acute) (subacute) 506.0
    chronic 506.4
    due to fumes or vapors (acute) (subacute) 506.0
      chronic 506.4
  chronic 491.9
    with
      tracheitis (chronic) 491.8
    asthmatic 493.2
    catarrhal 491.0
    chemical (due to fumes and vapors) 506.4

Bronchitis (*Continued*)
  chronic (*Continued*)
    due to
      fumes or vapors (chemical) (inhalation) 506.4
      radiation 508.8
      tobacco smoking 491.0
    mucopurulent 491.1
    obstructive 491.20
      with ◀▥
        acute bronchitis 491.22 ◀
        exacerbation (acute) 491.21 ◀
    purulent 491.1
    simple 491.0
    specified type NEC 491.8
  croupous 466.0
    with bronchospasm or obstruction 466.0
    due to fumes or vapors 506.0
  emphysematous 491.20
    with ◀▥
      acute bronchitis 491.22 ◀
      exacerbation (acute) 491.21 ◀
  exudative 466.0
  fetid (chronic) (recurrent) 491.1
  fibrinous, acute or subacute 466.0
    with bronchospasm or obstruction 466.0
  grippal 487.1
  influenzal 487.1
  membranous, acute or subacute 466.0
    with bronchospasm or obstruction 466.0
  moulders' 502
  mucopurulent (chronic) (recurrent) 491.1
    acute or subacute 466.0
  obliterans 491.8
  obstructive (chronic) 491.20
    with ◀▥
      acute bronchitis 491.22 ◀
      exacerbation (acute) 491.21 ◀
  pituitous 491.1
  plastic (inflammatory) 466.0
  pneumococcal, acute or subacute 466.0
    with bronchospasm or obstruction 466.0
  pseudomembranous 466.0
  purulent (chronic) (recurrent) 491.1
    acute or subacute 466.0
      with bronchospasm or obstruction 466.0
  putrid 491.1
  scrofulous (*see also* Tuberculosis) 011.3
  senile 491.9
  septic, acute or subacute 466.0
    with bronchospasm or obstruction 466.0
  smokers' 491.0
  spirochetal 104.8
  suffocative, acute or subacute 466.0
  summer (*see also* Asthma) 493.9
  suppurative (chronic) 491.1
    acute or subacute 466.0
  tuberculous (*see also* Tuberculosis) 011.3
  ulcerative 491.8
    Vincent's 101
  Vincent's 101

◀ **New**   ◀▥ **Revised**

Bronchitis (*Continued*)
viral, acute or subacute 466.0
with bronchospasm or obstruction 466.0
Bronchoalveolitis 485
Bronchoaspergillosis 117.3
Bronchocele
meaning
dilatation of bronchus 519.1
goiter 240.9
Bronchogenic carcinoma 162.9
Bronchohemisporosis 117.9
Broncholithiasis 518.89
tuberculous (*see also* Tuberculosis) 011.3
Bronchomalacia 748.3
Bronchomoniliasis 112.89
Bronchomycosis 112.89
Bronchonocardiosis 039.1
Bronchopleuropneumonia - *see* Pneumonia, broncho-
Bronchopneumonia - *see* Pneumonia, broncho-
Bronchopneumonitis - *see* Pneumonia, broncho-
Bronchopulmonary - *see* Condition
Bronchopulmonitis - *see* Pneumonia, broncho-
Bronchorrhagia 786.3
newborn 770.3
tuberculous (*see also* Tuberculosis) 011.3
Bronchorrhea (chronic) (purulent) 491.0
acute 466.0
Bronchospasm 519.1
with
asthma - *see* Asthma
bronchiolitis, acute 466.19
due to respiratory syncytial virus 466.11
bronchitis - *see* Bronchitis
chronic obstructive pulmonary disease (COPD) 496
emphysema - *see* Emphysema
due to external agent - *see* Condition, respiratory, acute, due to
exercise induced 493.81
Bronchospirochetosis 104.8
Bronchostenosis 519.1
Bronchus - *see* Condition
Bronze, bronzed
diabetes 275.0
disease (Addison's) (skin) 255.4
tuberculous (*see also* Tuberculosis) 017.6
Brooke's disease or tumor (M8100/0) - *see* Neoplasm, skin, benign
Brown's tendon sheath syndrome 378.61
Brown enamel of teeth (hereditary) 520.5
Brown-Séquard's paralysis (syndrome) 344.89
Brow presentation complicating delivery 652.4
Brucella, brucellosis (infection) 023.9
abortus 023.1
canis 023.3
dermatitis, skin 023.9
melitensis 023.0
mixed 023.8
suis 023.2

Bruck's disease 733.99
Bruck-de Lange disease or syndrome (Amsterdam dwarf, mental retardation, and brachycephaly) 759.89
Brugada syndrome 746.89
Brug's filariasis 125.1
Brugsch's syndrome (acropachyderma) 757.39
Bruhl's disease (splenic anemia with fever) 285.8
Bruise (skin surface intact) - *see also* Contusion
with
fracture - *see* Fracture, by site
open wound - *see* Wound, open, by site
internal organ (abdomen, chest, or pelvis) - *see* Injury, internal, by site
umbilical cord 663.6
affecting fetus or newborn 762.6
Bruit 785.9
arterial (abdominal) (carotid) 785.9
supraclavicular 785.9
Brushburn - *see* Injury, superficial, by site
Bruton's X-linked agammaglobulinemia 279.04
Bruxism 306.8
Bubbly lung syndrome 770.7
Bubo 289.3
blennorrhagic 098.89
chancroidal 099.0
climatic 099.1
due to Hemophilus ducreyi 099.0
gonococcal 098.89
indolent NEC 099.8
inguinal NEC 099.8
chancroidal 099.0
climatic 099.1
due to H. ducreyi 099.0
scrofulous (*see also* Tuberculosis) 017.2
soft chancre 099.0
suppurating 683
syphilitic 091.0
congenital 090.0
tropical 099.1
venereal NEC 099.8
virulent 099.0
Bubonic plague 020.0
Bubonocele - *see* Hernia, inguinal
Buccal - *see* Condition
Buchanan's disease (juvenile osteochondrosis of iliac crest) 732.1
Buchem's syndrome (hyperostosis corticalis) 733.3
Buchman's disease (osteochondrosis, juvenile) 732.1
Bucket handle fracture (semilunar cartilage) (*see also* Tear, meniscus) 836.2
Budd-Chiari syndrome (hepatic vein thrombosis) 453.0
Budgerigar-fanciers' disease of lung 495.2
Büdinger-Ludloff-Läwen disease 717.89
Buerger's disease (thromboangiitis obliterans) 443.1
Bulbar - *see* Condition
Bulbus cordis 745.9
persistent (in left ventricle) 745.8
Bulging fontanels (congenital) 756.0
Bulimia 783.6
nervosa 307.51
nonorganic origin 307.51

Bulky uterus 621.2
Bulla(e) 709.8
lung (emphysematous) (solitary) 492.0
Bullet wound - *see also* Wound, open, by site
fracture - *see* Fracture, by site, open
internal organ (abdomen, chest, or pelvis) - *see* Injury, internal, by site, with open wound
intracranial - *see* Laceration, brain, with open wound
Bullis fever 082.8
Bullying (*see also* Disturbance, conduct) 312.0
Bundle
branch block (complete) (false) (incomplete) 426.50
bilateral 426.53
left (*see also* Block, bundle branch, left) 426.3
hemiblock 426.2
right (*see also* Block, bundle branch, right) 426.4
of His - *see* Condition
of Kent syndrome (anomalous atrioventricular excitation) 426.7
Bungpagga 040.81
Bunion 727.1
Bunionette 727.1
Bunyamwera fever 066.3
Buphthalmia, buphthalmos (congenital) 743.20
associated with
keratoglobus, congenital 743.22
megalocornea 743.22
ocular anomalies NEC 743.22
isolated 743.21
simple 743.21
Bürger-Grütz disease or syndrome (essential familial hyperlipemia) 272.3
Buried roots 525.3
Burke's syndrome 577.8
Burkitt's
tumor (M9750/3) 200.2
type (malignant, lymphoma, lymphoblastic, or undifferentiated) (M9750/3) 200.2
Burn (acid) (cathode ray) (caustic) (chemical) (electric heating appliance) (electricity) (fire) (flame) (hot liquid or object) (irradiation) (lime) (radiation) (steam) (thermal) (x-ray) 949.0

ICD-9-CM

B

Vol.

Note   Use the following fifth-digit subclassification with category 948 to indicate the percent of body surface with third degree burn:

0	less than 10 percent or unspecified
1	10-19 percent
2	20-29 percent
3	30-39 percent
4	40-49 percent
5	50-59 percent
6	60-69 percent
7	70-79 percent
8	80-89 percent
9	90 percent or more of body surface

Burn (*Continued*)
with
blisters - *see* Burn, by site, second degree
erythema - *see* Burn, by site, first degree
skin loss (epidermal) - *see also* Burn, by site, second degree
full thickness - *see also* Burn, by site, third degree
with necrosis of underlying tissues - *see* Burn, by site, third degree, deep
first degree - *see* Burn, by site, first degree
second degree - *see* Burn, by site, second degree
third degree - *see also* Burn, by site, third degree
deep - *see* Burn, by site, third degree, deep
abdomen, abdominal (muscle) (wall) 942.03
with
trunk - *see* Burn, trunk, multiple sites
first degree 942.13
second degree 942.23
third degree 942.33
deep 942.43
with loss of body part 942.53
ankle 945.03
with
lower limb(s) - *see* Burn, leg, multiple sites
first degree 945.13
second degree 945.23
third degree 945.33
deep 945.43
with loss of body part 945.53
anus - *see* Burn, trunk, specified site NEC
arm(s) 943.00
first degree 943.10
second degree 943.20
third degree 943.30
deep 943.40
with loss of body part 943.50
lower - *see* Burn, forearm(s)
multiple sites, except hand(s) or wrist(s) 943.09
first degree 943.19
second degree 943.29
third degree 943.39
deep 943.49
with loss of body part 943.59
upper 943.03
first degree 943.13
second degree 943.23
third degree 943.33
deep 943.43
with loss of body part 943.53
auditory canal (external) - *see* Burn, ear
auricle (ear) - *see* Burn, ear
axilla 943.04
with
upper limb(s), except hand(s) or wrist(s) - *see* Burn, arm(s), multiple sites

Burn (*Continued*)
axilla (*Continued*)
first degree 943.14
second degree 943.24
third degree 943.34
deep 943.44
with loss of body part 943.54
back 942.04
with
trunk - *see* Burn, trunk, multiple sites
first degree 942.14
second degree 942.24
third degree 942.34
deep 942.44
with loss of body part 942.54
biceps
brachii - *see* Burn, arm(s), upper
femoris - *see* Burn, thigh
breast(s) 942.01
with
trunk - *see* Burn, trunk, multiple sites
first degree 942.11
second degree 942.21
third degree 942.31
deep 942.41
with loss of body part 942.51
brow - *see* Burn, forehead
buttock(s) - *see* Burn, back
canthus (eye) 940.1
chemical 940.0
cervix (uteri) 947.4
cheek (cutaneous) 941.07
with
face or head - *see* Burn, head, multiple sites
first degree 941.17
second degree 941.27
third degree 941.37
deep 941.47
with loss of body part 941.57
chest wall (anterior) 942.02
with
trunk - *see* Burn, trunk, multiple sites
first degree 942.12
second degree 942.22
third degree 942.32
deep 942.42
with loss of body part 942.52
chin 941.04
with
face or head - *see* Burn, head, multiple sites
first degree 941.14
second degree 941.24
third degree 941.34
deep 941.44
with loss of body part 941.54
clitoris - *see* Burn, genitourinary organs, external
colon 947.3
conjunctiva (and cornea) 940.4
chemical
acid 940.3
alkaline 940.2
cornea (and conjunctiva) 940.4
chemical
acid 940.3
alkaline 940.2
costal region - *see* Burn, chest wall

Burn (*Continued*)
due to ingested chemical agent - *see* Burn, internal organs
ear (auricle) (canal) (drum) (external) 941.01
with
face or head - *see* Burn, head, multiple sites
first degree 941.11
second degree 941.21
third degree 941.31
deep 941.41
with loss of a body part 941.51
elbow 943.02
with
hand(s) and wrist(s) - *see* Burn, multiple specified sites
upper limb(s), except hand(s) or wrist(s) - *see also* Burn, arm(s), multiple sites
first degree 943.12
second degree 943.22
third degree 943.32
deep 943.42
with loss of body part 943.52
electricity, electric current - *see* Burn, by site
entire body - *see* Burn, multiple, specified sites
epididymis - *see* Burn, genitourinary organs, external
epigastric region - *see* Burn, abdomen
epiglottis 947.1
esophagus 947.2
extent (percent of body surface)
less than 10 percent 948.0
10-19 percent 948.1
20-29 percent 948.2
30-39 percent 948.3
40-49 percent 948.4
50-59 percent 948.5
60-69 percent 948.6
70-79 percent 948.7
80-89 percent 948.8
90 percent or more 948.9
extremity
lower - *see* Burn, leg
upper - *see* Burn, arm(s)
eye(s) (and adnexa) (only) 940.9
with
face, head, or neck 941.02
first degree 941.12
second degree 941.22
third degree 941.32
deep 941.42
with loss of body part 941.52
other sites (classifiable to more than one category in 940-945) - *see* Burn, multiple, specified sites
resulting rupture and destruction of eyeball 940.5
specified part - *see* Burn, by site
eyeball - *see also* Burn, eye
with resulting rupture and destruction of eyeball 940.5
eyelid(s) 940.1
chemical 940.0
face - *see* Burn, head
finger (nail) (subungual) 944.01

◀ **New**   ◀▥ **Revised**

Burn (*Continued*)
  finger (*Continued*)
    with
      hand(s) - *see* Burn, hand(s), multiple sites
      other sites - *see* Burn, multiple, specified sites
      thumb 944.04
        first degree 944.14
        second degree 944.24
        third degree 944.34
          deep 944.44
            with loss of body part 944.54
      first degree 944.11
      second degree 944.21
      third degree 944.31
        deep 944.41
          with loss of body part 944.51
      multiple (digits) 944.03
        with thumb - *see* Burn, finger, with thumb
        first degree 944.13
        second degree 944.23
        third degree 944.33
          deep 944.43
            with loss of body part 944.53
  flank - *see* Burn, abdomen
  foot 945.02
    with
      lower limb(s) - *see* Burn, leg, multiple sites
    first degree 945.12
    second degree 945.22
    third degree 945.32
      deep 945.42
        with loss of body part 945.52
  forearm(s) 943.01
    with
      upper limb(s), except hand(s) or wrist(s) - *see* Burn, arm(s), multiple sites
    first degree 943.11
    second degree 943.21
    third degree 943.31
      deep 943.41
        with loss of body part 943.51
  forehead 941.07
    with
      face or head - *see* Burn, head, multiple sites
    first degree 941.17
    second degree 941.27
    third degree 941.37
      deep 941.47
        with loss of body part 941.57
  fourth degree - *see* Burn, by site, third degree, deep
  friction - *see* Injury, superficial, by site
  from swallowing caustic or corrosive substance NEC - *see* Burn, internal organs
  full thickness - *see* Burn, by site, third degree
  gastrointestinal tract 947.3
  genitourinary organs
    external 942.05
      with
        trunk - *see* Burn, trunk, multiple sites
      first degree 942.15
      second degree 942.25

Burn (*Continued*)
  genitourinary organs (*Continued*)
    external (*Continued*)
      third degree 942.35
        deep 942.45
          with loss of body part 942.55
      internal 947.8
  globe (eye) - *see* Burn, eyeball
  groin - *see* Burn, abdomen
  gum 947.0
  hand(s) (phalanges) (and wrist) 944.00
    first degree 944.10
    second degree 944.20
    third degree 944.30
      deep 944.40
        with loss of body part 944.50
    back (dorsal surface) 944.06
      first degree 944.16
      second degree 944.26
      third degree 944.36
        deep 944.46
          with loss of body part 944.56
    multiple sites 944.08
      first degree 944.18
      second degree 944.28
      third degree 944.38
        deep 944.48
          with loss of body part 944.58
  head (and face) 941.00
    eye(s) only 940.9
      specified part - *see* Burn, by site
    first degree 941.10
    second degree 941.20
    third degree 941.30
      deep 941.40
        with loss of body part 941.50
    multiple sites 941.09
      with eyes - *see* Burn, eyes, with face, head, or neck
      first degree 941.19
      second degree 941.29
      third degree 941.39
        deep 941.49
          with loss of body part 941.59
  heel - *see* Burn, foot
  hip - *see* Burn, trunk, specified site NEC
  iliac region - *see* Burn, trunk, specified site NEC
  infected 958.3
  inhalation (*see also* Burn, internal organs) 947.9
  internal organs 947.9
    from caustic or corrosive substance (swallowing) NEC 947.9
    specified NEC (*see also* Burn, by site) 947.8
  interscapular region - *see* Burn, back
  intestine (large) (small) 947.3
  iris - *see* Burn, eyeball
  knee 945.05
    with
      lower limb(s) - *see* Burn, leg, multiple sites
    first degree 945.15
    second degree 945.25
    third degree 945.35
      deep 945.45
        with loss of body part 945.55
  labium (majus) (minus) - *see* Burn, genitourinary organs, external

Burn (*Continued*)
  lacrimal apparatus, duct, gland, or sac 940.1
    chemical 940.0
  larynx 947.1
  late effect - *see* Late, effects (of), burn
  leg 945.00
    first degree 945.10
    second degree 945.20
    third degree 945.30
      deep 945.40
        with loss of body part 945.50
    lower 945.04
      with other part(s) of lower limb(s) - *see* Burn, leg, multiple sites
      first degree 945.14
      second degree 945.24
      third degree 945.34
        deep 945.44
          with loss of body part 945.54
    multiple sites 945.09
      first degree 945.19
      second degree 945.29
      third degree 945.39
        deep 945.49
          with loss of body part 945.59
    upper - *see* Burn, thigh
  lightning - *see* Burn, by site
  limb(s)
    lower (including foot or toe(s)) - *see* Burn, leg
    upper (except wrist and hand) - *see* Burn, arm(s)
  lip(s) 941.03
    with
      face or head - *see* Burn, head, multiple sites
    first degree 941.13
    second degree 941.23
    third degree 941.33
      deep 941.43
        with loss of body part 941.53
  lumbar region - *see* Burn, back
  lung 947.1
  malar region - *see* Burn, cheek
  mastoid region - *see* Burn, scalp
  membrane, tympanic - *see* Burn, ear
  midthoracic region - *see* Burn, chest wall
  mouth 947.0
  multiple (*see also* Burn, unspecified) 949.0
    specified sites classifiable to more than one category in 940-945 946.0
      first degree 946.1
      second degree 946.2
      third degree 946.3
        deep 946.4
          with loss of body part 946.5
  muscle, abdominal - *see* Burn, abdomen
  nasal (septum) - *see* Burn, nose
  neck 941.08
    with
      face or head - *see* Burn, head, multiple sites
    first degree 941.18
    second degree 941.28

ICD-9-CM
B
Vol. 2

Burn (*Continued*)
  neck (*Continued*)
    third degree 941.38
      deep 941.48
        with loss of body part 941.58
    nose (septum) 941.05
      with
        face or head - *see* Burn, head, multiple sites
      first degree 941.15
      second degree 941.25
      third degree 941.35
        deep 941.45
          with loss of body part 941.55
    occipital region - *see* Burn, scalp
    orbit region 940.1
      chemical 940.0
    oronasopharynx 947.0
    palate 947.0
    palm(s) 944.05
      with
        hand(s) and wrist(s) - *see* Burn, hand(s), multiple sites
      first degree 944.15
      second degree 944.25
      third degree 944.35
        deep 944.45
          with loss of a body part 944.55
    parietal region - *see* Burn, scalp
    penis - *see* Burn, genitourinary organs, external
    perineum - *see* Burn, genitourinary organs, external
    periocular area 940.1
      chemical 940.0
    pharynx 947.0
    pleura 947.1
    popliteal space - *see* Burn, knee
    prepuce - *see* Burn, genitourinary organs, external
    pubic region - *see* Burn, genitourinary organs, external
    pudenda - *see* Burn, genitourinary organs, external
    rectum 947.3
    sac, lacrimal 940.1
      chemical 940.0
    sacral region - *see* Burn, back
    salivary (ducts) (glands) 947.0
    scalp 941.06
      with
        face or neck - *see* Burn, head, multiple sites
      first degree 941.16
      second degree 941.26
      third degree 941.36
        deep 941.46
          with loss of body part 941.56
    scapular region 943.06
      with
        upper limb(s), except hand(s) or wrist(s) - *see* Burn, arm(s), multiple sites
      first degree 943.16
      second degree 943.26
      third degree 943.36
        deep 943.46
          with loss of body part 943.56
    sclera - *see* Burn, eyeball
    scrotum - *see* Burn, genitourinary organs, external
    septum, nasal - *see* Burn, nose
    shoulder(s) 943.05

Burn (*Continued*)
  shoulder(s) (*Continued*)
    with
      hand(s) and wrist(s) - *see* Burn, multiple, specified sites
      upper limb(s), except hand(s) or wrist(s) - *see* Burn, arm(s), multiple sites
    first degree 943.15
    second degree 943.25
    third degree 943.35
      deep 943.45
        with loss of body part 943.55
  skin NEC (*see also* Burn, unspecified) 949.0
  skull - *see* Burn, head
  small intestine 947.3
  sternal region - *see* Burn, chest wall
  stomach 947.3
  subconjunctival - *see* Burn, conjunctiva
  subcutaneous - *see* Burn, by site, third degree
  submaxillary region - *see* Burn, head
  submental region - *see* Burn, chin
  sun - *see* Sunburn
  supraclavicular fossa - *see* Burn, neck
  supraorbital - *see* Burn, forehead
  temple - *see* Burn, scalp
  temporal region - *see* Burn, scalp
  testicle - *see* Burn, genitourinary organs, external
  testis - *see* Burn, genitourinary organs, external
  thigh 945.06
    with
      lower limb(s) - *see* Burn, leg, multiple sites
    first degree 945.16
    second degree 945.26
    third degree 945.36
      deep 945.46
        with loss of body part 945.56
  thorax (external) - *see* Burn, chest wall
  throat 947.0
  thumb(s) (nail) (subungual) 944.02
    with
      finger(s) - *see* Burn, finger, with other sites, thumb
      hand(s) and wrist(s) - *see* Burn, hand(s), multiple sites
    first degree 944.12
    second degree 944.22
    third degree 944.32
      deep 944.42
        with loss of body part 944.52
  toe (nail) (subungual) 945.01
    with
      lower limb(s) - *see* Burn, leg, multiple sites
    first degree 945.11
    second degree 945.21
    third degree 945.31
      deep 945.41
        with loss of body part 945.51
  tongue 947.0
  tonsil 947.0
  trachea 947.1
  trunk 942.00
    first degree 942.10
    second degree 942.20
    third degree 942.30
      deep 942.40
        with loss of body part 942.50

Burn (*Continued*)
  trunk (*Continued*)
    multiple sites 942.09
      first degree 942.19
      second degree 942.29
      third degree 942.39
        deep 942.49
          with loss of body part 942.59
    specified site NEC 942.09
      first degree 942.19
      second degree 942.29
      third degree 942.39
        deep 942.49
          with loss of body part 942.59
    tunica vaginalis - *see* Burn, genitourinary organs, external
    tympanic membrane - *see* Burn, ear
    tympanum - *see* Burn, ear
    ultraviolet 692.82
    unspecified site (multiple) 949.0
      with extent of body surface involved specified
        less than 10 percent 948.0
        10-19 percent 948.1
        20-29 percent 948.2
        30-39 percent 948.3
        40-49 percent 948.4
        50-59 percent 948.5
        60-69 percent 948.6
        70-79 percent 948.7
        80-89 percent 948.8
        90 percent or more 948.9
      first degree 949.1
      second degree 949.2
      third degree 949.3
        deep 949.4
          with loss of body part 949.5
    uterus 947.4
    uvula 947.0
    vagina 947.4
    vulva - *see* Burn, genitourinary organs, external
    wrist(s) 944.07
      with
        hand(s) - *see* Burn, hand(s), multiple sites
      first degree 944.17
      second degree 944.27
      third degree 944.37
        deep 944.47
          with loss of body part 944.57
Burnett's syndrome (milk-alkali) 275.42
Burnier's syndrome (hypophyseal dwarfism) 253.3
Burning
  feet syndrome 266.2
  sensation (*see also* Disturbance, sensation) 782.0
  tongue 529.6
Burns' disease (osteochondrosis, lower ulna) 732.3
Bursa - *see also* condition
  pharynx 478.29
Bursitis NEC 727.3
  Achilles tendon 726.71
  adhesive 726.90
    shoulder 726.0
  ankle 726.79
  buttock 726.5
  calcaneal 726.79
  collateral ligament
    fibular 726.63
    tibial 726.62

◀ **New**   ◀▥ **Revised**

Bursitis NEC (*Continued*)
  Duplay's 726.2
  elbow 726.33
  finger 726.8
  foot 726.79
  gonococcal 098.52
  hand 726.4
  hip 726.5
  infrapatellar 726.69
  ischiogluteal 726.5
  knee 726.60
  occupational NEC 727.2
  olecranon 726.33
  pes anserinus 726.61
  pharyngeal 478.29
  popliteal 727.51
  prepatellar 726.65
  radiohumeral 727.3
  scapulohumeral 726.19
    adhesive 726.0

Bursitis NEC (*Continued*)
  shoulder 726.10
    adhesive 726.0
  subacromial 726.19
    adhesive 726.0
  subcoracoid 726.19
  subdeltoid 726.19
    adhesive 726.0
  subpatellar 726.69
  syphilitic 095.7
  Thornwaldt's, Tornwaldt's (pharyngeal) 478.29
  toe 726.79
  trochanteric area 726.5
  wrist 726.4
Burst stitches or sutures (complication of surgery) 998.32
  internal 998.31
Buruli ulcer 031.1

Bury's disease (erythema elevatum diutinum) 695.89
Buschke's disease or scleredema (adultorum) 710.1
Busquet's disease (osteoperiostitis) (*see also* Osteomyelitis) 730.1
Busse-Buschke disease (cryptococcosis) 117.5
Buttock - *see* condition
Button
  Biskra 085.1
  Delhi 085.1
  oriental 085.1
Buttonhole hand (intrinsic) 736.21
Bwamba fever (encephalitis) 066.3
Byssinosis (occupational) 504
Bywaters' syndrome 958.5

ICD-9-CM

B

Vol. 2

C

Cacergasia 300.9
Cachexia 799.4
  cancerous (M8000/3) 199.1
  cardiac - *see* Disease, heart
  dehydration 276.5
    with
      hypernatremia 276.0
      hyponatremia 276.1
  due to malnutrition 261
  exophthalmic 242.0
  heart - *see* Disease, heart
  hypophyseal 253.2
  hypopituitary 253.2
  lead 984.9
    specified type of lead - *see* Table of
      Drugs and Chemicals
  malaria 084.9
  malignant (M8000/3) 199.1
  marsh 084.9
  nervous 300.5
  old age 797
  pachydermic - *see* Hypothyroidism
  paludal 084.9
  pituitary (postpartum) 253.2
  renal (*see also* Disease, renal) 593.9
  saturnine 984.9
    specified type of lead - *see* Table of
      Drugs and Chemicals
  senile 797
  Simmonds' (pituitary cachexia) 253.2
  splenica 289.59
  strumipriva (*see also* Hypothyroidism)
    244.9
  tuberculous NEC (*see also* Tuberculo-
    sis) 011.9
Café au lait spots 709.09
Caffey's disease or syndrome (infantile
  cortical hyperostosis) 756.59
Caisson disease 993.3
Caked breast (puerperal, postpartum)
  676.2
Cake kidney 753.3
Calabar swelling 125.2
Calcaneal spur 726.73
Calcaneoapophysitis 732.5
Calcaneonavicular bar 755.67
Calcareous - *see* condition
Calcicosis (occupational) 502
Calciferol (vitamin D) deficiency
  268.9
  with
    osteomalacia 268.2
    rickets (*see also* Rickets) 268.0
Calcification
  adrenal (capsule) (gland) 255.4
    tuberculous (*see also* Tuberculosis)
      017.6
  aorta 440.0
  artery (annular) - *see* Arteriosclerosis
  auricle (ear) 380.89
  bladder 596.8
    due to S. hematobium 120.0
  brain (cortex) - *see* Calcification, cere-
    bral
  bronchus 519.1
  bursa 727.82
  cardiac (*see also* Degeneration, myocar-
    dial) 429.1
  cartilage (postinfectional) 733.99
  cerebral (cortex) 348.8
    artery 437.0
  cervix (uteri) 622.8

Calcification (*Continued*)
  choroid plexus 349.2
  conjunctiva 372.54
  corpora cavernosa (penis) 607.89
  cortex (brain) - *see* Calcification, cere-
    bral
  dental pulp (nodular) 522.2
  dentinal papilla 520.4
  disc, intervertebral 722.90
    cervical, cervicothoracic 722.91
    lumbar, lumbosacral 722.93
    thoracic, thoracolumbar 722.92
  fallopian tube 620.8
  falx cerebri - *see* Calcification, cerebral
  fascia 728.89
  gallbladder 575.8
  general 275.40
  heart (*see also* Degeneration, myocar-
    dial) 429.1
    valve - *see* Endocarditis
  intervertebral cartilage or disc (postin-
    fectional) 722.90
    cervical, cervicothoracic 722.91
    lumbar, lumbosacral 722.93
    thoracic, thoracolumbar 722.92
  intracranial - *see* Calcification, cerebral
  intraspinal ligament 728.89
  joint 719.80
    ankle 719.87
    elbow 719.82
    foot 719.87
    hand 719.84
    hip 719.85
    knee 719.86
    multiple sites 719.89
    pelvic region 719.85
    shoulder (region) 719.81
    specified site NEC 719.88
    wrist 719.83
  kidney 593.89
    tuberculous (*see also* Tuberculosis)
      016.0
  larynx (senile) 478.79
  lens 366.8
  ligament 728.89
    intraspinal 728.89
    knee (medial collateral) 717.89
  lung 518.89
    active 518.89
    postinfectional 518.89
    tuberculous (*see also* Tuberculosis,
      pulmonary) 011.9
  lymph gland or node (postinfectional)
    289.3
    tuberculous (*see also* Tuberculosis,
      lymph gland) 017.2
  massive (paraplegic) 728.10
  medial (*see also* Arteriosclerosis, ex-
    tremities) 440.20
  meninges (cerebral) 349.2
  metastatic 275.40
  Mönckeberg's - *see* Arteriosclerosis
  muscle 728.10
    heterotopic, postoperative 728.13
  myocardium, myocardial (*see also* De-
    generation, myocardial) 429.1
  ovary 620.8
  pancreas 577.8
  penis 607.89
  periarticular 728.89
  pericardium (*see also* Pericarditis) 423.8
  pineal gland 259.8
  pleura 511.0
    postinfectional 518.89

Calcification (*Continued*)
  pleura (*Continued*)
    tuberculous (*see also* Tuberculosis,
      pleura) 012.0
  pulp (dental) (nodular) 522.2
  renal 593.89
  Rider's bone 733.99
  sclera 379.16
  semilunar cartilage 717.89
  spleen 289.59
  subcutaneous 709.3
  suprarenal (capsule) (gland) 255.4
  tendon (sheath) 727.82
    with bursitis, synovitis or tenosyno-
      vitis 727.82
  trachea 519.1
  ureter 593.89
  uterus 621.8
  vitreous 379.29
Calcified - *see also* Calcification
  hematoma NEC 959.9
Calcinosis (generalized) (interstitial) (tu-
  moral) (universalis) 275.49
  circumscripta 709.3
  cutis 709.3
  intervertebralis 275.49 [722.90]
  Raynaud's phenomenon sclerodactyly-
    telangiectasis (CRST) 710.1
Calcium
  blood
    high (*see also* Hypercalcemia) 275.42
    low (*see also* Hypocalcemia) 275.41
  deposits - *see also* Calcification, by site
    in bursa 727.82
    in tendon (sheath) 727.82
      with bursitis, synovitis or teno-
        synovitis 727.82
  salts or soaps in vitreous 379.22
Calciuria 791.9
Calculi - *see* Calculus
Calculosis, intrahepatic - *see* Choledocholithiasis
Calculus, calculi, calculous 592.9
  ampulla of Vater - *see* Choledocholi-
    thiasis
  anuria (impacted) (recurrent) 592.0
  appendix 543.9
  bile duct (any) - *see* Choledocholithiasis
  biliary - *see* Cholelithiasis
  bilirubin, multiple - *see* Cholelithiasis
  bladder (encysted) (impacted) (uri-
    nary) 594.1
    diverticulum 594.0
  bronchus 518.89
  calyx (kidney) (renal) 592.0
    congenital 753.3
  cholesterol (pure) (solitary) - *see* Chole-
    lithiasis
  common duct (bile) - *see* Choledocho-
    lithiasis
  conjunctiva 372.54
  cystic 594.1
    duct - *see* Cholelithiasis
  dental 523.6
    subgingival 523.6
    supragingival 523.6
  epididymis 608.89
  gallbladder - *see also* Cholelithiasis
    congenital 751.69
  hepatic (duct) - *see* Choledocholithiasis
  intestine (impaction) (obstruction)
    560.39
  kidney (impacted) (multiple) (pelvis)
    (recurrent) (staghorn) 592.0

Calculus, calculi, calculous (Continued)
  kidney (Continued)
    congenital 753.3
    lacrimal (passages) 375.57
    liver (impacted) - see Choledocholithiasis
    lung 518.89
    nephritic (impacted) (recurrent) 592.0
    nose 478.1
    pancreas (duct) 577.8
    parotid gland 527.5
    pelvis, encysted 592.0
    prostate 602.0
    pulmonary 518.89
    renal (impacted) (recurrent) 592.0
      congenital 753.3
    salivary (duct) (gland) 527.5
    seminal vesicle 608.89
    staghorn 592.0
    Stensen's duct 527.5
    sublingual duct or gland 527.5
      congenital 750.26
    submaxillary duct, gland, or region 527.5
    suburethral 594.8
    tonsil 474.8
    tooth, teeth 523.6
    tunica vaginalis 608.89
    ureter (impacted) (recurrent) 592.1
    urethra (impacted) 594.2
    urinary (duct) (impacted) (passage)
      (tract) 592.9
      lower tract NEC 594.9
        specified site 594.8
    vagina 623.8
    vesicle (impacted) 594.1
    Wharton's duct 527.5
Caliectasis 593.89
California
  disease 114.0
  encephalitis 062.5
Caligo cornea 371.03
Callositas, callosity (infected) 700
Callus (infected) 700
  bone 726.91
  excessive, following fracture - see also
    Late, effect (of), fracture
Calvé (-Perthes) disease (osteochon-
    drosis, femoral capital) 732.1
Calvities (see also Alopecia) 704.00
Cameroon fever (see also Malaria) 084.6
Camptocormia 300.11
Camptodactyly (congenital) 755.59
Camurati-Engelmann disease (diaphy-
    seal sclerosis) 756.59
Canal - see condition
Canaliculitis (lacrimal) (acute) 375.31
  Actinomyces 039.8
  chronic 375.41
Canavan's disease 330.0
Cancer (M8000/3)-see also Neoplasm, by
    site, malignant

Note   The term "cancer" when modified by an adjective or adjectival
phrase indicating a morphological
type should be coded in the same
manner as "carcinoma" with that adjective or phrase. Thus, "squamous-
cell cancer" should be coded in the
same manner as "squamous-cell carcinoma," which appears in the list
under "Carcinoma."

  bile duct type (M8160/3), liver 155.1
  hepatocellular (M8170/3) 155.0

Cancerous (M8000/3) - see Neoplasm, by
    site, malignant
Cancerphobia 300.29
Cancrum oris 528.1
Candidiasis, candidal 112.9
  with pneumonia 112.4
  balanitis 112.2
  congenital 771.7
  disseminated 112.5
  endocarditis 112.81
  esophagus 112.84
  intertrigo 112.3
  intestine 112.85
  lung 112.4
  meningitis 112.83
  mouth 112.0
  nails 112.3
  neonatal 771.7
  onychia 112.3
  otitis externa 112.82
  otomycosis 112.82
  paronychia 112.3
  perionyxis 112.3
  pneumonia 112.4
  pneumonitis 112.4
  skin 112.3
  specified site NEC 112.89
  systemic 112.5
  urogenital site NEC 112.2
  vagina 112.1
  vulva 112.1
  vulvovaginitis 112.1
Candidiosis - see Candidiasis
Candiru infection or infestation 136.8
Canities (premature) 704.3
  congenital 757.4
Canker (mouth) (sore) 528.2
  rash 034.1
Cannabinosis 504
Canton fever 081.9
Cap
  cradle 690.11
Capillariasis 127.5
Capillary - see condition
Caplan's syndrome 714.81
Caplan-Colinet syndrome 714.81
Capsule - see condition
Capsulitis (joint) 726.90
  adhesive (shoulder) 726.0
  hip 726.5
  knee 726.60
  labyrinthine 387.8
  thyroid 245.9
  wrist 726.4
Caput
  crepitus 756.0
  medusae 456.8
  succedaneum 767.19
Carapata disease 087.1
Carate - see Pinta
Carboxyhemoglobinemia 986
Carbuncle 680.9
  abdominal wall 680.2
  ankle 680.6
  anus 680.5
  arm (any part, above wrist) 680.3
  auditory canal, external 680.0
  axilla 680.3
  back (any part) 680.2
  breast 680.2
  buttock 680.5
  chest wall 680.2
  corpus cavernosum 607.2
  ear (any part) (external) 680.0

Carbuncle (Continued)
  eyelid 373.13
  face (any part, except eye) 680.0
  finger (any) 680.4
  flank 680.2
  foot (any part) 680.7
  forearm 680.3
  genital organ (male) 608.4
  gluteal (region) 680.5
  groin 680.2
  hand (any part) 680.4
  head (any part, except face) 680.8
  heel 680.7
  hip 680.6
  kidney (see also Abscess, kidney) 590.2
  knee 680.6
  labia 616.4
  lacrimal
    gland (see also Dacryoadenitis) 375.00
    passages (duct) (sac) (see also Dac-
      ryocystitis) 375.30
  leg, any part except foot 680.6
  lower extremity, any part except foot
    680.6
  malignant 022.0
  multiple sites 680.9
  neck 680.1
  nose (external) (septum) 680.0
  orbit, orbital 376.01
  partes posteriores 680.5
  pectoral region 680.2
  penis 607.2
  perineum 680.2
  pinna 680.0
  scalp (any part) 680.8
  scrotum 608.4
  seminal vesicle 608.0
  shoulder 680.3
  skin NEC 680.9
  specified site NEC 680.8
  spermatic cord 608.4
  temple (region) 680.0
  testis 608.4
  thigh 680.6
  thumb 680.4
  toe (any) 680.7
  trunk 680.2
  tunica vaginalis 608.4
  umbilicus 680.2
  upper arm 680.3
  urethra 597.0
  vas deferens 608.4
  vulva 616.4
  wrist 680.4
Carbunculus (see also Carbuncle) 680.9
Carcinoid (tumor) (M8240/1) - see also
    Neoplasm, by site, uncertain behavior
    and struma ovarii (M9091/1) 236.2
  argentaffin (M8241/1) - see Neoplasm,
    by site, uncertain behavior
    malignant (M8241/3) - see Neo-
      plasm, by site, malignant
  benign (M9091/0) 220
  composite (M8244/3) - see Neoplasm,
    by site, malignant
  goblet cell (M8243/3) - see Neoplasm,
    by site, malignant
  malignant (M8240/3) - see Neoplasm,
    by site, malignant
  nonargentaffin (M8242/1) - see also Ne-
    oplasm, by site, uncertain behavior
    malignant (M8242/3) - see Neo-
      plasm, by site, malignant
  strumal (M9091/1) 236.2

ICD-9-CM

C

Vol. 2

Carcinoid *(Continued)*
  syndrome (intestinal) (metastatic) 259.2
  type bronchial adenoma (M8240/3) - *see* Neoplasm, lung, malignant
Carcinoidosis 259.2
Carcinoma (M8010/3) - *see also* Neoplasm, by site, malignant

> Note Except where otherwise indicated, the morphological varieties of carcinoma in the list below should be coded by site as for "Neoplasm, malignant."

  with
    apocrine metaplasia (M8573/3)
    cartilaginous (and osseous) metaplasia (M8571/3)
    osseous (and cartilaginous) metaplasia (M8571/3)
    productive fibrosis (M8141/3)
    spindle cell metaplasia (M8572/3)
    squamous metaplasia (M8570/3)
  acidophil (M8280/3)
    specified site - *see* Neoplasm, by site, malignant
    unspecified site 194.3
  acidophil-basophil, mixed (M8281/3)
    specified site - *see* Neoplasm, by site, malignant
    unspecified site 194.3
  acinar (cell) (M8550/3)
  acinic cell (M8550/3)
  adenocystic (M8200/3)
  adenoid
    cystic (M8200/3)
    squamous cell (M8075/3)
  adenosquamous (M8560/3)
  adnexal (skin) (M8390/3) - *see* Neoplasm, skin, malignant
  adrenal cortical (M8370/3) 194.0
  alveolar (M8251/3)
    cell (M8250/3) - *see* Neoplasm, lung, malignant
  anaplastic type (M8021/3)
  apocrine (M8401/3)
    breast - *see* Neoplasm, breast, malignant
    specified site NEC - *see* Neoplasm, skin, malignant
    unspecified site 173.9
  basal cell (pigmented) (M8090/3) - *see also* Neoplasm, skin, malignant
    fibro-epithelial type (M8093/3) - *see* Neoplasm, skin, malignant
    morphea type (M8092/3) - *see* Neoplasm, skin, malignant
    multicentric (M8091/3) - *see* Neoplasm, skin, malignant
  basaloid (M8123/3)
  basal-squamous cell, mixed (M8094/3) - *see* Neoplasm, skin, malignant
  basophil (M8300/3)
    specified site - *see* Neoplasm, by site, malignant
    unspecified site 194.3
  basophil-acidophil, mixed (M8281/3)
    specified site - *see* Neoplasm, by site, malignant
    unspecified site 194.3
  basosquamous (M8094/3) - *see* Neoplasm, skin, malignant

Carcinoma *(Continued)*
  bile duct type (M8160/3)
    and hepatocellular, mixed (M8180/3) 155.0
    liver 155.1
    specified site NEC - *see* Neoplasm, by site, malignant
    unspecified site 155.1
  branchial or branchiogenic 146.8
  bronchial or bronchogenic - *see* Neoplasm, lung, malignant
  bronchiolar (terminal) (M8250/3) - *see* Neoplasm, lung, malignant
  bronchiolo-alveolar (M8250/3) - *see* Neoplasm, lung, malignant
  bronchogenic (epidermoid) 162.9
  C cell (M8510/3)
    specified site - *see* Neoplasm, by site, malignant
    unspecified site 193
  ceruminous (M8420/3) 173.2
  chorionic (M9100/3)
    specified site - *see* Neoplasm, by site, malignant
    unspecified site
      female 181
      male 186.9
  chromophobe (M8270/3)
    specified site - *see* Neoplasm, by site, malignant
    unspecified site 194.3
  clear cell (mesonephroid type) (M8310/3)
  cloacogenic (M8124/3)
    specified site - *see* Neoplasm, by site, malignant
    unspecified site 154.8
  colloid (M8480/3)
  cribriform (M8201/3)
  cylindroid type (M8200/3)
  diffuse type (M8145/3)
    specified site - *see* Neoplasm, by site, malignant
    unspecified site 151.9
  duct (cell) (M8500/3)
    with Paget's disease (M8541/3) - *see* Neoplasm, breast, malignant
    infiltrating (M8500/3)
      specified site - *see* Neoplasm, by site, malignant
      unspecified site 174.9
  ductal (M8500/3)
  ductular, infiltrating (M8521/3)
  embryonal (M9070/3)
    and teratoma, mixed (M9081/3)
    combined with choriocarcinoma (M9101/3) - *see* Neoplasm, by site, malignant
    infantile type (M9071/3)
    liver 155.0
    polyembryonal type (M9072/3)
  endometrioid (M8380/3)
  eosinophil (M8280/3)
    specified site - *see* Neoplasm, by site, malignant
    unspecified site 194.3
  epidermoid (M8070/3) - *see also* Carcinoma, squamous cell
    and adenocarcinoma, mixed (M8560/3)
    in situ, Bowen's type (M8081/2) - *see* Neoplasm, skin, in situ
    intradermal - *see* Neoplasm, skin, in situ

Carcinoma *(Continued)*
  fibroepithelial type basal cell (M8093/3) - *see* Neoplasm, skin, malignant
  follicular (M8330/3)
    and papillary (mixed) (M8340/3) 193
    moderately differentiated type (M8332/3) 193
    pure follicle type (M8331/3) 193
    specified site - *see* Neoplasm, by site, malignant
    trabecular type (M8332/3) 193
    unspecified site 193
    well differentiated type (M8331/3) 193
  gelatinous (M8480/3)
  giant cell (M8031/3)
    and spindle cell (M8030/3)
  granular cell (M8320/3)
  granulosa cell (M8620/3) 183.0
  hepatic cell (M8170/3) 155.0
  hepatocellular (M8170/3) 155.0
    and bile duct, mixed (M8180/3) 155.0
  hepatocholangiolitic (M8180/3) 155.0
  Hürthle cell (thyroid) 193
  hypernephroid (M8311/3)
  in
    adenomatous
      polyp (M8210/3)
      polyposis coli (M8220/3) 153.9
    pleomorphic adenoma (M8940/3)
    polypoid adenoma (M8210/3)
    situ (M8010/3) - *see* Carcinoma, in situ
    tubular adenoma (M8210/3)
    villous adenoma (M8261/3)
  infiltrating duct (M8500/3)
    with Paget's disease (M8541/3) - *see* Neoplasm, breast, malignant
    specified site - *see* Neoplasm, by site, malignant
    unspecified site 174.9
  inflammatory (M8530/3)
    specified site - *see* Neoplasm, by site, malignant
    unspecified site 174.9
  in situ (M8010/2) - *see also* Neoplasm, by site, in situ
    epidermoid (M8070/2) - *see also* Neoplasm, by site, in situ
      with questionable stromal invasion (M8076/2)
      specified site - *see* Neoplasm, by site, in situ
      unspecified site 233.1
    Bowen's type (M8081/2) - *see* Neoplasm, skin, in situ
    intraductal (M8500/2)
      specified site - *see* Neoplasm, by site, in situ
      unspecified site 233.0
    lobular (M8520/2)
      specified site - *see* Neoplasm, by site, in situ
      unspecified site 233.0
    papillary (M8050/2) - *see* Neoplasm, by site, in situ
    squamous cell (M8070/2) - *see also* Neoplasm, by site, in situ
      with questionable stromal invasion (M8076/2)
      specified site - *see* Neoplasm, by site, in situ
      unspecified site 233.1

Carcinoma *(Continued)*
  in situ *(Continued)*
    transitional cell (M8120/2) - *see*
        Neoplasm, by site, in situ
    intestinal type (M8144/3)
      specified site - *see* Neoplasm, by site,
          malignant
      unspecified site 151.9
    intraductal (noninfiltrating)
        (M8500/2)
      papillary (M8503/2)
        specified site - *see* Neoplasm, by
            site, in situ
        unspecified site 233.0
      specified site - *see* Neoplasm, by site,
          in situ
      unspecified site 233.0
    intraepidermal (M8070/2) - *see also*
        Neoplasm, skin, in situ
      squamous cell, Bowen's type
          (M8081/2) - *see* Neoplasm, skin,
          in situ
    intraepithelial (M8010/2) - *see also*
        Neoplasm, by site, in situ
      squamous cell (M8072/2) - *see* Neo-
          plasm, by site, in situ
  intraosseous (M9270/3) 170.1
    upper jaw (bone) 170.0
  islet cell (M8150/3)
    and exocrine, mixed (M8154/3)
      specified site - *see* Neoplasm, by
          site, malignant
      unspecified site 157.9
    pancreas 157.4
    specified site NEC - *see* Neoplasm,
        by site, malignant
    unspecified site 157.4
  juvenile, breast (M8502/3) - *see* Neo-
      plasm, breast, malignant
  Kulchitsky's cell (carcinoid tumor of
      intestine) 259.2
  large cell (M8012/3)
    squamous cell, non-keratinizing type
        (M8072/3)
  Leydig cell (testis) (M8650/3)
    specified site - *see* Neoplasm, by site,
        malignant
    unspecified site 186.9
      female 183.0
      male 186.9
  liver cell (M8170/3) 155.0
  lobular (infiltrating) (M8520/3)
    noninfiltrating (M8520/3)
      specified site - *see* Neoplasm, by
          site, in situ
      unspecified site 233.0
    specified site - *see* Neoplasm, by site,
        malignant
    unspecified site 174.9
  lymphoepithelial (M8082/3)
  medullary (M8510/3)
    with
      amyloid stroma (M8511/3)
        specified site - *see* Neoplasm, by
            site, malignant
        unspecified site 193
      lymphoid stroma (M8512/3)
        specified site - *see* Neoplasm, by
            site, malignant
        unspecified site 174.9
  mesometanephric (M9110/3)
  mesonephric (M9110/3)
  metastatic (M8010/6) - *see* Metastasis,
      cancer

Carcinoma *(Continued)*
  metatypical (M8095/3) - *see* Neoplasm,
      skin, malignant
  morphea type basal cell (M8092/3) -
      see Neoplasm, skin, malignant
  mucinous (M8480/3)
  mucin-producing (M8481/3)
  mucin-secreting (M8481/3)
  mucoepidermoid (M8430/3)
  mucoid (M8480/3)
    cell (M8300/3)
      specified site - *see* Neoplasm, by
          site, malignant
      unspecified site 194.3
  mucous (M8480/3)
  nonencapsulated sclerosing (M8350/3)
      193
  noninfiltrating
    intracystic (M8504/2) - *see* Neo-
        plasm, by site, in situ
    intraductal (M8500/2)
      papillary (M8503/2)
        specified site - *see* Neoplasm, by
            site, in situ
        unspecified site 233.0
      specified site - *see* Neoplasm, by
          site, in situ
      unspecified site 233.0
    lobular (M8520/2)
      specified site - *see* Neoplasm, by
          site, in situ
      unspecified site 233.0
  oat cell (M8042/3)
    specified site - *see* Neoplasm, by site,
        malignant
    unspecified site 162.9
  odontogenic (M9270/3) 170.1
    upper jaw (bone) 170.0
  oncocytic (M8290/3)
  oxyphilic (M8290/3)
  papillary (M8050/3)
    and follicular (mixed) (M8340/3) 193
    epidermoid (M8052/3)
    intraductal (noninfiltrating) (M8503/2)
      specified site - *see* Neoplasm, by
          site, in situ
      unspecified site 233.0
    serous (M8460/3)
      specified site - *see* Neoplasm, by
          site, malignant
      surface (M8461/3)
        specified site - *see* Neoplasm, by
            site, malignant
        unspecified site 183.0
      unspecified site 183.0
    squamous cell (M8052/3)
    transitional cell (M8130/3)
  papillocystic (M8450/3)
    specified site - *see* Neoplasm, by site,
        malignant
    unspecified site 183.0
  parafollicular cell (M8510/3)
    specified site - *see* Neoplasm, by site,
        malignant
    unspecified site 193
  pleomorphic (M8022/3)
  polygonal cell (M8034/3)
  prickle cell (M8070/3)
  pseudoglandular, squamous cell
      (M8075/3)
  pseudomucinous (M8470/3)
    specified site - *see* Neoplasm, by site,
        malignant
    unspecified site 183.0

Carcinoma *(Continued)*
  pseudosarcomatous (M8033/3)
  regaud type (M8082/3) - *see* Neo-
      plasm, nasopharynx, malignant
  renal cell (M8312/3) 189.0
  reserve cell (M8041/3)
  round cell (M8041/3)
  Schmincke (M8082/3) - *see* Neoplasm,
      nasopharynx, malignant
  Schneiderian (M8121/3)
    specified site - *see* Neoplasm, by site,
        malignant
    unspecified site 160.0
  scirrhous (M8141/3)
  sebaceous (M8410/3) - *see* Neoplasm,
      skin, malignant
  secondary (M8010/6) - *see* Neoplasm,
      by site, malignant, secondary
  secretory, breast (M8502/3) - *see* Neo-
      plasm, breast, malignant
  serous (M8441/3)
    papillary (M8460/3)
      specified site - *see* Neoplasm, by
          site, malignant
      unspecified site 183.0
    surface, papillary (M8461/3)
      specified site - *see* Neoplasm, by
          site, malignant
      unspecified site 183.0
  Sertoli cell (M8640/3)
    specified site - *see* Neoplasm, by site,
        malignant
    unspecified site 186.9
  signet ring cell (M8490/3)
    metastatic (M8490/6) - *see* Neo-
        plasm, by site, secondary
  simplex (M8231/3)
  skin appendage (M8390/3) - *see* Neo-
      plasm, skin, malignant
  small cell (M8041/3)
    fusiform cell type (M8043/3)
    squamous cell, nonkeratinizing type
        (M8073/3)
  solid (M8230/3)
    with amyloid stroma (M8511/3)
      specified site - *see* Neoplasm, by
          site, malignant
      unspecified site 193
  spheroidal cell (M8035/3)
  spindle cell (M8032/3)
    and giant cell (M8030/3)
  spinous cell (M8070/3)
  squamous (cell) (M8070/3)
    adenoid type (M8075/3)
    and adenocarcinoma, mixed
        (M8560/3)
    intraepidermal, Bowen's type - *see*
        Neoplasm, skin, in situ
    keratinizing type (large cell)
        (M8071/3)
    large cell, nonkeratinizing type
        (M8072/3)
    microinvasive (M8076/3)
      specified site - *see* Neoplasm, by
          site, malignant
      unspecified site 180.9
    nonkeratinizing type (M8072/3)
    papillary (M8052/3)
    pseudoglandular (M8075/3)
    small cell, nonkeratinizing type
        (M8073/3)
    spindle cell type (M8074/3)
    verrucous (M8051/3)
  superficial spreading (M8143/3)

ICD-9-CM

c

Vol. 2

Carcinoma (Continued)
sweat gland (M8400/3) - see Neoplasm, skin, malignant
theca cell (M8600/3) 183.0
thymic (M8580/3) 164.0
trabecular (M8190/3)
transitional (cell) (M8120/3)
papillary (M8130/3)
spindle cell type (M8122/3)
tubular (M8211/3)
undifferentiated type (M8020/3)
urothelial (M8120/3)
ventriculi 151.9
verrucous (epidermoid) (squamous
cell) (M8051/3)
villous (M8262/3)
water-clear cell (M8322/3) 194.1
wolffian duct (M9110/3)
Carcinomaphobia 300.29
Carcinomatosis
peritonei (M8010/6) 197.6
specified site NEC (M8010/3) - see
Neoplasm, by site, malignant
unspecified site (M8010/6) 199.0
Carcinosarcoma (M8980/3) - see also
Neoplasm, by site, malignant
embryonal type (M8981/3) - see Neoplasm, by site, malignant
Cardia, cardial - see condition
Cardiac - see also condition
death - see Disease, heart
device
defibrillator, automatic implantable
V45.02
in situ NEC V45.00
pacemaker
cardiac
fitting or adjustment V53.31
in situ V45.01
carotid sinus
fitting or adjustment V53.39
in situ V45.09
pacemaker - see Cardiac, device, pacemaker
tamponade 423.9
Cardialgia (see also Pain, precordial) 786.51
Cardiectasis - see Hypertrophy, cardiac
Cardiochalasia 530.81
Cardiomalacia (see also Degeneration,
myocardial) 429.1
Cardiomegalia glycogenica diffusa 271.0
Cardiomegaly (see also Hypertrophy, cardiac) 429.3
congenital 746.89
glycogen 271.0
hypertensive (see also Hypertension,
heart) 402.90
idiopathic 425.4
Cardiomyoliposis (see also Degeneration,
myocardial) 429.1
Cardiomyopathy (congestive) (constrictive) (familial) (infiltrative) (obstructive) (restrictive) (sporadic) 425.4
alcoholic 425.5
amyloid 277.3 [425.7]
beriberi 265.0 [425.7]
cobalt-beer 425.5
congenital 425.3
due to
amyloidosis 277.3 [425.7]
beriberi 265.0 [425.7]
cardiac glycogenosis 271.0 [425.7]
Chagas' disease 086.0
Friedreich's ataxia 334.0 [425.8]

Cardiomyopathy (Continued)
due to (Continued)
hypertension - see Hypertension,
with, heart involvement
mucopolysaccharidosis 277.5 [425.7]
myotonia atrophica 359.2 [425.8]
progressive muscular dystrophy
359.1 [425.8]
sarcoidosis 135 [425.8]
glycogen storage 271.0 [425.7]
hypertensive - see Hypertension, with,
heart involvement
hypertrophic
nonobstructive 425.4
obstructive 425.1
congenital 746.84
idiopathic (concentric) 425.4
in
Chagas' disease 086.0
sarcoidosis 135 [425.8]
ischemic 414.8
metabolic NEC 277.9 [425.7]
amyloid 277.3 [425.7]
thyrotoxic (see also Thyrotoxicosis)
242.9 [425.7]
thyrotoxicosis (see also Thyrotoxicosis) 242.9 [425.7]
nutritional 269.9 [425.7]
beriberi 265.0 [425.7]
obscure of Africa 425.2
peripartum 674.5
postpartum 674.5
primary 425.4
secondary 425.9
thyrotoxic (see also Thyrotoxicosis)
242.9 [425.7]
toxic NEC 425.9
tuberculous (see also Tuberculosis)
017.9 [425.8]
Cardionephritis - see Hypertension, cardiorenal
Cardionephropathy - see Hypertension,
cardiorenal
Cardionephrosis - see Hypertension, cardiorenal
Cardioneurosis 306.2
Cardiopathia nigra 416.0
Cardiopathy (see also Disease, heart) 429.9
hypertensive (see also Hypertension,
heart) 402.90
idiopathic 425.4
mucopolysaccharidosis 277.5 [425.7]
Cardiopericarditis (see also Pericarditis)
423.9
Cardiophobia 300.29
Cardioptosis 746.87
Cardiorenal - see condition
Cardiorrhexis (see also Infarct, myocar-
dium) 410.9
Cardiosclerosis - see Arteriosclerosis, cor-
onary
Cardiosis - see Disease, heart
Cardiospasm (esophagus) (reflex) (stom-
ach) 530.0
congenital 750.7
Cardiostenosis - see Disease, heart
Cardiosymphysis 423.1
Cardiothyrotoxicosis - see Hyperthyroidism
Cardiovascular - see condition
Carditis (acute) (bacterial) (chronic) (sub-
acute) 429.89
Coxsackie 074.20
hypertensive (see also Hypertension,
heart) 402.90

Carditis (Continued)
meningococcal 036.40
rheumatic - see Disease, heart, rheumatic
rheumatoid 714.2
Care (of)
child (routine) V20.1
convalescent following V66.9
chemotherapy V66.2
medical NEC V66.5
psychotherapy V66.3
radiotherapy V66.1
surgery V66.0
surgical NEC V66.0
treatment (for) V66.5
combined V66.6
fracture V66.4
mental disorder NEC V66.3
specified type NEC V66.5
end-of-life V66.7
family member (handicapped) (sick)
creating problem for family
V61.49
provided away from home for holiday relief V60.5
unavailable, due to
absence (person rendering care)
(sufferer) V60.4
inability (any reason) of person
rendering care V60.4
holiday relief V60.5
hospice V66.7
lack of (at or after birth) (infant)
(child) 995.52
adult 995.84
lactation of mother V24.1
palliative V66.7
postpartum
immediately after delivery V24.0
routine follow-up V24.2
prenatal V22.1
first pregnancy V22.0
high-risk pregnancy V23.9
specified problem NEC V23.8
terminal V66.7
unavailable, due to
absence of person rendering care
V60.4
inability (any reason) of person rendering care V60.4
well baby V20.1
Caries (bone) (see also Tuberculosis,
bone) 015.9 [730.8]
arrested 521.04
cementum 521.03
cerebrospinal (tuberculous) 015.0 [730.88]
dental (acute) (chronic) (incipient)
(infected) 521.00   ◄▥
with pulp exposure 521.03
extending to
dentine 521.02
pulp 521.03
other specified NEC 521.09
pit and fissure 521.06   ◄
root surface 521.08   ◄
smooth surface 521.07   ◄
dentin (acute) (chronic) 521.02
enamel (acute) (chronic) (incipient)
521.01
external meatus 380.89
hip (see also Tuberculosis) 015.1 [730.85]
initial 521.01   ◄
knee 015.2 [730.86]
labyrinth 386.8

◄ **New**   ◄▥ **Revised**

Caries (Continued)
limb NEC 015.7 [730.88]
mastoid (chronic) (process) 383.1
middle ear 385.89
nose 015.7 [730.88]
orbit 015.7 [730.88]
ossicle 385.24
petrous bone 383.20
sacrum (tuberculous) 015.0 [730.88]
spine, spinal (column) (tuberculous)
015.0 [730.88]
syphilitic 095.5
congenital 090.0 [730.8]
teeth (internal) 521.00
initial 521.01
vertebra (column) (tuberculous) 015.0
[730.88]
Carini's syndrome (ichthyosis congenita)
757.1
Carious teeth 521.00
Carneous mole 631
Carnosinemia 270.5
Carotid body or sinus syndrome 337.0
Carotidynia 337.0
Carotinemia (dietary) 278.3
Carotinosis (cutis) (skin) 278.3
Carpal tunnel syndrome 354.0
Carpenter's syndrome 759.89
Carpopedal spasm (see also Tetany) 781.7
Carpoptosis 736.05
Carrier (suspected) of
amebiasis V02.2
bacterial disease (meningococcal,
staphylococcal) NEC V02.59
cholera V02.0
cystic fibrosis gene V83.81
defective gene V83.89
diphtheria V02.4
dysentery (bacillary) V02.3
amebic V02.2
Entamoeba histolytica V02.2
gastrointestinal pathogens NEC
V02.3
genetic defect V83.89
gonorrhea V02.7
group B streptococcus V02.51
HAA (hepatitis Australian-antigen)
V02.61
hemophilia A (asymptomatic) V83.01
symptomatic V83.02
hepatitis V02.60
Australian-antigen (HAA) V02.61
B V02.61
C V02.62
specified type NEC V02.69
serum V02.61
viral V02.60
infective organism NEC V02.9
malaria V02.9
paratyphoid V02.3
Salmonella V02.3
typhosa V02.1
serum hepatitis V02.61
Shigella V02.3
Staphylococcus NEC V02.59
Streptococcus NEC V02.52
group B V02.51
typhoid V02.1
venereal disease NEC V02.8
Carrión's disease (Bartonellosis) 088.0
Car sickness 994.6
Carter's
relapsing fever (Asiatic) 087.0
Cartilage - see condition

Caruncle (inflamed)
abscess, lacrimal (see also Dacryocystitis) 375.30
conjunctiva 372.00
acute 372.00
eyelid 373.00
labium (majus) (minus) 616.8
lacrimal 375.30
urethra (benign) 599.3
vagina (wall) 616.8
Cascade stomach 537.6
Caseation lymphatic gland (see also Tuberculosis) 017.2
Caseous
bronchitis - see Tuberculosis, pulmonary
meningitis 013.0
pneumonia - see Tuberculosis, pulmonary
Cassidy (-Scholte) **syndrome** (malignant
carcinoid) 259.2
Castellani's bronchitis 104.8
Castleman's tumor or lymphoma (mediastinal lymph node hyperplasia) 785.6
Castration, traumatic 878.2
complicated 878.3
Casts in urine 791.7
Cat's ear 744.29
Catalepsy 300.11
catatonic (acute) (see also Schizophrenia) 295.2
hysterical 300.11
schizophrenic (see also Schizophrenia)
295.2
Cataphasia 307.0
Cataplexy (idiopathic) (see also
Narcolepsy) ◀▥
Cataract (anterior cortical) (anterior polar) (black) (capsular) (central) (cortical) (hypermature) (immature) (incipient) (mature) 366.9
anterior
and posterior axial embryonal 743.33
pyramidal 743.31
subcapsular polar
infantile, juvenile, or presenile 366.01
senile 366.13
associated with
calcinosis 275.40 [366.42]
craniofacial dysostosis 756.0 [366.44]
galactosemia 271.1 [366.44]
hypoparathyroidism 252.1 [366.42]
myotonic disorders 359.2 [366.43]
neovascularization 366.33
blue dot 743.39
cerulean 743.39
complicated NEC 366.30
congenital 743.30
capsular or subcapsular 743.31
cortical 743.32
nuclear 743.33
specified type NEC 743.39
total or subtotal 743.34
zonular 743.32
coronary (congenital) 743.39
acquired 366.12
cupuliform 366.14
diabetic 250.5 [366.41]
drug-induced 366.45
due to
chalcosis 360.24 [366.34]
chronic choroiditis (see also Choroiditis) 363.20 [366.32]
degenerative myopia 360.21 [366.34]
glaucoma (see also Glaucoma) 365.9
[366.31]

Cataract (Continued)
due to (Continued)
infection, intraocular NEC 366.32
inflammatory ocular disorder NEC
366.32
iridocyclitis, chronic 364.10 [366.33]
pigmentary retinal dystrophy 362.74
[366.34]
radiation 366.46
electric 366.46
glassblowers' 366.46
heat ray 366.46
heterochromic 366.33
in eye disease NEC 366.30
infantile (see also Cataract, juvenile)
366.00
intumescent 366.12
irradiational 366.46
juvenile 366.00
anterior subcapsular polar 366.01
combined forms 366.09
cortical 366.03
lamellar 366.03
nuclear 366.04
posterior subcapsular polar 366.02
specified NEC 366.09
zonular 366.03
lamellar 743.32
infantile juvenile, or presenile 366.03
morgagnian 366.18
myotonic 359.2 [366.43]
myxedema 244.9 [366.44]
nuclear 366.16
posterior, polar (capsular) 743.31
infantile, juvenile, or presenile
366.02
senile 366.14
presenile (see also Cataract, juvenile)
366.00
punctate
acquired 366.12
congenital 743.39
secondary (membrane) 366.50
obscuring vision 366.53
specified type, not obscuring vision
366.52
senile 366.10
anterior subcapsular polar 366.13
combined forms 366.19
cortical 366.15
hypermature 366.18
immature 366.12
incipient 366.12
mature 366.17
nuclear 366.16
posterior subcapsular polar 366.14
specified NEC 366.19
total or subtotal 366.17
snowflake 250.5 [366.41]
specified NEC 366.8
subtotal (senile) 366.17
congenital 743.34
sunflower 360.24 [366.34]
tetanic NEC 252.1 [366.42]
total (mature) (senile) 366.17
congenital 743.34
localized 366.21
traumatic 366.22
toxic 366.45
traumatic 366.20
partially resolved 366.23
total 366.22
zonular (perinuclear) 743.32
infantile, juvenile, or presenile 366.03

ICD-9-CM

C

Vol. 2

Cataracta 366.10
brunescens 366.16
cerulea 743.39
complicata 366.30
congenita 743.30
coralliformis 743.39
coronaria (congenital) 743.39
acquired 366.12
diabetic 250.5 [366.41]
floriformis 360.24 [366.34]
membranacea
accreta 366.50
congenita 743.39
nigra 366.16
Catarrh, catarrhal (inflammation) (see also
condition) 460
acute 460
asthma, asthmatic (see also Asthma) 493.9
Bostock's (see also Fever, hay) 477.9
bowel - see Enteritis
bronchial 490
acute 466.0
chronic 491.0
subacute 466.0
cervix, cervical (canal) (uteri) - see Cervicitis
chest (see also Bronchitis) 490
chronic 472.0
congestion 472.0
conjunctivitis 372.03
due to syphilis 095.9
congenital 090.0
enteric - see Enteritis
epidemic 487.1
Eustachian 381.50
eye (acute) (vernal) 372.03
fauces (see also Pharyngitis) 462
febrile 460
fibrinous acute 466.0
gastroenteric - see Enteritis
gastrointestinal - see Enteritis
gingivitis 523.0
hay (see also Fever, hay) 477.9
infectious 460
intestinal - see Enteritis
larynx (see also Laryngitis, chronic) 476.0
liver 070.1
with hepatic coma 070.0
lung (see also Bronchitis) 490
acute 466.0
chronic 491.0
middle ear (chronic) - see Otitis media,
chronic
mouth 528.0
nasal (chronic) (see also Rhinitis) 472.0
acute 460
nasobronchial 472.2
nasopharyngeal (chronic) 472.2
acute 460
nose - see Catarrh, nasal
ophthalmia 372.03
pneumococcal, acute 466.0
pulmonary (see also Bronchitis) 490
acute 466.0
chronic 491.0
spring (eye) 372.13
suffocating (see also Asthma) 493.9
summer (hay) (see also Fever, hay) 477.9
throat 472.1
tracheitis 464.10
with obstruction 464.11
tubotympanal 381.4
acute (see also Otitis media, acute,
nonsuppurative) 381.00

Catarrh, catarrhal (Continued)
tubotympanal (Continued)
chronic 381.10
vasomotor (see also Fever, hay) 477.9
vesical (bladder) - see Cystitis
Catarrhus aestivus (see also Fever, hay)
477.9
Catastrophe, cerebral (see also Disease,
cerebrovascular, acute) 436
Catatonia, catatonic (acute) 781.99
with
affective psychosis - see Psychosis,
affective
agitation 295.2
Churg-Strauss syndrome 446.4
dementia (praecox) 295.2
due to or associated with physical
condition 293.89
excitation 295.2
excited type 295.2
in conditions classified elsewhere
293.89 ◀
schizophrenia 295.2
stupor 295.2
Cat-scratch - see also Injury, superficial
disease or fever 078.3
Cauda equina - see also condition
syndrome 344.60
Cauliflower ear 738.7
Caul over face 768.9
Causalgia 355.9
lower limb 355.71
upper limb 354.4
Cause
external, general effects NEC 994.9
not stated 799.9
unknown 799.9
Caustic burn - see also Burn, by site
from swallowing caustic or corrosive
substance - see Burn, internal organs
Cavare's disease (familial periodic paralysis) 359.3
Cave-in, injury
crushing (severe) (see also Crush, by
site) 869.1
suffocation 994.7
Cavernitis (penis) 607.2
lymph vessel - see Lymphangioma
Cavernositis 607.2
Cavernous - see condition
Cavitation of lung (see also Tuberculosis)
011.2
nontuberculous 518.89
primary, progressive 010.8
Cavity
lung - see Cavitation of lung
optic papilla 743.57
pulmonary - see Cavitation of lung
teeth 521.00
vitreous (humor) 379.21
Cavovarus foot, congenital 754.59
Cavus foot (congenital) 754.71
acquired 736.73
Cazenave's
disease (pemphigus) NEC 694.4
lupus (erythematosus) 695.4
Cecitis - see Appendicitis
Cecocele - see Hernia
Cecum - see condition
Celiac
artery compression syndrome 447.4
disease 579.0
infantilism 579.0
Cell, cellular - see also condition
anterior chamber (eye) (positive aqueous ray) 364.04

Cellulitis (diffuse) (with lymphangitis)
(see also Abscess) 682.9
abdominal wall 682.2
anaerobic (see also Gas gangrene) 040.0
ankle 682.6
anus 566
areola 611.0
arm (any part, above wrist) 682.3
auditory canal (external) 380.10
axilla 682.3
back (any part) 682.2
breast 611.0
postpartum 675.1
broad ligament (see also Disease, pelvis,
inflammatory) 614.4
acute 614.3
buttock 682.5
cervical (neck region) 682.1
cervix (uteri) (see also Cervicitis) 616.0
cheek, external 682.0
internal 528.3
chest wall 682.2
chronic NEC 682.9
colostomy 569.61
corpus cavernosum 607.2
digit 681.9
Douglas' cul-de-sac or pouch (chronic)
(see also Disease, pelvis, inflammatory) 614.4
acute 614.3
drainage site (following operation) 998.59
ear, external 380.10
enterostomy 569.61
erysipelar (see also Erysipelas) 035
esophagostomy 530.86 ◀
eyelid 373.13
face (any part, except eye) 682.0
finger (intrathecal) (periosteal) (subcutaneous) (subcuticular) 681.00
flank 682.2
foot (except toe) 682.7
forearm 682.3
gangrenous (see also Gangrene) 785.4
genital organ NEC
female - see Abscess, genital organ,
female
male 608.4
glottis 478.71
gluteal (region) 682.5
gonococcal NEC 098.0
groin 682.2
hand (except finger or thumb) 682.4
head (except face) NEC 682.8
heel 682.7
hip 682.6
jaw (region) 682.0
knee 682.6
labium (majus) (minus) (see also Vulvitis) 616.10
larynx 478.71
leg, except foot 682.6
lip 528.5
mammary gland 611.0
mouth (floor) 528.3
multiple sites NEC 682.9
nasopharynx 478.21
navel 682.2
newborn NEC 771.4
neck (region) 682.1
nipple 611.0
nose 478.1
external 682.0
orbit, orbital 376.01
palate (soft) 528.3

Cellulitis (*Continued*)
   pectoral (region) 682.2
   pelvis, pelvic
      with
         abortion - *see* Abortion, by type,
            with sepsis
         ectopic pregnancy (*see also* categories 633.0-633.9) 639.0
         molar pregnancy (*see also* categories 630-632) 639.0
      female (*see also* Disease, pelvis, inflammatory) 614.4
         acute 614.3
      following
         abortion 639.0
         ectopic or molar pregnancy 639.0
      male (*see also* Abscess, peritoneum) 567.2
      puerperal, postpartum, childbirth 670
   penis 607.2
   perineal, perineum 682.2
   perirectal 566
   peritonsillar 475
   periurethral 597.0
   periuterine (*see also* Disease, pelvis, inflammatory) 614.4
      acute 614.3
   pharynx 478.21
   phlegmonous NEC 682.9
   rectum 566
   retromammary 611.0
   retroperitoneal (*see also* Peritonitis) 567.2
   round ligament (*see also* Disease, pelvis, inflammatory) 614.4
      acute 614.3
   scalp (any part) 682.8
      dissecting 704.8
   scrotum 608.4
   seminal vesicle 608.0
   septic NEC 682.9
   shoulder 682.3
   specified sites NEC 682.8
   spermatic cord 608.4
   submandibular (region) (space) (triangle) 682.0
      gland 527.3
   submaxillary 528.3
      gland 527.3
   submental (pyogenic) 682.0
      gland 527.3
   suppurative NEC 682.9
   testis 608.4
   thigh 682.6
   thumb (intrathecal) (periosteal) (subcutaneous) (subcuticular) 681.00
   toe (intrathecal) (periosteal) (subcutaneous) (subcuticular) 681.10
   tonsil 475
   trunk 682.2
   tuberculous (primary) (*see also* Tuberculosis) 017.0
   tunica vaginalis 608.4
   umbilical 682.2
      newborn NEC 771.4
   vaccinal 999.3
   vagina - *see* Vaginitis
   vas deferens 608.4
   vocal cords 478.5
   vulva (*see also* Vulvitis) 616.10
   wrist 682.4
Cementoblastoma, benign (M9273/0) 213.1
   upper jaw (bone) 213.0

Cementoma (M9273/0) 213.1
   gigantiform (M9276/0) 213.1
      upper jaw (bone) 213.0
   upper jaw (bone) 213.0
Cementoperiostitis 523.4
Cephalgia, cephalgia (*see also* Headache) 784.0
   histamine 346.2
   nonorganic origin 307.81
   psychogenic 307.81
   tension 307.81
Cephalhematocele, cephalematocele
   due to birth injury 767.19
   fetus or newborn 767.19
   traumatic (*see also* Contusion, head) 920
Cephalhematoma, cephalematoma (calcified)
   due to birth injury 767.19
   fetus or newborn 767.19
   traumatic (*see also* Contusion, head) 920
Cephalic - *see* condition
Cephalitis - *see* Encephalitis
Cephalocele 742.0
Cephaloma - *see* Neoplasm, by site, malignant
Cephalomenia 625.8
Cephalopelvic - *see* condition
Cercomoniasis 007.3
Cerebellitis - *see* Encephalitis
Cerebellum (cerebellar) - *see* condition
Cerebral - *see* condition
Cerebritis - *see* Encephalitis
Cerebrohepatorenal syndrome 759.89
Cerebromacular degeneration 330.1
Cerebromalacia (*see also* Softening, brain) 434.9
Cerebrosidosis 272.7
Cerebrospasticity - *see* Palsy, cerebral
Cerebrospinal - *see* condition
Cerebrum - *see* condition
Ceroid storage disease 272.7
Cerumen (accumulation) (impacted) 380.4
Cervical - *see also* condition
   auricle 744.43
   high risk human papillomavirus (HPV) DNA test positive 795.05 ◄
   low risk human papillomavirus (HPV) DNA test positive 795.09 ◄
   rib 756.2
Cervicalgia 723.1
Cervicitis (acute) (chronic) (nonvenereal) (subacute) (with erosion or ectropion) 616.0
   with
      abortion - *see* Abortion, by type, with sepsis
      ectopic pregnancy (*see also* categories 633.0-633.9) 639.0
      molar pregnancy (*see also* categories 630-632) 639.0
      ulceration 616.0
   chlamydial 099.53
   complicating pregnancy or puerperium 646.6
      affecting fetus or newborn 760.8
   following
      abortion 639.0
      ectopic or molar pregnancy 639.0
   gonococcal (acute) 098.15
      chronic or duration of 2 months or more 098.35
   senile (atrophic) 616.0
   syphilitic 095.8
   trichomonal 131.09

Cervicitis (*Continued*)
   tuberculous (*see also* Tuberculosis) 016.7
Cervicoaural fistula 744.49
Cervicocolpitis (emphysematosa) (*see also* Cervicitis) 616.0
Cervix - *see* condition
Cesarean delivery, operation or section NEC 669.7
   affecting fetus or newborn 763.4
   post mortem, affecting fetus or newborn 761.6
   previous, affecting management of pregnancy 654.2
Céstan's syndrome 344.89
Céstan-Chenais paralysis 344.89
Céstan-Raymond syndrome 433.8
Cestode infestation NEC 123.9
   specified type NEC 123.8
Cestodiasis 123.9
Chabert's disease 022.9
Chacaleh 266.2
Chafing 709.8
Chagas' disease (*see also* Trypanosomiasis, American) 086.2
   with heart involvement 086.0
Chagres fever 084.0
Chalasia (cardiac sphincter) 530.81
Chalazion 373.2
Chalazoderma 757.39
Chalcosis 360.24
   cornea 371.15
   crystalline lens 360.24 [366.34]
   retina 360.24
Chalicosis (occupational) (pulmonum) 502
Chancre (any genital site) (hard) (indurated) (infecting) (primary) (recurrent) 091.0
   congenital 090.0
   conjunctiva 091.2
   Ducrey's 099.0
   extragenital 091.2
   eyelid 091.2
   Hunterian 091.0
   lip (syphilis) 091.2
   mixed 099.8
   nipple 091.2
   Nisbet's 099.0
   of
      carate 103.0
      pinta 103.0
      yaws 102.0
   palate, soft 091.2
   phagedenic 099.0
   Ricord's 091.0
   Rollet's (syphilitic) 091.0
   seronegative 091.0
   seropositive 091.0
   simple 099.0
   soft 099.0
      bubo 099.0
   urethra 091.0
   yaws 102.0
Chancriform syndrome 114.1
Chancroid 099.0
   anus 099.0
   penis (Ducrey's bacillus) 099.0
   perineum 099.0
   rectum 099.0
   scrotum 099.0
   urethra 099.0
   vulva 099.0
Chandipura fever 066.8
Chandler's disease (osteochondritis dissecans, hip) 732.7

ICD-9-CM

C

Vol. 2

Change(s) (of) - *see also* Removal of
arteriosclerotic - *see* Arteriosclerosis
battery
  cardiac pacemaker V53.31
bone 733.90
  diabetic 250.8 [731.8]
  in disease, unknown cause 733.90
bowel habits 787.99
cardiorenal (vascular) (*see also* Hypertension, cardiorenal) 404.90
cardiovascular - *see* Disease, cardiovascular
circulatory 459.9
cognitive or personality change of other type, nonpsychotic 310.1
color, teeth, tooth
  during formation 520.8
  extrinsic 523.6 ◄
  intrinsic posteruptive 521.7 ◄◄◄
contraceptive device V25.42
cornea, corneal
  degenerative NEC 371.40
  membrane NEC 371.30
  senile 371.41
coronary (*see also* Ischemia, heart) 414.9
degenerative
  chamber angle (anterior) (iris) 364.56
  ciliary body 364.57
  spine or vertebra (*see also* Spondylosis) 721.90
dental pulp, regressive 522.2
dressing V58.3
fixation device V54.89
  external V54.89
  internal V54.01
heart - *see also* Disease, heart
hip joint 718.95
hyperplastic larynx 478.79
hypertrophic
  nasal sinus (*see also* Sinusitis) 473.9
  turbinate, nasal 478.0
  upper respiratory tract 478.9
inflammatory - *see* Inflammation
joint (*see also* Derangement, joint) 718.90
  sacroiliac 724.6
Kirschner wire V54.89
knee 717.9
macular, congenital 743.55
malignant (M----/3) - *see also* Neoplasm, by site, malignant

> Note For malignant change occurring in a neoplasm, use the appropriate M code with behavior digit/3 e.g., malignant change in uterine fibroid-M8890/3. For malignant change occurring in a nonneoplastic condition (e.g., gastric ulcer) use the M code M8000/3.

mental (status) NEC 780.99
  due to or associated with physical condition - *see* Syndrome, brain
myocardium, myocardial - *see* Degeneration, myocardial
of life (*see also* Menopause) 627.2
pacemaker battery (cardiac) V53.31
peripheral nerve 355.9
personality (nonpsychotic) NEC 310.1
plaster cast V54.89
refractive, transient 367.81
regressive, dental pulp 522.2
retina 362.9

Change(s) (of) (*Continued*)
retina (*Continued*)
  myopic (degenerative) (malignant) 360.21
  vascular appearance 362.13
sacroiliac joint 724.6
scleral 379.19
  degenerative 379.16
senile (*see also* Senility) 797
sensory (*see also* Disturbance, sensation) 782.0
skin texture 782.8
spinal cord 336.9
splint, external V54.89
subdermal implantable contraceptive V25.5
suture V58.3
traction device V54.89
trophic 355.9
  arm NEC 354.9
  leg NEC 355.8
  lower extremity NEC 355.8
  upper extremity NEC 354.9
vascular 459.9
vasomotor 443.9
voice 784.49
  psychogenic 306.1
Changing sleep-work schedule, affecting sleep 307.45
Changuinola fever 066.0
Chapping skin 709.8
Character
depressive 301.12
Charcôt's
arthropathy 094.0 [713.5]
cirrhosis - *see* Cirrhosis, biliary
disease 094.0
  spinal cord 094.0
fever (biliary) (hepatic) (intermittent) - *see* Choledocholithiasis
joint (disease) 094.0 [713.5]
  diabetic 250.6 [713.5]
  syringomyelic 336.0 [713.5]
syndrome (intermittent claudication) 443.9
  due to atherosclerosis 440.21
Charcôt-Marie-Tooth disease, paralysis, or syndrome 356.1
CHARGE association (syndrome) 759.89 ◄
Charleyhorse (quadriceps) 843.8
muscle, except quadriceps - *see* Sprain, by site
Charlouis' disease (*see also* Yaws) 102.9
Chauffeur's fracture - *see* Fracture, ulna, lower end
Cheadle (-Möller) (-Barlow) disease or syndrome (infantile scurvy) 267
Checking (of)
contraceptive device (intrauterine) V25.42
device
  fixation V54.89
    external V54.89
    internal V54.09
  traction V54.89
Kirschner wire V54.89
plaster cast V54.89
splint, external V54.89
Checkup
following treatment - *see* Examination
health V70.0
infant (not sick) V20.2
pregnancy (normal) V22.1
  first V22.0
  high-risk pregnancy V23.9
    specified problem NEC V23.8

Chédiak-Higashi (-Steinbrinck) anomaly, disease, or syndrome (congenital gigantism of peroxidase granules) 288.2
Cheek - *see also* condition
biting 528.9
Cheese itch 133.8
Cheese washers' lung 495.8
Cheilitis 528.5
actinic (due to sun) 692.72
  chronic NEC 692.74
    due to radiation, except from sun 692.82
  due to radiation, except from sun 692.82
acute 528.5
angular 528.5
catarrhal 528.5
chronic 528.5
exfoliative 528.5
gangrenous 528.5
glandularis apostematosa 528.5
granulomatosa 351.8
infectional 528.5
membranous 528.5
Miescher's 351.8
suppurative 528.5
ulcerative 528.5
vesicular 528.5
Cheilodynia 528.5
Cheilopalatoschisis (*see also* Cleft, palate, with cleft lip) 749.20
Cheilophagia 528.9
Cheiloschisis (*see also* Cleft, lip) 749.10
Cheilosis 528.5
with pellagra 265.2
angular 528.5
due to
  dietary deficiency 266.0
  vitamin deficiency 266.0
Cheiromegaly 729.89
Cheiropompholyx 705.81
Cheloid (*see also* Keloid) 701.4
Chemical burn - *see also* Burn, by site
from swallowing chemical - *see* Burn, internal organs
Chemodectoma (M8693/1) - *see* Paraganglioma, nonchromaffin
Chemoprophylaxis NEC V07.39
Chemosis, conjunctiva 372.73
Chemotherapy
convalescence V66.2
encounter (for) V58.1
maintenance V58.1
prophylactic NEC V07.39
  fluoride V07.31
Cherubism 526.89
Chest - *see* condition
Cheyne-Stokes respiration (periodic) 786.04
Chiari's
disease or syndrome (hepatic vein thrombosis) 453.0
malformation
  type I 348.4
  type II (*see also* Spina bifida) 741.0
  type III 742.0
  type IV 742.2
  network 746.89
Chiari-Frommel syndrome 676.6
Chicago disease (North American blastomycosis) 116.0

◄ **New**   ◄◄◄ **Revised**

Chickenpox (*see also* Varicella) 052.9 ◀
   exposure to V01.71
   vaccination and inoculation (prophylactic) V05.4
Chiclero ulcer 085.4
Chiggers 133.8
Chignon 111.2
   fetus or newborn (from vacuum extraction) 767.19
Chigoe disease 134.1
Chikungunya fever 066.3
Chilaiditi's syndrome (subphrenic displacement, colon) 751.4
Chilblains 991.5
   lupus 991.5
Child
   behavior causing concern V61.20
Childbed fever 670
Childbirth - *see also* Delivery
   puerperal complications - *see* Puerperal
Childhood, period of rapid growth V21.0
Chill(s) 780.99
   with fever 780.6
   congestive 780.99
      in malarial regions 084.6
   septic - *see* Septicemia
   urethral 599.84
Chilomastigiasis 007.8
Chin - *see* condition
Chinese dysentery 004.9
Chiropractic dislocation (*see also* Lesion, nonallopathic, by site) 739.9
Chitral fever 066.0
Chlamydia, chlamydial - *see* condition
Chloasma 709.09
   cachecticorum 709.09
   eyelid 374.52
      congenital 757.33
      hyperthyroid 242.0
   gravidarum 646.8
   idiopathic 709.09
   skin 709.09
   symptomatic 709.09
Chloroma (M9930/3) 205.3
Chlorosis 280.9
   Egyptian (*see also* Ancylostomiasis) 126.9
   miners' (*see also* Ancylostomiasis) 126.9
Chlorotic anemia 280.9
Chocolate cyst (ovary) 617.1
Choked
   disk or disc - *see* Papilledema
   on food, phlegm, or vomitus NEC (*see also* Asphyxia, food) 933.1
   phlegm 933.1
   while vomiting NEC (*see also* Asphyxia, food) 933.1
Chokes (resulting from bends) 993.3
Choking sensation 784.9
Cholangiectasis (*see also* Disease, gallbladder) 575.8
Cholangiocarcinoma (M8160/3)
   and hepatocellular carcinoma, combined (M8180/3) 155.0
   liver 155.1
   specified site NEC - *see* Neoplasm, by site, malignant
   unspecified site 155.1
Cholangiohepatitis 575.8
   due to fluke infestation 121.1
Cholangiohepatoma (M8180/3) 155.0

Cholangiolitis (acute) (chronic) (extrahepatic) (gangrenous) 576.1
   intrahepatic 575.8
   paratyphoidal (*see also* Fever, paratyphoid) 002.9
   typhoidal 002.0
Cholangioma (M8160/0) 211.5
   malignant - *see* Cholangiocarcinoma
Cholangitis (acute) (ascending) (catarrhal) (chronic) (infective) (malignant) (primary) (recurrent) (sclerosing) (secondary) (stenosing) (suppurative) 576.1
   chronic nonsuppurative destructive 571.6
   nonsuppurative destructive (chronic) 571.6
Cholecystdocholithiasis - *see* Choledocholithiasis
Cholecystitis 575.10
   with
      calculus, stones in
         bile duct (common) (hepatic) -see Choledocholithiasis
         gallbladder - *see* Cholelithiasis
   acute 575.0
   acute and chronic 575.12
   chronic 575.11
   emphysematous (acute) (*see also* Cholecystitis, acute) 575.0
   gangrenous (*see also* Cholecystitis, acute) 575.0
   paratyphoidal, current (*see also* Fever, paratyphoid) 002.9
   suppurative (*see also* Cholecystitis, acute) 575.0
   typhoidal 002.0
Choledochitis (suppurative) 576.1
Choledocholith - *see* Choledocholithiasis
Choledocholithiasis 574.5

Note	Use the following fifth-digit subclassification with category 574:
0	without mention of obstruction
1	with obstruction

   with
      cholecystitis 574.4
         acute 574.3
         chronic 574.4
      cholelithiasis 574.9
         with
            cholecystitis 574.7
               acute 574.6
                  and chronic 574.8
               chronic 574.7
Cholelithiasis (impacted) (multiple) 574.2

Note	Use the following fifth-digit subclassification with category 574:
0	without mention of obstruction
1	with obstruction

   with
      cholecystitis 574.1
         acute 574.0
         chronic 574.1
      choledocholithiasis 574.9
         with
            cholecystitis 574.7
               acute 574.6
                  and chronic 574.8
               chronic cholecystitis 574.7

Cholemia (*see also* Jaundice) 782.4
   familial 277.4
   Gilbert's (familial nonhemolytic) 277.4
Cholemic gallstone - *see* Cholelithiasis
Choleperitoneum, choleperitonitis (*see also* Disease, gallbladder) 567.8
Cholera (algid) (Asiatic) (asphyctic) (epidemic) (gravis) (Indian) (malignant) (morbus) (pestilential) (spasmodic) 001.9
   antimonial 985.4
   carrier (suspected) of V02.0
   classical 001.0
   contact V01.0
   due to
      Vibrio
         cholerae (Inaba, Ogawa, Hikojima serotypes) 001.0
            el Tor 001.1
   el Tor 001.1
   exposure to V01.0
   vaccination, prophylactic (against) V03.0
Cholerine (*see also* Cholera) 001.9
Cholestasis 576.8
Cholesteatoma (ear) 385.30
   attic (primary) 385.31
   diffuse 385.35
   external ear (canal) 380.21
   marginal (middle ear) 385.32
      with involvement of mastoid cavity 385.33
      secondary (with middle ear involvement) 385.33
   mastoid cavity 385.30
   middle ear (secondary) 385.32
      with involvement of mastoid cavity 385.33
   postmastoidectomy cavity (recurrent) 383.32
   primary 385.31
   recurrent, postmastoidectomy cavity 383.32
   secondary (middle ear) 385.32
      with involvement of mastoid cavity 385.33
Cholesteatosis (middle ear) (*see also* Cholesteatoma) 385.30
   diffuse 385.35
Cholesteremia 272.0
Cholesterin
   granuloma, middle ear 385.82
   in vitreous 379.22
Cholesterol
   deposit
      retina 362.82
      vitreous 379.22
   imbibition of gallbladder (*see also* Disease, gallbladder) 575.6
Cholesterolemia 272.0
   essential 272.0
   familial 272.0
   hereditary 272.0
Cholesterosis, cholesterolosis (gallbladder) 575.6
   with
      cholecystitis - *see* Cholecystitis
      cholelithiasis - *see* Cholelithiasis
   middle ear (*see also* Cholesteatoma) 385.30
Cholocolic fistula (*see also* Fistula, gallbladder) 575.5
Choluria 791.4

ICD-9-CM
c
Vol. 2

Chondritis (purulent) 733.99 ◄
  auricle 380.03
  costal 733.6
    Tietze's 733.6
  patella, posttraumatic 717.7
  pinna 380.03 ◄
  posttraumatica patellae 717.7
  tuberculous (active) (see also Tuberculosis) 015.9
    intervertebral 015.0 [730.88]
Chondroangiopathia calcarea seu punctate 756.59
Chondroblastoma (M9230/0) - see also Neoplasm, bone, benign
  malignant (M9230/3) - see Neoplasm, bone, malignant
Chondrocalcinosis (articular) (crystal deposition) (dihydrate) (see also Arthritis, due to, crystals) 275.49 [712.3]
  due to
    calcium pyrophosphate 275.49 [712.2]
    dicalcium phosphate crystals 275.49 [712.1]
    pyrophosphate crystals 275.49 [712.2]
Chondrodermatitis nodularis helicis 380.00
Chondrodysplasia 756.4
  angiomatose 756.4
  calcificans congenita 756.59
  epiphysialis punctata 756.59
  hereditary deforming 756.4
  rhizomelic punctata 277.86 ◄
Chondrodystrophia (fetalis) 756.4
  calcarea 756.4
  calcificans congenita 756.59
  fetalis hypoplastica 756.59
  hypoplastica calcinosa 756.59
  punctata 756.59
  tarda 277.5
Chondrodystrophy (familial) (hypoplastic) 756.4
Chondroectodermal dysplasia 756.55
Chondrolysis 733.99
Chondroma (M9220/0) - see also Neoplasm, cartilage, benign
  juxtacortical (M9221/0) - see Neoplasm, bone, benign
  periosteal (M9221/0) - see Neoplasm, bone, benign
Chondromalacia 733.92
  epiglottis (congenital) 748.3
  generalized 733.92
  knee 717.7
  larynx (congenital) 748.3
  localized, except patella 733.92
  patella, patellae 717.7
  systemic 733.92
  tibial plateau 733.92
  trachea (congenital) 748.3
Chondromatosis (M9220/1) - see Neoplasm, cartilage, uncertain behavior
Chondromyxosarcoma (M9220/3) - see Neoplasm, cartilage, malignant
Chondro-osteodysplasia (Morquio-Brailsford type) 277.5
Chondro-osteodystrophy 277.5
Chondro-osteoma (M9210/0) - see Neoplasm, bone, benign
Chondropathia tuberosa 733.6
Chondrosarcoma (M9220/3) - see also Neoplasm, cartilage, malignant
  juxtacortical (M9221/3) - see Neoplasm, bone, malignant
  mesenchymal (M9240/3) - see Neoplasm, connective tissue, malignant

Chordae tendineae rupture (chronic) 429.5
Chordee (nonvenereal) 607.89
  congenital 752.63
  gonococcal 098.2
Chorditis (fibrinous) (nodosa) (tuberosa) 478.5
Chordoma (M9370/3) - see Neoplasm, by site, malignant
Chorea (gravis) (minor) (spasmodic) 333.5
  with
    heart involvement - see Chorea with rheumatic heart disease
    rheumatic heart disease (chronic, inactive, or quiescent) (conditions classifiable to 393-398) - see rheumatic heart condition involved
      active or acute (conditions classifiable to 391) 392.0
  acute - see Chorea, Sydenham's
  apoplectic (see also Disease, cerebrovascular, acute) 436
  chronic 333.4
  electric 049.8
  gravidarum - see Eclampsia, pregnancy
  habit 307.22
  hereditary 333.4
  Huntington's 333.4
  posthemiplegic 344.89
  pregnancy - see Eclampsia, pregnancy
  progressive 333.4
    chronic 333.4
    hereditary 333.4
  rheumatic (chronic) 392.9
    with heart disease or involvement - see Chorea, with rheumatic heart disease
  senile 333.5
  Sydenham's 392.9
    with heart involvement - see Chorea, with rheumatic heart disease
    nonrheumatic 333.5
  variabilis 307.23
Choreoathetosis (paroxysmal) 333.5
Chorioadenoma (destruens) (M9100/1) 236.1
Chorioamnionitis 658.4
  affecting fetus or newborn 762.7
Chorioangioma (M9120/0) 219.8
Choriocarcinoma (M9100/3)
  combined with
    embryonal carcinoma (M9101/3) - see Neoplasm, by site, malignant
    teratoma (M9101/3) - see Neoplasm, by site, malignant
  specified site - see Neoplasm, by site, malignant
  unspecified site
    female 181
    male 186.9
Chorioencephalitis, lymphocytic (acute) (serous) 049.0
Chorioepithelioma (M9100/3) - see Choriocarcinoma
Choriomeningitis (acute) (benign) (lymphocytic) (serous) 049.0
Chorionepithelioma (M9100/3) - see Choriocarcinoma
Chorionitis (see also Scleroderma) 710.1

Chorioretinitis 363.20
  disseminated 363.10
    generalized 363.13
    in
      neurosyphilis 094.83
      secondary syphilis 091.51
    peripheral 363.12
    posterior pole 363.11
    tuberculous (see also Tuberculosis) 017.3 [363.13]
  due to
    histoplasmosis (see also Histoplasmosis) 115.92
    toxoplasmosis (acquired) 130.2
      congenital (active) 771.2
  focal 363.00
    juxtapapillary 363.01
    peripheral 363.04
    posterior pole NEC 363.03
  juxtapapillaris, juxtapapillary 363.01
  progressive myopia (degeneration) 360.21
  syphilitic (secondary) 091.51
    congenital (early) 090.0 [363.13]
    late 090.5 [363.13]
    late 095.8 [363.13]
  tuberculous (see also Tuberculosis) 017.3 [363.13]
Choristoma - see Neoplasm, by site, benign
Choroid - see condition
Choroideremia, choroidermia (initial stage) (late stage) (partial or total atrophy) 363.55
Choroiditis (see also Chorioretinitis) 363.20
  leprous 030.9 [363.13]
  senile guttate 363.41
  sympathetic 360.11
  syphilitic (secondary) 091.51
    congenital (early) 090.0 [363.13]
    late 090.5 [363.13]
    late 095.8 [363.13]
  Tay's 363.41
  tuberculous (see also Tuberculosis) 017.3 [363.13]
Choroidopathy NEC 363.9
  degenerative (see also Degeneration, choroid) 363.40
  hereditary (see also Dystrophy, choroid) 363.50
  specified type NEC 363.8
Choroidoretinitis - see Chorioretinitis
Choroidosis, central serous 362.41
Choroidretinopathy, serous 362.41
Christian's syndrome (chronic histiocytosis X) 277.89
Christian-Weber disease (nodular nonsuppurative panniculitis) 729.30
Christmas disease 286.1
Chromaffinoma (M8700/0) - see also Neoplasm, by site, benign
  malignant (M8700/3) - see Neoplasm, by site, malignant
Chromatopsia 368.59
Chromhidrosis, chromidrosis 705.89
Chromoblastomycosis 117.2
Chromomycosis 117.2
Chromophytosis 111.0
Chromotrichomycosis 111.8
Chronic - see condition
Chyle cyst, mesentery 457.8
Chylocele (nonfilarial) 457.8
  filarial (see also Infestation, filarial) 125.9

Chylocele *(Continued)*
  tunica vaginalis (nonfilarial) 608.84
    filarial *(see also* Infestation, filarial)
      125.9
Chylomicronemia (fasting) (with hyper-
    prebetalipoproteinemia) 272.3
Chylopericardium (acute) 420.90
Chylothorax (nonfilarial) 457.8
  filarial *(see also* Infestation, filarial)
    125.9
Chylous
  ascites 457.8
  cyst of peritoneum 457.8
  hydrocele 603.9
  hydrothorax (nonfilarial) 457.8
    filarial *(see also* Infestation, filarial)
      125.9
Chyluria 791.1
  bilharziasis 120.0
  due to
    Brugia (malayi) 125.1
    Wuchereria (bancrofti) 125.0
      malayi 125.1
  filarial *(see also* Infestation, filarial)
    125.9
  filariasis *(see also* Infestation, filarial)
    125.9
  nonfilarial 791.1
Cicatricial (deformity) - *see* Cicatrix
Cicatrix (adherent) (contracted) (painful)
    (vicious) 709.2
  adenoid 474.8
  alveolar process 525.8
  anus 569.49
  auricle 380.89
  bile duct *(see also* Disease, biliary)
    576.8
  bladder 596.8
  bone 733.99
  brain 348.8
  cervix (postoperative) (postpartal)
    622.3
    in pregnancy or childbirth 654.6
      causing obstructed labor 660.2
  chorioretinal 363.30
    disseminated 363.35
    macular 363.32
    peripheral 363.34
    posterior pole NEC 363.33
  choroid - *see* Cicatrix, chorioretinal
  common duct *(see also* Disease, biliary)
    576.8
  congenital 757.39
  conjunctiva 372.64
  cornea 371.00
    tuberculous *(see also* Tuberculosis)
      017.3 [371.05]
  duodenum (bulb) 537.3
  esophagus 530.3
  eyelid 374.46
    with
      ectropion - *see* Ectropion
      entropion - *see* Entropion
  hypopharynx 478.29
  knee, semilunar cartilage 717.5
  lacrimal
    canaliculi 375.53
    duct
      acquired 375.56
      neonatal 375.55
    punctum 375.52
    sac 375.54
  larynx 478.79
  limbus (cystoid) 372.64

Cicatrix *(Continued)*
  lung 518.89
  macular 363.32
    disseminated 363.35
    peripheral 363.34
  middle ear 385.89
  mouth 528.9
  muscle 728.89
  nasolacrimal duct
    acquired 375.56
    neonatal 375.55
  nasopharynx 478.29
  palate (soft) 528.9
  penis 607.89
  prostate 602.8
  rectum 569.49
  retina 363.30
    disseminated 363.35
    macular 363.32
    peripheral 363.34
    posterior pole NEC 363.33
  semilunar cartilage - *see* Derangement,
    meniscus
  seminal vesicle 608.89
  skin 709.2
    infected 686.8
    postinfectional 709.2
    tuberculous *(see also* Tuberculosis)
      017.0
  specified site NEC 709.2
  throat 478.29
  tongue 529.8
  tonsil (and adenoid) 474.8
  trachea 478.9
  tuberculous NEC *(see also* Tuberculo-
    sis) 011.9
  ureter 593.89
  urethra 599.84
  uterus 621.8
  vagina 623.4
    in pregnancy or childbirth 654.7
      causing obstructed labor 660.2
  vocal cord 478.5
  wrist, constricting (annular) 709.2
**CIN I [cervical intraepithelial neoplasia
  I]** 622.11 ◄▥
**CIN II [cervical intraepithelial neopla-
  sia II]** 622.12 ◄▥
**CIN III [cervical intraepithelial neopla-
  sia III]** 233.1
Cinchonism
  correct substance properly adminis-
    tered 386.9
  overdose or wrong substance given or
    taken 961.4
Circine herpes 110.5
Circle of Willis - *see* condition
Circular - *see also* condition
  hymen 752.49
Circulating anticoagulants 286.5
  following childbirth 666.3
  postpartum 666.3
Circulation
  collateral (venous), any site 459.89
  defective 459.9
    congenital 747.9
    lower extremity 459.89
  embryonic 747.9
  failure 799.89
    fetus or newborn 779.89
    peripheral 785.59
  fetal, persistent 747.83
  heart, incomplete 747.9
Circulatory system - *see* condition

Circulus senilis 371.41
Circumcision
  in absence of medical indication
    V50.2
  ritual V50.2
  routine V50.2
Circumscribed - *see* condition
Circumvallata placenta - *see* Placenta,
  abnormal
Cirrhosis, cirrhotic 571.5
  with alcoholism 571.2
  alcoholic (liver) 571.2
  atrophic (of liver) - *see* Cirrhosis, por-
    tal
  Baumgarten-Cruveilhier 571.5
  biliary (cholangiolitic) (cholangitic)
    (cholestatic) (extrahepatic) (hyper-
    trophic) (intrahepatic) (nonob-
    structive) (obstructive) (pericho-
    langiolitic) (posthepatic) (primary)
    (secondary) (xanthomatous) 571.6
    due to
      clonorchiasis 121.1
      flukes 121.3
  brain 331.9
  capsular - *see* Cirrhosis, portal
  cardiac 571.5
    alcoholic 571.2
  central (liver) - *see* Cirrhosis, liver
  Charcôt's 571.6
  cholangiolitic - *see* Cirrhosis, biliary
  cholangitic - *see* Cirrhosis, biliary
  cholestatic - *see* Cirrhosis, biliary
  clitoris (hypertrophic) 624.2
  coarsely nodular 571.5
  congestive (liver) - *see* Cirrhosis, car-
    diac
  Cruveilhier-Baumgarten 571.5
  cryptogenic (of liver) 571.5
    alcoholic 571.2
  dietary *(see also* Cirrhosis, portal)
    571.5
  due to
    bronzed diabetes 275.0
    congestive hepatomegaly - *see* Cir-
      rhosis, cardiac
    cystic fibrosis 277.00
    hemochromatosis 275.0
    hepatolenticular degeneration 275.1
    passive congestion (chronic) - *see*
      Cirrhosis, cardiac
    Wilson's disease 275.1
    xanthomatosis 272.2
  extrahepatic (obstructive) - *see* Cirrho-
    sis, biliary
  fatty 571.8
    alcoholic 571.0
  florid 571.2
  Glisson's - *see* Cirrhosis, portal
  Hanot's (hypertrophic) - *see* Cirrhosis,
    biliary
  hepatic - *see* Cirrhosis, liver
  hepatolienal - *see* Cirrhosis, liver
  hobnail - *see* Cirrhosis, portal
  hypertrophic - *see also* Cirrhosis, liver
    biliary - *see* Cirrhosis, biliary
    Hanot's - *see* Cirrhosis, biliary
  infectious NEC - *see* Cirrhosis, portal
  insular - *see* Cirrhosis, portal
  intrahepatic (obstructive) (primary)
    (secondary) - *see* Cirrhosis, biliary
  juvenile *(see also* Cirrhosis, portal)
    571.5
  kidney *(see also* Sclerosis, renal) 587

Cirrhosis, cirrhotic *(Continued)*
   Laennec's (of liver) 571.2
      nonalcoholic 571.5
   liver (chronic) (hepatolienal) (hypertrophic) (nodular) (splenomegalic) (unilobar) 571.5
      with alcoholism 571.2
      alcoholic 571.2
      congenital (due to failure of obliteration of umbilical vein) 777.8
      cryptogenic 571.5
         alcoholic 571.2
      fatty 571.8
         alcoholic 571.0
      macronodular 571.5
         alcoholic 571.2
      micronodular 571.5
         alcoholic 571.2
      nodular, diffuse 571.5
         alcoholic 571.2
      pigmentary 275.0
      portal 571.5
         alcoholic 571.2
      postnecrotic 571.5
         alcoholic 571.2
      syphilitic 095.3
   lung (chronic) *(see also* Fibrosis, lung) 515
   macronodular (of liver) 571.5
      alcoholic 571.2
   malarial 084.9
   metabolic NEC 571.5
   micronodular (of liver) 571.5
      alcoholic 571.2
   monolobular - *see* Cirrhosis, portal
   multilobular - *see* Cirrhosis, portal
   nephritis *(see also* Sclerosis, renal) 587
   nodular - *see* Cirrhosis, liver
   nutritional (fatty) 571.5
   obstructive (biliary) (extrahepatic) (intrahepatic) - *see* Cirrhosis, biliary
   ovarian 620.8
   paludal 084.9
   pancreas (duct) 577.8
   pericholangiolitic - *see* Cirrhosis, biliary
   periportal - *see* Cirrhosis, portal
   pigment, pigmentary (of liver) 275.0
   portal (of liver) 571.5
      alcoholic 571.2
   posthepatitic *(see also* Cirrhosis, postnecrotic) 571.5
   postnecrotic (of liver) 571.5
      alcoholic 571.2
   primary (intrahepatic) - *see* Cirrhosis, biliary
   pulmonary *(see also* Fibrosis, lung) 515
   renal *(see also* Sclerosis, renal) 587
   septal *(see also* Cirrhosis, postnecrotic) 571.5
   spleen 289.51
   splenomegalic (of liver) - *see* Cirrhosis, liver
   stasis (liver) - *see* Cirrhosis, liver
   stomach 535.4
   Todd's *(see also* Cirrhosis, biliary) 571.6
   toxic (nodular) - *see* Cirrhosis, postnecrotic
   trabecular - *see* Cirrhosis, postnecrotic
   unilobar - *see* Cirrhosis, liver
   vascular (of liver) - *see* Cirrhosis, liver

Cirrhosis, cirrhotic *(Continued)*
   xanthomatous (biliary) *(see also* Cirrhosis, biliary) 571.6
      due to xanthomatosis (familial) (metabolic) (primary) 272.2
Cistern, subarachnoid 793.0
Citrullinemia 270.6
Citrullinuria 270.6
Ciuffini-Pancoast tumor (M8010/3) (carcinoma, pulmonary apex) 162.3
Civatte's disease or poikiloderma 709.09
Clam diggers' itch 120.3
Clap - *see* Gonorrhea
Clark's paralysis 343.9
Clarke-Hadfield syndrome (pancreatic infantilism) 577.8
Clastothrix 704.2
Claude's syndrome 352.6
Claude Bernard-Horner syndrome *(see also* Neuropathy, peripheral, autonomic) 337.9
Claudication, intermittent 443.9
   cerebral (artery) *(see also* Ischemia, cerebral, transient) 435.9
   due to atherosclerosis 440.21
   spinal cord (arteriosclerotic) 435.1
      syphilitic 094.89
   spinalis 435.1
   venous (axillary) 453.8
Claudicatio venosa intermittens 453.8
Claustrophobia 300.29
Clavus (infected) 700
Clawfoot (congenital) 754.71
   acquired 736.74
Clawhand (acquired) 736.06
   congenital 755.59
Clawtoe (congenital) 754.71
   acquired 735.5
Clay eating 307.52
Clay shovelers' fracture - *see* Fracture, vertebra, cervical
Cleansing of artificial opening *(see also* Attention to artificial opening) V55.9
Cleft (congenital) - *see also* Imperfect, closure
   alveolar process 525.8
   branchial (persistent) 744.41
      cyst 744.42
   clitoris 752.49
   cricoid cartilage, posterior 748.3
   facial *(see also* Cleft, lip) 749.10
   lip 749.10
      with cleft palate 749.20
         bilateral (lip and palate) 749.24
            with unilateral lip or palate 749.25
            complete 749.23
            incomplete 749.24
         unilateral (lip and palate) 749.22
            with bilateral lip or palate 749.25
            complete 749.21
            incomplete 749.22
      bilateral 749.14
         with cleft palate, unilateral 749.25
         complete 749.13
         incomplete 749.14
      unilateral 749.12
         with cleft palate, bilateral 749.25
         complete 749.11
         incomplete 749.12
   nose 748.1

Cleft *(Continued)*
   palate 749.00
      with cleft lip 749.20
         bilateral (lip and palate) 749.24
            with unilateral lip or palate 749.25
            complete 749.23
            incomplete 749.24
         unilateral (lip and palate) 749.22
            with bilateral lip or palate 749.25
            complete 749.21
            incomplete 749.22
      bilateral 749.04
         with cleft lip, unilateral 749.25
         complete 749.03
         incomplete 749.04
      unilateral 749.02
         with cleft lip, bilateral 749.25
         complete 749.01
         incomplete 749.02
   penis 752.69
   posterior, cricoid cartilage 748.3
   scrotum 752.89
   sternum (congenital) 756.3
   thyroid cartilage (congenital) 748.3
   tongue 750.13
   uvula 749.02
      with cleft lip *(see also* Cleft, lip, with cleft palate) 749.20
   water 366.12
Cleft hand (congenital) 755.58
Cleidocranial dysostosis 755.59
Cleidotomy, fetal 763.89
Cleptomania 312.32
Clérambault's syndrome 297.8
   erotomania 302.89
Clergyman's sore throat 784.49
Click, clicking
   systolic syndrome 785.2
Clifford's syndrome (postmaturity) 766.22
Climacteric *(see also* Menopause) 627.2
   arthritis NEC *(see also* Arthritis, climacteric) 716.3
   depression *(see also* Psychosis, affective) 296.2
   disease 627.2
      recurrent episode 296.3
      single episode 296.2
   female (symptoms) 627.2
   male (symptoms) (syndrome) 608.89
   melancholia *(see also* Psychosis, affective) 296.2
      recurrent episode 296.3
      single episode 296.2
   paranoid state 297.2
   paraphrenia 297.2
   polyarthritis NEC 716.39
      male 608.89
   symptoms (female) 627.2
Clinical research investigation (control) (participant) V70.7
Clinodactyly 755.59
Clitoris - *see* condition
Cloaca, persistent 751.5
Clonorchiasis 121.1
Clonorchiosis 121.1
Clonorchis infection, liver 121.1
Clonus 781.0
Closed bite 524.20
Closed surgical procedure converted to open procedure
   arthroscopic V64.43
   laparoscopic V64.41
   thoracoscopic V64.42
Closure
   artificial opening *(see also* Attention to artificial opening) V55.9

◄ **New**   ◄▥▥ **Revised**

Closure (*Continued*)
  congenital, nose 748.0
  cranial sutures, premature 756.0
  defective or imperfect NEC - *see* Imperfect, closure
  fistula, delayed - *see* Fistula
  fontanelle, delayed 756.0
  foramen ovale, imperfect 745.5
  hymen 623.3
  interauricular septum, defective 745.5
  interventricular septum, defective 745.4
  lacrimal duct 375.56
    congenital 743.65
    neonatal 375.55
  nose (congenital) 748.0
    acquired 738.0
  vagina 623.2
  valve - *see* Endocarditis
  vulva 624.8
Clot (blood)
  artery (obstruction) (occlusion) (*see also* Embolism) 444.9
  bladder 596.7
  brain (extradural or intradural) (*see also* Thrombosis, brain) 434.0
    late effect - *see* Late effect(s) (of) cerebrovascular disease
  circulation 444.9
  heart (*see also* Infarct, myocardium) 410.9
  vein (*see also* Thrombosis) 453.9
Clotting defect NEC (*see also* Defect, coagulation) 286.9
Clouded state 780.09
  epileptic (*see also* Epilepsy) 345.9
  paroxysmal (idiopathic) (*see also* Epilepsy) 345.9
Clouding
  corneal graft 996.51
Cloudy
  antrum, antra 473.0
  dialysis effluent 792.5
Clouston's (hidrotic) ectodermal dysplasia 757.31
Clubbing of fingers 781.5
Clubfinger 736.29
  acquired 736.29
  congenital 754.89
Clubfoot (congenital) 754.70
  acquired 736.71
  equinovarus 754.51
  paralytic 736.71
Club hand (congenital) 754.89
  acquired 736.07
Clubnail (acquired) 703.8
  congenital 757.5
Clump kidney 753.3
Clumsiness 781.3
  syndrome 315.4
Cluttering 307.0
Clutton's joints 090.5
Coagulation, intravascular (diffuse) (disseminated) (*see also* Fibrinolysis) 286.6
  newborn 776.2
Coagulopathy (*see also* Defect, coagulation) 286.9
  consumption 286.6
  intravascular (disseminated) NEC 286.6
    newborn 776.2
Coalition
  calcaneoscaphoid 755.67
  calcaneus 755.67
  tarsal 755.67
Coal miners'
  elbow 727.2
  lung 500

Coal workers' lung or pneumoconiosis 500
Coarctation
  aorta (postductal) (preductal) 747.10
  pulmonary artery 747.3
Coated tongue 529.3
Coats' disease 362.12
Cocainism (*see also* Dependence) 304.2
Coccidioidal granuloma 114.3
Coccidioidomycosis 114.9
  with pneumonia 114.0
  cutaneous (primary) 114.1
  disseminated 114.3
  extrapulmonary (primary) 114.1
  lung 114.5
    acute 114.0
    chronic 114.4
    primary 114.0
  meninges 114.2
  primary (pulmonary) 114.0
    acute 114.0
  prostate 114.3
  pulmonary 114.5
    acute 114.0
    chronic 114.4
    primary 114.0
  specified site NEC 114.3
Coccidioidosis 114.9
  lung 114.5
    acute 114.0
    chronic 114.4
    primary 114.0
  meninges 114.2
Coccidiosis (colitis) (diarrhea) (dysentery) 007.2
Cocciuria 791.9
Coccus in urine 791.9
Coccydynia 724.79
Coccygodynia 724.79
Coccyx - *see* condition
Cochin-China
  diarrhea 579.1
    anguilluliasis 127.2
  ulcer 085.1
Cock's peculiar tumor 706.2
Cockayne's disease or syndrome (microcephaly and dwarfism) 759.89
Cockayne-Weber syndrome (epidermolysis bullosa) 757.39
Cocked-up toe 735.2
Codman's tumor (benign chondroblastoma) (M9230/0) - *see* Neoplasm, bone, benign
Coenurosis 123.8
Coffee workers' lung 495.8
Cogan's syndrome 370.52
  congenital oculomotor apraxia 379.51
  nonsyphilitic interstitial keratitis 370.52
Coiling, umbilical cord - *see* Complications, umbilical cord
Coitus, painful (female) 625.0
  male 608.89
  psychogenic 302.76
Cold 460
  with influenza, flu, or grippe 487.1
  abscess - *see also* Tuberculosis, abscess
    articular - *see* Tuberculosis, joint
  agglutinin
    disease (chronic) or syndrome 283.0
    hemoglobinuria 283.0
      paroxysmal (cold) (nocturnal) 283.2
  allergic (*see also* Fever, hay) 477.9
  bronchus or chest - *see* Bronchitis
    with grippe or influenza 487.1

Cold (*Continued*)
  common (head) 460
    vaccination, prophylactic (against) V04.7
  deep 464.10
  effects of 991.9
    specified effect NEC 991.8
  excessive 991.9
    specified effect NEC 991.8
  exhaustion from 991.8
  exposure to 991.9
    specified effect NEC 991.8
  grippy 487.1
  head 460
  injury syndrome (newborn) 778.2
  intolerance 780.99
  on lung - *see* Bronchitis
  rose 477.0
  sensitivity, autoimmune 283.0
  virus 460
Coldsore (*see also* Herpes, simplex) 054.9
Colibacillosis 041.4
  generalized 038.42
Colibacilluria 791.9
Colic (recurrent) 789.0
  abdomen 789.0
    psychogenic 307.89
  appendicular 543.9
  appendix 543.9
  bile duct - *see* Choledocholithiasis
  biliary - *see* Cholelithiasis
  bilious - *see* Cholelithiasis
  common duct - *see* Choledocholithiasis
  Devonshire NEC 984.9
    specified type of lead - *see* Table of Drugs and Chemicals
  flatulent 787.3
  gallbladder or gallstone - *see* Cholelithiasis
  gastric 536.8
  hepatic (duct) - *see* Choledocholithiasis
  hysterical 300.11
  infantile 789.0
  intestinal 789.0
  kidney 788.0
  lead NEC 984.9
    specified type of lead - *see* Table of Drugs and Chemicals
  liver (duct) - *see* Choledocholithiasis
  mucous 564.9
    psychogenic 316 [564.9]
  nephritic 788.0
  Painter's NEC 984.9
  pancreas 577.8
  psychogenic 306.4
  renal 788.0
  saturnine NEC 984.9
    specified type of lead - *see* Table of Drugs and Chemicals
  spasmodic 789.0
  ureter 788.0
  urethral 599.84
    due to calculus 594.2
  uterus 625.8
    menstrual 625.3
  vermicular 543.9
  virus 460
  worm NEC 128.9
Colicystitis (*see also* Cystitis) 595.9
Colitis (acute) (catarrhal) (croupous) (cystica superficialis) (exudative) (hemorrhagic) (noninfectious) (phlegmonous) (presumed noninfectious) 558.9

ICD-9-CM
c
Vol. 2

Colitis (*Continued*)
  adaptive 564.9
  allergic 558.3
  amebic (*see also* Amebiasis) 006.9
    nondysenteric 006.2
  anthrax 022.2
  bacillary (*see also* Infection, Shigella)
    004.9
  balantidial 007.0
  chronic 558.9
    ulcerative (*see also* Colitis, ulcerative)
      556.9
  coccidial 007.2
  dietetic 558.9
  due to radiation 558.1
  functional 558.9
  gangrenous 009.0
  giardial 007.1
  granulomatous 555.1
  gravis (*see also* Colitis, ulcerative) 556.9
  infectious (*see also* Enteritis, due to,
    specific organism) 009.0
    presumed 009.1
  ischemic 557.9
    acute 557.0
    chronic 557.1
    due to mesenteric artery insuffi-
      ciency 557.1
  membranous 564.9
    psychogenic 316 [564.9]
  mucous 564.9
    psychogenic 316 [564.9]
  necrotic 009.0
  polyposa (*see also* Colitis, ulcerative)
    556.9
  protozoal NEC 007.9
  pseudomembranous 008.45
  pseudomucinous 564.9
  regional 555.1
  segmental 555.1
  septic (*see also* Enteritis, due to, specific
    organism) 009.0
  spastic 564.9
    psychogenic 316 [564.9]
  Staphylococcus 008.41
    food 005.0
  thromboulcerative 557.0
  toxic 558.2
  transmural 555.1
  trichomonal 007.3
  tuberculous (ulcerative) 014.8
  ulcerative (chronic) (idiopathic) (non-
    specific) 556.9
    entero- 556.0
    fulminant 557.0
    ileo- 556.1
    left-sided 556.5
    procto- 556.2
    proctosigmoid 556.3
    psychogenic 316 [556]
    specified NEC 556.8
    universal 556.6
Collagen disease NEC 710.9
  nonvascular 710.9
  vascular (allergic) (*see also* Angiitis, hy-
    persensitivity) 446.20
Collagenosis (*see also* Collagen disease)
  710.9
  cardiovascular 425.4
  mediastinal 519.3
Collapse 780.2
  adrenal 255.8
  cardiorenal (*see also* Hypertension, car-
    diorenal) 404.90

Collapse (*Continued*)
  cardiorespiratory 785.51
    fetus or newborn 779.89
  cardiovascular (*see also* Disease, heart)
    785.51
    fetus or newborn 779.89
  circulatory (peripheral) 785.59
    with
      abortion - see Abortion, by type,
        with shock
      ectopic pregnancy (*see also* catego-
        ries 633.0-633.9) 639.5
      molar pregnancy (*see also* catego-
        ries 630-632) 639.5
    during or after labor and delivery
      669.1
    fetus or newborn 779.89
    following
      abortion 639.5
      ectopic or molar pregnancy
        639.5
  during or after labor and delivery
    669.1
    fetus or newborn 779.89
  external ear canal 380.50
    secondary to
      inflammation 380.53
      surgery 380.52
      trauma 380.51
  general 780.2
  heart - see Disease, heart
  heat 992.1
  hysterical 300.11
  labyrinth, membranous (congenital)
    744.05
  lung (massive) (*see also* Atelectasis)
    518.0
    pressure, during labor 668.0
  myocardial - see Disease, heart
  nervous (*see also* Disorder, mental,
    nonpsychotic) 300.9
  neurocirculatory 306.2
  nose 738.0
  postoperative (cardiovascular) 998.0
  pulmonary (*see also* Atelectasis) 518.0
    fetus or newborn 770.5
      partial 770.5
      primary 770.4
  thorax 512.8
    iatrogenic 512.1
    postoperative 512.1
  trachea 519.1
  valvular - see Endocarditis
  vascular (peripheral) 785.59
    with
      abortion - see Abortion, by type,
        with shock
      ectopic pregnancy (*see also* catego-
        ries 633.0-633.9) 639.5
      molar pregnancy (*see also* catego-
        ries 630-632) 639.5
    cerebral (*see also* Disease, cerebrovas-
      cular, acute) 436
    during or after labor and delivery
      669.1
    fetus or newborn 779.89
    following
      abortion 639.5
      ectopic or molar pregnancy 639.5
  vasomotor 785.59
  vertebra 733.13
Collateral - *see also* condition
  circulation (venous) 459.89
  dilation, veins 459.89

Colles' fracture (closed) (reversed) (separation) 813.41
  open 813.51
Collet's syndrome 352.6
Collet-Sicard syndrome 352.6
Colliculitis urethralis (*see also* Urethritis)
  597.89
Colliers'
  asthma 500
  lung 500
  phthisis (*see also* Tuberculosis)
    011.4
Collodion baby (ichthyosis congenita)
  757.1
Colloid milium 709.3
Coloboma NEC 743.49
  choroid 743.59
  fundus 743.52
  iris 743.46
  lens 743.36
  lids 743.62
  optic disc (congenital) 743.57
    acquired 377.23
  retina 743.56
  sclera 743.47
Coloenteritis - see Enteritis
Colon - *see* condition
Coloptosis 569.89
Color
  amblyopia NEC 368.59
    acquired 368.55
  blindness NEC (congenital) 368.59
    acquired 368.55
Colostomy
  attention to V55.3
  fitting or adjustment V55.3
  malfunctioning 569.62
  status V44.3
Colpitis (*see also* Vaginitis) 616.10
Colpocele 618.6
Colpocystitis (*see also* Vaginitis)
  616.10
Colporrhexis 665.4
Colpospasm 625.1
Column, spinal, vertebral - *see* condition
Coma 780.01
  apoplectic (*see also* Disease, cerebrovas-
    cular, acute) 436
  diabetic (with ketoacidosis) 250.3
    hyperosmolar 250.2
  eclamptic (*see also* Eclampsia) 780.39
  epileptic 345.3
  hepatic 572.2
  hyperglycemic 250.2
  hyperosmolar (diabetic) (nonketotic)
    250.2
  hypoglycemic 251.0
    diabetic 250.3
  insulin 250.3
    hyperosmolar 250.2
    nondiabetic 251.0
    organic hyperinsulinism 251.0
  Kussmaul's (diabetic) 250.3
  liver 572.2
  newborn 779.2
  prediabetic 250.2
  uremic - see Uremia
Combat fatigue (*see also* Reaction, stress,
  acute) 308.9
Combined - *see* condition
Comedo 706.1
Comedocarcinoma (M8501/3) - *see also*
  Neoplasm, breast, malignant
  noninfiltrating (M8501/2)

Comedocarcinoma (*Continued*)
  noninfiltrating (*Continued*)
    specified site - *see* Neoplasm, by site, in situ
    unspecified site 233.0
Comedomastitis 610.4
Comedones 706.1
  lanugo 757.4
Comma bacillus, carrier (suspected) of V02.3
Comminuted fracture - *see* Fracture, by site
Common
  aortopulmonary trunk 745.0
  atrioventricular canal (defect) 745.69
  atrium 745.69
  cold (head) 460
    vaccination, prophylactic (against) V04.7
  truncus (arteriosus) 745.0
  ventricle 745.3
Commotio (current)
  cerebri (*see also* Concussion, brain) 850.9
    with skull fracture - *see* Fracture, skull, by site
  retinae 921.3
  spinalis - *see* Injury, spinal, by site
Commotion (current)
  brain (without skull fracture) (*see also* Concussion, brain) 850.9
    with skull fracture - *see* Fracture, skull, by site
  spinal cord - *see* Injury, spinal, by site
Communication
  abnormal - *see also* Fistula
    between
      base of aorta and pulmonary artery 745.0
      left ventricle and right atrium 745.4
      pericardial sac and pleural sac 748.8
      pulmonary artery and pulmonary vein 747.3
    congenital, between uterus and anterior abdominal wall 752.3
      bladder 752.3
      intestine 752.3
      rectum 752.3
  left ventricular-right atrial 745.4
  pulmonary artery-pulmonary vein 747.3
Compensation
  broken - *see* Failure, heart
  failure - *see* Failure, heart
  neurosis, psychoneurosis 300.11
Complaint - *see also* Disease
  bowel, functional 564.9
    psychogenic 306.4
  intestine, functional 564.9
    psychogenic 306.4
  kidney (*see also* Disease, renal) 593.9
  liver 573.9
  miners' 500
Complete - *see* condition
Complex
  cardiorenal (*see also* Hypertension, cardiorenal) 404.90
  castration 300.9
  Costen's 524.60
  ego-dystonic homosexuality 302.0
  Eisenmenger's (ventricular septal defect) 745.4
  homosexual, ego-dystonic 302.0
  hypersexual 302.89
  inferiority 301.9

Complex (*Continued*)
  jumped process
    spine - *see* Dislocation, vertebra
  primary, tuberculosis (*see also* Tuberculosis) 010.0
  Taussig-Bing (transposition, aorta and overriding pulmonary artery) 745.11
Complications
  abortion NEC - *see* categories 634-639
  accidental puncture or laceration during a procedure 998.2
  amputation stump (late) (surgical) 997.60
    traumatic - *see* Amputation, traumatic
  anastomosis (and bypass) - *see also* Complications, due to (presence of) any device, implant, or graft classified to 996.0-996.5 NEC
    hemorrhage NEC 998.11
    intestinal (internal) NEC 997.4
      involving urinary tract 997.5
    mechanical - *see* Complications, mechanical, graft
    urinary tract (involving intestinal tract) 997.5
  anesthesia, anesthetic NEC (*see also* Anesthesia, complication) 995.2
    in labor and delivery 668.9
      affecting fetus or newborn 763.5
      cardiac 668.1
      central nervous system 668.2
      pulmonary 668.0
      specified type NEC 668.8
  aortocoronary (bypass) graft 996.03
    atherosclerosis - *see* Arteriosclerosis, coronary
    embolism 996.72
    occlusion NEC 996.72
    thrombus 996.72
  arthroplasty 996.4
  artificial opening
    cecostomy 569.60
    colostomy 569.60
    cystostomy 997.5
    enterostomy 569.60
    esophagostomy   ◀
      infection 530.86   ◀
      mechanical 530.87   ◀
    gastrostomy 536.40
    ileostomy 569.60
    jejunostomy 569.60
    nephrostomy 997.5
    tracheostomy 519.00
    ureterostomy 997.5
    urethrostomy 997.5
  bariatric surgery 997.4   ◀
  bile duct implant (prosthetic) NEC 996.79
    infection or inflammation 996.69
    mechanical 996.59
  bleeding (intraoperative) (postoperative) 998.11
  blood vessel graft 996.1
    aortocoronary 996.03
      atherosclerosis - *see* Arteriosclerosis, coronary
      embolism 996.72
      occlusion NEC 996.72
      thrombus 996.72
    atherosclerosis - *see* Arteriosclerosis, extremities
    embolism 996.74

Complications (*Continued*)
  blood vessel graft (*Continued*)
    occlusion NEC 996.74
    thrombus 996.74
  bone growth stimulator NEC 996.78
    infection or inflammation 996.67
  bone marrow transplant 996.85
  breast implant (prosthetic) NEC 996.79
    infection or inflammation 996.69
    mechanical 996.54
  bypass - *see also* Complications, anastomosis
    aortocoronary 996.03
      atherosclerosis - *see* Arteriosclerosis, coronary
      embolism 996.72
      occlusion NEC 996.72
      thrombus 996.72
    carotid artery 996.1
      atherosclerosis - *see* Arteriosclerosis, coronary
      embolism 996.74
      occlusion NEC 996.74
      thrombus 996.74
  cardiac (*see also* Disease, heart) 429.9
    device, implant, or graft NEC 996.72
      infection or inflammation 996.61
      long-term effect 429.4
      mechanical (*see also* Complications, mechanical, by type) 996.00
      valve prosthesis 996.71
        infection or inflammation 996.61
    postoperative NEC 997.1
      long-term effect 429.4
  cardiorenal (*see also* Hypertension, cardiorenal) 404.90
  carotid artery bypass graft 996.1
    atherosclerosis - *see* Arteriosclerosis, coronary
    embolism 996.74
    occlusion NEC 996.74
    thrombus 996.74
  cataract fragments in eye 998.82
  catheter device NEC - *see also* Complications, due to (presence of) any device, implant, or graft classified to 996.0-996.5 NEC
    mechanical - *see* Complications, mechanical, catheter
  cecostomy 569.60
  cesarean section wound 674.3
  chin implant (prosthetic) NEC 996.79
    infection or inflammation 996.69
    mechanical 996.59
  colostomy (enterostomy) 569.60
    specified type NEC 569.69
  contraceptive device, intrauterine NEC 996.76
    infection 996.65
    inflammation 996.65
    mechanical 996.32
  cord (umbilical) - *see* Complications, umbilical cord
  cornea
    due to
      contact lens 371.82
  coronary (artery) bypass (graft) NEC 996.03
    atherosclerosis - *see* Arteriosclerosis, coronary
    embolism 996.72
    infection or inflammation 996.61
    mechanical 996.03
    occlusion NEC 996.72

ICD-9-CM

C

Vol. 2

Complications (*Continued*)
coronary (artery) bypass (graft) NEC
(*Continued*)
specified type NEC 996.72
thrombus 996.72
cystostomy 997.5
delivery 669.9
procedure (instrumental) (manual)
(surgical) 669.4
specified type NEC 669.8
dialysis (hemodialysis) (peritoneal) (renal) NEC 999.9
catheter NEC - *see also* Complications, due to (presence of) any
device, implant, or graft classified to 996.0-996.5 NEC
infection or inflammation 996.62
peritoneal 996.68
mechanical 996.1
peritoneal 996.56
due to (presence of) any device, implant, or graft classified to 996.0-
996.5 NEC 996.70
with infection or inflammation - *see*
Complications, infection or inflammation, due to (presence of)
any device, implant, or graft
classified to 996.0-996.5 NEC
arterial NEC 996.74
coronary NEC 996.03
atherosclerosis - *see* Arteriosclerosis, coronary
embolism 996.72
occlusion NEC 996.72
specified type NEC 996.72
thrombus 996.72
renal dialysis 996.73
arteriovenous fistula or shunt NEC
996.74
bone growth stimulator 996.78
breast NEC 996.79
cardiac NEC 996.72
defibrillator 996.72
pacemaker 996.72
valve prosthesis 996.71
catheter NEC 996.79
spinal 996.75
urinary, indwelling 996.76
vascular NEC 996.74
renal dialysis 996.73
ventricular shunt 996.75
coronary (artery) bypass (graft) NEC
996.03
atherosclerosis - *see* Arterioscle-
sis, coronary
embolism 996.72
occlusion NEC 996.72
thrombus 996.72
electrodes
brain 996.75
heart 996.72
gastrointestinal NEC 996.79
genitourinary NEC 996.76
heart valve prosthesis NEC 996.71
infusion pump 996.74
internal
joint prosthesis 996.77
orthopedic NEC 996.78
specified type NEC 996.79
insulin pump 996.57   ◀▥
intrauterine contraceptive device
NEC 996.76
joint prosthesis, internal NEC 996.77
mechanical - *see* Complications, mechanical

Complications (*Continued*)
due to (presence of) any device, implant, or graft classified to (*Continued*)
nervous system NEC 996.75
ocular lens NEC 996.79
orbital NEC 996.79
orthopedic NEC 996.78
joint, internal 996.77
renal dialysis 996.73
specified type NEC 996.79
urinary catheter, indwelling 996.76
vascular NEC 996.74
ventricular shunt 996.75
during dialysis NEC 999.9
ectopic or molar pregnancy NEC 639.9
electroshock therapy NEC 999.9
enterostomy 569.60
specified type NEC 569.69   ◀▥
esophagostomy   ◀
infection 530.86   ◀
mechanical 530.87   ◀
external (fixation) device with internal
component(s) NEC 996.78
infection or inflammation 996.67
mechanical 996.4
extracorporeal circulation NEC 999.9
eye implant (prosthetic) NEC 996.79
infection or inflammation 996.69
mechanical
ocular lens 996.53
orbital globe 996.59
gastrointestinal, postoperative NEC
(*see also* Complications, surgical
procedures) 997.4
gastrostomy 536.40
specified type NEC 536.49
genitourinary device, implant or graft
NEC 996.76
infection or inflammation 996.65
urinary catheter, indwelling 996.64
mechanical (*see also* Complications,
mechanical, by type) 996.30
specified NEC 996.39
graft (bypass) (patch) - *see also* Complications, due to (presence of) any
device, implant, or graft classified
to 996.0-996.5 NEC
bone marrow 996.85
corneal NEC 996.79
infection or inflammation 996.69
rejection or reaction 996.51
mechanical - *see* Complications, mechanical, graft
organ (immune or nonimmune
cause) (partial) (total) 996.80
bone marrow 996.85
heart 996.83
intestines 996.87
kidney 996.81
liver 996.82
lung 996.84
pancreas 996.86
specified NEC 996.89
skin NEC 996.79
infection or inflammation 996.69
rejection 996.52
artificial 996.55
decellularized allodermis 996.55
heart - *see also* Disease, heart transplant (immune or nonimmune
cause) 996.83
hematoma (intraoperative) (postoperative) 998.12
hemorrhage (intraoperative) (postoperative) 998.11

Complications (*Continued*)
hyperalimentation therapy NEC 999.9
immunization (procedure) - *see* Complications, vaccination
implant - *see also* Complications, due
to (presence of) any device, implant, or graft classified to 996.0-
996.5 NEC
mechanical - *see* Complications, mechanical, implant
infection and inflammation
due to (presence of) any device, implant or graft classified to 996.0-
996.5 NEC 996.60
arterial NEC 996.62
coronary 996.61
renal dialysis 996.62
arteriovenous fistula or shunt 996.62
artifical heart 996.61
bone growth stimulator 996.67
breast 996.69
cardiac 996.61
catheter NEC 996.69
peritoneal 996.68
spinal 996.63
urinary, indwelling 996.64
vascular NEC 996.62
ventricular shunt 996.63
coronary artery bypass 996.61
electrodes
brain 996.63
heart 996.61
gastrointestinal NEC 996.69
genitourinary NEC 996.65
indwelling urinary catheter 996.64
heart assist device 996.61
heart valve 996.61
infusion pump 996.62
insulin pump 996.69
intrauterine contraceptive device
996.65
joint prosthesis, internal 996.66
ocular lens 996.69
orbital (implant) 996.69
orthopedic NEC 996.67
joint, internal 996.66
specified type NEC 996.69
urinary catheter, indwelling 996.64
ventricular shunt 996.63
infusion (procedure) 999.9
blood - *see* Complications, transfusion
infection NEC 999.3
sepsis NEC 999.3
inhalation therapy NEC 999.9
injection (procedure) 999.9
drug reaction (*see also* Reaction,
drug) 995.2
infection NEC 999.3
sepsis NEC 999.3
serum (prophylactic) (therapeutic) -
see Complications, vaccination
vaccine (any) - *see* Complications,
vaccination
inoculation (any) - *see* Complications,
vaccination
insulin pump 996.57   ◀▥
internal device (catheter) (electronic)
(fixation) (prosthetic) - *see also*
Complications, due to (presence
of) any device, implant, or graft
classified to 996.0-996.5 NEC
mechanical - *see* Complications, mechanical
intestinal transplant (immune or nonimmune cause) 996.87

Complications (*Continued*)

intraoperative bleeding or hemorrhage 998.11

intrauterine contraceptive device (*see also* Complications, contraceptive device) 996.76

   with fetal damage affecting management of pregnancy 655.8

   infection or inflammation 996.65

jejunostomy 569.60

kidney transplant (immune or nonimmune cause) 996.81

labor 669.9

   specified condition NEC 669.8

liver transplant (immune or nonimmune cause) 996.82

lumbar puncture 349.0

mechanical

   anastomosis - *see* Complications, mechanical, graft

   artifical heart 996.09 ◄▥▥

   bypass - *see* Complications, mechanical, graft

   catheter NEC 996.59

     cardiac 996.09

     cystostomy 996.39

     dialysis (hemodialysis) 996.1

       peritoneal 996.56

     during a procedure 998.2

     urethral, indwelling 996.31

   colostomy 569.62

   device NEC 996.59

     balloon (counterpulsation), intra-aortic 996.1

     cardiac 996.00

       automatic implantable defibrillator 996.04

       long-term effect 429.4

       specified NEC 996.09

     contraceptive, intrauterine 996.32

     counterpulsation, intra-aortic 996.1

     fixation, external, with internal components 996.4

     fixation, internal (nail, rod, plate) 996.4

     genitourinary 996.30

       specified NEC 996.39

     insulin pump 996.57

     nervous system 996.2

     orthopedic, internal 996.4

     prosthetic NEC 996.59

     umbrella, vena cava 996.1

     vascular 996.1

   dorsal column stimulator 996.2

   electrode NEC 996.59

     brain 996.2

     cardiac 996.01

     spinal column 996.2

   enterostomy 569.62

   esophagostomy 530.87 ◄▥▥

   fistula, arteriovenous, surgically created 996.1

   gastrostomy 536.42

   graft NEC 996.52

     aortic (bifurcation) 996.1

     aortocoronary bypass 996.03

     blood vessel NEC 996.1

     bone 996.4

     cardiac 996.00

     carotid artery bypass 996.1

     cartilage 996.4

     corneal 996.51

     coronary bypass 996.03

     decellularized allodermis 996.55

     genitourinary 996.30

       specified NEC 996.39

Complications (*Continued*)

mechanical (*Continued*)

   graft NEC (*Continued*)

     muscle 996.4

     nervous system 996.2

     organ (immune or nonimmune cause) 996.80

       heart 996.83

       intestines 996.87

       kidney 996.81

       liver 996.82

       lung 996.84

       pancreas 996.86

       specified NEC 996.89

     orthopedic, internal 996.4

     peripheral nerve 996.2

     prosthetic NEC 996.59

     skin 996.52

       artificial 996.55

     specified NEC 996.59

     tendon 996.4

     tissue NEC 996.52

     tooth 996.59

     ureter, without mention of resection 996.39

     vascular 996.1

   heart valve prosthesis 996.02

     long-term effect 429.4

   implant NEC 996.59

     cardiac 996.00

       automatic implantable defibrillator 996.04

       long-term effect 429.4

       specified NEC 996.09

     electrode NEC 996.59

       brain 996.2

       cardiac 996.01

       spinal column 996.2

     genitourinary 996.30

     nervous system 996.2

     orthopedic, internal 996.4

     prosthetic NEC 996.59

       in

         bile duct 996.59

         breast 996.54

         chin 996.59

         eye

           ocular lens 996.53

           orbital globe 996.59

     vascular 996.1

   insulin pump 996.57 ◄▥▥

   nonabsorbable surgical material 996.59

   pacemaker NEC 996.59

     brain 996.2

     cardiac 996.01

     nerve (phrenic) 996.2

   patch - *see* Complications, mechanical, graft

   prosthesis NEC 996.59

     bile duct 996.59

     breast 996.54

     chin 996.59

     ocular lens 996.53

     reconstruction, vas deferens 996.39

   reimplant NEC 996.59

     extremity (*see also* Complications, reattached, extremity) 996.90

     organ (*see also* Complications, transplant, organ, by site) 996.80

   repair - *see* Complications, mechanical, graft

   shunt NEC 996.59

     arteriovenous, surgically created 996.1

     ventricular (communicating) 996.2

Complications (*Continued*)

mechanical (*Continued*)

   stent NEC 996.59

   tracheostomy 519.02

   vas deferens reconstruction 996.39

medical care NEC 999.9

   cardiac NEC 997.1

   gastrointestinal NEC 997.4

   nervous system NEC 997.00

   peripheral vascular NEC 997.2

   respiratory NEC 997.3

   urinary NEC 997.5

   vascular

     mesenteric artery 997.71

     other vessels 997.79

     peripheral vessels 997.2

     renal artery 997.72

nephrostomy 997.5

nervous system

   device, implant, or graft NEC 349.1

     mechanical 996.2

   postoperative NEC 997.00

obstetric 669.9

   procedure (instrumental) (manual) (surgical) 669.4

   specified NEC 669.8

   surgical wound 674.3

ocular lens implant NEC 996.79

   infection or inflammation 996.69

   mechanical 996.53

organ transplant - *see* Complications, transplant, organ, by site

orthopedic device, implant, or graft

   internal (fixation) (nail) (plate) (rod) NEC 996.78

   infection or inflammation 996.67

   joint prosthesis 996.77

     infection or inflammation 996.66

   mechanical 996.4

pacemaker (cardiac) 996.72

   infection or inflammation 996.61

   mechanical 996.01

pancreas transplant (immune or nonimmune cause) 996.86

perfusion NEC 999.9

perineal repair (obstetrical) 674.3

   disruption 674.2

pessary (uterus) (vagina) - *see* Complications, contraceptive device

phototherapy 990

postcystoscopic 997.5

postmastoidectomy NEC 383.30

postoperative - *see* Complications, surgical procedures

pregnancy NEC 646.9

   affecting fetus or newborn 761.9

prosthetic device, internal - *see also* Complications, due to (presence of) any device, implant or graft classified to 996.0-996.5 NEC

   mechanical NEC (*see also* Complications, mechanical) 996.59

puerperium NEC (*see also* Puerperal) 674.9

puncture, spinal 349.0

pyelogram 997.5

radiation 990

radiotherapy 990

reattached

   body part, except extremity 996.99

   extremity (infection) (rejection) 996.90

     arm(s) 996.94

     digit(s) (hand) 996.93

       foot 996.95

ICD-9-CM

C

Vol. 2

Complications *(Continued)*
  reattached *(Continued)*
    extremity (infection) (rejection)
      (Continued)
        finger(s) 996.93
        foot 996.95
        forearm 996.91
        hand 996.92
        leg 996.96
        lower NEC 996.96
        toe(s) 996.95
        upper NEC 996.94
    reimplant NEC - *see also* Complications, due to (presence of) any device, implant, or graft classified to 996.0-996.5 NEC
      bone marrow 996.85
      extremity (*see also* Complications, reattached, extremity) 996.90
        due to infection 996.90
      mechanical - *see* Complications, mechanical, reimplant
      organ (immune or nonimmune cause) (partial) (total) (*see also* Complications, transplant, organ, by site) 996.80
    renal allograft 996.81
    renal dialysis - *see* Complications, dialysis
    respiratory 519.9
      device, implant or graft NEC 996.79
        infection or inflammation 996.69
        mechanical 996.59
      distress syndrome, adult, following trauma or surgery 518.5
      insufficiency, acute, postoperative 518.5
      postoperative NEC 997.3
      therapy NEC 999.9
    sedation during labor and delivery 668.9
      affecting fetus or newborn 763.5
      cardiac 668.1
      central nervous system 668.2
      pulmonary 668.0
      specified type NEC 668.8
    seroma (intraoperative) (postoperative) (noninfected) 998.13
      infected 998.51
    shunt - *see also* Complications, due to (presence of) any device, implant, or graft classified to 996.0-996.5 NEC
      mechanical - *see* Complications, mechanical, shunt
    specified body system NEC
      device, implant, or graft - *see* Complications, due to (presence of) any device, implant, or graft classified to 996.0-996.5 NEC
      postoperative NEC 997.99
    spinal puncture or tap 349.0
    stoma, external
      gastrointestinal tract
        colostomy 569.60
        enterostomy 569.60
        esophagostomy ◀
          infection 530.86 ◀
          mechanical 530.87 ◀
        gastrostomy 536.40
      urinary tract 997.5
    stomach banding 997.4 ◀
    stomach stapling 997.4 ◀
    surgical procedures 998.9
      accidental puncture or laceration 998.2
      amputation stump (late) 997.60
      anastomosis - *see* Complications, anastomosis

Complications *(Continued)*
  surgical procedures *(Continued)*
    burst stitches or sutures (external) 998.32
      internal 998.31
    cardiac 997.1
      long-term effect following cardiac surgery 429.4
    catheter device - *see* Complications, catheter device
    cataract fragments in eye 998.82
    cecostomy malfunction 569.62
    colostomy malfunction 569.62
    cystostomy malfunction 997.5
    dehiscence (of incision) (external) 998.32
      internal 998.31
    dialysis NEC (*see also* Complications, dialysis) 999.9
    disruption
      anastomosis (internal) - *see* Complications, mechanical, graft
      internal suture (line) 998.31
      wound (external) 998.32
        internal 998.31
    dumping syndrome (postgastrectomy) 564.2
    elephantiasis or lymphedema 997.99
      postmastectomy 457.0
    emphysema (surgical) 998.81
    enterostomy malfunction 569.62
    esophagostomy malfunction 530.87 ◀
    evisceration 998.32
    fistula (persistent postoperative) 998.6
    foreign body inadvertently left in wound (sponge) (suture) (swab) 998.4
    from nonabsorbable surgical material (Dacron) (mesh) (permanent suture) (reinforcing) (Teflon) - *see* Complications due to (presence of) any device, implant, or graft classified to 996.0-996.5 NEC
    gastrointestinal NEC 997.4
    gastrostomy malfunction 536.42
    hematoma 998.12
    hemorrhage 998.11
    ileostomy malfunction 569.62
    internal prosthetic device NEC (*see also* Complications, internal device) 996.70
      hemolytic anemia 283.19
      infection or inflammation 996.60
      malfunction - *see* Complications, mechanical
      mechanical complication - *see* Complications, mechanical
      thrombus 996.70
    jejunostomy malfunction 569.62
    nervous system NEC 997.00
    obstruction, internal anastomosis - *see* Complications, mechanical, graft
    other body system NEC 997.99
    peripheral vascular NEC 997.2
    postcardiotomy syndrome 429.4
    postcholecystectomy syndrome 576.0
    postcommissurotomy syndrome 429.4
    postgastrectomy dumping syndrome 564.2
    postmastectomy lymphedema syndrome 457.0
    postmastoidectomy 383.30
      cholesteatoma, recurrent 383.32
      cyst, mucosal 383.31
      granulation 383.33
      inflammation, chronic 383.33
    postvagotomy syndrome 564.2

Complications *(Continued)*
  surgical procedures *(Continued)*
    postvalvulotomy syndrome 429.4
    reattached extremity (infection) (rejection) (*see also* Complications, reattached, extremity) 996.90
    respiratory NEC 997.3
    seroma 998.13
    shock (endotoxic) (hypovolemic) (septic) 998.0
    shunt, prosthetic (thrombus) - *see also* Complications, due to (presence of) any device, implant, or graft classified to 996.0-996.5 NEC
      hemolytic anemia 283.19
    specified complication NEC 998.89
    stitch abscess 998.59
    transplant - *see* Complications, graft
    ureterostomy malfunction 997.5
    urethrostomy malfunction 997.5
    urinary NEC 997.5
    vascular
      mesenteric artery 997.71
      other vessels 997.79
      peripheral vessels 997.2
      renal artery 997.72
    wound infection 998.59
  therapeutic misadventure NEC 999.9
    surgical treatment 998.9
  tracheostomy 519.00
  transfusion (blood) (lymphocytes) (plasma) NEC 999.8
    atrophy, liver, yellow, subacute (within 8 months of administration) - *see* Hepatitis, viral
    bone marrow 996.85
    embolism
      air 999.1
      thrombus 999.2
    hemolysis NEC 999.8
      bone marrow 996.85
    hepatitis (serum) (type B) (within 8 months after administration) - *see* Hepatitis, viral
    incompatibility reaction (ABO) (blood group) 999.6
      Rh (factor) 999.7
    infection 999.3
    jaundice (serum) (within 8 months after administration) - *see* Hepatitis, viral
    sepsis 999.3
    shock or reaction NEC 999.8
      bone marrow 996.85
    subacute yellow atrophy of liver (within 8 months after administration) - *see* Hepatitis, viral
    thromboembolism 999.2
  transplant NEC - *see also* Complications, due to (presence of) any device, implant, or graft classified to 996.0-996.5 NEC
    bone marrow 996.85
    organ (immune or nonimmune cause) (partial) (total) 996.80
      bone marrow 996.85
      heart 996.83
      intestines 996.87
      kidney 996.81
      liver 996.82
      lung 996.84
      pancreas 996.86
      specified NEC 996.89
  trauma NEC (early) 958.8
  ultrasound therapy NEC 999.9
  umbilical cord
    affecting fetus or newborn 762.6

◀ **New**   ◀▥ **Revised**

Complications *(Continued)*
umbilical cord *(Continued)*
complicating delivery 663.9
affecting fetus or newborn 762.6
specified type NEC 663.8
urethral catheter NEC 996.76
infection or inflammation 996.64
mechanical 996.31
urinary, postoperative NEC 997.5
vaccination 999.9
anaphylaxis NEC 999.4
cellulitis 999.3
encephalitis or encephalomyelitis
323.5
hepatitis (serum) (type B) (within 8
months after administration) -
see Hepatitis, viral
infection (general) (local) NEC 999.3
jaundice (serum) (within 8 months
after administration) - *see* Hepatitis, viral
meningitis 997.09 *[321.8]*
myelitis 323.5
protein sickness 999.5
reaction (allergic) 999.5
Herxheimer's 995.0
serum 999.5
sepsis 999.3
serum intoxication, sickness, rash, or
other serum reaction NEC
999.5
shock (allergic) (anaphylactic) 999.4
subacute yellow atrophy of liver
(within 8 months after administration) - *see* Hepatitis, viral
vaccinia (generalized) 999.0
localized 999.3
vascular
device, implant, or graft NEC 996.74
infection or inflammation 996.62
mechanical NEC 996.1
cardiac (*see also* Complications,
mechanical, by type) 996.00
following infusion, perfusion, or
transfusion 999.2
postoperative NEC 997.2
mesenteric artery 997.71
other vessels 997.79
peripheral vessels 997.2
renal artery 997.72
ventilation therapy NEC 999.9
**Compound presentation, complicating
delivery** 652.8
causing obstructed labor 660.0
Compressed air disease 993.3
Compression
with injury - *see* specific injury
arm NEC 354.9
artery 447.1
celiac, syndrome 447.4
brachial plexus 353.0
brain (stem) 348.4
due to
contusion, brain - *see* Contusion,
brain
injury NEC - *see also* Hemorrhage,
brain, traumatic
birth - *see* Birth, injury, brain
laceration, brain - *see* Laceration,
brain
osteopathic 739.0
bronchus 519.1
by cicatrix - *see* Cicatrix
cardiac 423.9

Compression *(Continued)*
cauda equina 344.60
with neurogenic bladder 344.61
celiac (artery) (axis) 447.4
cerebral - *see* Compression, brain
cervical plexus 353.2
cord (umbilical) - *see* Compression,
umbilical cord
cranial nerve 352.9
second 377.49
third (partial) 378.51
total 378.52
fourth 378.53
fifth 350.8
sixth 378.54
seventh 351.8
divers' squeeze 993.3
duodenum (external) (*see also* Obstruction, duodenum) 537.3
during birth 767.9
esophagus 530.3
congenital, external 750.3
Eustachian tube 381.63
facies (congenital) 754.0
fracture - *see* Fracture, by site
heart - *see* Disease, heart
intestine (*see also* Obstruction, intestine) 560.9
with hernia - *see* Hernia, by site,
with obstruction
laryngeal nerve, recurrent 478.79
leg NEC 355.8
lower extremity NEC 355.8
lumbosacral plexus 353.1
lung 518.89
lymphatic vessel 457.1
medulla - *see* Compression, brain
nerve NEC - *see also* Disorder, nerve
arm NEC 354.9
autonomic nervous system (*see also*
Neuropathy, peripheral, autonomic) 337.9
axillary 353.0
cranial NEC 352.9
due to displacement of intervertebral
disc 722.2
with myelopathy 722.70
cervical 722.0
with myelopathy 722.71
lumbar, lumbosacral 722.10
with myelopathy 722.73
thoracic, thoracolumbar 722.11
with myelopathy 722.72
iliohypogastric 355.79
ilioinguinal 355.79
leg NEC 355.8
lower extremity NEC 355.8
median (in carpal tunnel) 354.0
obturator 355.79
optic 377.49
plantar 355.6
posterior tibial (in tarsal tunnel)
355.5
root (by scar tissue) NEC 724.9
cervical NEC 723.4
lumbar NEC 724.4
lumbosacral 724.4
thoracic 724.4
saphenous 355.79
sciatic (acute) 355.0
sympathetic 337.9
traumatic - *see* Injury, nerve
ulnar 354.2
upper extremity NEC 354.9

Compression *(Continued)*
peripheral - *see* Compression, nerve
spinal (cord) (old or nontraumatic)
336.9
by displacement of intervertebral
disc - *see* Displacement, intervertebral disc
nerve
root NEC 724.9
postoperative 722.80
cervical region 722.81
lumbar region 722.83
thoracic region 722.82
traumatic - *see* Injury, nerve,
spinal
traumatic - *see* Injury, nerve, spinal
spondylogenic 721.91
cervical 721.1
lumbar, lumbosacral 721.42
thoracic 721.41
traumatic - *see also* Injury, spinal, by
site
with fracture, vertebra - *see* Fracture, vertebra, by site, with
spinal cord injury
spondylogenic - *see* Compression, spinal cord, spondylogenic
subcostal nerve (syndrome) 354.8
sympathetic nerve NEC 337.9
syndrome 958.5
thorax 512.8
iatrogenic 512.1
postoperative 512.1
trachea 519.1
congenital 748.3
ulnar nerve (by scar tissue) 354.2
umbilical cord
affecting fetus or newborn 762.5
cord prolapsed 762.4
complicating delivery 663.2
cord around neck 663.1
cord prolapsed 663.0
upper extremity NEC 354.9
ureter 593.3
urethra - *see* Stricture, urethra
vein 459.2
vena cava (inferior) (superior) 459.2
vertebral NEC - *see* Compression, spinal (cord)
Compulsion, compulsive
eating 307.51
neurosis (obsessive) 300.3
personality 301.4
states (mixed) 300.3
swearing 300.3
in Gilles de la Tourette's syndrome
307.23
tics and spasms 307.22
water drinking NEC (syndrome) 307.9
Concato's disease (pericardial polyserositis) 423.2
peritoneal 568.82
pleural - *see* Pleurisy
Concavity, chest wall 738.3
Concealed
hemorrhage NEC 459.0
penis 752.65
Concentric fading 368.12
Concern (normal) about sick person in
family V61.49
Concrescence (teeth) 520.2
Concretio cordis 423.1
rheumatic 393

Concretion - *see also* Calculus
 appendicular 543.9
 canaliculus 375.57
 clitoris 624.8
 conjunctiva 372.54
 eyelid 374.56
 intestine (impaction) (obstruction)
  560.39
 lacrimal (passages) 375.57
 prepuce (male) 605
  female (clitoris) 624.8
 salivary gland (any) 527.5
 seminal vesicle 608.89
 stomach 537.89
 tonsil 474.8
Concussion (current) 850.9
 with
  loss of consciousness 850.5
   brief (less than one hour)
    30 minutes or less 850.11
    31–59 minutes 850.12
   moderate (1-24 hours) 850.2
   prolonged (more than 24 hours)
    (with complete recovery)
    (with return to pre-existing
     conscious level) 850.3
    without return to pre-existing
     conscious level 850.4
  mental confusion or disorientation
   (without loss of consciousness)
   850.0
  with loss of consciousness - *see*
   Concussion, with, loss of consciousness
 without loss of consciousness 850.0
 blast (air) (hydraulic) (immersion) (underwater) 869.0
  with open wound into cavity 869.1
  abdomen or thorax - *see* Injury, internal, by site
  brain - *see* Concussion, brain
  ear (acoustic nerve trauma) 951.5
   with perforation, tympanic mem-
    brane - *see* Wound, open, ear
    drum
  thorax - *see* Injury, internal, intrathoracic organs NEC
 brain or cerebral (without skull fracture) 850.9
  with
   loss of consciousness 850.5
    brief (less than one hour)
     30 minutes or less 850.11
     31–59 minutes 850.12
    moderate (1-24 hours) 850.2
    prolonged (more than 24 hours)
     (with complete recovery)
     (with return to pre-existing
      conscious level) 850.3
     without return to pre-existing
      conscious level 850.4
   mental confusion or disorientation
    (without loss of conscious-
    ness) 850.0
   with loss of consciousness - *see*
    Concussion, brain, with,
    loss of consciousness
   skull fracture - *see* Fracture, skull,
    by site
  without loss of consciousness 850.0
 cauda equina 952.4
 cerebral - *see* Concussion, brain
 conus medullaris (spine) 952.4
 hydraulic - *see* Concussion, blast
 internal organs - *see* Injury, internal, by
  site

Concussion *(Continued)*
 labyrinth - *see* Injury, intracranial
 ocular 921.3
 osseous labyrinth - *see* Injury, intracranial
 spinal (cord) - *see also* Injury, spinal,
  by site
  due to
   broken
    back - *see* Fracture, vertebra,
     by site, with spinal cord
     injury
    neck - *see* Fracture, vertebra,
     cervical, with spinal cord
     injury
   fracture, fracture dislocation, or
    compression fracture of spine
    or vertebra - *see* Fracture, ver-
    tebra, by site, with spinal
    cord injury
  syndrome 310.2
  underwater blast - *see* Concussion,
   blast
Condition - *see also* Disease
 psychiatric 298.9
 respiratory NEC 519.9
  acute or subacute NEC 519.9
   due to
    external agent 508.9
     specified type NEC 508.8
    fumes or vapors (chemical) (in-
     halation) 506.3
    radiation 508.0
  chronic NEC 519.9
   due to
    external agent 508.9
     specified type NEC 508.8
    fumes or vapors (chemical) (in-
     halation) 506.4
    radiation 508.1
   due to
    external agent 508.9
     specified type NEC 508.8
    fumes or vapors (chemical) inhala-
     tion 506.9
Conduct disturbance *(see also* Disturbance, conduct) 312.9
 adjustment reaction 309.3
 hyperkinetic 314.2
Condyloma NEC 078.10
 acuminatum 078.11
 gonorrheal 098.0
 latum 091.3
 syphilitic 091.3
  congenital 090.0
 venereal, syphilitic 091.3
Confinement - *see* Delivery
Conflagration - *see also* Burn, by site
 asphyxia (by inhalation of smoke,
  gases, fumes, or vapors) 987.9
  specified agent - *see* Table of Drugs
   and Chemicals
Conflict
 family V61.9
  specified circumstance NEC V61.8
 interpersonal NEC V62.81
 marital V61.10
  involving divorce or estrangement
   V61.0
 parent-child V61.20
 partner V61.10
Confluent - *see* condition
Confusion, confused (mental) (state) *(see
 also* State, confusional) 298.9

Confusion, confused *(Continued)*
 acute 293.0
  epileptic 293.0
  postoperative 293.9
  psychogenic 298.2
  reactive (from emotional stress, psychological trauma) 298.2
  subacute 293.1
Congelation 991.9
Congenital - *see also* condition
 aortic septum 747.29
 intrinsic factor deficiency 281.0
 malformation - *see* Anomaly
Congestion, congestive (chronic) (passive)
 asphyxia, newborn 768.9
 bladder 596.8
 bowel 569.89
 brain *(see also* Disease, cerebrovascular
  NEC) 437.8
  malarial 084.9
 breast 611.79
 bronchi 519.1
 bronchial tube 519.1
 catarrhal 472.0
 cerebral - *see* Congestion, brain
 cerebrospinal - *see* Congestion, brain
 chest 514
 chill 780.99
  malarial *(see also* Malaria) 084.6
 circulatory NEC 459.9
 conjunctiva 372.71
 due to disturbance of circulation
  459.9
 duodenum 537.3
 enteritis - *see* Enteritis
 eye 372.71
 fibrosis syndrome (pelvic) 625.5
 gastroenteritis - *see* Enteritis
 general 799.89
 glottis 476.0
 heart *(see also* Failure, heart) 428.0
 hepatic 573.0
 hypostatic (lung) 514
 intestine 569.89
 intracranial - *see* Congestion, brain
 kidney 593.89
 labyrinth 386.50
 larynx 476.0
 liver 573.0
 lung 514
  active or acute *(see also* Pneumonia)
   486
   congenital 770.0
  chronic 514
  hypostatic 514
  idiopathic, acute 518.5
  passive 514
 malaria, malarial (brain) (fever) *(see
  also* Malaria) 084.6
 medulla - *see* Congestion, brain
 nasal 478.1
 orbit, orbital 376.33
  inflammatory (chronic) 376.10
   acute 376.00
 ovary 620.8
 pancreas 577.8
 pelvic, female 625.5
 pleural 511.0
 prostate (active) 602.1
 pulmonary - *see* Congestion, lung
 renal 593.89
 retina 362.89
 seminal vesicle 608.89
 spinal cord 336.1

◀ **New**   ◀▥ **Revised**

Congestion, congestive (Continued)
spleen 289.51
chronic 289.51
stomach 537.89
trachea 464.11
urethra 599.84
uterus 625.5
with subinvolution 621.1
viscera 799.89
Congestive - see Congestion
Conical
cervix 622.6
cornea 371.60
teeth 520.2
Conjoined twins 759.4
causing disproportion (fetopelvic) 653.7
Conjugal maladjustment V61.10
involving divorce or estrangement V61.0
Conjunctiva - see condition
Conjunctivitis (exposure) (infectious) (nondiphtheritic) (pneumococcal) (pustular) (staphylococcal) (streptococcal) NEC 372.30
actinic 370.24
acute 372.00
atopic 372.05
contagious 372.03
follicular 372.02
hemorrhagic (viral) 077.4
adenoviral (acute) 077.3
allergic (chronic) 372.14
with hay fever 372.05
anaphylactic 372.05
angular 372.03
Apollo (viral) 077.4
atopic 372.05
blennorrhagic (neonatorum) 098.40
catarrhal 372.03
chemical 372.05
chlamydial 077.98
due to
Chlamydia trachomatis - see Trachoma
paratrachoma 077.0
chronic 372.10
allergic 372.14
follicular 372.12
simple 372.11
specified type NEC 372.14
vernal 372.13
diphtheritic 032.81
due to
dust 372.05
enterovirus type 70 077.4
erythema multiforme 695.1 [372.33]
filariasis (see also Filariasis) 125.9 [372.15]
mucocutaneous
disease NEC 372.33
leishmaniasis 085.5 [372.15]
Reiter's disease 099.3 [372.33]
syphilis 095.8 [372.10]
toxoplasmosis (acquired) 130.1
congenital (active) 771.2
trachoma - see Trachoma
dust 372.05
eczematous 370.31
epidemic 077.1
hemorrhagic 077.4
follicular (acute) 372.02
adenoviral (acute) 077.3
chronic 372.12
glare 370.24
gonococcal (neonatorum) 098.40

Conjunctivitis (Continued)
granular (trachomatous) 076.1
late effect 139.1
hemorrhagic (acute) (epidemic) 077.4
herpetic (simplex) 054.43
zoster 053.21
inclusion 077.0
infantile 771.6
influenzal 372.03
Koch-Weeks 372.03
light 372.05
medicamentosa 372.05
membranous 372.04
meningococcic 036.89
Morax-Axenfeld 372.02
mucopurulent NEC 372.03
neonatal 771.6
gonococcal 098.40
Newcastle's 077.8
nodosa 360.14
of Beal 077.3
parasitic 372.15
filariasis (see also Filariasis) 125.9 [372.15]
mucocutaneous leishmaniasis 085.5 [372.15]
Parinaud's 372.02
petrificans 372.39
phlyctenular 370.31
pseudomembranous 372.04
diphtheritic 032.81
purulent 372.03
Reiter's 099.3 [372.33]
rosacea 695.3 [372.31]
serous 372.01
viral 077.99
simple chronic 372.11
specified NEC 372.39
sunlamp 372.04
swimming pool 077.0
trachomatous (follicular) 076.1
acute 076.0
late effect 139.1
traumatic NEC 372.39
tuberculous (see also Tuberculosis) 017.3 [370.31]
tularemic 021.3
tularensis 021.3
vernal 372.13
limbar 372.13 [370.32]
viral 077.99
acute hemorrhagic 077.4
specified NEC 077.8
Conjunctivochalasis 372.81
Conjunctoblepharitis - see Conjunctivitis
Conn (-Louis) syndrome (primary aldosteronism) 255.12
Connective tissue - see condition
Conradi (-Hünermann) syndrome or disease (chondrodysplasia calcificans congenita) 756.59
Consanguinity V19.7
Consecutive - see condition
Consolidated lung (base) - see Pneumonia, lobar
Constipation 564.00
atonic 564.09
drug induced
correct substance properly administered 564.09
overdose or wrong substance given or taken 977.9
specified drug - see Table of Drugs and Chemicals
neurogenic 564.09

Constipation (Continued)
other specified NEC 564.09
outlet dysfunction 564.02
psychogenic 306.4
simple 564.00
slow transit 564.01
spastic 564.09
Constitutional - see also condition
arterial hypotension (see also Hypotension) 458.9
obesity 278.00
morbid 278.01
psychopathic state 301.9
short stature in childhood 783.43
state, developmental V21.9
specified development NEC V21.8
substandard 301.6
Constitutionally substandard 301.6
Constriction
anomalous, meningeal bands or folds 742.8
aortic arch (congenital) 747.10
asphyxiation or suffocation by 994.7
bronchus 519.1
canal, ear (see also Stricture, ear canal, acquired) 380.50
duodenum 537.3
gallbladder (see also Obstruction, gallbladder) 575.2
congenital 751.69
intestine (see also Obstruction, intestine) 560.9
larynx 478.74
congenital 748.3
meningeal bands or folds, anomalous 742.8
organ or site, congenital NEC - see Atresia
prepuce (congenital) 605
pylorus 537.0
adult hypertrophic 537.0
congenital or infantile 750.5
newborn 750.5
ring (uterus) 661.4
affecting fetus or newborn 763.7
spastic - see also Spasm
ureter 593.3
urethra - see Stricture, urethra
stomach 537.89
ureter 593.3
urethra - see Stricture, urethra
visual field (functional) (peripheral) 368.45
Constrictive - see condition
Consultation V65.9
medical - see also Counseling, medical
specified reason NEC V65.8
without complaint or sickness V65.9
feared complaint unfounded V65.5
specified reason NEC V65.8
Consumption - see Tuberculosis
Contact
with
AIDS virus V01.79 ◀
anthrax V01.81
cholera V01.0
communicable disease V01.9
specified type NEC V01.89
viral NEC V01.79 ◀▥
Escherichia coli (E. coli) V01.83 ◀
German measles V01.4
gonorrhea V01.6
HIV V01.79 ◀▥
human immunodeficiency virus V01.79 ◀▥
meningococcus V01.84 ◀
parasitic disease NEC V01.89

ICD-9-CM

C

Vol. 2

Contact (*Continued*)
  with (*Continued*)
    poliomyelitis V01.2
    rabies V01.5
    rubella V01.4
    SARS-associated coronavirus V01.82
    smallpox V01.3
    syphilis V01.6
    tuberculosis V01.1
    varicella V01.71   ◀
    venereal disease V01.6
    viral disease NEC V01.79   ◀▥
  dermatitis - *see* Dermatitis
Contamination, food (*see also* Poisoning, food) 005.9
Contraception, contraceptive
  advice NEC V25.09
    family planning V25.09
    fitting of diaphragm V25.02
    prescribing or use of
      oral contraceptive agent V25.01
      specified agent NEC V25.02
  counseling NEC V25.09
    emergency V25.03
    family planning V25.09
    fitting of diaphragm V25.02
    prescribing or use of
      oral contraceptive agent V25.01
        emergency V25.03
        postcoital V25.03
      specified agent NEC V25.02
  device (in situ) V45.59
    causing menorrhagia 996.76
    checking V25.42
    complications 996.32
    insertion V25.1
    intrauterine V45.51
    reinsertion V25.42
    removal V25.42
    subdermal V45.52
  fitting of diaphragm V25.02
  insertion
    intrauterine contraceptive device V25.1
    subdermal implantable V25.5
  maintenance V25.40
    examination V25.40
      intrauterine device V25.42
      oral contraceptive V25.41
      specified method NEC V25.49
      subdermal implantable V25.43
    intrauterine device V25.42
    oral contraceptive V25.41
    specified method NEC V25.49
    subdermal implantable V25.43
  management NEC V25.49
  prescription
    oral contraceptive agent V25.01
      emergency V25.03
      postcoital V25.03
      repeat V25.41
    specified agent NEC V25.02
      repeat V25.49
  sterilization V25.2
  surveillance V25.40
    intrauterine device V25.42
    oral contraceptive agent V25.41
    specified method NEC V25.49
    subdermal implantable V25.43
Contraction, contracture, contracted
  Achilles tendon (*see also* Short, tendon, Achilles) 727.81
  anus 564.89
  axilla 729.9
  bile duct (*see also* Disease, biliary) 576.8
  bladder 596.8
    neck or sphincter 596.0
  bowel (*see also* Obstruction, intestine) 560.9
  Braxton Hicks 644.1

Contraction, contracture, contracted
  (*Continued*)
  bronchus 519.1
  burn (old) - *see* Cicatrix
  cecum (*see also* Obstruction, intestine) 560.9
  cervix (*see also* Stricture, cervix) 622.4
    congenital 752.49
  cicatricial - *see* Cicatrix
  colon (*see also* Obstruction, intestine) 560.9
  conjunctiva, trachomatous, active 076.1
    late effect 139.1
  Dupuytren's 728.6
  eyelid 374.41
  eye socket (after enucleation) 372.64
  face 729.9
  fascia (lata) (postural) 728.89
    Dupuytren's 728.6
    palmar 728.6
    plantar 728.71
  finger NEC 736.29
    congenital 755.59
    joint (*see also* Contraction, joint) 718.44
  flaccid, paralytic
    joint (*see also* Contraction, joint) 718.4
    muscle 728.85
      ocular 378.50
  gallbladder (*see also* Obstruction, gall-bladder) 575.2
  hamstring 728.89
    tendon 727.81
  heart valve - *see* Endocarditis
  Hicks' 644.1
  hip (*see also* Contraction, joint) 718.4
  hourglass
    bladder 596.8
      congenital 753.8
    gallbladder (*see also* Obstruction, gallbladder) 575.2
      congenital 751.69
    stomach 536.8
      congenital 750.7
      psychogenic 306.4
    uterus 661.4
      affecting fetus or newborn 763.7
  hysterical 300.11
  infantile (*see also* Epilepsy) 345.6
  internal os (*see also* Stricture, cervix) 622.4
  intestine (*see also* Obstruction, intestine) 560.9
  joint (abduction) (acquired) (adduction) (flexion) (rotation) 718.40
    ankle 718.47
    congenital NEC 755.8
      generalized or multiple 754.89
        lower limb joints 754.89
      hip (*see also* Subluxation, congenital, hip) 754.32
      lower limb (including pelvic girdle) not involving hip 754.89
      upper limb (including shoulder girdle) 755.59
    elbow 718.42
    foot 718.47
    hand 718.44
    hip 718.45
    hysterical 300.11
    knee 718.46
    multiple sites 718.49
    pelvic region 718.45
    shoulder (region) 718.41
    specified site NEC 718.48
    wrist 718.43

Contraction, contracture, contracted
  (*Continued*)
  kidney (granular) (secondary) (*see also* Sclerosis, renal) 587
    congenital 753.3
    hydronephritic 591
    pyelonephritic (*see also* Pyelitis, chronic) 590.00
    tuberculous (*see also* Tuberculosis) 016.0
  ligament 728.89
    congenital 756.89
  liver - *see* Cirrhosis, liver
  muscle (postinfectional) (postural) NEC 728.85
    congenital 756.89
      sternocleidomastoid 754.1
    extraocular 378.60
    eye (extrinsic) (*see also* Strabismus) 378.9
      paralytic (*see also* Strabismus, paralytic) 378.50
    flaccid 728.85
    hysterical 300.11
    ischemic (Volkmann's) 958.6
    paralytic 728.85
    posttraumatic 958.6
    psychogenic 306.0
      specified as conversion reaction 300.11
  myotonic 728.85
  neck (*see also* Torticollis) 723.5
    congenital 754.1
    psychogenic 306.0
  ocular muscle (*see also* Strabismus) 378.9
    paralytic (*see also* Strabismus, paralytic) 378.50
  organ or site, congenital NEC - *see* Atresia
  outlet (pelvis) - *see* Contraction, pelvis
  palmar fascia 728.6
  paralytic
    joint (*see also* Contraction, joint) 718.4
    muscle 728.85
      ocular (*see also* Strabismus, paralytic) 378.50
  pelvis (acquired) (general) 738.6
    affecting fetus or newborn 763.1
    complicating delivery 653.1
      causing obstructed labor 660.1
    generally contracted 653.1
      causing obstructed labor 660.1
    inlet 653.2
      causing obstructed labor 660.1
    midpelvic 653.8
      causing obstructed labor 660.1
    midplane 653.8
      causing obstructed labor 660.1
    outlet 653.3
      causing obstructed labor 660.1
  plantar fascia 728.71
  premature
    atrial 427.61
    auricular 427.61
    auriculoventricular 427.61
    heart (junctional) (nodal) 427.60
    supraventricular 427.61
    ventricular 427.69
  prostate 602.8
  pylorus (*see also* Pylorospasm) 537.81
  rectosigmoid (*see also* Obstruction, intestine) 560.9
  rectum, rectal (sphincter) 564.89
    psychogenic 306.4

◀ **New**   ◀▥ **Revised**

Contraction, contracture, contracted
(*Continued*)
ring (Bandl's) 661.4
  affecting fetus or newborn 763.7
scar - *see* Cicatrix
sigmoid (*see also* Obstruction, intestine)
  560.9
socket, eye 372.64
spine (*see also* Curvature, spine) 737.9
stomach 536.8
  hourglass 536.8
    congenital 750.7
    psychogenic 306.4
  psychogenic 306.4
tendon (sheath) (*see also* Short, tendon)
  727.81
toe 735.8
ureterovesical orifice (postinfectional)
  593.3
urethra 599.84
uterus 621.8
  abnormal 661.9
    affecting fetus or newborn 763.7
  clonic, hourglass or tetanic 661.4
    affecting fetus or newborn 763.7
  dyscoordinate 661.4
    affecting fetus or newborn 763.7
  hourglass 661.4
    affecting fetus or newborn 763.7
  hypotonic NEC 661.2
    affecting fetus or newborn 763.7
  incoordinate 661.4
    affecting fetus or newborn 763.7
  inefficient or poor 661.2
    affecting fetus or newborn 763.7
  irregular 661.2
    affecting fetus or newborn 763.7
  tetanic 661.4
    affecting fetus or newborn 763.7
vagina (outlet) 623.2
vesical 596.8
  neck or urethral orifice 596.0
visual field, generalized 368.45
Volkmann's (ischemic) 958.6
Contusion (skin surface intact) 924.9
with
  crush injury - *see* Crush
  dislocation - *see* Dislocation, by site
  fracture - *see* Fracture, by site
  internal injury - *see also* Injury, internal, by site
    heart - *see* Contusion, cardiac
    kidney - *see* Contusion, kidney
    liver - *see* Contusion, liver
    lung - *see* Contusion, lung
    spleen - *see* Contusion, spleen
  intracranial injury - *see* Injury, intracranial
  nerve injury - *see* Injury, nerve
  open wound - *see* Wound, open, by site
abdomen, abdominal (muscle) (wall)
  922.2
  organ(s) NEC 868.00
adnexa, eye NEC 921.9
ankle 924.21
  with other parts of foot 924.20
arm 923.9
  lower (with elbow) 923.10
  upper 923.03
    with shoulder or axillary region 923.09
auditory canal (external) (meatus) (and other part(s) of neck, scalp, or face, except eye) 920

Contusion (*Continued*)
auricle, ear, (and other part(s) of neck, scalp, or face except eye) 920
axilla 923.02
  with shoulder or upper arm 923.09
back 922.31
bone NEC 924.9
brain (cerebral) (membrane) (with hemorrhage) 851.8

> Note Use the following fifth-digit subclassification with categories 851-854:
>
> 0   unspecified state of consciousness
> 1   with no loss of consciousness
> 2   with brief [less than one hour] loss of consciousness
> 3   with moderate [1-24 hours] loss of consciousness
> 4   with prolonged [more than 24 hours] loss of consciousness and return to pre-existing conscious level
> 5   with prolonged [more than 24 hours] loss of consciousness, without return to pre-existing conscious level
>
> Use fifth-digit 5 to designate when a patient is unconscious and dies before regaining consciousness, regardless of the duration of the loss of consciousness
>
> 6   with loss of consciousness of unspecified duration
> 9   with concussion, unspecified

  with
    open intracranial wound 851.9
    skull fracture - *see* Fracture, skull, by site
  cerebellum 851.4
    with open intracranial wound 851.5
  cortex 851.0
    with open intracranial wound 851.1
  occipital lobe 851.4
    with open intracranial wound 851.5
  stem 851.4
    with open intracranial wound 851.5
breast 922.0
brow (and other part(s) of neck, scalp, or face, except eye) 920
buttock 922.32
canthus 921.1
cardiac 861.01
  with open wound into thorax 861.11
cauda equina (spine) 952.4
cerebellum - *see* Contusion, brain, cerebellum
cerebral - *see* Contusion, brain
cheek(s) (and other part(s) of neck, scalp, or face, except eye) 920
chest (wall) 922.1
chin (and other part(s) of neck, scalp, or face, except eye) 920
clitoris 922.4
conjunctiva 921.1
conus medullaris (spine) 952.4
cornea 921.3

Contusion (*Continued*)
corpus cavernosum 922.4
cortex (brain) (cerebral) - *see* Contusion, brain, cortex
costal region 922.1
ear (and other part(s) of neck, scalp, or face except eye) 920
elbow 923.11
  with forearm 923.10
epididymis 922.4
epigastric region 922.2
eye NEC 921.9
eyeball 921.3
eyelid(s) (and periocular area) 921.1
face (and neck, or scalp, any part, except eye) 920
femoral triangle 922.2
fetus or newborn 772.6
finger(s) (nail) (subungual) 923.3
flank 922.2
foot (with ankle) (excluding toe(s)) 924.20
forearm (and elbow) 923.10
forehead (and other part(s) of neck, scalp, or face, except eye) 920
genital organs, external 922.4
globe (eye) 921.3
groin 922.2
gum(s) (and other part(s) of neck, scalp, or face, except eye) 920
hand(s) (except fingers alone) 923.20
head (any part, except eye) (and face) (and neck) 920
heart - *see* Contusion, cardiac
heel 924.20
hip 924.01
  with thigh 924.00
iliac region 922.2
inguinal region 922.2
internal organs (abdomen, chest, or pelvis) NEC - *see* Injury, internal, by site
interscapular region 922.33
iris (eye) 921.3
kidney 866.01
  with open wound into cavity 866.11
knee 924.11
  with lower leg 924.10
labium (majus) (minus) 922.4
lacrimal apparatus, gland, or sac 921.1
larynx (and other part(s) of neck, scalp, or face, except eye) 920
late effect - *see* Late, effects (of), contusion
leg 924.5
  lower (with knee) 924.10
lens 921.3
lingual (and other part(s) of neck, scalp, or face, except eye) 920
lip(s) (and other part(s) of neck, scalp, or face, except eye) 920
liver 864.01
  with
    laceration - *see* Laceration, liver
    open wound into cavity 864.11
lower extremity 924.5
  multiple sites 924.4
lumbar region 922.31
lung 861.21
  with open wound into thorax 861.31
malar region (and other part(s) of neck, scalp, or face, except eye) 920

ICD-9-CM

C

Vol. 2

Contusion (*Continued*)
- mandibular joint (and other part(s) of neck, scalp, or face, except eye) 920
- mastoid region (and other part(s) of neck, scalp, or face, except eye) 920
- membrane, brain - *see* Contusion, brain
- midthoracic region 922.1
- mouth (and other part(s) of neck, scalp, or face, except eye) 920
- multiple sites (not classifiable to same three-digit category) 924.8
  - lower limb 924.4
  - trunk 922.8
  - upper limb 923.8
- muscle NEC 924.9
- myocardium - *see* Contusion, cardiac
- nasal (septum) (and other part(s) of neck, scalp, or face, except eye) 920
- neck (and scalp, or face, any part, except eye) 920
- nerve - *see* Injury, nerve, by site
- nose (and other part(s) of neck, scalp, or face, except eye) 920
- occipital region (scalp) (and neck or face, except eye) 920
  - lobe - *see* Contusion, brain, occipital lobe
- orbit (region) (tissues) 921.2
- palate (soft) (and other part(s) of neck, scalp, or face, except eye) 920
- parietal region (scalp) (and neck, or face, except eye) 920
  - lobe - *see* Contusion, brain
- penis 922.4
- pericardium - *see* Contusion, cardiac
- perineum 922.4
- periocular area 921.1
- pharynx (and other part(s) of neck, scalp, or face, except eye) 920
- popliteal space (*see also* Contusion, knee) 924.11
- prepuce 922.4
- pubic region 922.4
- pudenda 922.4
- pulmonary - *see* Contusion, lung
- quadriceps femoralis 924.00
- rib cage 922.1
- sacral region 922.32
- salivary ducts or glands (and other part(s) of neck, scalp, or face, except eye) 920
- scalp (and neck, or face, any part, except eye) 920
- scapular region 923.01
  - with shoulder or upper arm 923.09
- sclera (eye) 921.3
- scrotum 922.4
- shoulder 923.00
  - with upper arm or axillary regions 923.09
- skin NEC 924.9
- skull 920
- spermatic cord 922.4
- spinal cord - *see also* Injury, spinal, by site
  - cauda equina 952.4
  - conus medullaris 952.4
- spleen 865.01
  - with open wound into cavity 865.11
- sternal region 922.1
- stomach - *see* Injury, internal, stomach
- subconjunctival 921.1

Contusion (*Continued*)
- subcutaneous NEC 924.9
- submaxillary region (and other part(s) of neck, scalp, or face, except eye) 920
- submental region (and other part(s) of neck, scalp, or face, except eye) 920
- subperiosteal NEC 924.9
- supraclavicular fossa (and other part(s) of neck, scalp, or face, except eye) 920
- supraorbital (and other part(s) of neck, scalp, or face, except eye) 920
- temple (region) (and other part(s) of neck, scalp, or face, except eye) 920
- testis 922.4
- thigh (and hip) 924.00
- thorax 922.1
  - organ - *see* Injury, internal, intrathoracic
- throat (and other part(s) of neck, scalp, or face, except eye) 920
- thumb(s) (nail) (subungual) 923.3
- toe(s) (nail) (subungual) 924.3
- tongue (and other part(s) of neck, scalp, or face, except eye) 920
- trunk 922.9
  - multiple sites 922.8
  - specified site - *see* Contusion, by site
- tunica vaginalis 922.4
- tympanum (membrane) (and other part(s) of neck, scalp, or face, except eye) 920
- upper extremity 923.9
  - multiple sites 923.8
- uvula (and other part(s) of neck, scalp, or face, except eye) 920
- vagina 922.4
- vocal cord(s) (and other part(s) of neck, scalp, or face, except eye) 920
- vulva 922.4
- wrist 923.21
  - with hand(s), except finger(s) alone 923.20

Conus (any type) (congenital) 743.57
- acquired 371.60
- medullaris syndrome 336.8

Convalescence (following) V66.9
- chemotherapy V66.2
- medical NEC V66.5
- psychotherapy V66.3
- radiotherapy V66.1
- surgery NEC V66.0
- treatment (for) NEC V66.5
  - combined V66.6
  - fracture V66.4
  - mental disorder NEC V66.3
  - specified disorder NEC V66.5

Conversion
- closed surgical procedure to open procedure
  - arthroscopic V64.43
  - laparoscopic V64.41
  - thoracoscopic V64.42
- hysteria, hysterical, any type 300.11
- neurosis, any 300.11
- reaction, any 300.11

Converter, tuberculosis (test reaction) 795.5

Convulsions (idiopathic) 780.39
- apoplectiform (*see also* Disease, cerebrovascular, acute) 436
- brain 780.39

Convulsions (*Continued*)
- cerebral 780.39
- cerebrospinal 780.39
- due to trauma NEC - *see* Injury, intracranial
- eclamptic (*see also* Eclampsia) 780.39
- epileptic (*see also* Epilepsy) 345.9
- epileptiform (*see also* Seizure, epileptiform) 780.39
- epileptoid (*see also* Seizure, epileptiform) 780.39
- ether
  - anesthetic
    - correct substance properly administered 780.39
    - overdose or wrong substance given 968.2
  - other specified type - *see* Table of Drugs and Chemicals
- febrile 780.31
- generalized 780.39
- hysterical 300.11
- infantile 780.39
  - epilepsy - *see* Epilepsy
- internal 780.39
- jacksonian (*see also* Epilepsy) 345.5
- myoclonic 333.2
- newborn 779.0
- paretic 094.1
- pregnancy (nephritic) (uremic) - *see* Eclampsia, pregnancy
- psychomotor (*see also* Epilepsy) 345.4
- puerperal, postpartum - *see* Eclampsia, pregnancy
- recurrent 780.39
  - epileptic - *see* Epilepsy
- reflex 781.0
- repetitive 780.39
  - epileptic - *see* Epilepsy
- salaam (*see also* Epilepsy) 345.6
- scarlatinal 034.1
- spasmodic 780.39
- tetanus, tetanic (*see also* Tetanus) 037
- thymic 254.8
- uncinate 780.39
- uremic 586

Convulsive - *see also* Convulsions
- disorder or state 780.39
  - epileptic - *see* Epilepsy
- equivalent, abdominal (*see also* Epilepsy) 345.5

Cooke-Apert-Gallais syndrome (adrenogenital) 255.2

Cooley's anemia (erythroblastic) 282.49

Coolie itch 126.9

Cooper's
- disease 610.1
- hernia - *see* Hernia, Cooper's

Coordination disturbance 781.3

Copper wire arteries, retina 362.13

Copra itch 133.8

Coprolith 560.39

Coprophilia 302.89

Coproporphyria, hereditary 277.1

Coprostasis 560.39
- with hernia - *see also* Hernia, by site, with obstruction
  - gangrenous - *see* Hernia, by site, with gangrene

Cor
- biloculare 745.7
- bovinum - *see* Hypertrophy, cardiac
- bovis - *see* Hypertrophy, cardiac
- pulmonale (chronic) 416.9
  - acute 415.0

Cor (Continued)
triatriatum, triatrium 746.82
triloculare 745.8
biatriatum 745.3
biventriculare 745.69
Corbus' disease 607.1
Cord - see also condition
around neck (tightly) (with compression)
affecting fetus or newborn 762.5
complicating delivery 663.1
without compression 663.3
affecting fetus or newborn 762.6
bladder NEC 344.61
tabetic 094.0
prolapse
affecting fetus or newborn 762.4
complicating delivery 663.0
Cord's angiopathy (see also Tuberculosis) 017.3 [362.18]
Cordis ectopia 746.87
Corditis (spermatic) 608.4
Corectopia 743.46
Cori type glycogen storage disease - see Disease, glycogen storage
Cork-handlers' disease or lung 495.3
Corkscrew esophagus 530.5
Corlett's pyosis (impetigo) 684
Corn (infected) 700
Cornea - see also condition
donor V59.5
guttata (dystrophy) 371.57
plana 743.41
Cornelia de Lange's syndrome (Amsterdam dwarf, mental retardation, and brachycephaly) 759.89
Cornual gestation or pregnancy - see Pregnancy, cornual
Cornu cutaneum 702.8
Coronary (artery) - see also condition
arising from aorta or pulmonary trunk 746.85
Corpora - see also condition
amylacea (prostate) 602.8
cavernosa - see condition
Corpulence (see Obesity)
Corpus - see condition
Corrigan's disease - see Insufficiency, aortic
Corrosive burn - see Burn, by site
Corsican fever (see also Malaria) 084.6
Cortical - see also condition
blindness 377.75
necrosis, kidney (bilateral) 583.6
Corticoadrenal - see condition
Corticosexual syndrome 255.2
Coryza (acute) 460
with grippe or influenza 487.1
syphilitic 095.8
congenital (chronic) 090.0
Costen's syndrome or complex 524.60
Costiveness (see also Constipation) 564.00
Costochondritis 733.6
Cotard's syndrome (paranoia) 297.1
Cot death 798.0
Cotungo's disease 724.3
Cough 786.2
with hemorrhage (see also Hemoptysis) 786.3
affected 786.2
bronchial 786.2
with grippe or influenza 487.1
chronic 786.2
epidemic 786.2
functional 306.1
hemorrhagic 786.3
hysterical 300.11

Cough (Continued)
laryngeal, spasmodic 786.2
nervous 786.2
psychogenic 306.1
smokers' 491.0
tea tasters' 112.89
Counseling NEC V65.40
without complaint or sickness V65.49
abuse victim NEC V62.89
child V61.21
partner V61.11
spouse V61.11
child abuse, maltreatment, or neglect V61.21
contraceptive NEC V25.09
device (intrauterine) V25.02
maintenance V25.40
intrauterine contraceptive device V25.42
oral contraceptive (pill) V25.41
specified type NEC V25.49
subdermal implantable V25.43
management NEC V25.9
oral contraceptive (pill) V25.01
emergency V25.03
postcoital V25.30
prescription NEC V25.02
oral contraceptive (pill) V25.01
emergency V25.03
postcoital V25.30
repeat prescription V25.41
repeat prescription V25.40
subdermal implantable V25.43
surveillance NEC V25.40
dietary V65.3
exercise V65.41
expectant mother, pediatric pre-birth visit V65.11
explanation of
investigation finding NEC V65.49
medication NEC V65.49
family planning V25.09
for nonattending third party V65.19
genetic V26.3
gonorrhea V65.45
health (advice) (education) (instruction) NEC V65.49
HIV V65.44
human immunodeficiency virus V65.44
injury prevention V65.43
insulin pump training V65.46
marital V61.10
medical (for) V65.9
boarding school resident V60.6
condition not demonstrated V65.5
feared complaint and no disease found V65.5
institutional resident V60.6
on behalf of another V65.19
person living alone V60.3
parent-child conflict V61.20
specified problem NEC V61.29
partner abuse
perpetrator V61.12
victim V61.11
pediatric pre-birth visit for expectant mother V65.11
perpetrator of
child abuse V62.83
parental V61.22
partner abuse V61.12
spouse abuse V61.12
procreative V65.49
sex NEC V65.49
transmitted disease NEC V65.45
HIV V65.44
specified reason NEC V65.49

Counseling NEC (Continued)
spousal abuse
perpetrator V61.12
victim V61.11
substance use and abuse V65.42
syphilis V65.45
victim (of)
abuse NEC V62.89
child abuse V61.21
partner abuse V61.11
spousal abuse V61.11
Coupled rhythm 427.89
Couvelaire uterus (complicating delivery) - see Placenta, separation
Cowper's gland - see condition
Cowperitis (see also Urethritis) 597.89
gonorrheal (acute) 098.0
chronic or duration of 2 months or over 098.2
Cowpox (abortive) 051.0
due to vaccination 999.0
eyelid 051.0 [373.5]
postvaccination 999.0 [373.5]
Coxa
plana 732.1
valga (acquired) 736.31
congenital 755.61
late effect of rickets 268.1
vara (acquired) 736.32
congenital 755.62
late effect of rickets 268.1
Coxae malum senilis 715.25
Coxalgia (nontuberculous) 719.45
tuberculous (see also Tuberculosis) 015.1 [730.85]
Coxalgic pelvis 736.30
Coxitis 716.65
Coxsackie (infection) (virus) 079.2
central nervous system NEC 048
endocarditis 074.22
enteritis 008.67
meningitis (aseptic) 047.0
myocarditis 074.23
pericarditis 074.21
pharyngitis 074.0
pleurodynia 074.1
specific disease NEC 074.8
Crabs, meaning pubic lice 132.2
Crack baby 760.75
Cracked nipple 611.2
puerperal, postpartum 676.1
Cradle cap 690.11
Craft neurosis 300.89
Craigiasis 007.8
Cramp(s) 729.82
abdominal 789.0
bathing 994.1
colic 789.0
psychogenic 306.4
due to immersion 994.1
extremity (lower) (upper) NEC 729.82
fireman 992.2
heat 992.2
hysterical 300.11
immersion 994.1
intestinal 789.0
psychogenic 306.4
linotypists' 300.89
organic 333.84
muscle (extremity) (general) 729.82
due to immersion 994.1
hysterical 300.11
occupational (hand) 300.89
organic 333.84
psychogenic 307.89
salt depletion 276.1
stoker 992.2

ICD-9-CM

C

Vol.

Cramp(s) (*Continued*)
  stomach 789.0
  telegraphers' 300.89
    organic 333.84
  typists' 300.89
    organic 333.84
  uterus 625.8
    menstrual 625.3
  writers' 333.84
    organic 333.84
    psychogenic 300.89
Cranial - *see* condition
Cranioclasis, fetal 763.89
Craniocleidodysostosis 755.59
Craniofenestria (skull) 756.0
Craniolacunia (skull) 756.0
Craniopagus 759.4
Craniopathy, metabolic 733.3
Craniopharyngeal - *see* condition
Craniopharyngioma (M9350/1) 237.0
Craniorachischisis (totalis) 740.1
Cranioschisis 756.0
Craniostenosis 756.0
Craniosynostosis 756.0
Craniotabes (cause unknown) 733.3
  rachitic 268.1
  syphilitic 090.5
Craniotomy, fetal 763.89
Cranium - *see* condition
Craw-craw 125.3
Creaking joint 719.60
  ankle 719.67
  elbow 719.62
  foot 719.67
  hand 719.64
  hip 719.65
  knee 719.66
  multiple sites 719.69
  pelvic region 719.65
  shoulder (region) 719.61
  specified site NEC 719.68
  wrist 719.63
Creeping
  eruption 126.9
  palsy 335.21
  paralysis 335.21
Crenated tongue 529.8
Creotoxism 005.9
Crepitus
  caput 756.0
  joint 719.60
    ankle 719.67
    elbow 719.62
    foot 719.67
    hand 719.64
    hip 719.65
    knee 719.66
    multiple sites 719.69
    pelvic region 719.65
    shoulder (region) 719.61
    specified site NEC 719.68
    wrist 719.63
Crescent or conus choroid, congenital 743.57
Cretin, cretinism (athyrotic) (congenital) (endemic) (metabolic) (nongoitrous) (sporadic) 243
  goitrous (sporadic) 246.1
  pelvis (dwarf type) (male type) 243
    with disproportion (fetopelvic) 653.1
      affecting fetus or newborn 763.1
      causing obstructed labor 660.1
        affecting fetus or newborn 763.1
  pituitary 253.3

Cretinoid degeneration 243
Creutzfeldt-Jakob disease (syndrome) 046.1
  with dementia
    with behavioral disturbance 046.1 [294.11]
    without behavioral disturbance 046.1 [294.10]
Crib death 798.0
Cribriform hymen 752.49
Cri-du-chat syndrome 758.31
Crigler-Najjar disease or syndrome (congenital hyperbilirubinemia) 277.4
Crimean hemorrhagic fever 065.0
Criminalism 301.7
Crisis
  abdomen 789.0
  addisonian (acute adrenocortical insufficiency) 255.4
  adrenal (cortical) 255.4
  asthmatic - *see* Asthma
  brain, cerebral (*see also* Disease, cerebrovascular, acute) 436
  celiac 579.0
  Dietl's 593.4
  emotional NEC 309.29
    acute reaction to stress 308.0
    adjustment reaction 309.9
    specific to childhood or adolescence 313.9
  gastric (tabetic) 094.0
  glaucomatocyclitic 364.22
  heart (*see also* Failure, heart) 428.9
  hypertensive - *see* Hypertension
  nitritoid
    correct substance properly administered 458.29
    overdose or wrong substance given or taken 961.1
  oculogyric 378.87
    psychogenic 306.7
  Pel's 094.0
  psychosexual identity 302.6
  rectum 094.0
  renal 593.81
  sickle cell 282.62
  stomach (tabetic) 094.0
  tabetic 094.0
  thyroid (*see also* Thyrotoxicosis) 242.9
  thyrotoxic (*see also* Thyrotoxicosis) 242.9
  vascular - *see* Disease, cerebrovascular, acute
Crocq's disease (acrocyanosis) 443.89
Crohn's disease (*see also* Enteritis, regional) 555.9
Cronkhite-Canada syndrome 211.3
Crooked septum, nasal 470
Cross
  birth (of fetus) complicating delivery 652.3
    with successful version 652.1
    causing obstructed labor 660.0
  bite, anterior or posterior 524.20
  eye (*see also* Esotropia) 378.00
Crossed ectopia of kidney 753.3
Crossfoot 754.50
Croup, croupous (acute) (angina) (catarrhal) (infective) (inflammatory) (laryngeal) (membranous) (nondiphtheritic) (pseudomembranous) 464.4
  asthmatic (*see also* Asthma) 493.9
  bronchial 466.0
  diphtheritic (membranous) 032.3
  false 478.75
  spasmodic 478.75
    diphtheritic 032.3

Croup, croupous (*Continued*)
  stridulous 478.75
    diphtheritic 032.3
Crouzon's disease (craniofacial dysostosis) 756.0
Crowding, teeth 524.31
CRST syndrome (cutaneous systemic sclerosis) 710.1
Cruchet's disease (encephalitis lethargica) 049.8
Cruelty in children (*see also* Disturbance, conduct) 312.9
Crural ulcer (*see also* Ulcer, lower extremity) 707.10
Crush, crushed, crushing (injury) 929.9
  with
    fracture - *see* Fracture, by site
  abdomen 926.19
    internal - *see* Injury, internal, abdomen
  ankle 928.21
    with other parts of foot 928.20
  arm 927.9
    lower (and elbow) 927.10
    upper 927.03
      with shoulder or axillary region 927.09
  axilla 927.02
    with shoulder or upper arm 927.09
  back 926.11
  breast 926.19
  buttock 926.12
  cheek 925.1
  chest - *see* Injury, internal, chest
  ear 925.1
  elbow 927.11
    with forearm 927.10
  face 925.1
  finger(s) 927.3
    with hand(s) 927.20
    and wrist(s) 927.21
  flank 926.19
  foot, excluding toe(s) alone (with ankle) 928.20
  forearm (and elbow) 927.10
  genitalia, external (female) (male) 926.0
    internal - *see* Injury, internal, genital organ NEC
  hand, except finger(s) alone (and wrist) 927.20
  head - *see* Fracture, skull, by site
  heel 928.20
  hip 928.01
    with thigh 928.00
  internal organ (abdomen, chest, or pelvis) - *see* Injury, internal, by site
  knee 928.11
    with leg, lower 928.10
  labium (majus) (minus) 926.0
  larynx 925.2
  late effect - *see* Late, effects (of), crushing
  leg 928.9
    lower 928.10
      and knee 928.11
    upper 928.00
  limb
    lower 928.9
      multiple sites 928.8
    upper 927.9
      multiple sites 927.8
  multiple sites NEC 929.0
  neck 925.2
  nerve - *see* Injury, nerve, by site

◀ **New**   ◀◀◀ **Revised**

Crush, crushed, crushing (Continued)
nose 802.0
open 802.1
penis 926.0
pharynx 925.2
scalp 925.1
scapular region 927.01
with shoulder or upper arm 927.09
scrotum 926.0
shoulder 927.00
with upper arm or axillary region 927.09
skull or cranium - see Fracture, skull, by site
spinal cord - see Injury, spinal, by site
syndrome (complication of trauma) 958.5
testis 926.0
thigh (with hip) 928.00
throat 925.2
thumb(s) (and fingers) 927.3
toe(s) 928.3
with foot 928.20
and ankle 928.21
tonsil 925.2
trunk 926.9
chest - see Injury, internal, intrathoracic organs NEC
internal organ - see Injury, internal, by site
multiple sites 926.8
specified site NEC 926.19
vulva 926.0
wrist 927.21
with hand(s), except fingers alone 927.20
Crusta lactea 690.11
Crusts 782.8
Crutch paralysis 953.4
Cruveilhier's disease 335.21
Cruveilhier-Baumgarten cirrhosis, disease, or syndrome 571.5
Cruz-Chagas disease (see also Trypanosomiasis) 086.2
Cryoglobulinemia (mixed) 273.2
Crypt (anal) (rectal) 569.49
Cryptitis (anal) (rectal) 569.49
Cryptococcosis (European) (pulmonary) (systemic) 117.5
Cryptococcus 117.5
epidermicus 117.5
neoformans, infection by 117.5
Cryptopapillitis (anus) 569.49
Cryptophthalmos (eyelid) 743.06
Cryptorchid, cryptorchism, cryptorchidism 752.51
Cryptosporidiosis 007.4
Cryptotia 744.29
Crystallopathy
calcium pyrophosphate (see also Arthritis) 275.49 [712.2]
dicalcium phosphate (see also Arthritis) 275.49 [712.1]
gouty 274.0
pyrophosphate NEC (see also Arthritis) 275.49 [712.2]
uric acid 274.0
Crystalluria 791.9
Csillag's disease (lichen sclerosus et atrophicus) 701.0
Cuban itch 050.1
Cubitus
valgus (acquired) 736.01
congenital 755.59
late effect of rickets 268.1

Cubitus (Continued)
varus (acquired) 736.02
congenital 755.59
late effect of rickets 268.1
Cultural deprivation V62.4
Cupping of optic disc 377.14
Curling's ulcer - see Ulcer, duodenum
Curling esophagus 530.5
Curschmann (-Batten) (-Steinert) disease or syndrome 359.2
Curvature
organ or site, congenital NEC - see Distortion
penis (lateral) 752.69
Pott's (spinal) (see also Tuberculosis) 015.0 [737.43]
radius, idiopathic, progressive (congenital) 755.54
spine (acquired) (angular) (idiopathic) (incorrect) (postural) 737.9
congenital 754.2
due to or associated with
Charcôt-Marie-Tooth disease 356.1 [737.40]
mucopolysaccharidosis 277.5 [737.40]
neurofibromatosis 237.71 [737.40]
osteitis
deformans 731.0 [737.40]
fibrosa cystica 252.01 [737.40] ◀▥
osteoporosis (see also Osteoporosis) 733.00 [737.40]
poliomyelitis (see also Poliomyelitis) 138 [737.40]
tuberculosis (Pott's curvature) (see also Tuberculosis) 015.0 [737.43]
kyphoscoliotic (see also Kyphoscoliosis) 737.30
kyphotic (see also Kyphosis) 737.10
late effect of rickets 268.1 [737.40]
Pott's 015.0 [737.40]
scoliotic (see also Scoliosis) 737.30
specified NEC 737.8
tuberculous 015.0 [737.40]
Cushing's
basophilism, disease, or syndrome (iatrogenic) (idiopathic) (pituitary basophilism) (pituitary dependent) 255.0
ulcer - see Ulcer, peptic
Cushingoid due to steroid therapy
correct substance properly administered 255.0
overdose or wrong substance given or taken 962.0
Cut (external) - see Wound, open, by site
Cutaneous - see also condition
hemorrhage 782.7
horn (cheek) (eyelid) (mouth) 702.8
larva migrans 126.9
Cutis - see also condition
hyperelastic 756.83
acquired 701.8
laxa 756.83
senilis 701.8
marmorata 782.61
osteosis 709.3
pendula 756.83
acquired 701.8
rhomboidalis nuchae 701.8

Cutis (Continued)
verticis gyrata 757.39
acquired 701.8
Cyanopathy, newborn 770.83
Cyanosis 782.5
autotoxic 289.7
common atrioventricular canal 745.69
congenital 770.83
conjunctiva 372.71
due to
endocardial cushion defect 745.60
nonclosure, foramen botalli 745.5
patent foramen botalli 745.5
persistent foramen ovale 745.5
enterogenous 289.7
fetus or newborn 770.83
ostium primum defect 745.61
paroxysmal digital 443.0
retina, retinal 362.10
Cycle
anovulatory 628.0
menstrual, irregular 626.4
Cyclencephaly 759.89
Cyclical vomiting 536.2
psychogenic 306.4
Cyclitic membrane 364.74
Cyclitis (see also Iridocyclitis) 364.3
acute 364.00
primary 364.01
recurrent 364.02
chronic 364.10
in
sarcoidosis 135 [364.11]
tuberculosis (see also Tuberculosis) 017.3 [364.11]
Fuchs' heterochromic 364.21
granulomatous 364.10
lens induced 364.23
nongranulomatous 364.00
posterior 363.21
primary 364.01
recurrent 364.02
secondary (noninfectious) 364.04
infectious 364.03
subacute 364.00
primary 364.01
recurrent 364.02
Cyclokeratitis - see Keratitis
Cyclophoria 378.44
Cyclopia, cyclops 759.89
Cycloplegia 367.51
Cyclospasm 367.53
Cyclosporiasis 007.5
Cyclothymia 301.13
Cyclothymic personality 301.13
Cyclotropia 378.33
Cyesis - see Pregnancy
Cylindroma (M8200/3) - see also Neoplasm, by site, malignant
eccrine dermal (M8200/0) - see Neoplasm, skin, benign
skin (M8200/0) - see Neoplasm, skin, benign
Cylindruria 791.7
Cyllosoma 759.89
Cynanche
diphtheritic 032.3
tonsillaris 475
Cynorexia 783.6
Cyphosis - see Kyphosis
Cyprus fever (see also Brucellosis) 023.9
Cyriax's syndrome (slipping rib) 733.99
Cyst (mucous) (retention) (serous) (simple)

ICD-9-CM

C

Vol.

Cyst *(Continued)*

> **Note** In general, cysts are not neo-plastic and are classified to the appropriate category for disease of the specified anatomical site. This generalization does not apply to certain types of cysts which are neoplastic in nature, for example, dermoid, nor does it apply to cysts of certain structures, for example, branchial cleft, which are classified as developmental anomalies.
>
> The following listing includes some of the most frequently reported sites of cysts as well as qualifiers which indicate the type of cyst. The latter qualifiers usually are not repeated under the anatomical sites. Since the code assignment for a given site may vary depending upon the type of cyst, the coder should refer to the listings under the specified type of cyst before consideration is given to the site.

accessory, fallopian tube 752.11
adenoid (infected) 474.8
adrenal gland 255.8
  congenital 759.1
air, lung 518.89
allantoic 753.7
alveolar process (jaw bone) 526.2
amnion, amniotic 658.8
anterior chamber (eye) 364.60
  exudative 364.62
  implantation (surgical) (traumatic) 364.61
  parasitic 360.13
anterior nasopalatine 526.1
antrum 478.1
anus 569.49
apical (periodontal) (tooth) 522.8
appendix 543.9
arachnoid, brain 348.0
arytenoid 478.79
auricle 706.2
Baker's (knee) 727.51
  tuberculous (*see also* Tuberculosis) 015.2
Bartholin's gland or duct 616.2
bile duct (*see also* Disease, biliary) 576.8
bladder (multiple) (trigone) 596.8
Blessig's 362.62
blood, endocardial (*see also* Endocarditis) 424.90
blue dome 610.0
bone (local) 733.20
  aneurysmal 733.22
  jaw 526.2
    developmental (odontogenic) 526.0
    fissural 526.1
    latent 526.89
  solitary 733.21
  unicameral 733.21
brain 348.0
  congenital 742.4
  hydatid (*see also* Echinococcus) 122.9
  third ventricle (colloid) 742.4
branchial (cleft) 744.42
branchiogenic 744.42

Cyst *(Continued)*

breast (benign) (blue dome) (pedunculated) (solitary) (traumatic) 610.0
  involution 610.4
  sebaceous 610.8
broad ligament (benign) 620.8
  embryonic 752.11
bronchogenic (mediastinal) (sequestration) 518.89
  congenital 748.4
buccal 528.4
bulbourethral gland (Cowper's) 599.89
bursa, bursal 727.49
  pharyngeal 478.26
calcifying odontogenic (M9301/0) 213.1
  upper jaw (bone) 213.0
canal of Nuck (acquired) (serous) 629.1
  congenital 752.41
canthus 372.75
carcinomatous (M8010/3) - *see* Neoplasm, by site, malignant
cartilage (joint) - *see* Derangement, joint
cauda equina 336.8
cavum septi pellucidi NEC 348.0
celomic (pericardium) 746.89
cerebellopontine (angle) - *see* Cyst, brain
cerebellum - *see* Cyst, brain
cerebral - *see* Cyst, brain
cervical lateral 744.42
cervix 622.8
  embryonal 752.41
  nabothian (gland) 616.0
chamber, anterior (eye) 364.60
  exudative 364.62
  implantation (surgical) (traumatic) 364.61
  parasitic 360.13
chiasmal, optic NEC (*see also* Lesion, chiasmal) 377.54
chocolate (ovary) 617.1
choledochal (congenital) 751.69
  acquired 576.8
choledochus 751.69
chorion 658.8
choroid plexus 348.0
chyle, mesentery 457.8
ciliary body 364.60
  exudative 364.64
  implantation 364.61
  primary 364.63
clitoris 624.8
coccyx (*see also* Cyst, bone) 733.20
colloid
  third ventricle (brain) 742.4
  thyroid gland - *see* Goiter
colon 569.89
common (bile) duct (*see also* Disease, biliary) 576.8
congenital NEC 759.89
  adrenal glands 759.1
  epiglottis 748.3
  esophagus 750.4
  fallopian tube 752.11
  kidney 753.10
    multiple 753.19
    single 753.11
  larynx 748.3
  liver 751.62
  lung 748.4
  mediastinum 748.8
  ovary 752.0
  oviduct 752.11

Cyst *(Continued)*

congenital NEC *(Continued)*
  pancreas 751.7
  periurethral (tissue) 753.8
  prepuce NEC 752.69
    penis 752.69
  sublingual 750.26
  submaxillary gland 750.26
  thymus (gland) 759.2
  tongue 750.19
  ureterovesical orifice 753.4
  vulva 752.41
conjunctiva 372.75
cornea 371.23
corpora quadrigemina 348.0
corpus
  albicans (ovary) 620.2
  luteum (ruptured) 620.1
Cowper's gland (benign) (infected) 599.89
cranial meninges 348.0
craniobuccal pouch 253.8
craniopharyngeal pouch 253.8
cystic duct (*see also* Disease, gallbladder) 575.8
Cysticercus (any site) 123.1
Dandy-Walker 742.3
  with spina bifida (*see also* Spina bifida) 741.0
dental 522.8
  developmental 526.0
  eruption 526.0
  lateral periodontal 526.0
  primordial (keratocyst) 526.0
  root 522.8
dentigerous 526.0
  mandible 526.0
  maxilla 526.0
dermoid (M9084/0) - *see also* Neoplasm, by site, benign
  with malignant transformation (M9084/3) 183.0
  implantation
    external area or site (skin) NEC 709.8
    iris 364.61
    skin 709.8
    vagina 623.8
    vulva 624.8
  mouth 528.4
  oral soft tissue 528.4
  sacrococcygeal 685.1
    with abscess 685.0
developmental of ovary, ovarian 752.0
dura (cerebral) 348.0
  spinal 349.2
ear (external) 706.2
echinococcal (*see also* Echinococcus) 122.9
embryonal
  cervix uteri 752.41
  genitalia, female external 752.41
  uterus 752.3
  vagina 752.41
endometrial 621.8
  ectopic 617.9
endometrium (uterus) 621.8
  ectopic - *see* Endometriosis
enteric 751.5
enterogenous 751.5
epidermal (inclusion) (*see also* Cyst, skin) 706.2
epidermoid (inclusion) (*see also* Cyst, skin) 706.2

Cyst *(Continued)*
 epidermoid *(Continued)*
  mouth 528.4
  not of skin - *see* Cyst, by site
  oral soft tissue 528.4
 epididymis 608.89
 epiglottis 478.79
 epiphysis cerebri 259.8
 epithelial (inclusion) *(see also* Cyst, skin) 706.2
 epoophoron 752.11
 eruption 526.0
 esophagus 530.89
 ethmoid sinus 478.1
 eye (retention) 379.8
  congenital 743.03
  posterior segment, congenital 743.54
 eyebrow 706.2
 eyelid (sebaceous) 374.84
  infected 373.13
  sweat glands or ducts 374.84
 falciform ligament (inflammatory) 573.8
 fallopian tube 620.8
 female genital organs NEC 629.8
 fimbrial (congenital) 752.11
 fissural (oral region) 526.1
 follicle (atretic) (graafian) (ovarian) 620.0
  nabothian (gland) 616.0
 follicular (atretic) (ovarian) 620.0
  dentigerous 526.0
 frontal sinus 478.1
 gallbladder or duct 575.8
 ganglion 727.43
 Gartner's duct 752.11
 gas, of mesentery 568.89
 gingiva 523.8
 gland of moll 374.84
 globulomaxillary 526.1
 graafian follicle 620.0
 granulosal lutein 620.2
 hemangiomatous (M9121/0) *(see also* Hemangioma) 228.00
 hydatid *(see also* Echinococcus) 122.9
  fallopian tube (Morgagni) 752.11
  liver NEC 122.8
  lung NEC 122.9
  Morgagni 752.89
   fallopian tube 752.11
  specified site NEC 122.9
 hymen 623.8
  embryonal 752.41
 hypopharynx 478.26
 hypophysis, hypophyseal (duct) (recurrent) 253.8
  cerebri 253.8
 implantation (dermoid)
  anterior chamber (eye) 364.61
  external area or site (skin) NEC 709.8
  iris 364.61
  vagina 623.8
  vulva 624.8
 incisor, incisive canal 526.1
 inclusion (epidermal) (epithelial) (epidermoid) (mucous) (squamous) *(see also* Cyst, skin) 706.2
  not of skin - *see* Neoplasm, by site, benign
 intestine (large) (small) 569.89
 intracranial - *see* Cyst, brain

Cyst *(Continued)*
 intraligamentous 728.89
  knee 717.89
 intrasellar 253.8
 iris (idiopathic) 364.60
  exudative 364.62
  implantation (surgical) (traumatic) 364.61
  miotic pupillary 364.55
  parasitic 360.13
 Iwanoff's 362.62
 jaw (bone) (aneurysmal) (extravasation) (hemorrhagic) (traumatic) 526.2
  developmental (odontogenic) 526.0
  fissural 526.1
 keratin 706.2
 kidney (congenital) 753.10
  acquired 593.2
  calyceal *(see also* Hydronephrosis) 591
  multiple 753.19
  pyelogenic *(see also* Hydronephrosis) 591
  simple 593.2
  single 753.11
  solitary (not congenital) 593.2
 labium (majus) (minus) 624.8
  sebaceous 624.8
 lacrimal
  apparatus 375.43
  gland or sac 375.12
 larynx 478.79
 lens 379.39
  congenital 743.39
 lip (gland) 528.5
 liver 573.8
  congenital 751.62
  hydatid *(see also* Echinococcus) 122.8
   granulosis 122.0
   multilocularis 122.5
 lung 518.89
  congenital 748.4
  giant bullous 492.0
 lutein 620.1
 lymphangiomatous (M9173/0) 228.1
 lymphoepithelial
  mouth 528.4
  oral soft tissue 528.4
 macula 362.54
 malignant (M8000/3) - *see* Neoplasm, by site, malignant
 mammary gland (sweat gland) *(see also* Cyst, breast) 610.0
 mandible 526.2
  dentigerous 526.0
  radicular 522.8
 maxilla 526.2
  dentigerous 526.0
  radicular 522.8
 median
  anterior maxillary 526.1
  palatal 526.1
 mediastinum (congenital) 748.8
 meibomian (gland) (retention) 373.2
  infected 373.12
 membrane, brain 348.0
 meninges (cerebral) 348.0
  spinal 349.2
 meniscus knee 717.5
 mesentery, mesenteric (gas) 568.89
  chyle 457.8
  gas 568.89

Cyst *(Continued)*
 mesonephric duct 752.89
 mesothelial
  peritoneum 568.89
  pleura (peritoneal) 568.89
 milk 611.5
 miotic pupillary (iris) 364.55
 Morgagni (hydatid) 752.89
  fallopian tube 752.11
 mouth 528.4
 mullerian duct 752.89
 multilocular (ovary) (M8000/1) 239.5
 myometrium 621.8
 nabothian (follicle) (ruptured) 616.0
 nasal sinus 478.1
 nasoalveolar 528.4
 nasolabial 528.4
 nasopalatine (duct) 526.1
  anterior 526.1
 nasopharynx 478.26
 neoplastic (M8000/1) - *see also* Neoplasm, by site, unspecified nature
  benign (M8000/0) - *see* Neoplasm, by site, benign
   uterus 621.8
 nervous system - *see* Cyst, brain
 neuroenteric 742.59
 neuroepithelial ventricle 348.0
 nipple 610.0
 nose 478.1
  skin of 706.2
 odontogenic, developmental 526.0
 omentum (lesser) 568.89
  congenital 751.8
 oral soft tissue (dermoid) (epidermoid) (lymphoepithelial) 528.4
 ora serrata 361.19
 orbit 376.81
 ovary, ovarian (twisted) 620.2
  adherent 620.2
  chocolate 617.1
  corpus
   albicans 620.2
   luteum 620.1
  dermoid (M9084/0) 220
  developmental 752.0
  due to failure of involution NEC 620.2
  endometrial 617.1
  follicular (atretic) (graafian) (hemorrhagic) (mesothelial) 620.0
  hemorrhagic 620.2
  in pregnancy or childbirth 654.4
   affecting fetus or newborn 763.89
   causing obstructed labor 660.2
    affecting fetus or newborn 763.1
  multilocular (M8000/1) 239.5
  pseudomucinous (M8470/0) 220
  retention 620.2
  serous 620.2
  theca lutein 620.2
  tuberculous *(see also* Tuberculosis) 016.6
  unspecified 620.2
 oviduct 620.8
 palatal papilla (jaw) 526.1
 palate 526.1
  fissural 526.1
  median (fissural) 526.1
 palatine, of papilla 526.1
 pancreas, pancreatic 577.2
  congenital 751.7

ICD-9-CM

C

Vol. 2

Cyst *(Continued)*
  pancreas, pancreatic *(Continued)*
    false 577.2
    hemorrhagic 577.2
    true 577.2
  paranephric 593.2
  paraovarian 752.11
  paraphysis, cerebri 742.4
  parasitic NEC 136.9
  parathyroid (gland) 252.8
  paratubal (fallopian) 620.8
  paraurethral duct 599.89
  paroophoron 752.11
  parotid gland 527.6
    mucous extravasation or retention
      527.6
  parovarian 752.11
  pars planus 364.60
    exudative 364.64
    primary 364.63
  pelvis, female
    in pregnancy or childbirth 654.4
      affecting fetus or newborn 763.89
      causing obstructed labor 660.2
        affecting fetus or newborn
          763.1
  penis (sebaceous) 607.89
  periapical 522.8
  pericardial (congenital) 746.89
    acquired (secondary) 423.8
  pericoronal 526.0
  perineural (Tarlov's) 355.9
  periodontal 522.8
    lateral 526.0
  peripancreatic 577.2
  peripelvic (lymphatic) 593.2
  peritoneum 568.89
    chylous 457.8
  pharynx (wall) 478.26
  pilonidal (infected) (rectum) 685.1
    with abscess 685.0
    malignant (M9084/3) 173.5
  pituitary (duct) (gland) 253.8
  placenta (amniotic) - *see* Placenta, ab-
    normal
  pleura 519.8
  popliteal 727.51
  porencephalic 742.4
    acquired 348.0
  postanal (infected) 685.1
    with abscess 685.0
  posterior segment of eye, congenital
    743.54
  postmastoidectomy cavity 383.31
  preauricular 744.47
  prepuce 607.89
    congenital 752.69
  primordial (jaw) 526.0
  prostate 600.3   ◄▥
  pseudomucinous (ovary) (M8470/0)
    220
  pudenda (sweat glands) 624.8
  pupillary, miotic 364.55
    sebaceous 624.8
  radicular (residual) 522.8
  radiculodental 522.8
  ranular 527.6
  Rathke's pouch 253.8
  rectum (epithelium) (mucous) 569.49
  renal - *see* Cyst, kidney
  residual (radicular) 522.8
  retention (ovary) 620.2
  retina 361.19
    macular 362.54

Cyst *(Continued)*
  retina *(Continued)*
    parasitic 360.13
    primary 361.13
    secondary 361.14
  retroperitoneal 568.89
  sacrococcygeal (dermoid) 685.1
    with abscess 685.0
  salivary gland or duct 527.6
    mucous extravasation or retention
      527.6
  Sampson's 617.1
  sclera 379.19
  scrotum (sebaceous) 706.2
    sweat glands 706.2
  sebaceous (duct) (gland) 706.2
    breast 610.8
    eyelid 374.84
    genital organ NEC
      female 629.8
      male 608.89
    scrotum 706.2
  semilunar cartilage (knee) (multiple)
    717.5
  seminal vesicle 608.89
  serous (ovary) 620.2
  sinus (antral) (ethmoidal) (frontal)
    (maxillary) (nasal) (sphenoidal)
    478.1
  Skene's gland 599.89
  skin (epidermal) (epidermoid, inclu-
    sion) (epithelial) (inclusion) (reten-
    tion) (sebaceous) 706.2
    breast 610.8
    eyelid 374.84
    genital organ NEC
      female 629.8
      male 608.89
    neoplastic 216.3
    scrotum 706.2
    sweat gland or duct 705.89
  solitary
    bone 733.21
    kidney 593.2
  spermatic cord 608.89
  sphenoid sinus 478.1
  spinal meninges 349.2
  spine (*see also* Cyst, bone) 733.20
  spleen NEC 289.59
    congenital 759.0
    hydatid (*see also* Echinococcus)
      122.9
  spring water (pericardium) 746.89
  subarachnoid 348.0
    intrasellar 793.0
  subdural (cerebral) 348.0
    spinal cord 349.2
  sublingual gland 527.6
    mucous extravasation or retention
      527.6
  submaxillary gland 527.6
    mucous extravasation or retention
      527.6
  suburethral 599.89
  suprarenal gland 255.8
  suprasellar - *see* Cyst, brain
  sweat gland or duct 705.89
  sympathetic nervous system 337.9
  synovial 727.40
    popliteal space 727.51
  Tarlov's 355.9
  tarsal 373.2
  tendon (sheath) 727.42
  testis 608.89

Cyst *(Continued)*
  thecalutein (ovary) 620.2
  Thornwaldt's, Tornwaldt's
    478.26
  thymus (gland) 254.8
  thyroglossal (duct) (infected) (persist-
    ent) 759.2
  thyroid (gland) 246.2
    adenomatous - *see* Goiter, nodular
    colloid (*see also* Goiter) 240.9
  thyrolingual duct (infected) (persistent)
    759.2
  tongue (mucous) 529.8
  tonsil 474.8
  tooth (dental root) 522.8
  tubo-ovarian 620.8
    inflammatory 614.1
  tunica vaginalis 608.89
  turbinate (nose) (*see also* Cyst, bone)
    733.20
  Tyson's gland (benign) (infected)
    607.89
  umbilicus 759.89
  urachus 753.7
  ureter 593.89
  ureterovesical orifice 593.89
    congenital 753.4
  urethra 599.84
  urethral gland (Cowper's) 599.89
  uterine
    ligament 620.8
      embryonic 752.11
    tube 620.8
  uterus (body) (corpus) (recurrent)
    621.8
    embryonal 752.3
  utricle (ear) 386.8
    prostatic 599.89
  utriculus masculinus 599.89
  vagina, vaginal (squamous cell) (wall)
    623.8
    embryonal 752.41
    implantation 623.8
    inclusion 623.8
  vallecula, vallecular 478.79
  ventricle, neuroepithelial 348.0
  verumontanum 599.89
  vesical (orifice) 596.8
  vitreous humor 379.29
  vulva (sweat glands) 624.8
    congenital 752.41
    implantation 624.8
    inclusion 624.8
    sebaceous gland 624.8
  vulvovaginal gland 624.8
  wolffian 752.89
Cystadenocarcinoma (M8440/3) - *see also*
  Neoplasm, by site, malignant
  bile duct type (M8161/3) 155.1
  endometrioid (M8380/3) - *see* Neo-
    plasm, by site, malignant
  mucinous (M8470/3)
    papillary (M8471/3)
      specified site - *see* Neoplasm, by
        site, malignant
      unspecified site 183.0
    specified site - *see* Neoplasm, by site,
      malignant
    unspecified site 183.0
  papillary (M8450/3)
    mucinous (M8471/3)
      specified site - *see* Neoplasm, by
        site, malignant
      unspecified site 183.0

◄ **New**   ◄▥ **Revised**

Cystadenocarcinoma *(Continued)*
  papillary *(Continued)*
    pseudomucinous (M8471/3)
      specified site - *see* Neoplasm, by
        site, malignant
      unspecified site 183.0
    serous (M8460/3)
      specified site - *see* Neoplasm, by
        site, malignant
      unspecified site 183.0
    specified site - *see* Neoplasm, by site,
      malignant
    unspecified 183.0
  pseudomucinous (M8470/3)
    papillary (M8471/3)
      specified site - *see* Neoplasm, by
        site, malignant
      unspecified site 183.0
    specified site - *see* Neoplasm, by site,
      malignant
    unspecified site 183.0
  serous (M8441/3)
    papillary (M8460/3)
      specified site - *see* Neoplasm, by
        site, malignant
      unspecified site 183.0
    specified site - *see* Neoplasm, by site,
      malignant
    unspecified site 183.0
Cystadenofibroma (M9013/0)
  clear cell (M8313/0) - *see* Neoplasm,
    by site, benign
  endometrioid (M8381/0) 220
    borderline malignancy (M8381/1)
      236.2
    malignant (M8381/3) 183.0
  mucinous (M9015/0)
    specified site - *see* Neoplasm, by site,
      benign
    unspecified site 220
  serous (M9014/0)
    specified site - *see* Neoplasm, by site,
      benign
    unspecified site 220
  specified site - *see* Neoplasm, by site,
    benign
  unspecified site 220
Cystadenoma (M8440/0) - *see also* Neoplasm, by site, benign
  bile duct (M8161/0) 211.5
  endometrioid (M8380/0) - *see also*
    Neoplasm, by site, benign
    borderline malignancy (M8380/1) -
      see Neoplasm, by site, uncertain
      behavior
  malignant (M8440/3) - *see* Neoplasm,
    by site, malignant
  mucinous (M8470/0)
    borderline malignancy (M8470/1)
      specified site - *see* Neoplasm, by
        site, uncertain behavior
      unspecified site 236.2
    papillary (M8471/0)
      borderline malignancy (M8471/1)
        specified site - *see* Neoplasm, by
          site, uncertain behavior
        unspecified site 236.2
      specified site - *see* Neoplasm, by
        site, benign
      unspecified site 220
    specified site - *see* Neoplasm, by site,
      benign
    unspecified site 220
  papillary (M8450/0)

Cystadenoma *(Continued)*
  papillary *(Continued)*
    borderline malignancy (M8450/1)
      specified site - *see* Neoplasm, by
        site, uncertain behavior
      unspecified site 236.2
    lymphomatosum (M8561/0) 210.2
    mucinous (M8471/0)
      borderline malignancy (M8471/1)
        specified site - *see* Neoplasm, by
          site, uncertain behavior
        unspecified site 236.2
      specified site - *see* Neoplasm, by
        site, benign
      unspecified site 220
    pseudomucinous (M8471/0)
      borderline malignancy (M8471/1)
        specified site - *see* Neoplasm, by
          site, uncertain behavior
        unspecified site 236.2
      specified site - *see* Neoplasm, by
        site, benign
      unspecified site 220
    serous (M8460/0)
      borderline malignancy (M8460/1)
        specified site - *see* Neoplasm, by
          site, uncertain behavior
        unspecified site 236.2
      specified site - *see* Neoplasm, by
        site, benign
      unspecified site 220
    specified site - *see* Neoplasm, by site,
      benign
    unspecified site 220
  pseudomucinous (M8470/0)
    borderline malignancy (M8470/1)
      specified site - *see* Neoplasm, by
        site, uncertain behavior
      unspecified site 236.2
    papillary (M8471/0)
      borderline malignancy (M8471/1)
        specified site - *see* Neoplasm, by
          site, uncertain behavior
        unspecified site 236.2
      specified site - *see* Neoplasm, by
        site, benign
      unspecified site 220
    specified site - *see* Neoplasm, by site,
      benign
    unspecified site 220
  serous (M8441/0)
    borderline malignancy (M8441/1)
      specified site - *see* Neoplasm, by
        site, uncertain behavior
      unspecified site 236.2
    papillary (M8460/0)
      borderline malignancy (M8460/1)
        specified site - *see* Neoplasm, by
          site, uncertain behavior
        unspecified site 236.2
      specified site - *see* Neoplasm, by
        site, benign
      unspecified site 220
    specified site - *see* Neoplasm, by site,
      benign
    unspecified site 220
  thyroid 226
Cystathioninemia 270.4
Cystathioninuria 270.4
Cystic - *see also* condition
  breast, chronic 610.1
  corpora lutea 620.1
  degeneration, congenital
    brain 742.4

Cystic *(Continued)*
  degeneration, congenital *(Continued)*
    kidney (*see also* Cystic, disease, kid-
      ney) 753.10
  disease
    breast, chronic 610.1
    kidney, congenital 753.10
      medullary 753.16
      multiple 753.19
      polycystic - *see* Polycystic, kidney
      single 753.11
      specified NEC 753.19
    liver, congenital 751.62
    lung 518.89
      congenital 748.4
    pancreas, congenital 751.7
    semilunar cartilage 717.5
  duct - *see* condition
  eyeball, congenital 743.03
  fibrosis (pancreas) 277.00
    with
      manifestions
        gastrointestinal 277.03
        pulmonary 277.02
        specified NEC 277.09
      meconium ileus 277.01
      pulmonary exacerbation 277.02
  hygroma (M9173/0) 228.1
  kidney, congenital 753.10
    medullary 753.16
    multiple 753.19
    polycystic - *see* Polycystic, kidney
    single 753.11
    specified NEC 753.19
  liver, congenital 751.62
  lung 518.89
    congenital 748.4
  mass - *see* Cyst
  mastitis, chronic 610.1
  ovary 620.2
  pancreas, congenital 751.7
Cysticerciasis 123.1
Cysticercosis (mammary) (subretinal)
  123.1
Cysticercus 123.1
  cellulosae infestation 123.1
Cystinosis (malignant) 270.0
Cystinuria 270.0
Cystitis (bacillary) (colli) (diffuse) (exudative) (hemorrhagic) (purulent) (recurrent) (septic) (suppurative) (ulcerative) 595.9
  with
    abortion - *see* Abortion, by type,
      with urinary tract infection
    ectopic pregnancy (*see also* categories
      633.0-633.9) 639.8
    fibrosis 595.1
    leukoplakia 595.1
    malakoplakia 595.1
    metaplasia 595.1
    molar pregnancy (*see also* categories
      630-632) 639.8
  actinomycotic 039.8 *[595.4]*
  acute 595.0
    of trigone 595.3
  allergic 595.89
  amebic 006.8 *[595.4]*
  bilharzial 120.9 *[595.4]*
  blennorrhagic (acute) 098.11
    chronic or duration of 2 months or
      more 098.31
  bullous 595.89
  calculous 594.1
  chlamydial 099.53

ICD-9-CM

C

Vol. 2

Cystitis *(Continued)*
  chronic 595.2
    interstitial 595.1
    of trigone 595.3
  complicating pregnancy, childbirth, or
    puerperium 646.6
    affecting fetus or newborn 760.1
  cystic(a) 595.81
  diphtheritic 032.84
  echinococcal
    glanulosus 122.3 *[595.4]*
    multilocularis 122.6 *[595.4]*
  emphysematous 595.89
  encysted 595.81
  follicular 595.3
  following
    abortion 639.8
    ectopic or molar pregnancy 639.8
  gangrenous 595.89
  glandularis 595.89
  gonococcal (acute) 098.11
    chronic or duration of 2 months or
      more 098.31
  incrusted 595.89
  interstitial 595.1
  irradiation 595.82
  irritation 595.89
  malignant 595.89
  monilial 112.2
  of trigone 595.3
  panmural 595.1
  polyposa 595.89
  prostatic 601.3
  radiation 595.82
  Reiter's (abacterial) 099.3
  specified NEC 595.89

Cystitis *(Continued)*
  subacute 595.2
  submucous 595.1
  syphilitic 095.8
  trichomoniasis 131.09
  tuberculous *(see also* Tuberculosis)
    016.1
  ulcerative 595.1
Cystocele (-rectocele)
  female (without uterine prolapse)
    618.01 ◂▥
    lateral 618.02 ◂
    midline 618.01 ◂
    paravaginal 618.02 ◂
    with uterine prolapse 618.4
      complete 618.3
      incomplete 618.2
  in pregnancy or childbirth 654.4
    affecting fetus or newborn
      763.89
    causing obstructed labor 660.2
      affecting fetus or newborn
        763.1
  male 596.8
Cystoid
  cicatrix limbus 372.64
  degeneration, macula 362.53
Cystolithiasis 594.1
Cystoma (M8440/0) - *see also* Neoplasm,
  by site, benign
  endometrial, ovary 617.1
  mucinous (M8470/0)
    specified site - *see* Neoplasm, by site,
      benign
    unspecified site 220

Cystoma *(Continued)*
  serous (M8441/0)
    specified site - *see* Neoplasm, by site,
      benign
    unspecified site 220
  simple (ovary) 620.2
Cystoplegia 596.53
Cystoptosis 596.8
Cystopyelitis *(see also* Pyelitis) 590.80
Cystorrhagia 596.8
Cystosarcoma phyllodes (M9020/1)
  238.3
  benign (M9020/0) 217
  malignant (M9020/3) - *see* Neoplasm,
    breast, malignant
Cystostomy status V44.50
  with complication 997.5
  appendico-vesicostomy V44.52
  cutaneous-vesicostomy V44.51
  specified type NEC V44.59
Cystourethritis *(see also* Urethritis)
  597.89
Cystourethrocele *(see also* Cystocele)
  female (without uterine prolapse)
    618.09 ◂▥
    with uterine prolapse 618.4
      complete 618.3
      incomplete 618.2
  male 596.8
Cytomegalic inclusion disease 078.5
  congenital 771.1
Cytomycosis, reticuloendothelial *(see
  also* Histoplasmosis, American)
  115.00
Cytopenia 289.9 ◂

D

Daae (-Finsen) disease (epidemic pleuro-dynia) 074.1
Dabney's grip 074.1
Da Costa's syndrome (neurocirculatory asthenia) 306.2
Dacryoadenitis, dacryadenitis 375.00
 acute 375.01
 chronic 375.02
Dacryocystitis 375.30
 acute 375.32
 chronic 375.42
 neonatal 771.6
 phlegmonous 375.33
 syphilitic 095.8
  congenital 090.0
 trachomatous, active 076.1
  late effect 139.1
 tuberculous (*see also* Tuberculosis) 017.3
Dacryocystoblenorrhea 375.42
Dacryocystocele 375.43
Dacryolith, dacryolithiasis 375.57
Dacryoma 375.43
Dacryopericystitis (acute) (subacute) 375.32
 chronic 375.42
Dacryops 375.11
Dacryosialadenopathy, atrophic 710.2
Dacryostenosis 375.56
 congenital 743.65
Dactylitis 686.9
 bone (*see also* Osteomyelitis) 730.2
 sickle-cell 282.61
 syphilitic 095.5
 tuberculous (*see also* Tuberculosis) 015.5
Dactylolysis spontanea 136.0
Dactylosymphysis (*see also* Syndactylism) 755.10
Damage
 arteriosclerotic - *see* Arteriosclerosis
 brain 348.9
  anoxic, hypoxic 348.1
   during or resulting from a procedure 997.01
  child NEC 343.9
  due to birth injury 767.0
  minimal (child) (*see also* Hyperkinesia) 314.9
  newborn 767.0
 cardiac - *see also* Disease, heart
 cardiorenal (vascular) (*see also* Hypertension, cardiorenal) 404.90
 central nervous system - *see* Damage, brain
 cerebral NEC - *see* Damage, brain
 coccyx, complicating delivery 665.6
 coronary (*see also* Ischemia, heart) 414.9
 eye, birth injury 767.8
 heart - *see also* Disease, heart
  valve - *see* Endocarditis
 hypothalamus NEC 348.9
 liver 571.9
  alcoholic 571.3
 myocardium (*see also* Degeneration, myocardial) 429.1
 pelvic
  joint or ligament, during delivery 665.6

Damage (*Continued*)
 pelvic (*Continued*)
  organ NEC
   with
    abortion - *see* Abortion, by type, with damage to pelvic organs
    ectopic pregnancy (*see also* categories 633.0-633.9) 639.2
    molar pregnancy (*see also* categories 630-632) 639.2
   during delivery 665.5
   following
    abortion 639.2
    ectopic or molar pregnancy 639.2
 renal (*see also* Disease, renal) 593.9
 skin, solar 692.79
  acute 692.72
  chronic 692.74
 subendocardium, subendocardial (*see also* Degeneration, myocardial) 429.1
 vascular 459.9
Dameshek's syndrome (erythroblastic anemia) 282.49
Dana-Putnam syndrome (subacute combined sclerosis with pernicious anemia) 281.0 [336.2]
Danbolt (-Closs) syndrome (acrodermatitis enteropathica) 686.8
Dandruff 690.18
Dandy fever 061
Dandy-Walker deformity or syndrome (atresia, foramen of Magendie) 742.3
 with spina bifida (*see also* Spina bifida) 741.0
Dangle foot 736.79
Danielssen's disease (anesthetic leprosy) 030.1
Danlos' syndrome 756.83
Darier's disease (congenital) (keratosis follicularis) 757.39
 due to vitamin A deficiency 264.8
 meaning erythema annulare centrifugum 695.0
Darier-Roussy sarcoid 135
Darling's
 disease (*see also* Histoplasmosis, American) 115.00
 histoplasmosis (*see also* Histoplasmosis, American) 115.00
Dartre 054.9
Darwin's tubercle 744.29
Davidson's anemia (refractory) 284.9
Davies' disease 425.0
Davies-Colley syndrome (slipping rib) 733.99
Dawson's encephalitis 046.2
Day blindness (*see also* Blindness, day) 368.60
Dead
 fetus
  retained (in utero) 656.4
   early pregnancy (death before 22 completed weeks' gestation) 632
   late (death after 22 completed weeks' gestation) 656.4
  syndrome 641.3
 labyrinth 386.50
 ovum, retained 631
Deaf and dumb NEC 389.7

Deaf mutism (acquired) (congenital) NEC 389.7
 endemic 243
 hysterical 300.11
 syphilitic, congenital 090.0
Deafness (acquired) (bilateral) (both ears) (complete) (congenital) (hereditary) (middle ear) (partial) (unilateral) 389.9
 with blue sclera and fragility of bone 756.51
 auditory fatigue 389.9
 aviation 993.0
  nerve injury 951.5
 boilermakers' 951.5
 central 389.14
  with conductive hearing loss 389.2
 conductive (air) 389.00
  with sensorineural hearing loss 389.2
  combined types 389.08
  external ear 389.01
  inner ear 389.04
  middle ear 389.03
  multiple types 389.08
  tympanic membrane 389.02
 emotional (complete) 300.11
 functional (complete) 300.11
 high frequency 389.8
 hysterical (complete) 300.11
 injury 951.5
 low frequency 389.8
 mental 784.69
 mixed conductive and sensorineural 389.2
 nerve 389.12
  with conductive hearing loss 389.2
 neural 389.12
  with conductive hearing loss 389.2
 noise-induced 388.12
  nerve injury 951.5
 nonspeaking 389.7
 perceptive 389.10
  with conductive hearing loss 389.2
  central 389.14
  combined types 389.18
  multiple types 389.18
  neural 389.12
  sensory 389.11
 psychogenic (complete) 306.7
 sensorineural (*see also* Deafness, perceptive) 389.10
 sensory 389.11
  with conductive hearing loss 389.2
 specified type NEC 389.8
 sudden NEC 388.2
 syphilitic 094.89
 transient ischemic 388.02
 transmission - *see* Deafness, conductive
 traumatic 951.5
 word (secondary to organic lesion) 784.69
  developmental 315.31
Death
 after delivery (cause not stated) (sudden) 674.9
 anesthetic
  due to
   correct substance properly administered 995.4
   overdose or wrong substance given 968.4
   specified anesthetic - *see* Table of Drugs and Chemicals
  during delivery 668.9

ICD-9-CM

D

Vol. 2

Death *(Continued)*
  brain 348.8
  cardiac - *see* Disease, heart
  cause unknown 798.2
  cot (infant) 798.0
  crib (infant) 798.0
  fetus, fetal (cause not stated) (intra-
    uterine) 779.9
    early, with retention (before 22 com-
      pleted weeks' gestation) 632
    from asphyxia or anoxia (before la-
      bor) 768.0
      during labor 768.1
    late, affecting management of preg-
      nancy (after 22 completed
      weeks' gestation) 656.4
  from pregnancy NEC 646.9
  instantaneous 798.1
  intrauterine (*see also* Death, fetus) 779.9
    complicating pregnancy 656.4
  maternal, affecting fetus or newborn
    761.6
  neonatal NEC 779.9
  sudden (cause unknown) 798.1
    during delivery 669.9
      under anesthesia NEC 668.9
    infant, syndrome (SIDS) 798.0
    puerperal, during puerperium 674.9
  unattended (cause unknown) 798.9
  under anesthesia NEC
    due to
      correct substance properly admin-
        istered 995.4
      overdose or wrong substance
        given 968.4
        specified anesthetic - *see* Table
          of Drugs and Chemicals
    during delivery 668.9
  violent 798.1
de Beurmann-Gougerot disease (sporotrichosis) 117.1
Debility (general) (infantile) (postinfectional) 799.3
  with nutritional difficulty 269.9
  congenital or neonatal NEC 779.9
  nervous 300.5
  old age 797
  senile 797
Débove's disease (splenomegaly) 789.2
Decalcification
  bone (*see also* Osteoporosis) 733.00
  teeth 521.8
Decapitation 874.9
  fetal (to facilitate delivery) 763.89
Decapsulation, kidney 593.89
Decay
  dental 521.00
  senile 797
  tooth, teeth 521.00
Decensus, uterus - *see* Prolapse, uterus
Deciduitis (acute)
  with
    abortion - *see* Abortion, by type,
      with sepsis
    ectopic pregnancy (*see also* categories
      633.0-633.9) 639.0
    molar pregnancy (*see also* categories
      630-632) 639.0
  affecting fetus or newborn 760.8
  following
    abortion 639.0
    ectopic or molar pregnancy 639.0
  in pregnancy 646.6
  puerperal, postpartum 670

Deciduoma malignum (M9100/3) 181
Deciduous tooth (retained) 520.6
Decline (general) (*see also* Debility) 799.3
Decompensation
  cardiac (acute) (chronic) (*see also* Dis-
    ease, heart) 429.9
    failure - *see* Failure, heart
  cardiorenal (*see also* Hypertension, car-
    diorenal) 404.90
  cardiovascular (*see also* Disease, cardio-
    vascular) 429.2
  heart (*see also* Disease, heart) 429.9
    failure - *see* Failure, heart
  hepatic 572.2
  myocardial (acute) (chronic) (*see also*
    Disease, heart) 429.9
    failure - *see* Failure, heart
  respiratory 519.9
Decompression sickness 993.3
Decrease, decreased
  blood
    platelets (*see also* Thrombocytopenia)
      287.5
    pressure 796.3
      due to shock following
        injury 958.4
        operation 998.0
  cardiac reserve - *see* Disease, heart
  estrogen 256.39
    postablative 256.2
  fetal movements 655.7
  fragility of erythrocytes 289.89
  function
    adrenal (cortex) 255.4
      medulla 255.5
    ovary in hypopituitarism 253.4
    parenchyma of pancreas 577.8
    pituitary (gland) (lobe) (anterior) 253.2
      posterior (lobe) 253.8
  functional activity 780.99
  glucose 790.29
  haptoglobin (serum) NEC 273.8
  libido 799.81
  platelets (*see also* Thrombocytopenia)
    287.5
  pulse pressure 785.9
  respiration due to shock following in-
    jury 958.4
  sexual desire 799.81
  tear secretion NEC 375.15
  tolerance
    fat 579.8
    salt and water 276.9
  vision NEC 369.9
Decubial gangrene 707.00 [785.4] ◀▦
Decubiti (*see also* Decubitus) 707.00 ◀▦
Decubitus (ulcer) 707.00 ◀▦
  with gangrene 707.00 [785.4] ◀▦
  ankle 707.06 ◀
  back ◀
    lower 707.03 ◀
    upper 707.02 ◀
  buttock 707.05 ◀
  elbow 707.01 ◀
  head 707.09 ◀
  heel 707.07 ◀
  hip 707.04 ◀
  other site 707.09 ◀
  sacrum 707.03 ◀
  shoulder blades 707.02 ◀
Deepening acetabulum 718.85
Defect, defective 759.9
  3-beta-hydroxysteroid dehydrogenase
    255.2

Defect, defective *(Continued)*
  11-hydroxylase 255.2
  21-hydroxylase 255.2
  abdominal wall, congenital 756.70
  aorticopulmonary septum 745.0
  aortic septal 745.0
  atrial septal (ostium secundum type)
    745.5
    acquired 429.71
    ostium primum type 745.61
    sinus venosus 745.8
  atrioventricular
    canal 745.69
    septum 745.4
      acquired 429.71
  atrium secundum 745.5
    acquired 429.71
  auricular septal 745.5
    acquired 429.71
  bilirubin excretion 277.4
  biosynthesis, testicular androgen
    257.2
  bulbar septum 745.0
  butanol-insoluble iodide 246.1
  chromosome - *see* Anomaly, chromo-
    some
  circulation (acquired) 459.9
    congenital 747.9
    newborn 747.9
  clotting NEC (*see also* Defect, coagula-
    tion) 286.9
  coagulation (factor) (*see also* Deficiency,
    coagulation factor) 286.9
    with
      abortion - *see* Abortion, by type,
        with hemorrhage
      ectopic pregnancy (*see also* catego-
        ries 634-638) 639.1
      molar pregnancy (*see also* catego-
        ries 630-632) 639.1
    acquired (any) 286.7
    antepartum or intrapartum 641.3
      affecting fetus or newborn 762.1
    causing hemorrhage of pregnancy or
      delivery 641.3
    due to
      liver disease 286.7
      vitamin K deficiency 286.7
    newborn, transient 776.3
    postpartum 666.3
    specified type NEC 286.3
  conduction (heart) 426.9
    bone (*see also* Deafness, conductive)
      389.00
  congenital, organ or site NEC - *see also*
    Anomaly
    circulation 747.9
    Descemet's membrane 743.9
      specified type NEC 743.49
    diaphragm 756.6
    ectodermal 757.9
    esophagus 750.9
    pulmonic cusps - *see* Anomaly, heart
      valve
    respiratory system 748.9
      specified type NEC 748.8
  cushion endocardial 745.60
  dentin (hereditary) 520.5
  Descemet's membrane (congenital) 743.9
    acquired 371.30
    specific type NEC 743.49
  deutan 368.52
  developmental - *see also* Anomaly, by
    site

◀ **New**   ◀▦ **Revised**

Defect, defective (Continued)

developmental (Continued)

cauda equina 742.59

left ventricle 746.9

with atresia or hypoplasia of aortic orifice or valve, with hypoplasia of ascending aorta 746.7

in hypoplastic left heart syndrome 746.7

testis 752.9

vessel 747.9

diaphragm

with elevation, eventration, or hernia - see Hernia, diaphragm

congenital 756.6

with elevation, eventration, or hernia 756.6

gross (with elevation, eventration, or hernia) 756.6

ectodermal, congenital 757.9

Eisenmenger's (ventricular septal defect) 745.4

endocardial cushion 745.60

specified type NEC 745.69

esophagus, congenital 750.9

extensor retinaculum 728.9

fibrin polymerization (see also Defect, coagulation) 286.3

filling

biliary tract 793.3

bladder 793.5

gallbladder 793.3

kidney 793.5

stomach 793.4

ureter 793.5

fossa ovalis 745.5

gene, carrier (suspected) of V83.89

Gerbode 745.4

glaucomatous, without elevated tension 365.89

Hageman (factor) (see also Defect, coagulation) 286.3

hearing (see also Deafness) 389.9

high grade 317

homogentisic acid 270.2

interatrial septal 745.5

acquired 429.71

interauricular septal 745.5

acquired 429.71

interventricular septal 745.4

with pulmonary stenosis or atresia, dextraposition of aorta, and hypertrophy of right ventricle 745.2

acquired 429.71

in tetralogy of Fallot 745.2

iodide trapping 246.1

iodotyrosine dehalogenase 246.1

kynureninase 270.2

learning, specific 315.2

mental (see also Retardation, mental) 319

osteochondral NEC 738.8

ostium

primum 745.61

secundum 745.5

pericardium 746.89

peroxidase-binding 246.1

placental blood supply - see Placenta, insufficiency

platelet (qualitative) 287.1

constitutional 286.4

postural, spine 737.9

Defect, defective (Continued)

protan 368.51

pulmonic cusps, congenital 746.00

renal pelvis 753.9

obstructive 753.29

specified type NEC 753.3

respiratory system, congenital 748.9

specified type NEC 748.8

retina, retinal 361.30

with detachment (see also Detachment, retina, with retinal defect) 361.00

multiple 361.33

with detachment 361.02

nerve fiber bundle 362.85

single 361.30

with detachment 361.01

septal (closure) (heart) NEC 745.9

acquired 429.71

atrial 745.5

specified type NEC 745.8

speech NEC 784.5

developmental 315.39

secondary to organic lesion 784.5

Taussig-Bing (transposition, aorta and overriding pulmonary artery) 745.11

teeth, wedge 521.20 ◄⃫

thyroid hormone synthesis 246.1

tritan 368.53

ureter 753.9

obstructive 753.29

vascular (acquired) (local) 459.9

congenital (peripheral) NEC 747.60

gastrointestinal 747.61

lower limb 747.64

renal 747.62

specified NEC 747.69

spinal 747.82

upper limb 747.63

ventricular septal 745.4

with pulmonary stenosis or atresia, dextraposition of aorta, and hypertrophy of right ventricle 745.2

acquired 429.71

atrioventricular canal type 745.69

between infundibulum and anterior portion 745.4

in tetralogy of Fallot 745.2

isolated anterior 745.4

vision NEC 369.9

visual field 368.40

arcuate 368.43

heteronymous, bilateral 368.47

homonymous, bilateral 368.46

localized NEC 368.44

nasal step 368.44

peripheral 368.44

sector 368.43

voice 784.40

wedge, teeth (abrasion) 521.20 ◄⃫

Defeminization syndrome 255.2

Deferentitis 608.4

gonorrheal (acute) 098.14

chronic or duration of 2 months or over 098.34

Defibrination syndrome (see also Fibrinolysis) 286.6

Deficiency, deficient

3-beta-hydroxysteroid dehydrogenase 255.2

6-phosphogluconic dehydrogenase (anemia) 282.2

11-beta-hydroxylase 255.2

Deficiency, deficient (Continued)

17-alpha-hydroxylase 255.2

18-hydroxysteroid dehydrogenase 255.2

20-alpha-hydroxylase 255.2

21-hydroxylase 255.2

AAT (alpha-1 antitrypsin) 273.4 ◄

abdominal muscle syndrome 756.79

accelerator globulin (Ac G) (blood) (see also Defect, coagulation) 286.3

AC globulin (congenital) (see also Defect, coagulation) 286.3

acquired 286.7

activating factor (blood) (see also Defect, coagulation) 286.3

adenohypophyseal 253.2

adenosine deaminase 277.2

aldolase (hereditary) 271.2

alpha-1-antitrypsin 273.4 ◄⃫

alpha-1-trypsin inhibitor 273.4 ◄⃫

alpha-fucosidase 271.8

alpha-lipoprotein 272.5

alpha-mannosidase 271.8

amino acid 270.9

anemia - see Anemia, deficiency

aneurin 265.1

with beriberi 265.0

antibody NEC 279.00

antidiuretic hormone 253.5

antihemophilic

factor (A) 286.0

B 286.1

C 286.2

globulin (AHG) NEC 286.0

antithrombin III 289.81

antitrypsin 273.4 ◄⃫

argininosuccinate synthetase or lyase 270.6

ascorbic acid (with scurvy) 267

autoprothrombin

I (see also Defect, coagulation) 286.3

II 286.1

C (see also Defect, coagulation) 286.3

bile salt 579.8

biotin 266.2

biotinidase 277.6

bradykinase-1 277.6

brancher enzyme (amylopectinosis) 271.0

calciferol 268.9

with

osteomalacia 268.2

rickets (see also Rickets) 268.0

calcium 275.40

dietary 269.3

calorie, severe 261

carbamyl phosphate synthetase 270.6

cardiac (see also Insufficiency, myocardial) 428.0

carnitine 277.81

due to

hemodialysis 277.83

inborn errors of metabolism 277.82

valproic acid therapy 277.83

iatrogenic 277.83

palmitoyltransferase (CPT1, CPT2) 277.85 ◄

palmityl transferase (CPT1, CPT2) 277.85 ◄⃫

primary 277.81

secondary 277.84

carotene 264.9

Carr factor (see also Defect, coagulation) 286.9

ICD-9-CM

D

Vol. 2

Deficiency, deficient *(Continued)*
  central nervous system 349.9
  ceruloplasmin 275.1
  cevitamic acid (with scurvy) 267
  choline 266.2
  Christmas factor 286.1
  chromium 269.3
  citrin 269.1
  clotting (blood) *(see also* Defect, coagulation) 286.9
  coagulation factor NEC 286.9
    with
      abortion - *see* Abortion, by type, with hemorrhage
      ectopic pregnancy *(see also* categories 634-638) 639.1
      molar pregnancy *(see also* categories 630-632) 639.1
    acquired (any) 286.7
    antepartum or intrapartum 641.3
      affecting fetus or newborn 762.1
    due to
      liver disease 286.7
      vitamin K deficiency 286.7
    newborn, transient 776.3
    postpartum 666.3
    specified type NEC 286.3
  color vision (congenital) 368.59
    acquired 368.55
  combined, two or more coagulation factors *(see also* Defect, coagulation) 286.9
  complement factor NEC 279.8
  contact factor *(see also* Defect, coagulation) 286.3
  copper NEC 275.1
  corticoadrenal 255.4
  craniofacial axis 756.0
  cyanocobalamin (vitamin B_{12}) 266.2
  debrancher enzyme (limit dextrinosis) 271.0
  desmolase 255.2
  diet 269.9
  dihydrofolate reductase 281.2
  dihydropteridine reductase 270.1
  disaccharidase (intestinal) 271.3
  disease NEC 269.9
  ear(s) V48.8
  edema 262
  endocrine 259.9
  enzymes, circulating NEC *(see also* Deficiency, by specific enzyme) 277.6
  ergosterol 268.9
    with
      osteomalacia 268.2
      rickets *(see also* Rickets) 268.0
  erythrocytic glutathione (anemia) 282.2
  eyelid(s) V48.8
  factor *(see also* Defect, coagulation) 286.9
    I (congenital) (fibrinogen) 286.3
      antepartum or intrapartum 641.3
        affecting fetus or newborn 762.1
      newborn, transient 776.3
      postpartum 666.3
    II (congenital) (prothrombin) 286.3
    V (congenital) (labile) 286.3
    VII (congenital) (stable) 286.3
    VIII (congenital) (functional) 286.0
      with
        functional defect 286.0
        vascular defect 286.4

Deficiency, deficient *(Continued)*
  factor *(Continued)*
    IX (Christmas) (congenital) (functional) 286.1
    X (congenital) (Stuart-Prower) 286.3
    XI (congenital) (plasma thromboplastin antecedent) 286.2
    XII (congenital) (Hageman) 286.3
    XIII (congenital) (fibrin stabilizing) 286.3
    Hageman 286.3
    multiple (congenital) 286.9
      acquired 286.7
    fibrinase *(see also* Defect, coagulation) 286.3
    fibrinogen (congenital) *(see also* Defect, coagulation) 286.3
      acquired 286.6
    fibrin-stabilizing factor (congenital) *(see also* Defect, coagulation) 286.3
      acquired 286.7
    finger - *see* Absence, finger
    fletcher factor *(see also* Defect, coagulation) 286.9
    fluorine 269.3
    folate, anemia 281.2
    folic acid (vitamin B_C) 266.2
      anemia 281.2
    follicle-stimulating hormone (FSH) 253.4
    fructokinase 271.2
    fructose-1, 6-diphosphate 271.2
    fructose-1-phosphate aldolase 271.2
    FSH (follicle-stimulating hormone) 253.4
    fucosidase 271.8
    galactokinase 271.1
    galactose-1-phosphate uridyl transferase 271.1
    gamma globulin in blood 279.00
    glass factor *(see also* Defect, coagulation) 286.3
    glucocorticoid 255.4
    glucose-6-phosphatase 271.0
    glucose-6-phosphate dehydrogenase anemia 282.2
    glucuronyl transferase 277.4
    glutathione-reductase (anemia) 282.2
    glycogen synthetase 271.0
    growth hormone 253.3
    Hageman factor (congenital) *(see also* Defect, coagulation) 286.3
    head V48.0
    hemoglobin *(see also* Anemia) 285.9
    hepatophosphorylase 271.0
    hexose monophosphate (HMP) shunt 282.2
    hGH (human growth hormone) 253.3
    HG-PRT 277.2
    homogentisic acid oxidase 270.2
    hormone - *see also* Deficiency, by specific hormone
      anterior pituitary (isolated) (partial) NEC 253.4
        growth (human) 253.3
      follicle-stimulating 253.4
      growth (human) (isolated) 253.3
      human growth 253.3
      interstitial cell-stimulating 253.4
      luteinizing 253.4
      melanocyte-stimulating 253.4
      testicular 257.2
    human growth hormone 253.3

Deficiency, deficient *(Continued)*
  humoral 279.00
    with
      hyper-IgM 279.05
        autosomal recessive 279.05
        X-linked 279.05
      increased IgM 279.05
    congenital hypogammaglobulinemia 279.04
    non-sex-linked 279.06
    selective immunoglobulin NEC 279.03
      IgA 279.01
      IgG 279.03
      IgM 279.02
        increased 279.05
    specified NEC 279.09
  hydroxylase 255.2
  hypoxanthine-guanine phosphoribosyltransferase (HG-PRT) 277.2
  ICSH (interstitial cell-stimulating hormone) 253.4
  immunity NEC 279.3
    cell-mediated 279.10
      with
        hyperimmunoglobulinemia 279.2
        thrombocytopenia and eczema 279.12
      specified NEC 279.19
    combined (severe) 279.2
      syndrome 279.2
    common variable 279.06
    humoral NEC 279.00
    IgA (secretory) 279.01
    IgG 279.03
    IgM 279.02
  immunoglobulin, selective NEC 279.03
    IgA 279.01
    IgG 279.03
    IgM 279.02
  inositol (B complex) 266.2
  interferon 279.4
  internal organ V47.0
  interstitial cell-stimulating hormone (ICSH) 253.4
  intrinsic factor (Castle's) (congenital) 281.0
  intrinsic (urethral) sphincter (ISD) 599.82
  invertase 271.3
  iodine 269.3
  iron, anemia 280.9
  labile factor (congenital) *(see also* Defect, coagulation) 286.3
    acquired 286.7
  lacrimal fluid (acquired) 375.15
    congenital 743.64
  lactase 271.3
  Laki-Lorand factor *(see also* Defect, coagulation) 286.3
  lecithin-cholesterol acyltranferase 272.5
  LH (luteinizing hormone) 253.4
  limb V49.0
    lower V49.0
      congenital *(see also* Deficiency, lower limb, congenital) 755.30
    upper V49.0
      congenital *(see also* Deficiency, upper limb, congenital) 755.20
  lipocaic 577.8
  lipoid (high-density) 272.5
  lipoprotein (familial) (high-density) 272.5

◀ **New**   ◀▥ **Revised**

Deficiency, deficient (Continued)
liver phosphorylase 271.0
long chain 3-hydroxyacyl CoA dehydrogenase (LCHAD) 277.85 ◀
long chain/very long chain acyl CoA
   dehydrogenase (LCAD, VLCAD)
   277.85 ◀
lower limb V49.0
  congenital 755.30
    with complete absence of distal el-
      ements 755.31
    longitudinal (complete) (partial)
      (with distal deficiencies, in-
      complete) 755.32
      with complete absence of distal
        elements 755.31
      combined femoral, tibial, fibular
        (incomplete) 755.33
      femoral 755.34
      fibular 755.37
      metatarsal(s) 755.38
      phalange(s) 755.39
        meaning all digits 755.31
      tarsal(s) 755.38
      tibia 755.36
      tibiofibular 755.35
      transverse 755.31
luteinizing hormone (LH) 253.4
lysosomal alpha-1, 4 glucosidase 271.0
magnesium 275.2
mannosidase 271.8
medium chain acyl CoA dehydrogenase (MCAD) 277.85 ◀
melanocyte-stimulating hormone
   (MSH) 253.4
menadione (vitamin K) 269.0
  newborn 776.0
mental (familial) (hereditary) (see also
   Retardation, mental) 319
mineral NEC 269.3
molybdenum 269.3
moral 301.7
multiple, syndrome 260
myocardial (see also Insufficiency, myocardial) 428.0
myophosphorylase 271.0
NADH (DPNH)-methemoglobin-reduc-
   tase (congenital) 289.7
NADH diaphorase or reductase (congenital) 289.7
neck V48.1
niacin (amide) (-tryptophan) 265.2
nicotinamide 265.2
nicotinic acid (amide) 265.2
nose V48.8
number of teeth (see also Anodontia)
   520.0
nutrition, nutritional 269.9
  specified NEC 269.8
ornithine transcarbamylase 270.6
ovarian 256.39
oxygen (see also Anoxia) 799.0
pantothenic acid 266.2
parathyroid (gland) 252.1
phenylalanine hydroxylase 270.1
phosphoenolpyruvate carboxykinase
   271.8 ◀
phosphofructokinase 271.2
phosphoglucomutase 271.0
phosphohexosisomerase 271.0
phosphorylase kinase, liver 271.0
pituitary (anterior) 253.2
  posterior 253.5
placenta - see Placenta, insufficiency

Deficiency, deficient (Continued)
plasma
  cell 279.00
  protein (paraproteinemia) (pyroglob-
    ulinemia) 273.8
    gamma globulin 279.00
  thromboplastin
    antecedent (PTA) 286.2
    component (PTC) 286.1
platelet NEC 287.1
  constitutional 286.4
polyglandular 258.9
potassium (K) 276.8
proaccelerin (congenital) (see also Defect, congenital) 286.3
  acquired 286.7
proconvertin factor (congenital) (see
   also Defect, coagulation) 286.3
  acquired 286.7
prolactin 253.4
protein 260
  anemia 281.4
  C 289.81
  plasma - see Deficiency, plasma, pro-
    tein
  S 289.81
prothrombin (congenital) (see also Defect, coagulation) 286.3
  acquired 286.7
Prower factor (see also Defect, coagulation) 286.3
PRT 277.2
pseudocholinesterase 289.89
psychobiological 301.6
PTA 286.2
PTC 286.1
purine nucleoside phosphorylase
   277.2
pyracin (alpha) (beta) 266.1
pyridoxal 266.1
pyridoxamine 266.1
pyridoxine (derivatives) 266.1
pyruvate carboxylase 271.8 ◀
pyruvate dehydrogenase 271.8 ◀
pyruvate kinase (PK) 282.3
riboflavin (vitamin B$_2$) 266.0
saccadic eye movements 379.57
salivation 527.7
salt 276.1
secretion
  ovary 256.39
  salivary gland (any) 527.7
  urine 788.5
selenium 269.3
serum
  antitrypsin, familial 273.4 ◀⫶
  protein (congenital) 273.8
short chain acyl CoA dehydrogenase
   (SCAD) 277.85 ◀
smooth pursuit movements (eye)
   379.58
sodium (Na) 276.1
SPCA (see also Defect, coagulation)
   286.3
specified NEC 269.8
stable factor (congenital) (see also Defect, coagulation) 286.3
  acquired 286.7
Stuart (-Prower) factor (see also Defect,
   coagulation) 286.3
sucrase 271.3
sucrase-isomaltase 271.3
sulfite oxidase 270.0
syndrome, multiple 260

Deficiency, deficient (Continued)
thiamine, thiaminic (chloride) 265.1
thrombokinase (see also Defect, coagulation) 286.3
  newborn 776.0
thrombopoieten 287.3
thymolymphatic 279.2
thyroid (gland) 244.9
tocopherol 269.1
toe - see Absence, toe
tooth bud (see also Anodontia) 520.0
trunk V48.1
UDPG-glycogen transferase 271.0
upper limb V49.0
  congenital 755.20
    with complete absence of distal el-
      ements 755.21
    longitudinal (complete) (partial)
      (with distal deficiencies, in-
      complete) 755.22
      carpal(s) 755.28
      combined humeral, radial, ulnar
        (incomplete) 755.23
      humeral 755.24
      metacarpal(s) 755.28
      phalange(s) 755.29
        meaning all digits 755.21
      radial 755.26
      radioulnar 755.25
      ulnar 755.27
    transverse (complete) (partial)
      755.21
vascular 459.9
vasopressin 253.5
viosterol (see also Deficiency, calciferol)
   268.9
vitamin (multiple) NEC 269.2
  A 264.9
    with
      Bitôt's spot 264.1
        corneal 264.2
          with corneal ulceration 264.3
      keratomalacia 264.4
      keratosis, follicular 264.8
      night blindness 264.5
      scar of cornea, xerophthalmic
        264.6
      specified manifestation NEC
        264.8
        ocular 264.7
      xeroderma 264.8
      xerophthalmia 264.7
      xerosis
        conjunctival 264.0
          with Bitôt's spot 264.1
        corneal 264.2
          with corneal ulceration
            264.3
  B (complex) NEC 266.9
    with
      beriberi 265.0
      pellagra 265.2
    specified type NEC 266.2
  B$_1$ NEC 265.1
    beriberi 265.0
  B$_2$ 266.0
  B$_6$ 266.1
  B$_{12}$ 266.2
  B$_C$ (folic acid) 266.2
  C (ascorbic acid) (with scurvy) 267
  D (calciferol) (ergosterol) 268.9
    with
      osteomalacia 268.2
      rickets (see also Rickets) 268.0

ICD-9-CM

Vol. 2

Deficiency, deficient *(Continued)*
  vitamin (multiple) NEC *(Continued)*
    E 269.1
    folic acid 266.2
    G 266.0
    H 266.2
    K 269.0
      of newborn 776.0
    nicotinic acid 265.2
    P 269.1
    PP 265.2
    specified NEC 269.1
    zinc 269.3
Deficient - *see also* Deficiency
  blink reflex 374.45
  craniofacial axis 756.0
  number of teeth *(see also* Anodontia) 520.0
  secretion of urine 788.5
Deficit
  neurologic NEC 781.99
    due to
      cerebrovascular lesion *(see also* Disease, cerebrovascular, acute)* 436
        late effect - *see* Late effect(s) (of) cerebrovascular disease
      transient ischemic attack 435.9
  oxygen 799.0
Deflection
  radius 736.09
  septum (acquired) (nasal) (nose) 470
  spine - *see* Curvature, spine
  turbinate (nose) 470
Defluvium
  capillorum *(see also* Alopecia) 704.00
  ciliorum 374.55
  unguium 703.8
Deformity 738.9
  abdomen, congenital 759.9
  abdominal wall
    acquired 738.8
    congenital 756.70
    muscle deficiency syndrome 756.79
  acquired (unspecified site) 738.9
    specified site NEC 738.8
  adrenal gland (congenital) 759.1
  alimentary tract, congenital 751.9
    lower 751.5
    specified type NEC 751.8
    upper (any part, except tongue) 750.9
      specified type NEC 750.8
      tongue 750.10
        specified type NEC 750.19
  ankle (joint) (acquired) 736.70
    abduction 718.47
    congenital 755.69
    contraction 718.47
    specified NEC 736.79
  anus (congenital) 751.5
    acquired 569.49
  aorta (congenital) 747.20
    acquired 447.8
    arch 747.21
      acquired 447.8
    coarctation 747.10
  aortic
    arch 747.21
      acquired 447.8
    cusp or valve (congenital) 746.9
      acquired *(see also* Endocarditis, aortic) 424.1
    ring 747.21

Deformity *(Continued)*
  appendix 751.5
  arm (acquired) 736.89
    congenital 755.50
  arteriovenous (congenital) (peripheral) NEC 747.60
    gastrointestinal 747.61
    lower limb 747.64
    renal 747.62
    specified NEC 747.69
    spinal 747.82
    upper limb 747.63
  artery (congenital) (peripheral) NEC *(see also* Deformity, vascular) 747.60
    acquired 447.8
    cerebral 747.81
    coronary (congenital) 746.85
      acquired *(see also* Ischemia, heart) 414.9
    retinal 743.9
    umbilical 747.5
  atrial septal (congenital) (heart) 745.5
  auditory canal (congenital) (external) *(see also* Deformity, ear) 744.3
    acquired 380.50
  auricle
    ear (congenital) *(see also* Deformity, ear) 744.3
      acquired 380.32
    heart (congenital) 746.9
  back (acquired) - *see* Deformity, spine
  Bartholin's duct (congenital) 750.9
  bile duct (congenital) 751.60
    acquired 576.8
      with calculus, choledocholithiasis, or stones - *see* Choledocholithiasis
  biliary duct or passage (congenital) 751.60
    acquired 576.8
      with calculus, choledocholithiasis, or stones - *see* Choledocholithiasis
  bladder (neck) (sphincter) (trigone) (acquired) 596.8
    congenital 753.9
  bone (acquired) NEC 738.9
    congenital 756.9
    turbinate 738.0
  boutonniere (finger) 736.21
  brain (congenital) 742.9
    acquired 348.8
    multiple 742.4
    reduction 742.2
    vessel (congenital) 747.81
  breast (acquired) 611.8
    congenital 757.9
  bronchus (congenital) 748.3
    acquired 519.1
  bursa, congenital 756.9
  canal of Nuck 752.9
  canthus (congenital) 743.9
    acquired 374.89
  capillary (acquired) 448.9
    congenital NEC *(see also* Deformity, vascular) 747.60
  cardiac - *see* Deformity, heart
  cardiovascular system (congenital) 746.9
  caruncle, lacrimal (congenital) 743.9
    acquired 375.69

Deformity *(Continued)*
  cascade, stomach 537.6
  cecum (congenital) 751.5
    acquired 569.89
  cerebral (congenital) 742.9
    acquired 348.8
  cervix (acquired) (uterus) 622.8
    congenital 752.40
  cheek (acquired) 738.19
    congenital 744.9
  chest (wall) (acquired) 738.3
    congenital 754.89
    late effect of rickets 268.1
  chin (acquired) 738.19
    congenital 744.9
  choroid (congenital) 743.9
    acquired 363.8
    plexus (congenital) 742.9
      acquired 349.2
  cicatricial - *see* Cicatrix
  cilia (congenital) 743.9
    acquired 374.89
  circulatory system (congenital) 747.9
  clavicle (acquired) 738.8
    congenital 755.51
  clitoris (congenital) 752.40
    acquired 624.8
  clubfoot - *see* Clubfoot
  coccyx (acquired) 738.6
    congenital 756.10
  colon (congenital) 751.5
    acquired 569.89
  concha (ear) (congenital) *(see also* Deformity, ear) 744.3
    acquired 380.32
  congenital, organ or site not listed *(see also* Anomaly) 759.9
  cornea (congenital) 743.9
    acquired 371.70
  coronary artery (congenital) 746.85
    acquired *(see also* Ischemia, heart) 414.9
  cranium (acquired) 738.19
    congenital *(see also* Deformity, skull, congenital) 756.0
  cricoid cartilage (congenital) 748.3
    acquired 478.79
  cystic duct (congenital) 751.60
    acquired 575.8
  Dandy-Walker 742.3
    with spina bifida *(see also* Spina bifida) 741.0
  diaphragm (congenital) 756.6
    acquired 738.8
  digestive organ(s) or system (congenital) NEC 751.9
    specified type NEC 751.8
  ductus arteriosus 747.0
  duodenal bulb 537.89
  duodenum (congenital) 751.5
    acquired 537.89
  dura (congenital) 742.9
    brain 742.4
      acquired 349.2
    spinal 742.59
      acquired 349.2
  ear (congenital) 744.3
    acquired 380.32
    auricle 744.3
      causing impairment of hearing 744.02
    causing impairment of hearing 744.00
    external 744.3

◀ **New**   ◀▥ **Revised**

Deformity (*Continued*)
ear (*Continued*)
external (*Continued*)
causing impairment of hearing 744.02
internal 744.05
lobule 744.3
middle 744.03
ossicles 744.04
ossicles 744.04
ectodermal (congenital) NEC 757.9
specified type NEC 757.8
ejaculatory duct (congenital) 752.9
acquired 608.89
elbow (joint) (acquired) 736.00
congenital 755.50
contraction 718.42
endocrine gland NEC 759.2
epididymis (congenital) 752.9
acquired 608.89
torsion 608.2
epiglottis (congenital) 748.3
acquired 478.79
esophagus (congenital) 750.9
acquired 530.89
Eustachian tube (congenital) NEC 744.3
specified type NEC 744.24
extremity (acquired) 736.9
congenital, except reduction deformity 755.9
lower 755.60
upper 755.50
reduction - *see* Deformity, reduction
eye (congenital) 743.9
acquired 379.8
muscle 743.9
eyebrow (congenital) 744.89
eyelid (congenital) 743.9
acquired 374.89
specified type NEC 743.62
face (acquired) 738.19
congenital (any part) 744.9
due to intrauterine malposition and pressure 754.0
fallopian tube (congenital) 752.10
acquired 620.8
femur (acquired) 736.89
congenital 755.60
fetal
with fetopelvic disproportion 653.7
affecting fetus or newborn 763.1
causing obstructed labor 660.1
affecting fetus or newborn 763.1
known or suspected, affecting management of pregnancy 655.9
finger (acquired) 736.20
boutonniere type 736.21
congenital 755.50
flexion contracture 718.44
swan neck 736.22
flexion (joint) (acquired) 736.9
congenital NEC 755.9
hip or thigh (acquired) 736.39
congenital (*see also* Subluxation, congenital, hip) 754.32
foot (acquired) 736.70
cavovarus 736.75
congenital 754.59
congenital NEC 754.70
specified type NEC 754.79
valgus (acquired) 736.79
congenital 754.60
specified type NEC 754.69

Deformity (*Continued*)
foot (*Continued*)
varus (acquired) 736.79
congenital 754.50
specified type NEC 754.59
forearm (acquired) 736.00
congenital 755.50
forehead (acquired) 738.19
congenital (*see also* Deformity, skull, congenital) 756.0
frontal bone (acquired) 738.19
congenital (*see also* Deformity, skull, congenital) 756.0
gallbladder (congenital) 751.60
acquired 575.8
gastrointestinal tract (congenital) NEC 751.9
acquired 569.89
specified type NEC 751.8
genitalia, genital organ(s) or system NEC
congenital 752.9
female (congenital) 752.9
acquired 629.8
external 752.40
internal 752.9
male (congenital) 752.9
acquired 608.89
globe (eye) (congenital) 743.9
acquired 360.89
gum (congenital) 750.9
acquired 523.9
gunstock 736.02
hand (acquired) 736.00
claw 736.06
congenital 755.50
minus (and plus) (intrinsic) 736.09
pill roller (intrinsic) 736.09
plus (and minus) (intrinsic) 736.09
swan neck (intrinsic) 736.09
head (acquired) 738.10
congenital (*see also* Deformity, skull, congenital) 756.0
specified NEC 738.19
heart (congenital) 746.9
auricle (congenital) 746.9
septum 745.9
auricular 745.5
specified type NEC 745.8
ventricular 745.4
valve (congenital) NEC 746.9
acquired - *see* Endocarditis
pulmonary (congenital) 746.00
specified type NEC 746.89
ventricle (congenital) 746.9
heel (acquired) 736.76
congenital 755.67
hepatic duct (congenital) 751.60
acquired 576.8
with calculus, choledocholithiasis, or stones - *see* Choledocholithiasis
hip (joint) (acquired) 736.30
congenital NEC 755.63
flexion 718.45
congenital (*see also* Subluxation, congenital, hip) 754.32
hourglass - *see* Contraction, hourglass
humerus (acquired) 736.89
congenital 755.50
hymen (congenital) 752.40
hypophyseal (congenital) 759.2
ileocecal (coil) (valve) (congenital) 751.5
acquired 569.89

Deformity (*Continued*)
ileum (intestine) (congenital) 751.5
acquired 569.89
ilium (acquired) 738.6
congenital 755.60
integument (congenital) 757.9
intervertebral cartilage or disc (acquired) - *see also* Displacement, intervertebral disc
congenital 756.10
intestine (large) (small) (congenital) 751.5
acquired 569.89
iris (acquired) 364.75
congenital 743.9
prolapse 364.8
ischium (acquired) 738.6
congenital 755.60
jaw (acquired) (congenital) NEC 524.9
due to intrauterine malposition and pressure 754.0
joint (acquired) NEC 738.8
congenital 755.9
contraction (abduction) (adduction) (extension) (flexion) - *see* Contraction, joint
kidney(s) (calyx) (pelvis) (congenital) 753.9
acquired 593.89
vessel 747.62
acquired 459.9
Klippel-Feil (brevicollis) 756.16
knee (acquired) NEC 736.6
congenital 755.64
labium (majus) (minus) (congenital) 752.40
acquired 624.8
lacrimal apparatus or duct (congenital) 743.9
acquired 375.69
larynx (muscle) (congenital) 748.3
acquired 478.79
web (glottic) (subglottic) 748.2
leg (lower) (upper) (acquired) NEC 736.89
congenital 755.60
reduction - *see* Deformity, reduction, lower limb
lens (congenital) 743.9
acquired 379.39
lid (fold) (congenital) 743.9
acquired 374.89
ligament (acquired) 728.9
congenital 756.9
limb (acquired) 736.9
congenital, except reduction deformity 755.9
lower 755.60
reduction (*see also* Deformity, reduction, lower limb) 755.30
upper 755.50
reduction (*see also* Deformity, reduction, lower limb) 755.20
specified NEC 736.89
lip (congenital) NEC 750.9
acquired 528.5
specified type NEC 750.26
liver (congenital) 751.60
acquired 573.8
duct (congenital) 751.60
acquired 576.8
with calculus, choledocholithiasis, or stones - *see* Choledocholithiasis

ICD-9-CM

Vol. 2

Deformity *(Continued)*
lower extremity - *see* Deformity, leg
lumbosacral (joint) (region) (congenital) 756.10
  acquired 738.5
lung (congenital) 748.60
  acquired 518.89
  specified type NEC 748.69
lymphatic system, congenital 759.9
Madelung's (radius) 755.54
maxilla (acquired) (congenital) 524.9
meninges or membrane (congenital) 742.9
  brain 742.4
    acquired 349.2
  spinal (cord) 742.59
    acquired 349.2
mesentery (congenital) 751.9
  acquired 568.89
metacarpus (acquired) 736.00
  congenital 755.50
metatarsus (acquired) 736.70
  congenital 754.70
middle ear, except ossicles (congenital) 744.03
  ossicles 744.04
mitral (leaflets) (valve) (congenital) 746.9
  acquired - *see* Endocarditis, mitral
  Ebstein's 746.89
  parachute 746.5
  specified type NEC 746.89
  stenosis, congenital 746.5
mouth (acquired) 528.9
  congenital NEC 750.9
    specified type NEC 750.26
multiple, congenital NEC 759.7
  specified type NEC 759.89
muscle (acquired) 728.9
  congenital 756.9
    specified type NEC 756.89
    sternocleidomastoid (due to intra-uterine malposition and pressure) 754.1
musculoskeletal system, congenital NEC 756.9
  specified type NEC 756.9
nail (acquired) 703.9
  congenital 757.9
nasal - *see* Deformity, nose
neck (acquired) NEC 738.2
  congenital (any part) 744.9
    sternocleidomastoid 754.1
nervous system (congenital) 742.9
nipple (congenital) 757.9
  acquired 611.8
nose, nasal (cartilage) (acquired) 738.0
  bone (turbinate) 738.0
  congenital 748.1
    bent 754.0
    squashed 754.0
  saddle 738.0
    syphilitic 090.5
  septum 470
    congenital 748.1
  sinus (wall) (congenital) 748.1
    acquired 738.0
  syphilitic (congenital) 090.5
    late 095.8
ocular muscle (congenital) 743.9
  acquired 378.60
opticociliary vessels (congenital) 743.9

Deformity *(Continued)*
orbit (congenital) (eye) 743.9
  acquired NEC 376.40
    associated with craniofacial deformities 376.44
    due to
      bone disease 376.43
      surgery 376.47
      trauma 376.47
organ of Corti (congenital) 744.05
ovary (congenital) 752.0
  acquired 620.8
oviduct (congenital) 752.10
  acquired 620.8
palate (congenital) 750.9
  acquired 526.89
  cleft (congenital) (*see also* Cleft, palate) 749.00
  hard, acquired 526.89
  soft, acquired 528.9
pancreas (congenital) 751.7
  acquired 577.8
parachute, mitral.valve 746.5
parathyroid (gland) 759.2
parotid (gland) (congenital) 750.9
  acquired 527.8
patella (acquired) 736.6
  congenital 755.64
pelvis, pelvic (acquired) (bony) 738.6
  with disproportion (fetopelvic) 653.0
    affecting fetus or newborn 763.1
    causing obstructed labor 660.1
      affecting fetus or newborn 763.1
  congenital 755.60
  rachitic (late effect) 268.1
penis (glans) (congenital) 752.9
  acquired 607.89
pericardium (congenital) 746.9
  acquired - *see* Pericarditis
pharynx (congenital) 750.9
  acquired 478.29
Pierre Robin (congenital) 756.0
pinna (acquired) 380.32
  congenital 744.3
pituitary (congenital) 759.2
pleural folds (congenital) 748.8
portal vein (congenital) 747.40
posture - *see* Curvature, spine
prepuce (congenital) 752.9
  acquired 607.89
prostate (congenital) 752.9
  acquired 602.8
pulmonary valve - *see* Endocarditis, pulmonary
pupil (congenital) 743.9
  acquired 364.75
pylorus (congenital) 750.9
  acquired 537.89
rachitic (acquired), healed or old 268.1
radius (acquired) 736.00
  congenital 755.50
  reduction - *see* Deformity, reduction, upper limb
rectovaginal septum (congenital) 752.40
  acquired 623.8
rectum (congenital) 751.5
  acquired 569.49
reduction (extremity) (limb) 755.4
  brain 742.2
  lower limb 755.30
    with complete absence of distal elements 755.31

Deformity *(Continued)*
reduction *(Continued)*
  lower limb *(Continued)*
    longitudinal (complete) (partial) (with distal deficiencies, incomplete) 755.32
    with complete absence of distal elements 755.31
    combined femoral, tibial, fibular (incomplete) 755.33
    femoral 755.34
    fibular 755.37
    metatarsal(s) 755.38
    phalange(s) 755.39
      meaning all digits 755.31
    tarsal(s) 755.38
    tibia 755.36
    tibiofibular 755.35
    transverse 755.31
  upper limb 755.20
    with complete absence of distal elements 755.21
    longitudinal (complete) (partial) (with distal deficiencies, incomplete) 755.22
    with complete absence of distal elements 755.21
    carpal(s) 755.28
    combined humeral, radial, ulnar (incomplete) 755.23
    humeral 755.24
    metacarpal(s) 755.28
    phalange(s) 755.29
      meaning all digits 755.21
    radial 755.26
    radioulnar 755.25
    ulnar 755.27
    transverse (complete) (partial) 755.21
  renal - *see* Deformity, kidney
  respiratory system (congenital) 748.9
    specified type NEC 748.8
  rib (acquired) 738.3
    congenital 756.3
    cervical 756.2
  rotation (joint) (acquired) 736.9
    congenital 755.9
    hip or thigh 736.39
      congenital (*see also* Subluxation, congenital, hip) 754.32
  sacroiliac joint (congenital) 755.69
    acquired 738.5
  sacrum (acquired) 738.5
    congenital 756.10
  saddle
    back 737.8
    nose 738.0
      syphilitic 090.5
  salivary gland or duct (congenital) 750.9
    acquired 527.8
  scapula (acquired) 736.89
    congenital 755.50
  scrotum (congenital) 752.9
    acquired 608.89
  sebaceous gland, acquired 706.8
  seminal tract or duct (congenital) 752.9
    acquired 608.89
  septum (nasal) (acquired) 470
    congenital 748.1
  shoulder (joint) (acquired) 736.89
    congenital 755.50
    specified type NEC 755.59
    contraction 718.41

◀ **New**   ◀▥ **Revised**

Deformity (Continued)
sigmoid (flexure) (congenital) 751.5
  acquired 569.89
sinus of Valsalva 747.29
skin (congenital) 757.9
  acquired NEC 709.8
skull (acquired) 738.19
  congenital 756.0
    with
      anencephalus 740.0
      encephalocele 742.0
      hydrocephalus 742.3
        with spina bifida (see also
          Spina bifida) 741.0
      microcephalus 742.1
    due to intrauterine malposition
      and pressure 754.0
soft parts, organs or tissues (of pelvis)
  in pregnancy or childbirth NEC
    654.9
    affecting fetus or newborn
      763.89
    causing obstructed labor 660.2
      affecting fetus or newborn
        763.1
spermatic cord (congenital) 752.9
  acquired 608.89
    torsion 608.2
spinal
  column - see Deformity, spine
  cord (congenital) 742.9
    acquired 336.8
    vessel (congenital) 747.82
  nerve root (congenital) 742.9
    acquired 724.9
spine (acquired) NEC 738.5
  congenital 756.10
    due to intrauterine malposition
      and pressure 754.2
  kyphoscoliotic (see also Kyphosco-
    liosis) 737.30
  kyphotic (see also Kyphosis)
    737.10
  lordotic (see also Lordosis) 737.20
  rachitic 268.1
  scoliotic (see also Scoliosis)
    737.30
spleen
  acquired 289.59
  congenital 759.0
Sprengel's (congenital) 755.52
sternum (acquired) 738.3
  congenital 756.3
stomach (congenital) 750.9
  acquired 537.89
submaxillary gland (congenital)
  750.9
  acquired 527.8
swan neck (acquired)
  finger 736.22
  hand 736.09
talipes - see Talipes
teeth, tooth NEC 520.9
testis (congenital) 752.9
  acquired 608.89
    torsion 608.2
thigh (acquired) 736.89
  congenital 755.60
thorax (acquired) (wall) 738.3
  congenital 754.89
  late effect of rickets 268.1
thumb (acquired) 736.20
  congenital 755.50
thymus (tissue) (congenital) 759.2

Deformity (Continued)
thyroid (gland) (congenital) 759.2
  cartilage 748.3
    acquired 478.79
tibia (acquired) 736.89
  congenital 755.60
  saber 090.5
toe (acquired) 735.9
  congenital 755.66
  specified NEC 735.8
tongue (congenital) 750.10
  acquired 529.8
tooth, teeth NEC 520.9
trachea (rings) (congenital) 748.3
  acquired 519.1
transverse aortic arch (congenital) 747.21
tricuspid (leaflets) (valve) (congenital)
  746.9
  acquired - see Endocarditis, tricuspid
  atresia or stenosis 746.1
  specified type NEC 746.89
trunk (acquired) 738.3
  congenital 759.9
ulna (acquired) 736.00
  congenital 755.50
upper extremity - see Deformity, arm
urachus (congenital) 753.7
ureter (opening) (congenital) 753.9
  acquired 593.89
urethra (valve) (congenital) 753.9
  acquired 599.84
urinary tract or system (congenital)
  753.9
  urachus 753.7
uterus (congenital) 752.3
  acquired 621.8
uvula (congenital) 750.9
  acquired 528.9
vagina (congenital) 752.40
  acquired 623.8
valve, valvular (heart) (congenital)
  746.9
  acquired - see Endocarditis
  pulmonary 746.00
  specified type NEC 746.89
vascular (congenital) (peripheral) NEC
  747.60
  acquired 459.9
  gastrointestinal 747.61
  lower limb 747.64
  renal 747.62
  specified site NEC 747.69
  spinal 747.82
  upper limb 747.63
vas deferens (congenital) 752.9
  acquired 608.89
vein (congenital) NEC (see also Deformity, vascular) 747.60
  brain 747.81
  coronary 746.9
  great 747.40
vena cava (inferior) (superior) (congenital) 747.40
vertebra - see Deformity, spine
vesicourethral orifice (acquired) 596.8
  congenital NEC 753.9
    specified type NEC 753.8
vessels of optic papilla (congenital)
  743.9
visual field (contraction) 368.45
vitreous humor (congenital) 743.9
  acquired 379.29
vulva (congenital) 752.40
  acquired 624.8

Deformity (Continued)
wrist (joint) (acquired) 736.00
  congenital 755.50
  contraction 718.43
  valgus 736.03
    congenital 755.59
  varus 736.04
    congenital 755.59
Degeneration, degenerative
adrenal (capsule) (gland) 255.8
  with hypofunction 255.4
  fatty 255.8
  hyaline 255.8
  infectional 255.8
  lardaceous 277.3
amyloid (any site) (general) 277.3
anterior cornua, spinal cord 336.8
aorta, aortic 440.0
  fatty 447.8
  valve (heart) (see also Endocarditis,
    aortic) 424.1
arteriovascular - see Arteriosclerosis
artery, arterial (atheromatous) (calcareous) - see also Arteriosclerosis
  amyloid 277.3
  lardaceous 277.3
  medial NEC (see also Arteriosclerosis,
    extremities) 440.20
articular cartilage NEC (see also Disorder, cartilage, articular) 718.0
  elbow 718.02
  knee 717.5
  patella 717.7
  shoulder 718.01
  spine (see also Spondylosis) 721.90
atheromatous - see Arteriosclerosis
bacony (any site) 277.3
basal nuclei or ganglia NEC 333.0
bone 733.90
brachial plexus 353.0
brain (cortical) (progressive) 331.9
  arteriosclerotic 437.0
  childhood 330.9
    specified type NEC 330.8
  congenital 742.4
  cystic 348.0
    congenital 742.4
  familial NEC 331.89
  grey matter 330.8
  heredofamilial NEC 331.89
  in
    alcoholism 303.9 [331.7]
    beriberi 265.0 [331.7]
    cerebrovascular disease 437.9
      [331.7]
    congenital hydrocephalus 742.3
      [331.7]
      with spina bifida (see also Spina
        bifida) 741.0 [331.7]
    Fabry's disease 272.7 [330.2]
    Gaucher's disease 272.7 [330.2]
    Hunter's disease or syndrome
      277.5 [330.3]
    lipidosis
      cerebral [330.1]
      generalized 272.7 [330.2]
    mucopolysaccharidosis 277.5 [330.3]
    myxedema (see also Myxedema)
      244.9 [331.7]
    neoplastic disease NEC (M8000/1)
      239.9 [331.7]
    Niemann-Pick disease 272.7 [330.2]
    sphingolipidosis 272.7 [330.2]
    vitamin B_{12} deficiency 266.2 [331.7]

ICD-9-CM

Vol. 2

Degeneration, degenerative (*Continued*)
brain (*Continued*)
  motor centers 331.89
  senile 331.2
  specified type NEC 331.89
breast - *see* Disease, breast
Bruch's membrane 363.40
bundle of His 426.50
  left 426.3
  right 426.4
calcareous NEC 275.49
capillaries 448.9
  amyloid 277.3
  fatty 448.9
  lardaceous 277.3
cardiac (brown) (calcareous) (fatty) (fibrous) (hyaline) (mural) (muscular) (pigmentary) (senile) (with arteriosclerosis) (*see also*
  Degeneration, myocardial) 429.1
  valve, valvular - *see* Endocarditis
cardiorenal (*see also* Hypertension, cardiorenal) 404.90
cardiovascular (*see also* Disease, cardiovascular) 429.2
  renal (*see also* Hypertension, cardiorenal) 404.90
cartilage (joint) - *see* Derangement, joint
cerebellar NEC 334.9
  primary (hereditary) (sporadic) 334.2
cerebral - *see* Degeneration, brain
cerebromacular 330.1
cerebrovascular 437.1
  due to hypertension 437.2
  late effect - *see* Late effect(s) (of)
    cerebrovascular disease
cervical plexus 353.2
cervix 622.8
  due to radiation (intended effect)
    622.8
    adverse effect or misadventure
      622.8
changes, spine or vertebra (*see also*
  Spondylosis) 721.90
chitinous 277.3
chorioretinal 363.40
  congenital 743.53
  hereditary 363.50
choroid (colloid) (drusen) 363.40
  hereditary 363.50
  senile 363.41
    diffuse secondary 363.42
cochlear 386.8
collateral ligament (knee) (medial)
  717.82
  lateral 717.81
combined (spinal cord) (subacute)
  266.2 [336.2]
  with anemia (pernicious) 281.0
    [336.2]
    due to dietary deficiency 281.1
      [336.2]
    due to vitamin B$_{12}$ deficiency anemia
      (dietary) 281.1 [336.2]
conjunctiva 372.50
  amyloid 277.3 [372.50]
cornea 371.40
  calcerous 371.44
  familial (hereditary) (*see also* Dystro-
    phy, cornea) 371.50
    macular 371.55
    reticular 371.54
  hyaline (of old scars) 371.41
  marginal (Terrien's) 371.48

Degeneration, degenerative (*Continued*)
cornea (*Continued*)
  mosaic (shagreen) 371.41
  nodular 371.46
  peripheral 371.48
  senile 371.41
cortical (cerebellar) (parenchymatous)
  334.2
  alcoholic 303.9 [334.4]
  diffuse, due to arteriopathy 437.0
corticostriatal-spinal 334.8
cretinoid 243
cruciate ligament (knee) (posterior)
  717.84
  anterior 717.83
cutis 709.3
  amyloid 277.3
dental pulp 522.2
disc disease - *see* Degeneration, intervertebral disc
dorsolateral (spinal cord) - *see* Degeneration, combined
endocardial 424.90
extrapyramidal NEC 333.90
eye NEC 360.40
  macular (*see also* Degeneration, mac-
    ula) 362.50
  congenital 362.75
  hereditary 362.76
fatty (diffuse) (general) 272.8
  liver 571.8
    alcoholic 571.0
  localized site - *see* Degeneration, by
    site, fatty
  placenta - *see* Placenta, abnormal
globe (eye) NEC 360.40
  macular - *see* Degeneration, macula
grey matter 330.8
heart (brown) (calcareous) (fatty) (fibrous) (hyaline) (mural) (muscular) (pigmentary) (senile) (with arteriosclerosis) (*see also*
  Degeneration, myocardial) 429.1
  amyloid 277.3 [425.7]
  atheromatous - *see* Arteriosclerosis,
    coronary
  gouty 274.82
  hypertensive (*see also* Hypertension,
    heart) 402.90
  ischemic 414.9
  valve, valvular - *see* Endocarditis
hepatolenticular (Wilson's) 275.1
hepatorenal 572.4
heredofamilial
  brain NEC 331.89
  spinal cord NEC 336.8
hyaline (diffuse) (generalized) 728.9
  localized (*see also* Degeneration, by site
    cornea 371.41
    keratitis 371.41
hypertensive vascular - *see* Hypertension
infrapatellar fat pad 729.31
internal semilunar cartilage 717.3
intervertebral disc 722.6
  with myelopathy 722.70
  cervical, cervicothoracic 722.4
    with myelopathy 722.71
  lumbar, lumbosacral 722.52
    with myelopathy 722.73
  thoracic, thoracolumbar 722.51
    with myelopathy 722.72
intestine 569.89
  amyloid 277.3
  lardaceous 277.3

Degeneration, degenerative (*Continued*)
iris (generalized) (*see also* Atrophy, iris)
  364.59
  pigmentary 364.53
  pupillary margin 364.54
ischemic - *see* Ischemia
joint disease (*see also* Osteoarthrosis)
  715.9
  multiple sites 715.09
  spine (*see also* Spondylosis) 721.90
kidney (*see also* Sclerosis, renal) 587
  amyloid 277.3 [583.81]
  cyst, cystic (multiple) (solitary) 593.2
    congenital (*see also* Cystic, disease,
      kidney) 753.10
  fatty 593.89
  fibrocystic (congenital) 753.19
  lardaceous 277.3 [583.81]
  polycystic (congenital) 753.12
    adult type (APKD) 753.13
    autosomal dominant 753.13
    autosomal recessive 753.14
    childhood type (CPKD) 753.14
    infantile type 753.14
  waxy 277.3 [583.81]
Kuhnt-Junius (retina) 362.52
labyrinth, osseous 386.8
lacrimal passages, cystic 375.12
lardaceous (any site) 277.3
lateral column (posterior), spinal cord
  (*see also* Degeneration, combined)
  266.2 [336.2]
lattice 362.63
lens 366.9
  infantile, juvenile, or presenile 366.00
  senile 366.10
lenticular (familial) (progressive) (Wilson's) (with cirrhosis of liver)
  275.1
  striate artery 437.0
lethal ball, prosthetic heart valve 996.02
ligament
  collateral (knee) (medial) 717.82
    lateral 717.81
  cruciate (knee) (posterior) 717.84
    anterior 717.83
liver (diffuse) 572.8
  amyloid 277.3
  congenital (cystic) 751.62
  cystic 572.8
    congenital 751.62
  fatty 571.8
    alcoholic 571.0
  hypertrophic 572.8
  lardaceous 277.3
  parenchymatous, acute or subacute
    (*see also* Necrosis, liver) 570
  pigmentary 572.8
  toxic (acute) 573.8
  waxy 277.3
lung 518.89
lymph gland 289.3
  hyaline 289.3
  lardaceous 277.3
macula (acquired) (senile) 362.50
  atrophic 362.51
  Best's 362.76
  congenital 362.75
  cystic 362.54
  cystoid 362.53
  disciform 362.52
  dry 362.51
  exudative 362.52
  familial pseudoinflammatory 362.77

◀ **New**   ◀▥ **Revised**

Degeneration, degenerative (Continued)
macula (Continued)
hereditary 362.76
hole 362.54
juvenile (Stargardt's) 362.75
nonexudative 362.51
pseudohole 362.54
wet 362.52
medullary - see Degeneration, brain
membranous labyrinth, congenital (causing impairment of hearing) 744.05
meniscus - see Derangement, joint
microcystoid 362.62
mitral - see Insufficiency, mitral
Mönckeberg's (see also Arteriosclerosis, extremities) 440.20
moral 301.7
motor centers, senile 331.2
mural (see also Degeneration, myocardial) 429.1
heart, cardiac (see also Degeneration, myocardial) 429.1
myocardium, myocardial (see also Degeneration, myocardial) 429.1
muscle 728.9
fatty 728.9
fibrous 728.9
heart (see also Degeneration, myocardial) 429.1
hyaline 728.9
muscular progressive 728.2
myelin, central nervous system NEC 341.9
myocardium, myocardial (brown) (calcareous) (fatty) (fibrous) (hyaline) (mural) (muscular) (pigmentary) (senile) (with arteriosclerosis) 429.1
with rheumatic fever (conditions classifiable to 390) 398.0
active, acute, or subacute 391.2
with chorea 392.0
inactive or quiescent (with chorea) 398.0
amyloid 277.3 [425.7]
congenital 746.89
fetus or newborn 779.89
gouty 274.82
hypertensive (see also Hypertension, heart) 402.90
ischemic 414.8
rheumatic (see also Degeneration, myocardium, with rheumatic fever) 398.0
syphilitic 093.82
nasal sinus (mucosa) (see also Sinusitis) 473.9
frontal 473.1
maxillary 473.0
nerve - see Disorder, nerve
nervous system 349.89
amyloid 277.3 [357.4]
autonomic (see also Neuropathy, peripheral, autonomic) 337.9
fatty 349.89
peripheral autonomic NEC (see also Neuropathy, peripheral, autonomic) 337.9
nipple 611.9
nose 478.1
oculoacousticocerebral, congenital (progressive) 743.8

Degeneration, degenerative (Continued)
olivopontocerebellar (familial) (hereditary) 333.0
osseous labyrinth 386.8
ovary 620.8
cystic 620.2
microcystic 620.2
pallidal, pigmentary (progressive) 333.0
pancreas 577.8
tuberculous (see also Tuberculosis) 017.9
papillary muscle 429.81
paving stone 362.61
penis 607.89
peritoneum 568.89
pigmentary (diffuse) (general)
localized - see Degeneration, by site
pallidal (progressive) 333.0
secondary 362.65
pineal gland 259.8
pituitary (gland) 253.8
placenta (fatty) (fibrinoid) (fibroid) - see Placenta, abnormal
popliteal fat pad 729.31
posterolateral (spinal cord) (see also Degeneration, combined) 266.2 [336.2]
pulmonary valve (heart) (see also Endocarditis, pulmonary) 424.3
pulp (tooth) 522.2
pupillary margin 364.54
renal (see also Sclerosis, renal) 587
fibrocystic 753.19
polycystic 753.12
adult type (APKD) 753.13
autosomal dominant 753.13
autosomal recessive 753.14
childhood type (CPKD) 753.14
infantile type 753.14
reticuloendothelial system 289.89
retina (peripheral) 362.60
with retinal defect (see also Detachment, retina, with retinal defect) 361.00
cystic (senile) 362.50
cystoid 362.53
hereditary (see also Dystrophy, retina) 362.70
cerebroretinal 362.71
congenital 362.75
juvenile (Stargardt's) 362.75
macula 362.76
Kuhnt-Junius 362.52
lattice 362.63
macular (see also Degeneration, macula) 362.50
microcystoid 362.62
palisade 362.63
paving stone 362.61
pigmentary (primary) 362.74
secondary 362.65
posterior pole (see also Degeneration, macula) 362.50
secondary 362.66
senile 362.60
cystic 362.53
reticular 362.64
saccule, congenital (causing impairment of hearing) 744.05
sacculocochlear 386.8
senile 797
brain 331.2
cardiac, heart, or myocardium (see also Degeneration, myocardial) 429.1
motor centers 331.2

Degeneration, degenerative (Continued)
senile (Continued)
reticule 362.64
retina, cystic 362.50
vascular - see Arteriosclerosis
silicone rubber poppet (prosthetic valve) 996.02
sinus (cystic) (see also Sinusitis) 473.9
polypoid 471.1
skin 709.3
amyloid 277.3
colloid 709.3
spinal (cord) 336.8
amyloid 277.3
column 733.90
combined (subacute) (see also Degeneration, combined) 266.2 [336.2]
with anemia (pernicious) 281.0 [336.2]
dorsolateral (see also Degeneration, combined) 266.2 [336.2]
familial NEC 336.8
fatty 336.8
funicular (see also Degeneration, combined) 266.2 [336.2]
heredofamilial NEC 336.8
posterolateral (see also Degeneration, combined) 266.2 [336.2]
subacute combined - see Degeneration, combined
tuberculous (see also Tuberculosis) 013.8
spine 733.90
spleen 289.59
amyloid 277.3
lardaceous 277.3
stomach 537.89
lardaceous 277.3
strionigral 333.0
sudoriparous (cystic) 705.89
suprarenal (capsule) (gland) 255.8
with hypofunction 255.4
sweat gland 705.89
synovial membrane (pulpy) 727.9
tapetoretinal 362.74
adult or presenile form 362.50
testis (postinfectional) 608.89
thymus (gland) 254.8
fatty 254.8
lardaceous 277.3
thyroid (gland) 246.8
tricuspid (heart) (valve) - see Endocarditis, tricuspid
tuberculous NEC (see also Tuberculosis) 011.9
turbinate 733.90
uterus 621.8
cystic 621.8
vascular (senile) - see also Arteriosclerosis
hypertensive - see Hypertension
vitreoretinal (primary) 362.73
secondary 362.66
vitreous humor (with infiltration) 379.21
wallerian NEC - see Disorder, nerve
waxy (any site) 277.3
Wilson's hepatolenticular 275.1
Deglutition
paralysis 784.9
hysterical 300.11
pneumonia 507.0
Degos' disease or syndrome 447.8
Degradation disorder, branched-chain amino-acid 270.3

ICD-9-CM

Vol. 2

Dehiscence
anastomosis - *see* Complications, anastomosis
cesarean wound 674.1
episiotomy 674.2
operation wound 998.32
internal 998.31
perineal wound (postpartum) 674.2
postoperative 998.32
abdomen 998.32
internal 998.31
internal 998.31
uterine wound 674.1
Dehydration (cachexia) 276.5
with
hypernatremia 276.0
hyponatremia 276.1
newborn 775.5
Deiters' nucleus syndrome 386.19
Déjérine's disease 356.0
Déjérine-Klumpke paralysis 767.6
Déjérine-Roussy syndrome 348.8
Déjérine-Sottas disease or neuropathy
(hypertrophic) 356.0
Déjérine-Thomas atrophy or syndrome
333.0
de Lange's syndrome (Amsterdam
dwarf, mental retardation, and
brachycephaly) 759.89
Delay, delayed
adaptation, cones or rods 368.63
any plane in pelvis
affecting fetus or newborn 763.1
complicating delivery 660.1
birth or delivery NEC 662.1
affecting fetus or newborn 763.9
second twin, triplet, or multiple
mate 662.3
closure - *see also* Fistula
cranial suture 756.0
fontanel 756.0
coagulation NEC 790.92
conduction (cardiac) (ventricular) 426.9
delivery NEC 662.1
second twin, triplet, etc. 662.3
affecting fetus or newborn 763.89
development
in childhood 783.40
physiological 783.40
intellectual NEC 315.9
learning NEC 315.2
reading 315.00
sexual 259.0
speech 315.39
associated with hyperkinesis 314.1
spelling 315.09
gastric emptying 536.8
menarche 256.39
due to pituitary hypofunction 253.4
menstruation (cause unknown) 626.8
milestone in childhood 783.42
motility - *see* Hypomotility
passage of meconium (newborn) 777.1
primary respiration 768.9
puberty 259.0
separation of umbilical cord 779.83
sexual maturation, female 259.0
Del Castillo's syndrome (germinal aplasia) 606.0
Deleage's disease 359.89
Deletion syndrome ◄
5p 758.31 ◄
22q11.2 758.32 ◄
autosomal NEC 758.39 ◄

Delhi (boil) (button) (sore) 085.1
Delinquency (juvenile) 312.9
group (*see also* Disturbance, conduct)
312.2
neurotic 312.4
Delirium, delirious 780.09
acute (psychotic) 293.0
alcoholic 291.0
acute 291.0
chronic 291.1
alcoholicum 291.0
chronic (*see also* Psychosis) 293.89
due to or associated with physical
condition - *see* Psychosis, organic
drug-induced 292.81
due to conditions classified elsewhere
293.0 ◄
eclamptic (*see also* Eclampsia) 780.39
exhaustion (*see also* Reaction, stress,
acute) 308.9
hysterical 300.11
in
presenile dementia 290.11
senile dementia 290.3
induced by drug 292.81
manic, maniacal (acute) (*see also* Psychosis, affective) 296.0
recurrent episode 296.1
single episode 296.0
puerperal 293.9
senile 290.3
subacute (psychotic) 293.1
thyroid (*see also* Thyrotoxicosis) 242.9
traumatic - *see also* Injury, intracranial
with
lesion, spinal cord - *see* Injury, spinal, by site
shock, spinal - *see* Injury, spinal,
by site
tremens (impending) 291.0
uremic - *see* Uremia
withdrawal
alcoholic (acute) 291.0
chronic 291.1
drug 292.0
Delivery

Note   Use the following fifth-digit
subclassification with categories 640-
648, 651-676:

0   unspecified as to episode of
      care
1   delivered, with or without
      mention of antepartum condition
2   delivered, with mention of
      postpartum complication
3   antepartum condition or complication
4   postpartum condition or complication

breech (assisted) (buttocks) (complete)
(frank) (spontaneous) 652.2
affecting fetus or newborn 763.0
extraction NEC 669.6
cesarean (for) 669.7
abnormal
cervix 654.6
pelvic organs of tissues 654.9
pelvis (bony) (major) NEC 653.0
presentation or position 652.9
in multiple gestation 652.6

Delivery (*Continued*)
cesarean (for) (*Continued*)
abnormal (*Continued*)
size, fetus 653.5
soft parts (of pelvis) 654.9
uterus, congenital 654.0
vagina 654.7
vulva 654.8
abruptio placentae 641.2
acromion presentation 652.8
affecting fetus or newborn 763.4
anteversion, cervix or uterus 654.4
atony, uterus 666.1
bicornis or bicornuate uterus 654.0
breech presentation (buttocks) (complete) (frank) 652.2
brow presentation 652.4
cephalopelvic disproportion (normally formed fetus) 653.4
chin presentation 652.4
cicatrix of cervix 654.6
contracted pelvis (general) 653.1
inlet 653.2
outlet 653.3
cord presentation or prolapse 663.0
cystocele 654.4
deformity (acquired) (congenital)
pelvic organs or tissues NEC 654.9
pelvis (bony) NEC 653.0
displacement, uterus NEC 654.4
disproportion NEC 653.9
distress
fetal 656.8
maternal 669.0
eclampsia 642.6
face presentation 652.4
failed
forceps 660.7
trial of labor NEC 660.6
vacuum extraction 660.7
ventouse 660.7
fetal deformity 653.7
fetal-maternal hemorrhage 656.0
fetus, fetal
distress 656.8
prematurity 656.8
fibroid (tumor) (uterus) 654.1
footling 652.8
with successful version 652.1
hemorrhage (antepartum) (intrapartum) NEC 641.9
hydrocephalic fetus 653.6
incarceration of uterus 654.3
incoordinate uterine action 661.4
inertia, uterus 661.2
primary 661.0
secondary 661.1
lateroversion, uterus or cervix 654.4
mal lie 652.9
malposition
fetus 652.9
in multiple gestation 652.6
pelvic organs or tissues NEC 654.9
uterus NEC or cervix 654.4
malpresentation NEC 652.9
in multiple gestation 652.6
maternal
diabetes mellitus 648.0
heart disease NEC 648.6
meconium in liquor 656.8
staining only 792.3
oblique presentation 652.3
oversize fetus 653.5
pelvic tumor NEC 654.9

Delivery *(Continued)*
  cesarean (for) *(Continued)*
    placental insufficiency 656.5
    placenta previa 641.0
      with hemorrhage 641.1
    poor dilation, cervix 661.0
    pre-eclampsia 642.4
      severe 642.5
    previous
      cesarean delivery, section 654.2
      surgery (to)
        cervix 654.6
        gynecological NEC 654.9
        rectum 654.8 ◄
        uterus NEC 654.9
          previous cesarean delivery, section 654.2
        vagina 654.7
    prolapse
      arm or hand 652.7
      uterus 654.4
    prolonged labor 662.1
    rectocele 654.4
    retroversion, uterus or cervix 654.3
    rigid
      cervix 654.6
      pelvic floor 654.4
      perineum 654.8
      vagina 654.7
      vulva 654.8
    sacculation, pregnant uterus 654.4
    scar(s)
      cervix 654.6
      cesarean delivery, section 654.2
      uterus NEC 654.9
        due to previous cesarean delivery, section 654.2
    Shirodkar suture in situ 654.5
    shoulder presentation 652.8
    stenosis or stricture, cervix 654.6
    transverse presentation or lie 652.3
    tumor, pelvic organs or tissues NEC 654.4
    umbilical cord presentation or prolapse 663.0
  completely normal case - *see* category 650
  complicated (by) NEC 669.9
    abdominal tumor, fetal 653.7
      causing obstructed labor 660.1
    abnormal, abnormality of
      cervix 654.6
        causing obstructed labor 660.2
      forces of labor 661.9
      formation of uterus 654.0
      pelvic organs or tissues 654.9
        causing obstructed labor 660.2
      pelvis (bony) (major) NEC 653.0
        causing obstructed labor 660.1
      presentation or position NEC 652.9
        causing obstructed labor 660.0
      size, fetus 653.5
        causing obstructed labor 660.1
      soft parts (of pelvis) 654.9
        causing obstructed labor 660.2
      uterine contractions NEC 661.9
      uterus (formation) 654.0
        causing obstructed labor 660.2
      vagina 654.7
        causing obstructed labor 660.2
    abnormally formed uterus (any type) (congenital) 654.0
      causing obstructed labor 660.2

Delivery *(Continued)*
  complicated (by) NEC *(Continued)*
    acromion presentation 652.8
      causing obstructed labor 660.0
    adherent placenta 667.0
      with hemorrhage 666.0
    adhesions, uterus (to abdominal wall) 654.4
    advanced maternal age NEC 659.6
      multigravida 659.6
      primigravida 659.5
    air embolism 673.0
    amnionitis 658.4
    amniotic fluid embolism 673.1
    anesthetic death 668.9
    annular detachment, cervix 665.3
    antepartum hemorrhage - *see* Delivery, complicated, hemorrhage
    anteversion, cervix or uterus 654.4
      causing obstructed labor 660.2
    apoplexy 674.0
      placenta 641.2
    arrested active phase 661.1
    asymmetrical pelvis bone 653.0
      causing obstructed labor 660.1
    atony, uterus (hypotonic) (inertia) 666.1
      hypertonic 661.4
    Bandl's ring 661.4
    Battledore placenta - *see* Placenta, abnormal
    bicornis or bicornuate uterus 654.0
      causing obstructed labor 660.2
    birth injury to mother NEC 665.9
    bleeding (*see also* Delivery, complicated, hemorrhage) 641.9
    breech presentation (assisted) (buttocks) (complete) (frank) (spontaneous) 652.2
      with successful version 652.1
    brow presentation 652.4
    cephalopelvic disproportion (normally formed fetus) 653.4
      causing obstructed labor 660.1
    cerebral hemorrhage 674.0
    cervical dystocia 661.0
    chin presentation 652.4
      causing obstructed labor 660.0
    cicatrix
      cervix 654.6
        causing obstructed labor 660.2
      vagina 654.7
        causing obstructed labor 660.2
    colporrhexis 665.4
      with perineal laceration 664.0
    compound presentation 652.8
      causing obstructed labor 660.0
    compression of cord (umbilical) 663.2
      around neck 663.1
      cord prolapsed 663.0
    contraction, contracted pelvis 653.1
      causing obstructed labor 660.1
      general 653.1
        causing obstructed labor 660.1
      inlet 653.2
        causing obstructed labor 660.1
      midpelvic 653.8
        causing obstructed labor 660.1
      midplane 653.8
        causing obstructed labor 660.1
      outlet 653.3
        causing obstructed labor 660.1

Delivery *(Continued)*
  complicated (by) NEC *(Continued)*
    contraction ring 661.4
    cord (umbilical) 663.9
      around neck, tightly or with compression 663.1
        without compression 663.3
      bruising 663.6
      complication NEC 663.9
        specified type NEC 663.8
      compression NEC 663.2
      entanglement NEC 663.3
        with compression 663.2
      forelying 663.0
      hematoma 663.6
      marginal attachment 663.8
      presentation 663.0
      prolapse (complete) (occult) (partial) 663.0
      short 663.4
      specified complication NEC 663.8
      thrombosis (vessels) 663.6
      vascular lesion 663.6
      velamentous insertion 663.8
    Couvelaire uterus 641.2
    cretin pelvis (dwarf type) (male type) 653.1
      causing obstructed labor 660.1
    crossbirth 652.3
      with successful version 652.1
      causing obstructed labor 660.0
    cyst (Gartner's duct) 654.7
    cystocele 654.4
      causing obstructed labor 660.2
    death of fetus (near term) 656.4
      early (before 22 completed weeks' gestation) 632
    deformity (acquired) (congenital)
      fetus 653.7
        causing obstructed labor 660.1
      pelvic organs or tissues NEC 654.9
        causing obstructed labor 660.2
      pelvis (bony) NEC 653.0
        causing obstructed labor 660.1
    delay, delayed
      delivery in multiple pregnancy 662.3
        due to locked mates 660.5
      following rupture of membranes (spontaneous) 658.2
        artificial 658.3
    depressed fetal heart tones 656.7
    diastasis recti 665.8
    dilatation
      bladder 654.4
        causing obstructed labor 660.2
      cervix, incomplete, poor or slow 661.0
    diseased placenta 656.7
    displacement uterus NEC 654.4
      causing obstructed labor 660.2
    disproportion NEC 653.9
      causing obstructed labor 660.1
    disruptio uteri - *see* Delivery, complicated, rupture, uterus
    distress
      fetal 656.8
      maternal 669.0
    double uterus (congenital) 654.0
      causing obstructed labor 660.2
    dropsy amnion 657
    dysfunction, uterus 661.9
      hypertonic 661.4

ICD-9-CM

Vol. 2

Delivery *(Continued)*
  complicated (by) NEC *(Continued)*
    dysfunction, uterus *(Continued)*
      hypotonic 661.2
        primary 661.0
        secondary 661.1
      incoordinate 661.4
    dystocia
      cervical 661.0
      fetal - *see* Delivery, complicated, abnormal, presentation
      maternal - *see* Delivery, complicated, prolonged labor
      pelvic - *see* Delivery, complicated, contraction pelvis
      positional 652.8
      shoulder girdle 660.4
    eclampsia 642.6
    ectopic kidney 654.4
      causing obstructed labor 660.2
    edema, cervix 654.6
      causing obstructed labor 660.2
    effusion, amniotic fluid 658.1
    elderly multigravida 659.6
    elderly primigravida 659.5
    embolism (pulmonary) 673.2
      air 673.0
      amniotic fluid 673.1
      blood-clot 673.2
      cerebral 674.0
      fat 673.8
      pyemic 673.3
      septic 673.3
    entanglement, umbilical cord 663.3
      with compression 663.2
      around neck (with compression) 663.1
    eversion, cervix or uterus 665.2
    excessive
      fetal growth 653.5
        causing obstructed labor 660.1
      size of fetus 653.5
        causing obstructed labor 660.1
    face presentation 652.4
      causing obstructed labor 660.0
      to pubes 660.3
    failure, fetal head to enter pelvic brim 652.5
      causing obstructed labor 660.0
    fetal
      acid-base balance 656.8
      death (near term) NEC 656.4
        early (before 22 completed weeks' gestation) 632
      deformity 653.7
        causing obstructed labor 660.1
      distress 656.8
      heart rate or rhythm 659.7
    fetopelvic disproportion 653.4
      causing obstructed labor 660.1
    fever during labor 659.2
    fibroid (tumor) (uterus) 654.1
      causing obstructed labor 660.2
    fibromyomata 654.1
      causing obstructed labor 660.2
    forelying umbilical cord 663.0
    fracture of coccyx 665.6
    hematoma 664.5
      broad ligament 665.7
      ischial spine 665.7
      pelvic 665.7
      perineum 664.5

Delivery *(Continued)*
  complicated (by) NEC *(Continued)*
    hematoma *(Continued)*
      soft tissues 665.7
      subdural 674.0
      umbilical cord 663.6
      vagina 665.7
      vulva or perineum 664.5
    hemorrhage (uterine) (antepartum) (intrapartum) (pregnancy) 641.9
      accidental 641.2
      associated with
        afibrinogenemia 641.3
        coagulation defect 641.3
          hyperfibrinolysis 641.3
          hypofibrinogenemia 641.3
      cerebral 674.0
      due to
        low-lying placenta 641.1
        placenta previa 641.1
        premature separation of placenta (normally implanted) 641.2
        retained placenta 666.0
        trauma 641.8
        uterine leiomyoma 641.8
      marginal sinus rupture 641.2
      placenta NEC 641.9
      postpartum (atonic) (immediate) (within 24 hours) 666.1
        with retained or trapped placenta 666.0
        delayed 666.2
        secondary 666.2
        third stage 666.0
    hourglass contraction, uterus 661.4
    hydramnios 657
    hydrocephalic fetus 653.6
      causing obstructed labor 660.1
    hydrops fetalis 653.7
      causing obstructed labor 660.1
    hypertension - *see* Hypertension, complicating pregnancy
    hypertonic uterine dysfunction 661.4
    hypotonic uterine dysfunction 661.2
    impacted shoulders 660.4
    incarceration, uterus 654.3
      causing obstructed labor 660.2
    incomplete dilation (cervix) 661.0
    incoordinate uterus 661.4
    indication NEC 659.9
      specified type NEC 659.8
    inertia, uterus 661.2
      hypertonic 661.4
      hypotonic 661.2
      primary 661.0
      secondary 661.1
    infantile
      genitalia 654.4
        causing obstructed labor 660.2
      uterus (os) 654.4
        causing obstructed labor 660.2
    injury (to mother) NEC 665.9
    intrauterine fetal death (near term) NEC 656.4
      early (before 22 completed weeks' gestation) 632
    inversion, uterus 665.2
    kidney, ectopic 654.4
      causing obstructed labor 660.2
    knot (true), umbilical cord 663.2
    labor, premature (before 37 completed weeks' gestation) 644.2

Delivery *(Continued)*
  complicated (by) NEC *(Continued)*
    laceration 664.9
      anus (sphincter) 664.2
        with mucosa 664.3
      bladder (urinary) 665.5
      bowel 665.5
      central 664.4
      cervix (uteri) 665.3
      fourchette 664.0
      hymen 664.0
      labia (majora) (minora) 664.0
      pelvic
        floor 664.1
        organ NEC 665.5
      perineum, perineal 664.4
        first degree 664.0
        second degree 664.1
        third degree 664.2
        fourth degree 664.3
        central 664.4
        extensive NEC 664.4
        muscles 664.1
        skin 664.0
        slight 664.0
      peritoneum 665.5
      periurethral tissue 665.5
      rectovaginal (septum) (without perineal laceration) 665.4
        with perineum 664.2
          with anal or rectal mucosa 664.3
      skin (perineum) 664.0
      specified site or type NEC 664.8
      sphincter ani 664.2
        with mucosa 664.3
      urethra 665.5
      uterus 665.1
        before labor 665.0
      vagina, vaginal (deep) (high) (sulcus) (wall) (without perineal laceration) 665.4
        with perineum 664.0
        muscles, with perineum 664.1
      vulva 664.0
    lateroversion, uterus or cervix 654.4
      causing obstructed labor 660.2
    locked mates 660.5
    low implantation of placenta - *see* Delivery, complicated, placenta, previa
    mal lie 652.9
    malposition
      fetus NEC 652.9
        causing obstructed labor 660.0
      pelvic organs or tissues NEC 654.9
        causing obstructed labor 660.2
      placenta 641.1
        without hemorrhage 641.0
      uterus NEC or cervix 654.4
        causing obstructed labor 660.2
    malpresentation 652.9
      causing obstructed labor 660.0
    marginal sinus (bleeding) (rupture) 641.2
    maternal hypotension syndrome 669.2
    meconium in liquor 656.8
    membranes, retained - *see* Delivery, complicated, placenta, retained
    mentum presentation 652.4
      causing obstructed labor 660.0
    metrorrhagia (myopathia) - *see* Delivery, complicated, hemorrhage

◀ **New**　　　⬅ **Revised**

Delivery *(Continued)*
 complicated (by) NEC *(Continued)*
  metrorrhexis - *see* Delivery, complicated, rupture, uterus
  multiparity (grand) 659.4
  myelomeningocele, fetus 653.7
   causing obstructed labor 660.1
  Nägele's pelvis 653.0
   causing obstructed labor 660.1
  nonengagement, fetal head 652.5
   causing obstructed labor 660.0
  oblique presentation 652.3
   causing obstructed labor 660.0
  obstetric
   shock 669.1
   trauma NEC 665.9
  obstructed labor 660.9
   due to
    abnormality of pelvic organs or
     tissues (conditions classifia-
     ble to 654.0-654.9) 660.2
    deep transverse arrest 660.3
    impacted shoulders 660.4
    locked twins 660.5
    malposition and malpresenta-
     tion of fetus (conditions
     classifiable to 652.0-652.9)
     660.0
    persistent occipitoposterior
     660.3
    shoulder dystocia 660.4
  occult prolapse of umbilical cord
   663.0
  oversize fetus 653.5
   causing obstructed labor 660.1
  pathological retraction ring, uterus
   661.4
  pelvic
   arrest (deep) (high) (of fetal head)
    (transverse) 660.3
   deformity (bone) - *see also* Defor-
    mity, pelvis, with dispropor-
    tion
    soft tissue 654.9
     causing obstructed labor 660.2
   tumor NEC 654.9
    causing obstructed labor 660.2
  penetration, pregnant uterus by instrument 665.1
  perforation - *see* Delivery, complicated, laceration
  persistent
   hymen 654.8
    causing obstructed labor 660.2
   occipitoposterior 660.3
  placenta, placental
   ablatio 641.2
   abnormality 656.7
    with hemorrhage 641.2
   abruptio 641.2
   accreta 667.0
    with hemorrhage 666.0
   adherent (without hemorrhage)
    667.0
    with hemorrhage 666.0
   apoplexy 641.2
   Battledore - see Placenta, abnor-
    mal
   detachment (premature) 641.2
   disease 656.7
   hemorrhage NEC 641.9
   increta (without hemorrhage)
    667.0
    with hemorrhage 666.0

Delivery *(Continued)*
 complicated (by) NEC *(Continued)*
  placenta, placental *(Continued)*
   low (implantation) 641.1
    without hemorrhage 641.0
   malformation 656.7
    with hemorrhage 641.2
   malposition 641.1
    without hemorrhage 641.0
   marginal sinus rupture 641.2
   percreta 667.0
    with hemorrhage 666.0
   premature separation 641.2
   previa (central) (lateral) (marginal)
    (partial) 641.1
    without hemorrhage 641.0
   retained (with hemorrhage) 666.0
    without hemorrhage 667.0
   rupture of marginal sinus 641.2
   separation (premature) 641.2
   trapped 666.0
    without hemorrhage 667.0
   vicious insertion 641.1
  polyhydramnios 657
  polyp, cervix 654.6
   causing obstructed labor 660.2
  precipitate labor 661.3
  premature
   labor (before 37 completed weeks'
    gestation) 644.2
   rupture, membranes 658.1
    delayed delivery following 658.2
  presenting umbilical cord 663.0
  previous
   cesarean delivery, section 654.2
   surgery
    cervix 654.6
     causing obstructed labor 660.2
    gynecological NEC 654.9
     causing obstructed labor 660.2
    perineum 654.8
    rectum 654.8   ◄
    uterus NEC 654.9
     due to previous cesarean de-
      livery, section 654.2
    vagina 654.7
     causing obstructed labor 660.2
    vulva 654.8
  primary uterine inertia 661.0
  primipara, elderly or old 659.5
  prolapse
   arm or hand 652.7
    causing obstructed labor 660.0
   cord (umbilical) 663.0
   fetal extremity 652.8
   foot or leg 652.8
    causing obstructed labor 660.0
   umbilical cord (complete) (occult)
    (partial) 663.0
   uterus 654.4
    causing obstructed labor 660.2
  prolonged labor 662.1
   first stage 662.0
   second stage 662.2
   active phase 661.2
   due to
    cervical dystocia 661.0
    contraction ring 661.4
    tetanic uterus 661.4
    uterine inertia 661.2
     primary 661.0
     secondary 661.1
   latent phase 661.0
  pyrexia during labor 659.2

Delivery *(Continued)*
 complicated (by) NEC *(Continued)*
  rachitic pelvis 653.2
   causing obstructed labor 660.1
  rectocele 654.4
   causing obstructed labor 660.2
  retained membranes or portions of
   placenta 666.2
   without hemorrhage 667.1
  retarded (prolonged) birth 662.1
  retention secundines (with hemorrhage) 666.2
   without hemorrhage 667.1
  retroversion, uterus or cervix 654.3
   causing obstructed labor 660.2
  rigid
   cervix 654.6
    causing obstructed labor 660.2
   pelvic floor 654.4
    causing obstructed labor 660.2
   perineum or vulva 654.8
    causing obstructed labor 660.2
   vagina 654.7
    causing obstructed labor 660.2
  Robert's pelvis 653.0
   causing obstructed labor 660.1
  rupture - *see also* Delivery, complicated, laceration
   bladder (urinary) 665.5
   cervix 665.3
   marginal sinus 641.2
   membranes, premature 658.1
   pelvic organ NEC 665.5
   perineum (without mention of
    other laceration) - *see* Deliv-
    ery, complicated, laceration,
    perineum
   peritoneum 665.5
   urethra 665.5
   uterus (during labor) 665.1
    before labor 665.0
  sacculation, pregnant uterus
   654.4
  sacral teratomas, fetal 653.7
   causing obstructed labor 660.1
  scar(s)
   cervix 654.6
    causing obstructed labor 660.2
   cesarean delivery, section 654.2
    causing obstructed labor 660.2
   perineum 654.8
    causing obstructed labor 660.2
   uterus NEC 654.9
    causing obstructed labor 660.2
    due to previous cesarean deliv-
     ery, section 654.2
   vagina 654.7
    causing obstructed labor 660.2
   vulva 654.8
    causing obstructed labor 660.2
  scoliotic pelvis 653.0
   causing obstructed labor 660.1
  secondary uterine inertia 661.1
  secundines, retained - *see* Delivery,
   complicated, placenta, retained
  separation
   placenta (premature) 641.2
   pubic bone 665.6
   symphysis pubis 665.6
  septate vagina 654.7
   causing obstructed labor 660.2
  shock (birth) (obstetric) (puerperal)
   669.1
  short cord syndrome 663.4

ICD-9-CM

Vol. 2

Delivery (*Continued*)
  complicated (by) NEC (*Continued*)
    shoulder
      girdle dystocia 660.4
      presentation 652.8
        causing obstructed labor 660.0
    Siamese twins 653.7
      causing obstructed labor 660.1
    slow slope active phase 661.2
    spasm
      cervix 661.4
      uterus 661.4
    spondylolisthesis, pelvis 653.3
      causing obstructed labor 660.1
    spondylolysis (lumbosacral) 653.3
      causing obstructed labor 660.1
    spondylosis 653.0
      causing obstructed labor 660.1
    stenosis or stricture
      cervix 654.6
        causing obstructed labor 660.2
      vagina 654.7
        causing obstructed labor 660.2
    sudden death, unknown cause 669.9
    tear (pelvic organ) (*see also* Delivery,
        complicated, laceration) 664.9
    teratomas, sacral, fetal 653.7
      causing obstructed labor 660.1
    tetanic uterus 661.4
    tipping pelvis 653.0
      causing obstructed labor 660.1
    transverse
      arrest (deep) 660.3
      presentation or lie 652.3
        with successful version 652.1
        causing obstructed labor 660.0
    trauma (obstetrical) NEC 665.9
    tumor
      abdominal, fetal 653.7
        causing obstructed labor 660.1
      pelvic organs or tissues NEC 654.9
        causing obstructed labor 660.2
    umbilical cord (*see also* Delivery,
        complicated, cord) 663.9
      around neck tightly, or with com-
          pression 663.1
      entanglement NEC 663.3
        with compression 663.2
      prolapse (complete) (occult) (par-
          tial) 663.0
    unstable lie 652.0
      causing obstructed labor 660.0
    uterine
      inertia (*see also* Delivery, compli-
          cated, inertia, uterus) 661.2
        spasm 661.4
    vasa previa 663.5
    velamentous insertion of cord 663.8
    young maternal age 659.8
  delayed NEC 662.1
    following rupture of membranes
        (spontaneous) 658.2
      artificial 658.3
    second twin, triplet, etc. 662.3
  difficult NEC 669.9
    previous, affecting management of
        pregnancy or childbirth V23.49
    specified type NEC 669.8
  early onset (spontaneous) 644.2
  footling 652.8
    with successful version 652.1
  forceps NEC 669.5
    affecting fetus or newborn 763.2
  missed (at or near term) 656.4

Delivery (*Continued*)
  multiple gestation NEC 651.9
    with fetal loss and retention of one
        or more fetus(es) 651.6
    specified type NEC 651.8
      with fetal loss and retention of
          one or more fetus(es)
          651.6
  nonviable infant 656.4
  normal - *see* category 650
  precipitate 661.3
    affecting fetus or newborn 763.6
  premature NEC (before 37 completed
      weeks' gestation) 644.2
    previous, affecting management of
        pregnancy V23.41
  quadruplet NEC 651.2
    with fetal loss and retention of one
        or more fetus(es) 651.5
  quintuplet NEC 651.8
    with fetal loss and retention of one
        or more fetus(es) 651.6
  sextuplet NEC 651.8
    with fetal loss and retention of one
        or more fetus(es) 651.6
  specified complication NEC 669.8
  stillbirth (near term) NEC 656.4
    early (before 22 completed weeks'
        gestation) 632
  term pregnancy (live birth) NEC - *see*
      category 650
    stillbirth NEC 656.4
  threatened premature 644.2
  triplets NEC 651.1
    with fetal loss and retention of one
        or more fetus(es) 651.4
    delayed delivery (one or more
        mates) 662.3
    locked mates 660.5
  twins NEC 651.0
    with fetal loss and retention of one
        fetus 651.3
    delayed delivery (one or more
        mates) 662.3
    locked mates 660.5
  uncomplicated - *see* category 650
  vacuum extractor NEC 669.5
    affecting fetus or newborn 763.3
  ventouse NEC 669.5
    affecting fetus or newborn 763.3
Dellen, cornea 371.41
Delusions (paranoid) 297.9
  grandiose 297.1
  parasitosis 300.29
  systematized 297.1
Dementia 294.8
  alcohol-induced persisting (*see also*
      Psychosis, alcoholic) 291.2 ◀▮▮
  Alzheimer's - *see* Alzheimer's, demen-
      tia
  arteriosclerotic (simple type) (uncom-
      plicated) 290.40
    with
      acute confusional state 290.41
      delirium 290.41
      delusions 290.42 ◀▮▮
      depressed mood 290.43 ◀▮▮
    depressed type 290.43
    paranoid type 290.42
  Binswanger's 290.12
  catatonic (acute) (*see also* Schizophre-
      nia) 295.2
  congenital (*see also* Retardation, men-
      tal) 319

Dementia (*Continued*)
  degenerative 290.9
    presenile-onset - *see* Dementia, pre-
        senile
    senile-onset - *see* Dementia, senile
  developmental (*see also* Schizophrenia)
      295.9
  dialysis 294.8
    transient 293.9
  drug-induced persisting (*see also* Psy-
      chosis, drug) 292.82 ◀
  due to or associated with condition(s)
      classified elsewhere
    Alzheimer's
      with behavioral disturbance 331.0
          [294.11]
      without behavioral disturbance
          331.0 [294.10]
    cerebral lipidoses
      with behavioral disturbance 330.1
          [294.11]
      without behavioral disturbance
          330.1 [294.10]
    epilepsy
      with behavioral disturbance 345.9
          [294.11]
      without behavioral disturbance
          345.9 [294.10]
    hepatolenticular degeneration
      with behavioral disturbance 275.1
          [294.11]
      without behavioral disturbance
          275.1 [294.10]
    HIV
      with behavioral disturbance 042
          [294.11]
      without behavioral disturbance
          042 [294.10]
    Huntington's chorea
      with behavioral disturbance 333.4
          [294.11]
      without behavioral disturbance
          333.4 [294.10]
    Jakob-Creutzfeldt disease
      with behavioral disturbance 046.1
          [294.11]
      without behavioral disturbance
          046.1 [294.10]
    Lewy bodies
      with behavioral disturbance 331.82
          [294.11]
      without behavioral disturbance
          331.82 [294.10]
    multiple sclerosis
      with behavioral disturbance 340
          [294.11]
      without behavioral disturbance
          340 [294.10]
    neurosyphilis
      with behavioral disturbance 094.9
          [294.11]
      without behavioral disturbance
          094.9 [294.10]
    Pelizaeus-Merzbacher disease
      with behavioral disturbance 333.0
          [294.11]
      without behavioral disturbance
          333.0 [294.10]
    Parkinsonism
      with behavioral disturbance 331.82
          [294.11]
      without behavioral disturbance
          331.82 [294.10]

Dementia (*Continued*)
due to or associated with condition(s)
classified elsewhere (*Continued*)
Pick's disease
with behavioral disturbance 331.11
[294.11]
without behavioral disturbance
331.11 [294.10]
polyarteritis nodosa
with behavioral disturbance 446.0
[294.11]
without behavioral disturbance
446.0 [294.10]
syphilis
with behavioral disturbance 094.1
[294.11]
without behavioral disturbance
094.1 [294.10]
Wilson's disease
with behavioral disturbance 275.1
[294.11]
without behavioral disturbance
275.1 [294.10]
frontal 333.19
with behavioral disturbance 331.19
[294.11]
without behavioral disturbance
331.19 [294.10]
frontotemporal 333.19
with behavioral disturbance 331.19
[294.11]
without behavioral disturbance
331.19 [294.10]
hebephrenic (acute) 295.1
Heller's (infantile psychosis) (*see also*
Psychosis, childhood) 299.1
idiopathic 290.9
presenile-onset - *see* Dementia, presenile
senile-onset - *see* Dementia, senile
in
arteriosclerotic brain disease 290.40
senility 290.0
induced by drug 292.82
infantile, infantilia (*see also* Psychosis,
childhood) 299.0
Lewy body 331.82
with behavioral disturbance 331.82
[294.11]
without behavioral disturbance
331.82 [294.10]
multi-infarct (cerebrovascular) (*see also*
Dementia, arteriosclerotic) 290.40
old age 290.0
paralytica, paralytic 094.1
juvenilis 090.40
syphilitic 094.1
congenital 090.40
tabetic form 094.1
paranoid (*see also* Schizophrenia) 295.3
paraphrenic (*see also* Schizophrenia)
295.3
paretic 094.1
praecox (*see also* Schizophrenia) 295.9
presenile 290.10
with
acute confusional state 290.11
delirium 290.11
delusional features 290.12
depressive features 290.13
depressed type 290.13
paranoid type 290.12
simple type 290.10
uncomplicated 290.10

Dementia (*Continued*)
primary (acute) (*see also* Schizophrenia)
295.0
progressive, syphilitic 094.1
puerperal - *see* Psychosis, puerperal
schizophrenic (*see also* Schizophrenia)
295.9
senile 290.0
with
acute confusional state 290.3
delirium 290.3
delusional features 290.20
depressive features 290.21
depressed type 290.21
exhaustion 290.0
paranoid type 290.20
simple type (acute) (*see also* Schizophrenia) 295.0
simplex (acute) (*see also* Schizophrenia)
295.0
syphilitic 094.1
uremic - *see* Uremia
vascular 290.40
with ◄
delirium 290.41 ◄
delusions 290.42 ◄
depressed mood 290.43 ◄
Demerol dependence (*see also* Dependence) 304.0
Demineralization, ankle (*see also* Osteoporosis) 733.00
Demodex folliculorum (infestation) 133.8
de Morgan's spots (senile angiomas) 448.1
Demyelinating
polyneuritis, chronic inflammatory
357.81
Demyelination, demyelinization
central nervous system 341.9
specified NEC 341.8
corpus callosum (central) 341.8
global 340
Dengue (fever) 061
sandfly 061
vaccination, prophylactic (against) V05.1
virus hemorrhagic fever 065.4
Dens
evaginatus 520.2
in dente 520.2
invaginatus 520.2
Density
increased, bone (disseminated) (generalized) (spotted) 733.99
lung (nodular) 518.89
Dental - *see also* condition
examination only V72.2
Dentia praecox 520.6
Denticles (in pulp) 522.2
Dentigerous cyst 526.0
Dentin
irregular (in pulp) 522.3
opalescent 520.5
secondary (in pulp) 522.3
sensitive 521.8
Dentinogenesis imperfecta 520.5
Dentinoma (M9271/0) 213.1
upper jaw (bone) 213.0
Dentition 520.7
abnormal 520.6
anomaly 520.6
delayed 520.6
difficult 520.7
disorder of 520.6
precocious 520.6
retarded 520.6

Denture sore (mouth) 528.9
Dependence

Note   Use the following fifth-digit subclassification with category 304:
0   unspecified
1   continuous
2   episodic
3   in remission

with
withdrawal symptoms
alcohol 291.81
drug 292.0
14-hydroxy-dihydromorphinone 304.0
absinthe 304.6
acemorphan 304.0
acetanilid(e) 304.6
acetophenetidin 304.6
acetorphine 304.0
acetyldihydrocodeine 304.0
acetyldihydrocodeinone 304.0
Adalin 304.1
Afghanistan black 304.3
agrypnal 304.1
alcohol, alcoholic (ethyl) (methyl)
(wood) 303.9
maternal, with suspected fetal damage affecting management of
pregnancy 655.4
allobarbitone 304.1
allonal 304.1
allylisopropylacetylurea 304.1
alphaprodine (hydrochloride) 304.0
Alurate 304.1
Alvodine 304.0
amethocaine 304.6
amidone 304.0
amidopyrine 304.6
aminopyrine 304.6
amobarbital 304.1
amphetamine(s) (type) (drugs classifiable to 969.7) 304.4
amylene hydrate 304.6
amylobarbitone 304.1
amylocaine 304.6
Amytal (sodium) 304.1
analgesic (drug) NEC 304.6
synthetic with morphine-like effect
304.0
anesthetic (agent) (drug) (gas) (general) (local) NEC 304.6
Angel dust 304.6
anileridine 304.0
antipyrine 304.6
anxiolytic 304.1 ◄
aprobarbital 304.1
aprobarbitone 304.1
atropine 304.6
Avertin (bromide) 304.6
barbenyl 304.1
barbital(s) 304.1
barbitone 304.1
barbiturate(s) (compounds) (drugs
classifiable to 967.0) 304.1
barbituric acid (and compounds) 304.1
benzedrine 304.4
benzylmorphine 304.0
Beta-chlor 304.1
bhang 304.3
blue velvet 304.0
Brevital 304.1
bromal (hydrate) 304.1
bromide(s) NEC 304.1

Dependence (Continued)

bromine compounds NEC 304.1
bromisovalum 304.1
bromoform 304.1
Bromo-seltzer 304.1
bromural 304.1
butabarbital (sodium) 304.1
butabarpal 304.1
butallylonal 304.1
butethal 304.1
buthalitone (sodium) 304.1
Butisol 304.1
butobarbitone 304.1
butyl chloral (hydrate) 304.1
caffeine 304.4
cannabis (indica) (sativa) (resin) (deriv-
    atives) (type) 304.3
carbamazepine 304.6
Carbrital 304.1
carbromal 304.1
carisoprodol 304.6
Catha (edulis) 304.4
chloral (betaine) (hydrate) 304.1
chloralamide 304.1
chloralformamide 304.1
chloralose 304.1
chlordiazepoxide 304.1
Chloretone 304.1
chlorobutanol 304.1
chlorodyne 304.1
chloroform 304.6
Cliradon 304.0
coca (leaf) and derivatives 304.2
cocaine 304.2
    hydrochloride 304.2
    salt (any) 304.2
codeine 304.0
combination of drugs (excluding mor-
    phine or opioid type drug) NEC
    304.8
    morphine or opioid type drug with
        any other drug 304.7
croton-chloral 304.1
cyclobarbital 304.1
cyclobarbitone 304.1
dagga 304.3
Delvinal 304.1
Demerol 304.0
desocodeine 304.0
desomorphine 304.0
desoxyephedrine 304.4
DET 304.5
dexamphetamine 304.4
dexedrine 304.4
dextromethorphan 304.0
dextromoramide 304.0
dextronorpseudoephedrine 304.4
dextrorphan 304.0
diacetylmorphine 304.0
Dial 304.1
diallylbarbituric acid 304.1
diamorphine 304.0
diazepam 304.1
dibucaine 304.6
dichloroethane 304.6
diethyl barbituric acid 304.1
diethylsulfone-diethylmethane 304.1
difencloxazine 304.6
dihydrocodeine 304.0
dihydrocodeinone 304.0
dihydrohydroxycodeinone 304.0
dihydroisocodeine 304.0
dihydromorphine 304.0
dihydromorphinone 304.0

Dependence (Continued)

dihydroxcodeinone 304.0
Dilaudid 304.0
dimenhydrinate 304.6
dimethylmeperidine 304.0
dimethyltriptamine 304.5
Dionin 304.0
diphenoxylate 304.6
dipipanone 304.0
d-lysergic acid diethylamide 304.5
DMT 304.5
Dolophine 304.0
DOM 304.2
doriden 304.1
dormiral 304.1
Dormison 304.1
Dromoran 304.0
drug NEC 304.9
    analgesic NEC 304.6
    combination (excluding morphine or
        opioid type drug) NEC 304.8
    morphine or opioid type drug
        with any other drug 304.7
    complicating pregnancy, childbirth,
        or puerperium 648.3
        affecting fetus or newborn 779.5
    hallucinogenic 304.5
    hypnotic NEC 304.1
    narcotic NEC 304.9
    psychostimulant NEC 304.4
    sedative 304.1
    soporific NEC 304.1
    specified type NEC 304.6
    suspected damage to fetus affecting
        management of pregnancy 655.5
    synthetic, with morphine-like effect
        304.0
    tranquilizing 304.1
duboisine 304.6
ectylurea 304.1
Endocaine 304.6
Equanil 304.1
Eskabarb 304.1
ethchlorvynol 304.1
ether (ethyl) (liquid) (vapor) (vinyl)
    304.6
ethidene 304.6
ethinamate 304.1
ethoheptazine 304.6
ethyl
    alcohol 303.9
    bromide 304.6
    carbamate 304.6
    chloride 304.6
    morphine 304.0
ethylene (gas) 304.6
    dichloride 304.6
ethylidene chloride 304.6
etilfen 304.1
etorphine 304.0
etoval 304.1
eucodal 304.0
euneryl 304.1
Evipal 304.1
Evipan 304.1
fentanyl 304.0
ganja 304.3
gardenal 304.1
gardenpanyl 304.1
gelsemine 304.6
Gelsemium 304.6
Gemonil 304.1
glucochloral 304.1
glue (airplane) (sniffing) 304.6

Dependence (Continued)

glutethimide 304.1
hallucinogenics 304.5
hashish 304.3
headache powder NEC 304.6
Heavenly Blue 304.5
hedonal 304.1
hemp 304.3
heptabarbital 304.1
Heptalgin 304.0
heptobarbitone 304.1
heroin 304.0
    salt (any) 304.0
hexethal (sodium) 304.1
hexobarbital 304.1
Hycodan 304.0
hydrocodone 304.0
hydromorphinol 304.0
hydromorphinone 304.0
hydromorphone 304.0
hydroxycodeine 304.0
hypnotic NEC 304.1
Indian hemp 304.3
inhalant 304.6   ◀
intranarcon 304.1
Kemithal 304.1
ketobemidone 304.0
khat 304.4
kif 304.3
Lactuca (virosa) extract 304.1
lactucarium 304.1
laudanum 304.0
Lebanese red 304.3
Leritine 304.0
lettuce opium 304.1
Levanil 304.1
Levo-Dromoran 304.0
levo-iso-methadone 304.0
levorphanol 304.0
Librium 304.1
Lomotil 304.6
Lotusate 304.1
LSD (-25) (and derivatives) 304.5
Luminal 304.1
lysergic acid 304.5
    amide 304.5
maconha 304.3
magic mushroom 304.5
marihuana 304.3
MDA (methylene dioxyamphetamine)
    304.4
Mebaral 304.1
Medinal 304.1
Medomin 304.1
megahallucinogenics 304.5
meperidine 304.0
mephobarbital 304.1
meprobamate 304.1
mescaline 304.5
methadone 304.0
methamphetamine(s) 304.4
methaqualone 304.1
metharbital 304.1
methitural 304.1
methobarbitone 304.1
methohexital 304.1
methopholine 304.6
methyl
    alcohol 303.9
    bromide 304.6
    morphine 304.0
    sulfonal 304.1
methylated spirit 303.9
methylbutinol 304.6

Dependence *(Continued)*
methyldihydromorphinone 304.0
methylene
chloride 304.6
dichloride 304.6
dioxyamphetamine (MDA) 304.4
methylparafynol 304.1
methylphenidate 304.4
methyprylone 304.1
metopon 304.0
Miltown 304.1
morning glory seeds 304.5,
morphinan(s) 304.0
morphine (sulfate) (sulfite) (type) (drugs
classifiable to 965.00-965.09) 304.0
morphine or opioid type drug (drugs
classifiable to 965.00-965.09) with
any other drug 304.7
morphinol(s) 304.0
morphinon 304.0
morpholinylethylmorphine 304.0
mylomide 304.1
myristicin 304.5
narcotic (drug) NEC 304.9
nealbarbital 304.1
nealbarbitone 304.1
Nembutal 304.1
Neonal 304.1
Neraval 304.1
Neravan 304.1
neurobarb 304.1
nicotine 305.1
Nisentil 304.0
nitrous oxide 304.6
Noctec 304.1
Noludar 304.1
nonbarbiturate sedatives and tranquilizers with similar effect 304.1
noptil 304.1
normorphine 304.0
noscapine 304.0
Novocaine 304.6
Numorphan 304.0
nunol 304.1
Nupercaine 304.6
Oblivon 304.1
on
aspirator V46.0
hyperbaric chamber V46.8
iron lung V46.11 ◀━
machine (enabling) V46.9
specified type NEC V46.8
Possum (patient-operated-selector-
mechanism) V46.8
renal dialysis machine V45.1
respirator V46.11 ◀━
encounter during power failure
V46.12 ◀
supplemental oxygen V46.2
opiate 304.0
opioids 304.0
opioid type drug 304.0
with any other drug 304.7
opium (alkaloids) (derivatives) (tinc-
ture) 304.0
ortal 304.1
Oxazepam 304.1
oxycodone 304.0
oxymorphone 304.0
Palfium 304.0
Panadol 304.6
pantopium 304.0
pantopon 304.0
papaverine 304.0

Dependence *(Continued)*
paracetamol 304.6
paracodin 304.0
paraldehyde 304.1
paregoric 304.0
Parzone 304.0
PCP (phencyclidine) 304.6
Pearly Gates 304.5
pentazocine 304.0
pentobarbital 304.1
pentobarbitone (sodium) 304.1
Pentothal 304.1
Percaine 304.6
Percodan 304.0
Perichlor 304.1
Pernocton 304.1
Pernoston 304.1
peronine 304.0
pethidine (hydrochloride) 304.0
petrichloral 304.1
peyote 304.5
Phanodorn 304.1
phenacetin 304.6
phenadoxone 304.0
phenaglycodol 304.1
phenazocine 304.0
phencyclidine 304.6
phenmetrazine 304.4
phenobal 304.1
phenobarbital 304.1
phenobarbitone 304.1
phenomorphan 304.0
phenonyl 304.1
phenoperidine 304.0
pholcodine 304.0
piminodine 304.0
Pipadone 304.0
Pitkin's solution 304.6
Placidyl 304.1
polysubstance 304.8
Pontocaine 304.6
pot 304.3
potassium bromide 304.1
Preludin 304.4
Prinadol 304.0
probarbital 304.1
procaine 304.6
propanal 304.1
propoxyphene 304.6
psilocibin 304.5
psilocin 304.5
psilocybin 304.5
psilocyline 304.5
psilocyn 304.5
psychedelic agents 304.5
psychostimulant NEC 304.4
psychotomimetic agents 304.5
pyrahexyl 304.3
Pyramidon 304.6
quinalbarbitone 304.1
racemoramide 304.0
racemorphan 304.0
Rela 304.6
scopolamine 304.6
secobarbital 304.1
seconal 304.1
sedative NEC 304.1
nonbarbiturate with barbiturate effect 304.1
Sedormid 304.1
sernyl 304.1
sodium bromide 304.1
Soma 304.6
Somnal 304.1

Dependence *(Continued)*
Somnos 304.1
Soneryl 304.1
soporific (drug) NEC 304.1
specified drug NEC 304.6
speed 304.4
spinocaine 304.6
stovaine 304.6
STP 304.5
stramonium 304.6
Sulfonal 304.1
sulfonethylmethane 304.1
sulfonmethane 304.1
Surital 304.1
synthetic drug with morphine-like effect 304.0
talbutal 304.1
tetracaine 304.6
tetrahydrocannabinol 304.3
tetronal 304.1
THC 304.3
thebacon 304.0
thebaine 304.0
thiamil 304.1
thiamylal 304.1
thiopental 304.1
tobacco 305.1
toluene, toluol 304.6
tranquilizer NEC 304.1
nonbarbiturate with barbiturate effect 304.1
tribromacetaldehyde 304.6
tribromethanol 304.6
tribromomethane 304.6
trichloroethanol 304.6
trichoroethyl phosphate 304.1
triclofos 304.1
Trional 304.1
Tuinal 304.1
Turkish green 304.3
urethan(e) 304.6
Valium 304.1
Valmid 304.1
veganin 304.0
veramon 304.1
Veronal 304.1
versidyne 304.6
vinbarbital 304.1
vinbarbitone 304.1
vinyl bitone 304.1
vitamin B$_6$ 266.1
wine 303.9
Zactane 304.6
Dependency
passive 301.6
reactions 301.6
Depersonalization (episode, in neurotic
state) (neurotic) (syndrome) 300.6
Depletion
carbohydrates 271.9
complement factor 279.8
extracellular fluid 276.5
plasma 276.5
potassium 276.8
nephropathy 588.89 ◀━
salt or sodium 276.1
causing heat exhaustion or prostration 992.4
nephropathy 593.9
volume 276.5
extracellular fluid 276.5
plasma 276.5
Deposit
argentous, cornea 371.16

Deposit (*Continued*)
bone, in Boeck's sarcoid 135
calcareous, calcium - *see* Calcification
cholesterol
  retina 362.82
  skin 709.3
  vitreous (humor) 379.22
conjunctival 372.56
cornea, corneal NEC 371.10
  argentous 371.16
  in
    cystinosis 270.0 [371.15]
    mucopolysaccharidosis 277.5
      [371.15]
crystalline, vitreous (humor) 379.22
hemosiderin, in old scars of cornea
  371.11
metallic, in lens 366.45
skin 709.3
teeth, tooth (betel) (black) (green) (materia alba) (orange) (soft) (tobacco)
  523.6
urate, in kidney (*see also* Disease, renal) 593.9
Depraved appetite 307.52
Depression 311
acute (*see also* Psychosis, affective) 296.2
  recurrent episode 296.3
  single episode 296.2
agitated (*see also* Psychosis, affective)
  296.2
  recurrent episode 296.3
  single episode 296.2
anaclitic 309.21
anxiety 300.4
arches 734
  congenital 754.61
autogenous (*see also* Psychosis, affective) 296.2
  recurrent episode 296.3
  single episode 296.2
basal metabolic rate (BMR) 794.7
bone marrow 289.9
central nervous system 799.1
  newborn 779.2
cerebral 331.9
  newborn 779.2
cerebrovascular 437.8
  newborn 779.2
chest wall 738.3
endogenous (*see also* Psychosis, affective) 296.2
  recurrent episode 296.3
  single episode 296.2
functional activity 780.99
hysterical 300.11
involutional, climacteric, or menopausal
  (*see also* Psychosis, affective) 296.2
  recurrent episode 296.3
  single episode 296.2
manic (*see also* Psychosis, affective)
  296.80
medullary 348.8
  newborn 779.2
mental 300.4
metatarsal heads - see Depression,
  arches
metatarsus - see Depression, arches
monopolar (*see also* Psychosis, affective) 296.2
  recurrent episode 296.3
  single episode 296.2
nervous 300.4
neurotic 300.4

Depression (*Continued*)
nose 738.0
postpartum 648.4
psychogenic 300.4
  reactive 298.0
psychoneurotic 300.4
psychotic (*see also* Psychosis, affective)
  296.2
  reactive 298.0
  recurrent episode 296.3
  single episode 296.2
reactive 300.4
  neurotic 300.4
  psychogenic 298.0
  psychoneurotic 300.4
  psychotic 298.0
recurrent 296.3
respiratory center 348.8
  newborn 770.89
scapula 736.89
senile 290.21
situational (acute) (brief) 309.0
  prolonged 309.1
skull 754.0
sternum 738.3
visual field 368.40
Depressive reaction - *see also* Reaction,
  depressive
acute (transient) 309.0
  with anxiety 309.28
prolonged 309.1
situational (acute) 309.0
  prolonged 309.1
Deprivation
cultural V62.4
emotional V62.89
  affecting
    adult 995.82
    infant or child 995.51
food 994.2
  specific substance NEC 269.8
protein (familial) (kwashiorkor)
  260
sleep V69.4 ◄
social V62.4
  affecting
    adult 995.82
    infant or child 995.51
symptoms, syndrome
  alcohol 291.81
  drug 292.0
vitamins (*see also* Deficiency, vitamin)
  269.2
water 994.3
de Quervain's
disease (tendon sheath) 727.04
thyroiditis (subacute granulomatous
  thyroiditis) 245.1
Derangement
ankle (internal) 718.97
  current injury (*see also* Dislocation,
    ankle) 837.0
  recurrent 718.37
cartilage (articular) NEC (*see also* Disorder, cartilage, articular) 718.0
  knee 717.9
    recurrent 718.36
  recurrent 718.3
collateral ligament (knee) (medial) (tibial) 717.82
  current injury 844.1
    lateral (fibular) 844.0
  lateral (fibular) 717.81
    current injury 844.0

Derangement (*Continued*)
cruciate ligament (knee) (posterior)
  717.84
  anterior 717.83
    current injury 844.2
  current injury 844.2
elbow (internal) 718.92
  current injury (*see also* Dislocation,
    elbow) 832.00
  recurrent 718.32
gastrointestinal 536.9
heart - see Disease, heart
hip (joint) (internal) (old) 718.95
  current injury (*see also* Dislocation,
    hip) 835.00
  recurrent 718.35
intervertebral disc - see Displacement,
  intervertebral disc
joint (internal) 718.90
  ankle 718.97
  current injury - *see also* Dislocation,
    by site
    knee, meniscus or cartilage (*see
      also* Tear, meniscus) 836.2
  elbow 718.92
  foot 718.97
  hand 718.94
  hip 718.95
  knee 717.9
  multiple sites 718.99
  pelvic region 718.95
  recurrent 718.30
    ankle 718.37
    elbow 718.32
    foot 718.37
    hand 718.34
    hip 718.35
    knee 718.36
    multiple sites 718.39
    pelvic region 718.35
    shoulder (region) 718.31
    specified site NEC 718.38
    temporomandibular (old) 524.69
    wrist 718.33
  shoulder (region) 718.91
  specified site NEC 718.98
  spine NEC 724.9
  temporomandibular 524.69
  wrist 718.93
knee (cartilage) (internal) 717.9
  current injury (*see also* Tear, meniscus) 836.2
  ligament 717.89
    capsular 717.85
    collateral - *see* Derangement, collateral ligament
    cruciate - *see* Derangement, cruciate ligament
    specified NEC 717.85
  recurrent 718.36
low back NEC 724.9
meniscus NEC (knee) 717.5
  current injury (*see also* Tear, meniscus) 836.2
  lateral 717.40
    anterior horn 717.42
    posterior horn 717.43
    specified NEC 717.49
  medial 717.3
    anterior horn 717.1
    posterior horn 717.2
  recurrent 718.3
  site other than knee - see Disorder,
    cartilage, articular

Derangement (Continued)
  mental (see also Psychosis) 298.9
  rotator cuff (recurrent) (tear) 726.10
    current 840.4
  sacroiliac (old) 724.6
    current - see Dislocation, sacroiliac
  semilunar cartilage (knee) 717.5
    current injury 836.2
      lateral 836.1
      medial 836.0
    recurrent 718.3
  shoulder (internal) 718.91
    current injury (see also Dislocation,
      shoulder) 831.00
    recurrent 718.31
  spine (recurrent) NEC 724.9
    current - see Dislocation, spine
  temporomandibular (internal) (joint)
    (old) 524.69
    current - see Dislocation, jaw
Dercum's disease or syndrome (adiposis
    dolorosa) 272.8
Derealization (neurotic) 300.6
Dermal - see condition
Dermaphytid - see Dermatophytosis
Dermatergosis - see Dermatitis
Dermatitis (allergic) (contact) (occupa-
    tional) (venenata) 692.9
  ab igne 692.82
  acneiform 692.9
  actinic (due to sun) 692.70
    acute 692.72
    chronic NEC 692.74
    other than from sun NEC 692.82
  ambustionis
    due to
      burn or scald - see Burn, by site
      sunburn (see also Sunburn)
        692.71
  amebic 006.6
  ammonia 691.0
  anaphylactoid NEC 692.9
  arsenical 692.4
  artefacta 698.4
    psychogenic 316 [698.4]
  asthmatic 691.8
  atopic (allergic) (intrinsic) 691.8
    psychogenic 316 [691.8]
  atrophicans 701.8
    diffusa 701.8
    maculosa 701.3
  berlock, berloque 692.72
  blastomycetic 116.0
  blister beetle 692.89
  Brucella NEC 023.9
  bullosa 694.9
    striata pratensis 692.6
  bullous 694.9
    mucosynechial, atrophic 694.60
      with ocular involvement 694.61
    seasonal 694.8
  calorica
    due to
      burn or scald - see Burn, by site
      cold 692.89
      sunburn (see also Sunburn)
        692.71
  caterpillar 692.89
  cercarial 120.3
  combustionis
    due to
      burn or scald - see Burn, by site
      sunburn (see also Sunburn)
        692.71

Dermatitis (Continued)
  congelationis 991.5
  contusiformis 695.2
  diabetic 250.8
  diaper 691.0
  diphtheritica 032.85
  due to
    acetone 692.2
    acids 692.4
    adhesive plaster 692.4
    alcohol (skin contact) (substances
      classifiable to 980.0-980.9) 692.4
      taken internally 693.8
    alkalis 692.4
    allergy NEC 692.9
    ammonia (household) (liquid) 692.4 ◄
    animal   ◄
      dander (cat) (dog) 692.84   ◄
      hair (cat) (dog) 692.84   ◄
    arnica 692.3
    arsenic 692.4
      taken internally 693.8
    blister beetle 692.89
    cantharides 692.3
    carbon disulphide 692.2
    caterpillar 692.89
    caustics 692.4
    cereal (ingested) 693.1
      contact with skin 692.5
    chemical(s) NEC 692.4
      internal 693.8
      irritant NEC 692.4
      taken internally 693.8
    chlorocompounds 692.2
    coffee (ingested) 693.1
      contact with skin 692.5
    cold weather 692.89
    cosmetics 692.81
    cyclohexanes 692.2
    dander, animal (cat) (dog) 692.84 ◄
    deodorant 692.81
    detergents 692.0
    dichromate 692.4
    drugs and medicinals (correct sub-
      stance properly administered)
      (internal use) 693.0
      external (in contact with skin) 692.3
        wrong substance given or taken
          976.9
          specified substance - see Table
            of Drugs and Chemicals
      wrong substance given or taken
        977.9
        specified substance - see Table
          of Drugs and Chemicals
    dyes 692.89
      hair 692.89
    epidermophytosis - see Dermatophy-
      tosis
    esters 692.2
    external irritant NEC 692.9
      specified agent NEC 692.89
    eye shadow 692.81
    fish (ingested) 693.1
      contact with skin 692.5
    flour (ingested) 693.1
      contact with skin 692.5
    food (ingested) 693.1
      in contact with skin 692.5
    fruit (ingested) 693.1
      contact with skin 692.5
    fungicides 692.3
    furs 692.84   ◄▥
    glycols 692.2

Dermatitis (Continued)
  due to (Continued)
    greases NEC 692.1
    hair, animal (cat) (dog) 692.84   ◄
    hair dyes 692.89
    hot
      objects and materials - see Burn,
        by site
      weather or places 692.89
    hydrocarbons 692.2
    infrared rays, except from sun 692.82
      solar NEC (see also Dermatitis, due
        to, sun) 692.70
    ingested substance 693.9
      drugs and medicinals (see also
        Dermatitis, due to, drugs and
        medicinals) 693.0
      food 693.1
      specified substance NEC 693.8
    ingestion or injection of
      chemical 693.8
      drug (correct substance properly
        administered) 693.0
        wrong substance given or taken
          977.9
          specified substance - see
            Table of Drugs and
            Chemicals
    insecticides 692.4
    internal agent 693.9
      drugs and medicinals (see also
        Dermatitis, due to, drugs and
        medicinals) 693.0
      food (ingested) 693.1
        in contact with skin 692.5
      specified agent NEC 693.8
    iodine 692.3
    iodoform 692.3
    irradiation 692.82
    jewelry 692.83
    keratolytics 692.3
    ketones 692.2
    lacquer tree (Rhus verniciflua) 692.6
    light (sun) NEC (see also Dermatitis,
      due to, sun) 692.70
      other 692.82
    low temperature 692.89
    mascara 692.81
    meat (ingested) 693.1
      contact with skin 692.5
    mercury, mercurials 692.3
    metals 692.83
    milk (ingested) 693.1
      contact with skin 692.5
    Neomycin 692.3
    nylon 692.4
    oils NEC 692.1
    paint solvent 692.2
    pediculocides 692.3
    petroleum products (substances clas-
      sifiable to 981) 692.4
    phenol 692.3
    photosensitiveness, photosensitivity
      (sun) 692.72
      other light 692.82
    plants NEC 692.6
    plasters, medicated (any) 692.3
    plastic 692.4
    poison
      ivy (Rhus toxicodendron) 692.6
      oak (Rhus diversiloba) 692.6
      plant or vine 692.6
      sumac (Rhus venenata) 692.6
      vine (Rhus radicans) 692.6

ICD-9-CM

Vol. 2

Dermatitis *(Continued)*
due to *(Continued)*
preservatives 692.89
primrose (primula) 692.6
primula 692.6
radiation 692.82
sun NEC *(see also* Dermatitis, due to, sun) 692.70
tanning bed 692.82
radioactive substance 692.82
radium 692.82
ragweed (Senecio jacobae) 692.6
Rhus (diversiloba) (radicans) (toxicodendron) (venenata) (verniciflua) 692.6
rubber 692.4
scabicides 692.3
Senecio jacobae 692.6
solar radiation - *see* Dermatitis, due to, sun
solvents (any) (substances classifiable to (982.0-982.8) 692.2
chlorocompound group 692.2
cyclohexane group 692.2
ester group 692.2
glycol group 692.2
hydrocarbon group 692.2
ketone group 692.2
paint 692.2
specified agent NEC 692.89
sun 692.70
acute 692.72
chronic NEC 692.74
specified NEC 692.79
sunburn *(see also* Sunburn) 692.71
sunshine NEC *(see also* Dermatitis, due to, sun) 692.70
tanning bed 692.82
tetrachlorethylene 692.2
toluene 692.2
topical medications 692.3
turpentine 692.2
ultraviolet rays, except from sun 692.82
sun NEC *(see also* Dermatitis, due to, sun) 692.70
vaccine or vaccination (correct substance properly administered) 693.0
wrong substance given or taken
bacterial vaccine 978.8
specified - *see* Table of Drugs and Chemicals
other vaccines NEC 979.9
specified - *see* Table of Drugs and Chemicals
varicose veins *(see also* Varicose, vein, inflamed or infected) 454.1
x-rays 692.82
dyshydrotic 705.81
dysmenorrheica 625.8
eczematoid NEC 692.9
infectious 690.8
eczematous NEC 692.9
epidemica 695.89
erysipelatosa 695.81
escharotica - *see* Burn, by site
exfoliativa, exfoliative 695.89
generalized 695.89
infantum 695.81
neonatorum 695.81
eyelid 373.31
allergic 373.32
contact 373.32

Dermatitis *(Continued)*
eyelid *(Continued)*
eczematous 373.31
herpes (zoster) 053.20
simplex 054.41
infective 373.5
due to
actinomycosis 039.3 *[373.5]*
herpes
simplex 054.41
zoster 053.20
impetigo 684 *[373.5]*
leprosy *(see also* Leprosy) 030.0 *[373.4]*
lupus vulgaris (tuberculous) *(see also* Tuberculosis) 017.0 *[373.4]*
mycotic dermatitis *(see also* Dermatomycosis) 111.9 *[373.5]*
vaccinia 051.0 *[373.5]*
postvaccination 999.0 *[373.5]*
yaws *(see also* Yaws) 102.9 *[373.4]*
facta, factitia 698.4
psychogenic 316 *[698.4]*
ficta 698.4
psychogenic 316 *[698.4]*
flexural 691.8
follicularis 704.8
friction 709.8
fungus 111.9
specified type NEC 111.8
gangrenosa, gangrenous (infantum) *(see also* Gangrene) 785.4
gestationis 646.8
gonococcal 098.89
gouty 274.89
harvest mite 133.8
heat 692.89
herpetiformis (bullous) (erythematous) (pustular) (vesicular) 694.0
juvenile 694.2
senile 694.5
hiemalis 692.89
hypostatic, hypostatica 454.1
with ulcer 454.2
impetiginosa 684
infantile (acute) (chronic) (intertriginous) (intrinsic) (seborrheic) 690.12
infectiosa eczematoides 690.8
infectious (staphylococcal) (streptococcal) 686.9
eczematoid 690.8
infective eczematoid 690.8
Jacquet's (diaper dermatitis) 691.0
leptus 133.8
lichenified NEC 692.9
lichenoid, chronic 701.0
lichenoides purpurica pigmentosa 709.1
meadow 692.6
medicamentosa (correct substance properly administered) (internal use) *(see also* Dermatitis, due to, drugs or medicinals) 693.0
due to contact with skin 692.3
mite 133.8
multiformis 694.0
juvenile 694.2
senile 694.5
napkin 691.0
neuro 698.3
neurotica 694.0
nummular NEC 692.9
osteatosis, osteatotic 706.8
papillaris capillitii 706.1

Dermatophytosis *(Continued)*
pellagrous 265.2
perioral 695.3
perstans 696.1
photosensitivity (sun) 692.72
other light 692.82
pigmented purpuric lichenoid 709.1
polymorpha dolorosa 694.0
primary irritant 692.9
pruriginosa 694.0
pruritic NEC 692.9
psoriasiform nodularis 696.2
psychogenic 316
purulent 686.00
pustular contagious 051.2
pyococcal 686.00
pyocyaneus 686.09
pyogenica 686.00
radiation 692.82
repens 696.1
Ritter's (exfoliativa) 695.81
Schamberg's (progressive pigmentary dermatosis) 709.09
schistosome 120.3
seasonal bullous 694.8
seborrheic 690.10
infantile 690.12
sensitization NEC 692.9
septic *(see also* Septicemia) 686.00
gonococcal 098.89
solar, solare NEC *(see also* Dermatitis, due to, sun) 692.70
stasis 459.81
due to
postphlebitic syndrome 459.12
with ulcer 459.13
varicose veins - *see* Varicose
ulcerated or with ulcer (varicose) 454.2
sunburn *(see also* Sunburn) 692.71
suppurative 686.00
traumatic NEC 709.8
trophoneurotica 694.0
ultraviolet, except from sun 692.82
due to sun NEC *(see also* Dermatitis, due to, sun) 692.70
varicose 454.1
with ulcer 454.2
vegetans 686.8
verrucosa 117.2
xerotic 706.8
Dermatoarthritis, lipoid 272.8 *[713.0]*
Dermatochalasia, dermatochalasis 374.87
Dermatofibroma (lenticulare) (M8832/0) - *see also* Neoplasm, skin, benign
protuberans (M8832/1) - *see* Neoplasm, skin, uncertain behavior
Dermatofibrosarcoma (protuberans) (M8832/3) - *see* Neoplasm, skin, malignant
Dermatographia 708.3
Dermatolysis (congenital) (exfoliativa) 757.39
acquired 701.8
eyelids 374.34
palpebrarum 374.34
senile 701.8
Dermatomegaly NEC 701.8
Dermatomucomyositis 710.3
Dermatomycosis 111.9
furfuracea 111.0
specified type NEC 111.8
Dermatomyositis (acute) (chronic) 710.3
Dermatoneuritis of children 985.0
Dermatophiliasis 134.1

Dermatophytide - *see* Dermatophytosis
Dermatophytosis (Epidermophyton) (infection) (microsporum) (tinea) (Trichophyton) 110.9
  beard 110.0
  body 110.5
  deep seated 110.6
  fingernails 110.1
  foot 110.4
  groin 110.3
  hand 110.2
  nail 110.1
  perianal (area) 110.3
  scalp 110.0
  scrotal 110.8
  specified site NEC 110.8
  toenails 110.1
  vulva 110.8
Dermatopolyneuritis 985.0
Dermatorrhexis 756.83
  acquired 701.8
Dermatosclerosis (*see also* Scleroderma) 710.1
  localized 701.0
Dermatosis 709.9
  Andrews' 686.8
  atopic 691.8
  Bowen's (M8081/2) - *see* Neoplasm, skin, in situ
  bullous 694.9
    specified type NEC 694.8
  erythematosquamous 690.8
  exfoliativa 695.89
  factitial 698.4
  gonococcal 098.89
  herpetiformis 694.0
    juvenile 694.2
    senile 694.5
  hysterical 300.11
  Linear IgA 694.8
  menstrual NEC 709.8
  neutrophilic, acute febrile 695.89
  occupational (*see also* Dermatitis) 692.9
  papulosa nigra 709.8
  pigmentary NEC 709.00
    progressive 709.09
    Schamberg's 709.09
    Siemens-Bloch 757.33
  progressive pigmentary 709.09
  psychogenic 316
  pustular subcorneal 694.1
  Schamberg's (progressive pigmentary) 709.09
  senile NEC 709.3
  specified NEC 702.8
  Unna's (seborrheic dermatitis) 690.10
Dermographia 708.3
Dermographism 708.3
Dermoid (cyst) (M9084/0) - *see also* Neoplasm, by site, benign
  with malignant transformation (M9084/3) 183.0
Dermopathy
  infiltrative, with thyrotoxicosis 242.0
  senile NEC 709.3
Dermophytosis - *see* Dermatophytosis
Descemet's membrane - *see* condition
Descemetocele 371.72
Descending - *see* condition
Descensus uteri (complete) (incomplete) (partial) (without vaginal wall prolapse) 618.1
  with mention of vaginal wall prolapse - *see* Prolapse, uterovaginal

Desensitization to allergens V07.1
Desert
  rheumatism 114.0
  sore (*see also* Ulcer, skin) 707.9
Desertion (child) (newborn) 995.52
  adult 995.84
Desmoid (extra-abdominal) (tumor) (M8821/1) - *see also* Neoplasm, connective tissue, uncertain behavior
  abdominal (M8822/1) - *see* Neoplasm, connective tissue, uncertain behavior
Despondency 300.4
Desquamative dermatitis NEC 695.89
Destruction
  articular facet (*see also* Derangement, joint) 718.9
    vertebra 724.9
  bone 733.90
    syphilitic 095.5
  joint (*see also* Derangement, joint) 718.9
    sacroiliac 724.6
  kidney 593.89
  live fetus to facilitate birth NEC 763.89
  ossicles (ear) 385.24
  rectal sphincter 569.49
  septum (nasal) 478.1
  tuberculous NEC (*see also* Tuberculosis) 011.9
  tympanic membrane 384.82
  tympanum 385.89
  vertebral disc - *see* Degeneration, intervertebral disc
Destructiveness (*see also* Disturbance, conduct) 312.9
  adjustment reaction 309.3
Detachment
  cartilage - *see also* Sprain, by site
    knee - *see* Tear, meniscus
  cervix, annular 622.8
    complicating delivery 665.3
  choroid (old) (postinfectional) (simple) (spontaneous) 363.70
    hemorrhagic 363.72
    serous 363.71
  knee, medial meniscus (old) 717.3
    current injury 836.0
  ligament - *see* Sprain, by site
  placenta (premature) - *see* Placenta, separation
  retina (recent) 361.9
    with retinal defect (rhegmatogenous) 361.00
      giant tear 361.03
      multiple 361.02
      partial
        with
          giant tear 361.03
          multiple defects 361.02
          retinal dialysis (juvenile) 361.04
          single defect 361.01
      retinal dialysis (juvenile) 361.04
      single 361.01
      subtotal 361.05
      total 361.05
    delimited (old) (partial) 361.06
    old
      delimited 361.06
      partial 361.06
      total or subtotal 361.07
    pigment epithelium (RPE) (serous) 362.42
      exudative 362.42
      hemorrhagic 362.43
    rhegmatogenous (*see also* Detachment, retina, with retinal defect) 361.00

Detachment (*Continued*)
  retina (recent) (*Continued*)
    serous (without retinal defect) 361.2
    specified type NEC 361.89
    traction (with vitreoretinal organization) 361.81
  vitreous humor 379.21
Detergent asthma 507.8
Deterioration
  epileptic
    with behavioral disturbance 345.9 [294.11]
    without behavioral disturbance 345.9 [294.10]
  heart, cardiac (*see also* Degeneration, myocardial) 429.1
  mental (*see also* Psychosis) 298.9
  myocardium, myocardial (*see also* Degeneration, myocardial) 429.1
  senile (simple) 797
  transplanted organ - *see* Complications, transplant, organ, by site
de Toni-Fanconi syndrome (cystinosis) 270.0
Deuteranomaly 368.52
Deuteranopia (anomalous trichromat) (complete) (incomplete) 368.52
Deutschländer's disease - *see* Fracture, foot
Development
  abnormal, bone 756.9
  arrested 783.40
    bone 733.91
    child 783.40
    due to malnutrition (protein-calorie) 263.2
    fetus or newborn 764.9
    tracheal rings (congenital) 748.3
  defective, congenital - *see also* Anomaly
    cauda equina 742.59
    left ventricle 746.9
      with atresia or hypoplasia of aortic orifice or valve with hypoplasia of ascending aorta 746.7
      in hypoplastic left heart syndrome 746.7
  delayed (*see also* Delay, development) 783.40
    arithmetical skills 315.1
    language (skills) 315.31
      expressive 315.31
      mixed receptive-expressive 315.32
    learning skill, specified NEC 315.2
    mixed skills 315.5
    motor coordination 315.4
    reading 315.00
    specified
      learning skill NEC 315.2
      type NEC, except learning 315.8
    speech 315.39
      associated with hyperkinesia 314.1
      phonological 315.39
    spelling 315.09
    written expression 315.2
  imperfect, congenital - *see also* Anomaly
    heart 746.9
    lungs 748.60
  improper (fetus or newborn) 764.9
  incomplete (fetus or newborn) 764.9
    affecting management of pregnancy 656.5
    bronchial tree 748.3
    organ or site not listed - *see* Hypoplasia
    respiratory system 748.9

ICD-9-CM

Vol. 2

Development *(Continued)*
 sexual, precocious NEC 259.1
 tardy, mental *(see also* Retardation,
   mental) 319
Developmental - *see* condition
Devergie's disease (pityriasis rubra pilaris) 696.4
Deviation
 conjugate (eye) 378.87
  palsy 378.81
  spasm, spastic 378.82
 esophagus 530.89
 eye, skew 378.87
 mandible, opening and closing 524.53◄
 midline (jaw) (teeth) 524.29 ◄═
  specified site NEC - *see* Malposition
 occlusal plane 524.76 ◄
 organ or site, congenital NEC - *see*
   Malposition, congenital
 septum (acquired) (nasal) 470
  congenital 754.0
 sexual 302.9
  bestiality 302.1
  coprophilia 302.89
  ego-dystonic
   homosexuality 302.0
   lesbianism 302.0
  erotomania 302.89
   Clérambault's 297.8
  exhibitionism (sexual) 302.4
  fetishism 302.81
   transvestic 302.3
  frotteurism 302.89
  homosexuality, ego-dystonic 302.0
   pedophilic 302.2
  lesbianism, ego-dystonic 302.0
  masochism 302.83
  narcissism 302.89
  necrophilia 302.89
  nymphomania 302.89
  pederosis 302.2
  pedophilia 302.2
  sadism 302.84
  sadomasochism 302.84
  satyriasis 302.89
  specified type NEC 302.89
  transvestic fetishism 302.3
  transvestism 302.3
  voyeurism 302.82
  zoophilia (erotica) 302.1
 teeth, midline 524.29 ◄═
 trachea 519.1
 ureter (congenital) 753.4
Devic's disease 341.0
Device
 cerebral ventricle (communicating) in
   situ V45.2
 contraceptive - *see* Contraceptive, device
 drainage, cerebrospinal fluid V45.2
Devil's
 grip 074.1
 pinches (purpura simplex) 287.2
Devitalized tooth 522.9
Devonshire colic 984.9
 specified type of lead - *see* Table of
   Drugs and Chemicals
Dextraposition, aorta 747.21
 with ventricular septal defect, pulmonary stenosis or atresia, and hypertrophy of right ventricle 745.2
 in tetralogy of Fallot 745.2
Dextratransposition, aorta 745.11
Dextrinosis, limit (debrancher enzyme
   deficiency) 271.0

Dextrocardia (corrected) (false) (isolated)
   (secondary) (true) 746.87
 with
  complete transposition of viscera
    759.3
  situs inversus 759.3
Dextroversion, kidney (left) 753.3
Dhobie itch 110.3
Diabetes, diabetic (brittle) (congenital)
   (familial) (mellitus) (poorly controlled) (severe) (slight) (without
   complication) 250.0

Note   Use the following fifth-digit
subclassification with category 250:

0   type II or unspecified type, not
    stated as uncontrolled ◄═

    Fifth-digit 0 is for use for type
    II patients, even if the patient
    requires insulin ◄═

1   type I [juvenile type], not
    stated as uncontrolled ◄═

2   type II or unspecified type,
    uncontrolled

    Fifth-digit 2 is for use for type
    II patients, even if the patient
    requires insulin ◄═

3   type I [juvenile type],
    uncontrolled ◄═

---

 with
  coma (with ketoacidosis) 250.3
   hyperosmolar (nonketotic) 250.2
  complication NEC 250.9
   specified NEC 250.8
  gangrene 250.7 *[785.4]*
  hyperosmolarity 250.2
  ketosis, ketoacidosis 250.1
  osteomyelitis 250.8 *[731.8]*
  specified manifestations NEC
    250.8
 acetonemia 250.1
 acidosis 250.1
 amyotrophy 250.6 *[358.1]*
 angiopathy, peripheral 250.7 *[443.81]*
 asymptomatic 790.29
 autonomic neuropathy (peripheral)
   250.6 *[337.1]*
 bone change 250.8 *[731.8]*
 bronze, bronzed 275.0
 cataract 250.5 *[366.41]*
 chemical 790.29
  complicating pregnancy, childbirth,
    or puerperium 648.8
 coma (with ketoacidosis) 250.3
  hyperglycemic 250.3
  hyperosmolar (nonketotic) 250.2
  hypoglycemic 250.3
  insulin 250.3
 complicating pregnancy, childbirth, or
   puerperium (maternal) 648.0
  affecting fetus or newborn 775.0
 complication NEC 250.9
  specified NEC 250.8
 dorsal sclerosis 250.6 *[340]*
 dwarfism-obesity syndrome 258.1
 gangrene 250.7 *[785.4]*
 gastroparesis 250.6 *[536.3]*
 gestational 648.8
  complicating pregnancy, childbirth,
    or puerperium 648.8
 glaucoma 250.5 *[365.44]*

Diabetes, diabetic *(Continued)*
 glomerulosclerosis (intercapillary)
   250.4 *[581.81]*
 glycogenosis, secondary 250.8 *[259.8]*
 hemochromatosis 275.0
 hyperosmolar coma 250.2
 hyperosmolarity 250.2
 hypertension-nephrosis syndrome
   250.4 *[581.81]*
 hypoglycemia 250.8
 hypoglycemic shock 250.8
 insipidus 253.5
  nephrogenic 588.1
  pituitary 253.5
  vasopressin-resistant 588.1
 intercapillary glomerulosclerosis 250.4
   [581.81]
 iritis 250.5 *[364.42]*
 ketosis, ketoacidosis 250.1
 Kimmelstiel (-Wilson) disease or syndrome (intercapillary glomerulosclerosis) 250.4 *[581.81]*
 Lancereaux's (diabetes mellitus with
   marked emaciation) 250.8 *[261]*
 latent (chemical) 790.29
  complicating pregnancy, childbirth,
    or puerperium 648.8
 lipoidosis 250.8 *[272.7]*
 macular edema 250.5 *[362.01]*
 maternal
  with manifest disease in the infant
    775.1
  affecting fetus or newborn 775.0
 microaneurysms, retinal 250.5 *[362.01]*
 mononeuropathy 250.6 *[355.9]*
 neonatal, transient 775.1
 nephropathy 250.4 *[583.81]*
 nephrosis (syndrome) 250.4 *[581.81]*
 neuralgia 250.6 *[357.2]*
 neuritis 250.6 *[357.2]*
 neurogenic arthropathy 250.6 *[713.5]*
 neuropathy 250.6 *[357.2]*
 nonclinical 790.29
 osteomyelitis 250.8 *[731.8]*
 peripheral autonomic neuropathy 250.6
   [337.1]
 phosphate 275.3
 polyneuropathy 250.6 *[357.2]*
 renal (true) 271.4
 retinal
  edema 250.5 *[362.01]*
  hemorrhage 250.5 *[362.01]*
  microaneurysms 250.5 *[362.01]*
 retinitis 250.5 *[362.01]*
 retinopathy 250.5 *[362.01]*
  background 250.5 *[362.01]*
  proliferative 250.5 *[362.02]*
 steroid induced
  correct substance properly adminis-
    tered 251.8
  overdose or wrong substance given
    or taken 962.0
 stress 790.29
 subclinical 790.29
 subliminal 790.29
 sugar 250.0
 ulcer (skin) 250.8 *[707.9]*
  lower extremity 250.8 *[707.10]*
   ankle 250.8 *[707.13]*
   calf 250.8 *[707.12]*
   foot 250.8 *[707.15]*
   heel 250.8 *[707.14]*
   knee 250.8 *[707.19]*
   specified site NEC 250.8 *[707.19]*

Diabetes, diabetic *(Continued)*
  ulcer *(Continued)*
    lower extremity *(Continued)*
      thigh 250.8 *[707.11]*
      toes 250.8 *[707.15]*
    specified site NEC 250.8 *[707.8]*
    xanthoma 250.8 *[272.2]*
Diacyclothrombopathia 287.1
Diagnosis deferred 799.9
Dialysis (intermittent) (treatment)
  anterior retinal (juvenile) (with detachment) 361.04
  extracorporeal V56.0
  peritoneal V56.8
  renal V56.0
    status only V45.1
  specified type NEC V56.8
Diamond-Blackfan anemia or syndrome (congenital hypoplastic anemia) 284.0
Diamond-Gardener syndrome (autoerythrocyte sensitization) 287.2
Diaper rash 691.0
Diaphoresis (excessive) NEC *(see also* Hyperhidrosis) 780.8 ◀▥
Diaphragm - *see* condition
Diaphragmalgia 786.52
Diaphragmitis 519.4
Diaphyseal aclasis 756.4
Diaphysitis 733.99
Diarrhea, diarrheal (acute) (autumn) (bilious) (bloody) (catarrhal) (choleraic) (chronic) (gravis) (green) (infantile) (lienteric) (noninfectious) (presumed noninfectious) (putrefactive) (secondary) (sporadic) (summer) (symptomatic) (thermic) 787.91
  achlorhydric 536.0
  allergic 558.3
  amebic *(see also* Amebiasis) 006.9
    with abscess - *see* Abscess, amebic
    acute 006.0
    chronic 006.1
    nondysenteric 006.2
  bacillary - *see* Dysentery, bacillary
  bacterial NEC 008.5
  balantidial 007.0
  bile salt-induced 579.8
  cachectic NEC 787.91
  chilomastix 007.8
  choleriformis 001.1
  coccidial 007.2
  Cochin-China 579.1
    anguilluliasis 127.2
    psilosis 579.1
  Dientamoeba 007.8
  dietetic 787.91
  due to
    achylia gastrica 536.8
    Aerobacter aerogenes 008.2
    Bacillus coli - *see* Enteritis, E. coli
    bacteria NEC 008.5
    bile salts 579.8
    Capillaria
      hepatica 128.8
      philippinensis 127.5
    Clostridium perfringens (C) (F) 008.46
    Enterobacter aerogenes 008.2
    enterococci 008.49
    Escherichia coli - *see* Enteritis, E. coli
    Giardia lamblia 007.1
    Heterophyes heterophyes 121.6
    irritating foods 787.91
    Metagonimus yokogawai 121.5
    Necator americanus 126.1

Diarrhea, diarrheal *(Continued)*
  due to *(Continued)*
    Paracolobactrum arizonae 008.1
    Paracolon bacillus NEC 008.47
      Arizona 008.1
    Proteus (bacillus) (mirabilis) (Morganii) 008.3
    Pseudomonas aeruginosa 008.42
    S. japonicum 120.2
    specified organism NEC 008.8
      bacterial 008.49
      viral NEC 008.69
    Staphylococcus 008.41
    Streptococcus 008.49
      anaerobic 008.46
    Strongyloides stercoralis 127.2
    Trichuris trichiuria 127.3
    virus NEC *(see also* Enteritis, viral) 008.69
  dysenteric 009.2
    due to specified organism NEC 008.8
  dyspeptic 787.91
  endemic 009.3
    due to specified organism NEC 008.8
  epidemic 009.2
    due to specified organism NEC 008.8
  fermentative 787.91
  flagellate 007.9
  Flexner's (ulcerative) 004.1
  functional 564.5
    following gastrointestinal surgery 564.4
    psychogenic 306.4
  giardial 007.1
  Giardia lamblia 007.1
  hill 579.1
  hyperperistalsis (nervous) 306.4
  infectious 009.2
    due to specified organism NEC 008.8
    presumed 009.3
  inflammatory 787.91
    due to specified organism NEC 008.8
  malarial *(see also* Malaria) 084.6
  mite 133.8
  mycotic 117.9
  nervous 306.4
  neurogenic 564.5
  parenteral NEC 009.2
  postgastrectomy 564.4
  postvagotomy 564.4
  prostaglandin induced 579.8
  protozoal NEC 007.9
  psychogenic 306.4
  septic 009.2
    due to specified organism NEC 008.8
  specified organism NEC 008.8
    bacterial 008.49
    viral NEC 008.69
  Staphylococcus 008.41
  Streptococcus 008.49
    anaerobic 008.46
  toxic 558.2
  travelers' 009.2
    due to specified organism NEC 008.8
  trichomonal 007.3
  tropical 579.1
  tuberculous 014.8
  ulcerative (chronic) *(see also* Colitis, ulcerative) 556.9
  viral *(see also* Enteritis, viral) 008.8
  zymotic NEC 009.2
Diastasis
  cranial bones 733.99
    congenital 756.0
  joint (traumatic) - *see* Dislocation, by site

Diastasis *(Continued)*
  muscle 728.84
    congenital 756.89
  recti (abdomen) 728.84
    complicating delivery 665.8
    congenital 756.79
Diastema, teeth, tooth 524.30 ◀▥
Diastematomyelia 742.51
Diataxia, cerebral, infantile 343.0
Diathesis
  allergic V15.09
  bleeding (familial) 287.9
  cystine (familial) 270.0
  gouty 274.9
  hemorrhagic (familial) 287.9
    newborn NEC 776.0
  oxalic 271.8
  scrofulous *(see also* Tuberculosis) 017.2
  spasmophilic *(see also* Tetany) 781.7
  ulcer 536.9
  uric acid 274.9
Diaz's disease or osteochondrosis 732.5
Dibothriocephaliasis 123.4
  larval 123.5
Dibothriocephalus (infection) (infestation) (latus) 123.4
  larval 123.5
Dicephalus 759.4
Dichotomy, teeth 520.2
Dichromat, dichromata (congenital) 368.59
Dichromatopsia (congenital) 368.59
Dichuchwa 104.0
Dicroceliasis 121.8
Didelphys, didelphic *(see also* Double uterus) 752.2
Didymitis *(see also* Epididymitis) 604.90
Died - *see also* Death
  without
    medical attention (cause unknown) 798.9
    sign of disease 798.2
Dientamoeba diarrhea 007.8
Dietary
  inadequacy or deficiency 269.9
  surveillance and counseling V65.3
Dietl's crisis 593.4
Dieulafoy lesion (hemorrhagic)
  of
    duodenum 537.84
    intestine 569.86
    stomach 537.84
Dieulafoy's ulcer - *see* Ulcer, stomach
Difficult
  birth, affecting fetus or newborn 763.9
  delivery NEC 669.9
Difficulty
  feeding 783.3
    breast 676.8
    newborn 779.3
    nonorganic (infant) NEC 307.59
  mechanical, gastroduodenal stoma 537.89
  reading 315.00
  specific, spelling 315.09
  swallowing *(see also* Dysphagia) 787.2
  walking 719.7
Diffuse - *see* condition
Diffused ganglion 727.42
Di George's syndrome (thymic hypoplasia) 279.11
Digestive - *see* condition
Di Guglielmo's disease or syndrome (M9841/3) 207.0
Diktyoma (M9051/3) - *see* Neoplasm, by site, malignant
Dilaceration, tooth 520.4

ICD-9-CM

Vol. 2

Dilatation
anus 564.89
  venule - *see* Hemorrhoids
aorta (focal) (general) (*see also* Aneurysm, aorta) 441.9
  congenital 747.29
  infectional 093.0
  ruptured 441.5
  syphilitic 093.0
appendix (cystic) 543.9
artery 447.8
bile duct (common) (cystic) (congenital) 751.69
  acquired 576.8
bladder (sphincter) 596.8
  congenital 753.8
  in pregnancy or childbirth 654.4
    causing obstructed labor 660.2
      affecting fetus or newborn 763.1
blood vessel 459.89
bronchus, bronchi 494.0
  with acute exacerbation 494.1
calyx (due to obstruction) 593.89
capillaries 448.9
cardiac (acute) (chronic) (*see also* Hypertrophy, cardiac) 429.3
  congenital 746.89
    valve NEC 746.89
      pulmonary 746.09
  hypertensive (*see also* Hypertension, heart) 402.90
cavum septi pellucidi 742.4
cecum 564.89
  psychogenic 306.4
cervix (uteri) - *see also* Incompetency, cervix
incomplete, poor, slow
  affecting fetus or newborn 763.7
  complicating delivery 661.0
    affecting fetus or newborn 763.7
colon 564.7
  congenital 751.3
  due to mechanical obstruction 560.89
  psychogenic 306.4
common bile duct (congenital) 751.69
  acquired 576.8
    with calculus, choledocholithiasis, or stones - *see* Choledocholithiasis
cystic duct 751.69
  acquired (any bile duct) 575.8
duct, mammary 610.4
duodenum 564.89
esophagus 530.89
  congenital 750.4
  due to
    achalasia 530.0
    cardiospasm 530.0
Eustachian tube, congenital 744.24
fontanel 756.0
gallbladder 575.8
  congenital 751.69
gastric 536.8
  acute 536.1
  psychogenic 306.4
heart (acute) (chronic) (*see also* Hypertrophy, cardiac) 429.3
  congenital 746.89
  hypertensive (*see also* Hypertension, heart) 402.90
  valve - *see also* Endocarditis
    congenital 746.89
ileum 564.89
  psychogenic 306.4
inguinal rings - *see* Hernia, inguinal

Dilatation (*Continued*)
jejunum 564.89
  psychogenic 306.4
kidney (calyx) (collecting structures) (cystic) (parenchyma) (pelvis) 593.89
lacrimal passages 375.69
lymphatic vessel 457.1
mammary duct 610.4
Meckel's diverticulum (congenital) 751.0
meningeal vessels, congenital 742.8
myocardium (acute) (chronic) (*see also* Hypertrophy, cardiac) 429.3
organ or site, congenital NEC - *see* Distortion
pancreatic duct 577.8
pelvis, kidney 593.89
pericardium - *see* Pericarditis
pharynx 478.29
prostate 602.8
pulmonary
  artery (idiopathic) 417.8
    congenital 747.3
  valve, congenital 746.09
pupil 379.43
rectum 564.89
renal 593.89
saccule vestibularis, congenital 744.05
salivary gland (duct) 527.8
sphincter ani 564.89
stomach 536.8
  acute 536.1
  psychogenic 306.4
submaxillary duct 527.8
trachea, congenital 748.3
ureter (idiopathic) 593.89
  congenital 753.20
  due to obstruction 593.5
urethra (acquired) 599.84
vasomotor 443.9
vein 459.89
ventricular, ventricle (acute) (chronic) (*see also* Hypertrophy, cardiac) 429.3
  cerebral, congenital 742.4
  hypertensive (*see also* Hypertension, heart) 402.90
venule 459.89
  anus - *see* Hemorrhoids
vesical orifice 596.8
Dilated, dilation - *see* Dilatation
Diminished
hearing (acuity) (*see also* Deafness) 389.9
pulse pressure 785.9
vision NEC 369.9
vital capacity 794.2
Diminuta taenia 123.6
Diminution, sense or sensation (cold) (heat) (tactile) (vibratory) (*see also* Disturbance, sensation) 782.0
Dimitri-Sturge-Weber disease (encephalocutaneous angiomatosis) 759.6
Dimple
parasacral 685.1
  with abscess 685.0
pilonidal 685.1
  with abscess 685.0
postanal 685.1
  with abscess 685.0
Dioctophyma renale (infection) (infestation) 128.8
Dipetalonemiasis 125.4
Diphallus 752.69
Diphtheria, diphtheritic (gangrenous) (hemorrhagic) 032.9
carrier (suspected) of V02.4

Diphtheria, diphtheritic (*Continued*)
cutaneous 032.85
cystitis 032.84
faucial 032.0
infection of wound 032.85
inoculation (anti) (not sick) V03.5
laryngeal 032.3
myocarditis 032.82
nasal anterior 032.2
nasopharyngeal 032.1
neurological complication 032.89
peritonitis 032.83
specified site NEC 032.89
Diphyllobothriasis (intestine) 123.4
larval 123.5
Diplacusis 388.41
Diplegia (upper limbs) 344.2
brain or cerebral 437.8
congenital 343.0
facial 351.0
  congenital 352.6
infantile or congenital (cerebral) (spastic) (spinal) 343.0
lower limbs 344.1
syphilitic, congenital 090.49
Diplococcus, diplococcal - *see* condition
Diplomyelia 742.59
Diplopia 368.2
refractive 368.15
Dipsomania (*see also* Alcoholism) 303.9
with psychosis (*see also* Psychosis, alcoholic) 291.9
Dipylidiasis 123.8
intestine 123.8
Direction, teeth, abnormal 524.30
Dirt-eating child 307.52
Disability
heart - *see* Disease, heart
learning NEC 315.2
special spelling 315.09
Disarticulation (*see also* Derangement, joint) 718.9
meaning
  amputation
    status - *see* Absence, by site
    traumatic - *see* Amputation, traumatic
  dislocation, traumatic or congenital - *see* Dislocation
Disaster, cerebrovascular (*see also* Disease, cerebrovascular, acute) 436
Discharge
anal NEC 787.99
breast (female) (male) 611.79
conjunctiva 372.89
continued locomotor idiopathic (*see also* Epilepsy) 345.5
diencephalic autonomic idiopathic (*see also* Epilepsy) 345.5
ear 388.60
  blood 388.69
  cerebrospinal fluid 388.61
excessive urine 788.42
eye 379.93
nasal 478.1
nipple 611.79
patterned motor idiopathic (*see also* Epilepsy) 345.5
penile 788.7
postnasal - *see* Sinusitis
sinus, from mediastinum 510.0
umbilicus 789.9
urethral 788.7
  bloody 599.84
vaginal 623.5

Discitis 722.90
cervical, cervicothoracic 722.91
lumbar, lumbosacral 722.93
thoracic, thoracolumbar 722.92
Discogenic syndrome - *see* Displacement, intervertebral disc
Discoid
kidney 753.3
meniscus, congenital 717.5
semilunar cartilage 717.5
Discoloration
mouth 528.9
nails 703.8
teeth 521.7
due to
drugs 521.7
metals (copper) (silver) 521.7
pulpal bleeding 521.7
during formation 520.8
extrinsic 523.6 ◀
intrinsic posteruptive 521.7 ◀▥
Discomfort
chest 786.59
visual 368.13
Discomycosis - *see* Actinomycosis
Discontinuity, ossicles, ossicular chain 385.23
Discrepancy
centric occlusion maximum intercuspation 524.55 ◀
leg length (acquired) 736.81
congenital 755.30
uterine size-date 646.8
Discrimination
political V62.4
racial V62.4
religious V62.4
sex V62.4
Disease, diseased - *see also* Syndrome
Abrami's (acquired hemolytic jaundice) 283.9
absorbent system 459.89
accumulation - *see* Thesaurismosis
acid-peptic 536.8
Acosta's 993.2
Adams-Stokes (-Morgagni) (syncope with heart block) 426.9
Addison's (bronze) (primary adrenal insufficiency) 255.4
anemia (pernicious) 281.0
tuberculous (*see also* Tuberculosis) 017.6
Addison-Gull - *see* Xanthoma
adenoids (and tonsils) (chronic) 474.9
adrenal (gland) (capsule) (cortex) 255.9
hyperfunction 255.3
hypofunction 255.4
specified type NEC 255.8
ainhum (dactylolysis spontanea) 136.0
akamushi (scrub typhus) 081.2
Akureyri (epidemic neuromyasthenia) 049.8
Albarrán's (colibacilluria) 791.9
Albers-Schönberg's (marble bones) 756.52
Albert's 726.71
Albright (-Martin) (-Bantam) 275.49
Alibert's (mycosis fungoides) (M9700/3) 202.1
Alibert-Bazin (M9700/3) 202.1
alimentary canal 569.9
alligator skin (ichthyosis congenita) 757.1
acquired 701.1
Almeida's (Brazilian blastomycosis) 116.1
Alpers' 330.8

Disease, diseased (*Continued*)
alpine 993.2
altitude 993.2
alveoli, teeth 525.9
Alzheimer's - *see* Alzheimer's
amyloid (any site) 277.3
anarthritic rheumatoid 446.5
Anders' (adiposis tuberosa simplex) 272.8
Andersen's (glycogenosis IV) 271.0
Anderson's (angiokeratoma corporis diffusum) 272.7
Andes 993.2
Andrews' (bacterid) 686.8
angiopastic, angiospasmodic 443.9
cerebral 435.9
with transient neurologic deficit 435.9
vein 459.89
anterior
chamber 364.9
horn cell 335.9
specified type NEC 335.8
antral (chronic) 473.0
acute 461.0
anus NEC 569.49
aorta (nonsyphilitic) 447.9
syphilitic NEC 093.89
aortic (heart) (valve) (*see also* Endocarditis, aortic) 424.1
apollo 077.4
aponeurosis 726.90
appendix 543.9
aqueous (chamber) 364.9
arc-welders' lung 503
Armenian 277.3
Arnold-Chiari (*see also* Spina bifida) 741.0
arterial 447.9
occlusive (*see also* Occlusion, by site) 444.22
with embolus or thrombus - *see* Occlusion, by site
due to stricture or stenosis 447.1
specified type NEC 447.8
arteriocardiorenal (*see also* Hypertension, cardiorenal) 404.90
arteriolar (generalized) (obliterative) 447.90
specified type NEC 447.8
arteriorenal - *see* Hypertension, kidney
arteriosclerotic - *see also* Arteriosclerosis
cardiovascular 429.2
coronary - *see* Arteriosclerosis, coronary
heart - *see* Arteriosclerosis, coronary
vascular - *see* Arteriosclerosis
artery 447.9
cerebral 437.9
coronary - *see* Arteriosclerosis, coronary
specified type NEC 447.8
arthropod-borne NEC 088.9
specified type NEC 088.89
Asboe-Hansen's (incontinentia pigmenti) 757.33
atticoantral, chronic (with posterior or superior marginal perforation of ear drum) 382.2
auditory canal, ear 380.9
Aujeszky's 078.89
auricle, ear NEC 380.30
Australian X 062.4

Disease, diseased (*Continued*)
autoimmune NEC 279.4
hemolytic (cold type) (warm type) 283.0
parathyroid 252.1
thyroid 245.2
aviators' (*see also* Effect, adverse, high altitude) 993.2
ax(e)-grinders' 502
Ayala's 756.89
Ayerza's (pulmonary artery sclerosis with pulmonary hypertension) 416.0
Azorean (of the nervous system) 334.8
Babington's (familial hemorrhagic telangiectasia) 448.0
back bone NEC 733.90
bacterial NEC 040.89
zoonotic NEC 027.9
specified type NEC 027.8
Baehr-Schiffrin (thrombotic thrombocytopenic purpura) 446.6
Baelz's (cheilitis glandularis apostematosa) 528.5
Baerensprung's (eczema marginatum) 110.3
Balfour's (chloroma) 205.3
balloon (*see also* Effect, adverse, high altitude) 993.2
Baló's 341.1
Bamberger (-Marie) (hypertrophic pulmonary osteoarthropathy) 731.2
Bang's (Brucella abortus) 023.1
Bannister's 995.1
Banti's (with cirrhosis) (with portal hypertension) - *see* Cirrhosis, liver
Barcoo (*see also* Ulcer, skin) 707.9
barium lung 503
Barlow (-Möller) (infantile scurvy) 267
barometer makers' 985.0
Barraquer (-Simons) (progressive lipodystrophy) 272.6
basal ganglia 333.90
degenerative NEC 333.0
specified NEC 333.89
Basedow's (exophthalmic goiter) 242.0
basement membrane NEC 583.89
with
pulmonary hemorrhage (Goodpasture's syndrome) 446.21
[583.81]
Bateman's 078.0
purpura (senile) 287.2
Batten's 330.1 [362.71]
Batten-Mayou (retina) 330.1 [362.71]
Batten-Steinert 359.2
Battey 031.0
Baumgarten-Cruveilhier (cirrhosis of liver) 571.5
bauxite-workers' 503
Bayle's (dementia paralytica) 094.1
Bazin's (primary) (*see also* Tuberculosis) 017.1
Beard's (neurasthenia) 300.5
Beau's (*see also* Degeneration, myocardial) 429.1
Bechterew's (ankylosing spondylitis) 720.0
Becker's (idiopathic mural endomyocardial disease) 425.2
Begbie's (exophthalmic goiter) 242.0
Behr's 362.50
Beigel's (white piedra) 111.2

ICD-9-CM

◻

Vol. 2

Disease, diseased (*Continued*)
Bekhterev's (ankylosing spondylitis) 720.0
Bell's (*see also* Psychosis, affective) 296.0
Bennett's (leukemia) 208.9
Benson's 379.22
Bergeron's (hysteroepilepsy) 300.11
Berlin's 921.3
Bernard-Soulier (thrombopathy) 287.1
Bernhardt (-Roth) 355.1
beryllium 503
Besnier-Boeck (-Schaumann) (sarcoidosis) 135
Best's 362.76
Beurmann's (sporotrichosis) 117.1
Bielschowsky (-Jansky) 330.1
Biermer's (pernicious anemia) 281.0
Biett's (discoid lupus erythematosus) 695.4
bile duct (*see also* Disease, biliary) 576.9
biliary (duct) (tract) 576.9
with calculus, choledocholithiasis, or stones - *see* Choledocholithiasis
Billroth's (meningocele) (*see also* Spina bifida) 741.9
Binswanger's 290.12
Bird's (oxaluria) 271.8
bird fanciers' 495.2
black lung 500
bladder 596.9
specified NEC 596.8
bleeder's 286.0
Bloch-Sulzberger (incontinentia pigmenti) 757.33
Blocq's (astasia-abasia) 307.9
blood (-forming organs) 289.9
specified NEC 289.89
vessel 459.9
Bloodgood's 610.1
Blount's (tibia vara) 732.4
blue 746.9
Bodechtel-Guttmann (subacute sclerosing panencephalitis) 046.2
Boeck's (sarcoidosis) 135
bone 733.90
fibrocystic NEC 733.29
jaw 526.2
marrow 289.9
Paget's (osteitis deformans) 731.0
specified type NEC 733.99
von Recklinghausen's (osteitis fibrosa cystica) 252.01
Bonfils' - *see* Disease, Hodgkin's
Borna 062.9
Bornholm (epidemic pleurodynia) 074.1
Bostock's (*see also* Fever, hay) 477.9
Bouchard's (myopathic dilatation of the stomach) 536.1
Bouillaud's (rheumatic heart disease) 391.9
Bourneville (-Brissaud) (tuberous sclerosis) 759.5
Bouveret (-Hoffmann) (paroxysmal tachycardia) 427.2
bowel 569.9
functional 564.9
psychogenic 306.4
Bowen's (M8081/2) - *see* Neoplasm, skin, in situ
Bozzolo's (multiple myeloma) (M9730/3) 203.0
Bradley's (epidemic vomiting) 078.82
Brailsford's 732.3
radius, head 732.3
tarsal, scaphoid 732.5

Disease, diseased (*Continued*)
Brailsford-Morquio (mucopolysaccharidosis IV) 277.5
brain 348.9
Alzheimer's 331.0
with dementia - *see* Alzheimer's, dementia
arterial, artery 437.9
arteriosclerotic 437.0
congenital 742.9
degenerative - *see* Degeneration, brain
inflammatory - *see also* Encephalitis
late effect - *see* category 326
organic 348.9
arteriosclerotic 437.0
parasitic NEC 123.9
Pick's 331.11
with dementia
with behavioral disturbance 331.11 *[294.11]*
without behavioral disturbance 331.11 *[294.10]*
senile 331.2
braziers' 985.8
breast 611.9
cystic (chronic) 610.1
fibrocystic 610.1
inflammatory 611.0
Paget's (M8540/3) 174.0
puerperal, postpartum NEC 676.3
specified NEC 611.8
Breda's (*see also* Yaws) 102.9
Breisky's (kraurosis vulvae) 624.0
Bretonneau's (diphtheritic malignant angina) 032.0
Bright's (*see also* Nephritis) 583.9
arteriosclerotic (*see also* Hypertension, kidney) 403.90
Brill's (recrudescent typhus) 081.1
flea-borne 081.0
louse-borne 081.1
Brill-Symmers (follicular lymphoma) (M9690/3) 202.0
Brill-Zinsser (recrudescent typhus) 081.1
Brinton's (leather bottle stomach) (M8142/3) 151.9
Brion-Kayser (*see also* Fever, paratyphoid) 002.9
broad
beta 272.2
ligament, noninflammatory 620.9
specified NEC 620.8
Brocq's 691.8
meaning
atopic (diffuse) neurodermatitis 691.8
dermatitis herpetiformis 694.0
lichen simplex chronicus 698.3
parapsoriasis 696.2
prurigo 698.2
Brocq-Duhring (dermatitis herpetiformis) 694.0
Brodie's (joint) (*see also* Osteomyelitis) 730.1
bronchi 519.1
bronchopulmonary 519.1
bronze (Addison's) 255.4
tuberculous (*see also* Tuberculosis) 017.6
Brown-Séquard 344.89
Bruck's 733.99
Bruck-de Lange (Amsterdam dwarf, mental retardation, and brachycephaly) 759.89

Disease, diseased (*Continued*)
Bruhl's (splenic anemia with fever) 285.8
Bruton's (X-linked agammaglobulinemia) 279.04
buccal cavity 528.9
Buchanan's (juvenile osteochondrosis, iliac crest) 732.1
Buchman's (osteochondrosis juvenile) 732.1
Budgerigar-Fanciers' 495.2
Budinger-Ludloff-Läwen 717.89
Büerger's (thromboangiitis obliterans) 443.1
Burger-Grütz (essential familial hyperlipemia) 272.3
Burns' (lower ulna) 732.3
bursa 727.9
Bury's (erythema elevatum diutinum) 695.89
Buschke's 710.1
Busquet's (*see also* Osteomyelitis) 730.1
Busse-Buschke (cryptococcosis) 117.5
C₂ (*see also* Alcoholism) 303.9
Caffey's (infantile cortical hyperostosis) 756.59
caisson 993.3
calculous 592.9
California 114.0
Calvé (-Perthes) (osteochondrosis, femoral capital) 732.1
Camurati-Engelmann (diaphyseal sclerosis) 756.59
Canavan's 330.0
capillaries 448.9
Carapata 087.1
cardiac - *see* Disease, heart
cardiopulmonary, chronic 416.9
cardiorenal (arteriosclerotic) (hepatic) (hypertensive) (vascular) (*see also* Hypertension, cardiorenal) 404.90
cardiovascular (arteriosclerotic) 429.2
congenital 746.9
hypertensive (*see also* Hypertension, heart) 402.90
benign 402.10
malignant 402.00
renal (*see also* Hypertension, cardiorenal) 404.90
syphilitic (asymptomatic) 093.9
carotid gland 259.8
Carrión's (Bartonellosis) 088.0
cartilage NEC 733.90
specified NEC 733.99
Castellani's 104.8
cat-scratch 078.3
Cavare's (familial periodic paralysis) 359.3
Cazenave's (pemphigus) 694.4
cecum 569.9
celiac (adult) 579.0
infantile 579.0
cellular tissue NEC 709.9
central core 359.0
cerebellar, cerebellum - *see* Disease, brain
cerebral (*see also* Disease, brain) 348.9
arterial, artery 437.9
degenerative - *see* Degeneration, brain
cerebrospinal 349.9
cerebrovascular NEC 437.9
acute 436
embolic - *see* Embolism, brain
late effect - *see* Late effect(s) (of) cerebrovascular disease

◀ New   ◀▓ Revised

Disease, diseased (*Continued*)
cerebrovascular NEC (*Continued*)
  acute (*Continued*)
    puerperal, postpartum, childbirth 674.0
    thrombotic - *see* Thrombosis, brain
  arteriosclerotic 437.0
  embolic - *see* Embolism, brain
  ischemic, generalized NEC 437.1
  late effect - *see* Late effect(s) (of) cerebrovascular disease
  occlusive 437.1
  puerperal, postpartum, childbirth 674.0
  specified type NEC 437.8
  thrombotic - *see* Thrombosis, brain
ceroid storage 272.7
cervix (uteri)
  inflammatory 616.9
    specified NEC 616.8
  noninflammatory 622.9
    specified NEC 622.8
Chabert's 022.9
Chagas' (*see also* Trypanosomiasis, American) 086.2
Chandler's (osteochondritis dissecans, hip) 732.7
Charcôt's (joint) 094.0 [713.5]
  spinal cord 094.0
Charcôt-Marie-Tooth 356.1
Charlouis' (*see also* Yaws) 102.9
Cheadle (-Möller) (-Barlow) (infantile scurvy) 267
Chédiak-Steinbrinck (-Higashi) (congenital gigantism of peroxidase granules) 288.2
cheek, inner 528.9
chest 519.9
Chiari's (hepatic vein thrombosis) 453.0
Chicago (North American blastomycosis) 116.0
chignon (white piedra) 111.2
chigoe, chigo (jigger) 134.1
childhood granulomatous 288.1
Chinese liver fluke 121.1
chlamydial NEC 078.88
cholecystic (*see also* Disease, gallbladder) 575.9
choroid 363.9
  degenerative (*see also* Degeneration, choroid) 363.40
  hereditary (*see also* Dystrophy, choroid) 363.50
  specified type NEC 363.8
Christian's (chronic histiocytosis X) 277.89
Christian-Weber (nodular nonsuppurative panniculitis) 729.30
Christmas 286.1
ciliary body 364.9
circulatory (system) NEC 459.9
  chronic, maternal, affecting fetus or newborn 760.3
  specified NEC 459.89
  syphilitic 093.9
    congenital 090.5
Civatte's (poikiloderma) 709.09
climacteric 627.2
  male 608.89
coagulation factor deficiency (congenital) (*see also* Defect, coagulation) 286.9
Coats' 362.12

Disease, diseased (*Continued*)
coccidioidal pulmonary 114.5
  acute 114.0
  chronic 114.4
  primary 114.0
  residual 114.4
Cockayne's (microcephaly and dwarfism) 759.89
Cogan's 370.52
cold
  agglutinin 283.0
    or hemoglobinuria 283.0
      paroxysmal (cold) (nocturnal) 283.2
  hemagglutinin (chronic) 283.0
collagen NEC 710.9
  nonvascular 710.9
  specified NEC 710.8
  vascular (allergic) (*see also* Angiitis, hypersensitivity) 446.20
colon 569.9
  functional 564.9
    congenital 751.3
  ischemic 557.0
combined system (of spinal cord) 266.2 [336.2]
  with anemia (pernicious) 281.0 [336.2]
compressed air 993.3
Concato's (pericardial polyserositis) 423.2
  peritoneal 568.82
  pleural - *see* Pleurisy
congenital NEC 799.89
conjunctiva 372.9
  chlamydial 077.98
    specified NEC 077.8
  specified type NEC 372.89
  viral 077.99
    specified NEC 077.8
connective tissue, diffuse (*see also* Disease, collagen) 710.9
Conor and Bruch's (boutonneuse fever) 082.1
Conradi (-Hünermann) 756.59
Cooley's (erythroblastic anemia) 282.49
Cooper's 610.1
Corbus' 607.1
cork-handlers' 495.3
cornea (*see also* Keratopathy) 371.9
coronary (*see also* Ischemia, heart) 414.9
  congenital 746.85
  ostial, syphilitic 093.20
    aortic 093.22
    mitral 093.21
    pulmonary 093.24
    tricuspid 093.23
Corrigan's - *see* Insufficiency, aortic
Cotugno's 724.3
Coxsackie (virus) NEC 074.8
cranial nerve NEC 352.9
Creutzfeldt-Jakob 046.1
  with dementia
    with behavioral disturbance 046.1 [294.11]
    without behavioral disturbance 046.1 [294.10]
Crigler-Najjar (congenital hyperbilirubinemia) 277.4
Crocq's (acrocyanosis) 443.89
Crohn's (intestine) (*see also* Enteritis, regional) 555.9
Crouzon's (craniofacial dysostosis) 756.0
Cruchet's (encephalitis lethargica) 049.8
Cruveilhier's 335.21

Disease, diseased (*Continued*)
Cruz-Chagas (*see also* Trypanosomiasis, American) 086.2
crystal deposition (*see also* Arthritis, due to, crystals) 712.9
Csillag's (lichen sclerosus et atrophicus) 701.0
Curschmann's 359.2
Cushing's (pituitary basophilism) 255.0
cystic
  breast (chronic) 610.1
  kidney, congenital (*see also* Cystic, disease, kidney) 753.10
  liver, congenital 751.62
  lung 518.89
    congenital 748.4
  pancreas 577.2
    congenital 751.7
  renal, congenital (*see also* Cystic, disease, kidney) 753.10
  semilunar cartilage 717.5
cysticercus 123.1
cystine storage (with renal sclerosis) 270.0
cytomegalic inclusion (generalized) 078.5
  with
    pneumonia 078.5 [484.1]
  congenital 771.1
Daae (-Finsen) (epidemic pleurodynia) 074.1
dancing 297.8
Danielssen's (anesthetic leprosy) 030.1
Darier's (congenital) (keratosis follicularis) 757.39
  erythema annulare centrifugum 695.0
  vitamin A deficiency 264.8
Darling's (histoplasmosis) (*see also* Histoplasmosis, American) 115.00
Davies' 425.0
de Beurmann-Gougerot (sporotrichosis) 117.1
Débove's (splenomegaly) 789.2
deer fly (*see also* Tularemia) 021.9
deficiency 269.9
degenerative - *see also* Degeneration
  disc - *see* Degeneration, intervertebral disc
Degos' 447.8
Déjérine (-Sottas) 356.0
Déleage's 359.89
demyelinating, demyelinizating (brain stem) (central nervous system) 341.9
  multiple sclerosis 340
  specified NEC 341.8
de Quervain's (tendon sheath) 727.04
  thyroid (subacute granulomatous thyroiditis) 245.1
Dercum's (adiposis dolorosa) 272.8
Deutschländer's - *see* Fracture, foot
Devergie's (pityriasis rubra pilaris) 696.4
Devic's 341.0
diaphorase deficiency 289.7
diaphragm 519.4
diarrheal, infectious 009.2
diatomaceous earth 502
Diaz's (osteochondrosis astragalus) 732.5
digestive system 569.9
Di Guglielmo's (erythemic myelosis) (M9841/3) 207.0
Dimitri-Sturge-Weber (encephalocutaneous angiomatosis) 759.6
disc, degenerative - *see* Degeneration, intervertebral disc

ICD-9-CM

Vol. 2

Disease, diseased (*Continued*)

discogenic (*see also* Disease, intervertebral disc) 722.90
diverticular - *see* Diverticula
Down's (mongolism) 758.0
Dubini's (electric chorea) 049.8
Dubois' (thymus gland) 090.5
Duchenne's 094.0
  locomotor ataxia 094.0
  muscular dystrophy 359.1
  paralysis 335.22
  pseudohypertrophy, muscles 359.1
Duchenne-Griesinger 359.1
ductless glands 259.9
Duhring's (dermatitis herpetiformis) 694.0
Dukes (-Filatov) 057.8
duodenum NEC 537.9
  specified NEC 537.89
Duplay's 726.2
Dupré's (meningism) 781.6
Dupuytren's (muscle contracture) 728.6
Durand-Nicolas-Favre (climatic bubo) 099.1
Duroziez's (congenital mitral stenosis) 746.5
Dutton's (trypanosomiasis) 086.9
Eales' 362.18
ear (chronic) (inner) NEC 388.9
  middle 385.9
    adhesive (*see also* Adhesions, middle ear) 385.10
    specified NEC 385.89
Eberth's (typhoid fever) 002.0
Ebstein's
  heart 746.2
  meaning diabetes 250.4 *[581.81]*
Echinococcus (*see also* Echinococcus) 122.9
ECHO virus NEC 078.89
Economo's (encephalitis lethargica) 049.8
Eddowes' (brittle bones and blue sclera) 756.51
Edsall's 992.2
Eichstedt's (pityriasis versicolor) 111.0
Ellis-van Creveld (chondroectodermal dysplasia) 756.55
endocardium - *see* Endocarditis
endocrine glands or system NEC 259.9
  specified NEC 259.8
endomyocardial, idiopathic mural 425.2
Engel-von Recklinghausen (osteitis fibrosa cystica) 252.01 ◄▥
Engelmann's (diaphyseal sclerosis) 756.59
English (rickets) 268.0
Engman's (infectious eczematoid dermatitis) 690.8
enteroviral, enterovirus NEC 078.89
  central nervous system NEC 048
epidemic NEC 136.9
epididymis 608.9
epigastric, functional 536.9
  psychogenic 306.4
Erb (-Landouzy) 359.1
Erb-Goldflam 358.00
Erichsen's (railway spine) 300.16
esophagus 530.9
  functional 530.5
  psychogenic 306.4
Eulenburg's (congenital paramyotonia) 359.2
Eustachian tube 381.9
Evans' (thrombocytopenic purpura) 287.3
external auditory canal 380.9

Disease, diseased (*Continued*)

extrapyramidal NEC 333.90
eye 379.90
  anterior chamber 364.9
  inflammatory NEC 364.3
  muscle 378.9
eyeball 360.9
eyelid 374.9
eyeworm of Africa 125.2
Fabry's (angiokeratoma corporis diffusum) 272.7
facial nerve (seventh) 351.9
  newborn 767.5
Fahr-Volhard (malignant nephrosclerosis) 403.00
fallopian tube, noninflammatory 620.9
  specified NEC 620.8
familial periodic 277.3
  paralysis 359.3
Fanconi's (congenital pancytopenia) 284.0
Farber's (disseminated lipogranulomatosis) 272.8
fascia 728.9
  inflammatory 728.9
Fauchard's (periodontitis) 523.4
Favre-Durand-Nicolas (climatic bubo) 099.1
Favre-Racouchot (elastoidosis cutanea nodularis) 701.8
Fede's 529.0
Feer's 985.0
Felix's (juvenile osteochondrosis, hip) 732.1
Fenwick's (gastric atrophy) 537.89
Fernels' (aortic aneurysm) 441.9
fibrocaseous, of lung (*see also* Tuberculosis, pulmonary) 011.9
fibrocystic - *see also* Fibrocystic, disease
  newborn 277.01
Fiedler's (leptospiral jaundice) 100.0
fifth 057.0
Filatoff's (infectious mononucleosis) 075
Filatov's (infectious mononucleosis) 075
file-cutters' 984.9
  specified type of lead - *see* Table of Drugs and Chemicals
filterable virus NEC 078.89
fish skin 757.1
  acquired 701.1
Flajani (-Basedow) (exophthalmic goiter) 242.0
Flatau-Schilder 341.1
flax-dressers' 504
Fleischner's 732.3
flint 502
fluke - *see* Infestation, fluke
Følling's (phenylketonuria) 270.1
foot and mouth 078.4
foot process 581.3
Forbes' (glycogenosis III) 271.0
Fordyce's (ectopic sebaceous glands) (mouth) 750.26
Fordyce-Fox (apocrine miliaria) 705.82
Fothergill's
  meaning scarlatina anginosa 034.1
  neuralgia (*see also* Neuralgia, trigeminal) 350.1
Fournier's 608.83
fourth 057.8
Fox (-Fordyce) (apocrine miliaria) 705.82
Francis' (*see also* Tularemia) 021.9
Franklin's (heavy chain) 273.2
Frei's (climatic bubo) 099.1

Disease, diseased (*Continued*)

Freiberg's (flattening metatarsal) 732.5
Friedländer's (endarteritis obliterans) - *see* Arteriosclerosis
Friedreich's
  combined systemic or ataxia 334.0
  facial hemihypertrophy 756.0
  myoclonia 333.2
Fröhlich's (adiposogenital dystrophy) 253.8
Frommel's 676.6
frontal sinus (chronic) 473.1
  acute 461.1
Fuller's earth 502
fungus, fungous NEC 117.9
Gaisböck's (polycythemia hypertonica) 289.0
gallbladder 575.9
  congenital 751.60
Gamna's (siderotic splenomegaly) 289.51
Gamstorp's (adynamia episodica hereditaria) 359.3
Gandy-Nanta (siderotic splenomegaly) 289.51
Gannister (occupational) 502
Garré's (*see also* Osteomyelitis) 730.1
gastric (*see also* Disease, stomach) 537.9
gastrointestinal (tract) 569.9
  amyloid 277.3
  functional 536.9
    psychogenic 306.4
Gaucher's (adult) (cerebroside lipidosis) (infantile) 272.7
Gayet's (superior hemorrhagic polioencephalitis) 265.1
Gee (-Herter) (-Heubner) (-Thaysen) (nontropical sprue) 579.0
generalized neoplastic (M8000/6) 199.0
genital organs NEC
  female 629.9
    specified NEC 629.8
  male 608.9
Gerhardt's (erythromelalgia) 443.89
Gerlier's (epidemic vertigo) 078.81
Gibert's (pityriasis rosea) 696.3
Gibney's (perispondylitis) 720.9
Gierke's (glycogenosis I) 271.0
Gilbert's (familial nonhemolytic jaundice) 277.4
Gilchrist's (North American blastomycosis) 116.0
Gilford (-Hutchinson) (progeria) 259.8
Gilles de la Tourette's (motor-verbal tic) 307.23
Giovannini's 117.9
gland (lymph) 289.9
Glanzmann's (hereditary hemorrhagic thrombasthenia) 287.1
glassblowers' 527.1
Glénard's (enteroptosis) 569.89
Glisson's (*see also* Rickets) 268.0
glomerular
  membranous, idiopathic 581.1
  minimal change 581.3
glycogen storage (Andersen's) (Cori types 1-7) (Forbes') (McArdle-Schmid-Pearson) (Pompe's) (types I-VII) 271.0
  cardiac 271.0 *[425.7]*
  generalized 271.0
  glucose-6-phosphatase deficiency 271.0
  heart 271.0 *[425.7]*
  hepatorenal 271.0
  liver and kidneys 271.0

◄ **New** ◄▥ **Revised**

Disease, diseased *(Continued)*
glycogen storage *(Continued)*
myocardium 271.0 *[425.7]*
von Gierke's (glycogenosis I) 271.0
Goldflam-Erb 358.00
Goldscheider's (epidermolysis bullosa)
757.39
Goldstein's (familial hemorrhagic telangiectasia) 448.0
gonococcal NEC 098.0
Goodall's (epidemic vomiting) 078.82
Gordon's (exudative enteropathy)
579.8
Gougerot's (trisymptomatic) 709.1
Gougerot-Carteaud (confluent reticulate papillomatosis) 701.8
Gougerot-Hailey-Hailey (benign familial chronic pemphigus) 757.39
graft-versus-host (bone marrow) 996.85
due to organ transplant NEC - *see*
Complications, transplant, organ
grain-handlers' 495.8
Grancher's (splenopneumonia) - *see*
Pneumonia
granulomatous (childhood) (chronic)
288.1
graphite lung 503
Graves' (exophthalmic goiter) 242.0
Greenfield's 330.0
green monkey 078.89
Griesinger's *(see also* Ancylostomiasis)
126.9
grinders' 502
Grisel's 723.5
Gruby's (tinea tonsurans) 110.0
Guertin's (electric chorea) 049.8
Guillain-Barré 357.0
Guinon's (motor-verbal tic) 307.23
Gull's (thyroid atrophy with myx-
edema) 244.8
Gull and Sutton's - *see* Hypertension,
kidney
gum NEC 523.9
Günther's (congenital erythropoietic
porphyria) 277.1
gynecological 629.9
specified NEC 629.8
H 270.0
Haas' 732.3
Habermann's (acute parapsoriasis var-
ioliformis) 696.2
Haff 985.1
Hageman (congenital factor XII defi-
ciency) *(see also* Defect, congenital)
286.3
Haglund's (osteochondrosis os tibiale
externum) 732.5
Hagner's (hypertrophic pulmonary osteoarthropathy) 731.2
Hailey-Hailey (benign familial chronic
pemphigus) 757.39
hair (follicles) NEC 704.9
specified type NEC 704.8
Hallervorden-Spatz 333.0
Hallopeau's (lichen sclerosus et atrophicus) 701.0
Hamman's (spontaneous mediastinal
emphysema) 518.1
hand, foot, and mouth 074.3
Hand-Schüller-Christian (chronic histiocytosis X) 277.89
Hanot's - *see* Cirrhosis, biliary
Hansen's (leprosy) 030.9
benign form 030.1
malignant form 030.0

Disease, diseased *(Continued)*
Harada's 363.22
Harley's (intermittent hemoglobinuria)
283.2
Hart's (pellagra-cerebellar ataxia-renal
aminoaciduria) 270.0
Hartnup (pellagra-cerebellar ataxia-renal aminoaciduria) 270.0
Hashimoto's (struma lymphomatosa)
245.2
Hb - *see* Disease, hemoglobin
heart (organic) 429.9
with
acute pulmonary edema *(see also*
Failure, ventricular, left) 428.1
hypertensive 402.91
with renal failure 404.92
benign 402.11
with renal failure 404.12
malignant 402.01
with renal failure 404.02
kidney disease - *see* Hypertension, cardiorenal
rheumatic fever (conditions classifiable to 390)
active 391.9
with chorea 392.0
inactive or quiescent (with
chorea) 398.90
amyloid 277.3 *[425.7]*
aortic (valve) *(see also* Endocarditis,
aortic) 424.1
arteriosclerotic or sclerotic (minimal)
(senile) - *see* Arteriosclerosis,
coronary
artery, arterial - *see* Arteriosclerosis,
coronary
atherosclerotic - *see* Arteriosclerosis,
coronary
beer drinkers' 425.5
beriberi 265.0 *[425.7]*
black 416.0
congenital NEC 746.9
cyanotic 746.9
maternal, affecting fetus or newborn 760.3
specified type NEC 746.89
congestive *(see also* Failure, heart
428.0
coronary 414.9
cryptogenic 429.9
due to
amyloidosis 277.3 *[425.7]*
beriberi 265.0 *[425.7]*
cardiac glycogenosis 271.0 *[425.7]*
Friedreich's ataxia 334.0 *[425.8]*
gout 274.82
mucopolysaccharidosis 277.5 *[425.7]*
myotonia atrophica 359.2 *[425.8]*
progressive muscular dystrophy
359.1 *[425.8]*
sarcoidosis 135 *[425.8]*
fetal 746.9
inflammatory 746.89
fibroid *(see also* Myocarditis) 429.0
functional 427.9
postoperative 997.1
psychogenic 306.2
glycogen storage 271.0 *[425.7]*
gonococcal NEC 098.85
gouty 274.82
hypertensive *(see also* Hypertension,
heart) 402.90
benign 402.10
malignant 402.00

Disease, diseased *(Continued)*
heart *(Continued)*
hyperthyroid *(see also* Hyperthyroidism) 242.9 *[425.7]*
incompletely diagnosed - *see* Disease, heart
ischemic (chronic) *(see also* Ischemia,
heart) 414.9
acute *(see also* Infarct, myocardium) 410.9
without myocardial infarction
411.89
with coronary (artery) occlusion 411.81
asymptomatic 412
diagnosed on ECG or other special
investigation but currently presenting no symptoms 412
kyphoscoliotic 416.1
mitral *(see also* Endocarditis, mitral)
394.9
muscular *(see also* Degeneration,
myocardial) 429.1
postpartum 674.8
psychogenic (functional) 306.2
pulmonary (chronic) 416.9
acute 415.0
specified NEC 416.8
rheumatic (chronic) (inactive) (old)
(quiescent) (with chorea) 398.90
active or acute 391.9
with chorea (active) (rheumatic)
(Sydenham's) 392.0
specified type NEC 391.8
maternal, affecting fetus or newborn 760.3
rheumatoid - *see* Arthritis, rheumatoid
sclerotic - *see* Arteriosclerosis, coronary
senile *(see also* Myocarditis) 429.0
specified type NEC 429.89
syphilitic 093.89
aortic 093.1
aneurysm 093.0
asymptomatic 093.89
congenital 090.5
thyroid (gland) *(see also* Hyperthyroidism) 242.9 *[425.7]*
thyrotoxic *(see also* Thyrotoxicosis)
242.9 *[425.7]*
tuberculous *(see also* Tuberculosis)
017.9 *[425.8]*
valve, valvular (obstructive) (regurgitant) - *see also* Endocarditis
congenital NEC *(see also* Anomaly,
heart, valve) 746.9
pulmonary 746.00
specified type NEC 746.89
vascular - *see* Disease, cardiovascular
heavy-chain (gamma G) 273.2
Heberden's 715.04
Hebra's
dermatitis exfoliativa 695.89
erythema multiforme exudativum
695.1
pityriasis
maculata et circinata 696.3
rubra 695.89
pilaris 696.4
prurigo 698.2
Heerfordt's (uveoparotitis) 135
Heidenhain's 290.10
with dementia 290.10
Heilmeyer-Schöner (M9842/3) 207.1

ICD-9-CM

Vol. 2

Disease, diseased *(Continued)*
  Heine-Medin *(see also* Poliomyelitis)
    045.9
  Heller's *(see also* Psychosis, childhood)
    299.1
  Heller-Döhle (syphilitic aortitis) 093.1
  hematopoietic organs 289.9
  hemoglobin (Hb) 282.7
    with thalassemia 282.49
    abnormal (mixed) NEC 282.7
      with thalassemia 282.49
    AS genotype 282.5
    Bart's 282.7
    C (Hb-C) 282.7
      with other abnormal hemoglobin
        NEC 282.7
      elliptocytosis 282.7
      Hb-S (without crisis) 282.63
        with
          crisis 282.64
          vaso-occlusive pain 282.64
      sickle-cell (without crisis) 282.63
        with
          crisis 282.64
          vaso-occlusive pain 282.64
      thalassemia 282.49
    constant spring 282.7
    D (Hb-D) 282.7
      with other abnormal hemoglobin
        NEC 282.7
      Hb-S (without crisis) 282.68
        with crisis 282.69
      sickle-cell (without crisis) 282.68
        with crisis 282.69
      thalassemia 282.49
    E (Hb-E) 282.7
      with other abnormal hemoglobin
        NEC 282.7
      Hb-S (without crisis) 282.68
        with crisis 282.69
      sickle-cell (without crisis) 282.68
        with crisis 282.69
      thalassemia 282.49
    elliptocytosis 282.7
    F (Hb-F) 282.7
    G (Hb-G) 282.7
    H (Hb-H) 282.49
    hereditary persistence, fetal (HPFH)
      ("Swiss variety") 282.7
    high fetal gene 282.7
    I thalassemia 282.49
    M 289.7
    S - *see also* Disease, sickle-cell,
      Hb-S
      thalassemia (without crisis)
        282.41
        with
          crisis 282.42
          vaso-occlusive pain 282.42
    spherocytosis 282.7
    unstable, hemolytic 282.7
    Zurich (Hb-Zurich) 282.7
  hemolytic (fetus) (newborn) 773.2
    autoimmune (cold type) (warm
      type) 283.0
    due to or with
      incompatibility
        ABO (blood group) 773.1
        blood (group) (Duffy) (Kell)
          (Kidd) (Lewis) (M) (S) NEC
          773.2
        Rh (blood group) (factor) 773.0
        Rh negative mother 773.0
    unstable hemoglobin 282.7

Disease, diseased *(Continued)*
  hemorrhagic 287.9
    newborn 776.0
  Henoch (-Schönlein) (purpura nervosa)
    287.0
  hepatic - *see* Disease, liver
  hepatolenticular 275.1
  heredodegenerative NEC
    brain 331.89
    spinal cord 336.8
  Hers' (glycogenosis VI) 271.0
  Herter (-Gee) (-Heubner) (nontropical
    sprue) 579.0
  Herxheimer's (diffuse idiopathic cuta-
    neous atrophy) 701.8
  Heubner's 094.89
  Heubner-Herter (nontropical sprue)
    579.0
  high fetal gene or hemoglobin thalas-
    semia 282.49
  Hildenbrand's (typhus) 081.9
  hip (joint) NEC 719.95
    congenital 755.63
    suppurative 711.05
    tuberculous *(see also* Tuberculosis)
      015.1 *[730.85]*
  Hippel's (retinocerebral angiomatosis)
    759.6
  Hirschfeld's (acute diabetes mellitus)
    (see also Diabetes) 250.0
  Hirschsprung's (congenital megacolon)
    751.3
  His (-Werner) (trench fever) 083.1
  HIV 042
  Hodgkin's (M9650/3) 201.9

  > Note   Use the following fifth-digit
  > subclassification with category 201:
  >
  > 0   unspecified site
  > 1   lymph nodes of head, face, and
  >   neck
  > 2   intrathoracic lymph nodes
  > 3   intra-abdominal lymph nodes
  > 4   lymph nodes of axilla and up-
  >   per limb
  > 5   lymph nodes of inguinal re-
  >   gion and lower limb
  > 6   intrapelvic lymph nodes
  > 7   spleen
  > 8   lymph nodes of multiple sites

    lymphocytic
      depletion (M9653/3) 201.7
        diffuse fibrosis (M9654/3) 201.7
        reticular type (M9655/3) 201.7
      predominance (M9651/3) 201.4
    lymphocytic-histiocytic predomi-
      nance (M9651/3) 201.4
    mixed cellularity (M9652/3) 201.6
    nodular sclerosis (M9656/3) 201.5
      cellular phase (M9657/3) 201.5
  Hodgson's 441.9
    ruptured 441.5
  Hoffa (-Kastert) (liposynovitis prepa-
    tellaris) 272.8
  Holla *(see also* Spherocytosis) 282.0
  homozygous-Hb-S 282.61
  hoof and mouth 078.4
  hookworm *(see also* Ancylostomiasis)
    126.9
  Horton's (temporal arteritis) 446.5
  host-versus-graft (immune or nonim-
    mune cause) 996.80
    bone marrow 996.85
    heart 996.83

Disease, diseased *(Continued)*
  host-versus-graft *(Continued)*
    intestines 996.87
    kidney 996.81
    liver 996.82
    lung 996.84
    pancreas 996.86
    specified NEC 996.89
  HPFH (hereditary persistence of fetal
    hemoglobin) ("Swiss variety")
    282.7
  Huchard's (continued arterial hyper-
    tension) 401.9
  Huguier's (uterine fibroma) 218.9
  human immunodeficiency (virus) 042
  hunger 251.1
  Hunt's
    dyssynergia cerebellaris myoclonica
      334.2
    herpetic geniculate ganglionitis 053.11
  Huntington's 333.4
  Huppert's (multiple myeloma)
    (M9730/3) 203.0
  Hurler's (mucopolysaccharidosis I) 277.5
  Hutchinson's, meaning
    angioma serpiginosum 709.1
    cheiropompholyx 705.81
    prurigo estivalis 692.72
  Hutchinson-Boeck (sarcoidosis) 135
  Hutchinson-Gilford (progeria) 259.8
  hyaline (diffuse) (generalized) 728.9
    membrane (lung) (newborn) 769
  hydatid *(see also* Echinococcus) 122.9
  Hyde's (prurigo nodularis) 698.3
  hyperkinetic *(see also* Hyperkinesia) 314.9
    heart 429.82
  hypertensive *(see also* Hypertension)
    401.9
  hypophysis 253.9
    hyperfunction 253.1
    hypofunction 253.2
  Iceland (epidemic neuromyasthenia)
    049.8
  I cell 272.7
  ill-defined 799.89
  immunologic NEC 279.9
  immunoproliferative 203.8
  inclusion 078.5
    salivary gland 078.5
  infancy, early NEC 779.9
  infective NEC 136.9
  inguinal gland 289.9
  internal semilunar cartilage, cystic 717.5
  intervertebral disc 722.90
    with myelopathy 722.70
    cervical, cervicothoracic 722.91
      with myelopathy 722.71
    lumbar, lumbosacral 722.93
      with myelopathy 722.73
    thoracic, thoracolumbar 722.92
      with myelopathy 722.72
  intestine 569.9
    functional 564.9
      congenital 751.3
      psychogenic 306.4
    lardaceous 277.3
    organic 569.9
    protozoal NEC 007.9
  iris 364.9
  iron
    metabolism 275.0
    storage 275.0
  Isambert's *(see also* Tuberculosis, lar-
    ynx) 012.3

Disease, diseased (*Continued*)
  Iselin's (osteochondrosis, fifth metatarsal) 732.5
  island (scrub typhus) 081.2
  itai-itai 985.5
  Jadassohn's (maculopapular erythroderma) 696.2
  Jadassohn-Pellizari's (anetoderma) 701.3
  Jakob-Creutzfeldt 046.1
    with dementia
      with behavioral disturbance 046.1 [294.11]
      without behavioral disturbance 046.1 [294.10]
  Jaksch (-Luzet) (pseudoleukemia infantum) 285.8
  Janet's 300.89
  Jansky-Bielschowsky 330.1
  jaw NEC 526.9
    fibrocystic 526.2
  Jensen's 363.05
  Jeune's (asphyxiating thoracic dystrophy) 756.4
  jigger 134.1
  Johnson-Stevens (erythema multiforme exudativum) 695.1
  joint NEC 719.9
    ankle 719.97
    Charcôt 094.0 [713.5]
    degenerative (*see also* Osteoarthrosis) 715.9
      multiple 715.09
      spine (*see also* Spondylosis) 721.90
    elbow 719.92
    foot 719.97
    hand 719.94
    hip 719.95
    hypertrophic (chronic) (degenerative) (*see also* Osteoarthrosis) 715.9
      spine (*see also* Spondylosis) 721.90
    knee 719.96
    Luschka 721.90
    multiple sites 719.99
    pelvic region 719.95
    sacroiliac 724.6
    shoulder (region) 719.91
    specified site NEC 719.98
    spine NEC 724.9
      pseudarthrosis following fusion 733.82
      sacroiliac 724.6
    wrist 719.93
  Jourdain's (acute gingivitis) 523.0
  Jüngling's (sarcoidosis) 135
  Kahler (-Bozzolo) (multiple myeloma) (M9730/3) 203.0
  Kalischer's 759.6
  Kaposi's 757.33
    lichen ruber 697.8
      acuminatus 696.4
      moniliformis 697.8
    xeroderma pigmentosum 757.33
  Kaschin-Beck (endemic polyarthritis) 716.00
    ankle 716.07
    arm 716.02
      lower (and wrist) 716.03
      upper (and elbow) 716.02
    foot (and ankle) 716.07
    forearm (and wrist) 716.03
    hand 716.04
    leg 716.06
      lower 716.06
      upper 716.05

Disease, diseased (*Continued*)
  Kaschin-Beck (*Continued*)
    multiple sites 716.09
    pelvic region (hip) (thigh) 716.05
    shoulder region 716.01
    specified site NEC 716.08
  Katayama 120.2
  Kawasaki 446.1
  Kedani (scrub typhus) 081.2
  kidney (functional) (pelvis) (*see also* Disease, renal) 593.9
    cystic (congenital) 753.10
      multiple 753.19
      single 753.11
      specified NEC 753.19
    fibrocystic (congenital) 753.19
    in gout 274.10
    polycystic (congenital) 753.12
      adult type (APKD) 753.13
      autosomal dominant 753.13
      autosomal recessive 753.14
      childhood type (CPKD) 753.14
      infantile type 753.14
  Kienböck's (carpal lunate) (wrist) 732.3
  Kimmelstiel (-Wilson) (intercapillary glomerulosclerosis) 250.4 [581.81]
  Kinnier Wilson's (hepatolenticular degeneration) 275.1
  kissing 075
  Kleb's (*see also* Nephritis) 583.9
  Klinger's 446.4
  Klippel's 723.8
  Klippel-Feil (brevicollis) 756.16
  Knight's 911.1
  Köbner's (epidermolysis bullosa) 757.39
  Koenig-Wichmann (pemphigus) 694.4
  Köhler's
    first (osteoarthrosis juvenilis) 732.5
    second (Freiberg's infraction, metatarsal head) 732.5
    patellar 732.4
    tarsal navicular (bone) (osteoarthrosis juvenilis) 732.5
  Köhler-Freiberg (infraction, metatarsal head) 732.5
  Köhler-Mouchet (osteoarthrosis juvenilis) 732.5
  Köhler-Pellegrini-Stieda (calcification, knee joint) 726.62
  Kok 759.89   ◀
  König's (osteochondritis dissecans) 732.7
  Korsakoff's (nonalcoholic) 294.0
    alcoholic 291.1
  Kostmann's (infantile genetic agranulocytosis) 288.0
  Krabbe's 330.0
  Kraepelin-Morel (*see also* Schizophrenia) 295.9
  Kraft-Weber-Dimitri 759.6
  Kufs' 330.1
  Kugelberg-Welander 335.11
  Kuhnt-Junius 362.52
  Kümmell's (-Verneuil) (spondylitis) 721.7
  Kundrat's (lymphosarcoma) 200.1
  kuru 046.0
  Kussmaul (-Meier) (polyarteritis nodosa) 446.0
  Kyasanur Forest 065.2
  Kyrle's (hyperkeratosis follicularis in cutem penetrans) 701.1

Disease, diseased (*Continued*)
  labia
    inflammatory 616.9
      specified NEC 616.8
    noninflammatory 624.9
      specified NEC 624.8
  labyrinth, ear 386.8
  lacrimal system (apparatus) (passages) 375.9
    gland 375.00
    specified NEC 375.89
  Lafora's 333.2
  Lagleyze-von Hippel (retinocerebral angiomatosis) 759.6
  Lancereaux-Mathieu (leptospiral jaundice) 100.0
  Landry's 357.0
  Lane's 569.89
  lardaceous (any site) 277.3
  Larrey-Weil (leptospiral jaundice) 100.0
  Larsen (-Johansson) (juvenile osteopathia patellae) 732.4
  larynx 478.70
  Lasègue's (persecution mania) 297.9
  Leber's 377.16
  Lederer's (acquired infectious hemolytic anemia) 283.19
  Legg's (capital femoral osteochondrosis) 732.1
  Legg-Calvé-Perthes (capital femoral osteochondrosis) 732.1
  Legg-Calvé-Waldenström (femoral capital osteochondrosis) 732.1
  Legg-Perthes (femoral capital osteochrondosis) 732.1
  Legionnaires' 482.84
  Leigh's 330.8
  Leiner's (exfoliative dermatitis) 695.89
  Leloir's (lupus erythematosus) 695.4
  Lenegre's 426.0
  lens (eye) 379.39
  Leriche's (osteoporosis, posttraumatic) 733.7
  Letterer-Siwe (acute histiocytosis X) (M9722/3) 202.5
  Lev's (acquired complete heart block) 426.0
  Lewandowski's (*see also* Tuberculosis) 017.0
  Lewandowski-Lutz (epidermodysplasia verruciformis) 078.19
  Lewy body 331.82
    with dementia
      with behavioral disturbance 331.82 [294.11]
      without behavioral disturbance 331.82 [294.10]
  Leyden's (periodic vomiting) 536.2
  Libman-Sacks (verrucous endocarditis) 710.0 [424.91]
  Lichtheim's (subacute combined sclerosis with pernicious anemia) 281.0 [336.2]
  ligament 728.9
  light chain 203.0
  Lightwood's (renal tubular acidosis) 588.89   ◀▥
  Lignac's (cystinosis) 270.0
  Lindau's (retinocerebral angiomatosis) 759.6
  Lindau-von Hippel (angiomatosis retinocerebellosa) 759.6
  lip NEC 528.5
  lipidosis 272.7
  lipoid storage NEC 272.7

ICD-9-CM
Vol. 2

Disease, diseased (*Continued*)
Lipschütz's 616.50
Little's - *see* Palsy, cerebral
liver 573.9
  alcoholic 571.3
    acute 571.1
    chronic 571.3
  chronic 571.9
    alcoholic 571.3
  cystic, congenital 751.62
  drug-induced 573.3
  due to
    chemicals 573.3
    fluorinated agents 573.3
    hypersensitivity drugs 573.3
    isoniazids 573.3
  fibrocystic (congenital) 751.62
  glycogen storage 271.0
  organic 573.9
  polycystic (congenital) 751.62
Lobo's (keloid blastomycosis) 116.2
Lobstein's (brittle bones and blue
  sclera) 756.51
locomotor system 334.9
Lorain's (pituitary dwarfism) 253.3
Lou Gehrig's 335.20
Lucas-Championnière (fibrinous bronchitis) 466.0
Ludwig's (submaxillary cellulitis) 528.3
luetic - *see* Syphilis
lumbosacral region 724.6
lung NEC 518.89
  black 500
  congenital 748.60
  cystic 518.89
    congenital 748.4
  fibroid (chronic) (*see also* Fibrosis,
    lung) 515
  fluke 121.2
    Oriental 121.2
  in
    amyloidosis 277.3 [517.8]
    polymyositis 710.4 [517.8]
    sarcoidosis 135 [517.8]
    Sjögren's syndrome 710.2 [517.8]
    syphilis 095.1
    systemic lupus erythematosus
      710.0 [517.8]
    systemic sclerosis 710.1 [517.2]
  interstitial (chronic) 515
    acute 136.3
  nonspecific, chronic 496
  obstructive (chronic) (COPD) 496
    with
      acute ◀▥
        bronchitis 491.22 ◀
        exacerbation NEC 491.21 ◀
      alveolitis, allergic (*see also* Al-
        veolitis, allergic) 495.9
      asthma (chronic) (obstructive)
        493.2
      bronchiectasis 494.0
        with acute exacerbation 494.1
      bronchitis (chronic) 491.20
        with ◀▥
          acute bronchitis 491.22 ◀
          exacerbation (acute) 491.21◀
      emphysema NEC 492.8
      diffuse (with fibrosis) 496
    polycystic 518.89
      asthma (chronic) (obstructive) 493.2
      congenital 748.4
  purulent (cavitary) 513.0
  restrictive 518.89

Disease, diseased (*Continued*)
lung NEC (*Continued*)
  rheumatoid 714.81
    diffuse interstitial 714.81
  specified NEC 518.89
Lutembacher's (atrial septal defect
  with mitral stenosis) 745.5
Lutz-Miescher (elastosis perforans serpiginosa) 701.1
Lutz-Splendore-de Almeida (Brazilian
  blastomycosis) 116.1
Lyell's (toxic epidermal necrolysis)
  695.1
  due to drug
    correct substance properly admin-
      istered 695.1
    overdose or wrong substance
      given or taken 977.9
      specific drug - *see* Table of
        Drugs and Chemicals
Lyme 088.81
lymphatic (gland) (system) 289.9
  channel (noninfective) 457.9
  vessel (noninfective) 457.9
    specified NEC 457.8
lymphoproliferative (chronic) (M9970/
  1) 238.7
Machado-Joseph 334.8
Madelung's (lipomatosis) 272.8
Madura (actinomycotic) 039.9
  mycotic 117.4
Magitot's 526.4
Majocchi's (purpura annularis telangiectodes) 709.1
malarial (*see also* Malaria) 084.6
Malassez's (cystic) 608.89
Malibu 919.8
  infected 919.9
malignant (M8000/3) - *see also* Neoplasm, by site, malignant
  previous, affecting management of
    pregnancy V23.8
Manson's 120.1
maple bark 495.6
maple syrup (urine) 270.3
Marburg (virus) 078.89
Marchiafava (-Bignami) 341.8
Marfan's 090.49
  congenital syphilis 090.49
  meaning Marfan's syndrome 759.82
Marie-Bamberger (hypertrophic pulmonary osteoarthropathy) (secondary) 731.2
  primary or idiopathic (acropachy-
    derma) 757.39
  pulmonary (hypertrophic osteoar-
    thropathy) 731.2
Marie-Strümpell (ankylosing spondylitis) 720.0
Marion's (bladder neck obstruction)
  596.0
Marsh's (exophthalmic goiter) 242.0
Martin's 715.27
mast cell 757.33
  systemic (M9741/3) 202.6
mastoid (*see also* Mastoiditis) 383.9
  process 385.9
maternal, unrelated to pregnancy
  NEC, affecting fetus or newborn
  760.9
Mathieu's (leptospiral jaundice) 100.0
Mauclaire's 732.3
Mauriac's (erythema nodosum syphili-
  ticum) 091.3

Disease, diseased (*Continued*)
Maxcy's 081.0
McArdle (-Schmid-Pearson) (glycogenosis V) 271.0
mediastinum NEC 519.3
Medin's (*see also* Poliomyelitis) 045.9
Mediterranean (with hemoglobinopathy) 282.49
medullary center (idiopathic) (respiratory) 348.8
Meige's (chronic hereditary edema)
  757.0
Meleda 757.39
Ménétrier's (hypertrophic gastritis)
  535.2
Méniére's (active) 386.00
  cochlear 386.02
  cochleovestibular 386.01
  inactive 386.04
  in remission 386.04
  vestibular 386.03
meningeal - *see* Meningitis
mental (*see also* Psychosis) 298.9
Merzbacher-Pelizaeus 330.0
mesenchymal 710.9
mesenteric embolic 557.0
metabolic NEC 277.9
metal polishers' 502
metastatic - *see* Metastasis
Mibelli's 757.39
microdrepanocytic 282.49
microvascular 413.9
Miescher's 709.3
Mikulicz's (dryness of mouth, absent
  or decreased lacrimation) 527.1
Milkman (-Looser) (osteomalacia with
  pseudofractures) 268.2
Miller's (osteomalacia) 268.2
Mills' 335.29
Milroy's (chronic hereditary edema)
  757.0
Minamata 985.0
Minor's 336.1
Minot's (hemorrhagic disease, new-
  born) 776.0
Minot-von Willebrand-Jürgens (an-
  giohemophilia) 286.4
Mitchell's (erythromelalgia) 443.89
mitral - *see* Endocarditis, mitral
Mljet (mal de Meleda) 757.39
Möbius', Moebius' 346.8
Möeller's 267
Möller (-Barlow) (infantile scurvy) 267
Mönckeberg's (*see also* Arteriosclerosis,
  extremities) 440.20
Mondor's (thrombophlebitis of breast)
  451.89
Monge's 993.2
Morel-Kraepelin (*see also* Schizophre-
  nia) 295.9
Morgagni's (syndrome) (hyperostosis
  frontalis interna) 733.3
Morgagni-Adams-Stokes (syncope with
  heart block) 426.9
Morquio (-Brailsford) (-Ullrich) (muco-
  polysaccharidosis IV) 277.5
Morton's (with metatarsalgia) 355.6
Morvan's 336.0
motor neuron (bulbar) (mixed type)
  335.20
Mouchet's (juvenile osteochondrosis,
  foot) 732.5
mouth 528.9
Moyamoya 437.5

◀ **New** ◀▥ **Revised**

Disease, diseased (*Continued*)
  Mucha's (acute parapsoriasis varioli-
    formis) 696.2
  mu-chain 273.2
  mucolipidosis (I) (II) (III) 272.7
  Münchmeyer's (exostosis luxurians)
    728.11
  Murri's (intermittent hemoglobinuria)
    283.2
  muscle 359.9
    inflammatory 728.9
    ocular 378.9
  musculoskeletal system 729.9
  mushroom workers' 495.5
  Myà's (congenital dilation, colon) 751.3
  mycotic 117.9
  myeloproliferative (chronic) (M9960/1)
    238.7
  myocardium, myocardial (*see also* De-
    generation, myocardial) 429.1
    hypertensive (*see also* Hypertension,
      heart) 402.90
    primary (idiopathic) 425.4
  myoneural 358.9
  Naegeli's 287.1
  nail 703.9
    specified type NEC 703.8
  Nairobi sheep 066.1
  nasal 478.1
    cavity NEC 478.1
    sinus (chronic) - *see* Sinusitis
  navel (newborn) NEC 779.89
    delayed separation of umbilical cord
      779.83
  nemaline body 359.0
  neoplastic, generalized (M8000/6)
    199.0
  nerve - *see* Disorder, nerve
  nervous system (central) 349.9
    autonomic, peripheral (*see also* Neu-
      ropathy, peripheral, autonomic)
      337.9
    congenital 742.9
    inflammatory - *see* Encephalitis
    parasympathetic (*see also* Neuropathy,
      peripheral, autonomic) 337.9
    peripheral NEC 355.9
    specified NEC 349.89
    sympathetic (*see also* Neuropathy,
      peripheral, autonomic) 337.9
    vegetative (*see also* Neuropathy, pe-
      ripheral, autonomic) 337.9
  Nettleship's (urticaria pigmentosa)
    757.33
  Neumann's (pemphigus vegetans)
    694.4
  neurologic (central) NEC (*see also* Dis-
    ease, nervous system) 349.9
    peripheral NEC 355.9
  neuromuscular system NEC 358.9
  Newcastle 077.8
  Nicolas (-Durand) -Favre (climatic
    bubo) 099.1
  Niemann-Pick (lipid histiocytosis)
    272.7
  nipple 611.9
    Paget's (M8540/3) 174.0
  Nishimoto (-Takeuchi) 437.5
  nonarthropod-borne NEC 078.89
    central nervous system NEC 049.9
    enterovirus NEC 078.89
  nonautoimmune hemolytic NEC 283.10
  Nonne-Milroy-Meige (chronic heredi-
    tary edema) 757.0

Disease, diseased (*Continued*)
  Norrie's (congenital progressive ocu-
    loacousticocerebral degeneration)
    743.8
  nose 478.1
  nucleus pulposus - *see* Disease, inter-
    vertebral disc
  nutritional 269.9
    maternal, affecting fetus or newborn
      760.4
  oasthouse, urine 270.2
  obliterative vascular 447.1
  Odelberg's (juvenile osteochondrosis)
    732.1
  Oguchi's (retina) 368.61
  Ohara's (*see also* Tularemia) 021.9
  Ollier's (chondrodysplasia) 756.4
  Opitz's (congestive splenomegaly)
    289.51
  Oppenheim's 358.8
  Oppenheim-Urbach (necrobiosis li-
    poidica diabeticorum) 250.8 [709.3]
  optic nerve NEC 377.49
  orbit 376.9
    specified NEC 376.89
  Oriental liver fluke 121.1
  Oriental lung fluke 121.2
  Ormond's 593.4
  Osgood's tibia (tubercle) 732.4
  Osgood-Schlatter 732.4
  Osler (-Vaquez) (polycythemia vera)
    (M9950/1) 238.4
  Osler-Rendu (familial hemorrhagic tel-
    angiectasia) 448.0
  osteofibrocystic 252.01 ◀▥
  Otto's 715.35
  outer ear 380.9
  ovary (noninflammatory) NEC 620.9
    cystic 620.2
    polycystic 256.4
    specified NEC 620.8
  Owren's (congenital) (*see also* Defect,
    coagulation) 286.3
  Paas' 756.59
  Paget's (osteitis deformans) 731.0
    with infiltrating duct carcinoma of
      the breast (M8541/3) - *see* Neo-
      plasm, breast, malignant
    bone 731.0
      osteosarcoma in (M9184/3) - *see*
        Neoplasm, bone, malignant
    breast (M8540/3) 174.0
    extramammary (M8542/3) - *see also*
      Neoplasm, skin, malignant
      anus 154.3
        skin 173.5
    malignant (M8540/3)
      breast 174.0
      specified site NEC (M8542/3) - *see*
        Neoplasm, skin, malignant
      unspecified site 174.0
    mammary (M8540/3) 174.0
    nipple (M8540/3) 174.0
  palate (soft) 528.9
  Paltauf-Sternberg 201.9
  pancreas 577.9
    cystic 577.2
      congenital 751.7
    fibrocystic 277.00
  Panner's 732.3
    capitellum humeri 732.3
    head of humerus 732.3
    tarsal navicular (bone) (osteochon-
      drosis) 732.5
  panvalvular - *see* Endocarditis, mitral

Disease, diseased (*Continued*)
  parametrium 629.9
  parasitic NEC 136.9
    cerebral NEC 123.9
    intestinal NEC 129
    mouth 112.0
    skin NEC 134.9
    specified type - *see* Infestation
    tongue 112.0
  parathyroid (gland) 252.9
    specified NEC 252.8
  Parkinson's 332.0
  parodontal 523.9
  Parrot's (syphilitic osteochondritis)
    090.0
  Parry's (exophthalmic goiter) 242.0
  Parson's (exophthalmic goiter) 242.0
  Pavy's 593.6
  Paxton's (white piedra) 111.2
  Payr's (splenic flexure syndrome) 569.89
  pearl-workers' (chronic osteomyelitis)
    (*see also* Osteomyelitis) 730.1
  Pel-Ebstein - *see* Disease, Hodgkin's
  Pelizaeus-Merzbacher 330.0
    with dementia
      with behavioral disturbance 330.0
        [294.11]
      without behavioral disturbance
        330.0 [294.10]
  Pellegrini-Stieda (calcification, knee
    joint) 726.62
  pelvis, pelvic
    female NEC 629.9
      specified NEC 629.8
    gonococcal (acute) 098.19
      chronic or duration of 2 months
        or over 098.39
    infection (*see also* Disease, pelvis,
      inflammatory) 614.9
    inflammatory (female) (PID) 614.9
      with
        abortion - *see* Abortion, by type,
          with sepsis
        ectopic pregnancy (*see also* cate-
          gories 633.0-633.9) 639.0
        molar pregnancy (*see also* cate-
          gories 630-632) 639.0
      acute 614.3
      chronic 614.4
      complicating pregnancy 646.6
        affecting fetus or newborn 760.8
      following
        abortion 639.0
        ectopic or molar pregnancy 639.0
      peritonitis (acute) 614.5
        chronic NEC 614.7
      puerperal, postpartum, childbirth
        670
      specified NEC 614.8
    organ, female NEC 629.9
      specified NEC 629.8
    peritoneum, female NEC 629.9
      specified NEC 629.8
  penis 607.9
    inflammatory 607.2
  peptic NEC 536.9
    acid 536.8
  periapical tissues NEC 522.9
  pericardium 423.9
    specified type NEC 423.8
  perineum
    female
      inflammatory 616.9
        specified NEC 616.8

ICD-9-CM

▢

Vol. 2

Disease, diseased *(Continued)*
  perineum *(Continued)*
    female *(Continued)*
      noninflammatory 624.9
        specified NEC 624.8
      male (inflammatory) 682.2
    periodic (familial) (Reimann's) NEC
      277.3
      paralysis 359.3
    periodontal NEC 523.9
      specified NEC 523.8
    periosteum 733.90
    peripheral
      arterial 443.9
      autonomic nervous system (*see also*
        Neuropathy, autonomic) 337.9
      nerve NEC (*see also* Neuropathy)
        356.9
        multiple - *see* Polyneuropathy
      vascular 443.9
        specified type NEC 443.89
    peritoneum 568.9
      pelvic, female 629.9
      specified NEC 629.8
    Perrin-Ferraton (snapping hip) 719.65
    persistent mucosal (middle ear) (with
      posterior or superior marginal
      perforation of ear drum) 382.2
    Perthes' (capital femoral osteochon-
      drosis) 732.1
    Petit's (*see also* Hernia, lumbar) 553.8
    Peutz-Jeghers 759.6
    Peyronie's 607.85
    Pfeiffer's (infectious mononucleosis) 075
    pharynx 478.20
    Phocas' 610.1
    photochromogenic (acid-fast bacilli)
      (pulmonary) 031.0
      nonpulmonary 031.9
    Pick's
      brain 331.11
        with dementia
          with behavioral disturbance
            331.11 [294.11]
          without behavioral disturbance
            331.11 [294.10]
      cerebral atrophy 331.11
        with dementia
          with behavioral disturbance
            331.11 [294.11]
          without behavioral disturbance
            331.11 [294.10]
      lipid histiocytosis 272.7
      liver (pericardial pseudocirrhosis of
        liver) 423.2
      pericardium (pericardial pseudocir-
        rhosis of liver) 423.2
      polyserositis (pericardial pseudocir-
        rhosis of liver) 423.2
    Pierson's (osteochondrosis) 732.1
    pigeon fanciers' or breeders' 495.2
    pineal gland 259.8
    pink 985.0
    Pinkus' (lichen nitidus) 697.1
    pinworm 127.4
    pituitary (gland) 253.9
      hyperfunction 253.1
      hypofunction 253.2
    pituitary snuff-takers' 495.8
    placenta
      affecting fetus or newborn 762.2
      complicating pregnancy or childbirth
        656.7
    pleura (cavity) (*see also* Pleurisy) 511.0
    Plummer's (toxic nodular goiter) 242.3

Disease, diseased *(Continued)*
  pneumatic
    drill 994.9
    hammer 994.9
  policeman's 729.2
  Pollitzer's (hidradenitis suppurativa)
    705.83
  polycystic (congenital) 759.89
    kidney or renal 753.12
      adult type (APKD) 753.13
      autosomal dominant 753.13
      autosomal recessive 753.14
      childhood type (CPKD) 753.14
      infantile type 753.14
    liver or hepatic 751.62
    lung or pulmonary 518.89
      congenital 748.4
    ovary, ovaries 256.4
    spleen 759.0
  Pompe's (glycogenosis II) 271.0
  Poncet's (tuberculous rheumatism) (*see
    also* Tuberculosis) 015.9
  Posada-Wernicke 114.9
  Potain's (pulmonary edema) 514
  Pott's (*see also* Tuberculosis) 015.0
    [730.88]
    osteomyelitis 015.0 [730.88]
    paraplegia 015.0 [730.88]
    spinal curvature 015.0 [737.43]
    spondylitis 015.0 [720.81]
  Potter's 753.0
  Poulet's 714.2
  pregnancy NEC (*see also* Pregnancy)
    646.9
  Preiser's (osteoporosis) 733.09
  Pringle's (tuberous sclerosis) 759.5
  Profichet's 729.9
  prostate 602.9
    specified type NEC 602.8
  protozoal NEC 136.8
    intestine, intestinal NEC 007.9
  pseudo-Hurler's (mucolipidosis III)
    272.7
  psychiatric (*see also* Psychosis) 298.9
  psychotic (*see also* Psychosis) 298.9
  Puente's (simple glandular cheilitis) 528.5
  puerperal NEC (*see also* Puerperal) 674.9
  pulmonary - *see also* Disease, lung
    amyloid 277.3 [517.8]
    artery 417.9
    circulation, circulatory 417.9
      specified NEC 417.8
    diffuse obstructive (chronic) 496
      with
        acute bronchitis 491.22 ◄
        asthma (chronic) (obstructive)
          493.2 ◄
        exacerbation NEC (acute) 491.21
    heart (chronic) 416.9
      specified NEC 416.8
    hypertensive (vascular) 416.0
      cardiovascular 416.0
    obstructive diffuse (chronic) 496
      with
        acute bronchitis 491.22 ◄
        asthma (chronic) (obstructive)
          493.2
        bronchitis (chronic) 491.20
          with
            exacerbation (acute) 491.21◄
            exacerbation NEC (acute)
              491.21 ◄
        acute 491.22 ◄
        exacerbation NEC (acute)
          491.21 ◄
    valve (*see also* Endocarditis, pulmo-
      nary) 424.3

Disease, diseased *(Continued)*
  pulp (dental) NEC 522.9
  pulseless 446.7
  Putnam's (subacute combined sclerosis
    with pernicious anemia) 281.0
    [336.2]
  Pyle (-Cohn) (craniometaphyseal dys-
    plasia) 756.89
  pyramidal tract 333.90
  Quervain's
    tendon sheath 727.04
    thyroid (subacute granulomatous
      thyroiditis) 245.1
  Quincke's - *see* Edema, angioneurotic
  Quinquaud (acne decalvans) 704.09
  rag sorters' 022.1
  Raynaud's (paroxysmal digital cyano-
    sis) 443.0
  reactive airway - *see* Asthma
  Recklinghausen's (M9540/1) 237.71
    bone (osteitis fibrosa cystica)   ◄▦
      252.01
  Recklinghausen-Applebaum (hemo-
    chromatosis) 275.0
  Reclus' (cystic) 610.1
  rectum NEC 569.49
  Refsum's (heredopathia atactica poly-
    neuritiformis) 356.3
  Reichmann's (gastrosuccorrhea) 536.8
  Reimann's (periodic) 277.3
  Reiter's 099.3
  renal (functional) (pelvis) 593.9
    with
      edema (*see also* Nephrosis) 581.9
      exudative nephritis 583.89
      lesion of interstitial nephritis 583.89
      stated generalized cause - *see* Ne-
        phritis
    acute - *see* Nephritis, acute
    basement membrane NEC 583.89
      with
        pulmonary hemorrhage (Good-
          pasture's syndrome) 446.21
          [583.81]
    chronic 593.9
    complicating pregnancy or puerpe-
      rium NEC 646.2
      with hypertension - *see* Toxemia,
        of pregnancy
      affecting fetus or newborn 760.1
    cystic, congenital (*see also* Cystic, dis-
      ease, kidney) 753.10
    diabetic 250.4 [583.81]
    due to
      amyloidosis 277.3 [583.81]
      diabetes mellitus 250.4 [583.81]
      systemic lupus erythematosis
        710.0 [583.81]
    end-stage 585
    exudative 583.89
    fibrocystic (congenital) 753.19
    gonococcal 098.19 [583.81]
    gouty 274.10
    hypertensive (*see also* Hypertension,
      kidney) 403.90
    immune complex NEC 583.89
    interstitial (diffuse) (focal) 583.89
    lupus 710.0 [583.81]
    maternal, affecting fetus or newborn
      760.1
      hypertensive 760.0
    phosphate-losing (tubular) 588.0
    polycystic (congenital) 753.12
      adult type (APKD) 753.13
      autosomal dominant 753.13

◄ **New**   ◄▦ **Revised**

Disease, diseased *(Continued)*
  renal *(Continued)*
    polycystic *(Continued)*
      autosomal recessive 753.14
      childhood type (CPKD) 753.14
      infantile type 753.14
      specified lesion or cause NEC *(see also* Glomerulonephritis) 583.89
    subacute 581.9
    syphilitic 095.4
    tuberculous *(see also* Tuberculosis) 016.0 *[583.81]*
    tubular *(see also* Nephrosis, tubular) 584.5
  Rendu-Osler-Weber (familial hemorrhagic telangiectasia) 448.0
  renovascular (arteriosclerotic) *(see also* Hypertension, kidney) 403.90
  respiratory (tract) 519.9
    acute or subacute (upper) NEC 465.9
      due to fumes or vapors 506.3
      multiple sites NEC 465.8
      noninfectious 478.9
      streptococcal 034.0
    chronic 519.9
      arising in the perinatal period 770.7
      due to fumes or vapors 506.4
    due to
      aspiration of liquids or solids 508.9
      external agents NEC 508.9
        specified NEC 508.8
      fumes or vapors 506.9
        acute or subacute NEC 506.3
        chronic 506.4
    fetus or newborn NEC 770.9
    obstructive 496
    specified type NEC 519.8
    upper (acute) (infectious) NEC 465.9
      multiple sites NEC 465.8
      noninfectious NEC 478.9
      streptococcal 034.0
  retina, retinal NEC 362.9
    Batten's or Batten-Mayou 330.1 *[362.71]*
    degeneration 362.89
    vascular lesion 362.17
  rheumatic *(see also* Arthritis) 716.8
    heart - *see* Disease, heart, rheumatic
  rheumatoid (heart) - *see* Arthritis, rheumatoid
  rickettsial NEC 083.9
    specified type NEC 083.8
  Riedel's (ligneous thyroiditis) 245.3
  Riga (-Fede) (cachectic aphthae) 529.0
  Riggs' (compound periodontitis) 523.4
  Ritter's 695.81
  Rivalta's (cervicofacial actinomycosis) 039.3
  Robles' (onchocerciasis) 125.3 *[360.13]*
  Roger's (congenital interventricular septal defect) 745.4
  Rokitansky's *(see also* Necrosis, liver) 570
  Romberg's 349.89
  Rosenthal's (factor XI deficiency) 286.2
  Rossbach's (hyperchlorhydria) 536.8
    psychogenic 306.4
  Roth (-Bernhardt) 355.1
  Runeberg's (progressive pernicious anemia) 281.0
  Rust's (tuberculous spondylitis) *(see also* Tuberculosis) 015.0 *[720.81]*
  Rustitskii's (multiple myeloma) (M9730/3) 203.0
  Ruysch's (Hirschsprung's disease) 751.3
  Sachs (-Tay) 330.1

Disease, diseased *(Continued)*
  sacroiliac NEC 724.6
  salivary gland or duct NEC 527.9
    inclusion 078.5
      streptococcal 034.0
    virus 078.5
  Sander's (paranoia) 297.1
  Sandhoff's 330.1
  sandworm 126.9
  Savill's (epidemic exfoliative dermatitis) 695.89
  Schamberg's (progressive pigmentary dermatosis) 709.09
  Schaumann's (sarcoidosis) 135
  Schenck's (sporotrichosis) 117.1
  Scheuermann's (osteochondrosis) 732.0
  Schilder (-Flatau) 341.1
  Schimmelbusch's 610.1
  Schlatter's tibia (tubercle) 732.4
  Schlatter-Osgood 732.4
  Schmorl's 722.30
    cervical 722.39
    lumbar, lumbosacral 722.32
    specified region NEC 722.39
    thoracic, thoracolumbar 722.31
  Scholz's 330.0
  Schönlein (-Henoch) (purpura rheumatica) 287.0
  Schottmüller's *(see also* Fever, paratyphoid) 002.9
  Schüller-Christian (chronic histiocytosis X) 277.89
  Schultz's (agranulocytosis) 288.0
  Schwalbe-Ziehen-Oppenheimer 333.6
  Schweninger-Buzzi (macular atrophy) 701.3
  sclera 379.19
  scrofulous *(see also* Tuberculosis) 017.2
  scrotum 608.9
  sebaceous glands NEC 706.9
  Secretan's (posttraumatic edema) 782.3
  semilunar cartilage, cystic 717.5
  seminal vesicle 608.9
  Senear-Usher (pemphigus erythematosus) 694.4
  serum NEC 999.5
  Sever's (osteochondrosis calcaneum) 732.5
  Sézary's (reticulosis) (M9701/3) 202.2
  Shaver's (bauxite pneumoconiosis) 503
  Sheehan's (postpartum pituitary necrosis) 253.2
  shimamushi (scrub typhus) 081.2
  shipyard 077.1
  sickle-cell 282.60
    with
      crisis 282.62
      Hb-S disease 282.61
      other abnormal hemoglobin (Hb-D) (Hb-E) (Hb-G) (Hb-J) (Hb-K) (Hb-O) (Hb-P) (high fetal gene) (without crisis) 282.68
        with crisis 282.69
    elliptocytosis 282.60
    Hb-C (without crisis) 282.63
      with
        crisis 282.64
        vaso-occlusive pain 282.64
    Hb-S 282.61
      with
        crisis 282.62
        Hb-C (without crisis) 282.63
          with
            crisis 282.64
            vaso-occlusive pain 282.64

Disease, diseased *(Continued)*
  sickle-cell *(Continued)*
    Hb *(Continued)*
      with *(Continued)*
        other abnormal hemoglobin (Hb-D) (Hb-E) (Hb-G) (Hb-J) (Hb-K) (Hb-O) (Hb-P) (high fetal gene) (without crisis) 282.68
          with crisis 282.69
    spherocytosis 282.60
    thalassemia (without crisis) 282.41
      with
        crisis 282.44
        vaso-occlusive pain 282.42
  Siegal-Cattan-Mamou (periodic) 277.3
  silo fillers' 506.9
  Simian B 054.3
  Simmonds' (pituitary cachexia) 253.2
  Simons' (progressive lipodystrophy) 272.6
  Sinding-Larsen (juvenile osteopathia patellae) 732.4
  sinus - *see also* Sinusitis
    brain 437.9
    specified NEC 478.1
  Sirkari's 085.0
  sixth 057.8
  Sjögren (-Gougerot) 710.2
    with lung involvement 710.2 *[517.8]*
  Skevas-Zerfus 989.5
  skin NEC 709.9
    due to metabolic disorder 277.9
    specified type NEC 709.8
  sleeping *(see also* Narcolepsy) 347.00 ◄▦
    meaning sleeping sickness *(see also* Trypanosomiasis) 086.5
  small vessel 443.9
  Smith-Strang (oasthouse urine) 270.2
  Sneddon-Wilkinson (subcorneal pustular dermatosis) 694.1
  South African creeping 133.8
  Spencer's (epidemic vomiting) 078.82
  Spielmeyer-Stock 330.1
  Spielmeyer-Vogt 330.1
  spine, spinal 733.90
    combined system *(see also* Degeneration, combined) 266.2 *[336.2]*
      with pernicious anemia 281.0 *[336.2]*
    cord NEC 336.9
      congenital 742.9
    demyelinating NEC 341.8
    joint *(see also* Disease, joint, spine) 724.9
    tuberculous 015.0 *[730.8]*
  spinocerebellar 334.9
    specified NEC 334.8
  spleen (organic) (postinfectional) 289.50
    amyloid 277.3
    lardaceous 277.3
    polycystic 759.0
    specified NEC 289.59
  sponge divers' 989.5
  Stanton's (melioidosis) 025
  Stargardt's 362.75
  Startle 759.89 ◄
  Steinert's 359.2
  Sternberg's - *see* Disease, Hodgkin's
  Stevens-Johnson (erythema multiforme exudativum) 695.1
  Sticker's (erythema infectiosum) 057.0
  Stieda's (calcification, knee joint) 726.62
  Still's (juvenile rheumatoid arthritis) 714.30

Disease, diseased (Continued)
  Stiller's (asthenia) 780.79
  Stokes' (exophthalmic goiter) 242.0
  Stokes-Adams (syncope with heart block) 426.9
  Stokvis (-Talma) (enterogenous cyanosis) 289.7
  stomach NEC (organic) 537.9
    functional 536.9
      psychogenic 306.4
    lardaceous 277.3
  stonemasons' 502
  storage
    glycogen (see also Disease, glycogen storage) 271.0
    lipid 272.7
    mucopolysaccharide 277.5
  striatopallidal system 333.90
    specified NEC 333.89
  Strümpell-Marie (ankylosing spondylitis) 720.0
  Stuart's (congenital factor X deficiency) (see also Defect, coagulation) 286.3
  Stuart-Prower (congenital factor X deficiency) (see also Defect, coagulation) 286.3
  Sturge (-Weber) (-Dimitri) (encephalocutaneous angiomatosis) 759.6
  Stuttgart 100.89
  Sudeck's 733.7
  supporting structures of teeth NEC 525.9
  suprarenal (gland) (capsule) 255.9
    hyperfunction 255.3
    hypofunction 255.4
  Sutton's 709.09
  Sutton and Gull's - see Hypertension, kidney
  sweat glands NEC 705.9
    specified type NEC 705.89
  sweating 078.2
  Sweeley-Klionsky 272.4
  Swift (-Feer) 985.0
  swimming pool (bacillus) 031.1
  swineherd's 100.89
  Sylvest's (epidemic pleurodynia) 074.1
  Symmers (follicular lymphoma) (M9690/3) 202.0
  sympathetic nervous system (see also Neuropathy, peripheral, autonomic) 337.9
  synovium 727.9
  syphilitic - see Syphilis
  systemic tissue mast cell (M9741/3) 202.6
  Taenzer's 757.4
  Takayasu's (pulseless) 446.7
  Talma's 728.85
  Tangier (familial high-density lipoprotein deficiency) 272.5
  Tarral-Besnier (pityriasis rubra pilaris) 696.4
  Tay-Sachs 330.1
  Taylor's 701.8
  tear duct 375.69
  teeth, tooth 525.9
    hard tissues NEC 521.9
    pulp NEC 522.9
  tendon 727.9
    inflammatory NEC 727.9
  terminal vessel 443.9
  testis 608.9
  Thaysen-Gee (nontropical sprue) 579.0

Disease, diseased (Continued)
  Thomsen's 359.2
  Thomson's (congenital poikiloderma) 757.33
  Thornwaldt's, Tornwaldt's (pharyngeal bursitis) 478.29
  throat 478.20
    septic 034.0
  thromboembolic (see also Embolism) 444.9
  thymus (gland) 254.9
    specified NEC 254.8
  thyroid (gland) NEC 246.9
    heart (see also Hyperthyroidism) 242.9 [425.7]
    lardaceous 277.3
    specified NEC 246.8
  Tietze's 733.6
  Tommaselli's
    correct substance properly administered 599.7
    overdose or wrong substance given or taken 961.4
  tongue 529.9
  tonsils, tonsillar (and adenoids) (chronic) 474.9
    specified NEC 474.8
  tooth, teeth 525.9
    hard tissues NEC 521.9
    pulp NEC 522.9
  Tornwaldt's (pharyngeal bursitis) 478.29
  Tourette's 307.23
  trachea 519.1
  tricuspid - see Endocarditis, tricuspid
  triglyceride-storage, type I, II, III 272.7
  triple vessel - see Arteriosclerosis, coronary
  trisymptomatic, Gougerot's 709.1
  trophoblastic (see also Hydatidiform mole) 630
    previous, affecting management of pregnancy V23.1
  tsutsugamushi (scrub typhus) 081.2
  tube (fallopian), noninflammatory 620.9
    specified NEC 620.8
  tuberculous NEC (see also Tuberculosis) 011.9
  tubo-ovarian
    inflammatory (see also Salpingo-oophoritis) 614.2
    noninflammatory 620.9
      specified NEC 620.8
  tubotympanic, chronic (with anterior perforation of ear drum) 382.1
  tympanum 385.9
  Uhl's 746.84
  umbilicus (newborn) NEC 779.89
    delayed separation 779.83
  Underwood's (sclerema neonatorum) 778.1
  undiagnosed 799.9
  Unna's (seborrheic dermatitis) 690.18
  unstable hemoglobin hemolytic 282.7
  Unverricht (-Lundborg) 333.2
  Urbach-Oppenheim (necrobiosis lipoidica diabeticorum) 250.8 [709.3]
  Urbach-Wiethe (lipoid proteinosis) 272.8
  ureter 593.9
  urethra 599.9
    specified type NEC 599.84
  urinary (tract) 599.9
    bladder 596.9
      specified NEC 596.8
    maternal, affecting fetus or newborn 760.1

Disease, diseased (Continued)
  Usher-Senear (pemphigus erythematosus) 694.4
  uterus (organic) 621.9
    infective (see also Endometritis) 615.9
    inflammatory (see also Endometritis) 615.9
    noninflammatory 621.9
      specified type NEC 621.8
  uveal tract
    anterior 364.9
    posterior 363.9
  vagabonds' 132.1
  vagina, vaginal
    inflammatory 616.9
      specified NEC 616.8
    noninflammatory 623.9
      specified NEC 623.8
  Valsuani's (progressive pernicious anemia, puerperal) 648.2
    complicating pregnancy or puerperium 648.2
  valve, valvular - see Endocarditis
  van Bogaert-Nijssen (-Peiffer) 330.0
  van Creveld-von Gierke (glycogenosis I) 271.0
  van den Bergh's (enterogenous cyanosis) 289.7
  van Neck's (juvenile osteochondrosis) 732.1
  Vaquez (-Osler) (polycythemia vera) (M9950/1) 238.4
  vascular 459.9
    arteriosclerotic - see Arteriosclerosis
    hypertensive - see Hypertension
    obliterative 447.1
      peripheral 443.9
    occlusive 459.9
    peripheral (occlusive) 443.9
      in diabetes mellitus 250.7 [443.81]
      specified type NEC 443.89
  vas deferens 608.9
  vasomotor 443.9
  vasospastic 443.9
  vein 459.9
  venereal 099.9
    chlamydial NEC 099.50
      anus 099.52
      bladder 099.53
      cervix 099.53
      epididymis 099.54
      genitourinary NEC 099.55
        lower 099.53
        specified NEC 099.54
      pelvic inflammatory disease 099.54
      perihepatic 099.56
      peritoneum 099.56
      pharynx 099.51
      rectum 099.52
      specified site NEC 099.59
      testis 099.54
      vagina 099.53
      vulva 099.53
    fifth 099.1
    sixth 099.1
    complicating pregnancy, childbirth, or puerperium 647.2
    specified nature or type NEC 099.8
      chlamydial - see Disease, venereal, chlamydial
  Verneuil's (syphilitic bursitis) 095.7
  Verse's (calcinosis intervertebralis) 275.49 [722.90]

◀ New   ◀◀◀ Revised

Disease, diseased (*Continued*)
vertebra, vertebral NEC 733.90
  disc - *see* Disease, Intervertebral disc
vibration NEC 994.9
Vidal's (lichen simplex chronicus) 698.3
Vincent's (trench mouth) 101
Virchow's 733.99
virus (filterable) NEC 078.89
  arbovirus NEC 066.9
  arthropod-borne NEC 066.9
  central nervous system NEC 049.9
    specified type NEC 049.8
  complicating pregnancy, childbirth,
    or puerperium 647.6
  contact (with) V01.79 ◀▥
    varicella V01.71 ◀
  exposure to V01.79 ◀▥
    varicella V01.71 ◀
  Marburg 078.89
  maternal
    with fetal damage affecting man-
      agement of pregnancy 655.3
  nonarthropod-borne NEC 078.89
    central nervous system NEC 049.9
      specified NEC 049.8
  vaccination, prophylactic (against)
    V04.89
vitreous 379.29
vocal cords NEC 478.5
Vogt's (Cecile) 333.7
Vogt-Spielmeyer 330.1
Volhard-Fahr (malignant nephrosclerosis) 403.00
Volkmann's
  acquired 958.6
von Bechterew's (ankylosing spondylitis) 720.0
von Economo's (encephalitis lethargica) 049.8
von Eulenburg's (congenital paramyotonia) 359.2
von Gierke's (glycogenosis I) 271.0
von Graefe's 378.72
von Hippel's (retinocerebral angiomatosis) 759.6
von Hippel-Lindau (angiomatosis retinocerebellosa) 759.6
von Jaksch's (pseudoleukemia infantum) 285.8
von Recklinghausen's (M9540/1)
  237.71
  bone (osteitis fibrosa cystica)
    252.01 ◀▥
von Recklinghausen-Applebaum (hemochromatosis) 275.0
von Willebrand (-Jürgens) (angiohemophilia) 286.4
von Zambusch's (lichen sclerosus et
  atrophicus) 701.0
Voorhoeve's (dyschondroplasia) 756.4
Vrolik's (osteogenesis imperfecta)
  756.51
vulva
  noninflammatory 624.9
  specified NEC 624.8
Wagner's (colloid milium) 709.3
Waldenström's (osteochondrosis capital femoral) 732.1
Wallgren's (obstruction of splenic vein
  with collateral circulation) 459.89
Wardrop's (with lymphangitis) 681.9
  finger 681.02
  toe 681.11
Wassilieff's (leptospiral jaundice)
  100.0

Disease, diseased (*Continued*)
wasting NEC 799.4
  due to malnutrition 261
  paralysis 335.21
Waterhouse-Friderichsen 036.3
waxy (any site) 277.3
Weber-Christian (nodular nonsuppura-
  tive panniculitis) 729.30
Wegner's (syphilitic osteochondritis)
  090.0
Weil's (leptospiral jaundice) 100.0
  of lung 100.0
Weir Mitchell's (erythromelalgia) 443.89
Werdnig-Hoffmann 335.0
Werlhof's (*see also* Purpura, thrombo-
  cytopenic) 287.3
Wermer's 258.0
Werner's (progeria adultorum) 259.8
Werner-His (trench fever) 083.1
Werner-Schultz (agranulocytosis) 288.0
Wernicke's (superior hemorrhagic po-
  lioencephalitis) 265.1
Wernicke-Posadas 114.9
Whipple's (intestinal lipodystrophy)
  040.2
whipworm 127.3
white
  blood cell 288.9
    specified NEC 288.8
  spot 701.0
White's (congenital) (keratosis follicu-
  laris) 757.39
Whitmore's (melioidosis) 025
Widal-Abrami (acquired hemolytic
  jaundice) 283.9
Wilkie's 557.1
Wilkinson-Sneddon (subcorneal pustu-
  lar dermatosis) 694.1
Willis' (diabetes mellitus) (*see also* Diabetes) 250.0
Wilson's (hepatolenticular degeneration) 275.1
Wilson-Brocq (dermatitis exfoliativa)
  695.89
winter vomiting 078.82
Wise's 696.2
Wohlfart-Kugelberg-Welander 335.11
Woillez's (acute idiopathic pulmonary
  congestion) 518.5
Wolman's (primary familial xanthoma-
  tosis) 272.7
wool-sorters' 022.1
Zagari's (xerostomia) 527.7
Zahorsky's (exanthem subitum)
  057.8
Ziehen-Oppenheim 333.6
zoonotic, bacterial NEC 027.9
  specified type NEC 027.8
Disfigurement (due to scar) 709.2
head V48.6
limb V49.4
neck V48.7
trunk V48.7
Disgerminoma - *see* Dysgerminoma
Disinsertion, retina 361.04
Disintegration, complete, of the body
  799.89
traumatic 869.1
Disk kidney 753.3
Dislocatable hip, congenital (*see also*
  Dislocation, hip, congenital) 754.30
Dislocation (articulation) (closed) (displacement) (simple) (subluxation)
  839.8

Note

"Closed" includes simple, complete,
partial, uncomplicated, and unspecified dislocation.

"Open" includes dislocation specified
as infected or compound and dislocation with foreign body.

"Chronic," "habitual," "old," or "recurrent" dislocations should be coded
as indicated under the entry "Dislocation, recurrent"; and "pathological"
as indicated under the entry "Dislocation, pathological."

For late effect of dislocation see Late,
effect, dislocation.

with fracture - *see* Fracture, by site
acromioclavicular (joint) (closed)
  831.04
  open 831.14
anatomical site (closed)
  specified NEC 839.69
    open 839.79
  unspecified or ill-defined 839.8
    open 839.9
ankle (scaphoid bone) (closed) 837.0
  open 837.1
arm (closed) 839.8
  open 839.9
astragalus (closed) 837.0
  open 837.1
atlanto-axial (closed) 839.01
  open 839.11
atlas (closed) 839.01
  open 839.11
axis (closed) 839.02
  open 839.12
back (closed) 839.8
  open 839.9
Bell-Dally 723.8
breast bone (closed) 839.61
  open 839.71
capsule, joint - *see* Dislocation, by site
carpal (bone) - *see* Dislocation, wrist
carpometacarpal (joint) (closed) 833.04
  open 833.14
cartilage (joint) - *see also* Dislocation,
  by site
  knee - *see* Tear, meniscus
cervical, cervicodorsal, or cervicothoracic (spine) (vertebra) - *see* Dislocation, vertebra, cervical
chiropractic (*see also* Lesion, nonallopathic) 739.9
chondrocostal - *see* Dislocation, costochondral
chronic - *see* Dislocation, recurrent
clavicle (closed) 831.04
  open 831.14
coccyx (closed) 839.41
  open 839.51
collar bone (closed) 831.04
  open 831.14
compound (open) NEC 839.9
congenital NEC 755.8
  hip (*see also* Dislocation, hip, congen-
    ital) 754.30
  lens 743.37
  rib 756.3
  sacroiliac 755.69
  spine NEC 756.19
  vertebra 756.19

ICD-9-CM
▯
Vol. 2

Dislocation (*Continued*)
coracoid (closed) 831.09
  open 831.19
costal cartilage (closed) 839.69
  open 839.79
costochondral (closed) 839.69
  open 839.79
cricoarytenoid articulation (closed)
  839.69
  open 839.79
cricothyroid (cartilage) articulation
  (closed) 839.69
  open 839.79
dorsal vertebrae (closed) 839.21
  open 839.31
ear ossicle 385.23
elbow (closed) 832.00
  anterior (closed) 832.01
    open 832.11
  congenital 754.89
  divergent (closed) 832.09
    open 832.19
  lateral (closed) 832.04
    open 832.14
  medial (closed) 832.03
    open 832.13
  open 832.10
  posterior (closed) 832.02
    open 832.12
  recurrent 718.32
  specified type NEC 832.09
    open 832.19
eye 360.81
  lateral 376.36
eyeball 360.81
  lateral 376.36
femur
  distal end (closed) 836.50
    anterior 836.52
      open 836.62
    lateral 836.53
      open 836.63
    medial 836.54
      open 836.64
    open 836.60
    posterior 836.51
      open 836.61
  proximal end (closed) 835.00
    anterior (pubic) 835.03
      open 835.13
    obturator 835.02
      open 835.12
    open 835.10
    posterior 835.01
      open 835.11
fibula
  distal end (closed) 837.0
    open 837.1
  proximal end (closed) 836.59
    open 836.69
finger(s) (phalanx) (thumb) (closed)
  834.00
  interphalangeal (joint) 834.02
    open 834.12
  metacarpal (bone), distal end 834.01
    open 834.11
  metacarpophalangeal (joint) 834.01
    open 834.11
  open 834.10
  recurrent 718.34
foot (closed) 838.00
  open 838.10
  recurrent 718.37
forearm (closed) 839.8
  open 839.9

Dislocation (*Continued*)
fracture - *see* Fracture, by site
glenoid (closed) 831.09
  open 831.19
habitual - *see* Dislocation, recurrent
hand (closed) 839.8
  open 839.9
hip (closed) 835.00
  anterior 835.03
    obturator 835.02
      open 835.12
    open 835.13
  congenital (unilateral) 754.30
    with subluxation of other hip 754.35
    bilateral 754.31
  developmental 718.75
  open 835.10
  posterior 835.01
    open 835.11
  recurrent 718.35
humerus (closed) 831.00
  distal end (*see also* Dislocation, el-
    bow) 832.00
  open 831.10
  proximal end (closed) 831.00
    anterior (subclavicular) (subcora-
      coid) (subglenoid) (closed)
      831.01
      open 831.11
    inferior (closed) 831.03
      open 831.13
    open 831.10
    posterior (closed) 831.02
      open 831.12
implant - *see* Complications, mechanical
incus 385.23
infracoracoid (closed) 831.01
  open 831.11
innominate (pubic junction) (sacral
  junction) (closed) 839.69
  acetabulum (*see also* Dislocation, hip)
    835.00
  open 839.79
interphalangeal (joint)
  finger or hand (closed) 834.02
    open 834.12
  foot or toe (closed) 838.06
    open 838.16
jaw (cartilage) (meniscus) (closed)
  830.0
  open 830.1
  recurrent 524.69
joint NEC (closed) 839.8
  developmental 718.7
  open 839.9
  pathological - *see* Dislocation, patho-
    logical
  recurrent - *see* Dislocation, recurrent
knee (closed) 836.50
  anterior 836.51
    open 836.61
  congenital (with genu recurvatum)
    754.41
  habitual 718.36
  lateral 836.54
    open 836.64
  medial 836.53
    open 836.63
  old 718.36
  open 836.60
  posterior 836.52
    open 836.62
  recurrent 718.36
  rotatory 836.59
    open 836.69

Dislocation (*Continued*)
lacrimal gland 375.16
leg (closed) 839.8
  open 839.9
lens (crystalline) (complete) (partial)
  379.32
  anterior 379.33
  congenital 743.37
  ocular implant 996.53
  posterior 379.34
  traumatic 921.3
ligament - *see* Dislocation, by site
lumbar (vertebrae) (closed) 839.20
  open 839.30
lumbosacral (vertebrae) (closed) 839.20
  congenital 756.19
  open 839.30
mandible (closed) 830.0
  open 830.1
maxilla (inferior) (closed) 830.0
  open 830.1
meniscus (knee) - *see also* Tear, meniscus
  other sites - *see* Dislocation, by site
metacarpal (bone)
  distal end (closed) 834.01
    open 834.11
  proximal end (closed) 833.05
    open 833.15
metacarpophalangeal (joint) (closed)
  834.01
  open 834.11
metatarsal (bone) (closed) 838.04
  open 838.14
metatarsophalangeal (joint) (closed)
  838.05
  open 838.15
midcarpal (joint) (closed) 833.03
  open 833.13
midtarsal (joint) (closed) 838.02
  open 838.12
Monteggia's - *see* Dislocation, hip
multiple locations (except fingers only
  or toes only) (closed) 839.8
  open 839.9
navicular (bone) foot (closed) 837.0
  open 837.1
neck (*see also* Dislocation, vertebra, cervical) 839.00
Nélaton's - *see* Dislocation, ankle
nontraumatic (joint) - *see* Dislocation,
  pathological
nose (closed) 839.69
  open 839.79
not recurrent, not current injury - *see*
  Dislocation, pathological
occiput from atlas (closed) 839.01
  open 839.11
old - *see* Dislocation, recurrent
open (compound) NEC 839.9
ossicle, ear 385.23
paralytic (flaccid) (spastic) - *see* Dislocation, pathological
patella (closed) 836.3
  congenital 755.64
  open 836.4
pathological NEC 718.20
  ankle 718.27
  elbow 718.22
  foot 718.27
  hand 718.24
  hip 718.25
  knee 718.26
  lumbosacral joint 724.6

◀ **New**   ◀▥ **Revised**

Dislocation (*Continued*)
  pathological NEC (*Continued*)
    multiple sites 718.29
    pelvic region 718.25
    sacroiliac 724.6
    shoulder (region) 718.21
    specified site NEC 718.28
    spine 724.8
      sacroiliac 724.6
    wrist 718.23
  pelvis (closed) 839.69
    acetabulum (*see also* Dislocation, hip) 835.00
    open 839.79
  phalanx
    foot or toe (closed) 838.09
      open 838.19
    hand or finger (*see also* Dislocation, finger) 834.00
  postpoliomyelitic - *see* Dislocation, pathological
  prosthesis, internal - *see* Complications, mechanical
  radiocarpal (joint) (closed) 833.02
    open 833.12
  radioulnar (joint)
    distal end (closed) 833.01
      open 833.11
    proximal end (*see also* Dislocation, elbow) 832.00
  radius
    distal end (closed) 833.00
      open 833.10
    proximal end (closed) 832.01
      open 832.11
  recurrent (*see also* Derangement, joint, recurrent) 718.3
    elbow 718.32
    hip 718.35
    joint NEC 718.38
    knee 718.36
    lumbosacral (joint) 724.6
    patella 718.36
    sacroiliac 724.6
    shoulder 718.31
    temporomandibular 524.69
  rib (cartilage) (closed) 839.69
    congenital 756.3
    open 839.79
  sacrococcygeal (closed) 839.42
    open 839.52
  sacroiliac (joint) (ligament) (closed) 839.42
    congenital 755.69
    open 839.52
    recurrent 724.6
  sacrum (closed) 839.42
    open 839.52
  scaphoid (bone)
    ankle or foot (closed) 837.0
      open 837.1
    wrist (closed) (*see also* Dislocation, wrist) 833.00
      open 833.10
  scapula (closed) 831.09
    open 831.19
  semilunar cartilage, knee - *see* Tear, meniscus
  septal cartilage (nose) (closed) 839.69
    open 839.79
  septum (nasal) (old) 470
  sesamoid bone - *see* Dislocation, by site
  shoulder (blade) (ligament) (closed) 831.00

Dislocation (*Continued*)
  shoulder (*Continued*)
    anterior (subclavicular) (subcoracoid) (subglenoid) (closed) 831.01
      open 831.11
    chronic 718.31
    inferior 831.03
      open 831.13
    open 831.10
    posterior (closed) 831.02
      open 831.12
    recurrent 718.31
  skull - *see* Injury, intracranial
  Smith's - *see* Dislocation, foot
  spine (articular process) (*see also* Dislocation, vertebra) (closed) 839.40
    atlanto-axial (closed) 839.01
      open 839.11
      recurrent 723.8
    cervical, cervicodorsal, cervicothoracic (closed) (*see also* Dislocation, vertebrae, cervical) 839.00
      open 839.10
      recurrent 723.8
    coccyx 839.41
      open 839.51
    congenital 756.19
    due to birth trauma 767.4
    open 839.50
    recurrent 724.9
    sacroiliac 839.42
      recurrent 724.6
    sacrum (sacrococcygeal) (sacroiliac) 839.42
      open 839.52
  spontaneous - *see* Dislocation, pathological
  sternoclavicular (joint) (closed) 839.61
    open 839.71
  sternum (closed) 839.61
    open 839.71
  subastragalar - *see* Dislocation, foot
  subglenoid (closed) 831.01
    open 831.11
  symphysis
    jaw (closed) 830.0
      open 830.1
    mandibular (closed) 830.0
      open 830.1
    pubis (closed) 839.69
      open 839.79
  tarsal (bone) (joint) 838.01
    open 838.11
  tarsometatarsal (joint) 838.03
    open 838.13
  temporomandibular (joint) (closed) 830.0
    open 830.1
    recurrent 524.69
  thigh
    distal end (*see also* Dislocation, femur, distal end) 836.50
    proximal end (*see also* Dislocation, hip) 835.00
  thoracic (vertebrae) (closed) 839.21
    open 839.31
  thumb(s) (*see also* Dislocation, finger) 834.00
  thyroid cartilage (closed) 839.69
    open 839.79
  tibia
    distal end (closed) 837.0
      open 837.1

Dislocation (*Continued*)
  tibia (*Continued*)
    proximal end (closed) 836.50
      anterior 836.51
        open 836.61
      lateral 836.54
        open 836.64
      medial 836.53
        open 836.63
      open 836.60
      posterior 836.52
        open 836.62
      rotatory 836.59
        open 836.69
  tibiofibular
    distal (closed) 837.0
      open 837.1
    superior (closed) 836.59
      open 836.69
  toe(s) (closed) 838.09
    open 838.19
  trachea (closed) 839.69
    open 839.79
  ulna
    distal end (closed) 833.09
      open 833.19
    proximal end - *see* Dislocation, elbow
  vertebra (articular process) (body) (closed) 839.40
    cervical, cervicodorsal or cervicothoracic (closed) 839.00
      first (atlas) 839.01
        open 839.11
      second (axis) 839.02
        open 839.12
      third 839.03
        open 839.13
      fourth 839.04
        open 839.14
      fifth 839.05
        open 839.15
      sixth 839.06
        open 839.16
      seventh 839.07
        open 839.17
      congenital 756.19
      multiple sites 839.08
        open 839.18
      open 839.10
    congenital 756.19
    dorsal 839.21
      open 839.31
      recurrent 724.9
    lumbar, lumbosacral 839.20
      open 839.30
    open NEC 839.50
    recurrent 724.9
    specified region NEC 839.49
      open 839.59
    thoracic 839.21
      open 839.31
  wrist (carpal bone) (scaphoid) (semilunar) (closed) 833.00
    carpometacarpal (joint) 833.04
      open 833.14
    metacarpal bone, proximal end 833.05
      open 833.15
    midcarpal (joint) 833.03
      open 833.13
    open 833.10
    radiocarpal (joint) 833.02
      open 833.12
    radioulnar (joint) 833.01
      open 833.11

ICD-9-CM

D

Vol. 2

Dislocation (*Continued*)
  wrist (*Continued*)
    recurrent 718.33
    specified site NEC 833.09
      open 833.19
  xiphoid cartilage (closed) 839.61
    open 839.71
Dislodgement
  artificial skin graft 996.55
  decellularized allodermis graft 996.55
Disobedience, hostile (covert) (overt)
  (*see also* Disturbance, conduct) 312.0
Disorder - *see also* Disease
  academic underachievement, child-
    hood and adolescence 313.83
  accommodation 367.51
    drug-induced 367.89
    toxic 367.89
  adjustment (*see also* Reaction, adjust-
    ment) 309.9
    with ◄
      anxiety 309.24 ◄
      anxiety and depressed mood
        309.23 ◄
      depressed mood 309.0 ◄
      disturbance of conduct 309.3 ◄
      disturbance of emotions and con-
        duct 309.4
  adrenal (capsule) (cortex) (gland) 255.9
    specified type NEC 255.8
  adrenogenital 255.2
  affective (*see also* Psychosis, affective)
    296.90
    atypical 296.81
  aggressive, unsocialized (*see also* Dis-
    turbance, conduct) 312.0
  alcohol, alcoholic (*see also* Alcohol) 291.9
  allergic - *see* Allergy
  amino acid (metabolic) (*see also* Distur-
    bance, metabolism, amino acid)
    270.9
    albinism 270.2
    alkaptonuria 270.2
    argininosuccinicaciduria 270.6
    beta-amino-isobutyricaciduria 277.2
    cystathioninuria 270.4
    cystinosis 270.0
    cystinuria 270.0
    glycinuria 270.0
    homocystinuria 270.4
    imidazole 270.5
    maple syrup (urine) disease 270.3
    neonatal, transitory 775.8
    oasthouse urine disease 270.2
    ochronosis 270.2
    phenylketonuria 270.1
    phenylpyruvic oligophrenia 270.1
    purine NEC 277.2
    pyrimidine NEC 277.2
    renal transport NEC 270.0
    specified type NEC 270.8
    transport NEC 270.0
      renal 270.0
    xanthinuria 277.2
  amnestic (*see also* Amnestic syndrome)
    294.8 ◄▥
    alcohol-induced persisting 291.1 ◄
    drug-induced persisting 292.83 ◄
    in conditions classified elsewhere
      294.0 ◄
  anaerobic glycolysis with anemia 282.3
  anxiety (*see also* Anxiety) 300.00
    due to or associated with physical
      condition 293.84

Disorder (*Continued*)
  arteriole 447.9
    specified type NEC 447.8
  artery 447.9
    specified type NEC 447.8
  articulation - *see* Disorder, joint
  Asperger's 299.8
  attachment of infancy or early child-
    hood 313.89 ◄▥
  attention deficit 314.00
    with hyperactivity 314.01
    predominantly
      combined hyperactive/inattentive
        314.01
      hyperactive/impulsive 314.01
      inattentive 314.00
    residual type 314.8
  autistic 299.0
  autoimmune NEC 279.4
    hemolytic (cold type) (warm type)
      283.0
    parathyroid 252.1
    thyroid 245.2
  avoidant, childhood or adolescence
    313.21
  balance
    acid-base 276.9
      mixed (with hypercapnia) 276.4
    electrolyte 276.9
    fluid 276.9
  behavior NEC (*see also* Disturbance,
    conduct) 312.9
    disruptive 312.9 ◄
  bilirubin excretion 277.4
  bipolar (affective) (alternating)
    296.80 ◄▥

Note Use the following fifth-digit subclassification with category 296.0–296.6: ◄
0 unspecified ◄
1 mild ◄
2 moderate ◄
3 severe, without mention of psychotic behavior
4 severe, specified as with psychotic behavior
5 in partial or unspecified remission ◄
6 in full remission ◄

    atypical 296.7
    currently
      depressed 296.5
      hypomanic 296.4
      manic 296.4
      mixed 296.6
    specified type NEC 296.89 ◄
    type 1 296.7 ◄
      most recent episode (or current)◄▥
        depressed 296.5 ◄
        hypomanic 296.4 ◄
        manic 296.4 ◄
        mixed 296.6 ◄
        unspecified 296.7 ◄
      single manic episode 296.0 ◄
    type II (recurrent major depressive
      episodes with hypomania)
      296.89 ◄▥
  bladder 596.9
    functional NEC 596.59
    specified NEC 596.8
  bone NEC 733.90
    specified NEC 733.99
  brachial plexus 353.0

Disorder (*Continued*)
  branched-chain amino-acid degrada-
    tion 270.3
  breast 611.9
    puerperal, postpartum 676.3
    specified NEC 611.8
  Briquet's 300.81
  bursa 727.9
    shoulder region 726.10
  carbohydrate metabolism, congenital
    271.9
  cardiac, functional 427.9
    postoperative 997.1
    psychogenic 306.2
  cardiovascular, psychogenic 306.2
  cartilage NEC 733.90
    articular 718.00
      ankle 718.07
      elbow 718.02
      foot 718.07
      hand 718.04
      hip 718.05
      knee 717.9
      multiple sites 718.09
      pelvic region 718.05
      shoulder region 718.01
      specified
        site NEC 718.08
        type NEC 733.99
      wrist 718.03
  catatonic—*see* Catatonia
  cervical region NEC 723.9
  cervical root (nerve) NEC 353.2
  character NEC (*see also* Disorder, per-
    sonality) 301.9
  coagulation (factor) (*see also* Defect, co-
    agulation) 286.9
    factor VIII (congenital) (functional)
      286.0
    factor IX (congenital) (functional) 286.1
    neonatal, transitory 776.3
  coccyx 724.70
    specified NEC 724.79
  cognitive 294.9
  colon 569.9
    functional 564.9
      congenital 751.3
  communication 307.9 ◄
  conduct (*see also* Disturbance, conduct)
    312.9
    adjustment reaction 309.3
    adolescent onset type 312.82
    childhood onset type 312.81
    compulsive 312.30
      specified type NEC 312.39
    hyperkinetic 314.2
    onset unspecified 312.89 ◄
    socialized (type) 312.20
      aggressive 312.23
      unaggressive 312.21
    specified NEC 312.89
  conduction, heart 426.9
    specified NEC 426.89
  conflict ◄
    sexual orientation 302.0 ◄
  convulsive (secondary) (*see also* Con-
    vulsions) 780.39
    due to injury at birth 767.0
    idiopathic 780.39
  coordination 781.3
  cornea NEC 371.89
    due to contact lens 371.82
  corticosteroid metabolism NEC 255.2
  cranial nerve - *see* Disorder, nerve, cra-
    nial

◄ **New**   ◄▥ **Revised**

Disorder *(Continued)*
  cyclothymic 301.13
  degradation, branched-chain amino
      acid 270.3
  delusional 297.1 ◀▥
  dentition 520.6
  depersonalization 300.6 ◀
  depressive NEC 311
    atypical 296.82
    major *(see also* Psychosis, affective)
        296.2
      recurrent episode 296.3
      single episode 296.2
  development, specific 315.9
    associated with hyperkinesia 314.1
    coordination 315.4 ◀
    language 315.31
    learning 315.2
      arithmetical 315.1
      reading 315.00
    mixed 315.5
    motor coordination 315.4
    specified type NEC 315.8
    speech 315.39
  diaphragm 519.4
  digestive 536.9
    fetus or newborn 777.9
      specified NEC 777.8
    psychogenic 306.4
  disintegrative childhood 299.1 ◀▥
  dissociative 300.15 ◀▥
    identity 300.14
    nocturnal 307.47 ◀
  drug-related 292.9 ◀
  dysmorphic body 300.7
  dysthymic 300.4
  ear 388.9
    degenerative NEC 388.00
    external 380.9
      specified 380.89
    pinna 380.30
    specified type NEC 388.8
    vascular NEC 388.00
  eating NEC 307.50
  electrolyte NEC 276.9
    with
      abortion - *see* Abortion, by type,
          with metabolic disorder
      ectopic pregnancy *(see also* catego-
          ries 633.0-633.9) 639.4
      molar pregnancy *(see also* catego-
          ries 630-632) 639.4
    acidosis 276.2
      metabolic 276.2
      respiratory 276.2
    alkalosis 276.3
      metabolic 276.3
      respiratory 276.3
    following
      abortion 639.4
      ectopic or molar pregnancy 639.4
    neonatal, transitory NEC 775.5
  emancipation as adjustment reaction
      309.22
  emotional *(see also* Disorder, mental,
      nonpsychotic) V40.9
  endocrine 259.9
    specified type NEC 259.8
  esophagus 530.9
    functional 530.5
    psychogenic 306.4
  explosive
    intermittent 312.34
    isolated 312.35

Disorder *(Continued)*
  expressive language 315.31
  eye 379.90
    globe - *see* Disorder, globe
    ill-defined NEC 379.99
    limited duction NEC 378.63
    specified NEC 379.8
  eyelid 374.9
    degenerative 374.50
    sensory 374.44
    specified type NEC 374.89
    vascular 374.85
  factitious (with combined psychologi-
      cal and physical signs and symp-
      toms) (with predominantly physi-
      cal signs and symptoms)
      300.19 ◀▥
    with predominantly psychological
        signs and symptoms 300.16 ◀
  factor, coagulation *(see also* Defect, co-
      agulation) 286.9
    VIII (congenital) (functional) 286.0
    IX (congenital) (functional) 286.1
  fascia 728.9
  fatty acid oxidation 277.85 ◀
  feeding - *see* Feeding
  female sexual arousal 302.72
  fluid NEC 276.9
  gastric (functional) 536.9
    motility 536.8
    psychogenic 306.4
    secretion 536.8
  gastrointestinal (functional) NEC
      536.9
    newborn (neonatal) 777.9
      specified NEC 777.8
    psychogenic 306.4
  gender (child) 302.6
    adolescents 302.85 ◀
    adults (-life) 302.85 ◀▥
  gender identity (childhood) 302.6
    adult-life 302.85
  genitourinary system, psychogenic
      306.50
  globe 360.9
    degenerative 360.20
      specified NEC 360.29
    specified type NEC 360.89
  hearing - *see also* Deafness
    conductive type (air) *(see also* Deaf-
        ness, conductive) 389.00
    mixed conductive and sensorineural
        389.2
    nerve 389.12
    perceptive *(see also* Deafness, percep-
        tive) 389.10
    sensorineural type NEC *(see also*
        Deafness, perceptive) 389.10
  heart action 427.9
    postoperative 997.1
  hematological, transient neonatal 776.9
    specified type NEC 776.8
  hematopoietic organs 289.9
  hemorrhagic NEC 287.9
    due to intrinsic circulating anticoag-
        ulants 286.5 ◀▥
    specified type NEC 287.8
  hemostasis *(see also* Defect, coagula-
      tion) 286.9
  homosexual conflict 302.0
  hypomanic (chronic) 301.11
  identity
    childhood and adolescence 313.82
    gender 302.6

Disorder *(Continued)*
  immune mechanism (immunity) 279.9
    single complement (C_1-C_9) 279.8
    specified type NEC 279.8
  impulse control *(see also* Disturbance,
      conduct, compulsive) 312.30
  infant sialic acid storage 271.8
  integument, fetus or newborn 778.9
    specified type NEC 778.8
  interactional psychotic (childhood) *(see
      also* Psychosis, childhood) 299.1
  intermittent explosive 312.34
  intervertebral disc 722.90
    cervical, cervicothoracic 722.91
    lumbar, lumbosacral 722.93
    thoracic, thoracolumbar 722.92
  intestinal 569.9
    functional NEC 564.9
      congenital 751.3
      postoperative 564.4
    psychogenic 306.4
  introverted, of childhood and adoles-
      cence 313.22
  iron, metabolism 275.0
  isolated explosive 312.35
  joint NEC 719.90
    ankle 719.97
    elbow 719.92
    foot 719.97
    hand 719.94
    hip 719.95
    knee 719.96
    multiple sites 719.99
    pelvic region 719.95
    psychogenic 306.0
    shoulder (region) 719.91
    specified site NEC 719.98
    temporomandibular 524.60
      sounds on opening or closing
          524.64 ◀
      specified NEC 524.69
    wrist 719.93
  kidney 593.9
    functional 588.9
      specified NEC 588.89 ◀▥
  labyrinth, labyrinthine 386.9
    specified type NEC 386.8
  lactation 676.9
  language (developmental) (expressive)
      315.31
    mixed receptive-expressive 315.32 ◀▥
  learning 315.9 ◀
  ligament 728.9
  ligamentous attachments, peripheral -
      see also Enthesopathy
    spine 720.1
  limb NEC 729.9
    psychogenic 306.0
  lipid
    metabolism, congenital 272.9
    storage 272.7
  lipoprotein deficiency (familial) 272.5
  low back NEC 724.9
    psychogenic 306.0
  lumbosacral
    plexus 353.1
    root (nerve) NEC 353.4
  lymphoproliferative (chronic) NEC
      (M9970/1) 238.7
  major depressive *(see also* Psychosis, af-
      fective) 296.2
    recurrent episode 296.3
    single episode 296.2
  male erectile 302.72
    organic origin 607.84

ICD-9-CM

▢

Vol. 2

Disorder *(Continued)*
  manic *(see also* Psychosis, affective) 296.0
    atypical 296.81
  mathematics 315.1
  meniscus NEC *(see also* Disorder, carti-
    lage, articular) 718.0
  menopausal 627.9
    specified NEC 627.8
  menstrual 626.9
    psychogenic 306.52
    specified NEC 626.8
  mental (nonpsychotic) 300.9
    affecting management of pregnancy,
      childbirth, or puerperium 648.4
    drug-induced 292.9
      hallucinogen persisting perception
        292.89
      specified type NEC 292.89
    due to or associated with
      alcoholism 291.9
      drug consumption NEC 292.9
        specified type NEC 292.89
      physical condition NEC 293.9
    induced by drug 292.9
      specified type NEC 292.89
    neurotic *(see also* Neurosis) 300.9
    of infancy, childhood or adolescence
      313.9 ◀
    persistent ◀
      other ◀
        due to conditions classified else-
          where 294.8 ◀
      unspecified ◀
        due to conditions classified else-
          where 294.9 ◀
    presenile 310.1
      psychotic NEC 290.10
    previous, affecting management of
      pregnancy V23.8
    psychoneurotic *(see also* Neurosis)
      300.9
    psychotic *(see also* Psychosis) 298.9
      brief 298.8 ◀
      senile 290.20
    specific, following organic brain
      damage 310.9
      cognitive or personality change of
        other type 310.1
      frontal lobe syndrome 310.0
      postconcussional syndrome 310.2
      specified type NEC 310.8 ◀
    transient ◀
      in conditions classified elsewhere
        293.9 ◀
  metabolism NEC 277.9
    with
      abortion - *see* Abortion, by type,
        with metabolic disorder
      ectopic pregnancy *(see also* catego-
        ries 633.0-633.9) 639.4
      molar pregnancy *(see also* catego-
        ries 630-632) 639.4
    alkaptonuria 270.2
    amino acid *(see also* Disorder, amino
      acid) 270.9
      specified type NEC 270.8
    ammonia 270.6
    arginine 270.6
    argininosuccinic acid 270.6
    basal 794.7
    bilirubin 277.4
    calcium 275.40
    carbohydrate 271.9
      specified type NEC 271.8

Disorder *(Continued)*
  metabolism NEC *(Continued)*
    cholesterol 272.9
    citrulline 270.6
    copper 275.1
    corticosteroid 255.2
    cystine storage 270.0
    cystinuria 270.0
    fat 272.9
      fatty acid oxidation 277.85 ◀
    following
      abortion 639.4
      ectopic or molar pregnancy 639.4
    fructosemia 271.2
    fructosuria 271.2
    fucosidosis 271.8
    galactose-1-phosphate uridyl trans-
      ferase 271.1
    glutamine 270.7
    glycine 270.7
    glycogen storage NEC 271.0
      hepatorenal 271.0
    hemochromatosis 275.0
    in labor and delivery 669.0
    iron 275.0
    lactose 271.3
    lipid 272.9
      specified type NEC 272.8
      storage 272.7
    lipoprotein - *see also* Hyperlipemia
      deficiency (familial) 272.5
    lysine 270.7
    magnesium 275.2
    mannosidosis 271.8
    mineral 275.9
      specified type NEC 275.8
      mitochondrial 277.87 ◀
    mucopolysaccharide 277.5
    nitrogen 270.9
    ornithine 270.6
    oxalosis 271.8
    pentosuria 271.8
    phenylketonuria 270.1
    phosphate 275.3
    phosphorus 275.3
    plasma protein 273.9
      specified type NEC 273.8
    porphyrin 277.1
    purine 277.2
    pyrimidine 277.2
    serine 270.7
    sodium 276.9
    specified type NEC 277.89
    steroid 255.2
    threonine 270.7
    urea cycle 270.6
    xylose 271.8
  micturition NEC 788.69
    psychogenic 306.53
  misery and unhappiness, of childhood
    and adolescence 313.1
  mitochondrial metabolism 277.87 ◀
  mitral valve 424.0
  mood *(see also* Disorder, bipolar)
    296.90 ◀▥
    episodic 296.90 ◀
      specified NEC 296.99 ◀
    in conditions classified elsewhere
      293.83 ◀
  motor tic 307.20
    chronic 307.22
    transient (childhood) 307.21 ◀▥
  movement NEC 333.90
    hysterical 300.11
    periodic limb 780.58 ◀

Disorder *(Continued)*
  movement NEC *(Continued)*
    sleep related 780.58 ◀
    specified type NEC 333.99
    stereotypic 307.3
  mucopolysaccharide 277.5
  muscle 728.9
    psychogenic 306.0
    specified type NEC 728.3
  muscular attachments, peripheral - *see*
    also Enthesopathy
    spine 720.1
  musculoskeletal system NEC 729.9
    psychogenic 306.0
  myeloproliferative (chronic) NEC
    (M9960/1) 238.7
  myoneural 358.9
    due to lead 358.2
    specified type NEC 358.8
    toxic 358.2
  myotonic 359.2
  neck region NEC 723.9
  nerve 349.9
    abducens NEC 378.54
    accessory 352.4
    acoustic 388.5
    auditory 388.5
    auriculotemporal 350.8
    axillary 353.0
    cerebral - *see* Disorder, nerve, cranial
    cranial 352.9
      first 352.0
      second 377.49
      third
        partial 378.51
        total 378.52
      fourth 378.53
      fifth 350.9
      sixth 378.54
      seventh NEC 351.9
      eighth 388.5
      ninth 352.2
      tenth 352.3
      eleventh 352.4
      twelfth 352.5
      multiple 352.6
    entrapment - *see* Neuropathy, en-
      trapment
    facial 351.9
      specified NEC 351.8
    femoral 355.2
    glossopharyngeal NEC 352.2
    hypoglossal 352.5
    iliohypogastric 355.79
    ilioinguinal 355.79
    intercostal 353.8
    lateral
      cutaneous of thigh 355.1
      popliteal 355.3
    lower limb NEC 355.8
    medial, popliteal 355.4
    median NEC 354.1
    obturator 355.79
    oculomotor
      partial 378.51
      total 378.52
    olfactory 352.0
    optic 377.49
      ischemic 377.41
      nutritional 377.33
      toxic 377.34
    peroneal 355.3
    phrenic 354.8
    plantar 355.6

Disorder (*Continued*)
  nerve (*Continued*)
    pneumogastric 352.3
    posterior tibial 355.5
    radial 354.3
    recurrent laryngeal 352.3
    root 353.9
      specified NEC 353.8
    saphenous 355.79
    sciatic NEC 355.0
    specified NEC 355.9
      lower limb 355.79
      upper limb 354.8
    spinal 355.9
    sympathetic NEC 337.9
    trigeminal 350.9
      specified NEC 350.8
    trochlear 378.53
    ulnar 354.2
    upper limb NEC 354.9
    vagus 352.3
  nervous system NEC 349.9
    autonomic (peripheral) (*see also* Neuropathy, peripheral, autonomic) 337.9
    cranial 352.9
    parasympathetic (*see also* Neuropathy, peripheral, autonomic) 337.9
    specified type NEC 349.89
    sympathetic (*see also* Neuropathy, peripheral, autonomic) 337.9
    vegetative (*see also* Neuropathy, peripheral, autonomic) 337.9
  neurohypophysis NEC 253.6
  neurological NEC 781.99
    peripheral NEC 355.9
  neuromuscular NEC 358.9
    hereditary NEC 359.1
    specified NEC 358.8
    toxic 358.2
  neurotic 300.9
    specified type NEC 300.89
  neutrophil, polymorphonuclear (functional) 288.1
  nightmare 307.47   ◀
  night terror 307.46   ◀
  obsessive-compulsive 300.3
  oppositional defiant childhood and adolescence 313.81   ⬅▥
  optic
    chiasm 377.54
      associated with
        inflammatory disorders 377.54
        neoplasm NEC 377.52
          pituitary 377.51
        pituitary disorders 377.51
        vascular disorders 377.53
    nerve 377.49
    radiations 377.63
    tracts 377.63
  orbit 376.9
    specified NEC 376.89
  orgasmic   ◀
    female 302.73   ◀
    male 302.74   ◀
  overanxious, of childhood and adolescence 313.0
  oxidation, fatty acid 277.85   ◀
  pancreas, internal secretion (other than diabetes mellitus) 251.9
    specified type NEC 251.8
  panic 300.01
    with agoraphobia 300.21
  papillary muscle NEC 429.81

Disorder (*Continued*)
  paranoid 297.9
    induced 297.3
    shared 297.3
  parathyroid 252.9
    specified type NEC 252.8
  paroxysmal, mixed 780.39
  pentose phosphate pathway with anemia 282.2
  periodic limb movement 780.58   ◀
  peroxisomal 277.86   ◀
  personality 301.9
    affective 301.10
    aggressive 301.3
    amoral 301.7
    anancastic, anankastic 301.4
    antisocial 301.7
    asocial 301.7
    asthenic 301.6
    avoidant 301.82   ◀
    borderline 301.83
    compulsive 301.4
    cyclothymic 301.13
    dependent-passive 301.6
    dyssocial 301.7
    emotional instability 301.59
    epileptoid 301.3
    explosive 301.3
    following organic brain damage 310.1
    histrionic 301.50
    hyperthymic 301.11
    hypomanic (chronic) 301.11
    hypothymic 301.12
    hysterical 301.50
    immature 301.89
    inadequate 301.6
    introverted 301.21
    labile 301.59
    moral deficiency 301.7
    narcissistic 301.81   ◀
    obsessional 301.4
    obsessive-compulsive 301.4   ⬅▥
    overconscientious 301.4
    paranoid 301.0
    passive (-dependent) 301.6
    passive-aggressive 301.84
    pathological NEC 301.9
    pseudosocial 301.7
    psychopathic 301.9
    schizoid 301.20
      introverted 301.21
      schizotypal 301.22
    schizotypal 301.22
    seductive 301.59
    type A 301.4
    unstable 301.59
  pervasive developmental 299.9   ⬅▥
    childhood-onset 299.8   ◀
    specified NEC 299.8   ◀
  pigmentation, choroid (congenital) 743.53
  phonological 315.39   ◀
  pinna 380.30
    specified type NEC 380.39
  pituitary, thalamic 253.9
    anterior NEC 253.4
    iatrogenic 253.7
    postablative 253.7
    specified NEC 253.8
  pityriasis-like NEC 696.8
  platelets (blood) 287.1
  polymorphonuclear neutrophils (functional) 288.1

Disorder (*Continued*)
  porphyrin metabolism 277.1
  postmenopausal 627.9
    specified type NEC 627.8
  posttraumatic stress 309.81
    acute 309.81   ⬅▥
    brief 309.81   ⬅▥
    chronic 309.81
  premenstrual dysphoric (PMDD) 625.4
  psoriatic-like NEC 696.8
  psychic, with diseases classified elsewhere 316
  psychogenic NEC (*see also* condition) 300.9
    allergic NEC
      respiratory 306.1
    anxiety 300.00
      atypical 300.00
      generalized 300.02
    appetite 307.50
    articulation, joint 306.0
    asthenic 300.5
    blood 306.8
    cardiovascular (system) 306.2
    compulsive 300.3
    cutaneous 306.3
    depressive 300.4
    digestive (system) 306.4
    dysmenorrheic 306.52
    dyspneic 306.1
    eczematous 306.3
    endocrine (system) 306.6
    eye 306.7
    feeding 307.59
    functional NEC 306.9
    gastric 306.4
    gastrointestinal (system) 306.4
    genitourinary (system) 306.50
    heart (function) (rhythm) 306.2
    hemic 306.8
    hyperventilatory 306.1
    hypochondriacal 300.7
    hysterical 300.10
    intestinal 306.4
    joint 306.0
    learning 315.2
    limb 306.0
    lymphatic (system) 306.8
    menstrual 306.52
    micturition 306.53
    monoplegic NEC 306.0
    motor 307.9
    muscle 306.0
    musculoskeletal 306.0
    neurocirculatory 306.2
    obsessive 300.3
    occupational 300.89
    organ or part of body NEC 306.9
    organs of special sense 306.7
    paralytic NEC 306.0
    phobic 300.20
    physical NEC 306.9
    pruritic 306.3
    rectal 306.4
    respiratory (system) 306.1
    rheumatic 306.0
    sexual (function) 302.70
      specified type NEC 302.79
    sexual orientation conflict 302.0   ◀
    skin (allergic) (eczematous) (pruritic) 306.3

ICD-9-CM

Vol. 2

Disorder *(Continued)*
  psychogenic NEC *(Continued)*
    sleep 307.40
      initiation or maintenance 307.41
        persistent 307.42
        transient 307.41
      movement 780.58 ◄
      sleep terror 307.46 ◄
      specified type NEC 307.49
    specified part of body NEC 306.8
    stomach 306.4
  psychomotor NEC 307.9
    hysterical 300.11
  psychoneurotic *(see also* Neurosis) 300.9
    mixed NEC 300.89
  psychophysiologic *(see also* Disorder, psychosomatic) 306.9
  psychosexual identity (childhood) 302.6
    adult-life 302.85
  psychosomatic NEC 306.9
    allergic NEC
      respiratory 306.1
    articulation, joint 306.0
    cardiovascular (system) 306.2
    cutaneous 306.3
    digestive (system) 306.4
    dysmenorrheic 306.52
    dyspneic 306.1
    endocrine (system) 306.6
    eye 306.7
    gastric 306.4
    gastrointestinal (system) 306.4
    genitourinary (system) 306.50
    heart (functional) (rhythm) 306.2
    hyperventilatory 306.1
    intestinal 306.4
    joint 306.0
    limb 306.0
    lymphatic (system) 306.8
    menstrual 306.52
    micturition 306.53
    monoplegic NEC 306.0
    muscle 306.0
    musculoskeletal 306.0
    neurocirculatory 306.2
    organs of special sense 306.7
    paralytic NEC 306.0
    pruritic 306.3
    rectal 306.4
    respiratory (system) 306.1
    rheumatic 306.0
    sexual (function) 302.70
      specified type NEC 302.79
    skin 306.3
    specified part of body NEC 306.8
    stomach 306.4
  psychotic - *(see also* Psychosis) 298.9 ◄▥
    brief 298.8 ◄
  purine metabolism NEC 277.2
  pyrimidine metabolism NEC 277.2
  reactive attachment of infancy or early childhood 313.89 ◄▥
  reading, developmental 315.00
  reflex 796.1
  renal function, impaired 588.9
    specified type NEC 588.89 ◄▥
  renal transport NEC 588.89 ◄▥
  respiration, respiratory NEC 519.9
    due to
      aspiration of liquids or solids 508.9
      inhalation of fumes or vapors 506.9
    psychogenic 306.1
  retina 362.9
    specified type NEC 362.89
  rumination 307.53 ◄

Disorder *(Continued)*
  sacroiliac joint NEC 724.6
  sacrum 724.6
  schizo-affective *(see also* Schizophrenia) 295.7
  schizoid, childhood or adolescence 313.22
  schizophreniform 295.4
  schizotypal personality 301.22
  secretion, thyrocalcitonin 246.0
  seizure 780.39
    recurrent 780.39
      epileptic - *see* Epilepsy
  sense of smell 781.1
    psychogenic 306.7
  separation anxiety 309.21
  sexual *(see also* Deviation, sexual) 302.9
    aversion 302.79 ◄
    desire, hypoactive 302.71 ◄
    function, psychogenic 302.70
  shyness, of childhood and adolescence 313.21
  single complement (C_1-C_9) 279.8
  skin NEC 709.9
    fetus or newborn 778.9
      specified type 778.8
    psychogenic (allergic) (eczematous) (pruritic) 306.3
    specified type NEC 709.8
    vascular 709.1
  sleep 780.50
    with apnea - *see* Apnea, sleep
    arousal 307.46 ◄
    circadian rhythm 307.45
    initiation or maintenance *(see also* Insomnia) 780.52
      nonorganic origin (transient) 307.41
      persistent 307.42
    nonorganic origin 307.40
      specified type NEC 307.49
    specified NEC 780.59
  social, of childhood and adolescence 313.22
    specified NEC 780.59
  soft tissue 729.9
  somatization 300.81
  somatoform (atypical) (undifferentiated) 300.82
    severe 300.81
    specified type NEC 300.89 ◄
  speech NEC 784.5
    nonorganic origin 307.9
  spine NEC 724.9
    ligamentous or muscular attachments, peripheral 720.1
  steroid metabolism NEC 255.2
  stomach (functional) *(see also* Disorder, gastric) 536.9
    psychogenic 306.4
  storage, iron 275.0
  stress *(see also* Reaction, stress, acute) 308.3 ◄▥
    posttraumatic
      acute 309.81 ◄▥
      brief 309.81 ◄▥
      chronic (motor or vocal) 309.81
  substitution 300.11
  suspected - *see* Observation
  synovium 727.9
  temperature regulation, fetus or newborn 778.4
  temporomandibular joint NEC 524.60

Disorder *(Continued)*
  temporomandibular joint NEC *(Continued)*
    sounds on opening or closing 524.64 ◄
    specified NEC 524.69
  tendon 727.9
    shoulder region 726.10
  thoracic root (nerve) NEC 353.3
  thyrocalcitonin secretion 246.0
  thyroid (gland) NEC 246.9
    specified type NEC 246.8
  tic 307.20
    chronic (motor or vocal) 307.22
    motor-verbal 307.23
    organic origin 333.1
    transient (of childhood) 307.21 ◄▥
  tooth NEC 525.9
    development NEC 520.9
      specified type NEC 520.8
    eruption 520.6
    specified type NEC 525.8
  Tourette's 307.23 ◄
  transport, carbohydrate 271.9
    specified type NEC 271.8
  tubular, phosphate-losing 588.0
  tympanic membrane 384.9
  unaggressive, unsocialized *(see also* Disturbance, conduct) 312.1
  undersocialized, unsocialized *(see also* Disturbance, conduct)
    aggressive (type) 312.0
    unaggressive (type) 312.1
  vision, visual NEC 368.9
    binocular NEC 368.30
    cortex 377.73
      associated with
        inflammatory disorders 377.73
        neoplasms 377.71
        vascular disorders 377.72
    pathway NEC 377.63
      associated with
        inflammatory disorders 377.63
        neoplasms 377.61
        vascular disorders 377.62
  vocal tic ◄
    chronic 307.22 ◄
  wakefulness *(see also* Hypersomnia) 780.54
    nonorganic origin (transient) 307.43
      persistent 307.44
  written expression 315.2 ◄
Disorganized globe 360.29
Displacement, displaced

> Note   For acquired displacement of bones, cartilage, joints, tendons, due to injury, *see also* Dislocation.
>
> Displacements at ages under one year should be considered congenital, provided there is no indication the condition was acquired after birth.

  acquired traumatic of bone, cartilage, joint, tendon NEC (without fracture) *(see also* Dislocation) 839.8
    with fracture - *see* Fracture, by site
  adrenal gland (congenital) 759.1
  alveolus and teeth, vertical 524.75 ◄
  appendix, retrocecal (congenital) 751.5
  auricle (congenital) 744.29
  bladder (acquired) 596.8
    congenital 753.8
  brachial plexus (congenital) 742.8

Displacement, displaced (*Continued*)
brain stem, caudal 742.4
canaliculus lacrimalis 743.65
cardia, through esophageal hiatus 750.6
cerebellum, caudal 742.4
cervix (*see also* Malposition, uterus) 621.6
colon (congenital) 751.4
device, implant, or graft - *see* Complications, mechanical
epithelium
  columnar of cervix 622.10 ◀▥
  cuboidal, beyond limits of external os (uterus) 752.49
esophageal mucosa into cardia of stomach, congenital 750.4
esophagus (acquired) 530.89
  congenital 750.4
eyeball (acquired) (old) 376.36
  congenital 743.8
  current injury 871.3
  lateral 376.36
fallopian tube (acquired) 620.4
  congenital 752.19
  opening (congenital) 752.19
gallbladder (congenital) 751.69
gastric mucosa 750.7
  into
    duodenum 750.7
    esophagus 750.7
    Meckel's diverticulum, congenital 750.7
globe (acquired) (lateral) (old) 376.36
  current injury 871.3
graft
  artificial skin graft 996.55
  decellularized allodermis graft 996.55
heart (congenital) 746.87
  acquired 429.89
hymen (congenital) (upward) 752.49
internal prosthesis NEC - *see* Complications, mechanical
intervertebral disc (with neuritis, radiculitis, sciatica, or other pain) 722.2
  with myelopathy 722.70
  cervical, cervicodorsal, cervicothoracic 722.0
    with myelopathy 722.71
    due to major trauma - *see* Dislocation, vertebra, cervical
  due to major trauma - *see* Dislocation, vertebra
  lumbar, lumbosacral 722.10
    with myelopathy 722.73
    due to major trauma - *see* Dislocation, vertebra, lumbar
  thoracic, thoracolumbar 722.11
    with myelopathy 722.72
    due to major trauma - *see* Dislocation, vertebra, thoracic
intrauterine device 996.32
kidney (acquired) 593.0
  congenital 753.3
lacrimal apparatus or duct (congenital) 743.65
macula (congenital) 743.55
Meckel's diverticulum (congenital) 751.0
nail (congenital) 757.5
  acquired 703.8
opening of Wharton's duct in mouth 750.26
organ or site, congenital NEC - *see* Malposition, congenital

Displacement, displaced (*Continued*)
ovary (acquired) 620.4
  congenital 752.0
  free in peritoneal cavity (congenital) 752.0
  into hernial sac 620.4
oviduct (acquired) 620.4
  congenital 752.19
parathyroid (gland) 252.8
parotid gland (congenital) 750.26
punctum lacrimale (congenital) 743.65
sacroiliac (congenital) (joint) 755.69
  current injury - *see* Dislocation, sacroiliac
  old 724.6
spine (congenital) 756.19
spleen, congenital 759.0
stomach (congenital) 750.7
  acquired 537.89
subglenoid (closed) 831.01
sublingual duct (congenital) 750.26
teeth, tooth 524.30 ◀▥
  horizontal 524.33 ◀
  vertical 524.34 ◀
tongue (congenital) (downward) 750.19
trachea (congenital) 748.3
ureter or ureteric opening or orifice (congenital) 753.4
uterine opening of oviducts or fallopian tubes 752.19
uterus, uterine (*see also* Malposition, uterus) 621.6
  congenital 752.3
ventricular septum 746.89
  with rudimentary ventricle 746.89
xyphoid bone (process) 738.3
Disproportion 653.9
affecting fetus or newborn 763.1
caused by
  conjoined twins 653.7
  contraction, pelvis (general) 653.1
    inlet 653.2
    midpelvic 653.8
    midplane 653.8
    outlet 653.3
  fetal
    ascites 653.7
    hydrocephalus 653.6
    hydrops 653.7
    meningomyelocele 653.7
    sacral teratoma 653.7
    tumor 653.7
  hydrocephalic fetus 653.6
  pelvis, pelvic, abnormality (bony) NEC 653.0
  unusually large fetus 653.5
causing obstructed labor 660.1
cephalopelvic, normally formed fetus 653.4
  causing obstructed labor 660.1
fetal NEC 653.5
  causing obstructed labor 660.1
fetopelvic, normally formed fetus 653.4
  causing obstructed labor 660.1
mixed maternal and fetal origin, normally, formed fetus 653.4
pelvis, pelvic (bony) NEC 653.1
  causing obstructed labor 660.1
specified type NEC 653.8
Disruption
cesarean wound 674.1
family V61.0
gastrointestinal anastomosis 997.4

Disruption (*Continued*)
ligament(s) - *see also* Sprain
  knee
    current injury - *see* Dislocation, knee
    old 717.89
      capsular 717.85
      collateral (medial) 717.82
        lateral 717.81
      cruciate (posterior) 717.84
        anterior 717.83
      specified site NEC 717.85
marital V61.10
  involving divorce or estrangement V61.0
operation wound (external) 998.32
  internal 998.31
organ transplant, anastomosis site - *see* Complications, transplant, organ, by site
ossicles, ossicular chain 385.23
  traumatic - *see* Fracture, skull, base
parenchyma
  liver (hepatic) - *see* Laceration, liver, major
  spleen - *see* Laceration, spleen, parenchyma, massive
phase-shift, of 24-hour sleep-wake cycle 780.55
  nonorganic origin 307.45
sleep-wake cycle (24-hour) 780.55
  circadian rhythm 307.45
  nonorganic origin 307.45
suture line (external) 998.32
  internal 998.31
wound
  cesarean operation 674.1
  episiotomy 674.2
  operation 998.32
    cesarean 674.1
    internal 998.31
  perineal (obstetric) 674.2
  uterine 674.1
Disruptio uteri - *see also* Rupture, uterus
complicating delivery - *see* Delivery, complicated, rupture, uterus
Dissatisfaction with
employment V62.2
school environment V62.3
Dissecting - *see* condition
Dissection
aorta 441.00
  abdominal 441.02
  thoracic 441.01
  thoracoabdominal 441.03
artery 1 arterial
  carotid 443.21
  coronary 414.12
  iliac 443.22
  renal 443.23
  specified NEC 443.29
  vertebral 443.24
vascular 459.9
wound - *see* Wound, open, by site
Disseminated - *see* condition
Dissociated personality NEC 300.15
Dissociation
auriculoventricular or atrioventricular (any degree) (AV) 426.89
  with heart block 426.0
interference 426.89
isorhythmic 426.89
rhythm
  atrioventricular (AV) 426.89
  interference 426.89

ICD-9-CM ▯ **Vol. 2**

Dissociative
  identity disorder 300.14
  reaction NEC 300.15
Dissolution, vertebra (*see also* Osteoporosis) 733.00
Distention
  abdomen (gaseous) 787.3
  bladder 596.8
  cecum 569.89
  colon 569.89
  gallbladder 575.8
  gaseous (abdomen) 787.3
  intestine 569.89
  kidney 593.89
  liver 573.9
  seminal vesicle 608.89
  stomach 536.8
    acute 536.1
    psychogenic 306.4
  ureter 593.5
  uterus 621.8
Distichia, distichiasis (eyelid) 743.63
Distoma hepaticum infestation 121.3
Distomiasis 121.9
  bile passages 121.3
    due to Clonorchis sinensis 121.1
  hemic 120.9
  hepatic (liver) 121.3
    due to Clonorchis sinensis (clonorchiasis) 121.1
  intestinal 121.4
  liver 121.3
    due to Clonorchis sinensis 121.1
  lung 121.2
  pulmonary 121.2
Distomolar (fourth molar) 520.1
  causing crowding 524.31 ◀▦
Disto-occlusion (division I) (division II) 524.22 ◀
Distortion (congenital)
  adrenal (gland) 759.1
  ankle (joint) 755.69
  anus 751.5
  aorta 747.29
  appendix 751.5
  arm 755.59
  artery (peripheral) NEC (*see also* Distortion, peripheral vascular system) 747.60
    cerebral 747.81
    coronary 746.85
    pulmonary 747.3
    retinal 743.58
    umbilical 747.5
  auditory canal 744.29
    causing impairment of hearing 744.02
  bile duct or passage 751.69
  bladder 753.8
  brain 742.4
  bronchus 748.3
  cecum 751.5
  cervix (uteri) 752.49
  chest (wall) 756.3
  clavicle 755.51
  clitoris 752.49
  coccyx 756.19
  colon 751.5
  common duct 751.69
  cornea 743.41
  cricoid cartilage 748.3
  cystic duct 751.69
  duodenum 751.5

Distortion (*Continued*)
  ear 744.29
    auricle 744.29
      causing impairment of hearing 744.02
      causing impairment of hearing 744.09
    external 744.29
      causing impairment of hearing 744.02
    inner 744.05
    middle, except ossicles 744.03
      ossicles 744.04
    ossicles 744.04
  endocrine (gland) NEC 759.2
  epiglottis 748.3
  Eustachian tube 744.24
  eye 743.8
    adnexa 743.69
  face bone(s) 756.0
  fallopian tube 752.19
  femur 755.69
  fibula 755.69
  finger(s) 755.59
  foot 755.67
  gallbladder 751.69
  genitalia, genital organ(s)
    female 752.89
      external 752.49
      internal NEC 752.89
    male 752.89
      penis 752.69
  glottis 748.3
  gyri 742.4
  hand bone(s) 755.59
  heart (auricle) (ventricle) 746.89
    valve (cusp) 746.89
  hepatic duct 751.69
  humerus 755.59
  hymen 752.49
  ileum 751.5
  intestine (large) (small) 751.5
    with anomalous adhesions, fixation or malrotation 751.4
  jaw NEC 524.89 ◀▦
  jejunum 751.5
  kidney 753.3
  knee (joint) 755.64
  labium (majus) (minus) 752.49
  larynx 748.3
  leg 755.69
  lens 743.36
  liver 751.69
  lumbar spine 756.19
    with disproportion (fetopelvic) 653.0
      affecting fetus or newborn 763.1
      causing obstructed labor 660.1
  lumbosacral (joint) (region) 756.19
  lung (fissures) (lobe) 748.69
  nerve 742.8
  nose 748.1
  organ
    of Corti 744.05
    of site not listed - *see* Anomaly, specified type NEC
  ossicles, ear 744.04
  ovary 752.0
  oviduct 752.19
  pancreas 751.7
  parathyroid (gland) 759.2
  patella 755.64
  peripheral vascular system NEC 747.60
    gastrointestinal 747.61

Distortion (*Continued*)
  peripheral vascular system NEC (*Continued*)
    lower limb 747.64
    renal 747.62
    spinal 747.82
    upper limb 747.63
  pituitary (gland) 759.2
  radius 755.59
  rectum 751.5
  rib 756.3
  sacroiliac joint 755.69
  sacrum 756.19
  scapula 755.59
  shoulder girdle 755.59
  site not listed - *see* Anomaly, specified type NEC
  skull bone(s) 756.0
    with
      anencephalus 740.0
      encephalocele 742.0
      hydrocephalus 742.3
        with spina bifida (*see also* Spina bifida) 741.0
      microcephalus 742.1
  spinal cord 742.59
  spine 756.19
  spleen 759.0
  sternum 756.3
  thorax (wall) 756.3
  thymus (gland) 759.2
  thyroid (gland) 759.2
    cartilage 748.3
  tibia 755.69
  toe(s) 755.66
  tongue 750.19
  trachea (cartilage) 748.3
  ulna 755.59
  ureter 753.4
    causing obstruction 753.20
  urethra 753.8
    causing obstruction 753.6
  uterus 752.3
  vagina 752.49
  vein (peripheral) NEC (*see also* Distortion, peripheral vascular system) 747.60
    great 747.49
    portal 747.49
    pulmonary 747.49
  vena cava (inferior) (superior) 747.49
  vertebra 756.19
  visual NEC 368.15
    shape or size 368.14
  vulva 752.49
  wrist (bones) (joint) 755.59
Distress
  abdomen 789.0
  colon 789.0
  emotional V40.9
  epigastric 789.0
  fetal (syndrome) 768.4
    affecting management of pregnancy or childbirth 656.8
    liveborn infant 768.4
    first noted
      before onset of labor 768.2
      during labor or delivery 768.3
    stillborn infant (death before onset of labor) 768.0
      death during labor 768.1
  gastrointestinal (functional) 536.9
    psychogenic 306.4
  intestinal (functional) NEC 564.9
    psychogenic 306.4

Distress (Continued)

  intrauterine - *see* Distress, fetal

  leg 729.5

  maternal 669.0

  mental V40.9

  respiratory 786.09

    acute (adult) 518.82

    adult syndrome (following shock, surgery, or trauma) 518.5

      specified NEC 518.82

    fetus or newborn 770.89

    syndrome (idiopathic) (newborn) 769

  stomach 536.9

    psychogenic 306.4

Distribution vessel, atypical NEC 747.60

  coronary artery 746.85

  spinal 747.82

Districhiasis 704.2

Disturbance - *see also* Disease

  absorption NEC 579.9

    calcium 269.3

    carbohydrate 579.8

    fat 579.8

    protein 579.8

    specified type NEC 579.8

    vitamin (*see also* Deficiency, vitamin) 269.2

  acid-base equilibrium 276.9

  activity and attention, simple, with hyperkinesis 314.01

  amino acid (metabolic) (*see also* Disorder, amino acid) 270.9

    imidazole 270.5

    maple syrup (urine) disease 270.3

    transport 270.0

  assimilation, food 579.9

  attention, simple 314.00

    with hyperactivity 314.01

  auditory, nerve, except deafness 388.5

  behavior (*see also* Disturbance, conduct) 312.9

  blood clotting (hypoproteinemia) (mechanism) (*see also* Defect, coagulation) 286.9

  central nervous system NEC 349.9

  cerebral nerve NEC 352.9

  circulatory 459.9

  conduct 312.9

> Note   Use the following fifth-digit subclassification with categories 312.0-312.2:
>
> 0   unspecified
> 1   mild
> 2   moderate
> 3   severe

    adjustment reaction 309.3

    adolescent onset type 312.82

    childhood onset type 312.81

    compulsive 312.30

      intermittent explosive disorder 312.34

      isolated explosive disorder 312.35

      kleptomania 312.32

      pathological gambling 312.31

      pyromania 312.33

    hyperkinetic 314.2

    intermittent explosive 312.34

    isolated explosive 312.35

    mixed with emotions 312.4

    socialized (type) 312.20

      aggressive 312.23

      unaggressive 312.21

Disturbance (Continued)

  conduct (Continued)

    specified type NEC 312.89

    undersocialized, unsocialized

      aggressive (type) 312.0

      unaggressive (type) 312.1

  coordination 781.3

  cranial nerve NEC 352.9

  deep sensibility - *see* Disturbance, sensation

  digestive 536.9

    psychogenic 306.4

  electrolyte - *see* Imbalance, electrolyte

  emotions specific to childhood or adolescence 313.9

    with

      academic underachievement 313.83

      anxiety and fearfulness 313.0

      elective mutism 313.23

      identity disorder 313.82

      jealousy 313.3

      misery and unhappiness 313.1

      oppositional defiant disorder 313.81

      overanxiousness 313.0

      sensitivity 313.21

      shyness 313.21

      social withdrawal 313.22

      withdrawal reaction 313.22

    involving relationship problems 313.3

    mixed 313.89

    specified type NEC 313.89

  endocrine (gland) 259.9

    neonatal, transitory 775.9

      specified NEC 775.8

  equilibrium 780.4

  feeding (elderly) (infant) 783.3

    newborn 779.3

    nonorganic origin NEC 307.59

    psychogenic NEC 307.59

  fructose metabolism 271.2

  gait 781.2

    hysterical 300.11

  gastric (functional) 536.9

    motility 536.8

    psychogenic 306.4

    secretion 536.8

  gastrointestinal (functional) 536.9

    psychogenic 306.4

  habit, child 307.9

  hearing, except deafness 388.40

  heart, functional (conditions classifiable to 426, 427, 428)

    due to presence of (cardiac) prosthesis 429.4

    postoperative (immediate) 997.1

      long-term effect of cardiac surgery 429.4

    psychogenic 306.2

  hormone 259.9

  innervation uterus, sympathetic, parasympathetic 621.8

  keratinization NEC

    gingiva 523.1

    lip 528.5

    oral (mucosa) (soft tissue) 528.79 ◀▥

      residual ridge mucosa ◀

        excessive 528.72 ◀

        minimal 528.71 ◀

    tongue 528.79 ◀▥

  labyrinth, labyrinthine (vestibule) 386.9

  learning, specific NEC 315.2

Disturbance (Continued)

  memory (*see also* Amnesia) 780.93

    mild, following organic brain damage 310.8 ◀▥

  mental (*see also* Disorder, mental) 300.9

    associated with diseases classified elsewhere 316

  metabolism (acquired) (congenital) (*see also* Disorder, metabolism) 277.9

    with

      abortion - *see* Abortion, by type, with metabolic disorder

      ectopic pregnancy (*see also* categories 633.0-633.9) 639.4

      molar pregnancy (*see also* categories 630-632) 639.4

    amino acid (*see also* Disorder, amino acid) 270.9

      aromatic NEC 270.2

      branched-chain 270.3

      specified type NEC 270.8

      straight-chain NEC 270.7

      sulfur-bearing 270.4

      transport 270.0

    ammonia 270.6

    arginine 270.6

    argininosuccinic acid 270.6

    carbohydrate NEC 271.9

    cholesterol 272.9

    citrulline 270.6

    cystathionine 270.4

    fat 272.9

    following

      abortion 639.4

      ectopic or molar pregnancy 639.4

    general 277.9

      carbohydrate 271.9

      iron 275.0

      phosphate 275.3

      sodium 276.9

    glutamine 270.7

    glycine 270.7

    histidine 270.5

    homocystine 270.4

    in labor or delivery 669.0

    iron 275.0

    isoleucine 270.3

    leucine 270.3

    lipoid 272.9

      specified type NEC 272.8

    lysine 270.7

    methionine 270.4

    neonatal, transitory 775.9

      specified type NEC 775.8

    nitrogen 788.9

    ornithine 270.6

    phosphate 275.3

    phosphatides 272.7

    serine 270.7

    sodium NEC 276.9

    threonine 270.7

    tryptophan 270.2

    tyrosine 270.2

    urea cycle 270.6

    valine 270.3

  motor 796.1

  nervous functional 799.2

  neuromuscular mechanism (eye) due to syphilis 094.84

  nutritional 269.9

    nail 703.8

  ocular motion 378.87

    psychogenic 306.7

  oculogyric 378.87

    psychogenic 306.7

ICD-9-CM

▢

Vol. 2

Disturbance (Continued)
oculomotor NEC 378.87
psychogenic 306.7
olfactory nerve 781.1
optic nerve NEC 377.49
oral epithelium, including tongue
528.79 ◀▥
residual ridge mucosa ◀
excessive 528.72 ◀
minimal 528.71 ◀
personality (pattern) (trait) (see also
Disorder, personality) 301.9
following organic brain damage
310.1
polyglandular 258.9
psychomotor 307.9
pupillary 379.49
reflex 796.1
rhythm, heart 427.9
postoperative (immediate) 997.1
long-term effect of cardiac surgery
429.4
psychogenic 306.2
salivary secretion 527.7
sensation (cold) (heat) (localization)
(tactile discrimination localization)
(texture) (vibratory) NEC 782.0
hysterical 300.11
skin 782.0
smell 781.1
taste 781.1
sensory (see also Disturbance, sensation) 782.0
innervation 782.0
situational (transient) (see also Reaction,
adjustment) 309.9
acute 308.3
sleep 780.50
with apnea - see Apnea, sleep
initiation or maintenance (see also Insomnia) 780.52
nonorganic origin 307.41
nonorganic origin 307.40
specified type NEC 307.49
specified NEC 780.59
nonorganic origin 307.49
wakefulness (see also Hypersomnia)
780.54
nonorganic origin 307.43
sociopathic 301.7
speech NEC 784.5
developmental 315.39
associated with hyperkinesis 314.1
secondary to organic lesion 784.5
stomach (functional) (see also Disturbance, gastric) 536.9
sympathetic (nerve) (see also Neuropathy, peripheral, autonomic) 337.9
temperature sense 782.0
hysterical 300.11
tooth
eruption 520.6
formation 520.4
structure, hereditary NEC 520.5
touch (see also Disturbance, sensation)
782.0
vascular 459.9
arteriosclerotic - see Arteriosclerosis
vasomotor 443.9
vasospastic 443.9
vestibular labyrinth 386.9
vision, visual NEC 368.9
psychophysical 368.16
specified NEC 368.8
subjective 368.10

Disturbance (Continued)
voice 784.40
wakefulness (initiation or maintenance)
(see also Hypersomnia) 780.54
nonorganic origin 307.43
**Disulfiduria, beta-mercaptolactate-cyste-
ine** 270.0
Disuse atrophy, bone 733.7
Ditthomska syndrome 307.81
Diuresis 788.42
Divers'
palsy or paralysis 993.3
squeeze 993.3
Diverticula, diverticulosis, diverticulum
(acute) (multiple) (perforated) (ruptured) 562.10
with diverticulitis 562.11
aorta (Kommerell's) 747.21
appendix (noninflammatory) 543.9
bladder (acquired) (sphincter) 596.3
congenital 753.8
broad ligament 620.8
bronchus (congenital) 748.3
acquired 494.0
with acute exacerbation 494.1
calyx, calyceal (kidney) 593.89
cardia (stomach) 537.1
cecum 562.10
with
diverticulitis 562.11
with hemorrhage 562.13
hemorrhage 562.12
congenital 751.5
colon (acquired) 562.10
with
diverticulitis 562.11
with hemorrhage 562.13
hemorrhage 562.12
congenital 751.5
duodenum 562.00
with
diverticulitis 562.01
with hemorrhage 562.03
hemorrhage 562.02
congenital 751.5
epiphrenic (esophagus) 530.6
esophagus (congenital) 750.4
acquired 530.6
epiphrenic 530.6
pulsion 530.6
traction 530.6
Zenker's 530.6
Eustachian tube 381.89
fallopian tube 620.8
gallbladder (congenital) 751.69
gastric 537.1
heart (congenital) 746.89
ileum 562.00
with
diverticulitis 562.01
with hemorrhage 562.03
hemorrhage 562.02
intestine (large) 562.10
with
diverticulitis 562.11
with hemorrhage 562.13
hemorrhage 562.12
congenital 751.5
small 562.00
with
diverticulitis 562.01
with hemorrhage 562.03
hemorrhage 562.02
congenital 751.5

Diverticula, diverticulosis, diverticulum
(Continued)
jejunum 562.00
with
diverticulitis 562.01
with hemorrhage 562.03
hemorrhage 562.02
kidney (calyx) (pelvis) 593.89
with calculus 592.0
Kommerell's 747.21
laryngeal ventricle (congenital) 748.3
Meckel's (displaced) (hypertrophic)
751.0
midthoracic 530.6
organ or site, congenital NEC - see Distortion
pericardium (congenital) (cyst) 746.89
acquired (true) 423.8
pharyngoesophageal (pulsion) 530.6
pharynx (congenital) 750.27
pulsion (esophagus) 530.6
rectosigmoid 562.10
with
diverticulitis 562.11
with hemorrhage 562.13
hemorrhage 562.12
congenital 751.5
rectum 562.10
with
diverticulitis 562.11
with hemorrhage 562.13
hemorrhage 562.12
renal (calyces) (pelvis) 593.89
with calculus 592.0
Rokitansky's 530.6
seminal vesicle 608.0
sigmoid 562.10
with
diverticulitis 562.11
with hemorrhage 562.13
hemorrhage 562.12
congenital 751.5
small intestine 562.00
with
diverticulitis 562.01
with hemorrhage 562.03
hemorrhage 562.02
stomach (cardia) (juxtacardia) (juxtapy-
loric) (acquired) 537.1
congenital 750.7
subdiaphragmatic 530.6
trachea (congenital) 748.3
acquired 519.1
traction (esophagus) 530.6
ureter (acquired) 593.89
congenital 753.4
ureterovesical orifice 593.89
urethra (acquired) 599.2
congenital 753.8
ventricle, left (congenital) 746.89
vesical (urinary) 596.3
congenital 753.8
Zenker's (esophagus) 530.6
Diverticulitis (acute) (see also Diverticula) 562.11
with hemorrhage 562.13
bladder (urinary) 596.3
cecum (perforated) 562.11
with hemorrhage 562.13
colon (perforated) 562.11
with hemorrhage 562.13
duodenum 562.01
with hemorrhage 562.03
esophagus 530.6

◀ **New**   ◀▥ **Revised**

Diverticulitis (Continued)
ileum (perforated) 562.01
  with hemorrhage 562.03
intestine (large) (perforated) 562.11
  with hemorrhage 562.13
  small 562.01
    with hemorrhage 562.03
jejunum (perforated) 562.01
  with hemorrhage 562.03
Meckel's (perforated) 751.0
pharyngoesophageal 530.6
rectosigmoid (perforated) 562.11
  with hemorrhage 562.13
rectum 562.11
  with hemorrhage 562.13
sigmoid (old) (perforated) 562.11
  with hemorrhage 562.13
small intestine (perforated) 562.01
  with hemorrhage 562.03
vesical (urinary) 596.3
Diverticulosis - see Diverticula
Division
cervix uteri 622.8
  external os into two openings by fre-
    num 752.49
external (cervical) into two openings
  by frenum 752.49
glans penis 752.69
hymen 752.49
labia minora (congenital) 752.49
ligament (partial or complete) (current)
  - see also Sprain, by site
  with open wound - see Wound,
    open, by site
muscle (partial or complete) (current) -
  see also Sprain, by site
  with open wound - see Wound,
    open, by site
nerve - see Injury, nerve, by site
penis glans 752.69
spinal cord - see Injury, spinal, by site
vein 459.9
  traumatic - see Injury, vascular, by
    site
Divorce V61.0
Dix-Hallpike neurolabyrinthitis 386.12
Dizziness 780.4
hysterical 300.11
psychogenic 306.9
Doan-Wiseman syndrome (primary
  splenic neutropenia) 288.0
Dog bite - see Wound, open, by site
Döhle-Heller aortitis 093.1
Döhle body-panmyelopathic syndrome
  288.2
Dolichocephaly, dolichocephalus 754.0
Dolichocolon 751.5
Dolichostenomelia 759.82
Donohue's syndrome (leprechaunism)
  259.8
Donor
blood V59.01
  other blood components V59.09
  stem cells V59.02
  whole blood V59.01
bone V59.2
  marrow V59.3
cornea V59.5
heart V59.8
kidney V59.4
liver V59.6
lung V59.8
lymphocyte V59.8
organ V59.9
  specified NEC V59.8

Donor (Continued)
potential, examination of V70.8
skin V59.1
specified organ or tissue NEC V59.8
sperm V59.8 ◄
stem cells V59.02
tissue V59.9
  specified type NEC V59.8
Donovanosis (granuloma venereum)
  099.2
DOPS (diffuse obstructive pulmonary
  syndrome) 496
Double
albumin 273.8
aortic arch 747.21
auditory canal 744.29
auricle (heart) 746.82
bladder 753.8
external (cervical) os 752.49
kidney with double pelvis (renal) 753.3
larynx 748.3
meatus urinarius 753.8
organ or site NEC - see Accessory
orifice
  heart valve NEC 746.89
    pulmonary 746.09
outlet, right ventricle 745.11
pelvis (renal) with double ureter 753.4
penis 752.69
tongue 750.13
ureter (one or both sides) 753.4
  with double pelvis (renal) 753.4
urethra 753.8
urinary meatus 753.8
uterus (any degree) 752.2
  with doubling of cervix and vagina
    752.2
  in pregnancy or childbirth 654.0
    affecting fetus or newborn 763.89
vagina 752.49
  with doubling of cervix and uterus
    752.2
vision 368.2
vocal cords 748.3
vulva 752.49
whammy (syndrome) 360.81
Douglas' pouch, cul-de-sac - see condition
Down's disease or syndrome (mongolism) 758.0
Down-growth, epithelial (anterior chamber) 364.61
Dracontiasis 125.7
Dracunculiasis 125.7
Dracunculosis 125.7
Drainage
abscess (spontaneous) - see Abscess
anomalous pulmonary veins to hepatic
  veins or right atrium 747.41
stump (amputation) (surgical) 997.62
suprapubic, bladder 596.8
Dream state, hysterical 300.13
Drepanocytic anemia (see also Disease,
  sickle cell) 282.60
Dresbach's syndrome (elliptocytosis)
  282.1
Dreschlera (infection) 118
hawaiiensis 117.8
Dressler's syndrome (postmyocardial infarction) 411.0
Dribbling (post-void) 788.35
Drift, ulnar 736.09
Drinking (alcohol) - see also Alcoholism
excessive, to excess NEC (see also Abuse,
  drugs, nondependent) 305.0
bouts, periodic 305.0

Drinking (Continued)
excessive, to excess NEC (Continued)
  continual 303.9
  episodic 305.0
  habitual 303.9
  periodic 305.0
Drip, postnasal (chronic) - see Sinusitis
Drivers' license examination V70.3
Droop
Cooper's 611.8
facial 781.94
Drop
finger 736.29
foot 736.79
hematocrit (precipitous) 790.01
toe 735.8
wrist 736.05
Dropped
dead 798.1
heart beats 426.6
Dropsy, dropsical (see also Edema) 782.3
abdomen 789.5
amnion (see also Hydramnios) 657
brain - see Hydrocephalus
cardiac (see also Failure, heart)
  428.0
cardiorenal (see also Hypertension, cardiorenal) 404.90
chest 511.9
fetus or newborn 778.0
  due to isoimmunization 773.3
gangrenous (see also Gangrene) 785.4
heart (see also Failure, heart) 428.0
hepatic - see Cirrhosis, liver
infantile - see Hydrops, fetalis
kidney (see also Nephrosis) 581.9
liver - see Cirrhosis, liver
lung 514
malarial (see also Malaria) 084.9
neonatorum - see Hydrops, fetalis
nephritic 581.9
newborn - see Hydrops, fetalis
nutritional 269.9
ovary 620.8
pericardium (see also Pericarditis) 423.9
renal (see also Nephrosis) 581.9
uremic - see Uremia
Drowned, drowning 994.1
lung 518.5
Drowsiness 780.09
Drug - see also condition
addiction (see also Dependence) 304.9
adverse effect NEC, correct substance
  properly administered 995.2
dependence (see also Dependence)
  304.9
habit (see also Dependence) 304.9
induced   ◄
  mental disorder 292.9   ◄
    anxiety 292.89   ◄
    mood 292.84   ◄
    sexual 292.89   ◄
    sleep 292.89   ◄
    specified type 292.89   ◄
  persisting   ◄
    amnestic disorder 292.83   ◄
    dementia 292.82   ◄
  psychotic disorder   ◄
    with   ◄
      delusions 292.11   ◄
      hallucinations 292.12   ◄
intoxication 292.89   ◄
overdose - see Table of Drugs and
  Chemicals

ICD-9-CM

Vol. 2

Drug (Continued)
poisoning - see Table of Drugs and Chemicals
therapy (maintenance) status NEC V58.1
 long-term (current) use V58.69
  antibiotics V58.62
  anticoagulants V58.61 ◀▥
  anti-inflammatories, non-steroidal (NSAID) V58.64
  antiplatelets V58.63 ◀▥
  antithrombotics V58.63 ◀▥
  aspirin V58.66 ◀
  insulin V58.67 ◀
  steroids V58.65
 wrong substance given or taken in error - see Table of Drugs and Chemicals
Drunkenness (see also Abuse, drugs, nondependent) 305.0
 acute in alcoholism (see also Alcoholism) 303.0
 chronic (see also Alcoholism) 303.9
 pathologic 291.4
 simple (acute) 305.0
  in alcoholism 303.0
 sleep 307.47
Drusen
 optic disc or papilla 377.21
 retina (colloid) (hyaloid degeneration) 362.57
  hereditary 362.77
Drusenfieber 075
Dry, dryness - see also condition
 eye 375.15
  syndrome 375.15
 larynx 478.79
 mouth 527.7
 nose 478.1
 skin syndrome 701.1
 socket (teeth) 526.5
 throat 478.29
DSAP (disseminated superficial actinic porokeratosis) 692.75
Duane's retraction syndrome 378.71
Duane-Stilling-Türk syndrome (ocular retraction syndrome) 378.71
Dubin-Johnson disease or syndrome 277.4
Dubini's disease (electric chorea) 049.8
Dubois' abscess or disease 090.5
Duchenne's
 disease 094.0
  locomotor ataxia 094.0
  muscular dystrophy 359.1
  pseudohypertrophy, muscles 359.1
 paralysis 335.22
 syndrome 335.22
Duchenne-Aran myelopathic, muscular atrophy (nonprogressive) (progressive) 335.21
Duchenne-Griesinger disease 359.1
Ducrey's
 bacillus 099.0
 chancre 099.0
 disease (chancroid) 099.0
Duct, ductus - see condition
Duengero 061
Duhring's disease (dermatitis herpetiformis) 694.0
Dukes (-Filatov) disease 057.8
Dullness
 cardiac (decreased) (increased) 785.3
Dumb ague (see also Malaria) 084.6
Dumbness (see also Aphasia) 784.3
Dumdum fever 085.0

Dumping syndrome (postgastrectomy) 564.2
 nonsurgical 536.8
Duodenitis (nonspecific) (peptic) 535.60
 with hemorrhage 535.61
 due to
  strongyloides stercoralis 127.2
Duodenocholangitis 575.8
Duodenum, duodenal - see condition
Duplay's disease, periarthritis, or syndrome 726.2
Duplex - see also Accessory
 kidney 753.3
 placenta - see Placenta, abnormal
 uterus 752.2
Duplication - see also Accessory
 anus 751.5
 aortic arch 747.21
 appendix 751.5
 biliary duct (any) 751.69
 bladder 753.8
 cecum 751.5
  and appendix 751.5
 clitoris 752.49
 cystic duct 751.69
 digestive organs 751.8
 duodenum 751.5
 esophagus 750.4
 fallopian tube 752.19
 frontonasal process 756.0
 gallbladder 751.69
 ileum 751.5
 intestine (large) (small) 751.5
 jejunum 751.5
 kidney 753.3
 liver 751.69
 nose 748.1
 pancreas 751.7
 penis 752.69
 respiratory organs NEC 748.9
 salivary duct 750.22
 spinal cord (incomplete) 742.51
 stomach 750.7
 ureter 753.4
 vagina 752.49
 vas deferens 752.89
 vocal cords 748.3
Dupré's disease or syndrome (meningism) 781.6
Dupuytren's
 contraction 728.6
 disease (muscle contracture) 728.6
 fracture (closed) 824.4
  ankle (closed) 824.4
   open 824.5
  fibula (closed) 824.4
   open 824.5
  open 824.5
  radius (closed) 813.42
   open 813.52
 muscle contracture 728.6
Durand-Nicolas-Favre disease (climatic bubo) 099.1
Duroziez's disease (congenital mitral stenosis) 746.5
Dust
 conjunctivitis 372.05
 reticulation (occupational) 504
Dutton's
 disease (trypanosomiasis) 086.9
 relapsing fever (West African) 087.1
Dwarf, dwarfism 259.4
 with infantilism (hypophyseal) 253.3
 achondroplastic 756.4
 Amsterdam 759.89

Dwarf, dwarfism (Continued)
 bird-headed 759.89
 congenital 259.4
 constitutional 259.4
 hypophyseal 253.3
 infantile 259.4
 Levi type 253.3
 Lorain-Levi (pituitary) 253.3
 Lorain type (pituitary) 253.3
 metatropic 756.4
 nephrotic-glycosuric, with hypophosphatemic rickets 270.0
 nutritional 263.2
 ovarian 758.6
 pancreatic 577.8
 pituitary 253.3
 polydystrophic 277.5
 primordial 253.3
 psychosocial 259.4
 renal 588.0
  with hypertension - see Hypertension, kidney
 Russell's (uterine dwarfism and craniofacial dysostosis) 759.89
Dyke-Young anemia or syndrome (acquired macrocytic hemolytic anemia) (secondary) (symptomatic) 283.9
Dynia abnormality (see also Defect, coagulation) 286.9
Dysacousis 388.40
Dysadrenocortism 255.9
 hyperfunction 255.3
 hypofunction 255.4
Dysarthria 784.5
Dysautonomia (see also Neuropathy, peripheral, autonomic) 337.9
 familial 742.8
Dysbarism 993.3
Dysbasia 719.7
 angiosclerotica intermittens 443.9
  due to atherosclerosis 440.21
 hysterical 300.11
 lordotica (progressiva) 333.6
 nonorganic origin 307.9
 psychogenic 307.9
Dysbetalipoproteinemia (familial) 272.2
Dyscalculia 315.1
Dyschezia (see also Constipation) 564.00
Dyschondroplasia (with hemangiomata) 756.4
 Voorhoeve's 756.4
Dyschondrosteosis 756.59
Dyschromia 709.00
Dyscollagenosis 710.9
Dyscoria 743.41
Dyscraniopyophalangy 759.89
Dyscrasia
 blood 289.9
  with antepartum hemorrhage 641.3
  fetus or newborn NEC 776.9
  hemorrhage, subungual 287.8
  puerperal, postpartum 666.3
 ovary 256.8
 plasma cell 273.9
 pluriglandular 258.9
 polyglandular 258.9
Dysdiadochokinesia 781.3
Dysectasia, vesical neck 596.8
Dysendocrinism 259.9
Dysentery, dysenteric (bilious) (catarrhal) (diarrhea) (epidemic) (gangrenous) (hemorrhagic) (infectious) (sporadic) (tropical) (ulcerative) 009.0
 abscess, liver (see also Abscess, amebic) 006.3

◀ **New** ◀▥ **Revised**

Dysentery, dysenteric (*Continued*)
  amebic (*see also* Amebiasis) 006.9
    with abscess - *see* Abscess, amebic
    acute 006.0
    carrier (suspected) of V02.2
    chronic 006.1
  arthritis (*see also* Arthritis, due to, dys-
      entery) 009.0 *[711.3]*
    bacillary 004.9 *[711.3]*
    Boyd 004.2
    Flexner 004.1
    Schmitz (-Stutzer) 004.0
    Shiga 004.0
    Shigella 004.9
      group A 004.0
      group B 004.1
      group C 004.2
      group D 004.3
      specified type NEC 004.8
    Sonne 004.3
    specified type NEC 004.8
  bacterium 004.9
  balantidial 007.0
  Balantidium coli 007.0
  Boyd's 004.2
  Chilomastix 007.8
  Chinese 004.9
  choleriform 001.1
  coccidial 007.2
  Dientamoeba fragilis 007.8
  due to specified organism NEC - *see*
      Enteritis, due to, by organism
  Embadomonas 007.8
  Endolimax nana - *see* Dysentery, amebic
  Entamoba, entamebic - *see* Dysentery,
      amebic
  Flexner's 004.1
  Flexner-Boyd 004.2
  giardial 007.1
  Giardia lamblia 007.1
  Hiss-Russell 004.1
  lamblia 007.1
  leishmanial 085.0
  malarial (*see also* Malaria) 084.6
  metazoal 127.9
  Monilia 112.89
  protozoal NEC 007.9
  Russell's 004.8
  salmonella 003.0
  schistosomal 120.1
  Schmitz (-Stutzer) 004.0
  Shiga 004.0
  Shigella NEC (*see also* Dysentery, bacil-
      lary) 004.9
    boydii 004.2
    dysenteriae 004.0
      Schmitz 004.0
      Shiga 004.0
    flexneri 004.1
    group A 004.0
    group B 004.1
    group C 004.2
    group D 004.3
    Schmitz 004.0
    Shiga 004.0
    Sonnei 004.3
  Sonne 004.3
  strongyloidiasis 127.2
  trichomonal 007.3
  tuberculous (*see also* Tuberculosis)
      014.8
  viral (*see also* Enteritis, viral) 008.8

Dysequilibrium 780.4
Dysesthesia 782.0
  hysterical 300.11
Dysfibrinogenemia (congenital) (*see also*
    Defect, coagulation) 286.3
Dysfunction
  adrenal (cortical) 255.9
    hyperfunction 255.3
    hypofunction 255.4
  associated with sleep stages or arousal
      from sleep 780.56
    nonorganic origin 307.47
  bladder NEC 596.59
  bleeding, uterus 626.8
  brain, minimal (*see also* Hyperkinesia)
      314.9
  cerebral 348.30
  colon 564.9
    psychogenic 306.4
  colostomy or enterostomy 569.62
  cystic duct 575.8
  diastolic 429.9
    with heart failure - *see* Failure, heart
    due to
      cardiomyopathy - *see* Cardiomy-
          opathy
      hypertension - *see* Hypertension,
          heart
  endocrine NEC 259.9
  endometrium 621.8
  enteric stoma 569.62
  enterostomy 569.62
  esophagostomy 530.87 ◄
  Eustachian tube 381.81
  gallbladder 575.8
  gastrointestinal 536.9
  gland, glandular NEC 259.9
  heart 427.9
    postoperative (immediate) 997.1
      long-term effect of cardiac surgery
          429.4
  hemoglobin 288.8
  hepatic 573.9
  hepatocellular NEC 573.9
  hypophysis 253.9
    hyperfunction 253.1
    hypofunction 253.2
    posterior lobe 253.6
      hypofunction 253.5
  kidney (*see also* Disease, renal) 593.9
  labyrinthine 386.50
    specified NEC 386.58
  liver 573.9
    constitutional 277.4
  minimal brain (child) (*see also* Hyperki-
      nesia) 314.9
  ovary, ovarian 256.9
    hyperfunction 256.1
      estrogen 256.0
    hypofunction 256.39
      postablative 256.2
    postablative 256.2
    specified NEC 256.8
  papillary muscle 429.81
    with myocardial infarction 410.8
  parathyroid 252.8
    hyperfunction 252.00 ◄▥
    hypofunction 252.1
  pineal gland 259.8
  pituitary (gland) 253.9
    hyperfunction 253.1
    hypofunction 253.2
    posterior 253.6
      hypofunction 253.5

Dysfunction (*Continued*)
  placental - *see* Placenta, insufficiency
  platelets (blood) 287.1
  polyglandular 258.9
    specified NEC 258.8
  psychosexual 302.70
    with
      dyspareunia (functional) (psycho-
          genic) 302.76
      frigidity 302.72
      impotence 302.72
      inhibition
        orgasm
          female 302.73
          male 302.74
        sexual
          desire 302.71
          excitement 302.72
      premature ejaculation 302.75
      sexual aversion 302.79
      specified disorder NEC 302.79
      vaginismus 306.51
  pylorus 537.9
  rectum 564.9
    psychogenic 306.4
  segmental (*see also* Dysfunction, so-
      matic) 739.9
  senile 797
  sexual 302.70 ◄
  sinoatrial node 427.81
  somatic 739.9
    abdomen 739.9
    acromioclavicular 739.7
    cervical 739.1
    cervicothoracic 739.1
    costochondral 739.8
    costovertebral 739.8
    extremities
      lower 739.6
      upper 739.7
    head 739.0
    hip 739.5
    lumbar, lumbosacral 739.3
    occipitocervical 739.0
    pelvic 739.5
    pubic 739.5
    rib cage 739.8
    sacral 739.4
    sacrococcygeal 739.4
    sacroiliac 739.4
    specified site NEC 739.9
    sternochondral 739.8
    sternoclavicular 739.7
    temporomandibular 739.0
    thoracic, thoracolumbar 739.2
  stomach 536.9
    psychogenic 306.4
  suprarenal 255.9
    hyperfunction 255.3
    hypofunction 255.4
  symbolic NEC 784.60
    specified type NEC 784.69
  temporomandibular (joint) (joint-pain-
      syndrome) NEC 524.60
    sounds on opening or closing
        524.64 ◄
    specified NEC 524.69
  testicular 257.9
    hyperfunction 257.0
    hypofunction 257.2
    specified type NEC 257.8
  thymus 254.9
  thyroid 246.9
    complicating pregnancy, childbirth,
        or puerperium 648.1

ICD-9-CM
Vol. 2

Dysfunction (Continued)
  thyroid (Continued)
    hyperfunction - see Hyperthyroidism
    hypofunction - see Hypothyroidism
  uterus, complicating delivery 661.9
    affecting fetus or newborn 763.7
    hypertonic 661.4
    hypotonic 661.2
      primary 661.0
      secondary 661.1
  velopharyngeal (acquired) 528.9
    congenital 750.29
  ventricular 429.9
    with congestive heart failure (see also
      Failure, heart) 428.0
    due to
      cardiomyopathy - see Cardiomy-
        opathy
      hypertension - see Hypertension,
        heart
  vesicourethral NEC 596.59
  vestibular 386.50
    specified type NEC 386.58
Dysgammaglobulinemia 279.06
Dysgenesis
  gonadal (due to chromosomal anom-
    aly) 758.6
    pure 752.7
  kidney(s) 753.0
  ovarian 758.6
  renal 753.0
  reticular 279.2
  seminiferous tubules 758.6
  tidal platelet 287.3
Dysgerminoma (M9060/3)
  specified site - see Neoplasm, by site,
    malignant
  unspecified site
    female 183.0
    male 186.9
Dysgeusia 781.1
Dysgraphia 781.3
Dyshidrosis 705.81
Dysidrosis 705.81
Dysinsulinism 251.8
Dyskaryotic cervical smear 795.09
Dyskeratosis (see also Keratosis) 701.1
  bullosa hereditaria 757.39
  cervix 622.10   ◄▥
  congenital 757.39
  follicularis 757.39
    vitamin A deficiency 264.8
  gingiva 523.8
  oral soft tissue NEC 528.79   ◄▥
  tongue 528.79   ◄▥
  uterus NEC 621.8
Dyskinesia 781.3
  biliary 575.8
  esophagus 530.5
  hysterical 300.11
  intestinal 564.89
  nonorganic origin 307.9
  orofacial 333.82
  psychogenic 307.9
  tardive (oral) 333.82
Dyslalia 784.5
  developmental 315.39
Dyslexia 784.61
  developmental 315.02
  secondary to organic lesion 784.61
Dyslipidemia 272.4   ◄
Dysmaturity (see also Immaturity) 765.1
  lung 770.4
  pulmonary 770.4

Dysmenorrhea (essential) (exfoliative)
  (functional) (intrinsic) (membranous)
  (primary) (secondary) 625.3
  psychogenic 306.52
Dysmetabolic syndrome X 277.7
Dysmetria 781.3
**Dysmorodystrophia mesodermalis con-
  genita** 759.82
Dysnomia 784.3
Dysorexia 783.0
  hysterical 300.11
Dysostosis
  cleidocranial, cleidocranialis 755.59
  craniofacial 756.0
  Fairbank's (idiopathic familial general-
    ized osteophytosis) 756.50
  mandibularis 756.0
  mandibulofacial, incomplete 756.0
  multiplex 277.5
  orodigitofacial 759.89
Dyspareunia (female) 625.0
  male 608.89
  psychogenic 302.76
Dyspepsia (allergic) (congenital) (fermentative) (flatulent) (functional)
  (gastric) (gastrointestinal) (neurogenic) (occupational) (reflex)
  536.8
  acid 536.8
  atonic 536.3
    psychogenic 306.4
  diarrhea 787.91
    psychogenic 306.4
  intestinal 564.89
    psychogenic 306.4
  nervous 306.4
  neurotic 306.4
  psychogenic 306.4
Dysphagia 787.2
  functional 300.11
  hysterical 300.11
  nervous 300.11
  psychogenic 306.4
  sideropenic 280.8
  spastica 530.5
Dysphagocytosis, congenital 288.1
Dysphasia 784.5
Dysphonia 784.49
  clericorum 784.49
  functional 300.11
  hysterical 300.11
  psychogenic 306.1
  spastica 478.79
Dyspigmentation - see also Pigmentation
  eyelid (acquired) 374.52
Dyspituitarism 253.9
  hyperfunction 253.1
  hypofunction 253.2
  posterior lobe 253.6
Dysplasia - see also Anomaly
  artery
    fibromuscular NEC 447.8
      carotid 447.8
      renal 447.3
  bladder 596.8
  bone (fibrous) NEC 733.29
    diaphyseal, progressive 756.59
    jaw 526.89
    monostotic 733.29
    polyostotic 756.54
    solitary 733.29
  brain 742.9
  bronchopulmonary, fetus or newborn
    770.7

Dysplasia (Continued)
  cervix (uteri) 622.10   ◄▥
    cervical intraepithelial neoplasia I
      [CIN I] 622.11   ◄▥
    cervical intraepithelial neoplasia II
      [CIN II] 622.12   ◄▥
    cervical intraepithelial neoplasia III
      [CIN III] 233.1
    CIN I 622.11   ◄▥
    CIN II 622.12   ◄▥
    CIN III 233.1
    mild 622.11   ◄
    moderate 622.12   ◄
    severe 233.1   ◄
  chondroectodermal 756.55
  chondromatose 756.4
  craniocarpotarsal 759.89
  craniometaphyseal 756.89
  dentinal 520.5
  diaphyseal, progressive 756.59
  ectodermal (anhidrotic) (Bason) (Clous-
    ton's) (congenital) (Feinmesser)
    (hereditary) (hidrotic) (Marshall)
    (Robinson's) 757.31
  epiphysealis 756.9
    multiplex 756.56
    punctata 756.59
  epiphysis 756.9
    multiple 756.56
  epithelial
    epiglottis 478.79
    uterine cervix 622.10   ◄▥
  erythroid NEC 289.89
  eye (see also Microphthalmos) 743.10
  familial metaphyseal 756.89
  fibromuscular, artery NEC 447.8
    carotid 447.8
    renal 447.3
  fibrous
    bone NEC 733.29
    diaphyseal, progressive 756.59
    jaw 526.89
    monostotic 733.29
    polyostotic 756.54
    solitary 733.29
  hip (congenital) 755.63
    with dislocation (see also Dislocation,
      hip, congenital) 754.30
  hypohidrotic ectodermal 757.31
  joint 755.8
  kidney 753.15
  leg 755.69
  linguofacialis 759.89
  lung 748.5
  macular 743.55
  mammary (benign) (gland) 610.9
    cystic 610.1
    specified type NEC 610.8
  metaphyseal 756.9
    familial 756.89
  monostotic fibrous 733.29
  muscle 756.89
  myeloid NEC 289.89
  nervous system (general) 742.9
  neuroectodermal 759.6
  oculoauriculovertebral 756.0
  oculodentodigital 759.89
  olfactogenital 253.4
  osteo-onycho-arthro (hereditary)
    756.89
  periosteum 733.99
  polyostotic fibrous 756.54
  progressive diaphyseal 756.59
  prostate 602.3

◄ **New**   ◄▥ **Revised**

Dysplasia (Continued)
  prostate (Continued)
    intraepithelial neoplasia I [PIN I]
      602.3
    intraepithelial neoplasia II [PIN II]
      602.3
    intraepithelial neoplasia III [PIN III]
      233.4
  renal 753.15
  renofacialis 753.0
  retinal NEC 743.56
  retrolental 362.21
  spinal cord 742.9
  thymic, with immunodeficiency 279.2
  vagina 623.0
  vocal cord 478.5
  vulva 624.8
    intraepithelial neoplasia I [VIN I]
      624.8
    intraepithelial neoplasia II [VIN II]
      624.8
    intraepithelial neoplasia III [VIN III]
      233.3
    VIN I 624.8
    VIN II 624.8
    VIN III 233.3
Dyspnea (nocturnal) (paroxysmal)
  786.09
  asthmatic (bronchial) (see also Asthma)
    493.9
    with bronchitis (see also Asthma)
      493.9
      chronic 493.2
  cardiac (see also Failure, ventricular,
    left) 428.1
  cardiac (see also Failure, ventricular,
    left) 428.1
  functional 300.11
  hyperventilation 786.01
  hysterical 300.11
  Monday morning 504
  newborn 770.89
  psychogenic 306.1
  uremic - see Uremia
Dyspraxia 781.3
  syndrome 315.4
Dysproteinemia 273.8
  transient with copper deficiency
    281.4
Dysprothrombinemia (constitutional)
  (see also Defect, coagulation) 286.3
Dysreflexia, autonomic 337.3
Dysrhythmia
  cardiac 427.9
    postoperative (immediate) 997.1
      long-term effect of cardiac surgery
        429.4
    specified type NEC 427.89
  cerebral or cortical 348.30
Dyssecretosis, mucoserous 710.2
Dyssocial reaction, without manifest
  psychiatric disorder
  adolescent V71.02
  adult V71.01
  child V71.02
Dyssomnia NEC 780.56
  nonorganic origin 307.47
Dyssplenism 289.4
Dyssynergia
  biliary (see also Disease, biliary) 576.8
  cerebellaris myoclonica 334.2
  detrusor sphincter (bladder) 596.55
  ventricular 429.89
Dystasia, hereditary areflexic 334.3

Dysthymia 300.4
Dysthymic disorder 300.4
Dysthyroidism 246.9
Dystocia 660.9
  affecting fetus or newborn 763.1
  cervical 661.0
    affecting fetus or newborn 763.7
  contraction ring 661.4
    affecting fetus or newborn 763.7
  fetal 660.9
    abnormal size 653.5
    affecting fetus or newborn 763.1
    deformity 653.7
  maternal 660.9
    affecting fetus or newborn 763.1
  positional 660.0
    affecting fetus or newborn 763.1
  shoulder (girdle) 660.4
    affecting fetus or newborn 763.1
  uterine NEC 661.4
    affecting fetus or newborn 763.7
Dystonia
  deformans progressiva 333.6
  due to drugs 333.7
  lenticularis 333.6
  musculorum deformans 333.6
  torsion (idiopathic) 333.6
    fragments (of) 333.89
    symptomatic 333.7
Dystonic
  movements 781.0
Dystopia kidney 753.3
Dystrophy, dystrophia 783.9
  adiposogenital 253.8
  asphyxiating thoracic 756.4
  Becker's type 359.1
  brevicollis 756.16
  Bruch's membrane 362.77
  cervical (sympathetic) NEC 337.0
  chondro-osseus with punctate epiphys-
    eal dysplasia 756.59
  choroid (hereditary) 363.50
    central (areolar) (partial) 363.53
      total (gyrate) 363.54
    circinate 363.53
    circumpapillary (partial) 363.51
      total 363.52
    diffuse
      partial 363.56
      total 363.57
    generalized
      partial 363.56
      total 363.57
    gyrate
      central 363.54
      generalized 363.57
    helicoid 363.52
    peripapillary - see Dystrophy, cho-
      roid, circumpapillary
    serpiginous 363.54
  cornea (hereditary) 371.50
    anterior NEC 371.52
    Cogan's 371.52
    combined 371.57
    crystalline 371.56
    endothelial (Fuchs') 371.57
    epithelial 371.50
      juvenile 371.51
      microscopic cystic 371.52
    granular 371.53
    lattice 371.54
    macular 371.55
    marginal (Terrien's) 371.48
    Meesman's 371.51

Dystrophy, dystrophia (Continued)
  cornea (Continued)
    microscopic cystic (epithelial)
      371.52
    nodular, Salzmann's 371.46
    polymorphous 371.58
    posterior NEC 371.58
    ring-like 371.52
    Salzmann's nodular 371.46
    stromal NEC 371.56
  dermatochondrocorneal 371.50
  Duchenne's 359.1
  due to malnutrition 263.9
  Erb's 359.1
  familial
    hyperplastic periosteal 756.59
    osseous 277.5
  foveal 362.77
  Fuchs', cornea 371.57
  Gowers' muscular 359.1
  hair 704.2
  hereditary, progressive muscular 359.1
  hypogenital, with diabetic tendency
    759.81
  Landouzy-Déjérine 359.1
  Leyden-Möbius 359.1
  mesodermalis congenita 759.82
  muscular 359.1
    congenital (hereditary) 359.0
      myotonic 359.2
    distal 359.1
    Duchenne's 359.1
    Erb's 359.1
    fascioscapulohumeral 359.1
    Gowers' 359.1
    hereditary (progressive) 359.1
    Landouzy-Déjérine 359.1
    limb-girdle 359.1
    myotonic 359.2
    progressive (hereditary) 359.1
      Charcôt-Marie-Tooth 356.1
    pseudohypertrophic (infantile) 359.1
  myocardium, myocardial (see also De-
    generation, myocardial) 429.1
  myotonic 359.2
  myotonica 359.2
  nail 703.8
    congenital 757.5
  neurovascular (traumatic) (see also
    Neuropathy, peripheral, auto-
    nomic) 337.9
  nutritional 263.9
  ocular 359.1
  oculocerebrorenal 270.8
  oculopharyngeal 359.1
  ovarian 620.8
  papillary (and pigmentary) 701.1
  pelvicrural atrophic 359.1
  pigmentary (see also Acanthosis) 701.2
  pituitary (gland) 253.8
  polyglandular 258.8
  posttraumatic sympathetic - see Dys-
    trophy, sympathic
  progressive ophthalmoplegic 359.1
  retina, retinal (hereditary) 362.70
    albipunctate 362.74
    Bruch's membrane 362.77
    cone, progressive 362.75
    hyaline 362.77
    in
      Bassen-Kornzweig syndrome 272.5
      [362.72]
      cerebroretinal lipidosis 330.1
      [362.71]

ICD-9-CM

Vol. 2

Dystrophy, dystrophia *(Continued)*
retina, retinal *(Continued)*
in *(Continued)*
Refsum's disease 356.3 *[362.72]*
systemic lipidosis 272.7 *[362.71]*
juvenile (Stargardt's) 362.75
pigmentary 362.74
pigment epithelium 362.76
progressive cone (-rod) 362.75
pseudoinflammatory foveal 362.77
rod, progressive 362.75
sensory 362.75
vitelliform 362.76

Dystrophy, dystrophia *(Continued)*
Salzmann's nodular 371.46
scapuloperoneal 359.1
skin NEC 709.9
sympathetic (posttraumatic) (reflex) 337.20
lower limb 337.22
specified site NEC 337.29
upper limb 337.21
tapetoretinal NEC 362.74

Dystrophy, dystrophia *(Continued)*
thoracic asphyxiating 756.4
unguium 703.8
congenital 757.5
vitreoretinal (primary) 362.73
secondary 362.66
vulva 624.0
Dysuria 788.1
psychogenic 306.53

◀ New   ◀▥ Revised

E

Eagle-Barrett syndrome 756.71
Eales' disease (syndrome) 362.18
Ear - *see also* condition
  ache 388.70
    otogenic 388.71
    referred 388.72
  lop 744.29
  piercing V50.3
  swimmers' acute 380.12
  tank 380.12
  tropical 111.8 *[380.15]*
  wax 380.4
Earache 388.70
  otogenic 388.71
  referred 388.72
Early satiety 780.94
Eaton-Lambert syndrome (*see also* Neoplasm, by site, malignant) 199.1 *[358.1]*
Eberth's disease (typhoid fever) 002.0
Ebstein's
  anomaly or syndrome (downward displacement, tricuspid valve into right ventricle) 746.2
  disease (diabetes) 250.4 *[581.81]*
Eccentro-osteochondrodysplasia 277.5
Ecchondroma (M9210/0) - *see* Neoplasm, bone, benign
Ecchondrosis (M9210/1) 238.0
Ecchordosis physaliphora 756.0
Ecchymosis (multiple) 459.89
  conjunctiva 372.72
  eye (traumatic) 921.0
  eyelids (traumatic) 921.1
  newborn 772.6
  spontaneous 782.7
  traumatic - *see* Contusion
Echinococciasis - *see* Echinococcus
Echinococcosis - *see* Echinococcus
Echinococcus (infection) 122.9
  granulosus 122.4
    liver 122.0
    lung 122.1
    orbit 122.3 *[376.13]*
    specified site NEC 122.3
    thyroid 122.2
  liver NEC 122.8
    granulosus 122.0
    multilocularis 122.5
  lung NEC 122.9
    granulosus 122.1
    multilocularis 122.6
  multilocularis 122.7
    liver 122.5
    specified site NEC 122.6
  orbit 122.9 *[376.13]*
    granulosus 122.3 *[376.13]*
    multilocularis 122.6 *[376.13]*
  specified site NEC 122.9
    granulosus 122.3
    multilocularis 122.6 *[376.13]*
  thyroid NEC 122.9
    granulosus 122.2
    multilocularis 122.6
Echinorhynchiasis 127.7
Echinostomiasis 121.8
Echolalia 784.69
ECHO virus infection NEC 079.1
Eclampsia, eclamptic (coma) (convulsions) (delirium) 780.39
  female, child-bearing age NEC - *see* Eclampsia, pregnancy

Eclampsia, eclamptic (*Continued*)
  gravidarum - *see* Eclampsia, pregnancy
  male 780.39
  not associated with pregnancy or childbirth 780.39
  pregnancy, childbirth, or puerperium 642.6
    with pre-existing hypertension 642.7
    affecting fetus or newborn 760.0
  uremic 586
Eclipse blindness (total) 363.31
Economic circumstance affecting care V60.9
  specified type NEC V60.8
Economo's disease (encephalitis lethargica) 049.8
Ectasia, ectasis
  aorta (*see also* Aneurysm, aorta) 441.9
    ruptured 441.5
  breast 610.4
  capillary 448.9
  cornea (marginal) (postinfectional) 371.71
  duct (mammary) 610.4
  kidney 593.89
  mammary duct (gland) 610.4
  papillary 448.9
  renal 593.89
  salivary gland (duct) 527.8
  scar, cornea 371.71
  sclera 379.11
Ecthyma 686.8
  contagiosum 051.2
  gangrenosum 686.09
  infectiosum 051.2
Ectocardia 746.87
Ectodermal dysplasia, congenital 757.31
Ectodermosis erosiva pluriorificialis 695.1
Ectopic, ectopia (congenital) 759.89
  abdominal viscera 751.8
    due to defect in anterior abdominal wall 756.79
  ACTH syndrome 255.0
  adrenal gland 759.1
  anus 751.5
  auricular beats 427.61
  beats 427.60
  bladder 753.5
  bone and cartilage in lung 748.69
  brain 742.4
  breast tissue 757.6
  cardiac 746.87
  cerebral 742.4
  cordis 746.87
  endometrium 617.9
  gallbladder 751.69
  gastric mucosa 750.7
  gestation - *see* Pregnancy, ectopic
  heart 746.87
  hormone secretion NEC 259.3
  hyperparathyroidism 259.3
  kidney (crossed) (intrathoracic) (pelvis) 753.3
    in pregnancy or childbirth 654.4
    causing obstructed labor 660.2
  lens 743.37
  lentis 743.37
  mole - *see* Pregnancy, ectopic
  organ or site NEC - *see* Malposition, congenital
  ovary 752.0
  pancreas, pancreatic tissue 751.7
  pregnancy - *see* Pregnancy, ectopic

Ectopic, ectopia (*Continued*)
  pupil 364.75
  renal 753.3
  sebaceous glands of mouth 750.26
  secretion
    ACTH 255.0
    adrenal hormone 259.3
    adrenalin 259.3
    adrenocorticotropin 255.0
    antidiuretic hormone (ADH) 259.3
    epinephrine 259.3
    hormone NEC 259.3
    norepinephrine 259.3
    pituitary (posterior) 259.3
  spleen 759.0
  testis 752.51
  thyroid 759.2
  ureter 753.4
  ventricular beats 427.69
  vesicae 753.5
Ectrodactyly 755.4
  finger (*see also* Absence, finger, congenital) 755.29
  toe (*see also* Absence, toe, congenital) 755.39
Ectromelia 755.4
  lower limb 755.30
  upper limb 755.20
Ectropion 374.10
  anus 569.49
  cervix 622.0
    with mention of cervicitis 616.0
  cicatricial 374.14
  congenital 743.62
  eyelid 374.10
    cicatricial 374.14
    congenital 743.62
    mechanical 374.12
    paralytic 374.12
    senile 374.11
    spastic 374.13
  iris (pigment epithelium) 364.54
  lip (congenital) 750.26
    acquired 528.5
  mechanical 374.12
  paralytic 374.12
  rectum 569.49
  senile 374.11
  spastic 374.13
  urethra 599.84
  uvea 364.54
Eczema (acute) (allergic) (chronic) (erythematous) (fissum) (occupational) (rubrum) (squamous) 692.9
  asteatotic 706.8
  atopic 691.8
  contact NEC 692.9
  dermatitis NEC 692.9
  due to specified cause - *see* Dermatitis, due to
  dyshidrotic 705.81
  external ear 380.22
  flexural 691.8
  gouty 274.89
  herpeticum 054.0
  hypertrophicum 701.8
  hypostatic - *see* Varicose, vein
  impetiginous 684
  infantile (acute) (chronic) (due to any substance) (intertriginous) (seborrheic) 690.12
  intertriginous NEC 692.9
    infantile 690.12
  intrinsic 691.8

Eczema *(Continued)*
lichenified NEC 692.9
marginatum 110.3
nummular 692.9
pustular 686.8
seborrheic 690.18
infantile 690.12
solare 692.72
stasis (lower extremity) 454.1
ulcerated 454.2
vaccination, vaccinatum 999.0
varicose (lower extremity) - *see* Varicose, vein
verrucosum callosum 698.3
Eczematoid, exudative 691.8
Eddowes' syndrome (brittle bones and blue sclera) 756.51
Edema, edematous 782.3
with nephritis (*see also* Nephrosis) 581.9
allergic 995.1
angioneurotic (allergic) (any site) (with urticaria) 995.1
hereditary 277.6
angiospastic 443.9
Berlin's (traumatic) 921.3
brain 348.5
due to birth injury 767.8
fetus or newborn 767.8
cardiac (*see also* Failure, heart) 428.0
cardiovascular (*see also* Failure, heart) 428.0
cerebral - *see* Edema, brain
cerebrospinal vessel - *see* Edema, brain
cervix (acute) (uteri) 622.8
puerperal, postpartum 674.8
chronic hereditary 757.0
circumscribed, acute 995.1
hereditary 277.6
complicating pregnancy (gestational) 646.1
with hypertension - *see* Toxemia, of pregnancy
conjunctiva 372.73
connective tissue 782.3
cornea 371.20
due to contact lenses 371.24
idiopathic 371.21
secondary 371.22
cystoid macular 362.53
due to
lymphatic obstruction - *see* Edema, lymphatic
salt retention 276.0
epiglottis - *see* Edema, glottis
essential, acute 995.1
hereditary 277.6
extremities, lower - *see* Edema, legs
eyelid NEC 374.82
familial, hereditary (legs) 757.0
famine 262
fetus or newborn 778.5
genital organs
female 629.8
male 608.86
gestational 646.1
with hypertension - *see* Toxemia, of pregnancy
glottis, glottic, glottides (obstructive) (passive) 478.6
allergic 995.1
hereditary 277.6
due to external agent - *see* Condition, respiratory, acute, due to specified agent

Edema, edematous *(Continued)*
heart (*see also* Failure, heart) 428.0
newborn 779.89
heat 992.7
hereditary (legs) 757.0
inanition 262
infectious 782.3
intracranial 348.5
due to injury at birth 767.8
iris 364.8
joint (*see also* Effusion, joint) 719.0
larynx (*see also* Edema, glottis) 478.6
legs 782.3
due to venous obstruction 459.2
hereditary 757.0
localized 782.3
due to venous obstruction 459.2
lower extremity 459.2
lower extremities - *see* Edema, legs
lung 514
acute 518.4
with heart disease or failure (*see also* Failure, ventricular, left) 428.1
congestive 428.0
chemical (due to fumes or vapors) 506.1
due to
external agent(s) NEC 508.9
specified NEC 508.8
fumes and vapors (chemical) (inhalation) 506.1
radiation 508.0
chemical (acute) 506.1
chronic 506.4
chronic 514
chemical (due to fumes or vapors) 506.4
due to
external agent(s) NEC 508.9
specified NEC 508.8
fumes or vapors (chemical) (inhalation) 506.4
radiation 508.1
due to
external agent 508.9
specified NEC 508.8
high altitude 993.2
near drowning 994.1
postoperative 518.4
terminal 514
lymphatic 457.1
due to mastectomy operation 457.0
macula 362.83
cystoid 362.53
diabetic 250.5 *[362.01]*
malignant (*see also* Gangrene, gas) 040.0
Milroy's 757.0
nasopharynx 478.25
neonatorum 778.5
nutritional (newborn) 262
with dyspigmentation, skin and hair 260
optic disc or nerve - *see* Papilledema
orbit 376.33
circulatory 459.89
palate (soft) (hard) 528.9
pancreas 577.8
penis 607.83
periodic 995.1
hereditary 277.6
pharynx 478.25
pitting 782.3

Edema, edematous *(Continued)*
pulmonary - *see* Edema, lung
Quincke's 995.1
hereditary 277.6
renal (*see also* Nephrosis) 581.9
retina (localized) (macular) (peripheral) 362.83
cystoid 362.53
diabetic 250.5 *[362.01]*
salt 276.0
scrotum 608.86
seminal vesicle 608.86
spermatic cord 608.86
spinal cord 336.1
starvation 262
stasis - *see* Hypertension, venous 459.30
subconjunctival 372.73
subglottic (*see also* Edema, glottis) 478.6
supraglottic (*see also* Edema, glottis) 478.6
testis 608.86
toxic NEC 782.3
traumatic NEC 782.3
tunica vaginalis 608.86
vas deferens 608.86
vocal cord - *see* Edema, glottis
vulva (acute) 624.8
Edentia (complete) (partial) (*see also* Absence, tooth) 520.0
acquired 525.10
due to
caries 525.13
extraction 525.10
periodontal disease 525.12
specified NEC 525.19
trauma 525.11
causing malocclusion 524.30 ◄━
congenital (deficiency of tooth buds) 520.0
Edentulism 525.10
Edsall's disease 992.2
Educational handicap V62.3
Edwards' syndrome 758.2
Effect, adverse NEC
abnormal gravitational (G) forces or states 994.9
air pressure - *see* Effect, adverse, atmospheric pressure
altitude (high) - *see* Effect, adverse, high altitude
anesthetic
in labor and delivery NEC 668.9
affecting fetus or newborn 763.5
antitoxin - *see* Complications, vaccination
atmospheric pressure 993.9
due to explosion 993.4
high 993.3
low - *see* Effect, adverse, high altitude
specified effect NEC 993.8
biological, correct substance properly administered (*see also* Effect, adverse, drug) 995.2
blood (derivatives) (serum) (transfusion) - *see* Complications, transfusion
chemical substance NEC 989.9
specified - *see* Table of Drugs and Chemicals
cobalt, radioactive (*see also* Effect, adverse, radioactive substance) 990

◄ New   ◄━ Revised

Effect, adverse NEC *(Continued)*
  cold (temperature) (weather) 991.9
    chilblains 991.5
    frostbite - *see* Frostbite
    specified effect NEC 991.8
  drugs and medicinals NEC 995.2
    correct substance properly administered 995.2
    overdose or wrong substance given or taken 977.9
      specified drug - *see* Table of Drugs and Chemicals
  electric current (shock) 994.8
    burn - *see* Burn, by site
  electricity (electrocution) (shock) 994.8
    burn - *see* Burn, by site
  exertion (excessive) 994.5
  exposure 994.9
    exhaustion 994.4
  external cause NEC 994.9
  fallout (radioactive) NEC 990
  fluoroscopy NEC 990
  foodstuffs
    allergic reaction (*see also* Allergy, food) 693.1
      anaphylactic shock due to food NEC 995.60
    noxious 988.9
      specified type NEC (*see also* Poisoning, by name of noxious foodstuff) 988.8
  gases, fumes, or vapors - *see* Table of Drugs and Chemicals
  glue (airplane) sniffing 304.6
  heat - *see* Heat
  high altitude NEC 993.2
    anoxia 993.2
    on
      ears 993.0
      sinuses 993.1
    polycythemia 289.0
  hot weather - *see* Heat
  hunger 994.2
  immersion, foot 991.4
  immunization - *see* Complications, vaccination
  immunological agents - *see* Complications, vaccination
  implantation (removable) of isotope or radium NEC 990
  infrared (radiation) (rays) NEC 990
    burn - *see* Burn, by site
    dermatitis or eczema 692.82
  infusion - *see* Complications, infusion
  ingestion or injection of isotope (therapeutic) NEC 990
  irradiation NEC (*see also* Effect, adverse, radiation) 990
  isotope (radioactive) NEC 990
  lack of care (child) (infant) (newborn) 995.52
    adult 995.84
  lightning 994.0
    burn - *see* Burn, by site
  Lirugin - *see* Complications, vaccination
  medicinal substance, correct, properly administered (*see also* Effect, adverse, drugs) 995.2
  mesothorium NEC 990
  motion 994.6
  noise, inner ear 388.10
  overheated places - *see* Heat
  polonium NEC 990

Effect, adverse NEC *(Continued)*
  psychosocial, of work environment V62.1
  radiation (diagnostic) (fallout) (infrared) (natural source) (therapeutic) (tracer) (ultraviolet) (x-ray) NEC 990
    with pulmonary manifestations
      acute 508.0
      chronic 508.1
    dermatitis or eczema 692.82
      due to sun NEC (*see also* Dermatitis, due to, sun) 692.70
    fibrosis of lungs 508.1
    maternal with suspected damage to fetus affecting management of pregnancy 655.6
    pneumonitis 508.0
  radioactive substance NEC 990
    dermatitis or eczema 692.82
  radioactivity NEC 990
  radiotherapy NEC 990
    dermatitis or eczema 692.82
  radium NEC 990
  reduced temperature 991.9
    frostbite - *see* Frostbite
    immersion, foot (hand) 991.4
    specified effect NEC 991.8
  roentgenography NEC 990
  roentgenoscopy NEC 990
  roentgen rays NEC 990
  serum (prophylactic) (therapeutic) NEC 999.5
  specified NEC 995.89
    external cause NEC 994.9
  strangulation 994.7
  submersion 994.1
  teletherapy NEC 990
  thirst 994.3
  transfusion - *see* Complications, transfusion
  ultraviolet (radiation) (rays) NEC 990
    burn - *see also* Burn, by site
      from sun (*see also* Sunburn) 692.71
    dermatitis or eczema 692.82
      due to sun NEC (*see also* Dermatitis, due to, sun) 692.70
  uranium NEC 990
  vaccine (any) - *see* Complications, vaccination
  weightlessness 994.9
  whole blood - *see also* Complications, transfusion
    overdose or wrong substance given (*see also* Table of Drugs and Chemicals) 964.7
  working environment V62.1
  x-rays NEC 990
    dermatitis or eczema 692.82
Effect, remote
  of cancer-*see* condition
Effects, late - *see* Late, effect (of)
Effluvium, telogen 704.02
Effort
  intolerance 306.2
  syndrome (aviators) (psychogenic) 306.2
Effusion
  amniotic fluid (*see also* Rupture, membranes, premature) 658.1
  brain (serous) 348.5
  bronchial (*see also* Bronchitis) 490
  cerebral 348.5

Effusion *(Continued)*
  cerebrospinal (*see also* Meningitis) 322.9
    vessel 348.5
  chest - *see* Effusion, pleura
  intracranial 348.5
  joint 719.00
    ankle 719.07
    elbow 719.02
    foot 719.07
    hand 719.04
    hip 719.05
    knee 719.06
    multiple sites 719.09
    pelvic region 719.05
    shoulder (region) 719.01
    specified site NEC 719.08
    wrist 719.03
  meninges (*see also* Meningitis) 322.9
  pericardium, pericardial (*see also* Pericarditis) 423.9
    acute 420.90
  peritoneal (chronic) 568.82
  pleura, pleurisy, pleuritic, pleuropericardial 511.9
    bacterial, nontuberculous 511.1
    fetus or newborn 511.9
    malignant 197.2
    nontuberculous 511.9
      bacterial 511.1
    pneumococcal 511.1
    staphylococcal 511.1
    streptococcal 511.1
    traumatic 862.29
      with open wound 862.39
    tuberculous (*see also* Tuberculosis, pleura) 012.0
      primary progressive 010.1
  pulmonary - *see* Effusion, pleura
  spinal (*see also* Meningitis) 322.9
  thorax, thoracic - *see* Effusion, pleura
Eggshell nails 703.8
  congenital 757.5
Ego-dystonic
  homosexuality 302.0
  lesbianism 302.0
  sexual orientation 302.0 ◀
Egyptian splenomegaly 120.1
Ehlers-Danlos syndrome 756.83
Ehrlichiosis 082.40
  chaffeensis 082.41
  specified type NEC 082.49
Eichstedt's disease (pityriasis versicolor) 111.0
Eisenmenger's complex or syndrome (ventricular septal defect) 745.4
Ejaculation, semen
  painful 608.89
    psychogenic 306.59
  premature 302.75
  retrograde 608.87
Ekbom syndrome (restless legs) 333.99
Ekman's syndrome (brittle bones and blue sclera) 756.51
Elastic skin 756.83
  acquired 701.8
Elastofibroma (M8820/0) - *see* Neoplasm, connective tissue, benign
Elastoidosis
  cutanea nodularis 701.8
  cutis cystica et comedonica 701.8
Elastoma 757.39
  juvenile 757.39
  Miescher's (elastosis perforans serpiginosa) 701.1

ICD-9-CM

Vol.

Elastomyofibrosis 425.3
Elastosis 701.8
  atrophicans 701.8
  perforans serpiginosa 701.1
  reactive perforating 701.1
  senilis 701.8
  solar (actinic) 692.74
Elbow - *see* condition
Electric
  current, electricity, effects (concussion)
    (fatal) (nonfatal) (shock) 994.8
    burn - *see* Burn, by site
  feet (foot) syndrome 266.2
Electrocution 994.8
Electrolyte imbalance 276.9
  with
    abortion - *see* Abortion, by type,
      with metabolic disorder
    ectopic pregnancy (*see also* categories
      633.0-633.9) 639.4
    hyperemesis gravidarum (before 22
      completed weeks' gestation)
      643.1
    molar pregnancy (*see also* categories
      630-632) 639.4
    following
      abortion 639.4
      ectopic or molar pregnancy 639.4
Elephant man syndrome 237.71
Elephantiasis (nonfilarial) 457.1
  arabicum (*see also* Infestation, filarial)
    125.9
  congenita hereditaria 757.0
  congenital (any site) 757.0
  due to
    Brugia (malayi) 125.1
    mastectomy operation 457.0
    Wuchereria (bancrofti) 125.0
      malayi 125.1
  eyelid 374.83
  filarial (*see also* Infestation, filarial)
    125.9
  filariensis (*see also* Infestation, filarial)
    125.9
  gingival 523.8
  glandular 457.1
  graecorum 030.9
  lymphangiectatic 457.1
  lymphatic vessel 457.1
    due to mastectomy operation 457.0
  neuromatosa 237.71
  postmastectomy 457.0
  scrotum 457.1
  streptococcal 457.1
  surgical 997.99
    postmastectomy 457.0
  telangiectodes 457.1
  vulva (nonfilarial) 624.8
Elevated - *see* Elevation
Elevation
  17-ketosteroids 791.9
  acid phosphatase 790.5
  alkaline phosphatase 790.5
  amylase 790.5
  antibody titers 795.79
  basal metabolic rate (BMR) 794.7
  blood pressure (*see also* Hypertension)
    401.9
    reading (incidental) (isolated) (non-
      specific), no diagnosis of hyper-
      tension 796.2
  body temperature (of unknown origin)
    (*see also* Pyrexia) 780.6
  conjugate, eye 378.81

Elevation (*Continued*)
  C-reactive protein (CRP) 790.95 ◄
  CRP (C-reactive protein) 790.95 ◄
  diaphragm, congenital 756.6
  glucose
    fasting 790.21
    tolerance test 790.22
  immunoglobulin level 795.79
  indolacetic acid 791.9
  lactic acid dehydrogenase (LDH) level
    790.4
  lipase 790.5
  prostate specific antigen (PSA) 790.93
  renin 790.99
    in hypertension (*see also* Hyperten-
      sion, renovascular) 405.91
  Rh titer 999.7
  scapula, congenital 755.52
  sedimentation rate 790.1
  SGOT 790.4
  SGPT 790.4
  transaminase 790.4
  vanillylmandelic acid 791.9
  venous pressure 459.89
  VMA 791.9
Elliptocytosis (congenital) (hereditary) 282.1
  Hb-C (disease) 282.7
  hemoglobin disease 282.7
  sickle-cell (disease) 282.60
  trait 282.5
Ellis-van Creveld disease or syndrome
  (chondroectodermal dysplasia) 756.55
Ellison-Zollinger syndrome
  (gastric hypersecretion with pancreatic
    islet cell tumor) 251.5
Elongation, elongated (congenital) - *see*
  also Distortion
  bone 756.9
  cervix (uteri) 752.49
    acquired 622.6
    hypertrophic 622.6
  colon 751.5
  common bile duct 751.69
  cystic duct 751.69
  frenulum, penis 752.69
  labia minora, acquired 624.8
  ligamentum patellae 756.89
  petiolus (epiglottidis) 748.3
  styloid bone (process) 733.99
  tooth, teeth 520.2
  uvula 750.26
    acquired 528.9
Elschnig bodies or pearls 366.51
El Tor cholera 001.1
Emaciation (due to malnutrition) 261
Emancipation disorder 309.22
Embadomoniasis 007.8
Embarrassment heart, cardiac - *see* Disease, heart
Embedded tooth, teeth 520.6
  root only 525.3
Embolic - *see* condition
Embolism 444.9
  with
    abortion - *see* Abortion, by type,
      with embolism
    ectopic pregnancy (*see also* categories
      633.0-633.9) 639.6
    molar pregnancy (*see also* categories
      630-632) 639.6
  air (any site) 958.0
    with
      abortion - *see* Abortion, by type,
        with embolism

Embolism (*Continued*)
  air (*Continued*)
    with (*Continued*)
      ectopic pregnancy (*see also* catego-
        ries 633.0-633.9) 639.6
      molar pregnancy (*see also* catego-
        ries 630-632) 639.6
    due to implanted device - *see* Com-
      plications, due to (presence of)
      any device, implant, or graft
      classified to 996.0-996.5 NEC
    following
      abortion 639.6
      ectopic or molar pregnancy 639.6
      infusion, perfusion, or transfusion
        999.1
    in pregnancy, childbirth, or puerpe-
      rium 673.0
    traumatic 958.0
  amniotic fluid (pulmonary) 673.1
    with
      abortion - *see* Abortion, by type,
        with embolism
      ectopic pregnancy (*see also* catego-
        ries 633.0-633.9) 639.6
      molar pregnancy (*see also* catego-
        ries 630-632) 639.6
    following
      abortion 639.6
      ectopic or molar pregnancy 639.6
  aorta, aortic 444.1
    abdominal 444.0
    bifurcation 444.0
    saddle 444.0
    thoracic 444.1
  artery 444.9
    auditory, internal 433.8
    basilar (*see also* Occlusion, artery,
      basilar) 433.0
    bladder 444.89
    carotid (common) (internal) (*see also*
      Occlusion, artery, carotid) 433.1
    cerebellar (anterior inferior) (poste-
      rior inferior) (superior) 433.8
    cerebral (*see also* Embolism, brain)
      434.1
    choroidal (anterior) 433.8
    communicating posterior 433.8
    coronary (*see also* Infarct, myocar-
      dium) 410.9
      without myocardial infarction
        411.81
    extremity 444.22
      lower 444.22
      upper 444.21
    hypophyseal 433.8
    mesenteric (with gangrene) 557.0
    ophthalmic (*see also* Occlusion, ret-
      ina) 362.30
    peripheral 444.22
    pontine 433.8
    precerebral NEC - *see* Occlusion, ar-
      tery, precerebral
    pulmonary - *see* Embolism, pulmo-
      nary
    renal 593.81
    retinal (*see also* Occlusion, retina)
      362.30
    specified site NEC 444.89
    vertebral (*see also* Occlusion, artery,
      vertebral) 433.2
  auditory, internal 433.8
  basilar (artery) (*see also* Occlusion, ar-
    tery, basilar) 433.0

◄ **New**   ◄▦ **Revised**

Embolism (*Continued*)
birth, mother - *see* Embolism, obstetrical
blood-clot
with
abortion - *see* Abortion, by type, with embolism
ectopic pregnancy (*see also* categories 633.0-633.9) 639.6
molar pregnancy (*see also* categories 630-632) 639.6
following
abortion 639.6
ectopic or molar pregnancy 639.6
in pregnancy, childbirth, or puerperium 673.2
brain 434.1
with
abortion - *see* Abortion, by type, with embolism
ectopic pregnancy (*see also* categories 633.0-633.9) 639.6
molar pregnancy (*see also* categories 630-632) 639.6
following
abortion 639.6
ectopic or molar pregnancy 639.6
late effect - *see* Late effect(s) (of) cerebrovascular disease
puerperal, postpartum, childbirth 674.0
capillary 448.9
cardiac (*see also* Infarct, myocardium) 410.9
carotid (artery) (common) (internal) (*see also* Occlusion, artery, carotid) 433.1
cavernous sinus (venous) - *see* Embolism, intracranial venous sinus
cerebral (*see also* Embolism, brain) 434.1
cholesterol - *see* Atheroembolism
choroidal (anterior) (artery) 433.8
coronary (artery or vein) (systemic) (*see also* Infarct, myocardium) 410.9
without myocardial infarction 411.81
due to (presence of) any device, implant, or graft classifiable to 996.0-996.5 - *see* Complications, due to (presence of) any device, implant, or graft classified to 996.0-996.5 NEC
encephalomalacia (*see also* Embolism, brain) 434.1
extremities 444.22
lower 444.22
upper 444.21
eye 362.30
fat (cerebral) (pulmonary) (systemic) 958.1
with
abortion - *see* Abortion, by type, with embolism
ectopic pregnancy (*see also* categories 633.0-633.9) 639.6
molar pregnancy (*see also* categories 630-632) 639.6
complicating delivery or puerperium 673.8
following
abortion 639.6
ectopic or molar pregnancy 639.6

Embolism (*Continued*)
fat (*Continued*)
in pregnancy, childbirth, or the puerperium 673.8
femoral (artery) 444.22
vein 453.8
deep 453.41 ◀
following
abortion 639.6
ectopic or molar pregnancy 639.6
infusion, perfusion, or transfusion
air 999.1
thrombus 999.2
heart (fatty) (*see also* Infarct, myocardium) 410.9
hepatic (vein) 453.0
iliac (artery) 444.81
iliofemoral 444.81
in pregnancy, childbirth, or puerperium (pulmonary) - *see* Embolism, obstetrical
intestine (artery) (vein) (with gangrene) 557.0
intracranial (*see also* Embolism, brain) 434.1
venous sinus (any) 325
late effect - *see* category 326
nonpyogenic 437.6
in pregnancy or puerperium 671.5
kidney (artery) 593.81
lateral sinus (venous) - *see* Embolism, intracranial venous sinus
longitudinal sinus (venous) - *see* Embolism, intracranial venous sinus
lower extremity 444.22
lung (massive) - *see* Embolism, pulmonary
meninges (*see also* Embolism, brain) 434.1
mesenteric (artery) (with gangrene) 557.0
multiple NEC 444.9
obstetrical (pulmonary) 673.2
air 673.0
amniotic fluid (pulmonary) 673.1
blood-clot 673.2
cardiac 674.8
fat 673.8
heart 674.8
pyemic 673.3
septic 673.3
specified NEC 674.8
ophthalmic (*see also* Occlusion, retina) 362.30
paradoxical NEC 444.9
penis 607.82
peripheral arteries NEC 444.22
lower 444.22
upper 444.21
pituitary 253.8
popliteal (artery) 444.22
portal (vein) 452
postoperative NEC 997.2
cerebral 997.02
mesenteric artery 997.71
other vessels 997.79
peripheral vascular 997.2
pulmonary 415.11
renal artery 997.72
precerebral artery (*see also* Occlusion, artery, precerebral) 433.9
puerperal - *see* Embolism, obstetrical

Embolism (*Continued*)
pulmonary (artery) (vein) 415.19
with
abortion - *see* Abortion, by type, with embolism
ectopic pregnancy (*see also* categories 633.0-633.9) 639.6
molar pregnancy (*see also* categories 630-632) 639.6
following
abortion 639.6
ectopic or molar pregnancy 639.6
iatrogenic 415.11
in pregnancy, childbirth, or puerperium - *see* Embolism, obstetrical
postoperative 415.11
pyemic (multiple) 038.9
with
abortion - *see* Abortion, by type, with embolism
ectopic pregnancy (*see also* categories 633.0-633.9) 639.6
molar pregnancy (*see also* categories 630-632) 639.6
Aerobacter aerogenes 038.49
enteric gram-negative bacilli 038.40
Enterobacter aerogenes 038.49
Escherichia coli 038.42
following
abortion 639.6
ectopic or molar pregnancy 639.6
Hemophilus influenzae 038.41
pneumococcal 038.2
Proteus vulgaris 038.49
Pseudomonas (aeruginosa) 038.43
puerperal, postpartum, childbirth (any organism) 673.3
Serratia 038.44
specified organism NEC 038.8
staphylococcal 038.10
aureus 038.11
specified organism NEC 038.19
streptococcal 038.0
renal (artery) 593.81
vein 453.3
retina, retinal (*see also* Occlusion, retina) 362.30
saddle (aorta) 444.0
septicemic - *see* Embolism, pyemic
sinus - *see* Embolism, intracranial venous sinus
soap
with
abortion - *see* Abortion, by type, with embolism
ectopic pregnancy (*see also* categories 633.0-633.9) 639.6
molar pregnancy (*see also* categories 630-632) 639.6
following
abortion 639.6
ectopic or molar pregnancy 639.6
spinal cord (nonpyogenic) 336.1
in pregnancy or puerperium 671.5
pyogenic origin 324.1
late effect - *see* category 326
spleen, splenic (artery) 444.89
thrombus (thromboembolism) following infusion, perfusion, or transfusion 999.2
upper extremity 444.21
vein 453.9
with inflammation or phlebitis - *see* Thrombophlebitis

ICD-9-CM

Vol. 2

Embolism (Continued)
vein (Continued)
cerebral (see also Embolism, brain)
434.1
coronary (see also Infarct, myocardium) 410.9
without myocardial infarction
411.81
hepatic 453.0
lower extremity 453.8 ◄
deep 453.40 ◄
calf 453.42 ◄
distal (lower leg) 453.42 ◄
femoral 453.41 ◄
iliac 453.41 ◄
lower leg 453.42 ◄
peroneal 453.42 ◄
popliteal 453.41 ◄
proximal (upper leg) 453.41 ◄
thigh 453.41 ◄
tibial 453.42 ◄
mesenteric (with gangrene) 557.0
portal 452
pulmonary - see Embolism, pulmonary
renal 453.3
specified NEC 453.8
with inflammation or phlebitis -
see Thrombophlebitis
vena cava (inferior) (superior) 453.2
vessels of brain (see also Embolism,
brain) 434.1
Embolization - see Embolism
Embolus - see Embolism
Embryoma (M9080/1) - see also Neoplasm, by site, uncertain behavior
benign (M9080/0) - see Neoplasm, by
site, benign
kidney (M8960/3) 189.0
liver (M8970/3) 155.0
malignant (M9080/3) - see also Neoplasm, by site, malignant
kidney (M8960/3) 189.0
liver (M8970/3) 155.0
testis (M9070/3) 186.9
undescended 186.0
testis (M9070/3) 186.9
undescended 186.0
Embryonic
circulation 747.9
heart 747.9
vas deferens 752.89
Embryopathia NEC 759.9
Embryotomy, fetal 763.89
Embryotoxon 743.43
interfering with vision 743.42
Emesis - see also Vomiting
gravidarum - see Hyperemesis, gravidarum
Emissions, nocturnal (semen) 608.89
Emotional
crisis - see Crisis, emotional
disorder (see also Disorder, mental)
300.9
instability (excessive) 301.3
overlay - see Reaction, adjustment
upset 300.9
Emotionality, pathological 301.3
Emotogenic disease (see also Disorder,
psychogenic) 306.9
Emphysema (atrophic) (centriacinar)
(centrilobular) (chronic) (diffuse) (essential) (hypertrophic) (interlobular)
(lung) (obstructive) (panlobular)

Emphysema (Continued)
(paracicatricial) (paracinar) (postural)
(pulmonary) (senile) (subpleural)
(traction) (unilateral) (unilobular)
(vesicular) 492.8
with bronchitis
chronic 491.20
with ◄▥
acute bronchitis 491.22 ◄
exacerbation (acute) 491.21 ◄
bullous (giant) 492.0
cellular tissue 958.7
surgical 998.81
compensatory 518.2
congenital 770.2
conjunctiva 372.89
connective tissue 958.7
surgical 998.81
due to fumes or vapors 506.4
eye 376.89
eyelid 374.85
surgical 998.81
traumatic 958.7
fetus or newborn (interstitial) (mediastinal) (unilobular) 770.2
heart 416.9
interstitial 518.1
congenital 770.2
fetus or newborn 770.2
laminated tissue 958.7
surgical 998.81
mediastinal 518.1
fetus or newborn 770.2
newborn (interstitial) (mediastinal)
(unilobular) 770.2
obstructive diffuse with fibrosis 492.8
orbit 376.89
subcutaneous 958.7
due to trauma 958.7
nontraumatic 518.1
surgical 998.81
surgical 998.81
thymus (gland) (congenital)
254.8
traumatic 958.7
tuberculous (see also Tuberculosis, pulmonary) 011.9
Employment examination (certification)
V70.5
Empty sella (turcica) syndrome 253.8
Empyema (chest) (diaphragmatic) (double) (encapsulated) (general) (interlobar) (lung) (medial) (necessitatis)
(perforating chest wall) (pleura)
(pneumococcal) (residual) (sacculated) (streptococcal) (supradiaphragmatic) 510.9
with fistula 510.0
accessory sinus (chronic) (see also Sinusitis) 473.9
acute 510.9
with fistula 510.0
antrum (chronic) (see also Sinusitis,
maxillary) 473.0
brain (any part) (see also Abscess,
brain) 324.0
ethmoidal (sinus) (chronic) (see also Sinusitis, ethmoidal) 473.2
extradural (see also Abscess, extradural)
324.9
frontal (sinus) (chronic) (see also Sinusitis, frontal) 473.1
gallbladder (see also Cholecystitis,
acute) 575.0

Empyema (Continued)
mastoid (process) (acute) (see also Mastoiditis, acute) 383.00
maxilla, maxillary 526.4
sinus (chronic) (see also Sinusitis,
maxillary) 473.0
nasal sinus (chronic) (see also Sinusitis)
473.9
sinus (accessory) (nasal) (see also Sinusitis) 473.9
sphenoidal (chronic) (sinus) (see also Sinusitis, sphenoidal) 473.3
subarachnoid (see also Abscess, extradural) 324.9
subdural (see also Abscess, extradural)
324.9
tuberculous (see also Tuberculosis,
pleura) 012.0
ureter (see also Ureteritis) 593.89
ventricular (see also Abscess, brain)
324.0
Enameloma 520.2
Encephalitis (bacterial) (chronic) (hemorrhagic) (idiopathic) (nonepidemic)
(spurious) (subacute) 323.9
acute - see also Encephalitis, viral
disseminated (postinfectious) NEC
136.9 [323.6]
postimmunization or postvaccination 323.5
inclusional 049.8
inclusion body 049.8
necrotizing 049.8
arboviral, arbovirus NEC 064
arthropod-borne (see also Encephalitis,
viral, arthropod-borne) 064
Australian X 062.4
Bwamba fever 066.3
California (virus) 062.5
Central European 063.2
Czechoslovakian 063.2
Dawson's (inclusion body) 046.2
diffuse sclerosing 046.2
due to
actinomycosis 039.8 [323.4]
cat-scratch disease 078.3 [323.0]
infectious mononucleosis 075
[323.0]
malaria (see also Malaria) 084.6
[323.2]
Negishi virus 064
ornithosis 073.7 [323.0]
prophylactic inoculation against
smallpox 323.5
rickettsiosis (see also Rickettsiosis)
083.9 [323.1]
rubella 056.01
toxoplasmosis (acquired) 130.0
congenital (active) 771.2 [323.4]
typhus (fever) (see also Typhus) 081.9
[323.1]
vaccination (smallpox) 323.5
Eastern equine 062.2
endemic 049.8
epidemic 049.8
equine (acute) (infectious) (viral)
062.9
eastern 062.2
Venezuelan 066.2
western 062.1
Far Eastern 063.0
following vaccination or other immunization procedure 323.5
herpes 054.3

◄ **New**   ◄▥ **Revised**

Encephalitis *(Continued)*
  Ilheus (virus) 062.8
  inclusion body 046.2
  infectious (acute) (virus) NEC 049.8
  influenzal 487.8 *[323.4]*
    lethargic 049.8
  Japanese (B type) 062.0
  La Crosse 062.5
  Langat 063.8
  late effect - *see* Late, effect, encephalitis
  lead 984.9 *[323.7]*
  lethargic (acute) (infectious) (influenzal) 049.8
  lethargica 049.8
  louping ill 063.1
  lupus 710.0 *[323.8]*
  lymphatica 049.0
  Mengo 049.8
  meningococcal 036.1
  mumps 072.2
  Murray Valley 062.4
  myoclonic 049.8
  Negishi virus 064
  otitic NEC 382.4 *[323.4]*
  parasitic NEC 123.9 *[323.4]*
  periaxialis (concentrica) (diffusa) 341.1
  postchickenpox 052.0
  postexanthematous NEC 057.9 *[323.6]*
  postimmunization 323.5
  postinfectious NEC 136.9 *[323.6]*
  postmeasles 055.0
  posttraumatic 323.8
  postvaccinal (smallpox) 323.5
  postvaricella 052.0
  postviral NEC 079.99 *[323.6]*
    postexanthematous 057.9 *[323.6]*
      specified NEC 057.8 *[323.6]*
  Powassan 063.8
  progressive subcortical (Binswanger's) 290.12
  Rio Bravo 049.8
  rubella 056.01
  Russian
    autumnal 062.0
    spring-summer type (taiga) 063.0
  saturnine 984.9 *[323.7]*
  Semliki Forest 062.8
  serous 048
  slow-acting virus NEC 046.8
  specified cause NEC 323.8
  St. Louis type 062.3
  subacute sclerosing 046.2
  subcorticalis chronica 290.12
  summer 062.0
  suppurative 324.0
  syphilitic 094.81
    congenital 090.41
  tick-borne 063.9
  torula, torular 117.5 *[323.4]*
  toxic NEC 989.9 *[323.7]*
  toxoplasmic (acquired) 130.0
    congenital (active) 771.2 *[323.4]*
  trichinosis 124 *[323.4]*
  Trypanosomiasis (*see also* Trypanosomiasis) 086.9 *[323.2]*
  tuberculous (*see also* Tuberculosis) 013.6
  type B (Japanese) 062.0
  type C 062.3
  van Bogaert's 046.2
  Venezuelan 066.2
  Vienna type 049.8

Encephalitis *(Continued)*
  viral, virus 049.9
    arthropod-borne NEC 064
      mosquito-borne 062.9
        Australian X disease 062.4
        California virus 062.5
        Eastern equine 062.2
        Ilheus virus 062.8
        Japanese (B type) 062.0
        Murray Valley 062.4
        specified type NEC 062.8
        St. Louis 062.3
        type B 062.0
        type C 062.3
        Western equine 062.1
      tick-borne 063.9
        biundulant 063.2
        Central European 063.2
        Czechoslovakian 063.2
        diphasic meningoencephalitis 063.2
        Far Eastern 063.0
        Langat 063.8
        louping ill 063.1
        Powassan 063.8
        Russian spring-summer (taiga) 063.0
        specified type NEC 063.8
      vector unknown 064
    slow acting NEC 046.8
    specified type NEC 049.8
    vaccination, prophylactic (against) V05.0
  von Economo's 049.8
  Western equine 062.1
  West Nile type 066.41 ◀▥
Encephalocele 742.0
  orbit 376.81
Encephalocystocele 742.0
Encephalomalacia (brain) (cerebellar) (cerebral) (cerebrospinal) (*see also* Softening, brain) 434.9
  due to
    hemorrhage (*see also* Hemorrhage, brain) 431
    recurrent spasm of artery 435.9
  embolic (cerebral) (*see also* Embolism, brain) 434.1
  subcorticalis chronicus arteriosclerotica 290.12
  thrombotic (*see also* Thrombosis, brain) 434.0
Encephalomeningitis - *see* Meningoencephalitis
Encephalomeningocele 742.0
Encephalomeningomyelitis - *see* Meningoencephalitis
Encephalomeningopathy (*see also* Meningoencephalitis) 349.9
Encephalomyelitis (chronic) (granulomatous) (hemorrhagic necrotizing, acute) (myalgic, benign) (*see also* Encephalitis) 323.9
  abortive disseminated 049.8
  acute disseminated (postinfectious) 136.9 *[323.6]*
    postimmunization 323.5
  due to or resulting from vaccination (any) 323.5
  equine (acute) (infectious) 062.9
    eastern 062.2
    Venezuelan 066.2
    western 062.1

Encephalomyelitis *(Continued)*
  funicularis infectiosa 049.8
  late effect - *see* Late, effect, encephalitis
  Munch-Peterson's 049.8
  postchickenpox 052.0
  postimmunization 323.5
  postmeasles 055.0
  postvaccinal (smallpox) 323.5
  rubella 056.01
  specified cause NEC 323.8
  syphilitic 094.81
  West Nile 066.41 ◀
Encephalomyelocele 742.0
Encephalomyelomeningitis - *see* Meningoencephalitis
Encephalomyeloneuropathy 349.9
Encephalomyelopathy 349.9
  subacute necrotizing (infantile) 330.8
Encephalomyeloradiculitis (acute) 357.0
Encephalomyeloradiculoneuritis (acute) 357.0
Encephalomyeloradiculopathy 349.9
Encephalomyocarditis 074.23
Encephalopathia hyperbilirubinemica, newborn 774.7
  due to isoimmunization (conditions classifiable to 773.0-773.2) 773.4
Encephalopathy (acute) 348.30
  alcoholic 291.2
  anoxic - *see* Damage, brain, anoxic
  arteriosclerotic 437.0
    late effect - *see* Late effect(s) (of) cerebrovascular disease
  bilirubin, newborn 774.7
    due to isoimmunization 773.4
  congenital 742.9
  demyelinating (callosal) 341.8
  due to
    birth injury (intracranial) 767.8
    dialysis 294.8
      transient 293.9
    hyperinsulinism - *see* Hyperinsulinism
    influenza (virus) 487.8
    lack of vitamin (*see also* Deficiency, vitamin) 269.2
    nicotinic acid deficiency 291.2
    serum (nontherapeutic) (therapeutic) 999.5
    syphilis 094.81
    trauma (postconcussional) 310.2
      current (*see also* Concussion, brain) 850.9
        with skull fracture - *see* Fracture, skull, by site, with intracranial injury
    vaccination 323.5
  hepatic 572.2
  hyperbilirubinemic, newborn 774.7
    due to isoimmunization (conditions classifiable to 773.0-773.2) 773.4
  hypertensive 437.2
  hypoglycemic 251.2
  hypoxic - *see* Damage, brain, anoxic
  infantile cystic necrotizing (congenital) 341.8
  lead 984.9 *[323.7]*
  leukopolio 330.0
  metabolic - *see also* Delirium 348.31
    toxic 349.82
  necrotizing, subacute 330.8
    other specified type NEC 348.39
  pellagrous 265.2

ICD-9-CM

Ⅱ

Vol. 2

◄ **New**   ◄‖‖ **Revised**

Endocarditis (Continued)
  pulmonary (Continued)
    rheumatic (chronic) (inactive) (with chorea) 397.1
      active or acute 391.1
        with chorea (acute) (rheumatic) (Sydenham's) 392.0
  syphilitic 093.24
  purulent (acute) (any valve) (chronic) (subacute) 421.0
  rheumatic (chronic) (inactive) (with chorea) 397.9
    active or acute (aortic) (mitral) (pulmonary) (tricuspid) 391.1
      with chorea (acute) (rheumatic) (Sydenham's) 392.0
  septic (acute) (any valve) (chronic) (subacute) 421.0
  specified cause, except rheumatic 424.99
  streptococcal (acute) (any valve) (chronic) (subacute) 421.0
  subacute - see Endocarditis, acute
  suppurative (any valve) (acute) (chronic) (subacute) 421.0
  syphilitic NEC 093.20
  toxic (see also Endocarditis, acute) 421.9
  tricuspid (chronic) (heart) (inactive) (rheumatic) (valve) (with chorea) 397.0
    with
      rheumatic fever (conditions classifiable to 390)
        active - see Endocarditis, acute, rheumatic
        inactive or quiescent (with chorea) 397.0
      active or acute 391.1
        with chorea (acute) (rheumatic) (Sydenham's) 392.0
    arteriosclerotic 424.2
    congenital 746.89
    hypertensive 424.2
    nonrheumatic 424.2
      acute or subacute 421.9
    specified cause, except rheumatic 424.2
    syphilitic 093.23
  tuberculous (see also Tuberculosis) 017.9 [424.91]
  typhoid 002.0 [421.1]
  ulcerative (acute) (any valve) (chronic) (subacute) 421.0
  vegetative (acute) (any valve) (chronic) (subacute) 421.0
  verrucous (acute) (any valve) (chronic) (subacute) NEC 710.0 [424.91]
    nonbacterial 710.0 [424.91]
    nonrheumatic 710.0 [424.91]
Endocardium, endocardial - see also condition
  cushion defect 745.60
    specified type NEC 745.69
Endocervicitis (see also Cervicitis) 616.0
  due to
    intrauterine (contraceptive) device 996.65
  gonorrheal (acute) 098.15
    chronic or duration of 2 months or over 098.35
  hyperplastic 616.0
  syphilitic 095.8

Endocervicitis (Continued)
  trichomonal 131.09
  tuberculous (see also Tuberculosis) 016.7
Endocrine - see condition
Endocrinopathy, pluriglandular 258.9
Endodontitis 522.0
Endomastoiditis (see also Mastoiditis) 383.9
Endometrioma 617.9
Endometriosis 617.9
  appendix 617.5
  bladder 617.8
  bowel 617.5
  broad ligament 617.3
  cervix 617.0
  colon 617.5
  cul-de-sac (Douglas') 617.3
  exocervix 617.0
  fallopian tube 617.2
  female genital organ NEC 617.8
  gallbladder 617.8
  in scar of skin 617.6
  internal 617.0
  intestine 617.5
  lung 617.8
  myometrium 617.0
  ovary 617.1
  parametrium 617.3
  pelvic peritoneum 617.3
  peritoneal (pelvic) 617.3
  rectovaginal septum 617.4
  rectum 617.5
  round ligament 617.3
  skin 617.6
  specified site NEC 617.8
  stromal (M8931/1) 236.0
  umbilicus 617.8
  uterus 617.0
    internal 617.0
  vagina 617.4
  vulva 617.8
Endometritis (nonspecific) (purulent) (septic) (suppurative) 615.9
  with
    abortion - see Abortion, by type, with sepsis
    ectopic pregnancy (see also categories 633.0-633.9) 639.0
    molar pregnancy (see also categories 630-632) 639.0
  acute 615.0
  blennorrhagic 098.16
    acute 098.16
    chronic or duration of 2 months or over 098.36
  cervix, cervical (see also Cervicitis) 616.0
    hyperplastic 616.0
  chronic 615.1
  complicating pregnancy 646.6
    affecting fetus or newborn 760.8
  decidual 615.9
  following
    abortion 639.0
    ectopic or molar pregnancy 639.0
  gonorrheal (acute) 098.16
    chronic or duration of 2 months or over 098.36
  hyperplastic (see also Hyperplasia, endometrium) 621.30 ◀▥
    cervix 616.0
  polypoid - see Endometritis, hyperplastic

Endometritis (Continued)
  puerperal, postpartum, childbirth 670
  senile (atrophic) 615.9
  subacute 615.0
  tuberculous (see also Tuberculosis) 016.7
Endometrium - see condition
Endomyocardiopathy, South African 425.2
Endomyocarditis - see Endocarditis
Endomyofibrosis 425.0
Endomyometritis (see also Endometritis) 615.9
Endopericarditis - see Endocarditis
Endoperineuritis - see Disorder, nerve
Endophlebitis (see also Phlebitis) 451.9
  leg 451.2
    deep (vessels) 451.19
    superficial (vessels) 451.0
  portal (vein) 572.1
  retina 362.18
  specified site NEC 451.89
  syphilitic 093.89
Endophthalmia (see also Endophthalmitis) 360.00
  gonorrheal 098.42
Endophthalmitis (globe) (infective) (metastatic) (purulent) (subacute) 360.00
  acute 360.01
  chronic 360.03
  parasitic 360.13
  phacoanaphylactic 360.19
  specified type NEC 360.19
  sympathetic 360.11
Endosalpingioma (M9111/1) 236.2
Endosteitis - see Osteomyelitis
Endothelioma, bone (M9260/3) - see Neoplasm, bone, malignant
Endotheliosis 287.8
  hemorrhagic infectional 287.8
Endotoxic shock 785.52
Endotrachelitis (see also Cervicitis) 616.0
Enema rash 692.89
Engel-von Recklinghausen disease or syndrome (osteitis fibrosa cystica) 252.01 ◀▥
Engelmann's disease (diaphyseal sclerosis) 756.59
English disease (see also Rickets) 268.0
Engman's disease (infectious eczematoid dermatitis) 690.8
Engorgement
  breast 611.79
    newborn 778.7
    puerperal, postpartum 676.2
  liver 573.9
  lung 514
  pulmonary 514
  retina, venous 362.37
  stomach 536.8
  venous, retina 362.37
Enlargement, enlarged - see also Hypertrophy
  abdomen 789.3
  adenoids 474.12
    and tonsils 474.10
  alveolar process or ridge 525.8
  apertures of diaphragm (congenital) 756.6
  blind spot, visual field 368.42
  gingival 523.8
  heart, cardiac (see also Hypertrophy, cardiac) 429.3

ICD-9-CM
Vol. 2

Enlargement, enlarged (*Continued*)
lacrimal gland, chronic 375.03
liver (*see also* Hypertrophy, liver)
789.1
lymph gland or node 785.6
orbit 376.46
organ or site, congenital NEC - *see*
Anomaly, specified type NEC
parathyroid (gland) 252.01
pituitary fossa 793.0
prostate, (simple) (soft) 600.00
with urinary retention 600.01
sella turcica 793.0
spleen (*see also* Splenomegaly) 789.2
congenital 759.0
thymus (congenital) (gland) 254.0
thyroid (gland) (*see also* Goiter)
240.9
tongue 529.8
tonsils 474.11
and adenoids 474.10
uterus 621.2
Enophthalmos 376.50
due to
atrophy of orbital tissue 376.51
surgery 376.52
trauma 376.52
Enostosis 526.89
Entamebiasis - *see* Amebiasis
Entamebic - *see* Amebiasis
Entanglement, umbilical cord(s)
663.3
with compression 663.2
affecting fetus or newborn 762.5
around neck with compression 663.1
twins in monoamniotic sac 663.2
Enteralgia 789.0
Enteric - *see* condition
Enteritis (acute) (catarrhal) (choleraic)
(chronic) (congestive) (diarrheal) (exudative) (follicular) (hemorrhagic)
(infantile) (lienteric) (noninfectious)
(perforative) (phlegmonous) (presumed noninfectious) (pseudomembranous) 558.9
adaptive 564.9
aertrycke infection 003.0
allergic 558.3
amebic (*see also* Amebiasis) 006.9
with abscess - *see* Abscess, amebic
acute 006.0
with abscess - *see* Abscess, amebic
nondysenteric 006.2
chronic 006.1
with abscess - *see* Abscess, amebic
nondysenteric 006.2
nondysenteric 006.2
anaerobic (cocci) (gram-negative)
(gram-positive) (mixed) NEC
008.46
bacillary NEC 004.9
bacterial NEC 008.5
specified NEC 008.49
Bacteroides (fragilis) (melaninogenicus) (oralis) 008.46
Butyrivibrio (fibriosolvens) 008.46
Campylobacter 008.43
Candida 112.85
Chilomastix 007.8
choleriformis 001.1
chronic 558.9
ulcerative (*see also* Colitis, ulcerative)
556.9
cicatrizing (chronic) 555.0

Enteritis (*Continued*)
Clostridium
botulinum 005.1
difficile 008.45
haemolyticum 008.46
novyi 008.46
perfringens (C) (F) 008.46
specified type NEC 008.46
coccidial 007.2
dietetic 558.9
due to
achylia gastrica 536.8
adenovirus 008.62
Aerobacter aerogenes 008.2
anaerobes (*see also* Enteritis, anaerobic) 008.46
Arizona (bacillus) 008.1
astrovirus 008.66
Bacillus coli - *see* Enteritis, E. coli
bacteria NEC 008.5
specified NEC 008.49
Bacteroides (*see also* Enteritis, Bacteroides) 008.46
Butyrivibrio (fibriosolvens) 008.46
Calcivirus 008.65
Campylobacter 008.43
Clostridium - *see* Enteritis, Clostrid-
ium
Cockle agent 008.64
Coxsackie (virus) 008.67
Ditchling agent 008.64
ECHO virus 008.67
Enterobacter aerogenes 008.2
enterococci 008.49
enterovirus NEC 008.67
Escherichia coli - *see* Enteritis, E. coli
Eubacterium 008.46
Fusobacterium (nucleatum)
008.46
gram-negative bacteria NEC
008.47
anaerobic NEC 008.46
Hawaii agent 008.63
irritating foods 558.9
Klebsiella aerogenes 008.47
Marin County agent 008.66
Montgomery County agent 008.63
Norwalk-like agent 008.63
Norwalk virus 008.63
Otofuke agent 008.63
Paracolobactrum arizonae 008.1
paracolon bacillus NEC 008.47
Arizona 008.1
Paramatta agent 008.64
Peptococcus 008.46
Peptostreptococcus 008.46
Proprionibacterium 008.46
Proteus (bacillus) (mirabilis) (mor-
ganii) 008.3
Pseudomonas aeruginosa 008.42
Rotavirus 008.61
Sapporo agent 008.63
small round virus (SRV) NEC
008.64
featureless NEC 008.63
structured NEC 008.63
Snow Mountain (SM) agent
008.63
specified
bacteria NEC 008.49
organism, nonbacterial NEC
008.8
virus NEC 008.69
Staphylococcus 008.41

Enteritis (*Continued*)
due to (*Continued*)
Streptococcus 008.49
anaerobic 008.46
Taunton agent 008.63
Torovirus 008.69
Treponema 008.46
Veillonella 008.46
virus 008.8
specified type NEC 008.69
Wollan (W) agent 008.64
Yersinia enterocolitica 008.44
dysentery - *see* Dysentery
E. coli 008.00
enterohemorrhagic 008.04
enteroinvasive 008.03
enteropathogenic 008.01
enterotoxigenic 008.02
specified type NEC 008.09
El Tor 001.1
embadomonial 007.8
epidemic 009.0
Eubacterium 008.46
fermentative 558.9
fulminant 557.0
Fusobacterium (nucleatum) 008.46
gangrenous (*see also* Enteritis, due to,
by organism) 009.0
giardial 007.1
gram-negative bacteria NEC 008.47
anaerobic NEC 008.46
infectious NEC (*see also* Enteritis, due
to, by organism) 009.0
presumed 009.1
influenzal 487.8
ischemic 557.9
acute 557.0
chronic 557.1
due to mesenteric artery insufficiency 557.1
membranous 564.9
mucous 564.9
myxomembranous 564.9
necrotic (*see also* Enteritis, due to, by
organism) 009.0
necroticans 005.2
necrotizing of fetus or newborn 777.5
neurogenic 564.9
newborn 777.8
necrotizing 777.5
parasitic NEC 129
paratyphoid (fever) (*see also* Fever, paratyphoid) 002.9
Peptococcus 008.46
Peptostreptococcus 008.46
Proprionibacterium 008.46
protozoal NEC 007.9
radiation 558.1
regional (of) 555.9
intestine
large (bowel, colon, or rectum)
555.1
with small intestine 555.2
small (duodenum, ileum, or jejunum) 555.0
with large intestine 555.2
Salmonella infection 003.0
salmonellosis 003.0
segmental (*see also* Enteritis, regional)
555.9
septic (*see also* Enteritis, due to, by organism) 009.0
Shigella 004.9
simple 558.9

◀ **New**   ◀▉▉ **Revised**

Enteritis (Continued)
spasmodic 564.9
spastic 564.9
staphylococcal 008.41
due to food 005.0
streptococcal 008.49
anaerobic 008.46
toxic 558.2
Treponema (denticola) (macrodentium) 008.46
trichomonal 007.3
tuberculous (see also Tuberculosis) 014.8
typhosa 002.0
ulcerative (chronic) (see also Colitis, ulcerative) 556.9
Veillonella 008.46
viral 008.8
adenovirus 008.62
enterovirus 008.67
specified virus NEC 008.69
Yersinia enterocolitica 008.44
zymotic 009.0
Enteroarticular syndrome 099.3
Enterobiasis 127.4
Enterobius vermicularis 127.4
Enterocele (see also Hernia) 553.9
pelvis, pelvic (acquired) (congenital) 618.6
vagina, vaginal (acquired) (congenital) 618.6
Enterocolitis - see also Enteritis
fetus or newborn 777.8
necrotizing 777.5
fulminant 557.0
granulomatous 555.2
hemorrhagic (acute) 557.0
chronic 557.1
necrotizing (acute) (membranous) 557.0
primary necrotizing 777.5
pseudomembranous 008.45
radiation 558.1
newborn 777.5
ulcerative 556.0
Enterocystoma 751.5
Enterogastritis - see Enteritis
Enterogenous cyanosis 289.7
Enterolith, enterolithiasis (impaction) 560.39
with hernia - see also Hernia, by site, with obstruction
gangrenous - see Hernia, by site, with gangrene
Enteropathy 569.9
exudative (of Gordon) 579.8
gluten 579.0
hemorrhagic, terminal 557.0
protein-losing 579.8
Enteroperitonitis (see also Peritonitis) 567.9
Enteroptosis 569.89
Enterorrhagia 578.9
Enterospasm 564.9
psychogenic 306.4
Enterostenosis (see also Obstruction, intestine) 560.9
Enterostomy status V44.4
with complication 569.60
Enthesopathy 726.90
ankle and tarsus 726.70
elbow region 726.30
specified NEC 726.39
hip 726.5

Enthesopathy (Continued)
knee 726.60
peripheral NEC 726.8
shoulder region 726.10
adhesive 726.0
spinal 720.1
wrist and carpus 726.4
Entrance, air into vein - see Embolism, air
Entrapment, nerve - see Neuropathy, entrapment
Entropion (eyelid) 374.00
cicatricial 374.04
congenital 743.62
late effect of trachoma (healed) 139.1
mechanical 374.02
paralytic 374.02
senile 374.01
spastic 374.03
Enucleation of eye (current) (traumatic) 871.3
Enuresis 788.30
habit disturbance 307.6
nocturnal 788.36
psychogenic 307.6
nonorganic origin 307.6
psychogenic 307.6
Enzymopathy 277.9
Eosinopenia 288.0
Eosinophilia 288.3
allergic 288.3
hereditary 288.3
idiopathic 288.3
infiltrative 518.3
Loeffler's 518.3
myalgia syndrome 710.5
pulmonary (tropical) 518.3
secondary 288.3
tropical 518.3
Eosinophilic - see also condition
fasciitis 728.89
granuloma (bone) 277.89
infiltration lung 518.3
Ependymitis (acute) (cerebral) (chronic) (granular) (see also Meningitis) 322.9
Ependymoblastoma (M9392/3)
specified site - see Neoplasm, by site, malignant
unspecified site 191.9
Ependymoma (epithelial) (malignant) (M9391/3)
anaplastic type (M9392/3)
specified site - see Neoplasm, by site, malignant
unspecified site 191.9
benign (M9391/0)
specified site - see Neoplasm, by site, benign
unspecified site 225.0
myxopapillary (M9394/1) 237.5
papillary (M9393/1) 237.5
specified site - see Neoplasm, by site, malignant
unspecified site 191.9
Ependymopathy 349.2
spinal cord 349.2
Ephelides, ephelis 709.09
Ephemeral fever (see also Pyrexia) 780.6
Epiblepharon (congenital) 743.62
Epicanthus, epicanthic fold (congenital) (eyelid) 743.63
Epicondylitis (elbow) (lateral) 726.32
medial 726.31
Epicystitis (see also Cystitis) 595.9

Epidemic - see condition
Epidermidalization, cervix - see condition
Epidermidization, cervix - see condition
Epidermis, epidermal - see condition
Epidermization, cervix - see condition
Epidermodysplasia verruciformis 078.19
Epidermoid
cholesteatoma - see Cholesteatoma
inclusion (see also Cyst, skin) 706.2
Epidermolysis
acuta (combustiformis) (toxica) 695.1
bullosa 757.39
necroticans combustiformis 695.1
due to drug
correct substance properly administered 695.1
overdose or wrong substance given or taken 977.9
specified drug - see Table of Drugs and Chemicals
Epidermophytid - see Dermatophytosis
Epidermophytosis (infected) - see Dermatophytosis
Epidermosis, ear (middle) (see also Cholesteatoma) 385.30
Epididymis - see condition
Epididymitis (nonvenereal) 604.90
with abscess 604.0
acute 604.99
blennorrhagic (acute) 098.0
chronic or duration of 2 months or over 098.2
caseous (see also Tuberculosis) 016.4
chlamydial 099.54
diphtheritic 032.89 [604.91]
filarial 125.9 [604.91]
gonococcal (acute) 098.0
chronic or duration of 2 months or over 098.2
recurrent 604.99
residual 604.99
syphilitic 095.8 [604.91]
tuberculous (see also Tuberculosis) 016.4
Epididymo-orchitis (see also Epididymitis) 604.90
with abscess 604.0
chlamydial 099.54
gonococcal (acute) 098.13
chronic or duration of 2 months or over 098.33
Epidural - see condition
Epigastritis (see also Gastritis) 535.5
Epigastrium, epigastric - see condition
Epigastrocele (see also Hernia, epigastric) 553.29
Epiglottiditis (acute) 464.30
with obstruction 464.31
chronic 476.1
viral 464.30
with obstruction 464.31
Epiglottis - see condition
Epiglottitis (acute) 464.30
with obstruction 464.31
chronic 476.1
viral 464.30
with obstruction 464.31
Epignathus 759.4
Epilepsia
partialis continua (see also Epilepsy) 345.7
procursiva (see also Epilepsy) 345.8

ICD-9-CM
Vol. 2

Epilepsy, epileptic (idiopathic) 345.9

> Note use the following fifth-digit
> subclassifications with categories
> 345.0, 345.1, 345.4-345.9
>
> 0 without mention of intractable
>   epilepsy
> 1 with intractable epilepsy

abdominal 345.5
absence (attack) 345.0
akinetic 345.0
   psychomotor 345.4
automatism 345.4
autonomic diencephalic 345.5
brain 345.9
Bravais-Jacksonian 345.5
cerebral 345.9
climacteric 345.9
clonic 345.1
clouded state 345.9
coma 345.3
communicating 345.4
congenital 345.9
convulsions 345.9
cortical (focal) (motor) 345.5
cursive (running) 345.8
cysticercosis 123.1
deterioration
   with behavioral disturbance 345.9
      [294.11]
   without behavioral disturbance 345.9
      [294.10]
due to syphilis 094.89
equivalent 345.5
fit 345.9
focal (motor) 345.5
gelastic 345.8
generalized 345.9
   convulsive 345.1
   flexion 345.1
   nonconvulsive 345.0
grand mal (idiopathic) 345.1
Jacksonian (motor) (sensory) 345.5
Kojevnikoff's, Kojevnikov's, Kojewnikoff's 345.7
laryngeal 786.2
limbic system 345.4
major (motor) 345.1
minor 345.0
mixed (type) 345.9
motor partial 345.5
musicogenic 345.1
myoclonus, myoclonic 345.1
   progressive (familial) 333.2
nonconvulsive, generalized 345.0
parasitic NEC 123.9
partial (focalized) 345.5
   with
      impairment of consciousness 345.4
      memory and ideational distur-
         bances 345.4
   abdominal type 345.5
   motor type 345.5
   psychomotor type 345.4
   psychosensory type 345.4
   secondarily generalized 345.4
   sensory type 345.5
   somatomotor type 345.5
   somatosensory type 345.5
   temporal lobe type 345.4
   visceral type 345.5
   visual type 345.5
peripheral 345.9

Epilepsy, epileptic *(Continued)*
petit mal 345.0
photokinetic 345.8
progressive myoclonic (familial)
   33.2
psychic equivalent 345.5
psychomotor 345.4
psychosensory 345.4
reflex 345.1
seizure 345.9
senile 345.9
sensory-induced 345.5
sleep (see also Narcolepsy) 347.00 ◀▦
somatomotor type 345.5
somatosensory 345.5
specified type NEC 345.8
status (grand mal) 345.3
   focal motor 345.7
   petit mal 345.2
   psychomotor 345.7
   temporal lobe 345.7
symptomatic 345.9
temporal lobe 345.4
tonic (-clonic) 345.1
traumatic (injury unspecified) 907.0
   injury specified - see Late, effect
      (of) specified injury
twilight 293.0
uncinate (gyrus) 345.4
Unverricht (-Lundborg) (familial myoclonic) 333.2
visceral 345.5
visual 345.5
Epileptiform
convulsions 780.39
seizure 780.39
Epiloia 759.5
Epimenorrhea 626.2
Epipharyngitis (see also Nasopharyngitis)
   460
Epiphora 375.20
due to
   excess lacrimation 375.21
   insufficient drainage 375.22
Epiphyseal arrest 733.91
femoral head 732.2
Epiphyseolysis, epiphysiolysis (see also
   Osteochondrosis) 732.9
Epiphysitis (see also Osteochondrosis)
   732.9
juvenile 732.6
marginal (Scheuermann's) 732.0
os calcis 732.5
syphilitic (congenital) 090.0
vertebral (Scheuermann's) 732.0
Epiplocele (see also Hernia) 553.9
Epiploitis (see also Peritonitis) 567.9
Epiplosarcomphalocele (see also Hernia,
   umbilicus) 553.1
Episcleritis 379.00
gouty 274.89 [379.09]
nodular 379.02
periodica fugax 379.01
   angioneurotic - see Edema, angio-
      neurotic
specified NEC 379.09
staphylococcal 379.00
suppurative 379.00
syphilitic 095.0
tuberculous (see also Tuberculosis)
   017.3 [379.09]
Episode
brain (see also Disease, cerebrovascular,
   acute) 436

Episode *(Continued)*
cerebral (see also Disease, cerebrovascular, acute) 436
depersonalization (in neurotic state)
   300.6
hyporesponsive 780.09
psychotic (see also Psychosis) 298.9
   organic, transient 293.9
schizophrenic (acute) NEC (see also
   Schizophrenia) 295.4
Epispadias
female 753.8
male 752.62
Episplenitis 289.59
Epistaxis (multiple) 784.7
hereditary 448.0
vicarious menstruation 625.8
Epithelioma (malignant) (M8011/3) - see
   also Neoplasm, by site, malignant
adenoides cysticum (M8100/0) - see
   Neoplasm, skin, benign
basal cell (M8090/3) - see Neoplasm,
   skin, malignant
benign (M8011/0) - see Neoplasm, by
   site, benign
Bowen's (M8081/2) - see Neoplasm,
   skin, in situ
calcifying (benign) (Malherbe's)
   (M8110/0) - see Neoplasm, skin,
   benign
external site - see Neoplasm, skin, malignant
intraepidermal, Jadassohn (M8096/0) -
   see Neoplasm, skin, benign
squamous cell (M8070/3) - see Neoplasm, by site, malignant
Epitheliopathy
pigment, retina 363.15
posterior multifocal placoid (acute)
   363.15
Epithelium, epithelial - see condition
Epituberculosis (allergic) (with atelectasis) (see also Tuberculosis)
   010.8
Eponychia 757.5
Epstein's
nephrosis or syndrome (see also Nephrosis) 581.9
pearl (mouth) 528.4
Epstein-Barr infection (viral) 075
chronic 780.79 [139.8]
Epulis (giant cell) (gingiva) 523.8
Equinia 024
Equinovarus (congenital) 754.51
acquired 736.71
Equivalent
convulsive (abdominal) (see also Epilepsy) 345.5
epileptic (psychic) (see also Epilepsy)
   345.5
Erb's
disease 359.1
palsy, paralysis (birth) (brachial) (newborn) 767.6
spinal (spastic) syphilitic 094.89
pseudohypertrophic muscular dystrophy 359.1
Erb (-Duchenne) paralysis (birth injury)
   (newborn) 767.6
Erb-Goldflam disease or syndrome
   358.00
Erdheim's syndrome (acromegalic macrospondylitis) 253.0
Erection, painful (persistent) 607.3

◀ **New**   ◀▦ **Revised**

Ergosterol deficiency (vitamin D) 268.9
  with
    osteomalacia 268.2
    rickets (*see also* Rickets) 268.0
Ergotism (ergotized grain) 988.2
  from ergot used as drug (migraine
    therapy)
      correct substance properly adminis-
        tered 349.82
      overdose or wrong substance given
        or taken 975.0
Erichsen's disease (railway spine)
  300.16
Erlacher-Blount syndrome (tibia vara)
  732.4
Erosio interdigitalis blastomycetica
  112.3
Erosion
  arteriosclerotic plaque - *see* Arterioscle-
    rosis, by site
  artery NEC 447.2
    without rupture 447.8
  bone 733.99
  bronchus 519.1
  cartilage (joint) 733.99
  cervix (uteri) (acquired) (chronic) (con-
    genital) 622.0
    with mention of cervicitis 616.0
  cornea (recurrent) (*see also* Keratitis)
    371.42
    traumatic 918.1
  dental (idiopathic) (occupational)
    521.30 ◀▥
    extending into ◀
      dentine 521.32 ◀
      pulp 521.33 ◀
    generalized 521.35 ◀
    limited to enamel 521.31 ◀
    localized 521.34 ◀
  duodenum, postpyloric - *see* Ulcer, du-
    odenum
  esophagus 530.89
  gastric 535.4
  intestine 569.89
  lymphatic vessel 457.8
  pylorus, pyloric (ulcer) 535.4
  sclera 379.16
  spine, aneurysmal 094.89
  spleen 289.59
  stomach 535.4
  teeth (idiopathic) (occupational) (*see
    also* Erosion, dental) 521.30 ◀▥
    due to
      medicine 521.30 ◀▥
      persistent vomiting 521.30 ◀▥
  urethra 599.84
  uterus 621.8
  vertebra 733.99
Erotomania 302.89
  Clerambault's 297.8
Error
  in diet 269.9
  refractive 367.9
    astigmatism (*see also* Astigmatism)
      367.20
    drug-induced 367.89
    hypermetropia 367.0
    hyperopia 367.0
    myopia 367.1
    presbyopia 367.4
    toxic 367.89
Eructation 787.3
  nervous 306.4
  psychogenic 306.4

Eruption
  creeping 126.9
  drug - *see* Dermatitis, due to, drug
  Hutchinson, summer 692.72
  Kaposi's varicelliform 054.0
  napkin (psoriasiform) 691.0
  polymorphous
    light (sun) 692.72
      other source 692.82
  psoriasiform, napkin 691.0
  recalcitrant pustular 694.8
  ringed 695.89
  skin (*see also* Dermatitis) 782.1
    creeping (meaning hookworm) 126.9
    due to
      chemical(s) NEC 692.4
        internal use 693.8
      drug - *see* Dermatitis, due to, drug
      prophylactic inoculation or vacci-
        nation against disease - *see*
        Dermatitis, due to, vaccine
      smallpox vaccination NEC - *see*
        Dermatitis, due to, vaccine
    erysipeloid 027.1
    feigned 698.4
    Hutchinson, summer 692.72
    Kaposi's, varicelliform 054.0
      vaccinia 999.0
    lichenoid, axilla 698.3
    polymorphous, due to light 692.72
    toxic NEC 695.0
    vesicular 709.8
  teeth, tooth
    accelerated 520.6
    delayed 520.6
    difficult 520.6
    disturbance of 520.6
    in abnormal sequence 520.6
    incomplete 520.6
    late 520.6
    natal 520.6
    neonatal 520.6
    obstructed 520.6
    partial 520.6
    persistent primary 520.6
    premature 520.6
  vesicular 709.8
Erysipelas (gangrenous) (infantile) (newborn) (phlegmonous) (suppurative)
  035
  external ear 035 [380.13]
  puerperal, postpartum, childbirth 670
Erysipelatoid (Rosenbach's) 027.1
Erysipeloid (Rosenbach's) 027.1
Erythema, erythematous (generalized)
  695.9
  ab igne - *see* Burn, by site, first degree
  annulare (centrifugum) (rheumaticum)
    695.0
  arthriticum epidemicum 026.1
  brucellum (*see also* Brucellosis) 023.9
  bullosum 695.1
  caloricum - *see* Burn, by site, first de-
    gree
  chronicum migrans 088.81
  circinatum 695.1
  diaper 691.0
  due to
    chemical (contact) NEC 692.4
      internal 693.8
    drug (internal use) 693.0
      contact 692.3
  elevatum diutinum 695.89
  endemic 265.2

Erythema, erythematous (*Continued*)
  epidemic, arthritic 026.1
  figuratum perstans 695.0
  gluteal 691.0
  gyratum (perstans) (repens) 695.1
  heat - *see* Burn, by site, first degree
  ichthyosiforme congenitum 757.1
  induratum (primary) (scrofulosorum)
    (*see also* Tuberculosis) 017.1
    nontuberculous 695.2
  infantum febrile 057.8
  infectional NEC 695.9
  infectiosum 057.0
  inflammation NEC 695.9
  intertrigo 695.89
  iris 695.1
  lupus (discoid) (localized) (*see also* Lu-
    pus, erythematosus) 695.4
  marginatum 695.0
    rheumaticum - *see* Fever, rheumatic
  medicamentosum - *see* Dermatitis, due
    to, drug
  migrans 529.1
    chronicum 088.81
  multiforme 695.1
    bullosum 695.1
    conjunctiva 695.1
    exudativum (Hebra) 695.1
    pemphigoides 694.5
  napkin 691.0
  neonatorum 778.8
  nodosum 695.2
    tuberculous (*see also* Tuberculosis)
      017.1
  nummular, nummulare 695.1
  palmar 695.0
  palmaris hereditarium 695.0
  pernio 991.5
  perstans solare 692.72
  rash, newborn 778.8
  scarlatiniform (exfoliative) (recurrent)
    695.0
  simplex marginatum 057.8
  solare (*see also* Sunburn) 692.71
  streptogenes 696.5
  toxic, toxicum NEC 695.0
    newborn 778.8
  tuberculous (primary) (*see also* Tuber-
    culosis) 017.0
  venenatum 695.0
Erythematosus - *see* condition
Erythematous - *see* condition
Erythermalgia (primary) 443.89
Erythralgia 443.89
Erythrasma 039.0
Erythredema 985.0
  polyneuritica 985.0
  polyneuropathy 985.0
Erythremia (acute) (M9841/3) 207.0
  chronic (M9842/3) 207.1
  secondary 289.0
Erythroblastopenia (acquired) 284.8
  congenital 284.0
Erythroblastophthisis 284.0
Erythroblastosis (fetalis) (newborn)
  773.2
  due to
    ABO
      antibodies 773.1
      incompatibility, maternal/fetal
        773.1
      isoimmunization 773.1
    Rh
      antibodies 773.0

ICD-9-CM

E

Vol. 2

Erythroblastosis (Continued)
  due to (Continued)
    Rh (Continued)
      incompatibility, maternal/fetal
        773.0
      isoimmunization 773.0
Erythrocyanosis (crurum) 443.89
Erythrocythemia - see Erythremia
Erythrocytopenia 285.9
Erythrocytosis (megalosplenic)
  familial 289.6
  oval, hereditary (see also Elliptocytosis)
    282.1
  secondary 289.0
  stress 289.0
Erythroderma (see also Erythema) 695.9
  desquamativa (in infants) 695.89
  exfoliative 695.89
  ichthyosiform, congenital 757.1
  infantum 695.89
  maculopapular 696.2
  neonatorum 778.8
  psoriaticum 696.1
  secondary 695.9
Erythrogenesis imperfecta 284.0
Erythroleukemia (M9840/3) 207.0
Erythromelalgia 443.89
Erythromelia 701.8
Erythropenia 285.9
Erythrophagocytosis 289.9
Erythrophobia 300.23
Erythroplakia
  oral mucosa 528.79   ◄▥
  tongue 528.79   ◄▥
Erythroplasia (Queyrat) (M8080/2)
  specified site - see Neoplasm, skin, in situ
  unspecified site 233.5
Erythropoiesis, idiopathic ineffective
  285.0
Escaped beats, heart 427.60
  postoperative 997.1
Esoenteritis - see Enteritis
Esophagalgia 530.89
Esophagectasis 530.89
  due to cardiospasm 530.0
Esophagismus 530.5
Esophagitis (alkaline) (chemical)
  (chronic) (infectional) (necrotic)
  (peptic) (postoperative) (regurgitant)
  530.10
  acute 530.12
  candidal 112.84
  reflux 530.11
  specified NEC 530.19
  tuberculous (see also Tuberculosis)
    017.8
  ulcerative 530.19
Esophagocele 530.6
Esophagodynia 530.89
Esophagomalacia 530.89
Esophagoptosis 530.89
Esophagospasm 530.5
Esophagostenosis 530.3
Esophagostomiasis 127.7
Esophagostomy   ◄
  complication   ◄
    infection 530.86   ◄
    malfunctioning 530.87   ◄
    mechanical 530.87   ◄
Esophagotracheal - see condition
Esophagus - see condition
Esophoria 378.41
  convergence, excess 378.84
  divergence, insufficiency 378.85

Esotropia (nonaccommodative) 378.00
  accommodative 378.35
  alternating 378.05
    with
      A pattern 378.06
      specified noncomitancy NEC
        378.08
      V pattern 378.07
      X pattern 378.08
      Y pattern 378.08
    intermittent 378.22
  intermittent 378.20
    alternating 378.22
    monocular 378.21
  monocular 378.01
    with
      A pattern 378.02
      specified noncomitancy NEC
        378.04
      V pattern 378.03
      X pattern 378.04
      Y pattern 378.04
    intermittent 378.21
Espundia 085.5
Essential - see condition
Esterapenia 289.89
Esthesioneuroblastoma (M9522/3) 160.0
Esthesioneurocytoma (M9521/3) 160.0
Esthesioneuroepithelioma (M9523/3)
  160.0
Esthiomene 099.1
Estivo-autumnal
  fever 084.0
  malaria 084.0
Estrangement V61.0
Estriasis 134.0
Ethanolaminuria 270.8
Ethanolism (see also Alcoholism) 303.9
Ether dependence, dependency (see also
  Dependence) 304.6
Etherism (see also Dependence) 304.6
Ethmoid, ethmoidal - see condition
Ethmoiditis (chronic) (nonpurulent) (pu-
  rulent) (see also Sinusitis, ethmoidal)
  473.2
  influenzal 487.1
  Woakes' 471.1
Ethylism (see also Alcoholism) 303.9
Eulenburg's disease (congenital paramy-
  otonia) 359.2
Eunuchism 257.2
Eunuchoidism 257.2
  hypogonadotropic 257.2
European blastomycosis 117.5
Eustachian - see condition
Euthyroid sick syndrome 790.94
Euthyroidism 244.9
Evaluation
  fetal lung maturity 659.8
  for suspected condition (see also Obser-
    vation) V71.9
    abuse V71.81
    exposure
      anthrax 471.82
      biological agent NEC 471.83
      SARS V71.83
    neglect V71.81
    newborn - see Observation, sus-
      pected, condition, newborn
    specified condition NEC V71.89
  mental health V70.2
  requested by authority V70.1
  nursing care V63.8
  social service V63.8

Evan's syndrome (thrombocytopenic
  purpura) 287.3
Eventration
  colon into chest - see Hernia, dia-
    phragm
  diaphragm (congenital) 756.6
Eversion
  bladder 596.8
  cervix (uteri) 622.0
    with mention of cervicitis 616.0
  foot NEC 736.79
    congenital 755.67
  lacrimal punctum 375.51
  punctum lacrimale (postinfectional)
    (senile) 375.51
  ureter (meatus) 593.89
  urethra (meatus) 599.84
  uterus 618.1
    complicating delivery 665.2
      affecting fetus or newborn 763.89
    puerperal, postpartum 674.8
Evidence   ◄
  of malignancy   ◄
    cytologic   ◄
      without histologic confirmation
        795.04   ◄
Evisceration
  birth injury 767.8
  bowel (congenital) - see Hernia, ventral
  congenital (see also Hernia, ventral)
    553.29
  operative wound 998.32
  traumatic NEC 869.1
    eye 871.3
Evulsion - see Avulsion
Ewing's
  angioendothelioma (M9260/3) - see
    Neoplasm, bone, malignant
  sarcoma (M9260/3) - see Neoplasm,
    bone, malignant
  tumor (M9260/3) - see Neoplasm,
    bone, malignant
Exaggerated lumbosacral angle (with
  impinging spine) 756.12
Examination (general) (routine) (of) (for)
  V70.9
  allergy V72.7
  annual V70.0
  cardiovascular preoperative V72.81
  cervical Papanicolaou smear V76.2
    as a part of routine gynecological
      examination V72.31   ◄▥
    to confirm findings of recent normal
      smear following initial abnor-
      mal smear V72.32   ◄
  child care (routine) V20.2
  clinical research investigation (normal
    control patient) (participant) V70.7
  dental V72.2
  developmental testing (child) (infant)
    V20.2
  donor (potential) V70.8
  ear V72.1
  eye V72.0
  following
    accident (motor vehicle) V71.4
    alleged rape or seduction (victim or
      culprit) V71.5
    inflicted injury (victim or culprit)
      NEC V71.6
    rape or seduction, alleged (victim or
      culprit) V71.5
    treatment (for) V67.9
      combined V67.6

◄ **New**   ◄▥ **Revised**

Examination *(Continued)*
following *(Continued)*
treatment *(Continued)*
fracture V67.4
involving high-risk medication NEC V67.51
mental disorder V67.3
specified condition NEC V67.59
follow-up (routine) (following) V67.9
cancer chemotherapy V67.2
chemotherapy V67.2
disease NEC V67.59
high-risk medication NEC V67.51
injury NEC V67.59
population survey V70.6
postpartum V24.2
psychiatric V67.3
psychotherapy V67.3
radiotherapy V67.1
specified surgery NEC V67.09
surgery V67.00
vaginal pap smear V67.01
gynecological V72.31 ◀▥
for contraceptive maintenance V25.40
intrauterine device V25.42
pill V25.41
specified method NEC V25.49
health (of)
armed forces personnel V70.5
checkup V70.0
child, routine V20.2
defined subpopulation NEC V70.5
inhabitants of institutions V70.5
occupational V70.5
pre-employment screening V70.5
preschool children V70.5
for admission to school V70.3
prisoners V70.5
for entrance into prison V70.3
prostitutes V70.5
refugees V70.5
school children V70.5
students V70.5
hearing V72.1
infant V20.2
laboratory V72.6
lactating mother V24.1
medical (for) (of) V70.9
administrative purpose NEC V70.3
admission to
old age home V70.3
prison V70.3
school V70.3
adoption V70.3
armed forces personnel V70.5
at health care facility V70.0
camp V70.3
child, routine V20.2
clinical research investigation, (control) (normal comparison) (participant) V70.7
defined subpopulation NEC V70.5
donor (potential) V70.8
driving license V70.3
general V70.9
routine V70.0
specified reason NEC V70.8
immigration V70.3
inhabitants of institutions V70.5
insurance certification V70.3
marriage V70.3
medicolegal reasons V70.4
naturalization V70.3

Examination *(Continued)*
medical *(Continued)*
occupational V70.5
population survey V70.6
pre-employment V70.5
preschool children V70.5
for admission to school V70.3
prison V70.3
prisoners V70.5
for entrance into prison V70.3
prostitutes V70.5
refugees V70.5
school children V70.5
specified reason NEC V70.8
sport competition V70.3
students V70.5
medicolegal reason V70.4
pelvic (annual) (periodic) V72.31 ◀▥
periodic (annual) (routine) V70.0
postpartum
immediately after delivery V24.0
routine follow-up V24.2
pregnancy (unconfirmed) (possible) V72.40 ◀▥
negative result V72.41 ◀
prenatal V22.1
first pregnancy V22.0
high-risk pregnancy V23.9
specified problem NEC V23.8
preoperative V72.84
cardiovascular V72.81
respiratory V72.82
specified NEC V72.83
psychiatric V70.2
follow-up not needing further care V67.3
requested by authority V70.1
radiological NEC V72.5
respiratory preoperative V72.82
screening - *see* Screening
sensitization V72.7
skin V72.7
hypersensitivity V72.7
special V72.9
specified type or reason NEC V72.85
preoperative V72.83
specified NEC V72.83
teeth V72.2
vaginal Papanicolaou smear V76.47
following hysterectomy for malignant condition V67.01
victim or culprit following
alleged rape or seduction V71.5
inflicted injury NEC V71.6
vision V72.0
well baby V20.2
Exanthem, exanthema *(see also* Rash) 782.1
Boston 048
epidemic, with meningitis 048
lichenoid psoriasiform 696.2
subitum 057.8
viral, virus NEC 057.9
specified type NEC 057.8
Excess, excessive, excessively
alcohol level in blood 790.3
carbohydrate tissue, localized 278.1
carotene (dietary) 278.3
cold 991.9
specified effect NEC 991.8
convergence 378.84
crying of infant (baby) 780.92
development, breast 611.1
diaphoresis *(see also* Hyperhidrosis) 780.8 ◀▥

Excess, excessive, excessively *(Continued)*
distance, interarch 524.28 ◀
divergence 378.85
drinking (alcohol) NEC *(see also* Abuse, drugs, nondependent) 305.0
continual *(see also* Alcoholism) 303.9
habitual *(see also* Alcoholism) 303.9
eating 783.6
eyelid fold (congenital) 743.62
fat 278.00
in heart *(see also* Degeneration, myocardial) 429.1
tissue, localized 278.1
foreskin 605
gas 787.3
gastrin 251.5
glucagon 251.4
heat *(see also* Heat) 992.9
horizontal overlap 524.26 ◀
interarch distance 524.28 ◀
interocclusal distance of teeth 524.37 ◀
large
colon 564.7
congenital 751.3
fetus or infant 766.0
with obstructed labor 660.1
affecting management of pregnancy 656.6
causing disproportion 653.5
newborn (weight of 4500 grams or more) 766.0
organ or site, congenital NEC - *see* Anomaly, specified type NEC
lid fold (congenital) 743.62
long
colon 751.5
organ or site, congenital NEC - *see* Anomaly, specified type NEC
umbilical cord (entangled)
affecting fetus or newborn 762.5
in pregnancy or childbirth 663.3
with compression 663.2
menstruation 626.2
number of teeth 520.1
causing crowding 524.31 ◀▥
nutrients (dietary) NEC 783.6
potassium (K) 276.7
salivation *(see also* Ptyalism) 527.7
secretion - *see also* Hypersecretion
milk 676.6
sputum 786.4
sweat *(see also* Hyperhidrosis) 780.8 ◀▥
short
organ or site, congenital NEC - *see* Anomaly, specified type NEC
umbilical cord
affecting fetus or newborn 762.6
in pregnancy or childbirth 663.4
skin NEC 701.9
eyelid 743.62
acquired 374.30
sodium (Na) 276.0
spacing of teeth 524.32 ◀
sputum 786.4
sweating *(see also* Hyperhidrosis) 780.8 ◀▥
tearing (ducts) (eye) *(see also* Epiphora) 375.20
thirst 783.5
due to deprivation of water 994.3 ◀
tuberosity 524.07 ◀

ICD-9-CM
Ш
Vol. 2

Excess, excessive, excessively (Continued)
  vitamin
    A (dietary) 278.2
      administered as drug (chronic)
        (prolonged excessive intake)
        278.2
        reaction to sudden overdose
          963.5
    D (dietary) 278.4
      administered as drug (chronic)
        (prolonged excessive intake)
        278.4
        reaction to sudden overdose
          963.5
  weight 278.00
    gain 783.1
      of pregnancy 646.1
    loss 783.21
Excitability, abnormal, under minor stress 309.29
Excitation
  catatonic (see also Schizophrenia) 295.2
  psychogenic 298.1
  reactive (from emotional stress, psychological trauma) 298.1
Excitement
  manic (see also Psychosis, affective) 296.0
    recurrent episode 296.1
    single episode 296.0
  mental, reactive (from emotional stress, psychological trauma) 298.1
  state, reactive (from emotional stress, psychological trauma) 298.1
Excluded pupils 364.76
Excoriation (traumatic) (see also Injury, superficial, by site) 919.8
  neurotic 698.4
Excyclophoria 378.44
Excyclotropia 378.33
Exencephalus, exencephaly 742.0
Exercise
  breathing V57.0
  remedial NEC V57.1
  therapeutic NEC V57.1
Exfoliation, teeth due to systemic causes 525.0
Exfoliative - see also condition
  dermatitis 695.89
Exhaustion, exhaustive (physical NEC) 780.79
  battle (see also Reaction, stress, acute) 308.9
  cardiac (see also Failure, heart) 428.9
  delirium (see also Reaction, stress, acute) 308.9
  due to
    cold 991.8
    excessive exertion 994.5
    exposure 994.4
  fetus or newborn 779.89
  heart (see also Failure, heart) 428.9
  heat 992.5
    due to
      salt depletion 992.4
      water depletion 992.3
  manic (see also Psychosis, affective) 296.0
    recurrent episode 296.1
    single episode 296.0
  maternal, complicating delivery 669.8
    affecting fetus or newborn 763.89
  mental 300.5

Exhaustion, exhaustive (Continued)
  myocardium, myocardial (see also Failure, heart) 428.9
  nervous 300.5
  old age 797
  postinfectional NEC 780.79
  psychogenic 300.5
  psychosis (see also Reaction, stress, acute) 308.9
  senile 797
    dementia 290.0
Exhibitionism (sexual) 302.4
Exomphalos 756.79
Exophoria 378.42
  convergence, insufficiency 378.83
  divergence, excess 378.85
Exophthalmic
  cachexia 242.0
  goiter 242.0
  ophthalmoplegia 242.0 [376.22]
Exophthalmos 376.30
  congenital 743.66
  constant 376.31
  endocrine NEC 259.9 [376.22]
  hyperthyroidism 242.0 [376.21]
  intermittent NEC 376.34
  malignant 242.0 [376.21]
  pulsating 376.35
    endocrine NEC 259.9 [376.22]
  thyrotoxic 242.0 [376.21]
Exostosis 726.91
  cartilaginous (M9210/0) - see Neoplasm, bone, benign
  congenital 756.4
  ear canal, external 380.81
  gonococcal 098.89
  hip 726.5
  intracranial 733.3
  jaw (bone) 526.81
  luxurians 728.11
  multiple (cancellous) (congenital) (hereditary) 756.4
  nasal bones 726.91
  orbit, orbital 376.42
  osteocartilaginous (M9210/0) - see Neoplasm, bone, benign
  spine 721.8
    with spondylosis - see Spondylosis
  syphilitic 095.5
  wrist 726.4
Exotropia 378.10
  alternating 378.15
    with
      A pattern 378.16
      specified noncomitancy NEC 378.18
      V pattern 378.17
      X pattern 378.18
      Y pattern 378.18
      intermittent 378.24
  intermittent 378.20
    alternating 378.24
    monocular 378.23
  monocular 378.11
    with
      A pattern 378.12
      specified noncomitancy NEC 378.14
      V pattern 378.13
      X pattern 378.14
      Y pattern 378.14
      intermittent 378.23
Explanation of
  investigation finding V65.4
  medication V65.4

Exposure 994.9
  cold 991.9
    specified effect NEC 991.8
  effects of 994.9
  exhaustion due to 994.4
  to
    AIDS virus V01.79 ◀▥
    anthrax V01.81
    asbestos V15.84
    body fluids (hazardous) V15.85
    Escherichia coli (E. coli) V01.83 ◀
    cholera V01.0
    communicable disease V01.9
      specified type NEC V01.89
    German measles V01.4
    gonorrhea V01.6
    hazardous body fluids V15.85
    HIV V01.79 ◀▥
    human immunodeficiency virus V01.79 ◀▥
    lead V15.86
    meningococcus V01.84 ◀
    parasitic disease V01.89
    poliomyelitis V01.2
    potentially hazardous body fluids V15.85
    rabies V01.5
    rubella V01.4
    SARS-associated coronavirus V01.82
    smallpox V01.3
    syphilis V01.6
    tuberculosis V01.1
    varicella V01.71 ◀
    venereal disease V01.6
    viral disease NEC V01.79 ◀▥
      varicella V01.71 ◀
Exsanguination, fetal 772.0
Exstrophy
  abdominal content 751.8
  bladder (urinary) 753.5
Extensive - see condition
Extra - see also Accessory
  rib 756.3
    cervical 756.2
Extraction
  with hook 763.89
  breech NEC 669.6
    affecting fetus or newborn 763.0
  cataract postsurgical V45.61
  manual NEC 669.8
    affecting fetus or newborn 763.89
Extrasystole 427.60
  atrial 427.61
  postoperative 997.1
  ventricular 427.69
Extrauterine gestation or pregnancy - see Pregnancy, ectopic
Extravasation
  blood 459.0
    lower extremity 459.0
  chyle into mesentery 457.8
  pelvicalyceal 593.4
  pyelosinus 593.4
  urine 788.8
    from ureter 788.8
Extremity - see condition
Extrophy - see Exstrophy
Extroversion
  bladder 753.5
  uterus 618.1
    complicating delivery 665.2
      affecting fetus or newborn 763.89
    postpartal (old) 618.1

◀ **New**   ◀▥ **Revised**

Extrusion
  alveolus and teeth 524.75 ◀
  breast implant (prosthetic) 996.54
  device, implant, or graft - *see* Complications, mechanical
  eye implant (ball) (globe) 996.59
  intervertebral disc - *see* Displacement, intervertebral disc

Extrusion *(Continued)*
  lacrimal gland 375.43
  mesh (reinforcing) 996.59
  ocular lens implant 996.53
  prosthetic device NEC - *see* Complications, mechanical
  vitreous 379.26

Exudate, pleura - *see* Effusion, pleura
Exudates, retina 362.82
Exudative - *see* condition
Eye, eyeball, eyelid - *see* condition
Eyestrain 368.13
Eyeworm disease of Africa 125.2

ICD-9-CM

Vol. 2

F

Faber's anemia or syndrome (achlorhydric anemia) 280.9
Fabry's disease (angiokeratoma corporis diffusum) 272.7
Face, facial - *see* condition
Facet of cornea 371.44
Faciocephalalgia, autonomic (*see also* Neuropathy, peripheral, autonomic) 337.9
Facioscapulohumeral myopathy 359.1
Factitious disorder, illness - *see* Illness, factitious
Factor
  deficiency - *see* Deficiency, factor
  psychic, associated with diseases classified elsewhere 316
  risk-see problem
Fahr-Volhard disease (malignant nephrosclerosis) 403.00
Failure, failed
  adenohypophyseal 253.2
  attempted abortion (legal) (*see also* Abortion, failed) 638.9
  bone marrow (anemia) 284.9
    acquired (secondary) 284.8
    congenital 284.0
    idiopathic 284.9
  cardiac (*see also* Failure, heart) 428.9
    newborn 779.89
  cardiorenal (chronic) 428.9
    hypertensive (*see also* Hypertension, cardiorenal) 404.93
  cardiorespiratory 799.1
    specified during or due to a procedure 997.1
      long-term effect of cardiac surgery 429.4
  cardiovascular (chronic) 428.9
  cerebrovascular 437.8
  cervical dilatation in labor 661.0
    affecting fetus or newborn 763.7
  circulation, circulatory 799.89
    fetus or newborn 779.89
    peripheral 785.50
  compensation - *see* Disease, heart
  congestive (*see also* Failure, heart) 428.0
  coronary (*see also* Insufficiency, coronary) 411.89
  descent of head (at term) 652.5
    affecting fetus or newborn 763.1
    in labor 660.0
      affecting fetus or newborn 763.1
  device, implant, or graft - *see* Complications, mechanical
  engagement of head NEC 652.5
    in labor 660.0
  extrarenal 788.9
  fetal head to enter pelvic brim 652.5
    affecting fetus or newborn 763.1
    in labor 660.0
      affecting fetus or newborn 763.1
  forceps NEC 660.7
    affecting fetus or newborn 763.1
  fusion (joint) (spinal) 996.4
  growth in childhood 783.43
  heart (acute) (sudden) 428.9
    with
      abortion - *see* Abortion, by type, with specified complication NEC

Failure, failed (*Continued*)
  heart (*Continued*)
    with (*Continued*)
      acute pulmonary edema (*see also* Failure, ventricular, left) 428.1
        with congestion (*see also* Failure, heart) 428.0
      decompensation (*see also* Failure, heart) 428.0
      dilation - *see* Disease, heart
      ectopic pregnancy (*see also* categories 633.0-633.9) 639.8
      molar pregnancy (*see also* categories 630-632) 639.8
    arteriosclerotic 440.9
    combined left-right sided 428.0
    combined systolic and diastolic 428.40
      acute 428.41
      acute on chronic 428.23
      chronic 428.42
    compensated (*see also* Failure, heart) 428.0
    complicating
      abortion - *see* Abortion, by type, with specified complication NEC
      delivery (cesarean) (instrumental) 669.4
      ectopic pregnancy (*see also* categories 633.0-633.9) 639.8
      molar pregnancy (*see also* categories 630-632) 639.8
      obstetric anesthesia or sedation 668.1
      surgery 997.1
    congestive (compensated) (decompensated) (*see also* Failure, heart) 428.0
      with rheumatic fever (conditions classifiable to 390)
        active 391.8
        inactive or quiescent (with chorea) 398.91
      fetus or newborn 779.89
      hypertensive (*see also* Hypertension, heart) 402.91
        with renal disease (*see also* Hypertension, cardiorenal) 404.91
          with renal failure 404.93
        benign 402.11
        malignant 402.01
      rheumatic (chronic) (inactive) (with chorea) 398.91
        active or acute 391.8
          with chorea (Sydenham's) 392.0
    decompensated (*see also* Failure, heart) 428.0
    degenerative (*see also* Degeneration, myocardial) 429.1
    diastolic 428.30
      acute 428.31
      acute on chronic 428.33
      chronic 428.32
    due to presence of (cardiac) prosthesis 429.4
    fetus or newborn 779.89
    following
      abortion 639.8
      cardiac surgery 429.4
      ectopic or molar pregnancy 639.8
    high output NEC 428.9

Failure, failed (*Continued*)
  heart (*Continued*)
    hypertensive (*see also* Hypertension, heart) 402.91
      with renal disease (*see also* Hypertension, cardiorenal) 404.91
        with renal failure 404.93
      benign 402.11
      malignant 402.01
    left (ventricular) (*see also* Failure, ventricular, left) 428.1
      with right-sided failure (*see also* Failure, heart) 428.0
    low output (syndrome) NEC 428.9
    organic - *see* Disease, heart
    postoperative (immediate) 997.1
      long term effect of cardiac surgery 429.4
    rheumatic (chronic) (congestive) (inactive) 398.91
    right (secondary to left heart failure, conditions classifiable to 428.1) (ventricular) (*see also* Failure, heart) 428.0
    senile 797
    specified during or due to a procedure 997.1
      long-term effect of cardiac surgery 429.4
    systolic 428.20
      acute 428.21
      acute on chronic 428.23
      chronic 428.22
    thyrotoxic (*see also* Thyrotoxicosis) 242.9 [425.7]
    valvular - *see* Endocarditis
  hepatic 572.8
    acute 570
    due to a procedure 997.4
  hepatorenal 572.4
  hypertensive heart (*see also* Hypertension, heart) 402.91
    benign 402.11
    malignant 402.01
  induction (of labor) 659.1
    abortion (legal) (*see also* Abortion, failed) 638.9
    affecting fetus or newborn 763.89
    by oxytocic drugs 659.1
    instrumental 659.0
    mechanical 659.0
    medical 659.1
    surgical 659.0
  initial alveolar expansion, newborn 770.4
  involution, thymus (gland) 254.8
  kidney - *see* Failure, renal
  lactation 676.4
  Leydig's cell, adult 257.2
  liver 572.8
    acute 570
  medullary 799.89
  mitral - *see* Endocarditis, mitral
  myocardium, myocardial (*see also* Failure, heart) 428.9
    chronic (*see also* Failure, heart) 428.0
    congestive (*see also* Failure, heart) 428.0
  ovarian (primary) 256.39
    iatrogenic 256.2
    postablative 256.2
    postirradiation 256.2
    postsurgical 256.2
  ovulation 628.0

◀ **New**   ◀▥ **Revised**

Failure, failed (*Continued*)
prerenal 788.9
renal 586
  with
    abortion - *see* Abortion, by type,
      with renal failure
    ectopic pregnancy (*see also* catego-
      ries 633.0-633.9) 639.3
    edema (*see also* Nephrosis) 581.9
    hypertension (*see also* Hyperten-
      sion, kidney) 403.91
    hypertensive heart disease (condi-
      tions classifiable to 402) 404.92
      with heart failure 404.93
      benign 404.12
        with heart failure 404.13
      malignant 404.02
        with heart failure 404.03
    molar pregnancy (*see also* catego-
      ries 630-632) 639.3
    tubular necrosis (acute) 584.5
  acute 584.9
    with lesion of
      necrosis
        cortical (renal) 584.6
        medullary (renal) (papillary)
          584.7
        tubular 584.5
      specified pathology NEC 584.8
  chronic 585
    hypertensive or with hypertension
      (*see also* Hypertension, kid-
      ney) 403.91
  due to a procedure 997.5
  following
    abortion 639.3
    crushing 958.5
    ectopic or molar pregnancy 639.3
    labor and delivery (acute) 669.3
  hypertensive (*see also* Hypertension,
    kidney) 403.91
  puerperal, postpartum 669.3
respiration, respiratory 518.81
  acute 518.81
  acute and chronic 518.84
  center 348.8
    newborn 770.84
  chronic 518.83
  due to trauma, surgery or shock 518.5
  newborn 770.84
rotation
  cecum 751.4
  colon 751.4
  intestine 751.4
  kidney 753.3
segmentation - *see also* Fusion
  fingers (*see also* Syndactylism, fin-
    gers) 755.11
  toes (*see also* Syndactylism, toes)
    755.13
seminiferous tubule, adult 257.2
senile (general) 797
  with psychosis 290.20
testis, primary (seminal) 257.2
to progress 661.2
to thrive
  adult 783.7
  child 783.41
transplant 996.80
  bone marrow 996.85
  organ (immune or nonimmune
    cause) 996.80
    bone marrow 996.85
    heart 996.83

Failure, failed (*Continued*)
transplant (*Continued*)
  organ (*Continued*)
    intestines 996.87
    kidney 996.81
    liver 996.82
    lung 996.84
    pancreas 996.86
    specified NEC 996.89
  skin 996.52
    artificial 996.55
    decellularized allodermis 996.55
    temporary allograft or pigskin
      graft - omit code
trial of labor NEC 660.6
  affecting fetus or newborn 763.1
tubal ligation 998.89 ◀
urinary 586
vacuum extraction
  abortion - *see* Abortion, failed
  delivery NEC 660.7
    affecting fetus or newborn 763.1
vasectomy 998.89 ◀
ventouse NEC 660.7
  affecting fetus or newborn 763.1
ventricular (*see also* Failure, heart) 428.9
  left 428.1
    with rheumatic fever (conditions
      classifiable to 390)
      active 391.8
        with chorea 392.0
      inactive or quiescent (with cho-
        rea) 398.91
    hypertensive (*see also* Hyperten-
      sion, heart) 402.91
      benign 402.11
      malignant 402.01
    rheumatic (chronic) (inactive)
      (with chorea) 398.91
      active or acute 391.8
        with chorea 392.0
  right (*see also* Failure, heart) 428.0
vital centers, fetus or newborn 779.8
weight gain
  in childhood 783.41
Fainting (fit) (spell) 780.2
Falciform hymen 752.49
**Fall, maternal, affecting fetus or new-
  born** 760.5
Fallen arches 734
Falling, any organ or part - *see* Prolapse
Fallopian
insufflation
  fertility testing V26.21
  following sterilization reversal V26.22
tube - *see* condition
Fallot's
pentalogy 745.2
tetrad or tetralogy 745.2
triad or trilogy 746.09
Fallout, radioactive (adverse effect) NEC
  990
False - *see also* condition
bundle branch block 426.50
bursa 727.89
croup 478.75
joint 733.82
labor (pains) 644.1
opening, urinary, male 752.69
passage, urethra (prostatic) 599.4
positive
  serological test for syphilis 795.6
  Wassermann reaction 795.6
pregnancy 300.11

Family, familial - *see also* condition
disruption V61.0
Li-Fraumeni (syndrome) V84.01 ◀
planning advice V25.09
problem V61.9
  specified circumstance NEC V61.8
retinoblastoma (syndrome) 190.5 ◀
Famine 994.2
edema 262
Fanconi's anemia (congenital pancytopenia) 284.0
Fanconi (-de Toni) (-Debré) syndrome
  (cystinosis) 270.0
Farber (-Uzman) syndrome or disease (disseminated lipogranulomatosis) 272.8
Farcin 024
Farcy 024
Farmers'
lung 495.0
skin 692.74
Farsightedness 367.0
Fascia - *see* condition
Fasciculation 781.0
Fasciculitis optica 377.32
Fasciitis 729.4
eosinophilic 728.89
necrotizing 728.86
nodular 728.79
perirenal 593.4
plantar 728.71
pseudosarcomatous 728.79
traumatic (old) NEC 728.79
  current - *see* Sprain, by site
Fasciola hepatica infestation 121.3
Fascioliasis 121.3
Fasciolopsiasis (small intestine) 121.4
Fasciolopsis (small intestine) 121.4
Fast pulse 785.0
Fat
embolism (cerebral) (pulmonary) (systemic) 958.1
  with
    abortion - *see* Abortion, by type,
      with embolism
    ectopic pregnancy (*see also* catego-
      ries 633.0-633.9) 639.6
    molar pregnancy (*see also* catego-
      ries 630-632) 639.6
  complicating delivery or puerperium
    673.8
  following
    abortion 639.6
    ectopic or molar pregnancy 639.6
  in pregnancy, childbirth, or the pu-
    erperium 673.8
excessive 278.00
  in heart (*see also* Degeneration,
    myocardial) 429.1
general 278.00
hernia, herniation 729.30
  eyelid 374.34
  knee 729.31
  orbit 374.34
  retro-orbital 374.34
  retropatellar 729.31
  specified site NEC 729.39
indigestion 579.8
in stool 792.1
localized (pad) 278.1
  heart (*see also* Degeneration, myocar-
    dial) 429.1
  knee 729.31
  retropatellar 729.31
necrosis - *see also* Fatty, degeneration
  breast (aseptic) (segmental) 611.3

ICD-9-CM

Vol. 2

Fat (*Continued*)
  necrosis (*Continued*)
    mesentery 567.8
    omentum 567.8
  pad 278.1
Fatal syncope 798.1
Fatigue 780.79
  auditory deafness (*see also* Deafness) 389.9
  chronic, syndrome 780.71
  combat (*see also* Reaction, stress, acute) 308.9
  during pregnancy 646.8
  general 780.79
    psychogenic 300.5
  heat (transient) 992.6
  muscle 729.89
  myocardium (*see also* Failure, heart) 428.9
  nervous 300.5
  neurosis 300.5
  operational 300.89
  postural 729.89
  posture 729.89
  psychogenic (general) 300.5
  senile 797
  syndrome NEC 300.5
    chronic 780.71
  undue 780.79
  voice 784.49
Fatness 278.00
Fatty - *see also* condition
  apron 278.1
  degeneration (diffuse) (general) NEC 272.8
    localized - *see* Degeneration, by site, fatty
    placenta - *see* Placenta, abnormal
  heart (enlarged) (*see also* Degeneration, myocardial) 429.1
  infiltration (diffuse) (general) (*see also* Degeneration, by site, fatty) 272.8
    heart (enlarged) (*see also* Degeneration, myocardial) 429.1
  liver 571.8
    alcoholic 571.0
  necrosis - *see* Degeneration, fatty
  phanerosis 272.8
Fauces - *see* condition
Fauchard's disease (periodontitis) 523.4
Faucitis 478.29
Faulty - *see also* condition
  position of teeth 524.30 ◄▥
Favism (anemia) 282.2
Favre-Racouchot disease (elastoidosis cutanea nodularis) 701.8
Favus 110.9
  beard 110.0
  capitis 110.0
  corporis 110.5
  eyelid 110.8
  foot 110.4
  hand 110.2
  scalp 110.0
  specified site NEC 110.8
Fear, fearfulness (complex) (reaction) 300.20
  child 313.0
  of
    animals 300.29
    closed spaces 300.29
    crowds 300.29
    eating in public 300.23
    heights 300.29

Fear, fearfulness (*Continued*)
  of (*Continued*)
    open spaces 300.22
      with panic attacks 300.21
    public speaking 300.23
    streets 300.22
      with panic attacks 300.21
    travel 300.22
      with panic attacks 300.21
    washing in public 300.23
  transient 308.0
Feared complaint unfounded V65.5
Febricula (continued) (simple) (*see also* Pyrexia) 780.6
Febrile (*see also* Pyrexia) 780.6
  convulsion 780.31
  seizure 780.31
Febris (*see also* Fever) 780.6
  aestiva (*see also* Fever, hay) 477.9
  flava (*see also* Fever, yellow) 060.9
  melitensis 023.0
  pestis (*see also* Plague) 020.9
  puerperalis 672
  recurrens (*see also* Fever, relapsing) 087.9
    pediculo vestimenti 087.0
  rubra 034.1
  typhoidea 002.0
  typhosa 002.0
Fecal - *see* condition
Fecalith (impaction) 560.39
  with hernia - *see also* Hernia, by site, with obstruction
    gangrenous - *see* Hernia, by site, with gangrene
  appendix 543.9
  congenital 777.1
Fede's disease 529.0
Feeble-minded 317
Feeble rapid pulse due to shock following injury 958.4
Feeding
  faulty (elderly) (infant) 783.3
    newborn 779.3
  formula check V20.2
  improper (elderly) (infant) 783.3
    newborn 779.3
  problem (elderly) 783.3 ◄▥
    infancy or early childhood 307.59 ◄
    newborn 779.3
    nonorganic origin 307.59
Feer's disease 985.0
Feet - *see* condition
Feigned illness V65.2
Feil-Klippel syndrome (brevicollis) 756.16
Feinmesser's (hidrotic) ectodermal dysplasia 757.31
Felix's disease (juvenile osteochondrosis, hip) 732.1
Felon (any digit) (with lymphangitis) 681.01
  herpetic 054.6
Felty's syndrome (rheumatoid arthritis with splenomegaly and leukopenia) 714.1
Feminism in boys 302.6
Feminization, testicular 257.8
  with pseudohermaphroditism, male 257.8
Femoral hernia - *see* Hernia, femoral
Femora vara 736.32
Femur, femoral - *see* condition
Fenestrata placenta - *see* Placenta, abnormal

Fenestration, fenestrated - *see also* Imperfect, closure
  aorta-pulmonary 745.0
  aorticopulmonary 745.0
  aortopulmonary 745.0
  cusps, heart valve NEC 746.89
    pulmonary 746.09
  hymen 752.49
  pulmonic cusps 746.09
Fenwick's disease 537.89
Fermentation (gastric) (gastrointestinal) (stomach) 536.8
  intestine 564.89
    psychogenic 306.4
  psychogenic 306.4
Fernell's disease (aortic aneurysm) 441.9
Fertile eunuch syndrome 257.2
Fertility, meaning multiparity - *see* Multiparity
Fetal alcohol syndrome 760.71
Fetalis uterus 752.3
Fetid
  breath 784.9
  sweat 705.89
Fetishism 302.81
  transvestic 302.3
Fetomaternal hemorrhage
  affecting management of pregnancy 656.0
  fetus or newborn 772.0
Fetus, fetal - *see also* condition
  papyraceous 779.89
  type lung tissue 770.4
Fever 780.6
  with chills 780.6
    in malarial regions (*see also* Malaria) 084.6
  abortus NEC 023.9
  aden 061
  African tick-borne 087.1
  American
    mountain tick 066.1
    spotted 082.0
  and ague (*see also* Malaria) 084.6
  aphthous 078.4
  arbovirus hemorrhagic 065.9
  Assam 085.0
  Australian A or Q 083.0
  Bangkok hemorrhagic 065.4
  biliary, Charcôt's intermittent - *see* Choledocholithiasis
  bilious, hemoglobinuric 084.8
  blackwater 084.8
  blister 054.9
  Bonvale Dam 780.79
  boutonneuse 082.1
  brain 323.9
    late effect - *see* category 326
  breakbone 061
  Bullis 082.8
  Bunyamwera 066.3
  Burdwan 085.0
  Bwamba (encephalitis) 066.3
  Cameroon (*see also* Malaria) 084.6
  Canton 081.9
  catarrhal (acute) 460
    chronic 472.0
  cat-scratch 078.3
  cerebral 323.9
    late effect - *see* category 326
  cerebrospinal (meningococcal) (*see also* Meningitis, cerebrospinal) 036.0
  Chagres 084.0

◄ **New**   ◄▥ **Revised**

Fever *(Continued)*
  Chandipura 066.8
  changuinola 066.0
  Charcôt's (biliary) (hepatic) (intermittent) *see* Choledocholithiasis
  Chikungunya (viral) 066.3
    hemorrhagic 065.4
  childbed 670
  Chitral 066.0
  Colombo (*see also* Fever, paratyphoid) 002.9
  Colorado tick (virus) 066.1
  congestive
    malarial (*see also* Malaria) 084.6
    remittent (*see also* Malaria) 084.6
  Congo virus 065.0
  continued 780.6
    malarial 084.0
  Corsican (*see also* Malaria) 084.6
  Crimean hemorrhagic 065.0
  Cyprus (*see also* Brucellosis) 023.9
  dandy 061
  deer fly (*see also* Tularemia) 021.9
  dehydration, newborn 778.4
  dengue (virus) 061
    hemorrhagic 065.4
  desert 114.0
  due to heat 992.0
  Dumdum 085.0
  enteric 002.0
  ephemeral (of unknown origin) (*see also* Pyrexia) 780.6
  epidemic, hemorrhagic of the Far East 065.0
  erysipelatous (*see also* Erysipelas) 035
  estivo-autumnal (malarial) 084.0
  etiocholanolone 277.3
  famine - *see also* Fever, relapsing
    meaning typhus - *see* Typhus
  Far Eastern hemorrhagic 065.0
  five day 083.1
  Fort Bragg 100.89
  gastroenteric 002.0
  gastromalarial (*see also* Malaria) 084.6
  Gibraltar (*see also* Brucellosis) 023.9
  glandular 075
  Guama (viral) 066.3
  Haverhill 026.1
  hay (allergic) (with rhinitis) 477.9
    with
      asthma (bronchial) (*see also* Asthma) 493.0
    due to
      dander, animal (cat) (dog) 477.2 ◄▥
      dust 477.8
      fowl 477.8
      hair, animal (cat) (dog) 477.2 ◄
      pollen, any plant or tree 477.0
      specified allergen other than pollen 477.8
  heat (effects) 992.0
  hematuric, bilious 084.8
  hemoglobinuric (malarial) 084.8
    bilious 084.8
  hemorrhagic (arthropod-borne) NEC 065.9
    with renal syndrome 078.6
    arenaviral 078.7
    Argentine 078.7
    Bangkok 065.4
    Bolivian 078.7
    Central Asian 065.0
    chikungunya 065.4
    Crimean 065.0
    dengue (virus) 065.4

Fever *(Continued)*
  hemorrhagic *(Continued)*
    Ebola 065.8
    epidemic 078.6
      of Far East 065.0
    Far Eastern 065.0
    Junin virus 078.7
    Korean 078.6
    Kyasanur forest 065.2
    Machupo virus 078.7
    mite-borne NEC 065.8
    mosquito-borne 065.4
    Omsk 065.1
    Philippine 065.4
    Russian (Yaroslav) 078.6
    Singapore 065.4
    Southeast Asia 065.4
    Thailand 065.4
    tick-borne NEC 065.3
  hepatic (*see also* Cholecystitis) 575.8
    intermittent (Charcôt's) - *see* Choledocholithiasis
  herpetic (*see also* Herpes) 054.9
  hyalomma tick 065.0
  icterohemorrhagic 100.0
  inanition 780.6
    newborn 778.4
  infective NEC 136.9
  intermittent (bilious) (*see also* Malaria) 084.6
    hepatic (Charcôt) - *see* Choledocholithiasis
    of unknown origin (*see also* Pyrexia) 780.6
    pernicious 084.0
  iodide
    correct substance properly administered 780.6
    overdose or wrong substance given or taken 975.5
  Japanese river 081.2
  jungle yellow 060.0
  Junin virus, hemorrhagic 078.7
  Katayama 120.2
  Kedani 081.2
  Kenya 082.1
  Korean hemorrhagic 078.6
  Lassa 078.89
  Lone Star 082.8
  lung - *see* Pneumonia
  Machupo virus, hemorrhagic 078.7
  malaria, malarial (*see also* Malaria) 084.6
  Malta (*see also* Brucellosis) 023.9
  Marseilles 082.1
  marsh (*see also* Malaria) 084.6
  Mayaro (viral) 066.3
  Mediterranean (*see also* Brucellosis) 023.9
    familial 277.3
    tick 082.1
  meningeal - *see* Meningitis
  metal fumes NEC 985.8
  Meuse 083.1
  Mexican - *see* Typhus, Mexican
  Mianeh 087.1
  miasmatic (*see also* Malaria) 084.6
  miliary 078.2
  milk, female 672
  mill 504
  mite-borne hemorrhagic 065.8
  Monday 504
  mosquito-borne NEC 066.3
    hemorrhagic NEC 065.4

Fever *(Continued)*
  mountain 066.1
    meaning
      Rocky Mountain spotted 082.0
      undulant fever (*see also* Brucellosis) 023.9
    tick (American) 066.1
  Mucambo (viral) 066.3
  mud 100.89
  Neapolitan (*see also* Brucellosis) 023.9
  neutropenic 288.0
  nine-mile 083.0
  nonexanthematous tick 066.1
  North Asian tick-borne typhus 082.2
  Omsk hemorrhagic 065.1
  O'nyong nyong (viral) 066.3
  Oropouche (viral) 066.3
  Oroya 088.0
  paludal (*see also* Malaria) 084.6
  Panama 084.0
  pappataci 066.0
  paratyphoid 002.9
    A 002.1
    B (Schottmüller's) 002.2
    C (Hirschfeld) 002.3
  parrot 073.9
  periodic 277.3
  pernicious, acute 084.0
  persistent (of unknown origin) (*see also* Pyrexia) 780.6
  petechial 036.0
  pharyngoconjunctival 077.2
    adenoviral type 3 077.2
  Philippine hemorrhagic 065.4
  phlebotomus 066.0
  Piry 066.8
  Pixuna (viral) 066.3
  Plasmodium ovale 084.3
  pleural (*see also* Pleurisy) 511.0
  pneumonic - *see* Pneumonia
  polymer fume 987.8
  postoperative 998.89
    due to infection 998.59
  pretibial 100.89
  puerperal, postpartum 672
  putrid - *see* Septicemia
  pyemic - *see* Septicemia
  Q 083.0
    with pneumonia 083.0 [484.8]
  quadrilateral 083.0
  quartan (malaria) 084.2
  Queensland (coastal) 083.0
    seven-day 100.89
  Quintan (A) 083.1
  quotidian 084.0
  rabbit (*see also* Tularemia) 021.9
  rat-bite 026.9
    due to
      Spirillum minor or minus 026.0
      Spirochaeta morsus muris 026.0
      Streptobacillus moniliformis 026.1
  recurrent - *see* Fever, relapsing
  relapsing 087.9
    Carter's (Asiatic) 087.0
    Dutton's (West African) 087.1
    Koch's 087.9
    louse-borne (epidemic) 087.0
    Novy's (American) 087.1
    Obermeyer's (European) 087.0
    spirillum NEC 087.9
    tick-borne (endemic) 087.1
  remittent (bilious) (congestive) (gastric) (*see also* Malaria) 084.6

ICD-9-CM
ㄴ
Vol. 2

Fever (Continued)
  rheumatic (active) (acute) (chronic)
    (subacute) 390
    with heart involvement 391.9
      carditis 391.9
      endocarditis (aortic) (mitral) (pul-
        monary) (tricuspid) 391.1
      multiple sites 391.8
      myocarditis 391.2
      pancarditis, acute 391.8
      pericarditis 391.0
      specified type NEC 391.8
      valvulitis 391.1
    inactive or quiescent with
      cardiac hypertrophy 398.99
      carditis 398.90
      endocarditis 397.9
        aortic (valve) 395.9
          with mitral (valve) disease
            396.9
        mitral (valve) 394.9
          with aortic (valve) disease
            396.9
        pulmonary (valve) 397.1
        tricuspid (valve) 397.0
      heart conditions (classifiable to
        429.3, 429.6, 429.9) 398.99
      failure (congestive) (conditions
        classifiable to 428.0, 428.9)
        398.91
      left ventricular failure (conditions
        classifiable to 428.1) 398.91
      myocardial degeneration (conditions
        classifiable to 429.1) 398.0
      myocarditis (conditions classifiable
        to 429.0) 398.0
      pancarditis 398.99
      pericarditis 393
  Rift Valley (viral) 066.3
  Rocky Mountain spotted 082.0
  rose 477.0
  Ross river (viral) 066.3
  Russian hemorrhagic 078.6
  sandfly 066.0
  San Joaquin (valley) 114.0
  São Paulo 082.0
  scarlet 034.1
  septic - see Septicemia
  seven-day 061
    Japan 100.89
    Queensland 100.89
  shin bone 083.1
  Singapore hemorrhagic 065.4
  solar 061
  sore 054.9
  South African tick-bite 087.1
  Southeast Asia hemorrhagic 065.4
  spinal - see Meningitis
  spirillary 026.0
  splenic (see also Anthrax) 022.9
  spotted (Rocky Mountain) 082.0
    American 082.0
    Brazilian 082.0
    Colombian 082.0
    meaning
      cerebrospinal meningitis 036.0
      typhus 082.9
  spring 309.23
  steroid
    correct substance properly adminis-
      tered 780.6
    overdose or wrong substance given
      or taken 962.0
  streptobacillary 026.1
  subtertian 084.0
  Sumatran mite 081.2

Fever (Continued)
  sun 061
  swamp 100.89
  sweating 078.2
  swine 003.8
  sylvatic yellow 060.0
  Tahyna 062.5
  tertian - see Malaria, tertian
  Thailand hemorrhagic 065.4
  thermic 992.0
  three day 066.0
    with Coxsackie exanthem 074.8
  tick
    American mountain 066.1
    Colorado 066.1
    Kemerovo 066.1
    Mediterranean 082.1
    mountain 066.1
    nonexanthematous 066.1
    Quaranfil 066.1
  tick-bite NEC 066.1
  tick-borne NEC 066.1
    hemorrhagic NEC 065.3
  transitory of newborn 778.4
  trench 083.1
  tsutsugamushi 081.2
  typhogastric 002.0
  typhoid (abortive) (ambulant) (any site)
    (hemorrhagic) (infection) (intermit-
    tent) (malignant) (rheumatic) 002.0
  typhomalarial (see also Malaria) 084.6
  typhus - see Typhus
  undulant (see also Brucellosis) 023.9
  unknown origin (see also Pyrexia) 780.6
  uremic - see Uremia
  uveoparotid 135
  valley (Coccidioidomycosis) 114.0
  Venezuelan equine 066.2
  Volhynian 083.1
  Wesselsbron (viral) 066.3
  West
    African 084.8
    Nile (viral) 066.40 ◀━
      with ◀
        cranial nerve disorders 066.42 ◀
        encephalitis 066.41 ◀
        optic neuritis 066.42 ◀
        other complications 066.49 ◀
        other neurologic manifesta-
          tions 066.42 ◀
        polyradiculitis 066.42 ◀
  Whitmore's 025
  Wolhynian 083.1
  worm 128.9
  Yaroslav hemorrhagic 078.6
  yellow 060.9
    jungle 060.0
    sylvatic 060.0
    urban 060.1
    vaccination, prophylactic (against)
      V04.4
  Zika (viral) 066.3
Fibrillation
  atrial (established) (paroxysmal) 427.31
  auricular (atrial) (established) 427.31
  cardiac (ventricular) 427.41
  coronary (see also Infarct, myocardium)
    410.9
  heart (ventricular) 427.41
  muscular 728.9
  postoperative 997.1
  ventricular 427.41
Fibrin
  ball or bodies, pleural (sac) 511.0
  chamber, anterior (eye) (gelatinous ex-
    udate) 364.04

Fibrinogenolysis (hemorrhagic) - see Fibrinolysis
Fibrinogenopenia (congenital) (hereditary) (see also Defect, coagulation)
  286.3
  acquired 286.6
Fibrinolysis (acquired) (hemorrhagic)
  (pathologic) 286.6
  with
    abortion - see Abortion, by type,
      with hemorrhage, delayed or
      excessive
    ectopic pregnancy (see also categories
      633.0-633.9) 639.1
    molar pregnancy (see also categories
      630-632) 639.1
  antepartum or intrapartum 641.3
    affecting fetus or newborn 762.1
  following
    abortion 639.1
    ectopic or molar pregnancy 639.1
  newborn, transient 776.2
  postpartum 666.3
Fibrinopenia (hereditary) (see also Defect,
  coagulation) 286.3
  acquired 286.6
Fibrinopurulent - see condition
Fibrinous - see condition
Fibroadenoma (M9010/0)
  cellular intracanalicular (M9020/0) 217
  giant (intracanalicular) (M9020/0) 217
  intracanalicular (M9011/0)
    cellular (M9020/0) 217
    giant (M9020/0) 217
    specified site - see Neoplasm, by site,
      benign
    unspecified site 217
  juvenile (M9030/0) 217
  pericanicular (M9012/0)
    specified site - see Neoplasm, by site,
      benign
    unspecified site 217
  phyllodes (M9020/0) 217
  prostate 600.20
    with urinary retention 600.21
  specified site - see Neoplasm, by site,
    benign
  unspecified site 217
Fibroadenosis, breast (chronic) (cystic)
  (diffuse) (periodic) (segmental) 610.2
Fibroangioma (M9160/0) - see also Neoplasm, by site, benign
  juvenile (M9160/0)
    specified site - see Neoplasm, by site,
      benign
    unspecified site 210.7
Fibrocellulitis progressiva ossificans 728.11
Fibrochondrosarcoma (M9220/3) - see
  Neoplasm, cartilage, malignant
Fibrocystic
  disease 277.00
    bone NEC 733.29
    breast 610.1
    jaw 526.2
    kidney (congenital) 753.19
    liver 751.62
    lung 518.89
      congenital 748.4
    pancreas 277.00
  kidney (congenital) 753.19
Fibrodysplasia ossificans multiplex
  (progressiva) 728.11
Fibroelastosis (cordis) (endocardial) (en-
  domyocardial) 425.3
Fibroid (tumor) (M8890/0) - see also Ne-
  oplasm, connective tissue, benign

◀ **New**   ◀━ **Revised**

Fibroid (Continued)
  disease, lung (chronic) (see also Fibrosis, lung) 515
  heart (disease) (see also Myocarditis) 429.0
  induration, lung (chronic) (see also Fibrosis, lung) 515
  in pregnancy or childbirth 654.1
    affecting fetus or newborn 763.89
    causing obstructed labor 660.2
      affecting fetus or newborn 763.1
  liver - see Cirrhosis, liver
  lung (see also Fibrosis, lung) 515
  pneumonia (chronic) (see also Fibrosis, lung) 515
  uterus (M8890/0) (see also Leiomyoma, uterus) 218.9
Fibrolipoma (M8851/0) (see also Lipoma, by site) 214.9
Fibroliposarcoma (M8850/3) - see- Neoplasm, connective tissue, malignant
Fibroma (M8810/0) - see also Neoplasm, connective tissue, benign
  ameloblastic (M9330/0) 213.1
    upper jaw (bone) 213.0
  bone (nonossifying) 733.99
    ossifying (M9262/0) - see Neoplasm, bone, benign
  cementifying (M9274/0) - see Neoplasm, bone, benign
  chondromyxoid (M9241/0) - see Neoplasm, bone, benign
  desmoplastic (M8823/1) - see Neoplasm, connective tissue, uncertain behavior
  facial (M8813/0) - see Neoplasm, connective tissue, benign
  invasive (M8821/1) - see Neoplasm, connective tissue, uncertain behavior
  molle (M8851/0) (see also Lipoma, by site) 214.9
  myxoid (M8811/0) - see Neoplasm, connective tissue, benign
  nasopharynx, nasopharyngeal (juvenile) (M9160/0) 210.7
  nonosteogenic (nonossifying) - see Dysplasia, fibrous
  odontogenic (M9321/0) 213.1
    upper jaw (bone) 213.0
  ossifying (M9262/0) - see Neoplasm, bone, benign
  periosteal (M8812/0) - see Neoplasm, bone, benign
  prostate 600.20
    with urinary retention 600.21
  soft (M8851/0) (see also Lipoma, by site) 214.9
Fibromatosis
  abdominal (M8822/1) - see Neoplasm, connective tissue, uncertain behavior
  aggressive (M8821/1) - see Neoplasm, connective tissue, uncertain behavior
  Dupuytren's 728.6
  gingival 523.8
  plantar fascia 728.71
  proliferative 728.79
  pseudosarcomatous (proliferative) (subcutaneous) 728.79
  subcutaneous pseudosarcomatous (proliferative) 728.79
Fibromyalgia 729.1

Fibromyoma (M8890/0) - see also Neoplasm, connective tissue, benign
  uterus (corpus) (see also Leiomyoma, uterus) 218.9
  in pregnancy or childbirth 654.1
    affecting fetus or newborn 763.89
    causing obstructed labor 660.2
      affecting fetus or newborn 763.1
Fibromyositis (see also Myositis) 729.1
  scapulohumeral 726.2
Fibromyxolipoma (M8852/0) (see also Lipoma, by site) 214.9
Fibromyxoma (M8811/0) - see Neoplasm, connective tissue, benign
Fibromyxosarcoma (M8811/3) - see Neoplasm, connective tissue, malignant
Fibro-odontoma, ameloblastic (M9290/0) 213.1
  upper jaw (bone) 213.0
Fibro-osteoma (M9262/0) - see Neoplasm, bone, benign
Fibroplasia, retrolental 362.21
Fibropurulent - see condition
Fibrosarcoma (M8810/3) - see also Neoplasm, connective tissue, malignant
  ameloblastic (M9330/3) 170.1
    upper jaw (bone) 170.0
  congenital (M8814/3) - see Neoplasm, connective tissue, malignant
  fascial (M8813/3) - see Neoplasm, connective tissue, malignant
  infantile (M8814/3) - see Neoplasm, connective tissue, malignant
  odontogenic (M9330/3) 170.1
    upper jaw (bone) 170.0
  periosteal (M8812/3) - see Neoplasm, bone, malignant
Fibrosclerosis
  breast 610.3
  corpora cavernosa (penis) 607.89
  familial multifocal NEC 710.8
  multifocal (idiopathic) NEC 710.8
  penis (corpora cavernosa) 607.89
Fibrosis, fibrotic
  adrenal (gland) 255.8
  alveolar (diffuse) 516.3
  amnion 658.8
  anal papillae 569.49
  anus 569.49
  appendix, appendiceal, noninflammatory 543.9
  arteriocapillary - see Arteriosclerosis
  bauxite (of lung) 503
  biliary 576.8
    due to Clonorchis sinensis 121.1
  bladder 596.8
    interstitial 595.1
    localized submucosal 595.1
    panmural 595.1
  bone, diffuse 756.59
  breast 610.3
  capillary - see also Arteriosclerosis
    lung (chronic) (see also Fibrosis, lung) 515
  cardiac (see also Myocarditis) 429.0
  cervix 622.8
  chorion 658.8
  corpus cavernosum 607.89
  cystic (of pancreas) 277.00
    with
      manifestations
        gastrointestinal 277.03
        pulmonary 277.02
        specified NEC 277.09
      meconium ileus 277.01

Fibrosis, fibrotic (Continued)
  cystic (Continued)
    with (Continued)
      pulmonary exacerbation 277.02
    due to (presence of) any device, implant, or graft - see Complications, due to (presence of) any device, implant, or graft classified to 996.0-996.5 NEC
    ejaculatory duct 608.89
    endocardium (see also Endocarditis) 424.90
    endomyocardial (African) 425.0
    epididymis 608.89'
    eye muscle 378.62
    graphite (of lung) 503
    heart (see also Myocarditis) 429.0
    hepatic - see also Cirrhosis, liver
      due to Clonorchis sinensis 121.1
    hepatolienal - see Cirrhosis, liver
    hepatosplenic - see Cirrhosis, liver
    infrapatellar fat pad 729.31
    interstitial pulmonary, newborn 770.7
    intrascrotal 608.89
    kidney (see also Sclerosis, renal) 587
    liver - see Cirrhosis, liver
    lung (atrophic) (capillary) (chronic) (confluent) (massive) (perialveolar) (peribronchial) 515
      with
        anthracosilicosis (occupational) 500
        anthracosis (occupational) 500
        asbestosis (occupational) 501
        bagassosis (occupational) 495.1
        bauxite 503
        berylliosis (occupational) 503
        byssinosis (occupational) 504
        calcicosis (occupational) 502
        chalicosis (occupational) 502
        dust reticulation (occupational) 504
        farmers' lung 495.0
        gannister disease (occupational) 502
        graphite 503
        pneumonoconiosis (occupational) 505
        pneumosiderosis (occupational) 503
        siderosis (occupational) 503
        silicosis (occupational) 502
        tuberculosis (see also Tuberculosis) 011.4
      diffuse (idiopathic) (interstitial) 516.3
      due to
        bauxite 503
        fumes or vapors (chemical) (inhalation) 506.4
        graphite 503
      following radiation 508.1
      postinflammatory 515
      silicotic (massive) (occupational) 502
      tuberculous (see also Tuberculosis) 011.4
    lymphatic gland 289.3
    median bar 600.90
      with urinary retention 600.91
    mediastinum (idiopathic) 519.3
    meninges 349.2
    muscle NEC 728.2
      iatrogenic (from injection) 999.9
    myocardium, myocardial (see also Myocarditis) 429.0
    oral submucous 528.8

ICD-9-CM

Vol. 2

◄ **New**   ◄ **Revised**

Findings, abnormal, without diagnosis
  (Continued)
  function study NEC *(Continued)*
    kidney 794.4
    liver 794.8
    nervous system
      central 794.00
      peripheral 794.19
    oculomotor 794.14
    pancreas 794.9
    placenta 794.9
    pulmonary 794.2
    retina 794.11
    special senses 794.19
    spleen 794.9
    vestibular 794.16
  gallbladder, nonvisualization 793.3
  glucose 790.29
    elevated
      fasting 790.21
      tolerance test 790.22
  glycosuria 791.5
  heart
    shadow 793.2
    sounds 785.3
  hematinuria 791.2
  hematocrit
    drop (precipitous) 790.01
    elevated 282.7
    low 285.9
  hematologic NEC 790.99
  hematuria 599.7
  hemoglobin
    elevated 282.7
    low 285.9
  hemoglobinuria 791.2
  histological NEC 795.4
  hormones 259.9
  immunoglobulins, elevated 795.79
  indolacetic acid, elevated 791.9
  iron 790.6
  karyotype 795.2
  ketonuria 791.6
  lactic acid dehydrogenase (LDH) 790.4
  lipase 790.5
  lipids NEC 272.9
  lithium, blood 790.6
  lung field (coin lesion) (shadow) 793.1
  magnesium, blood 790.6
  mammogram 793.80
    microcalcification 793.81
  mediastinal shift 793.2
  melanin, urine 791.9
  microbiologic NEC 795.39
  mineral, blood NEC 790.6
  myoglobinuria 791.3
  nitrogen derivatives, blood 790.6
  nasal swab, anthrax 795.31
  neonatal screening 796.6 ◄
  nonvisualization of gallbladder 793.3
  nose culture, positive 795.39
  odor of urine (unusual) NEC 791.9
  oxygen saturation 790.91
  Papanicolaou (smear) 795.1
    cervix 795.00 ◄
      with
        atypical squamous cells ◄◄◄
          cannot exclude high grade
            squamous intraepithelial
            lesion (ASC-H) 795.01 ◄◄◄
          of undetermined significance
            (ASC-US) 795.02 ◄◄◄
        high grade squamous intraepithe-
          lial lesion (HGSIL) 795.04 ◄
        low grade squamous intraepithe-
          lial lesion (LGSIL) 795.03 ◄

Findings, abnormal, without diagnosis
  (Continued)
  Papanicolaou *(Continued)*
    cervix *(Continued)*
      dyskaryotic 795.09
      nonspecific finding NEC 795.09
    other site 795.1
  peritoneal fluid 792.9
  phonocardiogram 794.39
  phosphorus 275.3
  pleural fluid 792.9
  pneumoencephalogram 793.0
  PO_2-oxygen ratio 790.91
  poikilocytosis 790.09
  potassium
    deficiency 276.8
    excess 276.7
  PPD 795.5
  prostate specific antigen (PSA) 790.93
  protein, serum NEC 790.99
  proteinuria 791.0
  prothrombin time (prolonged) (partial)
    (PT) (PTT) 790.92
  pyuria 791.9
  radiologic (x-ray) 793.9
    abdomen 793.6
    biliary tract 793.3
    breast 793.89
      abnormal mammogram NOS
        793.80
      mammographic microcalcification
        793.81
    gastrointestinal tract 793.4
    genitourinary organs 793.5
    head 793.0
    intrathoracic organs NEC 793.2
    lung 793.1
    musculoskeletal 793.7
    placenta 793.9
    retroperitoneum 793.6
    skin 793.9
    skull 793.0
    subcutaneous tissue 793.9
  red blood cell 790.09
    count 790.09
    morphology 790.09
    sickling 790.09
    volume 790.09
  saliva 792.4
  scan NEC 794.9
    bladder 794.9
    bone 794.9
    brain 794.09
    kidney 794.4
    liver 794.8
    lung 794.2
    pancreas 794.9
    placental 794.9
    spleen 794.9
    thyroid 794.5
  sedimentation rate, elevated 790.1
  semen 792.2
  serological (for)
    human immunodeficiency virus (HIV)
      inconclusive 795.71
      positive V08
    syphilis - *see* Findings, serology for
      syphilis
  serology for syphilis
    false positive 795.6
    positive 097.1
      false 795.6
      follow-up of latent syphilis - *see*
        Syphilis, latent
      only finding - *see* Syphilis, latent

Findings, abnormal, without diagnosis
  (Continued)
  serum 790.99
    blood NEC 790.99
    enzymes NEC 790.5
    proteins 790.99
  SGOT 790.4
  SGPT 790.4
  sickling of red blood cells 790.09
  skin test, positive 795.79
    tuberculin (without active tuberculo-
      sis) 795.5
  sodium 790.6
    deficiency 276.1
    excess 276.0
  spermatozoa 792.2
  spinal fluid 792.0
    culture, positive 792.0
  sputum culture, positive 795.39
    for acid-fast bacilli 795.39
  stool NEC 792.1
    bloody 578.1
      occult 792.1
    color 792.1
    culture, positive 792.1
    occult blood 792.1
  stress test 794.39
  structure, body (echogram) (thermogram)
    (ultrasound) (x-ray) NEC 793.9
    abdomen 793.6
    breast 793.89
      abnormal mammogram NOS 793.80
      mammographic microcalcification
        793.81
    gastrointestinal tract 793.4
    genitourinary organs 793.5
    head 793.0
      echogram (ultrasound) 794.01
    intrathoracic organs NEC 793.2
    lung 793.1
    musculoskeletal 793.7
    placenta 793.9
    retroperitoneum 793.6
    skin 793.9
    subcutaneous tissue NEC 793.9
  synovial fluid 792.9
  thermogram - *see* Findings, abnormal,
    structure
  throat culture, positive 795.39
  thyroid (function) 794.5
    metabolism (rate) 794.5
    scan 794.5
    uptake 794.5
  total proteins 790.99
  toxicology (drugs) (heavy metals) 796.0
  transaminase (level) 790.4
  triglycerides 272.9
  tuberculin skin test (without active tu-
    berculosis) 795.5
  ultrasound - *see also* Findings, abnor-
    mal, structure
    cardiogram 793.2
  uric acid, blood 790.6
  urine, urinary constituents 791.9
    acetone 791.6
    albumin 791.0
    bacteria 791.9
    bile 791.4
    blood 599.7
    casts or cells 791.7
    chyle 791.1
    culture, positive 791.9
    glucose 791.5
    hemoglobin 791.2
    ketone 791.6
    protein 791.0

ICD-9-CM

Vol. 2

Findings, abnormal, without diagnosis
(*Continued*)
  urine, urinary constitutents (*Continued*)
    pus 791.9
    sugar 791.5
  vaginal fluid 792.9
  vanillylmandelic acid, elevated 791.9
  vectorcardiogram (VCG) 794.39
  ventriculogram (cerebral) 793.0
  VMA, elevated 791.9
  Wassermann reaction
    false positive 795.6
    positive 097.1
      follow-up of latent syphilis - *see*
        Syphilis, latent
      only finding - *see* Syphilis, latent
  white blood cell 288.9
    count 288.9
      elevated 288.8
      low 288.0
    differential 288.9
    morphology 288.9
  wound culture 795.39
  xerography 793.89
  zinc, blood 790.6
Finger - *see* condition
Fire, St. Anthony's (*see also* Erysipelas) 035
Fish
  hook stomach 537.89
  meal workers' lung 495.8
Fisher's syndrome 357.0
Fissure, fissured
  abdominal wall (congenital) 756.79
  anus, anal 565.0
    congenital 751.5
  buccal cavity 528.9
  clitoris (congenital) 752.49
  ear, lobule (congenital) 744.29
  epiglottis (congenital) 748.3
  larynx 478.79
    congenital 748.3
  lip 528.5
    congenital (*see also* Cleft, lip) 749.10
  nipple 611.2
    puerperal, postpartum 676.1
  palate (congenital) (*see also* Cleft, palate) 749.00
  postanal 565.0
  rectum 565.0
  skin 709.8
    streptococcal 686.9
  spine (congenital) (*see also* Spina bifida) 741.9
  sternum (congenital) 756.3
  tongue (acquired) 529.5
    congenital 750.13
Fistula (sinus) 686.9
  abdomen (wall) 569.81
    bladder 596.2
    intestine 569.81
    ureter 593.82
    uterus 619.2
  abdominorectal 569.81
  abdominosigmoidal 569.81
  abdominothoracic 510.0
  abdominouterine 619.2
    congenital 752.3
  abdominovesical 596.2
  accessory sinuses (*see also* Sinusitis) 473.9
  actinomycotic - *see* Actinomycosis
  alveolar
    antrum (*see also* Sinusitis, maxillary) 473.0
    process 522.7
  anorectal 565.1

Fistula (*Continued*)
  antrobuccal (*see also* Sinusitis, maxillary) 473.0
  antrum (*see also* Sinusitis, maxillary) 473.0
  anus, anal (infectional) (recurrent) 565.1
    congenital 751.5
    tuberculous (*see also* Tuberculosis) 014.8
  aortic sinus 747.29
  aortoduodenal 447.2
  appendix, appendicular 543.9
  arteriovenous (acquired) 447.0
    brain 437.3
      congenital 747.81
        ruptured (*see also* Hemorrhage, subarachnoid) 430
      ruptured (*see also* Hemorrhage, subarachnoid) 430
    cerebral 437.3
      congenital 747.81
    congenital (peripheral) 747.60
      brain - *see* Fistula, arteriovenous, brain, congenital
      coronary 746.85
      gastrointestinal 747.61
      lower limb 747.64
      pulmonary 747.3
      renal 747.62
      specified site NEC 747.69
      upper limb 747.63
    coronary 414.19
      congenital 746.85
    heart 414.19
    pulmonary (vessels) 417.0
      congenital 747.3
    surgically created (for dialysis) V45.1
      complication NEC 996.73
        atherosclerosis - *see* Arteriosclerosis, extremities
        embolism 996.74
        infection or inflammation 996.62
        mechanical 996.1
        occlusion NEC 996.74
        thrombus 996.74
      traumatic - *see* Injury, blood vessel, by site
  artery 447.2
  aural 383.81
    congenital 744.49
  auricle 383.81
    congenital 744.49
  Bartholin's gland 619.8
  bile duct (*see also* Fistula, biliary) 576.4
  biliary (duct) (tract) 576.4
    congenital 751.69
  bladder (neck) (sphincter) 596.2
    into seminal vesicle 596.2
  bone 733.99
  brain 348.8
    arteriovenous - *see* Fistula, arteriovenous, brain
  branchial (cleft) 744.41
  branchiogenous 744.41
  breast 611.0
    puerperal, postpartum 675.1
  bronchial 510.0
  bronchocutaneous, bronchomediastinal, bronchopleural, bronchopleuromediastinal (infective) 510.0
  tuberculous (*see also* Tuberculosis) 011.3
  bronchoesophageal 530.84
    congenital 750.3

Fistula (*Continued*)
  buccal cavity (infective) 528.3
  canal, ear 380.89
  carotid-cavernous
    congenital 747.81
      with hemorrhage 430
    traumatic 900.82
      with hemorrhage (*see also* Hemorrhage, brain, traumatic) 853.0
      late effect 908.3
  cecosigmoidal 569.81
  cecum 569.81
  cerebrospinal (fluid) 349.81
  cervical, lateral (congenital) 744.41
  cervicoaural (congenital) 744.49
  cervicosigmoidal 619.1
  cervicovesical 619.0
  cervix 619.8
  chest (wall) 510.0
  cholecystocolic (*see also* Fistula, gallbladder) 575.5
  cholecystocolonic (*see also* Fistula, gallbladder) 575.5
  cholecystoduodenal (*see also* Fistula, gallbladder) 575.5
  cholecystoenteric (*see also* Fistula, gallbladder) 575.5
  cholecystogastric (*see also* Fistula, gallbladder) 575.5
  cholecystointestinal (*see also* Fistula, gallbladder) 575.5
  choledochoduodenal 576.4
  cholocolic (*see also* Fistula, gallbladder) 575.5
  coccyx 685.1
    with abscess 685.0
  colon 569.81
  colostomy 569.69
  colovaginal (acquired) 619.1
  common duct (bile duct) 576.4
  congenital, NEC - *see* Anomaly, specified type NEC
  cornea, causing hypotony 360.32
  coronary, arteriovenous 414.19
    congenital 746.85
  costal region 510.0
  cul-de-sac, Douglas' 619.8
  cutaneous 686.9
  cystic duct (*see also* Fistula, gallbladder) 575.5
    congenital 751.69
  dental 522.7
  diaphragm 510.0
    bronchovisceral 510.0
    pleuroperitoneal 510.0
    pulmonoperitoneal 510.0
  duodenum 537.4
  ear (canal) (external) 380.89
  enterocolic 569.81
  enterocutaneous 569.81
  enteroenteric 569.81
  entero-uterine 619.1
    congenital 752.3
  enterovaginal 619.1
    congenital 752.49
  enterovesical 596.1
  epididymis 608.89
    tuberculous (*see also* Tuberculosis) 016.4
  esophagobronchial 530.89
    congenital 750.3
  esophagocutaneous 530.89
  esophagopleurocutaneous 530.89

Fistula (*Continued*)
  esophagotracheal 530.84
    congenital 750.3
  esophagus 530.89
    congenital 750.4
  ethmoid (*see also* Sinusitis, ethmoidal)
    473.2
  eyeball (cornea) (sclera) 360.32
  eyelid 373.11
  fallopian tube (external) 619.2
  fecal 569.81
    congenital 751.5
  from periapical lesion 522.7
  frontal sinus (*see also* Sinusitis, frontal)
    473.1
  gallbladder 575.5
    with calculus, cholelithiasis, stones
      (*see also* Cholelithiasis)
      574.2
    congenital 751.69
  gastric 537.4
  gastrocolic 537.4
    congenital 750.7
    tuberculous (*see also* Tuberculosis)
      014.8
  gastroenterocolic 537.4
  gastroesophageal 537.4
  gastrojejunal 537.4
  gastrojejunocolic 537.4
  genital
    organs
      female 619.9
        specified site NEC 619.8
      male 608.89
    tract-skin (female) 619.2
  hepatopleural 510.0
  hepatopulmonary 510.0
  horseshoe 565.1
  ileorectal 569.81
  ileosigmoidal 569.81
  ileostomy 569.69
  ileovesical 596.1
  ileum 569.81
  in ano 565.1
    tuberculous (*see also* Tuberculosis)
      014.8
  inner ear (*see also* Fistula, labyrinth)
    386.40
  intestine 569.81
  intestinocolonic (abdominal) 569.81
  intestinoureteral 593.82
  intestinouterine 619.1
  intestinovaginal 619.1
    congenital 752.49
  intestinovesical 596.1
  involving female genital tract 619.9
    digestive-genital 619.1
    genital tract-skin 619.2
    specified site NEC 619.8
    urinary-genital 619.0
  ischiorectal (fossa) 566
  jejunostomy 569.69
  jejunum 569.81
  joint 719.80
    ankle 719.87
    elbow 719.82
    foot 719.87
    hand 719.84
    hip 719.85
    knee 719.86
    multiple sites 719.89
    pelvic region 719.85
    shoulder (region) 719.81
    specified site NEC 719.88

Fistula (*Continued*)
  joint (*Continued*)
    tuberculous - *see* Tuberculosis, joint
    wrist 719.83
  kidney 593.89
  labium (majus) (minus) 619.8
  labyrinth, labyrinthine NEC 386.40
    combined sites 386.48
    multiple sites 386.48
    oval window 386.42
    round window 386.41
    semicircular canal 386.43
  lacrimal, lachrymal (duct) (gland) (sac)
    375.61
  lacrimonasal duct 375.61
  laryngotracheal 748.3
  larynx 478.79
  lip 528.5
    congenital 750.25
  lumbar, tuberculous (*see also* Tuberculosis) 015.0 [730.8]
  lung 510.0
  lymphatic (node) (vessel) 457.8
  mamillary 611.0
  mammary (gland) 611.0
    puerperal, postpartum 675.1
  mastoid (process) (region) 383.1
  maxillary (*see also* Sinusitis, maxillary)
    473.0
  mediastinal 510.0
  mediastinobronchial 510.0
  mediastinocutaneous 510.0
  middle ear 385.89
  mouth 528.3
  nasal 478.1
    sinus (*see also* Sinusitis) 473.9
  nasopharynx 478.29
  nipple - *see* Fistula, breast
  nose 478.1
  oral (cutaneous) 528.3
    maxillary (*see also* Sinusitis, maxillary) 473.0
    nasal (with cleft palate) (*see also* Cleft, palate) 749.00
  orbit, orbital 376.10
  oro-antral (*see also* Sinusitis, maxillary)
    473.0
  oval window (internal ear) 386.42
  oviduct (external) 619.2
  palate (hard) 526.89
    soft 528.9
  pancreatic 577.8
  pancreaticoduodenal 577.8
  parotid (gland) 527.4
    region 528.3
  pelvoabdominointestinal 569.81
  penis 607.89
  perianal 565.1
  pericardium (pleura) (sac) (*see also* Pericarditis) 423.8
  pericecal 569.81
  perineal - *see* Fistula, perineum
  perineorectal 569.81
  perineosigmoidal 569.81
  perineo-urethroscrotal 608.89
  perineum, perineal (with urethral involvement) NEC 599.1
    tuberculous (*see also* Tuberculosis)
      017.9
    ureter 593.82
  perirectal 565.1
    tuberculous (*see also* Tuberculosis)
      014.8
  peritoneum (*see also* Peritonitis) 567.2

Fistula (*Continued*)
  periurethral 599.1
  pharyngo-esophageal 478.29
  pharynx 478.29
    branchial cleft (congenital) 744.41
  pilonidal (infected) (rectum) 685.1
    with abscess 685.0
  pleura, pleural, pleurocutaneous, pleuroperitoneal 510.0
    stomach 510.0
    tuberculous (*see also* Tuberculosis)
      012.0
  pleuropericardial 423.8
  postauricular 383.81
  postoperative, persistent 998.6
  preauricular (congenital) 744.46
  prostate 602.8
  pulmonary 510.0
    arteriovenous 417.0
      congenital 747.3
    tuberculous (*see also* Tuberculosis, pulmonary) 011.9
  pulmonoperitoneal 510.0
  rectolabial 619.1
  rectosigmoid (intercommunicating)
    569.81
  rectoureteral 593.82
  rectourethral 599.1
    congenital 753.8
  rectouterine 619.1
    congenital 752.3
  rectovaginal 619.1
    congenital 752.49
    old, postpartal 619.1
    tuberculous (*see also* Tuberculosis)
      014.8
  rectovesical 596.1
    congenital 753.8
  rectovesicovaginal 619.1
  rectovulvar 619.1
    congenital 752.49
  rectum (to skin) 565.1
    tuberculous (*see also* Tuberculosis)
      014.8
  renal 593.89
  retroauricular 383.81
  round window (internal ear) 386.41
  salivary duct or gland 527.4
    congenital 750.24
  sclera 360.32
  scrotum (urinary) 608.89
    tuberculous (*see also* Tuberculosis)
      016.5
  semicircular canals (internal ear) 386.43
  sigmoid 569.81
    vesicoabdominal 596.1
  sigmoidovaginal 619.1
    congenital 752.49
  skin 686.9
    ureter 593.82
    vagina 619.2
  sphenoidal sinus (*see also* Sinusitis, sphenoidal) 473.3
  splenocolic 289.59
  stercoral 569.81
  stomach 537.4
  sublingual gland 527.4
    congenital 750.24
  submaxillary
    gland 527.4
      congenital 750.24
    region 528.3
  thoracic 510.0
    duct 457.8

ICD-9-CM

Vol.

Fistula (Continued)
thoracicoabdominal 510.0
thoracicogastric 510.0
thoracicointestinal 510.0
thoracoabdominal 510.0
thoracogastric 510.0
thorax 510.0
thyroglossal duct 759.2
thyroid 246.8
trachea (congenital) (external) (internal) 748.3
tracheoesophageal 530.84
 congenital 750.3
 following tracheostomy 519.09
traumatic
 arteriovenous (see also Injury, blood vessel, by site) 904.9
 brain - see Injury, intracranial
tuberculous - see Tuberculosis, by site
typhoid 002.0
umbilical 759.89
umbilico-urinary 753.8
urachal, urachus 753.7
ureter (persistent) 593.82
ureteroabdominal 593.82
ureterocervical 593.82
ureterorectal 593.82
ureterosigmoido-abdominal 593.82
ureterovaginal 619.0
ureterovesical 596.2
urethra 599.1
 congenital 753.8
 tuberculous (see also Tuberculosis) 016.3
urethroperineal 599.1
urethroperineovesical 596.2
urethrorectal 599.1
 congenital 753.8
urethroscrotal 608.89
urethrovaginal 619.0
urethrovesical 596.2
urethrovesicovaginal 619.0
urinary (persistent) (recurrent) 599.1
uteroabdominal (anterior wall) 619.2
 congenital 752.3
uteroenteric 619.1
uterofecal 619.1
uterointestinal 619.1
 congenital 752.3
uterorectal 619.1
 congenital 752.3
uteroureteric 619.0
uterovaginal 619.8
uterovesical 619.0
 congenital 752.3
uterus 619.8
vagina (wall) 619.8
 postpartal, old 619.8
vaginocutaneous (postpartal) 619.2
vaginoileal (acquired) 619.1
vaginoperineal 619.2
vesical NEC 596.2
vesicoabdominal 596.2
vesicocervicovaginal 619.0
vesicocolic 596.1
vesicocutaneous 596.2
vesicoenteric 596.1
vesicointestinal 596.1
vesicometrorectal 619.1
vesicoperineal 596.2
vesicorectal 596.1
 congenital 753.8
vesicosigmoidal 596.1
vesicosigmoidovaginal 619.1
vesicoureteral 596.2

Fistula (Continued)
vesicoureterovaginal 619.0
vesicourethral 596.2
vesicourethrorectal 596.1
vesicouterine 619.0
 congenital 752.3
vesicovaginal 619.0
vulvorectal 619.1
 congenital 752.49
Fit 780.39
apoplectic (see also Disease, cerebrovascular, acute) 436
 late effect - see Late effect(s) (of) cerebrovascular disease
epileptic (see also Epilepsy) 345.9
fainting 780.2
hysterical 300.11
newborn 779.0
Fitting (of)
artificial
 arm (complete) (partial) V52.0
 breast V52.4
 eye(s) V52.2
 leg(s) (complete) (partial) V52.1
brain neuropacemaker V53.02
cardiac pacemaker V53.31
carotid sinus pacemaker V53.39
cerebral ventricle (communicating) shunt V53.01
colostomy belt V53.5
contact lenses V53.1
cystostomy device V53.6
defibrillator, automatic implantable cardiac V53.32
dentures V52.3
device, unspecified type V53.90
 abdominal V53.5
 cardiac
  defibrillator, automatic implantable V53.32
  pacemaker V53.31
  specified NEC V53.39
 cerebral ventricle (communicating) shunt V53.01
 insulin pump V53.91
 intrauterine contraceptive V25.1
 nervous system V53.09
 orthodontic V53.4
 orthoptic V53.1
 other device V53.99
 prosthetic V52.9
  breast V52.4
  dental V52.3
  eye V52.2
  specified type NEC V52.8
 special senses V53.09
 substitution
  auditory V53.09
  nervous system V53.09
  visual V53.09
 urinary V53.6
diaphragm (contraceptive) V25.02
glasses (reading) V53.1
growth rod V54.02
hearing aid V53.2
ileostomy device V55.2
intestinal appliance or device NEC V53.5
intrauterine contraceptive device V25.1
neuropacemaker (brain) (peripheral nerve) (spinal cord) V53.02
orthodontic device V53.4
orthopedic (device) V53.7
 brace V53.7
 cast V53.7
 corset V53.7
 shoes V53.7

Fitting (Continued)
pacemaker (cardiac) V53.31
 brain V53.02
 carotid sinus V53.39
 peripheral nerve V53.02
 spinal cord V53.02
prosthesis V52.9
 arm (complete) (partial) V52.0
 breast V52.4
 dental V52.3
 eye V52.2
 leg (complete) (partial) V52.1
 specified type NEC V52.8
spectacles V53.1
wheelchair V53.8
Fitz's syndrome (acute hemorrhagic pancreatitis) 577.0
Fitz-Hugh and Curtis syndrome 098.86
due to:
 Chlamydia trachomatis 099.56
 Neisseria gonorrhoeae (gonococcal peritonitis) 098.86
Fixation
joint - see Ankylosis
larynx 478.79
pupil 364.76
stapes 385.22
 deafness (see also Deafness, conductive) 389.04
uterus (acquired) - see Malposition, uterus
vocal cord 478.5
Flaccid - see also condition
foot 736.79
forearm 736.09
palate, congenital 750.26
Flail
chest 807.4
 newborn 767.3
joint (paralytic) 718.80
 ankle 718.87
 elbow 718.82
 foot 718.87
 hand 718.84
 hip 718.85
 knee 718.86
 multiple sites 718.89
 pelvic region 718.85
 shoulder (region) 718.81
 specified site NEC 718.88
 wrist 718.83
Flajani (-Basedow) syndrome or disease (exophthalmic goiter) 242.0
Flap, liver 572.8
Flare, anterior chamber (aqueous) (eye) 364.04
Flashback phenomena (drug) (hallucinogenic) 292.89
Flat
chamber (anterior) (eye) 360.34
chest, congenital 754.89
electroencephalogram (EEG) 348.8
foot (acquired) (fixed type) (painful) (postural) (spastic) 734
 congenital 754.61
  rocker bottom 754.61
  vertical talus 754.61
 rachitic 268.1
 rocker bottom (congenital) 754.61
 vertical talus, congenital 754.61
organ or site, congenital NEC - see Anomaly, specified type NEC
pelvis 738.6
 with disproportion (fetopelvic) 653.2
  affecting fetus or newborn 763.1
  causing obstructed labor 660.1
   affecting fetus or newborn 763.1

Flat *(Continued)*
  pelvis *(Continued)*
    congenital 755.69
Flatau-Schilder disease 341.1
Flattening
  head, femur 736.39
  hip 736.39
  lip (congenital) 744.89
  nose (congenital) 754.0
    acquired 738.0
Flatulence 787.3
Flatus 787.3
  vaginalis 629.8
Flax dressers' disease 504
Flea bite - *see* Injury, superficial, by site
Fleischer (-Kayser) ring (corneal pigmentation) 275.1 *[371.14]*
Fleischner's disease 732.3
Fleshy mole 631
Flexibilitas cerea *(see also* Catalepsy) 300.11
Flexion
  cervix *(see also* Malposition, uterus) 621.6
  contracture, joint *(see also* Contraction, joint) 718.4
  deformity, joint *(see also* Contraction, joint) 718.4
    hip, congenital *(see also* Subluxation, congenital, hip) 754.32
  uterus *(see also* Malposition, uterus) 621.6
Flexner's
  bacillus 004.1
  diarrhea (ulcerative) 004.1
  dysentery 004.1
Flexner-Boyd dysentery 004.2
Flexure - *see* condition
Floater, vitreous 379.24
Floating
  cartilage (joint) *(see also* Disorder, cartilage, articular) 718.0
    knee 717.6
  gallbladder (congenital) 751.69
  kidney 593.0
    congenital 753.3
  liver (congenital) 751.69
  rib 756.3
  spleen 289.59
Flooding 626.2
Floor - *see* condition
Floppy
  infant NEC 781.99
  valve syndrome (mitral) 424.0
Flu - *see also* Influenza
  gastric NEC 008.8
Fluctuating blood pressure 796.4
Fluid
  abdomen 789.5
  chest *(see also* Pleurisy, with effusion) 511.9
  heart *(see also* Failure, heart) 428.0
  joint *(see also* Effusion, joint) 719.0
  loss (acute) 276.5
    with
      hypernatremia 276.0
      hyponatremia 276.1
  lung - *see also* Edema, lung
    encysted 511.8
  peritoneal cavity 789.5
  pleural cavity *(see also* Pleurisy, with effusion) 511.9
  retention 276.6
Flukes NEC *(see also* Infestation, fluke) 121.9
  blood NEC *(see also* Infestation, Schistosoma) 120.9
  liver 121.3

Fluor (albus) (vaginalis) 623.5
  trichomonal (Trichomonas vaginalis) 131.00
Fluorosis (dental) (chronic) 520.3
Flushing 782.62
  menopausal 627.2
Flush syndrome 259.2
Flutter
  atrial or auricular 427.32
  heart (ventricular) 427.42
    atrial 427.32
  impure 427.32
  postoperative 997.1
  ventricular 427.42
Flux (bloody) (serosanguineous) 009.0
Focal - *see* condition
Fochier's abscess - *see* Abscess, by site
Focus, Assmann's *(see also* Tuberculosis) 011.0
Fogo selvagem 694.4
Foix-Alajouanine syndrome 336.1
Folds, anomalous - *see also* Anomaly, specified type NEC
  Bowman's membrane 371.31
  Descemet's membrane 371.32
  epicanthic 743.63
  heart 746.89
  posterior segment of eye, congenital 743.54
Folie deux 297.3
Follicle
  cervix (nabothian) (ruptured) 616.0
  graafian, ruptured, with hemorrhage 620.0
  nabothian 616.0
Folliclis (primary) *(see also* Tuberculosis) 017.0
Follicular - *see also* condition
  cyst (atretic) 620.0
Folliculitis 704.8
  abscedens et suffodiens 704.8
  decalvans 704.09
  gonorrheal (acute) 098.0
    chronic or duration of 2 months or more 098.2
  keloid, keloidalis 706.1
  pustular 704.8
  ulerythematosa reticulata 701.8
Folliculosis, conjunctival 372.02
Foølling's disease (phenylketonuria) 270.1
Follow-up (examination) (routine) (following) V67.9
  cancer chemotherapy V67.2
  chemotherapy V67.2
  fracture V67.4
  high-risk medication V67.51
  injury NEC V67.59
  postpartum
    immediately after delivery V24.0
    routine V24.2
  psychiatric V67.3
  psychotherapy V67.3
  radiotherapy V67.1
  specified condition NEC V67.59
  specified surgery NEC V67.09
  surgery V67.00
    vaginal pap smear V67.01
  treatment V67.9
    combined NEC V67.6
    fracture V67.4
    involving high-risk medication NEC V67.51
    mental disorder V67.3
    specified NEC V67.59

Fong's syndrome (hereditary osteoonychodysplasia) 756.89
Food
  allergy 693.1
  anaphylactic shock - *see* Anaphylactic shock, due to food
  asphyxia (from aspiration or inhalation) *(see also* Asphyxia, food) 933.1
  choked on *(see also* Asphyxia, food) 933.1
  deprivation 994.2
    specified kind of food NEC 269.8
  intoxication *(see also* Poisoning, food) 005.9
  lack of 994.2
  poisoning *(see also* Poisoning, food) 005.9
  refusal or rejection NEC 307.59
  strangulation or suffocation *(see also* Asphyxia, food) 933.1
  toxemia *(see also* Poisoning, food) 005.9
Foot - *see also* condition
  and mouth disease 078.4
  process disease 581.3
Foramen ovale (nonclosure) (patent) (persistent) 745.5
Forbes' (glycogen storage) disease 271.0
Forbes-Albright syndrome (nonpuerperal amenorrhea and lactation associated with pituitary tumor) 253.1
Forced birth or delivery NEC 669.8
  affecting fetus or newborn NEC 763.89
Forceps
  delivery NEC 669.5
    affecting fetus or newborn 763.2
Fordyce's disease (ectopic sebaceous glands) (mouth) 750.26
Fordyce-Fox disease (apocrine miliaria) 705.82
Forearm - *see* condition
Foreign body

Note For foreign body with open wound or other injury, see Wound, open, or the type of injury specified.

  accidentally left during a procedure 998.4
  anterior chamber (eye) 871.6
    magnetic 871.5
      retained or old 360.51
    retained or old 360.61
  ciliary body (eye) 871.6
    magnetic 871.5
      retained or old 360.52
    retained or old 360.62
  entering through orifice (current) (old)
    accessory sinus 932
    air passage (upper) 933.0
      lower 934.8
    alimentary canal 938
    alveolar process 935.0
    antrum (Highmore) 932
    anus 937
    appendix 936
    asphyxia due to *(see also* Asphyxia, food) 933.1
    auditory canal 931
    auricle 931
    bladder 939.0
    bronchioles 934.8
    bronchus (main) 934.1
    buccal cavity 935.0

ICD-9-CM

Vol. 2

Foreign body *(Continued)*
entering through orifice *(Continued)*
canthus (inner) 930.1
cecum 936
cervix (canal) uterine 939.1
coil, ileocecal 936
colon 936
conjunctiva 930.1
conjunctival sac 930.1
cornea 930.0
digestive organ or tract NEC 938
duodenum 936
ear (external) 931
esophagus 935.1
eye (external) 930.9
combined sites 930.8
intraocular - *see* Foreign body, by site
specified site NEC 930.8
eyeball 930.8
intraocular - *see* Foreign body, intraocular
eyelid 930.1
retained or old 374.86
frontal sinus 932
gastrointestinal tract 938
genitourinary tract 939.9
globe 930.8
penetrating 871.6
magnetic 871.5
retained or old 360.50
retained or old 360.60
gum 935.0
Highmore's antrum 932
hypopharynx 933.0
ileocecal coil 936
ileum 936
inspiration (of) 933.1
intestine (large) (small) 936
lacrimal apparatus, duct, gland, or sac 930.2
larynx 933.1
lung 934.8
maxillary sinus 932
mouth 935.0
nasal sinus 932
nasopharynx 933.0
nose (passage) 932
nostril 932
oral cavity 935.0
palate 935.0
penis 939.3
pharynx 933.0
pyriform sinus 933.0
rectosigmoid 937
junction 937
rectum 937
respiratory tract 934.9
specified part NEC 934.8
sclera 930.1
sinus 932
accessory 932
frontal 932
maxillary 932
nasal 932
pyriform 933.0
small intestine 936
stomach (hairball) 935.2
suffocation by (*see also* Asphyxia, food) 933.1
swallowed 938
tongue 933.0
tear ducts or glands 930.2
throat 933.0

Foreign body *(Continued)*
entering through orifice *(Continued)*
tongue 935.0
swallowed 933.0
tonsil, tonsillar 933.0
fossa 933.0
trachea 934.0
ureter 939.0
urethra 939.0
uterus (any part) 939.1
vagina 939.2
vulva 939.2
wind pipe 934.0
granuloma (old) 728.82
bone 733.99
in operative wound (inadvertently left) 998.4
due to surgical material intentionally left - *see* Complications, due to (presence of) any device, implant, or graft classified to 996.0-996.5 NEC
muscle 728.82
skin 709.4
soft tissue NEC 709.4
subcutaneous tissue 709.4
in
bone (residual) 733.99
open wound - *see* Wound, open, by site complicated
soft tissue (residual) 729.6
inadvertently left in operation wound (causing adhesions, obstruction, or perforation) 998.4
ingestion, ingested NEC 938
inhalation or inspiration (*see also* Asphyxia, food) 933.1
internal organ, not entering through an orifice - *see* Injury, internal, by site, with open wound
intraocular (nonmagnetic) 871.6
combined sites 871.6
magnetic 871.5
retained or old 360.59
retained or old 360.69
magnetic 871.5
retained or old 360.50
retained or old 360.60
specified site NEC 871.6
magnetic 871.5
retained or old 360.59
retained or old 360.69
iris (nonmagnetic) 871.6
magnetic 871.5
retained or old 360.52
retained or old 360.62
lens (nonmagnetic) 871.6
magnetic 871.5
retained or old 360.53
retained or old 360.63
lid, eye 930.1
ocular muscle 870.4
retained or old 376.6
old or residual
bone 733.99
eyelid 374.86
middle ear 385.83
muscle 729.6
ocular 376.6
retrobulbar 376.6
skin 729.6
with granuloma 709.4
soft tissue 729.6
with granuloma 709.4

Foreign body *(Continued)*
old or residual *(Continued)*
subcutaneous tissue 729.6
with granuloma 709.4
operation wound, left accidentally 998.4
orbit 870.4
retained or old 376.6
posterior wall, eye 871.6
magnetic 871.5
retained or old 360.55
retained or old 360.65
respiratory tree 934.9
specified site NEC 934.8
retained (old) (nonmagnetic) (in)
anterior chamber (eye) 360.61
magnetic 360.51
ciliary body 360.62
magnetic 360.52
eyelid 374.86
globe 360.60
magnetic 360.50
intraocular 360.60
magnetic 360.50
specified site NEC 360.69
magnetic 360.59
iris 360.62
magnetic 360.52
lens 360.63
magnetic 360.53
muscle 729.6
orbit 376.6
posterior wall of globe 360.65
magnetic 360.55
retina 360.65
magnetic 360.55
retrobulbar 376.6
skin 729.6
with granuloma 709.4
soft tissue 729.6
with granuloma 709.4
subcutaneous tissue 729.6
with granuloma 709.4
vitreous 360.64
magnetic 360.54
retina 871.6
magnetic 871.5
retained or old 360.55
retained or old 360.65
superficial, without major open wound (*see also* Injury, superficial, by site) 919.6
swallowed NEC 938
vitreous (humor) 871.6
magnetic 871.5
retained or old 360.54
retained or old 360.64
Forking, aqueduct of Sylvius 742.3
with spina bifida (*see also* Spina bifida) 741.0
Formation
bone in scar tissue (skin) 709.3
connective tissue in vitreous 379.25
Elschnig pearls (postcataract extraction) 366.51
hyaline in cornea 371.49
sequestrum in bone (due to infection) (*see also* Osteomyelitis) 730.1
valve
colon, congenital 751.5
ureter (congenital) 753.29
Formication 782.0
Fort Bragg fever 100.89
Fossa - *see also* condition
pyriform - *see* condition

◀ **New**   ◀▥ **Revised**

Foster-Kennedy syndrome 377.04

Fothergill's

disease, meaning scarlatina anginosa 034.1

neuralgia (*see also* Neuralgia, trigeminal) 350.1

Foul breath 784.9

Found dead (cause unknown) 798.9

Foundling V20.0

Fournier's disease (idiopathic gangrene) 608.83

Fourth

cranial nerve - *see* condition

disease 057.8

molar 520.1

Foville's syndrome 344.89

Fox's

disease (apocrine miliaria) 705.82

impetigo (contagiosa) 684

Fox-Fordyce disease (apocrine miliaria) 705.82

Fracture (abduction) (adduction) (avulsion) (compression) (crush) (dislocation) (oblique) (separation) (closed) 829.0

Note For fracture of any of the following sites with fracture of other bones, *see* Fracture, multiple.

"Closed" includes the following descriptions of fractures, with or without delayed healing, unless they are specified as open or compound:

comminuted
depressed
elevated
fissured
greenstick
impacted
linear
simple
slipped epiphysis
spiral
unspecified

"Open" includes the following descriptions of fractures, with or without delayed healing:

compound
infected
missile
puncture
with foreign body

For late effect of fracture, *see* Late, effect, fracture, by site.

---

with

internal injuries in same region (conditions classifiable to 860-869) - *see also* Injury, internal, by site

pelvic region - *see* Fracture, pelvis

acetabulum (with visceral injury) (closed) 808.0

open 808.1

acromion (process) (closed) 811.01

open 811.11

alveolus (closed) 802.8

open 802.9

ankle (malleolus) (closed) 824.8

bimalleolar (Dupuytren's) (Pott's) 824.4

open 824.5

Fracture (*Continued*)

ankle (*Continued*)

bone 825.21

open 825.31

lateral malleolus only (fibular) 824.2

open 824.3

medial malleolus only (tibial) 824.0

open 824.1

open 824.9

pathologic 733.16

talus 825.21

open 825.31

trimalleolar 824.6

open 824.7

antrum - *see* Fracture, skull, base

arm (closed) 818.0

and leg(s) (any bones) 828.0

open 828.1

both (any bones) (with rib(s)) (with sternum) 819.0

open 819.1

lower 813.80

open 813.90

open 818.1

upper - *see* Fracture, humerus

astragalus (closed) 825.21

open 825.31

atlas - *see* Fracture, vertebra, cervical, first

axis - *see* Fracture, vertebra, cervical, second

back - *see* Fracture, vertebra, by site

Barton's - *see* Fracture, radius, lower end

basal (skull) - *see* Fracture, skull, base

Bennett's (closed) 815.01

open 815.11

bimalleolar (closed) 824.4

open 824.5

bone (closed) NEC 829.0

birth injury NEC 767.3

open 829.1

pathological NEC (*see also* Fracture, pathologic) 733.10

stress NEC (*see also* Fracture, stress) 733.95

boot top - *see* Fracture, fibula

boxers' - *see* Fracture, metacarpal bone(s)

breast bone - *see* Fracture, sternum

bucket handle (semilunar cartilage) - *see* Tear, meniscus

bursting - *see* Fracture, phalanx, hand, distal

calcaneus (closed) 825.0

open 825.1

capitate (bone) (closed) 814.07

open 814.17

capitellum (humerus) (closed) 812.49

open 812.59

carpal bone(s) (wrist NEC) (closed) 814.00

open 814.10

specified site NEC 814.09

open 814.19

cartilage, knee (semilunar) - *see* Tear, meniscus

cervical - *see* Fracture, vertebra, cervical

chauffeur's - *see* Fracture, ulna, lower end

chisel - *see* Fracture, radius, upper end

clavicle (interligamentous part) (closed) 810.00

acromial end 810.03

open 810.13

Fracture (*Continued*)

clavicle (*Continued*)

due to birth trauma 767.2

open 810.10

shaft (middle third) 810.02

open 810.12

sternal end 810.01

open 810.11

clayshovelers' - *see* Fracture, vertebra, cervical

coccyx - *see also* Fracture, vertebra, coccyx

complicating delivery 665.6

collar bone - *see* Fracture, clavicle

Colles' (reversed) (closed) 813.41

open 813.51

comminuted - *see* Fracture, by site

compression - *see also* Fracture, by site

nontraumatic - *see* Fracture, pathologic

congenital 756.9

coracoid process (closed) 811.02

open 811.12

coronoid process (ulna) (closed) 813.02

mandible (closed) 802.23

open 802.33

open 813.12

corpus cavernosum penis 959.13

costochondral junction - *see* Fracture, rib

costosternal junction - *see* Fracture, rib

cranium - *see* Fracture, skull, by site

cricoid cartilage (closed) 807.5

open 807.6

cuboid (ankle) (closed) 825.23

open 825.33

cuneiform

foot (closed) 825.24

open 825.34

wrist (closed) 814.03

open 814.13

due to

birth injury - *see* Birth injury, fracture

gunshot - *see* Fracture, by site, open

neoplasm - *see* Fracture, pathologic

osteoporosis - *see* Fracture, pathologic

Dupuytren's (ankle) (fibula) (closed) 824.4

open 824.5

radius 813.42

open 813.52

Duverney's - *see* Fracture, ilium

elbow - *see also* Fracture, humerus, lower end

olecranon (process) (closed) 813.01

open 813.11

supracondylar (closed) 812.41

open 812.51

ethmoid (bone) (sinus) - *see* Fracture, skull, base

face bone(s) (closed) NEC 802.8

with

other bone(s) - *see* Fracture, multiple, skull

skull - *see also* Fracture, skull

involving other bones - *see* Fracture, multiple, skull

open 802.9

fatigue - *see* Fracture, march

femur, femoral (closed) 821.00

cervicotrochanteric 820.03

open 820.13

condyles, epicondyles 821.21

open 821.31

distal end - *see* Fracture, femur, lower end

ICD-9-CM

F

Vol. 2

Fracture *(Continued)*
femur, femoral *(Continued)*
  epiphysis (separation)
    capital 820.01
      open 820.11
    head 820.01
      open 820.11
    lower 821.22
      open 821.32
    trochanteric 820.01
      open 820.11
    upper 820.01
      open 820.11
  head 820.09
    open 820.19
  lower end or extremity (distal end)
    (closed) 821.20
    condyles, epicondyles 821.21
      open 821.31
    epiphysis (separation) 821.22
      open 821.32
    multiple sites 821.29
      open 821.39
    open 821.30
    specified site NEC 821.29
      open 821.39
    supracondylar 821.23
      open 821.33
    T-shaped 821.21
      open 821.31
  neck (closed) 820.8
    base (cervicotrochanteric) 820.03
      open 820.13
    extracapsular 820.20
      open 820.30
    intertrochanteric (section)
        820.21
      open 820.31
    intracapsular 820.00
      open 820.10
    intratrochanteric 820.21
      open 820.31
    midcervical 820.02
      open 820.12
    open 820.9
    pathologic 733.14
      specified part NEC 733.15
    specified site NEC 820.09
      open 820.19
    transcervical 820.02
      open 820.12
    transtrochanteric 820.20
      open 820.30
  open 821.10
  pathologic 733.14
    specified part NEC 733.15
  peritrochanteric (section) 820.20
    open 820.30
  shaft (lower third) (middle third)
      (upper third) 821.01
    open 821.11
  subcapital 820.09
    open 820.19
  subtrochanteric (region) (section)
      820.22
    open 820.32
  supracondylar 821.23
    open 821.33
  transepiphyseal 820.01
    open 820.11
  trochanter (greater) (lesser) (*see also*
      Fracture, femur, neck, by site)
      820.20
    open 820.30

Fracture *(Continued)*
femur, femoral *(Continued)*
  T-shaped, into knee joint 821.21
    open 821.31
  upper end 820.8
    open 820.9
fibula (closed) 823.81
  with tibia 823.82
    open 823.92
  distal end 824.8
    open 824.9
  epiphysis
    lower 824.8
      open 824.9
    upper - *see* Fracture, fibula, upper
      end
  head - *see* Fracture, fibula, upper end
  involving ankle 824.2
    open 824.3
  lower end or extremity 824.8
    open 824.9
  malleolus (external) (lateral) 824.2
    open 824.3
  open NEC 823.91
  pathologic 733.16
  proximal end - *see* Fracture, fibula,
    upper end
  shaft 823.21
    with tibia 823.22
      open 823.32
    open 823.31
  stress 733.93
  torus 823.41
    with tibia 823.42
  upper end or extremity (epiphysis)
      (head) (proximal end) (styloid)
      823.01
    with tibia 823.02
      open 823.12
    open 823.11
finger(s), of one hand (closed) (*see also*
    Fracture, phalanx, hand) 816.00
  with
    metacarpal bone(s), of same hand
        817.0
      open 817.1
    thumb of same hand 816.03
      open 816.13
  open 816.10
foot, except toe(s) alone (closed) 825.20
  open 825.30
forearm (closed) NEC 813.80
  lower end (distal end) (lower epiph-
      ysis) 813.40
    open 813.50
  open 813.90
  shaft 813.20
    open 813.30
  upper end (proximal end) (upper
      epiphysis) 813.00
    open 813.10
fossa, anterior, middle, or posterior -
    see Fracture, skull, base
frontal (bone) - *see also* Fracture, skull,
    vault
  sinus - *see* Fracture, skull, base
Galeazzi's - *see* Fracture, radius, lower
    end
glenoid (cavity) (fossa) (scapula)
    (closed) 811.03
  open 811.13
Gosselin's - *see* Fracture, ankle
greenstick - *see* Fracture, by site
grenade-throwers' - *see* Fracture, hu-
    merus, shaft

Fracture *(Continued)*
gutter - *see* Fracture, skull, vault
hamate (closed) 814.08
  open 814.18
hand, one (closed) 815.00
  carpals 814.00
    open 814.10
    specified site NEC 814.09
      open 814.19
  metacarpals 815.00
    open 815.10
  multiple, bones of one hand
      817.0
    open 817.1
  open 815.10
  phalanges (*see also* Fracture, phalanx,
      hand) 816.00
    open 816.10
healing
  aftercare (*see also* - Aftercare, frac-
      ture) V54.89
  change of cast V54.89
  complications - *see* condition
  convalescence V66.4
  removal of
    cast V54.89
    fixation device
      external V54.89
      internal V54.01
heel bone (closed) 825.0
  open 825.1
hip (closed) (*see also* Fracture, femur,
    neck) 820.8
  open 820.9
  pathologic 733.14
humerus (closed) 812.20
  anatomical neck 812.02
    open 812.12
  articular process (*see also* Fracture
      humerus, condyle(s)) 812.44
    open 812.54
  capitellum 812.49
    open 812.59
  condyle(s) 812.44
    lateral (external) 812.42
      open 812.52
    medial (internal epicondyle)
        812.43
      open 812.53
    open 812.54
  distal end - *see* Fracture, humerus,
    lower end
  epiphysis
    lower (*see also* Fracture, humerus,
        condyle(s)) 812.44
      open 812.54
    upper 812.09
      open 812.19
  external condyle 812.42
    open 812.52
  great tuberosity 812.03
    open 812.13
  head 812.09
    open 812.19
  internal epicondyle 812.43
    open 812.53
  lesser tuberosity 812.09
    open 812.19
  lower end or extremity (distal end)
      (*see also* Fracture, humerus, by
      site) 812.40
  multiple sites NEC 812.49
    open 812.59
  open 812.50

◀ **New**　　　　⬅**||||** **Revised**

Fracture (*Continued*)
  humerus (*Continued*)
    lower end or extremity (*Continued*)
      specified site NEC 812.49
        open 812.59
      neck 812.01
        open 812.11
      open 812.30
      pathologic 733.11
      proximal end - *see* Fracture, humerus, upper end
      shaft 812.21
        open 812.31
      supracondylar 812.41
        open 812.51
      surgical neck 812.01
        open 812.11
      trochlea 812.49
        open 812.59
      T-shaped 812.44
        open 812.54
      tuberosity - *see* Fracture, humerus, upper end
      upper end or extremity (proximal end) (*see also* Fracture, humerus, by site) 812.00
        open 812.10
      specified site NEC 812.09
        open 812.19
  hyoid bone (closed) 807.5
    open 807.6
  hyperextension - *see* Fracture, radius, lower end
  ilium (with visceral injury) (closed) 808.41
    open 808.51
  impaction, impacted - *see* Fracture, by site
  incus - *see* Fracture, skull, base
  innominate bone (with visceral injury) (closed) 808.49
    open 808.59
  instep, of one foot (closed) 825.20
    with toe(s) of same foot 827.0
      open 827.1
    open 825.30
  internal
    ear - *see* Fracture, skull, base
    semilunar cartilage, knee - *see* Tear, meniscus, medial
  intertrochanteric - *see* Fracture, femur, neck, intertrochanteric
  ischium (with visceral injury) (closed) 808.42
    open 808.52
  jaw (bone) (lower) (closed) (*see also* Fracture, mandible) 802.20
    angle 802.25
      open 802.35
    open 802.30
    upper - *see* Fracture, maxilla
  knee
    cap (closed) 822.0
      open 822.1
    cartilage (semilunar) - *see* Tear, meniscus
  labyrinth (osseous) - *see* Fracture, skull, base
  larynx (closed) 807.5
    open 807.6
  late effect - *see* Late, effects (of), fracture
  Le Fort's - *see* Fracture, maxilla
  leg (closed) 827.0
    with rib(s) or sternum 828.0
      open 828.1

Fracture (*Continued*)
  leg (*Continued*)
    both (any bones) 828.0
      open 828.1
    lower - *see* Fracture, tibia
      open 827.1
    upper - *see* Fracture, femur
  limb
    lower (multiple) (closed) NEC 827.0
      open 827.1
    upper (multiple) (closed) NEC 818.0
      open 818.1
  long bones, due to birth trauma - *see* Birth injury, fracture
  lumbar - *see* Fracture, vertebra, lumbar
  lunate bone (closed) 814.02
    open 814.12
  malar bone (closed) 802.4
    open 802.5
  Malgaigne's (closed) 808.43
    open 808.53
  malleolus (closed) 824.8
    bimalleolar 824.4
      open 824.5
    lateral 824.2
      and medial - *see also* Fracture, malleolus, bimalleolar
        with lip of tibia - *see* Fracture, malleolus, trimalleolar
      open 824.3
    medial (closed) 824.0
      and lateral - *see also* Fracture, malleolus, bimalleolar
        with lip of tibia - *see* Fracture, malleolus, trimalleolar
      open 824.1
    open 824.9
    trimalleolar (closed) 824.6
      open 824.7
  malleus - *see* Fracture, skull, base
  malunion 733.81
  mandible (closed) 802.20
    angle 802.25
      open 802.35
    body 802.28
      alveolar border 802.27
        open 802.37
      open 802.38
      symphysis 802.26
        open 802.36
    condylar process 802.21
      open 802.31
    coronoid process 802.23
      open 802.33
    multiple sites 802.29
      open 802.39
    open 802.30
    ramus NEC 802.24
      open 802.34
    subcondylar 802.22
      open 802.32
  manubrium - *see* Fracture, sternum
  march 733.95
    fibula 733.93
    metatarsals 733.94
    tibia 733.93
  maxilla, maxillary (superior) (upper jaw) (closed) 802.4
    inferior - *see* Fracture, mandible
    open 802.5
  meniscus, knee - *see* Tear, meniscus
  metacarpus, metacarpal (bone(s)), of one hand (closed) 815.00

Fracture (*Continued*)
  metacarpus (*Continued*)
    with phalanx, phalanges, hand (finger(s)) (thumb) of same hand 817.0
      open 817.1
    base 815.02
      first metacarpal 815.01
        open 815.11
      open 815.12
      thumb 815.01
        open 815.11
    multiple sites 815.09
      open 815.19
    neck 815.04
      open 815.14
    open 815.10
    shaft 815.03
      open 815.13
  metatarsus, metatarsal (bone(s)), of one foot (closed) 825.25
    with tarsal bone(s) 825.29
      open 825.39
    open 825.35
  Monteggia's (closed) 813.03
    open 813.13
  Moore's - *see* Fracture, radius, lower end multangular bone (closed)
    larger 814.05
      open 814.15
    smaller 814.06
      open 814.16
  multiple (closed) 829.0

> Note Multiple fractures of sites classifiable to the same three- or four-digit category are coded to that category, except for sites classifiable to 810-818 or 820-827 in different limbs.
>
> Multiple fractures of sites classifiable to different fourth-digit subdivisions within the same three-digit category should be dealt with according to coding rules.
>
> Multiple fractures of sites classifiable to different three-digit categories (identifiable from the listing under "Fracture"), and of sites classifiable to 810-818 or 820-827 in different limbs should be coded according to the following list, which should be referred to in the following priority order: skull or face bones, pelvis or vertebral column, legs, arms.

ICD-9-CM

F

Vol. 2

---

    arm (multiple bones in same arm except in hand alone) (sites classifiable to 810-817 with sites classifiable to a different three-digit category in 810-817 in same arm) (closed) 818.0
      open 818.1
    arms, both or arm(s) with rib(s) or sternum (sites classifiable to 810-818 with sites classifiable to same range of categories in other limb or to 807) (closed) 819.0
      open 819.1
    bones of trunk NEC (closed) 809.0
      open 809.1
    hand, metacarpal bone(s) with phalanx or phalanges of same hand (sites classifiable to 815 with sites classifiable to 816 in same hand) (closed) 817.0
      open 817.1

Fracture (*Continued*)
  multiple (*Continued*)
    leg (multiple bones in same leg)
      (sites classifiable to 820-826 with
      sites classifiable to a different
      three-digit category in that
      range in same leg) (closed) 827.0
      open 827.1
    legs, both or leg(s) with arm(s),
      rib(s), or sternum (sites classifia-
      ble to 820-827 with sites classifi-
      able to same range of categories
      in other leg or to 807 or 810-
      819) (closed) 828.0
      open 828.1
    open 829.1
    pelvis with other bones except skull
      or face bones (sites classifiable
      to 808 with sites classifiable to
      805-807 or 810-829) (closed)
      809.0
      open 809.1
    skull, specified or unspecified bones,
      or face bone(s) with any other
      bone(s) (sites classifiable to 800-
      803 with sites classifiable to 805-
      829) (closed) 804.0

Note   Use the following fifth-digit
subclassification with categories 800,
801, 803, and 804:

  0   unspecified state of conscious-
       ness
  1   with no loss of consciousness
  2   with brief [less than one hour]
       loss of consciousness
  3   with moderate [1-24 hours]
       loss of consciousness
  4   with prolonged [more than 24
       hours] loss of consciousness
       and return to pre-existing con-
       scious level
  5   with prolonged [more than 24
       hours] loss of consciousness,
       without return to pre-existing
       conscious level

Use fifth-digit 5 to designate when a
patient is unconscious and dies before regaining consciousness, regardless of the duration of the loss of consciousness

  6   with loss of consciousness of
       unspecified duration
  9   with concussion, unspecified

---

  with
    contusion, cerebral 804.1
    epidural hemorrhage 804.2
    extradural hemorrhage 804.2
    hemorrhage (intracranial) NEC
      804.3
    intracranial injury NEC 804.4
    laceration, cerebral 804.1
    subarachnoid hemorrhage 804.2
    subdural hemorrhage 804.2
  open 804.5
    with
      contusion, cerebral 804.6
      epidural hemorrhage 804.7
      extradural hemorrhage 804.7
      hemorrhage (intracranial) NEC
        804.8

Fracture (*Continued*)
  multiple (*Continued*)
    open (*Continued*)
      with (*Continued*)
        intracranial injury NEC 804.9
        laceration, cerebral 804.6
        subarachnoid hemorrhage 804.7
        subdural hemorrhage 804.7
    vertebral column with other bones, ex-
      cept skull or face bones (sites clas-
      sifiable to 805 or 806 with sites
      classifiable to 807-808 or 810-829)
      (closed) 809.0
      open 809.1
  nasal (bone(s)) (closed) 802.0
    open 802.1
    sinus - *see* Fracture, skull, base
  navicular
    carpal (wrist) (closed) 814.01
      open 814.11
    tarsal (ankle) (closed) 825.22
      open 825.32
  neck - *see* Fracture, vertebra, cervical
  neural arch - *see* Fracture, vertebra, by
    site
  nonunion 733.82
  nose, nasal, (bone) (septum) (closed)
    802.0
    open 802.1
  occiput - *see* Fracture, skull, base
  odontoid process - *see* Fracture, verte-
    bra, cervical
  olecranon (process) (ulna) (closed)
    813.01
    open 813.11
  open 829.1
  orbit, orbital (bone) (region) (closed)
    802.8
    floor (blow-out) 802.6
      open 802.7
    open 802.9
    roof - *see* Fracture, skull, base
    specified part NEC 802.8
      open 802.9
  os
    calcis (closed) 825.0
      open 825.1
    magnum (closed) 814.07
      open 814.17
    pubis (with visceral injury) (closed)
      808.2
      open 808.3
    triquetrum (closed) 814.03
      open 814.13
  osseous
    auditory meatus - *see* Fracture, skull,
      base
    labyrinth - *see* Fracture, skull, base
  ossicles, auditory (incus) (malleus)
    (stapes) - *see* Fracture, skull, base
  osteoporotic - *see* Fracture, pathologic
  palate (closed) 802.8
    open 802.9
  paratrooper - *see* Fracture, tibia, lower
    end
  parietal bone - *see* Fracture, skull, vault
  parry - *see* Fracture, Monteggia's
  patella (closed) 822.0
    open 822.1
  pathologic (cause unknown) 733.10
    ankle 733.16
    femur (neck) 733.14
      specified NEC 733.15
    fibula 733.16
    hip 733.14

Fracture (*Continued*)
  pathologic (*Continued*)
    humerus 733.11
    radius (distal) 733.12
    specified site NEC 733.19
    tibia 733.16
    ulna 733.12
    vertebrae (collapse) 733.13
    wrist 733.12
  pedicle (of vertebral arch) - *see* Frac-
    ture, vertebra, by site
  pelvis, pelvic (bone(s)) (with visceral
    injury) (closed) 808.8
    multiple (with disruption of pelvic
      circle) 808.43
      open 808.53
    open 808.9
    rim (closed) 808.49
      open 808.59
  peritrochanteric (closed) 820.20
    open 820.30
  phalanx, phalanges, of one
    foot (closed) 826.0
      with bone(s) of same lower limb
        827.0
        open 827.1
      open 826.1
    hand (closed) 816.00
      with metacarpal bone(s) of same
        hand 817.0
        open 817.1
      distal 816.02
        open 816.12
      middle 816.01
        open 816.11
      multiple sites NEC 816.03
        open 816.13
      open 816.10
      proximal 816.01
        open 816.11
  pisiform (closed) 814.04
    open 814.14
  pond - *see* Fracture, skull, vault
  Pott's (closed) 824.4
    open 824.5
  prosthetic device, internal - *see* Com-
    plications, mechanical
  pubis (with visceral injury) (closed)
    808.2
    open 808.3
  Quervain's (closed) 814.01
    open 814.11
  radius (alone) (closed) 813.81
    with ulna NEC 813.83
      open 813.93
    distal end - *see* Fracture, radius,
      lower end
    epiphysis
      lower - *see* Fracture, radius, lower
        end
      upper - *see* Fracture, radius, upper
        end
    head - *see* Fracture, radius, upper
      end
    lower end or extremity (distal end)
      (lower epiphysis) 813.42
      with ulna (lower end) 813.44
        open 813.54
      torus 813.45
      open 813.52
    neck - *see* Fracture, radius, upper
      end
    open NEC 813.91
    pathologic 733.12

Fracture *(Continued)*
  radius *(Continued)*
    proximal end - *see* Fracture, radius,
      upper end
    shaft (closed) 813.21
      with ulna (shaft) 813.23
        open 813.33
      open 813.31
    upper end 813.07
      with ulna (upper end) 813.08
        open 813.18
      epiphysis 813.05
        open 813.15
      head 813.05
        open 813.15
      multiple sites 813.07
        open 813.17
      neck 813.06
        open 813.16
      open 813.17
      specified site NEC 813.07
        open 813.17
  ramus
    inferior or superior (with visceral in-
      jury) (closed) 808.2
      open 808.3
    ischium - *see* Fracture, ischium
    mandible 802.24
      open 802.34
  rib(s) (closed) 807.0

> Note   Use the following fifth-digit
> subclassification with categories
> 807.0-807.1:
>
> 0   rib(s), unspecified
> 1   one rib
> 2   two ribs
> 3   three ribs
> 4   four ribs
> 5   five ribs
> 6   six ribs
> 7   seven ribs
> 8   eight or more ribs
> 9   multiple ribs, unspecified

    with flail chest (open) 807.4
      open 807.1
  root, tooth 873.63
    complicated 873.73
  sacrum - *see* Fracture, vertebra, sacrum
  scaphoid
    ankle (closed) 825.22
      open 825.32
    wrist (closed) 814.01
      open 814.11
  scapula (closed) 811.00
    acromial, acromion (process) 811.01
      open 811.11
    body 811.09
      open 811.19
    coracoid process 811.02
      open 811.12
    glenoid (cavity) (fossa) 811.03
      open 811.13
    neck 811.03
      open 811.13
    open 811.10
  semilunar
    bone, wrist (closed) 814.02
      open 814.12
    cartilage (interior) (knee) - *see* Tear,
      meniscus
  sesamoid bone - *see* Fracture, by site
  Shepherd's (closed) 825.21
    open 825.31

Fracture *(Continued)*
  shoulder - *see also* Fracture, humerus,
    upper end
    blade - *see* Fracture, scapula
  silverfork - *see* Fracture, radius, lower
    end
  sinus (ethmoid) (frontal) (maxillary)
    (nasal) (sphenoidal) - *see* Fracture,
    skull, base
  Skillern's - *see* Fracture, radius, shaft
  skull (multiple NEC) (with face bones)
    (closed) 803.0

> Note   Use the following fifth-digit
> subclassification with categories 800,
> 801, 803, and 804:
>
> 0   unspecified state of conscious-
>   ness
> 1   with no loss of consciousness
> 2   with brief [less than one hour]
>   loss of consciousness
> 3   with moderate [1-24 hours]
>   loss of consciousness
> 4   with prolonged [more than 24
>   hours] loss of consciousness
>   and return to pre-existing con-
>   scious level
> 5   with prolonged [more than 24
>   hours] loss of consciousness,
>   without return to pre-existing
>   conscious level
>
> Use fifth-digit 5 to designate when a
> patient is unconscious and dies be-
> fore regaining consciousness, regard-
> less of the duration of the loss of con-
> sciousness
>
> 6   with loss of consciousness of
>   unspecified duration
> 9   with concussion, unspecified

    with
      contusion, cerebral 803.1
      epidural hemorrhage 803.2
      extradural hemorrhage 803.2
      hemorrhage (intracranial) NEC
        803.3
      intracranial injury NEC 803.4
      laceration, cerebral 803.1
      other bones - *see* Fracture, multi-
        ple, skull
      subarachnoid hemorrhage 803.2
      subdural hemorrhage 803.2
    base (antrum) (ethmoid bone) (fossa)
      (internal ear) (nasal sinus) (occi-
      put) (sphenoid) (temporal bone)
      (closed) 801.0
      with
        contusion, cerebral 801.1
        epidural hemorrhage 801.2
        extradural hemorrhage 801.2
        hemorrhage (intracranial) NEC
          801.3
        intracranial injury NEC 801.4
        laceration, cerebral 801.1
        subarachnoid hemorrhage 801.2
        subdural hemorrhage 801.2
      open 801.5
        with
          contusion, cerebral 801.6
          epidural hemorrhage 801.7
          extradural hemorrhage 801.7
          hemorrhage (intracranial)
            NEC 801.8

Fracture *(Continued)*
  skull *(Continued)*
    open *(Continued)*
      with *(Continued)*
        intracranial injury NEC 801.9
        laceration, cerebral 801.6
        subarachnoid hemorrhage
          801.7
        subdural hemorrhage 801.7
    birth injury 767.3
    face bones - *see* Fracture, face bones
    open 803.5
      with
        contusion, cerebral 803.6
        epidural hemorrhage 803.7
        extradural hemorrhage 803.7
        hemorrhage (intracranial) NEC
          803.8
        intracranial injury NEC 803.9
        laceration, cerebral 803.6
        subarachnoid hemorrhage 803.7
        subdural hemorrhage 803.7
    vault (frontal bone) (parietal bone)
      (vertex) (closed) 800.0
      with
        contusion, cerebral 800.1
        epidural hemorrhage 800.2
        extradural hemorrhage 800.2
        hemorrhage (intracranial) NEC
          800.3
        intracranial injury NEC 800.4
        laceration, cerebral 800.1
        subarachnoid hemorrhage 800.2
        subdural hemorrhage 800.2
      open 800.5
        with
          contusion, cerebral 800.6
          epidural hemorrhage 800.7
          extradural hemorrhage 800.7
          hemorrhage (intracranial)
            NEC 800.8
          intracranial injury NEC 800.9
          laceration, cerebral 800.6
          subarachnoid hemorrhage
            800.7
          subdural hemorrhage 800.7
  Smith's 813.41
    open 813.51
  sphenoid (bone) (sinus) - *see* Fracture,
    skull, base
  spine - *see also* Fracture, vertebra, by
    site due to birth trauma 767.4
  spinous process - *see* Fracture, verte-
    bra, by site
  spontaneous - *see* Fracture, pathologic
  sprinters' - *see* Fracture, ilium
  stapes - *see* Fracture, skull, base
  stave - *see also* Fracture, metacarpus,
    metacarpal bone(s)
    spine - *see* Fracture, tibia, upper end
  sternum (closed) 807.2
    with flail chest (open) 807.4
    open 807.3
  Stieda's - *see* Fracture, femur, lower
    end
  stress 733.95
    fibula 733.93
    metatarsals 733.94
    specified site NEC 733.95
    tibia 733.93
  styloid process
    metacarpal (closed) 815.02
      open 815.12
    radius - *see* Fracture, radius, lower
      end

ICD-9-CM

Vol. 2

Fracture (*Continued*)
  styloid process (*Continued*)
    temporal bone - *see* Fracture, skull, base
    ulna - *see* Fracture, ulna, lower end
  supracondylar, elbow 812.41
    open 812.51
  symphysis pubis (with visceral injury) (closed) 808.2
    open 808.3
  talus (ankle bone) (closed) 825.21
    open 825.31
  tarsus, tarsal bone(s) (with metatarsus) of one foot (closed) NEC 825.29
    open 825.39
  temporal bone (styloid) - *see* Fracture, skull, base
  tendon - *see* Sprain, by site
  thigh - *see* Fracture, femur, shaft
  thumb (and finger(s)) of one hand (closed) (*see also* Fracture, phalanx, hand) 816.00
    with metacarpal bone(s) of same hand 817.0
      open 817.1
    metacarpal(s) - *see* Fracture, metacarpus
    open 816.10
  thyroid cartilage (closed) 807.5
    open 807.6
  tibia (closed) 823.80
    with fibula 823.82
      open 823.92
    condyles - *see* Fracture, tibia, upper end
    distal end 824.8
      open 824.9
    epiphysis
      lower 824.8
        open 824.9
      upper - *see* Fracture, tibia, upper end
    head (involving knee joint) - *see* Fracture, tibia, upper end
    intercondyloid eminence - *see* Fracture, tibia, upper end
    involving ankle 824.0
      open 824.1
    lower end or extremity (anterior lip) (posterior lip) 824.8
      open 824.9
    malleolus (internal) (medial) 824.0
      open 824.1
    open NEC 823.90
    pathologic 733.16
    proximal end - *see* Fracture, tibia, upper end
    shaft 823.20
      with fibula 823.22
        open 823.32
      open 823.30
    spine - *see* Fracture, tibia, upper end
    stress 733.93
    torus 823.40
      with tibia 823.42
    tuberosity - *see* Fracture, tibia, upper end
    upper end or extremity (condyle) (epiphysis) (head) (spine) (proximal end) (tuberosity) 823.00
      with fibula 823.02
        open 823.12
      open 823.10

Fracture (*Continued*)
  toe(s), of one foot (closed) 826.0
    with bone(s) of same lower limb 827.0
      open 827.1
    open 826.1
  tooth (root) 873.63
    complicated 873.73
  torus
    fibula 823.41
      with tibia 823.42
    radius 813.45
    tibia 823.40
      with fibula 823.42
  trachea (closed) 807.5
    open 807.6
  transverse process - *see* Fracture, vertebra, by site
  trapezium (closed) 814.05
    open 814.15
  trapezoid bone (closed) 814.06
    open 814.16
  trimalleolar (closed) 824.6
    open 824.7
  triquetral (bone) (closed) 814.03
    open 814.13
  trochanter (greater) (lesser) (closed) (*see also* Fracture, femur, neck, by site) 820.20
    open 820.30
  trunk (bones) (closed) 809.0
    open 809.1
  tuberosity (external) - *see* Fracture, by site
  ulna (alone) (closed) 813.82
    with radius NEC 813.83
      open 813.93
    coronoid process (closed) 813.02
      open 813.12
    distal end - *see* Fracture, ulna, lower end
    epiphysis
      lower - *see* Fracture, ulna, lower end
      upper - *see* Fracture, ulna, upper, end
    head - *see* Fracture, ulna, lower end
    lower end (distal end) (head) (lower epiphysis) (styloid process) 813.43
      with radius (lower end) 813.44
        open 813.54
      open 813.53
    olecranon process (closed) 813.01
      open 813.11
    open NEC 813.92
    pathologic 733.12
    proximal end - *see* Fracture, ulna, upper end
    shaft 813.22
      with radius (shaft) 813.23
        open 813.33
      open 813.32
    styloid process - *see* Fracture, ulna, lower end
    transverse - *see* Fracture, ulna, by site
    upper end (epiphysis) 813.04
      with radius (upper end) 813.08
        open 813.18
      multiple sites 813.04
        open 813.14
      open 813.14
      specified site NEC 813.04
        open 813.14
  unciform (closed) 814.08
    open 814.18

Fracture (*Continued*)
  vertebra, vertebral (back) (body) (column) (neural arch) (pedicle) (spine) (spinous process) (transverse process) (closed) 805.8
    with
      hematomyelia - *see* Fracture, vertebra, by site, with spinal cord injury
      injury to
        cauda equina - *see* Fracture, vertebra, sacrum, with spinal cord injury
        nerve - *see* Fracture, vertebra, by site, with spinal cord injury
      paralysis - *see* Fracture, vertebra, by site, with spinal cord injury
      paraplegia - *see* Fracture, vertebra, by site, with spinal cord injury
      quadriplegia - *see* Fracture, vertebra, by site, with spinal cord injury
      spinal concussion - *see* Fracture, vertebra, by site, with spinal cord injury
      spinal cord injury (closed) NEC 806.8

> **Note** Use the following fifth-digit subclassification with categories 806.0-806.3:
>
> C_1-C_4 or unspecified level and D_1-D_6 (T_1-T_6) or unspecified level with:
>
>   0   unspecified spinal cord injury
>   1   complete lesion of cord
>   2   anterior cord syndrome
>   3   central cord syndrome
>   4   specified injury NEC
>
> level and D_1-D_{12} level with:
>
>   5   unspecified spinal cord injury
>   6   complete lesion of cord
>   7   anterior cord syndrome
>   8   central cord syndrome
>   9   specified injury NEC

        cervical 806.0
          open 806.1
        dorsal, dorsolumbar 806.2
          open 806.3
        open 806.9
        thoracic, thoracolumbar 806.2
          open 806.3
    atlanto-axial - *see* Fracture, vertebra, cervical
    cervical (hangman) (teardrop) (closed) 805.00
      with spinal cord injury - *see* Fracture, vertebra, with spinal cord injury, cervical
      first (atlas) 805.01
        open 805.11
      second (axis) 805.02
        open 805.12
      third 805.03
        open 805.13
      fourth 805.04
        open 805.14
      fifth 805.05
        open 805.15
      sixth 805.06
        open 805.16

Fracture (*Continued*)
  vertebra (*Continued*)
    cervical (*Continued*)
      seventh 805.07
        open 805.17
      multiple sites 805.08
        open 805.18
      open 805.10
    coccyx (closed) 805.6
    with spinal cord injury (closed) 806.60
      cauda equina injury 806.62
        complete lesion 806.61
          open 806.71
        open 806.72
      open 806.70
        specified type NEC 806.69
      open 806.79
      open 805.7
    collapsed 733.13
    compression, not due to trauma 733.13
    dorsal (closed) 805.2
    with spinal cord injury -
      see Fracture, vertebra, with
      spinal cord injury,
      dorsal
    open 805.3
    dorsolumbar (closed) 805.2
    with spinal cord injury - *see* Fracture, vertebra, with spinal cord injury, dorsal
    open 805.3
    due to osteoporosis 733.13
    fetus or newborn 767.4
    lumbar (closed) 805.4
    with spinal cord injury (closed) 806.4
      open 806.5
      open 805.5
    nontraumatic 733.13
    open NEC 805.9
    pathologic (any site) 733.13
    sacrum (closed) 805.6
    with spinal cord injury 806.60
      cauda equina injury 806.62
        complete lesion 806.61
          open 806.71
        open 806.72
      open 806.70
        specified type NEC 806.69
        open 806.79
      open 805.7
    site unspecified (closed) 805.8
    with spinal cord injury (closed) 806.8
      open 806.9
      open 805.9
    stress (any site) 733.95
    thoracic (closed) 805.2
    with spinal cord injury - *see* Fracture, vertebra, with spinal cord injury, thoracic
    open 805.3
  vertex - *see* Fracture, skull, vault
  vomer (bone) 802.0
    open 802.1
  Wagstaffe's - *see* Fracture, ankle
  wrist (closed) 814.00
    open 814.10
    pathologic 733.12
  xiphoid (process) - *see* Fracture, sternum
  zygoma (zygomatic arch) (closed) 802.4
    open 802.5
Fragile X syndrome 759.83

Fragilitas
  crinium 704.2
  hair 704.2
  ossium 756.51
    with blue sclera 756.51
  unguium 703.8
    congenital 757.5
Fragility
  bone 756.51
    with deafness and blue sclera 756.51
  capillary (hereditary) 287.8
  hair 704.2
  nails 703.8
Fragmentation - *see* Fracture, by site
Frambesia, frambesial (tropica) (*see also* Yaws) 102.9
  initial lesion or ulcer 102.0
  primary 102.0
Frambeside
  gummatous 102.4
  of early yaws 102.2
Frambesioma 102.1
Franceschetti's syndrome (mandibulofacial dysostosis) 756.0
Francis' disease (*see also* Tularemia) 021.9
Frank's essential thrombocytopenia (*see also* Purpura, thrombocytopenic) 287.3
Franklin's disease (heavy chain) 273.2
Fraser's syndrome 759.89
Freckle 709.09
  malignant melanoma in (M8742/3) - *see* Melanoma
  melanotic (of Hutchinson) (M8742/2) - *see* Neoplasm, skin, in situ
Freeman-Sheldon syndrome 759.89
Freezing 991.9
  specified effect NEC 991.8
Frei's disease (climatic bubo) 099.1
Freiberg's
  disease (osteochondrosis, second metatarsal) 732.5
  infraction of metatarsal head 732.5
  osteochondrosis 732.5
Fremitus, friction, cardiac 785.3
Frenulum linguae 750.0
Frenum
  external os 752.49
  tongue 750.0
Frequency (urinary) NEC 788.41
  micturition 788.41
  nocturnal 788.43
  polyuria 788.42
  psychogenic 306.53
Frey's syndrome (auriculotemporal syndrome) 705.22 ◀▥
Friction
  burn (*see also* Injury, superficial, by site) 919.0
  fremitus, cardiac 785.3
  precordial 785.3
  sounds, chest 786.7
Friderichsen-Waterhouse syndrome or disease 036.3
Friedländer's
  B (bacillus) NEC (*see also* condition) 041.3
  sepsis or septicemia 038.49
  disease (endarteritis obliterans) - *see* Arteriosclerosis
Friedreich's
  ataxia 334.0
  combined systemic disease 334.0
  disease 333.2
    combined systemic 334.0

Friedreich's (*Continued*)
  myoclonia 333.2
  sclerosis (spinal cord) 334.0
Friedrich-Erb-Arnold syndrome (acropachyderma) 757.39
Frigidity 302.72
  psychic or psychogenic 302.72
Fröhlich's disease or syndrome (adiposogenital dystrophy) 253.8
Froin's syndrome 336.8
Frommel's disease 676.6
Frommel-Chiari syndrome 676.6
Frontal - *see also* condition
  lobe syndrome 310.0
Frostbite 991.3
  face 991.0
  foot 991.2
  hand 991.1
  specified site NEC 991.3
Frotteurism 302.89
Frozen 991.9
  pelvis 620.8
  shoulder 726.0
Fructosemia 271.2
Fructosuria (benign) (essential) 271.2
Fuchs'
  black spot (myopic) 360.21
  corneal dystrophy (endothelial) 371.57
  heterochromic cyclitis 364.21
Fucosidosis 271.8
Fugue 780.99
  dissociative 300.13 ◀
  hysterical (dissociative) 300.13
  reaction to exceptional stress (transient) 308.1
Fukuhara syndrome 277.87 ◀
Fuller Albright's syndrome (osteitis fibrosa disseminata) 756.59
Fuller's earth disease 502
Fulminant, fulminating - *see* condition
Functional - *see* condition
Fundus - *see also* condition
  flavimaculatus 362.76
Fungemia 117.9
Fungus, fungous
  cerebral 348.8
  disease NEC 117.9
  infection - *see* Infection, fungus
  testis (*see also* Tuberculosis) 016.5
    [608.81]
Funiculitis (acute) 608.4
  chronic 608.4
  endemic 608.4
  gonococcal (acute) 098.14
    chronic or duration of 2 months or over 098.34
  tuberculous (*see also* Tuberculosis) 016.5
FUO (*see also* Pyrexia) 780.6
Funnel
  breast (acquired) 738.3
    congenital 754.81
    late effect of rickets 268.1
  chest (acquired) 738.3
    congenital 754.81
    late effect of rickets 268.1
  pelvis (acquired) 738.6
    with disproportion (fetopelvic) 653.3
      affecting fetus or newborn 763.1
      causing obstructed labor 660.1
        affecting fetus or newborn 763.1
    congenital 755.69
    tuberculous (*see also* Tuberculosis) 016.9

ICD-9-CM

F

Vol. 2

Furfur 690.18
  microsporon 111.0
Furor, paroxysmal (idiopathic) (*see also* Epilepsy) 345.8
Furriers' lung 495.8
Furrowed tongue 529.5
  congenital 750.13
Furrowing nail(s) (transverse) 703.8
  congenital 757.5
Furuncle 680.9
  abdominal wall 680.2
  ankle 680.6
  anus 680.5
  arm (any part, above wrist) 680.3
  auditory canal, external 680.0
  axilla 680.3
  back (any part) 680.2
  breast 680.2
  buttock 680.5
  chest wall 680.2
  corpus cavernosum 607.2
  ear (any part) 680.0
  eyelid 373.13
  face (any part, except eye) 680.0
  finger (any) 680.4
  flank 680.2
  foot (any part) 680.7
  forearm 680.3
  gluteal (region) 680.5
  groin 680.2
  hand (any part) 680.4
  head (any part, except face) 680.8
  heel 680.7
  hip 680.6
  kidney (*see also* Abscess, kidney) 590.2
  knee 680.6
  labium (majus) (minus) 616.4
  lacrimal
    gland (*see also* Dacryoadenitis) 375.00
    passages (duct) (sac) (*see also* Dacryocystitis) 375.30
  leg, any part except foot 680.6
  malignant 022.0
  multiple sites 680.9
  neck 680.1
  nose (external) (septum) 680.0
  orbit 376.01
  partes posteriores 680.5
  pectoral region 680.2
  penis 607.2

Furuncle (*Continued*)
  perineum 680.2
  pinna 680.0
  scalp (any part) 680.8
  scrotum 608.4
  seminal vesicle 608.0
  shoulder 680.3
  skin NEC 680.9
  specified site NEC 680.8
  spermatic cord 608.4
  temple (region) 680.0
  testis 604.90
  thigh 680.6
  thumb 680.4
  toe (any) 680.7
  trunk 680.2
  tunica vaginalis 608.4
  umbilicus 680.2
  upper arm 680.3
  vas deferens 608.4
  vulva 616.4
  wrist 680.4
Furunculosis (*see also* Furuncle) 680.9
  external auditory meatus 680.0
    [380.13]
Fusarium (infection) 118
Fusion, fused (congenital)
  anal (with urogenital canal) 751.5
  aorta and pulmonary artery 745.0
  astragaloscaphoid 755.67
  atria 745.5
  atrium and ventricle 745.69
  auditory canal 744.02
  auricles, heart 745.5
  binocular, with defective stereopsis 368.33
  bone 756.9
  cervical spine - *see* Fusion, spine
  choanal 748.0
  commissure, mitral valve 746.5
  cranial sutures, premature 756.0
  cusps, heart valve NEC 746.89
    mitral 746.5
    tricuspid 746.89
  ear ossicles 744.04
  fingers (*see also* Syndactylism, fingers) 755.11
  hymen 752.42
  hymeno-urethral 599.89
    causing obstructed labor 660.1
      affecting fetus or newborn 763.1

Fusion, fused (*Continued*)
  joint (acquired) - *see also* Ankylosis
    congenital 755.8
  kidneys (incomplete) 753.3
  labium (majus) (minus) 752.49
  larynx and trachea 748.3
  limb 755.8
    lower 755.69
    upper 755.59
  lobe, lung 748.5
  lumbosacral (acquired) 724.6
    congenital 756.15
    surgical V45.4
  nares (anterior) (posterior) 748.0
  nose, nasal 748.0
  nostril(s) 748.0
  organ or site NEC - *see* Anomaly, specified type NEC
  ossicles 756.9
    auditory 744.04
  pulmonary valve segment 746.02
  pulmonic cusps 746.02
  ribs 756.3
  sacroiliac (acquired) (joint) 724.6
    congenital 755.69
    surgical V45.4
  skull, imperfect 756.0
  spine (acquired) 724.9
    arthrodesis status V45.4
    congenital (vertebra) 756.15
    postoperative status V45.4
  sublingual duct with submaxillary duct at opening in mouth 750.26
  talonavicular (bar) 755.67
  teeth, tooth 520.2
  testes 752.89
  toes (*see also* Syndactylism, toes) 755.13
  trachea and esophagus 750.3
  twins 759.4
  urethral-hymenal 599.89
  vagina 752.49
  valve cusps - *see* Fusion, cusps, heart valve
  ventricles, heart 745.4
  vertebra (arch) - *see* Fusion, spine
  vulva 752.49
Fusospirillosis (mouth) (tongue) (tonsil) 101
Fussy infant (baby) 780.91

G

Gafsa boil 085.1
Gain, weight (abnormal) (excessive) (see also Weight, gain) 783.1
Gaisböck's disease or syndrome (polycythemia hypertonica) 289.0
Gait
  abnormality 781.2
    hysterical 300.11
  ataxic 781.2
    hysterical 300.11
  disturbance 781.2
    hysterical 300.11
  paralytic 781.2
  scissor 781.2
  spastic 781.2
  staggering 781.2
    hysterical 300.11
Galactocele (breast) (infected) 611.5
  puerperal, postpartum 676.8
Galactophoritis 611.0
  puerperal, postpartum 675.2
Galactorrhea 676.6
  not associated with childbirth 611.6
Galactosemia (classic) (congenital) 271.1
Galactosuria 271.1
Galacturia 791.1
  bilharziasis 120.0
Galen's vein - see condition
Gallbladder - see also condition
  acute (see also Disease, gallbladder) 575.0
Gall duct - see condition
Gallop rhythm 427.89
Gallstone (cholemic) (colic) (impacted) - see also Cholelithiasis
  causing intestinal obstruction 560.31
Gambling, pathological 312.31
Gammaloidosis 277.3
Gammopathy 273.9
  macroglobulinemia 273.3
  monoclonal (benign) (essential) (idiopathic) (with lymphoplasmacytic dyscrasia) 273.1
Gamna's disease (siderotic splenomegaly) 289.51
Gampsodactylia (congenital) 754.71
Gamstorp's disease (adynamia episodica hereditaria) 359.3
Gandy-Nanta disease (siderotic splenomegaly) 289.51
Gang activity, without manifest psychiatric disorder V71.09
  adolescent V71.02
  adult V71.01
  child V71.02
Gangliocytoma (M9490/0) - see Neoplasm, connective tissue, benign
Ganglioglioma (M9505/1) - see Neoplasm, by site, uncertain behavior
Ganglion 727.43
  joint 727.41
  of yaws (early) (late) 102.6
  periosteal (see also Periostitis) 730.3
  tendon sheath (compound) (diffuse) 727.42
  tuberculous (see also Tuberculosis) 015.9
Ganglioneuroblastoma (M9490/3) - see Neoplasm, connective tissue, malignant

Ganglioneuroma (M9490/0) - see also Neoplasm, connective tissue, benign
  malignant (M9490/3) - see Neoplasm, connective tissue, malignant
Ganglioneuromatosis (M9491/0) - see Neoplasm, connective tissue, benign
Ganglionitis
  fifth nerve (see also Neuralgia, trigeminal) 350.1
  gasserian 350.1
  geniculate 351.1
    herpetic 053.11
    newborn 767.5
  herpes zoster 053.11
  herpetic geniculate (Hunt's syndrome) 053.11
Gangliosidosis 330.1
Gangosa 102.5
Gangrene, gangrenous (anemia) (artery) (cellulitis) (dermatitis) (dry) (infective) (moist) (pemphigus) (septic) (skin) (stasis) (ulcer) 785.4
  with
    arteriosclerosis (native artery) 440.24
      bypass graft 440.30
        autologous vein 440.31
        nonautologous biological 440.32
    diabetes (mellitus) 250.7 [785.4]
  abdomen (wall) 785.4
  adenitis 683
  alveolar 526.5
  angina 462
    diphtheritic 032.0
  anus 569.49
  appendices epiploicae - see Gangrene, mesentery
  appendix - see Appendicitis, acute
  arteriosclerotic - see Arteriosclerosis, with, gangrene
  auricle 785.4
  Bacillus welchii (see also Gangrene, gas) 040.0
  bile duct (see also Cholangitis) 576.8
  bladder 595.89
  bowel - see Gangrene, intestine
  cecum - see Gangrene, intestine
  Clostridium perfringens or welchii (see also Gangrene, gas) 040.0
  colon - see Gangrene, intestine
  connective tissue 785.4
  cornea 371.40
  corpora cavernosa (infective) 607.2
    noninfective 607.89
  cutaneous, spreading 785.4
  decubital (see also Decubitus) 707.00 [785.4] ◀▥
  diabetic (any site) 250.7 [785.4]
  dropsical 785.4
  emphysematous (see also Gangrene, gas) 040.0
  epidemic (ergotized grain) 988.2
  epididymis (infectional) (see also Epididymitis) 604.99
  erysipelas (see also Erysipelas) 035
  extremity (lower) (upper) 785.4
  gallbladder or duct (see also Cholecystitis, acute) 575.0
  gas (bacillus) 040.0
    with
      abortion - see Abortion, by type, with sepsis
      ectopic pregnancy (see also categories 633.0-633.9) 639.0

Gangrene, gangrenous (Continued)
  gas (Continued)
    with (Continued)
      molar pregnancy (see also categories 630-632) 639.0
      following
        abortion 639.0
        ectopic or molar pregnancy 639.0
      puerperal, postpartum, childbirth 670
  glossitis 529.0
  gum 523.8
  hernia - see Hernia, by site, with gangrene
  hospital noma 528.1
  intestine, intestinal (acute) (hemorrhagic) (massive) 557.0
    with
      hernia - see Hernia, by site, with gangrene
      mesenteric embolism or infarction 557.0
      obstruction (see also Obstruction, intestine) 560.9
  laryngitis 464.00
    with obstruction 464.01
  liver 573.8
  lung 513.0
    spirochetal 104.8
  lymphangitis 457.2
  Meleney's (cutaneous) 686.09
  mesentery 557.0
    with
      embolism or infarction 557.0
      intestinal obstruction (see also Obstruction, intestine) 560.9
  mouth 528.1
  noma 528.1
  orchitis 604.90
  ovary (see also Salpingo-oophoritis) 614.2
  pancreas 577.0
  penis (infectional) 607.2
    noninfective 607.89
  perineum 785.4
  pharynx 462
    septic 034.0
  pneumonia 513.0
  Pott's 440.24
  presenile 443.1
  pulmonary 513.0
  pulp, tooth 522.1
  quinsy 475
  Raynaud's (symmetric gangrene) 443.0 [785.4]
  rectum 569.49
  retropharyngeal 478.24
  rupture - see Hernia, by site, with gangrene
  scrotum 608.4
    noninfective 608.83
  senile 440.24
  sore throat 462
  spermatic cord 608.4
    noninfective 608.89
  spine 785.4
  spirochetal NEC 104.8
  spreading cutaneous 785.4
  stomach 537.89
  stomatitis 528.1
  symmetrical 443.0 [785.4]
  testis (infectional) (see also Orchitis) 604.99
    noninfective 608.89

ICD-9-CM

Vol. 2

Gangrene, gangrenous (*Continued*)
  throat 462
    diphtheritic 032.0
  thyroid (gland) 246.8
  tonsillitis (acute) 463
  tooth (pulp) 522.1
  tuberculous NEC (*see also* Tuberculosis) 011.9
  tunica vaginalis 608.4
    noninfective 608.89
  umbilicus 785.4
  uterus (*see also* Endometritis) 615.9
  uvulitis 528.3
  vas deferens 608.4
    noninfective 608.89
  vulva (*see also* Vulvitis) 616.10
Gannister disease (occupational) 502
  with tuberculosis - *see* Tuberculosis, pulmonary
Ganser's syndrome, hysterical 300.16
Gardner-Diamond syndrome (autoerythrocyte sensitization) 287.2
Gargoylism 277.5
Garré's
  disease (*see also* Osteomyelitis) 730.1
  osteitis (sclerosing) (*see also* Osteomyelitis) 730.1
  osteomyelitis (*see also* Osteomyelitis) 730.1
Garrod's pads, knuckle 728.79
Gartner's duct
  cyst 752.11
  persistent 752.11
Gas
  asphyxia, asphyxiation, inhalation, poisoning, suffocation NEC 987.9
    specified gas - *see* Table of Drugs and Chemicals
  bacillus gangrene or infection - *see* Gas, gangrene
  cyst, mesentery 568.89
  excessive 787.3
  gangrene 040.0
    with
      abortion - *see* Abortion, by type, with sepsis
      ectopic pregnancy (*see also* categories 633.0-633.9) 639.0
      molar pregnancy (*see also* categories 630-632) 639.0
    following
      abortion 639.0
      ectopic or molar pregnancy 639.0
    puerperal, postpartum, childbirth 670
  on stomach 787.3
  pains 787.3
Gastradenitis 535.0
Gastralgia 536.8
  psychogenic 307.89
Gastrectasis, gastrectasia 536.1
  psychogenic 306.4
Gastric - *see* condition
Gastrinoma (M8153/1)
  malignant (M8153/3)
    pancreas 157.4
    specified site NEC - *see* Neoplasm, by site, malignant
    unspecified site 157.4
  specified site - *see* Neoplasm, by site, uncertain behavior
  unspecified site 235.5

Gastritis 535.5

> Note Use the following fifth-digit subclassification for category 535:
>
> 0   without mention of hemorrhage
> 1   with hemorrhage

  acute 535.0
  alcoholic 535.3
  allergic 535.4
  antral 535.4
  atrophic 535.1
  atrophic-hyperplastic 535.1
  bile-induced 535.4
  catarrhal 535.0
  chronic (atrophic) 535.1
  cirrhotic 535.4
  corrosive (acute) 535.4
  dietetic 535.4
  due to diet deficiency 269.9 [535.4]
  eosinophilic 535.4
  erosive 535.4
  follicular 535.4
    chronic 535.1
  giant hypertrophic 535.2
  glandular 535.4
    chronic 535.1
  hypertrophic (mucosa) 535.2
    chronic giant 211.1
  irritant 535.4
  nervous 306.4
  phlegmonous 535.0
  psychogenic 306.4
  sclerotic 535.4
  spastic 536.8
  subacute 535.0
  superficial 535.4
  suppurative 535.0
  toxic 535.4
  tuberculous (*see also* Tuberculosis) 017.9
Gastrocarcinoma (M8010/3) 151.9
Gastrocolic - *see* condition
Gastrocolitis - *see* Enteritis
Gastrodisciasis 121.8
Gastroduodenitis (*see also* Gastritis) 535.5
  catarrhal 535.0
  infectional 535.0
  virus, viral 008.8
    specified type NEC 008.69
Gastrodynia 536.8
Gastroenteritis (acute) (catarrhal) (congestive) (hemorrhagic) (noninfectious) (*see also* Enteritis) 558.9
  aertrycke infection 003.0
  allergic 558.3
  chronic 558.9
    ulcerative (*see also* Colitis, ulcerative) 556.9
  dietetic 558.9
  due to
    food poisoning (*see also* Poisoning, food) 005.9
    radiation 558.1
  epidemic 009.0
  functional 558.9
  infectious (*see also* Enteritis, due to, by organism) 009.0
    presumed 009.1
  salmonella 003.0
  septic (*see also* Enteritis, due to, by organism) 009.0
  toxic 558.2
  tuberculous (*see also* Tuberculosis) 014.8

Gastroenteritis (*Continued*)
  ulcerative (*see also* Colitis, ulcerative) 556.9
  viral NEC 008.8
    specified type NEC 008.69
  zymotic 009.0
Gastroenterocolitis - *see* Enteritis
Gastroenteropathy, protein-losing 579.8
Gastroenteroptosis 569.89
Gastroesophageal laceration-hemorrhage syndrome 530.7
Gastroesophagitis 530.19
Gastrohepatitis (*see also* Gastritis) 535.5
Gastrointestinal - *see* condition
Gastrojejunal - *see* condition
Gastrojejunitis (*see also* Gastritis) 535.5
Gastrojejunocolic - *see* condition
Gastroliths 537.89
Gastromalacia 537.89
Gastroparalysis 536.3 ◄▥
  diabetic 250.6 [536.3]
Gastroparesis 536.3
  diabetic 250.6 [536.3]
Gastropathy, exudative 579.8
Gastroptosis 537.5
Gastrorrhagia 578.0
Gastrorrhea 536.8
  psychogenic 306.4
Gastroschisis (congenital) 756.79
  acquired 569.89
Gastrospasm (neurogenic) (reflex) 536.8
  neurotic 306.4
  psychogenic 306.4
Gastrostaxis 578.0
Gastrostenosis 537.89
Gastrostomy
  attention to V55.1
  complication 536.40
    specified type 536.49
  infection 536.41
  malfunctioning 536.42
  status V44.1
Gastrosuccorrhea (continuous) (intermittent) 536.8
  neurotic 306.4
  psychogenic 306.4
Gaucher's
  disease (adult) (cerebroside lipidosis) (infantile) 272.7
  hepatomegaly 272.7
  splenomegaly (cerebroside lipidosis) 272.7
Gayet's disease (superior hemorrhagic polioencephalitis) 265.1
Gayet-Wernicke's syndrome (superior hemorrhagic polioencephalitis) 265.1
Gee (-Herter) (-Heubner) (-Thaysen) disease or syndrome (nontropical sprue) 579.0
Gélineau's syndrome (*see also* Narcolepsy) 347.00 ◄▥
Gemination, teeth 520.2
Gemistocytoma (M9411/3)
  specified site - *see* Neoplasm, by site, malignant
  unspecified site 191.9
General, generalized - *see* condition
Genetic ◄
  susceptibility to ◄
    neoplasm ◄
      malignant, of ◄
        breast V84.01 ◄
        endometrium V84.04 ◄
        other V84.09 ◄
        ovary V84.02 ◄
        prostate V84.03 ◄
      other disease V84.8 ◄

◄ **New**   ◄▥ **Revised**

Genital - *see* condition
  warts 078.19
Genito-anorectal syndrome 099.1
Genitourinary system - *see* condition
Genu
  congenital 755.64
  extrorsum (acquired) 736.42
    congenital 755.64
    late effects of rickets 268.1
  introrsum (acquired) 736.41
    congenital 755.64
    late effects of rickets 268.1
  rachitic (old) 268.1
  recurvatum (acquired) 736.5
    congenital 754.40
      with dislocation of knee 754.41
    late effects of rickets 268.1
  valgum (acquired) (knock-knee) 736.41
    congenital 755.64
    late effects of rickets 268.1
  varum (acquired) (bowleg) 736.42
    congenital 755.64
    late effect of rickets 268.1
Geographic tongue 529.1
Geophagia 307.52
Geotrichosis 117.9
  intestine 117.9
  lung 117.9
  mouth 117.9
Gephyrophobia 300.29
Gerbode defect 745.4
Gerhardt's
  disease (erythromelalgia) 443.89
  syndrome (vocal cord paralysis) 478.30
Gerlier's disease (epidemic vertigo) 078.81
German measles 056.9
  exposure to V01.4
Germinoblastoma (diffuse) (M9614/3) 202.8
  follicular (M9692/3) 202.0
Germinoma (M9064/3) - *see* Neoplasm,
  by site, malignant
Gerontoxon 371.41
Gerstmann's syndrome (finger agnosia)
  784.69
Gestation (period) - *see also* Pregnancy
  ectopic NEC (*see also* Pregnancy, ec-
    topic) 633.90
    with intrauterine pregnancy 633.91
Gestational proteinuria 646.2
  with hypertension - *see* Toxemia, of
    pregnancy
Ghon tubercle primary infection (*see*
  also Tuberculosis) 010.0
Ghost
  teeth 520.4
  vessels, cornea 370.64
Ghoul hand 102.3
Giant
  cell
    epulis 523.8
    peripheral (gingiva) 523.8
    tumor, tendon sheath 727.02
  colon (congenital) 751.3
  esophagus (congenital) 750.4
  kidney 753.3
  urticaria 995.1
    hereditary 277.6
Giardia lamblia infestation 007.1
Giardiasis 007.1
Gibert's disease (pityriasis rosea) 696.3
Gibraltar fever - *see* Brucellosis
Giddiness 780.4
  hysterical 300.11
  psychogenic 306.9

Gierke's disease (glycogenosis I) 271.0
Gigantism (cerebral) (hypophyseal) (pituitary) 253.0
Gilbert's disease or cholemia (familial
  nonhemolytic jaundice) 277.4
Gilchrist's disease (North American
  blastomycosis) 116.0
Gilford (-Hutchinson) disease or syndrome (progeria) 259.8
Gilles de la Tourette's disease (motor-
  verbal tic) 307.23
Gillespie's syndrome (dysplasia oculodentodigitalis) 759.89
Gingivitis 523.1
  acute 523.0
    necrotizing 101
  catarrhal 523.0
  chronic 523.1
  desquamative 523.1
  expulsiva 523.4
  hyperplastic 523.1
  marginal, simple 523.1
  necrotizing, acute 101
  pellagrous 265.2
  ulcerative 523.1
    acute necrotizing 101
  Vincent's 101
Gingivoglossitis 529.0
Gingivopericementitis 523.4
Gingivosis 523.1
Gingivostomatitis 523.1
  herpetic 054.2
Giovannini's disease 117.9
GISA (glycopeptide intermediate staphylococcus aureus) V09.8 ◀
Gland, glandular - *see* condition
Glanders 024
Glanzmann (-Naegeli) disease or thrombasthenia 287.1
Glassblowers' disease 527.1
Glaucoma (capsular) (inflammatory)
  (noninflammatory) (primary)
  365.9
  with increased episcleral venous pres-
    sure 365.82
  absolute 360.42
  acute 365.22
    narrow angle 365.22
    secondary 365.60
  angle closure 365.20
    acute 365.22
    chronic 365.23
    intermittent 365.21
    interval 365.21
    residual stage 365.24
    subacute 365.21
  borderline 365.00
  chronic 365.11
    noncongestive 365.11
    open angle 365.11
    simple 365.11
  closed angle - *see* Glaucoma, angle clo-
    sure
  congenital 743.20
    associated with other eye anomalies
      743.22
    simple 743.21
  congestive - *see* Glaucoma, narrow an-
    gle
  corticosteroid-induced (glaucomatous
    stage) 365.31
    residual stage 365.32
  hemorrhagic 365.60
  hypersecretion 365.81

Glaucoma (*Continued*)
  in or with
    aniridia 743.45 [365.42]
    Axenfeld's anomaly 743.44 [365.41]
    concussion of globe 921.3 [365.65]
    congenital syndromes NEC 759.89
      [365.44]
    dislocation of lens
      anterior 379.33 [365.59]
      posterior 379.34 [365.59]
    disorder of lens NEC [365.59]
    epithelial down-growth 364.61
      [365.64]
    glaucomatocyclitic crisis 364.22
      [365.62]
    hypermature cataract 366.18 [365.51]
    hyphema 364.41 [365.63]
    inflammation, ocular 365.62
    iridocyclitis 364.3 [365.62]
    iris
      anomalies NEC 743.46 [365.42]
      atrophy, essential 364.51 [365.42]
      bombé 364.74 [365.61]
      rubeosis 364.42 [365.63]
    microcornea 743.41 [365.43]
    neurofibromatosis 237.71 [365.44]
    ocular
      cysts NEC 365.64
      disorders NEC 365.60
      trauma 365.65
      tumors NEC 365.64
    postdislocation of lens
      anterior 379.33 [365.59]
      posterior 379.34 [365.59]
    pseudoexfoliation of capsule 366.11
      [365.52]
    pupillary block or seclusion 364.74
      [365.61]
    recession of chamber angle 364.77
      [365.65]
    retinal vein occlusion 362.35 [365.63]
    Rieger's anomaly or syndrome
      743.44 [365.41]
    rubeosis of iris 364.42 [365.63]
    seclusion of pupil 364.74 [365.61]
    spherophakia 743.36 [365.59]
    Sturge-Weber (-Dimitri) syndrome
      759.6 [365.44]
  systemic syndrome NEC 365.44
  tumor of globe 365.64
  vascular disorders NEC 365.63
  infantile 365.14
  congenital 743.20
    associated with other eye anoma-
      lies 743.22
    simple 743.21
  juvenile 365.14
  low tension 365.12
  malignant 365.83
  narrow angle (primary) 365.20
    acute 365.22
    chronic 365.23
    intermittent 365.21
    interval 365.21
    residual stage 365.24
    subacute 365.21
  newborn 743.20
    associated with other eye anomalies
      743.22
    simple 743.21
  noncongestive (chronic) 365.11
  nonobstructive (chronic) 365.11
  obstructive 365.60
    due to lens changes 365.59

ICD-9-CM

G

Vol. 2

Glaucoma (*Continued*)
open angle 365.10
  with
    borderline intraocular pressure 365.01
    cupping of optic discs 365.01
    primary 365.11
    residual stage 365.15
phacolytic 365.51
  with hypermature cataract 366.18 *[365.51]*
pigmentary 365.13
postinfectious 365.60
pseudoexfoliation 365.52
  with pseudoexfoliation of capsule 366.11 *[365.52]*
secondary NEC 365.60
simple (chronic) 365.11
simplex 365.11
steroid responders 365.03
suspect 365.00
syphilitic 095.8
traumatic NEC 365.65
  newborn 767.8
tuberculous (*see also* Tuberculosis) 017.3 *[365.62]*
wide angle (*see also* Glaucoma, open angle) 365.10
Glaucomatous flecks (subcapsular) 366.31
Glazed tongue 529.4
Gleet 098.2
Glénard's disease or syndrome (enteroptosis) 569.89
Glinski-Simmonds syndrome (pituitary cachexia) 253.2
Glioblastoma (multiforme) (M9440/3)
with sarcomatous component (M9442/3)
  specified site - *see* Neoplasm, by site, malignant
  unspecified site 191.9
giant cell (M9441/3)
  specified site - *see* Neoplasm, by site, malignant
  unspecified site 191.9
specified site - *see* Neoplasm, by site, malignant
unspecified site 191.9
Glioma (malignant) (M9380/3)
astrocytic (M9400/3)
  specified site - *see* Neoplasm, by site, malignant
  unspecified site 191.9
mixed (M9382/3)
  specified site - *see* Neoplasm, by site, malignant
  unspecified site 191.9
nose 748.1
specified site NEC - *see* Neoplasm, by site, malignant
subependymal (M9383/1) 237.5
unspecified site 191.9
Gliomatosis cerebri (M9381/3) 191.0
Glioneuroma (M9505/1) - *see* Neoplasm, by site, uncertain behavior
Gliosarcoma (M9380/3)
specified site - *see* Neoplasm, by site, malignant
unspecified site 191.9
Gliosis (cerebral) 349.89
spinal 336.0
Glisson's
cirrhosis - *see* Cirrhosis, portal
disease (*see also* Rickets) 268.0
Glissonitis 573.3

Globinuria 791.2
Globus 306.4
hystericus 300.11
Glomangioma (M8712/0) (*see also* Hemangioma) 228.00
Glomangiosarcoma (M8710/3) - *see* Neoplasm, connective tissue, malignant
Glomerular nephritis (*see also* Nephritis) 583.9
Glomerulitis (*see also* Nephritis) 583.9
Glomerulonephritis (*see also* Nephritis) 583.9
with
  edema (*see also* Nephrosis) 581.9
  lesion of
    exudative nephritis 583.89
    interstitial nephritis (diffuse) (focal) 583.89
    necrotizing glomerulitis 583.4
      acute 580.4
      chronic 582.4
    renal necrosis 583.9
      cortical 583.6
      medullary 583.7
    specified pathology NEC 583.89
      acute 580.89
      chronic 582.89
  necrosis, renal 583.9
    cortical 583.6
    medullary (papillary) 583.7
  specified pathology or lesion NEC 583.89
acute 580.9
  with
    exudative nephritis 580.89
    interstitial nephritis (diffuse) (focal) 580.89
    necrotizing glomerulitis 580.4
    extracapillary with epithelial crescents 580.4
    poststreptococcal 580.0
    proliferative (diffuse) 580.0
    rapidly progressive 580.4
    specified pathology NEC 580.89
arteriolar (*see also* Hypertension, kidney) 403.90
arteriosclerotic (*see also* Hypertension, kidney) 403.90
ascending (*see also* Pyelitis) 590.80
basement membrane NEC 583.89
  with
    pulmonary hemorrhage (Goodpasture's syndrome) 446.21 *[583.81]*
chronic 582.9
  with
    exudative nephritis 582.89
    interstitial nephritis (diffuse) (focal) 582.89
    necrotizing glomerulitis 582.4
    specified pathology or lesion NEC 582.89
  endothelial 582.2
  extracapillary with epithelial crescents 582.4
  hypocomplementemic persistent 582.2
  lobular 582.2
  membranoproliferative 582.2
  membranous 582.1
    and proliferative (mixed) 582.2
    sclerosing 582.1
  mesangiocapillary 582.2
  mixed membranous and proliferative 582.2

Glomerulonephritis (*Continued*)
chronic (*Continued*)
  proliferative (diffuse) 582.0
  rapidly progressive 582.4
  sclerosing 582.1
cirrhotic - *see* Sclerosis, renal
desquamative - *see* Nephrosis
due to or associated with
  amyloidosis 277.3 *[583.81]*
    with nephrotic syndrome 277.3 *[581.81]*
    chronic 277.3 *[582.81]*
  diabetes mellitus 250.4 *[583.81]*
    with nephrotic syndrome 250.4 *[581.81]*
  diphtheria 032.89 *[580.81]*
  gonococcal infection (acute) 098.19 *[583.81]*
    chronic or duration of 2 months or over 098.39 *[583.81]*
  infectious hepatitis 070.9 *[580.81]*
  malaria (with nephrotic syndrome) 084.9 *[581.81]*
  mumps 072.79 *[580.81]*
  polyarteritis (nodosa) (with nephrotic syndrome) 446.0 *[581.81]*
  specified pathology NEC 583.89
    acute 580.89
    chronic 582.89
  streptotrichosis 039.8 *[583.81]*
  subacute bacterial endocarditis 421.0 *[580.81]*
  syphilis (late) 095.4
    congenital 090.5 *[583.81]*
    early 091.69 *[583.81]*
  systemic lupus erythematosus 710.0 *[583.81]*
    with nephrotic syndrome 710.0 *[581.81]*
    chronic 710.0 *[582.81]*
  tuberculosis (*see also* Tuberculosis) 016.0 *[583.81]*
  typhoid fever 002.0 *[580.81]*
extracapillary with epithelial crescents 583.4
  acute 580.4
  chronic 582.4
exudative 583.89
  acute 580.89
  chronic 582.89
focal (*see also* Nephritis) 583.9
  embolic 580.4
granular 582.89
granulomatous 582.89
hydremic (*see also* Nephrosis) 581.9
hypocomplementemic persistent 583.2
  with nephrotic syndrome 581.2
  chronic 582.2
immune complex NEC 583.89
infective (*see also* Pyelitis) 590.80
interstitial (diffuse) (focal) 583.89
  with nephrotic syndrome 581.89
  acute 580.89
  chronic 582.89
latent or quiescent 582.9
lobular 583.2
  with nephrotic syndrome 581.2
  chronic 582.2
membranoproliferative 583.2
  with nephrotic syndrome 581.2
  chronic 582.2
membranous 583.1
  with nephrotic syndrome 581.1

Glomerulonephritis (Continued)
  membranous (Continued)
    and proliferative (mixed) 583.2
      with nephrotic syndrome 581.2
      chronic 582.2
    chronic 582.1
    sclerosing 582.1
      with nephrotic syndrome 581.1
    mesangiocapillary 583.2
      with nephrotic syndrome 581.2
      chronic 582.2
  minimal change 581.3
  mixed membranous and proliferative 583.2
      with nephrotic syndrome 581.2
      chronic 582.2
  necrotizing 583.4
    acute 580.4
    chronic 582.4
  nephrotic (see also Nephrosis) 581.9
  old - see Glomerulonephritis, chronic
  parenchymatous 581.89
  poststreptococcal 580.0
  proliferative (diffuse) 583.0
    with nephrotic syndrome 581.0
    acute 580.0
    chronic 582.0
  purulent (see also Pyelitis) 590.80
  quiescent - see Nephritis, chronic
  rapidly progressive 583.4
    acute 580.4
    chronic 582.4
  sclerosing membranous (chronic) 582.1
    with nephrotic syndrome 581.1
  septic (see also Pyelitis) 590.80
  specified pathology or lesion NEC 583.89
    with nephrotic syndrome 581.89
    acute 580.89
    chronic 582.89
  suppurative (acute) (disseminated) (see also Pyelitis) 590.80
  toxic - see Nephritis, acute
  tubal, tubular - see Nephrosis, tubular
  type II (Ellis) - see Nephrosis
  vascular - see Hypertension, kidney
Glomerulosclerosis (see also Sclerosis, renal) 587
  focal 582.1
    with nephrotic syndrome 581.1
  intercapillary (nodular) (with diabetes) 250.4 [581.81]
Glossagra 529.6
Glossalgia 529.6
Glossitis 529.0
  areata exfoliativa 529.1
  atrophic 529.4
  benign migratory 529.1
  gangrenous 529.0
  Hunter's 529.4
  median rhomboid 529.2
  Moeller's 529.4
  pellagrous 265.2
Glossocele 529.8
Glossodynia 529.6
  exfoliativa 529.4
Glossoncus 529.8
Glossophytia 529.3
Glossoplegia 529.8
Glossoptosis 529.8
Glossopyrosis 529.6
Glossotrichia 529.3
Glossy skin 701.9
Glottis - see condition
Glottitis - see Glossitis

Glucagonoma (M8152/0)
  malignant (M8152/3)
    pancreas 157.4
    specified site NEC - see Neoplasm, by site, malignant
    unspecified site 157.4
  pancreas 211.7
  specified site NEC - see Neoplasm, by site, benign
  unspecified site 211.7
Glucoglycinuria 270.7
Glue ear syndrome 381.20
Glue sniffing (airplane glue) (see also Dependence) 304.6
Glycinemia (with methylmalonic acidemia) 270.7
Glycinuria (renal) (with ketosis) 270.0
Glycogen
  infiltration (see also Disease, glycogen storage) 271.0
  storage disease (see also Disease, glycogen storage) 271.0
Glycogenosis (see also Disease, glycogen storage) 271.0
  cardiac 271.0 [425.7]
  Cori, types I-VII 271.0
  diabetic, secondary 250.8 [259.8]
  diffuse (with hepatic cirrhosis) 271.0
  generalized 271.0
  glucose-6-phosphatase deficiency 271.0
  hepatophosphorylase deficiency 271.0
  hepatorenal 271.0
  myophosphorylase deficiency 271.0
Glycopenia 251.2
Glycopeptide ◄
  intermediate staphylococcus aureus (GISA) V09.8 ◄
  resistant ◄
    enterococcus V09.8 ◄
    staphylococcus aureus (GRSA) V09.8 ◄
Glycoprolinuria 270.8
Glycosuria 791.5
  renal 271.4
Gnathostoma (spinigerum) (infection) (infestation) 128.1
  wandering swellings from 128.1
Gnathostomiasis 128.1
Goiter (adolescent) (colloid) (diffuse) (dipping) (due to iodine deficiency) (endemic) (euthyroid) (heart) (hyperplastic) (internal) (intrathoracic) (juvenile) (mixed type) (nonendemic) (parenchymatous) (plunging) (sporadic) (subclavicular) (substernal) 240.9
  with
    hyperthyroidism (recurrent) (see also Goiter, toxic) 242.0
    thyrotoxicosis (see also Goiter, toxic) 242.0
  adenomatous (see also Goiter, nodular) 241.9
  cancerous (M8000/3) 193
  complicating pregnancy, childbirth, or puerperium 648.1
  congenital 246.1
  cystic (see also Goiter, nodular) 241.9
  due to enzyme defect in synthesis of thyroid hormone (butane-insoluble iodine) (coupling) (deiodinase) (iodide trapping or organification) (iodotyrosine dehalogenase) (peroxidase) 246.1
  dyshormonogenic 246.1

Goiter (Continued)
  exophthalmic (see also Goiter, toxic) 242.0
  familial (with deaf-mutism) 243
  fibrous 245.3
  lingual 759.2
  lymphadenoid 245.2
  malignant (M8000/3) 193
  multinodular (nontoxic) 241.1
    toxic or with hyperthyroidism (see also Goiter, toxic) 242.2
  nodular (nontoxic) 241.9
    with
      hyperthyroidism (see also Goiter, toxic) 242.3
      thyrotoxicosis (see also Goiter, toxic) 242.3
    endemic 241.9
    exophthalmic (diffuse) (see also Goiter, toxic) 242.0
    multinodular (nontoxic) 241.1
    sporadic 241.9
    toxic (see also Goiter, toxic) 242.3
    uninodular (nontoxic) 241.0
  nontoxic (nodular) 241.9
    multinodular 241.1
    uninodular 241.0
  pulsating (see also Goiter, toxic) 242.0
  simple 240.0
  toxic 242.0

Note	Use the following fifth-digit subclassification with category 242:
0	without mention of thyrotoxic crisis or storm
1	with mention of thyrotoxic crisis or storm

    adenomatous 242.3
      multinodular 242.2
      uninodular 242.1
    multinodular 242.2
    nodular 242.3
      multinodular 242.2
      uninodular 242.1
    uninodular 242.1
  uninodular (nontoxic) 241.0
    toxic or with hyperthyroidism (see also Goiter, toxic) 242.1
Goldberg (-Maxwell) (-Morris) syndrome (testicular feminization) 257.8
Goldblatt's
  hypertension 440.1
  kidney 440.1
Goldenhar's syndrome (oculoauriculovertebral dysplasia) 756.0
Goldflam-Erb disease or syndrome 358.00
Goldscheider's disease (epidermolysis bullosa) 757.39
Goldstein's disease (familial hemorrhagic telangiectasia) 448.0
Golfer's elbow 726.32
Goltz-Gorlin syndrome (dermal hypoplasia) 757.39
Gonadoblastoma (M9073/1)
  specified site - see Neoplasm, by site, uncertain behavior
  unspecified site
    female 236.2
    male 236.4
Gonecystitis (see also Vesiculitis) 608.0
Gongylonemiasis 125.6
  mouth 125.6
Goniosynechiae 364.73
Gonococcemia 098.89

ICD-9-CM

Vol. 2

Gonococcus, gonococcal (disease) (infection) (*see also* condition) 098.0
  anus 098.7
  bursa 098.52
  chronic NEC 098.2
  complicating pregnancy, childbirth, or puerperium 647.1
    affecting fetus or newborn 760.2
  conjunctiva, conjunctivitis (neonatorum) 098.40
  dermatosis 098.89
  endocardium 098.84
  epididymo-orchitis 098.13
    chronic or duration of 2 months or over 098.33
  eye (newborn) 098.40
  fallopian tube (chronic) 098.37
    acute 098.17
  genitourinary (acute) (organ) (system) (tract) (*see also* Gonorrhea) 098.0
    lower 098.0
      chronic 098.2
    upper 098.10
      chronic 098.30
  heart NEC 098.85
  joint 098.50
  keratoderma 098.81
  keratosis (blennorrhagica) 098.81
  lymphatic (gland) (node) 098.89
  meninges 098.82
  orchitis (acute) 098.13
    chronic or duration of 2 months or over 098.33
  pelvis (acute) 098.19
    chronic or duration of 2 months or over 098.39
  pericarditis 098.83
  peritonitis 098.86
  pharyngitis 098.6
  pharynx 098.6
  proctitis 098.7
  pyosalpinx (chronic) 098.37
    acute 098.17
  rectum 098.7
  septicemia 098.89
  skin 098.89
  specified site NEC 098.89
  synovitis 098.51
  tendon sheath 098.51
  throat 098.6
  urethra (acute) 098.0
    chronic or duration of 2 months or over 098.2
  vulva (acute) 098.0
    chronic or duration of 2 months or over 098.2
Gonocytoma (M9073/1)
  specified site - *see* Neoplasm, by site, uncertain behavior
  unspecified site
    female 236.2
    male 236.4
Gonorrhea 098.0
  acute 098.0
  Bartholin's gland (acute) 098.0
    chronic or duration of 2 months or over 098.2
  bladder (acute) 098.11
    chronic or duration of 2 months or over 098.31
  carrier (suspected of) V02.7
  cervix (acute) 098.15
    chronic or duration of 2 months or over 098.35

Gonorrhea (*Continued*)
  chronic 098.2
  complicating pregnancy, childbirth, or puerperium 647.1
    affecting fetus or newborn 760.2
  conjunctiva, conjunctivitis (neonatorum) 098.40
  contact V01.6
  Cowper's gland (acute) 098.0
    chronic or duration of 2 months or over 098.2
  duration of 2 months or over 098.2
  exposure to V01.6
  fallopian tube (chronic) 098.37
    acute 098.17
  genitourinary (acute) (organ) (system) (tract) 098.0
    chronic 098.2
    duration of 2 months or over 098.2
  kidney (acute) 098.19
    chronic or duration of 2 months or over 098.39
  ovary (acute) 098.19
    chronic or duration of 2 months or over 098.39
  pelvis (acute) 098.19
    chronic or duration of 2 months or over 098.39
  penis (acute) 098.0
    chronic or duration of 2 months or over 098.2
  prostate (acute) 098.12
    chronic or duration of 2 months or over 098.32
  seminal vesicle (acute) 098.14
    chronic or duration of 2 months or over 098.34
  specified site NEC - *see* Gonococcus
  spermatic cord (acute) 098.14
    chronic or duration of 2 months or over 098.34
  urethra (acute) 098.0
    chronic or duration of 2 months or over 098.2
  vagina (acute) 098.0
    chronic or duration of 2 months or over 098.2
  vas deferens (acute) 098.14
    chronic or duration of 2 months or over 098.34
  vulva (acute) 098.0
    chronic or duration of 2 months or over 098.2
Goodpasture's syndrome (pneumorenal) 446.21
Good's syndrome 279.06 ◀
Gopalan's syndrome (burning feet) 266.2
Gordon's disease (exudative enteropathy) 579.8
Gorlin-Chaudhry-Moss syndrome 759.89
Gougerot's syndrome (trisymptomatic) 709.1
Gougerot-Blum syndrome (pigmented purpuric lichenoid dermatitis) 709.1
Gougerot-Carteaud disease or syndrome (confluent reticulate papillomatosis) 701.8
Gougerot-Hailey-Hailey disease (benign familial chronic pemphigus) 757.39
Gougerot (-Houwer)-Sjögren syndrome (keratoconjunctivitis sicca) 710.2
Gouley's syndrome (constrictive pericarditis) 423.2
Goundou 102.6

Gout, gouty 274.9
  with specified manifestations NEC 274.89
  arthritis (acute) 274.0
  arthropathy 274.0
  degeneration, heart 274.82
  diathesis 274.9
  eczema 274.89
  episcleritis 274.89 [379.09]
  external ear (tophus) 274.81
  glomerulonephritis 274.10
  iritis 274.89 [364.11]
  joint 274.0
  kidney 274.10
  lead 984.9
    specified type of lead - *see* Table of Drugs and Chemicals
  nephritis 274.10
  neuritis 274.89 [357.4]
  phlebitis 274.89 [451.9]
  rheumatic 714.0
  saturnine 984.9
    specified type of lead - *see* Table of Drugs and Chemicals
  spondylitis 274.0
  synovitis 274.0
  syphilitic 095.8
  tophi 274.0
    ear 274.81
    heart 274.82
    specified site NEC 274.82
Gowers'
  muscular dystrophy 359.1
  syndrome (vasovagal attack) 780.2
Gowers-Paton-Kennedy syndrome 377.04
Gradenigo's syndrome 383.02
Graft-versus-host disease (bone marrow) 996.85
  due to organ transplant NEC - *see* Complications, transplant, organ
Graham Steell's murmur (pulmonic regurgitation) (*see also* Endocarditis, pulmonary) 424.3
Grain-handlers' disease or lung 495.8
Grain mite (itch) 133.8
Grand
  mal (idiopathic) (*see also* Epilepsy) 345.1
    hysteria of Charcôt 300.11
    nonrecurrent or isolated 780.39
  multipara
    affecting management of labor and delivery 659.4
    status only (not pregnant) V61.5
Granite workers' lung 502
Granular - *see also* condition
  inflammation, pharynx 472.1
  kidney (contracting) (*see also* Sclerosis, renal) 587
  liver - *see* Cirrhosis, liver
  nephritis - *see* Nephritis
Granulation tissue, abnormal - *see also* Granuloma
  abnormal or excessive 701.5
  postmastoidectomy cavity 383.33
  postoperative 701.5
  skin 701.5
Granulocytopenia, granulocytopenic (primary) 288.0
  malignant 288.0
Granuloma NEC 686.1
  abdomen (wall) 568.89
    skin (pyogenicum) 686.1
      from residual foreign body 709.4

Granuloma NEC *(Continued)*
annulare 695.89
anus 569.49
apical 522.6
appendix 543.9
aural 380.23
beryllium (skin) 709.4
  lung 503
bone *(see also* Osteomyelitis) 730.1
  eosinophilic 277.89
  from residual foreign body 733.99
canaliculus lacrimalis 375.81
cerebral 348.8
cholesterin, middle ear 385.82
coccidioidal (progressive) 114.3
  lung 114.4
  meninges 114.2
  primary (lung) 114.0
colon 569.89
conjunctiva 372.61
dental 522.6
ear, middle (cholesterin) 385.82
  with otitis media - *see* Otitis media
eosinophilic 277.89
  bone 277.89
  lung 277.89
  oral mucosa 528.9
exuberant 701.5
eyelid 374.89
facial
  lethal midline 446.3
  malignant 446.3
faciale 701.8
fissuratum (gum) 523.8
foot NEC 686.1
foreign body (in soft tissue) NEC
  728.82
  bone 733.99
  in operative wound 998.4
  muscle 728.82
  skin 709.4
  subcutaneous tissue 709.4
fungoides 202.1
gangraenescens 446.3
giant cell (central) (jaw) (reparative)
  526.3
  gingiva 523.8
  peripheral (gingiva) 523.8
gland (lymph) 289.3
Hodgkin's (M9661/3) 201.1
ileum 569.89
infectious NEC 136.9
inguinale (Donovan) 099.2
  venereal 099.2
intestine 569.89
iridocyclitis 364.10
jaw (bone) 526.3
  reparative giant cell 526.3
kidney *(see also* Infection, kidney) 590.9
lacrimal sac 375.81
larynx 478.79
lethal midline 446.3
lipid 277.89
lipoid 277.89
liver 572.8
lung (infectious) *(see also* Fibrosis,
  lung) 515
  coccidioidal 114.4
  eosinophilic 277.89
lymph gland 289.3
Majocchi's 110.6
malignant, face 446.3
mandible 526.3
mediastinum 519.3

Granuloma NEC *(Continued)*
midline 446.3
monilial 112.3
muscle 728.82
  from residual foreign body 728.82
nasal sinus *(see also* Sinusitis) 473.9
operation wound 998.59
  foreign body 998.4
  stitch (external) 998.89
    internal wound 998.89
  talc 998.7
oral mucosa, eosinophilic or pyogenic
  528.9
orbit, orbital 376.11
paracoccidioidal 116.1
penis, venereal 099.2
periapical 522.6
peritoneum 568.89
  due to ova of helminths NEC *(see*
    also Helminthiasis) 128.9
postmastoidectomy cavity 383.33
postoperative - *see* Granuloma, operation wound
prostate 601.8
pudendi (ulcerating) 099.2
pudendorum (ulcerative) 099.2
pulp, internal (tooth) 521.49 ◄▥
pyogenic, pyogenicum (skin) 686.1
  maxillary alveolar ridge 522.6
  oral mucosa 528.9
rectum 569.49
reticulohistiocytic 277.89
rubrum nasi 705.89
sarcoid 135
Schistosoma 120.9
septic (skin) 686.1
silica (skin) 709.4
sinus (accessory) (infectional) (nasal)
  (see also Sinusitis) 473.9
skin (pyogenicum) 686.1
  from foreign body or material 709.4
sperm 608.89
spine
  syphilitic (epidural) 094.89
  tuberculous *(see also* Tuberculosis)
    015.0 *[730.88]*
stitch (postoperative) 998.89
  internal wound 998.89
suppurative (skin) 686.1
suture (postoperative) 998.89
  internal wound 998.89
swimming pool 031.1
talc 728.82
  in operation wound 998.7
telangiectaticum (skin) 686.1
trichophyticum 110.6
tropicum 102.4
umbilicus 686.1
  newborn 771.4
urethra 599.84
uveitis 364.10
vagina 099.2
venereum 099.2
vocal cords 478.5
Wegener's (necrotizing respiratory
  granulomatosis) 446.4
Granulomatosis NEC 686.1
disciformis chronica et progressiva
  709.3
infantiseptica 771.2
lipoid 277.89
lipophagic, intestinal 040.2
miliary 027.0
necrotizing, respiratory 446.4

Granulomatosis NEC *(Continued)*
progressive, septic 288.1
Wegener's (necrotizing respiratory)
  446.4
Granulomatous tissue - *see* Granuloma
Granulosis rubra nasi 705.89
Graphite fibrosis (of lung) 503
Graphospasm 300.89
organic 333.84
Grating scapula 733.99
Gravel (urinary) *(see also* Calculus)
  592.9
Graves' disease (exophthalmic goiter)
  (see also Goiter, toxic) 242.0
Gravis - *see* condition
Grawitz's tumor (hypernephroma)
  (M8312/3) 189.0
Grayness, hair (premature) 704.3
congenital 757.4
Gray or grey syndrome (chlorampheni-
  col) (newborn) 779.4
Greenfield's disease 330.0
Green sickness 280.9
Greenstick fracture - *see* Fracture, by site
Greig's syndrome (hypertelorism) 756.0
Griesinger's disease *(see also* Ancylosto-
  miasis) 126.9
Grinders'
asthma 502
lung 502
phthisis *(see also* Tuberculosis) 011.4
Grinding, teeth 306.8
Grip
Dabney's 074.1
devil's 074.1
Grippe, grippal - *see also* Influenza
Balkan 083.0
intestinal 487.8
summer 074.8
Grippy cold 487.1
Grisel's disease 723.5
Groin - *see* condition
Grooved
nails (transverse) 703.8
tongue 529.5
  congenital 750.13
Ground itch 126.9
Growing pains, children 781.99
Growth (fungoid) (neoplastic) (new)
  (M8000/1) - *see also* Neoplasm, by
  site, unspecified nature
adenoid (vegetative) 474.12
benign (M8000/0) - *see* Neoplasm, by
  site, benign
fetal, poor 764.9
  affecting management of pregnancy
    656.5
malignant (M8000/3) - *see* Neoplasm,
  by site, malignant
rapid, childhood V21.0
secondary (M8000/6) - *see* Neoplasm,
  by site, malignant, secondary
GRSA (glycopeptide resistant staphylococcus aurerus) V09.8 ◄
Gruber's hernia - *see* Hernia, Gruber's
Gruby's disease (tinea tonsurans) 110.0
G-trisomy 758.0
Guama fever 066.3
Gubler (-Millard) paralysis or syndrome
  344.89
Guérin-Stern syndrome (arthrogryposis
  multiplex congenita) 754.89
Guertin's disease (electric chorea)
  049.8

ICD-9-CM

G

Vol. 2

Guillain-Barré disease or syndrome
357.0
Guinea worms (infection) (infestation)
125.7
Guinon's disease (motor-verbal tic)
307.23
Gull's disease (thyroid atrophy with
myxedema) 244.8
Gull and Sutton's disease - see Hypertension, kidney
Gum - see condition
Gumboil 522.7
Gumma (syphilitic) 095.9
artery 093.89
cerebral or spinal 094.89
bone 095.5
of yaws (late) 102.6
brain 094.89
cauda equina 094.89
central nervous system NEC 094.9
ciliary body 095.8 [364.11]
congenital 090.5
testis 090.5
eyelid 095.8 [373.5]
heart 093.89
intracranial 094.89
iris 095.8 [364.11]
kidney 095.4
larynx 095.8

Gumma (Continued)
leptomeninges 094.2
liver 095.3
meninges 094.2
myocardium 093.82
nasopharynx 095.8
neurosyphilitic 094.9
nose 095.8
orbit 095.8
palate (soft) 095.8
penis 095.8
pericardium 093.81
pharynx 095.8
pituitary 095.8
scrofulous (see also Tuberculosis) 017.0
skin 095.8
specified site NEC 095.8
spinal cord 094.89
tongue 095.8
tonsil 095.8
trachea 095.8
tuberculous (see also Tuberculosis)
017.0
ulcerative due to yaws 102.4
ureter 095.8
yaws 102.4
bone 102.6
Gunn's syndrome (jaw-winking syndrome) 742.8

Gunshot wound - see also Wound, open,
by site
fracture - see Fracture, by site, open
internal organs (abdomen, chest, or
pelvis) - see Injury, internal, by
site, with open wound
intracranial - see Laceration, brain,
with open intracranial wound
Günther's disease or syndrome (congenital erythropoietic porphyria)
277.1
Gustatory hallucination 780.1
Gynandrism 752.7
Gynandroblastoma (M8632/1)
specified site - see Neoplasm, by site,
uncertain behavior
unspecified site
female 236.2
male 236.4
Gynandromorphism 752.7
Gynandromorphism 752.7
Gynatresia (congenital) 752.49
Gynecoid pelvis, male 738.6
Gynecological examination
V72.31
for contraceptive maintenance
V25.40
Gynecomastia 611.1
Gynephobia 300.29
Gyrate scalp 757.39

H

Haas' disease (osteochondrosis head of humerus) 732.3

Habermann's disease (acute parapsoriasis varioliformis) 696.2

Habit, habituation
chorea 307.22
disturbance, child 307.9
drug (see also Dependence) 304.9
laxative (see also Abuse, drugs, nondependent) 305.9
spasm 307.20
  chronic 307.22
  transient (of childhood) 307.21 ◀▥
tic 307.20
  chronic 307.22
  transient (of childhood) 307.21 ◀▥
use of
  nonprescribed drugs (see also Abuse, drugs, nondependent) 305.9
  patent medicines (see also Abuse, drugs, nondependent) 305.9
vomiting 536.2

Hadfield-Clarke syndrome (pancreatic infantilism) 577.8

Haff disease 985.1

Hag teeth, tooth 524.39 ◀▥

Hageman factor defect, deficiency, or disease (see also Defect, coagulation) 286.3

Haglund's disease (osteochondrosis os tibiale externum) 732.5

Haglund-Läwen-Fründ syndrome 717.89

Hagner's disease (hypertrophic pulmonary osteoarthropathy) 731.2

Hailey-Hailey disease (benign familial chronic pemphigus) 757.39

Hair - see also condition
plucking 307.9

Hairball in stomach 935.2

Hairy black tongue 529.3

Half vertebra 756.14

Halitosis 784.9

Hallermann-Streiff syndrome 756.0

Hallervorden-Spatz disease or syndrome 333.0

Hallopeau's
acrodermatitis (continua) 696.1
disease (lichen sclerosis et atrophicus) 701.0

Hallucination (auditory) (gustatory) (olfactory) (tactile) 780.1
alcohol-induced 291.3 ◀▥
drug-induced 292.12
visual 368.16

Hallucinosis 298.9
alcohol-induced (acute) 291.3 ◀▥
drug-induced 292.12

Hallus - see Hallux

Hallux 735.9
malleus (acquired) 735.3
rigidus (acquired) 735.2
  congenital 755.66
  late effects of rickets 268.1
valgus (acquired) 735.0
  congenital 755.66
varus (acquired) 735.1
  congenital 755.66

Halo, visual 368.15

Hamartoblastoma 759.6

Hamartoma 759.6
epithelial (gingival), odontogenic, central, or peripheral (M9321/0) 213.1
  upper jaw (bone) 213.0
vascular 757.32

Hamartosis, hamartoses NEC 759.6

Hamman's disease or syndrome (spontaneous mediastinal emphysema) 518.1

Hamman-Rich syndrome (diffuse interstitial pulmonary fibrosis) 516.3

Hammer toe (acquired) 735.4
congenital 755.66
late effects of rickets 268.1

Hand - see condition

Hand-Schüller-Christian disease or syndrome (chronic histiocytosis X) 277.89

Hand-foot syndrome 282.61

Hanging (asphyxia) (strangulation) (suffocation) 994.7

Hangnail (finger) (with lymphangitis) 681.02

Hangover (alcohol) (see also Abuse, drugs, nondependent) 305.0

Hanot's cirrhosis or disease - see Cirrhosis, biliary

Hanot-Chauffard (-Troisier) syndrome (bronze diabetes) 275.0

Hansen's disease (leprosy) 030.9
benign form 030.1
malignant form 030.0

Harada's disease or syndrome 363.22

Hard chancre 091.0

Hard firm prostate 600.10
with urinary retention 600.11

Hardening
artery - see Arteriosclerosis
brain 348.8
liver 571.8

Hare's syndrome (M8010/3) (carcinoma, pulmonary apex) 162.3

Harelip (see also Cleft, lip) 749.10

Harkavy's syndrome 446.0

Harlequin (fetus) 757.1
color change syndrome 779.89

Harley's disease (intermittent hemoglobinuria) 283.2

Harris'
lines 733.91
syndrome (organic hyperinsulinism) 251.1

Hart's disease or syndrome (pellagra-cerebellar ataxia-renal aminoaciduria) 270.0

Hartmann's pouch (abnormal sacculation of gallbladder neck) 575.8
of intestine V44.3
  attention to V55.3

Hartnup disease (pellagra-cerebellar ataxia-renal aminoaciduria) 270.0

Harvester lung 495.0

Hashimoto's disease or struma (struma lymphomatosa) 245.2

Hassall-Henle bodies (corneal warts) 371.41

Haut mal (see also Epilepsy) 345.1

Haverhill fever 026.1

Hawaiian wood rose dependence 304.5

Hawkins' keloid 701.4

Hay
asthma (see also Asthma) 493.0
fever (allergic) (with rhinitis) 477.9
  with asthma (bronchial) (see also Asthma) 493.0
  allergic, due to grass, pollen, ragweed, or tree 477.0

Hay (Continued)
fever (Continued)
  conjunctivitis 372.05
  due to
    dander, animal (cat) (dog) 477.2 ◀▥
    dust 477.8
    fowl 477.8
    hair, animal (cat) (dog) 477.2 ◀
    pollen 477.0
    specified allergen other than pollen 477.8

Hayem-Faber syndrome (achlorhydric anemia) 280.9

Hayem-Widal syndrome (acquired hemolytic jaundice) 283.9

Haygarth's nodosities 715.04

Hazard-Crile tumor (M8350/3) 193

Hb (abnormal)
disease - see Disease, hemoglobin
trait - see Trait

H disease 270.0

Head - see also condition
banging 307.3

Headache 784.0
allergic 346.2
cluster 346.2
due to
  loss, spinal fluid 349.0
  lumbar puncture 349.0
  saddle block 349.0
emotional 307.81
histamine 346.2
lumbar puncture 349.0
menopausal 627.2
migraine 346.9
nonorganic origin 307.81
postspinal 349.0
psychogenic 307.81
psychophysiologic 307.81
sick 346.1
spinal 349.0
  complicating labor and delivery 668.8
  postpartum 668.8
spinal fluid loss 349.0
tension 307.81
vascular 784.0
  migraine type 346.9
vasomotor 346.9

Health
advice V65.4
audit V70.0
checkup V70.0
education V65.4
hazard (see also History of) V15.9
  specified cause NEC V15.89
instruction V65.4
services provided because (of)
  boarding school residence V60.6
  holiday relief for person providing home care V60.5
  inadequate
    housing V60.1
    resources V60.2
  lack of housing V60.0
  no care available in home V60.4
  person living alone V60.3
  poverty V60.3
  residence in institution V60.6
  specified cause NEC V60.8
  vacation relief for person providing home care V60.5

Healthy
donor (see also Donor) V59.9
infant or child
  accompanying sick mother V65.0

ICD-9-CM

≡

Vol. 2

Healthy *(Continued)*
  infant or child *(Continued)*
    receiving care V20.1
  person
    accompanying sick relative V65.0
    admitted for sterilization V25.2
    receiving prophylactic inoculation or
      vaccination *(see also* Vaccination,
      prophylactic) V05.9
Hearing examination V72.1
Heart - *see* condition
Heartburn 787.1
  psychogenic 306.4
Heat (effects) 992.9
  apoplexy 992.0
  burn - *see also* Burn, by site
    from sun *(see also* Sunburn) 692.71
  collapse 992.1
  cramps 992.2
  dermatitis or eczema 692.89
  edema 992.7
  erythema - *see* Burn, by site
  excessive 992.9
    specified effect NEC 992.8
  exhaustion 992.5
    anhydrotic 992.3
    due to
      salt (and water) depletion 992.4
      water depletion 992.3
  fatigue (transient) 992.6
  fever 992.0
  hyperpyrexia 992.0
  prickly 705.1
  prostration - *see* Heat, exhaustion
  pyrexia 992.0
  rash 705.1
  specified effect NEC 992.8
  stroke 992.0
  sunburn *(see also* Sunburn) 692.71
  syncope 992.1
Heavy-chain disease 273.2
Heavy-for-dates (fetus or infant) 766.1
  4500 grams or more 766.0
  exceptionally 766.0
Hebephrenia, hebephrenic (acute) *(see
    also* Schizophrenia) 295.1
  dementia (praecox) *(see also* Schizo-
    phrenia) 295.1
  schizophrenia *(see also* Schizophrenia) 295.1
Heberden's
  disease or nodes 715.04
  syndrome (angina pectoris) 413.9
Hebra's disease
  dermatitis exfoliativa 695.89
  erythema multiforme exudativum 695.1
  pityriasis 695.89
    maculata et circinata 696.3
    rubra 695.89
      pilaris 696.4
  prurigo 698.2
Hebra, nose 040.1
Hedinger's syndrome (malignant carci-
    noid) 259.2
Heel - *see* condition
Heerfordt's disease or syndrome (uveo-
    parotitis) 135
Hegglin's anomaly or syndrome 288.2
Heidenhain's disease 290.10
  with dementia 290.10
Heilmeyer-Schoner disease (M9842/3)
    207.1
Heine-Medin disease *(see also* Poliomye-
    litis) 045.9
Heinz-body anemia, congenital 282.7

Heller's disease or syndrome (infantile
    psychosis) *(see also* Psychosis, child-
    hood) 299.1
H.E.L.L.P 642.5
Helminthiasis *(see also* Infestation, by
    specific parasite) 128.9
  Ancylostoma *(see also* Ancylostoma)
    126.9
  intestinal 127.9
    mixed types (types classifiable to
      more than one of the categories
      120.0-127.7) 127.8
    specified type 127.7
  mixed types (intestinal) (types classifi-
    able to more than one of the cate-
    gories 120.0-127.7) 127.8
  Necator americanus 126.1
  specified type NEC 128.8
  Trichinella 124
Heloma 700
Hemangioblastoma (M9161/1) - *see also*
    Neoplasm, connective tissue, uncer-
    tain behavior
  malignant (M9161/3) - *see* Neoplasm,
    connective tissue, malignant
Hemangioblastomatosis, cerebelloretinal
    759.6
Hemangioendothelioma (M9130/1) - *see
    also* Neoplasm, by site, uncertain be-
    havior
  benign (M9130/0) 228.00
  bone (diffuse) (M9130/3) - *see* Neo-
    plasm, bone, malignant
  malignant (M9130/3) - *see* Neoplasm,
    connective tissue, malignant
  nervous system (M9130/0) 228.09
Hemangioendotheliosarcoma (M9130/3)
  - *see* Neoplasm, connective tissue,
    malignant
Hemangiofibroma (M9160/0) - *see* Neo-
    plasm, by site, benign
Hemangiolipoma (M8861/0) - *see* Lipoma
Hemangioma (M9120/0) 228.00
  arteriovenous (M9123/0) - *see* Heman-
    gioma, by site
  brain 228.02
  capillary (M9131/0) - *see* Hemangioma,
    by site
  cavernous (M9121/0) - *see* Heman-
    gioma, by site
  central nervous system NEC 228.09
  choroid 228.09
  heart 228.09
  infantile (M9131/0) - *see* Hemangioma,
    by site
  intra-abdominal structures 228.04
  intracranial structures 228.02
  intramuscular (M9132/0) - *see* Heman-
    gioma, by site
  iris 228.09
  juvenile (M9131/0) - *see* Hemangioma,
    by site
  malignant (M9120/3) - *see* Neoplasm,
    connective tissue, malignant
  meninges 228.09
    brain 228.02
    spinal cord 228.09
  peritoneum 228.04
  placenta - *see* Placenta, abnormal
  plexiform (M9131/0) - *see* Heman-
    gioma, by site
  racemose (M9123/0) - *see* Heman-
    gioma, by site
  retina 228.03
  retroperitoneal tissue 228.04

Hemangioma *(Continued)*
  sclerosing (M8832/0) - *see* Neoplasm,
    skin, benign
  simplex (M9131/0) - *see* Hemangioma,
    by site
  skin and subcutaneous tissue 228.01
  specified site NEC 228.09
  spinal cord 228.09
  venous (M9122/0) - *see* Hemangioma,
    by site
  verrucous keratotic (M9142/0) - *see*
    Hemangioma, by site
Hemangiomatosis (systemic) 757.32
  involving single site - *see* Hemangioma
Hemangiopericytoma (M9150/1) - *see
    also* Neoplasm, connective tissue, un-
    certain behavior
  benign (M9150/0) - *see* Neoplasm, con-
    nective tissue, benign
  malignant (M9150/3) - *see* Neoplasm,
    connective tissue, malignant
Hemangiosarcoma (M9120/3) - *see* Neo-
    plasm, connective tissue, malignant
Hemarthrosis (nontraumatic) 719.10
  ankle 719.17
  elbow 719.12
  foot 719.17
  hand 719.14
  hip 719.15
  knee 719.16
  multiple sites 719.19
  pelvic region 719.15
  shoulder (region) 719.11
  specified site NEC 719.18
  traumatic - *see* Sprain, by site
  wrist 719.13
Hematemesis 578.0
  with ulcer - *see* Ulcer, by site, with
    hemorrhage
  due to S. japonicum 120.2
  Goldstein's (familial hemorrhagic tel-
    angiectasia) 448.0
  newborn 772.4
    due to swallowed maternal blood
      777.3
Hematidrosis 705.89
Hematinuria *(see also* Hemoglobinuria)
    791.2
  malarial 084.8
  paroxysmal 283.2
Hematite miners' lung 503
Hematobilia 576.8
Hematocele (congenital) (diffuse) (idio-
    pathic) 608.83
  broad ligament 620.7
  canal of Nuck 629.0
  cord, male 608.83
  fallopian tube 620.8
  female NEC 629.0
  ischiorectal 569.89
  male NEC 608.83
  ovary 629.0
  pelvis, pelvic
    female 629.0
      with ectopic pregnancy *(see also*
        Pregnancy, ectopic) 633.90
        with intrauterine pregnancy
          633.91
    male 608.83
  periuterine 629.0
  retrouterine 629.0
  scrotum 608.83
  spermatic cord (diffuse) 608.83
  testis 608.84
  traumatic - *see* Injury, internal, pelvis

◀ **New**   ◀▥ **Revised**

Hematocele (*Continued*)
 tunica vaginalis 608.83
 uterine ligament 629.0
 uterus 621.4
 vagina 623.6
 vulva 624.5
Hematocephalus 742.4
Hematochezia (*see also* Melena) 578.1
Hematochyluria (*see also* Infestation, filarial) 125.9
Hematocolpos 626.8
Hematocornea 371.12
Hematogenous - *see* condition
Hematoma (skin surface intact) (traumatic) - *see also* Contusion

Note   Hematomas are coded according to origin and the nature and site of the hematoma or the accompanying injury. Hematomas of unspecified origin are coded as injuries of the sites involved, except:

 (a) hematomas of genital organs which are coded as diseases of the organ involved unless they complicate pregnancy or delivery
 (b) hematomas of the eye which are coded as diseases of the eye.

For late effect of hematoma classifiable to 920-924 *see* Late, effect, contusion.

with
  crush injury - *see* Crush
  fracture - *see* Fracture, by site
  injury of internal organs - *see also*
    Injury, internal, by site
    kidney - *see* Hematoma, kidney,
      traumatic
    liver - *see* Hematoma, liver, traumatic
    spleen - *see* Hematoma, spleen
  nerve injury - *see* Injury, nerve
  open wound - *see* Wound, open, by
    site
  skin surface intact - *see* Contusion
 abdomen (wall) - *see* Contusion, abdomen
 amnion 658.8
 aorta, dissecting 441.00
  abdominal 441.02
  thoracic 441.01
  thoracoabdominal 441.03
 arterial (complicating trauma) 904.9
  specified site - *see* Injury, blood vessel, by site
 auricle (ear) 380.31
 birth injury 767.8
  skull 767.19
 brain (traumatic) 853.0

Note   Use the following fifth-digit subclassification with categories 851-854:

 0   unspecified state of consciousness
 1   with no loss of consciousness
 2   with brief [less than one hour]
   loss of consciousness
 3   with moderate [1-24 hours]
   loss of consciousness

Hematoma (*Continued*)
 4   with prolonged [more than 24
   hours] loss of consciousness
   and return to pre-existing conscious level
 5   with prolonged [more than 24
   hours] loss of consciousness,
   without return to pre-existing
   conscious level

Use fifth-digit 5 to designate when a patient is unconscious and dies before regaining consciousness, regardless of the duration of the loss of consciousness

 6   with loss of consciousness of
   unspecified duration
 9   with concussion, unspecified

 with
  cerebral
   contusion - *see* Contusion, brain
   laceration - *see* Laceration, brain
  open intracranial wound 853.1
  skull fracture - *see* Fracture, skull,
   by site
 extradural or epidural 852.4
  with open intracranial wound 852.5
  fetus or newborn 767.0
  nontraumatic 432.0
 fetus or newborn NEC 767.0
 nontraumatic (*see also* Hemorrhage,
   brain) 431
  epidural or extradural 432.0
  newborn NEC 772.8
  subarachnoid, arachnoid, or meningeal (*see also* Hemorrhage,
   subarachnoid) 430
  subdural (*see also* Hemorrhage,
   subdural) 432.1
 subarachnoid, arachnoid, or meningeal 852.0
  with open intracranial wound 852.1
  fetus or newborn 772.2
  nontraumatic (*see also* Hemorrhage, subarachnoid) 430
 subdural 852.2
  with open intracranial wound 852.3
  fetus or newborn (localized) 767.0
  nontraumatic (*see also* Hemorrhage, subdural) 432.1
 breast (nontraumatic) 611.8
 broad ligament (nontraumatic) 620.7
  complicating delivery 665.7
  traumatic - *see* Injury, internal, broad
   ligament
 calcified NEC 959.9
 capitis 920
  due to birth injury 767.19
  newborn 767.19
 cerebral - *see* Hematoma, brain
 cesarean section wound 674.3
 chorion - *see* Placenta, abnormal
 complicating delivery (perineum)
   (vulva) 664.5
  pelvic 665.7
  vagina 665.7
 corpus
  cavernosum (nontraumatic) 607.82
  luteum (nontraumatic) (ruptured)
   620.1
 dura (mater) - *see* Hematoma, brain,
   subdural
 epididymis (nontraumatic) 608.83

Hematoma (*Continued*)
 epidural (traumatic) - *see also* Hematoma, brain, extradural
  spinal - *see* Injury, spinal, by site
 episiotomy 674.3
 external ear 380.31
 extradural - *see also* Hematoma, brain,
   extradural
  fetus or newborn 767.0
  nontraumatic 432.0
   fetus or newborn 767.0
 fallopian tube 620.8
 genital organ (nontraumatic)
  female NEC 629.8
  male NEC 608.83
  traumatic (external site) 922.4
   internal - *see* Injury, internal, genital organ
 graafian follicle (ruptured) 620.0
 internal organs (abdomen, chest, or
   pelvis) - *see also* Injury, internal,
   by site
  kidney - *see* Hematoma, kidney,
   traumatic
  liver - *see* Hematoma, liver, traumatic
  spleen - *see* Hematoma, spleen
 intracranial - *see* Hematoma, brain
 kidney, cystic 593.81
  traumatic 866.01
   with open wound into cavity
    866.11
 labia (nontraumatic) 624.5
 lingual (and other parts of neck, scalp,
   or face, except eye) 920
 liver (subcapsular) 573.8
  birth injury 767.8
  fetus or newborn 767.8
  traumatic NEC 864.01
   with
    laceration - *see* Laceration, liver
    open wound into cavity 864.11
 mediastinum - *see* Injury, internal, mediastinum
 meninges, meningeal (brain) - *see also*
   Hematoma, brain, subarachnoid
  spinal - *see* Injury, spinal, by site
 mesosalpinx (nontraumatic) 620.8
  traumatic - *see* Injury, internal, pelvis
 muscle (traumatic) - *see* Contusion, by
   site
 nasal (septum) (and other part(s) of
   neck, scalp, or face, except eye)
   920
 obstetrical surgical wound 674.3
 orbit, orbital (nontraumatic) 376.32
  traumatic 921.2
 ovary (corpus luteum) (nontraumatic)
   620.1
  traumatic - *see* Injury, internal,
   ovary
 pelvis (female) (nontraumatic) 629.8
  complicating delivery 665.7
  male 608.83
  traumatic - *see also* Injury, internal,
   pelvis
   specified organ NEC (*see also* Injury, internal, pelvis) 867.6
 penis (nontraumatic) 607.82
 pericranial (and neck, or face any part,
   except eye) 920
  due to injury at birth 767.19
 perineal wound (obstetrical) 674.3
  complicating delivery 664.5

ICD-9-CM

H

Vol. 2

Hematoma *(Continued)*
  perirenal, cystic 593.81
  pinna 380.31
  placenta - *see* Placenta, abnormal
  postoperative 998.12
  retroperitoneal (nontraumatic) 568.81
    traumatic - *see* Injury, internal, retro-
      peritoneum
  retropubic, male 568.81
  scalp (and neck, or face any part, ex-
    cept eye) 920
    fetus or newborn 767.19
  scrotum (nontraumatic) 608.83
    traumatic 922.4
  seminal vesicle (nontraumatic) 608.83
    traumatic - *see* Injury, internal, semi-
      nal, vesicle
  spermatic cord - *see also* Injury, inter-
    nal, spermatic cord
    nontraumatic 608.83
  spinal (cord) (meninges) - *see also* In-
    jury, spinal, by site
    fetus or newborn 767.4
    nontraumatic 336.1
  spleen 865.01
    with
      laceration - *see* Laceration, spleen
      open wound into cavity 865.11
  sternocleidomastoid, birth injury
    767.8
  sternomastoid, birth injury 767.8
  subarachnoid - *see also* Hematoma,
    brain, subarachnoid
    fetus or newborn 772.2
    nontraumatic (*see also* Hemorrhage,
      subarachnoid) 430
      newborn 772.2
  subdural - *see also* Hematoma, brain,
    subdural
    fetus or newborn (localized) 767.0
    nontraumatic (*see also* Hemorrhage,
      subdural) 432.1
  subperiosteal (syndrome) 267
    traumatic - *see* Hematoma, by site
  superficial, fetus or newborn 772.6
  syncytium - *see* Placenta, abnormal
  testis (nontraumatic) 608.83
    birth injury 767.8
    traumatic 922.4
  tunica vaginalis (nontraumatic) 608.83
  umbilical cord 663.6
    affecting fetus or newborn 762.6
  uterine ligament (nontraumatic) 620.7
    traumatic - *see* Injury, internal, pelvis
  uterus 621.4
    traumatic - *see* Injury, internal, pelvis
  vagina (nontraumatic) (ruptured) 623.6
    complicating delivery 665.7
    traumatic 922.4
  vas deferens (nontraumatic) 608.83
    traumatic - *see* Injury, internal, vas
      deferens
  vitreous 379.23
  vocal cord 920
  vulva (nontraumatic) 624.5
    complicating delivery 664.5
    fetus or newborn 767.8
    traumatic 922.4
Hematometra 621.4
Hematomyelia 336.1
  with fracture of vertebra (*see also* Frac-
    ture, vertebra, by site, with spinal
    cord injury) 806.8
  fetus or newborn 767.4

Hematomyelitis 323.9
  late effect - *see* category 326
Hematoperitoneum (*see also* Hemoperitoneum) 568.81
Hematopneumothorax (*see also* Hemothorax) 511.8
Hematoporphyria (acquired) (congenital)
  277.1
Hematoporphyrinuria (acquired) (congenital) 277.1
Hematorachis, hematorrhachis 336.1
  fetus or newborn 767.4
Hematosalpinx 620.8
  with
    ectopic pregnancy (*see also* categories
      633.0-633.9) 639.2
    molar pregnancy (*see also* categories
      630-632) 639.2
  infectional (*see also* Salpingo-oophori-
    tis) 614.2
Hematospermia 608.82
Hematothorax (*see also* Hemothorax)
  511.8
Hematotympanum 381.03
Hematuria (benign) (essential) (idiopathic) 599.7
  due to S. hematobium 120.0
  endemic 120.0
  intermittent 599.7
  malarial 084.8
  paroxysmal 599.7
  sulfonamide
    correct substance properly adminis-
      tered 599.7
    overdose or wrong substance given
      or taken 961.0
  tropical (bilharziasis) 120.0
  tuberculous (*see also* Tuberculosis)
    016.9
Hematuric bilious fever 084.8
Hemeralopia 368.10
Hemiabiotrophy 799.89
Hemi-akinesia 781.8
Hemianalgesia (*see also* Disturbance, sensation) 782.0
Hemianencephaly 740.0
Hemianesthesia (*see also* Disturbance,
  sensation) 782.0
Hemianopia, hemianopsia (altitudinal)
  (homonymous) 368.46
  binasal 368.47
  bitemporal 368.47
  heteronymous 368.47
  syphilitic 095.8
Hemiasomatognosia 307.9
Hemiathetosis 781.0
Hemiatrophy 799.89
  cerebellar 334.8
  face 349.89
    progressive 349.89
  fascia 728.9
  leg 728.2
  tongue 529.8
Hemiballism(us) 333.5
Hemiblock (cardiac) (heart) (left) 426.2
Hemicardia 746.89
Hemicephalus, hemicephaly 740.0
Hemichorea 333.5
Hemicrania 346.9
  congenital malformation 740.0
Hemidystrophy - *see* Hemiatrophy
Hemiectromelia 755.4
Hemihypalgesia (*see also* Disturbance,
  sensation) 782.0

Hemihypertrophy (congenital) 759.89
  cranial 756.0
Hemihypesthesia (*see also* Disturbance,
  sensation) 782.0
Hemi-inattention 781.8
Hemimelia 755.4
  lower limb 755.30
    paraxial (complete) (incomplete) (in-
      tercalary) (terminal) 755.32
      fibula 755.37
      tibia 755.36
    transverse (complete) (partial) 755.31
  upper limb 755.20
    paraxial (complete) (incomplete) (in-
      tercalary) (terminal) 755.22
      radial 755.26
      ulnar 755.27
    transverse (complete) (partial) 755.21
Hemiparalysis (*see also* Hemiplegia)
  342.9
Hemiparesis (*see also* Hemiplegia) 342.9
Hemiparesthesia (*see also* Disturbance,
  sensation) 782.0
Hemiplegia 342.9
  acute (*see also* Disease, cerebrovascular,
    acute) 436
  alternans facialis 344.89
  apoplectic (*see also* Disease, cerebrovas-
    cular, acute) 436
    late effect or residual
      affecting
        dominant side 438.21
        nondominant side 438.22
        unspecified side 438.20
  arteriosclerotic 437.0
    late effect or residual
      affecting
        dominant side 438.21
        nondominant side 438.22
        unspecified side 438.20
  ascending (spinal) NEC 344.89
  attack (*see also* Disease, cerebrovascu-
    lar, acute) 436
  brain, cerebral (current episode) 437.8
    congenital 343.1
  cerebral - *see* Hemiplegia, brain
  congenital (cerebral) (spastic) (spinal)
    343.1
  conversion neurosis (hysterical) 300.11
  cortical - *see* Hemiplegia, brain
  due to
    arteriosclerosis 437.0
      late effect or residual
        affecting
          dominant side 438.21
          nondominant side 438.22
          unspecified side 438.20
    cerebrovascular lesion (*see also* Dis-
      ease, cerebrovascular, acute) 436
      late effect
        affecting
          dominant side 438.21
          nondominant side 438.22
          unspecified side 438.20
  embolic (current) (*see also* Embolism,
    brain) 434.1
    late effect
      affecting
        dominant side 438.21
        nondominant side 438.22
        unspecified side 438.20
  flaccid 342.0
  hypertensive (current episode) 437.8
  infantile (postnatal) 343.4

◀ **New**   ◀▥ **Revised**

Hemiplegia (Continued)
late effect
birth injury, intracranial or spinal
343.4
cerebrovascular lesion - see Late effect(s) (of) cerebrovascular disease
viral encephalitis 139.0
middle alternating NEC 344.89
newborn NEC 767.0
seizure (current episode) (see also Disease, cerebrovascular, acute) 436
spastic 342.1
congenital or infantile 343.1
specified NEC 342.8
thrombotic (current) (see also Thrombosis, brain) 434.0
late effect - see Late effect(s) (of) cerebrovascular disease
Hemisection, spinal cord - see Fracture, vertebra, by site, with spinal cord injury
Hemispasm 781.0
facial 781.0
Hemispatial neglect 781.8
Hemisporosis 117.9
Hemitremor 781.0
Hemivertebra 756.14
Hemobilia 576.8
Hemocholecyst 575.8
Hemochromatosis (acquired) (diabetic) (hereditary) (liver) (myocardium) (primary idiopathic) (secondary) 275.0
with refractory anemia 285.0
Hemodialysis V56.0
Hemoglobin - see also condition
abnormal (disease) - see Disease, hemoglobin
AS genotype 282.5
fetal, hereditary persistence 282.7
high-oxygen-affinity 289.0
low NEC 285.9
S (Hb-S), heterozygous 282.5
Hemoglobinemia 283.2
due to blood transfusion NEC 999.8
bone marrow 996.85
paroxysmal 283.2
Hemoglobinopathy (mixed) (see also Disease, hemoglobin) 282.7
with thalassemia 282.49
sickle-cell 282.60
with thalassemia (without crisis) 282.41
with
crisis 282.42
vaso-occlusive pain 282.42
Hemoglobinuria, hemoglobinuric 791.2
with anemia, hemolytic, acquired (chronic) NEC 283.2
cold (agglutinin) (paroxysmal) (with Raynaud's syndrome) 283.2
due to
exertion 283.2
hemolysis (from external causes) NEC 283.2
exercise 283.2
fever (malaria) 084.8
infantile 791.2
intermittent 283.2
malarial 084.8
march 283.2
nocturnal (paroxysmal) 283.2
paroxysmal (cold) (nocturnal) 283.2
Hemolymphangioma (M9175/0) 228.1

Hemolysis
fetal - see Jaundice, fetus or newborn
intravascular (disseminated) NEC 286.6
with
abortion - see Abortion, by type, with hemorrhage, delayed or excessive
ectopic pregnancy (see also categories 633.0-633.9) 639.1
hemorrhage of pregnancy 641.3
affecting fetus or newborn 762.1
molar pregnancy (see also categories 630-632) 639.1
acute 283.2
following
abortion 639.1
ectopic or molar pregnancy 639.1
neonatal - see Jaundice, fetus or newborn
transfusion NEC 999.8
bone marrow 996.85
Hemolytic - see also condition
anemia - see Anemia, hemolytic
uremic syndrome 283.11
Hemometra 621.4
Hemopericardium (with effusion) 423.0
newborn 772.8
traumatic (see also Hemothorax, traumatic) 860.2
with open wound into thorax 860.3
Hemoperitoneum 568.81
infectional (see also Peritonitis) 567.2
traumatic - see Injury, internal, peritoneum
Hemophilia (familial) (hereditary) 286.0
A 286.0
carrier (asymptomatic) V83.01
symptomatic V83.02
acquired 286.5
B (Leyden) 286.1
C 286.2
calcipriva (see also Fibrinolysis) 286.7
classical 286.0
nonfamilial 286.7
secondary 286.5 ◀
vascular 286.4
Hemophilus influenzae NEC 041.5
arachnoiditis (basic) (brain) (spinal) 320.0
late effect - see category 326
bronchopneumonia 482.2
cerebral ventriculitis 320.0
late effect - see category 326
cerebrospinal inflammation 320.0
late effect - see category 326
infection NEC 041.5
leptomeningitis 320.0
late effect - see category 326
meningitis (cerebral) (cerebrospinal) (spinal) 320.0
late effect - see category 326
meningomyelitis 320.0
late effect - see category 326
pachymeningitis (adhesive) (fibrous) (hemorrhagic) (hypertrophic) (spinal) 320.0
late effect - see category 326
pneumonia (broncho-) 482.2
Hemophthalmos 360.43
Hemopneumothorax (see also Hemothorax) 511.8
traumatic 860.4
with open wound into thorax 860.5
Hemoptysis 786.3
due to Paragonimus (westermani) 121.2
newborn 770.3
tuberculous (see also Tuberculosis, pulmonary) 011.9

Hemorrhage, hemorrhagic (nontraumatic) 459.0
abdomen 459.0
accidental (antepartum) 641.2
affecting fetus or newborn 762.1
adenoid 474.8
adrenal (capsule) (gland) (medulla) 255.4
newborn 772.5
after labor - see Hemorrhage, postpartum
alveolar
lung, newborn 770.3
process 525.8
alveolus 525.8
amputation stump (surgical) 998.11
secondary, delayed 997.69
anemia (chronic) 280.0
acute 285.1
antepartum - see Hemorrhage, pregnancy
anus (sphincter) 569.3
apoplexy (stroke) 432.9
arachnoid - see Hemorrhage, subarachnoid
artery NEC 459.0
brain (see also Hemorrhage, brain) 431
middle meningeal - see Hemorrhage, subarachnoid
basilar (ganglion) (see also Hemorrhage, brain) 431
bladder 596.8
blood dyscrasia 289.9
bowel 578.9
newborn 772.4
brain (miliary) (nontraumatic) 431
with
birth injury 767.0
arachnoid - see Hemorrhage, subarachnoid
due to
birth injury 767.0
rupture of aneurysm (congenital) (see also Hemorrhage, subarachnoid) 430
mycotic 431
syphilis 094.89
epidural or extradural - see Hemorrhage, extradural
fetus or newborn (anoxic) (hypoxic) (due to birth trauma) (nontraumatic) 767.0
intraventricular 772.10
grade I 772.11
grade II 772.12
grade III 772.13
grade IV 772.14
iatrogenic 997.02
postoperative 997.02
puerperal, postpartum, childbirth 674.0
stem 431
subarachnoid, arachnoid, or meningeal - see Hemorrhage, subarachnoid
subdural - see Hemorrhage, subdural
traumatic NEC 853.0

Note Use the following fifth-digit subclassification with categories 851-854:

0 unspecified state of consciousness

1 with no loss of consciousness

Hemorrhage, hemorrhagic (*Continued*)

> 2   with brief [less than one hour] loss of consciousness
> 3   with moderate [1-24 hours] loss of consciousness
> 4   with prolonged [more than 24 hours] loss of consciousness and return to pre-existing conscious level
> 5   with prolonged [more than 24 hours] loss of consciousness, without return to pre-existing conscious level
>
> Use fifth-digit 5 to designate when a patient is unconscious and dies before regaining consciousness, regardless of the duration of the loss of consciousness
>
> 6   with loss of consciousness of unspecified duration
> 9   with concussion, unspecified

   with
      cerebral
         contusion - *see* Contusion, brain
         laceration - *see* Laceration, brain
      open intracranial wound 853.1
      skull fracture - *see* Fracture, skull, by site
   extradural or epidural 852.4
      with open intracranial wound 852.5
   subarachnoid 852.0
      with open intracranial wound 852.1
   subdural 852.2
      with open intracranial wound 852.3
breast 611.79
bronchial tube - *see* Hemorrhage, lung
bronchopulmonary - *see* Hemorrhage, lung
bronchus (cause unknown) (*see also* Hemorrhage, lung) 786.3
bulbar (*see also* Hemorrhage, brain) 431
bursa 727.89
capillary 448.9
   primary 287.8
capsular - *see* Hemorrhage, brain
cardiovascular 429.89
cecum 578.9
cephalic (*see also* Hemorrhage, brain) 431
cerebellar (*see also* Hemorrhage, brain) 431
cerebellum (*see also* Hemorrhage, brain) 431
cerebral (*see also* Hemorrhage, brain) 431
   fetus or newborn (anoxic) (traumatic) 767.0
cerebromeningeal (*see also* Hemorrhage, brain) 431
cerebrospinal (*see also* Hemorrhage, brain) 431
cerebrum (*see also* Hemorrhage, brain) 431
cervix (stump) (uteri) 622.8
cesarean section wound 674.3
chamber, anterior (eye) 364.41
childbirth - *see* Hemorrhage, complicating, delivery
choroid 363.61
   expulsive 363.62

Hemorrhage, hemorrhagic (*Continued*)

ciliary body 364.41
cochlea 386.8
colon - *see* Hemorrhage, intestine
complicating
   delivery 641.9
      affecting fetus or newborn 762.1
      associated with
         afibrinogenemia 641.3
            affecting fetus or newborn 763.89
         coagulation defect 641.3
            affecting fetus or newborn 763.89
         hyperfibrinolysis 641.3
            affecting fetus or newborn 763.89
         hypofibrinogenemia 641.3
            affecting fetus or newborn 763.89
      due to
         low-lying placenta 641.1
            affecting fetus or newborn 762.0
         placenta previa 641.1
            affecting fetus or newborn 762.0
         premature separation of placenta 641.2
            affecting fetus or newborn 762.1
         retained
            placenta 666.0
            secundines 666.2
         trauma 641.8
            affecting fetus or newborn 763.89
         uterine leiomyoma 641.8
            affecting fetus or newborn 763.89
   surgical procedure 998.11
concealed NEC 459.0
congenital 772.9
conjunctiva 372.72
   newborn 772.8
cord, newborn 772.0
   slipped ligature 772.3
   stump 772.3
corpus luteum (ruptured) 620.1
cortical (*see also* Hemorrhage, brain) 431
cranial 432.9
cutaneous 782.7
   newborn 772.6
cyst, pancreas 577.2
cystitis - *see* Cystitis
delayed
   with
      abortion - *see* Abortion, by type, with hemorrhage, delayed or excessive
      ectopic pregnancy (*see also* categories 633.0-633.9) 639.1
      molar pregnancy (*see also* categories 630-632) 639.1
   following
      abortion 639.1
      ectopic or molar pregnancy 639.1
   postpartum 666.2
diathesis (familial) 287.9
   newborn 776.0
disease 287.9
   newborn 776.0
   specified type NEC 287.8
disorder 287.9

Hemorrhage, hemorrhagic (*Continued*)

disorder (*Continued*)
   due to intrinsic circulating anticoagulants 286.5 ◀▥
   specified type NEC 287.8
due to
   any device, implant, or graft (presence of) classifiable to 996.0-996.5 - *see* Complications, due to (presence of) any device, implant, or graft classified to 996.0-996.5 NEC
   intrinsic circulating anticoagulant 286.5 ◀▥
duodenum, duodenal 537.89
   ulcer - *see* Ulcer, duodenum, with hemorrhage
dura mater - *see* Hemorrhage, subdural
endotracheal - *see* Hemorrhage, lung
epicranial subaponeurotic (massive) 767.11
epidural - *see* Hemorrhage, extradural
episiotomy 674.3
esophagus 530.82
   varix (*see also* Varix, esophagus, bleeding) 456.0
excessive
   with
      abortion - *see* Abortion, by type, with hemorrhage, delayed or excessive
      ectopic pregnancy (*see also* categories 633.0-633.9) 639.1
      molar pregnancy (*see also* categories 630-632) 639.1
   following
      abortion 639.1
      ectopic or molar pregnancy 639.1
external 459.0
extradural (traumatic) - *see also* Hemorrhage, brain, traumatic, extradural
   birth injury 767.0
   fetus or newborn (anoxic) (traumatic) 767.0
   nontraumatic 432.0
eye 360.43
   chamber (anterior) (aqueous) 364.41
   fundus 362.81
eyelid 374.81
fallopian tube 620.8
fetomaternal 772.0
   affecting management of pregnancy or puerperium 656.0
fetus, fetal 772.0
   from
      cut end of co-twin's cord 772.0
      placenta 772.0
      ruptured cord 772.0
      vasa previa 772.0
   into
      co-twin 772.0
      mother's circulation 772.0
         affecting management of pregnancy or puerperium 656.0
fever (*see also* Fever, hemorrhagic) 065.9
   with renal syndrome 078.6
   arthropod-borne NEC 065.9
   Bangkok 065.4
   Crimean 065.0
   dengue virus 065.4
   epidemic 078.6
   Junin virus 078.7
   Korean 078.6
   Machupo virus 078.7
   mite-borne 065.8
   mosquito-borne 065.4

◀ **New**   ◀▥ **Revised**

Hemorrhage, hemorrhagic *(Continued)*
 fever *(Continued)*
  Philippine 065.4
  Russian (Yaroslav) 078.6
  Singapore 065.4
  Southeast Asia 065.4
  Thailand 065.4
  tick-borne NEC 065.3
 fibrinogenolysis *(see also Fibrinolysis)* 286.6
 fibrinolytic (acquired) *(see also Fibrinolysis)* 286.6
 fontanel 767.19
 from tracheostomy stoma 519.09
 fundus, eye 362.81
 funis
  affecting fetus or newborn 772.0
  complicating delivery 663.8
 gastric *(see also Hemorrhage, stomach)* 578.9
 gastroenteric 578.9
  newborn 772.4
 gastrointestinal (tract) 578.9
  newborn 772.4
 genitourinary (tract) NEC 599.89
 gingiva 523.8
 globe 360.43
 gravidarum - *see* Hemorrhage, pregnancy
 gum 523.8
 heart 429.89
 hypopharyngeal (throat) 784.8
 intermenstrual 626.6
  irregular 626.6
  regular 626.5
 internal (organs) 459.0
  capsule *(see also Hemorrhage brain)* 431
  ear 386.8
  newborn 772.8
 intestine 578.9
  congenital 772.4
  newborn 772.4
 into
  bladder wall 596.7
  bursa 727.89
  corpus luysii *(see also Hemorrhage, brain)* 431
 intra-abdominal 459.0
  during or following surgery 998.11
 intra-alveolar, newborn (lung) 770.3
 intracerebral *(see also Hemorrhage, brain)* 431
 intracranial NEC 432.9
  puerperal, postpartum, childbirth 674.0
  traumatic - *see* Hemorrhage, brain, traumatic
 intramedullary NEC 336.1
 intraocular 360.43
 intraoperative 998.11
 intrapartum - *see* Hemorrhage, complicating, delivery
 intrapelvic
  female 629.8
  male 459.0
 intraperitoneal 459.0
 intrapontine *(see also Hemorrhage, brain)* 431
 intrauterine 621.4
  complicating delivery - *see* Hemorrhage, complicating, delivery
  in pregnancy or childbirth - *see* Hemorrhage, pregnancy

Hemorrhage, hemorrhagic *(Continued)*
 intrauterine *(Continued)*
  postpartum *(see also Hemorrhage, postpartum)* 666.1
 intraventricular *(see also Hemorrhage, brain)* 431
  fetus or newborn (anoxic) (traumatic) 772.10
   grade I 772.11
   grade II 772.12
   grade III 772.13
   grade IV 772.14
 intravesical 596.7
 iris (postinfectional) (postinflammatory) (toxic) 364.41
 joint (nontraumatic) 719.10
  ankle 719.17
  elbow 719.12
  foot 719.17
  forearm 719.13
  hand 719.14
  hip 719.15
  knee 719.16
  lower leg 719.16
  multiple sites 719.19
  pelvic region 719.15
  shoulder (region) 719.11
  specified site NEC 719.18
  thigh 719.15
  upper arm 719.12
  wrist 719.13
 kidney 593.81
 knee (joint) 719.16
 labyrinth 386.8
 leg NEC 459.0
 lenticular striate artery *(see also Hemorrhage, brain)* 431
 ligature, vessel 998.11
 liver 573.8
 lower extremity NEC 459.0
 lung 786.3
  newborn 770.3
  tuberculous *(see also Tuberculosis, pulmonary)* 011.9
 malaria 084.8
 marginal sinus 641.2
 massive subaponeurotic, birth injury 767.11
 maternal, affecting fetus or newborn 762.1
 mediastinum 786.3
 medulla *(see also Hemorrhage, brain)* 431
 membrane (brain) *(see also Hemorrhage, subarachnoid)* 430
  spinal cord - *see* Hemorrhage, spinal cord
 meninges, meningeal (brain) (middle) *(see also Hemorrhage, subarachnoid)* 430
  spinal cord - *see* Hemorrhage, spinal cord
 mesentery 568.81
 metritis 626.8
 midbrain *(see also Hemorrhage, brain)* 431
 mole 631
 mouth 528.9
 mucous membrane NEC 459.0
  newborn 772.8
 muscle 728.89
 nail (subungual) 703.8
 nasal turbinate 784.7
  newborn 772.8
 nasopharynx 478.29

Hemorrhage, hemorrhagic *(Continued)*
 navel, newborn 772.3
 newborn 772.9
  adrenal 772.5
  alveolar (lung) 770.3
  brain (anoxic) (hypoxic) (due to birth trauma) 767.0
  cerebral (anoxic) (hypoxic) (due to birth trauma) 767.0
  conjunctiva 772.8
  cutaneous 772.6
  diathesis 776.0
  due to vitamin K deficiency 776.0
  epicranial subaponeurotic (massive) 767.11
  gastrointestinal 772.4
  internal (organs) 772.8
  intestines 772.4
  intra-alveolar (lung) 770.3
  intracranial (from any perinatal cause) 767.0
  intraventricular (from any perinatal cause) 772.10
   grade I 772.11
   grade II 772.12
   grade III 772.13
   grade IV 772.14
  lung 770.3
  pulmonary (massive) 770.3
  spinal cord, traumatic 767.4
  stomach 772.4
  subaponeurotic (massive) 767.11
  subarachnoid (from any perinatal cause) 772.2
  subconjunctival 772.8
  subgaleal 767.11
  umbilicus 772.0
   slipped ligature 772.3
   vasa previa 772.0
 nipple 611.79
 nose 784.7
  newborn 772.8
 obstetrical surgical wound 674.3
 omentum 568.89
  newborn 772.4
 optic nerve (sheath) 377.42
 orbit 376.32
 ovary 620.1
 oviduct 620.8
 pancreas 577.8
 parathyroid (gland) (spontaneous) 252.8
 parturition - *see* Hemorrhage, complicating, delivery
 penis 607.82
 pericardium, pericarditis 423.0
 perineal wound (obstetrical) 674.3
 peritoneum, peritoneal 459.0
 peritonsillar tissue 474.8
  after operation on tonsils 998.11
  due to infection 475
 petechial 782.7
 pituitary (gland) 253.8
 placenta NEC 641.9
  affecting fetus or newborn 762.1
  from surgical or instrumental damage 641.8
   affecting fetus or newborn 762.1
  previa 641.1
   affecting fetus or newborn 762.0
 pleura - *see* Hemorrhage, lung
 polioencephalitis, superior 265.1
 polymyositis - *see* Polymyositis
 pons *(see also Hemorrhage, brain)* 431
 pontine *(see also Hemorrhage, brain)* 431
 popliteal 459.0

ICD-9-CM

I

Vol. 2

Hemorrhage, hemorrhagic (*Continued*)

postcoital 626.7
postextraction (dental) 998.11
postmenopausal 627.1
postnasal 784.7
postoperative 998.11
postpartum (atonic) (following delivery of placenta) 666.1
  delayed or secondary (after 24 hours) 666.2
  retained placenta 666.0
  third stage 666.0
pregnancy (concealed) 641.9
  accidental 641.2
    affecting fetus or newborn 762.1
  affecting fetus or newborn 762.1
  before 22 completed weeks' gestation 640.9
    affecting fetus or newborn 762.1
  due to
    abruptio placentae 641.2
      affecting fetus or newborn 762.1
    afibrinogenemia or other coagulation defect (conditions classifiable to 286.0-286.9) 641.3
      affecting fetus or newborn 762.1
    coagulation defect 641.3
      affecting fetus or newborn 762.1
    hyperfibrinolysis 641.3
      affecting fetus or newborn 762.1
    hypofibrinogenemia 641.3
      affecting fetus or newborn 762.1
    leiomyoma, uterus 641.8
      affecting fetus or newborn 762.1
    low-lying placenta 641.1
      affecting fetus or newborn 762.1
    marginal sinus (rupture) 641.2
      affecting fetus or newborn 762.1
    placenta previa 641.1
      affecting fetus or newborn 762.0
    premature separation of placenta (normally implanted) 641.2
      affecting fetus or newborn 762.1
    threatened abortion 640.0
      affecting fetus or newborn 762.1
    trauma 641.8
      affecting fetus or newborn 762.1
  early (before 22 completed weeks' gestation) 640.9
    affecting fetus or newborn 762.1
  previous, affecting management of pregnancy or childbirth V23.49
  unavoidable - *see* Hemorrhage, pregnancy, due to placenta previa
prepartum (mother) - *see* Hemorrhage, pregnancy
preretinal, cause unspecified 362.81
prostate 602.1
puerperal (*see also* Hemorrhage, postpartum) 666.1
pulmonary - *see also* Hemorrhage, lung
  newborn (massive) 770.3
  renal syndrome 446.21
purpura (primary) (*see also* Purpura, thrombocytopenic) 287.3
rectum (sphincter) 569.3
recurring, following initial hemorrhage at time of injury 958.2
renal 593.81
  pulmonary syndrome 446.21
respiratory tract (*see also* Hemorrhage, lung) 786.3

Hemorrhage, hemorrhagic (*Continued*)

retina, retinal (deep) (superficial) (vessels) 362.81
  diabetic 250.5 [362.01]
  due to birth injury 772.8
retrobulbar 376.89
retroperitoneal 459.0
retroplacental (*see also* Placenta, separation) 641.2
scalp 459.0
  due to injury at birth 767.19
scrotum 608.83
secondary (nontraumatic) 459.0
  following initial hemorrhage at time of injury 958.2
seminal vesicle 608.83
skin 782.7
  newborn 772.6
spermatic cord 608.83
spinal (cord) 336.1
  aneurysm (ruptured) 336.1
    syphilitic 094.89
  due to birth injury 767.4
  fetus or newborn 767.4
spleen 289.59
spontaneous NEC 459.0
  petechial 782.7
stomach 578.9
  newborn 772.4
  ulcer - *see* Ulcer, stomach, with hemorrhage
subaponeurotic, newborn 767.11
  massive (birth injury) 767.11
subarachnoid (nontraumatic) 430
  fetus or newborn (anoxic) (traumatic) 772.2
  puerperal, postpartum, childbirth 674.0
  traumatic - *see* Hemorrhage, brain, traumatic, subarachnoid
subconjunctival 372.72
  due to birth injury 772.8
  newborn 772.8
subcortical (*see also* Hemorrhage, brain) 431
subcutaneous 782.7
subdiaphragmatic 459.0
subdural (nontraumatic) 432.1
  due to birth injury 767.0
  fetus or newborn (anoxic) (hypoxic) (due to birth trauma) 767.0
  puerperal, postpartum, childbirth 674.0
  spinal 336.1
  traumatic - *see* Hemorrhage, brain, traumatic, subdural
subgaleal 767.11
subhyaloid 362.81
subperiosteal 733.99
subretinal 362.81
subtentorial (*see also* Hemorrhage, subdural) 432.1
subungual 703.8
  due to blood dyscrasia 287.8
suprarenal (capsule) (gland) 255.4
  fetus or newborn 772.5
tentorium (traumatic) - *see also* Hemorrhage, brain, traumatic
  fetus or newborn 767.0
  nontraumatic - *see* Hemorrhage, subdural
testis 608.83
thigh 459.0
third stage 666.0

Hemorrhage, hemorrhagic (*Continued*)

thorax - *see* Hemorrhage, lung
throat 784.8
thrombocythemia 238.7
thymus (gland) 254.8
thyroid (gland) 246.3
  cyst 246.3
tongue 529.8
tonsil 474.8
  postoperative 998.11
tooth socket (postextraction) 998.11
trachea - *see* Hemorrhage, lung
traumatic - *see also* nature of injury
  brain - *see* Hemorrhage, brain, traumatic
  recurring or secondary (following initial hemorrhage at time of injury) 958.2
tuberculous NEC (*see also* Tuberculosis, pulmonary) 011.9
tunica vaginalis 608.83
ulcer - *see* Ulcer, by site, with hemorrhage
umbilicus, umbilical cord 772.0
  after birth, newborn 772.3
  complicating delivery 663.8
    affecting fetus or newborn 772.0
  slipped ligature 772.3
  stump 772.3
unavoidable (due to placenta previa) 641.1
  affecting fetus or newborn 762.0
upper extremity 459.0
urethra (idiopathic) 599.84
uterus, uterine (abnormal) 626.9
  climacteric 627.0
  complicating delivery - *see* Hemorrhage, complicating, delivery
  due to
    intrauterine contraceptive device 996.76
      perforating uterus 996.32
  functional or dysfunctional 626.8
  in pregnancy - *see* Hemorrhage, pregnancy
  intermenstrual 626.6
    irregular 626.6
    regular 626.5
  postmenopausal 627.1
  postpartum (*see also* Hemorrhage, postpartum) 666.1
  prepubertal 626.8
  pubertal 626.3
  puerperal (immediate) 666.1
vagina 623.8
vasa previa 663.5
  affecting fetus or newborn 772.0
vas deferens 608.83
ventricular (*see also* Hemorrhage, brain) 431
vesical 596.8
viscera 459.0
  newborn 772.8
vitreous (humor) (intraocular) 379.23
vocal cord 478.5
vulva 624.8

Hemorrhoids (anus) (rectum) (without complication) 455.6
bleeding, prolapsed, strangulated, or ulcerated NEC 455.8
  external 455.5
  internal 455.2
complicated NEC 455.8
complicating pregnancy and puerperium 671.8

◄ New   ◄▥ Revised

Hemorrhoids (Continued)
external 455.3
  with complication NEC 455.5
    bleeding, prolapsed, strangulated, or ulcerated 455.5
    thrombosed 455.4
internal 455.0
  with complication NEC 455.2
    bleeding, prolapsed, strangulated, or ulcerated 455.2
    thrombosed 455.1
residual skin tag 455.9
sentinel pile 455.9
thrombosed NEC 455.7
  external 455.4
  internal 455.1
Hemosalpinx 620.8
Hemosiderosis 275.0
dietary 275.0
pulmonary (idiopathic) 275.0 [516.1]
transfusion NEC 999.8
  bone marrow 996.85
Hemospermia 608.82
Hemothorax 511.8
bacterial, nontuberculous 511.1
newborn 772.8
nontuberculous 511.8
  bacterial 511.1
pneumococcal 511.1
postoperative 998.11
staphylococcal 511.1
streptococcal 511.1
traumatic 860.2
  with
    open wound into thorax 860.3
    pneumothorax 860.4
      with open wound into thorax 860.5
tuberculous (see also Tuberculosis, pleura) 012.0
Hemotympanum 385.89
Hench-Rosenberg syndrome (palindromic arthritis) (see also Rheumatism, palindromic) 719.3
Henle's warts 371.41
Henoch (-Schönlein)
disease or syndrome (allergic purpura) 287.0
purpura (allergic) 287.0
Henpue, henpuye 102.6
Heparitinuria 277.5
Hepar lobatum 095.3
Hepatalgia 573.8
Hepatic - see also condition
flexure syndrome 569.89
Hepatitis 573.3
acute (see also Necrosis, liver) 570
  alcoholic 571.1
  infective 070.1
    with hepatic coma 070.0
alcoholic 571.1
amebic - see Abscess, liver, amebic
anicteric (acute) - see Hepatitis, viral
antigen-associated (HAA) - see Hepatitis, viral, type B
Australian antigen (positive) - see Hepatitis, viral, type B
catarrhal (acute) 070.1
  with hepatic coma 070.0
  chronic 571.40
  newborn 070.1
    with hepatic coma 070.0
chemical 573.3
cholangiolitic 573.8
cholestatic 573.8

Hepatitis (Continued)
chronic 571.40
  active 571.49
    viral - see Hepatitis, viral
  aggressive 571.49
  persistent 571.41
  viral - see Hepatitis, viral
cytomegalic inclusion virus 078.5 [573.1]
diffuse 573.3
"dirty needle" - see Hepatitis, viral
drug-induced 573.3
due to
  Coxsackie 074.8 [573.1]
  cytomegalic inclusion virus 078.5 [573.1]
  infectious mononucleosis 075 [573.1]
  malaria 084.9 [573.2]
  mumps 072.71
  secondary syphilis 091.62
  toxoplasmosis (acquired) 130.5
    congenital (active) 771.2
epidemic - see Hepatitis, viral, type A
fetus or newborn 774.4
fibrous (chronic) 571.49
  acute 570
from injection, inoculation, or transfusion (blood) (other substance) (plasma) (serum) (onset within 8 months after administration) - see Hepatitis, viral
fulminant (viral) (see also Hepatitis, viral) 070.9
  with hepatic coma 070.6
  type A 070.1
    with hepatic coma 070.0
  type B - see Hepatitis, viral, type B
giant cell (neonatal) 774.4
hemorrhagic 573.8
homologous serum - see Hepatitis, viral
hypertrophic (chronic) 571.49
  acute 570
infectious, infective (acute) (chronic) (subacute) 070.1
  with hepatic coma 070.0
inoculation - see Hepatitis, viral
interstitial (chronic) 571.49
  acute 570
lupoid 571.49
malarial 084.9 [573.2]
malignant (see also Necrosis, liver) 570
neonatal (toxic) 774.4
newborn 774.4
parenchymatous (acute) (see also Necrosis, liver) 570
peliosis 573.3
persistent, chronic 571.41
plasma cell 571.49
postimmunization - see Hepatitis, viral
postnecrotic 571.49
posttransfusion - see Hepatitis, viral
recurrent 571.49
septic 573.3
serum - see Hepatitis, viral
  carrier (suspected of) V02.61
subacute (see also Necrosis, liver) 570
suppurative (diffuse) 572.0
syphilitic (late) 095.3
  congenital (early) 090.0 [573.2]
    late 090.5 [573.2]
  secondary 091.62
toxic (noninfectious) 573.3
  fetus or newborn 774.4
tuberculous (see also Tuberculosis) 017.9

Hepatitis (Continued)
viral (acute) (anicteric) (cholangiolitic) (cholestatic) (chronic) (subacute) 070.9
  with hepatic coma 070.6
  AU-SH type virus - see Hepatitis, viral, type B
  Australia antigen - see Hepatitis, viral, type B
  B-antigen - see Hepatitis, viral, type B
  Coxsackie 074.8 [573.1]
  cytomegalic inclusion 078.5 [573.1]
  IH (virus) - see Hepatitis, viral, type A
  infectious hepatitis virus - see Hepatitis, viral, type A
  serum hepatitis virus - see Hepatitis, viral, type B
  SH - see Hepatitis, viral, type B
  specified type NEC 070.59
    with hepatic coma 070.49
  type A 070.1
    with hepatic coma 070.0
  type B (acute) 070.30
    with
      hepatic coma 070.20
        with hepatitis delta 070.21
      hepatitis delta 070.31
        with hepatic coma 070.21
    carrier status V02.61
    chronic 070.32
      with
        hepatic coma 070.22
          with hepatitis delta 070.23
        hepatitis delta 070.33
          with hepatic coma 070.23
  type C ◀▥
    with hepatic coma 070.41
    acute 070.51 ◀
      with hepatic coma 070.41 ◀
    carrier status V02.62
    chronic 070.54
      with hepatic coma 070.44 ◀
    unspecified 070.70
      with hepatic coma 070.71 ◀
  type delta (with hepatitis B carrier state) 070.52
    with
      active hepatitis B disease - see Hepatitis, viral, type B
      hepatic coma 070.42
  type E 070.53
    with hepatic coma 070.43
  vaccination and inoculation (prophylactic) V05.3
Waldenström's (lupoid hepatitis) 571.49
Hepatization, lung (acute) - see also Pneumonia, lobar
chronic (see also Fibrosis, lung) 515
Hepatoblastoma (M8970/3) 155.0
Hepatocarcinoma (M8170/3) 155.0
Hepatocholangiocarcinoma (M8180/3) 155.0
Hepatocholangioma, benign (M8180/0) 211.5
Hepatocholangitis 573.8
Hepatocystitis (see also Cholecystitis) 575.10
Hepatodystrophy 570
Hepatolenticular degeneration 275.1
Hepatolithiasis - see Choledocholithiasis
Hepatoma (malignant) (M8170/3) 155.0
benign (M8170/0) 211.5
congenital (M8970/3) 155.0
embryonal (M8970/3) 155.0

ICD-9-CM

H

Vol. 2

Hepatomegalia glycogenica diffusa 271.0
Hepatomegaly (*see also* Hypertrophy,
    liver) 789.1
  congenital 751.69
    syphilitic 090.0
  due to Clonorchis sinensis 121.1
  Gaucher's 272.7
  syphilitic (congenital) 090.0
Hepatoptosis 573.8
Hepatorrhexis 573.8
Hepatosis, toxic 573.8
Hepatosplenomegaly 571.8
  due to S. japonicum 120.2
  hyperlipemic (Burger-Grutz type) 272.3
Herald patch 696.3
Hereditary - *see* condition
Heredodegeneration 330.9
  macular 362.70
Heredopathia atactica polyneuritiformis
  356.3
Heredosyphilis (*see also* Syphilis, congenital) 090.9
Hermaphroditism (true) 752.7
  with specified chromosomal anomaly -
    see Anomaly, chromosomes, sex
Hernia, hernial (acquired) (recurrent)
  553.9
  with
    gangrene (obstructed) NEC 551.9
    obstruction NEC 552.9
      and gangrene 551.9
  abdomen (wall) - *see* Hernia, ventral
  abdominal, specified site NEC 553.8
    with
      gangrene (obstructed) 551.8
      obstruction 552.8
        and gangrene 551.8
  appendix 553.8
    with
      gangrene (obstructed) 551.8
      obstruction 552.8
        and gangrene 551.8
  bilateral (inguinal) - *see* Hernia, inguinal
  bladder (sphincter)
    congenital (female) (male) 756.71
    female (*see also* Cystocele, female)
      618.01 ◀▥
    618.0
    male 596.8
  brain 348.4
    congenital 742.0
  broad ligament 553.8
  cartilage, vertebral - *see* Displacement,
    intervertebral disc
  cerebral 348.4
    congenital 742.0
    endaural 742.0
  ciliary body 364.8
    traumatic 871.1
  colic 553.9
    with
      gangrene (obstructed) 551.9
      obstruction 552.9
        and gangrene 551.9
  colon 553.9
    with
      gangrene (obstructed) 551.9
      obstruction 552.9
        and gangrene 551.9
  colostomy (stoma) 569.69
  Cooper's (retroperitoneal) 553.8
    with
      gangrene (obstructed) 551.8
      obstruction 552.8
        and gangrene 551.8

Hernia, hernial (*Continued*)
  crural - *see* Hernia, femoral
  diaphragm, diaphragmatic 553.3
    with
      gangrene (obstructed) 551.3
      obstruction 552.3
        and gangrene 551.3
    congenital 756.6
    due to gross defect of diaphragm
      756.6
    traumatic 862.0
      with open wound into cavity 862.1
  direct (inguinal) - *see* Hernia, inguinal
  disc, intervertebral - *see* Displacement,
    intervertebral disc
  diverticulum, intestine 553.9
    with
      gangrene (obstructed) 551.9
      obstruction 552.9
        and gangrene 551.9
  double (inguinal) - *see* Hernia, inguinal
  duodenojejunal 553.8
    with
      gangrene (obstructed) 551.8
      obstruction 552.8
        and gangrene 551.8
  en glissade - *see* Hernia, inguinal
  enterostomy (stoma) 569.69
  epigastric 553.29
    with
      gangrene (obstruction) 551.29
      obstruction 552.29
        and gangrene 551.29
    recurrent 553.21
      with
        gangrene (obstructed) 551.21
        obstruction 552.21
          and gangrene 551.21
  esophageal hiatus (sliding) 553.3
    with
      gangrene (obstructed) 551.3
      obstruction 552.3
        and gangrene 551.3
    congenital 750.6
  external (inguinal) - *see* Hernia, inguinal
  fallopian tube 620.4
  fascia 728.89
  fat 729.30
    eyelid 374.34
    orbital 374.34
    pad 729.30
      eye, eyelid 374.34
      knee 729.31
      orbit 374.34
      popliteal (space) 729.31
      specified site NEC 729.39
  femoral (unilateral) 553.00
    with
      gangrene (obstructed) 551.00
      obstruction 552.00
        with gangrene 551.00
    bilateral 553.02
      gangrenous (obstructed) 551.02
      obstructed 552.02
        with gangrene 551.02
      recurrent 553.03
        gangrenous (obstructed) 551.03
        obstructed 552.03
          with gangrene 551.03
    recurrent (unilateral) 553.01
      bilateral 553.03
        gangrenous (obstructed) 551.03
        obstructed 552.03
          with gangrene 551.03

Hernia, hernial (*Continued*)
  femoral (*Continued*)
    recurrent (*Continued*)
      gangrenous (obstructed) 551.01
      obstructed 552.01
        with gangrene 551.01
  foramen
    Bochdalek 553.3
      with
        gangrene (obstructed) 551.3
        obstruction 552.3
          and gangrene 551.3
      congenital 756.6
    magnum 348.4
    Morgagni, morgagnian 553.3
      with
        gangrene 551.3
        obstruction 552.3
          and gangrene 551.3
      congenital 756.6
  funicular (umbilical) 553.1
    with
      gangrene (obstructed) 551.1
      obstruction 552.1
        and gangrene 551.1
    spermatic cord - *see* Hernia, inguinal
  gangrenous - *see* Hernia, by site, with
    gangrene
  gastrointestinal tract 553.9
    with
      gangrene (obstructed) 551.9
      obstruction 552.9
        and gangrene 551.9
  gluteal - *see* Hernia, femoral
  Gruber's (internal mesogastric) 553.8
    with
      gangrene (obstructed) 551.8
      obstruction 552.8
        and gangrene 551.8
  Hesselbach's 553.8
    with
      gangrene (obstructed) 551.8
      obstruction 552.8
        and gangrene 551.8
  hiatal (esophageal) (sliding) 553.3
    with
      gangrene (obstructed) 551.3
      obstruction 552.3
        and gangrene 551.3
    congenital 750.6
  incarcerated (*see also* Hernia, by site,
    with obstruction) 552.9
    gangrenous (*see also* Hernia, by site,
      with gangrene) 551.9
  incisional 553.21
    with
      gangrene (obstructed) 551.21
      obstruction 552.21
        and gangrene 551.21
  lumbar - *see* Hernia, lumbar
    recurrent 553.21
      with
        gangrene (obstructed) 551.21
        obstruction 552.21
          and gangrene 551.21
  indirect (inguinal) - *see* Hernia, ingui-
    nal
  infantile - *see* Hernia, inguinal
  infrapatellar fat pad 729.31
  inguinal (direct) (double) (encysted)
    (external) (funicular) (indirect) (in-
    fantile) (internal) (interstitial)
    (oblique) (scrotal) (sliding)
    550.9

Hernia, hernial (*Continued*)
inguinal (*Continued*)

> Note   Use the following fifth-digit
> subclassification with category 550:
>
> 0   unilateral or unspecified (not
>   specified as recurrent)
> 1   unilateral or unspecified, recur-
>   rent
> 2   bilateral (not specified as re-
>   current)
> 3   bilateral, recurrent

  with
    gangrene (obstructed) 550.0
    obstruction 550.1
      and gangrene 550.0
  internal 553.8
    with
      gangrene (obstructed) 551.8
      obstruction 552.8
        and gangrene 551.8
    inguinal - *see* Hernia, inguinal
  interstitial 553.9
    with
      gangrene (obstructed) 551.9
      obstruction 552.9
        and gangrene 551.9
    inguinal - *see* Hernia, inguinal
  intervertebral cartilage or disc - *see*
      Displacement, intervertebral disc
  intestine, intestinal 553.9
    with
      gangrene (obstructed) 551.9
      obstruction 552.9
        and gangrene 551.9
  intra-abdominal 553.9
    with
      gangrene (obstructed) 551.9
      obstruction 552.9
        and gangrene 551.9
  intraparietal 553.9
    with
      gangrene (obstructed) 551.9
      obstruction 552.9
        and gangrene 551.9
  iris 364.8
    traumatic 871.1
  irreducible (*see also* Hernia, by site,
      with obstruction) 552.9
    gangrenous (with obstruction) (*see
        also* Hernia, by site, with gan-
        grene) 551.9
  ischiatic 553.8
    with
      gangrene (obstructed) 551.8
      obstruction 552.8
        and gangrene 551.8
  ischiorectal 553.8
    with
      gangrene (obstructed) 551.8
      obstruction 552.8
        and gangrene 551.8
  lens 379.32
    traumatic 871.1
  linea
    alba - *see* Hernia, epigastric
    semilunaris - *see* Hernia, spigelian
  Littre's (diverticular) 553.9
    with
      gangrene (obstructed) 551.9
      obstruction 552.9
        and gangrene 551.9
  lumbar 553.8
    with
      gangrene (obstructed) 551.8

Hernia, hernial (*Continued*)
  lumbar (*Continued*)
    with (*Continued*)
      obstruction 552.8
        and gangrene 551.8
    intervertebral disc 722.10
  lung (subcutaneous) 518.89
    congenital 748.69
  mediastinum 519.3
  mesenteric (internal) 553.8
    with
      gangrene (obstructed) 551.8
      obstruction 552.8
        and gangrene 551.8
  mesocolon 553.8
    with
      gangrene (obstructed) 551.8
      obstruction 552.8
        and gangrene 551.8
  muscle (sheath) 728.89
  nucleus pulposus - *see* Displacement,
      intervertebral disc
  oblique (inguinal) - *see* Hernia, ingui-
      nal
  obstructive (*see also* Hernia, by site,
      with obstruction) 552.9
    gangrenous (with obstruction) (*see
        also* Hernia, by site, with gan-
        grene) 551.9
  obturator 553.8
    with
      gangrene (obstructed) 551.8
      obstruction 552.8
        and gangrene 551.8
  omental 553.8
    with
      gangrene (obstructed) 551.8
      obstruction 552.8
        and gangrene 551.8
  orbital fat (pad) 374.34
  ovary 620.4
  oviduct 620.4
  paracolostomy (stoma) 569.69
  paraduodenal 553.8
    with
      gangrene (obstructed) 551.8
      obstruction 552.8
        and gangrene 551.8
  paraesophageal 553.3
    with
      gangrene (obstructed) 551.3
      obstruction 552.3
        and gangrene 551.3
    congenital 750.6
  parahiatal 553.3
    with
      gangrene (obstructed) 551.3
      obstruction 552.3
        and gangrene 551.3
  paraumbilical 553.1
    with
      gangrene (obstructed) 551.1
      obstruction 552.1
        and gangrene 551.1
  parietal 553.9
    with
      gangrene (obstructed) 551.9
      obstruction 552.9
        and gangrene 551.9
  perineal 553.8
    with
      gangrene (obstructed) 551.8
      obstruction 552.8
        and gangrene 551.8

Hernia, hernial (*Continued*)
  peritoneal sac, lesser 553.8
    with
      gangrene (obstructed) 551.8
      obstruction 552.8
        and gangrene 551.8
  popliteal fat pad 729.31
  postoperative 553.21
    with
      gangrene (obstructed) 551.21
      obstruction 552.21
        and gangrene 551.21
  pregnant uterus 654.4
  prevesical 596.8
  properitoneal 553.8
    with
      gangrene (obstructed) 551.8
      obstruction 552.8
        and gangrene 551.8
  pudendal 553.8
    with
      gangrene (obstructed) 551.8
      obstruction 552.8
        and gangrene 551.8
  rectovaginal 618.6
  retroperitoneal 553.8
    with
      gangrene (obstructed) 551.8
      obstruction 552.8
        and gangrene 551.8
  Richter's (parietal) 553.9
    with
      gangrene (obstructed) 551.9
      obstruction 552.9
        and gangrene 551.9
  Rieux's, Riex's (retrocecal) 553.8
    with
      gangrene (obstructed) 551.8
      obstruction 552.8
        and gangrene 551.8
  sciatic 553.8
    with
      gangrene (obstructed) 551.8
      obstruction 552.8
        and gangrene 551.8
  scrotum, scrotal - *see* Hernia, inguinal
  sliding (inguinal) - *see also* Hernia, in-
      guinal
    hiatus - *see* Hernia, hiatal
  spigelian 553.29
    with
      gangrene (obstructed) 551.29
      obstruction 552.29
        and gangrene 551.29
  spinal (*see also* Spina bifida) 741.9
    with hydrocephalus 741.0
  strangulated (*see also* Hernia, by site,
      with obstruction) 552.9
    gangrenous (with obstruction) (*see
        also* Hernia, by site, with gan-
        grene) 551.9
  supraumbilicus (linea alba) - *see* Her-
      nia, epigastric
  tendon 727.9
  testis (nontraumatic) 550.9
    meaning
      scrotal hernia 550.9
      symptomatic late syphillis
        095.8
  Treitz's (fossa) 553.8
    with
      gangrene (obstructed) 551.8
      obstruction 552.8
        and gangrene 551.8

ICD-9-CM

II

Vol. 2

◀ **New**　　　◀▥ **Revised**

High (Continued)
output failure (cardiac) (see also Failure, heart) 428.9
oxygen-affinity hemoglobin 289.0
palate 750.26
risk
behavior - see problem
cervical, human papillomavirus (HPV) DNA test positive 795.05 ◄
family situation V61.9
specified circumstance NEC V61.8
individual NEC V62.89
infant NEC V20.1
patient taking drugs (prescribed) V67.51
nonprescribed (see also Abuse, drugs, nondependent) 305.9
pregnancy V23.9
inadequate prenatal care V23.7
specified problem NEC V23.8
temperature (of unknown origin) (see also Pyrexia) 780.6
thoracic rib 756.3
Hildenbrand's disease (typhus) 081.9
Hilger's syndrome 337.0
Hill diarrhea 579.1
Hilliard's lupus (see also Tuberculosis) 017.0
Hilum - see condition
Hip - see condition
Hippel's disease (retinocerebral angiomatosis) 759.6
Hippus 379.49
Hirschfeld's disease (acute diabetes mellitus) (see also Diabetes) 250.0
Hirschsprung's disease or megacolon (congenital) 751.3
Hirsuties (see also Hypertrichosis) 704.1
Hirsutism (see also Hypertrichosis) 704.1
Hirudiniasis (external) (internal) 134.2
His-Werner disease (trench fever) 083.1
Hiss-Russell dysentery 004.1
Histamine cephalgia 346.2
Histidinemia 270.5
Histidinuria 270.5
Histiocytoma (M8832/0) - (see also Neoplasm, skin, benign)
fibrous (M8830/0) - (see also Neoplasm, skin, benign)
atypical (M8830/1) - see Neoplasm, connective tissue, uncertain behavior
malignant (M8830/3) - see Neoplasm, connective tissue, malignant
Histiocytosis (acute) (chronic) (subacute) 277.89
acute differentiated progressive (M9722/3) 202.5
cholesterol 277.89
essential 277.89
lipid, lipoid (essential) 272.7
lipochrome (familial) 288.1
malignant (M9720/3) 202.3
X (chronic) 277.89
acute (progressive) (M9722/3) 202.5
Histoplasmosis 115.90
with
endocarditis 115.94
meningitis 115.91
pericarditis 115.93
pneumonia 115.95
retinitis 115.92
specified manifestation NEC 115.99
African (due to Histoplasma duboisii) 115.10

Histoplasmosis (Continued)
African (Continued)
with
endocarditis 115.14
meningitis 115.11
pericarditis 115.13
pneumonia 115.15
retinitis 115.12
specified manifestation NEC 115.19
American (due to Histoplasma capsulatum) 115.00
with
endocarditis 115.04
meningitis 115.01
pericarditis 115.03
pneumonia 115.05
retinitis 115.02
specified manifestation NEC 115.09
Darling's - see Histoplasmosis, American
large form (see also Histoplasmosis, African) 115.10
lung 115.05
small form (see also Histoplasmosis, American) 115.00
History (personal) of
abuse
emotional V15.42
neglect V15.42
physical V15.41
sexual V15.41
affective psychosis V11.1
alcoholism V11.3
specified as drinking problem (see also Abuse, drugs, nondependent) 305.0
allergy to
analgesic agent NEC V14.6
anesthetic NEC V14.4
antibiotic agent NEC V14.1
penicillin V14.0
anti-infective agent NEC V14.3
diathesis V15.09
drug V14.9
specified type NEC V14.8
eggs V15.03
food additives V15.05
insect bite V15.06
latex V15.07
medicinal agents V14.9
specified type NEC V14.8
milk products V15.02
narcotic agent NEC V14.5
nuts V15.05
peanuts V15.01
penicillin V14.0
radiographic dye V15.08
seafood V15.04
serum V14.7
specified food NEC V15.05
specified nonmedicinal agents NEC V15.09
spider bite V15.06
sulfa V14.2
sulfonamides V14.2
therapeutic agent NEC V15.09
vaccine V14.7
anemia V12.3
arthritis V13.4
benign neoplasm of brain V12.41
blood disease V12.3
calculi, urinary V13.01
cardiovascular disease V12.50
myocardial infarction 412
child abuse V15.41
cigarette smoking V15.82

History (personal) of (Continued)
circulatory system disease V12.50
myocardial infarction 412
congenital malformation V13.69
contraception V15.7
diathesis, allergic V15.09
digestive system disease V12.70
peptic ulcer V12.71
polyps, colonic V12.72
specified NEC V12.79
disease (of) V13.9
blood V12.3
blood-forming organs V12.3
cardiovascular system V12.50
circulatory system V12.50
digestive system V12.70
peptic ulcer V12.71
polyps, colonic V12.72
specified NEC V12.79
infectious V12.00
malaria V12.03
poliomyelitis V12.02
specified NEC V12.09
tuberculosis V12.01
parasitic V12.00
specified NEC V12.09
respiratory system V12.6
skin V13.3
specified site NEC V13.8
subcutaneous tissue V13.3
trophoblastic V13.1
affecting management of pregnancy V23.1
disorder (of) V13.9
endocrine V12.2
genital system V13.29
hematological V12.3
immunity V12.2
mental V11.9
affective type V11.1
manic-depressive V11.1
neurosis V11.2
schizophrenia V11.0
specified type NEC V11.8
metabolic V12.2
musculoskeletal NEC V13.5
nervous system V12.40
specified type NEC V12.49
obstetric V13.29
affecting management of current pregnancy V23.49
pre-term labor V23.41
pre-term labor V13.21
sense organs V12.40
specified type NEC V12.49
specified site NEC V13.8
urinary system V13.00
calculi V13.01
specified NEC V13.09
drug use
nonprescribed (see also Abuse, drugs, nondependent) 305.9
patent (see also Abuse, drugs, nondependent) 305.9
effect NEC of external cause V15.89
embolism (pulmonary) V12.51
emotional abuse V15.42
endocrine disorder V12.2
extracorporeal membrane oxygenation (ECMO) V15.87
family
allergy V19.6
anemia V18.2
arteriosclerosis V17.4
arthritis V17.7
asthma V17.5
blindness V19.0

ICD-9-CM

Vol.

History (personal) of *(Continued)*
  family *(Continued)*
    blood disorder NEC V18.3
    cardiovascular disease V17.4
    cerebrovascular disease V17.1
    chronic respiratory condition NEC
      V17.6
    congenital anomalies V19.5
    consanguinity V19.7
    coronary artery disease V17.3
    cystic fibrosis V18.1
    deafness V19.2
    diabetes mellitus V18.0
    digestive disorders V18.5
    disease or disorder (of)
      allergic V19.6
      blood NEC V18.3
      cardiovascular NEC V17.4
      cerebrovascular V17.1
      coronary artery V17.3
      digestive V18.5
      ear NEC V19.3
      endocrine V18.1
      eye NEC V19.1
      genitourinary NEC V18.7
      hypertensive V17.4
      infectious V18.8
      ischemic heart V17.3
      kidney V18.69
        polycystic V18.61
      mental V17.0
      metabolic V18.1
      musculoskeletal NEC V17.8
      neurological NEC V17.2
      parasitic V18.8
      psychiatric condition V17.0
      skin condition V19.4
    ear disorder NEC V19.3
    endocrine disease V18.1
    epilepsy V17.2
    eye disorder NEC V19.1
    genitourinary disease NEC V18.7
    glomerulonephritis V18.69
    gout V18.1
    hay fever V17.6
    hearing loss V19.2
    hematopoietic neoplasia V16.7
    Hodgkin's disease V16.7
    Huntington's chorea V17.2
    hydrocephalus V19.5
    hypertension V17.4
    hypospadias V13.61
    infectious disease V18.8
    ischemic heart disease V17.3
    kidney disease V18.69
      polycystic V18.61
    leukemia V16.6
    lymphatic malignant neoplasia NEC
      V16.7
    malignant neoplasm (of) NEC V16.9
      anorectal V16.0
      anus V16.0
      appendix V16.0
      bladder V16.59
      bone V16.8
      brain V16.8
      breast V16.3
        male V16.8
      bronchus V16.1
      cecum V16.0
      cervix V16.49
      colon V16.0
      duodenum V16.0
      esophagus V16.0

History (personal) of *(Continued)*
  family *(Continued)*
    malignant neoplasm (of) NEC *(Continued)*
      eye V16.8
      gallbladder V16.0
      gastrointestinal tract V16.0
      genital organs V16.40
      hemopoietic NEC V16.7
      ileum V16.0
      ilium V16.8
      intestine V16.0
      intrathoracic organs NEC V16.2
      kidney V16.51
      larynx V16.2
      liver V16.0
      lung V16.1
      lymphatic NEC V16.7
      ovary V16.41
      oviduct V16.41
      pancreas V16.0
      penis V16.49
      prostate V16.42
      rectum V16.0
      respiratory organs NEC V16.2
      skin V16.8
      specified site NEC V16.8
      stomach V16.0
      testis V16.43
      trachea V16.1
      ureter V16.59
      urethra V16.59
      urinary organs V16.59
      uterus V16.49
      vagina V16.49
      vulva V16.49
    mental retardation V18.4
    metabolic disease NEC V18.1
    mongolism V19.5
    multiple myeloma V16.7
    musculoskeletal disease NEC
      V17.8
    nephritis V18.69
    nephrosis V18.69
    parasitic disease V18.8
    polycystic kidney disease V18.61
    psychiatric disorder V17.0
    psychosis V17.0
    retardation, mental V18.4
    retinitis pigmentosa V19.1
    schizophrenia V17.0
    skin conditions V19.4
    specified condition NEC V19.8
    stroke (cerebrovascular) V17.1
    visual loss V19.0
  genital system disorder V13.29
    pre-term labor V13.21
  health hazard V15.9
    specified cause NEC V15.89
  Hodgkin's disease V10.72
  immunity disorder V12.2
  infectious disease V12.00
    malaria V12.03
    poliomyelitis V12.02
    specified NEC V12.09
    tuberculosis V12.01
  injury NEC V15.5
  insufficient prenatal care V23.7
  irradiation V15.3
  leukemia V10.60
    lymphoid V10.61
    monocytic V10.63
    myeloid V10.62
    specified type NEC V10.69

History (personal) of *(Continued)*
  little or no prenatal care V23.7
  low birth weight (*see also* Status, low
    birth weight) V21.30
  lymphosarcoma V10.71
  malaria V12.03
  malignant neoplasm (of) V10.9
    accessory sinus V10.22
    adrenal V10.88
    anus V10.06
    bile duct V10.09
    bladder V10.51
    bone V10.81
    brain V10.85
    breast V10.3
    bronchus V10.11
    cervix uteri V10.41
    colon V10.05
    connective tissue NEC V10.89
    corpus uteri V10.42
    digestive system V10.00
      specified part NEC V10.09
    duodenum V10.09
    endocrine gland NEC V10.88
    epididymis V10.48
    esophagus V10.03
    eye V10.84
    fallopian tube V10.44
    female genital organ V10.40
      specified site NEC V10.44
    gallbladder V10.09
    gastrointestinal tract V10.00
    gum V10.02
    hematopoietic NEC V10.79
    hypopharynx V10.02
    ileum V10.09
    intrathoracic organs NEC V10.20
    jejunum V10.09
    kidney V10.52
    large intestine V10.05
    larynx V10.21
    lip V10.02
    liver V10.07
    lung V10.11
    lymphatic NEC V10.79
    lymph glands or nodes NEC V10.79
    male genital organ V10.45
      specified site NEC V10.49
    mediastinum V10.29
    melanoma (of skin) V10.82
    middle ear V10.22
    mouth V10.02
      specified part NEC V10.02
    nasal cavities V10.22
    nasopharynx V10.02
    nervous system NEC V10.86
    nose V10.22
    oropharynx V10.02
    ovary V10.43
    pancreas V10.09
    parathyroid V10.88
    penis V10.49
    pharynx V10.02
    pineal V10.88
    pituitary V10.88
    placenta V10.44
    pleura V10.29
    prostate V10.46
    rectosigmoid junction V10.06
    rectum V10.06
    renal pelvis V10.53
    respiratory organs NEC V10.20
    salivary gland V10.02
    skin V10.83
      melanoma V10.82

History (personal) of (*Continued*)
  malignant neoplasm (*Continued*)
    small intestine NEC V10.09
    soft tissue NEC V10.89
    specified site NEC V10.89
    stomach V10.04
    testis V10.47
    thymus V10.29
    thyroid V10.87
    tongue V10.01
    trachea V10.12
    ureter V10.59
    urethra V10.59
    urinary organ V10.50
    uterine adnexa V10.44
    uterus V10.42
    vagina V10.44
    vulva V10.44
  manic-depressive psychosis V11.1
  mental disorder V11.9
    affective type V11.1
    manic-depressive V11.1
    neurosis V11.2
    schizophrenia V11.0
    specified type NEC V11.8
  metabolic disorder V12.2
  musculoskeletal disorder NEC V13.5
  myocardial infarction 412
  neglect (emotional) V15.42
  nervous system disorder V12.40
    specified type NEC V12.49
  neurosis V11.2
  noncompliance with medical treatment V15.81
  nutritional deficiency V12.1
  obstetric disorder V13.29
    affecting management of current pregnancy V23.49
      pre-term labor V23.41
    pre-term labor V13.41
  parasitic disease V12.00
    specified NEC V12.09
  perinatal problems V13.7
    low birth weight (*see also* Status, low birth weight) V21.30
  physical abuse V15.41
  poisoning V15.6
  poliomyelitis V12.02
  polyps, colonic V12.72
  poor obstetric V13.49
    affecting management of current pregnancy V23.49
      pre-term labor V23.41
    pre-term labor V13.41
  psychiatric disorder V11.9
    affective type V11.1
    manic-depressive V11.1
    neurosis V11.2
    schizophrenia V11.0
    specified type NEC V11.8
  psychological trauma V15.49
    emotional abuse V15.42
    neglect V15.42
    physical abuse V15.41
    rape V15.41
  psychoneurosis V11.2
  radiation therapy V15.3
  rape V15.41
  respiratory system disease V12.6
  reticulosarcoma V10.71
  schizophrenia V11.0
  skin disease V13.3
  smoking (tobacco) V15.82
  subcutaneous tissue disease V13.3

History (personal) of (*Continued*)
  surgery (major) to
    great vessels V15.1
    heart V15.1
    major organs NEC V15.2
  thrombophlebitis V12.52
  thrombosis V12.51
  tobacco use V15.82
  trophoblastic disease V13.1
    affecting management of pregnancy V23.1
  tuberculosis V12.01
  ulcer, peptic V12.71
  urinary system disorder V13.00
    calculi V13.01
    specified NEC V13.09
HIV infection (disease) (illness) - *see* Human immunodeficiency virus (disease) (illness) (infection)
Hives (bold) (*see also* Urticaria) 708.9
Hoarseness 784.49
Hobnail liver - *see* Cirrhosis, portal
Hobo, hoboism V60.0
Hodgkin's
  disease (M9650/3) 201.9
    lymphocytic
      depletion (M9653/3) 201.7
        diffuse fibrosis (M9654/3) 201.7
        reticular type (M9655/3) 201.7
      predominance (M9651/3) 201.4
    lymphocytic-histiocytic predominance (M9651/3) 201.4
    mixed cellularity (M9652/3) 201.6
    nodular sclerosis (M9656/3) 201.5
      cellular phase (M9657/3) 201.5
  granuloma (M9661/3) 201.1
  lymphogranulomatosis (M9650/3) 201.9
  lymphoma (M9650/3) 201.9
  lymphosarcoma (M9650/3) 201.9
  paragranuloma (M9660/3) 201.0
  sarcoma (M9662/3) 201.2
Hodgson's disease (aneurysmal dilatation of aorta) 441.9
  ruptured 441.5
Hodi-potsy 111.0
Hoffa (-Kastert) disease or syndrome (liposynovitis prepatellaris) 272.8
Hoffmann's syndrome 244.9 *[359.5]*
Hoffmann-Bouveret syndrome (paroxysmal tachycardia) 427.2
Hole
  macula 362.54
  optic disc, crater-like 377.22
  retina (macula) 362.54
    round 361.31
      with detachment 361.01
Holla disease (*see also* Spherocytosis) 282.0
Holländer-Simons syndrome (progressive lipodystrophy) 272.6
Hollow foot (congenital) 754.71
  acquired 736.73
Holmes' syndrome (visual disorientation) 368.16
Holoprosencephaly 742.2
  due to
    trisomy 13 758.1
    trisomy 18 758.2
Holthouse's hernia - *see* Hernia, inguinal
Homesickness 309.89
Homocystinemia 270.4
Homocystinuria 270.4
Homologous serum jaundice (prophylactic) (therapeutic) - *see* Hepatitis, viral

Homosexuality - omit code
  ego-dystonic 302.0
  pedophilic 302.2
  problems with 302.0
Homozygous Hb-S disease 282.61
Honeycomb lung 518.89
  congenital 748.4
Hong Kong ear 117.3
HOOD (hereditary osteo-onychodysplasia) 756.89
Hooded
  clitoris 752.49
  penis 752.69
Hookworm (anemia) (disease) (infestation) - *see* Ancylostomiasis
Hoppe-Goldflam syndrome 358.00
Hordeolum (external) (eyelid) 373.11
  internal 373.12
Horn
  cutaneous 702.8
    cheek 702.8
    eyelid 702.8
    penis 702.8
  iliac 756.89
  nail 703.8
    congenital 757.5
  papillary 700
Horner's
  syndrome (*see also* Neuropathy, peripheral, autonomic) 337.9
    traumatic 954.0
  teeth 520.4
Horseshoe kidney (congenital) 753.3
Horton's
  disease (temporal arteritis) 446.5
  headache or neuralgia 346.2
Hospice care V66.7
Hospitalism (in children) NEC 309.83
Hourglass contraction, contracture
  bladder 596.8
  gallbladder 575.2
    congenital 751.69
  stomach 536.8
    congenital 750.7
    psychogenic 306.4
  uterus 661.4
    affecting fetus or newborn 763.7
Household circumstance affecting care V60.9
  specified type NEC V60.8
Housemaid's knee 727.2
Housing circumstance affecting care V60.9
  specified type NEC V60.8
Huchard's disease (continued arterial hypertension) 401.9
Hudson-Stähli lines 371.11
Huguier's disease (uterine fibroma) 218.9
Hum, venous - omit code
Human bite (open wound) - (*see also* Wound, open, by site)
  intact skin surface - *see* Contusion
Human immunodeficiency virus (disease) (illness) 042
  infection V08
    with symptoms, symptomatic 042
Human immunodeficiency virus-2 infection 079.53
Human immunovirus (disease) (illness) (infection) - *see* Human immunodeficiency virus (disease) (illness) (infection)
Human papillomavirus 079.4 ◄
  cervical
    high risk, DNA test positive 795.05 ◄
    low risk, DNA test positive 795.09 ◄

ICD-9-CM

Ξ

Vol. 2

Human T-cell lymphotrophic virus I infection 079.51
Human T-cell lymphotrophic virus II infection 079.52
Human T-cell lymphotropic virus-III (disease) (illness) (infection) - *see* Human immunodeficiency virus (disease) (illness) (infection)
HTLV-I infection 079.51
HTLV-II infection 079.52
HTLV-III (disease) (illness) (infection) - *see* Human immunodeficiency virus (disease) (illness) (infection)
HTLV-III/LAV (disease) (illness) (infection) - *see* Human immunodeficiency virus (disease) (illness) (infection)
Humpback (acquired) 737.9
    congenital 756.19
Hunchback (acquired) 737.9
    congenital 756.19
Hunger 994.2
    air, psychogenic 306.1
    disease 251.1
Hunner's ulcer (*see also* Cystitis) 595.1
Hunt's
    neuralgia 053.11
    syndrome (herpetic geniculate ganglionitis) 053.11
        dyssynergia cerebellaris myoclonica 334.2
Hunter's glossitis 529.4
Hunter (-Hurler) syndrome (mucopolysaccharidosis II) 277.5
Hunterian chancre 091.0
Huntington's
    chorea 333.4
    disease 333.4
Huppert's disease (multiple myeloma) (M9730/3) 203.0
Hurler (-Hunter) disease or syndrome (mucopolysaccharidosis II) 277.5
Hürthle cell
    adenocarcinoma (M8290/3) 193
    adenoma (M8290/0) 226
    carcinoma (M8290/3) 193
    tumor (M8290/0) 226
Hutchinson's
    disease meaning
        angioma serpiginosum 709.1
        cheiropompholyx 705.81
        prurigo estivalis 692.72
        summer eruption, or summer prurigo 692.72
    incisors 090.5
    melanotic freckle (M8742/2) - *see also* Neoplasm, skin, in situ
        malignant melanoma in (M8742/3) - *see* Melanoma
    teeth or incisors (congenital syphilis) 090.5
Hutchinson-Boeck disease or syndrome (sarcoidosis) 135
Hutchinson-Gilford disease or syndrome (progeria) 259.8
Hyaline
    degeneration (diffuse) (generalized) 728.9
        localized - *see* Degeneration, by site
    membrane (disease) (lung) (newborn) 769
Hyalinosis cutis et mucosae 272.8
Hyalin plaque, sclera, senile 379.16
Hyalitis (asteroid) 379.22
    syphilitic 095.8
Hydatid
    cyst or tumor - *see also* Echinococcus
        fallopian tube 752.11

Hydatid (*Continued*)
    mole - *see* Hydatidiform mole
    Morgagni (congenital) 752.89
        fallopian tube 752.11
Hydatidiform mole (benign) (complicating pregnancy) (delivered) (undelivered) 630
    invasive (M9100/1) 236.1
    malignant (M9100/1) 236.1
    previous, affecting management of pregnancy V23.1
Hydatidosis - *see* Echinococcus
Hyde's disease (prurigo nodularis) 698.3
Hydradenitis 705.83
Hydradenoma (M8400/0) - *see* Hidradenoma
Hydralazine lupus or syndrome
    correct substance properly administered 695.4
    overdose or wrong substance given or taken 972.6
Hydramnios 657
    affecting fetus or newborn 761.3
Hydrancephaly 742.3
    with spina bifida (*see also* Spina bifida) 741.0
Hydranencephaly 742.3
    with spina bifida (*see also* Spina bifida) 741.0
Hydrargyrism NEC 985.0
Hydrarthrosis (*see also* Effusion, joint) 719.0
    gonococcal 098.50
    intermittent (*see also* Rheumatism, palindromic) 719.3
    of yaws (early) (late) 102.6
    syphilitic 095.8
        congenital 090.5
Hydremia 285.9
Hydrencephalocele (congenital) 742.0
Hydrencephalomeningocele (congenital) 742.0
Hydroa 694.0
    aestivale 692.72
    gestationis 646.8
    herpetiformis 694.0
    pruriginosa 694.0
    vacciniforme 692.72
Hydroadenitis 705.83
Hydrocalycosis (*see also* Hydronephrosis) 591
    congenital 753.29
Hydrocalyx (*see also* Hydronephrosis) 591
Hydrocele (calcified) (chylous) (idiopathic) (infantile) (inguinal canal) (recurrent) (senile) (spermatic cord) (testis) (tunica vaginalis) 603.9
    canal of Nuck (female) 629.1
        male 603.9
    congenital 778.6
    encysted 603.0
        congenital 778.6
    female NEC 629.8
    infected 603.1
    round ligament 629.8
    specified type NEC 603.8
        congenital 778.6
    spinalis (*see also* Spina bifida) 741.9
    vulva 624.8
Hydrocephalic fetus
    affecting management or pregnancy 655.0
    causing disproportion 653.6
        with obstructed labor 660.1
            affecting fetus or newborn 763.1

Hydrocephalus (acquired) (external) (internal) (malignant) (noncommunicating) (obstructive) (recurrent) 331.4
    aqueduct of Sylvius stricture 742.3
        with spina bifida (*see also* Spina bifida) 741.0
    chronic 742.3
        with spina bifida (*see also* Spina bifida) 741.0
    communicating 331.3
    congenital (external) (internal) 742.3
        with spina bifida (*see also* Spina bifida) 741.0
    due to
        stricture of aqueduct of Sylvius 742.3
            with spina bifida (*see also* Spina bifida) 741.0
        toxoplasmosis (congenital) 771.2
    fetal affecting management of pregnancy 655.0
    foramen Magendie block (acquired) 331.3
        congenital 742.3
            with spina bifida (*see also* Spina bifida) 741.0
    newborn 742.3
        with spina bifida (*see also* Spina bifida) 741.0
    otitic 331.4
    syphilitic, congenital 090.49
    tuberculous (*see also* Tuberculosis) 013.8
Hydrocolpos (congenital) 623.8
Hydrocystoma (M8404/0) - *see* Neoplasm, skin, benign
Hydroencephalocele (congenital) 742.0
Hydroencephalomeningocele (congenital) 742.0
Hydrohematopneumothorax (*see also* Hemothorax) 511.8
Hydromeningitis - *see* Meningitis
Hydromeningocele (spinal) (*see also* Spina bifida) 741.9
    cranial 742.0
Hydrometra 621.8
Hydrometrocolpos 623.8
Hydromicrocephaly 742.1
Hydromphalus (congenital) (since birth) 757.39
Hydromyelia 742.53
Hydromyelocele (*see also* Spina bifida) 741.9
Hydronephrosis 591
    atrophic 591
    congenital 753.29
    due to S. hematobium 120.0
    early 591
    functionless (infected) 591
    infected 591
    intermittent 591
    primary 591
    secondary 591
    tuberculous (*see also* Tuberculosis) 016.0
Hydropericarditis (*see also* Pericarditis) 423.9
Hydropericardium (*see also* Pericarditis) 423.9
Hydroperitoneum 789.5
Hydrophobia 071
Hydrophthalmos (*see also* Buphthalmia) 743.20
Hydropneumohemothorax (*see also* Hemothorax) 511.8
Hydropneumopericarditis (*see also* Pericarditis) 423.9

Hydropneumopericardium (*see also* Pericarditis) 423.9
Hydropneumothorax 511.8
  nontuberculous 511.8
    bacterial 511.1
    pneumococcal 511.1
    staphylococcal 511.1
    streptococcal 511.1
  traumatic 860.0
    with open wound into thorax 860.1
  tuberculous (*see also* Tuberculosis, pleura) 012.0
Hydrops 782.3
  abdominis 789.5
  amnii (complicating pregnancy) (*see also* Hydramnios) 657
  articulorum intermittens (*see also* Rheumatism, palindromic) 719.3
  cardiac (*see also* Failure, heart) 428.0
  congenital - *see* Hydrops, fetalis
  endolymphatic (*see also* Disease, Meniere's) 386.00
  fetal(is) or newborn 778.0
    due to isoimmunization 773.3
    not due to isoimmunization 778.0
  gallbladder 575.3
  idiopathic (fetus or newborn) 778.0
  joint (*see also* Effusion, joint) 719.0
  labyrinth (*see also* Disease, Meniere's) 386.00
  meningeal NEC 331.4
  nutritional 262
  pericardium - *see* Pericarditis
  pleura (*see also* Hydrothorax) 511.8
  renal (*see also* Nephrosis) 581.9
  spermatic cord (*see also* Hydrocele) 603.9
Hydropyonephrosis (*see also* Pyelitis) 590.80
  chronic 590.00
Hydrorachis 742.53
Hydrorrhea (nasal) 478.1
  gravidarum 658.1
  pregnancy 658.1
Hydrosadenitis 705.83
Hydrosalpinx (fallopian tube) (follicularis) 614.1
Hydrothorax (double) (pleural) 511.8
  chylous (nonfilarial) 457.8
    filaria (*see also* Infestation, filarial) 125.9
  nontuberculous 511.8
    bacterial 511.1
    pneumococcal 511.1
    staphylococcal 511.1
    streptococcal 511.1
  traumatic 862.29
    with open wound into thorax 862.39
  tuberculous (*see also* Tuberculosis, pleura) 012.0
Hydroureter 593.5
  congenital 753.22
Hydroureteronephrosis (*see also* Hydronephrosis) 591
Hydrourethra 599.84
Hydroxykynureninuria 270.2
Hydroxyprolinemia 270.8
Hydroxyprolinuria 270.8
Hygroma (congenital) (cystic) (M9173/0) 228.1
  prepatellar 727.3
  subdural - *see* Hematoma, subdural
Hymen - *see* condition

Hymenolepiasis (diminuta) (infection) (infestation) (nana) 123.6
Hymenolepsis (diminuta) (infection) (infestation) (nana) 123.6
Hypalgesia (*see also* Disturbance, sensation) 782.0
Hyperabduction syndrome 447.8
Hyperacidity, gastric 536.8
  psychogenic 306.4
Hyperactive, hyperactivity
  basal cell, uterine cervix 622.10 ◀▬
  bladder 596.51
  bowel (syndrome) 564.9
    sounds 787.5
  cervix epithelial (basal) 622.10 ◀▬
  child 314.01
  colon 564.9
  gastrointestinal 536.8
    psychogenic 306.4
  intestine 564.9
  labyrinth (unilateral) 386.51
    with loss of labyrinthine reactivity 386.58
    bilateral 386.52
  nasal mucous membrane 478.1
  stomach 536.8
  thyroid (gland) (*see also* Thyrotoxicosis) 242.9
Hyperacusis 388.42
Hyperadrenalism (cortical) 255.3
  medullary 255.6
Hyperadrenocorticism 255.3
  congenital 255.2
  iatrogenic
    correct substance properly administered 255.3
    overdose or wrong substance given or taken 962.0
Hyperaffectivity 301.11
Hyperaldosteronism (atypical) (hyperplastic) (normoaldosteronal) (normotensive) (primary) 255.10
  seconday 255.14
Hyperalgesia (*see also* Disturbance, sensation) 782.0
Hyperalimentation 783.6
  carotene 278.3
  specified NEC 278.8
  vitamin A 278.2
  vitamin D 278.4
Hyperaminoaciduria 270.9
  arginine 270.6
  citrulline 270.6
  cystine 270.0
  glycine 270.0
  lysine 270.7
  ornithine 270.6
  renal (types I, II, III) 270.0
Hyperammonemia (congenital) 270.6
Hyperamnesia 780.9
Hyperamylasemia 790.5
Hyperamnesia 780.99
Hyperaphia 782.0
Hyperazotemia 791.9
Hyperbetalipoproteinemia (acquired) (essential) (familial) (hereditary) (primary) (secondary) 272.0
  with prebetalipoproteinemia 272.2
Hyperbilirubinemia 782.4
  congenital 277.4
  constitutional 277.4
  neonatal (transient) (*see also* Jaundice, fetus or newborn) 774.6
  of prematurity 774.2

Hyperbilirubinemica encephalopathia, newborn 774.7
  due to isoimmunization 773.4
Hypercalcemia, hypercalcemic (idiopathic) 275.42
  nephropathy 588.89 ◀▬
Hypercalcinuria 275.40
Hypercapnia 786.09
  with mixed acid-base disorder 276.4
  fetal, affecting newborn 770.89
Hypercarotinemia 278.3
Hypercementosis 521.5
Hyperchloremia 276.9
Hyperchlorhydria 536.8
  neurotic 306.4
  psychogenic 306.4
Hypercholesterinemia - *see* Hypercholesterolemia
Hypercholesterolemia 272.0
  with hyperglyceridemia, endogenous 272.2
  essential 272.0
  familial 272.0
  hereditary 272.0
  primary 272.0
  pure 272.0
Hypercholesterolosis 272.0
Hyperchylia gastrica 536.8
  psychogenic 306.4
Hyperchylomicronemia (familial) (with hyperbetalipoproteinemia) 272.3
Hypercoagulation syndrome (primary) 289.81
  secondary 289.82
Hypercorticosteronism
  correct substance properly administered 255.3
  overdose or wrong substance given or taken 962.0
Hypercortisonism
  correct substance properly administered 255.3
  overdose or wrong substance given or taken 962.0
Hyperdynamic beta-adrenergic state or syndrome (circulatory) 429.82
Hyperekplexia 759.89 ◀
Hyperelectrolytemia 276.9
Hyperemesis 536.2
  arising during pregnancy - *see* Hyperemesis, gravidarum
  gravidarum (mild) (before 22 completed weeks' gestation) 643.0
    with
      carbohydrate depletion 643.1
      dehydration 643.1
      electrolyte imbalance 643.1
      metabolic disturbance 643.1
    affecting fetus or newborn 761.8
    severe (with metabolic disturbance) 643.1
  psychogenic 306.4
Hyperemia (acute) 780.99
  anal mucosa 569.49
  bladder 596.7
  cerebral 437.8
  conjunctiva 372.71
  ear, internal, acute 386.30
  enteric 564.89
  eye 372.71
  eyelid (active) (passive) 374.82
  intestine 564.89
  iris 364.41
  kidney 593.81
  labyrinth 386.30
  liver (active) (passive) 573.8

ICD-9-CM

II

Vol. 2

Hyperemia (Continued)
  lung 514
  ovary 620.8
  passive 780.99
  pulmonary 514
  renal 593.81
  retina 362.89
  spleen 289.59
  stomach 537.89
Hyperesthesia (body surface) (see also
    Disturbance, sensation) 782.0
  larynx (reflex) 478.79
    hysterical 300.11
  pharynx (reflex) 478.29
Hyperestrinism 256.0
Hyperestrogenism 256.0
Hyperestrogenosis 256.0
Hyperextension, joint 718.80
  ankle 718.87
  elbow 718.82
  foot 718.87
  hand 718.84
  hip 718.85
  knee 718.86
  multiple sites 718.89
  pelvic region 718.85
  shoulder (region) 718.81
  specified site NEC 718.88
  wrist 718.83
Hyperexplexia 759.89 ◀
Hyperfibrinolysis - see Fibrinolysis
Hyperfolliculinism 256.0
Hyperfructosemia 271.2
Hyperfunction
  adrenal (cortex) 255.3
    androgenic, acquired benign 255.3
    medulla 255.6
    virilism 255.2
  corticoadrenal NEC 255.3
  labyrinth - see Hyperactive, labyrinth
  medulloadrenal 255.6
  ovary 256.1
    estrogen 256.0
  pancreas 577.8
  parathyroid (gland) 252.00 ◀═
  pituitary (anterior) (gland) (lobe) 253.1
  testicular 257.0
Hypergammaglobulinemia 289.89
  monoclonal, benign (BMH) 273.1
  polyclonal 273.0
  Waldenström's 273.0
Hyperglobulinemia 273.8
Hyperglycemia 790.6
  maternal
    affecting fetus or newborn 775.0
    manifest diabetes in infant 775.1
  postpancreatectomy (complete) (par-
    tial) 251.3
Hyperglyceridemia 272.1
  endogenous 272.1
  essential 272.1
  familial 272.1
  hereditary 272.1
  mixed 272.3
  pure 272.1
Hyperglycinemia 270.7
Hypergonadism
  ovarian 256.1
  testicular (infantile) (primary) 257.0
Hyperheparinemia (see also Circulating
    anticoagulants) 286.5
Hyperhidrosis, hyperidrosis 705.21 ◀═
  axilla 705.21 ◀
  face 705.21 ◀

Hyperhidrosis, hyperidrosis (Continued)
  focal (localized) 705.21 ◀
    primary 705.21 ◀
      axilla 705.21 ◀
      face 705.21 ◀
      palms 705.21 ◀
      soles 705.21 ◀
    secondary 705.22 ◀
      axilla 705.22 ◀
      face 705.22 ◀
      palms 705.22 ◀
      soles 705.22 ◀
  generalized 780.8 ◀
  palms 705.21 ◀
  psychogenic 306.3
  secondary 780.8 ◀
  soles 705.21 ◀
Hyperhistidinemia 270.5
Hyperinsulinism (ectopic) (functional)
    (organic) NEC 251.1
  iatrogenic 251.0
  reactive 251.2
  spontaneous 251.2
  therapeutic misadventure (from ad-
    ministration of insulin) 962.3
Hyperiodemia 276.9
Hyperirritability (cerebral), in newborn
    779.1
Hyperkalemia 276.7
Hyperkeratosis (see also Keratosis) 701.1 ◀═
  cervix 622.10
  congenital 757.39
  cornea 371.89
  due to yaws (early) (late) (palmar or
    plantar) 102.3
  eccentrica 757.39
  figurata centrifuga atrophica 757.39
  follicularis 757.39
    in cutem penetrans 701.1
  limbic (cornea) 371.89
  palmoplantaris climacterica 701.1
  pinta (carate) 103.1
  senile (with pruritus) 702.0
  tongue 528.79 ◀═
  universalis congenita 757.1
  vagina 623.1
  vocal cord 478.5
  vulva 624.0
Hyperkinesia, hyperkinetic (disease) (re-
    action) (syndrome) 314.9
  with
    attention deficit - see Disorder, atten-
      tion deficit
    conduct disorder 314.2
    developmental delay 314.1
    simple disturbance of activity and
      attention 314.01
    specified manifestation NEC 314.8
  heart (disease) 429.82
  of childhood or adolescence NEC 314.9
Hyperlacrimation (see also Epiphora)
    375.20
Hyperlipemia (see also Hyperlipidemia)
    272.4
Hyperlipidemia 272.4
  carbohydrate-induced 272.1
  combined 272.4
  endogenous 272.1
  exogenous 272.3
  fat-induced 272.3
  group
    A 272.0
    B 272.1
    C 272.2
    D 272.3

Hyperlipidemia (Continued)
  mixed 272.2
  specified type NEC 272.4
Hyperlipidosis 272.7
  hereditary 272.7
Hyperlipoproteinemia (acquired) (essen-
    tial) (familial) (hereditary) (primary)
    (secondary) 272.4
  Fredrickson type
    I 272.3
    IIA 272.0
    IIB 272.2
    III 272.2
    IV 272.1
    V 272.3
  low-density-lipoid-type (LDL) 272.0
  very-low-density-lipoid-type [VLDL]
    272.1
Hyperlucent lung, unilateral 492.8
Hyperluteinization 256.1
Hyperlysinemia 270.7
Hypermagnesemia 275.2
  neonatal 775.5
Hypermaturity (fetus or newborn)
  post-term infant 766.21 ◀═
  prolonged gestation infant 766.22
Hypermenorrhea 626.2
Hypermetabolism 794.7
Hypermethioninemia 270.4
Hypermetropia (congenital) 367.0
Hypermobility
  cecum 564.9
  coccyx 724.71
  colon 564.9
    psychogenic 306.4
  ileum 564.89
  joint (acquired) 718.80
    ankle 718.87
    elbow 718.82
    foot 718.87
    hand 718.84
    hip 718.85
    knee 718.86
    multiple sites 718.89
    pelvic region 718.85
    shoulder (region) 718.81
    specified site NEC 718.88
    wrist 718.83
  kidney, congenital 753.3
  meniscus (knee) 717.5
  scapula 718.81
  stomach 536.8
    psychogenic 306.4
  syndrome 728.5
  testis, congenital 752.52
  urethral 599.81
Hypermotility
  gastrointestinal 536.8
  intestine 564.9
    psychogenic 306.4
  stomach 536.8
Hypernasality 784.49
Hypernatremia 276.0
  with water depletion 276.0
Hypernephroma (M8312/3) 189.0
Hyperopia 367.0
Hyperorexia 783.6
Hyperornithinemia 270.6
Hyperosmia (see also Disturbance, sensa-
    tion) 781.1
Hyperosmolality 276.0
Hyperosteogenesis 733.99
Hyperostosis 733.99
  calvarial 733.3

◀ **New**   ◀═ **Revised**

Hyperostosis *(Continued)*
cortical 733.3
infantile 756.59
frontal, internal of skull 733.3
interna frontalis 733.3
monomelic 733.99
skull 733.3
congenital 756.0
vertebral 721.8
with spondylosis - *see* Spondylosis
ankylosing 721.6
Hyperovarianism 256.1
Hyperovarism, hyperovaria 256.1
Hyperoxaluria (primary) 271.8
Hyperoxia 987.8
Hyperparathyroidism 252.00
ectopic 259.3
other 252.08
primary 252.01
secondary (of renal origin) 588.81
non-renal 252.02
tertiary 252.08
Hyperpathia (*see also* Disturbance, sensation) 782.0
psychogenic 307.80
Hyperperistalsis 787.4
psychogenic 306.4
Hyperpermeability, capillary 448.9
Hyperphagia 783.6
Hyperphenylalaninemia 270.1
Hyperphoria 378.40
alternating 378.45
Hyperphosphatemia 275.3
Hyperpiesia (*see also* Hypertension) 401.9
Hyperpiesis (*see also* Hypertension) 401.9
Hyperpigmentation - *see* Pigmentation
Hyperpinealism 259.8
Hyperpipecolatemia 270.7
Hyperpituitarism 253.1
Hyperplasia, hyperplastic
adenoids (lymphoid tissue) 474.12
and tonsils 474.10
adrenal (capsule) (cortex) (gland) 255.8
with
sexual precocity (male) 255.2
virilism, adrenal 255.2
virilization (female) 255.2
congenital 255.2
due to excess ACTH (ectopic) (pituitary) 255.0
medulla 255.8
alpha cells (pancreatic)
with
gastrin excess 251.5
glucagon excess 251.4
appendix (lymphoid) 543.0
artery, fibromuscular NEC 447.8
carotid 447.8
renal 447.3
bone 733.99
marrow 289.9
breast (*see also* Hypertrophy, breast) 611.1
carotid artery 447.8
cementation, cementum (teeth) (tooth) 521.5
cervical gland 785.6
cervix (uteri) 622.10
basal cell 622.10
congenital 752.49
endometrium 622.10
polypoid 622.10
chin 524.05
clitoris, congenital 752.49
dentin 521.5

Hyperplasia, hyperplastic *(Continued)*
endocervicitis 616.0
endometrium, endometrial (adenomatous) (atypical) (cystic) (glandular) (polypoid) (uterus) 621.30
with atypia 621.33
without atypia
complex 621.32
simple 621.31
cervix 622.10
epithelial 709.8
focal, oral, including tongue 528.79
mouth (focal) 528.79
nipple 611.8
skin 709.8
tongue (focal) 528.79
vaginal wall 623.0
erythroid 289.9
fascialis ossificans (progressiva) 728.11
fibromuscular, artery NEC 447.8
carotid 447.8
renal 447.3
genital
female 629.8
male 608.89
gingiva 523.8
glandularis
cystica uteri 621.30
endometrium (uterus) 621.30
interstitialis uteri 621.30
granulocytic 288.8
gum 523.8
hymen, congenital 752.49
islands of Langerhans 251.1
islet cell (pancreatic) 251.9
alpha cells
with excess
gastrin 251.5
glucagon 251.4
beta cells 251.1
juxtaglomerular (complex) (kidney) 593.89
kidney (congenital) 753.3
liver (congenital) 751.69
lymph node (gland) 785.6
lymphoid (diffuse) (nodular) 785.6
appendix 543.0
intestine 569.89
mandibular 524.02
alveolar 524.72
unilateral condylar 526.89
Marchand multiple nodular (liver) - *see* Cirrhosis, postnecrotic
maxillary 524.01
alveolar 524.71
medulla, adrenal 255.8
myometrium, myometrial 621.2
nose (lymphoid) (polypoid) 478.1
oral soft tissue (inflammatory) (irritative) (mucosa) NEC 528.9
gingiva 523.8
tongue 529.8
organ or site, congenital NEC - *see* Anomaly, specified type NEC
ovary 620.8
palate, papillary 528.9
pancreatic islet cells 251.9
alpha
with excess
gastrin 251.5
glucagon 251.4
beta 251.1
parathyroid (gland) 252.01
persistent, vitreous (primary) 743.51

Hyperplasia, hyperplastic *(Continued)*
pharynx (lymphoid) 478.29
prostate 600.90
with urinary retention 600.91
adenofibromatous 600.20
with urinary retention 600.21
nodular 600.10
with urinary retention 600.11
renal artery (fibromuscular) 447.3
reticuloendothelial (cell) 289.9
salivary gland (any) 527.1
Schimmelbusch's 610.1
suprarenal (capsule) (gland) 255.8
thymus (gland) (persistent) 254.0
thyroid (*see also* Goiter) 240.9
primary 242.0
secondary 242.2
tonsil (lymphoid tissue) 474.11
and adenoids 474.10
urethrovaginal 599.89
uterus, uterine (myometrium) 621.2
endometrium (*see also* Hyperplasia, endometrium) 621.30
vitreous (humor), primary persistent 743.51
vulva 624.3
zygoma 738.11
Hyperpnea (*see also* Hyperventilation) 786.01
Hyperpotassemia 276.7
Hyperprebetalipoproteinemia 272.1
with chylomicronemia 272.3
familial 272.1
Hyperprolactinemia 253.1
Hyperprolinemia 270.8
Hyperproteinemia 273.8
Hyperprothrombinemia 289.89
Hyperpselaphesia 782.0
Hyperpyrexia 780.6
heat (effects of) 992.0
malarial (*see also* Malaria) 084.6
malignant, due to anesthetic 995.86
rheumatic - *see* Fever, rheumatic
unknown origin (*see also* Pyrexia) 780.6
Hyperreactor, vascular 780.2
Hyperreflexia 796.1
bladder, autonomic 596.54
with cauda equina 344.61
detrusor 344.61
Hypersalivation (*see also* Ptyalism) 527.7
Hypersarcosinemia 270.8
Hypersecretion
ACTH 255.3
androgens (ovarian) 256.1
calcitonin 246.0
corticoadrenal 255.3
cortisol 255.0
estrogen 256.0
gastric 536.8
psychogenic 306.4
gastrin 251.5
glucagon 251.4
hormone
ACTH 255.3
anterior pituitary 253.1
growth NEC 253.0
ovarian androgen 256.1
testicular 257.0
thyroid stimulating 242.8
insulin - *see* Hyperinsulinism
lacrimal glands (*see also* Epiphora) 375.20
medulloadrenal 255.6
milk 676.6

ICD-9-CM

Vol. 2

	Malignant	Benign	Unspecified
Hypertension, hypertensive (arterial) (arteriolar) (crisis) (degeneration) (disease) (essential) (fluctuating) (idiopathic) (intermittent) (labile) (low renin) (orthostatic) (paroxysmal) (primary) (systemic) (uncontrolled) (vascular)	401.0	401.1	401.9
with			
heart involvement (conditions classifiable to 429.0-429.3, 429.8, 429.9 due to hypertension) (*see also* Hypertension, heart)	402.00	402.10	402.90 ◀▥
with kidney involvement-*see* Hypertension, cardiorenal			
renal involvement (only conditions classifiable to 585, 586, 587) (excludes conditions classifiable to 584) (*see also* Hypertension, kidney)	403.00	403.10	403.90
with heart involvement-*see* Hypertension, cardiorenal			
failure (and sclerosis) (*see also* Hypertension, kidney)	403.01	403.11	403.91
sclerosis without failure (*see also* Hypertension, kidney)	403.00	403.10	403.90
accelerated (*see also* Hypertension, by type, malignant)	401.0	-	-
antepartum-see Hypertension, complicating pregnancy, childbirth, or the puerperium			
cardiorenal (disease)	404.00	404.10	404.90
with			
heart failure	404.01	404.11	404.91
and renal failure	404.03	404.13	404.93
renal failure	404.02	404.12	404.92
and heart failure	404.03	404.13	404.93
cardiovascular disease (arteriosclerotic) (sclerotic)	402.00	402.10	402.90
with			
heart failure	402.01	402.11	402.91
renal involvement (conditions classifiable to 403) (*see also* Hypertension, cardiorenal)	404.00	404.10	404.90
cardiovascular renal (disease) (sclerosis) (*see also* Hypertension, cardiorenal)	404.00	404.10	404.90
cerebrovascular disease NEC	437.2	437.2	437.2
complicating pregnancy, childbirth, or the puerperium	642.2	642.0	642.9
with			
albuminuria (and edema) (mild)	-	-	642.4
severe	-	-	642.5
edema (mild)	-	-	642.4
severe	-	-	642.5
heart disease	642.2	642.2	642.2
and renal disease	642.2	642.2	642.2
renal disease	642.2	642.2	642.2
and heart disease	642.2	642.2	642.2
chronic	642.2	642.0	642.0
with pre-eclampsia or eclampsia	642.7	642.7	642.7
fetus or newborn	760.0	760.0	760.0
essential	-	642.0	642.0
with pre-eclampsia or eclampsia	-	642.7	642.7
fetus or newborn	760.0	760.0	760.0
fetus or newborn	760.0	760.0	760.0
gestational	-	-	642.3
pre-existing	642.2	642.0	642.0
with pre-eclampsia or eclampsia	642.7	642.7	642.7
fetus or newborn	760.0	760.0	760.0
secondary to renal disease	642.1	642.1	642.1
with pre-eclampsia or eclampsia	642.7	642.7	642.7
fetus or newborn	760.0	760.0	760.0
transient	-	-	642.3
due to			
aldosteronism, primary	405.09	405.19	405.99
brain tumor	405.09	405.19	405.99
bulbar poliomyelitis	405.09	405.19	405.99
calculus			
kidney	405.09	405.19	405.99
ureter	405.09	405.19	405.99
coarctation, aorta	405.09	405.19	405.99
Cushing's disease	405.09	405.19	405.99
glomerulosclerosis (*see also* Hypertension, kidney)	403.00	403.10	403.90
periarteritis nodosa	405.09	405.19	405.99
pheochromocytoma	405.09	405.19	405.99
polycystic kidney(s)	405.09	405.19	405.99
polycythemia	405.09	405.19	405.99
porphyria	405.09	405.19	405.99
pyelonephritis	405.09	405.19	405.99
renal (artery)			
aneurysm	405.01	405.11	405.91
anomaly	405.01	405.11	405.91
embolism	405.01	405.11	405.91
fibromuscular hyperplasia	405.01	405.11	405.91
occlusion	405.01	405.11	405.91

◀ New   ◀▥ Revised

	Malignant	Benign	Unspecified
Hypertension *(Continued)*			
due to *(Continued)*			
renal *(Continued)*			
stenosis	405.01	405.11	405.91
thrombosis	405.01	405.11	405.91
encephalopathy	437.2	437.2	437.2
gestational (transient) NEC	-	-	642.3
Goldblatt's	440.1	440.1	440.1
heart (disease) (conditions classifiable to 429.0-429.3, 429.8, 429.9 due to hypertension)	402.00	402.10	402.90 ◀▥
with			
heart failure	402.01	402.11	402.91
hypertensive kidney disease (conditions classifiable to 403) (*see also* Hypertension, cardiorenal)	404.00	404.10	404.90
renal sclerosis (*see also* Hypertension, cardiorenal)	404.00	404.10	404.90
intracranial, benign	-	348.2	-
intraocular	-	-	365.04
kidney	403.00	403.10	403.90
with			
heart involvement (conditions classifiable to 429.0-429.3, 429.8, 429.9 due to hypertension) (*see also* Hypertension, cardiorenal)	404.00	404.10	404.90 ◀▥
hypertensive heart (disease) (conditions classifiable to 402) (*see also* Hypertension, cardiorenal)	404.00	404.10	404.90
renal failure (conditions classifiable to 585, 586)	403.01	403.11	403.91
lesser circulation	-	-	416.0
necrotizing	401.0	-	-
ocular	-	-	365.04
portal (due to chronic liver disease)	-	-	572.3
postoperative			997.91
psychogenic	-	-	306.2
puerperal, postpartum-			
see Hypertension, complicating pregnancy, childbirth, or the puerperium			
pulmonary (artery)	-	-	416.8
with cor pulmonale (chronic)	-	-	416.8
acute	-	-	415.0
idiopathic	-	-	416.0
primary	-	-	416.0
of newborn	-	-	747.83
secondary	-	-	416.8
renal (disease) (*see also* Hypertension, kidney)	403.00	403.10	403.90
renovascular NEC	405.01	405.11	405.91
secondary NEC	405.09	405.19	405.99
due to			
aldosteronism, primary	405.09	405.19	405.99
brain tumor	405.09	405.19	405.99
bulbar poliomyelitis	405.09	405.19	405.99
calculus			
kidney	405.09	405.19	405.99
ureter	405.09	405.19	405.99
coarctation, aorta	405.09	405.19	405.99
Cushing's disease	405.09	405.19	405.99
glomerulosclerosis (*see also* Hypertension, kidney)	403.00	403.10	403.90
periarteritis nodosa	405.09	405.19	405.99
pheochromocytoma	405.09	405.19	405.99
polycystic kidney(s)	405.09	405.19	405.99
polycythemia	405.09	405.19	405.99
porphyria	405.09	405.19	405.99
pyelonephritis	405.09	405.19	405.99
renal (artery)			
aneurysm	405.01	405.11	405.91
anomaly	405.01	405.11	405.91
embolism	405.01	405.11	405.91
fibromuscular hyperplasia	405.01	405.11	405.91
occlusion	405.01	405.11	405.91
stenosis	405.01	405.11	405.91
thrombosis	405.01	405.11	405.91
transient	-	-	796.2
of pregnancy			642.3
venous, chronic (asymptomatic) (idiopathic)	-	-	459.30
due to			
deep vein thrombosis (*see also* Syndrome, postphlebitic)	-	-	459.10
with			
complication, NEC	-	-	459.39
inflammation	-	-	459.32
with ulcer	-	-	459.33
ulcer	-	-	459.31
with inflammation	-	-	459.33

ICD-9-CM

Vol. 2

Hypersecretion (Continued)
ovarian androgens 256.1
pituitary (anterior) 253.1
salivary gland (any) 527.7
testicular hormones 257.0
thyrocalcitonin 246.0
upper respiratory 478.9
Hypersegmentation, hereditary 288.2
eosinophils 288.2
neutrophil nuclei 288.2
Hypersensitive, hypersensitiveness, hypersensitivity - see also Allergy
angiitis 446.20
specified NEC 446.29
carotid sinus 337.0
colon 564.9
psychogenic 306.4
DNA (deoxyribonucleic acid) NEC 287.2
drug (see also Allergy, drug) 995.2
esophagus 530.89
insect bites - see Injury, superficial, by site
labyrinth 386.58
pain (see also Disturbance, sensation)
782.0
pneumonitis NEC 495.9
reaction (see also Allergy) 995.3
upper respiratory tract NEC 478.8
stomach (allergic) (nonallergic) 536.8
psychogenic 306.4
Hypersomatotropism (classic) 253.0
Hypersomnia 780.54
with sleep apnea 780.53
nonorganic origin 307.43
persistent (primary) 307.44
transient 307.43
Hypersplenia 289.4
Hypersplenism 289.4
Hypersteatosis 706.3
Hyperstimulation, ovarian 256.1
Hypersuprarenalism 255.3
Hypersusceptibility - see Allergy
Hyper-TBG-nemia 246.8
Hypertelorism 756.0
orbit, orbital 376.41
Hyperthecosis, ovary 256.8
Hyperthermia (of unknown origin) (see also Pyrexia) 780.6
malignant (due to anesthesia) 995.86
newborn 778.4
Hyperthymergasia (see also Psychosis, affective) 296.0
reactive (from emotional stress, psychological trauma) 298.1
recurrent episode 296.1
single episode 296.0
Hyperthymism 254.8
Hyperthyroid (recurrent) - see Hyperthyroidism
Hyperthyroidism (latent) (preadult) (recurrent) (without goiter) 242.9

Note   Use the following fifth-digit
subclassification with category 242:

0	without mention of thyrotoxic crisis or storm
1	with mention of thyrotoxic crisis or storm

with
goiter (diffuse) 242.0
adenomatous 242.3
multinodular 242.2
uninodular 242.1

Hyperthyroidism (Continued)
with (Continued)
goiter (Continued)
nodular 242.3
multinodular 242.2
uninodular 242.1
thyroid nodule 242.1
complicating pregnancy, childbirth, or puerperium 648.1
neonatal (transient) 775.3
Hypertonia - see Hypertonicity
Hypertonicity
bladder 596.51
fetus or newborn 779.89
gastrointestinal (tract) 536.8
infancy 779.89
due to electrolyte imbalance 779.89
muscle 728.85
stomach 536.8
psychogenic 306.4
uterus, uterine (contractions) 661.4
affecting fetus or newborn 763.7
Hypertony - see Hypertonicity
Hypertransaminemia 790.4
Hypertrichosis 704.1
congenital 757.4
eyelid 374.54
lanuginosa 757.4
acquired 704.1
Hypertriglyceridemia, essential 272.1
Hypertrophy, hypertrophic
adenoids (infectional) 474.12
and tonsils (faucial) (infective) (lingual) (lymphoid) 474.10
adrenal 255.8
alveolar process or ridge 525.8
anal papillae 569.49
apocrine gland 705.82
artery NEC 447.8
carotid 447.8
congenital (peripheral) NEC 747.60
gastrointestinal 747.61
lower limb 747.64
renal 747.62
specified NEC 747.69
spinal 747.82
upper limb 747.63
renal 447.3
arthritis (chronic) (see also Osteoarthrosis) 715.9
spine (see also Spondylosis) 721.90
arytenoid 478.79
asymmetrical (heart) 429.9
auricular - see Hypertrophy, cardiac
Bartholin's gland 624.8
bile duct 576.8
bladder (sphincter) (trigone) 596.8
blind spot, visual field 368.42
bone 733.99
brain 348.8
breast 611.1
cystic 610.1
fetus or newborn 778.7
fibrocystic 610.1
massive pubertal 611.1
puerperal, postpartum 676.3
senile (parenchymatous) 611.1
cardiac (chronic) (idiopathic) 429.3
with
rheumatic fever (conditions classifiable to 390)
active 391.8
with chorea 392.0
inactive or quiescent (with chorea) 398.99

Hypertrophy, hypertrophic (Continued)
cardiac (Continued)
congenital NEC 746.89
fatty (see also Degeneration, myocardial) 429.1
hypertensive (see also Hypertension, heart) 402.90
rheumatic (with chorea) 398.99
active or acute 391.8
with chorea 392.0
valve (see also Endocarditis) 424.90
congenital NEC 746.89
cartilage 733.99
cecum 569.89
cervix (uteri) 622.6
congenital 752.49
elongation 622.6
clitoris (cirrhotic) 624.2
congenital 752.49
colon 569.89
congenital 751.3
conjunctiva, lymphoid 372.73
cornea 371.89
corpora cavernosa 607.89
duodenum 537.89
endometrium (uterus) (see also Hyperplasia, endometrium) 621.30 ◀▥
cervix 622.6
epididymis 608.89
esophageal hiatus (congenital) 756.6
with hernia - see Hernia, diaphragm
eyelid 374.30
falx, skull 733.99
fat pad 729.30
infrapatellar 729.31
knee 729.31
orbital 374.34
popliteal 729.31
prepatellar 729.31
retropatellar 729.31
specified site NEC 729.39
foot (congenital) 755.67
frenum, frenulum (tongue) 529.8
linguae 529.8
lip 528.5
gallbladder or cystic duct 575.8
gastric mucosa 535.2
gingiva 523.8
gland, glandular (general) NEC 785.6
gum (mucous membrane) 523.8
heart (idiopathic) - see also Hypertrophy, cardiac
valve - see also Endocarditis
congenital NEC 746.89
hemifacial 754.0
hepatic - see Hypertrophy, liver
hiatus (esophageal) 756.6
hilus gland 785.6
hymen, congenital 752.49
ileum 569.89
infrapatellar fat pad 729.31
intestine 569.89
jejunum 569.89
kidney (compensatory) 593.1
congenital 753.3
labial frenulum 528.5
labium (majus) (minus) 624.3
lacrimal gland, chronic 375.03
ligament 728.9
spinal 724.8
linguae frenulum 529.8
lingual tonsil (infectional) 474.11
lip (frenum) 528.5
congenital 744.81

◀ **New**   ◀▥ **Revised**

Hypertrophy, hypertrophic *(Continued)*
　liver 789.1
　　acute 573.8
　　cirrhotic - *see* Cirrhosis, liver
　　congenital 751.69
　　fatty - *see* Fatty, liver
　lymph gland 785.6
　　tuberculous - *see* Tuberculosis,
　　　lymph gland
　mammary gland - *see* Hypertrophy,
　　breast
　maxillary frenulum 528.5
　Meckel's diverticulum (congenital)
　　751.0
　medial meniscus, acquired 717.3
　median bar 600.90
　　with urinary retention 600.91
　mediastinum 519.3
　meibomian gland 373.2
　meniscus, knee, congenital 755.64
　metatarsal head 733.99
　metatarsus 733.99
　mouth 528.9
　mucous membrane
　　alveolar process 523.8
　　nose 478.1
　　turbinate (nasal) 478.0
　muscle 728.9
　muscular coat, artery NEC 447.8
　　carotid 447.8
　　renal 447.3
　myocardium (*see also* Hypertrophy,
　　cardiac) 429.3
　　idiopathic 425.4
　myometrium 621.2
　nail 703.8
　　congenital 757.5
　nasal 478.1
　　alae 478.1
　　bone 738.0
　　cartilage 478.1
　　mucous membrane (septum) 478.1
　　sinus (*see also* Sinusitis) 473.9
　　turbinate 478.0
　nasopharynx, lymphoid (infectional)
　　(tissue) (wall) 478.29
　neck, uterus 622.6
　nipple 611.1
　normal aperture diaphragm (congeni-
　　tal) 756.6
　nose (*see also* Hypertrophy, nasal) 478.1
　orbit 376.46
　organ or site, congenital NEC - *see*
　　Anomaly, specified type NEC
　osteoarthropathy (pulmonary) 731.2
　ovary 620.8
　palate (hard) 526.89
　　soft 528.9
　pancreas (congenital) 751.7
　papillae
　　anal 569.49
　　tongue 529.3
　parathyroid (gland) 252.01 ◄▪▪▪
　parotid gland 527.1
　penis 607.89
　phallus 607.89
　　female (clitoris) 624.2
　pharyngeal tonsil 474.12
　pharyngitis 472.1
　pharynx 478.29
　　lymphoid (infectional) (tissue) (wall)
　　　478.29
　pituitary (fossa) (gland) 253.8
　popliteal fat pad 729.31

Hypertrophy, hypertrophic *(Continued)*
　preauricular (lymph) gland (Hamp-
　　stead) 785.6
　prepuce (congenital) 605
　　female 624.2
　prostate (asymptomatic) (early) (recur-
　　rent) 600.90
　　with urinary retention 600.91
　　　adenofibromatous 600.20
　　　　with urinary retention 600.21
　　　benign 600.00
　　　　with urinary retention 600.01
　　　congenital 752.89
　pseudoedematous hypodermal
　　757.0
　pseudomuscular 359.1
　pylorus (muscle) (sphincter) 537.0
　　congenital 750.5
　　infantile 750.5
　rectal sphincter 569.49
　rectum 569.49
　renal 593.1
　rhinitis (turbinate) 472.0
　salivary duct or gland 527.1
　　congenital 750.26
　scaphoid (tarsal) 733.99
　scar 701.4
　scrotum 608.89
　sella turcica 253.8
　seminal vesicle 608.89
　sigmoid 569.89
　skin condition NEC 701.9
　spermatic cord 608.89
　spinal ligament 724.8
　spleen - *see* Splenomegaly
　spondylitis (spine) (*see also* Spondy-
　　losis) 721.90
　stomach 537.89
　subaortic stenosis (idiopathic) 425.1
　sublingual gland 527.1
　　congenital 750.26
　submaxillary gland 527.1
　suprarenal (gland) 255.8
　tendon 727.9
　testis 608.89
　　congenital 752.89
　thymic, thymus (congenital) (gland)
　　254.0
　thyroid (gland) (*see also* Goiter) 240.9
　　primary 242.0
　　secondary 242.2
　toe (congenital) 755.65
　　acquired 735.8
　tongue 529.8
　　congenital 750.15
　　frenum 529.8
　　papillae (foliate) 529.3
　tonsil (faucial) (infective) (lingual)
　　(lymphoid) 474.11
　　with
　　　adenoiditis 474.01
　　　tonsillitis 474.00
　　　　and adenoiditis 474.02
　　　and adenoids 474.10
　tunica vaginalis 608.89
　turbinate (mucous membrane) 478.0
　ureter 593.89
　urethra 599.84
　uterus 621.2
　　puerperal, postpartum 674.8
　uvula 528.9
　vagina 623.8
　vas deferens 608.89
　vein 459.89

Hypertrophy, hypertrophic *(Continued)*
　ventricle, ventricular (heart) (left)
　　(right) - *see also* Hypertrophy, car-
　　diac
　　congenital 746.89
　　due to hypertension (left) (right) (*see*
　　　also Hypertension, heart) 402.90
　　　benign 402.10
　　　malignant 402.00
　　right with ventricular septal defect,
　　　pulmonary stenosis or atresia,
　　　and dextraposition of aorta
　　　745.2
　verumontanum 599.89
　vesical 596.8
　vocal cord 478.5
　vulva 624.3
　　stasis (nonfilarial) 624.3
Hypertropia (intermittent) (periodic)
　378.31
Hypertyrosinemia 270.2
Hyperuricemia 790.6
Hypervalinemia 270.3
Hyperventilation (tetany) 786.01
　hysterical 300.11
　psychogenic 306.1
　syndrome 306.1
Hyperviscidosis 277.00
Hyperviscosity (of serum) (syndrome)
　NEC 273.3
　polycythemic 289.0
　sclerocythemic 282.8
Hypervitaminosis (dietary) NEC 278.8
　A (dietary) 278.2
　D (dietary) 278.4
　from excessive administration or use
　　of vitamin preparations (chronic)
　　278.8
　　reaction to sudden overdose 963.5
　　vitamin A 278.2
　　　reaction to sudden overdose 963.5
　　vitamin D 278.4
　　　reaction to sudden overdose 963.5
　　vitamin K
　　　correct substance properly admin-
　　　　istered 278.8
　　　overdose or wrong substance
　　　　given or taken 964.3
Hypervolemia 276.6
Hypesthesia (*see also* Disturbance, sensa-
　tion) 782.0
　cornea 371.81
Hyphema (anterior chamber) (ciliary
　body) (iris) 364.41
　traumatic 921.3
Hyphemia - *see* Hyphema
Hypoacidity, gastric 536.8
　psychogenic 306.4
Hypoactive labyrinth (function) - *see*
　Hypofunction, labyrinth
Hypoadrenalism 255.4
　tuberculous (*see also* Tuberculosis) 017.6
Hypoadrenocorticism 255.4
　pituitary 253.4
Hypoalbuminemia 273.8
Hypoalphalipoproteinemia 272.5
Hypobarism 993.2
Hypobaropathy 993.2
Hypobetalipoproteinemia (familial) 272.5
Hypocalcemia 275.41
　cow's milk 775.4
　dietary 269.3
　neonatal 775.4
　phosphate-loading 775.4

ICD-9-CM

II

Vol. 2

Hypocalcification, teeth 520.4
Hypochloremia 276.9
Hypochlorhydria 536.8
  neurotic 306.4
  psychogenic 306.4
Hypocholesteremia 272.5
Hypochondria (reaction) 300.7
Hypochondriac 300.7
Hypochondriasis 300.7
Hypochromasia blood cells 280.9
Hypochromic anemia 280.9
  due to blood loss (chronic) 280.0
    acute 285.1
  microcytic 280.9
Hypocoagulability (see also Defect, coagulation) 286.9
Hypocomplementemia 279.8
Hypocythemia (progressive) 284.9
Hypodontia (see also Anodontia) 520.0
Hypoeosinophilia 288.8
Hypoesthesia (see also Disturbance, sensation) 782.0
  cornea 371.81
  tactile 782.0
Hypoestrinism 256.39
Hypoestrogenism 256.39
Hypoferremia 280.9
  due to blood loss (chronic) 280.0
Hypofertility
  female 628.9
  male 606.1
Hypofibrinogenemia 286.3
  acquired 286.6
  congenital 286.3
Hypofunction
  adrenal (gland) 255.4
    cortex 255.4
    medulla 255.5
    specified NEC 255.5
  cerebral 331.9
  corticoadrenal NEC 255.4
  intestinal 564.89
  labyrinth (unilateral) 386.53
    with loss of labyrinthine reactivity 386.55
    bilateral 386.54
      with loss of labyrinthine reactivity 386.56
  Leydig cell 257.2
  ovary 256.39
    postablative 256.2
  pituitary (anterior) (gland) (lobe) 253.2
    posterior 253.5
  testicular 257.2
    iatrogenic 257.1
    postablative 257.1
    postirradiation 257.1
    postsurgical 257.1
Hypogammaglobulinemia 279.00
  acquired primary 279.06
  non-sex-linked, congenital 279.06
  sporadic 279.06
  transient of infancy 279.09
Hypogenitalism (congenital) (female) (male) 752.89
  penis 752.69
Hypoglycemia (spontaneous) 251.2
  coma 251.0
    diabetic 250.3
  diabetic 250.8
  due to insulin 251.0
    therapeutic misadventure 962.3
  familial (idiopathic) 251.2
  following gastrointestinal surgery 579.3

Hypoglycemia (Continued)
  infantile (idiopathic) 251.2
  in infant of diabetic mother 775.0
  leucine-induced 270.3
  neonatal 775.6
  reactive 251.2
  specified NEC 251.1
Hypoglycemic shock 251.0
  diabetic 250.8
  due to insulin 251.0
  functional (syndrome) 251.1
Hypogonadism
  female 256.39
  gonadotrophic (isolated) 253.4
  hypogonadotropic (isolated) (with anosmia) 253.4
  isolated 253.4
  male 257.2
  ovarian (primary) 256.39
  pituitary (secondary) 253.4
  testicular (primary) (secondary) 257.2
Hypohidrosis 705.0
Hypohidrotic ectodermal dysplasia 757.31
Hypoidrosis 705.0
Hypoinsulinemia, postsurgical 251.3
  postpancreatectomy (complete) (partial) 251.3
Hypokalemia 276.8
Hypokinesia 780.99
Hypoleukia splenica 289.4
Hypoleukocytosis 288.8
Hypolipidemia 272.5
Hypolipoproteinemia 272.5
Hypomagnesemia 275.2
  neonatal 775.4
Hypomania, hypomanic reaction (see also Psychosis, affective) 296.0
  recurrent episode 296.1
  single episode 296.0
Hypomastia (congenital) 757.6
Hypomenorrhea 626.1
Hypometabolism 783.9
Hypomotility
  gastrointestinal tract 536.8
    psychogenic 306.4
  intestine 564.89
    psychogenic 306.4
  stomach 536.8
    psychogenic 306.4
Hyponasality 784.49
Hyponatremia 276.1
Hypo-ovarianism 256.39
Hypo-ovarism 256.39
Hypoparathyroidism (idiopathic) (surgically induced) 252.1
  neonatal 775.4
Hypopharyngitis 462
Hypophoria 378.40
Hypophosphatasia 275.3
Hypophosphatemia (acquired) (congenital) (familial) 275.3
  renal 275.3
Hypophyseal, hypophysis - see also condition
  dwarfism 253.3
  gigantism 253.0
  syndrome 253.8
Hypophyseothalamic syndrome 253.8
Hypopiesis - see Hypotension
Hypopigmentation 709.00
  eyelid 374.53
Hypopinealism 259.8

Hypopituitarism (juvenile) (syndrome) 253.2
  due to
    hormone therapy 253.7
    hypophysectomy 253.7
    radiotherapy 253.7
  postablative 253.7
  postpartum hemorrhage 253.2
Hypoplasia, hypoplasis 759.89
  adrenal (gland) 759.1
  alimentary tract 751.8
    lower 751.2
    upper 750.8
  anus, anal (canal) 751.2
  aorta 747.22
  aortic
    arch (tubular) 747.10
    orifice or valve with hypoplasia of ascending aorta and defective development of left ventricle (with mitral valve atresia) 746.7
  appendix 751.2
  areola 757.6
  arm (see also Absence, arm, congenital) 755.20
  artery (congenital) (peripheral) 747.60
    brain 747.81
    cerebral 747.81
    coronary 746.85
    gastrointestinal 747.61
    lower limb 747.64
    pulmonary 747.3
    renal 747.62
    retinal 743.58
    specified NEC 747.69
    spinal 747.82
    umbilical 747.5
    upper limb 747.63
  auditory canal 744.29
    causing impairment of hearing 744.02
  biliary duct (common) or passage 751.61
  bladder 753.8
  bone NEC 756.9
    face 756.0
    malar 756.0
    mandible 524.04
      alveolar 524.74
    marrow 284.9
      acquired (secondary) 284.8
      congenital 284.0
      idiopathic 284.9
    maxilla 524.03
      alveolar 524.73
    skull (see also Hypoplasia, skull) 756.0
  brain 742.1
    gyri 742.2
    specified part 742.2
  breast (areola) 757.6
  bronchus (tree) 748.3
  cardiac 746.89
    valve - see Hypoplasia, heart, valve
    vein 746.89
  carpus (see also Absence, carpal, congenital) 755.28
  cartilaginous 756.9
  cecum 751.2
  cementum 520.4
    hereditary 520.5
  cephalic 742.1
  cerebellum 742.2
  cervix (uteri) 752.49

◀ **New**　　◀▥ **Revised**

Hypoplasia, hypoplasis (*Continued*)
- chin 524.06
- clavicle 755.51
- coccyx 756.19
- colon 751.2
- corpus callosum 742.2
- cricoid cartilage 748.3
- dermal, focal (Goltz) 757.39
- digestive organ(s) or tract NEC 751.8
  - lower 751.2
  - upper 750.8
- ear 744.29
  - auricle 744.23
  - lobe 744.29
  - middle, except ossicles 744.03
    - ossicles 744.04
  - ossicles 744.04
- enamel of teeth (neonatal) (postnatal) (prenatal) 520.4
  - hereditary 520.5
- endocrine (gland) NEC 759.2
- endometrium 621.8
- epididymis 752.89
- epiglottis 748.3
- erythroid, congenital 284.0
- erythropoietic, chronic acquired 284.8
- esophagus 750.3
- Eustachian tube 744.24
- eye (*see also* Microphthalmos) 743.10
  - lid 743.62
- face 744.89
  - bone(s) 756.0
- fallopian tube 752.19
- femur (*see also* Absence, femur, congenital) 755.34
- fibula (*see also* Absence, fibula, congenital) 755.37
- finger (*see also* Absence, finger, congenital) 755.29
- focal dermal 757.39
- foot 755.31
- gallbladder 751.69
- genitalia, genital organ(s)
  - female 752.89
    - external 752.49
    - internal NEC 752.89
  - in adiposogenital dystrophy 253.8
  - male 752.89
    - penis 752.69
- glottis 748.3
- hair 757.4
- hand 755.21
- heart 746.89
  - left (complex) (syndrome) 746.7
  - valve NEC 746.89
    - pulmonary 746.01
- humerus (*see also* Absence, humerus, congenital) 755.24
- hymen 752.49
- intestine (small) 751.1
  - large 751.2
- iris 743.46
- jaw 524.09
- kidney(s) 753.0
- labium (majus) (minus) 752.49
- labyrinth, membranous 744.05
- lacrimal duct (apparatus) 743.65
- larynx 748.3
- leg (*see also* Absence, limb, congenital, lower) 755.30
- limb 755.4
  - lower (*see also* Absence, limb, congenital, lower) 755.30

Hypoplasia, hypoplasis (*Continued*)
- limb (*Continued*)
  - upper (*see also* Absence, limb, congenital, upper) 755.20
- liver 751.69
- lung (lobe) 748.5
- mammary (areolar) 757.6
- mandibular 524.04
  - alveolar 524.74
  - unilateral condylar 526.89
- maxillary 524.03
  - alveolar 524.73
- medullary 284.9
- megakaryocytic 287.3
- metacarpus (*see also* Absence, metacarpal, congenital) 755.28
- metatarsus (*see also* Absence, metatarsal, congenital) 755.38
- muscle 756.89
  - eye 743.69
- myocardium (congenital) (Uhl's anomaly) 746.84
- nail(s) 757.5
- nasolacrimal duct 743.65
- nervous system NEC 742.8
- neural 742.8
- nose, nasal 748.1
- ophthalmic (*see also* Microphthalmos) 743.10
- organ
  - of Corti 744.05
  - or site NEC - *see* Anomaly, by site
- osseous meatus (ear) 744.03
- ovary 752.0
- oviduct 752.19
- pancreas 751.7
- parathyroid (gland) 759.2
- parotid gland 750.26
- patella 755.64
- pelvis, pelvic girdle 755.69
- penis 752.69
- peripheral vascular system (congenital) NEC 747.60
  - gastrointestinal 747.61
  - lower limb 747.64
  - renal 747.62
  - specified NEC 747.69
  - spinal 747.82
  - upper limb 747.63
- pituitary (gland) 759.2
- pulmonary 748.5
  - arteriovenous 747.3
  - artery 747.3
  - valve 746.01
- punctum lacrimale 743.65
- radioulnar (*see also* Absence, radius, congenital, with ulna) 755.25
- radius (*see also* Absence, radius, congenital) 755.26
- rectum 751.2
- respiratory system NEC 748.9
- rib 756.3
- sacrum 756.19
- scapula 755.59
- shoulder girdle 755.59
- skin 757.39
- skull (bone) 756.0
  - with
    - anencephalus 740.0
    - encephalocele 742.0
    - hydrocephalus 742.3
      - with spina bifida (*see also* Spina bifida) 741.0
    - microcephalus 742.1

Hypoplasia, hypoplasis (*Continued*)
- spinal (cord) (ventral horn cell) 742.59
  - vessel 747.82
- spine 756.19
- spleen 759.0
- sternum 756.3
- tarsus (*see also* Absence, tarsal, congenital) 755.38
- testis, testicle 752.89
- thymus (gland) 279.11
- thyroid (gland) 243
  - cartilage 748.3
- tibiofibular (*see also* Absence, tibia, congenital, with fibula) 755.35
- toe (*see also* Absence, toe, congenital) 755.39
- tongue 750.16
- trachea (cartilage) (rings) 748.3
- Turner's (tooth) 520.4
- ulna (*see also* Absence, ulna, congenital) 755.27
- umbilical artery 747.5
- ureter 753.29
- uterus 752.3
- vagina 752.49
- vascular (peripheral) NEC (*see also* Hypoplasia, peripheral vascular system) 747.60
  - brain 747.81
- vein(s) (peripheral) NEC (*see also* Hypoplasia, peripheral vascular system) 747.60
  - brain 747.81
  - cardiac 746.89
  - great 747.49
  - portal 747.49
  - pulmonary 747.49
- vena cava (inferior) (superior) 747.49
- vertebra 756.19
- vulva 752.49
- zonule (ciliary) 743.39
- zygoma 738.12

Hypopotassemia 276.8
Hypoproaccelerinemia (*see also* Defect, coagulation) 286.3
Hypoproconvertinemia (congenital) (*see also* Defect, coagulation) 286.3
Hypoproteinemia (essential) (hypermetabolic) (idiopathic) 273.8
Hypoproteinosis 260
Hypoprothrombinemia (congenital) (hereditary) (idiopathic) (*see also* Defect, coagulation) 286.3
- acquired 286.7
- newborn 776.3
Hypopselaphesia 782.0
Hypopyon (anterior chamber) (eye) 364.05
- iritis 364.05
- ulcer (cornea) 370.04
Hypopyrexia 780.99
Hyporeflex 796.1
Hyporeninemia, extreme 790.99
- in primary aldosteronism 255.10
Hyporesponsive episode 780.09
Hyposecretion
- ACTH 253.4
- ovary 256.39
  - postablative 256.2
- salivary gland (any) 527.7
Hyposegmentation of neutrophils, hereditary 288.2
Hyposiderinemia 280.9

ICD-9-CM

H

Vol. 2

Hyposmolality 276.1
  syndrome 276.1
Hyposomatotropism 253.3
Hyposomnia (see also Insomnia)
    780.52
Hypospadias (male) 752.61
  female 753.8
Hypospermatogenesis 606.1
Hyposphagma 372.72
Hyposplenism 289.59
Hypostasis, pulmonary 514
Hypostatic - see condition
Hyposthenuria 593.89
Hyposuprarenalism 255.4
Hypo-TBG-nemia 246.8
Hypotension (arterial) (constitutional)
    458.9
  chronic 458.1
  iatrogenic 458.29
  maternal, syndrome (following labor
    and delivery) 669.2
  of hemodialysis 458.21
  orthostatic (chronic) 458.0
    dysautonomic-dyskinetic syndrome
      333.0
  permanent idiopathic 458.1
  postoperative 458.29
  postural 458.0
  specified type NEC 458.8
  transient 796.3
Hypothermia (accidental) 991.6
  anesthetic 995.89
  newborn NEC 778.3
  not associated with low environmental
    temperature 780.99
Hypothymergasia (see also Psychosis, af-
    fective) 296.2
  recurrent episode 296.3
  single episode 296.2
Hypothyroidism (acquired) 244.9
  complicating pregnancy, childbirth, or
    puerperium 648.1

Hypothyroidism (Continued)
  congenital 243
  due to
    ablation 244.1
      radioactive iodine 244.1
      surgical 244.0
    iodine (administration) (ingestion)
      244.2
      radioactive 244.1
    irradiation therapy 244.1
    p-aminosalicylic acid (PAS)
      244.3
    phenylbutazone 244.3
    resorcinol 244.3
    specified cause NEC 244.8
    surgery 244.0
  goitrous (sporadic) 246.1
  iatrogenic NEC 244.3
  iodine 244.2
  pituitary 244.8
  postablative NEC 244.1
  postsurgical 244.0
  primary 244.9
  secondary NEC 244.8
  specified cause NEC 244.8
  sporadic goitrous 246.1
Hypotonia, hypotonicity, hypotony
    781.3
  benign congenital 358.8
  bladder 596.4
  congenital 779.89
    benign 358.8
  eye 360.30
    due to
      fistula 360.32
      ocular disorder NEC 360.33
    following loss of aqueous or vitre-
      ous 360.33
    primary 360.31
  infantile muscular (benign)
    359.0
  muscle 728.9

Hypotonia, hypotonicity, hypotony
    (Continued)
  uterus, uterine (contractions) - see Iner-
    tia, uterus
Hypotrichosis 704.09
  congenital 757.4
  lid (congenital) 757.4
    acquired 374.55
  postinfectional NEC 704.09
Hypotropia 378.32
Hypoventilation 786.09
Hypovitaminosis (see also Deficiency, vi-
    tamin) 269.2
Hypovolemia 276.5
  surgical shock 998.0
  traumatic (shock) 958.4
Hypoxemia (see also Anoxia) 799.0
Hypoxia (see also Anoxia) 799.0
  cerebral 348.1
    during or resulting from a proce-
      dure 997.01
    newborn 768.9
      mild or moderate 768.6
      severe 768.5
  fetal, affecting newborn 768.9
  intrauterine - see Distress, fetal
  myocardial (see also Insufficiency, coro-
    nary) 411.89
    arteriosclerotic - see Arteriosclerosis,
      coronary
  newborn 768.9
Hypsarrhythmia (see also Epilepsy) 345.6
Hysteralgia, pregnant uterus 646.8
Hysteria, hysterical 300.10
  anxiety 300.20
  Charcôt's gland 300.11
  conversion (any manifestation) 300.11
  dissociative type NEC 300.15
  psychosis, acute 298.1
Hysteroepilepsy 300.11
**Hysterotomy, affecting fetus or new-
    born** 763.89

◄ **New**　◄▬ **Revised**

I

Iatrogenic syndrome of excess cortisol 255.0
Iceland disease (epidemic neuromyasthenia) 049.8
Ichthyosis (congenita) 757.1
  acquired 701.1
  fetalis gravior 757.1
  follicularis 757.1
  hystrix 757.39
  lamellar 757.1
  lingual 528.6
  palmaris and plantaris 757.39
  simplex 757.1
  vera 757.1
  vulgaris 757.1
Ichthyotoxism 988.0
  bacterial (*see also* Poisoning, food) 005.9
Icteroanemia, hemolytic (acquired) 283.9
  congenital (*see also* Spherocytosis) 282.0
Icterus (*see also* Jaundice) 782.4
  catarrhal - *see* Icterus, infectious
  conjunctiva 782.4
    newborn 774.6
  epidemic - *see* Icterus, infectious
  febrilis - *see* Icterus, infectious
  fetus or newborn - *see* Jaundice, fetus
    or newborn
  gravis (*see also* Necrosis, liver) 570
    complicating pregnancy 646.7
      affecting fetus or newborn 760.8
    fetus or newborn NEC 773.0
    obstetrical 646.7
      affecting fetus or newborn 760.8
  hematogenous (acquired) 283.9
  hemolytic (acquired) 283.9
    congenital (*see also* Spherocytosis)
      282.0
  hemorrhagic (acute) 100.0
    leptospiral 100.0
    newborn 776.0
    spirochetal 100.0
  infectious 070.1
    with hepatic coma 070.0
    leptospiral 100.0
    spirochetal 100.0
  intermittens juvenilis 277.4
  malignant (*see also* Necrosis, liver) 570
  neonatorum (*see also* Jaundice, fetus or
    newborn) 774.6
  pernicious (*see also* Necrosis, liver) 570
  spirochetal 100.0
Ictus solaris, solis 992.0
Identity disorder 313.82
  dissociative 300.14
  gender role (child) 302.6
    adult 302.85
  psychosexual (child) 302.6
    adult 302.85
Idioglossia 307.9
Idiopathic - *see* condition
Idiosyncrasy (*see also* Allergy) 995.3
  drug, medicinal substance, and biological - *see* Allergy, drug
Idiot, idiocy (congenital) 318.2
  amaurotic (Bielschowsky) (-Jansky)
    (family) (infantile (late)) (juvenile
    (late)) (Vogt-Spielmeyer) 330.1
  microcephalic 742.1
  mongolian 758.0
  oxycephalic 756.0
Id reaction (due to bacteria) 692.89
IgE asthma 493.0

Ileitis (chronic) (*see also* Enteritis) 558.9
  infectious 009.0
  noninfectious 558.9
  regional (ulcerative) 555.0
    with large intestine 555.2
  segmental 555.0
    with large intestine 555.2
  terminal (ulcerative) 555.0
    with large intestine 555.2
Ileocolitis (*see also* Enteritis) 558.9
  infectious 009.0
  regional 555.2
  ulcerative 556.1
Ileostomy status V44.2
  with complication 569.60
Ileotyphus 002.0
Ileum - *see* condition
Ileus (adynamic) (bowel) (colon) (inhibitory) (intestine) (neurogenic) (paralytic) 560.1
  arteriomesenteric duodenal 537.2
  due to gallstone (in intestine) 560.31
  duodenal, chronic 537.2
  following gastrointestinal surgery 997.4
  gallstone 560.31
  mechanical (*see also* Obstruction, intestine) 560.9
  meconium 777.1
    due to cystic fibrosis 277.01
  myxedema 564.89
  postoperative 997.4
  transitory, newborn 777.4
Iliac - *see* condition
Iliotibial band friction syndrome 728.89
Ill, louping 063.1
Illegitimacy V61.6
Illness - *see also* Disease
  factitious 300.19
    with
      combined psychological and physical signs and symptoms
        300.19   ◀▥
      physical symptoms 300.19
      predominantly   ◀
        physical signs and symptoms
          300.19   ◀
        psychological symptoms
          300.16   ◀
      psychological symptoms 300.16
    chronic (with physical symptoms)
      301.51
  heart - *see* Disease, heart
  manic-depressive (*see also* Psychosis,
    affective) 296.80
  mental (*see also* Disorder, mental) 300.9
Imbalance 781.2
  autonomic (*see also* Neuropathy, peripheral, autonomic) 337.9
  electrolyte 276.9
    with
      abortion - *see* Abortion, by type,
        with metabolic disorder
      ectopic pregnancy (*see also* categories 633.0-633.9) 639.4
      hyperemesis gravidarum (before
        22 completed weeks' gestation) 643.1
      molar pregnancy (*see also* categories 630-632) 639.4
    following
      abortion 639.4
      ectopic or molar pregnancy 639.4
    neonatal, transitory NEC 775.5
  endocrine 259.9
  eye muscle NEC 378.9
    heterophoria - *see* Heterophoria

Imbalance (*Continued*)
  glomerulotubular NEC 593.89
  hormone 259.9
  hysterical (*see also* Hysteria) 300.10
  labyrinth NEC 386.50
  posture 729.9
  sympathetic (*see also* Neuropathy, peripheral, autonomic) 337.9
Imbecile, imbecility 318.0
  moral 301.7
  old age 290.9
  senile 290.9
  specified IQ - *see* IQ
  unspecified IQ 318.0
Imbedding, intrauterine device 996.32
Imbibition, cholesterol (gallbladder)
  575.6
Imerslund (-Gräsbeck) **syndrome** (anemia due to familial selective vitamin
  B_{12} malabsorption) 281.1
Iminoacidopathy 270.8
Iminoglycinuria, familial 270.8
Immature - *see also* Immaturity
  personality 301.89
Immaturity 765.1
  extreme 765.0
  fetus or infant light-for-dates - *see*
    Light-for-dates
  lung, fetus or newborn 770.4
  organ or site NEC - *see* Hypoplasia
  pulmonary, fetus or newborn 770.4
  reaction 301.89
  sexual (female) (male) 259.0
Immersion 994.1
  foot 991.4
  hand 991.4
Immobile, immobility
  intestine 564.89
  joint - *see* Ankylosis
  syndrome (paraplegic) 728.3
Immunization
  ABO
    affecting management of pregnancy
      656.2
    fetus or newborn 773.1
  complication - *see* Complications, vaccination
  Rh factor
    affecting management of pregnancy
      656.1
    fetus or newborn 773.0
    from transfusion 999.7
Immunodeficiency 279.3
  with
    adenosine-deaminase deficiency
      279.2
    defect, predominant
      B-cell 279.00
      T-cell 279.10
    hyperimmunoglobulinemia 279.2
    lymphopenia, hereditary 279.2
    thrombocytopenia and eczema
      279.12
    thymic
      aplasia 279.2
      dysplasia 279.2
  autosomal recessive, Swiss-type 279.2
  common variable 279.06
  severe combined (SCID) 279.2
  to Rh factor
    affecting management of pregnancy
      656.1
    fetus or newborn 773.0
  X-linked, with increased IgM 279.05

ICD-9-CM

—

Vol. 2

Immunotherapy, prophylactic
V07.2
Impaction, impacted
bowel, colon, rectum 560.30
with hernia - *see also* Hernia, by site,
with, obstruction
gangrenous - *see* Hernia, by site,
with gangrene
by
calculus 560.39
gallstone 560.31
fecal 560.39
specified type NEC 560.39
calculus - *see* Calculus
cerumen (ear) (external) 380.4
cuspid 520.6
dental 520.6
fecal, feces 560.39
with hernia - *see also* Hernia, by site,
with obstruction
gangrenous - *see* Hernia, by site,
with gangrene
fracture - *see* Fracture, by site
gallbladder - *see* Cholelithiasis
gallstone(s) - *see* Cholelithiasis
in intestine (any part) 560.31
intestine(s) 560.30
with hernia - *see also* Hernia, by site,
with obstruction
gangrenous - *see* Hernia, by site,
with gangrene
by
calculus 560.39
gallstone 560.31
fecal 560.39
specified type NEC 560.39
intrauterine device (IUD) 996.32
molar 520.6
shoulder 660.4
affecting fetus or newborn 763.1
tooth, teeth 520.6
turbinate 733.99
Impaired, impairment (function)
arm V49.1
movement, involving
musculoskeletal system V49.1
nervous system V49.2
auditory discrimination 388.43
back V48.3
body (entire) V49.89
glucose
fasting 790.21
tolerance test (oral) 790.22
hearing (*see also* Deafness) 389.9
heart - *see* Disease, heart
kidney (*see also* Disease, renal)
593.9
disorder resulting from 588.9
specified NEC 588.89 ◀▥
leg V49.1
movement, involving
musculoskeletal system
V49.1
nervous system V49.2
limb V49.1
movement, involving
musculoskeletal system
V49.1
nervous system V49.2
liver 573.8
mastication 524.9
mobility
ear ossicles NEC 385.22

Impaired, impairment (*Continued*)
mobility (*Continued*)
incostapedial joint 385.22
malleus 385.21
myocardium, myocardial (*see also* Insufficiency, myocardial) 428.0
neuromusculoskeletal NEC V49.89
back V48.3
head V48.2
limb V49.2
neck V48.3
spine V48.3
trunk V48.3
rectal sphincter 787.99
renal (*see also* Disease, renal) 593.9
disorder resulting from 588.9
specified NEC 588.89 ◀▥
spine V48.3
vision NEC 369.9
both eyes NEC 369.3
moderate 369.74
both eyes 369.25
with impairment of lesser eye
(specified as)
blind, not further specified
369.15
low vision, not further specified 369.23
near-total 369.17
profound 369.18
severe 369.24
total 369.16
one eye 369.74
with vision of other eye (specified as)
near-normal 369.75
normal 369.76
near-total 369.64
both eyes 369.04
with impairment of lesser eye
(specified as)
blind, not further specified
369.02
total 369.03
one eye 369.64
with vision of other eye (specified as)
near-normal 369.65
normal 369.66
one eye 369.60
with low vision of other eye
369.10
profound 369.67
both eyes 369.08
with impairment of lesser eye
(specified as)
blind, not further specified
369.05
near-total 369.07
total 369.06
one eye 369.67
with vision of other eye (specified as)
near-normal 369.68
normal 369.69
severe 369.71
both eyes 369.22
with impairment of lesser eye
(specified as)
blind, not further specified
369.11
low vision, not further specified 369.21
near-total 369.13

Impaired, impairment (*Continued*)
vision NEC (*Continued*)
severe (*Continued*)
both eyes (*Continued*)
with impairment of lesser eye
(*Continued*)
profound 369.14
total 369.12
one eye 369.71
with vision of other eye (specified as)
near-normal 369.72
normal 369.73
total
both eyes 369.01
one eye 369.61
with vision of other eye (specified as)
near-normal 369.62
normal 369.63
Impaludism - *see* Malaria
Impediment, speech NEC 784.5
psychogenic 307.9
secondary to organic lesion 784.5
Impending
cerebrovascular accident or attack
435.9
coronary syndrome 411.1
delirium tremens 291.0
myocardial infarction 411.1
Imperception, auditory (acquired) (congenital) 389.9
Imperfect
aeration, lung (newborn) 770.5
closure (congenital)
alimentary tract NEC 751.8
lower 751.5
upper 750.8
atrioventricular ostium 745.69
atrium (secundum) 745.5
primum 745.61
branchial cleft or sinus 744.41
choroid 743.59
cricoid cartilage 748.3
cusps, heart valve NEC 746.89
pulmonary 746.09
ductus
arteriosus 747.0
Botallo 747.0
ear drum 744.29
causing impairment of hearing
744.03
endocardial cushion 745.60
epiglottis 748.3
esophagus with communication to
bronchus or trachea 750.3
eustachian valve 746.89
eyelid 743.62
face, facial (*see also* Cleft, lip) 749.10
foramen
Botallo 745.5
ovale 745.5
genitalia, genital organ(s) or system
female 752.89
external 752.49
internal NEC 752.89
uterus 752.3
male 752.89
penis 752.69
glottis 748.3
heart valve (cusps) NEC 746.89
interatrial ostium or septum 745.5
interauricular ostium or septum
745.5

◀ **New**   ◀▥ **Revised**

Imperfect (*Continued*)
closure (*Continued*)
interventricular ostium or septum
745.4
iris 743.46
kidney 753.3
larynx 748.3
lens 743.36
lip (*see also* Cleft, lip) 749.10
nasal septum or sinus 748.1
nose 748.1
omphalomesenteric duct 751.0
optic nerve entry 743.57
organ or site NEC - *see* Anomaly,
specified type, by site
ostium
interatrial 745.5
interauricular 745.5
interventricular 745.4
palate (*see also* Cleft, palate) 749.00
preauricular sinus 744.46
retina 743.56
roof of orbit 742.0
sclera 743.47
septum
aortic 745.0
aorticopulmonary 745.0
atrial (secundum) 745.5
primum 745.61
between aorta and pulmonary artery 745.0
heart 745.9
interatrial (secundum) 745.5
primum 745.61
interauricular (secundum) 745.5
primum 745.61
interventricular 745.4
with pulmonary stenosis or
atresia, dextraposition of
aorta, and hypertrophy of
right ventricle 745.2
in tetralogy of Fallot 745.2
nasal 748.1
ventricular 745.4
with pulmonary stenosis or
atresia, dextraposition of
aorta, and hypertrophy of
right ventricle 745.2
in tetralogy of Fallot 745.2
skull 756.0
with
anencephalus 740.0
encephalocele 742.0
hydrocephalus 742.3
with spina bifida (*see also*
Spina bifida) 741.0
microcephalus 742.1
spine (with meningocele) (*see also*
Spina bifida) 741.90
thyroid cartilage 748.3
trachea 748.3
tympanic membrane 744.29
causing impairment of hearing
744.03
uterus (with communication to bladder, intestine, or rectum) 752.3
uvula 749.02
with cleft lip (*see also* Cleft, palate,
with cleft lip) 749.20
vitelline duct 751.0
development - *see* Anomaly, by site
erection 607.84
fusion - *see* Imperfect, closure
inflation lung (newborn) 770.5

Imperfect (*Continued*)
intestinal canal 751.5
poise 729.9
rotation - *see* Malrotation
septum, ventricular 745.4
Imperfectly descended testis 752.51
Imperforate (congenital) - *see also* Atresia
anus 751.2
bile duct 751.61
cervix (uteri) 752.49
esophagus 750.3
hymen 752.42
intestine (small) 751.1
large 751.2
jejunum 751.1
pharynx 750.29
rectum 751.2
salivary duct 750.23
urethra 753.6
urinary meatus 753.6
vagina 752.49
Impervious (congenital) - *see also* Atresia
anus 751.2
bile duct 751.61
esophagus 750.3
intestine (small) 751.1
large 751.5
rectum 751.2
urethra 753.6
Impetiginization of other dermatoses 684
Impetigo (any organism) (any site) (bullous) (circinate) (contagiosa) (neonatorum) (simplex) 684
Bockhart's (superficial folliculitis) 704.8
external ear 684 [380.13]
eyelid 684 [373.5]
Fox's (contagiosa) 684
furfuracea 696.5
herpetiformis 694.3
nonobstetrical 694.3
staphylococcal infection 684
ulcerative 686.8
vulgaris 684
Impingement, soft tissue between teeth
524.89 ◀▥
anterior 524.81 ◀
posterior 524.82 ◀
Implant, endometrial 617.9
Implantation
anomalous - *see also* Anomaly, specified type, by site
ureter 753.4
cyst
external area or site (skin) NEC
709.8
iris 364.61
vagina 623.8
vulva 624.8
dermoid (cyst)
external area or site (skin) NEC
709.8
iris 364.61
vagina 623.8
vulva 624.8
placenta, low or marginal - *see* Placenta previa
Impotence (sexual) (psychogenic) 302.72
organic origin NEC 607.84
Impoverished blood 285.9
Impression, basilar 756.0
Imprisonment V62.5
Improper
development, infant 764.9
Improperly tied umbilical cord (causing
hemorrhage) 772.3

Impulses, obsessional 300.3
Impulsive neurosis 300.3
Inaction, kidney (*see also* Disease, renal)
593.9
Inactive - *see* condition
Inadequate, inadequacy
biologic 301.6
cardiac and renal - *see* Hypertension,
cardiorenal
constitutional 301.6
development
child 783.40
fetus 764.9
affecting management of pregnancy 656.5
genitalia
after puberty NEC 259.0
congenital - *see* Hypoplasia, genitalia
lungs 748.5
organ or site NEC - *see* Hypoplasia,
by site
dietary 269.9
distance, interarch 524.28 ◀
education V62.3
environment
economic problem V60.2
household condition NEC V60.1
poverty V60.2
unemployment V62.0
functional 301.6
household care, due to
family member
handicapped or ill V60.4
temporarily away from home V60.4
on vacation V60.5
technical defects in home V60.1
temporary absence from home of
person rendering care V60.4
housing (heating) (space) V60.1
interarch distance 524.28 ◀
material resources V60.2
mental (*see also* Retardation, mental) 319
nervous system 799.2
personality 301.6
prenatal care in current pregnancy
V23.7
pulmonary
function 786.09
newborn 770.89
ventilation, newborn 770.89
respiration 786.09
newborn 770.89
sample, Papanicolaou smear 795.08 ◀
social 301.6
Inanition 263.9
with edema 262
due to
deprivation of food 994.2
malnutrition 263.9
fever 780.6
Inappropriate secretion
ACTH 255.0
antidiuretic hormone (ADH) (excessive) 253.6
deficiency 253.5
ectopic hormone NEC 259.3
pituitary (posterior) 253.6
Inattention after or at birth 995.52
Inborn errors of metabolism - *see* Disorder, metabolism
Incarceration, incarcerated
bubonocele - *see also* Hernia, inguinal,
with obstruction
gangrenous - *see* Hernia, inguinal,
with gangrene

ICD-9-CM

—

Vol. 2

Incarceration, incarcerated (Continued)
colon (by hernia) - see also Hernia, by
site with obstruction
gangrenous - see Hernia, by site,
with gangrene
enterocele 552.9
gangrenous 551.9
epigastrocele 552.29
gangrenous 551.29
epiplocele 552.9
gangrenous 551.9
exomphalos 552.1
gangrenous 551.1
fallopian tube 620.8
hernia - see also Hernia, by site, with
obstruction
gangrenous - see Hernia, by site,
with gangrene
iris, in wound 871.1
lens, in wound 871.1
merocele (see also Hernia, femoral,
with obstruction) 552.00
omentum (by hernia) - see also Hernia,
by site, with obstruction
gangrenous - see Hernia, by site,
with gangrene
omphalocele 756.79
rupture (meaning hernia) (see also Hernia, by site, with obstruction) 552.9
gangrenous (see also Hernia, by site,
with gangrene) 551.9
sarcoepiplocele 552.9
gangrenous 551.9
sarcoepiplomphalocele 552.1
with gangrene 551.1
uterus 621.8
gravid 654.3
causing obstructed labor 660.2
affecting fetus or newborn 763.1
Incident, cerebrovascular (see also Disease, cerebrovascular, acute) 436
Incineration (entire body) (from fire,
conflagration, electricity, or lightning) - see Burn, multiple, specified
sites
Incised wound
external - see Wound, open, by site
internal organs (abdomen, chest, or
pelvis) - see Injury, internal, by
site, with open wound
Incision, incisional
hernia - see Hernia, incisional
surgical, complication - see Complications, surgical procedures
traumatic
external - see Wound, open, by site
internal organs (abdomen, chest, or
pelvis) - see Injury, internal, by
site, with open wound
Inclusion
azurophilic leukocytic 288.2
blennorrhea (neonatal) (newborn) 771.6
cyst - see Cyst, skin
gallbladder in liver (congenital) 751.69
Incompatibility
ABO
affecting management of pregnancy
656.2
fetus or newborn 773.1
infusion or transfusion reaction 999.6
blood (group) (Duffy) (E) (K(ell)) (Kidd)
(Lewis) (M) (N) (P) (S) NEC
affecting management of pregnancy
656.2

Incompatibility (Continued)
blood (Continued)
fetus or newborn 773.2
infusion or transfusion reaction 999.6
marital V61.10
involving divorce or estrangement
V61.0
Rh (blood group) (factor)
affecting management of pregnancy
656.1
fetus or newborn 773.0
infusion or transfusion reaction 999.7
Rhesus - see Incompatibility, Rh
**Incompetency, incompetence, incompe-
tent**
annular
aortic (valve) (see also Insufficiency,
aortic) 424.1
mitral (valve) - (see also Insufficiency,
mitral) 424.0
pulmonary valve (heart) (see also Endocarditis, pulmonary) 424.3
aortic (valve) (see also Insufficiency,
aortic) 424.1
syphilitic 093.22
cardiac (orifice) 530.0
valve - see Endocarditis
cervix, cervical (os) 622.5
in pregnancy 654.5
affecting fetus or newborn 761.0
esophagogastric (junction) (sphincter)
530.0
heart valve, congenital 746.89
mitral (valve) - see Insufficiency, mitral
papillary muscle (heart) 429.81
pelvic fundus ◄▥
pubocervical tissue 618.81 ◄
rectovaginal tissue 618.82 ◄
pulmonary valve (heart) (see also Endocarditis, pulmonary) 424.3
congenital 746.09
tricuspid (annular) (rheumatic) (valve) (see
also Endocarditis, tricuspid) 397.0
valvular - see Endocarditis
vein, venous (saphenous) (varicose)
(see also Varicose, vein) 454.9
velopharyngeal (closure)
acquired 528.9
congenital 750.29
Incomplete - see also condition
bladder emptying 788.21
expansion lungs (newborn) 770.5
gestation (liveborn) - see Immaturity
rotation - see Malrotation
Incontinence 788.30
without sensory awareness 788.34
anal sphincter 787.6
continuous leakage 788.37
feces 787.6
due to hysteria 300.11
nonorganic origin 307.7
hysterical 300.11
mixed (male) (female) (urge and stress)
788.33
overflow 788.38 ◄▥
paradoxical 788.39
rectal 787.6
specified NEC 788.39
stress (female) 625.6
male NEC 788.32
urethral sphincter 599.84
urge 788.31
and stress (male) (female) 788.33
urine 788.30

Incontinence (Continued)
urine (Continued)
active 788.30
male 788.30
stress 788.32
and urge 788.33
neurogenic 788.39
nonorganic origin 307.6
stress (female) 625.6
male NEC 788.32
urge 788.31
and stress 788.33
Incontinentia pigmenti 757.33
Incoordinate
uterus (action) (contractions) 661.4
affecting fetus or newborn 763.7
Incoordination
esophageal-pharyngeal (newborn)
787.2
muscular 781.3
papillary muscle 429.81
Increase, increased
abnormal, in development 783.9
androgens (ovarian) 256.1
anticoagulants (antithrombin) (anti-VIIIa)
(anti-IXa) (anti-Xa) (anti-XIa) 286.5
postpartum 666.3
cold sense (see also Disturbance, sensation) 782.0
estrogen 256.0
function
adrenal (cortex) 255.3
medulla 255.6
pituitary (anterior) (gland) (lobe)
253.1
posterior 253.6
heat sense (see also Disturbance, sensation) 782.0
intracranial pressure 781.99
injury at birth 767.8
light reflex of retina 362.13
permeability, capillary 448.9
pressure
intracranial 781.99
injury at birth 767.8
intraocular 365.00
pulsations 785.9
pulse pressure 785.9
sphericity, lens 743.36
splenic activity 289.4
venous pressure 459.89
portal 572.3
Incrustation, cornea, lead, or zinc
930.0
Incyclophoria 378.44
Incyclotropia 378.33
Indeterminate sex 752.7
India rubber skin 756.83
Indicanuria 270.2
Indigestion (bilious) (functional) 536.8
acid 536.8
catarrhal 536.8
due to decomposed food NEC 005.9
fat 579.8
nervous 306.4
psychogenic 306.4
Indirect - see condition
Indolent bubo NEC 099.8
Induced
abortion - see Abortion, induced
birth, affecting fetus or newborn
763.89
delivery - see Delivery
labor - see Delivery

◄ **New**   ◄▥ **Revised**

Induration, indurated
brain 348.8
breast (fibrous) 611.79
puerperal, postpartum 676.3
broad ligament 620.8
chancre 091.0
anus 091.1
congenital 090.0
extragenital NEC 091.2
corpora cavernosa (penis) (plastic) 607.89
liver (chronic) 573.8
acute 573.8
lung (black) (brown) (chronic) (fibroid) (see also Fibrosis, lung) 515
essential brown 275.0 [516.1]
penile 607.89
phlebitic - see Phlebitis
skin 782.8
stomach 537.89
Induratio penis plastica 607.89
Industrial - see condition
Inebriety (see also Abuse, drugs, nondependent) 305.0
Inefficiency
kidney (see also Disease, renal) 593.9
thyroid (acquired) (gland) 244.9
Inelasticity, skin 782.8
Inequality, leg (acquired) (length) 736.81
congenital 755.30
Inertia
bladder 596.4
neurogenic 596.54
with cauda equina syndrome 344.61
stomach 536.8
psychogenic 306.4
uterus, uterine 661.2
affecting fetus or newborn 763.7
primary 661.0
secondary 661.1
vesical 596.4
neurogenic 596.54
with cauda equina syndrome 344.61
Infant - see also condition
excessive crying of 780.92
fussy (baby) 780.91
held for adoption V68.89
newborn - see Newborn
post-term (gestation period over 40 completed weeks to 42 completed weeks) 766.21
prolonged gestation of (period over 42 completed weeks) 766.22
syndrome of diabetic mother 775.0
"Infant Hercules" syndrome 255.2
Infantile - see also condition
genitalia, genitals 259.0
in pregnancy or childbirth NEC 654.4
affecting fetus or newborn 763.89
causing obstructed labor 660.2
affecting fetus or newborn 763.1
heart 746.9
kidney 753.3
lack of care 995.52
macula degeneration 362.75
melanodontia 521.05
os, uterus (see also Infantile, genitalia) 259.0
pelvis 738.6
with disproportion (fetopelvic) 653.1
affecting fetus or newborn 763.1
causing obstructed labor 660.1
affecting fetus or newborn 763.1
penis 259.0
testis 257.2
uterus (see also Infantile, genitalia) 259.0

Infantile (Continued)
vulva 752.49
Infantilism 259.9
with dwarfism (hypophyseal) 253.3
Brissaud's (infantile myxedema) 244.9
celiac 579.0
Herter's (nontropical sprue) 579.0
hypophyseal 253.3
hypothalamic (with obesity) 253.8
idiopathic 259.9
intestinal 579.0
pancreatic 577.8
pituitary 253.3
renal 588.0
sexual (with obesity) 259.0
Infants, healthy liveborn - see Newborn
Infarct, infarction
adrenal (capsule) (gland) 255.4
amnion 658.8
anterior (with contiguous portion of intraventricular septum) NEC (see also Infarct, myocardium) 410.1
appendices epiploicae 557.0
bowel 557.0
brain (stem) 434.91
embolic (see also Embolism, brain) 434.11
healed or old, without residuals V12.59
iatrogenic 997.02
lacunar 434.91
postoperative 997.02
puerperal, postpartum, childbirth 674.0
thrombotic (see also Thrombosis, brain) 434.01
breast 611.8
Brewer's (kidney) 593.81
cardiac (see also Infarct, myocardium) 410.9
cerebellar (see also Infarct, brain) 434.91
embolic (see also Embolism, brain) 434.11
cerebral (see also Infarct, brain) 434.91
embolic (see also Embolism, brain) 434.11
thrombotic (see also Infarct, brain) 434.01 ◄
chorion 658.8
colon (acute) (agnogenic) (embolic) (hemorrhagic) (nonocclusive) (nonthrombotic) (occlusive) (segmental) (thrombotic) (with gangrene) 557.0
coronary artery (see also Infarct, myocardium) 410.9
cortical 434.91 ◄
embolic (see also Embolism) 444.9
fallopian tube 620.8
gallbladder 575.8
heart (see also Infarct, myocardium) 410.9
hepatic 573.4
hypophysis (anterior lobe) 253.8
impending (myocardium) 411.1
intestine (acute) (agnogenic) (embolic) (hemorrhagic) (nonocclusive) (nonthrombotic) (occlusive) (thrombotic) (with gangrene) 557.0
kidney 593.81
lacunar 434.91
liver 573.4
lung (embolic) (thrombotic) 415.19
with
abortion - see Abortion, by type, with, embolism
ectopic pregnancy (see also categories 633.0-633.9) 639.6
molar pregnancy (see also categories 630-632) 639.6

Infarct, infarction (Continued)
lung (Continued)
following
abortion 639.6
ectopic or molar pregnancy 639.6
iatrogenic 415.11
in pregnancy, childbirth, or puerperium - see Embolism, obstetrical
postoperative 415.11
lymph node or vessel 457.8
medullary (brain) - see Infarct, brain
meibomian gland (eyelid) 374.85
mesentery, mesenteric (embolic) (thrombotic) (with gangrene) 557.0
midbrain - see Infarct, brain
myocardium, myocardial (acute or with a stated duration of 8 weeks or less) (with hypertension) 410.9

Note   Use the following fifth-digit subclassification with category 410:
0   episode unspecified
1   initial episode
2   subsequent episode without recurrence

with symptoms after 8 weeks from date of infarction 414.8
anterior (wall) (with contiguous portion of intraventricular septum) NEC 410.1
anteroapical (with contiguous portion of intraventricular septum) 410.1
anterolateral (wall) 410.0
anteroseptal (with contiguous portion of intraventricular septum) 410.1
apical-lateral 410.5
atrial 410.8
basal-lateral 410.5
chronic (with symptoms after 8 weeks from date of infarction) 414.8
diagnosed on ECG, but presenting no symptoms 412
diaphragmatic wall (with contiguous portion of intraventricular septum) 410.4
healed or old, currently presenting no symptoms 412
high lateral 410.5
impending 411.1
inferior (wall) (with contiguous portion of intraventricular septum) 410.4
inferolateral (wall) 410.2
inferoposterior wall 410.3
lateral wall 410.5
nontransmural 410.7
papillary muscle 410.8
past (diagnosed on ECG or other special investigation, but currently presenting no symptoms) 412
with symptoms NEC 414.8
posterior (strictly) (true) (wall) 410.6
posterobasal 410.6
posteroinferior 410.3
posterolateral 410.5
previous, currently presenting no symptoms 412
septal 410.8
specified site NEC 410.8
subendocardial 410.7
syphilitic 093.82

ICD-9-CM

—

Vol. 2

Infarct, infarction (Continued)
nontransmural 410.7
omentum 557.0
ovary 620.8
pancreas 577.8
papillary muscle (see also Infarct, myocardium) 410.8
parathyroid gland 252.8
pituitary (gland) 253.8
placenta (complicating pregnancy) 656.7
   affecting fetus or newborn 762.2
pontine - see Infarct, brain
posterior NEC (see also Infarct, myocardium) 410.6
prostate 602.8
pulmonary (artery) (hemorrhagic) (vein) 415.19
  with
    abortion - see Abortion, by type, with embolism
    ectopic pregnancy (see also categories 633.0-633.9) 639.6
    molar pregnancy (see also categories 630-632) 639.6
  following
    abortion 639.6
    ectopic or molar pregnancy 639.6
  iatrogenic 415.11
  in pregnancy, childbirth, or puerperium - see Embolism, obstetrical
  postoperative 415.11
renal 593.81
  embolic or thrombotic 593.81
retina, retinal 362.84
  with occlusion - see Occlusion, retina
spinal (acute) (cord) (embolic) (nonembolic) 336.1
spleen 289.59
  embolic or thrombotic 444.89
subchorionic - see Infarct, placenta
subendocardial (see also Infarct, myocardium) 410.7
suprarenal (capsule) (gland) 255.4
syncytium - see Infarct, placenta
testis 608.83
thrombotic (see also Thrombosis) 453.9
  artery, arterial - see Embolism
thyroid (gland) 246.3
ventricle (heart) (see also Infarct, myocardium) 410.9
Infecting - see condition
Infection, infected, infective (opportunistic) 136.9
with lymphangitis - see Lymphangitis
abortion - see Abortion, by type, with, sepsis
abscess (skin) - see Abscess, by site
Absidia 117.7
Acanthocheilonema (perstans) 125.4
  streptocerca 125.6
accessory sinus (chronic) (see also Sinusitis) 473.9
Achorion - see Dermatophytosis
Acremonium falciforme 117.4
acromioclavicular (joint) 711.91
Actinobacillus
  lignieresii 027.8
  mallei 024
  muris 026.1
Actinomadura - see Actinomycosis
Actinomyces (israelii) - see also Actinomycosis
  muris-ratti 026.1

Infection, infected, infective (Continued)
Actinomycetales (Actinomadura) (Actinomyces) (Nocardia) (Streptomyces) - see Actinomycosis
actinomycotic NEC (see also Actinomycosis) 039.9
adenoid (chronic) 474.01
  acute 463
  and tonsil (chronic) 474.02
    acute or subacute 463
adenovirus NEC 079.0
  in diseases classified elsewhere - see category 079
  unspecified nature or site 079.0
Aerobacter aerogenes NEC 041.85
  enteritis 008.2
Aerogenes capsulatus (see also Gangrene, gas) 040.0
aertrycke (see also Infection, Salmonella) 003.9
Ajellomyces dermatitidis 116.0
alimentary canal NEC (see also Enteritis, due to, by organism) 009.0
Allescheria boydii 117.6
Alternaria 118
alveolus, alveolar (process) (pulpal origin) 522.4
ameba, amebic (histolytica) (see also Amebiasis) 006.9
  acute 006.0
  chronic 006.1
  free-living 136.2
  hartmanni 007.8
  specified
    site NEC 006.8
    type NEC 007.8
amniotic fluid or cavity 658.4
  affecting fetus or newborn 762.7
anaerobes (cocci) (gram-negative) (gram-positive) (mixed) NEC 041.84
anal canal 569.49
Ancylostoma braziliense 126.2
Angiostrongylus cantonensis 128.8
anisakiasis 127.1
Anisakis larva 127.1
anthrax (see also Anthrax) 022.9
antrum (chronic) (see also Sinusitis, maxillary) 473.0
anus (papillae) (sphincter) 569.49
arbor virus NEC 066.9
arbovirus NEC 066.9
argentophil-rod 027.0
Ascaris lumbricoides 127.0
ascomycetes 117.4
Aspergillus (flavus) (fumigatus) (terreus) 117.3
atypical
  acid-fast (bacilli) (see also Mycobacterium, atypical) 031.9
  mycobacteria (see also Mycobacterium, atypical) 031.9
auditory meatus (circumscribed) (diffuse) (external) (see also Otitis, externa) 380.10
auricle (ear) (see also Otitis, externa) 380.10
axillary gland 683
babesiasis 088.82
babesiosis 088.82
Bacillus NEC 041.89
  abortus 023.1
  anthracis (see also Anthrax) 022.9
  cereus (food poisoning) 005.89

Infection, infected, infective (Continued)
Bacillus NEC (Continued)
  coli - see Infection, Escherichia coli
  coliform NEC 041.85
  Ducrey's (any location) 099.0
  Flexner's 004.1
  Friedländer's NEC 041.3
  fusiformis 101
  gas (gangrene) (see also Gangrene, gas) 040.0
  mallei 024
  melitensis 023.0
  paratyphoid, paratyphosus 002.9
    A 002.1
    B 002.2
    C 002.3
  Schmorl's 040.3
  Shiga 004.0
  suipestifer (see also Infection, Salmonella) 003.9
  swimming pool 031.1
  typhosa 002.0
  welchii (see also Gangrene, gas) 040.0
  Whitmore's 025
bacterial NEC 041.9
  specified NEC 041.89
    anaerobic NEC 041.84
    gram-negative NEC 041.85
      anaerobic NEC 041.84
Bacterium
  paratyphosum 002.9
    A 002.1
    B 002.2
    C 002.3
  typhosum 002.9
Bacteroides (fragilis) (melaninogenicus) (oralis) NEC 041.82 ◀▥
Balantidium coli 007.0
Bartholin's gland 616.8
Basidiobolus 117.7
Bedsonia 079.98
  specified NEC 079.88
bile duct 576.1
bladder (see also Cystitis) 595.9
Blastomyces, blastomycotic 116.0
  brasiliensis 116.1
  dermatitidis 116.0
  European 117.5
  loboi 116.2
  North American 116.0
  South American 116.1
blood stream - see Septicemia
bone 730.9
  specified - see Osteomyelitis
Bordetella 033.9
  bronchiseptica 033.8
  parapertussis 033.1
  pertussis 033.0
Borrelia
  bergdorfi 088.81
  vincentii (mouth) (pharynx) (tonsil) 101
brain (see also Encephalitis) 323.9
  late effect - see category 326
  membranes - (see also Meningitis) 322.9
  septic 324.0
    late effect - see category 326
  meninges (see also Meningitis) 320.9
branchial cyst 744.42
breast 611.0

◀ New   ◀▥ Revised

Infection, infected, infective (*Continued*)
  breast (*Continued*)
    puerperal, postpartum 675.2
      with nipple 675.9
        specified type NEC 675.8
      nonpurulent 675.2
      purulent 675.1
  bronchus (*see also* Bronchitis) 490
    fungus NEC 117.9
  Brucella 023.9
    abortus 023.1
    canis 023.3
    melitensis 023.0
    mixed 023.8
    suis 023.2
  Brugia (Wuchereria) malayi 125.1
  bursa - *see* Bursitis
  buttocks (skin) 686.9
  Candida (albicans) (tropicalis) (*see also*
    Candidiasis) 112.9
    congenital 771.7
  Candiru 136.8
  Capillaria
    hepatica 128.8
    philippinensis 127.5
  cartilage 733.99
  cat liver fluke 121.0
  cellulitis - *see* Cellulitis, by site
  Cephalosporum falciforme 117.4
  Cercomonas hominis (intestinal) 007.3
  cerebrospinal (*see also* Meningitis) 322.9
    late effect - *see* category 326
  cervical gland 683
  cervix (*see also* Cervicitis) 616.0
  cesarean section wound 674.3
  Chilomastix (intestinal) 007.8
  Chlamydia 079.98
    specified NEC 079.88
  Cholera (*see also* Cholera) 001.9
  chorionic plate 658.8
  Cladosporium
    bantianum 117.8
    carrionii 117.2
    mansonii 111.1
    trichoides 117.8
    werneckii 111.1
  Clonorchis (sinensis) (liver) 121.1
  Clostridium (haemolyticum) (novyi)
    NEC 041.84
    botulinum 005.1
    histolyticum (*see also* Gangrene, gas)
      040.0
    oedematiens (*see also* Gangrene, gas)
      040.0
    perfringens 041.83
      due to food 005.2
    septicum (*see also* Gangrene, gas)
      040.0
    sordellii (*see also* Gangrene, gas)
      040.0
    welchii (*see also* Gangrene, gas)
      040.0
      due to food 005.2
  Coccidioides (immitis) (*see also* Coccid-
    ioidomycosis) 114.9
  coccus NEC 041.89
  colon (*see also* Enteritis, due to, by or-
    ganism) 009.0
    bacillus - *see* Infection, Escherichia coli
  colostomy or enterostomy 569.61
  common duct 576.1
  complicating pregnancy, childbirth, or
    puerperium NEC 647.9
    affecting fetus or newborn 760.2

Infection, infected, infective (*Continued*)
  Condiobolus 117.7
  congenital NEC 771.89
    Candida albicans 771.7
    chronic 771.2
    cytomegalovirus 771.1
    hepatitis, viral 771.2
    herpes simplex 771.2
    listeriosis 771.2
    malaria 771.2
    poliomyelitis 771.2
    rubella 771.0
    toxoplasmosis 771.2
    tuberculosis 771.2
    urinary (tract) 771.82
    vaccinia 771.2
  Conidiobolus 117.7
  coronavirus 079.89
    SARS-associated 079.82
  corpus luteum (*see also* Salpingo-
    oophoritis) 614.2
  Corynebacterium diphtheriae - *see*
    Diphtheria
  Coxsackie (*see also* Coxsackie) 079.2
    endocardium 074.22
    heart NEC 074.20
    in diseases classified elsewhere - *see*
      category 079
    meninges 047.0
    myocardium 074.23
    pericardium 074.21
    pharynx 074.0
    specified disease NEC 074.8
    unspecified nature or site 079.2
  Cryptococcus neoformans 117.5
  Cryptosporidia 007.4
  Cunninghamella 117.7
  cyst - *see* Cyst
  Cysticercus cellulosae 123.1
  cytomegalovirus 078.5
    congenital 771.1
  dental (pulpal origin) 522.4
  deuteromycetes 117.4
  Dicrocoelium dendriticum 121.8
  Dipetalonema (perstans) 125.4
    streptocerca 125.6
  diphtherial - *see* Diphtheria
  Diphyllobothrium (adult) (latum) (pa-
    cificum) 123.4
    larval 123.5
  Diplogonoporus (grandis) 123.8
  Dipylidium (caninum) 123.8
  Dirofilaria 125.6
  dog tapeworm 123.8
  Dracunculus medinensis 125.7
  Dreschlera 118
    hawaiiensis 117.8
  Ducrey's bacillus (any site) 099.0
  due to or resulting from
    device, implant, or graft (any) (pres-
      ence of) - *see* Complications, in-
      fection and inflammation, due
      to (presence of) any device, im-
      plant, or graft classified to
      996.0-996.5 NEC
    injection, inoculation, infusion,
      transfusion, or vaccination
      (prophylactic) (therapeutic)
      999.3
    injury NEC - *see* Wound, open, by
      site, complicated
    surgery 998.59
  duodenum 535.6

Infection, infected, infective (*Continued*)
  ear - *see also* Otitis
    external (*see also* Otitis, externa)
      380.10
    inner (*see also* Labyrinthitis) 386.30
    middle - *see* Otitis, media
  Eaton's agent NEC 041.81
  Eberthella typhosa 002.0
  Ebola 065.8
  echinococcosis 122.9
  Echinococcus (*see also* Echinococcus)
    122.9
  Echinostoma 121.8
  ECHO virus 079.1
    in diseases classified elsewhere - *see*
      category 079
    unspecified nature or site 079.1
  Ehrlichiosis 082.40
    chaffeensis 082.41
    specified type NEC 082.49
  Endamoeba - *see* Infection, ameba
  endocardium (*see also* Endocarditis) 421.0
  endocervix (*see also* Cervicitis) 616.0
  Entamoeba - *see* Infection, ameba
  enteric (*see also* Enteritis, due to, by
    organism) 009.0
  Enterobacter aerogenes NEC 041.85
  Enterobius vermicularis 127.4
  enterococcus NEC 041.04
  enterovirus NEC 079.89
    central nervous system NEC 048
    enteritis 008.67
    meningitis 047.9
  Entomophthora 117.7
  Epidermophyton - *see* Dermatophytosis
  epidermophytosis - *see* Dermatophytosis
  episiotomy 674.3
  Epstein-Barr virus 075
    chronic 780.79 [139.8]
  erysipeloid 027.1
  Erysipelothrix (insidiosa) (rhusiopa-
    thiae) 027.1
  erythema infectiosum 057.0
  Escherichia coli NEC 041.4
    enteritis - *see* Enteritis, E. coli
    generalized 038.42
    intestinal - *see* Enteritis, E. coli
  esophagostomy 530.86   ◄
  ethmoidal (chronic) (sinus) (*see also* Si-
    nusitis, ethmoidal) 473.2
  Eubacterium 041.84
  Eustachian tube (ear) 381.50
    acute 381.51
    chronic 381.52
  exanthema subitum 057.8
  external auditory canal (meatus) (*see*
    also Otitis, externa) 380.10
  eye NEC 360.00
  eyelid 373.9
    specified NEC 373.8
  fallopian tube (*see also* Salpingo-
    oophoritis) 614.2
  fascia 728.89
  Fasciola
    gigantica 121.3
    hepatica 121.3
  Fasciolopsis (buski) 121.4
  fetus (intra-amniotic) - *see* Infection,
    congenital
  filarial - *see* Infestation, filarial
  finger (skin) 686.9
    abscess (with lymphangitis) 681.00
      pulp 681.01
    cellulitis (with lymphangitis) 681.00

Infection, infected, infective (Continued)
finger (Continued)
distal closed space (with lymphangitis) 681.00
nail 681.02
fungus 110.1
fish tapeworm 123.4
larval 123.5
flagellate, intestinal 007.9
fluke - see Infestation, fluke
focal
teeth (pulpal origin) 522.4
tonsils 474.00
and adenoids 474.02
Fonsecaea
compactum 117.2
pedrosoi 117.2
food (see also Poisoning, food) 005.9
foot (skin) 686.9
fungus 110.4
Francisella tularensis (see also Tularemia) 021.9
frontal sinus (chronic) (see also Sinusitis, frontal) 473.1
fungus NEC 117.9
beard 110.0
body 110.5
dematiaceous NEC 117.8
foot 110.4
groin 110.3
hand 110.2
nail 110.1
pathogenic to compromised host only 118
perianal (area) 110.3
scalp 110.0
scrotum 110.8
skin 111.9
foot 110.4
hand 110.2
toenails 110.1
trachea 117.9
Fusarium 118
Fusobacterium 041.84
gallbladder (see also Cholecystitis, acute) 575.0
Gardnerella vaginalis 041.89
gas bacillus (see also Gas, gangrene) 040.0
gastric (see also Gastritis) 535.5
Gastrodiscoides hominis 121.8
gastroenteric (see also Enteritis, due to, by organism) 009.0
gastrointestinal (see also Enteritis, due to, by organism) 009.0
gastrostomy 536.41
generalized NEC (see also Septicemia) 038.9
genital organ or tract NEC
female 614.9
with
abortion - see Abortion, by type, with sepsis
ectopic pregnancy (see also categories 633.0-633.9) 639.0
molar pregnancy (see also categories 630-632) 639.0
complicating pregnancy 646.6
affecting fetus or newborn 760.8
following
abortion 639.0
ectopic or molar pregnancy 639.0
puerperal, postpartum, childbirth 670
minor or localized 646.6
affecting fetus or newborn 760.8

Infection, infected, infective (Continued)
genital organ or tract NEC (Continued)
male 608.4
genitourinary tract NEC 599.0
Ghon tubercle, primary (see also Tuberculosis) 010.0
Giardia lamblia 007.1
gingival (chronic) 523.1
acute 523.0
Vincent's 101
glanders 024
Glenosporopsis amazonica 116.2
Gnathostoma spinigerum 128.1
Gongylonema 125.6
gonococcal NEC (see also Gonococcus) 098.0
gram-negative bacilli NEC 041.85
anaerobic 041.84
guinea worm 125.7
gum (see also Infection, gingival) 523.1
Hantavirus 079.81
heart 429.89
Helicobactor pylori 041.86
helminths NEC 128.9
intestinal 127.9
mixed (types classifiable to more than one category in 120.0-127.7) 127.8
specified type NEC 127.7
specified type NEC 128.8
Hemophilus influenzae NEC 041.5
generalized 038.41
herpes (simplex) (see also Herpes, simplex) 054.9
congenital 771.2
zoster (see also Herpes, zoster) 053.9
eye NEC 053.29
Heterophyes heterophyes 121.6
Histoplasma (see also Histoplasmosis) 115.90
capsulatum (see also Histoplasmosis, American) 115.00
duboisii (see also Histoplasmosis, African) 115.10
HIV V08
with symptoms, symptomatic 042
hookworm (see also Ancylostomiasis) 126.9
human immunodeficiency virus V08
with symptoms, symptomatic 042
human papillomavirus 079.4
hydrocele 603.1
hydronephrosis 591
Hymenolepis 123.6
hypopharynx 478.29
inguinal glands 683
due to soft chancre 099.0
intestine, intestinal (see also Enteritis, due to, by organism) 009.0
intrauterine (see also Endometritis) 615.9
complicating delivery 646.6
Isospora belli or hominis 007.2
Japanese B encephalitis 062.0
jaw (bone) (acute) (chronic) (lower) (subacute) (upper) 526.4
joint - see Arthritis, infectious or infective
kidney (cortex) (hematogenous) 590.9
with
abortion - see Abortion, by type, with urinary tract infection
calculus 592.0
ectopic pregnancy (see also categories 633.0-633.9) 639.8

Infection, infected, infective (Continued)
kidney (Continued)
with (Continued)
molar pregnancy (see also categories 630-632) 639.8
complicating pregnancy or puerperium 646.6
affecting fetus or newborn 760.1
following
abortion 639.8
ectopic or molar pregnancy 639.8
pelvis and ureter 590.3
Klebsiella pneumoniae NEC 041.3
knee (skin) NEC 686.9
joint - see Arthritis, infectious
Koch's (see also Tuberculosis, pulmonary) 011.9
labia (majora) (minora) (see also Vulvitis) 616.10
lacrimal
gland (see also Dacryoadenitis) 375.00
passages (duct) (sac) (see also Dacryocystitis) 375.30
larynx NEC 478.79
leg (skin) NEC 686.9
Leishmania (see also Leishmaniasis) 085.9
braziliensis 085.5
donovani 085.0
Ethiopica 085.3
furunculosa 085.1
infantum 085.0
mexicana 085.4
tropica (minor) 085.1
major 085.2
Leptosphaeria senegalensis 117.4
Leptospira (see also Leptospirosis) 100.9
australis 100.89
bataviae 100.89
pyrogenes 100.89
specified type NEC 100.89
leptospirochetal NEC (see also Leptospirosis) 100.9
Leptothrix - see Actinomycosis
Listeria monocytogenes (listeriosis) 027.0
congenital 771.2
liver fluke - see Infestation, fluke, liver
Loa loa 125.2
eyelid 125.2 [373.6]
Loboa loboi 116.2
local, skin (staphylococcal) (streptococcal) NEC 686.9
abscess - see Abscess, by site
cellulitis - see Cellulitis, by site
ulcer (see also Ulcer, skin) 707.9
Loefflerella
mallei 024
whitmori 025
lung 518.89
atypical mycobacterium 031.0
tuberculous (see also Tuberculosis, pulmonary) 011.9
basilar 518.89
chronic 518.89
fungus NEC 117.9
spirochetal 104.8
virus - see Pneumonia, virus
lymph gland (axillary) (cervical) (inguinal) 683
mesenteric 289.2
lymphoid tissue, base of tongue or posterior pharynx, NEC 474.00
Madurella
grisea 117.4
mycetomii 117.4

◀ **New**   ◀▥ **Revised**

Infection, infected, infective (*Continued*)
major
with
abortion - *see* Abortion, by type,
with sepsis
ectopic pregnancy (*see also* categories 633.0-633.9) 639.0
molar pregnancy (*see also* categories 630-632) 639.0
following
abortion 639.0
ectopic or molar pregnancy 639.0
puerperal, postpartum, childbirth
670
malarial - *see* Malaria
Malassezia furfur 111.0
Malleomyces
mallei 024
pseudomallei 025
mammary gland 611.0
puerperal, postpartum 675.2
Mansonella (ozzardi) 125.5
mastoid (suppurative) - *see* Mastoiditis
maxilla, maxillary 526.4
sinus (chronic) (*see also* Sinusitis,
maxillary) 473.0
mediastinum 519.2
medina 125.7
meibomian
cyst 373.12
gland 373.12
melioidosis 025
meninges (*see also* Meningitis) 320.9
meningococcal (*see also* condition) 036.9
brain 036.1
cerebrospinal 036.0
endocardium 036.42
generalized 036.2
meninges 036.0
meningococcemia 036.2
specified site NEC 036.89
mesenteric lymph nodes or glands
NEC 289.2
Metagonimus 121.5
metatarsophalangeal 711.97
microorganism resistant to drugs - *see*
Resistance (to), drugs by microorganisms
Microsporidia 136.8
Microsporum, microsporic - *see* Dermatophytosis
mima polymorpha NEC 041.85
mixed flora NEC 041.89
Monilia (*see also* Candidiasis) 112.9
neonatal 771.7
monkeypox 057.8
Monosporium apiospermum 117.6
mouth (focus) NEC 528.9
parasitic 112.0
Mucor 117.7
muscle NEC 728.89
mycelium NEC 117.9
mycetoma
actinomycotic NEC (*see also* Actinomycosis) 039.9
mycotic NEC 117.4
Mycobacterium, mycobacterial (*see also*
Mycobacterium) 031.9
mycoplasma NEC 041.81
mycotic NEC 117.9
pathogenic to compromised host
only 118
skin NEC 111.9
systemic 117.9

Infection, infected, infective (*Continued*)
myocardium NEC 422.90
nail (chronic) (with lymphangitis)
681.9
finger 681.02
fungus 110.1
ingrowing 703.0
toe 681.11
fungus 110.1
nasal sinus (chronic) (*see also* Sinusitis)
473.9
nasopharynx (chronic) 478.29
acute 460
navel 686.9
newborn 771.4
Neisserian - *see* Gonococcus
Neotestudina rosatii 117.4
newborn, generalized 771.89
nipple 611.0
puerperal, postpartum 675.0
with breast 675.9
specified type NEC 675.8
Nocardia - *see* Actinomycosis
nose 478.1
nostril 478.1
obstetrical surgical wound 674.3
Oesophagostomum (apiostomum)
127.7
Oestrus ovis 134.0
Oidium albicans (*see also* Candidiasis)
112.9
Onchocerca (volvulus) 125.3
eye 125.3 [360.13]
eyelid 125.3 [373.6]
operation wound 998.59
Opisthorchis (felineus) (tenuicollis) (viverrini) 121.0
orbit 376.00
chronic 376.10
ovary (*see also* Salpingo-oophoritis)
614.2
Oxyuris vermicularis 127.4
pancreas 577.0
Paracoccidioides brasiliensis 116.1
Paragonimus (westermani) 121.2
parainfluenza virus 079.89
parameningococcus NEC 036.9
with meningitis 036.0
parasitic NEC 136.9
paratyphoid 002.9
type A 002.1
type B 002.2
type C 002.3
paraurethral ducts 597.89
parotid gland 527.2
Pasteurella NEC 027.2
multocida (cat-bite) (dog-bite) 027.2
pestis (*see also* Plague) 020.9
pseudotuberculosis 027.2
septica (cat-bite) (dog-bite) 027.2
tularensis (*see also* Tularemia) 021.9
pelvic, female (*see also* Disease, pelvis,
inflammatory) 614.9
penis (glans) (retention) NEC 607.2
herpetic 054.13
Peptococcus 041.84
Peptostreptococcus 041.84
periapical (pulpal origin) 522.4
peridental 523.3
perineal wound (obstetrical) 674.3
periodontal 523.3
periorbital 376.00
chronic 376.10
perirectal 569.49

Infection, infected, infective (*Continued*)
perirenal (*see also* Infection, kidney)
590.9
peritoneal (*see also* Peritonitis) 567.9
periureteral 593.89
periurethral 597.89
Petriellidium boydii 117.6
pharynx 478.29
Coxsackie virus 074.0
phlegmonous 462
posterior, lymphoid 474.00
Phialophora
gougerotii 117.8
jeanselmei 117.8
verrucosa 117.2
Piedraia hortai 111.3
pinna, acute 380.11
pinta 103.9
intermediate 103.1
late 103.2
mixed 103.3
primary 103.0
pinworm 127.4
Pityrosporum furfur 111.0
pleuropneumonia-like organisms NEC
(PPLO) 041.81
pneumococcal NEC 041.2
generalized (purulent) 038.2
Pneumococcus NEC 041.2
postoperative wound 998.59
posttraumatic NEC 958.3
postvaccinal 999.3
prepuce NEC 607.1
Propionibacterium 041.84
prostate (capsule) (*see also* Prostatitis)
601.9
Proteus (mirabilis) (morganii) (vulgaris) NEC 041.6
enteritis 008.3
protozoal NEC 136.8
intestinal NEC 007.9
Pseudomonas NEC 041.7
mallei 024
pneumonia 482.1
pseudomallei 025
psittacosis 073.9
puerperal, postpartum (major) 670
minor 646.6
pulmonary - *see* Infection, lung
purulent - *see* Abscess
putrid, generalized - *see* Septicemia
pyemic - *see* Septicemia
Pyrenochaeta romeroi 117.4
Q fever 083.0
rabies 071
rectum (sphincter) 569.49
renal (*see also* Infection, kidney) 590.9
pelvis and ureter 590.3
resistant to drugs - *see* Resistance (to),
drugs by microorganisms
respiratory 519.8
chronic 519.8
influenzal (acute) (upper) 487.1
lung 518.89
rhinovirus 460
syncytial virus 079.6
upper (acute) (infectious) NEC 465.9
with flu, grippe, or influenza 487.1
influenzal 487.1
multiple sites NEC 465.8
streptococcal 034.0
viral NEC 465.9
respiratory syncytial virus (RSV)
079.6

ICD-9-CM

—

Vol. 2

Infection, infected, infective *(Continued)*
  resulting from presence of shunt or
      other internal prosthetic device -
      see Complications, infection and
      inflammation, due to (presence of)
      any device, implant, or graft clas-
      sified to 996.0-996.5 NEC
  retrovirus 079.50
      human immunodeficiency virus type
          2 [HIV 2] 079.53
      human T-cell lymphotrophic virus
          type I [HTLV-I] 079.51
      human T-cell lymphotrophic virus
          type II [HTLV-II] 079.52
      specified NEC 079.59
  Rhinocladium 117.1
  Rhinosporidium (seeberi) 117.0,
  rhinovirus
      in diseases classified elsewhere - *see*
          category 079
      unspecified nature or site 079.3
  Rhizopus 117.7
  rickettsial 083.9
  rickettsialpox 083.2
  rubella (*see also* Rubella) 056.9
      congenital 771.0
  Saccharomyces (*see also* Candidiasis)
      112.9
  Saksenaea 117.7
  salivary duct or gland (any) 527.2
  Salmonella (aertrycke) (callinarum)
      (choleraesuis) (enteritidis) (suipes-
      tifer) (typhimurium) 003.9
      with
          arthritis 003.23
          gastroenteritis 003.0
          localized infection 003.20
              specified type NEC 003.29
          meningitis 003.21
          osteomyelitis 003.24
          pneumonia 003.22
          septicemia 003.1
          specified manifestation NEC 003.8
      due to food (poisoning) (any sero-
          type) (*see also* Poisoning, food,
          due to, Salmonella)
      hirschfeldii 002.3
      localized 003.20
          specified type NEC 003.29
      paratyphi 002.9
          A 002.1
          B 002.2
          C 002.3
      schottmuelleri 002.2
      specified type NEC 003.8
      typhi 002.0
      typhosa 002.0
  saprophytic 136.8
  Sarcocystis, lindemanni 136.5
  SARS-associated coronavirus 079.82
  scabies 133.0
  Schistosoma - *see* Infestation, Schisto-
      soma
  Schmorl's bacillus 040.3
  scratch or other superficial injury - *see*
      Injury, superficial, by site
  scrotum (acute) NEC 608.4
  secondary, burn or open wound (dislo-
      cation) (fracture) 958.3
  seminal vesicle (*see also* Vesiculitis) 608.0
  septic
      generalized - *see* Septicemia
      localized, skin (*see also* Abscess)
          682.9

Infection, infected, infective *(Continued)*
  septicemic - *see* Septicemia
  seroma 998.51
  Serratia (marcescens) 041.85
      generalized 038.44
  sheep liver fluke 121.3
  Shigella 004.9
      boydii 004.2
      dysenteriae 004.0
      Flexneri 004.1
      group
          A 004.0
          B 004.1
          C 004.2
          D 004.3
      Schmitz (-Stutzer) 004.0
      Schmitzii 004.0
      Shiga 004.0
      Sonnei 004.3
      specified type NEC 004.8
  Sin Nombre virus 079.81
  sinus (*see also* Sinusitis) 473.9
      pilonidal 685.1
          with abscess 685.0
      skin NEC 686.9
  Skene's duct or gland (*see also* Urethri-
      tis) 597.89
  skin (local) (staphylococcal) (strepto-
      coccal) NEC 686.9
      abscess - *see* Abscess, by site
      cellulitis - *see* Cellulitis, by site
      due to fungus 111.9
          specified type NEC 111.8
      mycotic 111.9
          specified type NEC 111.8
      ulcer (*see also* Ulcer, skin) 707.9
  slow virus 046.9
      specified condition NEC 046.8
  Sparganum (mansoni) (proliferum) 123.5
  spermatic cord NEC 608.4
  sphenoidal (chronic) (sinus) (*see also* Si-
      nusitis, sphenoidal) 473.3
  Spherophorus necrophorus 040.3
  spinal cord NEC (*see also* Encephalitis)
      323.9
      abscess 324.1
          late effect - *see* category 326
      late effect - *see* category 326
      meninges - *see* Meningitis
      streptococcal 320.2
  Spirillum
      minus or minor 026.0
      morsus muris 026.0
      obermeieri 087.0
  spirochetal NEC 104.9
      lung 104.8
      specified nature or site NEC 104.8
  spleen 289.59
  Sporothrix schenckii 117.1
  Sporotrichum (schenckii) 117.1
  Sporozoa 136.8
  staphylococcal NEC 041.10
      aureus 041.11
      food poisoning 005.0
      generalized (purulent) 038.10
          aureus 038.11
          specified organism NEC 038.19
      pneumonia 482.40
          aureus 482.41
          specified type NEC 482.49
      septicemia 038.10
          aureus 038.11
          specified organism NEC 038.19
      specified NEC 041.19

Infection, infected, infective *(Continued)*
  steatoma 706.2
  Stellantchasmus falcatus 121.6
  Streptobacillus moniliformis 026.1
  streptococcal NEC 041.00
      generalized (purulent) 038.0
      group
          A 041.01
          B 041.02
          C 041.03
          D [enterococcus] 041.04
          G 041.05
      pneumonia - *see* Pneumonia, strepto-
          coccal
      septicemia 038.0
      sore throat 034.0
      specified NEC 041.09
  Streptomyces - *see* Actinomycosis
  streptotrichosis - *see* Actinomycosis
  Strongyloides (stercoralis) 127.2
  stump (amputation) (posttraumatic)
      (surgical) 997.62
      traumatic - *see* Amputation, trau-
          matic, by site, complicated
  subcutaneous tissue, local NEC 686.9
  submaxillary region 528.9
  suipestifer (*see also* Infection, Salmo-
      nella) 003.9
  swimming pool bacillus 031.1
  syphilitic - *see* Syphilis
  systemic - *see* Septicemia
  Taenia - *see* Infestation, Taenia
  Taeniarhynchus saginatus 123.2
  tapeworm - *see* Infestation, tapeworm
  tendon (sheath) 727.89
  Ternidens diminutus 127.7
  testis (*see also* Orchitis) 604.90
  thigh (skin) 686.9
  threadworm 127.4
  throat 478.29
      pneumococcal 462
      staphylococcal 462
      streptococcal 034.0
      viral NEC (*see also* Pharyngitis) 462
  thumb (skin) 686.9
      abscess (with lymphangitis) 681.00
          pulp 681.01
      cellulitis (with lymphangitis)
          681.00
      nail 681.02
  thyroglossal duct 529.8
  toe (skin) 686.9
      abscess (with lymphangitis) 681.10
      cellulitis (with lymphangitis)
          681.10
      nail 681.11
          fungus 110.1
  tongue NEC 529.0
      parasitic 112.0
  tonsil (faucial) (lingual) (pharyngeal)
      474.00
      acute or subacute 463
      and adenoid 474.02
      tag 474.00
  tooth, teeth 522.4
      periapical (pulpal origin) 522.4
      peridental 523.3
      periodontal 523.3
      pulp 522.0
      socket 526.5
  Torula histolytica 117.5
  Toxocara (cani) (cati) (felis) 128.0
  Toxoplasma gondii (*see also* Toxoplas-
      mosis) 130.9

◀ **New**   ◀▦ **Revised**

Infection, infected, infective (Continued)
  trachea, chronic 491.8
    fungus 117.9
  traumatic NEC 958.3
  trematode NEC 121.9
  trench fever 083.1
  Treponema
    denticola 041.84
    macrodenticum 041.84
    pallidum (see also Syphilis) 097.9
  Trichinella (spiralis) 124
  Trichomonas 131.9
    bladder 131.09
    cervix 131.09
    hominis 007.3
    intestine 007.3
    prostate 131.03
    specified site NEC 131.8
    urethra 131.02
    urogenitalis 131.00
    vagina 131.01
    vulva 131.01
  Trichophyton, trichophytid - see Dermatophytosis
  Trichosporon (beigelii) cutaneum 111.2
  Trichostrongylus 127.6
  Trichuris (trichuria) 127.3
  Trombicula (irritans) 133.8
  Trypanosoma (see also Trypanosomiasis) 086.9
    cruzi 086.2
  tubal (see also Salpingo-oophoritis) 614.2
  tuberculous NEC (see also Tuberculosis) 011.9
  tubo-ovarian (see also Salpingo-oophoritis) 614.2
  tunica vaginalis 608.4
  tympanic membrane - see Myringitis
  typhoid (abortive) (ambulant) (bacillus) 002.0
  typhus 081.9
    flea-borne (endemic) 081.0
    louse-borne (epidemic) 080
    mite-borne 081.2
    recrudescent 081.1
    tick-borne 082.9
      African 082.1
      North Asian 082.2
  umbilicus (septic) 686.9
    newborn NEC 771.4
  ureter 593.89
  urethra (see also Urethritis) 597.80
  urinary (tract) NEC 599.0
    with
      abortion - see Abortion, by type, with urinary tract infection
      ectopic pregnancy (see also categories 633.0-633.9) 639.8
      molar pregnancy (see also categories 630-632) 639.8
    candidal 112.2
    complicating pregnancy, childbirth, or puerperium 646.6
      affecting fetus or newborn 760.1
      asymptomatic 646.5
        affecting fetus or newborn 760.1
    diplococcal (acute) 098.0
      chronic 098.2
    due to Trichomonas (vaginalis) 131.00
    following
      abortion 639.8
      ectopic or molar pregnancy 639.8

Infection, infected, infective (Continued)
  urinary (tract) NEC (Continued)
    gonococcal (acute) 098.0
      chronic or duration of 2 months or over 098.2
    newborn 771.82
    trichomonal 131.00
    tuberculous (see also Tuberculosis) 016.3
  uterus, uterine (see also Endometritis) 615.9
  utriculus masculinus NEC 597.89
  vaccination 999.3
  vagina (granulation tissue) (wall) (see also Vaginitis) 616.10
  varicella 052.9
  varicose veins - see Varicose, veins
  variola 050.9
    major 050.0
    minor 050.1
  vas deferens NEC 608.4
  Veillonella 041.84
  verumontanum 597.89
  vesical (see also Cystitis) 595.9
  Vibrio
    cholerae 001.0
    el Tor 001.1
    parahaemolyticus (food poisoning) 005.4
    vulnificus 041.85
  Vincent's (gums) (mouth) (tonsil) 101
  virus, viral 079.99
    adenovirus
      in diseases classified elsewhere - see category 079
      unspecified nature or site 079.0
    central nervous system NEC 049.9
      enterovirus 048
        meningitis 047.9
          specified type NEC 047.8
      slow virus 046.9
        specified condition NEC 046.8
    chest 519.8
    conjunctivitis 077.99
      specified type NEC 077.89
    coronavirus 079.89
      SARS-associated 079.82
    Coxsackie (see also Infection, Coxsackie) 079.2
    Ebola 065.8
    ECHO
      in diseases classified elsewhere - see category 079
      unspecified nature or site 079.1
    encephalitis 049.9
      arthropod-borne NEC 064
      tick-borne 063.9
        specified type NEC 063.8
    enteritis NEC (see also Enteritis, viral) 008.8
    exanthem NEC 057.9
    Hantavirus 079.81
    human papilloma 079.4
    in diseases classified elsewhere - see category 079
    intestine (see also Enteritis, viral) 008.8
    lung - see Pneumonia, viral
    respiratory syncytial (RSV) 079.6
    Retrovirus 079.50
    rhinovirus
      in diseases classified elsewhere - see category 079
      unspecified nature or site 079.3
    salivary gland disease 078.5

Infection, infected, infective (Continued)
  virus, viral (Continued)
    slow 046.9
      specified condition NEC 046.8
    specified type NEC 079.89
      in diseases classified elsewhere - see category 079
    unspecified nature or site 079.99
    warts NEC 078.10
  vulva (see also Vulvitis) 616.10
  whipworm 127.3
  Whitmore's bacillus 025
  wound (local) (posttraumatic) NEC 958.3
    with
      dislocation - see Dislocation, by site, open
      fracture - see Fracture, by site, open
      open wound - see Wound, open, by site, complicated
    postoperative 998.59
    surgical 998.59
  Wuchereria 125.0
    bancrofti 125.0
    malayi 125.1
  yaws - see Yaws
  yeast (see also Candidiasis) 112.9
  yellow fever (see also Fever, yellow) 060.9
  Yersinia pestis (see also Plague) 020.9
  Zeis' gland 373.12
  zoonotic bacterial NEC 027.9
  Zopfia senegalensis 117.4
Infective, infectious - see condition
Inferiority complex 301.9
  constitutional psychopathic 301.9
Infertility
  female 628.9
    associated with
      adhesions, peritubal 614.6 [628.2]
      anomaly
        cervical mucus 628.4
        congenital
          cervix 628.4
          fallopian tube 628.2
          uterus 628.3
          vagina 628.4
      anovulation 628.0
      dysmucorrhea 628.4
      endometritis, tuberculous (see also Tuberculosis) 016.7 [628.3]
      Stein-Leventhal syndrome 256.4 [628.0]
    due to
      adiposogenital dystrophy 253.8 [628.1]
      anterior pituitary disorder NEC 253.4 [628.1]
        hyperfunction 253.1 [628.1]
      cervical anomaly 628.4
      fallopian tube anomaly 628.2
      ovarian failure 256.39 [628.0]
      Stein-Leventhal syndrome 256.4 [628.0]
      uterine anomaly 628.3
      vaginal anomaly 628.4
    nonimplantation 628.3
    origin
      cervical 628.4
      pituitary-hypothalamus NEC 253.8 [628.1]
        anterior pituitary NEC 253.4 [628.1]
          hyperfunction NEC 253.1 [628.1]
        dwarfism 253.3 [628.1]
        panhypopituitarism 253.2 [628.1]

ICD-9-CM

—

Vol. 2

◀ **New**   ◀▥ **Revised**

Infestation (Continued)
  pediculus 132.9
    capitis (humanus) (any site) 132.0
    corporis (humanus) (any site) 132.1
    eyelid 132.0 [373.6]
    mixed (classifiable to more than one
      category in 132.0-132.2) 132.3
    pubis (any site) 132.2
  phthirus (pubis) (any site) 132.2
    with any infestation classifiable to
      132.0 and 132.1 132.3
  pinworm 127.4
  pork tapeworm (adult) 123.0
  protozoal NEC 136.8
  pubic louse 132.2
  rat tapeworm 123.6
  red bug 133.8
  roundworm (large) NEC 127.0
  sand flea 134.1
  saprophytic NEC 136.8
  Sarcoptes scabiei 133.0
  scabies 133.0
  Schistosoma 120.9
    bovis 120.8
    cercariae 120.3
    hematobium 120.0
    intercalatum 120.8
    japonicum 120.2
    mansoni 120.1
    mattheii 120.8
    specified
      site - see Schistosomiasis
      type NEC 120.8
    spindale 120.8
  screw worms 134.0
  skin NEC 134.9
  Sparganum (mansoni) (proliferum)
    123.5
    larval 123.5
  specified type NEC 134.8
  Spirometra larvae 123.5
  Sporozoa NEC 136.8
  Stellantchasmus falcatus 121.6
  Strongyloides 127.2
  Strongylus (gibsoni) 127.7
  Taenia 123.3
    diminuta 123.6
    Echinococcus (see also Echinococcus)
      122.9
    mediocanellata 123.2
    nana 123.6
    saginata (mediocanellata) 123.2
    solium (intestinal form) 123.0
      larval form 123.1
  Taeniarhynchus saginatus 123.2
  tapeworm 123.9
    beef 123.2
    broad 123.4
      larval 123.5
    dog 123.8
    dwarf 123.6
    fish 123.4
      larval 123.5
    pork 123.0
    rat 123.6
  Ternidens diminutus 127.7
  Tetranychus molestissimus 133.8
  threadworm 127.4
  tongue 112.0
  Toxocara (cani) (cati) (felis) 128.0
  trematode(s) NEC 121.9
  Trichina spiralis 124
  Trichinella spiralis 124
  Trichocephalus 127.3

Infestation (Continued)
  Trichomonas 131.9
    bladder 131.09
    cervix 131.09
    intestine 007.3
    prostate 131.03
    specified site NEC 131.8
    urethra (female) (male) 131.02
    urogenital 131.00
    vagina 131.01
    vulva 131.01
  Trichophyton - see Dermatophytosis
  Trichostrongylus instabilis 127.6
  Trichuris (trichiuria) 127.3
  Trombicula (irritans) 133.8
  Trypanosoma - see Trypanosomiasis
  Tunga penetrans 134.1
  Uncinaria americana 126.1
  whipworm 127.3
  worms NEC 128.9
    intestinal 127.9
  Wuchereria 125.0
    bancrofti 125.0
    malayi 125.1
Infiltrate, infiltration
  with an iron compound 275.0
  amyloid (any site) (generalized) 277.3
  calcareous (muscle) NEC 275.49
    localized - see Degeneration, by site
  calcium salt (muscle) 275.49
  corneal (see also Edema, cornea) 371.20
  eyelid 373.9
  fatty (diffuse) (generalized) 272.8
    localized - see Degeneration, by site,
      fatty
  glycogen, glycogenic (see also Disease,
    glycogen storage) 271.0
  heart, cardiac
    fatty (see also Degeneration, myocar-
      dial) 429.1
    glycogenic 271.0 [425.7]
  inflammatory in vitreous 379.29
  kidney (see also Disease, renal) 593.9
  leukemic (M9800/3) - see Leukemia
  liver 573.8
    fatty - see Fatty, liver
    glycogen (see also Disease, glycogen
      storage) 271.0
  lung (see also Infiltrate, pulmonary)
    518.3
    eosinophilic 518.3
    x-ray finding only 793.1
  lymphatic (see also Leukemia, lym-
    phatic) 204.9
    gland, pigmentary 289.3
  muscle, fatty 728.9
  myelogenous (see also Leukemia, mye-
    loid) 205.9
  myocardium, myocardial
    fatty (see also Degeneration, myocar-
      dial) 429.1
    glycogenic 271.0 [425.7]
  pulmonary 518.3
    with
      eosinophilia 518.3
      pneumonia - see Pneumonia, by
        type
    x-ray finding only 793.1
  Ranke's primary (see also Tuberculosis)
    010.0
  skin, lymphocytic (benign) 709.8
  thymus (gland) (fatty) 254.8
  urine 788.8
  vitreous humor 379.29

Infirmity 799.89
  senile 797
Inflammation, inflamed, inflammatory
    (with exudation)
  abducens (nerve) 378.54
  accessory sinus (chronic) (see also Si-
    nusitis) 473.9
  adrenal (gland) 255.8
  alimentary canal - see Enteritis
  alveoli (teeth) 526.5
    scorbutic 267
  amnion - see Amnionitis
  anal canal 569.49
  antrum (chronic) (see also Sinusitis,
    maxillary) 473.0
  anus 569.49
  appendix (see also Appendicitis) 541
  arachnoid - see Meningitis
  areola 611.0
    puerperal, postpartum 675.0
  areolar tissue NEC 686.9
  artery - see Arteritis
  auditory meatus (external) (see also Oti-
    tis, externa) 380.10
  Bartholin's gland 616.8
  bile duct or passage 576.1
  bladder (see also Cystitis) 595.9
  bone - see Osteomyelitis
  bowel (see also Enteritis) 558.9
  brain (see also Encephalitis) 323.9
    late effect - see category 326
    membrane - see Meningitis
  breast 611.0
    puerperal, postpartum 675.2
  broad ligament (see also Disease, pelvis,
    inflammatory) 614.4
    acute 614.3
  bronchus - see Bronchitis
  bursa - see Bursitis
  capsule
    liver 573.3
    spleen 289.59
  catarrhal (see also Catarrh) 460
    vagina 616.10
  cecum (see also Appendicitis) 541
  cerebral (see also Encephalitis) 323.9
    late effect - see category 326
    membrane - see Meningitis
  cerebrospinal (see also Meningitis)
    322.9
    late effect - see category 326
    meningococcal 036.0
    tuberculous (see also Tuberculosis)
      013.6
  cervix (uteri) (see also Cervicitis) 616.0
  chest 519.9
  choroid NEC (see also Choroiditis)
    363.20
  cicatrix (tissue) - see Cicatrix
  colon (see also Enteritis) 558.9
    granulomatous 555.1
    newborn 558.9
  connective tissue (diffuse) NEC 728.9
  cornea (see also Keratitis) 370.9
    with ulcer (see also Ulcer, cornea)
      370.00
  corpora cavernosa (penis) 607.2
  cranial nerve - see Disorder, nerve, cra-
    nial
  diarrhea - see Diarrhea
  disc (intervertebral) (space) 722.90
    cervical, cervicothoracic 722.91
    lumbar, lumbosacral 722.93
    thoracic, thoracolumbar 722.92

ICD-9-CM

—

Vol. 2

Inflammation, inflamed, inflammatory
(Continued)
Douglas' cul-de-sac or pouch (chronic)
(*see also* Disease, pelvis, inflammatory) 614.4
acute 614.3
due to (presence of) any device, implant, or graft classifiable to 996.0-996.5 - *see* Complications, infection and inflammation, due to (presence of) any device, implant, or graft classified to 996.0-996.5 NEC
duodenum 535.6
dura mater - *see* Meningitis
ear - *see also* Otitis
external (*see also* Otitis, externa) 380.10
inner (*see also* Labyrinthitis) 386.30
middle - *see* Otitis media
esophagus 530.10
ethmoidal (chronic) (sinus) (*see also* Sinusitis, ethmoidal) 473.2
eustachian tube (catarrhal) 381.50
acute 381.51
chronic 381.52
extrarectal 569.49
eye 379.99
eyelid 373.9
specified NEC 373.8
fallopian tube (*see also* Salpingo-oophoritis) 614.2
fascia 728.9
fetal membranes (acute) 658.4
affecting fetus or newborn 762.7
follicular, pharynx 472.1
frontal (chronic) (sinus) (*see also* Sinusitis, frontal) 473.1
gallbladder (*see also* Cholecystitis, acute) 575.0
gall duct (*see also* Cholecystitis) 575.10
gastrointestinal (*see also* Enteritis) 558.9
genital organ (diffuse) (internal)
female 614.9
with
abortion - *see* Abortion, by type, with sepsis
ectopic pregnancy (*see also* categories 633.0-633.9) 639.0
molar pregnancy (*see also* categories 630-632) 639.0
complicating pregnancy, childbirth, or puerperium 646.6
affecting fetus or newborn 760.8
following
abortion 639.0
ectopic or molar pregnancy 639.0
male 608.4
gland (lymph) (*see also* Lymphadenitis) 289.3
glottis (*see also* Laryngitis) 464.00
with obstruction 464.01
granular, pharynx 472.1
gum 523.1
heart (*see also* Carditis) 429.89
hepatic duct 576.8
hernial sac - *see* Hernia, by site
ileum (*see also* Enteritis) 558.9
terminal or regional 555.0
with large intestine 555.2
intervertebral disc 722.90
cervical, cervicothoracic 722.91
lumbar, lumbosacral 722.93
thoracic, thoracolumbar 722.92
intestine (*see also* Enteritis) 558.9

Inflammation, inflamed, inflammatory
(Continued)
jaw (acute) (bone) (chronic) (lower) (suppurative) (upper) 526.4
jejunum - *see* Enteritis
joint NEC (*see also* Arthritis) 716.9
sacroiliac 720.2
kidney (*see also* Nephritis) 583.9
knee (joint) 716.66
tuberculous (active) (*see also* Tuberculosis) 015.2
labium (majus) (minus) (*see also* Vulvitis) 616.10
lacrimal
gland (*see also* Dacryoadenitis) 375.00
passages (duct) (sac) (*see also* Dacryocystitis) 375.30
larynx (*see also* Laryngitis) 464.00
with obstruction 464.01
diphtheritic 032.3
leg NEC 686.9
lip 528.5
liver (capsule) (*see also* Hepatitis) 573.3
acute 570
chronic 571.40
suppurative 572.0
lung (acute) (*see also* Pneumonia) 486
chronic (interstitial) 518.89
lymphatic vessel (*see also* Lymphangitis) 457.2
lymph node or gland (*see also* Lymphadenitis) 289.3
mammary gland 611.0
puerperal, postpartum 675.2
maxilla, maxillary 526.4
sinus (chronic) (*see also* Sinusitis, maxillary) 473.0
membranes of brain or spinal cord - *see* Meningitis
meninges - *see* Meningitis
mouth 528.0
muscle 728.9
myocardium (*see also* Myocarditis) 429.0
nasal sinus (chronic) (*see also* Sinusitis) 473.9
nasopharynx - *see* Nasopharyngitis
navel 686.9
newborn NEC 771.4
nerve NEC 729.2
nipple 611.0
puerperal, postpartum 675.0
nose 478.1
suppurative 472.0
oculomotor nerve 378.51
optic nerve 377.30
orbit (chronic) 376.10
acute 376.00
chronic 376.10
ovary (*see also* Salpingo-oophoritis) 614.2
oviduct (*see also* Salpingo-oophoritis) 614.2
pancreas - *see* Pancreatitis
parametrium (chronic) (*see also* Disease, pelvis, inflammatory) 614.4
acute 614.3
parotid region 686.9
gland 527.2
pelvis, female (*see also* Disease, pelvis, inflammatory) 614.9
penis (corpora cavernosa) 607.2
perianal 569.49
pericardium (*see also* Pericarditis) 423.9
perineum (female) (male) 686.9

Inflammation, inflamed, inflammatory
(Continued)
perirectal 569.49
peritoneum (*see also* Peritonitis) 567.9
periuterine (*see also* Disease, pelvis, inflammatory) 614.9
perivesical (*see also* Cystitis) 595.9
petrous bone (*see also* Petrositis) 383.20
pharynx (*see also* Pharyngitis) 462
follicular 472.1
granular 472.1
pia mater - *see* Meningitis
pleura - *see* Pleurisy
postmastoidectomy cavity 383.30
chronic 383.33
prostate (*see also* Prostatitis) 601.9
rectosigmoid - *see* Rectosigmoiditis
rectum (*see also* Proctitis) 569.49
respiratory, upper (*see also* Infection, respiratory, upper) 465.9
chronic, due to external agent - *see* Condition, respiratory, chronic, due to, external agent
due to
fumes or vapors (chemical) (inhalation) 506.2
radiation 508.1
retina (*see also* Retinitis) 363.20
retrocecal (*see also* Appendicitis) 541
retroperitoneal (*see also* Peritonitis) 567.9
salivary duct or gland (any) (suppurative) 527.2
scorbutic, alveoli, teeth 267
scrotum 608.4
sigmoid - *see* Enteritis
sinus (*see also* Sinusitis) 473.9
Skene's duct or gland (*see also* Urethritis) 597.89
skin 686.9
spermatic cord 608.4
sphenoidal (sinus) (*see also* Sinusitis, sphenoidal) 473.3
spinal
cord (*see also* Encephalitis) 323.9
late effect - *see* category 326
membrane - *see* Meningitis
nerve - *see* Disorder, nerve
spine (*see also* Spondylitis) 720.9
spleen (capsule) 289.59
stomach - *see* Gastritis
stricture, rectum 569.49
subcutaneous tissue NEC 686.9
suprarenal (gland) 255.8
synovial (fringe) (membrane) - *see* Bursitis
tendon (sheath) NEC 726.90
testis (*see also* Orchitis) 604.90
thigh 686.9
throat (*see also* Sore throat) 462
thymus (gland) 254.8
thyroid (gland) (*see also* Thyroiditis) 245.9
tongue 529.0
tonsil - *see* Tonsillitis
trachea - *see* Tracheitis
trochlear nerve 378.53
tubal (*see also* Salpingo-oophoritis) 614.2
tuberculous NEC (*see also* Tuberculosis) 011.9
tubo-ovarian (*see also* Salpingo-oophoritis) 614.2
tunica vaginalis 608.4

Inflammation, inflamed, inflammatory
(*Continued*)
tympanic membrane - *see* Myringitis
umbilicus, umbilical 686.9
newborn NEC 771.4
uterine ligament (*see also* Disease, pelvis, inflammatory) 614.4
acute 614.3
uterus (catarrhal) (*see also* Endometritis) 615.9
uveal tract (anterior) (*see also* Iridocyclitis) 364.3
posterior - *see* Chorioretinitis
sympathetic 360.11
vagina (*see also* Vaginitis) 616.10
vas deferens 608.4
vein (*see also* Phlebitis) 451.9
thrombotic 451.9
cerebral (*see also* Thrombosis, brain) 434.0
leg 451.2
deep (vessels) NEC 451.19
superficial (vessels) 451.0
lower extremity 451.2
deep (vessels) NEC 451.19
superficial (vessels) 451.0
vocal cord 478.5
vulva (*see also* Vulvitis) 616.10
Inflation, lung imperfect (newborn) 770.5
Influenza, influenzal 487.1
with
bronchitis 487.1
bronchopneumonia 487.0
cold (any type) 487.1
digestive manifestations 487.8
hemoptysis 487.1
involvement of
gastrointestinal tract 487.8
nervous system 487.8
laryngitis 487.1
manifestations NEC 487.8
respiratory 487.1
pneumonia 487.0
pharyngitis 487.1
pneumonia (any form classifiable to 480-483, 485-486) 487.0
respiratory manifestations NEC 487.1
sinusitis 487.1
sore throat 487.1
tonsillitis 487.1
tracheitis 487.1
upper respiratory infection (acute) 487.1
abdominal 487.8
Asian 487.1
bronchial 487.1
bronchopneumonia 487.0
catarrhal 487.1
epidemic 487.1
gastric 487.8
intestinal 487.8
laryngitis 487.1
maternal affecting fetus or newborn 760.2
manifest influenza in infant 771.2
pharyngitis 487.1
pneumonia (any form) 487.0
respiratory (upper) 487.1
stomach 487.8
vaccination, prophylactic (against) V04.81
Influenza-like disease 487.1

Infraction, Freiberg's (metatarsal head) 732.5
Infraeruption, teeth 524.34 ◀
Infusion complication, misadventure, or reaction - *see* Complication, infusion
Ingestion
chemical - *see* Table of Drugs and Chemicals
drug or medicinal substance
overdose or wrong substance given or taken 977.9
specified drug - *see* Table of Drugs and Chemicals
foreign body NEC (*see also* Foreign body) 938
Ingrowing
hair 704.8
nail (finger) (toe) (infected) 703.0
Inguinal - *see also* condition
testis 752.51
Inhalation
carbon monoxide 986
flame
mouth 947.0
lung 947.1
food or foreign body (*see also* Asphyxia, food or foreign body) 933.1
gas, fumes, or vapor (noxious) 987.9
specified agent - *see* Table of Drugs and Chemicals
liquid or vomitus (*see also* Asphyxia, food or foreign body) 933.1
lower respiratory tract NEC 934.9
meconium (fetus or newborn) 770.1
mucus (*see also* Asphyxia, mucus) 933.1
oil (causing suffocation) (*see also* Asphyxia, food or foreign body) 933.1
pneumonia - *see* Pneumonia, aspiration
smoke 987.9
steam 987.9
stomach contents or secretions (*see also* Asphyxia, food or foreign body) 933.1
in labor and delivery 668.0
Inhibition, inhibited
academic as adjustment reaction 309.23
orgasm
female 302.73
male 302.74
sexual
desire 302.71
excitement 302.72
work as adjustment reaction 309.23
Inhibitor, systemic lupus erythematosus (presence of) 286.5
Iniencephalus, iniencephaly 740.2
Injected eye 372.74
Injury 959.9

Note   For abrasion, insect bite (nonvenomous), blister, or scratch, *see* Injury, superficial.

For laceration, traumatic rupture, tear, or penetrating wound of internal organs, such as heart, lung, liver, kidney, pelvic organs, whether or not accompanied by open wound in the same region, *see* Injury, internal.

For nerve injury, *see* Injury, nerve.

For late effect of injuries classifiable to 850-854, 860-869, 900-919, 950-959, *see* Late, effect, injury, by type.

Injury (*Continued*)
abdomen, abdominal (viscera) - *see also* Injury, internal, abdomen
muscle or wall 959.12
acoustic, resulting in deafness 951.5
adenoid 959.09
adrenal (gland) - *see* Injury, internal, adrenal
alveolar (process) 959.09
ankle (and foot) (and knee) (and leg, except thigh) 959.7
anterior chamber, eye 921.3
anus 959.19
aorta (thoracic) 901.0
abdominal 902.0
appendix - *see* Injury, internal, appendix
arm, upper (and shoulder) 959.2
artery (complicating trauma) (*see also* Injury, blood vessel, by site) 904.9
cerebral or meningeal (*see also* Hemorrhage, brain, traumatic, subarachnoid) 852.0
auditory canal (external) (meatus) 959.09
auricle, auris, ear 959.09
axilla 959.2
back 959.19
bile duct - *see* Injury, internal, bile duct
birth - *see also* Birth, injury
canal NEC, complicating delivery 665.9
bladder (sphincter) - *see* Injury, internal, bladder
blast (air) (hydraulic) (immersion) (underwater) NEC 869.0
with open wound into cavity NEC 869.1
abdomen or thorax - *see* Injury, internal, by site
brain - *see* Concussion, brain
ear (acoustic nerve trauma) 951.5
with perforation of tympanic membrane - *see* Wound, open, ear, drum
blood vessel NEC 904.9
abdomen 902.9
multiple 902.87
specified NEC 902.89
aorta (thoracic) 901.0
abdominal 902.0
arm NEC 903.9
axillary 903.00
artery 903.1
vein 903.02
azygos vein 901.89
basilic vein 903.1
brachial (artery) (vein) 903.1
bronchial 901.89
carotid artery 900.00
common 900.01
external 900.02
internal 900.03
celiac artery 902.20
specified branch NEC 902.24
cephalic vein (arm) 903.1
colica dextra 902.26
cystic
artery 902.24
vein 902.39
deep plantar 904.6
digital (artery) (vein) 903.5
due to accidental puncture or laceration during procedure 998.2

ICD-9-CM
—
Vol. 2

Injury (*Continued*)
  blood vessel NEC (*Continued*)
    extremity
      lower 904.8
        multiple 904.7
        specified NEC 904.7
      upper 903.9
        multiple 903.8
        specified NEC 903.8
    femoral
      artery (superficial) 904.1
        above profunda origin 904.0
        common 904.0
      vein 904.2
    gastric
      artery 902.21
      vein 902.39
    head 900.9
      intracranial - *see* Injury, intracranial
      multiple 900.82
      specified NEC 900.89
    hemiazygos vein 901.89
    hepatic
      artery 902.22
      vein 902.11
    hypogastric 902.59
      artery 902.51
      vein 902.52
    ileocolic
      artery 902.26
      vein 902.31
    iliac 902.50
      artery 902.53
      specified branch NEC 902.59
      vein 902.54
    innominate
      artery 901.1
      vein 901.3
    intercostal (artery) (vein) 901.81
    jugular vein (external) 900.81
      internal 900.1
    leg NEC 904.8
    mammary (artery) (vein) 901.82
    mesenteric
      artery 902.20
        inferior 902.27
        specified branch NEC 902.29
        superior (trunk) 902.25
          branches, primary 902.26
      vein 902.39
        inferior 902.32
        superior (and primary subdivisions) 902.31
    neck 900.9
      multiple 900.82
      specified NEC 900.89
    ovarian 902.89
      artery 902.81
      vein 902.82
    palmar artery 903.4
    pelvis 902.9
      multiple 902.87
      specified NEC 902.89
    plantar (deep) (artery) (vein) 904.6
    popliteal 904.40
      artery 904.41
      vein 904.42
    portal 902.33
    pulmonary 901.40
      artery 901.41
      vein 901.42
    radial (artery) (vein) 903.2
    renal 902.40

Injury (*Continued*)
  blood vessel NEC (*Continued*)
    renal (*Continued*)
      artery 902.41
      specified NEC 902.49
      vein 902.42
    saphenous
      artery 904.7
      vein (greater) (lesser) 904.3
    splenic
      artery 902.23
      vein 902.34
    subclavian
      artery 901.1
      vein 901.3
    suprarenal 902.49
    thoracic 901.9
      multiple 901.83
      specified NEC 901.89
    tibial 904.50
      artery 904.50
        anterior 904.51
        posterior 904.53
      vein 904.50
        anterior 904.52
        posterior 904.54
    ulnar (artery) (vein) 903.3
    uterine 902.59
      artery 902.55
      vein 902.56
    vena cava
      inferior 902.10
        specified branches NEC 902.19
      superior 901.2
  brachial plexus 953.4
    newborn 767.6
  brain NEC (*see also* Injury, intracranial) 854.0
  breast 959.19
  broad ligament - *see* Injury, internal, broad ligament
  bronchus, bronchi - *see* Injury, internal, bronchus
  brow 959.09
  buttock 959.19
  canthus, eye 921.1
  cathode ray 990
  cauda equina 952.4
    with fracture, vertebra - *see* Fracture, vertebra, sacrum
  cavernous sinus (*see also* Injury, intracranial) 854.0
  cecum - *see* Injury, internal, cecum
  celiac ganglion or plexus 954.1
  cerebellum (*see also* Injury, intracranial) 854.0
  cervix (uteri) - *see* Injury, internal, cervix
  cheek 959.09
  chest - *see* Injury, internal, chest
    wall 959.11
  childbirth - *see also* Birth, injury
    maternal NEC 665.9
  chin 959.09
  choroid (eye) 921.3
  clitoris 959.14
  coccyx 959.19
    complicating delivery 665.6
  colon - *see* Injury, internal, colon
  common duct - *see* Injury, internal, common duct
  conjunctiva 921.1
    superficial 918.2

Injury (*Continued*)
  cord
    spermatic - *see* Injury, internal, spermatic cord
    spinal - *see* Injury, spinal, by site
  cornea 921.3
    abrasion 918.1
      due to contact lens 371.82
    penetrating - *see* Injury, eyeball, penetrating
    superficial 918.1
      due to contact lens 371.82
  cortex (cerebral) (*see also* Injury, intracranial) 854.0
    visual 950.3
  costal region 959.11
  costochondral 959.11
  cranial
    bones - *see* Fracture, skull, by site
    cavity (*see also* Injury, intracranial) 854.0
    nerve - *see* Injury, nerve, cranial
  crushing - *see* Crush
  cutaneous sensory nerve
    lower limb 956.4
    upper limb 955.5
  delivery - *see also* Birth, injury
    maternal NEC 665.9
  Descemet's membrane - *see* Injury, eyeball, penetrating
  diaphragm - *see* Injury, internal, diaphragm
  duodenum - *see* Injury, internal, duodenum
  ear (auricle) (canal) (drum) (external) 959.09
  elbow (and forearm) (and wrist) 959.3
  epididymis 959.14
  epigastric region 959.12
  epiglottis 959.09
  epiphyseal, current - *see* Fracture, by site
  esophagus - *see* Injury, internal, esophagus
  eustachian tube 959.09
  extremity (lower) (upper) NEC 959.8
  eye 921.9
    penetrating eyeball - *see* Injury, eyeball, penetrating
    superficial 918.9
  eyeball 921.3
    penetrating 871.7
      with
        partial loss (of intraocular tissue) 871.2
        prolapse or exposure (of intraocular tissue) 871.1
      without prolapse 871.0
      foreign body (nonmagnetic) 871.6
        magnetic 871.5
    superficial 918.9
  eyebrow 959.09
  eyelid(s) 921.1
    laceration - *see* Laceration, eyelid
    superficial 918.0
  face (and neck) 959.09
  fallopian tube - *see* Injury, internal, fallopian tube
  fingers(s) (nail) 959.5
  flank 959.19
  foot (and ankle) (and knee) (and leg, except thigh) 959.7
  forceps NEC 767.9
    scalp 767.19
  forearm (and elbow) (and wrist) 959.3

◀ **New**   ◀▥ **Revised**

Injury (Continued)
  forehead 959.09
  gallbladder - see Injury, internal, gall-
      bladder
  gasserian ganglion 951.2
  gastrointestinal tract - see Injury, inter-
      nal, gastrointestinal tract
  genital organ(s)
      with
          abortion - see Abortion, by type,
              with, damage to pelvic organs
          ectopic pregnancy (see also catego-
              ries 633.0-633.9) 639.2
          molar pregnancy (see also catego-
              ries 630-632) 639.2
      external 959.14
      fracture of corpus cavernosum penis
          959.13
      following
          abortion 639.2
          ectopic or molar pregnancy 639.2
      internal - see Injury, internal, genital
          organs
      obstetrical trauma NEC 665.9
          affecting fetus or newborn 763.89
  gland
      lacrimal 921.1
          laceration 870.8
      parathyroid 959.09
      salivary 959.09
      thyroid 959.09
  globe (eye) (see also Injury, eyeball) 921.3
  grease gun - see Wound, open, by site,
      complicated
  groin 959.19
  gum 959.09
  hand(s) (except fingers) 959.4
  head NEC 959.01
      with
          loss of consciousness 850.5
          skull fracture - see Fracture, skull,
              by site
  heart - see Injury, internal, heart
  heel 959.7
  hip (and thigh) 959.6
  hymen 959.14
  hyperextension (cervical) (vertebra)
      847.0
  ileum - see Injury, internal, ileum
  iliac region 959.19
  infrared rays NEC 990
  instrumental (during surgery) 998.2
      birth injury - see Birth, injury
      nonsurgical (see also Injury, by site)
          959.9
      obstetrical 665.9
          affecting fetus or newborn 763.89
          bladder 665.5
          cervix 665.3
          high vaginal 665.4
          perineal NEC 664.9
          urethra 665.5
          uterus 665.5
  internal 869.0

Note For injury of internal organ(s)
by foreign body entering through a
natural orifice (e.g., inhaled, ingested,
or swallowed)-see Foreign body, entering through orifice.

For internal injury of any of the following sites with internal injury of
any other of the sites-see Injury, internal, multiple.

Injury (Continued)
  internal (Continued)
      with
          fracture
              pelvis - see Fracture, pelvis
              specified site, except pelvis - see
                  Injury, internal, by site
          open wound into cavity 869.1
      abdomen, abdominal (viscera) NEC
          868.00
          with
              fracture, pelvis - see Fracture,
                  pelvis
              open wound into cavity 868.10
          specified site NEC 868.09
              with open wound into cavity
                  868.19
      adrenal (gland) 868.01
          with open wound into cavity
              868.11
      aorta (thoracic) 901.0
          abdominal 902.0
      appendix 863.85
          with open wound into cavity
              863.95
      bile duct 868.02
          with open wound into cavity
              868.12
      bladder (sphincter) 867.0
          with
              abortion - see Abortion, by type,
                  with, damage to pelvic or-
                  gans
              ectopic pregnancy (see also cate-
                  gories 633.0-633.9) 639.2
              molar pregnancy (see also cate-
                  gories 630-632) 639.2
              open wound into cavity 867.1
          following
              abortion 639.2
              ectopic or molar pregnancy
                  639.2
          obstetrical trauma 665.5
              affecting fetus or newborn
                  763.89
      blood vessel - see Injury, blood ves-
          sel, by site
      broad ligament 867.6
          with open wound into cavity
              867.7
      bronchus, bronchi 862.21
          with open wound into cavity
              862.31
      cecum 863.89
          with open wound into cavity
              863.99
      cervix (uteri) 867.4
          with
              abortion - see Abortion, by type,
                  with damage to pelvic or-
                  gans
              ectopic pregnancy (see also cate-
                  gories 633.0-633.9) 639.2
              molar pregnancy (see also cate-
                  gories 630-632) 639.2
              open wound into cavity 867.5
          following
              abortion 639.2
              ectopic or molar pregnancy 639.2
          obstetrical trauma 665.3
              affecting fetus or newborn
                  763.89
      chest (see also Injury, internal, in-
          trathoracic organs) 862.8

Injury (Continued)
  internal (Continued)
      chest (Continued)
          with open wound into cavity
              862.9
      colon 863.40
          with
              open wound into cavity 863.50
              rectum 863.46
                  with open wound into cavity
                      863.56
          ascending (right) 863.41
              with open wound into cavity
                  863.51
          descending (left) 863.43
              with open wound into cavity
                  863.53
          multiple sites 863.46
              with open wound into cavity
                  863.56
          sigmoid 863.44
              with open wound into cavity
                  863.54
          specified site NEC 863.49
              with open wound into cavity
                  863.59
          transverse 863.42
              with open wound into cavity
                  863.52
      common duct 868.02
          with open wound into cavity
              868.12
      complicating delivery 665.9
          affecting fetus or newborn
              763.89
      diaphragm 862.0
          with open wound into cavity
              862.1
      duodenum 863.21
          with open wound into cavity
              863.31
      esophagus (intrathoracic) 862.22
          with open wound into cavity
              862.32
          cervical region 874.4
          complicated 874.5
      fallopian tube 867.6
          with open wound into cavity
              867.7
      gallbladder 868.02
          with open wound into cavity
              868.12
      gastrointestinal tract NEC 863.80
          with open wound into cavity
              863.90
      genital organ NEC 867.6
          with open wound into cavity
              867.7
      heart 861.00
          with open wound into thorax
              861.10
      ileum 863.29
          with open wound into cavity
              863.39
      intestine NEC 863.89
          with open wound into cavity
              863.99
          large NEC 863.40
              with open wound into cavity
                  863.50
          small NEC 863.20
              with open wound into cavity
                  863.30
      intra-abdominal (organ) 868.00

ICD-9-CM

—

Vol. 2

Injury *(Continued)*
  internal *(Continued)*
    intra-abdominal *(Continued)*
      with open wound into cavity 868.10
      multiple sites 868.09
        with open wound into cavity 868.19
      specified site NEC 868.09
        with open wound into cavity 868.19
    intrathoracic organs (multiple) 862.8
      with open wound into cavity 862.9
      diaphragm (only) - *see* Injury, internal, diaphragm
      heart (only) - *see* Injury, internal, heart
      lung (only) - *see* Injury, internal, lung
      specified site NEC 862.29
        with open wound into cavity 862.39
    intrauterine *(see also* Injury, internal, uterus) 867.4
      with open wound into cavity 867.5
    jejunum 863.29
      with open wound into cavity 863.39
    kidney (subcapsular) 866.00
      with
        disruption of parenchyma (complete) 866.03
          with open wound into cavity 866.13
        hematoma (without rupture of capsule) 866.01
          with open wound into cavity 866.11
        laceration 866.02
          with open wound into cavity 866.12
      open wound into cavity 866.10
    liver 864.00
      with
        contusion 864.01
          with open wound into cavity 864.11
        hematoma 864.01
          with open wound into cavity 864.11
        laceration 864.05
          with open wound into cavity 864.15
        major (disruption of hepatic parenchyma) 864.04
          with open wound into cavity 864.14
        minor (capsule only) 864.02
          with open wound into cavity 864.12
        moderate (involving parenchyma) 864.03
          with open wound into cavity 864.13
        multiple 864.04
        stellate 864.04
          with open wound into cavity 864.14
      open wound into cavity 864.10
    lung 861.20
      with open wound into thorax 861.30

Injury *(Continued)*
  internal *(Continued)*
    lung *(Continued)*
      hemopneumothorax - *see* Hemopneumothorax, traumatic
      hemothorax - *see* Hemothorax, traumatic
      pneumohemothorax - *see* Pneumohemothorax, traumatic
      pneumothorax - *see* Pneumothorax, traumatic
    mediastinum 862.29
      with open wound into cavity 862.39
    mesentery 863.89
      with open wound into cavity 863.99
    mesosalpinx 867.6
      with open wound into cavity 867.7
    multiple 869.0

> Note Multiple internal injuries of sites classifiable to the same three- or four-digit category should be classified to that category.
>
> Multiple injuries classifiable to different fourth-digit subdivisions of 861.- (heart and lung injuries) should be dealt with according to coding rules.

      internal 869.0
        with open wound into cavity 869.1
      intra-abdominal organ (sites classifiable to 863-868)
        with
          intrathoracic organ(s) (sites classifiable to 861-862) 869.0
            with open wound into cavity 869.1
          other intra-abdominal organ(s) (sites classifiable to 863-868, except where classifiable to the same three-digit category) 868.09
            with open wound into cavity 868.19
      intrathoracic organ (sites classifiable to 861-862)
        with
          intra-abdominal organ(s) (sites classifiable to 863-868) 869.0
            with open wound into cavity 869.1
          other intrathoracic organs(s) (sites classifiable to 861-862, except where classifiable to the same three-digit category) 862.8
        with open wound into cavity 862.9
    myocardium - *see* Injury, internal, heart
    ovary 867.6
      with open wound into cavity 867.7
    pancreas (multiple sites) 863.84
      with open wound into cavity 863.94
      body 863.82
        with open wound into cavity 863.92

Injury *(Continued)*
  internal *(Continued)*
    pancreas *(Continued)*
      head 863.81
        with open wound into cavity 863.91
      tail 863.83
        with open wound into cavity 863.93
    pelvis, pelvic (organs) (viscera) 867.8
      with
        fracture, pelvis - *see* Fracture, pelvis
        open wound into cavity 867.9
      specified site NEC 867.6
        with open wound into cavity 867.7
    peritoneum 868.03
      with open wound into cavity 868.13
    pleura 862.29
      with open wound into cavity 862.39
    prostate 867.6
      with open wound into cavity 867.7
    rectum 863.45
      with
        colon 863.46
          with open wound into cavity 863.56
        open wound into cavity 863.55
    retroperitoneum 868.04
      with open wound into cavity 868.14
    round ligament 867.6
      with open wound into cavity 867.7
    seminal vesicle 867.6
      with open wound into cavity 867.7
    spermatic cord 867.6
      with open wound into cavity 867.7
    scrotal - *see* Wound, open, spermatic cord
    spleen 865.00
      with
        disruption of parenchyma (massive) 865.04
          with open wound into cavity 865.14
        hematoma (without rupture of capsule) 865.01
          with open wound into cavity 865.11
        open wound into cavity 865.10
        tear, capsular 865.02
          with open wound into cavity 865.12
          extending into parenchyma 865.03
            with open wound into cavity 865.13
    stomach 863.0
      with open wound into cavity 863.1
    suprarenal gland (multiple) 868.01
      with open wound into cavity 868.11
    thorax, thoracic (cavity) (organs) (multiple) *(see also* Injury, internal, intrathoracic organs) 862.8
      with open wound into cavity 862.9

◄ **New**   ◄▪▪ **Revised**

Injury (*Continued*)
  internal (*Continued*)
    thymus (gland) 862.29
      with open wound into cavity
        862.39
    trachea (intrathoracic) 862.29
      with open wound into cavity
        862.39
      cervical region (*see also* Wound,
        open, trachea) 874.02
    ureter 867.2
      with open wound into cavity 867.3
    urethra (sphincter) 867.0
      with
        abortion - *see* Abortion, by type,
          with, damage to pelvic or-
          gans
        ectopic pregnancy (*see also* cate-
          gories 633.0-633.9) 639.2
        molar pregnancy (*see also* cate-
          gories 630-632) 639.2
        open wound into cavity 867.1
      following
        abortion 639.2
        ectopic or molar pregnancy 639.2
      obstetrical trauma 665.5
        affecting fetus or newborn
          763.89
    uterus 867.4
      with
        abortion - *see* Abortion, by type,
          with, damage to pelvic or-
          gans
        ectopic pregnancy (*see also* cate-
          gories 633.0-633.9) 639.2
        molar pregnancy (*see also* cate-
          gories 630-632) 639.2
        open wound into cavity 867.5
      following
        abortion 639.2
        ectopic or molar pregnancy
          639.2
      obstetrical trauma NEC 665.5
        affecting fetus or newborn -
          763.89
    vas deferens 867.6
      with open wound into cavity 867.7
    vesical (sphincter) 867.0
      with open wound into cavity 867.1
    viscera (abdominal) (*see also* Injury,
      internal, multiple) 868.00
      with
        fracture, pelvis - *see* Fracture,
          pelvis
        open wound into cavity 868.10
      thoracic NEC (*see also* Injury, inter-
        nal, intrathoracic organs) 862.8
        with open wound into cavity
          862.9
  interscapular region 959.19
  intervertebral disc 959.19
  intestine - *see* Injury, internal, intestine
  intra-abdominal (organs) NEC - *see* In-
    jury, internal, intra-abdominal
  intracranial 854.0

Note   Use the following fifth-digit
subclassification with categories 851-
854:

  0   unspecified state of conscious-
       ness
  1   with no loss of consciousness
  2   with brief [less than one hour]
       loss of consciousness

Injury (*Continued*)
  intracranial (*Continued*)
    3   with moderate [1-24 hours]
         loss of consciousness
    4   with prolonged [more than 24
         hours] loss of consciousness
         and return to pre-existing con-
         scious level
    5   with prolonged [more than 24
         hours] loss of consciousness,
         without return to pre-existing
         conscious level

Use fifth-digit 5 to designate when a
patient is unconscious and dies before regaining consciousness, regardless of the duration of the loss of consciousness

    6   with loss of consciousness of
         unspecified duration
    9   with concussion, unspecified

    with
      open intracranial wound 854.1
      skull fracture - *see* Fracture, skull,
        by site
    contusion 851.8
      with open intracranial wound 851.9
      brain stem 851.4
        with open intracranial wound
          851.5
      cerebellum 851.4
        with open intracranial wound
          851.5
      cortex (cerebral) 851.0
        with open intracranial wound
          851.2
    hematoma - *see* Injury, intracra-
      nial, hemorrhage
    hemorrhage 853.0
      with
        laceration - *see* Injury, intra-
          cranial, laceration
        open intracranial wound 853.1
      extradural 852.4
        with open intracranial wound
          852.5
      subarachnoid 852.0
        with open intracranial wound
          852.1
      subdural 852.2
        with open intracranial wound
          852.3
    laceration 851.8
      with open intracranial wound
        851.9
      brain stem 851.6
        with open intracranial wound
          851.7
      cerebellum 851.6
        with open intracranial wound
          851.7
      cortex (cerebral) 851.2
        with open intracranial wound
          851.3
    intraocular - *see* Injury, eyeball, pene-
      trating
    intrathoracic organs (multiple) - *see* In-
      jury, internal, intrathoracic organs
    intrauterine - *see* Injury, internal, intra-
      uterine
    iris 921.3
      penetrating - *see* Injury, eyeball,
        penetrating

Injury (*Continued*)
  jaw 959.09
  jejunum - *see* Injury, internal, jejunum
  joint NEC 959.9
    old or residual 718.80
      ankle 718.87
      elbow 718.82
      foot 718.87
      hand 718.84
      hip 718.85
      knee 718.86
      multiple sites 718.89
      pelvic region 718.85
      shoulder (region) 718.81
      specified site NEC 718.88
      wrist 718.83
  kidney - *see* Injury, internal, kidney
  knee (and ankle) (and foot) (and leg,
    except thigh) 959.7
  labium (majus) (minus) 959.14
  labyrinth, ear 959.09
  lacrimal apparatus, gland, or sac 921.1
    laceration 870.8
  larynx 959.09
  late effect - *see* Late, effects (of), injury
  leg, except thigh (and ankle) (and foot)
    (and knee) 959.7
    upper or thigh 959.6
  lens, eye 921.3
    penetrating - *see* Injury, eyeball, pen-
      etrating
  lid, eye - *see* Injury, eyelid
  lip 959.09
  liver - *see* Injury, internal, liver
  lobe, parietal - *see* Injury, intracranial
  lumbar (region) 959.19
    plexus 953.5
  lumbosacral (region) 959.19
    plexus 953.5
  lung - *see* Injury, internal, lung
  malar region 959.09
  mastoid region 959.09
  maternal, during pregnancy, affecting
    fetus or newborn 760.5
  maxilla 959.09
  mediastinum - *see* Injury, internal, me-
    diastinum
  membrane
    brain (*see also* Injury, intracranial)
      854.0
    tympanic 959.09
  meningeal artery - *see* Hemorrhage,
    brain, traumatic, subarachnoid
  meninges (cerebral) - *see* Injury, intra-
    cranial
  mesenteric
    artery - *see* Injury, blood vessel, mes-
      enteric, artery
    plexus, inferior 954.1
    vein - *see* Injury, blood vessel, mes-
      enteric, vein
  mesentery - *see* Injury, internal, mesen-
    tery
  mesosalpinx - *see* Injury, internal, me-
    sosalpinx
  middle ear 959.09
  midthoracic region 959.11
  mouth 959.09
  multiple (sites not classifiable to the
    same four-digit category in 959.0-
    959.7) 959.8
    internal 869.0
      with open wound into cavity 869.1
  musculocutaneous nerve 955.4

ICD-9-CM

—

Vol. 2

Injury *(Continued)*
  nail
    finger 959.5
    toe 959.7
  nasal (septum) (sinus) 959.09
  nasopharynx 959.09
  neck (and face) 959.09
  nerve 957.9
    abducens 951.3
    abducent 951.3
    accessory 951.6
    acoustic 951.5
    ankle and foot 956.9
    anterior crural, femoral 956.1
    arm (*see also* Injury, nerve, upper
      limb) 955.9
    auditory 951.5
    axillary 955.0
    brachial plexus 953.4
    cervical sympathetic 954.0
    cranial 951.9
      first or olfactory 951.8
      second or optic 950.0
      third or oculomotor 951.0
      fourth or trochlear 951.1
      fifth or trigeminal 951.2
      sixth or abducens 951.3
      seventh or facial 951.4
      eighth, acoustic, or auditory 951.5
      ninth or glossopharyngeal 951.8
      tenth, pneumogastric, or vagus
        951.8
      eleventh or accessory 951.6
      twelfth or hypoglossal 951.7
      newborn 767.7
    cutaneous sensory
      lower limb 956.4
      upper limb 955.5
    digital (finger) 955.6
      toe 956.5
    facial 951.4
      newborn 767.5
    femoral 956.1
    finger 955.9
    foot and ankle 956.9
    forearm 955.9
    glossopharyngeal 951.8
    hand and wrist 955.9
    head and neck, superficial 957.0
    hypoglossal 951.7
    involving several parts of body 957.8
    leg (*see also* Injury, nerve, lower
      limb) 956.9
    lower limb 956.9
      multiple 956.8
      specified site NEC 956.5
    lumbar plexus 953.5
    lumbosacral plexus 953.5
    median 955.1
      forearm 955.1
      wrist and hand 955.1
    multiple (in several parts of body)
        (sites not classifiable to the same
        three-digit category) 957.8
    musculocutaneous 955.4
    musculospiral 955.3
      upper arm 955.3
    oculomotor 951.0
    olfactory 951.8
    optic 950.0
    pelvic girdle 956.9
      multiple sites 956.8
      specified site NEC 956.5
    peripheral 957.9

Injury *(Continued)*
  nerve *(Continued)*
    peripheral *(Continued)*
      multiple (in several regions) (sites
        not classifiable to the same
        three-digit category) 957.8
      specified site NEC 957.1
    peroneal 956.3
      ankle and foot 956.3
      lower leg 956.3
    plantar 956.5
    plexus 957.9
      celiac 954.1
      mesenteric, inferior 954.1
      spinal 953.9
        brachial 953.4
        lumbosacral 953.5
        multiple sites 953.8
      sympathetic NEC 954.1
    pneumogastric 951.8
    radial 955.3
      wrist and hand 955.3
    sacral plexus 953.5
    sciatic 956.0
      thigh 956.0
    shoulder girdle 955.9
      multiple 955.8
      specified site NEC 955.7
    specified site NEC 957.1
    spinal 953.9
      plexus - *see* Injury, nerve, plexus,
        spinal
      root 953.9
        cervical 953.0
        dorsal 953.1
        lumbar 953.2
        multiple sites 953.8
        sacral 953.3
      splanchnic 954.1
      sympathetic NEC 954.1
        cervical 954.0
    thigh 956.9
    tibial 956.5
      ankle and foot 956.2
      lower leg 956.5
      posterior 956.2
    toe 956.9
    trigeminal 951.2
    trochlear 951.1
    trunk, excluding shoulder and pelvic
        girdles 954.9
      specified site NEC 954.8
      sympathetic NEC 954.1
    ulnar 955.2
      forearm 955.2
      wrist (and hand) 955.2
    upper limb 955.9
      multiple 955.8
      specified site NEC 955.7
    vagus 951.8
    wrist and hand 955.9
  nervous system, diffuse 957.8
  nose (septum) 959.09
  obstetrical NEC 665.9
    affecting fetus or newborn
      763.89
  occipital (region) (scalp) 959.09
    lobe (*see also* Injury, intracranial)
      854.0
  optic 950.9
    chiasm 950.1
    cortex 950.3
    nerve 950.0
    pathways 950.2

Injury *(Continued)*
  orbit, orbital (region) 921.2
    penetrating 870.3
      with foreign body 870.4
  ovary - *see* Injury, internal, ovary
  paint-gun - *see* Wound, open, by site,
    complicated
  palate (soft) 959.09
  pancreas - *see* Injury, internal, pancreas
  parathyroid (gland) 959.09
  parietal (region) (scalp) 959.09
    lobe - *see* Injury, intracranial
  pelvic
    floor 959.19
      complicating delivery 664.1
        affecting fetus or newborn
          763.89
    joint or ligament, complicating deliv-
      ery 665.6
      affecting fetus or newborn 763.89
    organs - *see also* Injury, internal, pel-
      vis
      with
        abortion - *see* Abortion, by type,
          with damage to pelvic or-
          gans
        ectopic pregnancy (*see also* cate-
          gories 633.0-633.9) 639.2
        molar pregnancy (*see also* cate-
          gories 633.0-633.9) 639.2
      following
        abortion 639.2
        ectopic or molar pregnancy 639.2
      obstetrical trauma 665.5
        affecting fetus or newborn
          763.89
  pelvis 959.19
  penis 959.14
    fracture of corpus cavernosum
      959.13
  perineum 959.14
  peritoneum - *see* Injury, internal, peri-
    toneum
  periurethral tissue
    with
      abortion - *see* Abortion, by type,
        with damage to pelvic organs
      ectopic pregnancy (*see also* catego-
        ries 633.0-633.9) 639.2
      molar pregnancy (*see also* catego-
        ries 630-632) 639.2
    complicating delivery 665.5
      affecting fetus or newborn 763.89
    following
      abortion 639.2
      ectopic or molar pregnancy 639.2
  phalanges
    foot 959.7
    hand 959.5
  pharynx 959.09
  pleura - *see* Injury, internal, pleura
  popliteal space 959.7
  prepuce 959.14
  prostate - *see* Injury, internal, prostate
  pubic region 959.19
  pudenda 959.14
  radiation NEC 990
  radioactive substance or radium NEC
    990
  rectovaginal septum 959.14
  rectum - *see* Injury, internal, rectum
  retina 921.3
    penetrating - *see* Injury, eyeball, pen-
      etrating

◀ **New**   ◀▥ **Revised**

Injury *(Continued)*
retroperitoneal - *see* Injury, internal, retroperitoneum
roentgen rays NEC 990
round ligament - *see* Injury, internal, round ligament
sacral (region) 959.19
plexus 953.5
sacroiliac ligament NEC 959.19
sacrum 959.19
salivary ducts or glands 959.09
scalp 959.09
due to birth trauma 767.19
fetus or newborn 767.19
scapular region 959.2
sclera 921.3
penetrating - *see* Injury, eyeball, penetrating
superficial 918.2
scrotum 959.14
seminal vesicle - *see* Injury, internal, seminal vesicle
shoulder (and upper arm) 959.2
sinus
cavernous (*see also* Injury, intracranial) 854.0
nasal 959.09
skeleton NEC, birth injury 767.3
skin NEC 959.9
skull - *see* Fracture, skull, by site
soft tissue (of external sites) (severe) - *see* Wound, open, by site
specified site NEC 959.8
spermatic cord - *see* Injury, internal, spermatic cord
spinal (cord) 952.9
with fracture, vertebra - *see* Fracture, vertebra, by site, with spinal cord injury
cervical (C$_1$-C$_4$) 952.00
with
anterior cord syndrome 952.02
central cord syndrome 952.03
complete lesion of cord 952.01
incomplete lesion NEC 952.04
posterior cord syndrome 952.04
C$_5$-C$_7$ level 952.05
with
anterior cord syndrome 952.07
central cord syndrome 952.08
complete lesion of cord 952.06
incomplete lesion NEC 952.09
posterior cord syndrome 952.09
specified type NEC 952.09
specified type NEC 952.04
dorsal (D$_1$-D$_6$) (T$_1$-T$_6$) (thoracic) 952.10
with
anterior cord syndrome 952.12
central cord syndrome 952.13
complete lesion of cord 952.11
incomplete lesion NEC 952.14
posterior cord syndrome 952.14
D$_7$-D$_{12}$ level (T$_7$-T$_{12}$) 952.15
with
anterior cord syndrome 952.17
central cord syndrome 952.18
complete lesion of cord 952.16
incomplete lesion NEC 952.19
posterior cord syndrome 952.19
specified type NEC 952.19
specified type NEC 952.14

Injury *(Continued)*
spinal *(Continued)*
lumbar 952.2
multiple sites 952.8
nerve (root) NEC - *see* Injury, nerve, spinal, root
plexus 953.9
brachial 953.4
lumbosacral 953.5
multiple sites 953.8
sacral 952.3
thoracic (*see also* Injury, spinal, dorsal) 952.10
spleen - *see* Injury, internal, spleen
stellate ganglion 954.1
sternal region 959.11
stomach - *see* Injury, internal, stomach
subconjunctival 921.1
subcutaneous 959.9
subdural - *see* Injury, intracranial
submaxillary region 959.09
submental region 959.09
subungual
fingers 959.5
toes 959.7
superficial 919

Note   Use the following fourth-digit subdivisions with categories 910-919:

.0   abrasion or friction burn without mention of infection
.1   abrasion or friction burn, infected
.2   blister without mention of infection
.3   blister, infected
.4   insect bite, nonvenomous, without mention of infection
.5   insect bite, nonvenomous, infected
.6   superficial foreign body (splinter) without major open wound and without mention of infection
.7   superficial foreign body (splinter) without major open wound, infected
.8   other and unspecified superficial injury without mention of infection
.9   other and unspecified superficial injury, infected

For late effects of superficial injury, *see* category 906.2.

---

abdomen, abdominal (muscle) (wall) (and other part(s) of trunk) 911
ankle (and hip, knee, leg, or thigh) 916
anus (and other part(s) of trunk) 911
arm 913
upper (and shoulder) 912
auditory canal (external) (meatus) (and other part(s) of face, neck, or scalp, except eye) 910
axilla (and upper arm) 912
back (and other part(s) of trunk) 911
breast (and other part(s) of trunk) 911
brow (and other part(s) of face, neck, or scalp, except eye) 910
buttock (and other part(s) of trunk) 911

Injury *(Continued)*
superficial *(Continued)*
canthus, eye 918.0
cheek(s) (and other part(s) of face, neck, or scalp, except eye) 910
chest wall (and other part(s) of trunk) 911
chin (and other part(s) of face, neck, or scalp, except eye) 910
clitoris (and other part(s) of trunk) 911
conjunctiva 918.2
cornea 918.1
due to contact lens 371.82
costal region (and other part(s) of trunk) 911
ear(s) (auricle) (canal) (drum) (external) (and other part(s) of face, neck, or scalp, except eye) 910
elbow (and forearm) (and wrist) 913
epididymis (and other part(s) of trunk) 911
epigastric region (and other part(s) of trunk) 911
epiglottis (and other part(s) of face, neck, or scalp, except eye) 910
eye(s) (and adnexa) NEC 918.9
eyelid(s) (and periocular area) 918.0
face (any part), except eye (and neck or scalp) 910
finger(s) (nail) (any) 915
flank (and other part(s) of trunk) 911
foot (phalanges) (and toe(s)) 917
forearm (and elbow) (and wrist) 913
forehead (and other part(s) of face, neck, or scalp, except eye) 910
globe (eye) 918.9
groin (and other part(s) of trunk) 911
gum(s) (and other part(s) of face, neck, or scalp, except eye) 910
hand(s) (except fingers alone) 914
head (and other part(s) of face, neck, or scalp, except eye) 910
heel (and foot or toe) 917
hip (and ankle, knee, leg, or thigh) 916
iliac region (and other part(s) of trunk) 911
interscapular region (and other part(s) of trunk) 911
iris 918.9
knee (and ankle, hip, leg, or thigh) 916
labium (majus) (minus) (and other part(s) of trunk) 911
lacrimal (apparatus) (gland) (sac) 918.0
leg (lower) (upper) (and ankle, hip, knee, or thigh) 916
lip(s) (and other part(s) of face, neck, or scalp, except eye) 910
lower extremity (except foot) 916
lumbar region (and other part(s) of trunk) 911
malar region (and other part(s) of face, neck, or scalp, except eye) 910
mastoid region (and other part(s) of face, neck, or scalp, except eye) 910
midthoracic region (and other part(s) of trunk) 911

ICD-9-CM
—
Vol. 2

Injury (Continued)
  superficial (Continued)
    mouth (and other part(s) of face, neck, or scalp, except eye) 910
    multiple sites (not classifiable to the same three-digit category) 919
    nasal (septum) (and other part(s) of face, neck, or scalp, except eye) 910
    neck (and face or scalp, any part(s), except eye) 910
    nose (septum) (and other part(s) of face, neck, or scalp, except eye) 910
    occipital region (and other part(s) of face, neck, or scalp, except eye) 910
    orbital region 918.0
    palate (soft) (and other part(s) of face, neck, or scalp, except eye) 910
    parietal region (and other part(s) of face, neck, or scalp, except eye) 910
    penis (and other part(s) of trunk) 911
    perineum (and other part(s) of trunk) 911
    periocular area 918.0
    pharynx (and other part(s) of face, neck, or scalp, except eye) 910
    popliteal space (and ankle, hip, leg, or thigh) 916
    prepuce (and other part(s) of trunk) 911
    pubic region (and other part(s) of trunk) 911
    pudenda (and other part(s) of trunk) 911
    sacral region (and other part(s) of trunk) 911
    salivary (ducts) (glands) (and other part(s) of face, neck, or scalp, except eye) 910
    scalp (and other part(s) of face or neck, except eye) 910
    scapular region (and upper arm) 912
    sclera 918.2
    scrotum (and other part(s) of trunk) 911
    shoulder (and upper arm) 912
    skin NEC 919
    specified site(s) NEC 919
    sternal region (and other part(s) of trunk) 911
    subconjunctival 918.2
    subcutaneous NEC 919
    submaxillary region (and other part(s) of face, neck, or scalp, except eye) 910
    submental region (and other part(s) of face, neck, or scalp, except eye) 910
    supraclavicular fossa (and other part(s) of face, neck, or scalp, except eye) 910
    supraorbital 918.0
    temple (and other part(s) of face, neck, or scalp, except eye) 910
    temporal region (and other part(s) of face, neck, or scalp, except eye) 910

Injury (Continued)
  superficial (Continued)
    testis (and other part(s) of trunk) 911
    thigh (and ankle, hip, knee, or leg) 916
    thorax, thoracic (external) (and other part(s) of trunk) 911
    throat (and other part(s) of face, neck, or scalp, except eye) 910
    thumb(s) (nail) 915
    toe(s) (nail) (subungual) (and foot) 917
    tongue (and other part(s) of face, neck, or scalp, except eye) 910
    tooth, teeth (see also Abrasion, dental) 521.20 ◄▬▬
    trunk (any part(s)) 911
    tunica vaginalis (and other part(s) of trunk) 911
    tympanum, tympanic membrane (and other part(s) of face, neck, or scalp, except eye) 910
    upper extremity NEC 913
    uvula (and other part(s) of face, neck, or scalp, except eye) 910
    vagina (and other part(s) of trunk) 911
    vulva (and other part(s) of trunk) 911
    wrist (and elbow) (and forearm) 913
  supraclavicular fossa 959.19
  supraorbital 959.09
  surgical complication (external or internal site) 998.2
  symphysis pubis 959.19
    complicating delivery 665.6
      affecting fetus or newborn 763.89
  temple 959.09
  temporal region 959.09
  testis 959.14
  thigh (and hip) 959.6
  thorax, thoracic (external) 959.11
    cavity - see Injury, internal, thorax
    internal - see Injury, internal, intra-thoracic organs
  throat 959.09
  thumb(s) (nail) 959.5
  thymus - see Injury, internal, thymus
  thyroid (gland) 959.09
  toe (nail) (any) 959.7
  tongue 959.09
  tonsil 959.09
  tooth NEC 873.63
    complicated 873.73
  trachea - see Injury, internal, trachea
  trunk 959.19
  tunica vaginalis 959.14 ◄▬▬
  tympanum, tympanic membrane 959.09
  ultraviolet rays NEC 990
  ureter - see Injury, internal, ureter
  urethra (sphincter) - see Injury, internal, urethra
  uterus - see Injury, internal, uterus
  uvula 959.09
  vagina 959.14
  vascular - see Injury, blood vessel
  vas deferens - see Injury, internal, vas deferens
  vein (see also Injury, blood vessel, by site) 904.9
  vena cava
    inferior 902.10
    superior 901.2

Injury (Continued)
  vesical (sphincter) - see Injury, internal, vesical
  viscera (abdominal) - see Injury, internal, viscera
    with fracture, pelvis - see Fracture, pelvis
  visual 950.9
    cortex 950.3
  vitreous (humor) 871.2
  vulva 959.14
  whiplash (cervical spine) 847.0
  wringer - see Crush, by site
  wrist (and elbow) (and forearm) 959.3
  x-ray NEC 990
Inoculation - see also Vaccination
  complication or reaction - see Complication, vaccination
Insanity, insane (see also Psychosis) 298.9
  adolescent (see also Schizophrenia) 295.9
  alternating (see also Psychosis, affective, circular) 296.7
  confusional 298.9
    acute 293.0
    subacute 293.1
  delusional 298.9
  paralysis, general 094.1
    progressive 094.1
  paresis, general 094.1
  senile 290.20
Insect
  bite - see Injury, superficial, by site
  venomous, poisoning by 989.5
Insemination, artificial V26.1
Insertion
  cord (umbilical) lateral or velamentous 663.8
    affecting fetus or newborn 762.6
  intrauterine contraceptive device V25.1
  placenta, vicious - see Placenta, previa
  subdermal implantable contraceptive V25.5
  velamentous, umbilical cord 663.8
    affecting fetus or newborn 762.6
Insolation 992.0
  meaning sunstroke 992.0
Insomnia 780.52
  with sleep apnea 780.51
  nonorganic origin 307.41
    persistent (primary) 307.42
    transient 307.41
  subjective complaint 307.49
Inspiration
  food or foreign body (see also Asphyxia, food or foreign body) 933.1
  mucus (see also Asphyxia, mucus) 933.1
Inspissated bile syndrome, newborn 774.4
Instability
  detrusor 596.59
  emotional (excessive) 301.3
  joint (posttraumatic) 718.80
    ankle 718.87
    elbow 718.82
    foot 718.87
    hand 718.84
    hip 718.85
    knee 718.86
    lumbosacral 724.6
    multiple sites 718.89
    pelvic region 718.85
    sacroiliac 724.6

◄ **New**   ◄▬▬ **Revised**

ICD-9-CM

Vol. 2

Insufficiency, insufficient (*Continued*)
  vascular (*Continued*)
    peripheral 443.9
    renal (*see also* Hypertension, kidney)
      403.90
    velopharyngeal
      acquired 528.9
      congenital 750.29
    venous (peripheral) 459.81
    ventricular - *see* Insufficiency, myocar-
      dial
    vertebral artery 435.1
    vertebrobasilar artery 435.3
    weight gain during pregnancy 646.8
    zinc 269.3
Insufflation
  fallopian
    fertility testing V26.21
    following sterilization reversal
      V26.22
  meconium 770.1
Insular - *see* condition
Insulinoma (M8151/0)
  malignant (M8151/3)
    pancreas 157.4
    specified site - *see* Neoplasm, by site,
      malignant
    unspecified site 157.4
  pancreas 211.7
  specified site - *see* Neoplasm, by site,
    benign
  unspecified site 211.7
Insuloma - *see* Insulinoma
Insult
  brain 437.9
    acute 436
  cerebral 437.9
    acute 436
  cerebrovascular 437.9
    acute 436
  vascular NEC 437.9
    acute 436
Insurance examination (certification) V70.3
Intemperance (*see also* Alcoholism) 303.9
Interception of pregnancy (menstrual
  extraction) V25.3
Intermenstrual
  bleeding 626.6
    irregular 626.6
    regular 626.5
  hemorrhage 626.6
    irregular 626.6
    regular 626.5
  pain(s) 625.2
Intermittent - *see* condition
Internal - *see* condition
Interproximal wear 521.10 ◄▦
Interruption
  aortic arch 747.11
  bundle of His 426.50
  fallopian tube (for sterilization) V25.2
  phase-shift, sleep cycle 307.45
  repeated REM-sleep 307.48
  sleep
    due to perceived environmental
      disturbances 307.48
    phase-shift, of 24-hour sleep-wake
      cycle 307.45
    repeated REM-sleep type 307.48
  vas deferens (for sterilization) V25.2
Intersexuality 752.7
Interstitial - *see* condition
Intertrigo 695.89
  labialis 528.5

Intervertebral disc - *see* condition
Intestine, intestinal - *see also* condition
  flu 487.8
Intolerance
  carbohydrate NEC 579.8
  cardiovascular exercise, with pain (at
    rest) (with less than ordinary ac-
    tivity) (with ordinary activity)
    V47.2
  cold 780.99
  dissacharide (hereditary) 271.3
  drug
    correct substance properly adminis-
      tered 995.2
    wrong substance given or taken in
      error 977.9
      specified drug - *see* Table of Drugs
        and Chemicals
  effort 306.2
  fat NEC 579.8
  foods NEC 579.8
  fructose (hereditary) 271.2
  glucose (-galactose) (congenital) 271.3
  gluten 579.0
  lactose (hereditary) (infantile) 271.3
  lysine (congenital) 270.7
  milk NEC 579.8
  protein (familial) 270.7
  starch NEC 579.8
  sucrose (-isomaltose) (congenital) 271.3
Intoxicated NEC (*see also* Alcoholism)
  305.0
Intoxication
  acid 276.2
  acute
    alcoholic 305.0
      with alcoholism 303.0
      hangover effects 305.0
    caffeine 305.9
    hallucinogenic (*see also* Abuse,
      drugs, nondependent) 305.3
  alcohol (acute) 305.0
    with alcoholism 303.0
    hangover effects 305.0
    idiosyncratic 291.4
    pathological 291.4
  alimentary canal 558.2
  ammonia (hepatic) 572.2
  caffeine 305.9   ◄
  chemical - *see also* Table of Drugs and
    Chemicals
  via placenta or breast milk 760.70
    alcohol 760.71
    anti-infective agents 760.74
    cocaine 760.75
    "crack" 760.75
    hallucinogenic agents NEC 760.73
    medicinal agents NEC 760.79
    narcotics 760.72
    obstetric anesthetic or analgesic
      drug 763.5
    specified agent NEC 760.79
    suspected, affecting management
      of pregnancy 655.5
  cocaine, through placenta or breast
    milk 760.75
  delirium
    alcohol 291.0
    drug 292.81
  drug 292.9   ◄▦
    with delirium 292.81
    correct substance properly adminis-
      tered (*see also* Allergy, drug)
      995.2

Intoxication (*Continued*)
  drug (*Continued*)
    newborn 779.4
    obstetric anesthetic or sedation 668.9
      affecting fetus or newborn 763.5
    overdose or wrong substance given
      or taken - *see* Table of Drugs
      and Chemicals
    pathologic 292.2
    specific to newborn 779.4
    via placenta or breast milk 760.70
      alcohol 760.71
      anti-infective agents 760.74
      cocaine 760.75
      "crack" 760.75
      hallucinogenic agents 760.73
      medicinal agents NEC 760.79
      narcotics 760.72
      obstetric anesthetic or analgesic
        drug 763.5
      specified agent NEC 760.79
      suspected, affecting management
        of pregnancy 655.5
  enteric - *see* Intoxication, intestinal
  fetus or newborn, via placenta or
    breast milk 760.70
    alcohol 760.71
    anti-infective agents 760.74
    cocaine 760.75
    "crack" 760.75
    hallucinogenic agents 760.73
    medicinal agents NEC 760.79
    narcotics 760.72
    obstetric anesthetic or analgesic drug
      763.5
    specified agent NEC 760.79
    suspected, affecting management of
      pregnancy 655.5
  food - *see* Poisoning, food
  gastrointestinal 558.2
  hallucinogenic (acute) 305.3
  hepatocerebral 572.2
  idiosyncratic alcohol 291.4
  intestinal 569.89
    due to putrefaction of food 005.9
  methyl alcohol (*see also* Alcoholism)
    305.0
    with alcoholism 303.0
  pathologic 291.4
    drug 292.2
  potassium (K) 276.7
  septic
    with
      abortion - *see* Abortion, by type,
        with sepsis
      ectopic pregnancy (*see also* catego-
        ries 633.0-633.9) 639.0
      molar pregnancy (*see also* catego-
        ries 630-632) 639.0
    during labor 659.3
    following
      abortion 639.0
      ectopic or molar pregnancy 639.0
    generalized - *see* Septicemia
    puerperal, postpartum, childbirth 670
  serum (prophylactic) (therapeutic) 999.5
  uremic - *see* Uremia
  water 276.6
Intracranial - *see* condition
Intrahepatic gallbladder 751.69
Intraligamentous - *see also* condition
  pregnancy - *see* Pregnancy, cornual
Intraocular - *see also* condition
  sepsis 360.00

Intrathoracic - *see also* condition
  kidney 753.3
  stomach - *see* Hernia, diaphragm
Intrauterine contraceptive device
  checking V25.42
  insertion V25.1
  in situ V45.51
  management V25.42
  prescription V25.02
    repeat V25.42
  reinsertion V25.42
  removal V25.42
Intraventricular - *see* condition
Intrinsic deformity - *see* Deformity
Intrusion, repetitive, of sleep (due to
  environmental disturbances) (with
  atypical polysomnographic features)
  307.48
Intumescent, lens (eye) NEC 366.9
  senile 366.12
Intussusception (colon) (enteric) (intestine) (rectum) 560.0
  appendix 543.9
  congenital 751.5
  fallopian tube 620.8
  ileocecal 560.0
  ileocolic 560.0
  ureter (obstruction) 593.4
Invagination
  basilar 756.0
  colon or intestine 560.0
Invalid (since birth) 799.89
Invalidism (chronic) 799.89
Inversion
  albumin-globulin (A-G) ratio 273.8
  bladder 596.8
  cecum (*see also* Intussusception) 560.0
  cervix 622.8
  nipple 611.79
    congenital 757.6
    puerperal, postpartum 676.3
  optic papilla 743.57
  organ or site, congenital NEC - *see*
    Anomaly, specified type NEC
  sleep rhythm 780.55
    nonorganic origin 307.45
  testis (congenital) 752.51
  uterus (postinfectional) (postpartal,
    old) 621.7
    chronic 621.7
    complicating delivery 665.2
      affecting fetus or newborn 763.89
  vagina - *see* Prolapse, vagina
Investigation
  allergens V72.7
  clinical research (control) (normal com-
    parison) (participant) V70.7
Inviability - *see* Immaturity
Involuntary movement, abnormal 781.0
Involution, involutional - *see also* condition
  breast, cystic or fibrocystic 610.1
  depression (*see also* Psychosis, affec-
    tive) 296.2
    recurrent episode 296.3
    single episode 296.2
  melancholia (*see also* Psychosis, affec-
    tive) 296.2
    recurrent episode 296.3
    single episode 296.2
  ovary, senile 620.3
  paranoid state (reaction) 297.2
  paraphrenia (climacteric) (menopause)
    297.2

Involution, involutional (*Continued*)
  psychosis 298.8
  thymus failure 254.8
IQ
  under 20 318.2
  20-34 318.1
  35-49 318.0
  50-70 317
IRDS 769
Irideremia 743.45
Iridis rubeosis 364.42
  diabetic 250.5 [364.42]
Iridochoroiditis (panuveitis) 360.12
Iridocyclitis NEC 364.3
  acute 364.00
    primary 364.01
    recurrent 364.02
  chronic 364.10
    in
      lepromatous leprosy 030.0 [364.11]
      sarcoidosis 135 [364.11]
      tuberculosis (*see also* Tuberculosis)
        017.3 [364.11]
  due to allergy 364.04
  endogenous 364.01
  gonococcal 098.41
  granulomatous 364.10
  herpetic (simplex) 054.44
    zoster 053.22
  hypopyon 364.05
  lens induced 364.23
  nongranulomatous 364.00
  primary 364.01
  recurrent 364.02
  rheumatic 364.10
  secondary 364.04
    infectious 364.03
    noninfectious 364.04
  subacute 364.00
    primary 364.01
    recurrent 364.02
  sympathetic 360.11
  syphilitic (secondary) 091.52
  tuberculous (chronic) (*see also* Tubercu-
    losis) 017.3 [364.11]
Iridocyclochoroiditis (panuveitis) 360.12
Iridodialysis 364.76
Iridodonesis 364.8
Iridoplegia (complete) (partial) (reflex)
  379.49
Iridoschisis 364.52
Iris - *see* condition
Iritis 364.3
  acute 364.00
    primary 364.01
    recurrent 364.02
  chronic 364.10
    in
      sarcoidosis 135 [364.11]
      tuberculosis (*see also* Tuberculosis)
        017.3 [364.11]
  diabetic 250.5 [364.42]
  due to
    allergy 364.04
    herpes simplex 054.44
    leprosy 030.0 [364.11]
  endogenous 364.01
  gonococcal 098.41
  gouty 274.89 [364.11]
  granulomatous 364.10
  hypopyon 364.05
  lens induced 364.23
  nongranulomatous 364.00
  papulosa 095.8 [364.11]

Iritis (*Continued*)
  primary 364.01
  recurrent 364.02
  rheumatic 364.10
  secondary 364.04
    infectious 364.03
    noninfectious 364.04
  subacute 364.00
    primary 364.01
    recurrent 364.02
  sympathetic 360.11
  syphilitic (secondary) 091.52
    congenital 090.0 [364.11]
    late 095.8 [364.11]
  tuberculous (*see also* Tuberculosis)
    017.3 [364.11]
  uratic 274.89 [364.11]
Iron
  deficiency anemia 280.9
  metabolism disease 275.0
  storage disease 275.0
Iron-miners' lung 503
Irradiated enamel (tooth, teeth) 521.8
Irradiation
  burn - *see* Burn, by site
  effects, adverse 990
Irreducible, irreducibility - *see* condition
Irregular, irregularity
  action, heart 427.9
  alveolar process 525.8
  bleeding NEC 626.4
  breathing 786.09
  colon 569.89
  contour of cornea 743.41
    acquired 371.70
  dentin in pulp 522.3
  eye movements NEC 379.59
  menstruation (cause unknown) 626.4
  periods 626.4
  prostate 602.9
  pupil 364.75
  respiratory 786.09
  septum (nasal) 470
  shape, organ or site, congenital NEC -
    see Distortion
  sleep-wake rhythm (non-24-hour)
    780.55
    nonorganic origin 307.45
  vertebra 733.99
Irritability (nervous) 799.2
  bladder 596.8
    neurogenic 596.54
      with cauda equina syndrome
        344.61
  bowel (syndrome) 564.1
  bronchial (*see also* Bronchitis) 490
  cerebral, newborn 779.1
  colon 564.1
    psychogenic 306.4
  duodenum 564.89
  heart (psychogenic) 306.2
  ileum 564.89
  jejunum 564.89
  myocardium 306.2
  rectum 564.89
  stomach 536.9
    psychogenic 306.4
  sympathetic (nervous system) (*see also*
    Neuropathy, peripheral, auto-
    nomic) 337.9
  urethra 599.84
  ventricular (heart) (psychogenic)
    306.2
Irritable - *see* Irritability

ICD-9-CM

Vol. 2

Irritation
anus 569.49
axillary nerve 353.0
bladder 596.8
brachial plexus 353.0
brain (traumatic) (*see also* Injury, intracranial) 854.0
  nontraumatic - *see* Encephalitis
bronchial (*see also* Bronchitis) 490
cerebral (traumatic) (*see also* Injury, intracranial) 854.0
  nontraumatic - *see* Encephalitis
cervical plexus 353.2
cervix (*see also* Cervicitis) 616.0
choroid, sympathetic 360.11
cranial nerve - *see* Disorder, nerve, cranial
digestive tract 536.9
  psychogenic 306.4
gastric 536.9
  psychogenic 306.4
gastrointestinal (tract) 536.9
  functional 536.9
  psychogenic 306.4
globe, sympathetic 360.11
intestinal (bowel) 564.9
labyrinth 386.50
lumbosacral plexus 353.1
meninges (traumatic) (*see also* Injury, intracranial) 854.0
  nontraumatic - *see* Meningitis
myocardium 306.2
nerve - *see* Disorder, nerve
nervous 799.2
nose 478.1
penis 607.89
perineum 709.9
peripheral
  autonomic nervous system (*see also* Neuropathy, peripheral, autonomic) 337.9
  nerve - *see* Disorder, nerve
peritoneum (*see also* Peritonitis) 567.9
pharynx 478.29
plantar nerve 355.6
spinal (cord) (traumatic) - *see also* Injury, spinal, by site
  nerve - *see also* Disorder, nerve
    root NEC 724.9
    traumatic - *see* Injury, nerve, spinal
  nontraumatic - *see* Myelitis
stomach 536.9
  psychogenic 306.4
sympathetic nerve NEC (*see also* Neuropathy, peripheral, autonomic) 337.9
ulnar nerve 354.2
vagina 623.9
Isambert's disease 012.3
Ischemia, ischemic 459.9
basilar artery (with transient neurologic deficit) 435.0
bone NEC 733.40
bowel (transient) 557.9
  acute 557.0
  chronic 557.1
  due to mesenteric artery insufficiency 557.1
brain - *see also* Ischemia, cerebral
  recurrent focal 435.9
cardiac (*see also* Ischemia, heart) 414.9

Ischemia, ischemic (*Continued*)
cardiomyopathy 414.8
carotid artery (with transient neurologic deficit) 435.8
cerebral (chronic) (generalized) 437.1
  arteriosclerotic 437.0
  intermittent (with transient neurologic deficit) 435.9
  puerperal, postpartum, childbirth 674.0
  recurrent focal (with transient neurologic deficit) 435.9
  transient (with transient neurologic deficit) 435.9
colon 557.9
  acute 557.0
  chronic 557.1
  due to mesenteric artery insufficiency 557.1
coronary (chronic) (*see also* Ischemia, heart) 414.9
heart (chronic or with a stated duration of over 8 weeks) 414.9
  acute or with a stated duration of 8 weeks or less (*see also* Infarct, myocardium) 410.9
    without myocardial infarction 411.89
    with coronary (artery) occlusion 411.81
  subacute 411.89
intestine (transient) 557.9
  acute 557.0
  chronic 557.1
  due to mesenteric artery insufficiency 557.1
kidney 593.81
labyrinth 386.50
muscles, leg 728.89
myocardium, myocardial (chronic or with a stated duration of over 8 weeks) 414.8
  acute (*see also* Infarct, myocardium) 410.9
    without myocardial infarction 411.89
    with coronary (artery) occlusion 411.81
renal 593.81
retina, retinal 362.84
small bowel 557.9
  acute 557.0
  chronic 557.1
  due to mesenteric artery insufficiency 557.1
spinal cord 336.1
subendocardial (*see also* Insufficiency, coronary) 411.89
vertebral artery (with transient neurologic deficit) 435.1
Ischialgia (*see also* Sciatica) 724.3
Ischiopagus 759.4
Ischium, ischial - *see* condition
Ischomenia 626.8
Ischuria 788.5
Iselin's disease or osteochondrosis 732.5
Islands of
parotid tissue in
  lymph nodes 750.26
  neck structures 750.26

Islands of (*Continued*)
submaxillary glands in
  fascia 750.26
  lymph nodes 750.26
  neck muscles 750.26
Islet cell tumor, pancreas (M8150/0) 211.7
Isoimmunization NEC (*see also* Incompatibility) 656.2
fetus or newborn 773.2
  ABO blood groups 773.1
  rhesus (Rh) factor 773.0
Isolation V07.0
social V62.4
Isosporosis 007.2
Issue
medical certificate NEC V68.0
  cause of death V68.0
  fitness V68.0
  incapacity V68.0
repeat prescription NEC V68.1
  appliance V68.1
  contraceptive V25.40
    device NEC V25.49
      intrauterine V25.42
      specified type NEC V25.49
    pill V25.41
  glasses V68.1
  medicinal substance V68.1
Itch (*see also* Pruritus) 698.9
bakers' 692.89
barbers' 110.0
bricklayers' 692.89
cheese 133.8
clam diggers' 120.3
coolie 126.9
copra 133.8
Cuban 050.1
dew 126.9
dhobie 110.3
eye 379.99
filarial (*see also* Infestation, filarial) 125.9
grain 133.8
grocers' 133.8
ground 126.9
harvest 133.8
jock 110.3
Malabar 110.9
  beard 110.0
  foot 110.4
  scalp 110.0
meaning scabies 133.0
Norwegian 133.0
perianal 698.0
poultrymen's 133.8
sarcoptic 133.0
scrub 134.1
seven year V61.10
  meaning scabies 133.0
straw 133.8
swimmers' 120.3
washerwoman's 692.4
water 120.3
winter 698.8
Itsenko-Cushing syndrome (pituitary basophilism) 255.0
Ivemark's syndrome (asplenia with congenital heart disease) 759.0
Ivory bones 756.52
Ixodes 134.8
Ixodiasis 134.8

J

Jaccoud's nodular fibrositis, chronic
(Jaccoud's syndrome) 714.4
Jackson's
membrane 751.4
paralysis or syndrome 344.89
veil 751.4
Jacksonian
epilepsy (*see also* Epilepsy) 345.5
seizures (focal) (*see also* Epilepsy)
345.5
Jacob's ulcer (M8090/3) - *see* Neoplasm,
skin, malignant, by site
Jacquet's dermatitis (diaper dermatitis)
691.0
Jadassohn's
blue nevus (M8780/0) - *see* Neoplasm,
skin, benign
disease (maculopapular erythroderma)
696.2
intraepidermal epithelioma
(M8096/0) - *see* Neoplasm, skin,
benign
Jadassohn-Lewandowski syndrome
(pachyonychia congenita) 757.5
Jadassohn-Pellizari's disease (anetoderma) 701.3
Jadassohn-Tièche nevus (M8780/0) - *see*
Neoplasm, skin, benign
Jaffe-Lichtenstein (-Uehlinger) syndrome
252.01 ◄▥
Jahnke's syndrome (encephalocutaneous
angiomatosis) 759.6
Jakob-Creutzfeldt disease or syndrome
046.1
with dementia
with behavioral disturbance 046.1
[294.11]
without behavioral disturbance 046.1
[294.10]
Jaksch (-Luzet) disease or syndrome
(pseudoleukemia infantum) 285.8
Jamaican
neuropathy 349.82
paraplegic tropical ataxic-spastic syndrome 349.82
Janet's disease (psychasthenia) 300.89
Janiceps 759.4
**Jansky-Bielschowsky amaurotic familial
idiocy** 330.1
Japanese
B-type encephalitis 062.0
river fever 081.2
seven-day fever 100.89
Jaundice (yellow) 782.4
acholuric (familial) (splenomegalic) (*see
also* Spherocytosis) 282.0
acquired 283.9
breast milk 774.39
catarrhal (acute) 070.1
with hepatic coma 070.0
chronic 571.9
epidemic - *see* Jaundice, epidemic
cholestatic (benign) 782.4
chronic idiopathic 277.4
epidemic (catarrhal) 070.1
with hepatic coma 070.0
leptospiral 100.0
spirochetal 100.0
febrile (acute) 070.1
with hepatic coma 070.0

Jaundice (*Continued*)
febrile (*Continued*)
leptospiral 100.0
spirochetal 100.0
fetus or newborn 774.6
due to or associated with
ABO
antibodies 773.1
incompatibility, maternal/fetal
773.1
isoimmunization 773.1
absence or deficiency of enzyme
system for bilirubin conjugation (congenital) 774.39
blood group incompatibility NEC
773.2
breast milk inhibitors to conjugation 774.39
associated with preterm delivery 774.2
bruising 774.1
Crigler-Najjar syndrome 277.4
[774.31]
delayed conjugation 774.30
associated with preterm delivery 774.2
development 774.39
drugs or toxins transmitted from
mother 774.1
G-6-PD deficiency 282.2 [774.0]
galactosemia 271.1 [774.5]
Gilbert's syndrome 277.4 [774.31]
hepatocellular damage 774.4
hereditary hemolytic anemia (*see
also* Anemia, hemolytic) 282.9
[774.0]
hypothyroidism, congenital 243
[774.31]
incompatibility, maternal/fetal
NEC 773.2
infection 774.1
inspissated bile syndrome 774.4
isoimmunization NEC 773.2
mucoviscidosis 277.01 [774.5]
obliteration of bile duct, congenital 751.61 [774.5]
polycythemia 774.1
preterm delivery 774.2
red cell defect 282.9 [774.0]
Rh
antibodies 773.0
incompatibility, maternal/fetal
773.0
isoimmunization 773.0
spherocytosis (congenital) 282.0
[774.0]
swallowed maternal blood 774.1
physiological NEC 774.6
from injection, inoculation, infusion, or
transfusion (blood) (plasma) (serum) (other substance) (onset
within 8 months after administration) - *see* Hepatitis, viral
Gilbert's (familial nonhemolytic) 277.4
hematogenous 283.9
hemolytic (acquired) 283.9
congenital (*see also* Spherocytosis)
282.0
hemorrhagic (acute) 100.0
leptospiral 100.0
newborn 776.0
spirochetal 100.0

Jaundice (*Continued*)
hepatocellular 573.8
homologous (serum) - *see* Hepatitis, viral
idiopathic, chronic 277.4
infectious (acute) (subacute) 070.1
with hepatic coma 070.0
leptospiral 100.0
spirochetal 100.0
leptospiral 100.0
malignant (*see also* Necrosis, liver)
570
newborn (physiological) (*see also* Jaundice, fetus or newborn) 774.6
nonhemolytic, congenital familial (Gilbert's) 277.4
nuclear, newborn (*see also* Kernicterus
of newborn) 774.7
obstructive NEC (*see also* Obstruction,
biliary) 576.8
postimmunization - *see* Hepatitis, viral
posttransfusion - *see* Hepatitis, viral
regurgitation (*see also* Obstruction, biliary) 576.8
serum (homologous) (prophylactic)
(therapeutic) - *see* Hepatitis, viral
spirochetal (hemorrhagic) 100.0
symptomatic 782.4
newborn 774.6
Jaw - *see* condition
Jaw-blinking 374.43
congenital 742.8
Jaw-winking phenomenon or syndrome
742.8
Jealousy
alcoholic 291.5
childhood 313.3
sibling 313.3
Jejunitis (*see also* Enteritis) 558.9
Jejunostomy status V44.4
Jejunum, jejunal - *see* condition
Jensen's disease 363.05
Jericho boil 085.1
Jerks, myoclonic 333.2
Jeune's disease or syndrome (asphyxi-
ating thoracic dystrophy) 756.4
Jigger disease 134.1
Job's syndrome (chronic granulomatous
disease) 288.1
Jod-Basedow phenomenon 242.8
Johnson-Stevens disease (erythema mul-
tiforme exudativum) 695.1
Joint - *see also* condition
Charcôt's 094.0 [713.5]
false 733.82
flail - *see* Flail, joint
mice - *see* Loose, body, joint, by site
sinus to bone 730.9
von Gies' 095.8
Jordan's anomaly or syndrome 288.2
Josephs-Diamond-Blackfan anemia
(congenital hypoplastic) 284.0
Joubert 759.89
Jumpers' knee 727.2
Jungle yellow fever 060.0
Jungling's disease (sarcoidosis) 135
Junin virus hemorrhagic fever 078.7
Juvenile - *see also* condition
delinquent 312.9
group (*see also* Disturbance, conduct)
312.2
neurotic 312.4

ICD-9-CM

Vol. 2

K

Kabuki syndrome 759.89 ◄
Kahler (-Bozzolo) disease (multiple myeloma) (M9730/3) 203.0
Kakergasia 300.9
Kakke 265.0
Kala-azar (Indian) (infantile) (Mediterranean) (Sudanese) 085.0
Kalischer's syndrome (encephalocutaneous angiomatosis) 759.6
Kallmann's syndrome (hypogonadotropic hypogonadism with anosmia) 253.4
Kanner's syndrome (autism) (see also Psychosis, childhood) 299.0
Kaolinosis 502
Kaposi's
  disease 757.33
    lichen ruber 696.4
      acuminatus 696.4
      moniliformis 697.8
    xeroderma pigmentosum 757.33
  sarcoma (M9140/3) 176.9
    adipose tissue 176.1
    aponeurosis 176.1
    artery 176.1
    blood vessel 176.1
    bursa 176.1
    connective tissue 176.1
    external genitalia 176.8
    fascia 176.1
    fatty tissue 176.1
    fibrous tissue 176.1
    gastrointestinal tract NEC 176.3
    ligament 176.1
    lung 176.4
    lymph
      gland(s) 176.5
      node(s) 176.5
    lymphatic(s) NEC 176.1
    muscle (skeletal) 176.1
    oral cavity NEC 176.8
    palate 176.2
    scrotum 176.8
    skin 176.0
    soft tissue 176.1
    specified site NEC 176.8
    subcutaneous tissue 176.1
    synovia 176.1
    tendon (sheath) 176.1
    vein 176.1
    vessel 176.1
    viscera NEC 176.9
    vulva 176.8
  varicelliform eruption 054.0
    vaccinia 999.0
Kartagener's syndrome or triad (sinusitis, bronchiectasis, situs inversus) 759.3
Kasabach-Merritt syndrome (capillary hemangioma associated with thrombocytopenic purpura) 287.3
Kaschin-Beck disease (endemic polyarthritis) - see Disease, Kaschin-Beck
Kast's syndrome (dyschondroplasia with hemangiomas) 756.4
Katatonia- see Catatonia
Katayama disease or fever 120.2
Kathisophobia 781.0
Kawasaki disease 446.1
Kayser-Fleischer ring (cornea) (pseudosclerosis) 275.1 [371.14]
Kaznelson's syndrome (congenital hypoplastic anemia) 284.0

Kearns-Sayre syndrome 277.87 ◄
Kedani fever 081.2
Kelis 701.4
Kelly (-Paterson) syndrome (sideropenic dysphagia) 280.8
Keloid, cheloid 701.4
  Addison's (morphea) 701.0
  cornea 371.00
  Hawkins' 701.4
  scar 701.4
Keloma 701.4
Kenya fever 082.1
Keratectasia 371.71
  congenital 743.41
Keratitis (nodular) (nonulcerative) (simple) (zonular) NEC 370.9
  with ulceration (see also Ulcer, cornea) 370.00
  actinic 370.24
  arborescens 054.42
  areolar 370.22
  bullosa 370.8
  deep - see Keratitis, interstitial
  dendritic(a) 054.42
  desiccation 370.34
  diffuse interstitial 370.52
  disciform(is) 054.43
    varicella 052.7 [370.44]
  epithelialis vernalis 372.13 [370.32]
  exposure 370.34
  filamentary 370.23
  gonococcal (congenital) (prenatal) 098.43
  herpes, herpetic (simplex) NEC 054.43
    zoster 053.21
  hypopyon 370.04
  in
    chickenpox 052.7 [370.44]
    exanthema (see also Exanthem) 057.9 [370.44]
    paravaccinia (see also Paravaccinia) 051.9 [370.44]
    smallpox (see also Smallpox) 050.9 [370.44]
    vernal conjunctivitis 372.13 [370.32]
  interstitial (nonsyphilitic) 370.50
    with ulcer (see also Ulcer, cornea) 370.00
    diffuse 370.52
    herpes, herpetic (simplex) 054.43
      zoster 053.21
    syphilitic (congenital) (hereditary) 090.3
    tuberculous (see also Tuberculosis) 017.3 [370.59]
  lagophthalmic 370.34
  macular 370.22
  neuroparalytic 370.35
  neurotrophic 370.35
  nummular 370.22
  oyster-shuckers' 370.8
  parenchymatous - see Keratitis, interstitial
  petrificans 370.8
  phlyctenular 370.31
  postmeasles 055.71
  punctata, punctate 370.21
    leprosa 030.0 [370.21]
    profunda 090.3
    superficial (Thygeson's) 370.21
  purulent 370.8
  pustuliformis profunda 090.3
  rosacea 695.3 [370.49]
  sclerosing 370.54
  specified type NEC 370.8

Keratitis (Continued)
  stellate 370.22
  striate 370.22
  superficial 370.20
    with conjunctivitis (see also Keratoconjunctivitis) 370.40
    punctate (Thygeson's) 370.21
  suppurative 370.8
  syphilitic (congenital) (prenatal) 090.3
  trachomatous 076.1
    late effect 139.1
  tuberculous (phlyctenular) (see also Tuberculosis) 017.3 [370.31]
  ulcerated (see also Ulcer, cornea) 370.00
  vesicular 370.8
  welders' 370.24
  xerotic (see also Keratomalacia) 371.45
    vitamin A deficiency 264.4
Keratoacanthoma 238.2
Keratocele 371.72
Keratoconjunctivitis (see also Keratitis) 370.40
  adenovirus type 8 077.1
  epidemic 077.1
  exposure 370.34
  gonococcal 098.43
  herpetic (simplex) 054.43
    zoster 053.21
  in
    chickenpox 052.7 [370.44]
    exanthema (see also Exanthem) 057.9 [370.44]
    paravaccinia (see also Paravaccinia) 051.9 [370.44]
    smallpox (see also Smallpox) 050.9 [370.44]
  infectious 077.1
  neurotrophic 370.35
  phlyctenular 370.31
  postmeasles 055.71
  shipyard 077.1
  sicca (Sjögren's syndrome) 710.2
    not in Sjögren's syndrome 370.33
  specified type NEC 370.49
  tuberculous (phlyctenular) (see also Tuberculosis) 017.3 [370.31]
Keratoconus 371.60
  acute hydrops 371.62
  congenital 743.41
  stable 371.61
Keratocyst (dental) 526.0
Keratoderma, keratodermia (congenital) (palmaris et plantaris) (symmetrical) 757.39
  acquired 701.1
  blennorrhagica 701.1
    gonococcal 098.81
  climacterium 701.1
  eccentrica 757.39
  gonorrheal 098.81
  punctata 701.1
  tylodes, progressive 701.1
Keratodermatocele 371.72
Keratoglobus 371.70
  congenital 743.41
    associated with buphthalmos 743.22
Keratohemia 371.12
Keratoiritis (see also Iridocyclitis) 364.3
  syphilitic 090.3
  tuberculous (see also Tuberculosis) 017.3 [364.11]

◄ New   ◄■■ Revised

Keratolysis exfoliativa (congenital) 757.39
  acquired 695.89
  neonatorum 757.39
Keratoma 701.1
  congenital 757.39
  malignum congenitale 757.1
  palmaris et plantaris hereditarium 757.39
  senile 702.0
Keratomalacia 371.45
  vitamin A deficiency 264.4
Keratomegaly 743.41
Keratomycosis 111.1
  nigricans (palmaris) 111.1
Keratopathy 371.40
  band (*see also* Keratitis) 371.43
  bullous (*see also* Keratitis) 371.23
  degenerative (*see also* Degeneration, cornea) 371.40
    hereditary (*see also* Dystrophy, cornea) 371.50
  discrete colliquative 371.49
Keratoscleritis, tuberculous (*see also* Tuberculosis) 017.3 [370.31]
Keratosis 701.1
  actinic 702.0
  arsenical 692.4
  blennorrhagica 701.1
    gonococcal 098.81
  congenital (any type) 757.39
  ear (middle) (*see also* Cholesteatoma) 385.30
  female genital (external) 629.8
  follicular, vitamin A deficiency 264.8
  follicularis 757.39
    acquired 701.1
    congenital (acneiformis) (Siemens') 757.39
    spinulosa (decalvans) 757.39
    vitamin A deficiency 264.8
  gonococcal 098.81
  larynx, laryngeal 478.79
  male genital (external) 608.89
  middle ear (*see also* Cholesteatoma) 385.30
  nigricans 701.2
    congenital 757.39
  obturans 380.21
  oral epithelium ◄
    residual ridge mucosa ◄
      excessive 528.72 ◄
      minimal 528.71 ◄
  palmaris et plantaris (symmetrical) 757.39
  penile 607.89
  pharyngeus 478.29
  pilaris 757.39
    acquired 701.1
  punctata (palmaris et plantaris) 701.1
  scrotal 608.89
  seborrheic 702.19
    inflamed 702.11
  senilis 702.0
  solar 702.0
  suprafollicularis 757.39
  tonsillaris 478.29
  vagina 623.1
  vegetans 757.39
  vitamin A deficiency 264.8
Kerato-uveitis (*see also* Iridocyclitis) 364.3
Keraunoparalysis 994.0
Kerion (celsi) 110.0
Kernicterus of newborn (not due to isoimmunization) 774.7
  due to isoimmunization (conditions classifiable to 773.0-773.2) 773.4

Ketoacidosis 276.2
  diabetic 250.1
Ketonuria 791.6
  branched-chain, intermittent 270.3
Ketosis 276.2
  diabetic 250.1
Kidney - *see* condition
Kienböck's
  disease 732.3
    adult 732.8
  osteochondrosis 732.3
Kimmelstiel (-Wilson) disease or syndrome (intercapillary glomerulosclerosis) 250.4 [581.81]
Kink, kinking
  appendix 543.9
  artery 447.1
  cystic duct, congenital 751.61
  hair (acquired) 704.2
  ileum or intestine (*see also* Obstruction, intestine) 560.9
  Lane's (*see also* Obstruction, intestine) 560.9
  organ or site, congenital NEC - *see* Anomaly, specified type NEC, by site
  ureter (pelvic junction) 593.3
    congenital 753.20
  vein(s) 459.2
    caval 459.2
    peripheral 459.2
Kinnier Wilson's disease (hepatolenticular degeneration) 275.1
Kissing
  osteophytes 721.5
  spine 721.5
  vertebra 721.5
Klauder's syndrome (erythema multiforme exudativum) 695.1
Klebs' disease (*see also* Nephritis) 583.9
Klein-Waardenburg syndrome (ptosis-epicanthus) 270.2
Kleine-Levin syndrome 349.89
Kleptomania 312.32
Klinefelter's syndrome 758.7
Klinger's disease 446.4
Klippel's disease 723.8
Klippel-Feil disease or syndrome (brevicollis) 756.16
Klippel-Trenaunay syndrome 759.89
Klumpke (-Déjérine) palsy, paralysis (birth) (newborn) 767.6
Kluver-Bucy (-Terzian) syndrome 310.0
Knee - *see* condition
Knifegrinders' rot (*see also* Tuberculosis) 011.4
Knock-knee (acquired) 736.41
  congenital 755.64
Knot
  intestinal, syndrome (volvulus) 560.2
  umbilical cord (true) 663.2
    affecting fetus or newborn 762.5
Knots, surfer 919.8
  infected 919.9
Knotting (of)
  hair 704.2
  intestine 560.2
Knuckle pads (Garrod's) 728.79
Köbner's disease (epidermolysis bullosa) 757.39
Koch's
  infection (*see also* Tuberculosis, pulmonary) 011.9
  relapsing fever 087.9

Koch-Weeks conjunctivitis 372.03
Koenig-Wichman disease (pemphigus) 694.4
Köhler's disease (osteochondrosis) 732.5
  first (osteochondrosis juvenilis) 732.5
  second (Freiburg's infarction, metatarsal head) 732.5
  patellar 732.4
  tarsal navicular (bone) (osteoarthosis juvenilis) 732.5
Köhler-Mouchet disease (osteoarthrosis juvenilis) 732.5
Köhler-Pellegrini-Stieda disease or syndrome (calcification, knee joint) 726.62
Koilonychia 703.8
  congenital 757.5
Kojevnikov's, Kojewnikoff's epilepsy (*see also* Epilepsy) 345.7
König's
  disease (osteochondritis dissecans) 732.7
  syndrome 564.89
Koniophthisis (*see also* Tuberculosis) 011.4
Koplik's spots 055.9
Kopp's asthma 254.8
Korean hemorrhagic fever 078.6
Korsakoff (-Wernicke) disease, psychosis, or syndrome (nonalcoholic) 294.0
  alcoholic 291.1
Korsakov's disease - *see* Korsakoff's disease
Korsakow's disease - *see* Korsakoff's disease
Kostmann's disease or syndrome (infantile genetic agranulocytosis) 288.0
Krabbe's
  disease (leukodystrophy) 330.0
  syndrome
    congenital muscle hypoplasia 756.89
    cutaneocerebral angioma 759.6
Kraepelin-Morel disease (*see also* Schizophrenia) 295.9
Kraft-Weber-Dimitri disease 759.6
Kraurosis
  ani 569.49
  penis 607.0
  vagina 623.8
  vulva 624.0
Kreotoxism 005.9
Krukenberg's
  spindle 371.13
  tumor (M8490/6) 198.6
Kufs' disease 330.1
Kugelberg-Welander disease 335.11
Kuhnt-Junius degeneration or disease 362.52
Kulchitsky's cell carcinoma (carcinoid tumor of intestine) 259.2
Kummell's disease or spondylitis 721.7
Kundrat's disease (lymphosarcoma) 200.1
Kunekune - *see* Dermatophytosis
Kunkel syndrome (lupoid hepatitis) 571.49
Kupffer cell sarcoma (M9124/3) 155.0
Kuru 046.0
Kussmaul's
  coma (diabetic) 250.3
  disease (polyarteritis nodosa) 446.0
  respiration (air hunger) 786.09
Kwashiorkor (marasmus type) 260
Kyasanur Forest disease 065.2

ICD-9-CM

K

Vol. 2

Kyphoscoliosis, kyphoscoliotic (acquired) (*see also* Scoliosis) 737.30
  congenital 756.19
  due to radiation 737.33
  heart (disease) 416.1
  idiopathic 737.30
    infantile
      progressive 737.32
      resolving 737.31
  late effect of rickets 268.1 [737.43]
  specified NEC 737.39
  thoracogenic 737.34
  tuberculous (*see also* Tuberculosis)
    015.0 [737.43]
Kyphosis, kyphotic (acquired) (postural)
  737.10
  adolescent postural 737.0

Kyphosis, kyphotic (*Continued*)
  congenital 756.19
  dorsalis juvenilis 732.0
  due to or associated with
    Charcôt-Marie-Tooth disease 356.1
      [737.41]
    mucopolysaccharidosis 277.5
      [737.41]
    neurofibromatosis 237.71 [737.41]
    osteitis
      deformans 731.0 [737.41]
      fibrosa cystica 252.01 [737.41] ◄▬
    osteoporosis (*see also* Osteoporosis)
      733.0 [737.41]
    poliomyelitis (*see also* Poliomyelitis)
      138 [737.41]
    radiation 737.11

Kyphosis, kyphotic (*Continued*)
  due to or associated with (*Continued*)
    tuberculosis (*see also* Tuberculosis)
      015.0 [737.41]
    Kümmell's 721.7
    late effect of rickets 268.1 [737.41]
    Morquio-Brailsford type (spinal) 277.5
      [737.41]
    pelvis 738.6
    postlaminectomy 737.12
    specified cause NEC 737.19
    syphilitic, congenital 090.5 [737.41]
    tuberculous (*see also* Tuberculosis)
      015.0 [737.41]
Kyrle's disease (hyperkeratosis follicularis in cutem penetrans) 701.1

◄ **New**   ◄▬ **Revised**

L

Labia, labium - *see* condition
Labiated hymen 752.49
Labile
  blood pressure 796.2
  emotions, emotionality 301.3
  vasomotor system 443.9
Labioglossal paralysis 335.22
Labium leporinum (*see also* Cleft, lip)
  749.10
Labor (*see also* Delivery)
  with complications - *see* Delivery, complicated
  abnormal NEC 661.9
    affecting fetus or newborn 763.7
  arrested active phase 661.1
    affecting fetus or newborn 763.7
  desultory 661.2
    affecting fetus or newborn 763.7
  dyscoordinate 661.4
    affecting fetus or newborn 763.7
  early onset (22-36 weeks gestation) 644.2
  failed
    induction 659.1
      mechanical 659.0
      medical 659.1
      surgical 659.0
    trial (vaginal delivery) 660.6
  false 644.1
  forced or induced, affecting fetus or newborn 763.89
  hypertonic 661.4
    affecting fetus or newborn 763.7
  hypotonic 661.2
    affecting fetus or newborn 763.7
    primary 661.0
      affecting fetus or newborn 763.7
    secondary 661.1
      affecting fetus or newborn 763.7
  incoordinate 661.4
    affecting fetus or newborn 763.7
  irregular 661.2
    affecting fetus or newborn 763.7
  long - *see* Labor, prolonged
  missed (at or near term) 656.4
  obstructed NEC 660.9
    affecting fetus or newborn 763.1
    specified cause NEC 660.8
      affecting fetus or newborn 763.1
  pains, spurious 644.1
  precipitate 661.3
    affecting fetus or newborn 763.6
  premature 644.2
    threatened 644.0
  prolonged or protracted 662.1
    affecting fetus or newborn 763.89
    first stage 662.0
      affecting fetus or newborn 763.89
    second stage 662.2
      affecting fetus or newborn 763.89
  threatened NEC 644.1
  undelivered 644.1
Labored breathing (*see also* Hyperventilation) 786.09
Labyrinthitis (inner ear) (destructive) (latent) 386.30
  circumscribed 386.32
  diffuse 386.31
  focal 386.32
  purulent 386.33

Labyrinthitis (Continued)
  serous 386.31
  suppurative 386.33
  syphilitic 095.8
  toxic 386.34
  viral 386.35
Laceration - *see also* Wound, open, by site
  accidental, complicating surgery 998.2
  Achilles tendon 845.09
    with open wound 892.2
  anus (sphincter) 879.6
    with
      abortion - *see* Abortion, by type, with damage to pelvic organs
      ectopic pregnancy (*see also* categories 633.0-633.9) 639.2
      molar pregnancy (*see also* categories 630-632) 639.2
    complicated 879.7
    complicating delivery 664.2
      with laceration of anal or rectal mucosa 664.3
    following
      abortion 639.2
      ectopic or molar pregnancy 639.2
    nontraumatic, nonpuerperal 565.0
  bladder (urinary)
    with
      abortion - *see* Abortion, by type, with damage to pelvic organs
      ectopic pregnancy (*see also* categories 633.0-633.9) 639.2
      molar pregnancy (*see also* categories 630-632) 639.2
    following
      abortion 639.2
      ectopic or molar pregnancy 639.2
    obstetrical trauma 665.5
  blood vessel - *see* Injury, blood vessel, by site
  bowel
    with
      abortion - *see* Abortion, by type, with damage to pelvic organs
      ectopic pregnancy (*see also* categories 633.0-633.9) 639.2
      molar pregnancy (*see also* categories 630-632) 639.2
    following
      abortion 639.2
      ectopic or molar pregnancy 639.2
    obstetrical trauma 665.5
  brain (cerebral) (membrane) (with hemorrhage) 851.8

Note Use the following fifth-digit subclassification with categories 851-854:

  0 unspecified state of consciousness
  1 with no loss of consciousness
  2 with brief [less than one hour] loss of consciousness
  3 with moderate [1-24 hours] loss of consciousness
  4 with prolonged [more than 24 hours] loss of consciousness and return to pre-existing conscious level
  5 with prolonged [more than 24 hours] loss of consciousness, without return to pre-existing conscious level

Laceration (Continued)
  brain (Continued)

Use fifth-digit 5 to designate when a patient is unconscious and dies before regaining consciousness, regardless of the duration of the loss of consciousness

  6 with loss of consciousness of unspecified duration
  9 with concussion, unspecified

    with
      open intracranial wound 851.9
      skull fracture - *see* Fracture, skull, by site
    cerebellum 851.6
      with open intracranial wound 851.7
    cortex 851.2
      with open intracranial wound 851.3
    during birth 767.0
    stem 851.6
      with open intracranial wound 851.7
  broad ligament
    with
      abortion - *see* Abortion, by type, with damage to pelvic organs
      ectopic pregnancy (*see also* categories 633.0-633.9) 639.2
      molar pregnancy (*see also* categories 630-632) 639.2
    following
      abortion 639.2
      ectopic or molar pregnancy 639.2
    nontraumatic 620.6
    obstetrical trauma 665.6
    syndrome (nontraumatic) 620.6
  capsule, joint - *see* Sprain, by site
  cardiac - *see* Laceration, heart
  causing eversion of cervix uteri (old) 622.0
  central, complicating delivery 664.4
  cerebellum - *see* Laceration, brain, cerebellum
  cerebral - *see also* Laceration, brain
    during birth 767.0
  cervix (uteri)
    with
      abortion - *see* Abortion, by type, with damage to pelvic organs
      ectopic pregnancy (*see also* categories 633.0-633.9) 639.2
      molar pregnancy (*see also* categories 630-632) 639.2
    following
      abortion 639.2
      ectopic or molar pregnancy 639.2
    nonpuerperal, nontraumatic 622.3
    obstetrical trauma (current) 665.3
    old (postpartal) 622.3
    traumatic - *see* Injury, internal, cervix
  chordae heart 429.5
  complicated 879.9
  cornea - *see* Laceration, eyeball
    superficial 918.1
  cortex (cerebral) - *see* Laceration, brain, cortex
  esophagus 530.89
  eye(s) - *see* Laceration, ocular
  eyeball NEC 871.4
    with prolapse or exposure of intraocular tissue 871.1
    penetrating - *see* Penetrating wound, eyeball

Laceration *(Continued)*
  eyeball NEC *(Continued)*
    specified as without prolapse of intraocular tissue 871.0
  eyelid NEC 870.8
    full thickness 870.1
      involving lacrimal passages 870.2
    skin (and periocular area) 870.0
      penetrating - *see* Penetrating wound, orbit
  fourchette
    with
      abortion - *see* Abortion, by type, with damage to pelvic organs
      ectopic pregnancy (*see also* categories 633.0-633.9) 639.2
      molar pregnancy (*see also* categories 630-632) 639.2
    complicating delivery 664.0
    following
      abortion 639.2
      ectopic or molar pregnancy 639.2
  heart (without penetration of heart chambers) 861.02
    with
      open wound into thorax 861.12
      penetration of heart chambers 861.03
        with open wound into thorax 861.13
  hernial sac - *see* Hernia, by site
  internal organ (abdomen) (chest) (pelvis) NEC - *see* Injury, internal, by site
  kidney (parenchyma) 866.02
    with
      complete disruption of parenchyma (rupture) 866.03
        with open wound into cavity 866.13
      open wound into cavity 866.12
  labia
    complicating delivery 664.0
  ligament - *see also* Sprain, by site
    with open wound - *see* Wound, open, by site
  liver 864.05
    with open wound into cavity 864.15
    major (disruption of hepatic parenchyma) 864.04
      with open wound into cavity 864.14
    minor (capsule only) 864.02
      with open wound into cavity 864.12
    moderate (involving parenchyma without major disruption) 864.03
      with open wound into cavity 864.13
    multiple 864.04
      with open wound into cavity 864.14
    stellate 864.04
      with open wound into cavity 864.14
  lung 861.22
    with open wound into thorax 861.32
  meninges - *see* Laceration, brain
  meniscus (knee) (*see also* Tear, meniscus) 836.2
    old 717.5
    site other than knee - *see also* Sprain, by site
      old NEC (*see also* Disorder, cartilage, articular) 718.0

Laceration *(Continued)*
  muscle - *see also* Sprain, by site
    with open wound - *see* Wound, open, by site
  myocardium - *see* Laceration, heart
  nerve - *see* Injury, nerve, by site
  ocular NEC (*see also* Laceration, eyeball) 871.4
    adnexa NEC 870.8
      penetrating 870.3
        with foreign body 870.4
  orbit (eye) 870.8
    penetrating 870.3
      with foreign body 870.4
  pelvic
    floor (muscles)
      with
        abortion - *see* Abortion, by type, with damage to pelvic organs
        ectopic pregnancy (*see also* categories 633.0-633.9) 639.2
        molar pregnancy (*see also* categories 630-632) 639.2
      complicating delivery 664.1
      following
        abortion 639.2
        ectopic or molar pregnancy 639.2
      nonpuerperal 618.7
      old (postpartal) 618.7
    organ NEC
      with
        abortion - *see* Abortion, by type, with damage to pelvic organs
        ectopic pregnancy (*see also* categories 633.0-633.9) 639.2
        molar pregnancy (*see also* categories 630-632) 639.2
      complicating delivery 665.5
        affecting fetus or newborn 763.89
      following
        abortion 639.2
        ectopic or molar pregnancy 639.2
      obstetrical trauma 665.5
  perineum, perineal (old) (postpartal) 618.7
    with
      abortion - *see* Abortion, by type, with damage to pelvic floor
      ectopic pregnancy (*see also* categories 633.0-633.9) 639.2
      molar pregnancy (*see also* categories 630-632) 639.2
    complicating delivery 664.4
      first degree 664.0
      second degree 664.1
      third degree 664.2
      fourth degree 664.3
      central 664.4
      involving
        anal sphincter 664.2
        fourchette 664.0
        hymen 664.0
        labia 664.0
        pelvic floor 664.1
        perineal muscles 664.1
        rectovaginal with septum 664.2
          with anal mucosa 664.3
        skin 664.0
        sphincter (anal) 664.2
          with anal mucosa 664.3
        vagina 664.0

Laceration *(Continued)*
  perineum, perineal *(Continued)*
    complicating delivery *(Continued)*
      involving *(Continued)*
        vaginal muscles 664.1
        vulva 664.0
      secondary 674.2
    following
      abortion 639.2
      ectopic or molar pregnancy 639.2
    male 879.6
      complicated 879.7
    muscles, complicating delivery 664.1
    nonpuerperal, current injury 879.6
      complicated 879.7
    secondary (postpartal) 674.2
  peritoneum
    with
      abortion - *see* Abortion, by type, with damage to pelvic organs
      ectopic pregnancy (*see also* categories 633.0-633.9) 639.2
      molar pregnancy (*see also* categories 630-632) 639.2
    following
      abortion 639.2
      ectopic or molar pregnancy 639.2
    obstetrical trauma 665.5
  periurethral tissue
    with
      abortion - *see* Abortion, by type, with damage to pelvic organs
      ectopic pregnancy (*see also* categories 633.0-633.9) 639.2
      molar pregnancy (*see also* categories 630-632) 639.2
    following
      abortion 639.2
      ectopic or molar pregnancy 639.2
    obstetrical trauma 665.5
  rectovaginal (septum)
    with
      abortion - *see* Abortion, by type, with damage to pelvic organs
      ectopic pregnancy (*see also* categories 633.0-633.9) 639.2
      molar pregnancy (*see also* categories 630-632) 639.2
    complicating delivery 665.4
      with perineum 664.2
        involving anal or rectal mucosa 664.3
    following
      abortion 639.2
      ectopic or molar pregnancy 639.2
    nonpuerperal 623.4
    old (postpartal) 623.4
  spinal cord (meninges) - *see also* Injury, spinal, by site
    due to injury at birth 767.4
    fetus or newborn 767.4
  spleen 865.09
    with
      disruption of parenchyma (massive) 865.04
        with open wound into cavity 865.14
      open wound into cavity 865.19
    capsule (without disruption of parenchyma) 865.02
      with open wound into cavity 865.12
    parenchyma 865.03

◀ **New**   ◀||| **Revised**

Laceration (Continued)
  spleen (Continued)
    parenchyma (Continued)
      with open wound into cavity 865.13
      massive disruption (rupture) 865.04
        with open wound into cavity 865.14
  tendon 848.9
    with open wound - see Wound, open, by site
    Achilles 845.09
      with open wound 892.2
    lower limb NEC 844.9
      with open wound NEC 894.2
    upper limb NEC 840.9
      with open wound NEC 884.2
  tentorium cerebelli - see Laceration, brain, cerebellum
  tongue 873.64
    complicated 873.74
  urethra
    with
      abortion - see Abortion, by type, with damage to pelvic organs
      ectopic pregnancy (see also categories 633.0-633.9) 639.2
      molar pregnancy (see also categories 630-632) 639.2
    following
      abortion 639.2
      ectopic or molar pregnancy 639.2
    nonpuerperal, nontraumatic 599.84
    obstetrical trauma 665.5
  uterus
    with
      abortion - see Abortion, by type, with damage to pelvic organs
      ectopic pregnancy (see also categories 633.0-633.9) 639.2
      molar pregnancy (see also categories 630-632) 639.2
    following
      abortion 639.2
      ectopic or molar pregnancy 639.2
    nonpuerperal, nontraumatic 621.8
    obstetrical trauma NEC 665.5
    old (postpartal) 621.8
  vagina
    with
      abortion - see Abortion, by type, with damage to pelvic organs
      ectopic pregnancy (see also categories 633.0-633.9) 639.2
      molar pregnancy (see also categories 630-632) 639.2
      perineal involvement, complicating delivery 664.0
    complicating delivery 665.4
      first degree 664.0
      second degree 664.1
      third degree 664.2
      fourth degree 664.3
      high 665.4
      muscles 664.1
      sulcus 665.4
      wall 665.4
    following
      abortion 639.2
      ectopic or molar pregnancy 639.2
    nonpuerperal, nontraumatic 623.4
    old (postpartal) 623.4
  valve, heart - see Endocarditis

Laceration (Continued)
  vulva
    with
      abortion - see Abortion, by type, with damage to pelvic organs
      ectopic pregnancy (see also categories 633.0-633.9) 639.2
      molar pregnancy (see also categories 630-632) 639.2
    complicating delivery 664.0
    following
      abortion 639.2
      ectopic or molar pregnancy 639.2
    nonpuerperal, nontraumatic 624.4
    old (postpartal) 624.4
Lachrymal - see condition
Lachrymonasal duct - see condition
Lack of
  appetite (see also Anorexia) 783.0
  care
    in home V60.4
    of adult 995.84
    of infant (at or after birth) 995.52
  coordination 781.3
  development - see also Hypoplasia
    physiological in childhood 783.40
  education V62.3
  energy 780.79
  financial resources V60.2
  food 994.2
    in environment V60.8
  growth in childhood 783.43
  heating V60.1
  housing (permanent) (temporary) V60.0
    adequate V60.1
  material resources V60.2
  medical attention 799.89
  memory (see also Amnesia) 780.93
    mild, following organic brain damage 310.1
  ovulation 628.0
  person able to render necessary care V60.4
  physical exercise V69.0
  physiologic development in childhood 783.40
  posterior occlusal support 524.57 ◀
  prenatal care in current pregnancy V23.7
  shelter V60.0
  sleep V69.4 ◀
  water 994.3
Lacrimal - see condition
Lacrimation, abnormal (see also Epiphora) 375.20
Lacrimonasal duct - see condition
Lactation, lactating (breast) (puerperal) (postpartum)
  defective 676.4
  disorder 676.9
    specified type NEC 676.8
  excessive 676.6
  failed 676.4
  mastitis NEC 675.2
  mother (care and/or examination) V24.1
  nonpuerperal 611.6
  suppressed 676.5
Lacticemia 271.3
  excessive 276.2
Lactosuria 271.3
Lacunar skull 756.0
Laennec's cirrhosis (alcoholic) 571.2
  nonalcoholic 571.5
Lafora's disease 333.2
Lag, lid (nervous) 374.41
Lagleyze-von Hippel disease (retinocerebral angiomatosis) 759.6

Lagophthalmos (eyelid) (nervous) 374.20
  cicatricial 374.23
  keratitis (see also Keratitis) 370.34
  mechanical 374.22
  paralytic 374.21
La grippe - see Influenza
Lahore sore 085.1
Lakes, venous (cerebral) 437.8
Laki-Lorand factor deficiency (see also Defect, coagulation) 286.3
Lalling 307.9
Lambliasis 007.1
Lame back 724.5
Lancereaux's (diabetes, diabetes mellitus with marked emaciation) 250.8 [261]
Landouzy-Déjérine dystrophy (fascioscapulohumeral atrophy) 359.1
Landry's disease or paralysis 357.0
Landry-Guillain-Barré syndrome 357.0
Lane's
  band 751.4
  disease 569.89
  kink (see also Obstruction, intestine) 560.9
Langdon Down's syndrome (mongolism) 758.0
Language abolition 784.69
Lanugo (persistent) 757.4
Laparoscopic surgical procedure converted to open procedure V64.41
Lardaceous
  degeneration (any site) 277.3
  disease 277.3
  kidney 277.3 [583.81]
  liver 277.3
Large
  baby (regardless of gestational age) 766.1
    exceptionally (weight of 4500 grams or more) 766.0
    of diabetic mother 775.0
  ear 744.22
  fetus - see also Oversize, fetus
    causing disproportion 653.5
      with obstructed labor 660.1
  for dates
    fetus or newborn (regardless of gestational age) 766.1
      affecting management of pregnancy 656.6
      exceptionally (weight of 4500 grams or more) 766.0
  physiological cup 743.57
  stature 783.9 ◀
  waxy liver 277.3
  white kidney - see Nephrosis
Larsen's syndrome (flattened facies and multiple congenital dislocations) 755.8
Larsen-Johansson disease (juvenile osteopathia patellae) 732.4
Larva migrans
  cutaneous NEC 126.9
    ancylostoma 126.9
  of Diptera in vitreous 128.0
  visceral NEC 128.0
Laryngeal - see also condition
  syncope 786.2
Laryngismus (acute) (infectious) (stridulous) 478.75
  congenital 748.3
  diphtheritic 032.3
Laryngitis (acute) (edematous) (fibrinous) (gangrenous) (infective) (infiltrative) (malignant) (membranous) (phlegmonous) (pneumococcal)

Laryngitis (Continued)
 (pseudomembranous) (septic) (subglottic) (suppurative) (ulcerative) (viral) 464.00
 with
  influenza, flu, or grippe 487.1
  obstruction 464.01
  tracheitis (see also Laryngotracheitis) 464.20
   with obstruction 464.21
   acute 464.20
    with obstruction 464.21
   chronic 476.1
 atrophic 476.0
 Borrelia vincentii 101
 catarrhal 476.0
 chronic 476.0
  with tracheitis (chronic) 476.1
  due to external agent - see Condition, respiratory, chronic, due to
 diphtheritic (membranous) 032.3
 due to external agent - see Inflammation, respiratory, upper, due to
 H. influenzae 464.00
  with obstruction 464.01
 Hemophilus influenzae 464.00
  with obstruction 464.01
 hypertrophic 476.0
 influenzal 487.1
 pachydermic 478.79
 sicca 476.0
 spasmodic 478.75
  acute 464.00
   with obstruction 464.01
 streptococcal 034.0
 stridulous 478.75
 syphilitic 095.8
  congenital 090.5
 tuberculous (see also Tuberculosis, larynx) 012.3
 Vincent's 101
Laryngocele (congenital) (ventricular) 748.3
Laryngofissure 478.79
 congenital 748.3
Laryngomalacia (congenital) 748.3
Laryngopharyngitis (acute) 465.0
 chronic 478.9
  due to external agent - see Condition, respiratory, chronic, due to
 due to external agent - see Inflammation, respiratory, upper, due to
 septic 034.0
Laryngoplegia (see also Paralysis, vocal cord) 478.30
Laryngoptosis 478.79
Laryngospasm 478.75
 due to external agent - see Condition, respiratory, acute, due to
Laryngostenosis 478.74
 congenital 748.3
Laryngotracheitis (acute) (infectional) (viral) (see also Laryngitis) 464.20
 with obstruction 464.21
 atrophic 476.1
 Borrelia vincentii 101
 catarrhal 476.1
 chronic 476.1
  due to external agent - see Condition, respiratory, chronic, due to
 diphtheritic (membranous) 032.3
 due to external agent - see Inflammation, respiratory, upper, due to
 H. influenzae 464.20
  with obstruction 464.21

Laryngotracheitis (Continued)
 hypertrophic 476.1
 influenzal 487.1
 pachydermic 478.75
 sicca 476.1
 spasmodic 478.75
  acute 464.20
   with obstruction 464.21
 streptococcal 034.0
 stridulous 478.75
 syphilitic 095.8
  congenital 090.5
 tuberculous (see also Tuberculosis, larynx) 012.3
 Vincent's 101
Laryngotracheobronchitis (see also Bronchitis) 490
 acute 466.0
 chronic 491.8
 viral 466.0
Laryngotracheobronchopneumonitis - see Pneumonia, broncho-
Larynx, laryngeal - see condition
Lasègue's disease (persecution mania) 297.9
Lassa fever 078.89
Lassitude (see also Weakness) 780.79
Late - see also condition
 effect(s) (of) - see also condition
  abscess
   intracranial or intraspinal (conditions classifiable to 324) - see category 326
  adverse effect of drug, medicinal or biological substance 909.5
  allergic reaction 909.9
  amputation
   postoperative (late) 997.60
   traumatic (injury classifiable to 885-887 and 895-897) 905.9
  burn (injury classifiable to 948-949) 906.9
   extremities NEC (injury classifiable to 943 or 945) 906.7
   hand or wrist (injury classifiable to 944) 906.6
   eye (injury classifiable to 940) 906.5
   face, head, and neck (injury classifiable to 941) 906.5
   specified site NEC (injury classifiable to 942 and 946-947) 906.8
  cerebrovascular disease (conditions classifiable to 430-437) 438.9
   with
    alteration of sensations 438.6
    aphasia 438.11
    apraxia 438.81
    ataxia 438.84
    cognitive deficits 438.0
    disturbances of vision 438.7
    dysphagia 438.82
    dysphasia 438.12
    facial droop 438.83
    facial weakness 438.83
    hemiplegia/hemiparesis
     affecting
      dominant side 438.21
      nondominant side 438.22
      unspecified side 438.20
    monoplegia of lower limb
     affecting
      dominant side 438.41
      nondominant side 438.42
      unspecified side 438.40

Late (Continued)
 effect(s) (Continued)
  cerebrovascular disease (Continued)
   with (Continued)
    monoplegia of upper limb
     affecting
      dominant side 438.31
      nondominant side 438.32
      unspecified side 438.30
    paralytic syndrome NEC
     affecting
      bilateral 438.53
      dominant side 438.51
      nondominant side 438.52
      unspecified side 438.50
    speech and language deficit 438.10
     specified type NEC 438.19
    specified type NEC 438.89
    vertigo 438.85
  childbirth complication(s) 677
  complication(s) of
   childbirth 677
   delivery 677
   pregnancy 677
   puerperium 677
   surgical and medical care (conditions classifiable to 996-999) 909.3
   trauma (conditions classifiable to 958) 908.6
  contusion (injury classifiable to 920-924) 906.3
  crushing (injury classifiable to 925-929) 906.4
  delivery complication(s) 677
  dislocation (injury classifiable to 830-839) 905.6
  encephalitis or encephalomyelitis (conditions classifiable to 323) - see category 326
   in infectious diseases 139.8
    viral (conditions classifiable to 049.8, 049.9, 062-064) 139.0
  external cause NEC (conditions classifiable to 995) 909.9
   certain conditions classifiable to categories 991-994 909.4
  foreign body in orifice (injury classifiable to 930-939) 908.5
  fracture (multiple) (injury classifiable to 828-829) 905.5
   extremity
    lower (injury classifiable to 821-827) 905.4
     neck of femur (injury classifiable to 820) 905.3
    upper (injury classifiable to 810-819) 905.2
   face and skull (injury classifiable to 800-804) 905.0
   skull and face (injury classifiable to 800-804) 905.0
   spine and trunk (injury classifiable to 805 and 807-809) 905.1
    with spinal cord lesion (injury classifiable to 806) 907.2
  infection
   pyogenic, intracranial - see category 326
  infectious diseases (conditions classifiable to 001-136) NEC 139.8
  injury (injury classifiable to 959) 908.9
   blood vessel 908.3

◀ **New**   ◀▥ **Revised**

Late *(Continued)*
  effect(s) *(Continued)*
    injury *(Continued)*
      blood vessel *(Continued)*
        abdomen and pelvis (injury classifiable to 902) 908.4
        extremity (injury classifiable to 903-904) 908.3
        head and neck (injury classifiable to 900) 908.3
        intracranial (injury classifiable to 850-854) 907.0
          with skull fracture 905.0
        thorax (injury classifiable to 901) 908.4
      internal organ NEC (injury classifiable to 867 and 869) 908.2
        abdomen (injury classifiable to 863-866 and 868) 908.1
        thorax (injury classifiable to 860-862) 908.0
        intracranial (injury classifiable to 850-854) 907.0
          with skull fracture (injury classifiable to 800-801 and 803-804) 905.0
      nerve NEC (injury classifiable to 957) 907.9
        cranial (injury classifiable to 950-951) 907.1
        peripheral NEC (injury classifiable to 957) 907.9
          lower limb and pelvic girdle (injury classifiable to 956) 907.5
          upper limb and shoulder girdle (injury classifiable to 955) 907.4
        roots and plexus(es), spinal (injury classifiable to 953) 907.3
        trunk (injury classifiable to 954) 907.3
      spinal
        cord (injury classifiable to 806 and 952) 907.2
        nerve root(s) and plexus(es) (injury classifiable to 953) 907.3
      superficial (injury classifiable to 910-919) 906.2
      tendon (tendon injury classifiable to 840-848, 880-884 with .2, and 890-894 with .2) 905.8
    meningitis
      bacterial (conditions classifiable to 320) - *see* category 326
      unspecified cause (conditions classifiable to 322) - *see* category 326
    myelitis (*see also* Late, effect(s) (of), encephalitis) - *see* category 326
    parasitic diseases (conditions classifiable to 001-136 NEC) 139.8
    phlebitis or thrombophlebitis of intracranial venous sinuses (conditions classifiable to 325) - *see* category 326
    poisoning due to drug, medicinal or biological substance (conditions classifiable to 960-979) 909.0
    poliomyelitis, acute (conditions classifiable to 045) 138
    pregnancy complication(s) 677
    puerperal complication(s) 677
    radiation (conditions classifiable to 990) 909.2
    rickets 268.1

Late *(Continued)*
  effect(s) *(Continued)*
    sprain and strain without mention of tendon injury (injury classifiable to 840-848, except tendon injury) 905.7
      tendon involvement 905.8
    toxic effect of
      drug, medicinal or biological substance (conditions classifiable to 960-979) 909.0
      nonmedical substance (conditions classifiable to 980-989) 909.1
    trachoma (conditions classifiable to 076) 139.1
    tuberculosis 137.0
      bones and joints (conditions classifiable to 015) 137.3
      central nervous system (conditions classifiable to 013) 137.1
      genitourinary (conditions classifiable to 016) 137.2
      pulmonary (conditions classifiable to 010-012) 137.0
      specified organs NEC (conditions classifiable to 014, 017-018) 137.4
    viral encephalitis (conditions classifiable to 049.8, 049.9, 062-064) 139.0
    wound, open
      extremity (injury classifiable to 880-884 and 890-894, except .2) 906.1
        tendon (injury classifiable to 880-884 with .2 and 890-894 with .2) 905.8
      head, neck, and trunk (injury classifiable to 870-879) 906.0
    infant
      post-term (gestation period over 40 completed weeks to 42 completed weeks) 766.21
      prolonged gestation (period over 42 completed weeks) 766.22
Latent - *see* condition
Lateral - *see* condition
Laterocession - *see* Lateroversion
Lateroflexion - *see* Lateroversion
Lateroversion
  cervix - *see* Lateroversion, uterus
  uterus, uterine (cervix) (postinfectional) (postpartal, old) 621.6
    congenital 752.3
    in pregnancy or childbirth 654.4
      affecting fetus or newborn 763.89
Lathyrism 988.2
Launois' syndrome (pituitary gigantism) 253.0
Launois-Bensaude's lipomatosis 272.8
Launois-Cleret syndrome (adiposogenital dystrophy) 253.8
Laurence-Moon-Biedl syndrome (obesity, polydactyly, and mental retardation) 759.89
LAV (disease) (illness) (infection) - *see* Human immunodeficiency virus (disease) (illness) (infection)
LAV/HTLV-III (disease) (illness) (infection) - *see* Human immunodeficiency virus (disease) (illness) (infection)
Lawford's syndrome (encephalocutaneous angiomatosis) 759.6
Lax, laxity - *see also* Relaxation
  ligament 728.4
  skin (acquired) 701.8
    congenital 756.83

Laxative habit (*see also* Abuse, drugs, nondependent) 305.9
Lazy leukocyte syndrome 288.0
LCAD (long chain/very long chain acyl CoA dehydrogenase deficiency, VLCAD) 277.85 ◄
LCHAD (long chain 3-hydroxyacyl CoA dehydrogenase deficiency) 277.85 ◄
Lead - *see also* condition
  exposure to V15.86
  incrustation of cornea 371.15
  poisoning 984.0
    specified type of lead - *see* Table of Drugs and Chemicals
Lead miners' lung 503
Leakage
  amniotic fluid 658.1
    with delayed delivery 658.2
    affecting fetus or newborn 761.1
  bile from drainage tube (T tube) 997.4
  blood (microscopic), fetal, into maternal circulation 656.0
    affecting management of pregnancy or puerperium 656.0
  device, implant, or graft - *see* Complications, mechanical
  spinal fluid at lumbar puncture site 997.09
  urine, continuous 788.37
Leaky heart - *see* Endocarditis
Learning defect, specific NEC (strephosymbolia) 315.2
Leather bottle stomach (M8142/3) 151.9
Leber's
  congenital amaurosis 362.76
  optic atrophy (hereditary) 377.16
Lederer's anemia or disease (acquired infectious hemolytic anemia) 283.19
Lederer-Brill syndrome (acquired infectious hemolytic anemia) 283.19
Leeches (aquatic) (land) 134.2
Left-sided neglect 781.8
Leg - *see* condition
Legal investigation V62.5
Legg (-Calvé)-Perthes disease or syndrome (osteochondrosis, femoral capital) 732.1
Legionnaires' disease 482.84
Leigh's disease 330.8
Leiner's disease (exfoliative dermatitis) 695.89
Leiofibromyoma (M8890/0) - *see also* Leiomyoma
  uterus (cervix) (corpus) (*see also* Leiomyoma, uterus) 218.9
Leiomyoblastoma (M8891/1) - *see* Neoplasm, connective tissue, uncertain behavior
Leiomyofibroma (M8890/0) - *see also* Neoplasm, connective tissue, benign
  uterus (cervix) (corpus) (*see also* Leiomyoma, uterus) 218.9
Leiomyoma (M8890/0) - *see also* Neoplasm, connective tissue, benign
  bizarre (M8893/0) - *see* Neoplasm, connective tissue, benign
  cellular (M8892/1) - *see* Neoplasm, connective tissue, uncertain behavior
  epithelioid (M8891/1) - *see* Neoplasm, connective tissue, uncertain behavior
  prostate (polypoid) 600.20
    with urinary retention 600.21
  uterus (cervix) (corpus) 218.9
    interstitial 218.1
    intramural 218.1
    submucous 218.0
    subperitoneal 218.2
    subserous 218.2
  vascular (M8894/0) - *see* Neoplasm, connective tissue, benign

Leiomyomatosis (intravascular) (M8890/
1) - *see* Neoplasm, connective tissue,
uncertain behavior
Leiomyosarcoma (M8890/3) - *see also*
Neoplasm, connective tissue, malignant
epithelioid (M8891/3) - *see* Neoplasm,
connective tissue, malignant
Leishmaniasis 085.9
American 085.5
cutaneous 085.4
mucocutaneous 085.5
Asian desert 085.2
Brazilian 085.5
cutaneous 085.9
acute necrotizing 085.2
American 085.4
Asian desert 085.2
diffuse 085.3
dry form 085.1
Ethiopian 085.3
eyelid 085.5 [373.6]
late 085.1
lepromatous 085.3
recurrent 085.1
rural 085.2
ulcerating 085.1
urban 085.1
wet form 085.2
zoonotic form 085.2
dermal - *see also* Leishmaniasis, cutaneous
post kala-azar 085.0
eyelid 085.5 [373.6]
infantile 085.0
Mediterranean 085.0
mucocutaneous (American) 085.5
naso-oral 085.5
nasopharyngeal 085.5
Old World 085.1
tegumentaria diffusa 085.4
vaccination, prophylactic (against)
V05.2
visceral (Indian) 085.0
Leishmanoid, dermal - *see also* Leishmaniasis, cutaneous
post kala-azar 085.0
Leloir's disease 695.4
Lemiere syndrome 451.89   ◄
Lenegre's disease 426.0
Lengthening, leg 736.81
Lennox-Gastaut syndrome 345.0   ◄
with tonic seizures 345.1   ◄
Lennox's syndrome (*see also* Epilepsy)
345.0
Lens - *see* condition
Lenticonus (anterior) (posterior) (congenital) 743.36
Lenticular degeneration, progressive
275.1
Lentiglobus (posterior) (congenital)
743.36
Lentigo (congenital) 709.09
juvenile 709.09
maligna (M8742/2) - *see also* Neoplasm, skin, in situ
melanoma (M8742/3) - *see* Melanoma
senile 709.09
Leonine leprosy 030.0
Leontiasis
ossium 733.3
syphilitic 095.8
congenital 090.5
Léopold-Lévi's syndrome (paroxysmal
thyroid instability) 242.9

Lepore hemoglobin syndrome 282.49
Lepothrix 039.0
Lepra 030.9
Willan's 696.1
Leprechaunism 259.8
Lepromatous leprosy 030.0
Leprosy 030.9
anesthetic 030.1
beriberi 030.1
borderline (group B) (infiltrated) (neuritic) 030.3
cornea (*see also* Leprosy, by type) 030.9
[371.89]
dimorphous (group B) (infiltrated)
(lepromatous) (neuritic) (tuberculoid) 030.3
eyelid 030.0 [373.4]
indeterminate (group I) (macular)
(neuritic) (uncharacteristic) 030.2
leonine 030.0
lepromatous (diffuse) (infiltrated)
(macular) (neuritic) (nodular)
(type L) 030.0
macular (early) (neuritic) (simple) 030.2
maculoanesthetic 030.1
mixed 030.0
neuro 030.1
nodular 030.0
primary neuritic 030.3
specified type or group NEC 030.8
tubercular 030.1
tuberculoid (macular) (maculoanesthetic) (major) (minor) (neuritic)
(type T) 030.1
Leptocytosis, hereditary 282.49
Leptomeningitis (chronic) (circumscribed) (hemorrhagic) (nonsuppurative) (*see also* Meningitis) 322.9
aseptic 047.9
adenovirus 049.1
Coxsackie virus 047.0
ECHO virus 047.1
enterovirus 047.9
lymphocytic choriomeningitis 049.0
epidemic 036.0
late effect - *see* category 326
meningococcal 036.0
pneumococcal 320.1
syphilitic 094.2
tuberculous (*see also* Tuberculosis, meninges) 013.0
Leptomeningopathy (*see also* Meningitis)
322.9
Leptospiral - *see* condition
Leptospirochetal - *see* condition
Leptospirosis 100.9
autumnalis 100.89
canicula 100.89
grippotyphosa 100.89
hebdomadis 100.89
icterohemorrhagica 100.0
nanukayami 100.89
pomona 100.89
Weil's disease 100.0
Leptothricosis - *see* Actinomycosis
Leptothrix infestation - *see* Actinomycosis
Leptotricosis - *see* Actinomycosis
Leptus dermatitis 133.8
Léris pleonosteosis 756.89
Léri-Weill syndrome 756.59
Leriche's syndrome (aortic bifurcation
occlusion) 444.0
Lermoyez's syndrome (*see also* Disease,
Ménière's) 386.00

Lesbianism - *omit code*
ego-dystonic 302.0
problems with 302.0
Lesch-Nyhan syndrome (hypoxanthine-
guanine-phosphoribosyltransferase
deficiency) 277.2
Lesion
abducens nerve 378.54
alveolar process 525.8
anorectal 569.49
aortic (valve) - *see* Endocarditis, aortic
auditory nerve 388.5
basal ganglion 333.90
bile duct (*see also* Disease, biliary) 576.8
bladder 596.9
bone 733.90
brachial plexus 353.0
brain 348.8
congenital 742.9
vascular (*see also* Lesion, cerebrovascular) 437.9
degenerative 437.1
healed or old without residuals
V12.59
hypertensive 437.2
late effect - *see* Late effect(s) (of)
cerebrovascular disease
buccal 528.9
calcified - *see* Calcification
canthus 373.9
carate - *see* Pinta, lesions
cardia 537.89
cardiac - *see also* Disease, heart
congenital 746.9
valvular - *see* Endocarditis
cauda equina 344.60
with neurogenic bladder 344.61
cecum 569.89
cerebral - *see* Lesion, brain
cerebrovascular (*see also* Disease, cerebrovascular NEC) 437.9
degenerative 437.1
healed or old without residuals
V12.59
hypertensive 437.2
specified type NEC 437.8
cervical root (nerve) NEC 353.2
chiasmal 377.54
associated with
inflammatory disorders 377.54
neoplasm NEC 377.52
pituitary 377.51
pituitary disorders 377.51
vascular disorders 377.53
chorda tympani 351.8
coin, lung 793.1
colon 569.89
congenital - *see* Anomaly
conjunctiva 372.9
coronary artery (*see also* Ischemia,
heart) 414.9
cranial nerve 352.9
first 352.0
second 377.49
third
partial 378.51
total 378.52
fourth 378.53
fifth 350.9
sixth 378.54
seventh 351.9
eighth 388.5
ninth 352.2
tenth 352.3

Lesion (*Continued*)
  cranial nerve (*Continued*)
    eleventh 352.4
    twelfth 352.5
  cystic - *see* Cyst
  degenerative - *see* Degeneration
  dermal (skin) 709.9
  Dieulafoy (hemorrhagic)
    of
      duodenum 537.84
      intestine 569.86
      stomach 537.84
  duodenum 537.89
    with obstruction 537.3
  eyelid 373.9
  gasserian ganglion 350.8
  gastric 537.89
  gastroduodenal 537.89
  gastrointestinal 569.89
  glossopharyngeal nerve 352.2
  heart (organic) - *see also* Disease, heart
    vascular - *see* Disease, cardiovascular
  helix (ear) 709.9
  hyperchromic, due to pinta (carate)
    103.1
  hyperkeratotic (*see also* Hyperkeratosis)
    701.1
  hypoglossal nerve 352.5
  hypopharynx 478.29
  hypothalamic 253.9
  ileocecal coil 569.89
  ileum 569.89
  iliohypogastric nerve 355.79
  ilioinguinal nerve 355.79
  in continuity - *see* Injury, nerve, by site
  inflammatory - *see* Inflammation
  intestine 569.89
  intracerebral - *see* Lesion, brain
  intrachiasmal (optic) (*see also* Lesion,
    chiasmal) 377.54
  intracranial, space-occupying NEC
    784.2
  joint 719.90
    ankle 719.97
    elbow 719.92
    foot 719.97
    hand 719.94
    hip 719.95
    knee 719.96
    multiple sites 719.99
    pelvic region 719.95
    sacroiliac (old) 724.6
    shoulder (region) 719.91
    specified site NEC 719.98
    wrist 719.93
  keratotic (*see also* Keratosis) 701.1
  kidney (*see also* Disease, renal) 593.9
  laryngeal nerve (recurrent) 352.3
  leonine 030.0
  LGSIL (low grade squamous intraepi-
    thelial dysplasia 622.1
  lip 528.5
  liver 573.8
  lumbosacral
    plexus 353.1
    root (nerve) NEC 353.4
  lung 518.89
    coin 793.1
  maxillary sinus 473.0
  mitral - *see* Endocarditis, mitral
  motor cortex 348.8
  nerve (*see also* Disorder, nerve) 355.9
  nervous system 349.9
    congenital 742.9

Lesion (*Continued*)
  nonallopathic NEC 739.9
    in region (of)
      abdomen 739.9
      acromioclavicular 739.7
      cervical, cervicothoracic 739.1
      costochondral 739.8
      costovertebral 739.8
      extremity
        lower 739.6
        upper 739.7
      head 739.0
      hip 739.5
      lower extremity 739.6
      lumbar, lumbosacral 739.3
      occipitocervical 739.0
      pelvic 739.5
      pubic 739.5
      rib cage 739.8
      sacral, sacrococcygeal, sacroiliac
        739.4
      sternochondral 739.8
      sternoclavicular 739.7
      thoracic, thoracolumbar 739.2
      upper extremity 739.7
  nose (internal) 478.1
  obstructive - *see* Obstruction
  obturator nerve 355.79
  occlusive
    artery - *see* Embolism, artery
  organ or site NEC - *see* Disease, by site
  osteolytic 733.90
  paramacular, of retina 363.32
  peptic 537.89
  periodontal, due to traumatic occlusion
    523.8
  perirectal 569.49
  peritoneum (granulomatous)
    568.89
  pigmented (skin) 709.00
  pinta - *see* Pinta, lesions
  polypoid - *see* Polyp
  prechiasmal (optic) (*see also* Lesion,
    chiasmal) 377.54
  primary - *see also* Syphilis, primary
    carate 103.0
    pinta 103.0
    yaws 102.0
  pulmonary 518.89
    valve (*see also* Endocarditis, pulmo-
      nary) 424.3
  pylorus 537.89
  radiation NEC 990
  radium NEC 990
  rectosigmoid 569.89
  retina, retinal - *see also* Retinopathy
    vascular 362.17
  retroperitoneal 568.89
  romanus 720.1
  sacroiliac (joint) 724.6
  salivary gland 527.8
    benign lymphoepithelial 527.8
  saphenous nerve 355.79
  secondary - *see* Syphilis, secondary
  sigmoid 569.89
  sinus (accessory) (nasal) (*see also* Sinus-
    itis) 473.9
  skin 709.9
    suppurative 686.00
  SLAP (superior glenoid labrum) 840.7
  space-occupying, intracranial NEC
    784.2
  spinal cord 336.9
    congenital 742.9

Lesion (*Continued*)
  spinal cord (*Continued*)
    traumatic (complete) (incomplete)
      (transverse) - *see also* Injury, spi-
      nal, by site
      with
        broken
          back - *see* Fracture, vertebra,
            by site, with spinal cord
            injury
          neck - *see* Fracture, vertebra,
            cervical, with spinal cord
            injury
        fracture, vertebra - *see* Fracture,
          vertebra, by site, with spi-
          nal cord injury
  spleen 289.50
  stomach 537.89
  superior glenoid labrum (SLAP) 840.7
  syphilitic - *see* Syphilis
  tertiary - *see* Syphilis, tertiary
  thoracic root (nerve) 353.3
  tonsillar fossa 474.9
  tooth, teeth 525.8
    white spot 521.01
  traumatic NEC (*see also* nature and site
    of injury) 959.9
  tricuspid (valve) - *see* Endocarditis, tri-
    cuspid
  trigeminal nerve 350.9
  ulcerated or ulcerative - *see* Ulcer
  uterus NEC 621.9
  vagina 623.8
  vagus nerve 352.3
  valvular - *see* Endocarditis
  vascular 459.9
    affecting central nervous system (*see
      also* Lesion, cerebrovascular)
      437.9
    following trauma (*see also* Injury,
      blood vessel, by site) 904.9
    retina 362.17
    traumatic - *see* Injury, blood vessel,
      by site
    umbilical cord 663.6
      affecting fetus or newborn 762.6
  visual
    cortex NEC (*see also* Disorder, visual,
      cortex) 377.73
    pathway NEC (*see also* Disorder, vis-
      ual, pathway) 377.63
  warty - *see* Verruca
  white spot, on teeth 521.01
  x-ray NEC 990
Lethargic - *see* condition
Lethargy 780.79
Letterer-Siwe disease (acute histiocytosis
  X) (M9722/3) 202.5
Leucinosis 270.3
Leucocoria 360.44
Leucosarcoma (M9850/3) 207.8
Leukasmus 270.2
Leukemia, leukemic (congenital)
  (M9800/3) 208.9

Note Use the following fifth-digit
subclassification for categories 203-
208:

  0   without mention of remission
  1   with remission

acute NEC (M9801/3) 208.0
aleukemic NEC (M9804/3) 208.8
  granulocytic (M9864/3) 205.8

Leukemia, leukemic (*Continued*)
basophilic (M9870/3) 205.1
blast (cell) (M9801/3) 208.0
blastic (M9801/3) 208.0
granulocytic (M9861/3) 205.0
chronic NEC (M9803/3) 208.1
compound (M9810/3) 207.8
eosinophilic (M9880/3) 205.1
giant cell (M9910/3) 207.2
granulocytic (M9860/3) 205.9
acute (M9861/3) 205.0
aleukemic (M9864/3) 205.8
blastic (M9861/3) 205.0
chronic (M9863/3) 205.1
subacute (M9862/3) 205.2
subleukemic (M9864/3) 205.8
hairy cell (M9940/3) 202.4
hemoblastic (M9801/3) 208.0
histiocytic (M9890/3) 206.9
lymphatic (M9820/3) 204.9
acute (M9821/3) 204.0
aleukemic (M9824/3) 204.8
chronic (M9823/3) 204.1
subacute (M9822/3) 204.2
subleukemic (M9824/3) 204.8
lymphoblastic (M9821/3) 204.0
lymphocytic (M9820/3) 204.9
acute (M9821/3) 204.0
aleukemic (M9824/3) 204.8
chronic (M9823/3) 204.1
subacute (M9822/3) 204.2
subleukemic (M9824/3) 204.8
lymphogenous (M9820/3) - *see* Leukemia, lymphoid
lymphoid (M9820/3) 204.9
acute (M9821/3) 204.0
aleukemic (M9824/3) 204.8
blastic (M9821/3) 204.0
chronic (M9823/3) 204.1
subacute (M9822/3) 204.2
subleukemic (M9824/3) 204.8
lymphosarcoma cell (M9850/3) 207.8
mast cell (M9900/3) 207.8
megakaryocytic (M9910/3) 207.2
megakaryocytoid (M9910/3) 207.2
mixed (cell) (M9810/3) 207.8
monoblastic (M9891/3) 206.0
monocytic (Schilling-type) (M9890/3) 206.9
acute (M9891/3) 206.0
aleukemic (M9894/3) 206.8
chronic (M9893/3) 206.1
Naegeli-type (M9863/3) 205.1
subacute (M9892/3) 206.2
subleukemic (M9894/3) 206.8
monocytoid (M9890/3) 206.9
acute (M9891/3) 206.0
aleukemic (M9894/3) 206.8
chronic (M9893/3) 206.1
myelogenous (M9863/3) 205.1
subacute (M9892/3) 206.2
subleukemic (M9894/3) 206.8
monomyelocytic (M9860/3) - *see* Leukemia, myelomonocytic
myeloblastic (M9861/3) 205.0
myelocytic (M9863/3) 205.1
acute (M9861/3) 205.0
myelogenous (M9860/3) 205.9
acute (M9861/3) 205.0
aleukemic (M9864/3) 205.8
chronic (M9863/3) 205.1
monocytoid (M9863/3) 205.1
subacute (M9862/3) 205.2
subleukemic (M9864) 205.8
myeloid (M9860/3) 205.9

Leukemia, leukemic (*Continued*)
myeloid (M9860/3) (*Continued*)
acute (M9861/3) 205.0
aleukemic (M9864/3) 205.8
chronic (M9863/3) 205.1
subacute (M9862/3) 205.2
subleukemic (M9864/3) 205.8
myelomonocytic (M9860/3) 205.9
acute (M9861/3) 205.0
chronic (M9863/3) 205.1
Naegeli-type monocytic (M9863/3) 205.1
neutrophilic (M9865/3) 205.1
plasma cell (M9830/3) 203.1
plasmacytic (M9830/3) 203.1
prolymphocytic (M9825/3) - *see* Leukemia, lymphoid
promyelocytic, acute (M9866/3) 205.0
Schilling-type monocytic (M9890/3) - *see* Leukemia, monocytic
stem cell (M9801/3) 208.0
subacute NEC (M9802/3) 208.2
subleukemic NEC (M9804/3) 208.8
thrombocytic (M9910/3) 207.2
undifferentiated (M9801/3) 208.0
Leukemoid reaction (lymphocytic) (monocytic) (myelocytic) 288.8
Leukoclastic vasculitis 446.29
Leukocoria 360.44
Leukocythemia - *see* Leukemia
Leukocytosis 288.8
basophilic 288.8
eosinophilic 288.3
lymphocytic 288.8
monocytic 288.8
neutrophilic 288.8
Leukoderma 709.09
syphilitic 091.3
late 095.8
Leukodermia (*see also* Leukoderma) 709.09
Leukodystrophy (cerebral) (globoid cell) (metachromatic) (progressive) (sudanophilic) 330.0
Leukoedema, mouth or tongue 528.79 ◀▥
Leukoencephalitis
acute hemorrhagic (postinfectious) NEC 136.9 *[323.6]*
postimmunization or postvaccinal 323.5
subacute sclerosing 046.2
van Bogaert's 046.2
van Bogaert's (sclerosing) 046.2
Leukoencephalopathy (*see also* Encephalitis) 323.9
acute necrotizing hemorrhagic (postinfectious) 136.9 *[323.6]*
postimmunization or postvaccinal 323.5
metachromatic 330.0
multifocal (progressive) 046.3
progressive multifocal 046.3
Leukoerythroblastosis 289.0
Leukoerythrosis 289.0
Leukokeratosis (*see also* Leukoplakia) 702.8
mouth 528.6
nicotina palati 528.79 ◀▥
tongue 528.6
Leukokoria 360.44
Leukokraurosis vulva, vulvae 624.0
Leukolymphosarcoma (M9850/3) 207.8
Leukoma (cornea) (interfering with central vision) 371.03
adherent 371.04
Leukomalacia, periventricular 779.7
Leukomelanopathy, hereditary 288.2

Leukonychia (punctata) (striata) 703.8
congenital 757.5
Leukopathia
unguium 703.8
congenital 757.5
Leukopenia 288.0
cyclic 288.0
familial 288.0
malignant 288.0
periodic 288.0
transitory neonatal 776.7
Leukopenic - *see* condition
Leukoplakia 702.8
anus 569.49
bladder (postinfectional) 596.8
buccal 528.6
cervix (uteri) 622.2
esophagus 530.83
gingiva 528.6
kidney (pelvis) 593.89
larynx 478.79
lip 528.6
mouth 528.6
oral soft tissue (including tongue) (mucosa) 528.6
palate 528.6
pelvis (kidney) 593.89
penis (infectional) 607.0
rectum 569.49
syphilitic 095.8
tongue 528.6
tonsil 478.29
ureter (postinfectional) 593.89
urethra (postinfectional) 599.84
uterus 621.8
vagina 623.1
vesical 596.8
vocal cords 478.5
vulva 624.0
Leukopolioencephalopathy 330.0
Leukorrhea (vagina) 623.5
due to Trichomonas (vaginalis) 131.00
trichomonal (Trichomonas vaginalis) 131.00
Leukosarcoma (M9850/3) 207.8
Leukosis (M9800/3) - *see* Leukemia
Lev's disease or syndrome (acquired complete heart block) 426.0
Levi's syndrome (pituitary dwarfism) 253.3
Levocardia (isolated) 746.87
with situs inversus 759.3
Levulosuria 271.2
Lewandowski's disease (primary) (*see also* Tuberculosis) 017.0
Lewandowski-Lutz disease (epidermodysplasia verruciformis) 078.19
Lewy body dementia 331.82
Lewy body disease 331.82
Leyden's disease (periodic vomiting) 536.2
Leyden-Möbius dystrophy 359.1
Leydig cell
carcinoma (M8650/3)
specified site - *see* Neoplasm, by site, malignant
unspecified site
female 183.0
male 186.9
tumor (M8650/1)
benign (M8650/0)
specified site - *see* Neoplasm, by site, benign
unspecified site
female 220
male 222.0

◀ New   ◀▥ Revised

Leydig cell (*Continued*)
  tumor (*Continued*)
    malignant (M8650/3)
      specified site - *see* Neoplasm, by
        site, malignant
      unspecified site
        female 183.0
        male 186.9
    specified site - *see* Neoplasm, by site,
      uncertain behavior
    unspecified site
      female 236.2
      male 236.4
Leydig-Sertoli cell tumor (M8631/0)
  specified site - *see* Neoplasm, by site,
    benign
  unspecified site
    female 220
    male 222.0
LGSIL (low grade squamous intraepithelial lesion) 795.03 ◀▬
Liar, pathologic 301.7
Libman-Sacks disease or syndrome
  710.0 [424.91]
Lice (infestation) 132.9
  body (pediculus corporis) 132.1
  crab 132.2
  head (pediculus capitis) 132.0
  mixed (classifiable to more than one of
    the categories 132.0-132.2) 132.3
  pubic (pediculus pubis) 132.2
Lichen 697.9
  albus 701.0
  annularis 695.89
  atrophicus 701.0
  corneus obtusus 698.3
  myxedematous 701.8
  nitidus 697.1
  pilaris 757.39
    acquired 701.1
  planopilaris 697.0
  planus (acute) (chronicus) (hyper-
    trophic) (verrucous) 697.0
    morphoeicus 701.0
    sclerosus (et atrophicus) 701.0
  ruber 696.4
    acuminatus 696.4
    moniliformis 697.8
    obtusus corneus 698.3
    of Wilson 697.0
    planus 697.0
  sclerosus (et atrophicus) 701.0
  scrofulosus (primary) (*see also* Tubercu-
    losis) 017.0
  simplex (Vidal's) 698.3
    chronicus 698.3
    circumscriptus 698.3
  spinulosus 757.39
    mycotic 117.9
  striata 697.8
  urticatus 698.2
Lichenification 698.3
  nodular 698.3
Lichenoides tuberculosis (primary) (*see
  also* Tuberculosis) 017.0
Lichtheim's disease or syndrome (subacute combined sclerosis with pernicious anemia) 281.0 [336.2]
Lien migrans 289.59
Lientery (*see also* Diarrhea) 787.91
  infectious 009.2
Life circumstance problem NEC V62.89
Li-Fraumeni cancer syndrome V84.01 ◀▬
Ligament - *see* condition

Light-for-dates (infant) 764.0
  with signs of fetal malnutrition 764.1
  affecting management of pregnancy
    656.5
Light-headedness 780.4
Lightning (effects) (shock) (stroke)
  (struck by) 994.0
  burn - *see* Burn, by site
  foot 266.2
Lightwood's disease or syndrome (renal
  tubular acidosis) 588.89 ◀▬
Lignac's disease (cystinosis) 270.0
Lignac (-de Toni) (-Fanconi) (-Debré)
  syndrome (cystinosis) 270.0
Lignac (-Fanconi) syndrome (cystinosis)
  270.0
Ligneous thyroiditis 245.3
Likoff's syndrome (angina in meno-
  pausal women) 413.9
Limb - *see* condition
Limitation of joint motion (*see also* Stiff-
  ness, joint) 719.5
  sacroiliac 724.6
Limit dextrinosis 271.0
Limited
  cardiac reserve - *see* Disease, heart
  duction, eye NEC 378.63
  mandibular range of motion 524.52 ◀
Lindau's disease (retinocerebral angio-
  matosis) 759.6
Lindau (-von Hippel) disease (angio-
  matosis retinocerebellosa) 759.6
Linea corneae senilis 371.41
Lines
  Beau's (transverse furrows on finger-
    nails) 703.8
  Harris' 733.91
  Hudson-Stähli 371.11
  Stähli's 371.11
Lingua
  geographical 529.1
  nigra (villosa) 529.3
  plicata 529.5
    congenital 750.13
  tylosis 528.6
Lingual (tongue) - *see also* condition
  thyroid 759.2
Linitis (gastric) 535.4
  plastica (M8142/3) 151.9
Lioderma essentialis (cum melanosis et
  telangiectasia) 757.33
Lip - *see also* condition
  biting 528.9
Lipalgia 272.8
Lipedema - *see* Edema
Lipemia (*see also* Hyperlipidemia)
  272.4
  retina, retinalis 272.3
Lipidosis 272.7
  cephalin 272.7
  cerebral (infantile) (juvenile) (late) 330.1
  cerebroretinal 330.1 [362.71]
  cerebroside 272.7
  cerebrospinal 272.7
  chemically induced 272.7
  cholesterol 272.7
  diabetic 250.8 [272.7]
  dystopic (hereditary) 272.7
  glycolipid 272.7
  hepatosplenomegalic 272.3
  hereditary, dystopic 272.7
  sulfatide 330.0
Lipoadenoma (M8324/0 - *see* Neoplasm,
  by site, benign

Lipoblastoma (M8881/0) - *see* Lipoma,
  by site
Lipoblastomatosis (M8881/0) - *see* Li-
  poma, by site
Lipochondrodystrophy 277.5
Lipochrome histiocytosis (familial) 288.1
Lipodystrophia progressiva 272.6
Lipodystrophy (progressive) 272.6
  insulin 272.6
  intestinal 040.2
Lipofibroma (M8851/0) - *see* Lipoma, by
  site
Lipoglycoproteinosis 272.8
Lipogranuloma, sclerosing 709.8
Lipogranulomatosis (disseminated) 272.8
  kidney 272.8
Lipoid - *see also* condition
  histiocytosis 272.7
    essential 272.7
  nephrosis (*see also* Nephrosis) 581.3
  proteinosis of Urbach 272.8
Lipoidemia (*see also* Hyperlipidemia) 272.4
Lipoidosis (*see also* Lipidosis) 272.7
Lipoma (M8850/0) 214.9
  breast (skin) 214.1
  face 214.0
  fetal (M8881/0) - *see also* Lipoma, by
    site
    fat cell (M8880/0) - *see* Lipoma, by
      site
  infiltrating (M8856/0) - *see* Lipoma, by
    site
  intra-abdominal 214.3
  intramuscular (M8856/0) - *see* Lipoma,
    by site
  intrathoracic 214.2
  kidney 214.3
  mediastinum 214.2
  muscle 214.8
  peritoneum 214.3
  retroperitoneum 214.3
  skin 214.1
    face 214.0
  spermatic cord 214.4
  spindle cell (M8857/0) - *see* Lipoma,
    by site
  stomach 214.3
  subcutaneous tissue 214.1
    face 214.0
  thymus 214.2
  thyroid gland 214.2
Lipomatosis (dolorosa) 272.8
  epidural 214.8
  fetal (M8881/0) - *see* Lipoma, by site
  Launois-Bensaude's 272.8
Lipomyohemangioma (M8860/0)
  specified site - *see* Neoplasm, connec-
    tive tissue, benign
  unspecified site 223.0
Lipomyoma (M8860/0)
  specified site - *see* Neoplasm, connec-
    tive tissue, benign
  unspecified site 223.0
Lipomyxoma (M8852/0) - *see* Lipoma, by
  site
Lipomyxosarcoma (M8852/3) - *see* Neoplasm, connective tissue, malignant
Lipophagocytosis 289.89
Lipoproteinemia (alpha) 272.4
  broad-beta 272.2
  floating-beta 272.2
  hyper-pre-beta 272.1
Lipoproteinosis (Rossle-Urbach-Wiethe)
  272.8

Liposarcoma (M8850/3) - *see also* Neoplasm, connective tissue, malignant
  differentiated type (M8851/3) - *see* Neoplasm, connective tissue, malignant
  embryonal (M8852/3) - *see* Neoplasm, connective tissue, malignant
  mixed type (M8855/3) - *see* Neoplasm, connective tissue, malignant
  myxoid (M8852/3) - *see* Neoplasm, connective tissue, malignant
  pleomorphic (M8854/3) - *see* Neoplasm, connective tissue, malignant
  round cell (M8853/3) - *see* Neoplasm, connective tissue, malignant
  well differentiated type (M8851/3) - *see* Neoplasm, connective tissue, malignant
Liposynovitis prepatellaris 272.8
Lipping
  cervix 622.0
  spine (*see also* Spondylosis) 721.90
  vertebra (*see also* Spondylosis) 721.90
Lip pits (mucus), congenital 750.25
Lipschütz disease or ulcer 616.50
Lipuria 791.1
  bilharziasis 120.0
Liquefaction, vitreous humor 379.21
Lisping 307.9
Lissauer's paralysis 094.1
Lissencephalia, lissencephaly 742.2
Listerellose 027.0
Listeriose 027.0
Listeriosis 027.0
  congenital 771.2
  fetal 771.2
  suspected fetal damage affecting management of pregnancy 655.4
Listlessness 780.79
Lithemia 790.6
Lithiasis - *see also* Calculus
  hepatic (duct) - *see* Choledocholithiasis
  urinary 592.9
Lithopedion 779.9
  affecting management of pregnancy 656.8
Lithosis (occupational) 502
  with tuberculosis - *see* Tuberculosis, pulmonary
Lithuria 791.9
Litigation V62.5
Little
  league elbow 718.82
  stroke syndrome 435.9
Little's disease - *see* Palsy, cerebral
Littre's
  gland - *see* condition
  hernia - *see* Hernia, Littre's
Littritis (*see also* Urethritis) 597.89
Livedo 782.61
  annularis 782.61
  racemose 782.61
  reticularis 782.61
Live flesh 781.0
Liver - *see also* condition
  donor V59.6
Livida, asphyxia
  newborn 768.6
Living
  alone V60.3
    with handicapped person V60.4
Lloyd's syndrome 258.1
Loa loa 125.2
Loasis 125.2
Lobe, lobar - *see* condition
Lobo's disease or blastomycosis 116.2
Lobomycosis 116.2

Lobotomy syndrome 310.0
Lobstein's disease (brittle bones and blue sclera) 756.51
Lobster-claw hand 755.58
Lobulation (congenital) - *see also* Anomaly, specified type NEC, by site
  kidney, fetal 753.3
  liver, abnormal 751.69
  spleen 759.0
Lobule, lobular - *see* condition
Local, localized - *see* condition
Locked bowel or intestine (*see also* Obstruction, intestine) 560.9
Locked-in state 344.81
Locked twins 660.5
  affecting fetus or newborn 763.1
Locking
  joint (*see also* Derangement, joint) 718.90
  knee 717.9
Lockjaw (*see also* Tetanus) 037
Locomotor ataxia (progressive) 094.0
Löffler's
  endocarditis 421.0
  eosinophilia or syndrome 518.3
  pneumonia 518.3
  syndrome (eosinophilic pneumonitis) 518.3
Löfgren's syndrome (sarcoidosis) 135
Loiasis 125.2
  eyelid 125.2 [373.6]
Loneliness V62.89
Lone Star fever 082.8
Long labor 662.1
  affecting fetus or newborn 763.89
  first stage 662.0
  second stage 662.2
Longitudinal stripes or grooves, nails 703.8
  congenital 757.5
Long-term (current) drug use V58.69
  antibiotics V58.62
  anticoagulants V58.61
  anti-inflammatories, non-steroidal (NSAID) V58.64
  antiplatelets/antithrombotics V58.63
  aspirin V58.66 ◀▦
    steroids V58.65
  insulin V58.67 ◀
Loop
  intestine (*see also* Volvulus) 560.2
  intrascleral nerve 379.29
  vascular on papilla (optic) 743.57
Loose - *see also* condition
  body
    in tendon sheath 727.82
    joint 718.10
      ankle 718.17
      elbow 718.12
      foot 718.17
      hand 718.14
      hip 718.15
      knee 717.6
      multiple sites 718.19
      pelvic region 718.15
      prosthetic implant - *see* Complications, mechanical
      shoulder (region) 718.11
      specified site NEC 718.18
      wrist 718.13
    cartilage (joint) (*see also* Loose, body, joint) 718.1
      knee 717.6
    facet (vertebral) 724.9
    prosthetic implant - *see* Complications, mechanical

Loose (Continued)
  sesamoid, joint (*see also* Loose, body, joint) 718.1
  tooth, teeth 525.8
Loosening epiphysis 732.9
Looser (-Debray)-Milkman syndrome (osteomalacia with pseudofractures) 268.2
Lop ear (deformity) 744.29
Lorain's disease or syndrome (pituitary dwarfism) 253.3
Lorain-Levi syndrome (pituitary dwarfism) 253.3
Lordosis (acquired) (postural) 737.20
  congenital 754.2
  due to or associated with
    Charcôt-Marie-Tooth disease 356.1 [737.42]
    mucopolysaccharidosis 277.5 [737.42]
    neurofibromatosis 237.71 [737.42]
    osteitis
      deformans 731.0 [737.42]
      fibrosa cystica 252.01 [737.42] ◀▦
    osteoporosis (*see also* Osteoporosis) 733.00 [737.42]
    poliomyelitis (*see also* Poliomyelitis) 138 [737.42]
    tuberculosis (*see also* Tuberculosis) 015.0 [737.42]
  late effect of rickets 268.1 [737.42]
  postlaminectomy 737.21
  postsurgical NEC 737.22
  rachitic 268.1 [737.42]
  specified NEC 737.29
  tuberculous (*see also* Tuberculosis) 015.0 [737.42]
Loss
  appetite 783.0
    hysterical 300.11
    nonorganic origin 307.59
    psychogenic 307.59
  blood - *see* Hemorrhage
  central vision 368.41
  consciousness 780.09
    transient 780.2
  control, sphincter, rectum 787.6
    nonorganic origin 307.7
  ear ossicle, partial 385.24
  elasticity, skin 782.8
  extremity or member, traumatic, current - *see* Amputation, traumatic
  fluid (acute) 276.5
    with
      hypernatremia 276.0
      hyponatremia 276.1
    fetus or newborn 775.5
  hair 704.00
  hearing - *see also* Deafness
    central 389.14
    conductive (air) 389.00
      with sensorineural hearing loss 389.2
      combined types 389.08
      external ear 389.01
      inner ear 389.04
      middle ear 389.03
      multiple types 389.08
      tympanic membrane 389.02
    mixed type 389.2
    nerve 389.12
    neural 389.12
    noise-induced 388.12
    perceptive NEC (*see also* Loss, hearing, sensorineural) 389.10
    sensorineural 389.10
      with conductive hearing loss 389.2
      central 389.14

◀ **New**   ◀▦ **Revised**

Loss *(Continued)*
  hearing *(Continued)*
    sensorineural *(Continued)*
      combined types 389.18
      multiple types 389.18
      neural 389.12
      sensory 389.11
    sensory 389.11
    specified type NEC 389.8
    sudden NEC 388.2
  height 781.91
  labyrinthine reactivity (unilateral) 386.55
    bilateral 386.56
  memory *(see also* Amnesia) 780.93
    mild, following organic brain damage 310.1
  mind *(see also* Psychosis) 298.9
  occusal vertical dimension 524.37 ◄
  organ or part - *see* Absence, by site, acquired
  sensation 782.0
  sense of
    smell *(see also* Disturbance, sensation) 781.1
    taste *(see also* Disturbance, sensation) 781.1
    touch *(see also* Disturbance, sensation) 781.1
  sight (acquired) (complete) (congenital) - *see* Blindness
  spinal fluid
    headache 349.0
  substance of
    bone *(see also* Osteoporosis) 733.00
    cartilage 733.99
    ear 380.32
    vitreous (humor) 379.26
  tooth, teeth
    acquired 525.10
      due to
        caries 525.13
        extraction 525.10
        periodontal disease 525.12
        specified NEC 525.19
        trauma 525.11
  vision, visual *(see also* Blindness) 369.9
    both eyes *(see also* Blindness, both eyes) 369.3
    complete *(see also* Blindness, both eyes) 369.00
    one eye 369.8
    sudden 368.11
    transient 368.12
  vitreous 379.26
  voice *(see also* Aphonia) 784.41
  weight (cause unknown) 783.21
Lou Gehrig's disease 335.20
Louis-Bar syndrome (ataxia-telangiectasia) 334.8
Louping ill 063.1
Lousiness - *see* Lice
Low
  back syndrome 724.2
  basal metabolic rate (BMR) 794.7
  birthweight 765.1
    extreme (less than 1000 grams) 765.0
    for gestational age 764.0
    status *(see also* Status, low birth weight) V21.30
  bladder compliance 596.52
  blood pressure *(see also* Hypotension) 458.9
    reading (incidental) (isolated) (nonspecific) 796.3
  cardiac reserve - *see* Disease, heart

Low *(Continued)*
  compliance bladder 596.52
  frequency deafness - *see* Disorder, hearing
  function - *see also* Hypofunction
    kidney *(see also* Disease, renal) 593.9
    liver 573.9
  hemoglobin 285.9
  implantation, placenta - *see* Placenta, previa
  insertion, placenta - *see* Placenta, previa
  lying
    kidney 593.0
    organ or site, congenital - *see* Malposition, congenital
    placenta - *see* Placenta, previa
  output syndrome (cardiac) *(see also* Failure, heart) 428.9
  platelets (blood) *(see also* Thrombocytopenia) 287.5
  reserve, kidney *(see also* Disease, renal) 593.9 ◄
  risk
    cervical, human papillomavirus (HPV) ◄
      DNA test positive 795.09 ◄
  salt syndrome 593.9
  tension glaucoma 365.12
  vision 369.9
    both eyes 369.20
    one eye 369.70
Lowe (-Terry-MacLachlan) syndrome (oculocerebrorenal dystrophy) 270.8
Lower extremity - *see* condition
Lown (-Ganong)-Levine syndrome (short P-R interval, normal QRS complex, and paroxysmal supraventricular tachycardia) 426.81
LSD reaction *(see also* Abuse, drugs, nondependent) 305.3
L-shaped kidney 753.3
Lucas-Championnière disease (fibrinous bronchitis) 466.0
Lucey-Driscoll syndrome (jaundice due to delayed conjugation) 774.30
Ludwig's
  angina 528.3
  disease (submaxillary cellulitis) 528.3
Lues (venerea), luetic - *see* Syphilis
Luetscher's syndrome (dehydration) 276.5
Lumbago 724.2
  due to displacement, intervertebral disc 722.10
Lumbalgia 724.2
  due to displacement, intervertebral disc 722.10
Lumbar - *see* condition
Lumbarization, vertebra 756.15
Lumbermen's itch 133.8
Lump - *see also* Mass
  abdominal 789.3
  breast 611.72
  chest 786.6
  epigastric 789.3
  head 784.2
  kidney 753.3
  liver 789.1
  lung 786.6
  mediastinal 786.6
  neck 784.2
  nose or sinus 784.2
  pelvic 789.3
  skin 782.2
  substernal 786.6
  throat 784.2
  umbilicus 789.3
Lunacy *(see also* Psychosis) 298.9

Lunatomalacia 732.3
Lung - *see also* condition
  donor V59.8
  drug addict's 417.8
  mainliners' 417.8
  vanishing 492.0
Lupoid (miliary) of Boeck 135
Lupus 710.0
  anticoagulant 289.81
  Cazenave's (erythematosus) 695.4
  discoid (local) 695.4
  disseminated 710.0
  erythematodes (discoid) (local) 695.4
  erythematosus (discoid) (local) 695.4
    disseminated 710.0
    eyelid 373.34
    systemic 710.0
      with
        encephalitis 710.0 *[323.8]*
        lung involvement 710.0 *[517.8]*
      inhibitor (presence of) 286.5
  exedens 017.0
  eyelid *(see also* Tuberculosis) 017.0 *[373.4]*
  Hilliard's 017.0
  hydralazine
    correct substance properly administered 695.4
    overdose or wrong substance given or taken 972.6
  miliaris disseminatus faciei 017.0
  nephritis 710.0 *[583.81]*
    acute 710.0 *[580.81]*
    chronic 710.0 *[582.81]*
  nontuberculous, not disseminated 695.4
  pernio (Besnier) 135
  tuberculous *(see also* Tuberculosis) 017.0
    eyelid *(see also* Tuberculosis) 017.0 *[373.4]*
  vulgaris 017.0
Luschka's joint disease 721.90
Luteinoma (M8610/0) 220
Lutembacher's disease or syndrome (atrial septal defect with mitral stenosis) 745.5
Luteoma (M8610/0) 220
Lutz-Miescher disease (elastosis perforans serpiginosa) 701.1
Lutz-Splendore-de Almeida disease (Brazilian blastomycosis) 116.1
Luxatio
  bulbi due to birth injury 767.8
  coxae congenita *(see also* Dislocation, hip, congenital) 754.30
  erecta - *see* Dislocation, shoulder
  imperfecta - *see* Sprain, by site
  perinealis - *see* Dislocation, hip
Luxation - *see also* Dislocation, by site
  eyeball 360.81
    due to birth injury 767.8
    lateral 376.36
  genital organs (external) NEC - *see* Wound, open, genital organs
  globe (eye) 360.81
    lateral 376.36
  lacrimal gland (postinfectional) 375.16
  lens (old) (partial) 379.32
    congenital 743.37
      syphilitic 090.49 *[379.32]*
    Marfan's disease 090.49
    spontaneous 379.32
  penis - *see* Wound, open, penis
  scrotum - *see* Wound, open, scrotum
  testis - *see* Wound, open, testis
L-xyloketosuria 271.8
Lycanthropy *(see also* Psychosis) 298.9

Lyell's disease or syndrome (toxic epidermal necrolysis) 695.1
  due to drug
    correct substance properly administered 695.1
    overdose or wrong substance given or taken 977.9
      specified drug - *see* Table of Drugs and Chemicals
Lyme disease 088.81
Lymph
  gland or node - *see* condition
  scrotum (*see also* Infestation, filarial) 125.9
Lymphadenitis 289.3
  with
    abortion - *see* Abortion, by type, with sepsis
    ectopic pregnancy (*see also* categories 633.0-633.9) 639.0
    molar pregnancy (*see also* categories 630-632) 639.0
  acute 683
    mesenteric 289.2
  any site, except mesenteric 289.3
    acute 683
    chronic 289.1
    mesenteric (acute) (chronic) (nonspecific) (subacute) 289.2
    subacute 289.1
      mesenteric 289.2
  breast, puerperal, postpartum 675.2
  chancroidal (congenital) 099.0
  chronic 289.1
    mesenteric 289.2
  dermatopathic 695.89
  due to
    anthracosis (occupational) 500
    Brugia (Wuchereria) malayi 125.1
    diphtheria (toxin) 032.89
    lymphogranuloma venereum 099.1
    Wuchereria bancrofti 125.0
  following
    abortion 639.0
    ectopic or molar pregnancy 639.0
  generalized 289.3
  gonorrheal 098.89
  granulomatous 289.1
  infectional 683
  mesenteric (acute) (chronic) (nonspecific) (subacute) 289.2
    due to Bacillus typhi 002.0
    tuberculous (*see also* Tuberculosis) 014.8
  mycobacterial 031.8
  purulent 683
  pyogenic 683
  regional 078.3
  septic 683
  streptococcal 683
  subacute, unspecified site 289.1
  suppurative 683
  syphilitic (early) (secondary) 091.4
    late 095.8
  tuberculous - *see* Tuberculosis, lymph gland
  venereal 099.1
Lymphadenoid goiter 245.2
Lymphadenopathy (general) 785.6
  due to toxoplasmosis (acquired) 130.7
    congenital (active) 771.2
Lymphadenopathy-associated virus (disease) (illness) (infection) - *see* Human immunodeficiency virus (disease) (illness) (infection)

Lymphadenosis 785.6
  acute 075
Lymphangiectasis 457.1
  conjunctiva 372.89
  postinfectional 457.1
  scrotum 457.1
Lymphangiectatic elephantiasis, nonfilarial 457.1
Lymphangioendothelioma (M9170/0) 228.1
  malignant (M9170/3) - *see* Neoplasm, connective tissue, malignant
Lymphangioma (M9170/0) 228.1
  capillary (M9171/0) 228.1
  cavernous (M9172/0) 228.1
  cystic (M9173/0) 228.1
  malignant (M9170/3) - *see* Neoplasm, connective tissue, malignant
Lymphangiomyoma (M9174/0) 228.1
Lymphangiomyomatosis (M9174/1) - *see* Neoplasm, connective tissue, uncertain behavior
Lymphangiosarcoma (M9170/3) - *see* Neoplasm, connective tissue, malignant
Lymphangitis 457.2
  with
    abortion - *see* Abortion, by type, with sepsis
    abscess - *see* Abscess, by site
    cellulitis - *see* Abscess, by site
    ectopic pregnancy (*see also* categories 633.0-633.9) 639.0
    molar pregnancy (*see also* categories 630-632) 639.0
  acute (with abscess or cellulitis) 682.9
    specified site - *see* Abscess, by site
  breast, puerperal, postpartum 675.2
  chancroidal 099.0
  chronic (any site) 457.2
  due to
    Brugia (Wuchereria) malayi 125.1
    Wuchereria bancrofti 125.0
  following
    abortion 639.0
    ectopic or molar pregnancy 639.0
  gangrenous 457.2
  penis
    acute 607.2
    gonococcal (acute) 098.0
      chronic or duration of 2 months or more 098.2
  puerperal, postpartum, childbirth 670
  strumous, tuberculous (*see also* Tuberculosis) 017.2
  subacute (any site) 457.2
  tuberculous - *see* Tuberculosis, lymph gland
Lymphatic (vessel) - *see* condition
Lymphatism 254.8
  scrofulous (*see also* Tuberculosis) 017.2
Lymphectasia 457.1
Lymphedema (*see also* Elephantiasis) 457.1
  acquired (chronic) 457.1
  chronic hereditary 757.0
  congenital 757.0
  idiopathic hereditary 757.0
  praecox 457.1
  secondary 457.1
  surgical NEC 997.99
    postmastectomy (syndrome) 457.0
Lymph-hemangioma (M9120/0) - *see* Hemangioma, by site

Lymphoblastic - *see* condition
Lymphoblastoma (diffuse) (M9630/3) 200.1
  giant follicular (M9690/3) 202.0
  macrofollicular (M9690/3) 202.0
Lymphoblastosis, acute benign 075
Lymphocele 457.8
Lymphocythemia 288.8
Lymphocytic - *see also* condition
  chorioencephalitis (acute) (serous) 049.0
  choriomeningitis (acute) (serous) 049.0
Lymphocytoma (diffuse) (malignant) (M9620/3) 200.1
Lymphocytomatosis (M9620/3) 200.1
Lymphocytopenia 288.8
Lymphocytosis (symptomatic) 288.8
  infectious (acute) 078.89
Lymphoepithelioma (M8082/3) - *see* Neoplasm, by site, malignant
Lymphogranuloma (malignant) (M9650/3) 201.9
  inguinale 099.1
  venereal (any site) 099.1
    with stricture of rectum 099.1
  venereum 099.1
Lymphogranulomatosis (malignant) (M9650/3) 201.9
  benign (Boeck's sarcoid) (Schaumann's) 135
  Hodgkin's (M9650/3) 201.9
Lymphoid - *see* condition
Lympholeukoblastoma (M9850/3) 207.8
Lympholeukosarcoma (M9850/3) 207.8
Lymphoma (malignant) (M9590/3) 202.8

Note   Use the following fifth-digit subclassification with categories 200-202:

0	unspecified site
1	lymph nodes of head, face, and neck
2	intrathoracic lymph nodes
3	intra-abdominal lymph nodes
4	lymph nodes of axilla and upper limb
5	lymph nodes of inguinal region and lower limb
6	intrapelvic lymph nodes
7	spleen
8	lymph nodes of multiple sites

---

  benign (M9590/0) - *see* Neoplasm, by site, benign
  Burkitt's type (lymphoblastic) (undifferentiated) (M9750/3) 200.2
  Castleman's (mediastinal lymph node hyperplasia) 785.6
  centroblastic-centrocytic
    diffuse (M9614/3) 202.8
    follicular (M9692/3) 202.0
  centroblastic type (diffuse) (M9632/3) 202.8
    follicular (M9697/3) 202.0
  centrocytic (M9622/3) 202.8
  compound (M9613/3) 200.8
  convoluted cell type (lymphoblastic) (M9602/3) 202.8
  diffuse NEC (M9590/3) 202.8
  follicular (giant) (M9690/3) 202.0
    center cell (diffuse) (M9615/3) 202.8
      cleaved (diffuse) (M9623/3) 202.8
        follicular (M9695/3) 202.0

◀ **New**   ◀▥ **Revised**

Lymphoma (Continued)
  follicular (Continued)
    center cell (Continued)
      non-cleaved (diffuse) (M9633/3)
        202.8
        follicular (M9698/3) 202.0
      centroblastic-centrocytic (M9692/3)
        202.0
      centroblastic type (M9697/3) 202.0
      lymphocytic
        intermediate differentiation
          (M9694/3) 202.0
        poorly differentiated (M9696/3)
          202.0
      mixed (cell type) (lymphocytic-histi-
        ocytic) (small cell and large cell)
        (M9691/3) 202.0
    germinocytic (M9622/3) 202.8
    giant, follicular or follicle (M9690/3)
      202.0
    histiocytic (diffuse) (M9640/3) 200.0
      nodular (M9642/3) 200.0
      pleomorphic cell type (M9641/3)
        200.0
    Hodgkin's (M9650/3) (see also Disease,
      Hodgkin's) 201.9
    immunoblastic (type) (M9612/3) 200.8
    large cell (M9640/3) 200.0
      nodular (M9642/3) 200.0
      pleomorphic cell type (M9641/3)
        200.0
    lymphoblastic (diffuse) (M9630/3) 200.1
      Burkitt's type (M9750/3) 200.2
      convoluted cell type (M9602/3)
        202.8
    lymphocytic (cell type) (diffuse)
      (M9620/3) 200.1
      with plasmacytoid differentiation,
        diffuse (M9611/3) 200.8
      intermediate differentiation (diffuse)
        (M9621/3) 200.1
        follicular (M9694/3) 202.0
        nodular (M9694/3) 202.0
      nodular (M9690/3) 202.0
      poorly differentiated (diffuse)
        (M9630/3) 200.1

Lymphoma (Continued)
  lymphocytic (Continued)
    poorly differentiated (Continued)
      follicular (M9696/3) 202.0
      nodular (M9696/3) 202.0
    well differentiated (diffuse) (M9620/
      3) 200.1
      follicular (M9693/3) 202.0
      nodular (M9693/3) 202.0
    lymphocytic-histiocytic, mixed (diffuse)
      (M9613/3) 200.8
      follicular (M9691/3) 202.0
      nodular (M9691/3) 202.0
    lymphoplasmacytoid type (M9611/3)
      200.8
    lymphosarcoma type (M9610/3) 200.1
    macrofollicular (M9690/3) 202.0
    mixed cell type (diffuse) (M9613/3)
      200.8
      follicular (M9691/3) 202.0
      nodular (M9691/3) 202.0
    nodular (M9690/3) 202.0
      histiocytic (M9642/3) 200.0
      lymphocytic (M9690/3) 202.0
        intermediate differentiation
          (M9694/3) 202.0
        poorly differentiated (M9696/3)
          202.0
      mixed (cell type) (lymphocytic-histi-
        ocytic) (small cell and large cell)
        (M9691/3) 202.0
    non-Hodgkin's type NEC (M9591/3)
      202.8
    reticulum cell (type) (M9640/3) 200.0
    small cell and large cell, mixed (dif-
      fuse) (M9613/3) 200.8
      follicular (M9691/3) 202.0
      nodular (9691/3) 202.0
    stem cell (type) (M9601/3) 202.8
    T-cell 202.1
    undifferentiated (cell type) (non-Burk-
      itt's) (M9600/3) 202.8
      Burkitt's type (M9750/3) 200.2
Lymphomatosis (M9590/3) - see also
  Lymphoma
  granulomatous 099.1

Lymphopathia
  venereum 099.1
  veneris 099.1
Lymphopenia 288.8
  familial 279.2
Lymphoreticulosis, benign (of inoculation) 078.3
Lymphorrhea 457.8
Lymphosarcoma (M9610/3) 200.1
  diffuse (M9610/3) 200.1
    with plasmacytoid differentiation
      (M9611/3) 200.8
    lymphoplasmacytic (M9611/3)
      200.8
  follicular (giant) (M9690/3) 202.0
    lymphoblastic (M9696/3) 202.0
    lymphocytic, intermediate differenti-
      ation (M9694/3) 202.0
    mixed cell type (M9691/3) 202.0
  giant follicular (M9690/3) 202.0
  Hodgkin's (M9650/3) 201.9
  immunoblastic (M9612/3) 200.8
  lymphoblastic (diffuse) (M9630/3)
    200.1
    follicular (M9696/3) 202.0
    nodular (M9696/3) 202.0
  lymphocytic (diffuse) (M9620/3)
    200.1
    intermediate differentiation (diffuse)
      (M9621/3) 200.1
      follicular (M9694/3) 202.0
      nodular (M9694/3) 202.0
    mixed cell type (diffuse) (M9613/3)
      200.8
      follicular (M9691/3) 202.0
      nodular (M9691/3) 202.0
  nodular (M9690/3) 202.0
    lymphoblastic (M9696/3) 202.0
    lymphocytic, intermediate differenti-
      ation (M9694/3) 202.0
    mixed cell type (M9691/3) 202.0
  prolymphocytic (M9631/3) 200.1
  reticulum cell (M9640/3) 200.0
Lymphostasis 457.8
Lypemania (see also Melancholia) 296.2
Lyssa 071

M

Macacus ear 744.29
Maceration
  fetus (cause not stated) 779.9
  wet feet, tropical (syndrome) 991.4
Machado-Joseph disease 334.8
Machupo virus hemorrhagic fever 078.7
Macleod's syndrome (abnormal trans-
    radiancy, one lung) 492.8
Macrocephalia, macrocephaly 756.0
Macrocheilia (congenital) 744.81
Macrochilia (congenital) 744.81
Macrocolon (congenital) 751.3
Macrocornea 743.41
  associated with buphthalmos 743.22
Macrocytic - *see* condition
Macrocytosis 289.89
Macrodactylia, macrodactylism (fingers)
    (thumbs) 755.57
  toes 755.65
Macrodontia 520.2
Macroencephaly 742.4
Macrogenia 524.05
Macrogenitosomia (female) (male) (prae-
    cox) 255.2
Macrogingivae 523.8
Macroglobulinemia (essential) (idio-
    pathic) (monoclonal) (primary) (syn-
    drome) (Waldenström's) 273.3
Macroglossia (congenital) 750.15
  acquired 529.8
Macrognathia, macrognathism (congeni-
    tal) 524.00
  mandibular 524.02
    alveolar 524.72
  maxillary 524.01
    alveolar 524.71
Macrogyria (congenital) 742.4
Macrohydrocephalus (*see also* Hydro-
    cephalus) 331.4
Macromastia (*see also* Hypertrophy,
    breast) 611.1
Macropsia 368.14
Macrosigmoid 564.7
  congenital 751.3
Macrospondylitis, acromegalic 253.0
Macrostomia (congenital) 744.83
Macrotia (external ear) (congenital)
    744.22
Macula
  cornea, corneal
    congenital 743.43
      interfering with vision 743.42
    interfering with central vision
      371.03
    not interfering with central vision
      371.02
  degeneration (*see also* Degeneration,
    macula) 362.50
    hereditary (*see also* Dystrophy, ret-
      ina) 362.70
  edema, cystoid 362.53
Maculae ceruleae 132.1
Macules and papules 709.8
Maculopathy, toxic 362.55
Madarosis 374.55
Madelung's
  deformity (radius) 755.54
  disease (lipomatosis) 272.8
  lipomatosis 272.8
Madness (*see also* Psychosis) 298.9
  myxedema (acute) 293.0
    subacute 293.1

Madura
  disease (actinomycotic) 039.9
    mycotic 117.4
  foot (actinomycotic) 039.4
    mycotic 117.4
Maduromycosis (actinomycotic) 039.9
  mycotic 117.4
Maffucci's syndrome (dyschondroplasia
    with hemangiomas) 756.4
Magenblase syndrome 306.4
Main en griffe (acquired) 736.06
  congenital 755.59
Maintenance
  chemotherapy regimen or treatment
    V58.1
  dialysis regimen or treatment
    extracorporeal (renal) V56.0
    peritoneal V56.8
    renal V56.0
  drug therapy or regimen V58.1
  external fixation NEC V54.89
  radiotherapy V58.0
  traction NEC V54.89
Majocchi's
  disease (purpura annularis telangiecto-
    des) 709.1
  granuloma 110.6
Major - *see* condition
Mal
  cerebral (idiopathic) (*see also* Epilepsy)
    345.9
  comital (*see also* Epilepsy) 345.9
  de los pintos (*see also* Pinta) 103.9
  de Meleda 757.39
  de mer 994.6
  lie - *see* Presentation, fetal
  perforant (*see also* Ulcer, lower extrem-
    ity) 707.15
Malabar itch 110.9
  beard 110.0
  foot 110.4
  scalp 110.0
Malabsorption 579.9
  calcium 579.8
  carbohydrate 579.8
  disaccharide 271.3
  drug-induced 579.8
  due to bacterial overgrowth 579.8
  fat 579.8
  folate, congenital 281.2
  galactose 271.1
  glucose-galactose (congenital) 271.3
  intestinal 579.9
  isomaltose 271.3
  lactose (hereditary) 271.3
  methionine 270.4
  monosaccharide 271.8
  postgastrectomy 579.3
  postsurgical 579.3
  protein 579.8
  sucrose (-isomaltose) (congenital) 271.3
  syndrome 579.9
    postgastrectomy 579.3
    postsurgical 579.3
Malacia, bone 268.2
  juvenile (*see also* Rickets) 268.0
  Kienböck's (juvenile) (lunate) (wrist)
    732.3
    adult 732.8
Malacoplakia
  bladder 596.8
  colon 569.89
  pelvis (kidney) 593.89
  ureter 593.89

Malacoplakia (*Continued*)
  urethra 599.84
Malacosteon 268.2
  juvenile (*see also* Rickets) 268.0
Maladaptation - *see* Maladjustment
Maladie de Roger 745.4
Maladjustment
  conjugal V61.10
    involving divorce or estrangement
      V61.0
  educational V62.3
  family V61.9
    specified circumstance NEC V61.8
  marital V61.10
    involving divorce or estrangement
      V61.0
  occupational V62.2
  simple, adult (*see also* Reaction, adjust-
    ment) 309.9
  situational acute (*see also* Reaction, ad-
    justment) 309.9
  social V62.4
Malaise 780.79
Malakoplakia - *see* Malacoplakia
Malaria, malarial (fever) 084.6
  algid 084.9
  any type, with
    algid malaria 084.9
    blackwater fever 084.8
    fever
      blackwater 084.8
      hemoglobinuric (bilious) 084.8
    hemoglobinuria, malarial 084.8
    hepatitis 084.9 [573.2]
    nephrosis 084.9 [581.81]
    pernicious complication NEC 084.9
      cardiac 084.9
      cerebral 084.9
  cardiac 084.9
  carrier (suspected) of V02.9
  cerebral 084.9
  complicating pregnancy, childbirth, or
    puerperium 647.4
  congenital 771.2
  congestion, congestive 084.6
    brain 084.9
  continued 084.0
  estivo-autumnal 084.0
  falciparum (malignant tertian) 084.0
  hematinuria 084.8
  hematuria 084.8
  hemoglobinuria 084.8
  hemorrhagic 084.6
  induced (therapeutically) 084.7
    accidental - *see* Malaria, by type
  liver 084.9 [573.2]
  malariae (quartan) 084.2
  malignant (tertian) 084.0
  mixed infections 084.5
  monkey 084.4
  ovale 084.3
  pernicious, acute 084.0
  Plasmodium, P.
    falciparum 084.0
    malariae 084.2
    ovale 084.3
    vivax 084.1
  quartan 084.2
  quotidian 084.0
  recurrent 084.6
    induced (therapeutically) 084.7
      accidental - *see* Malaria, by type
  remittent 084.6
  specified types NEC 084.4

◄ **New**   ◄▦ **Revised**

Malaria, malarial (Continued)
spleen 084.6
subtertian 084.0
tertian (benign) 084.1
malignant 084.0
tropical 084.0
typhoid 084.6
vivax (benign tertian) 084.1
Malassez's disease (testicular cyst) 608.89
Malassimilation 579.9
Maldescent, testis 752.51
Maldevelopment - see also Anomaly, by
site
brain 742.9
colon 751.5
hip (joint) 755.63
congenital dislocation (see also Dislocation, hip, congenital) 754.30
mastoid process 756.0
middle ear, except ossicles 744.03
ossicles 744.04
newborn (not malformation) 764.9
ossicles, ear 744.04
spine 756.10
toe 755.66
Male type pelvis 755.69
with disproportion (fetopelvic) 653.2
affecting fetus or newborn 763.1
causing obstructed labor 660.1
affecting fetus or newborn 763.1
Malformation (congenital) - see also
Anomaly
bone 756.9
bursa 756.9
Chiari
type I 348.4
type II (see also Spina bifida) 741.0
type III 742.0
type IV 742.2
circulatory system NEC 747.9
specified type NEC 747.89
cochlea 744.05
digestive system NEC 751.9
lower 751.5
specified type NEC 751.8
upper 750.9
eye 743.9
gum 750.9
heart NEC 746.9
specified type NEC 746.89
valve 746.9
internal ear 744.05
joint NEC 755.9
specified type NEC 755.8
Mondini's (congenital) (malformation,
cochlea) 744.05
muscle 756.9
nervous system (central) 742.9
pelvic organs or tissues
in pregnancy or childbirth 654.9
affecting fetus or newborn
763.89
causing obstructed labor 660.2
affecting fetus or newborn 763.1
placenta (see also Placenta, abnormal)
656.7
respiratory organs 748.9
specified type NEC 748.8
Rieger's 743.44
sense organs NEC 742.9
specified type NEC 742.8
skin 757.9
specified type NEC 757.8
spinal cord 742.9
teeth, tooth NEC 520.9

Malformation (Continued)
tendon 756.9
throat 750.9
umbilical cord (complicating delivery)
663.9
affecting fetus or newborn 762.6
umbilicus 759.9
urinary system NEC 753.9
specified type NEC 753.8
Malfunction - see also Dysfunction
arterial graft 996.1
cardiac pacemaker 996.01
catheter device - see Complications,
mechanical, catheter
colostomy 569.62
cystostomy 997.5
device, implant, or graft NEC - see
Complications, mechanical
enteric stoma 569.62
enterostomy 569.62
esophagostomy 530.87   ◄
gastroenteric 536.8
gastrostomy 536.42
nephrostomy 997.5
pacemaker - see Complications, mechanical, pacemaker
prosthetic device, internal - see Complications, mechanical
tracheostomy 519.02
vascular graft or shunt 996.1
Malgaigne's fracture (closed) 808.43
open 808.53
Malherbe's
calcifying epithelioma (M8110/0) - see
Neoplasm, skin, benign
tumor (M8110/0) - see Neoplasm, skin,
benign
Malibu disease 919.8
infected 919.9
Malignancy (M8000/3) - see Neoplasm,
by site, malignant
Malignant - see condition
Malingerer, malingering V65.2
Mallet, finger (acquired) 736.1
congenital 755.59
late effect of rickets 268.1
Malleus 024
Mallory's bodies 034.1
Mallory-Weiss syndrome 530.7
Malnutrition (calorie) 263.9
complicating pregnancy 648.9
degree
first 263.1
second 263.0
third 262
mild 263.1
moderate 263.0
severe 261
protein-calorie 262
fetus 764.2
"light-for-dates" 764.1
following gastrointestinal surgery 579.3
intrauterine or fetal 764.2
fetus or infant "light-for-dates" 764.1
lack of care, or neglect (child) (infant)
995.52
adult 995.84
malignant 260
mild 263.1
moderate 263.0
protein 260
protein-calorie 263.9
severe 262
specified type NEC 263.8
severe 261
protein-calorie NEC 262

Malocclusion (teeth) 524.4
due to
abnormal swallowing 524.59   ◄▤
accessory teeth (causing crowding)
524.31   ◄▤
dentofacial abnormality NEC
524.89   ◄▤
impacted teeth (causing crowding)
520.6   ◄▤
missing teeth 524.30   ◄▤
mouth breathing 524.59   ◄▤
sleep postures 524.59   ◄
supernumerary teeth (causing
crowding) 524.31   ◄▤
thumb sucking 524.59   ◄▤
tongue, lip, or finger habits 524.59 ◄▤
temporomandibular (joint) 524.69
Malposition
cardiac apex (congenital) 746.87
cervix - see Malposition, uterus
congenital
adrenal (gland) 759.1
alimentary tract 751.8
lower 751.5
upper 750.8
aorta 747.21
appendix 751.5
arterial trunk 747.29
artery (peripheral) NEC (see also
Malposition, congenital, peripheral vascular system) 747.60
coronary 746.85
pulmonary 747.3
auditory canal 744.29
causing impairment of hearing
744.02
auricle (ear) 744.29
causing impairment of hearing
744.02
cervical 744.43
biliary duct or passage 751.69
bladder (mucosa) 753.8
exteriorized or extroverted 753.5
brachial plexus 742.8
brain tissue 742.4
breast 757.6
bronchus 748.3
cardiac apex 746.87
cecum 751.5
clavicle 755.51
colon 751.5
digestive organ or tract NEC 751.8
lower 751.5
upper 750.8
ear (auricle) (external) 744.29
ossicles 744.04
endocrine (gland) NEC 759.2
epiglottis 748.3
eustachian tube 744.24
eye 743.8
facial features 744.89
fallopian tube 752.19
finger(s) 755.59
supernumerary 755.01
foot 755.67
gallbladder 751.69
gastrointestinal tract 751.8
genitalia, genital organ(s) or tract
female 752.89
external 752.49
internal NEC 752.89
male 752.89
penis 752.69
scrotal transposition 752.81

ICD-9-CM

M

Vol. 2

Malposition (*Continued*)
congenital (*Continued*)
glottis 748.3
hand 755.59
heart 746.87
dextrocardia 746.87
with complete transposition of viscera 759.3
hepatic duct 751.69
hip (joint) (*see also* Dislocation, hip, congenital) 754.30
intestine (large) (small) 751.5
with anomalous adhesions, fixation, or malrotation 751.4
joint NEC 755.8
kidney 753.3
larynx 748.3
limb 755.8
lower 755.69
upper 755.59
liver 751.69
lung (lobe) 748.69
nail(s) 757.5
nerve 742.8
nervous system NEC 742.8
nose, nasal (septum) 748.1
organ or site NEC - *see* Anomaly, specified type NEC, by site
ovary 752.0
pancreas 751.7
parathyroid (gland) 759.2
patella 755.64
peripheral vascular system 747.60
gastrointestinal 747.61
lower limb 747.64
renal 747.62
specified NEC 747.69
spinal 747.82
upper limb 747.63
pituitary (gland) 759.2
respiratory organ or system NEC 748.9
rib (cage) 756.3
supernumerary in cervical region 756.2
scapula 755.59
shoulder 755.59
spinal cord 742.59
spine 756.19
spleen 759.0
sternum 756.3
stomach 750.7
symphysis pubis 755.69
testis (undescended)752.51
thymus (gland) 759.2
thyroid (gland) (tissue) 759.2
cartilage 748.3
toe(s) 755.66
supernumerary 755.02
tongue 750.19
trachea 748.3
uterus 752.3
vein(s) (peripheral) NEC (*see also* Malposition, congenital, peripheral vascular system) 747.60
great 747.49
portal 747.49
pulmonary 747.49
vena cava (inferior) (superior) 747.49
device, implant, or graft - *see* Complications, mechanical
fetus NEC (*see also* Presentation, fetal) 652.9
with successful version 652.1
affecting fetus or newborn 763.1

Malposition (*Continued*)
fetus NEC (*Continued*)
before labor, affecting fetus or newborn 761.7
causing obstructed labor 660.0
in multiple gestation (one fetus or more) 652.6
with locking 660.5
causing obstructed labor 660.0
gallbladder (*see also* Disease, gallbladder) 575.8
gastrointestinal tract 569.89
congenital 751.8
heart (*see also* Malposition, congenital, heart) 746.87
intestine 569.89
congenital 751.5
pelvic organs or tissues
in pregnancy or childbirth 654.4
affecting fetus or newborn 763.89
causing obstructed labor 660.2
affecting fetus or newborn 763.1
placenta - *see* Placenta, previa
stomach 537.89
congenital 750.7
tooth, teeth 524.30 ◀▥
with impaction 520.6 ◀
uterus or cervix (acquired) (acute) (adherent) (any degree) (asymptomatic) (postinfectional) (postpartal, old) 621.6
anteflexion or anteversion (*see also* Anteversion, uterus) 621.6
congenital 752.3
flexion 621.6
lateral (*see also* Lateroversion, uterus) 621.6
in pregnancy or childbirth 654.4
affecting fetus or newborn 763.89
causing obstructed labor 660.2
affecting fetus or newborn 763.1
inversion 621.6
lateral (flexion) (version) (*see also* Lateroversion, uterus) 621.6
lateroflexion (*see also* Lateroversion, uterus) 621.6
lateroversion (*see also* Lateroversion, uterus) 621.6
retroflexion or retroversion (*see also* Retroversion, uterus) 621.6
Malposture 729.9
Malpresentation, fetus (*see also* Presentation, fetal) 652.9
Malrotation
cecum 751.4
colon 751.4
intestine 751.4
kidney 753.3
Malta fever (*see also* Brucellosis) 023.9
Maltosuria 271.3
Maltreatment (of)
adult 995.80
emotional 995.82
multiple forms 995.85
neglect (nutritional) 995.84
physical 995.81
psychological 995.82
sexual 995.83
child 995.50
emotional 995.51
multiple forms 995.59
neglect (nutritional) 995.52
physical 995.54
shaken infant syndrome 995.55

Maltreatment (*Continued*)
child (*Continued*)
psychological 995.51
sexual 995.53
spouse 995.80 (*see also* Maltreatment, adult)
Malt workers' lung 495.4
Malum coxae senilis 715.25
Malunion, fracture 733.81
Mammillitis (*see also* Mastitis) 611.0
puerperal, postpartum 675.2
Mammitis (*see also* Mastitis) 611.0
puerperal, postpartum 675.2
Mammographic microcalcification 793.81
Mammoplasia 611.1
Management
contraceptive V25.9
specified type NEC V25.8
procreative V26.9
specified type NEC V26.8
Mangled NEC (*see also* nature and site of injury) 959.9
Mania (monopolar) (*see also* Psychosis, affective) 296.0
alcoholic (acute) (chronic) 291.9
Bell's - *see* Mania, chronic
chronic 296.0
recurrent episode 296.1
single episode 296.0
compulsive 300.3
delirious (acute) 296.0
recurrent episode 296.1
single episode 296.0
epileptic (*see also* Epilepsy) 345.4
hysterical 300.10
inhibited 296.89
puerperal (after delivery) 296.0
recurrent episode 296.1
single episode 296.0
recurrent episode 296.1
senile 290.8
single episode 296.0
stupor 296.89
stuporous 296.89
unproductive 296.89
Manic-depressive insanity, psychosis, reaction, or syndrome (*see also* Psychosis, affective) 296.80
circular (alternating) 296.7
currently
depressed 296.5
episode unspecified 296.7
hypomanic, previously depressed 296.4
manic 296.4
mixed 296.6
depressed (type), depressive 296.2
atypical 296.82
recurrent episode 296.3
single episode 296.2
hypomanic 296.0
recurrent episode 296.1
single episode 296.0
manic 296.0
atypical 296.81
recurrent episode 296.1
single episode 296.0
mixed NEC 296.89
perplexed 296.89
stuporous 296.89
Manifestations, rheumatoid
lungs 714.81
pannus - *see* Arthritis, rheumatoid

Manifestations, rheumatoid (Continued)
  subcutaneous nodules - see Arthritis, rheumatoid
Mankowsky's syndrome (familial dysplastic osteopathy) 731.2
Mannoheptulosuria 271.8
Mannosidosis 271.8
Manson's
  disease (schistosomiasis) 120.1
  pyosis (pemphigus contagiosus) 684
  schistosomiasis 120.1
Mansonellosis 125.5
Manual - see condition
Maple bark disease 495.6
Maple bark-strippers' lung 495.6
Maple syrup (urine) disease or syndrome 270.3
Marable's syndrome (celiac artery compression) 447.4
Marasmus 261
  brain 331.9
  due to malnutrition 261
  intestinal 569.89
  nutritional 261
  senile 797
  tuberculous NEC (see also Tuberculosis) 011.9
Marble
  bones 756.52
  skin 782.61
Marburg disease (virus) 078.89
March
  foot 733.94
  hemoglobinuria 283.2
Marchand multiple nodular hyperplasia (liver) 571.5
Marchesani (-Weill) syndrome (brachymorphism and ectopia lentis) 759.89
Marchiafava (-Bignami) disease or syndrome 341.8
Marchiafava-Micheli syndrome (paroxysmal nocturnal hemoglobinuria) 283.2
Marcus Gunn's syndrome (jaw-winking syndrome) 742.8
Marfan's
  congenital syphilis 090.49
  disease 090.49
  syndrome (arachnodactyly) 759.82
    meaning congenital syphilis 090.49
    with luxation of lens 090.49
      [379.32]
Marginal
  implantation, placenta - see Placenta, previa
  placenta - see Placenta, previa
  sinus (hemorrhage) (rupture) 641.2
    affecting fetus or newborn 762.1
Marie's
  cerebellar ataxia 334.2
  syndrome (acromegaly) 253.0
Marie-Bamberger disease or syndrome (hypertrophic) (pulmonary) (secondary) 731.2
  idiopathic (acropachyderma) 757.39
  primary (acropachyderma) 757.39
Marie-Charcôt-Tooth neuropathic atrophy, muscle 356.1
Marie-Strümpell arthritis or disease (ankylosing spondylitis) 720.0
Marihuana, marijuana
  abuse (see also Abuse, drugs, nondependent) 305.2

Marihuana, marijuana (Continued)
  dependence (see also Dependence) 304.3
Marion's disease (bladder neck obstruction) 596.0
Marital conflict V61.10
Mark
  port wine 757.32
  raspberry 757.32
  strawberry 757.32
  stretch 701.3
  tattoo 709.09
Maroteaux-Lamy syndrome (mucopolysaccharidosis VI) 277.5
Marriage license examination V70.3
Marrow (bone)
  arrest 284.9
  megakaryocytic 287.3
  poor function 289.9
Marseilles fever 082.1
Marsh's disease (exophthalmic goiter) 242.0
Marshall's (hidrotic) ectodermal dysplasia 757.31
Marsh fever (see also Malaria) 084.6
Martin's disease 715.27
Martin-Albright syndrome (pseudohypoparathyroidism) 275.49
Martorell-Fabre syndrome (pulseless disease) 446.7
Masculinization, female, with adrenal hyperplasia 255.2
Masculinovoblastoma (M8670/0) 220
Masochism 302.83
Masons' lung 502
Mass
  abdominal 789.3
  anus 787.99
  bone 733.90
  breast 611.72
  cheek 784.2
  chest 786.6
  cystic - see Cyst
  ear 388.8
  epigastric 789.3
  eye 379.92
  female genital organ 625.8
  gum 784.2
  head 784.2
  intracranial 784.2
  joint 719.60
    ankle 719.67
    elbow 719.62
    foot 719.67
    hand 719.64
    hip 719.65
    knee 719.66
    multiple sites 719.69
    pelvic region 719.65
    shoulder (region) 719.61
    specified site NEC 719.68
    wrist 719.63
  kidney (see also Disease, kidney) 593.9
  lung 786.6
  lymph node 785.6
  malignant (M8000/3) - see Neoplasm, by site, malignant
  mediastinal 786.6
  mouth 784.2
  muscle (limb) 729.89
  neck 784.2
  nose or sinus 784.2
  palate 784.2
  pelvis, pelvic 789.3

Mass (Continued)
  penis 607.89
  perineum 625.8
  rectum 787.99
  scrotum 608.89
  skin 782.2
  specified organ NEC - see Disease of specified organ or site
  splenic 789.2
  substernal 786.6
    thyroid (see also Goiter) 240.9
  superficial (localized) 782.2
  testes 608.89
  throat 784.2
  tongue 784.2
  umbilicus 789.3
  uterus 625.8
  vagina 625.8
  vulva 625.8
Massive - see condition
Mastalgia 611.71
  psychogenic 307.89
Mast cell
  disease 757.33
    systemic (M9741/3) 202.6
  leukemia (M9900/3) 207.8
  sarcoma (M9742/3) 202.6
  tumor (M9740/1) 238.5
    malignant (M9740/3) 202.6
Masters-Allen syndrome 620.6
Mastitis (acute) (adolescent) (diffuse) (interstitial) (lobular) (nonpuerperal) (nonsuppurative) (parenchymatous) (phlegmonous) (simple) (subacute) (suppurative) 611.0
  chronic (cystic) (fibrocystic) 610.1
  cystic 610.1
    Schimmelbusch's type 610.1
  fibrocystic 610.1
  infective 611.0
  lactational 675.2
  lymphangitis 611.0
  neonatal (noninfective) 778.7
    infective 771.5
  periductal 610.4
  plasma cell 610.4
  puerperal, postpartum, (interstitial) (nonpurulent) (parenchymatous) 675.2
    purulent 675.1
    stagnation 676.2
  puerperalis 675.2
  retromammary 611.0
    puerperal, postpartum 675.1
  submammary 611.0
    puerperal, postpartum 675.1
Mastocytoma (M9740/1) 238.5
  malignant (M9740/3) 202.6
Mastocytosis 757.33
  malignant (M9741/3) 202.6
  systemic (M9741/3) 202.6
Mastodynia 611.71
  psychogenic 307.89
Mastoid - see condition
Mastoidalgia (see also Otalgia) 388.70
Mastoiditis (coalescent) (hemorrhagic) (pneumococcal) (streptococcal) (suppurative) 383.9
  acute or subacute 383.00
    with
      Gradenigo's syndrome 383.02
      petrositis 383.02
      specified complication NEC 383.02
      subperiosteal abscess 383.01

Mastoiditis (*Continued*)
   chronic (necrotic) (recurrent) 383.1
   tuberculous (*see also* Tuberculosis) 015.6
Mastopathy, mastopathia 611.9
   chronica cystica 610.1
   diffuse cystic 610.1
   estrogenic 611.8
   ovarian origin 611.8
Mastoplasia 611.1
Masturbation 307.9
Maternal condition, affecting fetus or newborn
   acute yellow atrophy of liver 760.8
   albuminuria 760.1
   anesthesia or analgesia 763.5
   blood loss 762.1
   chorioamnionitis 762.7
   circulatory disease, chronic (conditions classifiable to 390-459, 745-747) 760.3
   congenital heart disease (conditions classifiable to 745-746) 760.3
   cortical necrosis of kidney 760.1
   death 761.6
   diabetes mellitus 775.0
      manifest diabetes in the infant 775.1
   disease NEC 760.9
      circulatory system, chronic (conditions classifiable to 390-459, 745-747) 760.3
      genitourinary system (conditions classifiable to 580-599) 760.1
      respiratory (conditions classifiable to 490-519, 748) 760.3
   eclampsia 760.0
   hemorrhage NEC 762.1
   hepatitis acute, malignant, or subacute 760.8
   hyperemesis (gravidarum) 761.8
   hypertension (arising during pregnancy) (conditions classifiable to 642) 760.0
   infection
      disease classifiable to 001-136 760.2
      genital tract NEC 760.8
      urinary tract 760.1
   influenza 760.2
      manifest influenza in the infant 771.2
   injury (conditions classifiable to 800-996) 760.5
   malaria 760.2
      manifest malaria in infant or fetus 771.2
   malnutrition 760.4
   necrosis of liver 760.8
   nephritis (conditions classifiable to 580-583) 760.1
   nephrosis (conditions classifiable to 581) 760.1
   noxious substance transmitted via breast milk or placenta 760.70
      alcohol 760.71
      anti-infective agents 760.74
      cocaine 760.75
      "crack" 760.75
      diethylstilbestrol [DES] 760.76
      hallucinogenic agents 760.73
      medicinal agents NEC 760.79
      narcotics 760.72
      obstetric anesthetic or analgesic drug 760.72
      specified agent NEC 760.79
   nutritional disorder (conditions classifiable to 260-269) 760.4

Maternal condition, affecting fetus or newborn (*Continued*)
   operation unrelated to current delivery 760.6
   pre-eclampsia 760.0
   pyelitis or pyelonephritis, arising during pregnancy (conditions classifiable to 590) 760.1
   renal disease or failure 760.1
   respiratory disease, chronic (conditions classifiable to 490-519, 748) 760.3
   rheumatic heart disease (chronic) (conditions classifiable to 393-398) 760.3
   rubella (conditions classifiable to 056) 760.2
      manifest rubella in the infant or fetus 771.0
   surgery unrelated to current delivery 760.6
      to uterus or pelvic organs 763.89
   syphilis (conditions classifiable to 090-097) 760.2
      manifest syphilis in the infant or fetus 090.0
   thrombophlebitis 760.3
   toxemia (of pregnancy) 760.0
      pre-eclamptic 760.0
   toxoplasmosis (conditions classifiable to 130) 760.2
      manifest toxoplasmosis in the infant or fetus 771.2
   transmission of chemical substance through the placenta 760.70
      alcohol 760.71
      anti-infective 760.74
      cocaine 760.75
      "crack" 760.75
      diethylstilbestrol [DES] 760.76
      hallucinogenic agents 760.73
      narcotics 760.72
      specified substance NEC 760.79
   uremia 760.1
   urinary tract conditions (conditions classifiable to 580-599) 760.1
   vomiting (pernicious) (persistent) (vicious) 761.8
Maternity - *see* Delivery
Matheiu's disease (leptospiral jaundice) 100.0
Mauclaire's disease or osteochondrosis 732.3
Maxcy's disease 081.0
Maxilla, maxillary - *see* condition
May (-Hegglin) anomaly or syndrome 288.2
Mayaro fever 066.3
Mazoplasia 610.8
MBD (minimal brain dysfunction), child (*see also* Hyperkinesia) 314.9
MCAD (medium chain acyl CoA dehydrogenase deficiency) 277.85 ◀
McArdle (-Schmid-Pearson) disease or syndrome (glycogenosis V) 271.0
McCune-Albright syndrome (osteitis fibrosa disseminata) 756.59
MCLS (mucocutaneous lymph node syndrome) 446.1
McQuarrie's syndrome (idiopathic familial hypoglycemia) 251.2
Measles (black) (hemorrhagic) (suppressed) 055.9
   with
      encephalitis 055.0
      keratitis 055.71
      keratoconjunctivitis 055.71

Measles (*Continued*)
   with (*Continued*)
      otitis media 055.2
      pneumonia 055.1
   complication 055.8
      specified type NEC 055.79
   encephalitis 055.0
   French 056.9
   German 056.9
   keratitis 055.71
   keratoconjunctivitis 055.71
   liberty 056.9
   otitis media 055.2
   pneumonia 055.1
   specified complications NEC 055.79
   vaccination, prophylactic (against) V04.2
Meatitis, urethral (*see also* Urethritis) 597.89
Meat poisoning - *see* Poisoning, food
Meatus, meatal - *see* condition
Meat-wrappers' asthma 506.9
Meckel's
   diverticulitis 751.0
   diverticulum (displaced) (hypertrophic) 751.0
Meconium
   aspiration 770.1
   delayed passage in newborn 777.1
   ileus 777.1
      due to cystic fibrosis 277.01
   in liquor 792.3
      noted during delivery 656.8
   insufflation 770.1
   obstruction
      fetus or newborn 777.1
         in mucoviscidosis 277.01
   passage of 792.3
      noted during delivery - omit code
   peritonitis 777.6
   plug syndrome (newborn) NEC 777.1
Median - *see also* condition
   arcuate ligament syndrome 447.4
   bar (prostate) 600.90
      with urinary retention 600.91
      vesical orifice 600.90
         with urinary retention 600.91
   rhomboid glossitis 529.2
Mediastinal shift 793.2
Mediastinitis (acute) (chronic) 519.2
   actinomycotic 039.8
   syphilitic 095.8
   tuberculous (*see also* Tuberculosis) 012.8
Mediastinopericarditis (*see also* Pericarditis) 423.9
   acute 420.90
   chronic 423.8
      rheumatic 393
   rheumatic, chronic 393
Mediastinum, mediastinal - *see* condition
Medical services provided for - *see* Health, services provided because (of)
Medicine poisoning (by overdose) (wrong substance given or taken in error) 977.9
   specified drug or substance - *see* Table of Drugs and Chemicals
Medin's disease (poliomyelitis) 045.9
Mediterranean
   anemia (with other hemoglobinopathy) 282.49
   disease or syndrome (hemipathic) 282.49
   fever (*see also* Brucellosis) 023.9
      familial 277.3

◀ **New**   ◀▥ **Revised**

Mediterranean *(Continued)*
  kala-azar 085.0
  leishmaniasis 085.0
  tick fever 082.1
Medulla - *see* condition
Medullary
  cystic kidney 753.16
  sponge kidney 753.17
Medullated fibers
  optic (nerve) 743.57
  retina 362.85
Medulloblastoma (M9470/3)
  desmoplastic (M9471/3) 191.6
  specified site - *see* Neoplasm, by site, malignant
  unspecified site 191.6
Medulloepithelioma (M9501/3) - *see also* Neoplasm, by site, malignant
  teratoid (M9502/3) - *see* Neoplasm, by site, malignant
Medullomyoblastoma (M9472/3)
  specified site - *see* Neoplasm, by site, malignant
  unspecified site 191.6
Meekeren-Ehlers-Danlos syndrome 756.83
Megacaryocytic - *see* condition
Megacolon (acquired) (functional) (not Hirschsprung's disease) 564.7
  aganglionic 751.3
  congenital, congenitum 751.3
  Hirschsprung's (disease) 751.3
  psychogenic 306.4
  toxic (*see also* Colitis, ulcerative) 556.9
Megaduodenum 537.3
Megaesophagus (functional) 530.0
  congenital 750.4
Megakaryocytic - *see* condition
Megalencephaly 742.4
Megalerythema (epidermicum) (infectiosum) 057.0
Megalia, cutis et ossium 757.39
Megaloappendix 751.5
Megalocephalus, megalocephaly NEC 756.0
Megalocornea 743.41
  associated with buphthalmos 743.22
Megalocytic anemia 281.9
Megalodactylia (fingers) (thumbs) 755.57
  toes 755.65
Megaloduodenum 751.5
Megaloesophagus (functional) 530.0
  congenital 750.4
Megalogastria (congenital) 750.7
Megalomania 307.9
Megalophthalmos 743.8
Megalopsia 368.14
Megalosplenia (*see also* Splenomegaly) 789.2
Megaloureter 593.89
  congenital 753.22
Megarectum 569.49
Megasigmoid 564.7
  congenital 751.3
Megaureter 593.89
  congenital 753.22
Megrim 346.9
Meibomian
  cyst 373.2
    infected 373.12
  gland - *see* condition
  infarct (eyelid) 374.85
  stye 373.11
Meibomitis 373.12

Meige
  -Milroy disease (chronic hereditary edema) 757.0
  syndrome (blepharospasm-oromandibular dystonia) 333.82
Melalgia, nutritional 266.2
Melancholia (*see also* Psychosis, affective) 296.90
  climacteric 296.2
    recurrent episode 296.3
    single episode 296.2
  hypochondriac 300.7
  intermittent 296.2
    recurrent episode 296.3
    single episode 296.2
  involutional 296.2
    recurrent episode 296.3
    single episode 296.2
  menopausal 296.2
    recurrent episode 296.3
    single episode 296.2
  puerperal 296.2
  reactive (from emotional stress, psychological trauma) 298.0
  recurrent 296.3
  senile 290.21
  stuporous 296.2
    recurrent episode 296.3
    single episode 296.2
Melanemia 275.0
Melanoameloblastoma (M9363/0) - *see* Neoplasm, bone, benign
Melanoblastoma (M8720/3) - *see* Melanoma
Melanoblastosis
  Block-Sulzberger 757.33
  cutis linearis sive systematisata 757.33
Melanocarcinoma (M8720/3) - *see* Melanoma
Melanocytoma, eyeball (M8726/0) 224.0
Melanoderma, melanodermia 709.09
  Addison's (primary adrenal insufficiency) 255.4
Melanodontia, infantile 521.05
Melanodontoclasia 521.05
Melanoepithelioma (M8720/3) - *see* Melanoma
Melanoma (malignant) (M8720/3) 172.9

Note   Except where otherwise indicated, the morphological varieties of melanoma in the list below should be coded by site as for "Melanoma (malignant)." Internal sites should be coded to malignant neoplasm of those sites.

  abdominal wall 172.5
  ala nasi 172.3
  amelanotic (M8730/3) - *see* Melanoma, by site
  ankle 172.7
  anus, anal 154.3
    canal 154.2
  arm 172.6
  auditory canal (external) 172.2
  auricle (ear) 172.2
  auricular canal (external) 172.2
  axilla 172.5
  axillary fold 172.5
  back 172.5
  balloon cell (M8722/3) - *see* Melanoma, by site

Melanoma *(Continued)*
  benign (M8720/0) - *see* Neoplasm, skin, benign
  breast (female) (male) 172.5
  brow 172.3
  buttock 172.5
  canthus (eye) 172.1
  cheek (external) 172.3
  chest wall 172.5
  chin 172.3
  choroid 190.6
  conjunctiva 190.3
  ear (external) 172.2
  epithelioid cell (M8771/3) - *see also* Melanoma, by site
    and spindle cell, mixed (M8775/3) - *see* Melanoma, by site
  external meatus (ear) 172.2
  eye 190.9
  eyebrow 172.3
  eyelid (lower) (upper) 172.1
  face NEC 172.3
  female genital organ (external) NEC 184.4
  finger 172.6
  flank 172.5
  foot 172.7
  forearm 172.6
  forehead 172.3
  foreskin 187.1
  gluteal region 172.5
  groin 172.5
  hand 172.6
  heel 172.7
  helix 172.2
  hip 172.7
  in
    giant pigmented nevus (M8761/3) - *see* Melanoma, by site
    Hutchinson's melanotic freckle (M8742/3) - *see* Melanoma, by site
    junctional nevus (M8740/3) - *see* Melanoma, by site
    precancerous melanosis (M8741/3) - *see* Melanoma, by site
  interscapular region 172.5
  iris 190.0
  jaw 172.3
  juvenile (M8770/0) - *see* Neoplasm, skin, benign
  knee 172.7
  labium
    majus 184.1
    minus 184.2
  lacrimal gland 190.2
  leg 172.7
  lip (lower) (upper) 172.0
  liver 197.7
  lower limb NEC 172.7
  male genital organ (external) NEC 187.9
  meatus, acoustic (external) 172.2
  meibomian gland 172.1
  metastatic
    of or from specified site - *see* Melanoma, by site
    site not of skin - *see* Neoplasm, by site, malignant, secondary
    to specified site - *see* Neoplasm, by site, malignant, secondary
    unspecified site 172.9
  nail 172.9
    finger 172.6
    toe 172.7
  neck 172.4

Melanoma (Continued)
nodular (M8721/3) - see Melanoma, by site
nose, external 172.3
orbit 190.1
penis 187.4
perianal skin 172.5
perineum 172.5
pinna 172.2
popliteal (fossa) (space) 172.7
prepuce 187.1
pubes 172.5
pudendum 184.4
retina 190.5
scalp 172.4
scrotum 187.7
septum nasal (skin) 172.3
shoulder 172.6
skin NEC 172.8
spindle cell (M8772/3) - see also Melanoma, by site
type A (M8773/3) 190.0
type B (M8774/3) 190.0
submammary fold 172.5
superficial spreading (M8743/3) - see Melanoma, by site
temple 172.3
thigh 172.7
toe 172.7
trunk NEC 172.5
umbilicus 172.5
upper limb NEC 172.6
vagina vault 184.0
vulva 184.4
Melanoplakia 528.9
Melanosarcoma (M8720/3) - see also Melanoma
epithelioid cell (M8771/3) - see Melanoma
Melanosis 709.09
addisonian (primary adrenal insufficiency) 255.4
tuberculous (see also Tuberculosis) 017.6
adrenal 255.4
colon 569.89
conjunctiva 372.55
congenital 743.49
corii degenerativa 757.33
cornea (presenile) (senile) 371.12
congenital 743.43
interfering with vision 743.42
prenatal 743.43
interfering with vision 743.42
eye 372.55
congenital 743.49
jute spinners' 709.09
lenticularis progressiva 757.33
liver 573.8
precancerous (M8741/2) - see also Neoplasm, skin, in situ
malignant melanoma in (M8741/3) - see Melanoma
Riehl's 709.09
sclera 379.19
congenital 743.47
suprarenal 255.4
tar 709.09
toxic 709.09
Melanuria 791.9
MELAS syndrome (mitochondrial encephalopathy, lactic acidosis and stroke-like episodes) 277.87 ◀▦

Melasma 709.09
adrenal (gland) 255.4
suprarenal (gland) 255.4
Melena 578.1
due to
swallowed maternal blood 777.3
ulcer - see Ulcer, by site, with hemorrhage
newborn 772.4
due to swallowed maternal blood 777.3
Meleney's
gangrene (cutaneous) 686.09
ulcer (chronic undermining) 686.09
Melioidosis 025
Melitensis, febris 023.0
Melitococcosis 023.0
Melkersson (-Rosenthal) syndrome 351.8
Mellitus, diabetes - see Diabetes
Melorheostosis (bone) (leri) 733.99
Meloschisis 744.83
Melotia 744.29
Membrana
capsularis lentis posterior 743.39
epipapillaris 743.57
Membranacea placenta - see Placenta, abnormal
Membranaceous uterus 621.8
Membrane, membranous - see also condition
folds, congenital - see Web
Jackson's 751.4
over face (causing asphyxia), fetus or newborn 768.9
premature rupture - see Rupture, membranes, premature
pupillary 364.74
persistent 743.46
retained (complicating delivery) (with hemorrhage) 666.2
without hemorrhage 667.1
secondary (eye) 366.50
unruptured (causing asphyxia) 768.9
vitreous humor 379.25
Membranitis, fetal 658.4
affecting fetus or newborn 762.7
Memory disturbance, loss or lack (see also Amnesia) 780.93
mild, following organic brain damage 310.1
Menadione (vitamin K) deficiency 269.0
Menarche, precocious 259.1
Mendacity, pathologic 301.7
Mende's syndrome (ptosis-epicanthus) 270.2
Mendelson's syndrome (resulting from a procedure) 997.3
obstetric 668.0
Ménétrier's disease or syndrome (hypertrophic gastritis) 535.2
Ménière's disease, syndrome, or vertigo 386.00
cochlear 386.02
cochleovestibular 386.01
inactive 386.04
in remission 386.04
vestibular 386.03
Meninges, meningeal - see condition
Meningioma (M9530/0) - see also Neoplasm, meninges, benign
angioblastic (M9535/0) - see Neoplasm, meninges, benign
angiomatous (M9534/0) - see Neoplasm, meninges, benign
endotheliomatous (M9531/0) - see Neoplasm, meninges, benign

Meningioma (Continued)
fibroblastic (M9532/0) - see Neoplasm, meninges, benign
fibrous (M9532/0) - see Neoplasm, meninges, benign
hemangioblastic (M9535/0) - see Neoplasm, meninges, benign
hemangiopericytic (M9536/0) - see Neoplasm, meninges, benign
malignant (M9530/3) - see Neoplasm, meninges, malignant
meningiothelial (M9531/0) - see Neoplasm, meninges, benign
meningotheliomatous (M9531/0) - see Neoplasm, meninges, benign
mixed (M9537/0) - see Neoplasm, meninges, benign
multiple (M9530/1) 237.6
papillary (M9538/1) 237.6
psammomatous (M9533/0) - see Neoplasm, meninges, benign
syncytial (M9531/0) - see Neoplasm, meninges, benign
transitional (M9537/0) - see Neoplasm, meninges, benign
Meningiomatosis (diffuse) (M9530/1) 237.6
Meningism (see also Meningismus) 781.6
Meningismus (infectional) (pneumococcal) 781.6
due to serum or vaccine 997.09 [321.8]
influenzal NEC 487.8
Meningitis (basal) (basic) (basilar) (brain) (cerebral) (cervical) (congestive) (diffuse) (hemorrhagic) (infantile) (membranous) (metastatic) (nonspecific) (pontine) (progressive) (simple) (spinal) (subacute) (sympathetica) (toxic) 322.9
abacterial NEC (see also Meningitis, aseptic) 047.9
actinomycotic 039.8 [320.7]
adenoviral 049.1
Aerobacter aerogenes 320.82
anaerobes (cocci) (gram-negative) (gram-positive) (mixed) (NEC) 320.81
arbovirus NEC 066.9 [321.2]
specified type NEC 066.8 [321.2]
aseptic (acute) NEC 047.9
adenovirus 049.1
Coxsackie virus 047.0
due to
adenovirus 049.1
Coxsackie virus 047.0
echo virus 047.1
enterovirus 047.9
mumps 072.1
poliovirus (see also Poliomyelitis) 045.2 [321.2]
echo virus 047.1
herpes (simplex) virus 054.72
zoster 053.0
leptospiral 100.81
lymphocytic choriomeningitis 049.0
noninfective 322.0
Bacillus pyocyaneus 320.89
bacterial NEC 320.9
anaerobic 320.81
gram-negative 320.82
anaerobic 320.81
Bacteroides (fragilis) (oralis) (melaninogenicus) 320.81
cancerous (M8000/6) 198.4

ICD-9-CM

M

Vol.

Meningitis *(Continued)*
  candidal 112.83
  carcinomatous (M8010/6) 198.4
  caseous *(see also* Tuberculosis, meninges) 013.0
  cerebrospinal (acute) (chronic) (diplococcal) (endemic) (epidemic) (fulminant) (infectious) (malignant) (meningococcal) (sporadic) 036.0
    carrier (suspected) of V02.59
  chronic NEC 322.2
  clear cerebrospinal fluid NEC 322.0
  Clostridium (haemolyticum) (novyi) NEC 320.81
  coccidioidomycosis 114.2
  Coxsackie virus 047.0
  cryptococcal 117.5 *[321.0]*
  diplococcal 036.0
    gram-negative 036.0
    gram-positive 320.1
  Diplococcus pneumoniae 320.1
  due to
    actinomycosis 039.8 *[320.7]*
    adenovirus 049.1
    coccidiomycosis 114.2
    enterovirus 047.9
      specified NEC 047.8
    histoplasmosis *(see also* Histoplasmosis) 115.91
    listerosis 027.0 *[320.7]*
    Lyme disease 088.81 *[320.7]*
    moniliasis 112.83
    mumps 072.1
    neurosyphilis 094.2
    nonbacterial organisms NEC 321.8
    oidiomycosis 112.83
    poliovirus *(see also* Poliomyelitis) 045.2 *[321.2]*
    preventive immunization, inoculation, or vaccination 997.09 *[321.8]*
    sarcoidosis 135 *[321.4]*
    sporotrichosis 117.1 *[321.1]*
    syphilis 094.2
      acute 091.81
      congenital 090.42
      secondary 091.81
    trypanosomiasis *(see also* Trypanosomiasis) 086.9 *[321.3]*
    whooping cough 033.9 *[320.7]*
  E. coli 320.82
  ECHO virus 047.1
  endothelial-leukocytic, benign, recurrent 047.9
  Enterobacter aerogenes 320.82
  enteroviral 047.9
    specified type NEC 047.8
  enterovirus 047.9
    specified NEC 047.8
  eosinophilic 322.1
  epidemic NEC 036.0
  Escherichia coli (E. coli) 320.82
  Eubacterium 320.81
  fibrinopurulent NEC 320.9
    specified type NEC 320.89
  Friedländer (bacillus) 320.82
  fungal NEC 117.9 *[321.1]*
  Fusobacterium 320.81
  gonococcal 098.82
  gram-negative bacteria NEC 320.82
    anaerobic 320.81
    cocci 036.0
      specified NEC 320.82
  gram-negative cocci NEC 036.0

Meningitis *(Continued)*
  gram-negative cocci NEC *(Continued)*
    specified NEC 320.82
  gram-positive cocci NEC 320.9
  H. influenzae 320.0
  herpes (simplex) virus 054.72
    zoster 053.0
  infectious NEC 320.9
  influenzal 320.0
  Klebsiella pneumoniae 320.82
  late effect - *see* Late, effect, meningitis
  leptospiral (aseptic) 100.81
  Listerella (monocytogenes) 027.0 *[320.7]*
  Listeria monocytogenes 027.0 *[320.7]*
  lymphocytic (acute) (benign) (serous) 049.0
    choriomeningitis virus 049.0
  meningococcal (chronic) 036.0
  Mima polymorpha 320.82
  Mollaret's 047.9
  monilial 112.83
  mumps (virus) 072.1
  mycotic NEC 117.9 *[321.1]*
  Neisseria 036.0
  neurosyphilis 094.2
  nonbacterial NEC *(see also* Meningitis, aseptic) 047.9
  nonpyogenic NEC 322.0
  oidiomycosis 112.83
  ossificans 349.2
  Peptococcus 320.81
  Peptostreptococcus 320.81
  pneumococcal 320.1
  poliovirus *(see also* Poliomyelitis) 045.2 *[321.2]*
  Propionibacterium 320.81
  Proteus morganii 320.82
  Pseudomonas (aeruginosa) (pyocyaneus) 320.82
  purulent NEC 320.9
    specified organism NEC 320.89
  pyogenic NEC 320.9
    specified organism NEC 320.89
  Salmonella 003.21
  septic NEC 320.9
    specified organism NEC 320.89
  serosa circumscripta NEC 322.0
  serous NEC *(see also* Meningitis, aseptic) 047.9
    lymphocytic 049.0
    syndrome 348.2
  Serratia (marcescens) 320.82
  specified organism NEC 320.89
  sporadic cerebrospinal 036.0
  sporotrichosis 117.1 *[321.1]*
  staphylococcal 320.3
  sterile 997.09
  streptococcal (acute) 320.2
  suppurative 320.9
    specified organism NEC 320.89
  syphilitic 094.2
    acute 091.81
    congenital 090.42
    secondary 091.81
  torula 117.5 *[321.0]*
  traumatic (complication of injury) 958.8
  Treponema (denticola) (macrodenticum) 320.81
  trypanosomiasis 086.1 *[321.3]*
  tuberculous *(see also* Tuberculosis, meninges) 013.0
  typhoid 002.0 *[320.7]*

Meningitis *(Continued)*
  Veillonella 320.81
  Vibrio vulnificus 320.82
  viral, virus NEC *(see also* Meningitis, aseptic) 047.9
  Wallgren's *(see also* Meningitis, aseptic) 047.9
Meningocele (congenital) (spinal) *(see also* Spina bifida) 741.9
  acquired (traumatic) 349.2
  cerebral 742.0
  cranial 742.0
Meningocerebritis - *see* Meningoencephalitis
Meningococcemia (acute) (chronic) 036.2
Meningococcus, meningococcal *(see also* condition) 036.9
  adrenalitis, hemorrhagic 036.3
  carditis 036.40
  carrier (suspected) of V02.59
  cerebrospinal fever 036.0
  encephalitis 036.1
  endocarditis 036.42
  exposure to V01.84   ◀
  infection NEC 036.9
  meningitis (cerebrospinal) 036.0
  myocarditis 036.43
  optic neuritis 036.81
  pericarditis 036.41
  septicemia (chronic) 036.2
Meningoencephalitis *(see also* Encephalitis) 323.9
  acute NEC 048
  bacterial, purulent, pyogenic, or septic - *see* Meningitis
  chronic NEC 094.1
  diffuse NEC 094.1
  diphasic 063.2
  due to
    actinomycosis 039.8 *[320.7]*
    blastomycosis NEC *(see also* Blastomycosis) 116.0 *[323.4]*
    free-living amebae 136.2
    Listeria monocytogenes 027.0 *[320.7]*
    Lyme disease 088.81 *[320.7]*
    mumps 072.2
    Naegleria (amebae) (gruberi) (organisms) 136.2
    rubella 056.01
    sporotrichosis 117.1 *[321.1]*
    toxoplasmosis (acquired) 130.0
      congenital (active) 771.2 *[323.4]*
    Trypanosoma 086.1 *[323.2]*
  epidemic 036.0
  herpes 054.3
  herpetic 054.3
  H. influenzae 320.0
  infectious (acute) 048
  influenzal 320.0
  late effect - *see* category 326
  Listeria monocytogenes 027.0 *[320.7]*
  lymphocytic (serous) 049.0
  mumps 072.2
  parasitic NEC 123.9 *[323.4]*
  pneumococcal 320.1
  primary amebic 136.2
  rubella 056.01
  serous 048
    lymphocytic 049.0
  specific 094.2
  staphylococcal 320.3
  streptococcal 320.2
  syphilitic 094.2
  toxic NEC 989.9 *[323.7]*

Meningoencephalitis (*Continued*)
 toxic NEC (*Continued*)
  due to
   carbon tetrachloride 987.8
    [323.7]
   hydroxyquinoline derivatives poi-
    soning 961.3 [323.7]
   lead 984.9 [323.7]
   mercury 985.0 [323.7]
   thallium 985.8 [323.7]
  toxoplasmosis (acquired) 130.0
  trypanosomic 086.1 [323.2]
  tuberculous (*see also* Tuberculosis, meninges) 013.0
  virus NEC 048
Meningoencephalocele 742.0
 syphilitic 094.89
  congenital 090.49
Meningoencephalomyelitis (*see also* Meningoencephalitis) 323.9
 acute NEC 048
  disseminated (postinfectious) 136.9
   [323.6]
   postimmunization or postvaccina-
    tion 323.5
 due to
  actinomycosis 039.8 [320.7]
  torula 117.5 [323.4]
  toxoplasma or toxoplasmosis (acquired) 130.0
   congenital (active) 771.2 [323.4]
 late effect - *see* category 326
Meningoencephalomyelopathy (*see also*
  Meningoencephalomyelitis) 349.9
Meningoencephalopathy (*see also* Meningoencephalitis) 348.39
Meningoencephalopoliomyelitis (*see also*
  Poliomyelitis, bulbar) 045.0
 late effect 138
Meningomyelitis (*see also* Meningoencephalitis) 323.9
 blastomycotic NEC (*see also* Blastomycosis) 116.0 [323.4]
 due to
  actinomycosis 039.8 [320.7]
  blastomycosis (*see also* Blastomycosis) 116.0 [323.4]
  Meningococcus 036.0
  sporotrichosis 117.1 [323.4]
  torula 117.5 [323.4]
 late effect - *see* category 326
 lethargic 049.8
 meningococcal 036.0
 syphilitic 094.2
 tuberculous (*see also* Tuberculosis, meninges) 013.0
Meningomyelocele (*see also* Spina bifida)
  741.9
 syphilitic 094.89
Meningomyeloneuritis - *see* Meningoencephalitis
Meningoradiculitis - *see* Meningitis
Meningovascular - *see* condition
Meniscocytosis 282.60
Menkes' syndrome - *see* Syndrome,
  Menkes'
Menolipsis 626.0
Menometrorrhagia 626.2
Menopause, menopausal (symptoms)
  (syndrome) 627.2
 arthritis (any site) NEC 716.3
 artificial 627.4
 bleeding 627.0
 crisis 627.2

Menopause, menopausal (*Continued*)
 depression (*see also* Psychosis, affective) 296.2
  agitated 296.2
   recurrent episode 296.3
   single episode 296.2
  psychotic 296.2
   recurrent episode 296.3
   single episode 296.2
  recurrent episode 296.3
  single episode 296.2
 melancholia (*see also* Psychosis, affective) 296.2
  recurrent episode 296.3
  single episode 296.2
 paranoid state 297.2
 paraphrenia 297.2
 postsurgical 627.4
 premature 256.31
  postirradiation 256.2
  postsurgical 256.2
 psychoneurosis 627.2
 psychosis NEC 298.8
 surgical 627.4
 toxic polyarthritis NEC 716.39
Menorrhagia (primary) 626.2
 climacteric 627.0
 menopausal 627.0
 postclimacteric 627.1
 postmenopausal 627.1
 preclimacteric 627.0
 premenopausal 627.0
 puberty (menses retained) 626.3
Menorrhalgia 625.3
Menoschesis 626.8
Menostaxis 626.2
Menses, retention 626.8
Menstrual - *see also* Menstruation
 cycle, irregular 626.4
 disorders NEC 626.9
 extraction V25.3
 fluid, retained 626.8
 molimen 625.4
 period, normal V65.5
 regulation V25.3
Menstruation
 absent 626.0
 anovulatory 628.0
 delayed 626.8
 difficult 625.3
 disorder 626.9
  psychogenic 306.52
  specified NEC 626.8
 during pregnancy 640.8
 excessive 626.2
 frequent 626.2
 infrequent 626.1
 irregular 626.4
 latent 626.8
 membranous 626.8
 painful (primary) (secondary) 625.3
  psychogenic 306.52
 passage of clots 626.2
 precocious 626.8
 protracted 626.8
 retained 626.8
 retrograde 626.8
 scanty 626.1
 suppression 626.8
 vicarious (nasal) 625.8
Mentagra (*see also* Sycosis) 704.8
Mental - *see also* condition
 deficiency (*see also* Retardation, mental)
  319

Mental (*Continued*)
 deterioration (*see also* Psychosis) 298.9
 disorder (*see also* Disorder, mental)
  300.9
 exhaustion 300.5
 insufficiency (congenital) (*see also* Retardation, mental) 319
 observation without need for further
  medical care NEC V71.09
 retardation (*see also* Retardation, mental) 319
 subnormality (*see also* Retardation,
  mental) 319
  mild 317
  moderate 318.0
  profound 318.2
  severe 318.1
 upset (*see also* Disorder, mental) 300.9
Meralgia paresthetica 355.1
Mercurial - *see* condition
Mercurialism NEC 985.0
Merergasia 300.9
MERFF 758.89
Merkel cell tumor - *see* Neoplasm, by
  site, malignant
Merocele (*see also* Hernia, femoral) 553.00
Meromelia 755.4
 lower limb 755.30
  intercalary 755.32
   femur 755.34
    tibiofibular (complete) (incom-
     plete) 755.33
   fibula 755.37
   metatarsal(s) 755.38
   tarsal(s) 755.38
   tibia 755.36
   tibiofibular 755.35
  terminal (complete) (partial) (transverse) 755.31
   longitudinal 755.32
    metatarsal(s) 755.38
    phalange(s) 755.39
    tarsal(s) 755.38
   transverse 755.31
 upper limb 755.20
  intercalary 755.22
   carpal(s) 755.28
   humeral 755.24
    radioulnar (complete) (incom-
     plete) 755.23
   metacarpal(s) 755.28
   phalange(s) 755.29
   radial 755.26
   radioulnar 755.25
   ulnar 755.27
  terminal (complete) (partial) (transverse) 755.21
   longitudinal 755.22
    carpal(s) 755.28
    metacarpal(s) 755.28
    phalange(s) 755.29
   transverse 755.21
Merosmia 781.1
MERRF syndrome (myoclonus with epilepsy and with ragged red fibers)
  277.87   ◄
Merycism - *see also* Vomiting
 psychogenic 307.53
Merzbacher-Pelizaeus disease 330.0
Mesaortitis - *see* Aortitis
Mesarteritis - *see* Arteritis
Mesencephalitis (*see also* Encephalitis)
  323.9
 late effect - *see* category 326

◄ **New**   ◄▥ **Revised**

Mesenchymoma (M8990/1) - *see also* Neoplasm, connective tissue, uncertain behavior
  benign (M8990/0) - *see* Neoplasm, connective tissue, benign
  malignant (M8990/3) - *see* Neoplasm, connective tissue, malignant
Mesentery, mesenteric - *see* condition
Mesiodens, mesiodentes 520.1
  causing crowding 524.31 ◀▥
Mesio-occlusion 524.23 ◀▥
Mesocardia (with asplenia) 746.87
Mesocolon - *see* condition
Mesonephroma (malignant) (M9110/3) - *see also* Neoplasm, by site, malignant
  benign (M9110/0) - *see* Neoplasm, by site, benign
Mesophlebitis - *see* Phlebitis
Mesostromal dysgenesis 743.51
Mesothelioma (malignant) (M9050/3) - *see also* Neoplasm, by site, malignant
  benign (M9050/0) - *see* Neoplasm, by site, benign
  biphasic type (M9053/3) - *see also* Neoplasm, by site, malignant
    benign (M9053/0) - *see* Neoplasm, by site, benign
  epithelioid (M9052/3) - *see also* Neoplasm, by site, malignant
    benign (M9052/0) - *see* Neoplasm, by site, benign
  fibrous (M9051/3) - *see also* Neoplasm, by site, malignant
    benign (M9051/0) - *see* Neoplasm, by site, benign
Metabolic syndrome 277.7 ◀
Metabolism disorder 277.9
  specified type NEC 277.89
Metagonimiasis 121.5
Metagonimus infestation (small intestine) 121.5
Metal
  pigmentation (skin) 709.00
  polishers' disease 502
Metalliferous miners' lung 503
Metamorphopsia 368.14
Metaplasia
  bone, in skin 709.3
  breast 611.8
  cervix - omit code
  endometrium (squamous) 621.8
  esophagus 530.85
  intestinal, of gastric mucosa 537.89
  kidney (pelvis) (squamous) (*see also* Disease, renal) 593.89
  myelogenous 289.89
  myeloid (agnogenic) (megakaryocytic) 289.89
  spleen 289.59
  squamous cell
    amnion 658.8
    bladder 596.8
    cervix - *see* condition
    trachea 519.1
    tracheobronchial tree 519.1
    uterus 621.8
    cervix - *see* condition
Metastasis, metastatic
  abscess - *see* Abscess
  calcification 275.40
  cancer, neoplasm, or disease
    from specified site (M8000/3) - *see* Neoplasm, by site, malignant
    to specified site (M8000/6) - *see* Neoplasm, by site, secondary

Metastasis, metastatic (*Continued*)
  deposits (in) (M8000/6) - *see* Neoplasm, by site, secondary
  pneumonia 038.8 [484.8]
  spread (to) (M8000/6) - *see* Neoplasm, by site, secondary
Metatarsalgia 726.70
  anterior 355.6
  due to Freiberg's disease 732.5
  Morton's 355.6
Metatarsus, metatarsal - *see also* condition
  abductus varus (congenital) 764.60
  adductus valgus (congenital) 754.53
  primus varus 754.52
  valgus (adductus) (congenital) 754.60
  varus (abductus) (congenital) 754.53
    primus 754.52
Methemoglobinemia 289.7
  acquired (with sulfhemoglobinemia) 289.7
  congenital 289.7
  enzymatic 289.7
  Hb-M disease 289.7
  hereditary 289.7
  toxic 289.7
Methemoglobinuria (*see also* Hemoglobinuria) 791.2
Methicillin-resistant staphylococcus aureus (MRSA) V09.0 ◀
Methioninemia 270.4
Metritis (catarrhal) (septic) (suppurative) (*see also* endometritis) 615.9
  blennorrhagic 098.16
    chronic or duration of 2 months or over 098.36
  cervical (*see also* Cervicitis) 616.0
  gonococcal 098.16
    chronic or duration of 2 months or over 098.36
  hemorrhagic 626.8
  puerperal, postpartum, childbirth 670
  tuberculous (*see also* Tuberculosis) 016.7
Metropathia hemorrhagica 626.8
Metroperitonitis (*see also* Peritonitis, pelvic, female) 614.5
Metrorrhagia 626.6
  arising during pregnancy - *see* Hemorrhage, pregnancy
  postpartum NEC 666.2
  primary 626.6
  psychogenic 306.59
  puerperal 666.2
Metrorrhexis - *see* Rupture, uterus
Metrosalpingitis (*see also* Salpingooophoritis) 614.2
Metrostaxis 626.6
Metrovaginitis (*see also* Endometritis) 615.9
  gonococcal (acute) 098.16
    chronic or duration of 2 months or over 098.36
Mexican fever - *see* Typhus, Mexican
Meyenburg-Altherr-Uehlinger syndrome 733.99
Meyer-Schwickerath and Weyers syndrome (dysplasia oculodentodigitalis) 759.89
Meynert's amentia (nonalcoholic) 294.0
  alcoholic 291.1
Mibelli's disease 757.39
Mice, joint (*see also* Loose, body, joint) 718.1
  knee 717.6
Micheli-Rietti syndrome (thalassemia minor) 282.49

Michotte's syndrome 721.5
Micrencephalon, micrencephaly 742.1
Microaneurysm, retina 362.14
  diabetic 250.5 [362.01]
Microangiopathy 443.9
  diabetic (peripheral) 250.7 [443.81]
    retinal 250.5 [362.01]
  peripheral 443.9
    diabetic 250.7 [443.81]
  retinal 362.18
    diabetic 250.5 [362.01]
  thrombotic 446.6
    Moschcowitz's (thrombotic thrombocytopenic purpura) 446.6
Microcalcification, mammographic 793.81
Microcephalus, microcephalic, microcephaly 742.1
  due to toxoplasmosis (congenital) 771.2
Microcheilia 744.82
Microcolon (congenital) 751.5
Microcornea (congenital) 743.41
Microcytic - *see* condition
Microdeletions NEC 758.33 ◀
Microdontia 520.2
Microdrepanocytosis (thalassemia-Hb-S disease) 282.49
Microembolism
  atherothrombotic - *see* Atheroembolism
  retina 362.33
Microencephalon 742.1
Microfilaria streptocerca infestation 125.3
Microgastria (congenital) 750.7
Microgenia 524.06
Microgenitalia (congenital) 752.89
  penis 752.64
Microglioma (M9710/3)
  specified site - *see* Neoplasm, by site, malignant
  unspecified site 191.9
Microglossia (congenital) 750.16
Micrognathia, micrognathism (congenital) 524.00
  mandibular 524.04
    alveolar 524.74
  maxillary 524.03
    alveolar 524.73
Microgyria (congenital) 742.2
Microinfarct, heart (*see also* Insufficiency, coronary) 411.89
Microlithiasis, alveolar, pulmonary 516.2
Micromyelia (congenital) 742.59
Micropenis 752.64
Microphakia (congenital) 743.36
Microphthalmia (congenital) (*see also* Microphthalmos) 743.10
Microphthalmos (congenital) 743.10
  associated with eye and adnexal anomalies NEC 743.12
  due to toxoplasmosis (congenital) 771.2
  isolated 743.11
  simple 743.11
  syndrome 759.89
Micropsia 368.14
Microsporidiosis 136.8
Microsporosis (*see also* Dermatophytosis) 110.9
  nigra 111.1
Microsporum furfur infestation 111.0
Microstomia (congenital) 744.84
Microthelia 757.6
Microthromboembolism - *see* Embolism
Microtia (congenital) (external ear) 744.23

ICD-9-CM
M
Vol. 2

Microtropia 378.34
Micturition
  disorder NEC 788.69
    psychogenic 306.53
  frequency 788.41
    psychogenic 306.53
  nocturnal 788.43
  painful 788.1
    psychogenic 306.53
Middle
  ear - *see* condition
  lobe (right) syndrome 518.0
Midplane - *see* condition
Miescher's disease 709.3
  cheilitis 351.8
  granulomatosis disciformis 709.3
**Miescher-Leder syndrome or granulom-
atosis** 709.3
Mieten's syndrome 759.89
Migraine (idiopathic) 346.9
  with aura 346.0
  abdominal (syndrome) 346.2
  allergic (histamine) 346.2
  atypical 346.1
  basilar 346.2
  classical 346.0
  common 346.1
  hemiplegic 346.8
  lower-half 346.2
  menstrual 625.4
  ophthalmic 346.8
  ophthalmoplegic 346.8
  retinal 346.2
  variant 346.2
Migrant, social V60.0
Migratory, migrating - *see also* condition
  person V60.0
  testis, congenital 752.52
Mikulicz's disease or syndrome (dryness of mouth, absent or decreased
lacrimation) 527.1
Milian atrophia blanche 701.3
Miliaria (crystallina) (rubra) (tropicalis)
705.1
  apocrine 705.82
Miliary - *see* condition
Milium (*see also* Cyst, sebaceous) 706.2
  colloid 709.3
  eyelid 374.84
Milk
  crust 690.11
  excess secretion 676.6
  fever, female 672
  poisoning 988.8
  retention 676.2
  sickness 988.8
  spots 423.1
Milkers' nodes 051.1
Milk-leg (deep vessels) 671.4
  complicating pregnancy 671.3
  nonpuerperal 451.19
  puerperal, postpartum, childbirth 671.4
Milkman (-Looser) disease or syndrome
(osteomalacia with pseudofractures)
268.2
Milky urine (*see also* Chyluria) 791.1
Millar's asthma (laryngismus stridulus)
478.75
Millard-Gubler paralysis or syndrome
344.89
Millard-Gubler-Foville paralysis 344.89
Miller-Dieker syndrome 758.33 ◄
Miller's disease (osteomalacia) 268.2
Miller Fisher's syndrome 357.0

Milles' syndrome (encephalocutaneous
angiomatosis) 759.6
Mills' disease 335.29
Millstone makers' asthma or lung 502
Milroy's disease (chronic hereditary
edema) 757.0
Miners' - *see also* condition
  asthma 500
  elbow 727.2
  knee 727.2
  lung 500
  nystagmus 300.89
  phthisis (*see also* Tuberculosis) 011.4
  tuberculosis (*see also* Tuberculosis)
011.4
Minkowski-Chauffard syndrome (*see
also* Spherocytosis) 282.0
Minor - *see* condition
Minor's disease 336.1
Minot's disease (hemorrhagic disease,
newborn) 776.0
Minot-von Willebrand (-Jurgens) disease
or syndrome (angiohemophilia)
286.4
Minus (and plus) hand (intrinsic)
736.09
Miosis (persistent) (pupil) 379.42
Mirizzi's syndrome (hepatic duct stenosis) (*see also* Obstruction, biliary)
576.2
  with calculus, cholelithiasis, or stones -
see Choledocholithiasis
Mirror writing 315.09
  secondary to organic lesion 784.69
Misadventure (prophylactic) (therapeutic) (*see also* Complications) 999.9
  administration of insulin 962.3
  infusion - *see* Complications, infusion
  local applications (of fomentations,
plasters, etc.) 999.9
    burn or scald - *see* Burn, by site
  medical care (early) (late) NEC 999.9
    adverse effect of drugs or chemicals
- *see* Table of Drugs and Chemicals
    burn or scald - *see* Burn, by site
  radiation NEC 990
  radiotherapy NEC 990
  surgical procedure (early) (late) - *see*
Complications, surgical procedure
  transfusion - *see* Complications, transfusion
  vaccination or other immunological
procedure - *see* Complications,
vaccination
Misanthropy 301.7
Miscarriage - *see* Abortion, spontaneous
Mischief, malicious, child (*see also* Disturbance, conduct) 312.0
Misdirection
  aqueous 365.83
Mismanagement, feeding 783.3
Misplaced, misplacement
  kidney (*see also* Disease, renal) 593.0
    congenital 753.3
  organ or site, congenital NEC - *see*
Malposition, congenital
Missed
  abortion 632
  delivery (at or near term) 656.4
  labor (at or near term) 656.4
Missing - *see also* Absence
  teeth (acquired) 525.10
    congenital (*see also* Anodontia) 520.0

Missing (*Continued*)
  teeth (*Continued*)
    due to
      caries 525.13
      extraction 525.10
      periodontal disease 525.12
      specified NEC 525.19
      trauma 525.11
  vertebrae (congenital) 756.13
Misuse of drugs NEC (*see also* Abuse,
drug, nondependent) 305.9
Mitchell's disease (erythromelalgia) 443.89
Mite(s)
  diarrhea 133.8
  grain (itch) 133.8
  hair follicle (itch) 133.8
  in sputum 133.8
**Mitochondrial encephalopathy, lactic
acidosis and stroke-like episodes**
(MELAS syndrome) 277.87 ◄
**Mitochondrial neurogastrointestinal en-
cephalopathy syndrome** (MNGIE)
277.87 ◄
Mitral - *see* condition
Mittelschmerz 625.2
Mixed - *see* condition
Mljet disease (mal de Meleda) 757.39
Mobile, mobility
  cecum 751.4
  coccyx 733.99
  excessive - *see* Hypermobility
  gallbladder 751.69
  kidney 593.0
    congenital 753.3
  organ or site, congenital NEC - *see*
Malposition, congenital
  spleen 289.59
Mobitz heart block (atrioventricular)
426.10
  type I (Wenckebach's) 426.13
  type II 426.12
Möbius'
  disease 346.8
  syndrome
    congenital oculofacial paralysis 352.6
    ophthalmoplegic migraine 346.8
Moeller (-Barlow) disease (infantile
scurvy) 267
  glossitis 529.4
Mohr's syndrome (types I and II) 759.89
Mola destruens (M9100/1) 236.1
Molarization, premolars 520.2
Molar pregnancy 631
  hydatidiform (delivered) (undelivered)
630
Mold(s) in vitreous 117.9
Molding, head (during birth) - *omit
code*
Mole (pigmented) (M8720/0) - *see also*
Neoplasm, skin, benign
  blood 631
  Breus' 631
  cancerous (M8720/3) - *see* Melanoma
  carneous 631
  destructive (M9100/1) 236.1
  ectopic - *see* Pregnancy, ectopic
  fleshy 631
  hemorrhagic 631
  hydatid, hydatidiform (benign) (complicating pregnancy) (delivered)
(undelivered) (*see also* Hydatidiform mole) 630
    invasive (M9100/1) 236.1
    malignant (M9100/1) 236.1

◄ **New**   ◄◼ **Revised**

Mole *(Continued)*
hydatid, hydatidiform *(Continued)*
previous, affecting management of pregnancy V23.1
invasive (hydatidiform) (M9100/1) 236.1
malignant
meaning
malignant hydatidiform mole (9100/1) 236.1
melanoma (M8720/3) - *see* Melanoma
nonpigmented (M8730/0) - *see* Neoplasm, skin, benign
pregnancy NEC 631
skin (M8720/0) - *see* Neoplasm, skin, benign
tubal - *see* Pregnancy, tubal
vesicular (*see also* Hydatidiform mole) 630
Molimen, molimina (menstrual) 625.4
Mollaret's meningitis 047.9
Mollities (cerebellar) (cerebral) 437.8
ossium 268.2
Molluscum
contagiosum 078.0
epitheliale 078.0
fibrosum (M8851/0) - *see* Lipoma, by site
pendulum (M8851/0) - *see* Lipoma, by site
Mönckeberg's arteriosclerosis, degeneration, disease, or sclerosis (*see also* Arteriosclerosis, extremities) 440.20
Monday fever 504
Monday morning dyspnea or asthma 504
Mondini's malformation (cochlea) 744.05
Mondor's disease (thrombophlebitis of breast) 451.89
Mongolian, mongolianism, mongolism, mongoloid 758.0
spot 757.33
Monilethrix (congenital) 757.4
Monilia infestation - *see* Candidiasis
Moniliasis - *see also* Candidiasis
neonatal 771.7
vulvovaginitis 112.1
Monkeypox 057.8
Monoarthritis 716.60
ankle 716.67
arm 716.62
lower (and wrist) 716.63
upper (and elbow) 716.62
foot (and ankle) 716.67
forearm (and wrist) 716.63
hand 716.64
leg 716.66
lower 716.66
upper 716.65
pelvic region (hip) (thigh) 716.65
shoulder (region) 716.61
specified site NEC 716.68
Monoblastic - *see* condition
Monochromatism (cone) (rod) 368.54
Monocytic - *see* condition
Monocytosis (symptomatic) 288.8
Monofixation syndrome 378.34
Monomania (*see also* Psychosis) 298.9
Mononeuritis 355.9
cranial nerve - *see* Disorder, nerve, cranial
femoral nerve 355.2
lateral
cutaneous nerve of thigh 355.1
popliteal nerve 355.3

Mononeuritis *(Continued)*
lower limb 355.8
specified nerve NEC 355.79
medial popliteal nerve 355.4
median nerve 354.1
multiplex 354.5
plantar nerve 355.6
posterior tibial nerve 355.5
radial nerve 354.3
sciatic nerve 355.0
ulnar nerve 354.2
upper limb 354.9
specified nerve NEC 354.8
vestibular 388.5
Mononeuropathy (*see also* Mononeuritis) 355.9
diabetic NEC 250.6 *[355.9]*
lower limb 250.6 *[355.8]*
upper limb 250.6 *[354.9]*
iliohypogastric nerve 355.79
ilioinguinal nerve 355.79
obturator nerve 355.79
saphenous nerve 355.79
Mononucleosis, infectious 075
with hepatitis 075 *[573.1]*
Monoplegia 344.5
brain (current episode) (*see also* Paralysis, brain) 437.8
fetus or newborn 767.8
cerebral (current episode) (*see also* Paralysis, brain) 437.8
congenital or infantile (cerebral) (spastic) (spinal) 343.3
embolic (current) (*see also* Embolism, brain) 434.1
late effect - *see* Late effect(s) (of) cerebrovascular disease
infantile (cerebral) (spastic) (spinal) 343.3
lower limb 344.30
affecting
dominant side 344.31
nondominant side 344.32
due to late effect of cerebrovascular accident - *see* Late effect(s) (of) cerebrovascular accident
newborn 767.8
psychogenic 306.0
specified as conversion reaction 300.11
thrombotic (current) (*see also* Thrombosis, brain) 434.0
late effect - *see* Late effect(s) (of) cerebrovascular disease
transient 781.4
upper limb 344.40
affecting
dominant side 344.41
nondominant side 344.42
due to late effect of cerebrovascular accident - *see* Late effect(s) (of) cerebrovascular accident
Monorchism, monorchidism 752.89
Monteggia's fracture (closed) 813.03
open 813.13
Mood swings
brief compensatory 296.99
rebound 296.99
Moore's syndrome (*see also* Epilepsy) 345.5
Mooren's ulcer (cornea) 370.07
Mooser-Neill reaction 081.0
Mooser bodies 081.0
Moral
deficiency 301.7
imbecility 301.7

Morax-Axenfeld conjunctivitis 372.03
Morbilli (*see also* Measles) 055.9
Morbus
anglicus, anglorum 268.0
Beigel 111.2
caducus (*see also* Epilepsy) 345.9
caeruleus 746.89
celiacus 579.0
comitialis (*see also* Epilepsy) 345.9
cordis - *see also* Disease, heart
valvulorum - *see* Endocarditis
coxae 719.95
tuberculous (*see also* Tuberculosis) 015.1
hemorrhagicus neonatorum 776.0
maculosus neonatorum 772.6
renum 593.0
senilis (*see also* Osteoarthrosis) 715.9
Morel-Kraepelin disease (*see also* Schizophrenia) 295.9
Morel-Moore syndrome (hyperostosis frontalis interna) 733.3
Morel-Morgagni syndrome (hyperostosis frontalis interna) 733.3
Morgagni
cyst, organ, hydatid, or appendage 752.89
fallopian tube 752.11
disease or syndrome (hyperostosis frontalis interna) 733.3
Morgagni-Adams-Stokes syndrome (syncope with heart block) 426.9
Morgagni-Stewart-Morel syndrome (hyperostosis frontalis interna) 733.3
Moria (*see also* Psychosis) 298.9
Morning sickness 643.0
Moron 317
Morphea (guttate) (linear) 701.0
Morphine dependence (*see also* Dependence) 304.0
Morphinism (*see also* Dependence) 304.0
Morphinomania (*see also* Dependence) 304.0
Morphoea 701.0
Morquio (-Brailsford) (-Ullrich) disease or syndrome (mucopolysaccharidosis IV) 277.5
kyphosis 277.5
Morris syndrome (testicular feminization) 257.8
Morsus humanus (open wound) - *see also* Wound, open, by site
skin surface intact - *see* Contusion
Mortification (dry) (moist) (*see also* Gangrene) 785.4
Morton's
disease 355.6
foot 355.6
metatarsalgia (syndrome) 355.6
neuralgia 355.6
neuroma 355.6
syndrome (metatarsalgia) (neuralgia) 355.6
toe 355.6
Morvan's disease 336.0
Mosaicism, mosaic (chromosomal) 758.9
autosomal 758.5
sex 758.81
Moschcowitz's syndrome (thrombotic thrombocytopenic purpura) 446.6
Mother yaw 102.0
Motion sickness (from travel, any vehicle) (from roundabouts or swings) 994.6

ICD-9-CM

M

Vol. 2

Mottled teeth (enamel) (endemic) (non-endemic) 520.3
Mottling enamel (endemic) (nonendemic) (teeth) 520.3
Mouchet's disease 732.5
Mould(s) (in vitreous) 117.9
Moulders'
  bronchitis 502
  tuberculosis (see also Tuberculosis) 011.4
Mounier-Kuhn syndrome 494.0
  with acute exacerbation 494.1
Mountain
  fever - see Fever, mountain
  sickness 993.2
    with polycythemia, acquired 289.0
    acute 289.0
  tick fever 066.1
Mouse, joint (see also Loose, body, joint) 718.1
  knee 717.6
Mouth - see condition
Movable
  coccyx 724.71
  kidney (see also Disease, renal) 593.0
    congenital 753.3
  organ or site, congenital NEC - see Malposition, congenital
  spleen 289.59
Movement
  abnormal (dystonic) (involuntary) 781.0
  decreased fetal 655.7
  paradoxical facial 374.43
Moya Moya disease 437.5
Mozart's ear 744.29
MRSA (methicillin-resistant staphylococcus aureus) V09.0 ◄
Mucha's disease (acute parapsoriasis varioliformis) 696.2
Mucha-Haberman syndrome (acute parapsoriasis varioliformis) 696.2
Mu-chain disease 273.2
Mucinosis (cutaneous) (papular) 701.8
Mucocele
  appendix 543.9
  buccal cavity 528.9
  gallbladder (see also Disease, gallbladder) 575.3
  lacrimal sac 375.43
  orbit (eye) 376.81
  salivary gland (any) 527.6
  sinus (accessory) (nasal) 478.1
  turbinate (bone) (middle) (nasal) 478.1
  uterus 621.8
Mucocutaneous lymph node syndrome (acute) (febrile) (infantile) 446.1
Mucoenteritis 564.9
Mucolipidosis I, II, III 272.7
Mucopolysaccharidosis (types 1-6) 277.5
  cardiopathy 277.5 [425.7]
Mucormycosis (lung) 117.7
Mucositis - see also Inflammation, by site
  necroticans agranulocytica 288.0
Mucous - see also condition
  patches (syphilitic) 091.3
    congenital 090.0
Mucoviscidosis 277.00
  with meconium obstruction 277.01
Mucus
  asphyxia or suffocation (see also Asphyxia, mucus) 933.1
    newborn 770.1
  in stool 792.1

Mucus (Continued)
  plug (see also Asphyxia, mucus) 933.1
    aspiration, of newborn 770.1
      tracheobronchial 519.1
    newborn 770.1
Muguet 112.0
Mulberry molars 090.5
Mullerian mixed tumor (M8950/3) - see Neoplasm, by site, malignant
Multicystic kidney 753.19
Multilobed placenta - see Placenta, abnormal
Multinodular prostate 600.10
  with urinary retention 600.11
Multiparity V61.5
  affecting
    fetus or newborn 763.89
    management of
      labor and delivery 659.4
      pregnancy V23.3
  requiring contraceptive management (see also Contraception) V25.9
Multipartita placenta - see Placenta, abnormal
Multiple, multiplex - see also condition
  birth
    affecting fetus or newborn 761.5
    healthy liveborn - see Newborn, multiple
  digits (congenital) 755.00
    fingers 755.01
    toes 755.02
  organ or site NEC - see Accessory
  personality 300.14
  renal arteries 747.62
Mumps 072.9
  with complication 072.8
    specified type NEC 072.79
  encephalitis 072.2
  hepatitis 072.71
  meningitis (aseptic) 072.1
  meningoencephalitis 072.2
  oophoritis 072.79
  orchitis 072.0
  pancreatitis 072.3
  polyneuropathy 072.72
  vaccination, prophylactic (against) V04.6
Mumu (see also Infestation, filarial) 125.9
Münchausen syndrome 301.51
Münchmeyer's disease or syndrome (exostosis luxurians) 728.11
Mural - see condition
Murmur (cardiac) (heart) (nonorganic) (organic) 785.2
  abdominal 787.5
  aortic (valve) (see also Endocarditis, aortic) 424.1
  benign - omit code
  cardiorespiratory 785.2
  diastolic - see condition
  Flint (see also Endocarditis, aortic) 424.1
  functional - omit code
  Graham Steell (pulmonic regurgitation) (see also Endocarditis, pulmonary) 424.3
  innocent - omit code
  insignificant - omit code
  midsystolic 785.2
  mitral (valve) - see Stenosis
  physiologic - see condition
  presystolic, mitral - see Insufficiency, mitral
  pulmonic (valve) (see also Endocarditis, pulmonary) 424.3

Mumur (Continued)
  Still's (vibratory) - omit code
  systolic (valvular) - see condition
  tricuspid (valve) - see Endocarditis, tricuspid
  undiagnosed 785.2
  valvular - see condition
  vibratory - omit code
Murri's disease (intermittent hemoglobinuria) 283.2
Muscae volitantes 379.24
Muscle, muscular - see condition
Musculoneuralgia 729.1
Mushrooming hip 718.95
Mushroom workers' (pickers') lung 495.5
Mutation
  factor V leiden 289.81
  prothrombin gene 289.81
Mutism (see also Aphasia) 784.3
  akinetic 784.3
  deaf (acquired) (congenital) 389.7
  selective (elective) 313.23 ◄|||
    adjustment reaction 309.83
  hysterical 300.11
Myà's disease (congenital dilation, colon) 751.3
Myalgia (intercostal) 729.1
  eosinophilia syndrome 710.5
  epidemic 074.1
    cervical 078.89
  psychogenic 307.89
  traumatic NEC 959.9
Myasthenia 358.00 ◄|||
Myasthenic 728.87 ◄
  cordis - see Failure, heart
  gravis 358.00
    with exacerbation (acute) 358.01
    in crisis 358.01
    neonatal 775.2
    pseudoparalytica 358.00
  stomach 536.8
    psychogenic 306.4
  syndrome
    in
      botulism 005.1 [358.1]
      diabetes mellitus 250.6 [358.1]
      hypothyroidism (see also Hypothyroidism) 244.9 [358.1]
      malignant neoplasm NEC 199.1 [358.1]
      pernicious anemia 281.0 [358.1]
      thyrotoxicosis (see also Thyrotoxicosis) 242.9 [358.1]
Mycelium infection NEC 117.9
Mycetismus 988.1
Mycetoma (actinomycotic) 039.9
  bone 039.8
    mycotic 117.4
  foot 039.4
    mycotic 117.4
  madurae 039.9
    mycotic 117.4
  maduromycotic 039.9
    mycotic 117.4
  mycotic 117.4
  nocardial 039.9
Mycobacteriosis - see Mycobacterium
Mycobacterium, mycobacterial (infection) 031.9
  acid-fast (bacilli) 031.9
  anonymous (see also Mycobacterium, atypical) 031.9

Mycobacterium, mycobacterial
(*Continued*)
atypical (acid-fast bacilli) 031.9
cutaneous 031.1
pulmonary 031.0
tuberculous (*see also* Tuberculosis, pulmonary) 011.9
specified site NEC 031.8
avium 031.0
intracellulare complex bacteremia (MAC) 031.2
balnei 031.1
Battey 031.0
cutaneous 031.1
disseminated 031.2
avium-intracellulare complex (DMAC) 031.2
fortuitum 031.0
intracellulare (Battey bacillus) 031.0
kakerifu 031.8
kansasii 031.0
kasongo 031.8
leprae - *see* Leprosy
luciflavum 031.0
marinum 031.1
pulmonary 031.0
tuberculous (*see also* Tuberculosis, pulmonary) 011.9
scrofulaceum 031.1
tuberculosis (human, bovine) - *see also* Tuberculosis
avian type 031.0
ulcerans 031.1
xenopi 031.0
Mycosis, mycotic 117.9
cutaneous NEC 111.9
ear 111.8 [380.15]
fungoides (M9700/3) 202.1
mouth 112.0
pharynx 117.9
skin NEC 111.9
stomatitis 112.0
systemic NEC 117.9
tonsil 117.9
vagina, vaginitis 112.1
Mydriasis (persistent) (pupil) 379.43
Myelatelia 742.59
Myelinoclasis, perivascular, acute (post-infectious) NEC 136.9 [323.6]
postimmunization or postvaccinal 323.5
Myelinosis, central pontine 341.8
Myelitis (acute) (ascending) (cerebellar) (childhood) (chronic) (descending) (diffuse) (disseminated) (pressure) (progressive) (spinal cord) (subacute) (transverse) (*see also* Encephalitis) 323.9
late effect - *see* category 326
optic neuritis in 341.0
postchickenpox 052.7
postvaccinal 323.5
syphilitic (transverse) 094.89
tuberculous (*see also* Tuberculosis) 013.6
virus 049.9
Myeloblastic - *see* condition
Myelocele (*see also* Spina bifida) 741.9
with hydrocephalus 741.0
Myelocystocele (*see also* Spina bifida) 741.9
Myelocytic - *see* condition
Myelocytoma 205.1

Myelodysplasia (spinal cord) 742.59
meaning myelodysplastic syndrome - *see* Syndrome, myelodysplastic
Myeloencephalitis - *see* Encephalitis
Myelofibrosis (osteosclerosis) 289.89
Myelogenous - *see* condition
Myeloid - *see* condition
Myelokathexis 288.0
Myeloleukodystrophy 330.0
Myelolipoma (M8870/0) - *see* Neoplasm, by site, benign
Myeloma (multiple) (plasma cell) (plasmacytic) (M9730/3) 203.0
monostotic (M9731/1) 238.6
solitary (M9731/1) 238.6
Myelomalacia 336.8
Myelomata, multiple (M9730/3) 203.0
Myelomatosis (M9730/3) 203.0
Myelomeningitis - *see* Meningoencephalitis
Myelomeningocele (spinal cord) (*see also* Spina bifida) 741.9
fetal, causing fetopelvic disproportion 653.7
Myelo-osteo-musculodysplasia hereditaria 756.89
Myelopathic - *see* condition
Myelopathy (spinal cord) 336.9
cervical 721.1
diabetic 250.6 [336.3]
drug-induced 336.8
due to or with
carbon tetrachloride 987.8 [323.7]
degeneration or displacement, intervertebral disc 722.70
cervical, cervicothoracic 722.71
lumbar, lumbosacral 722.73
thoracic, thoracolumbar 722.72
hydroxyquinoline derivatives 961.3 [323.7]
infection - *see* Encephalitis
intervertebral disc disorder 722.70
cervical, cervicothoracic 722.71
lumbar, lumbosacral 722.73
thoracic, thoracolumbar 722.72
lead 984.9 [323.7]
mercury 985.0 [323.7]
neoplastic disease (*see also* Neoplasm, by site) 239.9 [336.3]
pernicious anemia 281.0 [336.3]
spondylosis 721.91
cervical 721.1
lumbar, lumbosacral 721.42
thoracic 721.41
thallium 985.8 [323.7]
lumbar, lumbosacral 721.42
necrotic (subacute) 336.1
radiation-induced 336.8
spondylogenic NEC 721.91
cervical 721.1
lumbar, lumbosacral 721.42
thoracic 721.41
thoracic 721.41
toxic NEC 989.9 [323.7]
transverse (*see also* Encephalitis) 323.9
vascular 336.1
Myeloproliferative disease (M9960/1) 238.7
Myeloradiculitis (*see also* Polyneuropathy) 357.0
Myeloradiculodysplasia (spinal) 742.59
Myelosarcoma (M9930/3) 205.3

Myelosclerosis 289.89
with myeloid metaplasia (M9961/1) 238.7
disseminated, of nervous system 340
megakaryocytic (M9961/1) 238.7
Myelosis (M9860/3) (*see also* Leukemia, myeloid) 205.9
acute (M9861/3) 205.0
aleukemic (M9864/3) 205.8
chronic (M9863/3) 205.1
erythremic (M9840/3) 207.0
acute (M9841/3) 207.0
megakaryocytic (M9920/3) 207.2
nonleukemic (chronic) 288.8
subacute (M9862/3) 205.2
Myesthenia - *see* Myasthenia
Myiasis (cavernous) 134.0
orbit 134.0 [376.13]
Myoadenoma, prostate 600.20
with urinary retention 600.21
Myoblastoma
granular cell (M9580/0) - *see also* Neoplasm, connective tissue, benign
malignant (M9580/3) - *see* Neoplasm, connective tissue, malignant
tongue (M9580/0) 210.1
Myocardial - *see* condition
Myocardiopathy (congestive) (constrictive) (familial) (hypertrophic nonobstructive) (idiopathic) (infiltrative) (obstructive) (primary) (restrictive) (sporadic) 425.4
alcoholic 425.5
amyloid 277.3 [425.7]
beriberi 265.0 [425.7]
cobalt-beer 425.5
due to
amyloidosis 277.3 [425.7]
beriberi 265.0 [425.7]
cardiac glycogenosis 271.0 [425.7]
Chagas' disease 086.0
Friedreich's ataxia 334.0 [425.8]
influenza 487.8 [425.8]
mucopolysaccharidosis 277.5 [425.7]
myotonia atrophica 359.2 [425.8]
progressive muscular dystrophy 359.1 [425.8]
sarcoidosis 135 [425.8]
glycogen storage 271.0 [425.7]
hypertrophic obstructive 425.1
metabolic NEC 277.9 [425.7]
nutritional 269.9 [425.7]
obscure (African) 425.2
peripartum 674.5
postpartum 674.5
secondary 425.9
thyrotoxic (*see also* Thyrotoxicosis) 242.9 [425.7]
toxic NEC 425.9
Myocarditis (fibroid) (interstitial) (old) (progressive) (senile) (with arteriosclerosis) 429.0
with
rheumatic fever (conditions classifiable to 390) 398.0
active (*see also* Myocarditis, acute, rheumatic) 391.2
inactive or quiescent (with chorea) 398.0
active (nonrheumatic) 422.90
rheumatic 391.2
with chorea (acute) (rheumatic) (Sydenham's) 392.0

ICD-9-CM

M

Vol. 2

Myocarditis (Continued)
acute or subacute (interstitial) 422.90
due to Streptococcus (beta-hemo-lytic) 391.2
idiopathic 422.91
rheumatic 391.2
with chorea (acute) (rheumatic) (Sydenham's) 392.0
specified type NEC 422.99
aseptic of newborn 074.23
bacterial (acute) 422.92
chagasic 086.0
chronic (interstitial) 429.0
congenital 746.89
constrictive 425.4
Coxsackie (virus) 074.23
diphtheritic 032.82
due to or in
Coxsackie (virus) 074.23
diphtheria 032.82
epidemic louse-borne typhus 080 [422.0]
influenza 487.8 [422.0]
Lyme disease 088.81 [422.0]
scarlet fever 034.1 [422.0]
toxoplasmosis (acquired) 130.3
tuberculosis (see also Tuberculosis) 017.9 [422.0]
typhoid 002.0 [422.0]
typhus NEC 081.9 [422.0]
eosinophilic 422.91
epidemic of newborn 074.23
Fiedler's (acute) (isolated) (subacute) 422.91
giant cell (acute) (subacute) 422.91
gonococcal 098.85
granulomatous (idiopathic) (isolated) (nonspecific) 422.91
hypertensive (see also Hypertension, heart) 402.90
idiopathic 422.91
granulomatous 422.91
infective 422.92
influenzal 487.8 [422.0]
isolated (diffuse) (granulomatous) 422.91
malignant 422.99
meningococcal 036.43
nonrheumatic, active 422.90
parenchymatous 422.90
pneumococcal (acute) (subacute) 422.92
rheumatic (chronic) (inactive) (with chorea) 398.0
active or acute 391.2
with chorea (acute) (rheumatic) (Sydenham's) 392.0
septic 422.92
specific (giant cell) (productive) 422.91
staphylococcal (acute) (subacute) 422.92
suppurative 422.92
syphilitic (chronic) 093.82
toxic 422.93
rheumatic (see also Myocarditis, acute rheumatic) 391.2
tuberculous (see also Tuberculosis) 017.9 [422.0]
typhoid 002.0 [422.0]
valvular - see Endocarditis
viral, except Coxsackie 422.91
Coxsackie 074.23
of newborn (Coxsackie) 074.23
Myocardium, myocardial - see condition

Myocardosis (see also Cardiomyopathy) 425.4
Myoclonia (essential) 333.2
epileptica 333.2
Friedrich's 333.2
massive 333.2
Myoclonic
epilepsy, familial (progressive) 333.2
jerks 333.2
Myoclonus (familial essential) (multifo-cal) (simplex) 333.2
with epilepsy and with ragged red fi-bers (MERRF syndrome) 277.87 ◄
facial 351.8
massive (infantile) 333.2
pharyngeal 478.29
Myodiastasis 728.84
Myoendocarditis - see also Endocarditis
acute or subacute 421.9
Myoepithelioma (M8982/0) - see Neo-plasm, by site, benign
Myofascitis (acute) 729.1
low back 724.2
Myofibroma (M8890/0) - see also Neo-plasm, connective tissue, benign
uterus (cervix) (corpus) (see also Leio-myoma) 218.9
Myofibrosis 728.2
heart (see also Myocarditis) 429.0
humeroscapular region 726.2
scapulohumeral 726.2
Myofibrositis (see also Myositis) 729.1
scapulohumeral 726.2
Myogelosis (occupational) 728.89
Myoglobinuria 791.3
Myoglobulinuria, primary 791.3
Myokymia - see also Myoclonus
facial 351.8
Myolipoma (M8860/0)
specified site - see Neoplasm, connec-tive tissue, benign
unspecified site 223.0
Myoma (M8895/0) - see also Neoplasm, connective tissue, benign
cervix (stump) (uterus) (see also Leio-myoma) 218.9
malignant (M8895/3) - see Neoplasm, connective tissue, malignant
prostate 600.20
with urinary retention 600.21
uterus (cervix) (corpus) (see also Leio-myoma) 218.9
in pregnancy or childbirth 654.1
affecting fetus or newborn 763.89
causing obstructed labor 660.2
affecting fetus or newborn 763.1
Myomalacia 728.9
cordis, heart (see also Degeneration, myocardial) 429.1
Myometritis (see also Endometritis) 615.9
Myometrium - see condition
Myonecrosis, clostridial 040.0
Myopathy 359.9
alcoholic 359.4
amyloid 277.3 [359.6]
benign, congenital 359.0
central core 359.0
centronuclear 359.0
congenital (benign) 359.0
critical illness 359.81
distal 359.1
due to drugs 359.4
endocrine 259.9 [359.5]
specified type NEC 259.8 [359.5]

Myopathy (Continued)
extraocular muscles 376.82
facioscapulohumeral 359.1
in
Addison's disease 255.4 [359.5]
amyloidosis 277.3 [359.6]
cretinism 243 [359.5]
Cushing's syndrome 255.0 [359.5]
disseminated lupus erythematosus 710.0 [359.6]
giant cell arteritis 446.5 [359.6]
hyperadrenocorticism NEC 255.3 [359.5]
hyperparathyroidism 252.01 [359.5] ◄■
hypopituitarism 253.2 [359.5]
hypothyroidism (see also Hypothy-roidism) 244.9 [359.5]
malignant neoplasm NEC (M8000/3) 199.1 [359.6]
myxedema (see also Myxedema) 244.9 [359.5]
polyarteritis nodosa 446.0 [359.6]
rheumatoid arthritis 714.0 [359.6]
sarcoidosis 135 [359.6]
scleroderma 710.1 [359.6]
Sjögren's disease 710.2 [359.6]
thyrotoxicosis (see also Thyrotoxico-sis) 242.9 [359.5]
inflammatory 359.89
intensive care (ICU) 359.81
limb-girdle 359.1
myotubular 359.0
necrotizing, acute 359.81
nemaline 359.0
ocular 359.1
oculopharyngeal 359.1
of critical illness 359.81
primary 359.89
progressive NEC 359.89
quadriplegic, acute 359.81
rod body 359.0
scapulohumeral 359.1
specified type NEC 359.89
toxic 359.4
Myopericarditis (see also Pericarditis) 423.9
Myopia (axial) (congenital) (increased curvature or refraction, nucleus of lens) 367.1
degenerative, malignant 360.21
malignant 360.21
progressive high (degenerative) 360.21
Myosarcoma (M8895/3) - see Neoplasm, connective tissue, malignant
Myosis (persistent) 379.42
stromal (endolymphatic) (M8931/1) 236.0
Myositis 729.1
clostridial 040.0
due to posture 729.1
epidemic 074.1
fibrosa or fibrous (chronic) 728.2
Volkmann's (complicating trauma) 958.6
infective 728.0
interstitial 728.81
multiple - see Polymyositis
occupational 729.1
orbital, chronic 376.12
ossificans 728.12
circumscribed 728.12
progressive 728.11
traumatic 728.12
progressive fibrosing 728.11

◄ New   ◄■ Revised

Myositis (*Continued*)
purulent 728.0
rheumatic 729.1
rheumatoid 729.1
suppurative 728.0
syphilitic 095.6
traumatic (old) 729.1
Myospasia impulsiva 307.23
Myotonia (acquisita) (intermittens)
728.85
atrophica 359.2
congenita 359.2
dystrophica 359.2
Myotonic pupil 379.46
Myriapodiasis 134.1
Myringitis
with otitis media - *see* Otitis media
acute 384.00
specified type NEC 384.09
bullosa hemorrhagica 384.01

Myringitis (*Continued*)
bullous 384.01
chronic 384.1
Mysophobia 300.29
Mytilotoxism 988.0
Myxadenitis labialis 528.5
Myxedema (adult) (idiocy) (infantile) (juvenile) (thyroid gland) (*see also* Hypothyroidism) 244.9
circumscribed 242.9
congenital 243
cutis 701.8
localized (pretibial) 242.9
madness (acute) 293.0
subacute 293.1
papular 701.8
pituitary 244.8
postpartum 674.8
pretibial 242.9
primary 244.9

Myxochondrosarcoma (M9220/3) - *see* Neoplasm, cartilage, malignant
Myxofibroma (M8811/0) - *see also* Neoplasm, connective tissue, benign
odontogenic (M9320/0) 213.1
upper jaw (bone) 213.0
Myxofibrosarcoma (M8811/3) - *see* Neoplasm, connective tissue, malignant
Myxolipoma (M8852/0) (*see also* Lipoma, by site) 214.9
Myxoliposarcoma (M8852/3) - *see* Neoplasm, connective tissue, malignant
Myxoma (M8840/0) - *see also* Neoplasm, connective tissue, benign
odontogenic (M9320/0) 213.1
upper jaw (bone) 213.0
Myxosarcoma (M8840/3) - *see* Neoplasm, connective tissue, malignant

ICD-9-CM

M

Vol. 2

N

Naegeli's
disease (hereditary hemorrhagic thrombasthenia 287.1
leukemia, monocytic (M9863/3) 205.1
syndrome (incontinentia pigmenti) 757.33
Naffziger's syndrome 353.0
Naga sore (*see also* Ulcer, skin) 707.9
Nägele's pelvis 738.6
with disproportion (fetopelvic) 653.0
affecting fetus or newborn 763.1
causing obstructed labor 660.1
affecting fetus or newborn 763.1
Nager-de Reynier syndrome (dysostosis mandibularis) 756.0
Nail - *see also* condition
biting 307.9
patella syndrome (hereditary osteoonychodysplasia) 756.89
Nanism, nanosomia (*see also* Dwarfism) 259.4
hypophyseal 253.3
pituitary 253.3
renis, renalis 588.0
Nanukayami 100.89
Napkin rash 691.0
Narcissism 301.81
Narcolepsy 347.00 ◀▥
with cataplexy 347.01 ◀
in conditions classified elsewhere 347.10 ◀
with cataplexy 347.11 ◀
Narcosis
carbon dioxide (respiratory) 786.09
due to drug
correct substance properly administered 780.09
overdose or wrong substance given or taken 977.9
specified drug - *see* Table of Drugs and Chemicals
Narcotism (chronic) (*see also* Dependence) 304.9
acute
correct substance properly administered 349.82
overdose or wrong substance given or taken 967.8
specified drug - *see* Table of Drugs and Chemicals
Narrow
anterior chamber angle 365.02
pelvis (inlet) (outlet) - *see* Contraction, pelvis
Narrowing
artery NEC 447.1
auditory, internal 433.8
basilar 433.0
with other precerebral artery 433.3
bilateral 433.3
carotid 433.1
with other precerebral artery 433.3
bilateral 433.3
cerebellar 433.8
choroidal 433.8
communicating posterior 433.8
coronary - *see also* Arteriosclerosis, coronary
congenital 746.85
due to syphilis 090.5
hypophyseal 433.8
pontine 433.8

Narrowing (*Continued*)
artery NEC (*Continued*)
precerebral NEC 433.9
multiple or bilateral 433.3
specified NEC 433.8
vertebral 433.2
with other precerebral artery 433.3
bilateral 433.3
auditory canal (external) (*see also* Stricture, ear canal, acquired) 380.50
cerebral arteries 437.0
cicatricial - *see* Cicatrix
congenital - *see* Anomaly, congenital
coronary artery - *see* Narrowing, artery, coronary
ear, middle 385.22
Eustachian tube (*see also* Obstruction, Eustachian tube) 381.60
eyelid 374.46
congenital 743.62
intervertebral disc or space NEC - *see* Degeneration, intervertebral disc
joint space, hip 719.85
larynx 478.74
lids 374.46
congenital 743.62
mesenteric artery (with gangrene) 557.0
palate 524.89 ◀▥
palpebral fissure 374.46
retinal artery 362.13
ureter 593.3
urethra (*see also* Stricture, urethra) 598.9
Narrowness, abnormal, eyelid 743.62
Nasal - *see* condition
Nasolacrimal - *see* condition
Nasopharyngeal - *see also* condition
bursa 478.29
pituitary gland 759.2
torticollis 723.5
Nasopharyngitis (acute) (infective) (subacute) 460
chronic 472.2
due to external agent - *see* Condition, respiratory, chronic, due to
due to external agent - *see* Condition, respiratory, due to
septic 034.0
streptococcal 034.0
suppurative (chronic) 472.2
ulcerative (chronic) 472.2
Nasopharynx, nasopharyngeal - *see* condition
Natal tooth, teeth 520.6
Nausea (*see also* Vomiting) 787.02
with vomiting 787.01
epidemic 078.82
gravidarum - *see* Hyperemesis, gravidarum
marina 994.6
Naval - *see* condition
Neapolitan fever (*see also* Brucellosis) 023.9
Nearsightedness 367.1
Near-syncope 780.2
Nebécourt's syndrome 253.3
Nebula, cornea (eye) 371.01
congenital 743.43
interfering with vision 743.42
Necator americanus infestation 126.1
Necatoriasis 126.1

Neck - *see* condition
Necrencephalus (*see also* Softening, brain) 437.8
Necrobacillosis 040.3
Necrobiosis 799.89
brain or cerebral (*see also* Softening, brain) 437.8
lipoidica 709.3
diabeticorum 250.8 [709.3]
Necrodermolysis 695.1
Necrolysis, toxic epidermal 695.1
due to drug
correct substance properly administered 695.1
overdose or wrong substance given or taken 977.9
specified drug - *see* Table of Drugs and Chemicals
Neuropathy, ataxia and retinitis pigmentosa (NARP syndrome) 277.87 ◀
Necrophilia 302.89
Necrosis, necrotic
adrenal (capsule) (gland) 255.8
antrum, nasal sinus 478.1
aorta (hyaline) (*see also* Aneurysm, aorta) 441.9
cystic medial 441.00
abdominal 441.02
thoracic 441.01
thoracoabdominal 441.03
ruptured 441.5
arteritis 446.0
artery 447.5
aseptic, bone 733.40
femur (head) (neck) 733.42
medial condyle 733.43
humoral head 733.41
medial femoral condyle 733.43
specific site NEC 733.49
talus 733.44
avascular, bone NEC (*see also* Necrosis, aseptic, bone) 733.40
bladder (aseptic) (sphincter) 596.8
bone (*see also* Osteomyelitis) 730.1
acute 730.0
aseptic or avascular 733.40
femur (head) (neck) 733.42
medial condyle 733.43
humoral head 733.41
medial femoral condyle 733.43
specified site NEC 733.49
talus 733.44
ethmoid 478.1
ischemic 733.40
jaw 526.4
marrow 289.89
Paget's (osteitis deformans) 731.0
tuberculous - *see* Tuberculosis, bone
brain (softening) (*see also* Softening, brain) 437.8
breast (aseptic) (fat) (segmental) 611.3
bronchus, bronchi 519.1
central nervous system NEC (*see also* Softening, brain) 437.8
cerebellar (*see also* Softening, brain) 437.8
cerebral (softening) (*see also* Softening, brain) 437.8
cerebrospinal (softening) (*see also* Softening, brain) 437.8
cornea (*see also* Keratitis) 371.40
cortical, kidney 583.6
cystic medial (aorta) 441.00
abdominal 441.02

◀ New   ◀▥ Revised

Necrosis, necrotic (*Continued*)
  cystic medial (*Continued*)
    thoracic 441.01
    thoracoabdominal 441.03
  dental 521.09
    pulp 522.1
  due to swallowing corrosive substance
    - *see* Burn, by site
  ear (ossicle) 385.24
  esophagus 530.89
  ethmoid (bone) 478.1
  eyelid 374.50
  fat, fatty (generalized) (*see also* Degeneration, fatty) 272.8
    abdominal wall 567.8 ◄
    breast (aseptic) (segmental) 611.3
    intestine 569.89
    localized - *see* Degeneration, by site, fatty
    mesentery 567.8
    omentum 567.8
    pancreas 577.8
    peritoneum 567.8
    skin (subcutaneous) 709.3
      newborn 778.1
  femur (aseptic) (avascular) 733.42
    head 733.42
    medial condyle 733.43
    neck 733.42
  gallbladder (*see also* Cholecystitis, acute) 575.0
  gangrenous 785.4
  gastric 537.89
  glottis 478.79
  heart (myocardium) - *see* Infarct, myocardium
  hepatic (*see also* Necrosis, liver) 570
  hip (aseptic) (avascular) 733.42
  intestine (acute) (hemorrhagic) (massive) 557.0
  ischemic 785.4
  jaw 526.4
  kidney (bilateral) 583.9
    acute 584.9
    cortical 583.6
      acute 584.6
        with
          abortion - *see* Abortion, by type, with renal failure
          ectopic pregnancy (*see also* categories 633.0-633.9) 639.3
          molar pregnancy (*see also* categories 630-632) 639.3
        complicating pregnancy 646.2
          affecting fetus or newborn 760.1
        following labor and delivery 669.3
    medullary (papillary) (*see also* Pyelitis) 590.80
      in
        acute renal failure 584.7
        nephritis, nephropathy 583.7
    papillary (*see also* Pyelitis) 590.80
      in
        acute renal failure 584.7
        nephritis, nephropathy 583.7
    tubular 584.5
      with

Necrosis, necrotic (*Continued*)
  kidney (*Continued*)
    tubular (*Continued*)
      with (*Continued*)
        abortion - *see* Abortion, by type, with renal failure
        ectopic pregnancy (*see also* categories 633.0-633.9) 639.3
        molar pregnancy (*see also* categories 630-632) 639.3
      complicating
        abortion 639.3
        ectopic or molar pregnancy 639.3
        pregnancy 646.2
          affecting fetus or newborn 760.1
      following labor and delivery 669.3
      traumatic 958.5
  larynx 478.79
  liver (acute) (congenital) (diffuse) (massive) (subacute) 570
    with
      abortion - *see* Abortion, by type, with specified complication NEC
      ectopic pregnancy (*see also* categories 633.0-633.9) 639.8
      molar pregnancy (*see also* categories 630-632) 639.8
      complicating pregnancy 646.7
        affecting fetus or newborn 760.8
      following
        abortion 639.8
        ectopic or molar pregnancy 639.8
      obstetrical 646.7
      postabortal 639.8
      puerperal, postpartum 674.8
      toxic 573.3
  lung 513.0
  lymphatic gland 683
  mammary gland 611.3
  mastoid (chronic) 383.1
  mesentery 557.0
    fat 567.8
  mitral valve - *see* Insufficiency, mitral
  myocardium, myocardial - *see* Infarct, myocardium
  nose (septum) 478.1
  omentum 557.0
    with mesenteric infarction 557.0
    fat 567.8
  orbit, orbital 376.10
  ossicles, ear (aseptic) 385.24
  ovary (*see also* Salpingo-oophoritis) 614.2
  pancreas (aseptic) (duct) (fat) 577.8
    acute 577.0
    infective 577.0
  papillary, kidney (*see also* Pyelitis) 590.80
  peritoneum 557.0
    with mesenteric infarction 557.0
    fat 567.8
  pharynx 462
    in granulocytopenia 288.0
  phosphorus 983.9
  pituitary (gland) (postpartum) (Sheehan) 253.2

Necrosis, necrotic (*Continued*)
  placenta (*see also* Placenta, abnormal) 656.7
  pneumonia 513.0
  pulmonary 513.0
  pulp (dental) 522.1
  pylorus 537.89
  radiation - *see* Necrosis, by site
  radium - *see* Necrosis, by site
  renal - *see* Necrosis, kidney
  sclera 379.19
  scrotum 608.89
  skin or subcutaneous tissue 709.8
    due to burn - *see* Burn, by site
    gangrenous 785.4
  spine, spinal (column) 730.18
    acute 730.18
    cord 336.1
  spleen 289.59
  stomach 537.89
  stomatitis 528.1
  subcutaneous fat 709.3
    fetus or newborn 778.1
  subendocardial - *see* Infarct, myocardium
  suprarenal (capsule) (gland) 255.8
  teeth, tooth 521.09
  testis 608.89
  thymus (gland) 254.8
  tonsil 474.8
  trachea 519.1
  tuberculous NEC - *see* Tuberculosis
  tubular (acute) (anoxic) (toxic) 584.5
    due to a procedure 997.5
  umbilical cord, affecting fetus or newborn 762.6
  vagina 623.8
  vertebra (lumbar) 730.18
    acute 730.18
    tuberculous (*see also* Tuberculosis) 015.0 [730.8]
  vesical (aseptic) (bladder) 596.8
  x-ray - *see* Necrosis, by site
Necrospermia 606.0
Necrotizing angiitis 446.0
Negativism 301.7
Neglect (child) (newborn) NEC 995.52
  adult 995.84
  after or at birth 995.52
  hemispatial 781.8
  left-sided 781.8
  sensory 781.8
  visuospatial 781.8
Negri bodies 071
  Neill-Dingwall syndrome (microcephaly and dwarfism) 759.89
Neisserian infection NEC - *see* Gonococcus
Nematodiasis NEC (*see also* Infestation, Nematode) 127.9
  ancylostoma (*see also* Ancylostomiasis) 126.9
Neoformans cryptococcus infection 117.5
Neonatal - *see also* condition
  adrenoleukodystrophy 277.86 ◄
  teeth, tooth 520.6
Neonatorum - *see* condition

ICD-9-CM

N

Vol.

	Malignant					
	Primary	**Secondary**	**Ca in situ**	**Benign**	**Uncertain Behavior**	**Unspecified**
Neoplasm, neoplastic	199.1	199.1	234.9	229.9	238.9	239.9

Notes — *1. The list below gives the code numbers for neoplasms by anatomical site. For each site there are six possible code numbers according to whether the neoplasm in question is malignant, benign, in situ, of uncertain behavior, or of unspecified nature. The description of the neoplasm will often indicate which of the six columns is appropriate; e.g., malignant melanoma of skin, benign fibroadenoma of breast, carcinoma in situ of cervix uteri.*

Where such descriptors are not present, the remainder of the Index should be consulted where guidance is given to the appropriate column for each morphological (histological) variety listed; e.g., Mesonephroma—see Neoplasm, malignant; Embryoma—see also Neoplasm, uncertain behavior; Disease, Bowen's—see Neoplasm, skin, in situ. However, the guidance in the Index can be overridden if one of the descriptors mentioned above is present; e.g., malignant adenoma of colon is coded to 153.9 and not to 211.3 as the adjective "malignant" overrides the Index entry "Adenoma—see also Neoplasm, benign."

2. Sites marked with the sign * (e.g., face NEC*) should be classified to malignant neoplasm of skin of these sites if the variety of neoplasm is a squamous cell carcinoma or an epidermoid carcinoma and to benign neoplasm of skin of these sites if the variety of neoplasm is a papilloma (any type).

	Primary	Secondary	Ca in situ	Benign	Uncertain Behavior	Unspecified
abdomen, abdominal	195.2	198.89	234.8	229.8	238.8	239.8
cavity	195.2	198.89	234.8	229.8	238.8	239.8
organ	195.2	198.89	234.8	229.8	238.8	239.8
viscera	195.2	198.89	234.8	229.8	238.8	239.8
wall	173.5	198.2	232.5	216.5	238.2	239.2
connective tissue	171.5	198.89	—	215.5	238.1	239.2
abdominopelvic	195.8	198.89	234.8	229.8	238.8	239.8
accessory sinus-see Neoplasm, sinus						
acoustic nerve	192.0	198.4	—	225.1	237.9	239.7
acromion (process)	170.4	198.5	—	213.4	238.0	239.2
adenoid (pharynx) (tissue)	147.1	198.89	230.0	210.7	235.1	239.0
adipose tissue (see also Neoplasm, connective tissue)	171.9	198.89	—	215.9	238.1	239.2
adnexa (uterine)	183.9	198.82	233.3	221.8	236.3	239.5
adrenal (cortex) (gland) (medulla)	194.0	198.7	234.8	227.0	237.2	239.7
ala nasi (external)	173.3	198.2	232.3	216.3	238.2	239.2
alimentary canal or tract NEC	159.9	197.8	230.9	211.9	235.5	239.0
alveolar	143.9	198.89	230.0	210.4	235.1	239.0
mucosa	143.9	198.89	230.0	210.4	235.1	239.0
lower	143.1	198.89	230.0	210.4	235.1	239.0
upper	143.0	198.89	230.0	210.4	235.1	239.0
ridge or process	170.1	198.5	—	213.1	238.0	239.2
carcinoma	143.9	—	—	—	—	—
lower	143.1	—	—	—	—	—
upper	143.0	—	—	—	—	—
lower	170.1	198.5	—	213.1	238.0	239.2
mucosa	143.9	198.89	230.0	210.4	235.1	239.0
lower	143.1	198.89	230.0	210.4	235.1	239.0
upper	143.0	198.89	230.0	210.4	235.1	239.0
upper	170.0	198.5	—	213.0	238.0	239.2
sulcus	145.1	198.89	230.0	210.4	235.1	239.0
alveolus	143.9	198.89	230.0	210.4	235.1	239.0
lower	143.1	198.89	230.0	210.4	235.1	239.0
upper	143.0	198.89	230.0	210.4	235.1	239.0
ampulla of Vater	156.2	197.8	230.8	211.5	235.3	239.0
ankle NEC*	195.5	198.89	232.7	229.8	238.8	239.8
anorectum, anorectal (junction)	154.8	197.5	230.7	211.4	235.2	239.0
antecubital fossa or space*	195.4	198.89	232.6	229.8	238.8	239.8
antrum (Highmore) (maxillary)	160.2	197.3	231.8	212.0	235.9	239.1
pyloric	151.2	197.8	230.2	211.1	235.2	239.0
tympanicum	160.1	197.3	231.8	212.0	235.9	239.1
anus, anal	154.3	197.5	230.6	211.4	235.5	239.0
canal	154.2	197.5	230.5	211.4	235.5	239.0
contiguous sites with rectosigmoid junction or rectum	154.8	—	—	—	—	—
margin	173.5	198.2	232.5	216.5	238.2	239.2
skin	173.5	198.2	232.5	216.5	238.2	239.2
sphincter	154.2	197.5	230.5	211.4	235.5	239.0
aorta (thoracic)	171.4	198.89	—	215.4	238.1	239.2
abdominal	171.5	198.89	—	215.5	238.1	239.2
aortic body	194.6	198.89	—	227.6	237.3	239.7
aponeurosis	171.9	198.89	—	215.9	238.1	239.2
palmar	171.2	198.89	—	215.2	238.1	239.2
plantar	171.3	198.89	—	215.3	238.1	239.2

◄ New   ◀▥ Revised

	Malignant					
	Primary	Secondary	Ca in situ	Benign	Uncertain Behavior	Unspecified
Neoplasm *(Continued)*						
appendix	153.5	197.5	230.3	211.3	235.2	239.0
arachnoid (cerebral)	192.1	198.4	—	225.2	237.6	239.7
spinal	192.3	198.4	—	225.4	237.6	239.7
areola (female)	174.0	198.81	233.0	217	238.3	239.3
male	175.0	198.81	233.0	217	238.3	239.3
arm NEC*	195.4	198.89	232.6	229.8	238.8	239.8
artery-*see* Neoplasm, connective tissue						
aryepiglottic fold	148.2	198.89	230.0	210.8	235.1	239.0
hypopharyngeal aspect	148.2	198.89	230.0	210.8	235.1	239.0
laryngeal aspect	161.1	197.3	231.0	212.1	235.6	239.1
marginal zone	148.2	198.89	230.0	210.8	235.1	239.0
arytenoid (cartilage)	161.3	197.3	231.0	212.1	235.6	239.1
fold-*see* Neoplasm, aryepiglottic						
atlas	170.2	198.5	—	213.2	238.0	239.2
atrium, cardiac	164.1	198.89	—	212.7	238.8	239.8
auditory						
canal (external) (skin)	173.2	198.2	232.2	216.2	238.2	239.2
internal	160.1	197.3	231.8	212.0	235.9	239.1
nerve	192.0	198.4	—	225.1	237.9	239.7
tube	160.1	197.3	231.8	212.0	235.9	239.1
opening	147.2	198.89	230.0	210.7	235.1	239.0
auricle, ear	173.2	198.2	232.2	216.2	238.2	239.2
cartilage	171.0	198.89	—	215.0	238.1	239.2
auricular canal (external)	173.2	198.2	232.2	216.2	238.2	239.2
internal	160.1	197.3	231.8	212.0	235.9	239.1
autonomic nerve or nervous system NEC	171.9	198.89	—	215.9	238.1	239.2
axilla, axillary	195.1	198.89	234.8	229.8	238.8	239.8
fold	173.5	198.2	232.5	216.5	238.2	239.2
back NEC*	195.8	198.89	232.5	229.8	238.8	239.8
Bartholin's gland	184.1	198.82	233.3	221.2	236.3	239.5
basal ganglia	191.0	198.3	—	225.0	237.5	239.6
basis pedunculi	191.7	198.3	—	225.0	237.5	239.6
bile or biliary (tract)	156.9	197.8	230.8	211.5	235.3	239.0
canaliculi (biliferi) (intrahepatic)	155.1	197.8	230.8	211.5	235.3	239.0
canals, interlobular	155.1	197.8	230.8	211.5	235.3	239.0
contiguous sites	156.8	—	—	—	—	—
duct or passage (common) (cystic) (extrahepatic)	156.1	197.8	230.8	211.5	235.3	239.0
contiguous sites						
with gallbladder	156.8	—	—	—	—	—
interlobular	155.1	197.8	230.8	211.5	235.3	239.0
intrahepatic	155.1	197.8	230.8	211.5	235.3	239.0
and extrahepatic	156.9	197.8	230.8	211.5	235.3	239.0
bladder (urinary)	188.9	198.1	233.7	223.3	236.7	239.4
contiguous sites	188.8	—	—	—	—	—
dome	188.1	198.1	233.7	223.3	236.7	239.4
neck	188.5	198.1	233.7	223.3	236.7	239.4
orifice	188.9	198.1	233.7	223.3	236.7	239.4
ureteric	188.6	198.1	233.7	223.3	236.7	239.4
urethral	188.5	198.1	233.7	223.3	236.7	239.4
sphincter	188.8	198.1	233.7	223.3	236.7	239.4
trigone	188.0	198.1	233.7	223.3	236.7	239.4
urachus	188.7	—	233.7	223.3	236.7	239.4
wall	188.9	198.1	233.7	223.3	236.7	239.4
anterior	188.3	198.1	233.7	223.3	236.7	239.4
lateral	188.2	198.1	233.7	223.3	236.7	239.4
posterior	188.4	198.1	233.7	223.3	236.7	239.4
blood vessel-*see* Neoplasm, connective tissue						
bone (periosteum)	170.9	198.5	—	213.9	238.0	239.2

Note-Carcinomas and adenocarcinomas, of any type other than intraosseous or odontogenic, of the sites listed under "Neoplasm, bone" should be considered as constituting metastatic spread from an unspecified primary site and coded to 198.5 for morbidity coding and to 199.1 for underlying cause of death coding.

acetabulum	170.6	198.5	—	213.6	238.0	239.2

ICD-9-CM

N

Vol. 2

	Malignant					
	Primary	Secondary	Ca in situ	Benign	Uncertain Behavior	Unspecified
Neoplasm *(Continued)*						
bone *(Continued)*						
acromion (process)	170.4	198.5	—	213.4	238.0	239.2
ankle	170.8	198.5	—	213.8	238.0	239.2
arm NEC	170.4	198.5	—	213.4	238.0	239.2
astragalus	170.8	198.5	—	213.8	238.0	239.2
atlas	170.2	198.5	—	213.2	238.0	239.2
axis	170.2	198.5	—	213.2	238.0	239.2
back NEC	170.2	198.5	—	213.2	238.0	239.2
calcaneus	170.8	198.5	—	213.8	238.0	239.2
calvarium	170.0	198.5	—	213.0	238.0	239.2
carpus (any)	170.5	198.5	—	213.5	238.0	239.2
cartilage NEC	170.9	198.5	—	213.9	238.0	239.2
clavicle	170.3	198.5	—	213.3	238.0	239.2
clivus	170.0	198.5	—	213.0	238.0	239.2
coccygeal vertebra	170.6	198.5	—	213.6	238.0	239.2
coccyx	170.6	198.5	—	213.6	238.0	239.2
costal cartilage	170.3	198.5	—	213.3	238.0	239.2
costovertebral joint	170.3	198.5	—	213.3	238.0	239.2
cranial	170.0	198.5	—	213.0	238.0	239.2
cuboid	170.8	198.5	—	213.8	238.0	239.2
cuneiform	170.9	198.5	—	213.9	238.0	239.2
ankle	170.8	198.5	—	213.8	238.0	239.2
wrist	170.5	198.5	—	213.5	238.0	239.2
digital	170.9	198.5	—	213.9	238.0	239.2
finger	170.5	198.5	—	213.5	238.0	239.2
toe	170.8	198.5	—	213.8	238.0	239.2
elbow	170.4	198.5	—	213.4	238.0	239.2
ethmoid (labyrinth)	170.0	198.5	—	213.0	238.0	239.2
face	170.0	198.5	—	213.0	238.0	239.2
lower jaw	170.1	198.5	—	213.1	238.0	239.2
femur (any part)	170.7	198.5	—	213.7	238.0	239.2
fibula (any part)	170.7	198.5	—	213.7	238.0	239.2
finger (any)	170.5	198.5	—	213.5	238.0	239.2
foot	170.8	198.5	—	213.8	238.0	239.2
forearm	170.4	198.5	—	213.4	238.0	239.2
frontal	170.0	198.5	—	213.0	238.0	239.2
hand	170.5	198.5	—	213.5	238.0	239.2
heel	170.8	198.5	—	213.8	238.0	239.2
hip	170.6	198.5	—	213.6	238.0	239.2
humerus (any part)	170.4	198.5	—	213.4	238.0	239.2
hyoid	170.0	198.5	—	213.0	238.0	239.2
ilium	170.6	198.5	—	213.6	238.0	239.2
innominate	170.6	198.5	—	213.6	238.0	239.2
intervertebral cartilage or disc	170.2	198.5	—	213.2	238.0	239.2
ischium	170.6	198.5	—	213.6	238.0	239.2
jaw (lower)	170.1	198.5	—	213.1	238.0	239.2
upper	170.0	198.5	—	213.0	238.0	239.2
knee	170.7	198.5	—	213.7	238.0	239.2
leg NEC	170.7	198.5	—	213.7	238.0	239.2
limb NEC	170.9	198.5	—	213.9	238.0	239.2
lower (long bones)	170.7	198.5	—	213.7	238.0	239.2
short bones	170.8	198.5	—	213.8	238.0	239.2
upper (long bones)	170.4	198.5	—	213.4	238.0	239.2
short bones	170.5	198.5	—	213.5	238.0	239.2
long	170.9	198.5	—	213.9	238.0	239.2
lower limbs NEC	170.7	198.5	—	213.7	238.0	239.2
upper limbs NEC	170.4	198.5	—	213.4	238.0	239.2
malar	170.0	198.5	—	213.0	238.0	239.2
mandible	170.1	198.5	—	213.1	238.0	239.2
marrow NEC	202.9	198.5	—	—	—	238.7
mastoid	170.0	198.5	—	213.0	238.0	239.2
maxilla, maxillary (superior)	170.0	198.5	—	213.0	238.0	239.2
inferior	170.1	198.5	—	213.1	238.0	239.2

◄ New   ◄▦ Revised

	Malignant					
	Primary	Secondary	Ca in stiu	Benign	Uncertain Behavior	Unspecified
Neoplasm *(Continued)*						
bone *(Continued)*						
metacarpus (any)	170.5	198.5	—	213.5	238.0	239.2
metatarsus (any)	170.8	198.5	—	213.8	238.0	239.2
navicular (ankle)	170.8	198.5	—	213.8	238.0	239.2
hand	170.5	198.5	—	213.5	238.0	239.2
nose, nasal	170.0	198.5	—	213.0	238.0	239.2
occipital	170.0	198.5	—	213.0	238.0	239.2
orbit	170.0	198.5	—	213.0	238.0	239.2
parietal	170.0	198.5	—	213.0	238.0	239.2
patella	170.8	198.5	—	213.8	238.0	239.2
pelvic	170.6	198.5	—	213.6	238.0	239.2
phalanges	170.9	198.5	—	213.9	238.0	239.2
foot	170.8	198.5	—	213.8	238.0	239.2
hand	170.5	198.5	—	213.5	238.0	239.2
pubic	170.6	198.5	—	213.6	238.0	239.2
radius (any part)	170.4	198.5	—	213.4	238.0	239.2
rib	170.3	198.5	—	213.3	238.0	239.2
sacral vertebra	170.6	198.5	—	213.6	238.0	239.2
sacrum	170.6	198.5	—	213.6	238.0	239.2
scaphoid (of hand)	170.5	198.5	—	213.5	238.0	239.2
of ankle	170.8	198.5	—	213.8	238.0	239.2
scapula (any part)	170.4	198.5	—	213.4	238.0	239.2
sella turcica	170.0	198.5	—	213.0	238.0	239.2
short	170.9	198.5	—	213.9	238.0	239.2
lower limb	170.8	198.5	—	213.8	238.0	239.2
upper limb	170.5	198.5	—	213.5	238.0	239.2
shoulder	170.4	198.5	—	213.4	238.0	239.2
skeleton, skeletal NEC	170.9	198.5	—	213.9	238.0	239.2
skull	170.0	198.5	—	213.0	238.0	239.2
sphenoid	170.0	198.5	—	213.0	238.0	239.2
spine, spinal (column)	170.2	198.5	—	213.2	238.0	239.2
coccyx	170.6	198.5	—	213.6	238.0	239.2
sacrum	170.6	198.5	—	213.6	238.0	239.2
sternum	170.3	198.5	—	213.3	238.0	239.2
tarsus (any)	170.8	198.5	—	213.8	238.0	239.2
temporal	170.0	198.5	—	213.0	238.0	239.2
thumb	170.5	198.5	—	213.5	238.0	239.2
tibia (any part)	170.7	198.5	—	213.7	238.0	239.2
toe (any)	170.8	198.5	—	213.8	238.0	239.2
trapezium	170.5	198.5	—	213.5	238.0	239.2
trapezoid	170.5	198.5	—	213.5	238.0	239.2
turbinate	170.0	198.5	—	213.0	238.0	239.2
ulna (any part)	170.4	198.5	—	213.4	238.0	239.2
unciform	170.5	198.5	—	213.5	238.0	239.2
vertebra (column)	170.2	198.5	—	213.2	238.0	239.2
coccyx	170.6	198.5	—	213.6	238.0	239.2
sacrum	170.6	198.5	—	213.6	238.0	239.2
vomer	170.0	198.5	—	213.0	238.0	239.2
wrist	170.5	198.5	—	213.5	238.0	239.2
xiphoid process	170.3	198.5	—	213.3	238.0	239.2
zygomatic	170.0	198.5	—	213.0	238.0	239.2
book-leaf (mouth)	145.8	198.89	230.0	210.4	235.1	239.0
bowel - *see* Neoplasm, intestine						
brachial plexus	171.2	198.89	—	215.2	238.1	239.2
brain NEC	191.9	198.3	—	225.0	237.5	239.6
basal ganglia	191.0	198.3	—	225.0	237.5	239.6
cerebellopontine angle	191.6	198.3	—	225.0	237.5	239.6
cerebellum NOS	191.6	198.3	—	225.0	237.5	239.6
cerebrum	191.0	198.3	—	225.0	237.5	239.6
choroid plexus	191.5	198.3	—	225.0	237.5	239.6
contiguous sites	191.8	—	—	—	—	—
corpus callosum	191.8	198.3	—	225.0	237.5	239.6
corpus striatum	191.0	198.3	—	225.0	237.5	239.6

	Malignant					
	Primary	Secondary	Ca in stiu	Benign	Uncertain Behavior	Unspecified
Neoplasm *(Continued)*						
brain *(Continued)*						
cortex (cerebral)	191.0	198.3	—	225.0	237.5	239.6
frontal lobe	191.1	198.3	—	225.0	237.5	239.6
globus pallidus	191.0	198.3	—	225.0	237.5	239.6
hippocampus	191.2	198.3	—	225.0	237.5	239.6
hypothalamus	191.0	198.3	—	225.0	237.5	239.6
internal capsule	191.0	198.3	—	225.0	237.5	239.6
medulla oblongata	191.7	198.3	—	225.0	237.5	239.6
meninges	192.1	198.4	—	225.2	237.6	239.7
midbrain	191.7	198.3	—	225.0	237.5	239.6
occipital lobe	191.4	198.3	—	225.0	237.5	239.6
parietal lobe	191.3	198.3	—	225.0	237.5	239.6
peduncle	191.7	198.3	—	225.0	237.5	239.6
pons	191.7	198.3	—	225.0	237.5	239.6
stem	191.7	198.3	—	225.0	237.5	239.6
tapetum	191.8	198.3	—	225.0	237.5	239.6
temporal lobe	191.2	198.3	—	225.0	237.5	239.6
thalamus	191.0	198.3	—	225.0	237.5	239.6
uncus	191.2	198.3	—	225.0	237.5	239.6
ventricle (floor)	191.5	198.3	—	225.0	237.5	239.6
branchial (cleft) (vestiges)	146.8	198.89	230.0	210.6	235.1	239.0
breast (connective tissue) (female) (glandular tissue) (soft parts)	174.9	198.81	233.0	217	238.3	239.3
areola	174.0	198.81	233.0	217	238.3	239.3
male	175.0	198.81	233.0	217	238.3	239.3
axillary tail	174.6	198.81	233.0	217	238.3	239.3
central portion	174.1	198.81	233.0	217	238.3	239.3
contiguous sites	174.8	—	—	—	—	—
ectopic sites	174.8	198.81	233.0	217	238.3	239.3
inner	174.8	198.81	233.0	217	238.3	239.3
lower	174.8	198.81	233.0	217	238.3	239.3
lower-inner quadrant	174.3	198.81	233.0	217	238.3	239.3
lower-outer quadrant	174.5	198.81	233.0	217	238.3	239.3
male	175.9	198.81	233.0	217	238.3	239.3
areola	175.0	198.81	233.0	217	238.3	239.3
ectopic tissue	175.9	198.81	233.0	217	238.3	239.3
nipple	175.0	198.81	233.0	217	238.3	239.3
mastectomy site (skin)	173.5	198.2	—	—	—	—
specified as breast tissue	174.8	198.81	—	—	—	—
midline	174.8	198.81	233.0	217	238.3	239.3
nipple	174.0	198.81	233.0	217	238.3	239.3
male	175.0	198.81	233.0	217	238.3	239.3
outer	174.8	198.81	233.0	217	238.3	239.3
skin	173.5	198.2	232.5	216.5	238.2	239.2
tail (axillary)	174.6	198.81	233.0	217	238.3	239.3
upper	174.8	198.81	233.0	217	238.3	239.3
upper-inner quadrant	174.2	198.81	233.0	217	238.3	239.3
upper-outer quadrant	174.4	198.81	233.0	217	238.3	239.3
broad ligament	183.3	198.82	233.3	221.0	236.3	239.5
bronchiogenic, bronchogenic (lung)	162.9	197.0	231.2	212.3	235.7	239.1
bronchiole	162.9	197.0	231.2	212.3	235.7	239.1
bronchus	162.9	197.0	231.2	212.3	235.7	239.1
carina	162.2	197.0	231.2	212.3	235.7	239.1
contiguous sites with lung or trachea	162.8	—	—	—	—	—
lower lobe of lung	162.5	197.0	231.2	212.3	235.7	239.1
main	162.2	197.0	231.2	212.3	235.7	239.1
middle lobe of lung	162.4	197.0	231.2	212.3	235.7	239.1
upper lobe of lung	162.3	197.0	231.2	212.3	235.7	239.1
brow	173.3	198.2	232.3	216.3	238.2	239.2
buccal (cavity)	145.9	198.89	230.0	210.4	235.1	239.0
commissure	145.0	198.89	230.0	210.4	235.1	239.0
groove (lower) (upper)	145.1	198.89	230.0	210.4	235.1	239.0
mucosa	145.0	198.89	230.0	210.4	235.1	239.0
sulcus (lower) (upper)	145.1	198.89	230.0	210.4	235.1	239.0

◄ New   ◄ Revised

	Malignant					
	Primary	Secondary	Ca in stiu	Benign	Uncertain Behavior	Unspecified
Neoplasm *(Continued)*						
bulbourethral gland	189.3	198.1	233.9	223.81	236.99	239.5
bursa-*see* Neoplasm, connective tissue						
buttock NEC*	195.3	198.89	232.5	229.8	238.8	239.8
calf*	195.5	198.89	232.7	229.8	238.8	239.8
calvarium	170.0	198.5	—	213.0	238.0	239.2
calyx, renal	189.1	198.0	233.9	223.1	236.91	239.5
canal						
anal	154.2	197.5	230.5	211.4	235.5	239.0
auditory (external)	173.2	198.2	232.2	216.2	238.2	239.2
auricular (external)	173.2	198.2	232.2	216.2	238.2	239.2
canaliculi, biliary (biliferi) (intrahepatic)	155.1	197.8	230.8	211.5	235.3	239.0
canthus (eye) (inner) (outer)	173.1	198.2	232.1	216.1	238.2	239.2
capillary-*see* Neoplasm, connective tissue						
caput coli	153.4	197.5	230.3	211.3	235.2	239.0
cardia (gastric)	151.0	197.8	230.2	211.1	235.2	239.0
cardiac orifice (stomach)	151.0	197.8	230.2	211.1	235.2	239.0
cardio-esophageal junction	151.0	197.8	230.2	211.1	235.2	239.0
cardio-esophagus	151.0	197.8	230.2	211.1	235.2	239.0
carina (bronchus) (trachea)	162.2	197.0	231.2	212.3	235.7	239.1
carotid (artery)	171.0	198.89	—	215.0	238.1	239.2
body	194.5	198.89	—	227.5	237.3	239.7
carpus (any bone)	170.5	198.5	—	213.5	238.0	239.2
cartilage (articular) (joint) NEC-*see also* Neoplasm, bone	170.9	198.5	—	213.9	238.0	239.2
arytenoid	161.3	197.3	231.0	212.1	235.6	239.1
auricular	171.0	198.89	—	215.0	238.1	239.2
bronchi	162.2	197.3	—	212.3	235.7	239.1
connective tissue-*see* Neoplasm, connective tissue						
costal	170.3	198.5	—	213.3	238.0	239.2
cricoid	161.3	197.3	231.0	212.1	235.6	239.1
cuneiform	161.3	197.3	231.0	212.1	235.6	239.1
ear (external)	171.0	198.89	—	215.0	238.1	239.2
ensiform	170.3	198.5	—	213.3	238.0	239.2
epiglottis	161.1	197.3	231.0	212.1	235.6	239.1
anterior surface	146.4	198.89	230.0	210.6	235.1	239.0
eyelid	171.0	198.89	—	215.0	238.1	239.2
intervertebral	170.2	198.5	—	213.2	238.0	239.2
larynx, laryngeal	161.3	197.3	231.0	212.1	235.6	239.1
nose, nasal	160.0	197.3	231.8	212.0	235.9	239.1
pinna	171.0	198.89	—	215.0	238.1	239.2
rib	170.3	198.5	—	213.3	238.0	239.2
semilunar (knee)	170.7	198.5	—	213.7	238.0	239.2
thyroid	161.3	197.3	231.0	212.1	235.6	239.1
trachea	162.0	197.3	231.1	212.2	235.7	239.1
cauda equina	192.2	198.3	—	225.3	237.5	239.7
cavity						
buccal	145.9	198.89	230.0	210.4	235.1	239.0
nasal	160.0	197.3	231.8	212.0	235.9	239.1
oral	145.9	198.89	230.0	210.4	235.1	239.0
peritoneal	158.9	197.6	—	211.8	235.4	239.0
tympanic	160.1	197.3	231.8	212.0	235.9	239.1
cecum	153.4	197.5	230.3	211.3	235.2	239.0
central nervous system-*see* Neoplasm, white matter	191.0	198.3	—	225.0	237.5	239.6
cerebellopontine (angle)	191.6	198.3	—	225.0	237.5	239.6
cerebellum, cerebellar	191.6	198.3	—	225.0	237.5	239.6
cerebrum, cerebral (cortex) (hemisphere) (white matter)	191.0	198.3	—	225.0	237.5	239.6
meninges	192.1	198.4	—	225.2	237.6	239.7
peduncle	191.7	198.3	—	225.0	237.5	239.6
ventricle (any)	191.5	198.3	—	225.0	237.5	239.6
cervical region	195.0	198.89	234.8	229.8	238.8	239.8
cervix (cervical) (uteri) (uterus)	180.9	198.82	233.1	219.0	236.0	239.5

ICD-9-CM

N

Vol. 2

◀ New   ◀◼◼◼ Revised

	Malignant					
	Primary	Secondary	Ca in situ	Benign	Uncertain Behavior	Unspecified
Neoplasm *(Continued)*						
cervix *(Continued)*						
canal	180.0	198.82	233.1	219.0	236.0	239.5
contiguous sites	180.8	—	—	—	—	—
endocervix (canal) (gland)	180.0	198.82	233.1	219.0	236.0	239.5
exocervix	180.1	198.82	233.1	219.0	236.0	239.5
external os	180.1	198.82	233.1	219.0	236.0	239.5
internal os	180.0	198.82	233.1	219.0	236.0	239.5
nabothian gland	180.0	198.82	233.1	219.0	236.0	239.5
squamocolumnar junction	180.8	198.82	233.1	219.0	236.0	239.5
stump	180.8	198.82	233.1	219.0	236.0	239.5
cheek	195.0	198.89	234.8	229.8	238.8	239.8
external	173.3	198.2	232.3	216.3	238.2	239.2
inner aspect	145.0	198.89	230.0	210.4	235.1	239.0
internal	145.0	198.89	230.0	210.4	235.1	239.0
mucosa	145.0	198.89	230.0	210.4	235.1	239.0
chest (wall) NEC	195.1	198.89	234.8	229.8	238.8	239.8
chiasma opticum	192.0	198.4	—	225.1	237.9	239.7
chin	173.3	198.2	232.3	216.3	238.2	239.2
choana	147.3	198.89	230.0	210.7	235.1	239.0
cholangiole	155.1	197.8	230.8	211.5	235.3	239.0
choledochal duct	156.1	197.8	230.8	211.5	235.3	239.0
choroid	190.6	198.4	234.0	224.6	238.8	239.8
plexus	191.5	198.3	—	225.0	237.5	239.6
ciliary body	190.0	198.4	234.0	224.0	238.8	239.8
clavicle	170.3	198.5	—	213.3	238.0	239.2
clitoris	184.3	198.82	233.3	221.2	236.3	239.5
clivus	170.0	198.5	—	213.0	238.0	239.2
cloacogenic zone	154.8	197.5	230.7	211.4	235.5	239.0
coccygeal						
body or glomus	194.6	198.89	—	227.6	237.3	239.7
vertebra	170.6	198.5	—	213.6	238.0	239.2
coccyx	170.6	198.5	—	213.6	238.0	239.2
colon-*see also* Neoplasm, intestine, large and rectum	154.0	197.5	230.4	211.4	235.2	239.0
column, spinal-*see* Neoplasm, spine						
columnella	173.3	198.2	232.3	216.3	238.2	239.2
commissure						
labial, lip	140.6	198.89	230.0	210.4	235.1	239.0
laryngeal	161.0	197.3	231.0	212.1	235.6	239.1
common (bile) duct	156.1	197.8	230.8	211.5	235.3	239.0
concha	173.2	198.2	232.2	216.2	238.2	239.2
nose	160.0	197.3	231.8	212.0	235.9	239.1
conjunctiva	190.3	198.4	234.0	224.3	238.8	239.8
connective tissue NEC	171.9	198.89	—	215.9	238.1	239.2

Note-For neoplasms of connective tissue (blood vessel, bursa, fascia, ligament, muscle, peripheral nerves, sympathetic and parasympathetic nerves and ganglia, synovia, tendon, etc.) or of morphological types that indicate connective tissue, code according to the list under "Neoplasm, connective tissue;" for sites that do not appear in this list, code to neoplasm of that site; e.g.,

liposarcoma, shoulder 171.2
leiomyosarcoma, stomach 151.9
neurofibroma, chest wall 215.4

Morphological types that indicate connective tissue appear in their proper place in the alphabetic index with the instruction "see Neoplasm, connective tissue ...."

abdomen	171.5	198.89	—	215.5	238.1	239.2
abdominal wall	171.5	198.89	—	215.5	238.1	239.2
ankle	171.3	198.89	—	215.3	238.1	239.2
antecubital fossa or space	171.2	198.89	—	215.2	238.1	239.2
arm	171.2	198.89	—	215.2	238.1	239.2
auricle (ear)	171.0	198.89	—	215.0	238.1	239.2
axilla	171.4	198.89	—	215.4	238.1	239.2
back	171.7	198.89	—	215.7	238.1	239.2
breast (female) (*see also* Neoplasm, breast)	174.9	198.81	233.0	217	238.3	239.3
male	175.9	198.81	233.0	217	238.3	239.3
buttock	171.6	198.89	—	215.6	238.1	239.2

◀ New   ◀▥▥ Revised

	Malignant					
	Primary	Secondary	Ca in situ	Benign	Uncertain Behavior	Unspecified
Neoplasm *(Continued)*						
connective tissue NEC *(Continued)*						
calf	171.3	198.89	—	215.3	238.1	239.2
cervical region	171.0	198.89	—	215.0	238.1	239.2
cheek	171.0	198.89	—	215.0	238.1	239.2
chest (wall)	171.4	198.89	—	215.4	238.1	239.2
chin	171.0	198.89	—	215.0	238.1	239.2
contiguous sites	171.8	—	—	—	—	—
diaphragm	171.4	198.89	—	215.4	238.1	239.2
ear (external)	171.0	198.89	—	215.0	238.1	239.2
elbow	171.2	198.89	—	215.2	238.1	239.2
extrarectal	171.6	198.89	—	215.6	238.1	239.2
extremity	171.8	198.89	—	215.8	238.1	239.2
lower	171.3	198.89	—	215.3	238.1	239.2
upper	171.2	198.89	—	215.2	238.1	239.2
eyelid	171.0	198.89	—	215.0	238.1	239.2
face	171.0	198.89	—	215.0	238.1	239.2
finger	171.2	198.89	—	215.2	238.1	239.2
flank	171.7	198.89	—	215.7	238.1	239.2
foot	171.3	198.89	—	215.3	238.1	239.2
forearm	171.2	198.89	—	215.2	238.1	239.2
forehead	171.0	198.89	—	215.0	238.1	239.2
gastric	171.5	198.89	—	215.5	238.1	—
gastrointestinal	171.5	198.89	—	215.5	238.1	—
gluteal region	171.6	198.89	—	215.6	238.1	239.2
great vessels NEC	171.4	198.89	—	215.4	238.1	239.2
groin	171.6	198.89	—	215.6	238.1	239.2
hand	171.2	198.89	—	215.2	238.1	239.2
head	171.0	198.89	—	215.0	238.1	239.2
heel	171.3	198.89	—	215.3	238.1	239.2
hip	171.3	198.89	—	215.3	238.1	239.2
hypochondrium	171.5	198.89	—	215.5	238.1	239.2
iliopsoas muscle	171.6	198.89	—	215.5	238.1	239.2
infraclavicular region	171.4	198.89	—	215.4	238.1	239.2
inguinal (canal) (region)	171.6	198.89	—	215.6	238.1	239.2
intestine	171.5	198.89	—	215.5	238.1	—
intrathoracic	171.4	198.89	—	215.4	238.1	239.2
ischiorectal fossa	171.6	198.89	—	215.6	238.1	239.2
jaw	143.9	198.89	230.0	210.4	235.1	239.0
knee	171.3	198.89	—	215.3	238.1	239.2
leg	171.3	198.89	—	215.3	238.1	239.2
limb NEC	171.9	198.89	—	215.8	238.1	239.2
lower	171.3	198.89	—	215.3	238.1	239.2
upper	171.2	198.89	—	215.2	238.1	239.2
nates	171.6	198.89	—	215.6	238.1	239.2
neck	171.0	198.89	—	215.0	238.1	239.2
orbit	190.1	198.4	234.0	224.1	238.8	239.8
pararectal	171.6	198.89	—	215.6	238.1	239.2
para-urethral	171.6	198.89	—	215.6	238.1	239.2
paravaginal	171.6	198.89	—	215.6	238.1	239.2
pelvis (floor)	171.6	198.89	—	215.6	238.1	239.2
pelvo-abdominal	171.8	198.89	—	215.8	238.1	239.2
perineum	171.6	198.89	—	215.6	238.1	239.2
perirectal (tissue)	171.6	198.89	—	215.6	238.1	239.2
periurethral (tissue)	171.6	198.89	—	215.6	238.1	239.2
popliteal fossa or space	171.3	198.89	—	215.3	238.1	239.2
presacral	171.6	198.89	—	215.6	238.1	239.2
psoas muscle	171.5	198.89	—	215.5	238.1	239.2
pterygoid fossa	171.0	198.89	—	215.0	238.1	239.2
rectovaginal septum or wall	171.6	198.89	—	215.6	238.1	239.2
rectovesical	171.6	198.89	—	215.6	238.1	239.2
retroperitoneum	158.0	197.6	—	211.8	235.4	239.0
sacrococcygeal region	171.6	198.89	—	215.6	238.1	239.2
scalp	171.0	198.89	—	215.0	238.1	239.2
scapular region	171.4	198.89	—	215.4	238.1	239.2

	Malignant					
	Primary	Secondary	Ca in situ	Benign	Uncertain Behavior	Unspecified
Neoplasm (Continued)						
connective tissue NEC (Continued)						
shoulder	171.2	198.89	—	215.2	238.1	239.2
skin (dermis) NEC	173.9	198.2	232.9	216.9	238.2	239.2
stomach	171.5	198.89	—	215.5	238.1	—
submental	171.0	198.89	—	215.0	238.1	239.2
supraclavicular region	171.0	198.89	—	215.0	238.1	239.2
temple	171.0	198.89	—	215.0	238.1	239.2
temporal region	171.0	198.89	—	215.0	238.1	239.2
thigh	171.3	198.89	—	215.3	238.1	239.2
thoracic (duct) (wall)	171.4	198.89	—	215.4	238.1	239.2
thorax	171.4	198.89	—	215.4	238.1	239.2
thumb	171.2	198.89	—	215.2	238.1	239.2
toe	171.3	198.89	—	215.3	238.1	239.2
trunk	171.7	198.89	—	215.7	238.1	239.2
umbilicus	171.5	198.89	—	215.5	238.1	239.2
vesicorectal	171.6	198.89	—	215.6	238.1	239.2
wrist	171.2	198.89	—	215.2	238.1	239.2
conus medullaris	192.2	198.3	—	225.3	237.5	239.7
cord (true) (vocal)	161.0	197.3	231.0	212.1	235.6	239.1
false	161.1	197.3	231.0	212.1	235.6	239.1
spermatic	187.6	198.82	233.6	222.8	236.6	239.5
spinal (cervical) (lumbar) (thoracic)	192.2	198.3	—	225.3	237.5	239.7
cornea (limbus)	190.4	198.4	234.0	224.4	238.8	239.8
corpus						
albicans	183.0	198.6	233.3	220	236.2	239.5
callosum, brain	191.8	198.3	—	225.0	237.5	239.6
cavernosum	187.3	198.82	233.5	222.1	236.6	239.5
gastric	151.4	197.8	230.2	211.1	235.2	239.0
penis	187.3	198.82	233.5	222.1	236.6	239.5
striatum, cerebrum	191.0	198.3	—	225.0	237.5	239.6
uteri	182.0	198.82	233.2	219.1	236.0	239.5
isthmus	182.1	198.82	233.2	219.1	236.0	239.5
cortex						
adrenal	194.0	198.7	234.8	227.0	237.2	239.7
cerebral	191.0	198.3	—	225.0	237.5	239.6
costal cartilage	170.3	198.5	—	213.3	238.0	239.2
costovertebral joint	170.3	198.5	—	213.3	238.0	239.2
Cowper's gland	189.3	198.1	233.9	223.81	236.99	239.5
cranial (fossa, any)	191.9	198.3	—	225.0	237.5	239.6
meninges	192.1	198.4	—	225.2	237.6	239.7
nerve (any)	192.0	198.4	—	225.1	237.9	239.7
craniobuccal pouch	194.3	198.89	234.8	227.3	237.0	239.7
craniopharyngeal (duct) (pouch)	194.3	198.89	234.8	227.3	237.0	239.7
cricoid	148.0	198.89	230.0	210.8	235.1	239.0
cartilage	161.3	197.3	231.0	212.1	235.6	239.1
cricopharynx	148.0	198.89	230.0	210.8	235.1	239.0
crypt of Morgagni	154.8	197.5	230.7	211.4	235.2	239.0
crystalline lens	190.0	198.4	234.0	224.0	238.8	239.8
cul-de-sac (Douglas')	158.8	197.6	—	211.8	235.4	239.0
cuneiform cartilage	161.3	197.3	231.0	212.1	235.6	239.1
cutaneous-see Neoplasm, skin						
cutis-see Neoplasm, skin						
cystic (bile) duct (common)	156.1	197.8	230.8	211.5	235.3	239.0
dermis-see Neoplasm, skin						
diaphragm	171.4	198.89	—	215.4	238.1	239.2
digestive organs, system, tube, or tract NEC	159.9	197.8	230.9	211.9	235.5	239.0
contiguous sites with peritoneum	159.8	—	—	—	—	—
disc, intervertebral	170.2	198.5	—	213.2	238.0	239.2
disease, generalized	199.0	199.0	234.9	229.9	238.9	199.0
disseminated	199.0	199.0	234.9	229.9	238.9	199.0
Douglas' cul-de-sac or pouch	158.8	197.6	—	211.8	235.4	239.0
duodenojejunal junction	152.8	197.4	230.7	211.2	235.2	239.0
duodenum	152.0	197.4	230.7	211.2	235.2	239.0
dura (cranial) (mater)	192.1	198.4	—	225.2	237.6	239.7

◀ New   ◀▥ Revised

	Malignant					
	Primary	Secondary	Ca in stiu	Benign	Uncertain Behavior	Unspecified
Neoplasm *(Continued)*						
dura *(Continued)*						
cerebral	192.1	198.4	—	225.2	237.6	239.7
spinal	192.3	198.4	—	225.4	237.6	239.7
ear (external)	173.2	198.2	232.2	216.2	238.2	239.2
auricle or auris	173.2	198.2	232.2	216.2	238.2	239.2
canal, external	173.2	198.2	232.2	216.2	238.2	239.2
cartilage	171.0	198.89	—	215.0	238.1	239.2
external meatus	173.2	198.2	232.2	216.2	238.2	239.2
inner	160.1	197.3	231.8	212.0	235.9	239.8
lobule	173.2	198.2	232.2	216.2	238.2	239.2
middle	160.1	197.3	231.8	212.0	235.9	239.8
contiguous sites with accessory sinuses or nasal cavities	160.8	—	—	—	—	—
skin	173.2	198.2	232.2	216.2	238.2	239.2
earlobe	173.2	198.2	232.2	216.2	238.2	239.2
ejaculatory duct	187.8	198.82	233.6	222.8	236.6	239.5
elbow NEC*	195.4	198.89	232.6	229.8	238.8	239.8
endocardium	164.1	198.89	—	212.7	238.8	239.8
endocervix (canal) (gland)	180.0	198.82	233.1	219.0	236.0	239.5
endocrine gland NEC	194.9	198.89	—	227.9	237.4	239.7
pluriglandular NEC	194.8	198.89	234.8	227.8	237.4	239.7
endometrium (gland) (stroma)	182.0	198.82	233.2	219.1	236.0	239.5
ensiform cartilage	170.3	198.5	—	213.3	238.0	239.2
enteric-*see* Neoplasm, intestine						
ependyma (brain)	191.5	198.3	—	225.0	237.5	239.6
epicardium	164.1	198.89	—	212.7	238.8	239.8
epididymis	187.5	198.82	233.6	222.3	236.6	239.5
epidural	192.9	198.4	—	225.9	237.9	239.7
epiglottis	161.1	197.3	231.0	212.1	235.6	239.1
anterior aspect or surface	146.4	198.89	230.0	210.6	235.1	239.0
cartilage	161.3	197.3	231.0	212.1	235.6	239.1
free border (margin)	146.4	198.89	230.0	210.6	235.1	239.0
junctional region	146.5	198.89	230.0	210.6	235.1	239.0
posterior (laryngeal) surface	161.1	197.3	231.0	212.1	235.6	239.1
suprahyoid portion	161.1	197.3	231.0	212.1	235.6	239.1
esophagogastric junction	151.0	197.8	230.2	211.1	235.2	239.0
esophagus	150.9	197.8	230.1	211.0	235.5	239.0
abdominal	150.2	197.8	230.1	211.0	235.5	239.0
cervical	150.0	197.8	230.1	211.0	235.5	239.0
contiguous sites	150.8	—	—	—	—	—
distal (third)	150.5	197.8	230.1	211.0	235.5	239.0
lower (third)	150.5	197.8	230.1	211.0	235.5	239.0
middle (third)	150.4	197.8	230.1	211.0	235.5	239.0
proximal (third)	150.3	197.8	230.1	211.0	235.5	239.0
specified part NEC	150.8	197.8	230.1	211.0	235.5	239.0
thoracic	150.1	197.8	230.1	211.0	235.5	239.0
upper (third)	150.3	197.8	230.1	211.0	235.5	239.0
ethmoid (sinus)	160.3	197.3	231.8	212.0	235.9	239.1
bone or labyrinth	170.0	198.5	—	213.0	238.0	239.2
Eustachian tube	160.1	197.3	231.8	212.0	235.9	239.1
exocervix	180.1	198.82	233.1	219.0	236.0	239.5
external						
meatus (ear)	173.2	198.2	232.2	216.2	238.2	239.2
os, cervix uteri	180.1	198.82	233.1	219.0	236.0	239.5
extradural	192.9	198.4	—	225.9	237.9	239.7
extrahepatic (bile) duct	156.1	197.8	230.8	211.5	235.3	239.0
contiguous sites with gallbladder	156.8	—	—	—	—	—
extraocular muscle	190.1	198.4	234.0	224.1	238.8	239.8
extrarectal	195.3	198.89	234.8	229.8	238.8	239.8
extremity*	195.8	198.89	232.8	229.8	238.8	239.8
lower*	195.5	198.89	232.7	229.8	238.8	239.8
upper*	195.4	198.89	232.6	229.8	238.8	239.8
eye NEC	190.9	198.4	234.0	224.9	238.8	239.8

| | Malignant | | | | | |
	Primary	Secondary	Ca in situ	Benign	Uncertain Behavior	Unspecified
Neoplasm *(Continued)*						
eye NEC *(Continued)*						
contiguous sites	190.8	—	—	—	—	—
specified sites NEC	190.8	198.4	234.0	224.8	238.8	239.8
eyeball	190.0	198.4	234.0	224.0	238.8	239.8
eyebrow	173.3	198.2	232.3	216.3	238.2	239.2
eyelid (lower) (skin) (upper)	173.1	198.2	232.1	216.1	238.2	239.2
cartilage	171.0	198.89	—	215.0	238.1	239.2
face NEC*	195.0	198.89	232.3	229.8	238.8	239.8
Fallopian tube (accessory)	183.2	198.82	233.3	221.0	236.3	239.5
falx (cerebella) (cerebri)	192.1	198.4	—	225.2	237.6	239.7
fascia-*see also* Neoplasm, connective tissue						
palmar	171.2	198.89	—	215.2	238.1	239.2
plantar	171.3	198.89	—	215.3	238.1	239.2
fatty tissue-*see* Neoplasm, connective tissue						
fauces, faucial NEC	146.9	198.89	230.0	210.6	235.1	239.0
pillars	146.2	198.89	230.0	210.6	235.1	239.0
tonsil	146.0	198.89	230.0	210.5	235.1	239.0
femur (any part)	170.7	198.5	—	213.7	238.0	239.2
fetal membrane	181	198.82	233.2	219.8	236.1	239.5
fibrous tissue-*see* Neoplasm, connective tissue						
fibula (any part)	170.7	198.5	—	213.7	238.0	239.2
filum terminale	192.2	198.3	—	225.3	237.5	239.7
finger NEC*	195.4	198.89	232.6	229.8	238.8	239.8
flank NEC*	195.8	198.89	232.5	229.8	238.8	239.8
follicle, nabothian	180.0	198.82	233.1	219.0	236.0	239.5
foot NEC*	195.5	198.89	232.7	229.8	238.8	239.8
forearm NEC*	195.4	198.89	232.6	229.8	238.8	239.8
forehead (skin)	173.3	198.2	232.3	216.3	238.2	239.2
foreskin	187.1	198.82	233.5	222.1	236.6	239.5
fornix						
pharyngeal	147.3	198.89	230.0	210.7	235.1	239.0
vagina	184.0	198.82	233.3	221.1	236.3	239.5
fossa (of)						
anterior (cranial)	191.9	198.3	—	225.0	237.5	239.6
cranial	191.9	198.3	—	225.0	237.5	239.6
ischiorectal	195.3	198.89	234.8	229.8	238.8	239.8
middle (cranial)	191.9	198.3	—	225.0	237.5	239.6
pituitary	194.3	198.89	234.8	227.3	237.0	239.7
posterior (cranial)	191.9	198.3	—	225.0	237.5	239.6
pterygoid	171.0	198.89	—	215.0	238.1	239.2
pyriform	148.1	198.89	230.0	210.8	235.1	239.0
Rosenmüller	147.2	198.89	230.0	210.7	235.1	239.0
tonsillar	146.1	198.89	230.0	210.6	235.1	239.0
fourchette	184.4	198.82	233.3	221.2	236.3	239.5
frenulum						
labii-*see* Neoplasm, lip, internal						
linguae	141.3	198.89	230.0	210.1	235.1	239.0
frontal						
bone	170.0	198.5	—	213.0	238.0	239.2
lobe, brain	191.1	198.3	—	225.0	237.5	239.6
meninges	192.1	198.4	—	225.2	237.6	239.7
pole	191.1	198.3	—	225.0	237.5	239.6
sinus	160.4	197.3	231.8	212.0	235.9	239.1
fundus						
stomach	151.3	197.8	230.2	211.1	235.2	239.0
uterus	182.0	198.82	233.2	219.1	236.0	239.5
gall duct (extrahepatic)	156.1	197.8	230.8	211.5	235.3	239.0
intrahepatic	155.1	197.8	230.8	211.5	235.3	239.0
gallbladder	156.0	197.8	230.8	211.5	235.3	239.0
contiguous sites with extrahepatic bile ducts	156.8	—	—	—	—	—
ganglia (*see also* Neoplasm, connective tissue)	171.9	198.89	—	215.9	238.1	239.2
basal	191.0	198.3	—	225.0	237.5	239.6

◀ New   ◀▥ Revised

	Malignant					
	Primary	Secondary	Ca in stiu	Benign	Uncertain Behavior	Unspecified
Neoplasm *(Continued)*						
ganglion (*see also* Neoplasm, connective tissue)	171.9	198.89	—	215.9	238.1	239.2
cranial nerve	192.0	198.4	—	225.1	237.9	239.7
Gartner's duct	184.0	198.82	233.3	221.1	236.3	239.5
gastric-*see* Neoplasm, stomach						
gastrocolic	159.8	197.8	230.9	211.9	235.5	239.0
gastroesophageal junction	151.0	197.8	230.2	211.1	235.2	239.0
gastrointestinal (tract) NEC	159.9	197.8	230.9	211.9	235.5	239.0
generalized	199.0	199.0	234.9	229.9	238.9	199.0
genital organ or tract						
female NEC	184.9	198.82	233.3	221.9	236.3	239.5
contiguous sites	184.8					
specified site NEC	184.8	198.82	233.3	221.8	236.3	239.5
male NEC	187.9	198.82	233.6	222.9	236.6	239.5
contiguous sites	187.8	—	—	—	—	—
specified site NEC	187.8	198.82	233.6	222.8	236.6	239.5
genitourinary tract						
female	184.9	198.82	233.3	221.9	236.3	239.5
male	187.9	198.82	233.6	222.9	236.6	239.5
gingiva (alveolar) (marginal)	143.9	198.89	230.0	210.4	235.1	239.0
lower	143.1	198.89	230.0	210.4	235.1	239.0
mandibular	143.1	198.89	230.0	210.4	235.1	239.0
maxillary	143.0	198.89	230.0	210.4	235.1	239.0
upper	143.0	198.89	230.0	210.4	235.1	239.0
gland, glandular (lymphatic) (system)-*see also* Neoplasm, lymph gland						
endocrine NEC	194.9	198.89	—	227.9	237.4	239.7
salivary-*see* Neoplasm, salivary, gland						
glans penis	187.2	198.82	233.5	222.1	236.6	239.5
globus pallidus	191.0	198.3	—	225.0	237.5	239.6
glomus						
coccygeal	194.6	198.89	—	227.6	237.3	239.7
jugularis	194.6	198.89	—	227.6	237.3	239.7
glosso-epiglottic fold(s)	146.4	198.89	230.0	210.6	235.1	239.0
glossopalatine fold	146.2	198.89	230.0	210.6	235.1	239.0
glossopharyngeal sulcus	146.1	198.89	230.0	210.6	235.1	239.0
glottis	161.0	197.3	231.0	212.1	235.6	239.1
gluteal region*	195.3	198.89	232.5	229.8	238.8	239.8
great vessels NEC	171.4	198.89	—	215.4	238.1	239.2
groin NEC	195.3	198.89	232.5	229.8	238.8	239.8
gum	143.9	198.89	230.0	210.4	235.1	239.0
contiguous sites	143.8	—	—	—	—	—
lower	143.1	198.89	230.0	210.4	235.1	239.0
upper	143.0	198.89	230.0	210.4	235.1	239.0
hand NEC*	195.4	198.89	232.6	229.8	238.8	239.8
head NEC*	195.0	198.89	232.4	229.8	238.8	239.8
heart	164.1	198.89	—	212.7	238.8	239.8
contiguous sites with mediastinum or thymus	164.8	—	—	—	—	—
heel NEC*	195.5	198.89	232.7	229.8	238.8	239.8
helix	173.2	198.2	232.2	216.2	238.2	239.2
hematopoietic, hemopoietic tissue NEC	202.8	198.89	—	—	—	238.7
hemisphere, cerebral	191.0	198.3	—	225.0	237.5	239.6
hemorrhoidal zone	154.2	197.5	230.5	211.4	235.5	239.0
hepatic	155.2	197.7	230.8	211.5	235.3	239.0
duct (bile)	156.1	197.8	230.8	211.5	235.3	239.0
flexure (colon)	153.0	197.5	230.3	211.3	235.2	239.0
primary	155.0	—	—	—	—	—
hilus of lung	162.2	197.0	231.2	212.3	235.7	239.1
hip NEC*	195.5	198.89	232.7	229.8	238.8	239.8
hippocampus, brain	191.2	198.3	—	225.0	237.5	239.6
humerus (any part)	170.4	198.5	—	213.4	238.0	239.2
hymen	184.0	198.82	233.3	221.1	236.3	239.5
hypopharynx, hypopharyngeal NEC	148.9	198.89	230.0	210.8	235.1	239.0
contiguous sites	148.8	—	—	—	—	—

ICD-9-CM

N

Vol. 2

	Malignant					
	Primary	Secondary	Ca in stiu	Benign	Uncertain Behavior	Unspecified
Neoplasm *(Continued)*						
hypopharynx, hypopharyngeal NEC *(Continued)*						
postcricoid region	148.0	198.89	230.0	210.8	235.1	239.0
posterior wall	148.3	198.89	230.0	210.8	235.1	239.0
pyriform fossa (sinus)	148.1	198.89	230.0	210.8	235.1	239.0
specified site NEC	148.8	198.89	230.0	210.8	235.1	239.0
wall	148.9	198.89	230.0	210.8	235.1	239.0
posterior	148.3	198.89	230.0	210.8	235.1	239.0
hypophysis	194.3	198.89	234.8	227.3	237.0	239.7
hypothalamus	191.0	198.3	—	225.0	237.5	239.6
ileocecum, ileocecal (coil) (junction) (valve)	153.4	197.5	230.3	211.3	235.2	239.0
ileum	152.2	197.4	230.7	211.2	235.2	239.0
ilium	170.6	198.5	—	213.6	238.0	239.2
immunoproliferative NEC	203.8	—	—	—	—	—
infraclavicular (region)*	195.1	198.89	232.5	229.8	238.8	239.8
inguinal (region)*	195.3	198.89	232.5	229.8	238.8	239.8
insula	191.0	198.3	—	225.0	237.5	239.6
insular tissue (pancreas)	157.4	197.8	230.9	211.7	235.5	239.0
brain	191.0	198.3	—	225.0	237.5	239.6
interarytenoid fold	148.2	198.89	230.0	210.8	235.1	239.0
hypopharyngeal aspect	148.2	198.89	230.0	210.8	235.1	239.0
laryngeal aspect	161.1	197.3	231.0	212.1	235.6	239.1
marginal zone	148.2	198.89	230.0	210.8	235.1	239.0
interdental papillae	143.9	198.89	230.0	210.4	235.1	239.0
lower	143.1	198.89	230.0	210.4	235.1	239.0
upper	143.0	198.89	230.0	210.4	235.1	239.0
internal						
capsule	191.0	198.3	—	225.0	237.5	239.6
os (cervix)	180.0	198.82	233.1	219.0	236.0	239.5
intervertebral cartilage or disc	170.2	198.5	—	213.2	238.0	239.2
intestine, intestinal	159.0	197.8	230.7	211.9	235.2	239.0
large	153.9	197.5	230.3	211.3	235.2	239.0
appendix	153.5	197.5	230.3	211.3	235.2	239.0
caput coli	153.4	197.5	230.3	211.3	235.2	239.0
cecum	153.4	197.5	230.3	211.3	235.2	239.0
colon	153.9	197.5	230.3	211.3	235.2	239.0
and rectum	154.0	197.5	230.4	211.4	235.2	239.0
ascending	153.6	197.5	230.3	211.3	235.2	239.0
caput	153.4	197.5	230.3	211.3	235.2	239.0
contiguous sites	153.8	—	—	—	—	—
descending	153.2	197.5	230.3	211.3	235.2	239.0
distal	153.2	197.5	230.3	211.3	235.2	239.0
left	153.2	197.5	230.3	211.3	235.2	239.0
pelvic	153.3	197.5	230.3	211.3	235.2	239.0
right	153.6	197.5	230.3	211.3	235.2	239.0
sigmoid (flexure)	153.3	197.5	230.3	211.3	235.2	239.0
transverse	153.1	197.5	230.3	211.3	235.2	239.0
contiguous sites	153.8	—	—	—	—	—
hepatic flexure	153.0	197.5	230.3	211.3	235.2	239.0
ileocecum, ileocecal (coil) (valve)	153.4	197.5	230.3	211.3	235.2	239.0
sigmoid flexure (lower) (upper)	153.3	197.5	230.3	211.3	235.2	239.0
splenic flexure	153.7	197.5	230.3	211.3	235.2	239.0
small	152.9	197.4	230.7	211.2	235.2	239.0
contiguous sites	152.8	—	—	—	—	—
duodenum	152.0	197.4	230.7	211.2	235.2	239.0
ileum	152.2	197.4	230.7	211.2	235.2	239.0
jejunum	152.1	197.4	230.7	211.2	235.2	239.0
tract NEC	159.0	197.8	230.7	211.9	235.2	239.0
intra-abdominal	195.2	198.89	234.8	229.8	238.8	239.8
intracranial NEC	191.9	198.3	—	225.0	237.5	239.6
intrahepatic (bile) duct	155.1	197.8	230.8	211.5	235.3	239.0
intraocular	190.0	198.4	234.0	224.0	238.8	239.8
intraorbital	190.1	198.4	234.0	224.1	238.8	239.8

◀ New   ◀▥ Revised

	Malignant					
	Primary	Secondary	Ca in situ	Benign	Uncertain Behavior	Unspecified
Neoplasm *(Continued)*						
intrasellar	194.3	198.89	234.8	227.3	237.0	239.7
intrathoracic (cavity) (organs NEC)	195.1	198.89	234.8	229.8	238.8	239.8
contiguous sites with respiratory organs	165.8	—	—	—	—	—
iris	190.0	198.4	234.0	224.0	238.8	239.8
ischiorectal (fossa)	195.3	198.89	234.8	229.8	238.8	239.8
ischium	170.6	198.5	—	213.6	238.0	239.2
island of Reil	191.0	198.3	—	225.0	237.5	239.6
islands or islets of Langerhans	157.4	197.8	230.9	211.7	235.5	239.0
isthmus uteri	182.1	198.82	233.2	219.1	236.0	239.5
jaw	195.0	198.89	234.8	229.8	238.8	239.8
bone	170.1	198.5	—	213.1	238.0	239.2
carcinoma	143.9	—	—	—	—	—
lower	143.1	—	—	—	—	—
upper	143.0	—	—	—	—	—
lower	170.1	198.5	—	213.1	238.0	239.2
upper	170.0	198.5	—	213.0	238.0	239.2
carcinoma (any type) (lower) (upper)	195.0	—	—	—	—	—
skin	173.3	198.2	232.3	216.3	238.2	239.2
soft tissues	143.9	198.89	230.0	210.4	235.1	239.0
lower	143.1	198.89	230.0	210.4	235.1	239.0
upper	143.0	198.89	230.0	210.4	235.1	239.0
jejunum	152.1	197.4	230.7	211.2	235.2	239.0
joint NEC *(see also* Neoplasm, bone)	170.9	198.5	—	213.9	238.0	239.2
acromioclavicular	170.4	198.5	—	213.4	238.0	239.2
bursa or synovial membrane-*see* Neoplasm, connective tissue						
costovertebral	170.3	198.5	—	213.3	238.0	239.2
sternocostal	170.3	198.5	—	213.3	238.0	239.2
temporomandibular	170.1	198.5	—	213.1	238.0	239.2
junction						
anorectal	154.8	197.5	230.7	211.4	235.5	239.0
cardioesophageal	151.0	197.8	230.2	211.1	235.2	239.0
esophagogastric	151.0	197.8	230.2	211.1	235.2	239.0
gastroesophageal	151.0	197.8	230.2	211.1	235.2	239.0
hard and soft palate	145.5	198.89	230.0	210.4	235.1	239.0
ileocecal	153.4	197.5	230.3	211.3	235.2	239.0
pelvirectal	154.0	197.5	230.4	211.4	235.2	239.0
pelviureteric	189.1	198.0	233.9	223.1	236.91	239.5
rectosigmoid	154.0	197.5	230.4	211.4	235.2	239.0
squamocolumnar, of cervix	180.8	198.82	233.1	219.0	236.0	239.5
kidney (parenchymal)	189.0	198.0	233.9	223.0	236.91	239.5
calyx	189.1	198.0	233.9	223.1	236.91	239.5
hilus	189.1	198.0	233.9	223.1	236.91	239.5
pelvis	189.1	198.0	233.9	223.1	236.91	239.5
knee NEC*	195.5	198.89	232.7	229.8	238.8	239.8
labia (skin)	184.4	198.82	233.3	221.2	236.3	239.5
majora	184.1	198.82	233.3	221.2	236.3	239.5
minora	184.2	198.82	233.3	221.2	236.3	239.5
labial-*see also* Neoplasm, lip sulcus (lower) (upper)	145.1	198.89	230.0	210.4	235.1	239.0
labium (skin)	184.4	198.82	233.3	221.2	236.3	239.5
majus	184.1	198.82	233.3	221.2	236.3	239.5
minus	184.2	198.82	233.3	221.2	236.3	239.5
lacrimal						
canaliculi	190.7	198.4	234.0	224.7	238.8	239.8
duct (nasal)	190.7	198.4	234.0	224.7	238.8	239.8
gland	190.2	198.4	234.0	224.2	238.8	239.8
punctum	190.7	198.4	234.0	224.7	238.8	239.8
sac	190.7	198.4	234.0	224.7	238.8	239.8
Langerhans, islands or islets	157.4	197.8	230.9	211.7	235.5	239.0
laryngopharynx	148.9	198.89	230.0	210.8	235.1	239.0
larynx, laryngeal NEC	161.9	197.3	231.0	212.1	235.6	239.1
aryepiglottic fold	161.1	197.3	231.0	212.1	235.6	239.1
cartilage (arytenoid) (cricoid) (cuneiform) (thyroid)	161.3	197.3	231.0	212.1	235.6	239.1

ICD-9-CM

N

Vol. 2

	Malignant					
	Primary	Secondary	Ca in stiu	Benign	Uncertain Behavior	Unspecified
Neoplasm *(Continued)*						
larynx, laryngeal NEC *(Continued)*						
commissure (anterior) (posterior)	161.0	197.3	231.0	212.1	235.6	239.1
contiguous sites	161.8	—	—	—	—	—
extrinsic NEC	161.1	197.3	231.0	212.1	235.6	239.1
meaning hypopharynx	148.9	198.89	230.0	210.8	235.1	239.0
interarytenoid fold	161.1	197.3	231.0	212.1	235.6	239.1
intrinsic	161.0	197.3	231.0	212.1	235.6	239.1
ventricular band	161.1	197.3	231.0	212.1	235.6	239.1
leg NEC*	195.5	198.89	232.7	229.8	238.8	239.8
lens, crystalline	190.0	198.4	234.0	224.0	238.8	239.8
lid (lower) (upper)	173.1	198.2	232.1	216.1	238.2	239.2
ligament-*see also* Neoplasm, connective tissue						
broad	183.3	198.82	233.3	221.0	236.3	239.5
Mackenrodt's	183.8	198.82	233.3	221.8	236.3	239.5
non-uterine-*see* Neoplasm, connective tissue						
round	183.5	198.82	—	221.0	236.3	239.5
sacro-uterine	183.4	198.82	—	221.0	236.3	239.5
uterine	183.4	198.82	—	221.0	236.3	239.5
utero-ovarian	183.8	198.82	233.3	221.8	236.3	239.5
uterosacral	183.4	198.82	—	221.0	236.3	239.5
limb*	195.8	198.89	232.8	229.8	238.8	239.8
lower*	195.5	198.89	232.7	229.8	238.8	239.8
upper*	195.4	198.89	232.6	229.8	238.8	239.8
limbus of cornea	190.4	198.4	234.0	224.4	238.8	239.8
lingual NEC (*see also* Neoplasm, tongue)	141.9	198.89	230.0	210.1	235.1	239.0
lingula, lung	162.3	197.0	231.2	212.3	235.7	239.1
lip (external) (lipstick area) (vermillion border)	140.9	198.89	230.0	210.0	235.1	239.0
buccal aspect-*see* Neoplasm, lip, internal						
commissure	140.6	198.89	230.0	210.4	235.1	239.0
contiguous sites	140.8	—	—	—	—	—
with oral cavity or pharynx	149.8	—	—	—	—	—
frenulum-*see* Neoplasm, lip, internal						
inner aspect-*see* Neoplasm, lip, internal						
internal (buccal) (frenulum) (mucosa) (oral)	140.5	198.89	230.0	210.0	235.1	239.0
lower	140.4	198.89	230.0	210.0	235.1	239.0
upper	140.3	198.89	230.0	210.0	235.1	239.0
lower	140.1	198.89	230.0	210.0	235.1	239.0
internal (buccal) (frenulum) (mucosa) (oral)	140.4	198.89	230.0	210.0	235.1	239.0
mucosa-*see* Neoplasm, lip, internal						
oral aspect-*see* Neoplasm, lip, internal						
skin (commissure) (lower) (upper)	173.0	198.2	232.0	216.0	238.2	239.2
upper	140.0	198.89	230.0	210.0	235.1	239.0
internal (buccal) (frenulum) (mucosa) (oral)	140.3	198.89	230.0	210.0	235.1	239.0
liver	155.2	197.7	230.8	211.5	235.3	239.0
primary	155.0	—	—	—	—	—
lobe						
azygos	162.3	197.0	231.2	212.3	235.7	239.1
frontal	191.1	198.3	—	225.0	237.5	239.6
lower	162.5	197.0	231.2	212.3	235.7	239.1
middle	162.4	197.0	231.2	212.3	235.7	239.1
occipital	191.4	198.3	—	225.0	237.5	239.6
parietal	191.3	198.3	—	225.0	237.5	239.6
temporal	191.2	198.3	—	225.0	237.5	239.6
upper	162.3	197.0	231.2	212.3	235.7	239.1
lumbosacral plexus	171.6	198.4	—	215.6	238.1	239.2
lung	162.9	197.0	231.2	212.3	235.7	239.1
azygos lobe	162.3	197.0	231.2	212.3	235.7	239.1
carina	162.2	197.0	231.2	212.3	235.7	239.1
contiguous sites with bronchus or trachea	162.8	—	—	—	—	—
hilus	162.2	197.0	231.2	212.3	235.7	239.1
lingula	162.3	197.0	231.2	212.3	235.7	239.1
lobe NEC	162.9	197.0	231.2	212.3	235.7	239.1

◀ New ◀▥ Revised

	Malignant					
	Primary	Secondary	Ca in stiu	Benign	Uncertain Behavior	Unspecified
Neoplasm *(Continued)*						
lung *(Continued)*						
lower lobe	162.5	197.0	231.2	212.3	235.7	239.1
main bronchus	162.2	197.0	231.2	212.3	235.7	239.1
middle lobe	162.4	197.0	231.2	212.3	235.7	239.1
upper lobe	162.3	197.0	231.2	212.3	235.7	239.1
lymph, lymphatic channel NEC *(see also* Neoplasm, connective tissue)	171.9	198.89	—	215.9	238.1	239.2
gland (secondary)	—	196.9	—	229.0	238.8	239.8
abdominal	—	196.2	—	229.0	238.8	239.8
aortic	—	196.2	—	229.0	238.8	239.8
arm	—	196.3	—	229.0	238.8	239.8
auricular (anterior) (posterior)	—	196.0	—	229.0	238.8	239.8
axilla, axillary	—	196.3	—	229.0	238.8	239.8
brachial	—	196.3	—	229.0	238.8	239.8
bronchial	—	196.1	—	229.0	238.8	239.8
bronchopulmonary	—	196.1	—	229.0	238.8	239.8
celiac	—	196.2	—	229.0	238.8	239.8
cervical	—	196.0	—	229.0	238.8	239.8
cervicofacial	—	196.0	—	229.0	238.8	239.8
Cloquet	—	196.5	—	229.0	238.8	239.8
colic	—	196.2	—	229.0	238.8	239.8
common duct	—	196.2	—	229.0	238.8	239.8
cubital	—	196.3	—	229.0	238.8	239.8
diaphragmatic	—	196.1	—	229.0	238.8	239.8
epigastric, inferior	—	196.6	—	229.0	238.8	239.8
epitrochlear	—	196.3	—	229.0	238.8	239.8
esophageal	—	196.1	—	229.0	238.8	239.8
face	—	196.0	—	229.0	238.8	239.8
femoral	—	196.5	—	229.0	238.8	239.8
gastric	—	196.2	—	229.0	238.8	239.8
groin	—	196.5	—	229.0	238.8	239.8
head	—	196.0	—	229.0	238.8	239.8
hepatic	—	196.2	—	229.0	238.8	239.8
hilar (pulmonary)	—	196.1	—	229.0	238.8	239.8
splenic	—	196.2	—	229.0	238.8	239.8
hypogastric	—	196.6	—	229.0	238.8	239.8
ileocolic	—	196.2	—	229.0	238.8	239.8
iliac	—	196.6	—	229.0	238.8	239.8
infraclavicular	—	196.3	—	229.0	238.8	239.8
inguina, inguinal	—	196.5	—	229.0	238.8	239.8
innominate	—	196.1	—	229.0	238.8	239.8
intercostal	—	196.1	—	229.0	238.8	239.8
intestinal	—	196.2	—	229.0	238.8	239.8
intrabdominal	—	196.2	—	229.0	238.8	239.8
intrapelvic	—	196.6	—	229.0	238.8	239.8
intrathoracic	—	196.1	—	229.0	238.8	239.9
jugular	—	196.0	—	229.0	238.8	239.8
leg	—	196.5	—	229.0	238.8	239.8
limb						
lower	—	196.5	—	229.0	238.8	239.8
upper	—	196.3	—	229.0	238.8	239.8
lower limb	—	196.5	—	229.0	238.8	239.9
lumbar	—	196.2	—	229.0	238.8	239.8
mandibular	—	196.0	—	229.0	238.8	239.8
mediastinal	—	196.1	—	229.0	238.8	239.8
mesenteric (inferior) (superior)	—	196.2	—	229.0	238.8	239.8
midcolic	—	196.2	—	229.0	238.8	239.8
multiple sites in categories 196.0-196.6	—	196.8	—	229.0	238.8	239.8
neck	—	196.0	—	229.0	238.8	239.8
obturator	—	196.6	—	229.0	238.8	239.8
occipital	—	196.0	—	229.0	238.8	239.8
pancreatic	—	196.2	—	229.0	238.8	239.8
para-aortic	—	196.2	—	229.0	238.8	239.8

ICD-9-CM

N

Vol. 2

| | Malignant | | | | | |
	Primary	Secondary	Ca in stiu	Benign	Uncertain Behavior	Unspecified
Neoplasm *(Continued)*						
lymph, lymphatic channel NEC *(Continued)*						
gland *(Continued)*						
paracervical	—	196.6	—	229.0	238.8	239.8
parametrial	—	196.6	—	229.0	238.8	239.8
parasternal	—	196.1	—	229.0	238.8	239.8
parotid	—	196.0	—	229.0	238.8	239.8
pectoral	—	196.3	—	229.0	238.8	239.8
pelvic	—	196.6	—	229.0	238.8	239.8
peri-aortic	—	196.2	—	229.0	238.8	239.8
peripancreatic	—	196.2	—	229.0	238.8	239.8
popliteal	—	196.5	—	229.0	238.8	239.8
porta hepatis	—	196.2	—	229.0	238.8	239.8
portal	—	196.2	—	229.0	238.8	239.8
preauricular	—	196.0	—	229.0	238.8	239.8
prelaryngeal	—	196.0	—	229.0	238.8	239.8
presymphysial	—	196.6	—	229.0	238.8	239.8
pretracheal	—	196.0	—	229.0	238.8	239.8
primary (any site) NEC	202.9	—	—	—	—	—
pulmonary (hiler)	—	196.1	—	229.0	238.8	239.8
pyloric	—	196.2	—	229.0	238.8	239.8
retroperitoneal	—	196.2	—	229.0	238.8	239.8
retropharyngeal	—	196.0	—	229.0	238.8	239.8
Rosenmüller's	—	196.5	—	229.0	238.8	239.8
sacral	—	196.6	—	229.0	238.8	239.8
scalene	—	196.0	—	229.0	238.8	239.8
site NEC	—	196.9	—	229.0	238.8	239.8
splenic (hilar)	—	196.2	—	229.0	238.8	239.8
subclavicular	—	196.3	—	229.0	238.8	239.8
subinguinal	—	196.5	—	229.0	238.8	239.8
sublingual	—	196.0	—	229.0	238.8	239.8
submandibular	—	196.0	—	229.0	238.8	239.8
submaxillary	—	196.0	—	229.0	238.8	239.8
submental	—	196.0	—	229.0	238.8	239.8
subscapular	—	196.3	—	229.0	238.8	239.8
supraclavicular	—	196.0	—	229.0	238.8	239.8
thoracic	—	196.1	—	229.0	238.8	239.8
tibial	—	196.5	—	229.0	238.8	239.8
tracheal		196.1	—	229.0	238.8	239.8
tracheobronchial	—	196.1	—	229.0	238.8	239.8
upper limb	—	196.3	—	229.0	238.8	239.8
Virchow's	—	196.0	—	229.0	238.8	239.8
node-*see also* Neoplasm, lymph gland primary NEC	202.9	—	—	—	—	—
vessel (*see also* Neoplasm, connective tissue)	171.9	198.89	—	215.9	238.1	239.2
Mackenrodt's ligament	183.8	198.82	233.3	221.8	236.3	239.5
malar region-*see* Neoplasm, cheek	170.0	198.5	—	213.0	238.0	239.2
mammary gland-*see* Neoplasm, breast						
mandible	170.1	198.5	—	213.1	238.0	239.2
alveolar						
mucosa	143.1	198.89	230.0	210.4	235.1	239.0
ridge or process	170.1	198.5	—	213.1	238.0	239.2
carcinoma	143.1	—	—	—	—	—
carcinoma	143.1	—	—	—	—	—
marrow (bone) NEC	202.9	198.5	—	—	—	238.7
mastectomy site (skin)	173.5	198.2	—	—	—	—
specified as breast tissue	174.8	198.81	—	—	—	—
mastoid (air cells) (antrum) (cavity)	160.1	197.3	231.8	212.0	235.9	239.1
bone or process	170.0	198.5	—	213.0	238.0	239.2
maxilla, maxillary (superior)	170.0	198.5	—	213.0	238.0	239.2
alveolar						
mucosa	143.0	198.89	230.0	210.4	235.1	239.0
ridge or process	170.0	198.5	—	213.0	238.0	239.2
carcinoma	143.0	—	—	—	—	—

◀ New   ◀▦ Revised

	Malignant					
	Primary	Secondary	Ca in situ	Benign	Uncertain Behavior	Unspecified
Neoplasm *(Continued)*						
maxilla, maxillary *(Continued)*						
antrum	160.2	197.3	231.8	212.0	235.9	239.1
carcinoma	143.0	—	—	—	—	—
inferior-*see* Neoplasm, mandible						
sinus	160.2	197.3	231.8	212.0	235.9	239.1
meatus						
external (ear)	173.2	198.2	232.2	216.2	238.2	239.2
Meckel's diverticulum	152.3	197.4	230.7	211.2	235.2	239.0
mediastinum, mediastinal	164.9	197.1	—	212.5	235.8	239.8
anterior	164.2	197.1	—	212.5	235.8	239.8
contiguous sites with heart and thymus	164.8	—	—	—	—	—
posterior	164.3	197.1	—	212.5	235.8	239.8
medulla						
adrenal	194.0	198.7	234.8	227.0	237.2	239.7
oblongata	191.7	198.3	—	225.0	237.5	239.6
meibomian gland	173.1	198.2	232.1	216.1	238.2	239.2
melanoma-*see* Melanoma						
meninges (brain) (cerebral) (cranial) (intracranial)	192.1	198.4	—	225.2	237.6	239.7
spinal (cord)	192.3	198.4	—	225.4	237.6	239.7
meniscus, knee joint (lateral) (medial)	170.7	198.5	—	213.7	238.0	239.2
mesentery, mesenteric	158.8	197.6	—	211.8	235.4	239.0
mesoappendix	158.8	197.6	—	211.8	235.4	239.0
mesocolon	158.8	197.6	—	211.8	235.4	239.0
mesopharynx-*see* Neoplasm, oropharynx						
mesosalpinx	183.3	198.82	233.3	221.0	236.3	239.5
mesovarium	183.3	198.82	233.3	221.0	236.3	239.5
metacarpus (any bone)	170.5	198.5	—	213.5	238.0	239.2
metastatic NEC-*see also* Neoplasm, by site, secondary	—	199.1	—	—	—	—
metatarsus (any bone)	170.8	198.5	—	213.8	238.0	239.2
midbrain	191.7	198.3	—	225.0	237.5	239.6
milk duct-*see* Neoplasm, breast						
mons						
pubis	184.4	198.82	233.3	221.2	236.3	239.5
veneris	184.4	198.82	233.3	221.2	236.3	239.5
motor tract	192.9	198.4	—	225.9	237.9	239.7
brain	191.9	198.3	—	225.0	237.5	239.6
spinal	192.2	198.3	—	225.3	237.5	239.7
mouth	145.9	198.89	230.0	210.4	235.1	239.0
contiguous sites	145.8	—	—	—	—	—
floor	144.9	198.89	230.0	210.3	235.1	239.0
anterior portion	144.0	198.89	230.0	210.3	235.1	239.0
contiguous sites	144.8	—	—	—	—	—
lateral portion	144.1	198.89	230.0	210.3	235.1	239.0
roof	145.5	198.89	230.0	210.4	235.1	239.0
specified part NEC	145.8	198.89	230.0	210.4	235.1	239.0
vestibule	145.1	198.89	230.0	210.4	235.1	239.0
mucosa						
alveolar (ridge or process)	143.9	198.89	230.0	210.4	235.1	239.0
lower	143.1	198.89	230.0	210.4	235.1	239.0
upper	143.0	198.89	230.0	210.4	235.1	239.0
buccal	145.0	198.89	230.0	210.4	235.1	239.0
cheek	145.0	198.89	230.0	210.4	235.1	239.0
lip-*see* Neoplasm, lip, internal						
nasal	160.0	197.3	231.8	212.0	235.9	239.1
oral	145.0	198.89	230.0	210.4	235.1	239.0
Müllerian duct						
female	184.8	198.82	233.3	221.8	236.3	239.5
male	187.8	198.82	233.6	222.8	236.6	239.5
multiple sites NEC	199.0	199.0	234.9	229.9	238.9	199.0
muscle-*see also* Neoplasm, connective tissue extraocular	190.1	198.4	234.0	224.1	238.8	239.8
myocardium	164.1	198.89	—	212.7	238.8	239.8
myometrium	182.0	198.82	233.2	219.1	236.0	239.5

ICD-9-CM

N

Vol. 2

	Malignant					
	Primary	Secondary	Ca in situ	Benign	Uncertain Behavior	Unspecified
Neoplasm *(Continued)*						
myopericardium	164.1	198.89	—	212.7	238.8	239.8
nabothian gland (follicle)	180.0	198.82	233.1	219.0	236.0	239.5
nail	173.9	198.2	232.9	216.9	238.2	239.2
finger	173.6	198.2	232.6	216.6	238.2	239.2
toe	173.7	198.2	232.7	216.7	238.2	239.2
nares, naris (anterior) (posterior)	160.0	197.3	231.8	212.0	235.9	239.1
nasal-*see* Neoplasm, nose						
nasolabial groove	173.3	198.2	232.3	216.3	238.2	239.2
nasolacrimal duct	190.7	198.4	234.0	224.7	238.8	239.8
nasopharynx, nasopharyngeal	147.9	198.89	230.0	210.7	235.1	239.0
contiguous sites	147.8	—	—	—	—	—
floor	147.3	198.89	230.0	210.7	235.1	239.0
roof	147.0	198.89	230.0	210.7	235.1	239.0
specified site NEC	147.8	198.89	230.0	210.7	235.1	239.0
wall	147.9	198.89	230.0	210.7	235.1	239.0
anterior	147.3	198.89	230.0	210.7	235.1	239.0
lateral	147.2	198.89	230.0	210.7	235.1	239.0
posterior	147.1	198.89	230.0	210.7	235.1	239.0
superior	147.0	198.89	230.0	210.7	235.1	239.0
nates	173.5	198.2	232.5	216.5	238.2	239.2
neck NEC*	195.0	198.89	234.8	229.8	238.8	239.8
nerve (autonomic) (parasympathetic) (peripheral) (sympathetic) - *see also* Neoplasm, connective tissue						
abducens	192.0	198.4	—	225.1	237.9	239.7
accessory (spinal)	192.0	198.4	—	225.1	237.9	239.7
acoustic	192.0	198.4	—	225.1	237.9	239.7
auditory	192.0	198.4	—	225.1	237.9	239.7
brachial	171.2	198.89	—	215.2	238.1	239.2
cranial (any)	192.0	198.4	—	225.1	237.9	239.7
facial	192.0	198.4	—	225.1	237.9	239.7
femoral	171.3	198.89	—	215.3	238.1	239.2
glossopharyngeal	192.0	198.4	—	225.1	237.9	239.7
hypoglossal	192.0	198.4	—	225.1	237.9	239.7
intercostal	171.4	198.89	—	215.4	238.1	239.2
lumbar	171.7	198.89	—	215.7	238.1	239.2
median	171.2	198.89	—	215.2	238.1	239.2
obturator	171.3	198.89	—	215.3	238.1	239.2
oculomotor	192.0	198.4	—	225.1	237.9	239.7
olfactory	192.0	198.4	—	225.1	237.9	239.7
optic	192.0	198.4	—	225.1	237.9	239.7
peripheral NEC	171.9	198.89	—	215.9	238.1	239.2
radial	171.2	198.89	—	215.2	238.1	239.2
sacral	171.6	198.89	—	215.6	238.1	239.2
sciatic	171.3	198.89	—	215.3	238.1	239.2
spinal NEC	171.9	198.89	—	215.9	238.1	239.2
trigeminal	192.0	198.4	—	225.1	237.9	239.7
trochlear	192.0	198.4	—	225.1	237.9	239.7
ulnar	171.2	198.89	—	215.2	238.1	239.2
vagus	192.0	198.4	—	225.1	237.9	239.7
nervous system (central) NEC	192.9	198.4	—	225.9	237.9	239.7
autonomic NEC	171.9	198.89	—	215.9	238.1	239.2
brain-*see also* Neoplasm, brain membrane or meninges	192.1	198.4	—	225.2	237.6	239.7
contiguous sites	192.8	—	—	—	—	—
parasympathetic NEC	171.9	198.89	—	215.9	238.1	239.2
sympathetic NEC	171.9	198.89	—	215.9	238.1	239.2
nipple (female)	174.0	198.81	233.0	217	238.3	239.3
male	175.0	198.81	233.0	217	238.3	239.3
nose, nasal	195.0	198.89	234.8	229.8	238.8	239.8
ala (external)	173.3	198.2	232.3	216.3	238.2	239.2
bone	170.0	198.5	—	213.0	238.0	239.2
cartilage	160.0	197.3	231.8	212.0	235.9	239.1
cavity	160.0	197.3	231.8	212.0	235.9	239.1
contiguous sites with accessory sinuses or middle ear	160.8	—	—	—	—	—

◀ **New**   ◀⫸ **Revised**

	Malignant					
	Primary	Secondary	Ca in situ	Benign	Uncertain Behavior	Unspecified
Neoplasm *(Continued)*						
nose, nasal *(Continued)*						
choana	147.3	198.89	230.0	210.7	235.1	239.0
external (skin)	173.3	198.2	232.3	216.3	238.2	239.2
fossa	160.0	197.3	231.8	212.0	235.9	239.1
internal	160.0	197.3	231.8	212.0	235.9	239.1
mucosa	160.0	197.3	231.8	212.0	235.9	239.1
septum	160.0	197.3	231.8	212.0	235.9	239.1
posterior margin	147.3	198.89	230.0	210.7	235.1	239.0
sinus-*see* Neoplasm, sinus						
skin	173.3	198.2	232.3	216.3	238.2	239.2
turbinate (mucosa)	160.0	197.3	231.8	212.0	235.9	239.1
bone	170.0	198.5	—	2130	238.0	239.2
vestibule	160.0	197.3	231.8	212.0	235.9	239.1
nostril	160.0	197.3	231.8	212.0	235.9	239.1
nucleus pulposus	170.2	198.5	—	213.2	238.0	230.2
occipital						
bone	170.0	198.5	—	213.0	238.0	239.2
lobe or pole, brain	191.4	198.3	—	225.0	237.5	239.6
odontogenic-*see* Neoplasm, jaw bone						
oesophagus-*see* Neoplasm, esophagus						
olfactory nerve or bulb	192.0	198.4	—	225.1	237.9	239.7
olive (brain)	191.7	198.3	—	225.0	237.5	239.6
omentum	158.8	197.6	—	211.8	235.4	239.0
operculum (brain)	191.0	198.3	—	225.0	237.5	239.6
optic nerve, chiasm, or tract	192.0	198.4	—	225.1	237.9	239.7
oral (cavity)	145.9	198.89	230.0	210.4	235.1	239.0
contiguous sites with lip or pharynx	149.8	—	—	—	—	—
ill-defined	149.9	198.89	230.0	210.4	235.1	239.0
mucosa	145.9	198.89	230.0	210.4	235.1	239.0
orbit	190.1	198.4	234.0	224.1	238.8	239.8
bone	170.0	198.5	—	213.0	238.0	239.2
eye	190.1	198.4	234.0	224.1	238.8	239.8
soft parts	190.1	198.4	234.0	224.1	238.8	239.8
organ of Zuckerkandl	194.6	198.89	—	227.6	237.3	239.7
oropharynx	146.9	198.89	230.0	210.6	235.1	239.0
branchial cleft (vestige)	146.8	198.89	230.0	210.6	235.1	239.0
contiguous sites	146.8	—	—	—	—	—
junctional region	146.5	198.89	230.0	210.6	235.1	239.0
lateral wall	146.6	198.89	230.0	210.6	235.1	239.0
pillars of fauces	146.2	198.89	230.0	210.6	235.1	239.0
posterior wall	146.7	198.89	230.0	210.6	235.1	239.0
specified part NEC	146.8	198.89	230.0	210.6	235.1	239.0
vallecula	146.3	198.89	230.0	210.6	235.1	239.0
os						
external	180.1	198.82	233.1	219.0	236.0	239.5
internal	180.0	198.82	233.1	219.0	236,0	239.5
ovary	183.0	198.6	233.3	220	236.2	239.5
oviduct	183.2	198.82	233.3	221.0	236.3	239.5
palate	145.5	198.89	230.0	210.4	235.1	239.0
hard	145.2	198.89	230.0	210.4	235.1	239.0
junction of hard and soft palate	145.5	198.89	230.0	210.4	235.1	239.0
soft	145.3	198.89	230.0	210.4	235.1	239.0
nasopharyngeal surface	147.3	198.89	230.0	210.7	235.1	239.0
posterior surface	147.3	198.89	230.0	210.7	235.1	239.0
superior surface	147.3	198.89	230.0	210.7	235.1	239.0
palatoglossal arch	146.2	198.89	230.0	210.6	235.1	239.0
palatopharyngeal arch	146.2	198.89	230.0	210.6	235.1	239.0
pallium	191.0	198.3	—	225.0	237.5	239.6
palpebra	173.1	198.2	232.1	216.1	238.2	239.2
pancreas	157.9	197.8	230.9	211.6	235.5	239.0
body	157.1	197.8	230.9	211.6	235.5	239.0
contiguous sites	157.8	—	—	—	—	—

ICD-9-CM

N

Vol. 2

| | Malignant | | | | | |
	Primary	Secondary	Ca in situ	Benign	Uncertain Behavior	Unspecified
Neoplasm *(Continued)*						
pancreas *(Continued)*						
duct (of Santorini) (of Wirsung)	157.3	197.8	230.9	211.6	235.5	239.0
ectopic tissue	157.8	197.8				
head	157.0	197.8	230.9	211.6	235.5	239.0
islet cells	157.4	197.8	230.9	211.7	235.5	239.0
neck	157.8	197.8	230.9	211.6	235.5	239.0
tail	157.2	197.8	230.9	211.6	235.5	239.0
para-aortic body	194.6	198.89	—	227.6	237.3	239.7
paraganglion NEC	194.6	198.89	—	227.6	237.3	239.7
parametrium	183.4	198.82	—	221.0	236.3	239.5
paranephric	158.0	197.6	—	211.8	235.4	239.0
pararectal	195.3	198.89	—	229.8	238.8	239.8
parasagittal (region)	195.0	198.89	234.8	229.8	238.8	239.8
parasellar	192.9	198.4	—	225.9	237.9	239.7
parathyroid (gland)	194.1	198.89	234.8	227.1	237.4	239.7
paraurethral	195.3	198.89	—	229.8	238.8	239.8
gland	189.4	198.1	233.9	223.89	236.99	239.5
paravaginal	195.3	198.89	—	229.8	238.8	239.8
parenchyma, kidney	189.0	198.0	233.9	223.0	236.91	239.5
parietal						
bone	170.0	198.5	—	213.0	238.0	239.2
lobe, brain	191.3	198.3	—	225.0	237.5	239.6
paroophoron	183.3	198.82	233.3	221.0	236.3	239.5
parotid (duct) (gland)	142.0	198.89	230.0	210.2	235.0	239.0
parovarium	183.3	198.82	233.3	221.0	236.3	239.5
patella	170.8	198.5	—	213.8	238.0	239.2
peduncle, cerebral	191.7	198.3	—	225.0	237.5	239.6
pelvirectal junction	154.0	197.5	230.4	211.4	235.2	239.0
pelvis, pelvic	195.3	198.89	234.8	229.8	238.8	239.8
bone	170.6	198.5	—	213.6	238.0	239.2
floor	195.3	198.89	234.8	229.8	238.8	239.8
renal	189.1	198.0	233.9	223.1	236.91	239.5
viscera	195.3	198.89	234.8	229.8	238.8	239.8
wall	195.3	198.89	234.8	229.8	238.8	239.8
pelvo-abdominal	195.8	198.89	234.8	229.8	238.8	239.8
penis	187.4	198.82	233.5	222.1	236.6	239.5
body	187.3	198.82	233.5	222.1	236.6	239.5
corpus (cavernosum)	187.3	198.82	233.5	222.1	236.6	239.5
glans	187.2	198.82	233.5	222.1	236.6	239.5
skin NEC	187.4	198.82	233.5	222.1	236.6	239.5
periadrenal (tissue)	158.0	197.6	—	211.8	235.4	239.0
perianal (skin)	173.5	198.2	232.5	216.5	238.2	239.2
pericardium	164.1	198.89	—	212.7	238.8	239.8
perinephric	158.0	197.6	—	211.8	235.4	239.0
perineum	195.3	198.89	234.8	229.8	238.8	239.8
periodontal tissue NEC	143.9	198.89	230.0	210.4	235.1	239.0
periosteum-*see* Neoplasm, bone						
peripancreatic	158.0	197.6	—	211.8	235.4	239.0
peripheral nerve NEC	171.9	198.89	—	215.9	238.1	239.2
perirectal (tissue)	195.3	198.89	—	229.8	238.8	239.8
perirenal (tissue)	158.0	197.6	—	211.8	235.4	239.0
peritoneum, peritoneal (cavity)	158.9	197.6	—	211.8	235.4	239.0
contiguous sites	158.8	—	—	—	—	—
with digestive organs	159.8	—	—	—	—	—
parietal	158.8	197.6	—	211.8	235.4	239.0
pelvic	158.8	197.6	—	211.8	235.4	239.0
specified part NEC	158.8	197.6	—	211.8	235.4	239.0
peritonsillar (tissue)	195.0	198.89	234.8	229.8	238.8	239.8
periurethral tissue	195.3	198.89	—	229.8	238.8	239.8
phalanges	170.9	198.5	—	213.9	238.0	239.2
foot	170.8	198.5	—	213.8	238.0	239.2
hand	170.5	198.5	—	213.5	238.0	239.2

◄ New   ◄▮▮ Revised

	Malignant					
	Primary	Secondary	Ca in stiu	Benign	Uncertain Behavior	Unspecified
Neoplasm *(Continued)*						
pharynx, pharyngeal	149.0	198.89	230.0	210.9	235.1	239.0
bursa	147.1	198.89	230.0	210.7	235.1	239.0
fornix	147.3	198.89	230.0	210.7	235.1	239.0
recess	147.2	198.89	230.0	210.7	235.1	239.0
region	149.0	198.89	230.0	210.9	235.1	239.0
tonsil	147.1	198.89	230.0	210.7	235.1	239.0
wall (lateral) (posterior)	149.0	198.89	230.0	210.9	235.1	239.0
pia mater (cerebral) (cranial)	192.1	198.4	—	225.2	237.6	239.7
spinal	192.3	198.4	—	225.4	237.6	239.7
pillars of fauces	146.2	198.89	230.0	210.6	235.1	239.0
pineal (body) (gland)	194.4	198.89	234.8	227.4	237.1	239.7
pinna (ear) NEC	173.2	198.2	232.2	216.2	238.2	239.2
cartilage	171.0	198.89	—	215.0	238.1	239.2
piriform fossa or sinus	148.1	198.89	230.0	210.8	235.1	239.0
pituitary (body) (fossa) (gland) (lobe)	194.3	198.89	234.8	227.3	237.0	239.7
placenta	181	198.82	233.2	219.8	236.1	239.5
pleura, pleural (cavity)	163.9	197.2	—	212.4	235.8	239.1
contiguous sites	163.8	—	—	—	—	—
parietal	163.0	197.2	—	212.4	235.8	239.1
visceral	163.1	197.2	—	212.4	235.8	239.1
plexus						
brachial	171.2	198.89	—	215.2	238.1	239.2
cervical	171.0	198.89	—	215.0	238.1	239.2
choroid	191.5	198.3	—	225.0	237.5	239.6
lumbosacral	171.6	198.89	—	215.6	238.1	239.2
sacral	171.6	198.89	—	215.6	238.1	239.2
pluri-endocrine	194.8	198.89	234.8	227.8	237.4	239.7
pole						
frontal	191.1	198.3	—	225.0	237.5	239.6
occipital	191.4	198.3	—	225.0	237.5	239.6
pons (varolii)	191.7	198.3	—	225.0	237.5	239.6
popliteal fossa or space*	195.5	198.89	234.8	229.8	238.8	239.8
postcricoid (region)	148.0	198.89	230.0	210.8	235.1	239.0
posterior fossa (cranial)	191.6	198.3	—	225.0	237.5	239.6
postnasal space	147.9	198.89	230.0	210.7	235.1	239.0
prepuce	187.1	198.82	233.5	222.1	236.6	239.5
prepylorus	151.1	197.8	230.2	211.1	235.2	239.0
presacral (region)	195.3	198.89	—	229.8	238.8	239.8
prostate (gland)	185	198.82	233.4	222.2	236.5	239.5
utricle	189.3	198.1	233.9	223.81	236.99	239.5
pterygoid fossa	171.0	198.89	—	215.0	238.1	239.2
pubic bone	170.6	198.5	—	213.6	238.0	239.2
pudenda, pudendum (female)	184.4	198.82	233.3	221.2	236.3	239.5
pulmonary	162.9	197.0	231.2	212.3	235.7	239.1
putamen	191.0	198.3	—	225.0	237.5	239.6
pyloric						
antrum	151.2	197.8	230.2	211.1	235.2	239.0
canal	151.1	197.8	230.2	211.1	235.2	239.0
pylorus	151.1	197.8	230.2	211.1	235.2	239.0
pyramid (brain)	191.7	198.3	—	225.0	237.5	239.6
pyriform fossa or sinus	148.1	198.89	230.0	210.8	235.1	239.0
radius (any part)	170.4	198.5	—	213.4	238.0	239.2
Rathke's pouch	194.3	198.89	234.8	227.3	237.0	239.7
rectosigmoid (colon) (junction)	154.0	197.5	230.4	211.4	235.2	239.0
contiguous sites with anus or rectum	154.8	—	—	—	—	—
rectouterine pouch	158.8	197.6	—	211.8	235.4	239.0
rectovaginal septum or wall	195.3	198.89	234.8	229.8	238.8	239.8
rectovesical septum	195.3	198.89	234.8	229.8	238.8	239.8
rectum (ampulla)	154.1	197.5	230.4	211.4	235.2	239.0
and colon	154.0	197.5	230.4	211.4	235.2	239.0
contiguous sites with anus or rectosigmoid junction	154.8	—	—	—	—	—
renal	189.0	198.0	233.9	223.0	236.91	239.5

ICD-9-CM
N
Vol. 2

	Malignant					
	Primary	Secondary	Ca in situ	Benign	Uncertain Behavior	Unspecified
Neoplasm *(Continued)*						
renal *(Continued)*						
calyx	189.1	198.0	233.9	223.1	236.91	239.5
hilus	189.1	198.0	233.9	223.1	236.91	239.5
parenchyma	189.0	198.0	233.9	223.0	236.91	239.5
pelvis	189.1	198.0	233.9	223.1	236.91	239.5
respiratory						
organs or system NEC	165.9	197.3	231.9	212.9	235.9	239.1
contiguous sites with intrathoracic organs	165.8	—	—	—	—	—
specified sites NEC	165.8	197.3	231.8	212.8	235.9	239.1
tract NEC	165.9	197.3	231.9	212.9	235.9	239.1
upper	165.0	197.3	231.9	212.9	235.9	239.1
retina	190.5	198.4	234.0	224.5	238.8	239.8
retrobulbar	190.1	198.4	—	224.1	238.8	239.8
retrocecal	158.0	197.6	—	211.8	235.4	239.0
retromolar (area) (triangle) (trigone)	145.6	198.89	230.0	210.4	235.1	239.0
retro-orbital	195.0	198.89	234.8	229.8	238.8	239.8
retroperitoneal (space) (tissue)	158.0	197.6	—	211.8	235.4	239.0
contiguous sites	158.8	—	—	—	—	—
retroperitoneum	158.0	197.6	—	211.8	235.4	239.0
contiguous sites	158.8	—	—	—	—	—
retropharyngeal	149.0	198.89	230.0	210.9	235.1	239.0
retrovesical (septum)	195.3	198.89	234.8	229.8	238.8	239.8
rhinencephalon	191.0	198.3	—	225.0	237.5	239.6
rib	170.3	198.5	—	213.3	238.0	239.2
Rosenmüller's fossa	147.2	198.89	230.0	210.7	235.1	239.0
round ligament	183.5	198.82	—	221.0	236.3	239.5
sacrococcyx, sacrococcygeal	170.6	198.5	—	213.6	238.0	239.2
region	195.3	198.89	234.8	229.8	238.8	239.8
sacrouterine ligament	183.4	198.82	—	221.0	236.3	239.5
sacrum, sacral (vertebra)	170.6	198.5	—	213.6	238.0	239.2
salivary gland or duct (major)	142.9	198.89	230.0	210.2	235.0	239.0
contiguous sites	142.8	—	—	—	—	—
minor NEC	145.9	198.89	230.0	210.4	235.1	239.0
parotid	142.0	198.89	230.0	210.2	235.0	239.0
pluriglandular	142.8	198.89	230.0	210.2	235.0	239.0
sublingual	142.2	198.89	230.0	210.2	235.0	239.0
submandibular	142.1	198.89	230.0	210.2	235.0	239.0
submaxillary	142.1	198.89	230.0	210.2	235.0	239.0
salpinx (uterine)	183.2	198.82	233.3	221.0	236.3	239.5
Santorini's duct	157.3	197.8	230.9	211.6	235.5	239.0
scalp	173.4	198.2	232.4	216.4	238.2	239.2
scapula (any part)	170.4	198.5	—	213.4	238.0	239.2
scapular region	195.1	198.89	234.8	229.8	238.8	239.8
scar NEC (*see also* Neoplasm, skin)	173.9	198.2	232.9	216.9	238.2	239.2
sciatic nerve	171.3	198.89	—	215.3	238.1	239.2
sclera	190.0	198.4	234.0	224.0	238.8	239.8
scrotum (skin)	187.7	198.82	233.6	222.4	236.6	239.5
sebaceous gland-*see* Neoplasm, skin						
sella turcica	194.3	198.89	234.8	227.3	237.0	239.7
bone	170.0	198.5	—	213.0	238.0	239.2
semilunar cartilage (knee)	170.7	198.5	—	213.7	238.0	239.2
seminal vesicle	187.8	198.82	233.6	222.8	236.6	239.5
septum						
nasal	160.0	197.3	231.8	212.0	235.9	239.1
posterior margin	147.3	198.89	230.0	210.7	235.1	239.0
rectovaginal	195.3	198.89	234.8	229.8	238.8	239.8
rectovesical	195.3	198.89	234.8	229.8	238.8	239.8
urethrovaginal	184.9	198.82	233.3	221.9	236.3	239.5
vesicovaginal	184.9	198.82	233.3	221.9	236.3	239.5
shoulder NEC*	195.4	198.89	232.6	229.8	238.8	239.8
sigmoid flexure (lower) (upper)	153.3	197.5	230.3	211.3	235.2	239.0
sinus (accessory)	160.9	197.3	231.8	212.0	235.9	239.1
bone (any)	170.0	198.5	—	213.0	238.0	239.2

◄ New   ◄▩ Revised

	Malignant					
	Primary	Secondary	Ca in stiu	Benign	Uncertain Behavior	Unspecified
Neoplasm *(Continued)*						
sinus *(Continued)*						
contiguous sites with middle ear or nasal cavities	160.8	—	—	—	—	—
ethmoidal	160.3	197.3	231.8	212.0	235.9	239.1
frontal	160.4	197.3	231.8	212.0	235.9	239.1
maxillary	160.2	197.3	231.8	212.0	235.9	239.1
nasal, paranasal NEC	160.9	197.3	231.8	212.0	235.9	239.1
pyriform	148.1	198.89	230.0	210.8	235.1	239.0
sphenoidal	160.5	197.3	231.8	212.0	235.9	239.1
skeleton, skeletal NEC	170.9	198.5	—	213.9	238.0	239.2
Skene's gland	189.4	198.1	233.9	223.89	236.99	239.5
skin NEC	173.9	198.2	232.9	216.9	238.2	239.2
abdominal wall	173.5	198.2	232.5	216.5	238.2	239.2
ala nasi	173.3	198.2	232.3	216.3	238.2	239.2
ankle	173.7	198.2	232.7	216.7	238.2	239.2
antecubital space	173.6	198.2	232.6	216.6	238.2	239.2
anus	173.5	198.2	232.5	216.5	238.2	239.2
arm	173.6	198.2	232.6	216.6	238.2	239.2
auditory canal (external)	173.2	198.2	232.2	216.2	238.2	239.2
auricle (ear)	173.2	198.2	232.2	216.2	238.2	239.2
auricular canal (external)	173.2	198.2	232.2	216.2	238.2	239.2
axilla, axillary fold	173.5	198.2	232.5	216.5	238.2	239.2
back	173.5	198.2	232.5	216.5	238.2	239.2
breast	173.5	198.2	232.5	216.5	238.2	239.2
brow	173.3	198.2	232.3	216.3	238.2	239.2
buttock	173.5	198.2	232.5	216.5	238.2	239.2
calf	173.7	198.2	232.7	216.7	238.2	239.2
canthus (eye) (inner) (outer)	173.1	198.2	232.1	216.1	238.2	239.2
cervical region	173.4	198.2	232.4	216.4	238.2	239.2
cheek (external)	173.3	198.2	232.3	216.3	238.2	239.2
chest (wall)	173.5	198.2	232.5	216.5	238.2	239.2
chin	173.3	198.2	232.3	216.3	238.2	239.2
clavicular area	173.5	198.2	232.5	216.5	238.2	239.2
clitoris	184.3	198.82	233.3	221.2	236.3	239.5
columnella	173.3	198.2	232.3	216.3	238.2	239.2
concha	173.2	198.2	232.2	216.2	238.2	239.2
contiguous sites	173.8	—	—	—	—	—
ear (external)	173.2	198.2	232.2	216.2	238.2	239.2
elbow	173.6	198.2	232.6	216.6	238.2	239.2
eyebrow	173.3	198.2	232.3	216.3	238.2	239.2
eyelid	173.1	198.2	232.1	216.1	238.2	239.2
face NEC	173.3	198.2	232.3	216.3	238.2	239.2
female genital organs (external)	184.4	198.82	233.3	221.2	236.3	239.5
clitoris	184.3	198.82	233.3	221.2	236.3	239.5
labium NEC	184.4	198.82	233.3	221.2	236.3	239.5
majus	184.1	198.82	233.3	221.2	236.3	239.5
minus	184.2	198.82	233.3	221.2	236.3	239.5
pudendum	184.4	198.82	233.3	221.2	236.3	239.5
vulva	184.4	198.82	233.3	221.2	236.3	239.5
finger	173.6	198.2	232.6	216.6	238.2	239.2
flank	173.5	198.2	232.5	216.5	238.2	239.2
foot	173.7	198.2	232.7	216.7	238.2	239.2
forearm	173.6	198.2	232.6	216.6	238.2	239.2
forehead	173.3	198.2	232.3	216.3	238.2	239.2
glabella	173.3	198.2	232.3	216.3	238.2	239.2
gluteal region	173.5	198.2	232.5	216.5	238.2	239.2
groin	173.5	198.2	232.5	216.5	238.2	239.2
hand	173.6	198.2	232.6	216.6	238.2	239.2
head NEC	173.4	198.2	232.4	216.4	238.2	239.2
heel	173.7	198.2	232.7	216.7	238.2	239.2
helix	173.2	198.2	232.2	216.2	238.2	239.2
hip	173.7	198.2	232.7	216.7	238.2	239.2
infraclavicular region	173.5	198.2	232.5	216.5	238.2	239.2

ICD-9-CM

N

Vol. 2

	Malignant					
	Primary	Secondary	Ca in stiu	Benign	Uncertain Behavior	Unspecified
Neoplasm *(Continued)*						
skin NEC *(Continued)*						
inguinal region	173.5	198.2	232.5	216.5	238.2	239.2
jaw	173.3	198.2	232.3	216.3	238.2	239.2
knee	173.7	198.2	232.7	216.7	238.2	239.2
labia						
majora	184.1	198.82	233.3	221.2	236.3	239.5
minora	184.2	198.82	233.3	221.2	236.3	239.5
leg	173.7	198.2	232.7	216.7	238.2	239.2
lid (lower) (upper)	173.1	198.2	232.1	216.1	238.2	239.2
limb NEC	173.9	198.2	232.9	216.9	238.2	239.5
lower	173.7	198.2	232.7	216.7	238.2	239.2
upper	173.6	198.2	232.6	216.6	238.2	239.2
lip (lower) (upper)	173.0	198.2	232.0	216.0	238.2	239.2
male genital organs	187.9	198.82	233.6	222.9	236.6	239.5
penis	187.4	198.82	233.5	222.1	236.6	239.5
prepuce	187.1	198.82	233.5	222.1	236.6	239.5
scrotum	187.7	198.82	233.6	222.4	236.6	239.5
mastectomy site	173.5	198.2	—	—	—	—
specified as breast tissue	174.8	198.81	—	—	—	—
meatus, acoustic (external)	173.2	198.2	232.2	216.2	238.2	239.2
nates	173.5	198.2	232.5	216.5	238.2	239.2
neck	173.4	198.2	232.4	216.4	238.2	239.2
nose (external)	173.3	198.2	232.3	216.3	238.2	239.2
palm	173.6	198.2	232.6	216.6	238.2	239.2
palpebra	173.1	198.2	232.1	216.1	238.2	239.2
penis NEC	187.4	198.82	233.5	222.1	236.6	239.5
perianal	173.5	198.2	232.5	216.5	238.2	239.2
perineum	173.5	198.2	232.5	216.5	238.2	239.2
pinna	173.2	198.2	232.2	216.2	238.2	239.2
plantar	173.7	198.2	232.7	216.7	238.2	239.2
popliteal fossa or space	173.7	198.2	232.7	216.7	238.2	239.2
prepuce	187.1	198.82	233.5	222.1	236.6	239.5
pubes	173.5	198.2	232.5	216.5	238.2	239.2
sacrococcygeal region	173.5	198.2	232.5	216.5	238.2	239.2
scalp	173.4	198.2	232.4	216.4	238.2	239.2
scapular region	173.5	198.2	232.5	216.5	238.2	239.2
scrotum	187.7	198.82	233.6	222.4	236.6	239.5
shoulder	173.6	198.2	232.6	216.6	238.2	239.2
sole (foot)	173.7	198.2	232.7	216.7	238.2	239.2
specified sites NEC	173.8	198.2	232.8	216.8	232.8	239.2
submammary fold	173.5	198.2	232.5	216.5	238.2	239.2
supraclavicular region	173.4	198.2	232.4	216.4	238.2	239.2
temple	173.3	198.2	232.3	216.3	238.2	239.2
thigh	173.7	198.2	232.7	216.7	238.2	239.2
thoracic wall	173.5	198.2	232.5	216.5	238.2	239.2
thumb	173.6	198.2	232.6	216.6	238.2	239.2
toe	173.7	198.2	232.7	216.7	238.2	239.2
tragus	173.2	198.2	232.2	216.2	238.2	239.2
trunk	173.5	198.2	232.5	216.5	238.2	239.2
umbilicus	173.5	198.2	232.5	216.5	238.2	239.2
vulva	184.4	198.82	233.3	221.2	236.3	239.5
wrist	173.6	198.2	232.6	216.6	238.2	239.2
skull	170.0	198.5	—	213.0	238.0	239.2
soft parts or tissues-*see* Neoplasm, connective tissue						
specified site NEC	195.8	198.89	234.8	229.8	238.8	239.8
spermatic cord	187.6	198.82	233.6	222.8	236.6	239.5
sphenoid	160.5	197.3	231.8	212.0	235.9	239.1
bone	170.0	198.5	—	213.0	238.0	239.2
sinus	160.5	197.3	231.8	212.0	235.9	239.1
sphincter						
anal	154.2	197.5	230.5	211.4	235.5	239.0
of Oddi	156.1	197.8	230.8	211.5	235.3	239.0

◀ **New**   ◀ **Revised**

	Malignant					
	Primary	Secondary	Ca in situ	Benign	Uncertain Behavior	Unspecified
Neoplasm *(Continued)*						
spine, spinal (column)	170.2	198.5	—	213.2	238.0	239.2
bulb	191.7	198.3	—	225.0	237.5	239.6
coccyx	170.6	198.5	—	213.6	238.0	239.2
cord (cervical) (lumbar) (sacral) (thoracic)	192.2	198.3	—	225.3	237.5	239.7
dura mater	192.3	198.4	—	225.4	237.6	239.7
lumbosacral	170.2	198.5	—	213.2	238.0	239.2
membrane	192.3	198.4	—	225.4	237.6	239.7
meninges	192.3	198.4	—	225.4	237.6	239.7
nerve (root)	171.9	198.89	—	215.9	238.1	239.2
pia mater	192.3	198.4	—	225.4	237.6	239.7
root	171.9	198.89	—	215.9	238.1	239.2
sacrum	170.6	198.5	—	213.6	238.0	239.2
spleen, splenic NEC	159.1	197.8	230.9	211.9	235.5	239.0
flexure (colon)	153.7	197.5	230.3	211.3	235.2	239.0
stem, brain	191.7	198.3	—	225.0	237.5	239.6
Stensen's duct	142.0	198.89	230.0	210.2	235.0	239.0
sternum	170.3	198.5	—	213.3	238.0	239.2
stomach	151.9	197.8	230.2	211.1	235.2	239.0
antrum (pyloric)	151.2	197.8	230.2	211.1	235.2	239.0
body	151.4	197.8	230.2	211.1	235.2	239.0
cardia	151.0	197.8	230.2	211.1	235.2	239.0
cardiac orifice	151.0	197.8	230.2	211.1	235.2	239.0
contiguous sites	151.8	—	—	—	—	—
corpus	151.4	197.8	230.2	211.1	235.2	239.0
fundus	151.3	197.8	230.2	211.1	235.2	239.0
greater curvature NEC	151.6	197.8	230.2	211.1	235.2	239.0
lesser curvature NEC	151.5	197.8	230.2	211.1	235.2	239.0
prepylorus	151.1	197.8	230.2	211.1	235.2	239.0
pylorus	151.1	197.8	230.2	211.1	235.2	239.0
wall NEC	151.9	197.8	230.2	211.1	235.2	239.0
anterior NEC	151.8	197.8	230.2	211.1	235.2	239.0
posterior NEC	151.8	197.8	230.2	211.1	235.2	239.0
stroma, endometrial	182.0	198.82	233.2	219.1	236.0	239.5
stump, cervical	180.8	198.82	233.1	219.0	236.0	239.5
subcutaneous (nodule) (tissue) NEC-*see* Neoplasm, connective tissue						
subdural	192.1	198.4	—	225.2	237.6	239.7
subglottis, subglottic	161.2	197.3	231.0	212.1	235.6	239.1
sublingual	144.9	198.89	230.0	210.3	235.1	239.0
gland or duct	142.2	198.89	230.0	210.2	235.0	239.0
submandibular gland	142.1	198.89	230.0	210.2	235.0	239.0
submaxillary gland or duct	142.1	198.89	230.0	210.2	235.0	239.0
submental	195.0	198.89	234.8	229.8	238.8	239.8
subpleural	162.9	197.0	—	212.3	235.7	239.1
substernal	164.2	197.1	—	212.5	235.8	239.8
sudoriferous, sudoriparous gland, site unspecified	173.9	198.2	232.9	216.9	238.2	239.2
specified site-*see* Neoplasm, skin						
supraclavicular region	195.0	198.89	234.8	229.8	238.8	239.8
supraglottis	161.1	197.3	231.0	212.1	235.6	239.1
suprarenal (capsule) (cortex) (gland) (medulla)	194.0	198.7	234.8	227.0	237.2	239.7
suprasellar (region)	191.9	198.3	—	225.0	237.5	239.6
sweat gland (apocrine) (eccrine), site unspecified	173.9	198.2	232.9	216.9	238.2	239.2
specified site-*see* Neoplasm, skin						
sympathetic nerve or nervous system NEC	171.9	198.89	—	215.9	238.1	239.2
symphysis pubis	170.6	198.5	—	213.6	238.0	239.2
synovial membrane-*see* Neoplasm, connective tissue						
tapetum, brain	191.8	198.3	—	225.0	237.5	239.6
tarsus (any bone)	170.8	198.5	—	213.8	238.0	239.2
temple (skin)	173.3	198.2	232.3	216.3	238.2	239.2
temporal						
bone	170.0	198.5	—	213.0	238.0	239.2
lobe or pole	191.2	198.3	—	225.0	237.5	239.6
region	195.0	198.89	234.8	229.8	238.8	239.8
skin	173.3	198.2	232.3	216.3	238.2	239.2

ICD-9-CM

N

Vol.

	Malignant					
	Primary	Secondary	Ca in stiu	Benign	Uncertain Behavior	Unspecified
Neoplasm *(Continued)*						
tendon (sheath)-*see* Neoplasm, connective tissue						
tentorium (cerebelli)	192.1	198.4	—	225.2	237.6	239.7
testis, testes (descended) (scrotal)	186.9	198.82	233.6	222.0	236.4	239.5
ectopic	186.0	198.82	233.6	222.0	236.4	239.5
retained	186.0	198.82	233.6	222.0	236.4	239.5
undescended	186.0	198.82	233.6	222.0	236.4	239.5
thalamus	191.0	198.3	—	225.0	237.5	239.6
thigh NEC*	195.5	198.89	234.8	229.8	238.8	239.8
thorax, thoracic (cavity) (organs NEC)	195.1	198.89	234.8	229.8	238.8	239.8
duct	171.4	198.89	—	215.4	238.1	239.2
wall NEC	195.1	198.89	234.8	229.8	238.8	239.8
throat	149.0	198.89	230.0	210.9	235.1	239.0
thumb NEC*	195.4	198.89	232.6	229.8	238.8	239.8
thymus (gland)	164.0	198.89	—	212.6	235.8	239.8
contiguous sites with heart and mediastinum	164.8	—	—	—	—	—
thyroglossal duct	193	198.89	234.8	226	237.4	239.7
thyroid (gland)	193	198.89	234.8	226	237.4	239.7
cartilage	161.3	197.3	231.0	212.1	235.6	239.1
tibia (any part)	170.7	198.5	—	213.7	238.0	239.2
toe NEC*	195.5	198.89	232.7	229.8	238.8	239.8
tongue	141.9	198.89	230.0	210.1	235.1	239.0
anterior (two-thirds) NEC	141.4	198.89	230.0	210.1	235.1	239.0
dorsal surface	141.1	198.89	230.0	210.1	235.1	239.0
ventral surface	141.3	198.89	230.0	210.1	235.1	239.0
base (dorsal surface)	141.0	198.89	230.0	210.1	235.1	239.0
border (lateral)	141.2	198.89	230.0	210.1	235.1	239.0
contiguous sites	141.8	—	—	—	—	—
dorsal surface NEC	141.1	198.89	230.0	210.1	235.1	239.0
fixed part NEC	141.0	198.89	230.0	210.1	235.1	239.0
foramen cecum	141.1	198.89	230.0	210.1	235.1	239.0
frenulum linguae	141.3	198.89	230.0	210.1	235.1	239.0
junctional zone	141.5	198.89	230.0	210.1	235.1	239.0
margin (lateral)	141.2	198.89	230.0	210.1	235.1	239.0
midline NEC	141.1	198.89	230.0	210.1	235.1	239.0
mobile part NEC	141.4	198.89	230.0	210.1	235.1	239.0
posterior (third)	141.0	198.89	230.0	210.1	235.1	239.0
root	141.0	198.89	230.0	210.1	235.1	239.0
surface (dorsal)	141.1	198.89	230.0	210.1	235.1	239.0
base	141.0	198.89	230.0	210.1	235.1	239.0
ventral	141.3	198.89	230.0	210.1	235.1	239.0
tip	141.2	198.89	230.0	210.1	235.1	239.0
tonsil	141.6	198.89	230.0	210.1	235.1	239.0
tonsil	146.0	198.89	230.0	210.5	235.1	239.0
fauces, faucial	146.0	198.89	230.0	210.5	235.1	239.0
lingual	141.6	198.89	230.0	210.1	235.1	239.0
palatine	146.0	198.89	230.0	210.5	235.1	239.0
pharyngeal	147.1	198.89	230.0	210.7	235.1	239.0
pillar (anterior) (posterior)	146.2	198.89	230.0	210.6	235.1	239.0
tonsillar fossa	146.1	198.89	230.0	210.6	235.1	239.0
tooth socket NEC	143.9	198.89	230.0	210.4	235.1	239.0
trachea (cartilage) (mucosa)	162.0	197.3	231.1	212.2	235.7	239.1
contiguous sites with bronchus or lung	162.8	—	—	—	—	—
tracheobronchial	162.8	197.3	231.1	212.2	235.7	239.1
contiguous sites with lung	162.8	—	—	—	—	—
tragus	173.2	198.2	232.2	216.2	238.2	239.2
trunk NEC*	195.8	198.89	232.5	229.8	238.8	239.8
tubo-ovarian	183.8	198.82	233.3	221.8	236.3	239.5
tunica vaginalis	187.8	198.82	233.6	222.8	236.6	239.5
turbinate (bone)	170.0	198.5	—	213.0	238.0	239.2
nasal	160.0	197.3	231.8	212.0	235.9	239.1
tympanic cavity	160.1	197.3	231.8	212.0	235.9	239.1
ulna (any part)	170.4	198.5	—	213.4	238.0	239.2

◀ New   ◀▥ Revised

| | Malignant | | | | | |
	Primary	Secondary	Ca in situ	Benign	Uncertain Behavior	Unspecified
Neoplasm *(Continued)*						
umbilicus, umbilical	173.5	198.2	232.5	216.5	238.2	239.2
uncus, brain	191.2	198.3	—	225.0	237.5	239.6
unknown site or unspecified	199.1	199.1	234.9	229.9	238.9	239.9
urachus	188.7	198.1	233.7	223.3	236.7	239.4
ureter, ureteral	189.2	198.1	233.9	223.2	236.91	239.5
orifice (bladder)	188.6	198.1	233.7	223.3	236.7	239.4
ureter-bladder (junction)	188.6	198.1	233.7	223.3	236.7	239.4
urethra, urethral (gland)	189.3	198.1	233.9	223.81	236.99	239.5
orifice, internal	188.5	198.1	233.7	223.3	236.7	239.4
urethrovaginal (septum)	184.9	198.82	233.3	221.9	236.3	239.5
urinary organ or system NEC	189.9	198.1	233.9	223.9	236.99	239.5
bladder-*see* Neoplasm, bladder						
contiguous sites	189.8	—	—	—	—	—
specified sites NEC	189.8	198.1	233.9	223.89	236.99	239.5
utero-ovarian	183.8	198.82	233.3	221.8	236.3	239.5
ligament	183.3	198.82	—	221.0	236.3	239.5
uterosacral ligament	183.4	198.82	—	221.0	236.3	239.5
uterus, uteri, uterine	179	198.82	233.2	219.9	236.0	239.5
adnexa NEC	183.9	198.82	233.3	221.8	236.3	239.5
contiguous sites	183.8	—	—	—	—	—
body	182.0	198.82	233.2	219.1	236.0	239.5
contiguous sites	182.8	—	—	—	—	—
cervix	180.9	198.82	233.1	219.0	236.0	239.5
cornu	182.0	198.82	233.2	219.1	236.0	239.5
corpus	182.0	198.82	233.2	219.1	236.0	239.5
endocervix (canal) (gland)	180.0	198.82	233.1	219.0	236.0	239.5
endometrium	182.0	198.82	233.2	219.1	236.0	239.5
exocervix	180.1	198.82	233.1	219.0	236.0	239.5
external os	180.1	198.82	233.1	219.0	236.0	239.5
fundus	182.0	198.82	233.2	219.1	236.0	239.5
internal os	180.0	198.82	233.1	219.0	236.0	239.5
isthmus	182.1	198.82	233.2	219.1	236.0	239.5
ligament	183.4	198.82	—	221.0	236.3	239.5
broad	183.3	198.82	233.3	221.0	236.3	239.5
round	183.5	198.82	—	221.0	236.3	239.5
lower segment	182.1	198.82	233.2	219.1	236.0	239.5
myometrium	182.0	198.82	233.2	219.1	236.0	239.5
squamocolumnar junction	180.8	198.82	233.1	219.0	236.0	239.5
tube	183.2	198.82	233.3	221.0	236.3	239.5
utricle, prostatic	189.3	198.1	233.9	223.81	236.99	239.5
uveal tract	190.0	198.4	234.0	224.0	238.8	239.8
uvula	145.4	198.89	230.0	210.4	235.1	239.0
vagina, vaginal (fornix) (vault) (wall)	184.0	198.82	233.3	221.1	236.3	239.5
vaginovesical	184.9	198.82	233.3	221.9	236.3	239.5
septum	194.9	198.82	233.3	221.9	236.3	239.5
vallecula (epiglottis)	146.3	198.89	230.0	210.6	235.1	239.0
vascular-*see* Neoplasm, connective tissue						
vas deferens	187.6	198.82	233.6	222.8	236.6	239.5
Vater's ampulla	156.2	197.8	230.8	211.5	235.3	239.0
vein, venous-*see* Neoplasm, connective tissue						
vena cava (abdominal) (inferior)	171.5	198.89	—	215.5	238.1	239.2
superior	171.4	198.89	—	215.4	238.1	239.2
ventricle (cerebral) (floor) (fourth) (lateral) (third)	191.5	198.3	—	225.0	237.5	239.6
cardiac (left) (right)	164.1	198.89	—	212.7	238.8	239.8
ventricular band of larynx	161.1	197.3	231.0	212.1	235.6	239.1
ventriculus-*see* Neoplasm, stomach						
vermillion border-*see* Neoplasm, lip						
vermis, cerebellum	191.6	198.3	—	225.0	237.5	239.6
vertebra (column)	170.2	198.5	—	213.2	238.0	239.2
coccyx	170.6	198.5	—	213.6	238.0	239.2
sacrum	170.6	198.5	—	213.6	238.0	239.2
vesical-*see* Neoplasm, bladder						

ICD-9-CM

N

Vol.

	Malignant					
	Primary	Secondary	Ca in situ	Benign	Uncertain Behavior	Unspecified
Neoplasm *(Continued)*						
vesicle, seminal	187.8	198.82	233.6	222.8	236.6	239.5
vesicocervical tissue	184.9	198.82	233.3	221.9	236.3	239.5
vesicorectal	195.3	198.89	234.8	229.8	238.8	239.8
vesicovaginal	184.9	198.82	233.3	221.9	236.3	239.5
septum	184.9	198.82	233.3	221.9	236.3	239.5
vessel (blood)-*see* Neoplasm, connective tissue						
vestibular gland, greater	184.1	198.82	233.3	221.2	236.3	239.5
vestibule						
mouth	145.1	198.89	230.0	210.4	235.1	239.0
nose	160.0	197.3	231.8	212.0	235.9	239.1
Virchow's gland	—	196.0	—	229.0	238.8	239.8
viscera NEC	195.8	198.89	234.8	229.8	238.8	239.8
vocal cords (true)	161.0	197.3	231.0	212.1	235.6	239.1
false	161.1	197.3	231.0	212.1	235.6	239.1
vomer	170.0	198.5	—	213.0	238.0	239.2
vulva	184.4	198.82	233.3	221.2	236.3	239.5
vulvovaginal gland	184.4	198.82	233.3	221.2	236.3	239.5
Waldeyer's ring	149.1	198.89	230.0	210.9	235.1	239.0
Wharton's duct	142.1	198.89	230.0	210.2	235.0	239.0
white matter (central) (cerebral)	191.0	198.3	—	225.0	237.5	239.6
windpipe	162.0	197.3	231.1	212.2	235.7	239.1
Wirsung's duct	157.3	197.8	230.9	211.6	235.5	239.0
wolffian (body) (duct)						
female	184.8	198.82	233.3	221.8	236.3	239.5
male	187.8	198.82	233.6	222.8	236.6	239.5
womb-*see* Neoplasm, uterus						
wrist NEC*	195.4	198.89	232.6	229.8	238.8	239.8
xiphoid process	170.3	198.5	—	213.3	238.0	239.2
Zuckerkandl's organ	194.6	198.89	—	227.6	237.3	239.7

◄ New   ◄▦ Revised

Neovascularization
choroid 362.16
ciliary body 364.42
cornea 370.60
deep 370.63
localized 370.61
iris 364.42
retina 362.16
subretinal 362.16
Nephralgia 788.0
Nephritis, nephritic (albuminuric) (azotemic) (congenital) (degenerative) (diffuse) (disseminated) (epithelial) (familial) (focal) (granulomatous) (hemorrhagic) (infantile) (nonsuppurative, excretory) (uremic) 583.9
with
edema - *see* Nephrosis
lesion of
glomerulonephritis
hypocomplementemic persistent 583.2
with nephrotic syndrome 581.2
chronic 582.2
lobular 583.2
with nephrotic syndrome 581.2
chronic 582.2
membranoproliferative 583.2
with nephrotic syndrome 581.2
chronic 582.2
membranous 583.1
with nephrotic syndrome 581.1
chronic 582.1
mesangiocapillary 583.2
with nephrotic syndrome 581.2
chronic 582.2
mixed membranous and proliferative 583.2
with nephrotic syndrome 581.2
chronic 582.2
proliferative (diffuse) 583.0
with nephrotic syndrome 581.0
acute 580.0
chronic 582.0
rapidly progressive 583.4
acute 580.4
chronic 582.4
interstitial nephritis (diffuse) (focal) 583.89
with nephrotic syndrome 581.89
acute 580.89
chronic 582.89
necrotizing glomerulitis 583.4
acute 580.4
chronic 582.4
renal necrosis 583.9
cortical 583.6
medullary 583.7
specified pathology NEC 583.89
with nephrotic syndrome 581.89
acute 580.89
chronic 582.89
necrosis, renal 583.9
cortical 583.6
medullary (papillary) 583.7

Nephritis, nephritic (*Continued*)
with (*Continued*)
nephrotic syndrome (*see also* Nephrosis) 581.9
papillary necrosis 583.7
specified pathology NEC 583.89
acute 580.9
extracapillary with epithelial crescents 580.4
hypertensive (*see also* Hypertension, kidney) 403.90
necrotizing 580.4
poststreptococcal 580.0
proliferative (diffuse) 580.0
rapidly progressive 580.4
specified pathology NEC 580.89
amyloid 277.3 [583.81]
chronic 277.3 [582.81]
arteriolar (*see also* Hypertension, kidney) 403.90
arteriosclerotic (*see also* Hypertension, kidney) 403.90
ascending (*see also* Pyelitis) 590.80
atrophic 582.9
basement membrane NEC 583.89
with pulmonary hemorrhage (Goodpasture's syndrome) 446.21 [583.81]
calculous, calculus 592.0
cardiac (*see also* Hypertension, kidney) 403.90
cardiovascular (*see also* Hypertension, kidney) 403.90
chronic 582.9
arteriosclerotic (*see also* Hypertension, kidney) 403.90
hypertensive (*see also* Hypertension, kidney) 403.90
cirrhotic (*see also* Sclerosis, renal) 587
complicating pregnancy, childbirth, or puerperium 646.2
with hypertension 642.1
affecting fetus or newborn 760.0
affecting fetus or newborn 760.1
croupous 580.9
desquamative - *see* Nephrosis
due to
amyloidosis 277.3 [583.81]
chronic 277.3 [582.81]
arteriosclerosis (*see also* Hypertension, kidney) 403.90
diabetes mellitus 250.4 [583.81]
with nephrotic syndrome 250.4 [581.81]
diphtheria 032.89 [580.81]
gonococcal infection (acute) 098.19 [583.81]
chronic or duration of 2 months or over 098.39 [583.81]
gout 274.10
infectious hepatitis 070.9 [580.81]
mumps 072.79 [580.81]
specified kidney pathology NEC 583.89
acute 580.89
chronic 582.89
streptotrichosis 039.8 [583.81]
subacute bacterial endocarditis 421.0 [580.81]
systemic lupus erythematosus 710.0 [583.81]
chronic 710.0 [582.81]
typhoid fever 002.0 [580.81]
endothelial 582.2

Nephritis, nephritic (*Continued*)
end state (chronic) (terminal) NEC 585
epimembranous 581.1
exudative 583.89
with nephrotic syndrome 581.89
acute 580.89
chronic 582.89
gonococcal (acute) 098.19 [583.81]
chronic or duration of 2 months or over 098.39 [583.81]
gouty 274.10
hereditary (Alport's syndrome) 759.89
hydremic - *see* Nephrosis
hypertensive (*see also* Hypertension, kidney) 403.90
hypocomplementemic persistent 583.2
with nephrotic syndrome 581.2
chronic 582.2
immune complex NEC 583.89
infective (*see also* Pyelitis) 590.80
interstitial (diffuse) (focal) 583.89
with nephrotic syndrome 581.89
acute 580.89
chronic 582.89
latent or quiescent - *see* Nephritis, chronic
lead 984.9
specified type of lead - *see* Table of Drugs and Chemicals
lobular 583.2
with nephrotic syndrome 581.2
chronic 582.2
lupus 710.0 [583.81]
acute 710.0 [580.81]
chronic 710.0 [582.81]
membranoproliferative 583.2
with nephrotic syndrome 581.2
chronic 582.2
membranous 583.1
with nephrotic syndrome 581.1
chronic 582.1
mesangiocapillary 583.2
with nephrotic syndrome 581.2
chronic 582.2
minimal change 581.3
mixed membranous and proliferative 583.2
with nephrotic syndrome 581.2
chronic 582.2
necrotic, necrotizing 583.4
acute 580.4
chronic 582.4
nephrotic - *see* Nephrosis
old - *see* Nephritis, chronic
parenchymatous 581.89
polycystic 753.12
adult type (APKD) 753.13
autosomal dominant 753.13
autosomal recessive 753.14
childhood type (CPKD) 753.14
infantile type 753.14
poststreptococcal 580.0
pregnancy - *see* Nephritis, complicating pregnancy
proliferative 583.0
with nephrotic syndrome 581.0
acute 580.0
chronic 582.0
purulent (*see also* Pyelitis) 590.80
rapidly progressive 583.4
acute 580.4
chronic 582.4
salt-losing or salt-wasting (*see also* Disease, renal) 593.9

ICD-9-CM

N

Vol. 2

Nephritis, nephritic *(Continued)*
  saturnine 584.9
    specified type of lead - *see* Table of Drugs and Chemicals
  septic *(see also* Pyelitis) 590.80
  specified pathology NEC 583.89
    acute 580.89
    chronic 582.89
  staphylococcal *(see also* Pyelitis) 590.80
  streptotrichosis 039.8 *[583.81]*
  subacute *(see also* Nephrosis) 581.9
  suppurative *(see also* Pyelitis) 590.80
  syphilitic (late) 095.4
    congenital 090.5 *[583.81]*
    early 091.69 *[583.81]*
  terminal (chronic) (end-stage) NEC 585
  toxic - *see* Nephritis, acute
  tubal, tubular - *see* Nephrosis, tubular
  tuberculous *(see also* Tuberculosis) 016.0 *[583.81]*
  type II (Ellis) - *see* Nephrosis
  vascular - *see also* Hypertension, kidney
  war 580.9
Nephroblastoma (M8960/3) 189.0
  epithelial (M8961/3) 189.0
  mesenchymal (M8962/3) 189.0
Nephrocalcinosis 275.49
Nephrocystitis, pustular *(see also* Pyelitis) 590.80
Nephrolithiasis (congenital) (pelvis) (recurrent) 592.0
  uric acid 274.11
Nephroma (M8960/3) 189.0
  mesoblastic (M8960/1) 236.9
Nephronephritis *(see also* Nephrosis) 581.9
Nephronopthisis 753.16
Nephropathy *(see also* Nephritis) 583.9
  with
    exudative nephritis 583.89
    interstitial nephritis (diffuse) (focal) 583.89
    medullary necrosis 583.7
    necrosis 583.9
      cortical 583.6
      medullary or papillary 583.7
    papillary necrosis 583.7
    specified lesion or cause NEC 583.89
  analgesic 583.89
    with medullary necrosis, acute 584.7
  arteriolar *(see also* Hypertension, kidney) 403.90
  arteriosclerotic *(see also* Hypertension, kidney) 403.90
  complicating pregnancy 646.2
  diabetic 250.4 *[583.81]*
  gouty 274.10
    specified type NEC 274.19
  hypercalcemic 588.89   ◀▥
  hypertensive *(see also* Hypertension, kidney) 403.90
  hypokalemic (vacuolar) 588.89   ◀▥
  IgA 583.9   ◀
  obstructive 593.89
    congenital 753.20
  phenacetin 584.7
  phosphate-losing 588.0
  potassium depletion 588.89   ◀▥
  proliferative *(see also* Nephritis, proliferative) 583.0
  protein-losing 588.89   ◀▥
  salt-losing or salt-wasting *(see also* Disease, renal) 593.9
  sickle-cell *(see also* Disease, sickle-cell) 282.60 *[583.81]*

Nephropathy *(Continued)*
  toxic 584.5
  vasomotor 584.5
  water-losing 588.89   ◀▥
Nephroptosis *(see also* Disease, renal) 593.0
  congenital (displaced) 753.3
Nephropyosis *(see also* Abscess, kidney) 590.2
Nephrorrhagia 593.81
Nephrosclerosis (arteriolar) (arteriosclerotic) (chronic) (hyaline) *(see also* Hypertension, kidney) 403.90
  gouty 274.10
  hyperplastic (arteriolar) *(see also* Hypertension, kidney) 403.90
  senile *(see also* Sclerosis, renal) 587
Nephrosis, nephrotic (Epstein's) (syndrome) 581.9
  with
    lesion of
      focal glomerulosclerosis 581.1
      glomerulonephritis
        endothelial 581.2
        hypocomplementemic persistent 581.2
        lobular 581.2
        membranoproliferative 581.2
        membranous 581.1
        mesangiocapillary 581.2
        minimal change 581.3
        mixed membranous and proliferative 581.2
        proliferative 581.0
      segmental hyalinosis 581.1
      specified pathology NEC 581.89
  acute - *see* Nephrosis, tubular
  anoxic - *see* Nephrosis, tubular
  arteriosclerotic *(see also* Hypertension, kidney) 403.90
  chemical - *see* Nephrosis, tubular
  cholemic 572.4
  complicating pregnancy, childbirth, or puerperium - *see* Nephritis, complicating pregnancy
  diabetic 250.4 *[581.81]*
  hemoglobinuric - *see* Nephrosis, tubular
  in
    amyloidosis 277.3 *[581.81]*
    diabetes mellitus 250.4 *[581.81]*
    epidemic hemorrhagic fever 078.6
    malaria 084.9 *[581.81]*
    polyarteritis 446.0 *[581.81]*
    systemic lupus erythematosus 710.0 *[581.81]*
  ischemic - *see* Nephrosis, tubular
  lipoid 581.3
  lower nephron - *see* Nephrosis, tubular
  lupoid 710.0 *[581.81]*
  lupus 710.0 *[581.81]*
  malarial 084.9 *[581.81]*
  minimal change 581.3
  necrotizing - *see* Nephrosis, tubular
  osmotic (sucrose) 588.89   ◀▥
  polyarteritic 446.0 *[581.81]*
  radiation 581.9
  specified lesion or cause NEC 581.89
  syphilitic 095.4
  toxic - *see* Nephrosis, tubular
  tubular (acute) 584.5

Nephrosis, nephrotic *(Continued)*
  tubular *(Continued)*
    due to a procedure 997.5
    radiation 581.9
Nephrosonephritis hemorrhagic (endemic) 078.6
Nephrostomy status V44.6
  with complication 997.5
Nerve - *see* condition
Nerves 799.2
Nervous *(see also* condition) 799.2
  breakdown 300.9
  heart 306.2
  stomach 306.4
  tension 799.2
Nervousness 799.2
Nesidioblastoma (M8150/0)
  pancreas 211.7
  specified site NEC - *see* Neoplasm, by site, benign
  unspecified site 211.7
Netherton's syndrome (ichthyosiform erythroderma) 757.1
Nettle rash 708.8
Nettleship's disease (urticaria pigmentosa) 757.33
Neumann's disease (pemphigus vegetans) 694.4
Neuralgia, neuralgic (acute) *(see also* Neuritis) 729.2
  accessory (nerve) 352.4
  acoustic (nerve) 388.5
  ankle 355.8
  anterior crural 355.8
  anus 787.99
  arm 723.4
  auditory (nerve) 388.5
  axilla 353.0
  bladder 788.1
  brachial 723.4
  brain - *see* Disorder, nerve, cranial
  broad ligament 625.9
  cerebral - *see* Disorder, nerve, cranial
  ciliary 346.2
  cranial nerve - *see also* Disorder, nerve, cranial
    fifth or trigeminal *(see also* Neuralgia, trigeminal) 350.1
  ear 388.71
    middle 352.1
  facial 351.8
  finger 354.9
  flank 355.8
  foot 355.8
  forearm 354.9
  Fothergill's *(see also* Neuralgia, trigeminal) 350.1
    postherpetic 053.12
  glossopharyngeal (nerve) 352.1
  groin 355.8
  hand 354.9
  heel 355.8
  Horton's 346.2
  Hunt's 053.11
  hypoglossal (nerve) 352.5
  iliac region 355.8
  infraorbital *(see also* Neuralgia, trigeminal) 350.1
  inguinal 355.8
  intercostal (nerve) 353.8
    postherpetic 053.19
  jaw 352.1
  kidney 788.0
  knee 355.8

Neuralgia, neuralgic (*Continued*)
  loin 355.8
  malarial (*see also* Malaria) 084.6
  mastoid 385.89
  maxilla 352.1
  median thenar 354.1
  metatarsal 355.6
  middle ear 352.1
  migrainous 346.2
  Morton's 355.6
  nerve, cranial - *see* Disorder, nerve,
    cranial
  nose 352.0
  occipital 723.8
  olfactory (nerve) 352.0
  ophthalmic 377.30
    postherpetic 053.19
  optic (nerve) 377.30
  penis 607.9
  perineum 355.8
  pleura 511.0
  postherpetic NEC 053.19
    geniculate ganglion 053.11
    ophthalmic 053.19
    trifacial 053.12
    trigeminal 053.12
  pubic region 355.8
  radial (nerve) 723.4
  rectum 787.99
  sacroiliac joint 724.3
  sciatic (nerve) 724.3
  scrotum 608.9
  seminal vesicle 608.9
  shoulder 354.9
  sluder's 337.0
  specified nerve NEC - *see* Disorder,
    nerve
  spermatic cord 608.9
  sphenopalatine (ganglion) 337.0
  subscapular (nerve) 723.4
  suprascapular (nerve) 723.4
  testis 608.89
  thenar (median) 354.1
  thigh 355.8
  tongue 352.5
  trifacial (nerve) (*see also* Neuralgia, tri-
    geminal) 350.1
  trigeminal (nerve) 350.1
    postherpetic 053.12
  tympanic plexus 388.71
  ulnar (nerve) 723.4
  vagus (nerve) 352.3
  wrist 354.9
  writers' 300.89
    organic 333.84
Neurapraxia - *see* Injury, nerve, by site
Neurasthenia 300.5
  cardiac 306.2
  gastric 306.4
  heart 306.2
  postfebrile 780.79
  postviral 780.79
Neurilemmoma (M9560/0) - *see also* Ne-
    oplasm, connective tissue, benign
  acoustic (nerve) 225.1
  malignant (M9560/3) - *see also* Neo-
    plasm, connective tissue, malignant
    acoustic (nerve) 192.0
Neurilemmosarcoma (M9560/3) - *see*
    Neoplasm, connective tissue, malig-
    nant
Neurilemoma - *see* Neurilemmoma
Neurinoma (M9560/0) - *see* Neurilem-
    moma

Neurinomatosis (M9560/1) - *see also* Ne-
    oplasm, connective tissue, uncertain
    behavior
  centralis 759.5
Neuritis (*see also* Neuralgia) 729.2
  abducens (nerve) 378.54
  accessory (nerve) 352.4
  acoustic (nerve) 388.5
    syphilitic 094.86
  alcoholic 357.5
    with psychosis 291.1
  amyloid, any site 277.3 [357.4]
  anterior crural 355.8
  arising during pregnancy 646.4
  arm 723.4
  ascending 355.2
  auditory (nerve) 388.5
  brachial (nerve) NEC 723.4
    due to displacement, intervertebral
      disc 722.0
  cervical 723.4
  chest (wall) 353.8
  costal region 353.8
  cranial nerve - *see also* Disorder, nerve,
    cranial
    first or olfactory 352.0
    second or optic 377.30
    third or oculomotor 378.52
    fourth or trochlear 378.53
    fifth or trigeminal (*see also* Neural-
      gia, trigeminal) 350.1
    sixth or abducens 378.54
    seventh or facial 351.8
      newborn 767.5
    eighth or acoustic 388.5
    ninth or glossopharyngeal 352.1
    tenth or vagus 352.3
    eleventh or accessory 352.4
    twelfth or hypoglossal 352.5
  Déjérine-Sottas 356.0
  diabetic 250.6 [357.2]
  diphtheritic 032.89 [357.4]
  due to
    beriberi 265.0 [357.4]
    displacement, prolapse, protrusion,
      or rupture of intervertebral disc
      722.2
      cervical 722.0
      lumbar, lumbosacral 722.10
      thoracic, thoracolumbar 722.11
    herniation, nucleus pulposus 722.2
      cervical 722.0
      lumbar, lumbosacral 722.10
      thoracic, thoracolumbar 722.11
  endemic 265.0 [357.4]
  facial (nerve) 351.8
    newborn 767.5
  general - *see* Polyneuropathy
  geniculate ganglion 351.1
    due to herpes 053.11
  glossopharyngeal (nerve) 352.1
  gouty 274.89 [357.4]
  hypoglossal (nerve) 352.5
  ilioinguinal (nerve) 355.8
  in diseases classified elsewhere - *see*
    Polyneuropathy, in
  infectious (multiple) 357.0
  intercostal (nerve) 353.8
  interstitial hypertrophic progressive
    NEC 356.9
  leg 355.8
  lumbosacral NEC 724.4
  median (nerve) 354.1
    thenar 354.1

Neuritis (*Continued*)
  multiple (acute) (infective) 356.9
    endemic 265.0 [357.4]
  multiplex endemica 265.0 [357.4]
  nerve root (*see also* Radiculitis) 729.2
  oculomotor (nerve) 378.52
  olfactory (nerve) 352.0
  optic (nerve) 377.30
    in myelitis 341.0
    meningococcal 036.81
  pelvic 355.8
  peripheral (nerve) - *see also* Neuropa-
    thy, peripheral
    complicating pregnancy or puerpe-
      rium 646.4
    specified nerve NEC - *see* Mononeu-
      ritis
  pneumogastric (nerve) 352.3
  postchickenpox 052.7
  postherpetic 053.19
  progressive hypertrophic interstitial
    NEC 356.9
  puerperal, postpartum 646.4
  radial (nerve) 723.4
  retrobulbar 377.32
    syphilitic 094.85
  rheumatic (chronic) 729.2
  sacral region 355.8
  sciatic (nerve) 724.3
    due to displacement of intervertebral
      disc 722.10
  serum 999.5
  specified nerve NEC - *see* Disorder,
    nerve
  spinal (nerve) 355.9
    root (*see also* Radiculitis) 729.2
  subscapular (nerve) 723.4
  suprascapular (nerve) 723.4
  syphilitic 095.8
  thenar (median) 354.1
  thoracic NEC 724.4
  toxic NEC 357.7
  trochlear (nerve) 378.53
  ulnar (nerve) 723.4
  vagus (nerve) 352.3
Neuroangiomatosis, encephalofacial
    759.6
Neuroastrocytoma (M9505/1) - *see* Neo-
    plasm, by site, uncertain behavior
Neuro-avitaminosis 269.2
Neuroblastoma (M9500/3)
  olfactory (M9522/3) 160.0
  specified site - *see* Neoplasm, by site,
    malignant
  unspecified site 194.0
Neurochorioretinitis (*see also* Chorioreti-
    nitis) 363.20
Neurocirculatory asthenia 306.2
Neurocytoma (M9506/0) - *see* Neoplasm,
    by site, benign
Neurodermatitis (circumscribed) (cir-
    cumscripta) (local) 698.3
  atopic 691.8
  diffuse (Brocq) 691.8
  disseminated 691.8
  nodulosa 698.3
Neuroencephalomyelopathy, optic 341.0
Neuroepithelioma (M9503/3) - *see also*
    Neoplasm, by site, malignant
  olfactory (M9521/3) 160.0
Neurofibroma (M9540/0) - *see also* Neo-
    plasm, connective tissue, benign
  melanotic (M9541/0) - *see* Neoplasm,
    connective tissue, benign

ICD-9-CM

Vol. 2

Neurofibroma *(Continued)*
  multiple (M9540/1) 237.70
    type 1 237.71
    type 2 237.72
  plexiform (M9550/0) - *see* Neoplasm,
    connective tissue, benign
Neurofibromatosis (multiple) (M9540/1)
  237.70
  acoustic 237.72
  malignant (M9540/3) - *see* Neoplasm,
    connective tissue, malignant
  type 1 237.71
  type 2 237.72
  von Recklinghausen's 237.71
Neurofibrosarcoma (M9540/3) - *see* Neoplasm, connective tissue, malignant
Neurogenic - *see also* condition
  bladder (atonic) (automatic) (auto-
    nomic) (flaccid) (hypertonic) (hy-
    potonic) (inertia) (infranuclear) (ir-
    ritable) (motor) (nonreflex)
    (nuclear) (paralysis) (reflex) (sen-
    sory) (spastic) (supranuclear) (un-
    inhibited) 596.54
    with cauda equina syndrome 344.61
  bowel 564.81
  heart 306.2
Neuroglioma (M9505/1) - *see* Neoplasm,
  by site, uncertain behavior
Neurolabyrinthitis (of Dix and Hallpike)
  386.12
Neurolathyrism 988.2
Neuroleprosy 030.1
Neuroleptic malignant syndrome 333.92
Neurolipomatosis 272.8
Neuroma (M9570/0) - *see also* Neoplasm,
  connective tissue, benign
  acoustic (nerve) (M9560/0) 225.1
  amputation (traumatic) - *see also* In-
    jury, nerve, by site
    surgical complication (late) 997.61
  appendix 211.3
  auditory nerve 225.1
  digital 355.6
    toe 355.6
  interdigital (toe) 355.6
  intermetatarsal 355.6
  Morton's 355.6
  multiple 237.70
    type 1 237.71
    type 2 237.72
  nonneoplastic 355.9
    arm NEC 354.9
    leg NEC 355.8
    lower extremity NEC 355.8
    specified site NEC - *see* Mononeuri-
      tis, by site
    upper extremity NEC 354.9
  optic (nerve) 225.1
  plantar 355.6
  plexiform (M9550/0) - *see* Neoplasm,
    connective tissue, benign
  surgical (nonneoplastic) 355.9
    arm NEC 354.9
    leg NEC 355.8
    lower extremity NEC 355.8
    upper extremity NEC 354.9
  traumatic - *see also* Injury, nerve, by site
    old-see Neuroma, nonneoplastic
Neuromyalgia 729.1
Neuromyasthenia (epidemic) 049.8
Neuromyelitis 341.8
  ascending 357.0
  optica 341.0
Neuromyopathy NEC 358.9

Neuromyositis 729.1
Neuronevus (M8725/0) - *see* Neoplasm,
  skin, benign
Neuronitis 357.0
  ascending (acute) 355.2
  vestibular 386.12
Neuroparalytic - *see* condition
Neuropathy, neuropathic (*see also* Disorder, nerve) 355.9
  acute motor 357.82
  alcoholic 357.5
    with psychosis 291.1
  arm NEC 354.9
  ataxia and retinitis pigmentosa (NARP
    syndrome) 277.87 ◀
  autonomic (peripheral) - *see* Neuropa-
    thy, peripheral, autonomic
  axillary nerve 353.0
  brachial plexus 353.0
  cervical plexus 353.2
  chronic
    progressive segmentally demyelinat-
      ing 357.89
    relapsing demyelinating 357.89
  congenital sensory 356.2
  Déjérine-Sottas 356.0
  diabetic 250.6 *[357.2]*
  entrapment 355.9
    iliohypogastric nerve 355.79
    ilioinguinal nerve 355.79
    lateral cutaneous nerve of thigh
      355.1
    median nerve 354.0
    obturator nerve 355.79
    peroneal nerve 355.3
    posterior tibial nerve 355.5
    saphenous nerve 355.79
    ulnar nerve 354.2
  facial nerve 351.9
  hereditary 356.9
    peripheral 356.0
    sensory (radicular) 356.2
  hypertrophic
    Charcôt-Marie-Tooth 356.1
    Déjérine-Sottas 356.0
    interstitial 356.9
    Refsum 356.3
  intercostal nerve 354.8
  ischemic - *see* Disorder, nerve
  Jamaican (ginger) 357.7
  leg NEC 355.8
  lower extremity NEC 355.8
  lumbar plexus 353.1
  median nerve 354.1
  motor
    acute 357.82
  multiple (acute) (chronic) (*see also*
    Polyneuropathy) 356.9
  optic 377.39
    ischemic 377.41
    nutritional 377.33
    toxic 377.34
  peripheral (nerve) (*see also* Polyneurop-
    athy) 356.9
    arm NEC 354.9
    autonomic 337.9
      amyloid 277.3 *[337.1]*
      idiopathic 337.0
      in
        amyloidosis 277.3 *[337.1]*
        diabetes (mellitus) 250.6 *[337.1]*
        diseases classified elsewhere
          337.1
        gout 274.89 *[337.1]*
        hyperthyroidism 242.9 *[337.1]*

Neuropathy, neuropathic *(Continued)*
  peripheral *(Continued)*
    due to
      antitetanus serum 357.6
      arsenic 357.7
      drugs 357.6
      lead 357.7
      organophosphate compounds
        357.7
      toxic agent NEC 357.7
    hereditary 356.0
    idiopathic 356.9
      progressive 356.4
      specified type NEC 356.8
    in diseases classified elsewhere - *see*
      Polyneuropathy, in
    leg NEC 355.8
    lower extremity NEC 355.8
    upper extremity NEC 354.9
  plantar nerves 355.6
  progressive hypertrophic interstitial
    356.9
  radicular NEC 729.2
    brachial 723.4
    cervical NEC 723.4
    hereditary sensory 356.2
    lumbar 724.4
    lumbosacral 724.4
    thoracic NEC 724.4
  sacral plexus 353.1
  sciatic 355.0
  spinal nerve NEC 355.9
    root (*see also* Radiculitis) 729.2
  toxic 357.7
  trigeminal sensory 350.8
  ulnar nerve 354.2
  upper extremity NEC 354.9
  uremic 585 *[357.4]*
  vitamin B$_{12}$ 266.2 *[357.4]*
    with anemia (pernicious) 281.0 *[357.4]*
      due to dietary deficiency 281.1
        [357.4]
Neurophthisis - *see also* Disorder, nerve
  peripheral 356.9
  diabetic 250.6 *[357.2]*
Neuropraxia - *see* Injury, nerve
Neuroretinitis 363.05
  syphilitic 094.85
Neurosarcoma (M9540/3) - *see* Neoplasm, connective tissue, malignant
Neurosclerosis - *see* Disorder, nerve
Neurosis, neurotic 300.9
  accident 300.16
  anancastic, anankastic 300.3
  anxiety (state) 300.00
    generalized 300.02
    panic type 300.01
  asthenic 300.5
  bladder 306.53
  cardiac (reflex) 306.2
  cardiovascular 306.2
  climacteric, unspecified type 627.2
  colon 306.4
  compensation 300.16
  compulsive, compulsion 300.3
  conversion 300.11
  craft 300.89
  cutaneous 306.3
  depersonalization 300.6
  depressive (reaction) (type) 300.4
  endocrine 306.6
  environmental 300.89
  fatigue 300.5
  functional (*see also* Disorder, psychoso-
    matic) 306.9

◀ **New**   ⬅️ **Revised**

Neurosis, neurotic (Continued)
gastric 306.4
gastrointestinal 306.4
genitourinary 306.50
heart 306.2
hypochondriacal 300.7
hysterical 300.10
conversion type 300.11
dissociative type 300.15
impulsive 300.3
incoordination 306.0
larynx 306.1
vocal cord 306.1
intestine 306.4
larynx 306.1
hysterical 300.11
sensory 306.1
menopause, unspecified type 627.2
mixed NEC 300.89
musculoskeletal 306.0
obsessional 300.3
phobia 300.3
obsessive-compulsive 300.3
occupational 300.89
ocular 306.7
oral 307.0
organ (see also Disorder, psychosomatic) 306.9
pharynx 306.1
phobic 300.20
posttraumatic (acute) (situational) 309.81 ◄▥▥
chronic 309.81
psychasthenic (type) 300.89
railroad 300.16
rectum 306.4
respiratory 306.1
rumination 306.4
senile 300.89
sexual 302.70
situational 300.89
specified type NEC 300.89
state 300.9
with depersonalization episode 300.6
stomach 306.4
vasomotor 306.2
visceral 306.4
war 300.16
Neurospongioblastosis diffusa 759.5
Neurosyphilis (arrested) (early) (inactive) (late) (latent) (recurrent) 094.9
with ataxia (cerebellar) (locomotor) (spastic) (spinal) 094.0
acute meningitis 094.2
aneurysm 094.89
arachnoid (adhesive) 094.2
arteritis (any artery) 094.89
asymptomatic 094.3
congenital 090.40
dura (mater) 094.89
general paresis 094.1
gumma 094.9
hemorrhagic 094.9
juvenile (asymptomatic) (meningeal) 090.40
leptomeninges (aseptic) 094.2
meningeal 094.2
meninges (adhesive) 094.2
meningovascular (diffuse) 094.2
optic atrophy 094.84
parenchymatous (degenerative) 094.1
paresis (see also Paresis, general) 094.1

Neurosyphilis (Continued)
paretic (see also Paresis, general) 094.1
relapse 094.9
remission in (sustained) 094.9
serological 094.3
specified nature or site NEC 094.89
tabes (dorsalis) 094.0
juvenile 090.40
tabetic 094.0
juvenile 090.40
taboparesis 094.1
juvenile 090.40
thrombosis 094.89
vascular 094.89
Neurotic (see also Neurosis) 300.9
excoriation 698.4
psychogenic 306.3
Neurotmesis - see Injury, nerve, by site
Neurotoxemia - see Toxemia
Neuroclusion 524.2
Neutro-occlusion 524.21 ◄
Neutropenia, neutropenic (chronic) (cyclic) (drug-induced) (genetic) (idiopathic) (immune) (infantile) (malignant) (periodic) (pernicious) (primary) (splenic) (splenomegaly) (toxic) 288.0
chronic hypoplastic 288.0
congenital (nontransient) 288.0
fever 288.0
neonatal, transitory (isoimmune) (maternal transfer) 776.7
Neutrophilia, hereditary giant 288.2
Nevocarcinoma (M8720/3) - see Melanoma
Nevus (M8720/0) - see also Neoplasm, skin, benign

> Note   Except where otherwise indicated, varieties of nevus in the list below that are followed by a morphology code number (M-/0) should be coded by site as for "Neoplasm, skin, benign."

acanthotic 702.8
achromic (M8730/0)
amelanotic (M8730/0)
anemic, anemicus 709.09
angiomatous (M9120/0) (see also Hemangioma) 228.00
araneus 448.1
avasculosus 709.09
balloon cell (M8722/0)
bathing trunk (M8761/1) 238.2
blue (M8780/0)
cellular (M8790/0)
giant (M8790/0)
Jadassohn's (M8780/0)
malignant (M8780/3) - see Melanoma
capillary (M9131/0) (see also Hemangioma) 228.00
cavernous (M9121/0) (see also Hemangioma) 228.00
cellular (M8720/0)
blue (M8790/0)
comedonicus 757.33
compound (M8760/0)
conjunctiva (M8720/0) 224.3
dermal (8750/0)
and epidermal (M8760/0)
epithelioid cell (and spindle cell) (M8770/0)

Nevus (Continued)
flammeus 757.32
osteohypertrophic 759.89
hairy (M8720/0)
halo (M8723/0)
hemangiomatous (M9120/0) (see also Hemangioma) 228.00
intradermal (M8750/0)
intraepidermal (M8740/0)
involuting (M8724/0)
Jadassohn's (blue) (M8780/0)
junction, junctional (M8740/0)
malignant melanoma in (M8740/3) - see Melanoma
juvenile (M8770/0)
lymphatic (M9170/0) 228.1
magnocellular (M8726/0)
specified site - see Neoplasm, by site, benign
unspecified site 224.0
malignant (M8720/3) - see Melanoma
meaning hemangioma (M9120/0) (see also Hemangioma) 228.00
melanotic (pigmented) (M8720/0)
multiplex 759.5
nonneoplastic 448.1
nonpigmented (M8730/0)
nonvascular (M8720/0)
oral mucosa, white sponge 750.26
osteohypertrophic, flammeus 759.89
papillaris (M8720/0)
papillomatosus (M8720/0)
pigmented (M8720/0)
giant (M8761/1) - see also Neoplasm, skin, uncertain behavior
malignant melanoma in (M8761/3) - see Melanoma
systematicus 757.33
pilosus (M8720/0)
port wine 757.32
sanguineous 757.32
sebaceous (senile) 702.8
senile 448.1
spider 448.1
spindle cell (and epithelioid cell) (M8770/0)
stellar 448.1
strawberry 757.32
syringocystadenomatous papilliferous (M8406/0)
unius lateris 757.33
Unna's 757.32
vascular 757.32
verrucous 757.33
white sponge (oral mucosa) 750.26
Newborn (infant) (liveborn)
affected by maternal abuse of drugs (gestational) (via placenta) (via breast milk) 760.70
gestation
24 completed weeks 765.22
25–26 completed weeks 765.23
27–28 completed weeks 765.24
29–30 completed weeks 765.25
31–32 completed weeks 765.26
33–34 completed weeks 765.27
35–36 completed weeks 765.28
37 or more completed weeks 765.29
less than 24 completed weeks 765.21
unspecified completed weeks 765.20
multiple NEC
born in hospital (without mention of cesarean delivery or section) V37.00

ICD-9-CM

N

Vol. 2

Newborn *(Continued)*
  multiple NEC *(Continued)*
    born in hospital *(Continued)*
      with cesarean delivery or section V37.01
    born outside hospital
      hospitalized V37.1
      not hospitalized V37.2
    mates all liveborn
      born in hospital (without mention of cesarean delivery or section) V34.00
        with cesarean delivery or section V34.01
      born outside hospital
        hospitalized V34.1
        not hospitalized V34.2
    mates all stillborn
      born in hospital (without mention of cesarean delivery or section) V35.00
        with cesarean delivery or section V35.01
      born outside hospital
        hospitalized V35.1
        not hospitalized V35.2
    mates liveborn and stillborn
      born in hospital (without mention of cesarean delivery or section) V36.00
        with cesarean delivery or section V36.01
      born outside hospital
        hospitalized V36.1
        not hospitalized V36.2
  single
    born in hospital (without mention of cesarean delivery or section) V30.00
      with cesarean delivery or section V30.01
    born outside hospital
      hospitalized V30.1
      not hospitalized V30.2
  twin NEC
    born in hospital (without mention of cesarean delivery or section) V33.00
      with cesarean delivery or section V33.01
    born outside hospital
      hospitalized V33.1
      not hospitalized V33.2
    mate liveborn
      born in hospital V31.0
      born outside hospital
        hospitalized V31.1
        not hospitalized V31.2
    mate stillborn
      born in hospital V32.0
      born outside hospital
        hospitalized V32.1
        not hospitalized V32.2
  unspecified as to single or multiple birth
    born in hospital (without mention of cesarean delivery or section) V39.00
      with cesarean delivery or section V39.01
    born outside hospital
      hospitalized V39.1
      not hospitalized V39.2
Newcastle's conjunctivitis or disease 077.8

Nezelof's syndrome (pure alymphocytosis) 279.13
Niacin (amide) deficiency 265.2
Nicolas-Durand-Favre disease (climatic bubo) 099.1
Nicolas-Favre disease (climatic bubo) 099.1
Nicotinic acid (amide) deficiency 265.2
Niemann-Pick disease (lipid histiocytosis) (splenomegaly) 272.7
Night
  blindness (*see also* Blindness, night) 368.60
    congenital 368.61
    vitamin A deficiency 264.5
  cramps 729.82
  sweats 780.8
  terrors, child 307.46
Nightmare 307.47
  REM-sleep type 307.47
Nipple - *see* condition
Nisbet's chancre 099.0
Nishimoto (-Takeuchi) disease 437.5
Nitritoid crisis or reaction - *see* Crisis, nitritoid
Nitrogen retention, extrarenal 788.9
Nitrosohemoglobinemia 289.89
Njovera 104.0
No
  diagnosis 799.9
  disease (found) V71.9
  room at the inn V65.0
Nocardiasis - *see* Nocardiosis
Nocardiosis 039.9
  with pneumonia 039.1
  lung 039.1
  specified type NEC 039.8
Nocturia 788.43
  psychogenic 306.53
Nocturnal - *see also* condition
  dyspnea (paroxysmal) 786.09
  emissions 608.89
  enuresis 788.36
    psychogenic 307.6
  frequency (micturition) 788.43
    psychogenic 306.53
Nodal rhythm disorder 427.89
Nodding of head 781.0
Node(s) - *see also* Nodules
  Heberden's 715.04
  larynx 478.79
  lymph - *see* condition
  milkers' 051.1
  Osler's 421.0
  rheumatic 729.89
  Schmorl's 722.30
    lumbar, lumbosacral 722.32
    specified region NEC 722.39
    thoracic, thoracolumbar 722.31
  singers' 478.5
  skin NEC 782.2
  tuberculous - *see* Tuberculosis, lymph gland
  vocal cords 478.5
Nodosities, Haygarth's 715.04
Nodule(s), nodular
  actinomycotic (*see also* Actinomycosis) 039.9
  arthritic - *see* Arthritis, nodosa
  cutaneous 782.2
  Haygarth's 715.04
  inflammatory - *see* Inflammation
  juxta-articular 102.7
    syphilitic 095.7
    yaws 102.7

Nodule(s) *(Continued)*
  larynx 478.79
  lung, solitary 518.89
    emphysematous 492.8
  milkers' 051.1
  prostate 600.10
    with urinary retention 600.11
  rheumatic 729.89
  rheumatoid - *see* Arthritis rheumatoid
  scrotum (inflammatory) 608.4
  singers' 478.5
  skin NEC 782.2
  solitary, lung 518.89
    emphysematous 492.8
  subcutaneous 782.2
  thyroid (gland) (nontoxic) (uninodular) 241.0
    with
      hyperthyroidism 242.1
      thyrotoxicosis 242.1
    toxic or with hyperthyroidism 242.1
  vocal cords 478.5
Noma (gangrenous) (hospital) (infective) 528.1
  auricle (*see also* Gangrene) 785.4
  mouth 528.1
  pudendi (*see also* Vulvitis) 616.10
  vulvae (*see also* Vulvitis) 616.10
Nomadism V60.0
Non-adherence
  artificial skin graft 996.55
  decellularized allodermis graft 996.55
Non-autoimmune hemolytic anemia NEC 283.10
Nonclosure - *see also* Imperfect, closure
  ductus
    arteriosus 747.0
    Botalli 747.0
  Eustachian valve 746.89
  foramen
    Botalli 745.5
    ovale 745.5
Noncompliance with medical treatment V15.81
Nondescent (congenital) - *see also* Malposition, congenital
  cecum 751.4
  colon 751.4
  testis 752.51
Nondevelopment
  brain 742.1
    specified part 742.2
  heart 746.89
  organ or site, congenital NEC - *see* Hypoplasia
Nonengagement
  head NEC 652.5
    in labor 660.1
      affecting fetus or newborn 763.1
Nonexanthematous tick fever 066.1
Nonexpansion, lung (newborn) NEC 770.4
Nonfunctioning
  cystic duct (*see also* Disease, gallbladder) 575.8
  gallbladder (*see also* Disease, gallbladder) 575.8
  kidney (*see also* Disease, renal) 593.9
  labyrinth 386.58
Nonhealing
  stump (surgical) 997.69
  wound, surgical 998.83
Nonimplantation of ovum, causing infertility 628.3
Noninsufflation, fallopian tube 628.2

◀ **New**　　　◀▪▪ **Revised**

Nonne-Milroy-Meige syndrome (chronic hereditary edema) 757.0
Nonovulation 628.0
Nonpatent fallopian tube 628.2
Nonpneumatization, lung NEC 770.4
Nonreflex bladder 596.54
  with cauda equina 344.61
Nonretention of food - *see* Vomiting
Nonrotation - *see* Malrotation
Nonsecretion, urine (*see also* Anuria) 788.5
  newborn 753.3
Nonunion
  fracture 733.82
  organ or site, congenital NEC - *see* Imperfect, closure
  symphysis pubis, congenital 755.69
  top sacrum, congenital 756.19
Nonviability 765.0
Nonvisualization, gallbladder 793.3
Nonvitalized tooth 522.9
Non-working side interference 524.56 ◀
Normal
  delivery - *see* category 650
  menses V65.5
  state (feared complaint unfounded) V65.5
Normoblastosis 289.89
Normocytic anemia (infectional) 285.9
  due to blood loss (chronic) 280.0
    acute 285.1
Norrie's disease (congenital) (progressive oculoacousticocerebral degeneration) 743.8
North American blastomycosis 116.0
Norwegian itch 133.0
Nose, nasal - *see* condition
Nosebleed 784.7

Nosomania 298.9
Nosophobia 300.29
Nostalgia 309.89
Notch of iris 743.46
Notched lip, congenital (*see also* Cleft, lip) 749.10
Notching nose, congenital (tip) 748.1
Nothnagel's
  syndrome 378.52
  vasomotor acroparesthesia 443.89
Novy's relapsing fever (American) 087.1
Noxious
  foodstuffs, poisoning by
    fish 988.0
    fungi 988.1
    mushrooms 988.1
    plants (food) 988.2
    shellfish 988.0
    specified type NEC 988.8
    toadstool 988.1
  substances transmitted through placenta or breast milk (affecting fetus or newborn) 760.70 ◀━
    alcohol 760.71
    anti-infective agents 760.74
    cocaine 760.75
    "crack" 760.75
    diethylstilbestrol (DES) 760.76
    hallucinogenic agents NEC 760.73
    medicinal agents NEC 760.79
    narcotics 760.72
    obstetric anesthetic or analgesic 763.5
    specified agent NEC 760.79
    suspected, affecting management of pregnancy 655.5
Nuchal hitch (arm) 652.8

Nucleus pulposus - *see* condition
Numbness 782.0
Nuns' knee 727.2
Nursemaid's
  elbow 832.0
  shoulder 831.0
Nutmeg liver 573.8
Nutrition, deficient or insufficient (particular kind of food) 269.9
  due to
    insufficient food 994.2
    lack of
      care (child) (infant) 995.52
        adult 995.84
      food 994.2
Nyctalopia (*see also* Blindness, night) 368.60
  vitamin A deficiency 264.5
Nycturia 788.43
  psychogenic 306.53
Nymphomania 302.89
Nystagmus 379.50
  associated with vestibular system disorders 379.54
  benign paroxysmal positional 386.11
  central positional 386.2
  congenital 379.51
  deprivation 379.53
  dissociated 379.55
  latent 379.52
  miners' 300.89
  positional
    benign paroxysmal 386.11
    central 386.2
  specified NEC 379.56
  vestibular 379.54
  visual deprivation 379.53

ICD-9-CM

N

Vol. 2

O

Oasthouse urine disease 270.2
Obermeyer's relapsing fever (European) 087.0
Obesity (constitutional) (exogenous) (familial) (nutritional) (simple) 278.00
  adrenal 255.8
  due to hyperalimentation 278.00
  endocrine NEC 259.9
  endogenous 259.9
  Fröhlich's (adiposogenital dystrophy) 253.8
  glandular NEC 259.9
  hypothyroid (see also Hypothyroidism) 244.9
  morbid 278.01
  of pregnancy 646.1
  pituitary 253.8
  severe 278.01
  thyroid (see also Hypothyroidism) 244.9
Oblique - see also condition
  lie before labor, affecting fetus or newborn 761.7
Obliquity, pelvis 738.6
Obliteration
  abdominal aorta 446.7
  appendix (lumen) 543.9
  artery 447.1
  ascending aorta 446.7
  bile ducts 576.8
    with calculus, choledocholithiasis, or stones - see Choledocholithiasis
    congenital 751.61
      jaundice from 751.61 [774.5]
  common duct 576.8
    with calculus, choledocholithiasis, or stones - see Choledocholithiasis
    congenital 751.61
  cystic duct 575.8
    with calculus, choledocholithiasis, or stones - see Choledocholithiasis
  disease, arteriolar 447.1
  endometrium 621.8
  eye, anterior chamber 360.34
  fallopian tube 628.2
  lymphatic vessel 457.1
    postmastectomy 457.0
  organ or site, congenital NEC - see Atresia
  placental blood vessels - see Placenta, abnormal
  supra-aortic branches 446.7
  ureter 593.89
  urethra 599.84
  vein 459.9
  vestibule (oral) 525.8
Observation (for) V71.9
  without need for further medical care V71.9
  accident NEC V71.4
    at work V71.3
  criminal assault V71.6
  deleterious agent ingestion V71.89
  disease V71.9
    cardiovascular V71.7
    heart V71.7
    mental V71.09
    specified condition NEC V71.89
  foreign body ingestion V71.89
  growth and development variations V21.8
  injuries (accidental) V71.4
    inflicted NEC V71.6
      during alleged rape or seduction V71.5

Observation (Continued)
  malignant neoplasm, suspected V71.1
  postpartum
    immediately after delivery V24.0
    routine follow-up V24.2
  pregnancy
    high-risk V23.9
      specified problem NEC V23.8
    normal (without complication) V22.1
      with nonobstetric complication V22.2
      first V22.0
  rape or seduction, alleged V71.5
    injury during V71.5
  suicide attempt, alleged V71.89
  suspected (undiagnosed) (unproven) V71.81
    abuse V71.81
    cardiovascular disease V71.7
    child or wife battering victim V71.6
    concussion (cerebral) V71.6
    condition NEC V71.89
      infant - see Observation, suspected, condition, newborn
      newborn V29.9
        cardiovascular disease V29.8
        congenital anomaly V29.8
        genetic V29.3
        infectious V29.0
        ingestion foreign object V29.8
        injury V29.8
        metabolic V29.3
        neoplasm V29.8
        neurological V29.1
        poison, poisoning V29.8
        respiratory V29.2
        specified NEC V29.8
    exposure
      anthrax V71.82
      biologic agent NEC V71.83
      SARS V71.81
    infectious disease not requiring isolation V71.89
    malignant neoplasm V71.1
    mental disorder V71.09
    neglect V71.81
    neoplasm
      benign V71.89
      malignant V71.1
    specified condition NEC V71.89
    tuberculosis V71.2
  tuberculosis, suspected V71.2
Obsession, obsessional 300.3
  ideas and mental images 300.3
  impulses 300.3
  neurosis 300.3
  phobia 300.3
  psychasthenia 300.3
  ruminations 300.3
  state 300.3
  syndrome 300.3
Obsessive-compulsive 300.3
  neurosis 300.3
  personality 301.4 ◄
  reaction 300.3
Obstetrical trauma NEC (complicating delivery) 665.9
  with
    abortion - see Abortion, by type, with damage to pelvic organs
    ectopic pregnancy (see also categories 633.0-633.9) 639.2
    molar pregnancy (see also categories 630-632) 639.2
  affecting fetus or newborn 763.89
  following
    abortion 639.2
    ectopic or molar pregnancy 639.2

Obstipation (see also Constipation) 564.00
  psychogenic 306.4
Obstruction, obstructed, obstructive
  airway NEC 519.8
    with
      allergic alveolitis NEC 495.9
      asthma NEC (see also Asthma) 493.9
      bronchiectasis 494.0
        with acute exacerbation 494.1
      bronchitis (chronic) (see also Bronchitis, obstructive) 491.20
      emphysema NEC 492.8
    chronic 496
      with
        allergic alveolitis NEC 495.5
        asthma NEC (see also Asthma) 493.2
        bronchiectasis 494.0
          with acute exacerbation 494.1
        bronchitis (chronic) (see also Bronchitis, chronic, obstructive) 491.20
        emphysema NEC 492.8
    due to
      bronchospasm 519.1
      foreign body 934.9
      inhalation of fumes or vapors 506.9
      laryngospasm 478.75
  alimentary canal (see also Obstruction, intestine) 560.9
  ampulla of Vater 576.2
    with calculus, cholelithiasis, or stones - see Choledocholithiasis
  aortic (heart) (valve) (see also Stenosis, aortic) 424.1
    rheumatic (see also Stenosis, aortic, rheumatic) 395.0
  aortoiliac 444.0
  aqueduct of Sylvius 331.4
    congenital 742.3
      with spina bifida (see also Spina bifida) 741.0
  Arnold-Chiari (see also Spina bifida) 741.0
  artery (see also Embolism, artery) 444.9
    basilar (complete) (partial) (see also Occlusion, artery, basilar) 433.0
    carotid (complete) (partial) (see also Occlusion, artery, carotid) 433.1
    precerebral - see Occlusion, artery, precerebral NEC
    retinal (central) (see also Occlusion, retina) 362.30
    vertebral (complete) (partial) (see also Occlusion, artery, vertebral) 433.2
  asthma (chronic) (with obstructive pulmonary disease) 493.2
  band (intestinal) 560.81
  bile duct or passage (see also Obstruction, biliary) 576.2
    congenital 751.61
      jaundice from 751.61 [774.5]
  biliary (duct) (tract) 576.2
    with calculus 574.51
      with cholecystitis (chronic) 574.41
        acute 574.31
    congenital 751.61
      jaundice from 751.61 [774.5]
    gallbladder 575.2
      with calculus 574.21
        with cholecystitis (chronic) 574.11
          acute 574.01

◄ **New**   ⬅▥ **Revised**

Obstruction, obstructed, obstructive
(Continued)
bladder neck (acquired) 596.0
  congenital 753.6
bowel (*see also* Obstruction, intestine)
  560.9
bronchus 519.1
canal, ear (*see also* Stricture, ear canal,
  acquired) 380.50
cardia 537.89
caval veins (inferior) (superior) 459.2
cecum (*see also* Obstruction, intestine)
  560.9
circulatory 459.9
colon (*see also* Obstruction, intestine)
  560.9
  sympathicotonic 560.89
common duct (*see also* Obstruction, biliary) 576.2
  congenital 751.61
coronary (artery) (heart) - *see also* Arteriosclerosis, coronary
  acute (*see also* Infarct, myocardium)
    410.9
    without myocardial infarction
      411.81
cystic duct (*see also* Obstruction, gallbladder) 575.2
  congenital 751.61
device, implant, or graft - *see* Complications, due to (presence of) any
  device, implant, or graft classified
  to 996.0-996.5 NEC
due to foreign body accidentally left in
  operation wound 998.4
duodenum 537.3
  congenital 751.1
  due to
    compression NEC 537.3
    cyst 537.3
    intrinsic lesion or disease NEC 537.3
    scarring 537.3
    torsion 537.3
    ulcer 532.91
    volvulus 537.3
ejaculatory duct 608.89
endocardium 424.90
  arteriosclerotic 424.99
  specified cause, except rheumatic
    424.99
esophagus 530.3
Eustachian tube (complete) (partial)
  381.60
  cartilaginous
    extrinsic 381.63
    intrinsic 381.62
  due to
    cholesteatoma 381.61
    osseous lesion NEC 381.61
    polyp 381.61
  osseous 381.61
fallopian tube (bilateral) 628.2
fecal 560.39
  with hernia - *see also* Hernia, by site,
    with obstruction
    gangrenous - *see* Hernia, by site,
      with gangrene
foramen of Monro (congenital) 742.3
  with spina bifida (*see also* Spina bi-
    fida) 741.0
foreign body - *see* Foreign body
gallbladder 575.2
  with calculus, cholelithiasis, or
    stones 574.21

Obstruction, obstructed, obstructive
(Continued)
gallbladder *(Continued)*
  with calculus, cholelithiasis, or
    stones *(Continued)*
    with cholecystitis (chronic) 574.11
      acute 574.01
  congenital 751.69
    jaundice from 751.69 *[774.5]*
gastric outlet 537.0
gastrointestinal (*see also* Obstruction,
  intestine) 560.9
glottis 478.79
hepatic 573.8
  duct (*see also* Obstruction, biliary)
    576.2
    congenital 751.61
icterus (*see also* Obstruction, biliary)
  576.8
  congenital 751.61
ileocecal coil (*see also* Obstruction, intestine) 560.9
ileum (*see also* Obstruction, intestine)
  560.9
iliofemoral (artery) 444.81
internal anastomosis - *see* Complications, mechanical, graft
intestine (mechanical) (neurogenic)
  (paroxysmal) (postinfectional) (reflex) 560.9
  with
    adhesions (intestinal) (peritoneal)
      560.81
    hernia - *see also* Hernia, by site,
      with obstruction
      gangrenous - *see* Hernia, by site,
        with gangrene
  adynamic (*see also* Ileus) 560.1
  by gallstone 560.31
  congenital or infantile (small) 751.1
    large 751.2
  due to
    Ascaris lumbricoides 127.0
    mural thickening 560.89
    procedure 997.4
      involving urinary tract 997.5
  impaction 560.39
  infantile - *see* Obstruction, intestine,
    congenital
  newborn
    due to
      fecaliths 777.1
      inspissated milk 777.2
      meconium (plug) 777.1
        in mucoviscidosis 277.01
      transitory 777.4
  specified cause NEC 560.89
  transitory, newborn 777.4
  volvulus 560.2
intracardiac ball valve prosthesis 996.02
jaundice (*see also* Obstruction, biliary)
  576.8
  congenital 751.61
jejunum (*see also* Obstruction, intestine)
  560.9
kidney 593.89
labor 660.9
  affecting fetus or newborn 763.1
  by
    bony pelvis (conditions classifiable
      to 653.0-653.9) 660.1
    deep transverse arrest 660.3
    impacted shoulder 660.4
    locked twins 660.5

Obstruction, obstructed, obstructive
(Continued)
labor *(Continued)*
  by *(Continued)*
    malposition (fetus) (conditions clas-
      sifiable to 652.0-652.9) 660.0
      head during labor 660.3
    persistent occipitoposterior posi-
      tion 660.3
    soft tissue, pelvic (conditions clas-
      sifiable to 654.0-654.9) 660.2
lacrimal
  canaliculi 375.53
    congenital 743.65
  punctum 375.52
  sac 375.54
lacrimonasal duct 375.56
  congenital 743.65
  neonatal 375.55
lacteal, with steatorrhea 579.2
laryngitis (*see also* Laryngitis) 464.01
larynx 478.79
  congenital 748.3
liver 573.8
  cirrhotic (*see also* Cirrhosis, liver) 571.5
lung 518.89
  with
    asthma - *see* Asthma
    bronchitis (chronic) 491.20
    emphysema NEC 492.8
  airway, chronic 496
  chronic NEC 496
    with
      asthma (chronic) (obstructive)
        493.2
  disease, chronic 496
    with
      asthma (chronic) (obstructive)
        493.2
  emphysematous 492.8
lymphatic 457.1
meconium
  fetus or newborn 777.1
    in mucoviscidosis 277.01
  newborn due to fecaliths 777.1
mediastinum 519.3
mitral (rheumatic) - *see* Stenosis, mitral
nasal 478.1
  duct 375.56
    neonatal 375.55
  sinus - *see* Sinusitis
nasolacrimal duct 375.56
  congenital 743.65
  neonatal 375.55
nasopharynx 478.29
nose 478.1
organ or site, congenital NEC - *see*
  Atresia
pancreatic duct 577.8
parotid gland 527.8
pelviureteral junction (*see also* Obstruction, ureter) 593.4
pharynx 478.29
portal (circulation) (vein) 452
prostate 600.90
  with urinary retention 600.91
  valve (urinary) 596.0
pulmonary
  valve (heart) (*see also* Endocarditis,
    pulmonary) 424.3
  vein, isolated 747.49
pyemic - *see* Septicemia
pylorus (acquired) 537.0
  congenital 750.5
  infantile 750.5

ICD-9-CM

Vol. 2

Obstruction, obstructed, obstructive
(*Continued*)
rectosigmoid (*see also* Obstruction, intestine) 560.9
rectum 569.49
renal 593.89
respiratory 519.8
  chronic 496
retinal (artery) (vein) (central) (*see also* Occlusion, retina) 362.30
salivary duct (any) 527.8
  with calculus 527.5
sigmoid (*see also* Obstruction, intestine) 560.9
sinus (accessory) (nasal) (*see also* Sinusitis) 473.9
Stensen's duct 527.8
stomach 537.89
  acute 536.1
  congenital 750.7
submaxillary gland 527.8
  with calculus 527.5
thoracic duct 457.1
thrombotic - *see* Thrombosis
tooth eruption 520.6
trachea 519.1
tracheostomy airway 519.09
tricuspid - *see* Endocarditis, tricuspid
upper respiratory, congenital 748.8
ureter (functional) 593.4
  congenital 753.20
  due to calculus 592.1
ureteropelvic junction, congenital 753.21
ureterovesical junction, congenital 753.22
urethra 599.6
  congenital 753.6
urinary (moderate) 599.6
  organ or tract (lower) 599.6
  prostatic valve 596.0
uropathy 599.6
uterus 621.8
vagina 623.2
valvular - *see* Endocarditis
vascular graft or shunt 996.1
  atherosclerosis - *see* Arteriosclerosis, coronary
  embolism 996.74
  occlusion NEC 996.74
  thrombus 996.74
vein, venous 459.2
  caval (inferior) (superior) 459.2
  thrombotic - *see* Thrombosis
vena cava (inferior) (superior) 459.2
ventricular shunt 996.2
vesical 596.0
vesicourethral orifice 596.0
vessel NEC 459.9
Obturator - *see* condition
Occlusal ◀▥
plane deviation 524.76 ◀
wear, teeth 521.10 ◀
Occlusion
anus 569.49
  congenital 751.2
  infantile 751.2
aortoiliac (chronic) 444.0
aqueduct of Sylvius 331.4
  congenital 742.3
    with spina bifida (*see also* Spina bifida) 741.0
arteries of extremities, lower 444.22
  without thrombus or embolus (*see also* Arteriosclerosis, extremities) 440.20

Occlusion (*Continued*)
arteries of extremities, lower (*Continued*)
  due to stricture or stenosis 447.1
  upper 444.21
    without thrombus or embolus (*see also* Arteriosclerosis, extremities) 440.20
    due to stricture or stenosis 447.1
artery NEC (*see also* Embolism, artery) 444.9
  auditory, internal 433.8
  basilar 433.0
    with other precerebral artery 433.3
    bilateral 433.3
  brain or cerebral (*see also* Infarct, brain) 434.9
  carotid 433.1
    with other precerebral artery 433.3
    bilateral 433.3
  cerebellar (anterior inferior) (posterior inferior) (superior) 433.8
  cerebral (*see also* Infarct, brain) 434.9
  choroidal (anterior) 433.8
  communicating posterior 433.8
  coronary (acute) (thrombotic) (*see also* Infarct, myocardium) 410.9
    without myocardial infarction 411.81
    healed or old 412
  hypophyseal 433.8
  iliac 444.81
  mesenteric (embolic) (thrombotic) (with gangrene) 557.0
  pontine 433.8
  precerebral NEC 433.9
    late effect - *see* Late effect(s) (of) cerebrovascular disease
    multiple or bilateral 433.3
    puerperal, postpartum, childbirth 674.0
    specified NEC 433.8
  renal 593.81
  retinal - *see* Occlusion, retina, artery
  spinal 433.8
  vertebral 433.2
    with other precerebral artery 433.3
    bilateral 433.3
basilar (artery) - *see* Occlusion, artery, basilar
bile duct (any) (*see also* Obstruction, biliary) 576.2
bowel (*see also* Obstruction, intestine) 560.9
brain (artery) (vascular) (*see also* Infarct, brain) 434.9
breast (duct) 611.8
carotid (artery) (common) (internal) - *see* Occlusion, artery, carotid
cerebellar (anterior inferior) (artery) (posterior inferior) (superior) 433.8
cerebral (artery) (*see also* Infarct, brain) 434.9
cerebrovascular (*see also* Infarct, brain) 434.9
  diffuse 437.0
cervical canal (*see also* Stricture, cervix) 622.4
  by falciparum malaria 084.0
cervix (uteri) (*see also* Stricture, cervix) 622.4
choanal 748.0
choroidal (artery) 433.8
colon (*see also* Obstruction, intestine) 560.9

Occlusion (*Continued*)
communicating posterior artery 433.8
coronary (artery) (thrombotic) (*see also* Infarct, myocardium) 410.9
  acute 410.9
    without myocardial infarction 411.81
  healed or old 412
    without myocardial infarction 411.81
cystic duct (*see also* Obstruction, gallbladder) 575.2
  congenital 751.69
disto ◀
  division I 524.22 ◀
  division II 524.22 ◀
embolic - *see* Embolism
fallopian tube 628.2
  congenital 752.19
gallbladder (*see also* Obstruction, gallbladder) 575.2
  congenital 751.69
    jaundice from 751.69 [744.5]
gingiva, traumatic 523.8
hymen 623.3
  congenital 752.42
hypophyseal (artery) 433.8
iliac (artery) 444.81
intestine (*see also* Obstruction, intestine) 560.9
kidney 593.89
lacrimal apparatus - *see* Stenosis, lacrimal
lung 518.89
lymph or lymphatic channel 457.1
mammary duct 611.8
mesenteric artery (embolic) (thrombotic) (with gangrene) 557.0
nose 478.1
  congenital 748.0
organ or site, congenital NEC - *see* Atresia
oviduct 628.2
  congenital 752.19
periodontal, traumatic 523.8
peripheral arteries (lower extremity) 444.22
  without thrombus or embolus (*see also* Arteriosclerosis, extremities) 440.20
  due to stricture or stenosis 447.1
  upper extremity 444.21
    without thrombus or embolus (*see also* Arteriosclerosis, extremities) 440.20
    due to stricture or stenosis 447.1
pontine (artery) 433.8
posterior lingual, of mandibular teeth 524.29 ◀▥
precerebral artery - *see* Occlusion, artery, precerebral NEC
puncta lacrimalia 375.52
pupil 364.74
pylorus (*see also* Stricture, pylorus) 537.0
renal artery 593.81
retina, retinal (vascular) 362.30
  artery, arterial 362.30
    branch 362.32
    central (total) 362.31
    partial 362.33
    transient 362.34
    tributary 362.32
  vein 362.30
    branch 362.36
    central (total) 362.35
    incipient 362.37
    partial 362.37
    tributary 362.36

Occlusion *(Continued)*
  spinal artery 433.8
  stent
    coronary 996.72
    teeth (mandibular) (posterior lingual) 524.29 ◀▥
  thoracic duct 457.1
  tubal 628.2
  ureter (complete) (partial) 593.4
    congenital 753.29
  urethra *(see also* Stricture, urethra) 598.9
    congenital 753.6
  uterus 621.8
  vagina 623.2
  vascular NEC 459.9
  vein - *see* Thrombosis
  vena cava (inferior) (superior) 453.2
  ventricle (brain) NEC 331.4
  vertebral (artery) - *see* Occlusion, artery, vertebral
  vessel (blood) NEC 459.9
  vulva 624.8
Occlusio pupillae 364.74
Occupational
  problems NEC V62.2
  therapy V57.21
Ochlophobia 300.29
Ochronosis (alkaptonuric) (congenital) (endogenous) 270.2
  with chloasma of eyelid 270.2
Ocular muscle - *see also* condition
  myopathy 359.1
  torticollis 781.93
Oculoauriculovertebral dysplasia 756.0
Oculogyric
  crisis or disturbance 378.87
    psychogenic 306.7
Oculomotor syndrome 378.81
Oddi's sphincter spasm 576.5
Odelberg's disease (juvenile osteochondrosis) 732.1
Odontalgia 525.9
Odontoameloblastoma (M9311/0) 213.1
  upper jaw (bone) 213.0
Odontoclasia 521.05
Odontoclasis 873.63
  complicated 873.73
Odontodysplasia, regional 520.4
Odontogenesis imperfecta 520.5
Odontoma (M9280/0) 213.1
  ameloblastic (M9311/0) 213.1
    upper jaw (bone) 213.0
  calcified (M9280/0) 213.1
    upper jaw (bone) 213.0
  complex (M9282/0) 213.1
    upper jaw (bone) 213.0
  compound (M9281/0) 213.1
    upper jaw (bone) 213.0
  fibroameloblastic (M9290/0) 213.1
    upper jaw (bone) 213.0
  follicular 526.0
    upper jaw (bone) 213.0
Odontomyelitis (closed) (open) 522.0
Odontonecrosis 521.09
Odontorrhagia 525.8
Odontosarcoma, ameloblastic (M9290/3) 170.1
  upper jaw (bone) 170.0
Odynophagia 787.2
Oesophagostomiasis 127.7
Oesophagostomum infestation 127.7
Oestriasis 134.0
Ogilvie's syndrome (sympathicotonic colon obstruction) 560.89

Oguchi's disease (retina) 368.61
Ohara's disease *(see also* Tularemia) 021.9
Oidiomycosis *(see also* Candidiasis) 112.9
Oidiomycotic meningitis 112.83
Oidium albicans infection *(see also* Candidiasis) 112.9
Old age 797
  dementia (of) 290.0
Olfactory - *see* condition
Oligemia 285.9
Oligergasia *(see also* Retardation, mental) 319
Oligoamnios 658.0
  affecting fetus or newborn 761.2
Oligoastrocytoma, mixed (M9382/3)
  specified site - *see* Neoplasm, by site, malignant
  unspecified site 191.9
Oligocythemia 285.9
Oligodendroblastoma (M9460/3)
  specified site - *see* Neoplasm, by site, malignant
  unspecified site 191.9
Oligodendroglioma (M9450/3)
  anaplastic type (M9451/3)
    specified site - *see* Neoplasm, by site, malignant
    unspecified site 191.9
  specified site - *see* Neoplasm, by site, malignant
  unspecified site 191.9
Oligodendroma - *see* Oligodendroglioma
Oligodontia *(see also* Anodontia) 520.0
Oligoencephalon 742.1
Oligohydramnios 658.0
  affecting fetus or newborn 761.2
  due to premature rupture of membranes 658.1
    affecting fetus or newborn 761.2
Oligohydrosis 705.0
Oligomenorrhea 626.1
Oligophrenia *(see also* Retardation, mental) 319
  phenylpyruvic 270.1
Oligospermia 606.1
Oligotrichia 704.09
  congenita 757.4
Oliguria 788.5
  with
    abortion - *see* Abortion, by type, with renal failure
    ectopic pregnancy *(see also* categories 633.0-633.9) 639.3
    molar pregnancy *(see also* categories 630-632) 639.3
  complicating
    abortion 639.3
    ectopic or molar pregnancy 639.3
    pregnancy 646.2
      with hypertension - *see* Toxemia, of pregnancy
  due to a procedure 997.5
  following labor and delivery 669.3
  heart or cardiac - *see* Failure, heart
  puerperal, postpartum 669.3
  specified due to a procedure 997.5
Ollier's disease (chondrodysplasia) 756.4
Omentitis *(see also* Peritonitis) 567.9
Omentocele *(see also* Hernia, omental) 553.8
Omentum, omental - *see* condition
Omphalitis (congenital) (newborn) 771.4
  not of newborn 686.9
  tetanus 771.3

Omphalocele 756.79
Omphalomesenteric duct, persistent 751.0
Omphalorrhagia, newborn 772.3
Omsk hemorrhagic fever 065.1
Onanism 307.9
Onchocerciasis 125.3
  eye 125.3 [360.13]
Onchocercosis 125.3
Oncocytoma (M8290/0) - *see* Neoplasm, by site, benign
Ondine's curse 348.8
Oneirophrenia *(see also* Schizophrenia) 295.4
Onychauxis 703.8
  congenital 757.5
Onychia (with lymphangitis) 681.9
  dermatophytic 110.1
  finger 681.02
  toe 681.11
Onychitis (with lymphangitis) 681.9
  finger 681.02
  toe 681.11
Onychocryptosis 703.0
Onychodystrophy 703.8
  congenital 757.5
Onychogryphosis 703.8
Onychogryposis 703.8
Onycholysis 703.8
Onychomadesis 703.8
Onychomalacia 703.8
Onychomycosis 110.1
  finger 110.1
  toe 110.1
Onycho-osteodysplasia 756.89
Onychophagy 307.9
Onychoptosis 703.8
Onychorrhexis 703.8
  congenital 757.5
Onychoschizia 703.8
Onychotrophia *(see also* Atrophy, nail) 703.8
O'Nyong Nyong fever 066.3
Onyxis (finger) (toe) 703.0
Onyxitis (with lymphangitis) 681.9
  finger 681.02
  toe 681.11
Oophoritis (cystic) (infectional) (interstitial) *(see also* Salpingo-oophoritis) 614.2
  complicating pregnancy 646.6
  fetal (acute) 752.0
  gonococcal (acute) 098.19
    chronic or duration of 2 months or over 098.39
  tuberculous *(see also* Tuberculosis) 016.6
Opacity, opacities
  cornea 371.00
    central 371.03
    congenital 743.43
      interfering with vision 743.42
    degenerative *(see also* Degeneration, cornea) 371.40
    hereditary *(see also* Dystrophy, cornea) 371.50
    inflammatory *(see also* Keratitis) 370.9
    late effect of trachoma (healed) 139.1
    minor 371.01
    peripheral 371.02
  enamel (fluoride) (nonfluoride) (teeth) 520.3
  lens *(see also* Cataract) 366.9
  snowball 379.22
  vitreous (humor) 379.24
    congenital 743.51

ICD-9-CM

O

Vol. 2

Opalescent dentin (hereditary) 520.5
Open, opening
  abnormal, organ or site, congenital - see Imperfect, closure
  angle with
    borderline intraocular pressure 365.01
    cupping of discs 365.01
  bite (anterior) (posterior) 524.29 ◀▥
  false - see Imperfect, closure
  wound - see Wound, open, by site
Operation
  causing mutilation of fetus 763.89
  destructive, on live fetus, to facilitate birth 763.89
  for delivery, fetus or newborn 763.89
  maternal, unrelated to current delivery, affecting fetus or newborn 760.6
Operational fatigue 300.89
Operative - see condition
Operculitis (chronic) 523.4
  acute 523.3
Operculum, retina 361.32
  with detachment 361.01
Ophiasis 704.01
Ophthalmia (see also Conjunctivitis) 372.30
  actinic rays 370.24
  allergic (acute) 372.05
    chronic 372.14
  blennorrhagic (neonatorum) 098.40
  catarrhal 372.03
  diphtheritic 032.81
  Egyptian 076.1
  electric, electrica 370.24
  gonococcal (neonatorum) 098.40
  metastatic 360.11
  migraine 346.8
  neonatorum, newborn 771.6
    gonococcal 098.40
  nodosa 360.14
  phlyctenular 370.31
    with ulcer (see also Ulcer, cornea) 370.00
  sympathetic 360.11
Ophthalmitis - see Ophthalmia
Ophthalmocele (congenital) 743.66
Ophthalmoneuromyelitis 341.0
Ophthalmopathy, infiltrative with thyrotoxicosis 242.0
Ophthalmoplegia (see also Strabismus) 378.9
  anterior internuclear 378.86
  ataxia-areflexia syndrome 357.0
  bilateral 378.9
  diabetic 250.5 [378.86]
  exophthalmic 242.0 [376.22]
  external 378.55
    progressive 378.72
    total 378.56
  internal (complete) (total) 367.52
  internuclear 378.86
  migraine 346.8
  painful 378.55
  Parinaud's 378.81
  progressive external 378.72
  supranuclear, progressive 333.0
  total (external) 378.56
    internal 367.52
  unilateral 378.9
Opisthognathism 524.00
Opisthorchiasis (felineus) (tenuicollis) (viverrini) 121.0
Opisthotonos, opisthotonus 781.0

Opitz's disease (congestive splenomegaly) 289.51
Opiumism (see also Dependence) 304.0
Oppenheim's disease 358.8
Oppenheim-Urbach disease or syndrome (necrobiosis lipoidica diabeticorum) 250.8 [709.3]
Opsoclonia 379.59
Optic nerve - see condition
Orbit - see condition
Orchioblastoma (M9071/3) 186.9
Orchitis (nonspecific) (septic) 604.90
  with abscess 604.0
  blennorrhagic (acute) 098.13
    chronic or duration of 2 months or over 098.33
  diphtheritic 032.89 [604.91]
  filarial 125.9 [604.91]
  gangrenous 604.99
  gonococcal (acute) 098.13
    chronic or duration of 2 months or over 098.33
  mumps 072.0
  parotidea 072.0
  suppurative 604.99
  syphilitic 095.8 [604.91]
  tuberculous (see also Tuberculosis) 016.5 [608.81]
Orf 051.2
Organic - see also condition
  heart - see Disease, heart
  insufficiency 799.89
Oriental
  bilharziasis 120.2
  schistosomiasis 120.2
  sore 085.1
Orientation ◀
  ego-dystonic sexual 302.0 ◀
Orifice - see condition
Origin, both great vessels from right ventricle 745.11
Ormond's disease or syndrome 593.4
Ornithosis 073.9
  with
    complication 073.8
      specified NEC 073.7
    pneumonia 073.0
    pneumonitis (lobular) 073.0
Orodigitofacial dysostosis 759.89
Oropouche fever 066.3
Orotaciduria, oroticaciduria (congenital) (hereditary) (pyrimidine deficiency) 281.4
Oroya fever 088.0
Orthodontics V58.5
  adjustment V53.4
  aftercare V58.5
  fitting V53.4
Orthopnea 786.02
Os, uterus - see condition
Osgood-Schlatter
  disease 732.4
  osteochondrosis 732.4
Osler's
  disease (M9950/1) (polycythemia vera) 238.4
  nodes 421.0
Osler-Rendu disease (familial hemorrhagic telangiectasia) 448.0
Osler-Vaquez disease (M9950/1) (polycythemia vera) 238.4
Osler-Weber-Rendu syndrome (familial hemorrhagic telangiectasia) 448.0
Osmidrosis 705.89

Osseous - see condition
Ossification
  artery - see Arteriosclerosis
  auricle (ear) 380.39
  bronchus 519.1
  cardiac (see also Degeneration, myocardial) 429.1
  cartilage (senile) 733.99
  coronary - see Arteriosclerosis, coronary
  diaphragm 728.10
  ear 380.39
    middle (see also Otosclerosis) 387.9
  falx cerebri 349.2
  fascia 728.10
  fontanel
    defective or delayed 756.0
    premature 756.0
  heart (see also Degeneration, myocardial) 429.1
    valve - see Endocarditis
  larynx 478.79
  ligament
    posterior longitudinal 724.8
      cervical 723.7
  meninges (cerebral) 349.2
    spinal 336.8
  multiple, eccentric centers 733.99
  muscle 728.10
    heterotopic, postoperative 728.13
  myocardium, myocardial (see also Degeneration, myocardial) 429.1
  penis 607.81
  periarticular 728.89
  sclera 379.16
  tendon 727.82
  trachea 519.1
  tympanic membrane (see also Tympanosclerosis) 385.00
  vitreous (humor) 360.44
Osteitis (see also Osteomyelitis) 730.2
  acute 730.0
  alveolar 526.5
  chronic 730.1
  condensans (ilii) 733.5
  deformans (Paget's) 731.0
    due to or associated with malignant neoplasm (see also Neoplasm, bone, malignant) 170.9 [731.1]
  due to yaws 102.6
  fibrosa NEC 733.29
    cystica (generalisata) 252.01 ◀▥
    disseminata 756.59
    osteoplastica 252.01 ◀▥
  fragilitans 756.51
  Garré's (sclerosing) 730.1
  infectious (acute) (subacute) 730.0
    chronic or old 730.1
  jaw (acute) (chronic) (lower) (neonatal) (suppurative) (upper) 526.4
  parathyroid 252.01 ◀▥
  petrous bone (see also Petrositis) 383.20
  pubis 733.5
  sclerotic, nonsuppurative 730.1
  syphilitic 095.5
  tuberculosa
    cystica (of Jüngling) 135
    multiplex cystoides 135
Osteoarthritica spondylitis (spine) (see also Spondylosis) 721.90
Osteoarthritis (see also Osteoarthrosis) 715.9
  distal interphalangeal 715.9
  hyperplastic 731.2
  interspinalis (see also Spondylosis) 721.90

◀ New   ◀▥ Revised

Osteoarthritis *(Continued)*
spine, spinal NEC *(see also* Spondylosis) 721.90
Osteoarthropathy *(see also* Osteoarthrosis) 715.9
chronic idiopathic hypertrophic 757.39
familial idiopathic 757.39
hypertrophic pulmonary 731.2
secondary 731.2
idiopathic hypertrophic 757.39
primary hypertrophic 731.2
pulmonary hypertrophic 731.2
secondary hypertrophic 731.2
Osteoarthrosis (degenerative) (hypertrophic) (rheumatoid) 715.9

> Note   Use the following fifth-digit
> subclassification with category 715:
>
> 0   site unspecified
> 1   shoulder region
> 2   upper arm
> 3   forearm
> 4   hand
> 5   pelvic region and thigh
> 6   lower leg
> 7   ankle and foot
> 8   other specified sites except
>   spine
> 9   multiple sites

deformans alkaptonurica 270.2
generalized 715.09
juvenilis (Köhler's) 732.5
localized 715.3
idiopathic 715.1
primary 715.1
secondary 715.2
multiple sites, not specified as generalized 715.89
polyarticular 715.09
spine *(see also* Spondylosis) 721.90
temporomandibular joint 524.69
Osteoblastoma (M9200/0) - *see* Neoplasm, bone, benign
Osteochondritis *(see also* Osteochondrosis) 732.9
dissecans 732.7
hip 732.7
ischiopubica 732.1
multiple 756.59
syphilitic (congenital) 090.0
Osteochondrodermodysplasia 756.59
Osteochondrodystrophy 277.5
deformans 277.5
familial 277.5
fetalis 756.4
Osteochondrolysis 732.7
Osteochondroma (M9210/0) - *see also*
Neoplasm, bone, benign
multiple, congenital 756.4
Osteochondromatosis (M9210/1) 238.0
synovial 727.82
Osteochondromyxosarcoma (M9180/3) -
see Neoplasm, bone, malignant
Osteochondropathy NEC 732.9
Osteochondrosarcoma (M9180/3) - *see*
Neoplasm, bone, malignant
Osteochondrosis 732.9
acetabulum 732.1
adult spine 732.8
astragalus 732.5
Blount's 732.4
Buchanan's (juvenile osteochondrosis
of iliac crest) 732.1

Osteochondrosis *(Continued)*
Buchman's (juvenile osteochondrosis)
732.1
Burns' 732.3
calcaneus 732.5
capitular epiphysis (femur) 732.1
carpal
lunate (wrist) 732.3
scaphoid 732.3
coxae juvenilis 732.1
deformans juvenilis (coxae) (hip) 732.1
scheuermann's 732.0
spine 732.0
tibia 732.4
vertebra 732.0
Diaz's (astragalus) 732.5
dissecans (knee) (shoulder) 732.7
femoral capital epiphysis 732.1
femur (head) (juvenile) 732.1
foot (juvenile) 732.5
Freiberg's (disease) (second metatarsal)
732.5
Haas' 732.3
Haglund's (os tibiale externum) 732.5
hand (juvenile) 732.3
head of
femur 732.1
humerus (juvenile) 732.3
hip (juvenile) 732.1
humerus (juvenile) 732.3
iliac crest (juvenile) 732.1
ilium (juvenile) 732.1
ischiopubic synchondrosis 732.1
Iselin's (osteochondrosis fifth metatarsal) 732.5
juvenile, juvenilis 732.6
arm 732.3
capital femoral epiphysis 732.1
capitellum humeri 732.3
capitular epiphysis 732.1
carpal scaphoid 732.3
clavicle, sternal epiphysis 732.6
coxae 732.1
deformans 732.1
foot 732.5
hand 732.3
hip and pelvis 732.1
lower extremity, except foot 732.4
lunate, wrist 732.3
medial cuneiform bone 732.5
metatarsal (head) 732.5
metatarsophalangeal 732.5
navicular, ankle 732.5
patella 732.4
primary patellar center (of Köhler)
732.4
specified site NEC 732.6
spine 732.0
tarsal scaphoid 732.5
tibia (epiphysis) (tuberosity) 732.4
upper extremity 732.3
vertebra (body) (Calvé) 732.0
epiphyseal plates (of Scheuermann) 732.0
Kienböck's (disease) 732.3
Köhler's (disease) (navicular, ankle)
732.5
patellar 732.4
tarsal navicular 732.5
Legg-Calvé-Perthes (disease) 732.1
lower extremity (juvenile) 732.4
lunate bone 732.3
Mauclaire's 732.3
metacarpal heads (of Mauclaire) 732.3

Osteochondrosis *(Continued)*
metatarsal (fifth) (head) (second) 732.5
navicular, ankle 732.5
os calcis 732.5
Osgood-Schlatter 732.4
os tibiale externum 732.5
Panner's 732.3
patella (juvenile) 732.4
patellar center
primary (of Köhler) 732.4
secondary (of Sinding-Larsen) 732.4
pelvis (juvenile) 732.1
Pierson's 732.1
radial head (juvenile) 732.3
Scheuermann's 732.0
Sever's (calcaneum) 732.5
Sinding-Larsen (secondary patellar
center) 732.4
spine (juvenile) 732.0
adult 732.8
symphysis pubis (of Pierson) (juvenile)
732.1
syphilitic (congenital) 090.0
tarsal (navicular) (scaphoid) 732.5
tibia (proximal) (tubercle) 732.4
tuberculous - *see* Tuberculosis, bone
ulna 732.3
upper extremity (juvenile) 732.3
van Neck's (juvenile osteochondrosis)
732.1
vertebral (juvenile) 732.0
adult 732.8
Osteoclastoma (M9250/1) 238.0
malignant (M9250/3) - *see* Neoplasm,
bone, malignant
Osteocopic pain 733.90
Osteodynia 733.90
Osteodystrophy
azotemic 588.0
chronica deformans hypertrophica
731.0
congenital 756.50
specified type NEC 756.59
deformans 731.0
fibrosa localisata 731.0
parathyroid 252.01   ◀▥▥
renal 588.0
Osteofibroma (M9262/0) - *see* Neoplasm,
bone, benign
Osteofibrosarcoma (M9182/3) - *see* Neoplasm, bone, malignant
Osteogenesis imperfecta 756.51
Osteogenic - *see* condition
Osteoma (M9180/0) - *see also* Neoplasm,
bone, benign
osteoid (M9191/0) - *see also* Neoplasm,
bone, benign
giant (M9200/0) - *see* Neoplasm,
bone, benign
Osteomalacia 268.2
chronica deformans hypertrophica
731.0
due to vitamin D deficiency 268.2
infantile *(see also* Rickets) 268.0
juvenile *(see also* Rickets) 268.0
pelvis 268.2
vitamin D-resistant 275.3
Osteomalacic bone 268.2
Osteomalacosis 268.2
Osteomyelitis (general) (infective) (localized) (neonatal) (purulent) (pyo-
genic) (septic) (staphylococcal)
(streptococcal) (suppurative) (with
periostitis) 730.2

ICD-9-CM

O

Vol. 2

Osteomyelitis (*Continued*)

Note	Use the following fifth-digit

subclassification with category 730:

0   site unspecified
1   shoulder region
2   upper arm
3   forearm
4   hand
5   pelvic region and thigh
6   lower leg
7   ankle and foot
8   other specified sites
9   multiple sites

acute or subacute 730.0
chronic or old 730.1
due to or associated with
    diabetes mellitus 250.8 *[731.8]*
    tuberculosis (*see also* Tuberculosis,
        bone) 015.9 *[730.8]*
        limb bones 015.5 *[730.8]*
        specified bones NEC 015.7 *[730.8]*
        spine 015.0 *[730.8]*
        typhoid 002.0 *[730.8]*
Garré's 730.1
jaw (acute) (chronic) (lower) (neonatal)
    (suppurative) (upper) 526.4
nonsuppurating 730.1
orbital 376.03
petrous bone (*see also* Petrositis) 383.20
Salmonella 003.24
sclerosing, nonsuppurative 730.1
sicca 730.1
syphilitic 095.5
    congenital 090.0 *[730.8]*
tuberculous - *see* Tuberculosis, bone
typhoid 002.0 *[730.8]*
Osteomyelofibrosis 289.89
Osteomyelosclerosis 289.89
Osteonecrosis 733.40
    meaning osteomyelitis 730.1
Osteo-onycho-arthro dysplasia 756.89
Osteo-onychodysplasia, hereditary 756.89
Osteopathia
    condensans disseminata 756.53
    hyperostotica multiplex infantilis 756.59
    hypertrophica toxica 731.2
    striata 756.4
Osteopathy resulting from poliomyelitis
    (*see also* Poliomyelitis) 045.9 *[730.7]*
    familial dysplastic 731.2
Osteopecilia 756.53
Osteopenia 733.90
Osteoperiostitis (*see also* Osteomyelitis)
    730.2
    ossificans toxica 731.2
    toxica ossificans 731.2
Osteopetrosis (familial) 756.52
Osteophyte - *see* Exostosis
Osteophytosis - *see* Exostosis
Osteopoikilosis 756.53
Osteoporosis (generalized) 733.00
    circumscripta 731.0
    disuse 733.03
    drug-induced 733.09
    idiopathic 733.02
    postmenopausal 733.01
    posttraumatic 733.7
    screening V82.81
    senile 733.01
    specified type NEC 733.09
Osteoporosis-osteomalacia syndrome
    268.2

Osteopsathyrosis 756.51
Osteoradionecrosis, jaw 526.89
Osteosarcoma (M9180/3) - *see also* Neo-
    plasm, bone, malignant
    chondroblastic (M9181/3) - *see* Neo-
        plasm, bone, malignant
    fibroblastic (M9182/3) - *see* Neoplasm,
        bone, malignant
    in Paget's disease of bone (M9184/3) -
        see Neoplasm, bone, malignant
    juxtacortical (M9190/3) - *see* Neo-
        plasm, bone malignant
    parosteal (M9190/3) - *see* Neoplasm,
        bone, malignant
    telangiectatic (M9183/3) - *see* Neo-
        plasm, bone, malignant
Osteosclerosis 756.52
    fragilis (generalisata) 756.52
    myelofibrosis 289.89
Osteosclerotic anemia 289.89
Osteosis
    acromegaloid 757.39
    cutis 709.3
    parathyroid 252.01   ◀▥
    renal fibrocystic 588.0
Österreicher-Turner syndrome 756.89
Ostium
    atrioventriculare commune 745.69
    primum (arteriosum) (defect) (persist-
        ent) 745.61
    secundum (arteriosum) (defect) (pat-
        ent) (persistent) 745.5
Ostrum-Furst syndrome 756.59
Otalgia 388.70
    otogenic 388.71
    referred 388.72
Othematoma 380.31
Otitic hydrocephalus 348.2
Otitis 382.9
    with effusion 381.4
        purulent 382.4
        secretory 381.4
        serous 381.4
        suppurative 382.4
    acute 382.9
    adhesive (*see also* Adhesions, middle
        ear) 385.10
    chronic 382.9
        with effusion 381.3
        mucoid, mucous (simple) 381.20
        purulent 382.3
        secretory 381.3
        serous 381.10
        suppurative 382.3
    diffuse parasitic 136.8
    externa (acute) (diffuse) (hemorrhag-
        ica) 380.10
        actinic 380.22
        candidal 112.82
        chemical 380.22
        chronic 380.23
            mycotic - *see* Otitis, externa, mycotic
            specified type NEC 380.23
        circumscribed 380.10
        contact 380.22
        due to
            erysipelas 035 *[380.13]*
            impetigo 684 *[380.13]*
            seborrheic dermatitis 690.10
                [380.13]
        eczematoid 380.22
        furuncular 680.0 *[380.13]*
        infective 380.10
            chronic 380.16

Otitis (*Continued*)
    externa (*Continued*)
        malignant 380.14
        mycotic (chronic) 380.15
            due to
                aspergillosis 117.3 *[380.15]*
                moniliasis 112.82
                otomycosis 111.8 *[380.15]*
        reactive 380.22
        specified type NEC 380.22
        tropical 111.8 *[380.15]*
    insidiosa (*see also* Otosclerosis) 387.9
    interna (*see also* Labyrinthitis) 386.30
    media (hemorrhagic) (staphylococcal)
        (streptococcal) 382.9
        acute 382.9
            with effusion 381.00
            allergic 381.04
                mucoid 381.05
                sanguineous 381.06
                serous 381.04
            catarrhal 381.00
            exudative 381.00
            mucoid 381.02
                allergic 381.05
            necrotizing 382.00
                with spontaneous rupture of ear
                    drum 382.01
                in
                    influenza 487.8 *[382.02]*
                    measles 055.2
                    scarlet fever 034.1 *[382.02]*
            nonsuppurative 381.00
            purulent 382.00
                with spontaneous rupture of ear
                    drum 382.01
            sanguineous 381.03
                allergic 381.06
            secretory 381.01
            seromucinous 381.02
            serous 381.01
                allergic 381.04
            suppurative 382.00
                with spontaneous rupture of ear
                    drum 382.01
                due to
                    influenza 487.8 *[382.02]*
                    scarlet fever 034.1 *[382.02]*
            transudative 381.00
        adhesive (*see also* Adhesions, middle
            ear) 385.10
        allergic 381.4
            acute 381.04
                mucoid 381.05
                sanguineous 381.06
                serous 381.04
            chronic 381.3
        catarrhal 381.4
            acute 381.00
            chronic (simple) 381.10
        chronic 382.9
            with effusion 381.3
            adhesive (*see also* Adhesions, mid-
                dle ear) 385.10
            allergic 381.3
            atticoantral, suppurative (with
                posterior or superior margin-
                al perforation of ear drum)
                382.2
            benign suppurative (with anterior
                perforation of ear drum) 382.1
            catarrhal 381.10
            exudative 381.3
            mucinous 381.20

◀ **New**   ◀▥ **Revised**

ICD-9-CM

Vol. 2

P

Pacemaker syndrome 429.4
Pachyderma, pachydermia 701.8
  laryngis 478.5
  laryngitis 478.79
  larynx (verrucosa) 478.79
Pachydermatitis 701.8
Pachydermatocele (congenital) 757.39
  acquired 701.8
Pachydermatosis 701.8
Pachydermoperiostitis
  secondary 731.2
Pachydermoperiostosis
  primary idiopathic 757.39
  secondary 731.2
Pachymeningitis (adhesive) (basal)
    (brain) (cerebral) (cervical) (chronic)
    (circumscribed) (external) (fibrous)
    (hemorrhagic) (hypertrophic) (inter-
    nal) (purulent) (spinal) (suppurative)
    (see also Meningitis) 322.9
  gonococcal 098.82
Pachyonychia (congenital) 757.5
  acquired 703.8
Pachyperiosteodermia
  primary or idiopathic 757.39
  secondary 731.2
Pachyperiostosis
  primary or idiopathic 757.39
  secondary 731.2
Pacinian tumor (M9507/0) - see Neo-
    plasm, skin, benign
Pads, knuckle or Garrod's 728.79
Paget's disease (osteitis deformans)
    731.0
  with infiltrating duct carcinoma of the
      breast (M8541/3) - see Neoplasm,
      breast, malignant
  bone 731.0
    osteosarcoma in (M9184/3) - see Ne-
        oplasm, bone, malignant
  breast (M8540/3) 174.0
  extramammary (M8542/3) - see also
      Neoplasm, skin, malignant
    anus 154.3
    skin 173.5
  malignant (M8540/3)
    breast 174.0
    specified site NEC (M8542/3) - see
        Neoplasm, skin, malignant
    unspecified site 174.0
  mammary (M8540/3) 174.0
  necrosis of bone 731.0
  nipple (M8540/3) 174.0
  osteitis deformans 731.0
Paget-Schroetter syndrome (intermittent
    venous claudication) 453.8
Pain(s)
  abdominal 789.0
  adnexa (uteri) 625.9
  alimentary, due to vascular insuffi-
      ciency 557.9
  anginoid (see also Pain, precordial)
      786.51
  anus 569.42
  arch 729.5
  arm 729.5
  back (postural) 724.5
    low 724.2
    psychogenic 307.89
  bile duct 576.9
  bladder 788.9
  bone 733.90

Pain(s) (Continued)
  breast 611.71
    psychogenic 307.89
  broad ligament 625.9
  cartilage NEC 733.90
  cecum 789.0
  cervicobrachial 723.3
  chest (central) 786.50
    atypical 786.59
    midsternal 786.51
    musculoskeletal 786.59
    noncardiac 786.59
    substernal 786.51
    wall (anterior) 786.52
  coccyx 724.79
  colon 789.0
  common duct 576.9
  coronary - see Angina
  costochondral 786.52
  diaphragm 786.52
  due to (presence of) any device, im-
      plant, or graft classifiable to 996.0-
      996.5 - see Complications, due to
      (presence of) any device, implant,
      or graft classified to 996.0-996.5
      NEC
  ear (see also Otalgia) 388.70
  epigastric, epigastrium 789.06
  extremity (lower) (upper) 729.5
  eye 379.91
  face, facial 784.0
    atypical 350.2
    nerve 351.8
  false (labor) 644.1
  female genital organ NEC 625.9
    psychogenic 307.89
  finger 729.5
  flank 789.0
  foot 729.5
  gallbladder 575.9
  gas (intestinal) 787.3
  gastric 536.8
  generalized 780.99
  genital organ
    female 625.9
    male 608.9
    psychogenic 307.89
  groin 789.0
  growing 781.99
  hand 729.5
  head (see also Headache) 784.0
  heart (see also Pain, precordial) 786.51
  infraorbital (see also Neuralgia, trigemi-
      nal) 350.1
  intermenstrual 625.2
  jaw 526.9
  joint 719.40
    ankle 719.47
    elbow 719.42
    foot 719.47
    hand 719.44
    hip 719.45
    knee 719.46
    multiple sites 719.49
    pelvic region 719.45
    psychogenic 307.89
    shoulder (region) 719.41
    specified site NEC 719.48
    wrist 719.43
  kidney 788.0
  labor, false or spurious 644.1
  laryngeal 784.1
  leg 729.5
  limb 729.5

Pain(s) (Continued)
  low back 724.2
  lumbar region 724.2
  mastoid (see also Otalgia) 388.70
  maxilla 526.9
  metacarpophalangeal (joint) 719.44
  metatarsophalangeal (joint) 719.47
  mouth 528.9
  muscle 729.1
    intercostal 786.59
  nasal 478.1
  nasopharynx 478.29
  neck NEC 723.1
    psychogenic 307.89
  nerve NEC 729.2
  neuromuscular 729.1
  nose 478.1
  ocular 379.91
  ophthalmic 379.91
  orbital region 379.91
  osteocopic 733.90
  ovary 625.9
    psychogenic 307.89
  over heart (see also Pain, precordial)
      786.51
  ovulation 625.2
  pelvic (female) 625.9
    male NEC 789.0
      psychogenic 307.89
    psychogenic 307.89
  penis 607.9
    psychogenic 307.89
  pericardial (see also Pain, precordial)
      786.51
  perineum
    female 625.9
    male 608.9
  pharynx 478.29
  pleura, pleural, pleuritic 786.52
  postoperative - see Pain, by site
  preauricular 388.70
  precordial (region) 786.51
    psychogenic 307.89
  psychogenic 307.80
    cardiovascular system 307.89
    gastrointestinal system 307.89
    genitourinary system 307.89
    heart 307.89
    musculoskeletal system 307.89
    respiratory system 307.89
    skin 306.3
  radicular (spinal) (see also Radiculitis)
      729.2
  rectum 569.42
  respiration 786.52
  retrosternal 786.51
  rheumatic NEC 729.0
    muscular 729.1
  rib 786.50
  root (spinal) (see also Radiculitis) 729.2
  round ligament (stretch) 625.9
  sacroiliac 724.6
  sciatic 724.3
  scrotum 608.9
    psychogenic 307.89
  seminal vesicle 608.9
  sinus 478.1
  skin 782.0
  spermatic cord 608.9
  spinal root (see also Radiculitis) 729.2
  stomach 536.8
    psychogenic 307.89
  substernal 786.51
  temporomandibular (joint) 524.62

◀ New   ◀▥ Revised

Pain(s) *(Continued)*
  temporomaxillary joint 524.62
  testis 608.9
    psychogenic 307.89
  thoracic spine 724.1
    with radicular and visceral pain
        724.4
  throat 784.1
  tibia 733.90
  toe 729.5
  tongue 529.6
  tooth 525.9
  trigeminal *(see also* Neuralgia, trigeminal) 350.1
  umbilicus 789.05
  ureter 788.0
  urinary (organ) (system) 788.0
  uterus 625.9
    psychogenic 307.89
  vagina 625.9
  vertebrogenic (syndrome) 724.5
  vesical 788.9
  vulva 625.9
  xiphoid 733.90
Painful - *see also* Pain
  arc syndrome 726.19
  coitus
    female 625.0
    male 608.89
      psychogenic 302.76
  ejaculation (semen) 608.89
    psychogenic 302.79
  erection 607.3
  feet syndrome 266.2
  menstruation 625.3
    psychogenic 306.52
  micturition 788.1
  ophthalmoplegia 378.55
  respiration 786.52
  scar NEC 709.2
  urination 788.1
  wire sutures 998.89
Painters' colic 984.9
  specified type of lead - *see* Table of
      Drugs and Chemicals
Palate - *see* condition
Palatoplegia 528.9
Palatoschisis *(see also* Cleft, palate)
    749.00
Palilalia 784.69
Palindromic arthritis *(see also* Rheumatism, palindromic) 719.3
Palliative care V66.7
Pallor 782.61
  temporal, optic disc 377.15
Palmar - *see also* condition
  fascia - *see* condition
Palpable
  cecum 569.89
  kidney 593.89
  liver 573.9
  lymph nodes 785.6
  ovary 620.8
  prostate 602.9
  spleen *(see also* Splenomegaly) 789.2
  uterus 625.8
Palpitation (heart) 785.1
  psychogenic 306.2
Palsy *(see also* Paralysis) 344.9
  atrophic diffuse 335.20
  Bell's 351.0
    newborn 767.5
  birth 767.7
  brachial plexus 353.0
    fetus or newborn 767.6

Palsy *(Continued)*
  brain - *see also* Palsy, cerebral
    noncongenital or noninfantile 344.89
      late effects - *see* Late effect(s) (of)
          cerebrovascular disease
    syphilitic 094.89
      congenital 090.49
  bulbar (chronic) (progressive) 335.22
    pseudo NEC 335.23
    supranuclear NEC 344.89
  cerebral (congenital) (infantile) (spastic) 343.9
    athetoid 333.7
    diplegic 343.0
      late effects - *see* Late effect(s) (of)
          cerebrovascular disease
    hemiplegic 343.1
    monoplegic 343.3
    noncongenital or noninfantile 437.8
      late effects - *see* Late effect(s) (of)
          cerebrovascular disease
    paraplegic 343.0
    quadriplegic 343.2
    spastic, not congenital or infantile
        344.89
    syphilitic 094.89
      congenital 090.49
    tetraplegic 343.2
  cranial nerve - *see also* Disorder, nerve,
      cranial
    multiple 352.6
  creeping 335.21
  divers' 993.3
  erb's (birth injury) 767.6
  facial 351.0
    newborn 767.5
  glossopharyngeal 352.2
  Klumpke (-Déjérine) 767.6
  lead 984.9
    specified type of lead - *see* Table of
        Drugs and Chemicals
  median nerve (tardy) 354.0
  peroneal nerve (acute) (tardy) 355.3
  progressive supranuclear 333.0
  pseudobulbar NEC 335.23
  radial nerve (acute) 354.3
  seventh nerve 351.0
    newborn 767.5
  shaking *(see also* Parkinsonism) 332.0
  spastic (cerebral) (spinal) 343.9
    hemiplegic 343.1
  specified nerve NEC - *see* Disorder, nerve
  supranuclear NEC 356.8
    progressive 333.0
  ulnar nerve (tardy) 354.2
  wasting 335.21
Paltauf-Sternberg disease 201.9
Paludism - *see* Malaria
Panama fever 084.0
Panaris (with lymphangitis) 681.9
  finger 681.02
  toe 681.11
Panaritium (with lymphangitis) 681.9
  finger 681.02
  toe 681.11
Panarteritis (nodosa) 446.0
  brain or cerebral 437.4
Pancake heart 793.2
  with cor pulmonale (chronic) 416.9
Pancarditis (acute) (chronic) 429.89
  with
    rheumatic
      fever (active) (acute) (chronic)
          (subacute) 391.8
        inactive or quiescent 398.99
  rheumatic, acute 391.8
    chronic or inactive 398.99

Pancoast's syndrome or tumor (carcinoma, pulmonary apex) (M8010/3)
    162.3
Pancoast-Tobias syndrome (M8010/3)
    (carcinoma, pulmonary apex) 162.3
Pancolitis 556.6
Pancreas, pancreatic - *see* condition
Pancreatitis 577.0
  acute (edematous) (hemorrhagic) (recurrent) 577.0
  annular 577.0
  apoplectic 577.0
  calcereous 577.0
  chronic (infectious) 577.1
    recurrent 577.1
  cystic 577.2
  fibrous 577.8
  gangrenous 577.0
  hemorrhagic (acute) 577.0
  interstitial (chronic) 577.1
    acute 577.0
  malignant 577.0
  mumps 072.3
  painless 577.1
  recurrent 577.1
  relapsing 577.1
  subacute 577.0
  suppurative 577.0
  syphilitic 095.8
Pancreatolithiasis 577.8
Pancytolysis 289.9
Pancytopenia (acquired) 284.8
  with malformations 284.0
  congenital 284.0
Panencephalitis - *see also* Encephalitis
  subacute, sclerosing 046.2
Panhematopenia 284.8
  congenital 284.0
  constitutional 284.0
  splenic, primary 289.4
Panhemocytopenia 284.8
  congenital 284.0
  constitutional 284.0
Panhypogonadism 257.2
Panhypopituitarism 253.2
  prepubertal 253.3
Panic (attack) (state) 300.01
  reaction to exceptional stress (transient) 308.1
Panmyelopathy, familial constitutional
    284.0
Panmyelophthisis 284.9
  acquired (secondary) 284.8
  congenital 284.0
  idiopathic 284.9
Panmyelosis (acute) (M9951/1) 238.7
Panner's disease 732.3
  capitellum humeri 732.3
  head of humerus 732.3
  tarsal navicular (bone) (osteochondrosis) 732.5
Panneuritis endemica 265.0 [357.4]
Panniculitis 729.30
  back 724.8
  knee 729.31
  neck 723.6
  nodular, nonsuppurative 729.30
  sacral 724.8
  specified site NEC 729.39
Panniculus adiposus (abdominal) 278.1
Pannus 370.62
  allergic eczematous 370.62
  degenerativus 370.62
  keratic 370.62

ICD-9-CM

P.

Vol. 2

Pannus (*Continued*)
rheumatoid - *see* Arthritis, rheumatoid
trachomatosus, trachomatous (active)
076.1 [370.62]
late effect 139.1
Panophthalmitis 360.02
Panotitis - *see* Otitis media
Pansinusitis (chronic) (hyperplastic)
(nonpurulent) (purulent) 473.8
acute 461.8
due to fungus NEC 117.9
tuberculous (*see also* Tuberculosis) 012.8
Panuveitis 360.12
sympathetic 360.11
Panvalvular disease - *see* Endocarditis,
mitral
Papageienkrankheit 073.9
Papanicolaou smear
cervix (screening test) V76.2
as part of gynecological examination
V72.31
for suspected malignant neoplasm
V76.2
no disease found V71.1
inadequate sample 795.08 ◄
nonspecific abnormal finding 795.00 ◄
with
atypical squamous cell changes
of undetermined
significance ◄▥
cannot exclude high grade
squamous intraepithelial
lesion (ASC-H) 795.01 ◄▥
of undetermined significance
(ASC-US) 795.02 ◄▥
high grade squamous intraepithelial lesion (HGSIL)
795.04 ◄
low grade squamous intraepithelial lesion (LGSIL)
795.03 ◄
favor benign (ASCUS favor benign) 795.01
favor dysplasia (ASCUS favor
dysplasia) 795.02
nonspecific findings NEC 795.09
to confirm findings of recent normal smear following initial
abnormal smear V72.32 ◄
unsatisfactory 795.08 ◄▥
other specified site - *see also* Screening,
malignant neoplasm
for suspected malignant neoplasm -
see also Screening, malignant neoplasm
no disease found V71.1
nonspecific abnormal finding 795.1
vagina V76.47
following hysterectomy for malignant condition V67.01
Papilledema 377.00
associated with
decreased ocular pressure 377.02
increased intracranial pressure 377.01
retinal disorder 377.03
choked disc 377.00
infectional 377.00
Papillitis 377.31
anus 569.49
chronic lingual 529.4
necrotizing, kidney 584.7
optic 377.31
rectum 569.49
renal, necrotizing 584.7
tongue 529.0

Papilloma (M8050/0) - *see also* Neoplasm, by site, benign

Note Except where otherwise indicated, the morphological varieties of
papilloma in the list below should be
coded by site as for "Neoplasm, benign".

Acuminatum (female) (male) 078.11
bladder (urinary) (transitional cell)
(M8120/1) 236.7
benign (M8120/0) 223.3
choroid plexus (M9390/0) 225.0
anaplastic type (M9390/3) 191.5
malignant (M9390/3) 191.5
ductal (M8503/0)
dyskeratotic (M8052/0)
epidermoid (M8052/0)
hyperkeratotic (M8052/0)
intracystic (M8504/0)
intraductal (M8503/0)
inverted (M8053/0)
keratotic (M8052/0)
parakeratotic (M8052/0)
pinta (primary) 103.0
renal pelvis (transitional cell) (M8120/
1) 236.99
benign (M8120/0) 223.1
Schneiderian (M8121/0)
specified site - *see* Neoplasm, by site,
benign
unspecified site 212.0
serous surface (M8461/0)
borderline malignancy (M8461/1)
specified site - *see* Neoplasm, by
site, uncertain behavior
unspecified site 236.2
specified site - *see* Neoplasm, by site,
benign
unspecified site 220
squamous (cell) (M8052/0)
transitional (cell) (M8120/0)
bladder (urinary) (M8120/1) 236.7
inverted type (M8121/1) - *see* Neoplasm, by site, uncertain behavior
renal pelvis (M8120/1) 236.91
ureter (M8120/1) 236.91
ureter (transitional cell) (M8120/1) 236.91
benign (M8120/0) 223.2
urothelial (M8120/1) - *see* Neoplasm,
by site, uncertain behavior
verrucous (M8051/0)
villous (M8261/1) - *see* Neoplasm, by
site, uncertain behavior
yaws, plantar or palmar 102.1
Papillomata, multiple, of yaws 102.1
Papillomatosis (M8060/0) - *see also* Neoplasm, by site, benign
confluent and reticulate 701.8
cutaneous 701.8
ductal, breast 610.1
Gougerot-Carteaud (confluent reticulate) 701.8
intraductal (diffuse) (M8505/0) - *see*
Neoplasm, by site, benign
subareolar duct (M8506/0) 217
Papillon-Léage and Psaume syndrome
(orodigitofacial dysostosis) 759.89
Papyraceous fetus 779.89
Papule 709.8
carate (primary) 103.0
fibrous, of nose (M8724/0) 216.3
pinta (primary) 103.0

Papulosis, malignant 447.8
Papyraceous fetus 779.8
complicating pregnancy 646.0
Paracephalus 759.7
Parachute mitral valve 746.5
Paracoccidioidomycosis 116.1
mucocutaneous-lymphangitic
116.1
pulmonary 116.1
visceral 116.1
Paracoccidiomycosis - *see* Paracoccidioidomycosis
Paracusis 388.40
Paradentosis 523.5
Paradoxical facial movements
374.43
Paraffinoma 999.9
Paraganglioma (M8680/1)
adrenal (M8700/0) 227.0
malignant (M8700/3) 194.0
aortic body (M8691/1) 237.3
malignant (M8691/3) 194.6
carotid body (M8692/1) 237.3
malignant (M8692/3) 194.5
chromaffin (M8700/0) - *see also* Neoplasm, by site, benign
malignant (M8700/3) - *see* Neoplasm, by site, malignant
extra-adrenal (M8693/1)
malignant (M8693/3)
specified site - *see* Neoplasm, by
site, malignant
unspecified site 194.6
specified site - *see* Neoplasm, by site,
uncertain behavior
unspecified site 237.3
glomus jugulare (M8690/1) 237.3
malignant (M8690/3) 194.6
jugular (M8690/1) 237.3
malignant (M8680/3)
specified site - *see* Neoplasm, by site,
malignant
unspecified site 194.6
nonchromaffin (M8693/1)
malignant (M8693/3)
specified site - *see* Neoplasm, by
site, malignant
unspecified site 194.6
specified site - *see* Neoplasm, by site,
uncertain behavior
unspecified site 237.3
parasympathetic (M8682/1)
specified site - *see* Neoplasm, by site,
uncertain behavior
unspecified site 237.3
specified site - *see* Neoplasm, by site,
uncertain behavior
sympathetic (M8681/1)
specified site - *see* Neoplasm, by site,
uncertain behavior
unspecified site 237.3
unspecified site 237.3
Parageusia 781.1
psychogenic 306.7
Paragonimiasis 121.2
Paragranuloma, Hodgkin's (M9660/3)
201.0
Parahemophilia (*see also* Defect, coagulation) 286.3
Parakeratosis 690.8
psoriasiformis 696.2
variegata 696.2
Paralysis, paralytic (complete) (incomplete) 344.9

◄ **New** ◄▥ **Revised**

Paralysis, paralytic (*Continued*)
with
  broken
    back - *see* Fracture, vertebra, by
      site, with spinal cord injury
    neck - *see* Fracture, vertebra, cervi-
      cal, with spinal cord injury
    fracture, vertebra - *see* Fracture, ver-
      tebra, by site, with spinal cord
      injury
  syphilis 094.89
abdomen and back muscles 355.9
abdominal muscles 355.9
abducens (nerve) 378.54
abductor 355.9
  lower extremity 355.8
  upper extremity 354.9
accessory nerve 352.4
accommodation 367.51
  hysterical 300.11
acoustic nerve 388.5
agitans 332.0
  arteriosclerotic 332.0
alternating 344.89
  oculomotor 344.89
amyotrophic 335.20
ankle 355.8
anterior serratus 355.9
anus (sphincter) 569.49
apoplectic (current episode) (*see also*
  Disease, cerebrovascular, acute)
  436
  late effect - *see* Late effect(s) (of)
    cerebrovascular disease
arm 344.40
  affecting
    dominant side 344.41
    nondominant side 344.42
  both 344.2
  hysterical 300.11
  late effect - *see* Late effect(s) (of)
    cerebrovascular disease
  psychogenic 306.0
  transient 781.4
    traumatic NEC (*see also* Injury,
      nerve, upper limb) 955.9
  arteriosclerotic (current episode)
    437.0
    late effect - *see* Late effect(s) (of)
      cerebrovascular disease
ascending (spinal), acute 357.0
associated, nuclear 344.89
asthenic bulbar 358.00
ataxic NEC 334.9
  general 094.1
athetoid 333.7
atrophic 356.9
  infantile, acute (*see also* Poliomyelitis,
    with paralysis) 045.1
  muscle NEC 355.9
  progressive 335.21
  spinal (acute) (*see also* Poliomyelitis,
    with paralysis) 045.1
attack (*see also* Disease, cerebrovascular, acute) 436
axillary 353.0
Babinski-Nageotte's 344.89
Bell's 351.0
  newborn 767.5
Benedikt's 344.89
birth (injury) 767.7
  brain 767.0
  intracranial 767.0
  spinal cord 767.4

Paralysis, paralytic (*Continued*)
bladder (sphincter) 596.53
  neurogenic 596.54
    with cauda equina syndrome
      344.61
  puerperal, postpartum, childbirth
    665.5
  sensory 596.54
    with cauda equina 344.61
  spastic 596.54
    with cauda equina 344.61
bowel, colon, or intestine (*see also* Ileus) 560.1
brachial plexus 353.0
  due to birth injury 767.6
  newborn 767.6
brain
  congenital - *see* Palsy, cerebral
  current episode 437.8
  diplegia 344.2
    late effect - *see* Late effect(s) (of)
      cerebrovascular disease
  hemiplegia 342.9
    late effect - *see* Late effect(s) (of)
      cerebrovascular disease
  infantile - *see* Palsy, cerebral
  monoplegia - *see also* Monoplegia
    late effect - *see* Late effect(s) (of)
      cerebrovascular disease
  paraplegia 344.1
  quadriplegia - *see* Quadriplegia
  syphilitic, congenital 090.49
  triplegia 344.89
bronchi 519.1
Brown-Séquard's 344.89
bulbar (chronic) (progressive) 335.22
  infantile (*see also* Poliomyelitis, bul-
    bar) 045.0
  poliomyelitic (*see also* Poliomyelitis,
    bulbar) 045.0
  pseudo 335.23
  supranuclear 344.89
bulbospinal 358.00
cardiac (*see also* Failure, heart) 428.9
cerebral
  current episode 437.8
  spastic, infantile - *see* Palsy, cerebral
cerebrocerebellar 437.8
  diplegic infantile 343.0
cervical
  plexus 353.2
  sympathetic NEC 337.0
Céstan-Chenais 344.89
Charcôt-Marie-Tooth type 356.1
childhood - *see* Palsy, cerebral
Clark's 343.9
colon (*see also* Ileus) 560.1
compressed air 993.3
compression
  arm NEC 354.9
  cerebral - *see* Paralysis, brain
  leg NEC 355.8
  lower extremity NEC 355.8
  upper extremity NEC 354.9
congenital (cerebral) (spastic) (spinal) -
  see Palsy, cerebral
conjugate movement (of eye) 378.81
  cortical (nuclear) (supranuclear)
    378.81
convergence 378.83
cordis (*see also* Failure, heart) 428.9
cortical (*see also* Paralysis, brain) 437.8
cranial or cerebral nerve (*see also* Disorder, nerve, cranial) 352.9

Paralysis, paralytic (*Continued*)
creeping 335.21
crossed leg 344.89
crutch 953.4
deglutition 784.9
  hysterical 300.11
dementia 094.1
descending (spinal) NEC 335.9
diaphragm (flaccid) 519.4
  due to accidental section of
    phrenic nerve during procedure
    998.2
digestive organs NEC 564.89
diplegic - *see* Diplegia
divergence (nuclear) 378.85
divers' 993.3
Duchenne's 335.22
due to intracranial or spinal birth injury - *see* Palsy, cerebral
embolic (current episode) (*see also* Embolism, brain) 434.1
  late effect - *see* Late effect(s) (of)
    cerebrovascular disease
enteric (*see also* Ileus) 560.1
  with hernia - *see* Hernia, by site,
    with obstruction
Erb's syphilitic spastic spinal 094.89
Erb (-Duchenne) (birth) (newborn)
  767.6
esophagus 530.89
essential, infancy (*see also* Poliomyelitis) 045.9
extremity
  lower - *see* Paralysis, leg
    spastic (hereditary) 343.3
      noncongenital or noninfantile
        344.1
    transient (cause unknown) 781.4
  upper - *see* Paralysis, arm
eye muscle (extrinsic) 378.55
  intrinsic 367.51
facial (nerve) 351.0
  birth injury 767.5
  congenital 767.5
  following operation NEC 998.2
  newborn 767.5
familial 359.3
  periodic 359.3
  spastic 334.1
fauces 478.29
finger NEC 354.9
foot NEC 355.8
gait 781.2
gastric nerve 352.3
gaze 378.81
general 094.1
  ataxic 094.1
  insane 094.1
  juvenile 090.40
  progressive 094.1
  tabetic 094.1
glossopharyngeal (nerve) 352.2
glottis (*see also* Paralysis, vocal cord)
  478.30
gluteal 353.4
Gubler (-Millard) 344.89
hand 354.9
  hysterical 300.11
  psychogenic 306.0
heart (*see also* Failure, heart) 428.9
hemifacial, progressive 349.89
hemiplegic - *see* Hemiplegia
hyperkalemic periodic (familial) 359.3
hypertensive (current episode) 437.8

Paralysis, paralytic (*Continued*)
    hypoglossal (nerve) 352.5
    hypokalemic periodic 359.3
    Hyrtl's sphincter (rectum) 569.49
    hysterical 300.11
    ileus (*see also* Ileus) 560.1
    infantile (*see also* Poliomyelitis) 045.9
        atrophic acute 045.1
        bulbar 045.0
        cerebral - *see* Palsy, cerebral
            paralytic 045.1
        progressive acute 045.9
        spastic - *see* Palsy, cerebral
        spinal 045.9
    infective (*see also* Poliomyelitis) 045.9
    inferior nuclear 344.9
    insane, general or progressive 094.1
    internuclear 378.86
    interosseous 355.9
    intestine (*see also* Ileus) 560.1
    intracranial (current episode) (*see also* Paralysis, brain) 437.8
        due to birth injury 767.0
    iris 379.49
        due to diphtheria (toxin) 032.81
            [379.49]
    ischemic, Volkmann's (complicating trauma) 958.6
    Jackson's 344.89
    jake 357.7
    Jamaica ginger (jake) 357.7
    juvenile general 090.40
    Klumpke (-Déjérine) (birth) (newborn) 767.6
    labioglossal (laryngeal) (pharyngeal) 335.22
    Landry's 357.0
    laryngeal nerve (recurrent) (superior) (*see also* Paralysis, vocal cord) 478.30
    larynx (*see also* Paralysis, vocal cord) 478.30
        due to diphtheria (toxin) 032.3
    late effect
        due to
            birth injury, brain or spinal (cord) - *see* Palsy, cerebral
            edema, brain or cerebral - *see* Paralysis, brain
            lesion
                cerebrovascular - *see* Late effect(s) (of) cerebrovascular disease
                spinal (cord) - *see* Paralysis, spinal
    lateral 335.24
    lead 984.9
        specified type of lead - *see* Table of Drugs and Chemicals
    left side - *see* Hemiplegia
    leg 344.30
        affecting
            dominant side 344.31
            nondominant side 344.32
        both (*see also* Paraplegia) 344.1
        crossed 344.89
        hysterical 300.11
        psychogenic 306.0
        transient or transitory 781.4
            traumatic NEC (*see also* Injury, nerve, lower limb) 956.9
    levator palpebrae superioris 374.31
    limb NEC 344.5
        all four - *see* Quadriplegia
        quadriplegia - *see* Quadriplegia
    lip 528.5

Paralysis, paralytic (*Continued*)
    Lissauer's 094.1
    local 355.9
    lower limb - *see also* Paralysis, leg
        both (*see also* Paraplegia) 344.1
    lung 518.89
        newborn 770.89
    median nerve 354.1
    medullary (tegmental) 344.89
    mesencephalic NEC 344.89
        tegmental 344.89
    middle alternating 344.89
    Millard-Gubler-Foville 344.89
    monoplegic - *see* Monoplegia
    motor NEC 344.9
        cerebral - *see* Paralysis, brain
        spinal - *see* Paralysis, spinal
    multiple
        cerebral - *see* Paralysis, brain
        spinal - *see* Paralysis, spinal
    muscle (flaccid) 359.9
        due to nerve lesion NEC 355.9
        eye (extrinsic) 378.55
            intrinsic 367.51
            oblique 378.51
        iris sphincter 364.8
        ischemic (complicating trauma) (Volkmann's) 958.6
        pseudohypertrophic 359.1
    muscular (atrophic) 359.9
        progressive 335.21
    musculocutaneous nerve 354.9
    musculospiral 354.9
    nerve - *see also* Disorder, nerve
        third or oculomotor (partial) 378.51
            total 378.52
        fourth or trochlear 378.53
        sixth or abducens 378.54
        seventh or facial 351.0
            birth injury 767.5
            due to
                injection NEC 999.9
                operation NEC 997.09
            newborn 767.5
        accessory 352.4
        auditory 388.5
        birth injury 767.7
        cranial or cerebral (*see also* Disorder, nerve, cranial) 352.9
        facial 351.0
            birth injury 767.5
            newborn 767.5
        laryngeal (*see also* Paralysis, vocal cord) 478.30
        newborn 767.7
        phrenic 354.8
            newborn 767.7
        radial 354.3
            birth injury 767.6
            newborn 767.6
        syphilitic 094.89
        traumatic NEC (*see also* Injury, nerve, by site) 957.9
        trigeminal 350.9
        ulnar 354.2
    newborn NEC 767.0
    normokalemic periodic 359.3
    obstetrical, newborn 767.7
    ocular 378.9
    oculofacial, congenital 352.6
    oculomotor (nerve) (partial) 378.51
        alternating 344.89
        external bilateral 378.55
        total 378.52

Paralysis, paralytic (*Continued*)
    olfactory nerve 352.0
    palate 528.9
    palatopharyngolaryngeal 352.6
    paratrigeminal 350.9
    periodic (familial) (hyperkalemic) (hypokalemic) (normokalemic) (secondary) 359.3
    peripheral
        autonomic nervous system - *see* Neuropathy, peripheral, autonomic
        nerve NEC 355.9
    peroneal (nerve) 355.3
    pharynx 478.29
    phrenic nerve 354.8
    plantar nerves 355.6
    pneumogastric nerve 352.3
    poliomyelitis (current) (*see also* Poliomyelitis, with paralysis) 045.1
        bulbar 045.0
    popliteal nerve 355.3
    pressure (*see also* Neuropathy, entrapment) 355.9
    progressive 335.21
        atrophic 335.21
        bulbar 335.22
        general 094.1
        hemifacial 349.89
        infantile, acute (*see also* Poliomyelitis) 045.9
        multiple 335.20
    pseudobulbar 335.23
    pseudohypertrophic 359.1
        muscle 359.1
    psychogenic 306.0
    pupil, pupillary 379.49
    quadriceps 355.8
    quadriplegic (*see also* Quadriplegia) 344.0
    radial nerve 354.3
        birth injury 767.6
    rectum (sphincter) 569.49
    rectus muscle (eye) 378.55
    recurrent laryngeal nerve (*see also* Paralysis, vocal cord) 478.30
    respiratory (muscle) (system) (tract) 786.09
        center NEC 344.89
            fetus or newborn 770.89
        congenital 768.9
        newborn 768.9
    right side - *see* Hemiplegia
    Saturday night 354.3
    saturnine 984.9
        specified type of lead - *see* Table of Drugs and Chemicals
    sciatic nerve 355.0
    secondary - *see* Paralysis, late effect
    seizure (cerebral) (current episode) (*see also* Disease, cerebrovascular, acute) 436
        late effect - *see* Late effect(s) (of) cerebrovascular disease
    senile NEC 344.9
    serratus magnus 355.9
    shaking (*see also* Parkinsonism) 332.0
    shock (*see also* Disease, cerebrovascular, acute) 436
        late effect - *see* Late effect(s) (of) cerebrovascular disease
    shoulder 354.9
    soft palate 528.9
    spasmodic - *see* Paralysis, spastic
    spastic 344.9

◄ **New**   ◄■■ **Revised**

Paralysis, paralytic (*Continued*)
  spastic (*Continued*)
    cerebral infantile - *see* Palsy, cerebral
    congenital (cerebral) - *see* Palsy, cerebral
    familial 334.1
    hereditary 334.1
    infantile 343.9
    noncongenital or noninfantile, cerebral 344.9
    syphilitic 094.0
      spinal 094.89
  sphincter, bladder (*see also* Paralysis, bladder) 596.53
  spinal (cord) NEC 344.1
    accessory nerve 352.4
    acute (*see also* Poliomyelitis) 045.9
    ascending acute 357.0
    atrophic (acute) (*see also* Poliomyelitis, with paralysis) 045.1
      spastic, syphilitic 094.89
    congenital NEC 343.9
    hemiplegic - *see* Hemiplegia
    hereditary 336.8
    infantile (*see also* Poliomyelitis) 045.9
    late effect NEC 344.89
    monoplegic - *see* Monoplegia
    nerve 355.9
    progressive 335.10
    quadriplegic - *see* Quadriplegia
    spastic NEC 343.9
    traumatic - *see* Injury, spinal, by site
  sternomastoid 352.4
  stomach 536.3
    diabetic 250.6 [536.3]
    nerve 352.3
  stroke (current episode) - *see* Infarct, brain ◀▥
    late effect - *see* Late effect(s) (of) cerebrovascular disease
  subscapularis 354.8
  superior nuclear NEC 334.9
  supranuclear 356.8
  sympathetic
    cervical NEC 337.0
    nerve NEC (*see also* Neuropathy, peripheral, autonomic) 337.9
    nervous system - *see* Neuropathy, peripheral, autonomic
  syndrome 344.9
    specified NEC 344.89
  syphilitic spastic spinal (Erb's) 094.89
  tabetic general 094.1
  thigh 355.8
  throat 478.29
    diphtheritic 032.0
    muscle 478.29
  thrombotic (current episode) (*see also* Thrombosis, brain) 434.0
    old - *see* Late effect(s) (of) cerebrovascular disease
  thumb NEC 354.9
  tick (-bite) 989.5
  Todd's (postepileptic transitory paralysis) 344.89
  toe 355.6
  tongue 529.8
  transient
    arm or leg NEC 781.4
    traumatic NEC (*see also* Injury, nerve, by site) 957.9
  trapezius 352.4
  traumatic, transient NEC (*see also* Injury, nerve, by site) 957.9

Paralysis, paralytic (*Continued*)
  trembling (*see also* Parkinsonism) 332.0
  triceps brachii 354.9
  trigeminal nerve 350.9
  trochlear nerve 378.53
  ulnar nerve 354.2
  upper limb - *see also* Paralysis, arm
    both (*see also* Diplegia) 344.2
  uremic - *see* Uremia
  uveoparotitic 135
  uvula 528.9
    hysterical 300.11
    postdiphtheritic 032.0
  vagus nerve 352.3
  vasomotor NEC 337.9
  velum palati 528.9
  vesical (*see also* Paralysis, bladder) 596.53
  vestibular nerve 388.5
  visual field, psychic 368.16
  vocal cord 478.30
    bilateral (partial) 478.33
      complete 478.34
    complete (bilateral) 478.34
    unilateral (partial) 478.31
      complete 478.32
  Volkmann's (complicating trauma) 958.6
  wasting 335.21
  Weber's 344.89
  wrist NEC 354.9
Paramedial orifice, urethrovesical 753.8
Paramenia 626.9
Parametritis (chronic) (*see also* Disease, pelvis, inflammatory) 614.4
  acute 614.3
  puerperal, postpartum, childbirth 670
Parametrium, parametric - *see* condition
Paramnesia (*see also* Amnesia) 780.93
Paramolar 520.1
  causing crowding 524.31 ◀▥
Paramyloidosis 277.3
Paramyoclonus multiplex 333.2
Paramyotonia 359.2
  congenita 359.2
Paraneoplastic syndrome - *see* condition
Parangi (*see also* Yaws) 102.9
Paranoia 297.1
  alcoholic 291.5
  querulans 297.8
  senile 290.20
Paranoid
  dementia (*see also* Schizophrenia) 295.3
    praecox (acute) 295.3
    senile 290.20
  personality 301.0
  psychosis 297.9
    alcoholic 291.5
    climacteric 297.2
    drug-induced 292.11
    involutional 297.2
    menopausal 297.2
    protracted reactive 298.4
    psychogenic 298.4
      acute 298.3
    senile 290.20
  reaction (chronic) 297.9
    acute 298.3
  schizophrenia (acute) (*see also* Schizophrenia) 295.3
  state 297.9
    alcohol-induced 291.5
    climacteric 297.2
    drug-induced 292.11

Paranoid (*Continued*)
  state (*Continued*)
    due to or associated with
      arteriosclerosis (cerebrovascular) 290.42
      presenile brain disease 290.12
      senile brain disease 290.20
    involutional 297.2
    menopausal 297.2
    senile 290.20
    simple 297.0
    specified type NEC 297.8
  tendencies 301.0
  traits 301.0
  trends 301.0
  type, psychopathic personality 301.0
Paraparesis (*see also* Paralysis) 344.9
Paraphasia 784.3
Paraphilia (*see also* Deviation, sexual) 302.9
Paraphimosis (congenital) 605
  chancroidal 099.0
Paraphrenia, paraphrenic (late) 297.2
  climacteric 297.2
  dementia (*see also* Schizophrenia) 295.3
  involutional 297.2
  menopausal 297.2
  schizophrenia (acute) (*see also* Schizophrenia) 295.3
Paraplegia 344.1
  with
    broken back - *see* Fracture, vertebra, by site, with spinal cord injury
    fracture, vertebra - *see* Fracture, vertebra, by site, with spinal cord injury
  ataxic - *see* Degeneration, combined, spinal cord
  brain (current episode) (*see also* Paralysis, brain) 437.8
  cerebral (current episode) (*see also* Paralysis, brain) 437.8
  congenital or infantile (cerebral) (spastic) (spinal) 343.0
  cortical - *see* Paralysis, brain
  familial spastic 334.1
  functional (hysterical) 300.11
  hysterical 300.11
  infantile 343.0
  late effect 344.1
  Pott's (*see also* Tuberculosis) 015.0 [730.88]
  psychogenic 306.0
  spastic
    Erb's spinal 094.89
    hereditary 334.1
    not infantile or congenital 344.1
  spinal (cord)
    traumatic NEC - *see* Injury, spinal, by site
  syphilitic (spastic) 094.89
  traumatic NEC - *see* Injury, spinal, by site
Paraproteinemia 273.2
  benign (familial) 273.1
  monoclonal 273.1
  secondary to malignant or inflammatory disease 273.1
Parapsoriasis 696.2
  en plaques 696.2
  guttata 696.2
  lichenoides chronica 696.2
  retiformis 696.2
  varioliformis (acuta) 696.2

ICD-9-CM

P

Vol. 2

Parascarlatina 057.8
Parasitic - *see also* condition
  disease NEC (*see also* Infestation, para-
    sitic) 136.9
    contact V01.89
    exposure to V01.89
    intestinal NEC 129
    skin NEC 134.9
  stomatitis 112.0
  sycosis 110.0
    beard 110.0
    scalp 110.0
  twin 759.4
Parasitism NEC 136.9
  intestinal NEC 129
  skin NEC 134.9
  specified - *see* Infestation
Parasitophobia 300.29
Parasomnia 780.59
  nonorganic origin 307.47
Paraspadias 752.69
Paraspasm facialis 351.8
Parathyroid gland - *see* condition
Parathyroiditis (autoimmune) 252.1
Parathyroprival tetany 252.1
Paratrachoma 077.0
Paratyphilitis (*see also* Appendicitis) 541
Paratyphoid (fever) - *see* Fever, paraty-
  phoid
Paratyphus - *see* Fever, paratyphoid
Paraurethral duct 753.8
Para-urethritis 597.89
  gonococcal (acute) 098.0
    chronic or duration of 2 months or
      over 098.2
Paravaccinia NEC 051.9
  milkers' node 051.1
Paravaginitis (*see also* Vaginitis) 616.10
Parencephalitis (*see also* Encephalitis)
  323.9
  late effect - *see* category 326
Parergasia 298.9
Paresis (*see also* Paralysis) 344.9
  accommodation 367.51
  bladder (spastic) (sphincter) (*see also*
    Paralysis, bladder) 596.53
    tabetic 094.0
  bowel, colon, or intestine (*see also* Il-
    eus) 560.1
  brain or cerebral - *see* Paralysis, brain
  extrinsic muscle, eye 378.55
  general 094.1
    arrested 094.1
    brain 094.1
    cerebral 094.1
    insane 094.1
    juvenile 090.40
      remission 090.49
    progressive 094.1
    remission (sustained) 094.1
    tabetic 094.1
  heart (*see also* Failure, heart) 428.9
  infantile (*see also* Poliomyelitis) 045.9
  insane 094.1
  juvenile 090.40
  late effect - *see* Paralysis, late effect
  luetic (general) 094.1
  peripheral progressive 356.9
  pseudohypertrophic 359.1
  senile NEC 344.9
  stomach 536.3
    diabetic 250.6 [536.3]
  syphilitic (general) 094.1
    congenital 090.40

Paresis (*Continued*)
  transient, limb 781.4
  vesical (sphincter) NEC 596.53
Paresthesia (*see also* Disturbance, sensation) 782.0
  Berger's (paresthesia of lower limb)
    782.0
  Bernhardt 355.1
  Magnan's 782.0
Paretic - *see* condition
Parinaud's
  conjunctivitis 372.02
  oculoglandular syndrome 372.02
  ophthalmoplegia 378.81
  syndrome (paralysis of conjugate up-
    ward gaze) 378.81
Parkes Weber and Dimitri syndrome
  (encephalocutaneous angiomatosis)
  759.6
Parkinson's disease, syndrome, or
  tremor - *see* Parkinsonism
Parkinsonism (arteriosclerotic) (idiopathic) (primary) 332.0
  associated with orthostatic hypotension
    (idiopathic) (symptomatic) 333.0
  due to drugs 332.1
  secondary 332.1
  syphilitic 094.82
Parodontitis 523.4
Parodontosis 523.5
Paronychia (with lymphangitis) 681.9
  candidal (chronic) 112.3
  chronic 681.9
    candidal 112.3
    finger 681.02
    toe 681.11
  finger 681.02
  toe 681.11
  tuberculous (primary) (*see also* Tuber-
    culosis) 017.0
Parorexia NEC 307.52
  hysterical 300.11
Parosmia 781.1
  psychogenic 306.7
Parotid gland - *see* condition
Parotiditis (*see also* Parotitis) 527.2
  epidemic 072.9
  infectious 072.9
Parotitis 527.2
  allergic 527.2
  chronic 527.2
  epidemic (*see also* Mumps) 072.9
  infectious (*see also* Mumps) 072.9
  noninfectious 527.2
  nonspecific toxic 527.2
  not mumps 527.2
  postoperative 527.2
  purulent 527.2
  septic 527.2
  suppurative (acute) 527.2
  surgical 527.2
  toxic 527.2
Paroxysmal - *see also* condition
  dyspnea (nocturnal) 786.09
Parrot's disease (syphilitic osteochondritis) 090.0
Parrot fever 073.9
Parry's disease or syndrome (exophthalmic goiter) 242.0
Parry-Romberg syndrome 349.89
Parson's disease (exophthalmic goiter)
  242.0
Parsonage-Aldren-Turner syndrome
  353.5

Parsonage-Turner syndrome 353.5
Pars planitis 363.21
Particolored infant 757.39
Parturition - *see* Delivery
Passage
  false, urethra 599.4
  of sounds or bougies (*see also* Atten-
    tion to artificial opening) V55.9
Passive - *see* condition
Pasteurella septica 027.2
Pasteurellosis (*see also* Infection, Pasteu-
  rella) 027.2
PAT (paroxysmal atrial tachycardia)
  427.0
Patau's syndrome (trisomy D$_1$) 758.1
Patch
  herald 696.3
Patches
  mucous (syphilitic) 091.3
    congenital 090.0
  smokers' (mouth) 528.6
Patellar - *see* condition
Patellofemoral syndrome 719.46
Patent - *see also* Imperfect closure
  atrioventricular ostium 745.69
  canal of Nuck 752.41
  cervix 622.5
    complicating pregnancy 654.5
      affecting fetus or newborn 761.0
  ductus arteriosus or Botalli 747.0
  Eustachian
    tube 381.7
    valve 746.89
  foramen
    Botalli 745.5
    ovale 745.5
  interauricular septum 745.5
  interventricular septum 745.4
  omphalomesenteric duct 751.0
  os (uteri) - *see* Patent, cervix
  ostium secundum 745.5
  urachus 753.7
  vitelline duct 751.0
Paternity testing V70.4
Paterson's syndrome (sideropenic dysphagia) 280.8
Paterson (-Brown) (-Kelly) **syndrome**
  (sideropenic dysphagia) 280.8
Paterson-Kelly syndrome or web (sideropenic dysphagia) 280.8
Pathologic, pathological - *see also* condition
  asphyxia 799.0
  drunkenness 291.4
  emotionality 301.3
  fracture - *see* Fracture, pathologic
  liar 301.7
  personality 301.9
  resorption, tooth 521.40 ◀▥
    external 521.42 ◀
    internal 521.41 ◀
    specified NEC 521.49 ◀
  sexuality (*see also* Deviation, sexual)
    302.9
Pathology (of) - *see* Disease
Patterned motor discharge, idiopathic
  (*see also* Epilepsy) 345.5
Patulous - *see also* Patent
  anus 569.49
  Eustachian tube 381.7
Pause, sinoatrial 427.81
Pavor nocturnus 307.46
Pavy's disease 593.6
Paxton's disease (white piedra) 111.2

Payr's disease or syndrome (splenic flexure syndrome) 569.89
Pearls
  Elschnig 366.51
  enamel 520.2
Pearl-workers' disease (chronic osteomyelitis) (*see also* Osteomyelitis) 730.1
Pectenitis 569.49
Pectenosis 569.49
Pectoral - *see* condition
Pectus
  carinatum (congenital) 754.82
    acquired 738.3
    rachitic (*see also* Rickets) 268.0
  excavatum (congenital) 754.81
    acquired 738.3
    rachitic (*see also* Rickets) 268.0
  recurvatum (congenital) 754.81
    acquired 738.3
Pedatrophia 261
Pederosis 302.2
Pediculosis (infestation) 132.9
  capitis (head louse) (any site) 132.0
  corporis (body louse) (any site) 132.1
  eyelid 132.0 [373.6]
  mixed (classifiable to more than one category in 132.0-132.2) 132.3
  pubis (pubic louse) (any site) 132.2
  vestimenti 132.1
  vulvae 132.2
Pediculus (infestation) - *see* Pediculosis
Pedophilia 302.2
Peg-shaped teeth 520.2
Pel's crisis 094.0
Pel-Ebstein disease - *see* Disease, Hodgkin's
Pelade 704.01
Pelger-Huët anomaly or syndrome (hereditary hyposegmentation) 288.2
Peliosis (rheumatica) 287.0
Pelizaeus-Merzbacher
  disease 330.0
  sclerosis, diffuse cerebral 330.0
Pellagra (alcoholic or with alcoholism) 265.2
  with polyneuropathy 265.2 [357.4]
Pellagra-cerebellar-ataxia-renal aminoaciduria syndrome 270.0
Pellegrini's disease (calcification, knee joint) 726.62
Pellegrini (-Stieda) disease or syndrome (calcification, knee joint) 726.62
Pellizzi's syndrome (pineal) 259.8
Pelvic - *see also* condition
  congestion-fibrosis syndrome 625.5
  kidney 753.3
Pelvioectasis 591
Pelviolithiasis 592.0
Pelviperitonitis
  female (*see also* Peritonitis, pelvic, female) 614.5
  male (*see also* Peritonitis) 567.2
Pelvis, pelvic - *see also* condition or type
  infantile 738.6
  Nägele's 738.6
  obliquity 738.6
  Robert's 755.69
Pemphigoid 694.5
  benign, mucous membrane 694.60
    with ocular involvement 694.61
  bullous 694.5
  cicatricial 694.60
    with ocular involvement 694.61
  juvenile 694.2

Pemphigus 694.4
  benign 694.5
    chronic familial 757.39
  Brazilian 694.4
  circinatus 694.0
  congenital, traumatic 757.39
  conjunctiva 694.61
  contagiosus 684
  erythematodes 694.4
  erythematosus 694.4
  foliaceus 694.4
  frambesiodes 694.4
  gangrenous (*see also* Gangrene) 785.4
  malignant 694.4
  neonatorum, newborn 684
  ocular 694.61
  papillaris 694.4
  seborrheic 694.4
  South American 694.4
  syphilitic (congenital) 090.0
  vegetans 694.4
  vulgaris 694.4
  wildfire 694.4
Pendred's syndrome (familial goiter with deaf-mutism) 243
Pendulous
  abdomen 701.9
    in pregnancy or childbirth 654.4
      affecting fetus or newborn 763.89
  breast 611.8
Penetrating wound - *see also* Wound, open, by site
  with internal injury - *see* Injury, internal, by site, with open wound
  eyeball 871.7
    with foreign body (nonmagnetic) 871.6
      magnetic 871.5
  ocular (*see also* Penetrating wound, eyeball) 871.7
    adnexa 870.3
      with foreign body 870.4
  orbit 870.3
    with foreign body 870.4
Penetration, pregnant uterus by instrument
  with
    abortion - *see* Abortion, by type, with damage to pelvic organs
    ectopic pregnancy (*see also* categories 633.0-633.9) 639.2
    molar pregnancy (*see also* categories 630-632) 639.2
  complication of delivery 665.1
    affecting fetus or newborn 763.89
  following
    abortion 639.2
    ectopic or molar pregnancy 639.2
Penfield's syndrome (*see also* Epilepsy) 345.5
Penicilliosis of lung 117.3
Penis - *see* condition
Penitis 607.2
Penta X syndrome 758.81
Pentalogy (of Fallot) 745.2
Pentosuria (benign) (essential) 271.8
Peptic acid disease 536.8
Peregrinating patient V65.2
Perforated - *see* Perforation
Perforation, perforative (nontraumatic)
  antrum (*see also* Sinusitis, maxillary) 473.0
  appendix 540.0
    with peritoneal abscess 540.1

Perforation, perforative (*Continued*)
  atrial septum, multiple 745.5
  attic, ear 384.22
    healed 384.81
  bile duct, except cystic (*see also* Disease, biliary) 576.3
    cystic 575.4
  bladder (urinary) 596.6
    with
      abortion - *see* Abortion, by type, with damage to pelvic organs
      ectopic pregnancy (*see also* categories 633.0-633.9) 639.2
      molar pregnancy (*see also* categories 630-632) 639.2
    following
      abortion 639.2
      ectopic or molar pregnancy 639.2
    obstetrical trauma 665.5
  bowel 569.83
    with
      abortion - *see* Abortion, by type, with damage to pelvic organs
      ectopic pregnancy (*see also* categories 633.0-633.9) 639.2
      molar pregnancy (*see also* categories 630-632) 639.2
    fetus or newborn 777.6
    following
      abortion 639.2
      ectopic or molar pregnancy 639.2
    obstetrical trauma 665.5
  broad ligament
    with
      abortion - *see* Abortion, by type, with damage to pelvic organs
      ectopic pregnancy (*see also* categories 633.0-633.9) 639.2
      molar pregnancy (*see also* categories 630-632) 639.2
    following
      abortion 639.2
      ectopic or molar pregnancy 639.2
    obstetrical trauma 665.6
  by
    device, implant, or graft - *see* Complications, mechanical
    foreign body left accidentally in operation wound 998.4
    instrument (any) during a procedure, accidental 998.2
  cecum 540.0
    with peritoneal abscess 540.1
  cervix (uteri) - *see also* Injury, internal, cervix
    with
      abortion - *see* Abortion, by type, with damage to pelvic organs
      ectopic pregnancy (*see also* categories 633.0-633.9) 639.2
      molar pregnancy (*see also* categories 630-632) 639.2
    following
      abortion 639.2
      ectopic or molar pregnancy 639.2
    obstetrical trauma 665.3
  colon 569.83
  common duct (bile) 576.3
  cornea (*see also* Ulcer, cornea) 370.00
    due to ulceration 370.06
  cystic duct 575.4
  diverticulum (*see also* Diverticula) 562.10
    small intestine 562.00

ICD-9-CM

P

Vol. 2

Perforation, perforative (Continued)

duodenum, duodenal (ulcer) - see Ulcer, duodenum, with perforation

ear drum - see Perforation, tympanum

enteritis - see Enteritis

esophagus 530.4

ethmoidal sinus (see also Sinusitis, ethmoidal) 473.2

foreign body (external site) - see also Wound, open, by site, complicated internal site, by ingested object - see Foreign body

frontal sinus (see also Sinusitis, frontal) 473.1

gallbladder or duct (see also Disease, gallbladder) 575.4

gastric (ulcer) - see Ulcer, stomach, with perforation

heart valve - see Endocarditis

ileum (see also Perforation, intestine) 569.83

instrumental

external - see Wound, open, by site

pregnant uterus, complicating delivery 665.9

surgical (accidental) (blood vessel) (nerve) (organ) 998.2

intestine 569.83

with

abortion - see Abortion, by type, with damage to pelvic organs

ectopic pregnancy (see also categories 633.0-633.9) 639.2

molar pregnancy (see also categories 630-632) 639.2

fetus or newborn 777.6

obstetrical trauma 665.5

ulcerative NEC 569.83

jejunum, jejunal 569.83

ulcer - see Ulcer, gastrojejunal, with perforation

mastoid (antrum) (cell) 383.89

maxillary sinus (see also Sinusitis, maxillary) 473.0

membrana tympani - see Perforation, tympanum

nasal

septum 478.1

congenital 748.1

syphilitic 095.8

sinus (see also Sinusitis) 473.9

congenital 748.1

palate (hard) 526.89

soft 528.9

syphilitic 095.8

syphilitic 095.8

palatine vault 526.89

syphilitic 095.8

congenital 090.5

pelvic

floor

with

abortion - see Abortion, by type, with damage to pelvic organs

ectopic pregnancy (see also categories 633.0-633.9) 639.2

molar pregnancy (see also categories 630-632) 639.2

obstetrical trauma 664.1

organ

with

abortion - see Abortion, by type, with damage to pelvic organs

Perforation, perforative (Continued)

pelvic (Continued)

organ (Continued)

with (Continued)

ectopic pregnancy (see also categories 633.0-633.9) 639.2

molar pregnancy (see also categories 630-632) 639.2

following

abortion 639.2

ectopic or molar pregnancy 639.2

obstetrical trauma 665.5

perineum - see Laceration, perineum

periurethral tissue

with

abortion - see Abortion, by type, with damage to pelvic organs

ectopic pregnancy (see also categories 630-632) 639.2

molar pregnancy (see also categories 630-632) 639.2

pharynx 478.29

pylorus, pyloric (ulcer) - see Ulcer, stomach, with perforation

rectum 569.49

sigmoid 569.83

sinus (accessory) (chronic) (nasal) (see also Sinusitis) 473.9

sphenoidal sinus (see also Sinusitis, sphenoidal) 473.3

stomach (due to ulcer) - see Ulcer, stomach, with perforation

surgical (accidental) (by instrument) (blood vessel) (nerve) (organ) 998.2

traumatic

external - see Wound, open, by site

eye (see also Penetrating wound, ocular) 871.7

internal organ - see Injury, internal, by site

tympanum (membrane) (persistent posttraumatic) (postinflammatory) 384.20

with

otitis media - see Otitis media

attic 384.22

central 384.21

healed 384.81

marginal NEC 384.23

multiple 384.24

pars flaccida 384.22

total 384.25

traumatic - see Wound, open, ear, drum

typhoid, gastrointestinal 002.0

ulcer - see Ulcer, by site, with perforation

ureter 593.89

urethra

with

abortion - see Abortion, by type, with damage to pelvic organs

ectopic pregnancy (see also categories 633.0-633.9) 639.2

molar pregnancy (see also categories 630-632) 639.2

following

abortion 639.2

ectopic or molar pregnancy 639.2

obstetrical trauma 665.5

Perforation, perforative (Continued)

uterus - see also Injury, internal, uterus

with

abortion - see Abortion, by type, with damage to pelvic organs

ectopic pregnancy (see also categories 633.0-633.9) 639.2

molar pregnancy (see also categories 630-632) 639.2

by intrauterine contraceptive device 996.32

following

abortion 639.2

ectopic or molar pregnancy 639.2

obstetrical trauma - see Injury, internal, uterus, obstetrical trauma

uvula 528.9

syphilitic 095.8

vagina - see Laceration, vagina

viscus NEC 799.89

traumatic 868.00

with open wound into cavity 868.10

Periadenitis mucosa necrotica recurrens 528.2

Periangiitis 446.0

Periantritis 535.4

Periappendicitis (acute) (see also Appendicitis) 541

Periarteritis (disseminated) (infectious) (necrotizing) (nodosa) 446.0

Periarthritis (joint) 726.90

Duplay's 726.2

gonococcal 098.50

humeroscapularis 726.2

scapulohumeral 726.2

shoulder 726.2

wrist 726.4

Periarthrosis (angioneural) - see Periarthritis

Peribronchitis 491.9

tuberculous (see also Tuberculosis) 011.3

Pericapsulitis, adhesive (shoulder) 726.0

Pericarditis (granular) (with decompensation) (with effusion) 423.9

with

rheumatic fever (conditions classifiable to 390)

active (see also Pericarditis, rheumatic) 391.0

inactive or quiescent 393

actinomycotic 039.8 [420.0]

acute (nonrheumatic) 420.90

with chorea (acute) (rheumatic) (Sydenham's) 392.0

bacterial 420.99

benign 420.91

hemorrhagic 420.90

idiopathic 420.91

infective 420.90

nonspecific 420.91

rheumatic 391.0

with chorea (acute) (rheumatic) (Sydenham's) 392.0

sicca 420.90

viral 420.91

adhesive or adherent (external) (internal) 423.1

acute - see Pericarditis, acute

rheumatic (external) (internal) 393

amebic 006.8 [420.0]

bacterial (acute) (subacute) (with serous or seropurulent effusion) 420.99

calcareous 423.2

Pericarditis *(Continued)*
  cholesterol (chronic) 423.8
    acute 420.90
  chronic (nonrheumatic) 423.8
    rheumatic 393
  constrictive 423.2
  Coxsackie 074.21
  due to
    actinomycosis 039.8 *[420.0]*
    amebiasis 006.8 *[420.0]*
    Coxsackie (virus) 074.21
    histoplasmosis *(see also* Histoplasmosis) 115.93
    nocardiosis 039.8 *[420.0]*
    tuberculosis *(see also* Tuberculosis) 017.9 *[420.0]*
  fibrinocaseous *(see also* Tuberculosis) 017.9 *[420.0]*
  fibrinopurulent 420.99
  fibrinous - *see* Pericarditis, rheumatic
  fibropurulent 420.99
  fibrous 423.1
  gonococcal 098.83
  hemorrhagic 423.0
  idiopathic (acute) 420.91
  infective (acute) 420.90
  meningococcal 036.41
  neoplastic (chronic) 423.8
    acute 420.90
  nonspecific 420.91
  obliterans, obliterating 423.1
  plastic 423.1
  pneumococcal (acute) 420.99
  postinfarction 411.0
  purulent (acute) 420.99
  rheumatic (active) (acute) (with effusion) (with pneumonia) 391.0
    with chorea (acute) (rheumatic) (Sydenham's) 392.0
    chronic or inactive (with chorea) 393
  septic (acute) 420.99
  serofibrinous - *see* Pericarditis, rheumatic
  staphylococcal (acute) 420.99
  streptococcal (acute) 420.99
  suppurative (acute) 420.99
  syphilitic 093.81
  tuberculous (acute) (chronic) *(see also* Tuberculosis) 017.9 *[420.0]*
  uremic 585 *[420.0]*
  viral (acute) 420.91
Pericardium, pericardial - *see* condition
Pericellulitis *(see also* Cellulitis) 682.9
Pericementitis 523.4
  acute 523.3
  chronic (suppurative) 523.4
Pericholecystitis *(see also* Cholecystitis) 575.10
Perichondritis
  auricle 380.00
    acute 380.01
    chronic 380.02
  bronchus 491.9
  ear (external) 380.00
    acute 380.01
    chronic 380.02
  larynx 478.71
    syphilitic 095.8
    typhoid 002.0 *[478.71]*
  nose 478.1
  pinna 380.00
    acute 380.01
    chronic 380.02
  trachea 478.9
Periclasia 523.5

Pericolitis 569.89
Pericoronitis (chronic) 523.4
  acute 523.3
Pericystitis *(see also* Cystitis) 595.9
Pericytoma (M9150/1) - *see also* Neoplasm, connective tissue, uncertain behavior
  benign (M9150/0) - *see* Neoplasm, connective tissue, benign
  malignant (M9150/3) - *see* Neoplasm, connective tissue, malignant
Peridacryocystitis, acute 375.32
Peridiverticulitis *(see also* Diverticulitis) 562.11
Periduodenitis 535.6
Periendocarditis *(see also* Endocarditis) 424.90
  acute or subacute 421.9
Periepididymitis *(see also* Epididymitis) 604.90
Perifolliculitis (abscedens) 704.8
  capitis, abscedens et suffodiens 704.8
  dissecting, scalp 704.8
  scalp 704.8
  superficial pustular 704.8
Perigastritis (acute) 535.0
Perigastrojejunitis (acute) 535.0
Perihepatitis (acute) 573.3
  chlamydial 099.56
  gonococcal 098.86
Peri-ileitis (subacute) 569.89
Perilabyrinthitis (acute) - *see* Labyrinthitis
Perimeningitis - *see* Meningitis
Perimetritis *(see also* Endometritis) 615.9
Perimetrosalpingitis *(see also* Salpingo-oophoritis) 614.2
Perineocele 618.05 ◄
Perinephric - *see* condition
Perinephritic - *see* condition
Perinephritis *(see also* Infection, kidney) 590.9
  purulent *(see also* Abscess, kidney) 590.2
Perineum, perineal - *see* condition
Perineuritis NEC 729.2
Periodic - *see also* condition
  disease (familial) 277.3
  edema 995.1
    hereditary 277.6
  fever 277.3
  limb movement disorder 780.58 ◄
  paralysis (familial) 359.3
  peritonitis 277.3
  polyserositis 277.3
  somnolence *(see also* Narcolepsy) 347.00 ◄◄◄
Periodontal
  cyst 522.8
  pocket 523.8
Periodontitis (chronic) (complex) (compound) (local) (simplex) 523.4
  acute 523.3
  apical 522.6
    acute (pulpal origin) 522.4
Periodontoclasia 523.5
Periodontosis 523.5
Periods - *see also* Menstruation
  heavy 626.2
  irregular 626.4
Perionychia (with lymphangitis) 681.9
  finger 681.02
  toe 681.11
Perioophoritis *(see also* Salpingo-oophoritis) 614.2

Periorchitis *(see also* Orchitis) 604.90
Periosteum, periosteal - *see* condition
Periostitis (circumscribed) (diffuse) (infective) 730.3

> Note   Use the following fifth-digit subclassification with category 730:
>
> 0   site unspecified
> 1   shoulder region
> 2   upper arm
> 3   forearm
> 4   hand
> 5   pelvic region and thigh
> 6   lower leg
> 7   ankle and foot
> 8   other specified sites
> 9   multiple sites

  with osteomyelitis *(see also* Osteomyelitis) 730.2
    acute or subacute 730.0
    chronic or old 730.1
  albuminosa, albuminosus 730.3
  alveolar 526.5
  alveolodental 526.5
  dental 526.5
  gonorrheal 098.89
  hyperplastica, generalized 731.2
  jaw (lower) (upper) 526.4
  monomelic 733.99
  orbital 376.02
  syphilitic 095.5
    congenital 090.0 *[730.8]*
    secondary 091.61
  tuberculous *(see also* Tuberculosis, bone) 015.9 *[730.8]*
  yaws (early) (hypertrophic) (late) 102.6
Periostosis *(see also* Periostitis) 730.3
  with osteomyelitis *(see also* Osteomyelitis) 730.2
    acute or subacute 730.0
    chronic or old 730.1
  hyperplastic 756.59
Peripartum cardiomyopathy 674.5
Periphlebitis *(see also* Phlebitis) 451.9
  lower extremity 451.2
    deep (vessels) 451.19
    superficial (vessels) 451.0
  portal 572.1
  retina 362.18
  superficial (vessels) 451.0
  tuberculous *(see also* Tuberculosis) 017.9
    retina 017.3 *[362.18]*
Peripneumonia - *see* Pneumonia
Periproctitis 569.49
Periprostatitis *(see also* Prostatitis) 601.9
Perirectal - *see* condition
Perirenal - *see* condition
Perisalpingitis *(see also* Salpingo-oophoritis) 614.2
Perisigmoiditis 569.89
Perisplenitis (infectional) 289.59
Perispondylitis - *see* Spondylitis
Peristalsis reversed or visible 787.4
Peritendinitis *(see also* Tenosynovitis) 726.90
  adhesive (shoulder) 726.0
Perithelioma (M9150/1) - *see* Pericytoma
Peritoneum, peritoneal - *see also* condition
  equilibration test V56.32
Peritonitis (acute) (adhesive) (fibrinous) (hemorrhagic) (idiopathic) (localized) (perforative) (primary) (with adhesions) (with effusion) 567.9

Peritonitis *(Continued)*
  with or following
    abortion - *see* Abortion, by type,
        with sepsis
    abscess 567.2
    appendicitis 540.0
        with peritoneal abscess 540.1
    ectopic pregnancy *(see also* categories
        633.0-633.9) 639.0
    molar pregnancy *(see also* categories
        630-632) 639.0
  aseptic 998.7
  bacterial 567.2
  bile, biliary 567.8
  chemical 998.7
  chlamydial 099.56
  chronic proliferative 567.8
  congenital NEC 777.6
  diaphragmatic 567.2
  diffuse NEC 567.2
  diphtheritic 032.83
  disseminated NEC 567.2
  due to
    bile 567.8
    foreign
      body or object accidentally left
          during a procedure (instru-
          ment) (sponge) (swab) 998.4
      substance accidentally left during
          a procedure (chemical) (pow-
          der) (talc) 998.7
    talc 998.7
    urine 567.8
  fibrinopurulent 567.2
  fibrinous 567.2
  fibrocaseous *(see also* Tuberculosis) 014.0
  fibropurulent 567.2
  general, generalized (acute) 567.2
  gonococcal 098.86
  in infective disease NEC 136.9 *[567.0]*
  meconium (newborn) 777.6
  pancreatic 577.8
  paroxysmal, benign 277.3
  pelvic
    female (acute) 614.5
      chronic NEC 614.7
        with adhesions 614.6
      puerperal, postpartum, childbirth
          670
    male (acute) 567.2
  periodic (familial) 277.3
  phlegmonous 567.2
  pneumococcal 567.1
  postabortal 639.0
  proliferative, chronic 567.8
  puerperal, postpartum, childbirth 670
  purulent 567.2
  septic 567.2
  staphylococcal 567.2
  streptococcal 567.2
  subdiaphragmatic 567.2
  subphrenic 567.2
  suppurative 567.2
  syphilitic 095.2
    congenital 090.0 *[567.0]*
  talc 998.7
  tuberculous *(see also* Tuberculosis) 014.0
  urine 567.8
Peritonsillar - *see* condition
Peritonsillitis 475
Perityphlitis *(see also* Appendicitis) 541
Periureteritis 593.89
Periurethral - *see* condition
Periurethritis (gangrenous) 597.89

Periuterine - *see* condition
Perivaginitis *(see also* Vaginitis) 616.10
Perivasculitis, retinal 362.18
Perivasitis (chronic) 608.4
Periventricular leukomalacia 779.7
Perivesiculitis (seminal) *(see also* Vesicu-
    litis) 608.0
Perlèche 686.8
  due to
    moniliasis 112.0
    riboflavin deficiency 266.0
Pernicious - *see* condition
Pernio, perniosis 991.5
Persecution
  delusion 297.9
  social V62.4
Perseveration (tonic) 784.69
Persistence, persistent (congenital)
    759.89
  anal membrane 751.2
  arteria stapedia 744.04
  atrioventricular canal 745.69
  bloody ejaculate 792.2
  branchial cleft 744.41
  bulbus cordis in left ventricle 745.8
  canal of Cloquet 743.51
  capsule (opaque) 743.51
  cilioretinal artery or vein 743.51
  cloaca 751.5
  communication - *see* Fistula, congenital
  convolutions
    aortic arch 747.21
    fallopian tube 752.19
    oviduct 752.19
    uterine tube 752.19
  double aortic arch 747.21
  ductus
    arteriosus 747.0
    Botalli 747.0
  fetal
    circulation 747.83
    form of cervix (uteri) 752.49
    hemoglobin (hereditary) ("Swiss va-
        riety") 282.7
    pulmonary hypertension 747.83
  foramen
    Botalli 745.5
    ovale 745.5
  Gartner's duct 752.11
  hemoglobin, fetal (hereditary) (HPFH)
      282.7
  hyaloid
    artery (generally incomplete) 743.51
    system 743.51
  hymen (tag)
    in pregnancy or childbirth 654.8
      causing obstructed labor 660.2
  lanugo 757.4
  left
    posterior cardinal vein 747.49
    root with right arch of aorta 747.21
    superior vena cava 747.49
  Meckel's diverticulum 751.0
  mesonephric duct 752.89
    fallopian tube 752.11
  mucosal disease (middle ear) (with
      posterior or superior marginal
      perforation of ear drum) 382.2
  nail(s), anomalous 757.5
  occiput, anterior or posterior 660.3
    fetus or newborn 763.1
  omphalomesenteric duct 751.0
  organ or site NEC - *see* Anomaly, spec-
      ified type NEC

Persistence, persistent *(Continued)*
  ostium
    atrioventriculare commune 745.69
    primum 745.61
    secundum 745.5
  ovarian rests in fallopian tube 752.19
  pancreatic tissue in intestinal tract
      751.5
  primary (deciduous)
    teeth 520.6
    vitreous hyperplasia 743.51
  pulmonary hypertension 747.83
  pupillary membrane 743.46
    iris 743.46
    Rhesus (Rh) titer 999.7
  right aortic arch 747.21
  sinus
    urogenitalis 752.89
    venosus with imperfect incorpora-
        tion in right auricle 747.49
  thymus (gland) 254.8
    hyperplasia 254.0
  thyroglossal duct 759.2
  thyrolingual duct 759.2
  truncus arteriosus or communis 745.0
  tunica vasculosa lentis 743.39
  umbilical sinus 753.7
  urachus 753.7
  vegetative state 780.03
  vitelline duct 751.0
  wolffian duct 752.89
Person (with)
  admitted for clinical research, as par-
      ticipant or control subject V70.7
  awaiting admission to adequate facility
      elsewhere V63.2
    undergoing social agency investiga-
        tion V63.8
  concern (normal) about sick person in
      family V61.49
  consulting on behalf of another V65.19
    pediatric pre-birth visit for expectant
        mother V65.11
  feared
    complaint in whom no diagnosis
        was made V65.5
    condition not demonstrated V65.5
  feigning illness V65.2
  healthy, accompanying sick person V65.0
  living (in)
    alone V60.3
    boarding school V60.6
    residence remote from hospital or
        medical care facility V63.0
    residential institution V60.6
    without
      adequate
        financial resources V60.2
        housing (heating) (space) V60.1
      housing (permanent) (temporary)
          V60.0
      material resources V60.2
      person able to render necessary
          care V60.4
      shelter V60.0
  medical services in home not available
      V63.1
  on waiting list V63.2
    undergoing social agency investiga-
        tion V63.8
  sick or handicapped in family V61.49
  "worried well" V65.5
Personality
  affective 301.10

Personality (*Continued*)
aggressive 301.3
amoral 301.7
anancastic, anankastic 301.4
antisocial 301.7
asocial 301.7
asthenic 301.6
avoidant 301.82
borderline 301.83
change 310.1
compulsive 301.4
cycloid 301.13
cyclothymic 301.13
dependent 301.6
depressive (chronic) 301.12
disorder, disturbance NEC 301.9
  with
    antisocial disturbance 301.7
    pattern disturbance NEC 301.9
    sociopathic disturbance 301.7
    trait disturbance 301.9
dual 300.14
dyssocial 301.7
eccentric 301.89
  "haltlose" type 301.89
emotionally unstable 301.59
epileptoid 301.3
explosive 301.3
fanatic 301.0
histrionic 301.50
hyperthymic 301.11
hypomanic 301.11
hypothymic 301.12
hysterical 301.50
immature 301.89
inadequate 301.6
labile 301.59
masochistic 301.89
morally defective 301.7
multiple 300.14
narcissistic 301.81
obsessional 301.4
obsessive-compulsive 301.4 ◀▥
overconscientious 301.4
paranoid 301.0
passive (-dependent) 301.6
passive-aggressive 301.84
pathologic NEC 301.9
pattern defect or disturbance 301.9
pseudosocial 301.7
psychoinfantile 301.59
psychoneurotic NEC 301.89
psychopathic 301.9
  with
    amoral trend 301.7
    antisocial trend 301.7
    asocial trend 301.7
    pathologic sexuality (*see also* Deviation, sexual) 302.9
  mixed types 301.9
schizoid 301.20
  introverted 301.21
  schizotypal 301.22
  with sexual deviation (*see also* Deviation, sexual) 302.9
  antisocial 301.7
  dyssocial 301.7
type A 301.4
unstable (emotional) 301.59
Perthes' disease (capital femoral osteochondrosis) 732.1
Pertussis (*see also* Whooping cough) 033.9
vaccination, prophylactic (against) V03.6

Peruvian wart 088.0
Perversion, perverted
appetite 307.52
  hysterical 300.11
function
  pineal gland 259.8
  pituitary gland 253.9
    anterior lobe
      deficient 253.2
      excessive 253.1
    posterior lobe 253.6
  placenta - *see* Placenta, abnormal
sense of smell or taste 781.1
  psychogenic 306.7
sexual (*see also* Deviation, sexual) 302.9
Pervious, congenital - *see also* Imperfect, closure
ductus arteriosus 747.0
Pes (congenital) (*see also* Talipes) 754.70
abductus (congenital) 754.60
  acquired 736.79
acquired NEC 736.79
  planus 734
adductus (congenital) 754.79
  acquired 736.79
cavus 754.71
  acquired 736.73
planovalgus (congenital) 754.69
  acquired 736.79
planus (acquired) (any degree) 734
  congenital 754.61
  rachitic 268.1
valgus (congenital) 754.61
  acquired 736.79
varus (congenital) 754.50
  acquired 736.79
Pest (*see also* Plague) 020.9
Pestis (*see also* Plague) 020.9
bubonica 020.0
fulminans 020.0
minor 020.8
pneumonica - *see* Plague, pneumonic
Petechia, petechiae 782.7
fetus or newborn 772.6
Petechial
fever 036.0
typhus 081.9
Petges-Cléjat or Petges-Clégat syndrome (poikilodermatomyositis) 710.3
Petit's
disease (*see also* Hernia, lumbar) 553.8
Petit mal (idiopathic) (*see also* Epilepsy) 345.0
status 345.2
Petrellidosis 117.6
Petrositis 383.20
acute 383.21
chronic 383.22
Peutz-Jeghers disease or syndrome 759.6
Peyronie's disease 607.85
Pfeiffer's disease 075
Phacentocele 379.32
traumatic 921.3
Phacoanaphylaxis 360.19
Phacocele (old) 379.32
traumatic 921.3
Phaehyphomycosis 117.8
Phagedena (dry) (moist) (*see also* Gangrene) 785.4
arteriosclerotic 440.24
geometric 686.09
penis 607.89
senile 440.24
sloughing 785.4

Phagedena (*Continued*)
tropical (*see also* Ulcer, skin) 707.9
vulva 616.50
Phagedenic - *see also* condition
abscess - *see also* Abscess
  chancroid 099.0
bubo NEC 099.8
chancre 099.0
ulcer (tropical) (*see also* Ulcer, skin) 707.9
Phagomania 307.52
Phakoma 362.89
Phantom limb (syndrome) 353.6
Pharyngeal - *see also* condition
arch remnant 744.41
pouch syndrome 279.11
Pharyngitis (acute) (catarrhal) (gangrenous) (infective) (malignant) (membranous) (phlegmonous) (pneumococcal) (pseudomembranous) (simple) (staphylococcal) (subacute) (suppurative) (ulcerative) (viral) 462
with influenza, flu, or grippe 487.1
aphthous 074.0
atrophic 472.1
chlamydial 099.51
chronic 472.1
Coxsackie virus 074.0
diphtheritic (membranous) 032.0
follicular 472.1
fusospirochetal 101
gonococcal 098.6
granular (chronic) 472.1
herpetic 054.79
hypertrophic 472.1
infectional, chronic 472.1
influenzal 487.1
lymphonodular, acute 074.8
septic 034.0
streptococcal 034.0
tuberculous (*see also* Tuberculosis) 012.8
vesicular 074.0
Pharyngoconjunctival fever 077.2
Pharyngoconjunctivitis, viral 077.2
Pharyngolaryngitis (acute) 465.0
chronic 478.9
septic 034.0
Pharyngoplegia 478.29
Pharyngotonsillitis 465.8
tuberculous 012.8
Pharyngotracheitis (acute) 465.8
chronic 478.9
Pharynx, pharyngeal - *see* condition
Phase of life problem NEC V62.89
Phenomenon
Arthus' - *see* Arthus' phenomenon
flashback (drug) 292.89
jaw-winking 742.8
Jod-Basedow 242.8
L. E. cell 710.0
lupus erythematosus cell 710.0
Pelger-Huët (hereditary hyposegmentation) 288.2
Raynaud's (paroxysmal digital cyanosis) (secondary) 443.0
Reilly's (*see also* Neuropathy, peripheral, autonomic) 337.9
vasomotor 780.2
vasospastic 443.9
vasovagal 780.2
Wenckebach's, heart block (second degree) 426.13
Phenylketonuria (PKU) 270.1

ICD-9-CM
P
Vol. 2

Phenylpyruvicaciduria 270.1
Pheochromoblastoma (M8700/3)
  specified site - *see* Neoplasm, by site,
    malignant
  unspecified site 194.0
Pheochromocytoma (M8700/0)
  malignant (M8700/3)
    specified site - *see* Neoplasm, by site,
      malignant
    unspecified site 194.0
  specified site - *see* Neoplasm, by site,
    benign
  unspecified site 227.0
Phimosis (congenital) 605
  chancroidal 099.0
  due to infection 605
Phlebectasia (*see also* Varicose, vein) 454.9
  congenital NEC 747.60
  esophagus (*see also* Varix, esophagus)
    456.1
    with hemorrhage (*see also* Varix,
      esophagus, bleeding) 456.0
Phlebitis (infective) (pyemic) (septic)
  (suppurative) 451.9
  antecubital vein 451.82
  arm NEC 451.84
    axillary vein 451.89
    basilic vein 451.82
    deep 451.83
    superficial 451.82
  basilic vein 451.82
  blue 451.9
  brachial vein 451.83
  breast, superficial 451.89
  cavernous (venous) sinus - *see* Phlebi-
    tis, intracranial sinus
  cephalic vein 451.82
  cerebral (venous) sinus - *see* Phlebitis,
    intracranial sinus
  chest wall, superficial 451.89
  complicating pregnancy or puerperium
    671.9
    affecting fetus or newborn 760.3
  cranial (venous) sinus - *see* Phlebitis,
    intracranial sinus
  deep (vessels) 451.19
    femoral vein 451.11
    specified vessel NEC 451.19
  due to implanted device - *see* Compli-
    cations, due to (presence of) any
    device, implant, or graft classified
    to 996.0-996.5 NEC
  during or resulting from a procedure
    997.2
  femoral vein (deep) (superficial) 451.11
  femoropopliteal 451.19
  following infusion, perfusion, or trans-
    fusion 999.2
  gouty 274.89 [*451.9*]
  hepatic veins 451.89
  iliac vein 451.81
  iliofemoral 451.11
  intracranial sinus (any) (venous) 325
    late effect - *see* category 326
    nonpyogenic 437.6
      in pregnancy or puerperium 671.5
  jugular vein 451.89
  lateral (venous) sinus - *see* Phlebitis,
    intracranial sinus
  leg 451.2
    deep (vessels) 451.19
      specified vessel NEC 451.19
    superficial (vessels) 451.0
      femoral vein 451.11

Phlebitis (*Continued*)
  longitudinal sinus - *see* Phlebitis, intra-
    cranial sinus
  lower extremity 451.2
    deep (vessels) 451.19
      femoral vein 451.11
      specified vessel NEC 451.19
    superficial (vessels) 451.0
      femoral vein 451.11
  migrans, migrating (superficial) 453.1
  pelvic
    with
      abortion - *see* Abortion, by type,
        with sepsis
      ectopic pregnancy (*see also* catego-
        ries 633.0-633.9) 639.0
      molar pregnancy (*see also* catego-
        ries 630-632) 639.0
    following
      abortion 639.0
      ectopic or molar pregnancy 639.0
    puerperal, postpartum 671.4
  popliteal vein 451.19
  portal (vein) 572.1
  postoperative 997.2
  pregnancy 671.9
    deep 671.3
    specified type NEC 671.5
    superficial 671.2
  puerperal, postpartum, childbirth 671.9
    deep 671.4
    lower extremities 671.2
    pelvis 671.4
    specified site NEC 671.5
    superficial 671.2
  radial vein 451.83
  retina 362.18
  saphenous (great) (long) 451.0
    accessory or small 451.0
  sinus (meninges) - *see* Phlebitis, intra-
    cranial sinus
  specified site NEC 451.89
  subclavian vein 451.89
  syphilitic 093.89
  tibial vein 451.19
  ulcer, ulcerative 451.9
    leg 451.2
      deep (vessels) 451.19
        femoral vein 451.11
        specified vessel NEC 451.19
      superficial (vessels) 451.0
        femoral vein 451.11
    lower extremity 451.2
      deep (vessels) 451.19
        femoral vein 451.11
        specified vessel NEC 451.19
      superficial (vessels) 451.0
  ulnar vein 451.83
  umbilicus 451.89
  upper extremity - *see* Phlebitis, arm
    deep (veins) 451.83
      brachial vein 451.83
      radial vein 451.83
      ulnar vein 451.83
    superficial (veins) 451.82
      antecubital vein 451.82
      basilic vein 451.82
      cephalic vein 451.82
  uterus (septic) (*see also* Endometritis)
    615.9
  varicose (leg) (lower extremity) (*see
    also* Varicose, vein) 454.1
Phlebofibrosis 459.89
Phleboliths 459.89

Phlebosclerosis 459.89
Phlebothrombosis - *see* Thrombosis
Phlebotomus fever 066.0
Phlegm, choked on 933.1
Phlegmasia
  alba dolens (deep vessels) 451.19
    complicating pregnancy 671.3
    nonpuerperal 451.19
    puerperal, postpartum, childbirth
      671.4
  cerulea dolens 451.19
Phlegmon (*see also* Abscess) 682.9
  erysipelatous (*see also* Erysipelas) 035
  iliac 682.2
    fossa 540.1
  throat 478.29
Phlegmonous - *see* condition
Phlyctenulosis (allergic) (keratoconjunctivitis) (nontuberculous) 370.31
  cornea 370.31
    with ulcer (*see also* Ulcer, cornea) 370.00
  tuberculous (*see also* Tuberculosis)
    017.3 [*370.31*]
Phobia, phobic (reaction) 300.20
  animal 300.29
  isolated NEC 300.29
  obsessional 300.3
  simple NEC 300.29
  social 300.23
  specified NEC 300.29
  state 300.20
Phocas' disease 610.1
Phocomelia 755.4
  lower limb 755.32
    complete 755.33
    distal 755.35
    proximal 755.34
  upper limb 755.22
    complete 755.23
    distal 755.25
    proximal 755.24
Phoria (*see also* Heterophoria) 378.40
Phosphate-losing tubular disorder 588.0
Phosphatemia 275.3
Phosphaturia 275.3
Photoallergic response 692.72
Photocoproporphyria 277.1
Photodermatitis (sun) 692.72
  light other than sun 692.82
Photokeratitis 370.24
Photo-ophthalmia 370.24
Photophobia 368.13
Photopsia 368.15
Photoretinitis 363.31
Photoretinopathy 363.31
Photosensitiveness (sun) 692.72
  light other than sun 692.82
Photosensitization skin (sun) 692.72
  light other than sun 692.82
Phototoxic response 692.72
Phrenitis 323.9
Phrynoderma 264.8
Phthiriasis (pubis) (any site) 132.2
  with any infestation classifiable to
    132.0 and 132.1 132.3
Phthirus infestation - *see* Phthiriasis
Phthisis (*see also* Tuberculosis) 011.9
  bulbi (infectional) 360.41
  colliers' 011.4
  cornea 371.05
  eyeball (due to infection) 360.41
  millstone makers' 011.4
  miners' 011.4
  potters' 011.4

◀ **New**   ◀▥ **Revised**

Phthisis (*Continued*)
sandblasters' 011.4
stonemasons' 011.4
Phycomycosis 117.7
Physalopteriasis 127.7
Physical therapy NEC V57.1
breathing exercises V57.0
Physiological cup, optic papilla
borderline, glaucoma suspect 365.00
enlarged 377.14
glaucomatous 377.14
Phytobezoar 938
intestine 936
stomach 935.2
Pian (*see also* Yaws) 102.9
Pianoma 102.1
Piarhemia, piarrhemia (*see also* Hyperlipemia) 272.4
bilharziasis 120.9
Pica 307.52
hysterical 300.11
Pick's
cerebral atrophy 331.11
with dementia
with behavioral disturbance 331.11
[294.11]
without behavioral disturbance
331.11 [294.10]
disease
brain 331.11
dementia in
with behavioral disturbance
331.11 [294.11]
without behavioral disturbance
331.11 [294.10]
lipid histiocytosis 272.7
liver (pericardial pseudocirrhosis of
liver) 423.2
pericardium (pericardial pseudocirrhosis of liver) 423.2
polyserositis (pericardial pseudocirrhosis of liver) 423.2
syndrome
heart (pericardial pseudocirrhosis of
liver) 423.2
liver (pericardial pseudocirrhosis of
liver) 423.2
tubular adenoma (M8640/0)
specified site - *see* Neoplasm, by site,
benign
unspecified site
female 220
male 222.0
Pick-Herxheimer syndrome (diffuse idiopathic cutaneous atrophy) 701.8
Pick-Niemann disease (lipid histiocytosis) 272.7
Pickwickian syndrome (cardiopulmonary obesity) 278.8
Piebaldism, classic 709.09
Piedra 111.2
beard 111.2
black 111.3
white 111.2
black 111.3
scalp 111.3
black 111.3
white 111.2
white 111.2
Pierre Marie's syndrome (pulmonary
hypertrophic osteoarthropathy) 731.2
Pierre Marie-Bamberger syndrome (hypertrophic pulmonary osteoarthropathy) 731.2

Pierre Mauriac's syndrome (diabetes-
dwarfism-obesity) 258.1
Pierre Robin deformity or syndrome
(congenital) 756.0
Pierson's disease or osteochondrosis 732.1
Pigeon
breast or chest (acquired) 738.3
congenital 754.82
rachitic (*see also* Rickets) 268.0
breeders' disease or lung 495.2
fanciers' disease or lung 495.2
toe 735.8
Pigmentation (abnormal) 709.00
anomalies NEC 709.00
congenital 757.33
specified NEC 709.09
conjunctiva 372.55
cornea 371.10
anterior 371.11
posterior 371.13
stromal 371.12
lids (congenital) 757.33
acquired 374.52
limbus corneae 371.10
metals 709.00
optic papilla, congenital 743.57
retina (congenital) (grouped) (nevoid)
743.53
acquired 362.74
scrotum, congenital 757.33
Piles - *see* Hemorrhoids
Pili
annulati or torti (congenital) 757.4
incarnati 704.8
Pill roller hand (intrinsic) 736.09
Pilomatrixoma (M8110/0) - *see* Neoplasm, skin, benign
Pilonidal - *see* condition
Pimple 709.8
**PIN I (prostatic intraepithelial neo-
plasia I)** 602.3
**PIN II (prostatic intraepithelial neo-
plasia II)** 602.3
**PIN III (prostatic intraepithelial neo-
plasia III)** 233.4
Pinched nerve - *see* Neuropathy, entrap-
ment
Pineal body or gland - *see* condition
Pinealoblastoma (M9362/3) 194.4
Pinealoma (M9360/1) 237.1
malignant (M9360/3) 194.4
Pineoblastoma (M9362/3) 194.4
Pineocytoma (M9361/1) 237.1
Pinguecula 372.51
Pinhole meatus (*see also* Stricture, urethra) 598.9
Pink
disease 985.0
eye 372.03
puffer 492.8
Pinkus' disease (lichen nitidus) 697.1
Pinpoint
meatus (*see also* Stricture, urethra) 598.9
os (uteri) (*see also* Stricture, cervix) 622.4
Pinselhaare (congenital) 757.4
Pinta 103.9
cardiovascular lesions 103.2
chancre (primary) 103.0
erythematous plaques 103.1
hyperchromic lesions 103.1
hyperkeratosis 103.1
lesions 103.9
cardiovascular 103.2
hyperchromic 103.1

Pinta (*Continued*)
lesions (*Continued*)
intermediate 103.1
late 103.2
mixed 103.3
primary 103.0
skin (achromic) (cicatricial) (dyschromic) 103.2
hyperchromic 103.1
mixed (achromic and hyperchromic) 103.3
papule (primary) 103.0
skin lesions (achromic) (cicatricial)
(dyschromic) 103.2
hyperchromic 103.1
mixed (achromic and hyperchromic)
103.3
vitiligo 103.2
Pintid 103.0
Pinworms (disease) (infection) (infestation) 127.4
Piry fever 066.8
Pistol wound - *see* Gunshot wound
Pit, lip (mucus), congenital 750.25
Pitchers' elbow 718.82
Pithecoid pelvis 755.69
with disproportion (fetopelvic) 653.2
affecting fetus or newborn 763.1
causing obstructed labor 660.1
Pithiatism 300.11
Pitted - *see also* Pitting
teeth 520.4
Pitting (edema) (*see also* Edema) 782.3
lip 782.3
nail 703.8
congenital 757.5
Pituitary gland - *see* condition
Pituitary snuff-takers' disease 495.8
Pityriasis 696.5
alba 696.5
capitis 690.11
circinata (et maculata) 696.3
Hebra's (exfoliative dermatitis)
695.89
lichenoides et varioliformis 696.2
maculata (et circinata) 696.3
nigra 111.1
pilaris 757.39
acquired 701.1
Hebra's 696.4
rosea 696.3
rotunda 696.3
rubra (Hebra) 695.89
pilaris 696.4
sicca 690.18
simplex 690.18
specified type NEC 696.5
streptogenes 696.5
versicolor 111.0
scrotal 111.0
Placenta, placental
ablatio 641.2
affecting fetus or newborn 762.1
abnormal, abnormality 656.7
with hemorrhage 641.8
affecting fetus or newborn 762.1
affecting fetus or newborn 762.2
abruptio 641.2
affecting fetus or newborn 762.1
accessory lobe - *see* Placenta, abnormal
accreta (without hemorrhage) 667.0
with hemorrhage 666.0
adherent (without hemorrhage) 667.0
with hemorrhage 666.0

ICD-9-CM

P

Vol. 2

Placenta, placental *(Continued)*
  apoplexy - *see* Placenta, separation
  battledore - *see* Placenta, abnormal
  bilobate - *see* Placenta, abnormal
  bipartita - *see* Placenta, abnormal
  carneous mole 631
  centralis - *see* Placenta, previa
  circumvallata - *see* Placenta, abnormal
  cyst (amniotic) - *see* Placenta, abnormal
  deficiency - *see* Placenta, insufficiency
  degeneration - *see* Placenta, insufficiency
  detachment (partial) (premature) (with hemorrhage) 641.2
    affecting fetus or newborn 762.1
  dimidiata - *see* Placenta, abnormal
  disease 656.7
    affecting fetus or newborn 762.2
  duplex - *see* Placenta, abnormal
  dysfunction - *see* Placenta, insufficiency
  fenestrata - *see* Placenta, abnormal
  fibrosis - *see* Placenta, abnormal
  fleshy mole 631
  hematoma - *see* Placenta, abnormal
  hemorrhage NEC - *see* Placenta, separation
  hormone disturbance or malfunction - *see* Placenta, abnormal
  hyperplasia - *see* Placenta, abnormal
  increta (without hemorrhage) 667.0
    with hemorrhage 666.0
  infarction 656.7
    affecting fetus or newborn 762.2
  insertion, vicious - *see* Placenta, previa
  insufficiency
    affecting
      fetus or newborn 762.2
      management of pregnancy 656.5
  lateral - *see* Placenta, previa
  low implantation or insertion - *see* Placenta, previa
  low-lying - *see* Placenta, previa
  malformation - *see* Placenta, abnormal
  malposition - *see* Placenta, previa
  marginalis, marginata - *see* Placenta, previa
  marginal sinus (hemorrhage) (rupture) 641.2
    affecting fetus or newborn 762.1
  membranacea - *see* Placenta, abnormal
  multilobed - *see* Placenta, abnormal
  multipartita - *see* Placenta, abnormal
  necrosis - *see* Placenta, abnormal
  percreta (without hemorrhage) 667.0
    with hemorrhage 666.0
  polyp 674.4
  previa (central) (centralis) (complete) (lateral) (marginal) (marginalis) (partial) (partialis) (total) (with hemorrhage) 641.1
    affecting fetus or newborn 762.0
    noted
      before labor, without hemorrhage (with cesarean delivery) 641.0
      during pregnancy (without hemorrhage) 641.0
    without hemorrhage (before labor and delivery) (during pregnancy) 641.0
  retention (with hemorrhage) 666.0
    fragments, complicating puerperium (delayed hemorrhage) 666.2
      without hemorrhage 667.1
    postpartum, puerperal 666.2
    without hemorrhage 667.0

Placenta, placental *(Continued)*
  separation (normally implanted) (partial) (premature) (with hemorrhage) 641.2
    affecting fetus or newborn 762.1
  septuplex - *see* Placenta, abnormal
  small - *see* Placenta, insufficiency
  softening (premature) - *see* Placenta, abnormal
  spuria - *see* Placenta, abnormal
  succenturiata - *see* Placenta, abnormal
  syphilitic 095.8
  transfusion syndromes 762.3
  transmission of chemical substance - *see* Absorption, chemical, through placenta
  trapped (with hemorrhage) 666.0
    without hemorrhage 667.0
  trilobate - *see* Placenta, abnormal
  tripartita - *see* Placenta, abnormal
  triplex - *see* Placenta, abnormal
  varicose vessel - *see* Placenta, abnormal
  vicious insertion - *see* Placenta, previa
Placentitis
  affecting fetus or newborn 762.7
  complicating pregnancy 658.4
Plagiocephaly (skull) 754.0
Plague 020.9
  abortive 020.8
  ambulatory 020.8
  bubonic 020.0
  cellulocutaneous 020.1
  lymphatic gland 020.0
  pneumonic 020.5
    primary 020.3
    secondary 020.4
  pulmonary - *see* Plague, pneumonic
  pulmonic - *see* Plague, pneumonic
  septicemic 020.2
  tonsillar 020.9
    septicemic 020.2
  vaccination, prophylactic (against) V03.3
Planning, family V25.09
  contraception V25.9
  procreation V26.4
Plaque
  artery, arterial - *see* Arteriosclerosis
  calcareous - *see* Calcification
  Hollenhorst's (retinal) 362.33
  tongue 528.6
Plasma cell myeloma 203.0
Plasmacytoma, plasmocytoma (solitary) (M9731/1) 238.6
  benign (M9731/0) - *see* Neoplasm, by site, benign
  malignant (M9731/3) 203.8
Plasmacytosis 288.8
Plaster ulcer (*see also* Decubitus) 707.00 ◀▬
Platybasia 756.0
Platyonychia (congenital) 757.5
  acquired 703.8
Platypelloid pelvis 738.6
  with disproportion (fetopelvic) 653.2
    affecting fetus or newborn 763.1
    causing obstructed labor 660.1
      affecting fetus or newborn 763.1
  congenital 755.69
Platyspondylia 756.19
Plethora 782.62
  newborn 776.4
Pleura, pleural - *see* condition
Pleuralgia 786.52

Pleurisy (acute) (adhesive) (chronic) (costal) (diaphragmatic) (double) (dry) (fetid) (fibrinous) (fibrous) (interlobar) (latent) (lung) (old) (plastic) (primary) (residual) (sicca) (sterile) (subacute) (unresolved) (with adherent pleura) 511.0
  with
    effusion (without mention of cause) 511.9
      bacterial, nontuberculous 511.1
      nontuberculous NEC 511.9
        bacterial 511.1
      pneumococcal 511.1
      specified type NEC 511.8
      staphylococcal 511.1
      streptococcal 511.1
      tuberculous (*see also* Tuberculosis, pleura) 012.0
        primary, progressive 010.1
    influenza, flu, or grippe 487.1
    tuberculosis - *see* Pleurisy, tuberculous
  encysted 511.8
  exudative (*see also* Pleurisy, with effusion) 511.9
    bacterial, nontuberculous 511.1
  fibrinopurulent 510.9
    with fistula 510.0
  fibropurulent 510.9
    with fistula 510.0
  hemorrhagic 511.8
  influenzal 487.1
  pneumococcal 511.0
    with effusion 511.1
  purulent 510.9
    with fistula 510.0
  septic 510.9
    with fistula 510.0
  serofibrinous (*see also* Pleurisy, with effusion) 511.9
    bacterial, nontuberculous 511.1
  seropurulent 510.9
    with fistula 510.0
  serous (*see also* Pleurisy, with effusion) 511.9
    bacterial, nontuberculous 511.1
  staphylococcal 511.0
    with effusion 511.1
  streptococcal 511.0
    with effusion 511.1
  suppurative 510.9
    with fistula 510.0
  traumatic (post) (current) 862.29
    with open wound into cavity 862.39
  tuberculous (with effusion) (*see also* Tuberculosis, pleura) 012.0
    primary, progressive 010.1
Pleuritis sicca - *see* Pleurisy
Pleurobronchopneumonia (*see also* Pneumonia, broncho-) 485
Pleurodynia 786.52
  epidemic 074.1
  viral 074.1
Pleurohepatitis 573.8
Pleuropericarditis (*see also* Pericarditis) 423.9
  acute 420.90
Pleuropneumonia (acute) (bilateral) (double) (septic) (*see also* Pneumonia) 486
  chronic (*see also* Fibrosis, lung) 515
Pleurorrhea (*see also* Hydrothorax) 511.8
Plexitis, brachial 353.0

◀ **New**   ◀▬ **Revised**

Plica
knee 727.83
polonica 132.0
tonsil 474.8
Plicae dysphonia ventricularis 784.49
Plicated tongue 529.5
congenital 750.13
Plug
bronchus NEC 519.1
meconium (newborn) NEC 777.1
mucus - *see* Mucus, plug
Plumbism 984.9
specified type of lead - *see* Table of
Drugs and Chemicals
Plummer's disease (toxic nodular goiter)
242.3
Plummer-Vinson syndrome (sideropenic
dysphagia) 280.8
Pluricarential syndrome of infancy 260
Plurideficiency syndrome of infancy 260
Plus (and minus) hand (intrinsic) 736.09
PMDD (premenstrual dysphoric disor-
der) 625.4
PMS 625.4
Pneumathemia - *see* Air, embolism, by type
Pneumatic drill or hammer disease 994.9
Pneumatocele (lung) 518.89
intracranial 348.8
tension 492.0
Pneumatosis
cystoides intestinalis 569.89
peritonei 568.89
pulmonum 492.8
Pneumaturia 599.84
Pneumoblastoma (M8981/3) - *see* Neoplasm, lung, malignant
Pneumocephalus 348.8
Pneumococcemia 038.2
Pneumococcus, pneumococcal - *see* condition
Pneumoconiosis (due to) (inhalation of)
505
aluminum 503
asbestos 501
bagasse 495.1
bauxite 503
beryllium 503
carbon electrode makers' 503
coal
miners' (simple) 500
workers' (simple) 500
cotton dust 504
diatomite fibrosis 502
dust NEC 504
inorganic 503
lime 502
marble 502
organic NEC 504
fumes or vapors (from silo) 506.9
graphite 503
hard metal 503
mica 502
moldy hay 495.0
rheumatoid 714.81
silica NEC 502
and carbon 500
silicate NEC 502
talc 502
Pneumocystis carinii pneumonia 136.3
Pneumocystosis 136.3
with pneumonia 136.3
Pneumoenteritis 025
Pneumohemopericardium (*see also* Pericarditis) 423.9

Pneumohemothorax (*see also* Hemothorax) 511.8
traumatic 860.4
with open wound into thorax 860.5
Pneumohydropericardium (*see also* Pericarditis) 423.9
Pneumohydrothorax (*see also* Hydrothorax) 511.8
Pneumomediastinum 518.1
congenital 770.2
fetus or newborn 770.2
Pneumomycosis 117.9
Pneumonia (acute) (Alpenstich) (benign)
(bilateral) (brain) (cerebral) (circumscribed) (congestive) (creeping) (delayed resolution) (double) (epidemic)
(fever) (flash) (fulminant) (fungoid)
(granulomatous) (hemorrhagic) (incipient) (infantile) (infectious) (infiltration) (insular) (intermittent) (latent) (lobe) (migratory) (newborn)
(organized) (overwhelming) (primary) (progressive) (pseudolobar)
(purulent) (resolved) (secondary) (senile) (septic) (suppurative) (terminal)
(true) (unresolved) (vesicular) 486
with influenza, flu, or grippe 487.0
adenoviral 480.0
adynamic 514
alba 090.0
allergic 518.3
alveolar - *see* Pneumonia, lobar
anaerobes 482.81
anthrax 022.1 [484.5]
apex, apical - *see* Pneumonia, lobar
ascaris 127.0 [484.8]
aspiration 507.0
due to
aspiration of microorganisms
bacterial 482.9
specified type NEC 482.89
specified organism NEC 483.8
bacterial NEC 482.89
viral 480.9
specified type NEC 480.8
food (regurgitated) 507.0
gastric secretions 507.0
milk 507.0
oils, essences 507.1
solids, liquids NEC 507.8
vomitus 507.0
newborn 770.1
asthenic 514
atypical (disseminated) (focal) (primary) 486
with influenza 487.0
bacillus 482.9
specified type NEC 482.89
bacterial 482.9
specified type NEC 482.89
Bacteroides (fragilis) (oralis) (melaninogenicus) 482.81
basal, basic, basilar - *see* Pneumonia,
lobar
broncho-, bronchial (confluent) (croupous) (diffuse) (disseminated)
(hemorrhagic) (involving lobes)
(lobar) (terminal) 485
with influenza 487.0
allergic 518.3
aspiration (*see also* Pneumonia, aspiration) 507.0
bacterial 482.9
specified type NEC 482.89

Pneumonia (*Continued*)
broncho-, bronchial (*Continued*)
capillary 466.19
with bronchospasm or obstruction
466.19
chronic (*see also* Fibrosis, lung) 515
congenital (infective) 770.0
diplococcal 481
Eaton's agent 483.0
Escherichia coli (E. coli) 482.82
Friedlander's bacillus 482.0
Haemophilus influenzae 482.2
hiberno-vernal 083.0 [484.8]
hypostatic 514
influenzal 487.0
inhalation (*see also* Pneumonia, aspiration) 507.0
due to fumes or vapors (chemical)
506.0
Klebsiella 482.0
lipid 507.1
endogenous 516.8
Mycoplasma (pneumoniae) 483.0
ornithosis 073.0
pleuropneumonia-like organisms
(PPLO) 483.0
pneumococcal 481
Proteus 482.83
Pseudomonas 482.1
specified organism NEC 483.8
bacterial NEC 482.89
staphylococcal 482.40
aureus 482.41
specified type NEC 482.49
streptococcal - *see* Pneumonia, streptococcal
typhoid 002.0 [484.8]
viral, virus (*see also* Pneumonia, viral) 480.9
butyrivibirio (fibriosolvens) 482.81
candida 112.4
capillary 466.19
with bronchospasm or obstruction
466.19
caseous (*see also* Tuberculosis) 011.6
catarrhal - *see* Pneumonia, broncho-
central - *see* Pneumonia, lobar
chlamydia, chlamydial 483.1
pneumoniae 483.1
psittaci 073.0
specified type NEC 483.1
trachomatis 483.1
cholesterol 516.8
chronic (*see also* Fibrosis, lung) 515
cirrhotic (chronic) (*see also* Fibrosis,
lung) 515
clostridium (haemolyticum) (novyi)
NEC 482.81
confluent - *see* Pneumonia, broncho-
congenital (infective) 770.0
aspiration 770.1
croupous - *see* Pneumonia, lobar
cytomegalic inclusion 078.5 [484.1]
deglutition (*see also* Pneumonia, aspiration) 507.0
desquamative interstitial 516.8
diffuse - *see* Pneumonia, broncho-
diplococcal, diplococcus (broncho-) (lobar) 481
disseminated (focal) - *see* Pneumonia,
broncho-
due to
adenovirus 480.0
anaerobes 482.81

Pneumonia (*Continued*)
  due to (*Continued*)
    Bacterium anitratum 482.83
    Chlamydia, chlamydial 483.1
      pneumoniae 483.1
      psittaci 073.0
      specified type NEC 483.1
      trachomatis 483.1
    coccidioidomycosis 114.0
    Diplococcus (pneumoniae) 481
    Eaton's agent 483.0
    Escherichia coli (E. coli) 482.82
    Friedlander's bacillus 482.0
    fumes or vapors (chemical) (inhalation) 506.0
    fungus NEC 117.9 *[484.7]*
      coccidioidomycosis 114.0
    Haemophilus influenzae (H. influenzae) 482.2
    Herellea 482.83
    influenza 487.0
    Klebsiella pneumoniae 482.0
    Mycoplasma (pneumoniae) 483.0
    parainfluenza virus 480.2
    pleuropneumonia-like organism (PPLO) 483.0
    Pneumococcus 481
    Pneumocystis carinii 136.3
    Proteus 482.83
    Pseudomonas 482.1
    respiratory syncytial virus 480.1
    rickettsia 083.9 *[484.8]*
    SARS-associated coronavirus 480.3
    specified
      bacteria NEC 482.89
      organism NEC 483.8
      virus NEC 480.8
    Staphylococcus 482.40
      aureus 482.41
      specified type NEC 482.49
    Streptococcus - *see also* Pneumonia, streptococcal
      pneumoniae 481
    virus (*see also* Pneumonia, viral) 480.9
  Eaton's agent 483.0
  embolic, embolism (*see* Embolism, pulmonary) 415.19
  eosinophilic 518.3
  Escherichia coli (E. coli) 482.82
  eubacterium 482.81
  fibrinous - *see* Pneumonia, lobar
  fibroid (chronic) (*see also* Fibrosis, lung) 515
  fibrous (*see also* Fibrosis, lung) 515
  Friedländer's bacillus 482.0
  fusobacterium (nucleatum) 482.81
  gangrenous 513.0
  giant cell (*see also* Pneumonia, viral) 480.9
  gram-negative bacteria NEC 482.83
    anaerobic 482.81
  grippal 487.0
  hemophilus influenzae (bronchial) (lobar) 482.2
  hypostatic (broncho-) (lobar) 514
  in
    actinomycosis 039.1
    anthrax 022.1 *[484.5]*
    aspergillosis 117.3 *[484.6]*
    candidiasis 112.4
    coccidioidomycosis 114.0
    cytomegalic inclusion disease 078.5 *[484.1]*
    histoplasmosis (*see also* Histoplasmosis) 115.95

Pneumonia (*Continued*)
  in (*Continued*)
    infectious disease NEC 136.9 *[484.8]*
    measles 055.1
    mycosis, systemic NEC 117.9 *[484.7]*
    nocardiasis, nocardiosis 039.1
    ornithosis 073.0
    pneumocystosis 136.3
    psittacosis 073.0
    Q fever 083.0 *[484.8]*
    salmonellosis 003.22
    toxoplasmosis 130.4
    tularemia 021.2
    typhoid (fever) 002.0 *[484.8]*
    varicella 052.1
    whooping cough (*see also* Whooping cough) 033.9 *[484.3]*
  infective, acquired prenatally 770.0
  influenzal (broncho) (lobar) (virus) 487.0
  inhalation (*see also* Pneumonia, aspiration) 507.0
    fumes or vapors (chemical) 506.0
  interstitial 516.8
    with influenzal 487.0
    acute 136.3
    chronic (*see also* Fibrosis, lung) 515
    desquamative 516.8
    hypostatic 514
    lipoid 507.1
    lymphoid 516.8
    plasma cell 136.3
    Pseudomonas 482.1
  intrauterine (infective) 770.0
    aspiration 770.1
  Klebsiella pneumoniae 482.0
  Legionnaires' 482.84
  lipid, lipoid (exogenous) (interstitial) 507.1
    endogenous 516.8
  lobar (diplococcal) (disseminated) (double) (interstitial) (pneumococcal, any type) 481
    with influenza 487.0
    bacterial 482.9
      specified type NEC 482.89
    chronic (*see also* Fibrosis, lung) 515
    Escherichia coli (E. coli) 482.82
    Friedländer's bacillus 482.0
    hemophilus influenzae (H. influenzae) 482.2
    hypostatic 514
    influenzal 487.0
    klebsiella 482.0
    ornithosis 073.0
    proteus 482.83
    Pseudomonas 482.1
    psittacosis 073.0
    specified organism NEC 483.8
      bacterial NEC 482.89
    staphylococcal 482.40
      aureus 482.41
      specified type NEC 482.49
    streptococcal - *see* Pneumonia, streptococcal
    viral, virus (*see also* Pneumonia, viral) 480.9
  lobular (confluent) - *see* Pneumonia, broncho-
  Löffler's 518.3
  massive - *see* Pneumonia, lobar
  meconium 770.1
  metastatic NEC 038.8 *[484.8]*
  mycoplasma (pneumoniae) 483.0
  necrotic 513.0

Pneumonia (*Continued*)
  nitrogen dioxide 506.9
  orthostatic 514
  parainfluenza virus 480.2
  parenchymatous (*see also* Fibrosis, lung) 515
  passive 514
  patchy - *see* Pneumonia, broncho
  Peptococcus 482.81
  Peptostreptococcus 482.81
  plasma cell 136.3
  pleurolobar - *see* Pneumonia, lobar
  pleuropneumonia-like organism (PPLO) 483.0
  pneumococcal (broncho) (lobar) 481
  Pneumocystis (carinii) 136.3
  postinfectional NEC 136.9 *[484.8]*
  postmeasles 055.1
  postoperative 997.3
  primary atypical 486
  Proprionibacterium 482.81
  Proteus 482.83
  Pseudomonas 482.1
  psittacosis 073.0
  radiation 508.0
  respiratory syncytial virus 480.1
  resulting from a procedure 997.3
  rheumatic 390 *[517.1]*
  Salmonella 003.22
  SARS-associated coronavirus 480.3
  segmented, segmental - *see* Pneumonia, broncho-
  Serratia (marcascens) 482.83
  specified
    bacteria NEC 482.89
    organism NEC 483.8
    virus NEC 480.8
  spirochetal 104.8 *[484]*
  staphylococcal (broncho) (lobar) 482.40
    aureus 482.41
    specified type NEC 482.49
  static, stasis 514
  streptococcal (broncho) (lobar) NEC 482.30
    Group
      A 482.31
      B 482.32
      specified NEC 482.39
    pneumoniae 481
    specified type NEC 482.39
  Streptococcus pneumoniae 481
  traumatic (complication) (early) (secondary) 958.8
  tuberculous (any) (*see also* Tuberculosis) 011.6
  tularemic 021.2
  TWAR agent 483.1
  varicella 052.1
  Veillonella 482.81
  viral, virus (broncho) (interstitial) (lobar) 480.9
    with influenza, flu, or grippe 487.0
    adenoviral 480.0
    parainfluenza 480.2
    respiratory syncytial 480.1
    SARS-associated coronavirus 480.3
    specified type NEC 480.8
  white (congenital) 090.0
Pneumonic - *see* condition
Pneumonitis (acute) (primary) (*see also* Pneumonia) 486
  allergic 495.9
    specified type NEC 495.8

Pneumonitis (Continued)
  aspiration 507.0
    due to fumes or gases 506.0
    newborn 770.1
    obstetric 668.0
  chemical 506.0
    due to fumes or gases 506.0
  cholesterol 516.8
  chronic (see also Fibrosis, lung) 515
  congenital rubella 771.0
  crack 506.0 ◀
  due to
    crack (cocaine) 506.0 ◀
    fumes or vapors 506.0
    inhalation
      food (regurgitated), milk, vomitus 507.0
      oils, essences 507.1
      saliva 507.0
      solids, liquids NEC 507.8
    toxoplasmosis (acquired) 130.4
      congenital (active) 771.2 [484.8]
  eosinophilic 518.3
  fetal aspiration 770.1
  hypersensitivity 495.9
  interstitial (chronic) (see also Fibrosis, lung) 515
    lymphoid 516.8
  lymphoid, interstitial 516.8
  meconium 770.1
  postanesthetic
    correct substance properly administered 507.0
    obstetric 668.0
    overdose or wrong substance given 968.4
      specified anesthetic - see Table of Drugs and Chemicals
  postoperative 997.3
    obstetric 668.0
  radiation 508.0
  rubella, congenital 771.0
  "ventilation" 495.7
  wood-dust 495.8
Pneumonoconiosis - see Pneumoconiosis
Pneumoparotid 527.8
Pneumopathy NEC 518.89
  alveolar 516.9
    specified NEC 516.8
    due to dust NEC 504
  parietoalveolar 516.9
    specified condition NEC 516.8
Pneumopericarditis (see also Pericarditis) 423.9
  acute 420.90
Pneumopericardium - see also Pericarditis
  congenital 770.2
  fetus or newborn 770.2
  traumatic (post) (see also Pneumothorax, traumatic) 860.0
    with open wound into thorax 860.1
Pneumoperitoneum 568.89
  fetus or newborn 770.2
Pneumophagia (psychogenic) 306.4
Pneumopleurisy, pneumopleuritis (see also Pneumonia) 486
Pneumopyopericardium 420.99
Pneumopyothorax (see also Pyopneumothorax) 510.9
  with fistula 510.0
Pneumorrhagia 786.3
  newborn 770.3
  tuberculous (see also Tuberculosis, pulmonary) 011.9

Pneumosiderosis (occupational) 503
Pneumothorax (acute) (chronic) 512.8
  congenital 770.2
  due to operative injury of chest wall or lung 512.1
    accidental puncture or laceration 512.1
  fetus or newborn 770.2
  iatrogenic 512.1
  postoperative 512.1
  spontaneous 512.8
    fetus or newborn 770.2
    tension 512.0
  sucking 512.8
    iatrogenic 512.1
    postoperative 512.1
  tense valvular, infectional 512.0
  tension 512.0
    iatrogenic 512.1
    postoperative 512.1
    spontaneous 512.0
  traumatic 860.0
    with
      hemothorax 860.4
        with open wound into thorax 860.5
      open wound into thorax 860.1
  tuberculous (see also Tuberculosis) 011.7
Pocket(s)
  endocardial (see also Endocarditis) 424.90
  periodontal 523.8
Podagra 274.9
Podencephalus 759.89
Poikilocytosis 790.09
Poikiloderma 709.09
  Civatte's 709.09
  congenital 757.33
  vasculare atrophicans 696.2
Poikilodermatomyositis 710.3
Pointed ear 744.29
Poise imperfect 729.9
Poisoned - see Poisoning
Poisoning (acute) - see also Table of Drugs and Chemicals
  Bacillus, B.
    aertrycke (see also Infection, Salmonella) 003.9
    botulinus 005.1
    cholerae (suis) (see also Infection, Salmonella) 003.9
    paratyphosus (see also Infection, Salmonella) 003.9
    suipestifer (see also Infection, Salmonella) 003.9
  bacterial toxins NEC 005.9
  berries, noxious 988.2
  blood (general) - see Septicemia
  botulism 005.1
  bread, moldy, mouldy - see Poisoning, food
  damaged meat - see Poisoning, food
  death-cap (Amanita phalloides) (Amanita verna) 988.1
  decomposed food - see Poisoning, food
  diseased food - see Poisoning, food
  drug - see Table of Drugs and Chemicals
  epidemic, fish, meat, or other food - see Poisoning, food
  fava bean 282.2
  fish (bacterial) - see also Poisoning, food
    noxious 988.0
  food (acute) (bacterial) (diseased) (infected) NEC 005.9

Poisoning (Continued)
  food (Continued)
    due to
      bacillus
        aertrycke (see also Poisoning, food, due to Salmonella) 003.9
        botulinus 005.1
        cereus 005.89
        choleraesuis (see also Poisoning, food, due to Salmonella) 003.9
        paratyphosus (see also Poisoning, food, due to Salmonella) 003.9
        suipestifer (see also Poisoning, food, due to Salmonella) 003.9
      Clostridium 005.3
        botulinum 005.1
        perfringens 005.2
        welchii 005.2
      Salmonella (aertrycke) (callinarum) (choleraesuis) (enteritidis) (paratyphi) (suipestifer) 003.9
        with
          gastroenteritis 003.0
          localized infection(s) (see also Infection, Salmonella) 003.20
          septicemia 003.1
          specified manifestation NEC 003.8
      specified bacterium NEC 005.89
      Staphylococcus 005.0
      Streptococcus 005.0
      Vibrio parahaemolyticus 005.4
      Vibrio vulnificus 005.81
    noxious or naturally toxic 988.0
      berries 988.2
      fish 988.0
      mushroom 988.1
      plants NEC 988.2
  ice cream - see Poisoning, food
  ichthyotoxism (bacterial) 005.9
  kreotoxism, food 005.9
  malarial - see Malaria
  meat - see Poisoning, food
  mushroom (noxious) 988.1
  mussel - see also Poisoning, food
    noxious 988.0
  noxious foodstuffs (see also Poisoning, food, noxious) 988.9
    specified type NEC 988.8
  plants, noxious 988.2
  pork - see also Poisoning, food
    specified NEC 988.8
    Trichinosis 124
  ptomaine - see Poisoning, food
  putrefaction, food - see Poisoning, food
  radiation 508.0
  Salmonella (see also Infection, Salmonella) 003.9
  sausage - see also Poisoning, food
    Trichinosis 124
  saxitoxin 988.0
  shellfish - see also Poisoning, food
    noxious 988.0
  Staphylococcus, food 005.0
  toxic, from disease NEC 799.89
  truffles - see Poisoning, food
  uremic - see Uremia
  uric acid 274.9
Poison ivy, oak, sumac or other plant dermatitis 692.6

ICD-9-CM

P

Vol.

Poker spine 720.0
Policeman's disease 729.2
Polioencephalitis (acute) (bulbar) (*see also* Poliomyelitis, bulbar) 045.0
  inferior 335.22
  influenzal 487.8
  superior hemorrhagic (acute) (Wernicke's) 265.1
  Wernicke's (superior hemorrhagic) 265.1
Polioencephalomyelitis (acute) (anterior) (bulbar) (*see also* Polioencephalitis) 045.0
Polioencephalopathy, superior hemorrhagic 265.1
  with
    beriberi 265.0
    pellagra 265.2
Poliomeningoencephalitis - *see* Meningoencephalitis
Poliomyelitis (acute) (anterior) (epidemic) 045.9

Note   Use the following fifth-digit subclassification with category 045:

0   poliovirus, unspecified type
1   poliovirus, type I
2   poliovirus, type II
3   poliovirus, type III

  with
    paralysis 045.1
      bulbar 045.0
  abortive 045.2
  ascending 045.9
    progressive 045.9
  bulbar 045.0
  cerebral 045.0
  chronic 335.21
  congenital 771.2
  contact V01.2
  deformities 138
  exposure to V01.2
  late effect 138
  nonepidemic 045.9
  nonparalytic 045.2
  old with deformity 138
  posterior, acute 053.19
  residual 138
  sequelae 138
  spinal, acute 045.9
  syphilitic (chronic) 094.89
  vaccination, prophylactic (against) V04.0
Poliosis (eyebrow) (eyelashes) 704.3
  circumscripta (congenital) 757.4
    acquired 704.3
  congenital 757.4
Pollakiuria 788.41
  psychogenic 306.53
Pollinosis 477.0
Pollitzer's disease (hidradenitis suppurativa) 705.83
Polyadenitis (*see also* Adenitis) 289.3
  malignant 020.0
Polyalgia 729.9
Polyangiitis (essential) 446.0
Polyarteritis (nodosa) (renal) 446.0
Polyarthralgia 719.49
  psychogenic 306.0
Polyarthritis, polyarthropathy NEC 716.59
  due to or associated with other specified conditions - *see* Arthritis, due to or associated with
  endemic (*see also* Disease, Kaschin-Beck) 716.0

Polyarthritis, polyarthropathy NEC
  (*Continued*)
  inflammatory 714.9
    specified type NEC 714.89
  juvenile (chronic) 714.30
    acute 714.31
  migratory - *see* Fever, rheumatic
  rheumatic 714.0
    fever (acute) - *see* Fever, rheumatic
Polycarential syndrome of infancy 260
Polychondritis (atrophic) (chronic) (relapsing) 733.99
Polycoria 743.46
Polycystic (congenital) (disease) 759.89
  degeneration, kidney - *see* Polycystic, kidney
  kidney (congenital) 753.12
    adult type (APKD) 753.13
    autosomal dominant 753.13
    autosomal recessive 753.14
    childhood type (CPKD) 753.14
    infantile type 753.14
  liver 751.62
  lung 518.89
    congenital 748.4
  ovary, ovaries 256.4
  spleen 759.0
Polycythemia (primary) (rubra) (vera) (M9950/1) 238.4
  acquired 289.0
  benign 289.0
    familial 289.6
  due to
    donor twin 776.4
    fall in plasma volume 289.0
    high altitude 289.0
    maternal-fetal transfusion 776.4
    stress 289.0
  emotional 289.0
  erythropoietin 289.0
  familial (benign) 289.6
  Gaisböck's (hypertonica) 289.0
  high altitude 289.0
  hypertonica 289.0
  hypoxemic 289.0
  neonatorum 776.4
  nephrogenous 289.0
  relative 289.0
  secondary 289.0
  spurious 289.0
  stress 289.0
Polycytosis cryptogenica 289.0
Polydactylism, polydactyly 755.00
  fingers 755.01
  toes 755.02
Polydipsia 783.5
Polydystrophic oligophrenia 277.5
Polyembryoma (M9072/3) - *see* Neoplasm, by site, malignant
Polygalactia 676.6
Polyglandular
  deficiency 258.9
  dyscrasia 258.9
  dysfunction 258.9
  syndrome 258.8
Polyhydramnios (*see also* Hydramnios) 657
Polymastia 757.6
Polymenorrhea 626.2
Polymicrogyria 742.2
Polymyalgia 725
  arteritica 446.5
  rheumatica 725

Polymyositis (acute) (chronic) (hemorrhagic) 710.4
  with involvement of
    lung 710.4 [517.8]
    skin 710.3
  ossificans (generalisata) (progressiva) 728.19
  Wagner's (dermatomyositis) 710.3
Polyneuritis, polyneuritic (*see also* Polyneuropathy) 356.9
  alcoholic 357.5
    with psychosis 291.1
  cranialis 352.6
  demyelinating, chronic inflammatory 357.81
  diabetic 250.6 [357.2]
  due to lack of vitamin NEC 269.2 [357.4]
  endemic 265.0 [357.4]
  erythredema 985.0
  febrile 357.0
  hereditary ataxic 356.3
  idiopathic, acute 357.0
  infective (acute) 357.0
  nutritional 269.9 [357.4]
  postinfectious 357.0
Polyneuropathy (peripheral) 356.9
  alcoholic 357.5
  amyloid 277.3 [357.4]
  arsenical 357.7
  critical illness 357.82
  diabetic 250.6 [357.2]
  due to
    antitetanus serum 357.6
    arsenic 357.7
    drug or medicinal substance 357.6
      correct substance properly administered 357.6
      overdose or wrong substance given or taken 977.9
      specified drug - *see* Table of Drugs and Chemicals
    lack of vitamin NEC 269.2 [357.4]
    lead 357.7
    organophosphate compounds 357.7
    pellagra 265.2 [357.4]
    porphyria 277.1 [357.4]
    serum 357.6
    toxic agent NEC 357.7
  hereditary 356.0
  idiopathic 356.9
    progressive 356.4
  in
    amyloidosis 277.3 [357.4]
    avitaminosis 269.2 [357.4]
      specified NEC 269.1 [357.4]
    beriberi 265.0 [357.4]
    collagen vascular disease NEC 710.9 [357.1]
    deficiency
      B-complex NEC 266.2 [357.4]
      vitamin B 266.9 [357.4]
      vitamin B_6 266.1 [357.4]
    diabetes 250.6 [357.2]
    diphtheria (*see also* Diphtheria) 032.89 [357.4]
    disseminated lupus erythematosus 710.0 [357.1]
    herpes zoster 053.13
    hypoglycemia 251.2 [357.4]
    malignant neoplasm (M8000/3) NEC 199.1 [357.3]
    mumps 072.72
    pellagra 265.2 [357.4]

◄ **New**   ◄▥ **Revised**

Polyneuropathy (Continued)
  in (Continued)
    polyarteritis nodosa 446.0 [357.1]
    porphyria 277.1 [357.4]
    rheumatoid arthritis 714.0 [357.1]
    sarcoidosis 135 [357.4]
    uremia 585 [357.4]
  lead 357.7
  nutritional 269.9 [357.4]
    specified NEC 269.8 [357.4]
  postherpetic 053.13
  progressive 356.4
  sensory (hereditary) 356.2
Polyonychia 757.5
Polyopia 368.2
  refractive 368.15
Polyorchism, polyorchidism (three testes) 752.89
Polyorrhymenitis (peritoneal) (see also Polyserositis) 568.82
  pericardial 423.2
Polyostotic fibrous dysplasia 756.54
Polyotia 744.1
Polyp, polypus

> Note   Polyps of organs or sites that do not appear in the list below should be coded to the residual category for diseases of the organ or site concerned.

  accessory sinus 471.8
  adenoid tissue 471.0
  adenomatous (M8210/0) - see also Neoplasm, by site, benign
    adenocarcinoma in (M8210/3) - see Neoplasm, by site, malignant
    carcinoma in (M8210/3) - see Neoplasm, by site, malignant
    multiple (M8221/0) - see Neoplasm, by site, benign
  antrum 471.8
  anus, anal (canal) (nonadenomatous) 569.0
    adenomatous 211.4
  Bartholin's gland 624.6
  bladder (M8120/1) 236.7
  broad ligament 620.8
  cervix (uteri) 622.7
    adenomatous 219.0
    in pregnancy or childbirth 654.6
      affecting fetus or newborn 763.89
      causing obstructed labor 660.2
    mucous 622.7
    nonneoplastic 622.7
  choanal 471.0
  cholesterol 575.6
  clitoris 624.6
  colon (M8210/0) (see also Polyp, adenomatous) 211.3
  corpus uteri 621.0
  dental 522.0
  ear (middle) 385.30
  endometrium 621.0
  ethmoidal (sinus) 471.8
  fallopian tube 620.8
  female genital organs NEC 624.8
  frontal (sinus) 471.8
  gallbladder 575.6
  gingiva 523.8
  gum 523.8
  labia 624.6
  larynx (mucous) 478.4

Polyp, polypus (Continued)
  malignant (M8000/3) - see Neoplasm, by site, malignant
  maxillary (sinus) 471.8
  middle ear 385.30
  myometrium 621.0
  nares
    anterior 471.9
    posterior 471.0
  nasal (mucous) 471.9
    cavity 471.0
    septum 471.9
  nasopharyngeal 471.0
  neoplastic (M8210/0) - see Neoplasm, by site, benign
  nose (mucous) 471.9
  oviduct 620.8
  paratubal 620.8
  pharynx 478.29
    congenital 750.29
  placenta, placental 674.4
  prostate 600.20
    with urinary retention 600.21
  pudenda 624.6
  pulp (dental) 522.0
  rectosigmoid 211.4
  rectum (nonadenomatous) 569.0
    adenomatous 211.4
  septum (nasal) 471.9
  sinus (accessory) (ethmoidal) (frontal) (maxillary) (sphenoidal) 471.8
  sphenoidal (sinus) 471.8
  stomach (M8210/0) 211.1
  tube, fallopian 620.8
  turbinate, mucous membrane 471.8
  ureter 593.89
  urethra 599.3
  uterine
    ligament 620.8
    tube 620.8
  uterus (body) (corpus) (mucous) 621.0
    in pregnancy or childbirth 654.1
      affecting fetus or newborn 763.89
      causing obstructed labor 660.2
  vagina 623.7
  vocal cord (mucous) 478.4
  vulva 624.6
Polyphagia 783.6
Polypoid - see condition
Polyposis - see also Polyp
  coli (adenomatous) (M8220/0) 211.3
    adenocarcinoma in (M8220/3) 153.9
    carcinoma in (M8220/3) 153.9
  familial (M8220/0) 211.3
  intestinal (adenomatous) (M8220/0) 211.3
  multiple (M8221/0) - see Neoplasm, by site, benign
Polyradiculitis (acute) 357.0
Polyradiculoneuropathy (acute) (segmentally demyelinating) 357.0
Polysarcia 278.00
Polyserositis (peritoneal) 568.82
  due to pericarditis 423.2
  paroxysmal (familial) 277.3
  pericardial 423.2
  periodic 277.3
  pleural - see Pleurisy
  recurrent 277.3
  tuberculous (see also Tuberculosis, polyserositis) 018.9
Polysialia 527.7
Polysplenia syndrome 759.0
Polythelia 757.6

Polytrichia (see also Hypertrichosis) 704.1
Polyunguia (congenital) 757.5
  acquired 703.8
Polyuria 788.42
Pompe's disease (glycogenosis II) 271.0
Pompholyx 705.81
Poncet's disease (tuberculous rheumatism) (see also Tuberculosis) 015.9
Pond fracture - see Fracture, skull, vault
Ponos 085.0
Pons, pontine - see condition
Poor
  contractions, labor 661.2
    affecting fetus or newborn 763.7
  fetal growth NEC 764.9
    affecting management of pregnancy 656.5
  incorporation
    artificial skin graft 996.55
    decellularized allodermis graft 996.55
  obstetrical history V13.49
    affecting management of current pregnancy V23.49
      pre-term labor V23.41
    pre-term labor V13.41
  sucking reflex (newborn) 796.1
  vision NEC 369.9
Poradenitis, nostras 099.1
Porencephaly (congenital) (developmental) (true) 742.4
  acquired 348.0
  nondevelopmental 348.0
  traumatic (post) 310.2
Porocephaliasis 134.1
Porokeratosis 757.39
  disseminated superficial actinic (DSAP) 692.75
Poroma, eccrine (M8402/0) - see Neoplasm, skin, benign
Porphyria (acute) (congenital) (constitutional) (erythropoietic) (familial) (hepatica) (idiopathic) (idiosyncratic) (intermittent) (latent) (mixed hepatic) (photosensitive) (South African genetic) (Swedish) 277.1
  acquired 277.1
  cutaneatarda
    hereditaria 277.1
    symptomatica 277.1
  due to drugs
    correct substance properly administered 277.1
    overdose or wrong substance given or taken 977.9
      specified drug - see Table of Drugs and Chemicals
  secondary 277.1
  toxic NEC 277.1
  variegata 277.1
Porphyrinuria (acquired) (congenital) (secondary) 277.1
Porphyruria (acquired) (congenital) 277.1
Portal - see condition
Port wine nevus or mark 757.32
Posadas-Wernicke disease 114.9
Position
  fetus, abnormal (see also Presentation, fetal) 652.9
  teeth, faulty (see also Anomaly, position tooth) 524.30 ◀▬
Positive
  culture (nonspecific) 795.39
    AIDS virus V08

ICD-9-CM

P

Vol. 2

Positive (Continued)
 culture (Continued)
  blood 790.7
  HIV V08
  human immunodeficiency virus V08
  nose 795.39
  skin lesion NEC 795.39
  spinal fluid 792.0
  sputum 795.39
  stool 792.1
  throat 795.39
  urine 791.9
  wound 795.39
 findings, anthrax 795.31
 HIV V08
 human immunodeficiency virus (HIV)
   V08
 PPD 795.5
 serology
  AIDS virus V08
   inconclusive 795.71
  HIV V08
   inconclusive 795.71
  human immunodeficiency virus V08
   inconclusive 795.71
  syphilis 097.1
   with signs or symptoms - see
     Syphilis, by site and stage
   false 795.6
 skin test 795.7
  tuberculin (without active tuberculo-
    sis) 795.5
 VDRL 097.1
  with signs or symptoms - see Syphi-
    lis, by site and stage
  false 795.6
 Wassermann reaction 097.1
  false 795.6
Postcardiotomy syndrome 429.4
Postcaval ureter 753.4
Postcholecystectomy syndrome 576.0
Postclimacteric bleeding 627.1
Postcommissurotomy syndrome 429.4
Postconcussional syndrome 310.2
Postcontusional syndrome 310.2
Postcricoid region - see condition
Post-dates (pregnancy) - see Pregnancy
Postencephalitic - see also condition
 syndrome 310.8
Posterior - see condition
Posterolateral sclerosis (spinal cord) - see
   Degeneration, combined
Postexanthematous - see condition
Postfebrile - see condition
Postgastrectomy dumping syndrome
 564.2
Posthemiplegic chorea 344.89
Posthemorrhagic anemia (chronic) 280.0
 acute 285.1
 newborn 776.5
Posthepatitis syndrome 780.79
Postherpetic neuralgia (intercostal) (syn-
   drome) (zoster) 053.19
 geniculate ganglion 053.11
 ophthalmica 053.19
 trigeminal 053.12
Posthitis 607.1
**Postimmunization complication or reac-
 tion** - see Complications, vaccination
Postinfectious - see condition
Postinfluenzal syndrome 780.79
Postlaminectomy syndrome 722.80
 cervical, cervicothoracic 722.81
 kyphosis 737.12

Postlaminectomy syndrome (Continued)
 lumbar, lumbosacral 722.83
 thoracic, thoracolumbar 722.82
Postleukotomy syndrome 310.0
Postlobectomy syndrome 310.0
Postmastectomy lymphedema (syndrome) 457.0
Postmaturity, postmature (fetus or newborn) (gestation period over 42 completed weeks) 766.22
 affecting management of pregnancy
  post-term pregnancy 645.1 ◀▦
  prolonged pregnancy 645.2
 syndrome 766.22
Postmeasles - see also condition
 complication 055.8
  specified NEC 055.79
Postmenopausal
 endometrium (atrophic) 627.8
  suppurative (see also Endometritis) 615.9
 hormone replacement therapy V07.4
 status (age related) (natural) V49.81
Postnasal drip - see Sinusitis
Postnatal - see condition
Postoperative - see also condition
 confusion state 293.9
 psychosis 293.9
 status NEC (see also Status (post)) V45.89
Postpancreatectomy hyperglycemia 251.3
Postpartum - see also condition
 anemia 648.2
  cardiomyopathy 674.5
 observation
  immediately after delivery V24.0
  routine follow-up V24.2
Postperfusion syndrome NEC 999.8
 bone marrow 996.85
Postpoliomyelitic - see condition
Postsurgery status NEC (see also Status
 (post)) V45.89
Post-term (pregnancy) 645.1 ◀▦
 infant (gestation period over 40 com-
  pleted weeks to 42 completed
  weeks) 766.21
Posttraumatic - see condition
**Posttraumatic brain syndrome, nonpsy-
 chotic** 310.2
Post-typhoid abscess 002.0
Postures, hysterical 300.11
Postvaccinal reaction or complication -
 see Complications, vaccination
Postvagotomy syndrome 564.2
Postvalvulotomy syndrome 429.4
Postvasectomy sperm count V25.8
Potain's disease (pulmonary edema) 514
Potain's syndrome (gastrectasis with
 dyspepsia) 536.1
Pott's
 curvature (spinal) (see also Tuberculosis) 015.0 [737.43]
 disease or paraplegia (see also Tuberculosis) 015.0 [730.88]
 fracture (closed) 824.4
  open 824.5
 gangrene 440.24
 osteomyelitis (see also Tuberculosis)
  015.0 [730.88]
 spinal curvature (see also Tuberculosis)
  015.0 [737.43]
 tumor, puffy (see also Osteomyelitis)
  730.2
Potter's
 asthma 502
 disease 753.0

Potter's (Continued)
 facies 754.0
 lung 502
 syndrome (with renal agenesis)
  753.0
Pouch
 bronchus 748.3
 Douglas' - see condition
 esophagus, esophageal (congenital)
  750.4
  acquired 530.6
 gastric 537.1
 Hartmann's (abnormal sacculation of
  gallbladder neck) 575.8
  of intestine V44.3
   attention to V55.3
 pharynx, pharyngeal (congenital)
  750.27
Poulet's disease 714.2
Poultrymen's itch 133.8
Poverty V60.2
Prader-Labhart-Willi-Fanconi syndrome
 (hypogenital dystrophy with diabetic
 tendency) 759.81
Prader-Willi syndrome (hypogenital dystrophy with diabetic tendency)
 759.81
Preachers' voice 784.49
Pre-AIDS - see Human immunodeficiency virus (disease) (illness) (infection)
Preauricular appendage 744.1
Prebetalipoproteinemia (acquired) (essential) (familial) (hereditary) (primary) (secondary) 272.1
 with chylomicronemia 272.3
Precipitate labor 661.3
 affecting fetus or newborn 763.6
Preclimacteric bleeding 627.0
 menorrhagia 627.0
Precocious
 adrenarche 259.1
 menarche 259.1
 menstruation 626.8
 pubarche 259.1
 puberty NEC 259.1
 sexual development NEC 259.1
 thelarche 259.1
Precocity, sexual (constitutional) (cryptogenic) (female) (idiopathic) (male)
 NEC 259.1
 with adrenal hyperplasia 255.2
Precordial pain 786.51
 psychogenic 307.89
Predeciduous teeth 520.2
Prediabetes, prediabetic 790.29
 complicating pregnancy, childbirth, or
  puerperium 648.8
 fetus or newborn 775.8
Predislocation status of hip, at birth (see
 also Subluxation, congenital, hip)
 754.32
Pre-eclampsia (mild) 642.4
 with pre-existing hypertension 642.7
 affecting fetus or newborn 760.0
 severe 642.5
 superimposed on pre-existing hypertensive disease 642.7
Preeruptive color change, teeth, tooth
 520.8
Preexcitation 426.7
 atrioventricular conduction 426.7
 ventricular 426.7
Preglaucoma 365.00

Pregnancy (single) (uterine) (without sickness) V22.2

> Note Use the following fifth-digit subclassification with categories 640-648, 651-676:
>
> 0   unspecified as to episode of care
> 1   delivered, with or without mention of antepartum condition
> 2   delivered, with mention of postpartum complication
> 3   antepartum condition or complication
> 4   postpartum condition or complication

abdominal (ectopic) 633.00
  with intrauterine pregnancy 633.01
  affecting fetus or newborn 761.4
abnormal NEC 646.9
ampullar - *see* Pregnancy, tubal
broad ligament - *see* Pregnancy, cornual
cervical - *see* Pregnancy, cornual
combined (extrauterine and intrauterine) - *see* Pregnancy, cornual
complicated (by) 646.9
  abnormal, abnormality NEC 646.9
    cervix 654.6
    cholelithiasis 646.8
    cord (umbilical) 663.9
    gallbladder disease 646.8
    glucose tolerance (conditions classifiable to 790.21-790.29) 648.8
    pelvic organs or tissues NEC 654.9
    pelvis (bony) 653.0
    perineum or vulva 654.8
    placenta, placental (vessel) 656.7
    position
      cervix 654.4
      placenta 641.1
        without hemorrhage 641.0
      uterus 654.4
    size, fetus 653.5
    uterus (congenital) 654.0
  abscess or cellulitis
    bladder 646.6
    genitourinary tract (conditions classifiable to 590, 595, 597, 599.0, 614.0-614.5, 614.7-614.9, 615) 646.6
    kidney 646.6
    urinary tract NEC 646.6
  adhesion, pelvic peritoneal 648.9
  air embolism 673.0
  albuminuria 646.2
    with hypertension - *see* Toxemia, of pregnancy
  amnionitis 658.4
  amniotic fluid embolism 673.1
  anemia (conditions classifiable to 280-285) 648.2
  atrophy, yellow (acute) (liver) (subacute) 646.7
  bacilluria, asymptomatic 646.5
  bacteriuria, asymptomatic 646.5
  bicornis or bicornuate uterus 654.0
  biliary problems 646.8 ◀
  bone and joint disorders (conditions classifiable to 720-724 or conditions affecting lower limbs classifiable to 711-719, 725-738) 648.7

Pregnancy *(Continued)*
  complicated *(Continued)*
    breech presentation 652.2
      with successful version 652.1
    cardiovascular disease (conditions classifiable to 390-398, 410-429) 648.6
      congenital (conditions classifiable to 745-747) 648.5
    cerebrovascular disorders (conditions classifiable to 430-434, 436-437) 674.0
    cervicitis (conditions classifiable to 616.0) 646.6
    chloasma (gravidarum) 646.8
    chorea (gravidarum) - *see* Eclampsia, pregnancy
    contraction, pelvis (general) 653.1
      inlet 653.2
      outlet 653.3
    convulsions (eclamptic) (uremic) 642.6
      with pre-existing hypertension 642.7
    current disease or condition (nonobstetric)
      abnormal glucose tolerance 648.8
      anemia 648.2
      bone and joint (lower limb) 648.7
      cardiovascular 648.6
      congenital 648.5
      cerebrovascular 674.0
      diabetic 648.0
      drug dependence 648.3
      genital organ or tract 646.6
      gonorrheal 647.1
      hypertensive 642.2
        renal 642.1
      infectious 647.9
        specified type NEC 647.8
      liver 646.7
      malarial 647.4
      nutritional deficiency 648.9
      parasitic NEC 647.8
      periodontal disease 648.9 ◀
      renal 646.2
        hypertensive 642.1
      rubella 647.5
      specified condition NEC 648.9
      syphilitic 647.0
      thyroid 648.1
      tuberculous 647.3
      urinary 646.6
      venereal 647.2
      viral NEC 647.6
    cystitis 646.6
    cystocele 654.4
    death of fetus (near term) 656.4
      early pregnancy (before 22 completed weeks' gestation) 632
    deciduitis 646.6
    decreased fetal movements 655.7
    diabetes (mellitus) (conditions classifiable to 250) 648.0
    disorders of liver 646.7
    displacement, uterus NEC 654.4
    disproportion - *see* Disproportion
    double uterus 654.0
    drug dependence (conditions classifiable to 304) 648.3
    dysplasia, cervix 654.6
    early onset of delivery (spontaneous) 644.2

Pregnancy *(Continued)*
  complicated *(Continued)*
    eclampsia, eclamptic (coma) (convulsions) (delirium) (nephritis) (uremia) 642.6
      with pre-existing hypertension 642.7
    edema 646.1
      with hypertension - *see* Toxemia, of pregnancy
    effusion, amniotic fluid 658.1
      delayed delivery following 658.2
    embolism
      air 673.0
      amniotic fluid 673.1
      blood-clot 673.2
      cerebral 674.0
      pulmonary NEC 673.2
      pyemic 673.3
      septic 673.3
    emesis (gravidarum) - *see* Pregnancy, complicated, vomiting
    endometritis (conditions classifiable to 615.0-615.9) 646.6
      decidual 646.6
    excessive weight gain NEC 646.1
    face presentation 652.4
    failure, fetal head to enter pelvic brim 652.5
    false labor (pains) 644.1
    fatigue 646.8
    fatty metamorphosis of liver 646.7
    fetal
      death (near term) 656.4
        early (before 22 completed weeks' gestation) 632
      deformity 653.7
      distress 656.8
    fibroid (tumor) (uterus) 654.1
    footling presentation 652.8
      with successful version 652.1
    goiter 648.1
    gonococcal infection (conditions classifiable to 098) 647.1
    gonorrhea (conditions classifiable to 098) 647.1
    hemorrhage 641.9
      accidental 641.2
      before 22 completed weeks' gestation NEC 640.9
      cerebrovascular 674.0
      due to
        afibrinogenemia or other coagulation defect (conditions classifiable to 286.0-286.9) 641.3
        leiomyoma, uterine 641.8
        marginal sinus (rupture) 641.2
        premature separation, placenta 641.2
        trauma 641.8
      early (before 22 completed weeks' gestation) 640.9
      threatened abortion 640.0
      unavoidable 641.1
    hepatitis (acute) (malignant) (subacute) 646.7
      viral 647.6
    herniation of uterus 654.4
    high head at term 652.5
    hydatidiform mole (delivered) (undelivered) 630
    hydramnios 657
    hydrocephalic fetus 653.6
    hydrops amnii 657
    hydrorrhea 658.1

ICD-9-CM

P

Vol. 2

Pregnancy *(Continued)*
  complicated *(Continued)*
    hyperemesis (gravidarum) - *see* Hy-
        peremesis, gravidarum
    hypertension - *see* Hypertension,
        complicating pregnancy
    hypertensive
      heart and renal disease 642.2
      heart disease 642.2
      renal disease 642.2
    hyperthyroidism 648.1
    hypothyroidism 648.1
    hysteralgia 646.8
    icterus gravis 646.7
    incarceration, uterus 654.3
    incompetent cervix (os) 654.5
    infection 647.9
      amniotic fluid 658.4
      bladder 646.6
      genital organ (conditions classifia-
          ble to 614.0-614.5, 614.7-614.9,
          615) 646.6
      kidney (conditions classifiable to
          590.0-590.9) 646.6
      urinary (tract) 646.6
        asymptomatic 646.5
    infective and parasitic diseases NEC
        647.8
    inflammation
      bladder 646.6
      genital organ (conditions classifia-
          ble to 614.0-614.5, 614.7-614.9,
          615) 646.6
      urinary tract NEC 646.6
    injury 648.9
      obstetrical NEC 665.9
    insufficient weight gain 646.8
    intrauterine fetal death (near term)
        NEC 656.4
      early (before 22 completed weeks'
          gestation) 632
    malaria (conditions classifiable to
        084) 647.4
    malformation, uterus (congenital)
        654.0
    malnutrition (conditions classifiable
        to 260-269) 648.9
    malposition
      fetus - *see* Pregnancy, complicated,
          malpresentation
      uterus or cervix 654.4
    malpresentation 652.9
      with successful version 652.1
      in multiple gestation 652.6
      specified type NEC 652.8
    marginal sinus hemorrhage or rup-
        ture 641.2
    maternal obesity syndrome 646.1
    menstruation 640.8
    mental disorders (conditions classifi-
        able to 290-303, 305-316, 317-
        319) 648.4
    mentum presentation 652.4
    missed
      abortion 632
      delivery (at or near term) 656.4
      labor (at or near term) 656.4
    necrosis
      genital organ or tract (conditions
          classifiable to 614.0-614.5,
          614.7-614.9, 615) 646.6
      liver (conditions classifiable to
          570) 646.7
      renal, cortical 646.2

Pregnancy *(Continued)*
  complicated *(Continued)*
    nephritis or nephrosis (conditions
        classifiable to 580-589) 646.2
      with hypertension 642.1
    nephropathy NEC 646.2
    neuritis (peripheral) 646.4
    nutritional deficiency (conditions
        classifiable to 260-269) 648.9
    oblique lie or presentation 652.3
      with successful version 652.1
    obstetrical trauma NEC 665.9
    oligohydramnios NEC 658.0
    onset of contractions before 37
        weeks 644.0
    oversize fetus 653.5
    papyraceous fetus 646.0
    patent cervix 654.5
    pelvic inflammatory disease (condi-
        tions classifiable to 614.0-614.5,
        614.7-614.9, 615) 646.6
    pelvic peritoneal adhesion 648.9
    placenta, placental
      abnormality 656.7
      abruptio or ablatio 641.2
      detachment 641.2
      disease 656.7
      infarct 656.7
      low implantation 641.1
        without hemorrhage 641.0
      malformation 656.7
      malposition 641.1
        without hemorrhage 641.0
      marginal sinus hemorrhage 641.2
      previa 641.1
        without hemorrhage 641.0
      separation (premature) (undeliv-
          ered) 641.2
    placentitis 658.4
    polyhydramnios 657
    postmaturity
      post-term 645.1   ◀▥
      prolonged 645.2
    prediabetes 648.8
    pre-eclampsia (mild) 642.4
      severe 642.5
      superimposed on pre-existing hy-
          pertensive disease 642.7
    premature rupture of membranes
        658.1
      with delayed delivery 658.2
    previous
      infertility V23.0
      nonobstetric condition V23.8
      poor obstetrical history V23.49
      premature delivery V23.41
      trophoblastic disease (conditions
          classifiable to 630) V23.1
    prolapse, uterus 654.4
    proteinuria (gestational) 646.2
      with hypertension - *see* Toxemia,
          of pregnancy
    pruritus (neurogenic) 646.8
    psychosis or psychoneurosis 648.4
    ptyalism 646.8
    pyelitis (conditions classifiable to
        590.0-590.9) 646.6
    renal disease or failure NEC 646.2
      with secondary hypertension 642.1
      hypertensive 642.2
    retention, retained dead ovum 631
    retroversion, uterus 654.3
    Rh immunization, incompatibility, or
        sensitization 656.1

Pregnancy *(Continued)*
  complicated *(Continued)*
    rubella (conditions classifiable to
        056) 647.5
    rupture
      amnion (premature) 658.1
        with delayed delivery 658.2
      marginal sinus (hemorrhage)
          641.2
      membranes (premature) 658.1
        with delayed delivery 658.2
      uterus (before onset of labor)
          665.0
    salivation (excessive) 646.8
    salpingo-oophoritis (conditions clas-
        sifiable to 614.0-614.2) 646.6
    septicemia (conditions classifiable to
        038.0-038.9) 647.8
      postpartum 670
      puerperal 670
    spasms, uterus (abnormal) 646.8
    specified condition NEC 646.8
    spurious labor pains 644.1
    superfecundation 651.9
    superfetation 651.9
    syphilis (conditions classifiable to
        090-097) 647.0
    threatened
      abortion 640.0
      premature delivery 644.2
      premature labor 644.0
    thrombophlebitis (superficial) 671.2
      deep 671.3
    thrombosis 671.9
      venous (superficial) 671.2
        deep 671.3
    thyroid dysfunction (conditions clas-
        sifiable to 240-246) 648.1
    thyroiditis 648.1
    thyrotoxicosis 648.1
    torsion of uterus 654.4
    toxemia - *see* Toxemia, of pregnancy
    transverse lie or presentation
        652.3
      with successful version 652.1
    trauma 648.9
      obstetrical 665.9
    tuberculosis (conditions classifiable
        to 010-018) 647.3
    tumor
      cervix 654.6
      ovary 654.4
      pelvic organs or tissue NEC 654.4
      uterus (body) 654.1
        cervix 654.6
      vagina 654.7
      vulva 654.8
    unstable lie 652.0
    uremia - *see* Pregnancy, complicated,
        renal disease
    urethritis 646.6
    vaginitis or vulvitis (conditions clas-
        sifiable to 616.1) 646.6
    varicose
      placental vessels 656.7
      veins (legs) 671.0
        perineum 671.1
        vulva 671.1
    varicosity, labia or vulva 671.1
    venereal disease NEC (conditions
        classifiable to 099) 647.2
    viral disease NEC (conditions classi-
        fiable to 042, 050-055, 057-079)
        647.6

◀ **New**   ◀▥ **Revised**

Pregnancy (*Continued*)
  complicated (*Continued*)
    vomiting (incoercible) (pernicious)
        (persistent) (uncontrollable) (vi-
        cious) 643.9
      due to organic disease or other
          cause 643.8
      early - *see* Hyperemesis, gravida-
          rum
      late (after 22 completed weeks
          gestation) 643.2
    young maternal age 659.8
  complications NEC 646.9
  cornual 633.80
    with intrauterine pregnancy 633.81
    affecting fetus or newborn 761.4
  death, maternal NEC 646.9
  delivered - *see* Delivery
  ectopic (ruptured) NEC 633.90
    with intrauterine pregnancy 633.91
    abdominal - *see* Pregnancy, abdomi-
        nal
    affecting fetus or newborn 761.4
    combined (extrauterine and intra-
        uterine) - *see* Pregnancy, cornual
    ovarian - *see* Pregnancy, ovarian
    specified type NEC 633.80
      with intrauterine pregnancy 633.81
      affecting fetus or newborn 761.4
    tubal - *see* Pregnancy, tubal
  examination, pregnancy   ◀▥
    negative result V72.41   ◀
    not confirmed V72.40   ◀
  extrauterine - *see* Pregnancy, ectopic
  fallopian - *see* Pregnancy, tubal
  false 300.11
    labor (pains) 644.1
  fatigue 646.8
  illegitimate V61.6
  incidental finding V22.2
  in double uterus 654.0
  interstitial - *see* Pregnancy, cornual
  intraligamentous - *see* Pregnancy, cor-
      nual
  intramural - *see* Pregnancy, cornual
  intraperitoneal - *see* Pregnancy, ab-
      dominal
  isthmian - *see* Pregnancy, tubal
  management affected by
    abnormal, abnormality
      fetus (suspected) 655.9
        specified NEC 655.8
      placenta 656.7
    advanced maternal age NEC 659.6
      multigravida 659.6
      primigravida 659.5
    antibodies (maternal)
      anti-c 656.1
      anti-d 656.1
      anti-e 656.1
      blood group (ABO) 656.2
        rh(esus) 656.1
    elderly multigravida 659.6
    elderly primigravida 659.5
    fetal (suspected)
      abnormality 655.9
        acid-base balance 656.8
        heart rate or rhythm 659.7
        specified NEC 655.8
      acidemia 656.3
      anencephaly 655.0
      bradycardia 659.7
      central nervous system malforma-
          tion 655.0

Pregnancy (*Continued*)
  management affected by (*Continued*)
    fetal (*Continued*)
      chromosomal abnormalities (con-
          ditions classifiable to 758.0-
          758.9) 655.1
      damage from
        drugs 655.5
          obstetric, anesthetic, or seda-
              tive 655.5
        environmental toxins 655.8
        intrauterine contraceptive device
            655.8
        maternal
          alcohol addiction 655.4
          disease NEC 655.4
          drug use 655.5
          listeriosis 655.4
          rubella 655.3
          toxoplasmosis 655.4
          viral infection 655.3
        radiation 655.6
      death (near term) 656.4
        early (before 22 completed
            weeks' gestation) 632
      distress 656.8
      excessive growth 656.6
      growth retardation 656.5
      hereditary disease 655.2
      hydrocephalus 655.0
      intrauterine death 656.4
      poor growth 656.5
      spina bifida (with myelomeningo-
          cele) 655.0
    fetal-maternal hemorrhage
        656.0
    hereditary disease in family (possi-
        bly) affecting fetus 655.2
    incompatibility, blood groups (ABO)
        656.2
      Rh(esus) 656.1
    insufficient prenatal care V23.7
    intrauterine death 656.4
    isoimmunization (ABO) 656.2
      Rh(esus) 656.1
    large-for-dates fetus 656.6
    light-for-dates fetus 656.5
    meconium in liquor 656.8
    mental disorder (conditions classifia-
        ble to 290-303, 305-316, 317-319)
        648.4
    multiparity (grand) 659.4
    poor obstetric history V23.49
      pre-term labor V25.41
    postmaturity
      post-term 645.1   ◀▥
      prolonged 645.2
    post-term pregnancy 645.1   ◀▥
    possible, not (yet) confirmed
        V72.40   ◀
    previous
      abortion V23.2
        habitual 646.3
      cesarean delivery 654.2
      difficult delivery V23.49
      forceps delivery V23.49
      habitual abortions 646.3
      hemorrhage, antepartum or post-
          partum V23.49
      hydatidiform mole V23.1
      infertility V23.0
      malignancy NEC V23.8
      nonobstetrical conditions V23.8
      premature delivery V23.41

Pregnancy (*Continued*)
  management affected by (*Continued*)
    previous (*Continued*)
      trophoblastic disease (conditions
          in 630) V23.1
      vesicular mole V23.1
    prolonged pregnancy 645.2
    small-for-dates fetus 656.5
    young maternal age 659.8
  maternal death NEC 646.9
  mesometric (mural) - *see* Pregnancy,
      cornual
  molar 631
    hydatidiform (*see also* Hydatidiform
        mole) 630
      previous, affecting management of
          pregnancy V23.1
      previous, affecting management of
          pregnancy V23.49
    multiple NEC 651.9
      with fetal loss and retention of one
          or more fetus(es) 651.6
      affecting fetus or newborn 761.5
      specified type NEC 651.8
        with fetal loss and retention of
            one or more fetus(es) 651.6
    mural - *see* Pregnancy, cornual
    observation NEC V22.1
      first pregnancy V22.0
      high-risk V23.9
        specified problem NEC V23.8
    ovarian 633.20
      with intrauterine pregnancy
          633.21
      affecting fetus or newborn 761.4
    postmature
      post-term 645.1   ◀▥
      prolonged 645.2
    post-term 645.1   ◀▥
    prenatal care only V22.1
      first pregnancy V22.0
      high-risk V23.9
        specified problem NEC V23.8
    prolonged 645.2
    quadruplet NEC 651.2
      with fetal loss and retention of one
          or more fetus(es) 651.5
      affecting fetus or newborn 761.5
    quintuplet NEC 651.8
      with fetal loss and retention of one
          or more fetus(es) 651.6
      affecting fetus or newborn 761.5
    sextuplet NEC 651.8
      with fetal loss and retention of one
          or more fetus(es) 651.6
      affecting fetus or newborn 761.5
    spurious 300.11
    superfecundation NEC 651.9
      with fetal loss and retention of one
          or more fetus(es) 651.6
    superfetation NEC 651.9
      with fetal loss and retention of one
          or more fetus(es) 651.6
    supervision (of) (for) - *see also*-
        Pregnancy, management affected
        by elderly
      multigravida V23.82
      primigravida V23.81
    high-risk V23.9
      insufficient prenatal care V23.7
      specified problem NEC V23.8
    multiparity V23.3
    normal NEC V22.1
      first V22.0

ICD-9-CM

P

Vol. 2

Pregnancy (*Continued*)
  supervision (*Continued*)
    poor
      obstetric history V23.49
        pre-term labor V23.41
      reproductive history V23.5
    previous
      abortion V23.2
      hydatidiform mole V23.1
      infertility V23.0
      neonatal death V23.5
      stillbirth V23.5
      trophoblastic disease V23.1
      vesicular mole V23.1
    specified problem NEC V23.8
    young
      multigravida V23.84
      primigravida V23.83
  triplet NEC 651.1
    with fetal loss and retention of one
      or more fetus(es) 651.4
    affecting fetus or newborn 761.5
  tubal (with rupture) 633.10
    with intrauterine pregnancy 633.11
    affecting fetus or newborn 761.4
  twin NEC 651.0
    with fetal loss and retention of one
      fetus 651.3
    affecting fetus or newborn 761.5
  unconfirmed V72.40   ◀▥
  undelivered (no other diagnosis)
    V22.2
    with false labor 644.1
    high-risk V23.9
      specified problem NEC V23.8
  unwanted NEC V61.7
Pregnant uterus - *see* condition
Preiser's disease (osteoporosis) 733.09
Prekwashiorkor 260
Preleukemia 238.7
Preluxation of hip, congenital (*see also*
    Subluxation, congenital, hip)
    754.32
Premature - *see also* condition
  beats (nodal) 427.60
    atrial 427.61
    auricular 427.61
    postoperative 997.1
    specified type NEC 427.69
    supraventricular 427.61
    ventricular 427.69
  birth NEC 765.1
  closure
    cranial suture 756.0
    fontanel 756.0
    foramen ovale 745.8
  contractions 427.60
    atrial 427.61
    auricular 427.61
    auriculoventricular 427.61
    heart (extrasystole) 427.60
    junctional 427.60
    nodal 427.60
    postoperative 997.1
    ventricular 427.69
  ejaculation 302.75
  infant NEC 765.1
    excessive 765.0
    light-for-dates - *see* Light-for-dates
  labor 644.2
    threatened 644.0
  lungs 770.4
  menopause 256.31
  puberty 259.1

Premature (*Continued*)
  rupture of membranes or amnion 658.1
    affecting fetus or newborn 761.1
    delayed delivery following 658.2
  senility (syndrome) 259.8
  separation, placenta (partial) - *see* Pla-
    centa, separation
  ventricular systole 427.69
Prematurity NEC 765.1
  extreme 765.0
Premenstrual syndrome 625.4
Premenstrual tension 625.4
Premolarization, cuspids 520.2
Premyeloma 273.1
Prenatal
  care, normal pregnancy V22.1
    first V22.0
  death, cause unknown - *see* Death, fetus
  screening - *see* Antenatal, screening
Prepartum - *see* condition
Preponderance, left or right ventricular
    429.3
Prepuce - *see* condition
Presbycardia 797
  hypertensive (*see also* Hypertension,
    heart) 402.90
Presbycusis 388.01
Presbyesophagus 530.89
Presbyophrenia 310.1
Presbyopia 367.4
Prescription of contraceptives NEC
    V25.02
  diaphragm V25.02
  oral (pill) V25.01
    emergency V25.03
    postcoital V25.03
    repeat V25.41
  repeat V25.40
    oral (pill) V25.41
Presenile - *see also* condition
  aging 259.8
  dementia (*see also* Dementia, presenile)
    290.10
Presenility 259.8
Presentation, fetal
  abnormal 652.9
    with successful version 652.1
    before labor, affecting fetus or new-
      born 761.7
    causing obstructed labor 660.0
      affecting fetus or newborn, any,
        except breech 763.1
    in multiple gestation (one or more)
      652.6
    specified NEC 652.8
  arm 652.7
    causing obstructed labor 660.0
  breech 652.2
    with successful version 652.1
      before labor, affecting fetus or
        newborn 761.7
    before labor, affecting fetus or new-
      born 761.7
  brow 652.4
    causing obstructed labor 660.0
  buttocks 652.2
  chin 652.4
  complete 652.2
  compound 652.8
  cord 663.0
  extended head 652.4
  face 652.4
    to pubes 652.8
  footling 652.8

Presentation, fetal (*Continued*)
  frank 652.2
  hand, leg, or foot NEC 652.8
  incomplete 652.8
  mentum 652.4
  multiple gestation (one fetus or more)
    652.6
  oblique 652.3
    with successful version 652.1
  shoulder 652.8
    affecting fetus or newborn 763.1
  transverse 652.3
    with successful version 652.1
  umbilical cord 663.0
  unstable 652.0
Prespondylolisthesis (congenital) (lum-
    bosacral) 756.11
Pressure
  area, skin ulcer (*see also* Decubitus)
    707.00   ◀▥
  atrophy, spine 733.99
  birth, fetus or newborn NEC 767.9
  brachial plexus 353.0
  brain 348.4
    injury at birth 767.0
  cerebral - *see* Pressure, brain
  chest 786.59
  cone, tentorial 348.4
    injury at birth 767.0
  funis - *see* Compression, umbilical cord
  hyposystolic (*see also* Hypotension)
    458.9
  increased
    intracranial 781.99
      due to
        benign intracranial hypertension
          348.2
        hydrocephalus - *see* hydrocepha-
          lus
        injury at birth 767.8
    intraocular 365.00
  lumbosacral plexus 353.1
  mediastinum 519.3
  necrosis (chronic) (skin) (*see also* Decu-
    bitus) 707.00   ◀▥
  nerve - *see* Compression, nerve
  paralysis (*see also* Neuropathy, entrap-
    ment) 355.9
  sore (chronic) (*see also* Decubitus)
    707.00   ◀▥
  spinal cord 336.9
  ulcer (chronic) (*see also* Decubitus)
    707.00   ◀▥
  umbilical cord - *see* Compression, um-
    bilical cord
  venous, increased 459.89
Pre-syncope 780.2
Preterm infant NEC 765.1
  extreme 765.0
Priapism (penis) 607.3
Prickling sensation (*see also* Disturbance,
    sensation) 782.0
Prickly heat 705.1
Primary - *see* condition
Primigravida, elderly
  affecting
    fetus or newborn 763.89
    management of pregnancy, labor,
      and delivery 659.5
Primipara, old
  affecting
    fetus or newborn 763.89
    management of pregnancy, labor,
      and delivery 659.5

◀ **New**   ◀▥ **Revised**

Primula dermatitis 692.6
Primus varus (bilateral) (metatarsus) 754.52
P.R.I.N.D. 436
Pringle's disease (tuberous sclerosis) 759.5
Prinzmetal's angina 413.1
Prinzmetal-Massumi syndrome (anterior chest wall) 786.52
Prizefighter ear 738.7
Problem (with) V49.9
  academic V62.3
  acculturation V62.4
  adopted child V61.29
  aged
    in-law V61.3
    parent V61.3
    person NEC V61.8
  alcoholism in family V61.41
  anger reaction (see also Disturbance, conduct) 312.0
  behavior, child 312.9
  behavioral V40.9
    specified NEC V40.3
  betting V69.3
  cardiorespiratory NEC V47.2
  care of sick or handicapped person in family or household V61.49
  career choice V62.2
  communication V40.1
  conscience regarding medical care V62.6
  delinquency (juvenile) 312.9
  diet, inappropriate V69.1
  digestive NEC V47.3
  ear NEC V41.3
  eating habits, inappropriate V69.1
  economic V60.2
    affecting care V60.9
      specified type NEC V60.8
  educational V62.3
  enuresis, child 307.6
  exercise, lack of V69.0
  eye NEC V41.1
  family V61.9
    specified circumstance NEC V61.8
  fear reaction, child 313.0
  feeding (elderly) (infant) 783.3
    newborn 779.3
    nonorganic 307.50
  fetal, affecting management of pregnancy 656.9
    specified type NEC 656.8
  financial V60.2
  foster child V61.29
    specified NEC V41.8
  functional V41.9
    specified type NEC V41.8
  gambling V69.3
  genital NEC V47.5
  head V48.9
    deficiency V48.0
    disfigurement V48.6
    mechanical V48.2
    motor V48.2
    movement of V48.2
    sensory V48.4
    specified condition NEC V48.8
  hearing V41.2
  high-risk sexual behavior V69.2
  identity 313.82 ◄
  influencing health status NEC V49.89
  internal organ NEC V47.9
    deficiency V47.0
    mechanical or motor V47.1

Problem (Continued)
  interpersonal NEC V62.81
  jealousy, child 313.3
  learning V40.0
  legal V62.5
  life circumstance NEC V62.89
  lifestyle V69.9
    specified NEC V69.8
  limb V49.9
    deficiency V49.0
    disfigurement V49.4
    mechanical V49.1
    motor V49.2
    movement, involving
      musculoskeletal system V49.1
      nervous system V49.2
    sensory V49.3
    specified condition NEC V49.5
  litigation V62.5
  living alone V60.3
  loneliness NEC V62.89
  marital V61.10
    involving
      divorce V61.0
      estrangement V61.0
      psychosexual disorder 302.9
      sexual function V41.7
  mastication V41.6
  medical care, within family V61.49
  mental V40.9
    specified NEC V40.2
  mental hygiene, adult V40.9
  multiparity V61.5
  nail biting, child 307.9
  neck V48.9
    deficiency V48.1
    disfigurement V48.7
    mechanical V48.3
    motor V48.3
    movement V48.3
    sensory V48.5
    specified condition NEC V48.8
  neurological NEC 781.99
  none (feared complaint unfounded) V65.5
  occupational V62.2
  parent-child V61.20
  partner V61.10
  personal NEC V62.89
    interpersonal conflict NEC V62.81
  personality (see also Disorder, personality) 301.9
  phase of life V62.89
  placenta, affecting management of pregnancy 656.9
    specified type NEC 656.8
  poverty V60.2
  presence of sick or handicapped person in family or household V61.49
  psychiatric 300.9
  psychosocial V62.9
    specified type NEC V62.89
  relational NEC V62.81
  relationship, childhood 313.3
  religious or spiritual belief
    other than medical care V62.89
    regarding medical care V62.6
  self-damaging behavior V69.8
  sexual
    behavior, high-risk V69.2
    function NEC V41.7
  sibling relational V61.8
  sight V41.0
  sleep disorder, child 307.40

Problem (Continued)
  sleep, lack of V69.4 ◄
  smell V41.5
  speech V40.1
  spite reaction, child (see also Disturbance, conduct 312.0
  spoiled child reaction (see also Disturbance, conduct) 312.1
  swallowing V41.6
  tantrum, child (see also Disturbance, conduct) 312.1
  taste V41.5
  thumb sucking, child 307.9
  tic (child) 307.21 ◄▥
  trunk V48.9
    deficiency V48.1
    disfigurement V48.7
    mechanical V48.3
    motor V48.3
    movement V48.3
    sensory V48.5
    specified condition NEC V48.8
  unemployment V62.0
  urinary NEC V47.4
  voice production V41.4
Procedure (surgical) not done NEC V64.3
  because of
    contraindication V64.1
    patient's decision V64.2
      for reasons of conscience or religion V62.6
    specified reason NEC V64.3
Procidentia
  anus (sphincter) 569.1
  rectum (sphincter) 569.1
  stomach 537.89
  uteri 618.1
Proctalgia 569.42
  fugax 564.6
  spasmodic 564.6
    psychogenic 307.89
Proctitis 569.49
  amebic 006.8
  chlamydial 099.52
  gonococcal 098.7
  granulomatous 555.1
  idiopathic 556.2
    with ulcerative sigmoiditis 556.3
  tuberculous (see also Tuberculosis) 014.8
  ulcerative (chronic) (nonspecific) 556.2
    with ulcerative sigmoiditis 556.3
Proctocele
  female (without uterine prolapse) 618.04 ◄▥
    with uterine prolapse 618.4
      complete 618.3
      incomplete 618.2
  male 569.49
Proctocolitis, idiopathic 556.2
  with ulcerative sigmoiditis 556.3
Proctoptosis 569.1
Proctosigmoiditis 569.89
  ulcerative (chronic) 556.3
Proctospasm 564.6
  psychogenic 306.4
Prodromal-AIDS - see Human immunodeficiency virus (disease) (illness) (infection)
Profichet's disease or syndrome 729.9
Progeria (adultorum) (syndrome) 259.8
Prognathism (mandibular) (maxillary) 524.00

ICD-9-CM

Vol. 2

Progonoma (melanotic) (M9363/0) - *see* Neoplasm, by site, benign

Progressive - *see* condition

Prolapse, prolapsed
  anus, anal (canal) (sphincter) 569.1
  arm or hand, complicating delivery 652.7
    causing obstructed labor 660.0
      affecting fetus or newborn 763.1
    fetus or newborn 763.1
  bladder (acquired) (mucosa) (sphincter)
    congenital (female) (male) 756.71
    female (*see also* Cystocele, female) 618.01 ◀▥
    male 596.8
  breast implant (prosthetic) 996.54
  cecostomy 569.69
  cecum 569.89
  cervix, cervical (stump) (hypertrophied) 618.1
    anterior lip, obstructing labor 660.2
      affecting fetus or newborn 763.1
    congenital 752.49
    postpartal (old) 618.1
  ciliary body 871.1
  colon (pedunculated) 569.89
  colostomy 569.69
  conjunctiva 372.73
  cord - *see* Prolapse, umbilical cord
  disc (intervertebral) - *see* Displacement, intervertebral disc
  duodenum 537.89
  eye implant (orbital) 996.59
    lens (ocular) 996.53
  fallopian tube 620.4
  fetal extremity, complicating delivery 652.8
    causing obstructed labor 660.0
    fetus or newborn 763.1
  funis - *see* Prolapse, umbilical cord
  gastric (mucosa) 537.89
  genital, female 618.9
    specified NEC 618.89 ◀▥
  globe 360.81
  ileostomy bud 569.69
  intervertebral disc - *see* Displacement, intervertebral disc
  intestine (small) 569.89
  iris 364.8
    traumatic 871.1
  kidney (*see also* Disease, renal) 593.0
    congenital 753.3
  laryngeal muscles or ventricle 478.79
  leg, complicating delivery 652.8
    causing obstructed labor 660.0
    fetus or newborn 763.1
  liver 573.8
  meatus urinarius 599.5
  mitral valve 424.0
  ocular lens implant 996.53
  organ or site, congenital NEC - *see* Malposition, congenital
  ovary 620.4
  pelvic (floor), female 618.89 ◀▥
  perineum, female 618.89 ◀▥
  pregnant uterus 654.4
  rectum (mucosa) (sphincter) 569.1
    due to Trichuris trichiuria 127.3
  spleen 289.59
  stomach 537.89
  umbilical cord
    affecting fetus or newborn 762.4
    complicating delivery 663.0

Prolapse, prolapsed (*Continued*)
  ureter 593.89
    with obstruction 593.4
  ureterovesical orifice 593.89
  urethra (acquired) (infected) (mucosa) 599.5
    congenital 753.8
  uterovaginal 618.4
    complete 618.3
    incomplete 618.2
    specified NEC 618.89 ◀▥
  uterus (first degree) (second degree) (third degree) (complete) (without vaginal wall prolapse) 618.1
    with mention of vaginal wall prolapse - *see* Prolapse, uterovaginal
    congenital 752.3
    in pregnancy or childbirth 654.4
      affecting fetus or newborn 763.1
      causing obstructed labor 660.2
        affecting fetus or newborn 763.1
    postpartal (old) 618.1
  uveal 871.1
  vagina (anterior) (posterior) (vault) (wall) (without uterine prolapse) 618.00 ◀▥
    with uterine prolapse 618.4
      complete 618.3
      incomplete 618.2
    paravaginal 618.02 ◀▥
    posthysterectomy 618.5
    specified NEC 618.09 ◀
  vitreous (humor) 379.26
    traumatic 871.1
  womb - *see* Prolapse, uterus

Prolapsus, female 618.9

Proliferative - *see* condition

Prolinemia 270.8

Prolinuria 270.8

Prolonged, prolongation
  bleeding time (*see also* Defect, coagulation) 790.92
    "idiopathic" (in von Willebrand's disease) 286.4
  coagulation time (*see also* Defect, coagulation) 790.92
  gestation syndrome 766.22
  labor 662.1
    affecting fetus or newborn 763.89
    first stage 662.0
    second stage 662.2
  pregnancy 645.2
  PR interval 426.11
  prothrombin time (*see also* Defect, coagulation) 790.92
  rupture of membranes (24 hours or more prior to onset of labor) 658.2
  uterine contractions in labor 661.4
    affecting fetus or newborn 763.7

Prominauris 744.29

Prominence
  auricle (ear) (congenital) 744.29
    acquired 380.32
  ischial spine or sacral promontory
    with disproportion (fetopelvic) 653.3
      affecting fetus or newborn 763.1
      causing obstructed labor 660.1
        affecting fetus or newborn 763.1
  nose (congenital) 748.1
    acquired 738.0

Pronation
  ankle 736.79
  foot 736.79
    congenital 755.67

Prophylactic
  administration of
    antibiotics V07.39
    antitoxin, any V07.2
    antivenin V07.2
    chemotherapeutic agent NEC V07.39
      fluoride V07.31
    diphtheria antitoxin V07.2
    gamma globulin V07.2
    immune sera (gamma globulin) V07.2
    RhoGAM V07.2
    tetanus antitoxin V07.2
  chemotherapy NEC V07.39
    fluoride V07.31
  hormone replacement (postmenopausal) V07.4 ◀
  immunotherapy V07.2
  measure V07.9
    specified type NEC V07.8
  postmenopausal hormone replacement V07.4
  sterilization V25.2

Proptosis (ocular) (*see also* Exophthalmos) 376.30
  thyroid 242.0

Propulsion
  eyeball 360.81

Prosecution, anxiety concerning V62.5

Prostate, prostatic - *see* condition

Prostatism 600.90
  with urinary retention 600.91

Prostatitis (congestive) (suppurative) 601.9
  acute 601.0
  cavitary 601.8
  chlamydial 099.54
  chronic 601.1
  diverticular 601.8
  due to Trichomonas (vaginalis) 131.03
  fibrous 600.90
    with urinary retention 600.91
  gonococcal (acute) 098.12
    chronic or duration of 2 months or over 098.32
  granulomatous 601.8
  hypertrophic 600.00
    with urinary retention 600.01
  specified type NEC 601.8
  subacute 601.1
  trichomonal 131.03
  tuberculous (*see also* Tuberculosis) 016.5 [601.4]

Prostatocystitis 601.3

Prostatorrhea 602.8

Prostatoseminovesiculitis, trichomonal 131.03

Prostration 780.79
  heat 992.5
    anhydrotic 992.3
    due to
      salt (and water) depletion 992.4
      water depletion 992.3
  nervous 300.5
  newborn 779.89
  senile 797

Protanomaly 368.51

Protanopia (anomalous trichromat) (complete) (incomplete) 368.51

Protein
  deficiency 260
  malnutrition 260
  sickness (prophylactic) (therapeutic) 999.5

Proteinemia 790.99

◀ **New**   ◀▥ **Revised**

Proteinosis
  alveolar, lung or pulmonary 516.0
  lipid 272.8
  lipoid (of Urbach) 272.8
Proteinuria (*see also* Albuminuria) 791.0
  Bence-Jones NEC 791.0
  gestational 646.2
    with hypertension - *see* Toxemia, of
      pregnancy
  orthostatic 593.6
  postural 593.6
Proteolysis, pathologic 286.6
Protocoproporphyria 277.1
Protoporphyria (erythrohepatic) (erythropoietic) 277.1
Protrusio acetabuli 718.65
Protrusion
  acetabulum (into pelvis) 718.65
  device, implant, or graft - *see* Compli-
    cations, mechanical
  ear, congenital 744.29
  intervertebral disc - *see* Displacement,
    intervertebral disc
  nucleus pulposus - *see* Displacement,
    intervertebral disc
Proud flesh 701.5
Prune belly (syndrome) 756.71
Prurigo (ferox) (gravis) (Hebra's) (he-
  brae) (mitis) (simplex) 698.2
  agria 698.3
  asthma syndrome 691.8
  Besnier's (atopic dermatitis) (infantile
    eczema) 691.8
  eczematodes allergicum 691.8
  estivalis (Hutchinson's) 692.72
  Hutchinson's 692.72
  nodularis 698.3
  psychogenic 306.3
Pruritus, pruritic 698.9
  ani 698.0
    psychogenic 306.3
  conditions NEC 698.9
    psychogenic 306.3
  due to Onchocerca volvulus 125.3
  ear 698.9
  essential 698.9
  genital organ(s) 698.1
    psychogenic 306.3
  gravidarum 646.8
  hiemalis 698.8
  neurogenic (any site) 306.3
  perianal 698.0
  psychogenic (any site) 306.3
  scrotum 698.1
    psychogenic 306.3
  senile, senilis 698.8
  trichomonas 131.9
  vulva, vulvae 698.1
    psychogenic 306.3
Psammocarcinoma (M8140/3) - *see* Neoplasm, by site, malignant
Pseudarthrosis, pseudoarthrosis (bone)
  733.82
  joint following fusion V45.4
Pseudoacanthosis
  nigricans 701.8
Pseudoaneurysm - *see* Aneurysm
Pseudoangina (pectoris) - *see* Angina
Pseudoangioma 452
Pseudo-Argyll-Robertson pupil 379.45
Pseudoarteriosus 747.89
Pseudoarthrosis - *see* Pseudarthrosis
Pseudoataxia 799.89
Pseudobursa 727.89

Pseudocholera 025
Pseudochromidrosis 705.89
Pseudocirrhosis, liver, pericardial 423.2
Pseudocoarctation 747.21
Pseudocowpox 051.1
Pseudocoxalgia 732.1
Pseudocroup 478.75
Pseudocyesis 300.11
Pseudocyst
  lung 518.89
  pancreas 577.2
  retina 361.19
Pseudodementia 300.16
Pseudoelephantiasis neuroarthritica
  757.0
Pseudoemphysema 518.89
Pseudoencephalitis
  superior (acute) hemorrhagic 265.1
Pseudoerosion cervix, congenital
  752.49
Pseudoexfoliation, lens capsule 366.11
Pseudofracture (idiopathic) (multiple)
  (spontaneous) (symmetrical)
  268.2
Pseudoglanders 025
Pseudoglioma 360.44
Pseudogout - *see* Chondrocalcinosis
Pseudohallucination 780.1
Pseudohemianesthesia 782.0
Pseudohemophilia (Bernuth's) (heredi-
  tary) (type B) 286.4
  type A 287.8
  vascular 287.8
Pseudohermaphroditism 752.7
  with chromosomal anomaly - *see*
    Anomaly, chromosomal
  adrenal 255.2
  female (without adrenocortical disor-
    der) 752.7
    with adrenocortical disorder 255.2
    adrenal 255.2
  male (without gonadal disorder) 752.7
    with
      adrenocortical disorder 255.2
      cleft scrotum 752.7
      feminizing testis 257.8
      gonadal disorder 257.9
    adrenal 255.2
Pseudohole, macula 362.54
Pseudo-Hurler's disease (mucolipidosis
  III) 272.7
Pseudohydrocephalus 348.2
**Pseudohypertrophic muscular dystro-
  phy** (Erb's) 359.1
Pseudohypertrophy, muscle 359.1
Pseudohypoparathyroidism 275.49
Pseudoinfluenza 487.1
Pseudoinsomnia 307.49
Pseudoleukemia 288.8
  infantile 285.8
Pseudomembranous - *see* condition
Pseudomeningocele (cerebral) (infective)
  (surgical) 349.2
  spinal 349.2
Pseudomenstruation 626.8
Pseudomucinous
  cyst (ovary) (M8470/0) 220
  peritoneum 568.89
Pseudomyeloma 273.1
Pseudomyxoma peritonei (M8480/6) 197.6
Pseudoneuritis optic (nerve) 377.24
  papilla 377.24
  congenital 743.57
Pseudoneuroma - *see* Injury, nerve, by site

Pseudo-obstruction
  intestine (chronic) (idiopathic) (inter-
    mittent secondary) (primary)
    564.89 ◀▥
    acute 560.89 ◀
Pseudopapilledema 377.24
Pseudoparalysis
  arm or leg 781.4
  atonic, congenital 358.8
Pseudopelade 704.09
Pseudophakia V43.1
Pseudopolycythemia 289.0
Pseudopolyposis, colon 556.4
Pseudoporencephaly 348.0
Pseudopseudohypoparathyroidism
  275.49
Pseudopsychosis 300.16
Pseudopterygium 372.52
Pseudoptosis (eyelid) 374.34
Pseudorabies 078.89
Pseudoretinitis, pigmentosa 362.65
Pseudorickets 588.0
  senile (Pozzi's) 731.0
Pseudorubella 057.8
Pseudoscarlatina 057.8
Pseudosclerema 778.1
Pseudosclerosis (brain)
  Jakob's 046.1
  of Westphal (-Strümpell) (hepatolenti-
    cular degeneration) 275.1
  spastic 046.1
    with dementia
      with behavioral disturbance
        046.1 [294.11]
      without behavioral disturbance
        046.1 [294.10]
Pseudoseizure 780.39
  non-psychiatric 780.39
  psychiatric 300.11
Pseudotabes 799.89
  diabetic 250.6 [337.1]
Pseudotetanus (*see also* Convulsions)
  780.39
Pseudotetany 781.7
  hysterical 300.11
Pseudothalassemia 285.0
Pseudotrichinosis 710.3
Pseudotruncus arteriosus 747.29
Pseudotuberculosis, pasteurella (infection) 027.2
Pseudotumor
  cerebri 348.2
  orbit (inflammatory) 376.11
Pseudo-Turner's syndrome 759.89
Pseudoxanthoma elasticum 757.39
Psilosis (sprue) (tropical) 579.1
  Monilia 112.89
  nontropical 579.0
  not sprue 704.00
Psittacosis 073.9
Psoitis 728.89
Psora NEC 696.1
Psoriasis 696.1
  any type, except arthropathic
    696.1
  arthritic, arthropathic 696.0
  buccal 528.6
  flexural 696.1
  follicularis 696.1
  guttate 696.1
  inverse 696.1
  mouth 528.6
  nummularis 696.1
  psychogenic 316 [696.1]

ICD-9-CM

P

Vol. 2

Psoriasis (*Continued*)
  punctata 696.1
  pustular 696.1
  rupioides 696.1
  vulgaris 696.1
Psorospermiasis 136.4
Psorospermosis 136.4
  follicularis (vegetans) 757.39
Psychalgia 307.80
Psychasthenia 300.89
  compulsive 300.3
  mixed compulsive states 300.3
  obsession 300.3
Psychiatric disorder or problem NEC
    300.9
Psychogenic - *see also* condition
  factors associated with physical condi-
      tions 316
Psychoneurosis, psychoneurotic (*see also*
    Neurosis) 300.9
  anxiety (state) 300.00
  climacteric 627.2
  compensation 300.16
  compulsion 300.3
  conversion hysteria 300.11
  depersonalization 300.6
  depressive type 300.4
  dissociative hysteria 300.15
  hypochondriacal 300.7
  hysteria 300.10
    conversion type 300.11
    dissociative type 300.15
  mixed NEC 300.89
  neurasthenic 300.5
  obsessional 300.3
  obsessive-compulsive 300.3
  occupational 300.89
  personality NEC 301.89
  phobia 300.20
  senile NEC 300.89
Psychopathic - *see also* condition
  constitution, posttraumatic 310.2
    with psychosis 293.9
  personality 301.9
    amoral trends 301.7
    antisocial trends 301.7
    asocial trends 301.7
    mixed types 301.7
  state 301.9
Psychopathy, sexual (*see also* Deviation,
    sexual) 302.9
Psychophysiologic, psychophysiological
    condition - *see* Reaction, psycho-
    physiologic
Psychose passionelle 297.8
Psychosexual identity disorder 302.6
  adult-life 302.85
  childhood 302.6
Psychosis 298.9
  acute hysterical 298.1
  affecting management of pregnancy,
      childbirth, or puerperium 648.4
  affective (*see also* Disorder, mood)
      296.90 ◄▥
    drug-induced 292.84
    due to or associated with physical
        condition 293.83

  Note   Use the following fifth-digit
  subclassification with categories
  296.0-296.6:

  0   unspecified
  1   mild
  2   moderate

Psychosis (*Continued*)
  3   severe, without mention of
      psychotic behavior
  4   severe, specified as with psy-
      chotic behavior
  5   in partial or unspecified remis-
      sion
  6   in full remission

  involutional 296.2
    recurrent episode 296.3
    single episode 296.2
  manic-depressive 296.80
    circular (alternating) 296.7
      currently depressed 296.5
      currently manic 296.4
    depressed type 296.2
      atypical 296.82
      recurrent episode 296.3
      single episode 296.2
    manic 296.0
      atypical 296.81
      recurrent episode 296.1
      single episode 296.0
    mixed type NEC 296.89
    specified type NEC 296.89
  senile 290.21
  specified type NEC 296.99
  alcoholic 291.9
    with
      anxiety 291.89
      delirium tremens 291.0
      delusions 291.5
      dementia 291.2
      hallucinosis 291.3
      jealousy 291.5
      mood disturbance 291.89
      paranoia 291.5
      persisting amnesia 291.1
      sexual dysfunction 291.89
      sleep disturbance 291.89
    amnestic confabulatory 291.1
    delirium tremens 291.0
    hallucinosis 291.3
    Korsakoff's, Korsakov's, Korsakow's
        291.1
    paranoid type 291.5
    pathological intoxication 291.4
    polyneuritic 291.1
    specified type NEC 291.89
  alternating (*see also* Psychosis, manic-
      depressive, circular) 296.7
  anergastic (*see also* Psychosis, organic)
      294.9
  arteriosclerotic 290.40
    with
      acute confusional state 290.41
      delirium 290.41
      delusions 290.42 ◄▥
      depressed mood 290.43 ◄▥
    depressed type 290.43
    paranoid type 290.42
    simple type 290.40
    uncomplicated 290.40
  atypical 298.9
    depressive 296.82
    manic 296.81
  borderline (schizophrenia) (*see also*
      Schizophrenia) 295.5
    of childhood (*see also* Psychosis,
        childhood) 299.8
      prepubertal 299.8
  brief reactive 298.8
  childhood, with origin specific to 299.9

Psychosis (*Continued*)

  Note   Use the following fifth-digit
  subclassification with category 299:

  0   current or active state
  1   residual state

  atypical 299.8
    specified type NEC 299.8
  circular (*see also* Psychosis, manic-de-
      pressive, circular) 296.7
  climacteric (*see also* Psychosis, involu-
      tional) 298.8
  confusional 298.9
    acute 293.0
    reactive 298.2
    subacute 293.1
  depressive (*see also* Psychosis, affective)
      296.2
    atypical 296.82
    involutional 296.2
      with hypomania (bipolar II) 296.89
      recurrent episode 296.3
      single episode 296.2
    psychogenic 298.0
    reactive (emotional stress) (psycho-
        logical trauma) 298.0
    recurrent episode 296.3
      with hypomania (bipolar II) 296.89
    single episode 296.2
  disintegrative childhood (*see also* Psy-
      chosis, childhood) 299.1   ◄▥
  drug 292.9
    with
      affective syndrome 292.84
      amnestic syndrome 292.83
      anxiety 292.89
      delirium 292.81
        withdrawal 292.0
      delusions 292.11   ◄▥
      dementia 292.82
      depressive state 292.84
      hallucinations 282.12   ◄
      hallucinosis 292.12
      mood disorder 292.84   ◄
      mood disturbance 292.84
      organic personality syndrome
          NEC 292.89
      sexual dysfunction 292.89
      sleep disturbance 292.89
      withdrawal syndrome (and delir-
          ium) 292.0
    affective syndrome 292.84
    delusions 292.11   ◄▥
    hallucinatory state 292.12
    hallucinosis 292.12
    paranoid state 292.11
    specified type NEC 292.89
    withdrawal syndrome (and delir-
        ium) 292.0
  due to or associated with physical con-
      dition (*see also* Psychosis, organic)
      293.9
  epileptic NEC 294.8
  excitation (psychogenic) (reactive)
      298.1
  exhaustive (*see also* Reaction, stress,
      acute) 308.9
  hypomanic (*see also* Psychosis, affec-
      tive) 296.0
    recurrent episode 296.1
    single episode 296.0
  hysterical 298.8
    acute 298.1

Psychosis (*Continued*)
  incipient 298.8
    schizophrenic (*see also* Schizophrenia) 295.5
  induced 297.3
  infantile (*see also* Psychosis, childhood) 299.0
  infective 293.9
    acute 293.0
    subacute 293.1
  in ◀▥
    conditions classified elsewhere ◀
      with ◀
        delusions 293.81 ◀
        hallucinations 293.82 ◀
      pregnancy, childbirth, or puerperium 648.4 ◀
  interactional (childhood) (*see also* Psychosis, childhood) 299.1
  involutional 298.8
    depressive (*see also* Psychosis, affective) 296.2
      recurrent episode 296.3
      single episode 296.2
    melancholic 296.2
      recurrent episode 296.3
      single episode 296.2
    paranoid state 297.2
    paraphrenia 297.2
  Korsakoff's, Korakov's, Korsakow's (nonalcoholic) 294.0
    alcoholic 291.1
  mania (phase) (*see also* Psychosis, affective) 296.0
    recurrent episode 296.1
    single episode 296.0
  manic (*see also* Psychosis, affective) 296.0
    atypical 296.81
    recurrent episode 296.1
    single episode 296.0
  manic-depressive 296.80
    circular 296.7
      currently
        depressed 296.5
        manic 296.4
        mixed 296.6
    depressive 296.2
      recurrent episode 296.3
        with hypomania (bipolar II) 296.89
      single episode 296.2
    hypomanic 296.0
      recurrent episode 296.1
      single episode 296.0
    manic 296.0
      atypical 296.81
      recurrent episode 296.1
      single episode 296.0
    mixed NEC 296.89
    perplexed 296.89
    stuporous 296.89
  menopausal (*see also* Psychosis, involutional) 298.8
  mixed schizophrenic and affective (*see also* Schizophrenia) 295.7
  multi-infarct (cerebrovascular) (*see also* Psychosis, arteriosclerotic) 290.40
  organic NEC 294.9
    due to or associated with
      addiction
        alcohol (*see also* Psychosis, alcoholic) 291.9

Psychosis (*Continued*)
  organic NEC (*Continued*)
    due to or associated with (*Continued*)
      addiction (*Continued*)
        drug (*see also* Psychosis, drug) 292.9
      alcohol intoxication, acute (*see also* Psychosis, alcoholic) 291.9
      alcoholism (*see also* Psychosis, alcoholic) 291.9
      arteriosclerosis (cerebral) (*see also* Psychosis, arteriosclerotic) 290.40
      cerebrovascular disease
        acute (psychosis) 293.0
        arteriosclerotic (*see also* Psychosis, arteriosclerotic) 290.40
      childbirth - *see* Psychosis, puerperal
      dependence
        alcohol (*see also* Psychosis, alcoholic) 291.9
        drug 292.9
      disease
        alcoholic liver (*see also* Psychosis, alcoholic) 291.9
        brain
          arteriosclerotic (*see also* Psychosis, arteriosclerotic) 290.40
          cerebrovascular
            acute (psychosis) 293.0
            arteriosclerotic (*see also* Psychosis, arteriosclerotic) 290.40
          endocrine or metabolic 293.9
            acute (psychosis) 293.0
            subacute (psychosis) 293.1
          Jakob-Creutzfeldt
            with behavioral disturbance 046.1 [294.11]
            without behavioral disturbance 046.1 [294.10]
          liver, alcoholic (*see also* Psychosis, alcoholic) 291.9
      disorder
        cerebrovascular
          acute (psychosis) 293.0
        endocrine or metabolic 293.9
          acute (psychosis) 293.0
          subacute (psychosis) 293.1
      epilepsy
        with behavioral disturbance 345.9 [294.11]
        without behavioral disturbance 345.9 [294.10]
        transient (acute) 293.0
      Huntington's chorea
        with behavioral disturbance 333.4 [294.11]
        without behavioral disturbance 333.4 [294.10]
      infection
        brain 293.9
          acute (psychosis) 293.0
          chronic 294.8
          subacute (psychosis) 293.1
        intracranial NEC 293.9
          acute (psychosis) 293.0
          chronic 294.8
          subacute (psychosis) 293.1
      intoxication
        alcoholic (acute) (*see also* Psychosis, alcoholic) 291.9
        pathological 291.4

Psychosis (*Continued*)
  organic (*Continued*)
    due to or associated with (*Continued*)
      intoxication (*Continued*)
        drug (*see also* Psychosis, drug) 292.9
      ischemia
        cerebrovascular (generalized) (*see also* Psychosis, arteriosclerotic) 290.40
      Jakob-Creutzfeldt disease or syndrome
        with behavioral disturbance 046.1 [294.11]
        without behavioral disturbance 046.1 [294.10]
      multiple sclerosis
        with behavioral disturbance 340 [294.11]
        without behavioral disturbance 340 [294.10]
      physical condition NEC 293.9
        with
          delusions 293.81
          hallucinations 293.82
      presenility 290.10
      puerperium - *see* Psychosis, puerperal
      sclerosis, multiple
        with behavioral disturbance 340 [294.11]
        without behavioral disturbance 340 [294.10]
      senility 290.20
      status epilepticus
        with behavioral disturbance 345.3 [294.11]
        without behavioral disturbance 345.3 [294.10]
      trauma
        brain (birth) (from electrical current) (surgical) 293.9
          acute (psychosis) 293.0
          chronic 294.8
          subacute (psychosis) 293.1
      unspecified physical condition 293.9
        with
          delusional 293.81
          hallucination 293.82
    infective 293.9
      acute (psychosis) 293.0
      subacute 293.1
    posttraumatic 293.9
      acute 293.0
      subacute 293.1
    specified type NEC 294.8
    transient 293.9
      with
        anxiety 293.84
        delusions 293.81
        depression 293.83
        hallucinations 293.82
      depressive type 293.83
      hallucinatory type 293.82
      paranoid type 293.81
      specified type NEC 293.89
  paranoic 297.1
  paranoid (chronic) 297.9
    alcoholic 291.5
    chronic 297.1
    climacteric 297.2
    involutional 297.2
    menopausal 297.2
    protracted reactive 298.4

ICD-9-CM

P

Vol. 2

Psychosis *(Continued)*
  paranoid *(Continued)*
    psychogenic 298.4
      acute 298.3
    schizophrenic *(see also* Schizophrenia) 295.3
    senile 290.20
  paroxysmal 298.9
    senile 290.20
  polyneuritic, alcoholic 291.1
  postoperative 293.9
  postpartum - *see* Psychosis, puerperal
  prepsychotic *(see also* Schizophrenia) 295.5
  presbyophrenic (type) 290.8
  presenile *(see also* Dementia, presenile) 290.10
  prison 300.16
  psychogenic 298.8
    depressive 298.0
    paranoid 298.4
      acute 298.3
  puerperal
    specified type - *see* categories 295-298
    unspecified type 293.89
      acute 293.0
      chronic 293.89
      subacute 293.1
  reactive (emotional stress) (psychological trauma) 298.8
    brief 298.8
    confusion 298.2
    depressive 298.0
    excitation 298.1
  schizo-affective (depressed) (excited) *(see also* Schizophrenia) 295.7
  schizophrenia, schizophrenic *(see also* Schizophrenia) 295.9
    borderline type 295.5
      of childhood *(see also* Psychosis, childhood) 299.8
    catatonic (excited) (withdrawn) 295.2
    childhood type *(see also* Psychosis, childhood) 299.9
    hebephrenic 295.1
    incipient 295.5
    latent 295.5
    paranoid 295.3
    prepsychotic 295.5
    prodromal 295.5
    pseudoneurotic 295.5
    pseudopsychopathic 295.5
    schizophreniform 295.4
    simple 295.0
    undifferentiated type 295.9 ◄
  schizophreniform 295.4
  senile NEC 290.20
    with
      delusional features 290.20
      depressive features 290.21
    depressed type 290.21
    paranoid type 290.20
    simple deterioration 290.20
    specified type - *see* categories 295-298
  shared 297.3
  situational (reactive) 298.8
  symbiotic (childhood) *(see also* Psychosis, childhood) 299.1
  toxic (acute) 293.9
Psychotic *(see also* condition) 298.9
  episode 298.9
    due to or associated with physical conditions *(see also* Psychosis, organic) 293.9

Pterygium (eye) 372.40
  central 372.43
  colli 744.5
  double 372.44
  peripheral (stationary) 372.41
    progressive 372.42
  recurrent 372.45
Ptilosis 374.55
Ptomaine (poisoning) *(see also* Poisoning, food) 005.9
Ptosis (adiposa) 374.30
  breast 611.8
  cecum 569.89
  colon 569.89
  congenital (eyelid) 743.61
    specified site NEC - *see* Anomaly, specified type NEC
  epicanthus syndrome 270.2
  eyelid 374.30
    congenital 743.61
    mechanical 374.33
    myogenic 374.32
    paralytic 374.31
  gastric 537.5
  intestine 569.89
  kidney *(see also* Disease, renal) 593.0
    congenital 753.3
  liver 573.8
  renal *(see also* Disease, renal) 593.0
    congenital 753.3
  splanchnic 569.89
  spleen 289.59
  stomach 537.5
  viscera 569.89
Ptyalism 527.7
  hysterical 300.11
  periodic 527.2
  pregnancy 646.8
  psychogenic 306.4
Ptyalolithiasis 527.5
Pubalgia 848.8
Pubarche, precocious 259.1
Pubertas praecox 259.1
Puberty V21.1
  abnormal 259.9
  bleeding 626.3
  delayed 259.0
  precocious (constitutional) (cryptogenic) (idiopathic) NEC 259.1
    due to
      adrenal
        cortical hyperfunction 255.2
        hyperplasia 255.2
      cortical hyperfunction 255.2
      ovarian hyperfunction 256.1
        estrogen 256.0
      pineal tumor 259.8
      testicular hyperfunction 257.0
  premature 259.1
    due to
      adrenal cortical hyperfunction 255.2
      pineal tumor 259.8
      pituitary (anterior) hyperfunction 253.1
Puckering, macula 362.56
Pudenda, pudendum - *see* condition
Puente's disease (simple glandular cheilitis) 528.5
Puerperal
  abscess
    areola 675.1
    Bartholin's gland 646.6
    breast 675.1
    cervix (uteri) 670
    fallopian tube 670

Puerperal *(Continued)*
  abscess *(Continued)*
    genital organ 670
    kidney 646.6
    mammary 675.1
    mesosalpinx 670
    nabothian 646.6
    nipple 675.0
    ovary, ovarian 670
    oviduct 670
    parametric 670
    para-uterine 670
    pelvic 670
    perimetric 670
    periuterine 670
    retro-uterine 670
    subareolar 675.1
    suprapelvic 670
    tubal (ruptured) 670
    tubo-ovarian 670
    urinary tract NEC 646.6
    uterine, uterus 670
    vagina (wall) 646.6
    vaginorectal 646.6
    vulvovaginal gland 646.6
  accident 674.9
  adnexitis 670
  afibrinogenemia, or other coagulation defect 666.3
  albuminuria (acute) (subacute) 646.2
    pre-eclamptic 642.4
  anemia (conditions classifiable to 280-285) 648.2
  anuria 669.3
  apoplexy 674.0
  asymptomatic bacteriuria 646.5
  atrophy, breast 676.3
  blood dyscrasia 666.3
  caked breast 676.2
  cardiomyopathy 674.5
  cellulitis - *see* Puerperal, abscess
  cerebrovascular disorder (conditions classifiable to 430-434, 436-437) 674.0
  cervicitis (conditions classifiable to 616.0) 646.6
  coagulopathy (any) 666.3
  complications 674.9
    specified type NEC 674.8
  convulsions (eclamptic) (uremic) 642.6
    with pre-existing hypertension 642.7
  cracked nipple 676.1
  cystitis 646.6
  cystopyelitis 646.6
  deciduitis (acute) 670
  delirium NEC 293.9
  diabetes (mellitus) (conditions classifiable to 250) 648.0
  disease 674.9
    breast NEC 676.3
    cerebrovascular (acute) 674.0
    nonobstetric NEC *(see also* Pregnancy, complicated, current disease or condition) 648.9
    pelvis inflammatory 670
    renal NEC 646.2
    tubo-ovarian 670
    Valsuani's (progressive pernicious anemia) 648.2
  disorder
    lactation 676.9
      specified type NEC 676.8
    nonobstetric NEC *(see also* Pregnancy, complicated, current disease or condition) 648.9

Puerperal (*Continued*)
disruption
  cesarean wound 674.1
  episiotomy wound 674.2
  perineal laceration wound 674.2
drug dependence (conditions classifiable to 304) 648.3
eclampsia 642.6
  with pre-existing hypertension 642.7
embolism (pulmonary) 673.2
  air 673.0
  amniotic fluid 673.1
  blood clot 673.2
  brain or cerebral 674.0
  cardiac 674.8
  fat 673.8
  intracranial sinus (venous) 671.5
  pyemic 673.3
  septic 673.3
  spinal cord 671.5
endometritis (conditions classifiable to 615.0-615.9) 670
endophlebitis - *see* Puerperal, phlebitis
endotrachelitis 646.6
engorgement, breasts 676.2
erysipelas 670
failure
  lactation 676.4
  renal, acute 669.3
fever 670
  meaning pyrexia (of unknown origin) 672
  meaning sepsis 670
fissure, nipple 676.1
fistula
  breast 675.1
  mammary gland 675.1
  nipple 675.0
galactophoritis 675.2
galactorrhea 676.6
gangrene
  gas 670
  uterus 670
gonorrhea (conditions classifiable to 098) 647.1
hematoma, subdural 674.0
hematosalpinx, infectional 670
hemiplegia, cerebral 674.0
hemorrhage 666.1
  brain 674.0
  bulbar 674.0
  cerebellar 674.0
  cerebral 674.0
  cortical 674.0
  delayed (after 24 hours) (uterine) 666.2
  extradural 674.0
  internal capsule 674.0
  intracranial 674.0
  intrapontine 674.0
  meningeal 674.0
  pontine 674.0
  subarachnoid 674.0
  subcortical 674.0
  subdural 674.0
  uterine, delayed 666.2
  ventricular 674.0
hemorrhoids 671.8
hepatorenal syndrome 674.8
hypertrophy
  breast 676.3
  mammary gland 676.3
induration breast (fibrous) 676.3
infarction
  lung - *see* Puerperal, embolism
  pulmonary - *see* Puerperal, embolism

Puerperal (*Continued*)
infection
  Bartholin's gland 646.6
  breast 675.2
    with nipple 675.9
      specified type NEC 675.8
  cervix 646.6
  endocervix 646.6
  fallopian tube 670
  generalized 670
  genital tract (major) 670
    minor or localized 646.6
  kidney (bacillus coli) 646.6
  mammary gland 675.2
    with nipple 675.9
      specified type NEC 675.8
  nipple 675.0
    with breast 675.9
      specified type NEC 675.8
  ovary 670
  pelvic 670
  peritoneum 670
  renal 646.6
  tubo-ovarian 670
  urinary (tract) NEC 646.6
    asymptomatic 646.5
  uterus, uterine 670
  vagina 646.6
inflammation - *see also* Puerperal, infection
  areola 675.1
  Bartholin's gland 646.6
  breast 675.2
  broad ligament 670
  cervix (uteri) 646.6
  fallopian tube 670
  genital organs 670
    localized 646.6
  mammary gland 675.2
  nipple 675.0
  ovary 670
  oviduct 670
  pelvis 670
  periuterine 670
  tubal 670
  vagina 646.6
  vein - *see* Puerperal, phlebitis
inversion, nipple 676.3
ischemia, cerebral 674.0
lymphangitis 670
  breast 675.2
malaria (conditions classifiable to 084) 647.4
malnutrition 648.9
mammillitis 675.0
mammitis 675.2
mania 296.0
  recurrent episode 296.1
  single episode 296.0
mastitis 675.2
  purulent 675.1
  retromammary 675.1
  submammary 675.1
melancholia 296.2
  recurrent episode 296.3
  single episode 296.2
mental disorder (conditions classifiable to 290-303, 305-316, 317-319) 648.4
metritis (septic) (suppurative) 670
metroperitonitis 670
metrorrhagia 666.2
metrosalpingitis 670
metrovaginitis 670
milk leg 671.4

Puerperal (*Continued*)
monoplegia, cerebral 674.0
necrosis
  kidney, tubular 669.3
  liver (acute) (subacute) (conditions classifiable to 570) 674.8
  ovary 670
  renal cortex 669.3
nephritis or nephrosis (conditions classifiable to 580-589) 646.2
  with hypertension 642.1
nutritional deficiency (conditions classifiable to 260-269) 648.9
occlusion, precerebral artery 674.0
oliguria 669.3
oophoritis 670
ovaritis 670
paralysis
  bladder (sphincter) 665.5
  cerebral 674.0
paralytic stroke 674.0
parametritis 670
paravaginitis 646.6
pelviperitonitis 670
perimetritis 670
perimetrosalpingitis 670
perinephritis 646.6
perioophoritis 670
periphlebitis - *see* Puerperal, phlebitis
perisalpingitis 670
peritoneal infection 670
peritonitis (pelvic) 670
perivaginitis 646.6
phlebitis 671.9
  deep 671.4
  intracranial sinus (venous) 671.5
  pelvic 671.4
  specified site NEC 671.5
  superficial 671.2
phlegmasia alba dolens 671.4
placental polyp 674.4
pneumonia, embolic - *see* Puerperal, embolism
prediabetes 648.8
pre-eclampsia (mild) 642.4
  with pre-existing hypertension 642.7
  severe 642.5
psychosis, unspecified (*see also* Psychosis, puerperal) 293.89
pyelitis 646.6
pyelocystitis 646.6
pyelohydronephrosis 646.6
pyelonephritis 646.6
pyelonephrosis 646.6
pyemia 670
pyocystitis 646.6
pyohemia 670
pyometra 670
pyonephritis 646.6
pyonephrosis 646.6
pyo-oophoritis 670
pyosalpingitis 670
pyosalpinx 670
pyrexia (of unknown origin) 672
renal
  disease NEC 646.2
  failure, acute 669.3
retention
  decidua (fragments) (with delayed hemorrhage) 666.2
    without hemorrhage 667.1
  placenta (fragments) (with delayed hemorrhage) 666.2
    without hemorrhage 667.1

ICD-9-CM

P

Vol. 2

Puerperal (*Continued*)
  retention (*Continued*)
    secundines (fragments) (with de-
      layed hemorrhage) 666.2
    without hemorrhage 667.1
  retracted nipple 676.0
  rubella (conditions classifiable to 056)
    647.5
  salpingitis 670
  salpingo-oophoritis 670
  salpingo-ovaritis 670
  salpingoperitonitis 670
  sapremia 670
  secondary perineal tear 674.2
  sepsis (pelvic) 670
  septicemia 670
  subinvolution (uterus) 674.8
  sudden death (cause unknown) 674.9
  suppuration - *see* Puerperal, abscess
  syphilis (conditions classifiable to 090-
    097) 647.0
  tetanus 670
  thelitis 675.0
  thrombocytopenia 666.3
  thrombophlebitis (superficial) 671.2
    deep 671.4
    pelvic 671.4
    specified site NEC 671.5
  thrombosis (venous) - *see* Thrombosis,
    puerperal
  thyroid dysfunction (conditions classi-
    fiable to 240-246) 648.1
  toxemia (*see also* Toxemia, of preg-
    nancy) 642.4
    eclamptic 642.6
      with pre-existing hypertension 642.7
    pre-eclamptic (mild) 642.4
      with
        convulsions 642.6
        pre-existing hypertension 642.7
      severe 642.5
  tuberculosis (conditions classifiable to
    010-018) 647.3
  uremia 669.3
  vaginitis (conditions classifiable to
    616.1) 646.6
  varicose veins (legs) 671.0
    vulva or perineum 671.1
  vulvitis (conditions classifiable to
    616.1) 646.6
  vulvovaginitis (conditions classifiable
    to 616.1) 646.6
  white leg 671.4
Pulled muscle - *see* Sprain, by site
Pulmolithiasis 518.89
Pulmonary - *see* condition
Pulmonitis (unknown etiology) 486
Pulpitis (acute) (anachoretic) (chronic)
  (hyperplastic) (putrescent) (suppurative) (ulcerative) 522.0
Pulpless tooth 522.9
Pulse
  alternating 427.89
    psychogenic 306.2
  bigeminal 427.89
  fast 785.0
  feeble, rapid, due to shock following
    injury 958.4
  rapid 785.0
  slow 427.89
  strong 785.9
  trigeminal 427.89
  water-hammer (*see also* Insufficiency,
    aortic) 424.1
  weak 785.9

Pulseless disease 446.7
Pulsus
  alternans or trigeminy 427.89
    psychogenic 306.2
Punch drunk 310.2
Puncta lacrimalia occlusion 375.52
Punctiform hymen 752.49
Puncture (traumatic) - *see also* Wound,
  open, by site
  accidental, complicating surgery 998.2
  bladder, nontraumatic 596.6
  by
    device, implant, or graft - *see* Com-
      plications, mechanical
    foreign body
      internal organs - *see also* Injury, in-
        ternal, by site
        by ingested object - *see* Foreign
          body
      left accidentally in operation
        wound 998.4
    instrument (any) during a proce-
      dure, accidental 998.2
  internal organs, abdomen, chest, or
    pelvis - *see* Injury, internal, by site
  kidney, nontraumatic 593.89
Pupil - *see* condition
Pupillary membrane 364.74
  persistent 743.46
Pupillotonia 379.46
  pseudotabetic 379.46
Purpura 287.2
  abdominal 287.0
  allergic 287.0
  anaphylactoid 287.0
  annularis telangiectodes 709.1
  arthritic 287.0
  autoerythrocyte sensitization 287.2
  autoimmune 287.0
  bacterial 287.0
  Bateman's (senile) 287.2
  capillary fragility (hereditary) (idio-
    pathic) 287.8
  cryoglobulinemic 273.2
  devil's pinches 287.2
  fibrinolytic (*see also* Fibrinolysis) 286.6
  fulminans, fulminous 286.6
  gangrenous 287.0
  hemorrhagic (*see also* Purpura, throm-
    bocytopenic) 287.3
    nodular 272.7
    nonthrombocytopenic 287.0
    thrombocytopenic 287.3
  Henoch's (purpura nervosa) 287.0
  Henoch-Schönlein (allergic) 287.0
  hypergammaglobulinemic (benign pri-
    mary) (Waldenström's) 273.0
  idiopathic 287.3
    nonthrombocytopenic 287.0
    thrombocytopenic 287.3
  infectious 287.0
  malignant 287.0
  neonatorum 772.6
  nervosa 287.0
  newborn NEC 772.6
  nonthrombocytopenic 287.2
    hemorrhagic 287.0
    idiopathic 287.0
  nonthrombopenic 287.2
  peliosis rheumatica 287.0
  pigmentaria, progressiva 709.09
  posttransfusion 287.4
  primary 287.0
  primitive 287.0

Purpura (*Continued*)
  red cell membrane sensitivity 287.2
  rheumatica 287.0
  Schönlein (-Henoch) (allergic) 287.0
  scorbutic 267
  senile 287.2
  simplex 287.2
  symptomatica 287.0
  telangiectasia annularis 709.1
  thrombocytopenic (congenital) (essential)
    (hereditary) (idiopathic) (primary)
    (*see also* Thrombocytopenia) 287.3
    neonatal, transitory (*see also* Throm-
      bocytopenia, neonatal transi-
      tory) 776.1
    puerperal, postpartum 666.3
    thrombotic 446.6
  thrombohemolytic (*see also* Fibrinoly-
    sis) 286.6
  thrombopenic (congenital) (essential)
    (*see also* Thrombocytopenia)
    287.3
  thrombotic 446.6
    thrombocytic 446.6
    thrombocytopenic 446.6
  toxic 287.0
  variolosa 050.0
  vascular 287.0
  visceral symptoms 287.0
  Werlhof's (*see also* Purpura, thrombo-
    cytopenic) 287.3
Purpuric spots 782.7
Purulent - *see* condition
Pus
  absorption, general - *see* Septicemia
  in
    stool 792.1
    urine 791.9
  tube (rupture) (*see also* Salpingooo-
    phoritis) 614.2
Pustular rash 782.1
Pustule 686.9
  malignant 022.0
  nonmalignant 686.9
Putnam's disease (subacute combined
  sclerosis with pernicious anemia)
  281.0 *[336.2]*
Putnam-Dana syndrome (subacute com-
  bined sclerosis with pernicious ane-
  mia) 281.0 *[336.2]*
Putrefaction, intestinal 569.89
Putrescent pulp (dental) 522.1
Pyarthritis - *see* Pyarthrosis
Pyarthrosis (*see also* Arthritis, pyogenic)
  711.0
  tuberculous - *see* Tuberculosis, joint
Pycnoepilepsy, pycnolepsy (idiopathic)
  (*see also* Epilepsy) 345.0
Pyelectasia 593.89
Pyelectasis 593.89
Pyelitis (congenital) (uremic) 590.80
  with
    abortion - *see* Abortion, by type, with
      specified complication NEC
    contracted kidney 590.00
    ectopic pregnancy (*see also* categories
      633.0-633.9) 639.8
    molar pregnancy (*see also* categories
      630-632) 639.8
  acute 590.10
    with renal medullary necrosis 590.11
  chronic 590.00
    with
      renal medullary necrosis 590.01

◀ **New**   ◀▥ **Revised**

Pyelitis (*Continued*)
  complicating pregnancy, childbirth, or puerperium 646.6
    affecting fetus or newborn 760.1
  cystica 590.3
  following
    abortion 639.8
    ectopic or molar pregnancy 639.8
  gonococcal 098.19
    chronic or duration of 2 months or over 098.39
  tuberculous (*see also* Tuberculosis) 016.0 [590.81]
Pyelocaliectasis 593.89
Pyelocystitis (*see also* Pyelitis) 590.80
Pyelohydronephrosis 591
Pyelonephritis (*see also* Pyelitis) 590.80
  acute 590.10
    with renal medullary necrosis 590.11
  chronic 590.00
  syphilitic (late) 095.4
  tuberculous (*see also* Tuberculosis) 016.0 [590.81]
Pyelonephrosis (*see also* Pyelitis) 590.80
  chronic 590.00
Pyelophlebitis 451.89
Pyelo-ureteritis cystica 590.3
Pyemia, pyemic (purulent) (*see also* Septicemia) 038.9
  abscess - *see* Abscess
  arthritis (*see also* Arthritis, pyogenic) 711.0
  Bacillus coli 038.42
  embolism - *see* Embolism, pyemic
  fever 038.9
  infection 038.9
  joint (*see also* Arthritis, pyogenic) 711.0
  liver 572.1
  meningococcal 036.2
  newborn 771.81
  phlebitis - *see* Phlebitis
  pneumococcal 038.2
  portal 572.1
  postvaccinal 999.3
  specified organism NEC 038.8
  staphylococcal 038.10
    aureus 038.11
    specified organism NEC 038.19
  streptococcal 038.0
  tuberculous - *see* Tuberculosis, miliary
Pygopagus 759.4

Pykno-epilepsy, pyknolepsy (idiopathic) (*see also* Epilepsy) 345.0
Pyle (-Cohn) disease (craniometaphyseal dysplasia) 756.89
Pylephlebitis (suppurative) 572.1
Pylethrombophlebitis 572.1
Pylethrombosis 572.1
Pyloritis (*see also* Gastritis) 535.5
Pylorospasm (reflex) 537.81
  congenital or infantile 750.5
  neurotic 306.4
  newborn 750.5
  psychogenic 306.4
Pylorus, pyloric - *see* condition
Pyoarthrosis - *see* Pyarthrosis
Pyocele
  mastoid 383.00
  sinus (accessory) (nasal) (*see also* Sinusitis) 473.9
  turbinate (bone) 473.9
  urethra (*see also* Urethritis) 597.0
Pyococcal dermatitis 686.00
Pyococcide, skin 686.00
Pyocolpos (*see also* Vaginitis) 616.10
Pyocyaneus dermatitis 686.09
Pyocystitis (*see also* Cystitis) 595.9
Pyoderma, pyodermia 686.00
  gangrenosum 686.01
  specified type NEC 686.09
  vegetans 686.8
Pyodermatitis 686.00
  vegetans 686.8
Pyogenic - *see* condition
Pyohemia - *see* Septicemia
Pyohydronephrosis (*see also* Pyelitis) 590.80
Pyometra 615.9
Pyometritis (*see also* Endometritis) 615.9
Pyometrium (*see also* Endometritis) 615.9
Pyomyositis 728.0
  ossificans 728.19
  tropical (bungpagga) 040.81
Pyonephritis (*see also* Pyelitis) 590.80
  chronic 590.00
Pyonephrosis (congenital) (*see also* Pyelitis) 590.80
  acute 590.10
Pyo-oophoritis (*see also* Salpingo-oophoritis) 614.2

Pyo-ovarium (*see also* Salpingo-oophoritis) 614.2
Pyopericarditis 420.99
Pyopericardium 420.99
Pyophlebitis - *see* Phlebitis
Pyopneumopericardium 420.99
Pyopneumothorax (infectional) 510.9
  with fistula 510.0
  subdiaphragmatic (*see also* Peritonitis) 567.2
  subphrenic (*see also* Peritonitis) 567.2
  tuberculous (*see also* Tuberculosis, pleura) 012.0
Pyorrhea (alveolar) (alveolaris) 523.4
  degenerative 523.5
Pyosalpingitis (*see also* Salpingo-oophoritis) 614.2
Pyosalpinx (*see also* Salpingo-oophoritis) 614.2
Pyosepticemia - *see* Septicemia
Pyosis
  Corlett's (impetigo) 684
  Manson's (pemphigus contagiosus) 684
Pyothorax 510.9
  with fistula 510.0
  tuberculous (*see also* Tuberculosis, pleura) 012.0
Pyoureter 593.89
  tuberculous (*see also* Tuberculosis) 016.2
Pyramidopallidonigral syndrome 332.0
Pyrexia (of unknown origin) (P.U.O.) 780.6
  atmospheric 992.0
  during labor 659.2
  environmentally-induced newborn 778.4
  heat 992.0
  newborn, environmentally-induced 778.4
  puerperal 672
Pyroglobulinemia 273.8
Pyromania 312.33
Pyrosis 787.1
Pyrroloporphyria 277.1
Pyuria (bacterial) 791.9

ICD-9-CM

P

Vol. 2

Q

Q fever 083.0
  with pneumonia 083.0 *[484.8]*
Quadricuspid aortic valve 746.89
Quadrilateral fever 083.0
Quadriparesis - *see* Quadriplegia
Quadriplegia 344.00
  with fracture, vertebra (process) - *see*
    Fracture, vertebra, cervical, with
    spinal cord injury
  brain (current episode) 437.8
  C_1-C_4
    complete 344.01
    incomplete 344.02
  C_5-C_7
    complete 344.03
    incomplete 344.04
  cerebral (current episode) 437.8
  congenital or infantile (cerebral) (spas-
    tic) (spinal) 343.2
  cortical 437.8
  embolic (current episode) (*see also* Em-
    bolism, brain) 434.1
  infantile (cerebral) (spastic) (spinal) 343.2

Quadriplegia *(Continued)*
  newborn NEC 767.0
  specified NEC 344.09
  thrombotic (current episode) (*see also*
    Thrombosis, brain) 434.0
  traumatic - *see* Injury, spinal, cervical
Quadruplet
  affected by maternal complications of
    pregnancy 761.5
  healthy liveborn - *see* Newborn, multi-
    ple
  pregnancy (complicating delivery)
    NEC 651.8
    with fetal loss and retention of one
      or more fetus(es) 651.5
Quarrelsomeness 301.3
Quartan
  fever 084.2
  malaria (fever) 084.2
Queensland fever 083.0
  coastal 083.0
  seven-day 100.89
Quervain's disease 727.04
  thyroid (subacute granulomatous thy-
    roiditis) 245.1

Queyrat's erythroplasia (M8080/2)
  specified site - *see* Neoplasm, skin, in
    situ
  unspecified site 233.5
Quincke's disease or edema - *see*
  Edema, angioneurotic
Quinquaud's disease (acne decalvans)
  704.09
Quinsy (gangrenous) 475
Quintan fever 083.1
Quintuplet
  affected by maternal complications of
    pregnancy 761.5
  healthy liveborn - *see* Newborn, multi-
    ple
  pregnancy (complicating delivery)
    NEC 651.2
    with fetal loss and retention of one
      or more fetus(es) 651.6
Quotidian
  fever 084.0
  malaria (fever) 084.0

◄ **New**   ◄▦ **Revised**

R

Rabbia 071
Rabbit fever (see also Tularemia) 021.9
Rabies 071
  contact V01.5
  exposure to V01.5
  inoculation V04.5
    reaction - see Complications, vacci-
      nation
  vaccination, prophylactic (against)
    V04.5
Rachischisis (see also Spina bifida) 741.9
Rachitic - see also condition
  deformities of spine 268.1
  pelvis 268.1
    with disproportion (fetopelvic) 653.2
      affecting fetus or newborn 763.1
    causing obstructed labor 660.1
      affecting fetus or newborn 763.1
Rachitis, rachitism - see also Rickets
  acute 268.0
  fetalis 756.4
  renalis 588.0
  tarda 268.0
Racket nail 757.5
Radial nerve - see condition
Radiation effects or sickness - see also
    Effect, adverse, radiation
  cataract 366.46
  dermatitis 692.82
    sunburn (see also Sunburn) 692.71
Radiculitis (pressure) (vertebrogenic)
    729.2
  accessory nerve 723.4
  anterior crural 724.4
  arm 723.4
  brachial 723.4
  cervical NEC 723.4
  due to displacement of intervertebral
    disc - see Neuritis, due to, dis-
    placement intervertebral disc
  leg 724.4
  lumbar NEC 724.4
  lumbosacral 724.4
  rheumatic 729.2
  syphilitic 094.89
  thoracic (with visceral pain) 724.4
Radiculomyelitis 357.0
  toxic, due to
    Clostridium tetani 037
    Corynebacterium diphtheriae 032.89
Radiculopathy (see also Radiculitis) 729.2
Radioactive substances, adverse effect -
    see Effect, adverse, radioactive sub-
    stance
Radiodermal burns (acute) (chronic) (oc-
    cupational) - see Burn, by site
Radiodermatitis 692.82
Radionecrosis - see Effect, adverse, radia-
    tion
Radiotherapy session V58.0
Radium, adverse effect - see Effect, ad-
    verse, radioactive substance
Raeder-Harbitz syndrome (pulseless dis-
    ease) 446.7
Rage (see also Disturbance, conduct)
    312.0
  meaning rabies 071
Rag sorters' disease 022.1
Raillietiniasis 123.8
Railroad neurosis 300.16
Railway spine 300.16
Raised - see Elevation

Raiva 071
Rake teeth, tooth 524.39 ◀▦
Rales 786.7
Ramifying renal pelvis 753.3
Ramsay Hunt syndrome (herpetic genic-
    ulate ganglionitis) 053.11
  meaning dyssynergia cerebellaris
    myoclonica 334.2
Ranke's primary infiltration (see also Tu-
    berculosis) 010.0
Ranula 527.6
  congenital 750.26
Rape - see Injury, by site 959.9
  alleged, observation or examination
    V71.5
Rapid
  feeble pulse, due to shock, following
    injury 958.4
  heart (beat) 785.0
    psychogenic 306.2
  respiration 786.06
    psychogenic 306.1
  second stage (delivery) 661.3
    affecting fetus or newborn 763.6
  time-zone change syndrome 307.45
Rarefaction, bone 733.99
Rash 782.1
  canker 034.1
  diaper 691.0
  drug (internal use) 693.0
    contact 692.3
  ECHO 9 virus 078.89
  enema 692.89
  food (see also Allergy, food) 693.1
  heat 705.1
  napkin 691.0
  nettle 708.8
  pustular 782.1
  rose 782.1
    epidemic 056.9
    of infants 057.8
  scarlet 034.1
  serum (prophylactic) (therapeutic)
    999.5
  toxic 782.1
  wandering tongue 529.1
Rasmussen's aneurysm (see also Tuber-
    culosis) 011.2
Rat-bite fever 026.9
  due to Streptobacillus moniliformis
    026.1
  spirochetal (morsus muris) 026.0
Rathke's pouch tumor (M9350/1)
    237.0
Raymond (-Céstan) syndrome 433.8
Raynaud's
  disease or syndrome (paroxysmal digi-
    tal cyanosis) 443.0
  gangrene (symmetric) 443.0 [785.4]
  phenomenon (paroxysmal digital cya-
    nosis) (secondary) 443.0
RDS 769
Reaction
  acute situational maladjustment (see
    also Reaction, adjustment) 309.9
  adaptation (see also Reaction, adjust-
    ment) 309.9
  adjustment 309.9
    with
      anxious mood 309.24
        with depressed mood 309.28
      conduct disturbance 309.3
        combined with disturbance of
          emotions 309.4

Reaction (Continued)
  adjustment (Continued)
    with (Continued)
      depressed mood 309.0
        brief 309.0
          with anxious mood 309.28
        prolonged 309.1
      elective mutism 309.83
      mixed emotions and conduct 309.4
      mutism, elective 309.83
      physical symptoms 309.82
      predominant disturbance (of)
        conduct 309.3
        emotions NEC 309.29
          mixed 309.28
        mixed, emotions and conduct
          309.4
      specified type NEC 309.89
      specific academic or work inhibi-
        tion 309.23
      withdrawal 309.83
    depressive 309.0
      with conduct disturbance 309.4
      brief 309.0
      prolonged 309.1
    specified type NEC 309.89
  adverse food NEC 995.7
  affective (see also Psychosis, affective)
    296.90
    specified type NEC 296.99
  aggressive 301.3
    unsocialized (see also Disturbance,
      conduct) 312.0
  allergic (see also Allergy) 995.3
    drug, medicinal substance, and bio-
      logical - see Allergy, drug
    food - see Allergy, food
    serum 999.5
  anaphylactic - see Shock, anaphylactic
  anesthesia - see Anesthesia, complica-
    tion
  anger 312.0
  antisocial 301.7
  antitoxin (prophylactic) (therapeutic) -
    see Complications, vaccination
  anxiety 300.00
  asthenic 300.5
  compulsive 300.3
  conversion (anesthetic) (autonomic)
    (hyperkinetic) (mixed paralytic)
    (paresthetic) 300.11
  deoxyribonuclease (DNA) (DNase) hy-
    persensitivity NEC 287.2
  depressive 300.4
    acute 309.0
    affective (see also Psychosis, affective)
      296.2
      recurrent episode 296.3
      single episode 296.2
    brief 309.0
    manic (see also Psychosis, affective)
      296.80
    neurotic 300.4
    psychoneurotic 300.4
    psychotic 298.0
  dissociative 300.15
  drug NEC (see also Table of Drugs and
    Chemicals) 995.2
    allergic - see Allergy, drug
    correct substance properly adminis-
      tered 995.2
    obstetric anesthetic or analgesic NEC
      668.9
      affecting fetus or newborn 763.5

ICD-9-CM

R

Vol. 2

Reaction *(Continued)*
  drug NEC *(Continued)*
    obstetric anesthetic or analgesic NEC *(Continued)*
      specified drug - *see* Table of Drugs and Chemicals
      overdose or poisoning 977.9
        specified drug - *see* Table of Drugs and Chemicals
      specific to newborn 779.4
      transmitted via placenta or breast milk - *see* Absorption, drug, through placenta
      withdrawal NEC 292.0
        infant of dependent mother 779.5
      wrong substance given or taken in error 977.9
        specified drug - *see* Table of Drugs and Chemicals
  dyssocial 301.7
  erysipeloid 027.1
  fear 300.20
    child 313.0
  fluid loss, cerebrospinal 349.0
  food - *see also* Allergy, food
    adverse NEC 995.7
    anaphylactic shock - *see* Anaphylactic shock, due to, food
  foreign
    body NEC 728.82
      in operative wound (inadvertently left) 998.4
        due to surgical material intentionally left - *see* Complications, due to (presence of) any device, implant, or graft classified to 996.0-996.5 NEC
    substance accidentally left during a procedure (chemical) (powder) (talc) 998.7
      body or object (instrument) (sponge) (swab) 998.4
  graft-versus-host (GVH) 996.85
  grief (acute) (brief) 309.0
    prolonged 309.1
  gross stress (*see also* Reaction, stress, acute) 308.9
  group delinquent (*see also* Disturbance, conduct) 312.2
  Herxheimer's 995.0
  hyperkinetic (*see also* Hyperkinesia) 314.9
  hypochondriacal 300.7
  hypoglycemic, due to insulin 251.0
    therapeutic misadventure 962.3
  hypomanic (*see also* Psychosis, affective) 296.0
    recurrent episode 296.1
    single episode 296.0
  hysterical 300.10
    conversion type 300.11
    dissociative 300.15
  id (bacterial cause) 692.89
  immaturity NEC 301.89
    aggressive 301.3
    emotional instability 301.59
  immunization - *see* Complications, vaccination
  incompatibility
    blood group (ABO) (infusion) (transfusion) 999.6
    Rh (factor) (infusion) (transfusion) 999.7
  inflammatory - *see* Infection
  infusion - *see* Complications, infusion

Reaction *(Continued)*
  inoculation (immune serum) - *see* Complications, vaccination
  insulin 995.2
  involutional
    paranoid 297.2
    psychotic (*see also* Psychosis, affective, depressive) 296.2
  leukemoid (lymphocytic) (monocytic) (myelocytic) 288.8
  LSD (*see also* Abuse, drugs, nondependent) 305.3
  lumbar puncture 349.0
  manic-depressive (*see also* Psychosis, affective) 296.80
    depressed 296.2
      recurrent episode 296.3
      single episode 296.2
    hypomanic 296.0
  neurasthenic 300.5
  neurogenic (*see also* Neurosis) 300.9
  neurotic NEC 300.9
  neurotic-depressive 300.4
  nitritoid - *see* Crisis, nitritoid
  obsessive (-compulsive) 300.3
  organic 293.9
    acute 293.0
    subacute 293.1
  overanxious, child or adolescent 313.0
  paranoid (chronic) 297.9
    acute 298.3
    climacteric 297.2
    involutional 297.2
    menopausal 297.2
    senile 290.20
    simple 297.0
  passive
    aggressive 301.84
    dependency 301.6
  personality (*see also* Disorder, personality) 301.9
  phobic 300.20
  postradiation - *see* Effect, adverse, radiation
  psychogenic NEC 300.9
  psychoneurotic (*see also* Neurosis) 300.9
    anxiety 300.00
    compulsive 300.3
    conversion 300.11
    depersonalization 300.6
    depressive 300.4
    dissociative 300.15
    hypochondriacal 300.7
    hysterical 300.10
      conversion type 300.11
      dissociative type 300.15
    neurasthenic 300.5
    obsessive 300.3
    obsessive-compulsive 300.3
    phobic 300.20
    tension state 300.9
  psychophysiologic NEC (*see also* Disorder, psychosomatic) 306.9
    cardiovascular 306.2
    digestive 306.4
    endocrine 306.6
    gastrointestinal 306.4
    genitourinary 306.50
    heart 306.2
    hemic 306.8
    intestinal (large) (small) 306.4
    laryngeal 306.1
    lymphatic 306.8

Reaction *(Continued)*
  psychophysiologic NEC *(Continued)*
    musculoskeletal 306.0
    pharyngeal 306.1
    respiratory 306.1
    skin 306.3
    special sense organs 306.7
  psychosomatic (*see also* Disorder, psychosomatic) 306.9
  psychotic (*see also* Psychosis) 298.9
    depressive 298.0
    due to or associated with physical condition (*see also* Psychosis, organic) 293.9
    involutional (*see also* Psychosis, affective) 296.2
      recurrent episode 296.3
      single episode 296.2
  pupillary (myotonic) (tonic) 379.46
  radiation - *see* Effect, adverse, radiation
  runaway - *see also* Disturbance, conduct
    socialized 312.2
    undersocialized, unsocialized 312.1
  scarlet fever toxin - *see* Complications, vaccination
  schizophrenic (*see also* Schizophrenia) 295.9
    latent 295.5
  serological for syphilis - *see* Serology for syphilis
  serum (prophylactic) (therapeutic) 999.5
    immediate 999.4
  situational (*see also* Reaction, adjustment) 309.9
    acute, to stress 308.3
    adjustment (*see also* Reaction, adjustment) 309.9
  somatization (*see also* Disorder, psychosomatic) 306.9
  spinal puncture 349.0
  spite, child (*see also* Disturbance, conduct) 312.0
  stress, acute 308.9
    with predominant disturbance (of)
      consciousness 308.1
      emotions 308.0
      mixed 308.4
      psychomotor 308.2
    bone or cartilage - *see* fracture stress
    specified type NEC 308.3
  surgical procedure - *see* Complications, surgical procedure
  tetanus antitoxin - *see* Complications, vaccination
  toxin-antitoxin - *see* Complications, vaccination
  transfusion (blood) (bone marrow) (lymphocytes) (allergic) - *see* Complications, transfusion
  tuberculin skin test, nonspecific (without active tuberculosis) 795.5
    positive (without active tuberculosis) 795.5
  ultraviolet - *see* Effect, adverse, ultraviolet
  undersocialized, unsocialized - *see also* Disturbance, conduct
    aggressive (type) 312.0
    unaggressive (type) 312.1
  vaccination (any) - *see* Complications, vaccination
  white graft (skin) 996.52

◄ **New**   ◄▬ **Revised**

Reaction *(Continued)*
　withdrawing, child or adolescent
　　313.22
　x-ray - *see* Effect, adverse, x-rays
Reactive depression *(see also* Reaction,
　depressive) 300.4
　neurotic 300.4
　psychoneurotic 300.4
　psychotic 298.0
Rebound tenderness 789.6
Recalcitrant patient V15.81
Recanalization, thrombus - *see* Throm-
　bosis
Recession, receding
　chamber angle (eye) 364.77
　chin 524.06
　gingival (post-infective) (postoperative)
　　523.20 ◀▥
　　generalized 523.25 ◀
　　localized 523.24 ◀
　　minimal 523.21 ◀
　　moderate 523.22 ◀
　　severe 523.23 ◀
Recklinghausen's disease (M9540/1)
　237.71
　bones (osteitis fibrosa cystica) 252.01 ◀▥
Recklinghausen-Applebaum disease
　(hemochromatosis) 275.0
Reclus' disease (cystic) 610.1
Recrudescent typhus (fever) 081.1
Recruitment, auditory 388.44
Rectalgia 569.42
Rectitis 569.49
Rectocele
　female (without uterine prolapse)
　　618.04 ◀▥
　　with uterine prolapse 618.4
　　　complete 618.3
　　　incomplete 618.2
　in pregnancy or childbirth 654.4
　　causing obstructed labor 660.2
　　　affecting fetus or newborn 763.1
　male 569.49
　vagina, vaginal (outlet) 618.04 ◀▥
Rectosigmoiditis 569.89
　ulcerative (chronic) 556.3
Rectosigmoid junction - *see* condition
Rectourethral - *see* condition
Rectovaginal - *see* condition
Rectovesical - *see* condition
Rectum, rectal - *see* condition
Recurrent - *see* condition
Red bugs 133.8
Red cedar asthma 495.8
Redness
　conjunctiva 379.93
　eye 379.93
　nose 478.1
Reduced ventilatory or vital capacity
　794.2
Reduction
　function
　　kidney *(see also* Disease, renal) 593.9
　　liver 573.8
　ventilatory capacity 794.2
　vital capacity 794.2
Redundant, redundancy
　abdomen 701.9
　anus 751.5
　cardia 537.89
　clitoris 624.2
　colon (congenital) 751.5
　foreskin (congenital) 605
　intestine 751.5
　labia 624.3

Redundant, redundancy *(Continued)*
　organ or site, congenital NEC - *see* Ac-
　　cessory
　panniculus (abdominal) 278.1
　prepuce (congenital) 605
　pylorus 537.89
　rectum 751.5
　scrotum 608.89
　sigmoid 751.5
　skin (of face) 701.9
　　eyelids 374.30
　stomach 537.89
　uvula 528.9
　vagina 623.8
Reduplication - *see* Duplication
Referral
　adoption (agency) V68.89
　nursing care V63.8
　patient without examination or treat-
　　ment V68.81
　social services V63.8
Reflex - *see also* condition
　blink, deficient 374.45
　hyperactive gag 478.29
　neurogenic bladder NEC 596.54
　　atonic 596.54
　　　with cauda equina syndrome
　　　　344.61
　vasoconstriction 443.9
　vasovagal 780.2
Reflux
　esophageal 530.81
　　with esophagitis 530.11
　esophagitis 530.11
　gastroesophageal 530.81
　mitral - *see* Insufficiency, mitral
　ureteral - *see* Reflux, vesicoureteral
　vesicoureteral 593.70
　　with
　　　reflux nephropathy 593.73
　　　　bilateral 593.72
　　　　unilateral 593.71
Reformed gallbladder 576.0
Reforming, artificial openings *(see also*
　Attention to, artificial, opening)
　V55.9
Refractive error *(see also* Error, refrac-
　tive) 367.9
Refsum's disease or syndrome (heredo-
　pathia atactica polyneuritiformis)
　356.3
Refusal of
　food 307.59
　　hysterical 300.11
　treatment because of, due to
　　patient's decision NEC V64.2
　　reason of conscience or religion
　　　V62.6
Regaud
　tumor (M8082/3) - *see* Neoplasm, na-
　　sopharynx, malignant
　type carcinoma (M8082/3) - *see* Neo-
　　plasm, nasopharynx, malignant
Regional - *see* condition
Regulation feeding (elderly) (infant)
　783.3
　newborn 779.3
Regurgitated
　food, choked on 933.1
　stomach contents, choked on 933.1
Regurgitation
　aortic (valve) *(see also* Insufficiency,
　　aortic) 424.1
　　congenital 746.4
　　syphilitic 093.22

Regurgitation *(Continued)*
　food - *see also* Vomiting
　　with reswallowing - *see* Rumination
　　newborn 779.3
　gastric contents - *see* Vomiting
　heart - *see* Endocarditis
　mitral (valve) - *see also* Insufficiency,
　　mitral
　　congenital 746.6
　myocardial - *see* Endocarditis
　pulmonary (heart) (valve) *(see also* En-
　　docarditis, pulmonary) 424.3
　stomach - *see* Vomiting
　tricuspid - *see* Endocarditis, tricuspid
　valve, valvular - *see* Endocarditis
　vesicoureteral - *see* Reflux, vesicoure-
　　teral
Rehabilitation V57.9
　multiple types V57.89
　occupational V57.21
　specified type NEC V57.89
　speech V57.3
　vocational V57.22
Reichmann's disease or syndrome (gas-
　trosuccorrhea) 536.8
Reifenstein's syndrome (hereditary fa-
　milial hypogonadism, male) 257.2
Reilly's syndrome or phenomenon *(see
　also* Neuropathy, peripheral, auto-
　nomic) 337.9
Reimann's periodic disease 277.3
Reinsertion, contraceptive device
　V25.42
**Reiter's disease, syndrome, or
　urethritis** 099.3 *[711.1]*
Rejection
　food, hysterical 300.11
　transplant 996.80
　　bone marrow 996.85
　　corneal 996.51
　　organ (immune or nonimmune
　　　cause) 996.80
　　　bone marrow 996.85
　　　heart 996.83
　　　intestines 996.87
　　　kidney 996.81
　　　liver 996.82
　　　lung 996.84
　　　pancreas 996.86
　　　specified NEC 996.89
　　skin 996.52
　　　artificial 996.55
　　　decellularized allodermis
　　　　996.55
Relapsing fever 087.9
　Carter's (Asiatic) 087.0
　Dutton's (West African) 087.1
　Koch's 087.9
　louse-borne (epidemic) 087.0
　Novy's (American) 087.1
　Obermeyer's (European) 087.0
　Spirillum 087.9
　tick-borne (endemic) 087.1
Relaxation
　anus (sphincter) 569.49
　　due to hysteria 300.11
　arch (foot) 734
　　congenital 754.61
　back ligaments 728.4
　bladder (sphincter) 596.59
　cardio-esophageal 530.89
　cervix *(see also* Incompetency, cervix)
　　622.5
　diaphragm 519.4
　inguinal rings - *see* Hernia, inguinal

ICD-9-CM

R

Vol. 2

Relaxation (Continued)
  joint (capsule) (ligament) (paralytic)
    (see also Derangement, joint) 718.90
    congenital 755.8
  lumbosacral joint 724.6
  pelvic floor 618.89 ◀▥
  pelvis 618.89 ◀▥
  perineum 618.89 ◀▥
  posture 729.9
  rectum (sphincter) 569.49
  sacroiliac (joint) 724.6
  scrotum 608.89
  urethra (sphincter) 599.84
  uterus (outlet) 618.89 ◀▥
  vagina (outlet) 618.89 ◀▥
  vesical 596.59
Remains
  canal of Cloquet 743.51
  capsule (opaque) 743.51
Remittent fever (malarial) 084.6
Remnant
  canal of Cloquet 743.51
  capsule (opaque) 743.51
  cervix, cervical stump (acquired) (post-
    operative) 622.8
  cystic duct, postcholecystectomy 576.0
  fingernail 703.8
    congenital 757.5
  meniscus, knee 717.5
  thyroglossal duct 759.2
  tonsil 474.8
    infected 474.00
  urachus 753.7
Remote effect of cancer - see condition
Removal (of)
  catheter (urinary) (indwelling) V53.6
    from artificial opening - see Atten-
      tion to, artificial, opening
    non-vascular V58.82
    vascular V58.81
  cerebral ventricle (communicating)
    shunt V53.01
  device - see also Fitting (of)
    contraceptive V25.42
    fixation
      external V54.89
      internal V54.01
    traction V54.89
  dressing V58.3
  ileostomy V55.2
  Kirschner wire V54.89
  non-vascular catheter V58.82
  pin V54.01
  plaster cast V54.89
  plate (fracture) V54.01
  rod V54.01
  screw V54.01
  splint, external V54.89
  subdermal implantable contraceptive
    V25.43
  suture V58.3
  traction device, external V54.89
  vascular catheter V58.81
Ren
  arcuatus 753.3
  mobile, mobilis (see also Disease, renal)
    593.0
    congenital 753.3
  unguliformis 753.3
Renal - see also condition
  glomerulohyalinosis-diabetic syndrome
    250.4 [581.81]
**Rendu-Osler-Weber disease or syn-
drome** (familial hemorrhagic telangiectasia) 448.0

Reninoma (M8361/1) 236.91
Rénon-Delille syndrome 253.8
Repair
  pelvic floor, previous, in pregnancy or
    childbirth 654.4
    affecting fetus or newborn
      763.89
  scarred tissue V51
**Replacement by artificial or mechanical
device or prosthesis of** (see also Fitting (of))
  artificial skin V43.83
  bladder V43.5
  blood vessel V43.4
  breast V43.82
  eye globe V43.0
  heart
    with
      assist device V43.21
      fully implantable artificial heart
        V43.22
    valve V43.3
  intestine V43.89
  joint V43.60
    ankle V43.66
    elbow V43.62
    finger V43.69
    hip (partial) (total) V43.64
    knee V43.65
    shoulder V43.61
    specified NEC V43.69
    wrist V43.63
  kidney V43.89
  larynx V43.81
  lens V43.1
  limb(s) V43.7
  liver V43.89
  lung V43.89
  organ NEC V43.89
  pancreas V43.89
  skin (artificial) V43.83
  tissue NEC V43.89
Reprogramming
  cardiac pacemaker V53.31
Request for expert evidence V68.2
Reserve, decreased or low
  cardiac - see Disease, heart
    kidney (see also Disease, renal) 593.9
Residual - see also condition
  bladder 596.8
  foreign body - see Retention, foreign body
  state, schizophrenic (see also Schizo-
    phrenia) 295.6
  urine 788.69
Resistance, resistant (to)
  activated protein C 289.81

> Note Use the following subclassifi-
> cation for categories V09.5, V09.7,
> V09.8, V09.9:
>
> 0   without mention of resistance
>   to multiple drugs
> 1   with resistance to multiple drugs
>   V09.5 quinolones and fluoro-
>   quinolones
>   V09.7 antimycobacterial agents
>   V09.8 specified drugs NEC
>   V09.9 unspecified drugs
> 9   multiple sites

  drugs by microorganisms V09.90
    amikacin V09.4
    aminoglycosides V09.4
    amodiaquine V09.5

Resistance, resistant (Continued)
  drugs by microorganisms (Continued)
    amoxicillin V09.0
    ampicillin V09.0
    antimycobacterial agents V09.7
    azithromycin V09.2
    azlocillin V09.0
    aztreonam V09.1
    B-lactam antibiotics V09.1
    bacampicillin V09.0
    bacitracin V09.8
    benznidazole V09.8
    capreomycin V09.7
    carbenicillin V09.0
    cefaclor V09.1
    cefadroxil V09.1
    cefamandole V09.1
    cefatetan V09.1
    cefazolin V09.1
    cefixime V09.1
    cefonicid V09.1
    cefoperazone V09.1
    ceforanide V09.1
    cefotaxime V09.1
    cefoxitin V09.1
    ceftazidine V09.1
    ceftizoxime V09.1
    ceftriaxone V09.1
    cefuroxime V09.1
    cephalexin V09.1
    cephaloglycin V09.1
    cephaloridine V09.1
    cephalosporins V09.1
    cephalothin V09.1
    cephapirin V09.1
    cephradine V09.1
    chloramphenicol V09.8
    chloraquine V09.5
    chlorguanide V09.8
    chlorproguanil V09.8
    chlortetracycline V09.3
    cinoxacin V09.5
    ciprofloxacin V09.5
    clarithromycin V09.2
    clindamycin V09.8
    clioquinol V09.5
    clofazimine V09.7
    cloxacillin V09.0
    cyclacillin V09.0
    cycloserine V09.7
    dapsone [Dz] V09.7
    demeclocycline V09.3
    dicloxacillin V09.0
    doxycycline V09.3
    enoxacin V09.5
    erythromycin V09.2
    ethambutol [Emb] V09.7
    ethionamide [Eta] V09.7
    fluoroquinolones NEC V09.5
    gentamicin V09.4
    halofantrine V09.8
    imipenem V09.1
    iodoquinol V09.5
    isoniazid [INH] V09.7
    kanamycin V09.4
    macrolides V09.2
    mafenide V09.6
    MDRO (multiple drug resistant or-
      ganisms) NOS V09.91 ◀
    mefloquine V09.8
    melarsoprol V09.8
    methicillin V09.0
    methacycline V09.3
    methenamine V09.8

◀ New   ◀▥ Revised

Resistance, resistant (Continued)
  drugs by microorganisms (Continued)
    metronidazole V09.8
    mezlocillin V09.0
    minocycline V09.3
    multiple drug resistant organisms
      NOS V09.91 ◀
    nafcillin V09.0
    nalidixic acid V09.5
    natamycin V09.2
    neomycin V09.4
    netilmicin V09.4
    nimorazole V09.8
    nitrofurantoin V09.8
    norfloxacin V09.5
    nystatin V09.2
    ofloxacin V09.5
    oleandomycin V09.2
    oxacillin V09.0
    oxytetracycline V09.3
    para-amino salicyclic acid [PAS]
      V09.7
    paromomycin V09.4
    penicillin (G) (V) (Vk) V09.0
    penicillins V09.0
    pentamidine V09.8
    piperacillin V09.0
    primaquine V09.5
    proguanil V09.8
    pyrazinamide [Pza] V09.7
    pyrimethamine/sulfalene V09.8
    pyrimethamine/sulfodoxine V09.8
    quinacrine V09.5
    quinidine V09.8
    quinine V09.8
    quinolones V09.5
    rifabutin V09.7
    rifampin [Rif] V09.7
    rifamycin V09.7
    rolitetracycline V09.3
    specified drugs NEC V09.8
    spectinomycin V09.8
    spiramycin V09.2
    streptomycin [Sm] V09.4
    sulfacetamide V09.6
    sulfacytine V09.6
    sulfadiazine V09.6
    sulfadoxine V09.6
    sulfamethoxazole V09.6
    sulfapyridine V09.6
    sulfasalizine V09.6
    sulfasoxazone V09.6
    sulfonamides V09.6
    sulfoxone V09.7
    tetracycline V09.3
    tetracyclines V09.3
    thiamphenicol V09.8
    ticarcillin V09.0
    tinidazole V09.8
    tobramycin V09.4
    triamphenicol V09.8
    trimethoprim V09.8
    vancomycin V09.8
  insulin 277.7 ◀

Resorption
  biliary 576.8
    purulent or putrid (see also Cholecystitis) 576.8
  dental (roots) 521.40 ◀━
    alveoli 525.8
    pathological ◀
      external 521.42 ◀
      internal 521.41 ◀
      specified NEC 521.49 ◀

Resorption (Continued)
  septic - see Septicemia
  teeth (roots) 521.40 ◀━
    pathological ◀
      external 521.42 ◀
      internal 521.41 ◀
      specified NEC 521.49 ◀

Respiration
  asymmetrical 786.09
  bronchial 786.09
  Cheyne-Stokes (periodic respiration)
    786.04
  decreased, due to shock following injury 958.4
  disorder of 786.00
    psychogenic 306.1
    specified NEC 786.09
  failure 518.81
    acute 518.81
    acute and chronic 518.84
    chronic 518.83
    newborn 770.84
  insufficiency 786.09
    acute 518.82
    newborn NEC 770.89
  Kussmaul (air hunger) 786.09
  painful 786.52
  periodic 786.09
  poor 786.09
    newborn NEC 770.89
  sighing 786.7
    psychogenic 306.1
  wheezing 786.07
Respiratory - see also condition
  distress 786.09
    acute 518.82
    fetus or newborn NEC 770.89
    syndrome (newborn) 769
      adult (following shock, surgery, or
        trauma) 518.5
      specified NEC 518.82
  failure 518.81
    acute 518.81
    acute and chronic 518.84
    chronic 518.83
Respiratory syncytial virus (RSV) 079.6
  bronchiolitis 466.11
  pneumonia 480.1
  vaccination, prophylactic (against)
    V04.82
Response
  photoallergic 692.72
  phototoxic 692.72
Rest, rests
  mesonephric duct 752.89
    fallopian tube 752.11
  ovarian, in fallopian tubes 752.19
  wolffian duct 752.89
Restless leg (syndrome) 333.99
Restlessness 799.2
**Restoration of organ continuity from
  previous sterilization** (tuboplasty)
  (vasoplasty) V26.0
Restriction of housing space V60.1
Restzustand, schizophrenic (see also
  Schizophrenia) 295.6
Retained - see Retention
Retardation
  development, developmental, specific
    (see also Disorder, development,
    specific) 315.9
    learning, specific 315.2
      arithmetical 315.1

Retardation (Continued)
  development, developmental, specific
    (Continued)
    learning, specific (Continued)
      language (skills) 315.31
        expressive 315.31
        mixed receptive-expressive
          315.32
      mathematics 315.1
      reading 315.00
        phonological 315.39
        written expression 315.2
    motor 315.4
  endochondral bone growth 733.91
  growth (physical) in childhood
    783.43
    due to malnutrition 263.2
    fetal (intrauterine) 764.9
      affecting management of pregnancy 656.5
  intrauterine growth 764.9
    affecting management of pregnancy
      656.5
  mental 319
    borderline V62.89
    mild, IQ 50-70 317
    moderate, IQ 35-49 318.0
    profound, IQ under 20 318.2
    severe, IQ 20-34 318.1
  motor, specific 315.4
  physical 783.43
    child 783.43
    due to malnutrition 263.2
    fetus (intrauterine) 764.9
      affecting management of pregnancy 656.5
  psychomotor NEC 307.9
  reading 315.00
Retching - see Vomiting
Retention, retained
  bladder (see also Retention, urine)
    788.20
    psychogenic 306.53
  carbon dioxide 276.2
  cyst - see Cyst
  dead
    fetus (after 22 completed weeks' gestation) 656.4
      early fetal death (before 22 completed weeks' gestation) 632
    ovum 631
  decidua (following delivery) (fragments) (with hemorrhage) 666.2
    without hemorrhage 667.1
  deciduous tooth 520.6
  dental root 525.3
  fecal (see also Constipation) 564.00
  fluid 276.6
  foreign body - see also Foreign body,
    retained
    bone 733.99
    current trauma - see Foreign body,
      by site or type
    middle ear 385.83
    muscle 729.6
    soft tissue NEC 729.6
  gastric 536.8
  membranes (following delivery) (with
    hemorrhage) 666.2
    with abortion - see Abortion, by type
    without hemorrhage 667.1
  menses 626.8
  milk (puerperal) 676.2
  nitrogen, extrarenal 788.9

ICD-9-CM

R

Vol. 2

Retention, retained (Continued)
placenta (total) (with hemorrhage)
666.0
with abortion - see Abortion, by type
portions or fragments 666.2
without hemorrhage 667.1
without hemorrhage 667.0
products of conception
early pregnancy (fetal death before
22 completed weeks' gestation)
632
following
abortion - see Abortion, by type
delivery 666.2
with hemorrhage 666.2
without hemorrhage 667.1
secundines (following delivery) (with
hemorrhage) 666.2
with abortion - see Abortion, by type
complicating puerperium (delayed
hemorrhage) 666.2
without hemorrhage 667.1
smegma, clitoris 624.8
urine NEC 788.20
bladder, incomplete emptying 788.21
psychogenic 306.53
specified NEC 788.29
water (in tissue) (see also Edema) 782.3
Reticulation, dust (occupational) 504
Reticulocytosis NEC 790.99
Reticuloendotheliosis
acute infantile (M9722/3) 202.5
leukemic (M9940/3) 202.4
malignant (M9720/3) 202.3
nonlipid (M9722/3) 202.5
Reticulohistiocytoma (giant cell) 277.89
Reticulohistiocytosis, multicentric 272.8
Reticulolymphosarcoma (diffuse)
(M9613/3) 200.8
follicular (M9691/3) 202.0
nodular (M9691/3) 202.0
Reticulosarcoma (M9640/3) 200.0
nodular (M9642/3) 200.0
pleomorphic cell type (M9641/3) 200.0
Reticulosis (skin)
acute of infancy (M9722/3) 202.5
histiocytic medullary (M9721/3) 202.3
lipomelanotic 695.89
malignant (M9720/3) 202.3
Sezary's (M9701/3) 202.2
Retina, retinal - see condition
Retinitis (see also Chorioretinitis) 363.20
albuminurica 585 [363.10]
arteriosclerotic 440.8 [362.13]
central angiospastic 362.41
Coat's 362.12
diabetic 250.5 [362.01]
disciformis 362.52
disseminated 363.10
metastatic 363.14
neurosyphilitic 094.83
pigment epitheliopathy 363.15
exudative 362.12
focal 363.00
in histoplasmosis 115.92
capsulatum 115.02
duboisii 115.12
juxtapapillary 363.05
macular 363.06
paramacular 363.06
peripheral 363.08
posterior pole NEC 363.07
gravidarum 646.8
hemorrhagica externa 362.12

Retinitis (Continued)
juxtapapillary (Jensen's) 363.05
luetic - see Retinitis, syphilitic
metastatic 363.14
pigmentosa 362.74
proliferans 362.29
proliferating 362.29
punctata albescens 362.76
renal 585 [363.13]
syphilitic (secondary) 091.51
congenital 090.0 [363.13]
early 091.51
late 095.8 [363.13]
syphilitica, central, recurrent 095.8
[363.13]
tuberculous (see also Tuberculosis)
017.3 [363.13]
Retinoblastoma (M9510/3) 190.5
differentiated type (M9511/3) 190.5
undifferentiated type (M9512/3) 190.5
Retinochoroiditis (see also Chorioretinitis) 363.20
central angiospastic 362.41
disseminated 363.10
metastatic 363.14
neurosyphilitic 094.83
pigment epitheliopathy 363.15
syphilitic 094.83
due to toxoplasmosis (acquired) (focal)
130.2
focal 363.00
in histoplasmosis 115.92
capsulatum 115.02
duboisii 115.12
juxtapapillary (Jensen's) 363.05
macular 363.06
paramacular 363.06
peripheral 363.08
posterior pole NEC 363.07
juxtapapillaris 363.05
syphilitic (disseminated) 094.83
Retinopathy (background) 362.10
arteriosclerotic 440.8 [362.13]
atherosclerotic 440.8 [362.13]
central serous 362.41
circinate 362.10
Coat's 362.12
diabetic 250.5 [362.01]
proliferative 250.5 [362.02]
exudative 362.12
hypertensive 362.11
of prematurity 362.21
pigmentary, congenital 362.74
proliferative 362.29
diabetic 250.5 [362.02]
sickle-cell 282.60 [362.29]
solar 363.31
Retinoschisis 361.10
bullous 361.12
congenital 743.56
flat 361.11
juvenile 362.73
Retractile testis 752.52
Retraction
cervix (see also Retroversion, uterus)
621.6
drum (membrane) 384.82
eyelid 374.41
finger 736.29
head 781.0
lid 374.41
lung 518.89
mediastinum 519.3
nipple 611.79

Retraction (Continued)
nipple (Continued)
congenital 757.6
puerperal, postpartum 676.0
palmar fascia 728.6
pleura (see also Pleurisy) 511.0
ring, uterus (Bandl's) (pathological)
661.4
affecting fetus or newborn 763.7
sternum (congenital) 756.3
acquired 738.3
during respiration 786.9
substernal 738.3
supraclavicular 738.8
syndrome (Duane's) 378.71
uterus (see also Retroversion, uterus)
621.6
valve (heart) - see Endocarditis
Retrobulbar - see condition
Retrocaval ureter 753.4
Retrocecal - see also condition
appendix (congenital) 751.5
Retrocession - see Retroversion
Retrodisplacement - see Retroversion
Retroflection, retroflexion - see Retroversion
Retrognathia, retrognathism (mandibular) (maxillary) 524.10
Retrograde
ejaculation 608.87
menstruation 626.8
Retroiliac ureter 753.4
Retroperineal - see condition
Retroperitoneal - see condition
Retroperitonitis (see also Peritonitis) 567.9
Retropharyngeal - see condition
Retroplacental - see condition
Retroposition - see Retroversion
Retrosternal thyroid (congenital) 759.2
Retroversion, retroverted
cervix (see also Retroversion, uterus)
621.6
female NEC (see also Retroversion,
uterus) 621.6
iris 364.70
testis (congenital) 752.51
uterus, uterine (acquired) (acute) (adherent) (any degree) (asymptomatic) (cervix) (postinfectional)
(postpartal, old) 621.6
congenital 752.3
in pregnancy or childbirth 654.3
affecting fetus or newborn 763.89
causing obstructed labor 660.2
affecting fetus or newborn 763.1
Retrusion, premaxilla (developmental)
524.04
Rett's syndrome 330.8
Reverse, reversed
peristalsis 787.4
Reye's syndrome 331.81
Reye-Sheehan syndrome (postpartum
pituitary necrosis) 253.2
Rh (factor)
hemolytic disease 773.0
incompatibility, immunization, or sensitization
affecting management of pregnancy
656.1
fetus or newborn 773.0
transfusion reaction 999.7
negative mother, affecting fetus or
newborn 773.0
titer elevated 999.7
transfusion reaction 999.7

◀ **New**   ⬅ **Revised**

Rhabdomyolysis (idiopathic) 728.88
Rhabdomyoma (M8900/0) - *see also* Neoplasm, connective tissue, benign
  adult (M8904/0) - *see* Neoplasm, connective tissue, benign
  fetal (M8903/0) - *see* Neoplasm, connective tissue, benign
  glycogenic (M8904/0) - *see* Neoplasm, connective tissue, benign
Rhabdomyosarcoma (M8900/3) - *see also* Neoplasm, connective tissue, malignant
  alveolar (M8920/3) - *see* Neoplasm, connective tissue, malignant
  embryonal (M8910/3) - *see* Neoplasm, connective tissue, malignant
  mixed type (M8902/3) - *see* Neoplasm, connective tissue, malignant
  pleomorphic (M8901/3) - *see* Neoplasm, connective tissue, malignant
Rhabdosarcoma (M8900/3) - *see* Rhabdomyosarcoma
Rhesus (factor) (Rh) incompatibility - *see* Rh, incompatibility
Rheumaticosis - *see* Rheumatism
Rheumatism, rheumatic (acute NEC) 729.0
  adherent pericardium 393
  arthritis
    acute or subacute - *see* Fever, rheumatic
    chronic 714.0
      spine 720.0
  articular (chronic) NEC (*see also* Arthritis) 716.9
    acute or subacute - *see* Fever, rheumatic
  back 724.9
  blennorrhagic 098.59
  carditis - *see* Disease, heart, rheumatic
  cerebral - *see* Fever, rheumatic
  chorea (acute) - *see* Chorea, rheumatic
  chronic NEC 729.0
  coronary arteritis 391.9
    chronic 398.99
  degeneration, myocardium (*see also* Degeneration, myocardium, with rheumatic fever) 398.0
  desert 114.0
  febrile - *see* Fever, rheumatic
  fever - *see* Fever, rheumatic
  gonococcal 098.59
  gout 274.0
  heart
    disease (*see also* Disease, heart, rheumatic) 398.90
    failure (chronic) (congestive) (inactive) 398.91
  hemopericardium - *see* Rheumatic, pericarditis
  hydropericardium - *see* Rheumatic, pericarditis
  inflammatory (acute) (chronic) (subacute) - *see* Fever, rheumatic
  intercostal 729.0
    meaning Tietze's disease 733.6
  joint (chronic) NEC (*see also* Arthritis) 716.9
    acute - *see* Fever, rheumatic
  mediastinopericarditis - *see* Rheumatic, pericarditis
  muscular 729.0
  myocardial degeneration (*see also* Degeneration, myocardium, with rheumatic fever) 398.0

Rheumatism, rheumatic (*Continued*)
  myocarditis (chronic) (inactive) (with chorea) 398.0
    active or acute 391.2
      with chorea (acute) (rheumatic) (Sydenham's) 392.0
  myositis 729.1
  neck 724.9
  neuralgic 729.0
  neuritis (acute) (chronic) 729.2
  neuromuscular 729.0
  nodose - *see* Arthritis, nodosa
  nonarticular 729.0
  palindromic 719.30
    ankle 719.37
    elbow 719.32
    foot 719.37
    hand 719.34
    hip 719.35
    knee 719.36
    multiple sites 719.39
    pelvic region 719.35
    shoulder (region) 719.31
    specified site NEC 719.38
    wrist 719.33
  pancarditis, acute 391.8
    with chorea (acute) (rheumatic) (Sydenham's) 392.0
    chronic or inactive 398.99
  pericarditis (active) (acute) (with effusion) (with pneumonia) 391.0
    with chorea (acute) (rheumatic) (Sydenham's) 392.0
    chronic or inactive 393
  pericardium - *see* Rheumatic, pericarditis
  pleuropericarditis - *see* Rheumatic, pericarditis
  pneumonia 390 [517.1]
  pneumonitis 390 [517.1]
  pneumopericarditis - *see* Rheumatic, pericarditis
  polyarthritis
    acute or subacute - *see* Fever, rheumatic
    chronic 714.0
  polyarticular NEC (*see also* Arthritis) 716.9
  psychogenic 306.0
  radiculitis 729.2
  sciatic 724.3
  septic - *see* Fever, rheumatic
  spine 724.9
  subacute NEC 729.0
  torticollis 723.5
  tuberculous NEC (*see also* Tuberculosis) 015.9
  typhoid fever 002.0
Rheumatoid - *see also* condition
  lungs 714.81
Rhinitis (atrophic) (catarrhal) (chronic) (croupous) (fibrinous) (hyperplastic) (hypertrophic) (membranous) (purulent) (suppurative) (ulcerative) 472.0
  with
    hay fever (*see also* Fever, hay) 477.9
      with asthma (bronchial) 493.0
    sore throat - *see* Nasopharyngitis
  acute 460
  allergic (nonseasonal) (seasonal) (*see also* Fever, hay) 477.9
    with asthma (*see also* Asthma) 493.0
    due to food 477.1
  granulomatous 472.0
  infective 460

Rhinitis (*Continued*)
  obstructive 472.0
  pneumococcal 460
  syphilitic 095.8
    congenital 090.0
  tuberculous (*see also* Tuberculosis) 012.8
  vasomotor (*see also* Fever, hay) 477.9
Rhinoantritis (chronic) 473.0
  acute 461.0
Rhinodacryolith 375.57
Rhinolalia (aperta) (clausa) (open) 784.49
Rhinolith 478.1
  nasal sinus (*see also* Sinusitis) 473.9
Rhinomegaly 478.1
Rhinopharyngitis (acute) (subacute) (*see also* Nasopharyngitis) 460
  chronic 472.2
  destructive ulcerating 102.5
  mutilans 102.5
Rhinophyma 695.3
Rhinorrhea 478.1
  cerebrospinal (fluid) 349.81
  paroxysmal (*see also* Fever, hay) 477.9
  spasmodic (*see also* Fever, hay) 477.9
Rhinosalpingitis 381.50
  acute 381.51
  chronic 381.52
Rhinoscleroma 040.1
Rhinosporidiosis 117.0
Rhinovirus infection 079.3
Rhizomelic chrondrodysplasia punctata 277.86 ◄
Rhizomelique, pseudopolyarthritic 446.5
Rhoads and Bomford anemia (refractory) 284.9
Rhus
  diversiloba dermatitis 692.6
  radicans dermatitis 692.6
  toxicodendron dermatitis 692.6
  venenata dermatitis 692.6
  verniciflua dermatitis 692.6
Rhythm
  atrioventricular nodal 427.89
  disorder 427.9
    coronary sinus 427.89
    ectopic 427.89
    nodal 427.89
  escape 427.89
  heart, abnormal 427.9
    fetus or newborn - *see* Abnormal, heart rate
  idioventricular 426.89
    accelerated 427.89
  nodal 427.89
  sleep, inversion 780.55
    nonorganic origin 307.45
Rhytidosis facialis 701.8
Rib - *see also* condition
  cervical 756.2
Riboflavin deficiency 266.0
Rice bodies (*see also* Loose, body, joint) 718.1
  knee 717.6
Richter's hernia - *see* Hernia, Richter's
Ricinism 988.2
Rickets (active) (acute) (adolescent) (adult) (chest wall) (congenital) (current) (infantile) (intestinal) 268.0
  celiac 579.0
  fetal 756.4
  hemorrhagic 267
  hypophosphatemic with nephrotic-glycosuric dwarfism 270.0
  kidney 588.0

ICD-9-CM
R
Vol. 2

Rickets (Continued)
late effect 268.1
renal 588.0
scurvy 267
vitamin D-resistant 275.3
Rickettsial disease 083.9
specified type NEC 083.8
Rickettsialpox 083.2
Rickettsiosis NEC 083.9
specified type NEC 083.8
tick-borne 082.9
specified type NEC 082.8
vesicular 083.2
Ricord's chancre 091.0
Riddoch's syndrome (visual disorientation) 368.16
Rider's
bone 733.99
chancre 091.0
Ridge, alveolus - see also condition
edentulous
atrophy 525.20 ◄
mandible 525.20 ◄
minimal 525.21 ◄
moderate 525.22 ◄
severe 525.23 ◄
maxilla 525.20 ◄
minimal 525.24 ◄
moderate 525.25 ◄
severe 525.26 ◄
flabby 525.20 ◄▥
Ridged ear 744.29
Riedel's
disease (ligneous thyroiditis) 245.3
lobe, liver 751.69
struma (ligneous thyroiditis) 245.3
thyroiditis (ligneous) 245.3
Rieger's anomaly or syndrome (mesodermal dysgenesis, anterior ocular
segment) 743.44
Riehl's melanosis 709.09
**Rietti-Greppi-Micheli anemia or syn-
drome** 282.49
Rieux's hernia - see Hernia, Rieux's
Rift Valley fever 066.3
Riga's disease (cachectic aphthae) 529.0
Riga-Fede disease (cachectic aphthae)
529.0
Riggs' disease (compound periodontitis)
523.4
Right middle lobe syndrome 518.0
Rigid, rigidity - see also condition
abdominal 789.4
articular, multiple congenital 754.89
back 724.8
cervix uteri
in pregnancy or childbirth 654.6
affecting fetus or newborn 763.89
causing obstructed labor 660.2
affecting fetus or newborn 763.1
hymen (acquired) (congenital) 623.3
nuchal 781.6
pelvic floor
in pregnancy or childbirth 654.4
affecting fetus or newborn 763.89
causing obstructed labor 660.2
affecting fetus or newborn 763.1
perineum or vulva
in pregnancy or childbirth 654.8
affecting fetus or newborn 763.89
causing obstructed labor 660.2
affecting fetus or newborn 763.1
spine 724.8
vagina

Rigid, rigidity (Continued)
vagina (Continued)
in pregnancy or childbirth 654.7
affecting fetus or newborn 763.89
causing obstructed labor 660.2
affecting fetus or newborn 763.1
Rigors 780.99
Riley-Day syndrome (familial dysautonomia) 742.8
Ring(s)
aorta 747.21
Bandl's, complicating delivery 661.4
affecting fetus or newborn 763.7
contraction, complicating delivery 661.4
affecting fetus or newborn 763.7
esophageal (congenital) 750.3
Fleischer (-Kayser) (cornea) 275.1
[371.14]
hymenal, tight (acquired) (congenital)
623.3
Kayser-Fleischer (cornea) 275.1 [371.14]
retraction, uterus, pathological 661.4
affecting fetus or newborn 763.7
Schatzki's (esophagus) (congenital)
(lower) 750.3
acquired 530.3
Soemmering's 366.51
trachea, abnormal 748.3
vascular (congenital) 747.21
Vossius' 921.3
late effect 366.21
Ringed hair (congenital) 757.4
Ringing in the ear (see also Tinnitus)
388.30
Ringworm 110.9
beard 110.0
body 110.5
burmese 110.9
corporeal 110.5
foot 110.4
groin 110.3
hand 110.2
honeycomb 110.0
nails 110.1
perianal (area) 110.3
scalp 110.0
specified site NEC 110.8
Tokelau 110.5
Rise, venous pressure 459.89
Risk
factor - see Problem
suicidal 300.9
Ritter's disease (dermatitis exfoliativa
neonatorum) 695.81
Rivalry, sibling 313.3
Rivalta's disease (cervicofacial actinomycosis) 039.3
River blindness 125.3 [360.13]
Robert's pelvis 755.69
with disproportion (fetopelvic) 653.0
affecting fetus or newborn 763.1
causing obstructed labor 660.1
affecting fetus or newborn 763.1
Robin's syndrome 756.0
Robinson's (hidrotic) ectodermal dyspla-
sia 757.31
Robles' disease (onchocerciasis) 125.3
[360.13]
Rochalimaea - see Rickettsial disease
Rocky Mountain fever (spotted) 082.0
Rodent ulcer (M8090/3) - see also Neoplasm, skin, malignant
cornea 370.07
Roentgen ray, adverse effect - see Effect,
adverse, x-ray

Roetheln 056.9
Roger's disease (congenital interventric-
ular septal defect) 745.4
Rokitansky's
disease (see also Necrosis, liver) 570
tumor 620.2
Rokitansky-Aschoff sinuses (mucosal
outpouching of gallbladder) (see also
Disease, gallbladder) 575.8
Rokitansky-Kuster-Hauser syndrome
(congenital absence of vagina) 752.49
Rollet's chancre (syphilitic) 091.0
Rolling of head 781.0
Romano-Ward syndrome (prolonged Q-
T interval) 794.31
Romanus lesion 720.1
Romberg's disease or syndrome 349.89
Roof, mouth - see condition
Rosacea 695.3
acne 695.3
keratitis 695.3 [370.49]
Rosary, rachitic 268.0
Rose
cold 477.0
fever 477.0
rash 782.1
epidemic 056.9
of infants 057.8
Rosen-Castleman-Liebow syndrome
(pulmonary proteinosis) 516.0
**Rosenbach's erysipelatoid or erysipe-
loid** 027.1
Rosenthal's disease (factor XI deficiency)
286.2
Roseola 057.8
infantum, infantilis 057.8
Rossbach's disease (hyperchlorhydria)
536.8
psychogenic 306.4
Rossle-Urbach-Wiethe lipoproteinosis
272.8
Ross river fever 066.3
Rostan's asthma (cardiac) (see also Failure, ventricular, left) 428.1
Rot
Barcoo (see also Ulcer, skin) 707.9
knife-grinders' (see also Tuberculosis)
011.4
Rot-Bernhardt disease 355.1
Rotation
anomalous, incomplete or insufficient -
see Malrotation
cecum (congenital) 751.4
colon (congenital) 751.4
manual, affecting fetus or newborn
763.89
spine, incomplete or insufficient 737.8
tooth, teeth 524.35 ◄▥
vertebra, incomplete or insufficient
737.8
Röteln 056.9
Roth's disease or meralgia 355.1
Roth-Bernhardt disease or syndrome
355.1
Rothmund (-Thomson) **syndrome** 757.33
Rotor's disease or syndrome (idiopathic
hyperbilirubinemia) 277.4
Rotundum ulcus - see Ulcer, stomach
Round
back (with wedging of vertebrae)
737.10
late effect of rickets 268.1
hole, retina 361.31
with detachment 361.01

◄ **New**   ◄▥ **Revised**

Round (Continued)
ulcer (stomach) - see Ulcer, stomach
worms (infestation) (large) NEC 127.0
Roussy-Lévy syndrome 334.3
Routine postpartum follow-up V24.2
Roy (-Jutras) syndrome (acropachyderma) 757.39
Rubella (German measles) 056.9
complicating pregnancy, childbirth, or
puerperium 647.5
complication 056.8
neurological 056.00
encephalomyelitis 056.01
specified type NEC 056.09
specified type NEC 056.79
congenital 771.0
contact V01.4
exposure to V01.4
maternal
with suspected fetal damage affecting management of pregnancy
655.3
affecting fetus or newborn 760.2
manifest rubella in infant 771.0
specified complications NEC 056.79
vaccination, prophylactic (against)
V04.3
Rubeola (measles) (see also Measles)
055.9
complicated 055.8
meaning rubella (see also Rubella) 056.9
scarlatinosis 057.8
Rubeosis iridis 364.42
diabetica 250.5 [364.42]
Rubinstein-Taybi's syndrome (brachydactylia, short stature and mental retardation) 759.89
Rud's syndrome (mental deficiency, epilepsy, and infantilism) 759.89
Rudimentary (congenital) - see also
Agenesis
arm 755.22
bone 756.9
cervix uteri 752.49
eye (see also Microphthalmos) 743.10
fallopian tube 752.19
leg 755.32
lobule of ear 744.21
patella 755.64
respiratory organs in thoracopagus
759.4
tracheal bronchus 748.3
uterine horn 752.3
uterus 752.3
in male 752.7
solid or with cavity 752.3
vagina 752.49
Ruiter-Pompen (-Wyers) syndrome (angiokeratoma corporis diffusum)
272.7
Ruled out condition (see also Observation, suspected) V71.9
Rumination - see also Vomiting
disorder 307.53   ◄
neurotic 300.3
obsessional 300.3
psychogenic 307.53
Runaway reaction - see also Disturbance,
conduct
socialized 312.2
undersocialized, unsocialized 312.1
Runeberg's disease (progressive pernicious anemia) 281.0
Runge's syndrome (postmaturity) 766.22

Rupia 091.3
congenital 090.0
tertiary 095.9
Rupture, ruptured 553.9
abdominal viscera NEC 799.89
obstetrical trauma 665.5
abscess (spontaneous) - see Abscess, by
site
amnion - see Rupture, membranes
aneurysm - see Aneurysm
anus (sphincter) - see Laceration, anus
aorta, aortic 441.5
abdominal 441.3
arch 441.1
ascending 441.1
descending 441.5
abdominal 441.3
thoracic 441.1
syphilitic 093.0
thoracoabdominal 441.6
thorax, thoracic 441.1
transverse 441.1
traumatic (thoracic) 901.0
abdominal 902.0
valve or cusp (see also Endocarditis,
aortic) 424.1
appendix (with peritonitis) 540.0
with peritoneal abscess 540.1
traumatic - see Injury, internal, gastrointestinal tract
arteriovenous fistula, brain (congenital)
430
artery 447.2
brain (see also Hemorrhage, brain)
431
coronary (see also Infarct, myocardium) 410.9
heart (see also Infarct, myocardium)
410.9
pulmonary 417.8
traumatic (complication) (see also Injury, blood vessel, by site) 904.9
bile duct, except cystic (see also Disease, biliary) 576.3
cystic 575.4
traumatic - see Injury, internal, intraabdominal
bladder (sphincter) 596.6
with
abortion - see Abortion, by type,
with damage to pelvic organs
ectopic pregnancy (see also categories 633.0-633.9) 639.2
molar pregnancy (see also categories 630-632) 639.2
following
abortion 639.2
ectopic or molar pregnancy 639.2
nontraumatic 596.6
obstetrical trauma 665.5
spontaneous 596.6
traumatic - see Injury, internal, bladder
blood vessel (see also Hemorrhage)
459.0
brain (see also Hemorrhage, brain)
431
heart (see also Infarct, myocardium)
410.9
traumatic (complication) (see also Injury, blood vessel, by site) 904.9
bone - see Fracture, by site
bowel 569.89
traumatic - see Injury, internal, intestine

Rupture, ruptured (Continued)
Bowman's membrane 371.31
brain
aneurysm (congenital) (see also Hemorrhage, subarachnoid) 430
late effect - see Late effect(s) (of)
cerebrovascular disease
syphilitic 094.87
hemorrhagic (see also Hemorrhage,
brain) 431
injury at birth 767.0
syphilitic 094.89
capillaries 448.9
cardiac (see also Infarct, myocardium)
410.9
cartilage (articular) (current) - see also
Sprain, by site
knee - see Tear, meniscus
semilunar - see Tear, meniscus
cecum (with peritonitis) 540.0
with peritoneal abscess 540.1
traumatic 863.89
with open wound into cavity
863.99
cerebral aneurysm (congenital) (see also
Hemorrhage, subarachnoid) 430
late effect - see Late effect(s) (of)
cerebrovascular disease
cervix (uteri)
with
abortion - see Abortion, by type,
with damage to pelvic organs
ectopic pregnancy (see also categories 633.0-633.9) 639.2
molar pregnancy (see also categories 630-632) 639.2
following
abortion 639.2
ectopic or molar pregnancy 639.2
obstetrical trauma 665.3
traumatic - see Injury, internal, cervix
chordae tendineae 429.5
choroid (direct) (indirect) (traumatic)
363.63
circle of Willis (see also Hemorrhage,
subarachnoid) 430
late effect - see Late effect(s) (of)
cerebrovascular disease
colon 569.89
traumatic - see Injury, internal, colon
cornea (traumatic) - see also Rupture,
eye
due to ulcer 370.00
coronary (artery) (thrombotic) (see also
Infarct, myocardium) 410.9
corpus luteum (infected) (ovary) 620.1
cyst - see Cyst
cystic duct (see also Disease, gallbladder) 575.4
Descemet's membrane 371.33
traumatic - see Rupture, eye
diaphragm - see also Hernia, diaphragm
traumatic - see Injury, internal, diaphragm
diverticulum
bladder 596.3
intestine (large) (see also Diverticula)
562.10
small 562.00
duodenal stump 537.89
duodenum (ulcer) - see Ulcer, duodenum, with perforation

ICD-9-CM

R

Vol. 2

Rupture, ruptured (*Continued*)
  ear drum (*see also* Perforation, tympanum) 384.20
    with otitis media - *see* Otitis media
    traumatic - *see* Wound, open, ear
  esophagus 530.4
    traumatic 862.22
      with open wound into cavity 862.32
      cervical region - *see* Wound, open, esophagus
  eye (without prolapse of intraocular tissue) 871.0
    with
      exposure of intraocular tissue 871.1
      partial loss of intraocular tissue 871.2
      prolapse of intraocular tissue 871.1
    due to burn 940.5
  fallopian tube 620.8
    due to pregnancy - *see* Pregnancy, tubal
    traumatic - *see* Injury, internal, fallopian tube
  fontanel 767.3
  free wall (ventricle) (*see also* Infarct, myocardium) 410.9
  gallbladder or duct (*see also* Disease, gallbladder) 575.4
    traumatic - *see* Injury, internal, gallbladder
  gastric (*see also* Rupture, stomach) 537.89
    vessel 459.0
  globe (eye) (traumatic) - *see* Rupture, eye
  graafian follicle (hematoma) 620.0
  heart (auricle) (ventricle) (*see also* Infarct, myocardium) 410.9
    infectional 422.90
    traumatic - *see* Rupture, myocardium, traumatic
  hymen 623.8
  internal
    organ, traumatic - *see also* Injury, internal, by site
      heart - *see* Rupture, myocardium, traumatic
      kidney - *see* Rupture, kidney
      liver - *see* Rupture, liver
      spleen - *see* Rupture, spleen, traumatic
      semilunar cartilage - *see* Tear, meniscus
    intervertebral disc - *see* Displacement, intervertebral disc
    traumatic (current) - *see* Dislocation, vertebra
  intestine 569.89
    traumatic - *see* Injury, internal, intestine
  intracranial, birth injury 767.0
  iris 364.76
    traumatic - *see* Rupture, eye
  joint capsule - *see* Sprain, by site
  kidney (traumatic) 866.03
    with open wound into cavity 866.13
    due to birth injury 767.8
    nontraumatic 593.89
  lacrimal apparatus (traumatic) 870.2
  lens (traumatic) 366.20
  ligament - *see also* Sprain, by site
    with open wound - *see* Wound, open, by site

Rupture, ruptured (*Continued*)
  ligament (*Continued*)
    old (*see also* Disorder, cartilage, articular) 718.0
  liver (traumatic) 864.04
    with open wound into cavity 864.14
    due to birth injury 767.8
    nontraumatic 573.8
  lymphatic (node) (vessel) 457.8
  marginal sinus (placental) (with hemorrhage) 641.2
    affecting fetus or newborn 762.1
  meaning hernia - *see* Hernia
  membrana tympani (*see also* Perforation, tympanum) 384.20
    with otitis media - *see* Otitis media
    traumatic - *see* Wound, open, ear
  membranes (spontaneous)
    artificial
      delayed delivery following 658.3
        affecting fetus or newborn 761.1
      fetus or newborn 761.1
    delayed delivery following 658.2
      affecting fetus or newborn 761.1
    premature (less than 24 hours prior to onset of labor) 658.1
      affecting fetus or newborn 761.1
    delayed delivery following 658.2
      affecting fetus or newborn 761.1
  meningeal artery (*see also* Hemorrhage, subarachnoid) 430
    late effect - *see* Late effect(s) (of) cerebrovascular disease
  meniscus (knee) - *see also* Tear, meniscus
    old (*see also* Derangement, meniscus) 717.5
      site other than knee - *see* Disorder, cartilage, articular
    site other than knee - *see* Sprain, by site
  mesentery 568.89
    traumatic - *see* Injury, internal, mesentery
  mitral - *see* Insufficiency, mitral
  muscle (traumatic) NEC - *see also* Sprain, by site
    with open wound - *see* Wound, open, by site
    nontraumatic 728.83
  musculotendinous cuff (nontraumatic) (shoulder) 840.4
  mycotic aneurysm, causing cerebral hemorrhage (*see also* Hemorrhage, subarachnoid) 430
    late effect - *see* Late effect(s) (of) cerebrovascular disease
  myocardium, myocardial (*see also* Infarct, myocardium) 410.9
    traumatic 861.03
      with open wound into thorax 861.13
  nontraumatic (meaning hernia) (*see also* Hernia, by site) 553.9
  obstructed (*see also* Hernia, by site, with obstruction) 552.9
  gangrenous (*see also* Hernia, by site, with gangrene) 551.9
  operation wound 998.32
    internal 998.31
  ovary, ovarian 620.8
    corpus luteum 620.1
    follicle (graafian) 620.0
  oviduct 620.8
    due to pregnancy - *see* Pregnancy, tubal

Rupture, ruptured (*Continued*)
  pancreas 577.8
    traumatic - *see* Injury, internal, pancreas
  papillary muscle (ventricular) 429.6
  pelvic
    floor, complicating delivery 664.1
    organ NEC - *see* Injury, pelvic, organs
  penis (traumatic) - *see* Wound, open, penis
  perineum 624.8
    during delivery (*see also* Laceration, perineum, complicating delivery) 664.4
  pharynx (nontraumatic) (spontaneous) 478.29
  pregnant uterus (before onset of labor) 665.0
  prostate (traumatic) - *see* Injury, internal, prostate
  pulmonary
    artery 417.8
    valve (heart) (*see also* Endocarditis, pulmonary) 424.3
    vein 417.8
    vessel 417.8
  pupil, sphincter 364.75
  pus tube (*see also* Salpingo-oophoritis) 614.2
  pyosalpinx (*see also* Salpingo-oophoritis) 614.2
  rectum 569.49
    traumatic - *see* Injury, internal, rectum
  retina, retinal (traumatic) (without detachment) 361.30
    with detachment (*see also* Detachment, retina, with retinal defect) 361.00
  rotator cuff (capsule) (traumatic) 840.4
    nontraumatic, complete 727.61
  sclera 871.0
  semilunar cartilage, knee (*see also* Tear, meniscus) 836.2
    old (*see also* Derangement, meniscus) 717.5
  septum (cardiac) 410.8
  sigmoid 569.89
    traumatic - *see* Injury, internal, colon, sigmoid
  sinus of Valsalva 747.29
  spinal cord - *see also* Injury, spinal, by site
    due to injury at birth 767.4
    fetus or newborn 767.4
    syphilitic 094.89
    traumatic - *see also* Injury, spinal, by site
      with fracture - *see* Fracture, vertebra, by site, with spinal cord injury
  spleen 289.59
    congenital 767.8
    due to injury at birth 767.8
    malarial 084.9
    nontraumatic 289.59
    spontaneous 289.59
    traumatic 865.04
      with open wound into cavity 865.14
  splenic vein 459.0
  stomach 537.89
    due to injury at birth 767.8

◀ **New**   ◀≡ **Revised**

Rupture, ruptured (*Continued*)
  stomach (*Continued*)
    traumatic - *see* Injury, internal, stomach
    ulcer - *see* Ulcer, stomach, with perforation
  synovium 727.50
    specified site NEC 727.59
  tendon (traumatic) - *see also* Sprain, by site
    with open wound - *see* Wound, open, by site
    Achilles 845.09
      nontraumatic 727.67
    ankle 845.09
      nontraumatic 727.68
    biceps (long bead) 840.8
      nontraumatic 727.62
    foot 845.10
      interphalangeal (joint) 845.13
      metatarsophalangeal (joint) 845.12
      nontraumatic 727.68
      specified site NEC 845.19
      tarsometatarsal (joint) 845.11
    hand 842.10
      carpometacarpal (joint) 842.11
      interphalangeal (joint) 842.13
      metacarpophalangeal (joint) 842.12
      nontraumatic 727.63
        extensors 727.63
        flexors 727.64
      specified site NEC 842.19
    nontraumatic 727.60
      specified site NEC 727.69
    patellar 844.8
      nontraumatic 727.66
    quadriceps 844.8
      nontraumatic 727.65
    rotator cuff (capsule) 840.4
      nontraumatic, complete 727.61
    wrist 842.00
      carpal (joint) 842.01
      nontraumatic 727.63
        extensors 727.63
        flexors 727.64
      radiocarpal (joint) (ligament) 842.02
      radioulnar (joint), distal 842.09
      specified site NEC 842.09
  testis (traumatic) 878.2
    complicated 878.3
    due to syphilis 095.8
  thoracic duct 457.8

Rupture, ruptured (*Continued*)
  tonsil 474.8
  traumatic
    with open wound - *see* Wound, open, by site
    aorta - *see* Rupture, aorta, traumatic
    ear drum - *see* Wound, open, ear, drum
    external site - *see* Wound, open, by site
    eye 871.2
    globe (eye) - *see* Wound, open, eyeball
    internal organ (abdomen, chest, or pelvis) - *see also* Injury, internal, by site
      heart - *see* Rupture, myocardium, traumatic
      kidney - *see* Rupture, kidney
      liver - *see* Rupture, liver
      spleen - *see* Rupture, spleen, traumatic
    ligament, muscle, or tendon - *see also* Sprain, by site
      with open wound - *see* Wound, open, by site
    meaning hernia - *see* Hernia
  tricuspid (heart) (valve) - *see* Endocarditis, tricuspid
  tube, tubal 620.8
    abscess (*see also* Salpingo-oophoritis) 614.2
    due to pregnancy - *see* Pregnancy, tubal
  tympanum, tympanic (membrane) (*see also* Perforation, tympanum) 384.20
    with otitis media - *see* Otitis media
    traumatic - *see* Wound, open, ear, drum
  umbilical cord 663.8
    fetus or newborn 772.0
  ureter (traumatic) (*see also* Injury, internal, ureter) 867.2
    nontraumatic 593.89
  urethra 599.84
    with
      abortion - *see* Abortion, by type, with damage to pelvic organs
      ectopic pregnancy (*see also* categories 633.0-633.9) 639.2
      molar pregnancy (*see also* categories 630-632) 639.2
    following
      abortion 639.2

Rupture, ruptured (*Continued*)
  urethra (*Continued*)
    following (*Continued*)
      ectopic or molar pregnancy 639.2
    obstetrical trauma 665.5
    traumatic - *see* Injury, internal urethra
  uterosacral ligament 620.8
  uterus (traumatic) - *see also* Injury, internal, uterus
    affecting fetus or newborn 763.89
    during labor 665.1
    nonpuerperal, nontraumatic 621.8
    nontraumatic 621.8
    pregnant (during labor) 665.1
      before labor 665.0
  vagina 878.6
    complicated 878.7
    complicating delivery - *see* Laceration, vagina, complicating delivery
  valve, valvular (heart) - *see* Endocarditis
  varicose vein - *see* Varicose, vein
  varix - *see* Varix
  vena cava 459.0
  ventricle (free wall) (left) (*see also* Infarct, myocardium) 410.9
  vesical (urinary) 596.6
    traumatic - *see* Injury, internal, bladder
  vessel (blood) 459.0
    pulmonary 417.8
  viscus 799.89
  vulva 878.4
    complicated 878.5
    complicating delivery 664.0
Russell's dwarf (uterine dwarfism and craniofacial dysostosis) 759.89
Russell's dysentery 004.8
Russell (-Silver) syndrome (congenital hemihypertrophy and short stature) 759.89
Russian spring-summer type encephalitis 063.0
Rust's disease (tuberculous spondylitis) 015.0 [720.81]
Rustitskii's disease (multiple myeloma) (M9730/3) 203.0
Ruysch's disease (Hirschsprung's disease) 751.3
Rytand-Lipsitch syndrome (complete atrioventricular block) 426.0

ICD-9-CM

R

Vol. 2

S

Saber
shin 090.5
tibia 090.5
Sac, lacrimal - *see* condition
Saccharomyces infection (*see also* Candidiasis) 112.9
Saccharopinuria 270.7
Saccular - *see* condition
Sacculation
aorta (nonsyphilitic) (*see also* Aneurysm, aorta) 441.9
ruptured 441.5
syphilitic 093.0
bladder 596.3
colon 569.89
intralaryngeal (congenital) (ventricular) 748.3
larynx (congenital) (ventricular) 748.3
organ or site, congenital - *see* Distortion
pregnant uterus, complicating delivery 654.4
affecting fetus or newborn 763.1
causing obstructed labor 660.2
affecting fetus or newborn 763.1
rectosigmoid 569.89
sigmoid 569.89
ureter 593.89
urethra 599.2
vesical 596.3
Sachs (-Tay) disease (amaurotic familial idiocy) 330.1
Sacks-Libman disease 710.0 [424.91]
Sacralgia 724.6
Sacralization
fifth lumbar vertebra 756.15
incomplete (vertebra) 756.15
Sacrodynia 724.6
Sacroiliac joint - *see* condition
Sacroiliitis NEC 720.2
Sacrum - *see* condition
Saddle
back 737.8
embolus, aorta 444.0
nose 738.0
congenital 754.0
due to syphilis 090.5
Sadism (sexual) 302.84
Saemisch's ulcer 370.04
Saenger's syndrome 379.46
Sago spleen 277.3
Sailors' skin 692.74
Saint
Anthony's fire (*see also* Erysipelas) 035
Guy's dance - *see* Chorea
Louis-type encephalitis 062.3
triad (*see also* Hernia, diaphragm) 553.3
Vitus' dance - *see* Chorea
Salicylism
correct substance properly administered 535.4
overdose or wrong substance given or taken 965.1
Salivary duct or gland - *see also* condition
virus disease 078.5
Salivation (excessive) (*see also* Ptyalism) 527.7
Salmonella (aertrycke) (choleraesuis) (enteritidis) (gallinarum) (suipestifer) (typhimurium) (*see also* Infection, Salmonella) 003.9

Salmonella (*Continued*)
arthritis 003.23
carrier (suspected) of V02.3
meningitis 003.21
osteomyelitis 003.24
pneumonia 003.22
septicemia 003.1
typhosa 002.0
carrier (suspected) of V02.1
Salmonellosis 003.0
with pneumonia 003.22
Salpingitis (catarrhal) (fallopian tube) (nodular) (pseudofollicular) (purulent) (septic) (*see also* Salpingo-oophoritis) 614.2
ear 381.50
acute 381.51
chronic 381.52
Eustachian (tube) 381.50
acute 381.51
chronic 381.52
follicularis 614.1
gonococcal (chronic) 098.37
acute 098.17
interstitial, chronic 614.1
isthmica nodosa 614.1
old - *see* Salpingo-oophoritis, chronic
puerperal, postpartum, childbirth 670
specific (chronic) 098.37
acute 098.17
tuberculous (acute) (chronic) (*see also* Tuberculosis) 016.6
venereal (chronic) 098.37
acute 098.17
Salpingocele 620.4
Salpingo-oophoritis (catarrhal) (purulent) (ruptured) (septic) (suppurative) 614.2
acute 614.0
with
abortion - *see* Abortion, by type, with sepsis
ectopic pregnancy (*see also* categories 633.0-633.9) 639.0
molar pregnancy (*see also* categories 630-632) 639.0
following
abortion 639.0
ectopic or molar pregnancy 639.0
gonococcal 098.17
puerperal, postpartum, childbirth 670
tuberculous (*see also* Tuberculosis) 016.6
chronic 614.1
gonococcal 098.37
tuberculous (*see also* Tuberculosis) 016.6
complicating pregnancy 646.6
affecting fetus or newborn 760.8
gonococcal (chronic) 098.37
acute 098.17
old - *see* Salpingo-oophoritis, chronic
puerperal 670
specific - *see* Salpingo-oophoritis, gonococcal
subacute (*see also* Salpingo-oophoritis, acute) 614.0
tuberculous (acute) (chronic) (*see also* Tuberculosis) 016.6
venereal - *see* Salpingo-oophoritis, gonococcal

Salpingo-ovaritis (*see also* Salpingo-oophoritis) 614.2
Salpingoperitonitis (*see also* Salpingo-oophoritis) 614.2
Salt-losing
nephritis (*see also* Disease, renal) 593.9
syndrome (*see also* Disease, renal) 593.9
Salt-rheum (*see also* Eczema) 692.9
Salzmann's nodular dystrophy 371.46
Sampson's cyst or tumor 617.1
Sandblasters'
asthma 502
lung 502
Sander's disease (paranoia) 297.1
Sandfly fever 066.0
Sandhoff's disease 330.1
Sanfilippo's syndrome (mucopolysaccharidosis III) 277.5
Sanger-Brown's ataxia 334.2
San Joaquin Valley fever 114.0
São Paulo fever or typhus 082.0
Saponification, mesenteric 567.8
Sapremia - *see* Septicemia
Sarcocele (benign)
syphilitic 095.8
congenital 090.5
Sarcoepiplocele (*see also* Hernia) 553.9
Sarcoepiplomphalocele (*see also* Hernia, umbilicus) 553.1
Sarcoid (any site) 135
with lung involvement 135 [517.8]
Boeck's 135
Darier-Roussy 135
Spiegler-Fendt 686.8
Sarcoidosis 135
cardiac 135 [425.8]
lung 135 [517.8]
Sarcoma (M8800/3) - *see also* Neoplasm, connective tissue, malignant
alveolar soft part (M9581/3) - *see* Neoplasm, connective tissue, malignant
ameloblastic (M9330/3) 170.1
upper jaw (bone) 170.0
botryoid (M8910/3) - *see* Neoplasm, connective tissue, malignant
botryoides (M8910/3) - *see* Neoplasm, connective tissue, malignant
cerebellar (M9480/3) 191.6
circumscribed (arachnoidal) (M9471/3) 191.6
circumscribed (arachnoidal) cerebellar (M9471/3) 191.6
clear cell, of tendons and aponeuroses (M9044/3) - *see* Neoplasm, connective tissue, malignant
embryonal (M8991/3) - *see* Neoplasm, connective tissue, malignant
endometrial (stromal) (M8930/3) 182.0
isthmus 182.1
endothelial (M9130/3) - *see also* Neoplasm, connective tissue, malignant
bone (M9260/3) - *see* Neoplasm, bone, malignant
epithelioid cell (M8804/3) - *see* Neoplasm, connective tissue, malignant
Ewing's (M9260/3) - *see* Neoplasm, bone, malignant
follicular dendritic cell 202.9
germinoblastic (diffuse) (M9632/3) 202.8
follicular (M9697/3) 202.0

◀ **New**   ◀▥ **Revised**

Sarcoma (*Continued*)
giant cell (M8802/3) - *see also* Neoplasm, connective tissue, malignant
  bone (M9250/3) - *see* Neoplasm, bone, malignant
glomoid (M8710/3) - *see* Neoplasm, connective tissue, malignant
granulocytic (M9930/3) 205.3
hemangioendothelial (M9130/3) - *see* Neoplasm, connective tissue, malignant
hemorrhagic, multiple (M9140/3) - *see* Kaposi's, sarcoma
Hodgkin's (M9662/3) 201.2
immunoblastic (M9612/3) 200.8
interdigitating dendritic cell 202.9
Kaposi's (M9140/3) - *see* Kaposi's, sarcoma
Kupffer cell (M9124/3) 155.0
Langerhans cell 202.9
leptomeningeal (M9530/3) - *see* Neoplasm, meninges, malignant
lymphangioendothelial (M9170/3) - *see* Neoplasm, connective tissue, malignant
lymphoblastic (M9630/3) 200.1
lymphocytic (M9620/3) 200.1
mast cell (M9740/3) 202.6
melanotic (M8720/3) - *see* Melanoma
meningeal (M9530/3) - *see* Neoplasm, meninges, malignant
meningothelial (M9530/3) - *see* Neoplasm, meninges, malignant
mesenchymal (M8800/3) - *see also* Neoplasm, connective tissue, malignant
  mixed (M8990/3) - *see* Neoplasm, connective tissue, malignant
mesothelial (M9050/3) - *see* Neoplasm, by site, malignant
monstrocellular (M9481/3)
  specified site - *see* Neoplasm, by site, malignant
  unspecified site 191.9
myeloid (M9930/3) 205.3
neurogenic (M9540/3) - *see* Neoplasm, connective tissue, malignant
odontogenic (M9270/3) 170.1
  upper jaw (bone) 170.0
osteoblastic (M9180/3) - *see* Neoplasm, bone, malignant
osteogenic (M9180/3) - *see also* Neoplasm, bone, malignant
  juxtacortical (M9190/3) - *see* Neoplasm, bone, malignant
  periosteal (M9190/3) - *see* Neoplasm, bone, malignant
periosteal (M8812/3) - *see also* Neoplasm, bone, malignant
  osteogenic (M9190/3) - *see* Neoplasm, bone, malignant
plasma cell (M9731/3) 203.8
pleomorphic cell (M8802/3) - *see* Neoplasm, connective tissue, malignant
reticuloendothelial (M9720/3) 202.3
reticulum cell (M9640/3) 200.0
  nodular (M9642/3) 200.0
    pleomorphic cell type (M9641/3) 200.0
round cell (M8803/3) - *see* Neoplasm, connective tissue, malignant
small cell (M8803/3) - *see* Neoplasm, connective tissue, malignant

Sarcoma (*Continued*)
spindle cell (M8801/3) - *see* Neoplasm, connective tissue, malignant
stromal (endometrial) (M8930/3) 182.0
  isthmus 182.1
synovial (M9040/3) - *see also* Neoplasm, connective tissue, malignant
  biphasic type (M9043/3) - *see* Neoplasm, connective tissue, malignant
  epithelioid cell type (M9042/3) - *see* Neoplasm, connective tissue, malignant
  spindle cell type (M9041/3) - *see* Neoplasm, connective tissue, malignant
Sarcomatosis
meningeal (M9539/3) - *see* Neoplasm, meninges, malignant
specified site NEC (M8800/3) - *see* Neoplasm, connective tissue, malignant
unspecified site (M8800/6) 171.9
Sarcosinemia 270.8
Sarcosporidiosis 136.5
Satiety, early 780.94
Saturnine - *see* condition
Saturnism 984.9
specified type of lead - *see* Table of Drugs and Chemicals
Satyriasis 302.89
Sauriasis - *see* Ichthyosis
Sauriderma 757.39
Sauriosis - *see* Ichthyosis
Savill's disease (epidemic exfoliative dermatitis) 695.89
SBE (subacute bacterial endocarditis) 421.0
Scabies (any site) 133.0
Scabs 782.8
Scaglietti-Dagnini syndrome (acromegalic macrospondylitis) 253.0
Scald, scalded - *see also* Burn, by site
skin syndrome 695.1
Scalenus anticus (anterior) syndrome 353.0
Scales 782.8
Scalp - *see* condition
Scaphocephaly 756.0
Scaphoiditis, tarsal 732.5
Scapulalgia 733.90
Scapulohumeral myopathy 359.1
Scar, scarring (*see also* Cicatrix) 709.2
adherent 709.2
atrophic 709.2
cervix
  in pregnancy or childbirth 654.6
    affecting fetus or newborn 763.89
    causing obstructed labor 660.2
      affecting fetus or newborn 763.1
cheloid 701.4
chorioretinal 363.30
  disseminated 363.35
  macular 363.32
  peripheral 363.34
  posterior pole NEC 363.33
choroid (*see also* Scar, chorioretinal) 363.30
compression, pericardial 423.9
congenital 757.39
conjunctiva 372.64
cornea 371.00
  xerophthalmic 264.6

Scar, scarring (*Continued*)
due to previous cesarean delivery, complicating pregnancy or childbirth 654.2
  affecting fetus or newborn 763.89
duodenal (bulb) (cap) 537.3
hypertrophic 701.4
keloid 701.4
labia 624.4
lung (base) 518.89
macula 363.32
  disseminated 363.35
  peripheral 363.34
muscle 728.89
myocardium, myocardial 412
painful 709.2
papillary muscle 429.81
posterior pole NEC 363.33
  macular - *see* Scar, macula
postnecrotic (hepatic) (liver) 571.9
psychic V15.49
retina (*see also* Scar, chorioretinal) 363.30
trachea 478.9
uterus 621.8
  in pregnancy or childbirth NEC 654.9
    affecting fetus or newborn 763.89
    from previous cesarean delivery 654.2
vulva 624.4
Scarabiasis 134.1
Scarlatina 034.1
anginosa 034.1
maligna 034.1
myocarditis, acute 034.1 [422.0]
old (*see also* Myocarditis) 429.0
otitis media 034.1 [382.02]
ulcerosa 034.1
Scarlatinella 057.8
Scarlet fever (albuminuria) (angina) (convulsions) (lesions of lid) (rash) 034.1
Schamberg's disease, dermatitis, or dermatosis (progressive pigmentary dermatosis) 709.09
Schatzki's ring (esophagus) (lower) (congenital) 750.3
acquired 530.3
Schaufenster krankheit 413.9
Schaumann's
benign lymphogranulomatosis 135
disease (sarcoidosis) 135
syndrome (sarcoidosis) 135
Scheie's syndrome (mucopolysaccharidosis IS) 277.5
Schenck's disease (sporotrichosis) 117.1
Scheuermann's disease or osteochondrosis 732.0
Scheuthauer-Marie-Sainton syndrome (cleidocranialis dysostosis) 755.59
Schilder (-Flatau) **disease** 341.1
Schilling-type monocytic leukemia (M9890/3) 206.9
Schimmelbusch's disease, cystic mastitis, or hyperplasia 610.1
Schirmer's syndrome (encephalocutaneous angiomatosis) 759.6
Schistocelia 756.79
Schistoglossia 750.13
Schistosoma infestation - *see* Infestation, Schistosoma

ICD-9-CM

S

Vol.

Schistosomiasis 120.9
Asiatic 120.2
bladder 120.0
chestermani 120.8
colon 120.1
cutaneous 120.3
due to
S. hematobium 120.0
S. japonicum 120.2
S. mansoni 120.1
S. mattheii 120.8
eastern 120.2
genitourinary tract 120.0
intestinal 120.1
lung 120.2
Manson's (intestinal) 120.1
Oriental 120.2
pulmonary 120.2
specified type NEC 120.8
vesical 120.0
Schizencephaly 742.4
Schizo-affective psychosis (*see also* Schizophrenia) 295.7
Schizodontia 520.2
Schizoid personality 301.20
introverted 301.21
schizotypal 301.22
Schizophrenia, schizophrenic (reaction) 295.9

> Note   Use the following fifth-digit subclassification with category 295:
>
> 0   unspecified
> 1   subchronic
> 2   chronic
> 3   subchronic with acute exacerbation
> 4   chronic with acute exacerbation
> 5   in remission

acute (attack) NEC 295.8
episode 295.4
atypical form 295.8
borderline 295.5
catalepsy 295.2
catatonic (type) (acute) (excited) (withdrawn) 295.2
childhood (type) (*see also* Psychosis, childhood) 299.9
chronic NEC 295.6
coenesthesiopathic 295.8
cyclic (type) 295.7
disorganized (type) 295.1
flexibilitas cerea 295.2
hebephrenic (type) (acute) 295.1
incipient 295.5
latent 295.5
paranoid (type) (acute) 295.3
paraphrenic (acute) 295.3
prepsychotic 295.5
primary (acute) 295.0
prodromal 295.5
pseudoneurotic 295.5
pseudopsychopathic 295.5
reaction 295.9
residual type (state) 295.6 ◀━
restzustand 295.6
schizo-affective (type) (depressed) (excited) 295.7
schizophreniform type 295.4
simple (type) (acute) 295.0
simplex (acute) 295.0
specified type NEC 295.8

Schizophrenia, schizophrenic (*Continued*)
syndrome of childhood NEC (*see also* Psychosis, childhood) 299.9
undifferentiated type 295.9 ◀━
acute 295.8
chronic 295.6
Schizothymia 301.20
introverted 301.21
schizotypal 301.22
Schlafkrankheit 086.5
Schlatter's tibia (osteochondrosis) 732.4
Schlatter-Osgood disease (osteochondrosis, tibial tubercle) 732.4
Schloffer's tumor (*see also* Peritonitis) 567.2
Schmidt's syndrome
sphallo-pharyngo-laryngeal hemiplegia 352.6
thyroid-adrenocortical insufficiency 258.1
vagoaccessory 352.6
Schmincke
carcinoma (M8082/3) - *see* Neoplasm, nasopharynx, malignant
tumor (M8082/3) - *see* Neoplasm, nasopharynx, malignant
Schmitz (-Stutzer) dysentery 004.0
Schmorl's disease or nodes 722.30
lumbar, lumbosacral 722.32
specified region NEC 722.39
thoracic, thoracolumbar 722.31
Schneider's syndrome 047.9
Schneiderian
carcinoma (M8121/3)
specified site - *see* Neoplasm, by site, malignant
unspecified site 160.0
papilloma (M8121/0)
specified site - *see* Neoplasm, by site, benign
unspecified site 212.0
Schnitzler syndrome 273.1 ◀
Schoffer's tumor (*see also* Peritonitis) 567.2
Scholte's syndrome (malignant carcinoid) 259.2
Scholz's disease 330.0
Scholz (-Bielschowsky-Henneberg) syndrome 330.0
Schönlein (-Henoch) disease (primary) (purpura) (rheumatic) 287.0
School examination V70.3
Schottmüller's disease (*see also* Fever, paratyphoid) 002.9
Schroeder's syndrome (endocrine-hypertensive) 255.3
Schüller-Christian disease or syndrome (chronic histiocytosis X) 277.89
Schultz's disease or syndrome (agranulocytosis) 288.0
Schultze's acroparesthesia, simple 443.89
Schwalbe-Ziehen-Oppenheimer disease 333.6
Schwannoma (M9560/0) - *see also* Neoplasm, connective tissue, benign
malignant (M9560/3) - *see* Neoplasm, connective tissue, malignant
Schwartz (-Jampel) syndrome 756.89
Schwartz-Bartter syndrome (inappropriate secretion of antidiuretic hormone) 253.6
Schweninger-Buzzi disease (macular atrophy) 701.3
Sciatic - *see* condition

Sciatica (infectional) 724.3
due to
displacement of intervertebral disc 722.10
herniation, nucleus pulposus 722.10
Scimitar syndrome (anomalous venous drainage, right lung to inferior vena cava) 747.49
Sclera - *see* condition
Sclerectasia 379.11
Scleredema
adultorum 710.1
Buschke's 710.1
newborn 778.1
Sclerema
adiposum (newborn) 778.1
adultorum 710.1
edematosum (newborn) 778.1
neonatorum 778.1
newborn 778.1
Scleriasis - *see* Scleroderma
Scleritis 379.00
with corneal involvement 379.05
anterior (annular) (localized) 379.03
brawny 379.06
granulomatous 379.09
posterior 379.07
specified NEC 379.09
suppurative 379.09
syphilitic 095.0
tuberculous (nodular) (*see also* Tuberculosis) 017.3 [379.09]
Sclerochoroiditis (*see also* Scleritis) 379.00
Scleroconjunctivitis (*see also* Scleritis) 379.00
Sclerocystic ovary (syndrome) 256.4
Sclerodactylia 701.0
Scleroderma, sclerodermia (acrosclerotic) (diffuse) (generalized) (progressive) (pulmonary) 710.1
circumscribed 701.0
linear 701.0
localized (linear) 701.0
newborn 778.1
Sclerokeratitis 379.05
meaning sclerosing keratitis 370.54
tuberculous (*see also* Tuberculosis) 017.3 [379.09]
Scleroma, trachea 040.1
Scleromalacia
multiple 731.0
perforans 379.04
Scleromyxedema 701.8
Scleroperikeratitis 379.05
Sclerose en plaques 340
Sclerosis, sclerotic
adrenal (gland) 255.8
Alzheimer's 331.0
with dementia - *see* Alzheimer's, dementia
amyotrophic (lateral) 335.20
annularis fibrosi
aortic 424.1
mitral 424.0
aorta, aortic 440.0
valve (*see also* Endocarditis, aortic) 424.1
artery, arterial, arteriolar, arteriovascular - *see* Arteriosclerosis
ascending multiple 340
Baló's (concentric) 341.1
basilar - *see* Sclerosis, brain

Sclerosis, sclerotic *(Continued)*
  bone (localized) NEC 733.99
  brain (general) (lobular) 341.9
    Alzheimer's - *see* Alzheimer's, dementia
    artery, arterial 437.0
    atrophic lobar 331.0
      with dementia
        with behavioral disturbance
          331.0 *[294.11]*
        without behavioral disturbance
          331.0 *[294.10]*
    diffuse 341.1
      familial (chronic) (infantile) 330.0
      infantile (chronic) (familial) 330.0
      Pelizaeus-Merzbacher type 330.0
    disseminated 340
    hereditary 334.2
    infantile (degenerative) (diffuse) 330.0
    insular 340
    Krabbe's 330.0
    miliary 340
    multiple 340
    Pelizaeus-Merzbacher 330.0
    progressive familial 330.0
    senile 437.0
    tuberous 759.5
  bulbar, progressive 340
  bundle of His 426.50
    left 426.3
    right 426.4
  cardiac - *see* Arteriosclerosis, coronary
  cardiorenal (*see also* Hypertension, cardiorenal) 404.90
  cardiovascular (*see also* Disease, cardiovascular) 429.2
    renal (*see also* Hypertension, cardiorenal) 404.90
  centrolobar, familial 330.0
  cerebellar - *see* Sclerosis, brain
  cerebral - *see* Sclerosis, brain
  cerebrospinal 340
    disseminated 340
    multiple 340
  cerebrovascular 437.0
  choroid 363.40
    diffuse 363.56
  combined (spinal cord) - *see also* Degeneration, combined
    multiple 340
  concentric, Baló's 341.1
  cornea 370.54
  coronary (artery) - *see* Arteriosclerosis, coronary
  corpus cavernosum
    female 624.8
    male 607.89
  Dewitzky's
    aortic 424.1
    mitral 424.0
  diffuse NEC 341.1
  disease, heart - *see* Arteriosclerosis, coronary
  disseminated 340
  dorsal 340
  dorsolateral (spinal cord) - *see* Degeneration, combined
  endometrium 621.8
  extrapyramidal 333.90
  eye, nuclear (senile) 366.16
  Friedreich's (spinal cord) 334.0
  funicular (spermatic cord) 608.89
  gastritis 535.4
  general (vascular) - *see* Arteriosclerosis

Sclerosis, sclerotic *(Continued)*
  gland (lymphatic) 457.8
  hepatic 571.9
  hereditary
    cerebellar 334.2
    spinal 334.0
  idiopathic cortical (Garré's) (*see also* Osteomyelitis) 730.1
  ilium, piriform 733.5
  insular 340
    pancreas 251.8
  Islands of Langerhans 251.8
  kidney - *see* Sclerosis, renal
  larynx 478.79
  lateral 335.24
    amyotrophic 335.20
    descending 335.24
    primary 335.24
    spinal 335.24
  liver 571.9
  lobar, atrophic (of brain) 331.0
    with dementia
      with behavioral disturbance
        331.0 *[294.11]*
      without behavioral disturbance
        331.0 *[294.10]*
  lung (*see also* Fibrosis, lung) 515
  mastoid 383.1
  mitral - *see* Endocarditis, mitral
  Mönckeberg's (medial) (*see also* Arteriosclerosis, extremities) 440.20
  multiple (brain stem) (cerebral) (generalized) (spinal cord) 340
  myocardium, myocardial - *see* Arteriosclerosis, coronary
  nuclear (senile), eye 366.16
  ovary 620.8
  pancreas 577.8
  penis 607.89
  peripheral arteries (*see also* Arteriosclerosis, extremities) 440.20
  plaques 340
  pluriglandular 258.8
  polyglandular 258.8
  posterior (spinal cord) (syphilitic) 094.0
  posterolateral (spinal cord) - *see* Degeneration, combined
  prepuce 607.89
  primary lateral 335.24
  progressive systemic 710.1
  pulmonary (*see also* Fibrosis, lung) 515
    artery 416.0
    valve (heart) (*see also* Endocarditis, pulmonary) 424.3
  renal 587
    with
      cystine storage disease 270.0
      hypertension (*see also* Hypertension, kidney) 403.90
      hypertensive heart disease (conditions classifiable to 402) (*see also* Hypertension, cardiorenal) 404.90
      arteriolar (hyaline) (*see also* Hypertension, kidney) 403.90
      hyperplastic (*see also* Hypertension, kidney) 403.90
  retina (senile) (vascular) 362.17
  rheumatic
    aortic valve 395.9
    mitral valve 394.9
  Schilder's 341.1
  senile - *see* Arteriosclerosis

Sclerosis, sclerotic *(Continued)*
  spinal (cord) (general) (progressive) (transverse) 336.8
    ascending 357.0
    combined - *see also* Degeneration, combined
      multiple 340
      syphilitic 094.89
    disseminated 340
    dorsolateral - *see* Degeneration, combined
    hereditary (Friedreich's) (mixed form) 334.0
    lateral (amyotrophic) 335.24
    multiple 340
    posterior (syphilitic) 094.0
  stomach 537.89
  subendocardial, congenital 425.3
  systemic (progressive) 710.1
    with lung involvement 710.1 *[517.2]*
  tricuspid (heart) (valve) - *see* Endocarditis, tricuspid
  tuberous (brain) 759.5
  tympanic membrane (*see also* Tympanosclerosis) 385.00
  valve, valvular (heart) - *see* Endocarditis
  vascular - *see* Arteriosclerosis
  vein 459.89
Sclerotenonitis 379.07
Sclerotitis (*see also* Scleritis) 379.00
  syphilitic 095.0
  tuberculous (*see also* Tuberculosis) 017.3 *[379.09]*
Scoliosis (acquired) (postural) 737.30
  congenital 754.2
  due to or associated with
    Charcôt-Marie-Tooth disease 356.1 *[737.43]*
    mucopolysaccharidosis 277.5 *[737.43]*
    neurofibromatosis 237.71 *[737.43]*
    osteitis
      deformans 731.0 *[737.43]*
      fibrosa cystica 252.01 *[737.43]* ◀═
    osteoporosis (*see also* Osteoporosis) 733.00 *[737.43]*
    poliomyelitis 138 *[737.43]*
    radiation 737.33
    tuberculosis (*see also* Tuberculosis) 015.0 *[737.43]*
  idiopathic 737.30
    infantile
      progressive 737.32
      resolving 737.31
  paralytic 737.39
  rachitic 268.1
  sciatic 724.3
  specified NEC 737.39
  thoracogenic 737.34
  tuberculous (*see also* Tuberculosis) 015.0 *[737.43]*
Scoliotic pelvis 738.6
  with disproportion (fetopelvic) 653.0
    affecting fetus or newborn 763.1
    causing obstructed labor 660.1
      affecting fetus or newborn 763.1
Scorbutus, scorbutic 267
  anemia 281.8
Scotoma (ring) 368.44
  arcuate 368.43
  Bjerrum 368.43
  blind spot area 368.42
  central 368.41
  centrocecal 368.41
  paracecal 368.42

ICD-9-CM

s

Vol. 2

Scotoma *(Continued)*
   paracentral 368.41
   scintillating 368.12
   Seidel 368.43
Scratch - *see* Injury, superficial, by site
Screening (for) V82.9
   alcoholism V79.1
   anemia, deficiency NEC V78.1
      iron V78.0
   anomaly, congenital V82.89
   antenatal V28.9
      alphafetoprotein levels
         V28.1
      based on amniocentesis V28.2
         chromosomal anomalies V28.0
         raised alphafetoprotein levels V28.1
      fetal growth retardation using ultra-
         sonics V28.4
      isoimmunization V28.5
      malformations using ultrasonics V28.3
      raised alphafetoprotein levels V28.1
      specified condition NEC V28.8
      Streptococcus B V28.6
   arterial hypertension V81.1
   arthropod-borne viral disease NEC V73.5
   asymptomatic bacteriuria V81.5
   bacterial
      conjunctivitis V74.4
      disease V74.9
         specified condition NEC V74.8
   bacteriuria, asymptomatic V81.5
   blood disorder NEC V78.9
      specified type NEC V78.8
   bronchitis, chronic V81.3
   brucellosis V74.8
   cancer - *see* Screening, malignant neo-
      plasm
   cardiovascular disease NEC V81.2
   cataract V80.2
   Chagas' disease V75.3
   chemical poisoning V82.5
   cholera V74.0
   cholesterol level V77.91
   chromosomal
      anomalies
         by amniocentesis, antenatal V28.0
         maternal postnatal V82.4
      athletes V70.3
   condition
      cardiovascular NEC V81.2
      eye NEC V80.2
      genitourinary NEC V81.6
      neurological V80.0
      respiratory NEC V81.4
      skin V82.0
      specified NEC V82.89
   congenital
      anomaly V82.89
         eye V80.2
      dislocation of hip V82.3
      eye condition or disease V80.2
   conjunctivitis, bacterial V74.4
   contamination NEC (*see also* Poisoning)
      V82.5
   coronary artery disease V81.0
   cystic fibrosis V77.6
   deficiency anemia NEC V78.1
      iron V78.0
   dengue fever V73.5
   depression V79.0
   developmental handicap V79.9
      in early childhood V79.3
      specified type NEC V79.8
   diabetes mellitus V77.1

Screening (for) *(Continued)*
   diphtheria V74.3
   disease or disorder V82.9
      bacterial V74.9
         specified NEC V74.8
      blood V78.9
         specified type NEC V78.8
      blood-forming organ V78.9
         specified type NEC V78.8
      cardiovascular NEC V81.2
         hypertensive V81.1
         ischemic V81.0
      Chagas' V75.3
      chlamydial V73.98
         specified NEC V73.88
      ear NEC V80.3
      endocrine NEC V77.99
      eye NEC V80.2
      genitourinary NEC V81.6
      heart NEC V81.2
         hypertensive V81.1
         ischemic V81.0
      immunity NEC V77.99
      infectious NEC V75.9
      lipoid NEC V77.91
      mental V79.9
         specified type NEC V79.8
      metabolic NEC V77.99
         inborn NEC V77.7
      neurological V80.0
      nutritional NEC V77.99
      rheumatic NEC V82.2
      rickettsial V75.0
      sickle-cell V78.2
         trait V78.2
      specified type NEC V82.89
      thyroid V77.0
      vascular NEC V81.2
         ischemic V81.0
      venereal V74.5
      viral V73.99
         arthropod-borne NEC V73.5
         specified type NEC V73.89
   dislocation of hip, congenital V82.3
   drugs in athletes V70.3
   emphysema (chronic) V81.3
   encephalitis, viral (mosquito- or tick-
      borne) V73.5
   endocrine disorder NEC V77.99
   eye disorder NEC V80.2
      congenital V80.2
   fever
      dengue V73.5
      hemorrhagic V73.5
      yellow V73.4
   filariasis V75.6
   galactosemia V77.4
   genitourinary condition NEC V81.6
   glaucoma V80.1
   gonorrhea V74.5
   gout V77.5
   Hansen's disease V74.2
   heart disease NEC V81.2
      hypertensive V81.1
      ischemic V81.0
   heavy metal poisoning V82.5
   helminthiasis, intestinal V75.7
   hematopoietic malignancy V76.89
   hemoglobinopathies NEC V78.3
   hemorrhagic fever V73.5
   Hodgkin's disease V76.89
   hormones in athletes V70.3
   hypercholesterolemia V77.91
   hyperlipidemia V77.91

Screening (for) *(Continued)*
   hypertension V81.1
   immunity disorder NEC V77.99
   inborn errors of metabolism NEC
      V77.7
   infection
      bacterial V74.9
         specified type NEC V74.8
      mycotic V75.4
      parasitic NEC V75.8
   infectious disease V75.9
      specified type NEC V75.8
   ingestion of radioactive substance V82.5
   intestinal helminthiasis V75.7
   iron deficiency anemia V78.0
   ischemic heart disease V81.0
   lead poisoning V82.5
   leishmaniasis V75.2
   leprosy V74.2
   leptospirosis V74.8
   leukemia V76.89
   lipoid disorder NEC V77.91
   lymphoma V76.89
   malaria V75.1
   malignant neoplasm (of) V76.9
      bladder V76.3
      blood V76.89
      breast V76.10
         mammogram NEC V76.12
            for high-risk patient V76.11
         specified type NEC V76.19
      cervix V76.2
      colon V76.51
      colorectal V76.51
      hematopoietic system V76.89
      intestine V76.50
         colon V76.51
         small V76.52
      lung V76.0
      lymph (glands) V76.89
      nervous system V76.81
      oral cavity V76.42
      other specified neoplasm NEC V76.89
      ovary V76.46
      prostate V76.44
      rectum V76.41
      respiratory organs V76.0
      skin V76.43
      specified sites NEC V76.49
      testis V76.45
      vagina V76.47
         following hysterectomy for
            malignant condition V67.01
   malnutrition V77.2
   mammogram NEC V76.12
      for high-risk patient V76.11
   maternal postnatal chromosomal
      anomalies V82.4
   measles V73.2
   mental
      disorder V79.9
         specified type NEC V79.8
      retardation V79.2
   metabolic disorder NEC V77.99
   metabolic errors, inborn V77.7
   mucoviscidosis V77.6
   multiphasic V82.6
   mycosis V75.4
   mycotic infection V75.4
   nephropathy V81.5
   neurological condition V80.0
   nutritional disorder NEC V77.99
   obesity V77.8
   osteoporosis V82.81

Screening (for) (*Continued*)
  parasitic infection NEC V75.8
  phenylketonuria V77.3
  plague V74.8
  poisoning
    chemical NEC V82.5
    contaminated water supply V82.5
    heavy metal V82.5
  poliomyelitis V73.0
  postnatal chromosomal anomalies maternal V82.4
  prenatal - *see* Screening, antenatal
  pulmonary tuberculosis V74.1
  radiation exposure V82.5
  renal disease V81.5
  respiratory condition NEC V81.4
  rheumatic disorder NEC V82.2
  rheumatoid arthritis V82.1
  rickettsial disease V75.0
  rubella V73.3
  schistosomiasis V75.5
  senile macular lesions of eye V80.2
  sickle-cell anemia, disease, or trait V78.2
  skin condition V82.0
  sleeping sickness V75.3
  smallpox V73.1
  special V82.9
    specified condition NEC V82.89
  specified type NEC V82.89
  spirochetal disease V74.9
    specified type NEC V74.8
  stimulants in athletes V70.3
  syphilis V74.5
  tetanus V74.8
  thyroid disorder V77.0
  trachoma V73.6
  trypanosomiasis V75.3
  tuberculosis, pulmonary V74.1
  venereal disease V74.5
  viral encephalitis
    mosquito-borne V73.5
    tick-borne V73.5
  whooping cough V74.8
  worms, intestinal V75.7
  yaws V74.6
  yellow fever V73.4
Scrofula (*see also* Tuberculosis) 017.2
Scrofulide (primary) (*see also* Tuberculosis) 017.0
Scrofuloderma, scrofulodermia (any site) (primary) (*see also* Tuberculosis) 017.0
Scrofulosis (universal) (*see also* Tuberculosis) 017.2
Scrofulosis lichen (primary) (*see also* Tuberculosis) 017.0
Scrofulous - *see* condition
Scrotal tongue 529.5
  congenital 750.13
Scrotum - *see* condition
Scurvy (gum) (infantile) (rickets) (scorbutic) 267
Sea-blue histiocyte syndrome 272.7
Seabright-Bantam syndrome (pseudohypoparathyroidism) 275.49
Seasickness 994.6
Seatworm 127.4
Sebaceous
  cyst (*see also* Cyst, sebaceous) 706.2
  gland disease NEC 706.9
Sebocystomatosis 706.2
Seborrhea, seborrheic 706.3
  adiposa 706.3
  capitis 690.11
  congestiva 695.4

Seborrhea, seborrheic (*Continued*)
  corporis 706.3
  dermatitis 690.10
    infantile 690.12
  diathesis in infants 695.89
  eczema 690.18
    infantile 690.12
  keratosis 702.19
    inflamed 702.11
  nigricans 759.89
  sicca 690.18
  wart 702.19
    inflamed 702.11
Seckel's syndrome 759.89
Seclusion pupil 364.74
Seclusiveness, child 313.22
Secondary - *see also* condition
  neoplasm - *see* Neoplasm, by site, malignant, secondary
Secretan's disease or syndrome (posttraumatic edema) 782.3
Secretion
  antidiuretic hormone, inappropriate (syndrome) 253.6
  catecholamine, by pheochromocytoma 255.6
  hormone
    antidiuretic, inappropriate (syndrome) 253.6
    by
      carcinoid tumor 259.2
      pheochromocytoma 255.6
    ectopic NEC 259.3
  urinary
    excessive 788.42
    suppression 788.5
Section
  cesarean
    affecting fetus or newborn 763.4
    post mortem, affecting fetus or newborn 761.6
    previous, in pregnancy or childbirth 654.2
      affecting fetus or newborn 763.89
  nerve, traumatic - *see* Injury, nerve, by site
Seeligmann's syndrome (ichthyosis congenita) 757.1
Segmentation, incomplete (congenital) - *see also* Fusion
  bone NEC 756.9
  lumbosacral (joint) 756.15
  vertebra 756.15
    lumbosacral 756.15
Seizure 780.39
  akinetic (idiopathic) (*see also* Epilepsy) 345.0
    psychomotor 345.4
  apoplexy, apoplectic (*see also* Disease, cerebrovascular, acute) 436
  atonic (*see also* Epilepsy) 345.0
  autonomic 300.11
  brain or cerebral (*see also* Disease, cerebrovascular, acute) 436
  convulsive (*see also* Convulsions) 780.39
  cortical (focal) (motor) (*see also* Epilepsy) 345.5
  epilepsy, epileptic (cryptogenic) (*see also* Epilepsy) 345.9
  epileptiform, epileptoid 780.39
    focal (*see also* Epilepsy) 345.5
  febrile 780.31
  heart - *see* Disease, heart
  hysterical 300.11

Seizure (*Continued*)
  Jacksonian (focal) (*see also* Epilepsy) 345.5
    motor type 345.5
    sensory type 345.5
  newborn 779.0
  paralysis (*see also* Disease, cerebrovascular, acute) 436
  recurrent 780.39
    epileptic - *see* Epilepsy
  repetitive 780.39
    epileptic - *see* Epilepsy
  salaam (*see also* Epilepsy) 345.6
  uncinate (*see also* Epilepsy) 345.4
Self-mutilation 300.9
Semicoma 780.09
Semiconsciousness 780.09
Seminal
  vesicle - *see* condition
  vesiculitis (*see also* Vesiculitis) 608.0
Seminoma (M9061/3)
  anaplastic type (M9062/3)
    specified site - *see* Neoplasm, by site, malignant
    unspecified site 186.9
  specified site - *see* Neoplasm, by site, malignant
  spermatocytic (M9063/3)
    specified site - *see* Neoplasm, by site, malignant
    unspecified site 186.9
  unspecified site 186.9
Semliki Forest encephalitis 062.8
Senear-Usher disease or syndrome (pemphigus erythematosus) 694.4
Senecio jacobae dermatitis 692.6
Senectus 797
Senescence 797
Senile (*see also* condition) 797
  cervix (atrophic) 622.8
  degenerative atrophy, skin 701.3
  endometrium (atrophic) 621.8
  fallopian tube (atrophic) 620.3
  heart (failure) 797
  lung 492.8
  ovary (atrophic) 620.3
  syndrome 259.8
  vagina, vaginitis (atrophic) 627.3
  wart 702.0
Senility 797
  with
    acute confusional state 290.3
    delirium 290.3
    mental changes 290.9
    psychosis NEC (*see also* Psychosis, senile) 290.20
  premature (syndrome) 259.8
Sensation
  burning (*see also* Disturbance, sensation) 782.0
    tongue 529.6
  choking 784.9
  loss of (*see also* Disturbance, sensation) 782.0
  prickling (*see also* Disturbance, sensation) 782.0
  tingling (*see also* Disturbance, sensation) 782.0
Sense loss (touch) (*see also* Disturbance, sensation) 782.0
  smell 781.1
  taste 781.1
Sensibility disturbance NEC (cortical) (deep) (vibratory) (*see also* Disturbance, sensation) 782.0

ICD-9-CM

S

Vol. 2

Sensitive dentine 521.8
Sensitiver Beziehungswahn 297.8
Sensitivity, sensitization - *see also* Allergy
  autoerythrocyte 287.2
  carotid sinus 337.0
  child (excessive) 313.21
  cold, autoimmune 283.0
  methemoglobin 289.7
  suxamethonium 289.89
  tuberculin, without clinical or radio-
    logical symptoms 795.5
Sensory
  extinction 781.8
  neglect 781.8
Separation
  acromioclavicular - *see* Dislocation,
    acromioclavicular
  anxiety, abnormal 309.21
  apophysis, traumatic - *see* Fracture, by
    site
  choroid 363.70
    hemorrhagic 363.72
    serous 363.71
  costochondral (simple) (traumatic) - *see*
    Dislocation, costochondral
  delayed
    umbilical cord 779.83
  epiphysis, epiphyseal
    nontraumatic 732.9
      upper femoral 732.2
    traumatic - *see* Fracture, by site
  fracture - *see* Fracture, by site
  infundibulum cardiac from right ven-
    tricle by a partition 746.83
  joint (current) (traumatic) - *see* Disloca-
    tion, by site
  placenta (normally implanted) - *see*
    Placenta, separation
  pubic bone, obstetrical trauma 665.6
  retina, retinal (*see also* Detachment, ret-
    ina) 361.9
    layers 362.40
      sensory (*see also* Retinoschisis) 361.10
      pigment epithelium (exudative) 362.42
        hemorrhagic 362.43
  sternoclavicular (traumatic) - *see* Dislo-
    cation, sternoclavicular
  symphysis pubis, obstetrical trauma
    665.6
  tracheal ring, incomplete (congenital)
    748.3
Sepsis (generalized) 995.91 ◄▥
  with
    abortion - *see* Abortion, by type,
      with sepsis
    ectopic pregnancy (*see also* categories
      633.0-633.9) 639.0
    molar pregnancy (*see also* categories
      630-632) 639.0
  buccal 528.3
  complicating labor 659.3
  dental (pulpal origin) 522.4
  female genital organ NEC 614.9
  fetus (intrauterine) 771.81
  following
    abortion 639.0
    ectopic or molar pregnancy 639.0
    infusion, perfusion, or transfusion
      999.3
  Friedländer's 038.49
  intraocular 360.00
  localized
    in operation wound 998.59
    skin (*see also* Abscess) 682.9
  malleus 024

Sepsis (*Continued*)
  nadir 038.9
  newborn (organism unspecified) NEC
    771.81
  oral 528.3
  puerperal, postpartum, childbirth (pel-
    vic) 670
  resulting from infusion, injection,
    transfusion, or vaccination 999.3
  severe 995.92
  skin, localized (*see also* Abscess) 682.9
  umbilical (newborn) (organism unspec-
    ified) 771.89
    tetanus 771.3
  urinary 599.0
    meaning sepsis 995.91 ◄▥
    meaning urinary tract infection
      599.0
Septate - *see also* Septum
Septic - *see also* condition
  adenoids 474.01
    and tonsils 474.02
  arm (with lymphangitis) 682.3
  embolus - *see* Embolism
  finger (with lymphangitis) 681.00
  foot (with lymphangitis) 682.7
  gallbladder (*see also* Cholecystitis) 575.8
  hand (with lymphangitis) 682.4
  joint (*see also* Arthritis, septic) 711.0
  kidney (*see also* Infection, kidney) 590.9
  leg (with lymphangitis) 682.6
  mouth 528.3
  nail 681.9
    finger 681.02
    toe 681.11
  shock (endotoxic) 785.52
  sore (*see also* Abscess) 682.9
    throat 034.0
      milk-borne 034.0
      streptococcal 034.0
  spleen (acute) 289.59
  teeth (pulpal origin) 522.4
  throat 034.0
  thrombus - *see* Thrombosis
  toe (with lymphangitis) 681.10
  tonsils 474.00
    and adenoids 474.02
  umbilical cord (newborn) (organism
    unspecified) 771.89
  uterus (*see also* Endometritis) 615.9
Septicemia, septicemic (generalized)
  (suppurative) 038.9
  with
    abortion - *see* Abortion, by type,
      with sepsis
    ectopic pregnancy (*see also* categories
      633.0-633.9) 639.0
    molar pregnancy (*see also* categories
      630-632) 639.0
  Aerobacter aerogenes 038.49
  anaerobic 038.3
  anthrax 022.3
  Bacillus coli 038.42
  Bacteroides 038.3
  Clostridium 038.3
  complicating labor 659.3
  cryptogenic 038.9
  enteric gram-negative bacilli 038.40
  Enterobacter aerogenes 038.49
  Erysipelothrix (insidiosa) (rhusiopa-
    thiae) 027.1
  Escherichia coli 038.42
  following
    abortion 639.0
    ectopic or molar pregnancy 639.0

Septicemia, septicemic (*Continued*)
  infusion, injection, transfusion, or
    vaccination 999.3
  Friedländer's (bacillus) 038.49
  gangrenous 038.9
  gonococcal 098.89
  gram-negative (organism) 038.40
    anaerobic 038.3
  Hemophilus influenzae 038.41
  herpes (simplex) 054.5
  herpetic 054.5
  Listeria monocytogenes 027.0
  meningeal - *see* Meningitis
  meningococcal (chronic) (fulminating)
    036.2
  navel, newborn (organism unspecified)
    771.89
  newborn (organism unspecified) 771.81
  plague 020.2
  pneumococcal 038.2
  postabortal 639.0
  postoperative 998.59
  Proteus vulgaris 038.49
  Pseudomonas (aeruginosa) 038.43
  puerperal, postpartum 670
  Salmonella (aertrycke) (choleraesuis)
    (enteritidis) (callinarum) (suipesti-
    fer) 003.1
  Serratia 038.44
  Shigella (*see also* Dysentery, bacillary)
    004.9
  specified organism NEC 038.8
  staphylococcal 038.10
    aureus 038.11
    specified organism NEC 038.19
  streptococcal (anaerobic) 038.0
  streptococcus pneumoniae 038.2
  suipestifer 003.1
  umbilicus, newborn (organism unspec-
    ified) 771.89
  viral 079.99
  Yersinia enterocolitica 038.49
Septum, septate (congenital) - *see also*
  Anomaly, specified type NEC
  anal 751.2
  aqueduct of Sylvius 742.3
    with spina bifida (*see also* Spina bi-
      fida) 741.0
  hymen 752.49
  uterus (*see also* Double, uterus) 752.2
  vagina 752.49
    in pregnancy or childbirth 654.7
      affecting fetus or newborn 763.89
      causing obstructed labor 660.2
        affecting fetus or newborn 763.1
Sequestration
  lung (congenital) (extralobar) (intralo-
    bar) 748.5
  orbit 376.10
  pulmonary artery (congenital) 747.3
  splenic 289.52
Sequestrum
  bone (*see also* Osteomyelitis) 730.1
    jaw 526.4
  dental 525.8
  jaw bone 526.4
  sinus (accessory) (nasal) (*see also* Sinus-
    itis) 473.9
    maxillary 473.0
Sequoiosis asthma 495.8
Serology for syphilis
  doubtful
    with signs or symptoms - *see* Syphi-
      lis, by site and stage
    follow-up of latent syphilis - *see*
      Syphilis, latent

◄ **New**   ◄▥ **Revised**

Serology for syphilis (*Continued*)
false positive 795.6
negative, with signs or symptoms - *see*
Syphilis, by site and stage
positive 097.1
with signs or symptoms - *see* Syphilis, by site and stage
false 795.6
follow-up of latent syphilis - *see*
Syphilis, latent
only finding - *see* Syphilis, latent
reactivated 097.1
Seroma - (postoperative) (non-infected)
998.13
infected 998.51
Seropurulent - *see* condition
Serositis, multiple 569.89
pericardial 423.2
peritoneal 568.82
pleural - *see* Pleurisy
Serotonin syndrome 333.99
Serous - *see* condition
Sertoli cell
adenoma (M8640/0)
specified site - *see* Neoplasm, by site, benign
unspecified site
female 220
male 222.0
carcinoma (M8640/3)
specified site - *see* Neoplasm, by site, malignant
unspecified site 186.9
syndrome (germinal aplasia) 606.0
tumor (M8640/0)
with lipid storage (M8641/0)
specified site - *see* Neoplasm, by site, benign
unspecified site
female 220
male 222.0
specified site - *see* Neoplasm, by site, benign
unspecified site
female 220
male 222.0
Sertoli-Leydig cell tumor (M8631/0)
specified site - *see* Neoplasm, by site, benign
unspecified site
female 220
male 222.0
Serum
allergy, allergic reaction 999.5
shock 999.4
arthritis 999.5 [713.6]
complication or reaction NEC 999.5
disease NEC 999.5
hepatitis 070.3
intoxication 999.5
jaundice (homologous) - *see* Hepatitis, viral, type B
neuritis 999.5
poisoning NEC 999.5
rash NEC 999.5
reaction NEC 999.5
sickness NEC 999.5
Sesamoiditis 733.99
Seven-day fever 061
of
Japan 100.89
Queensland 100.89
Sever's disease or osteochondrosis (calcaneum) 732.5

Sex chromosome mosaics 758.81
Sextuplet
affected by maternal complication of pregnancy 761.5
healthy liveborn - *see* Newborn, multiple
pregnancy (complicating delivery) NEC 651.8
with fetal loss and retention of one or more fetus(es) 651.6
Sexual
anesthesia 302.72
deviation (*see also* Deviation, sexual) 302.9
disorder (*see also* Deviation, sexual) 302.9
frigidity (female) 302.72
function, disorder of (psychogenic) 302.70
specified type NEC 302.79
immaturity (female) (male) 259.0
impotence (psychogenic) 302.72
organic origin NEC 607.84
precocity (constitutional) (cryptogenic) (female) (idiopathic) (male) NEC 259.1
with adrenal hyperplasia 255.2
sadism 302.84
Sexuality, pathological (*see also* Deviation, sexual) 302.9
Sézary's disease, reticulosis, or syndrome (M9701/3) 202.2
Shadow, lung 793.1
Shaken infant syndrome 995.55
Shaking
head (tremor) 781.0
palsy or paralysis (*see also* Parkinsonism) 332.0
Shallowness, acetabulum 736.39
Shaver's disease or syndrome (bauxite pneumoconiosis) 503
Shearing
artificial skin graft 996.55
decellularized allodermis graft 996.55
Sheath (tendon) - *see* condition
Shedding
nail 703.8
teeth, premature, primary (deciduous) 520.6
Sheehan's disease or syndrome (postpartum pituitary necrosis) 253.2
Shelf, rectal 569.49
Shell
shock (current) (*see also* Reaction, stress, acute) 308.9
lasting state 300.16
teeth 520.5
Shield kidney 753.3
Shift, mediastinal 793.2
Shifting
pacemaker 427.89
sleep-work schedule (affecting sleep) 307.45
Shiga's
bacillus 004.0
dysentery 004.0
Shigella (dysentery) (*see also* Dysentery, bacillary) 004.9
carrier (suspected) of V02.3
Shigellosis (*see also* Dysentery, bacillary) 004.9
Shingles (*see also* Herpes, zoster) 053.9
eye NEC 053.29
Shin splints 844.9
Shipyard eye or disease 077.1

Shirodkar suture, in pregnancy 654.5
Shock 785.50
with
abortion - *see* Abortion, by type, with shock
ectopic pregnancy (*see also* categories 633.0-633.9) 639.5
molar pregnancy (*see also* categories 630-632) 639.5
allergic - *see* Shock, anaphylactic
anaclitic 309.21
anaphylactic 995.0
chemical - *see* Table of Drugs and Chemicals
correct medicinal substance properly administered 995.0
drug or medicinal substance
correct substance properly administered 995.0
overdose or wrong substance given or taken 977.9
specified drug - *see* Table of Drugs and Chemicals
following sting(s) 989.5
food - *see* Anaphylactic shock, due to, food
immunization 999.4
serum 999.4
anaphylactoid - *see* Shock, anaphylactic
anesthetic
correct substance properly administered 995.4
overdose or wrong substance given 968.4
specified anesthetic - *see* Table of Drugs and Chemicals
birth, fetus or newborn NEC 779.89
cardiogenic 785.51
chemical substance - *see* Table of Drugs and Chemicals
circulatory 785.59
complicating
abortion - *see* Abortion, by type, with shock
ectopic pregnancy - *see also* categories 633.0-633.9) 639.5
labor and delivery 669.1
molar pregnancy (*see also* categories 630-632) 639.5
culture 309.29
due to
drug 995.0
correct substance properly administered 995.0
overdose or wrong substance given or taken 977.9
specified drug - *see* Table of Drugs and Chemicals
food - *see* Anaphylactic shock, due to, food
during labor and delivery 669.1
electric 994.8
endotoxic 785.52
due to surgical procedure 998.0
following
abortion 639.5
ectopic or molar pregnancy 639.5
injury (immediate) (delayed) 958.4
labor and delivery 669.1
gram-negative 785.52
hematogenic 785.59
hemorrhagic
due to
disease 785.59

ICD-9-CM
S
Vol. 2

Shock *(Continued)*
hemorrhagic *(Continued)*
due to *(Continued)*
surgery (intraoperative) (postoperative) 998.0
trauma 958.4
hypovolemic NEC 785.59
surgical 998.0
traumatic 958.4
insulin 251.0
therapeutic misadventure 962.3
kidney 584.5
traumatic (following crushing) 958.5
lightning 994.0
lung 518.5
nervous *(see also* Reaction, stress, acute) 308.9
obstetric 669.1
with
abortion - *see* Abortion, by type, with shock
ectopic pregnancy *(see also* categories 633.0-633.9) 639.5
molar pregnancy *(see also* categories 630-632) 639.5
following
abortion 639.5
ectopic or molar pregnancy 639.5
paralysis, paralytic *(see also* Disease, cerebrovascular, acute) 436
late effect - *see* Late effect(s) (of) cerebrovascular disease
pleural (surgical) 998.0
due to trauma 958.4
postoperative 998.0
with
abortion - *see* Abortion, by type, with shock
ectopic pregnancy *(see also* categories 633.0-633.9) 639.5
molar pregnancy *(see also* categories 630-632) 639.5
following
abortion 639.5
ectopic or molar pregnancy 639.5
psychic *(see also* Reaction, stress, acute) 308.9
past history (of) V15.49
psychogenic *(see also* Reaction, stress, acute) 308.9
septic 785.52
with
abortion - *see* Abortion, by type, with shock
ectopic pregnancy *(see also* categories 633.0-633.9) 639.5
molar pregnancy *(see also* categories 630-632) 639.5
due to
surgical procedure 998.0
transfusion NEC 999.8
bone marrow 996.85
following
abortion 639.5
ectopic or molar pregnancy 639.5
surgical procedure 998.0
transfusion NEC 999.8
bone marrow 996.85
spinal - *see also* Injury, spinal, by site
with spinal bone injury - *see* Fracture, vertebra, by site, with spinal cord injury
surgical 998.0
therapeutic misadventure NEC *(see also* Complications) 998.89
thyroxin 962.7

Shock *(Continued)*
toxic 040.82
transfusion - *see* Complications, transfusion
traumatic (immediate) (delayed) 958.4
Shoemakers' chest 738.3
Short, shortening, shortness
Achilles tendon (acquired) 727.81
arm 736.89
congenital 755.20
back 737.9
bowel syndrome 579.3
breath 786.05
chain acyl CoA dehydrogenase deficiency (SCAD) 277.85 ◄
common bile duct, congenital 751.69
cord (umbilical) 663.4
affecting fetus or newborn 762.6
cystic duct, congenital 751.69
esophagus (congenital) 750.4
femur (acquired) 736.81
congenital 755.34
frenulum linguae 750.0
frenum, lingual 750.0
hamstrings 727.81
hip (acquired) 736.39
congenital 755.63
leg (acquired) 736.81
congenital 755.30
metatarsus (congenital) 754.79
acquired 736.79
organ or site, congenital NEC - *see* Distortion
palate (congenital) 750.26
P-R interval syndrome 426.81
radius (acquired) 736.09
congenital 755.26
round ligament 629.8
sleeper 307.49
stature, constitutional (hereditary) 783.43
tendon 727.81
Achilles (acquired) 727.81
congenital 754.79
congenital 756.89
thigh (acquired) 736.81
congenital 755.34
tibialis anticus 727.81
umbilical cord 663.4
affecting fetus or newborn 762.6
urethra 599.84
uvula (congenital) 750.26
vagina 623.8
Shortsightedness 367.1
Shoshin (acute fulminating beriberi) 265.0
Shoulder - *see* condition
Shovel-shaped incisors 520.2
Shower, thromboembolic - *see* Embolism
Shunt (status)
aortocoronary bypass V45.81
arterial-venous (dialysis) V45.1
arteriovenous, pulmonary (acquired) 417.0
congenital 747.3
traumatic (complication) 901.40
cerebral ventricle (communicating) in situ V45.2
coronary artery bypass V45.81
surgical, prosthetic, with complications - *see* Complications, shunt
vascular NEC V45.89
Shutdown
renal 586
with
abortion - *see* Abortion, by type, with renal failure
ectopic pregnancy *(see also* categories 633.0-633.9) 639.3

Shutdown *(Continued)*
renal *(Continued)*
with *(Continued)*
molar pregnancy *(see also* categories 630-632) 639.3
complicating
abortion 639.3
ectopic or molar pregnancy 639.3
following labor and delivery 669.3
Shwachman's syndrome 288.0
Shy-Drager syndrome (orthostatic hypotension with multisystem degeneration) 333.0
Sialadenitis (any gland) (chronic) (suppurative) 527.2
epidemic - *see* Mumps
Sialadenosis, periodic 527.2
Sialaporia 527.7
Sialectasia 527.8
Sialitis 527.2
Sialoadenitis *(see also* Sialadenitis) 527.2
Sialoangitis 527.2
Sialodochitis (fibrinosa) 527.2
Sialodocholithiasis 527.5
Sialolithiasis 527.5
Sialorrhea *(see also* Ptyalism) 527.7
periodic 527.2
Sialosis 527.8
rheumatic 710.2
Siamese twin 759.4
Sicard's syndrome 352.6
Sicca syndrome (keratoconjunctivitis) 710.2
Sick 799.9
cilia syndrome 759.89
or handicapped person in family V61.49
Sickle-cell
anemia *(see also* Disease, sickle-cell) 282.60
disease *(see also* Disease, sickle-cell) 282.60
hemoglobin
C disease (without crisis) 282.63
with
crisis 282.64
vaso-occlusive pain 282.64
D disease (without crisis) 282.68
with crisis 282.69
E disease (without crisis) 282.68
with crisis 282.69
thalassemia (without crisis) 282.41
with
crisis 282.42
vaso-occlusive pain 282.42
trait 282.5
Sicklemia *(see also* Disease, sickle-cell) 282.60
trait 282.5
Sickness
air (travel) 994.6
airplane 994.6
alpine 993.2
altitude 993.2
Andes 993.2
aviators' 993.2
balloon 993.2
car 994.6
compressed air 993.3
decompression 993.3
green 280.9
harvest 100.89
milk 988.8
morning 643.0
motion 994.6
mountain 993.2
acute 289.0
protein *(see also* Complications, vaccination) 999.5

◄ **New**   ◄▥ **Revised**

Sickness *(Continued)*
  radiation NEC 990
  roundabout (motion) 994.6
  sea 994.6
  serum NEC 999.5
  sleeping (African) 086.5
    by Trypanosoma 086.5
      gambiense 086.3
      rhodesiense 086.4
    Gambian 086.3
    late effect 139.8
    Rhodesian 086.4
  sweating 078.2
  swing (motion) 994.6
  train (railway) (travel) 994.6
  travel (any vehicle) 994.6
Sick sinus syndrome 427.81
Sideropenia *(see also* Anemia, iron deficiency) 280.9
Siderosis (lung) (occupational) 503
  cornea 371.15
  eye (bulbi) (vitreous) 360.23
  lens 360.23
Siegal-Cattan-Mamou disease (periodic) 277.3
Siemens' syndrome
  ectodermal dysplasia 757.31
  keratosis follicularis spinulosa (decalvans) 757.39
Sighing respiration 786.7
Sigmoid
  flexure - *see* condition
  kidney 753.3
Sigmoiditis - *see* Enteritis
Silfverskiöld's syndrome 756.50
Silicosis, silicotic (complicated) (occupational) (simple) 502
  fibrosis, lung (confluent) (massive) (occupational) 502
  non-nodular 503
  pulmonum 502
Silicotuberculosis *(see also* Tuberculosis) 011.4
Silo fillers' disease 506.9
Silver's syndrome (congenital hemihypertrophy and short stature) 759.89
Silver wire arteries, retina 362.13
Silvestroni-Bianco syndrome (thalassemia minima) 282.49
Simian crease 757.2
Simmonds' cachexia or disease (pituitary cachexia) 253.2
Simons' disease or syndrome (progressive lipodystrophy) 272.6
Simple, simplex - *see* condition
Sinding-Larsen disease (juvenile osteopathia patellae) 732.4
Singapore hemorrhagic fever 065.4
Singers' node or nodule 478.5
Single
  atrium 745.69
  coronary artery 746.85
  umbilical artery 747.5
  ventricle 745.3
Singultus 786.8
  epidemicus 078.89
Sinus - *see also* Fistula
  abdominal 569.81
  arrest 426.6
  arrhythmia 427.89
  bradycardia 427.89
    chronic 427.81
  branchial cleft (external) (internal) 744.41
  coccygeal (infected) 685.1
    with abscess 685.0
  dental 522.7

Sinus *(Continued)*
  dermal (congenital) 685.1
    with abscess 685.0
  draining - *see* Fistula
  infected, skin NEC 686.9
  marginal, rupture or bleeding 641.2
    affecting fetus or newborn 762.1
  pause 426.6
  pericranii 742.0
  pilonidal (infected) (rectum) 685.1
    with abscess 685.0
  preauricular 744.46
  rectovaginal 619.1
  sacrococcygeal (dermoid) (infected) 685.1
    with abscess 685.0
  skin
    infected NEC 686.9
    noninfected- *see* Ulcer, skin
  tachycardia 427.89
  tarsi syndrome 726.79
  testis 608.89
  tract (postinfectional) - *see* Fistula
  urachus 753.7
Sinuses, Rokitansky-Aschoff *(see also* Disease, gallbladder) 575.8
Sinusitis (accessory) (chronic) (hyperplastic) (nasal) (nonpurulent) (purulent) 473.9
  with influenza, flu, or grippe 487.1
  acute 461.9
    ethmoidal 461.2
    frontal 461.1
    maxillary 461.0
    specified type NEC 461.8
    sphenoidal 461.3
  allergic *(see also* Fever, hay) 477.9
  antrum - *see* Sinusitis, maxillary
  due to
    fungus, any sinus 117.9
    high altitude 993.1
  ethmoidal 473.2
    acute 461.2
  frontal 473.1
    acute 461.1
  influenzal 478.1
  maxillary 473.0
    acute 461.0
  specified site NEC 473.8
  sphenoidal 473.3
    acute 461.3
  syphilitic, any sinus 095.8
  tuberculous, any sinus *(see also* Tuberculosis) 012.8
Sinusitis-bronchiectasis-situs inversus (syndrome) (triad) 759.3
Sipple's syndrome (medullary thyroid carcinoma-pheochromocytoma) 193
Sirenomelia 759.89
Siriasis 992.0
Sirkari's disease 085.0
SIRS systemic inflammatory response syndrome 995.90
  due to
    infectious process 995.91
      with organ dysfunction 995.92
    non-infectious process 995.93
      with organ dysfunction 995.94
Siti 104.0
Sitophobia 300.29
Situation, psychiatric 300.9
Situational
  disturbance (transient) *(see also* Reaction, adjustment) 309.9
    acute 308.3
  maladjustment, acute *(see also* Reaction, adjustment) 309.9

Situational *(Continued)*
  reaction *(see also* Reaction, adjustment) 309.9
    acute 308.3
Situs inversus or transversus 759.3
  abdominalis 759.3
  thoracis 759.3
Sixth disease 057.8
Sjögren (-Gougerot) syndrome or disease (keratoconjunctivitis sicca) 710.2
  with lung involvement 710.2 [517.8]
Sjögren-Larsson syndrome (ichthyosis congenita) 757.1
Skeletal - *see* condition
Skene's gland - *see* condition
Skenitis *(see also* Urethritis) 597.89
  gonorrheal (acute) 098.0
    chronic or duration of 2 months or over 098.2
Skerljevo 104.0
Skevas-Zerfus disease 989.5
Skin - *see also* condition
  donor V59.1
  hidebound 710.9
SLAP lesion (superior glenoid labrum) 840.7
Slate-dressers' lung 502
Slate-miners' lung 502
Sleep
  deprivation V69.4 ◄
  disorder 780.50
    with apnea - *see* Apnea, sleep
    child 307.40
    movement 780.58 ◄
    nonorganic origin 307.40
      specified type NEC 307.49
  disturbance 780.50
    with apnea - *see* Apnea, sleep
    nonorganic origin 307.40
      specified type NEC 307.49
  drunkenness 307.47
  movement disorder 780.58 ◄
  paroxysmal *(see also* Narcolepsy) 347.00 ◄▥
  related movement disorder 780.58 ◄
  rhythm inversion 780.55
    nonorganic origin 307.45
  walking 307.46
    hysterical 300.13
Sleeping sickness 086.5
  late effect 139.8
Sleeplessness *(see also* Insomnia) 780.52
  menopausal 627.2
  nonorganic origin 307.41
Slipped, slipping
  epiphysis (postinfectional) 732.9
    traumatic (old) 732.9
      current - *see* Fracture, by site
    upper femoral (nontraumatic) 732.2
  intervertebral disc - *see* Displacement, intervertebral disc
  ligature, umbilical 772.3
  patella 717.89
  rib 733.99
  sacroiliac joint 724.6
  tendon 727.9
  ulnar nerve, nontraumatic 354.2
  vertebra NEC *(see also* Spondylolisthesis) 756.12
Slocumb's syndrome 255.3
Sloughing (multiple) (skin) 686.9
  abscess - *see* Abscess, by site
  appendix 543.9
  bladder 596.8
  fascia 728.9
  graft - *see* Complications, graft
  phagedena *(see also* Gangrene) 785.4
  reattached extremity *(see also* Complications, reattached extremity) 996.90

ICD-9-CM

S

Vol. 2

Sloughing (*Continued*)
rectum 569.49
scrotum 608.89
tendon 727.9
transplanted organ (*see also* Rejection, transplant, organ, by site) 996.80
ulcer (*see also* Ulcer, skin) 707.9
Slow
feeding newborn 779.3
fetal, growth NEC 764.9
affecting management of pregnancy 656.5
Slowing
heart 427.89
urinary stream 788.62
Sluder's neuralgia or syndrome 337.0
Slurred, slurring, speech 784.5
Small, smallness
cardia reserve - *see* Disease, heart
for dates
fetus or newborn 764.0
with malnutrition 764.1
affecting management of pregnancy 656.5
infant, term 764.0
with malnutrition 764.1
affecting management of pregnancy 656.5
introitus, vagina 623.3
kidney, unknown cause 589.9
bilateral 589.1
unilateral 589.0
ovary 620.8
pelvis
with disproportion (fetopelvic) 653.1
affecting fetus or newborn 763.1
causing obstructed labor 660.1
affecting fetus or newborn 763.1
placenta - *see* Placenta, insufficiency
uterus 621.8
white kidney 582.9
Small-for-dates (*see also* Light-for-dates) 764.0
affecting management of pregnancy 656.5
Smallpox 050.9
contact V01.3
exposure to V01.3
hemorrhagic (pustular) 050.0
malignant 050.0
modified 050.2
vaccination
complications - *see* Complications, vaccination
prophylactic (against) V04.1
Smith's fracture (separation) (closed) 813.41
open 813.51
Smith-Lemli-Opitz syndrome (cerebrohepatorenal syndrome) 759.89
Smith-Magenis syndrome 758.33 ◀
Smith-Strang disease (oasthouse urine) 270.2
Smokers'
bronchitis 491.0
cough 491.0
syndrome (*see also* Abuse, drugs, nondependent) 305.1
throat 472.1
tongue 528.6
Smothering spells 786.09
Snaggle teeth, tooth 524.39 ◀═
Snapping
finger 727.05
hip 719.65

Snapping (*Continued*)
jaw 524.69
temporomandibular joint sounds on opening or closing 524.64 ◀
knee 717.9
thumb 727.05
Sneddon-Wilkinson disease or syndrome (subcorneal pustular dermatosis) 694.1
Sneezing 784.9
intractable 478.1
Sniffing
cocaine (*see also* Dependence) 304.2
ether (*see also* Dependence) 304.6
glue (airplane) (*see also* Dependence) 304.6
Snoring 786.09
Snow blindness 370.24
Snuffles (nonsyphilitic) 460
syphilitic (infant) 090.0
Social migrant V60.0
Sodoku 026.0
Soemmering's ring 366.51
Soft - *see also* condition
enlarged prostate 600.00
with urinary retention 600.01
nails 703.8
Softening
bone 268.2
brain (necrotic) (progressive) 434.9
arteriosclerotic 437.0
congenital 742.4
embolic (*see also* Embolism, brain) 434.1
hemorrhagic (*see also* Hemorrhage, brain) 431
occlusive 434.9
thrombotic (*see also* Thrombosis, brain) 434.0
cartilage 733.92
cerebellar - *see* Softening, brain
cerebral - *see* Softening, brain
cerebrospinal - *see* Softening, brain
myocardial, heart (*see also* Degeneration, myocardial) 429.1
nails 703.8
spinal cord 336.8
stomach 537.89
Solar fever 061
Soldier's
heart 306.2
patches 423.1
Solitary
cyst
bone 733.21
kidney 593.2
kidney (congenital) 753.0
tubercle, brain (*see also* Tuberculosis, brain) 013.2
ulcer, bladder 596.8
Somatization reaction, somatic reaction (*see also* Disorder, psychosomatic) 306.9
disorder 300.81
Somatoform disorder 300.82
atypical 300.82
severe 300.81
undifferentiated 300.82
Somnambulism 307.46
hysterical 300.13
Somnolence 780.09
nonorganic origin 307.43
periodic 349.89
Sonne dysentery 004.3
Soor 112.0
Sore
Delhi 085.1

Sore (*Continued*)
desert (*see also* Ulcer, skin) 707.9
eye 379.99
Lahore 085.1
mouth 528.9
canker 528.2
due to dentures 528.9
muscle 729.1
Naga (*see also* Ulcer, skin) 707.9
oriental 085.1
pressure (*see also* Decubitus) 707.00 ◀═
with gangrene (*see also* Decubitus) 707.00 [785.4] ◀═
skin NEC 709.9
soft 099.0
throat 462
with influenza, flu, or grippe 487.1
acute 462
chronic 472.1
clergyman's 784.49
Coxsackie (virus) 074.0
diphtheritic 032.0
epidemic 034.0
gangrenous 462
herpetic 054.79
influenzal 487.1
malignant 462
purulent 462
putrid 462
septic 034.0
streptococcal (ulcerative) 034.0
ulcerated 462
viral NEC 462
Coxsackie 074.0
tropical (*see also* Ulcer, skin) 707.9
veldt (*see also* Ulcer, skin) 707.9
Sotos' syndrome (cerebral gigantism) 253.0
Sounds
friction, pleural 786.7
succussion, chest 786.7
temporomandibular joint ◀
on opening or closing 524.64 ◀
South African cardiomyopathy syndrome 425.2
South American
blastomycosis 116.1
trypanosomiasis - *see* Trypanosomiasis
Southeast Asian hemorrhagic fever 065.4
Spacing, teeth, abnormal 524.30 ◀═
excessive 524.32 ◀
Spade-like hand (congenital) 754.89
Spading nail 703.8
congenital 757.5
Spanemia 285.9
Spanish collar 605
Sparganosis 123.5
Spasm, spastic, spasticity (*see also* condition) 781.0
accommodation 367.53
ampulla of Vater (*see also* Disease, gallbladder) 576.8
anus, ani (sphincter) (reflex) 564.6
psychogenic 306.4
artery NEC 443.9
basilar 435.0
carotid 435.8
cerebral 435.9
specified artery NEC 435.8
retinal (*see also* Occlusion, retinal, artery) 362.30
vertebral 435.1
vertebrobasilar 435.3
Bell's 351.0
bladder (sphincter, external or internal) 596.8
bowel 564.9
psychogenic 306.4

◀ **New**   ◀═ **Revised**

Spasm, spastic, spasticity (*Continued*)
 bronchus, bronchiole 519.1
 cardia 530.0
 cardiac - *see* Angina
 carpopedal (*see also* Tetany) 781.7
 cecum 564.9
  psychogenic 306.4
 cerebral (arteries) (vascular) 435.9
  specified artery NEC 435.8
 cerebrovascular 435.9
 cervix, complicating delivery 661.4
  affecting fetus or newborn 763.7
 ciliary body (of accommodation) 367.53
 colon 564.1
  psychogenic 306.4
 common duct (*see also* Disease, biliary)
  576.8
 compulsive 307.22
 conjugate 378.82
 convergence 378.84
 coronary (artery) - *see* Angina
 diaphragm (reflex) 786.8
  psychogenic 306.1
 duodenum, duodenal (bulb) 564.89
 esophagus (diffuse) 530.5
  psychogenic 306.4
 facial 351.8
 fallopian tube 620.8
 gait 781.2
 gastrointestinal (tract) 536.8
  psychogenic 306.4
 glottis 478.75
  hysterical 300.11
  psychogenic 306.1
   specified as conversion reaction
    300.11
  reflex through recurrent laryngeal
   nerve 478.75
 habit 307.20
  chronic 307.22
  transient (of childhood) 307.21 ◀▮▮▮
 heart - *see* Angina
 hourglass - *see* Contraction, hourglass
 hysterical 300.11
 infantile (*see also* Epilepsy) 345.6
 internal oblique, eye 378.51
 intestinal 564.9
  psychogenic 306.4
 larynx, laryngeal 478.75
  hysterical 300.11
  psychogenic 306.1
   specified as conversion reaction
    300.11
 levator palpebrae superioris 333.81
 lightning (*see also* Epilepsy) 345.6
 mobile 781.0
 muscle 728.85
  back 724.8
  psychogenic 306.0
 nerve, trigeminal 350.1
 nervous 306.0
 nodding 307.3
  infantile (*see also* Epilepsy) 345.6
 occupational 300.89
 oculogyric 378.87
 ophthalmic artery 362.30
 orbicularis 781.0
 perineal 625.8
 peroneo-extensor (*see also* Flat, foot) 734
 pharynx (reflex) 478.29
  hysterical 300.11
  psychogenic 306.1
   specified as conversion reaction
    300.11

Spasm, spastic, spasticity (*Continued*)
 pregnant uterus, complicating delivery
  661.4
 psychogenic 306.0
 pylorus 537.81
  adult hypertrophic 537.0
  congenital or infantile 750.5
  psychogenic 306.4
 rectum (sphincter) 564.6
  psychogenic 306.4
 retinal artery NEC (*see also* Occlusion,
  retina, artery) 362.30
 sacroiliac 724.6
 salaam (infantile) (*see also* Epilepsy) 345.6
 saltatory 781.0
 sigmoid 564.9
  psychogenic 306.4
 sphincter of Oddi (*see also* Disease,
  gallbladder) 576.5
 stomach 536.8
  neurotic 306.4
 throat 478.29
  hysterical 300.11
  psychogenic 306.1
   specified as conversion reaction
    300.11
 tic 307.20
  chronic 307.22
  transient (of childhood) 307.21 ◀▮▮▮
 tongue 529.8
 torsion 333.6
 trigeminal nerve 350.1
  postherpetic 053.12
 ureter 593.89
 urethra (sphincter) 599.84
 uterus 625.8
  complicating labor 661.4
   affecting fetus or newborn 763.7
 vagina 625.1
  psychogenic 306.51
 vascular NEC 443.9
 vasomotor NEC 443.9
 vein NEC 459.89
 vesical (sphincter, external or internal)
  596.8
 viscera 789.0
Spasmodic - *see* condition
Spasmophilia (*see also* Tetany) 781.7
Spasmus nutans 307.3
Spastic - *see also* Spasm
 child 343.9
Spasticity - *see also* Spasm
 cerebral, child 343.9
Speakers' throat 784.49
Specific, specified - *see* condition
Speech
 defect, disorder, disturbance, impediment NEC 784.5
 psychogenic 307.9
 therapy V57.3
Spells 780.39
 breath-holding 786.9
Spencer's disease (epidemic vomiting)
 078.82
Spens' syndrome (syncope with heart
 block) 426.9
Spermatic cord - *see* condition
Spermatocele 608.1
 congenital 752.89
Spermatocystitis 608.4
Spermatocytoma (M9063/3)
 specified site - *see* Neoplasm, by site,
  malignant
 unspecified site 186.9

Spermatorrhea 608.89
Sperm counts
 fertility testing V26.21
 following sterilization reversal
  V26.22
 postvasectomy V25.8
Sphacelus (*see also* Gangrene) 785.4
Sphenoidal - *see* condition
Sphenoiditis (chronic) (*see also* Sinusitis,
  sphenoidal) 473.3
Sphenopalatine ganglion neuralgia 337.0
Sphericity, increased, lens 743.36
Spherocytosis (congenital) (familial) (he-
  reditary) 282.0
 hemoglobin disease 282.7
 sickle-cell (disease) 282.60
Spherophakia 743.36
Sphincter - *see* condition
Sphincteritis, sphincter of Oddi (*see also*
  Cholecystitis) 576.8
Sphingolipidosis 272.7
Sphingolipodystrophy 272.7
Sphingomyelinosis 272.7
Spicule tooth 520.2
Spider
 finger 755.59
 nevus 448.1
 vascular 448.1
Spiegler-Fendt sarcoid 686.8
Spielmeyer-Stock disease 330.1
Spielmeyer-Vogt disease 330.1
Spina bifida (aperta) 741.9

Note   Use the following fifth-digit subclassification with category 741:
0   unspecified region
1   cervical region
2   dorsal [thoracic] region
3   lumbar region

 with hydrocephalus 741.0
  fetal (suspected), affecting manage-
   ment of pregnancy 655.0
 occulta 756.17
Spindle, Krukenberg's 371.13
Spine, spinal - *see* condition
Spiradenoma (eccrine) (M8403/0) - *see*
 Neoplasm, skin, benign
Spirillosis NEC (*see also* Fever, relaps-
 ing) 087.9
Spirillum minus 026.0
Spirillum obermeieri infection 087.0
Spirochetal - *see* condition
Spirochetosis 104.9
 arthritic, arthritica 104.9 [711.8]
 bronchopulmonary 104.8
 icterohemorrhagica 100.0
 lung 104.8
Spitting blood (*see also* Hemoptysis)
 786.3
Splanchnomegaly 569.89
Splanchnoptosis 569.89
Spleen, splenic - *see also* condition
 agenesis 759.0
 flexure syndrome 569.89
 neutropenia syndrome 288.0
 sequestration syndrome 289.52
Splenectasis (*see also* Splenomegaly)
 789.2
Splenitis (interstitial) (malignant) (nonspecific) 289.59
 malarial (*see also* Malaria) 084.6
 tuberculous (*see also* Tuberculosis)
  017.7

ICD-9-CM

S

Vol. 2

Splenocele 289.59
Splenomegalia - *see* Splenomegaly
Splenomegalic - *see* condition
Splenomegaly 789.2
  Bengal 789.2
  cirrhotic 289.51
  congenital 759.0
  congestive, chronic 289.51
  cryptogenic 789.2
  Egyptian 120.1
  Gaucher's (cerebroside lipidosis) 272.7
  idiopathic 789.2
  malarial (*see also* Malaria) 084.6
  neutropenic 288.0
  Niemann-Pick (lipid histiocytosis) 272.7
  siderotic 289.51
  syphilitic 095.8
    congenital 090.0
  tropical (Bengal) (idiopathic) 789.2
Splenopathy 289.50
Splenopneumonia - *see* Pneumonia
Splenoptosis 289.59
Splinter - *see* Injury, superficial, by site
Split, splitting
  heart sounds 427.89
  lip, congenital (*see also* Cleft, lip) 749.10
  nails 703.8
  urinary stream 788.61
Spoiled child reaction (*see also* Disturbance, conduct) 312.1
Spondylarthritis (*see also* Spondylosis) 721.90
Spondylarthrosis (*see also* Spondylosis) 721.90
Spondylitis 720.9
  ankylopoietica 720.0
  ankylosing (chronic) 720.0
  atrophic 720.9
    ligamentous 720.9
  chronic (traumatic) (*see also* Spondylosis) 721.90
  deformans (chronic) (*see also* Spondylosis) 721.90
  gonococcal 098.53
  gouty 274.0
  hypertrophic (*see also* Spondylosis) 721.90
  infectious NEC 720.9
  juvenile (adolescent) 720.0
  Kummell's 721.7
  Marie-Strümpell (ankylosing) 720.0
  muscularis 720.9
  ossificans ligamentosa 721.6
  osteoarthritica (*see also* Spondylosis) 721.90
  posttraumatic 721.7
  proliferative 720.0
  rheumatoid 720.0
  rhizomelica 720.0
  sacroiliac NEC 720.2
  senescent (*see also* Spondylosis) 721.90
  senile (*see also* Spondylosis) 721.90
  static (*see also* Spondylosis) 721.90
  traumatic (chronic) (*see also* Spondylosis) 721.90
  tuberculous (*see also* Tuberculosis) 015.0 *[720.81]*
  typhosa 002.0 *[720.81]*
Spondyloarthrosis (*see also* Spondylosis) 721.90
Spondylolisthesis (congenital) (lumbosacral) 756.12

Spondylolisthesis (*Continued*)
  with disproportion (fetopelvic) 653.3
    affecting fetus or newborn 763.1
    causing obstructed labor 660.1
      affecting fetus or newborn 763.1
  acquired 738.4
  degenerative 738.4
  traumatic 738.4
    acute (lumbar) - *see* Fracture, vertebra, lumbar
    site other than lumbosacral - *see* Fracture, vertebra, by site
Spondylolysis (congenital) 756.11
  acquired 738.4
  cervical 756.19
  lumbosacral region 756.11
    with disproportion (fetopelvic) 653.3
    affecting fetus or newborn 763.1
    causing obstructed labor 660.1
      affecting fetus or newborn 763.1
Spondylopathy
  inflammatory 720.9
    specified type NEC 720.89
  traumatic 721.7
Spondylose rhizomelique 720.0
Spondylosis 721.90
  with
    disproportion 653.3
      affecting fetus or newborn 763.1
      causing obstructed labor 660.1
        affecting fetus or newborn 763.1
    myelopathy NEC 721.91
  cervical, cervicodorsal 721.0
    with myelopathy 721.1
  inflammatory 720.9
  lumbar, lumbosacral 721.3
    with myelopathy 721.42
  sacral 721.3
    with myelopathy 721.42
  thoracic 721.2
    with myelopathy 721.41
  traumatic 721.7
Sponge
  divers' disease 989.5
  inadvertently left in operation wound 998.4
  kidney (medullary) 753.17
Spongioblastoma (M9422/3)
  multiforme (M9440/3)
    specified site - *see* Neoplasm, by site, malignant
    unspecified site 191.9
  polare (M9423/3)
    specified site - *see* Neoplasm, by site, malignant
    unspecified site 191.9
  primitive polar (M9443/3)
    specified site - *see* Neoplasm, by site, malignant
    unspecified site 191.9
  specified site - *see* Neoplasm, by site, malignant
  unspecified site 191.9
Spongiocytoma (M9400/3)
  specified site - *see* Neoplasm, by site, malignant
  unspecified site 191.9
Spongioneuroblastoma (M9504/3) - *see* Neoplasm, by site, malignant
Spontaneous - *see also* condition
  fracture - *see* Fracture, pathologic
Spoon nail 703.8
  congenital 757.5
Sporadic - *see* condition

Sporotrichosis (bones) (cutaneous) (disseminated) (epidermal) (lymphatic) (lymphocutaneous) (mucous membranes) (pulmonary) (skeletal) (visceral) 117.1
Sporotrichum schenckii infection 117.1
Spots, spotting
  atrophic (skin) 701.3
  Bitôt's (in the young child) 264.1
  café au lait 709.09
  cayenne pepper 448.1
  cotton wool (retina) 362.83
  de Morgan's (senile angiomas) 448.1
  Fúchs' black (myopic) 360.21
  intermenstrual
    irregular 626.6
    regular 626.5
  interpalpebral 372.53
  Koplik's 055.9
  liver 709.09
  Mongolian (pigmented) 757.33
  of pregnancy 641.9
  purpuric 782.7
  ruby 448.1
Spotted fever - *see* Fever, spotted
Sprain, strain (joint) (ligament) (muscle) (tendon) 848.9
  abdominal wall (muscle) 848.8
  Achilles tendon 845.09
  acromioclavicular 840.0
  ankle 845.00
    and foot 845.00
  anterior longitudinal, cervical 847.0
  arm 840.9
    upper 840.9
      and shoulder 840.9
  astragalus 845.00
  atlanto-axial 847.0
  atlanto-occipital 847.0
  atlas 847.0
  axis 847.0
  back (*see also* Sprain, spine) 847.9
  breast bone 848.40
  broad ligaments - *see* Injury, internal, broad ligament
  calcaneofibular 845.02
  carpal 842.01
  carpometacarpal 842.11
  cartilage
    costal, without mention of injury to sternum 848.3
      involving sternum 848.42
    ear 848.8
    knee 844.9
      with current tear (*see also* Tear, meniscus) 836.2
    semilunar (knee) 844.8
      with current tear (*see also* Tear, meniscus) 836.2
    septal, nose 848.0
    thyroid region 848.2
    xiphoid 848.49
  cervical, cervicodorsal, cervicothoracic 847.0
  chondrocostal, without mention of injury to sternum 848.3
    involving sternum 848.42
  chondrosternal 848.42
  chronic (joint) - *see* Derangement, joint
  clavicle 840.9
  coccyx 847.4
  collar bone 840.9
  collateral, knee (medial) (tibial) 844.1
    lateral (fibular) 844.0

Sprain, strain (Continued)
  collateral, knee (Continued)
    recurrent or old 717.89
      lateral 717.81
      medial 717.82
  coracoacromial 840.8
  coracoclavicular 840.1
  coracohumeral 840.2
  coracoid (process) 840.9
  coronary, knee 844.8
  costal cartilage, without mention of in-
      jury to sternum 848.3
    involving sternum 848.42
  cricoarytenoid articulation 848.2
  cricothyroid articulation 848.2
  cruciate
    knee 844.2
    old 717.89
      anterior 717.83
      posterior 717.84
  deltoid
    ankle 845.01
    shoulder 840.8
  dorsal (spine) 847.1
  ear cartilage 848.8
  elbow 841.9
    and forearm 841.9
    specified site NEC 841.8
  femur (proximal end) 843.9
    distal end 844.9
  fibula (proximal end) 844.9
    distal end 845.00
  fibulocalcaneal 845.02
  finger(s) 842.10
  foot 845.10
    and ankle 845.00
  forearm 841.9
    and elbow 841.9
    specified site NEC 841.8
  glenoid (shoulder) (see also SLAP
      lesion) 840.8
  hand 842.10
  hip 843.9
    and thigh 843.9
  humerus (proximal end) 840.9
    distal end 841.9
  iliofemoral 843.0
  infraspinatus 840.3
  innominate
    acetabulum 843.9
    pubic junction 848.5
    sacral junction 846.1
  internal
    collateral, ankle 845.01
    semilunar cartilage 844.8
      with current tear (see also Tear,
          meniscus) 836.2
      old 717.5
  interphalangeal
    finger 842.13
    toe 845.13
  ischiocapsular 843.1
  jaw (cartilage) (meniscus) 848.1
    old 524.69
  knee 844.9
    and leg 844.9
    old 717.5
      collateral
        lateral 717.81
        medial 717.82
      cruciate
        anterior 717.83
        posterior 717.84
  late effect - see Late, effects (of), sprain

Sprain, strain (Continued)
  lateral collateral, knee 844.0
    old 717.81
  leg 844.9
    and knee 844.9
  ligamentum teres femoris 843.8
  low back 846.9
  lumbar (spine) 847.2
  lumbosacral 846.0
    chronic or old 724.6
  mandible 848.1
    old 524.69
  maxilla 848.1
  medial collateral, knee 844.1
    old 717.82
  meniscus
    jaw 848.1
      old 524.69
    knee 844.8
      with current tear (see also Tear,
          meniscus) 836.2
      old 717.5
    mandible 848.1
      old 524.69
    specified site NEC 848.8
  metacarpal 842.10
    distal 842.12
    proximal 842.11
  metacarpophalangeal 842.12
  metatarsal 845.10
  metatarsophalangeal 845.12
  midcarpal 842.19
  midtarsal 845.19
  multiple sites, except fingers alone or
      toes alone 848.8
  neck 847.0
  nose (septal cartilage) 848.0
  occiput from atlas 847.0
  old - see Derangement, joint
  orbicular, hip 843.8
  patella(r) 844.8
    old 717.89
  pelvis 848.5
  phalanx
    finger 842.10
    toe 845.10
  radiocarpal 842.02
  radiohumeral 841.2
  radioulnar 841.9
    distal 842.09
  radius, radial (proximal end) 841.9
    and ulna 841.9
      distal 842.09
    collateral 841.0
    distal end 842.00
  recurrent - see Sprain, by site
  rib (cage), without mention of injury
      to sternum 848.3
    involving sternum 848.42
  rotator cuff (capsule) 840.4
  round ligament - see also Injury, inter-
      nal, round ligament
    femur 843.8
  sacral (spine) 847.3
  sacrococcygeal 847.3
  sacroiliac (region) 846.9
    chronic or old 724.6
    ligament 846.1
    specified site NEC 846.8
  sacrospinatus 846.2
  sacrospinous 846.2
  sacrotuberous 846.3
  scaphoid bone, ankle 845.00
  scapula(r) 840.9

Sprain, strain (Continued)
  semilunar cartilage (knee) 844.8
    with current tear (see also Tear, me-
        niscus) 836.2
    old 717.5
  septal cartilage (nose) 848.0
  shoulder 840.9
    and arm, upper 840.9
    blade 840.9
  specified site NEC 848.8
  spine 847.9
    cervical 847.0
    coccyx 847.4
    dorsal 847.1
    lumbar 847.2
    lumbosacral 846.0
      chronic or old 724.6
    sacral 847.3
    sacroiliac (see also Sprain, sacroiliac)
        846.9
      chronic or old 724.6
    thoracic 847.1
  sternoclavicular 848.41
  sternum 848.40
  subglenoid (see also SLAP lesion)
      840.8
  subscapularis 840.5
  supraspinatus 840.6
  symphysis
    jaw 848.1
      old 524.69
    mandibular 848.1
      old 524.69
    pubis 848.5
  talofibular 845.09
  tarsal 845.10
  tarsometatarsal 845.11
  temporomandibular 848.1
    old 524.69
  teres
    ligamentum femoris 843.8
    major or minor 840.8
  thigh (proximal end) 843.9
    and hip 843.9
    distal end 844.9
  thoracic (spine) 847.1
  thorax 848.8
  thumb 842.10
  thyroid cartilage or region 848.2
  tibia (proximal end) 844.9
    distal end 845.00
  tibiofibular
    distal 845.03
    superior 844.3
  toe(s) 845.10
  trachea 848.8
  trapezoid 840.8
  ulna, ulnar (proximal end) 841.9
    collateral 841.1
    distal end 842.00
  ulnohumeral 841.3
  vertebrae (see also Sprain, spine) 847.9
    cervical, cervicodorsal, cervicothora-
        cic 847.0
  wrist (cuneiform) (scaphoid) (semilu-
      nar) 842.00
  xiphoid cartilage 848.49
Sprengel's deformity (congenital) 755.52
Spring fever 309.23
Sprue 579.1
  celiac 579.0
  idiopathic 579.0
  meaning thrush 112.0
  nontropical 579.0

ICD-9-CM

S

Vol. 2

Sprue *(Continued)*
  tropical 579.1
Spur - *see also* Exostosis
  bone 726.91
    calcaneal 726.73
  calcaneal 726.73
  iliac crest 726.5
  nose (septum) 478.1
    bone 726.91
  septal 478.1
Spuria placenta - *see* Placenta, abnormal
Spurway's syndrome (brittle bones and
    blue sclera) 756.51
Sputum, abnormal (amount) (color) (ex-
    cessive) (odor) (purulent) 786.4
  bloody 786.3
Squamous - *see also* condition
  cell metaplasia
    bladder 596.8
    cervix - *see* condition
  epithelium in
    cervical canal (congenital) 752.49
    uterine mucosa (congenital) 752.3
  metaplasia
    bladder 596.8
    cervix - *see* condition
Squashed nose 738.0
  congenital 754.0
Squeeze, divers' 993.3
Squint (*see also* Strabismus) 378.9
  accommodative (*see also* Esotropia)
    378.00
  concomitant (*see also* Heterotropia)
    378.30
Stab - *see also* Wound, open, by site
  internal organs - *see* Injury, internal, by
    site, with open wound
Staggering gait 781.2
  hysterical 300.11
Staghorn calculus 592.0
Stähl's
  ear 744.29
  pigment line (cornea) 371.11
Stähli's pigment lines (cornea) 371.11
Stain
  port wine 757.32
  tooth, teeth (hard tissues) 521.7
    due to
      accretions 523.6
      deposits (betel) (black) (green)
        (materia alba) (orange) (to-
        bacco) 523.6
      metals (copper) (silver) 521.7
      nicotine 523.6
      pulpal bleeding 521.7
      tobacco 523.6
Stammering 307.0
Standstill
  atrial 426.6
  auricular 426.6
  cardiac (*see also* Arrest, cardiac) 427.5
  sinoatrial 426.6
  sinus 426.6
  ventricular (*see also* Arrest, cardiac) 427.5
Stannosis 503
Stanton's disease (melioidosis) 025
Staphylitis (acute) (catarrhal) (chronic)
    (gangrenous) (membranous) (suppu-
    rative) (ulcerative) 528.3
Staphylococcemia 038.10
  aureus 038.11
  specified organism NEC 038.19
Staphylococcus, staphylococcal - *see* con-
    dition

Staphyloderma (skin) 686.00
Staphyloma 379.11
  anterior, localized 379.14
  ciliary 379.11
  cornea 371.73
  equatorial 379.13
  posterior 379.12
  posticum 379.12
  ring 379.15
  sclera NEC 379.11
Starch eating 307.52
Stargardt's disease 362.75
Starvation (inanition) (due to lack of
    food) 994.2
  edema 262
  voluntary NEC 307.1
Stasis
  bile (duct) (*see also* Disease, biliary) 576.8
  bronchus (*see also* Bronchitis) 490
  cardiac (*see also* Failure, heart) 428.0
  cecum 564.89
  colon 564.89
  dermatitis (*see also* Varix, with stasis
    dermatitis) 454.1
  duodenal 536.8
  eczema (*see also* Varix, with stasis der-
    matitis) 454.1
  edema (*see also* Hypertension, venous)
    459.30
  foot 991.4
  gastric 536.3
  ileocecal coil 564.89
  ileum 564.89
  intestinal 564.89
  jejunum 564.89
  kidney 586
  liver 571.9
    cirrhotic - *see* Cirrhosis, liver
  lymphatic 457.8
  pneumonia 514
  portal 571.9
  pulmonary 514
  rectal 564.89
  renal 586
    tubular 584.5
  stomach 536.3
  ulcer
    with varicose veins 454.0
    without varicose veins 459.81
  urine NEC (*see also* Retention, urine)
    788.20
  venous 459.81
State
  affective and paranoid, mixed, organic
    psychotic 294.8
  agitated 307.9
    acute reaction to stress 308.2
  anxiety (neurotic) (*see also* Anxiety) 300.00
    specified type NEC 300.09
  apprehension (*see also* Anxiety) 300.00
    specified type NEC 300.09
  climacteric, female 627.2
    following induced menopause 627.4
  clouded
    epileptic (*see also* Epilepsy) 345.9
    paroxysmal (idiopathic) (*see also* Epi-
      lepsy) 345.9
  compulsive (mixed) (with obsession)
    300.3
  confusional 298.9
    acute 293.0
      with
        arteriosclerotic dementia 290.41
        presenile brain disease 290.11
        senility 290.3

State *(Continued)*
  confusional *(Continued)*
    acute *(Continued)*
      alcoholic 291.0
      drug-induced 292.81
    epileptic 293.0
    postoperative 293.9
    reactive (emotional stress) (psycho-
      logical trauma) 298.2
    subacute 293.1
  constitutional psychopathic 301.9
  convulsive (*see also* Convulsions) 780.39
  depressive NEC 311
    induced by drug 292.84
    neurotic 300.4
  dissociative 300.15
  hallucinatory 780.1
    induced by drug 292.12
  hypercoagulable (primary) 289.81
    secondary 289.82
  hyperdynamic beta-adrenergic circula-
    tory 429.82
  locked-in 344.81
  menopausal 627.2
    artificial 627.4
    following induced menopause 627.4
  neurotic NEC 300.9
    with depersonalization episode 300.6
  obsessional 300.3
  oneiroid (*see also* Schizophrenia) 295.4
  panic 300.01
  paranoid 297.9
    alcohol-induced 291.5
    arteriosclerotic 290.42
    climacteric 297.2
    drug-induced 292.11
    in
      presenile brain disease 290.12
      senile brain disease 290.20
    involutional 297.2
    menopausal 297.2
    senile 290.20
    simple 297.0
  postleukotomy 310.0
  pregnant (*see also* Pregnancy) V22.2
  psychogenic, twilight 298.2
  psychotic, organic (*see also* Psychosis,
    organic) 294.9
    mixed paranoid and affective 294.8
    senile or presenile NEC 290.9
    transient NEC 293.9
      with
        anxiety 293.84
        delusions 293.81
        depression 293.83
        hallucinations 293.82
  residual schizophrenic (*see also* Schizo-
    phrenia) 295.6
  tension (*see also* Anxiety) 300.9
  transient organic psychotic 293.9
    anxiety type 293.84
    depressive type 293.83
    hallucinatory type 293.83
    paranoid type 293.81
    specified type NEC 293.89
  twilight
    epileptic 293.0
    psychogenic 298.2
  vegetative (persistent) 780.03
Status (post)
  absence
    epileptic (*see also* Epilepsy) 345.2
    of organ, acquired (postsurgical) -
      see Absence, by site, acquired

◀ **New**   ◀▥▥ **Revised**

Status (post) *(Continued)*
  anastomosis of intestine (for bypass)
    V45.3
  anginosus 413.9
  angioplasty, percutaneous transluminal
    coronary V45.82
  ankle prosthesis V43.66
  aortocoronary bypass or shunt V45.81
  arthrodesis V45.4
  artificially induced condition NEC
    V45.89
  artificial opening (of) V44.9
    gastrointestinal tract NEC V44.4
    specified site NEC V44.8
    urinary tract NEC V44.6
    vagina V44.7
  aspirator V46.0
  asthmaticus (*see also* Asthma) 493.9
  awaiting organ transplant V49.83 ◄
  breast implant removal V45.83
  cardiac
    device (in situ) V45.00
      carotid sinus V45.09
        fitting or adjustment V53.39
      defibrillator, automatic implanta-
        ble V45.02
      pacemaker V45.01
        fitting or adjustment V53.31
  carotid sinus stimulator V45.09
  cataract extraction V45.61
  chemotherapy V66.2
    current V58.69
  circumcision, female 629.20 ◄
  clitorectomy (female genital mutilation
    type I) 629.21 ◄
    with excision of labia minora (fe-
      male genital mutiliation type II)
      629.22 ◄
  colostomy V44.3
  contraceptive device V45.59
    intrauterine V45.51
    subdermal V45.52
  convulsivus idiopathicus (*see also* Epi-
    lepsy) 345.3
  coronary artery bypass or shunt V45.81
  cystostomy V44.50
    appendico-vesicostomy V44.52
    cutaneous-vesicostomy V44.51
    specified type NEC V44.59
  defibrillator, automatic implantable
    cardiac V45.02
  dental crowns V45.84
  dental fillings V45.84
  dental restoration V45.84
  dental sealant V49.82
  dialysis V45.1
  donor V59.9
  drug therapy or regimen V67.59
    high-risk medication NEC V67.51
  elbow prosthesis V43.62
  enterostomy V44.4
  epileptic, epilepticus (absence) (grand
    mal) (*see also* Epilepsy) 345.3
    focal motor 345.7
    partial 345.7
    petit mal 345.2
    psychomotor 345.7
    temporal lobe 345.7
  eye (adnexa) surgery V45.69
  female genital mutilation 629.20 ◄
    type I 629.21 ◄
    type II 629.22 ◄
    type III 629.23 ◄

Status (post) *(Continued)*
  filtering bleb (eye) (postglaucoma)
    V45.69
    with rupture or complication 997.99
    postcataract extraction (complica-
      tion) 997.99
  finger joint prosthesis V43.69
  gastrostomy V44.1
  grand mal 345.3
  heart valve prosthesis V43.3
  hip prosthesis (joint) (partial) (total)
    V43.64
  ileostomy V44.2
  infibulation (female genital mutilation
    type III) 629.23 ◄
  insulin pump V45.85
  intestinal bypass V45.3
  intrauterine contraceptive device V45.51
  jejunostomy V44.4
  knee joint prosthesis V43.65
  lacunaris 437.8
  lacunosis 437.8
  low birth weight V21.30
    less than 500 grams V21.31
    500–999 grams V21.32
    1000–1499 grams V21.33
    1500–1999 grams V21.34
    2000–2500 grams V21.35
  lymphaticus 254.8
  malignant neoplasm, ablated or ex-
    cised - *see* History, malignant neo-
    plasm
  marmoratus 333.7
  multilation, female 629.20 ◄
    type I 629.21 ◄
    type II 629.22 ◄
    type III 629.23 ◄
  nephrostomy V44.6
  neuropacemaker NEC V45.89
    brain V45.89
    carotid sinus V45.09
    neurologic NEC V45.89
  organ replacement
    by artificial or mechanical device or
      prosthesis of
      artery V43.4
      artificial skin V43.83
      bladder V43.5
      blood vessel V43.4
      breast V43.82
      eye globe V43.0
      heart
        assist device V43.21
        fully implantable artificial heart
          V43.22
        valve V43.3
      intestine V43.89
      joint V43.60
        ankle V43.66
        elbow V43.62
        finger V43.69
        hip (partial) (total) V43.64
        knee V43.65
        shoulder V43.61
        specified NEC V43.69
        wrist V43.63
      kidney V43.89
      larynx V43.81
      lens V43.1
      limb(s) V43.7
      liver V43.89
      lung V43.89
      organ NEC V43.89
      pancreas V43.89
      skin (artificial) V43.83

Status (post) *(Continued)*
  organ replacement *(Continued)*
    by artificial or mechanical device or
      prosthesis of *(Continued)*
      tissue NEC V43.89
      vein V43.4
    by organ transplant (heterologous)
      (homologous) - *see* Status, trans-
      plant
  pacemaker
    brain V45.89
    cardiac V45.01
    carotid sinus V45.09
    neurologic NEC V45.89
    specified site NEC V45.89
  percutaneous transluminal coronary
    angioplasty V45.82
  petit mal 345.2
  postcommotio cerebri 310.2
  postmenopausal (age related) (natural)
    V49.81
  postoperative NEC V45.89
  postpartum NEC V24.2
    care immediately following delivery
      V24.0
    routine follow-up V24.2
  postsurgical NEC V45.89
  renal dialysis V45.1
  respirator V46.11 ◄▥
    encounter during power failure
      V46.12 ◄
  reversed jejunal transposition (for by-
    pass) V45.3
  shoulder prosthesis V43.61
  shunt
    aortocoronary bypass V45.81
    arteriovenous (for dialysis) V45.1
    cerebrospinal fluid V45.2
    vascular NEC V45.89
      aortocoronary (bypass) V45.81
    ventricular (communicating) (for
      drainage) V45.2
  sterilization
    tubal ligation V26.51
    vasectomy V26.52
  subdermal contraceptive device V45.52
  thymicolymphaticus 254.8
  thymicus 254.8
  thymolymphaticus 254.8
  tooth extraction 525.10
  tracheostomy V44.0
  transplant
    blood vessel V42.89
    bone V42.4
      marrow V42.81
    cornea V42.5
    heart V42.1
      valve V42.2
    intestine V42.84
    kidney V42.0
    liver V42.7
    lung V42.6
    organ V42.9
      specified site NEC V42.89
    pancreas V42.83
    peripheral stem cells V42.82
    skin V42.3
    stem cells, peripheral V42.82
    tissue V42.9
      specified type NEC V42.89
    vessel, blood V42.89
  tubal ligation V26.51
  ureterostomy V44.6
  urethrostomy V44.6
  vagina, artificial V44.7

ICD-9-CM

S

Vol. 2

Status (post) *(Continued)*
  vascular shunt NEC V45.89
    aortocoronary (bypass) V45.81
  vasectomy V26.52
  ventilator V46.11 ◀▥
    encounter during power failure
      V46.12 ◀
  wrist prosthesis V43.63
Stave fracture - *see* Fracture, metacarpus,
  metacarpal bone(s)
Steal
  subclavian artery 435.2
  vertebral artery 435.1
Stealing, solitary, child problem *(see also*
  Disturbance, conduct) 312.1
Steam burn - *see* Burn, by site
Steatocystoma multiplex 706.2
Steatoma (infected) 706.2
  eyelid (cystic) 374.84
    infected 373.13
Steatorrhea (chronic) 579.8
  with lacteal obstruction 579.2
  idiopathic 579.0
    adult 579.0
    infantile 579.0
  pancreatic 579.4
  primary 579.0
  secondary 579.8
  specified cause NEC 579.8
  tropical 579.1
Steatosis 272.8
  heart *(see also* Degeneration, myocar-
    dial) 429.1
  kidney 593.89
  liver 571.8
Steele-Richardson (-Olszewski) syndrome 333.0
Stein's syndrome (polycystic ovary) 256.4
Stein-Leventhal syndrome (polycystic
  ovary) 256.4
Steinbrocker's syndrome *(see also* Neuropathy, peripheral, autonomic) 337.9
Steinert's disease 359.2
Stenocardia *(see also* Angina) 413.9
Stenocephaly 756.0
Stenosis (cicatricial) - *see also* Stricture
  ampulla of Vater 576.2
    with calculus, cholelithiasis, or
      stones - *see* Choledocholithiasis
  anus, anal (canal) (sphincter) 569.2
    congenital 751.2
  aorta (ascending) 747.22
    arch 747.10
    arteriosclerotic 440.0
    calcified 440.0
  aortic (valve) 424.1
    with
      mitral (valve)
        insufficiency or incompetence
          396.2
        stenosis or obstruction 396.0
    atypical 396.0
    congenital 746.3
    rheumatic 395.0
      with
        insufficiency, incompetency or
          regurgitation 395.2
        with mitral (valve) disease
          396.8
        mitral (valve)
          disease (stenosis) 396.0
          insufficiency or incompetence
            396.2
          stenosis or obstruction 396.0

Stenosis *(Continued)*
  aorta *(Continued)*
    specified cause, except rheumatic
      424.1
    syphilitic 093.22
  aqueduct of Sylvius (congenital) 742.3
    with spina bifida *(see also* Spina
      bifida) 741.0
    acquired 331.4
  artery NEC 447.1
    basilar - *see* Narrowing, artery, basilar
    carotid (common) (internal) - *see*
      Narrowing, artery, carotid
    celiac 447.4
    cerebral 437.0
      due to
        embolism *(see also* Embolism,
          brain) 434.1
        thrombus *(see also* Thrombosis,
          brain) 434.0
    precerebral - *see* Narrowing, artery,
      precerebral
    pulmonary (congenital) 747.3
      acquired 417.8
    renal 440.1
    vertebral - *see* Narrowing, artery,
      vertebral
  bile duct or biliary passage *(see also*
    Obstruction, biliary) 576.2
    congenital 751.61
  bladder neck (acquired) 596.0
    congenital 753.6
  brain 348.8
  bronchus 519.1
    syphilitic 095.8
  cardia (stomach) 537.89
    congenital 750.7
  cardiovascular *(see also* Disease, cardio-
    vascular) 429.2
  carotid artery - *see* Narrowing, artery,
    carotid
  cervix, cervical (canal) 622.4
    congenital 752.49
    in pregnancy or childbirth 654.6
      affecting fetus or newborn 763.89
      causing obstructed labor 660.2
        affecting fetus or newborn 763.1
  colon *(see also* Obstruction, intestine)
    560.9
    congenital 751.2
  colostomy 569.62
  common bile duct *(see also* Obstruction,
    biliary) 576.2
    congenital 751.61
  coronary (artery) - *see* Arteriosclerosis,
    coronary
  cystic duct *(see also* Obstruction, gall-
    bladder) 575.2
    congenital 751.61
  due to (presence of) any device, implant,
    or graft classifiable to 996.0-996.5 -
    see Complications, due to (presence
    of) any device, implant, or graft
    classified to 996.0-996.5 NEC
  duodenum 537.3
    congenital 751.1
  ejaculatory duct NEC 608.89
  endocervical os - *see* Stenosis, cervix
  enterostomy 569.62
  esophagostomy 530.87 ◀
  esophagus 530.3
    congenital 750.3
    syphilitic 095.8
      congenital 090.5

Stenosis *(Continued)*
  external ear canal 380.50
    secondary to
      inflammation 380.53
      surgery 380.52
      trauma 380.51
  gallbladder *(see also* Obstruction, gall-
    bladder) 575.2
  glottis 478.74
  heart valve (acquired) - *see also* Endo-
    carditis
    congenital NEC 746.89
      aortic 746.3
      mitral 746.5
      pulmonary 746.02
      tricuspid 746.1
  hepatic duct *(see also* Obstruction, bili-
    ary) 576.2
  hymen 623.3
  hypertrophic subaortic (idiopathic) 425.1
  infundibulum cardiac 746.83
  intestine *(see also* Obstruction, intes-
    tine) 560.9
    congenital (small) 751.1
    large 751.2
  lacrimal
    canaliculi 375.53
    duct 375.56
      congenital 743.65
    punctum 375.52
      congenital 743.65
    sac 375.54
      congenital 743.65
  lacrimonasal duct 375.56
    congenital 743.65
    neonatal 375.55
  larynx 478.74
    congenital 748.3
    syphilitic 095.8
      congenital 090.5
  mitral (valve) (chronic) (inactive)
    394.0
    with
      aortic (valve)
        disease (insufficiency) 396.1
        insufficiency or incompetence
          396.1
        stenosis or obstruction 396.0
      incompetency, insufficiency or re-
        gurgitation 394.2
        with aortic valve disease 396.8
    active or acute 391.1
      with chorea (acute) (rheumatic)
        (Sydenham's) 392.0
    congenital 746.5
    specified cause, except rheumatic
      424.0
    syphilitic 093.21
  myocardium, myocardial *(see also* De-
    generation, myocardial) 429.1
    hypertrophic subaortic (idiopathic)
      425.1
  nares (anterior) (posterior) 478.1
    congenital 748.0
  nasal duct 375.56
    congenital 743.65
  nasolacrimal duct 375.56
    congenital 743.65
    neonatal 375.55
  organ or site, congenital NEC - *see*
    Atresia
  papilla of Vater 576.2
    with calculus, cholelithiasis, or
      stones - *see* Choledocholithiasis

Stenosis (*Continued*)
  pulmonary (artery) (congenital) 747.3
    with ventricular septal defect, dextraposition of aorta and hypertrophy of right ventricle 745.2
    acquired 417.8
    infundibular 746.83
    in tetralogy of Fallot 745.2
    subvalvular 746.83
    valve (*see also* Endocarditis, pulmonary) 424.3
      congenital 746.02
    vein 747.49
      acquired 417.8
    vessel NEC 417.8
  pulmonic (congenital) 746.02
    infundibular 746.83
    subvalvular 746.83
  pylorus (hypertrophic) 537.0
    adult 537.0
    congenital 750.5
    infantile 750.5
  rectum (sphincter) (*see also* Stricture, rectum) 569.2
  renal artery 440.1
  salivary duct (any) 527.8
  sphincter of Oddi (*see also* Obstruction, biliary) 576.2
  spinal 724.00
    cervical 723.0
    lumbar, lumbosacral 724.02
    nerve (root) NEC 724.9
    specified region NEC 724.09
    thoracic, thoracolumbar 724.01
  stomach, hourglass 537.6
  subaortic 746.81
    hypertrophic (idiopathic) 425.1
  supra (valvular)-aortic 747.22
  trachea 519.1
    congenital 748.3
    syphilitic 095.8
    tuberculous (*see also* Tuberculosis) 012.8
  tracheostomy 519.02
  tricuspid (valve) (*see also* Endocarditis, tricuspid) 397.0
    congenital 746.1
    nonrheumatic 424.2
  tubal 628.2
  ureter (*see also* Stricture, ureter) 593.3
    congenital 753.29
  urethra (*see also* Stricture, urethra) 598.9
  vagina 623.2
    congenital 752.49
    in pregnancy or childbirth 654.7
      affecting fetus or newborn 763.89
      causing obstructed labor 660.2
        affecting fetus or newborn 763.1
  valve (cardiac) (heart) (*see also* Endocarditis) 424.90
    congenital NEC 746.89
      aortic 746.3
      mitral 746.5
      pulmonary 746.02
      tricuspid 746.1
      urethra 753.6
  valvular (*see also* Endocarditis) 424.90
    congenital NEC 746.89
    urethra 753.6
  vascular graft or shunt 996.1
    atherosclerosis - *see* Arteriosclerosis, extremities
    embolism 996.74
    occlusion NEC 996.74
    thrombus 996.74

Stenosis (*Continued*)
  vena cava (inferior) (superior) 459.2
    congenital 747.49
  ventricular shunt 996.2
  vulva 624.8
Stercolith (*see also* Fecalith) 560.39
  appendix 543.9
Stercoraceous, stercoral ulcer 569.82
  anus or rectum 569.41
Stereopsis, defective
  with fusion 368.33
  without fusion 368.32
Stereotypies NEC 307.3
Sterility
  female - *see* Infertility, female
  male (*see also* Infertility, male) 606.9
Sterilization, admission for V25.2
  status
    tubal ligation V26.51
    vasectomy V26.52
Sternalgia (*see also* Angina) 413.9
Sternopagus 759.4
Sternum bifidum 756.3
Sternutation 784.9
Steroid
  effects (adverse) (iatrogenic)
    cushingoid
      correct substance properly administered 255.0
      overdose or wrong substance given or taken 962.0
    diabetes
      correct substance properly administered 251.8
      overdose or wrong substance given or taken 962.0
    due to
      correct substance properly administered 255.8
      overdose or wrong substance given or taken 962.0
    fever
      correct substance properly administered 780.6
      overdose or wrong substance given or taken 962.0
    withdrawal
      correct substance properly administered 255.4
      overdose or wrong substance given or taken 962.0
  responder 365.03
Stevens-Johnson disease or syndrome (erythema multiforme exudativum) 695.1
Stewart-Morel syndrome (hyperostosis frontalis interna) 733.3
Sticker's disease (erythema infectiosum) 057.0
Sticky eye 372.03
Stieda's disease (calcification, knee joint) 726.62
Stiff
  back 724.8
  neck (*see also* Torticollis) 723.5
Stiff-baby 759.89 ◀
Stiff-man syndrome 333.91
Stiffness, joint NEC 719.50
  ankle 719.57
  back 724.8
  elbow 719.52
  finger 719.54
  hip 719.55
  knee 719.56

Stiffness, joint NEC (*Continued*)
  multiple sites 719.59
  sacroiliac 724.6
  shoulder 719.51
  specified site NEC 719.58
  spine 724.9
  surgical fusion V45.4
  wrist 719.53
Stigmata, congenital syphilis 090.5
Still's disease or syndrome 714.30
Still-Felty syndrome (rheumatoid arthritis with splenomegaly and leukopenia) 714.1
Stillbirth, stillborn NEC 779.9
Stiller's disease (asthenia) 780.79
Stilling-Türk-Duane syndrome (ocular retraction syndrome) 378.71
Stimulation, ovary 256.1
Sting (animal) (bee) (fish) (insect) (jellyfish) (Portuguese man-o-war) (wasp) (venomous) 989.5
  anaphylactic shock or reaction 989.5
  plant 692.6
Stippled epiphyses 756.59
Stitch
  abscess 998.59
  burst (in external operation wound) 998.32
    internal 998.31
  in back 724.5
Stojano's (subcostal) syndrome 098.86
Stokes' disease (exophthalmic goiter) 242.0
Stokes-Adams syndrome (syncope with heart block) 426.9
Stokvis' (-Talma) disease (enterogenous cyanosis) 289.7
Stomach - *see* condition
Stoma malfunction
  colostomy 569.62
  cystostomy 997.5
  enterostomy 569.62
  esophagostomy 530.87
  gastrostomy 536.42
  ileostomy 569.62
  nephrostomy 997.5
  tracheostomy 519.02
  ureterostomy 997.5
Stomatitis 528.0
  angular 528.5
    due to dietary or vitamin deficiency 266.0
  aphthous 528.2
  candidal 112.0
  catarrhal 528.0
  denture 528.9
  diphtheritic (membranous) 032.0
  due to
    dietary deficiency 266.0
    thrush 112.0
    vitamin deficiency 266.0
  epidemic 078.4
  epizootic 078.4
  follicular 528.0
  gangrenous 528.1
  herpetic 054.2
  herpetiformis 528.2
  malignant 528.0
  membranous acute 528.0
  monilial 112.0
  mycotic 112.0
  necrotic 528.1
    ulcerative 101
  necrotizing ulcerative 101
  parasitic 112.0

ICD-9-CM

S

Vol. 2

Stomatitis *(Continued)*
  septic 528.0
  spirochetal 101
  suppurative (acute) 528.0
  ulcerative 528.0
    necrotizing 101
  ulceromembranous 101
  vesicular 528.0
    with exanthem 074.3
  Vincent's 101
Stomatocytosis 282.8
Stomatomycosis 112.0
Stomatorrhagia 528.9
Stone(s) - *see also* Calculus
  bladder 594.1
    diverticulum 594.0
  cystine 270.0
  heart syndrome (*see also* Failure, ventricular, left) 428.1
  kidney 592.0
  prostate 602.0
  pulp (dental) 522.2
  renal 592.0
  salivary duct or gland (any) 527.5
  ureter 592.1
  urethra (impacted) 594.2
  urinary (duct) (impacted) (passage) 592.9
    bladder 594.1
      diverticulum 594.0
    lower tract NEC 594.9
    specified site 594.8
  xanthine 277.2
Stonecutters' lung 502
  tuberculous (*see also* Tuberculosis) 011.4
Stonemasons'
  asthma, disease, or lung 502
    tuberculous (*see also* Tuberculosis) 011.4
  phthisis (*see also* Tuberculosis) 011.4
Stoppage
  bowel (*see also* Obstruction, intestine) 560.9
  heart (*see also* Arrest, cardiac) 427.5
  intestine (*see also* Obstruction, intestine) 560.9
  urine NEC (*see also* Retention, urine) 788.20
Storm, thyroid (apathetic) (*see also* Thyrotoxicosis) 242.9
Strabismus (alternating) (congenital) (nonparalytic) 378.9
  concomitant (*see also* Heterotropia) 378.30
    convergent (*see also* Esotropia) 378.00
    divergent (*see also* Exotropia) 378.10
  convergent (*see also* Esotropia) 378.00
  divergent (*see also* Exotropia) 378.10
  due to adhesions, scars - *see* Strabismus, mechanical
  in neuromuscular disorder NEC 378.73
    intermittent 378.20
      vertical 378.31
  latent 378.40
    convergent (esophoria) 378.41
    divergent (exophoria) 378.42
    vertical 378.43
  mechanical 378.60
    due to
      Brown's tendon sheath syndrome 378.61
      specified musculofascial disorder NEC 378.62
  paralytic 378.50
    third or oculomotor nerve (partial) 378.51
      total 378.52

Strabismus *(Continued)*
  paralytic *(Continued)*
    fourth or trochlear nerve 378.53
    sixth or abducens nerve 378.54
  specified type NEC 378.73
  vertical (hypertropia) 378.31
Strain - *see also* Sprain, by site
  eye NEC 368.13
  heart - *see* Disease, heart
  meaning gonorrhea - *see* Gonorrhea
  physical NEC V62.89
  postural 729.9
  psychological NEC V62.89
Strands
  conjunctiva 372.62
  vitreous humor 379.25
Strangulation, strangulated 994.7
  appendix 543.9
  asphyxiation or suffocation by 994.7
  bladder neck 596.0
  bowel - *see* Strangulation, intestine
  colon - *see* Strangulation, intestine
  cord (umbilical) - *see* Compression, umbilical cord
  due to birth injury 767.8
  food or foreign body (*see also* Asphyxia, food) 933.1
  hemorrhoids 455.8
    external 455.5
    internal 455.2
  hernia - *see also* Hernia, by site, with obstruction
    gangrenous - *see* Hernia, by site, with gangrene
  intestine (large) (small) 560.2
    with hernia - *see also* Hernia, by site, with obstruction
      gangrenous - *see* Hernia, by site, with gangrene
    congenital (small) 751.1
      large 751.2
  mesentery 560.2
  mucus (*see also* Asphyxia, mucus) 933.1
    newborn 770.1
  omentum 560.2
  organ or site, congenital NEC - *see* Atresia
  ovary 620.8
    due to hernia 620.4
  penis 607.89
    foreign body 939.3
  rupture (*see also* Hernia, by site, with obstruction) 552.9
    gangrenous (*see also* Hernia, by site, with gangrene) 551.9
  stomach, due to hernia (*see also* Hernia, by site, with obstruction) 552.9
    with gangrene (*see also* Hernia, by site, with gangrene) 551.9
  umbilical cord - *see* Compression, umbilical cord
  vesicourethral orifice 596.0
Strangury 788.1
Strawberry
  gallbladder (*see also* Disease, gallbladder) 575.6
  mark 757.32
  tongue (red) (white) 529.3
Straw itch 133.8
Streak, ovarian 752.0
Strephosymbolia 315.01
  secondary to organic lesion 784.69
Streptobacillary fever 026.1
Streptobacillus moniliformis 026.1
Streptococcemia 038.0

Streptococcicosis - *see* Infection, streptococcal
Streptococcus, streptococcal - *see* condition
Streptoderma 686.00
Streptomycosis - *see* Actinomycosis
Streptothricosis - *see* Actinomycosis
Streptothrix - *see* Actinomycosis
Streptotrichosis - *see* Actinomycosis
Stress
  fracture - *see* Fracture, stress
  polycythemia 289.0
  reaction (gross) (*see also* Reaction, stress, acute) 308.9
Stretching, nerve - *see* Injury, nerve, by site
Striae (albicantes) (atrophicae) (cutis distensae) (distensae) 701.3
Striations of nails 703.8
Stricture (*see also* Stenosis) 799.89
  ampulla of Vater 576.2
    with calculus, cholelithiasis, or stones - *see* Choledocholithiasis
  anus (sphincter) 569.2
    congenital 751.2
    infantile 751.2
  aorta (ascending) 747.22
    arch 747.10
    arteriosclerotic 440.0
    calcified 440.0
  aortic (valve) (*see also* Stenosis, aortic) 424.1
    congenital 746.3
  aqueduct of Sylvius (congenital) 742.3
    with spina bifida (*see also* Spina bifida) 741.0
    acquired 331.4
  artery 447.1
    basilar - *see* Narrowing, artery, basilar
    carotid (common) (internal) - *see* Narrowing, artery, carotid
    celiac 447.4
    cerebral 437.0
      congenital 747.81
      due to
        embolism (*see also* Embolism, brain) 434.1
        thrombus (*see also* Thrombosis, brain) 434.0
    congenital (peripheral) 747.60
      cerebral 747.81
      coronary 746.85
      gastrointestinal 747.61
      lower limb 747.64
      renal 747.62
      retinal 743.58
      specified NEC 747.69
      spinal 747.82
      umbilical 747.5
      upper limb 747.63
    coronary - *see* Arteriosclerosis, coronary
      congenital 746.85
    precerebral - *see* Narrowing, artery, precerebral NEC
    pulmonary (congenital) 747.3
      acquired 417.8
    renal 440.1
    vertebral - *see* Narrowing, artery, vertebral
  auditory canal (congenital) (external) 744.02
    acquired (*see also* Stricture, ear canal, acquired) 380.50

◀ **New**   ◀▥ **Revised**

Stricture (Continued)

bile duct or passage (any) (postoperative) (see also Obstruction, biliary) 576.2
  congenital 751.61
bladder 596.8
  congenital 753.6
  neck 596.0
    congenital 753.6
bowel (see also Obstruction, intestine) 560.9
brain 348.8
bronchus 519.1
  syphilitic 095.8
cardia (stomach) 537.89
  congenital 750.7
cardiac - see also Disease, heart orifice (stomach) 537.89
cardiovascular (see also Disease, cardiovascular) 429.2
carotid artery - see Narrowing, artery, carotid
cecum (see also Obstruction, intestine) 560.9
cervix, cervical (canal) 622.4
  congenital 752.49
  in pregnancy or childbirth 654.6
    affecting fetus or newborn 763.89
    causing obstructed labor 660.2
      affecting fetus or newborn 763.1
colon (see also Obstruction, intestine) 560.9
  congenital 751.2
colostomy 569.62
common bile duct (see also Obstruction, biliary) 576.2
  congenital 751.61
coronary (artery) - see Arteriosclerosis, coronary
  congenital 746.85
cystic duct (see also Obstruction, gallbladder) 575.2
  congenital 751.61
cystostomy 997.5
digestive organs NEC, congenital 751.8
duodenum 537.3
  congenital 751.1
ear canal (external) (congenital) 744.02
  acquired 380.50
    secondary to
      inflammation 380.53
      surgery 380.52
      trauma 380.51
ejaculatory duct 608.85
enterostomy 569.62
esophagostomy 530.87 ◄
esophagus (corrosive) (peptic) 530.3
  congenital 750.3
  syphilitic 095.8
    congenital 090.5
Eustachian tube (see also Obstruction, Eustachian tube) 381.60
  congenital 744.24
fallopian tube 628.2
  gonococcal (chronic) 098.37
    acute 098.17
  tuberculous (see also Tuberculosis) 016.6
gallbladder (see also Obstruction, gallbladder) 575.2
  congenital 751.69
glottis 478.74
heart - see also Disease, heart
  congenital NEC 746.89

Stricture (Continued)

heart (Continued)
  valve - see also Endocarditis
    congenital NEC 746.89
      aortic 746.3
      mitral 746.5
      pulmonary 746.02
      tricuspid 746.1
hepatic duct (see also Obstruction, biliary) 576.2
hourglass, of stomach 537.6
hymen 623.3
hypopharynx 478.29
intestine (see also Obstruction, intestine) 560.9
  congenital (small) 751.1
    large 751.2
  ischemic 557.1
lacrimal
  canaliculi 375.53
    congenital 743.65
  punctum 375.52
    congenital 743.65
  sac 375.54
    congenital 743.65
lacrimonasal duct 375.56
  congenital 743.65
  neonatal 375.55
larynx 478.79
  congenital 748.3
  syphilitic 095.8
    congenital 090.5
lung 518.89
meatus
  ear (congenital) 744.02
    acquired (see also Stricture, ear canal, acquired) 380.50
  osseous (congenital) (ear) 744.03
    acquired (see also Stricture, ear canal, acquired) 380.50
  urinarius (see also Stricture, urethra) 598.9
    congenital 753.6
mitral (valve) (see also Stenosis, mitral) 394.0
  congenital 746.5
  specified cause, except rheumatic 424.0
myocardium, myocardial (see also Degeneration, myocardial) 429.1
  hypertrophic subaortic (idiopathic) 425.1
nares (anterior) (posterior) 478.1
  congenital 748.0
nasal duct 375.56
  congenital 743.65
  neonatal 375.55
nasolacrimal duct 375.56
  congenital 743.65
  neonatal 375.55
nasopharynx 478.29
  syphilitic 095.8
nephrostomy 997.5
nose 478.1
  congenital 748.0
nostril (anterior) (posterior) 478.1
  congenital 748.0
organ or site, congenital NEC - see Atresia
osseous meatus (congenital) (ear) 744.03
  acquired (see also Stricture, ear canal, acquired) 380.50
os uteri (see also Stricture, cervix) 622.4
oviduct - see Stricture, fallopian tube
pelviureteric junction 593.3

Stricture (Continued)

pharynx (dilation) 478.29
prostate 602.8
pulmonary, pulmonic
  artery (congenital) 747.3
    acquired 417.8
    noncongenital 417.8
  infundibulum (congenital) 746.83
  valve (see also Endocarditis, pulmonary) 424.3
    congenital 746.02
  vein (congenital) 747.49
    acquired 417.8
  vessel NEC 417.8
punctum lacrimale 375.52
  congenital 743.65
pylorus (hypertrophic) 537.0
  adult 537.0
  congenital 750.5
  infantile 750.5
rectosigmoid 569.89
rectum (sphincter) 569.2
  congenital 751.2
  due to
    chemical burn 947.3
    irradiation 569.2
    lymphogranuloma venereum 099.1
  gonococcal 098.7
  inflammatory 099.1
  syphilitic 095.8
  tuberculous (see also Tuberculosis) 014.8
renal artery 440.1
salivary duct or gland (any) 527.8
sigmoid (flexure) (see also Obstruction, intestine) 560.9
spermatic cord 608.85
stoma (following) (of)
  colostomy 569.62
  cystostomy 997.5
  enterostomy 569.62
  esophagostomy 530.87
  gastrostomy 536.42
  ileostomy 569.62
  nephrostomy 997.5
  tracheostomy 519.02
  ureterostomy 997.5
stomach 537.89
  congenital 750.7
  hourglass 537.6
subaortic 746.81
  hypertrophic (acquired) (idiopathic) 425.1
subglottic 478.74
syphilitic NEC 095.8
tendon (sheath) 727.81
trachea 519.1
  congenital 748.3
  syphilitic 095.8
  tuberculous (see also Tuberculosis) 012.8
tracheostomy 519.02
tricuspid (valve) (see also Endocarditis, tricuspid) 397.0
  congenital 746.1
  nonrheumatic 424.2
tunica vaginalis 608.85
ureter (postoperative) 593.3
  congenital 753.29
  tuberculous (see also Tuberculosis) 016.2
ureteropelvic junction 593.3
  congenital 753.21
ureterovesical orifice 593.3
  congenital 753.22

◄

ICD-9-CM

S

Vol. 2

Stricture (Continued)
  urethra (anterior) (meatal) (organic)
    (posterior) (spasmodic) 598.9
    associated with schistosomiasis (see
      also Schistosomiasis) 120.9
      [598.01]
    congenital (valvular) 753.6
    due to
      infection 598.00
        syphilis 095.8 [598.01]
      trauma 598.1
    gonococcal 098.2 [598.01]
    gonorrheal 098.2 [598.01]
    infective 598.00
    late effect of injury 598.1
    postcatheterization 598.2
    postobstetric 598.1
    postoperative 598.2
    specified cause NEC 598.8
    syphilitic 095.8 [598.01]
    traumatic 598.1
    valvular, congenital 753.6
  urinary meatus (see also Stricture, ure-
    thra) 598.9
    congenital 753.6
  uterus, uterine 621.5
    os (external) (internal) - see Stricture,
      cervix
  vagina (outlet) 623.2
    congenital 752.49
  valve (cardiac) (heart) (see also Endo-
    carditis) 424.90
    congenital (cardiac) (heart) NEC
      746.89
      aortic 746.3
      mitral 746.5
      pulmonary 746.02
      tricuspid 746.1
      urethra 753.6
  valvular (see also Endocarditis) 424.90
  vascular graft or shunt 996.1
    vascular or shunt
      atherosclerosis - see Arteriosclero-
        sis, extremities
      embolism 996.74
      occlusion NEC 996.74
      thrombus 996.74
  vas deferens 608.85
    congenital 752.89
  vein 459.2
  vena cava (inferior) (superior) NEC 459.2
    congenital 747.49
  ventricular shunt 996.2
  vesicourethral orifice 596.0
    congenital 753.6
  vulva (acquired) 624.8
Stridor 786.1
  congenital (larynx) 748.3
Stridulous - see condition
Strippling of nails 703.8
Stroke 434.91 ◀▥
  apoplectic (see also Disease, cerebrovas-
    cular, acute) 436
  brain - see Infarct, brain ◀▥
  embolic 434.11 ◀
  epileptic - see Epilepsy
  healed or old V12.59
  heart - see Disease, heart
  heat 992.0
  iatrogenic 997.02
  in evolution 435.9
  ischemic 434.91 ◀
  late effect - see Late effect(s) (of) cere-
    brovascular disease

Stroke (Continued)
  lightning 994.0
  paralytic - see Infarct, brain ◀▥
  postoperative 997.02
  progressive 435.9
  thrombotic 434.01 ◀
Stromatosis, endometrial (M8931/1) 236.0
Strong pulse 785.9
Strongyloides stercoralis infestation
  127.2
Strongyloidiasis 127.2
Strongyloidosis 127.2
Strongylus (gibsoni) infestation 127.7
Strophulus (newborn) 779.89
  pruriginosus 698.2
Struck by lightning 994.0
Struma (see also Goiter) 240.9
  fibrosa 245.3
  Hashimoto (struma lymphomatosa)
    245.2
  lymphomatosa 245.2
  nodosa (simplex) 241.9
    endemic 241.9
    multinodular 241.1
    sporadic 241.9
    toxic or with hyperthyroidism 242.3
      multinodular 242.2
      uninodular 242.1
    toxicosa 242.3
      multinodular 242.2
      uninodular 242.1
    uninodular 241.0
  ovarii (M9090/0) 220
    and carcinoid (M9091/1) 236.2
    malignant (M9090/3) 183.0
  Riedel's (ligneous thyroiditis) 245.3
  scrofulous (see also Tuberculosis) 017.2
  tuberculous (see also Tuberculosis) 017.2
    abscess 017.2
    adenitis 017.2
    lymphangitis 017.2
    ulcer 017.2
Strumipriva cachexia (see also Hypothyroidism) 244.9
Strümpell-Marie disease or spine (ankylosing spondylitis) 720.0
Strümpell-Westphal pseudosclerosis
  (hepatolenticular degeneration) 275.1
Stuart's disease (congenital factor X deficiency) (see also Defect, coagulation)
  286.3
Stuart-Prower factor deficiency (congenital factor X deficiency) (see also Defect, coagulation) 286.3
Students' elbow 727.2
Stuffy nose 478.1
Stump - see also Amputation
  cervix, cervical (healed) 622.8
Stupor 780.09
  catatonic (see also Schizophrenia) 295.2
  circular (see also Psychosis, manic-
    depressive, circular) 296.7
  manic 296.89
  manic-depressive (see also Psychosis,
    affective) 296.89
  mental (anergic) (delusional) 298.9
  psychogenic 298.8
  reaction to exceptional stress (tran-
    sient) 308.2
  traumatic NEC - see also Injury, intra-
    cranial
    with spinal (cord)
      lesion - see Injury, spinal, by site
      shock - see Injury, spinal, by site

Sturge (-Weber) (-Dimitri) disease or
  syndrome (encephalocutaneous an-
  giomatosis) 759.6
Sturge-Kalischer-Weber syndrome (en-
  cephalocutaneous angiomatosis)
  759.6
Stuttering 307.0
Sty, stye 373.11
  external 373.11
  internal 373.12
  meibomian 373.12
Subacidity, gastric 536.8
  psychogenic 306.4
Subacute - see condition
Subarachnoid - see condition
Subclavian steal syndrome 435.2
Subcortical - see condition
Subcostal syndrome 098.86
  nerve compression 354.8
Subcutaneous, subcuticular - see condition
Subdelirium 293.1
Subdural - see condition
Subendocardium - see condition
Subependymoma (M9383/1) 237.5
Suberosis 495.3
Subglossitis - see Glossitis
Subhemophilia 286.0
Subinvolution (uterus) 621.1
  breast (postlactational) (postpartum)
    611.8
  chronic 621.1
  puerperal, postpartum 674.8
Sublingual - see condition
Sublinguitis 527.2
Subluxation - see also Dislocation, by site
  congenital NEC - see also Malposition,
    congenital
    hip (unilateral) 754.32
      with dislocation of other hip
        754.35
      bilateral 754.33
    joint
      lower limb 755.69
      shoulder 755.59
      upper limb 755.59
    lower limb (joint) 755.69
    shoulder (joint) 755.59
    upper limb (joint) 755.59
  lens 379.32
    anterior 379.33
    posterior 379.34
  rotary, cervical region of spine - see
    Fracture, vertebra, cervical
Submaxillary - see condition
Submersion (fatal) (nonfatal) 994.1
Submissiveness (undue), in child 313.0
Submucous - see condition
Subnormal, subnormality
  accommodation (see also Disorder, ac-
    commodation) 367.9
  mental (see also Retardation, mental)
    319
    mild 317
    moderate 318.0
    profound 318.2
    severe 318.1
  temperature (accidental) 991.6
    not associated with low environ-
      mental temperature 780.99
Subphrenic - see condition
Subscapular nerve - see condition
Subseptus uterus 752.3
Subsiding appendicitis 542
Substernal thyroid (see also Goiter) 240.9
  congenital 759.2

◀ **New** ◀▥ **Revised**

Substitution disorder 300.11
Subtentorial - *see* condition
Subtertian
  fever 084.0
  malaria (fever) 084.0
Subthyroidism (acquired) (*see also* Hypo-
  thyroidism) 244.9
  congenital 243
Succenturiata placenta - *see* Placenta, ab-
  normal
Succussion sounds, chest 786.7
Sucking thumb, child 307.9
Sudamen 705.1
Sudamina 705.1
Sudanese kala-azar 085.0
Sudden
  death, cause unknown (less than 24
    hours) 798.1
    during childbirth 669.9
    infant 798.0
    puerperal, postpartum 674.9
  hearing loss NEC 388.2
  heart failure (*see also* Failure, heart)
    428.9
  infant death syndrome 798.0
Sudeck's atrophy, disease, or syndrome
  733.7
SUDS (Sudden unexplained death) 798.2
Suffocation (*see also* Asphyxia) 799.0
  by
    bed clothes 994.7
    bunny bag 994.7
    cave-in 994.7
    constriction 994.7
    drowning 994.1
    inhalation
      food or foreign body (*see also* As-
        phyxia, food or foreign body)
        933.1
      oil or gasoline (*see also* Asphyxia,
        food or foreign body) 933.1
    overlying 994.7
    plastic bag 994.7
    pressure 994.7
    strangulation 994.7
  during birth 768.1
  mechanical 994.7
Sugar
  blood
    high 790.29
    low 251.2
  in urine 791.5
Suicide, suicidal (attempted)
  by poisoning - *see* Table of Drugs and
    Chemicals
  risk 300.9
  tendencies 300.9
  trauma NEC (*see also* nature and site
    of injury) 959.9
Suipestifer infection (*see also* Infection,
  Salmonella) 003.9
Sulfatidosis 330.0
**Sulfhemoglobinemia, sulphemoglobine-
  mia** (acquired) (congenital) 289.7
Sumatran mite fever 081.2
Summer - *see* condition
Sunburn 692.71
  dermatitis 692.71
  due to
    other ultraviolet radiation 692.82
      tanning bed 692.82
  first degree 692.71
  second degree 692.76
  third degree 692.77

Sunken
  acetabulum 718.85
  fontanels 756.0
Sunstroke 992.0
Superfecundation
  with fetal loss and retention of one or
    more fetus(es) 651.6
Superfetation 651.9
  with fetal loss and retention of one or
    more fetus(es) 651.6
Superinvolution uterus 621.8
Supernumerary (congenital)
  aortic cusps 746.89
  auditory ossicles 744.04
  bone 756.9
  breast 757.6
  carpal bones 755.56
  cusps, heart valve NEC 746.89
    mitral 746.5
    pulmonary 746.09
  digit(s) 755.00
    finger 755.01
    toe 755.02
  ear (lobule) 744.1
  fallopian tube 752.19
  finger 755.01
  hymen 752.49
  kidney 753.3
  lacrimal glands 743.64
  lacrimonasal duct 743.65
  lobule (ear) 744.1
  mitral cusps 746.5
  muscle 756.82
  nipples 757.6
  organ or site NEC - *see* Accessory
  ossicles, auditory 744.04
  ovary 752.0
  oviduct 752.19
  pulmonic cusps 746.09
  rib 756.3
    cervical or first 756.2
      syndrome 756.2
  roots (of teeth) 520.2
  spinal vertebra 756.19
  spleen 759.0
  tarsal bones 755.67
  teeth 520.1
    causing crowding 524.31 ◀▥
  testis 752.89
  thumb 755.01
  toe 755.02
  uterus 752.2
  vagina 752.49
  vertebra 756.19
Supervision (of)
  contraceptive method previously pre-
    scribed V25.40
    intrauterine device V25.42
    oral contraceptive (pill) V25.41
    specified type NEC V25.49
    subdermal implantable contraceptive
      V25.43
  dietary (for) V65.3
    allergy (food) V65.3
    colitis V65.3
    diabetes mellitus V65.3
    food allergy intolerance V65.3
    gastritis V65.3
    hypercholesterolemia V65.3
    hypoglycemia V65.3
    intolerance (food) V65.3
    obesity V65.3
    specified NEC V65.3
  lactation V24.1
  pregnancy - *see* Pregnancy, supervision
    of

Supplemental teeth 520.1
  causing crowding 524.31 ◀▥
Suppression
  binocular vision 368.31
  lactation 676.5
  menstruation 626.8
  ovarian secretion 256.39
  renal 586
  urinary secretion 788.5
  urine 788.5
Suppuration, suppurative - *see also* condition
  accessory sinus (chronic) (*see also* Si-
    nusitis) 473.9
  adrenal gland 255.8
  antrum (chronic) (*see also* Sinusitis,
    maxillary) 473.0
  bladder (*see also* Cystitis) 595.89
  bowel 569.89
  brain 324.0
    late effect 326
  breast 611.0
    puerperal, postpartum 675.1
  dental periosteum 526.5
  diffuse (skin) 686.00
  ear (middle) (*see also* Otitis media) 382.4
    external (*see also* Otitis, externa)
      380.10
    internal 386.33
  ethmoidal (sinus) (chronic) (*see also* Si-
    nusitis, ethmoidal) 473.2
  fallopian tube (*see also* Salpingo-
    oophoritis) 614.2
  frontal (sinus) (chronic) (*see also* Sinusi-
    tis, frontal) 473.1
  gallbladder (*see also* Cholecystitis,
    acute) 575.0
  gum 523.3
  hernial sac - *see* Hernia, by site
  intestine 569.89
  joint (*see also* Arthritis, suppurative)
    711.0
  labyrinthine 386.33
  lung 513.0
  mammary gland 611.0
    puerperal, postpartum 675.1
  maxilla, maxillary 526.4
    sinus (chronic) (*see also* Sinusitis,
      maxillary) 473.0
  muscle 728.0
  nasal sinus (chronic) (*see also* Sinusitis)
    473.9
  pancreas 577.0
  parotid gland 527.2
  pelvis, pelvic
    female (*see also* Disease, pelvis, in-
      flammatory) 614.4
      acute 614.3
    male (*see also* Peritonitis) 567.2
  pericranial (*see also* Osteomyelitis)
    730.2
  salivary duct or gland (any) 527.2
  sinus (nasal) (*see also* Sinusitis) 473.9
  sphenoidal (sinus) (chronic) (*see also* Si-
    nusitis, sphenoidal) 473.3
  thymus (gland) 254.1
  thyroid (gland) 245.0
  tonsil 474.8
  uterus (*see also* Endometritis) 615.9
  vagina 616.10
  wound - *see also* Wound, open, by site,
    complicated
    dislocation - *see* Dislocation, by site,
      compound

ICD-9-CM

S

Vol. 2

Suppuration, suppurative *(Continued)*
wound *(Continued)*
fracture - *see* Fracture, by site, open
scratch or other superficial injury -
see Injury, superficial, by site
Supraeruption, teeth 524.34 ◀
Supraglottitis 464.50
with obstruction 464.51
Suprapubic drainage 596.8
Suprarenal (gland) - *see* condition
Suprascapular nerve - *see* condition
Suprasellar - *see* condition
Supraspinatus syndrome 726.10
Surfer knots 919.8
infected 919.9
Surgery
cosmetic NEC V50.1
following healed injury or operation
V51
hair transplant V50.0
elective V50.9
breast augmentation or reduction
V50.1
circumcision, ritual or routine (in absence of medical indication)
V50.2
cosmetic NEC V50.1
ear piercing V50.3
face-lift V50.1
following healed injury or operation
V51
hair transplant V50.0
not done because of
contraindication V64.1
patient's decision V64.2
specified reason NEC V64.3
plastic
breast augmentation or reduction
V50.1
cosmetic V50.1
face-lift V50.1
following healed injury or operation
V51
repair of scarred tissue (following
healed injury or operation) V51
specified type NEC V50.8
previous, in pregnancy or childbirth
cervix 654.6
affecting fetus or newborn 763.89
causing obstructed labor 660.2
affecting fetus or newborn
763.1
pelvic soft tissues NEC 654.9
affecting fetus or newborn 763.89
causing obstructed labor 660.2
affecting fetus or newborn
763.1
perineum or vulva 654.8
uterus NEC 654.9
affecting fetus or newborn 763.89
causing obstructed labor 660.2
affecting fetus or newborn 763.1
from previous cesarean delivery
654.2
vagina 654.7
Surgical
abortion - *see* Abortion, legal
emphysema 998.81
kidney (*see also* Pyelitis) 590.80
operation NEC 799.9
procedures, complication or misadventure - *see* Complications, surgical
procedure
shock 998.0

Susceptibility ◀
genetic ◀
to ◀
neoplasm ◀
maglignant, of ◀
breast V84.01 ◀
endometrium V84.04 ◀
other V84.09 ◀
ovary V84.02 ◀
prostate V84.03 ◀
other disease V84.8 ◀
Suspected condition, ruled out (*see also*
Observation, suspected) V71.9
specified condition NEC V71.89
**Suspended uterus, in pregnancy or
childbirth** 654.4
affecting fetus or newborn 763.89
causing obstructed labor 660.2
affecting fetus or newborn 763.1
Sutton's disease 709.09
Sutton and Gull's disease (arteriolar
nephrosclerosis) (*see also* Hypertension, kidney) 403.90
Suture
burst (in external operation wound)
998.32
internal 998.31
inadvertently left in operation wound
998.4
removal V58.3
shirodkar, in pregnancy (with or without cervical incompetence) 654.5
**Swab inadvertently left in operation
wound** 998.4
Swallowed, swallowing
difficulty (*see also* Dysphagia) 787.2
foreign body NEC (*see also* Foreign
body) 938
Swamp fever 100.89
Swan neck hand (intrinsic) 736.09
Sweat(s), sweating
disease or sickness 078.2
excessive (*see also* Hyperhidrosis)
780.8 ◀▥
fetid 705.89
fever 078.2
gland disease 705.9
specified type NEC 705.89
miliary 078.2
night 780.8
Sweeley-Klionsky disease (angiokeratoma corporis diffusum) 272.7
Sweet's syndrome (acute febrile neutrophilic dermatosis) 695.89
Swelling
abdominal (not referable to specific organ) 789.3
adrenal gland, cloudy 255.8
ankle 719.07
anus 787.99
arm 729.81
breast 611.72
Calabar 125.2
cervical gland 785.6
cheek 784.2
chest 786.6
ear 388.8
epigastric 789.3
extremity (lower) (upper) 729.81
eye 379.92
female genital organ 625.8
finger 729.81
foot 729.81
glands 785.6
gum 784.2

Swelling *(Continued)*
hand 729.81
head 784.2
inflammatory - *see* Inflammation
joint (*see also* Effusion, joint) 719.0
tuberculous - *see* Tuberculosis, joint
kidney, cloudy 593.89
leg 729.81
limb 729.81
liver 573.8
lung 786.6
lymph nodes 785.6
mediastinal 786.6
mouth 784.2
muscle (limb) 729.81
neck 784.2
nose or sinus 784.2
palate 784.2
pelvis 789.3
penis 607.83
perineum 625.8
rectum 787.99
scrotum 608.86
skin 782.2
splenic (*see also* Splenomegaly) 789.2
substernal 786.6
superficial, localized (skin) 782.2
testicle 608.86
throat 784.2
toe 729.81
tongue 784.2
tubular (*see also* Disease, renal) 593.9
umbilicus 789.3
uterus 625.8
vagina 625.8
vulva 625.8
wandering, due to Gnathostoma (spinigerum) 128.1
white - *see* Tuberculosis, arthritis
Swift's disease 985.0
Swimmers'
ear (acute) 380.12
itch 120.3
Swimming in the head 780.4
Swollen - *see also* Swelling
glands 785.6
Swyer-James syndrome (unilateral hyperlucent lung) 492.8
Swyer's syndrome (XY pure gonadal
dysgenesis) 752.7
Sycosis 704.8
barbae (not parasitic) 704.8
contagiosa 110.0
lupoid 704.8
mycotic 110.0
parasitic 110.0
vulgaris 704.8
Sydenham's chorea - *see* Chorea, Sydenham's
Sylvatic yellow fever 060.0
Sylvest's disease (epidemic pleurodynia)
074.1
Symblepharon 372.63
congenital 743.62
Symonds' syndrome 348.2
Sympathetic - *see* condition
Sympatheticotonia (*see also* Neuropathy,
peripheral, autonomic) 337.9
Sympathicoblastoma (M9500/3)
specified site - *see* Neoplasm, by site,
malignant
unspecified site 194.0
Sympathicogonioma (M9500/3) - *see*
Sympathicoblastoma

◀ **New**   ◀▥ **Revised**

Sympathoblastoma (M9500/3) - *see* Sympathicoblastoma
Sympathogonioma (M9500/3) - *see* Sympathicoblastoma
Symphalangy (*see also* Syndactylism) 755.10
Symptoms, specified (general) NEC 780.99
  abdomen NEC 789.9
  bone NEC 733.90
  breast NEC 611.79
  cardiac NEC 785.9
  cardiovascular NEC 785.9
  chest NEC 786.9
  development NEC 783.9
  digestive system NEC 787.99
  eye NEC 379.99
  gastrointestinal tract NEC 787.99
  genital organs NEC
    female 625.9
    male 608.9
  head and neck NEC 784.9
  heart NEC 785.9
  joint NEC 719.60
    ankle 719.67
    elbow 719.62
    foot 719.67
    hand 719.64
    hip 719.65
    knee 719.66
    multiple sites 719.69
    pelvic region 719.65
    shoulder (region) 719.61
    specified site NEC 719.68
    wrist 719.63
  larynx NEC 784.9
  limbs NEC 729.89
  lymphatic system NEC 785.9
  menopausal 627.2
  metabolism NEC 783.9
  mouth NEC 528.9
  muscle NEC 728.9
  musculoskeletal NEC 781.99
    limbs NEC 729.89
  nervous system NEC 781.99
  neurotic NEC 300.9
  nutrition, metabolism, and development NEC 783.9
  pelvis NEC 789.9
    female 625.9
  peritoneum NEC 789.9
  respiratory system NEC 786.9
  skin and integument NEC 782.9
  subcutaneous tissue NEC 782.9
  throat NEC 784.9
  tonsil NEC 784.9
  urinary system NEC 788.9
  vascular NEC 785.9
Sympus 759.89
Synarthrosis 719.80
  ankle 719.87
  elbow 719.82
  foot 719.87
  hand 719.84
  hip 719.85
  knee 719.86
  multiple sites 719.89
  pelvic region 719.85
  shoulder (region) 719.81
  specified site NEC 719.88
  wrist 719.83
Syncephalus 759.4
Synchondrosis 756.9
  abnormal (congenital) 756.9
  ischiopubic (van Neck's) 732.1

Synchysis (senile) (vitreous humor) 379.21
  scintillans 379.22
Syncope (near) (pre-) 780.2
  anginosa 413.9
  bradycardia 427.89
  cardiac 780.2
  carotid sinus 337.0
  complicating delivery 669.2
  due to lumbar puncture 349.0
  fatal 798.1
  heart 780.2
  heat 992.1
  laryngeal 786.2
  tussive 786.2
  vasoconstriction 780.2
  vasodepressor 780.2
  vasomotor 780.2
  vasovagal 780.2
Syncytial infarct - *see* Placenta, abnormal
Syndactylism, syndactyly (multiple sites) 755.10
  fingers (without fusion of bone) 755.11
    with fusion of bone 755.12
  toes (without fusion of bone) 755.13
    with fusion of bone 755.14
Syndrome - *see also* Disease
  abdominal
    acute 789.0
    migraine 346.2
    muscle deficiency 756.79
  Abercrombie's (amyloid degeneration) 277.3
  abnormal innervation 374.43
  abstinence
    alcohol 291.81
    drug 292.0
  Abt-Letterer-Siwe (acute histiocytosis X) (M9722/3) 202.5
  Achard-Thiers (adrenogenital) 255.2
  acid pulmonary aspiration 997.3
    obstetric (Mendelson's) 668.0
  acquired immune deficiency 042
  acquired immunodeficiency 042
  acrocephalosyndactylism 755.55
  acute abdominal 789.0
  acute chest 517.3
  acute coronary 411.1
  Adair-Dighton (brittle bones and blue sclera, deafness) 756.51
  Adams-Stokes (-Morgagni) (syncope with heart block) 426.9
  Addisonian 255.4
  Adie (-Holmes) (pupil) 379.46
  adiposogenital 253.8
  adrenal
    hemorrhage 036.3
    meningococcic 036.3
  adrenocortical 255.3
  adrenogenital (acquired) (congenital) 255.2
    feminizing 255.2
    iatrogenic 760.79
    virilism (acquired) (congenital) 255.2
  affective organic NEC 293.89
    drug-induced 292.84
  afferent loop NEC 537.89
  African macroglobulinemia 273.3
  Ahumada-Del Castillo (nonpuerperal galactorrhea and amenorrhea) 253.1
  air blast concussion - *see* Injury, internal, by site
  Albright (-Martin) (pseudohypoparathyroidism) 275.49
  Albright-McCune-Sternberg (osteitis fibrosa disseminata) 756.59

Syndrome (*Continued*)
  alcohol withdrawal 291.81
  Alder's (leukocyte granulation anomaly) 288.2
  Aldrich (-Wiskott) (eczema-thrombocytopenia) 279.12
  Alibert-Bazin (mycosis fungoides) (M9700/3) 202.1
  Alice in Wonderland 293.89
  Allen-Masters 620.6
  Alligator baby (ichthyosis congenita) 757.1
  Alport's (hereditary hematuria-nephropathy-deafness) 759.89
  Alvarez (transient cerebral ischemia) 435.9
  alveolar capillary block 516.3
  Alzheimer's 331.0
    with dementia - *see* Alzheimer's, dementia
  amnestic (confabulatory) 294.0
    alcohol-induced persisting 291.1 ◀▥
    drug-induced 292.83
    posttraumatic 294.0
  amotivational 292.89
  amyostatic 275.1
  amyotrophic lateral sclerosis 335.20
  Angelman 759.89
  angina (*see also* Angina) 413.9
  ankyloglossia superior 750.0
  anterior
    chest wall 786.52
    compartment (tibial) 958.8
    spinal artery 433.8
      compression 721.1
    tibial (compartment) 958.8
  antibody deficiency 279.00
    agammaglobulinemic 279.00
    congenital 279.04
    hypogammaglobulinemic 279.00
  anticardiolipin antibody 795.79
  antimongolism 758.39 ◀▥
  antiphospholipid antibody 795.79
  Anton (-Babinski) (hemiasomatognosia) 307.9
  anxiety (*see also* Anxiety) 300.00
    organic 293.84
  aortic
    arch 446.7
    bifurcation (occlusion) 444.0
    ring 747.21
  Apert's (acrocephalosyndactyly) 755.55
  Apert-Gallais (adrenogenital) 255.2
  aphasia-apraxia-alexia 784.69
  "approximate answers" 300.16
  arcuate ligament (-celiac axis) 447.4
  arcus aortae 446.7
  arc welders' 370.24
  argentaffin, argentaffinoma 259.2
  Argonz-Del Castillo (nonpuerperal galactorrhea and amenorrhea) 253.1
  Argyll Robertson's (syphilitic) 094.89
    nonsyphilitic 379.45
  arm-shoulder (*see also* Neuropathy, peripheral, autonomic) 337.9
  Arnold-Chiari (*see also* Spina bifida) 741.0
    type I 348.4
    type II 741.0
    type III 742.0
    type IV 742.2
  Arrillaga-Ayerza (pulmonary artery sclerosis with pulmonary hypertension) 416.0

ICD-9-CM

S

Vol. 2

Syndrome *(Continued)*
arteriomesenteric duodenum occlusion 537.89
arteriovenous steal 996.73
arteritis, young female (obliterative brachiocephalic) 446.7
aseptic meningitis - *see* Meningitis, aseptic
Asherman's 621.5
Asperger's 299.8 ◀
asphyctic (*see also* Anxiety) 300.00
aspiration, of newborn, massive or meconium 770.1
ataxia-telangiectasia 334.8
Audry's (acropachyderma) 757.39
auriculotemporal 350.8
autosomal - *see also* Abnormal, autosomes NEC
  deletion 758.39 ◀▥
    5p 758.31 ◀
    22g11.2 758.32 ◀
Avellis' 344.89
Axenfeld's 743.44
Ayerza (-Arrillaga) (pulmonary artery sclerosis with pulmonary hypertension) 416.0
Baader's (erythema multiforme exudativum) 695.1
Baastrup's 721.5
Babinski (-Vaquez) (cardiovascular syphilis) 093.89
Babinski-Fröhlich (adiposogenital dystrophy) 253.8
Babinski-Nageotte 344.89
Bagratuni's (temporal arteritis) 446.5
Bakwin-Krida (craniometaphyseal dysplasia) 756.89
Balint's (psychic paralysis of visual disorientation) 368.16
Ballantyne (-Runge) (postmaturity) 766.22
ballooning posterior leaflet 424.0
Banti's - *see* Cirrhosis, liver
Bard-Pic's (carcinoma, head of pancreas) 157.0
Bardet-Biedl (obesity, polydactyly, and mental retardation) 759.89
Barlow's (mitral valve prolapse) 424.0
Barlow (-Möller) (infantile scurvy) 267
Baron Munchausen's 301.51
Barré-Guillain 357.0
Barré-Liéou (posterior cervical sympathetic) 723.2
Barrett's (chronic peptic ulcer of esophagus) 530.85
Bársony-Pólgar (corkscrew esophagus) 530.5
Bársony-Teschendorf (corkscrew esophagus) 530.5
Bartter's (secondary hyperaldosteronism with juxtaglomerular hyperplasia) 255.13
Basedow's (exophthalmic goiter) 242.0
basilar artery 435.0
basofrontal 377.04
Bassen-Kornzweig (abetalipoproteinemia) 272.5
Batten-Steinert 359.2
battered
  adult 995.81
  baby or child 995.54
  spouse 995.81
Baumgarten-Cruveilhier (cirrhosis of liver) 571.5

Syndrome *(Continued)*
Beals 759.82 ◀
Bearn-Kunkel (-Slater) (lupoid hepatitis) 571.49
Beau's (*see also* Degeneration, myocardial) 429.1
Bechterew-Strümpell-Marie (ankylosing spondylitis) 720.0
Beck's (anterior spinal artery occlusion) 433.8
Beckwith (-Wiedemann) 759.89
Behçet's 136.1
Bekhterev-Strümpell-Marie (ankylosing spondylitis) 720.0
Benedikt's 344.89
Béquez César (-Steinbrinck-Chédiak-Higashi) (congenital gigantism of peroxidase granules) 288.2
Bernard-Horner (*see also* Neuropathy, peripheral, autonomic) 337.9
Bernard-Sergent (acute adrenocortical insufficiency) 255.4
Bernhardt-Roth 355.1
Bernheim's (*see also* Failure, heart) 428.0
Bertolotti's (sacralization of fifth lumbar vertebra) 756.15
Besnier-Boeck-Schaumann (sarcoidosis) 135
Bianchi's (aphasia-apraxia-alexia syndrome) 784.69
Biedl-Bardet (obesity, polydactyly, and mental retardation) 759.89
Biemond's (obesity, polydactyly, and mental retardation) 759.89
big spleen 289.4
bilateral polycystic ovarian 256.4
Bing-Horton's 346.2
Biörck (-Thorson) (malignant carcinoid) 259.2
Blackfan-Diamond (congenital hypoplastic anemia) 284.0
black lung 500
black widow spider bite 989.5
bladder neck (*see also* Incontinence, urine) 788.30
blast (concussion) - *see* Blast, injury
blind loop (postoperative) 579.2
Block-Siemens (incontinentia pigmenti) 757.33
Bloch-Sulzberger (incontinentia pigmenti) 757.33
Bloom (-Machacek) (-Torre) 757.39
Blount-Barber (tibia vara) 732.4
blue
  bloater 491.20
    with ◀▥
      acute bronchitis 491.22 ◀
      exacerbation (acute) 491.21 ◀
  diaper 270.0
  drum 381.02
  sclera 756.51
  toe 445.02
Boder-Sedgwick (ataxia-telangiectasia) 334.8
Boerhaave's (spontaneous esophageal rupture) 530.4
Bonnevie-Ullrich 758.6
Bonnier's 386.19
Bouillaud's (rheumatic heart disease) 391.9
Bourneville (-Pringle) (tuberous sclerosis) 759.5
Bouveret (-Hoffmann) (paroxysmal tachycardia) 427.2

Syndrome *(Continued)*
brachial plexus 353.0
Brachman-de Lange (Amsterdam dwarf, mental retardation, and brachycephaly) 759.89
bradycardia-tachycardia 427.81
Brailsford-Morquio (dystrophy) (mucopolysaccharidosis IV) 277.5
brain (acute) (chronic) (nonpsychotic) (organic) (with behavioral reaction) (with neurotic reaction) 310.9
with
  presenile brain disease (*see also* Dementia, presenile) 290.10
  psychosis, psychotic reaction (*see also* Psychosis, organic) 294.9
chronic alcoholic 291.2
congenital (*see also* Retardation, mental) 319
postcontusional 310.2
posttraumatic
  nonpsychotic 310.2
  psychotic 293.9
    acute 293.0
    chronic (*see also* Psychosis, organic) 294.8
    subacute 293.1
psycho-organic (*see also* Syndrome, psycho-organic) 310.9
psychotic (*see also* Psychosis, organic) 294.9
senile (*see also* Dementia, senile) 290.0
branchial arch 744.41
Brandt's (acrodermatitis enteropathica) 686.8
Brennemann's 289.2
Briquet's 300.81
Brissaud-Meige (infantile myxedema) 244.9
broad ligament laceration 620.6
Brock's (atelectasis due to enlarged lymph nodes) 518.0
Brown's tendon sheath 378.61
Brown-Séquard 344.89
brown spot 756.59
Brugada 746.89
Brugsch's (acropachyderma) 757.39
bubbly lung 770.7
Buchem's (hyperostosis corticalis) 733.3
Budd-Chiari (hepatic vein thrombosis) 453.0
Büdinger-Ludloff-Läwen 717.89
bulbar 335.22
  lateral (*see also* Disease, cerebrovascular, acute) 436
Bullis fever 082.8
bundle of Kent (anomalous atrioventricular excitation) 426.7
Burger-Grutz (essential familial hyperlipemia) 272.3
Burke's (pancreatic insufficiency and chronic neutropenia) 577.8
Burnett's (milk-alkali) 275.42
Burnier's (hypophyseal dwarfism) 253.3
burning feet 266.2
Bywaters' 958.5
Caffey's (infantile cortical hyperostosis) 756.59
Calvé-Legg-Perthes (osteochrondrosis, femoral capital) 732.1
Caplan (-Colinet) syndrome 714.81
capsular thrombosis (*see also* Thrombosis, brain) 434.0
carcinogenic thrombophlebitis 453.1
carcinoid 259.2

Syndrome (*Continued*)
cardiac asthma (*see also* Failure, ventricular, left) 428.1
cardiacos negros 416.0
cardiopulmonary obesity 278.8
cardiorenal (*see also* Hypertension, cardiorenal) 404.90
cardiorespiratory distress (idiopathic), newborn 769
cardiovascular renal (*see also* Hypertension, cardiorenal) 404.90
cardiovasorenal 272.7
Carini's (ichthyosis congenita) 757.1
carotid
    artery (internal) 435.8
    body or sinus 337.0
carpal tunnel 354.0
Carpenter's 759.89
Cassidy (-Scholte) (malignant carcinoid) 259.2
cat-cry 758.31 ◀▥
cauda equina 344.60
causalgia 355.9
    lower limb 355.71
    upper limb 354.4
cavernous sinus 437.6
celiac 579.0
    artery compression 447.4
    axis 447.4
cerebellomedullary malformation (*see also* Spina bifida) 741.0
cerebral gigantism 253.0
cerebrohepatorenal 759.89
cervical (root) (spine) NEC 723.8
    disc 722.71
    posterior, sympathetic 723.2
    rib 353.0
    sympathetic paralysis 337.0
    traumatic (acute) NEC 847.0
cervicobrachial (diffuse) 723.3
cervicocranial 723.2
cervicodorsal outlet 353.2
Céstan's 344.89
Céstan (-Raymond) 433.8
Céstan-Chenais 344.89
chancriform 114.1
Charcôt's (intermittent claudication) 443.9
    angina cruris 443.9
    due to atherosclerosis 440.21
Charcôt-Marie-Tooth 356.1
Charcôt-Weiss-Baker 337.0
CHARGE association 759.89 ◀
Cheadle (-Möller) (-Barlow) (infantile scurvy) 267
Chédiak-Higashi (-Steinbrink) (congenital gigantism of peroxidase granules) 288.2
chest wall 786.52
Chiari's (hepatic vein thrombosis) 453.0
Chiari-Frommel 676.6
chiasmatic 368.41
Chilaiditi's (subphrenic displacement, colon) 751.4
chondroectodermal dysplasia 756.55
chorea-athetosis-agitans 275.1
Christian's (chronic histiocytosis X) 277.89
chromosome 4 short arm deletion 758.39 ◀▥
Churg-Strauss 446.4
Clarke-Hadfield (pancreatic infantilism) 577.8
Claude's 352.6

Syndrome (*Continued*)
Claude Bernard-Horner (*see also* Neuropathy, peripheral, autonomic) 337.9
Clérambault's
    automatism 348.8
    erotomania 297.8
Clifford's (postmaturity) 766.22
climacteric 627.2
Clouston's (hidrotic ectodermal dysplasia) 757.31
clumsiness 315.4
Cockayne's (microencephaly and dwarfism) 759.89
Cockayne-Weber (epidermolysis bullosa) 757.39
Coffin-Lowry 759.89
Cogan's (nonsyphilitic interstitial keratitis) 370.52
cold injury (newborn) 778.2
Collet (-Sicard) 352.6
combined immunity deficiency 279.2
compartment(al) (anterior) (deep) (posterior) (tibial) 958.8
    nontraumatic 729.9
compression 958.5
    cauda equina 344.60
        with neurogenic bladder 344.61
concussion 310.2
congenital
    affecting more than one system 759.7
        specified type NEC 759.89
    facial diplegia 352.6
    muscular hypertrophy-cerebral 759.89
congestion-fibrosis (pelvic) 625.5
conjunctivourethrosynovial 099.3
Conn (-Louis) (primary aldosteronism) 255.12
Conradi (-Hünermann) (chondrodysplasia calcificans congenita) 756.59
conus medullaris 336.8
Cooke-Apert-Gallais (adrenogenital) 255.2
Cornelia de Lange's (Amsterdam dwarf, mental retardation, and brachycephaly) 759.8
coronary insufficiency or intermediate 411.1
cor pulmonale 416.9
corticosexual 255.2
Costen's (complex) 524.60
costochondral junction 733.6
costoclavicular 353.0
costovertebral 253.0
Cotard's (paranoia) 297.1
Cowden 759.6
craniovertebral 723.2
Creutzfeldt-Jakob 046.1
    with dementia
        with behavioral disturbance 046.1 [294.11]
        without behavioral disturbance 046.1 [294.10]
crib death 798.0
cricopharyngeal 787.2
cri-du-chat 758.31 ◀▥
Crigler-Najjar (congenital hyperbilirubinemia) 277.4
crocodile tears 351.8
Cronkhite-Canada 211.3
croup 464.4
CRST (cutaneous systemic sclerosis) 710.1

Syndrome (*Continued*)
crush 958.5
crushed lung (*see also* Injury, internal, lung) 861.20
Cruveilhier-Baumgarten (cirrhosis of liver) 571.5
cubital tunnel 354.2
Cuiffini-Pancoast (M8010/3) (carcinoma, pulmonary apex) 162.3
Curschmann (-Batten) (-Steinert) 359.2
Cushing's (iatrogenic) (idiopathic) (pituitary basophilism) (pituitary-dependent) 255.0
    overdose or wrong substance given or taken 962.0
Cyriax's (slipping rib) 733.99
cystic duct stump 576.0
Da Costa's (neurocirculatory asthenia) 306.2
Dameshek's (erythroblastic anemia) 282.49
Dana-Putnam (subacute combined sclerosis with pernicious anemia) 281.0 [336.2]
Danbolt (-Closs) (acrodermatitis enteropathica) 686.8
Dandy-Walker (atresia, foramen of Magendie) 742.3
    with spina bifida (*see also* Spina bifida) 741.0
Danlos' 756.83
Davies-Colley (slipping rib) 733.99
dead fetus 641.3
defeminization 255.2
defibrination (*see also* Fibrinolysis) 286.6
Degos' 447.8
Deiters' nucleus 386.19
Déjérine-Roussy 348.8
Déjérine-Thomas 333.0
de Lange's (Amsterdam dwarf, mental retardation, and brachycephaly) (Cornelia) 759.89
Del Castillo's (germinal aplasia) 606.0
deletion chromosomes 758.39 ◀▥
delusional
    induced by drug 292.11
dementia-aphonia, of childhood (*see also* Psychosis, childhood) 299.1
demyelinating NEC 341.9
denial visual hallucination 307.9
depersonalization 300.6
Dercum's (adiposis dolorosa) 272.8
de Toni-Fanconi (-Debré) (cystinosis) 270.0
diabetes-dwarfism-obesity (juvenile) 258.1
diabetes mellitus-hypertension-nephrosis 250.4 [581.81]
diabetes mellitus in newborn infant 775.1
diabetes-nephrosis 250.4 [581.81]
diabetic amyotrophy 250.6 [358.1]
Diamond-Blackfan (congenital hypoplastic anemia) 284.0
Diamond-Gardner (autoerythrocyte sensitization) 287.2
DIC (diffuse or disseminated intravascular coagulopathy) (*see also* Fibrinolysis) 286.6
diencephalohypophyseal NEC 253.8
diffuse cervicobrachial 723.3
diffuse obstructive pulmonary 496
DiGeorge's (thymic hypoplasia) 279.11

ICD-9-CM
S
Vol. 2

Syndrome (*Continued*)

Dighton's 756.51

Di Guglielmo's (erythremic myelosis) (M9841/3) 207.0

disc - *see* Displacement, intervertebral disc

discogenic - *see* Displacement, intervertebral disc

disequilibrium 276.9

disseminated platelet thrombosis 446.6

Ditthomska 307.81

Doan-Wiseman (primary splenic neutropenia) 288.0

Döhle body-panmyelopathic 288.2

Donohue's (leprechaunism) 259.8

dorsolateral medullary (*see also* Disease, cerebrovascular, acute) 436

double whammy 360.81

Down's (mongolism) 758.0

Dresbach's (elliptocytosis) 282.1

Dressler's (postmyocardial infarction) 411.0

   hemoglobinuria 283.2

drug withdrawal, infant, of dependent mother 779.5

dry skin 701.1

   eye 375.15

DSAP (disseminated superficial actinic porokeratosis) 692.75

Duane's (retraction) 378.71

Duane-Stilling-Türk (ocular retraction syndrome) 378.71

Dubin-Johnson (constitutional hyperbilirubinemia) 277.4

Dubin-Sprinz (constitutional hyperbilirubinemia) 277.4

Duchenne's 335.22

due to abnormality

   autosomal NEC (*see also* Abnormal, autosomes NEC) 758.5

      13 758.1

      18 758.2

      21 or 22 758.0

      D₁ 758.1

      E₃ 758.2

      G 758.0

   chromosomal 758.89

      sex 758.81

dumping 564.2

   nonsurgical 536.8

Duplay's 726.2

Dupré's (meningism) 781.6

Dyke-Young (acquired macrocytic hemolytic anemia) 283.9

dyspraxia 315.4

dystocia, dystrophia 654.9

Eagle-Barret 756.71

Eales' 362.18

Eaton-Lambert (*see also* Neoplasm, by site, malignant) 199.1 *[358.1]*

Ebstein's (downward displacement, tricuspid valve into right ventricle) 746.2

ectopic ACTH secretion 255.0

eczema-thrombocytopenia 279.12

Eddowes' (brittle bones and blue sclera) 756.51

Edwards' 758.2

efferent loop 537.89

effort (aviators') (psychogenic) 306.2

Ehlers-Danlos 756.83

Eisenmenger's (ventricular septal defect) 745.4

Ekbom's (restless legs) 333.99

Syndrome (*Continued*)

Ekman's (brittle bones and blue sclera) 756.51

electric feet 266.2

Elephant man 237.71

Ellison-Zollinger (gastric hypersecretion with pancreatic islet cell tumor) 251.5

Ellis-van Creveld (chondroectodermal dysplasia) 756.55

embryonic fixation 270.2

empty sella (turcica) 253.8

endocrine-hypertensive 255.3

Engel-von Recklinghausen (osteitis fibrosa cystica) 252.01 ◀▥

enteroarticular 099.3

entrapment - *see* Neuropathy, entrapment

eosinophilia myalgia 710.5

epidemic vomiting 078.82

Epstein's - *see* Nephrosis

Erb (-Oppenheim)-Goldflam 358.00

Erdheim's (acromegalic macrospondylitis) 253.0

Erlacher-Blount (tibia vara) 732.4

erythrocyte fragmentation 283.19

euthyroid sick 790.94

Evans' (thrombocytopenic purpura) 287.3

excess cortisol, iatrogenic 255.0

exhaustion 300.5

extrapyramidal 333.90

eyelid-malar-mandible 756.0

eye retraction 378.71

Faber's (achlorhydric anemia) 280.9

Fabry (-Anderson) (angiokeratoma corporis diffusum) 272.7

facet 724.8

Fallot's 745.2

falx (*see also* Hemorrhage, brain) 431

familial eczema-thrombocytopenia 279.12

Fanconi's (anemia) (congenital pancytopenia) 284.0

Fanconi (-de Toni) (-Debré) (cystinosis) 270.0

Farber (-Uzman) (disseminated lipogranulomatosis) 272.8

fatigue NEC 300.5

   chronic 780.71

faulty bowel habit (idiopathic megacolon) 564.7

FDH (focal dermal hypoplasia) 757.39

fecal reservoir 560.39

Feil-Klippel (brevicollis) 756.16

Felty's (rheumatoid arthritis with splenomegaly and leukopenia) 714.1

fertile eunuch 257.2

fetal alcohol 760.71

   late effect 760.71

fibrillation-flutter 427.32

fibrositis (periarticular) 729.0

Fiedler's (acute isolated myocarditis) 422.91

Fiessinger-Leroy (-Reiter) 099.3

Fiessinger-Rendu (erythema multiforme exudativum) 695.1

first arch 756.0

Fisher's 357.0

Fitz's (acute hemorrhagic pancreatitis) 577.0

Fitz-Hugh and Curtis 098.86

   due to:

      Chlamydia trachomatis 099.56

      Neisseria gonorrhorea (gonococcal peritonitis) 098.86

Syndrome (*Continued*)

Flajani (-Basedow) (exophthalmic goiter) 242.0

floppy

   infant 781.99

   valve (mitral) 424.0

flush 259.2

Foix-Alajouanine 336.1

Fong's (hereditary osteo-onychodysplasia) 756.89

foramen magnum 348.4

Forbes-Albright (nonpuerperal amenorrhea and lactation associated with pituitary tumor) 253.1

Foster-Kennedy 377.04

Foville's (peduncular) 344.89

fragile X 759.83

Franceschetti's (mandibulofacial dysostosis) 756.0

Fraser's 759.89

Freeman-Sheldon 759.89

Frey's (auriculotemporal) 705.22 ◀▥

Friderichsen-Waterhouse 036.3

Friedrich-Erb-Arnold (acropachyderma) 757.39

Fröhlich's (adiposogenital dystrophy) 253.8

Froin's 336.8

Frommel-Chiari 676.6

frontal lobe 310.0

Fukuhara 277.87 ◀

Fuller Albright's (osteitis fibrosa disseminata) 756.59

functional

   bowel 564.9

   prepubertal castrate 752.89

Gaisbock's (polycythemia hypertonica) 289.0

ganglion (basal, brain) 333.90

   geniculi 351.1

Ganser's, hysterical 300.16

Gardner-Diamond (autoerythrocyte sensitization) 287.2

gastroesophageal junction 530.0

gastroesophageal laceration-hemorrhage 530.7

gastrojejunal loop obstruction 537.89

Gayet-Wernicke's (superior hemorrhagic polioencephalitis) 265.1

Gee-Herter-Heubner (nontropical sprue) 579.0

Gélineau's (*see also* Narcolepsy) 347.00 ◀▥

genito-anorectal 099.1

Gerhardt's (vocal cord paralysis) 478.30

Gerstmann's (finger agnosia) 784.69

Gilbert's 277.4

Gilford (-Hutchinson) (progeria) 259.8

Gilles de la Tourette's 307.23

Gillespie's (dysplasia oculodentodigitalis) 759.89

Glénard's (enteroptosis) 569.89

Glinski-Simmonds (pituitary cachexia) 253.2

glucuronyl transferase 277.4

glue ear 381.20

Goldberg (-Maxwell) (-Morris) (testicular feminization) 257.8

Goldenhar's (oculoauriculovertebral dysplasia) 756.0

Goldflam-Erb 358.00

Goltz-Gorlin (dermal hypoplasia) 757.39

Good's 279.06

Goodpasture's (pneumorenal) 446.21

Gopalan's (burning feet) 266.2

Syndrome *(Continued)*
  Gorlin-Chaudhry-Moss 759.89
  Gougerot (-Houwer)-Sjögren (kerato-
    conjunctivitis sicca) 710.2
  Gougerot-Blum (pigmented purpuric
    lichenoid dermatitis) 709.1
  Gougerot-Carteaud (confluent reticu-
    late papillomatosis) 701.8
  Gouley's (constrictive pericarditis) 423.2
  Gowers' (vasovagal attack) 780.2
  Gowers-Paton-Kennedy 377.04
  Gradenigo's 383.02
  Gray or grey (chloramphenicol) (new-
    born) 779.4
  Greig's (hypertelorism) 756.0
  Gubler-Millard 344.89
  Guérin-Stern (arthrogryposis multiplex
    congenita) 754.89
  Guillain-Barré (-Strohl) 357.0
  Gunn's (jaw-winking syndrome) 742.8
  Gunther's (congenital erythropoietic
    porphyria) 277.1
  gustatory sweating 350.8
  H₂O 759.81
  Hadfield-Clarke (pancreatic infantil-
    ism) 577.8
  Haglund-Läwen-Fründ 717.89
  hair tourniquet - *see also* Injury, super-
    ficial, by site
    finger 915.8
      infected 915.9
    penis 911.8
      infected 911.9
    toe 917.8
      infected 917.9
  hairless women 257.8
  Hallermann-Strieff 756.0
  Hallervorden-Spatz 333.0
  Hamman's (spontaneous mediastinal
    emphysema) 518.1
  Hamman-Rich (diffuse interstitial pul-
    monary fibrosis) 516.3
  Hand-Schüller-Christian (chronic his-
    tiocytosis X) 277.89
  hand-foot 282.61
  Hanot-Chauffard (-Troisier) (bronze di-
    abetes) 275.0
  Harada's 363.22
  Hare's (M8010/3) (carcinoma, pulmo-
    nary apex) 162.3
  Harkavy's 446.0
  harlequin color change 779.89
  Harris' (organic hyperinsulinism) 251.1
  Hart's (pellagra-cerebellar ataxia-renal
    aminoaciduria) 270.0
  Hayem-Faber (achlorhydric anemia) 280.9
  Hayem-Widal (acquired hemolytic
    jaundice) 283.9
  Heberden's (angina pectoris) 413.9
  Hedinger's (malignant carcinoid) 259.2
  Hegglin's 288.2
  Heller's (infantile psychosis) (*see also*
    Psychosis, childhood) 299.1
  H.E.L.L.P 642.5
  hemolytic-uremic (adult) (child) 283.11
  Hench-Rosenberg (palindromic arthri-
    tis) (*see also* Rheumatism, palin-
    dromic) 719.3
  Henoch-Schönlein (allergic purpura)
    287.0
  hepatic flexure 569.89
  hepatorenal 572.4
    due to a procedure 997.4
    following delivery 674.8

Syndrome *(Continued)*
  hepatourologic 572.4
  Herrick's (hemoglobin S disease) 282.61
  Herter (-Gee) (nontropical sprue) 579.0
  Heubner-Herter (nontropical sprue) 579.0
  Heyd's (hepatorenal) 572.4
  HHHO 759.81
  Hilger's 337.0
  Hoffa (-Kastert) (liposynovitis prepa-
    tellaris) 272.8
  Hoffmann's 244.9 *[359.5]*
  Hoffmann-Bouveret (paroxysmal
    tachycardia) 427.2
  Hoffmann-Werdnig 335.0
  Holländer-Simons (progressive lipo-
    dystrophy) 272.6
  Holmes' (visual disorientation) 368.16
  Holmes-Adie 379.46
  Hoppe-Goldflam 358.00
  Horner's (*see also* Neuropathy, periph-
    eral, autonomic) 337.9
    traumatic - *see* Injury, nerve, cervical
      sympathetic
  hospital addiction 301.51
  Hunt's (herpetic geniculate ganglioni-
    tis) 053.11
    dyssynergia cerebellaris myoclonica
      334.2
  Hunter (-Hurler) (mucopolysaccharido-
    sis II) 277.5
  hunterian glossitis 529.4
  Hurler (-Hunter) (mucopolysaccharido-
    sis II) 277.5
  Hutchinson's incisors or teeth 090.5
  Hutchinson-Boeck (sarcoidosis) 135
  Hutchinson-Gilford (progeria) 259.8
  hydralazine
    correct substance properly adminis-
      tered 695.4
    overdose or wrong substance given
      or taken 972.6
  hydraulic concussion (abdomen) (*see also*
    Injury, internal, abdomen) 868.00
  hyperabduction 447.8
  hyperactive bowel 564.9
  hyperaldosteronism with hypokalemic
    alkalosis (Bartter's) 255.13
  hypercalcemic 275.42
  hypercoagulation NEC 289.89
  hypereosinophilic (idiopathic) 288.3
  hyperkalemic 276.7
  hyperkinetic - *see also* Hyperkinesia,
    heart 429.82
  hyperlipemia-hemolytic anemia-icterus
    571.1
  hypermobility 728.5
  hypernatremia 276.0
  hyperosmolarity 276.0
  hypersomnia-bulimia 349.89
  hypersplenic 289.4
  hypersympathetic (*see also* Neuropathy,
    peripheral, autonomic) 337.9
  hypertransfusion, newborn 776.4
  hyperventilation, psychogenic 306.1
  hyperviscosity (of serum) NEC 273.3
    polycythemic 289.0
    sclerothymic 282.8
  hypoglycemic (familial) (neonatal) 251.2
    functional 251.1
  hypokalemic 276.8
  hypophyseal 253.8
  hypophyseothalamic 253.8
  hypopituitarism 253.2
  hypoplastic left heart 746.7
  hypopotassemia 276.8

Syndrome *(Continued)*
  hyposmolality 276.1
  hypotension, maternal 669.2
  hypotonia-hypomentia-hypogonadism-
    obesity 759.81
  ICF (intravascular coagulation-fibrinol-
    ysis) (*see also* Fibrinolysis) 286.6
  idiopathic cardiorespiratory distress,
    newborn 769
  idiopathic nephrotic (infantile) 581.9
  Imerslund (-Gräsbeck) (anemia due to
    familial selective vitamin B₁₂ mal-
    absorption) 281.1
  immobility (paraplegic) 728.3
  immunity deficiency, combined 279.2
  impending coronary 411.1
  impingement
    shoulder 726.2
    vertebral bodies 724.4
  inappropriate secretion of antidiuretic
    hormone (ADH) 253.6
  incomplete
    mandibulofacial 756.0
  infant
    death, sudden (SIDS) 798.0
    Hercules 255.2
    of diabetic mother 775.0
    shaken 995.55
  infantilism 253.3
  inferior vena cava 459.2
  influenza-like 487.1
  inspissated bile, newborn 774.4
  intermediate coronary (artery) 411.1
  internal carotid artery (*see also* Occlu-
    sion, artery, carotid) 433.1
  interspinous ligament 724.8
  intestinal
    carcinoid 259.2
    gas 787.3
    knot 560.2
  intravascular
    coagulation-fibrinolysis (ICF) (*see
      also* Fibrinolysis) 286.6
    coagulopathy (*see also* Fibrinolysis)
      286.6
  inverted Marfan's 759.89
  IRDS (idiopathic respiratory distress,
    newborn) 769
  irritable
    bowel 564.1
    heart 306.2
    weakness 300.5
  ischemic bowel (transient) 557.9
    chronic 557.1
    due to mesenteric artery insuffi-
      ciency 557.1
  Itsenko-Cushing (pituitary basophil-
    ism) 255.0
  IVC (intravascular coagulopathy) (*see
    also* Fibrinolysis) 286.6
  Ivemark's (asplenia with congenital
    heart disease) 759.0
  Jaccoud's 714.4
  Jackson's 344.89
  Jadassohn-Lewandowski (pachyo-
    nychia congenita) 757.5
  Jaffe-Lichtenstein (-Uehlinger) 252.01 ◀▦
  Jahnke's (encephalocutaneous angio-
    matosis) 759.6
  Jakob-Creutzfeldt 046.1
    with dementia
      with behavioral disturbance
        046.1 *[294.11]*
      without behavioral disturbance
        046.1 *[294.10]*

ICD-9-CM

S

Vol. 2

Syndrome *(Continued)*

Jaksch's (pseudoleukemia infantum) 285.8

Jaksch-Hayem (-Luzet) (pseudoleukemia infantum) 285.8

jaw-winking 742.8

jejunal 564.2

jet lag 307.45

Jeune's (asphyxiating thoracic dystrophy of newborn) 756.4

Job's (chronic granulomatous disease) 288.1

Jordan's 288.2

Joseph-Diamond-Blackfan (congenital hypoplastic anemia) 284.0

Joubert 759.89

jugular foramen 352.6

Kabuki 759.89 ◀

Kahler's (multiple myeloma) (M9730/3) 203.0

Kalischer's (encephalocutaneous angiomatosis) 759.6

Kallmann's (hypogonadotropic hypogonadism with anosmia) 253.4

Kanner's (autism) *(see also* Psychosis, childhood) 299.0

Kartagener's (sinusitis, bronchiectasis, situs inversus) 759.3

Kasabach-Merritt (capillary hemangioma associated with thrombocytopenic purpura) 287.3

Kast's (dyschondroplasia with hemangiomas) 756.4

Kaznelson's (congenital hypoplastic anemia) 284.0

Kearns-Sayre 277.87 ◀

Kelly's (sideropenic dysphagia) 280.8

Kimmelstiel-Wilson (intercapillary glomerulosclerosis) 250.4 [581.81]

Klauder's (erythema multiforme exudativum) 695.1

Klein-Waardenburg (ptosis-epicanthus) 270.2

Kleine-Levin 349.89

Klinefelter's 758.7

Klippel-Feil (brevicollis) 756.16

Klippel-Trenaunay 759.89

Klumpke (-Déjérine) (injury to brachial plexus at birth) 767.6

Klüver-Bucy (-Terzian) 310.0

Köhler-Pelligrini-Stieda (calcification, knee joint) 726.62

König's 564.89

Korsakoff's (nonalcoholic) 294.0
  alcoholic 291.1

Korsakoff (-Wernicke) (nonalcoholic) 294.0
  alcoholic 291.1

Kostmann's (infantile genetic agranulocytosis) 288.0

Krabbe's
  congenital muscle hypoplasia 756.89
  cutaneocerebral angioma 759.6

Kunkel (lupoid hepatitis) 571.49

labyrinthine 386.50

laceration, broad ligament 620.6

Langdon Down (mongolism) 758.0

Larsen's (flattened facies and multiple congenital dislocations) 755.8

lateral
  cutaneous nerve of thigh 355.1
  medullary *(see also* Disease, cerebrovascular, acute) 436

Launois' (pituitary gigantism) 253.0

Launois-Cléret (adiposogenital dystrophy) 253.8

Syndrome *(Continued)*

Laurence-Moon (-Bardet)-Biedl (obesity, polydactyly, and mental retardation) 759.89

Lawford's (encephalocutaneous angiomatosis) 759.6

lazy
  leukocyte 288.0
  posture 728.3

Lederer-Brill (acquired infectious hemolytic anemia) 283.19

Legg-Calvé-Perthes (osteochondrosis capital femoral) 732.1

Lemierre 451.89 ◀

Lennox's *(see also* Epilepsy) 345.0 ◀

Lennox-Gastaut 345.0 ◀
  with tonic seizures 345.1 ◀

lenticular 275.1

Leopold-Levi's (paroxysmal thyroid instability) 242.9

Lepore hemoglobin 282.49

Léri-Weill 756.59

Leriche's (aortic bifurcation occlusion) 444.0

Lermoyez's *(see also* Disease, Meniere's) 386.00

Lesch-Nyhan (hypoxanthine-guanine-phosphoribosyltransferase deficiency) 277.2

Lev's (acquired complete heart block) 426.0

Levi's (pituitary dwarfism) 253.3

Lévy-Roussy 334.3

Lichtheim's (subacute combined sclerosis with pernicious anemia) 281.0 [336.2]

Li-Fraumeni V84.01 ◀▥

Lightwood's (renal tubular acidosis) 588.89 ◀▥

Lignac (-de Toni) (-Fanconi) (-Debré) (cystinosis) 270.0

Likoff's (angina in menopausal women) 413.9

liver-kidney 572.4

Lloyd's 258.1

lobotomy 310.0

Löffler's (eosinophilic pneumonitis) 518.3

Löfgren's (sarcoidosis) 135

long arm 18 or 21 deletion 758.39 ◀▥

Looser (-Debray)-Milkman (osteomalacia with pseudofractures) 268.2

Lorain-Levi (pituitary dwarfism) 253.3

Louis-Bar (ataxia-telangiectasia) 334.8

low
  atmospheric pressure 993.2
  back 724.2
    psychogenic 306.0
  output (cardiac) *(see also* Failure, heart) 428.9

Lowe's (oculocerebrorenal dystrophy) 270.8

Lowe-Terrey-MacLachlan (oculocerebrorenal dystrophy) 270.8

lower radicular, newborn 767.4

Lown (-Ganong)-Levine (short P-R internal, normal QRS complex, and supraventricular tachycardia) 426.81

Lucey-Driscoll (jaundice due to delayed conjugation) 774.30

Luetscher's (dehydration) 276.5

lumbar vertebral 724.4

Lutembacher's (atrial septal defect with mitral stenosis) 745.5

Syndrome *(Continued)*

Lyell's (toxic epidermal necrolysis) 695.1
  due to drug
    correct substance properly administered 695.1
    overdose or wrong substance given or taken 977.9
    specified drug - *see* Table of Drugs and Chemicals

MacLeod's 492.8

macrogenitosomia praecox 259.8

macroglobulinemia 273.3

Maffucci's (dyschondroplasia with hemangiomas) 756.4

Magenblase 306.4

Mal de Debarquement 780.4

magnesium-deficiency 781.7

malabsorption 579.9
  postsurgical 579.3
  spinal fluid 331.3

malignant carcinoid 259.2

Mallory-Weiss 530.7

mandibulofacial dysostosis 756.0

manic-depressive *(see also* Psychosis, affective) 296.80

Mankowsky's (familial dysplastic osteopathy) 731.2

maple syrup (urine) 270.3

Marable's (celiac artery compression) 447.4

Marchesani (-Weill) (brachymorphism and ectopia lentis) 759.89

Marchiafava-Bignami 341.8

Marchiafava-Micheli (paroxysmal nocturnal hemoglobinuria) 283.2

Marcus Gunn's (jaw-winking syndrome) 742.8

Marfan's (arachnodactyly) 759.82
  meaning congenital syphilis 090.49
    with luxation of lens 090.49 [379.32]

Marie's (acromegaly) 253.0
  primary or idiopathic (acropachyderma) 757.39
  secondary (hypertrophic pulmonary osteoarthropathy) 731.2

Markus-Adie 379.46

Maroteaux-Lamy (mucopolysaccharidosis VI) 277.5

Martin's 715.27

Martin-Albright (pseudohypoparathyroidism) 275.49

Martorell-Fabré (pulseless disease) 446.7

massive aspiration of newborn 770.1

Masters-Allen 620.6

mastocytosis 757.33

maternal hypotension 669.2

maternal obesity 646.1

May (-Hegglin) 288.2

McArdle (-Schmid) (-Pearson) (glycogenosis V) 271.0

McCune-Albright (osteitis fibrosa disseminata) 756.59

McQuarrie's (idiopathic familial hypoglycemia) 251.2

meconium
  aspiration 770.1
  plug (newborn) NEC 777.1

median arcuate ligament 447.4

mediastinal fibrosis 519.3

Meekeren-Ehlers-Danlos 756.83

Meige (blepharospasm-oromandibular dystonia) 333.82

-Milroy (chronic hereditary edema) 757.0

Syndrome *(Continued)*
  MELAS (mitochondrial encephalopa-
    thy, lactic acidosis and stroke-like
    episodes) 277.87   ◀▥
  Melkersson (-Rosenthal) 351.8
  Mende's (ptosis-epicanthus) 270.2
  Mendelson's (resulting from a proce-
    dure) 997.3
    during labor 668.0
    obstetric 668.0
  Ménétrier's (hypertrophic gastritis)
    535.2
  Ménière's (*see also* Disease, Meniere's)
    386.00
  meningo-eruptive 047.1
  Menkes' 759.89
    glutamic acid 759.89
    maple syrup (urine) disease 270.3
  menopause 627.2
    postartificial 627.4
  menstruation 625.4
  MERRF (myoclonus with epilepsy and
    with ragged red fibers) 277.87 ◀▥
  mesenteric
    artery, superior 557.1
    vascular insufficiency (with gan-
      grene) 557.1
  metabolic 277.7   ◀
  metastatic carcinoid 259.2
  Meyenburg-Altherr-Uehlinger 733.99
  Meyer-Schwickerath and Weyers (dys-
    plasia oculodentodigitalis) 759.89
  Micheli-Rietti (thalassemia minor)
    282.49
  Michotte's 721.5
  micrognathia-glossoptosis 756.0
  microphthalmos (congenital) 759.89
  midbrain 348.8
  middle
    lobe (lung) (right) 518.0
    radicular 353.0
  Miescher's
    familial acanthosis nigricans 701.2
    granulomatosis disciformis 709.3
  Mieten's 759.89
  migraine 346.0
  Mikity-Wilson (pulmonary dysmatur-
    ity) 770.7
  Mikulicz's (dryness of mouth, absent
    or decreased lacrimation) 527.1
  milk alkali (milk drinkers') 275.42
  Milkman (-Looser) (osteomalacia with
    pseudofractures) 268.2
  Millard-Gubler 344.89
  Miller Fisher's 357.0
  Miller-Dieker 758.33   ◀
  Milles' (encephalocutaneous angioma-
    tosis) 759.6
  Minkowski-Chauffard (*see also* Sphe-
    rocytosis) 282.0
  Mirizzi's (hepatic duct stenosis) 576.2
    with calculus, cholelithiasis, or
      stones - *see* Choledocholithiasis
  mitochondrial neurogastrointestinal en-
    cephalopathy (MNGIE) 277.87   ◀
  mitral
    click (-murmur) 785.2
    valve prolapse 424.0
  MNGIE (mitochondrial neurogastroin-
    testinal encephalopathy) 277.87 ◀
  Möbius'
    congenital oculofacial paralysis 352.6
    ophthalmoplegic migraine 346.8
  Mohr's (types I and II) 759.89

Syndrome *(Continued)*
  monofixation 378.34
  Moore's (*see also* Epilepsy) 345.5
  Morel-Moore (hyperostosis frontalis in-
    terna) 733.3
  Morel-Morgagni (hyperostosis frontalis
    interna) 733.3
  Morgagni (-Stewart-Morel) (hyperosto-
    sis frontalis interna) 733.3
  Morgagni-Adams-Stokes (syncope with
    heart block) 426.9
  Morquio (-Brailsford) (-Ullrich) (muco-
    polysaccharidosis IV) 277.5
  Morris (testicular feminization) 257.8
  Morton's (foot) (metatarsalgia) (meta-
    tarsal neuralgia) (neuralgia) (neu-
    roma) (toe) 355.6
  Moschcowitz (-Singer-Symmers)
    (thrombotic thrombocytopenic
    purpura) 446.6
  Mounier-Kuhn 494.0
    with acute exacerbation 494.1
  Mucha-Haberman (acute parapsoriasis
    varioliformis) 696.2
  mucocutaneous lymph node (acute)
    (febrile) (infantile) (MCLS) 446.1
  multiple
    deficiency 260
    operations 301.51
  Munchausen's 301.51
  Munchmeyer's (exostosis luxurians)
    728.11
  Murchison-Sanderson - *see* Disease,
    Hodgkin's
  myasthenic - *see* Myasthenia, syndrome
  myelodysplastic 238.7
  myeloproliferative (chronic) (M9960/1)
    238.7
  myofascial pain NEC 729.1
  Naffziger's 353.0
  Nager-de Reynier (dysostosis mandib-
    ularis) 756.0
  nail-patella (hereditary osteo-onycho-
    dysplasia) 756.89
  NARP (neuropathy, ataxia and retinitis
    pigmentosa) 277.87   ◀
  Nebécourt's 253.3
  Neill Dingwall (microencephaly and
    dwarfism) 759.89
  nephrotic (*see also* Nephrosis) 581.9
    diabetic 250.4 [581.81]
  Netherton's (ichthyosiform erythro-
    derma) 757.1
  neurocutaneous 759.6
  neuroleptic malignant 333.92
  Nezelof's (pure alymphocytosis) 279.13
  Niemann-Pick (lipid histiocytosis)
    272.7
  Nonne-Milroy-Meige (chronic heredi-
    tary edema) 757.0
  nonsense 300.16
  Noonan's 759.89
  Nothnagel's
    ophthalmoplegia-cerebellar ataxia
      378.52
    vasomotor acroparesthesia 443.89
  nucleus ambiguous-hypoglossal 352.6
  OAV (oculoauriculovertebral dyspla-
    sia) 756.0
  obsessional 300.3
  oculocutaneous 364.24
  oculomotor 378.81
  oculourethroarticular 099.3
  Ogilvie's (sympathicotonic colon ob-
    struction) 560.89

Syndrome *(Continued)*
  ophthalmoplegia-cerebellar ataxia
    378.52
  Oppenheim-Urbach (necrobiosis li-
    poidica diabeticorum) 250.8 [709.3]
  oral-facial-digital 759.89
  organic
    affective NEC 293.83
      drug-induced 292.84
    anxiety 293.84
    delusional 293.81
      alcohol-induced 291.5
      drug-induced 292.11
      due to or associated with
        arteriosclerosis 290.42
        presenile brain disease 290.12
        senility 290.20
    depressive 293.83
      drug-induced 292.84
      due to or associated with
        arteriosclerosis 290.43
        presenile brain disease 290.13
        senile brain disease 290.21
    hallucinosis 293.82
      drug-induced 292.84
  organic affective 293.83
    induced by drug 292.84
  organic personality 310.1
    induced by drug 292.89
  Ormond's 593.4
  orodigitofacial 759.89
  orthostatic hypotensive-dysautonomic-
    dyskinetic 333.0
  Osler-Weber-Rendu (familial hemor-
    rhagic telangiectasia) 448.0
  osteodermopathic hyperostosis 757.39
  osteoporosis-osteomalacia 268.2
  Österreicher-Turner (hereditary osteo-
    onychodysplasia) 756.89
  Ostrum-Furst 756.59
  otolith 386.19
  otopalatodigital 759.89
  outlet (thoracic) 353.0
  ovarian remnant 620.8
  ovarian vein 593.4
  Owren's (*see also* Defect, coagulation)
    286.3
  OX 758.6
  pacemaker 429.4
  Paget-Schroetter (intermittent venous
    claudication) 453.8
  pain - *see* Pain
  painful
    apicocostal vertebral (M8010/3) 162.3
    arc 726.19
    bruising 287.2
    feet 266.2
  Pancoast's (carcinoma, pulmonary
    apex) (M8010/3) 162.3
  panhypopituitary (postpartum) 253.2
  papillary muscle 429.81
    with myocardial infarction 410.8
  Papillon-Léage and Psaume (orodigito-
    facial dysostosis) 759.89
  paraneoplastic- *see* condition
  parobiotic (transfusion)
    donor (twin) 772.0
    recipient (twin) 776.4
  paralysis agitans 332.0
  paralytic 344.9
    specified type NEC 344.89
  paraneoplastic - *see* Condition
  Parinaud's (paralysis of conjugate up-
    ward gaze) 378.81
    oculoglandular 372.02

ICD-9-CM

S

Vol. 2

Syndrome (Continued)

Parkes Weber and Dimitri (encephalocutaneous angiomatosis) 759.6

Parkinson's (see also Parkinsonism) 332.0

parkinsonian (see also Parkinsonism) 332.0

Parry's (exophthalmic goiter) 242.0

Parry-Romberg 349.89

Parsonage-Aldren-Turner 353.5

Parsonage-Turner 353.5

Patau's (trisomy D₁) 758.1

patellofemoral 719.46

Paterson (-Brown) (-Kelly) (sideropenic dysphagia) 280.8

Payr's (splenic flexure syndrome) 569.89

pectoral girdle 447.8

pectoralis minor 447.8

Pelger-Huët (hereditary hyposegmentation) 288.2

Pellagra-cerebellar ataxia-renal aminoaciduria 270.0

Pellegrini-Stieda 726.62

pellagroid 265.2

Pellizzi's (pineal) 259.8

pelvic congestion (-fibrosis) 625.5

Pendred's (familial goiter with deafmutism) 243

Penfield's (see also Epilepsy) 345.5

Penta X 758.81

peptic ulcer - see Ulcer, peptic 533.9

perabduction 447.8

periodic 277.3

periurethral fibrosis 593.4

persistent fetal circulation 747.83

Petges-Cléjat (poikilodermatomyositis) 710.3

Peutz-Jeghers 759.6

Pfeiffer (acrocephalosyndactyly) 755.55

phantom limb 353.6

pharyngeal pouch 279.11

Pick's (pericardial pseudocirrhosis of liver) 423.2

heart 423.2

liver 423.2

Pick-Herxheimer (diffuse idiopathic cutaneous atrophy) 701.8

Pickwickian (cardiopulmonary obesity) 278.8

PIE (pulmonary infiltration with eosinophilia 518.3

Pierre Marie-Bamberger (hypertrophic pulmonary osteoarthropathy) 731.2

Pierre Mauriac's (diabetes-dwarfismobesity) 258.1

Pierre Robin 756.0

pigment dispersion, iris 364.53

pineal 259.8

pink puffer 492.8

pituitary 253.0

placental

dysfunction 762.2

insufficiency 762.2

transfusion 762.3

plantar fascia 728.71

plica knee 727.83

Plummer-Vinson (sideropenic dysphagia) 280.8

pluricarential of infancy 260

plurideficiency of infancy 260

pluriglandular (compensatory) 258.8

polycarential of infancy 260

polyglandular 258.8

Syndrome (Continued)

polysplenia 759.0

pontine 433.8

popliteal

artery entrapment 447.8

web 756.89

postartificial menopause 627.4

postcardiotomy 429.4

postcholecystectomy 576.0

postcommissurotomy 429.4

postconcussional 310.2

postcontusional 310.2

postencephalitic 310.8

posterior

cervical sympathetic 723.2

fossa compression 348.4

inferior cerebellar artery (see also Disease, cerebrovascular, acute) 436

postgastrectomy (dumping) 564.2

post-gastric surgery 564.2

posthepatitis 780.79

posttherpetic (neuralgia) (zoster) 053.19

geniculate ganglion 053.11

ophthalmica 053.19

postimmunization - see Complications, vaccination

postinfarction 411.0

postinfluenza (asthenia) 780.79

postirradiation 990

postlaminectomy 722.80

cervical, cervicothoracic 722.81

lumbar, lumbosacral 722.83

thoracic, thoracolumbar 722.82

postleukotomy 310.0

postlobotomy 310.0

postmastectomy lymphedema 457.0

postmature (of newborn) 766.22

postmyocardial infarction 411.0

postoperative NEC 998.9

blind loop 579.2

postpartum panhypopituitary 253.2

postperfusion NEC 999.8

bone marrow 996.85

postpericardiotomy 429.4

postphlebitic 459.10

with

complications NEC 459.19

inflammation 459.12

and ulcer 459.13

stasis dermatitis 459.12

with ulcer 459.13

ulcer 459.11

with inflammation 459.13

postpolio (myelitis) 138

postvagotomy 564.2

postvalvulotomy 429.4

postviral (asthenia) NEC 780.7

Potain's (gastrectasis with dyspepsia) 536.1

potassium intoxication 276.7

Potter's 753.0

Prader (-Labhart)-Willi (-Fanconi) 759.81

preinfarction 411.1

preleukemic 238.7

premature senility 259.8

premenstrual 625.4

premenstrual tension 625.4

pre-ulcer 536.9

Prinzmetal-Massumi (anterior chest wall syndrome) 786.52

Profichet's 729.9

progeria 259.8

progressive pallidal degeneration 333.0

prolonged gestation 766.22

Syndrome (Continued)

Proteus (dermal hypoplasia 757.39

prune belly 756.71

prurigo-asthma 691.8

pseudocarpal tunnel (sublimis) 354.0

pseudohermaphroditism-virilism-hirsutism 255.2

pseudoparalytica 358.00

pseudo-Turner's 759.89

psycho-organic 293.9

acute 293.0

anxiety type 293.84

depressive type 293.83

hallucinatory type 293.82

nonpsychotic severity 310.1

specified focal (partial) NEC 310.8

paranoid type 293.81

specified type NEC 293.89

subacute 293.1

pterygolymphangiectasia 758.6

ptosis-epicanthus 270.2

pulmonary

arteriosclerosis 416.0

hypoperfusion (idiopathic) 769

renal (hemorrhagic) 446.21

pulseless 446.7

Putnam-Dana (subacute combined sclerosis with pernicious anemia) 281.0 [336.2]

pyloroduodenal 537.89

pyramidopallidonigral 332.0

pyriformis 355.0

Q-T interval prolongation 794.31

radicular NEC 729.2

lower limbs 724.4

upper limbs 723.4

newborn 767.4

Raeder-Harbitz (pulseless disease) 446.7

Ramsay Hunt's

dyssynergia cerebellaris myoclonica 334.2

herpetic geniculate ganglionitis 053.11

rapid time-zone change 307.45

Raymond (-Céstan) 433.8

Raynaud's (paroxysmal digital cyanosis) 443.0

RDS (respiratory distress syndrome, newborn) 769

Refsum's (heredopathia atactica polyneuritiformis) 356.3

Reichmann's (gastrosuccorrhea) 536.8

Reifenstein's (hereditary familial hypogonadism, male) 257.2

Reilly's (see also Neuropathy, peripheral, autonomic) 337.9

Reiter's 099.3

renal glomerulohyalinosis-diabetic 250.4 [581.81]

Rendu-Osler-Weber (familial hemorrhagic telangiectasia) 448.0

renofacial (congenital biliary fibroangiomatosis) 753.0

Rénon-Delille 253.8

respiratory distress (idiopathic) (newborn) 769

adult (following shock, surgery, or trauma) 518.5

specified NEC 518.82

restless leg 333.99 ◀

retinoblastoma (familial) 190.5

retraction (Duane's) 378.71

retroperitoneal fibrosis 593.4

Rett's 330.8

Reye's 331.81

Syndrome *(Continued)*

Reye-Sheehan (postpartum pituitary necrosis) 253.2

Riddoch's (visual disorientation) 368.16

Ridley's *(see also* Failure, ventricular, left) 428.1

Rieger's (mesodermal dysgenesis, anterior ocular segment) 743.44

Rietti-Greppi-Micheli (thalassemia minor) 282.49

right ventricular obstruction - *see* Failure, heart

Riley-Day (familial dysautonomia) 742.8

Robin's 756.0

Rokitansky-Kuster-Hauser (congenital absence, vagina) 752.49

Romano-Ward (prolonged Q-T interval) 794.31

Romberg's 349.89

Rosen-Castleman-Liebow (pulmonary proteinosis) 516.0

rotator cuff, shoulder 726.10

Roth's 355.1

Rothmund's (congenital poikiloderma) 757.33

Rotor's (idiopathic hyperbilirubinemia) 277.4

Roussy-Lévy 334.3

Roy (-Jutras) (acropachyderma) 757.39

rubella (congenital) 771.0

Rubinstein-Taybi's (brachydactylia, short stature, and mental retardation) 759.89

Rud's (mental deficiency, epilepsy, and infantilism) 759.89

Ruiter-Pompen (-Wyers) (angiokeratoma corporis diffusum) 272.7

Runge's (postmaturity) 766.22

Russell (-Silver) (congenital hemihypertrophy and short stature) 759.89

Rytand-Lipsitch (complete atrioventricular block) 426.0

sacralization-scoliosis-sciatica 756.15

sacroiliac 724.6

Saenger's 379.46

salt

depletion *(see also* Disease, renal) 593.9

due to heat NEC 992.8

causing heat exhaustion or prostration 992.4

low *(see also* Disease, renal) 593.9

salt-losing *(see also* Disease, renal) 593.9

Sanfilippo's (mucopolysaccharidosis III) 277.5

Scaglietti-Dagnini (acromegalic macrospondylitis) 253.0

scalded skin 695.1

scalenus anticus (anterior) 353.0

scapulocostal 354.8

scapuloperoneal 359.1

scapulovertebral 723.4

Schaumann's (sarcoidosis) 135

Scheie's (mucopolysaccharidosis IS) 277.5

Scheuthauer-Marie-Sainton (cleidocranialis dysostosis) 755.59

Schirmer's (encephalocutaneous angiomatosis) 759.6

schizophrenic, of childhood NEC *(see also* Psychosis, childhood) 299.9

Syndrome *(Continued)*

Schmidt's

sphallo-pharyngo-laryngeal hemiplegia 352.6

thyroid-adrenocortical insufficiency 258.1

vagoaccessory 352.6

Schneider's 047.9

Schnitzler 273.1 ◀

Scholte's (malignant carcinoid) 259.2

Scholz (-Bielschowsky-Henneberg) 330.0

Schroeder's (endocrine-hypertensive) 255.3

Schüller-Christian (chronic histiocytosis X) 277.89

Schultz's (agranulocytosis) 288.0

Schwachman's 288.0

Schwartz (-Jampel) 756.89

Schwartz-Bartter (inappropriate secretion of antidiuretic hormone) 253.6

scimitar (anomalous venous drainage, right lung to inferior vena cava) 747.49

sclerocystic ovary 256.4

sea-blue histiocyte 272.7

Seabright-Bantam (pseudohypoparathyroidism) 275.49

Seckel's 759.89

Secretan's (posttraumatic edema) 782.3

secretoinhibitor (keratoconjunctivitis sicca) 710.2

Seeligmann's (ichthyosis congenita) 757.1

Senear-Usher (pemphigus erythematosus) 694.4

senilism 259.8

serotonin 333.99

serous meningitis 348.2

Sertoli cell (germinal aplasia) 606.0

sex chromosome mosaic 758.81

Sézary's (reticulosis) (M9701/3) 202.2

shaken infant 995.55

Shaver's (bauxite pneumoconiosis) 503

Sheehan's (postpartum pituitary necrosis) 253.2

shock (traumatic) 040.82

kidney 584.5

following crush injury 958.5

lung 518.5

neurogenic 308.9

psychic 308.9

short

bowel 579.3

P-R interval 426.81

shoulder-arm *(see also* Neuropathy, peripheral, autonomic) 337.9

shoulder-girdle 723.4

shoulder-hand *(see also* Neuropathy, peripheral, autonomic) 337.9

Shwachman's 288.0

Shy-Drager (orthostatic hypotension with multisystem degeneration) 333.0

Sicard's 352.6

sicca (keratoconjunctivitis) 710.2

sick

cell 276.1

cilia 759.89

sinus 427.81

sideropenic 280.8

Siemens'

ectodermal dysplasia 757.31

keratosis follicularis spinulosa (decalvans) 757.39

Syndrome *(Continued)*

Silfverskiöld's (osteochondrodystrophy, extremities) 756.50

Silver's (congenital hemihypertrophy and short stature) 759.89

Silvestroni-Bianco (thalassemia minima) 282.49

Simons' (progressive lipodystrophy) 272.6

sinus tarsi 726.79

sinusitis-bronchiectasis-situs inversus 759.3

Sipple's (medullary thyroid carcinoma-pheochromocytoma) 193

Sjögren (-Gougerot) (keratoconjunctivitis sicca) 710.2

with lung involvement 710.2 *[517.8]*

Sjögren-Larsson (ichthyosis congenita) 757.1

Slocumb's 255.3

Sluder's 337.0

Smith-Lemli-Opitz (cerebrohepatorenal syndrome) 759.89

Smith-Magenis 758.33 ◀▥

smokers' 305.1

Sneddon-Wilkinson (subcorneal pustular dermatosis) 694.1

Sotos' (cerebral gigantism) 253.0

South African cardiomyopathy 425.2

spasmodic

upward movement, eye(s) 378.82

winking 307.20

Spens' (syncope with heart block) 426.9

spherophakia-brachymorphia 759.89

spinal cord injury - *see also* Injury, spinal, by site

with fracture, vertebra - *see* Fracture, vertebra, by site, with spinal cord injury

cervical - *see* Injury, spinal, cervical

fluid malabsorption (acquired) 331.3

splenic

agenesis 759.0

flexure 569.89

neutropenia 288.0

sequestration 289.52

Spurway's (brittle bones and blue sclera) 756.51

staphylococcal scalded skin 695.1

Stein's (polycystic ovary) 256.4

Stein-Leventhal (polycystic ovary) 256.4

Steinbrocker's *(see also* Neuropathy, peripheral, autonomic) 337.9

Stevens-Johnson (erythema multiforme exudativum) 695.1

Stewart-Morel (hyperostosis frontalis interna) 733.3

stiff-baby 759.89 ◀

stiff-man 333.91

Still's (juvenile rheumatoid arthritis) 714.30

Still-Felty (rheumatoid arthritis with splenomegaly and leukopenia) 714.1

Stilling-Türk-Duane (ocular retraction syndrome) 378.71

Stojano's (subcostal) 098.86

Stokes (-Adams) (syncope with heart block) 426.9

Stokvis-Talma (enterogenous cyanosis) 289.7

stone heart *(see also* Failure, ventricular, left) 428.1

ICD-9-CM

S

Vol. 2

Syndrome (*Continued*)
straight-back 756.19
stroke (*see also* Disease, cerebrovascular, acute) 436
little 435.9
Sturge-Kalischer-Weber (encephalotrigeminal angiomatosis) 759.6
Sturge-Weber (-Dimitri) (encephalocutaneous angiomatosis) 759.6
subclavian-carotid obstruction (chronic) 446.7
subclavian steal 435.2
subcoracoid-pectoralis minor 447.8
subcostal 098.86
nerve compression 354.8
subperiosteal hematoma 267
subphrenic interposition 751.4
sudden infant death (SIDS) 798.0
Sudeck's 733.7
Sudeck-Leriche 733.7
superior
cerebellar artery (*see also* Disease, cerebrovascular, acute) 436
mesenteric artery 557.1
pulmonary sulcus (tumor) (M8010/3) 162.3
vena cava 459.2
suprarenal cortical 255.3
supraspinatus 726.10
swallowed blood 777.3
sweat retention 705.1
Sweet's (acute febrile neutrophilic dermatosis) 695.89
Swyer-James (unilateral hyperlucent lung) 492.8
Swyer's (XY pure gonadal dysgenesis) 752.7
Symonds' 348.2
sympathetic
cervical paralysis 337.0
pelvic 625.5
syndactylic oxycephaly 755.55
syphilitic-cardiovascular 093.89
systemic
fibrosclerosing 710.8
inflammatory response (SIR) 995.90
due to infectious process 995.91
with organ dysfunction 995.92
non-infectious process 995.93
with organ dysfunction 995.94
systolic click (-murmur) 785.2
Tabagism 305.1
tachycardia-bradycardia 427.81
Takayasu (-Onishi) (pulseless disease) 446.7
Tapia's 352.6
tarsal tunnel 355.5
Taussig-Bing (transposition, aorta and overriding pulmonary artery) 745.11
Taybi's (otopalatodigital) 759.89
Taylor's 625.5
teething 520.7
tegmental 344.89
telangiectasis-pigmentation-cataract 757.33
temporal 383.02
lobectomy behavior 310.0
temporomandibular joint-pain-dysfunction [TMJ] NEC 524.60
specified NEC 524.69
Terry's 362.21

Syndrome (*Continued*)
testicular feminization 257.8
testis, nonvirilizing 257.8
tethered (spinal) cord 742.59
thalamic 348.8
Thibierge-Weissenbach (cutaneous systemic sclerosis) 710.1
Thiele 724.6
thoracic outlet (compression) 353.0
thoracogenous rheumatic (hypertrophic pulmonary osteoarthropathy) 731.2
Thorn's (*see also* Disease, renal) 593.9
Thorson-Biörck (malignant carcinoid) 259.2
thrombopenia-hemangioma 287.3
thyroid-adrenocortical insufficiency 258.1
Tietze's 733.6
time-zone change (rapid) 307.45
Tobias' (carcinoma, pulmonary apex) (M8010/3) 162.3
toilet seat 926.0
Tolosa-Hunt 378.55
Toni-Fanconi (cystinosis) 270.0
Touraine's (hereditary osteo-onychodysplasia) 756.89
Touraine-Solente-Golé (acropachyderma) 757.39
toxic
oil 710.5
shock 040.82
transfusion
fetal-maternal 772.0
twin
donor (infant) 772.0
recipient (infant) 776.4
Treacher Collins' (incomplete mandibulofacial dysostosis) 756.0
trigeminal plate 259.8
triplex X female 758.81
trisomy NEC 758.5
13 or D$_1$ 758.1
16-18 or E 758.2
18 or E$_3$ 758.2
20 758.5
21 or G (mongolism) 758.0
22 or G (mongolism) 758.0
G 758.0
Troisier-Hanot-Chauffard (bronze diabetes) 275.0
tropical wet feet 991.4
Trousseau's (thrombophlebitis migrans visceral cancer) 453.1
Türk's (ocular retraction syndrome) 378.71
Turner's 758.6
Turner-Varny 758.6
twin-to-twin transfusion 762.3
recipient twin 776.4
Uehlinger's (acropachyderma) 757.39
Ullrich (-Bonnevie) (-Turner) 758.6
Ullrich-Feichtiger 759.89
underwater blast injury (abdominal) (*see also* Injury, internal, abdomen) 868.00
universal joint, cervix 620.6
Unverricht (-Lundborg) 333.2
Unverricht-Wagner (dermatomyositis) 710.3
upward gaze 378.81
Urbach-Oppenheim (necrobiosis lipoidica diabeticorum) 250.8 [709.3]
Urbach-Wiethe (lipoid proteinosis) 272.8
uremia, chronic 585

Syndrome (*Continued*)
urethral 597.81
urethro-oculoarticular 099.3
urethro-oculosynovial 099.3
urohepatic 572.4
uveocutaneous 364.24
uveomeningeal, uveomeningitis 363.22
vagohypoglossal 352.6
vagovagal 780.2
van Buchem's (hyperostosis corticalis) 733.3
van der Hoeve's (brittle bones and blue sclera, deafness) 756.51
van der Hoeve-Halbertsma-Waardenburg (ptosis-epicanthus) 270.2
van der Hoeve-Waardenburg-Gualdi (ptosis-epicanthus) 270.2
vanishing twin 651.33
van Neck-Odelberg (juvenile osteochondrosis) 732.1
vascular splanchnic 557.0
vasomotor 443.9
vasovagal 780.2
VATER 759.89
Velo-cardio-facial 758.32 ◀▥
vena cava (inferior) (superior) (obstruction) 459.2
Verbiest's (claudicatio intermittens spinalis) 435.1
Vernet's 352.6
vertebral
artery 435.1
compression 721.1
lumbar 724.4
steal 435.1
vertebrogenic (pain) 724.5
vertiginous NEC 386.9
video display tube 723.8
Villaret's 352.6
Vinson-Plummer (sideropenic dysphagia) 280.8
virilizing adrenocortical hyperplasia, congenital 255.2
virus, viral 079.99
visceral larval migrans 128.0
visual disorientation 368.16
vitamin B$_6$ deficiency 266.1
vitreous touch 997.99
Vogt's (corpus striatum) 333.7
Vogt-Koyanagi 364.24
Volkmann's 958.6
von Bechterew-Strümpell (ankylosing spondylitis) 720.0
von Graefe's 378.72
von Hippel-Lindau (angiomatosis retinocerebellosa) 759.6
von Schroetter's (intermittent venous claudication) 453.8
von Willebrand (-Jürgens) (angiohemophilia) 286.4
Waardenburg-Klein (ptosis epicanthus) 270.2
Wagner (-Unverricht) (dermatomyositis) 710.3
Waldenström's (macroglobulinemia) 273.3
Waldenström-Kjellberg (sideropenic dysphagia) 280.8
Wallenberg's (posterior inferior cerebellar artery) (*see also* Disease, cerebrovascular, acute) 436
Waterhouse (-Friderichsen) 036.3
water retention 276.6
Weber's 344.89

◀ **New**   ◀▥ **Revised**

Syndrome *(Continued)*
  Weber-Christian (nodular nonsuppura-
    tive panniculitis) 729.30
  Weber-Cockayne (epidermolysis bul-
    losa) 757.39
  Weber-Dimitri (encephalocutaneous
    angiomatosis) 759.6
  Weber-Gubler 344.89
  Weber-Leyden 344.89
  Weber-Osler (familial hemorrhagic tel-
    angiectasia) 448.0
  Wegener's (necrotizing respiratory
    granulomatosis) 446.4
  Weill-Marchesani (brachymorphism
    and ectopia lentis) 759.89
  Weingarten's (tropical eosinophilia)
    518.3
  Weiss-Baker (carotid sinus syncope)
    337.0
  Weissenbach-Thibierge (cutaneous sys-
    temic sclerosis) 710.1
  Werdnig-Hoffmann 335.0
  Werlhof-Wichmann (*see also* Purpura,
    thrombocytopenic) 287.3
  Wermer's (polyendocrine adenomato-
    sis) 258.0
  Werner's (progeria adultorum) 259.8
  Wernicke's (nonalcoholic) (superior
    hemorrhagic polioencephalitis) 265.1
  Wernicke-Korsakoff (nonalcoholic) 294.0
    alcoholic 291.1
  Westphal-Strümpell (hepatolenticular
    degeneration) 275.1
  wet
    brain (alcoholic) 303.9
    feet (maceration) (tropical) 991.4
    lung
      adult 518.5
      newborn 770.6
  whiplash 847.0
  Whipple's (intestinal lipodystrophy) 040.2
  "whistling face" (craniocarpotarsal
    dystrophy) 759.89
  Widal (-Abrami) (acquired hemolytic
    jaundice) 283.9
  Wilkie's 557.1
  Wilkinson-Sneddon (subcorneal pustu-
    lar dermatosis) 694.1
  Willan-Plumbe (psoriasis) 696.1
  Willebrand (-Jürgens) (angiohemophi-
    lia) 286.4
  Willi-Prader (hypogenital dystrophy
    with diabetic tendency) 759.81
  Wilson's (hepatolenticular degenera-
    tion) 275.1
  Wilson-Mikity 770.7
  Wiskott-Aldrich (eczema-thrombocyto-
    penia) 279.12
  withdrawal
    alcohol 291.81
    drug 292.0
    infant of dependent mother 779.5
  Woakes' (ethmoiditis) 471.1
  Wolff-Parkinson-White (anomalous
    atrioventricular excitation) 426.7
  Wright's (hyperabduction) 447.8
  X
    cardiac 413.9
    dysmetabolic 277.7
  xiphoidalgia 733.99
  XO 758.6
  XXX 758.81
  XXXXY 758.81
  XXY 758.7

Syndrome *(Continued)*
  yellow vernix (placental dysfunction)
    762.2
  Zahorsky's 074.0
  Zellweger 277.86 ◀
  Zieve's (jaundice, hyperlipemia and
    hemolytic anemia) 571.1
  Zollinger-Ellison (gastric hypersecre-
    tion with pancreatic islet cell tu-
    mor) 251.5
  Zuelzer-Ogden (nutritional megalo-
    blastic anemia) 281.2
Synechia (iris) (pupil) 364.70
  anterior 364.72
    peripheral 364.73
  intrauterine (traumatic) 621.5
  posterior 364.71
  vulvae, congenital 752.49
Synesthesia (*see also* Disturbance, sensa-
  tion) 782.0
Synodontia 520.2
Synophthalmus 759.89
Synorchidism 752.89
Synorchism 752.89
Synostosis (congenital) 756.59
  astragaloscaphoid 755.67
  radioulnar 755.53
  talonavicular (bar) 755.67
  tarsal 755.67
Synovial - *see* condition
Synovioma (M9040/3) - *see also* Neoplasm, connective tissue, malignant
  benign (M9040/0) - *see* Neoplasm, con-
    nective tissue, benign
Synoviosarcoma (M9040/3) - *see* Neoplasm, connective tissue, malignant
Synovitis 727.00
  chronic crepitant, wrist 727.2
  due to crystals - *see* Arthritis, due to
    crystals
  gonococcal 098.51
  gouty 274.0
  syphilitic 095.7
    congenital 090.0
  traumatic, current - *see* Sprain, by site
  tuberculous - *see* Tuberculosis, synovi-
    tis
  villonodular 719.20
    ankle 719.27
    elbow 719.22
    foot 719.27
    hand 719.24
    hip 719.25
    knee 719.26
    multiple sites 719.29
    pelvic region 719.25
    shoulder (region) 719.21
    specified site NEC 719.28
    wrist 719.23
Syphilide 091.3
  congenital 090.0
  newborn 090.0
  tubercular 095.8
    congenital 090.0
Syphilis, syphilitic (acquired) 097.9
  with lung involvement 095.1
  abdomen (late) 095.2
  acoustic nerve 094.86
  adenopathy (secondary) 091.4
  adrenal (gland) 095.8
    with cortical hypofunction 095.8
  age under 2 years NEC (*see also* Syphi-
    lis, congenital) 090.9
    acquired 097.9

Syphilis, syphilitic *(Continued)*
  alopecia (secondary) 091.82
  anemia 095.8
  aneurysm (artery) (ruptured) 093.89
    aorta 093.0
    central nervous system 094.89
    congenital 090.5
  anus 095.8
    primary 091.1
    secondary 091.3
  aorta, aortic (arch) (abdominal) (insuf-
    ficiency) (pulmonary) (regurgita-
    tion) (stenosis) (thoracic) 093.89
    aneurysm 093.0
  arachnoid (adhesive) 094.2
  artery 093.89
    cerebral 094.89
    spinal 094.89
  arthropathy (neurogenic) (tabetic)
    094.0 [713.5]
  asymptomatic - *see* Syphilis, latent
  ataxia, locomotor (progressive) 094.0
  atrophoderma maculatum 091.3
  auricular fibrillation 093.89
  Bell's palsy 094.89
  bladder 095.8
  bone 095.5
    secondary 091.61
  brain 094.89
  breast 095.8
  bronchus 095.8
  bubo 091.0
  bulbar palsy 094.89
  bursa (late) 095.7
  cardiac decompensation 093.89
  cardiovascular (early) (late) (primary)
    (secondary) (tertiary) 093.9
    specified type and site NEC 093.89
  causing death under 2 years of age (*see
    also* Syphilis, congenital) 090.9
    stated to be acquired NEC 097.9
  central nervous system (any site)
    (early) (late) (latent) (primary) (re-
    current) (relapse) (secondary) (ter-
    tiary) 094.9
    with
      ataxia 094.0
      paralysis, general 094.1
        juvenile 090.40
      paresis (general) 094.1
        juvenile 090.40
      tabes (dorsalis) 094.0
        juvenile 090.40
      taboparesis 094.1
        juvenile 090.40
    aneurysm (ruptured) 094.87
    congenital 090.40
    juvenile 090.40
    remission in (sustained) 094.9
    serology doubtful, negative, or posi-
      tive 094.9
    specified nature or site NEC 094.89
    vascular 094.89
  cerebral 094.89
    meningovascular 094.2
    nerves 094.89
    sclerosis 094.89
    thrombosis 094.89
  cerebrospinal 094.89
    tabetic 094.0
  cerebrovascular 094.89
  cervix 095.8
  chancre (multiple) 091.0
    extragenital 091.2
    Rollet's 091.2

ICD-9-CM

S

Vol. 2

Syphilis, syphilitic (Continued)
Charcôt's joint 094.0 [713.5]
choked disc 094.89 [377.00]
chorioretinitis 091.51
  congenital 090.0 [363.13]
  late 094.83
choroiditis 091.51
  congenital 090.0 [363.13]
  late 094.83
  prenatal 090.0 [363.13]
choroidoretinitis (secondary) 091.51
  congenital 090.0 [363.13]
  late 094.83
ciliary body (secondary) 091.52
  late 095.8 [364.11]
colon (late) 095.8
combined sclerosis 094.89
complicating pregnancy, childbirth, or
  puerperium 647.0
  affecting fetus or newborn 760.2
condyloma (latum) 091.3
congenital 090.9
  with
    encephalitis 090.41
    paresis (general) 090.40
    tabes (dorsalis) 090.40
    taboparesis 090.40
  chorioretinitis, choroiditis 090.0
    [363.13]
  early or less than 2 years after birth
    NEC 090.2
    with manifestations 090.0
    latent (without manifestations)
      090.1
      negative spinal fluid test 090.1
      serology, positive 090.1
    symptomatic 090.0
    interstitial keratitis 090.3
  juvenile neurosyphilis 090.40
  late or 2 years or more after birth
    NEC 090.7
    chorioretinitis, choroiditis 090.5
      [363.13]
    interstitial keratitis 090.3
    juvenile neurosyphilis NEC 090.40
    latent (without manifestations)
      090.6
      negative spinal fluid test 090.6
      serology, positive 090.6
    symptomatic or with manifesta-
      tions NEC 090.5
      interstitial keratitis 090.3
conjugal 097.9
  tabes 094.0
conjunctiva 095.8 [372.10]
contact V01.6
cord, bladder 094.0
cornea, late 095.8 [370.59]
coronary (artery) 093.89
  sclerosis 093.89
coryza 095.8
  congenital 090.0
cranial nerve 094.89
cutaneous - see Syphilis, skin
dacryocystitis 095.8
degeneration, spinal cord 094.89
d'emblée 095.8
dementia 094.1
  paralytica 094.1
    juvenilis 090.40
destruction of bone 095.5
dilatation, aorta 093.0
due to blood transfusion 097.9
dura mater 094.89

Syphilis, syphilitic (Continued)
ear 095.8
  inner 095.8
    nerve (eighth) 094.86
    neurorecurrence 094.86
early NEC 091.0
  cardiovascular 093.9
  central nervous system 094.9
    paresis 094.1
    tabes 094.0
  latent (without manifestations) (less
    than 2 years after infection)
    092.9
    negative spinal fluid test 092.9
    serological relapse following treat-
      ment 092.0
    serology positive 092.9
  paresis 094.1
  relapse (treated, untreated) 091.7
  skin 091.3
  symptomatic NEC 091.89
    extragenital chancre 091.2
    primary, except extragenital chan-
      cre 091.0
    secondary (see also Syphilis, sec-
      ondary) 091.3
      relapse (treated, untreated) 091.7
  tabes 094.0
  ulcer 091.3
eighth nerve 094.86
endemic, nonvenereal 104.0
endocarditis 093.20
  aortic 093.22
  mitral 093.21
  pulmonary 093.24
  tricuspid 093.23
epididymis (late) 095.8
epiglottis 095.8
epiphysitis (congenital) 090.0
esophagus 095.8
Eustachian tube 095.8
exposure to V01.6
eye 095.8 [363.13]
  neuromuscular mechanism 094.85
eyelid 095.8 [373.5]
  with gumma 095.8 [373.5]
  ptosis 094.89
fallopian tube 095.8
fracture 095.5
gallbladder (late) 095.8
gastric 095.8
  crisis 094.0
  polyposis 095.8
general 097.9
  paralysis 094.1
    juvenile 090.40
genital (primary) 091.0
glaucoma 095.8
gumma (late) NEC 095.9
  cardiovascular system 093.9
  central nervous system 094.9
  congenital 090.5
  heart or artery 093.89
heart 093.89
  block 093.89
  decompensation 093.89
  disease 093.89
  failure 093.89
  valve (see also Syphilis, endocarditis)
    093.20
hemianesthesia 094.89
hemianopsia 095.8
hemiparesis 094.89
hemiplegia 094.89

Syphilis, syphilitic (Continued)
hepatic artery 093.89
hepatitis 095.3
hepatomegaly 095.3
  congenital 090.0
hereditaria tarda (see also Syphilis, congenital, late) 090.7
hereditary (see also Syphilis, congenital)
  090.9
  interstitial keratitis 090.3
Hutchinson's teeth 090.5
hyalitis 095.8
inactive - see Syphilis, latent
infantum NEC (see also Syphilis, congenital) 090.9
inherited - see Syphilis, congenital
internal ear 095.8
intestine (late) 095.8
iris, iritis (secondary) 091.52
  late 095.8 [364.11]
joint (late) 095.8
keratitis (congenital) (early) (interstitial) (late) (parenchymatous)
  (punctata profunda) 090.3
kidney 095.4
lacrimal apparatus 095.8
laryngeal paralysis 095.8
larynx 095.8
late 097.0
  cardiovascular 093.9
  central nervous system 094.9
  latent or 2 years or more after infec-
    tion (without manifestation) 096
    negative spinal fluid test 096
    serology positive 096
  paresis 094.1
  specified site NEC 095.8
  symptomatic or with symptoms
    095.9
  tabes 094.0
latent 097.1
  central nervous system 094.9
  date of infection unspecified 097.1
  early or less than 2 years after infec-
    tion 092.9
  late or 2 years or more after infec-
    tion 096
  serology
    doubtful
      follow-up of latent syphilis
        097.1
        central nervous system 094.9
        date of infection unspecified
          097.1
        early or less than 2 years after
          infection 092.9
        late or 2 years or more after
          infection 096
    positive, only finding 097.1
      date of infection unspecified
        097.1
      early or less than 2 years after
        infection 097.1
      late or 2 years or more after in-
        fection 097.1
lens 095.8
leukoderma 091.3
  late 095.8
lienis 095.8
lip 091.3
  chancre 091.2
  late 095.8
  primary 091.2
Lissauer's paralysis 094.1

◀ **New**   ◀▥▥ **Revised**

Syphilis, syphilitic *(Continued)*
liver 095.3
  secondary 091.62
locomotor ataxia 094.0
lung 095.1
lymphadenitis (secondary) 091.4
lymph gland (early) (secondary)
  091.4
  late 095.8
macular atrophy of skin 091.3
  striated 095.8
maternal, affecting fetus or newborn
  760.2
  manifest syphilis in newborn - *see*
    Syphilis, congenital
mediastinum (late) 095.8
meninges (adhesive) (basilar) (brain)
  (spinal cord) 094.2
meningitis 094.2
  acute 091.81
  congenital 090.42
meningoencephalitis 094.2
meningovascular 094.2
  congenital 090.49
mesarteritis 093.89
  brain 094.89
  spine 094.89
middle ear 095.8
mitral stenosis 093.21
monoplegia 094.89
mouth (secondary) 091.3
  late 095.8
mucocutaneous 091.3
  late 095.8
mucous
  membrane 091.3
    late 095.8
  patches 091.3
    congenital 090.0
mulberry molars 090.5
muscle 095.6
myocardium 093.82
myositis 095.6
nasal sinus 095.8
neonatorum NEC (*see also* Syphilis,
  congenital) 090.9
nerve palsy (any cranial nerve)
  094.89
nervous system, central 094.9
neuritis 095.8
  acoustic nerve 094.86
neurorecidive of retina 094.83
neuroretinitis 094.85
newborn (*see also* Syphilis, congenital)
  090.9
nodular superficial 095.8
nonvenereal, endemic 104.0
nose 095.8
  saddle back deformity 090.5
  septum 095.8
    perforated 095.8
occlusive arterial disease 093.89
ophthalmic 095.8 [363.13]
ophthalmoplegia 094.89
optic nerve (atrophy) (neuritis) (papilla) 094.84
orbit (late) 095.8
orchitis 095.8
organic 097.9
osseous (late) 095.5
osteochondritis (congenital) 090.0
osteoporosis 095.5
ovary 095.8
oviduct 095.8

Syphilis, syphilitic *(Continued)*
palate 095.8
  gumma 095.8
  perforated 090.5
pancreas (late) 095.8
pancreatitis 095.8
paralysis 094.89
  general 094.1
  juvenile 090.40
paraplegia 094.89
paresis (general) 094.1
  juvenile 090.40
paresthesia 094.89
Parkinson's disease or syndrome
  094.82
paroxysmal tachycardia 093.89
pemphigus (congenital) 090.0
penis 091.0
  chancre 091.0
  late 095.8
pericardium 093.81
perichondritis, larynx 095.8
periosteum 095.5
  congenital 090.0
  early 091.61
  secondary 091.61
peripheral nerve 095.8
petrous bone (late) 095.5
pharynx 095.8
  secondary 091.3
pituitary (gland) 095.8
placenta 095.8
pleura (late) 095.8
pneumonia, white 090.0
pontine (lesion) 094.89
portal vein 093.89
primary NEC 091.2
  anal 091.1
  and secondary (*see also* Syphilis, sec-
    ondary) 091.9
  cardiovascular 093.9
  central nervous system 094.9
  extragenital chancre NEC
    091.2
  fingers 091.2
  genital 091.0
  lip 091.2
  specified site NEC 091.2
  tonsils 091.2
prostate 095.8
psychosis (intracranial gumma)
  094.89
ptosis (eyelid) 094.89
pulmonary (late) 095.1
  artery 093.89
pulmonum 095.1
pyelonephritis 095.4
recently acquired, symptomatic NEC
  091.89
rectum 095.8
respiratory tract 095.8
retina
  late 094.83
  neurorecidive 094.83
retrobulbar neuritis 094.85
salpingitis 095.8
sclera (late) 095.0
sclerosis
  cerebral 094.89
  coronary 093.89
  multiple 094.89
  subacute 094.89
scotoma (central) 095.8
scrotum 095.8

Syphilis, syphilitic *(Continued)*
secondary (and primary) 091.9
  adenopathy 091.4
  anus 091.3
  bone 091.61
  cardiovascular 093.9
  central nervous system 094.9
  chorioretinitis, choroiditis 091.51
  hepatitis 091.62
  liver 091.62
  lymphadenitis 091.4
  meningitis, acute 091.81
  mouth 091.3
  mucous membranes 091.3
  periosteum 091.61
  periostitis 091.61
  pharynx 091.3
  relapse (treated) (untreated) 091.7
  skin 091.3
  specified form NEC 091.89
  tonsil 091.3
  ulcer 091.3
  viscera 091.69
  vulva 091.3
seminal vesicle (late) 095.8
seronegative
  with signs or symptoms - *see* Syphi-
    lis, by site and stage
seropositive
  with signs or symptoms - *see* syphi-
    lis, by site and stage
  follow-up of latent syphilis - *see*
    Syphilis, latent
  only finding - *see* Syphilis, latent
seventh nerve (paralysis) 094.89
sinus 095.8
sinusitis 095.8
skeletal system 095.5
skin (early) (secondary) (with ulceration) 091.3
  late or tertiary 095.8
small intestine 095.8
spastic spinal paralysis 094.0
spermatic cord (late) 095.8
spinal (cord) 094.89
  with
    paresis 094.1
    tabes 094.0
spleen 095.8
splenomegaly 095.8
spondylitis 095.5
staphyloma 095.8
stigmata (congenital) 090.5
stomach 095.8
synovium (late) 095.7
tabes dorsalis (early) (late) 094.0
  juvenile 090.40
tabetic type 094.0
  juvenile 090.40
taboparesis 094.1
  juvenile 090.40
tachycardia 093.89
tendon (late) 095.7
tertiary 097.0
  with symptoms 095.8
  cardiovascular 093.9
  central nervous system 094.9
  multiple NEC 095.8
  specified site NEC 095.8
testis 095.8
thorax 095.8
throat 095.8
thymus (gland) 095.8
thyroid (late) 095.8

ICD-9-CM

S

Vol. 2

Syphilis, syphilitic *(Continued)*
  tongue 095.8
  tonsil (lingual) 095.8
    primary 091.2
    secondary 091.3
  trachea 095.8
  tricuspid valve 093.23
  tumor, brain 094.89
  tunica vaginalis (late) 095.8
  ulcer (any site) (early) (secondary)
      091.3
    late 095.9
    perforating 095.9
      foot 094.0
  urethra (stricture) 095.8
  urogenital 095.8
  uterus 095.8
  uveal tract (secondary) 091.50
    late 095.8 [363.13]
  uveitis (secondary) 091.50
    late 095.8 [363.13]
  uvula (late) 095.8
    perforated 095.8
  vagina 091.0
    late 095.8
  valvulitis NEC 093.20
  vascular 093.89
    brain or cerebral 094.89

Syphilis, syphilitic *(Continued)*
  vein 093.89
    cerebral 094.89
  ventriculi 095.8
  vesicae urinariae 095.8
  viscera (abdominal) 095.2
    secondary 091.69
  vitreous (hemorrhage) (opacities) 095.8
  vulva 091.0
    late 095.8
    secondary 091.3
Syphiloma 095.9
  cardiovascular system 093.9
  central nervous system 094.9
  circulatory system 093.9
  congenital 090.5
Syphilophobia 300.29
Syringadenoma (M8400/0) - *see also*
      Neoplasm, skin, benign
  papillary (M8406/0) - *see* Neoplasm,
      skin, benign
Syringobulbia 336.0
Syringocarcinoma (M8400/3) - *see Neo-*
      plasm, skin, malignant
Syringocystadenoma (M8400/0) - *see also*
      Neoplasm, skin, benign
  papillary (M8406/0) - *see* Neoplasm,
      skin, benign

Syringocystoma (M8407/0) - *see* Neo-
      plasm, skin, benign
Syringoma (M8407/0) - *see also* Neo-
      plasm, skin, benign
  chondroid (M8940/0) - *see* Neoplasm,
      by site, benign
Syringomyelia 336.0
Syringomyelitis 323.9
  late effect - *see* category 326
Syringomyelocele (*see also* Spina bifida)
      741.9
Syringopontia 336.0
System, systemic - *see also condition*
  disease, combined - *see* Degeneration,
      combined
  fibrosclerosing syndrome 710.8
  inflammatory response (SIR)
      995.90
    due to
      infectious process 995.91
        with organ dysfunction
          995.92
      non-infectious process
          995.93
        with organ dysfunction
          995.94
  lupus erythematosus 710.0
    inhibitor 286.5

◀ **New**   ◀▥ **Revised**

T

Tab - *see* Tag
Tabacism 989.84
Tabacosis 989.84
Tabardillo 080
  flea-borne 081.0
  louse-borne 080
Tabes, tabetic
  with
    central nervous system syphilis
      094.0
    Charcôt's joint 094.0 [713.5]
    cord bladder 094.0
    crisis, viscera (any) 094.0
    paralysis, general 094.1
    paresis (general) 094.1
    perforating ulcer 094.0
  arthropathy 094.0 [713.5]
  bladder 094.0
  bone 094.0
  cerebrospinal 094.0
  congenital 090.40
  conjugal 094.0
  dorsalis 094.0
    neurosyphilis 094.0
  early 094.0
  juvenile 090.40
  latent 094.0
  mesenterica (*see also* Tuberculosis)
    014.8
  paralysis insane, general 094.1
  peripheral (nonsyphilitic) 799.89
  spasmodic 094.0
    not dorsal or dorsalis 343.9
  syphilis (cerebrospinal) 094.0
Taboparalysis 094.1
Taboparesis (remission) 094.1
  with
    Charcôt's joint 094.1 [713.5]
    cord bladder 094.1
    perforating ulcer 094.1
  juvenile 090.40
Tachyalimentation 579.3
Tachyarrhythmia, tachyrhythmia - *see
  also* Tachycardia
  paroxysmal with sinus bradycardia
    427.81
Tachycardia 785.0
  atrial 427.89
  auricular 427.89
  newborn 779.82
  nodal 427.89
    nonparoxysmal atrioventricular
      426.89
    nonparoxysmal atrioventricular (nodal)
      426.89
  paroxysmal 427.2
    with sinus bradycardia 427.81
    atrial (PAT) 427.0
      psychogenic 316 [427.0]
    atrioventricular (AV) 427.0
      psychogenic 316 [427.0]
    essential 427.2
    junctional 427.0
    nodal 427.0
    psychogenic 316 [427.2]
      atrial 316 [427.0]
      supraventricular 316 [427.0]
      ventricular 316 [427.1]
    supraventricular 427.0
      psychogenic 316 [427.0]
    ventricular 427.1
      psychogenic 316 [427.1]
  postoperative 997.1

Tachycardia *(Continued)*
  psychogenic 306.2
  sick sinus 427.81
  sinoauricular 427.89
  sinus 427.89
  supraventricular 427.89
  ventricular (paroxysmal) 427.1
    psychogenic 316 [427.1]
Tachypnea 786.06
  hysterical 300.11
  newborn (idiopathic) (transitory) 770.6
  psychogenic 306.1
  transitory, of newborn 770.6
Taenia (infection) (infestation) (*see also*
    Infestation, taenia) 123.3
  diminuta 123.6
  echinococcal infestation (*see also* Echi-
    nococcus) 122.9
  nana 123.6
  saginata infestation 123.2
  solium (intestinal form) 123.0
    larval form 123.1
Taeniasis (intestine) (*see also* Infestation,
    taenia) 123.3
  saginata 123.2
  solium 123.0
Taenzer's disease 757.4
Tag (hypertrophied skin) (infected)
    701.9
  adenoid 474.8
  anus 455.9
  endocardial (*see also* Endocarditis)
    424.90
  hemorrhoidal 455.9
  hymen 623.8
  perineal 624.8
  preauricular 744.1
  rectum 455.9
  sentinel 455.9
  skin 701.9
    accessory 757.39
    anus 455.9
    congenital 757.39
    preauricular 744.1
    rectum 455.9
  tonsil 474.8
  urethra, urethral 599.84
  vulva 624.8
Tahyna fever 062.5
Takayasu (-Onishi) disease or syndrome
    (pulseless disease) 446.7
Talc granuloma 728.82
Talcosis 502
Talipes (congenital) 754.70
  acquired NEC 736.79
    planus 734
  asymmetric 754.79
    acquired 736.79
  calcaneovalgus 754.62
    acquired 736.76
  calcaneovarus 754.59
    acquired 736.76
  calcaneus 754.79
    acquired 736.76
  cavovarus 754.59
    acquired 736.75
  cavus 754.71
    acquired 736.73
  equinovalgus 754.69
    acquired 736.72
  equinovarus 754.51
    acquired 736.71
  equinus 754.79
    acquired, NEC 736.72

Talipes *(Continued)*
  percavus 754.71
    acquired 736.73
  planovalgus 754.69
    acquired 736.79
  planus (acquired) (any degree) 734
    congenital 754.61
    due to rickets 268.1
  valgus 754.60
    acquired 736.79
  varus 754.50
    acquired 736.79
Talma's disease 728.85
Tamponade heart (Rose's) (*see also* Peri-
    carditis) 423.9
Tanapox 078.89
Tangier disease (familial high-density
    lipoprotein deficiency) 272.5
Tank ear 380.12
Tantrum (childhood) (*see also* Distur-
    bance, conduct) 312.1
Tapeworm (infection) (infestation) (*see
    also* Infestation, tapeworm) 123.9
Tapia's syndrome 352.6
Tarantism 297.8
Target-oval cell anemia 282.49
Tarlov's cyst 355.9
Tarral-Besnier disease (pityriasis rubra
    pilaris) 696.4
Tarsalgia 729.2
Tarsal tunnel syndrome 355.5
Tarsitis (eyelid) 373.00
  syphilitic 095.8 [373.00]
  tuberculous (*see also* Tuberculosis)
    017.0 [373.4]
Tartar (teeth) 523.6
Tattoo (mark) 709.09
Taurodontism 520.2
Taussig-Bing defect, heart, or syndrome
    (transposition, aorta and overriding
    pulmonary artery) 745.11
Tay's choroiditis 363.41
Tay-Sachs
  amaurotic familial idiocy 330.1
  disease 330.1
Taybi's syndrome (otopalatodigital)
    759.89
Taylor's
  disease (diffuse idiopathic cutaneous
    atrophy) 701.8
  syndrome 625.5
Tear, torn (traumatic) - *see also* Wound,
    open, by site
  anus, anal (sphincter) 863.89
    with open wound in cavity
      863.99
    complicating delivery 664.2
      with mucosa 664.3
    nontraumatic, nonpuerperal 565.0
  articular cartilage, old (*see also* Disor-
    der, cartilage, articular) 718.0
  bladder
    with
      abortion - *see* Abortion, by type,
        with damage to pelvic organs
      ectopic pregnancy (*see also* catego-
        ries 633.0-633.9) 639.2
      molar pregnancy (*see also* catego-
        ries 630-632) 639.2
    following
      abortion 639.2
      ectopic or molar pregnancy
        639.2
    obstetrical trauma 665.5

ICD-9-CM

I

Vol. 2

Tear, torn *(Continued)*
  bowel
    with
      abortion - *see* Abortion, by type, with damage to pelvic organs
      ectopic pregnancy *(see also* categories 633.0-633.9) 639.2
      molar pregnancy *(see also* categories 630-632) 639.2
    following
      abortion 639.2
      ectopic or molar pregnancy 639.2
    obstetrical trauma 665.5
  broad ligament
    with
      abortion - *see* Abortion, by type, with damage to pelvic organs
      ectopic pregnancy *(see also* categories 633.0-633.9) 639.2
      molar pregnancy *(see also* categories 630-632) 639.2
    following
      abortion 639.2
      ectopic or molar pregnancy 639.2
    obstetrical trauma 665.5
  bucket handle (knee) (meniscus) - *see* Tear, meniscus
  capsule
    joint - *see* Sprain, by site
    spleen - *see* Laceration, spleen, capsule
  cartilage - *see also* Sprain, by site
    articular, old *(see also* Disorder, cartilage, articular) 718.0
    knee - *see* Tear, meniscus
    semilunar (knee) (current injury) - *see* Tear, meniscus
  cervix
    with
      abortion - *see* Abortion, by type, with damage to pelvic organs
      ectopic pregnancy *(see also* categories 633.0-633.9) 639.2
      molar pregnancy *(see also* categories 630-632) 639.2
    following
      abortion 639.2
      ectopic or molar pregnancy 639.2
    obstetrical trauma (current) 665.3
    old 622.3
  internal organ (abdomen, chest, or pelvis) - *see* Injury, internal, by site
  ligament - *see also* Sprain, by site
    with open wound - *see* Wound, open, by site
  meniscus (knee) (current injury) 836.2
    bucket handle 836.0
      old 717.0
    lateral 836.1
      anterior horn 836.1
        old 717.42
      bucket handle 836.1
        old 717.41
      old 717.40
      posterior horn 836.1
        old 717.43
      specified site NEC 836.1
        old 717.49
    medial 836.0
      anterior horn 836.0
        old 717.1
      bucket handle 836.0
        old 717.0

Tear, torn *(Continued)*
  meniscus *(Continued)*
    medial *(Continued)*
      old 717.3
      posterior horn 836.0
        old 717.2
    old NEC 717.5
    site other than knee - *see* Sprain, by site
  muscle - *see also* Sprain, by site
    with open wound - *see* Wound, open, by site
  pelvic
    floor, complicating delivery 664.1
    organ NEC
      with
        abortion - *see* Abortion, by type, with damage to pelvic organs
        ectopic pregnancy *(see also* categories 633.0-633.9) 639.2
        molar pregnancy *(see also* categories 630-632) 639.2
      following
        abortion 639.2
        ectopic or molar pregnancy 639.2
      obstetrical trauma 665.5
  perineum - *see also* Laceration, perineum
    obstetrical trauma 665.5
  periurethral tissue
    with
      abortion - *see* Abortion, by type, with damage to pelvic organs
      ectopic pregnancy *(see also* categories 633.0-633.9) 639.2
      molar pregnancy *(see also* categories 630-632) 639.2
    following
      abortion 639.2
      ectopic or molar pregnancy 639.2
    obstetrical trauma 665.5
  rectovaginal septum - *see* Laceration, rectovaginal septum
  retina, retinal (recent) (with detachment) 361.00
    without detachment 361.30
    dialysis (juvenile) (with detachment) 361.04
    giant (with detachment) 361.03
    horseshoe (without detachment) 361.32
    multiple (with detachment) 361.02
      without detachment 361.33
    old
      delimited (partial) 361.06
      partial 361.06
      total or subtotal 361.07
    partial (without detachment)
      giant 361.03
      multiple defects 361.02
      old (delimited) 361.06
      single defect 361.01
    round hole (without detachment) 361.31
    single defect (with detachment) 361.01
    total or subtotal (recent) 361.05
      old 361.07
  rotator cuff (traumatic) 840.4
    current injury 840.4
    degenerative 726.10
    nontraumatic 727.61

Tear, torn *(Continued)*
  semilunar cartilage, knee *(see also* Tear, meniscus) 836.2
    old 717.5
  tendon - *see also* Sprain, by site
    with open wound - *see* Wound, open, by site
  tentorial, at birth 767.0
  umbilical cord
    affecting fetus or newborn 772.0
    complicating delivery 663.8
  urethra
    with
      abortion - *see* Abortion, by type, with damage to pelvic organs
      ectopic pregnancy *(see also* categories 633.0-663.9) 639.2
      molar pregnancy *(see also* categories 630-632) 639.2
    following
      abortion 639.2
      ectopic or molar pregnancy 639.2
    obstetrical trauma 665.5
  uterus - *see* Injury, internal, uterus
  vagina - *see* Laceration, vagina
  vessel, from catheter 998.2
  vulva, complicating delivery 664.0
Tear stone 375.57
Teeth, tooth - *see also* condition
  grinding 306.8
Teething 520.7
  syndrome 520.7
Tegmental syndrome 344.89
Telangiectasia, telangiectasis (verrucous) 448.9
  ataxic (cerebellar) 334.8
  familial 448.0
  hemorrhagic, hereditary (congenital) (senile) 448.0
  hereditary hemorrhagic 448.0
  retina 362.15
  spider 448.1
Telecanthus (congenital) 743.63
Telescoped bowel or intestine *(see also* Intussusception) 560.0
Teletherapy, adverse effect NEC 990
Telogen effluvium 704.02
Temperature
  body, high (of unknown origin) *(see also* Pyrexia) 780.6
  cold, trauma from 991.9
    newborn 778.2
    specified effect NEC 991.8
  high
    body (of unknown origin) *(see also* Pyrexia) 780.6
    trauma from - *see* Heat
Temper tantrum (childhood) *(see also* Disturbance, conduct) 312.1
Temple - *see* condition
Temporal - *see also* condition
  lobe syndrome 310.0
Temporomandibular joint-pain-dysfunction syndrome 524.60
Temporosphenoidal - *see* condition
Tendency
  bleeding *(see also* Defect, coagulation) 286.9
  homosexual, ego-dystonic 302.0
  paranoid 301.0
  suicide 300.9
Tenderness
  abdominal (generalized) (localized) 789.6

Tenderness (Continued)
  rebound 789.6
  skin 782.0
Tendinitis, tendonitis (see also Tenosynovitis) 726.90
  Achilles 726.71
  adhesive 726.90
    shoulder 726.0
  calcific 727.82
    shoulder 726.11
  gluteal 726.5
  patellar 726.64
  peroneal 726.79
  pes anserinus 726.61
  psoas 726.5
  tibialis (anterior) (posterior) 726.72
  trochanteric 726.5
Tendon - see condition
Tendosynovitis - see Tenosynovitis
Tendovaginitis - see Tenosynovitis
Tenesmus 787.99
  rectal 787.99
  vesical 788.9
Tenia - see Taenia
Teniasis - see Taeniasis
Tennis elbow 726.32
Tenonitis - see also Tenosynovitis
  eye (capsule) 376.04
Tenontosynovitis - see Tenosynovitis
Tenontothecitis - see Tenosynovitis
Tenophyte 727.9
Tenosynovitis 727.00
  adhesive 726.90
    shoulder 726.0
  ankle 727.06
  bicipital (calcifying) 726.12
  buttock 727.09
  due to crystals - see Arthritis, due to
    crystals
  elbow 727.09
  finger 727.05
  foot 727.06
  gonococcal 098.51
  hand 727.05
  hip 727.09
  knee 727.09
  radial styloid 727.04
  shoulder 726.10
    adhesive 726.0
  spine 720.1
  supraspinatus 726.10
  toe 727.06
  tuberculous - see Tuberculosis, teno-
    synovitis
  wrist 727.05
Tenovaginitis - see Tenosynovitis
Tension
  arterial, high (see also Hypertension)
    401.9
    without diagnosis of hypertension
      796.2
  headache 307.81
  intraocular (elevated) 365.00
  nervous 799.2
  ocular (elevated) 365.00
  pneumothorax 512.0
    iatrogenic 512.1
    postoperative 512.1
    spontaneous 512.0
  premenstrual 625.4
  state 300.9
Tentorium - see condition
Teratencephalus 759.89
Teratism 759.7

Teratoblastoma (malignant) (M9080/3) -
  see Neoplasm, by site, malignant
Teratocarcinoma (M9081/3) - see also
  Neoplasm, by site, malignant
  liver 155.0
Teratoma (solid) (M9080/1) - see also
  Neoplasm, by site, uncertain behavior
  adult (cystic) (M9080/0) - see Neo-
    plasm, by site, benign
  and embryonal carcinoma, mixed
    (M9081/3) - see Neoplasm, by site,
    malignant
  benign (M9080/0) - see Neoplasm, by
    site, benign
  combined with choriocarcinoma
    (M9101/3) - see Neoplasm, by site,
    malignant
  cystic (adult) (M9080/0) - see Neo-
    plasm, by site, benign
  differentiated type (M9080/0) - see
    Neoplasm, by site, benign
  embryonal (M9080/3) - see also Neo-
    plasm, by site, malignant
    liver 155.0
  fetal
    sacral, causing fetopelvic dispropor-
      tion 653.7
  immature (M9080/3) - see Neoplasm,
    by site, malignant
  liver (M9080/3) 155.0
    adult, benign, cystic, differentiated
      type, or mature (M9080/0) 211.5
  malignant (M9080/3) - see also Neo-
    plasm, by site, malignant
    anaplastic type (M9082/3) - see Neo-
      plasm, by site, malignant
    intermediate type (M9083/3) - see
      Neoplasm, by site, malignant
    liver (M9080/3) 155.0
    trophoblastic (M9102/3)
      specified site - see Neoplasm, by
        site, malignant
      unspecified site 186.9
    undifferentiated type (M9082/3) - see
      Neoplasm, by site, malignant
  mature (M9080/0) - see Neoplasm, by
    site, benign
  ovary (M9080/0) 220
    embryonal, immature, or malignant
      (M9080/3) 183.0
  suprasellar (M9080/3) - see Neoplasm,
    by site, malignant
  testis (M9080/3) 186.9
    adult, benign, cystic, differentiated
      type or mature (M9080/0) 222.0
    undescended 186.0
Terminal care V66.7
Termination
  anomalous - see also Malposition, con-
    genital
    portal vein 747.49
    right pulmonary vein 747.42
  pregnancy (legal) (therapeutic) (see
    Abortion, legal) 635.9
    fetus NEC 779.6
    illegal (see also Abortion, illegal)
      636.9
Ternidens diminutus infestation 127.7
Terrors, night (child) 307.46
Terry's syndrome 362.21
Tertiary - see condition
Tessellated fundus, retina (tigroid)
  362.89

Test(s)
  adequacy
    hemodialysis V56.31
    peritoneal dialysis V56.32
  AIDS virus V72.6
  allergen V72.7
  bacterial disease NEC (see also Screen-
    ing, by name of disease) V74.9
  basal metabolic rate V72.6
  blood-alcohol V70.4
  blood-drug V70.4
    for therapeutic drug monitoring
      V58.83
  developmental, infant or child V20.2
  Dick V74.8
  fertility V26.21
  genetic V26.3
  hearing V72.1
  HIV V72.6
  human immunodeficiency virus V72.6
  Kveim V82.89
  laboratory V72.6
    for medicolegal reason V70.4
  Mantoux (for tuberculosis) V74.1
  mycotic organism V75.4
  parasitic agent NEC V75.8
  paternity V70.4
  peritoneal equilibration V56.32
  pregnancy
    positive V22.1
      first pregnancy V22.0
    negative result V72.41   ◀
    unconfirmed V72.40   ◀▥
  preoperative V72.84
    cardiovascular V72.81
    respiratory V72.82
    specified NEC V72.83
  procreative management NEC V26.29
  sarcoidosis V82.89
  Schick V74.3
  Schultz-Charlton V74.8
  skin, diagnostic
    allergy V72.7
    bacterial agent NEC (see also Screen-
      ing, by name of disease) V74.9
    Dick V74.8
    hypersensitivity V72.7
    Kveim V82.89
    Mantoux V74.1
    mycotic organism V75.4
    parasitic agent NEC V75.8
    sarcoidosis V82.89
    Schick V74.3
    Schultz-Charlton V74.8
    tuberculin V74.1
  specified type NEC V72.85
  tuberculin V74.1
  vision V72.0
  Wassermann
    positive (see also Serology for syphi-
      lis, positive) 097.1
    false 795.6
Testicle, testicular, testis - see also condition
  feminization (syndrome) 257.8
Tetanus, tetanic (cephalic) (convulsions)
  037
  with
    abortion - see Abortion, by type,
      with sepsis
    ectopic pregnancy (see also categories
      633.0-633.9) 639.0
    molar pregnancy (see categories 630-
      632) 639.0
  following
    abortion 639.0
    ectopic or molar pregnancy 639.0

ICD-9-CM

T

Vol. 2

Tetanus, tetanic (Continued)
  inoculation V03.7
    reaction (due to serum) - see Complications, vaccination
  neonatorum 771.3
  puerperal, postpartum, childbirth 670
Tetany, tetanic 781.7
  alkalosis 276.3
  associated with rickets 268.0
  convulsions 781.7
    hysterical 300.11
  functional (hysterical) 300.11
  hyperkinetic 781.7
    hysterical 300.11
  hyperpnea 786.01
    hysterical 300.11
    psychogenic 306.1
  hyperventilation 786.01
    hysterical 300.11
    psychogenic 306.1
  hypocalcemic, neonatal 775.4
  hysterical 300.11
  neonatal 775.4
  parathyroid (gland) 252.1
  parathyroprival 252.1
  postoperative 252.1
  postthyroidectomy 252.1
  pseudotetany 781.7
    hysterical 300.11
  psychogenic 306.1
    specified as conversion reaction 300.11
Tetralogy of Fallot 745.2
Tetraplegia - see Quadriplegia
Thailand hemorrhagic fever 065.4
Thalassanemia 282.49
Thalassemia (alpha) (beta) (disease) (Hb-C) (Hb-D) (Hb-E) (Hb-H) (Hb-I) (Hb-S) (high fetal gene) (high fetal hemoglobin) (intermedia) (major) (minima) (minor) (mixed) (sickle-cell) (trait) (with other hemoglobinopathy) 282.49
  Hb-S (without crisis) 282.41
    with
      crisis 282.42
        vaso-occlusive pain 282.42
    sickle-cell (without crisis) 282.41
      with
        crisis 282.42
          vaso-occlusive pain 282.42
Thalassemic variants 282.49
Thaysen-Gee disease (nontropical sprue) 579.0
Thecoma (M8600/0) 220
  malignant (M8600/3) 183.0
Thelarche, precocious 259.1
Thelitis 611.0
  puerperal, postpartum 675.0
Therapeutic - see condition
Therapy V57.9
  blood transfusion, without reported diagnosis V58.2
  breathing V57.0
  chemotherapy V58.1
    fluoride V07.31
    prophylactic NEC V07.39
  dialysis (intermittent) (treatment)
    extracorporeal V56.0
    peritoneal V56.8
    renal V56.0
    specified type NEC V56.8
  exercise NEC V57.1
    breathing V57.0
  extracorporeal dialysis (renal) V56.0
  fluoride prophylaxis V07.31
  hemodialysis V56.0

Therapy (Continued)
  hormone replacement (postmenopausal) V07.4 ◀
  long term oxygen therapy V46.2
  occupational V57.21
  orthoptic V57.4
  orthotic V57.81
  peritoneal dialysis V56.8
  physical NEC V57.1
  postmenopausal hormone replacement V07.4
  radiation V58.0
  speech V57.3
  vocational V57.22
Thermalgesia 782.0
Thermalgia 782.0
Thermanalgesia 782.0
Thermanesthesia 782.0
Thermic - see condition
Thermography (abnormal) 793.9
  breast 793.89
Thermoplegia 992.0
Thesaurismosis
  amyloid 277.3
  bilirubin 277.4
  calcium 275.40
  cystine 270.0
  glycogen (see also Disease, glycogen storage) 271.0
  kerasin 272.7
  lipoid 272.7
  melanin 255.4
  phosphatide 272.7
  urate 274.9
Thiaminic deficiency 265.1
  with beriberi 265.0
Thibierge-Weissenbach syndrome (cutaneous systemic sclerosis) 710.1
Thickened endometrium 793.5
Thickening
  bone 733.99
    extremity 733.99
  breast 611.79
  hymen 623.3
  larynx 478.79
  nail 703.8
    congenital 757.5
  periosteal 733.99
  pleura (see also Pleurisy) 511.0
  skin 782.8
  subepiglottic 478.79
  tongue 529.8
  valve, heart - see Endocarditis
Thiele syndrome 724.6
Thigh - see condition
Thinning vertebra (see also Osteoporosis) 733.00
Thirst, excessive 783.5
  due to deprivation of water 994.3
Thomsen's disease 359.2
Thomson's disease (congenital poikiloderma) 757.33
Thoracic - see also condition
  kidney 753.3
  outlet syndrome 353.0
  stomach - see Hernia, diaphragm
Thoracogastroschisis (congenital) 759.89
Thoracopagus 759.4
Thoracoschisis 756.3
Thoracoscopic surgical procedure converted to open procedure V64.42
Thorax - see condition
Thorn's syndrome (see also Disease, renal) 593.9

Thornwaldt's, Tornwaldt's
  bursitis (pharyngeal) 478.29
  cyst 478.26
  disease (pharyngeal bursitis) 478.29
Thorson-Biörck syndrome (malignant carcinoid) 259.2
Threadworm (infection) (infestation) 127.4
Threatened
  abortion or miscarriage 640.0
    with subsequent abortion (see also Abortion, spontaneous) 634.9
    affecting fetus 762.1
  labor 644.1
    affecting fetus or newborn 761.8
    premature 644.0
  miscarriage 640.0
    affecting fetus 762.1
  premature
    delivery 644.2
      affecting fetus or newborn 761.8
    labor 644.0
      before 22 completed weeks of gestation 640.0
Three-day fever 066.0
Threshers' lung 495.0
Thrix annulata (congenital) 757.4
Throat - see condition
Thrombasthenia (Glanzmann's) (hemorrhagic) (hereditary) 287.1
Thromboangiitis 443.1
  obliterans (general) 443.1
    cerebral 437.1
    vessels
      brain 437.1
      spinal cord 437.1
Thromboarteritis - see Arteritis
Thromboasthenia (Glanzmann's) (hemorrhagic) (hereditary) 287.1
Thrombocytasthenia (Glanzmann's) 287.1
Thrombocythemia (essential) (hemorrhagic) (primary) (M9962/1) 238.7
  idiopathic (M9962/1) 238.7
Thrombocytopathy (dystrophic) (granulopenic) 287.1
Thrombocytopenia, thrombocytopenic 287.5
  with giant hemangioma 287.3
  amegakaryocytic, congenital 287.3
  congenital 287.3
  cyclic 287.3
  dilutional 287.4
  due to
    drugs 287.4
    extracorporeal circulation of blood 287.4
    massive blood transfusion 287.4
    platelet alloimmunization 287.4
  essential 287.3
  hereditary 287.3
  Kasabach-Merritt 287.3
  neonatal, transitory 776.1
    due to
      exchange transfusion 776.1
      idiopathic maternal thrombocytopenia 776.1
      isoimmunization 776.1
  primary 287.3
  puerperal, postpartum 666.3
  purpura (see also Purpura, thrombocytopenic) 287.3
    thrombotic 446.6
  secondary 287.4
  sex-linked 287.3
Thrombocytosis, essential 289.9
Thromboembolism - see Embolism

◀ **New**   ◀▥▥ **Revised**

Thrombopathy (Bernard-Soulier) 287.1
  constitutional 286.4
  Willebrand-Jürgens (angiohemophilia)
    286.4
Thrombopenia (*see also* Thrombocytopenia) 287.5
Thrombophlebitis 451.9
  antecubital vein 451.82
  antepartum (superficial) 671.2
    affecting fetus or newborn 760.3
    deep 671.3
  arm 451.89
    deep 451.83
    superficial 451.82
  breast, superficial 451.89
  cavernous (venous) sinus - *see* Thrombophlebitis, intracranial venous sinus
  cephalic vein 451.82
  cerebral (sinus) (vein) 325
    late effect - *see* category 326
    nonpyogenic 437.6
      in pregnancy or puerperium 671.5
      late effect - *see* Late effect(s) (of)
        cerebrovascular disease
  due to implanted device - *see* Complications, due to (presence of) any device, implant, or graft classified to 996.0-996.5 NEC
  during or resulting from a procedure NEC 997.2
  femoral 451.11
  femoropopliteal 451.19
  following infusion, perfusion, or transfusion 999.2
  hepatic (vein) 451.89
  idiopathic, recurrent 453.1
  iliac vein 451.81
  iliofemoral 451.11
  intracranial venous sinus (any) 325
    late effect - *see* category 326
    nonpyogenic 437.6
      in pregnancy or puerperium 671.5
      late effect - *see* Late effect(s) (of)
        cerebrovascular disease
  jugular vein 451.89
  lateral (venous) sinus - *see* Thrombophlebitis, intracranial venous sinus
  leg 451.2
    deep (vessels) 451.19
      femoral vein 451.11
      specified vessel NEC 451.19
    superficial (vessels) 451.0
      femoral vein 451.11
  longitudinal (venous) sinus - *see* Thrombophlebitis, intracranial venous sinus
  lower extremity 451.2
    deep (vessels) 451.19
      femoral vein 451.11
      specified vessel NEC 451.19
    superficial (vessels) 451.0
  migrans, migrating 453.1
  pelvic
    with
      abortion - *see* Abortion, by type, with sepsis
      ectopic pregnancy (*see also* categories 633.0-633.9) 639.0
      molar pregnancy (*see also* categories 630-632) 639.0
    following
      abortion 639.0
      ectopic or molar pregnancy 639.0
    puerperal 671.4
  popliteal vein 451.19

Thrombophlebitis (*Continued*)
  portal (vein) 572.1
  postoperative 997.2
  pregnancy (superficial) 671.2
    affecting fetus or newborn 760.3
    deep 671.3
  puerperal, postpartum, childbirth (extremities) (superficial) 671.2
    deep 671.4
    pelvic 671.4
    specified site NEC 671.5
  radial vein 451.82
  saphenous (greater) (lesser) 451.0
  sinus (intracranial) - *see* Thrombophlebitis, intracranial venous sinus
  specified site NEC 451.89
  tibial vein 451.19
Thrombosis, thrombotic (marantic)
    (multiple) (progressive) (septic)
    (vein) (vessel) 453.9
  with childbirth or during the puerperium - *see* Thrombosis, puerperal, postpartum
  antepartum - *see* Thrombosis, pregnancy
  aorta, aortic 444.1
    abdominal 444.0
    bifurcation 444.0
    saddle 444.0
    terminal 444.0
    thoracic 444.1
    valve - *see* Endocarditis, aortic
  apoplexy (*see also* Thrombosis, brain) 434.0
    late effect - *see* Late effect(s) (of) cerebrovascular disease
  appendix, septic - *see* Appendicitis, acute
  arteriolar-capillary platelet, disseminated 446.6
  artery, arteries (postinfectional) 444.9
    auditory, internal 433.8
    basilar (*see also* Occlusion, artery, basilar) 433.0
    carotid (common) (internal) (*see also* Occlusion, artery, carotid) 433.1
      with other precerebral artery 433.3
    cerebellar (anterior inferior) (posterior inferior) (superior) 433.8
    cerebral (*see also* Thrombosis, brain) 434.0
    choroidal (anterior) 433.8
    communicating posterior 433.8
    coronary (*see also* Infarct, myocardium) 410.9
      without myocardial infarction 411.81
      due to syphilis 093.89
      healed or specified as old 412
    extremities 444.22
      lower 444.22
      upper 444.21
    femoral 444.22
    hepatic 444.89
    hypophyseal 433.8
    meningeal, anterior or posterior 433.8
    mesenteric (with gangrene) 557.0
    ophthalmic (*see also* Occlusion, retina) 362.30
    pontine 433.8
    popliteal 444.22
    precerebral - *see* Occlusion, artery, precerebral NEC
    pulmonary 415.19
      iatrogenic 415.11
      postoperative 415.11

Thrombosis, thrombotic (*Continued*)
  artery, arteries (*Continued*)
    renal 593.81
    retinal (*see also* Occlusion, retina) 362.30
    specified site NEC 444.89
    spinal, anterior or posterior 433.8
    traumatic (complication) (early) (*see also* Injury, blood vessel, by site) 904.9
    vertebral (*see also* Occlusion, artery, vertebral) 433.2
      with other precerebral artery 433.3
  atrial (endocardial) 424.90
    due to syphilis 093.89
  auricular (*see also* Infarct, myocardium) 410.9
  axillary (vein) 453.8
  basilar (artery) (*see also* Occlusion, artery, basilar) 433.0
  bland NEC 453.9
  brain (artery) (stem) 434.0
    due to syphilis 094.89
    iatrogenic 997.02
    late effect - *see* Late effect(s) (of) cerebrovascular disease
    postoperative 997.02
    puerperal, postpartum, childbirth 674.0
    sinus (*see also* Thrombosis, intracranial venous sinus) 325
  capillary 448.9
    arteriolar, generalized 446.6
  cardiac (*see also* Infarct, myocardium) 410.9
    due to syphilis 093.89
    healed or specified as old 412
    valve - *see* Endocarditis
  carotid (artery) (common) (internal) (*see also* Occlusion, artery, carotid) 433.1
    with other precerebral artery 433.3
  cavernous sinus (venous) - *see* Thrombosis, intracranial venous sinus
  cerebellar artery (anterior inferior) (posterior inferior) (superior) 433.8
    late effect - *see* Late effect(s) (of) cerebrovascular disease
  cerebral (arteries) (*see also* Thrombosis, brain) 434.0
    late effect - *see* Late effect(s) (of) cerebrovascular disease
  coronary (artery) (*see also* Infarct, myocardium) 410.9
    without myocardial infarction 411.81
    due to syphilis 093.89
    healed or specified as old 412
  corpus cavernosum 607.82
  cortical (*see also* Thrombosis, brain) 434.0
  due to (presence of) any device, implant, or graft classifiable to 996.0-996.5 - *see* Complications, due to (presence of) any device, implant, or graft classified to 996.0-996.5 NEC
  effort 453.8
  endocardial - *see* Infarct, myocardium
  eye (*see also* Occlusion, retina) 362.30
  femoral (vein) 453.8   ◀━━
    with inflammation or phlebitis 451.11
    artery 444.22
    deep 453.41

Thrombosis, thrombotic (*Continued*)
  genital organ, male 608.83
  heart (chamber) (*see also* Infarct, myocardium) 410.9
  hepatic (vein) 453.0
    artery 444.89
    infectional or septic 572.1
  iliac (vein) 453.8
    with inflammation or phlebitis 451.81
    artery (common) (external) (internal) 444.81
  inflammation, vein - *see* Thrombophlebitis
  internal carotid artery (*see also* Occlusion, artery, carotid) 433.1
    with other precerebral artery 433.3
  intestine (with gangrene) 557.0
  intracranial (*see also* Thrombosis, brain) 434.0
    venous sinus (any) 325
      nonpyogenic origin 437.6
        in pregnancy or puerperium 671.5
  intramural (*see also* Infarct, myocardium) 410.9
    without
      cardiac condition 429.89
      coronary artery disease 429.89
      myocardial infarction 429.89
    healed or specified as old 412
  jugular (bulb) 453.8
  kidney 593.81
    artery 593.81
  lateral sinus (venous) - *see* Thrombosis, intracranial venous sinus
  leg 453.8
    with inflammation or phlebitis - *see* Thrombophlebitis
    deep (vessels) 453.40 ◀▥
      lower (distal) 453.42 ◀
      upper (proximal) 453.41 ◀
    superficial (vessels) 453.8
  liver (venous) 453.0
    artery 444.89
    infectional or septic 572.1
    portal vein 452
  longitudinal sinus (venous) - *see* Thrombosis, intracranial venous sinus
  lower extremity 453.8 ◀▥
    deep vessels 453.40 ◀
      calf 453.42 ◀
      distal (lower leg) 453.42 ◀
      femoral 453.41 ◀
      iliac 453.41 ◀
      lower leg 453.42 ◀
      peroneal 453.42 ◀
      popliteal 453.41 ◀
      proximal (upper leg) 453.41 ◀
      thigh 453.41 ◀
      tibial 453.42 ◀
  lung 415.19
    iatrogenic 415.11
    postoperative 415.11
  marantic, dural sinus 437.6
  meninges (brain) (*see also* Thrombosis, brain) 434.0
  mesenteric (artery) (with gangrene) 557.0
    vein (inferior) (superior) 557.0
  mitral - *see* Insufficiency, mitral
  mural (heart chamber) (*see also* Infarct, myocardium) 410.9
    without
      cardiac condition 429.89

Thrombosis, thrombotic (*Continued*)
  mural (*Continued*)
    without (*Continued*)
      coronary artery disease 429.89
      myocardial infarction 429.89
    due to syphilis 093.89
    following myocardial infarction 429.79
    healed or specified as old 412
  omentum (with gangrene) 557.0
  ophthalmic (artery) (*see also* Occlusion, retina) 362.30
  pampiniform plexus (male) 608.83
    female 620.8
  parietal (*see also* Infarct, myocardium) 410.9
  penis, penile 607.82
  peripheral arteries 444.22
    lower 444.22
    upper 444.21
  platelet 446.6
  portal 452
    due to syphilis 093.89
    infectional or septic 572.1
  precerebral artery - *see also* Occlusion, artery, precerebral NEC
  pregnancy 671.9
    deep (vein) 671.3
    superficial (vein) 671.2
  puerperal, postpartum, childbirth 671.9
    brain (artery) 674.0
      venous 671.5
    cardiac 674.8
    cerebral (artery) 674.0
      venous 671.5
    deep (vein) 671.4
    intracranial sinus (nonpyogenic) (venous) 671.5
    pelvic 671.4
    pulmonary (artery) 673.2
    specified site NEC 671.5
    superficial 671.2
  pulmonary (artery) (vein) 415.19
    iatrogenic 415.11
    postoperative 415.11
  renal (artery) 593.81
    vein 453.3
  resulting from presence of shunt or other internal prosthetic device - *see* Complications, due to (presence of) any device, implant, or graft classifiable to 996.0-996.5 NEC
  retina, retinal (artery) 362.30
    arterial branch 362.32
    central 362.31
    partial 362.33
    vein
      central 362.35
      tributary (branch) 362.36
  scrotum 608.83
  seminal vesicle 608.83
  sigmoid (venous) sinus (*see* Thrombosis, intracranial venous sinus) 325
  silent NEC 453.9
  sinus, intracranial (venous) (any) (*see also* Thrombosis, intracranial venous sinus) 325
  softening, brain (*see also* Thrombosis, brain) 434.0
  specified site NEC 453.8
  spermatic cord 608.83
  spinal cord 336.1
    due to syphilis 094.89
    in pregnancy or puerperium 671.5
    pyogenic origin 324.1
    late effect - *see* category 326

Thrombosis, thrombotic (*Continued*)
  spleen, splenic 289.59
    artery 444.89
  testis 608.83
  traumatic (complication) (early) (*see also* Injury, blood vessel, by site) 904.9
  tricuspid - *see* Endocarditis, tricuspid
  tunica vaginalis 608.83
  umbilical cord (vessels) 663.6
    affecting fetus or newborn 762.6
  vas deferens 608.83 ◀▥
  vein ◀
    deep 453.8 ◀
    lower extremity - *see* Thrombosis, lower extremity ◀
  vena cava (inferior) (superior) 453.2
Thrombus - *see* Thrombosis
Thrush 112.0
  newborn 771.7
Thumb - *see also* condition
  gamekeeper's 842.12
  sucking (child problem) 307.9
Thygeson's superficial punctate keratitis 370.21
Thymergasia (*see also* Psychosis, affective) 296.80
Thymitis 254.8
Thymoma (benign) (M8580/0) 212.6
  malignant (M8580/3) 164.0
Thymus, thymic (gland) - *see* condition
Thyrocele (*see also* Goiter) 240.9
Thyroglossal - *see also* condition
  cyst 759.2
  duct, persistent 759.2
Thyroid (body) (gland) - *see also* condition
  lingual 759.2
Thyroiditis 245.9
  acute (pyogenic) (suppurative) 245.0
    nonsuppurative 245.0
  autoimmune 245.2
  chronic (nonspecific) (sclerosing) 245.8
    fibrous 245.3
    lymphadenoid 245.2
    lymphocytic 245.2
    lymphoid 245.2
  complicating pregnancy, childbirth, or puerperium 648.1
  de Quervain's (subacute granulomatous) 245.1
  fibrous (chronic) 245.3
  giant (cell) (follicular) 245.1
  granulomatous (de Quervain's) (subacute) 245.1
  Hashimoto's (struma lymphomatosa) 245.2
  iatrogenic 245.4
  invasive (fibrous) 245.3
  ligneous 245.3
  lymphocytic (chronic) 245.2
  lymphoid 245.2
  lymphomatous 245.2
  pseudotuberculous 245.1
  pyogenic 245.0
  radiation 245.4
  Riedel's (ligneous) 245.3
  subacute 245.1
  suppurative 245.0
  tuberculous (*see also* Tuberculosis) 017.5
  viral 245.1
  woody 245.3
Thyrolingual duct, persistent 759.2
Thyromegaly 240.9

◀ **New**   ◀▥ **Revised**

Thyrotoxic
crisis or storm (see also Thyrotoxicosis) 242.9
heart failure (see also Thyrotoxicosis) 242.9 [425.7]
Thyrotoxicosis 242.9

> Note   Use the following fifth-digit subclassification with category 242:
>
> 0   without mention of thyrotoxic crisis or storm
> 1   with mention of thyrotoxic crisis or storm

with
goiter (diffuse) 242.0
adenomatous 242.3
multinodular 242.2
uninodular 242.1
nodular 242.3
multinodular 242.2
uninodular 242.1
infiltrative
dermopathy 242.0
ophthalmopathy 242.0
thyroid acropachy 242.0
complicating pregnancy, childbirth, or puerperium 648.1
due to
ectopic thyroid nodule 242.4
ingestion of (excessive) thyroid material 242.8
specified cause NEC 242.8
factitia 242.8
heart 242.9 [425.7]
neonatal (transient) 775.3
TIA (transient ischemic attack) 435.9
with transient neurologic deficit 435.9
late effect - see Late effect(s) (of) cerebrovascular disease
Tibia vara 732.4
Tic 307.20
breathing 307.20
child problem 307.21
compulsive 307.22
convulsive 307.20
degenerative (generalized) (localized) 333.3
facial 351.8
douloureux (see also Neuralgia, trigeminal) 350.1
atypical 350.2
habit 307.20
chronic (motor or vocal) 307.22
transient (of childhood) 307.21 ⬅
lid 307.20
transient (of childhood) 307.21 ⬅
motor-verbal 307.23
occupational 300.89
orbicularis 307.20
transient (of childhood) 307.21 ⬅
organic origin 333.3
postchoreic - see Chorea
psychogenic 307.20
compulsive 307.22
salaam 781.0
spasm 307.20
chronic (motor or vocal) 307.22
transient (of childhood) 307.21 ⬅
Tick (-borne) fever NEC 066.1
American mountain 066.1
Colorado 066.1
hemorrhagic NEC 065.3

Tick (Continued)
hemorrhagic NEC (Continued)
Crimean 065.0
Kyasanur Forest 065.2
Omsk 065.1
mountain 066.1
nonexanthematous 066.1
Tick-bite fever NEC 066.1
African 087.1
Colorado (virus) 066.1
Rocky Mountain 082.0
Tick paralysis 989.5
Tics and spasms, compulsive 307.22
Tietze's disease or syndrome 733.6
Tight, tightness
anus 564.89
chest 786.59
fascia (lata) 728.9
foreskin (congenital) 605
hymen 623.3
introitus (acquired) (congenital) 623.3
rectal sphincter 564.89
tendon 727.81
Achilles (heel) 727.81
urethral sphincter 598.9
Tilting vertebra 737.9
Timidity, child 313.21
Tinea (intersecta) (tarsi) 110.9
amiantacea 110.0
asbestina 110.0
barbae 110.0
beard 110.0
black dot 110.0
blanca 111.2
capitis 110.0
corporis 110.5
cruris 110.3
decalvans 704.09
flava 111.0
foot 110.4
furfuracea 111.0
imbricata (Tokelau) 110.5
lepothrix 039.0
manuum 110.2
microsporic (see also Dermatophytosis) 110.9
nigra 111.1
nodosa 111.2
pedis 110.4
scalp 110.0
specified site NEC 110.8
sycosis 110.0
tonsurans 110.0
trichophytic (see also Dermatophytosis) 110.9
unguium 110.1
versicolor 111.0
Tingling sensation (see also Disturbance, sensation) 782.0
Tin-miners' lung 503
Tinnitus (aurium) 388.30
audible 388.32
objective 388.32
subjective 388.31
Tipping ⬅
pelvis 738.6 ◀
with disproportion (fetopelvic) 653.0 ⬅
affecting fetus or newborn 763.1 ⬅
causing obstructed labor 660.1 ⬅
affecting fetus or newborn 763.1 ⬅
teeth 524.33 ◀

Tiredness 780.79
Tissue - see condition
Tobacco
abuse (affecting health) NEC (see also Abuse, drugs, nondependent) 305.1
heart 989.84
Tobias' syndrome (carcinoma, pulmonary apex) (M8010/3) 162.3
Tocopherol deficiency 269.1
Todd's
cirrhosis - see Cirrhosis, biliary
paralysis (postepileptic transitory paralysis) 344.89
Toe - see condition
Toilet, artificial opening (see also Attention to, artificial, opening) V55.9
Tokelau ringworm 110.5
Tollwut 071
Tolosa-Hunt syndrome 378.55
Tommaselli's disease
correct substance properly administered 599.7
overdose or wrong substance given or taken 961.4
Tongue - see also condition
worms 134.1
Tongue tie 750.0
Toni-Fanconi syndrome (cystinosis) 270.0
Tonic pupil 379.46
Tonsil - see condition
Tonsillitis (acute) (catarrhal) (croupous) (follicular) (gangrenous) (infective) (lacunar) (lingual) (malignant) (membranous) (phlegmonous) (pneumococcal) (pseudomembranous) (purulent) (septic) (staphylococcal) (subacute) (suppurative) (toxic) (ulcerative) (vesicular) (viral) 463
with influenza, flu, or grippe 487.1
chronic 474.00
diphtheritic (membranous) 032.0
hypertrophic 474.00
influenzal 487.1
parenchymatous 475
streptococcal 034.0
tuberculous (see also Tuberculosis) 012.8
Vincent's 101
Tonsillopharyngitis 465.8
Tooth, teeth - see condition
Toothache 525.9
Topagnosis 782.0
Tophi (gouty) 274.0
ear 274.81
heart 274.82
specified site NEC 274.82
Torn - see Tear, torn
Tornwaldt's bursitis (disease) (pharyngeal bursitis) 478.29
cyst 478.26
Torpid liver 573.9
Torsion
accessory tube 620.5
adnexa (female) 620.5
aorta (congenital) 747.29
acquired 447.1
appendix epididymis 608.2
bile duct 576.8
with calculus, choledocholithiasis or stones - see Choledocholithiasis
congenital 751.69
bowel, colon, or intestine 560.2

ICD-9-CM
T
Vol. 2

Torsion *(Continued)*
  cervix *(see also* Malposition, uterus)
    621.6
  duodenum 537.3
  dystonia - *see* Dystonia, torsion
  epididymis 608.2
    appendix 608.2
  fallopian tube 620.5
  gallbladder *(see also* Disease, gallbladder) 575.8
    congenital 751.69
  gastric 537.89
  hydatid of Morgagni (female) 620.5
  kidney (pedicle) 593.89
  Meckel's diverticulum (congenital) 751.0
  mesentery 560.2
  omentum 560.2
  organ or site, congenital NEC - *see* Anomaly, specified type NEC
  ovary (pedicle) 620.5
    congenital 752.0
  oviduct 620.5
  penis 607.89
    congenital 752.69
  renal 593.89
  spasm - *see* Dystonia, torsion
  spermatic cord 608.2
  spleen 289.59
  testicle, testis 608.2
  tibia 736.89
  umbilical cord - *see* Compression, umbilical cord
  uterus *(see also* Malposition, uterus) 621.6
Torticollis (intermittent) (spastic) 723.5
  congenital 754.1
    sternomastoid 754.1
  due to birth injury 767.8
  hysterical 300.11
  ocular 781.93
  psychogenic 306.0
    specified as conversion reaction 300.11
  rheumatic 723.5
  rheumatoid 714.0
  spasmodic 333.83
  traumatic, current NEC 847.0
Tortuous
  artery 447.1
  fallopian tube 752.19
  organ or site, congenital NEC - *see* Distortion
  renal vessel (congenital) 747.62
  retina vessel (congenital) 743.58
    acquired 362.17
  ureter 593.4
  urethra 599.84
  vein - *see* Varicose, vein
Torula, torular (infection) 117.5
  histolytica 117.5
  lung 117.5
Torulosis 117.5
Torus
  fracture
    fibula 823.41
      with tibia 823.42
    radius 813.45
    tibia 823.40
      with fibula 823.42
  mandibularis 526.81
  palatinus 526.81
Touch, vitreous 997.99
Touraine's syndrome (hereditary osteo-onychodysplasia) 756.89

Touraine-Solente-Golé syndrome (acro-pachyderma) 757.39
Tourette's disease (motor-verbal tic) 307.23
Tower skull 756.0
  with exophthalmos 756.0
Toxemia 799.89
  with
    abortion - *see* Abortion, by type, with toxemia
  bacterial - *see* Septicemia
  biliary *(see also* Disease, biliary) 576.8
  burn - *see* Burn, by site
  congenital NEC 779.89
  eclamptic 642.6
    with pre-existing hypertension 642.7
  erysipelatous *(see also* Erysipelas) 035
  fatigue 799.89
  fetus or newborn NEC 779.89
  food *(see also* Poisoning, food) 005.9
  gastric 537.89
  gastrointestinal 558.2
  intestinal 558.2
  kidney *(see also* Disease, renal) 593.9
  lung 518.89
  malarial NEC *(see also* Malaria) 084.6
  maternal (of pregnancy), affecting fetus or newborn 760.0
  myocardial - *see* Myocarditis, toxic
  of pregnancy (mild) (pre-eclamptic) 642.4
    with
      convulsions 642.6
      pre-existing hypertension 642.7
    affecting fetus or newborn 760.0
    severe 642.5
  pre-eclamptic - *see* Toxemia, of pregnancy
  puerperal, postpartum - *see* Toxemia, of pregnancy
  pulmonary 518.89
  renal *(see also* Disease, renal) 593.9
  septic *(see also* Septicemia) 038.9
  small intestine 558.2
  staphylococcal 038.10
    aureus 038.11
    due to food 005.0
    specified organism NEC 038.19
  stasis 799.89
  stomach 537.89
  uremic *(see also* Uremia) 586
  urinary 586
Toxemica cerebropathia psychica (nonalcoholic) 294.0
  alcoholic 291.1
Toxic (poisoning) - *see also* condition
  from drug or poison - *see* Table of Drugs and Chemicals
  oil syndrome 710.5
  shock syndrome 040.82
  thyroid (gland) *(see also* Thyrotoxicosis) 242.9
Toxicemia - *see* Toxemia
Toxicity
  dilantin
    asymptomatic 796.0
    symptomatic -*see* Table of Drugs and Chemicals
  drug
    asymptomatic 796.0
    symptomatic - *see* Table of Drugs and Chemicals
  fava bean 282.2

Toxicity *(Continued)*
  from drug or poison
    asymptomatic 796.0
    symptomatic - *see* Table of Drugs and Chemicals
Toxicosis *(see also* Toxemia) 799.89
  capillary, hemorrhagic 287.0
Toxinfection 799.89
  gastrointestinal 558.2
Toxocariasis 128.0
Toxoplasma infection, generalized 130.9
Toxoplasmosis (acquired) 130.9
  with pneumonia 130.4
  congenital, active 771.2
  disseminated (multisystemic) 130.8
  maternal
    with suspected damage to fetus affecting management of pregnancy 655.4
    affecting fetus or newborn 760.2
      manifest toxoplasmosis in fetus or newborn 771.2
  multiple sites 130.8
  multisystemic disseminated 130.8
  specified site NEC 130.7
Trabeculation, bladder 596.8
Trachea - *see* condition
Tracheitis (acute) (catarrhal) (infantile) (membranous) (plastic) (pneumococcal) (septic) (suppurative) (viral) 464.10
  with
    bronchitis 490
      acute or subacute 466.0
      chronic 491.8
      tuberculosis - *see* Tuberculosis, pulmonary
    laryngitis (acute) 464.20
      with obstruction 464.21
      chronic 476.1
      tuberculous *(see also* Tuberculosis, larynx) 012.3
    obstruction 464.11
  chronic 491.8
    with
      bronchitis (chronic) 491.8
      laryngitis (chronic) 476.1
    due to external agent - *see* Condition, respiratory, chronic, due to
  diphtheritic (membranous) 032.3
    due to external agent - *see* Inflammation, respiratory, upper, due to
  edematous 464.11
  influenzal 487.1
  streptococcal 034.0
  syphilitic 095.8
  tuberculous *(see also* Tuberculosis) 012.8
Trachelitis (nonvenereal) *(see also* Cervicitis) 616.0
  trichomonal 131.09
Tracheobronchial - *see* condition
Tracheobronchitis *(see also* Bronchitis) 490
  acute or subacute 466.0
    with bronchospasm or obstruction 466.0
  chronic 491.8
  influenzal 487.1
  senile 491.8
Tracheobronchomegaly (congenital) 748.3
Tracheobronchopneumonitis - *see* Pneumonia, broncho

◀ **New**   ◀▥ **Revised**

Tracheocele (external) (internal) 519.1
  congenital 748.3
Tracheomalacia 519.1
  congenital 748.3
Tracheopharyngitis (acute) 465.8
  chronic 478.9
    due to external agent - see Condition, respiratory, chronic, due to
  due to external agent - see Inflammation, respiratory, upper, due to
Tracheostenosis 519.1
  congenital 748.3
Tracheostomy
  attention to V55.0
  complication 519.00
  hemorrhage 519.09
  infection 519.01
  malfunctioning 519.02
  obstruction 519.09
  sepsis 519.01
  status V44.0
  stenosis 519.02
Trachoma, trachomatous 076.9
  active (stage) 076.1
  contraction of conjunctiva 076.1
  dubium 076.0
  healed or late effect 139.1
  initial (stage) 076.0
  Türck's (chronic catarrhal laryngitis) 476.0
Trachyphonia 784.49
Training
  insulin pump V65.46
  orthoptic V57.4
  orthotic V57.81
Train sickness 994.6
Trait
  hemoglobin
    abnormal NEC 282.7
      with thalassemia 282.49
    C (see also Disease, hemoglobin, C) 282.7
      with elliptocytosis 282.7
    S (Hb-S) 282.5
  Lepore 282.49
    with other abnormal hemoglobin NEC 282.49
  paranoid 301.0
  sickle-cell 282.5
    with
      elliptocytosis 282.5
      spherocytosis 282.5
Traits, paranoid 301.0
Tramp V60.0
Trance 780.09
  hysterical 300.13
Transaminasemia 790.4
Transfusion, blood
  donor V59.01
    stem cells V59.02
  incompatible 999.6
  reaction or complication - see Complications, transfusion
  syndrome
    fetomaternal 772.0
    twin-to-twin
      blood loss (donor twin) 772.0
      recipient twin 776.4
  without reported diagnosis V58.2
Transient - see also condition
  alteration of awareness 780.02
  blindness 368.12
  deafness (ischemic) 388.02
  global amnesia 437.7
  person (homeless) NEC V60.0

Transitional, lumbosacral joint of vertebra 756.19
Translocation
  autosomes NEC 758.5
    13-15 758.1
    16-18 758.2
    21 or 22 758.0
    balanced in normal individual 758.4
    D_1 758.1
    E_3 758.2
    G 758.0
  balanced autosomal in normal individual 758.4
  chromosomes NEC 758.89
  Down's syndrome 758.0
Translucency, iris 364.53
Transmission of chemical substances through the placenta (affecting fetus or newborn) 760.70
  alcohol 760.71
  anti-infective agents 760.74
  cocaine 760.75
  "crack" 760.75
  diethylstilbestrol [DES] 760.76
  hallucinogenic agents 760.73
  medicinal agents NEC 760.79
  narcotics 760.72
  obstetric anesthetic or analgesic drug 763.5
  specified agent NEC 760.79
  suspected, affecting management of pregnancy 655.5
Transplant (ed)
  bone V42.4
    marrow V42.81
  complication - see also Complications, due to (presence of) any device, implant, or graft classified to 996.0-996.5 NEC
    bone marrow 996.85
    corneal graft NEC 996.79
      infection or inflammation 996.69
      reaction 996.51
      rejection 996.51
    organ (failure) (immune or nonimmune cause) (infection) (rejection) 996.80
      bone marrow 996.85
      heart 996.83
      intestines 996.87
      kidney 996.81
      liver 996.82
      lung 996.84
      pancreas 996.86
      specified NEC 996.89
    skin NEC 996.79
      infection or inflammation 996.69
      rejection 996.52
      artificial 996.55
        decellularized allodermis 996.55
  cornea V42.5
  hair V50.0
  heart V42.1
    valve V42.2
  intestine V42.84
  kidney V42.0
  liver V42.7
  lung V42.6
  organ V42.9
    specified NEC V42.89
  pancreas V42.83
  peripheral stem cells V42.82
  skin V42.3
  stem cells, peripheral V42.82

Transplant (Continued)
  tissue V42.9
    specified NEC V42.89
Transplants, ovarian, endometrial 617.1
Transposed - see Transposition
Transposition (congenital) - see also Malposition, congenital
  abdominal viscera 759.3
  aorta (dextra) 745.11
  appendix 751.5
  arterial trunk 745.10
  colon 751.5
  great vessels (complete) 745.10
    both originating from right ventricle 745.11
    corrected 745.12
    double outlet right ventricle 745.11
    incomplete 745.11
    partial 745.11
    specified type NEC 745.19
  heart 746.87
    with complete transposition of viscera 759.3
  intestine (large) (small) 751.5
  pulmonary veins 747.49
  reversed jejunal (for bypass) (status) V45.3
  scrotal 752.81
  stomach 750.7
    with general transposition of viscera 759.3
  teeth, tooth 524.30
  vessels (complete) 745.10
    partial 745.11
  viscera (abdominal) (thoracic) 759.3
Trans-sexualism 302.50
  with
    asexual history 302.51
    heterosexual history 302.53
    homosexual history 302.52
Transverse - see also condition
  arrest (deep), in labor 660.3
    affecting fetus or newborn 763.1
  lie 652.3
    before labor, affecting fetus or newborn 761.7
    causing obstructed labor 660.0
      affecting fetus or newborn 763.1
    during labor, affecting fetus or newborn 763.1
Transvestism, transvestitism (transvestic fetishism) 302.3
Trapped placenta (with hemorrhage) 666.0
  without hemorrhage 667.0
Trauma, traumatism (see also Injury, by site) 959.9
  birth - see Birth, injury NEC
  causing hemorrhage of pregnancy or delivery 641.8
  complicating
    abortion - see Abortion, by type, with damage to pelvic organs
    ectopic pregnancy (see also categories 633.0-633.9) 639.2
    molar pregnancy (see also categories 630-632) 639.2
  during delivery NEC 665.9
  following
    abortion 639.2
    ectopic or molar pregnancy 639.2
  maternal, during pregnancy, affecting fetus or newborn 760.5
  neuroma - see Injury, nerve, by site

ICD-9-CM

I

Vol. 2

Trauma, traumatism (Continued)
  previous major, affecting management of pregnancy, childbirth, or puerperium V23.8
  psychic (current) - see also Reaction, adjustment
    previous (history) V15.49
  psychologic, previous (affecting health) V15.49
  transient paralysis - see Injury, nerve, by site
Traumatic - see condition
Treacher Collins' syndrome (incomplete facial dysostosis) 756.0
Treitz's hernia - see Hernia, Treitz's
Trematode infestation NEC 121.9
Trematodiasis NEC 121.9
Trembles 988.8
Trembling paralysis (see also Parkinsonism) 332.0
Tremor 781.0
  essential (benign) 333.1
  familial 333.1
  flapping (liver) 572.8
  hereditary 333.1
  hysterical 300.11
  intention 333.1
  mercurial 985.0
  muscle 728.85
  Parkinson's (see also Parkinsonism) 332.0
  psychogenic 306.0
    specified as conversion reaction 300.11
  senilis 797
  specified type NEC 333.1
Trench
  fever 083.1
  foot 991.4
  mouth 101
  nephritis - see Nephritis, acute
Treponema pallidum infection (see also Syphilis) 097.9
Treponematosis 102.9
  due to
    T. pallidum - see Syphilis
    T. pertenue (yaws) (see also Yaws) 102.9
Triad
  Kartagener's 759.3
  Reiter's (complete) (incomplete) 099.3
  Saint's (see also Hernia, diaphragm) 553.3
Trichiasis 704.2
  cicatricial 704.2
  eyelid 374.05
    with entropion (see also Entropion) 374.00
Trichinella spiralis (infection) (infestation) 124
Trichinelliasis 124
Trichinellosis 124
Trichiniasis 124
Trichinosis 124
Trichobezoar 938
  intestine 936
  stomach 935.2
Trichocephaliasis 127.3
Trichocephalosis 127.3
Trichocephalus infestation 127.3
Trichoclasis 704.2
Trichoepithelioma (M8100/0) - see also Neoplasm, skin, benign
  breast 217

Trichoepithelioma (Continued)
  genital organ NEC - see Neoplasm, by site, benign
  malignant (M8100/3) - see Neoplasm, skin, malignant
Trichofolliculoma (M8101/0) - see Neoplasm, skin, benign
Tricholemmoma (M8102/0) - see Neoplasm, skin, benign
Trichomatosis 704.2
Trichomoniasis 131.9
  bladder 131.09
  cervix 131.09
  intestinal 007.3
  prostate 131.03
  seminal vesicle 131.09
  specified site NEC 131.8
  urethra 131.02
  urogenitalis 131.00
  vagina 131.01
  vulva 131.01
  vulvovaginal 131.01
Trichomycosis 039.0
  axillaris 039.0
  nodosa 111.2
  nodularis 111.2
  rubra 039.0
Trichonocardiosis (axillaris) (palmellina) 039.0
Trichonodosis 704.2
Trichophytid, trichophyton infection (see also Dermatophytosis) 110.9
Trichophytide - see Dermatophytosis
Trichophytobezoar 938
  intestine 936
  stomach 935.2
Trichophytosis - see Dermatophytosis
Trichoptilosis 704.2
Trichorrhexis (nodosa) 704.2
Trichosporosis nodosa 111.2
Trichostasis spinulosa (congenital) 757.4
Trichostrongyliasis (small intestine) 127.6
Trichostrongylosis 127.6
Trichostrongylus (instabilis) infection 127.6
Trichotillomania 312.39
Trichromat, anomalous (congenital) 368.59
Trichromatopsia, anomalous (congenital) 368.59
Trichuriasis 127.3
Trichuris trichiura (any site) (infection) (infestation) 127.3
Tricuspid (valve) - see condition
Trifid - see also Accessory
  kidney (pelvis) 753.3
  tongue 750.13
Trigeminal neuralgia (see also Neuralgia, trigeminal) 350.1
Trigeminoencephaloangiomatosis 759.6
Trigeminy 427.89
  postoperative 997.1
Trigger finger (acquired) 727.03
  congenital 756.89
Trigonitis (bladder) (chronic) (pseudomembranous) 595.3
  tuberculous (see also Tuberculosis) 016.1
Trigonocephaly 756.0
Trihexosidosis 272.7
Trilobate placenta - see Placenta, abnormal
Trilocular heart 745.8

Tripartita placenta - see Placenta, abnormal
Triple - see also Accessory
  kidneys 753.3
  uteri 752.2
  X female 758.81
Triplegia 344.89
  congenital or infantile 343.8
Triplet
  affected by maternal complications of pregnancy 761.5
  healthy liveborn - see Newborn, multiple
  pregnancy (complicating delivery) NEC 651.1
    with fetal loss and retention of one or more fetus(es) 651.4
Triplex placenta - see Placenta, abnormal
Triplication - see Accessory
Trismus 781.0
  neonatorum 771.3
  newborn 771.3
Trisomy (syndrome) NEC 758.5
  13 (partial) 758.1
  16-18 758.2
  18 (partial) 758.2
  21 (partial) 758.0
  22 758.0
  autosomes NEC 758.5
  D_1 758.1
  E_3 758.2
  G (group) 758.0
  group D_1 758.1
  group E 758.2
  group G 758.0
Tritanomaly 368.53
Tritanopia 368.53
Troisier-Hanot-Chauffard syndrome (bronze diabetes) 275.0
Trombidiosis 133.8
Trophedema (hereditary) 757.0
  congenital 757.0
Trophoblastic disease (see also Hydatidiform mole) 630
  previous, affecting management of pregnancy V23.1
Tropholymphedema 757.0
Trophoneurosis NEC 356.9
  arm NEC 354.9
  disseminated 710.1
  facial 349.89
  leg NEC 355.8
  lower extremity NEC 355.8
  upper extremity NEC 354.9
Tropical - see also condition
  maceration feet (syndrome) 991.4
  wet foot (syndrome) 991.4
Trouble - see also Disease
  bowel 569.9
  heart - see Disease, heart
  intestine 569.9
  kidney (see also Disease, renal) 593.9
  nervous 799.2
  sinus (see also Sinusitis) 473.9
Trousseau's syndrome (thrombophlebitis migrans) 453.1
Truancy, childhood - see also Disturbance, conduct
  socialized 312.2
  undersocialized, unsocialized 312.1
Truncus
  arteriosus (persistent) 745.0
  common 745.0
  communis 745.0

◀ **New**   ◀▥ **Revised**

Trunk - *see* condition
Trychophytide - *see* Dermatophytosis
Trypanosoma infestation - *see* Trypanosomiasis
Trypanosomiasis 086.9
with meningoencephalitis 086.9
[323.2]
African 086.5
due to Trypanosoma 086.5
gambiense 086.3
rhodesiense 086.4
American 086.2
with
heart involvement 086.0
other organ involvement 086.1
without mention of organ involvement 086.2
Brazilian - *see* Trypanosomiasis, American
Chagas' - *see* Trypanosomiasis, American
due to Trypanosoma
cruzi - *see* Trypanosomiasis, American
gambiense 086.3
rhodesiense 086.4
gambiensis, Gambian 086.3
North American - *see* Trypanosomiasis,
American
rhodesiensis, Rhodesian 086.4
South American - *see* Trypanosomiasis,
American
T-shaped incisors 520.2
Tsutsugamushi fever 081.2
Tube, tubal, tubular - *see also* condition
ligation, admission for V25.2
Tubercle - *see also* Tuberculosis
brain, solitary 013.2
Darwin's 744.29
epithelioid noncaseating 135
Ghon, primary infection 010.0
Tuberculid, tuberculide (indurating)
(lichenoid) (miliary) (papulonecrotic)
(primary) (skin) (subcutaneous) (*see
also* Tuberculosis) 017.0
Tuberculoma - *see also* Tuberculosis
brain (any part) 013.2
meninges (cerebral) (spinal) 013.1
spinal cord 013.4
Tuberculosis, tubercular, tuberculous
(calcification) (calcified) (caseous)
(chromogenic acid-fast bacilli) (congenital) (degeneration) (disease) (fibrocaseous) (fistula) (gangrene) (interstitial) (isolated circumscribed
lesions) (necrosis) (parenchymatous)
(ulcerative) 011.9

Note   Use the following fifth-digit
subclassification with categories 010-
018:

0   unspecified
1   bacteriological or histological
examination not done
2   bacteriological or histological
examination unknown (at
present)
3   tubercle bacilli found (in sputum) by microscopy
4   tubercle bacilli not found (in
sputum) by microscopy, but
found by bacterial culture
5   tubercle bacilli not found by
bacteriological examination,

Tuberculosis, tubercular, tuberculous
(Continued)
but tuberculosis confirmed histologically
6   tubercle bacilli not found by
bacteriological or histological
examination, but tuberculosis
confirmed by other methods
[inoculation of animals]

For tuberculous conditions specified
as late effects or sequelae, *see* category 137.

abdomen 014.8
lymph gland 014.8
abscess 011.9
arm 017.9
bone (*see also* Osteomyelitis, due to,
tuberculosis) 015.9 *[730.8]*
hip 015.1 *[730.85]*
knee 015.2 *[730.86]*
sacrum 015.0 *[730.88]*
specified site NEC 015.7 *[730.88]*
spinal 015.0 *[730.88]*
vertebra 015.0 *[730.88]*
brain 013.3
breast 017.9
Cowper's gland 016.5
dura (mater) 013.8
brain 013.3
spinal cord 013.5
epidural 013.8
brain 013.3
spinal cord 013.5
frontal sinus - *see* Tuberculosis, sinus
genital organs NEC 016.9
female 016.7
male 016.5
genitourinary NEC 016.9
gland (lymphatic) - *see* Tuberculosis,
lymph gland
hip 015.1
iliopsoas 015.0 *[730.88]*
intestine 014.8
ischiorectal 014.8
joint 015.9
hip 015.1
knee 015.2
specified joint NEC 015.8
vertebral 015.0 *[730.88]*
kidney 016.0 *[590.81]*
knee 015.2
lumbar 015.0 *[730.88]*
lung 011.2
primary, progressive 010.8
meninges (cerebral) (spinal) 013.0
pelvic 016.9
female 016.7
male 016.5
perianal 014.8
fistula 014.8
perinephritic 016.0 *[590.81]*
perineum 017.9
perirectal 014.8
psoas 015.0 *[730.88]*
rectum 014.8
retropharyngeal 012.8
sacrum 015.0 *[730.88]*
scrofulous 017.2
scrotum 016.5
skin 017.0
primary 017.0
spinal cord 013.5
spine or vertebra (column) 015.0
[730.88]

Tuberculosis, tubercular, tuberculous
(Continued)
abscess *(Continued)*
strumous 017.2
subdiaphragmatic 014.8
testis 016.5
thigh 017.9
urinary 016.3
kidney 016.0 *[590.81]*
uterus 016.7
accessory sinus - *see* Tuberculosis, sinus
Addison's disease 017.6
adenitis (*see also* Tuberculosis, lymph
gland) 017.2
adenoids 012.8
adenopathy (*see also* Tuberculosis,
lymph gland) 017.2
tracheobronchial 012.1
primary progressive 010.8
adherent pericardium 017.9 *[420.0]*
adnexa (uteri) 016.7
adrenal (capsule) (gland) 017.6
air passage NEC 012.8
alimentary canal 014.8
anemia 017.9
ankle (joint) 015.8
bone 015.5 *[730.87]*
anus 014.8
apex (*see also* Tuberculosis, pulmonary)
011.9
apical (*see also* Tuberculosis, pulmonary) 011.9
appendicitis 014.8
appendix 014.8
arachnoid 013.0
artery 017.9
arthritis (chronic) (synovial) 015.9
[711.40]
ankle 015.8 *[730.87]*
hip 015.1 *[711.45]*
knee 015.2 *[711.46]*
specified site NEC 015.8 *[711.48]*
spine or vertebra (column) 015.0
[720.81]
wrist 015.8 *[730.83]*
articular - *see* Tuberculosis, joint
ascites 014.0
asthma (*see also* Tuberculosis, pulmonary) 011.9
axilla, axillary 017.2
gland 017.2
bilateral (*see also* Tuberculosis, pulmonary) 011.9
bladder 016.1
bone (*see also* Osteomyelitis, due to, tuberculosis) 015.9 *[730.8]*
hip 015.1 *[730.85]*
knee 015.2 *[730.86]*
limb NEC 015.5 *[730.88]*
sacrum 015.0 *[730.88]*
specified site NEC 015.7 *[730.88]*
spinal or vertebral column 015.0
[730.88]
bowel 014.8
miliary 018.9
brain 013.2
breast 017.9
broad ligament 016.7
bronchi, bronchial, bronchus 011.3
ectasia, ectasis 011.5
fistula 011.3
primary, progressive 010.8
gland 012.1
primary, progressive 010.8

ICD-9-CM

I

Vol. 2

Tuberculosis, tubercular, tuberculous
(Continued)
bronchi, bronchial, bronchus
(Continued)
isolated 012.2
lymph gland or node 012.1
primary, progressive 010.8
bronchiectasis 011.5
bronchitis 011.3
bronchopleural 012.0
bronchopneumonia, bronchopneumonic 011.6
bronchorrhagia 011.3
bronchotracheal 011.3
isolated 012.2
bronchus - see Tuberculosis, bronchi
bronze disease (Addison's) 017.6
buccal cavity 017.9
bulbourethral gland 016.5
bursa (see also Tuberculosis, joint) 015.9
cachexia NEC (see also Tuberculosis, pulmonary) 011.9
cardiomyopathy 017.9 [425.8]
caries (see also Tuberculosis, bone) 015.9 [730.8]
cartilage (see also Tuberculosis, bone) 015.9 [730.8]
intervertebral 015.0 [730.88]
catarrhal (see also Tuberculosis, pulmonary) 011.9
cecum 014.8
cellular tissue (primary) 017.0
cellulitis (primary) 017.0
central nervous system 013.9
specified site NEC 013.8
cerebellum (current) 013.2
cerebral (current) 013.2
meninges 013.0
cerebrospinal 013.6
meninges 013.0
cerebrum (current) 013.2
cervical 017.2
gland 017.2
lymph nodes 017.2
cervicitis (uteri) 016.7
cervix 016.7
chest (see also Tuberculosis, pulmonary) 011.9
childhood type or first infection 010.0
choroid 017.3 [363.13]
choroiditis 017.3 [363.13]
ciliary body 017.3 [364.11]
colitis 014.8
colliers' 011.4
colliquativa (primary) 017.0
colon 014.8
ulceration 014.8
complex, primary 010.0
complicating pregnancy, childbirth, or puerperium 647.3
affecting fetus or newborn 760.2
congenital 771.2
conjunctiva 017.3 [370.31]
connective tissue 017.9
bone - see Tuberculosis, bone
contact V01.1
converter (tuberculin skin test) (without disease) 795.5
cornea (ulcer) 017.3 [370.31]
Cowper's gland 016.5
coxae 015.1 [730.85]
coxalgia 015.1 [730.85]
cul-de-sac of Douglas 014.8
curvature, spine 015.0 [737.40]

Tuberculosis, tubercular, tuberculous
(Continued)
cutis (colliquativa) (primary) 017.0
cyst, ovary 016.6
cystitis 016.1
dacryocystitis 017.3 [375.32]
dactylitis 015.5
diarrhea 014.8
diffuse (see also Tuberculosis, miliary) 018.9
lung - see Tuberculosis, pulmonary
meninges 013.0
digestive tract 014.8
disseminated (see also Tuberculosis, miliary) 018.9
meninges 013.0
duodenum 014.8
dura (mater) 013.9
abscess 013.8
cerebral 013.3
spinal 013.5
dysentery 014.8
ear (inner) (middle) 017.4
bone 015.6
external (primary) 017.0
skin (primary) 017.0
elbow 015.8
emphysema - see Tuberculosis, pulmonary
empyema 012.0
encephalitis 013.6
endarteritis 017.9
endocarditis (any valve) 017.9 [424.91]
endocardium (any valve) 017.9 [424.91]
endocrine glands NEC 017.9
endometrium 016.7
enteric, enterica 014.8
enteritis 014.8
enterocolitis 014.8
epididymis 016.4
epididymitis 016.4
epidural abscess 013.8
brain 013.3
spinal cord 013.5
epiglottis 012.3
episcleritis 017.3 [379.00]
erythema (induratum) (nodosum) (primary) 017.1
esophagus 017.8
Eustachian tube 017.4
exposure to V01.1
exudative 012.0
primary, progressive 010.1
eye 017.3
glaucoma 017.3 [365.62]
eyelid (primary) 017.0
lupus 017.0 [373.4]
fallopian tube 016.6
fascia 017.9
fauces 012.8
finger 017.9
first infection 010.0
fistula, perirectal 014.8
Florida 011.6
foot 017.9
funnel pelvis 137.3
gallbladder 017.9
galloping (see also Tuberculosis, pulmonary) 011.9
ganglionic 015.9
gastritis 017.9
gastrocolic fistula 014.8
gastroenteritis 014.8
gastrointestinal tract 014.8

Tuberculosis, tubercular, tuberculous
(Continued)
general, generalized 018.9
acute 018.0
chronic 018.8
genital organs NEC 016.9
female 016.7
male 016.5
genitourinary NEC 016.9
genu 015.2
glandulae suprarenalis 017.6
glandular, general 017.2
glottis 012.3
grinders' 011.4
groin 017.2
gum 017.9
hand 017.9
heart 017.9 [425.8]
hematogenous - see Tuberculosis, miliary
hemoptysis (see also Tuberculosis, pulmonary) 011.9
hemorrhage NEC (see also Tuberculosis, pulmonary) 011.9
hemothorax 012.0
hepatitis 017.9
hilar lymph nodes 012.1
primary, progressive 010.8
hip (disease) (joint) 015.1
bone 015.1 [730.85]
hydrocephalus 013.8
hydropneumothorax 012.0
hydrothorax 012.0
hypoadrenalism 017.6
hypopharynx 012.8
ileocecal (hyperplastic) 014.8
ileocolitis 014.8
ileum 014.8
iliac spine (superior) 015.0 [730.88]
incipient NEC (see also Tuberculosis, pulmonary) 011.9
indurativa (primary) 017.1
infantile 010.0
infection NEC 011.9
without clinical manifestation 010.0
infraclavicular gland 017.2
inguinal gland 017.2
inguinalis 017.2
intestine (any part) 014.8
iris 017.3 [364.11]
iritis 017.3 [364.11]
ischiorectal 014.8
jaw 015.7 [730.88]
jejunum 014.8
joint 015.9
hip 015.1
knee 015.2
specified site NEC 015.8
vertebral 015.0 [730.88]
keratitis 017.3 [370.31]
interstitial 017.3 [370.59]
keratoconjunctivitis 017.3 [370.31]
kidney 016.0
knee (joint) 015.2
kyphoscoliosis 015.0 [737.43]
kyphosis 015.0 [737.41]
lacrimal apparatus, gland 017.3
laryngitis 012.3
larynx 012.3
leptomeninges, leptomeningitis (cerebral) (spinal) 013.0
lichenoides (primary) 017.0
linguae 017.9
lip 017.9

Tuberculosis, tubercular, tuberculous
(*Continued*)
liver 017.9
lordosis 015.0 [737.42]
lung - *see* Tuberculosis, pulmonary
luposa 017.0
  eyelid 017.0 [373.4]
lymphadenitis - *see* Tuberculosis, lymph gland
lymphangitis - *see* Tuberculosis, lymph gland
lymphatic (gland) (vessel) - *see* Tuberculosis, lymph gland
lymph gland or node (peripheral) 017.2
  abdomen 014.8
  bronchial 012.1
    primary, progressive 010.8
  cervical 017.2
  hilar 012.1
    primary, progressive 010.8
  intrathoracic 012.1
    primary, progressive 010.8
  mediastinal 012.1
    primary, progressive 010.8
  mesenteric 014.8
  peripheral 017.2
  retroperitoneal 014.8
  tracheobronchial 012.1
    primary, progressive 010.8
malignant NEC (*see also* Tuberculosis, pulmonary) 011.9
mammary gland 017.9
marasmus NEC (*see also* Tuberculosis, pulmonary) 011.9
mastoiditis 015.6
maternal, affecting fetus or newborn 760.2
mediastinal (lymph) gland or node 012.1
  primary, progressive 010.8
mediastinitis 012.8
  primary, progressive 010.8
mediastinopericarditis 017.9 [420.0]
mediastinum 012.8
  primary, progressive 010.8
medulla 013.9
  brain 013.2
  spinal cord 013.4
melanosis, Addisonian 017.6
membrane, brain 013.0
meninges (cerebral) (spinal) 013.0
meningitis (basilar) (brain) (cerebral) (cerebrospinal) (spinal) 013.0
meningoencephalitis 013.0
mesentery, mesenteric 014.8
  lymph gland or node 014.8
miliary (any site) 018.9
  acute 018.0
  chronic 018.8
  specified type NEC 018.8
millstone makers' 011.4
miners' 011.4
moulders' 011.4
mouth 017.9
multiple 018.9
  acute 018.0
  chronic 018.8
muscle 017.9
myelitis 013.6
myocarditis 017.9 [422.0]
myocardium 017.9 [422.0]
nasal (passage) (sinus) 012.8
nasopharynx 012.8
neck gland 017.2

Tuberculosis, tubercular, tuberculous
(*Continued*)
nephritis 016.0 [583.81]
nerve 017.9
nose (septum) 012.8
ocular 017.3
old NEC 137.0
  without residuals V12.01
omentum 014.8
oophoritis (acute) (chronic) 016.6
optic 017.3 [377.39]
  nerve trunk 017.3 [377.39]
  papilla, papillae 017.3 [377.39]
orbit 017.3
orchitis 016.5 [608.81]
organ, specified NEC 017.9
orificialis (primary) 017.0
osseous (*see also* Tuberculosis, bone) 015.9 [730.8]
osteitis (*see also* Tuberculosis, bone) 015.9 [730.8]
osteomyelitis (*see also* Tuberculosis, bone) 015.9 [730.8]
otitis (media) 017.4
ovaritis (acute) (chronic) 016.6
ovary (acute) (chronic) 016.6
oviducts (acute) (chronic) 016.6
pachymeningitis 013.0
palate (soft) 017.9
pancreas 017.9
papulonecrotic (primary) 017.0
parathyroid glands 017.9
paronychia (primary) 017.0
parotid gland or region 017.9
pelvic organ NEC 016.9
  female 016.7
  male 016.5
pelvis (bony) 015.7 [730.85]
penis 016.5
peribronchitis 011.3
pericarditis 017.9 [420.0]
pericardium 017.9 [420.0]
perichondritis, larynx 012.3
perineum 017.9
periostitis (*see also* Tuberculosis, bone) 015.9 [730.8]
periphlebitis 017.9
  eye vessel 017.3 [362.18]
  retina 017.3 [362.18]
perirectal fistula 014.8
peritoneal gland 014.8
peritoneum 014.0
peritonitis 014.0
pernicious NEC (*see also* Tuberculosis, pulmonary) 011.9
pharyngitis 012.8
pharynx 012.8
phlyctenulosis (conjunctiva) 017.3 [370.31]
phthisis NEC (*see also* Tuberculosis, pulmonary) 011.9
pituitary gland 017.9
placenta 016.7
pleura, pleural, pleurisy, pleuritis (fibrinous) (obliterative) (purulent) (simple plastic) (with effusion) 012.0
  primary, progressive 010.1
pneumonia, pneumonic 011.6
pneumothorax 011.7
polyserositis 018.9
  acute 018.0
  chronic 018.8
potters' 011.4
prepuce 016.5

Tuberculosis, tubercular, tuberculous
(*Continued*)
primary 010.9
  complex 010.0
  complicated 010.8
    with pleurisy or effusion 010.1
  progressive 010.8
    with pleurisy or effusion 010.1
  skin 017.0
proctitis 014.8
prostate 016.5 [601.4]
prostatitis 016.5 [601.4]
pulmonaris (*see also* Tuberculosis, pulmonary) 011.9
pulmonary (artery) (incipient) (malignant) (multiple round foci) (pernicious) (reinfection stage) 011.9
  cavitated or with cavitation 011.2
    primary, progressive 010.8
  childhood type or first infection 010.0
  chromogenic acid-fast bacilli 795.39
  fibrosis or fibrotic 011.4
  infiltrative 011.0
    primary, progressive 010.9
  nodular 011.1
  specified NEC 011.8
  sputum positive only 795.39
  status following surgical collapse of lung NEC 011.9
pyelitis 016.0 [590.81]
pyelonephritis 016.0 [590.81]
pyemia - *see* Tuberculosis, miliary
pyonephrosis 016.0
pyopneumothorax 012.0
pyothorax 012.0
rectum (with abscess) 014.8
  fistula 014.8
reinfection stage (*see also* Tuberculosis, pulmonary) 011.9
renal 016.0
renes 016.0
reproductive organ 016.7
respiratory NEC (*see also* Tuberculosis, pulmonary) 011.9
  specified site NEC 012.8
retina 017.3 [363.13]
retroperitoneal (lymph gland or node) 014.8
  gland 014.8
retropharyngeal abscess 012.8
rheumatism 015.9
rhinitis 012.8
sacroiliac (joint) 015.8
sacrum 015.0 [730.88]
salivary gland 017.9
salpingitis (acute) (chronic) 016.6
sandblasters' 011.4
sclera 017.3 [379.09]
scoliosis 015.0 [737.43]
scrofulous 017.2
scrotum 016.5
seminal tract or vesicle 016.5 [608.81]
senile NEC (*see also* Tuberculosis, pulmonary) 011.9
septic NEC (*see also* Tuberculosis, miliary) 018.9
shoulder 015.8
  blade 015.7 [730.8]
sigmoid 014.8
sinus (accessory) (nasal) 012.8
  bone 015.7 [730.88]
  epididymis 016.4
skeletal NEC (*see also* Osteomyelitis, due to tuberculosis) 015.9 [730.8]

ICD-9-CM

T

Vol. 2

Tuberculosis, tubercular, tuberculous
(Continued)
skin (any site) (primary) 017.0
small intestine 014.8
soft palate 017.9
spermatic cord 016.5
spinal
column 015.0 [730.88]
cord 013.4
disease 015.0 [730.88]
medulla 013.4
membrane 013.0
meninges 013.0
spine 015.0 [730.88]
spleen 017.7
splenitis 017.7
spondylitis 015.0 [720.81]
spontaneous pneumothorax - see Tuberculosis, pulmonary
sternoclavicular joint 015.8
stomach 017.9
stonemasons' 011.4
struma 017.2
subcutaneous tissue (cellular) (primary) 017.0
subcutis (primary) 017.0
subdeltoid bursa 017.9
submaxillary 017.9
region 017.9
supraclavicular gland 017.2
suprarenal (capsule) (gland) 017.6
swelling, joint (see also Tuberculosis, joint) 015.9
symphysis pubis 015.7 [730.88]
synovitis 015.9 [727.01]
hip 015.1 [727.01]
knee 015.2 [727.01]
specified site NEC 015.8 [727.01]
spine or vertebra 015.0 [727.01]
systemic - see Tuberculosis, miliary
tarsitis (eyelid) 017.0 [373.4]
ankle (bone) 015.5 [730.87]
tendon (sheath) - see Tuberculosis, tenosynovitis
tenosynovitis 015.9 [727.01]
hip 015.1 [727.01]
knee 015.2 [727.01]
specified site NEC 015.8 [727.01]
spine or vertebra 015.0 [727.01]
testis 016.5 [608.81]
throat 012.8
thymus gland 017.9
thyroid gland 017.5
toe 017.9
tongue 017.9
tonsil (lingual) 012.8
tonsillitis 012.8
trachea, tracheal 012.8
gland 012.1
primary, progressive 010.8
isolated 012.2
tracheobronchial 011.3
glandular 012.1
primary, progressive 010.8
isolated 012.2
lymph gland or node 012.1
primary, progressive 010.8
tubal 016.6
tunica vaginalis 016.5
typhlitis 014.8
ulcer (primary) (skin) 017.0
bowel or intestine 014.8
specified site NEC - see Tuberculosis, by site

Tuberculosis, tubercular, tuberculous
(Continued)
unspecified site - see Tuberculosis, pulmonary
ureter 016.2
urethra, urethral 016.3
urinary organ or tract 016.3
kidney 016.0
uterus 016.7
uveal tract 017.3 [363.13]
uvula 017.9
vaccination, prophylactic (against) V03.2
vagina 016.7
vas deferens 016.5
vein 017.9
verruca (primary) 017.0
verrucosa (cutis) (primary) 017.0
vertebra (column) 015.0 [730.88]
vesiculitis 016.5 [608.81]
viscera NEC 014.8
vulva 016.7 [616.51]
wrist (joint) 015.8
bone 015.5 [730.83]
Tuberculum
auriculae 744.29
occlusal 520.2
paramolare 520.2
Tuberous sclerosis (brain) 759.5
Tubo-ovarian - see condition
Tuboplasty, after previous sterilization V26.0
Tubotympanitis 381.10
Tularemia 021.9
with
conjunctivitis 021.3
pneumonia 021.2
bronchopneumonic 021.2
conjunctivitis 021.3
cryptogenic 021.1
disseminated 021.8
enteric 021.1
generalized 021.8
glandular 021.8
intestinal 021.1
oculoglandular 021.3
ophthalmic 021.3
pneumonia 021.2
pulmonary 021.2
specified NEC 021.8
typhoidal 021.1
ulceroglandular 021.0
vaccination, prophylactic (against) V03.4
Tularensis conjunctivitis 021.3
Tumefaction - see also Swelling
liver (see also Hypertrophy, liver) 789.1
Tumor (M8000/1) - see also Neoplasm, by site, unspecified nature
Abrikosov's (M9580/0) - see also Neoplasm, connective tissue, benign
malignant (M9580/3) - see Neoplasm, connective tissue, malignant
acinar cell (M8550/1) - see Neoplasm, by site, uncertain behavior
acinic cell (M8550/1) - see Neoplasm, by site, uncertain behavior
adenomatoid (M9054/0) - see also Neoplasm, by site, benign
odontogenic (M9300/0) 213.1
upper jaw (bone) 213.0
adnexal (skin) (M8390/0) - see Neoplasm, skin, benign

Tumor (Continued)
adrenal
cortical (benign) (M8370/0) 227.0
malignant (M8370/3) 194.0
rest (M8671/0) - see Neoplasm, by site, benign
alpha cell (M8152/0)
malignant (M8152/3)
pancreas 157.4
specified site NEC - see Neoplasm, by site, malignant
unspecified site 157.4
pancreas 211.7
specified site NEC - see Neoplasm, by site, benign
unspecified site 211.7
aneurysmal (see also Aneurysm) 442.9
aortic body (M8691/1) 237.3
malignant (M8691/3) 194.6
argentaffin (M8241/1) - see Neoplasm, by site, uncertain behavior
basal cell (M8090/1) - see also Neoplasm, skin, uncertain behavior
benign (M8000/0) - see Neoplasm, by site, benign
beta cell (M8151/0)
malignant (M8151/3)
pancreas 157.4
specified site - see Neoplasm, by site, malignant
unspecified site 157.4
pancreas 211.7
specified site NEC - see Neoplasm, by site, benign
unspecified site 211.7
blood - see Hematoma
Brenner (M9000/0) 220
borderline malignancy (M9000/1) 236.2
malignant (M9000/3) 183.0
proliferating (M9000/1) 236.2
Brooke's (M8100/0) - see Neoplasm, skin, benign
brown fat (M8880/0) - see Lipoma, by site
Burkitt's (M9750/3) 200.2
calcifying epithelial odontogenic (M9340/0) 213.1
upper jaw (bone) 213.0
carcinoid (M8240/1) - see Carcinoid
carotid body (M8692/1) 237.3
malignant (M8692/3) 194.5
Castleman's (mediastinal lymph node hyperplasia) 785.6
cells (M8001/1) - see also Neoplasm, by site, unspecified nature
benign (M8001/0) - see Neoplasm, by site, benign
malignant (M8001/3) - see Neoplasm, by site, malignant
uncertain whether benign or malignant (M8001/1) - see Neoplasm, by site, uncertain nature
cervix
in pregnancy or childbirth 654.6
affecting fetus or newborn 763.89
causing obstructed labor 660.2
affecting fetus or newborn 763.1
chondromatous giant cell (M9230/0) - see Neoplasm, bone, benign
chromaffin (M8700/0) - see also Neoplasm, by site, benign
malignant (M8700/3) - see Neoplasm, by site, malignant

Tumor *(Continued)*
  Cock's peculiar 706.2
  Codman's (benign chondroblastoma)
    (M9230/0) - *see* Neoplasm, bone,
    benign
  dentigerous, mixed (M9282/0) 213.1
    upper jaw (bone) 213.0
  dermoid (M9084/0) - *see* Neoplasm, by
    site, benign
    with malignant transformation
      (M9084/3) 183.0
  desmoid (extra-abdominal) (M8821/1)
    - *see also* Neoplasm, connective tis-
    sue, uncertain behavior
    abdominal (M8822/1) - *see* Neo-
      plasm, connective tissue, uncer-
      tain behavior
  embryonal (mixed) (M9080/1) - *see also*
    Neoplasm, by site, uncertain be-
    havior
    liver (M9080/3) 155.0
  endodermal sinus (M9071/3)
    specified site - *see* Neoplasm, by site,
      malignant
    unspecified site
      female 183.0
      male 186.9
  epithelial
    benign (M8010/0) - *see* Neoplasm,
      by site, benign
    malignant (M8010/3) - *see* Neo-
      plasm, by site, malignant
  Ewing's (M9260/3) - *see* Neoplasm,
    bone, malignant
  fatty - *see* Lipoma
  fetal, causing disproportion 653.7
    causing obstructed labor 660.1
  fibroid (M8890/0) - *see* Leiomyoma
  G cell (M8153/1)
    malignant (M8153/3)
      pancreas 157.4
      specified site NEC - *see* Neoplasm,
        by site, malignant
      unspecified site 157.4
    specified site - *see* Neoplasm, by site,
      uncertain behavior
    unspecified site 235.5
  giant cell (type) (M8003/1) - *see also*
    Neoplasm, by site, unspecified na-
    ture
    bone (M9250/1) 238.0
      malignant (M9250/3) - *see* Neo-
        plasm, bone, malignant
    chondromatous (M9230/0) - *see* Neo-
      plasm, bone, benign
    malignant (M8003/3) - *see* Neo-
      plasm, by site, malignant
    peripheral (gingiva) 523.8
    soft parts (M9251/1) - *see also* Neo-
      plasm, connective tissue, uncer-
      tain behavior
      malignant (M9251/3) - *see* Neo-
        plasm, connective tissue, ma-
        lignant
    tendon sheath 727.02
  glomus (M8711/0) - *see also* Heman-
    gioma, by site
    jugulare (M8690/1) 237.3
      malignant (M8690/3) 194.6
  gonadal stromal (M8590/1) - *see* Neo-
    plasm, by site, uncertain behavior
  granular cell (M9580/0) - *see also* Neo-
    plasm, connective tissue, benign
    malignant (M9580/3) - *see* Neoplasm,
      connective tissue, malignant

Tumor *(Continued)*
  granulosa cell (M8620/1) 236.2
    malignant (M8620/3) 183.0
  granulosa cell-theca cell (M8621/1)
    236.2
    malignant (M8621/3) 183.0
  Grawitz's (hypernephroma) (M8312/3)
    189.0
  hazard-crile (M8350/3) 193
  hemorrhoidal - *see* Hemorrhoids
  hilar cell (M8660/0) 220
  Hürthle cell (benign) (M8290/0) 226
    malignant (M8290/3) 193
  hydatid (*see also* Echinococcus) 122.9
  hypernephroid (M8311/1) - *see also*
    Neoplasm, by site, uncertain be-
    havior
  interstitial cell (M8650/1) - *see also*
    Neoplasm, by site, uncertain be-
    havior
    benign (M8650/0) - *see* Neoplasm,
      by site, benign
    malignant (M8650/3) - *see* Neo-
      plasm, by site, malignant
  islet cell (M8150/0)
    malignant (M8150/3)
      pancreas 157.4
      specified site - *see* Neoplasm, by
        site, malignant
      unspecified site 157.4
    pancreas 211.7
    specified site NEC - *see* Neoplasm,
      by site, benign
    unspecified site 211.7
  juxtaglomerular (M8361/1) 236.91
  Krukenberg's (M8490/6) 198.6
  Leydig cell (M8650/1)
    benign (M8650/0)
      specified site - *see* Neoplasm, by
        site, benign
      unspecified site
        female 220
        male 222.0
    malignant (M8650/3)
      specified site - *see* Neoplasm, by
        site, malignant
      unspecified site
        female 183.0
        male 186.9
    specified site - *see* Neoplasm, by site,
      uncertain behavior
    unspecified site
      female 236.2
      male 236.4
  lipid cell, ovary (M8670/0) 220
  lipoid cell, ovary (M8670/0) 220
  lymphomatous, benign (M9590/0) - *see*
    also Neoplasm, by site, benign
  Malherbe's (M8110/0) - *see* Neoplasm,
    skin, benign
  malignant (M8000/3) - *see also* Neo-
    plasm, by site, malignant
    fusiform cell (type) (M8004/3) - *see*
      Neoplasm, by site, malignant
    giant cell (type) (M8003/3) - *see*
      Neoplasm, by site, malignant
    mixed NEC (M8940/3) - *see* Neo-
      plasm, by site, malignant
    small cell (type) (M8002/3) - *see*
      Neoplasm, by site, malignant
    spindle cell (type) (M8004/3) - *see*
      Neoplasm, by site, malignant
  mast cell (M8740/1) 238.5
    malignant (M8740/3) 202.6

Tumor *(Continued)*
  melanotic, neuroectodermal (M9363/0)
    - *see* Neoplasm, by site, benign
  Merkel cell - *see* Neoplasm, by site,
    malignant
  mesenchymal
    malignant (M8800/3) - *see* Neo-
      plasm, connective tissue, malig-
      nant
    mixed (M8990/1) - *see* Neoplasm,
      connective tissue, uncertain be-
      havior
  mesodermal, mixed (M8951/3) - *see*
    also Neoplasm, by site, malignant
    liver 155.0
  mesonephric (M9110/1) - *see also*
    Neoplasm, by site, uncertain be-
    havior
    malignant (M9110/3) - *see* Neo-
      plasm, by site, malignant
  metastatic
    from specified site (M8000/3) - *see*
      Neoplasm, by site, malignant
    to specified site (M8000/6) - *see*
      Neoplasm, by site, malignant,
      secondary
  mixed NEC (M8940/0) - *see also* Neo-
    plasm, by site, benign
    malignant (M8940/3) - *see* Neo-
      plasm, by site, malignant
  mucocarcinoid, malignant (M8243/3) -
    see Neoplasm, by site, malignant
  mucoepidermoid (M8430/1) - *see* Neo-
    plasm, by site, uncertain behavior
  Mullerian, mixed (M8950/3) - *see* Neo-
    plasm, by site, malignant
  myoepithelial (M8982/0) - *see* Neo-
    plasm, by site, benign
  neurogenic olfactory (M9520/3) 160.0
  nonencapsulated sclerosing (M8350/3)
    193
  odontogenic (M9270/1) 238.0
    adenomatoid (M9300/0) 213.1
      upper jaw (bone) 213.0
    benign (M9270/0) 213.1
      upper jaw (bone) 213.0
    calcifying epithelial (M9340/0) 213.1
      upper jaw (bone) 213.0
    malignant (M9270/3) 170.1
      upper jaw (bone) 170.0
    squamous (M9312/0) 213.1
      upper jaw (bone) 213.0
  ovarian stromal (M8590/1) 236.2
  ovary
    in pregnancy or childbirth 654.4
      affecting fetus or newborn 763.89
      causing obstructed labor 660.2
        affecting fetus or newborn 763.1
  pacinian (M9507/0) - *see* Neoplasm,
    skin, benign
  Pancoast's (M8010/3) 162.3
  papillary - *see* Papilloma
  pelvic, in pregnancy or childbirth 654.9
    affecting fetus or newborn 763.89
    causing obstructed labor 660.2
      affecting fetus or newborn 763.1
  phantom 300.11
  plasma cell (M9731/1) 238.6
    benign (M9731/0) - *see* Neoplasm,
      by site, benign
    malignant (M9731/3) 203.8
  polyvesicular vitelline (M9071/3)
    specified site - *see* Neoplasm, by site,
      malignant

ICD-9-CM

T

Vol. 2

Tumor *(Continued)*
  polyvesiculvr vitelline *(Continued)*
    unspecified site
      female 183.0
      male 186.9
  Pott's puffy *(see also* Osteomyelitis) 730.2
  Rathke's pouch (M9350/1) 237.0
  Regaud's (M8082/3) - *see* Neoplasm, nasopharynx, malignant
  rete cell (M8140/0) 222.0
  retinal anlage (M9363/0) - *see* Neoplasm, by site, benign
  Rokitansky's 620.2
  salivary gland type, mixed (M8940/0) - *see also* Neoplasm, by site, benign
    malignant (M8940/3) - *see* Neoplasm, by site, malignant
  Sampson's 617.1
  Schloffer's *(see also* Peritonitis) 567.2
  Schmincke's (M8082/3) - *see* Neoplasm, nasopharynx, malignant
  sebaceous *(see also* Cyst, sebaceous) 706.2
  secondary (M8000/6) - *see* Neoplasm, by site, secondary
  Sertoli cell (M8640/0)
    with lipid storage (M8641/0)
      specified site - *see* Neoplasm, by site, benign
      unspecified site
        female 220
        male 222.0
    specified site - *see* Neoplasm, by site, benign
    unspecified site
      female 220
      male 222.0
  Sertoli-Leydig cell (M8631/0)
    specified site - *see* Neoplasm, by site, benign
    unspecified site
      female 220
      male 222.0
  sex cord (-stromal) (M8590/1) - *see* Neoplasm, by site, uncertain behavior
  skin appendage (M8390/0) - *see* Neoplasm, skin, benign
  soft tissue
    benign (M8800/0) - *see* Neoplasm, connective tissue, benign
    malignant (M8800/3) - *see* Neoplasm, connective tissue, malignant
  sternomastoid 754.1
  stromal
    gastric 238.1 ◄
      benign 215.8 ◄
      malignant 171.5 ◄
      uncertain behavior 238.1 ◄
    gastrointestinal 238.1 ◄
      benign 215.5 ◄
      malignant 171.5 ◄
      uncertain behavior 238.1 ◄
    intestine 238.1 ◄
      benign 215.5 ◄
      malignant 171.5 ◄
      uncertain behavior 238.1 ◄
    stomach 238.1 ◄
      benign 215.5 ◄
      malignant 171.5 ◄
      uncertain behavior 238.1 ◄
  superior sulcus (lung) (pulmonary) (syndrome) (M8010/3) 162.3

Tumor *(Continued)*
  suprasulcus (M8010/3) 162.3
  sweat gland (M8400/1) - *see also* Neoplasm, skin, uncertain behavior
    benign (M8400/0) - *see* Neoplasm, skin, benign
    malignant (M8400/3) - *see* Neoplasm, skin, malignant
  syphilitic brain 094.89
    congenital 090.49
  testicular stromal (M8590/1) 236.4
  theca cell (M8600/0) 220
  theca cell-granulosa cell (M8621/1) 236.2
  theca-lutein (M8610/0) 220
  turban (M8200/0) 216.4
  uterus
    in pregnancy or childbirth 654.1
      affecting fetus or newborn 763.89
      causing obstructed labor 660.2
        affecting fetus or newborn 763.1
  vagina
    in pregnancy or childbirth 654.7
      affecting fetus or newborn 763.89
      causing obstructed labor 660.2
        affecting fetus or newborn 763.1
  varicose *(see also* Varicose, vein) 454.9
  von Recklinghausen's (M9540/1) 237.71
  vulva
    in pregnancy or childbirth 654.8
      affecting fetus or newborn 763.89
      causing obstructed labor 660.2
        affecting fetus or newborn 763.1
  Warthin's (salivary gland) (M8561/0) 210.2
  white - *see also* Tuberculosis, arthritis
  White-Darier 757.39
  Wilms' (nephroblastoma) (M8960/3) 189.0
  yolk sac (M9071/3)
    specified site - *see* Neoplasm, by site, malignant
    unspecified site
      female 183.0
      male 186.9
Tumorlet (M8040/1) - *see* Neoplasm, by site, uncertain behavior
Tungiasis 134.1
Tunica vasculosa lentis 743.39
Tunnel vision 368.45
Turban tumor (M8200/0) 216.4
Türck's trachoma (chronic catarrhal laryngitis) 476.0
Türk's syndrome (ocular retraction syndrome) 378.71
Turner's
  hypoplasia (tooth) 520.4
  syndrome 758.6
  tooth 520.4
Turner-Kieser syndrome (hereditary osteo-onychodysplasia) 756.89
Turner-Varny syndrome 758.6
Turricephaly 756.0
Tussis convulsiva *(see also* Whooping cough) 033.9
Twin
  affected by maternal complications of pregnancy 761.5
  conjoined 759.4
  healthy liveborn - *see* Newborn, twin
  pregnancy (complicating delivery) NEC 651.0
    with fetal loss and retention of one fetus 651.3

Twinning, teeth 520.2
Twist, twisted
  bowel, colon, or intestine 560.2
  hair (congenital) 757.4
  mesentery 560.2
  omentum 560.2
  organ or site, congenital NEC - *see* Anomaly, specified type NEC
  ovarian pedicle 620.5
    congenital 752.0
  umbilical cord - *see* Compression, umbilical cord
Twitch 781.0
Tylosis 700
  buccalis 528.6
  gingiva 523.8
  linguae 528.6
  palmaris et plantaris 757.39
Tympanism 787.3
Tympanites (abdominal) (intestine) 787.3
Tympanitis - *see* Myringitis
Tympanosclerosis 385.00
  involving
    combined sites NEC 385.09
      with tympanic membrane 385.03
    tympanic membrane 385.01
      with ossicles 385.02
        and middle ear 385.03
Tympanum - *see* condition
Tympany
  abdomen 787.3
  chest 786.7
Typhlitis *(see also* Appendicitis) 541
Typhoenteritis 002.0
Typhogastric fever 002.0
Typhoid (abortive) (ambulant) (any site) (fever) (hemorrhagic) (infection) (intermittent) (malignant) (rheumatic) 002.0
  with pneumonia 002.0 *[484.8]*
  abdominal 002.0
  carrier (suspected) of V02.1
  cholecystitis (current) 002.0
  clinical (Widal and blood test negative) 002.0
  endocarditis 002.0 *[421.1]*
  inoculation reaction - *see* Complications, vaccination
  meningitis 002.0 *[320.7]*
  mesenteric lymph nodes 002.0
  myocarditis 002.0 *[422.0]*
  osteomyelitis *(see also* Osteomyelitis, due to, typhoid) 002.0 *[730.8]*
  perichondritis, larynx 002.0 *[478.71]*
  pneumonia 002.0 *[484.8]*
  spine 002.0 *[720.81]*
  ulcer (perforating) 002.0
  vaccination, prophylactic (against) V03.1
  Widal negative 002.0
Typhomalaria (fever) *(see also* Malaria) 084.6
Typhomania 002.0
Typhoperitonitis 002.0
Typhus (fever) 081.9
  abdominal, abdominalis 002.0
  African tick 082.1
  amarillic *(see also* Fever, yellow) 060.9
  brain 081.9
  cerebral 081.9
  classical 080
  endemic (flea-borne) 081.0
  epidemic (louse-borne) 080
  exanthematic NEC 080

◄ **New**   ◄▭ **Revised**

Typhus (*Continued*)
  exanthematicus SAI 080
    brillii SAI 081.1
    mexicanus SAI 081.0
    pediculo vestimenti causa 080
    typhus murinus 081.0
  flea-borne 081.0
  Indian tick 082.1
  Kenya tick 082.1
  louse-borne 080
  Mexican 081.0
    flea-borne 081.0
    louse-borne 080
    tabardillo 080

Typhus (*Continued*)
  mite-borne 081.2
  murine 081.0
  North Asian tick-borne 082.2
  petechial 081.9
  Queensland tick 082.3
  rat 081.0
  recrudescent 081.1
  recurrent (*see also* Fever, relapsing)
    087.9
  São Paulo 082.0
  scrub (China) (India) (Malaya) (New
    Guinea) 081.2

Typhus (*Continued*)
  shop (of Malaya) 081.0
  Siberian tick 082.2
  tick-borne NEC 082.9
  tropical 081.2
  vaccination, prophylactic (against)
    V05.8
Tyrosinemia 270.2
  neonatal 775.8
Tyrosinosis (Medes) (Sakai) 270.2
Tyrosinuria 270.2
Tyrosyluria 270.2

ICD-9-CM

Vol. 2

U

Uehlinger's syndrome (acropachyderma) 757.39

Uhl's anomaly or disease (hypoplasia of myocardium, right ventricle) 746.84

Ulcer, ulcerated, ulcerating, ulceration, ulcerative 707.9
  with gangrene 707.9 [785.4]
  abdomen (wall) (*see also* Ulcer, skin) 707.8
  ala, nose 478.1
  alveolar process 526.5
  amebic (intestine) 006.9
    skin 006.6
  anastomotic - *see* Ulcer, gastrojejunal
  anorectal 569.41
  antral - *see* Ulcer, stomach
  anus (sphincter) (solitary) 569.41
    varicose - *see* Varicose, ulcer, anus
  aphthous (oral) (recurrent) 528.2
    genital organ(s)
      female 616.8
      male 608.89
    mouth 528.2
  arm (*see also* Ulcer, skin) 707.8
  arteriosclerotic plaque - *see* Arteriosclerosis, by site
  artery NEC 447.2
    without rupture 447.8
  atrophic NEC - *see* Ulcer, skin
  Barrett's (chronic peptic ulcer of esophagus) 530.85
  bile duct 576.8
  bladder (solitary) (sphincter) 596.8
    bilharzial (*see also* Schistosomiasis) 120.9 [595.4]
    submucosal (*see also* Cystitis) 595.1
    tuberculous (*see also* Tuberculosis) 016.1
  bleeding NEC - *see* Ulcer, peptic, with hemorrhage
  bone 730.9
  bowel (*see also* Ulcer, intestine) 569.82
  breast 611.0
  bronchitis 491.8
  bronchus 519.1
  buccal (cavity) (traumatic) 528.9
  burn (acute) - *see* Ulcer, duodenum
  Buruli 031.1
  buttock (*see also* Ulcer, skin) 707.8
    decubitus (*see also* Ulcer, decubitus) 707.00
  cancerous (M8000/3) - *see* Neoplasm, by site, malignant
  cardia - *see* Ulcer, stomach
  cardio-esophageal (peptic) 530.20
    with bleeding 530.21
  cecum (*see also* Ulcer, intestine) 569.82
  cervix (uteri) (trophic) 622.0
    with mention of cervicitis 616.0
  chancroidal 099.0
  chest (wall) (*see also* Ulcer, skin) 707.8
  Chiclero 085.4
  chin (pyogenic) (*see also* Ulcer, skin) 707.8
  chronic (cause unknown) - *see also* Ulcer, skin
    penis 607.89
  Cochin-China 085.1
  colitis - *see* Colitis, ulcerative
  colon (*see also* Ulcer, intestine) 569.82
  conjunctiva (acute) (postinfectional) 372.00

Ulcer, ulcerated, ulcerating, ulceration, ulcerative (*Continued*)
  cornea (infectional) 370.00
    with perforation 370.06
    annular 370.02
    catarrhal 370.01
    central 370.03
    dendritic 054.42
    marginal 370.01
    mycotic 370.05
    phlyctenular, tuberculous (*see also* Tuberculosis) 017.3 [370.31]
    ring 370.02
    rodent 370.07
    serpent, serpiginous 370.04
    superficial marginal 370.01
    tuberculous (*see also* Tuberculosis) 017.3 [370.31]
  corpus cavernosum (chronic) 607.89
  crural - *see* Ulcer, lower extremity
  Curling's - *see* Ulcer, duodenum
  Cushing's - *see* Ulcer, peptic
  cystitis (interstitial) 595.1
  decubitus (unspecified site) 707.00 ◄▥
    with gangrene 707.00 [785.4] ◄▥
    ankle 707.06 ◄
    back ◄
      lower 707.03 ◄
      upper 707.02 ◄
    buttock 707.05 ◄
    elbow 707.01 ◄
    head 707.09 ◄
    heel 707.07 ◄
    hip 707.04 ◄
    other site 707.09 ◄
    sacrum 707.03 ◄
    shoulder blades 707.02 ◄
  dendritic 054.42
  diabetes, diabetic (mellitus) 250.8 [707.9]
    lower limb 250.8 [707.10]
      ankle 250.8 [707.13]
      calf 250.8 [707.12]
      foot 250.8 [707.15]
      heel 250.8 [707.14]
      knee 250.8 [707.19]
      specified site NEC 250.8 [707.19]
      thigh 250.8 [707.11]
      toes 250.8 [707.15]
    specified site NEC 250.8 [707.8]
  Dieulafoy - *see* Lesion, Dieulafoy
  due to
    infection NEC - *see* Ulcer, skin
    radiation, radium - *see* Ulcer, by site
    trophic disturbance (any region) - *see* Ulcer, skin
    x-ray - *see* Ulcer, by site
  duodenum, duodenal (eroded) (peptic) 532.9

> **Note** Use the following fifth-digit subclassification with categories 531-534:
>
> 0   without mention of obstruction
> 1   with obstruction

    with
      hemorrhage (chronic) 532.4
        and perforation 532.6
      perforation (chronic) 532.5
        and hemorrhage 532.6
    acute 532.3
      with

Ulcer, ulcerated, ulcerating, ulceration, ulcerative (*Continued*)
  duodenum, duodenal (*Continued*)
    acute (*Continued*)
      with (*Continued*)
        hemorrhage 532.0
          and perforation 532.2
        perforation 532.1
          and hemorrhage 532.2
    bleeding (recurrent) - *see* Ulcer, duodenum, with hemorrhage
    chronic 532.7
      with
        hemorrhage 532.4
          and perforation 532.6
        perforation 532.5
          and hemorrhage 532.6
    penetrating - *see* Ulcer, duodenum, with perforation
    perforating - *see* Ulcer, duodenum, with perforation
  dysenteric NEC 009.0
  elusive 595.1
  endocarditis (any valve) (acute) (chronic) (subacute) 421.0
  enteritis - *see* Colitis, ulcerative
  enterocolitis 556.0
  epiglottis 478.79
  esophagus (peptic) 530.20
    with bleeding 530.21
    due to ingestion
      aspirin 530.20
      chemicals 530.20
      medicinal agents 530.20
    fungal 530.20
    infectional 530.20
    varicose (*see also* Varix, esophagus) 456.1
      bleeding (*see also* Varix, esophagus, bleeding) 456.0
  eye NEC 360.00
    dendritic 054.42
  eyelid (region) 373.01
  face (*see also* Ulcer, skin) 707.8
  fauces 478.29
  Fenwick (-Hunner) (solitary) (*see also* Cystitis) 595.1
  fistulous NEC - *see* Ulcer, skin
  foot (indolent) (*see also* Ulcer, lower extremity) 707.15
    perforating 707.15
      leprous 030.1
      syphilitic 094.0
    trophic 707.15
    varicose 454.0
      inflamed or infected 454.2
  frambesial, initial or primary 102.0
  gallbladder or duct 575.8
  gall duct 576.8
  gangrenous (*see also* Gangrene) 785.4
  gastric - *see* Ulcer, stomach
  gastrocolic - *see* Ulcer, gastrojejunal
  gastroduodenal - *see* Ulcer, peptic
  gastroesophageal - *see* Ulcer, stomach
  gastrohepatic - *see* Ulcer, stomach
  gastrointestinal - *see* Ulcer, gastrojejunal
  gastrojejunal (eroded) (peptic) 534.9

> **Note** Use the following fifth-digit subclassification with categories 531-534:
>
> 0   without mention of obstruction
> 1   with obstruction

◄ **New**   ◄▥ **Revised**

Ulcer, ulcerated, ulcerating, ulceration, ulcerative (Continued)
gastrojejunal (Continued)
  with
    hemorrhage (chronic) 534.4
      and perforation 534.6
    perforation 534.5
      and hemorrhage 534.6
  acute 534.3
    with
      hemorrhage 534.0
        and perforation 534.2
      perforation 534.1
        and hemorrhage 534.2
  bleeding (recurrent) - see Ulcer, gas-
    trojejunal, with hemorrhage
  chronic 534.7
    with
      hemorrhage 534.4
        and perforation 534.6
      perforation 534.5
        and hemorrhage 534.6
  penetrating - see Ulcer, gastrojejunal,
    with perforation
  perforating - see Ulcer, gastrojejunal,
    with perforation
gastrojejunocolic - see Ulcer, gastrojejunal
genital organ
  female 629.8
  male 608.89
gingiva 523.8
gingivitis 523.1
glottis 478.79
granuloma of pudenda 099.2
groin (see also Ulcer, skin) 707.8
gum 523.8
gumma, due to yaws 102.4
hand (see also Ulcer, skin) 707.8
hard palate 528.9
heel (see also Ulcer, lower extremity)
  707.14
  decubitus (see also Ulcer, decubitus)
    707.07 ◀▥
hemorrhoids 455.8
  external 455.5
  internal 455.2
hip (see also Ulcer, skin) 707.8
  decubitus (see also Ulcer, decubitus)
    707.04 ◀▥
Hunner's 595.1
hypopharynx 478.29
hypopyon (chronic) (subacute)
  370.04
hypostaticum - see Ulcer, varicose
ileocolitis 556.1
ileum (see also Ulcer, intestine)
  569.82
intestine, intestinal 569.82
  with perforation 569.83
  amebic 006.9
  duodenal - see Ulcer, duodenum
  granulocytopenic (with hemorrhage)
    288.0
  marginal 569.82
  perforating 569.83
  small, primary 569.82
  stercoraceous 569.82
  stercoral 569.82
  tuberculous (see also Tuberculosis)
    014.8
  typhoid (fever) 002.0
  varicose 456.8

Ulcer, ulcerated, ulcerating, ulceration, ulcerative (Continued)
ischemic 707.9
  lower extremity (see also Ulcer, lower
    extremity) 707.10
    ankle 707.13
    calf 707.12
    foot 707.15
    heel 707.14
    knee 707.19
    specified site NEC 707.19
    thigh 707.11
    toes 707.15
jejunum, jejunal - see Ulcer, gastrojejunal
keratitis (see also Ulcer, cornea) 370.00
knee - see Ulcer, lower extremity
labium (majus) (minus) 616.50
laryngitis (see also Laryngitis) 464.00
  with obstruction 464.01
larynx (aphthous) (contact) 478.79
  diphtheritic 032.3
leg - see Ulcer, lower extremity
lip 528.5
Lipschütz's 616.50
lower extremity (atrophic) (chronic)
  (neurogenic) (perforating) (pyogenic) (trophic) (tropical) 707.10
  with gangrene (see also Ulcer, lower
    extremity) 707.10 [785.4]
  ankle 707.13
  arteriosclerotic 440.23
    with gangrene 440.24
  calf 707.12
  decubitus 707.00 ◀▥
    with gangrene 707.00 [785.4] ◀▥
    ankle 707.06 ◀
    buttock 707.05 ◀
    heel 707.07 ◀
    hip 707.04 ◀
  foot 707.15
  heel 707.14
  knee 707.19
  specified site NEC 707.19
  thigh 707.11
  toes 707.15
  varicose 454.0
    inflamed or infected 454.2
luetic - see Ulcer, syphilitic
lung 518.89
  tuberculous (see also Tuberculosis)
    011.2
malignant (M8000/3) - see Neoplasm,
  by site, malignant
marginal NEC - see Ulcer, gastrojejunal
meatus (urinarius) 597.89
Meckel's diverticulum 751.0
Meleney's (chronic undermining)
  686.09
Mooren's (cornea) 370.07
mouth (traumatic) 528.9
mycobacterial (skin) 031.1
nasopharynx 478.29
navel cord (newborn) 771.4
neck (see also Ulcer, skin) 707.8
  uterus 622.0
neurogenic NEC - see Ulcer, skin
nose, nasal (infectional) (passage)
  478.1
  septum 478.1
    varicose 456.8
  skin - see Ulcer, skin
  spirochetal NEC 104.8
oral mucosa (traumatic) 528.9
palate (soft) 528.9

Ulcer, ulcerated, ulcerating, ulceration, ulcerative (Continued)
penetrating NEC - see Ulcer, peptic,
  with perforation
penis (chronic) 607.89
peptic (site unspecified) 533.9

> Note Use the following fifth-digit
> subclassification with categories 531-
> 534:
>
> 0   without mention of obstruction
> 1   with obstruction

  with
    hemorrhage 533.4
      and perforation 533.6
    perforation (chronic) 533.5
      and hemorrhage 533.6
  acute 533.3
    with
      hemorrhage 533.0
        and perforation 533.2
      perforation 533.1
        and hemorrhage 533.2
  bleeding (recurrent) - see Ulcer, pep-
    tic, with hemorrhage
  chronic 533.7
    with
      hemorrhage 533.4
        and perforation 533.6
      perforation 533.5
        and hemorrhage 533.6
  penetrating - see Ulcer, peptic, with
    perforation
  perforating NEC (see also Ulcer, peptic,
    with perforation) 533.5
skin 707.9
perineum (see also Ulcer, skin) 707.8
peritonsillar 474.8
phagedenic (tropical) NEC - see Ulcer,
  skin
pharynx 478.29
phlebitis - see Phlebitis
plaster (see also Ulcer, decubitus)
  707.00 ◀▥
popliteal space - see Ulcer, lower extremity
postpyloric - see Ulcer, duodenum
prepuce 607.89
prepyloric - see Ulcer, stomach
pressure (see also Ulcer, decubitus)
  707.00 ◀▥
primary of intestine 569.82
  with perforation 569.83
proctitis 556.2
  with ulcerative sigmoiditis 556.3
prostate 601.8
pseudopeptic - see Ulcer, peptic
pyloric - see Ulcer, stomach
rectosigmoid 569.82
  with perforation 569.83
rectum (sphincter) (solitary) 569.41
  stercoraceous, stercoral 569.41
  varicose - see Varicose, ulcer, anus
retina (see also Chorioretinitis) 363.20
rodent (M8090/3) - see also Neoplasm,
  skin, malignant
  cornea 370.07
round - see Ulcer, stomach
sacrum (region) (see also Ulcer, skin)
  707.8
Saemisch's 370.04
scalp (see also Ulcer, skin) 707.8
sclera 379.09

Ulcer, ulcerated, ulcerating, ulceration, ulcerative *(Continued)*
scrofulous *(see also* Tuberculosis) 017.2
scrotum 608.89
tuberculous *(see also* Tuberculosis) 016.5
varicose 456.4
seminal vesicle 608.89
sigmoid 569.82
with perforation 569.83
skin (atrophic) (chronic) (neurogenic) (non-healing) (perforating) (pyogenic) (trophic) 707.9
with gangrene *(see also* Ulcer, lower extremity) 707.9 *[785.4]*
amebic 006.6
decubitus *(see also* Ulcer, decubitus) 707.00 ◀▥
with gangrene 707.00 *[785.4]* ◀▥
in granulocytopenia 288.0
lower extremity *(see also* Ulcer, lower extremity) 707.10
with gangrene 707.10 *[785.4]*
ankle 707.13
arteriosclerotic 440.24
arteriosclerotic 440.23
with gangrene 440.24
calf 707.12
foot 707.15
heel 707.14
knee 707.19
specified site NEC 707.19
thigh 707.11
toes 707.15
mycobacterial 031.1
syphilitic (early) (secondary) 091.3
tuberculous (primary) *(see also* Tuberculosis) 017.0
varicose - *see* Ulcer, varicose
sloughing NEC - *see* Ulcer, skin
soft palate 528.9
solitary, anus or rectum (sphincter) 569.41
sore throat 462
streptococcal 034.0
spermatic cord 608.89
spine (tuberculous) 015.0 *[730.88]*
stasis (leg) (venous) 454.0
inflamed or infected 454.2
without varicose vein 459.81
stercoral, stercoraceous 569.82
with perforation 569.83
anus or rectum 569.41
stoma, stomal - *see* Ulcer, gastrojejunal
stomach (eroded) (peptic) (round) 531.9

Note   Use the following fifth-digit subclassification with categories 531-534:
0   without mention of obstruction
1   with obstruction

with
hemorrhage 531.4
and perforation 531.6
perforation (chronic) 531.5
and hemorrhage 531.6
acute 531.3
with
hemorrhage 531.0
and perforation 531.2
perforation 531.1
and hemorrhage 531.2

Ulcer, ulcerated, ulcerating, ulceration, ulcerative *(Continued)*
stomach *(Continued)*
bleeding (recurrent) - *see* Ulcer, stomach, with hemorrhage
chronic 531.7
with
hemorrhage 531.4
and perforation 531.6
perforation 531.5
and hemorrhage 531.6
penetrating - *see* Ulcer, stomach, with perforation
perforating - *see* Ulcer, stomach, with perforation
stomatitis 528.0
stress - *see* Ulcer, peptic
strumous (tuberculous) *(see also* Tuberculosis) 017.2
submental *(see also* Ulcer, skin) 707.8
submucosal, bladder 595.1
syphilitic (any site) (early) (secondary) 091.3
late 095.9
perforating 095.9
foot 094.0
testis 608.89
thigh - *see* Ulcer, lower extremity
throat 478.29
diphtheritic 032.0
toe - *see* Ulcer, lower extremity
tongue (traumatic) 529.0
tonsil 474.8
diphtheritic 032.0
trachea 519.1
trophic - *see* Ulcer, skin
tropical NEC *(see also* Ulcer, skin) 707.9
tuberculous - *see* Tuberculosis, ulcer
tunica vaginalis 608.89
turbinate 730.9
typhoid (fever) 002.0
perforating 002.0
umbilicus (newborn) 771.4
unspecified site NEC - *see* Ulcer, skin
urethra (meatus) *(see also* Urethritis) 597.89
uterus 621.8
cervix 622.0
with mention of cervicitis 616.0
neck 622.0
with mention of cervicitis 616.0
vagina 616.8
valve, heart 421.0
varicose (lower extremity, any part) 454.0
anus - *see* Varicose, ulcer, anus
broad ligament 456.5
esophagus *(see also* Varix, esophagus) 456.1
bleeding *(see also* Varix, esophagus, bleeding) 456.0
inflamed or infected 454.2
nasal septum 456.8
perineum 456.6
rectum - *see* Varicose, ulcer, anus
scrotum 456.4
specified site NEC 456.8
sublingual 456.3
vulva 456.6
vas deferens 608.89
vesical *(see also* Ulcer, bladder) 596.8

Ulcer, ulcerated, ulcerating, ulceration, ulcerative *(Continued)*
vulva (acute) (infectional) 616.50
Behçet's syndrome 136.1 *[616.51]*
herpetic 054.12
tuberculous 016.7 *[616.51]*
vulvobuccal, recurring 616.50
x-ray - *see* Ulcer, by site
yaws 102.4
Ulcerosa scarlatina 034.1
Ulcus - *see also* Ulcer
cutis tuberculosum *(see also* Tuberculosis) 017.0
duodeni - *see* Ulcer, duodenum
durum 091.0
extragenital 091.2
gastrojejunale - *see* Ulcer, gastrojejunal
hypostaticum - *see* Ulcer, varicose
molle (cutis) (skin) 099.0
serpens corneae (pneumococcal) 370.04
ventriculi - *see* Ulcer, stomach
Ulegyria 742.4
Ulerythema
acneiforma 701.8
centrifugum 695.4
ophryogenes 757.4
Ullrich (-Bonnevie) (-Turner) syndrome 758.6
Ullrich-Feichtiger syndrome 759.89
Ulnar - *see* condition
Ulorrhagia 523.8
Ulorrhea 523.8
Umbilicus, umbilical - *see also* condition
cord necrosis, affecting fetus or newborn 762.6
Unavailability of medical facilities (at) V63.9
due to
investigation by social service agency V63.8
lack of services at home V63.1
remoteness from facility V63.0
waiting list V63.2
home V63.1
outpatient clinic V63.0
specified reason NEC V63.8
Uncinaria americana infestation 126.1
Uncinariasis *(see also* Ancylostomiasis) 126.9
Unconscious, unconsciousness 780.09
Underdevelopment - *see also* Undeveloped
sexual 259.0
Undernourishment 269.9
Undernutrition 269.9
Under observation - *see* Observation
Underweight 783.22
for gestational age - *see* Light-for-dates
Underwood's disease (sclerema neonatorum) 778.1
Undescended - *see also* Malposition, congenital
cecum 751.4
colon 751.4
testis 752.51
Undetermined diagnosis or cause 799.9
Undeveloped, undevelopment - *see also* Hypoplasia
brain (congenital) 742.1
cerebral (congenital) 742.1
fetus or newborn 764.9
heart 746.89
lung 748.5

◀ New   ◀▥ Revised

Undeveloped, undevelopment
   (Continued)
   testis 257.2
   uterus 259.0
Undiagnosed (disease) 799.9
Undulant fever *(see also* Brucellosis)
   023.9
Unemployment, anxiety concerning
   V62.0
Unequal leg (acquired) (length) 736.81
   congenital 755.30
Unerupted teeth, tooth 520.6
Unextracted dental root 525.3
Unguis incarnatus 703.0
Unicornis uterus 752.3
Unicorporeus uterus 752.3
Uniformis uterus 752.3
Unilateral - *see also* condition
   development, breast 611.8
   organ or site, congenital NEC - *see*
      Agenesis
   vagina 752.49
Unilateralis uterus 752.3
Unilocular heart 745.8
Uninhibited bladder 596.54
   with cauda equina syndrome
      344.61
   neurogenic *(see also* Neurogenic, blad-
      der) 596.54
Union, abnormal - *see also* Fusion
   divided tendon 727.89
   larynx and trachea 748.3
Universal
   joint, cervix 620.6
   mesentery 751.4
Unknown
   cause of death 799.9
   diagnosis 799.9
Unna's disease (seborrheic dermatitis)
   690.10
Unresponsiveness, adrenocorticotropin
   (ACTH) 255.4
Unsatisfactory smear 795.08   ◄
Unsoundness of mind *(see also* Psychosis) 298.9
Unspecified cause of death 799.9
Unstable
   back NEC 724.9
   colon 569.89
   joint - *see* Instability, joint
   lie 652.0
      affecting fetus or newborn (before
         labor) 761.7
      causing obstructed labor 660.0
         affecting fetus or newborn 763.1
   lumbosacral joint (congenital)
      756.19
      acquired 724.6
   sacroiliac 724.6
   spine NEC 724.9
Untruthfulness, child problem *(see also*
   Disturbance, conduct) 312.0
Unverricht (-Lundborg) disease, syndrome, or epilepsy 333.2
Unverricht-Wagner syndrome (dermatomyositis) 710.3
Upper respiratory - *see* condition
Upset
   gastric 536.8
      psychogenic 306.4
   gastrointestinal 536.8
      psychogenic 306.4
      virus *(see also* Enteritis, viral)
         008.8

Upset *(Continued)*
   intestinal (large) (small) 564.9
      psychogenic 306.4
   menstruation 626.9
   mental 300.9
   stomach 536.8
      psychogenic 306.4
Urachus - *see also* condition
   patent 753.7
   persistent 753.7
Uratic arthritis 274.0
Urbach's lipoid proteinosis 272.8
**Urbach-Oppenheim disease or syn-
   drome** (necrobiosis lipoidica diabeticorum) 250.8 *[709.3]*
Urbach-Wiethe disease or syndrome
   (lipoid proteinosis) 272.8
Urban yellow fever 060.1
Urea, blood, high - *see* Uremia
Uremia, uremic (absorption) (amaurosis)
   (amblyopia) (aphasia) (apoplexy)
   (coma) (delirium) (dementia)
   (dropsy) (dyspnea) (fever) (intoxication) (mania) (paralysis) (poisoning)
   (toxemia) (vomiting) 586
   with
      abortion - *see* Abortion, by type,
         with renal failure
      ectopic pregnancy *(see also* categories
         633.0-633.9) 639.3
      hypertension *(see also* Hypertension,
         kidney) 403.91
      molar pregnancy *(see also* categories
         630-632) 639.3
   chronic 585
   complicating
      abortion 639.3
      ectopic or molar pregnancy 639.3
      hypertension *(see also* Hypertension,
         kidney) 403.91
      labor and delivery 669.3
   congenital 779.89
   extrarenal 788.9
   hypertensive (chronic) *(see also* Hyper-
      tension, kidney) 403.91
   maternal NEC, affecting fetus or new-
      born 760.1
   neuropathy 585 *[357.4]*
   pericarditis 585 *[420.0]*
   prerenal 788.9
   pyelitic *(see also* Pyelitis) 590.80
Ureter, ureteral - *see* condition
Ureteralgia 788.0
Ureterectasis 593.89
Ureteritis 593.89
   cystica 590.3
   due to calculus 592.1
   gonococcal (acute) 098.19
      chronic or duration of 2 months or
         over 098.39
   nonspecific 593.89
Ureterocele (acquired) 593.89
   congenital 753.23
Ureterolith 592.1
Ureterolithiasis 592.1
Ureterostomy status V44.6
   with complication 997.5
Urethra, urethral - *see* condition
Urethralgia 788.9
Urethritis (abacterial) (acute) (allergic)
   (anterior) (chronic) (nonvenereal)
   (posterior) (recurrent) (simple) (subacute) (ulcerative) (undifferentiated)
   597.80

Urethritis *(Continued)*
   diplococcal (acute) 098.0
      chronic or duration of 2 months or
         over 098.2
   due to Trichomonas (vaginalis) 131.02
   gonococcal (acute) 098.0
      chronic or duration of 2 months or
         over 098.2
   nongonococcal (sexually transmitted)
      099.40
      Chlamydia trachomatis 099.41
      Reiter's 099.3
      specified organism NEC 099.49
   nonspecific (sexually transmitted) *(see
      also* Urethritis, nongonococcal)
      099.40
   not sexually transmitted 597.80
   Reiter's 099.3
   trichomonal or due to Trichomonas
      (vaginalis) 131.02
   tuberculous *(see also* Tuberculosis)
      016.3
   venereal NEC *(see also* Urethritis, non-
      gonococcal) 099.40
Urethrocele   ◄▥▥
   female 618.03
      with uterine prolapse 618.4
         complete 618.3
         incomplete 618.2
   male 599.5
Urethrolithiasis 594.2
Urethro-oculoarticular syndrome 099.3
Urethro-oculosynovial syndrome 099.3
Urethrorectal - *see* condition
Urethrorrhagia 599.84
Urethrorrhea 788.7
Urethrostomy status V44.6
   with complication 997.5
Urethrotrigonitis 595.3
Urethrovaginal - *see* condition
Urhidrosis, uridrosis 705.89
Uric acid
   diathesis 274.9
   in blood 790.6
Uricacidemia 790.6
Uricemia 790.6
Uricosuria 791.9
Urination
   frequent 788.41
   painful 788.1
   urgency 788.63
Urine, urinary - *see also* condition
   abnormality NEC 788.69
   blood in *(see also* Hematuria) 599.7
   discharge, excessive 788.42
   enuresis 788.30
      nonorganic origin 307.6
   extravasation 788.8
   frequency 788.41
   incontinence 788.30
      active 788.30
      female 788.30
         stress 625.6
            and urge 788.33
      male 788.30
         stress 788.32
            and urge 788.33
      mixed (stress and urge) 788.33
      neurogenic 788.39
      nonorganic origin 307.6
      overflow 788.38   ◄
      stress (female) 625.6
         male NEC 788.32
   intermittent stream 788.61

Urine, urinary (*Continued*)
  pus in 791.9
  retention or stasis NEC 788.20
    bladder, incomplete emptying 788.21
    psychogenic 306.53
    specified NEC 788.29
  secretion
    deficient 788.5
    excessive 788.42
    frequency 788.41
  stream
    intermittent 788.61
    slowing 788.62
    splitting 788.61
    weak 788.62
  urgency 788.63
Urinemia - *see* Uremia
Urinoma NEC 599.9
  bladder 596.8
  kidney 593.89
  renal 593.89
  ureter 593.89
  urethra 599.84
Uroarthritis, infectious 099.3
Urodialysis 788.5
Urolithiasis 592.9
Uronephrosis 593.89
Uropathy 599.9
  obstructive 599.6
Urosepsis 599.0
  meaning sepsis 995.91
  meaning urinary tract infection 599.0
Urticaria 708.9
  with angioneurotic edema 995.1
    hereditary 277.6
  allergic 708.0
  cholinergic 708.5
  chronic 708.8
  cold, familial 708.2
  dermatographic 708.3
  due to
    cold or heat 708.2
    drugs 708.0
    food 708.0

Urticaria (*Continued*)
  due to (*Continued*)
    inhalants 708.0
    plants 708.8
    serum 999.5
  factitial 708.3
  giant 995.1
    hereditary 277.6
  gigantea 995.1
    hereditary 277.6
  idiopathic 708.1
  larynx 995.1
    hereditary 277.6
  neonatorum 778.8
  nonallergic 708.1
  papulosa (Hebra) 698.2
  perstans hemorrhagica 757.39
  pigmentosa 757.33
  recurrent periodic 708.8
  serum 999.5
  solare 692.72
  specified type NEC 708.8
  thermal (cold) (heat) 708.2
  vibratory 708.4
Urticarioides acarodermatitis 133.9
Use of
  nonprescribed drugs (*see also* Abuse,
    drugs, nondependent) 305.9
  patent medicines (*see also* Abuse,
    drugs, nondependent) 305.9
Usher-Senear disease (pemphigus erythematosus) 694.4
Uta 085.5
Uterine size-date discrepancy 646.8
Uteromegaly 621.2
Uterovaginal - *see* condition
Uterovesical - *see* condition
Uterus - *see* condition
Utriculitis (utriculus prostaticus) 597.89
Uveal - *see* condition
Uveitis (anterior) (*see also* Iridocyclitis)
  364.3
  acute or subacute 364.00
    due to or associated with

Uveitis (*Continued*)
  acute or subacute (*Continued*)
    due to or associated with (*Continued*)
      gonococcal infection 098.41
      herpes (simplex) 054.44
      zoster 053.22
    primary 364.01
    recurrent 364.02
    secondary (noninfectious) 364.04
      infectious 364.03
  allergic 360.11
  chronic 364.10
    due to or associated with
      sarcoidosis 135 [364.11]
      tuberculosis (*see also* Tuberculosis)
        017.3 [364.11]
  due to
    operation 360.11
    toxoplasmosis (acquired) 130.2
      congenital (active) 771.2
  granulomatous 364.10
  heterochromic 364.21
  lens-induced 364.23
  nongranulomatous 364.00
  posterior 363.20
    disseminated - *see* Chorioretinitis,
      disseminated
    focal - *see* Chorioretinitis, focal
  recurrent 364.02
  sympathetic 360.11
  syphilitic (secondary) 091.50
    congenital 090.0 [363.13]
    late 095.8 [363.13]
  tuberculous (*see also* Tuberculosis)
    017.3 [364.11]
Uveoencephalitis 363.22
Uveokeratitis (*see also* Iridocyclitis)
  364.3
Uveoparotid fever 135
Uveoparotitis 135
Uvula - *see* condition
Uvulitis (acute) (catarrhal) (chronic)
  (gangrenous) (membranous) (suppurative) (ulcerative) 528.3

V

Vaccination

complication or reaction - *see* Complications, vaccination

not done (contraindicated) V64.0
  because of patient's decision V64.2

prophylactic (against) V05.9
  arthropod-borne viral
    disease NEC V05.1
    encephalitis V05.0
  chicken pox V05.4
  cholera (alone) V03.0
    with typhoid-paratyphoid
      (cholera + TAB) V06.0
  common cold V04.7
  diphtheria (alone) V03.5
    with
      poliomyelitis (DTP + polio)
        V06.3
      tetanus V06.5
        pertussis combined [DTP]
          [PTaP] V06.1
      typhoid-paratyphoid (DTP +
        TAB) V06.2
  disease (single) NEC V05.9
    bacterial NEC V03.9
      specified type NEC V03.89
    combination NEC V06.9
      specified type NEC V06.8
    specified type NEC V05.8
  encephalitis, viral, arthropod-borne
    V05.0
  Haemophilus influenzae, type B
    [Hib] V03.81
  hepatitis, viral V05.3
  influenza V04.81
    with
      Streptococcus pneumoniae
        [pneumococcus] V06.6
  leishmaniasis V05.2 ◄▬
  measles (alone) V04.2
    with mumps-rubella (MMR) V06.4
  mumps (alone) V04.6
    with measles and rubella (MMR)
      V06.4
  pertussis alone V03.6
  plague V03.3
  poliomyelitis V04.0
    with diphtheria-tetanus-pertussis
      (DTP + polio) V06.3
  rabies V04.5
  respiratory syncytial virus (RSV)
    V04.82
  rubella (alone) V04.3
    with measles and mumps (MMR)
      V06.4
  smallpox V04.1
  Streptococcus pneumoniae [pneumococcus] V03.82
    with
      influenza V06.6
  tetanus toxoid (alone) V03.7
    with diphtheria [Td] [DT] V06.5
      with
        pertussis (DTP) [DTaP] V06.1
          with poliomyelitis (DTP +
            polio) V06.3
  tuberculosis (BCG) V03.2
  tularemia V03.4
  typhoid-paratyphoid (TAB) (alone)
    V03.1
    with diphtheria-tetanus-pertussis
      (TAB DTP) V06.2

Vaccination *(Continued)*
  prophylactic *(Continued)*
    varicella V05.4
    viral
      disease NEC V04.89
      encephalitis, arthropod-borne
        V05.0
      hepatitis V05.3
      yellow fever V04.4

Vaccinia (generalized) 999.0
  congenital 771.2
  conjunctiva 999.3
  eyelids 999.0 *[373.5]*
  localized 999.3
  nose 999.3
  not from vaccination 051.0
    eyelid 051.0 *[373.5]*
  sine vaccinatione 051.0
  without vaccination 051.0

Vacuum
  extraction of fetus or newborn 763.3
  in sinus (accessory) (nasal) (*see also* Sinusitis) 473.9

Vagabond V60.0
Vagabondage V60.0
Vagabonds' disease 132.1
Vagina, vaginal - *see* condition
Vaginalitis (tunica) 608.4
Vaginismus (reflex) 625.1
  functional 306.51
  hysterical 300.11
  psychogenic 306.51
Vaginitis (acute) (chronic) (circumscribed)
  (diffuse) (emphysematous) (Haemophilus vaginalis) (nonspecific) (nonvenereal) (ulcerative) 616.10
  with
    abortion - *see* Abortion, by type,
      with sepsis
    ectopic pregnancy (*see also* categories
      633.0-633.9) 639.0
    molar pregnancy (*see also* categories
      630-632) 639.0
  adhesive, congenital 752.49
  atrophic, postmenopausal 627.3
  bacterial 616.10
  blennorrhagic (acute) 098.0
    chronic or duration of 2 months or
      over 098.2
  candidal 112.1
  chlamydial 099.53
  complicating pregnancy or puerperium
    646.6
    affecting fetus or newborn 760.8
  congenital (adhesive) 752.49
  due to
    C. albicans 112.1
    Trichomonas (vaginalis) 131.01
  following
    abortion 639.0
    ectopic or molar pregnancy 639.0
  gonococcal (acute) 098.0
    chronic or duration of 2 months or
      over 098.2
  granuloma 099.2
  Monilia 112.1
  mycotic 112.1
  pinworm 127.4 *[616.11]*
  postirradiation 616.10
  postmenopausal atrophic 627.3
  senile (atrophic) 627.3
  syphilitic (early) 091.0
    late 095.8
  trichomonal 131.01

Vaginitis *(Continued)*
  tuberculous (*see also* Tuberculosis)
    016.7
  venereal NEC 099.8
Vaginosis - *see* Vaginitis
Vagotonia 352.3
Vagrancy V60.0
Vallecula - *see* condition
Valley fever 114.0
Valsuani's disease (progressive pernicious anemia, puerperal) 648.2
Valve, valvular (formation) - *see also*
  condition
  cerebral ventricle (communicating) in
    situ V45.2
  cervix, internal os 752.49
  colon 751.5
  congenital NEC - *see* Atresia
  formation, congenital, NEC - *see* Atresia
  heart defect - *see* Anomaly, heart, valve
  ureter 753.29
    pelvic junction 753.21
    vesical orifice 753.22
  urethra 753.6
Valvulitis (chronic) (*see also* Endocarditis) 424.90
  rheumatic (chronic) (inactive) (with
    chorea) 397.9
    active or acute (aortic) (mitral) (pulmonary) (tricuspid) 391.1
  syphilitic NEC 093.20
    aortic 093.22
    mitral 093.21
    pulmonary 093.24
    tricuspid 093.23
Valvulopathy - *see* Endocarditis
van Bogaert's leukoencephalitis (sclerosing) (subacute) 046.2
van Bogaert-Nijssen (-Peiffer) **disease**
  330.0
van Buchem's syndrome (hyperostosis
  corticalis) 733.3
Vancomycin (glycopeptide) ◄
  intermediate staphylococcus aureus
    (VISA/GISA) V09.8 ◄
  resistant ◄
    enterococcus (VRE) V09.8 ◄
    staphylococcus aureus (VRSA/
      GRSA) V09.8 ◄
van Creveld-von Gierke disease (glycogenosis I) 271.0
van den Bergh's disease (enterogenous
  cyanosis) 289.7
van der Hoeve's syndrome (brittle bones
  and blue sclera, deafness) 756.51
van der Hoeve-Halbertsma-Waardenburg syndrome (ptosis-epicanthus)
  270.2
**van der Hoeve-Waardenburg-Gualdi
  syndrome** (ptosis-epicanthus)
  270.2
Vanillism 692.89
Vanishing lung 492.0
Vanishing twin 651.33
van Neck (-Odelberg) **disease or syndrome** (juvenile osteochondrosis)
  732.1
Vapor asphyxia or suffocation NEC
  987.9
  specified agent - *see* Table of Drugs
    and Chemicals
Vaquez's disease (M9950/1) 238.4
Vaquez-Osler disease (polycythemia
  vera) (M9950/1) 238.4

ICD-9-CM

\>

Vol. 2

Variance, lethal ball, prosthetic heart valve 996.02
Variants, thalassemic 282.49
Variations in hair color 704.3
Varicella 052.9
with
   complication 052.8
     specified NEC 052.7
   pneumonia 052.1
exposure to V01.71 ◄
vaccination and inoculation (against)
   (prophylactic) V05.4
Varices - *see* Varix
Varicocele (scrotum) (thrombosed)
   456.4
ovary 456.5
perineum 456.6
spermatic cord (ulcerated) 456.4
Varicose
aneurysm (ruptured) (*see also* Aneurysm) 442.9
dermatitis (lower extremity) - *see* Varicose, vein, inflamed or infected
eczema - *see* Varicose, vein
phlebitis - *see* Varicose, vein, inflamed or infected
placental vessel - *see* Placenta, abnormal
tumor - *see* Varicose, vein
ulcer (lower extremity, any part) 454.0
   anus 455.8
     external 455.5
     internal 455.2
   esophagus (*see also* Varix, esophagus) 456.1
     bleeding (*see also* Varix, esophagus, bleeding) 456.0
   inflamed or infected 454.2
   nasal septum 456.8
   perineum 456.6
   rectum - *see* Varicose, ulcer, anus
   scrotum 456.4
   specified site NEC 456.8
vein (lower extremity) (ruptured) (*see also* Varix) 454.9
   with
     complications NEC 454.8
     edema 454.8
     inflammation or infection 454.1
       ulcerated 454.2
     pain 454.8
     stasis dermatitis 454.1
       with ulcer 454.2
     swelling 454.8
     ulcer 454.0
       inflamed or infected 454.2
   anus - *see* Hemorrhoids
   broad ligament 456.5
   congenital (peripheral) 747.60
     gastrointestinal 747.61
     lower limb 747.64
     renal 747.62
     specified NEC 747.69
     upper limb 747.63
   esophagus (ulcerated (*see also* Varix, esophagus) 456.1
     bleeding (*see also* Varix, esophagus, bleeding) 456.0
   inflamed or infected 454.1
     with ulcer 454.2
   in pregnancy or puerperium 671.0
     vulva or perineum 671.1
   nasal septum (with ulcer) 456.8
   pelvis 456.5

Varicose (*Continued*)
vein (*Continued*)
   perineum 456.6
     in pregnancy, childbirth, or puerperium 671.1
   rectum - *see* Hemorrhoids
   scrotum (ulcerated) 456.4
   specified site NEC 456.8
   sublingual 456.3
   ulcerated 454.0
     inflamed or infected 454.2
   umbilical cord, affecting fetus or newborn 762.6
   urethra 456.8
   vulva 456.6
     in pregnancy, childbirth, or puerperium 671.1
vessel - *see also* Varix
   placenta - *see* Placenta, abnormal
Varicosis, varicosities, varicosity (*see also* Varix) 454.9
Variola 050.9
hemorrhagic (pustular) 050.0
major 050.0
minor 050.1
modified 050.2
Varioloid 050.2
Variolosa, purpura 050.0
Varix (lower extremity) (ruptured) 454.9
with
   complications NEC 454.8
   edema 454.8
   inflammation or infection 454.1
     with ulcer 454.2
   pain 454.8
   stasis dermatitis 454.1
     with ulcer 454.2
   swelling 454.8
   ulcer 454.0
     with inflammation or infection 454.2
aneurysmal (*see also* Aneurysm) 442.9
anus - *see* Hemorrhoids
arteriovenous (congenital) (peripheral) NEC 747.60
   gastrointestinal 747.61
   lower limb 747.64
   renal 747.62
   specified NEC 747.69
   spinal 747.82
   upper limb 747.63
bladder 456.5
broad ligament 456.5
congenital (peripheral) 747.60
esophagus (ulcerated) 456.1
   bleeding 456.0
     in
       cirrhosis of liver 571.5 [456.20]
       portal hypertension 572.3 [456.20]
   congenital 747.69
   in
     cirrhosis of liver 571.5 [456.21]
       with bleeding 571.5 [456.20]
     portal hypertension 572.3 [456.21]
       with bleeding 572.3 [456.20]
gastric 456.8
inflamed or infected 454.1
   ulcerated 454.2
in pregnancy or puerperium 671.0
   perineum 671.1
   vulva 671.1
labia (majora) 456.6

Varix (*Continued*)
orbit 456.8
   congenital 747.69
ovary 456.5
papillary 448.1
pelvis 456.5
perineum 456.6
   in pregnancy or puerperium 671.1
pharynx 456.8
placenta - *see* Placenta, abnormal
prostate 456.8
rectum - *see* Hemorrhoids
renal papilla 456.8
retina 362.17
scrotum (ulcerated) 456.4
sigmoid colon 456.8
specified site NEC 456.8
spinal (cord) (vessels) 456.8
spleen, splenic (vein) (with phlebolith) 456.8
sublingual 456.3
ulcerated 454.0
   inflamed or infected 454.2
umbilical cord, affecting fetus or newborn 762.6
uterine ligament 456.5
vocal cord 456.8
vulva 456.6
   in pregnancy, childbirth, or puerperium 671.1
Vasa previa 663.5
affecting fetus or newborn 762.6
hemorrhage from, affecting fetus or newborn 772.0
Vascular - *see also* condition
loop on papilla (optic) 743.57
sheathing, retina 362.13
spasm 443.9
spider 448.1
Vascularity, pulmonary, congenital 747.3
Vascularization
choroid 362.16
cornea 370.60
   deep 370.63
   localized 370.61
retina 362.16
subretinal 362.16
Vasculitis 447.6
allergic 287.0
cryoglobulinemic 273.2
disseminated 447.6
kidney 447.8
leukocytoclastic 446.29
nodular 695.2
retinal 362.18
rheumatic - *see* Fever, rheumatic
Vasculopathy
cardiac allograft 996.83
Vas deferens - *see* condition
Vas deferentitis 608.4
Vasectomy, admission for V25.2
Vasitis 608.4
nodosa 608.4
scrotum 608.4
spermatic cord 608.4
testis 608.4
tuberculous (*see also* Tuberculosis) 016.5
tunica vaginalis 608.4
vas deferens 608.4
Vasodilation 443.9
Vasomotor - *see* condition
Vasoplasty, after previous sterilization V26.0

◄ **New**   ◄▥ **Revised**

Vasoplegia, splanchnic (*see also* Neuropathy, peripheral, autonomic) 337.9
Vasospasm 443.9
  cerebral (artery) 435.9
    with transient neurologic deficit 435.9
  nerve
    arm NEC 354.9
    autonomic 337.9
    brachial plexus 353.0
    cervical plexus 353.2
    leg NEC 355.8
    lower extremity NEC 355.8
    peripheral NEC 335.9
    spinal NEC 355.9
    sympathetic 337.9
    upper extremity NEC 354.9
  peripheral NEC 443.9
  retina (artery) (*see also* Occlusion, retinal, artery) 362.30
Vasospastic - *see* condition
Vasovagal attack (paroxysmal) 780.2
  psychogenic 306.2
Vater's ampulla - *see* condition
VATER syndrome 759.89
Vegetation, vegetative
  adenoid (nasal fossa) 474.2
  consciousness (persistent) 780.03
  endocarditis (acute) (any valve) (chronic) (subacute) 421.0
  heart (mycotic) (valve) 421.0
  state (persistent) 780.03
Veil
  Jackson's 751.4
  over face (causing asphyxia) 768.9
Vein, venous - *see* condition
Veldt sore (*see also* Ulcer, skin) 707.9
Velo-cardio-facial syndrome 758.32 ◄
Velpeau's hernia - *see* Hernia, femoral
Venereal
  balanitis NEC 099.8
  bubo 099.1
  disease 099.9
    specified nature or type NEC 099.8
  granuloma inguinale 099.2
  lymphogranuloma (Durand-Nicolas-Favre), any site 099.1
  salpingitis 098.37
  urethritis (*see also* Urethritis, nongonococcal) 099.40
  vaginitis NEC 099.8
  warts 078.19
Vengefulness, in child (*see also* Disturbance, conduct) 312.0
Venofibrosis 459.89
Venom, venomous
  bite or sting (animal or insect) 989.5
  poisoning 989.5
Venous - *see* condition
Ventouse delivery NEC 669.5
  affecting fetus or newborn 763.3
Ventral - *see* condition
Ventricle, ventricular - *see also* condition
  escape 427.69
  standstill (*see also* Arrest, cardiac) 427.5
Ventriculitis, cerebral (*see also* Meningitis) 322.9
Ventriculostomy status V45.2
Verbiest's syndrome (claudicatio intermittens spinalis) 435.1
Vernet's syndrome 352.6
Verneuil's disease (syphilitic bursitis) 095.7

Verruca (filiformis) 078.10
  acuminata (any site) 078.11
  necrogenica (primary) (*see also* Tuberculosis) 017.0
  peruana 088.0
  peruviana 088.0
  plana (juvenilis) 078.19
  plantaris 078.19
  seborrheica 702.19
    inflamed 702.11
  senilis 702.0
  tuberculosa (primary) (*see also* Tuberculosis) 017.0
  venereal 078.19
  viral NEC 078.10
Verrucosities (*see also* Verruca) 078.10
Verrucous endocarditis (acute) (any valve) (chronic) (subacute) 710.0 [424.91]
  nonbacterial 710.0 [424.91]
Verruga
  peruana 088.0
  peruviana 088.0
Verse's disease (calcinosis intervertebralis) 275.49 [722.90]
Version
  before labor, affecting fetus or newborn 761.7
  cephalic (correcting previous malposition) 652.1
    affecting fetus or newborn 763.1
  cervix (*see also* Malposition, uterus) 621.6
  uterus (postinfectional) (postpartal, old) (*see also* Malposition, uterus) 621.6
    forward - *see* Anteversion, uterus
    lateral - *see* Lateroversion, uterus
Vertebra, vertebral - *see* condition
Vertigo 780.4
  auditory 386.19
  aural 386.19
  benign paroxysmal positional 386.11
  central origin 386.2
  cerebral 386.2
  Dix and Hallpike (epidemic) 386.12
  endemic paralytic 078.81
  epidemic 078.81
    Dix and Hallpike 386.12
    Gerlier's 078.81
    Pedersen's 386.12
    vestibular neuronitis 386.12
  epileptic - *see* Epilepsy
  Gerlier's (epidemic) 078.81
  hysterical 300.11
  labyrinthine 386.10
  laryngeal 786.2
  malignant positional 386.2
  Ménière's (*see also* Disease, Meniere's) 386.00
  menopausal 627.2
  otogenic 386.19
  paralytic 078.81
  paroxysmal positional, benign 386.11
  Pedersen's (epidemic) 386.12
  peripheral 386.10
    specified type NEC 386.19
  positional
    benign paroxysmal 386.11
    malignant 386.2
Verumontanitis (chronic) (*see also* Urethritis) 597.89
Vesania (*see also* Psychosis) 298.9

Vesical - *see* condition
Vesicle
  cutaneous 709.8
  seminal - *see* condition
  skin 709.8
Vesicocolic - *see* condition
Vesicoperineal - *see* condition
Vesicorectal - *see* condition
Vesicourethrorectal - *see* condition
Vesicovaginal - *see* condition
Vesicular - *see* condition
Vesiculitis (seminal) 608.0
  amebic 006.8
  gonorrheal (acute) 098.14
    chronic or duration of 2 months or over 098.34
  trichomonal 131.09
  tuberculous (*see also* Tuberculosis) 016.5 [608.81]
Vestibulitis (ear) (*see also* Labyrinthitis) 386.30
  nose (external) 478.1
  vulvar 616.10
Vestibulopathy, acute peripheral (recurrent) 386.12
Vestige, vestigial - *see also* Persistence
  branchial 744.41
  structures in vitreous 743.51
Vibriosis NEC 027.9
Vidal's disease (lichen simplex chronicus) 698.3
Video display tube syndrome 723.8
Vienna-type encephalitis 049.8
Villaret's syndrome 352.6
Villous - *see* condition
VIN I (vulvar intraepithelial neoplasia I) 624.8
VIN II (vulvar intraepithelial neoplasia I) 624.8
VIN III (vulvar intraepithelial neoplasia I) 233.3
Vincent's
  angina 101
  bronchitis 101
  disease 101
  gingivitis 101
  infection (any site) 101
  laryngitis 101
  stomatitis 101
  tonsillitis 101
Vinson-Plummer syndrome (sideropenic dysphagia) 280.8
Viosterol deficiency (*see also* Deficiency, calciferol) 268.9
Virchow's disease 733.99
Viremia 790.8
Virilism (adrenal) (female) NEC 255.2
  with
    3-beta-hydroxysteroid dehydrogenase defect 255.2
    11-hydroxylase defect 255.2
    21-hydroxylase defect 255.2
    adrenal
      hyperplasia 255.2
      insufficiency (congenital) 255.2
    cortical hyperfunction 255.2
Virilization (female) (suprarenal) (*see also* Virilism) 255.2
  isosexual 256.4
Virulent bubo 099.0
Virus, viral - *see also* condition
  infection NEC (*see also* Infection, viral) 079.99
  septicemia 079.99

ICD-9-CM

>

Vol. 2

VISA (vancomycin intermediate staphylococcus aureus) V09.8 ◄

Viscera, visceral - *see* condition

Visceroptosis 569.89

Visible peristalsis 787.4

Vision, visual
binocular, suppression 368.31
blurred, blurring 368.8
  hysterical 300.11
defect, defective (*see also* Impaired, vision) 369.9
disorientation (syndrome) 368.16
disturbance NEC (*see also* Disturbance, vision) 368.9
  hysterical 300.11
examination V72.0
field, limitation 368.40
fusion, with defective stereopsis 368.33
hallucinations 368.16
halos 368.16
loss 369.9
  both eyes (*see also* Blindness, both eyes) 369.3
    complete (*see also* Blindness, both eyes) 369.00
  one eye 369.8
  sudden 368.16
low (both eyes) 369.20
  one eye (other eye normal) (*see also* Impaired, vision) 369.70
    blindness, other eye 369.10
perception, simultaneous without fusion 368.32
tunnel 368.45

Vitality, lack or want of 780.79
newborn 779.89

Vitamin deficiency NEC (*see also* Deficiency, vitamin) 269.2

Vitelline duct, persistent 751.0

Vitiligo 709.01
due to pinta (carate) 103.2
eyelid 374.53
vulva 624.8

Vitium cordis - *see* Disease, heart

Vitreous - *see also* condition
touch syndrome 997.99

VLCAD (long chain/very long chain acyl CoA dehydrogenase deficiency, LCAD) 277.85 ◄

Vocal cord - *see* condition

Vocational rehabilitation V57.22

Vogt's (Cecile) disease or syndrome 333.7

Vogt-Koyanagi syndrome 364.24

Vogt-Spielmeyer disease (amaurotic familial idiocy) 330.1

Voice
change (*see also* Dysphonia) 784.49
loss (*see also* Aphonia) 784.41

Volhard-Fahr disease (malignant nephrosclerosis) 403.00

Volhynian fever 083.1

Volkmann's ischemic contracture or paralysis (complicating trauma) 958.6

Voluntary starvation 307.1

Volvulus (bowel) (colon) (intestine) 560.2
with
  hernia - *see also* Hernia, by site, with obstruction

Volvulus (*Continued*)
with (*Continued*)
  hernia (*Continued*)
    gangrenous - *see* Hernia, by site, with gangrene
  perforation 560.2
congenital 751.5
duodenum 537.3
fallopian tube 620.5
oviduct 620.5
stomach (due to absence of gastrocolic ligament) 537.89

Vomiting 787.03
with nausea 787.01
allergic 535.4
asphyxia 933.1
bilious (cause unknown) 787.0
  following gastrointestinal surgery 564.3
blood (*see also* Hematemesis) 578.0
causing asphyxia, choking, or suffocation (*see also* Asphyxia, food) 933.1
cyclical 536.2
  psychogenic 306.4
epidemic 078.82
fecal matter 569.89
following gastrointestinal surgery 564.3
functional 536.8
  psychogenic 306.4
habit 536.2
hysterical 300.11
nervous 306.4
neurotic 306.4
newborn 779.3
of or complicating pregnancy 643.9
  due to
    organic disease 643.8
    specific cause NEC 643.8
  early - *see* Hyperemesis, gravidarum
  late (after 22 completed weeks of gestation) 643.2
pernicious or persistent 536.2
  complicating pregnancy - *see* Hyperemesis, gravidarum
  psychogenic 306.4
physiological 787.0
psychic 306.4
psychogenic 307.54
stercoral 569.89
uncontrollable 536.2
  psychogenic 306.4
uremic - *see* Uremia
winter 078.82

von Bechterew (-Strümpell) disease or syndrome (ankylosing spondylitis) 720.0

von Bezold's abscess 383.01

von Economo's disease (encephalitis lethargica) 049.8

von Eulenburg's disease (congenital paramyotonia) 359.2

von Gierke's disease (glycogenosis I) 271.0

von Gies' joint 095.8

von Graefe's disease or syndrome 378.72

von Hippel (-Lindau) disease or syndrome (retinocerebral angiomatosis) 759.6

von Jaksch's anemia or disease (pseudoleukemia infantum) 285.8

von Recklinghausen's
disease or syndrome (nerves) (skin) (M9540/1) 237.71
bones (osteitis fibrosa cystica) 252.01 ◀▥▥
tumor (M9540/1) 237.71

von Recklinghausen-Applebaum disease (hemochromatosis) 275.0

von Schroetter's syndrome (intermittent venous claudication) 453.8

von Willebrand (-Jürgens) (-Minot) disease or syndrome (angiohemophilia) 286.4

von Zambusch's disease (lichen sclerosus et atrophicus) 701.0

Voorhoeve's disease or dyschondroplasia 756.4

Vossius' ring 921.3
late effect 366.21

Voyeurism 302.82

VRE (vancomycin resistant enterococcus) V09.8 ◄

Vrolik's disease (osteogenesis imperfecta) 756.51

VRSA (vancomycin resistant staphylococcus aureus) V09.8 ◄

Vulva - *see* condition

Vulvismus 625.1

Vulvitis (acute) (allergic) (aphthous) (chronic) (gangrenous) (hypertrophic) (intertriginous) 616.10
with
  abortion - *see* Abortion, by type, with sepsis
  ectopic pregnancy (*see also* categories 633.0-633.9) 639.0
  molar pregnancy (*see also* categories 630-632) 639.0
adhesive, congenital 752.49
blennorrhagic (acute) 098.0
  chronic or duration of 2 months or over 098.2
chlamydial 099.53
complicating pregnancy or puerperium 646.6
due to Ducrey's bacillus 099.0
following
  abortion 639.0
  ectopic or molar pregnancy 639.0
gonococcal (acute) 098.0
  chronic or duration of 2 months or over 098.2
herpetic 054.11
leukoplakic 624.0
monilial 112.1
puerperal, postpartum, childbirth 646.6
syphilitic (early) 091.0
  late 095.8
trichomonal 131.01

Vulvodynia 625.9

Vulvorectal - *see* condition

Vulvovaginitis (*see also* Vulvitis) 616.10
amebic 006.8
chlamydial 099.53
gonococcal (acute) 098.0
  chronic or duration of 2 months or over 098.2
herpetic 054.11
monilial 112.1
trichomonal (Trichomonas vaginalis) 131.01

W

Waardenburg's syndrome 756.89
  meaning ptosis-epicanthus 270.2
Waardenburg-Klein syndrome (ptosis-epicanthus) 270.2
Wagner's disease (colloid milium) 709.3
Wagner (-Unverricht) **syndrome** (dermatomyositis) 710.3
Waiting list, person on V63.2
  undergoing social agency investigation V63.8
Wakefulness disorder (see also Hypersomnia) 780.54
  nonorganic origin 307.43
Waldenström's
  disease (osteochondrosis, capital femoral) 732.1
  hepatitis (lupoid hepatitis) 571.49
  hypergammaglobulinemia 273.0
  macroglobulinemia 273.3
  purpura, hypergammaglobulinemic 273.0
  syndrome (macroglobulinemia) 273.3
Waldenström-Kjellberg syndrome (sideropenic dysphagia) 280.8
Walking
  difficulty 719.7
    psychogenic 307.9
  sleep 307.46
    hysterical 300.13
Wall, abdominal - see condition
Wallenberg's syndrome (posterior inferior cerebellar artery) (see also Disease, cerebrovascular, acute) 436
Wallgren's
  disease (obstruction of splenic vein with collateral circulation) 459.89
  meningitis (see also Meningitis, aseptic) 047.9
Wandering
  acetabulum 736.39
  gallbladder 751.69
  kidney, congenital 753.3
  organ or site, congenital NEC - see Malposition, congenital
  pacemaker (atrial) (heart) 427.89
  spleen 289.59
Wardrop's disease (with lymphangitis) 681.9
  finger 681.02
  toe 681.11
War neurosis 300.16
Wart (common) (digitate) (filiform) (infectious) (viral) 078.10
  external genital organs (venereal) 078.19
  fig 078.19
  Hassall-Henle's (of cornea) 371.41
  Henle's (of cornea) 371.41
  juvenile 078.19
  moist 078.10
  Peruvian 088.0
  plantar 078.19
  prosector (see also Tuberculosis) 017.0
  seborrheic 702.19
    inflamed 702.11
  senile 702.0
  specified NEC 078.19
  syphilitic 091.3
  tuberculous (see also Tuberculosis) 017.0
  venereal (female) (male) 078.19
Warthin's tumor (salivary gland) (M8561/0) 210.2
Washerwoman's itch 692.4

Wassilieff's disease (leptospiral jaundice) 100.0
Wasting
  disease 799.4
    due to malnutrition 261
  extreme (due to malnutrition) 261
  muscular NEC 728.2
  palsy, paralysis 335.21 ◄
  pelvic muscle 618.83
Water
  clefts 366.12
  deprivation of 994.3
  in joint (see also Effusion, joint) 719.0
  intoxication 276.6
  itch 120.3
  lack of 994.3
  loading 276.6
  on
    brain - see Hydrocephalus
    chest 511.8
  poisoning 276.6
Waterbrash 787.1
Water-hammer pulse (see also Insufficiency, aortic) 424.1
Waterhouse (-Friderichsen) **disease or syndrome** 036.3
Water-losing nephritis 588.89 ◄▥
Wax in ear 380.4
Waxy
  degeneration, any site 277.3
  disease 277.3
  kidney 277.3 [583.81]
  liver (large) 277.3
  spleen 277.3
Weak, weakness (generalized) 780.79
  arches (acquired) 734
    congenital 754.61
  bladder sphincter 596.59
  congenital 779.89
  eye muscle - see Strabismus
  facial 781.94
  foot (double) - see Weak, arches
  heart, cardiac (see also Failure, heart) 428.9
    congenital 746.9
  mind 317
  muscle 728.87
  myocardium (see also Failure, heart) 428.9
  newborn 779.89
  pelvic fundus ◄▥
    pubocervical tissue 618.81 ◄
    rectovaginal tissue 618.82 ◄
  pulse 785.9
  senile 797
  urinary stream 788.62
  valvular - see Endocarditis
Wear, worn, tooth, teeth (approximal) (hard tissues) (interproximal) (occlusal) - see also Attrition, teeth 521.10 ◄▥
Weather, weathered
  effects of
    cold NEC 991.9
      specified effect NEC 991.8
    hot (see also Heat) 992.9
  skin 692.74
Web, webbed (congenital) - see also Anomaly, specified type NEC
  canthus 743.63
  digits (see also Syndactylism) 755.10
  duodenal 751.5
  esophagus 750.3
  fingers (see also Syndactylism, fingers) 755.11

Web, webbed (Continued)
  larynx (glottic) (subglottic) 748.2
  neck (pterygium colli) 744.5
  Paterson-Kelly (sideropenic dysphagia) 280.8
  popliteal syndrome 756.89
  toes (see also Syndactylism, toes) 755.13
Weber's paralysis or syndrome 344.89
Weber-Christian disease or syndrome (nodular nonsuppurative panniculitis) 729.30
Weber-Cockayne syndrome (epidermolysis bullosa) 757.39
Weber-Dimitri syndrome 759.6
Weber-Gubler syndrome 344.89
Weber-Leyden syndrome 344.89
Weber-Osler syndrome (familial hemorrhagic telangiectasia) 448.0
Wedge-shaped or wedging vertebra (see also Osteoporosis) 733.00
Wegener's granulomatosis or syndrome 446.4
Wegner's disease (syphilitic osteochondritis) 090.0
Weight
  gain (abnormal) (excessive) 783.1
    during pregnancy 646.1
      insufficient 646.8
  less than 1000 grams at birth 765.0
  loss (cause unknown) 783.21
Weightlessness 994.9
Weil's disease (leptospiral jaundice) 100.0
Weill-Marchesani syndrome (brachymorphism and ectopia lentis) 759.89
Weingarten's syndrome (tropical eosinophilia) 518.3
Weir Mitchell's disease (erythromelalgia) 443.89
Weiss-Baker syndrome (carotid sinus syncope) 337.0
Weissenbach-Thibierge syndrome (cutaneous systemic sclerosis) 710.1
Wen (see also Cyst, sebaceous) 706.2
Wenckebach's phenomenon, heart block (second degree) 426.13
Werdnig-Hoffmann syndrome (muscular atrophy) 335.0
Werlhof's disease (see also Purpura, thrombocytopenic) 287.3
Werlhof-Wichmann syndrome (see also Purpura, thrombocytopenic) 287.3
Wermer's syndrome or disease (polyendocrine adenomatosis) 258.0
Werner's disease or syndrome (progeria adultorum) 259.8
Werner-His disease (trench fever) 083.1
Werner-Schultz disease (agranulocytosis) 288.0
Wernicke's encephalopathy, disease, or syndrome (superior hemorrhagic polioencephalitis) 265.1
Wernicke-Korsakoff syndrome or psychosis (nonalcoholic) 294.0
  alcoholic 291.1
Wernicke-Posadas disease (see also Coccidioidomycosis) 114.9
Wesselsbron fever 066.3
West African fever 084.8
West Nile ◄
  encephalitis 066.41 ◄
  encephalomyelitis 066.41 ◄

ICD-9-CM

W

Vol. 2

West Nile *(Continued)*
fever 066.40 ◄▦
with
cranial nerve disorders 066.42 ◄
encephalitis 066.41 ◄
optic neuritis 066.42 ◄
other complications 066.49 ◄
other neurologic manifestations 066.42 ◄
polyradiculitis 066.42 ◄
virus 066.40 ◄▦

Westphal-Strümpell syndrome (hepato-lenticular degeneration) 275.1

Wet
brain (alcoholic) *(see also* Alcoholism) 303.9
feet, tropical (syndrome) (maceration) 991.4
lung (syndrome)
adult 518.5
newborn 770.6

Wharton's duct - *see* condition
Wheal 709.8
Wheezing 786.07
Whiplash injury or syndrome 847.0
Whipple's disease or syndrome (intestinal lipodystrophy) 040.2
Whipworm 127.3
"Whistling face" syndrome (craniocarpotarsal dystrophy) 759.89
White - *see also* condition
kidney
large - *see* Nephrosis
small 582.9
leg, puerperal, postpartum, childbirth 671.4
nonpuerperal 451.19
mouth 112.0
patches of mouth 528.6
sponge nevus of oral mucosa 750.26
spot lesions, teeth 521.01
White's disease (congenital) (keratosis follicularis) 757.39
Whitehead 706.2
Whitlow (with lymphangitis) 681.01
herpetic 054.6
Whitmore's disease or fever (melioidosis) 025
Whooping cough 033.9
with pneumonia 033.9 *[484.3]*
due to
Bordetella
bronchoseptica 033.8
with pneumonia 033.8 *[484.3]*
parapertussis 033.1
with pneumonia 033.1 *[484.3]*
pertussis 033.0
with pneumonia 033.0 *[484.3]*
specified organism NEC 033.8
with pneumonia 033.8 *[484.3]*
vaccination, prophylactic (against) V03.6
Wichmann's asthma (laryngismus stridulus) 478.75
Widal (-Abrami) syndrome (acquired hemolytic jaundice) 283.9
Widening aorta *(see also* Aneurysm, aorta) 441.9
ruptured 441.5
Wilkie's disease or syndrome 557.1
Wilkinson-Sneddon disease or syndrome (subcorneal pustular dermatosis) 694.1
Willan's lepra 696.1

Willan-Plumbe syndrome (psoriasis) 696.1
Willebrand (-Jürgens) syndrome or thrombopathy (angiohemophilia) 286.4
Willi-Prader syndrome (hypogenital dystrophy with diabetic tendency) 759.81
Willis' disease (diabetes mellitus) *(see also* Diabetes) 250.0
Wilms' tumor or neoplasm (nephroblastoma) (M8960/3) 189.0
Wilson's
disease or syndrome (hepatolenticular degeneration) 275.1
hepatolenticular degeneration 275.1
lichen ruber 697.0
Wilson-Brocq disease (dermatitis exfoliativa) 695.89
Wilson-Mikity syndrome 770.7
Window - *see also* Imperfect, closure aorticopulmonary 745.0
Winged scapula 736.89
Winter - *see also* condition
vomiting disease 078.82
Wise's disease 696.2
Wiskott-Aldrich syndrome (eczema-thrombocytopenia) 279.12
Withdrawal symptoms, syndrome
alcohol 291.81
delirium (acute) 291.0
chronic 291.1
newborn 760.71
drug or narcotic 292.0
newborn, infant of dependent mother 779.5
steroid NEC
correct substance properly administered 255.4
overdose or wrong substance given or taken 962.0
Withdrawing reaction, child or adolescent 313.22
Witts' anemia (achlorhydric anemia) 280.9
Witzelsucht 301.9
Woakes' syndrome (ethmoiditis) 471.1
Wohlfart-Kugelberg-Welander disease 335.11
Woillez's disease (acute idiopathic pulmonary congestion) 518.5
Wolff-Parkinson-White syndrome (anomalous atrioventricular excitation) 426.7
Wolhynian fever 083.1
Wolman's disease (primary familial xanthomatosis) 272.7
Wood asthma 495.8
Woolly, wooly hair (congenital) (nevus) 757.4
Wool-sorters' disease 022.1
Word
blindness (congenital) (developmental) 315.01
secondary to organic lesion 784.61
deafness (secondary to organic lesion) 784.69
developmental 315.31
Worm(s) (colic) (fever) (infection) (infestation) *(see also* Infestation) 128.9
guinea 125.7
in intestine NEC 127.9
Worm-eaten soles 102.3
Worn out *(see also* Exhaustion) 780.79
"Worried well" V65.5

Wound, open (by cutting or piercing instrument) (by firearms) (cut) (dissection) (incised) (laceration) (penetration) (perforating) (puncture) (with initial hemorrhage, not internal) 879.8

> Note For fracture with open wound, see Fracture.
>
> For laceration, traumatic rupture, tear, or penetrating wound of internal organs, such as heart, lung, liver, kidney, pelvic organs, etc., whether or not accompanied by open wound or fracture in the same region, see Injury, internal.
> For contused wound, see Contusion. For crush injury, see Crush. For abrasion, insect bite (nonvenomous), blister, or scratch, see Injury, superficial.
>
> Complicated includes wounds with:
>
> delayed healing
> delayed treatment
> foreign body
> primary infection
>
> For late effect of open wound, see Late, effect, wound, open, by site.

abdomen, abdominal (external) (muscle) 879.2
complicated 879.3
wall (anterior) 879.2
complicated 879.3
lateral 879.4
complicated 879.5
alveolar (process) 873.62
complicated 873.72
ankle 891.0
with tendon involvement 891.2
complicated 891.1
anterior chamber, eye *(see also* Wound, open, intraocular) 871.9
anus 879.6
complicated 879.7
arm 884.0
with tendon involvement 884.2
complicated 884.1
forearm 881.00
with tendon involvement 881.20
complicated 881.10
multiple sites - *see* Wound, open, multiple, upper limb
upper 880.03
with tendon involvement 880.23
complicated 880.13
multiple sites (with axillary or shoulder regions) 880.09
with tendon involvement 880.29
complicated 880.19
artery - *see* Injury, blood vessel, by site
auditory
canal (external) (meatus) 872.02
complicated 872.12
ossicles (incus) (malleus) (stapes) 872.62
complicated 872.72
auricle, ear 872.01
complicated 872.11
axilla 880.02
with tendon involvement 880.22
complicated 880.12
with tendon involvement 880.29

◄ **New** ◄▦ **Revised**

Wound, open (*Continued*)
  axilla (*Continued*)
    involving other sites of upper arm
        880.09
      complicated 880.19
  back 876.0
    complicated 876.1
  bladder - *see* Injury, internal, bladder
  blood vessel - *see* Injury, blood vessel,
      by site
  brain - *see* Injury, intracranial, with
      open intracranial wound
  breast 879.0
    complicated 879.1
  brow 873.42
    complicated 873.52
  buccal mucosa 873.61
    complicated 873.71
  buttock 877.0
    complicated 877.1
  calf 891.0
    with tendon involvement 891.2
    complicated 891.1
  canaliculus lacrimalis 870.8
    with laceration of eyelid 870.2
  canthus, eye 870.8
    laceration - *see* Laceration, eyelid
  cavernous sinus - *see* Injury, intracra-
      nial
  cerebellum - *see* Injury, intracranial
  cervical esophagus 874.4
    complicated 874.5
  cervix - *see* Injury, internal, cervix
  cheek(s) (external) 873.41
    complicated 873.51
    internal 873.61
      complicated 873.71
  chest (wall) (external) 875.0
    complicated 875.1
  chin 873.44
    complicated 873.54
  choroid 363.63
  ciliary body (eye) (*see also* Wound,
      open, intraocular) 871.9
  clitoris 878.8
    complicated 878.9
  cochlea 872.64
    complicated 872.74
  complicated 879.9
  conjunctiva - *see* Wound, open, intra-
      ocular
  cornea (nonpenetrating) (*see also*
      Wound, open, intraocular) 871.9
  costal region 875.0
    complicated 875.1
  Descemet's membrane (*see also* Wound,
      open, intraocular) 871.9
  digit(s)
    foot 893.0
      with tendon involvement 893.2
      complicated 893.1
    hand 883.0
      with tendon involvement 883.2
      complicated 883.1
  drumhead, ear 872.61
    complicated 872.71
  ear 872.8
    canal 872.02
      complicated 872.12
    complicated 872.9
    drum 872.61
      complicated 872.71
    external 872.00
      complicated 872.10

Wound, open (*Continued*)
  ear (*Continued*)
    multiple sites 872.69
      complicated 872.79
    ossicles (incus) (malleus) (stapes)
        872.62
      complicated 872.72
    specified part NEC 872.69
      complicated 872.79
  elbow 881.01
    with tendon involvement 881.21
    complicated 881.11
  epididymis 878.2
    complicated 878.3
  epigastric region 879.2
    complicated 879.3
  epiglottis 874.01
    complicated 874.11
  esophagus (cervical) 874.4
    complicated 874.5
    thoracic - *see* Injury, internal, esophagus
  Eustachian tube 872.63
    complicated 872.73
  extremity
    lower (multiple) NEC 894.0
      with tendon involvement 894.2
      complicated 894.1
    upper (multiple) NEC 884.0
      with tendon involvement 884.2
      complicated 884.1
  eye(s) (globe) - *see* Wound, open, intra-
      ocular
  eyeball NEC 871.9
    laceration (*see also* Laceration, eye-
        ball) 871.4
    penetrating (*see also* Penetrating
        wound, eyeball) 871.7
  eyebrow 873.42
    complicated 873.52
  eyelid NEC 870.8
    laceration - *see* Laceration, eyelid
  face 873.40
    complicated 873.50
    multiple sites 873.49
      complicated 873.59
    specified part NEC 873.49
      complicated 873.59
  fallopian tube - *see* Injury, internal, fal-
      lopian tube
  finger(s) (nail) (subungual) 883.0
    with tendon involvement 883.2
    complicated 883.1
  flank 879.4
    complicated 879.5
  foot (any part, except toe(s) alone) 892.0
    with tendon involvement 892.2
    complicated 892.1
  forearm 881.00
    with tendon involvement 881.20
    complicated 881.10
  forehead 873.42
    complicated 873.52
  genital organs (external) NEC 878.8
    complicated 878.9
    internal - *see* Injury, internal, by site
  globe (eye) (*see also* Wound, open, eye-
      ball) 871.9
  groin 879.4
    complicated 879.5
  gum(s) 873.62
    complicated 873.72
  hand (except finger(s) alone) 882.0
    with tendon involvement 882.2
    complicated 882.1

Wound, open (*Continued*)
  head NEC 873.8
    with intracranial injury - *see* Injury,
        intracranial
    due to or associated with skull
        fracture - *see* Fracture, skull
    complicated 873.9
    scalp - *see* Wound, open, scalp
  heel 892.0
    with tendon involvement 892.2
    complicated 892.1
  high-velocity (grease gun) - *see*
      Wound, open, complicated, by site
  hip 890.0
    with tendon involvement 890.2
    complicated 890.1
  hymen 878.6
    complicated 878.7
  hypochondrium 879.4
    complicated 879.5
  hypogastric region 879.2
    complicated 879.3
  iliac (region) 879.4
    complicated 879.5
  incidental to
    dislocation - *see* Dislocation, open,
        by site
    fracture - *see* Fracture, open, by site
    intracranial injury - *see* Injury, intra-
        cranial, with open intracranial
        wound
    nerve injury - *see* Injury, nerve, by
        site
  inguinal region 879.4
    complicated 879.5
  instep 892.0
    with tendon involvement 892.2
    complicated 892.1
  interscapular region 876.0
    complicated 876.1
  intracranial - *see* Injury, intracranial,
      with open intracranial wound
  intraocular 871.9
    with
      partial loss (of intraocular tissue)
          871.2
      prolapse or exposure (of intraocu-
          lar tissue) 871.1
    laceration (*see also* Laceration, eye-
        ball) 871.4
    penetrating 871.7
      with foreign body (nonmagnetic)
          871.6
        magnetic 871.5
    without prolapse (of intraocular tis-
        sue) 871.0
  iris (*see also* Wound, open, eyeball)
      871.9
  jaw (fracture not involved) 873.44
    with fracture - *see* Fracture, jaw
    complicated 873.54
  knee 891.0
    with tendon involvement
        891.2
    complicated 891.1
  labium (majus) (minus) 878.4
    complicated 878.5
  lacrimal apparatus, gland, or sac
      870.8
    with laceration of eyelid 870.2
  larynx 874.01
    with trachea 874.00
      complicated 874.10
      complicated 874.11

ICD-9-CM

Ⅲ

Vol.

Wound, open *(Continued)*
leg (multiple) 891.0
  with tendon involvement 891.2
  complicated 891.1
  lower 891.0
    with tendon involvement 891.2
    complicated 891.1
  thigh 890.0
    with tendon involvement 890.2
    complicated 890.1
  upper 890.0
    with tendon involvement 890.2
    complicated 890.1
lens (eye) (alone) *(see also* Cataract, traumatic) 366.20
  with involvement of other eye structures - *see* Wound, open, eyeball
limb
  lower (multiple) NEC 894.0
    with tendon involvement 894.2
    complicated 894.1
  upper (multiple) NEC 884.0
    with tendon involvement 884.2
    complicated 884.1
lip 873.43
  complicated 873.53
loin 876.0
  complicated 876.1
lumbar region 876.0
  complicated 876.1
malar region 873.41
  complicated 873.51
mastoid region 873.49
  complicated 873.59
mediastinum - *see* Injury, internal, mediastinum
midthoracic region 875.0
  complicated 875.1
mouth 873.60
  complicated 873.70
  floor 873.64
    complicated 873.74
  multiple sites 873.69
    complicated 873.79
  specified site NEC 873.69
    complicated 873.79
multiple, unspecified site(s) 879.8

> Note Multiple open wounds of sites classifiable to the same four-digit category should be classified to that category unless they are in different limbs.
>
> Multiple open wounds of sites classifiable to different four-digit categories, or to different limbs, should be coded separately.

  complicated 879.9
  lower limb(s) (one or both) (sites classifiable to more than one three-digit category in 890-893) 894.0
    with tendon involvement 894.2
    complicated 894.1
  upper limb(s) (one or both) (sites classifiable to more than one three-digit category in 880-883) 884.0
    with tendon involvement 884.2
    complicated 884.1
muscle - *see* Sprain, by site

Wound, open *(Continued)*
nail
  finger(s) 883.0
    complicated 883.1
  thumb 883.0
    complicated 883.1
  toe(s) 893.0
    complicated 893.1
nape (neck) 874.8
  complicated 874.9
  specified part NEC 874.8
    complicated 874.9
nasal - *see also* Wound, open, nose
  cavity 873.22
    complicated 873.32
  septum 873.21
    complicated 873.31
  sinuses 873.23
    complicated 873.33
nasopharynx 873.22
  complicated 873.32
neck 874.8
  complicated 874.9
  nape 874.8
    complicated 874.9
  specified part NEC 874.8
    complicated 874.9
nerve - *see* Injury, nerve, by site
non-healing surgical 998.83
nose 873.20
  complicated 873.30
  multiple sites 873.29
    complicated 873.39
  septum 873.21
    complicated 873.31
  sinuses 873.23
    complicated 873.33
occipital region - *see* Wound, open, scalp
ocular NEC 871.9
  adnexa 870.9
    specified region NEC 870.8
  laceration *(see also* Laceration, ocular) 871.4
  muscle (extraocular) 870.3
    with foreign body 870.4
    eyelid 870.1
    intraocular - *see* Wound, open, eyeball
  penetrating *(see also* Penetrating wound, ocular) 871.7
orbit 870.8
  penetrating 870.3
    with foreign body 870.4
orbital region 870.9
ovary - *see* Injury, internal, pelvic organs
palate 873.65
  complicated 873.75
palm 882.0
  with tendon involvement 882.2
  complicated 882.1
parathyroid (gland) 874.2
  complicated 874.3
parietal region - *see* Wound, open, scalp
pelvic floor or region 879.6
  complicated 879.7
penis 878.0
  complicated 878.1
perineum 879.6
  complicated 879.7
periocular area 870.8
  laceration of skin 870.0

Wound, open *(Continued)*
pharynx 874.4
  complicated 874.5
pinna 872.01
  complicated 872.11
popliteal space 891.0
  with tendon involvement 891.2
  complicated 891.1
prepuce 878.0
  complicated 878.1
pubic region 879.2
  complicated 879.3
pudenda 878.8
  complicated 878.9
rectovaginal septum 878.8
  complicated 878.9
sacral region 877.0
  complicated 877.1
sacroiliac region 877.0
  complicated 877.1
salivary (ducts) (glands) 873.69
  complicated 873.79
scalp 873.0
  complicated 873.1
scalpel, fetus or newborn 767.8
scapular region 880.01
  with tendon involvement 880.21
  complicated 880.11
  involving other sites of upper arm 880.09
    with tendon involvement 880.29
    complicated 880.19
sclera *(see also* Wound, open, intraocular) 871.9
scrotum 878.2
  complicated 878.3
seminal vesicle - *see* Injury, internal, pelvic organs
shin 891.0
  with tendon involvement 891.2
  complicated 891.1
shoulder 880.00
  with tendon involvement 880.20
  complicated 880.10
  involving other sites of upper arm 880.09
    with tendon involvement 880.29
    complicated 880.19
skin NEC 879.8
  complicated 879.9
skull - *see also* Injury, intracranial, with open intracranial wound
  with skull fracture - *see* Fracture, skull
spermatic cord (scrotal) 878.2
  complicated 878.3
  pelvic region - *see* Injury, internal, spermatic cord
spinal cord - *see* Injury, spinal
sternal region 875.0
  complicated 875.1
subconjunctival - *see* Wound, open, intraocular
subcutaneous NEC 879.8
  complicated 879.9
submaxillary region 873.44
  complicated 873.54
submental region 873.44
  complicated 873.54
subungual
  finger(s) (thumb) - *see* Wound, open, finger
  toe(s) - *see* Wound, open, toe
supraclavicular region 874.8
  complicated 874.9

Wound, open (*Continued*)
supraorbital 873.42
    complicated 873.52
surgical, non-healing 998.83
temple 873.49
    complicated 873.59
temporal region 873.49
    complicated 873.59
testis 878.2
    complicated 878.3
thigh 890.0
    with tendon involvement 890.2
    complicated 890.1
thorax, thoracic (external) 875.0
    complicated 875.1
throat 874.8
    complicated 874.9
thumb (nail) (subungual) 883.0
    with tendon involvement 883.2
    complicated 883.1
thyroid (gland) 874.2
    complicated 874.3
toe(s) (nail) (subungual) 893.0
    with tendon involvement
        893.2
    complicated 893.1
tongue 873.64
    complicated 873.74
tonsil - *see* Wound, open, neck

Wound, open (*Continued*)
trachea (cervical region) 874.02
    with larynx 874.00
        complicated 874.10
    complicated 874.12
    intrathoracic - *see* Injury, internal,
        trachea
trunk (multiple) NEC 879.6
    complicated 879.7
    specified site NEC 879.6
        complicated 879.7
tunica vaginalis 878.2
    complicated 878.3
tympanic membrane 872.61
    complicated 872.71
tympanum 872.61
    complicated 872.71
umbilical region 879.2
    complicated 879.3
ureter - *see* Injury, internal, ureter
urethra - *see* Injury, internal,
    urethra
uterus - *see* Injury, internal, uterus
uvula 873.69
    complicated 873.79
vagina 878.6
    complicated 878.7
vas deferens - *see* Injury, internal, vas
    deferens

Wound, open (*Continued*)
vitreous (humor) 871.2
vulva 878.4
    complicated 878.5
wrist 881.02
    with tendon involvement 881.22
    complicated 881.12
Wright's syndrome (hyperabduction)
    447.8
    pneumonia 390 [517.1]
Wringer injury - *see* Crush injury,
    by site
Wrinkling of skin 701.8
Wrist - *see also* condition
    drop (acquired) 736.05
Wrong drug (given in error) NEC
    977.9
    specified drug or substance - *see* Table
        of Drugs and Chemicals
Wry neck - *see also* Torticollis
    congenital 754.1
Wuchereria infestation 125.0
    bancrofti 125.0
    Brugia malayi 125.1
    malayi 125.1
Wuchereriasis 125.0
Wuchereriosis 125.0
Wuchernde struma langhans (M8332/3)
    193

ICD-9-CM

W

Vol. 2

X

Xanthelasma 272.2
  eyelid 272.2 *[374.51]*
  palpebrarum 272.2 *[374.51]*
Xanthelasmatosis (essential) 272.2
Xanthelasmoidea 757.33
Xanthine stones 277.2
Xanthinuria 277.2
Xanthofibroma (M8831/0) - *see* Neoplasm, connective tissue, benign
Xanthoma(s), xanthomatosis 272.2
  with
    hyperlipoproteinemia
      type I 272.3
      type III 272.2
      type IV 272.1
      type V 272.3
  bone 272.7
  craniohypophyseal 277.89
  cutaneotendinous 272.7
  diabeticorum 250.8 *[272.2]*
  disseminatum 272.7
  eruptive 272.2
  eyelid 272.2 *[374.51]*
  familial 272.7
  hereditary 272.7
  hypercholesterinemic 272.0
  hypercholesterolemic 272.0

Xanthoma *(Continued)*
  hyperlipemic 272.4
  hyperlipidemic 272.4
  infantile 272.7
  joint 272.7
  juvenile 272.7
  multiple 272.7
  multiplex 272.7
  primary familial 272.7
  tendon (sheath) 272.7
  tuberosum 272.2
  tuberous 272.2
  tubo-eruptive 272.2
Xanthosis 709.09
  surgical 998.81
Xenophobia 300.29
Xeroderma (congenital) 757.39
  acquired 701.1
    eyelid 373.33
  eyelid 373.33
  pigmentosum 757.33
  vitamin A deficiency 264.8
Xerophthalmia 372.53
  vitamin A deficiency 264.7
Xerosis
  conjunctiva 372.53
    with Bitôt's spot 372.53
      vitamin A deficiency 264.1
    vitamin A deficiency 264.0

Xerosis *(Continued)*
  cornea 371.40
    with corneal ulceration 370.00
      vitamin A deficiency 264.3
    vitamin A deficiency 264.2
  cutis 706.8
  skin 706.8
Xerostomia 527.7
Xiphodynia 733.90
Xiphoidalgia 733.90
Xiphoiditis 733.99
Xiphopagus 759.4
XO syndrome 758.6
X-ray
  effects, adverse, NEC 990
  of chest
    for suspected tuberculosis V71.2
    routine V72.5
XXX syndrome 758.81
XXXXY syndrome 758.81
XXY syndrome 758.7
Xyloketosuria 271.8
Xylosuria 271.8
Xylulosuria 271.8
XYY syndrome 758.81

◀ **New**   ◀◢ **Revised**

Y

Yawning 786.09
  psychogenic 306.1
Yaws 102.9
  bone or joint lesions 102.6
  butter 102.1
  chancre 102.0
  cutaneous, less than five years after in-
      fection 102.2
  early (cutaneous) (macular)
      (maculopapular) (micropapular)
      (papular) 102.2
    frambeside 102.2
    skin lesions NEC 102.2
  eyelid 102.9 *[373.4]*
  ganglion 102.6
  gangosis, gangosa 102.5
  gumma, gummata 102.4
    bone 102.6
  gummatous
    frambeside 102.4
    osteitis 102.6
    periostitis 102.6
  hydrarthrosis 102.6
  hyperkeratosis (early) (late) (palmar)
      (plantar) 102.3
  initial lesions 102.0
  joint lesions 102.6

Yaws *(Continued)*
  juxta-articular nodules 102.7
  late nodular (ulcerated) 102.4
  latent (without clinical manifestations)
      (with positive serology) 102.8
  mother 102.0
  mucosal 102.7
  multiple papillomata 102.1
  nodular, late (ulcerated) 102.4
  osteitis 102.6
  papilloma, papillomata (palmar) (plan-
      tar) 102.1
  periostitis (hypertrophic) 102.6
  ulcers 102.4
  wet crab 102.1
Yeast infection (*see also* Candidiasis)
    112.9
Yellow
  atrophy (liver) 570
    chronic 571.8
    resulting from administration of
        blood, plasma, serum, or other
        biological substance (within 8
        months of administration) - *see*
        Hepatitis, viral
  fever - *see* Fever, yellow
  jack (*see also* Fever, yellow) 060.9
  jaundice (*see also* Jaundice) 782.4
Yersinia septica 027.8

Z

Zagari's disease (xerostomia) 527.7
Zahorsky's disease (exanthema subitum)
    057.8
  syndrome (herpangina) 074.0
Zellweger syndrome 277.86 ◀
Zenker's diverticulum (esophagus)
    530.6
Ziehen-Oppenheim disease 333.6
Zieve's syndrome (jaundice, hyper-
    lipemia, and hemolytic anemia)
    571.1
Zika fever 066.3
Zollinger-Ellison syndrome (gastric hy-
    persecretion with pancreatic islet cell
    tumor) 251.5
Zona (*see also* Herpes, zoster) 053.9
Zoophilia (erotica) 302.1
Zoophobia 300.29
Zoster (herpes) (*see also* Herpes, zoster)
    053.9
Zuelzer (-Ogden) anemia or syndrome
    (nutritional megaloblastic anemia)
    281.2
Zygodactyly (*see also* Syndactylism)
    755.10
Zygomycosis 117.7
Zymotic - *see* condition

SECTION II TABLE OF DRUGS AND CHEMICALS

ALPHABETIC INDEX TO POISONING AND EXTERNAL CAUSES OF ADVERSE EFFECTS OF DRUGS AND OTHER CHEMICAL SUBSTANCES

This table contains a classification of drugs and other chemical substances to identify poisoning states and external causes of adverse effects.

Each of the listed substances in the table is assigned a code according to the poisoning classification (960-989). These codes are used when there is a statement of poisoning, overdose, wrong substance given or taken, or intoxication.

The table also contains a listing of external causes of adverse effects. An adverse effect is a pathologic manifestation due to ingestion or exposure to drugs or other chemical substances (e.g., dermatitis, hypersensitivity reaction, aspirin gastritis). The adverse effect is to be identified by the appropriate code found in Section I, Index to Diseases and Injuries. An external cause code can then be used to identify the circumstances involved. The table headings pertaining to external causes are defined below:

Accidental poisoning (E850-E869)-accidental overdose of drug, wrong substance given or taken, drug taken inadvertently, accidents in the usage of drugs and biologicals in medical and surgical procedures, and to show external causes of poisonings classifiable to 980-989.

Therapeutic use (E930-E949)-a correct substance properly administered in therapeutic or prophylactic dosage as the external cause of adverse effects.

Suicide attempt (E950-E952)-instances in which self-inflicted injuries or poisonings are involved.

Assault (E961-E962)-injury or poisoning inflicted by another person with the intent to injure or kill.

Undetermined (E980-E982)-to be used when the intent of the poisoning or injury cannot be determined whether it was intentional or accidental.

The American Hospital Formulary Service (AHFS) list numbers are included in the table to help classify new drugs not identified in the table by name. The AHFS list numbers are keyed to the continually revised AHFS (American Hospital Formulary Service, 2 vol. Washington, D.C.: American Society of Hospital Pharmacists, 1959-). These listings are found in the table under the main term **Drug.**

Excluded from the table are radium and other radioactive substances. The classification of adverse effects and complications pertaining to these substances will be found in Index to Diseases and Injuries, and Index to External Causes of Injuries.

Although certain substances are indexed with one or more subentries, the majority are listed according to one use or state. It is recognized that many substances may be used in various ways, in medicine and in industry, and may cause adverse effects whatever the state of the agent (solid, liquid, or fumes arising from a liquid). In cases in which the reported data indicate a use or state not in the table, or which is clearly different from the one listed, an attempt should be made to classify the substance in the form which most nearly expresses the reported facts.

Substance	Poisoning	External Cause (E-Code)				
		Accident	Therapeutic Use	Suicide Attempt	Assault	Undetermined
1-propanol	980.3	E860.4	—	E950.9	E962.1	E980.9
2-propanol	980.2	E860.3	—	E950.9	E962.1	E980.9
2,4-D (dichlorophenoxyacetic acid)	989.4	E863.5	—	E950.6	E962.1	E980.7
2,4-toluene diisocyanate	983.0	E864.0	—	E950.7	E962.1	E980.6
2,4,5-T (trichlorophenoxyacetic acid)	989.2	E863.5	—	E950.6	E962.1	E980.7
14-hydroxydihydromorphinone	965.09	E850.2	E935.2	E950.0	E962.0	E980.0
ABOB	961.7	E857	E931.7	E950.4	E962.0	E980.4
Abrus (seed)	988.2	E865.3	—	E950.9	E962.1	E980.9
Absinthe	980.0	E860.1	—	E950.9	E962.1	E980.9
beverage	980.0	E860.0	—	E950.9	E962.1	E980.9
Acenocoumarin, acenocoumarol	964.2	E858.2	E934.2	E950.4	E962.0	E980.4
Acepromazine	969.1	E853.0	E939.1	E950.3	E962.0	E980.3
Acetal	982.8	E862.4	—	E950.9	E962.1	E980.9
Acetaldehyde (vapor)	987.8	E869.8	—	E952.8	E962.2	E982.8
liquid	989.89	E866.8	—	E950.9	E962.1	E980.9
Acetaminophen	965.4	E850.4	E935.4	E950.0	E962.0	E980.0
Acetaminosalol	965.1	E850.3	E935.3	E950.0	E962.0	E980.0
Acetanilid(e)	965.4	E850.4	E935.4	E950.0	E962.0	E980.0
Acetarsol, acetarsone	961.1	E857	E931.1	E950.4	E962.0	E980.4
Acetazolamide	974.2	E858.5	E944.2	E950.4	E962.0	E980.4
Acetic	—	—	—	—	—	—
acid	983.1	E864.1	—	E950.7	E962.1	E980.6
with sodium acetate (ointment)	976.3	E858.7	E946.3	E950.4	E962.0	E980.4
irrigating solution	974.5	E858.5	E944.5	E950.4	E962.0	E980.4
lotion	976.2	E858.7	E946.2	E950.4	E962.0	E980.4
anhydride	983.1	E864.1	—	E950.7	E962.1	E980.6
ether (vapor)	982.8	E862.4	—	E950.9	E962.1	E980.9
Acetohexamide	962.3	E858.0	E932.3	E950.4	E962.0	E980.4
Acetomenaphthone	964.3	E858.2	E934.3	E950.4	E962.0	E980.4
Acetomorphine	965.01	E850.0	E935.0	E950.0	E962.0	E980.0
Acetone (oils) (vapor)	982.8	E862.4	—	E950.9	E962.1	E980.9
Acetophenazine (maleate)	969.1	E853.0	E939.1	E950.3	E962.0	E980.3
Acetophenetidin	965.4	E850.4	E935.4	E950.0	E962.0	E980.0
Acetophenone	982.0	E862.4	—	E950.9	E962.1	E980.9
Acetorphine	965.09	E850.2	E935.2	E950.0	E962.0	E980.0
Acetosulfone (sodium)	961.8	E857	E931.8	E950.4	E962.0	E980.4
Acetrizoate (sodium)	977.8	E858.8	E947.8	E950.4	E962.0	E980.4
Acetylcarbromal	967.3	E852.2	E937.3	E950.2	E962.0	E980.2
Acetylcholine (chloride)	971.0	E855.3	E941.0	E950.4	E962.0	E980.4
Acetylcysteine	975.5	E858.6	E945.5	E950.4	E962.0	E980.4
Acetyldigitoxin	972.1	E858.3	E942.1	E950.4	E962.0	E980.4
Acetyldihydrocodeine	965.09	E850.2	E935.2	E950.0	E962.0	E980.0
Acetyldihydrocodeinone	965.09	E850.2	E935.2	E950.0	E962.0	E980.0
Acetylene (gas) (industrial)	987.1	E868.1	—	E951.8	E962.2	E981.8
incomplete combustion of - see Carbon monoxide, fuel, utility	—	—	—	—	—	—
tetrachloride (vapor)	982.3	E862.4	—	E950.9	E962.1	E980.9
Acetyliodosalicylic acid	965.1	E850.3	E935.3	E950.0	E962.0	E980.0
Acetylphenylhydrazine	965.8	E850.8	E935.8	E950.0	E962.0	E980.0
Acetylsalicylic acid	965.1	E850.3	E935.3	E950.0	E962.0	E980.0
Achromycin	960.4	E856	E930.4	E950.4	E962.0	E980.4
ophthalmic preparation	976.5	E858.7	E946.5	E950.4	E962.0	E980.4
topical NEC	976.0	E858.7	E946.0	E950.4	E962.0	E980.4
Acidifying agents	963.2	E858.1	E933.2	E950.4	E962.0	E980.4
Acids (corrosive) NEC	983.1	E864.1	—	E950.7	E962.1	E980.6
Aconite (wild)	988.2	E865.4	—	E950.9	E962.1	E980.9
Aconitine (liniment)	976.8	E858.7	E946.8	E950.4	E962.0	E980.4
Aconitum ferox	988.2	E865.4	—	E950.9	E962.1	E980.9
Acridine	983.0	E864.0	—	E950.7	E962.1	E980.6
vapor	987.8	E869.8	—	E952.8	E962.2	E982.8
Acriflavine	961.9	E857	E931.9	E950.4	E962.0	E980.4
Acrisorcin	976.0	E858.7	E946.0	E950.4	E962.0	E980.4

Substance	Poisoning	External Cause (E-Code)				
		Accident	Therapeutic Use	Suicide Attempt	Assault	Undetermined
Acrolein (gas)	987.8	E869.8	—	E952.8	E962.2	E982.8
liquid	989.89	E866.8	—	E950.9	E962.1	E980.9
Actaea spicata	988.2	E865.4	—	E950.9	E962.1	E980.9
Acterol	961.5	E857	E931.5	E950.4	E962.0	E980.4
ACTH	962.4	E858.0	E932.4	E950.4	E962.0	E980.4
Acthar	962.4	E858.0	E932.4	E950.4	E962.0	E980.4
Actinomycin (C) (D)	960.7	E856	E930.7	E950.4	E962.0	E980.4
Adalin (acetyl)	967.3	E852.2	E937.3	E950.2	E962.0	E980.2
Adenosine (phosphate)	977.8	E858.8	E947.8	E950.4	E962.0	E980.4
Adhesives	989.89	E866.6	—	E950.9	E962.1	E980.9
ADH	962.5	E858.0	E932.5	E950.4	E962.0	E980.4
Adicillin	960.0	E856	E930.0	E950.4	E962.0	E980.4
Adiphenine	975.1	E855.6	E945.1	E950.4	E962.0	E980.4
Adjunct, pharmaceutical	977.4	E858.8	E947.4	E950.4	E962.0	E980.4
Adrenal (extract, cortex or medulla) (glucocorticoids) (hormones) (mineralocorticoids)	962.0	E858.0	E932.0	E950.4	E962.0	E980.4
ENT agent	976.6	E858.7	E946.6	E950.4	E962.0	E980.4
ophthalmic preparation	976.5	E858.7	E946.5	E950.4	E962.0	E980.4
topical NEC	976.0	E858.7	E946.0	E950.4	E962.0	E980.4
Adrenalin	971.2	E855.5	E941.2	E950.4	E962.0	E980.4
Adrenergic blocking agents	971.3	E855.6	E941.3	E950.4	E962.0	E980.4
Adrenergics	971.2	E855.5	E941.2	E950.4	E962.0	E980.4
Adrenochrome (derivatives)	972.8	E858.3	E942.8	E950.4	E962.0	E980.4
Adrenocorticotropic hormone	962.4	E858.0	E932.4	E950.4	E962.0	E980.4
Adrenocorticotropin	962.4	E858.0	E932.4	E950.4	E962.0	E980.4
Adriamycin	960.7	E856	E930.7	E950.4	E962.0	E980.4
Aerosol spray - see Sprays	—	—	—	—	—	—
Aerosporin	960.8	E856	E930.8	E950.4	E962.0	E980.4
ENT agent	976.6	E858.7	E946.6	E950.4	E962.0	E980.4
ophthalmic preparation	976.5	E858.7	E946.5	E950.4	E962.0	E980.4
topical NEC	976.0	E858.7	E946.0	E950.4	E962.0	E980.4
Aethusa cynapium	988.2	E865.4	—	E950.9	E962.1	E980.9
Afghanistan black	969.6	E854.1	E939.6	E950.3	E962.0	E980.3
Aflatoxin	989.7	E865.9	—	E950.9	E962.1	E980.9
African boxwood	988.2	E865.4	—	E950.9	E962.1	E980.9
Agar (-agar)	973.3	E858.4	E943.3	E950.4	E962.0	E980.4
Agricultural agent NEC	989.89	E863.9	—	E950.6	E962.1	E980.7
Agrypnal	967.0	E851	E937.0	E950.1	E962.0	E980.1
Air contaminant(s), source or type not specified	—	—	—	—	—	—
specified type - see specific substance	987.9	E869.9	—	E952.9	E962.2	E982.9
Akee	988.2	E865.4	—	E950.9	E962.1	E980.9
Akrinol	976.0	E858.7	E946.0	E950.4	E962.0	E980.4
Alantolactone	961.6	E857	E931.6	E950.4	E962.0	E980.4
Albamycin	960.8	E856	E930.8	E950.4	E962.0	E980.4
Albumin (normal human serum)	964.7	E858.2	E934.7	E950.4	E962.0	E980.4
Albuterol	975.7	E858.6	E945.7	E950.4	E962.0	E980.4
Alcohol	980.9	E860.9	—	E950.9	E962.1	E980.9
absolute	980.0	E860.1	—	E950.9	E962.1	E980.9
beverage	980.0	E860.0	E947.8	E950.9	E962.1	E980.9
amyl	980.3	E860.4	—	E950.9	E962.1	E980.9
antifreeze	980.1	E860.2	—	E950.9	E962.1	E980.9
butyl	980.3	E860.4	—	E950.9	E962.1	E980.9
dehydrated	980.0	E860.1	—	E950.9	E862.1	E980.9
beverage	980.0	E860.0	E947.8	E950.9	E962.1	E980.9
denatured	980.0	E860.1	—	E950.9	E962.1	E980.9
deterrents	977.3	E858.8	E947.3	E950.4	E962.0	E980.4
diagnostic (gastric function)	977.8	E858.8	E947.8	E950.4	E962.0	E980.4
ethyl	980.0	E860.1	—	E950.9	E962.1	E980.9
beverage	980.0	E860.0	E947.8	E950.9	E962.1	E980.9
grain	980.0	E860.1	—	E950.9	E962.1	E980.9
beverage	980.0	E860.0	E947.8	E950.9	E962.1	E980.9
industrial	980.9	E860.9	—	E950.9	E962.1	E980.9

◄ New   ◄ Revised

Substance	Poisoning	External Cause (E-Code)				
		Accident	Therapeutic Use	Suicide Attempt	Assault	Undetermined
Alcohol (Continued)						
isopropyl	980.2	E860.3	—	E950.9	E962.1	E980.9
methyl	980.1	E860.2	—	E950.9	E962.1	E980.9
preparation for consumption	980.0	E860.0	E947.8	E950.9	E962.1	E980.9
propyl	980.3	E860.4	—	E950.9	E962.1	E980.9
secondary	980.2	E860.3	—	E950.9	E962.1	E980.9
radiator	980.1	E860.2	—	E950.9	E962.1	E980.9
rubbing	980.2	E860.3	—	E950.9	E962.1	E980.9
specified type NEC	980.8	E860.8	—	E950.9	E962.1	E980.9
surgical	980.9	E860.9	—	E950.9	E962.1	E980.9
vapor (from any type of alcohol)	987.8	E869.8	—	E952.8	E962.2	E982.8
wood	980.1	E860.2	—	E950.9	E962.1	E980.9
Alcuronium chloride	975.2	E858.6	E945.2	E950.4	E962.0	E980.4
Aldactone	974.4	E858.5	E944.4	E950.4	E962.0	E980.4
Aldicarb	989.3	E863.2	—	E950.6	E962.1	E980.7
Aldomet	972.6	E858.3	E942.6	E950.4	E962.0	E980.4
Aldosterone	962.0	E858.0	E932.0	E950.4	E962.0	E980.4
Aldrin (dust)	989.2	E863.0	—	E950.6	E962.1	E980.7
Aleve - see Naproxen	—	—	—	—	—	—
Algeldrate	973.0	E858.4	E943.0	E950.4	E962.0	E980.4
Alidase	963.4	E858.1	E933.4	E950.4	E962.0	E980.4
Aliphatic thiocyanates	989.0	E866.8	—	E950.9	E962.1	E980.9
Alkaline antiseptic solution (aromatic)	976.6	E858.7	E946.6	E950.4	E962.0	E980.4
Alkalinizing agents (medicinal)	963.3	E858.1	E933.3	E950.4	E962.0	E980.4
Alkalis, caustic	983.2	E864.2	—	E950.7	E962.1	E980.6
Alkalizing agents (medicinal)	963.3	E858.1	E933.3	E950.4	E962.0	E980.4
Alka-seltzer	965.1	E850.3	E935.3	E950.0	E962.0	E980.0
Alkavervir	972.6	E858.3	E942.6	E950.4	E962.0	E980.4
Allegron	969.0	E854.0	E939.0	E950.3	E962.0	E980.3
Allobarbital, allobarbitone	967.0	E851	E937.0	E950.1	E962.0	E980.1
Allopurinol	974.7	E858.5	E944.7	E950.4	E962.0	E980.4
Allylestrenol	962.2	E858.0	E932.2	E950.4	E962.0	E980.4
Allylisopropylacetylurea	967.8	E852.8	E937.8	E950.2	E962.0	E980.2
Allylisopropylmalonylurea	967.0	E851	E937.0	E950.1	E962.0	E980.1
Allyltribromide	967.3	E852.2	E937.3	E950.2	E962.0	E980.2
Aloe, aloes, aloin	973.1	E858.4	E943.1	E950.4	E962.0	E980.4
Alosetron	973.8	E858.4	E943.8	E950.4	E962.0	E980.4
Aloxidone	966.0	E855.0	E936.0	E950.4	E962.0	E980.4
Aloxiprin	965.1	E850.3	E935.3	E950.0	E962.0	E980.0
Alpha amylase	963.4	E858.1	E933.4	E950.4	E962.0	E980.4
Alphaprodine (hydrochloride)	965.09	E850.2	E935.2	E950.0	E962.0	E980.0
Alpha tocopherol	963.5	E858.1	E933.5	E950.4	E962.0	E980.4
Alseroxylon	972.6	E858.3	E942.6	E950.4	E962.0	E980.4
Alum (ammonium) (potassium)	983.2	E864.2	—	E950.7	E962.1	E980.6
medicinal (astringent) NEC	976.2	E858.7	E946.2	E950.4	E962.0	E980.4
Aluminium, aluminum (gel) (hydroxide)	973.0	E858.4	E943.0	E950.4	E962.0	E980.4
acetate solution	976.2	E858.7	E946.2	E950.4	E962.0	E980.4
aspirin	965.1	E850.3	E935.3	E950.0	E962.0	E980.0
carbonate	973.0	E858.4	E943.0	E950.4	E962.0	E980.4
glycinate	973.0	E858.4	E943.0	E950.4	E962.0	E980.4
nicotinate	972.2	E858.3	E942.2	E950.4	E962.0	E980.4
ointment (surgical) (topical)	976.3	E858.7	E946.3	E950.4	E962.0	E980.4
phosphate	973.0	E858.4	E943.0	E950.4	E962.0	E980.4
subacetate	976.2	E858.7	E946.2	E950.4	E962.0	E980.4
topical NEC	976.3	E858.7	E946.3	E950.4	E962.0	E980.4
Alurate	967.0	E851	E937.0	E950.1	E962.0	E980.1
Alverine (citrate)	975.1	E858.6	E945.1	E950.4	E962.0	E980.4
Alvodine	965.09	E850.2	E935.2	E950.0	E962.0	E980.0
Amanita phalloides	988.1	E865.5	—	E950.9	E962.1	E980.9
Amantadine (hydrochloride)	966.4	E855.0	E936.4	E950.4	E962.0	E980.4
Ambazone	961.9	E857	E931.9	E950.4	E962.0	E980.4
Ambenonium	971.0	E855.3	E941.0	E950.4	E962.0	E980.4

Substance	Poisoning	External Cause (E-Code)				
		Accident	Therapeutic Use	Suicide Attempt	Assault	Undetermined
Ambutonium bromide	971.1	E855.4	E941.1	E950.4	E962.0	E990.4
Ametazole	977.8	E858.8	E947.8	E950.4	E962.0	E980.4
Amethocaine (infiltration) (topical)	968.5	E855.2	E938.5	E950.4	E962.0	E980.4
nerve block (peripheral) (plexus)	968.6	E855.2	E938.6	E950.4	E962.0	E980.4
spinal	968.7	E855.2	E938.7	E950.4	E962.0	E980.4
Amethopterin	963.1	E858.1	E933.1	E950.4	E962.0	E980.4
Amfepramone	977.0	E858.8	E947.0	E950.4	E962.0	E980.4
Amidone	965.02	E850.1	E935.1	E950.0	E962.0	E980.0
Amidopyrine	965.5	E850.5	E935.5	E950.0	E962.0	E980.0
Aminacrine	976.0	E858.7	E946.0	E950.4	E962.0	E980.4
Aminitrozole	961.5	E857	E931.5	E950.4	E962.0	E980.4
Aminoacetic acid	974.5	E858.5	E944.5	E950.4	E962.0	E980.4
Amino acids	974.5	E858.5	E944.5	E950.4	E962.0	E980.4
Aminocaproic acid	964.4	E858.2	E934.4	E950.4	E962.0	E980.4
Aminoethylisothiourium	963.8	E858.1	E933.8	E950.4	E962.0	E980.4
Aminoglutethimide	966.3	E855.0	E936.3	E950.4	E962.0	E980.4
Aminometradine	974.3	E858.5	E944.3	E950.4	E962.0	E980.4
Aminopentamide	971.1	E855.4	E941.1	E950.4	E962.0	E980.4
Aminophenazone	965.5	E850.5	E935.5	E950.0	E962.0	E980.0
Aminophenol	983.0	E864.0	—	E950.7	E962.1	E980.6
Aminophenylpyridone	969.5	E853.8	E939.5	E950.3	E962.0	E980.3
Aminophylline	975.7	E858.6	E945.7	E950.4	E962.0	E980.4
Aminopterin	963.1	E858.1	E933.1	E950.4	E962.0	E980.4
Aminopyrine	965.5	E850.5	E935.5	E950.0	E962.0	E980.0
Aminosalicylic acid	961.8	E857	E931.8	E950.4	E962.0	E980.4
Amiphenazole	970.1	E854.3	E940.1	E950.4	E962.0	E980.4
Amiquinsin	972.6	E858.3	E942.6	E950.4	E962.0	E980.4
Amisometradine	974.3	E858.5	E944.3	E950.4	E962.0	E980.4
Amitriptyline	969.0	E854.0	E939.0	E950.3	E962.0	E980.3
Ammonia (fumes) (gas) (vapor)	987.8	E869.8	—	E952.8	E962.2	E982.8
liquid (household) NEC	983.2	E861.4	—	E950.7	E962.1	E980.6
spirit, aromatic	970.8	E854.3	E940.8	E950.4	E962.0	E980.4
Ammoniated mercury	976.0	E858.7	E946.0	E950.4	E962.0	E980.4
Ammonium	—	—	—	—	—	—
carbonate	983.2	E864.2	—	E950.7	E962.1	E980.6
chloride (acidifying agent)	963.2	E858.1	E933.2	E950.4	E962.0	E980.4
expectorant	975.5	E858.6	E945.5	E950.4	E962.0	E980.4
compounds (household) NEC	983.2	E861.4	—	E950.7	E962.1	E980.6
fumes (any usage)	987.8	E869.8	—	E952.8	E962.2	E982.8
industrial	983.2	E864.2	—	E950.7	E962.1	E980.6
ichthosulfonate	976.4	E858.7	E946.4	E950.4	E962.0	E980.4
mandelate	961.9	E857	E931.9	E950.4	E962.0	E980.4
Amobarbital	967.0	E851	E937.0	E950.1	E962.0	E980.1
Amodiaquin(e)	961.4	E857	E931.4	E950.4	E962.0	E980.4
Amopyroquin(e)	961.4	E857	E931.4	E950.4	E962.0	E980.4
Amphenidone	969.5	E853.8	E939.5	E950.3	E962.0	E980.3
Amphetamine	969.7	E854.2	E939.7	E950.3	E962.0	E980.3
Amphomycin	960.8	E856	E930.8	E950.4	E962.0	E980.4
Amphotericin B	960.1	E856	E930.1	E950.4	E962.0	E980.4
topical	976.0	E858.7	E946.0	E950.4	E962.0	E980.4
Ampicillin	960.0	E856	E930.0	E950.4	E962.0	E980.4
Amprotropine	971.1	E855.4	E941.1	E950.4	E962.0	E980.4
Amygdalin	977.8	E858.8	E947.8	E950.4	E962.0	E980.4
Amyl	—	—	—	—	—	—
acetate (vapor)	982.8	E862.4	—	E950.9	E962.1	E980.9
alcohol	980.3	E860.4	—	E950.9	E962.1	E980.9
nitrite (medicinal)	972.4	E858.3	E942.4	E950.4	E962.0	E980.4
Amylase (alpha)	963.4	E858.1	E933.4	E950.4	E962.0	E980.4
Amylene hydrate	980.8	E860.8	—	E950.9	E962.1	E980.9
Amylobarbitone	967.0	E851	E937.0	E950.1	E962.0	E980.1
Amylocaine	968.9	E855.2	E938.9	E950.4	E962.0	E980.4

◀ **New**   ◀▥ **Revised**

ICD-9-CM
Drugs
Vol. 2

Substance	Poisoning	External Cause (E-Code)				
		Accident	Therapeutic Use	Suicide Attempt	Assault	Undetermined
Amylocaine *(Continued)*						
infiltration (subcutaneous)	968.5	E855.2	E938.5	E950.4	E962.0	E980.4
nerve block (peripheral) (plexus)	968.6	E855.2	E938.6	E950.4	E962.0	E980.4
spinal	968.7	E855.2	E938.7	E950.4	E962.0	E980.4
topical (surface)	968.5	E855.2	E938.5	E950.4	E962.0	E980.4
Amytal (sodium)	967.0	E851	E937.0	E950.1	E962.0	E980.1
Analeptics	970.0	E854.3	E940.0	E950.4	E962.0	E980.4
Analgesics	965.9	E850.9	E935.9	E950.0	E962.0	E980.0
aromatic NEC	965.4	E850.4	E935.4	E950.0	E962.0	E980.0
non-narcotic NEC	965.7	E850.7	E935.7	E950.0	E962.0	E980.0
specified NEC	965.8	E850.8	E935.8	E950.0	E962.0	E980.0
Anamirta cocculus	988.2	E865.3	—	E950.9	E962.1	E980.9
Ancillin	960.0	E856	E930.0	E950.4	E962.0	E980.4
Androgens (anabolic congeners)	962.1	E858.0	E932.1	E950.4	E962.0	E980.4
Androstalone	962.1	E858.0	E932.1	E950.4	E962.0	E980.4
Androsterone	962.1	E858.0	E932.1	E950.4	E962.0	E980.4
Anemone pulsatilia	988.2	E865.4	—	E950.9	E962.1	E980.9
Anesthesia, anesthetic (general) NEC	968.4	E855.1	E938.4	E950.4	E962.0	E980.4
block (nerve) (plexus)	968.6	E855.2	E938.6	E950.4	E962.0	E980.4
gaseous NEC	968.2	E855.1	E938.2	E950.4	E962.0	E980.4
halogenated hydrocarbon derivatives NEC	968.2	E855.1	E938.2	E950.4	E962.0	E980.4
infiltration (intradermal) (subcutaneous) (submucosal)	968.5	E855.2	E938.5	E950.4	E962.0	E980.4
intravenous	968.3	E855.1	E938.3	E950.4	E962.0	E980.4
local NEC	968.9	E855.2	E938.9	E950.4	E962.0	E980.4
nerve blocking (peripheral) (plexus)	968.6	E855.2	E938.6	E950.4	E962.0	E980.4
rectal NEC	968.3	E855.1	E938.3	E950.4	E962.0	E980.4
spinal	968.7	E855.2	E938.7	E950.4	E962.0	E980.4
surface	968.5	E855.2	E938.5	E950.4	E962.0	E980.4
topical	968.5	E855.2	E938.5	E950.4	E962.0	E980.4
Aneurine	963.5	E858.1	E933.5	E950.4	E962.0	E980.4
Angio-Conray	977.8	E858.8	E947.8	E950.4	E962.0	E980.4
Angiotensin	971.2	E855.5	E941.2	E950.4	E962.0	E980.4
Anhydrohydroxyprogesterone	962.2	E858.0	E932.2	E950.4	E962.0	E980.4
Anhydron	974.3	E858.5	E944.3	E950.4	E962.0	E980.4
Anileridine	965.09	E850.2	E935.2	E950.0	E962.0	E980.0
Aniline (dye) (liquid)	983.0	E864.0	—	E950.7	E962.1	E980.6
analgesic	965.4	E850.4	E935.4	E950.0	E962.0	E980.0
derivatives, therapeutic NEC	965.4	E850.4	E935.4	E950.0	E962.0	E980.0
vapor	987.8	E869.8	—	E952.8	E962.2	E982.8
Aniscoropine	971.1	E855.4	E941.1	E950.4	E962.0	E980.4
Anisindione	964.2	E858.2	E934.2	E950.4	E962.0	E980.4
Anorexic agents	977.0	E858.8	E947.0	E950.4	E962.0	E980.4
Ant (bite) (sting)	989.5	E905.5	—	E950.9	E962.1	E980.9
Antabuse	977.3	E858.8	E947.3	E950.4	E962.0	E980.4
Antacids	973.0	E858.4	E943.0	E950.4	E962.0	E980.4
Antazoline	963.0	E858.1	E933.0	E950.4	E962.0	E980.4
Anthelmintics	961.6	E857	E931.6	E950.4	E962.0	E980.4
Anthralin	976.4	E858.7	E946.4	E950.4	E962.0	E980.4
Anthramycin	960.7	E856	E930.7	E950.4	E962.0	E980.4
Antiadrenergics	971.3	E855.6	E941.3	E950.4	E962.0	E980.4
Antiallergic agents	963.0	E858.1	E933.0	E950.4	E962.0	E980.4
Antianemic agents NEC	964.1	E858.2	E934.1	E950.4	E962.0	E980.4
Antiaris toxicaria	988.2	E865.4	—	E950.9	E962.1	E980.9
Antiarteriosclerotic agents	972.2	E858.3	E942.2	E950.4	E962.0	E980.4
Antiasthmatics	975.7	E858.6	E945.7	E950.4	E962.0	E980.4
Antibiotics	960.9	E856	E930.9	E950.4	E962.0	E980.4
antifungal	960.1	E856	E930.1	E950.4	E962.0	E980.4
antimycobacterial	960.6	E856	E930.6	E950.4	E962.0	E980.4
antineoplastic	960.7	E856	E930.7	E950.4	E962.0	E980.4
cephalosporin (group)	960.5	E856	E930.5	E950.4	E962.0	E980.4
chloramphenicol (group)	960.2	E856	E930.2	E950.4	E962.0	E980.4
macrolides	960.3	E856	E930.3	E950.4	E962.0	E980.4

Substance	Poisoning	External Cause (E-Code)				
		Accident	Therapeutic Use	Suicide Attempt	Assault	Undetermined
Antibiotics *(Continued)*						
specified NEC	960.8	E856	E930.8	E950.4	E962.0	E980.4
tetracycline (group)	960.4	E856	E930.4	E950.4	E962.0	E980.4
Anticancer agents NEC	963.1	E858.1	E933.1	E950.4	E962.0	E980.4
antibiotics	960.7	E856	E930.7	E950.4	E962.0	E980.4
Anticholinergics	971.1	E855.4	E941.1	E950.4	E962.0	E980.4
Anticholinesterase (organophosphorus) (reversible)	971.0	E855.3	E941.0	E950.4	E962.0	E980.4
Anticoagulants	964.2	E858.2	E934.2	E950.4	E962.0	E980.4
antagonists	964.5	E858.2	E934.5	E950.4	E962.0	E980.4
Anti-common cold agents NEC	975.6	E858.6	E945.6	E950.4	E962.0	E980.4
Anticonvulsants NEC	966.3	E855.0	E936.3	E950.4	E962.0	E980.4
Antidepressants	969.0	E854.0	E939.0	E950.3	E962.0	E980.3
Antidiabetic agents	962.3	E858.0	E932.3	E950.4	E962.0	E980.4
Antidiarrheal agents	973.5	E858.4	E943.5	E950.4	E962.0	E980.4
Antidiuretic hormone	962.5	E858.0	E932.5	E950.4	E962.0	E980.4
Antidotes NEC	977.2	E858.8	E947.2	E950.4	E962.0	E980.4
Antiemetic agents	963.0	E858.1	E933.0	E950.4	E962.0	E980.4
Antiepilepsy agent NEC	966.3	E855.0	E936.3	E950.4	E962.0	E980.4
Antifertility pills	962.2	E858.0	E932.2	E950.4	E962.0	E980.4
Antiflatulents	973.8	E858.4	E943.8	E950.4	E962.0	E980.4
Antifreeze	989.89	E866.8	—	E950.9	E962.1	E980.9
alcohol	980.1	E860.2	—	E950.9	E962.1	E980.9
ethylene glycol	982.8	E862.4	—	E950.9	E962.1	E980.9
Antifungals (nonmedicinal) (sprays)	989.4	E863.6	—	E950.6	E962.1	E980.7
medicinal NEC	961.9	E857	E931.9	E950.4	E962.0	E980.4
antibiotic	960.1	E856	E930.1	E950.4	E962.0	E980.4
topical	976.0	E858.7	E946.0	E950.4	E962.0	E980.4
Antigastric secretion agents	973.0	E858.4	E943.0	E950.4	E962.0	E980.4
Antihelmintics	961.6	E857	E931.6	E950.4	E962.0	E980.4
Antihemophilic factor (human)	964.7	E858.2	E934.7	E950.4	E962.0	E980.4
Antihistamine	963.0	E858.1	E933.0	E950.4	E962.0	E980.4
Antihypertensive agents NEC	972.6	E858.3	E942.6	E950.4	E962.0	E980.4
Anti-infectives NEC	961.9	E857	E931.9	E950.4	E962.0	E980.4
antibiotics	960.9	E856	E930.9	E950.4	E962.0	E980.4
specified NEC	960.8	E856	E930.8	E950.4	E962.0	E980.4
anthelmintic	961.6	E857	E931.6	E950.4	E962.0	E980.4
antimalarial	961.4	E857	E931.4	E950.4	E962.0	E980.4
antimycobacterial NEC	961.8	E857	E931.8	E950.4	E962.0	E980.4
antibiotics	960.6	E856	E930.6	E950.4	E962.0	E980.4
antiprotozoal NEC	961.5	E857	E931.5	E950.4	E962.0	E980.4
blood	961.4	E857	E931.4	E950.4	E962.0	E980.4
antiviral	961.7	E857	E931.7	E950.4	E962.0	E980.4
arsenical	961.1	E857	E931.1	E950.4	E962.0	E980.4
ENT agents	976.6	E858.7	E946.6	E950.4	E962.0	E980.4
heavy metals NEC	961.2	E857	E931.2	E950.4	E962.0	E980.4
local	976.0	E858.7	E946.0	E950.4	E962.0	E980.4
ophthalmic preparation	976.5	E858.7	E946.5	E950.4	E962.0	E980.4
topical NEC	976.0	E858.7	E946.0	E950.4	E962.0	E980.4
Anti-inflammatory agents (topical)	976.0	E858.7	E946.0	E950.4	E962.0	E980.4
Antiknock (tetraethyl lead)	984.1	E862.1	—	E950.9	E962.1	E980.9
Antilipemics	972.2	E858.3	E942.2	E950.4	E962.0	E980.4
Antimalarials	961.4	E857	E931.4	E950.4	E962.0	E980.4
Antimony (compounds) (vapor) NEC	985.4	E866.2	—	E950.9	E962.1	E980.9
anti-infectives	961.2	E857	E931.2	E950.4	E962.0	E980.4
pesticides (vapor)	985.4	E863.4	—	E950.6	E962.2	E980.7
potassium tartrate	961.2	E857	E931.2	E950.4	E962.0	E980.4
tartrated	961.2	E857	E931.2	E950.4	E962.0	E980.4
Antimuscarinic agents	971.1	E855.4	E941.1	E950.4	E962.0	E980.4
Antimycobacterials NEC	961.8	E857	E931.8	E950.4	E962.0	E980.4
antibiotics	960.6	E856	E930.6	E950.4	E962.0	E980.4
Antineoplastic agents	963.1	E858.1	E933.1	E950.4	E962.0	E980.4
antibiotics	960.7	E856	E930.7	E950.4	E962.0	E980.4
Anti-Parkinsonism agents	966.4	E855.0	E936.4	E950.4	E962.0	E980.4

Substance	Poisoning	External Cause (E-Code)				
		Accident	Therapeutic Use	Suicide Attempt	Assault	Undetermined
Antiphlogistics	965.69	E850.6	E935.6	E950.0	E962.0	E980.0
Antiprotozoals NEC	961.5	E857	E931.5	E950.4	E962.0	E980.4
blood	961.4	E857	E931.4	E950.4	E962.0	E980.4
Antipruritics (local)	976.1	E858.7	E946.1	E950.4	E962.0	E980.4
Antipsychotic agents NEC	969.3	E853.8	E939.3	E950.3	E962.0	E980.3
Antipyretics	965.9	E850.9	E935.9	E950.0	E962.0	E980.0
specified NEC	965.8	E850.8	E935.8	E950.0	E962.0	E980.0
Antipyrine	965.5	E850.5	E935.5	E950.0	E962.0	E980.0
Antirabies serum (equine)	979.9	E858.8	E949.9	E950.4	E962.0	E980.4
Antirheumatics	965.69	E850.6	E935.6	E950.0	E962.0	E980.0
Antiseborrheics	976.4	E858.7	E946.4	E950.4	E962.0	E980.4
Antiseptics (external) (medicinal)	976.0	E858.7	E946.0	E950.4	E962.0	E980.4
Antistine	963.0	E858.1	E933.0	E950.4	E962.0	E980.4
Antithyroid agents	962.8	E858.0	E932.8	E950.4	E962.0	E980.4
Antitoxin, any	979.9	E858.8	E949.9	E950.4	E962.0	E980.4
Antituberculars	961.8	E857	E931.8	E950.4	E962.0	E980.4
antibiotics	960.6	E856	E930.6	E950.4	E962.0	E980.4
Antitussives	975.4	E858.6	E945.4	E950.4	E962.0	E980.4
Antivaricose agents (sclerosing)	972.7	E858.3	E942.7	E950.4	E962.0	E980.4
Antivenin (crotaline) (spider-bite)	979.9	E858.8	E949.9	E950.4	E962.0	E980.4
Antivert	963.0	E858.1	E933.0	E950.4	E962.0	E980.4
Antivirals NEC	961.7	E857	E931.7	E950.4	E962.0	E980.4
Ant poisons - *see* Pesticides	—	—	—	—	—	—
Antrol	989.4	E863.4	—	E950.6	E962.1	E980.7
fungicide	989.4	E863.6	—	E950.6	E962.1	E980.7
Apomorphine hydrochloride (emetic)	973.6	E858.4	E943.6	E950.4	E962.0	E980.4
Appetite depressants, central	977.0	E858.8	E947.0	E950.4	E962.0	E980.4
Apresoline	972.6	E858.3	E942.6	E950.4	E962.0	E980.4
Aprobarbital, aprobarbitone	967.0	E851	E937.0	E950.1	E962.0	E980.1
Apronalide	967.8	E852.8	E937.8	E950.2	E962.0	E980.2
Aqua fortis	983.1	E864.1	—	E950.7	E962.1	E980.6
Arachis oil (topical)	976.3	E858.7	E946.3	E950.4	E962.0	E980.4
cathartic	973.2	E858.4	E943.2	E950.4	E962.0	E980.4
Aralen	961.4	E857	E931.4	E950.4	E962.0	E980.4
Arginine salts	974.5	E858.5	E944.5	E950.4	E962.0	E980.4
Argyrol	976.0	E858.7	E946.0	E950.4	E962.0	E980.4
ENT agent	976.6	E858.7	E946.6	E950.4	E962.0	E980.4
ophthalmic preparation	976.5	E858.7	E946.5	E950.4	E962.0	E980.4
Aristocort	962.0	E858.0	E932.0	E950.4	E962.0	E980.4
ENT agent	976.6	E858.7	E946.6	E950.4	E962.0	E980.4
ophthalmic preparation	976.5	E858.7	E946.5	E950.4	E962.0	E980.4
topical NEC	976.0	E858.7	E946.0	E950.4	E962.0	E980.4
Aromatics, corrosive	983.0	E864.0	—	E950.7	E962.1	E980.6
disinfectants	983.0	E861.4	—	E950.7	E962.1	E980.6
Arsenate of lead (insecticide)	985.1	E863.4	—	E950.8	E962.1	E980.8
herbicide	985.1	E863.5	—	E950.8	E962.1	E980.8
Arsenic, arsenicals (compounds) (dust) (fumes) (vapor) NEC	985.1	E866.3	—	E950.8	E962.1	E980.8
anti-infectives	961.1	E857	E931.1	E950.4	E962.0	E980.4
pesticide (dust) (fumes)	985.1	E863.4	—	E950.8	E962.1	E980.8
Arsine (gas)	985.1	E866.3	—	E950.8	E962.1	E980.8
Arsphenamine (silver)	961.1	E857	E931.1	E950.4	E962.0	E980.4
Arsthinol	961.1	E857	E931.1	E950.4	E962.0	E980.4
Artane	971.1	E855.4	E941.1	E950.4	E962.0	E980.4
Arthropod (venomous) NEC	989.5	E905.5	—	E950.9	E962.1	E980.9
Asbestos	989.81	E866.8	—	E950.9	E962.1	E980.9
Ascaridole	961.6	E857	E931.6	E950.4	E962.0	E980.4
Ascorbic acid	963.5	E858.1	E933.5	E950.4	E962.0	E980.4
Asiaticoside	976.0	E858.7	E946.0	E950.4	E962.0	E980.4
Aspidium (oleoresin)	961.6	E857	E931.6	E950.4	E962.0	E980.4
Aspirin	965.1	E850.3	E935.3	E950.0	E962.0	E980.0

Substance	Poisoning	External Cause (E-Code)				
		Accident	Therapeutic Use	Suicide Attempt	Assault	Undetermined
Astringents (local)	976.2	E858.7	E946.2	E950.4	E962.0	E980.4
Atabrine	961.3	E857	E931.3	E950.4	E962.0	E980.4
Ataractics	969.5	E853.8	E939.5	E950.3	E962.0	E980.3
Atonia drug, intestinal	973.3	E858.4	E943.3	E950.4	E962.0	E980.4
Atophan	974.7	E858.5	E944.7	E950.4	E962.0	E980.4
Atropine	971.1	E855.4	E941.1	E950.4	E962.0	E980.4
Attapulgite	973.5	E858.4	E943.5	E950.4	E962.0	E980.4
Attenuvax	979.4	E858.8	E949.4	E950.4	E962.0	E980.4
Aureomycin	960.4	E856	E930.4	E950.4	E962.0	E980.4
ophthalmic preparation	976.5	E858.7	E946.5	E950.4	E962.0	E980.4
topical NEC	976.0	E858.7	E946.0	E950.4	E962.0	E980.4
Aurothioglucose	965.69	E850.6	E935.6	E950.0	E962.0	E980.0
Aurothioglycanide	965.69	E850.6	E935.6	E950.0	E962.0	E980.0
Aurothiomalate	965.69	E850.6	E935.6	E950.0	E962.0	E980.0
Automobile fuel	981	E862.1	—	E950.9	E962.1	E980.9
Autonomic nervous system agents NEC	971.9	E855.9	E941.9	E950.4	E962.0	E980.4
Avlosulfon	961.8	E857	E931.8	E950.4	E962.0	E980.4
Avomine	967.8	E852.8	E937.8	E950.2	E962.0	E980.2
Azacyclonol	969.5	E853.8	E939.5	E950.3	E962.0	E980.3
Azapetine	971.3	E855.6	E941.3	E950.4	E962.0	E980.4
Azaribine	963.1	E858.1	E933.1	E950.4	E962.0	E980.4
Azaserine	960.7	E856	E930.7	E950.4	E962.0	E980.4
Azathioprine	963.1	E858.1	E933.1	E950.4	E962.0	E980.4
Azosulfamide	961.0	E857	E931.0	E950.4	E962.0	E980.4
Azulfidine	961.0	E857	E931.0	E950.4	E962.0	E980.4
Azuresin	977.8	E858.8	E947.8	E950.4	E962.0	E980.4
Bacimycin	976.0	E858.7	E946.0	E950.4	E962.0	E980.4
ophthalmic preparation	976.5	E858.7	E946.5	E950.4	E962.0	E980.4
Bacitracin	960.8	E856	E930.8	E950.4	E962.0	E980.4
ENT agent	976.6	E858.7	E946.6	E950.4	E962.0	E980.4
ophthalmic preparation	976.5	E858.7	E946.5	E950.4	E962.0	E980.4
topical NEC	976.0	E858.7	E946.0	E950.4	E962.0	E980.4
Baking soda	963.3	E858.1	E933.3	E950.4	E962.0	E980.4
BAL	963.8	E858.1	E933.8	E950.4	E962.0	E980.4
Bamethan (sulfate)	972.5	E858.3	E942.5	E950.4	E962.0	E980.4
Bamipine	963.0	E858.1	E933.0	E950.4	E962.0	E980.4
Baneberry	988.2	E865.4	—	E950.9	E962.1	E980.9
Banewort	988.2	E865.4	—	E950.9	E962.1	E980.9
Barbenyl	967.0	E851	E937.0	E950.1	E962.0	E980.1
Barbital, barbitone	967.0	E851	E937.0	E950.1	E962.0	E980.1
Barbiturates, barbituric acid	967.0	E851	E937.0	E950.1	E962.0	E980.1
anesthetic (intravenous)	968.3	E855.1	E938.3	E950.4	E962.0	E980.4
Barium (carbonate) (chloride) (sulfate)	985.8	E866.4	—	E950.9	E962.1	E980.9
diagnostic agent	977.8	E858.8	E947.8	E950.4	E962.0	E980.4
pesticide	985.8	E863.4	—	E950.6	E962.1	E980.7
rodenticide	985.8	E863.7	—	E950.6	E962.1	E980.7
Barrier cream	976.3	E858.7	E946.3	E950.4	E962.0	E980.4
Battery acid or fluid	983.1	E864.1	—	E950.7	E962.1	E980.6
Bay rum	980.8	E860.8	—	E950.9	E962.1	E980.9
BCG vaccine	978.0	E858.8	E948.0	E950.4	E962.0	E980.4
Bearsfoot	988.2	E865.4	—	E950.9	E962.1	E980.9
Beclamide	966.3	E855.0	E936.3	E950.4	E962.0	E980.4
Bee (sting) (venom)	989.5	E905.3	—	E950.9	E962.1	E980.9
Belladonna (alkaloids)	971.1	E855.4	E941.1	E950.4	E962.0	E980.4
Bemegride	970.0	E854.3	E940.0	E950.4	E962.0	E980.4
Benactyzine	969.8	E855.8	E939.8	E950.3	E962.0	E980.3
Benadryl	963.0	E858.1	E933.0	E950.4	E962.0	E980.4

◀ New   ◀▥ Revised

Substance	Poisoning	External Cause (E-Code)				
		Accident	Therapeutic Use	Suicide Attempt	Assault	Undetermined
Bendrofluazide	974.3	E858.5	E944.3	E950.4	E962.0	E980.4
Bendroflumethiazide	974.3	E858.5	E944.3	E950.4	E962.0	E980.4
Benemid	974.7	E858.5	E944.7	E950.4	E962.0	E980.4
Benethamine penicillin G	960.0	E856	E930.0	E950.4	E962.0	E980.4
Benisone	976.0	E858.7	E946.0	E950.4	E962.0	E980.4
Benoquin	976.8	E858.7	E946.8	E950.4	E962.0	E980.4
Benoxinate	968.5	E855.2	E938.5	E950.4	E962.0	E980.4
Bentonite	976.3	E858.7	E946.3	E950.4	E962.0	E980.4
Benzalkonium (chloride)	976.0	E858.7	E946.0	E950.4	E962.0	E980.4
ophthalmic preparation	976.5	E858.7	E946.5	E950.4	E962.0	E980.4
Benzamidosalicylate (calcium)	961.8	E857	E931.8	E950.4	E962.0	E980.4
Benzathine penicillin	960.0	E856	E930.0	E950.4	E962.0	E980.4
Benzcarbimine	963.1	E858.1	E933.1	E950.4	E962.0	E980.4
Benzedrex	971.2	E855.5	E941.2	E950.4	E962.0	E980.4
Benzedrine (amphetamine)	969.7	E854.2	E939.7	E950.3	E962.0	E980.3
Benzene (acetyl) (dimethyl) (methyl) (solvent) (vapor)	982.0	E862.4	—	E950.9	E962.1	E980.9
hexachloride (gamma) (insecticide) (vapor)	989.2	E863.0	—	E950.6	E962.1	E980.7
Benzethonium	976.0	E858.7	E946.0	E950.4	E962.0	E980.4
Benzhexol (chloride)	966.4	E855.0	E936.4	E950.4	E962.0	E980.4
Benzilonium	971.1	E855.4	E941.1	E950.4	E962.0	E980.4
Benzin(e) - see Ligroin	—	—	—	—	—	—
Benziodarone	972.4	E858.3	E942.4	E950.4	E962.0	E980.4
Benzocaine	968.5	E855.2	E938.5	E950.4	E962.0	E980.4
Benzodiapin	969.4	E853.2	E939.4	E950.3	E962.0	E980.3
Benzodiazepines (tranquilizers) NEC	969.4	E853.2	E939.4	E950.3	E962.0	E980.3
Benzoic acid (with salicylic acid) (anti-infective)	976.0	E858.7	E946.0	E950.4	E962.0	E980.4
Benzoin	976.3	E858.7	E946.3	E950.4	E962.0	E980.4
Benzol (vapor)	982.0	E862.4	—	E950.9	E962.1	E980.9
Benzomorphan	965.09	E850.2	E935.2	E950.0	E962.0	E980.0
Benzonatate	975.4	E858.6	E945.4	E950.4	E962.0	E980.4
Benzothiadiazides	974.3	E858.5	E944.3	E950.4	E962.0	E980.4
Benzoylpas	961.8	E857	E931.8	E950.4	E962.0	E980.4
Benzperidol	969.5	E853.8	E939.5	E950.3	E962.0	E980.3
Benzphetamine	977.0	E858.8	E947.0	E950.4	E962.0	E980.4
Benzpyrinium	971.0	E855.3	E941.0	E950.4	E962.0	E980.4
Benzquinamide	963.0	E858.1	E933.0	E950.4	E962.0	E980.4
Benzthiazide	974.3	E858.5	E944.3	E950.4	E962.0	E980.4
Benztropine	971.1	E855.4	E941.1	E950.4	E962.0	E980.4
Benzyl	—	—	—	—	—	—
acetate	982.8	E862.4	—	E950.9	E962.1	E980.9
benzoate (anti-infective)	976.0	E858.7	E946.0	E950.4	E962.0	E980.4
morphine	965.09	E850.2	E935.2	E950.0	E962.0	E980.0
penicillin	960.0	E856	E930.0	E950.4	E962.0	E980.4
Bephenium	—	—	—	—	—	—
hydroxynapthoate	961.6	E857	E931.6	E950.4	E962.0	E980.4
Bergamot oil	989.89	E866.8	—	E950.9	E962.1	E980.9
Berries, poisonous	988.2	E865.3	—	E950.9	E962.1	E980.9
Beryllium (compounds) (fumes)	985.3	E866.4	—	E950.9	E962.1	E980.9
Beta-carotene	976.3	E858.7	E946.3	E950.4	E962.0	E980.4
Beta-Chlor	967.1	E852.0	E937.1	E950.2	E962.0	E980.2
Betamethasone	962.0	E858.0	E932.0	E950.4	E962.0	E980.4
topical	976.0	E858.7	E946.0	E950.4	E962.0	E980.4
Betazole	977.8	E858.8	E947.8	E950.4	E962.0	E980.4
Bethanechol	971.0	E855.3	E941.0	E950.4	E962.0	E980.4
Bethanidine	972.6	E858.3	E942.6	E950.4	E962.0	E980.4
Betula oil	976.3	E858.7	E946.3	E950.4	E962.0	E980.4
Bhang	969.6	E854.1	E939.6	E950.3	E962.0	E980.3
Bialamicol	961.5	E857	E931.5	E950.4	E962.0	E980.4
Bichloride of mercury - see Mercury, chloride	—	—	—	—	—	—
Bichromates (calcium) (crystals) (potassium) (sodium)	983.9	E864.3	—	E950.7	E962.1	E980.6
fumes	987.8	E869.8	—	E952.8	E962.2	E982.8
Biguanide derivatives, oral	962.3	E858.0	E932.3	E950.4	E962.0	E980.4
Biligrafin	977.8	E858.8	E947.8	E950.4	E962.0	E980.4

Substance	Poisoning	External Cause (E-Code)				
		Accident	Therapeutic Use	Suicide Attempt	Assault	Undetermined
Bilopaque	977.8	E858.8	E947.8	E950.4	E962.0	E980.4
Bioflavonoids	972.8	E858.3	E942.8	E950.4	E962.0	E980.4
Biological substance NEC	979.9	E858.8	E949.9	E950.4	E962.0	E980.4
Biperiden	966.4	E855.0	E936.4	E950.4	E962.0	E980.4
Bisacodyl	973.1	E858.4	E943.1	E950.4	E962.0	E980.4
Bishydroxycoumarin	964.2	E858.2	E934.2	E950.4	E962.0	E980.4
Bismarsen	961.1	E857	E931.1	E950.4	E962.0	E980.4
Bismuth (compounds) NEC	985.8	E866.4	—	E950.9	E962.1	E980.9
anti-infectives	961.2	E857	E931.2	E950.4	E962.0	E980.4
subcarbonate	973.5	E858.4	E943.5	E950.4	E962.0	E980.4
sulfarsphenamine	961.1	E857	E931.1	E950.4	E962.0	E980.4
Bithionol	961.6	E857	E931.6	E950.4	E962.0	E980.4
Bitter almond oil	989.0	E866.8	—	E950.9	E962.1	E980.9
Bittersweet	988.2	E865.4	—	E950.9	E962.1	E930.9
Black	—	—	—	—	—	—
flag	989.4	E863.4	—	E950.6	E962.1	E980.7
henbane	988.2	E865.4	—	E950.9	E962.1	E980.9
leaf (40)	989.4	E863.4	—	E950.6	E962.1	E980.7
widow spider (bite)	989.5	E905.1	—	E950.9	E962.1	E980.9
antivenin	979.9	E858.8	E949.9	E950.4	E962.0	E980.4
Blast furnace gas (carbon monoxide from)	986	E868.8	—	E952.1	E962.2	E982.1
Bleach NEC	983.9	E864.3	—	E950.7	E962.1	E980.6
Bleaching solutions	983.9	E864.3	—	E950.7	E962.1	E980.6
Bleomycin (sulfate)	960.7	E856	E930.7	E950.4	E962.0	E980.4
Blockain	968.9	E855.2	E938.9	E950.4	E962.0	E980.4
infiltration (subcutaneous)	968.5	E855.2	E938.5	E950.4	E962.0	E980.4
nerve block (peripheral) (plexus)	968.6	E855.2	E938.6	E950.4	E962.0	E980.4
topical (surface)	968.5	E855.2	E938.5	E950.4	E962.0	E980.4
Blood (derivatives) (natural) (plasma) (whole)	964.7	E858.2	E934.7	E950.4	E962.0	E980.4
affecting agent	964.9	E858.2	E934.9	E950.4	E962.0	E980.4
specified NEC	964.8	E858.2	E934.8	E950.4	E962.0	E980.4
substitute (macromolecular)	964.8	E858.2	E934.8	E950.4	E962.0	E980.4
Blue velvet	965.09	E850.2	E935.2	E950.0	E962.0	E980.0
Bone meal	989.89	E866.5	—	E950.9	E962.1	E980.9
Bonine	963.0	E858.1	E933.0	E950.4	E962.0	E980.4
Boracic acid	976.0	E858.7	E946.0	E950.4	E962.0	E980.4
ENT agent	976.6	E858.7	E946.6	E950.4	E962.0	E980.4
ophthalmic preparation	976.5	E858.7	E946.5	E950.4	E962.0	E980.4
Borate (cleanser) (sodium)	989.6	E861.3	—	E950.9	E962.1	E980.9
Borax (cleanser)	989.6	E861.3	—	E950.9	E962.1	E980.9
Boric acid	976.0	E858.7	E946.0	E950.4	E962.0	E980.4
ENT agent	976.6	E858.7	E946.6	E950.4	E962.0	E980.4
ophthalmic preparation	976.5	E858.7	E946.5	E950.4	E962.0	E980.4
Boron hydride NEC	989.89	E866.8	—	E950.9	E962.1	E980.9
fumes or gas	987.8	E869.8	—	E952.8	E962.2	E982.8
Botox	975.3	E858.6	E945.3	E950.4	E962.0	E980.4
Brake fluid vapor	987.8	E869.8	—	E952.8	E962.2	E982.8
Brass (compounds) (fumes)	985.8	E866.4	—	E950.9	E962.1	E980.9
Brasso	981	E861.3	—	E950.9	E962.1	E980.9
Bretylium (tosylate)	972.6	E858.3	E942.6	E950.4	E962.0	E980.4
Brevital (sodium)	968.3	E855.1	E938.3	E950.4	E962.0	E980.4
British antilewisite	963.8	E858.1	E933.8	E950.4	E962.0	E980.4
Bromal (hydrate)	967.3	E852.2	E937.3	E950.2	E962.0	E980.2
Bromelains	963.4	E858.1	E933.4	E950.4	E962.0	E980.4
Bromides NEC	967.3	E852.2	E937.3	E950.2	E962.0	E980.2
Bromine (vapor)	987.8	E869.8	—	E952.8	E962.2	E982.8
compounds (medicinal)	967.3	E852.2	E937.3	E950.2	E962.0	E980.2
Bromisovalum	967.3	E852.2	E937.3	E950.2	E962.0	E980.2
Bromobenzyl cyanide	987.5	E869.3	—	E952.8	E962.2	E982.8
Bromodiphenhydramine	963.0	E858.1	E933.0	E950.4	E962.0	E980.4
Bromoform	967.3	E852.2	E937.3	E950.2	E962.0	E980.2
Bromophenol blue reagent	977.8	E858.8	E947.8	E950.4	E962.0	E980.4
Bromosalicylhydroxamic acid	961.8	E857	E931.8	E950.4	E962.0	E980.4

◀ New   ◀▥ Revised

Substance	Poisoning	Accident	Therapeutic Use	Suicide Attempt	Assault	Undetermined
Bromo-seltzer	965.4	E850.4	E935.4	E950.0	E962.0	E980.0
Brompheniramine	963.0	E858.1	E933.0	E950.4	E962.0	E980.4
Bromural	967.3	E852.2	E937.3	E950.2	E962.0	E980.2
Brown spider (bite) (venom)	989.5	E905.1	—	E950.9	E962.1	E980.9
Brucia	988.2	E865.3	—	E950.9	E962.1	E980.9
Brucine	989.1	E863.7	—	E950.6	E962.1	E980.7
Brunswick green - see Copper	—	—	—	—	—	—
Bruten - see Ibuprofen	—	—	—	—	—	—
Bryonia (alba) (dioica)	988.2	E865.4	—	E950.9	E962.1	E980.9
Buclizine	969.5	E853.8	E939.5	E950.3	E962.0	E980.3
Bufferin	965.1	E850.3	E935.3	E950.0	E962.0	E980.0
Bufotenine	969.6	E854.1	E939.6	E950.3	E962.0	E980.3
Buphenine	971.2	E855.5	E941.2	E950.4	E962.0	E980.4
Bupivacaine	968.9	E855.2	E938.9	E950.4	E962.0	E980.4
infiltration (subcutaneous)	968.5	E855.2	E938.5	E950.4	E962.0	E980.4
nerve block (peripheral) (plexus)	968.6	E855.2	E938.6	E950.4	E962.0	E980.4
Busulfan	963.1	E858.1	E933.1	E950.4	E962.0	E980.4
Butabarbital (sodium)	967.0	E851	E937.0	E950.1	E962.0	E980.1
Butabarbitone	967.0	E851	E937.0	E950.1	E962.0	E980.1
Butabarpal	967.0	E851	E937.0	E950.1	E962.0	E980.1
Butacaine	968.5	E855.2	E938.5	E950.4	E962.0	E980.4
Butallylonal	967.0	E851	E937.0	E950.1	E962.0	E980.1
Butane (distributed in mobile container)	987.0	E868.0	—	E951.1	E962.2	E981.1
distributed through pipes	987.0	E867	—	E951.0	E962.2	E981.0
incomplete combustion of - see Carbon monoxide, butane	—	—	—	—	—	—
Butanol	980.3	E860.4	—	E950.9	E962.1	E980.9
Butanone	982.8	E862.4	—	E950.9	E962.1	E980.9
Butaperazine	969.1	E853.0	E939.1	E950.3	E962.0	E980.3
Butazolidin	965.5	E850.5	E935.5	E950.0	E962.0	E980.0
Butethal	967.0	E851	E937.0	E950.1	E962.0	E980.1
Butethamate	971.1	E855.4	E941.1	E950.4	E962.0	E980.4
Buthalitone (sodium)	968.3	E855.1	E938.3	E950.4	E962.0	E980.4
Butisol (sodium)	967.0	E851	E937.0	E950.1	E962.0	E980.1
Butobarbital, butobarbitone	967.0	E851	E937.0	E950.1	E962.0	E980.1
Butriptyline	969.0	E854.0	E939.0	E950.3	E962.0	E980.3
Buttercups	988.2	E865.4	—	E950.9	E962.1	E980.9
Butter of antimony - see Antimony	—	—	—	—	—	—
Butyl	—	—	—	—	—	—
acetate (secondary)	982.8	E862.4	—	E950.9	E962.1	E980.9
alcohol	980.3	E860.4	—	E950.9	E962.1	E980.9
carbinol	980.8	E860.8	—	E950.9	E962.1	E980.9
carbitol	982.8	E862.4	—	E950.9	E962.1	E980.9
cellosolve	982.8	E862.4	—	E950.9	E962.1	E980.9
chloral (hydrate)	967.1	E852.0	E937.1	E950.2	E962.0	E980.2
formate	982.8	E862.4	—	E950.9	E962.1	E980.9
scopolammonium bromide	971.1	E855.4	E941.1	E950.4	E962.0	E980.4
Butyn	968.5	E855.2	E938.5	E950.4	E962.0	E980.4
Butyrophenone (-based tranquilizers)	969.2	E853.1	E939.2	E950.3	E962.0	E980.3
Cacodyl, cacodylic acid - see Arsenic	—	—	—	—	—	—
Cactinomycin	960.7	E856	E930.7	E950.4	E962.0	E980.4
Cade oil	976.4	E858.7	E946.4	E950.4	E962.0	E980.4
Cadmium (chloride) (compounds) (dust) (fumes) (oxide)	985.5	E866.4	—	E950.9	E962.1	E980.9
sulfide (medicinal) NEC	976.4	E858.7	E946.4	E950.4	E962.0	E980.4
Caffeine	969.7	E854.2	E939.7	E950.3	E962.0	E980.3
Calabar bean	988.2	E865.4	—	E950.9	E962.1	E980.9
Caladium seguinium	988.2	E865.4	—	E950.9	E962.1	E980.9
Calamine (liniment) (lotion)	976.3	E858.7	E946.3	E950.4	E962.0	E980.4
Calciferol	963.5	E858.1	E933.5	E950.4	E962.0	E980.4
Calcium (salts) NEC	974.5	E858.5	E944.5	E950.4	E962.0	E980.4
acetylsalicylate	965.1	E850.3	E935.3	E950.0	E962.0	E980.0
benzamidosalicylate	961.8	E857	E931.8	E950.4	E962.0	E980.4
carbaspirin	965.1	E850.3	E935.3	E950.0	E962.0	E980.0
carbimide (citrated)	977.3	E858.8	E947.3	E950.4	E962.0	E980.4

Substance	Poisoning	External Cause (E-Code)				
		Accident	Therapeutic Use	Suicide Attempt	Assault	Undetermined
Calcium *(Continued)*						
carbonate (antacid)	973.0	E858.4	E943.0	E950.4	E962.0	E980.4
cyanide (citrated)	977.3	E858.8	E947.3	E950.4	E962.0	E980.4
dioctyl sulfosuccinate	973.2	E858.4	E943.2	E950.4	E962.0	E980.4
disodium edathamil	963.8	E858.1	E933.8	E950.4	E962.0	E980.4
disodium edetate	963.8	E858.1	E933.8	E950.4	E962.0	E980.4
EDTA	963.8	E858.1	E933.8	E950.4	E962.0	E980.4
hydrate, hydroxide	983.2	E864.2	—	E950.7	E962.1	E980.6
mandelate	961.9	E857	E931.9	E950.4	E962.0	E980.4
oxide	983.2	E864.2	—	E950.7	E962.1	E980.6
Calomel - *see* Mercury, chloride	—	—	—	—	—	—
Caloric agents NEC	974.5	E858.5	E944.5	E950.4	E962.0	E980.4
Calusterone	963.1	E858.1	E933.1	E950.4	E962.0	E980.4
Camoquin	961.4	E857	E931.4	E950.4	E962.0	E980.4
Camphor (oil)	976.1	E858.7	E946.1	E950.4	E962.0	E980.4
Candeptin	976.0	E858.7	E946.0	E950.4	E962.0	E980.4
Candicidin	976.0	E858.7	E946.0	E950.4	E962.0	E980.4
Cannabinols	969.6	E854.1	E939.6	E950.3	E962.0	E980.3
Cannabis (derivatives) (indica) (sativa)	969.6	E854.1	E939.6	E950.3	E962.0	E980.3
Canned heat	980.1	E860.2	—	E950.9	E962.1	E980.9
Cantharides, cantharidin, cantharis	976.8	E858.7	E946.8	E950.4	E962.0	E980.4
Capillary agents	972.8	E858.3	E942.8	E950.4	E962.0	E980.4
Capreomycin	960.6	E856	E930.6	E950.4	E962.0	E980.4
Captodiame, captodiamine	969.5	E853.8	E939.5	E950.3	E962.0	E980.3
Caramiphen (hydrochloride)	971.1	E855.4	E941.1	E950.4	E962.0	E980.4
Carbachol	971.0	E855.3	E941.0	E950.4	E962.0	E980.4
Carbacrylamine resins	974.5	E858.5	E944.5	E950.4	E962.0	E980.4
Carbamate (sedative)	967.8	E852.8	E937.8	E950.2	E962.0	E980.2
herbicide	989.3	E863.5	—	E950.6	E962.1	E980.7
insecticide	989.3	E863.2	—	E950.6	E962.1	E980.7
Carbamazepine	966.3	E855.0	E936.3	E950.4	E962.0	E980.4
Carbamic esters	967.8	E852.8	E937.8	E950.2	E962.0	E980.2
Carbamide	974.4	E858.5	E944.4	E950.4	E962.0	E980.4
topical	976.8	E858.7	E946.8	E950.4	E962.0	E980.4
Carbamylcholine chloride	971.0	E855.3	E941.0	E950.4	E962.0	E980.4
Carbarsone	961.1	E857	E931.1	E950.4	E962.0	E980.4
Carbaryl	989.3	E863.2	—	E950.6	E962.1	E980.7
Carbaspirin	965.1	E850.3	E935.3	E950.0	E962.0	E980.0
Carbazochrome	972.8	E858.3	E942.8	E950.4	E962.0	E980.4
Carbenicillin	960.0	E856	E930.0	E950.4	E962.0	E980.4
Carbenoxolone	973.8	E858.4	E943.8	E950.4	E962.0	E980.4
Carbetapentane	975.4	E858.6	E945.4	E950.4	E962.0	E980.4
Carbimazole	962.8	E858.0	E932.8	E950.4	E962.0	E980.4
Carbinol	980.1	E860.2	—	E950.9	E962.1	E980.9
Carbinoxamine	963.0	E858.1	E933.0	E950.4	E962.0	E980.4
Carbitol	982.8	E862.4	—	E950.9	E962.1	E980.9
Carbocaine	968.9	E855.2	E938.9	E950.4	E962.0	E980.4
infiltration (subcutaneous)	968.5	E855.2	E938.5	E950.4	E962.0	E980.4
nerve block (peripheral) (plexus)	968.6	E855.2	E938.6	E950.4	E962.0	E980.4
topical (surface)	968.5	E855.2	E938.5	E950.4	E962.0	E980.4
Carbol-fuchsin solution	976.0	E858.7	E946.0	E950.4	E962.0	E980.4
Carbolic acid (*see also* Phenol)	983.0	E864.0	—	E950.7	E962.1	E980.6
Carbomycin	960.8	E856	E930.8	E950.4	E962.0	E980.4
Carbon	—	—	—	—	—	—
bisulfide (liquid) (vapor)	982.2	E862.4	—	E950.9	E962.1	E980.9
dioxide (gas)	987.8	E869.8	—	E952.8	E962.2	E982.8
disulfide (liquid) (vapor)	982.2	E862.4	—	E950.9	E962.1	E980.9
monoxide (from incomplete combustion of) (in) NEC	986	E868.9	—	E952.1	E962.2	E982.1
blast furnace gas	986	E868.8	—	E952.1	E962.2	E982.1
butane (distributed in mobile container)	986	E868.0	—	E951.1	E962.2	E981.1
distributed through pipes	986	E867	—	E951.0	E962.2	E981.0
charcoal fumes	986	E868.3	—	E952.1	E962.2	E982.1

◀ New   ◀▦ Revised

Substance	Poisoning	External Cause (E-Code)				
		Accident	Therapeutic Use	Suicide Attempt	Assault	Undetermined
Carbon *(Continued)*						
coal						
gas (piped)	986	E867	—	E951.0	E962.2	E981.0
solid (in domestic stoves, fireplaces)	986	E868.3	—	E952.1	E962.2	E982.1
coke (in domestic stoves, fireplaces)	986	E868.3	—	E952.1	E962.2	E982.1
exhaust gas (motor) not in transit	986	E868.2	—	E952.0	E962.2	E982.0
combustion engine, any not in watercraft	986	E868.2	—	E952.0	E962.2	E982.0
farm tractor, not in transit	986	E868.2	—	E952.0	E962.2	E982.0
gas engine	986	E868.2	—	E952.0	E962.2	E982.0
motor pump	986	E868.2	—	E952.0	E962.2	E982.0
motor vehicle, not in transit	986	E868.2	—	E952.0	E962.2	E982.0
fuel (in domestic use)	986	E868.3	—	E952.1	E962.2	E982.1
gas (piped)	986	E867	—	E951.0	E962.2	E981.0
in mobile container	986	E868.0	—	E951.1	E962.2	E981.1
utility	986	E868.1	—	E951.8	E962.2	E981.1
in mobile container	986	E868.0	—	E951.1	E962.2	E981.1
piped (natural)	986	E867	—	E951.0	E962.2	E981.0
illuminating gas	986	E868.1	—	E951.8	E962.2	E981.8
industrial fuels or gases, any	986	E868.8	—	E952.1	E962.2	E982.1
kerosene (in domestic stoves, fireplaces)	986	E868.3	—	E952.1	E962.2	E982.1
kiln gas or vapor	986	E868.8	—	E952.1	E962.2	E982.1
motor exhaust gas, not in transit	986	E868.2	—	E952.0	E962.2	E982.0
piped gas (manufactured) (natural)	986	E867	—	E951.0	E962.2	E981.0
producer gas	986	E868.8	—	E952.1	E962.2	E982.1
propane (distributed in mobile container)	986	E868.0	—	E951.1	E962.2	E981.1
distributed through pipes	986	E867	—	E951.0	E962.2	E981.0
specified source NEC	986	E868.8	—	E952.1	E962.2	E982.1
stove gas	986	E868.1	—	E951.8	E962.2	E981.8
piped	986	E867	—	E951.0	E962.2	E981.0
utility gas	986	E868.1	—	E951.8	E962.2	E981.8
piped	986	E867	—	E951.0	E962.2	E981.0
water gas	986	E868.1	—	E951.8	E962.2	E981.8
wood (in domestic stoves, fireplaces)	986	E868.3	—	E952.1	E962.2	E982.1
tetrachloride (vapor) NEC	987.8	E869.8	—	E952.8	E962.2	E982.8
liquid (cleansing agent) NEC	982.1	E861.3	—	E950.9	E962.1	E980.9
solvent	982.1	E862.4	—	E950.9	E962.1	E980.9
Carbonic acid (gas)	987.8	E869.8	—	E952.8	E962.2	E982.8
anhydrase inhibitors	974.2	E858.5	E944.2	E950.4	E962.0	E980.4
Carbowax	976.3	E858.7	E946.3	E950.4	E962.0	E980.4
Carbrital	967.0	E851	E937.0	E950.1	E962.0	E980.1
Carbromal (derivatives)	967.3	E852.2	E937.3	E950.2	E962.0	E980.2
Cardiac	—	—	—	—	—	—
depressants	972.0	E858.3	E942.0	E950.4	E962.0	E980.4
rhythm regulators	972.0	E858.3	E942.0	E950.4	E962.0	E980.4
Cardiografin	977.8	E858.8	E947.8	E950.4	E962.0	E980.4
Cardio-green	977.8	E858.8	E947.8	E950.4	E962.0	E980.4
Cardiotonic glycosides	972.1	E858.3	E942.1	E950.4	E962.0	E980.4
Cardiovascular agents NEC	972.9	E858.3	E942.9	E950.4	E962.0	E980.4
Cardrase	974.2	E858.5	E944.2	E950.4	E962.0	E980.4
Carfusin	976.0	E858.7	E946.0	E950.4	E962.0	E980.4
Carisoprodol	968.0	E855.1	E938.0	E950.4	E962.0	E980.4
Carmustine	963.1	E858.1	E933.1	E950.4	E962.0	E980.4
Carotene	963.5	E858.1	E933.5	E950.4	E962.0	E980.4
Carphenazine (maleate)	969.1	E853.0	E939.1	E950.3	E962.0	E980.3
Carter's Little Pills	973.1	E858.4	E943.1	E950.4	E962.0	E980.4
Cascara (sagrada)	973.1	E858.4	E943.1	E950.4	E962.0	E980.4
Cassava	988.2	E865.4	—	E950.9	E962.1	E980.9
Castellani's paint	976.0	E858.7	E946.0	E950.4	E962.0	E980.4
Castor	—	—	—	—	—	—
bean	988.2	E865.3	—	E950.9	E962.1	E980.9
oil	973.1	E858.4	E943.1	E950.4	E962.0	E980.4
Caterpillar (sting)	989.5	E905.5	—	E950.9	E962.1	E980.9
Catha (edulis)	970.8	E854.3	E940.8	E950.4	E962.0	E980.4

Substance	Poisoning	External Cause (E-Code)				
		Accident	Therapeutic Use	Suicide Attempt	Assault	Undetermined
Cathartics NEC	973.3	E858.4	E943.3	E950.4	E962.0	E980.4
contact	973.1	E858.4	E943.1	E950.4	E962.0	E980.4
emollient	973.2	E858.4	E943.2	E950.4	E962.0	E980.4
intestinal irritants	973.1	E858.4	E943.1	E950.4	E962.0	E980.4
saline	973.3	E858.4	E943.3	E950.4	E962.0	E980.4
Cathomycin	960.8	E856	E930.8	E950.4	E962.0	E980.4
Caustic(s)	983.9	E864.4	—	E950.7	E962.1	E980.6
alkali	983.2	E864.2	—	E950.7	E962.1	E980.6
hydroxide	983.2	E864.2	—	E950.7	E962.1	E980.6
potash	983.2	E864.2	—	E950.7	E962.1	E980.6
soda	983.2	E864.2	—	E950.7	E962.1	E980.6
specified NEC	983.9	E864.3	—	E950.7	E962.1	E980.6
Ceepryn	976.0	E858.7	E946.0	E950.4	E962.0	E980.4
ENT agent	976.6	E858.7	E946.6	E950.4	E962.0	E980.4
lozenges	976.6	E858.7	E946.6	E950.4	E962.0	E980.4
Celestone	962.0	E858.0	E932.0	E950.4	E962.0	E980.4
topical	976.0	E858.7	E946.0	E950.4	E962.0	E980.4
Cellosolve	982.8	E862.4	—	E950.9	E962.1	E980.9
Cell stimulants and proliferants	976.8	E858.7	E946.8	E950.4	E962.0	E980.4
Cellulose derivatives, cathartic	973.3	E858.4	E943.3	E950.4	E962.0	E980.4
nitrates (topical)	976.3	E858.7	E946.3	E950.4	E962.0	E980.4
Centipede (bite)	989.5	E905.4	—	E950.9	E962.1	E980.9
Central nervous system	—	—	—	—	—	—
depressants	968.4	E855.1	E938.4	E950.4	E962.0	E980.4
anesthetic (general) NEC	968.4	E855.1	E938.4	E950.4	E962.0	E980.4
gases NEC	968.2	E855.1	E938.2	E950.4	E962.0	E980.4
intravenous	968.3	E855.1	E938.3	E950.4	E962.0	E980.4
barbiturates	967.0	E851	E937.0	E950.1	E962.0	E980.1
bromides	967.3	E852.2	E937.3	E950.2	E962.0	E980.2
cannabis sativa	969.6	E854.1	E939.6	E950.3	E962.0	E980.3
chloral hydrate	967.1	E852.0	E937.1	E950.2	E962.0	E980.2
hallucinogenics	969.6	E854.1	E939.6	E950.3	E962.0	E980.3
hypnotics	967.9	E852.9	E937.9	E950.2	E962.0	E980.2
specified NEC	967.8	E852.8	E937.8	E950.2	E962.0	E980.2
muscle relaxants	968.0	E855.1	E938.0	E950.4	E962.0	E980.4
paraldehyde	967.2	E852.1	E937.2	E950.2	E962.0	E980.2
sedatives	967.9	E852.9	E937.9	E950.2	E962.0	E980.2
mixed NEC	967.6	E852.5	E937.6	E950.2	E962.0	E980.2
specified NEC	967.8	E852.8	E937.8	E950.2	E962.0	E980.2
muscle-tone depressants	968.0	E855.1	E938.0	E950.4	E962.0	E980.4
stimulants	970.9	E854.3	E940.9	E950.4	E962.0	E980.4
amphetamines	969.7	E854.2	E939.7	E950.3	E962.0	E980.3
analeptics	970.0	E854.3	E940.0	E950.4	E962.0	E980.4
antidepressants	969.0	E854.0	E939.0	E950.3	E962.0	E980.3
opiate antagonists	970.1	E854.3	E940.0	E950.4	E962.0	E980.4
specified NEC	970.8	E854.3	E940.8	E950.4	E962.0	E980.4
Cephalexin	960.5	E856	E930.5	E950.4	E962.0	E980.4
Cephaloglycin	960.5	E856	E930.5	E950.4	E962.0	E980.4
Cephaloridine	960.5	E856	E930.5	E950.4	E962.0	E980.4
Cephalosporins NEC	960.5	E856	E930.5	E950.4	E962.0	E980.4
N (adicillin)	960.0	E856	E930.0	E950.4	E962.0	E980.4
Cephalothin (sodium)	960.5	E856	E930.5	E950.4	E962.0	E980.4
Cerbera (odallam)	988.2	E865.4	—	E950.9	E962.1	E980.9
Cerberin	972.1	E858.3	E942.1	E950.4	E962.0	E980.4
Cerebral stimulants	970.9	E854.3	E940.9	E950.4	E962.0	E980.4
psychotherapeutic	969.7	E854.2	E939.7	E950.3	E962.0	E980.3
specified NEC	970.8	E854.3	E940.8	E950.4	E962.0	E980.4
Cetalkonium (chloride)	976.0	E858.7	E946.0	E950.4	E962.0	E980.4
Cetoxime	963.0	E858.1	E933.0	E950.4	E962.0	E980.4
Cetrimide	976.2	E858.7	E946.2	E950.4	E962.0	E980.4

◀ New ◀▥ Revised

Substance	Poisoning	External Cause (E-Code)				
		Accident	Therapeutic Use	Suicide Attempt	Assault	Undetermined
Cetylpyridinium	976.0	E858.7	E946.0	E950.4	E962.0	E980.4
ENT agent	976.6	E858.7	E946.6	E950.4	E962.0	E980.4
lozenges	976.6	E858.7	E946.6	E950.4	E962.0	E980.4
Cevadilla - see Sabadilla	—	—	—	—	—	—
Cevitamic acid	963.5	E858.1	E933.5	E950.4	E962.0	E980.4
Chalk, precipitated	973.0	E858.4	E943.0	E950.4	E962.0	E980.4
Charcoal	—	—	—	—	—	—
fumes (carbon monoxide)	986	E868.3	—	E952.1	E962.2	E982.1
industrial	986	E868.8	—	E952.1	E962.2	E982.1
medicinal (activated)	973.0	E858.4	E943.0	E950.4	E962.0	E980.4
Chelating agents NEC	977.2	E858.8	E947.2	E950.4	E962.0	E980.4
Chelidonium majus	988.2	E865.4	—	E950.9	E962.1	E980.9
Chemical substance	989.9	E866.9	—	E950.9	E962.1	E980.9
specified NEC	989.89	E866.8	—	E950.9	E962.1	E980.9
Chemotherapy, antineoplastic	963.1	E858.1	E933.1	E950.4	E962.0	E980.4
Chenopodium (oil)	961.6	E857	E931.6	E950.4	E962.0	E980.4
Cherry laurel	988.2	E865.4	—	E950.9	E962.1	E980.9
Chiniofon	961.3	E857	E931.3	E950.4	E962.0	E980.4
Chlophedianol	975.4	E858.6	E945.4	E950.4	E962.0	E980.4
Chloral (betaine) (formamide) (hydrate)	967.1	E852.0	E937.1	E950.2	E962.0	E980.2
Chloralamide	967.1	E852.0	E937.1	E950.2	E962.0	E980.2
Chlorambucil	963.1	E858.1	E933.1	E950.4	E962.0	E980.4
Chloramphenicol	960.2	E856	E930.2	E950.4	E962.0	E980.4
ENT agent	976.6	E858.7	E946.6	E950.4	E962.0	E980.4
ophthalmic preparation	976.5	E858.7	E946.5	E950.4	E962.0	E980.4
topical NEC	976.0	E858.7	E946.0	E950.4	E962.0	E980.4
Chlorate(s) (potassium) (sodium) NEC	983.9	E864.3	—	E950.7	E962.1	E980.6
herbicides	989.4	E863.5	—	E950.6	E962.1	E980.7
Chlorcyclizine	963.0	E858.1	E933.0	E950.4	E962.0	E980.4
Chlordan(e) (dust)	989.2	E863.0	—	E950.6	E962.1	E980.7
Chlordantoin	976.0	E858.7	E946.0	E950.4	E962.0	E980.4
Chlordiazepoxide	969.4	E853.2	E939.4	E950.3	E962.0	E980.3
Chloresium	976.8	E858.7	E946.8	E950.4	E962.0	E980.4
Chlorethiazol	967.1	E852.0	E937.1	E950.2	E962.0	E980.2
Chlorethyl - see Ethyl, chloride	—	—	—	—	—	—
Chloretone	967.1	E852.0	E937.1	E950.2	E962.0	E980.2
Chlorex	982.3	E862.4	—	E950.9	E962.1	E980.9
Chlorhexadol	967.1	E852.0	E937.1	E950.2	E962.0	E980.2
Chlorhexidine (hydrochloride)	976.0	E858.7	E946.0	E950.4	E962.0	E980.4
Chlorhydroxyquinolin	976.0	E858.7	E946.0	E950.4	E962.0	E980.4
Chloride of lime (bleach)	983.9	E864.3	—	E950.7	E962.1	E980.6
Chlorinated	—	—	—	—	—	—
camphene	989.2	E863.0	—	E950.6	E962.1	E980.7
diphenyl	989.89	E866.8	—	E950.9	E962.1	E980.9
hydrocarbons NEC	989.2	E863.0	—	E950.6	E962.1	E980.7
solvent	982.3	E862.4	—	E950.9	E962.1	E980.9
lime (bleach)	983.9	E864.3	—	E950.7	E962.1	E980.6
naphthalene - see Naphthalene	—	—	—	—	—	—
pesticides NEC	989.2	E863.0	—	E950.6	E962.1	E980.7
soda - see Sodium, hypochlorite	—	—	—	—	—	—
Chlorine (fumes) (gas)	987.6	E869.8	—	E952.8	E962.2	E982.8
bleach	983.9	E864.3	—	E950.7	E962.1	E980.6
compounds NEC	983.9	E864.3	—	E950.7	E962.1	E980.6
disinfectant	983.9	E861.4	—	E950.7	E962.1	E980.6
releasing agents NEC	983.9	E864.3	—	E950.7	E962.1	E980.6
Chlorisondamine	972.3	E858.3	E942.3	E950.4	E962.0	E980.4
Chlormadinone	962.2	E858.0	E932.2	E950.4	E962.0	E980.4
Chlormerodrin	974.0	E858.5	E944.0	E950.4	E962.0	E980.4
Chlormethiazole	967.1	E852.0	E937.1	E950.2	E962.0	E980.2
Chlormethylenecycline	960.4	E856	E930.4	E950.4	E962.0	E980.4
Chlormezanone	969.5	E853.8	E939.5	E950.3	E962.0	E980.3
Chloroacetophenone	987.5	E869.3	—	E952.8	E962.2	E982.8

Substance	Poisoning	External Cause (E-Code)				
		Accident	Therapeutic Use	Suicide Attempt	Assault	Undetermined
Chloroaniline	983.0	E864.0	—	E950.7	E962.1	E980.6
Chlorobenzene, chlorobenzol	982.0	E862.4	—	E950.9	E962.1	E980.9
Chlorobutanol	967.1	E852.0	E937.1	E950.2	E962.0	E980.2
Chlorodinitrobenzene	983.0	E864.0	—	E950.7	E962.1	E980.6
dust or vapor	987.8	E869.8	—	E952.8	E962.2	E982.8
Chloroethane - *see* Ethyl, chloride	—	—	—	—	—	—
Chloroform (fumes) (vapor)	987.8	E869.8	—	E952.8	E962.2	E982.8
anesthetic (gas)	968.2	E855.1	E938.2	E950.4	E962.0	E980.4
liquid NEC	968.4	E855.1	E938.4	E950.4	E962.0	E980.4
solvent	982.3	E862.4	—	E950.9	E962.1	E980.9
Chloroguanide	961.4	E857	E931.4	E950.4	E962.0	E980.4
Chloromycetin	960.2	E856	E930.2	E950.4	E962.0	E980.4
ENT agent	976.6	E858.7	E946.6	E950.4	E962.0	E980.4
ophthalmic preparation	976.5	E858.7	E946.5	E950.4	E962.0	E980.4
otic solution	976.6	E858.7	E946.6	E950.4	E962.0	E980.4
topical NEC	976.0	E858.7	E946.0	E950.4	E962.0	E980.4
Chloronitrobenzene	983.0	E864.0	—	E950.7	E962.1	E980.6
dust or vapor	987.8	E869.8	—	E952.8	E962.2	E982.8
Chlorophenol	983.0	E864.0	—	E950.7	E962.1	E980.6
Chlorophenothane	989.2	E863.0	—	E950.6	E962.1	E980.7
Chlorophyll (derivatives)	976.8	E858.7	E946.8	E950.4	E962.0	E980.4
Chloropicrin (fumes)	987.8	E869.8	—	E952.8	E962.2	E982.8
fumigant	989.4	E863.8	—	E950.6	E962.1	E980.7
fungicide	989.4	E863.6	—	E950.6	E962.1	E980.7
pesticide (fumes)	989.4	E863.4	—	E950.6	E962.1	E980.7
Chloroprocaine	968.9	E855.2	E938.9	E950.4	E962.0	E980.4
infiltration (subcutaneous)	968.5	E855.2	E938.5	E950.4	E962.0	E980.4
nerve block (peripheral) (plexus)	968.6	E855.2	E938.6	E950.4	E962.0	E980.4
Chloroptic	976.5	E858.7	E946.5	E950.4	E962.0	E980.4
Chloropurine	963.1	E858.1	E933.1	E950.4	E962.0	E980.4
Chloroquine (hydrochloride) (phosphate)	961.4	E857	E931.4	E950.4	E962.0	E980.4
Chlorothen	963.0	E858.1	E933.0	E950.4	E962.0	E980.4
Chlorothiazide	974.3	E858.5	E944.3	E950.4	E962.0	E980.4
Chlorotrianisene	962.2	E858.0	E932.2	E950.4	E962.0	E980.4
Chlorovinyldichloroarsine	985.1	E866.3	—	E950.8	E962.1	E980.8
Chloroxylenol	976.0	E858.7	E946.0	E950.4	E962.0	E980.4
Chlorphenesin (carbamate)	968.0	E855.1	E938.0	E950.4	E962.0	E980.4
topical (antifungal)	976.0	E858.7	E946.0	E950.4	E962.0	E980.4
Chlorpheniramine	963.0	E858.1	E933.0	E950.4	E962.0	E980.4
Chlorphenoxamine	966.4	E855.0	E936.4	E950.4	E962.0	E980.4
Chlorphentermine	977.0	E858.8	E947.0	E950.4	E962.0	E980.4
Chlorproguanil	961.4	E857	E931.4	E950.4	E962.0	E980.4
Chlorpromazine	969.1	E853.0	E939.1	E950.3	E962.0	E980.3
Chlorpropamide	962.3	E858.0	E932.3	E950.4	E962.0	E980.4
Chlorprothixene	969.3	E853.8	E939.3	E950.3	E962.0	E980.3
Chlorquinaldol	976.0	E858.7	E946.0	E950.4	E962.0	E980.4
Chlortetracycline	960.4	E856	E930.4	E950.4	E962.0	E980.4
Chlorthalidone	974.4	E858.5	E944.4	E950.4	E962.0	E980.4
Chlortrianisene	962.2	E858.0	E932.2	E950.4	E962.0	E980.4
Chlor-Trimeton	963.0	E858.1	E933.0	E950.4	E962.0	E980.4
Chlorzoxazone	968.0	E855.1	E938.0	E950.4	E962.0	E980.4
Choke damp	987.8	E869.8	—	E952.8	E962.2	E982.8
Cholebrine	977.8	E858.8	E947.8	E950.4	E962.0	E980.4
Cholera vaccine	978.2	E858.8	E948.2	E950.4	E962.0	E980.4
Cholesterol-lowering agents	972.2	E858.3	E942.2	E950.4	E962.0	E980.4
Cholestyramine (resin)	972.2	E858.3	E942.2	E950.4	E962.0	E980.4
Cholic acid	973.4	E858.4	E943.4	E950.4	E962.0	E980.4
Choline	—	—	—	—	—	—
dihydrogen citrate	977.1	E858.8	E947.1	E950.4	E962.0	E980.4
salicylate	965.1	E850.3	E935.3	E950.0	E962.0	E980.0
theophyllinate	974.1	E858.5	E944.1	E950.4	E962.0	E980.4

◀ New   ◀▥ Revised

Substance	Poisoning	External Cause (E-Code)				
		Accident	Therapeutic Use	Suicide Attempt	Assault	Undetermined
Cholinergics	971.0	E855.3	E941.0	E950.4	E962.0	E980.4
Cholografin	977.8	E858.8	E947.8	E950.4	E962.0	E980.4
Chorionic gonadotropin	962.4	E858.0	E932.4	E950.4	E962.0	E980.4
Chromates	983.9	E864.3	—	E950.7	E962.1	E980.6
dust or mist	987.8	E869.8	—	E952.8	E962.2	E982.8
lead	984.0	E866.0	—	E950.9	E962.1	E980.9
paint	984.0	E861.5	—	E950.9	E962.1	E980.9
Chromic acid	983.9	E864.3	—	E950.7	E962.1	E980.6
dust or mist	987.8	E869.8	—	E952.8	E962.2	E982.8
Chromium	985.6	E866.4	—	E950.9	E962.1	E980.9
compounds - see Chromates	—	—	—	—	—	—
Chromonar	972.4	E858.3	E942.4	E950.4	E962.0	E980.4
Chromyl chloride	983.9	E864.3	—	E950.7	E962.1	E980.6
Chrysarobin (ointment)	976.4	E858.7	E946.4	E950.4	E962.0	E980.4
Chrysazin	973.1	E858.4	E943.1	E950.4	E962.0	E980.4
Chymar	963.4	E858.1	E933.4	E950.4	E962.0	E980.4
ophthalmic preparation	976.5	E858.7	E946.5	E950.4	E962.0	E980.4
Chymotrypsin	963.4	E858.1	E933.4	E950.4	E962.0	E980.4
ophthalmic preparation	976.5	E858.7	E946.5	E950.4	E962.0	E980.4
Cicuta maculata or virosa	988.2	E865.4	—	E950.9	E962.1	E980.9
Cigarette lighter fluid	981	E862.1	—	E950.9	E962.1	E980.9
Cinchocaine (spinal)	968.7	E855.2	E938.7	E950.4	E962.0	E980.4
topical (surface)	968.5	E855.2	E938.5	E950.4	E962.0	E980.4
Cinchona	961.4	E857	E931.4	E950.4	E962.0	E980.4
Cinchonine alkaloids	961.4	E857	E931.4	E950.4	E962.0	E980.4
Cinchophen	974.7	E858.5	E944.7	E950.4	E962.0	E980.4
Cinnarizine	963.0	E858.1	E933.0	E950.4	E962.0	E980.4
Citanest	968.9	E855.2	E938.9	E950.4	E962.0	E980.4
infiltration (subcutaneous)	968.5	E855.2	E938.5	E950.4	E962.0	E980.4
nerve block (peripheral) (plexus)	968.6	E855.2	E938.6	E950.4	E962.0	E980.4
Citric acid	989.89	E866.8	—	E950.9	E962.1	E980.9
Citrovorum factor	964.1	E858.2	E934.1	E950.4	E962.0	E980.4
Claviceps purpurea	988.2	E865.4	—	E950.9	E962.1	E980.9
Cleaner, cleansing agent NEC	989.89	E861.3	—	E950.9	E962.1	E980.9
of paint or varnish	982.8	E862.9	—	E950.9	E962.1	E980.9
Clematis vitalba	988.2	E865.4	—	E950.9	E962.1	E980.9
Clemizole	963.0	E858.1	E933.0	E950.4	E962.0	E980.4
penicillin	960.0	E856	E930.0	E950.4	E962.0	E980.4
Clidinium	971.1	E855.4	E941.1	E950.4	E962.0	E980.4
Clindamycin	960.8	E856	E930.8	E950.4	E962.0	E980.4
Cliradon	965.09	E850.2	E935.2	E950.0	E962.0	E980.0
Clocortolone	962.0	E858.0	E932.0	E950.4	E962.0	E980.4
Clofedanol	975.4	E858.6	E945.4	E950.4	E962.0	E980.4
Clofibrate	972.2	E858.3	E942.2	E950.4	E962.0	E980.4
Clomethiazole	967.1	E852.0	E937.1	E950.2	E962.0	E980.2
Clomiphene	977.8	E858.8	E947.8	E950.4	E962.0	E980.4
Clonazepam	969.4	E853.2	E939.4	E950.3	E962.0	E980.3
Clonidine	972.6	E858.3	E942.6	E950.4	E962.0	E980.4
Clopamide	974.3	E858.5	E944.3	E950.4	E962.0	E980.4
Clorazepate	969.4	E853.2	E939.4	E950.3	E962.0	E980.3
Clorexolone	974.4	E858.5	E944.4	E950.4	E962.0	E980.4
Clorox (bleach)	983.9	E864.3	—	E950.7	E962.1	E980.6
Clortermine	977.0	E858.8	E947.0	E950.4	E962.0	E980.4
Clotrimazole	976.0	E858.7	E946.0	E950.4	E962.0	E980.4
Cloxacillin	960.0	E856	E930.0	E950.4	E962.0	E980.4
Coagulants NEC	964.5	E858.2	E934.5	E950.4	E962.0	E980.4
Coal (carbon monoxide from) - see also Carbon, monoxide, coal	—	—	—	—	—	—
oil - see Kerosene	—	—	—	—	—	—
tar NEC	983.0	E864.0	—	E950.7	E962.1	E980.6
fumes	987.8	E869.8	—	E952.8	E962.2	E982.8
medicinal (ointment)	976.4	E858.7	E946.4	E950.4	E962.0	E980.4

Substance	Poisoning	External Cause (E-Code)				
		Accident	Therapeutic Use	Suicide Attempt	Assault	Undetermined
Coal (Continued)						
analgesics NEC	965.5	E850.5	E935.5	E950.0	E962.0	E980.0
naphtha (solvent)	981	E862.0	—	E950.9	E962.1	E980.9
Cobalt (fumes) (industrial)	985.8	E866.4	—	E950.9	E962.1	E980.9
Cobra (venom)	989.5	E905.0	—	E950.9	E962.1	E980.9
Coca (leaf)	970.8	E854.3	E940.8	E950.4	E962.0	E980.4
Cocaine (hydrochloride) (salt)	970.8	E854.3	E940.8	E950.4	E962.0	E980.4
topical anesthetic	968.5	E855.2	E938.5	E950.4	E962.0	E980.4
Coccidioidin	977.8	E858.8	E947.8	E950.4	E962.0	E980.4
Cocculus indicus	988.2	E865.3	—	E950.9	E962.1	E980.9
Cochineal	989.89	E866.8	—	E950.9	E962.1	E980.9
medicinal products	977.4	E858.8	E947.4	E950.4	E962.0	E980.4
Codeine	965.09	E850.2	E935.2	E950.0	E962.0	E980.0
Coffee	989.89	E866.8	—	E950.9	E962.1	E980.9
Cogentin	971.1	E855.4	E941.1	E950.4	E962.0	E980.4
Coke fumes or gas (carbon monoxide)	986	E868.3	—	E952.1	E962.2	E982.1
industrial use	986	E868.8	—	E952.1	E962.2	E982.1
Colace	973.2	E858.4	E943.2	E950.4	E962.0	E980.4
Colchicine	974.7	E858.5	E944.7	E950.4	E962.0	E980.4
Colchicum	988.2	E865.3	—	E950.9	E962.1	E980.9
Cold cream	976.3	E858.7	E946.3	E950.4	E962.0	E980.4
Colestipol	972.2	E858.3	E942.2	E950.4	E962.0	E980.4
Colistimethate	960.8	E856	E930.8	E950.4	E962.0	E980.4
Colistin	960.8	E856	E930.8	E950.4	E962.0	E980.4
Collagen	977.8	E866.8	E947.8	E950.9	E962.1	E980.9
Collagenase	976.8	E858.7	E946.8	E950.4	E962.0	E980.4
Collodion (flexible)	976.3	E858.7	E946.3	E950.4	E962.0	E980.4
Colocynth	973.1	E858.4	E943.1	E950.4	E962.0	E980.4
Coloring matter - see Dye(s)	—	—	—	—	—	—
Combustion gas - see Carbon, monoxide	—	—	—	—	—	—
Compazine	969.1	E853.0	E939.1	E950.3	E962.0	E980.3
Compound	—	—	—	—	—	—
42 (warfarin)	989.4	E863.7	—	E950.6	E962.1	E980.7
269 (endrin)	989.2	E863.0	—	E950.6	E962.1	E980.7
497 (dieldrin)	989.2	E863.0	—	E950.6	E962.1	E980.7
1080 (sodium fluoroacetate)	989.4	E863.7	—	E950.6	E962.1	E980.7
3422 (parathion)	989.3	E863.1	—	E950.6	E962.1	E980.7
3911 (phorate)	989.3	E863.1	—	E950.6	E962.1	E980.7
3956 (toxaphene)	989.2	E863.0	—	E950.6	E962.1	E980.7
4049 (malathion)	989.3	E863.1	—	E950.6	E962.1	E980.7
4124 (dicapthon)	989.4	E863.4	—	E950.6	E962.1	E980.7
E (cortisone)	962.0	E858.0	E932.0	E950.4	E962.0	E980.4
F (hydrocortisone)	962.0	E858.0	E932.0	E950.4	E962.0	E980.4
Congo red	977.8	E858.8	E947.8	E950.4	E962.0	E980.4
Coniine, conine	965.7	E850.7	E935.7	E950.0	E962.0	E980.0
Conium (maculatum)	988.2	E865.4	—	E950.9	E962.1	E980.9
Conjugated estrogens (equine)	962.2	E858.0	E932.2	E950.4	E962.0	E980.4
Contac	975.6	E858.6	E945.6	E950.4	E962.0	E980.4
Contact lens solution	976.5	E858.7	E946.5	E950.4	E962.0	E980.4
Contraceptives (oral)	962.2	E858.0	E932.2	E950.4	E962.0	E980.4
vaginal	976.8	E858.7	E946.8	E950.4	E962.0	E980.4
Contrast media (roentgenographic)	977.8	E858.8	E947.8	E950.4	E962.0	E980.4
Convallaria majalis	988.2	E865.4	—	E950.9	E962.1	E980.9
Copper (dust) (fumes) (salts) NEC	985.8	E866.4	—	E950.9	E962.1	E980.9
arsenate, arsenite	985.1	E866.3	—	E950.8	E962.1	E980.8
insecticide	985.1	E863.4	—	E950.8	E962.1	E980.8
emetic	973.6	E858.4	E943.6	E950.4	E962.0	E980.4
fungicide	985.8	E863.6	—	E950.6	E962.1	E980.7
insecticide	985.8	E863.4	—	E950.6	E962.1	E980.7
oleate	976.0	E858.7	E946.0	E950.4	E962.0	E980.4
sulfate	983.9	E864.3	—	E950.7	E962.1	E980.6
fungicide	983.9	E863.6	—	E950.7	E962.1	E980.6

◀ New   ◀▥ Revised

ICD-9-CM

Drugs

Vol. 2

Substance	Poisoning	External Cause (E-Code)				
		Accident	Therapeutic Use	Suicide Attempt	Assault	Undetermined
Copper *(Continued)*						
cupric	973.6	E858.4	E943.6	E950.4	E962.0	E980.4
cuprous	983.9	E864.3	—	E950.7	E962.1	E980.6
Copperhead snake (bite) (venom)	989.5	E905.0	—	E950.9	E962.1	E980.9
Coral (sting)	989.5	E905.6	—	E950.9	E962.1	E980.9
snake (bite) (venom)	989.5	E905.0	—	E950.9	E962.1	E980.9
Cordran	976.0	E858.7	E946.0	E950.4	E962.0	E980.4
Corn cures	976.4	E858.7	E946.4	E950.4	E962.0	E980.4
Cornhusker's lotion	976.3	E858.7	E946.3	E950.4	E962.0	E980.4
Corn starch	976.3	E858.7	E946.3	E950.4	E962.0	E980.4
Corrosive	983.9	E864.4	—	E950.7	E962.1	E980.6
acids NEC	983.1	E864.1	—	E950.7	E962.1	E980.6
aromatics	983.0	E864.0	—	E950.7	E962.1	E980.6
disinfectant	983.0	E861.4	—	E950.7	E962.1	E980.6
fumes NEC	987.9	E869.9	—	E952.9	E962.2	E982.9
specified NEC	983.9	E864.3	—	E950.7	E962.1	E980.6
sublimate - *see* Mercury, chloride	—	—	—	—	—	—
Cortate	962.0	E858.0	E932.0	E950.4	E962.0	E980.4
Cort-Dome	962.0	E858.0	E932.0	E950.4	E962.0	E980.4
ENT agent	976.6	E858.7	E946.6	E950.4	E962.0	E980.4
ophthalmic preparation	976.5	E858.7	E946.5	E950.4	E962.0	E980.4
topical NEC	976.0	E858.7	E946.0	E950.4	E962.0	E980.4
Cortef	962.0	E858.0	E932.0	E950.4	E962.0	E980.4
ENT agent	976.6	E858.7	E946.6	E950.4	E962.0	E980.4
ophthalmic preparation	976.5	E858.7	E946.5	E950.4	E962.0	E980.4
topical NEC	976.0	E858.7	E946.0	E950.4	E962.0	E980.4
Corticosteroids (fluorinated)	962.0	E858.0	E932.0	E950.4	E962.0	E980.4
ENT agent	976.6	E858.7	E946.6	E950.4	E962.0	E980.4
ophthalmic preparation	976.5	E858.7	E946.5	E950.4	E962.0	E980.4
topical NEC	976.0	E858.7	E946.0	E950.4	E962.0	E980.4
Corticotropin	962.4	E858.0	E932.4	E950.4	E962.0	E980.4
Cortisol	962.0	E858.0	E932.0	E950.4	E962.0	E980.4
ENT agent	976.6	E858.7	E946.6	E950.4	E962.0	E980.4
ophthalmic preparation	976.5	E858.7	E946.5	E950.4	E962.0	E980.4
topical NEC	976.0	E858.7	E946.0	E950.4	E962.0	E980.4
Cortisone derivatives (acetate)	962.0	E858.0	E932.0	E950.4	E962.0	E980.4
ENT agent	976.6	E858.7	E946.6	E950.4	E962.0	E980.4
ophthalmic preparation	976.5	E858.7	E946.5	E950.4	E962.0	E980.4
topical NEC	976.0	E858.7	E946.0	E950.4	E962.0	E980.4
Cortogen	962.0	E858.0	E932.0	E950.4	E962.0	E980.4
ENT agent	976.6	E858.7	E946.6	E950.4	E962.0	E980.4
ophthalmic preparation	976.5	E858.7	E946.5	E950.4	E962.0	E980.4
Cortone	962.0	E858.0	E932.0	E950.4	E962.0	E980.4
ENT agent	976.6	E858.7	E946.6	E950.4	E962.0	E980.4
ophthalmic preparation	976.5	E858.7	E946.5	E950.4	E962.0	E980.4
Cortril	962.0	E858.0	E932.0	E950.4	E962.0	E980.4
ENT agent	976.6	E858.7	E946.6	E950.4	E962.0	E980.4
ophthalmic preparation	976.5	E858.7	E946.5	E950.4	E962.0	E980.4
topical NEC	976.0	E858.7	E946.0	E950.4	E962.0	E980.4
Cosmetics	989.89	E866.7	—	E950.9	E962.1	E980.9
Cosyntropin	977.8	E858.8	E947.8	E950.4	E962.0	E980.4
Cotarnine	964.5	E858.2	E934.5	E950.4	E962.0	E980.4
Cottonseed oil	976.3	E858.7	E946.3	E950.4	E962.0	E980.4
Cough mixtures (antitussives)	975.4	E858.6	E945.4	E950.4	E962.0	E980.4
containing opiates	965.09	E850.2	E935.2	E950.0	E962.0	E980.0
expectorants	975.5	E858.6	E945.5	E950.4	E962.0	E980.4
Coumadin	964.2	E858.2	E934.2	E950.4	E962.0	E980.4
rodenticide	989.4	E863.7	—	E950.6	E962.1	E980.7
Coumarin	964.2	E858.2	E934.2	E950.4	E962.0	E980.4
Coumetarol	964.2	E858.2	E934.2	E950.4	E962.0	E980.4
Cowbane	988.2	E865.4	—	E950.9	E962.1	E980.9
Cozyme	963.5	E858.1	E933.5	E950.4	E962.0	E980.4
Crack	970.8	E854.3	E940.8	E950.4	E962.0	E980.4

◀ New   ◀▥ Revised

Substance	Poisoning	External Cause (E-Code)				
		Accident	Therapeutic Use	Suicide Attempt	Assault	Undetermined
Creolin	983.0	E864.0	—	E950.7	E962.1	E980.6
disinfectant	983.0	E861.4	—	E950.7	E962.1	E980.6
Creosol (compound)	983.0	E864.0	—	E950.7	E962.1	E980.6
Creosote (beechwood) (coal tar)	983.0	E864.0	—	E950.7	E962.1	E980.6
medicinal (expectorant)	975.5	E858.6	E945.5	E950.4	E962.0	E980.4
syrup	975.5	E858.6	E945.5	E950.4	E962.0	E980.4
Cresol	983.0	E864.0	—	E950.7	E962.1	E980.6
disinfectant	983.0	E861.4	—	E950.7	E962.1	E980.6
Cresylic acid	983.0	E864.0	—	E950.7	E962.1	E980.6
Cropropamide	965.7	E850.7	E935.7	E950.0	E962.0	E980.0
with crotethamide	970.0	E854.3	E940.0	E950.4	E962.0	E980.4
Crotamiton	976.0	E858.7	E946.0	E950.4	E962.0	E980.4
Crotethamide	965.7	E850.7	E935.7	E950.0	E962.0	E980.0
with cropropamide	970.0	E854.3	E940.0	E950.4	E962.0	E980.4
Croton (oil)	973.1	E858.4	E943.1	E950.4	E962.0	E980.4
chloral	967.1	E852.0	E937.1	E950.2	E962.0	E980.2
Crude oil	981	E862.1	—	E950.9	E962.1	E980.9
Cryogenine	965.8	E850.8	E935.8	E950.0	E962.0	E980.0
Cryolite (pesticide)	989.4	E863.4	—	E950.6	E962.1	E980.7
Cryptenamine	972.6	E858.3	E942.6	E950.4	E962.0	E980.4
Crystal violet	976.0	E858.7	E946.0	E950.4	E962.0	E980.4
Cuckoopint	988.2	E865.4	—	E950.9	E962.1	E980.9
Cumetharol	964.2	E858.2	E934.2	E950.4	E962.0	E980.4
Cupric sulfate	973.6	E858.4	E943.6	E950.4	E962.0	E980.4
Cuprous sulfate	983.9	E864.3	—	E950.7	E962.1	E980.6
Curare, curarine	975.2	E858.6	E945.2	E950.4	E962.0	E980.4
Cyanic acid - see Cyanide(s)	—	—	—	—	—	—
Cyanide(s) (compounds) (hydrogen) (potassium) (sodium) NEC	989.0	E866.8	—	E950.9	E962.1	E980.9
dust or gas (inhalation) NEC	987.7	E869.8	—	E952.8	E962.2	E982.8
fumigant	989.0	E863.8	—	E950.6	E962.1	E980.7
mercuric - see Mercury	—	—	—	—	—	—
pesticide (dust) (fumes)	989.0	E863.4	—	E950.6	E962.1	E980.7
Cyanocobalamin	964.1	E858.2	E934.1	E950.4	E962.0	E980.4
Cyanogen (chloride) (gas)	—	—	—	—	—	—
NEC	987.8	E869.8	—	E952.8	E962.2	E982.8
Cyclaine	968.5	E855.2	E938.5	E950.4	E962.0	E980.4
Cyclamen europaeum	988.2	E865.4	—	E950.9	E962.1	E980.9
Cyclandelate	972.5	E858.3	E942.5	E950.4	E962.0	E980.4
Cyclazocine	965.09	E850.2	E935.2	E950.0	E962.0	E980.0
Cyclizine	963.0	E858.1	E933.0	E950.4	E962.0	E980.4
Cyclobarbital, cyclobarbitone	967.0	E851	E937.0	E950.1	E962.0	E980.1
Cycloguanil	961.4	E857	E931.4	E950.4	E962.0	E980.4
Cyclohexane	982.0	E862.4	—	E950.9	E962.1	E980.9
Cyclohexanol	980.8	E860.8	—	E950.9	E962.1	E980.9
Cyclohexanone	982.8	E862.4	—	E950.9	E962.1	E980.9
Cyclomethycaine	968.5	E855.2	E938.5	E950.4	E962.0	E980.4
Cyclopentamine	971.2	E855.5	E941.2	E950.4	E962.0	E980.4
Cyclopenthiazide	974.3	E858.5	E944.3	E950.4	E962.0	E980.4
Cyclopentolate	971.1	E855.4	E941.1	E950.4	E962.0	E980.4
Cyclophosphamide	963.1	E858.1	E933.1	E950.4	E962.0	E980.4
Cyclopropane	968.2	E855.1	E938.2	E950.4	E962.0	E980.4
Cycloserine	960.6	E856	E930.6	E950.4	E962.0	E980.4
Cyclothiazide	974.3	E858.5	E944.3	E950.4	E962.0	E980.4
Cycrimine	966.4	E855.0	E936.4	E950.4	E962.0	E980.4
Cymarin	972.1	E858.3	E942.1	E950.4	E962.0	E980.4
Cyproheptadine	963.0	E858.1	E933.0	E950.4	E962.0	E980.4
Cyprolidol	969.0	E854.0	E939.0	E950.3	E962.0	E980.3
Cytarabine	963.1	E858.1	E933.1	E950.4	E962.0	E980.4
Cytisus	—	—	—	—	—	—
laburnum	988.2	E865.4	—	E950.9	E962.1	E980.9
scoparius	988.2	E865.4	—	E950.9	E962.1	E980.9

◀ New ◀▥ Revised

		External Cause (E-Code)				
Substance	Poisoning	Accident	Therapeutic Use	Suicide Attempt	Assault	Undetermined
Cytomel	962.7	E858.0	E932.7	E950.4	E962.0	E980.4
Cytosine (antineoplastic)	963.1	E858.1	E933.1	E950.4	E962.0	E980.4
Cytoxan	963.1	E858.1	E933.1	E950.4	E962.0	E980.4
Dacarbazine	963.1	E858.1	E933.1	E950.4	E962.0	E980.4
Dactinomycin	960.7	E856	E930.7	E950.4	E962.0	E980.4
DADPS	961.8	E857	E931.8	E950.4	E962.0	E980.4
Dakin's solution (external)	976.0	E858.7	E946.0	E950.4	E962.0	E980.4
Dalmane	969.4	E853.2	E939.4	E950.3	E962.0	E980.3
DAM	977.2	E858.8	E947.2	E950.4	E962.0	E980.4
Danilone	964.2	E858.2	E934.2	E950.4	E962.0	E980.4
Danthron	973.1	E858.4	E943.1	E950.4	E962.0	E980.4
Dantrolene	975.2	E858.6	E945.2	E950.4	E962.0	E980.4
Daphne (gnidium) (mezereum)	988.2	E865.4	—	E950.9	E962.1	E980.9
berry	988.2	E865.3	—	E950.9	E962.1	E980.9
Dapsone	961.8	E857	E931.8	E950.4	E962.0	E980.4
Daraprim	961.4	E857	E931.4	E950.4	E962.0	E980.4
Darnel	988.2	E865.3		E950.9	E962.1	E980.9
Darvon	965.8	E850.8	E935.8	E950.0	E962.0	E980.0
Daunorubicin	960.7	E856	E930.7	E950.4	E962.0	E980.4
DBI	962.3	E858.0	E932.3	E950.4	E962.0	E980.4
D-Con (rodenticide)	989.4	E863.7	—	E950.6	E962.1	E980.7
DDS	961.8	E857	E931.8	E950.4	E962.0	E980.4
DDT	989.2	E863.0	—	E950.6	E962.1	E980.7
Deadly nightshade	988.2	E865.4	—	E950.9	E962.1	E980.9
berry	988.2	E865.3	—	E950.9	E962.1	E980.9
Deanol	969.7	E854.2	E939.7	E950.3	E962.0	E980.3
Debrisoquine	972.6	E858.3	E942.6	E950.4	E962.0	E980.4
Decaborane	989.89	E866.8	—	E950.9	E962.1	E980.9
fumes	987.8	E869.8	—	E952.8	E962.2	E982.8
Decadron	962.0	E858.0	E932.0	E950.4	E962.0	E980.4
ENT agent	976.6	E858.7	E946.6	E950.4	E962.0	E980.4
ophthalmic preparation	976.5	E858.7	E946.5	E950.4	E962.0	E980.4
topical NEC	976.0	E858.7	E946.0	E950.4	E962.0	E980.4
Decahydronaphthalene	982.0	E862.4	—	E950.9	E962.1	E980.9
Decalin	982.0	E862.4	—	E950.9	E962.1	E980.9
Decamethonium	975.2	E858.6	E945.2	E950.4	E962.0	E980.4
Decholin	973.4	E858.4	E943.4	E950.4	E962.0	E980.4
sodium (diagnostic)	977.8	E858.8	E947.8	E950.4	E962.0	E980.4
Declomycin	960.4	E856	E930.4	E950.4	E962.0	E980.4
Deferoxamine	963.8	E858.1	E933.8	E950.4	E962.0	E980.4
Dehydrocholic acid	973.4	E858.4	E943.4	E950.4	E962.0	E980.4
DeKalin	982.0	E862.4	—	E950.9	E962.1	E980.9
Delalutin	962.2	E858.0	E932.2	E950.4	E962.0	E980.4
Delphinium	988.2	E865.3	—	E950.9	E962.1	E980.9
Deltasone	962.0	E858.0	E932.0	E950.4	E962.0	E980.4
Deltra	962.0	E858.0	E932.0	E950.4	E962.0	E980.4
Delvinal	967.0	E851	E937.0	E950.1	E962.0	E980.1
Demecarium (bromide)	971.0	E855.3	E941.0	E950.4	E962.0	E980.4
Demeclocycline	960.4	E856	E930.4	E950.4	E962.0	E980.4
Demecolcine	963.1	E858.1	E933.1	E950.4	E962.0	E980.4
Demelanizing agents	976.8	E858.7	E946.8	E950.4	E962.0	E980.4
Demerol	965.09	E850.2	E935.2	E950.0	E962.0	E980.0
Demethylchlortetracycline	960.4	E856	E930.4	E950.4	E962.0	E980.4
Demethyltetracycline	960.4	E856	E930.4	E950.4	E962.0	E980.4
Demeton	989.3	E863.1	—	E950.6	E962.1	E980.7
Demulcents	976.3	E858.7	E946.3	E950.4	E962.0	E980.4
Demulen	962.2	E858.0	E932.2	E950.4	E962.0	E980.4
Denatured alcohol	980.0	E860.1	—	E950.9	E962.1	E980.9
Dendrid	976.5	E858.7	E946.5	E950.4	E962.0	E980.4
Dental agents, topical	976.7	E858.7	E946.7	E950.4	E962.0	E980.4
Deodorant spray (feminine hygiene)	976.8	E858.7	E946.8	E950.4	E962.0	E980.4

Substance	Poisoning	External Cause (E-Code)				
		Accident	Therapeutic Use	Suicide Attempt	Assault	Undetermined
Deoxyribonuclease	963.4	E858.1	E933.4	E950.4	E962.0	E980.4
Depressants	—	—	—	—	—	—
appetite, central	977.0	E858.8	E947.0	E950.4	E962.0	E980.4
cardiac	972.0	E858.3	E942.0	E950.4	E962.0	E980.4
central nervous system (anesthetic)	968.4	E855.1	E938.4	E950.4	E962.0	E980.4
psychotherapeutic	969.5	E853.9	E939.5	E950.3	E962.0	E980.3
Dequalinium	976.0	E858.7	E946.0	E950.4	E962.0	E980.4
Dermolate	976.2	E858.7	E946.2	E950.4	E962.0	E980.4
DES	962.2	E858.0	E932.2	E950.4	E962.0	E980.4
Desenex	976.0	E858.7	E946.0	E950.4	E962.0	E980.4
Deserpidine	972.6	E858.3	E942.6	E950.4	E962.0	E980.4
Desipramine	969.0	E854.0	E939.0	E950.3	E962.0	E980.3
Deslanoside	972.1	E858.3	E942.1	E950.4	E962.0	E980.4
Desocodeine	965.09	E850.2	E935.2	E950.0	E962.0	E980.0
Desomorphine	965.09	E850.2	E935.2	E950.0	E962.0	E980.0
Desonide	976.0	E858.7	E946.0	E950.4	E962.0	E980.4
Desoxycorticosterone derivatives	962.0	E858.0	E932.0	E950.4	E962.0	E980.4
Desoxyephedrine	969.7	E854.2	E939.7	E950.3	E962.0	E980.3
DET	969.6	E854.1	E939.6	E950.3	E962.0	E980.3
Detergents (ingested) (synthetic)	989.6	E861.0	—	E950.9	E962.1	E980.9
external medication	976.2	E858.7	E946.2	E950.4	E962.0	E980.4
Deterrent, alcohol	977.3	E858.8	E947.3	E950.4	E962.0	E980.4
Detrothyronine	962.7	E858.0	E932.7	E950.4	E962.0	E980.4
Dettol (external medication)	976.0	E858.7	E946.0	E950.4	E962.0	E980.4
Dexamethasone	962.0	E858.0	E932.0	E950.4	E962.0	E980.4
ENT agent	976.6	E858.7	E946.6	E950.4	E962.0	E980.4
ophthalmic preparation	976.5	E858.7	E946.5	E950.4	E962.0	E980.4
topical NEC	976.0	E858.7	E946.0	E950.4	E962.0	E980.4
Dexamphetamine	969.7	E854.2	E939.7	E950.3	E962.0	E980.3
Dexedrine	969.7	E854.2	E939.7	E950.3	E962.0	E980.3
Dexpanthenol	963.5	E858.1	E933.5	E950.4	E962.0	E980.4
Dextran	964.8	E858.2	E934.8	E950.4	E962.0	E980.4
Dextriferron	964.0	E858.2	E934.0	E950.4	E962.0	E980.4
Dextroamphetamine	969.7	E854.2	E939.7	E950.3	E962.0	E980.3
Dextro calcium pantothenate	963.5	E858.1	E933.5	E950.4	E962.0	E980.4
Dextromethorphan	975.4	E858.6	E945.4	E950.4	E962.0	E980.4
Dextromoramide	965.09	E850.2	E935.2	E950.0	E962.0	E980.0
Dextro pantothenyl alcohol	963.5	E858.1	E933.5	E950.4	E962.0	E980.4
topical	976.8	E858.7	E946.8	E950.4	E962.0	E980.4
Dextropropoxyphene (hydrochloride)	965.8	E850.8	E935.8	E950.0	E962.0	E980.0
Dextrorphan	965.09	E850.2	E935.2	E950.0	E962.0	E980.0
Dextrose NEC	974.5	E858.5	E944.5	E950.4	E962.0	E980.4
Dextrothyroxine	962.7	E858.0	E932.7	E950.4	E962.0	E980.4
DFP	971.0	E855.3	E941.0	E950.4	E962.0	E980.4
DHE-45	972.9	E858.3	E942.9	E950.4	E962.0	E980.4
Diabinese	962.3	E858.0	E932.3	E950.4	E962.0	E980.4
Diacetyl monoxime	977.2	E858.8	E947.2	E950.4	E962.0	E980.4
Diacetylmorphine	965.01	E850.0	E935.0	E950.0	E962.0	E980.0
Diagnostic agents	977.8	E858.8	E947.8	E950.4	E962.0	E980.4
Dial (soap)	976.2	E858.7	E946.2	E950.4	E962.0	E980.4
sedative	967.0	E851	E937.0	E950.1	E962.0	E980.1
Diallylbarbituric acid	967.0	E851	E937.0	E950.1	E962.0	E980.1
Diaminodiphenyisulfone	961.8	E857	E931.8	E950.4	E962.0	E980.4
Diamorphine	965.01	E850.0	E935.0	E950.0	E962.0	E980.0
Diamox	974.2	E858.5	E944.2	E950.4	E962.0	E980.4
Diamthazole	976.0	E858.7	E946.0	E950.4	E962.0	E980.4
Diaphenyisulfone	961.8	E857	E931.8	E950.4	E962.0	E980.4
Diasone (sodium)	961.8	E857	E931.8	E950.4	E962.0	E980.4
Diazepam	969.4	E853.2	E939.4	E950.3	E962.0	E980.3
Diazinon	989.3	E863.1	—	E950.6	E962.1	E980.7
Diazomethane (gas)	987.8	E869.8	—	E952.8	E962.2	E982.8

◀ **New**   ◀ **Revised**

Substance	Poisoning	External Cause (E-Code)				
		Accident	Therapeutic Use	Suicide Attempt	Assault	Undetermined
Diazoxide	972.5	E858.3	E942.5	E950.4	E962.0	E980.4
Dibenamine	971.3	E855.6	E941.3	E950.4	E962.0	E980.4
Dibenzheptropine	963.0	E858.1	E933.0	E950.4	E962.0	E980.4
Dibenzyline	971.3	E855.6	E941.3	E950.4	E962.0	E980.4
Diborane (gas)	987.8	E869.8	—	E952.8	E962.2	E982.8
Dibromomannitol	963.1	E858.1	E933.1	E950.4	E962.0	E980.4
Dibucaine (spinal)	968.7	E855.2	E938.7	E950.4	E962.0	E980.4
topical (surface)	968.5	E855.2	E938.5	E950.4	E962.0	E980.4
Dibunate sodium	975.4	E858.6	E945.4	E950.4	E962.0	E980.4
Dibutoline	971.1	E855.4	E941.1	E950.4	E962.0	E980.4
Dicapthon	989.4	E863.4	—	E950.6	E962.1	E980.7
Dichloralphenazone	967.1	E852.0	E937.1	E950.2	E962.0	E980.2
Dichlorodifluoromethane	987.4	E869.2	—	E952.8	E962.2	E982.8
Dichloroethane	982.3	E862.4	—	E950.9	E962.1	E980.9
Dichloroethylene	982.3	E862.4	—	E950.9	E962.1	E980.9
Dichloroethyl sulfide	987.8	E869.8	—	E952.8	E962.2	E982.8
Dichlorohydrin	982.3	E862.4	—	E950.9	E962.1	E980.9
Dichloromethane (solvent) (vapor)	982.3	E862.4	—	E950.9	E962.1	E980.9
Dichlorophen(e)	961.6	E857	E931.6	E950.4	E962.0	E980.4
Dichlorphenamide	974.2	E858.5	E944.2	E950.4	E962.0	E980.4
Dichlorvos	989.3	E863.1	—	E950.6	E962.1	E980.7
Diclofenac sodium	965.69	E850.6	E935.6	E950.0	E962.0	E980.0
Dicoumarin, dicumarol	964.2	E858.2	E934.2	E950.4	E962.0	E980.4
Dicyanogen (gas)	987.8	E869.8	—	E952.8	E962.2	E982.8
Dicyclomine	971.1	E855.4	E941.1	E950.4	E962.0	E980.4
Dieldrin (vapor)	989.2	E863.0	—	E950.6	E962.1	E980.7
Dienestrol	962.2	E858.0	E932.2	E950.4	E962.0	E980.4
Dietetics	977.0	E858.8	E947.0	E950.4	E962.0	E980.4
Diethazine	966.4	E855.0	E936.4	E950.4	E962.0	E980.4
Diethyl	—	—	—	—	—	—
barbituric acid	967.0	E851	E937.0	E950.1	E962.0	E980.1
carbamazine	961.6	E857	E931.6	E950.4	E962.0	E980.4
carbinol	980.8	E860.8	—	E950.9	E962.1	E980.9
carbonate	982.8	E862.4	—	E950.9	E962.1	E980.9
ether (vapor) - *see* Ether(s)	—	—	—	—	—	—
propion	977.0	E858.8	E947.0	E950.4	E962.0	E980.4
stilbestrol	962.2	E858.0	E932.2	E950.4	E962.0	E980.4
Diethylene	—	—	—	—	—	—
dioxide	982.8	E862.4	—	E950.9	E962.1	E980.9
glycol (monoacetate) (monoethyl ether)	982.8	E862.4	—	E950.9	E962.1	E980.9
Diethylsulfone-diethylmethane	967.8	E852.8	E937.8	E950.2	E962.0	E980.2
Difencloxazine	965.09	E850.2	E935.2	E950.0	E962.0	E980.0
Diffusin	963.4	E858.1	E933.4	E950.4	E962.0	E980.4
Diflos	971.0	E855.3	E941.0	E950.4	E962.0	E980.4
Digestants	973.4	E858.4	E943.4	E950.4	E962.0	E980.4
Digitalin(e)	972.1	E858.3	E942.1	E950.4	E962.0	E980.4
Digitalis glycosides	972.1	E858.3	E942.1	E950.4	E962.0	E980.4
Digitoxin	972.1	E858.3	E942.1	E950.4	E962.0	E980.4
Digoxin	972.1	E858.3	E942.1	E950.4	E962.0	E980.4
Dihydrocodeine	965.09	E850.2	E935.2	E950.0	E962.0	E980.0
Dihydrocodeinone	965.09	E850.2	E935.2	E950.0	E962.0	E980.0
Dihydroergocristine	972.9	E858.3	E942.9	E950.4	E962.0	E980.4
Dihydroergotamine	972.9	E858.3	E942.9	E950.4	E962.0	E980.4
Dihydroergotoxine	972.9	E858.3	E942.9	E950.4	E962.0	E980.4
Dihydrohydroxycodeinone	965.09	E850.2	E935.2	E950.0	E962.0	E980.0
Dihydrohydroxymorphinone	965.09	E850.2	E935.2	E950.0	E962.0	E980.0
Dihydroisocodeine	965.09	E850.2	E935.2	E950.0	E962.0	E980.0
Dihydromorphine	965.09	E850.2	E935.2	E950.0	E962.0	E980.0
Dihydromorphinone	965.09	E850.2	E935.2	E950.0	E962.0	E980.0
Dihydrostreptomycin	960.6	E856	E930.6	E950.4	E962.0	E980.4
Dihydrotachysterol	962.6	E858.0	E932.6	E950.4	E962.0	E980.4

Substance	Poisoning	External Cause (E-Code)				
		Accident	Therapeutic Use	Suicide Attempt	Assault	Undetermined
Dihydroxyanthraquinone	973.1	E858.4	E943.1	E950.4	E962.0	E980.4
Dihydroxycodeinone	965.09	E850.2	E935.2	E950.0	E962.0	E980.0
Diiodohydroxyquin	961.3	E857	E931.3	E950.4	E962.0	E980.4
topical	976.0	E858.7	E946.0	E950.4	E962.0	E980.4
Diiodohydroxyquinoline	961.3	E857	E931.3	E950.4	E962.0	E980.4
Dilantin	966.1	E855.0	E936.1	E950.4	E962.0	E980.4
Dilaudid	965.09	E850.2	E935.2	E950.0	E962.0	E980.0
Diloxanide	961.5	E857	E931.5	E950.4	E962.0	E980.4
Dimefline	970.0	E854.3	E940.0	E950.4	E962.0	E980.4
Dimenhydrinate	963.0	E858.1	E933.0	E950.4	E962.0	E980.4
Dimercaprol	963.8	E858.1	E933.8	E950.4	E962.0	E980.4
Dimercaptopropanol	963.8	E858.1	E933.8	E950.4	E962.0	E980.4
Dimetane	963.0	E858.1	E933.0	E950.4	E962.0	E980.4
Dimethicone	976.3	E858.7	E946.3	E950.4	E962.0	E980.4
Dimethindene	963.0	E858.1	E933.0	E950.4	E962.0	E980.4
Dimethisoquin	968.5	E855.2	E938.5	E950.4	E962.0	E980.4
Dimethisterone	962.2	E858.0	E932.2	E950.4	E962.0	E980.4
Dimethoxanate	975.4	E858.6	E945.4	E950.4	E962.0	E980.4
Dimethyl	—	—	—	—	—	—
arsine, arsinic acid - *see* Arsenic	—	—	—	—	—	—
carbinol	980.2	E860.3	—	E950.9	E962.1	E980.9
diguanide	962.3	E858.0	E932.3	E950.4	E962.0	E980.4
ketone	982.8	E862.4	—	E950.9	E962.1	E980.9
vapor	987.8	E869.8	—	E952.8	E962.2	E982.8
meperidine	965.09	E850.2	E935.2	E950.0	E962.0	E980.0
parathion	989.3	E863.1	—	E950.6	E962.1	E980.7
polysiloxane	973.8	E858.4	E943.8	E950.4	E962.0	E980.4
sulfate (fumes)	987.8	E869.8	—	E952.8	E962.2	E982.8
liquid	983.9	E864.3	—	E950.7	E962.1	E980.6
sulfoxide NEC	982.8	E862.4	—	E950.9	E962.1	E980.9
medicinal	976.4	E858.7	E946.4	E950.4	E962.0	E980.4
triptamine	969.6	E854.1	E939.6	E950.3	E962.0	E980.3
tubocurarine	975.2	E858.6	E945.2	E950.4	E962.0	E980.4
Dindevan	964.2	E858.2	E934.2	E950.4	E962.0	E980.4
Dinitro (-ortho-) cresol (herbicide) (spray)	989.4	E863.5	—	E950.6	E962.1	E980.7
insecticide	989.4	E863.4	—	E950.6	E962.1	E980.7
Dinitrobenzene	983.0	E864.0	—	E950.7	E962.1	E980.6
vapor	987.8	E869.8	—	E952.8	E962.2	E982.8
Dinitro-orthocresol (herbicide)	989.4	E863.5	—	E950.6	E962.1	E980.7
insecticide	989.4	E863.4	—	E950.6	E962.1	E980.7
Dinitrophenol (herbicide) (spray)	989.4	E863.5	—	E950.6	E962.1	E980.7
insecticide	989.4	E863.4	—	E950.6	E962.1	E980.7
Dinoprost	975.0	E858.6	E945.0	E950.4	E962.0	E980.4
Dioctyl sulfosuccinate (calcium) (sodium)	973.2	E858.4	E943.2	E950.4	E962.0	E980.4
Diodoquin	961.3	E857	E931.3	E950.4	E962.0	E980.4
Dione derivatives NEC	966.3	E855.0	E936.3	E950.4	E962.0	E980.4
Dionin	965.09	E850.2	E935.2	E950.0	E962.0	E980.0
Dioxane	982.8	E862.4	—	E950.9	E962.1	E980.9
Dioxin - *see* herbicide	—	—	—	—	—	—
Dioxyline	972.5	E858.3	E942.5	E950.4	E962.0	E980.4
Dipentene	982.8	E862.4	—	E950.9	E962.1	E980.9
Diphemanil	971.1	E855.4	E941.1	E950.4	E962.0	E980.4
Diphenadione	964.2	E858.2	E934.2	E950.4	E962.0	E980.4
Diphenhydramine	963.0	E858.1	E933.0	E950.4	E962.0	E980.4
Diphenidol	963.0	E858.1	E933.0	E950.4	E962.0	E980.4
Diphenoxylate	973.5	E858.4	E943.5	E950.4	E962.0	E980.4
Diphenylchlorarsine	985.1	E866.3	—	E950.8	E962.1	E980.8
Diphenylhydantoin (sodium)	966.1	E855.0	E936.1	E950.4	E962.0	E980.4
Diphenylpyraline	963.0	E858.1	E933.0	E950.4	E962.0	E980.4
Diphtheria	—	—	—	—	—	—
antitoxin	979.9	E858.8	E949.9	E950.4	E962.0	E980.4

◄ New   ◄═ Revised

Substance	Poisoning	External Cause (E-Code)				
		Accident	Therapeutic Use	Suicide Attempt	Assault	Undetermined
Diphtheria *(Continued)*						
toxoid	978.5	E858.8	E948.5	E950.4	E962.0	E980.4
with tetanus toxoid	978.9	E858.8	E948.9	E950.4	E962.0	E980.4
with pertussis component	978.6	E858.8	E948.6	E950.4	E962.0	E980.4
vaccine	978.5	E858.8	E948.5	E950.4	E962.0	E980.4
Dipipanone	965.09	E850.2	E935.2	E950.0	E962.0	E980.0
Diplovax	979.5	E858.8	E949.5	E950.4	E962.0	E980.4
Diprophylline	975.1	E858.6	E945.1	E950.4	E962.0	E980.4
Dipyridamole	972.4	E858.3	E942.4	E950.4	E962.0	E980.4
Dipyrone	965.5	E850.5	E935.5	E950.0	E962.0	E980.0
Diquat	989.4	E863.5	—	E950.6	E962.1	E980.7
Disinfectant NEC	983.9	E861.4	—	E950.7	E962.1	E980.6
alkaline	983.2	E861.4	—	E950.7	E962.1	E980.6
aromatic	983.0	E861.4	—	E950.7	E962.1	E980.6
Disipal	966.4	E855.0	E936.4	E950.4	E962.0	E980.4
Disodium edetate	963.8	E858.1	E933.8	E950.4	E962.0	E980.4
Disulfamide	974.4	E858.5	E944.4	E950.4	E962.0	E980.4
Disulfanilamide	961.0	E857	E931.0	E950.4	E962.0	E980.4
Disulfiram	977.3	E858.8	E947.3	E950.4	E962.0	E980.4
Dithiazanine	961.6	E857	E931.6	E950.4	E962.0	E980.4
Dithioglycerol	963.8	E858.1	E933.8	E950.4	E962.0	E980.4
Dithranol	976.4	E858.7	E946.4	E950.4	E962.0	E980.4
Diucardin	974.3	E858.5	E944.3	E950.4	E962.0	E980.4
Diupres	974.3	E858.5	E944.3	E950.4	E962.0	E980.4
Diuretics NEC	974.4	E858.5	E944.4	E950.4	E962.0	E980.4
carbonic acid anhydrase inhibitors	974.2	E858.5	E944.2	E950.4	E962.0	E980.4
mercurial	974.0	E858.5	E944.0	E950.4	E962.0	E980.4
osmotic	974.4	E858.5	E944.4	E950.4	E962.0	E980.4
purine derivatives	974.1	E858.5	E944.1	E950.4	E962.0	E980.4
saluretic	974.3	E858.5	E944.3	E950.4	E962.0	E980.4
Diuril	974.3	E858.5	E944.3	E950.4	E962.0	E980.4
Divinyl ether	968.2	E855.1	E938.2	E950.4	E962.0	E980.4
D-lysergic acid diethylamide	969.6	E854.1	E939.6	E950.3	E962.0	E980.3
DMCT	960.4	E856	E930.4	E950.4	E962.0	E980.4
DMSO	982.8	E862.4	—	E950.9	E962.1	E980.9
DMT	969.6	E854.1	E939.6	E950.3	E962.0	E980.3
DNOC	989.4	E863.5	—	E950.6	E962.1	E980.7
DOCA	962.0	E858.0	E932.0	E950.4	E962.0	E980.4
Dolophine	965.02	E850.1	E935.1	E950.0	E962.0	E980.0
Doloxene	965.8	E850.8	E935.8	E950.0	E962.0	E980.0
DOM	969.6	E854.1	E939.6	E950.3	E962.0	E980.3
Domestic gas - *see* Gas, utility	—	—	—	—	—	—
Domiphen (bromide) (lozenges)	976.6	E858.7	E946.6	E950.4	E962.0	E980.4
Dopa (levo)	966.4	E855.0	E936.4	E950.4	E962.0	E980.4
Dopamine	971.2	E855.5	E941.2	E950.4	E962.0	E980.4
Doriden	967.5	E852.4	E937.5	E950.2	E962.0	E980.2
Dormiral	967.0	E851	E937.0	E950.1	E962.0	E980.1
Dormison	967.8	E852.8	E937.8	E950.2	E962.0	E980.2
Dornase	963.4	E858.1	E933.4	E950.4	E962.0	E980.4
Dorsacaine	968.5	E855.2	E938.5	E950.4	E962.0	E980.4
Dothiepin hydrochloride	969.0	E854.0	E939.0	E950.3	E962.0	E980.3
Doxapram	970.0	E854.3	E940.0	E950.4	E962.0	E980.4
Doxepin	969.0	E854.0	E939.0	E950.3	E962.0	E980.3
Doxorubicin	960.7	E856	E930.7	E950.4	E962.0	E980.4
Doxycycline	960.4	E856	E930.4	E950.4	E962.0	E980.4
Doxylamine	963.0	E858.1	E933.0	E950.4	E962.0	E980.4
Dramamine	963.0	E858.1	E933.0	E950.4	E962.0	E980.4
Drano (drain cleaner)	983.2	E864.2	—	E950.7	E962.1	E980.6
Dromoran	965.09	E850.2	E935.2	E950.0	E962.0	E980.0
Dromostanolone	962.1	E858.0	E932.1	E950.4	E962.0	E980.4
Droperidol	969.2	E853.1	E939.2	E950.3	E962.0	E980.3
Drotrecogin alfa	964.2	E858.2	E934.2	E950.4	E962.0	E980.4

Substance	Poisoning	External Cause (E-Code)				
		Accident	Therapeutic Use	Suicide Attempt	Assault	Undetermined
Drug	977.9	E858.9	E947.9	E950.5	E962.0	E980.5
specified NEC	977.8	E858.8	E947.8	E950.4	E962.0	E980.4
AHFS List	—	—	—	—	—	—
4:00 antihistamine drugs	963.0	E858.1	E933.0	E950.4	E962.0	E980.4
8:04 amebacides	961.5	E857	E931.5	E950.4	E962.0	E980.4
arsenical anti-infectives	961.1	E857	E931.1	E950.4	E962.0	E980.4
quinoline derivatives	961.3	E857	E931.3	E950.4	E962.0	E980.4
8:08 anthelmintics	961.6	E857	E931.6	E950.4	E962.0	E980.4
quinoline derivatives	961.3	E857	E931.3	E950.4	E962.0	E980.4
8:12.04 antifungal antibiotics	960.1	E856	E930.1	E950.4	E962.0	E980.4
8:12.06 cephalosporins	960.5	E856	E930.5	E950.4	E962.0	E980.4
8:12.08 chloramphenicol	960.2	E856	E930.2	E950.4	E962.0	E980.4
8:12.12 erythromycins	960.3	E856	E930.3	E950.4	E962.0	E980.4
8:12.16 penicillins	960.0	E856	E930.0	E950.4	E962.0	E980.4
8:12.20 streptomycins	960.6	E856	E930.6	E950.4	E962.0	E980.4
8:12.24 tetracyclines	960.4	E856	E930.4	E950.4	E962.0	E980.4
8:12.28 other antibiotics	960.8	E856	E930.8	E950.4	E962.0	E980.4
antimycobacterial	960.6	E856	E930.6	E950.4	E962.0	E980.4
macrolides	960.3	E856	E930.3	E950.4	E962.0	E980.4
8:16 antituberculars	961.8	E857	E931.8	E950.4	E962.0	E980.4
antibiotics	960.6	E856	E930.6	E950.4	E962.0	E980.4
8:18 antivirals	961.7	E857	E931.7	E950.4	E962.0	E980.4
8:20 plasmodicides (antimalarials)	961.4	E857	E931.4	E950.4	E962.0	E980.4
8:24 sulfonamides	961.0	E857	E931.0	E950.4	E962.0	E980.4
8:26 sulfones	961.8	E857	E931.8	E950.4	E962.0	E980.4
8:28 treponemicides	961.2	E857	E931.2	E950.4	E962.0	E980.4
8:32 trichomonacides	961.5	E857	E931.5	E950.4	E962.0	E980.4
quinoline derivatives	961.3	E857	E931.3	E950.4	E962.0	E980.4
nitrofuran derivatives	961.9	E857	E931.9	E950.4	E962.0	E980.4
8:36 urinary germicides	961.9	E857	E931.9	E950.4	E962.0	E980.4
quinoline derivatives	961.3	E857	E931.3	E950.4	E962.0	E980.4
8:40 other anti-infectives	961.9	E857	E931.9	E950.4	E962.0	E980.4
10:00 antineoplastic agents	963.1	E858.1	E933.1	E950.4	E962.0	E980.4
antibiotics	960.7	E856	E930.7	E950.4	E962.0	E980.4
progestogens	962.2	E858.0	E932.2	E950.4	E962.0	E980.4
12:04 parasympathomimetic (cholinergic) agents	971.0	E855.3	E941.0	E950.4	E962.0	E980.4
12:08 parasympatholytic (cholinergic-blocking) agents	971.1	E855.4	E941.1	E950.4	E962.0	E980.4
12:12 sympathomimetic (adrenergic) agents	971.2	E855.5	E941.2	E950.4	E962.0	E980.4
12:16 sympatholytic (adrenergic-blocking) agents	971.3	E855.6	E941.3	E950.4	E962.0	E980.4
12:20 skeletal muscle relaxants	—	—	—	—	—	—
central nervous system muscle-tone depressants	968.0	E855.1	E938.0	E950.4	E962.0	E980.4
myoneural blocking agents	975.2	E858.6	E945.2	E950.4	E962.0	E980.4
16:00 blood derivatives	964.7	E858.2	E934.7	E950.4	E962.0	E980.4
20:04 antianemia drugs	964.1	E858.2	E934.1	E950.4	E962.0	E980.4
20:04.04 iron preparations	964.0	E858.2	E934.0	E950.4	E962.0	E980.4
20:04.08 liver and stomach preparations	964.1	E858.2	E934.1	E950.4	E962.0	E980.4
20:12.04 anticoagulants	964.2	E858.2	E934.2	E950.4	E962.0	E980.4
20:12.08 antiheparin agents	964.5	E858.2	E934.5	E950.4	E962.0	E980.4
20:12.12 coagulants	964.5	E858.2	E934.5	E950.4	E962.0	E980.4
20:12.16 hemostatics NEC	964.5	E858.2	E934.5	E950.4	E962.0	E980.4
capillary active drugs	972.8	E858.3	E942.8	E950.4	E962.0	E980.4
24:04 cardiac drugs	972.9	E858.3	E942.9	E950.4	E962.0	E980.4
cardiotonic agents	972.1	E858.3	E942.1	E950.4	E962.0	E980.4
rhythm regulators	972.0	E858.3	E942.0	E950.4	E962.0	E980.4
24:06 antilipemic agents	972.2	E858.3	E942.2	E950.4	E962.0	E980.4
thyroid derivatives	962.7	E858.0	E932.7	E950.4	E962.0	E980.4
24:08 hypotensive agents	972.6	E858.3	E942.6	E950.4	E962.0	E980.4
adrenergic blocking agents	971.3	E855.6	E941.3	E950.4	E962.0	E980.4
ganglion blocking agents	972.3	E858.3	E942.3	E950.4	E962.0	E980.4
vasodilators	972.5	E858.3	E942.5	E950.4	E962.0	E980.4

◀ New   ⬅▥ Revised

Substance	Poisoning	External Cause (E-Code)				
		Accident	Therapeutic Use	Suicide Attempt	Assault	Undetermined
Drug *(Continued)*						
24:12 vasodilating agents NEC	972.5	E858.3	E942.5	E950.4	E962.0	E980.4
coronary	972.4	E858.3	E942.4	E950.4	E962.0	E980.4
nicotinic acid derivatives	972.2	E858.3	E942.2	E950.4	E962.0	E980.4
24:16 sclerosing agents	972.7	E858.3	E942.7	E950.4	E962.0	E980.4
28:04 general anesthetics	968.4	E855.1	E938.4	E950.4	E962.0	E980.4
gaseous anesthetics	968.2	E855.1	E938.2	E950.4	E962.0	E980.4
halothane	968.1	E855.1	E938.1	E950.4	E962.0	E980.4
intravenous anesthetics	968.3	E855.1	E938.3	E950.4	E962.0	E980.4
28:08 analgesics and antipyretics	965.9	E850.9	E935.9	E950.0	E962.0	E980.0
antirheumatics	965.69	E850.6	E935.6	E950.0	E962.0	E980.0
aromatic analgesics	965.4	E850.4	E935.4	E950.0	E962.0	E980.0
non-narcotic NEC	965.7	E850.7	E935.7	E950.0	E962.0	E980.0
opium alkaloids	965.00	E850.2	E935.2	E950.0	E962.0	E980.0
heroin	965.01	E850.0	E935.0	E950.0	E962.0	E980.0
methadone	965.02	E850.1	E935.1	E950.0	E962.0	E980.0
specified type NEC	965.09	E850.2	E935.2	E950.0	E962.0	E980.0
pyrazole derivatives	965.5	E850.5	E935.5	E950.0	E962.0	E980.0
salicylates	965.1	E850.3	E935.3	E950.0	E962.0	E980.0
specified NEC	965.8	E850.8	E935.8	E950.0	E962.0	E980.0
28:10 narcotic antagonists	970.1	E854.3	E940.1	E950.4	E962.0	E980.4
28:12 anticonvulsants	966.3	E855.0	E936.3	E950.4	E962.0	E980.4
barbiturates	967.0	E851	E937.0	E950.1	E962.0	E980.1
benzodiazepine-based tranquilizers	969.4	E853.4	E939.4	E950.3	E962.0	E980.3
bromides	967.3	E852.2	E937.3	E950.2	E962.0	E980.2
hydantoin derivatives	966.1	E855.0	E936.1	E950.4	E962.0	E980.4
oxazolidine (derivatives)	966.0	E855.0	E936.0	E950.4	E962.0	E980.4
succinimides	966.2	E855.0	E936.2	E950.4	E962.0	E980.4
28:16.04 antidepressants	969.0	E854.0	E939.0	E950.3	E962.0	E980.3
28:16.08 tranquilizers	969.5	E853.9	E939.5	E950.3	E962.0	E980.3
benzodiazepine-based	969.4	E853.2	E939.4	E950.3	E962.0	E980.3
butyrophenone-based	969.2	E853.1	E939.2	E950.3	E962.0	E980.3
major NEC	969.3	E853.8	E939.3	E950.3	E962.0	E980.3
phenothiazine-based	969.1	E853.0	E939.1	E950.3	E962.0	E980.3
28:16.12 other psychotherapeutic agents	969.8	E855.8	E939.8	E950.3	E962.0	E980.3
28:20 respiratory and cerebral stimulants	970.9	E854.3	E940.9	E950.4	E962.0	E980.4
analeptics	970.0	E854.3	E940.0	E950.4	E962.0	E980.4
anorexigenic agents	977.0	E858.8	E947.0	E950.4	E962.0	E980.4
psychostimulants	969.7	E854.2	E939.7	E950.3	E962.0	E980.3
specified NEC	970.8	E854.3	E940.8	E950.4	E962.0	E980.4
28:24 sedatives and hypnotics	967.9	E852.9	E937.9	E950.2	E962.0	E980.2
barbiturates	967.0	E851	E937.0	E950.1	E962.0	E980.1
benzodiazepine-based tranquilizers	969.4	E853.2	E939.4	E950.3	E962.0	E980.3
chloral hydrate (group)	967.1	E852.0	E937.1	E950.2	E962.0	E980.2
glutethimide group	967.5	E852.4	E937.5	E950.2	E962.0	E980.2
intravenous anesthetics	968.3	E855.1	E938.3	E950.4	E962.0	E980.4
methaqualone (compounds)	967.4	E852.3	E937.4	E950.2	E962.0	E980.2
paraldehyde	967.2	E852.1	E937.2	E950.2	E962.0	E980.2
phenothiazine-based tranquilizers	969.1	E853.0	E939.1	E950.3	E962.0	E980.3
specified NEC	967.8	E852.8	E937.8	E950.2	E962.0	E980.2
thiobarbiturates	968.3	E855.1	E938.3	E950.4	E962.0	E980.4
tranquilizer NEC	969.5	E853.9	E939.5	E950.3	E962.0	E980.3
36:04 to 36:88 diagnostic agents	977.8	E858.8	E947.8	E950.4	E962.0	E980.4
40:00 electrolyte, caloric, and water balance agents NEC	974.5	E858.5	E944.5	E950.4	E962.0	E980.4
40:04 acidifying agents	963.2	E858.1	E933.2	E950.4	E962.0	E980.4
40:08 alkalinizing agents	963.3	E858.1	E933.3	E950.4	E962.0	E980.4
40:10 ammonia detoxicants	974.5	E858.5	E944.5	E950.4	E962.0	E980.4
40:12 replacement solutions	974.5	E858.5	E944.5	E950.4	E962.0	E980.4
plasma expanders	964.8	E858.2	E934.8	E950.4	E962.0	E980.4
40:16 sodium-removing resins	974.5	E858.5	E944.5	E950.4	E962.0	E980.4
40:18 potassium-removing resins	974.5	E858.5	E944.5	E950.4	E962.0	E980.4
40:20 caloric agents	974.5	E858.5	E944.5	E950.4	E962.0	E980.4

Substance	Poisoning	External Cause (E-Code)				
		Accident	Therapeutic Use	Suicide Attempt	Assault	Undetermined
Drug *(Continued)*						
40:24 salt and sugar substitutes	974.5	E858.5	E944.5	E950.4	E962.0	E980.4
40:28 diuretics NEC	974.4	E858.5	E944.4	E950.4	E962.0	E980.4
carbonic acid anhydrase inhibitors	974.2	E858.5	E944.2	E950.4	E962.0	E980.4
mercurials	974.0	E858.5	E944.0	E950.4	E962.0	E980.4
purine derivatives	974.1	E858.5	E944.1	E950.4	E962.0	E980.4
saluretics	974.3	E858.5	E944.3	E950.4	E962.0	E980.4
thiazides	974.3	E858.5	E944.3	E950.4	E962.0	E980.4
40:36 irrigating solutions	974.5	E858.5	E944.5	E950.4	E962.0	E980.4
40:40 uricosuric agents	974.7	E858.5	E944.7	E950.4	E962.0	E980.4
44:00 enzymes	963.4	E858.1	E933.4	E950.4	E962.0	E980.4
fibrinolysis-affecting agents	964.4	E858.2	E934.4	E950.4	E962.0	E980.4
gastric agents	973.4	E858.4	E943.4	E950.4	E962.0	E980.4
48:00 expectorants and cough preparations	—	—	—	—	—	—
antihistamine agents	963.0	E858.1	E933.0	E950.4	E962.0	E980.4
antitussives	975.4	E858.6	E945.4	E950.4	E962.0	E980.4
codeine derivatives	965.09	E850.2	E935.2	E950.0	E962.0	E980.0
expectorants	975.5	E858.6	E945.5	E950.4	E962.0	E980.4
narcotic agents NEC	965.09	E850.2	E935.2	E950.0	E962.0	E980.0
52:04 anti-infectives (EENT)	—	—	—	—	—	—
ENT agent	976.6	E858.7	E946.6	E950.4	E962.0	E980.4
ophthalmic preparation	976.5	E858.7	E946.5	E950.4	E962.0	E980.4
52:04.04 antibiotics (EENT)	—	—	—	—	—	—
ENT agent	976.6	E858.7	E946.6	E950.4	E962.0	E980.4
ophthalmic preparation	976.5	E858.7	E946.5	E950.4	E962.0	E980.4
52:04.06 antivirals (EENT)	—	—	—	—	—	—
ENT agent	976.6	E858.7	E946.6	E950.4	E962.0	E980.4
ophthalmic preparation	976.5	E858.7	E946.5	E950.4	E962.0	E980.4
2:04.08 sulfonamides (EENT)	—	—	—	—	—	—
ENT agent	976.6	E858.7	E946.6	E950.4	E962.0	E980.4
ophthalmic preparation	976.5	E858.7	E946.5	E950.4	E962.0	E980.4
52:04.12 miscellaneous anti-infectives (EENT)	—	—	—	—	—	—
ENT agent	976.6	E858.7	E946.6	E950.4	E962.0	E980.4
ophthalmic preparation	976.5	E858.7	E946.5	E950.4	E962.0	E980.4
52:08 anti-inflammatory agents (EENT)	—	—	—	—	—	—
ENT agent	976.6	E858.7	E946.6	E950.4	E962.0	E980.4
ophthalmic preparation	976.5	E858.7	E946.5	E950.4	E962.0	E980.4
52:10 carbonic anhydrase inhibitors	974.2	E858.5	E944.2	E950.4	E962.0	E980.4
52:12 contact lens solutions	976.5	E858.7	E946.5	E950.4	E962.0	E980.4
52:16 local anesthetics (EENT)	968.5	E855.2	E938.5	E950.4	E962.0	E980.4
52:20 miotics	971.0	E855.3	E941.0	E950.4	E962.0	E980.4
52:24 mydriatics	—	—	—	—	—	—
adrenergics	971.2	E855.5	E941.2	E950.4	E962.0	E980.4
anticholinergics	971.1	E855.4	E941.1	E950.4	E962.0	E980.4
antimuscarinics	971.1	E855.4	E941.1	E950.4	E962.0	E980.4
parasympatholytics	971.1	E855.4	E941.1	E950.4	E962.0	E980.4
spasmolytics	971.1	E855.4	E941.1	E950.4	E962.0	E980.4
sympathomimetics	971.2	E855.5	E941.2	E950.4	E962.0	E980.4
52:28 mouth washes and gargles	976.6	E858.7	E946.6	E950.4	E962.0	E980.4
52:32 vasoconstrictors (EENT)	971.2	E855.5	E941.2	E950.4	E962.0	E980.4
52:36 unclassified agents (EENT)	—	—	—	—	—	—
ENT agent	976.6	E858.7	E946.6	E950.4	E962.0	E980.4
ophthalmic preparation	976.5	E858.7	E946.5	E950.4	E962.0	E980.4
56:04 antacids and adsorbents	973.0	E858.4	E943.0	E950.4	E962.0	E980.4
56:08 antidiarrhea agents	973.5	E858.4	E943.5	E950.4	E962.0	E980.4
56:10 antiflatulents	973.8	E858.4	E943.8	E950.4	E962.0	E980.4
56:12 cathartics NEC	973.3	E858.4	E943.3	E950.4	E962.0	E980.4
emollients	973.2	E858.4	E943.2	E950.4	E962.0	E980.4
irritants	973.1	E858.4	E943.1	E950.4	E962.0	E980.4
56:16 digestants	973.4	E858.4	E943.4	E950.4	E962.0	E980.4
56:20 emetics and antiemetics	—	—	—	—	—	—
antiemetics	963.0	E858.1	E933.0	E950.4	E962.0	E980.4
emetics	973.6	E858.4	E943.6	E950.4	E962.0	E980.4

		External Cause (E-Code)				
Substance	**Poisoning**	**Accident**	**Therapeutic Use**	**Suicide Attempt**	**Assault**	**Undetermined**
Drug *(Continued)*						
56:24 lipotropic agents	977.1	E858.8	E947.1	E950.4	E962.0	E980.4
56:40 miscellaneous G.I. drugs	973.8	E858.4	E943.8	E950.4	E962.0	E980.4
60:00 gold compounds	965.69	E850.6	E935.6	E950.0	E962.0	E980.0
64:00 heavy metal antagonists	963.8	E858.1	E933.8	E950.4	E962.0	E980.4
68:04 adrenals	962.0	E858.0	E932.0	E950.4	E962.0	E980.4
68:08 androgens	962.1	E858.0	E932.1	E950.4	E962.0	E980.4
68:12 contraceptives, oral	962.2	E858.0	E932.2	E950.4	E962.0	E980.4
68:16 estrogens	962.2	E858.0	E932.2	E950.4	E962.0	E980.4
68:18 gonadotropins	962.4	E858.0	E932.4	E950.4	E962.0	E980.4
68:20 insulins and antidiabetic agents	962.3	E858.0	E932.3	E950.4	E962.0	E980.4
68:20.08 insulins	962.3	E858.0	E932.3	E950.4	E962.0	E980.4
68:24 parathyroid	962.6	E858.0	E932.6	E950.4	E962.0	E980.4
68:28 pituitary (posterior)	962.5	E858.0	E932.5	E950.4	E962.0	E980.4
anterior	962.4	E858.0	E932.4	E950.4	E962.0	E980.4
68:32 progestogens	962.2	E858.0	E932.2	E950.4	E962.0	E980.4
68:34 other corpus luteum hormones NEC	962.2	E858.0	E932.2	E950.4	E962.0	E980.4
68:36 thyroid and antithyroid	—	—	—	—	—	—
antithyroid	962.8	E858.0	E932.8	E950.4	E962.0	E980.4
thyroid (derivatives)	962.7	E858.0	E932.7	E950.4	E962.0	E980.4
72:00 local anesthetics NEC	968.9	E855.2	E938.9	E950.4	E962.0	E980.4
topical (surface)	968.5	E855.2	E938.5	E950.4	E962.0	E980.4
infiltration (intradermal) (subcutaneous) (submucosal)	968.5	E855.2	E938.5	E950.4	E962.0	E980.4
nerve blocking (peripheral) (plexus) (regional)	968.6	E855.2	E938.6	E950.4	E962.0	E980.4
spinal	968.7	E855.2	E938.7	E950.4	E962.0	E980.4
76:00 oxytocics	975.0	E858.6	E945.0	E950.4	E962.0	E980.4
78:00 radioactive agents	990	—	—	—	—	—
80:04 serums NEC	979.9	E858.8	E949.9	E950.4	E962.0	E980.4
immune gamma globulin (human)	964.6	E858.2	E934.6	E950.4	E962.0	E980.4
80:08 toxoids NEC	978.8	E858.8	E948.8	E950.4	E962.0	E980.4
diphtheria	978.5	E858.8	E948.5	E950.4	E962.0	E980.4
and tetanus	978.9	E858.8	E948.9	E950.4	E962.0	E980.4
with pertussis component	978.6	E858.8	E948.6	E950.4	E962.0	E980.4
tetanus	978.4	E858.8	E948.4	E950.4	E962.0	E980.4
and diphtheria	978.9	E858.8	E948.9	E950.4	E962.0	E980.4
with pertussis component	978.6	E858.8	E948.6	E950.4	E962.0	E980.4
80:12 vaccines	979.9	E858.8	E949.9	E950.4	E962.0	E980.4
bacterial NEC	978.8	E858.8	E948.8	E950.4	E962.0	E980.4
with	—	—	—	—	—	—
other bacterial components	978.9	E858.8	E948.9	E950.4	E962.0	E980.4
pertussis component	978.6	E858.8	E948.6	E950.4	E962.0	E980.4
viral and rickettsial components	979.7	E858.8	E949.7	E950.4	E962.0	E980.4
rickettsial NEC	979.6	E858.8	E949.6	E950.4	E962.0	E980.4
with	—	—	—	—	—	—
bacterial component	979.7	E858.8	E949.7	E950.4	E962.0	E980.4
pertussis component	978.6	E858.8	E948.6	E950.4	E962.0	E980.4
viral component	979.7	E858.8	E949.7	E950.4	E962.0	E980.4
viral NEC	979.6	E858.8	E949.6	E950.4	E962.0	E980.4
with	—	—	—	—	—	—
bacterial component	979.7	E858.8	E949.7	E950.4	E962.0	E980.4
pertussis component	978.6	E858.8	E948.6	E950.4	E962.0	E980.4
rickettsial component	979.7	E858.8	E949.7	E950.4	E962.0	E980.4
84:04.04 antibiotics (skin and mucous membrane)	976.0	E858.7	E946.0	E950.4	E962.0	E980.4
84:04.08 fungicides (skin and mucous membrane)	976.0	E858.7	E946.0	E950.4	E962.0	E980.4
84:04.12 scabicides and pediculicides (skin and mucous membrane)	976.0	E858.7	E946.0	E950.4	E962.0	E980.4
84:04.16 miscellaneous local anti-infectives (skin and mucous membrane)	976.0	E858.7	E946.0	E950.4	E962.0	E980.4
84:06 anti-inflammatory agents (skin and mucous membrane)	976.0	E858.7	E946.0	E950.4	E962.0	E980.4
84:08 antipruritics and local anesthetics	—	—	—	—	—	—
antipruritics	976.1	E858.7	E946.1	E950.4	E962.0	E980.4
local anesthetics	968.5	E855.2	E938.5	E950.4	E962.0	E980.4
84:12 astringents	976.2	E858.7	E946.2	E950.4	E962.0	E980.4
84:16 cell stimulants and proliferants	976.8	E858.7	E946.8	E950.4	E962.0	E980.4
84:20 detergents	976.2	E858.7	E946.2	E950.4	E962.0	E980.4

ICD-9-CM
Drugs
Vol.

Substance	Poisoning	External Cause (E-Code)				
		Accident	Therapeutic Use	Suicide Attempt	Assault	Undetermined
Drug *(Continued)*						
84:24 emollients, demulcents, and protectants	976.3	E858.7	E946.3	E950.4	E962.0	E980.4
84:28 keratolytic agents	976.4	E858.7	E946.4	E950.4	E962.0	E980.4
84:32 keratoplastic agents	976.4	E858.7	E946.4	E950.4	E962.0	E980.4
84:36 miscellaneous agents (skin and mucous membrane)	976.8	E858.7	E946.8	E950.4	E962.0	E980.4
86:00 spasmolytic agents	975.1	E858.6	E945.1	E950.4	E962.0	E980.4
antiasthmatics	975.7	E858.6	E945.7	E950.4	E962.0	E980.4
papaverine	972.5	E858.3	E942.5	E950.4	E962.0	E980.4
theophylline	974.1	E858.5	E944.1	E950.4	E962.0	E980.4
88:04 vitamin A	963.5	E858.1	E933.5	E950.4	E962.0	E980.4
88:08 vitamin B complex	963.5	E858.1	E933.5	E950.4	E962.0	E980.4
hematopoietic vitamin	964.1	E858.2	E934.1	E950.4	E962.0	E980.4
nicotinic acid derivatives	972.2	E858.3	E942.2	E950.4	E962.0	E980.4
88:12 vitamin C	963.5	E858.1	E933.5	E950.4	E962.0	E980.4
88:16 vitamin D	963.5	E858.1	E933.5	E950.4	E962.0	E980.4
88:20 vitamin E	963.5	E858.1	E933.5	E950.4	E962.0	E980.4
88:24 vitamin K activity	964.3	E858.2	E934.3	E950.4	E962.0	E980.4
88:28 multivitamin preparations	963.5	E858.1	E933.5	E950.4	E962.0	E980.4
92:00 unclassified therapeutic agents	977.8	E858.8	E947.8	E950.4	E962.0	E980.4
Duboisine	971.1	E855.4	E941.1	E950.4	E962.0	E980.4
Dulcolax	973.1	E858.4	E943.1	E950.4	E962.0	E980.4
Duponol (C) (EP)	976.2	E858.7	E946.2	E950.4	E962.0	E980.4
Durabolin	962.1	E858.0	E932.1	E950.4	E962.0	E980.4
Dyclone	968.5	E855.2	E938.5	E950.4	E962.0	E980.4
Dyclonine	968.5	E855.2	E938.5	E950.4	E962.0	E980.4
Dydrogesterone	962.2	E858.0	E932.2	E950.4	E962.0	E980.4
Dyes NEC	989.89	E866.8	—	E950.9	E962.1	E980.9
diagnostic agents	977.8	E858.8	E947.8	E950.4	E962.0	E980.4
pharmaceutical NEC	977.4	E858.8	E947.4	E950.4	E962.0	E980.4
Dyflos	971.0	E855.3	E941.0	E950.4	E962.0	E980.4
Dymelor	962.3	E858.0	E932.3	E950.4	E962.0	E980.4
Dynamite	989.89	E866.8	—	E950.9	E962.1	E980.9
fumes	987.8	E869.8	—	E952.8	E962.2	E982.8
Dyphylline	975.1	E858.6	E945.1	E950.4	E962.0	E980.4
Ear preparations	976.6	E858.7	E946.6	E950.4	E962.0	E980.4
Echothiopate, ecothiopate	971.0	E855.3	E941.0	E950.4	E962.0	E980.4
Ecstasy	969.7	E854.2	E939.7	E950.3	E962.0	E980.3
Ectylurea	967.8	E852.8	E937.8	E950.2	E962.0	E980.2
Edathamil disodium	963.8	E858.1	E933.8	E950.4	E962.0	E980.4
Edecrin	974.4	E858.5	E944.4	E950.4	E962.0	E980.4
Edetate, disodium (calcium)	963.8	E858.1	E933.8	E950.4	E962.0	E980.4
Edrophonium	971.0	E855.3	E941.0	E950.4	E962.0	E980.4
Elase	976.8	E858.7	E946.8	E950.4	E962.0	E980.4
Elaterium	973.1	E858.4	E943.1	E950.4	E962.0	E980.4
Elder	988.2	E865.4	—	E950.9	E962.1	E980.9
berry (unripe)	988.2	E865.3	—	E950.9	E962.1	E980.9
Electrolytes NEC	974.5	E858.5	E944.5	E950.4	E962.0	E980.4
Electrolytic agent NEC	974.5	E858.5	E944.5	E950.4	E962.0	E980.4
Embramine	963.0	E858.1	E933.0	E950.4	E962.0	E980.4
Emetics	973.6	E858.4	E943.6	E950.4	E962.0	E980.4
Emetine (hydrochloride)	961.5	E857	E931.5	E950.4	E962.0	E980.4
Emollients	976.3	E858.7	E946.3	E950.4	E962.0	E980.4
Emylcamate	969.5	E853.8	E939.5	E950.3	E962.0	E980.3
Encyprate	969.0	E854.0	E939.0	E950.3	E962.0	E980.3
Endocaine	968.5	E855.2	E938.5	E950.4	E962.0	E980.4
Endrin	989.2	E863.0	—	E950.6	E962.1	E980.7
Enflurane	968.2	E855.1	E938.2	E950.4	E962.0	E980.4
Enovid	962.2	E858.0	E932.2	E950.4	E962.0	E980.4
ENT preparations (anti-infectives)	976.6	E858.7	E946.6	E950.4	E962.0	E980.4
Enzodase	963.4	E858.1	E933.4	E950.4	E962.0	E980.4
Enzymes NEC	963.4	E858.1	E933.4	E950.4	E962.0	E980.4
Epanutin	966.1	E855.0	E936.1	E950.4	E962.0	E980.4
Ephedra (tincture)	971.2	E855.5	E941.2	E950.4	E962.0	E980.4

ICD-9-CM

Drugs

Vol. 2

Substance	Poisoning	External Cause (E-Code)				
		Accident	Therapeutic Use	Suicide Attempt	Assault	Undetermined
Ephedrine	971.2	E855.5	E941.2	E950.4	E962.0	E980.4
Epiestriol	962.2	E858.0	E932.2	E950.4	E962.0	E980.4
Epilim - see Sodium valproate	—	—	—	—	—	—
Epinephrine	971.2	E855.5	E941.2	E950.4	E962.0	E980.4
Epsom salt	973.3	E858.4	E943.3	E950.4	E962.0	E980.4
Equanil	969.5	E853.8	E939.5	E950.3	E962.0	E980.3
Equisetum (diuretic)	974.4	E858.5	E944.4	E950.4	E962.0	E980.4
Ergometrine	975.0	E858.6	E945.0	E950.4	E962.0	E980.4
Ergonovine	975.0	E858.6	E945.0	E950.4	E962.0	E980.4
Ergot NEC	988.2	E865.4	—	E950.9	E962.1	E980.9
medicinal (alkaloids)	975.0	E858.6	E945.0	E950.4	E962.0	E980.4
Ergotamine (tartrate) (for migraine) NEC	972.9	E858.3	E942.9	E950.4	E962.0	E980.4
Ergotrate	975.0	E858.6	E945.0	E950.4	E962.0	E980.4
Erythrityl tetranitrate	972.4	E858.3	E942.4	E950.4	E962.0	E980.4
Erythrol tetranitrate	972.4	E858.3	E942.4	E950.4	E962.0	E980.4
Erythromycin	960.3	E856	E930.3	E950.4	E962.0	E980.4
ophthalmic preparation	976.5	E858.7	E946.5	E950.4	E962.0	E980.4
topical NEC	976.0	E858.7	E946.0	E950.4	E962.0	E980.4
Eserine	971.0	E855.3	E941.0	E950.4	E962.0	E980.4
Eskabarb	967.0	E851	E937.0	E950.1	E962.0	E980.1
Eskalith	969.8	E855.8	E939.8	E950.3	E962.0	E980.3
Estradiol (cypionate) (dipropionate) (valerate)	962.2	E858.0	E932.2	E950.4	E962.0	E980.4
Estriol	962.2	E858.0	E932.2	E950.4	E962.0	E980.4
Estrogens (with progestogens)	962.2	E858.0	E932.2	E950.4	E962.0	E980.4
Estrone	962.2	E858.0	E932.2	E950.4	E962.0	E980.4
Etafedrine	971.2	E855.5	E941.2	E950.4	E962.0	E980.4
Ethacrynate sodium	974.4	E858.5	E944.4	E950.4	E962.0	E980.4
Ethacrynic acid	974.4	E858.5	E944.4	E950.4	E962.0	E980.4
Ethambutol	961.8	E857	E931.8	E950.4	E962.0	E980.4
Ethamide	974.2	E858.5	E944.2	E950.4	E962.0	E980.4
Ethamivan	970.0	E854.3	E940.0	E950.4	E962.0	E980.4
Ethamsylate	964.5	E858.2	E934.5	E950.4	E962.0	E980.4
Ethanol	980.0	E860.1	—	E950.9	E962.1	E980.9
beverage	980.0	E860.0	—	E950.9	E962.1	E980.9
Ethchlorvynol	967.8	E852.8	E937.8	E950.2	E962.0	E980.2
Ethebenecid	974.7	E858.5	E944.7	E950.4	E962.0	E980.4
Ether(s) (diethyl) (ethyl) (vapor)	987.8	E869.8	—	E952.8	E962.2	E982.8
anesthetic	968.2	E855.1	E938.2	E950.4	E962.0	E980.4
petroleum - see Ligroin solvent	982.8	E862.4	—	E950.9	E962.1	E980.9
Ethidine chloride (vapor)	987.8	E869.8	—	E952.8	E962.2	E982.8
liquid (solvent)	982.3	E862.4	—	E950.9	E962.1	E980.9
Ethinamate	967.8	E852.8	E937.8	E950.2	E962.0	E980.2
Ethinylestradiol	962.2	E858.0	E932.2	E950.4	E962.0	E980.4
Ethionamide	961.8	E857	E931.8	E950.4	E962.0	E980.4
Ethisterone	962.2	E858.0	E932.2	E950.4	E962.0	E980.4
Ethobral	967.0	E851	E937.0	E950.1	E962.0	E980.1
Ethocaine (infiltration) (topical)	968.5	E855.2	E938.5	E950.4	E962.0	E980.4
nerve block (peripheral) (plexus)	968.6	E855.2	E938.6	E950.4	E962.0	E980.4
spinal	968.7	E855.2	E938.7	E950.4	E962.0	E980.4
Ethoheptazine (citrate)	965.7	E850.7	E935.7	E950.0	E962.0	E980.0
Ethopropazine	966.4	E855.0	E936.4	E950.4	E962.0	E980.4
Ethosuximide	966.2	E855.0	E936.2	E950.4	E962.0	E980.4
Ethotoin	966.1	E855.0	E936.1	E950.4	E962.0	E980.4
Ethoxazene	961.9	E857	E931.9	E950.4	E962.0	E980.4
Ethoxzolamide	974.2	E858.5	E944.2	E950.4	E962.0	E980.4
Ethyl	—	—	—	—	—	—
acetate (vapor)	982.8	E862.4	—	E950.9	E962.1	E980.9
alcohol	980.0	E860.1	—	E950.9	E962.1	E980.9
beverage	980.0	E860.0	—	E950.9	E962.1	E980.9
aldehyde (vapor)	987.8	E869.8	—	E952.8	E962.2	E982.8
liquid	989.89	E866.8	—	E950.9	E962.1	E980.9
aminobenzoate	968.5	E855.2	E938.5	E950.4	E962.0	E980.4

Substance	Poisoning	External Cause (E-Code)				
		Accident	Therapeutic Use	Suicide Attempt	Assault	Undetermined
Ethyl *(Continued)*						
biscoumacetate	964.2	E858.2	E934.2	E950.4	E962.0	E980.4
bromide (anesthetic)	968.2	E855.1	E938.2	E950.4	E962.0	E980.4
carbamate (antineoplastic)	963.1	E858.1	E933.1	E950.4	E962.0	E980.4
carbinol	980.3	E860.4	—	E950.9	E962.1	E980.9
chaulmoograte	961.8	E857	E931.8	E950.4	E962.0	E980.4
chloride (vapor)	987.8	E869.8	—	E952.8	E962.2	E982.8
anesthetic (local)	968.5	E855.2	E938.5	E950.4	E962.0	E980.4
inhaled	968.2	E855.1	E938.2	E950.4	E962.0	E980.4
solvent	982.3	E862.4	—	E950.9	E962.1	E980.9
estranol	962.1	E858.0	E932.1	E950.4	E962.0	E980.4
ether - *see* Ether(s)	—	—	—	—	—	—
formate (solvent) NEC	982.8	E862.4	—	E950.9	E962.1	E980.9
iodoacetate	987.5	E869.3	—	E952.8	E962.2	E982.8
lactate (solvent) NEC	982.8	E862.4	—	E950.9	E962.1	E980.9
methylcarbinol	980.8	E860.8	—	E950.9	E962.1	E980.9
morphine	965.09	E850.2	E935.2	E950.0	E962.0	E980.0
Ethylene (gas)	987.1	E869.8	—	E952.8	E962.2	E982.8
anesthetic (general)	968.2	E855.1	E938.2	E950.4	E962.0	E980.4
chlorohydrin (vapor)	982.3	E862.4	—	E950.9	E962.1	E980.9
dichloride (vapor)	982.3	E862.4	—	E950.9	E962.1	E980.9
glycol(s) (any) (vapor)	982.8	E862.4	—	E950.9	E962.1	E980.9
Ethylidene	—	—	—	—	—	—
chloride NEC	982.3	E862.4	—	E950.9	E962.1	E980.9
diethyl ether	982.8	E862.4	—	E950.9	E962.1	E980.9
Ethynodiol	962.2	E858.0	E932.2	E950.4	E962.0	E980.4
Etidocaine	968.9	E855.2	E938.9	E950.4	E962.0	E980.4
infiltration (subcutaneous)	968.5	E855.2	E938.5	E950.4	E962.0	E980.4
nerve (peripheral) (plexus)	968.6	E855.2	E938.6	E950.4	E962.0	E980.4
Etilfen	967.0	E851	E937.0	E950.1	E962.0	E980.1
Etomide	965.7	E850.7	E935.7	E950.0	E962.0	E980.0
Etorphine	965.09	E850.2	E935.2	E950.0	E962.0	E980.0
Etoval	967.0	E851	E937.0	E950.1	E962.0	E980.1
Etryptamine	969.0	E854.0	E939.0	E950.3	E962.0	E980.3
Eucaine	968.5	E855.2	E938.5	E950.4	E962.0	E980.4
Eucalyptus (oil) NEC	975.5	E858.6	E945.5	E950.4	E962.0	E980.4
Eucatropine	971.1	E855.4	E941.1	E950.4	E962.0	E980.4
Eucodal	965.09	E850.2	E935.2	E950.0	E962.0	E980.0
Euneryl	967.0	E851	E937.0	E950.1	E962.0	E980.1
Euphthalmine	971.1	E855.4	E941.1	E950.4	E962.0	E980.4
Eurax	976.0	E858.7	E946.0	E950.4	E962.0	E980.4
Euresol	976.4	E858.7	E946.4	E950.4	E962.0	E980.4
Euthroid	962.7	E858.0	E932.7	E950.4	E962.0	E980.4
Evans blue	977.8	E858.8	E947.8	E950.4	E962.0	E980.4
Evipal	967.0	E851	E937.0	E950.1	E962.0	E980.1
sodium	968.3	E855.1	E938.3	E950.4	E962.0	E980.4
Evipan	967.0	E851	E937.0	E950.1	E962.0	E980.1
sodium	968.3	E855.1	E938.3	E950.4	E962.0	E980.4
Exalgin	965.4	E850.4	E935.4	E950.0	E962.0	E980.0
Excipients, pharmaceutical	977.4	E858.8	E947.4	E950.4	E962.0	E980.4
Exhaust gas - *see* Carbon, monoxide	—	—	—	—	—	—
Ex-Lax (phenolphthalein)	973.1	E858.4	E943.1	E950.4	E962.0	E980.4
Expectorants	975.5	E858.6	E945.5	E950.4	E962.0	E980.4
External medications (skin) (mucous membrane)	976.9	E858.7	E946.9	E950.4	E962.0	E980.4
dental agent	976.7	E858.7	E946.7	E950.4	E962.0	E980.4
ENT agent	976.6	E858.7	E946.6	E950.4	E962.0	E980.4
ophthalmic preparation	976.5	E858.7	E946.5	E950.4	E962.0	E980.4
specified NEC	976.8	E858.7	E946.8	E950.4	E962.0	E980.4
Eye agents (anti-infective)	976.5	E858.7	E946.5	E950.4	E962.0	E980.4
Factor IX complex (human)	964.5	E858.2	E934.5	E950.4	E962.0	E980.4
Fecal softeners	973.2	E858.4	E943.2	E950.4	E962.0	E980.4
Fenbutrazate	977.0	E858.8	E947.0	E950.4	E962.0	E980.4

◄ New   ◄▥ Revised

ICD-9-CM

Drugs

Vol.

Substance	Poisoning	External Cause (E-Code)				
		Accident	Therapeutic Use	Suicide Attempt	Assault	Undetermined
Fencamfamin	970.8	E854.3	E940.8	E950.4	E962.0	E980.4
Fenfluramine	977.0	E858.8	E947.0	E950.4	E962.0	E980.4
Fenoprofen	965.61	E850.6	E935.6	E950.0	E962.0	E980.0
Fentanyl	965.09	E850.2	E935.2	E950.0	E962.0	E980.0
Fentazin	969.1	E853.0	E939.1	E930.3	E962.0	E980.3
Fenticlor, fentichlor	976.0	E858.7	E946.0	E950.4	E962.0	E980.4
Fer de lance (bite) (venom)	989.5	E905.0	—	E950.9	E962.1	E980.9
Ferric - see Iron	—	—	—	—	—	—
Ferrocholinate	964.0	E858.2	E934.0	E950.4	E962.0	E980.4
Ferrous fumerate, gluconate, lactate, salt NEC, sulfate (medicinal)	964.0	E858.2	E934.0	E950.4	E962.0	E980.4
Ferrum - see Iron	—	—	—	—	—	—
Fertilizers NEC	989.89	E866.5	—	E950.9	E962.1	E980.4
with herbicide mixture	989.4	E863.5	—	E950.6	E962.1	E980.7
Fibrinogen (human)	964.7	E858.2	E934.7	E950.4	E962.0	E980.4
Fibrinolysin	964.4	E858.2	E934.4	E950.4	E962.0	E980.4
Fibrinolysis-affecting agents	964.4	E858.2	E934.4	E950.4	E962.0	E980.4
Filix mas	961.6	E857	E931.6	E950.4	E962.0	E980.4
Fiorinal	965.1	E850.3	E935.3	E950.0	E962.0	E980.0
Fire damp	987.1	E869.8	—	E952.8	E962.2	E982.8
Fish, nonbacterial or noxious	988.0	E865.2	—	E950.9	E962.1	E980.9
shell	988.0	E865.1	—	E950.9	E962.1	E980.9
Flagyl	961.5	E857	E931.5	E950.4	E962.0	E980.4
Flavoxate	975.1	E858.6	E945.1	E950.4	E962.0	E980.4
Flaxedil	975.2	E858.6	E945.2	E950.4	E962.0	E980.4
Flaxseed (medicinal)	976.3	E858.7	E946.3	E950.4	E962.0	E980.4
Florantyrone	973.4	E858.4	E943.4	E950.4	E962.0	E980.4
Floraquin	961.3	E857	E931.3	E950.4	E962.0	E980.4
Florinef	962.0	E858.0	E932.0	E950.4	E962.0	E980.4
ENT agent	976.6	E858.7	E946.6	E950.4	E962.0	E980.4
ophthalmic preparation	976.5	E858.7	E946.5	E950.4	E962.0	E980.4
topical NEC	976.0	E858.7	E946.0	E950.4	E962.0	E980.4
Flowers of sulfur	976.4	E858.7	E946.4	E950.4	E962.0	E980.4
Floxuridine	963.1	E858.1	E933.1	E950.4	E962.0	E980.4
Flucytosine	961.9	E857	E931.9	E950.4	E962.0	E980.4
Fludrocortisone	962.0	E858.0	E932.0	E950.4	E962.0	E980.4
ENT agent	976.6	E858.7	E946.6	E950.4	E962.0	E980.4
ophthalmic preparation	976.5	E858.7	E946.5	E950.4	E962.0	E980.4
topical NEC	976.0	E858.7	E946.0	E950.4	E962.0	E980.4
Flumethasone	976.0	E858.7	E946.0	E950.4	E962.0	E980.4
Flumethiazide	974.3	E858.5	E944.3	E950.4	E962.0	E980.4
Flumidin	961.7	E857	E931.7	E950.4	E962.0	E980.4
Flunitrazepam	969.4	E853.2	E939.4	E950.3	E962.0	E980.3
Fluocinolone	976.0	E858.7	E946.0	E950.4	E962.0	E980.4
Fluocortolone	962.0	E858.0	E932.0	E950.4	E962.0	E980.4
Fluohydrocortisone	962.0	E858.0	E932.0	E950.4	E962.0	E980.4
ENT agent	976.6	E858.7	E946.6	E950.4	E962.0	E980.4
ophthalmic preparation	976.5	E858.7	E946.5	E950.4	E962.0	E980.4
topical NEC	976.0	E858.7	E946.0	E950.4	E962.0	E980.4
Fluonid	976.0	E858.7	E946.0	E950.4	E962.0	E980.4
Fluopromazine	969.1	E853.0	E939.1	E950.3	E962.0	E980.3
Fluoracetate	989.4	E863.7	—	E950.6	E962.1	E980.7
Fluorescein (sodium)	977.8	E858.8	E947.8	E950.4	E962.0	E980.4
Fluoride(s) (pesticides) (sodium) NEC	989.4	E863.4	—	E950.6	E962.1	E980.7
hydrogen - see Hydrofluoric acid	—	—	—	—	—	—
medicinal	976.7	E858.7	E946.7	E950.4	E962.0	E980.4
not pesticide NEC	983.9	E864.4	—	E950.7	E962.1	E980.6
stannous	976.7	E858.7	E946.7	E950.4	E962.0	E980.4
Fluorinated corticosteroids	962.0	E858.0	E932.0	E950.4	E962.0	E980.4
Fluorine (compounds) (gas)	987.8	E869.8	—	E952.8	E962.2	E982.8
salt - see Fluoride(s)	—	—	—	—	—	—
Fluoristan	976.7	E858.7	E946.7	E950.4	E962.0	E980.4
Fluoroacetate	989.4	E863.7	—	E950.6	E962.1	E980.7
Fluorodeoxyuridine	963.1	E858.1	E933.1	E950.4	E962.0	E980.4

			External Cause (E-Code)			
Substance	Poisoning	Accident	Therapeutic Use	Suicide Attempt	Assault	Undetermined
Fluorometholone (topical) NEC	976.0	E858.7	E946.0	E950.4	E962.0	E980.4
ophthalmic preparation	976.5	E858.7	E946.5	E950.4	E962.0	E980.4
Fluorouracil	963.1	E858.1	E933.1	E950.4	E962.0	E980.4
Fluothane	968.1	E855.1	E938.1	E950.4	E962.0	E980.4
Fluoxetine hydrochloride	969.0	E854.0	E939.0	E950.3	E962.0	E980.3
Fluoxymesterone	962.1	E858.0	E932.1	E950.4	E962.0	E980.4
Fluphenazine	969.1	E853.0	E939.1	E950.3	E962.0	E980.3
Fluprednisolone	962.0	E858.0	E932.0	E950.4	E962.0	E980.4
Flurandrenolide	976.0	E858.7	E946.0	E950.4	E962.0	E980.4
Flurazepam (hydrochloride)	969.4	E853.2	E939.4	E950.3	E962.0	E980.3
Flurbiprofen	965.61	E850.6	E935.6	E950.0	E962.0	E980.0
Flurobate	976.0	E858.7	E946.0	E950.4	E962.0	E980.4
Flurothyl	969.8	E855.8	E939.8	E950.3	E962.0	E980.3
Fluroxene	968.2	E855.1	E938.2	E950.4	E962.0	E980.4
Folacin	964.1	E858.2	E934.1	E950.4	E962.0	E980.4
Folic acid	964.1	E858.2	E934.1	E950.4	E962.0	E980.4
Follicle stimulating hormone	962.4	E858.0	E932.4	E950.4	E962.0	E980.4
Food, foodstuffs, nonbacterial or noxious	988.9	E865.9	—	E950.9	E962.1	E980.9
berries, seeds	988.2	E865.3	—	E950.9	E962.1	E980.9
fish	988.0	E865.2	—	E950.9	E962.1	E980.9
mushrooms	988.1	E865.5	—	E950.9	E962.1	E980.9
plants	988.2	E865.9	—	E950.9	E962.1	E980.9
specified type NEC	988.2	E865.4	—	E950.9	E962.1	E980.9
shellfish	988.0	E865.1	—	E950.9	E962.1	E980.9
specified NEC	988.8	E865.8	—	E950.9	E962.1	E980.9
Fool's parsley	988.2	E865.4	—	E950.9	E962.1	E980.9
Formaldehyde (solution)	989.89	E861.4	—	E950.9	E962.1	E980.9
fungicide	989.4	E863.6	—	E950.6	E962.1	E980.7
gas or vapor	987.8	E869.8	—	E952.8	E962.2	E982.8
Formalin	989.89	E861.4	—	E950.9	E962.1	E980.9
fungicide	989.4	E863.6	—	E950.6	E962.1	E980.7
vapor	987.8	E869.8	—	E952.8	E962.2	E982.8
Formic acid	983.1	E864.1	—	E950.7	E962.1	E980.6
vapor	987.8	E869.8	—	E952.8	E962.2	E982.8
Fowler's solution	985.1	E866.3	—	E950.8	E962.1	E980.8
Foxglove	988.2	E865.4	—	E950.9	E962.1	E980.9
Fox green	977.8	E858.8	E947.8	E950.4	E962.0	E980.4
Framycetin	960.8	E856	E930.8	E950.4	E962.0	E980.4
Frangula (extract)	973.1	E858.4	E943.1	E950.4	E962.0	E980.4
Frei antigen	977.8	E858.8	E947.8	E950.4	E962.0	E980.4
Freons	987.4	E869.2	—	E952.8	E962.2	E982.8
Fructose	974.5	E858.5	E944.5	E950.4	E962.0	E980.4
Frusemide	974.4	E858.5	E944.4	E950.4	E962.0	E980.4
FSH	962.4	E858.0	E932.4	E950.4	E962.0	E980.4
Fuel	—	—	—	—	—	—
automobile	981	E862.1	—	E950.9	E962.1	E980.9
exhaust gas, not in transit	986	E868.2	—	E952.0	E962.2	E982.0
vapor NEC	987.1	E869.8	—	E952.8	E962.2	E982.8
gas (domestic use) - see also Carbon, monoxide, fuel	—	—	—	—	—	—
utility	987.1	E868.1	—	E951.8	E962.2	E981.8
incomplete combustion of - see Carbon, monoxide, fuel, utility	—	—	—	—	—	—
in mobile container	987.0	E868.0	—	E951.1	E962.2	E981.1
piped (natural)	987.1	E867	—	E951.0	E962.2	E981.0
industrial, incomplete combustion	986	E868.3	—	E952.1	E962.2	E982.1
Fugillin	960.8	E856	E930.8	E950.4	E962.0	E980.4
Fulminate of mercury	985.0	E866.1	—	E950.9	E962.1	E980.9
Fulvicin	960.1	E856	E930.1	E950.4	E962.0	E980.4
Fumadil	960.8	E856	E930.8	E950.4	E962.0	E980.4
Fumagillin	960.8	E856	E930.8	E950.4	E962.0	E980.4
Fumes (from)	987.9	E869.9	—	E952.9	E962.2	E982.9
carbon monoxide - see Carbon, monoxide	—	—	—	—	—	—
charcoal (domestic use)	986	E868.3	—	E952.1	E962.2	E982.1

◀ New   ◀█ Revised

Substance	Poisoning	External Cause (E-Code)				
		Accident	Therapeutic Use	Suicide Attempt	Assault	Undetermined
Fumes *(Continued)*						
chloroform - *see* Chloroform						
coke (in domestic stoves, fireplaces)	986	E868.3	—	E952.1	E962.2	E982.1
corrosive NEC	987.8	E869.8	—	E952.8	E962.2	E982.8
ether - *see* Ether(s)						
freons	987.4	E869.2	—	E952.8	E962.2	E982.8
hydrocarbons	987.1	E869.8	—	E952.8	E962.2	E982.8
petroleum (liquefied)	987.0	E868.0	—	E951.1	E962.2	E981.1
distributed through pipes (pure or mixed with air)	987.0	E867	—	E951.0	E962.2	E981.0
lead - *see* Lead	—	—	—	—	—	—
metals - *see* specified metal	—	—	—	—	—	—
nitrogen dioxide	987.2	E869.0	—	E952.8	E962.2	E982.8
pesticides - *see* Pesticides	—	—	—	—	—	—
petroleum (liquefied)	987.0	E868.0	—	E951.1	E962.2	E981.1
distributed through pipes (pure or mixed with air)	987.0	E867	—	E951.0	E962.2	E981.0
polyester	987.8	E869.8	—	E952.8	E962.2	E982.8
specified source, other (*see also* substance specified)	987.8	E869.8	—	E952.8	E962.2	E982.8
sulfur dioxide	987.3	E869.1	—	E952.8	E962.2	E982.8
Fumigants	989.4	E863.8	—	E950.6	E962.1	E980.7
Fungi, noxious, used as food	988.1	E865.5	—	E950.9	E962.1	E980.9
Fungicides (*see also* Antifungals)	989.4	E863.6	—	E950.6	E962.1	E980.7
Fungizone	960.1	E856	E930.1	E950.4	E962.0	E980.4
topical	976.0	E858.7	E946.0	E950.4	E962.0	E980.4
Furacin	976.0	E858.7	E946.0	E950.4	E962.0	E980.4
Furadantin	961.9	E857	E931.9	E950.4	E962.0	E980.4
Furazolidone	961.9	E857	E931.9	E950.4	E962.0	E980.4
Furnace (coal burning) (domestic), gas from	986	E868.3	—	E952.1	E962.2	E982.1
industrial	986	E868.8	—	E952.1	E962.2	E982.1
Furniture polish	989.89	E861.2	—	E950.9	E962.1	E980.9
Furosemide	974.4	E858.5	E944.4	E950.4	E962.0	E980.4
Furoxone	961.9	E857	E931.9	E950.4	E962.0	E980.4
Fusel oil (amyl) (butyl) (propyl)	980.3	E860.4	—	E950.9	E962.1	E980.9
Fusidic acid	960.8	E856	E930.8	E950.4	E962.0	E980.4
Gallamine	975.2	E858.6	E945.2	E950.4	E962.0	E980.4
Gallotannic acid	976.2	E858.7	E946.2	E950.4	E962.0	E980.4
Gamboge	973.1	E858.4	E943.1	E950.4	E962.0	E980.4
Gamimune	964.6	E858.2	E934.6	E950.4	E962.0	E980.4
Gamma-benzene hexachloride (vapor)	989.2	E863.0	—	E950.6	E962.1	E980.7
Gamma globulin	964.6	E858.2	E934.6	E950.4	E962.0	E980.4
Gamma hydroxy butyrate (GHB)	968.4	E855.1	E938.4	E950.4	E962.0	E980.4
Gamulin	964.6	E858.2	E934.6	E950.4	E962.0	E980.4
Ganglionic blocking agents	972.3	E858.3	E942.3	E950.4	E962.0	E980.4
Ganja	969.6	E854.1	E939.6	E950.3	E962.0	E980.3
Garamycin	960.8	E856	E930.8	E950.4	E962.0	E980.4
ophthalmic preparation	976.5	E858.7	E946.5	E950.4	E962.0	E980.4
topical NEC	976.0	E858.7	E946.0	E950.4	E962.0	E980.4
Gardenal	967.0	E851	E937.0	E950.1	E962.0	E980.1
Gardepanyl	967.0	E851	E937.0	E950.1	E962.0	E980.1
Gas	987.9	E869.9	—	E952.9	E962.2	E982.9
acetylene	987.1	E868.1	—	E951.8	E962.2	E981.8
incomplete combustion of - *see* Carbon, monoxide, fuel, utility	—	—	—	—	—	—
air contaminants, source or type not specified	987.9	E869.9	—	E952.9	E962.2	E982.9
anesthetic (general) NEC	968.2	E855.1	E938.2	E950.4	E962.0	E980.4
blast furnace	986	E868.8	—	E952.1	E962.2	E982.1
butane - *see* Butane	—	—	—	—	—	—
carbon monoxide - *see* Carbon, monoxide, chlorine	987.6	E869.8	—	E952.8	E962.2	E982.8
coal - *see* Carbon, monoxide, coal	—	—	—	—	—	—
cyanide	987.7	E869.8	—	E952.8	E962.2	E982.8
dicyanogen	987.8	E869.8	—	E952.8	E962.2	E982.8
domestic - *see* Gas, utility	—	—	—	—	—	—
exhaust - *see* Carbon, monoxide, exhaust gas	—	—	—	—	—	—
from wood- or coal-burning stove or fireplace	986	E868.3	—	E952.1	E962.2	E982.1

◀ New   ◀▥ Revised

Substance	Poisoning	External Cause (E-Code)				
		Accident	Therapeutic Use	Suicide Attempt	Assault	Undetermined
Gas (Continued)	—	—	—	—	—	—
fuel (domestic use) - see also Carbon, monoxide, fuel						
industrial use	986	E868.8	—	E952.1	E962.2	E982.1
utility	987.1	E868.1	—	E951.8	E962.2	E981.8
incomplete combustion of - see Carbon, monoxide, fuel, utility	—	—	—	—	—	—
in mobile container	987.0	E868.0	—	E951.1	E962.2	E981.1
piped (natural)	987.1	E867	—	E951.0	E962.2	E981.0
garage	986	E868.2	—	E952.0	E962.2	E982.0
hydrocarbon NEC	987.1	E869.8	—	E952.8	E962.2	E982.8
incomplete combustion of - see Carbon, monoxide, fuel, utility	—	—	—	—	—	—
liquefied (mobile container)	987.0	E868.0	—	E951.1	E962.2	E981.1
piped	987.0	E867	—	E951.0	E962.2	E981.0
hydrocyanic acid	987.7	E869.8	—	E952.8	E962.2	E982.8
illuminating - see Gas, utility	—	—	—	—	—	—
incomplete combustion, any - see Carbon, monoxide	—	—	—	—	—	—
kiln	986	E868.8	—	E952.1	E962.2	E982.1
lacrimogenic	987.5	E869.3	—	E952.8	E962.2	E982.8
marsh	987.1	E869.8	—	E952.8	E962.2	E982.8
motor exhaust, not in transit	986	E868.8	—	E952.1	E962.2	E982.1
mustard - see Mustard, gas	—	—	—	—	—	—
natural	987.1	E867	—	E951.0	E962.2	E981.0
nerve (war)	987.9	E869.9	—	E952.9	E962.2	E982.9
oils	981	E862.1	—	E950.9	E962.1	E980.9
petroleum (liquefied) (distributed in mobile containers)	987.0	E868.0	—	E951.1	E962.2	E981.1
piped (pure or mixed with air)	987.0	E867	—	E951.1	E962.2	E981.1
piped (manufactured) (natural) NEC	987.1	E867	—	E951.0	E962.2	E981.0
producer	986	E868.8	—	E952.1	E962.2	E982.1
propane - see Propane	—	—	—	—	—	—
refrigerant (freon)	987.4	E869.2	—	E952.8	E962.2	E982.8
not freon	987.9	E869.9	—	E952.9	E962.2	E982.9
sewer	987.8	E869.8	—	E952.8	E962.2	E982.8
specified source NEC (see also substance specified)	987.8	E869.8	—	E952.8	E962.2	E982.8
stove - see Gas, utility	—	—	—	—	—	—
tear	987.5	E869.3	—	E952.8	E962.2	E982.8
utility (for cooking, heating, or lighting) (piped) NEC	987.1	E868.1	—	E951.8	E962.2	E981.8
incomplete combustion of - see Carbon, monoxide, fuel, utilty	—	—	—	—	—	—
in mobile container	987.0	E868.0	—	E951.1	E962.2	E981.1
piped (natural)	987.1	E867	—	E951.0	E962.2	E981.0
water	987.1	E868.1	—	E951.8	E962.2	E981.8
incomplete combustion of - see Carbon, monoxide, fuel, utility	—	—	—	—	—	—
Gaseous substance - see Gas	—	—	—	—	—	—
Gasoline, gasolene	981	E862.1	—	E950.9	E962.1	E980.9
vapor	987.1	E869.8	—	E952.8	E962.2	E982.8
Gastric enzymes	973.4	E858.4	E943.4	E950.4	E962.0	E980.4
Gastrografin	977.8	E858.8	E947.8	E950.4	E962.0	E980.4
Gastrointestinal agents	973.9	E858.4	E943.9	E950.4	E962.0	E980.4
specified NEC	973.8	E858.4	E943.8	E950.4	E962.0	E980.4
Gaultheria procumbens	988.2	E865.4	—	E950.9	E962.1	E980.9
Gelatin (intravenous)	964.8	E858.2	E934.8	E950.4	E962.0	E980.4
absorbable (sponge)	964.5	E858.2	E934.5	E950.4	E962.0	E980.4
Gelfilm	976.8	E858.7	E946.8	E950.4	E962.0	E980.4
Gelfoam	964.5	E858.2	E934.5	E950.4	E962.0	E980.4
Gelsemine	970.8	E854.3	E940.8	E950.4	E962.0	E980.4
Gelsemium (sempervirens)	988.2	E865.4	—	E950.9	E962.1	E980.9
Gemonil	967.0	E851	E937.0	E950.1	E962.0	E980.1
Gentamicin	960.8	E856	E930.8	E950.4	E962.0	E980.4
ophthalmic preparation	976.5	E858.7	E946.5	E950.4	E962.0	E980.4
topical NEC	976.0	E858.7	E946.0	E950.4	E962.0	E980.4
Gentian violet	976.0	E858.7	E946.0	E950.4	E962.0	E980.4
Gexane	976.0	E858.7	E946.0	E950.4	E962.0	E980.4
Gila monster (venom)	989.5	E905.0	—	E950.9	E962.1	E980.9
Ginger, Jamaica	989.89	E866.8	—	E950.9	E962.1	E980.9
Gitalin	972.1	E858.3	E942.1	E950.4	E962.0	E980.4

◀ New   ◀▥ Revised

Substance	Poisoning	External Cause (E-Code)				
		Accident	Therapeutic Use	Suicide Attempt	Assault	Undetermined
Gitoxin	972.1	E858.3	E942.1	E950.4	E962.0	E980.4
Glandular extract (medicinal) NEC	977.9	E858.9	E947.9	E950.5	E962.0	E980.5
Glaucarubin	961.5	E857	E931.5	E950.4	E962.0	E980.4
Globin zinc insulin	962.3	E858.0	E932.3	E950.4	E962.0	E980.4
Glucagon	962.3	E858.0	E932.3	E950.4	E962.0	E980.4
Glucochloral	967.1	E852.0	E937.1	E950.2	E962.0	E980.2
Glucocorticoids	962.0	E858.0	E932.0	E950.4	E962.0	E980.4
Glucose	974.5	E858.5	E944.5	E950.4	E962.0	E980.4
oxidase reagent	977.8	E858.8	E947.8	E950.4	E962.0	E980.4
Glucosulfone sodium	961.8	E857	E931.8	E950.4	E962.0	E980.4
Glue(s)	989.89	E866.6	—	E950.9	E962.1	E980.9
Glutamic acid (hydrochloride)	973.4	E858.4	E943.4	E950.4	E962.0	E980.4
Glutaraldehyde	989.89	E861.4	—	E950.9	E962.1	E980.9
Glutathione	963.8	E858.1	E933.8	E950.4	E962.0	E980.4
Glutethimide (group)	967.5	E852.4	E937.5	E950.2	E962.0	E980.2
Glycerin (lotion)	976.3	E858.7	E946.3	E950.4	E962.0	E980.4
Glycerol (topical)	976.3	E858.7	E946.3	E950.4	E962.0	E980.4
Glyceryl	—	—	—	—	—	—
guaiacolate	975.5	E858.6	E945.5	E950.4	E962.0	E980.4
triacetate (topical)	976.0	E858.7	E946.0	E950.4	E962.0	E980.4
trinitrate	972.4	E858.3	E942.4	E950.4	E962.0	E980.4
Glycine	974.5	E858.5	E944.5	E950.4	E962.0	E980.4
Glycobiarsol	961.1	E857	E931.1	E950.4	E962.0	E980.4
Glycols (ether)	982.8	E862.4	—	E950.9	E962.1	E980.9
Glycopyrrolate	971.1	E855.4	E941.1	E950.4	E962.0	E980.4
Glymidine	962.3	E858.0	E932.3	E950.4	E962.0	E980.4
Gold (compounds) (salts)	965.69	E850.6	E935.6	E950.0	E962.0	E980.0
Golden sulfide of antimony	985.4	E866.2	—	E950.9	E962.1	E980.9
Goldylocks	988.2	E865.4	—	E950.9	E962.1	E980.9
Gonadal tissue extract	962.9	E858.0	E932.9	E950.4	E962.0	E980.4
female	962.2	E858.0	E932.2	E950.4	E962.0	E980.4
male	962.1	E858.0	E932.1	E950.4	E962.0	E980.4
Gonadotropin	962.4	E858.0	E932.4	E950.4	E962.0	E980.4
Grain alcohol	980.0	E860.1	—	E950.9	E962.1	E980.9
beverage	980.0	E860.0	—	E950.9	E962.1	E980.9
Gramicidin	960.8	E856	E930.8	E950.4	E962.0	E980.4
Gratiola officinalis	988.2	E865.4	—	E950.9	E962.1	E980.9
Grease	989.89	E866.8	—	E950.9	E962.1	E980.9
Green hellebore	988.2	E865.4	—	E950.9	E962.1	E980.9
Green soap	976.2	E858.7	E946.2	E950.4	E962.0	E980.4
Grifulvin	960.1	E856	E930.1	E950.4	E962.0	E980.4
Griseofulvin	960.1	E856	E930.1	E950.4	E962.0	E980.4
Growth hormone	962.4	E858.0	E932.4	E950.4	E962.0	E980.4
Guaiacol	975.5	E858.6	E945.5	E950.4	E962.0	E980.4
Giuaiac reagent	977.8	E858.8	E947.8	E950.4	E962.0	E980.4
Guaifenesin	975.5	E858.6	E945.5	E950.4	E962.0	E980.4
Guaiphenesin	975.5	E858.6	E945.5	E950.4	E962.0	E980.4
Guanatol	961.4	E857	E931.4	E950.4	E962.0	E980.4
Guanethidine	972.6	E858.3	E942.6	E950.4	E962.0	E980.4
Guano	989.89	E866.5	—	E950.9	E962.1	E980.9
Guanochlor	972.6	E858.3	E942.6	E950.4	E962.0	E980.4
Guanoctine	972.6	E858.3	E942.6	E950.4	E962.0	E980.4
Guanoxan	972.6	E858.3	E942.6	E950.4	E962.0	E980.4
Hair treatment agent NEC	976.4	E858.7	E946.4	E950.4	E962.0	E980.4
Halcinonide	976.0	E858.7	E946.0	E950.4	E962.0	E980.4
Halethazole	976.0	E858.7	E946.0	E950.4	E962.0	E980.4
Hallucinogens	969.6	E854.1	E939.6	E950.3	E962.0	E980.3
Haloperidol	969.2	E853.1	E939.2	E950.3	E962.0	E980.3
Haloprogin	976.0	E858.7	E946.0	E950.4	E962.0	E980.4
Halotex	976.0	E858.7	E946.0	E950.4	E962.0	E980.4
Halothane	968.1	E855.1	E938.1	E950.4	E962.0	E980.4
Halquinols	976.0	E858.7	E946.0	E950.4	E962.0	E980.4
Harmonyl	972.6	E858.3	E942.6	E950.4	E962.0	E980.4

Substance	Poisoning	External Cause (E-Code)				
		Accident	Therapeutic Use	Suicide Attempt	Assault	Undetermined
Hartmann's solution	974.5	E858.5	E944.5	E950.4	E962.0	E980.4
Hashish	969.6	E854.1	E939.6	E950.3	E962.0	E980.3
Hawaiian wood rose seeds	969.6	E854.1	E939.6	E950.3	E962.0	E980.3
Headache cures, drugs, powders NEC	977.9	E858.9	E947.9	E950.5	E962.0	E980.9
Heavenly Blue (morning glory)	969.6	E854.1	E939.6	E950.3	E962.0	E980.3
Heavy metal antagonists	963.8	E858.1	E933.8	E950.4	E962.0	E980.4
anti-infectives	961.2	E857	E931.2	E950.4	E962.0	E980.4
Hedaquinium	976.0	E858.7	E946.0	E950.4	E962.0	E980.4
Hedge hyssop	988.2	E865.4	—	E950.9	E962.1	E980.9
Heet	976.8	E858.7	E946.8	E950.4	E962.0	E980.4
Helenin	961.6	E857	E931.6	E950.4	E962.0	E980.4
Hellebore (black) (green) (white)	988.2	E865.4	—	E950.9	E962.1	E980.9
Hemlock	988.2	E865.4	—	E950.9	E962.1	E980.9
Hemostatics	964.5	E858.2	E934.5	E950.4	E962.0	E980.4
capillary active drugs	972.8	E858.3	E942.8	E950.4	E962.0	E980.4
Henbane	988.2	E865.4	—	E950.9	E962.1	E980.9
Heparin (sodium)	964.2	E858.2	E934.2	E950.4	E962.0	E980.4
Heptabarbital, heptabarbitone	967.0	E851	E937.0	E950.1	E962.0	E980.1
Heptachlor	989.2	E863.0	—	E950.6	E962.1	E980.7
Heptalgin	965.09	E850.2	E935.2	E950.0	E962.0	E980.0
Herbicides	989.4	E863.5	—	E950.6	E962.1	E980.7
Heroin	965.01	E850.0	E935.0	E950.0	E962.0	E980.0
Herplex	976.5	E858.7	E946.5	E950.4	E962.0	E980.4
HES	964.8	E858.2	E934.8	E950.4	E962.0	E980.4
Hetastarch	964.8	E858.2	E934.8	E950.4	E962.0	E980.7
Hexachlorocyclohexane	989.2	E863.0	—	E950.6	E962.1	E980.7
Hexachlorophene	976.2	E858.7	E946.2	E950.4	E962.0	E980.4
Hexadimethrine (bromide)	964.5	E858.2	E934.5	E950.4	E962.0	E980.4
Hexafluorenium	975.2	E858.6	E945.2	E950.4	E962.0	E980.4
Hexa-germ	976.2	E858.7	E946.2	E950.4	E962.0	E980.4
Hexahydrophenol	980.8	E860.8	—	E950.9	E962.1	E980.9
Hexalen	980.8	E860.8	—	E950.9	E962.1	E980.9
Hexamethonium	972.3	E858.3	E942.3	E950.4	E962.0	E980.4
Hexamethylenamine	961.9	E857	E931.9	E950.4	E962.0	E980.4
Hexamine	961.9	E857	E931.9	E950.4	E962.0	E980.4
Hexanone	982.8	E862.4	—	E950.9	E962.1	E980.9
Hexapropymate	967.8	E852.8	E937.8	E950.2	E962.0	E980.2
Hexestrol	962.2	E858.0	E932.2	E950.4	E962.0	E980.4
Hexethal (sodium)	967.0	E851	E937.0	E950.1	E962.0	E980.1
Hexetidine	976.0	E858.7	E946.0	E950.4	E962.0	E980.4
Hexobarbital, hexobarbitone	967.0	E851	E937.0	E950.1	E962.0	E980.1
sodium (anesthetic)	968.3	E855.1	E938.3	E950.4	E962.0	E980.4
soluble	968.3	E855.1	E938.3	E950.4	E962.0	E980.4
Hexocyclium	971.1	E855.4	E941.1	E950.4	E962.0	E980.4
Hexoestrol	962.2	E858.0	E932.2	E950.4	E962.0	E980.4
Hexone	982.8	E862.4	—	E950.9	E962.1	E980.9
Hexylcaine	968.5	E855.2	E938.5	E950.4	E962.0	E980.4
Hexylresorcinol	961.6	E857	E931.6	E950.4	E962.0	E980.4
Hinkle's pills	973.1	E858.4	E943.1	E950.4	E962.0	E980.4
Histalog	977.8	E858.8	E947.8	E950.4	E962.0	E980.4
Histamine (phosphate)	972.5	E858.3	E942.5	E950.4	E962.0	E980.4
Histoplasmin	977.8	E858.8	E947.8	E950.4	E962.0	E980.4
Holly berries	988.2	E865.3	—	E950.9	E962.1	E980.9
Homatropine	971.1	E855.4	E941.1	E950.4	E962.0	E980.4
Homo-tet	964.6	E858.2	E934.6	E950.4	E962.0	E980.4
Hormones (synthetic substitute) NEC	962.9	E858.0	E932.9	E950.4	E962.0	E980.4
adrenal cortical steroids	962.0	E858.0	E932.0	E950.4	E962.0	E980.4
antidiabetic agents	962.3	E858.0	E932.3	E950.4	E962.0	E980.4
follicle stimulating	962.4	E858.0	E932.4	E950.4	E962.0	E980.4
gonadotropic	962.4	E858.0	E932.4	E950.4	E962.0	E980.4
growth	962.4	E858.0	E932.4	E950.4	E962.0	E980.4

◄ New   ⬅ Revised

ICD-9-CM

Drugs

Vol. 2

Substance	Poisoning	External Cause (E-Code)				
		Accident	Therapeutic Use	Suicide Attempt	Assault	Undetermined
Hormones *(Continued)*						
ovarian (substitutes)	962.2	E858.0	E932.2	E950.4	E962.0	E980.4
parathyroid (derivatives)	962.6	E858.0	E932.6	E950.4	E962.0	E980.4
pituitary (posterior)	962.5	E858.0	E932.5	E950.4	E962.0	E980.4
anterior	962.4	E858.0	E932.4	E950.4	E962.0	E980.4
thyroid (derivative)	962.7	E858.0	E932.7	E950.4	E962.0	E980.4
Hornet (sting)	989.5	E905.3	—	E950.9	E962.1	E980.9
Horticulture agent NEC	989.4	E863.9	—	E950.6	E962.1	E980.7
Hyaluronidase	963.4	E858.1	E933.4	E950.4	E962.0	E980.4
Hyazyme	963.4	E858.1	E933.4	E950.4	E962.0	E980.4
Hycodan	965.09	E850.2	E935.2	E950.0	E962.0	E980.0
Hydantoin derivatives	966.1	E855.0	E936.1	E950.4	E962.0	E980.4
Hydeltra	962.0	E858.0	E932.0	E950.4	E962.0	E980.4
Hydergine	971.3	E855.6	E941.3	E950.4	E962.0	E980.4
Hydrabamine penicillin	960.0	E856	E930.0	E950.4	E962.0	E980.4
Hydralazine, hydrallazine	972.6	E858.3	E942.6	E950.4	E962.0	E980.4
Hydrargaphen	976.0	E858.7	E946.0	E950.4	E962.0	E980.4
Hydrazine	983.9	E864.3	—	E950.7	E962.1	E980.6
Hydriodic acid	975.5	E858.6	E945.5	E950.4	E962.0	E980.4
Hydrocarbon gas	987.1	E869.8	—	E952.8	E962.2	E982.8
incomplete combustion of - *see* Carbon, monoxide, fuel, utility	—	—	—	—	—	—
liquefied (mobile container)	987.0	E868.0	—	E951.1	E962.2	E981.1
piped (natural)	987.0	E867	—	E951.0	E962.2	E981.0
Hydrochloric acid (liquid)	983.1	E864.1	—	E950.7	E962.1	E980.6
medicinal	973.4	E858.4	E943.4	E950.4	E962.0	E980.4
vapor	987.8	E869.8	—	E952.8	E962.2	E982.8
Hydrochlorothiazide	974.3	E858.5	E944.3	E950.4	E962.0	E980.4
Hydrocodone	965.09	E850.2	E935.2	E950.0	E962.0	E980.0
Hydrocortisone	962.0	E858.0	E932.0	E950.4	E962.0	E980.4
ENT agent	976.6	E858.7	E946.6	E950.4	E962.0	E980.4
ophthalmic preparation	976.5	E858.7	E946.5	E950.4	E962.0	E980.4
topical NEC	976.0	E858.7	E946.0	E950.4	E962.0	E980.4
Hydrocortone	962.0	E858.0	E932.0	E950.4	E962.0	E980.4
ENT agent	976.6	E858.7	E946.6	E950.4	E962.0	E980.4
ophthalmic preparation	976.5	E858.7	E946.5	E950.4	E962.0	E980.4
topical NEC	976.0	E858.7	E946.0	E950.4	E962.0	E980.4
Hydrocyanic acid - *see* Cyanide(s)	—	—	—	—	—	—
Hydroflumethiazide	974.3	E858.5	E944.3	E950.4	E962.0	E980.4
Hydrofluoric acid (liquid)	983.1	E864.1	—	E950.7	E962.1	E980.6
vapor	987.8	E869.8	—	E952.8	E962.2	E982.8
Hydrogen	987.8	E869.8	—	E952.8	E962.2	E982.8
arsenide	985.1	E866.3	—	E950.8	E962.1	E980.8
arseniurated	985.1	E866.3	—	E950.8	E962.1	E980.8
cyanide (salts)	989.0	E866.8	—	E950.9	E962.1	E980.9
gas	987.7	E869.8	—	E952.8	E962.2	E982.8
fluoride (liquid)	983.1	E864.1	—	E950.7	E962.1	E980.6
vapor	987.8	E869.8	—	E952.8	E962.2	E982.8
peroxide (solution)	976.6	E858.7	E946.6	E950.4	E962.0	E980.4
phosphorated	987.8	E869.8	—	E952.8	E962.2	E982.8
sulfide (gas)	987.8	E869.8	—	E952.8	E962.2	E982.8
arseniurated	985.1	E866.3	—	E950.8	E962.1	E980.8
sulfureted	987.8	E869.8	—	E952.8	E962.2	E982.8
Hydromorphinol	965.09	E850.2	E935.2	E950.0	E962.0	E980.0
Hydromorphinone	965.09	E850.2	E935.2	E950.0	E962.0	E980.0
Hydromorphone	965.09	E850.2	E935.2	E950.0	E962.0	E980.0
Hydromox	974.3	E858.5	E944.3	E950.4	E962.0	E980.4
Hydrophilic lotion	976.3	E858.7	E946.3	E950.4	E962.0	E980.4
Hydroquinone	983.0	E864.0	—	E950.7	E962.1	E980.6
vapor	987.8	E869.8	—	E952.8	E962.2	E982.8
Hydrosulfuric acid (gas)	987.8	E869.8	—	E952.8	E962.2	E982.8
Hydrous wool fat (lotion)	976.3	E858.7	E946.3	E950.4	E962.0	E980.4
Hydroxide, caustic	983.2	E864.2	—	E950.7	E962.1	E980.6

Substance	Poisoning	External Cause (E-Code)				
		Accident	Therapeutic Use	Suicide Attempt	Assault	Undetermined
Hydroxocobalamin	964.1	E858.2	E934.1	E950.4	E962.0	E980.4
Hydroxyamphetamine	971.2	E855.5	E941.2	E950.4	E962.0	E980.4
Hydroxychloroquine	961.4	E857	E931.4	E950.4	E962.0	E980.4
Hydroxydihydrocodeinone	965.09	E850.2	E935.2	E950.0	E962.0	E980.0
Hydroxyethyl starch	964.8	E858.2	E934.8	E950.4	E962.0	E980.4
Hydroxyphenamate	969.5	E853.8	E939.5	E950.3	E962.0	E980.3
Hydroxyphenylbutazone	965.5	E850.5	E935.5	E950.0	E962.0	E980.0
Hydroxyprogesterone	962.2	E858.0	E932.2	E950.4	E962.0	E980.4
Hydroxyquinoline derivatives	961.3	E857	E931.3	E950.4	E962.0	E980.4
Hydroxystilbamidine	961.5	E857	E931.5	E950.4	E962.0	E980.4
Hydroxyurea	963.1	E858.1	E933.1	E950.4	E962.0	E980.4
Hydroxyzine	969.5	E853.8	E939.5	E950.3	E962.0	E980.3
Hyoscine (hydrobromide)	971.1	E855.4	E941.1	E950.4	E962.0	E980.4
Hyoscyamine	971.1	E855.4	E941.1	E950.4	E962.0	E980.4
Hyoscyamus (albus) (niger)	988.2	E865.4	—	E950.9	E962.1	E980.9
Hypaque	977.8	E858.8	E947.8	E950.4	E962.0	E980.4
Hypertussis	964.6	E858.2	E934.6	E950.4	E962.0	E980.4
Hypnotics NEC	967.9	E852.9	E937.9	E950.2	E962.0	E980.2
Hypochlorites - see Sodium, hypochlorite	—	—	—	—	—	—
Hypotensive agents NEC	972.6	E858.3	E942.6	E950.4	E962.0	E980.4
Ibufenac	965.69	E850.6	E935.6	E950.0	E962.0	E980.0
Ibuprofen	965.61	E850.6	E935.6	E950.0	E962.0	E980.0
ICG	977.8	E858.8	E947.8	E950.4	E962.0	E980.4
Ichthammol	976.4	E858.7	E946.4	E950.4	E962.0	E980.4
Ichthyol	976.4	E858.7	E946.4	E950.4	E962.0	E980.4
Idoxuridine	976.5	E858.7	E946.5	E950.4	E962.0	E980.4
IDU	976.5	E858.7	E946.5	E950.4	E962.0	E980.4
Iletin	962.3	E858.0	E932.3	E950.4	E962.0	E980.4
Ilex	988.2	E865.4	—	E950.9	E962.1	E980.9
Illuminating gas - see Gas, utility	—	—	—	—	—	—
Ilopan	963.5	E858.1	E933.5	E950.4	E962.0	E980.4
Ilotycin	960.3	E856	E930.3	E950.4	E962.0	E980.4
ophthalmic preparation	976.5	E858.7	E946.5	E950.4	E962.0	E980.4
topical NEC	976.0	E858.7	E946.0	E950.4	E962.0	E980.4
Imipramine	969.0	E854.0	E939.0	E950.3	E962.0	E980.3
Immu-G	964.6	E858.2	E934.6	E950.4	E962.0	E980.4
Immuglobin	964.6	E858.2	E934.6	E950.4	E962.0	E980.4
Immune serum globulin	964.6	E858.2	E934.6	E950.4	E962.0	E980.4
Immunosuppressive agents	963.1	E858.1	E933.1	E950.4	E962.0	E980.4
Immu-tetanus	964.6	E858.2	E934.6	E950.4	E962.0	E980.4
Indandione (derivatives)	964.2	E858.2	E934.2	E950.4	E962.0	E980.4
Inderal	972.0	E858.3	E942.0	E950.4	E962.0	E980.4
Indian	—	—	—	—	—	—
hemp	969.6	E854.1	E939.6	E950.3	E962.0	E980.3
tobacco	988.2	E865.4	—	E950.9	E962.1	E980.9
Indigo carmine	977.8	E858.8	E947.8	E950.4	E962.0	E980.4
Indocin	965.69	E850.6	E935.6	E950.0	E962.0	E980.0
Indocyanine green	977.8	E858.8	E947.8	E950.4	E962.0	E980.4
Indomethacin	965.69	E850.6	E935.6	E950.0	E962.0	E980.0
Industrial	—	—	—	—	—	—
alcohol	980.9	E860.9	—	E950.9	E962.1	E980.9
fumes	987.8	E869.8	—	E952.8	E962.2	E982.8
solvents (fumes) (vapors)	982.8	E862.9	—	E950.9	E962.1	E980.9
Influenza vaccine	979.6	E858.8	E949.6	E950.4	E962.0	E982.8
Ingested substances NEC	989.9	E866.9	—	E950.9	E962.1	E980.9
INH (isoniazid)	961.8	E857	E931.8	E950.4	E962.0	E980.4
Inhalation, gas (noxious) - see Gas	—	—	—	—	—	—
Ink	989.89	E866.8	—	E950.9	E962.1	E980.9
Innovar	967.6	E852.5	E937.6	E950.2	E962.0	E980.2
Inositol niacinate	972.2	E858.3	E942.2	E950.4	E962.0	E980.4
Inproquone	963.1	E858.1	E933.1	E950.4	E962.0	E980.4

◀ New   ⬅ Revised

Substance	Poisoning	External Cause (E-Code)				
		Accident	Therapeutic Use	Suicide Attempt	Assault	Undetermined
Insect (sting), venomous	989.5	E905.5	—	E950.9	E962.1	E980.9
Insecticides (see also Pesticides)	989.4	E863.4	—	E950.6	E962.1	E980.7
chlorinated	989.2	E863.0	—	E950.6	E962.1	E980.7
mixtures	989.4	E863.3	—	E950.6	E962.1	E980.7
organochlorine (compounds)	989.2	E863.0	—	E950.6	E962.1	E980.7
organophosphorus (compounds)	989.3	E863.1	—	E950.6	E962.1	E980.7
Insular tissue extract	962.3	E858.0	E932.3	E950.4	E962.0	E980.4
Insulin (amorphous) (globin) (isophane) (Lente) (NPH) (Protamine) (Semilente) (Ultralente) (zinc)	962.3	E858.0	E932.3	E950.4	E962.0	E980.4
Intranarcon	968.3	E855.1	E938.3	E950.4	E962.0	E980.4
Inulin	977.8	E858.8	E947.8	E950.4	E962.0	E980.4
Invert sugar	974.5	E858.5	E944.5	E950.4	E962.0	E980.4
Inza - see Naproxen	—	—	—	—	—	—
Iodide NEC (see also Iodine)	976.0	E858.7	E946.0	E950.4	E962.0	E980.4
mercury (ointment)	976.0	E858.7	E946.0	E950.4	E962.0	E980.4
methylate	976.0	E858.7	E946.0	E950.4	E962.0	E980.4
potassium (expectorant) NEC	975.5	E858.6	E945.5	E950.4	E962.0	E980.4
Iodinated glycerol	975.5	E858.6	E945.5	E950.4	E962.0	E980.4
Iodine (antiseptic, external) (tincture) NEC	976.0	E858.7	E946.0	E950.4	E962.0	E980.4
diagnostic	977.8	E858.8	E947.8	E950.4	E962.0	E980.4
for thyroid conditions (antithyroid)	962.8	E858.0	E932.8	E950.4	E962.0	E980.4
vapor	987.8	E869.8	—	E952.8	E962.2	E982.8
Iodized oil	977.8	E858.8	E947.8	E950.4	E962.0	E980.4
Iodobismitol	961.2	E857	E931.2	E950.4	E962.0	E980.4
Iodochlorhydroxyquin	961.3	E857	E931.3	E950.4	E962.0	E980.4
topical	976.0	E858.7	E946.0	E950.4	E962.0	E980.4
Iodoform	976.0	E858.7	E946.0	E950.4	E962.0	E980.4
Iodopanoic acid	977.8	E858.8	E947.8	E950.4	E962.0	E980.4
Iodophthalein	977.8	E858.8	E947.8	E950.4	E962.0	E980.4
Ion exchange resins	974.5	E858.5	E944.5	E950.4	E962.0	E980.4
Iopanoic acid	977.8	E858.8	E947.8	E950.4	E962.0	E980.4
Iophendylate	977.8	E858.8	E947.8	E950.4	E962.0	E980.4
Iothiouracil	962.8	E858.0	E932.8	E950.4	E962.0	E980.4
Ipecac	973.6	E858.4	E943.6	E950.4	E962.0	E980.4
Ipecacuanha	973.6	E858.4	E943.6	E950.4	E962.0	E980.4
Ipodate	977.8	E858.8	E947.8	E950.4	E962.0	E980.4
Ipral	967.0	E851	E937.0	E950.1	E962.0	E980.1
Ipratropium	975.1	E858.6	E945.1	E950.4	E962.0	E980.4
Iproniazid	969.0	E854.0	E939.0	E950.3	E962.0	E980.3
Iron (compounds) (medicinal) (preparations)	964.0	E858.2	E934.0	E950.4	E962.0	E980.4
dextran	964.0	E858.2	E934.0	E950.4	E962.0	E980.4
nonmedicinal (dust) (fumes) NEC	985.8	E866.4	—	E950.9	E962.1	E980.9
Irritant drug	977.9	E858.9	E947.9	E950.5	E962.0	E980.5
Ismelin	972.6	E858.3	E942.6	E950.4	E962.0	E980.4
Isoamyl nitrite	972.4	E858.3	E942.4	E950.4	E962.0	E980.4
Isobutyl acetate	982.8	E862.4	—	E950.9	E962.1	E980.9
Isocarboxazid	969.0	E854.0	E939.0	E950.3	E962.0	E980.3
Isoephedrine	971.2	E855.5	E941.2	E950.4	E962.0	E980.4
Isoetharine	971.2	E855.5	E941.2	E950.4	E962.0	E980.4
Isofluorophate	971.0	E855.3	E941.0	E950.4	E962.0	E980.4
Isoniazid (INH)	961.8	E857	E931.8	E950.4	E962.0	E980.4
Isopentaquine	961.4	E857	E931.4	E950.4	E962.0	E980.4
Isophane insulin	962.3	E858.0	E932.3	E950.4	E962.0	E980.4
Isopregnenone	962.2	E858.0	E932.2	E950.4	E962.0	E980.4
Isoprenaline	971.2	E855.5	E941.2	E950.4	E962.0	E980.4
Isopropamide	971.1	E855.4	E941.1	E950.4	E962.0	E980.4
Isopropanol	980.2	E860.3	—	E950.9	E962.1	E980.9
topical (germicide)	976.0	E858.7	E946.0	E950.4	E962.0	E980.4
Isopropyl	—	—	—	—	—	—
acetate	982.8	E862.4	—	E950.9	E962.1	E980.9
alcohol	980.2	E860.3	—	E950.9	E962.1	E980.9
topical (germicide)	976.0	E858.7	E946.0	E950.4	E962.0	E980.4
ether	982.8	E862.4	—	E950.9	E962.1	E980.9

Substance	Poisoning	External Cause (E-Code)				
		Accident	Therapeutic Use	Suicide Attempt	Assault	Undetermined
Isoproterenol	971.2	E855.5	E941.2	E950.4	E962.0	E980.4
Isosorbide dinitrate	972.4	E858.3	E942.4	E950.4	E962.0	E980.4
Isothipendyl	963.0	E858.1	E933.0	E950.4	E962.0	E980.4
Isoxazolyl penicillin	960.0	E856	E930.0	E950.4	E962.0	E980.4
Isoxsuprine hydrochloride	972.5	E858.3	E942.5	E950.4	E962.0	E980.4
l-thyroxine sodium	962.7	E858.0	E932.7	E950.4	E962.0	E980.4
Jaborandi (pilocarpus) (extract)	971.0	E855.3	E941.0	E950.4	E962.0	E980.4
Jalap	973.1	E858.4	E943.1	E950.4	E962.0	E980.4
Jamaica	—	—	—	—	—	—
dogwood (bark)	965.7	E850.7	E935.7	E950.0	E962.0	E980.0
ginger	989.89	E866.8	—	E950.9	E962.1	E980.9
Jatropha	988.2	E865.4	—	E950.9	E962.1	E980.9
curcas	988.2	E865.3	—	E950.9	E962.1	E980.9
Jectofer	964.0	E858.2	E934.0	E950.4	E962.0	E980.4
Jellyfish (sting)	989.5	E905.6	—	E950.9	E962.1	E980.9
Jequirity (bean)	988.2	E865.3	—	E950.9	E962.1	E980.9
Jimson weed	988.2	E865.4	—	E950.9	E962.1	E980.9
seeds	988.2	E865.3	—	E950.9	E962.1	E980.9
Juniper tar (oil) (ointment)	976.4	E858.7	E946.4	E950.4	E962.0	E980.4
Kallikrein	972.5	E858.3	E942.5	E950.4	E962.0	E980.4
Kanamycin	960.6	E856	E930.6	E950.4	E962.0	E980.4
Kantrex	960.6	E856	E930.6	E950.4	E962.0	E980.4
Kaolin	973.5	E858.4	E943.5	E950.4	E962.0	E980.4
Karaya (gum)	973.3	E858.4	E943.3	E950.4	E962.0	E980.4
Kemithal	968.3	E855.1	E938.3	E950.4	E962.0	E980.4
Kenacort	962.0	E858.0	E932.0	E950.4	E962.0	E980.4
Keratolytics	976.4	E858.7	E946.4	E950.4	E962.0	E980.4
Keratoplastics	976.4	E858.7	E946.4	E950.4	E962.0	E980.4
Kerosene, kerosine (fuel) (solvent) NEC	981	E862.1	—	E950.9	E962.1	E980.9
insecticide	981	E863.4	—	E950.6	E962.1	E980.7
vapor	987.1	E869.8	—	E952.8	E962.2	E982.8
Ketamine	968.3	E855.1	E938.3	E950.4	E962.0	E980.4
Ketobemidone	965.09	E850.2	E935.2	E950.0	E962.0	E980.0
Ketols	982.8	E862.4	—	E950.9	E962.1	E980.9
Ketone oils	982.8	E862.4	—	E950.9	E962.1	E980.9
Ketoprofen	965.61	E850.6	E935.6	E950.0	E962.0	E980.0
Kiln gas or vapor (carbon monoxide)	986	E868.8	—	E952.1	E962.2	E982.1
Konsyl	973.3	E858.4	E943.3	E950.4	E962.0	E980.4
Kosam seed	988.2	E865.3	—	E950.9	E962.1	E980.9
Krait (venom)	989.5	E905.0	—	E950.9	E962.1	E980.9
Kwell (insecticide)	989.2	E863.0	—	E950.6	E962.1	E980.7
anti-infective (topical)	976.0	E858.7	E946.0	E950.4	E962.0	E980.4
Laburnum (flowers) (seeds)	988.2	E865.3	—	E950.9	E962.1	E980.9
leaves	988.2	E865.4	—	E950.9	E962.1	E980.9
Lacquers	989.89	E861.6	—	E950.9	E962.1	E980.9
Lacrimogenic gas	987.5	E869.3	—	E952.8	E962.2	E982.8
Lactic acid	983.1	E864.1	—	E950.7	E962.1	E980.6
Lactobacillus acidophilus	973.5	E858.4	E943.5	E950.4	E962.0	E980.4
Lactoflavin	963.5	E858.1	E933.5	E950.4	E962.0	E980.4
Lactuca (virosa) (extract)	967.8	E852.8	E937.8	E950.2	E962.0	E980.2
Lactucarium	967.8	E852.8	E937.8	E950.2	E962.0	E980.2
Laevulose	974.5	E858.5	E944.5	E950.4	E962.0	E980.4
Lanatoside (C)	972.1	E858.3	E942.1	E950.4	E962.0	E980.4
Lanolin (lotion)	976.3	E858.7	E946.3	E950.4	E962.0	E980.4
Largactil	969.1	E853.0	E939.1	E950.3	E962.0	E980.3
Larkspur	988.2	E865.3	—	E950.9	E962.1	E980.9
Laroxyl	969.0	E854.0	E939.0	E950.3	E962.0	E980.3
Lasix	974.4	E858.5	E944.4	E950.4	E962.0	E980.4
Latex	989.82	E866.8	—	E950.9	E962.1	E980.9
Lathyrus (seed)	988.2	E865.3	—	E950.9	E962.1	E980.9
Laudanum	965.09	E850.2	E935.2	E950.0	E962.0	E980.0
Laudexium	975.2	E858.6	E945.2	E950.4	E962.0	E980.4

◀ New   ◀▥ Revised

ICD-9-CM

Drugs

Vol. 2

Substance	Poisoning	External Cause (E-Code)				
		Accident	Therapeutic Use	Suicide Attempt	Assault	Undetermined
Laurel, black or cherry	988.2	E865.4	—	E950.9	E962.1	E980.9
Laurolinium	976.0	E858.7	E946.0	E950.4	E962.0	E980.4
Lauryl sulfoacetate	976.2	E858.7	E946.2	E950.4	E962.0	E980.4
Laxatives NEC	973.3	E858.4	E943.3	E950.4	E962.0	E980.4
emollient	973.2	E858.4	E943.2	E950.4	E962.0	E980.4
L-dopa	966.4	E855.0	E936.4	E950.4	E962.0	E980.4
L-Tryptophan - *see* amino acid	—	—	—	—	—	—
Lead (dust) (fumes) (vapor) NEC	984.9	E866.0	—	E950.9	E962.1	E980.9
acetate (dust)	984.1	E866.0	—	E950.9	E962.1	E980.9
anti-infectives	961.2	E857	E931.2	E950.4	E962.0	E980.4
antiknock compound (tetra-ethyl)	984.1	E862.1	—	E950.9	E962.1	E980.9
arsenate, arsenite (dust) (insecticide) (vapor)	985.1	E863.4	—	E950.8	E962.1	E980.8
herbicide	985.1	E863.5	—	E950.8	E962.1	E980.8
carbonate	984.0	E866.0	—	E950.9	E962.1	E980.9
paint	984.0	E861.5	—	E950.9	E962.1	E980.9
chromate	984.0	E866.0	—	E950.9	E962.1	E980.9
paint	984.0	E861.5	—	E950.9	E962.1	E980.9
dioxide	984.0	E866.0	—	E950.9	E962.1	E980.9
inorganic (compound)	984.0	E866.0	—	E950.9	E962.1	E980.9
paint	984.0	E861.5	—	E950.9	E962.1	E980.9
iodide	984.0	E866.0	—	E950.9	E962.1	E980.9
pigment (paint)	984.0	E861.5	—	E950.9	E962.1	E980.9
monoxide (dust)	984.0	E866.0	—	E950.9	E962.1	E980.9
paint	984.0	E861.5	—	E950.9	E962.1	E980.9
organic	984.1	E866.0	—	E950.9	E962.1	E980.9
oxide	984.0	E866.0	—	E950.9	E962.1	E980.9
paint	984.0	E861.5	—	E950.9	E962.1	E980.9
paint	984.0	E861.5	—	E950.9	E962.1	E980.9
salts	984.0	E866.0	—	E950.9	E962.1	E980.9
specified compound NEC	984.8	E866.0	—	E950.9	E962.1	E980.9
tetra-ethyl	984.1	E862.1	—	E950.9	E962.1	E980.9
Lebanese red	969.6	E854.1	E939.6	E950.3	E962.0	E980.3
Lente Iletin (insulin)	962.3	E858.0	E932.3	E950.4	E962.0	E980.4
Leptazol	970.0	E854.3	E940.0	E950.4	E962.0	E980.4
Leritine	965.09	E850.2	E935.2	E950.0	E962.0	E980.0
Letter	962.7	E858.0	E932.7	E950.4	E962.0	E980.4
Lettuce opium	967.8	E852.8	E937.8	E950.2	E962.0	E980.2
Leucovorin (factor)	964.1	E858.2	E934.1	E950.4	E962.0	E980.4
Leukeran	963.1	E858.1	E933.1	E950.4	E962.0	E980.4
Levalbuterol	975.7	E858.6	E945.7	E950.4	E962.0	E980.4
Levallorphan	970.1	E854.3	E940.1	E950.4	E962.0	E980.4
Levanil	967.8	E852.8	E937.8	E950.2	E962.0	E980.2
Levarterenol	971.2	E855.5	E941.2	E950.4	E962.0	E980.4
Levodopa	966.4	E855.0	E936.4	E950.4	E962.0	E980.4
Levo-dromoran	965.09	E850.2	E935.2	E950.0	E962.0	E980.0
Levoid	962.7	E858.0	E932.7	E950.4	E962.0	E980.4
Levo-iso-methadone	965.02	E850.1	E935.1	E950.0	E962.0	E980.0
Levomepromazine	967.8	E852.8	E937.8	E950.2	E962.0	E980.2
Levoprome	967.8	E852.8	E937.8	E950.2	E962.0	E980.2
Levopropoxyphene	975.4	E858.6	E945.4	E950.4	E962.0	E980.4
Levorphan, levophanol	965.09	E850.2	E935.2	E950.0	E962.0	E980.0
Levothyroxine (sodium)	962.7	E858.0	E932.7	E950.4	E962.0	E980.4
Levsin	971.1	E855.4	E941.1	E950.4	E962.0	E980.4
Levulose	974.5	E858.5	E944.5	E950.4	E962.0	E980.4
Lewisite (gas)	985.1	E866.3	—	E950.8	E962.1	E980.8
Librium	969.4	E853.2	E939.4	E950.3	E962.0	E980.3
Lidex	976.0	E858.7	E946.0	E950.4	E962.0	E980.4
Lidocaine (infiltration) (topical)	968.5	E855.2	E938.5	E950.4	E962.0	E980.4
nerve block (peripheral) (plexus)	968.6	E855.2	E938.6	E950.4	E962.0	E980.4
spinal	968.7	E855.2	E938.7	E950.4	E962.0	E980.4
Lighter fluid	981	E862.1	—	E950.9	E962.1	E980.9

◀ New   ◀▦ Revised

Substance	Poisoning	External Cause (E-Code) Accident	Therapeutic Use	Suicide Attempt	Assault	Undetermined
Lignocaine (infiltration) (topical)	968.5	E855.2	E938.5	E950.4	E962.0	E980.4
nerve block (peripheral) (plexus)	968.6	E855.2	E938.6	E950.4	E962.0	E980.4
spinal	968.7	E855.2	E938.7	E950.4	E962.0	E980.4
Ligroin(e) (solvent)	981	E862.0	—	E950.9	E962.1	E980.9
vapor	987.1	E869.8	—	E952.8	E962.2	E982.8
Ligustrum vulgare	988.2	E865.3	—	E950.9	E962.1	E980.9
Lily of the valley	988.2	E865.4	—	E950.9	E962.1	E980.9
Lime (chloride)	983.2	E864.2	—	E950.7	E962.1	E980.6
solution, sulferated	976.4	E858.7	E946.4	E950.4	E962.0	E980.4
Limonene	982.8	E862.4	—	E950.9	E962.1	E980.9
Lincomycin	960.8	E856	E930.8	E950.4	E962.0	E980.4
Lindane (insecticide) (vapor)	989.2	E863.0	—	E950.6	E962.1	E980.7
anti-infective (topical)	976.0	E858.7	E946.0	E950.4	E962.0	E980.4
Liniments NEC	976.9	E858.7	E946.9	E950.4	E962.0	E980.4
Linoleic acid	972.2	E858.3	E942.2	E950.4	E962.0	E980.4
Liothyronine	962.7	E858.0	E932.7	E950.4	E962.0	E980.4
Liotrix	962.7	E858.0	E932.7	E950.4	E962.0	E980.4
Lipancreatin	973.4	E858.4	E943.4	E950.4	E962.0	E980.4
Lipo-Lutin	962.2	E858.0	E932.2	E950.4	E962.0	E980.4
Lipotropic agents	977.1	E858.8	E947.1	E950.4	E962.0	E980.4
Liquefied petroleum gases	987.0	E868.0	—	E951.1	E962.2	E981.1
piped (pure or mixed with air)	987.0	E867	—	E951.0	E962.2	E981.0
Liquid petrolatum	973.2	E858.4	E943.2	E950.4	E962.0	E980.4
substance	989.9	E866.9	—	E950.9	E962.1	E980.9
specified NEC	989.89	E866.8	—	E950.9	E962.1	E980.9
Lirugen	979.4	E858.8	E949.4	E950.4	E962.0	E980.4
Lithane	969.8	E855.8	E939.8	E950.3	E962.0	E980.3
Lithium	985.8	E866.4	—	E950.9	E962.1	E980.9
carbonate	969.8	E855.8	E939.8	E950.3	E962.0	E980.3
Lithonate	969.8	E855.8	E939.8	E950.3	E962.0	E980.3
Liver (extract) (injection) (preparations)	964.1	E858.2	E934.1	E950.4	E962.0	E980.4
Lizard (bite) (venom)	989.5	E905.0	—	E950.9	E962.1	E980.9
LMD	964.8	E858.2	E934.8	E950.4	E962.0	E980.4
Lobelia	988.2	E865.4	—	E950.9	E962.1	E980.9
Lobeline	970.0	E854.3	E940.0	E950.4	E962.0	E980.4
Locorten	976.0	E858.7	E946.0	E950.4	E962.0	E980.4
Lolium temulentum	988.2	E865.3	—	E950.9	E962.1	E980.9
Lomotil	973.5	E858.4	E943.5	E950.4	E962.0	E980.4
Lomustine	963.1	E858.1	E933.1	E950.4	E962.0	E980.4
Lophophora williamsii	969.6	E854.1	E939.6	E950.3	E962.0	E980.3
Lorazepam	969.4	E853.2	E939.4	E950.3	E962.0	E980.3
Lotions NEC	976.9	E858.7	E946.9	E950.4	E962.0	E980.4
Lotronex	973.8	E858.4	E943.8	E950.4	E962.0	E980.4
Lotusate	967.0	E851	E937.0	E950.1	E962.0	E980.1
Lowila	976.2	E858.7	E946.2	E950.4	E962.0	E980.4
Loxapine	969.3	E853.8	E939.3	E950.3	E962.0	E980.3
Lozenges (throat)	976.6	E858.7	E946.6	E950.4	E962.0	E980.4
LSD (25)	969.6	E854.1	E939.6	E950.3	E962.0	E980.3
Lubricating oil NEC	981	E862.2	—	E950.9	E962.1	E980.9
Lucanthone	961.6	E857	E931.6	E950.4	E962.0	E980.4
Luminal	967.0	E851	E937.0	E950.1	E962.0	E980.1
Lung irritant (gas) NEC	987.9	E869.9	—	E952.9	E962.2	E982.9
Lutocylol	962.2	E858.0	E932.2	E950.4	E962.0	E980.4
Lutromone	962.2	E858.0	E932.2	E950.4	E962.0	E980.4
Lututrin	975.0	E858.6	E945.0	E950.4	E962.0	E980.4
Lye (concentrated)	983.2	E864.2	—	E950.7	E962.1	E980.6
Lygranum (skin test)	977.8	E858.8	E947.8	E950.4	E962.0	E980.4
Lymecycline	960.4	E856	E930.4	E950.4	E962.0	E980.4
Lymphogranuloma venereum antigen	977.8	E858.8	E947.8	E950.4	E962.0	E980.4
Lynestrenol	962.2	E858.0	E932.2	E950.4	E962.0	E980.4
Lyovac Sodium Edecrin	974.4	E858.5	E944.4	E950.4	E962.0	E980.4
Lypressin	962.5	E858.0	E932.5	E950.4	E962.0	E980.4

Substance	Poisoning	External Cause (E-Code)				
		Accident	Therapeutic Use	Suicide Attempt	Assault	Undetermined
Lysergic acid (amide) (diethylamide)	969.6	E854.1	E939.6	E950.3	E962.0	E980.3
Lysergide	969.6	E854.1	E939.6	E950.3	E962.0	E980.3
Lysine vasopressin	962.5	E858.0	E932.5	E950.4	E962.0	E980.4
Lysol	983.0	E864.0	—	E950.7	E962.1	E980.6
Lytta (vitatta)	976.8	E858.7	E946.8	E950.4	E962.0	E980.4
Mace	987.5	E869.3	—	E952.8	E962.2	E982.8
Macrolides (antibiotics)	960.3	E856	E930.3	E950.4	E962.0	E980.4
Mafenide	976.0	E858.7	E946.0	E950.4	E962.0	E980.4
Magaldrate	973.0	E858.4	E943.0	E950.4	E962.0	E980.4
Magic mushroom	969.6	E854.1	E939.6	E950.3	E962.0	E980.3
Magnamycin	960.8	E856	E930.8	E950.4	E962.0	E980.4
Magnesia magma	973.0	E858.4	E943.0	E950.4	E962.0	E980.4
Magnesium (compounds) (fumes) NEC	985.8	E866.4	—	E950.9	E962.1	E980.9
antacid	973.0	E858.4	E943.0	E950.4	E962.0	E980.4
carbonate	973.0	E858.4	E943.0	E950.4	E962.0	E980.4
cathartic	973.3	E858.4	E943.3	E950.4	E962.0	E980.4
citrate	973.3	E858.4	E943.3	E950.4	E962.0	E980.4
hydroxide	973.0	E858.4	E943.0	E950.4	E962.0	E980.4
oxide	973.0	E858.4	E943.0	E950.4	E962.0	E980.4
sulfate (oral)	973.3	E858.4	E943.3	E950.4	E962.0	E980.4
intravenous	966.3	E855.0	E936.3	E950.4	E962.0	E980.4
trisilicate	973.0	E858.4	E943.0	E950.4	E962.0	E980.4
Malathion (insecticide)	989.3	E863.1	—	E950.6	E962.1	E980.7
Male fern (oleoresin)	961.6	E857	E931.6	E950.4	E962.0	E980.4
Mandelic acid	961.9	E857	E931.9	E950.4	E962.0	E980.4
Manganese compounds (fumes) NEC	985.2	E866.4	—	E950.9	E962.1	E980.9
Mannitol (diuretic) (medicinal) NEC	974.4	E858.5	E944.4	E950.4	E962.0	E980.4
hexanitrate	972.4	E858.3	E942.4	E950.4	E962.0	E980.4
mustard	963.1	E858.1	E933.1	E950.4	E962.0	E980.4
Mannomustine	963.1	E858.1	E933.1	E950.4	E962.0	E980.4
MAO inhibitors	969.0	E854.0	E939.0	E950.3	E962.0	E980.3
Mapharsen	961.1	E857	E931.1	E950.4	E962.0	E980.4
Marcaine	968.9	E855.2	E938.9	E950.4	E962.0	E980.4
infiltration (subcutaneous)	968.5	E855.2	E938.5	E950.4	E962.0	E980.4
nerve block (peripheral) (plexus)	968.6	E855.2	E938.6	E950.4	E962.0	E980.4
Marezine	963.0	E858.1	E933.0	E950.4	E962.0	E980.4
Marihuana, marijuana (derivatives)	969.6	E854.1	E939.6	E950.3	E962.0	E980.3
Marine animals or plants (sting)	989.5	E905.6	—	E950.9	E962.1	E980.9
Marplan	969.0	E854.0	E939.0	E950.3	E962.0	E980.3
Marsh gas	987.1	E869.8	—	E952.8	E962.2	E982.8
Marsilid	969.0	E854.0	E939.0	E950.3	E962.0	E980.3
Matulane	963.1	E858.1	E933.1	E950.4	E962.0	E980.4
Mazindol	977.0	E858.8	E947.0	E950.4	E962.0	E980.4
MDMA	969.7	E854.2	E939.7	E950.3	E962.0	E980.3
Meadow saffron	988.2	E865.3	—	E950.9	E962.1	E980.9
Measles vaccine	979.4	E858.8	E949.4	E950.4	E962.0	E980.4
Meat, noxious or nonbacterial	988.8	E865.0	—	E950.9	E962.1	E980.9
Mebanazine	969.0	E854.0	E939.0	E950.3	E962.0	E980.3
Mebaral	967.0	E851	E937.0	E950.1	E962.0	E980.1
Mebendazole	961.6	E857	E931.6	E950.4	E962.0	E980.4
Mebeverine	975.1	E858.6	E945.1	E950.4	E962.0	E980.4
Mebhydroline	963.0	E858.1	E933.0	E950.4	E962.0	E980.4
Mebrophenhydramine	963.0	E858.1	E933.0	E950.4	E962.0	E980.4
Mebutamate	969.5	E853.8	E939.5	E950.3	E962.0	E980.3
Mecamylamine (chloride)	972.3	E858.3	E942.3	E950.4	E962.0	E980.4
Mechlorethamine hydrochloride	963.1	E858.1	E933.1	E950.4	E962.0	E980.4
Meclizene (hydrochloride)	963.0	E858.1	E933.0	E950.4	E962.0	E980.4
Meclofenoxate	970.0	E854.3	E940.0	E950.4	E962.0	E980.4
Meclozine (hydrochloride)	963.0	E858.1	E933.0	E950.4	E962.0	E980.4
Medazepam	969.4	E853.2	E939.4	E950.3	E962.0	E980.3
Medicine, medicinal substance	977.9	E858.9	E947.9	E950.5	E962.0	E980.5
specified NEC	977.8	E858.8	E947.8	E950.4	E962.0	E980.4

Substance	Poisoning	External Cause (E-Code)				
		Accident	Therapeutic Use	Suicide Attempt	Assault	Undetermined
Medinal	967.0	E851	E937.0	E950.1	E962.0	E980.1
Medomin	967.0	E851	E937.0	E950.1	E962.0	E980.1
Medroxyprogesterone	962.2	E858.0	E932.2	E950.4	E962.0	E980.4
Medrysone	976.5	E858.7	E946.5	E950.4	E962.0	E980.4
Mefenamic acid	965.7	E850.7	E935.7	E950.0	E962.0	E980.0
Megahallucinogen	969.6	E854.1	E939.6	E950.3	E962.0	E980.3
Megestrol	962.2	E858.0	E932.2	E950.4	E962.0	E980.4
Meglumine	977.8	E858.8	E947.8	E950.4	E962.0	E980.4
Meladinin	976.3	E858.7	E946.3	E950.4	E962.0	E980.4
Melanizing agents	976.3	E858.7	E946.3	E950.4	E962.0	E980.4
Melarsoprol	961.1	E857	E931.1	E950.4	E962.0	E980.4
Melia azedarach	988.2	E865.3	—	E950.9	E962.1	E980.9
Mellaril	969.1	E853.0	E939.1	E950.3	E962.0	E980.3
Meloxine	976.3	E858.7	E946.3	E950.4	E962.0	E980.4
Melphalan	963.1	E858.1	E933.1	E950.4	E962.0	E980.4
Menadiol sodium diphosphate	964.3	E858.2	E934.3	E950.4	E962.0	E980.4
Menadione (sodium bisulfite)	964.3	E858.2	E934.3	E950.4	E962.0	E980.4
Menaphthone	964.3	E858.2	E934.3	E950.4	E962.0	E980.4
Meningococcal vaccine	978.8	E858.8	E948.8	E950.4	E962.0	E980.4
Menningovax-C	978.8	E858.8	E948.8	E950.4	E962.0	E980.4
Menotropins	962.4	E858.0	E932.4	E950.4	E962.0	E980.4
Menthol NEC	976.1	E858.7	E946.1	E950.4	E962.0	E980.4
Mepacrine	961.3	E857	E931.3	E950.4	E962.0	E980.4
Meparfynol	967.8	E852.8	E937.8	E950.2	E962.0	E980.2
Mepazine	969.1	E853.0	E939.1	E950.3	E962.0	E980.3
Mepenzolate	971.1	E855.4	E941.1	E950.4	E962.0	E980.4
Meperidine	965.09	E850.2	E935.2	E950.0	E962.0	E980.0
Mephenamin(e)	966.4	E855.0	E936.4	E950.4	E962.0	E980.4
Mephenesin (carbamate)	968.0	E855.1	E938.0	E950.4	E962.0	E980.4
Mephenoxalone	969.5	E853.8	E939.5	E950.3	E962.0	E980.3
Mephentermine	971.2	E855.5	E941.2	E950.4	E962.0	E980.4
Mephenytoin	966.1	E855.0	E936.1	E950.4	E962.0	E980.4
Mephobarbital	967.0	E851	E937.0	E950.1	E962.0	E980.1
Mepiperphenidol	971.1	E855.4	E941.1	E950.4	E962.0	E980.4
Mepivacaine	968.9	E855.2	E938.9	E950.4	E962.0	E980.4
infiltration (subcutaneous)	968.5	E855.2	E938.5	E950.4	E962.0	E980.4
nerve block (peripheral) (plexus)	968.6	E855.2	E938.6	E950.4	E962.0	E980.4
topical (surface)	968.5	E855.2	E938.5	E950.4	E962.0	E980.4
Meprednisone	962.0	E858.0	E932.0	E950.4	E962.0	E980.4
Meprobam	969.5	E853.8	E939.5	E950.3	E962.0	E980.3
Meprobamate	969.5	E853.8	E939.5	E950.3	E962.0	E980.3
Mepyramine (maleate)	963.0	E858.1	E933.0	E950.4	E962.0	E980.4
Meralluride	974.0	E858.5	E944.0	E950.4	E962.0	E980.4
Merbaphen	974.0	E858.5	E944.0	E950.4	E962.0	E980.4
Merbromin	976.0	E858.7	E946.0	E950.4	E962.0	E980.4
Mercaptomerin	974.0	E858.5	E944.0	E950.4	E962.0	E980.4
Mercaptopurine	963.1	E858.1	E933.1	E950.4	E962.0	E980.4
Mercumatilin	974.0	E858.5	E944.0	E950.4	E962.0	E980.4
Mercuramide	974.0	E858.5	E944.0	E950.4	E962.0	E980.4
Mercuranin	976.0	E858.7	E946.0	E950.4	E962.0	E980.4
Mercurochrome	976.0	E858.7	E946.0	E950.4	E962.0	E980.4
Mercury, mercuric, mercurous (compounds) (cyanide) (fumes) (nonmedicinal) (vapor) NEC	985.0	E866.1	—	E950.9	E962.1	E980.9
ammoniated	976.0	E858.7	E946.0	E950.4	E962.0	E980.4
anti-infective	961.2	E857	E931.2	E950.4	E962.0	E980.4
topical	976.0	E858.7	E946.0	E950.4	E962.0	E980.4
chloride (antiseptic) NEC	976.0	E858.7	E946.0	E950.4	E962.0	E980.4
fungicide	985.0	E863.6	—	E950.6	E962.1	E980.7
diuretic compounds	974.0	E858.5	E944.0	E950.4	E962.0	E980.4
fungicide	985.0	E863.6	—	E950.6	E962.1	E980.7
organic (fungicide)	985.0	E863.6	—	E950.6	E962.1	E980.7
Merethoxylline	974.0	E858.5	E944.0	E950.4	E962.0	E980.4

◀ New   ⬅ Revised

ICD-9-CM

Drugs

Vol. 2

Substance	Poisoning	External Cause (E-Code)				
		Accident	Therapeutic Use	Suicide Attempt	Assault	Undetermined
Mersalyl	974.0	E858.5	E944.0	E950.4	E962.0	E980.4
Merthiolate (topical)	976.0	E858.7	E946.0	E950.4	E962.0	E980.4
ophthalmic preparation	976.5	E858.7	E946.5	E950.4	E962.0	E980.4
Meruvax	979.4	E858.8	E949.4	E950.4	E962.0	E980.4
Mescal buttons	969.6	E854.1	E939.6	E950.3	E962.0	E980.3
Mescaline (salts)	969.6	E854.1	E939.6	E950.3	E962.0	E980.3
Mesoridazine besylate	969.1	E853.0	E939.1	E950.3	E962.0	E980.3
Mestanolone	962.1	E858.0	E932.1	E950.4	E962.0	E980.4
Mestranol	962.2	E858.0	E932.2	E950.4	E962.0	E980.4
Metactesylacetate	976.0	E858.7	E946.0	E950.4	E962.0	E980.4
Metaldehyde (snail killer) NEC	989.4	E863.4	—	E950.6	E962.1	E980.7
Metals (heavy) (nonmedicinal) NEC	985.9	E866.4	—	E950.9	E962.1	E980.9
dust, fumes, or vapor NEC	985.9	E866.4	—	E950.9	E962.1	E980.9
light NEC	985.9	E866.4	—	E950.9	E962.1	E980.9
dust, fumes, or vapor NEC	985.9	E866.4	—	E950.9	E962.1	E980.9
pesticides (dust) (vapor)	985.9	E863.4	—	E950.6	E962.1	E980.7
Metamucil	973.3	E858.4	E943.3	E950.4	E962.0	E980.4
Metaphen	976.0	E858.7	E946.0	E950.4	E962.0	E980.4
Metaproterenol	975.1	E858.6	E945.1	E950.4	E962.0	E980.4
Metaraminol	972.8	E858.3	E942.8	E950.4	E962.0	E980.4
Metaxalone	968.0	E855.1	E938.0	E950.4	E962.0	E980.4
Metformin	962.3	E858.0	E932.3	E950.4	E962.0	E980.4
Methacycline	960.4	E856	E930.4	E950.4	E962.0	E980.4
Methadone	965.02	E850.1	E935.1	E950.0	E962.0	E980.0
Methallenestril	962.2	E858.0	E932.2	E950.4	E962.0	E980.4
Methamphetamine	969.7	E854.2	E939.7	E950.3	E962.0	E980.3
Methandienone	962.1	E858.0	E932.1	E950.4	E962.0	E980.4
Methandriol	962.1	E858.0	E932.1	E950.4	E962.0	E980.4
Methandrostenolone	962.1	E858.0	E932.1	E950.4	E962.0	E980.4
Methane gas	987.1	E869.8	—	E952.8	E962.2	E982.8
Methanol	980.1	E860.2	—	E950.9	E962.1	E980.9
vapor	987.8	E869.8	—	E952.8	E962.2	E982.8
Methantheline	971.1	E855.4	E941.1	E950.4	E962.0	E980.4
Methaphenilene	963.0	E858.1	E933.0	E950.4	E962.0	E980.4
Methapyrilene	963.0	E858.1	E933.0	E950.4	E962.0	E980.4
Methaqualone (compounds)	967.4	E852.3	E937.4	E950.2	E962.0	E980.2
Metharbital, metharbitone	967.0	E851	E937.0	E950.1	E962.0	E980.1
Methazolamide	974.2	E858.5	E944.2	E950.4	E962.0	E980.4
Methdilazine	963.0	E858.1	E933.0	E950.4	E962.0	E980.4
Methedrine	969.7	E854.2	E939.7	E950.3	E962.0	E980.3
Methenamine (mandelate)	961.9	E857	E931.9	E950.4	E962.0	E980.4
Methenolone	962.1	E858.0	E932.1	E950.4	E962.0	E980.4
Methergine	975.0	E858.6	E945.0	E950.4	E962.0	E980.4
Methiacil	962.8	E858.0	E932.8	E950.4	E962.0	E980.4
Methicillin (sodium)	960.0	E856	E930.0	E950.4	E962.0	E980.4
Methimazole	962.8	E858.0	E932.8	E950.4	E962.0	E980.4
Methionine	977.1	E858.8	E947.1	E950.4	E962.0	E980.4
Methisazone	961.7	E857	E931.7	E950.4	E962.0	E980.4
Methitural	967.0	E851	E937.0	E950.1	E962.0	E980.1
Methixene	971.1	E855.4	E941.1	E950.4	E962.0	E980.4
Methobarbital, methobarbitone	967.0	E851	E937.0	E950.1	E962.0	E980.1
Methocarbamol	968.0	E855.1	E938.0	E950.4	E962.0	E980.4
Methohexital, methohexitone (sodium)	968.3	E855.1	E938.3	E950.4	E962.0	E980.4
Methoin	966.1	E855.0	E936.1	E950.4	E962.0	E980.4
Methopholine	965.7	E850.7	E935.7	E950.0	E962.0	E980.0
Methorate	975.4	E858.6	E945.4	E950.4	E962.0	E980.4
Methoserpidine	972.6	E858.3	E942.6	E950.4	E962.0	E980.4
Methotrexate	963.1	E858.1	E933.1	E950.4	E962.0	E980.4
Methotrimeprazine	967.8	E852.8	E937.8	E950.2	E962.0	E980.2
Methoxa-Dome	976.3	E858.7	E946.3	E950.4	E962.0	E980.4
Methoxamine	971.2	E855.5	E941.2	E950.4	E962.0	E980.4

Substance	Poisoning	External Cause (E-Code)				
		Accident	Therapeutic Use	Suicide Attempt	Assault	Undetermined
Methoxsalen	976.3	E858.7	E946.3	E950.4	E962.0	E980.4
Methoxybenzyl penicillin	960.0	E856	E930.0	E950.4	E962.0	E980.4
Methoxychlor	989.2	E863.0	—	E950.6	E962.1	E980.7
Methoxyflurane	968.2	E855.1	E938.2	E950.4	E962.0	E980.4
Methoxyphenamine	971.2	E855.5	E941.2	E950.4	E962.0	E980.4
Methoxypromazine	969.1	E853.0	E939.1	E950.3	E962.0	E980.3
Methoxypsoralen	976.3	E858.7	E946.3	E950.4	E962.0	E980.4
Methscopolamine (bromide)	971.1	E855.4	E941.1	E950.4	E962.0	E980.4
Methsuximide	966.2	E855.0	E936.2	E950.4	E962.0	E980.4
Methyclothiazide	974.3	E858.5	E944.3	E950.4	E962.0	E980.4
Methyl	—	—	—	—	—	—
acetate	982.8	E862.4	—	E950.9	E962.1	E980.9
acetone II	982.8	E862.4	—	E950.9	E962.1	E980.9
alcohol	980.1	E860.2	—	E950.9	E962.1	E980.9
amphetamine	969.7	E854.2	E939.7	E950.3	E962.0	E980.3
androstanolone	962.1	E858.0	E932.1	E950.4	E962.0	E980.4
atropine	971.1	E855.4	E941.1	E950.4	E962.0	E980.4
benzene	982.0	E862.4	—	E950.9	E962.1	E980.9
bromide (gas)	987.8	E869.8	—	E952.8	E962.2	E982.8
fumigant	987.8	E863.8	—	E950.6	E962.2	E980.7
butanol	980.8	E860.8	—	E950.9	E962.1	E980.9
carbinol	980.1	E860.2	—	E950.9	E962.1	E980.9
cellosolve	982.8	E862.4	—	E950.9	E962.1	E980.9
cellulose	973.3	E858.4	E943.3	E950.4	E961.0	E980.4
chloride (gas)	987.8	E869.8	—	E952.8	E962.2	E982.8
cyclohexane	982.8	E862.4	—	E950.9	E962.1	E980.9
cyclohexanone	982.8	E862.4	—	E950.9	E962.1	E980.9
dihydromorphinone	965.09	E850.2	E935.2	E950.0	E962.0	E980.0
ergometrine	975.0	E858.6	E945.0	E950.4	E962.0	E980.4
ergonovine	975.0	E858.6	E945.0	E950.4	E962.0	E980.4
ethyl ketone	982.8	E862.4	—	E950.9	E962.1	E980.9
hydrazine	983.9	E864.3	—	E950.7	E962.1	E980.6
isobutyl ketone	982.8	E862.4	—	E950.9	E962.1	E980.9
morphine NEC	965.09	E850.2	E935.2	E950.0	E962.0	E980.0
parafynol	967.8	E852.8	E937.8	E950.2	E962.0	E980.2
parathion	989.3	E863.1	—	E950.6	E962.1	E980.7
pentynol NEC	967.8	E852.8	E937.8	E950.2	E962.0	E980.2
peridol	969.2	E853.1	E939.2	E950.3	E962.0	E980.3
phenidate	969.7	E854.2	E939.7	E950.3	E962.0	E980.3
prednisolone	962.0	E858.0	E932.0	E950.4	E962.0	E980.4
ENT agent	976.6	E858.7	E946.6	E950.4	E962.0	E980.4
ophthalmic preparation	976.5	E858.7	E946.5	E950.4	E962.0	E980.4
topical NEC	976.0	E858.7	E946.0	E950.4	E962.0	E980.4
propylcarbinol	980.8	E860.8	—	E950.9	E962.1	E980.9
rosaniline NEC	976.0	E858.7	E946.0	E950.4	E962.0	E980.4
salicylate NEC	976.3	E858.7	E946.3	E950.4	E962.0	E980.4
sulfate (fumes)	987.8	E869.8	—	E952.8	E962.2	E982.8
liquid	983.9	E864.3	—	E950.7	E962.1	E980.6
sulfonal	967.8	E852.8	E937.8	E950.2	E962.0	E980.2
testosterone	962.1	E858.0	E932.1	E950.4	E962.0	E980.4
thiouracil	962.8	E858.0	E932.8	E950.4	E962.0	E980.4
Methylated spirit	980.0	E860.1	—	E950.9	E962.1	E980.9
Methyldopa	972.6	E858.3	E942.6	E950.4	E962.0	E980.4
Methylene blue	961.9	E857	E931.9	E950.4	E962.0	E980.4
chloride or dichloride (solvent) NEC	982.3	E862.4	—	E950.9	E962.1	E980.9
Methylhexabital	967.0	E851	E937.0	E950.1	E962.0	E980.1
Methylparaben (ophthalmic)	976.5	E858.7	E946.5	E950.4	E962.0	E980.4
Methyprylon	967.5	E852.4	E937.5	E950.2	E962.0	E980.2
Methysergide	971.3	E855.6	E941.3	E950.4	E962.0	E980.4
Metoclopramide	963.0	E858.1	E933.0	E950.4	E962.0	E980.4
Metofoline	965.7	E850.7	E935.7	E950.0	E962.0	E980.0

◀ New   ◀▥ Revised

ICD-9-CM

Drugs

Vol. 2

Substance	Poisoning	External Cause (E-Code)				
		Accident	Therapeutic Use	Suicide Attempt	Assault	Undetermined
Metopon	965.09	E850.2	E935.2	E950.0	E962.0	E980.0
Metronidazole	961.5	E857	E931.5	E950.4	E962.0	E980.4
Metycaine	968.9	E855.2	E938.9	E950.4	E962.0	E980.4
infiltration (subcutaneous)	968.5	E855.2	E938.5	E950.4	E962.0	E980.4
nerve block (peripheral) (plexus)	968.6	E855.2	E938.6	E950.4	E962.0	E980.4
topical (surface)	968.5	E855.2	E938.5	E950.4	E962.0	E980.4
Metyrapone	977.8	E858.8	E947.8	E950.4	E962.0	E980.4
Mevinphos	989.3	E863.1	—	E950.6	E962.1	E980.7
Mezereon (berries)	988.2	E865.3	—	E950.9	E962.1	E980.9
Micatin	976.0	E858.7	E946.0	E950.4	E962.0	E980.4
Miconazole	976.0	E858.7	E946.0	E950.4	E962.0	E980.4
Midol	965.1	E850.3	E935.3	E950.0	E962.0	E980.0
Mifepristone	962.9	E858.0	E932.9	E950.4	E962.0	E980.4
Milk of magnesia	973.0	E858.4	E943.0	E950.4	E962.0	E980.4
Millipede (tropical) (venomous)	989.5	E905.4	—	E950.9	E962.1	E980.9
Miltown	969.5	E853.8	E939.5	E950.3	E962.0	E980.3
Mineral	—	—	—	—	—	—
oil (medicinal)	973.2	E858.4	E943.2	E950.4	E962.0	E980.4
nonmedicinal	981	E862.1	—	E950.9	E962.1	E980.9
topical	976.3	E858.7	E946.3	E950.4	E962.0	E980.4
salts NEC	974.6	E858.5	E944.6	E950.4	E962.0	E980.4
spirits	981	E862.0	—	E950.9	E962.1	E980.9
Minocycline	960.4	E856	E930.4	E950.4	E962.0	E980.4
Mithramycin (antineoplastic)	960.7	E856	E930.7	E950.4	E962.0	E980.4
Mitobronitol	963.1	E858.1	E933.1	E950.4	E962.0	E980.4
Mitomycin (antineoplastic)	960.7	E856	E930.7	E950.4	E962.0	E980.4
Mitotane	963.1	E858.1	E933.1	E950.4	E962.0	E980.4
Moderil	972.6	E858.3	E942.6	E950.4	E962.0	E980.4
Mogadon - see Nitrazepam	—	—	—	—	—	—
Molindone	969.3	E853.8	E939.3	E950.3	E962.0	E980.3
Monistat	976.0	E858.7	E946.0	E950.4	E962.0	E980.4
Monkshood	988.2	E865.4	—	E950.9	E962.1	E980.9
Monoamine oxidase inhibitors	969.0	E854.0	E939.0	E950.3	E962.0	E980.3
Monochlorobenzene	982.0	E862.4	—	E950.9	E962.1	E980.9
Monosodium glutamate	989.89	E866.8	—	E950.9	E962.1	E980.9
Monoxide, carbon - see Carbon, monoxide	—	—	—	—	—	—
Moperone	969.2	E853.1	E939.2	E950.3	E962.0	E980.3
Morning glory seeds	969.6	E854.1	E939.6	E950.3	E962.0	E980.3
Moroxydine (hydrochloride)	961.7	E857	E931.7	E950.4	E962.0	E980.4
Morphazinamide	961.8	E857	E931.8	E950.4	E962.0	E980.4
Morphinans	965.09	E850.2	E935.2	E950.0	E962.0	E980.0
Morphine NEC	965.09	E850.2	E935.2	E950.0	E962.0	E980.0
antagonists	970.1	E854.3	E940.1	E950.4	E962.0	E980.4
Morpholinylethyl morphine	965.09	E850.2	E935.2	E950.0	E962.0	E980.0
Morrhuate sodium	972.7	E858.3	E942.7	E950.4	E962.0	E980.4
Moth balls (see also Pesticides)	989.4	E863.4	—	E950.6	E962.1	E980.7
naphthalene	983.0	E863.4	—	E950.7	E962.1	E980.6
Motor exhaust gas - see Carbon, monoxide, exhaust gas	—	—	—	—	—	—
Mouth wash	976.6	E858.7	E946.6	E950.4	E962.0	E980.4
Mucolytic agent	975.5	E858.6	E945.5	E950.4	E962.0	E980.4
Mucomyst	975.5	E858.6	E945.5	E950.4	E962.0	E980.4
Mucous membrane agents (external)	976.9	E858.7	E946.9	E950.4	E962.0	E980.4
specified NEC	976.8	E858.7	E946.8	E950.4	E962.0	E980.4
Mumps	—	—	—	—	—	—
immune globulin (human)	964.6	E858.2	E934.6	E950.4	E962.0	E980.4
skin test antigen	977.8	E858.8	E947.8	E950.4	E962.0	E980.4
vaccine	979.6	E858.8	E949.6	E950.4	E962.0	E980.4
Mumpsvax	979.6	E858.8	E949.6	E950.4	E962.0	E980.4
Muriatic acid - see Hydrochloric acid	—	—	—	—	—	—
Muscarine	971.0	E855.3	E941.0	E950.4	E962.0	E980.4
Muscle affecting agents NEC	975.3	E858.6	E945.3	E950.4	E962.0	E980.4
oxytocic	975.0	E858.6	E945.0	E950.4	E962.0	E980.4

Substance	Poisoning	External Cause (E-Code)				
		Accident	Therapeutic Use	Suicide Attempt	Assault	Undetermined
Muscle affecting agents NEC *(Continued)*						
relaxants	975.3	E858.6	E945.3	E950.4	E962.0	E980.4
central nervous system	968.0	E855.1	E938.0	E950.4	E962.0	E980.4
skeletal	975.2	E858.6	E945.2	E950.4	E962.0	E980.4
smooth	975.1	E858.6	E945.1	E950.4	E962.0	E980.4
Mushrooms, noxious	988.1	E865.5	—	E950.9	E962.1	E980.9
Mussel, noxious	988.0	E865.1	—	E950.9	E962.1	E980.9
Mustard (emetic)	973.6	E858.4	E943.6	E950.4	E962.0	E980.4
gas	987.8	E869.8	—	E952.8	E962.2	E982.8
nitrogen	963.1	E858.1	E933.1	E950.4	E962.0	E980.4
Mustine	963.1	E858.1	E933.1	E950.4	E962.0	E980.4
M-vac	979.4	E858.8	E949.4	E950.4	E962.0	E980.4
Mycifradin	960.8	E856	E930.8	E950.4	E962.0	E980.4
topical	976.0	E858.7	E946.0	E950.4	E962.0	E980.4
Mycitracin	960.8	E856	E930.8	E950.4	E962.0	E980.4
ophthalmic preparation	976.5	E858.7	E946.5	E950.4	E962.0	E980.4
Mycostatin	960.1	E856	E930.1	E950.4	E962.0	E980.4
topical	976.0	E858.7	E946.0	E950.4	E962.0	E980.4
Mydriacyl	971.1	E855.4	E941.1	E950.4	E962.0	E980.4
Myelobromal	963.1	E858.1	E933.1	E950.4	E962.0	E980.4
Myleran	963.1	E858.1	E933.1	E950.4	E962.0	E980.4
Myochrysin(e)	965.69	E850.6	E935.6	E950.0	E962.0	E980.0
Myoneural blocking agents	975.2	E858.6	E945.2	E950.4	E962.0	E980.4
Myristica fragrans	988.2	E865.3	—	E950.9	E962.1	E980.9
Myristicin	988.2	E865.3	—	E950.9	E962.1	E980.9
Mysoline	966.3	E855.0	E936.3	E950.4	E962.0	E980.4
Nafcillin (sodium)	960.0	E856	E930.0	E950.4	E962.0	E980.4
Nail polish remover	982.8	E862.4	—	E950.9	E962.1	E980.9
Nalidixic acid	961.9	E857	E931.9	E950.4	E962.0	E980.4
Nalorphine	970.1	E854.3	E940.1	E950.4	E962.0	E980.4
Naloxone	970.1	E854.3	E940.1	E950.4	E962.0	E980.4
Nandrolone (decanoate) (phenpropionate)	962.1	E858.0	E932.1	E950.4	E962.0	E980.4
Naphazoline	971.2	E855.5	E941.2	E950.4	E962.0	E980.4
Naphtha (painter's) (petroleum)	981	E862.0	—	E950.9	E962.1	E980.9
solvent	981	E862.0	—	E950.9	E962.1	E980.9
vapor	987.1	E869.8	—	E952.8	E962.2	E982.8
Naphthalene (chlorinated)	983.0	E864.0	—	E950.7	E962.1	E980.6
insecticide or moth repellent	983.0	E863.4	—	E950.7	E962.1	E980.6
vapor	987.8	E869.8	—	E952.8	E962.2	E982.8
Naphthol	983.0	E864.0	—	E950.7	E962.1	E980.6
Naphthylamine	983.0	E864.0	—	E950.7	E962.1	E980.6
Naprosyn - *see* Naproxen	—	—	—	—	—	—
Naproxen	965.61	E850.6	E935.6	E950.0	E962.0	E980.0
Narcotic (drug)	967.9	E852.9	E937.9	E950.2	E962.0	E980.2
analgesic NEC	965.8	E850.8	E935.8	E950.0	E962.0	E980.0
antagonist	970.1	E854.3	E940.1	E950.4	E962.0	E980.4
specified NEC	967.8	E852.8	E937.8	E950.2	E962.0	E980.2
Narcotine	975.4	E858.6	E945.4	E950.4	E962.0	E980.4
Nardil	969.0	E854.0	E939.0	E950.3	E962.0	E980.3
Natrium cyanide - *see* Cyanide(s)	—	—	—	—	—	—
Natural	—	—	—	—	—	—
blood (product)	964.7	E858.2	E934.7	E950.4	E962.0	E980.4
gas (piped)	987.1	E867	—	E951.0	E962.2	E981.0
incomplete combustion	986	E867	—	E951.0	E962.2	E981.0
Nealbarbital, nealbarbitone	967.0	E851	E937.0	E950.1	E962.0	E980.1
Nectadon	975.4	E858.6	E945.4	E950.4	E962.0	E980.4
Nematocyst (sting)	989.5	E905.6	—	E950.9	E962.1	E980.9
Nembutal	967.0	E851	E937.0	E950.1	E962.0	E980.1
Neoarsphenamine	961.1	E857	E931.1	E950.4	E962.0	E980.4
Neocinchophen	974.7	E858.5	E944.7	E950.4	E962.0	E980.4
Neomycin	960.8	E856	E930.8	E950.4	E962.0	E980.4
ENT agent	976.6	E858.7	E946.6	E950.4	E962.0	E980.4
ophthalmic preparation	976.5	E858.7	E946.5	E950.4	E962.0	E980.4

◀ New   ◀═ Revised

Substance	Poisoning	External Cause (E-Code)				
		Accident	Therapeutic Use	Suicide Attempt	Assault	Undetermined
Neomycin (Continued)						
topical NEC	976.0	E858.7	E946.0	E950.4	E962.0	E980.4
Neonal	967.0	E851	E937.0	E950.1	E962.0	E980.1
Neoprontosil	961.0	E857	E931.0	E950.4	E962.0	E980.4
Neosalvarsan	961.1	E857	E931.1	E950.4	E962.0	E980.4
Neosilversalvarsan	961.1	E857	E931.1	E950.4	E962.0	E980.4
Neosporin	960.8	E856	E930.8	E950.4	E962.0	E980.4
ENT agent	976.6	E858.7	E946.6	E950.4	E962.0	E980.4
ophthalmic preparation	976.5	E858.7	E946.5	E950.4	E962.0	E980.4
topical NEC	976.0	E858.7	E946.0	E950.4	E962.0	E980.4
Neostigmine	971.0	E855.3	E941.0	E950.4	E962.0	E980.4
Neraval	967.0	E851	E937.0	E950.1	E962.0	E980.1
Neravan	967.0	E851	E937.0	E950.1	E962.0	E980.1
Nerium oleander	988.2	E865.4	—	E950.9	E962.1	E980.9
Nerve gases (war)	987.9	E869.9	—	E952.9	E962.2	E982.9
Nesacaine	968.9	E855.2	E938.9	E950.4	E962.0	E980.4
infiltration (subcutaneous)	968.5	E855.2	E938.5	E950.4	E962.0	E980.4
nerve block (peripheral) (plexus)	968.6	E855.2	E938.6	E950.4	E962.0	E980.4
Neurobarb	967.0	E851	E937.0	E950.1	E962.0	E980.1
Neuroleptics NEC	969.3	E853.8	E939.3	E950.3	E962.0	E980.3
Neuroprotective agent	977.8	E858.8	E947.8	E950.4	E962.0	E980.4
Neutral spirits	980.0	E860.1	—	E950.9	E962.1	E980.9
beverage	980.0	E860.0	—	E950.9	E962.1	E980.9
Niacin, niacinamide	972.2	E858.3	E942.2	E950.4	E962.0	E980.4
Nialamide	969.0	E854.0	E939.0	E950.3	E962.0	E980.3
Nickle (carbonyl) (compounds) (fumes) (tetracarbonyl) (vapor)	985.8	E866.4	—	E950.9	E962.1	E980.9
Niclosamide	961.6	E857	E931.6	E950.4	E962.0	E980.4
Nicomorphine	965.09	E850.2	E935.2	E950.0	E962.0	E980.0
Nicotinamide	972.2	E858.3	E942.2	E950.4	E962.0	E980.4
Nicotine (insecticide) (spray) (sulfate) NEC	989.4	E863.4	—	E950.6	E962.1	E980.7
not insecticide	989.89	E866.8	—	E950.9	E962.1	E980.9
Nicotinic acid (derivatives)	972.2	E858.3	E942.2	E950.4	E962.0	E980.4
Nicotinyl alcohol	972.2	E858.3	E942.2	E950.4	E962.0	E980.4
Nicoumalone	964.2	E858.2	E934.2	E950.4	E962.0	E980.4
Nifenazone	965.5	E850.5	E935.5	E950.0	E962.0	E980.0
Nifuraldezone	961.9	E857	E931.9	E950.4	E962.0	E980.4
Nightshade (deadly)	988.2	E865.4	—	E950.9	E962.1	E980.9
Nikethamide	970.0	E854.3	E940.0	E950.4	E962.0	E980.4
Nilstat	960.1	E856	E930.1	E950.4	E962.0	E980.4
topical	976.0	E858.7	E946.0	E950.4	E962.0	E980.4
Nimodipine	977.8	E858.8	E947.8	E950.4	E962.0	E980.4
Niridazole	961.6	E857	E931.6	E950.4	E962.0	E980.4
Nisentil	965.09	E850.2	E935.2	E950.0	E962.0	E980.0
Nitrates	972.4	E858.3	E942.4	E950.4	E962.0	E980.4
Nitrazepam	969.4	E853.2	E939.4	E950.3	E962.0	E980.3
Nitric	—	—	—	—	—	—
acid (liquid)	983.1	E864.1	—	E950.7	E962.1	E980.6
vapor	987.8	E869.8	—	E952.8	E962.2	E982.8
oxide (gas)	987.2	E869.0	—	E952.8	E962.2	E982.8
Nitrite, amyl (medicinal) (vapor)	972.4	E858.3	E942.4	E950.4	E962.0	E980.4
Nitroaniline	983.0	E864.0	—	E950.7	E962.1	E980.6
vapor	987.8	E869.8	—	E952.8	E962.2	E982.8
Nitrobenzene, nitrobenzol	983.0	E864.0	—	E950.7	E962.1	E980.6
vapor	987.8	E869.8	—	E952.8	E962.2	E982.8
Nitrocellulose	976.3	E858.7	E946.3	E950.4	E962.0	E980.4
Nitrofuran derivatives	961.9	E857	E931.9	E950.4	E962.0	E980.4
Nitrofurantoin	961.9	E857	E931.9	E950.4	E962.0	E980.4
Nitrofurazone	976.0	E858.7	E946.0	E950.4	E962.0	E980.4
Nitrogen (dioxide) (gas) (oxide)	987.2	E869.0	—	E952.8	E962.2	E982.8
mustard (antineoplastic)	963.1	E858.1	E933.1	E950.4	E962.0	E980.4
Nitroglycerin, nitroglycerol (medicinal)	972.4	E858.3	E942.4	E950.4	E962.0	E980.4
nonmedicinal	989.89	E866.8	—	E950.9	E962.1	E980.9
fumes	987.8	E869.8	—	E952.8	E962.2	E982.8

ICD-9-CM

Drugs

Vol.

◀ New   ◀‖‖ Revised

Substance	Poisoning	External Cause (E-Code)				
		Accident	Therapeutic Use	Suicide Attempt	Assault	Undetermined
Nitrohydrochloric acid	983.1	E864.1	—	E950.7	E962.1	E980.6
Nitromersol	976.0	E858.7	E946.0	E950.4	E962.0	E980.4
Nitronaphthalene	983.0	E864.0	—	E950.7	E962.2	E980.6
Nitrophenol	983.0	E864.0	—	E950.7	E962.2	E980.6
Nitrothiazol	961.6	E857	E931.6	E950.4	E962.0	E980.4
Nitrotoluene, nitrotoluol	983.0	E864.0	—	E950.7	E962.1	E980.6
vapor	987.8	E869.8	—	E952.8	E962.2	E982.8
Nitrous	968.2	E855.1	E938.2	E950.4	E962.0	E980.4
acid (liquid)	983.1	E864.1	—	E950.7	E962.1	E980.6
fumes	987.2	E869.0	—	E952.8	E962.2	E982.8
oxide (anesthetic) NEC	968.2	E855.1	E938.2	E950.4	E962.0	E980.4
Nitrozone	976.0	E858.7	E946.0	E950.4	E962.0	E980.4
Noctec	967.1	E852.0	E937.1	E950.2	E962.0	E980.2
Noludar	967.5	E852.4	E937.5	E950.2	E962.0	E980.2
Noptil	967.0	E851	E937.0	E950.1	E962.0	E980.1
Noradrenalin	971.2	E855.5	E941.2	E950.4	E962.0	E980.4
Noramidopyrine	965.5	E850.5	E935.5	E950.0	E962.0	E980.0
Norepinephrine	971.2	E855.5	E941.2	E950.4	E962.0	E980.4
Norethandrolone	962.1	E858.0	E932.1	E950.4	E962.0	E980.4
Norethindrone	962.2	E858.0	E932.2	E950.4	E962.0	E980.4
Norethisterone	962.2	E858.0	E932.2	E950.4	E962.0	E980.4
Norethynodrel	962.2	E858.0	E932.2	E950.4	E962.0	E980.4
Norlestrin	962.2	E858.0	E932.2	E950.4	E962.0	E980.4
Norlutin	962.2	E858.0	E932.2	E950.4	E962.0	E980.4
Normison - see Benzodiazepines	—	—	—	—	—	—
Normorphine	965.09	E850.2	E935.2	E950.0	E962.0	E980.0
Nortriptyline	969.0	E854.0	E939.0	E950.3	E962.0	E980.3
Noscapine	975.4	E858.6	E945.4	E950.4	E962.0	E980.4
Nose preparations	976.6	E858.7	E946.6	E950.4	E962.0	E980.4
Novobiocin	960.8	E856	E930.8	E950.4	E962.0	E980.4
Novocain (infiltration) (topical)	968.5	E855.2	E938.5	E950.4	E962.0	E980.4
nerve block (peripheral) (plexus)	968.6	E855.2	E938.6	E950.4	E962.0	E980.4
spinal	968.7	E855.2	E938.7	E950.4	E962.0	E980.4
Noxythiolin	961.9	E857	E931.9	E950.4	E962.0	E980.4
NPH Iletin (insulin)	962.3	E858.0	E932.3	E950.4	E962.0	E980.4
Numorphan	965.09	E850.2	E935.2	E950.0	E962.0	E980.0
Nunol	967.0	E851	E937.0	E950.1	E962.0	E980.1
Nupercaine (spinal anesthetic)	968.7	E855.2	E938.7	E950.4	E962.0	E980.4
topical (surface)	968.5	E855.2	E938.5	E950.4	E962.0	E980.4
Nutmeg oil (liniment)	976.3	E858.7	E946.3	E950.4	E962.0	E980.4
Nux vomica	989.1	E863.7	—	E950.6	E962.1	E980.7
Nydrazid	961.8	E857	E931.8	E950.4	E962.0	E980.4
Nylidrin	971.2	E855.5	E941.2	E950.4	E962.0	E980.4
Nystatin	960.1	E856	E930.1	E950.4	E962.0	E980.4
topical	976.0	E858.7	E946.0	E950.4	E962.0	E980.4
Nytol	963.0	E858.1	E933.0	E950.4	E962.0	E980.4
Oblivion	967.8	E852.8	E937.8	E950.2	E962.0	E980.2
Octyl nitrite	972.4	E858.3	E942.4	E950.4	E962.0	E980.4
Oestradiol (cypionate) (dipropionate) (valerate)	962.2	E858.0	E932.2	E950.4	E962.0	E980.4
Oestriol	962.2	E858.0	E932.2	E950.4	E962.0	E980.4
Oestrone	962.2	E858.0	E932.2	E950.4	E962.0	E980.4
Oil (of) NEC	989.89	E866.8	—	E950.9	E962.1	E980.9
bitter almond	989.0	E866.8	—	E950.9	E962.1	E980.9
camphor	976.1	E858.7	E946.1	E950.4	E962.0	E980.4
colors	989.89	E861.6	—	E950.9	E962.1	E980.9
fumes	987.8	E869.8	—	E952.8	E962.2	E982.8
lubricating	981	E862.2	—	E950.9	E962.1	E980.9
specified source, other - see substance specified	—	—	—	—	—	—
vitriol (liquid)	983.1	E864.1	—	E950.7	E962.1	E980.6
fumes	987.8	E869.8	—	E952.8	E962.2	E982.8
wintergreen (bitter) NEC	976.3	E858.7	E946.3	E950.4	E962.0	E980.4

Substance	Poisoning	External Cause (E-Code)				
		Accident	Therapeutic Use	Suicide Attempt	Assault	Undetermined
Ointments NEC	976.9	E858.7	E946.9	E950.4	E962.0	E980.4
Oleander	988.2	E865.4	—	E950.9	E962.1	E980.9
Oleandomycin	960.3	E856	E930.3	E950.4	E962.0	E980.4
Oleovitamin A	963.5	E858.1	E933.5	E950.4	E962.0	E980.4
Oleum ricini	973.1	E858.4	E943.1	E950.4	E962.0	E980.4
Olive oil (medicinal) NEC	973.2	E858.4	E943.2	E950.4	E962.0	E980.4
OMPA	989.3	E863.1	—	E950.6	E962.1	E980.7
Oncovin	963.1	E858.1	E933.1	E950.4	E962.0	E980.4
Ophthaine	968.5	E855.2	E938.5	E950.4	E962.0	E980.4
Ophthetic	968.5	E855.2	E938.5	E950.4	E962.0	E980.4
Opiates, opioids, opium NEC	965.00	E850.2	E935.2	E950.0	E962.0	E980.0
antagonists	970.1	E854.3	E940.1	E950.4	E962.0	E980.4
Oracon	962.2	E858.0	E932.2	E950.4	E962.0	E980.4
Oragrafin	977.8	E858.8	E947.8	E950.4	E962.0	E980.4
Oral contraceptives	962.2	E858.0	E932.2	E950.4	E962.0	E980.4
Orciprenaline	975.1	E858.6	E945.1	E950.4	E962.0	E980.4
Organidin	975.5	E858.6	E945.5	E950.4	E962.0	E980.4
Organophosphates	989.3	E863.1	—	E950.6	E962.1	E980.7
Orimune	979.5	E858.8	E949.5	E950.4	E962.0	E980.4
Orinase	962.3	E858.0	E932.3	E950.4	E962.0	E980.4
Orphenadrine	966.4	E855.0	E936.4	E950.4	E962.0	E980.4
Ortal (sodium)	967.0	E851	E937.0	E950.1	E962.0	E980.1
Orthoboric acid	976.0	E858.7	E946.0	E950.4	E962.0	E980.4
ENT agent	976.6	E858.7	E946.6	E950.4	E962.0	E980.4
ophthalmic preparation	976.5	E858.7	E946.5	E950.4	E962.0	E980.4
Orthocaine	968.5	E855.2	E938.5	E950.4	E962.0	E980.4
Ortho-Novum	962.2	E858.0	E932.2	E950.4	E962.0	E980.4
Orthotolidine (reagent)	977.8	E858.8	E947.8	E950.4	E962.0	E980.4
Osmic acid (liquid)	983.1	E864.1	—	E950.7	E962.1	E980.6
fumes	987.8	E869.8	—	E952.8	E962.2	E982.8
Osmotic diuretics	974.4	E858.5	E944.4	E950.4	E962.0	E980.4
Ouabain	972.1	E858.3	E942.1	E950.4	E962.0	E980.4
Ovarian hormones (synthetic substitutes)	962.2	E858.0	E932.2	E950.4	E962.0	E980.4
Ovral	962.2	E858.0	E932.2	E950.4	E962.0	E980.4
Ovulation suppressants	962.2	E858.0	E932.2	E950.4	E962.0	E980.4
Ovulen	962.2	E858.0	E932.2	E950.4	E962.0	E980.4
Oxacillin (sodium)	960.0	E856	E930.0	E950.4	E962.0	E980.4
Oxalic acid	983.1	E864.1	—	E950.7	E962.1	E980.6
Oxanamide	969.5	E853.8	E939.5	E950.3	E962.0	E980.3
Oxandrolone	962.1	E858.0	E932.1	E950.4	E962.0	E980.4
Oxaprozin	965.61	E850.6	E935.6	E950.0	E962.0	E980.0
Oxazepam	969.4	E853.2	E939.4	E950.3	E962.0	E980.3
Oxazolidine derivatives	966.0	E855.0	E936.0	E950.4	E962.0	E980.4
Ox bile extract	973.4	E858.4	E943.4	E950.4	E962.0	E980.4
Oxedrine	971.2	E855.5	E941.2	E950.4	E962.0	E980.4
Oxeladin	975.4	E858.6	E945.4	E950.4	E962.0	E980.4
Oxethazaine NEC	968.5	E855.2	E938.5	E950.4	E962.0	E980.4
Oxidizing agents NEC	983.9	E864.3	—	E950.7	E962.1	E980.6
Oxolinic acid	961.3	E857	E931.3	E950.4	E962.0	E980.4
Oxophenarsine	961.1	E857	E931.1	E950.4	E962.0	E980.4
Oxsoralen	976.3	E858.7	E946.3	E950.4	E962.0	E980.4
Oxtriphylline	976.7	E858.6	E945.7	E950.4	E962.0	E980.4
Oxybuprocaine	968.5	E855.2	E938.5	E950.4	E962.0	E980.4
Oxybutynin	975.1	E858.6	E945.1	E950.4	E962.0	E980.4
Oxycodone	965.09	E850.2	E935.2	E950.0	E962.0	E980.0
Oxygen	987.8	E869.8	—	E952.8	E962.2	E982.8
Oxylone	976.0	E858.7	E946.0	E950.4	E962.0	E980.4
ophthalmic preparation	976.5	E858.7	E946.5	E950.4	E962.0	E980.4
Oxymesterone	962.1	E858.0	E932.1	E950.4	E962.0	E980.4
Oxymetazoline	971.2	E855.5	E941.2	E950.4	E962.0	E980.4
Oxymetholone	962.1	E858.0	E932.1	E950.4	E962.0	E980.4
Oxymorphone	965.09	E850.2	E935.2	E950.0	E962.0	E980.0

ICD-9-CM

Drugs

Vol. 2

Substance	Poisoning	External Cause (E-Code)				
		Accident	Therapeutic Use	Suicide Attempt	Assault	Undetermined
Oxypertine	969.0	E854.0	E939.0	E950.3	E962.0	E980.3
Oxyphenbutazone	965.5	E850.5	E935.5	E950.0	E962.0	E980.0
Oxyphencyclimine	971.1	E855.4	E941.1	E950.4	E962.0	E980.4
Oxyphenisatin	973.1	E858.4	E943.1	E950.4	E962.0	E980.4
Oxyphenonium	971.1	E855.4	E941.1	E950.4	E962.0	E980.4
Oxyquinoline	961.3	E857	E931.3	E950.4	E962.0	E980.4
Oxytetracycline	960.4	E856	E930.4	E950.4	E962.0	E980.4
Oxytocics	975.0	E858.6	E945.0	E950.4	E962.0	E980.4
Oxytocin	975.0	E858.6	E945.0	E950.4	E962.0	E980.4
Ozone	987.8	E869.8	—	E952.8	E962.2	E982.8
PABA	976.3	E858.7	E946.3	E950.4	E962.0	E980.4
Packed red cells	964.7	E858.2	E934.7	E950.4	E962.0	E980.4
Paint NEC	989.89	E861.6	—	E950.9	E962.1	E980.9
cleaner	982.8	E862.9	—	E950.9	E962.1	E980.9
fumes NEC	987.8	E869.8	—	E952.8	E962.1	E982.8
lead (fumes)	984.0	E861.5	—	E950.9	E962.1	E980.9
solvent NEC	982.8	E862.9	—	E950.9	E962.1	E980.9
stripper	982.8	E862.9	—	E950.9	E962.1	E980.9
Palfium	965.09	E850.2	E935.2	E950.0	E962.0	E980.0
Palivizumab	979.9	E858.8	E949.6	E950.4	E962.0	E980.4
Paludrine	961.4	E857	E931.4	E950.4	E962.0	E980.4
PAM	977.2	E855.8	E947.2	E950.4	E962.0	E980.4
Pamaquine (napthoate)	961.4	E857	E931.4	E950.4	E962.0	E980.4
Pamprin	965.1	E850.3	E935.3	E950.0	E962.0	E980.0
Panadol	965.4	E850.4	E935.4	E950.0	E962.0	E980.0
Pancreatic dornase (mucolytic)	963.4	E858.1	E933.4	E950.4	E962.0	E980.4
Pancreatin	973.4	E858.4	E943.4	E950.4	E962.0	E980.4
Pancrelipase	973.4	E858.4	E943.4	E950.4	E962.0	E980.4
Pangamic acid	963.5	E858.1	E933.5	E950.4	E962.0	E980.4
Panthenol	963.5	E858.1	E933.5	E950.4	E962.0	E980.4
topical	976.8	E858.7	E946.8	E950.4	E962.0	E980.4
Pantopaque	977.8	E858.8	E947.8	E950.4	E962.0	E980.4
Pantopon	965.00	E850.2	E935.2	E950.0	E962.0	E980.0
Pantothenic acid	963.5	E858.1	E933.5	E950.4	E962.0	E980.4
Panwarfin	964.2	E858.2	E934.2	E950.4	E962.0	E980.4
Papain	973.4	E858.4	E943.4	E950.4	E962.0	E980.4
Papaverine	972.5	E858.3	E942.5	E950.4	E962.0	E980.4
Para-aminobenzoic acid	976.3	E858.7	E946.3	E950.4	E962.0	E980.4
Para-aminophenol derivatives	965.4	E850.4	E935.4	E950.0	E962.0	E980.0
Para-aminosalicylic acid (derivatives)	961.8	E857	E931.8	E950.4	E962.0	E980.4
Paracetaldehyde (medicinal)	967.2	E852.1	E937.2	E950.2	E962.0	E980.2
Paracetamol	965.4	E850.4	E935.4	E950.0	E962.0	E980.0
Paracodin	965.09	E850.2	E935.2	E950.0	E962.0	E980.0
Paradione	966.0	E855.0	E936.0	E950.4	E962.0	E980.4
Paraffin(s) (wax)	981	E862.3	—	E950.9	E962.1	E980.9
liquid (medicinal)	973.2	E858.4	E943.2	E950.4	E962.0	E980.4
nonmedicinal (oil)	981	E962.1	—	E950.9	E962.1	E980.9
Paraldehyde (medicinal)	967.2	E852.1	E937.2	E950.2	E962.0	E980.2
Paramethadione	966.0	E855.0	E936.0	E950.4	E962.0	E980.4
Paramethasone	962.0	E858.0	E932.0	E950.4	E962.0	E980.4
Paraquat	989.4	E863.5	—	E950.6	E962.1	E980.7
Parasympatholytics	971.1	E855.4	E941.1	E950.4	E962.0	E980.4
Parasympathomimetics	971.0	E855.3	E941.0	E950.4	E962.0	E980.4
Parathion	989.3	E863.1	—	E950.6	E962.1	E980.7
Parathormone	962.6	E858.0	E932.6	E950.4	E962.0	E980.4
Parathyroid (derivatives)	962.6	E858.0	E932.6	E950.4	E962.0	E980.4
Paratyphoid vaccine	978.1	E858.8	E948.1	E950.4	E962.0	E980.4
Paredrine	971.2	E855.5	E941.2	E950.4	E962.0	E980.4
Paregoric	965.00	E850.2	E935.2	E950.0	E962.0	E980.0
Pargyline	972.3	E858.3	E942.3	E950.4	E962.0	E980.4
Paris green	985.1	E866.3	—	E950.8	E962.1	E980.8
insecticide	985.1	E863.4	—	E950.8	E962.1	E980.8

◀ New   ◀▥ Revised

Substance	Poisoning	External Cause (E-Code)				
		Accident	Therapeutic Use	Suicide Attempt	Assault	Undetermined
Parnate	969.0	E854.0	E939.0	E950.3	E962.0	E980.3
Paromomycin	960.8	E856	E930.8	E950.4	E962.0	E980.4
Paroxypropione	963.1	E858.1	E933.1	E950.4	E962.0	E980.4
Parzone	965.09	E850.2	E935.2	E950.0	E962.0	E980.0
PAS	961.8	E857	E931.8	E950.4	E962.0	E980.4
PCBs	981	E862.3	—	E950.9	E962.1	E980.9
PCP (pentachlorophenol)	989.4	E863.6	—	E950.6	E962.1	E980.7
herbicide	989.4	E863.5	—	E950.6	E962.1	E980.7
insecticide	989.4	E863.4	—	E950.6	E962.1	E980.7
phencyclidine	968.3	E855.1	E938.3	E950.4	E962.0	E980.4
Peach kernel oil (emulsion)	973.2	E858.4	E943.2	E950.4	E962.0	E980.4
Peanut oil (emulsion) NEC	973.2	E858.4	E943.2	E950.4	E962.0	E980.4
topical	976.3	E858.7	E946.3	E950.4	E962.0	E980.4
Pearly Gates (morning glory seeds)	969.6	E854.1	E939.6	E950.3	E962.0	E980.3
Pecazine	969.1	E853.0	E939.1	E950.3	E962.0	E980.3
Pecilocin	960.1	E856	E930.1	E950.4	E962.0	E980.4
Pectin (with kaolin) NEC	973.5	E858.4	E943.5	E950.4	E962.0	E980.4
Pelletierine tannate	961.6	E857	E931.6	E950.4	E962.0	E980.4
Pemoline	969.7	E854.2	E939.7	E950.3	E962.0	E980.3
Pempidine	972.3	E858.3	E942.3	E950.4	E962.0	E980.4
Penamecillin	960.0	E856	E930.0	E950.4	E962.0	E980.4
Penethamate hydriodide	960.0	E856	E930.0	E950.4	E962.0	E980.4
Penicillamine	963.8	E858.1	E933.8	E950.4	E962.0	E980.4
Penicillin (any type)	960.0	E856	E930.0	E950.4	E962.0	E980.4
Penicillinase	963.4	E858.1	E933.4	E950.4	E962.0	E980.4
Pentachlorophenol (fungicide)	989.4	E863.6	—	E950.6	E962.1	E980.7
herbicide	989.4	E863.5	—	E950.6	E962.1	E980.7
insecticide	989.4	E863.4	—	E950.6	E962.1	E980.7
Pentaerythritol	972.4	E858.3	E942.4	E950.4	E962.0	E980.4
chloral	967.1	E852.0	E937.1	E950.2	E962.0	E980.2
tetranitrate NEC	972.4	E858.3	E942.4	E950.4	E962.0	E980.4
Pentagastrin	977.8	E858.8	E947.8	E950.4	E962.0	E980.4
Pentalin	982.3	E862.4	—	E950.9	E962.1	E980.9
Pentamethonium (bromide)	972.3	E858.3	E942.3	E950.4	E962.0	E980.4
Pentamidine	961.5	E857	E931.5	E950.4	E962.0	E980.4
Pentanol	980.8	E860.8	—	E950.9	E962.1	E980.9
Pentaquine	961.4	E857	E931.4	E950.4	E962.0	E980.4
Pentazocine	965.8	E850.8	E935.8	E950.0	E962.0	E980.0
Penthienate	971.1	E855.4	E941.1	E950.4	E962.0	E980.4
Pentobarbital, pentobarbitone (sodium)	967.0	E851	E937.0	E950.1	E962.0	E980.1
Pentolinium (tartrate)	972.3	E858.3	E942.3	E950.4	E962.0	E980.4
Pentothal	968.3	E855.1	E938.3	E950.4	E962.0	E980.4
Pentylenetetrazol	970.0	E854.3	E940.0	E950.4	E962.0	E980.4
Pentylsalicylamide	961.8	E857	E931.8	E950.4	E962.0	E980.4
Pepsin	973.4	E858.4	E943.4	E950.4	E962.0	E980.4
Peptavlon	977.8	E858.8	E947.8	E950.4	E962.0	E980.4
Percaine (spinal)	968.7	E855.2	E938.7	E950.4	E962.0	E980.4
topical (surface)	968.5	E855.2	E938.5	E950.4	E962.0	E980.4
Perchloroethylene (vapor)	982.3	E862.4	—	E950.9	E962.1	E980.9
medicinal	961.6	E857	E931.6	E950.4	E962.0	E980.4
Percodan	965.09	E850.2	E935.2	E950.0	E962.0	E980.0
Percogesic	965.09	E850.2	E935.2	E950.0	E962.0	E980.0
Percorten	962.0	E858.0	E932.0	E950.4	E962.0	E980.4
Pergonal	962.4	E858.0	E932.4	E950.4	E962.0	E980.4
Perhexiline	972.4	E858.3	E942.4	E950.4	E962.0	E980.4
Periactin	963.0	E858.1	E933.0	E950.4	E962.0	E980.4
Periclor	967.1	E852.0	E937.1	E950.2	E962.0	E980.2
Pericyazine	969.1	E853.0	E939.1	E950.3	E962.0	E980.3
Peritrate	972.4	E858.3	E942.4	E950.4	E962.0	E980.4
Permanganates NEC	983.9	E864.3	—	E950.7	E962.1	E980.6
potassium (topical)	976.0	E858.7	E946.0	E950.4	E962.0	E980.4

Substance	Poisoning	External Cause (E-Code)				
		Accident	Therapeutic Use	Suicide Attempt	Assault	Undetermined
Pernocton	967.0	E851	E937.0	E950.1	E962.0	E980.1
Pernoston	967.0	E851	E937.0	E950.1	E962.0	E980.1
Peronin(e)	965.09	E850.2	E935.2	E950.0	E962.0	E980.0
Perphenazine	969.1	E853.0	E939.1	E950.3	E962.0	E980.3
Pertofrane	969.0	E854	E939.0	E950.3	E962.0	E980.3
Pertussis	—	—	—	—	—	—
immune serum (human)	964.6	E858.2	E934.6	E950.4	E962.0	E980.4
vaccine (with diphtheria toxoid) (with tetanus toxoid)	978.6	E858.8	E948.6	E950.4	E962.0	E980.4
Peruvian balsam	976.8	E858.7	E946.8	E950.4	E962.0	E980.4
Pesticides (dust) (fumes) (vapor)	989.4	E863.4	—	E950.6	E962.1	E980.7
arsenic	985.1	E863.4	—	E950.8	E962.1	E980.8
chlorinated	989.2	E863.0	—	E950.6	E962.1	E980.7
cyanide	989.0	E863.4	—	E950.6	E962.1	E980.7
kerosene	981	E863.4	—	E950.6	E962.1	E980.7
mixture (of compounds)	989.4	E863.3	—	E950.6	E962.1	E980.7
naphthalene	983.0	E863.4	—	E950.7	E962.1	E980.6
organochlorine (compounds)	989.2	E863.0	—	E950.6	E962.1	E980.7
petroleum (distillate) (products) NEC	981	E863.4	—	E950.6	E962.1	E980.7
specified ingredient NEC	989.4	E863.4	—	E950.6	E962.1	E980.7
strychnine	989.1	E863.4	—	E950.6	E962.1	E980.7
thallium	985.8	E863.7	—	E950.6	E962.1	E980.7
Pethidine (hydrochloride)	965.09	E850.2	E935.2	E950.0	E962.0	E980.0
Petrichloral	967.1	E852.0	E937.1	E950.2	E962.0	E980.2
Petrol	981	E862.1	—	E950.9	E962.1	E980.9
vapor	987.1	E869.8	—	E952.8	E962.2	E982.8
Petrolatum (jelly) (ointment)	976.3	E858.7	E946.3	E950.4	E962.0	E980.4
hydrophilic	976.3	E858.7	E946.3	E950.4	E962.0	E980.4
liquid	973.2	E858.4	E943.2	E950.4	E962.0	E980.4
topical	976.3	E858.7	E946.3	E950.4	E962.0	E980.4
nonmedicinal	981	E862.1	—	E950.9	E962.1	E980.9
Petroleum (cleaners) (fuels) (products) NEC	981	E862.1	—	E950.9	E962.1	E980.9
benzin(e) - see Ligroin	—	—	—	—	—	—
ether - see Ligroin	—	—	—	—	—	—
jelly - see Petrolatum	—	—	—	—	—	—
aphtha - see Ligroin	—	—	—	—	—	—
pesticide	981	E863.4	—	E950.6	E962.1	E980.7
solids	981	E862.3	—	E950.9	E962.1	E980.9
solvents	981	E862.0	—	E950.9	E962.1	E980.9
vapor	987.1	E869.8	—	E952.8	E962.2	E982.8
Peyote	969.6	E854.1	E939.6	E950.3	E962.0	E980.3
Phanodorm, phanodorn	967.0	E851	E937.0	E950.1	E962.0	E980.1
Phanquinone, phanquone	961.5	E857	E931.5	E950.4	E962.0	E980.4
Pharmaceutical excipient or adjunct	977.4	E858.8	E947.4	E950.4	E962.0	E980.4
Phenacemide	966.3	E855.0	E936.3	E950.4	E962.0	E980.4
Phenacetin	965.4	E850.4	E935.4	E950.0	E962.0	E980.0
Phenadoxone	965.09	E850.2	E935.2	E950.0	E962.0	E980.0
Phenaglycodol	969.5	E853.8	E939.5	E950.3	E962.0	E980.3
Phenantoin	966.1	E855.0	E936.1	E950.4	E962.0	E980.4
Phenaphthazine reagent	977.8	E858.8	E947.8	E950.4	E962.0	E980.4
Phenazocine	965.09	E850.2	E935.2	E950.0	E962.0	E980.0
Phenazone	965.5	E850.5	E935.5	E950.0	E962.0	E980.0
Phenazopyridine	976.1	E858.7	E946.1	E950.4	E962.0	E980.4
Phenbenicillin	960.0	E856	E930.0	E950.4	E962.0	E980.4
Phenbutrazate	977.0	E858.8	E947.0	E950.4	E962.0	E980.4
Phencyclidine	968.3	E855.1	E938.3	E950.4	E962.0	E980.4
Phendimetrazine	977.0	E858.8	E947.0	E950.4	E962.0	E980.4
Phenelzine	969.0	E854.0	E939.0	E950.3	E962.0	E980.3
Phenergan	967.8	E852.8	E937.8	E950.2	E962.0	E980.2
Phenethicillin (potassium)	960.0	E856	E930.0	E950.4	E962.0	E980.4
Phenetsal	965.1	E850.3	E935.3	E950.0	E962.0	E980.0
Pheneturide	966.3	E855.0	E936.3	E950.4	E962.0	E980.4

◀ New   ◀◀ Revised

Substance	Poisoning	External Cause (E-Code)				
		Accident	Therapeutic Use	Suicide Attempt	Assault	Undetermined
Phenformin	962.3	E858.0	E932.3	E950.4	E962.0	E980.4
Phenglutarimide	971.1	E855.4	E941.1	E950.4	E962.0	E980.4
Phenicarbazide	965.8	E850.8	E935.8	E950.0	E962.0	E980.0
Phenindamine (tartrate)	963.0	E858.1	E933.0	E950.4	E962.0	E980.4
Phenindione	964.2	E858.2	E934.2	E950.4	E962.0	E980.4
Pheniprazine	969.0	E854.0	E939.0	E950.3	E962.0	E980.3
Pheniramine (maleate)	963.0	E858.1	E933.0	E950.4	E962.0	E980.4
Phenmetrazine	977.0	E858.8	E947.0	E950.4	E962.0	E980.4
Phenobal	967.0	E851	E937.0	E950.1	E962.0	E980.1
Phenobarbital	967.0	E851	E937.0	E950.1	E962.0	E980.1
Phenobarbitone	967.0	E851	E937.0	E950.1	E962.0	E980.1
Phenoctide	976.0	E858.7	E946.0	E950.4	E962.0	E980.4
Phenol (derivatives) NEC	983.0	E864.0	—	E950.7	E962.1	E980.6
disinfectant	983.0	E864.0	—	E950.7	E962.1	E980.6
pesticide	989.4	E863.4		E950.6	E962.1	E980.7
red	977.8	E858.8	E947.8	E950.4	E962.0	E980.4
Phenolphthalein	973.1	E858.4	E943.1	E950.4	E962.0	E980.4
Phenolsulfonphthalein	977.8	E858.8	E947.8	E950.4	E962.0	E980.4
Phenomorphan	965.09	E850.2	E935.2	E950.0	E962.0	E980.0
Phenonyl	967.0	E851	E937.0	E950.1	E962.0	E980.1
Phenoperidine	965.09	E850.2	E935.2	E950.0	E962.0	E980.0
Phenoquin	974.7	E858.5	E944.7	E950.4	E962.0	E980.4
Phenothiazines (tranquilizers) NEC	969.1	E853.0	E939.1	E950.3	E962.0	E980.3
insecticide	989.3	E863.4	—	E950.6	E962.1	E980.7
Phenoxybenzamine	971.3	E855.6	E941.3	E950.4	E962.0	E980.4
Phenoxymethyl penicillin	960.0	E856	E930.0	E950.4	E962.0	E980.4
Phenprocoumon	964.2	E858.2	E934.2	E950.4	E962.0	E980.4
Phensuximide	966.2	E855.0	E936.2	E950.4	E962.0	E980.4
Phentermine	977.0	E858.8	E947.0	E950.4	E962.0	E980.4
Phentolamine	971.3	E855.6	E941.3	E950.4	E962.0	E980.4
Phenyl	—	—	—	—	—	—
butazone	965.5	E850.5	E935.5	E950.0	E962.0	E980.0
enediamine	983.0	E864.0	—	E950.7	E962.1	E980.6
hydrazine	983.0	E864.0	—	E950.7	E962.1	E980.6
antineoplastic	963.1	E858.1	E933.1	E950.4	E962.0	E980.4
mercuric compounds - see Mercury	—	—	—	—	—	—
salicylate	976.3	E858.7	E946.3	E950.4	E962.0	E980.4
Phenylephrine	971.2	E855.5	E941.2	E950.4	E962.0	E980.4
Phenylethylbiguanide	962.3	E858.0	E932.3	E950.4	E962.0	E980.4
Phenylpropanolamine	971.2	E855.5	E941.2	E950.4	E962.0	E980.4
Phenylsulfthion	989.3	E863.1	—	E950.6	E962.1	E980.7
Phenyramidol, phenyramidon	965.7	E850.7	E935.7	E950.0	E962.0	E980.0
Phenytoin	966.1	E855.0	E936.1	E950.4	E962.0	E980.4
pHisoHex	976.2	E858.7	E946.2	E950.4	E962.0	E980.4
Pholcodine	965.09	E850.2	E935.2	E950.0	E962.0	E980.0
Phorate	989.3	E863.1	—	E950.6	E962.1	E980.7
Phosdrin	989.3	E863.1	—	E950.6	E962.1	E980.7
Phosgene (gas)	987.8	E869.8	—	E952.8	E962.2	E982.8
Phosphate (tricresyl)	989.89	E866.8	—	E950.9	E962.1	E980.9
organic	989.3	E863.1	—	E950.6	E962.1	E980.7
solvent	982.8	E862.4	—	E950.9	E962.1	E980.9
Phosphine	987.8	E869.8	—	E952.8	E962.2	E982.8
fumigant	987.8	E863.8	—	E950.6	E962.2	E980.7
Phospholine	971.0	E855.3	E941.0	E950.4	E962.0	E980.4
Phosphoric acid	983.1	E864.1	—	E950.7	E962.1	E980.6
Phosphorus (compounds) NEC	983.9	E864.3	—	E950.7	E962.1	E980.6
rodenticide	983.9	E863.7	—	E950.7	E962.1	E980.6
Phthalimidoglutarimide	967.8	E852.8	E937.8	E950.2	E962.0	E980.2
Phthalylsulfathiazole	961.0	E857	E931.0	E950.4	E962.0	E980.4
Phylloquinone	964.3	E858.2	E934.3	E950.4	E962.0	E980.4
Physeptone	965.02	E850.1	E935.1	E950.0	E962.0	E980.0

Substance	Poisoning	External Cause (E-Code)				
		Accident	Therapeutic Use	Suicide Attempt	Assault	Undetermined
Physostigma venenosum	988.2	E865.4	—	E950.9	E962.1	E980.9
Physostigmine	971.0	E855.3	E941.0	E950.4	E962.0	E980.4
Phytolacca decandra	988.2	E865.4	—	E950.9	E962.1	E980.9
Phytomenadione	964.3	E858.2	E934.3	E950.4	E962.0	E980.4
Phytonadione	964.3	E858.2	E934.3	E950.4	E962.0	E980.4
Picric (acid)	983.0	E864.0	—	E950.7	E962.1	E980.6
Picrotoxin	970.0	E854.3	E940.0	E950.4	E962.0	E980.4
Pilocarpine	971.0	E855.3	E941.0	E950.4	E962.0	E980.4
Pilocarpus (jaborandi) extract	971.0	E855.3	E941.0	E950.4	E962.0	E980.4
Pimaricin	960.1	E856	E930.1	E950.4	E962.0	E980.4
Piminodine	965.09	E850.2	E935.2	E950.0	E962.0	E980.0
Pine oil, pinesol (disinfectant)	983.9	E861.4	—	E950.7	E962.1	E980.6
Pinkroot	961.6	E857	E931.6	E950.4	E962.0	E980.4
Pipadone	965.09	E850.2	E935.2	E950.0	E962.0	E980.0
Pipamazine	963.0	E858.1	E933.0	E950.4	E962.0	E980.4
Pipazethate	975.4	E858.6	E945.4	E950.4	E962.0	E980.4
Pipenzolate	971.1	E855.4	E941.1	E950.4	E962.0	E980.4
Piperacetazine	969.1	E853.0	E939.1	E950.3	E962.0	E980.3
Piperazine NEC	961.6	E857	E931.6	E950.4	E962.0	E980.4
estrone sulfate	962.2	E858.0	E932.2	E950.4	E962.0	E980.4
Piper cubeba	988.2	E865.4	—	E950.9	E962.1	E980.9
Piperidione	975.4	E858.6	E945.4	E950.4	E962.0	E980.4
Piperidolate	971.1	E855.4	E941.1	E950.4	E962.0	E980.4
Piperocaine	968.9	E855.2	E938.9	E950.4	E962.0	E980.4
infiltration (subcutaneous)	968.5	E855.2	E938.5	E950.4	E962.0	E980.4
nerve block (peripheral) (plexus)	968.6	E855.2	E938.6	E950.4	E962.0	E980.4
topical (surface)	968.5	E855.2	E938.5	E950.4	E962.0	E980.4
Pipobroman	963.1	E858.1	E933.1	E950.4	E962.0	E980.4
Pipradrol	970.8	E854.3	E940.8	E950.4	E962.0	E980.4
Piscidia (bark) (erythrina)	965.7	E850.7	E935.7	E950.0	E962.0	E980.0
Pitch	983.0	E864.0	—	E950.7	E962.1	E980.6
Pitkin's solution	968.7	E855.2	E938.7	E950.4	E962.0	E980.4
Pitocin	975.0	E858.6	E945.0	E950.4	E962.0	E980.4
Pitressin (tannate)	962.5	E858.0	E932.5	E950.4	E962.0	E980.4
Pituitary extracts (posterior)	962.5	E858.0	E932.5	E950.4	E962.0	E980.4
anterior	962.4	E858.0	E932.4	E950.4	E962.0	E980.4
Pituitrin	962.5	E858.0	E932.5	E950.4	E962.0	E980.4
Placental extract	962.9	E858.0	E932.9	E950.4	E962.0	E980.4
Placidyl	967.8	E852.8	E937.8	E950.2	E962.0	E980.2
Plague vaccine	978.3	E858.8	E948.3	E950.4	E962.0	E980.4
Plant foods or fertilizers NEC	989.89	E866.5	—	E950.9	E962.1	E980.9
mixed with herbicides	989.4	E863.5	—	E950.6	E962.1	E930.7
Plants, noxious, used as food	988.2	E865.9	—	E950.9	E962.1	E980.9
berries and seeds	988.2	E865.3	—	E950.9	E962.1	E980.9
specified type NEC	988.2	E865.4	—	E950.9	E962.1	E980.9
Plasma (blood)	964.7	E858.2	E934.7	E950.4	E962.0	E980.4
expanders	964.8	E858.2	E934.8	E950.4	E962.0	E980.4
Plasmanate	964.7	E858.2	E934.7	E950.4	E962.0	E980.4
Plegicil	969.1	E853.0	E939.1	E950.3	E962.0	E980.3
Podophyllin	976.4	E858.7	E946.4	E950.4	E962.0	E980.4
Podophyllum resin	976.4	E858.7	E946.4	E950.4	E962.0	E980.4
Poison NEC	989.9	E866.9	—	E950.9	E962.1	E980.9
Poisonous berries	988.2	E865.3	—	E950.9	E962.1	E980.9
Pokeweed (any part)	988.2	E865.4	—	E950.9	E962.1	E980.9
Poldine	971.1	E855.4	E941.1	E950.4	E962.0	E980.4
Poliomyelitis vaccine	979.5	E858.8	E949.5	E950.4	E962.0	E980.4
Poliovirus vaccine	979.5	E858.8	E949.5	E950.4	E962.0	E980.4
Polish (car) (floor) (furniture) (metal) (silver)	989.89	E861.2	—	E950.9	E962.1	E980.9
abrasive	989.89	E861.3	—	E950.9	E962.1	E980.9
porcelain	989.89	E861.3	—	E950.9	E962.1	E980.9
Poloxalkol	973.2	E858.4	E943.2	E950.4	E962.0	E980.4

◀ New   ◀▥▥▥ Revised

Substance	Poisoning	Accident	Therapeutic Use	Suicide Attempt	Assault	Undetermined
			External Cause (E-Code)			
Polyaminostyrene resins	974.5	E858.5	E944.5	E950.4	E962.0	E980.4
Polychlorinated biphenyl - see PCBs	—	—	—	—	—	—
Polycycline	960.4	E856	E930.4	E950.4	E962.0	E980.4
Polyester resin hardener	982.8	E862.4	—	E950.9	E962.1	E980.9
fumes	987.8	E869.8	—	E952.8	E962.2	E982.8
Polyestradiol (phosphate)	962.2	E858.0	E932.2	E950.4	E962.0	E980.4
Polyethanolamine alkyl sulfate	976.2	E858.7	E946.2	E950.4	E962.0	E980.4
Polyethylene glycol	976.3	E858.7	E946.3	E950.4	E962.0	E980.4
Polyferose	964.0	E858.2	E934.0	E950.4	E962.0	E980.4
Polymyxin B	960.8	E856	E930.8	E950.4	E962.0	E980.4
ENT agent	976.6	E858.7	E946.6	E950.4	E962.0	E980.4
ophthalmic preparation	976.5	E858.7	E946.5	E950.4	E962.0	E980.4
topical NEC	976.0	E858.7	E946.0	E950.4	E962.0	E980.4
Polynoxylin(e)	976.0	E858.7	E946.0	E950.4	E962.0	E980.4
Polyoxymethyleneurea	976.0	E858.7	E946.0	E950.4	E962.0	E980.4
Polytetrafluoroethylene (inhaled)	987.8	E869.8	—	E952.8	E962.2	E982.8
Polythiazide	974.3	E858.5	E944.3	E950.4	E962.0	E980.4
Polyvinylpyrrolidone	964.8	E858.2	E934.8	E950.4	E962.0	E980.4
Pontocaine (hydrochloride) (infiltration) (topical)	968.5	E855.2	E938.5	E950.4	E962.0	E980.4
nerve block (peripheral) (plexus)	968.6	E855.2	E938.6	E950.4	E962.0	E980.4
spinal	968.7	E855.2	E938.7	E950.4	E962.0	E980.4
Pot	969.6	E854.1	E939.6	E950.3	E962.0	E980.3
Potash (caustic)	983.2	E864.2	—	E950.7	E962.1	E980.6
Potassic saline injection (lactated)	974.5	E858.5	E944.5	E950.4	E962.0	E980.4
Potassium (salts) NEC	974.5	E858.5	E944.5	E950.4	E962.0	E980.4
aminosalicylate	961.8	E857	E931.8	E950.4	E962.0	E980.4
arsenite (solution)	985.1	E866.3	—	E950.8	E962.1	E980.8
bichromate	983.9	E864.3	—	E950.7	E962.1	E980.6
bisulfate	983.9	E864.3	—	E950.7	E962.1	E980.6
bromide (medicinal) NEC	967.3	E852.2	E937.3	E950.2	E962.0	E980.2
carbonate	983.2	E864.2	—	E950.7	E962.1	E980.6
chlorate NEC	983.9	E864.3	—	E950.7	E962.1	E980.6
cyanide - see Cyanide	—	—	—	—	—	—
hydroxide	983.2	E864.2	—	E950.7	E962.1	E980.6
iodide (expectorant) NEC	975.5	E858.6	E945.5	E950.4	E962.0	E980.4
nitrate	989.89	E866.8	—	E950.9	E962.1	E980.9
oxalate	983.9	E864.3	—	E950.7	E962.1	E980.6
perchlorate NEC	977.8	E858.8	E947.8	E950.4	E962.0	E980.4
antithyroid	962.8	E858.0	E932.8	E950.4	E962.0	E980.4
permanganate	976.0	E858.7	E946.0	E950.4	E962.0	E980.4
nonmedicinal	983.9	E864.3	—	E950.7	E962.1	E980.6
Povidone-iodine (anti-infective) NEC	976.0	E858.7	E946.0	E950.4	E962.0	E980.4
Practolol	972.0	E858.3	E942.0	E950.4	E962.0	E980.4
Pralidoxime (chloride)	977.2	E858.8	E947.2	E950.4	E962.0	E980.4
Pramoxine	968.5	E855.2	E938.5	E950.4	E962.0	E980.4
Prazosin	972.6	E858.3	E942.6	E950.4	E962.0	E980.4
Prednisolone	962.0	E858.0	E932.0	E950.4	E962.0	E980.4
ENT agent	976.6	E858.7	E946.6	E950.4	E962.0	E980.4
ophthalmic preparation	976.5	E858.7	E946.5	E950.4	E962.0	E980.4
topical NEC	976.0	E858.7	E946.0	E950.4	E962.0	E980.4
Prednisone	962.0	E858.0	E932.0	E950.4	E962.0	E980.4
Pregnanediol	962.2	E858.0	E932.2	E950.4	E962.0	E990.4
Pregneninolone	962.2	E858.0	E932.2	E950.4	E962.0	E980.4
Preludin	977.0	E858.8	E947.0	E950.4	E962.0	E980.4
Premarin	962.2	E858.0	E932.2	E950.4	E962.0	E980.4
Prenylamine	972.4	E858.3	E942.4	E950.4	E962.0	E980.4
Preparation H	976.8	E858.7	E946.8	E950.4	E962.0	E980.4
Preservatives	989.89	E866.8	—	E950.9	E962.1	E980.9
Pride of China	988.2	E865.3	—	E950.9	E962.1	E980.9
Prilocaine	968.9	E855.2	E938.9	E950.4	E962.0	E980.4
infiltration (subcutaneous)	968.5	E855.2	E938.5	E950.4	E962.0	E980.4
nerve block (peripheral) (plexus)	968.6	E855.2	E938.6	E950.4	E962.0	E980.4

Substance	Poisoning	External Cause (E-Code)				
		Accident	Therapeutic Use	Suicide Attempt	Assault	Undetermined
Primaquine	961.4	E857	E931.4	E950.4	E962.0	E980.4
Primidone	966.3	E855.0	E936.3	E950.4	E962.0	E980.4
Primula (veris)	988.2	E865.4	—	E950.9	E962.1	E980.9
Prinodol	965.09	E850.2	E935.2	E950.0	E962.0	E980.0
Priscol, Priscoline	971.3	E855.6	E941.3	E950.4	E962.0	E980.4
Privet	988.2	E865.4	—	E950.9	E962.1	E980.9
Privine	971.2	E855.5	E941.2	E950.4	E962.0	E980.4
Pro-Banthine	971.1	E855.4	E941.1	E950.4	E962.0	E980.4
Probarbital	967.0	E851	E937.0	E950.1	E962.0	E980.1
Probenecid	974.7	E858.5	E944.7	E950.4	E962.0	E990.4
Procainamide (hydrochloride)	972.0	E858.3	E942.0	E950.4	E962.0	E980.4
Procaine (hydrochloride) (infiltration) (topical)	968.5	E855.2	E938.5	E950.4	E962.0	E980.4
nerve block (periphreal) (plexus)	968.6	E855.2	E938.6	E950.4	E962.0	E980.4
penicillin G	960.0	E856	E930.0	E950.4	E962.0	E980.4
spinal	968.7	E855.2	E938.7	E950.4	E962.0	E980.4
Procalmidol	969.5	E853.8	E939.5	E950.3	E962.0	E980.3
Procarbazine	963.1	E858.1	E933.1	E950.4	E962.0	E980.4
Prochlorperazine	969.1	E853.0	E939.1	E950.3	E962.0	E980.3
Procyclidine	966.4	E855.0	E936.4	E950.4	E962.0	E980.4
Producer gas	986	E868.8	—	E952.1	E962.2	E982.1
Profenamine	966.4	E855.0	E936.4	E950.4	E962.0	E980.4
Profenil	975.1	E858.6	E945.1	E950.4	E962.0	E980.4
Progesterones	962.2	E858.0	E932.2	E950.4	E962.0	E980.4
Progestin	962.2	E858.0	E932.2	E950.4	E962.0	E980.4
Progestogens (with estrogens)	962.2	E858.0	E932.2	E950.4	E962.0	E980.4
Progestone	962.2	E858.0	E932.2	E950.4	E962.0	E980.4
Proguanil	961.4	E857	E931.4	E950.4	E962.0	E980.4
Prolactin	962.4	E858.0	E932.4	E950.4	E962.0	E980.4
Proloid	962.7	E858.0	E932.7	E950.4	E962.0	E980.4
Proluton	962.2	E858.0	E932.2	E950.4	E962.0	E980.4
Promacetin	961.8	E857	E931.8	E950.4	E962.0	E980.4
Promazine	969.1	E853.0	E939.1	E950.3	E962.0	E980.3
Promedrol	965.09	E850.2	E935.2	E950.0	E962.0	E980.0
Promethazine	967.8	E852.8	E937.8	E950.2	E962.0	E980.2
Promine	961.8	E857	E931.8	E950.4	E962.0	E980.4
Pronestyl (hydrochloride)	972.0	E858.3	E942.0	E950.4	E962.0	E980.4
Pronetalol, pronethalol	972.0	E858.3	E942.0	E950.4	E962.0	E980.4
Prontosil	961.0	E857	E931.0	E950.4	E962.0	E980.4
Propamidine isethionate	961.5	E857	E931.5	E950.4	E962.0	E980.4
Propanal (medicinal)	967.8	E852.8	E937.8	E950.2	E962.0	E980.2
Propane (gas) (distributed in mobile container)	987.0	E868.0	—	E951.1	E962.2	E981.1
distributed through pipes	987.0	E867	—	E951.0	E962.2	E981.0
incomplete combustion of - see Carbon monoxide, Propane	—	—	—	—	—	—
Propanidid	968.3	E855.1	E938.3	E950.4	E962.0	E980.4
Propanol	980.3	E860.4	—	E950.9	E962.1	E980.9
Propantheline	971.1	E855.4	E941.1	E950.4	E962.0	E980.4
Proparacaine	968.5	E855.2	E938.5	E950.4	E962.0	E980.4
Propatyl nitrate	972.4	E858.3	E942.4	E950.4	E962.0	E980.4
Propicillin	960.0	E856	E930.0	E950.4	E962.0	E980.4
Propiolactone (vapor)	987.8	E869.8	—	E952.8	E962.2	E982.8
Propiomazine	967.8	E852.8	E937.8	E950.2	E962.0	E980.2
Propionaldehyde (medicinal)	967.8	E852.8	E937.8	E950.2	E962.0	E980.2
Propionate compound	976.0	E858.7	E946.0	E950.4	E962.0	E980.4
Propion gel	976.0	E858.7	E946.0	E950.4	E962.0	E980.4
Propitocaine	968.9	E855.2	E938.9	E950.4	E962.0	E980.4
infiltration (subcutaneous)	968.5	E855.2	E938.5	E950.4	E962.0	E980.4
nerve block (peripheral) (plexus)	968.6	E855.2	E938.6	E950.4	E962.0	E980.4
Propoxur	989.3	E863.2	—	E950.6	E962.1	E980.7
Propoxycaine	968.9	E855.2	E938.9	E950.4	E962.0	E980.4
infiltration (subcutaneous)	968.5	E855.2	E938.5	E950.4	E962.0	E980.4
nerve block (peripheral) (plexus)	968.6	E855.2	E938.6	E950.4	E962.0	E980.4
topical (surface)	968.5	E855.2	E938.5	E950.4	E962.0	E980.4

◀ New   ◀◀ Revised

Substance	Poisoning	External Cause (E-Code)				
		Accident	Therapeutic Use	Suicide Attempt	Assault	Undetermined
Propoxyphene (hydrochloride)	965.8	E850.8	E935.8	E950.0	E962.0	E980.0
Propranolol	972.0	E858.3	E942.0	E950.4	E962.0	E980.4
Propyl	—	—	—	—	—	—
alcohol	980.3	E860.4	—	E950.9	E962.1	E980.9
carbinol	980.3	E860.4	—	E950.9	E962.1	E980.9
hexadrine	971.2	E855.5	E941.2	E950.4	E962.0	E980.4
iodone	977.8	E858.8	E947.8	E950.4	E962.0	E980.4
thiouracil	962.8	E858.0	E932.8	E950.4	E962.0	E980.4
Propylene	987.1	E869.8	—	E952.8	E962.2	E982.8
Propylparaben (ophthalmic)	976.5	E858.7	E946.5	E950.4	E962.0	E980.4
Proscillaridin	972.1	E858.3	E942.1	E950.4	E962.0	E980.4
Prostaglandins	975.0	E858.6	E945.0	E950.4	E962.0	E980.4
Prostigmin	971.0	E855.3	E941.0	E950.4	E962.0	E980.4
Protamine (sulfate)	964.5	E858.2	E934.5	E950.4	E962.0	E980.4
zinc insulin	962.3	E858.0	E932.3	E950.4	E962.0	E980.4
Protectants (topical)	976.3	E858.7	E946.3	E950.4	E962.0	E980.4
Protein hydrolysate	974.5	E858.5	E944.5	E950.4	E962.0	E980.4
Prothiaden - *see* Dothiepin hydrochloride	—	—	—	—	—	—
Prothionamide	961.8	E857	E931.8	E950.4	E962.0	E980.4
Prothipendyl	969.5	E853.8	E939.5	E950.3	E962.0	E980.3
Protokylol	971.2	E855.5	E941.2	E950.4	E962.0	E980.4
Protopam	977.2	E858.8	E947.2	E950.4	E962.0	E980.4
Protoveratrine(s) (A) (B)	972.6	E858.3	E942.6	E950.4	E962.0	E980.4
Protriptyline	969.0	E854.0	E939.0	E950.3	E962.0	E980.3
Provera	962.2	E858.0	E932.2	E950.4	E962.0	E980.4
Provitamin A	963.5	E858.1	E933.5	E950.4	E962.0	E980.4
Proxymetacaine	968.5	E855.2	E938.5	E950.4	E962.0	E980.4
Proxyphylline	975.1	E858.6	E945.1	E950.4	E962.0	E980.4
Prozac - *see* Fluoxetine hydrochloride	—	—	—	—	—	—
Prunus	—	—	—	—	—	—
laurocerasus	988.2	E865.4	—	E950.9	E962.1	E980.9
virginiana	988.2	E865.4	—	E950.9	E962.1	E980.9
Prussic acid	989.0	E866.8	—	E950.9	E962.1	E980.9
vapor	987.7	E869.8	—	E952.8	E962.2	E982.8
Pseudoephedrine	971.2	E855.5	E941.2	E950.4	E962.0	E980.4
Psilocin	969.6	E854.1	E939.6	E950.3	E962.0	E980.3
Psilocybin	969.6	E854.1	E939.6	E950.3	E962.0	E980.3
PSP	977.8	E858.8	E947.8	E950.4	E962.0	E980.4
Psychedelic agents	969.6	E854.1	E939.6	E950.3	E962.0	E980.3
Psychodysleptics	969.6	E854.1	E939.6	E950.3	E962.0	E980.3
Psychostimulants	969.7	E854.2	E939.7	E950.3	E962.0	E980.3
Psychotherapeutic agents	969.9	E855.9	E939.9	E950.3	E962.0	E980.3
antidepressants	969.0	E854.0	E939.0	E950.3	E962.0	E980.3
specified NEC	969.8	E855.8	E939.8	E950.3	E962.0	E980.3
tranquilizers NEC	969.5	E853.9	E939.5	E950.3	E962.0	E980.3
Psychotomimetic agents	969.6	E854.1	E939.6	E950.3	E962.0	E980.3
Psychotropic agents	969.9	E854.8	E939.9	E950.3	E962.0	E980.3
specified NEC	969.8	E854.8	E939.8	E950.3	E962.0	E980.3
Psyllium	973.3	E858.4	E943.3	E950.4	E962.0	E980.4
Pteroylglutamic acid	964.1	E858.2	E934.1	E950.4	E962.0	E980.4
Pteroyltriglutamate	963.1	E858.1	E933.1	E950.4	E962.0	E980.4
PTFE	987.8	E869.8	—	E952.8	E962.2	E982.8
Pulsatilla	988.2	E865.4	—	E950.9	E962.1	E980.9
Purex (bleach)	983.9	E864.3	—	E950.7	E962.1	E980.6
Purine diuretics	974.1	E858.5	E944.1	E950.4	E962.0	E980.4
Purinethol	963.1	E858.1	E933.1	E950.4	E962.0	E980.4
PVP	964.8	E858.2	E934.8	E950.4	E962.0	E980.4
Pyrabital	965.7	E850.7	E935.7	E950.0	E962.0	E980.0
Pyramidon	965.5	E850.5	E935.5	E950.0	E962.0	E980.0
Pyrantel (pamoate)	961.6	E857	E931.6	E950.4	E962.0	E980.4
Pyrathiazine	963.0	E858.1	E933.0	E950.4	E962.0	E980.4

ICD-9-CM

Drugs

Vol.

◀ New   ◀▥ Revised

Substance	Poisoning	External Cause (E-Code)				
		Accident	Therapeutic Use	Suicide Attempt	Assault	Undetermined
Pyrazinamide	961.8	E857	E931.8	E950.4	E962.0	E980.4
Pyrazinoic acid (amide)	961.8	E857	E931.8	E950.4	E962.0	E980.4
Pyrazole (derivatives)	965.5	E850.5	E935.5	E950.0	E962.0	E980.0
Pyrazolone (analgesics)	965.5	E850.5	E935.5	E950.0	E962.0	E980.0
Pyrethrins, pyrethrum	989.4	E863.4	—	E950.6	E962.1	E980.7
Pyribenzamine	963.0	E858.1	E933.0	E950.4	E962.0	E980.4
Pyridine (liquid) (vapor)	982.0	E862.4	—	E950.9	E962.1	E980.9
aldoxime chloride	977.2	E858.8	E947.2	E950.4	E962.0	E980.4
Pyridium	976.1	E858.7	E946.1	E950.4	E962.0	E980.4
Pyridostigmine	971.0	E855.3	E941.0	E950.4	E962.0	E980.4
Pyridoxine	963.5	E858.1	E933.5	E950.4	E962.0	E980.4
Pyrilamine	963.0	E858.1	E933.0	E950.4	E962.0	E980.4
Pyrimethamine	961.4	E857	E931.4	E950.4	E962.0	E980.4
Pyrogallic acid	983.0	E864.0	—	E950.7	E962.1	E980.6
Pyroxylin	976.3	E858.7	E946.3	E950.4	E962.0	E980.4
Pyrrobutamine	963.0	E858.1	E933.0	E950.4	E962.0	E980.4
Pyrrocitine	968.5	E855.2	E938.5	E950.4	E962.0	E980.4
Pyrvinium (pamoate)	961.6	E857	E931.6	E950.4	E962.0	E980.4
PZI	962.3	E858.0	E932.3	E950.4	E962.0	E980.4
Quaalude	967.4	E852.3	E937.4	E950.2	E962.0	E980.2
Quaternary ammonium derivatives	971.1	E855.4	E941.1	E950.4	E962.0	E980.4
Quicklime	983.2	E864.2	—	E950.7	E962.1	E980.6
Quinacrine	961.3	E857	E931.3	E950.4	E962.0	E980.4
Quinaglute	972.0	E858.3	E942.0	E950.4	E962.0	E980.4
Quinalbarbitone	967.0	E851	E937.0	E950.1	E962.0	E980.1
Quinestradiol	962.2	E858.0	E932.2	E950.4	E962.0	E980.4
Quinethazone	974.3	E858.5	E944.3	E950.4	E962.0	E980.4
Quinidine (gluconate) (polygalacturonate) (salts) (sulfate)	972.0	E858.3	E942.0	E950.4	E962.0	E980.4
Quinine	961.4	E857	E931.4	E950.4	E962.0	E980.4
Quiniobine	961.3	E857	E931.3	E950.4	E962.0	E980.4
Quinolines	961.3	E857	E931.3	E950.4	E962.0	E980.4
Quotane	968.5	E855.2	E938.5	E950.4	E962.0	E980.4
Rabies	—	—	—	—	—	—
immune globulin (human)	964.6	E858.2	E934.6	E950.4	E962.0	E980.4
vaccine	979.1	E858.8	E949.1	E950.4	E962.0	E980.4
Racemoramide	965.09	E850.2	E935.2	E950.0	E962.0	E980.0
Racemorphan	965.09	E850.2	E935.2	E950.0	E962.0	E980.0
Radiator alcohol	980.1	E860.2	—	E950.9	E962.1	E980.9
Radio-opaque (drugs) (materials)	977.8	E858.8	E947.8	E950.4	E962.0	E980.4
Ranunculus	988.2	E865.4	—	E950.9	E962.1	E980.9
Rat poison	989.4	E863.7	—	E950.6	E962.1	E980.7
Rattlesnake (venom)	989.5	E905.0	—	E950.9	E962.1	E980.9
Raudixin	972.6	E858.3	E942.6	E950.4	E962.0	E980.4
Rautensin	972.6	E858.3	E942.6	E950.4	E962.0	E980.4
Rautina	972.6	E858.3	E942.6	E950.4	E962.0	E980.4
Rautotal	972.6	E858.3	E942.6	E950.4	E962.0	E980.4
Rauwiloid	972.6	E858.3	E942.6	E950.4	E962.0	E980.4
Rauwoldin	972.6	E858.3	E942.6	E950.4	E962.0	E980.4
Rauwolfia (alkaloids)	972.6	E858.3	E942.6	E950.4	E962.0	E980.4
Realgar	985.1	E866.3	—	E950.8	E962.1	E980.8
Red cells, packed	964.7	E858.2	E934.7	E950.4	E962.0	E980.4
Reducing agents, industrial NEC	983.9	E864.3	—	E950.7	E962.1	E980.6
Refrigerant gas (freon)	987.4	E869.2	—	E952.8	E962.2	E982.8
not freon	987.9	E869.9	—	E952.9	E962.2	E982.9
Regroton	974.4	E858.5	E944.4	E950.4	E962.0	E980.4
Rela	968.0	E855.1	E938.0	E950.4	E962.0	E980.4
Relaxants, skeletal muscle (autonomic)	975.2	E858.6	E945.2	E950.4	E962.0	E980.4
central nervous system	968.0	E855.1	E938.0	E950.4	E962.0	E980.4
Renese	974.3	E858.5	E944.3	E950.4	E962.0	E980.4
Renografin	977.8	E858.8	E947.8	E950.4	E962.0	E980.4
Replacement solutions	974.5	E858.5	E944.5	E950.4	E962.0	E980.4

◀ New ◀ Revised

	External Cause (E-Code)					
Substance	**Poisoning**	**Accident**	**Therapeutic Use**	**Suicide Attempt**	**Assault**	**Undetermined**
Rescinnamine	972.6	E858.3	E942.6	E950.4	E962.0	E980.4
Reserpine	972.6	E858.3	E942.6	E950.4	E962.0	E980.4
Resorcin, resorcinol	976.4	E858.7	E946.4	E950.4	E962.0	E980.4
Respaire	975.5	E858.6	E945.5	E950.4	E962.0	E980.4
Respiratory agents NEC	975.8	E858.6	E945.8	E950.4	E962.0	E980.4
Retinoic acid	976.8	E858.7	E946.8	E950.4	E962.0	E980.4
Retinol	963.5	E858.1	E933.5	E950.4	E962.0	E980.4
Rh (D) immune globulin (human)	964.6	E858.2	E934.6	E950.4	E962.0	E980.4
Rhodine	965.1	E850.3	E935.3	E950.0	E962.0	E980.0
RhoGAM	964.6	E858.2	E934.6	E950.4	E962.0	E980.4
Riboflavin	963.5	E858.1	E933.5	E950.4	E962.0	E980.4
Ricin	989.89	E866.8	—	E950.9	E962.1	E980.9
Ricinus communis	988.2	E865.3	—	E950.9	E962.1	E980.9
Rickettsial vaccine NEC	979.6	E858.8	E949.6	E950.4	E962.0	E980.4
with viral and bacterial vaccine	979.7	E858.8	E949.7	E950.4	E962.0	E980.4
Rifampin	960.6	E856	E930.6	E950.4	E962.0	E980.4
Rimifon	961.8	E857	E931.8	E950.4	E962.0	E980.4
Ringer's injection (lactated)	974.5	E858.5	E944.5	E950.4	E962.0	E980.4
Ristocetin	960.8	E856	E930.8	E950.4	E962.0	E980.4
Ritalin	969.7	E854.2	E939.7	E950.3	E962.0	E980.3
Roach killers - *see* Pesticides	—	—	—	—	—	—
Rocky Mountain spotted fever vaccine	979.6	E858.8	E949.6	E950.4	E962.0	E980.4
Rodenticides	989.4	E863.7	—	E950.6	E962.1	E980.7
Rohypnol	969.4	E853.2	E939.4	E950.3	E962.0	E980.3
Rolaids	973.0	E858.4	E943.0	E950.4	E962.0	E980.4
Rolitetracycline	960.4	E856	E930.4	E950.4	E962.0	E980.4
Romilar	975.4	E858.6	E945.4	E950.4	E962.0	E980.4
Rose water ointment	976.3	E858.7	E946.3	E950.4	E962.0	E980.4
Rotenone	989.4	E863.7	—	E950.6	E962.1	E980.7
Rotoxamine	963.0	E858.1	E933.0	E950.4	E962.0	E980.4
Rough-on-rats	989.4	E863.7	—	E950.6	E962.1	E980.7
RU486	962.9	E858.0	E932.9	E950.4	E962.0	E980.4
Rubbing alcohol	980.2	E860.3	—	E950.9	E962.1	E980.9
Rubella virus vaccine	979.4	E858.8	E949.4	E950.4	E962.0	E980.4
Rubelogen	979.4	E858.8	E949.4	E950.4	E962.0	E980.4
Rubeovax	979.4	E858.8	E949.4	E950.4	E962.0	E980.4
Rubidomycin	960.7	E856	E930.7	E950.4	E962.0	E980.4
Rue	988.2	E865.4	—	E950.9	E962.1	E980.9
Ruta	988.2	E865.4	—	E950.9	E962.1	E980.9
Sabadilla (medicinal)	976.0	E858.7	E946.0	E950.4	E962.0	E980.4
pesticide	989.4	E863.4	—	E950.6	E962.1	E980.7
Sabin oral vaccine	979.5	E858.8	E949.5	E950.4	E962.0	E980.4
Saccharated iron oxide	964.0	E858.2	E934.0	E950.4	E962.0	E980.4
Saccharin	974.5	E858.5	E944.5	E950.4	E962.0	E980.4
Safflower oil	972.2	E858.3	E942.2	E950.4	E962.0	E980.4
Salbutamol sulfate	975.7	E858.6	E945.7	E950.4	E962.0	E980.4
Salicylamide	965.1	E850.3	E935.3	E950.0	E962.0	E980.0
Salicylate(s)	965.1	E850.3	E935.3	E950.0	E962.0	E980.0
methyl	976.3	E858.7	E946.3	E950.4	E962.0	E980.4
theobromine calcium	974.1	E858.5	E944.1	E950.4	E962.0	E980.4
Salicylazosulfapyridine	961.0	E857	E931.0	E950.4	E962.0	E980.4
Salicylhydroxamic acid	976.0	E858.7	E946.0	E950.4	E962.0	E980.4
Salicylic acid (keratolytic) NEC	976.4	E858.7	E946.4	E950.4	E962.0	E980.4
congeners	965.1	E850.3	E935.3	E950.0	E962.0	E980.0
salts	965.1	E850.3	E935.3	E950.0	E962.0	E980.0
Saliniazid	961.8	E857	E931.8	E950.4	E962.0	E980.4
Salol	976.3	E858.7	E946.3	E950.4	E962.0	E980.4
Salt (substitute) NEC	974.5	E858.5	E944.5	E950.4	E962.0	E980.4
Saluretics	974.3	E858.5	E944.3	E950.4	E962.0	E980.4
Saluron	974.3	E858.5	E944.3	E950.4	E962.0	E980.4
Salvarsan 606 (neosilver) (silver)	961.1	E857	E931.1	E950.4	E962.0	E980.4
Sambucus canadensis	988.2	E865.4	—	E950.9	E962.1	E980.9
berry	988.2	E865.3	—	E950.9	E962.1	E980.9

Substance	Poisoning	External Cause (E-Code)				
		Accident	Therapeutic Use	Suicide Attempt	Assault	Undetermined
Sandril	972.6	E858.3	E942.6	E950.4	E962.0	E980.4
Sanguinaria canadensis	988.2	E865.4	—	E950.9	E962.1	E980.9
Saniflush (cleaner)	983.9	E861.3	—	E950.7	E962.1	E980.6
Santonin	961.6	E857	E931.6	E950.4	E962.0	E980.4
Santyl	976.8	E858.7	E946.8	E950.4	E962.0	E980.4
Sarkomycin	960.7	E856	E930.7	E950.4	E962.0	E980.4
Saroten	969.0	E854.0	E939.0	E950.3	E962.0	E980.3
Saturnine - see Lead	—	—	—	—	—	—
Savin (oil)	976.4	E858.7	E946.4	E950.4	E962.0	E980.4
Scammony	973.1	E858.4	E943.1	E950.4	E962.0	E980.4
Scarlet red	976.8	E858.7	E946.8	E950.4	E962.0	E980.4
Scheele's green	985.1	E866.3	—	E950.8	E962.1	E980.8
insecticide	985.1	E863.4	—	E950.8	E962.1	E980.8
Schradan	989.3	E863.1	—	E950.6	E962.1	E980.7
Schweinfurt(h) green	985.1	E866.3	—	E950.8	E962.1	E980.8
insecticide	985.1	E863.4	—	E950.8	E962.1	E980.8
Scilla - see Squill	—	—	—	—	—	—
Sclerosing agents	972.7	E858.3	E942.7	E950.4	E962.0	E980.4
Scopolamine	971.1	E855.4	E941.1	E950.4	E962.0	E980.4
Scouring powder	989.89	E861.3	—	E950.9	E962.1	E980.9
Sea	—	—	—	—	—	—
anemone (sting)	989.5	E905.6	—	E950.9	E962.1	E980.9
cucumber (sting)	989.5	E905.6	—	E950.9	E962.1	E980.9
snake (bite) (venom)	989.5	E905.0	—	E950.9	E962.1	E980.9
urchin spine (puncture)	989.5	E905.6	—	E950.9	E962.1	E980.9
Secbutabarbital	967.0	E851	E937.0	E950.1	E962.0	E980.1
Secbutabarbitone	967.0	E851	E937.0	E950.1	E962.0	E980.1
Secobarbital	967.0	E851	E937.0	E950.1	E962.0	E980.1
Seconal	967.0	E851	E937.0	E950.1	E962.0	E980.1
Secretin	977.8	E858.8	E947.8	E950.4	E962.0	E980.4
Sedatives, nonbarbiturate	967.9	E852.9	E937.9	E950.2	E962.0	E980.2
specified NEC	967.8	E852.8	E937.8	E950.2	E962.0	E980.2
Sedormid	967.8	E852.8	E937.8	E950.2	E962.0	E980.2
Seed (plant)	988.2	E865.3	—	E950.9	E962.1	E980.9
disinfectant or dressing	989.89	E866.5	—	E950.9	E962.1	E980.9
Selenium (fumes) NEC	985.8	E866.4	—	E950.9	E962.1	E980.9
disulfide or sulfide	976.4	E858.7	E946.4	E950.4	E962.0	E980.4
Selsun	976.4	E858.7	E946.4	E950.4	E962.0	E980.4
Senna	973.1	E858.4	E943.1	E950.4	E962.0	E980.4
Septisol	976.2	E858.7	E946.2	E950.4	E962.0	E980.4
Serax	969.4	E853.2	E939.4	E950.3	E962.0	E980.3
Serenesil	967.8	E852.8	E937.8	E950.2	E962.0	E980.2
Serenium (hydrochloride)	961.9	E857	E931.9	E950.4	E962.0	E980.4
Serepax - see Oxazepam	—	—	—	—	—	—
Sernyl	968.3	E855.1	E938.3	E950.4	E962.0	E980.4
Serotonin	977.8	E858.8	E947.8	E950.4	E962.0	E980.4
Serpasil	972.6	E858.3	E942.6	E950.4	E962.0	E980.4
Sewer gas	987.8	E869.8	—	E952.8	E962.2	E982.8
Shampoo	989.6	E861.0	—	E950.9	E962.1	E980.9
Shellfish, nonbacterial or noxious	988.0	E865.1	—	E950.9	E962.1	E980.9
Silicones NEC	989.83	E866.8	E947.8	E950.9	E962.1	E980.9
Silvadene	976.0	E858.7	E946.0	E950.4	E962.0	E980.4
Silver (compound) (medicinal) NEC	976.0	E858.7	E946.0	E950.4	E962.0	E980.4
anti-infectives	976.0	E858.7	E946.0	E950.4	E962.0	E980.4
arsphenamine	961.1	E857	E931.1	E950.4	E962.0	E980.4
nitrate	976.0	E858.7	E946.0	E950.4	E962.0	E980.4
ophthalmic preparation	976.5	E858.7	E946.5	E950.4	E962.0	E980.4
toughened (keratolytic)	976.4	E858.7	E946.4	E950.4	E962.0	E980.4
nonmedicinal (dust)	985.8	E866.4	—	E950.9	E962.1	E980.9
protein (mild) (strong)	976.0	E858.7	E946.0	E950.4	E962.0	E980.4
salvarsan	961.1	E857	E931.1	E950.4	E962.0	E980.4

◄ New   ◄▬ Revised

Substance	Poisoning	Accident	Therapeutic Use	Suicide Attempt	Assault	Undetermined
Simethicone	973.8	E858.4	E943.8	E950.4	E962.0	E980.4
Sinequan	969.0	E854.0	E939.0	E950.3	E962.0	E980.3
Singoserp	972.6	E858.3	E942.6	E950.4	E962.0	E980.4
Sintrom	964.2	E858.2	E934.2	E950.4	E962.0	E980.4
Sitosterols	972.2	E858.3	E942.2	E950.4	E962.0	E980.4
Skeletal muscle relaxants	975.2	E858.6	E945.2	E950.4	E962.0	E980.4
Skin	—	—	—	—	—	—
agents (external)	976.9	E858.7	E946.9	E950.4	E962.0	E980.4
specified NEC	976.8	E858.7	E946.8	E950.4	E962.0	E980.4
test antigen	977.8	E858.8	E947.8	E950.4	E962.0	E980.4
Sleep-eze	963.0	E858.1	E933.0	E950.4	E962.0	E980.4
Sleeping draught (drug) (pill) (tablet)	967.9	E852.9	E937.9	E950.2	E962.0	E980.2
Smallpox vaccine	979.0	E858.8	E949.0	E950.4	E962.0	E980.4
Smelter fumes NEC	985.9	E866.4	—	E950.9	E962.1	E980.9
Smog	987.3	E869.1	—	E952.8	E962.2	E982.8
Smoke NEC	987.9	E869.9	—	E952.9	E962.2	E982.9
Smooth muscle relaxant	975.1	E858.6	E945.1	E950.4	E962.0	E980.4
Snail killer	989.4	E863.4	—	E950.6	E962.1	E980.7
Snake (bite) (venom)	989.5	E905.0	—	E950.9	E962.1	E980.9
Snuff	989.89	E866.8	—	E950.9	E962.1	E980.9
Soap (powder) (product)	989.6	E861.1	—	E950.9	E962.1	E980.9
medicinal, soft	976.2	E858.7	E946.2	E950.4	E962.0	E980.4
Soda (caustic)	983.2	E864.2	—	E950.7	E962.1	E980.6
bicarb	963.3	E858.1	E933.3	E950.4	E962.0	E980.4
chlorinated - *see* Sodium, hypochlorite	—	—	—	—	—	—
Sodium	—	—	—	—	—	—
acetosulfone	961.8	E857	E931.8	E950.4	E962.0	E980.4
acetrizoate	977.8	E858.8	E947.8	E950.4	E962.0	E980.4
amytal	967.0	E851	E937.0	E950.1	E962.0	E980.1
arsenate - *see* Arsenic	—	—	—	—	—	—
bicarbonate	963.3	E858.1	E933.3	E950.4	E962.0	E980.4
bichromate	983.9	E864.3	—	E950.7	E962.1	E980.6
biphosphate	963.2	E858.1	E933.2	E950.4	E962.0	E980.4
bisulfate	983.9	E864.3	—	E950.7	E962.1	E980.6
borate (cleanser)	989.6	E861.3	—	E950.9	E962.1	E980.9
bromide NEC	967.3	E852.2	E937.3	E950.2	E962.0	E980.2
cacodylate (nonmedicinal) NEC	978.8	E858.8	E948.8	E950.4	E962.0	E980.4
anti-infective	961.1	E857	E931.1	E950.4	E962.0	E980.4
herbicide	989.4	E863.5	—	E950.6	E962.1	E980.7
calcium edetate	963.8	E858.1	E933.8	E950.4	E962.0	E980.4
carbonate NEC	983.2	E864.2	—	E950.7	E962.1	E980.6
chlorate NEC	983.9	E864.3	—	E950.7	E962.1	E980.6
herbicide	983.9	E863.5	—	E950.7	E962.1	E980.6
chloride NEC	974.5	E858.5	E944.5	E950.4	E962.0	E980.4
chromate	983.9	E864.3	—	E950.7	E962.1	E980.6
citrate	963.3	E858.1	E933.3	E950.4	E962.0	E980.4
cyanide - *see* Cyanide(s)	—	—	—	—	—	—
cyclamate	974.5	E858.5	E944.5	E950.4	E962.0	E980.4
diatrizoate	977.8	E858.8	E947.8	E950.4	E962.0	E980.4
dibunate	975.4	E858.6	E945.4	E950.4	E962.0	E980.4
dioctyl sulfosuccinate	973.2	E858.4	E943.2	E950.4	E962.0	E980.4
edetate	963.8	E858.1	E933.8	E950.4	E962.0	E980.4
ethacrynate	974.4	E858.5	E944.4	E950.4	E962.0	E980.4
fluoracetate (dust) (rodenticide)	989.4	E863.7	—	E950.6	E962.1	E980.7
fluoride - *see* Fluoride(s)	—	—	—	—	—	—
free salt	974.5	E858.5	E944.5	E950.4	E962.0	E980.4
glucosulfone	961.8	E857	E931.8	E950.4	E962.0	E980.4
hydroxide	983.2	E864.2	—	E950.7	E962.1	E980.6
hypochlorite (bleach) NEC	983.9	E864.3	—	E950.7	E962.1	E980.6
disinfectant	983.9	E861.4	—	E950.7	E962.1	E980.6
medicinal (anti-infective) (external)	976.0	E858.7	E946.0	E950.4	E962.0	E980.4
vapor	987.8	E869.8	—	E952.8	E962.2	E982.8

ICD-9-CM

Drugs

Vol.

Substance	Poisoning	External Cause (E-Code)				
		Accident	Therapeutic Use	Suicide Attempt	Assault	Undetermined
Sodium *(Continued)*						
hyposulfite	976.0	E858.7	E946.0	E950.4	E962.0	E980.4
indigotindisulfonate	977.8	E858.8	E947.8	E950.4	E962.0	E980.4
iodide	977.8	E858.8	E947.8	E950.4	E962.0	E980.4
iothalamate	977.8	E858.8	E947.8	E950.4	E962.0	E980.4
iron edetate	964.0	E858.2	E934.0	E950.4	E962.0	E980.4
lactate	963.3	E858.1	E933.3	E950.4	E962.0	E980.4
lauryl sulfate	976.2	E858.7	E946.2	E950.4	E962.0	E980.4
L-triiodothyronine	962.7	E858.0	E932.7	E950.4	E962.0	E980.4
metrizoate	977.8	E858.8	E947.8	E950.4	E962.0	E980.4
monofluoracetate (dust) (rodenticide)	989.4	E863.7	—	E950.6	E962.1	E980.7
morrhuate	972.7	E858.3	E942.7	E950.4	E962.0	E980.4
nafcillin	960.0	E856	E930.0	E950.4	E962.0	E980.4
nitrate (oxidizing agent)	983.9	E864.3	—	E950.7	E962.1	E980.6
nitrite (medicinal)	972.4	E858.3	E942.4	E950.4	E962.0	E980.4
nitroferricyanide	972.6	E858.3	E942.6	E950.4	E962.0	E980.4
nitroprusside	972.6	E858.3	E942.6	E950.4	E962.0	E980.4
para-aminohippurate	977.8	E858.8	E947.8	E950.4	E962.0	E980.4
perborate (nonmedicinal) NEC	989.89	E866.8	—	E950.9	E962.1	E980.9
medicinal	976.6	E858.7	E946.6	E950.4	E962.0	E980.4
soap	989.6	E861.1	—	E950.9	E962.1	E980.9
percarbonate - *see* Sodium, perborate	—	—	—	—	—	—
phosphate	973.3	E858.4	E943.3	E950.4	E962.0	E980.4
polystyrene sulfonate	974.5	E858.5	E944.5	E950.4	E962.0	E980.4
propionate	976.0	E858.7	E946.0	E950.4	E962.0	E980.4
psylliate	972.7	E858.3	E942.7	E950.4	E962.0	E980.4
removing resins	974.5	E858.5	E944.5	E950.4	E962.0	E980.4
salicylate	965.1	E850.3	E935.3	E950.0	E962.0	E980.0
sulfate	973.3	E858.4	E943.3	E950.4	E962.0	E980.4
sulfoxone	961.8	E857	E931.8	E950.4	E962.0	E980.4
tetradecyl sulfate	972.7	E858.3	E942.7	E950.4	E962.0	E980.4
thiopental	968.3	E855.1	E938.3	E950.4	E962.0	E980.4
thiosalicylate	965.1	E850.3	E935.3	E950.0	E962.0	E980.0
thiosulfate	976.0	E858.7	E946.0	E950.4	E962.0	E980.4
tolbutamide	977.8	E858.8	E947.8	E950.4	E962.0	E980.4
tyropanoate	977.8	E858.8	E947.8	E950.4	E962.0	E980.4
valproate	966.3	E855.0	E936.3	E950.4	E962.0	E980.4
Solanine	977.8	E858.8	E947.8	E950.4	E962.0	E980.4
Solanum dulcamara	988.2	E865.4	—	E950.9	E962.1	E980.9
Solapsone	961.8	E857	E931.8	E950.4	E962.0	E980.4
Solasulfone	961.8	E857	E931.8	E950.4	E962.0	E980.4
Soldering fluid	983.1	E864.1	—	E950.7	E962.1	E980.6
Solid substance	989.9	E866.9	—	E950.9	E962.1	E980.9
specified NEC	989.9	E866.8	—	E950.9	E962.1	E980.9
Solvents, industrial	982.8	E862.9	—	E950.9	E962.1	E980.9
naphtha	981	E862.0	—	E950.9	E962.1	E980.9
petroleum	981	E862.0	—	E950.9	E962.1	E980.9
specified NEC	982.8	E862.4	—	E950.9	E962.1	E980.9
Soma	968.0	E855.1	E938.0	E950.4	E962.0	E980.4
Somatotropin	962.4	E858.0	E932.4	E950.4	E962.0	E980.4
Sominex	963.0	E858.1	E933.0	E950.4	E962.0	E980.4
Somnos	967.1	E852.0	E937.1	E950.2	E962.0	E980.2
Somonal	967.0	E851	E937.0	E950.1	E962.0	E980.1
Soneryl	967.0	E851	E937.0	E950.1	E962.0	E980.1
Soothing syrup	977.9	E858.9	E947.9	E950.5	E962.0	E980.5
Sopor	967.4	E852.3	E937.4	E950.2	E962.0	E980.2
Soporific drug	967.9	E852.9	E937.9	E950.2	E962.0	E980.2
specified type NEC	967.8	E852.8	E937.8	E950.2	E962.0	E980.2
Sorbitol NEC	977.4	E858.8	E947.4	E950.4	E962.0	E980.4
Sotradecol	972.7	E858.3	E942.7	E950.4	E962.0	E980.4
Spacoline	975.1	E858.6	E945.1	E950.4	E962.0	E980.4
Spanish fly	976.8	E858.7	E946.8	E950.4	E962.0	E980.4

◀ New   ◀▥ Revised

Substance	Poisoning	External Cause (E-Code)				
		Accident	Therapeutic Use	Suicide Attempt	Assault	Undetermined
Sparine	969.1	E853.0	E939.1	E950.3	E962.0	E980.3
Sparteine	975.0	E858.6	E945.0	E950.4	E962.0	E980.4
Spasmolytics	975.1	E858.6	E945.1	E950.4	E962.0	E980.4
anticholinergics	971.1	E855.4	E941.1	E950.4	E962.0	E980.4
Spectinomycin	960.8	E856	E930.8	E950.4	E962.0	E980.4
Speed	969.7	E854.2	E939.7	E950.3	E962.0	E980.3
Spermicides	976.8	E858.7	E946.8	E950.4	E962.0	E980.4
Spider (bite) (venom)	989.5	E905.1	—	E950.9	E962.1	E980.9
antivenin	979.9	E858.8	E949.9	E950.4	E962.0	E980.4
Spigelia (root)	961.6	E857	E931.6	E950.4	E962.0	E980.4
Spiperone	969.2	E853.1	E939.2	E950.3	E962.0	E980.3
Spiramycin	960.3	E856	E930.3	E950.4	E962.0	E980.4
Spirilene	969.5	E853.8	E939.5	E950.3	E962.0	E980.3
Spirit(s) (neutral) NEC	980.0	E860.1	—	E950.9	E962.1	E980.9
beverage	980.0	E860.0	—	E950.9	E962.1	E980.9
industrial	980.9	E860.9	—	E950.9	E962.1	E980.9
mineral	981	E862.0	—	E950.9	E962.1	E980.9
of salt - *see* Hydrochloric acid	—	—	—	—	—	—
surgical	980.9	E860.9	—	E950.9	E962.1	E980.9
Spironolactone	974.4	E858.5	E944.4	E950.4	E962.0	E980.4
Sponge, absorbable (gelatin)	964.5	E858.2	E934.5	E950.4	E962.0	E980.4
Sporostacin	976.0	E858.7	E946.0	E950.4	E962.0	E980.4
Sprays (aerosol)	989.89	E866.8	—	E950.9	E962.1	E980.9
cosmetic	989.89	E866.7	—	E950.9	E962.1	E980.9
medicinal NEC	977.9	E858.9	E947.9	E950.5	E962.0	E980.5
pesticides - *see* Pesticides	—	—	—	—	—	—
specified content - *see* substance specified	—	—	—	—	—	—
Spurge flax	988.2	E865.4	—	E950.9	E962.1	E980.9
Spurges	988.2	E865.4	—	E950.9	E962.1	E980.9
Squill (expectorant) NEC	975.5	E858.6	E945.5	E950.4	E962.0	E980.4
rat poison	989.4	E863.7	—	E950.6	E962.1	E980.7
Squirting cucumber (cathartic)	973.1	E858.4	E943.1	E950.4	E962.0	E980.4
Stains	989.89	E866.8	—	E950.9	E962.1	E980.9
Stannous - *see also* Tin fluoride	976.7	E858.7	E946.7	E950.4	E962.0	E980.4
Stanolone	962.1	E858.0	E932.1	E950.4	E962.0	E980.4
Stanozolol	962.1	E858.0	E932.1	E950.4	E962.0	E980.4
Staphisagria or stavesacre (pediculicide)	976.0	E858.7	E946.0	E950.4	E962.0	E980.4
Stelazine	969.1	E853.0	E939.1	E950.3	E962.0	E980.3
Stemetil	969.1	E853.0	E939.1	E950.3	E962.0	E980.3
Sterculia (cathartic) (gum)	973.3	E858.4	E943.3	E950.4	E962.0	E980.4
Sternutator gas	987.8	E869.8	—	E952.8	E962.2	E982.8
Steroids NEC	962.0	E858.0	E932.0	E950.4	E962.0	E980.4
ENT agent	976.6	E858.7	E946.6	E950.4	E962.0	E980.4
ophthalmic preparation	976.5	E858.7	E946.5	E950.4	E962.0	E980.4
topical NEC	976.0	E858.7	E946.0	E950.4	E962.0	E980.4
Stibine	985.8	E866.4	—	E950.9	E962.1	E980.9
Stibophen	961.2	E857	E931.2	E950.4	E962.0	E980.4
Stilbamide, stilbamidine	961.5	E857	E931.5	E950.4	E962.0	E980.4
Stilbestrol	962.2	E858.0	E932.2	E950.4	E962.0	E980.4
Stimulants (central nervous system)	970.9	E854.3	E940.9	E950.4	E962.0	E980.4
analeptics	970.0	E854.3	E940.0	E950.4	E962.0	E980.4
opiate antagonist	970.1	E854.3	E940.1	E950.4	E962.0	E980.4
psychotherapeutic NEC	969.0	E854.0	E939.0	E950.3	E962.0	E980.3
specified NEC	970.8	E854.3	E940.8	E950.4	E962.0	E980.4
Storage batteries (acid) (cells)	983.1	E864.1	—	E950.7	E962.1	E980.6
Stovaine	968.9	E855.2	E938.9	E950.4	E962.0	E980.4
infiltration (subcutaneous)	968.5	E855.2	E938.5	E950.4	E962.0	E980.4
nerve block (peripheral) (plexus)	968.6	E855.2	E938.6	E950.4	E962.0	E980.4
spinal	968.7	E855.2	E938.7	E950.4	E962.0	E980.4
topical (surface)	968.5	E855.2	E938.5	E950.4	E962.0	E980.4
Stovarsal	961.1	E857	E931.1	E950.4	E962.0	E980.4

Substance	Poisoning	External Cause (E-Code)				
		Accident	Therapeutic Use	Suicide Attempt	Assault	Undetermined
Stove gas - *see* Gas, utility	—	—	—	—	—	—
Stoxil	976.5	E858.7	E946.5	E950.4	E962.0	E980.4
STP	969.6	E854.1	E939.6	E950.3	E962.0	E980.3
Stramonium (medicinal) NEC	971.1	E855.4	E941.1	E950.4	E962.0	E980.4
natural state	988.2	E865.4	—	E950.9	E962.1	E980.9
Streptodornase	964.4	E858.2	E934.4	E950.4	E962.0	E980.4
Streptoduocin	960.6	E856	E930.6	E950.4	E962.0	E980.4
Streptokinase	964.4	E858.2	E934.4	E950.4	E962.0	E980.4
Streptomycin	960.6	E856	E930.6	E950.4	E962.0	E980.4
Streptozocin	960.7	E856	E930.7	E950.4	E962.0	E980.4
Stripper (paint) (solvent)	982.8	E862.9	—	E950.9	E962.1	E980.9
Strobane	989.2	E863.0	—	E950.6	E962.1	E980.7
Strophanthin	972.1	E858.3	E942.1	E950.4	E962.0	E980.4
Strophanthus hispidus or kombe	988.2	E865.4	—	E950.9	E962.1	E980.9
Strychnine (rodenticide) (salts)	989.1	E863.7	—	E950.6	E962.1	E980.7
medicinal NEC	970.8	E854.3	E940.8	E950.4	E962.0	E980.4
Strychnos (ignatii) - *see* Strychnine	—	—	—	—	—	—
Styramate	968.0	E855.1	E938.0	E950.4	E962.0	E980.4
Styrene	983.0	E864.0	—	E950.7	E962.1	E980.6
Succinimide (anticonvulsant)	966.2	E855.0	E936.2	E950.4	E962.0	E980.4
mercuric - *see* Mercury	—	—	—	—	—	—
Succinylcholine	975.2	E858.6	E945.2	E950.4	E962.0	E980.4
Succinylsulfathiazole	961.0	E857	E931.0	E950.4	E962.0	E980.4
Sucrose	974.5	E858.5	E944.5	E950.4	E962.0	E980.4
Sulfacetamide	961.0	E857	E931.0	E950.4	E962.0	E980.4
ophthalmic preparation	976.5	E858.7	E946.5	E950.4	E962.0	E980.4
Sulfachlorpyridazine	961.0	E857	E931.0	E950.4	E962.0	E980.4
Sulfacytine	961.0	E857	E931.0	E950.4	E962.0	E980.4
Sulfadiazine	961.0	E857	E931.0	E950.4	E962.0	E980.4
silver (topical)	976.0	E858.7	E946.0	E950.4	E962.0	E980.4
Sulfadimethoxine	961.0	E857	E931.0	E950.4	E962.0	E980.4
Sulfadimidine	961.0	E857	E931.0	E950.4	E962.0	E980.4
Sulfaethidole	961.0	E857	E931.0	E950.4	E962.0	E980.4
Sulfafurazole	961.0	E857	E931.0	E950.4	E962.0	E980.4
Sulfaguanidine	961.0	E857	E931.0	E950.4	E962.0	E980.4
Sulfamerazine	961.0	E857	E931.0	E950.4	E962.0	E980.4
Sulfameter	961.0	E857	E931.0	E950.4	E962.0	E980.4
Sulfamethizole	961.0	E857	E931.0	E950.4	E962.0	E980.4
Sulfamethoxazole	961.0	E857	E931.0	E950.4	E962.0	E980.4
Sulfamethoxydiazine	961.0	E857	E931.0	E950.4	E962.0	E980.4
Sulfamethoxypyridazine	961.0	E857	E931.0	E950.4	E962.0	E980.4
Sulfamethylthiazole	961.0	E857	E931.0	E950.4	E962.0	E980.4
Sulfamylon	976.0	E858.7	E946.0	E950.4	E962.0	E980.4
Sulfan blue (diagnostic dye)	977.8	E858.8	E947.8	E950.4	E962.0	E980.4
Sulfanilamide	961.0	E857	E931.0	E950.4	E962.0	E980.4
Sulfanilylguanidine	961.0	E857	E931.0	E950.4	E962.0	E980.4
Sulfaphenazole	961.0	E857	E931.0	E950.4	E962.0	E980.4
Sulfaphenylthiazole	961.0	E857	E931.0	E950.4	E962.0	E980.4
Sulfaproxyline	961.0	E857	E931.0	E950.4	E962.0	E980.4
Sulfapyridine	961.0	E857	E931.0	E950.4	E962.0	E980.4
Sulfapyrimidine	961.0	E857	E931.0	E950.4	E962.0	E980.4
Sulfarsphenamine	961.1	E857	E931.1	E950.4	E962.0	E980.4
Sulfasalazine	961.0	E857	E931.0	E950.4	E962.0	E980.4
Sulfasomizole	961.0	E857	E931.0	E950.4	E962.0	E980.4
Sulfasuxidine	961.0	E857	E931.0	E950.4	E962.0	E980.4
Sulfinpyrazone	974.7	E858.5	E944.7	E950.4	E962.0	E980.4
Sulfisoxazole	961.0	E857	E931.0	E950.4	E962.0	E980.4
ophthalmic preparation	976.5	E858.7	E946.5	E950.4	E962.0	E980.4
Sulfomyxin	960.8	E856	E930.8	E950.4	E962.0	E980.4
Sulfonal	967.8	E852.8	E937.8	E950.2	E962.0	E980.2
Sulfonamides (mixtures)	961.0	E857	E931.0	E950.4	E962.0	E980.4

◀ New   ◀▥ Revised

Substance	Poisoning	External Cause (E-Code)				
		Accident	Therapeutic Use	Suicide Attempt	Assault	Undetermined
Sulfones	961.8	E857	E931.8	E950.4	E962.0	E980.4
Sulfonethylmethane	967.8	E852.8	E937.8	E950.2	E962.0	E980.2
Sulfonmethane	967.8	E852.8	E937.8	E950.2	E962.0	E980.2
Sulfonphthal, sulfonphthol	977.8	E858.8	E947.8	E950.4	E962.0	E980.4
Sulfonylurea derivatives, oral	962.3	E858.0	E932.3	E950.4	E962.0	E980.4
Sulfoxone	961.8	E857	E931.8	E950.4	E962.0	E980.4
Sulfur, sulfureted, sulfuric, sulfurous, sulfuryl (compounds) NEC	989.89	E866.8	—	E950.9	E962.1	E980.9
acid	983.1	E864.1	—	E950.7	E962.1	E980.6
dioxide	987.3	E869.1	—	E952.8	E962.2	E982.8
ether - see Ether(s)	—	—	—			
hydrogen	987.8	E869.8	—	E952.8	E962.2	E982.8
medicinal (keratolytic) (ointment) NEC	976.4	E858.7	E946.4	E950.4	E962.0	E980.4
pesticide (vapor)	989.4	E863.4	—	E950.6	E962.1	E980.7
vapor NEC	987.8	E869.8	—	E952.8	E962.2	E982.8
Sulkowitch's reagent	977.8	E858.8	E947.8	E950.4	E962.0	E980.4
Sulph - see also Sulf-	—	—	—	—	—	—
Sulphadione	961.8	E857	E931.8	E950.4	E962.0	E980.4
Sulthiame, sultiame	966.3	E855.0	E936.3	E950.4	E962.0	E980.4
Superinone	975.5	E858.6	E945.5	E950.4	E962.0	E980.4
Suramin	961.5	E857	E931.5	E950.4	E962.0	E980.4
Surfacaine	968.5	E855.2	E938.5	E950.4	E962.0	E980.4
Surital	968.3	E855.1	E938.3	E950.4	E962.0	E980.4
Sutilains	976.8	E858.7	E946.8	E950.4	E962.0	E980.4
Suxamethonium (bromide) (chloride) (iodide)	975.2	E858.6	E945.2	E950.4	E962.0	E980.4
Suxethonium (bromide)	975.2	E858.6	E945.2	E950.4	E962.0	E980.4
Sweet oil (birch)	976.3	E858.7	E946.3	E950.4	E962.0	E980.4
Sym-dichloroethyl ether	982.3	E862.4	—	E950.9	E962.1	E980.9
Sympatholytics	971.3	E855.6	E941.3	E950.4	E962.0	E980.4
Sympathomimetics	971.2	E855.5	E941.2	E950.4	E962.0	E980.4
Synagis	979.6	E858.8	E949.6	E950.4	E962.0	E980.4
Synalar	976.0	E858.7	E946.0	E950.4	E962.0	E980.4
Synthroid	962.7	E858.0	E932.7	E950.4	E962.0	E980.4
Syntocinon	975.0	E858.6	E945.0	E950.4	E962.0	E950.4
Syrosingopine	972.6	E858.3	E942.6	E950.4	E962.0	E980.4
Systemic agents (primarily)	963.9	E858.1	E933.9	E950.4	E962.0	E980.4
specified NEC	963.8	E858.1	E933.8	E950.4	E962.0	E980.4
Tablets (see also specified substance)	977.9	E858.9	E947.9	E950.5	E962.0	E980.5
Tace	962.2	E858.0	E932.2	E950.4	E962.0	E980.4
Tacrine	971.0	E855.3	E941.0	E950.4	E962.0	E980.4
Talbutal	967.0	E851	E937.0	E950.1	E962.0	E980.1
Talc	976.3	E858.7	E946.3	E950.4	E962.0	E980.4
Talcum	976.3	E858.7	E946.3	E950.4	E962.0	E980.4
Tandearil, tanderil	965.5	E850.5	E935.5	E950.0	E962.0	E980.0
Tannic acid	983.1	E864.1	—	E950.7	E962.1	E980.6
medicinal (astringent)	976.2	E858.7	E946.2	E950.4	E962.0	E980.4
Tannin - see Tannic acid	—	—	—	—	—	—
Tansy	988.2	E865.4	—	E950.9	E962.1	E980.9
TAO	960.3	E856	E930.3	E950.4	E962.0	E980.4
Tapazole	962.8	E858.0	E932.8	E950.4	E962.0	E980.4
Tar NEC	983.0	E864.0	—	E950.7	E962.1	E980.6
camphor - see Naphthalene	—	—	—			
fumes	987.8	E869.8	—	E952.8	E962.2	E982.8
Taractan	969.3	E853.8	E939.3	E950.3	E962.0	E980.3
Tarantula (venomous)	989.5	E905.1	—	E950.9	E962.1	E980.9
Tartar emetic (anti-infective)	961.2	E857	E931.2	E950.4	E962.0	E980.4
Tartaric acid	983.1	E864.1	—	E950.7	E962.1	E980.6
Tartrated antimony (anti-infective)	961.2	E857	E931.2	E950.4	E962.0	E980.4
TCA - see Trichloroacetic acid	—	—	—			
TDI	983.0	E864.0	—	E950.7	E962.1	E980.6
vapor	987.8	E869.8	—	E952.8	E962.2	E982.8
Tear gas	987.5	E869.3	—	E952.8	E962.2	E982.8
Teclothiazide	974.3	E858.5	E944.3	E950.4	E962.0	E980.4

Substance	Poisoning	External Cause (E-Code)				
		Accident	Therapeutic Use	Suicide Attempt	Assault	Undetermined
Tegretol	966.3	E855.0	E936.3	E950.4	E962.0	E980.4
Telepaque	977.8	E858.8	E947.8	E950.4	E962.0	E980.4
Tellurium	985.8	E866.4	—	E950.9	E962.1	E980.9
fumes	985.8	E866.4	—	E950.9	E962.1	E980.9
TEM	963.1	E858.1	E933.1	E950.4	E962.0	E980.4
Temazepam - see Benzodiazepines	—	—	—	—	—	—
TEPA	963.1	E858.1	E933.1	E950.4	E962.0	E980.4
TEPP	989.3	E863.1	—	E950.6	E962.1	E980.7
Terbutaline	971.2	E855.5	E941.2	E950.4	E962.0	E980.4
Teroxalene	961.6	E857	E931.6	E950.4	E962.0	E980.4
Terpin hydrate	975.5	E858.6	E945.5	E950.4	E962.0	E980.4
Terramycin	960.4	E856	E930.4	E950.4	E962.0	E980.4
Tessalon	975.4	E858.6	E945.4	E950.4	E962.0	E980.4
Testosterone	962.1	E858.0	E932.1	E950.4	E962.0	E980.4
Tetanus (vaccine)	978.4	E858.8	E948.4	E950.4	E962.0	E980.4
antitoxin	979.9	E858.8	E949.9	E950.4	E962.0	E980.4
immune globulin (human)	964.6	E858.2	E934.6	E950.4	E962.0	E980.4
toxoid	978.4	E858.8	E948.4	E950.4	E962.0	E980.4
with diphtheria toxoid	978.9	E858.8	E948.9	E950.4	E962.0	E980.4
with pertussis	978.6	E858.8	E948.6	E950.4	E962.0	E980.4
Tetrabenazine	969.5	E853.8	E939.5	E950.3	E962.0	E980.3
Tetracaine (infiltration) (topical)	968.5	E855.2	E938.5	E950.4	E962.0	E980.4
nerve block (peripheral) (plexus)	968.6	E855.2	E938.6	E950.4	E962.0	E980.4
spinal	968.7	E855.2	E938.7	E950.4	E962.0	E980.4
Tetrachlorethvlene - see Tetrachloroethylene	—	—	—	—	—	—
Tetrachlormethiazide	974.3	E858.5	E944.3	E950.4	E962.0	E980.4
Tetrachloroethane (liquid) (vapor)	982.3	E862.4	—	E950.9	E962.1	E980.9
paint or varnish	982.3	E861.6	—	E950.9	E962.1	E980.9
Tetrachloroethylene (liquid) (vapor)	982.3	E862.4	—	E950.9	E962.1	E980.9
medicinal	961.6	E857	E931.6	E950.4	E962.0	E980.4
Tetrachloromethane - see Carbon, tetrachloride	—	—	—	—	—	—
Tetracycline	960.4	E856	E930.4	E950.4	E962.0	E980.4
ophthalmic preparation	976.5	E858.7	E946.5	E950.4	E962.0	E980.4
topical NEC	976.0	E858.7	E946.0	E950.4	E962.0	E980.4
Tetraethylammonium chloride	972.3	E858.3	E942.3	E950.4	E962.0	E980.4
Tetraethyl lead (antiknock compound)	984.1	E862.1	—	E950.9	E962.1	E980.9
Tetraethyl pyrophosphate	989.3	E863.1	—	E950.6	E962.1	E980.7
Tetraethylthiuram disulfide	977.3	E858.8	E947.3	E950.4	E962.0	E980.4
Tetrahydroaminoacridine	971.0	E855.3	E941.0	E950.4	E962.0	E980.4
Tetrahydrocannabinol	969.6	E854.1	E939.6	E950.3	E962.0	E980.3
Tetrahydronaphthalene	982.0	E862.4	—	E950.9	E962.1	E980.9
Tetrahydrozoline	971.2	E855.5	E941.2	E950.4	E962.0	E980.4
Tetralin	982.0	E862.4	—	E950.9	E962.1	E980.9
Tetramethylthiuram (disulfide) NEC	989.4	E863.6	—	E950.6	E962.1	E980.7
medicinal	976.2	E858.7	E946.2	E950.4	E962.0	E980.4
Tetronal	967.8	E852.8	E937.8	E950.2	E962.0	E980.2
Tetryl	983.0	E864.0	—	E950.7	E962.1	E980.6
Thalidomide	967.8	E852.8	E937.8	E950.2	E962.0	E980.2
Thallium (compounds) (dust) NEC	985.8	E866.4	—	E950.9	E962.1	E980.9
pesticide (rodenticide)	985.8	E863.7	—	E950.6	E962.1	E980.7
THC	969.6	E854.1	E939.6	E950.3	E962.0	E980.3
Thebacon	965.09	E850.2	E935.2	E950.0	E962.0	E980.0
Thebaine	965.09	E850.2	E935.2	E950.0	E962.0	E980.0
Theobromine (calcium salicylate)	974.1	E858.5	E944.1	E950.4	E962.0	E980.4
Theophylline (diuretic)	974.1	E858.5	E944.1	E950.4	E962.0	E980.4
ethylenediamine	975.7	E858.6	E945.7	E950.4	E962.0	E980.4
Thiabendazole	961.6	E857	E931.6	E950.4	E962.0	E980.4
Thialbarbital, thialbarbitone	968.3	E855.1	E938.3	E950.4	E962.0	E980.4
Thiamine	963.5	E858.1	E933.5	E950.4	E962.0	E980.4
Thiamylal (sodium)	968.3	E855.1	E938.3	E950.4	E962.0	E980.4
Thiazesim	969.0	E854.0	E939.0	E950.3	E962.0	E980.3

◀ New   ◀▦ Revised

ICD-9-CM

Drugs

Vol. 2

Substance	Poisoning	External Cause (E-Code)				
		Accident	Therapeutic Use	Suicide Attempt	Assault	Undetermined
Thiazides (diuretics)	974.3	E858.5	E944.3	E950.4	E962.0	E980.4
Thiethylperazine	963.0	E858.1	E933.0	E950.4	E962.0	E980.4
Thimerosal (topical)	976.0	E858.7	E946.0	E950.4	E962.0	E980.4
ophthalmic preparation	976.5	E858.7	E946.5	E950.4	E962.0	E980.4
Thioacetazone	961.8	E857	E931.8	E950.4	E962.0	E980.4
Thiobarbiturates	968.3	E855.1	E938.3	E950.4	E962.0	E980.4
Thiobismol	961.2	E857	E931.2	E950.4	E962.0	E980.4
Thiocarbamide	962.8	E858.0	E932.8	E950.4	E962.0	E980.4
Thiocarbarsone	961.1	E857	E931.1	E950.4	E962.0	E980.4
Thiocarlide	961.8	E857	E931.8	E950.4	E962.0	E980.4
Thioguanine	963.1	E858.1	E933.1	E950.4	E962.0	E980.4
Thiomercaptomerin	974.0	E858.5	E944.0	E950.4	E962.0	E980.4
Thiomerin	974.0	E858.5	E944.0	E950.4	E962.0	E980.4
Thiopental, thiopentone (sodium)	968.3	E855.1	E938.3	E950.4	E962.0	E980.4
Thiopropazate	969.1	E853.0	E939.1	E950.3	E962.0	E980.3
Thioproperazine	969.1	E853.0	E939.1	E950.3	E962.0	E980.3
Thioridazine	969.1	E853.0	E939.1	E950.3	E962.0	E980.3
Thio-TEPA, thiotepa	963.1	E858.1	E933.1	E950.4	E962.0	E980.4
Thiothixene	969.3	E853.8	E939.3	E950.3	E962.0	E980.3
Thiouracil	962.8	E858.0	E932.8	E950.4	E962.0	E980.4
Thiourea	962.8	E858.0	E932.8	E950.4	E962.0	E980.4
Thiphenamil	971.1	E855.4	E941.1	E950.4	E962.0	E980.4
Thiram NEC	989.4	E863.	—	E950.6	E962.1	E980.7
medicinal	976.2	E858.7	E946.2	E950.4	E962.0	E980.4
Thonzylamine	963.0	E858.1	E933.0	E950.4	E962.0	E980.4
Thorazine	969.1	E853.0	E939.1	E950.3	E962.0	E980.3
Thornapple	988.2	E865.4	—	E950.9	E962.1	E980.9
Throat preparation (lozenges) NEC	976.6	E858.7	E946.6	E950.4	E962.0	E980.4
Thrombin	964.5	E858.2	E934.5	E950.4	E962.0	E980.4
Thrombolysin	964.4	E858.2	E934.4	E950.4	E962.0	E980.4
Thymol	983.0	E864.0	—	E950.7	E962.1	E980.6
Thymus extract	962.9	E858.0	E932.9	E950.4	E962.0	E980.4
Thyroglobulin	962.7	E858.0	E932.7	E950.4	E962.0	E980.4
Thyroid (derivatives) (extract)	962.7	E858.0	E932.7	E950.4	E962.0	E980.4
Thyrolar	962.7	E858.0	E932.7	E950.4	E962.0	E980.4
Thyrotrophin, thyrotropin	977.8	E858.8	E947.8	E950.4	E962.0	E980.4
Thyroxin(e)	962.7	E858.0	E932.7	E950.4	E962.0	E980.4
Tigan	963.0	E858.1	E933.0	E950.4	E962.0	E980.4
Tigloidine	968.0	E855.1	E938.0	E950.4	E962.0	E980.4
Tin (chloride) (dust) (oxide) NEC	985.8	E866.4	—	E950.9	E962.1	E980.9
anti-infectives	961.2	E857	E931.2	E950.4	E962.0	E980.4
Tinactin	976.0	E858.7	E946.0	E950.4	E962.0	E980.4
Tincture, iodine - *see* Iodine	—	—	—	—	—	—
Tindal	969.1	E853.0	E939.1	E950.3	E962.0	E980.3
Titanium (compounds) (vapor)	985.8	E866.4	—	E950.9	E962.1	E980.9
ointment	976.3	E858.7	E946.3	E950.4	E962.0	E980.4
Titroid	962.7	E858.0	E932.7	E950.4	E962.0	E980.4
TMTD - *see* Tetramethylthiuram disulfide	—	—	—	—	—	—
TNT	989.89	E866.8	—	E950.9	E962.1	E980.9
fumes	987.8	E869.8	—	E952.8	E962.2	E982.8
Toadstool	988.1	E865.5	—	E950.9	E962.1	E980.9
Tobacco NEC	989.84	E866.8	—	E950.9	E962.1	E980.9
Indian	988.2	E865.4	—	E950.9	E962.1	E980.9
smoke, second-hand	987.8	E869.4	—	—	—	—
Tocopherol	963.5	E858.1	E933.5	E950.4	E962.0	E980.4
Tocosamine	975.0	E858.6	E945.0	E950.4	E962.0	E980.4
Tofranil	969.0	E854.0	E939.0	E950.3	E962.0	E980.3
Toilet deodorizer	989.89	E866.8	—	E950.9	E962.1	E980.9
Tolazamide	962.3	E858.0	E932.3	E950.4	E962.0	E980.4
Tolazoline	971.3	E855.6	E941.3	E950.4	E962.0	E980.4
Tolbutamide	962.3	E858.0	E932.3	E950.4	E962.0	E980.4
sodium	977.8	E858.8	E947.8	E950.4	E962.0	E980.4

Substance	Poisoning	External Cause (E-Code)				
		Accident	Therapeutic Use	Suicide Attempt	Assault	Undetermined
Tolmetin	965.69	E856.0	E935.6	E950.0	E962.0	E980.0
Tolnaftate	976.0	E858.7	E946.0	E950.4	E962.0	E980.4
Tolpropamine	976.1	E858.7	E946.1	E950.4	E962.0	E980.4
Tolserol	968.0	E855.1	E938.0	E950.4	E962.0	E980.4
Toluene (liquid) (vapor)	982.0	E862.4	—	E950.9	E962.1	E980.9
diisocyanate	983.0	E864.0	—	E950.7	E962.1	E980.6
Toluidine	983.0	E864.0	—	E950.7	E962.1	E980.6
vapor	987.8	E869.8	—	E952.8	E962.2	E982.8
Toluol (liquid) (vapor)	982.0	E862.4	—	E950.9	E962.1	E980.9
Tolylene-2,4-diisocyanate	983.0	E864.0	—	E950.7	E962.1	E980.6
Tonics, cardiac	972.1	E858.3	E942.1	E950.4	E962.0	E980.4
Toxaphene (dust) (spray)	989.2	E863.0	—	E950.6	E962.1	E980.7
Toxoids NEC	978.8	E858.8	E948.8	E950.4	E962.0	E980.4
Tractor fuel NEC	981	E862.1	—	E950.9	E962.1	E980.9
Tragacanth	973.3	E858.4	E943.3	E950.4	E962.0	E980.4
Tramazoline	971.2	E855.5	E941.2	E950.4	E962.0	E980.4
Tranquilizers	969.5	E853.9	E939.5	E950.3	E962.0	E980.3
benzodiazepine-based	969.4	E853.2	E939.4	E950.3	E962.0	E980.3
butyrophenone-based	969.2	E853.1	E939.2	E950.3	E962.0	E980.3
major NEC	969.3	E853.8	E939.3	E950.3	E962.0	E980.3
phenothiazine-based	969.1	E853.0	E939.1	E950.3	E962.0	E980.3
specified NEC	969.5	E853.8	E939.5	E950.3	E962.0	E980.3
Trantoin	961.9	E857	E931.9	E950.4	E962.0	E980.4
Tranxene	969.4	E853.2	E939.4	E950.3	E962.0	E980.3
Tranylcypromine (sulfate)	969.0	E854.0	E939.0	E950.3	E962.0	E980.3
Trasentine	975.1	E858.6	E945.1	E950.4	E962.0	E980.4
Travert	974.5	E858.5	E944.5	E950.4	E962.0	E980.4
Trecator	961.8	E857	E931.8	E950.4	E962.0	E980.4
Tretinoin	976.8	E858.7	E946.8	E950.4	E962.0	E980.4
Triacetin	976.0	E858.7	E946.0	E950.4	E962.0	E980.4
Triacetyloleandomycin	960.3	E856	E930.3	E950.4	E962.0	E980.4
Triamcinolone	962.0	E858.0	E932.0	E950.4	E962.0	E980.4
ENT agent	976.6	E858.7	E946.6	E950.4	E962.0	E980.4
ophthalmic preparation	976.5	E858.7	E946.5	E950.4	E962.0	E980.4
topical NEC	976.0	E858.7	E946.0	E950.4	E962.0	E980.4
Triamterene	974.4	E858.5	E944.4	E950.4	E962.0	E980.4
Triaziquone	963.1	E858.1	E933.1	E950.4	E962.0	E980.4
Tribromacetaldehyde	967.3	E852.2	E937.3	E950.2	E962.0	E980.2
Tribromoethanol	968.2	E855.1	E938.2	E950.4	E962.0	E980.4
Tribromomethane	967.3	E852.2	E937.3	E950.2	E962.0	E980.2
Trichlorethane	982.3	E862.4	—	E950.9	E962.1	E980.9
Trichlormethiazide	974.3	E858.5	E944.3	E950.4	E962.0	E980.4
Trichloroacetic acid	983.1	E864.1	—	E950.7	E962.1	E980.6
medicinal (keratolytic)	976.4	E858.7	E946.4	E950.4	E962.0	E980.4
Trichloroethanol	967.1	E852.0	E937.1	E950.2	E962.0	E980.2
Trichloroethylene (liquid) (vapor)	982.3	E862.4	—	E950.9	E962.1	E980.9
anesthetic (gas)	968.2	E855.1	E938.2	E950.4	E962.0	E980.4
Trichloroethyl phosphate	967.1	E852.0	E937.1	E950.2	E962.0	E980.2
Trichlorofluoromethane NEC	987.4	E869.2	—	E952.8	E962.2	E982.8
Trichlorotriethylamine	963.1	E858.1	E933.1	E950.4	E962.0	E980.4
Trichomonacides NEC	961.5	E857	E931.5	E950.4	E962.0	E980.4
Trichomycin	960.1	E856	E930.1	E950.4	E962.0	E980.4
Triclofos	967.1	E852.0	E937.1	E950.2	E962.0	E980.2
Tricresyl phosphate	989.89	E866.8	—	E950.9	E962.1	E980.9
solvent	982.8	E862.4	—	E950.9	E962.1	E980.9
Tricyclamol	966.4	E855.0	E936.4	E950.4	E962.0	E980.4
Tridesilon	976.0	E858.7	E946.0	E950.4	E962.0	E980.4
Tridihexethyl	971.1	E855.4	E941.1	E950.4	E962.0	E980.4
Tridione	966.0	E855.0	E936.0	E950.4	E962.0	E980.4

◀ New   ◀▥ Revised

ICD-9-CM

Drugs

Vol. 2

Substance	Poisoning	External Cause (E-Code)				
		Accident	Therapeutic Use	Suicide Attempt	Assault	Undetermined
Triethanolamine NEC	983.2	E864.2	—	E950.7	E962.1	E980.6
detergent	983.2	E861.0	—	E950.7	E962.1	E980.6
trinitrate	972.4	E858.3	E942.4	E950.4	E962.0	E980.4
Triethanomelamine	963.1	E858.1	E933.1	E950.4	E962.0	E980.4
Triethylene melamine	963.1	E858.1	E933.1	E950.4	E962.0	E980.4
Triethylenephosphoramide	963.1	E858.1	E933.1	E950.4	E962.0	E980.4
Triethylenethiophosphoramide	963.1	E858.1	E933.1	E950.4	E962.0	E980.4
Trifluoperazine	969.1	E853.0	E939.1	E950.3	E962.0	E980.3
Trifluperidol	969.2	E853.1	E939.2	E950.3	E962.0	E980.3
Triflupromazine	969.1	E853.0	E939.1	E950.3	E962.0	E980.3
Trihexyphenidyl	971.1	E855.4	E941.1	E950.4	E962.0	E980.4
Triiodothyronine	962.7	E858.0	E932.7	E950.4	E962.0	E980.4
Trilene	968.2	E855.1	E938.2	E950.4	E962.0	E980.4
Trimeprazine	963.0	E858.1	E933.0	E950.4	E962.0	E980.4
Trimetazidine	972.4	E858.3	E942.4	E950.4	E962.0	E980.4
Trimethadione	966.0	E855.0	E936.0	E950.4	E962.0	E980.4
Trimethaphan	972.3	E858.3	E942.3	E950.4	E962.0	E980.4
Trimethidinium	972.3	E858.3	E942.3	E950.4	E962.0	E980.4
Trimethobenzamide	963.0	E858.1	E933.0	E950.4	E962.0	E980.4
Trimethylcarbinol	980.8	E860.8	—	E950.9	E962.1	E980.9
Trimethylpsoralen	976.3	E858.7	E946.3	E950.4	E962.0	E980.4
Trimeton	963.0	E858.1	E933.0	E950.4	E962.0	E980.4
Trimipramine	969.0	E854.0	E939.0	E950.3	E962.0	E980.3
Trimustine	963.1	E858.1	E933.1	E950.4	E962.0	E980.4
Trinitrin	972.4	E858.3	E942.4	E950.4	E962.0	E980.4
Trinitrophenol	983.0	E864.0	—	E950.7	E962.1	E980.6
Trinitrotoluene	989.89	E866.8	—	E950.9	E962.1	E980.9
fumes	987.8	E869.8	—	E952.8	E962.2	E982.8
Trional	967.8	E852.8	E937.8	E950.2	E962.0	E980.2
Trioxide of arsenic - see Arsenic	—	—	—	—	—	—
Trioxsalen	976.3	E858.7	E946.3	E950.4	E962.0	E980.4
Tripelennamine	963.0	E858.1	E933.0	E950.4	E962.0	E980.4
Triperidol	969.2	E853.1	E939.2	E950.3	E962.0	E980.3
Triprolidine	963.0	E858.1	E933.0	E950.4	E962.0	E980.4
Trisoralen	976.3	E858.7	E946.3	E950.4	E962.0	E980.4
Troleandomycin	960.3	E856	E930.3	E950.4	E962.0	E980.4
Trolnitrate (phosphate)	972.4	E858.3	E942.4	E950.4	E962.0	E980.4
Trometamol	963.3	E858.1	E933.3	E950.4	E962.0	E980.4
Tromethamine	963.3	E858.1	E933.3	E950.4	E962.0	E980.4
Tronothane	968.5	E855.2	E938.5	E950.4	E962.0	E980.4
Tropicamide	971.1	E855.4	E941.1	E950.4	E962.0	E980.4
Troxidone	966.0	E855.0	E936.0	E950.4	E962.0	E980.4
Tryparsamide	961.1	E857	E931.1	E950.4	E962.0	E980.4
Trypsin	963.4	E858.1	E933.4	E950.4	E962.0	E980.4
Tryptizol	969.0	E854.0	E939.0	E950.3	E962.0	E980.3
Tuaminoheptane	971.2	E855.5	E941.2	E950.4	E962.0	E980.4
Tuberculin (old)	977.8	E858.8	E947.8	E950.4	E962.0	E980.4
Tubocurare	975.2	E858.6	E945.2	E950.4	E962.0	E980.4
Tubocurarine	975.2	E858.6	E945.2	E950.4	E962.0	E980.4
Turkish green	969.6	E854.1	E939.6	E950.3	E962.0	E980.3
Turpentine (spirits of) (liquid) (vapor)	982.8	E862.4	—	E950.9	E962.1	E980.9
Tybamate	969.5	E853.8	E939.5	E950.3	E962.0	E980.3
Tyloxapol	975.5	E858.6	E945.5	E950.4	E962.0	E980.4
Tymazoline	971.2	E855.5	E941.2	E950.4	E962.0	E980.4
Typhoid vaccine	978.1	E858.8	E948.1	E950.4	E962.0	E980.4
Typhus vaccine	979.2	E858.8	E949.2	E950.4	E962.0	E980.4
Tyrothricin	976.0	E858.7	E946.0	E950.4	E962.0	E980.4
ENT agent	976.6	E858.7	E946.6	E950.4	E962.0	E980.4
ophthalmic preparation	976.5	E858.7	E946.5	E950.4	E962.0	E980.4
Undecenoic acid	976.0	E858.7	E946.0	E950.4	E962.0	E980.4
Undecylenic acid	976.0	E858.7	E946.0	E950.4	E962.0	E980.4

Substance	Poisoning	External Cause (E-Code)				
		Accident	Therapeutic Use	Suicide Attempt	Assault	Undetermined
Unna's boot	976.3	E858.7	E946.3	E950.4	E962.0	E980.4
Uracil mustard	963.1	E858.1	E933.1	E950.4	E962.0	E980.4
Uramustine	963.1	E858.1	E933.1	E950.4	E962.0	E980.4
Urari	975.2	E858.6	E945.2	E950.4	E962.0	E980.4
Urea	974.4	E858.5	E944.4	E950.4	E962.0	E980.4
topical	976.8	E858.7	E946.8	E950.4	E962.0	E980.4
Urethan(e) (antineoplastic)	963.1	E858.1	E933.1	E950.4	E962.0	E980.4
Urginea (maritima) (scilla) - see Squill	—	—	—	—	—	—
Uric acid metabolism agents NEC	974.7	E858.5	E944.7	E950.4	E962.0	E980.4
Urokinase	964.4	E858.2	E934.4	E950.4	E962.0	E980.4
Urokon	977.8	E858.8	E947.8	E950.4	E962.0	E980.4
Urotropin	961.9	E857	E931.9	E950.4	E962.0	E980.4
Urtica	988.2	E865.4	—	E950.9	E962.1	E980.9
Utility gas - see Gas, utility	—	—	—	—	—	—
Vaccine NEC	979.9	E858.8	E949.9	E950.4	E962.0	E980.4
bacterial NEC	978.8	E858.8	E948.8	E950.4	E962.0	E980.4
with	—	—	—	—	—	—
other bacterial component	978.9	E858.8	E948.9	E950.4	E962.0	E980.4
pertussis component	978.6	E858.8	E948.6	E950.4	E962.0	E980.4
viral-rickettsial component	979.7	E858.8	E949.7	E950.4	E962.0	E980.4
mixed NEC	978.9	E858.8	E948.9	E950.4	E962.0	E980.4
BCG	978.0	E858.8	E948.0	E950.4	E962.0	E980.4
cholera	978.2	E858.8	E948.2	E950.4	E962.0	E980.4
diphtheria	978.5	E858.8	E948.5	E950.4	E962.0	E980.4
influenza	979.6	E858.8	E949.6	E950.4	E962.0	E980.4
measles	979.4	E858.8	E949.4	E950.4	E962.0	E980.4
meningococcal	978.8	E858.8	E948.8	E950.4	E962.0	E980.4
mumps	979.6	E858.8	E949.6	E950.4	E962.0	E980.4
paratyphoid	978.1	E858.8	E948.1	E950.4	E962.0	E980.4
pertussis (with diphtheria toxoid) (with tetanus toxoid)	978.6	E858.8	E948.6	E950.4	E962.0	E980.4
plague	978.3	E858.8	E948.3	E950.4	E962.0	E980.4
poliomyelitis	979.5	E858.8	E949.5	E950.4	E962.0	E980.4
poliovirus	979.5	E858.8	E949.5	E950.4	E962.0	E980.4
rabies	979.1	E858.8	E949.1	E950.4	E962.0	E980.4
respiratory syncytial virus	979.6	E858.8	E949.6	E950.4	E962.0	E980.4
rickettsial NEC	979.6	E858.8	E949.6	E950.4	E962.0	E980.4
with	—	—	—	—	—	—
bacterial component	979.7	E858.8	E949.7	E950.4	E962.0	E980.4
pertussis component	978.6	E858.8	E948.6	E950.4	E962.0	E980.4
viral component	979.7	E858.8	E949.7	E950.4	E962.0	E980.4
Rocky Mountain spotted fever	979.6	E858.8	E949.6	E950.4	E962.0	E980.4
rotavirus	979.6	E858.8	E949.6	E950.4	E962.0	E980.4
rubella virus	979.4	E858.8	E949.4	E950.4	E962.0	E980.4
sabin oral	979.5	E858.8	E949.5	E950.4	E962.0	E980.4
smallpox	979.0	E858.8	E949.0	E950.4	E962.0	E980.4
tetanus	978.4	E858.8	E948.4	E950.4	E962.0	E980.4
typhoid	978.1	E858.8	E948.1	E950.4	E962.0	E980.4
typhus	979.2	E858.8	E949.2	E950.4	E962.0	E980.4
viral NEC	979.6	E858.8	E949.6	E950.4	E962.0	E980.4
with	—	—	—	—	—	—
bacterial component	979.7	E858.8	E949.7	E950.4	E962.0	E980.4
pertussis component	978.6	E858.8	E948.6	E950.4	E962.0	E980.4
rickettsial component	979.7	E858.8	E949.7	E950.4	E962.0	E980.4
yellow fever	979.3	E858.8	E949.3	E950.4	E962.0	E980.4
Vaccinia immune globulin (human)	964.6	E858.2	E934.6	E950.4	E962.0	E980.4
Vaginal contraceptives	976.8	E858.7	E946.8	E950.4	E962.0	E980.4
Valethamate	971.1	E855.4	E941.1	E950.4	E962.0	E980.4
Valisone	976.0	E858.7	E946.0	E950.4	E962.0	E980.4
Valium	969.4	E853.2	E939.4	E950.3	E962.0	E980.3
Valmid	967.8	E852.8	E937.8	E950.2	E962.0	E980.2
Vanadium	985.8	E866.4	—	E950.9	E962.1	E980.9
Vancomycin	960.8	E856	E930.8	E950.4	E962.0	E980.4

◀ New   ◀▦ Revised

ICD-9-CM

Drugs

Vol. 2

		External Cause (E-Code)				
Substance	**Poisoning**	**Accident**	**Therapeutic Use**	**Suicide Attempt**	**Assault**	**Undetermined**
Vapor (*see also* Gas)	987.9	E869.9	—	E952.9	E962.2	E982.9
kiln (carbon monoxide)	986	E868.8	—	E952.1	E962.2	E982.1
lead - *see* Lead	—	—	—	—	—	—
specified source NEC - (*see also* specific substance)	987.8	E869.8	—	E952.8	E962.2	E982.8
Varidase	964.4	E858.2	E934.4	E950.4	E962.0	E980.4
Varnish	989.89	E861.6	—	E950.9	E962.1	E980.9
cleaner	982.8	E862.9	—	E950.9	E962.1	E980.9
Vaseline	976.3	E858.7	E946.3	E950.4	E962.0	E980.4
Vasodilan	972.5	E858.3	E942.5	E950.4	E962.0	E980.4
Vasodilators NEC	972.5	E858.3	E942.5	E950.4	E962.0	E980.4
coronary	972.4	E858.3	E942.4	E950.4	E962.0	E980.4
Vasopressin	962.5	E858.0	E932.5	E950.4	E962.0	E980.4
Vasopressor drugs	962.5	E858.0	E932.5	E950.4	E962.0	E980.4
Venom, venomous (bite) (sting)	989.5	E905.9	—	E950.9	E962.1	E980.9
arthropod NEC	989.5	E905.5	—	E950.9	E962.1	E980.9
bee	989.5	E905.3	—	E950.9	E962.1	E980.9
centipede	989.5	E905.4	—	E950.9	E962.1	E980.9
hornet	989.5	E905.3	—	E950.9	E962.1	E980.9
lizard	989.5	E905.0	—	E950.9	E962.1	E980.9
marine animals or plants	989.5	E905.6	—	E950.9	E962.1	E980.9
millipede (tropical)	989.5	E905.4	—	E950.9	E962.1	E980.9
plant NEC	989.5	E905.7	—	E950.9	E962.1	E980.9
marine	989.5	E905.6	—	E950.9	E962.1	E980.9
scorpion	989.5	E905.2	—	E950.9	E962.1	E980.9
snake	989.5	E905.0	—	E950.9	E962.1	E980.9
specified NEC	989.5	E905.8	—	E950.9	E962.1	E980.9
spider	989.5	E905.1	—	E950.9	E962.1	E980.9
wasp	989.5	E905.3	—	E950.9	E962.1	E980.9
Ventolin - *see* Salbutamol sulfate	—	—	—	—	—	—
Veramon	967.0	E851	E937.0	E950.1	E962.0	E980.1
Veratrum	—	—	—	—	—	—
album	988.2	E865.4	—	E950.9	E962.1	E980.9
alkaloids	972.6	E858.3	E942.6	E950.4	E962.0	E980.4
viride	988.2	E865.4	—	E950.9	E962.1	E980.9
Verdigris (*see also* Copper)	985.8	E866.4	—	E950.9	E962.1	E980.9
Veronal	967.0	E851	E937.0	E950.1	E962.0	E980.1
Veroxil	961.6	E857	E931.6	E950.4	E962.0	E980.4
Versidyne	965.7	E850.7	E935.7	E950.0	E962.0	E980.0
Viagra	972.5	E858.3	E942.5	E950.4	E962.0	E980.4
Vienna	—	—	—	—	—	—
green	985.1	E866.3	—	E950.8	E962.1	E980.8
insecticide	985.1	E863.4	—	E950.6	E962.1	E980.7
red	989.89	E866.8	—	E950.9	E962.1	E980.9
pharmaceutical dye	977.4	E858.8	E947.4	E950.4	E962.0	E980.4
Vinbarbital, vinbarbitone	967.0	E851	E937.0	E950.1	E962.0	E980.1
Vinblastine	963.1	E858.1	E933.1	E950.4	E962.0	E980.4
Vincristine	963.1	E858.1	E933.1	E950.4	E962.0	E980.4
Vinesthene, vinethene	968.2	E855.1	E938.2	E950.4	E962.0	E980.4
Vinyl	—	—	—	—	—	—
bital	967.0	E851	E937.0	E950.1	E962.0	E980.1
ether	968.2	E855.1	E938.2	E950.4	E962.0	E980.4
Vioform	961.3	E857	E931.3	E950.4	E962.0	E980.4
topical	976.0	E858.7	E946.0	E950.4	E962.0	E980.4
Viomycin	960.6	E856	E930.6	E950.4	E962.0	E980.4
Viosterol	963.5	E858.1	E933.5	E950.4	E962.0	E980.4
Viper (venom)	989.5	E905.0	—	E950.9	E962.1	E980.9
Viprynium (embonate)	961.6	E857	E931.6	E950.4	E962.0	E980.4
Virugon	961.7	E857	E931.7	E950.4	E962.0	E980.4
Visine	976.5	E858.7	E946.5	E950.4	E962.0	E980.4
Vitamins NEC	963.5	E858.1	E933.5	E950.4	E962.0	E980.4
B_{12}	964.1	E858.2	E934.1	E950.4	E962.0	E980.4

Substance	Poisoning	External Cause (E-Code)				
		Accident	Therapeutic Use	Suicide Attempt	Assault	Undetermined
Vitamins NEC *(Continued)*	—	—	—	—	—	—
hematopoietic	964.1	E858.2	E934.1	E950.4	E962.0	E980.4
K	964.3	E858.2	E934.3	E950.4	E962.0	E980.4
Vleminckx's solution	976.4	E858.7	E946.4	E950.4	E962.0	E980.4
Voltaren - *see* Diclofenac sodium	—	—	—	—	—	—
Warfarin (potassium) (sodium)	964.2	E858.2	E934.2	E950.4	E962.0	E980.4
rodenticide	989.4	E863.7	—	E950.6	E962.1	E980.7
Wasp (sting)	989.5	E905.3	—	E950.9	E962.1	E980.9
Water	—	—	—	—	—	—
balance agents NEC	974.5	E858.5	E944.5	E950.4	E962.0	E980.4
gas	987.1	E868.1	—	E951.8	E962.2	E981.8
incomplete combustion of - *see* Carbon, monoxide, fuel, utility	—	—	—	—	—	—
hemlock	988.2	E865.4	—	E950.9	E962.1	E980.9
moccasin (venom)	989.5	E905.0	—	E950.9	E962.1	E980.9
Wax (paraffin) (petroleum)	981	E862.3	—	E950.9	E962.1	E980.9
automobile	989.89	E861.2	—	E950.9	E962.1	E980.9
floor	981	E862.0	—	E950.9	E962.1	E980.9
Weed killers NEC	989.4	E863.5	—	E950.6	E962.1	E980.7
Welldorm	967.1	E852.0	E937.1	E950.2	E962.0	E980.2
White	—	—	—	—	—	—
arsenic - *see* Arsenic	—	—	—	—	—	—
hellebore	988.2	E865.4	—	E950.9	E962.1	E980.9
lotion (keratolytic)	976.4	E858.7	E946.4	E950.4	E962.0	E980.4
spirit	981	E862.0	—	E950.9	E962.1	E980.9
Whitewashes	989.89	E861.6	—	E950.9	E962.1	E980.9
Whole blood	964.7	E858.2	E934.7	E950.4	E962.0	E980.4
Wild	—	—	—	—	—	—
black cherry	988.2	E865.4	—	E950.9	E962.1	E980.9
poisonous plants NEC	988.2	E865.4	—	E950.9	E962.1	E980.9
Window cleaning fluid	989.89	E861.3	—	E950.9	E962.1	E980.9
Wintergreen (oil)	976.3	E858.7	E946.3	E950.4	E962.0	E980.4
Witch hazel	976.2	E858.7	E946.2	E950.4	E962.0	E980.4
Wood	—	—	—	—	—	—
alcohol	980.1	E860.2	—	E950.9	E962.1	E980.9
spirit	980.1	E860.2	—	E950.9	E962.1	E980.9
Woorali	975.2	E858.6	E945.2	E950.4	E962.0	E980.4
Wormseed, American	961.6	E857	E931.6	E950.4	E962.0	E980.4
Xanthine diuretics	974.1	E858.5	E944.1	E950.4	E962.0	E980.4
Xanthocillin	960.0	E856	E930.0	E950.4	E962.0	E980.4
Xanthotoxin	976.3	E858.7	E946.3	E950.4	E962.0	E980.4
Xigris	964.2	E858.2	E934.2	E950.4	E962.0	E980.4
Xylene (liquid) (vapor)	982.0	E862.4	—	E950.9	E962.1	E980.9
Xylocaine (infiltration) (topical)	968.5	E855.2	E938.5	E950.4	E962.0	E980.4
nerve block (peripheral) (plexus)	968.6	E855.2	E938.6	E950.4	E962.0	E980.4
spinal	968.7	E855.2	E938.7	E950.4	E962.0	E980.4
Xylol (liquid) (vapor)	982.0	E862.4	—	E950.9	E962.1	E980.9
Xylometazoline	971.2	E855.5	E941.2	E950.4	E962.0	E980.4
Yellow	—	—	—	—	—	—
fever vaccine	979.3	E858.8	E949.3	E950.4	E962.0	E980.4
jasmine	988.2	E865.4	—	E950.9	E962.1	E980.9
Yew	988.2	E865.4	—	E950.9	E962.1	E980.9
Zactane	965.7	E850.7	E935.7	E950.0	E962.0	E980.0
Zaroxolyn	974.3	E858.5	E944.3	E950.4	E962.0	E980.4
Zephiran (topical)	976.0	E858.7	E946.0	E950.4	E962.0	E980.4
ophthalmic preparation	976.5	E858.7	E946.5	E950.4	E962.0	E980.4
Zerone	980.1	E860.2	—	E950.9	E962.1	E980.9
Zinc (compounds) (fumes) (salts) (vapor) NEC	985.8	E866.4	—	E950.9	E962.1	E980.9
anti-infectives	976.0	E858.7	E946.0	E950.4	E962.0	E980.4
antivaricose	972.7	E858.3	E942.7	E950.4	E962.0	E980.4
bacitracin	976.0	E858.7	E946.0	E950.4	E962.0	E980.4
chloride	976.2	E858.7	E946.2	E950.4	E962.0	E980.4
gelatin	976.3	E858.7	E946.3	E950.4	E962.0	E980.4
oxide	976.3	E858.7	E946.3	E950.4	E962.0	E980.4

◄ New   ◄▦ Revised

Substance	Poisoning	External Cause (E-Code)				
		Accident	Therapeutic Use	Suicide Attempt	Assault	Undetermined
Zinc *(Continued)*						
peroxide	976.0	E858.7	E946.0	E950.4	E962.0	E980.4
pesticides	985.8	E863.4	—	E950.6	E962.1	E980.7
phosphide (rodenticide)	985.8	E863.7	—	E950.6	E962.1	E980.7
stearate	976.3	E858.7	E946.3	E950.4	E962.0	E980.4
sulfate (antivaricose)	972.7	E858.3	E942.7	E950.4	E962.0	E980.4
ENT agent	976.6	E858.7	E946.6	E950.4	E962.0	E980.4
ophthalmic solution	976.5	E858.7	E946.5	E950.4	E962.0	E980.4
topical NEC	976.0	E858.7	E946.0	E950.4	E962.0	E980.4
undecylenate	976.0	E858.7	E946.0	E950.4	E962.0	E980.4
Zovant	964.2	E858.2	E934.2	E950.4	E962.0	E980.4
Zoxazolamine	968.0	E855.1	E938.0	E950.4	E962.0	E980.4
Zygadenus (venenosus)	988.2	E865.4	—	E950.9	E962.1	E980.9

SECTION III

INDEX TO EXTERNAL CAUSES OF INJURY (E CODE)

This section contains the index to the codes which classify environmental events, circumstances, and other conditions as the cause of injury and other adverse effects. Where a code from the section Supplementary Classification of External Causes of Injury and Poisoning (E800-E998) is applicable, it is intended that the E code shall be used in addition to a code from the main body of the classification, Chapters 1 to 17.

The alphabetic index to the E codes is organized by main terms which describe the accident, circumstance, event, or specific agent which caused the injury or other adverse effect.

Note   Transport accidents (E800-E848) include accidents involving:

> aircraft and spacecraft (E840-E845)
> watercraft (E830-E838)
> motor vehicle (E810-E825)
> railway (E800-E807)
> other road vehicles (E826-E829)

For definitions and examples related to transport accidents - see Supplementary Classification of External Causes of Injury and Poisoning (E800-E999).

The fourth-digit subdivisions for use with categories E800-E848 to identify the injured person are found at the end of this section.

For identifying the place in which an accident or poisoning occurred (circumstances classifiable to categories E850-E869 and E880-E928) - see the listing in this section under "Accident, occurring."

See the Table of Drugs and Chemicals (Section 2 of this volume) for identifying the specific agent involved in drug overdose or a wrong substance given or taken in error, and for intoxication or poisoning by a drug or other chemical substance.

The specific adverse effect, reaction, or localized toxic effect of a correct drug or substance properly administered in therapeutic or prophylactic dosage should be classified according to the nature of the adverse effect (e.g., allergy, dermatitis, tachycardia) listed in Section I of this volume.

A

Abandonment

causing exposure to weather conditions - *see* Exposure

child, with intent to injure or kill E968.4

helpless person, infant, newborn E904.0

  with intent to injure or kill E968.4

Abortion, criminal, injury to child E968.8

Abuse (alleged) (suspected)

adult

  by

    child E967.4

    ex-partner E967.3

    ex-spouse E967.3

    father E967.0

    grandchild E967.7

    grandparent E967.6

    mother E967.2

    non-related caregiver E967.8

    other relative E967.7

    other specified person E967.1

    partner E967.3

    sibling E967.5

    spouse E967.3

    stepfather E967.0

    stepmother E967.2

    unspecified person E967.9

child

  by

    boyfriend of parent or guardian E967.0

    child E967.4

    father E967.0

    female partner of parent or guardian E967.2

    girlfriend of parent or guardian E967.2

    grandchild E967.7

    grandparent E967.6

    male partner of parent or guardian E967.0

    mother E967.2

    non-related caregiver E967.8

    other relative E967.7

    other specified person(s) E967.1

    sibling E967.5

    stepfather E967.0

    stepmother E967.2

    unspecified person E967.9

Accident (to) E928.9

aircraft (in transit) (powered) E841

  at landing, take-off E840

  due to, caused by cataclysm - *see* categories E908, E909

  late effect of E929.1

  unpowered (*see also* Collision, aircraft, unpowered) E842

  while alighting, boarding E843

amphibious vehicle

  on

    land - *see* Accident, motor vehicle

    water - *see* Accident, watercraft

animal, ridden NEC E828

animal-drawn vehicle NEC E827

balloon (*see also* Collision, aircraft, unpowered) E842

caused by, due to

  abrasive wheel (metalworking) E919.3

  animal NEC E906.9

Accident (*Continued*)

caused by, due to (*Continued*)

  animal NEC (*Continued*)

    being ridden (in sport or transport) E828

  avalanche NEC E909.2

  band saw E919.4

  bench saw E919.4

  bore, earth-drilling or mining (land) (seabed) E919.1

  bulldozer E919.7

  cataclysmic

    earth surface movement or eruption E909.9

    storm E908.9

  chain

    hoist E919.2

      agricultural operations E919.0

      mining operations E919.1

    saw E920.1

  circular saw E919.4

  cold (excessive) (*see also* Cold, exposure to) E901.9

  combine E919.0

    conflagration - *see* Conflagration

  corrosive liquid, substance NEC E924.1

  cotton gin E919.8

  crane E919.2

    agricultural operations E919.0

    mining operations E919.1

  cutting or piercing instrument (*see also* Cut) E920.9

  dairy equipment E919.8

  derrick E919.2

    agricultural operations E919.0

    mining operations E919.1

  drill E920.1

    earth (land) (seabed) E919.1

    hand (powered) E920.1

      not powered E920.4

    metalworking E919.3

    woodworking E919.4

  earth(-)

    drilling machine E919.1

    moving machine E919.7

    scraping machine E919.7

  electric

    current (*see also* Electric shock) E925.9

    motor - *see also* Accident, machine, by type of machine

      current (of) - *see* Electric shock

  elevator (building) (grain) E919.2

    agricultural operations E919.0

    mining operations E919.1

  environmental factors NEC E928.9

  excavating machine E919.7

  explosive material (*see also* Explosion) E923.9

  farm machine E919.0

  fire, flames - *see also* Fire

    conflagration - *see* Conflagration

  firearm missile - *see* Shooting

  forging (metalworking) machine E919.3

  forklift (truck) E919.2

    agricultural operations E919.0

    mining operations E919.1

  gas turbine E919.5

  harvester E919.0

  hay derrick, mower, or rake E919.0

  heat (excessive) (*see also* Heat) E900.9

Accident (*Continued*)

caused by, due to (*Continued*)

  hoist (*see also* Accident, caused by, due to, lift) E919.2

    chain - *see* Accident, caused by, due to, chain

    shaft E919.1

  hot

    liquid E924.0

      caustic or corrosive E924.1

    object (not producing fire or flames) E924.8

    substance E924.9

      caustic or corrosive E924.1

      liquid (metal) NEC E924.0

      specified type NEC E924.8

  human bite E928.3

  ignition - *see* Ignition E919.4

  internal combustion engine E919.5

  landslide NEC E909.2

  lathe (metalworking) E919.3

    turnings E920.8

    woodworking E919.4

  lift, lifting (appliances) E919.2

    agricultural operations E919.0

    mining operations E919.1

    shaft E919.1

  lightning NEC E907

  machine, machinery - *see also* Accident, machine

    drilling, metal E919.3

    manufacturing, for manufacture of steam

      beverages E919.8

      clothing E919.8

      foodstuffs E919.8

      paper E919.8

      textiles E919.8

    milling, metal E919.3

    moulding E919.4

    power press, metal E919.3

    printing E919.8

    rolling mill, metal E919.3

    sawing, metal E919.3

    specified type NEC E919.8

    spinning E919.8

    weaving E919.8

  natural factor NEC E928.9

  overhead plane E919.4

  plane E920.4

    overhead E919.4

  powered

    hand tool NEC E920.1

    saw E919.4

      hand E920.1

  printing machine E919.8

  pulley (block) E919.2

    agricultural operations E919.0

    mining operations E919.1

    transmission E919.6

  radial saw E919.4

  radiation - *see* Radiation

  reaper E919.0

  road scraper E919.7

    when in transport under its own power - *see* categories E810-E825

  roller coaster E919.8

  sander E919.4

  saw E920.4

    band E919.4

    bench E919.4

    chain E920.1

    circular E919.4

ICD-9-CM

E Codes

Vol.

Accident (*Continued*)
  caused by, due to (*Continued*)
    saw (*Continued*)
      hand (*Continued*)
        hand E920.4
          powered E920.1
        powered, except hand E919.4
        radial E919.4
      sawing machine, metal E919.3
      shaft
        hoist E919.1
        lift E919.1
        transmission E919.6
      shears E920.4
        hand E920.4
          powered E920.1
        mechanical E919.3
      shovel E920.4
        steam E919.7
      spinning machine E919.8
      steam - *see also* Burning, steam
        engine E919.5
        shovel E919.7
      thresher E919.0
      thunderbolt NEC E907
      tractor E919.0
        when in transport under its own
          power - *see* categories E810-
          E825
      transmission belt, cable, chain, gear,
        pinion, pulley, shaft E919.6
      turbine (gas) (water driven) E919.5
      under-cutter E919.1
      weaving machine E919.8
      winch E919.2
        agricultural operations E919.0
        mining operations E919.1
    diving E883.0
      with insufficient air supply E913.2
    glider (hang) (*see also* Collision, air-
      craft, unpowered) E842
    hovercraft
      on
        land - *see* Accident, motor vehicle
        water - *see* Accident, watercraft
    ice yacht (*see also* Accident, vehicle
      NEC) E848
    in
      medical, surgical procedure
      as, or due to misadventure - *see* Mis-
        adventure
      causing an abnormal reaction or
        later complication without men-
        tion of misadventure - *see* Reac-
        tion, abnormal
    kite carrying a person (*see also* Colli-
      sion, involving aircraft, unpow-
      ered) E842
    land yacht (*see also* Accident, vehicle
      NEC) E848
    late effect of - *see* Late effect
    launching pad E845
    machine, machinery (*see also* Accident,
      caused by, due to, by specific type
      of machine) E919.9
      agricultural including animal-pow-
        ered premises E919.0
      earth-drilling E919.1
      earth moving or scraping E919.7
      excavating E919.7
      involving transport under own
        power on highway or transport
        vehicle - *see* categories E810-
        E825, E840-E845

Accident (*Continued*)
  machine, machinery (*Continued*)
    lifting (appliances) E919.2
    metalworking E919.3
    mining E919.1
    prime movers, except electric motors
      E919.5
      electric motors - *see* Accident, ma-
        chine, by specific type of ma-
        chine
    recreational E919.8
    specified type NEC E919.8
    transmission E919.6
    watercraft (deck) (engine room) (gal-
      ley) (laundry) (loading) E836
    woodworking or forming E919.4
  motor vehicle (on public highway)
    (traffic) E819
    due to cataclysm - *see* categories
      E908, E909
    involving
      collision (*see also* Collision, motor
        vehicle) E812
      nontraffic, not on public highway -
        see categories E820-E825
      not involving collision - *see* catego-
        ries E816-E819
  nonmotor vehicle NEC E829
    nonroad - *see* Accident, vehicle NEC
    road, except pedal cycle, animal-
      drawn vehicle, or animal being
      ridden E829
  nonroad vehicle NEC - *see* Accident,
    vehicle NEC
  not elsewhere classifiable involving
    cable car (not on rails) E847
      on rails E829
    coal car in mine E846
    hand truck - *see* Accident, vehicle
      NEC
    logging car E846
    sled(ge), meaning snow or ice vehi-
      cle E848
    tram, mine or quarry E846
    truck
      mine or quarry E846
      self-propelled, industrial E846
      station baggage E846
    tub, mine or quarry E846
    vehicle NEC E848
      snow and ice E848
      used only on industrial premises
        E846
    wheelbarrow E848
  occurring (at) (in)
    apartment E849.0
    baseball field, diamond E849.4
    construction site, any E849.3
    dock E849.8
      yard E849.3
    dormitory E849.7
    factory (building) (premises) E849.3
    farm E849.1
      buildings E849.1
      house E849.0
    football field E849.4
    forest E849.8
    garage (place of work) E849.3
      private (home) E849.0
    gravel pit E849.2
    gymnasium E849.4
    highway E849.5
    home (private) (residential) E849.0
      institutional E849.7

Accident (*Continued*)
  occurring (*Continued*)
    hospital E849.7
    hotel E849.6
    house (private) (residential) E849.0
      movie E849.6
      public E849.6
    institution, residential E849.7
    jail E849.7
    mine E849.2
    motel E849.6
    movie house E849.6
    office (building) E849.6
    orphanage E849.7
    park (public) E849.4
      mobile home E849.8
      trailer E849.8
    parking lot or place E849.8
    place
      industrial NEC E849.3
      parking E849.8
      public E849.8
        specified place NEC E849.5
      recreational NEC E849.4
      sport NEC E849.4
    playground (park) (school) E849.4
    prison E849.6
    public building NEC E849.6
    quarry E849.2
    railway
      line NEC E849.8
      yard E849.3
    residence
      home (private) E849.0
    resort (beach) (lake) (mountain) (sea-
      shore) (vacation) E849.4
    restaurant E849.6
    sand pit E849.2
    school (building) (private) (public)
      (state) E849.6
      reform E849.7
      riding E849.4
    seashore E849.8
      resort E849.4
    shop (place of work) E849.3
      commercial E849.6
    skating rink E849.4
    sports palace E849.4
    stadium E849.4
    store E849.6
    street E849.5
    swimming pool (public) E849.4
      private home or garden E849.0
    tennis court E849.4 public
    theatre, theater E849.6
    trailer court E849.8
    tunnel E849.8
      under construction E849.2
    warehouse E849.3
    yard
      dock E849.3
      industrial E849.3
      private (home) E849.0
      railway E849.3
  off-road type motor vehicle (not on
    public highway) NEC E821
  on public highway - *see* categories
    E810-E819
  pedal cycle E826
  railway E807
    due to cataclysm - *see* categories
      E908, E909
    involving
      avalanche E909.2

◄ **New**   ◄▪▪ **Revised**

Accident *(Continued)*
  railway *(Continued)*
    involving *(Continued)*
      burning by engine, locomotive, train *(see also* Explosion, railway engine) E803
      collision *(see also* collision, railway) E800
      derailment *(see also* Derailment, railway) E802
      explosion *(see also* Explosion, railway engine) E803
      fall *(see also* Fall, from, railway rolling stock) E804
      fire *(see also* Explosion, railway engine) E803
      hitting by, being struck by
        object falling in, on, from, rolling stock, train, vehicle E806
        rolling stock, train, vehicle E805
      overturning, railway rolling stock, train, vehicle *(see also* Derailment, railway) E802
      running off rails, railway *(see also* Derailment, railway) E802
      specified circumstances NEC E806
      train or vehicle hit by
        avalanche E909.2
        falling object (earth, rock, tree) E806
          due to cataclysm - *see* categories E908, E909
        landslide E909.2
  roller skate E885.1
  scooter (nonmotorized) E885.0
  skateboard E885.2
  ski(ing) E885.3
    jump E884.9
    lift or tow (with chair or gondola) E847
  snow vehicle, motor driven (not on public highway) E820
    on public highway - *see* categories E810-E819
  snowboard E885.4
  spacecraft E845
  specified cause NEC E928.8
  street car E829
  traffic NEC E819
  vehicle NEC (with pedestrian) E848
    battery powered
      airport passenger vehicle E846
      truck (baggage) (mail) E846
    powered commercial or industrial (with other vehicle or object within commercial or industrial premises) E846
  watercraft E838
    with
      drowning or submersion resulting from
        accident other than to watercraft E832
        accident to watercraft E830
      injury, except drowning or submersion, resulting from
        accident other than to watercraft - *see* categories E833-E838
        accident to watercraft E831
    due to, caused by cataclysm - *see* categories E908, E909
    machinery E836
Acid throwing E961
Acosta syndrome E902.0
Aeroneurosis E902.1

Aero-otitis media - *see* Effects of, air pressure
Aerosinusitis - *see* Effects of, air pressure
After-effect, late - *see* Late effect
Air
  blast
    in
      terrorism E979.2
      war operations E993
  embolism (traumatic) NEC E928.9
    in
      infusion or transfusion E874.1
      perfusion E874.2
  sickness E903
Alpine sickness E902.0
Altitude sickness - *see* Effects of, air pressure
Anaphylactic shock, anaphylaxis *(see also* Table of Drugs and Chemicals) E947.9
  due to bite or sting (venomous) - *see* Bite, venomous
Andes disease E902.0
Apoplexy
  heat - *see* Heat
Arachnidism E905.1
Arson E968.0
Asphyxia, asphyxiation
  by
    chemical
      in
        terrorism E979.7
        war operations E997.2
    explosion - *see* Explosion
    food (bone) (regurgitated food) (seed) E911
    foreign object, except food E912
    fumes
      in
        terrorism (chemical weapons) E979.7
        war operations E997.2
    gas - *see also* Table of Drugs and Chemicals
      in
        terrorism E979.7
        war operations E997.2
      legal
        execution E978
        intervention (tear) E972
      tear E972
    mechanical means *(see also* Suffocation) E913.9
  from
    conflagration - *see* Conflagration
    fire - *see also* Fire E899
      in
        terrorism E979.3
        war operations E990.9
    ignition - *see* Ignition
Aspiration
  foreign body - *see* Foreign body, aspiration
  mucus, not of newborn (with asphyxia, obstruction respiratory passage, suffocation) E912
  phlegm (with asphyxia, obstruction respiratory passage, suffocation) E912
  vomitus (with asphyxia, obstruction respiratory passage, suffocation) (see also Foreign body, aspiration, food) E911
Assassination (attempt) *(see also* Assault) E968.9
Assault (homicidal) (by) (in) E968.9
  acid E961
    swallowed E962.1

Assault *(Continued)*
  air gun E968.6
  BB gun E968.6
  bite NEC E968.8
    of human being E968.7
  bomb ((placed in) car or house) E965.8
    antipersonnel E965.5
    letter E965.7
    petrol E965.6
  brawl (hand) (fists) (foot) E960.0
  burning, burns (by fire) E968.0
    acid E961
      swallowed E962.1
    caustic, corrosive substance E961
      swallowed E962.1
    chemical from swallowing caustic, corrosive substance NEC E962.1
    hot liquid E968.3
    scalding E968.3
    vitriol E961
      swallowed E962.1
  caustic, corrosive substance E961
    swallowed E962.1
  cut, any part of body E966
  dagger E966
  drowning E964
  explosives E965.9
    bomb *(see also* Assault, bomb) E965.8
    dynamite E965.8
  fight (hand) (fists) (foot) E960.0
    with weapon E968.9
      blunt or thrown E968.2
      cutting or piercing E966
      firearm - *see* Shooting, homicide
  fire E968.0
  firearm(s) - *see* Shooting, homicide
  garrotting E963
  gunshot (wound) - *see* Shooting, homicide
  hanging E963
  injury NEC E968.9
  knife E966
  late effect of E969
  ligature E963
  poisoning E962.9
    drugs or medicinals E962.0
    gas(es) or vapors, except drugs and medicinals E962.2
    solid or liquid substances, except drugs and medicinals E962.1
  puncture, any part of body E966
  pushing
    before moving object, train, vehicle E968.5
    from high place E968.1
  rape E960.1
  scalding E968.3
  shooting - *see* Shooting, homicide
  sodomy E960.1
  stab, any part of body E966
  strangulation E963
  submersion E964
  suffocation E963
  transport vehicle E968.5
  violence NEC E968.9
  vitriol E961
    swallowed E962.1
  weapon E968.9
    blunt or thrown E968.2
    cutting or piercing E966
    firearm - *see* Shooting, homicide
  wound E968.9
    cutting E966
    gunshot - *see* Shooting, homicide

ICD-9-CM

E Codes

Vol. 2

Assault *(Continued)*
 wound *(Continued)*
  knife E966
  piercing E966
  puncture E966
  stab E966
Attack by animal NEC E906.9
Avalanche E909.2
 falling on or hitting
  motor vehicle (in motion) (on public
   highway) E909.2
  railway train E909.2
Aviators' disease E902.1

B

**Barotitis, barodontalgia, barosinusitis,
 barotrauma** (otitic) (sinus) - *see* Effects of, air pressure
Battered
 baby or child (syndrome) - *see* Abuse,
  child; category E967
 person other than baby or child - *see*
  Assault
Bayonet wound (*see also* Cut, by bayonet) E920.3
 in
  legal intervention E974
  terrorism E979.8
  war operations E995
Bean in nose E912
Bed set on fire NEC E898.0
Beheading (by guillotine)
 homicide E966
 legal execution E978
Bending, injury in E927
Bends E902.0
Bite
 animal NEC E906.5
  other specified (except arthropod)
   E906.3
  venomous NEC E905.9
 arthropod (nonvenomous) NEC E906.4
  venomous - *see* Sting
 black widow spider E905.1
 cat E906.3
 centipede E905.4
 cobra E905.0
 copperhead snake E905.0
 coral snake E905.0
 dog E906.0
 fer de lance E905.0
 gila monster E905.0
 human being
  accidental E928.3
  assault E968.7
 insect (nonvenomous) E906.4
  venomous - *see* Sting
 krait E905.0
 late effect of - *see* Late effect
 lizard E906.2
  venomous E905.0
 mamba E905.0
 marine animal
  nonvenomous E906.3
   snake E906.2
  venomous E905.6
   snake E905.0
 millipede E906.4
  venomous E905.4
 moray eel E906.3
 rat E906.1
 rattlesnake E905.0

Bite *(Continued)*
 rodent, except rat E906.3
 serpent - *see* Bite, snake
 shark E906.3
 snake (venomous) E905.0
  nonvenomous E906.2
  sea E905.0
 spider E905.1
  nonvenomous E906.4
 tarantula (venomous) E905.1
 venomous NEC E905.9
  by specific animal - *see* category E905
 viper E905.0
 water moccasin E905.0
Blast (air)
 in
  terrorism E979.2
   from nuclear explosion E979.5
   underwater E979.0
  war operations E993
   from nuclear explosion E996
   underwater E992
Blizzard E908.3
Blow E928.9
 by law-enforcing agent, police (on
  duty) E975
  with blunt object (baton) (nightstick)
   (stave) (truncheon) E973
Blowing up (*see also* Explosion) E923.9
Brawl (hand) (fists) (foot) E960.0
Breakage (accidental)
 cable of cable car not on rails E847
 ladder (causing fall) E881.0
 part (any) of
  animal-drawn vehicle E827
  ladder (causing fall) E881.0
  motor vehicle
   in motion (on public highway)
    E818
   not on public highway E825
  nonmotor road vehicle, except animal-drawn vehicle or pedal cycle E829
  off-road type motor vehicle (not on
   public highway) NEC E821
   on public highway E818
  pedal cycle E826
  scaffolding (causing fall) E881.1
  snow vehicle, motor-driven (not on
   public highway) E820
   on public highway E818
  vehicle NEC - *see* Accident, vehicle
Broken
 glass,
  fall on E888.0
  injury by E920.8
 power line (causing electric shock) E925.1
Bumping against, into (accidentally)
 object (moving) E917.9
  caused by crowd E917.1
   with subsequent fall E917.6
  furniture E917.3
   with subsequent fall E917.7
  in
   running water E917.2
   sports E917.0
    with subsequent fall E917.5
  stationary E917.4
   with subsequent fall E917.8
 person(s) E917.9
  with fall E886.9
   in sports E886.0
  as, or caused by, a crowd E917.1
   with subsequent fall E917.6

Bumping, against, into *(Continued)*
 person(s) *(Continued)*
  in sports E917.0
  with fall E886.0
Burning, burns (accidental) (by) (from)
 (on) E899
 acid (any kind) E924.1
  swallowed - *see* Table of Drugs and
   Chemicals
 bedclothes (*see also* Fire, specified
  NEC) E898.0
 blowlamp (*see also* Fire, specified NEC)
  E898.1
 blowtorch (*see also* Fire, specified NEC)
  E898.1
 boat, ship, watercraft - *see* categories
  E830, E831, E837
 bonfire (controlled) E897
  uncontrolled E892
 candle (*see also* Fire, specified NEC)
  E898.1
 caustic liquid, substance E924.1
  swallowed - *see* Table of Drugs and
   Chemicals
 chemical E924.1
  from swallowing caustic, corrosive
   substance - *see* Table of Drugs
   and Chemicals
  in
   terrorism E979.7
   war operations E997.2
 cigar(s) or cigarette(s) (*see also* Fire,
  specified NEC) E898.1
 clothes, clothing, nightdress - *see* Ignition, clothes
  with conflagration - *see* Conflagration
 conflagration - *see* Conflagration
 corrosive liquid, substance E924.1
  swallowed - *see* Table of Drugs and
   Chemicals
 electric current (*see also* Electric shock)
  E925.9
 fire, flames (*see also* Fire) E899
 flare, Verey pistol E922.8
 heat
  from appliance (electrical) E924.8
  in local application, or packing during medical or surgical procedure E873.5
 homicide (attempt) (*see also* Assault,
  burning) E968.0
 hot
  liquid E924.0
   caustic or corrosive E924.1
  object (not producing fire or flames)
   E924.8
  substance E924.9
   caustic or corrosive E924.1
   liquid (metal) NEC E924.0
   specified type NEC E924.8
  tap water E924.2
 ignition - *see also* Ignition
  clothes, clothing, nightdress - *see also*
   Ignition, clothes
   with conflagration - *see* Conflagration
  highly inflammable material (benzine) (fat) (gasoline) (kerosene)
   (paraffin) (petrol) E894
 inflicted by other person
  stated as
   homicidal, intentional (*see also* Assault, burning) E968.0

Burning, burns *(Continued)*
 inflicted by other person *(Continued)*
  stated as *(Continued)*
   undetermined whether accidental or intentional *(see also Burn, stated as undetermined whether accidental or intentional)* E988.1
  internal, from swallowed caustic, corrosive liquid, substance - *see* Table of Drugs and Chemicals
 in
  terrorism E979.3
   from nuclear explosion E979.5
   petrol bomb E979.3
  war operations (from fire-producing device or conventional weapon) E990.9
   from nuclear explosion E996
   petrol bomb E990.0
  from nuclear explosion E996
  petrol bomb E990.0
 lamp *(see also Fire, specified NEC)* E898.1
 late effect of NEC E929.4
 lighter (cigar) (cigarette) *(see also Fire, specified NEC)* E898.1
 lightning E907
 liquid (boiling) (hot) (molten) E924.0
  caustic, corrosive (external) E924.1
   swallowed - *see* Table of Drugs and Chemicals
 local application of externally applied substance in medical or surgical care E873.5
 machinery - *see* Accident, machine
 matches *(see also Fire, specified NEC)* E898.1
 medicament, externally applied E873.5
 metal, molten E924.0
 object (hot) E924.8
  producing fire or flames - *see* Fire
 oven (electric) (gas) E924.8
 pipe (smoking) *(see also Fire, specified NEC)* E898.1
 radiation - *see* Radiation
 railway engine, locomotive, train *(see also Explosion, railway engine)* E803
 self-inflicted (unspecified whether accidental or intentional) E988.1
  caustic or corrosive substance NEC E988.7
  stated as intentional, purposeful E958.1
   caustic or corrosive substance NEC E958.7
  stated as undetermined whether accidental or intentional E988.1
   caustic or corrosive substance NEC E988.7
 steam E924.0
  pipe E924.8
 substance (hot) E924.9
  boiling or molten E924.0
  caustic, corrosive (external) E924.1
   swallowed - *see* Table of Drugs and Chemicals
 suicidal (attempt) NEC E958.1
  caustic substance E958.7
  late effect of E959
 tanning bed E926.2
 therapeutic misadventure
  overdose of radiation E873.2

Burning, burns *(Continued)*
 torch, welding *(see also Fire, specified NEC)* E898.1
 trash fire *(see also Burning, bonfire)* E897
 vapor E924.0
 vitriol E924.1
 x-rays E926.3
  in medical, surgical procedure - *see* Misadventure, failure, in dosage, radiation operations
Butted by animal E906.8

C

Cachexia, lead or saturnine E866.0
 from pesticide NEC *(see also Table of Drugs and Chemicals)* E863.4
Caisson disease E902.2
Capital punishment (any means) E978
Car sickness E903
Casualty (not due to war) NEC E928.9
 terrorism E979.8
 war *(see also War operations)* E995
Cat
 bite E906.3
 scratch E906.8
Cataclysmic (any injury)
 earth surface movement or eruption E909.9
  specified type NEC E909.8
 storm or flood resulting from storm E908.9
  specified type NEC E909.8
Catching fire - *see* Ignition
Caught
 between
  objects (moving) (stationary and moving) E918
   and machinery - *see* Accident, machine
 by cable car, not on rails E847
 in
  machinery (moving parts of) - *see* Accident, machine
  object E918
Cave-in (causing asphyxia, suffocation (by pressure)) *(see also Suffocation, due to, cave-in)* E913.3
 with injury other than asphyxia or suffocation E916
  with asphyxia or suffocation *(see also Suffocation, due to, cave-in)* E913.3
 struck or crushed by E916
  with asphyxia or suffocation *(see also Suffocation, due to, cave-in)* E913.3
Change(s) in air pressure - *see also* Effects of, air pressure
 sudden, in aircraft (ascent) (descent) (causing aeroneurosis or aviators' disease) E902.1
Chilblains E901.0
 due to manmade conditions E901.1
Choking (on) (any object except food or vomitus) E912
 apple E911
 bone E911
 food, any type (regurgitated) E911
 mucus or phlegm E912
 seed E911
Civil insurrection - *see* War operations

Cloudburst E908.8
Cold, exposure to (accidental) (excessive) (extreme) (place) E901.9
 causing chilblains or immersion foot E901.0
 due to
  manmade conditions E901.1
  specified cause NEC E901.8
  weather (conditions) E901.0
 late effect of NEC E929.5
 self-inflicted (undetermined whether accidental or intentional) E988.3
  suicidal E958.3
 suicide E958.3
Colic, lead, painters', or saturnine - *see* category E866
Collapse
 burning (uncontrolled fire) E891.8
  in terrorism E979.3
  private E890.8 higher
 dam E909.3
 due to heat - *see* Heat
 machinery - *see* Accident, machine or vehicle
 man-made structure E909.3
 postoperative NEC E878.9
 structure, burning NEC E891.8
  burning (uncontrolled fire)
   in terrorism E979.3
Collision (accidental)

> Note In the case of collisions between different types of vehicles, persons and objects, priority in classification is in the following order:
>
>   Aircraft
>   Watercraft
>   Motor vehicle
>   Railway vehicle
>   Pedal cycle
>   Animal-drawn vehicle
>   Animal being ridden
>   Streetcar or other nonmotor road vehicle
>   Other vehicle
>   Pedestrian or person using pedestrian conveyance
>   Object (except where falling from or set in motion by vehicle, etc. listed above)
>
> In the listing below, the combinations are listed only under the vehicle, etc., having priority. For definitions, *see* Supplementary Classification of External Causes of Injury and Poisoning (E800-E999).

 aircraft (with object or vehicle) (fixed)-entrance (on (movable) (moving)) E841
  with
   person (while landing, taking off) vehicle off the (without accident to aircraft) E844
   powered (in transit) (with unpowered aircraft) E841
   while landing, taking off E840
   unpowered E842
   while landing, taking off E840
 animal being ridden (in sport or transport) E828
  and
   animal (being ridden) (herded) (unattended) E828

Collision *(Continued)*
animal being ridden *(Continued)*
and *(Continued)*
nonmotor road vehicle, except
pedal cycle or animal-drawn
vehicle E828
object (fallen) (fixed) (movable)
(moving) not falling from or
set in motion by vehicle of
higher priority E828
pedestrian (conveyance or vehicle)
E828
animal-drawn vehicle E827
and
animal (being ridden) (herded)
(unattended) E827
nonmotor road vehicle, except
pedal cycle E827
object (fallen) (fixed) (movable)
(moving) not falling from or
set in motion by vehicle of
higher priority E827
pedestrian (conveyance or vehicle)
E827
streetcar E827
motor vehicle (on public highway)
(traffic accident) E812
after leaving, running off, public
highway (without antecedent
collision) (without re-entry)
E816
with antecedent collision on public highway - *see* categories
E810-E815
with re-entrance collision with another motor vehicle E811
and
abutment (bridge) (overpass) E815
animal (herded) (unattended) E815
carrying person, property E813
animal-drawn vehicle E813
another motor vehicle (abandoned) (disabled) (parked)
(stalled) (stopped) E812
with, involving re-entrance (on
same roadway) (across me-
dian strip) E811
any object, person, or vehicle off
the public highway resulting
from a noncollision motor vehicle nontraffic accident E816
avalanche, fallen or not moving
E815
falling E909.2
boundary fence E815
culvert E815
fallen
stone E815
tree E815
guard post or guard rail E815
inter-highway divider E815
landslide, fallen or not moving
E815
moving E909.2
machinery (road) E815
nonmotor road vehicle NEC E813
object (any object, person, or vehicle off the public highway resulting from a noncollision
motor vehicle nontraffic accident) E815
off, normally not on, public
highway resulting from a
noncollision motor vehicle
traffic accident E816

Collision *(Continued)*
motor vehicle *(Continued)*
and *(Continued)*
pedal cycle E813
pedestrian (conveyance) E814
person (using pedestrian conveyance) E814
post or pole (lamp) (light) (signal)
(telephone) (utility) E815
railway rolling stock, train, vehicle
E810
safety island E815
street car E813
traffic signal, sign, or marker
(temporary) E815
tree E815
tricycle E813
wall or cut made for road E815
due to cataclysm - *see* categories
E908, E909
not on public highway, nontraffic
accident E822
and
animal (carrying person, property) (herded) (unattended)
E822
animal-drawn vehicle E822
another motor vehicle (moving),
except off-road motor vehicle E822
stationary E823
avalanche, fallen, not moving
NEC E823
moving E909.2
landslide, fallen, not moving
E823
moving E909.2
nonmotor vehicle (moving) E822
stationary E823
object (fallen) ((normally)
(fixed)) (movable but not in
motion) (stationary) E823
moving, except when falling
from, set in motion by,
aircraft or cataclysm E822
pedal cycle (moving) E822
stationary E823
pedestrian (conveyance) E822
person (using pedestrian conveyance) E822
railway rolling stock, train, vehicle (moving) E822
stationary E823
road vehicle (any) (moving)
E822
stationary E823
tricycle (moving) E822
stationary E823
off-road type motor vehicle (not on
public highway) E821
and
animal (being ridden) (-drawn vehicle) E821
another off-road motor vehicle,
except snow vehicle E821
other motor vehicle, not on public
highway E821
other object or vehicle NEC, fixed
or movable, not set in motion
by aircraft, motor vehicle on
highway, or snow vehicle,
motor-driven E821
pedal cycle E821
pedestrian (conveyance) E821
railway train E821

Collision *(Continued)*
off-road type motor vehicle *(Continued)*
on public highway - *see* Collision,
motor vehicle
pedal cycle E826
and
animal (carrying person, property)
(herded) (unherded) E826
animal-drawn vehicle E826
another pedal cycle E826
nonmotor road vehicle E826
object (fallen) (fixed) (movable)
(moving) not falling from or
set in motion by aircraft, motor vehicle, or railway train
NEC E826
pedestrian (conveyance) E826
person (using pedestrian conveyance) E826
street car E826
pedestrian(s) (conveyance) E917.9
with fall E886.9
in sports E886.0
and
crowd, human stampede E917.1
with subsequent fall E917.6
furniture E917.3
with subsequent fall E917.7
machinery - *see* Accident, machine
object (fallen) (moving) not falling
from or NEC, fixed or set in
motion by any vehicle classifiable to E800-E848, E917.9
caused by a crowd E917.1
with subsequent fall E917.6
furniture E917.3
with subsequent fall E917.7
in
running water E917.2
with drowning or submer-
sion - *see* Submersion
sports E917.0
with subsequent fall E917.5
stationary E917.4
with subsequent fall E917.8
vehicle, nonmotor, nonroad E848
in
running water E917.2
with drowning or submersion -
see Submersion E829
sports E917.0
with fall E886.0
person(s) (using pedestrian conveyance) (*see also* Collision, pedestrian) E917.9
railway (rolling stock) (train) (vehicle)
(with (subsequent) derailment, explosion, fall or fire) E800
with antecedent derailment E802
and
animal (carrying person) (herded)
(unattended) E801
another railway train or vehicle
E800
buffers E801
fallen tree on railway E801
farm machinery, nonmotor (in
transport) (stationary) E801
gates E801
nonmotor vehicle E801
object (fallen) (fixed) (movable)
(movable) (moving) not falling from, set in motion by,
aircraft or motor vehicle NEC
E801

Collision (Continued)
  railway (Continued)
    and (Continued)
      pedal cycle E801
      pedestrian (conveyance) E805
      person (using pedestrian convey-
        ance) E805
      platform E801
      rock on railway E801
      street car E801
  snow vehicle, motor-driven (not on
    public highway) E820
    and
      animal (being ridden) (-drawn ve-
        hicle) E820
      another off-road motor vehicle
        E820
      other motor vehicle, not on public
        highway E820
      other object or vehicle NEC, fixed
        or movable, not set in motion
        by aircraft or motor vehicle
        on highway E820
      pedal cycle E820
      pedestrian (conveyance) E820
      railway train E820
  on public highway - see Collision,
    motor vehicle
  street car(s) E829
  and
    animal, herded, not being ridden,
      unattended E829
    nonmotor road vehicle NEC E829
    object (fallen) (fixed) (movable)
      (moving) not falling from or set
      in motion by aircraft, animal-
      drawn vehicle, animal being
      ridden, motor vehicle, pedal cy-
      cle, or railway train E829
    pedestrian (conveyance) E829
    person (using pedestrian convey-
      ance) E829
  vehicle
    animal-drawn - see Collision, animal-
      drawn vehicle
    motor - see Collision, motor vehicle
    nonmotor
      nonroad E848
      and
        another nonmotor, nonroad
          vehicle E848
        object (fallen) (fixed) (mov-
          able) (moving) not falling
          from or set in motion by
          aircraft, animal-drawn ve-
          hicle, animal being rid-
          den, motor vehicle, non-
          motor road vehicle, pedal
          cycle, railway train, or
          streetcar E848
      road, except animal being ridden,
        animal-drawn vehicle, or
        pedal cycle E829
      and
        animal, herded, not being rid-
          den, unattended E829
        another nonmotor road vehi-
          cle, except animal being
          ridden, animal-drawn ve-
          hicle, or pedal cycle E829
        object (fallen) (fixed) (mov-
          able) (moving) not falling
          from or set in motion by,
          aircraft, animal-drawn ve-
          hicle, animal being rid-

Collision (Continued)
  vehicle (Continued)
    nonmotor (Continued)
      road (Continued)
        and (Continued)
          den, motor vehicle, pedal
          cycle, or railway train
          E829
        pedestrian (conveyance) E829
        person (using pedestrian con-
          veyance) E829
        vehicle, nonmotor, nonroad
          E829
    watercraft E838
    and
      person swimming or water skiing
        E838
    causing
      drowning, submersion E830
      injury except drowning, submer-
        sion E831
Combustion, spontaneous - see Ignition
Complication of medical or surgical
  procedure or treatment
  as an abnormal reaction - see Reaction,
    abnormal
  delayed, without mention of misadven-
    ture - see Reaction, abnormal
  due to misadventure - see Misadventure
Compression
  divers' squeeze E902.2
  trachea by
    food E911
    foreign body, except food E912
Conflagration
  building or structure, except private
    dwelling (barn) (church) (conva-
    lescent or residential home) (fac-
    tory) (farm outbuilding) (hospital)
    (hotel) or (institution (educational)
    (dormitory) (residential)) (school)
    (shop) (store) (theatre) E891.9
    with or causing (injury due to)
      accident or injury NEC E891.9
        specified circumstance NEC
          E891.8
      burns, burning E891.3
      carbon monoxide E891.2
      fumes E891.2
      polyvinylchloride (PVC) or similar
        material E891.1
      smoke E891.2
    causing explosion E891.0
    in terrorism E979.3
  not in building or structure E892
  private dwelling (apartment) (boarding
    house) (camping place) (caravan)
    (farmhouse) (home (private))
    (house) (lodging house) (private
    garage) (rooming house) (tene-
    ment) E890.9
    with or causing (injury due to) acci-
      dent or injury NEC E890.9
        specified circumstance NEC
          E890.8
      burns, burning E890.3
      carbon monoxide E890.2
      fumes E890.2
        polyvinylchloride (PVC) or sim-
          ilar material E890.1
      smoke E890.2
    causing explosion E890.0
Constriction, external
  caused by
    hair E928.4
    other object E928.5

Contact with
  dry ice E901.1
  liquid air, hydrogen, nitrogen E901.1
Cramp(s)
  Heat - see Heat
  swimmers (see also category E910)
    E910.2
  not in recreation or sport E910.3
Cranking (car) (truck) (bus) (engine) injury by E917.9
Crash
  aircraft (in transit) (powered) E841
    at landing, take-off E840
    in
      terrorism E979.1
      war operations E994
    on runway NEC E840
    stated as
      homicidal E968.8
      suicidal E958.6
      undetermined whether accidental
        or intentional E988.6
    unpowered E842
  glider E842
  motor vehicle - see also Accident, mo-
    tor vehicle
    homicidal E968.5
    suicidal E958.5
    undetermined whether accidental or
      intentional E988.5
Crushed (accidentally) E928.9
  between
    boat(s), ship(s), watercraft (and dock
      or pier) (without accident to
      watercraft) E838
      after accident to, or collision, wa-
        tercraft E831
    objects (moving) (stationary and
      moving) E918
  by
    avalanche NEC E909.2
    boat, ship, watercraft after accident
      to, collision, watercraft E831
    cave-in E916
      with asphyxiation or suffocation
        (see also Suffocation, due to,
        cave-in) E913.3
    crowd, human stampede E917.1
    falling
      aircraft (see also Accident, aircraft)
        E841
      in
        terrorism E979.1
        war operations E994
      earth, material E916
      with asphyxiation or suffocation
        (see also Suffocation, due to,
        cave-in) E913.3
      object E916
      on ship, watercraft E838
      while loading, unloading water-
        craft E838
    landslide NEC E909.2
    lifeboat after abandoning ship E831
    machinery - see Accident, machine
    railway rolling stock, train, vehicle
      (part of) E805
    street car E829
    vehicle NEC - see Accident, vehicle
      NEC
  in
    machinery - see Accident, machine
    object E918
    transport accident - see categories
      E800-E848
  late effect of NEC E929.9

ICD-9-CM

E Codes

Vol. 2

Cut, cutting (any part of body) (accidental) E920.9
by
arrow E920.8
axe E920.4
bayonet (*see also* Bayonet wound) E920.3
blender E920.2
broken glass E920.8
following fall E888.0
can opener E920.4
powered E920.2
chisel E920.4
circular saw E919.4
cutting or piercing instrument - *see also* category E920
following fall E888.0
late effect of E929.8
dagger E920.3
dart E920.8
drill - *see* Accident, caused by drill
edge of stiff paper E920.8
electric
beater E920.2
fan E920.2
knife E920.2
mixer E920.2
fork E920.4
garden fork E920.4
hand saw or tool (not powered) E920.4
powered E920.1
hedge clipper E920.4
powered E920.1
hoe E920.4
ice pick E920.4
knife E920.3
electric E920.2
lathe turnings E920.8
lawn mower E920.4
powered E920.0
riding E919.8
machine - *see* Accident, machine
meat
grinder E919.8
slicer E919.8
nails E920.8
needle E920.4
hypodermic E920.5
object, edged, pointed, sharp - *see* category E920
following fall E888.0
paper cutter E920.4
piercing instrument - *see also* category E920
late effect of E929.8
pitchfork E920.4
powered
can opener E920.2
garden cultivator E920.1
riding E919.8
hand saw E920.1
hand tool NEC E920.1
hedge clipper E920.1
household appliance or implement E920.2
lawn mower (hand) E920.0
riding E919.8
rivet gun E920.1
staple gun E920.1
rake E920.4
saw
circular E919.4
hand E920.4

Cut, cutting (*Continued*)
by (*Continued*)
saw (*Continued*)
scissors E920.4
screwdriver E920.4
sewing machine (electric) (powered) E920.2
not powered E920.4
shears E920.4
shovel E920.4
spade E920.4
splinters E920.8
sword E920.3
tin can lid E920.8
wood slivers E920.8
homicide (attempt) E966
inflicted by other person
stated as
intentional, homicidal E966
undetermined whether accidental or intentional E986
late effect of NEC E929.8
legal
execution E978
intervention E974
self-inflicted (unspecified whether accidental or intentional) E986
stated as intentional, purposeful E956
stated as undetermined whether accidental or intentional E986
suicidal (attempt) E956
terrorism E979.8
war operations E995
Cyclone E908.1

D

Death due to injury occurring one year or more previous - *see* Late effect
Decapitation (accidental circumstances) NEC E928.9
homicidal E966
legal execution (by guillotine) E978
Deprivation - *see also* Privation E913.3
homicidal intent E968.4
Derailment (accidental)
railway (rolling stock) (train) (vehicle) (with subsequent collision) E802
with
collision (antecedent) (*see also* Collision, railway) E800
explosion (subsequent) (without antecedent collision) E802
antecedent collision E803
fall (without collision (antecedent)) E802
fire (without collision (antecedent)) E802
street car E829
Descent
parachute (voluntary) (without accident to aircraft) E844
due to accident to aircraft - *see* categories E840-E842
Desertion
child, with intent to injure or kill E968.4
helpless person, infant, newborn E904.0
with intent to injure or kill E968.4
Destitution - *see* Privation
Disability, late effect or sequela of injury - *see* Late effect

Disease
Andes E902.0
aviators' E902.1
caisson E902.2
range E902.0
Divers' disease, palsy, paralysis, squeeze E902.0
Dog bite E906.0
Dragged by
cable car (not on rails) E847
on rails E829
motor vehicle (on highway) E814
not on highway, nontraffic accident E825
street car E829
Drinking poison (accidental) - *see* Table of Drugs and Chemicals
Drowning - *see* Submersion
Dust in eye E914

E

Earth falling (on) (with asphyxia or suffocation (by pressure)) (*see also* Suffocation, due to, cave-in) E913.3
as, or due to, a cataclysm (involving any transport vehicle) - *see* categories E908, E909
not due to cataclysmic action E913.3
motor vehicle (in motion) (on public highway) E818
not on public highway E825
nonmotor road vehicle NEC E829
pedal cycle E826
railway rolling stock, train, vehicle E806
street car E829
struck or crushed by E916
with asphyxiation or suffocation E913.3
with injury other than asphyxia, suffocation E916
Earthquake (any injury) E909.0
Effect(s) (adverse) of
air pressure E902.9
at high altitude E902.9
in aircraft E902.1
residence or prolonged visit (causing conditions classifiable to E902.0) E902.0
due to
diving E902.2
specified cause NEC E902.8
in aircraft E902.1
cold, excessive (exposure to) (*see also* Cold, exposure to) E901.9
heat (excessive) (*see also* Heat) E900.9
hot
place - *see* Heat
weather E900.0
insulation - *see* Heat
late - *see* Late effect of
motion E903
nuclear explosion or weapon
in
terrorism E979.5
war operations (blast) (fireball) (heat) (radiation) (direct) (secondary) E996
radiation - *see* Radiation
terrorism, secondary E979.9
travel E903

Electric shock, electrocution (accidental) (from exposed wire, faulty appliance, high voltage cable, live rail, open socket) (by) (in) E925.9
appliance or wiring
  domestic E925.0
  factory E925.2
  farm (building) E925.8
    house E925.0
  home E925.0
  industrial (conductor) (control apparatus) (transformer) E925.2
  outdoors E925.8
  public building E925.8
  residential institution E925.8
  school E925.8
  specified place NEC E925.8
caused by other person
  stated as
    intentional, homicidal E968.8
    undetermined whether accidental or intentional E988.4
electric power generating plant, distribution station E925.1
homicidal (attempt) E968.8
legal execution E978
lightning E907
machinery E925.9
  domestic E925.0
  factory E925.2
  farm E925.8
  home E925.0
misadventure in medical or surgical procedure
  in electroshock therapy E873.4
self-inflicted (undetermined whether accidental or intentional) E988.4
stated as intentional E958.4
stated as undetermined whether accidental or intentional E988.4
suicidal (attempt) E958.4
transmission line E925.1
Electrocution - *see* Electric shock
Embolism
air (traumatic) NEC - *see* Air, embolism
Encephalitis
lead or saturnine E866.0
  from pesticide NEC E863.4
Entanglement
in
  bedclothes, causing suffocation E913.0
  wheel of pedal cycle E826
Entry of foreign body, material, any - *see* Foreign body
Execution, legal (any method) E978
Exhaustion
cold - *see* Cold, exposure to
due to excessive exertion E927
heat - *see* Heat
Explosion (accidental) (in) (of) (on) E923.9
acetylene E923.2
aerosol can E921.8
aircraft (in transit) (powered) E841
  at landing, take-off E840
  in
    terrorism E979.1
    war operations E994
  unpowered E842
air tank (compressed) (in machinery) E921.1
anesthetic gas in operating theatre E923.2

Explosion *(Continued)*
automobile tire NEC E921.8
  causing transport accident - *see* categories E810-E825
blasting (cap) (materials) E923.1
boiler (machinery), not on transport vehicle E921.0
  steamship - *see* Explosion, watercraft
bomb E923.8
  in
    terrorism E979.2
    war operations E993
      after cessation of hostilities E998
      atom, hydrogen or nuclear E996
      injury by fragments from E991.9
        antipersonnel bomb E991.3
butane E923.2
caused by
  other person
    stated as
      intentional, homicidal - *see* Assault, explosive
      undetermined whether accidental or homicidal E985.5
coal gas E923.2
detonator E923.1
dynamite E923.1
explosive (material) NEC E923.9
  gas(es) E923.2
  missile E923.8
    in
      terrorism E979.2
      war operations E993
        injury by fragments from E991.9
          antipersonnel bomb E991.3
  used in blasting operations E923.1
fire-damp E923.2
fireworks E923.0
gas E923.2
  cylinder (in machinery) E921.1
  pressure tank (in machinery) E921.1
gasoline (fumes) (tank) not in moving motor vehicle E923.2
grain store (military) (munitions) E923.8
grenade E923.8
  in
    terrorism E979.2
    war operations E993
      injury by fragments from E991.9
homicide (attempt) - *see* Assault, explosive
hot water heater, tank (in machinery) E921.0
in mine (of explosive gases) NEC E923.2
late effect of NEC E929.8
machinery - *see also* Accident, machine
pressure vessel - *see* Explosion, pressure vessel
methane E923.2
missile E923.8
  in
    terrorism E979.2
    war operations E993

Explosion *(Continued)*
missile *(Continued)*
  in *(Continued)*
    injury by fragments from E991.9
motor vehicle (part of)
  in motion (on public highway) E818
  not on public highway E825
munitions (dump) (factory) E923.8
  in
    terrorism E979.2
    war operations E993
  of mine E923.8
    in
      terrorism
        at sea or in harbor E979.0
        land E979.2
        marine E979.0
      war operations
        after cessation of hostilities E998
        at sea or in harbor E992
        land E993
          after cessation of hostilities E998
          injured by fragments from E991.9
        marine E992
own weapons
  in
    terrorism (*see also* Suicide) E979.2
    war operations E993
      injured by fragments from E991.9
        antipersonnel bomb E991.3
    injury by fragments from E991.9
      antipersonnel bomb E991.3
pressure
  cooker E921.8
  gas tank (in machinery) E921.1
  vessel (in machinery) E921.9
    on transport vehicle - *see* categories E800-E848
    specified type NEC E921.8
propane E923.2
railway engine, locomotive, train (boiler) (with subsequent collision, derailment, fall) E803
  with
    collision (antecedent) (*see also* Collision, railway) E800
    derailment (antecedent) E802
    fire (without antecedent collision or derailment) E803
secondary fire resulting from - *see* Fire
self-inflicted (unspecified whether accidental or intentional) E985.5
  stated as intentional, purposeful E955.5
shell (artillery) E923.8
  in
    terrorism E979.2
    war operations E993
      injury by fragments from E991.9
stated as undetermined whether caused accidentally or purposely inflicted E985.5
steam or water lines (in machinery) E921.0
suicide (attempted) E955.5
terrorism - *see* Terrorism, explosion

ICD-9-CM
F Codes
Vol.

Explosion (Continued)
  torpedo E923.8
  in
    terrorism E979.0
    war operations E992
  transport accident - see categories
    E800-E848
  war operations - see War operations,
    explosion
  watercraft (boiler) E837
    causing drowning, submersion (after
      jumping from watercraft) E830
Exposure (to) (conditions) (rain)
  (weather) (wind) E904.3
  with homicidal intent E968.4
  algae bloom E905.7 ◀
  excessive E904.3
    cold (see also Cold, exposure to)
      E901.9
      self-inflicted - see Cold, exposure
        to, self-inflicted
    heat (see also Heat) E900.9
  fire, see Fire
  helpless person, infant, newborn due
    to abandonment or neglect E904.0
  marine phytoplankton E905.7 ◀
  noise E928.1
  prolonged in deep-freeze unit or re-
    frigerator E901.1
  radiation - see Radiation
  red tide E905.7 ◀
  resulting from transport accident - see
    categories E800-E848
  smoke from, due to
    fire - see Fire
  tobacco, second-hand E869.4
  vibration E928.2

F

Fall, falling (accidental) E888.9
  building E916
    burning E891.8
      private E890.8
  down
    escalator E880.0
    ladder E881.0
      in boat, ship, watercraft E833
    staircase E880.9
    stairs, steps - see Fall, from, stairs
  earth (with asphyxia or suffocation (by
    pressure)) (see also Earth, falling)
    E913.3
  from, off
    aircraft (at landing, take-off) (in
      transit) (while alighting, board-
      ing) E843
      resulting from accident to aircraft
        - see categories E840-E842
    animal (in sport or transport) E828
    animal-drawn vehicle E827
    balcony E882
    bed E884.4
    bicycle E826
    boat, ship, watercraft (into water) E832
      after accident to, collision, fire on
        E830
        and subsequently struck by
          (part of) boat E831
        and subsequently struck by (part
          of) while alighting, boat E838
      burning, crushed, sinking E830
        and subsequently struck by
          (part of) boat E831

Fall, falling (Continued)
  from, off (Continued)
    bridge E882
    building E882
      burning (uncontrolled fire) E891.8
        in terrorism E979.3
        private E890.8
    bunk in boat, ship, watercraft E834
      due to accident to watercraft E831
    cable car (not on rails) E847
      on rails E829
    car - see Fall from motor vehicle
    chair E884.2
    cliff E884.1
    commode E884.6
    curb (sidewalk) E880.1
    elevation aboard ship E834
      due to accident to ship E831
    embankment E884.9
    escalator E880.0
    fire escape E882
    flagpole E882
    furniture NEC E884.5
    gangplank (into water) (see also Fall,
      from, boat) E832
      to deck, dock E834
    hammock on ship E834
      due to accident to watercraft E831
    haystack E884.9
    high place NEC E884.9
      stated as undetermined whether
        accidental or intentional - see
        Jumping, from, high place
    horse (in sport or transport) E828
    in-line skates E885.1
    ladder E881.0
      in boat, ship, watercraft E833
        due to accident to watercraft E831
    machinery - see also Accident, machine
      not in operation E884.9
    motor vehicle (in motion) (on public
      highway) E818
      not on public highway E825
        stationary, except while alight-
          ing, boarding, entering,
          leaving E884.9
        while alighting, boarding, enter-
          ing, leaving E824
      stationary, except while alighting,
        boarding, entering, leaving
        E884.9
      while alighting, boarding, enter-
        ing, leaving, except off-road
        type motor vehicle E817
      off-road type - see Fall, from,
        off-road type motor vehicle
    nonmotor road vehicle (while alight-
      ing, boarding) NEC E829
      stationary, except while alighting,
        boarding, entering, leaving
        E884.9
    off-road type motor vehicle (not on
      public highway) NEC E821
      on public highway E818
        while alighting, boarding, enter-
          ing, leaving E817
    snow vehicle - see Fall from snow
      vehicle, motor-driven
    one
      deck to another on ship E834
        due to accident to ship E831
      level to another NEC E884.9
        boat, ship, or watercraft E834
          due to accident to watercraft
          E831

Fall, falling (Continued)
  from, off (Continued)
    pedal cycle E826
    playground equipment E884.0
    railway rolling stock, train, vehicle
      (while alighting, boarding) E804
      with
        collision (see also Collision, rail-
          way) E800
        derailment (see also Derailment,
          railway) E802
        explosion (see also Explosion,
          railway engine) E803
    rigging (aboard ship) E834
      due to accident to watercraft E831
    roller skates E885.1
    scaffolding E881.1
    scooter (nonmotorized) E885.0
    sidewalk (curb) E880.1
      moving E885.9
    skateboard E885.2
    skis E885.3
    snow vehicle, motor-driven (not on
      public highway) E820
      on public highway E818
        while alighting, boarding, enter-
          ing, leaving E817
    snowboard E885.4
    stairs, steps E880.9
      boat, ship, watercraft E833
        due to accident to watercraft
          E831
      motor bus, motor vehicle - see
        Fall, from, motor vehicle,
        while alighting, boarding
      street car E829
    stationary vehicle NEC E884.9
    stepladder E881.0
    street car (while boarding, alighting)
      E829
      stationary, except while boarding
        or alighting E884.9
    structure NEC E882
      burning (uncontrolled fire)E891.8
        in terrorism E979.3
    table E884.9
    toilet E884.6
    tower E882
    tree E884.9
    turret E882
    vehicle NEC - see also Accident, ve-
      hicle NEC
      stationary E884.9
    viaduct E882
    wall E882
    wheelchair E884.3
    window E882
  in, on
    aircraft (at landing, take-off) (in
      transit) E843
      resulting from accident to aircraft
        - see categories E840-E842
    boat, ship, watercraft E835
      due to accident to watercraft E831
      one level to another NEC E834
      on ladder, stairs E833
    cutting or piercing instrument ma-
      chine E888.0
    deck (of boat, ship, watercraft) E835
      due to accident to watercraft E831
    escalator E880.0
    gangplank E835
    glass, broken E888.0
    knife E888.0

ICD-9-CM
E Codes
Vol. 2

Fall, falling (Continued)
 in, on (Continued)
  ladder E881.0
   in boat, ship, watercraft E833
    due to accident to watercraft E831
  object
   edged, pointed or sharp E888.0
   other E888.1
  pitchfork E888.0
  railway rolling stock, train, vehicle
    (while alighting, boarding) E804
   with
    collision (see also Collision, rail-
      way) E800
    derailment (see also Derailment,
      railway) E802
    explosion (see also Explosion,
      railway engine) E803
  scaffolding E881.1
  scissors E888.0
  staircase, stairs, steps (see also Fall,
    from, stairs) E880.9
  street car E829
  water transport (see also Fall, in,
    boat) E835
 into
  cavity E883.9
  dock E883.9
   from boat, ship, watercraft (see
     also Fall, from, boat) E832
  hold (of ship) E834
   due to accident to watercraft E831
  hole E883.9
  manhole E883.2
  moving part of machinery - see Acci-
    dent, machine
  opening in surface NEC E883.9
  pit E883.9
  quarry E883.9
  shaft E883.9
  storm drain E883.2
  tank E883.9
  water (with drowning or submer-
    sion) E910.9
  well E883.1
 late effect of NEC E929.3
 object (see also Hit by, object, falling)
   E916
 other E888.8
 over
  animal E885.9
  cliff E884.1
  embankment E884.9
  small object E885.9
 overboard (see also Fall, from, boat)
   E832
 resulting in striking against object
   E888.1
 sharp E888.0
 rock E916
 same level NEC E888.9
  aircraft (any kind) E843
   resulting from accident to aircraft
     - see categories E840-E842
  boat, ship, watercraft E835
   due to accident to, collision, wa-
     tercraft E831
  from
   collision, pushing, shoving, by or
     with other person(s) E886.9
    as, or caused by, a crowd
      E917.6
    in sports E886.0
   in-line skates E885.1

Fall, falling (Continued)
 same level NEC (Continued)
  from (Continued)
   roller skates E885.1
   scooter (nonmotorized) E885.0
   skateboard E885.2
   skis E885.3
   slipping, stumbling, tripping
     E885.9
   snowboard E885.4
  snowslide E916
   as avalanche E909.2
  stone E916
  through
   hatch (on ship) E834
    due to accident to watercraft E831
   roof E882
   window E882
  timber E916
  while alighting from, boarding, enter-
    ing, leaving
   aircraft (any kind) E843
   motor bus, motor vehicle - see Fall,
     from, motor vehicle, while
     alighting, boarding
   nonmotor road vehicle NEC E829
   railway train E804
   street car E829
Fallen on by
 animal (horse) (not being ridden)
   E906.8
  being ridden (in sport or transport)
    E828
**Fell or jumped from high place, so
 stated** - see Jumping, from, high
 place
Felo-de-se (see also Suicide) E958.9
Fever
 heat - see Heat
 thermic - see Heat
Fight (hand) (fist) (foot) (see also Assault,
 fight) E960.0
Fire (accidental) (caused by great heat
 from appliance (electrical), hot object
 or hot substance) (secondary, resulting from explosion) E899
 conflagration - see Conflagration
 controlled, normal (in brazier, fireplace, furnace, or stove) (charcoal)
   (coal) (coke) (electric) (gas) (wood)
  bonfire E897
  brazier, not in building or structure
    E897
  in building or structure, except pri-
    vate dwelling (barn) (church)
    (convalescent or residential
    home) (factory) (farm outbuild-
    ing) (hospital) (hotel) (institu-
    tion (educational) (dormitory)
    (residential)) (private garage)
    (school) (shop) (store) (theatre)
    E896
  in private dwelling (apartment)
    (boarding house) (camping
    place) (caravan) (farmhouse)
    (home (private)) (house) (lodg-
    ing house) (rooming house)
    (tenement) E895
   not in building or structure E897
  trash E897
 forest (uncontrolled) E892
 grass (uncontrolled) E892
 hay (uncontrolled) E892
 homicide (attempt) E968.0
  late effect of E969

Fire (Continued)
 in, of, on, starting in E892
  aircraft (in transit) (powered) E841
   at landing, take-off E840
   stationary E892
   unpowered (balloon) (glider) E842
  balloon E842
  boat, ship, watercraft - see categories
    E830, E831, E837
  building or structure, except private
    dwelling (barn) (church) (conva-
    lescent or residential home) (fac-
    tory) (farm outbuilding) (hospi-
    tal) (hotel) (institution)
    (educational) (dormitory) (resi-
    dential)) (school) (shop) (store)
    (theatre) (see also Conflagration,
    building or structure, except
    private dwelling) E891.9
  forest (uncontrolled) E892
  glider E842
  grass (uncontrolled) E892
  hay (uncontrolled) E892
  lumber (uncontrolled) E892
  machinery - see Accident, machine
  mine (uncontrolled) E892
  motor vehicle (in motion) (on public
    highway) E818
   not on public highway E825
   stationary E892
  prairie (uncontrolled) E892
  private dwelling (apartment) (board-
    ing house) (camping place) (car-
    avan) (farmhouse) (home (pri-
    vate)) (house) (lodging house)
    (private garage) (rooming house)
    (tenement) (see also Conflagra-
    tion, private dwelling) E890.9
  railway rolling stock, train, vehicle
    (see also Explosion, railway en-
    gine) E803
   stationary E892
  room NEC E898.1
  street car (in motion) E829
   stationary E892
  terrorism (by fire-producing device)
    E979.3
   fittings or furniture (burning
     buildings) (uncontrolled fire)
     E979.3
   from nuclear explosion E979.5
  transport vehicle, stationary NEC
    E892
  tunnel (uncontrolled) E892
  war operations (by fire-producing
    device or conventional weapon)
    E990.9
   from nuclear explosion E996
   petrol bomb E990.0
 late effect of NEC E929.4
 lumber (uncontrolled) E892
 mine (uncontrolled) E892
 prairie (uncontrolled) E892
 self-inflicted (unspecified whether accidental or intentional) E988.1
  stated as intentional, purposeful
    E958.1
 specified NEC E898.1
  with
   conflagration - see Conflagration
   ignition (of)
    clothing - see Ignition, clothes
    highly inflammable material
      (benzine) (fat) (gasoline)
      (kerosene) (paraffin) (petrol)
      E894

Fire *(Continued)*
started by other person
stated as
with intent to injure or kill E968.0
undetermined whether or not with
intent to injure or kill E988.1
suicide (attempted) E958.1
late effect of E959
tunnel (uncontrolled) E892
Fireball effects from nuclear explosion
in
terrorism E979.5
war operations E996
Fireworks (explosion) E923.0
Flash burns from explosion *(see also* Explosion) E923.9
Flood (any injury) (resulting from storm)
E908.2
caused by collapse of dam or manmade structure E909.3
Forced landing (aircraft) E840
Foreign body, object or material (entrance into (accidental))
air passage (causing injury) E915
with asphyxia, obstruction, suffocation E912
food or vomitus E911
nose (with asphyxia, obstruction, suffocation) E912
causing injury without asphyxia, obstruction, suffocation E915
alimentary canal (causing injury) (with obstruction) E915
with asphyxia, obstruction respiratory passage, suffocation E912
food E911
mouth E915
with asphyxia, obstruction, suffocation E912
food E911
pharynx E915
with asphyxia, obstruction, suffocation E912
food E911
aspiration (with asphyxia, obstruction respiratory passage, suffocation) E912
causing injury without asphyxia, obstruction respiratory passage, suffocation E915
food (regurgitated) (vomited) E911
causing injury without asphyxia, obstruction respiratory passage, suffocation E915
mucus (not of newborn) E912
phlegm E912
bladder (causing injury or obstruction) E915
bronchus, bronchi - *see* Foreign body, air passages
conjunctival sac E914
digestive system - *see* Foreign body, alimentary canal
ear (causing injury or obstruction) E915
esophagus (causing injury or obstruction) *(see also* Foreign body, alimentary canal) E915
eye (any part) E914
eyelid E914
hairball (stomach) (with obstruction) E915
ingestion - *see* Foreign body, alimentary canal

Foreign body, object or material *(Continued)*
inhalation - *see* Foreign body, aspiration
intestine (causing injury or obstruction) E915
iris E914
lacrimal apparatus E914
larynx - *see* Foreign body, air passage
late effect of NEC E929.8
lung - *see* Foreign body, air passage
mouth - *see* Foreign body, alimentary canal, mouth
nasal passage - *see* Foreign body, air passage, nose
nose - *see* Foreign body, air passage, nose
ocular muscle E914
operation wound (left in) - *see* Misadventure, foreign object
orbit E914
pharynx - *see* Foreign body, alimentary canal, pharynx
rectum (causing injury or obstruction) E915
stomach (hairball) (causing injury or obstruction) E915
tear ducts or glands E914
trachea - *see* Foreign body, air passage
urethra (causing injury or obstruction) E915
vagina (causing injury or obstruction) E915
Found dead, injured
from exposure (to) - *see* Exposure
on
public highway E819
railway right of way E807
Fracture (circumstances unknown or unspecified) E887
due to specified external means - *see* manner of accident
late effect of NEC E929.3
occurring in water transport NEC E835
Freezing - *see* Cold, exposure to
Frostbite E901.0
due to manmade conditions E901.1
Frozen - *see* Cold, exposure to

G

Garrotting, homicidal (attempted) E963
Gored E906.8
Gunshot wound *(see also* Shooting)
E922.9

H

Hailstones, injury by E904.3
Hairball (stomach) (with obstruction)
E915
Hanged himself *(see also* Hanging, self-inflicted) E983.0
Hang gliding E842
Hanging (accidental) E913.8
caused by other person
in accidental circumstances E913.8
stated as
intentional, homicidal E963
undetermined whether accidental or intentional E983.0
homicide (attempt) E963

Hanging *(Continued)*
in bed or cradle E913.0
legal execution E978
self-inflicted (unspecified whether accidental or intentional) E983.0
in accidental circumstances E913.8
stated as intentional, purposeful E953.0
stated as undetermined whether accidental or intentional E983.0
suicidal (attempt) E953.0
Heat (apoplexy) (collapse) (cramps) (effects of) (excessive) (exhaustion) (fever) (prostration) (stroke) E900.9
due to
manmade conditions (as listed in E900.1, except boat, ship, watercraft) E900.1
weather (conditions) E900.0
from
electric heating apparatus causing burning E924.8
nuclear explosion
in
terrorism E979.5
war operations E996
generated in, boiler, engine, evaporator, fire room of boat, ship, watercraft E838
inappropriate in local application or packing in medical or surgical procedure E873.5
late effect of NEC E989
Hemorrhage
delayed following medical or surgical treatment without mention of misadventure - *see* Reaction, abnormal
during medical or surgical treatment as misadventure - *see* Misadventure, cut
High
altitude, effects E902.9
level of radioactivity, effects - *see* Radiation
pressure effects - *see also* Effects of, air pressure
from rapid descent in water (causing caisson or divers' disease, palsy, or paralysis) E902.2
temperature, effects - *see* Heat
Hit, hitting (accidental) by
aircraft (propeller) (without accident to aircraft) E844
unpowered E842
avalanche E909.2
being thrown against object in or part of
motor vehicle (in motion) (on public highway) E818
not on public highway E825
nonmotor road vehicle NEC E829
street car E829
boat, ship, watercraft
after fall from watercraft E838
damaged, involved in accident E831
while swimming, water skiing E838
bullet *(see also* Shooting) E922.9
from air gun E922.4
in
terrorism E979.4
war operations E991.2
rubber E991.0
flare, Verey pistol *(see also* Shooting)
E922.8

◄ **New**   ◄⊪ **Revised**

Hit, hitting (*Continued*)
  hailstones E904.3
  landslide E909.2
  law-enforcing agent (on duty) E975
    with blunt object (baton) (night stick) (stave) (truncheon) E973
  machine - *see* Accident, machine
  missile
    firearm (*see also* Shooting) E922.9
    in
      terrorism - *see* Terrorism, missile
      war operations - *see* War operations, missile
  motor vehicle (on public highway) (traffic accident) E814
    not on public highway, nontraffic accident E822
  nonmotor road vehicle NEC E829
  object
    falling E916
      from, in, on
        aircraft E844
          due to accident to aircraft - *see* categories E840-E842
          unpowered E842
        boat, ship, watercraft E838
          due to accident to watercraft E831
        building E916
          burning E891.8
            in terrorism E979.3
            private E890.8
        cataclysmic
          earth surface movement or eruption E909.9
          storm E908.9
        cave-in E916
          with asphyxiation or suffocation (*see also* Suffocation, due to, cave-in) E913.3
        earthquake E909.0
        motor vehicle (in motion) (on public highway) E818
          not on public highway E825
          stationary E916
        nonmotor road vehicle NEC E829
        pedal cycle E826
        railway rolling stock, train, vehicle E806
        street car E829
        structure, burning NEC E891.8
        vehicle, stationary E916
    moving NEC - *see* Striking against, object
    projected NEC - *see* Striking against, object
    set in motion by
      compressed air or gas, spring, striking, throwing - *see* Striking against, object
      explosion - *see* Explosion
    thrown into, on, or towards
      motor vehicle (in motion) (on public highway) E818
        not on public highway E825
      nonmotor road vehicle NEC E829
      pedal cycle E826
      street car E829
  off-road type motor vehicle (not on public highway) E821
    on public highway E814

Hit, hitting (*Continued*)
  other person(s) E917.9
    with blunt or thrown object E917.9
      in sports E917.0
        with subsequent fall E917.5
      intentionally, homicidal E968.2
    as, or caused by, a crowd E917.1
      with subsequent fall E917.6
      in sports E917.0
  pedal cycle E826
  police (on duty) E975
    with blunt object (baton) (nightstick) (stave) (truncheon) E973
  railway, rolling stock, train, vehicle (part of) E805
  shot - *see* Shooting
  snow vehicle, motor-driven (not on public highway) E820
    on public highway E814
  street car E829
  vehicle NEC - *see* Accident, vehicle NEC
Homicide, homicidal (attempt) (justifiable) (*see also* Assault) E968.9
Hot
  liquid, object, substance, accident caused by - *see also* Accident, caused by, hot, by type of substance
    late effect of E929.8
  place, effects - *see* Heat
  weather, effects E900.0
Humidity, causing problem E904.3
Hunger E904.1
  resulting from
    abandonment or neglect E904.0
    transport accident - *see* categories E800-E848
Hurricane (any injury) E908.0
Hypobarism, hypobaropathy - *see* Effects of, air pressure
Hypothermia - *see* Cold, exposure to

I

Ictus
  caloris - *see* Heat
  solaris E900.0
Ignition (accidental)
  anesthetic gas in operating theatre E923.2
  bedclothes
    with
      conflagration - *see* Conflagration
      ignition (of)
        clothing - *see* Ignition, clothes
        highly inflammable material obstruction (benzine) (fat) (gasoline) (kerosene) (paraffin) (petrol) E894
  benzine E894
  clothes, clothing (from controlled fire) (in building) E893.9
    with conflagration - *see* Conflagration
    from
      bonfire E893.2
      highly inflammable material E894
      sources or material as listed in E893.8
      trash fire E893.2
      uncontrolled fire - *see* Conflagration

Ignition (*Continued*)
  clothes, clothing (*Continued*)
    in
      private dwelling E893.0
      specified building or structure, except of private dwelling E893.1
    not in building or structure E893.2
  explosive material - *see* Explosion
  fat E894
  gasoline E894
  kerosene E894
  material
    explosive - *see* Explosion
    highly inflammable E894
      with conflagration - *see* Conflagration
      with explosion E923.2
  nightdress - *see* Ignition, clothes
  paraffin E894
  petrol E894
Immersion - *see* Submersion
Implantation of quills of porcupine E906.8
Inanition (from) E904.9
  hunger - *see* Lack of, food
  resulting from homicidal intent E968.4
  thirst - *see* Lack of, water
Inattention after, at birth E904.0
  homicidal, infanticidal intent E968.4
Infanticide (*see also* Assault)
Ingestion
  foreign body (causing injury) (with obstruction) - *see* Foreign body, alimentary canal
  poisonous substance NEC - *see* Table of Drugs and Chemicals
Inhalation
  excessively cold substance, manmade E901.1
  foreign body - *see* Foreign body, aspiration
  liquid air, hydrogen, nitrogen E901.1
  mucus, not of newborn (with asphyxia, obstruction respiratory passage, suffocation) E912
  phlegm (with asphyxia, obstruction respiratory passage, suffocation) E912
  poisonous gas - *see* Table of Drugs and Chemicals
  smoke from, due to
    fire - *see* Fire
  tobacco, second-hand E869.4
  vomitus (with asphyxia, obstruction respiratory passage, suffocation) E911
Injury, injured (accidental(ly)) NEC E928.9
  by, caused by, from
    air rifle (B-B gun) E922.4
    animal (not being ridden) NEC E906.9
      being ridden (in sport or transport) E828
    assault (*see also* Assault) E968.9
    avalanche E909.2
    bayonet (*see also* Bayonet wound) E920.3
    being thrown against some part of, or object in
      motor vehicle (in motion) (on public highway) E818
        not on public highway E825
      nonmotor road vehicle NEC E829

ICD-9-CM

E Codes

Vol.

Injury, injured (*Continued*)
  by, caused by, from (*Continued*)
    being thrown against some part of (*Continued*)
      off-road motor vehicle NEC E821
      railway train E806
      snow vehicle, motor-driven E820
      street car E829
    bending E927
    bite, human E928.3
    broken glass E920.8
    bullet - *see* Shooting
    cave-in (*see also* Suffocation, due to, cave-in) E913.3
      earth surface movement or eruption E909.9
      storm E908.9
      without asphyxiation or suffocation E916
    cloudburst E908.8
    cutting or piercing instrument (*see also* Cut) E920.9
    cyclone E908.1
    earthquake E909.0
    electric current (*see also* Electric shock) E925.9
    explosion (*see also* Explosion) E923.9
    fire - *see* Fire
    flare, Verey pistol E922.8
    flood E908.2
    foreign body - *see* Foreign body
    hailstones E904.3
    hurricane E908.0
    landslide E909.2
    law-enforcing agent, police, in course of legal intervention - *see* Legal intervention
    lightning E907
    live rail or live wire - *see* Electric shock
    machinery - *see also* Accident, machine aircraft, without accident to aircraft E844
      boat, ship, watercraft (deck) (engine room) (galley) (laundry) (loading) E836
    missile
      explosive E923.8
      firearm - *see* Shooting
      in
        terrorism - *see* Terrorism, missile
        war operations - *see* War operations, missile
    moving part of motor vehicle (in motion) (on public highway) E818
      not on public highway, nontraffic accident E825
      while alighting, boarding, entering, leaving - *see* Fall, from, motor vehicle, while alighting, boarding
    nail E920.8
    needle (sewing) E920.4
      hypodermic E920.5
    noise E928.1
    object
      fallen on
        motor vehicle (in motion) (on public highway) E818
        not on public highway E825
      falling - *see* Hit by, object, failing
    paintball gun E922.5

Injury, injured (*Continued*)
  by, caused by, from (*Continued*)
    radiation - *see* Radiation
    railway rolling stock, train, vehicle (part of) E805
      door or window E806
    rotating propeller, aircraft E844
    rough landing of off-road type motor vehicle (after leaving ground or rough terrain) E821
      snow vehicle E820
    saber (*see also* Wound, saber) E920.3
    shot - *see* Shooting
    sound waves E928.1
    splinter or sliver, wood E920.8
    straining E927
    street car (door) E829
    suicide (attempt) E958.9
    sword E920.3
    terrorism - *see* Terrorism
    third rail - *see* Electric shock
    thunderbolt E907
    tidal wave E909.4
      caused by storm E908.0
    tornado E908.1
    torrential rain E908.2
    twisting E927
    vehicle NEC - *see* Accident, vehicle NEC
    vibration E928.2
    volcanic eruption E909.1
    weapon burst, in war operations E993
    weightlessness (in spacecraft, real or simulated) E928.0
    wood splinter or sliver E920.8
  due to
    civil insurrection - *see* War operations
      occurring after cessation of hostilities E998
    terrorism - *see* Terrorism
    war operations - *see* War operations
      occurring after cessation of hostilities E998
  homicidal (*see also* Assault) E968.9
  in, on
    civil insurrection - *see* War operations
    fight E960.0
    parachute descent (voluntary) (without accident to aircraft) E844
      with accident to aircraft - *see* categories E840-E842
    public highway E819
    railway right of way E807
    terrorism - *see* Terrorism
    war operations - *see* War operations
  inflicted (by)
    in course of arrest (attempted), suppression of disturbance, maintenance of order, by law enforcing agents - *see* Legal intervention
    law-enforcing agent (on duty) - *see* Legal intervention
    other person
      stated as
        accidental E928.9
        homicidal, intentional - *see* Assault
        undetermined whether accidental or intentional - *see* Injury, stated as undetermined

Injury, injured (*Continued*)
  inflicted (*Continued*)
    police (on duty) - *see* Legal intervention
    late effect of E929.9
    purposely (inflicted) by other person(s) - *see* Assault
    self-inflicted (unspecified whether accidental or intentional) E988.9
      stated as
        accidental E928.9
        intentionally, purposely E958.9
    specified cause NEC E928.8
    stated as
      undetermined whether accidentally or purposely inflicted (by) E988.9
        cut (any part of body) E986
        cutting or piercing instrument (classifiable to E920) E986
        drowning E984
        explosive(s) (missile) E985.5
        falling from high place E987.9
          manmade structure, except residential E987.1
          natural site E987.2
          residential premises E987.0
        hanging E983.0
        knife E986
        late effect of E989
        puncture (any part of body) E986
        shooting - *see* Shooting, stated as undetermined whether accidental or intentional
        specified means NEC E988.8
        stab (any part of body) E986
        strangulation - *see* Suffocation, stated as undetermined whether accidental or intentional
        submersion E984
        suffocation - *see* Suffocation, stated as undetermined whether accidental or intentional
    to child due to criminal abortion E968.8
Insufficient nourishment - *see also* Lack of, food
  homicidal intent E968.4
Insulation, effects - *see* Heat
Interruption of respiration by
  food lodged in esophagus E911
  foreign body, except food, in esophagus E912
Intervention, legal - *see* Legal intervention
Intoxication, drug or poison - *see* Table of Drugs and Chemicals
Irradiation - *see* Radiation

J

Jammed (accidentally)
  between objects (moving) (stationary and moving) E918
  in object E918
Jumped or fell from high place, so stated - *see* Jumping, from, high place, stated as
  in undetermined circumstances
Jumping
  before train, vehicle or other moving object (unspecified whether accidental or intentional) E988.0

Jumping (Continued)
  before train (Continued)
    stated as
      intentional, purposeful E958.0
      suicidal (attempt) E958.0
  from
    aircraft
      by parachute (voluntarily) (without accident to aircraft) E844
      due to accident to aircraft - see categories E840-E842
    boat, ship, watercraft (into water)
      after accident to, fire on, watercraft E830
        and subsequently struck by (part of) boat E831
      burning, crushed, sinking E830
        and subsequently struck by (part of) boat E831
      voluntarily, without accident (to boat) with injury other than drowning or submersion E883.0
    building see also Jumping, from, high place
      burning (uncontrolled fire) E891.8
        in terrorism E979.3
        private E890.8
    cable car (not on rails) E847
      on rails E829
    high place
      in accidental circumstances or in sport - see categories E880-E884
      stated as
        with intent to injure self E957.9
          man-made structures NEC E957.1
          natural sites E957.2
          residential premises E957.0
        in undetermined circumstances E987.9
          man-made structures NEC E987.1
          natural sites E987.2
          residential premises E987.0
        suicidal (attempt) E957.9
          man-made structures NEC E957.1
          natural sites E957.1
          residential premises E957.0
    motor vehicle (in motion) (on public highway) - see Fall, from, motor vehicle
    nonmotor road vehicle NEC E829
    street car E829
    structure - see also Jumping, from high places
      burning (uncontrolled fire) E891.8
        in terrorism E979.3
    into water
      with injury other than drowning or submersion E883.0
      drowning or submersion - see Submersion
    from, off, watercraft - see Jumping, from, boat
Justifiable homicide - see Assault

K

Kicked by
  animal E906.8

Kicked by (Continued)
  person(s) (accidentally) E917.9
    with intent to injure or kill E960.0
    as, or caused by a crowd E917.1
      with subsequent fall E917.6
    in fight E960.0
    in sports E917.0
      with subsequent fall E917.5
Kicking against
  object (moving) E917.9
    in sports E917.0
      with subsequent fall E917.5
    stationary E917.4
      with subsequent fall E917.8
  person - see Striking against, person
Killed, killing (accidentally) NEC (see also Injury) E928.9
  in
    action - see War operations
    brawl, fight (hand) (fists) (foot) E960.0
      by weapon - see also Assault
        cutting, piercing E966
        firearm - see Shooting, homicide
  self
    stated as
      accident E928.9
      suicide - see Suicide
    unspecified whether accidental or suicidal E988.9
Knocked down (accidentally) (by) NEC E928.9
  animal (not being ridden) E906.8
    being ridden (in sport or transport) E828
  blast from explosion (see also Explosion) E923.9
  crowd, human stampede E917.6
  late effect of - see Late effect
  person (accidentally) E917.9
    in brawl, fight E960.0
    in sports E917.5
  transport vehicle - see vehicle involved under Hit by
  while boxing E917.5

L

Laceration NEC E928.9
Lack of
  air (refrigerator or closed place), suffocation by E913.2
  care (helpless person) (infant) (newborn) E904.0
    homicidal intent E968.4
  food except as result of transport accident E904.1
    helpless person, infant, newborn due to abandonment or neglect E904.0
  water except as result of transport accident E904.2
    helpless person, infant, newborn due to abandonment or neglect E904.0
Landslide E909.2
  falling on, hitting
    motor vehicle (any) (in motion) (on or off public highway) E909.2
    railway rolling stock, train, vehicle E909.2
Late effect of
  accident NEC (accident classifiable to E928.9) E929.9
    specified NEC (accident classifiable to E910-E928.8) E929.8

Late effect of (Continued)
  assault E969
  fall, accidental (accident classifiable to E880-E888) E929.3
  fire, accident caused by (accident classifiable to E890-E899) E929.4
  homicide, attempt (any means) E969
  injury due to terrorism E999.1
  injury undetermined whether accidentally or purposely inflicted (injury classifiable to E980-E988) E989
  legal intervention (injury classifiable to E970-E976) E977
  medical or surgical procedure, test or therapy
    as, or resulting in, or from
      abnormal or delayed reaction or complication - see Reaction, abnormal
      misadventure - see Misadventure
  motor vehicle accident (accident classifiable to E810-E825) E929.0
  natural or environmental factor, accident due to (accident classifiable to E900-E909) E929.5
  poisoning, accidental (accident classifiable to E850-E858, E860-E869) E929.2
  suicide, attempt (any means) E959
  transport accident NEC (accident classifiable to E800-E807, E826-E838, E840-E848) E929.1
  war operations, injury due to (injury classifiable to E990-E998) E999.0
Launching pad accident E845
Legal
  execution, any method E978
  intervention (by) (injury from) E976
    baton E973
    bayonet E974
    blow E975
    blunt object (baton) (nightstick) (stave) (truncheon) E973
    cutting or piercing instrument E974
    dynamite E971
    execution, any method E973
    explosive(s) (shell) E971
    firearm(s) E970
    gas (asphyxiation) (poisoning) (tear) E972
    grenade E971
    late effect of E977
    machine gun E970
    manhandling E975
    mortar bomb E971
    nightstick E973
    revolver E970
    rifle E970
    specified means NEC E975
    stabbing E974
    stave E973
    truncheon E973
Lifting, injury in E927
Lightning (shock) (stroke) (struck by) E907
Liquid (noncorrosive) in eye E914
  corrosive E924.1
Loss of control
  motor vehicle (on public highway) (without antecedent collision) E816
    with
      antecedent collision on public highway - see Collision, motor vehicle

ICD-9-CM

E Codes

Vol. 2

Loss of control (Continued)
  motor vehicle (Continued)
    with (Continued)
      antecedent collision on public
        highway (Continued)
        involving any object, person or
          vehicle not on public high-
          way E816
        on public highway - see Colli-
          sion, motor vehicle
        not on public highway, non-
          traffic accident E825
          with antecedent collision - see
            Collision, motor vehicle,
            not on public highway
    off-road type motor vehicle (not on
      public highway) E821
    on public highway - see Loss of con-
      trol, motor vehicle
    snow vehicle, motor-driven (not on
      public highway) E820
    on public highway - see Loss of con-
      trol, motor vehicle
Lost at sea E832
  with accident to watercraft E830
  in war operations E995
Low
  pressure, effects - see Effects of, air
    pressure
  temperature, effects - see Cold expo-
    sure to
Lying before train, vehicle or other
  moving object (unspecified whether
  accidental or intentional) E988.0
  stated as intentional, purposeful, sui-
    cidal (attempt) E958.0
Lynching (see also Assault) E968.9

M

**Malfunction, atomic power plant in wa-
ter transport** E838
Mangled (accidentally) NEC E928.9
Manhandling (in brawl, fight)
  E960.0
  legal intervention E975
Manslaughter (nonaccidental) - see As-
  sault
Marble in nose E912
Mauled by animal E906.8
Medical procedure, complication of
  delayed or as an abnormal reaction
    without mention of misadventure
    - see Reaction, abnormal
  due to or as a result of misadventure -
    see Misadventure
Melting of fittings and furniture in
  burning
  in terrorism E979.3
Minamata disease E865.2
Misadventure(s) to patient(s) during
  surgical or medical care E876.9
  contaminated blood, fluid, drug or bio-
    logical substance (presence of
    agents and toxins as listed in
    E875) E875.9
    administered (by) NEC E875.9
      infusion E875.0
      injection E875.1
      specified means NEC E875.2
      transfusion E875.0
      vaccination E875.1

**Misadventure(s) to patient(s) during
surgical or medical care** (Continued)
  cut, cutting, puncture, perforation or
    hemorrhage (accidental) (inadver-
    tent) (inappropriate) (during) E870.9
    aspiration of fluid or tissue (by
      puncture or catheterization, ex-
      cept heart) E870.5
    biopsy E870.8
      needle (aspirating) E870.5
    blood sampling E870.5
    catheterization E870.5
      heart E870.6
    dialysis (kidney) E870.2
    endoscopic examination E870.4
    enema E870.7
    infusion E870.1
    injection E870.3
    lumbar puncture E870.5
    needle biopsy E870.5
    paracentesis, abdominal E870.5
    perfusion E870.2
    specified procedure NEC E870.8
    surgical operation E870.0
    thoracentesis E870.5
    transfusion E870.1
    vaccination E870.3
  excessive amount of blood or other
    fluid during transfusion or infu-
    sion E873.0
  failure
    in dosage E873.9
      electroshock therapy E873.4
      inappropriate temperature (too
        hot or too cold) in local appli-
        cation and packing E873.5
      infusion
        excessive amount of fluid E873.0
        incorrect dilution of fluid E873.1
      insulin-shock therapy E873.4
      nonadministration of necessary
        drug or medicinal E873.6
      overdose - see also Overdose
        radiation, in therapy E873.2
      radiation
        inadvertent exposure of patient
          (receiving radiation for test
          or therapy) E873.3
        not receiving radiation for test
          or therapy - see Radiation
        overdose E873.2
      specified procedure NEC E873.8
      transfusion
        excessive amount of blood
          E873.0
    mechanical, of instrument or appa-
      ratus (during procedure) E874.9
      aspiration of fluid or tissue (by
        puncture or catheterization,
        except of heart) E874.4
      biopsy E874.8
        needle (aspirating) E874.4
      blood sampling E874.4
      catheterization E874.4
        heart E874.5
      dialysis (kidney) E874.2
      endoscopic examination E874.3
      enema E874.8
      infusion E874.1
      injection E874.8
      lumbar puncture E874.4
      needle biopsy E874.4
      paracentesis, abdominal E874.4
      perfusion E874.2
      specified procedure NEC E874.8

**Misadventure(s) to patient(s) during
surgical or medical care** (Continued)
  failure (Continued)
    mechanical, of instrument or appa-
      ratus (Continued)
      surgical operation E874.0
      thoracentesis E874.4
      transfusion E874.1
      vaccination E874.8
    sterile precautions (during proce-
      dure) E872.9
      aspiration of fluid or tissue (by
        puncture or catheterization,
        except heart) E872.5
      biopsy E872.8
        needle (aspirating) E872.5
      blood sampling E872.5
      catheterization E872.5
        heart E872.6
      dialysis (kidney) E872.2
      endoscopic examination E872.4
      enema E872.8
      infusion E872.1
      injection E872.3
      lumbar puncture E872.5
      needle biopsy E872.5
      paracentesis, abdominal E872.5
      perfusion E872.2
      removal of catheter or packing
        E872.8
      specified procedure NEC
        E872.8
      surgical operation E872.0
      thoracentesis E872.5
      transfusion E872.1
      vaccination E872.3
    suture or ligature during surgical
      procedure E876.2
    to introduce or to remove tube or
      instrument E876.4
      foreign object left in body - see
        Misadventure, foreign object
  foreign object left in body (during pro-
    cedure) E871.9
    aspiration of fluid or tissue (by
      puncture or catheterization, ex-
      cept heart) E871.5
    biopsy E871.8
      needle (aspirating) E871.5
    blood sampling E871.5
    catheterization E871.5
      heart E871.6
    dialysis (kidney) E871.2
    endoscopic examination E871.4
    enema E871.8
    infusion E871.1
    injection E871.3
    lumbar puncture E871.5
    needle biopsy E871.5
    paracentesis, abdominal E871.5
    perfusion E871.2
    removal of catheter or packing
      E871.7
    specified procedure NEC E871.8
    surgical operation E871.0
    thoracentesis E871.5
    transfusion E871.1
    vaccination E871.3
  hemorrhage - see Misadventure, cut
  inadvertent exposure of patient to ra-
    diation (being received for test or
    therapy) E873.3
  inappropriate
    operation performed E876.5

Misadventure(s) to patient(s) during surgical or medical care *(Continued)*
inappropriate *(Continued)*
   temperature (too hot or too cold) in local application or packing E873.5
  infusion - *see also* Misadventure, by specific type, infusion
   excessive amount of fluid E873.0
   incorrect dilution of fluid E873.1
   wrong fluid E876.1
  mismatched blood in transfusion E876.0
  nonadministration of necessary drug or medicinal E873.6
  overdose - *see also* Overdose
  radiation, in therapy E873.2
  perforation - *see* Misadventure, cut
  performance of inappropriate operation E876.5
  puncture - *see* Misadventure, cut
  specified type NEC E876.8
  failure
   suture or ligature during surgical operation E876.2
   to introduce or to remove tube or instrument E876.4
    foreign object left in body E871.9
   infusion of wrong fluid E876.1
   performance of inappropriate operation E876.5
   transfusion of mismatched blood E876.0
   wrong
    fluid in infusion E876.1
    placement of endotracheal tube during anesthetic procedure E876.3
  transfusion - *see also* Misadventure, by specific type, transfusion
   excessive amount of blood E873.0
   mismatched blood E876.0
  wrong
   drug given in error - *see* Table of Drugs and Chemicals
   fluid in infusion E876.1
   placement of endotracheal tube during anesthetic procedure E876.3
Motion (effects) E903
  sickness E903
Mountain sickness E902.0
Mucus aspiration or inhalation, not of newborn (with asphyxia, obstruction respiratory passage, suffocation) E912
Mudslide of cataclysmic nature E909.2
Murder (attempt) (*see also* Assault) E968.9

N

Nail, injury by E920.8
Needlestick (sewing needle) E920.4
  hypodermic E920.5
Neglect - *see also* Privation
  criminal E968.4
  homicidal intent E968.4
Noise (causing injury) (pollution) E928.1

O

Object
  falling
   from, in, on, hitting
    aircraft E844
     due to accident to aircraft - *see* categories E840-E842
    machinery - *see also* Accident, machine
     not in operation E916
    motor vehicle (in motion) (on public highway) E818
     not on public highway E825
     stationary E916
    nonmotor road vehicle NEC E829
    pedal cycle E826
    person E916
    railway rolling stock, train, vehicle E806
    street car E829
    watercraft E838
     due to accident to watercraft E831
  set in motion by
   accidental explosion of pressure vessel - *see* category E921
   firearm - *see* category E922
   machine(ry) - *see* Accident, machine
   transport vehicle - *see* categories E800-E848
  thrown from, in, on, towards
   aircraft E844
   cable car (not on rails) E847
    on rails E829
   motor vehicle (in motion) (on public highway) E818
    not on public highway E825
   nonmotor road vehicle NEC E829
   pedal cycle E826
   street car E829
   vehicle NEC - *see* Accident, vehicle NEC
Obstruction
  air passages, larynx, respiratory passages
   by
    external means NEC - *see* Suffocation
    food, any type (regurgitated) (vomited) E911
    material or object, except food E912
    mucus E912
    phlegm E912
    vomitus E911
  digestive tract, except mouth or pharynx
   by
    food, any type E915
    foreign body (any) E915
  esophagus
   food E911
   foreign body, except food E912
   without asphyxia or obstruction of respiratory passage E915
  mouth or pharynx
   by
    food, any type E911
    material or object, except food E912
  respiration - *see* Obstruction, air passages

Oil in eye E914
Overdose
  anesthetic (drug) - *see* Table of Drugs and Chemicals
  drug - *see* Table of Drugs and Chemicals
Overexertion (lifting) (pulling) (pushing) E927
Overexposure (accidental) (to)
  cold (*see also* Cold, exposure to) E901.9
   due to manmade conditions E901.1
  heat (*see also* Heat) E900.9
  radiation - *see* Radiation
  radioactivity - *see* Radiation
  sun, except sunburn E900.0
  weather - *see* Exposure
  wind - *see* Exposure
Overheated (*see also* Heat) E900.9
Overlaid E913.0
Overturning (accidental)
  animal-drawn vehicle E827
  boat, ship, watercraft
   causing
    drowning, submersion E830
    injury except drowning, submersion E831
  machinery - *see* Accident, machine
  motor vehicle (*see also* Loss of control, motor vehicle) E816
   with antecedent collision on public highway - *see* Collision, motor vehicle
   not on public highway, nontraffic accident E825
    with antecedent collision - *see* Collision, motor vehicle, not on public highway
  nonmotor road vehicle NEC E829
  off-road type motor vehicle - *see* Loss of control, off-road type motor vehicle
  pedal cycle E826
  railway rolling stock, train, vehicle (*see also* Derailment, railway) E802
  street car E829
  vehicle NEC - *see* Accident, vehicle NEC

P

Palsy, divers' E902.2
Parachuting (voluntary) (without accident to aircraft) E844
  due to accident to aircraft - *see* categories E840-E842
Paralysis
  divers' E902.2
  lead or saturnine E866.0
   from pesticide NEC E863.4
Pecked by bird E906.8
Phlegm aspiration or inhalation (with asphyxia, obstruction respiratory passage, suffocation) E912
Piercing (*see also* Cut) E920.9
Pinched
  between objects (moving) (stationary and moving) E918
  in object E918
Pinned under
  machine(ry) - *see* Accident, machine
Place of occurrence of accident - *see* Accident (to), occurring (at) (in)
Plumbism E866.0
  from insecticide NEC E863.4

ICD-9-CM
E Codes
Vol. 2

Poisoning (accidental) (by) - *see also* Table of Drugs and Chemicals
  carbon monoxide
    generated by
      aircraft in transit E844
      motor vehicle
        in motion (on public highway) E818
          not on public highway E825
      watercraft (in transit) (not in transit) E838
  caused by injection of poisons or toxins into or through skin by plant thorns, spines, or other mechanism E905.7
    marine or sea plants E905.6
  fumes or smoke due to
    conflagration - *see* Conflagration
    explosion or fire - *see* Fire
    ignition - *see* Ignition
  gas
    in legal intervention E972
    legal execution, by E978
    on watercraft E838
    used as anesthetic - *see* Table of Drugs and Chemicals
  in
    terrorism (chemical weapons) E979.7
    war operations E997.2
  late effect of - *see* Late effect
  legal
    execution E978
    intervention
      by gas E972
Pressure, external, causing asphyxia, suffocation (*see also* Suffocation) E913.9
Privation E904.9
  food (*see also* Lack of, food) E904.1
  helpless person, infant, newborn due to abandonment or neglect E904.0
  late effect of NEC E929.5
  resulting from transport accident - *see* categories E800-E848
  water (*see also* Lack of, water) E904.2
Projected objects, striking against or struck by - *see* Striking against, object
Prolonged stay in
  high altitude (causing conditions as listed in E902.0) E902.0
  weightless environment E928.0
Prostration
  heat - *see* Heat
Pulling, injury in E927
Puncture, puncturing (*see also* Cut) E920.9
  by
    plant thorns or spines E920.8
      toxic reaction E905.7
        marine or sea plants E905.6
    sea-urchin spine E905.6
Pushing (injury in) (overexertion) E927
  by other person(s) (accidental) E917.9
    as, or caused by, a crowd, human stampede E917.1
      with subsequent fall E917.6
    before moving vehicle or object
      stated as
        intentional, homicidal E968.8
        undetermined whether accidental or intentional E988.8
    from
      high place
        in accidental circumstances - *see* categories E880-E884

Pushing (*Continued*)
  by other person(s) (*Continued*)
    from (*Continued*)
      high place (*Continued*)
        stated as
          intentional, homicidal E968.1
          undetermined whether accidental or intentional E987.9
          man-made structure, except residential E987.1
          natural site E987.2
          residential E987.0
      motor vehicle (*see also* Fall, from, motor vehicle) E818
        stated as
          intentional, homicidal E968.5
          undetermined whether accidental or intentional E988.8
      in sports E917.0
      with fall E886.0
    with fall E886.9
      in sports E886.0

R

Radiation (exposure to) E926.9
  abnormal reaction to medical test or therapy E879.2
  arc lamps E926.2
  atomic power plant (malfunction) NEC E926.9
    in water transport E838
  electromagnetic, ionizing E926.3
  gamma rays E926.3
  in
    terrorism (from or following nuclear explosion) (direct) (secondary) E979.5
      laser E979.8
    war operations (from or following nuclear explosion) (direct) (secondary) E996
      laser(s) E997.0
    water transport E838
  inadvertent exposure of patient (receiving test or therapy) E873.3
  infrared (heaters and lamps) E926.1
    excessive heat E900.1
  ionized, ionizing (particles, artificially accelerated) E926.8
    electromagnetic E926.3
  isotopes, radioactive - *see* Radiation, radioactive isotopes
  laser(s) E926.4
    in
      terrorism E979.8
      war operations E997.0
    misadventure in medical care - *see* Misadventure, failure, in dosage, radiation
  late effect of NEC E929.8
    excessive heat from - *see* Heat
  light sources (visible) (ultraviolet) E926.2
  misadventure in medical or surgical procedure - *see* Misadventure, failure, in dosage, radiation
  overdose (in medical or surgical pacemaker procedure) E873.2
  radar E926.0

Radiation (*Continued*)
  radioactive isotopes E926.5
    atomic power plant malfunction E926.5
    in water transport E838
    misadventure in medical or surgical treatment - *see* Misadventure, failure, in dosage, radiation
  radiobiologicals - *see* Radiation, radioactive isotopes
  radiofrequency E926.0
  radiopharmaceuticals - *see* Radiation, radioactive isotopes
  radium NEC E926.9
  sun E926.2
    excessive heat from E900.0
  tanning bed E926.2
  welding arc or torch E926.2
    excessive heat from E900.1
  x-rays (hard) (soft) E926.3
    misadventure in medical or surgical treatment - *see* Misadventure, failure, in dosage, radiation
Rape E960.1
Reaction, abnormal, to or following (medical or surgical procedure) E879.9
  amputation (of limbs) E878.5
  anastomosis (arteriovenous) (blood vessel) (gastrojejunal) (skin) (tendon) (natural, artificial material, tissue) E878.2
    external stoma, creation of E878.3
  aspiration (of fluid) E879.4
    tissue E879.8
  biopsy E879.8
  blood
    sampling E879.7
    transfusion
      procedure E879.8
  bypass - *see* Reaction, abnormal, anastomosis
  catheterization
    cardiac E879.0
    urinary E879.6
  colostomy E878.3
  cystostomy E878.3
  dialysis (kidney) E879.1
  drugs or biologicals - *see* Table of Drugs and Chemicals
  duodenostomy E878.3
  electroshock therapy E879.3
  formation of external stoma E878.3
  gastrostomy E878.3
  graft - *see* Reaction, abnormal, anastomosis
  hypothermia E879.8
  implant, implantation (of)
    artificial
      internal device (cardiac pacemaker) (electrodes in brain) (heart valve prosthesis) (orthopedic) E878.1
      material or tissue (for anastomosis or bypass) E878.2
        with creation of external stoma E878.3
      natural tissues (for anastomosis or bypass) E878.2
      as transplantion - *see* Reaction, abnormal, transplant
        with creation of external stoma E878.3

Reaction, abnormal, to or following
(Continued)
infusion
procedure E879.8
injection
procedure E879.8
insertion of gastric or duodenal sound E879.5
insulin-shock therapy E879.3
lumbar puncture E879.4
perfusion E879.1
procedures other than surgical operation (see also Reaction, abnormal, by specific type of procedure) E879.9
specified procedure NEC E879.8
radiological procedure or therapy E879.2
removal of organ (partial) (total) NEC E878.6
with
anastomosis, bypass or graft E878.2
formation of external stoma E878.3
implant of artificial internal device E878.1
transplant(ation)
partial organ E878.4
whole organ E878.0
sampling
blood E879.7
fluid NEC E879.4
tissue E879.8
shock therapy E879.3
surgical operation (see also Reaction, abnormal, by specified type of operation) E878.9
restorative NEC E878.4
with
anastomosis, bypass or graft E878.2
formation of external stoma E878.3
implant(ation) - see Reaction, abnormal, implant
transplantation - see Reaction, abnormal, transplant
specified operation NEC E878.8
thoracentesis E879.4
transfusion
procedure E879.8
transplant, transplantation (heart) (kidney) (liver) E878.0
partial organ E878.4
ureterostomy E878.3
vaccination E879.8
Reduction in
atmospheric pressure - see also Effects of, air pressure
while surfacing from
deep water diving causing caisson or divers' disease, palsy or paralysis E902.2
underground E902.8
Residual (effect) - see Late effect
Rock falling on or hitting (accidentally)
motor vehicle (in motion) (on public highway) E818
not on public highway E825
nonmotor road vehicle NEC E829
pedal cycle E826
person E916
railway rolling stock, train, vehicle E806

Running off, away
animal (being ridden) (in sport or transport) E828
not being ridden E906.8
animal-drawn vehicle E827
rails, railway (see also Derailment) E802
roadway
motor vehicle (without antecedent collision) E816
nontraffic accident E825
with antecedent collision - see Collision, motor vehicle, not on public highway
with
antecedent collision - see Collision, motor vehicle
subsequent collision
involving any object, person or vehicle not on public highway E816
on public highway E811
nonmotor road vehicle NEC E829
pedal cycle E826
Run over (accidentally) (by)
animal (not being ridden) E906.8
being ridden (in sport or transport) E828
animal-drawn vehicle E827
machinery - see Accident, machine
motor vehicle (on public highway) - see Hit by, motor vehicle
nonmotor road vehicle NEC E829
railway train E805
street car E829
vehicle NEC E848

S

Saturnism E866.0
from insecticide NEC E863.4
Scald, scalding (accidental) (by) (from) (in) E924.0
acid - see Scald, caustic
boiling tap water E924.2
caustic or corrosive liquid, substance E924.1
swallowed - see Table of Drugs and Chemicals
homicide (attempt) - see Assault, burning
inflicted by other person
stated as
intentional or homicidal E968.3
undetermined whether accidental or intentional E988.2
late effect of NEC E929.8
liquid (boiling) (hot) E924.0
local application of externally applied substance in medical or surgical care E873.5
molten metal E924.0
self-inflicted (unspecified whether accidental or intentional) E988.2
stated as intentional, purposeful E958.2
stated as undetermined whether accidental or intentional E988.2
steam E924.0
tap water (boiling) E924.2
transport accident - see categories E800-E848
vapor E924.0
Scratch, cat E906.8

Sea
sickness E903
Self-mutilation - see Suicide
Sequelae (of)
in
terrorism E999.1
war operations E999.0
Shock
anaphylactic (see also Table of Drugs and Chemicals) E947.9
due to
bite (venomous) - see Bite, venomous NEC
sting - see Sting
electric (see also Electric shock) E925.9
from electric appliance or current (see also Electric shock) E925.9
Shooting, shot (accidental(ly)) E922.9
air gun E922.4
BB gun E922.4
hand gun (pistol) (revolver) E922.0
himself (see also Shooting, self-inflicted) E985.4
hand gun (pistol) (revolver) E985.0
military firearm, except hand gun E985.3
hand gun (pistol) (revolver) E985.0
rifle (hunting) E985.2
military E985.3
shotgun (automatic) E985.1
specified firearm NEC E985.4
Verey pistol E985.4
homicide (attempt) E965.4
air gun E968.6
BB gun E968.6
hand gun (pistol) (revolver) E965.0
military firearm, except hand gun E965.3
hand gun (pistol) (revolver) E965.0
paintball gun E965.4
rifle (hunting) E965.2
military E965.3
shotgun (automatic) E965.1
specified firearm NEC E965.4
Verey pistol E965.4
inflicted by other person
in accidental circumstances E922.9
hand gun (pistol) (revolver) E922.0
military firearm, except hand gun E922.3
hand gun (pistol) (revolver) E922.0
rifle (hunting) E922.2
military E922.3
shotgun (automatic) E922.1
specified firearm NEC E922.8
Verey pistol E922.8
stated as
intentional, homicidal E965.4
hand gun (pistol) (revolver) E965
military firearm, except hand gun E965.3
hand gun (pistol) (revolver) E965.0
paintball gun E965.4
rifle (hunting) E965.2
military E965.3
shotgun (automatic) E965.1
specified firearm E965.4
Verey pistol E965.4
undetermined whether accidental or intentional E985.4
air gun E985.6

ICD-9-CM

E Codes

Vol.

Shooting, shot *(Continued)*
  inflicted by other person *(Continued)*
    stated as *(Continued)*
      undetermined whether accidental or intentional *(Continued)*
        BB gun E985.6
        hand gun (pistol) (revolver) E985.0
        military firearm, except hand gun E985.3
          hand gun (pistol) (revolver) E985.0
        paintball gun E985.7
        rifle (hunting) E985.2
        shotgun (automatic) E985.1
        specified firearm NEC E985.4
        Verey pistol E985.4
  in
    terrorism - *see* Terrorism, shooting
    war operations - *see* War operations, shooting
  legal
    execution E978
    intervention E970
  military firearm, except hand gun E922.3
    hand gun (pistol) (revolver) E922.0
  paintball gun E922.5
  rifle (hunting) E922.2
    military E922.3
  self-inflicted (unspecified whether accidental or intentional) E985.4
    air gun E985.6
    BB gun E985.6
    hand gun (pistol) (revolver) E985.0
    military firearm, except hand gun E985.3
      hand gun (pistol) (revolver) E985.0
    paintball gun E985.7
    rifle (hunting) E985.2
      military E985.3
    shotgun (automatic) E985.1
    specified firearm NEC E985.4
    stated as
      accidental E922.9
        hand gun (pistol) (revolver) E922.0
        military firearm, except hand gun E922.3
          hand gun (pistol) (revolver) E922.0
        paintball gun 922.5
        rifle (hunting) E922.2
          military E922.3
        shotgun (automatic) E922.1
        specified firearm NEC E922.8
        Verey pistol E922.8
      intentional, purposeful E955.4
        hand gun (pistol) (revolver) E955.0
        military firearm, except hand gun E955.3
          hand gun (pistol) (revolver) E955.0
        paintball gun E955.7
        rifle (hunting) E955.2
          military E955.3
        shotgun (automatic) E955.1
        specified firearm NEC E955.4
        Verey pistol E955.4
  shotgun (automatic) E922.1
  specified firearm NEC E922.8
  stated as undetermined whether accidental or intentional E985.4

Shooting, shot *(Continued)*
  stated as undetermined whether accidental or intentional *(Continued)*
    hand gun (pistol) (revolver) E985.0
    military firearm, except hand gun E985.3
      hand gun (pistol) (revolver) E985.0
    paintball gun E985.7
    rifle (hunting) E985.2
      military E985.3
    shotgun (automatic) E985.1
    specified firearm NEC E985.4
    Verey pistol E985.4
  suicidal (attempt) E955.4
    air gun E985.6
    BB gun E985.6
    hand gun (pistol) (revolver) E955.0
    military firearm, except hand gun E955.3
      hand gun (pistol) (revolver) E955.0
    paintball gun E955.7
    rifle (hunting) E955.2
      military E955.3
    shotgun (automatic) E955.1
    specified firearm NEC E955.4
    Verey pistol E955.4
  Verey pistol E922.8
Shoving (accidentally) by other person (*see also* Pushing by other person) E917.9
Sickness
  air E903
  alpine E902.0
  car E903
  motion E903
  mountain E902.0
  sea E903
  travel E903
Sinking (accidental)
  boat, ship, watercraft (causing drowning, submersion) E830
    causing injury except drowning, submersion E831
Siriasis E900.0
Skydiving E844
Slashed wrists (*see also* Cut, self-inflicted) E986
Slipping (accidental)
  on
    deck (of boat, ship, watercraft) (icy) (oily) (wet) E835
    ice E885.9
    ladder of ship E833
      due to accident to watercraft E831
    mud E885.9
    oil E885.9
    snow E885.9
    stairs of ship E833
      due to accident to watercraft E831
    surface
      slippery E885.9
      wet E885.9
Sliver, wood, injury by E920.8
Smothering, smothered (*see also* Suffocation) E913.9
Smouldering building or structure in terrorism E979.3
Sodomy (assault) E960.1
Solid substance in eye (any part) or adnexa E914
Sound waves (causing injury) E928.1
Splinter, injury by E920.8
Stab, stabbing E966
  accidental - *see* Cut

Starvation E904.1
  helpless person, infant, newborn - *see* Lack of food
  homicidal intent E968.4
  late effect of NEC E929.5
  resulting from accident connected with transport - *see* categories E800-E848
Stepped on
  by
    animal (not being ridden) E906.8
      being ridden (in sport or transport) E828
    crowd E917.1
    person E917.9
      in sports E917.0
  in sports E917.0
Stepping on
  object (moving) E917.9
    in sports E917.0
      with subsequent fall E917.5
    stationary E917.4
      with subsequent fall E917.8
  person E917.9
    as, or caused by a crowd E917.1
      with subsequent fall E917.6
    in sports E917.0
Sting E905.9
  ant E905.5
  bee E905.3
  caterpillar E905.5
  coral E905.6
  hornet E905.3
  insect NEC E905.5
  jelly fish E905.6
  marine animal or plant E905.6
  nematocysts E905.6
  scorpion E905.2
  sea anemone E905.6
  sea cucumber E905.6
  wasp E905.3
  yellow jacket E905.3
Storm E908.9
  specified type NEC E908.8
Straining, injury in E927
Strangling - *see* Suffocation
Strangulation - *see* Suffocation
Strenuous movements (in recreational or other activities) E927
Striking against
  bottom (when jumping or diving into water) E883.0
  object (moving) E917.9
    caused by crowd E917.1
      with subsequent fall E917.6
    furniture E917.3
      with subsequent fall E917.7
    in
      running water E917.2
        with drowning or submersion - *see* Submersion
      sports E917.0
        with subsequent fall E917.5
    stationary E917.4
      with subsequent fall E917.8
  person(s) E917.9
    with fall E886.9
      in sports E886.0
    as, or caused by, a crowd E917.1
      with subsequent fall E917.6
    in sports E917.0
      with fall E886.0
Stroke
  heat - *see* Heat
  lightning E907

Struck by - *see also* Hit by
  bullet
    in
      terrorism E979.4
      war operations E991.2
        rubber E991.0
  lightning E907
  missile
    in terrorism - *see* Terrorism, missile
  object
    falling
      from, in, on
        building
          burning (uncontrolled fire)
            in terrorism E979.3
  thunderbolt E907
Stumbling over animal, carpet, curb, rug or (small) object (with fall) E885.9
  without fall - *see* Striking against, object
Submersion (accidental) E910.8
  boat, ship, watercraft (causing drowning, submersion) E830
    causing injury except drowning, submersion E831
  by other person
    in accidental circumstances - *see* category E910
    intentional, homicidal E964
    stated as undetermined whether accidental or intentional E984
  due to
    accident
      machinery - *see* Accident, machine
      to boat, ship, watercraft E830
      transport - *see* categories E800-E848
    avalanche E909.2
    cataclysmic
      earth surface movement or eruption E909.9
      storm E908.9
    cloudburst E908.8
    cyclone E908.1
    fall
      from
        boat, ship, watercraft (not involved in accident) E832
        burning, crushed E830
        involved in accident, collision E830
        gangplank (into water) E832
      overboard NEC E832
    flood E908.2
    hurricane E908.0
    jumping into water E910.8
      from boat, ship, watercraft
        burning, crushed, sinking E830
        involved in accident, collision E830
        not involved in accident, for swim E910.2
      in recreational activity (without diving equipment) E910.2
        with or using diving equipment E910.1
      to rescue another person E910.3
  homicide (attempt) E964
  in
    bathtub E910.4
    specified activity, not sport, transport or recreational E910.3
    sport or recreational activity (without diving equipment) E910.2

Submersion (*Continued*)
  in (*Continued*)
    sport or recreational activity (*Continued*)
      with or using diving equipment E910.1
      water skiing E910.0
    swimming pool NEC E910.8
    terrorism E979.8
    war operations E995
    water transport E832
      due to accident to boat, ship, watercraft E830
  landslide E909.2
  overturning boat, ship, watercraft E909.2
  sinking boat, ship, watercraft E909.2
  submersion boat, ship, watercraft E909.2
  tidal wave E909.4
    caused by storm E908.0
  torrential rain E908.2
  late effect of NEC E929.8
  quenching tank E910.8
  self-inflicted (unspecified whether accidental or intentional) E984
    in accidental circumstances - *see* category E910
    stated as intentional, purposeful E954
  stated as undetermined whether accidental or intentional E984
  suicidal (attempted) E954
  while
    attempting rescue of another person E910.3
    engaged in
      marine salvage E910.3
      underwater construction or repairs E910.3
    fishing, not from boat E910.2
    hunting, not from boat E910.2
    ice skating E910.2
    pearl diving E910.3
    placing fishing nets E910.3
    playing in water E910.2
    scuba diving E910.1
      nonrecreational E910.3
    skin diving E910.1
    snorkel diving E910.2
    spear fishing underwater E910.1
    surfboarding E910.2
    swimming (swimming pool) E910.2
    wading (in water) E910.2
    water skiing E910.0
Sucked
  into
    jet (aircraft) E844
Suffocation (accidental) (by external means) (by pressure) (mechanical) E913.9
  caused by other person
    in accidental circumstances - *see* category E913
    stated as
      intentional, homicidal E963
      undetermined whether accidental or intentional E983.9
        by, in
          hanging E983.0
          plastic bag E983.1
          specified means NEC E983.8
  due to, by
    avalanche E909.2
    bedclothes E913.0

Suffocation (*Continued*)
  due to, by (*Continued*)
    bib E913.0
    blanket E913.0
    cave-in E913.3
      caused by cataclysmic earth surface movement or eruption E909.9
    conflagration - *see* Conflagration
    explosion - *see* Explosion
    falling earth, other substance E913.3
    fire - *see* Fire
    food, any type (ingestion) (inhalation) (regurgitated) (vomited) E911
    foreign body, except food (ingestion) (inhalation) E912
    ignition - *see* Ignition
    landslide E909.2
    machine(ry) - *see* Accident, machine
    material object except food entering by nose or mouth, ingested, inhaled E912
    mucus (aspiration) (inhalation), not of newborn E912
    phlegm (aspiration) (inhalation) E912
    pillow E913.0
    plastic bag - *see* Suffocation, in, plastic bag
    sheet (plastic) E913.0
    specified means NEC E913.8
    vomitus (aspiration) (inhalation) E911
  homicidal (attempt) E963
  in
    airtight enclosed place E913.2
    baby carriage E913.0
    bed E913.0
    closed place E913.2
    cot, cradle E913.0
    perambulator E913.0
    plastic bag (in accidental circumstances) E913.1
      homicidal, purposely inflicted by other person E963
      self-inflicted (unspecified whether accidental or intentional) E983.1
        in accidental circumstances E913.1
        intentional, suicidal E953.1
      stated as undetermined whether accidentally or purposely inflicted E983.1
      suicidal, purposely self-inflicted E953.1
    refrigerator E913.2
  self-inflicted - *see also* Suffocation, stated as undetermined whether accidental or intentional E953.9
    in accidental circumstances - *see* category E913
    stated as intentional, purposeful - *see* Suicide, suffocation
  stated as undetermined whether accidental or intentional E983.9
    by, in
      hanging E983.0
      plastic bag E983.1
      specified means NEC E983.8
  suicidal - *see* Suicide, suffocation
Suicide, suicidal (attempted) (by) E958.9
  burning, burns E958.1

Suicide, suicidal (Continued)
  caustic substance E958.7
    poisoning E950.7
    swallowed E950.7
  cold, extreme E958.3
  cut (any part of body) E956
  cutting or piercing instrument (classifiable to E920) E956
  drowning E954
  electrocution E958.4
  explosive(s) (classifiable to E923) E955.5
  fire E958.1
  firearm (classifiable to E922) - *see* Shooting, suicidal
  hanging E953.0
  jumping
    before moving object, train, vehicle E958.0
    from high place - *see* Jumping, from, high place, stated as, suicidal
  knife E956
  late effect of E959
  motor vehicle, crashing of E958.5
  poisoning - *see* Table of Drugs and Chemicals
  puncture (any part of body) E956
  scald E958.2
  shooting - *see* Shooting, suicidal
  specified means NEC E958.8
  stab (any part of body) E956
  strangulation - *see* Suicide, suffocation
  submersion E954
  suffocation E953.9
    by, in
      hanging E953.0
      plastic bag E953.1
      specified means NEC E953.8
  wound NEC E958.9
Sunburn E926.2
Sunstroke E900.0
Supersonic waves (causing injury) E928.1
Surgical procedure, complication of
  delayed or as an abnormal reaction without mention of misadventure, *see* Reaction, abnormal
  due to or as a result of misadventure - *see* Misadventure
Swallowed, swallowing
  foreign body - *see* Foreign body, alimentary canal
  poison - *see* Table of Drugs and Chemicals
  substance
    caustic - *see* Table of Drugs and Chemicals
    corrosive - *see* Table of Drugs and Chemicals
    poisonous - *see* Table of Drugs and Chemicals
Swimmers' cramp (*see also* category E910) E910.2
  not in recreation or sport E910.3
Syndrome, battered
  baby or child - *see* Abuse, child
  wife - *see* Assault

T

Tackle in sport E886.0
Terrorism (injury) (by) (in) E979.8
  air blast E979.2

Terrorism (Continued)
  aircraft burned, destroyed, exploded, shot down E979.1
    used as a weapon E979.1
  anthrax E979.6
  asphyxia from
    chemical (weapons) E979.7
    fire, conflagration (caused by fire-producing device) E979.3
      from nuclear explosion E979.5
    gas or fumes E979.7
  bayonet E979.8
  biological agents E979.6
  blast (air) (effects) E979.2
    from nuclear explosion E979.5
    underwater E979.0
  bomb (antipersonnel) (mortar) (explosion) (fragments) E979.2
  bullet(s) (from carbine, machine gun, pistol, rifle, shotgun) E979.4
  burn from
    chemical E979.7
    fire, conflagration (caused by fire-producing device) E979.3
      from nuclear explosion E979.5
    gas E979.7
  burning aircraft E979.1
  chemical E979.7
  cholera E979.6
  conflagration E979.3
  crushed by falling aircraft E979.1
  depth-charge E979.0
  destruction of aircraft E979.1
  disability, as sequelae one year or more after injury E999.1
  drowning E979.8
  effect
    of nuclear weapon (direct) (secondary) E979.5
    secondary NEC E979.9
    sequelae E999.1
  explosion (artillery shell) (breech-block) (cannon block) E979.2
    aircraft E979.1
    bomb (antipersonnel) (mortar) E979.2
      nuclear (atom) (hydrogen) E979.5
    depth-charge E979.0
    grenade E979.2
    injury by fragments from E979.2
    land-mine E979.2
    marine weapon E979.0
    mine (land) E979.2
      at sea or in harbor E979.0
      marine E979.0
    missile (explosive) NEC E979.2
    munitions (dump) (factory) E979.2
    nuclear (weapon) E979.5
      other direct or secondary effects of E979.5
    sea-based artillery shell E979.0
    torpedo E979.0
  exposure to ionizing radiation from nuclear explosion E979.5
  falling aircraft E979.1
  fire or fire-producing device E979.3
  firearms E979.4
  fireball effects from nuclear explosion E979.5
  fragments from artillery shell, bomb NEC, grenade, guided missile, land-mine, rocket, shell, shrapnel E979.2
  gas or fumes E979.7

Terrorism (Continued)
  grenade (explosion) (fragments) E979.2
  guided missile (explosion) (fragments) E979.2
    nuclear E979.5
  heat from nuclear explosion E979.5
  hot substances E979.3
  hydrogen cyanide E979.7
  land-mine (explosion) (fragments) E979.2
  laser(s) E979.8
  late effect of E999.1
  lewisite E979.9
  lung irritant (chemical) (fumes) (gas) E979.7
  marine mine E979.0
  mine E979.2
    at sea E979.0
    in harbor E979.0
    land (explosion) (fragments) E979.2
    marine E979.0
  missile (explosion) (fragments) (guided) E979.2
    marine E979.0
    nuclear E979.5
  mortar bomb (explosion) (fragments) (guided) E979.2
  mustard gas E979.7
  nerve gas E979.7
  nuclear weapons E979.5
  pellets (shotgun) E979.4
  petrol bomb E979.3
  piercing object E979.8
  phosgene E979.7
  poisoning (chemical) (fumes) (gas) E979.7
  radiation, ionizing from nuclear explosion E979.5
  rocket (explosion) (fragments) E979.2
  saber, sabre E979.8
  sarin E979.7
  screening smoke E979.7
  sequelae effect (of) E999.1
  shell (aircraft) (artillery) (cannon) (land-based) (explosion) (fragments) E979.2
    sea-based E979.0
  shooting E979.4
    bullet(s) E979.4
    pellet(s) (rifle) (shotgun) E979.4
  shrapnel E979.2
  smallpox E979.7
  stabbing object(s) E979.8
  submersion E979.8
  torpedo E979.0
  underwater blast E979.0
  vesicant (chemical) (fumes) (gas) E979.7
  weapon burst E979.2
Thermic fever E900.9
Thermoplegia E900.9
Thirst - *see also* Lack of water
  resulting from accident connected with transport - *see* categories E800-E848
Thrown (accidentally)
  against object in or part of vehicle
    by motion of vehicle
      aircraft E844
      boat, ship, watercraft E838
      motor vehicle (on public highway) E818
        not on public highway E825

◀ **New**   ⬰ **Revised**

Thrown (*Continued*)
  against object in or part of vehicle by motion of vehicle (*Continued*)
    by motion of vehicle (*Continued*)
      motor vehicle (*Continued*)
        off-road type (not on public highway) E821
          on public highway E818
        snow vehicle E820
          on public highway E818
      nonmotor road vehicle NEC E829
      railway rolling stock, train, vehicle E806
      street car E829
  from
    animal (being ridden) (in sport or transport) E828
    high place, homicide (attempt) E968.1
    machinery - *see* Accident, machine
    vehicle NEC - *see* Accident, vehicle NEC
  off - *see* Thrown, from
  overboard (by motion of boat, ship, watercraft) E832
    by accident to boat, ship, watercraft E830
Thunderbolt NEC E907
Tidal wave (any injury) E909.4
  caused by storm E908.0
Took
  overdose of drug - *see* Table of Drugs and Chemicals
  poison - *see* Table of Drugs and Chemicals
Tornado (any injury) E908.1
Torrential rain (any injury) E908.2
Traffic accident NEC E819
Trampled by animal E906.8
  being ridden (in sport or transport) E828
Trapped (accidentally)
  between
    objects (moving) (stationary and moving) E918
  by
    door of
      elevator E918
      motor vehicle (on public highway) (while alighting, boarding) - *see* Fall, from, motor vehicle, while alighting
    railway train (underground) E806
    street car E829
    subway train E806
  in object E918
Travel (effects) E903
  sickness E903
Tree
  falling on or hitting E916
    motor vehicle (in motion) (on public highway) E818
      not on public highway E825
    nonmotor road vehicle NEC E829
    pedal cycle E826
    person E916
    railway rolling stock, train, vehicle E806
    street car E829
Trench foot E901.0
Tripping over animal, carpet, curb, rug, or small object (with fall) E885.9
  without fall - *see* Striking against, object
Tsunami E909.4
Twisting, Injury in E927

V

Violence, nonaccidental (*see also* Assault) E968.9
Volcanic eruption (any injury) E909.1
Vomitus in air passages (with asphyxia, obstruction or suffocation) E911

W

War operations (during hostilities) (injury) (by) (in) E995
  after cessation of hostilities, injury due to E998
  air blast E993
  aircraft burned, destroyed, exploded, shot down E994
  asphyxia from
    chemical E997.2
    fire, conflagration (caused by fire-producing device or conventional weapon) E990.9
      from nuclear explosion E996
      petrol bomb E990.0
    fumes E997.2
    gas E997.2
  battle wound NEC E995
  bayonet E995
  biological warfare agents E997.1
  blast (air) (effects) E993
    from nuclear explosion E996
    underwater E992
  bomb (mortar) (explosion) E993
    after cessation of hostilities E998
    fragments, injury by E991.9
      antipersonnel E991.3
  bullet(s) (from carbine, machine gun, pistol, rifle, shotgun) E991.2
    rubber E991.0
  burn from
    chemical E997.2
    fire, conflagration (caused by fire-producing device or conventional weapon) E990.9
      from nuclear explosion E996
      petrol bomb E990.0
    gas E997.2
  burning aircraft E994
  chemical E997.2
  chlorine E997.2
  conventional warfare, specified form NEC E995
  crushing by falling aircraft E994
  depth charge E992
  destruction of aircraft E994
  disability as sequela one year or more after injury E999.0
  drowning E995
  effect (direct) (secondary) of nuclear weapon E996
  explosion (artillery shell) (breech block) (cannon shell) E993
    after cessation of hostilities of bomb, mine placed in war E998
    aircraft E994
    bomb (mortar) E993
      atom E996
      hydrogen E996
      injury by fragments from E991.9
        antipersonnel E991.3
      nuclear E996
    depth charge E992

War operations (*Continued*)
  explosion (*Continued*)
    injury by fragments from E991.9
      antipersonnel E991.3
    marine weapon E992
    mine
      at sea or in harbor E992
      land E993
        injury by fragments from E991.9
      marine E992
    munitions (accidental) (being used in war) (dump) (factory) E993
    nuclear (weapon) E996
    own weapons (accidental) E993
      injury by fragments from E991.9
        antipersonnel E991.3
    sea-based artillery shell E992
    torpedo E992
  exposure to ionizing radiation from nuclear explosion E996
  falling aircraft E994
  fire or fire-producing device E990.9
    petrol bomb E990.0
  fireball effects from nuclear explosion E996
  fragments from
    antipersonnel bomb E991.3
    artillery shell, bomb NEC, grenade, guided missile, land mine, rocket, shell, shrapnel E991.9
  fumes E997.2
  gas E997.2
  grenade (explosion) E993
    fragments, injury by E991.9
  guided missile (explosion) E993
    fragments, injury by E991.9
    nuclear E996
  heat from nuclear explosion E996
  injury due to, but occurring after cessation of hostilities E998
  lacrimator (gas) (chemical) E997.2
  land mine (explosion) E993
    after cessation of hostilities E998
    fragments, injury by E991.9
  laser(s) E997.0
  late effect of E999.0
  lewisite E997.2
  lung irritant (chemical) (fumes) (gas) E997.2
  marine mine E992
  mine
    after cessation of hostilities E998
    at sea E992
    in harbor E992
    land (explosion) E993
      fragments, injury by E991.9
    marine E992
  missile (guided) (explosion) E993
    fragments, injury by E991.9
    marine E992
    nuclear E996
  mortar bomb (explosion) E993
    fragments, injury by E991.9
  mustard gas E997.2
  nerve gas E997.2
  phosgene E997.2
  poisoning (chemical) (fumes) (gas) E997.2
  radiation, ionizing from nuclear explosion E996
  rocket (explosion) E993
    fragments, injury by E991.9
  saber, sabre E995
  screening smoke E997.8

ICD-9-CM

E Codes

Vol. 2

War operations *(Continued)*
  shell (aircraft) (artillery) (cannon) (land
      based) (explosion) E993
    fragments, injury by E991.9
    sea-based E992
  shooting E991.2
    after cessation of hostilities E998
    bullet(s) E991.2
      rubber E991.0
    pellet(s) (rifle) E991.1
    shrapnel E991.9
    submersion E995
    torpedo E992
    unconventional warfare, except by
        nuclear weapon E997.9
      biological (warfare) E997.1
      gas, fumes, chemicals E997.2

War operations *(Continued)*
    laser(s) E997.0
      specified type NEC E997.8
    underwater blast E992
    vesicant (chemical) (fumes) (gas)
        E997.2
    weapon burst E993
Washed
  away by flood - *see* Flood
  away by tidal wave - *see* Tidal wave
  off road by storm (transport vehicle)
      E908.9
  overboard E832
Weather exposure - *see also* Exposure
  cold E901.0
  hot E900.0

Weightlessness (causing injury) (effects
    of) (in spacecraft, real or simulated)
    E928.0
Wound (accidental) NEC (*see also* Injury)
    E928.9
  battle (*see also* War operations)
      E995
  bayonet E920.3
    in
      legal intervention E974
      war operations E995
  gunshot - *see* Shooting
  incised - *see* Cut
  saber, sabre E920.3
    in war operations E995

◀ **New**   ◀▥ **Revised**

PART III

Diseases: Tabular List Volume 1

1.   INFECTIOUS AND PARASITIC DISEASES (001–139)

Note: Categories for "late effects" of infectious and parasitic diseases are to be found at 137–139.

Includes: diseases generally recognized as communicable or transmissible as well as a few diseases of unknown but possibly infectious origin

Excludes   *acute respiratory infections (460–466)*
carrier or suspected carrier of infectious organism (V02.0–V02.9)
certain localized infections
influenza (487.0–487.8)

INTESTINAL INFECTIOUS DISEASES (001–009)

Excludes   *helminthiases (120.0–129)*

● **001   Cholera**

   001.0   Due to Vibrio cholerae

   001.1   Due to Vibrio cholerae el tor

   ❑ **001.9   Cholera, unspecified**

● **002   Typhoid and paratyphoid fevers**

   002.0   Typhoid fever
      Typhoid (fever) (infection) [any site]

   002.1   Paratyphoid fever A

   002.2   Paratyphoid fever B

   002.3   Paratyphoid fever C

   ❑ **002.9   Paratyphoid fever, unspecified**

● **003   Other salmonella infections**

   Includes: infection or food poisoning by Salmonella [any serotype]

   003.0   Salmonella gastroenteritis
      Salmonellosis

   003.1   Salmonella septicemia

● **003.2   Localized salmonella infections**

   ❑ **003.20   Localized salmonella infection, unspecified**

   003.21   Salmonella meningitis

   003.22   Salmonella pneumonia

   003.23   Salmonella arthritis

   003.24   Salmonella osteomyelitis

   ❑ **003.29   Other**

❑ **003.8   Other specified salmonella infections**

❑ **003.9   Salmonella infection, unspecified**

● **004   Shigellosis**

   Includes: bacillary dysentery

   004.0   Shigella dysenteriae
      Infection by group A Shigella (Schmitz) (Shiga)

   004.1   Shigella flexneri
      Infection by group B Shigella

   004.2   Shigella boydii
      Infection by group C Shigella

   004.3   Shigella sonnei
      Infection by group D Shigella

   ❑ **004.8   Other specified shigella infections**

   ❑ **004.9   Shigellosis, unspecified**

● **005   Other food poisoning (bacterial)**

   Excludes   *salmonella infections (003.0–003.9)*
toxic effect of:
food contaminants (989.7)
noxious foodstuffs (988.0–988.9)

   005.0   Staphylococcal food poisoning
      Staphylococcal toxemia specified as due to food

   005.1   Botulism
      Food poisoning due to Clostridium botulinum

   005.2   Food poisoning due to Clostridium perfringens [C. welchii]
      Enteritis necroticans

005.3   **Food poisoning due to other Clostridia**

005.4   **Food poisoning due to Vibrio parahaemolyticus**

● 005.8   **Other bacterial food poisoning**

    Excludes   *salmonella food poisoning (003.0–003.9)*

      005.81   **Food poisoning due to Vibrio vulnificus**

      ❏ 005.89   **Other bacterial food poisoning**
                Food poisoning due to Bacillus cereus

❏ 005.9   **Food poisoning, unspecified**

● 006   **Amebiasis**

    Includes: infection due to Entamoeba histolytica

    Excludes   *amebiasis due to organisms other than Ent-amoeba histolytica (007.8)*

006.0   **Acute amebic dysentery without mention of ab-scess**
       Acute amebiasis

006.1   **Chronic intestinal amebiasis without mention of abscess**
       Chronic:
         amebiasis
         amebic dysentery

006.2   **Amebic nondysenteric colitis**

006.3   **Amebic liver abscess**
       Hepatic amebiasis

006.4   **Amebic lung abscess**
       Amebic abscess of lung (and liver)

006.5   **Amebic brain abscess**
       Amebic abscess of brain (and liver) (and lung)

006.6   **Amebic skin ulceration**
       Cutaneous amebiasis

❏ 006.8   **Amebic infection of other sites**
       Amebic:
         appendicitis
         balanitis
         Ameboma

    Excludes   *specific infections by free-living amebae (136.2)*

❏ 006.9   **Amebiasis, unspecified**
       Amebiasis NOS

● 007   **Other protozoal intestinal diseases**

    Includes: protozoal:
          colitis
          diarrhea
          dysentery

007.0   **Balantidiasis**
       Infection by Balantidium coli

007.1   **Giardiasis**
       Infection by Giardia lamblia
       Lambliasis

007.2   **Coccidiosis**
       Infection by Isospora belli and Isospora hominis
       Isosporiasis

007.3   **Intestinal trichomoniasis**

007.4   **Cryptosporidiosis**

007.5   **Cyclosporiasis**

❏ 007.8   **Other specified protozoal intestinal diseases**
       Amebiasis due to organisms other than Ent-amoeba histolytica

❏ 007.9   **Unspecified protozoal intestinal disease**
       Flagellate diarrhea
       Protozoal dysentery NOS

Figure 1–1   *E. coli* particles.

Item 1–1   ***Escherichia coli [E. coli]*** **is a gram-negative bacterium found in the intestinal tracts of humans and animals and is usually nonpathogenic. Pathogenic strains can cause diarrhea or pyogenic (pus-producing) infections.**

● 008   **Intestinal infections due to other organisms**

    Includes: any condition classifiable to 009.0–009.3 with mention of the responsible organisms

    Excludes   *food poisoning by these organisms (005.0–005.9)*

● 008.0   **Escherichia coli [E. coli]**

      ❏ 008.00   **E. coli, unspecified**
              E. coli enteritis NOS

      008.01   **Enteropathogenic E. coli**

      008.02   **Enterotoxigenic E. coli**

      008.03   **Enteroinvasive E. coli**

      008.04   **Enterohemorrhagic E. coli**

      ❏ 008.09   **Other intestinal E. coli infections**

008.1   **Arizona group of paracolon bacilli**

008.2   **Aerobacter aerogenes**
       Enterobacter aerogenes

008.3   **Proteus (mirabilis) (morganii)**

● 008.4   **Other specified bacteria**

      008.41   **Staphylococcus**
              Staphylococcal enterocolitis

      008.42   **Pseudomonas**

      008.43   **Campylobacter**

      008.44   **Yersinia enterocolitica**

      008.45   **Clostridium difficile**
              Pseudomembranous colitis

      ❏ 008.46   **Other anaerobes**
              Anaerobic enteritis NOS
              Bacteroides (fragilis)
              Gram-negative anaerobes   ◀▦

      ❏ 008.47   **Other gram-negative bacteria**
              Gram-negative enteritis NOS

    Excludes   *gram-negative anaerobes (008.46)*

      ❏ 008.49   **Other**

❏ 008.5   **Bacterial enteritis, unspecified**

● **008.6 Enteritis due to specified virus**

   008.61 Rotavirus

   008.62 Adenovirus

   008.63 Norwalk virus
      Norwalk-like agent

☐ **008.64 Other small round viruses [SRVs]**
      Small round virus NOS

   008.65 Calcivirus

   008.66 Astrovirus

   008.67 Enterovirus NEC
      Coxsackie virus
      Echovirus

  Excludes | *poliovirus (045.0–045.9)*

☐ **008.69 Other viral enteritis**
      Torovirus

☐ **008.8 Other organism, not elsewhere classified**
    Viral:
      enteritis NOS
      gastroenteritis

  Excludes | *influenza with involvement of gastrointestinal*
      tract (487.8)

● **009 Ill-defined intestinal infections**

  Excludes | *diarrheal disease or intestinal infection due to*
     specified organism (001.0–008.8)
    diarrhea following gastrointestinal surgery
     (564.4)
    intestinal malabsorption (579.0–579.9)
    ischemic enteritis (557.0–557.9)
    other noninfectious gastroenteritis and colitis
     (558.1–558.9)
    regional enteritis (555.0–555.9)
    ulcerative colitis (556)

009.0 Infectious colitis, enteritis, and gastroenteritis
    Colitis (septic)
    Dysentery:
      NOS
      catarrhal
      hemorrhagic
    Enteritis (septic)
    Gastroenteritis (septic)

009.1 Colitis, enteritis, and gastroenteritis of presumed infectious origin

  Excludes | *colitis NOS (558.9)*
    enteritis NOS (558.9)
    gastroenteritis NOS (558.9)

009.2 Infectious diarrhea
    Diarrhea:
      dysenteric
      epidemic
    Infectious diarrheal disease NOS

009.3 Diarrhea of presumed infectious origin

  Excludes | *diarrhea NOS (787.91)*

ICD-9-CM
010-099
Vol. 1

Item 1–2 Tuberculosis is caused by the *Mycobacterium tuberculosis* organism. The first tuberculosis infection is called the **primary infection.** A **Ghon** lesion is the **initial lesion.** A **secondary lesion** occurs when the tubercle bacilli are carried to other areas.

TUBERCULOSIS (010–018)

Includes: infection by Mycobacterium tuberculosis (human) (bovine)

  Excludes | *congenital tuberculosis (771.2)*
    late effects of tuberculosis (137.0–137.4)

The following fifth-digit subclassification is for use with categories 010–018:

☐ **0** unspecified
  1 bacteriological or histological examination not done
  2 bacteriological or histological examination unknown (at present)
  3 tubercle bacilli found (in sputum) by microscopy
  4 tubercle bacilli not found (in sputum) by microscopy, but found by bacterial culture
  5 tubercle bacilli not found by bacteriological examination, but tuberculosis confirmed histologically
  6 tubercle bacilli not found by bacteriological or histological examination, but tuberculosis confirmed by other methods [inoculation of animals]

Figure 1–2 Far advanced bilateral pulmonary tuberculosis before and after 8 months of treatment with streptomycin, PAS, and isoniazid. (From Hinshaw HC, Garland LH: Diseases of the Chest, 2nd ed. Philadelphia, WB Saunders, 1963, p. 538.)

● **010   Primary tuberculous infection**

Requires fifth digit. See beginning of section 010–018 for codes and definitions.

  ● **010.0   Primary tuberculous infection**

     | Excludes | *nonspecific reaction to tuberculin skin test without active tuberculosis (795.5)*
                    positive PPD (795.5)
                    positive tuberculin skin test without active tuberculosis (795.5)

  ● **010.1   Tuberculous pleurisy in primary progressive tuberculosis**

  ● ❏ **010.8   Other primary progressive tuberculosis**

     | Excludes | *tuberculous erythema nodosum (017.1)*

  ● ❏ **010.9   Primary tuberculous infection, unspecified**

● **011   Pulmonary tuberculosis**

Requires fifth digit. See beginning of section 010–018 for codes and definitions.

Use additional code to identify any associated silicosis (502)

  ● **011.0   Tuberculosis of lung, infiltrative**

  ● **011.1   Tuberculosis of lung, nodular**

  ● **011.2   Tuberculosis of lung with cavitation**

  ● **011.3   Tuberculosis of bronchus**

     | Excludes | *isolated bronchial tuberculosis (012.2)*

  ● **011.4   Tuberculous fibrosis of lung**

  ● **011.5   Tuberculous bronchiectasis**

  ● **011.6   Tuberculous pneumonia [any form]**

  ● **011.7   Tuberculous pneumothorax**

  ● ❏ **011.8   Other specified pulmonary tuberculosis**

  ● ❏ **011.9   Pulmonary tuberculosis, unspecified**
     Respiratory tuberculosis NOS
     Tuberculosis of lung NOS

● **012   Other respiratory tuberculosis**

Requires fifth digit. See beginning of section 010–018 for codes and definitions.

     | Excludes | *respiratory tuberculosis, unspecified (011.9)*

  ● **012.0   Tuberculous pleurisy**
     Tuberculosis of pleura
     Tuberculous empyema
     Tuberculous hydrothorax

     | Excludes | *pleurisy with effusion without mention of cause (511.9)*
                    tuberculous pleurisy in primary progressive tuberculosis (010.1)

  ● **012.1   Tuberculosis of intrathoracic lymph nodes**
     Tuberculosis of lymph nodes:
       hilar
       mediastinal
       tracheobronchial
     Tuberculous tracheobronchial adenopathy

     | Excludes | *that specified as primary (010.0–010.9)*

  ● **012.2   Isolated tracheal or bronchial tuberculosis**

  ● **012.3   Tuberculous laryngitis**
     Tuberculosis of glottis

  ● ❏ **012.8   Other specified respiratory tuberculosis**
     Tuberculosis of:
       mediastinum
       nasopharynx
       nose (septum)
       sinus [any nasal]

● **013   Tuberculosis of meninges and central nervous system**

Requires fifth digit. See beginning of section 010–018 for codes and definitions.

  ● **013.0   Tuberculous meningitis**
     Tuberculosis of meninges (cerebral) (spinal)
     Tuberculous:
       leptomeningitis
       meningoencephalitis

     | Excludes | *tuberculoma of meninges (013.1)*

  ● **013.1   Tuberculoma of meninges**

  ● **013.2   Tuberculoma of brain**
     Tuberculosis of brain (current disease)

  ● **013.3   Tuberculous abscess of brain**

  ● **013.4   Tuberculoma of spinal cord**

  ● **013.5   Tuberculous abscess of spinal cord**

  ● **013.6   Tuberculous encephalitis or myelitis**

  ● ❏ **013.8   Other specified tuberculosis of central nervous system**

  ● ❏ **013.9   Unspecified tuberculosis of central nervous system**
     Tuberculosis of central nervous system NOS

● **014   Tuberculosis of intestines, peritoneum, and mesenteric glands**

Requires fifth digit. See beginning of section 010–018 for codes and definitions.

  ● **014.0   Tuberculous peritonitis**
     Tuberculous ascites

  ● ❏ **014.8   Other**
     Tuberculosis (of):
       anus
       intestine (large) (small)
       mesenteric glands
       rectum
       retroperitoneal (lymph nodes)
     Tuberculous enteritis

● **015   Tuberculosis of bones and joints**

Requires fifth digit. See beginning of section 010–018 for codes and definitions.

Use additional code to identify manifestation, as:
   tuberculous:
     arthropathy (711.4)
     necrosis of bone (730.8)
     osteitis (730.8)
     osteomyelitis (730.8)
     synovitis (727.01)
     tenosynovitis (727.01)

  ● **015.0   Vertebral column**
     Pott's disease
     Use additional code to identify manifestation, as:
       curvature of spine [Pott's] (737.4)
       kyphosis (737.4)
       spondylitis (720.81)

  ● **015.1   Hip**

  ● **015.2   Knee**

  ● **015.5   Limb bones**
     Tuberculous dactylitis

  ● **015.6   Mastoid**
     Tuberculous mastoiditis

  ● ❏ **015.7   Other specified bone**

  ● ❏ **015.8   Other specified joint**

  ● ❏ **015.9   Tuberculosis of unspecified bones and joints**

● 016 **Tuberculosis of genitourinary system**

Requires fifth digit. See beginning of section 010–018 for codes and definitions.

● 016.0 **Kidney**
Renal tuberculosis

Use additional code to identify manifestation, as:
tuberculous:
    nephropathy (583.81)
    pyelitis (590.81)
    pyelonephritis (590.81)

● 016.1 **Bladder**

● 016.2 **Ureter**

● ❑ 016.3 **Other urinary organs**

● 016.4 **Epididymis**

● ❑ 016.5 **Other male genital organs**
Use additional code to identify manifestation, as:
tuberculosis of:
    prostate (601.4)
    seminal vesicle (608.81)
    testis (608.81)

● 016.6 **Tuberculous oophoritis and salpingitis**

● ❑ 016.7 **Other female genital organs**
Tuberculous:
    cervicitis
    endometritis

● ❑ 016.9 **Genitourinary tuberculosis, unspecified**

● 017 **Tuberculosis of other organs**

Requires fifth digit. See beginning of section 010–018 for codes and definitions.

● 017.0 **Skin and subcutaneous cellular tissue**
Lupus: Tuberculosis:
  exedens   colliquativa
  vulgaris   cutis
  Scrofuloderma   lichenoides
                 papulonecrotica
                 verrucosa cutis

Excludes *lupus erythematosus (695.4)*
       disseminated (710.0)
    lupus NOS (710.0)
    nonspecific reaction to tuberculin skin test without active tuberculosis (795.5)
    positive PPD (795.5)
    positive tuberculin skin test without active tuberculosis (795.5)

● 017.1 **Erythema nodosum with hypersensitivity reaction in tuberculosis**
Bazin's disease
Erythema:
  induratum
  nodosum, tuberculous
Tuberculosis indurativa

Excludes *erythema nodosum NOS (695.2)*

● 017.2 **Peripheral lymph nodes**
Scrofula
Scrofulous abscess
Tuberculous adenitis

Excludes *tuberculosis of lymph nodes:*
    bronchial and mediastinal (012.1)
    mesenteric and retroperitoneal (014.8)
    tuberculous tracheobronchial adenopathy (012.1)

● 017.3 **Eye**
Use additional code to identify manifestation, as:
tuberculous:
    chorioretinitis, disseminated (363.13)
    episcleritis (379.09)
    interstitial keratitis (370.59)
    iridocyclitis, chronic (364.11)
    keratoconjunctivitis (phlyctenular) (370.31)

● 017.4 **Ear**
Tuberculosis of ear
Tuberculous otitis media

Excludes *tuberculous mastoiditis (015.6)*

● 017.5 **Thyroid gland**

● 017.6 **Adrenal glands**
Addison's disease, tuberculous

● 017.7 **Spleen**

● 017.8 **Esophagus**

● ❑ 017.9 **Other specified organs**
Use additional code to identify manifestation, as:
tuberculosis of:
    endocardium [any valve] (424.91)
    myocardium (422.0)
    pericardium (420.0)

● 018 **Miliary tuberculosis**

Requires fifth digit. See beginning of section 010–018 for codes and definitions.

Includes: tuberculosis:
    disseminated
    generalized
    miliary, whether of a single specified site, multiple sites, or unspecified site
    polyserositis

● 018.0 **Acute miliary tuberculosis**

● ❑ 018.8 **Other specified miliary tuberculosis**

● ❑ 018.9 **Miliary tuberculosis, unspecified**

ZOONOTIC BACTERIAL DISEASES (020–027)

● 020 **Plague**

Includes: infection by Yersinia [Pasteurella] pestis

020.0 **Bubonic**

020.1 **Cellulocutaneous**

020.2 **Septicemic**

020.3 **Primary pneumonic**

020.4 **Secondary pneumonic**

❑ 020.5 **Pneumonic, unspecified**

❑ 020.8 **Other specified types of plague**
Abortive plague
Ambulatory plague
Pestis minor

❑ 020.9 **Plague, unspecified**

● 021 **Tularemia**

Includes: deerfly fever
    infection by Francisella [Pasteurella] tularensis
    rabbit fever

021.0 **Ulceroglandular tularemia**

021.1 **Enteric tularemia**
Tularemia:
    cryptogenic
    intestinal
    typhoidal

021.2 **Pulmonary tularemia**
Bronchopneumonic tularemia

021.3 **Oculoglandular tularemia**

❑ 021.8 **Other specified tularemia**
Tularemia:
    generalized or disseminated
    glandular

❑ 021.9 **Unspecified tularemia**

ICD-9-CM

010-018

Vol. 1

Figure 1-3 Schematic summary of some major interactions between rickettsial organisms and their small animal hosts and arthropod vectors, the participation of domestic animals, and examples of the typical ambiance under which each rickettsial infection is contacted by humans. (From Strickland GT: Hunter's Tropical Medicine, 7th ed. Philadelphia, WB Saunders, 1991, p. 261. Courtesy of Dr. J. K. Frenkel, University of Kansas Medical Center, Kansas City, KS.)

● **022 Anthrax**

    022.0 Cutaneous anthrax
        Malignant pustule

    022.1 Pulmonary anthrax
        Respiratory anthrax
        Wool-sorters' disease

    022.2 Gastrointestinal anthrax

    022.3 Anthrax septicemia

    ☐**022.8 Other specified manifestations of anthrax**

    ☐**022.9 Anthrax, unspecified**

● **023 Brucellosis**

    Includes: fever:
        Malta
        Mediterranean
        undulant

    023.0 Brucella melitensis

    023.1 Brucella abortus

    023.2 Brucella suis

    023.3 Brucella canis

    ☐**023.8 Other brucellosis**
        Infection by more than one organism

    ☐**023.9 Brucellosis, unspecified**

    024 Glanders
        Infection by:
            Actinobacillus mallei
            Malleomyces mallei
            Pseudomonas mallei
            Farcy
            Malleus

    025 Melioidosis
        Infection by:
            Malleomyces pseudomallei
            Pseudomonas pseudomallei
            Whitmore's bacillus
        Pseudoglanders

● **026 Rat-bite fever**

    026.0 Spirillary fever
        Rat-bite fever due to Spirillum minor [S. minus]
        Sodoku

    026.1 Streptobacillary fever
        Epidemic arthritic erythema
        Haverhill fever
        Rat-bite fever due to Streptobacillus moniliformis

    ☐**026.9 Unspecified rat-bite fever**

● 027 Other zoonotic bacterial diseases

027.0 Listeriosis
Infection by Listeria monocytogenes
Septicemia by Listeria monocytogenes

Use additional code to identify manifestations, as meningitis (320.7)

Excludes congenital listeriosis (771.2)

027.1 Erysipelothrix infection
Erysipeloid (of Rosenbach)
Infection by Erysipelothrix insidiosa [E. rhusiopathiae]
Septicemia by Erysipelothrix insidiosa [E. rhusiopathiae]

027.2 Pasteurellosis
Pasteurella pseudotuberculosis infection by Pasteurella multocida [P. septica]
Mesenteric adenitis by Pasteurella multocida [P. septica]
Septic infection (cat bite) (dog bite) by Pasteurella multocida [P. septica]

Excludes infection by:
Francisella [Pasteurella] tularensis (021.0–021.9)
Yersinia [Pasteurella] pestis (020.0–020.9)

❏ 027.8 Other specified zoonotic bacterial diseases

❏ 027.9 Unspecified zoonotic bacterial disease

OTHER BACTERIAL DISEASES (030–041)

Excludes bacterial venereal diseases (098.0–099.9)
bartonellosis (088.0)

● 030 Leprosy

Includes: Hansen's disease
infection by Mycobacterium leprae

030.0 Lepromatous [type L]
Lepromatous leprosy (macular) (diffuse) (infiltrated) (nodular) (neuritic)

030.1 Tuberculoid [type T]
Tuberculoid leprosy (macular) (maculoanesthetic) (major) (minor) (neuritic)

030.2 Indeterminate [group I]
Indeterminate [uncharacteristic] leprosy (macular) (neuritic)

030.3 Borderline [group B]
Borderline or dimorphous leprosy (infiltrated) (neuritic)

❏ 030.8 Other specified leprosy

❏ 030.9 Leprosy, unspecified

● 031 Diseases due to other mycobacteria

031.0 Pulmonary
Battey disease
Infection by Mycobacterium:
avium
intracellulare [Battey bacillus]
kansasii

031.1 Cutaneous
Buruli ulcer
Infection by Mycobacterium:
marinum [M. balnei]
ulcerans

031.2 Disseminated
Disseminated mycobacterium avium-intracellulare complex (DMAC)
Mycobacterium avium-intracellulare complex (MAC) bacteremia

❏ 031.8 Other specified mycobacterial diseases

❏ 031.9 Unspecified diseases due to mycobacteria
Atypical mycobacterium infection NOS

● 032 Diphtheria

Includes: infection by Corynebacterium diphtheriae

032.0 Faucial diphtheria
Membranous angina, diphtheritic

032.1 Nasopharyngeal diphtheria

032.2 Anterior nasal diphtheria

032.3 Laryngeal diphtheria
Laryngotracheitis, diphtheritic

● 032.8 Other specified diphtheria

032.81 Conjunctival diphtheria
Pseudomembranous diphtheritic conjunctivitis

032.82 Diphtheritic myocarditis

032.83 Diphtheritic peritonitis

032.84 Diphtheritic cystitis

032.85 Cutaneous diphtheria

❏ 032.89 Other

❏ 032.9 Diphtheria, unspecified

● 033 Whooping cough

Includes: pertussis
Use additional code to identify any associated pneumonia (484.3)

033.0 Bordetella pertussis [B. pertussis]

033.1 Bordetella parapertussis [B. parapertussis]

❏ 033.8 Whooping cough due to other specified organism
Bordetella bronchiseptica [B. bronchiseptica]

❏ 033.9 Whooping cough, unspecified organism

● 034 Streptococcal sore throat and scarlet fever

034.0 Streptococcal sore throat
Septic:
angina
sore throat
Streptococcal:
angina
laryngitis
pharyngitis
tonsillitis

034.1 Scarlet fever
Scarlatina

Excludes parascarlatina (057.8)

035 Erysipelas
Excludes postpartum or puerperal erysipelas (670)

● 036 Meningococcal infection

036.0 Meningococcal meningitis
Cerebrospinal fever (meningococcal)
Meningitis:
cerebrospinal
epidemic

036.1 Meningococcal encephalitis

036.2 Meningococcemia
Meningococcal septicemia

036.3 Waterhouse-Friderichsen syndrome, meningococcal
Meningococcal hemorrhagic adrenalitis
Meningococcic adrenal syndrome
Waterhouse-Friderichsen syndrome NOS

ICD-9-CM

001–099

Vol. 1

● 036.4 **Meningococcal carditis**

   ❏ 036.40 **Meningococcal carditis, unspecified**

   036.41 **Meningococcal pericarditis**

   036.42 **Meningococcal endocarditis**

   036.43 **Meningococcal myocarditis**

● 036.8 **Other specified meningococcal infections**

   036.81 **Meningococcal optic neuritis**

   036.82 **Meningococcal arthropathy**

   ❏ 036.89 **Other**

   ❏ 036.9 **Meningococcal infection, unspecified**
   Meningococcal infection NOS

037 **Tetanus**

   Excludes tetanus:
   complicating:
   abortion (634–638 with .0, 639.0)
   ectopic or molar pregnancy (639.0)
   neonatorum (771.3)
   puerperal (670)

● 038 **Septicemia**

   Note: Use additional code for systemic inflammatory response syndrome (SIRS), 995.91-995.92

   Excludes bacteremia (790.7)
   septicemia (sepsis) of newborn (771.81)

   038.0 **Streptococcal septicemia**

● 038.1 **Staphylococcal septicemia**

   ❏ 038.10 **Staphylococcal septicemia, unspecified**

   038.11 **Staphylococcus aureus septicemia**

   ❏ 038.19 **Other staphylococcal septicemia**

   038.2 **Pneumococcal septicemia [Streptococcus pneumoniae septicemia]**

   038.3 **Septicemia due to anaerobes**
   Septicemia due to Bacteroides

   Excludes gas gangrene (040.0)
   that due to anaerobic streptococci (038.0)

● 038.4 **Septicemia due to other gram-negative organisms**

   ❏ 038.40 **Gram-negative organism, unspecified**
   Gram-negative septicemia NOS

   038.41 **Hemophilus influenzae [H. influenzae]**

   038.42 **Escherichia coli [E. coli]**

   038.43 **Pseudomonas**

   038.44 **Serratia**

   ❏ 038.49 **Other**

   ❏ 038.8 **Other specified septicemias**

   Excludes septicemia (due to):
   anthrax (022.3)
   gonococcal (098.89)
   herpetic (054.5)
   meningococcal (036.2)
   septicemic plague (020.2)

   ❏ 038.9 **Unspecified septicemia**
   Septicemia NOS

   Excludes bacteremia NOS (790.7)

● 039 **Actinomycotic infections**

   Includes: actinomycotic mycetoma
   infection by Actinomycetales, such as species
   of Actinomyces, Actinomadura, Nocardia,
   Streptomyces
   maduromycosis (actinomycotic)
   schizomycetoma (actinomycotic)

   039.0 **Cutaneous**
   Erythrasma
   Trichomycosis axillaris

   039.1 **Pulmonary**
   Thoracic actinomycosis

   039.2 **Abdominal**

   039.3 **Cervicofacial**

   039.4 **Madura foot**

   Excludes madura foot due to mycotic infection (117.4)

   ❏ 039.8 **Of other specified sites**

   ❏ 039.9 **Of unspecified site**
   Actinomycosis NOS
   Maduromycosis NOS
   Nocardiosis NOS

● 040 **Other bacterial diseases**

   Excludes bacteremia NOS (790.7)
   bacterial infection NOS (041.9)

   040.0 **Gas gangrene**
   Gas bacillus infection or gangrene
   Infection by Clostridium:
   histolyticum
   oedematiens
   perfringens [welchii]
   septicum
   sordellii
   Malignant edema
   Myonecrosis, clostridial
   Myositis, clostridial

   040.1 **Rhinoscleroma**

   040.2 **Whipple's disease**
   Intestinal lipodystrophy

   040.3 **Necrobacillosis**

● 040.8 **Other specified bacterial diseases**

   040.81 **Tropical pyomyositis**

   040.82 **Toxic shock syndrome**

   Use additional code to identify the organism

   ❏ 040.89 **Other**

● 041 **Bacterial infection in conditions classified elsewhere and
   of unspecified site**

   Note: This category is provided to be used as an additional
   code to identify the bacterial agent in diseases classified elsewhere. This category will also be used to classify bacterial infections of unspecified nature or site.

   Excludes bacteremia NOS (790.7)
   septicemia (038.0–038.9)

● 041.0 **Streptococcus**

   ❏ 041.00 **Streptococcus, unspecified**

   041.01 **Group A**

   041.02 **Group B**

   041.03 **Group C**

   041.04 **Group D [Enterococcus]**

   041.05 **Group G**

   ❏ 041.09 **Other Streptococcus**

● 041.1 **Staphylococcus**

   ❏ 041.10 **Staphylococcus, unspecified**

041.11   **Staphylococcus aureus**

041.19   **Other Staphylococcus**

041.2   **Pneumococcus**

041.3   **Friedländer's bacillus**
     Infection by Klebsiella pneumoniae

041.4   **Escherichia coli [E. coli]**

041.5   **Hemophilus influenzae [H. influenzae]**

041.6   **Proteus (mirabilis) (morganii)**

041.7   **Pseudomonas**

● 041.8   **Other specified bacterial infections**

     041.81   **Mycoplasma**
         Eaton's agent
         Pleuropneumonia-like organisms [PPLO]

     041.82   **Bacteroides fragilis** ◀▦

     041.83   **Clostridium perfringens**

     041.84   **Other anaerobes**
         Gram-negative anaerobes

     | **Excludes** | *Helicobacter pylori (041.86)* |

     041.85   **Other gram-negative organisms**
         Aerobacter aerogenes
         Gram-negative bacteria NOS
         Mima polymorpha
         Serratia

     | **Excludes** | *gram-negative anaerobes (041.84)* |

     041.86   **Helicobacter pylori (H. pylori)**

     041.89   **Other specified bacteria**

041.9   **Bacterial infection, unspecified**

Figure 1–3 Vesicular, pustular, scabby, and necrotic lesions in Kaposi's sarcoma. (From Debre R, Celers J: Clinical Virology—The Evaluation and Management of Human Viral Infections. Philadelphia, WB Saunders, 1970, p. 460.)

Item 1–3 AIDS (acquired immune deficiency syndrome) is caused by **HIV** (human immunodeficiency virus). HIV affects certain white blood cells (T-4 lymphocytes) and destroys the ability of the cells to fight infections, making patients susceptible to a host of infectious diseases, e.g., *Pneumocystis carinii* pneumonia (PCP), Kaposi's sarcoma, and **lymphoma. AIDS-related complex (ARC)** is an early stage of AIDS in which tests for HIV are positive but the symptoms are mild.

HUMAN IMMUNODEFICIENCY VIRUS (HIV) INFECTION (042)

042   **Human immunodeficiency virus [HIV] disease**
     Acquired immune deficiency syndrome
     Acquired immunodeficiency syndrome
     AIDS
     AIDS-like syndrome
     AIDS-related complex
     ARC
     HIV infection, symptomatic

Use additional code(s) to identify all manifestations of HIV

Use additional code to identify HIV-2 infection (079.53)

Excludes	*asymptomatic HIV infection status (V08)*
	exposure to HIV virus (V01.79)
	nonspecific serologic evidence of HIV (795.71)

◀▦   ICD-9-CM

009-100

Vol. 1

POLIOMYELITIS AND OTHER NON-ARTHROPOD-BORNE VIRAL DISEASES OF CENTRAL NERVOUS SYSTEM (045–049)

● 045   **Acute poliomyelitis**

     | **Excludes** | *late effects of acute poliomyelitis (138)* |

     The following fifth-digit subclassification is for use with category 045:
     0   **poliovirus, unspecified type**
     1   **poliovirus type I**
     2   **poliovirus type II**
     3   **poliovirus type III**

● 045.0   **Acute paralytic poliomyelitis specified as bulbar**
     Infantile paralysis (acute) specified as bulbar
     Poliomyelitis (acute) (anterior) specified as bulbar
     Polioencephalitis (acute) (bulbar)
     Polioencephalomyelitis (acute) (anterior) (bulbar)

● 045.1   **Acute poliomyelitis with other paralysis**
     Paralysis:
         acute atrophic, spinal
         infantile, paralytic
     Poliomyelitis (acute) with paralysis except bulbar
         anterior with paralysis except bulbar
         epidemic with paralysis except bulbar

● 045.2   **Acute nonparalytic poliomyelitis**
     Poliomyelitis (acute) specified as nonparalytic
         anterior specified as nonparalytic
         epidemic specified as nonparalytic

● 045.9   **Acute poliomyelitis, unspecified**
     Infantile paralysis unspecified whether paralytic or nonparalytic
     Poliomyelitis (acute) unspecified whether paralytic or nonparalytic
     anterior unspecified whether paralytic or nonparalytic
     epidemic unspecified whether paralytic or nonparalytic

● 046   **Slow virus infection of central nervous system**

     046.0   **Kuru**

     046.1   **Jakob-Creutzfeldt disease**
         Subacute spongiform encephalopathy

     046.2   **Subacute sclerosing panencephalitis**
         Dawson's inclusion body encephalitis
         Van Bogaert's sclerosing leukoencephalitis

     046.3   **Progressive multifocal leukoencephalopathy**
         Multifocal leukoencephalopathy NOS

     046.8   **Other specified slow virus infection of central nervous system**

     046.9   **Unspecified slow virus infection of central nervous system**

● 047   **Meningitis due to enterovirus**

    Includes: meningitis:
       abacterial
       aseptic
       viral

    | **Excludes** | *meningitis due to:*
       adenovirus (049.1)
       arthropod-borne virus (060.0–066.9)
       leptospira (100.81)
       virus of:
         herpes simplex (054.72)
         herpes zoster (053.0)
         lymphocytic choriomeningitis (049.0)
         mumps (072.1)
         poliomyelitis (045.0–045.9)
       any other infection specifically classified elsewhere

    047.0   Coxsackie virus

    047.1   ECHO virus
       Meningo-eruptive syndrome

    □ **047.8   Other specified viral meningitis**

    □ **047.9   Unspecified viral meningitis**
       Viral meningitis NOS

□ 048   **Other enterovirus diseases of central nervous system**
    Boston exanthem

● 049   **Other non-arthropod-borne viral diseases of central nervous system**

    | **Excludes** | *late effects of viral encephalitis (139.0)*

    049.0   Lymphocytic choriomeningitis
       Lymphocytic:
         meningitis (serous) (benign)
         meningoencephalitis (serous) (benign)

    049.1   Meningitis due to adenovirus

    □ **049.8   Other specified non-arthropod-borne viral diseases of central nervous system**
       Encephalitis:
         acute:
           inclusion body
           necrotizing
         epidemic
         lethargica
         Rio Bravo
       von Economo's disease

    □ **049.9   Unspecified non-arthropod-borne viral diseases of central nervous system**
       Viral encephalitis NOS

VIRAL DISEASES ACCOMPANIED BY EXANTHEM (050–057)

    | **Excludes** | *arthropod-borne viral diseases (060.0–066.9)*
       Boston exanthem (048)

● 050   **Smallpox**

    050.0   Variola major
       Hemorrhagic (pustular) smallpox
       Malignant smallpox
       Purpura variolosa

    050.1   Alastrim
       Variola minor

    050.2   Modified smallpox
       Varioloid

    □ **050.9   Smallpox, unspecified**

● 051   **Cowpox and paravaccinia**

    051.0   Cowpox
       Vaccinia not from vaccination

    | **Excludes** | *vaccinia (generalized) (from vaccination) (999.0)*

    051.1   Pseudocowpox
       Milkers' node

    051.2   Contagious pustular dermatitis
       Ecthyma contagiosum
       Orf

    □ **051.9   Paravaccinia, unspecified**

● 052   **Chickenpox**

    052.0   Postvaricella encephalitis
       Postchickenpox encephalitis

    052.1   Varicella (hemorrhagic) pneumonitis

    □ **052.7   With other specified complications**

    □ **052.8   With unspecified complication**

    052.9   Varicella without mention of complication
       Chickenpox NOS
       Varicella NOS

● 053   **Herpes zoster**

    Includes: shingles
       zona

    053.0   With meningitis

    ● **053.1   With other nervous system complications**

       □ **053.10   With unspecified nervous system complication**

       053.11   Geniculate herpes zoster
         Herpetic geniculate ganglionitis

       053.12   Postherpetic trigeminal neuralgia

       053.13   Postherpetic polyneuropathy

       □ **053.19   Other**

    ● **053.2   With ophthalmic complications**

       053.20   Herpes zoster dermatitis of eyelid
         Herpes zoster ophthalmicus

       053.21   Herpes zoster keratoconjunctivitis

       053.22   Herpes zoster iridocyclitis

       □ **053.29   Other**

Figure 1–5   Grouped outbursts of herpes vesicles on the face. (From Debre R, Celers J: Clinical Virology—The Evaluation and Management of Human Viral Infections. Philadelphia, WB Saunders, 1970, p. 460.)

Item 1-4 Herpes is a viral disease for which there is no cure. There are two types of the herpes simplex virus: Type I causes cold sores or fever blisters and Type II causes genital herpes. The virus can be spread from a sore on the lips to the genitals or from the genitals to the lips.

● 053.7 **With other specified complications**
  053.71 **Otitis externa due to herpes zoster**
 ❑053.79 **Other**

❑053.8 **With unspecified complication**

 053.9 **Herpes zoster without mention of complication**
  Herpes zoster NOS

● 054 **Herpes simplex**
 Excludes *congenital herpes simplex (771.2)*

 054.0 **Eczema herpeticum**
  Kaposi's varicelliform eruption

● 054.1 **Genital herpes**
 ❑054.10 **Genital herpes, unspecified**
  Herpes progenitalis
 054.11 **Herpetic vulvovaginitis**
 054.12 **Herpetic ulceration of vulva**
 054.13 **Herpetic infection of penis**
 ❑054.19 **Other**

 054.2 **Herpetic gingivostomatitis**

 054.3 **Herpetic meningoencephalitis**
  Herpes encephalitis
  Simian B disease

● 054.4 **With ophthalmic complications**
 ❑054.40 **With unspecified ophthalmic complication**
 054.41 **Herpes simplex dermatitis of eyelid**
 054.42 **Dendritic keratitis**
 054.43 **Herpes simplex disciform keratitis**
 054.44 **Herpes simplex iridocyclitis**
 ❑054.49 **Other**

 054.5 **Herpetic septicemia**

 054.6 **Herpetic whitlow**
  Herpetic felon

● 054.7 **With other specified complications**
 054.71 **Visceral herpes simplex**
 054.72 **Herpes simplex meningitis**
 054.73 **Herpes simplex otitis externa**
 ❑054.79 **Other**

❑054.8 **With unspecified complication**

 054.9 **Herpes simplex without mention of complication**

● 055 **Measles**
 Includes: morbilli
  rubeola

 055.0 **Postmeasles encephalitis**
 055.1 **Postmeasles pneumonia**
 055.2 **Postmeasles otitis media**

● 055.7 **With other specified complications**
 055.71 **Measles keratoconjunctivitis**
  Measles keratitis
 ❑055.79 **Other**

❑055.8 **With unspecified complication**

 055.9 **Measles without mention of complication**

● 056 **Rubella**
 Includes: German measles
 Excludes *congenital rubella (771.0)*

● 056.0 **With neurological complications**
 ❑056.00 **With unspecified neurological complication**
 056.01 **Encephalomyelitis due to rubella**
  Encephalitis due to rubella
  Meningoencephalitis due to rubella
 ❑056.09 **Other**

● 056.7 **With other specified complications**
 056.71 **Arthritis due to rubella**
 ❑056.79 **Other**

❑056.8 **With unspecified complications**

 056.9 **Rubella without mention of complication**

● 057 **Other viral exanthemata**
 057.0 **Erythema infectiosum [fifth disease]**
 ❑057.8 **Other specified viral exanthemata**
  Dukes (-Filatow) disease
  Exanthema subitum [sixth disease]
  Fourth disease
  Parascarlatina
  Pseudoscarlatina
  Roseola infantum
 ❑057.9 **Viral exanthem, unspecified**

ARTHROPOD-BORNE VIRAL DISEASES (060–066)

Use additional code to identify any associated meningitis (321.2)
 Excludes *late effects of viral encephalitis (139.0)*

● 060 **Yellow fever**
 060.0 **Sylvatic**
  Yellow fever:
   jungle
   sylvan
 060.1 **Urban**
 ❑060.9 **Yellow fever, unspecified**

 061 **Dengue**
  Breakbone fever
  Excludes *hemorrhagic fever caused by dengue virus (065.4)*

● 062 **Mosquito-borne viral encephalitis**
 062.0 **Japanese encephalitis**
  Japanese B encephalitis
 062.1 **Western equine encephalitis**
 062.2 **Eastern equine encephalitis**
  Excludes *Venezuelan equine encephalitis (066.2)*
 062.3 **St. Louis encephalitis**
 062.4 **Australian encephalitis**
  Australian arboencephalitis
  Australian X disease
  Murray Valley encephalitis
 062.5 **California virus encephalitis**
  Encephalitis:
   California
   La Crosse
   Tahyna fever

ICD-9-CM
060-100
Vol. 1

☐ **062.8 Other specified mosquito-borne viral encephalitis**
Encephalitis by Ilheus virus
Excludes *West Nile virus (066.40–066.49)* ◀▥

☐ **062.9 Mosquito-borne viral encephalitis, unspecified**

● **063 Tick-borne viral encephalitis**
Includes: diphasic meningoencephalitis

063.0 Russian spring-summer [taiga] encephalitis

063.1 Louping ill

063.2 Central European encephalitis

☐ **063.8 Other specified tick-borne viral encephalitis**
Langat encephalitis
Powassan encephalitis

☐ **063.9 Tick-borne viral encephalitis, unspecified**

064 Viral encephalitis transmitted by other and unspecified arthropods
Arthropod-borne viral encephalitis, vector unknown
Negishi virus encephalitis
Excludes *viral encephalitis NOS (049.9)*

● **065 Arthropod-borne hemorrhagic fever**

065.0 Crimean hemorrhagic fever [CHF Congo virus]
Central Asian hemorrhagic fever

065.1 Omsk hemorrhagic fever

065.2 Kyasanur Forest disease

☐ **065.3 Other tick-borne hemorrhagic fever**

065.4 Mosquito-borne hemorrhagic fever
Chikungunya hemorrhagic fever
Dengue hemorrhagic fever
Excludes *Chikungunya fever (066.3)*
dengue (061)
yellow fever (060.0–060.9)

☐ **065.8 Other specified arthropod-borne hemorrhagic fever**
Mite-borne hemorrhagic fever

☐ **065.9 Arthropod-borne hemorrhagic fever, unspecified**
Arbovirus hemorrhagic fever NOS

● **066 Other arthropod-borne viral diseases**

066.0 Phlebotomus fever
Changuinola fever
Sandfly fever

066.1 Tick-borne fever
Nairobi sheep disease
Tick fever:
American mountain
Colorado
Kemerovo
Quaranfil

066.2 Venezuelan equine fever
Venezuelan equine encephalitis

☐ **066.3 Other mosquito-borne fever**

Fever (viral):	Fever (viral):
Bunyamwera	Oropouche
Bwamba	Pixuna
Chikungunya	Rift valley
Guama	Ross river
Mayaro	Wesselsbron
Mucambo	Zika
O' Nyong-Nyong	

Excludes *dengue (061)*
yellow fever (060.0–060.9)

● **066.4 West Nile fever**

☐ **066.40 West Nile Fever, unspecified** ◀
West Nile fever NOS ◀
West Nile without complications ◀
West Nile virus NOS ◀

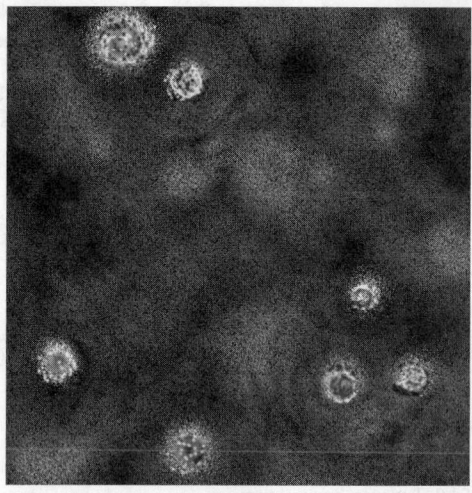

Figure 1–6   Hepatitis B virions (Dane particles).

Item 1–5 Hepatitis A (HAV) was formerly called epidemic, infectious, short-incubation, or acute catarrhal jaundice hepatitis. The primary transmission mode is the oral–fecal route.

Item 1–6 Hepatitis B (HBV) was formerly called long-incubation period, serum, or homologous serum hepatitis. Transmission modes are through body fluids and from mother to neonate.

Item 1–7 Hepatitis C, caused by the hepatitis C virus, is primarily transfusion associated.

Item 1–8 Hepatitis D, also called delta hepatitis, is caused by the hepatitis D virus in patients formerly or currently infected with hepatitis B.

Item 1–9 Hepatitis E is also called enterically transmitted non-A, non-B hepatitis. The primary transmission mode is the oral–fecal route, usually through contaminated water.

066.41 West Nile fever with encephalitis ◀
West Nile encephalitis ◀
West Nile encephalomyelitis ◀

066.42 West Nile fever with other neurologic manifestation ◀
Use additional code to specify the neurologic manifestation ◀

066.49 West Nile fever with other complications ◀
Use additional code to specify the other conditions ◀

☐ **066.8 Other specified arthropod-borne viral diseases**
Chandipura fever
Piry fever

☐ **066.9 Arthropod-borne viral disease, unspecified**
Arbovirus infection NOS

OTHER DISEASES DUE TO VIRUSES AND CHLAMYDIAE (070–079)

● **070 Viral hepatitis**
Includes: viral hepatitis (acute) (chronic)
Excludes *cytomegalic inclusion virus hepatitis (078.5)*

The following fifth-digit subclassification is for use with categories 070.2 and 070.3:

❑0 acute or unspecified, without mention of hepatitis delta

❑1 acute or unspecified, with hepatitis delta

2 chronic, without mention of hepatitis delta

3 chronic, with hepatitis delta

070.0 Viral hepatitis A with hepatic coma

070.1 Viral hepatitis A without mention of hepatic coma
Infectious hepatitis

● **070.2 Viral hepatitis B with hepatic coma**

● **070.3 Viral hepatitis B without mention of hepatic coma**
Serum hepatitis

● **070.4 Other specified viral hepatitis with hepatic coma**

❑ **070.41 Acute hepatitis C with hepatic coma**   ◀▥

070.42 Hepatitis delta without mention of active hepatitis B disease with hepatic coma
Hepatitis delta with hepatitis B carrier state

070.43 Hepatitis E with hepatic coma

070.44 Chronic hepatitis C with hepatic coma

❑ **070.49 Other specified viral hepatitis with hepatic coma**

● **070.5 Other specified viral hepatitis without mention of hepatic coma**

❑ **070.51 Acute hepatitis C without mention of hepatic coma**   ◀▥

070.52 Hepatitis delta without mention of active hepatitis B disease or hepatic coma

070.53 Hepatitis E without mention of hepatic coma

070.54 Chronic hepatitis C without mention of hepatic coma

❑ **070.59 Other specified viral hepatitis without mention of hepatic coma**

❑ **070.6 Unspecified viral hepatitis with hepatic coma**

Excludes *unspecified viral hepatitis C with hepatic coma (070.71)*   ◀

● **070.7 Unspecified viral hepatitis**   ◀

❑ **070.70 Unspecified viral hepatatis C without hepatic coma**   ◀
Unspecified viral hepatitis C NOS   ◀

❑ **070.71 Unspecified viral hepatitis C with hepatic coma**   ◀

❑ **070.9 Unspecified viral hepatitis without mention of hepatic coma**
Viral hepatitis NOS

Excludes *unspecified viral hepatitis C with hepatic coma (070.70)*   ◀

071 Rabies
Hydrophobia
Lyssa

● **072 Mumps**

072.0 Mumps orchitis

072.1 Mumps meningitis

072.2 Mumps encephalitis
Mumps meningoencephalitis

072.3 Mumps pancreatitis

● **072.7 Mumps with other specified complications**

072.71 Mumps hepatitis

072.72 Mumps polyneuropathy

❑ **072.79 Other**

❑ **072.8 Mumps with unspecified complication**

❑ **072.9 Mumps without mention of complication**
Epidemic parotitis
Infectious parotitis

● **073 Ornithosis**

Includes: parrot fever
psittacosis

073.0 With pneumonia
Lobular pneumonitis due to ornithosis

❑ **073.7 With other specified complications**

❑ **073.8 With unspecified complication**

❑ **073.9 Ornithosis, unspecified**

● **074 Specific diseases due to Coxsackie virus**

Excludes *Coxsackie virus:*
infection NOS (079.2)
meningitis (047.0)

074.0 Herpangina
Vesicular pharyngitis

074.1 Epidemic pleurodynia
Bornholm disease
Devil's grip
Epidemic:
myalgia
myositis

● **074.2 Coxsackie carditis**

❑ **074.20 Coxsackie carditis, unspecified**

074.21 Coxsackie pericarditis

074.22 Coxsackie endocarditis

074.23 Coxsackie myocarditis
Aseptic myocarditis of newborn

074.3 Hand, foot, and mouth disease
Vesicular stomatitis and exanthem

❑ **074.8 Other specified diseases due to Coxsackie virus**
Acute lymphonodular pharyngitis

075 Infectious mononucleosis
Glandular fever
Monocytic angina
Pfeiffer's disease

● **076 Trachoma**

Excludes *late effect of trachoma (139.1)*

076.0 Initial stage
Trachoma dubium

076.1 Active stage
Granular conjunctivitis (trachomatous)
Trachomatous:
follicular conjunctivitis
pannus

❑ **076.9 Trachoma, unspecified**
Trachoma NOS

● **077 Other diseases of conjunctiva due to viruses and Chlamydiae**

Excludes *ophthalmic complications of viral diseases classified elsewhere*

077.0 Inclusion conjunctivitis
Paratrachoma
Swimming pool conjunctivitis

Excludes *inclusion blennorrhea (neonatal) (771.6)*

077.1 Epidemic keratoconjunctivitis
Shipyard eye

077.2 Pharyngoconjunctival fever
Viral pharyngoconjunctivitis

ICD-9-CM

001-099

Vol. 1

❏ **077.3 Other adenoviral conjunctivitis**
Acute adenoviral follicular conjunctivitis

077.4 Epidemic hemorrhagic conjunctivitis
Apollo:
conjunctivitis
disease
Conjunctivitis due to enterovirus type 70
Hemorrhagic conjunctivitis (acute) (epidemic)

❏ **077.8 Other viral conjunctivitis**
Newcastle conjunctivitis

● **077.9 Unspecified diseases of conjunctiva due to viruses and Chlamydiae**

❏ **077.98 Due to Chlamydiae**

❏ **077.99 Due to viruses**
Viral conjunctivitis NOS

● **078 Other diseases due to viruses and Chlamydiae**

Excludes	*viral infection NOS (079.0–079.9)*
	viremia NOS (790.8)

078.0 Molluscum contagiosum

● **078.1 Viral warts**
Viral warts due to human papillomavirus

❏ **078.10 Viral warts, unspecified**
Condyloma NOS
Verruca NOS:
NOS
Vulgaris
Warts (infectious)

078.11 Condyloma acuminatum

❏ **078.19 Other specified viral warts**
Genital warts NOS
Verruca
plana
plantaris

078.2 Sweating fever
Miliary fever
Sweating disease

078.3 Cat-scratch disease
Benign lymphoreticulosis (of inoculation)
Cat-scratch fever

078.4 Foot and mouth disease
Aphthous fever
Epizootic:
aphthae
stomatitis

078.5 Cytomegaloviral disease
Cytomegalic inclusion disease
Salivary gland virus disease

Use additional code to identify manifestation, as:
cytomegalic inclusion virus:
hepatitis (573.1)
pneumonia (484.1)

Excludes	*congenital cytomegalovirus infection (771.1)*

078.6 Hemorrhagic nephrosonephritis
Hemorrhagic fever:
epidemic
Korean
Russian with renal syndrome

078.7 Arenaviral hemorrhagic fever
Hemorrhagic fever:
Argentine
Bolivian
Junin virus
Machupo virus

● **078.8 Other specified diseases due to viruses and Chlamydiae**

Excludes	*epidemic diarrhea (009.2)*
	lymphogranuloma venereum (099.1)

078.81 Epidemic vertigo

078.82 Epidemic vomiting syndrome
Winter vomiting disease

❏ **078.88 Other specified diseases due to Chlamydiae**

❏ **078.89 Other specified diseases due to viruses**
Epidemic cervical myalgia
Marburg disease
Tanapox

Item 1–10 Retrovirus develops by copying its RNA, genetic materials, into the DNA, which then produces new virus particles. It is from the Retroviridae virus family.
Human T-cell lymphotropic virus, Type I (HTLV-I) is also called human T-cell leukemia virus, Type I, and is a retrovirus thought to cause T-cell leukemia/lymphoma.
Human T-cell lymphotropic virus, Type II (HTLV-II), is also called human T-cell leukemia virus, Type II, and is a retrovirus associated with hematologic disorders.
HIV-2 is one of the serotypes of HIV and is usually confined to West Africa, whereas HIV-1 is found worldwide.

● **079 Viral and chlamydial infection in conditions classified elsewhere and of unspecified site**

Note: This category is provided to be used as an additional code to identify the viral agent in diseases classifiable elsewhere. This category will also be used to classify virus infection of unspecified nature or site.

079.0 Adenovirus

079.1 ECHO virus

079.2 Coxsackie virus

079.3 Rhinovirus

079.4 Human papillomavirus

● **079.5 Retrovirus**

Excludes	*human immunodeficiency virus, type 1 [HIV-1] (042)*
	human T-cell lymphotropic virus, type III [HTLV-III] (042)
	lymphadenopathy-associated virus [LAV] (042)

❏ **079.50 Retrovirus, unspecified**

079.51 Human T-cell lymphotropic virus, type I [HTLV-I]

079.52 Human T-cell lymphotropic virus, type II [HTLV-II]

079.53 Human immunodeficiency virus, type 2 [HIV-2]

❏ **079.59 Other specified retrovirus**

079.6 Respiratory syncytial virus (RSV)

● **079.8 Other specified viral and chlamydial infections**

079.81 Hantavirus

079.82 SARS-associated coronavirus

❏ **079.88 Other specified chlamydial infection**

❏ **079.89 Other specified viral infection**

● **079.9 Unspecified viral and chlamydial infections**

Excludes	*viremia NOS (790.8)*

❏ **079.98 Unspecified chlamydial infection**
Chlamydial infection NOS

❏ **079.99 Unspecified viral infection**
Viral infection NOS

Item 1–11 Rickettsioses are diseases spread from ticks, lice, fleas, or mites to humans. See Figure 1–3. **Typhus** is spread to humans chiefly by the fleas of rats. **Endemic** identifies a disease as being present in low numbers of humans at all times, whereas, **epidemic** identifies a disease as being present in high numbers of humans at a specific time. Morbidity (death) is higher in epidemic diseases.

Brill's disease, also known as **Brill-Zinsser disease,** is spread from human to human by body lice and also from the lice of flying squirrels. **Scrub typhus** is spread in the same ways as Brill's disease.

Malaria is spread to humans by mosquitos.

RICKETTSIOSES AND OTHER ARTHROPOD-BORNE DISEASES (080–088)

> **Excludes** *arthropod-borne viral diseases (060.0–066.9)*

080 Louse-borne [epidemic] typhus
Typhus (fever):
classical
epidemic
exanthematic NOS
louse-borne

● **081 Other typhus**

081.0 **Murine [endemic] typhus**
Typhus (fever):
endemic
flea-borne

081.1 **Brill's disease**
Brill-Zinsser disease
Recrudescent typhus (fever)

081.2 **Scrub typhus**
Japanese river fever
Kedani fever
Mite-borne typhus
Tsutsugamushi

❑081.9 **Typhus, unspecified**
Typhus (fever) NOS

● **082 Tick-borne rickettsioses**

082.0 **Spotted fevers**
Rocky mountain spotted fever
São Paulo fever

082.1 **Boutonneuse fever**
African tick typhus
India tick typhus
Kenya tick typhus
Marseilles fever
Mediterranean tick fever

082.2 **North Asian tick fever**
Siberian tick typhus

082.3 **Queensland tick typhus**

● 082.4 **Ehrlichiosis**

❑082.40 **Ehrlichiosis, unspecified**

082.41 **Ehrlichiosis chafeensis (E. chafeensis)**

❑082.49 **Other ehrlichiosis**

❑082.8 **Other specified tick-borne rickettsioses**
Lone star fever

❑082.9 **Tick-borne rickettsiosis, unspecified**
Tick-borne typhus NOS

● **083 Other rickettsioses**

083.0 **Q fever**

083.1 **Trench fever**
Quintan fever
Wolhynian fever

083.2 **Rickettsialpox**
Vesicular rickettsiosis

❑083.8 **Other specified rickettsioses**

❑083.9 **Rickettsiosis, unspecified**

● **084 Malaria**

Note: Subcategories 084.0–084.6 exclude the listed conditions with mention of pernicious complications (084.8–084.9).

> **Excludes** *congenital malaria (771.2)*

084.0 **Falciparum malaria [malignant tertian]**
Malaria (fever):
by Plasmodium falciparum
subtertian

084.1 **Vivax malaria [benign tertian]**
Malaria (fever) by Plasmodium vivax

084.2 **Quartan malaria**
Malaria (fever) by Plasmodium malariae
Malariae malaria

084.3 **Ovale malaria**
Malaria (fever) by Plasmodium ovale

❑084.4 **Other malaria**
Monkey malaria

084.5 **Mixed malaria**
Malaria (fever) by more than one parasite

❑084.6 **Malaria, unspecified**
Malaria (fever) NOS

084.7 **Induced malaria**
Therapeutically induced malaria

> **Excludes** *accidental infection from syringe, blood transfusion, etc. (084.0–084.6, above, according to parasite species)*
> *transmission from mother to child during delivery (771.2)*

084.8 **Blackwater fever**
Hemoglobinuric:
fever (bilious)
malaria
Malarial hemoglobinuria

❑084.9 **Other pernicious complications of malaria**
Algid malaria
Cerebral malaria

Use additional code to identify complication, as:
malarial:
hepatitis (573.2)
nephrosis (581.81)

● **085 Leishmaniasis**

085.0 **Visceral [kala-azar]**
Dumdum fever
Infection by Leishmania:
donovani
infantum
Leishmaniasis:
dermal, post-kala-azar
Mediterranean
visceral (Indian)

085.1 **Cutaneous, urban**
Aleppo boil
Baghdad boil
Delhi boil
Infection by Leishmania tropica (minor)
Leishmaniasis, cutaneous:
dry form
late
recurrent
ulcerating
Oriental sore

085.2 Cutaneous, Asian desert
Infection by Leishmania tropica major
Leishmaniasis, cutaneous:
    acute necrotizing
    rural
    wet form
    zoonotic form

085.3 Cutaneous, Ethiopian
Infection by Leishmania ethiopica
Leishmaniasis, cutaneous:
    diffuse
    lepromatous

085.4 Cutaneous, American
Chiclero ulcer
Infection by Leishmania mexicana
Leishmaniasis tegumentaria diffusa

085.5 Mucocutaneous (American)
Espundia
Infection by Leishmania braziliensis
Uta

❏ **085.9 Leishmaniasis, unspecified**

● **086 Trypanosomiasis**
Use additional code to identify manifestations, as:
trypanosomiasis:
    encephalitis (323.2)
    meningitis (321.3)

086.0 Chagas' disease with heart involvement
American trypanosomiasis with heart involvement
Infection by Trypanosoma cruzi with heart involvement
Any condition classifiable to 086.2 with heart involvement

086.1 Chagas' disease with other organ involvement
American trypanosomiasis with involvement of organ other than heart
Infection by Trypanosoma cruzi with involvement of organ other than heart
Any condition classifiable to 086.2 with involvement of organ other than heart

086.2 Chagas' disease without mention of organ involvement
American trypanosomiasis
Infection by Trypanosoma cruzi

086.3 Gambian trypanosomiasis
Gambian sleeping sickness
Infection by Trypanosoma gambiense

086.4 Rhodesian trypanosomiasis
Infection by Trypanosoma rhodesiense
Rhodesian sleeping sickness

❏ **086.5 African trypanosomiasis, unspecified**
Sleeping sickness NOS

❏ **086.9 Trypanosomiasis, unspecified**

● **087 Relapsing fever**
    Includes: recurrent fever

087.0 Louse-borne

087.1 Tick-borne

❏ **087.9 Relapsing fever, unspecified**

● **088 Other arthropod-borne diseases**

088.0 Bartonellosis
Carrión's disease
Oroya fever
Verruga peruana

● ❏ **088.8 Other specified arthropod-borne diseases**
088.81 Lyme disease
Erythema chronicum migrans
088.82 Babesiosis
Babesiasis
❏ **088.89 Other**
❏ **088.9 Arthropod-borne disease, unspecified**

Figure 1–7   Chancre. (From Delp MH, Manning RT: Major Physical Diagnosis, 8th ed. Philadelphia, WB Saunders, 1975, p. 613.)

Item 1–12 Syphilis, also known as lues, is the most serious of the venereal diseases caused by *Treponema pallidum.* The **primary** stage is characterized by an ulceration known as **chancre,** which usually appears on the genitals but can also develop on the anus, lips, tonsils, breasts, or fingers.
The **secondary** stage is characterized by a rash that can affect any area of the body. **Latent** syphilis is divided into **early,** which is diagnosed within two years of infection, and **late,** which is diagnosed two years or more after infection. **Congenital** syphilis is also labeled **early** or **late** based on the time of diagnosis.

SYPHILIS AND OTHER VENEREAL DISEASES (090–099)

Excludes   nonvenereal endemic syphilis (104.0)
                 urogenital trichomoniasis (131.0)

● **090 Congenital syphilis**

090.0 Early congenital syphilis, symptomatic
Congenital syphilitic:
    choroiditis
    coryza (chronic)
    hepatomegaly
    mucous patches
    periostitis
    splenomegaly
Syphilitic (congenital):
    epiphysitis
    osteochondritis
    pemphigus
Any congenital syphilitic condition specified as early or manifesting less than two years after birth

090.1 Early congenital syphilis, latent
Congenital syphilis without clinical manifestations, with positive serological reaction and negative spinal fluid test, less than two years after birth

❏090.2 **Early congenital syphilis, unspecified**
Congenital syphilis NOS, less than two years after birth

090.3 **Syphilitic interstitial keratitis**
Syphilitic keratitis:
parenchymatous
punctata profunda

> **Excludes** *interstitial keratitis NOS (370.50)*

● 090.4 **Juvenile neurosyphilis**

Use additional code to identify any associated mental disorder

❏090.40 **Juvenile neurosyphilis, unspecified**
Congenital neurosyphilis
Dementia paralytica juvenilis
Juvenile:
general paresis
tabes
taboparesis

090.41 **Congenital syphilitic encephalitis**

090.42 **Congenital syphilitic meningitis**

❏090.49 **Other**

❏090.5 **Other late congenital syphilis, symptomatic**
Gumma due to congenital syphilis
Hutchinson's teeth
Syphilitic saddle nose
Any congenital syphilitic condition specified as late or manifesting two years or more after birth

090.6 **Late congenital syphilis, latent**
Congenital syphilis without clinical manifestations, with positive serological reaction and negative spinal fluid test, two years or more after birth

❏090.7 **Late congenital syphilis, unspecified**
Congenital syphilis NOS, two years or more after birth

❏090.9 **Congenital syphilis, unspecified**

● 091 **Early syphilis, symptomatic**

> **Excludes** *early cardiovascular syphilis (093.0–093.9)*
> *early neurosyphilis (094.0–094.9)*

091.0 **Genital syphilis (primary)**
Genital chancre

091.1 **Primary anal syphilis**

❏091.2 **Other primary syphilis**
Primary syphilis of:
breast
fingers
lip
tonsils

091.3 **Secondary syphilis of skin or mucous membranes**
Condyloma latum
Secondary syphilis of:
anus
mouth
pharynx
skin
tonsils
vulva

091.4 **Adenopathy due to secondary syphilis**
Syphilitic adenopathy (secondary)
Syphilitic lymphadenitis (secondary)

● 091.5 **Uveitis due to secondary syphilis**

❏091.50 **Syphilitic uveitis, unspecified**

091.51 **Syphilitic chorioretinitis (secondary)**

091.52 **Syphilitic iridocyclitis (secondary)**

● 091.6 **Secondary syphilis of viscera and bone**

091.61 **Secondary syphilitic periostitis**

091.62 **Secondary syphilitic hepatitis**
Secondary syphilis of liver

❏091.69 **Other viscera**

091.7 **Secondary syphilis, relapse**
Secondary syphilis, relapse (treated) (untreated)

● 091.8 **Other forms of secondary syphilis**

091.81 **Acute syphilitic meningitis (secondary)**

091.82 **Syphilitic alopecia**

❏091.89 **Other**

❏091.9 **Unspecified secondary syphilis**

● 092 **Early syphilis, latent**

> **Includes:** syphilis (acquired) without clinical manifestations, with positive serological reaction and negative spinal fluid test, less than two years after infection

092.0 **Early syphilis, latent, serological relapse after treatment**

❏092.9 **Early syphilis, latent, unspecified**

● 093 **Cardiovascular syphilis**

093.0 **Aneurysm of aorta, specified as syphilitic**
Dilatation of aorta, specified as syphilitic

093.1 **Syphilitic aortitis**

● 093.2 **Syphilitic endocarditis**

❏093.20 **Valve, unspecified**
Syphilitic ostial coronary disease

093.21 **Mitral valve**

093.22 **Aortic valve**
Syphilitic aortic incompetence or stenosis

093.23 **Tricuspid valve**

093.24 **Pulmonary valve**

● 093.8 **Other specified cardiovascular syphilis**

093.81 **Syphilitic pericarditis**

093.82 **Syphilitic myocarditis**

❏093.89 **Other**

❏093.9 **Cardiovascular syphilis, unspecified**

● 094 **Neurosyphilis**

Use additional code to identify any associated mental disorder

094.0 **Tabes dorsalis**
Locomotor ataxia (progressive)
Posterior spinal sclerosis (syphilitic)
Tabetic neurosyphilis

Use additional code to identify manifestation, as:
neurogenic arthropathy [Charcot's joint disease] (713.5)

094.1 **General paresis**
Dementia paralytica
General paralysis (of the insane) (progressive)
Paretic neurosyphilis
Taboparesis

094.2 **Syphilitic meningitis**
Meningovascular syphilis

> **Excludes** *acute syphilitic meningitis (secondary) (091.81)*

094.3 **Asymptomatic neurosyphilis**

● 094.8 **Other specified neurosyphilis**

094.81 **Syphilitic encephalitis**

094.82 **Syphilitic Parkinsonism**

094.83 **Syphilitic disseminated retinochoroiditis**

094.84 **Syphilitic optic atrophy**

094.85 **Syphilitic retrobulbar neuritis**

094.86 **Syphilitic acoustic neuritis**

094.87 **Syphilitic ruptured cerebral aneurysm**

❏ 094.89 **Other**

❏ 094.9 **Neurosyphilis, unspecified**
Gumma (syphilitic) of central nervous system
NOS
Syphilis (early) (late) of central nervous system
NOS
Syphiloma of central nervous system NOS

● 095 **Other forms of late syphilis, with symptoms**

Includes: gumma (syphilitic)
tertiary, or unspecified stage

095.0 **Syphilitic episcleritis**

095.1 **Syphilis of lung**

095.2 **Syphilitic peritonitis**

095.3 **Syphilis of liver**

095.4 **Syphilis of kidney**

095.5 **Syphilis of bone**

095.6 **Syphilis of muscle**
Syphilitic myositis

095.7 **Syphilis of synovium, tendon, and bursa**
Syphilitic:
bursitis
synovitis

❏ 095.8 **Other specified forms of late symptomatic syphilis**

Excludes *cardiovascular syphilis (093.0–093.9)*
neurosyphilis (094.0–094.9)

❏ 095.9 **Late symptomatic syphilis, unspecified**

096 **Late syphilis, latent**
Syphilis (acquired) without clinical manifestations, with
positive serological reaction and negative spinal
fluid test, two years or more after infection

● 097 **Other and unspecified syphilis**

❏ 097.0 **Late syphilis, unspecified**

❏ 097.1 **Latent syphilis, unspecified**
Positive serological reaction for syphilis

❏ 097.9 **Syphilis, unspecified**
Syphilis (acquired) NOS

Excludes *syphilis NOS causing death under two years of*
age (090.9)

● 098 **Gonococcal infections**

098.0 **Acute, of lower genitourinary tract**
Gonococcal:
Bartholinitis (acute)
urethritis (acute)
vulvovaginitis (acute)
Gonorrhea (acute):
NOS
genitourinary (tract) NOS

● 098.1 **Acute, of upper genitourinary tract**

❏ 098.10 **Gonococcal infection (acute) of upper genitourinary tract, site unspecified**

098.11 **Gonococcal cystitis (acute)**
Gonorrhea (acute) of bladder

098.12 **Gonococcal prostatitis (acute)**

098.13 **Gonococcal epididymo-orchitis (acute)**
Gonococcal orchitis (acute)

098.14 **Gonococcal seminal vesiculitis (acute)**
Gonorrhea (acute) of seminal vesicle

098.15 **Gonococcal cervicitis (acute)**
Gonorrhea (acute) of cervix

098.16 **Gonococcal endometritis (acute)**
Gonorrhea (acute) of uterus

098.17 **Gonococcal salpingitis, specified as acute**

❏ 098.19 **Other**

098.2 **Chronic, of lower genitourinary tract**
Gonococcal specified as chronic or with duration
of two months or more:
Bartholinitis specified as chronic or with duration of two months or more
urethritis specified as chronic or with duration
of two months or more
vulvovaginitis specified as chronic or with duration of two months or more
Gonorrhea specified as chronic or with duration
of two months or more:
NOS specified as chronic or with duration of
two months or more
genitourinary (tract) specified as chronic or
with duration of two months or more
Any condition classifiable to 098.0 specified as
chronic or with duration of two months or
more

● 098.3 **Chronic, of upper genitourinary tract**
Includes: any condition classifiable to 098.1 stated
as chronic or with a duration of two months
or more

❏ 098.30 **Chronic gonococcal infection of upper genitourinary tract, site unspecified**

098.31 **Gonococcal cystitis, chronic**
Any condition classifiable to 098.11, specified as chronic
Gonorrhea of bladder, chronic

098.32 **Gonococcal prostatitis, chronic**
Any condition classifiable to 098.12, specified as chronic

098.33 **Gonococcal epididymo-orchitis, chronic**
Any condition classifiable to 098.13, specified as chronic
Chronic gonococcal orchitis

098.34 **Gonococcal seminal vesiculitis, chronic**
Any condition classifiable to 098.14, specified as chronic
Gonorrhea of seminal vesicle, chronic

098.35 **Gonococcal cervicitis, chronic**
Any condition classifiable to 098.15, specified as chronic
Gonorrhea of cervix, chronic

098.36 **Gonococcal endometritis, chronic**
Any condition classifiable to 098.16, specified as chronic

098.37 **Gonococcal salpingitis (chronic)**

❏ 098.39 **Other**

● 098.4 **Gonococcal infection of eye**

098.40 **Gonococcal conjunctivitis (neonatorum)**
Gonococcal ophthalmia (neonatorum)

098.41 **Gonococcal iridocyclitis**

098.42 **Gonococcal endophthalmia**

098.43 **Gonococcal keratitis**

❏ 098.49 **Other**

● **098.5 Gonococcal infection of joint**

     098.50 Gonococcal arthritis
         Gonococcal infection of joint NOS

     098.51 Gonococcal synovitis and tenosynovitis

     098.52 Gonococcal bursitis

     098.53 Gonococcal spondylitis

     ☐ **098.59 Other**
         Gonococcal rheumatism

098.6 Gonococcal infection of pharynx

098.7 Gonococcal infection of anus and rectum
     Gonococcal proctitis

● **098.8 Gonococcal infection of other specified sites**

     098.81 Gonococcal keratosis (blennorrhagica)

     098.82 Gonococcal meningitis

     098.83 Gonococcal pericarditis

     098.84 Gonococcal endocarditis

     ☐ **098.85 Other gonococcal heart disease**

     098.86 Gonococcal peritonitis

     ☐ **098.89 Other**
         Gonococcemia

● **099 Other venereal diseases**

099.0 Chancroid
     Bubo (inguinal):
         chancroidal
         due to Hemophilus ducreyi
     Chancre:
         Ducrey's simple soft
     Ulcus molle (cutis) (skin)

099.1 Lymphogranuloma venereum
     Climatic or tropical bubo
     (Durand-) Nicolas-Favre disease
     Esthiomene
     Lymphogranuloma inguinale

099.2 Granuloma inguinale
     Donovanosis
     Granuloma pudendi (ulcerating)
     Granuloma venereum
     Pudendal ulcer

099.3 Reiter's disease
     Reiter's syndrome

     Use additional code for associated:
         arthropathy (711.1)
         conjunctivitis (372.33)

● **099.4 Other nongonococcal urethritis [NGU]**

     ☐ **099.40 Unspecified**
         Nonspecific urethritis

     099.41 Chlamydia trachomatis

     ☐ **099.49 Other specified organism**

● **099.5 Other venereal diseases due to Chlamydia trachomatis**

     Excludes *Chlamydia trachomatis infection of conjunctiva (076.0–076.9, 077.0, 077.9)*
         Lymphogranuloma venereum (099.1)

     ☐ **099.50 Unspecified site**

     099.51 Pharynx

     099.52 Anus and rectum

     099.53 Lower genitourinary sites

     Excludes *urethra (099.41)*

     Use additional code to specify site of infection, such as:
         bladder (595.4)
         cervix (616.0)
         vagina and vulva (616.11)

☐ **099.54 Other genitourinary sites**

     Use additional code to specify site of infection, such as:
         pelvic inflammatory disease NOS (614.9)
         testis and epididymis (604.91)

☐ **099.55 Unspecified genitourinary site**

     099.56 Peritoneum
         Perihepatitis

☐ **099.59 Other specified site**

☐ **099.8 Other specified venereal diseases**

☐ **099.9 Venereal disease, unspecified**

OTHER SPIROCHETAL DISEASES (100–104)

● **100 Leptospirosis**

100.0 Leptospirosis icterohemorrhagica
     Leptospiral or spirochetal jaundice (hemorrhagic)
     Weil's disease

● **100.8 Other specified leptospiral infections**

     100.81 Leptospiral meningitis (aseptic)

     ☐ **100.89 Other**
         Fever:
             Fort Bragg
             pretibial
             swamp
         Infection by Leptospira:
             australis
             bataviae
             pyrogenes

☐ **100.9 Leptospirosis, unspecified**

101 Vincent's angina
     Acute necrotizing ulcerative:
         gingivitis
         stomatitis
     Fusospirochetal pharyngitis
     Spirochetal stomatitis
     Trench mouth
     Vincent's:
         gingivitis
         infection [any site]

● **102 Yaws**

     Includes: frambesia
                pian

     102.0 Initial lesions
         Chancre of yaws
         Frambesia, initial or primary
         Initial frambesial ulcer
         Mother yaw

     102.1 Multiple papillomata and wet crab yaws
         Butter yaws
         Frambesioma
         Pianoma
         Plantar or palmar papilloma of yaws

     ☐ **102.2 Other early skin lesions**
         Cutaneous yaws, less than five years after infection
         Early yaws (cutaneous) (macular) (papular) (maculopapular) (micropapular)
         Frambeside of early yaws

     102.3 Hyperkeratosis
         Ghoul hand
         Hyperkeratosis, palmar or plantar (early) (late) due to yaws
         Worm-eaten soles

ICD-9-CM

100-104

Vol. 1

102.4 Gummata and ulcers
Nodular late yaws (ulcerated)
Gummatous frambeside

102.5 Gangosa
Rhinopharyngitis mutilans

102.6 Bone and joint lesions
Goundou of yaws (late)
Gumma, bone of yaws (late)
Gummatous osteitis or periostitis of yaws (late)
Hydrarthrosis of yaws (early) (late)
Osteitis of yaws (early) (late)
Periostitis (hypertrophic) of yaws (early) (late)

❑ **102.7 Other manifestations**
Juxta-articular nodules of yaws
Mucosal yaws

102.8 Latent yaws
Yaws without clinical manifestations, with positive serology

❑ **102.9 Yaws, unspecified**

● **103 Pinta**

103.0 Primary lesions
Chancre (primary) of pinta [carate]
Papule (primary) of pinta [carate]
Pintid of pinta [carate]

103.1 Intermediate lesions
Erythematous plaques of pinta [carate]
Hyperchromic lesions of pinta [carate]
Hyperkeratosis of pinta [carate]

103.2 Late lesions
Cardiovascular lesions of pinta [carate]
Skin lesions of pinta [carate]:
  achromic of pinta [carate]
  cicatricial of pinta [carate]
  dyschromic of pinta [carate]
Vitiligo of pinta [carate]

103.3 Mixed lesions
Achromic and hyperchromic skin lesions of pinta [carate]

❑ **103.9 Pinta, unspecified**

● **104 Other spirochetal infection**

104.0 Nonvenereal endemic syphilis
Bejel
Njovera

❑ **104.8 Other specified spirochetal infections**
  Excludes *relapsing fever (087.0–087.9)*
               syphilis (090.0–097.9)

❑ **104.9 Spirochetal infection, unspecified**

MYCOSES (110–118)

Use additional code to identify manifestation, as:
arthropathy (711.6)
meningitis (321.0–321.1)
otitis externa (380.15)

  Excludes *infection by Actinomycetales, such as species of Actinomyces, Actinomadura, Nocardia, Streptomyces (039.0–039.9)*

● **110 Dermatophytosis**

Includes: infection by species of Epidermophyton, Microsporum, and Trichophyton
tinea, any type except those in 111

110.0 Of scalp and beard
Kerion
Sycosis, mycotic
Trichophytic tinea [black dot tinea], scalp

110.1 Of nail
Dermatophytic onychia
Onychomycosis
Tinea unguium

110.2 Of hand
Tinea manuum

110.3 Of groin and perianal area
Dhobie itch
Eczema marginatum
Tinea cruris

110.4 Of foot
Athlete's foot
Tinea pedis

110.5 Of the body
Herpes circinatus
Tinea imbricata [Tokelau]

110.6 Deep seated dermatophytosis
Granuloma trichophyticum
Majocchi's granuloma

❑ **110.8 Of other specified sites**

❑ **110.9 Of unspecified site**
Favus NOS
Microsporic tinea NOS
Ringworm NOS

● **111 Dermatomycosis, other and unspecified**

111.0 Pityriasis versicolor
Infection by Malassezia [Pityrosporum] furfur
Tinea flava
Tinea versicolor

111.1 Tinea nigra
Infection by Cladosporium species
Keratomycosis nigricans
Microsporosis nigra
Pityriasis nigra
Tinea palmaris nigra

111.2 Tinea blanca
Infection by Trichosporon (beigelii) cutaneum
White piedra

Figure 1–8 Oral candidiasis, also called thrush. (From Rippon JW: Medical Mycology, 3rd ed. Philadelphia, WB Saunders, 1988, p. 542.)

Item 1-13 Candidiasis, also called oidiomycosis or moniliasis, is a fungal infection. It most often appears on moist cutaneous areas of the body, but can also be responsible for a variety of systemic infections such as endocarditis, meningitis, arthritis, and myositis.

111.3 **Black piedra**
Infection by Piedraia hortai

☐ 111.8 **Other specified dermatomycoses**

☐ 111.9 **Dermatomycosis, unspecified**

● 112 **Candidiasis**
Includes: infection by Candida species
moniliasis
Excludes neonatal monilial infection (771.7)

112.0 **Of mouth**
Thrush (oral)

112.1 **Of vulva and vagina**
Candidal vulvovaginitis
Monilial vulvovaginitis

☐ 112.2 **Of other urogenital sites**
Candidal balanitis

112.3 **Of skin and nails**
Candidal intertrigo
Candidal onychia
Candidal perionyxis [paronychia]

112.4 **Of lung**
Candidal pneumonia

112.5 **Disseminated**
Systemic candidiasis

● 112.8 **Of other specified sites**

112.81 **Candidal endocarditis**

112.82 **Candidal otitis externa**
Otomycosis in moniliasis

112.83 **Candidal meningitis**

112.84 **Candidal esophagitis**

112.85 **Candidal enteritis**

☐ 112.89 **Other**

☐ 112.9 **Of unspecified site**

● 114 **Coccidioidomycosis**
Includes: infection by Coccidioides (immitis)
Posada-Wernicke disease

114.0 **Primary coccidioidomycosis (pulmonary)**
Acute pulmonary coccidioidomycosis
Coccidioidomycotic pneumonitis
Desert rheumatism
Pulmonary coccidioidomycosis
San Joaquin Valley fever

114.1 **Primary extrapulmonary coccidioidomycosis**
Chancriform syndrome
Primary cutaneous coccidioidomycosis

114.2 **Coccidioidal meningitis**

☐ 114.3 **Other forms of progressive coccidioidomycosis**
Coccidioidal granuloma
Disseminated coccidioidomycosis

114.4 **Chronic pulmonary coccidioidomycosis**

☐ 114.5 **Pulmonary coccidioidomycosis, unspecified**

☐ 114.9 **Coccidioidomycosis, unspecified**

● 115 **Histoplasmosis**
The following fifth-digit subclassification is for use with category 115:
0 **without mention of manifestation**
1 **meningitis**
2 **retinitis**
3 **pericarditis**
4 **endocarditis**
5 **pneumonia**
☐ 9 **other**

● 115.0 **Infection by Histoplasma capsulatum**
American histoplasmosis
Darling's disease
Reticuloendothelial cytomycosis
Small form histoplasmosis

● 115.1 **Infection by Histoplasma duboisii**
African histoplasmosis
Large form histoplasmosis

● ☐ 115.9 **Histoplasmosis, unspecified**
Histoplasmosis NOS

● 116 **Blastomycotic infection**

116.0 **Blastomycosis**
Blastomycotic dermatitis
Chicago disease
Cutaneous blastomycosis
Disseminated blastomycosis
Gilchrist's disease
Infection by Blastomyces [Ajellomyces] dermatitidis
North American blastomycosis
Primary pulmonary blastomycosis

116.1 **Paracoccidioidomycosis**
Brazilian blastomycosis
Infection by Paracoccidioides [Blastomyces] brasiliensis
Lutz-Splendore-Almeida disease
Mucocutaneous-lymphangitic paracoccidioidomycosis
Pulmonary paracoccidioidomycosis
South American blastomycosis
Visceral paracoccidioidomycosis

116.2 **Lobomycosis**
Infections by Loboa [Blastomyces] loboi
Keloidal blastomycosis
Lobo's disease

● 117 **Other mycoses**

117.0 **Rhinosporidiosis**
Infection by Rhinosporidium seeberi

117.1 **Sporotrichosis**
Cutaneous sporotrichosis
Disseminated sporotrichosis
Infection by Sporothrix [Sporotrichum] schenckii
Lymphocutaneous sporotrichosis
Pulmonary sporotrichosis
Sporotrichosis of the bones

117.2 **Chromoblastomycosis**
Chromomycosis
Infection by Cladosporidium carrionii, Fonsecaea compactum, Fonsecaea pedrosoi, Phialophora verrucosa

117.3 **Aspergillosis**
Infection by Aspergillus species, mainly A. fumigatus, A. flavus group, A. terreus group

ICD-9-CM
100-199
Vol. 1

117.4 Mycotic mycetomas
Infection by various genera and species of Ascomycetes and Deuteromycetes, such as Acremonium [Cephalosporium] falciforme, Neotestudina rosatii, Madurella grisea, Madurella
mycetomii, Pyrenochaeta romeroi, Zopfia
[Leptosphaeria] senegalensis
Madura foot, mycotic
Maduromycosis, mycotic

> **Excludes** *actinomycotic mycetomas (039.0–039.9)*

117.5 Cryptococcosis
Busse-Buschke's disease
European cryptococcosis
Infection by Cryptococcus neoformans
Pulmonary cryptococcosis
Systemic cryptococcosis
Torula

117.6 Allescheriosis [Petriellidosis]
Infections by Allescheria [Petriellidium] boydii
[Monosporium apiospermum]

> **Excludes** *mycotic mycetoma (117.4)*

117.7 Zygomycosis [Phycomycosis or Mucormycosis]
Infection by species of Absidia, Basidiobolus, Con-
idiobolus, Cunninghamella, Entomophthora,
Mucor, Rhizopus, Saksenaea

117.8 Infection by dematiacious fungi [Phaehyphomy-cosis]
Infection by dematiacious fungi, such as Cladosporium trichoides [bantianum], Dreschlera
hawaiiensis, Phialophora gougerotii, Phialophora jeanselmi

☐ **117.9 Other and unspecified mycoses**

118 Opportunistic mycoses
Infection of skin, subcutaneous tissues, and/or organs
by a wide variety of fungi generally considered to
be pathogenic to compromised hosts only (e.g., infection by species of Alternaria, Dreschlera, Fusarium)

HELMINTHIASES (120–129)

● **120 Schistosomiasis [bilharziasis]**

120.0 Schistosoma haematobium
Vesical schistosomiasis NOS

120.1 Schistosoma mansoni
Intestinal schistosomiasis NOS

120.2 Schistosoma japonicum
Asiatic schistosomiasis NOS
Katayama disease or fever

120.3 Cutaneous
Cercarial dermatitis
Infection by cercariae of Schistosoma
Schistosome dermatitis
Swimmers' itch

☐ **120.8 Other specified schistosomiasis**
Infection by Schistosoma:
bovis
intercalatum
mattheii
spindale
Schistosomiasis chestermani

☐ **120.9 Schistosomiasis, unspecified**
Blood flukes NOS
Hemic distomiasis

● **121 Other trematode infections**

121.0 Opisthorchiasis
Infection by:
cat liver fluke
Opisthorchis (felineus) (tenuicollis) (viverrini)

121.1 Clonorchiasis
Biliary cirrhosis due to clonorchiasis
Chinese liver fluke disease
Hepatic distomiasis due to Clonorchis sinensis
Oriental liver fluke disease

121.2 Paragonimiasis
Infection by Paragonimus
Lung fluke disease (oriental)
Pulmonary distomiasis

121.3 Fascioliasis
Infection by Fasciola:
gigantica
hepatica
Liver flukes NOS
Sheep liver fluke infection

121.4 Fasciolopsiasis
Infection by Fasciolopsis (buski)
Intestinal distomiasis

121.5 Metagonimiasis
Infection by Metagonimus yokogawai

121.6 Heterophyiasis
Infection by:
Heterophyes heterophyes
Stellantchasmus falcatus

☐ **121.8 Other specified trematode infections**
Infection by:
Dicrocoelium dendriticum
Echinostoma ilocanum
Gastrodiscoides hominis

☐ **121.9 Trematode infection, unspecified**
Distomiasis NOS
Fluke disease NOS

● **122 Echinococcosis**

> **Includes:** echinococciasis
> hydatid disease
> hydatidosis

122.0 Echinococcus granulosus infection of liver

122.1 Echinococcus granulosus infection of lung

122.2 Echinococcus granulosus infection of thyroid

☐ **122.3 Echinococcus granulosus infection, other**

☐ **122.4 Echinococcus granulosus infection, unspecified**

122.5 Echinococcus multilocularis infection of liver

☐ **122.6 Echinococcus multilocularis infection, other**

☐ **122.7 Echinococcus multilocularis infection, unspecified**

☐ **122.8 Echinococcosis, unspecified, of liver**

☐ **122.9 Echinococcosis, other and unspecified**

● **123 Other cestode infection**

123.0 Taenia solium infection, intestinal form
Pork tapeworm (adult) (infection)

123.1 Cysticercosis
Cysticerciasis
Infection by Cysticercus cellulosae [larval form of
Taenia solium]

123.2 Taenia saginata infection
Beef tapeworm (infection)
Infection by Taeniarhynchus saginatus

☐ **123.3 Taeniasis, unspecified**

123.4 Diphyllobothriasis, intestinal
Diphyllobothrium (adult) (latum) (pacificum) in-
fection
Fish tapeworm (infection)

123.5 Sparganosis [larval diphyllobothriasis]
Infection by:
     Diphyllobothrium larvae
     Sparganum (mansoni) (proliferum)
     Spirometra larvae

123.6 Hymenolepiasis
Dwarf tapeworm (infection)
Hymenolepis (diminuta) (nana) infection
Rat tapeworm (infection)

☐123.8 Other specified cestode infection
Diplogonoporus (grandis) infection
Dipylidium (caninum) infection
Dog tapeworm (infection)

☐123.9 Cestode infection, unspecified
Tapeworm (infection) NOS

124 Trichinosis
Trichinella spiralis infection
Trichinellosis
Trichiniasis

● 125 Filarial infection and dracontiasis

125.0 Bancroftian filariasis
Chyluria due to Wuchereria bancrofti
Elephantiasis due to Wuchereria bancrofti
Infection due to Wuchereria bancrofti
Lymphadenitis due to Wuchereria bancrofti
Lymphangitis due to Wuchereria bancrofti
Wuchereriasis

125.1 Malayan filariasis
Brugia filariasis due to Brugia [Wuchereria] malayi
Chyluria due to Brugia [Wuchereria] malayi
Elephantiasis due to Brugia [Wuchereria] malayi
Infection due to Brugia [Wuchereria] malayi
Lymphadenitis due to Brugia [Wuchereria] malayi
Lymphangitis due to Brugia [Wuchereria] malayi

125.2 Loiasis
Eyeworm disease of Africa
Loa loa infection

125.3 Onchocerciasis
Onchocerca volvulus infection
Onchocercosis

125.4 Dipetalonemiasis
Infection by:
     Acanthocheilonema perstans
     Dipetalonema perstans

125.5 Mansonella ozzardi infection
Filariasis ozzardi

☐125.6 Other specified filariasis
Dirofilaria infection
Infection by:
     Acanthocheilonema streptocerca
     Dipetalonema streptocerca

125.7 Dracontiasis
Guinea-worm infection
Infection by Dracunculus medinensis

☐125.9 Unspecified filariasis

●126 Ancylostomiasis and necatoriasis

     Includes: cutaneous larva migrans due to Ancylostoma
               hookworm (disease) (infection)
               uncinariasis

126.0 Ancylostoma duodenale

126.1 Necator americanus

126.2 Ancylostoma braziliense

126.3 Ancylostoma ceylanicum

☐126.8 Other specified Ancylostoma

☐126.9 Ancylostomiasis and necatoriasis, unspecified
Creeping eruption NOS
Cutaneous larva migrans NOS

● 127 Other intestinal helminthiases

127.0 Ascariasis
Ascaridiasis
Infection by Ascaris lumbricoides
Roundworm infection

127.1 Anisakiasis
Infection by Anisakis larva

127.2 Strongyloidiasis
Infection by Strongyloides stercoralis
    Excludes   *trichostrongyliasis (127.6)*

127.3 Trichuriasis
Infection by Trichuris trichiuria
Trichocephaliasis
Whipworm (disease) (infection)

127.4 Enterobiasis
Infection by Enterobius vermicularis
Oxyuriasis
Oxyuris vermicularis infection
Pinworm (disease) (infection)
Threadworm infection

127.5 Capillariasis
Infection by Capillaria philippinensis
    Excludes   *infection by Capillaria hepatica (128.8)*

127.6 Trichostrongyliasis
Infection by Trichostrongylus species

☐127.7 Other specified intestinal helminthiasis
Infection by:
     Oesophagostomum apiostomum and related
         species
     Ternidens diminutus
     Other specified intestinal helminth
Physalopteriasis

127.8 Mixed intestinal helminthiasis
Infection by intestinal helminths classified to more
     than one of the categories 120.0–127.7
Mixed helminthiasis NOS

☐127.9 Intestinal helminthiasis, unspecified

● 128 Other and unspecified helminthiases

128.0 Toxocariasis
Larva migrans visceralis
Toxocara (canis) (cati) infection
Visceral larva migrans syndrome

128.1 Gnathostomiasis
Infection by Gnathostoma spinigerum and related
     species

☐128.8 Other specified helminthiasis
Infection by:
     Angiostrongylus cantonensis
     Capillaria hepatica
     Other specified helminth

☐128.9 Helminth infection, unspecified
Helminthiasis NOS
Worms NOS

☐129 Intestinal parasitism, unspecified

ICD-9-CM

100-139

Vol. 1

Item 1-14 Toxoplasmosis is caused by the protozoa **Toxoplasma gondii,** of which the house cat can be a host. Human infection occurs when contact is made with materials containing the pathogen, such as feces or contaminated soil.

Infection can also occur with ingestion of lamb, goat, and pork meat, especially when the meat contains infected cysts.

OTHER INFECTIOUS AND PARASITIC DISEASES (130–136)

● 130 **Toxoplasmosis**

> **Includes:** infection by toxoplasma gondii
> toxoplasmosis (acquired)

> **Excludes** *congenital toxoplasmosis (771.2)*

130.0 **Meningoencephalitis due to toxoplasmosis**
Encephalitis due to acquired toxoplasmosis

130.1 **Conjunctivitis due to toxoplasmosis**

130.2 **Chorioretinitis due to toxoplasmosis**
Focal retinochoroiditis due to acquired toxoplasmosis

130.3 **Myocarditis due to toxoplasmosis**

130.4 **Pneumonitis due to toxoplasmosis**

130.5 **Hepatitis due to toxoplasmosis**

□ 130.7 **Toxoplasmosis of other specified sites**

130.8 **Multisystemic disseminated toxoplasmosis**
Toxoplasmosis of multiple sites

□ 130.9 **Toxoplasmosis, unspecified**

● 131 **Trichomoniasis**

> **Includes:** infection due to Trichomonas (vaginalis)

● 131.0 **Urogenital trichomoniasis**

□ 131.00 **Urogenital trichomoniasis, unspecified**
Fluor (vaginalis) trichomonal or due to Trichomonas (vaginalis)
Leukorrhea (vaginalis) trichomonal or due to Trichomonas (vaginalis)

131.01 **Trichomonal vulvovaginitis**
Vaginitis, trichomonal or due to Trichomonas (vaginalis)

131.02 **Trichomonal urethritis**

131.03 **Trichomonal prostatitis**

□ 131.09 **Other**

□ 131.8 **Other specified sites**

> **Excludes** *intestinal (007.3)*

□ 131.9 **Trichomoniasis, unspecified**

● 132 **Pediculosis and Phthirus infestation**

132.0 **Pediculus capitis [head louse]**

132.1 **Pediculus corporis [body louse]**

132.2 **Phthirus pubis [pubic louse]**
Pediculus pubis

132.3 **Mixed infestation**
Infestation classifiable to more than one of the categories 132.0–132.2

□ 132.9 **Pediculosis, unspecified**

● 133 **Acariasis**

133.0 **Scabies**
Infestation by Sarcoptes scabiei
Norwegian scabies
Sarcoptic itch

□ 133.8 **Other acariasis**
Chiggers
Infestation by:
Demodex folliculorum
Trombicula

□ 133.9 **Acariasis, unspecified**
Infestation by mites NOS

● 134 **Other infestation**

134.0 **Myiasis**
Infestation by:
Dermatobia (hominis)
fly larvae
Gasterophilus (intestinalis)
maggots
Oestrus ovis

□ 134.1 **Other arthropod infestation**
Infestation by:
chigoe
sand flea
Tunga penetrans
Jigger disease
Scarabiasis
Tungiasis

134.2 **Hirudiniasis**
Hirudiniasis (external) (internal)
Leeches (aquatic) (land)

□ 134.8 **Other specified infestations**

□ 134.9 **Infestation, unspecified**
Infestation (skin) NOS
Skin parasites NOS

135 **Sarcoidosis**
Besnier-Boeck-Schaumann disease
Lupoid (miliary) of Boeck
Lupus pernio (Besnier)
Lymphogranulomatosis, benign (Schaumann's)
Sarcoid (any site):
NOS
Boeck
Darier-Roussy
Uveoparotid fever

● 136 **Other and unspecified infectious and parasitic diseases**

136.0 **Ainhum**
Dactylolysis spontanea

136.1 **Behçet's syndrome**

136.2 **Specific infections by free-living amebae**
Meningoencephalitis due to Naegleria

136.3 **Pneumocystosis**
Pneumonia due to Pneumocystis carinii

136.4 **Psorospermiasis**

136.5 **Sarcosporidiosis**
Infection by Sarcocystis lindemanni

□ 136.8 **Other specified infectious and parasitic diseases**
Candiru infestation

□ 136.9 **Unspecified infectious and parasitic diseases**
Infectious disease NOS
Parasitic disease NOS

LATE EFFECTS OF INFECTIOUS AND PARASITIC DISEASES (137–139)

● 137 **Late effects of tuberculosis**

Note: This category is to be used to indicate conditions classifiable to 010–018 as the cause of late effects, which are themselves classified elsewhere. The "late effects" include those specified as such, as sequelae, or as due to old or inactive tuberculosis, without evidence of active disease.

❑ **137.0 Late effects of respiratory or unspecified tuberculosis**

❑ **137.1 Late effects of central nervous system tuberculosis**

❑ **137.2 Late effects of genitourinary tuberculosis**

❑ **137.3 Late effects of tuberculosis of bones and joints**

❑ **137.4 Late effects of tuberculosis of other specified organs**

138 **Late effects of acute poliomyelitis**

Note: This category is to be used to indicate conditions classifiable to 045 as the cause of late effects, which are themselves classified elsewhere. The "late effects" include conditions specified as such, or as sequelae, or as due to old or inactive poliomyelitis, without evidence of active disease.

● ❑ 139 **Late effects of other infectious and parasitic diseases**

Note: This category is to be used to indicate conditions classifiable to categories 001–009, 020–041, 046–136 as the cause of late effects, which are themselves classified elsewhere. The "late effects" include conditions specified as such; they also include sequelae of diseases classifiable to the above categories if there is evidence that the disease itself is no longer present.

139.0 **Late effects of viral encephalitis**
Late effects of conditions classifiable to 049.8–049.9, 062–064

❑ **139.1 Late effects of trachoma**
Late effects of conditions classifiable to 076

❑ **139.8 Late effects of other and unspecified infectious and parasitic diseases**

2. NEOPLASMS (140–239)

1. Content:
   This chapter contains the following broad groups:
   140–195 Malignant neoplasms, stated or presumed to be primary, of specified sites, except of lymphatic and hematopoietic tissue
   196–198 Malignant neoplasms, stated or presumed to be secondary, of specified sites
   199   Malignant neoplasms, without specification of site
   200–208 Malignant neoplasms, stated or presumed to be primary, of lymphatic and hematopoietic tissue
   210–229 Benign neoplasms
   230–234 Carcinoma in situ
   235–238 Neoplasms of uncertain behavior [see Note, at beginning of section 235–238]
   239   Neoplasms of unspecified nature

2. Functional activity
   All neoplasms are classified in this chapter, whether or not functionally active. An additional code from Chapter 3 may be used to identify such functional activity associated with any neoplasm, e.g.:
   catecholamine-producing malignant pheochromocytoma of adrenal:
   code 194.0, additional code 255.6
   basophil adenoma of pituitary with Cushing's syndrome:
   code 227.3, additional code 255.0

3. Morphology [Histology]
   For those wishing to identify the histological type of neoplasms, a comprehensive coded nomenclature, which comprises the morphology rubrics of the ICD-Oncology, is given after the E-code chapter.

4. Malignant neoplasms overlapping site boundaries
   Categories 140–195 are for the classification of primary malignant neoplasms according to their point of origin. A malignant neoplasm that overlaps two or more subcategories within a three-digit rubric and whose point of origin cannot be determined should be classified to the subcategory .8 "Other." For example, "carcinoma involving tip and ventral surface of tongue" should be assigned to 141.8. On the other hand, "carcinoma of tip of tongue, extending to involve the ventral surface" should be coded to 141.2, as the point of origin, the tip, is known. Three subcategories (149.8, 159.8, 165.8) have been provided for malignant neoplasms that overlap the boundaries of three-digit rubrics within certain systems. Overlapping malignant neoplasms that cannot be classified as indicated above should be assigned to the appropriate subdivision of category 195 (Malignant neoplasm of other and ill-defined sites).

MALIGNANT NEOPLASM OF LIP, ORAL CAVITY, AND PHARYNX (140–149)

> **Excludes** *carcinoma in situ (230.0)*

● **140 Malignant neoplasm of lip**

> **Excludes** *skin of lip (173.0)*

  140.0 Upper lip, vermilion border
   Upper lip: Upper lip:
   NOS   lipstick area
   external

  140.1 Lower lip, vermilion border
   Lower lip: Lower lip:
   NOS   lipstick area
   external

  140.3 Upper lip, inner aspect
   Upper lip: Upper lip:
   buccal aspect   mucosa
   frenulum   oral aspect

  140.4 Lower lip, inner aspect
   Lower lip: Lower lip:
   buccal aspect   mucosa
   frenulum   oral aspect

  ☐ **140.5 Lip, unspecified, inner aspect**
   Lip, not specified whether upper or lower:
   buccal aspect
   frenulum
   mucosa
   oral aspect

  140.6 Commissure of lip
   Labial commissure

  ☐ **140.8 Other sites of lip**
   Malignant neoplasm of contiguous or overlapping sites of lip whose point of origin cannot be determined

  ☐ **140.9 Lip, unspecified, vermilion border**
   Lip, not specified as upper or lower:
   NOS
   external
   lipstick area

● **141 Malignant neoplasm of tongue**

  141.0 Base of tongue
   Dorsal surface of base of tongue
   Fixed part of tongue NOS

  141.1 Dorsal surface of tongue
   Anterior two-thirds of tongue, dorsal surface
   Dorsal tongue NOS
   Midline of tongue

> **Excludes** *dorsal surface of base of tongue (141.0)*

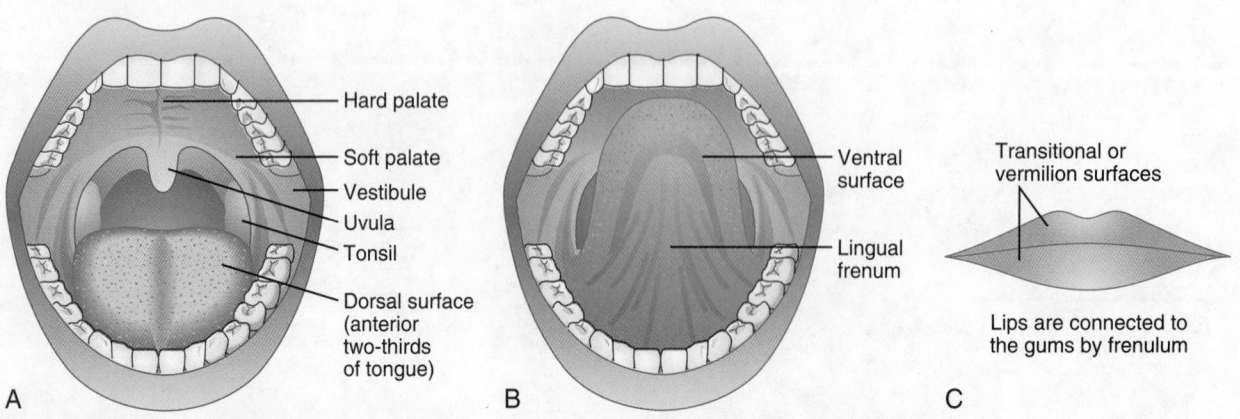

Figure 2-1 Anatomical structures of the mouth and lips. **A.** Dorsal surface. **B.** Ventral surface. **C.** Transitional or vermilion borders. Lips are connected to the gums by frenulum.

141.2 **Tip and lateral border of tongue**

141.3 **Ventral surface of tongue**
Anterior two-thirds of tongue, ventral surface
Frenulum linguae

❑141.4 **Anterior two-thirds of tongue, part unspecified**
Mobile part of tongue NOS

141.5 **Junctional zone**
Border of tongue at junction of fixed and mobile parts at insertion of anterior tonsillar pillar

141.6 **Lingual tonsil**

❑141.8 **Other sites of tongue**
Malignant neoplasm of contiguous or overlapping sites of tongue whose point of origin cannot be determined

❑141.9 **Tongue, unspecified**
Tongue NOS

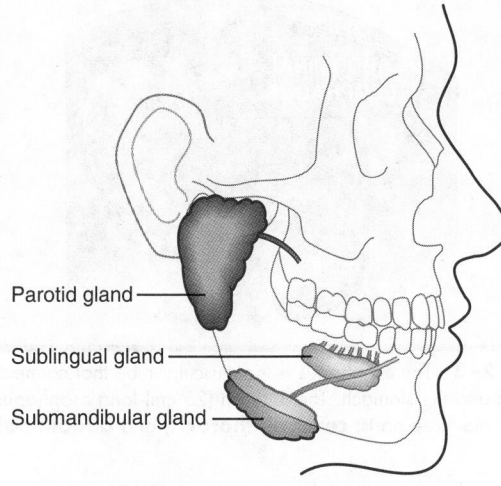

Parotid gland

Sublingual gland

Submandibular gland

Figure 2–2 Major salivary glands.

● 142 **Malignant neoplasm of major salivary glands**

Includes: salivary ducts

Excludes *malignant neoplasm of minor salivary glands:*
NOS (145.9)
buccal mucosa (145.0)
soft palate (145.3)
tongue (141.0–141.9)
tonsil, palatine (146.0)

142.0 **Parotid gland**

142.1 **Submandibular gland**
Submaxillary gland

142.2 **Sublingual gland**

❑142.8 **Other major salivary glands**
Malignant neoplasm of contiguous or overlapping sites of salivary glands and ducts whose point of origin cannot be determined

❑142.9 **Salivary gland, unspecified**
Salivary gland (major) NOS

● 143 **Malignant neoplasm of gum**

Includes: alveolar (ridge) mucosa
gingiva (alveolar) (marginal)
interdental papillae

Excludes *malignant odontogenic neoplasms (170.0–170.1)*

143.0 **Upper gum**

143.1 **Lower gum**

❑143.8 **Other sites of gum**
Malignant neoplasm of contiguous or overlapping sites of gum whose point of origin cannot be determined

❑143.9 **Gum, unspecified**

● 144 **Malignant neoplasm of floor of mouth**

144.0 **Anterior portion**
Anterior to the premolar-canine junction

144.1 **Lateral portion**

❑144.8 **Other sites of floor of mouth**
Malignant neoplasm of contiguous or overlapping sites of floor of mouth whose point of origin cannot be determined

❑144.9 **Floor of mouth, part unspecified**

● 145 **Malignant neoplasm of other and unspecified parts of mouth**

Excludes *mucosa of lips (140.0–140.9)*

145.0 **Cheek mucosa**
Buccal mucosa
Cheek, inner aspect

145.1 **Vestibule of mouth**
Buccal sulcus (upper) (lower)
Labial sulcus (upper) (lower)

145.2 **Hard palate**

145.3 **Soft palate**

Excludes *nasopharyngeal [posterior] [superior] surface of soft palate (147.3)*

145.4 **Uvula**

❑145.5 **Palate, unspecified**
Junction of hard and soft palate
Roof of mouth

145.6 **Retromolar area**

❑145.8 **Other specified parts of mouth**
Malignant neoplasm of contiguous or overlapping sites of mouth whose point of origin cannot be determined

❑145.9 **Mouth, unspecified**
Buccal cavity NOS
Minor salivary gland, unspecified site
Oral cavity NOS

● 146 **Malignant neoplasm of oropharynx**

146.0 **Tonsil**
Tonsil: Tonsil:
  NOS   palatine
  faucial

Excludes *lingual tonsil (141.6)*
pharyngeal tonsil (147.1)

146.1 **Tonsillar fossa**

146.2 **Tonsillar pillars (anterior) (posterior)**
Faucial pillar
Glossopalatine fold
Palatoglossal arch
Palatopharyngeal arch

146.3 **Vallecula**
Anterior and medial surface of the pharyngoepiglottic fold

146.4 **Anterior aspect of epiglottis**
Epiglottis, free border [margin]
Glossoepiglottic fold(s)

Excludes *epiglottis:*
NOS (161.1)
suprahyoid portion (161.1)

ICD-9-CM

100-199

Vol. 1

146.5 Junctional region
Junction of the free margin of the epiglottis, the aryepiglottic fold, and the pharyngoepiglottic fold

146.6 Lateral wall of oropharynx

146.7 Posterior wall of oropharynx

☐ **146.8 Other specified sites of oropharynx**
Branchial cleft
Malignant neoplasm of contiguous or overlapping sites of oropharynx whose point of origin cannot be determined

☐ **146.9 Oropharynx, unspecified**

● **147 Malignant neoplasm of nasopharynx**

147.0 Superior wall
Roof of nasopharynx

147.1 Posterior wall
Adenoid
Pharyngeal tonsil

147.2 Lateral wall
Fossa of Rosenmüller
Opening of auditory tube
Pharyngeal recess

147.3 Anterior wall
Floor of nasopharynx
Nasopharyngeal [posterior] [superior] surface of soft palate
Posterior margin of nasal septum and choanae

☐ **147.8 Other specified sites of nasopharynx**
Malignant neoplasm of contiguous or overlapping sites of nasopharynx whose point of origin cannot be determined

☐ **147.9 Nasopharynx, unspecified**
Nasopharyngeal wall NOS

● **148 Malignant neoplasm of hypopharynx**

148.0 Postcricoid region

148.1 Pyriform sinus
Pyriform fossa

148.2 Aryepiglottic fold, hypopharyngeal aspect
Aryepiglottic fold or interarytenoid fold:
NOS
marginal zone

> **Excludes** aryepiglottic fold or interarytenoid fold, laryngeal aspect (161.1)

148.3 Posterior hypopharyngeal wall

☐ **148.8 Other specified sites of hypopharynx**
Malignant neoplasm of contiguous or overlapping sites of hypopharynx whose point of origin cannot be determined

☐ **148.9 Hypopharynx, unspecified**
Hypopharyngeal wall NOS
Hypopharynx NOS

● **149 Malignant neoplasm of other and ill-defined sites within the lip, oral cavity, and pharynx**

☐ **149.0 Pharynx, unspecified**

149.1 Waldeyer's ring

☐ **149.8 Other**
Malignant neoplasms of lip, oral cavity, and pharynx whose point of origin cannot be assigned to any one of the categories 140–148

> **Excludes** "book leaf" neoplasm [ventral surface of tongue and floor of mouth] (145.8)

☐ **149.9 Ill-defined**

Figure 2–3 The esophagus is the muscular tube that connects the pharynx and the stomach. The 10 inch (25 cm) long esophagus is divided into three parts: **cervical, thoracic,** and **abdominal.**

MALIGNANT NEOPLASM OF DIGESTIVE ORGANS AND PERITONEUM (150–159)

> **Excludes** carcinoma in situ (230.1–230.9)

● **150 Malignant neoplasm of esophagus**

150.0 Cervical esophagus

150.1 Thoracic esophagus

150.2 Abdominal esophagus

> **Excludes** adenocarcinoma (151.0)
> cardioesophageal junction (151.0)

150.3 Upper third of esophagus
Proximal third of esophagus

150.4 Middle third of esophagus

150.5 Lower third of esophagus
Distal third of esophagus

> **Excludes** adenocarcinoma (151.0)
> cardioesophageal junction (151.0)

☐ **150.8 Other specified part**
Malignant neoplasm of contiguous or overlapping sites of esophagus whose point of origin cannot be determined

☐ **150.9 Esophagus, unspecified**

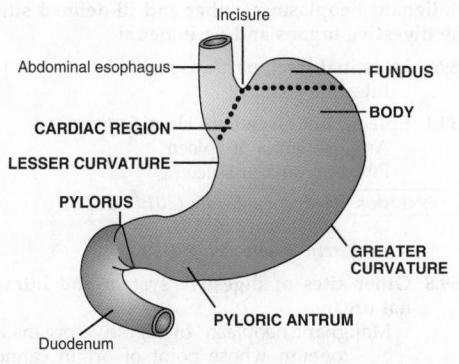

Figure 2-4 Parts of the stomach.

Item 2-1 The esophagus enters the stomach through the **cardiac orifice**, also called the **cardioesophageal junction**. The **cardia** is adjacent to the cardiac orifice. The stomach widens into the **greater** and **lesser curvatures**. The **pyloric antrum** precedes the **pylorus**, which connects to the duodenum.

● 151   Malignant neoplasm of stomach

  151.0   **Cardia**
          Cardiac orifice
          Cardioesophageal junction
          Excludes   *squamous cell carcinoma (150.2, 150.5)*

  151.1   **Pylorus**
          Prepylorus
          Pyloric canal

  151.2   **Pyloric antrum**
          Antrum of stomach NOS

  151.3   **Fundus of stomach**

  151.4   **Body of stomach**

  ❑ 151.5   **Lesser curvature, unspecified**
          Lesser curvature, not classifiable to 151.1–151.4

  ❑ 151.6   **Greater curvature, unspecified**
          Greater curvature, not classifiable to 151.0–151.4

  ❑ 151.8   **Other specified sites of stomach**
          Anterior wall, not classifiable to 151.0–151.4
          Posterior wall, not classifiable to 151.0–151.4
          Malignant neoplasm of contiguous or overlapping
              sites of stomach whose point of origin cannot
              be determined

  ❑ 151.9   **Stomach, unspecified**
          Carcinoma ventriculi
          Gastric cancer

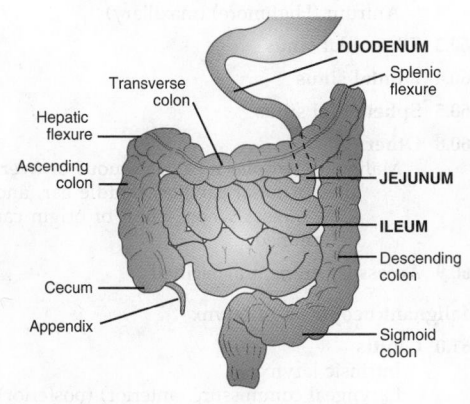

Figure 2-5 Small intestine and colon.

● 152   Malignant neoplasm of small intestine, including duodenum

  152.0   **Duodenum**

  152.1   **Jejunum**

  152.2   **Ileum**
          Excludes   *ileocecal valve (153.4)*

  152.3   **Meckel's diverticulum**

  ❑ 152.8   **Other specified sites of small intestine**
          Duodenojejunal junction
          Malignant neoplasm of contiguous or overlapping
              sites of small intestine whose point of origin
              cannot be determined

  ❑ 152.9   **Small intestine, unspecified**

● 153   Malignant neoplasm of colon

  153.0   **Hepatic flexure**

  153.1   **Transverse colon**

  153.2   **Descending colon**
          Left colon

  153.3   **Sigmoid colon**
          Sigmoid (flexure)
          Excludes   *rectosigmoid junction (154.0)*

  153.4   **Cecum**
          Ileocecal valve

  153.5   **Appendix**

  153.6   **Ascending colon**
          Right colon

  153.7   **Splenic flexure**

  ❑ 153.8   **Other specified sites of large intestine**
          Malignant neoplasm of contiguous or overlapping
              sites of colon whose point of origin cannot be
              determined
          Excludes   *ileocecal valve (153.4)*
                     rectosigmoid junction (154.0)

  ❑ 153.9   **Colon, unspecified**
          Large intestine NOS

● 154   Malignant neoplasm of rectum, rectosigmoid junction, and anus

  154.0   **Rectosigmoid junction**
          Colon with rectum
          Rectosigmoid (colon)

  154.1   **Rectum**
          Rectal ampulla

  154.2   **Anal canal**
          Anal sphincter
          Excludes   *skin of anus (172.5, 173.5)*

  ❑ 154.3   **Anus, unspecified**
          Excludes   *anus:*
                     margin (172.5, 173.5)
                     skin (172.5, 173.5)
                     perianal skin (172.5, 173.5)

  ❑ 154.8   **Other**
          Anorectum
          Cloacogenic zone
          Malignant neoplasm of contiguous or overlapping
              sites of rectum, rectosigmoid junction, and
              anus whose point of origin cannot be deter-
              mined

● 155   Malignant neoplasm of liver and intrahepatic bile ducts

  155.0   **Liver, primary**
          Carcinoma:
              liver, specified as primary
              hepatocellular
              liver cell
          Hepatoblastoma

ICD-9-CM

100-
100

Vol. 1

155.1 Intrahepatic bile ducts
Canaliculi biliferi
Interlobular:
    bile ducts
    biliary canals
Intrahepatic:
    biliary passages
    canaliculi
    gall duct
> Excludes | *hepatic duct (156.1)*

☐ **155.2 Liver, not specified as primary or secondary**

● **156 Malignant neoplasm of gallbladder and extrahepatic bile ducts**

156.0 Gallbladder

156.1 Extrahepatic bile ducts
Biliary duct or passage   Cystic duct
NOS   Hepatic duct
Common bile duct   Sphincter of Oddi

156.2 Ampulla of Vater

☐ **156.8 Other specified sites of gallbladder and extrahepatic bile ducts**
Malignant neoplasm of contiguous or overlapping sites of gallbladder and extrahepatic bile ducts whose point of origin cannot be determined

☐ **156.9 Biliary tract, part unspecified**
Malignant neoplasm involving both intrahepatic and extrahepatic bile ducts

● **157 Malignant neoplasm of pancreas**

157.0 Head of pancreas

157.1 Body of pancreas

157.2 Tail of pancreas

157.3 Pancreatic duct
Duct of:
    Santorini
    Wirsung

157.4 Islets of Langerhans
Islets of Langerhans, any part of pancreas

Use additional code to identify any functional activity

☐ **157.8 Other specified sites of pancreas**
Ectopic pancreatic tissue
Malignant neoplasm of contiguous or overlapping sites of pancreas whose point of origin cannot be determined

☐ **157.9 Pancreas, part unspecified**

● **158 Malignant neoplasm of retroperitoneum and peritoneum**

158.0 Retroperitoneum
Periadrenal tissue
Perinephric tissue
Perirenal tissue
Retrocecal tissue

☐ **158.8 Specified parts of peritoneum**
Cul-de-sac (of Douglas)
Mesentery
Mesocolon
Omentum
Peritoneum:
    parietal
    pelvic
Rectouterine pouch
Malignant neoplasm of contiguous or overlapping sites of retroperitoneum and peritoneum whose point of origin cannot be determined

☐ **158.9 Peritoneum, unspecified**

● **159 Malignant neoplasm of other and ill-defined sites within the digestive organs and peritoneum**

☐ **159.0 Intestinal tract, part unspecified**
Intestine NOS

☐ **159.1 Spleen, not elsewhere classified**
Angiosarcoma of spleen
Fibrosarcoma of spleen
> Excludes | *Hodgkin's disease (201.0–201.9)*
> *lymphosarcoma (200.1)*
> *reticulosarcoma (200.0)*

☐ **159.8 Other sites of digestive system and intra-abdominal organs**
Malignant neoplasm of digestive organs and peritoneum whose point of origin cannot be assigned to any one of the categories 150–158
> Excludes | *anus and rectum (154.8)*
> *cardioesophageal junction (151.0)*
> *colon and rectum (154.0)*

☐ **159.9 Ill-defined**
Alimentary canal or tract NOS
Gastrointestinal tract NOS
> Excludes | *abdominal NOS (195.2)*
> *intra-abdominal NOS (195.2)*

MALIGNANT NEOPLASM OF RESPIRATORY AND INTRATHORACIC ORGANS (160–165)

> Excludes | *carcinoma in situ (231.0–231.9)*

● **160 Malignant neoplasm of nasal cavities, middle ear, and accessory sinuses**

160.0 Nasal cavities
Cartilage of nose
Conchae, nasal
Internal nose
Septum of nose
Vestibule of nose
> Excludes | *nasal bone (170.0)*
> *nose NOS (195.0)*
> *olfactory bulb (192.0)*
> *posterior margin of septum and choanae (147.3)*
> *skin of nose (172.3, 173.3)*
> *turbinates (170.0)*

160.1 Auditory tube, middle ear, and mastoid air cells
Antrum tympanicum
Eustachian tube
Tympanic cavity
> Excludes | *auditory canal (external) (172.2, 173.2)*
> *bone of ear (meatus) (170.0)*
> *cartilage of ear (171.0)*
> *ear (external) (skin) (172.2, 173.2)*

160.2 Maxillary sinus
Antrum (Highmore) (maxillary)

160.3 Ethmoidal sinus

160.4 Frontal sinus

160.5 Sphenoidal sinus

☐ **160.8 Other**
Malignant neoplasm of contiguous or overlapping sites of nasal cavities, middle ear, and accessory sinuses whose point of origin cannot be determined

☐ **160.9 Accessory sinus, unspecified**

● **161 Malignant neoplasm of larynx**

161.0 Glottis
Intrinsic larynx
Laryngeal commissure (anterior) (posterior)
True vocal cord
Vocal cord NOS

161.1　Supraglottis
Aryepiglottic fold or interarytenoid fold, laryngeal aspect
Epiglottis (suprahyoid portion) NOS
Extrinsic larynx
False vocal cords
Posterior (laryngeal) surface of epiglottis
Ventricular bands

> **Excludes**　*anterior aspect of epiglottis (146.4)*
> *aryepiglottic fold or interarytenoid fold:*
>   *NOS (148.2)*
>   *hypopharyngeal aspect (148.2)*
>   *marginal zone (148.2)*

161.2　Subglottis

161.3　Laryngeal cartilages
Cartilage:　　　　　Cartilage:
　arytenoid　　　　　cuneiform
　cricoid　　　　　　thyroid

161.8　Other specified sites of larynx
Malignant neoplasm of contiguous or overlapping sites of larynx whose point of origin cannot be determined

161.9　Larynx, unspecified

● **162　Malignant neoplasm of trachea, bronchus, and lung**

162.0　Trachea
Cartilage of trachea
Mucosa of trachea

162.2　Main bronchus
Carina
Hilus of lung

162.3　Upper lobe, bronchus or lung

162.4　Middle lobe, bronchus or lung

162.5　Lower lobe, bronchus or lung

162.8　Other parts of bronchus or lung
Malignant neoplasm of contiguous or overlapping sites of bronchus or lung whose point of origin cannot be determined

162.9　Bronchus and lung, unspecified

● **163　Malignant neoplasm of pleura**

163.0　Parietal pleura

163.1　Visceral pleura

163.8　Other specified sites of pleura
Malignant neoplasm of contiguous or overlapping sites of pleura whose point of origin cannot be determined

163.9　Pleura, unspecified

● **164　Malignant neoplasm of thymus, heart, and mediastinum**

164.0　Thymus

164.1　Heart
Endocardium
Epicardium
Myocardium
Pericardium

> **Excludes**　*great vessels (171.4)*

164.2　Anterior mediastinum

164.3　Posterior mediastinum

164.8　Other
Malignant neoplasm of contiguous or overlapping sites of thymus, heart, and mediastinum whose point of origin cannot be determined

164.9　Mediastinum, part unspecified

● **165　Malignant neoplasm of other and ill-defined sites within the respiratory system and intrathoracic organs**

165.0　Upper respiratory tract, part unspecified

165.8　Other
Malignant neoplasm of respiratory and intrathoracic organs whose point of origin cannot be assigned to any one of the categories 160–164

165.9　Ill-defined sites within the respiratory system
Respiratory tract NOS

> **Excludes**　*intrathoracic NOS (195.1)*
> *thoracic NOS (195.1)*

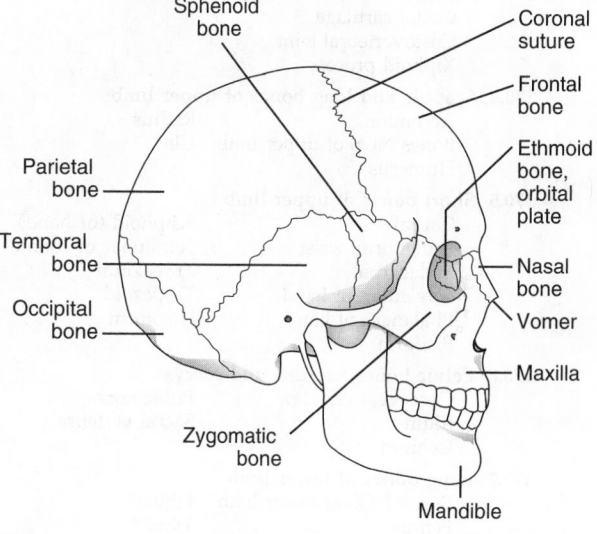

Figure 2–6　Bones of the skull and face.

MALIGNANT NEOPLASM OF BONE, CONNECTIVE TISSUE, SKIN, AND BREAST (170–176)

> **Excludes**　*carcinoma in situ:*
> *breast (233.0)*
> *skin (232.0–232.9)*

● **170　Malignant neoplasm of bone and articular cartilage**

Includes: cartilage (articular) (joint)
periosteum

> **Excludes**　*bone marrow NOS (202.9)*
> *cartilage:*
>   *ear (171.0)*
>   *eyelid (171.0)*
>   *larynx (161.3)*
>   *nose (160.0)*
> *synovia (171.0–171.9)*

170.0　Bones of skull and face, except mandible

Bone:　　　　　　Bone:
　ethmoid　　　　　sphenoid
　frontal　　　　　　temporal
　malar　　　　　　zygomatic
　nasal　　　　　　Maxilla (superior)
　occipital　　　　　Turbinate
　orbital　　　　　Upper jaw bone
　parietal　　　　　Vomer

> **Excludes**　*carcinoma, any type except intraosseous or odontogenic:*
> *maxilla, maxillary (sinus) (160.2)*
> *upper jaw bone (143.0)*
> *jaw bone (lower) (170.1)*

170.1 Mandible
Inferior maxilla
Jaw bone NOS
Lower jaw bone
Excludes | *carcinoma, any type except intraosseous or odon-*
togenic:
jaw bone NOS (143.9)
lower (143.1)
upper jaw bone (170.0)

170.2 Vertebral column, excluding sacrum and coccyx
Spinal column
Spine
Vertebra
Excludes | *sacrum and coccyx (170.6)*

170.3 Ribs, sternum, and clavicle
Costal cartilage
Costovertebral joint
Xiphoid process

170.4 Scapula and long bones of upper limb
Acromion   Radius
Bones NOS of upper limb   Ulna
Humerus

170.5 Short bones of upper limb
Carpal   Scaphoid (of hand)
Cuneiform, wrist   Semilunar or lunate
Metacarpal   Trapezium
Navicular, of hand   Trapezoid
Phalanges of hand   Unciform
Pisiform

170.6 Pelvic bones, sacrum, and coccyx
Coccygeal vertebra   Pubic bone
Ilium   Sacral vertebra
Ischium

170.7 Long bones of lower limb
Bones NOS of lower limb   Fibula
Femur   Tibia

170.8 Short bones of lower limb
Astragalus [talus]   Navicular (of ankle)
Calcaneus   Patella
Cuboid   Phalanges of foot
Cuneiform, ankle   Tarsal
Metatarsal

❑ **170.9 Bone and articular cartilage, site unspecified**

● **171 Malignant neoplasm of connective and other soft tissue**
Includes: blood vessel
bursa
fascia
fat
ligament, except uterine
muscle
peripheral, sympathetic, and parasympathetic
nerves and ganglia
synovia
tendon (sheath)
Excludes | *cartilage (of):*
articular (170.0–170.9)
larynx (161.3)
nose (160.0)
connective tissue:
breast (174.0–175.9)
internal organs - code to malignant neoplasm
of the site [e.g., leiomyosarcoma of stom-
ach, 151.9]
heart (164.1)
uterine ligament (183.4)

171.0 Head, face, and neck
Cartilage of:
ear
eyelid

171.2 Upper limb, including shoulder
Arm
Finger
Forearm
Hand

171.3 Lower limb, including hip
Foot
Leg
Popliteal space
Thigh
Toe

171.4 Thorax
Axilla
Diaphragm
Great vessels
Excludes | *heart (164.1)*
mediastinum (164.2–164.9)
thymus (164.0)

171.5 Abdomen
Abdominal wall
Hypochondrium
Excludes | *peritoneum (158.8)*
retroperitoneum (158.0)

171.6 Pelvis
Buttock
Groin
Inguinal region
Perineum
Excludes | *pelvic peritoneum (158.8)*
retroperitoneum (158.0)
uterine ligament, any (183.3–183.5)

❑ **171.7 Trunk, unspecified**
Back NOS
Flank NOS

❑ **171.8 Other specified sites of connective and other soft**
tissue
Malignant neoplasm of contiguous or overlapping
sites of connective tissue whose point of origin cannot be determined

❑ **171.9 Connective and other soft tissue, site unspecified**

● **172 Malignant melanoma of skin**
Includes: melanocarcinoma
melanoma (skin) NOS
Excludes | *skin of genital organs (184.0–184.9, 187.1–187.9)*
sites other than skin - code to malignant neo-
plasm of the site

172.0 Lip
Excludes | *vermilion border of lip (140.0–140.1, 140.9)*

172.1 Eyelid, including canthus

172.2 Ear and external auditory canal
Auricle (ear)
Auricular canal, external
External [acoustic] meatus
Pinna

❑ **172.3 Other and unspecified parts of face**
Cheek (external)
Chin
Eyebrow
Forehead
Nose, external
Temple

172.4 Scalp and neck

172.5 Trunk, except scrotum

Axilla	Perianal skin
Breast	Perineum
Buttock	Umbilicus
Groin	

> **Excludes** anal canal (154.2)
> anus NOS (154.3)
> scrotum (187.7)

172.6 Upper limb, including shoulder

Arm	Forearm
Finger	Hand

172.7 Lower limb, including hip

Ankle	Leg
Foot	Popliteal area
Heel	Thigh
Knee	Toe

☐ **172.8 Other specified sites of skin**
Malignant melanoma of contiguous or overlapping sites of skin whose point of origin cannot be determined

☐ **172.9 Melanoma of skin, site unspecified**

● **173 Other malignant neoplasm of skin**

Includes: malignant neoplasm of:
sebaceous glands
sudoriferous, sudoriparous glands
sweat glands

> **Excludes** Kaposi's sarcoma (176.0–176.9)
> malignant melanoma of skin (172.0–172.9)
> skin of genital organs (184.0–184.9, 187.1– 187.9)

173.0 Skin of lip

> **Excludes** vermilion border of lip (140.0–140.1, 140.9)

173.1 Eyelid, including canthus

> **Excludes** cartilage of eyelid (171.0)

173.2 Skin of ear and external auditory canal
Auricle (ear)
Auricular canal, external
External meatus
Pinna

> **Excludes** cartilage of ear (171.0)

☐ **173.3 Skin of other and unspecified parts of face**
Cheek, external
Chin
Eyebrow
Forehead
Nose, external
Temple

173.4 Scalp and skin of neck

173.5 Skin of trunk, except scrotum
Axillary fold
Perianal skin
Skin of:
abdominal wall
anus
back
breast
buttock
chest wall
groin
perineum
umbilicus

> **Excludes** anal canal (154.2)
> anus NOS (154.3)
> skin of scrotum (187.7)

173.6 Skin of upper limb, including shoulder
Arm
Finger
Forearm
Hand

173.7 Skin of lower limb, including hip
Ankle
Foot
Heel
Knee
Leg
Popliteal area
Thigh
Toe

☐ **173.8 Other specified sites of skin**
Malignant neoplasm of contiguous or overlapping sites of skin whose point of origin cannot be determined

☐ **173.9 Skin, site unspecified**

Figure 2–7 Female breast quadrants and axillary tail.

● **174 Malignant neoplasm of female breast**

Includes: breast (female)
connective tissue
soft parts
Paget's disease of:
breast
nipple

> **Excludes** skin of breast (172.5, 173.5)

174.0 Nipple and areola

174.1 Central portion

174.2 Upper-inner quadrant

174.3 Lower-inner quadrant

174.4 Upper-outer quadrant

174.5 Lower-outer quadrant

174.6 Axillary tail

☐ **174.8 Other specified sites of female breast**
Ectopic sites
Inner breast
Lower breast
Malignant neoplasm of contiguous or overlapping sites of breast whose point of origin cannot be determined
Midline of breast
Outer breast
Upper breast

◀ **New**   ◀▥ **Revised**   ● **Not a Principal Diagnosis**   ● **Use Additional Digit(s)**   ☐ **Nonspecific Code**

☐ **174.9 Breast (female), unspecified**

● **175 Malignant neoplasm of male breast**

> **Excludes** *skin of breast (172.5, 173.5)*

175.0 Nipple and areola

☐ **175.9 Other and unspecified sites of male breast**
Ectopic breast tissue, male

● **176 Kaposi's sarcoma**

176.0 Skin

176.1 Soft tissue

> **Includes:** Blood vessel ◀▥
> Connective tissue ◀▥
> Fascia ◀▥
> Ligament ◀▥
> Lymphatic(s) NEC ◀▥
> Muscle ◀▥

> **Excludes** *lymph glands and nodes (176.5)*

176.2 Palate

176.3 Gastrointestinal sites

176.4 Lung

176.5 Lymph nodes

☐ **176.8 Other specified sites**

> **Includes:** Oral cavity NEC ◀▥

☐ **176.9 Unspecified**
Viscera NOS

● **180 Malignant neoplasm of cervix uteri**

> **Includes:** invasive malignancy [carcinoma]
> **Excludes** *carcinoma in situ (233.1)*

180.0 Endocervix
Cervical canal NOS
Endocervical canal
Endocervical gland

180.1 Exocervix

☐ **180.8 Other specified sites of cervix**
Cervical stump
Squamocolumnar junction of cervix
Malignant neoplasm of contiguous or overlapping sites of cervix uteri whose point of origin cannot be determined

☐ **180.9 Cervix uteri, unspecified**

181 Malignant neoplasm of placenta
Choriocarcinoma NOS
Chorioepithelioma NOS

> **Excludes** *chorioadenoma (destruens) (236.1)*
> *hydatidiform mole (630)*
> *malignant (236.1)*
> *invasive mole (236.1)*
> *male choriocarcinoma NOS (186.0–186.9)*

● **182 Malignant neoplasm of body of uterus**

> **Excludes** *carcinoma in situ (233.2)*

182.0 Corpus uteri, except isthmus
Cornu
Endometrium
Fundus
Myometrium

182.1 Isthmus
Lower uterine segment

☐ **182.8 Other specified sites of body of uterus**
Malignant neoplasm of contiguous or overlapping sites of body of uterus whose point of origin cannot be determined

> **Excludes** *uterus NOS (179)*

● **183 Malignant neoplasm of ovary and other uterine adnexa**

> **Excludes** *Douglas' cul-de-sac (158.8)*

183.0 Ovary

Use additional code to identify any functional activity

183.2 Fallopian tube
Oviduct
Uterine tube

183.3 Broad ligament
Mesovarium
Parovarian region

183.4 Parametrium
Uterine ligament NOS
Uterosacral ligament

183.5 Round ligament

☐ **183.8 Other specified sites of uterine adnexa**
Tubo-ovarian
Utero-ovarian
Malignant neoplasm of contiguous or overlapping sites of ovary and other uterine adnexa whose point of origin cannot be determined

☐ **183.9 Uterine adnexa, unspecified**

● **184 Malignant neoplasm of other and unspecified female genital organs**

> **Excludes** *carcinoma in situ (233.3)*

184.0 Vagina
Gartner's duct
Vaginal vault

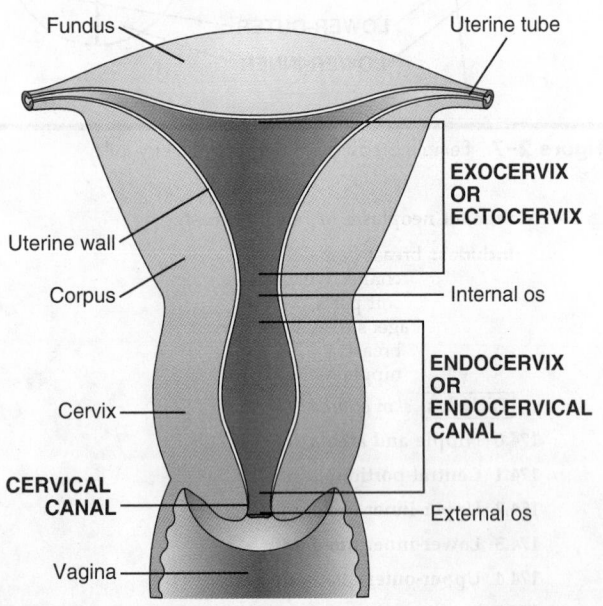

Fundus

Uterine tube

EXOCERVIX OR ECTOCERVIX

Uterine wall

Internal os

Corpus

ENDOCERVIX OR ENDOCERVICAL CANAL

Cervix

CERVICAL CANAL

External os

Vagina

Figure 2–8 Cervix uteri.

MALIGNANT NEOPLASM OF GENITOURINARY ORGANS (179–189)

> **Excludes** *carcinoma in situ (233.1–233.9)*

☐ **179 Malignant neoplasm of uterus, part unspecified**

◀ **New**   ◀▥ **Revised**   ● **Not a Principal Diagnosis**   ● **Use Additional Digit(s)**   ☐ **Nonspecific Code**

184.1 **Labia majora**
  Greater vestibular [Bartholin's] gland

184.2 **Labia minora**

184.3 **Clitoris**

❑ 184.4 **Vulva, unspecified**
  External female genitalia NOS
  Pudendum

❑ 184.8 **Other specified sites of female genital organs**
  Malignant neoplasm of contiguous or overlapping sites of female genital organs whose point of origin cannot be determined

❑ 184.9 **Female genital organ, site unspecified**
  Female genitourinary tract NOS

185 **Malignant neoplasm of prostate**
  Excludes *seminal vesicles (187.8)*

● 186 **Malignant neoplasm of testis**
  Use additional code to identify any functional activity

  186.0 **Undescended testis**
    Ectopic testis
    Retained testis

  ❑ 186.9 **Other and unspecified testis**
    Testis:
    NOS
    descended
    scrotal

● 187 **Malignant neoplasm of penis and other male genital organs**

  187.1 **Prepuce**
    Foreskin

  187.2 **Glans penis**

  187.3 **Body of penis**
    Corpus cavernosum

  ❑ 187.4 **Penis, part unspecified**
    Skin of penis NOS

  187.5 **Epididymis**

  187.6 **Spermatic cord**
    Vas deferens

  187.7 **Scrotum**
    Skin of scrotum

❑ 187.8 **Other specified sites of male genital organs**
  Seminal vesicle
  Tunica vaginalis
  Malignant neoplasm of contiguous or overlapping sites of penis and other male genital organs whose point of origin cannot be determined

❑ 187.9 **Male genital organ, site unspecified**
  Male genital organ or tract NOS

● 188 **Malignant neoplasm of bladder**
  Excludes *carcinoma in situ (233.7)*

  188.0 **Trigone of urinary bladder**

  188.1 **Dome of urinary bladder**

  188.2 **Lateral wall of urinary bladder**

  188.3 **Anterior wall of urinary bladder**

  188.4 **Posterior wall of urinary bladder**

  188.5 **Bladder neck**
    Internal urethral orifice

  188.6 **Ureteric orifice**

  188.7 **Urachus**

  ❑ 188.8 **Other specified sites of bladder**
    Malignant neoplasm of contiguous or overlapping sites of bladder whose point of origin cannot be determined

  ❑ 188.9 **Bladder, part unspecified**
    Bladder wall NOS

● 189 **Malignant neoplasm of kidney and other and unspecified urinary organs**

  189.0 **Kidney, except pelvis**
    Kidney NOS   Kidney parenchyma

  189.1 **Renal pelvis**
    Renal calyces   Ureteropelvic junction

  189.2 **Ureter**
    Excludes *ureteric orifice of bladder (188.6)*

  189.3 **Urethra**
    Excludes *urethral orifice of bladder (188.5)*

  189.4 **Paraurethral glands**

  ❑ 189.8 **Other specified sites of urinary organs**
    Malignant neoplasm of contiguous or overlapping sites of kidney and other urinary organs whose point of origin cannot be determined

  ❑ 189.9 **Urinary organ, site unspecified**
    Urinary system NOS

ICD-9-CM

100-199

Vol. 1

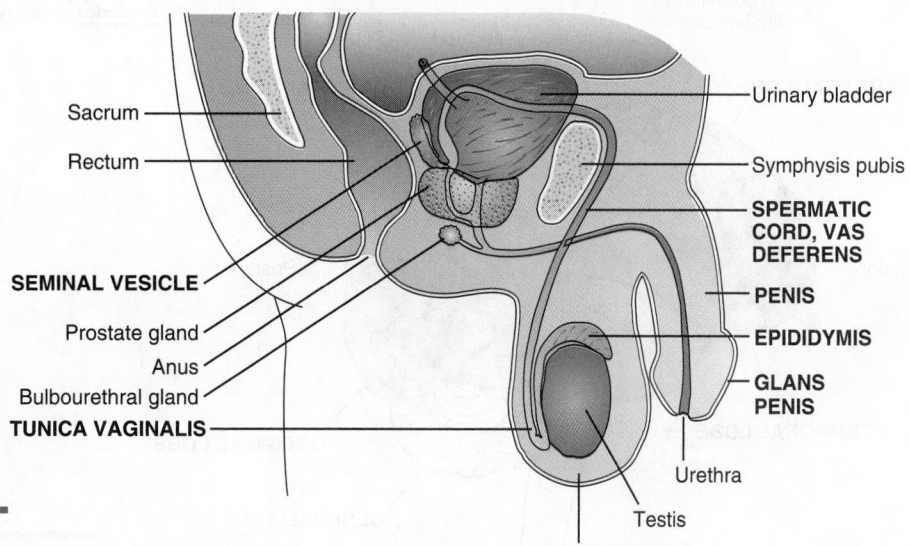

Figure 2-9 Penis and other male genital organs.

◀ **New**   ◀▥ **Revised**   ● **Not a Principal Diagnosis**   ● **Use Additional Digit(s)**   ❑ **Nonspecific Code**

MALIGNANT NEOPLASM OF OTHER AND UNSPECIFIED SITES (190–199)

> **Excludes** *carcinoma in situ (234.0–234.9)*

● **190 Malignant neoplasm of eye**

> **Excludes** *carcinoma in situ (234.0)*
> *eyelid (skin) (172.1, 173.1)*
>   *cartilage (171.0)*
> *optic nerve (192.0)*
> *orbital bone (170.0)*

190.0 Eyeball, except conjunctiva, cornea, retina, and choroid
     Ciliary body
     Crystalline lens
     Iris
     Sclera
     Uveal tract

190.1 Orbit
     Connective tissue of orbit
     Extraocular muscle
     Retrobulbar

> **Excludes** *bone of orbit (170.0)*

190.2 Lacrimal gland

190.3 Conjunctiva

190.4 Cornea

190.5 Retina

190.6 Choroid

190.7 Lacrimal duct
     Lacrimal sac
     Nasolacrimal duct

❏ **190.8 Other specified sites of eye**
     Malignant neoplasm of contiguous or overlapping sites of eye whose point of origin cannot be determined

❏ **190.9 Eye, part unspecified**

● **191 Malignant neoplasm of brain**

> **Excludes** *cranial nerves (192.0)*
> *retrobulbar area (190.1)*

191.0 Cerebrum, except lobes and ventricles
     Basal ganglia
     Cerebral cortex
     Corpus striatum
     Globus pallidus
     Hypothalamus
     Thalamus

191.1 Frontal lobe

191.2 Temporal lobe
     Hippocampus
     Uncus

191.3 Parietal lobe

191.4 Occipital lobe

191.5 Ventricles
     Choroid plexus
     Floor of ventricle

191.6 Cerebellum NOS
     Cerebellopontine angle

191.7 Brain stem
     Cerebral peduncle
     Medulla oblongata
     Midbrain
     Pons

❏ **191.8 Other parts of brain**
     Corpus callosum
     Tapetum
     Malignant neoplasm of contiguous or overlapping sites of brain whose point of origin cannot be determined

❏ **191.9 Brain, unspecified**
     Cranial fossa NOS

● **192 Malignant neoplasm of other and unspecified parts of nervous system**

> **Excludes** *peripheral, sympathetic, and parasympathetic nerves and ganglia (171.0–171.9)*

192.0 Cranial nerves
     Olfactory bulb

192.1 Cerebral meninges
     Dura (mater)
     Falx (cerebelli) (cerebri)
     Meninges NOS
     Tentorium

192.2 Spinal cord
     Cauda equina

192.3 Spinal meninges

❏ **192.8 Other specified sites of nervous system**
     Malignant neoplasm of contiguous or overlapping sites of other parts of nervous system whose point of origin cannot be determined

❏ **192.9 Nervous system, part unspecified**
     Nervous system (central) NOS

> **Excludes** *meninges NOS (192.1)*

FRONTAL LOBE   PARIETAL LOBE

Anterior   Posterior

TEMPORAL LOBE   OCCIPITAL LOBE

CEREBELLUM

Figure 2–10 The brain.

193 Malignant neoplasm of thyroid gland
Sipple's syndrome
Thyroglossal duct

Use additional code to identify any functional activity

● **194 Malignant neoplasm of other endocrine glands and related structures**

Use additional code to identify any functional activity

Excludes   *islets of Langerhans (157.4)*
ovary (183.0)
testis (186.0–186.9)
thymus (164.0)

194.0 Adrenal gland
Adrenal cortex
Adrenal medulla
Suprarenal gland

194.1 Parathyroid gland

194.3 Pituitary gland and craniopharyngeal duct
Craniobuccal pouch
Hypophysis
Rathke's pouch
Sella turcica

194.4 Pineal gland

194.5 Carotid body

194.6 Aortic body and other paraganglia
Coccygeal body
Glomus jugulare
Para-aortic body

❑ **194.8 Other**
Pluriglandular involvement NOS

Note: If the sites of multiple involvements are known, they should be coded separately.

❑ **194.9 Endocrine gland, site unspecified**

● **195 Malignant neoplasm of other and ill-defined sites**

Includes: malignant neoplasms of contiguous sites, not elsewhere classified, whose point of origin cannot be determined

Excludes   *malignant neoplasm:*
lymphatic and hematopoietic tissue (200.0–208.9)
secondary sites (196.0–198.8)
unspecified site (199.0–199.1)

195.0 Head, face, and neck
Cheek NOS
Jaw NOS
Nose NOS
Supraclavicular region NOS

195.1 Thorax
Axilla
Chest (wall) NOS
Intrathoracic NOS

195.2 Abdomen
Intra-abdominal NOS

195.3 Pelvis
Groin
Inguinal region NOS
Presacral region
Sacrococcygeal region
Sites overlapping systems within pelvis, as:
rectovaginal (septum)
rectovesical (septum)

195.4 Upper limb

195.5 Lower limb

❑ **195.8 Other specified sites**
Back NOS
Flank NOS
Trunk NOS

● **196 Secondary and unspecified malignant neoplasm of lymph nodes**

Excludes   *any malignant neoplasm of lymph nodes, specified as primary (200.0–202.9)*
Hodgkin's disease (201.0–201.9)
lymphosarcoma (200.1)
reticulosarcoma (200.0)
other forms of lymphoma (202.0–202.9)

196.0 Lymph nodes of head, face, and neck
Cervical   Scalene
Cervicofacial   Supraclavicular

196.1 Intrathoracic lymph nodes
Bronchopulmonary   Mediastinal
Intercostal   Tracheobronchial

196.2 Intra-abdominal lymph nodes
Intestinal   Retroperitoneal
Mesenteric

196.3 Lymph nodes of axilla and upper limb
Brachial   Infraclavicular
Epitrochlear   Pectoral

196.5 Lymph nodes of inguinal region and lower limb
Femoral   Popliteal
Groin   Tibial

196.6 Intrapelvic lymph nodes
Hypogastric   Obturator
Iliac   Parametrial

❑ **196.8 Lymph nodes of multiple sites**

❑ **196.9 Site unspecified**
Lymph nodes NOS

● **197 Secondary malignant neoplasm of respiratory and digestive systems**

Excludes   *lymph node metastasis (196.0–196.9)*

197.0 Lung
Bronchus

197.1 Mediastinum

197.2 Pleura

❑ **197.3 Other respiratory organs**
Trachea

197.4 Small intestine, including duodenum

197.5 Large intestine and rectum

197.6 Retroperitoneum and peritoneum

197.7 Liver, specified as secondary

❑ **197.8 Other digestive organs and spleen**

● **198 Secondary malignant neoplasm of other specified sites**
Excludes   *lymph node metastasis (196.0–196.9)*

198.0 Kidney

❑ **198.1 Other urinary organs**

198.2 Skin
Skin of breast

198.3 Brain and spinal cord

❑ **198.4 Other parts of nervous system**
Meninges (cerebral) (spinal)

198.5 Bone and bone marrow

198.6 Ovary

ICD-9-CM

200-299

Vol. 1

198.7 **Adrenal gland**
Suprarenal gland

● 198.8 **Other specified sites**

198.81 **Breast**

| Excludes | skin of breast (198.2)

198.82 **Genital organs**

❑ 198.89 **Other**

| Excludes | retroperitoneal lymph nodes (196.2)

● 199 **Malignant neoplasm without specification of site**

199.0 **Disseminated**
Carcinomatosis unspecified site (primary) (secondary)
Generalized:
cancer unspecified site (primary) (secondary)
malignancy unspecified site (primary) (secondary)
Multiple cancer unspecified site (primary) (secondary)

❑ 199.1 **Other**
Cancer unspecified site (primary) (secondary)
Carcinoma unspecified site (primary) (secondary)
Malignancy unspecified site (primary) (secondary)

MALIGNANT NEOPLASM OF LYMPHATIC AND HEMATOPOIETIC TISSUE (200–208)

| Excludes | secondary neoplasm of:
bone marrow (198.5)
spleen (197.8)
secondary and unspecified neoplasm of lymph nodes (196.0–196.9)

The following fifth-digit subclassification is for use with categories 200–202:
❑ 0 unspecified site, extranodal and solid organ sites
1 lymph nodes of head, face, and neck
2 intrathoracic lymph nodes
3 intra-abdominal lymph nodes
4 lymph nodes of axilla and upper limb
5 lymph nodes of inguinal region and lower limb
6 intrapelvic lymph nodes
7 spleen
8 lymph nodes of multiple sites

● 200 **Lymphosarcoma and reticulosarcoma**

Requires fifth digit. See note before section 200 for codes and definitions.

● 200.0 **Reticulosarcoma**
Lymphoma (malignant):
histiocytic (diffuse):
nodular
pleomorphic cell type
reticulum cell type
Reticulum cell sarcoma:
NOS
pleomorphic cell type

● 200.1 **Lymphosarcoma**
Lymphoblastoma (diffuse)
Lymphoma (malignant):
lymphoblastic (diffuse)
lymphocytic (cell type) (diffuse)
lymphosarcoma type
Lymphosarcoma:
NOS
diffuse NOS
lymphoblastic (diffuse)
lymphocytic (diffuse)
prolymphocytic

| Excludes | lymphosarcoma:
follicular or nodular (202.0)
mixed cell type (200.8)
lymphosarcoma cell leukemia (207.8)

● 200.2 **Burkitt's tumor or lymphoma**
Malignant lymphoma, Burkitt's type

● ❑ 200.8 **Other named variants**
Lymphoma (malignant):
lymphoplasmacytoid type
mixed lymphocytic-histiocytic (diffuse)
Lymphosarcoma, mixed cell type (diffuse)
Reticulolymphosarcoma (diffuse)

● 201 **Hodgkin's disease**

Requires fifth digit. See note before section 200 for codes and definitions.

● 201.0 **Hodgkin's paragranuloma**

● 201.1 **Hodgkin's granuloma**

● 201.2 **Hodgkin's sarcoma**

● 201.4 **Lymphocytic-histiocytic predominance**

● 201.5 **Nodular sclerosis**
Hodgkin's disease, nodular sclerosis:
NOS
cellular phase

● 201.6 **Mixed cellularity**

● 201.7 **Lymphocytic depletion**
Hodgkin's disease, lymphocytic depletion:
NOS
diffuse fibrosis
reticular type

● ❑ 201.9 **Hodgkin's disease, unspecified**
Hodgkin's:
disease NOS
lymphoma NOS
Malignant:
lymphogranuloma
lymphogranulomatosis

● 202 **Other malignant neoplasms of lymphoid and histiocytic tissue**

Requires fifth digit. See note before section 200 for codes and definitions.

● 202.0 **Nodular lymphoma**
Brill-Symmers disease
Lymphoma:
follicular (giant)
lymphocytic, nodular
Lymphosarcoma:
follicular (giant)
nodular
Reticulosarcoma, follicular or nodular

● 202.1 **Mycosis fungoides**

● 202.2 **Sézary's disease**

● 202.3 **Malignant histiocytosis**
Histiocytic medullary reticulosis
Malignant:
reticuloendotheliosis
reticulosis

● 202.4 **Leukemic reticuloendotheliosis**
Hairy-cell leukemia

● 202.5 **Letterer-Siwe disease**
Acute:
differentiated progressive histiocytosis
histiocytosis X (progressive)
infantile reticuloendotheliosis
reticulosis of infancy

| Excludes | Hand-Schüller-Christian disease (277.89)
histiocytosis (acute) (chronic) (277.89)
histiocytosis X (chronic) (277.89)

● **202.6 Malignant mast cell tumors**
  Malignant:
    mastocytoma
    mastocytosis
  Mast cell sarcoma
  Systemic tissue mast cell disease

  Excludes *mast cell leukemia (207.8)*

● ❏ **202.8 Other lymphomas**
  Lymphoma (malignant):
    NOS
    diffuse

  Excludes *benign lymphoma (229.0)*

● ❏ **202.9 Other and unspecified malignant neoplasms of lymphoid and histiocytic tissue**
  Follicular dendritic cell sarcoma
  Interdigitating dendritic cell sarcoma
  Langerhans cell sarcoma
  Malignant neoplasm of bone marrow NOS

● **203 Multiple myeloma and immunoproliferative neoplasms**

  The following fifth-digit subclassification is for use with category 203:
    0 without mention of remission
    1 in remission

● **203.0 Multiple myeloma**
  Kahler's disease   Myelomatosis

  Excludes *solitary myeloma (238.6)*

● **203.1 Plasma cell leukemia**
  Plasmacytic leukemia

● ❏ **203.8 Other immunoproliferative neoplasms**

● **204 Lymphoid leukemia**

  Includes: leukemia: leukemia:
    lymphatic   lymphocytic
    lymphoblastic   lymphogenous

  The following fifth-digit subclassification is for use with category 204:
    0 without mention of remission
    1 in remission

● **204.0 Acute**
  Excludes *acute exacerbation of chronic lymphoid leukemia (204.1)*

● **204.1 Chronic**

● **204.2 Subacute**

● ❏ **204.8 Other lymphoid leukemia**
  Aleukemic leukemia:
    lymphatic
    lymphocytic
    lymphoid

● ❏ **204.9 Unspecified lymphoid leukemia**

● **205 Myeloid leukemia**

  Includes: leukemia:
    granulocytic
    myeloblastic
    myelocytic
    myelogenous
    myelomonocytic
    myelosclerotic
    myelosis

  The following fifth-digit subclassification is for use with category 205:
    0 without mention of remission
    1 in remission

● **205.0 Acute**
  Acute promyelocytic leukemia

  Excludes *acute exacerbation of chronic myeloid leukemia (205.1)*

● **205.1 Chronic**
  Eosinophilic leukemia
  Neutrophilic leukemia

● **205.2 Subacute**

● **205.3 Myeloid sarcoma**
  Chloroma
  Granulocytic sarcoma

● ❏ **205.8 Other myeloid leukemia**
  Aleukemic leukemia:
    granulocytic
    myelogenous
    myeloid
  Aleukemic myelosis

● ❏ **205.9 Unspecified myeloid leukemia**

● **206 Monocytic leukemia**

  Includes: leukemia:
    histiocytic
    monoblastic
    monocytoid

  The following fifth-digit subclassification is for use with category 206:
    0 without mention of remission
    1 in remission

● **206.0 Acute**
  Excludes *acute exacerbation of chronic monocytic leukemia (206.1)*

● **206.1 Chronic**

● **206.2 Subacute**

● ❏ **206.8 Other monocytic leukemia**
  Aleukemic:
    monocytic leukemia
    monocytoid leukemia

● ❏ **206.9 Unspecified monocytic leukemia**

● **207 Other specified leukemia**

  Excludes *leukemic reticuloendotheliosis (202.4)*
  plasma cell leukemia (203.1)

  The following fifth-digit subclassification is for use with category 207:
    0 without mention of remission
    1 in remission

● **207.0 Acute erythremia and erythroleukemia**
  Acute erythremic myelosis
  Di Guglielmo's disease
  Erythremic myelosis

● **207.1 Chronic erythremia**
  Heilmeyer-Schöner disease

● **207.2 Megakaryocytic leukemia**
  Megakaryocytic myelosis
  Thrombocytic leukemia

● ❏ **207.8 Other specified leukemia**
  Lymphosarcoma cell leukemia

● **208 Leukemia of unspecified cell type**

  The following fifth-digit subclassification is for use with category 208:
    0 without mention of remission
    1 in remission

● ❏ **208.0 Acute**
  Acute leukemia NOS
  Blast cell leukemia
  Stem cell leukemia

  Excludes *acute exacerbation of chronic unspecified leukemia (208.1)*

ICD-9-CM
200-299
Vol. 1

● ❑ **208.1 Chronic**
Chronic leukemia NOS

● ❑ **208.2 Subacute**
Subacute leukemia NOS

● ❑ **208.8 Other leukemia of unspecified cell type**

● ❑ **208.9 Unspecified leukemia**
Leukemia NOS

BENIGN NEOPLASMS (210–229)

● **210 Benign neoplasm of lip, oral cavity, and pharynx**

Excludes *cyst (of):*
jaw (526.0–526.2, 526.89)
oral soft tissue (528.4)
radicular (522.8)

210.0 Lip
Frenulum labii
Lip (inner aspect) (mucosa) (vermilion border)

Excludes *labial commissure (210.4)*
skin of lip (216.0)

210.1 Tongue
Lingual tonsil

210.2 Major salivary glands
Gland:
parotid
sublingual
submandibular

Excludes *benign neoplasms of minor salivary glands:*
NOS (210.4)
buccal mucosa (210.4)
lips (210.0)
palate (hard) (soft) (210.4)
tongue (210.1)
tonsil, palatine (210.5)

210.3 Floor of mouth

❑ **210.4 Other and unspecified parts of mouth**
Gingiva
Gum (upper) (lower)
Labial commissure
Oral cavity NOS
Oral mucosa
Palate (hard) (soft)
Uvula

Excludes *benign odontogenic neoplasms of bone (213.0–*
213.1)
developmental odontogenic cysts (526.0)
mucosa of lips (210.0)
nasopharyngeal [posterior] [superior] surface of
soft palate (210.7)

210.5 Tonsil
Tonsil (faucial) (palatine)

Excludes *lingual tonsil (210.1)*
pharyngeal tonsil (210.7)
tonsillar:
fossa (210.6)
pillars (210.6)

❑ **210.6 Other parts of oropharynx**
Branchial cleft or vestiges
Epiglottis, anterior aspect
Fauces NOS
Mesopharynx NOS
Tonsillar:
fossa
pillars
Vallecula

Excludes *epiglottis:*
NOS (212.1)
suprahyoid portion (212.1)

210.7 Nasopharynx
Adenoid tissue   Pharyngeal tonsil
Lymphadenoid tissue   Posterior nasal septum

210.8 Hypopharynx
Arytenoid fold   Postcricoid region
Laryngopharynx   Pyriform fossa

❑ **210.9 Pharynx, unspecified**
Throat NOS

● **211 Benign neoplasm of other parts of digestive system**

211.0 Esophagus

211.1 Stomach
Body of stomach
Cardia of stomach
Fundus of stomach
Cardiac orifice
Pylorus

211.2 Duodenum, jejunum, and ileum
Small intestine NOS

Excludes *ampulla of Vater (211.5)*
ileocecal valve (211.3)

211.3 Colon
Appendix
Cecum
Ileocecal valve
Large intestine NOS

Excludes *rectosigmoid junction (211.4)*

211.4 Rectum and anal canal
Anal canal or sphincter
Anus NOS
Rectosigmoid junction

Excludes *anus:*
margin (216.5)
skin (216.5)
perianal skin (216.5)

211.5 Liver and biliary passages
Ampulla of Vater
Common bile duct
Cystic duct
Gallbladder
Hepatic duct
Sphincter of Oddi

211.6 Pancreas, except islets of Langerhans

211.7 Islets of Langerhans
Islet cell tumor

Use additional code to identify any functional activity

211.8 Retroperitoneum and peritoneum
Mesentery
Mesocolon
Omentum
Retroperitoneal tissue

❑ **211.9 Other and unspecified site**
Alimentary tract NOS
Digestive system NOS
Gastrointestinal tract NOS
Intestinal tract NOS
Intestine NOS
Spleen, not elsewhere classified

● 212 **Benign neoplasm of respiratory and intrathoracic organs**

    212.0 **Nasal cavities, middle ear, and accessory sinuses**
        Cartilage of nose
        Eustachian tube
        Nares
        Septum of nose
        Sinus: Sinus:
          ethmoidal   maxillary
          frontal   sphenoidal

      | **Excludes** | *auditory canal (external) (216.2)* |

        bone of:
          ear (213.0)
          nose [turbinates] (213.0)
        cartilage of ear (215.0)
        ear (external) (skin) (216.2)
        nose NOS (229.8)
          skin (216.3)
        olfactory bulb (225.1)
        polyp of:
          accessory sinus (471.8)
          ear (385.30–385.35)
          nasal cavity (471.0)
        posterior margin of septum and choanae (210.7)

    212.1 **Larynx**
        Cartilage:
          arytenoid
          cricoid
          cuneiform
          thyroid
        Epiglottis (suprahyoid portion) NOS
        Glottis
        Vocal cords (false) (true)

      | **Excludes** | *epiglottis, anterior aspect (210.6)* |
               polyp of vocal cord or larynx (478.4)

    212.2 **Trachea**

    212.3 **Bronchus and lung**
        Carina   Hilus of lung

    212.4 **Pleura**

    212.5 **Mediastinum**

    212.6 **Thymus**

    212.7 **Heart**
      | **Excludes** | *great vessels (215.4)* |

    ☐212.8 **Other specified sites**

    ☐212.9 **Site unspecified**
        Respiratory organ NOS
        Upper respiratory tract NOS

      | **Excludes** | *intrathoracic NOS (229.8)* |
               thoracic NOS (229.8)

● 213 **Benign neoplasm of bone and articular cartilage**

    Includes: cartilage (articular) (joint)
             periosteum

      | **Excludes** | *cartilage of:*   *cartilage of:* |
          ear (215.0)   *nose (212.0)*
          eyelid (215.0)   *exostosis NOS (726.91)*
          larynx (212.1)   *synovia (215.0–215.9)*

    213.0 **Bones of skull and face**
      | **Excludes** | *lower jaw bone (213.1)* |

    213.1 **Lower jaw bone**

    213.2 **Vertebral column, excluding sacrum and coccyx**

    213.3 **Ribs, sternum, and clavicle**

    213.4 **Scapula and long bones of upper limb**

    213.5 **Short bones of upper limb**

    213.6 **Pelvic bones, sacrum, and coccyx**

    213.7 **Long bones of lower limb**

    213.8 **Short bones of lower limb**

    ☐213.9 **Bone and articular cartilage, site unspecified**

● 214 **Lipoma**

    Includes: angiolipoma
             fibrolipoma
             hibernoma
             lipoma (fetal) (infiltrating) (intramuscular)
             myelolipoma
             myxolipoma

    214.0 **Skin and subcutaneous tissue of face**

    ☐214.1 **Other skin and subcutaneous tissue**

    214.2 **Intrathoracic organs**

    214.3 **Intra-abdominal organs**

    214.4 **Spermatic cord**

    ☐214.8 **Other specified sites**

    ☐214.9 **Lipoma, unspecified site**

● 215 **Other benign neoplasm of connective and other soft tissue**

    Includes: blood vessel
             bursa
             fascia
             ligament
             muscle
             peripheral, sympathetic, and parasympathetic
               nerves and ganglia
             synovia
             tendon (sheath)

      | **Excludes** | *cartilage:* |
          articular (213.0–213.9)
          larynx (212.1)
          nose (212.0)
         connective tissue of:
          breast (217)
          internal organ, except lipoma and hemangioma
            - code to benign neoplasm of the site
         lipoma (214.0–214.9)

    215.0 **Head, face, and neck**

    215.2 **Upper limb, including shoulder**

    215.3 **Lower limb, including hip**

    215.4 **Thorax**
      | **Excludes** | *heart (212.7)* |
                mediastinum (212.5)
                thymus (212.6)

    215.5 **Abdomen**
        Abdominal wall
        Hypochondrium

    215.6 **Pelvis**
        Buttock
        Groin
        Inguinal region
        Perineum

      | **Excludes** | *uterine:* |
          leiomyoma (218.0–218.9)
          ligament, any (221.0)

    ☐215.7 **Trunk, unspecified**
        Back NOS
        Flank NOS

    ☐215.8 **Other specified sites**

    ☐215.9 **Site unspecified**

ICD-9-CM

200-299

Vol. 1

◀ **New**   ← **Revised**   ● **Not a Principal Diagnosis**   ● **Use Additional Digit(s)**   ☐ **Nonspecific Code**

● **216 Benign neoplasm of skin**

Includes: blue nevus
         dermatofibroma
         hydrocystoma
         pigmented nevus
         syringoadenoma
         syringoma

Excludes *skin of genital organs (221.0–222.9)*

216.0 Skin of lip

Excludes *vermilion border of lip (210.0)*

216.1 Eyelid, including canthus

Excludes *cartilage of eyelid (215.0)*

216.2 Ear and external auditory canal
         Auricle (ear)
         Auricular canal, external
         External meatus
         Pinna

Excludes *cartilage of ear (215.0)*

☐ **216.3 Skin of other and unspecified parts of face**
         Cheek, external
         Eyebrow
         Nose, external
         Temple

216.4 Scalp and skin of neck

216.5 Skin of trunk, except scrotum
         Axillary fold
         Perianal skin
         Skin of:

abdominal wall	Skin of:
anus	chest wall
back	groin
breast	perineum
buttock	Umbilicus

Excludes *anal canal (211.4)*
         anus NOS (211.4)
         skin of scrotum (222.4)

216.6 Skin of upper limb, including shoulder

216.7 Skin of lower limb, including hip

☐ **216.8 Other specified sites of skin**

☐ **216.9 Skin, site unspecified**

● **217 Benign neoplasm of breast**
        Breast (male) (female)
         connective tissue
         glandular tissue
         soft parts

Excludes *adenofibrosis (610.2)*
         benign cyst of breast (610.0)
         fibrocystic disease (610.1)
         skin of breast (216.5)

● **218 Uterine leiomyoma**

Includes: fibroid (bleeding) (uterine)
         uterine:
           fibromyoma
           myoma

218.0 Submucous leiomyoma of uterus

218.1 Intramural leiomyoma of uterus
         Interstitial leiomyoma of uterus

218.2 Subserous leiomyoma of uterus
         Subperitoneal leiomyoma of uterus

☐ **218.9 Leiomyoma of uterus, unspecified**

● **219 Other benign neoplasm of uterus**

219.0 Cervix uteri

219.1 Corpus uteri

Endometrium	Myometrium
Fundus	

☐ **219.8 Other specified parts of uteru**

☐ **219.9 Uterus, part unspecified**

220 Benign neoplasm of ovary

Use additional code to identify any functional activity (256.0–256.1)

Excludes *cyst:*
         corpus albicans (620.2)
         corpus luteum (620.1)
         endometrial (617.1)
         follicular (atretic) (620.0)
         graafian follicle (620.0)
         ovarian NOS (620.2)
         retention (620.2)

● **221 Benign neoplasm of other female genital organs**

Includes: adenomatous polyp
         benign teratoma

Excludes *cyst:*
         epoophoron (752.11)
         fimbrial (752.11)
         Gartner's duct (752.11)
         parovarian (752.11)

221.0 Fallopian tube and uterine ligaments
         Oviduct
         Parametrium
         Uterine ligament (broad) (round) (uterosacral)
         Uterine tube

221.1 Vagina

221.2 Vulva
         Clitoris
         External female genitalia NOS
         Greater vestibular [Bartholin's] gland
         Labia (majora) (minora)
         Pudendum

Excludes *Bartholin's (duct) (gland) cyst (616.2)*

☐ **221.8 Other specified sites of female genital organs**

☐ **221.9 Female genital organ, site unspecified**
         Female genitourinary tract NOS

● **222 Benign neoplasm of male genital organs**

222.0 Testis

Use additional code to identify any functional activity

222.1 Penis
         Corpus cavernosum
         Glans penis
         Prepuce

222.2 Prostate

Excludes *adenomatous hyperplasia of prostate (600.20–*
          600.21)
         prostatic:
         adenoma (600.20–600.21)
         enlargement (600.00–600.01)
         hypertrophy (600.00–600.01)

222.3 Epididymis

222.4 Scrotum
         Skin of scrotum

☐ **222.8 Other specified sites of male genital organs**
         Seminal vesicle
         Spermatic cord

☐ **222.9 Male genital organ, site unspecified**
         Male genitourinary tract NOS

● **223 Benign neoplasm of kidney and other urinary organs**

    223.0 Kidney, except pelvis
        Kidney NOS
        Excludes *renal:*
            calyces (223.1)
            pelvis (223.1)

    223.1 Renal pelvis

    223.2 Ureter
        Excludes *ureteric orifice of bladder (223.3)*

    223.3 Bladder

● **223.8 Other specified sites of urinary organs**

      223.81 Urethra
        Excludes *urethral orifice of bladder (223.3)*

      ☐**223.89 Other**
        Paraurethral glands

  ☐**223.9 Urinary organ, site unspecified**
      Urinary system NOS

● **224 Benign neoplasm of eye**
    Excludes *cartilage of eyelid (215.0)*
        eyelid (skin) (216.1)
        optic nerve (225.1)
        orbital bone (213.0)

    224.0 Eyeball, except conjunctiva, cornea, retina, and choroid
      Ciliary body
      Iris
      Sclera
      Uveal tract

    224.1 Orbit
        Excludes *bone of orbit (213.0)*

    224.2 Lacrimal gland

    224.3 Conjunctiva

    224.4 Cornea

    224.5 Retina
        Excludes *hemangioma of retina (228.03)*

    224.6 Choroid

    224.7 Lacrimal duct
      Lacrimal sac
      Nasolacrimal duct

  ☐**224.8 Other specified parts of eye**

  ☐**224.9 Eye, part unspecified**

● **225 Benign neoplasm of brain and other parts of nervous system**
    Excludes *hemangioma (228.02)*
        neurofibromatosis (237.7)
        peripheral, sympathetic, and parasympathetic nerves and ganglia (215.0–215.9)
        retrobulbar (224.1)

    225.0 Brain

    225.1 Cranial nerves

    225.2 Cerebral meninges
      Meninges NOS
      Meningioma (cerebral)

    225.3 Spinal cord
      Cauda equina

    225.4 Spinal meninges
      Spinal meningioma

  ☐**225.8 Other specified sites of nervous system**

  ☐**225.9 Nervous system, part unspecified**
      Nervous system (central) NOS
      Excludes *meninges NOS (225.2)*

● **226 Benign neoplasm of thyroid glands**
    Use additional code to identify any functional activity

● **227 Benign neoplasm of other endocrine glands and related structures**
    Use additional code to identify any functional activity
    Excludes *ovary (220)*
        pancreas (211.6)
        testis (222.0)

    227.0 Adrenal gland
      Suprarenal gland

    227.1 Parathyroid gland

    227.3 Pituitary gland and craniopharyngeal duct (pouch)
      Craniobuccal pouch
      Hypophysis
      Rathke's pouch
      Sella turcica

    227.4 Pineal gland
      Pineal body

    227.5 Carotid body

    227.6 Aortic body and other paraganglia
      Coccygeal body
      Glomus jugulare
      Para-aortic body

  ☐**227.8 Other**

  ☐**227.9 Endocrine gland, site unspecified**

● **228 Hemangioma and lymphangioma, any site**
    Includes: angioma (benign) (cavernous) (congenital) NOS
      cavernous nevus
      glomus tumor
      hemangioma (benign) (congenital)
    Excludes *benign neoplasm of spleen, except hemangioma and lymphangioma (211.9)*
        glomus jugulare (227.6)
        nevus:
          NOS (216.0–216.9)
          blue or pigmented (216.0–216.9)
          vascular (757.32)

● **228.0 Hemangioma, any site**
    ☐**228.00 Of unspecified site**
    228.01 Of skin and subcutaneous tissue
    228.02 Of intracranial structures
    228.03 Of retina
    228.04 Of intra-abdominal structures
      Peritoneum
      Retroperitoneal tissue
    ☐**228.09 Of other sites**
      Systemic angiomatosis

    228.1 Lymphangioma, any site
      Congenital lymphangioma
      Lymphatic nevus

● **229 Benign neoplasm of other and unspecified sites**

    229.0 Lymph nodes
      Excludes *lymphangioma (228.1)*

  ☐**229.8 Other specified sites**
      Intrathoracic NOS
      Thoracic NOS

  ☐**229.9 Site unspecified**

ICD-9-CM
200-299
Vol. 1

CARCINOMA IN SITU (230–234)

Includes: Bowen's disease
erythroplasia
Queyrat's erythroplasia

Excludes leukoplakia - see Alphabetic Index

● **230 Carcinoma in situ of digestive organs**

230.0 Lip, oral cavity, and pharynx
Gingiva
Hypopharynx
Mouth [any part]
Nasopharynx
Oropharynx
Salivary gland or duct
Tongue

Excludes aryepiglottic fold or interarytenoid fold, laryngeal
aspect (231.0)
epiglottis:
NOS (231.0)
suprahyoid portion (231.0)
skin of lip (232.0)

230.1 Esophagus

230.2 Stomach
Body of stomach
Cardia of stomach
Fundus of stomach
Cardiac orifice
Pylorus

230.3 Colon
Appendix
Cecum
Ileocecal valve
Large intestine NOS

Excludes rectosigmoid junction (230.4)

230.4 Rectum
Rectosigmoid junction

230.5 Anal canal
Anal sphincter

❑ **230.6 Anus, unspecified**

Excludes anus:
margin (232.5)
skin (232.5)
perianal skin (232.5)

❑ **230.7 Other and unspecified parts of intestine**
Duodenum
Ileum
Jejunum
Small intestine NOS

Excludes ampulla of Vater (230.8)

230.8 Liver and biliary system
Ampulla of Vater
Common bile duct
Cystic duct
Gallbladder
Hepatic duct
Sphincter of Oddi

❑ **230.9 Other and unspecified digestive organs**
Digestive organ NOS
Gastrointestinal tract NOS
Pancreas
Spleen

● **231 Carcinoma in situ of respiratory system**

231.0 Larynx

Cartilage: Epiglottis:
arytenoid   NOS
cricoid   posterior surface
cuneiform   suprahyoid portion
thyroid   Vocal cords (false) (true)

Excludes aryepiglottic fold or interarytenoid fold:
NOS (230.0)
hypopharyngeal aspect (230.0)
marginal zone (230.0)

231.1 Trachea

231.2 Bronchus and lung
Carina
Hilus of lung

❑ **231.8 Other specified parts of respiratory system**
Accessory sinuses
Middle ear
Nasal cavities
Pleura

Excludes ear (external) (skin) (232.2)
nose NOS (234.8)
skin (232.3)

❑ **231.9 Respiratory system, part unspecified**
Respiratory organ NOS

● **232 Carcinoma in situ of skin**

Includes: pigment cells

232.0 Skin of lip

Excludes vermilion border of lip (230.0)

232.1 Eyelid, including canthus

232.2 Ear and external auditory canal

❑ **232.3 Skin of other and unspecified parts of face**

232.4 Scalp and skin of neck

232.5 Skin of trunk, except scrotum
Anus, margin   Skin of:
Axillary fold   breast
Perianal skin   buttock
Skin of: chest wall
abdominal wall   groin
anus   perineum
back   Umbilicus

Excludes anal canal (230.5)
anus NOS (230.6)
skin of genital organs (233.3, 233.5–233.6)

232.6 Skin of upper limb, including shoulder

232.7 Skin of lower limb, including hip

❑ **232.8 Other specified sites of skin**

❑ **232.9 Skin, site unspecified**

● **233 Carcinoma in situ of breast and genitourinary system**

233.0 Breast

Excludes Paget's disease (174.0–174.9)
skin of breast (232.5)

233.1 Cervix uteri
Cervical intraepithelial neoplasia III [CIN III] ◄
Severe dysplasia of cervix ◄

Excludes cervical intraepithelial neoplasia II [CIN II] ◄
(622.12)
cytologic evidence of malignancy without histo- ◄
logic confirmation (795.04)
high grade squamous intraepithelial lesion
(HGSIL) (795.04) ◄
moderate dysplasia of cervix (622.12) ◄

◄ **New**   ◄III **Revised**   ● **Not a Principal Diagnosis**   ● **Use Additional Digit(s)**   ❑ **Nonspecific Code**

☐ 233.2 **Other and unspecified parts of uterus**

☐ 233.3 **Other and unspecified female genital organs**

233.4 **Prostate**

233.5 **Penis**

☐ 233.6 **Other and unspecified male genital organs**

233.7 **Bladder**

☐ 233.9 **Other and unspecified urinary organs**

● 234 **Carcinoma in situ of other and unspecified sites**

234.0 **Eye**

Excludes	cartilage of eyelid (234.8)
	eyelid (skin) (232.1)
	optic nerve (234.8)
	orbital bone (234.8)

☐ 234.8 **Other specified sites**
Endocrine gland [any]

☐ 234.9 **Site unspecified**
Carcinoma in situ NOS

NEOPLASMS OF UNCERTAIN BEHAVIOR (235–238)

Note: Categories 235–238 classify by site certain histo-morphologically well-defined neoplasms, the subsequent behavior of which cannot be predicted from the present appearance.

● 235 **Neoplasm of uncertain behavior of digestive and respiratory systems**

235.0 **Major salivary glands**
Gland:
parotid
sublingual
submandibular

Excludes	minor salivary glands (235.1)

235.1 **Lip, oral cavity, and pharynx**
Gingiva
Hypopharynx
Minor salivary glands
Mouth
Nasopharynx
Oropharynx
Tongue

Excludes	aryepiglottic fold or interarytenoid fold, laryngeal
	aspect (235.6)
	epiglottis:
	NOS (235.6)
	suprahyoid portion (235.6)
	skin of lip (238.2)

235.2 **Stomach, intestines, and rectum**

235.3 **Liver and biliary passages**
Ampulla of Vater
Bile ducts [any]
Gallbladder
Liver

235.4 **Retroperitoneum and peritoneum**

☐ 235.5 **Other and unspecified digestive organs**
Anal:
canal
sphincter
Anus NOS
Esophagus
Pancreas
Spleen

Excludes	anus:
	margin (238.2)
	skin (238.2)
	perianal skin (238.2)

235.6 **Larynx**

Excludes	aryepiglottic fold or interarytenoid fold:
	NOS (235.1)
	hypopharyngeal aspect (235.1)
	marginal zone (235.1)

235.7 **Trachea, bronchus, and lung**

235.8 **Pleura, thymus, and mediastinum**

☐ 235.9 **Other and unspecified respiratory organs**
Accessory sinuses
Middle ear
Nasal cavities
Respiratory organ NOS

Excludes	ear (external) (skin) (238.2)
	nose (238.8)
	skin (238.2)

● 236 **Neoplasm of uncertain behavior of genitourinary organs**

236.0 **Uterus**

236.1 **Placenta**
Chorioadenoma (destruens)
Invasive mole
Malignant hydatid(iform) mole

236.2 **Ovary**

Use additional code to identify any functional activity

☐ 236.3 **Other and unspecified female genital organs**

236.4 **Testis**

Use additional code to identify any functional activity

236.5 **Prostate**

☐ 236.6 **Other and unspecified male genital organs**

236.7 **Bladder**

● 236.9 **Other and unspecified urinary organs**

☐ 236.90 **Urinary organ, unspecified**

236.91 **Kidney and ureter**

☐ 236.99 **Other**

● 237 **Neoplasm of uncertain behavior of endocrine glands and nervous system**

237.0 **Pituitary gland and craniopharyngeal duct**

Use additional code to identify any functional activity

237.1 **Pineal gland**

237.2 **Adrenal gland**
Suprarenal gland

Use additional code to identify any functional activity

237.3 **Paraganglia**
Aortic body
Carotid body
Coccygeal body
Glomus jugulare

☐ 237.4 **Other and unspecified endocrine glands**
Parathyroid gland
Thyroid gland

237.5 **Brain and spinal cord**

237.6 **Meninges**
Meninges:
NOS
cerebral
spinal

ICD-9-CM

200-299

Vol. 1

● 237.7 Neurofibromatosis
          von Recklinghausen's disease

☐ 237.70 Neurofibromatosis, unspecified

237.71 Neurofibromatosis, type 1 [von Reckling-
        hausen's disease]

237.72 Neurofibromatosis, type 2 [acoustic neurofi-
        bromatosis]

☐ 237.9 Other and unspecified parts of nervous system
          Cranial nerves

Excludes *peripheral, sympathetic, and parasympathetic*
          nerves and ganglia (238.1)

● 238 Neoplasm of uncertain behavior of other and unspecified
       sites and tissues

238.0 Bone and articular cartilage

Excludes *cartilage:*
          ear (238.1)
          eyelid (238.1)
          larynx (235.6)
          nose (235.9)
          synovia (238.1)

☐ 238.1 Connective and other soft tissue
          Peripheral, sympathetic, and parasympathetic
          nerves and ganglia

Excludes *cartilage (of):*
          articular (238.0)
          larynx (235.6)
          nose (235.9)
          connective tissue of breast (238.3)

238.2 Skin

Excludes *anus NOS (235.5)*
          skin of genital organs (236.3, 236.6)
          vermilion border of lip (235.1)

238.3 Breast

Excludes *skin of breast (238.2)*

238.4 Polycythemia vera

238.5 Histiocytic and mast cells
       Mast cell tumor NOS
       Mastocytoma NOS

238.6 Plasma cells
       Plasmacytoma NOS
       Solitary myeloma

☐ 238.7 Other lymphatic and hematopoietic tissues
          Disease:
             lymphoproliferative (chronic) NOS
             myeloproliferative (chronic) NOS
          Idiopathic thrombocythemia
          Megakaryocytic myelosclerosis
          Myelodysplastic syndrome
          Myelosclerosis with myeloid metaplasia
          Panmyelosis (acute)

Excludes *myelofibrosis (289.89)*
          myelosclerosis NOS (289.89)
          myelosis:
             NOS (205.9)
             megakaryocytic (207.2)

238.8 Other specified sites
       Eye
       Heart

Excludes *eyelid (skin) (238.2)*
          cartilage (238.1)

☐ 238.9 Site unspecified

NEOPLASMS OF UNSPECIFIED NATURE (239)

● 239 Neoplasms of unspecified nature

Note: Category 239 classifies by site neoplasms of unspeci-
      fied morphology and behavior. The term "mass,"
      unless otherwise stated, is not to be regarded as a
      neoplastic growth.

Includes: "growth" NOS
          neoplasm NOS
          new growth NOS
          tumor NOS

☐ 239.0 Digestive system

Excludes *anus:*
          margin (239.2)
          skin (239.2)
          perianal skin (239.2)

☐ 239.1 Respiratory system

☐ 239.2 Bone, soft tissue, and skin

Excludes *anal canal (239.0)*
          anus NOS (239.0)
          bone marrow (202.9)
          cartilage:
          larynx (239.1)
          nose (239.1)
          connective tissue of breast (239.3)
          skin of genital organs (239.5)
          vermilion border of lip (239.0)

☐ 239.3 Breast

Excludes *skin of breast (239.2)*

☐ 239.4 Bladder

☐ 239.5 Other genitourinary organs

☐ 239.6 Brain

Excludes *cerebral meninges (239.7)*
          cranial nerves (239.7)

☐ 239.7 Endocrine glands and other parts of nervous
          system

Excludes *peripheral, sympathetic, and parasympathetic*
          nerves and ganglia (239.2)

☐ 239.8 Other specified sites

Excludes *eyelid (skin) (239.2)*
          cartilage (239.2)
          great vessels (239.2)
          optic nerve (239.7)

☐ 239.9 Site unspecified

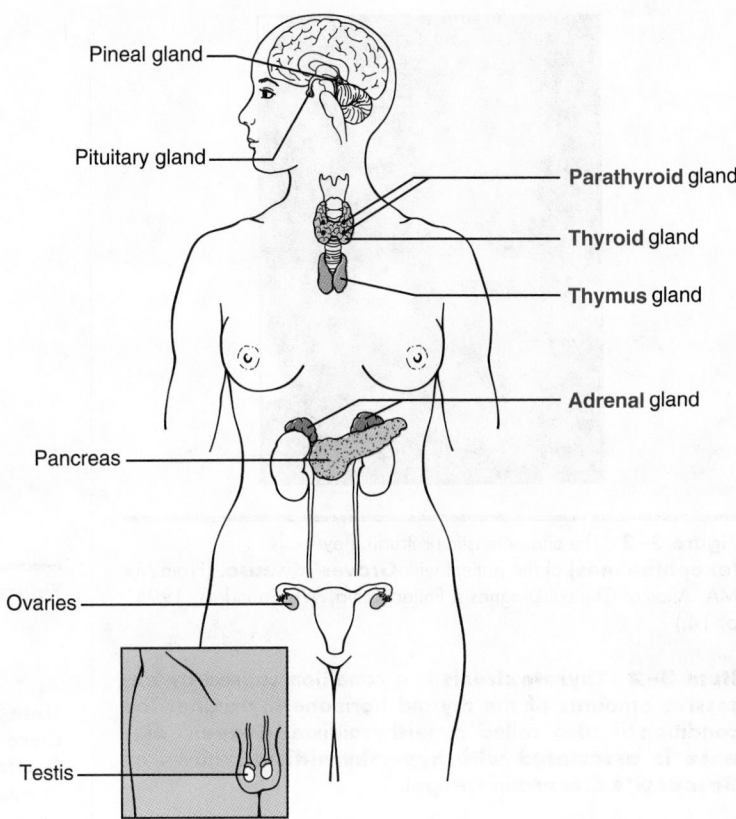

Figure 3-1 The endocrine system. (From Buck CJ: Step-by-Step Medical Coding, 2005 ed. Philadelphia, WBS, 2005.)

ICD-9-CM

200-

Vol.

Figure 3-2 **Goiter** is an enlargement of the thyroid gland.

Item 3-1 **Simple** indicates no nodules are present. The most common type of goiter is a **diffuse colloidal,** also called a **nontoxic** or **endemic** goiter. Goiters classifiable to 240.0 or 240.9 are those goiters without mention of nodules.

3. ENDOCRINE, NUTRITIONAL AND METABOLIC DISEASES, AND IMMUNITY DISORDERS (240–279)

> Excludes endocrine and metabolic disturbances specific to the fetus and newborn (775.0–775.9)

Note: All neoplasms, whether functionally active or not, are classified in Chapter 2. Codes in Chapter 3 (i.e., 242.8, 246.0, 251–253, 255–259) may be used to identify such functional activity associated with any neoplasm, or by ectopic endocrine tissue.

DISORDERS OF THYROID GLAND (240–246)

● **240   Simple and unspecified goiter**

    240.0   Goiter, specified as simple
       Any condition classifiable to 240.9, specified as simple

☐ **240.9   Goiter, unspecified**
       Enlargement of thyroid   Goiter or struma:
       Goiter or struma: hyperplastic
         NOS   nontoxic (diffuse)
         diffuse colloid   parenchymatous
         endemic   sporadic

> Excludes congenital (dyshormonogenic) goiter (246.1)

● **241   Nontoxic nodular goiter**

> Excludes adenoma of thyroid (226)
> cystadenoma of thyroid (226)

    241.0   Nontoxic uninodular goiter
       Thyroid nodule
       Uninodular goiter (nontoxic)

    241.1   Nontoxic multinodular goiter
       Multinodular goiter (nontoxic)

☐ **241.9   Unspecified nontoxic nodular goiter**
       Adenomatous goiter
       Nodular goiter (nontoxic) NOS
       Struma nodosa (simplex)

Figure 3-3 The characteristic protruding eyeballs **(exophthalmos)** of the patient with **Graves' disease.** (From Mir MA: Atlas of Clinical Diagnosis. Philadelphia, WB Saunders, 1995, p. 14.)

Figure 3-4   Myxedema is severe hypothyroidism.

Item 3-2   Thyrotoxicosis is a condition caused by excessive amounts of the thyroid hormone thyroxine. The condition is also called hyperthyroidism. **Graves' disease is associated with hyperthyroidism** (known as **Basedow's disease** in Europe).

● 242 Thyrotoxicosis with or without goiter

> ⎸Excludes⎹ *neonatal thyrotoxicosis (775.3)*

> The following fifth-digit subclassification is for use with category 242:
>   **0 without mention of thyrotoxic crisis or storm**
>   **1 with mention of thyrotoxic crisis or storm**

● 242.0 **Toxic diffuse goiter**
    Basedow's disease
    Exophthalmic or toxic goiter NOS
    Graves' disease
    Primary thyroid hyperplasia

● 242.1 **Toxic uninodular goiter**
    Thyroid nodule, toxic or with hyperthyroidism
    Uninodular goiter, toxic or with hyperthyroidism

● 242.2 **Toxic multinodular goiter**
    Secondary thyroid hyperplasia

● ❑ 242.3 **Toxic nodular goiter, unspecified**
    Adenomatous goiter, toxic or with hyperthyroidism
    Nodular goiter, toxic or with hyperthyroidism
    Struma nodosa, toxic or with hyperthyroidism
    Any condition classifiable to 241.9 specified as toxic or with hyperthyroidism

● 242.4 **Thyrotoxicosis from ectopic thyroid nodule**

● ❑ 242.8 **Thyrotoxicosis of other specified origin**
    Overproduction of thyroid-stimulating hormone [TSH]
    Thyrotoxicosis:
      factitia from ingestion of excessive thyroid material

    Use additional E code to identify cause, if drug-induced

● ❑ 242.9 **Thyrotoxicosis without mention of goiter or other cause**
    Hyperthyroidism NOS
    Thyrotoxicosis NOS

Item 3-3   Hypothyroidism is a condition in which there are insufficient levels of thyroxine.
Cretinism is congenital hypothyroidism, which can result in mental and physical retardation.

  243 Congenital hypothyroidism
    Congenital thyroid insufficiency
    Cretinism (athyrotic) (endemic)

    Use additional code to identify associated mental retardation

> ⎸Excludes⎹ *congenital (dyshormonogenic) goiter (246.1)*

● 244 Acquired hypothyroidism

    Includes: athyroidism (acquired)
             hypothyroidism (acquired)
             myxedema (adult) (juvenile)
             thyroid (gland) insufficiency (acquired)

    244.0 **Postsurgical hypothyroidism**

  ❑ 244.1 **Other postablative hypothyroidism**
    Hypothyroidism following therapy, such as irradiation

    244.2 **Iodine hypothyroidism**
    Hypothyroidism resulting from administration or ingestion of iodide

    Use additional E to identify drug

  ❑ 244.3 **Other iatrogenic hypothyroidism**
    Hypothyroidism resulting from:
      P-aminosalicylic acid [PAS]
      Phenylbutazone
      Resorcinol
    Iatrogenic hypothyroidism NOS

    Use additional E to identify drug

  ❑ 244.8 **Other specified acquired hypothyroidism**
    Secondary hypothyroidism NEC

  ❑ 244.9 **Unspecified hypothyroidism**
    Hypothyroidism, primary or NOS
    Myxedema, primary or NOS

● **245 Thyroiditis**

245.0 Acute thyroiditis
　　Abscess of thyroid
　　Thyroiditis:
　　　nonsuppurative, acute
　　　pyogenic
　　　suppurative

　　Use additional code to identify organism

245.1 Subacute thyroiditis
　　Thyroiditis:
　　　de Quervain's
　　　giant cell
　　　granulomatous
　　　viral

245.2 Chronic lymphocytic thyroiditis
　　Hashimoto's disease
　　Struma lymphomatosa
　　Thyroiditis:
　　　autoimmune
　　　lymphocytic (chronic)

245.3 Chronic fibrous thyroiditis
　　Struma fibrosa
　　Thyroiditis:
　　　invasive (fibrous)
　　　ligneous
　　　Riedel's

245.4 Iatrogenic thyroiditis
　　Use additional E to identify cause

❑ **245.8 Other and unspecified chronic thyroiditis**
　　Chronic thyroiditis:
　　　NOS
　　　nonspecific

❑ **245.9 Thyroiditis, unspecified**
　　Thyroiditis NOS

● **246 Other disorders of thyroid**

246.0 Disorders of thyrocalcitonin secretion
　　Hypersecretion of calcitonin or thyrocalcitonin

246.1 Dyshormonogenic goiter
　　Congenital (dyshormonogenic) goiter
　　Goiter due to enzyme defect in synthesis of thy-
　　　roid hormone
　　Goitrous cretinism (sporadic)

246.2 Cyst of thyroid
　　Excludes cystadenoma of thyroid (226)

246.3 Hemorrhage and infarction of thyroid

❑ **246.8 Other specified disorders of thyroid**
　　Abnormality of thyroid-binding globulin
　　Atrophy of thyroid
　　Hyper-TBG-nemia
　　Hypo-TBG-nemia

❑ **246.9 Unspecified disorder of thyroid**

DISEASES OF OTHER ENDOCRINE GLANDS (250–259)

● **250 Diabetes mellitus**

　　Excludes gestational diabetes (648.8)
　　　　　hyperglycemia NOS (790.6)
　　　　　neonatal diabetes mellitus (775.1)
　　　　　nonclinical diabetes (790.29)

The following fifth-digit subclassification is for use with category 250:

　0 **type II or unspecified type, not stated as uncon-**
　　trolled ◀▥

　　Fifth-digit 0 is for use for type II patients, even if
　　the patient requires insulin ◀▥

　　Use additional code, if applicable, for associated
　　long-term (current) insulin use V58.67 ◀

　1 **type I [juvenile type], not stated as uncontrolled** ◀▥

　2 **type II or unspecified type, uncontrolled** ◀▥

　　Fifth-digit 2 is for use for type II patients, even if
　　the patient requires insulin ◀▥

　　Use additional code, if applicable, for associated
　　long-term (current) insulin use V58.67 ◀

　3 **type I [insulin dependent type] [IDDM] [juvenile**
　　type], uncontrolled

● **250.0 Diabetes mellitus without mention of complication**
　　Diabetes mellitus without mention of complication
　　　or manifestation classifiable to 250.1–250.9
　　Diabetes (mellitus) NOS

● **250.1 Diabetes with ketoacidosis**
　　Diabetic:
　　　acidosis without mention of coma
　　　ketosis without mention of coma

● **250.2 Diabetes with hyperosmolarity**
　　Hyperosmolar (nonketotic) coma

● **250.3 Diabetes with other coma**
　　Diabetic coma (with ketoacidosis)
　　Diabetic hypoglycemic coma
　　Insulin coma NOS

　　Excludes diabetes with hyperosmolar coma (250.2)

● **250.4 Diabetes with renal manifestations**

　　Use additional code to identify manifestation, as:
　　diabetic:
　　　nephropathy NOS (583.81)
　　　nephrosis (581.81)
　　intercapillary glomerulosclerosis (581.81)
　　Kimmelstiel-Wilson syndrome (581.81)

● **250.5 Diabetes with ophthalmic manifestations**

　　Use additional code to identify manifestation, as:
　　diabetic:
　　　blindness (369.00–369.9)
　　　cataract (366.41)
　　　glaucoma (365.44)
　　　retinal edema (362.01)
　　　retinopathy (362.01–362.02)

● **250.6 Diabetes with neurological manifestations**

　　Use additional code to identify manifestation, as:
　　diabetic:
　　　amyotrophy (358.1)
　　　gastroparalysis (536.3) ◀
　　　gastroparesis (536.3) ◀
　　　mononeuropathy (354.0–355.9)
　　　neurogenic arthropathy (713.5)
　　　peripheral autonomic neuropathy (337.1)
　　　polyneuropathy (357.2)

● **250.7 Diabetes with peripheral circulatory disorders**

　　Use additional code to identify manifestation, as:
　　diabetic:
　　　gangrene (785.4)
　　　peripheral angiopathy (443.81)

ICD-9-CM

200-299

Vol. 1

● ❏ **250.8 Diabetes with other specified manifestations**
Diabetic hypoglycemia
Hypoglycemic shock

Use additional code to identify manifestation, as:
any associated ulceration (707.10–707.9)
diabetic bone changes (731.8)

Use additional E code to identify cause, if drug-
induced

● ❏ **250.9 Diabetes with unspecified complication**

● **251 Other disorders of pancreatic internal secretion**

251.0 Hypoglycemic coma
Iatrogenic hyperinsulinism
Non-diabetic insulin coma

Use additional E code to identify cause, if drug-
induced

Excludes *hypoglycemic coma in diabetes mellitus (250.3)*

❏ **251.1 Other specified hypoglycemia**
Hyperinsulinism:
  NOS
  ectopic
  functional
Hyperplasia of pancreatic islet beta cells NOS

Excludes *hypoglycemia in diabetes mellitus (250.8)*
hypoglycemia in infant of diabetic mother (775.0)
hypoglycemic coma (251.0)
neonatal hypoglycemia (775.6)

Use additional E code to identify cause, if drug-
induced

❏ **251.2 Hypoglycemia, unspecified**
Hypoglycemia:
  NOS
  reactive
  spontaneous

Excludes *hypoglycemia:*
with coma (251.0)
in diabetes mellitus (250.8)
leucine-induced (270.3)

251.3 Postsurgical hypoinsulinemia
Hypoinsulinemia following complete or partial
  pancreatectomy
Postpancreatectomy hyperglycemia

251.4 Abnormality of secretion of glucagon
Hyperplasia of pancreatic islet alpha cells with
  glucagon excess

251.5 Abnormality of secretion of gastrin
Hyperplasia of pancreatic alpha cells with gastrin
  excess
Zollinger-Ellison syndrome

❏ **251.8 Other specified disorders of pancreatic internal secretion**

❏ **251.9 Unspecified disorder of pancreatic internal secretion**
Islet cell hyperplasia NOS

Figure 3-5 Tetany caused by hypoparathyroidism.

Item 3-4 Hyperparathyroidism is an overactive parathyroid gland that secretes excessive parathormone,
causing increased levels of circulating calcium. This results in a loss of calcium in the bone.
Hypoparathyroidism is an underactive parathyroid
gland that results in decreased levels of circulating calcium. The primary manifestation is **tetany,** a continuous
muscle spasm.

● **252 Disorders of parathyroid gland**

● **252.0 Hyperparathyroidism**

Excludes *ectopic hyperparathyroidism (259.3)*

❏ **252.00 Hyperparathyroidism, unspecified** ◀

252.01 Primary hyperparathyroidism ◀
Hyperplasia of parathyroid ◀

252.02 Secondary hyperparathyroidism, non-renal ◀

Excludes *secondary hyperparathyroidism (of renal origin)* ◀
(588.81)

252.08 Other hyperparathyroidism ◀
Tertiary hyperparathyroidism ◀

252.1 Hypoparathyroidism
Parathyroiditis (autoimmune)
Tetany:
  parathyroid
  parathyroprival

Excludes *pseudohypoparathyroidism (275.4)*
pseudopseudohypoparathyroidism (275.4)
tetany NOS (781.7)
transitory neonatal hypoparathyroidism (775.4)

❏ **252.8 Other specified disorders of parathyroid gland**
Cyst of parathyroid gland
Hemorrhage of parathyroid gland

❏ **252.9 Unspecified disorder of parathyroid gland**

● **253 Disorders of the pituitary gland and its hypothalamic
control**

Includes: the listed conditions whether the disorder is
in the pituitary or the hypothalamus

Excludes *Cushing's syndrome (255.0)*

253.0 Acromegaly and gigantism
Overproduction of growth hormone

❏ **253.1 Other and unspecified anterior pituitary hyperfunction**
Forbes-Albright syndrome

Excludes *overproduction of:*
ACTH (255.3)
thyroid-stimulating hormone [TSH] (242.8)

253.2 Panhypopituitarism
Cachexia, pituitary
Necrosis of pituitary (postpartum)
Pituitary insufficiency NOS
Sheehan's syndrome
Simmonds' disease

Excludes *iatrogenic hypopituitarism (253.7)*

253.3 Pituitary dwarfism
Isolated deficiency of (human) growth hormone
  [HGH]
Lorain-Levi dwarfism

❏ **253.4 Other anterior pituitary disorders**
Isolated or partial deficiency of an anterior pitui-
  tary hormone, other than growth hormone
Prolactin deficiency

253.5 Diabetes insipidus
Vasopressin deficiency

Excludes *nephrogenic diabetes insipidus (588.1)*

❑253.6 **Other disorders of neurohypophysis**
Syndrome of inappropriate secretion of antidiuretic hormone [ADH]

Excludes ectopic antidiuretic hormone secretion (259.3)

253.7 **Iatrogenic pituitary disorders**
Hypopituitarism:
hormone-induced
hypophysectomy-induced
postablative
radiotherapy-induced

Use additional E code to identify cause

❑253.8 **Other disorders of the pituitary and other syndromes of diencephalohypophyseal origin**
Abscess of pituitary
Adiposogenital dystrophy
Cyst of Rathke's pouch
Fröhlich's syndrome

Excludes craniopharyngioma (237.0)

❑253.9 **Unspecified**
Dyspituitarism

● 254 **Diseases of thymus gland**

Excludes aplasia or dysplasia with immunodeficiency (279.2)
hypoplasia with immunodeficiency (279.2)
myasthenia gravis (358.00–358.01)

254.0 **Persistent hyperplasia of thymus**
Hypertrophy of thymus

254.1 **Abscess of thymus**

❑254.8 **Other specified diseases of thymus gland**
Atrophy of thymus
Cyst of thymus

Excludes thymoma (212.6)

❑254.9 **Unspecified disease of thymus gland**

Item 3-5 Hyperadrenalism is overactivity of the adrenal cortex, which secretes a variety of hormones. Excessive glucocorticoid hormone results in hyperglycemia (**Cushing's syndrome**), and excessive aldosterone results in **Conn's syndrome**. **Adrenogenital syndrome** is the result of excessive secretion of androgens, male hormones, which stimulates premature sexual development. **Hypoadrenalism, Addison's disease,** is a condition in which the adrenal glands atrophy.

● 255 **Disorders of adrenal glands**

Includes: the listed conditions whether the basic disorder is in the adrenals or is pituitary-induced

255.0 **Cushing's syndrome**
Adrenal hyperplasia due to excess ACTH
Cushing's syndrome:
NOS
iatrogenic
idiopathic
pituitary-dependent
Ectopic ACTH syndrome
Iatrogenic syndrome of excess cortisol
Overproduction of cortisol

Use additional E code to identify cause, if drug-induced

Excludes congenital adrenal hyperplasia (255.2)

● 255.1 **Hyperaldosteronism**

255.10 **Primary aldosteronism**
Aldosteronism NOS
Hyperaldosteronism, unspecified

Excludes Conn's syndrome (255.12) ◄

255.11 **Glucocorticoid-remediable aldosteronism**
Familial aldosteronism type I

Excludes Conn's syndrome (255.12) ◄

255.12 **Conn's syndrome**

255.13 **Bartter's syndrome**

❑255.14 **Other secondary aldosteronism**

255.2 **Adrenogenital disorders**
Achard-Thiers syndrome
Adrenogenital syndromes, virilizing or feminizing, whether acquired or associated with congenital adrenal hyperplasia consequent on inborn enzyme defects in hormone synthesis
Congenital adrenal hyperplasia
Female adrenal pseudohermaphroditism
Male:
macrogenitosomia praecox
sexual precocity with adrenal hyperplasia
Virilization (female) (suprarenal)

Excludes adrenal hyperplasia due to excess ACTH (255.0)
isosexual virilization (256.4)

ICD-9-CM

200-
Vol.

Figure 3-6 Cushing's syndrome, showing characteristic purple striae and abdominal obesity. (From Mir MA: Atlas of Clinical Diagnosis. Philadelphia, WB Saunders, 1995, p. 10.)

❑ **255.3 Other corticoadrenal overactivity**
Acquired benign adrenal androgenic overactivity
Overproduction of ACTH

255.4 Corticoadrenal insufficiency

Addisonian crisis
Addison's disease NOS
Adrenal:
  atrophy (autoimmune)
  calcification

Adrenal:
  crisis
  hemorrhage
  infarction
  insufficiency NOS

| Excludes | *tuberculous Addison's disease (017.6)* |

❑ **255.5 Other adrenal hypofunction**
Adrenal medullary insufficiency

| Excludes | *Waterhouse-Friderichsen syndrome (meningococcal) (036.3)* |

255.6 Medulloadrenal hyperfunction
Catecholamine secretion by pheochromocytoma

❑ **255.8 Other specified disorders of adrenal glands**
Abnormality of cortisol-binding globulin

❑ **255.9 Unspecified disorder of adrenal glands**

● **256 Ovarian dysfunction**

256.0 Hyperestrogenism

❑ **256.1 Other ovarian hyperfunction**
Hypersecretion of ovarian androgens

256.2 Postablative ovarian failure
Ovarian failure:
  iatrogenic
  postirradiation
  postsurgical

Use additional code for states associated with artificial menopause (627.4)

| Excludes | *acquired absence of ovary (V45.77)*
asymptomatic age-related (natural) postmenopausal status (V49.81) |

● **256.3 Other ovarian failure**

| Excludes | *asymptomatic age-related (natural) postmenopausal status (V49.81)* |

Use additional code for states associated with natural menopause (627.2)

256.31 Premature menopause

❑ **256.39 Other ovarian failure**
Delayed menarche
Ovarian hypofunction
Primary ovarian failure NOS

256.4 Polycystic ovaries
Isosexual virilization Stein-Leventhal syndrome

❑ **256.8 Other ovarian dysfunction**

❑ **256.9 Unspecified ovarian dysfunction**

● **257 Testicular dysfunction**

257.0 Testicular hyperfunction
Hypersecretion of testicular hormones

257.1 Postablative testicular hypofunction
Testicular hypofunction:
  iatrogenic
  postirradiation
  postsurgical

❑ **257.2 Other testicular hypofunction**
Defective biosynthesis of testicular androgen
Eunuchoidism:
  NOS
  hypogonadotropic
Failure:
  Leydig's cell, adult
  seminiferous tubule, adult
Testicular hypogonadism

| Excludes | *azoospermia (606.0)* |

❑ **257.8 Other testicular dysfunction**
Goldberg-Maxwell syndrome
Male pseudohermaphroditism with testicular feminization
Testicular feminization

❑ **257.9 Unspecified testicular dysfunction**

● **258 Polyglandular dysfunction and related disorders**

258.0 Polyglandular activity in multiple endocrine adenomatosis
Wermer's syndrome

❑ **258.1 Other combinations of endocrine dysfunction**
Lloyd's syndrome
Schmidt's syndrome

❑ **258.8 Other specified polyglandular dysfunction**

❑ **258.9 Polyglandular dysfunction, unspecified**

● **259 Other endocrine disorders**

259.0 Delay in sexual development and puberty, not elsewhere classified
Delayed puberty

259.1 Precocious sexual development and puberty, not elsewhere classified

Sexual precocity:
  NOS
  constitutional

Sexual precocity:
  cryptogenic
  idiopathic

259.2 Carcinoid syndrome
Hormone secretion by carcinoid tumors

259.3 Ectopic hormone secretion, not elsewhere classified
Ectopic:
  antidiuretic hormone secretion [ADH]
  hyperparathyroidism

| Excludes | *ectopic ACTH syndrome (255.0)* |

259.4 Dwarfism, not elsewhere classified
Dwarfism:
  NOS
  constitutional

| Excludes | *dwarfism:*
  achondroplastic (756.4)
  intrauterine (759.7)
  nutritional (263.2)
  pituitary (253.3)
  renal (588.0)
  progeria (259.8) |

❑ **259.8 Other specified endocrine disorders**
Pineal gland dysfunction
Progeria
Werner's syndrome

❑ **259.9 Unspecified endocrine disorder**
Disturbance:
  endocrine NOS
  hormone NOS
Infantilism NOS

NUTRITIONAL DEFICIENCIES (260–269)

| Excludes | *deficiency anemias (280.0–281.9)* |

260 Kwashiorkor
Nutritional edema with dyspigmentation of skin and hair

261 Nutritional marasmus
Nutritional atrophy
Severe calorie deficiency
Severe malnutrition NOS

❑ **262 Other severe protein-calorie malnutrition**
Nutritional edema without mention of dyspigmentation of skin and hair

● **263 Other and unspecified protein-calorie malnutrition**

263.0 Malnutrition of moderate degree

263.1 Malnutrition of mild degree

263.2 **Arrested development following protein-calorie malnutrition**
Nutritional dwarfism
Physical retardation due to malnutrition

☐263.8 **Other protein-calorie malnutrition**

☐263.9 **Unspecified protein-calorie malnutrition**
Dystrophy due to malnutrition
Malnutrition (calorie) NOS
Excludes *nutritional deficiency NOS (269.9)*

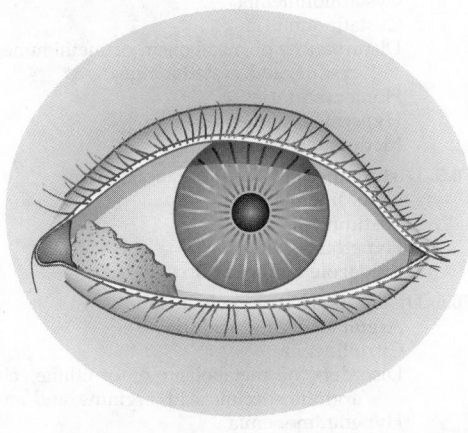

Figure 3–7 Bitot's spot on the conjunctiva.

Item 3-6 Bitot's spot is a gray, foamy erosion on the conjunctiva, usually associated with vitamin A deficiency. The disease may progress to **keratomalacia,** which can result in eventual prolapse of the iris and loss of the lens.

Figure 3–8 In chronic **pellagra,** the skin changes include thickening, scaling, pigmentation, and hyperkeratinization. (From Mir MA: Atlas of Clinical Diagnosis. Philadelphia, WB Saunders, 1995, p. 57.)

Item 3-7 Pellagra is associated with a deficiency of niacin and its precursor, **tryptophan.** Characteristics of the condition include dermatitis on exposed skin surfaces. **Beriberi** is associated with thiamin deficiency.

●264 **Vitamin A deficiency**
264.0 **With conjunctival xerosis**
264.1 **With conjunctival xerosis and Bitot's spot**
Bitot's spot in the young child
264.2 **With corneal xerosis**
264.3 **With corneal ulceration and xerosis**
264.4 **With keratomalacia**
264.5 **With night blindness**
264.6 **With xerophthalmic scars of cornea**
☐264.7 **Other ocular manifestations of vitamin A deficiency**
Xerophthalmia due to vitamin A deficiency
☐264.8 **Other manifestations of vitamin A deficiency**
Follicular keratosis due to vitamin A deficiency
Xeroderma due to vitamin A deficiency
☐264.9 **Unspecified vitamin A deficiency**
Hypovitaminosis A NOS

●265 **Thiamine and niacin deficiency states**
265.0 **Beriberi**
☐265.1 **Other and unspecified manifestations of thiamine deficiency**
Other vitamin B$_1$ deficiency states
265.2 **Pellagra**
Deficiency:
niacin (-tryptophan)
nicotinamide
nicotinic acid
vitamin PP
Pellagra (alcoholic)

●266 **Deficiency of B-complex components**
266.0 **Ariboflavinosis**
Riboflavin [vitamin B$_2$] deficiency
266.1 **Vitamin B$_6$ deficiency**
Deficiency:
pyridoxal
pyridoxamine
pyridoxine
Vitamin B$_6$ deficiency syndrome
Excludes *vitamin B$_6$-responsive sideroblastic anemia (285.0)*
☐266.2 **Other B-complex deficiencies**
Deficiency:
cyanocobalamin
folic acid
vitamin B$_{12}$
Excludes *combined system disease with anemia (281.0–281.1)*
deficiency anemias (281.0–281.9)
subacute degeneration of spinal cord with anemia (281.0–281.1)
☐266.9 **Unspecified vitamin B deficiency**

267 **Ascorbic acid deficiency**
Deficiency of vitamin C
Scurvy
Excludes *scorbutic anemia (281.8)*

●268 **Vitamin D deficiency**
Excludes *vitamin D-resistant:*
osteomalacia (275.3)
rickets (275.3)
268.0 **Rickets, active**
Excludes *celiac rickets (579.0)*
renal rickets (588.0)
☐268.1 **Rickets, late effect**
Any condition specified as due to rickets and stated to be a late effect or sequela of rickets
Use additional code to identify the nature of late effect

ICD-9-CM
200-299
Vol. 1

❏ **268.2 Osteomalacia, unspecified**

❏ **268.9 Unspecified vitamin D deficiency**
   Avitaminosis D

● **269 Other nutritional deficiencies**

   269.0 Deficiency of vitamin K

Excludes	*deficiency of coagulation factor due to vitamin K deficiency (286.7)*
	vitamin K deficiency of newborn (776.0)

   ❏ **269.1 Deficiency of other vitamins**
      Deficiency:
         vitamin E
         vitamin P

   ❏ **269.2 Unspecified vitamin deficiency**
      Multiple vitamin deficiency NOS

   269.3 Mineral deficiency, not elsewhere classified
      Deficiency:
         calcium, dietary
         iodine

Excludes	*deficiency:*
	calcium NOS (275.4)
	potassium (276.8)
	sodium (276.1)

   ❏ **269.8 Other nutritional deficiency**

Excludes	*adult failure to thrive (783.7)*
	failure to thrive in childhood (783.41)
	feeding problems (783.3)
	newborn (779.3)

   ❏ **269.9 Unspecified nutritional deficiency**

OTHER METABOLIC AND IMMUNITY DISORDERS (270–279)

Use additional code to identify any associated mental retardation

● **270 Disorders of amino-acid transport and metabolism**

Excludes	*abnormal findings without manifest disease (790.0–796.9)*
	disorders of purine and pyrimidine metabolism (277.1–277.2)
	gout (274.0–274.9)

   270.0 Disturbances of amino-acid transport
      Cystinosis
      Cystinuria
      Fanconi (-de Toni) (-Debré) syndrome
      Glycinuria (renal)
      Hartnup disease

   270.1 Phenylketonuria [PKU]
      Hyperphenylalaninemia

   ❏ **270.2 Other disturbances of aromatic amino-acid metabolism**
      Albinism
      Alkaptonuria
      Alkaptonuric ochronosis
      Disturbances of metabolism of tyrosine and tryptophan
      Homogentisic acid defects
      Hydroxykynureninuria
      Hypertyrosinemia
      Indicanuria
      Kynureninase defects
      Oasthouse urine disease
      Ochronosis
      Tyrosinosis
      Tyrosinuria
      Waardenburg syndrome

Excludes	*vitamin B₆-deficiency syndrome (266.1)*

   270.3 Disturbances of branched-chain amino-acid metabolism
      Disturbances of metabolism of leucine, isoleucine, and valine
      Hypervalinemia
      Intermittent branched-chain ketonuria
      Leucine-induced hypoglycemia
      Leucinosis
      Maple syrup urine disease

   270.4 Disturbances of sulphur-bearing amino-acid metabolism
      Cystathioninemia
      Cystathioninuria
      Disturbances of metabolism of methionine, homocystine, and cystathionine
      Homocystinuria
      Hypermethioninemia
      Methioninemia

   270.5 Disturbances of histidine metabolism
      Carnosinemia
      Histidinemia
      Hyperhistidinemia
      Imidazole aminoaciduria

   270.6 Disorders of urea cycle metabolism
      Argininosuccinic aciduria
      Citrullinemia
      Disorders of metabolism of ornithine, citrulline, argininosuccinic acid, arginine, and ammonia
      Hyperammonemia
      Hyperornithinemia

   ❏ **270.7 Other disturbances of straight-chain amino-acid metabolism**
      Glucoglycinuria
      Glycinemia (with methylmalonic acidemia)
      Hyperglycinemia
      Hyperlysinemia
      Pipecolic acidemia
      Saccharopinuria
      Other disturbances of metabolism of glycine, threonine, serine, glutamine, and lysine

   ❏ **270.8 Other specified disorders of amino-acid metabolism**
      Alaninemia
      Ethanolaminuria
      Glycoprolinuria
      Hydroxyprolinemia
      Hyperprolinemia
      Iminoacidopathy
      Prolinemia
      Prolinuria
      Sarcosinemia

   ❏ **270.9 Unspecified disorder of amino-acid metabolism**

● **271 Disorders of carbohydrate transport and metabolism**

Excludes	*abnormality of secretion of glucagon (251.4)*
	diabetes mellitus (250.0–250.9)
	hypoglycemia NOS (251.2)
	mucopolysaccharidosis (277.5)

   271.0 Glycogenosis
      Amylopectinosis
      Glucose-6-phosphatase deficiency
      Glycogen storage disease
      McArdle's disease
      Pompe's disease
      von Gierke's disease

   271.1 Galactosemia
      Galactose-1-phosphate uridyl transferase deficiency
      Galactosuria

   271.2 Hereditary fructose intolerance
      Essential benign fructosuria
      Fructosemia

271.3 Intestinal disaccharidase deficiencies and disaccharide malabsorption
Intolerance or malabsorption (congenital) (of):
glucose-galactose
lactose
sucrose-isomaltose

271.4 Renal glycosuria
Renal diabetes

☐ **271.8 Other specified disorders of carbohydrate transport and metabolism**
Essential benign pentosuria
Fucosidosis
Glycolic aciduria
Hyperoxaluria (primary)
Mannosidosis
Oxalosis
Xylosuria
Xylulosuria

☐ **271.9 Unspecified disorder of carbohydrate transport and metabolism**

● **272 Disorders of lipoid metabolism**

| **Excludes** | localized cerebral lipidoses (330.1) |

272.0 Pure hypercholesterolemia
Familial hypercholesterolemia
Fredrickson Type IIa hyperlipoproteinemia
Hyperbetalipoproteinemia
Hyperlipidemia, Group A
Low-density-lipoid-type [LDL] hyperlipoproteinemia

272.1 Pure hyperglyceridemia
Endogenous hyperglyceridemia
Fredrickson Type IV hyperlipoproteinemia
Hyperlipidemia, Group B
Hyperprebetalipoproteinemia
Hypertriglyceridemia, essential
Very-low-density-lipoid-type [VLDL] hyperlipoproteinemia

272.2 Mixed hyperlipidemia
Broad- or floating-betalipoproteinemia
Fredrickson Type IIb or III hyperlipoproteinemia
Hypercholesterolemia with endogenous hyperglyceridemia
Hyperbetalipoproteinemia with prebetalipoproteinemia
Tubo-eruptive xanthoma
Xanthoma tuberosum

272.3 Hyperchylomicronemia
Bürger-Grütz syndrome
Fredrickson type I or V hyperlipoproteinemia
Hyperlipidemia, Group D
Mixed hyperglyceridemia

☐ **272.4 Other and unspecified hyperlipidemia**
Alpha-lipoproteinemia
Combined hyperlipidemia
Hyperlipidemia NOS
Hyperlipoproteinemia NOS

272.5 Lipoprotein deficiencies
Abetalipoproteinemia
Bassen-Kornzweig syndrome
High-density lipoid deficiency
Hypoalphalipoproteinemia
Hypobetalipoproteinemia (familial)

272.6 Lipodystrophy
Barraquer-Simons disease
Progressive lipodystrophy

Use additional E code to identify cause, if iatrogenic

| **Excludes** | intestinal lipodystrophy (040.2) |

272.7 Lipidoses
Chemically induced lipidosis
Disease:
Anderson's
Fabry's
Gaucher's
I cell [mucolipidosis I]
lipoid storage NOS
Niemann-Pick
pseudo-Hurler's or mucolipidosis III
triglyceride storage, Type I or II
Wolman's or triglyceride storage, Type III
Mucolipidosis II
Primary familial xanthomatosis

| **Excludes** | cerebral lipidoses (330.1) |
| | Tay-Sachs disease (330.1) |

☐ **272.8 Other disorders of lipoid metabolism**
Hoffa's disease or liposynovitis prepatellaris
Launois-Bensaude's lipomatosis
Lipoid dermatoarthritis

☐ **272.9 Unspecified disorder of lipoid metabolism**

● **273 Disorders of plasma protein metabolism**

Excludes	agammaglobulinemia and hypogammaglobulinemia (279.0–279.2)
	coagulation defects (286.0–286.9)
	hereditary hemolytic anemias (282.0–282.9)

273.0 Polyclonal hypergammaglobulinemia
Hypergammaglobulinemic purpura:
benign primary
Waldenström's

273.1 Monoclonal paraproteinemia
Benign monoclonal hypergammaglobulinemia [BMH]
Monoclonal gammopathy:
NOS
associated with lymphoplasmacytic dyscrasias
benign
Paraproteinemia:
benign (familial)
secondary to malignant or inflammatory disease

☐ **273.2 Other paraproteinemias**
Cryoglobulinemic:
purpura
vasculitis
Mixed cryoglobulinemia

273.3 Macroglobulinemia
Macroglobulinemia (idiopathic) (primary)
Waldenström's macroglobulinemia

273.4 Alpha-1-antitrypsin deficiency ◀
AAT deficiency ◀

☐ **273.8 Other disorders of plasma protein metabolism**
Abnormality of transport protein
Bisalbuminemia

☐ **273.9 Unspecified disorder of plasma protein metabolism**

● **274 Gout**

| **Excludes** | lead gout (984.0–984.9) |

274.0 Gouty arthropathy

● **274.1 Gouty nephropathy**

☐ **274.10 Gouty nephropathy, unspecified**

274.11 Uric acid nephrolithiasis

☐ **274.19 Other**

● **274.8 Gout with other specified manifestations**

274.81 Gouty tophi of ear

☐ **274.82 Gouty tophi of other sites**
Gouty tophi of heart

ICD-9-CM
200-299
Vol. 1

❏ **274.89 Other**

     Use additional code to identify manifestations, as:
         gouty:
            iritis (364.11)
            neuritis (357.4)

❏ **274.9 Gout, unspecified**

● **275 Disorders of mineral metabolism**

     Excludes *abnormal findings without manifest disease (790.0–796.9)*

     275.0 Disorders of iron metabolism
         Bronzed diabetes
         Hemochromatosis
         Pigmentary cirrhosis (of liver)

         Excludes *anemia:*
            iron deficiency (280.0–280.9)
            sideroblastic (285.0)

     275.1 Disorders of copper metabolism
         Hepatolenticular degeneration
         Wilson's disease

     275.2 Disorders of magnesium metabolism
         Hypermagnesemia
         Hypomagnesemia

     275.3 Disorders of phosphorus metabolism
         Familial hypophosphatemia
         Hypophosphatasia
         Vitamin D-resistant:
            osteomalacia
            rickets

● **275.4 Disorders of calcium metabolism**

         Excludes *parathyroid disorders (252.00–252.9)* ◀▥
            vitamin D deficiency (268.0–268.9)

         ❏ **275.40 Unspecified disorder of calcium metabolism**

         275.41 Hypocalcemia

         275.42 Hypercalcemia

         ❏ **275.49 Other disorders of calcium metabolism**
            Nephrocalcinosis
            Pseudohypoparathyroidism
            Pseudopseudohypoparathyroidism

❏ **275.8 Other specified disorders of mineral metabolism**

❏ **275.9 Unspecified disorder of mineral metabolism**

● **276 Disorders of fluid, electrolyte, and acid-base balance**

     Excludes *diabetes insipidus (253.5)*
         familial periodic paralysis (359.3)

     276.0 Hyperosmolality and/or hypernatremia
         Sodium [Na] excess
         Sodium [Na] overload

     276.1 Hyposmolality and/or hyponatremia
         Sodium [Na] deficiency

     276.2 Acidosis
         Acidosis:
            NOS   metabolic
            lactic   respiratory

         Excludes *diabetic acidosis (250.1)*

     276.3 Alkalosis
         Alkalosis:
         NOS
         metabolic
         respiratory

     276.4 Mixed acid-base balance disorder
         Hypercapnia with mixed acid-base disorder

276.5 Volume depletion
     Dehydration
     Depletion of volume of plasma or extracellular fluid
     Hypovolemia

     Excludes *hypovolemic shock:*
         postoperative (998.0)
         traumatic (958.4)

276.6 Fluid overload
     Fluid retention

     Excludes *ascites (789.5)*
         localized edema (782.3)

276.7 Hyperpotassemia
     Hyperkalemia
     Potassium [K]:   Potassium [K]:
         excess   overload
         intoxication

276.8 Hypopotassemia
     Hypokalemia
     Potassium [K] deficiency

❏ **276.9 Electrolyte and fluid disorders not elsewhere classified**
     Electrolyte imbalance
     Hyperchloremia
     Hypochloremia

     Excludes *electrolyte imbalance:*
         associated with hyperemesis gravidarum (643.1)
         complicating labor and delivery (669.0)
         following abortion and ectopic or molar pregnancy (634–638 with .4, 639.4)

● **277 Other and unspecified disorders of metabolism**

● **277.0 Cystic fibrosis**
     Fibrocystic disease of the pancreas
     Mucoviscidosis

     277.00 Without mention of meconium ileus
         Cystic fibrosis NOS

     277.01 With meconium ileus
         Meconium:
            ileus (of newborn)
            obstruction of intestine in mucoviscidosis

     277.02 With pulmonary manifestations
         Cystic fibrosis with pulmonary exacerbation
         Use additional code to identify any infectious organism present, such as:
            pseudomonas (041.7)

     277.03 With gastrointestinal manifestations

     Excludes *with meconium ileus (277.01)*

❏ **277.09 With other manifestations**

     277.1 Disorders of porphyrin metabolism
         Hematoporphyria
         Hematoporphyrinuria
         Hereditary coproporphyria
         Porphyria
         Porphyrinuria
         Protocoproporphyria
         Protoporphyria
         Pyrroloporphyria

❏ **277.2 Other disorders of purine and pyrimidine metabolism**
     Hypoxanthine-guanine-phosphoribosyltransferase deficiency [HG-PRT deficiency]
     Lesch-Nyhan syndrome
     Xanthinuria

     Excludes *gout (274.0–274.9)*
         orotic aciduric anemia (281.4)

277.3 Amyloidosis
　　Amyloidosis:
　　　NOS
　　　inherited systemic
　　　nephropathic
　　　neuropathic (Portuguese) (Swiss)
　　　secondary
　　Benign paroxysmal peritonitis
　　Familial Mediterranean fever
　　Hereditary cardiac amyloidosis

277.4 Disorders of bilirubin excretion
　　Hyperbilirubinemia:　　　Syndrome:
　　　congenital　　　　　　　Crigler-Najjar
　　　constitutional　　　　　Dubin-Johnson
　　　　　　　　　　　　　　Gilbert's
　　　　　　　　　　　　　　Rotor's

　　| Excludes | *hyperbilirubinemias specific to the perinatal period (774.0–774.7)*

277.5 Mucopolysaccharidosis
　　Gargoylism
　　Hunter's syndrome
　　Hurler's syndrome
　　Lipochondrodystrophy
　　Maroteaux-Lamy syndrome
　　Morquio-Brailsford disease
　　Osteochondrodystrophy
　　Sanfilippo's syndrome
　　Scheie's syndrome

☐ **277.6 Other deficiencies of circulating enzymes**
　　Hereditary angioedema

277.7 Dysmetabolic syndrome X
　　Use additional code for associated manifestation, such as:
　　　cardiovascular disease (414.00–414.07)
　　　obesity (278.00–278.01)

● **277.8 Other specified disorders of metabolism**

　277.81 Primary carnitine deficiency

　277.82 Carnitine deficiency due to inborn errors of metabolism

　277.83 Iatrogenic carnitine deficiency
　　　Carnitine deficiency due to:
　　　　hemodialysis
　　　　valproic acid therapy

　277.84 Other secondary carnitine deficiency

　277.85 Disorders of fatty acid oxidation ◀
　　　Carnitine palmitoyltransferase deficiencies (CPT1, CPT2)
　　　Glutaric aciduria type II (type IIA, IIB, IIC) ◀
　　　Long chain 3-hydroxyacyl CoA dehydrogenase deficiency (LCHAD) ◀
　　　Long chain/very long chain acyl CoA dehydrogenase deficiency (LCAD, VLCAD) ◀
　　　Medium chain acyl CoA dehydrogenase deficiency (MCAD) ◀
　　　Short chain acyl CoA dehydrogenase deficiency (SCAD) ◀

　　| Excludes | *primary carnitine deficiency (277.81)* ◀

　277.86 Paroxysmal disorders ◀
　　　Adrenomyeloneuropathy ◀
　　　Neonatal adrenoleukodystrophy ◀
　　　Rhizomelic chondrodysplasia punctata ◀
　　　X-linked adrenoleukodystrophy ◀
　　　Zellweger syndrome ◀

　　| Excludes | *infantile Refsum disease (356.3)* ◀

277.87 Disorders of mitochondrial metabolism ◀
　　Kearns-Sayre syndrome
　　Mitochondrial Encephalopathy, Lactic Acidosis and Stroke-like episodes (MELAS syndrome) ◀
　　Mitochondrial Neurogastrointestinal Encephalopathy syndrome (MNGIE) ◀
　　Myoclonus with Epilepsy and with Ragged Red Fibers (MERRF syndrome) ◀
　　Neuropathy, Ataxi and Retinitis Pigmentosa (NARP syndrome) ◀
　　Use additional code for associated conditions ◀

　　| Excludes | *disorders of pyruvate metabolism (271.8)* ◀
　　　Leber's optic atrophy (377.16) ◀
　　　Leigh's subacute necrotizing encephalopathy (330.8) ◀
　　　Reye's syndrome (331.81) ◀

☐ **277.89 Other specified disorders of metabolism**
　　Hand-Schüller-Christian disease
　　Histiocytosis (acute) (chronic)
　　Histiocytosis X (chronic)

　　| Excludes | *histiocytosis:*
　　　acute differentiated progressive (202.5)
　　　X, acute (progressive) (202.5)

☐ **277.9 Unspecified disorder of metabolism**
　　Enzymopathy NOS

● **278 Obesity and other hyperalimentation**

　　| Excludes | *hyperalimentation NOS (783.6)*
　　　poisoning by vitamins NOS (963.5)
　　　polyphagia (783.6)

● **278.0 Obesity**

　　| Excludes | *adiposogenital dystrophy (253.8)*
　　　obesity of endocrine origin NOS (259.9)

　☐ **278.00 Obesity, unspecified**
　　　Obesity NOS

　278.01 Morbid obesity
　　　Severe obesity

278.1 Localized adiposity
　　Fat pad

278.2 Hypervitaminosis A

278.3 Hypercarotinemia

278.4 Hypervitaminosis D

☐ **278.8 Other hyperalimentation**

● **279 Disorders involving the immune mechanism**

　● **279.0 Deficiency of humoral immunity**

　☐ **279.00 Hypogammaglobulinemia, unspecified**
　　　Agammaglobulinemia NOS

　279.01 Selective IgA immunodeficiency

　279.02 Selective IgM immunodeficiency

　☐ **279.03 Other selective immunoglobulin deficiencies**
　　　Selective deficiency of IgG

　279.04 Congenital hypogammaglobulinemia
　　　Agammaglobulinemia:
　　　　Bruton's type
　　　　X-linked

　279.05 Immunodeficiency with increased IgM
　　　Immunodeficiency with hyper-IgM:
　　　　autosomal recessive
　　　　X-linked

ICD-9-CM

200-
___

Vol. ___

279.06　Common variable immunodeficiency
　　　　Dysgammaglobulinemia (acquired) (congenital) (primary)
　　　　Hypogammaglobulinemia:
　　　　　acquired primary
　　　　　congenital non-sex-linked
　　　　　sporadic

❑ **279.09　Other**
　　　　Transient hypogammaglobulinemia of infancy

● **279.1　Deficiency of cell-mediated immunity**

❑ **279.10　Immunodeficiency with predominant T-cell defect, unspecified**

279.11　DiGeorge's syndrome
　　　　Pharyngeal pouch syndrome
　　　　Thymic hypoplasia

279.12　Wiskott-Aldrich syndrome

279.13　Nezelof's syndrome
　　　　Cellular immunodeficiency with abnormal immunoglobulin deficiency

❑ **279.19　Other**
　　❘ **Excludes** ❘ *ataxia-telangiectasia (334.8)*

279.2　Combined immunity deficiency
　　　　Agammaglobulinemia:
　　　　　autosomal recessive
　　　　　Swiss-type
　　　　　X-linked recessive
　　　　Severe combined immunodeficiency [SCID]
　　　　Thymic:
　　　　　alymphoplasia
　　　　　aplasia or dysplasia with immunodeficiency
　　❘ **Excludes** ❘ *thymic hypoplasia (279.11)*

❑ **279.3　Unspecified immunity deficiency**

❑ **279.4　Autoimmune disease, not elsewhere classified**
　　　　Autoimmune disease NOS
　　❘ **Excludes** ❘ *transplant failure or rejection (996.80–996.89)*

❑ **279.8　Other specified disorders involving the immune mechanism**
　　　　Single complement $[C_1$-$C_9]$ deficiency or dysfunction

❑ **279.9　Unspecified disorder of immune mechanism**

4.   DISEASES OF THE BLOOD AND BLOOD-FORMING ORGANS (280–289)

Excludes *anemia complicating pregnancy or the puerperium (648.2)*

● **280   Iron deficiency anemias**

Includes: anemia:
   asiderotic
   hypochromic-microcytic
   sideropenic

Excludes *familial microcytic anemia (282.49)*

280.0   Secondary to blood loss (chronic)
   Normocytic anemia due to blood loss

Excludes *acute posthemorrhagic anemia (285.1)*

280.1   Secondary to inadequate dietary iron intake

❑ **280.8   Other specified iron deficiency anemias**
   Paterson-Kelly syndrome
   Plummer-Vinson syndrome
   Sideropenic dysphagia

❑ **280.9   Iron deficiency anemia, unspecified**
   Anemia:
      achlorhydric
      chlorotic
      idiopathic hypochromic
      iron [Fe] deficiency NOS

● **281   Other deficiency anemias**

281.0   Pernicious anemia
   Anemia:
      Addison's
      Biermer's
      congenital pernicious
   Congenital intrinsic factor [Castle's] deficiency

Excludes *combined system disease without mention of anemia (266.2)*
subacute degeneration of spinal cord without mention of anemia (266.2)

❑ **281.1   Other vitamin B$_{12}$ deficiency anemia**
   Anemia:
      vegan's
      vitamin B$_{12}$ deficiency (dietary)
      due to selective vitamin B$_{12}$ malabsorption with proteinuria
   Syndrome:
      Imerslund's
      Imerslund-Gräsbeck

Excludes *combined system disease without mention of anemia (266.2)*
subacute degeneration of spinal cord without mention of anemia (266.2)

281.2   Folate-deficiency anemia
   Congenital folate malabsorption
   Folate or folic acid deficiency anemia:
      NOS
      dietary
      drug-induced
   Goat's milk anemia
   Nutritional megaloblastic anemia (of infancy)

   Use additional E code to identify drug

❑ **281.3   Other specified megaloblastic anemias, not elsewhere classified**
   Combined B$_{12}$ and folate-deficiency anemia
   Refractory megaloblastic anemia

281.4   Protein-deficiency anemia
   Amino-acid-deficiency anemia

❑ **281.8   Anemia associated with other specified nutritional deficiency**
   Scorbutic anemia

❑ **281.9   Unspecified deficiency anemia**
   Anemia:
      dimorphic
      macrocytic
      megaloblastic NOS
      nutritional NOS
      simple chronic

● **282   Hereditary hemolytic anemias**

282.0   Hereditary spherocytosis
   Acholuric (familial) jaundice
   Congenital hemolytic anemia (spherocytic)
   Congenital spherocytosis
   Minkowski-Chauffard syndrome
   Spherocytosis (familial)

Excludes *hemolytic anemia of newborn (773.0–773.5)*

282.1   Hereditary elliptocytosis
   Elliptocytosis (congenital)
   Ovalocytosis (congenital) (hereditary)

282.2   Anemias due to disorders of glutathione metabolism
   Anemia:
      6-phosphogluconic dehydrogenase deficiency
      enzyme deficiency, drug-induced
      erythrocytic glutathione deficiency
      glucose-6-phosphate dehydrogenase [G-6-PD] deficiency
      glutathione-reductase deficiency
      hemolytic nonspherocytic (hereditary), type I
   Disorder of pentose phosphate pathway
   Favism

❑ **282.3   Other hemolytic anemias due to enzyme deficiency**
   Anemia:
      hemolytic nonspherocytic (hereditary), type II
      hexokinase deficiency
      pyruvate kinase [PK] deficiency
      triosephosphate isomerase deficiency

● **282.4   Thalassemias**

Excludes *sickle-cell:*
disease (282.60–282.69)
trait (282.5)

282.41   Sickle-cell thalassemia without crisis
   Sickle-cell thalassemia NOS
   Thalassemia Hb-S disease without crisis

282.42   Sickle-cell thalassemia with crisis
   Sickle-cell thalassemia with vasco-occlusive pain
   Thalassemia Hb-S disease with crisis

   Use additional code for types of crisis, such as:
      acute chest syndrome (517.3)
      splenic sequestration (289.52)

❑ **282.49   Other thalassemia**
   Cooley's anemia
   Hereditary leptocytosis
   Mediterranean anemia (with other hemoglobinopathy)
   Microdrepanocytosis
   Thalassemia (alpha) (beta) (intermedia) (major) (minima) (minor) (mixed) (trait) (with other hemoglobinopathy)
   Thalassemia NOS

282.5   Sickle-cell trait
   Hb-AS genotype
   Hemoglobin S [Hb-S] trait
   Heterozygous:
      hemoglobin S
      Hb-S

Excludes *that with other hemoglobinopathy (282.60–282.69)*
that with thalassemia (282.49)

ICD-9-CM
200-299
Vol. 1

● **282.6 Sickle-cell disease**
Sickle-cell anemia

> **Excludes** *sickle-cell thalassemia (282.41–282.42)*
> *sickle-cell trait (282.5)*

☐ **282.60 Sickle-cell disease, unspecified**
Sickle-cell anemia NOS

282.61 Hb-SS disease without crisis

282.62 Hb-SS disease with crisis
Hb-SS disease with vaso-occlusive pain

Use additional code for types of crisis, such as:
   acute chest syndrome (517.3)
   splenic sequestration (289.52)

282.63 Sickle-cell/Hb-C disease without crisis
Hb-S/Hb-C disease without crisis

282.64 Sickle-cell/Hb-C disease with crisis
Hb-S/Hb-C disease with crisis
Sickle-cell/Hb-C disease with vaso-occlusive pain

Use additional code for types of crisis, such as:
   acute chest syndrome (517.3)
   splenic sequestration (289.52)

282.68 Other sickle-cell disease without crisis
Hb-S/Hb-D disease without crisis
Hb-S/Hb-E disease without crisis
Sickle-cell/Hb-D disease without crisis
Sickle-cell/Hb-E disease without crisis

☐ **282.69 Other sickle-cell disease with crisis**
Hb-S/Hb-D disease with crisis
Hb-S/Hb-E disease with crisis
Other sickle-cell disease with vaso-occlusive pain
Sickle-cell/Hb-D disease with crisis
Sickle-cell/Hb-E disease with crisis

Use additional code for types of crisis, such as:
   acute chest syndrome (517.3)
   splenic sequestration (289.52)

☐ **282.7 Other hemoglobinopathies**
Abnormal hemoglobin NOS
Congenital Heinz-body anemia
Disease:
   Hb-Bart's
   hemoglobin C [Hb-C]
   hemoglobin D [Hb-D]
   hemoglobin E [Hb-E]
   hemoglobin Zurich [Hb-Zurich]
Hemoglobinopathy NOS
Hereditary persistence of fetal hemoglobin [HPFH]
Unstable hemoglobin hemolytic disease

> **Excludes** *familial polycythemia (289.6)*
> *hemoglobin M [Hb-M] disease (289.7)*
> *high-oxygen-affinity hemoglobin (289.0)*

☐ **282.8 Other specified hereditary hemolytic anemias**
Stomatocytosis

☐ **282.9 Hereditary hemolytic anemia, unspecified**
Hereditary hemolytic anemia NOS

● **283 Acquired hemolytic anemias**

283.0 Autoimmune hemolytic anemias
Autoimmune hemolytic disease (cold type) (warm type)
Chronic cold hemagglutinin disease
Cold agglutinin disease or hemoglobinuria
Hemolytic anemia:
   cold type (secondary) (symptomatic)
   drug-induced
   warm type (secondary) (symptomatic)

Use additional E code to identify cause, if drug-induced

> **Excludes** *Evans' syndrome (287.3)*
> *hemolytic disease of newborn (773.0–773.5)*

● **283.1 Non-autoimmune hemolytic anemias**

☐ **283.10 Non-autoimmune hemolytic anemia, unspecified**

283.11 Hemolytic-uremic syndrome

☐ **283.19 Other non-autoimmune hemolytic anemias**
Hemolytic anemia:
   mechanical
   microangiopathic
   toxic

Use additional E code to identify cause

283.2 Hemoglobinuria due to hemolysis from external causes
Acute intravascular hemolysis
Hemoglobinuria:
   from exertion
   march
   paroxysmal (cold) (nocturnal)
   due to other hemolysis
Marchiafava-Micheli syndrome

Use additional E code to identify cause

☐ **283.9 Acquired hemolytic anemia, unspecified**
Acquired hemolytic anemia NOS
Chronic idiopathic hemolytic anemia

● **284 Aplastic anemia**

☐ **284.0 Constitutional aplastic anemia**
Aplasia, (pure) red cell:
   congenital
   of infants
   primary
Blackfan-Diamond syndrome
Familial hypoplastic anemia
Fanconi's anemia
Pancytopenia with malformations

☐ **284.8 Other specified aplastic anemias**
Aplastic anemia (due to):
   chronic systemic disease
   drugs
   infection
   radiation
   toxic (paralytic)
Pancytopenia (acquired)
Red cell aplasia (acquired) (adult) (pure) (with thymoma)

Use additional E code to identify cause

☐ **284.9 Aplastic anemia, unspecified**
Anemia:
   aplastic (idiopathic) NOS
   aregenerative
   hypoplastic NOS
   nonregenerative
   refractory
Medullary hypoplasia

● 285 **Other and unspecified anemias**

285.0 **Sideroblastic anemia**
Anemia:
hypochromic with iron loading
sideroachrestic
sideroblastic
acquired
congenital
hereditary
primary
refractory
secondary (drug-induced) (due to disease)
sex-linked hypochromic
vitamin B$_6$-responsive
Pyridoxine-responsive (hypochromic) anemia

Use additional E code to identify cause, if drug-induced

285.1 **Acute posthemorrhagic anemia**
Anemia due to acute blood loss

Excludes | *anemia due to chronic blood loss (280.0)*
blood loss anemia NOS (280.0)

● 285.2 **Anemia in chronic illness**

285.21 **Anemia in end-stage renal disease**
Erythropoietin-resistant anemia (EPO resistant anemia)

285.22 **Anemia in neoplastic disease**

285.29 **Anemia of other chronic illness**

❑ 285.8 **Other specified anemias**
Anemia:
dyserythropoietic (congenital)
dyshematopoietic (congenital)
leukoerythroblastic
von Jaksch's
Infantile pseudoleukemia

❑ 285.9 **Anemia, unspecified**
Anemia:
NOS
essential
normocytic, not due to blood loss
profound
progressive
secondary
Oligocythemia

Excludes | *anemia (due to):*
blood loss:
acute (285.1)
chronic or unspecified (280.0)
iron deficiency (280.0–280.9)

● 286 **Coagulation defects**

286.0 **Congenital factor VIII disorder**
Antihemophilic globulin [AHG] deficiency
Factor VIII (functional) deficiency
Hemophilia:
NOS
A
classical
familial
hereditary
Subhemophilia

Excludes | *factor VIII deficiency with vascular defect*
(286.4)

286.1 **Congenital factor IX disorder**
Christmas disease
Deficiency:
factor IX (functional)
plasma thromboplastin component [PTC]
Hemophilia B

286.2 **Congenital factor XI deficiency**
Hemophilia C
Plasma thromboplastin antecedent [PTA] deficiency
Rosenthal's disease

❑ 286.3 **Congenital deficiency of other clotting factors**
Congenital afibrinogenemia
Deficiency:
AC globulin factor:
I [fibrinogen]
II [prothrombin]
V [labile]
VII [stable]
X [Stuart-Prower]
XII [Hageman]
XIII [fibrin stabilizing]
Laki-Lorand factor
proaccelerin
Disease:
Owren's
Stuart-Prower
Dysfibrinogenemia (congenital)
Dysprothrombinemia (constitutional)
Hypoproconvertinemia
Hypoprothrombinemia (hereditary)
Parahemophilia

286.4 **von Willebrand's disease**
Angiohemophilia (A) (B)
Constitutional thrombopathy
Factor VIII deficiency with vascular defect
Pseudohemophilia type B
Vascular hemophilia
von Willebrand's (-Jürgens') disease

Excludes | *factor VIII deficiency:*
NOS (286.0)
with functional defect (286.0)
hereditary capillary fragility (287.8)

286.5 **Hemorrhagic disorder due to intrinsic circulating anticoagulants** ◀▥
Antithrombinemia
Antithromboplastinemia
Antithromboplastinogenemia
Hyperheparinemia
Increase in:
anti-VIIIa
anti-IXa
anti-Xa
anti-XIa
antithrombin
Secondary hemophilia ◀
Systemic lupus erythematosus [SLE] inhibitor

286.6 **Defibrination syndrome**
Afibrinogenemia, acquired
Consumption coagulopathy
Diffuse or disseminated intravascular coagulation [DIC syndrome]
Fibrinolytic hemorrhage, acquired
Hemorrhagic fibrinogenolysis
Pathologic fibrinolysis
Purpura:
fibrinolytic
fulminans

Excludes | *that complicating:*
abortion (634–638 with .1, 639.1)
pregnancy or the puerperium (641.3, 666.3)
disseminated intravascular coagulation in newborn (776.2)

ICD-9-CM
200-
Vol.

286.7 Acquired coagulation factor deficiency
Deficiency of coagulation factor due to:
liver disease
vitamin K deficiency
Hypoprothrombinemia, acquired

> **Excludes** *vitamin K deficiency of newborn (776.0)*

Use additional E code to identify cause, if drug-induced

☐ **286.9 Other and unspecified coagulation defects**
Defective coagulation NOS
Deficiency, coagulation factor NOS
Delay, coagulation
Disorder:
coagulation
hemostasis

> **Excludes** *abnormal coagulation profile (790.92)*
> *hemorrhagic disease of newborn (776.0)*
> *that complicating:*
> *abortion (634–638 with .1, 639.1)*
> *pregnancy or the puerperium (641.3, 666.3)*

● **287 Purpura and other hemorrhagic conditions**

> **Excludes** *hemorrhagic thrombocythemia (238.7)*
> *purpura fulminans (286.6)*

287.0 Allergic purpura
Peliosis rheumatica
Purpura:
anaphylactoid
autoimmune
Henoch's
nonthrombocytopenic:
hemorrhagic
idiopathic
rheumatica
Schönlein-Henoch
vascular
Vasculitis, allergic

> **Excludes** *hemorrhagic purpura (287.3)*
> *purpura annularis telangiectodes (709.1)*

287.1 Qualitative platelet defects
Thrombasthenia (hemorrhagic) (hereditary)
Thrombocytasthenia
Thrombocytopathy (dystrophic)
Thrombopathy (Bernard-Soulier)

> **Excludes** *von Willebrand's disease (286.4)*

☐ **287.2 Other nonthrombocytopenic purpuras**
Purpura:
NOS
senile
simplex

287.3 Primary thrombocytopenia
Evans'syndrome
Megakaryocytic hypoplasia
Purpura, thrombocytopenic
congenital
hereditary
idiopathic
Thrombocytopenia:
congenital
hereditary
primary
Tidal platelet dysgenesis

> **Excludes** *thrombotic thrombocytopenic purpura (446.6)*
> *transient thrombocytopenia of newborn*
> *(776.1)*

287.4 Secondary thrombocytopenia
Posttransfusion purpura
Thrombocytopenia (due to):
dilutional
drugs
extracorporeal circulation of blood
massive blood transfusion
platelet alloimmunization

Use additional E code to identify cause

> **Excludes** *transient thrombocytopenia of newborn*
> *(776.1)*

☐ **287.5 Thrombocytopenia, unspecified**

☐ **287.8 Other specified hemorrhagic conditions**
Capillary fragility (hereditary)
Vascular pseudohemophilia

☐ **287.9 Unspecified hemorrhagic conditions**
Hemorrhagic diathesis (familial)

● **288 Diseases of white blood cells**

> **Excludes** *leukemia (204.0–208.9)*

288.0 Agranulocytosis
Infantile genetic agranulocytosis
Kostmann's syndrome
Neutropenia: Neutropenia:
NOS   immune
cyclic   periodic
drug-induced   toxic
Neutropenic splenomegaly

Use additional E code to identify drug or other cause

> **Excludes** *transitory neonatal neutropenia (776.7)*

288.1 Functional disorders of polymorphonuclear neutrophils
Chronic (childhood) granulomatous disease
Congenital dysphagocytosis
Job's syndrome
Lipochrome histiocytosis (familial)
Progressive septic granulomatosis

288.2 Genetic anomalies of leukocytes
Anomaly (granulation) (granulocyte) or syndrome:
Alder's (-Reilly)
Chédiak-Steinbrinck (-Higashi)
Jordan's
May-Hegglin
Pelger-Huet
Hereditary:
hypersegmentation
hyposegmentation
leukomelanopathy

288.3 Eosinophilia
Eosinophilia
allergic   idiopathic
hereditary   secondary
Eosinophilic leukocytosis

> **Excludes** *Löffler's syndrome (518.3)*
> *pulmonary eosinophilia (518.3)*

☐ **288.8 Other specified disease of white blood cells**
Leukemoid reaction
lymphocytic
monocytic
myelocytic
Leukocytosis
Lymphocytopenia
Lymphocytosis (symptomatic)
Lymphopenia
Monocytosis (symptomatic)
Plasmacytosis

> **Excludes** *immunity disorders (279.0–279.9)*

☐ **288.9 Unspecified disease of white blood cells**

● **289 Other diseases of blood and blood-forming organs**

289.0 Polycythemia, secondary
High-oxygen-affinity hemoglobin
Polycythemia:
   acquired
   benign
   due to:
      fall in plasma volume
      high altitude
   emotional
   erythropoietin
   hypoxemic
   nephrogenous
   relative
   spurious
   stress

Excludes	polycythemia:

   polycythemia:
      neonatal (776.4)
      primary (238.4)
      vera (238.4)

289.1 Chronic lymphadenitis
Chronic:
   adenitis any lymph node, except mesenteric
   lymphadenitis any lymph node, except mesen-
      teric

Excludes	acute lymphadenitis (683)

   acute lymphadenitis (683)
      mesenteric (289.2)
      enlarged glands NOS (785.6)

❑ **289.2 Nonspecific mesenteric lymphadenitis**
Mesenteric lymphadenitis (acute) (chronic)

❑ **289.3 Lymphadenitis, unspecified, except mesenteric**

289.4 Hypersplenism
"Big spleen" syndrome
Dyssplenism
Hypersplenia

Excludes	primary splenic neutropenia (288.0)

● **289.5 Other diseases of spleen**

❑ **289.50 Disease of spleen, unspecified**

289.51 Chronic congestive splenomegaly

289.52 Splenic sequestration
Code first sickle-cell disease in crisis (282.42, 282.62, 282.64, 282.69)

❑ **289.59 Other**

Lien migrans	Splenic:
Perisplenitis	fibrosis
Splenic:	infarction
abscess	rupture, nontraumatic
atrophy	Splenitis
cyst	Wandering spleen

Excludes	bilharzial splenic fibrosis (120.0–120.9)

   bilharzial splenic fibrosis (120.0–120.9)
   hepatolienal fibrosis (571.5)
   splenomegaly NOS (789.2)

289.6 Familial polycythemia
Familial:
   benign polycythemia
   erythrocytosis

289.7 Methemoglobinemia
Congenital NADH [DPNH]-methemoglobin-re-
   ductase deficiency
Hemoglobin M [Hb-M] disease
Methemoglobinemia:
   NOS
   acquired (with sulfhemoglobinemia)
   hereditary
   toxic
Stokvis' disease
Sulfhemoglobinemia

Use additional E code to identify cause

● **289.8 Other specified diseases of blood and blood-forming organs**

289.81 Primary hypercoagulable state
Activated protein C resistance
Antithrombin III deficiency
Factor V Leiden mutation
Lupus anticoagulant
Protein C deficiency
Protein S deficiency
Prothombin gene mutation

289.82 Secondary hypercoagulable state

❑ **289.89 Other specified disease of blood and blood-
forming organs**
Hypergammaglobulinemia
Myelofibrosis
Pseudocholinesterase deficiency

❑ **289.9 Unspecified diseases of blood and blood-forming
organs**
Blood dyscrasia NOS
Erythroid hyperplasia

ICD-9-CM

200-299

Vol. 1

5.   MENTAL DISORDERS (290–319)

PSYCHOSES (290–299)

Excludes	mental retardation (317–319)

ORGANIC PSYCHOTIC CONDITIONS (290–294)

Includes: psychotic organic brain syndrome

Excludes	nonpsychotic syndromes of organic etiology (310.0–310.9)
	psychoses classifiable to 295–298 and without impairment of orientation, comprehension, calculation, learning capacity, and judgment, but associated with physical disease, injury, or condition affecting the brain [e.g., following childbirth] (295.0–298.8)

● **290   Dementias** ◀▦

Code first the associated neurological condition

Excludes	dementia due to alcohol (291.0–291.2) ◀
	dementia due to drugs (292.82) ◀
	dementia not classified as senile, presenile, or arteriosclerotic (294.10–294.11)
	psychoses classifiable to 295–298 occurring in the senium without dementia or delirium (295.0–298.8)
	senility with mental changes of nonpsychotic severity (310.1)
	transient organic psychotic conditions (293.0–293.9)

290.0   Senile dementia, uncomplicated
     Senile dementia:
         NOS
         simple type

Excludes	mild memory disturbances, not amounting to dementia, associated with senile brain disease (310.1)
	senile dementia with:
	delirium or confusion (290.3)
	delusional [paranoid] features (290.20)
	depressive features (290.21)

● **290.1   Presenile dementia**
     Brain syndrome with presenile brain disease

Excludes	arteriosclerotic dementia (290.40–290.43)
	dementia associated with other cerebral conditions (294.10–294.11)

     290.10   Presenile dementia, uncomplicated
         Presenile dementia:
            NOS
            simple type

     290.11   Presenile dementia with delirium
         Presenile dementia with acute confusional state

     290.12   Presenile dementia with delusional features
         Presenile dementia, paranoid type

     290.13   Presenile dementia with depressive features
         Presenile dementia, depressed type

● **290.2   Senile dementia with delusional or depressive features**

Excludes	senile dementia:
	NOS (290.0)
	with delirium and/or confusion (290.3)

     290.20   Senile dementia with delusional features
         Senile dementia, paranoid type
         Senile psychosis NOS

     290.21   Senile dementia with depressive features

290.3   Senile dementia with delirium
     Senile dementia with acute confusional state

Excludes	senile:
	dementia NOS (290.0)
	psychosis NOS (290.20)

● **290.4   Vascular dementia** ◀▦
     Multi-infarct dementia or psychosis

     Use additional code to identify cerebral atherosclerosis (437.0)

Excludes	suspected cases with no clear evidence of arteriosclerosis (290.9)

     290.40   Vascular dementia, uncomplicated ◀▦
         Arteriosclerotic dementia:
            NOS
            simple type

     290.41   Vascular dementia with delirium ◀▦
         Arteriosclerotic dementia with acute confusional state

     290.42   Vascular dementia with delusions ◀▦
         Arteriosclerotic dementia, paranoid type

     290.43   Vascular dementia with depressed mood ◀▦
         Arteriosclerotic dementia, depressed type

❑ **290.8   Other specified senile psychotic conditions**
     Presbyophrenic psychosis

❑ **290.9   Unspecified senile psychotic condition**

● **291   Alcohol-induced mental disorders** ◀▦

Excludes	alcoholism without psychosis (303.0–303.9)

     291.0   Alcohol withdrawal delirium
         Alcoholic delirium
         Delirium tremens

Excludes	alcohol withdrawal (291.81)

     291.1   Alcohol-induced persisting amnestic disorder ◀▦
         Alcoholic polyneuritic psychosis
         Korsakoff's psychosis, alcoholic
         Wernicke-Korsakoff syndrome (alcoholic)

❑ **291.2   Alcohol-induced persisting dementia** ◀▦
     Alcoholic dementia NOS
     Alcoholism associated with dementia NOS
     Chronic alcoholic brain syndrome

     291.3   Alcohol-induced psychotic disorder with hallucinations ◀▦
         Alcoholic:
            hallucinosis (acute)
            psychosis with hallucinosis

Excludes	alcohol withdrawal with delirium (291.0)
	schizophrenia (295.0–295.9) and paranoid states (297.0–297.9) taking the form of chronic hallucinosis with clear consciousness in an alcoholic

     291.4   Idiosyncratic alcohol intoxication
         Pathologic:
            alcohol intoxication
            drunkenness

Excludes	acute alcohol intoxication (305.0)
	in alcoholism (303.0)
	simple drunkenness (305.0)

     291.5   Alcoholic-induced psychotic disorder with delusions ◀▦
         Alcoholic:
            paranoia
            psychosis, paranoid type

Excludes	nonalcoholic paranoid states (297.0–297.9)
	schizophrenia, paranoid type (295.3)

● **291.8 Other specified alcohol-induced mental disorders** ◄▥

    291.81 Alcohol withdrawal
        Alcohol:
            abstinence syndrome or symptoms
            withdrawal syndrome or symptoms

        | Excludes | *alcohol withdrawal:*
              delirium (291.0)
              hallucinosis (291.3)
              delirium tremens (291.0)

    □ **291.89 Other**
        Alcohol-induced anxiety disorder ◄
        Alcohol-induced mood disorder ◄
        Alcohol-induced sexual dysfunction ◄
        Alcohol-induced sleep disorder ◄

□ **291.9 Unspecified alcohol-induced mental disorders** ◄▥
    Alcohol-related disorder NOS ◄
    Alcoholic:
        mania NOS
        psychosis NOS
    Alcoholism (chronic) with psychosis

● **292 Drug-induced mental disorders** ◄▥

    Includes: organic brain syndrome associated with consumption of drugs

    Use additional code for any associated drug dependence (304.0–304.9)

    Use additional E code to identify drug

    292.0 Drug withdrawal ◄▥
        Drug:
            abstinence syndrome or symptoms
            withdrawal syndrome or symptoms

● **292.1 Drug-induced psychotic disorders** ◄▥

    292.11 Drug-induced psychotic disorder with delusions ◄▥
        Paranoid state induced by drugs

    292.12 Drug-induced psychotic disorder with hallucinations ◄▥
        Hallucinatory state induced by drugs

        | Excludes | *states following LSD or other hallucinogens, lasting only a few days or less ["bad trips"] (305.3)*

    292.2 Pathological drug intoxication
        Drug reaction: resulting in brief psychotic states
            NOS
            idiosyncratic
            pathologic

        | Excludes | *expected brief psychotic reactions to hallucinogens ["bad trips"] (305.3)*
              physiological side-effects of drugs (e.g., dystonias)

● **292.8 Other specified drug-induced mental disorders**

    292.81 Drug-induced delirium

    292.82 Drug-induced persisting dementia ◄▥

    292.83 Drug-induced persisting amnestic disorder ◄▥

    292.84 Drug-induced mood disorder ◄▥
        Depressive state induced by drugs

    □ **292.89 Other**
        Drug-induced anxiety disorder ◄
        Drug-induced organic personality syndrome
        Drug-induced sexual dysfunction ◄
        Drug-induced sleep disorder ◄
        Drug intoxication ◄

□ **292.9 Unspecified drug-induced mental disorder**
    Drug-related disorder NOS ◄
    Organic psychosis NOS due to or associated with drugs

● **293 Transient mental disorders due to conditions classified elsewhere** ◄▥

    Includes: transient organic mental disorders not associated with alcohol or drugs

    Code first the associated physical or neurological condition

        | Excludes | *confusional state or delirium superimposed on senile dementia (290.3)*
              dementia due to:
                alcohol (291.0–291.9)
                arteriosclerosis (290.40–290.43)
                drugs (292.82)
                senility (290.0)

    293.0 Delirium due to conditions classified elsewhere ◄▥
        Acute:
            confusional state
            infective psychosis
            organic reaction
            posttraumatic organic psychosis
            psycho-organic syndrome
        Acute psychosis associated with endocrine, metabolic, or cerebrovascular disorder
        Epileptic:
            confusional state
            twilight state

    293.1 Subacute delirium
        Subacute:
            confusional state
            infective psychosis
            organic reaction
            posttraumatic organic psychosis
            psycho-organic syndrome
            psychosis associated with endocrine or metabolic disorder

● **293.8 Other specified transient mental disorders due to conditions classified elsewhere** ◄▥

    293.81 Psychotic disorder with delusions in conditions classified elsewhere ◄▥
        Transient organic psychotic condition, paranoid type

    293.82 Psychotic disorder with hallucinations in conditions classified elsewhere ◄▥
        Transient organic psychotic condition, hallucinatory type

    293.83 Mood disorder in conditions classified elsewhere ◄▥
        Transient organic psychotic condition, depressive type

    293.84 Anxiety disorder in conditions classified elsewhere ◄▥

    □ **293.89 Other**
        Catatonic disorder in conditions classified elsewhere ◄

□ **293.9 Unspecified transient mental disorder in conditions classified elsewhere** ◄▥
    Organic psychosis:
        infective NOS
        posttraumatic NOS
        transient NOS
    Psycho-organic syndrome

ICD-9-CM

200-299

Vol. 1

● **294 Persistent mental disorders due to conditions classified elsewhere**

Includes: organic psychotic brain syndromes (chronic), not elsewhere classified

294.0 Amnestic disorder in conditions classified elsewhere
Korsakoff's psychosis or syndrome (nonalcoholic)

Code first underlying condition ◀

Excludes *alcoholic:*
amnestic syndrome (291.1)
Korsakoff's psychosis (291.1)

● **294.1 Dementia in conditions classified elsewhere**
Code first any underlying physical condition as:
dementia in:
Alzheimer's disease (331.0)
Cerebral lipidoses (330.1)
Dementia of the Alzheimer's type ◀
Dementia with Lewy bodies (331.82)
Dementia with Parkinsonism (331.82)
Epilepsy (345.0–345.9)
Frontal dementia (331.19)
Frontotemporal dementia (331.19)
General paresis [syphilis] (094.1)
Hepatolenticular degeneration (275.1)
Huntington's chorea (333.4)
Jakob-Creutzfeldt disease (046.1)
Multiple sclerosis (340)
Pick's disease of the brain (331.11)
Polyarteritis nodosa (446.0)
Syphilis (094.1)

Excludes *dementia:*
arteriosclerotic (290.40–290.43)
presenile (290.10–290.13)
senile (290.0)
epileptic psychosis NOS (294.8)

294.10 *Dementia in conditions classified elsewhere without behavioral disturbance*
Dementia in conditions classified elsewhere NOS

294.11 *Dementia in conditions classified elsewhere with behavioral disturbance*
Aggressive behavior
Combative behavior
Violent behavior
Wandering off

❑ **294.8 Other persistent mental disorders due to conditions classified elsewhere** ◀▦
Amnestic disorder NOS ◀
Dementia NOS ◀
Epileptic psychosis NOS
Mixed paranoid and affective organic psychotic states

Use additional code for associated epilepsy (345.0–345.9)

Excludes *mild memory disturbances, not amounting to dementia (310.1)*

❑ **294.9 Unspecified persistent mental disorders due to conditions classified elsewhere** ◀▦
Cognitive disorder NOS ◀
Organic psychosis (chronic)

OTHER PSYCHOSES (295–299)

Use additional code to identify any associated physical disease, injury, or condition affecting the brain with psychoses classifiable to 295–298

● **295 Schizophrenic disorders**

Includes: schizophrenia of the types described in 295.0–295.9 occurring in children

Excludes *childhood type schizophrenia (299.9)*
infantile autism (299.0)

The following fifth-digit subclassification is for use with category 295:
❑ 0 **unspecified**
1 **subchronic**
2 **chronic**
3 **subchronic with acute exacerbation**
4 **chronic with acute exacerbation**
5 **in remission**

● **295.0 Simple type**
Schizophrenia simplex

Excludes *latent schizophrenia (295.5)*

● **295.1 Disorganized type**
Hebephrenia
Hebephrenic type schizophrenia

● **295.2 Catatonic type**
Catatonic (schizophrenia):   Schizophrenic:
  agitation   catalepsy
  excitation   catatonia
  excited type   flexibilitas cerea
  stupor
  withdrawn type

● **295.3 Paranoid type**
Paraphrenic schizophrenia

Excludes *involutional paranoid state (297.2)*
paranoia (297.1)
paraphrenia (297.2)

● **295.4 Schizophreniform disorder** ◀▦
Oneirophrenia
Schizophreniform:
attack
psychosis, confusional type

Excludes *acute forms of schizophrenia of:*
catatonic type (295.2)
hebephrenic type (295.1)
paranoid type (295.3)
simple type (295.0)
undifferentiated type (295.8)

● **295.5 Latent schizophrenia**
Latent schizophrenic reaction
Schizophrenia:
borderline
incipient
prepsychotic
prodromal
pseudoneurotic
pseudopsychopathic

Excludes *schizoid personality (301.20–301.22)*

● **295.6 Residual type** ◀▦
Chronic undifferentiated schizophrenia
Restzustand (schizophrenic)
Schizophrenic residual state

● **295.7 Schizoaffective disorder** ◀▦
Cyclic schizophrenia
Mixed schizophrenic and affective psychosis
Schizo-affective psychosis
Schizophreniform psychosis, affective type

● ❑ **295.8 Other specified types of schizophrenia**
　　　　Acute (undifferentiated) schizophrenia
　　　　Atypical schizophrenia
　　　　Cenesthopathic schizophrenia
　　　　Excludes *infantile autism (299.0)*

● ❑ **295.9 Unspecified schizophrenia**
　　　　Schizophrenia:
　　　　　NOS
　　　　　mixed NOS
　　　　　undifferentiated type　　　　　　　◀
　　　　　undifferentiated NOS
　　　　Schizophrenic reaction NOS
　　　　Schizophreniform psychosis NOS

● **296 Episodic mood disorders**　　　　　　◀▥

　　　Includes: episodic affective disorders
　　　Excludes *neurotic depression (300.4)*
　　　　　　　　reactive depressive psychosis (298.0)
　　　　　　　　reactive excitation (298.1)

　　　The following fifth-digit subclassification is for use with
　　　categories 296.0–296.6:
❑ **0 unspecified**
　1 mild
　2 moderate
　3 severe, without mention of psychotic behavior
　4 severe, specified as with psychotic behavior
　5 in partial or unspecified remission
　6 in full remission

● **296.0 Bipolar I disorder, single manic episode**　　◀▥
　　　　Hypomania (mild) NOS single episode or unspe-
　　　　　cified
　　　　Hypomanic psychosis single episode or unspecified
　　　　Mania (monopolar) NOS single episode or unspe-
　　　　　cified
　　　　Manic-depressive psychosis or reaction, single epi-
　　　　　sode or unspecified:
　　　　　hypomanic, single episode or unspecified
　　　　　manic, single episode or unspecified
　　　　Excludes *circular type, if there was a previous attack of*
　　　　　　　　depression (296.4)

● **296.1 Manic disorder, recurrent episode**
　　　　Any condition classifiable to 296.0, stated to be
　　　　　recurrent
　　　　Excludes *circular type, if there was a previous attack of*
　　　　　　　　depression (296.4)

● **296.2 Major depressive disorder, single episode**
　　　　Depressive psychosis, single episode or unspeci-
　　　　　fied
　　　　Endogenous depression, single episode or unspe-
　　　　　cified
　　　　Involutional melancholia, single episode or unspe-
　　　　　cified
　　　　Manic-depressive psychosis or reaction, depressed
　　　　　type, single episode or unspecified
　　　　Monopolar depression, single episode or unspeci-
　　　　　fied
　　　　Psychotic depression, single episode or unspeci-
　　　　　fied
　　　　Excludes *circular type, if previous attack was of manic*
　　　　　　　　type (296.5)
　　　　　　　　depression NOS (311)
　　　　　　　　reactive depression (neurotic) (300.4)
　　　　　　　　psychotic (298.0)

● **296.3 Major depressive disorder, recurrent episode**
　　　　Any condition classifiable to 296.2, stated to be
　　　　　recurrent
　　　　Excludes *circular type, if previous attack was of manic*
　　　　　　　　type (296.5)
　　　　　　　　depression NOS (311)
　　　　　　　　reactive depression (neurotic) (300.4)
　　　　　　　　psychotic (298.0)

● **296.4 Bipolar I disorder, most recent episode (or current)
　　　　manic**　　　　　　　　　　　　◀▥
　　　　Bipolar disorder, now manic
　　　　Manic-depressive psychosis, circular type but cur-
　　　　　rently manic
　　　　Excludes *brief compensatory or rebound mood swings*
　　　　　　　　(296.99)

● **296.5 Bipolar I disorder, most recent episode (or current)
　　　　depressed**
　　　　Bipolar disorder, now depressed
　　　　Manic-depressive psychosis, circular type but cur-
　　　　　rently depressed
　　　　Excludes *brief compensatory or rebound mood swings*
　　　　　　　　(296.99)

● **296.6 Bipolar I disorder, most recent episode (or current)
　　　　mixed**　　　　　　　　　　　　◀▥
　　　　Manic-depressive psychosis, circular type, mixed

❑ **296.7 Bipolar I disorder, most recent episode (or current)
　　　　unspecified**　　　　　　　　　　◀▥
　　　　Atypical bipolar affective disorder NOS
　　　　Manic-depressive psychosis, circular type, current
　　　　　condition not specified as either manic or de-
　　　　　pressive

● **296.8 Other and unspecified bipolar disorders**　◀▥

❑ **296.80 Bipolar disorder, unspecified**
　　　　Bipolar disorder NOS　　　　　◀
　　　　Manic-depressive:
　　　　　reaction NOS
　　　　　syndrome NOS

296.81 Atypical manic disorder

296.82 Atypical depressive disorder

❑ **296.89 Other**
　　　　Bipolar II disorder　　　　　　◀
　　　　Manic-depressive psychosis, mixed type

● **296.9 Other and unspecified episodic mood disorder**　◀▥
　　　Excludes *psychogenic affective psychoses (298.0–298.8)*

❑ **296.90 Unspecified episodic mood disorder**　◀▥
　　　　Affective psychosis NOS
　　　　Melancholia NOS
　　　　Mood disorder NOS　　　　　　◀

❑ **296.99 Other specified episodic mood disorder**　◀▥
　　　　Mood swings:
　　　　　brief compensatory
　　　　　rebound

● **297 Delusional disorders**　　　　　　◀▥

　　　Includes: paranoid disorders
　　　Excludes *acute paranoid reaction (298.3)*
　　　　　　　　alcoholic jealousy or paranoid state (291.5)
　　　　　　　　paranoid schizophrenia (295.3)

297.0 Paranoid state, simple

297.1 Delusional disorder　　　　　　◀▥
　　　　Chronic paranoid psychosis
　　　　Sander's disease
　　　　Systematized delusions
　　　Excludes *paranoid personality disorder (301.0)*

297.2 Paraphrenia
　　　　Involutional paranoid state
　　　　Late paraphrenia
　　　　Paraphrenia (involutional)

297.3 Shared psychotic disorder　　　　◀▥
　　　　Folie à deux
　　　　Induced psychosis or paranoid disorder

ICD-9-CM
200-299
Vol. 1

☐ **297.8 Other specified paranoid states**
  Paranoia querulans
  Sensitiver Beziehungswahn

  Excludes   *acute paranoid reaction or state (298.3)*
              senile paranoid state (290.20)

☐ **297.9 Unspecified paranoid state**
  Paranoid:
    disorder NOS
    psychosis NOS
    reaction NOS
    state NOS

● **298 Other nonorganic psychoses**

  Includes: psychotic conditions due to or provoked by:
            emotional stress
            environmental factors as major part of etiology

  298.0 Depressive type psychosis
    Psychogenic depressive psychosis
    Psychotic reactive depression
    Reactive depressive psychosis

    Excludes   *manic-depressive psychosis, depressed type (296.2–296.3)*
                neurotic depression (300.4)
                reactive depression NOS (300.4)

  298.1 Excitative type psychosis
    Acute hysterical psychosis
    Psychogenic excitation
    Reactive excitation

    Excludes   *manic-depressive psychosis, manic type (296.0–296.1)*

  298.2 Reactive confusion
    Psychogenic confusion
    Psychogenic twilight state

    Excludes   *acute confusional state (293.0)*

  298.3 Acute paranoid reaction
    Acute psychogenic paranoid psychosis
    Bouffée délirante

    Excludes   *paranoid states (297.0–297.9)*

  298.4 Psychogenic paranoid psychosis
    Protracted reactive paranoid psychosis

☐ **298.8 Other and unspecified reactive psychosis**
    Brief psychotic disorder   ◄
    Brief reactive psychosis NOS
    Hysterical psychosis
    Psychogenic psychosis NOS
    Psychogenic stupor

    Excludes   *acute hysterical psychosis (298.1)*

☐ **298.9 Unspecified psychosis**
    Atypical psychosis
    Psychosis NOS
    Psychotic disorder NOS   ◄

● **299 Pervasive developmental disorders**   ◄▥

    Excludes   *adult type psychoses occurring in childhood, as:*
                affective disorders (296.0–296.9)
                manic-depressive disorders (296.0–296.9)
                schizophrenia (295.0–295.9)

  The following fifth-digit subclassification is for use with category 299:
    0 current or active state
    1 residual state

● **299.0 Autistic disorder**   ◄▥
    Childhood autism
    Infantile psychosis
    Kanner's syndrome

    Excludes   *disintegrative psychosis (299.1)*
                Heller's syndrome (299.1)
                schizophrenic syndrome of childhood (299.9)

● **299.1 Childhood disintegrative disorder**   ◄▥
    Heller's syndrome

    Use additional code to identify any associated neurological disorder

    Excludes   *infantile autism (299.0)*
                schizophrenic syndrome of childhood (299.9)

● ☐ **299.8 Other specified pervasive developmental disorders**   ◄▥
    Asperger's disorder   ◄
    Atypical childhood psychosis
    Borderline psychosis of childhood

    Excludes   *simple stereotypes without psychotic disturbance (307.3)*

● ☐ **299.9 Unspecified pervasive developmental disorder** ◄▥
    Child psychosis NOS
    Pervasive developmental disorder NOS   ◄
    Schizophrenia, childhood type NOS
    Schizophrenic syndrome of childhood NOS

    Excludes   *schizophrenia of adult type occurring in childhood (295.0–295.9)*

NEUROTIC DISORDERS, PERSONALITY DISORDERS, AND OTHER NONPSYCHOTIC MENTAL DISORDERS (300–316)

● **300 Anxiety, dissociative and somatoform disorders** ◄▥

  ● **300.0 Anxiety states**

    Excludes   *anxiety in:*
                acute stress reaction (308.0)
                transient adjustment reaction (309.24)
                neurasthenia (300.5)
                psychophysiological disorders (306.0–306.9)
                separation anxiety (309.21)

  ☐ **300.00 Anxiety state, unspecified**
    Anxiety:
      neurosis
      reaction
      state (neurotic)
    Atypical anxiety disorder

  300.01 Panic disorder without agoraphobia   ◄▥
    Panic:
      attack
      state

    Excludes   *panic disorder with agoraphobia (300.21)*   ◄

  300.02 Generalized anxiety disorder

  ☐ **300.09 Other**

  ● **300.1 Dissociative, conversion and factitious disorders**   ◄▥

    Excludes   *adjustment reaction (309.0–309.9)*
                anorexia nervosa (307.1)
                gross stress reaction (308.0–308.9)
                hysterical personality (301.50–301.59)
                psychophysiologic disorders (306.0–306.9)

  ☐ **300.10 Hysteria, unspecified**

  300.11 Conversion disorder
    Astasia-abasia, hysterical
    Conversion hysteria or reaction
    Hysterical:
      blindness
      deafness
      paralysis

  300.12 Dissociative amnesia   ◄▥
    Hysterical amnesia

  300.13 Dissociative fugue   ◄▥
    Hysterical fugue

300.14 **Dissociative identity disorder**   ◀▥

❏300.15 **Dissociative disorder or reaction, unspecified**

300.16 **Factitious disorder with predominantly psychological signs and symptoms** ◀▥
     Compensation neurosis
     Ganser's syndrome, hysterical

❏300.19 **Other and unspecified factitious illness**
     Factitious disorder (with combined psychological and physical signs and symptoms) (with predominantly physical signs and symptoms) NOS ◀▥

Excludes *multiple operations or hospital addiction syndrome (301.51)*

● **300.2 Phobic disorders**

Excludes *anxiety state not associated with a specific situation or object (300.00–300.09)*
obsessional phobias (300.3)

❏300.20 **Phobia, unspecified**
     Anxiety-hysteria NOS
     Phobia NOS

300.21 **Agoraphobia with panic disorder** ◀▥
     Fear of:
       open spaces with panic attacks
       streets with panic attacks
       travel with panic attacks
     Panic disorder with agoraphobia ◀

Excludes *agoraphobia without panic disorder (300.22)* ◀
panic disorder without agoraphobia (300.01) ◀

300.22 **Agoraphobia without mention of panic attacks**
     Any condition classifiable to 300.21 without mention of panic attacks

300.23 **Social phobia**
     Fear of:
       eating in public
       public speaking
       washing in public

❏300.29 **Other isolated or specific phobias** ◀▥
     Acrophobia
     Animal phobias
     Claustrophobia
     Fear of crowds

300.3 **Obsessive-compulsive disorders**
     Anancastic neurosis
     Compulsive neurosis
     Obsessional phobia [any]

Excludes *obsessive-compulsive symptoms occurring in:*
endogenous depression (296.2–296.3)
organic states (e.g., encephalitis)
schizophrenia (295.0–295.9)

300.4 **Dysthmic disorder** ◀▥
     Anxiety depression
     Depression with anxiety
     Depressive reaction
     Neurotic depressive state
     Reactive depression

Excludes *adjustment reaction with depressive symptoms (309.0–309.1)*
depression NOS (311)
manic-depressive psychosis, depressed type (296.2–296.3)
reactive depressive psychosis (298.0)

300.5 **Neurasthenia**
     Fatigue neurosis
     Nervous debility
     Psychogenic:
       asthenia
       general fatigue

Use additional code to identify any associated physical disorder

Excludes *anxiety state (300.00–300.09)*
neurotic depression (300.4)
psychophysiological disorders (306.0–306.9)
specific nonpsychotic mental disorders following organic brain damage (310.0–310.9)

300.6 **Depersonalization disorder** ◀▥
     Derealization (neurotic)
     Neurotic state with depersonalization episode

Excludes *depersonalization associated with:*
anxiety (300.00–300.09)
depression (300.4)
manic-depressive disorder or psychosis (296.0–296.9)
schizophrenia (295.0–295.9)

300.7 **Hypochondriasis**
     Body dysmorphic disorder

Excludes *hypochondriasis in:*
hysteria (300.10–300.19)
manic-depressive psychosis, depressed type (296.2–296.3)
neurasthenia (300.5)
obsessional disorder (300.3)
schizophrenia (295.0–295.9)

● **300.8 Somatoform disorders** ◀▥

300.81 **Somatization disorder**
     Briquet's disorder
     Severe somatoform disorder

300.82 **Undifferentiated somatoform disorder**
     Atypical somatoform disorder
     Somatoform disorder NOS

❏300.89 **Other somatoform disorders** ◀▥
     Occupational neurosis, including writers' cramp
     Psychasthenia
     Psychasthenic neurosis

❏300.9 **Unspecified nonpsychotic mental disorder** ◀▥
     Psychoneurosis NOS

● **301 Personality disorders**

Includes: character neurosis

Use additional code to identify any associated neurosis or psychosis, or physical condition

Excludes *nonpsychotic personality disorder associated with organic brain syndromes (310.0–310.9)*

301.0 **Paranoid personality disorder**
     Fanatic personality
     Paranoid personality (disorder)
     Paranoid traits

Excludes *acute paranoid reaction (298.3)*
alcoholic paranoia (291.5)
paranoid schizophrenia (295.3)
paranoid states (297.0–297.9)

● **301.1 Affective personality disorder**

Excludes *affective psychotic disorders (296.0–296.9)*
neurasthenia (300.5)
neurotic depression (300.4)

301.10 **Affective personality disorder, unspecified**

ICD-9-CM

300-399

Vol. 1

301.11 Chronic hypomanic personality disorder
Chronic hypomanic disorder
Hypomanic personality

301.12 Chronic depressive personality disorder
Chronic depressive disorder
Depressive character or personality

301.13 Cyclothymic disorder
Cycloid personality
Cyclothymia
Cyclothymic personality

● 301.2 Schizoid personality disorder

Excludes schizophrenia (295.0–295.9)

❏ **301.20 Schizoid personality disorder, unspecified**

301.21 Introverted personality

301.22 Schizotypal personality disorder ◀▦

301.3 Explosive personality disorder
Aggressive:
  personality
  reaction
Aggressiveness
Emotional instability (excessive)
Pathological emotionality
Quarrelsomeness

Excludes dyssocial personality (301.7)
  hysterical neurosis (300.10–300.19)

301.4 Obsessive-compulsive personality disorder ◀▦
Anancastic personality
Obsessional personality

Excludes obsessive-compulsive disorder (300.3)
  phobic state (300.20–300.29)

● 301.5 Histrionic personality disorder

Excludes hysterical neurosis (300.10–300.19)

❏ **301.50 Histrionic personality disorder, unspecified**
Hysterical personality NOS

301.51 Chronic factitious illness with physical symptoms
Hospital addiction syndrome
Multiple operations syndrome
Munchausen syndrome

❏ **301.59 Other histrionic personality disorder**
Personality:
  emotionally unstable
  labile
  psychoinfantile

301.6 Dependent personality disorder
Asthenic personality
Inadequate personality
Passive personality

Excludes neurasthenia (300.5)
  passive-aggressive personality (301.84)

301.7 Antisocial personality disorder
Amoral personality
Asocial personality
Dyssocial personality
Personality disorder with predominantly sociopathic or asocial manifestation

Excludes disturbance of conduct without specifiable personality disorder (312.0–312.9)
  explosive personality (301.3)

● 301.8 Other personality disorders

301.81 Narcissistic personality disorder ◀▦

301.82 Avoidant personality disorder ◀▦

301.83 Borderline personality disorder ◀▦

301.84 Passive-aggressive personality

❏ **301.89 Other**
Personality:
  eccentric
  "haltlose" type
  immature
  masochistic
  psychoneurotic

Excludes psychoinfantile personality (301.59)

❏ **301.9 Unspecified personality disorder**
Pathological personality NOS
Personality disorder NOS
Psychopathic:
  constitutional state
  personality (disorder)

● 302 Sexual and gender identity disorders ◀▦

Excludes sexual disorder manifest in:
  organic brain syndrome (290.0–294.9, 310.0–310.9)
  psychosis (295.0–298.9)

302.0 Ego-dystonic sexual orientation ◀▦
Ego-dystonic lesbianism
Sexual orientation conflict disorder ◀▦

Excludes homosexual pedophilia (302.2)

302.1 Zoophilia
Bestiality

302.2 Pedophilia

302.3 Transvestic fetishism ◀▦

Excludes trans-sexualism (302.5)

302.4 Exhibitionism

● 302.5 Trans-sexualism

Excludes transvestism (302.3)

❏ **302.50 With unspecified sexual history**

302.51 With asexual history

302.52 With homosexual history

302.53 With heterosexual history

302.6 Gender identity disorder in children ◀▦
Feminism in boys
Gender identity disorder NOS ◀

Excludes gender identity disorder in adult (302.85)
  trans-sexualism (302.50–302.53)
  transvestism (302.3)

● 302.7 Psychosexual dysfunction

Excludes impotence of organic origin (607.84)
  normal transient symptoms from ruptured hymen
  transient or occasional failures of erection due to fatigue, anxiety, alcohol, or drugs

❏ **302.70 Psychosexual dysfunction, unspecified** ◀
Sexual dysfunction NOS

302.71 Hypoactive sexual desire disorder ◀▦

Excludes decreased sexual desire NOS (799.81)

302.72 With inhibited sexual excitement
Female sexual arousal disorder ◀
Male erectile disorder ◀

302.73 Female orgasmic disorder ◀▦

302.74 Male orgasmic disorder ◀▦

302.75 Premature ejaculation ◀▦

302.76 Dyspareunia, psychogenic ◀▦

❏ **302.79 With other specified psychosexual dysfunctions**
Sexual aversion disorder ◀

- **302.8 Other specified psychosexual disorders**

    302.81 Fetishism

    302.82 Voyeurism

    302.83 Sexual masochism

    302.84 Sexual sadism

    302.85 Gender identity disorder in adolescents or adults ◀▥

    Excludes *gender identity disorder NOS (302.6)* ◀
    gender identity disorder in children (302.6) ◀

    ❏ **302.89 Other**
    Frotteurism ◀
    Nymphomania
    Satyriasis

    ❏ **302.9 Unspecified psychosexual disorder**
    Paraphilia NOS ◀
    Pathologic sexuality NOS
    Sexual deviation NOS
    Sexual disorder NOS ◀

- **303 Alcohol dependence syndrome**

    Use additional code to identify any associated condition, as:
    alcoholic psychoses (291.0–291.9)
    drug dependence (304.0–304.9)
    physical complications of alcohol, such as:
    cerebral degeneration (331.7)
    cirrhosis of liver (571.2)
    epilepsy (345.0–345.9)
    gastritis (535.3)
    hepatitis (571.1)
    liver damage NOS (571.3)

    Excludes *drunkenness NOS (305.0)*

    The following fifth-digit subclassification is for use with category 303:
    ❏ **0 unspecified**
    1 continuous
    2 episodic
    3 in remission

- **303.0 Acute alcoholic intoxication**
    Acute drunkenness in alcoholism

- ❏ **303.9 Other and unspecified alcohol dependence**
    Chronic alcoholism
    Dipsomania

- **304 Drug dependence**
    Excludes *nondependent abuse of drugs (305.1–305.9)*

    The following fifth-digit subclassification is for use with category 304:
    ❏ **0 unspecified**
    1 continuous
    2 episodic
    3 in remission

- **304.0 Opioid type dependence**
    Heroin
    Meperidine
    Methadone
    Morphine
    Opium
    Opium alkaloids and their derivatives
    Synthetics with morphine-like effects

- **304.1 Sedative, hypnotic or anxiolytic dependence** ◀▥
    Barbiturates
    Nonbarbiturate sedatives and tranquilizers with a similar effect:
    chlordiazepoxide
    diazepam
    glutethimide
    meprobamate
    methaqualone

- **304.2 Cocaine dependence**
    Coca leaves and derivatives

- **304.3 Cannabis dependence**
    Hashish
    Hemp
    Marihuana

- **304.4 Amphetamine and other psychostimulant dependence**
    Methylphenidate
    Phenmetrazine

- **304.5 Hallucinogen dependence**
    Dimethyltryptamine [DMT]
    Lysergic acid diethylamide [LSD] and derivatives
    Mescaline
    Psilocybin

- ❏ **304.6 Other specified drug dependence**
    Absinthe addiction
    Glue sniffing
    Inhalant dependence ◀
    Phencyclidine dependence ◀

    Excludes *tobacco dependence (305.1)*

- **304.7 Combinations of opioid type drug with any other**

- **304.8 Combinations of drug dependence excluding opioid type drug**

- ❏ **304.9 Unspecified drug dependence**
    Drug addiction NOS
    Drug dependence NOS

- **305 Nondependent abuse of drugs**

    Note: Includes cases where a person, for whom no other diagnosis is possible, has come under medical care because of the maladaptive effect of a drug on which he is not dependent and that he has taken on his own initiative to the detriment of his health or social functioning.

    Excludes *alcohol dependence syndrome (303.0–303.9)*
    drug dependence (304.0–304.9)
    drug withdrawal syndrome (292.0)
    poisoning by drugs or medicinal substances (960.0–979.9)

    The following fifth-digit subclassification is for use with codes 305.0, 305.2–305.9:
    ❏ **0 unspecified**
    1 continuous
    2 episodic
    3 in remission

- **305.0 Alcohol abuse**
    Drunkenness NOS
    Excessive drinking of alcohol NOS
    "Hangover" (alcohol)
    Inebriety NOS

    Excludes *acute alcohol intoxication in alcoholism (303.0)*
    alcoholic psychoses (291.0–291.9)

    305.1 Tobacco use disorder
    Tobacco dependence

    Excludes *history of tobacco use (V15.82)*

- **305.2 Cannabis abuse**

- **305.3 Hallucinogen abuse**
    Acute intoxication from hallucinogens ["bad trips"]
    LSD reaction

- **305.4 Sedative, hypnotic or anxiolytic abuse** ◀▥

- **305.5 Opioid abuse**

- **305.6 Cocaine abuse**

- **305.7 Amphetamine or related acting sympathomimetic abuse**

ICD-9-CM
300-399
Vol. 1

● 305.8 **Antidepressant type abuse**

● ☐ 305.9 **Other, mixed, or unspecified drug abuse**
        Caffeine intoxication ◄
        Inhalant abuse ◄
        "Laxative habit"
        Phencyclidine abuse ◄
        Misuse of drugs NOS
        Nonprescribed use of drugs or patent medicinals

● 306 **Physiological malfunction arising from mental factors**

     Includes: psychogenic:
                physical symptoms not involving tissue damage
                physiological manifestations not involving tissue damage

     Excludes hysteria (300.11–300.19)
        physical symptoms secondary to a psychiatric disorder classified elsewhere
        psychic factors associated with physical conditions involving tissue damage classified elsewhere (316)
        specific nonpsychotic mental disorders following organic brain damage (310.0–310.9)

   306.0 **Musculoskeletal**
        Psychogenic paralysis
        Psychogenic torticollis

     Excludes Gilles de la Tourette's syndrome (307.23)
        paralysis as hysterical or conversion reaction (300.11)
        tics (307.20–307.22)

   306.1 **Respiratory**
        Psychogenic: Psychogenic:
        air hunger   hyperventilation
        cough   yawning
        hiccough

     Excludes psychogenic asthma (316 and 493.9)

   306.2 **Cardiovascular**
        Cardiac neurosis
        Cardiovascular neurosis
        Neurocirculatory asthenia
        Psychogenic cardiovascular disorder

     Excludes psychogenic paroxysmal tachycardia (316 and 427.2)

   306.3 **Skin**
        Psychogenic pruritus

     Excludes psychogenic:
        alopecia (316 and 704.00)
        dermatitis (316 and 692.9)
        eczema (316 and 691.8 or 692.9)
        urticaria (316 and 708.0–708.9)

   306.4 **Gastrointestinal**
        Aerophagy
        Cyclical vomiting, psychogenic
        Diarrhea, psychogenic
        Nervous gastritis
        Psychogenic dyspepsia

     Excludes cyclical vomiting NOS (536.2)
        globus hystericus (300.11)
        mucous colitis (316 and 564.9)
        psychogenic:
        cardiospasm (316 and 530.0)
        duodenal ulcer (316 and 532.0–532.9)
        gastric ulcer (316 and 531.0–531.9)
        peptic ulcer NOS (316 and 533.0–533.9)
        vomiting NOS (307.54)

● 306.5 **Genitourinary**

     Excludes enuresis, psychogenic (307.6)
        frigidity (302.72)
        impotence (302.72)
        psychogenic dyspareunia (302.76)

☐ 306.50 **Psychogenic genitourinary malfunction, unspecified**

   306.51 **Psychogenic vaginismus**
        Functional vaginismus

   306.52 **Psychogenic dysmenorrhea**

   306.53 **Psychogenic dysuria**

☐ 306.59 **Other**

   306.6 **Endocrine**

   306.7 **Organs of special sense**

     Excludes hysterical blindness or deafness (300.11)
        psychophysical visual disturbances (368.16)

☐ 306.8 **Other specified psychophysiological malfunction**
        Bruxism
        Teeth grinding

☐ 306.9 **Unspecified psychophysiological malfunction**
        Psychophysiologic disorder NOS
        Psychosomatic disorder NOS

● 307 **Special symptoms or syndromes, not elsewhere classified**

     Note: This category is intended for use if the psychopathology is manifested by a single specific symptom or group of symptoms which are not part of an organic illness or other mental disorder classifiable elsewhere.

     Excludes those due to mental disorders classified elsewhere
        those of organic origin

   307.0 **Stuttering** ◀━

     Excludes dysphasia (784.5)
        lisping or lalling (307.9)
        retarded development of speech (315.31–315.39)

   307.1 **Anorexia nervosa**

     Excludes eating disturbance NOS (307.50)
        feeding problem (783.3)
        of nonorganic origin (307.59)
        loss of appetite (783.0)
        of nonorganic origin (307.59)

● 307.2 **Tics**

     Excludes nail-biting or thumb-sucking (307.9)
        stereotypes occurring in isolation (307.3)
        tics of organic origin (333.3)

☐ 307.20 **Tic disorder, unspecified**
        Tic disorder NOS ◀

   307.21 **Transient tic disorder** ◀━

   307.22 **Chronic motor or vocal tic disorder** ◀━

   307.23 **Tourette's disorder** ◀━
        Motor-verbal tic disorder

   307.3 **Stereotypic movement disorder** ◀━
        Body-rocking
        Head banging
        Spasmus nutans
        Stereotypes NOS

     Excludes tics (307.20–307.23)
        of organic origin (333.3)

● 307.4 **Specific disorders of sleep of nonorganic origin**

     Excludes narcolepsy (347.00–347.11) ◀━
        those of unspecified cause (780.50–780.59)

☐ 307.40 **Nonorganic sleep disorder, unspecified**

   307.41 **Transient disorder of initiating or maintaining sleep**
        Hyposomnia associated with acute or intermittent emotional reactions or conflicts
        Insomnia associated with acute or intermittent emotional reactions or conflicts
        Sleeplessness associated with acute or intermittent emotional reactions or conflicts

307.42 Persistent disorder of initiating or maintaining sleep
Hyposomnia, insomnia, or sleeplessness associated with:
anxiety
conditioned arousal
depression (major) (minor)
psychosis

307.43 Transient disorder of initiating or maintaining wakefulness
Hypersomnia associated with acute or intermittent emotional reactions or conflicts

307.44 Persistent disorder of initiating or maintaining wakefulness
Hypersomnia associated with depression (major) (minor)

307.45 Circadian rhythm sleep disorder ◄
Irregular sleep-wake rhythm, nonorganic origin
Jet lag syndrome
Rapid time-zone change
Shifting sleep-work schedule

307.46 Sleep arousal disorder ◄
Night terror disorder ◄
Night terrors ◄
Sleep terror disorder ◄
Sleepwalking ◄
Somnambulism ◄

❑ **307.47 Other dysfunctions of sleep stages or arousal from sleep**
Dyssomnia NOS ◄
Nightmare disorder ◄
Nightmares:
NOS
REM-sleep type
Parasomnia NOS ◄
Sleep drunkenness

307.48 Repetitive intrusions of sleep
Repetitive intrusions of sleep with:
atypical polysomnographic features
environmental disturbances
repeated REM-sleep interruptions

❑ **307.49 Other**
"Short-sleeper"
Subjective insomnia complaint

● **307.5 Other and unspecified disorders of eating**
Excludes anorexia:
nervosa (307.1)
of unspecified cause (783.0)
overeating, of unspecified cause (783.6)
vomiting:
NOS (787.0)
cyclical (536.2)
psychogenic (306.4)

❑ **307.50 Eating disorder, unspecified**
Eating disorder NOS ◄

307.51 Bulimia nervosa ◄
Overeating of nonorganic origin

307.52 Pica
Perverted appetite of nonorganic origin

307.53 Rumination disorder ◄
Regurgitation, of nonorganic origin, of food with reswallowing

Excludes obsessional rumination (300.3)

307.54 Psychogenic vomiting

❑ **307.59 Other**
Feeding disorder of infancy or early childhood ◄
Infantile feeding disturbances of nonorganic origin
Loss of appetite of nonorganic origin

307.6 Enuresis
Enuresis (primary) (secondary) of nonorganic origin
Excludes enuresis of unspecified cause (788.3)

307.7 Encopresis
Encopresis (continuous) (discontinuous) of nonorganic origin
Excludes encopresis of unspecified cause (787.6)

● **307.8 Pain disorders related to psychological factors** ◄

❑ **307.80 Psychogenic pain, site unspecified**

307.81 Tension headache
Excludes headache:
NOS (784.0)
migraine (346.0–346.9)

❑ **307.89 Other**
Code first to site of pain ◄
Excludes pain disorder exclusively attributed to psychological factors (307.80) ◄
psychogenic pain (307.80) ◄

❑ **307.9 Other and unspecified special symptoms or syndromes, not elsewhere classified**
Communication disorder NOS ◄
Hair plucking
Lalling
Lisping
Masturbation
Nail-biting
Thumb-sucking

● **308 Acute reaction to stress**
Includes: catastrophic stress
combat fatigue
gross stress reaction (acute)
transient disorders in response to exceptional physical or mental stress which usually subside within hours or days
Excludes adjustment reaction or disorder (309.0–309.9)
chronic stress reaction (309.1–309.9)

308.0 Predominant disturbance of emotions
Anxiety as acute reaction to exceptional [gross] stress
Emotional crisis as acute reaction to exceptional [gross] stress
Panic state as acute reaction to exceptional [gross] stress

308.1 Predominant disturbance of consciousness
Fugues as acute reaction to exceptional [gross] stress

308.2 Predominant psychomotor disturbance
Agitation states as acute reaction to exceptional [gross] stress
Stupor as acute reaction to exceptional [gross] stress

❑ **308.3 Other acute reactions to stress**
Acute situational disturbance
Acute stress disorder ◄
Excludes prolonged posttraumatic emotional disturbance (309.81)

308.4 Mixed disorders as reaction to stress

❑ **308.9 Unspecified acute reaction to stress**

ICD-9-CM
300-399
Vol. 1

● 309 Adjustment reaction

Includes: adjustment disorders
    reaction (adjustment) to chronic stress

Excludes *acute reaction to major stress (308.0–308.9)*
        neurotic disorders (300.0–300.9)

309.0 Adjustment disorder with depressed mood ◀▦
    Grief reaction

Excludes *affective psychoses (296.0–296.9)*
        neurotic depression (300.4)
        prolonged depressive reaction (309.1)
        psychogenic depressive psychosis (298.0)

309.1 Prolonged depressive reaction

Excludes *affective psychoses (296.0–296.9)*
        brief depressive reaction (309.0)
        neurotic depression (300.4)
        psychogenic depressive psychosis (298.0)

● 309.2 With predominant disturbance of other emotions

    309.21 Separation anxiety disorder

    309.22 Emancipation disorder of adolescence and
            early adult life

    309.23 Specific academic or work inhibition

    309.24 Adjustment disorder with anxiety ◀▦

    309.28 Adjustment disorder with mixed anxiety
            and depressed mood ◀▦
            Adjustment reaction with anxiety and de-
            pression

    ☐ 309.29 Other
            Culture shock

309.3 Adjustment disorder with disturbance of con-
       duct ◀▦
    Conduct disturbance as adjustment reaction
    Destructiveness as adjustment reaction

Excludes *destructiveness in child (312.9)*
        disturbance of conduct NOS (312.9)
        dyssocial behavior without manifest psychiatric
        *   disorder (V71.01–V71.02)*
        personality disorder with predominantly socio-
        *   pathic or asocial manifestations (301.7)*

309.4 Adjustment disorder with mixed disturbance of
       emotions and conduct ◀▦

● 309.8 Other specified adjustment reactions

    309.81 Posttraumatic stress disorder ◀▦
            Chronic posttraumatic stress disorder
            Concentration camp syndrome
            Posttraumatic stress disorder NOS ◀

    Excludes *acute stress disorder (308.3)* ◀
            posttraumatic brain syndrome:
            *   nonpsychotic (310.2)*
            *   psychotic (293.0–293.9)*

    309.82 Adjustment reaction with physical symp-
            toms

    309.83 Adjustment reaction with withdrawal
            Elective mutism as adjustment reaction
            Hospitalism (in children) NOS

    ☐ 309.89 Other

☐ 309.9 Unspecified adjustment reaction
    Adaptation reaction NOS
    Adjustment reaction NOS

● 310 Specific nonpsychotic mental disorders due to brain
       damage ◀▦

    Excludes *neuroses, personality disorders, or other nonpsy-*
            chotic conditions occurring in a form simi-
            lar to that seen with functional disorders
            but in association with a physical condition
            (300.0–300.9, 301.0–301.9)

310.0 Frontal lobe syndrome
    Lobotomy syndrome
    Postleucotomy syndrome [state]

Excludes *postcontusion syndrome (310.2)*

310.1 Personality change due to conditions classified
       elsewhere ◀▦
    Cognitive or personality change of other type, of
        nonpsychotic severity
    Organic psychosyndrome of nonpsychotic severity
    Presbyophrenia NOS
    Senility with mental changes of nonpsychotic se-
        verity

Excludes *memory loss of unknown cause (780.93)*

310.2 Postconcussion syndrome
    Postcontusion syndrome or encephalopathy
    Posttraumatic brain syndrome, nonpsychotic
    Status postcommotio cerebri

Excludes *any organic psychotic conditions following head*
        *   injury (293.0–294.0)*
        frontal lobe syndrome (310.0)
        postencephalitic syndrome (310.8)

☐ 310.8 Other specified nonpsychotic mental disorders fol-
         lowing organic brain damage
    Mild memory disturbance ◀
    Postencephalitic syndrome
    Other focal (partial) organic psychosyndromes

☐ 310.9 Unspecified nonpsychotic mental disorder follow-
         ing organic brain damage

311 Depressive disorder, not elsewhere classified
    Depressive disorder NOS   Depression NOS
    Depressive state NOS

Excludes *acute reaction to major stress with depressive*
        *   symptoms (308.0)*
        affective personality disorder (301.10–301.13)
        affective psychoses (296.0–296.9)
        brief depressive reaction (309.0)
        depressive states associated with stressful events
        *   (309.0–309.1)*
        disturbance of emotions specific to childhood and
        *   adolescence, with misery and unhappiness*
        *   (313.1)*
        mixed adjustment reaction with depressive symp-
        *   toms (309.4)*
        neurotic depression (300.4)
        prolonged depressive adjustment reaction (309.1)
        psychogenic depressive psychosis (298.0)

● 312 Disturbance of conduct, not elsewhere classified

    Excludes *adjustment reaction with disturbance of conduct*
            *   (309.3)*
            drug dependence (304.0–304.9)
            dyssocial behavior without manifest psychiatric
            *   disorder (V71.01–V71.02)*
            personality disorder with predominantly socio-
            *   pathic or asocial manifestations (301.7)*
            sexual deviations (302.0–302.9)

The following fifth-digit subclassification is for use with
categories 312.0–312.2:
☐ 0 unspecified
   1 mild
   2 moderate
   3 severe

● 312.0 Undersocialized conduct disorder, aggressive type
    Aggressive outburst
    Anger reaction
    Unsocialized aggressive disorder

● **312.1 Undersocialized conduct disorder, unaggressive type**
Childhood truancy, unsocialized
Solitary stealing
Tantrums

● **312.2 Socialized conduct disorder**
Childhood truancy, socialized
Group delinquency

Excludes   *gang activity without manifest psychiatric disor-der (V71.01)*

● **312.3 Disorders of impulse control, not elsewhere classified**

❏ **312.30 Impulse control disorder, unspecified**

312.31 Pathological gambling

312.32 Kleptomania

312.33 Pyromania

312.34 Intermittent explosive disorder

312.35 Isolated explosive disorder

❏ **312.39 Other**
Trichotillomania   ◀

312.4 Mixed disturbance of conduct and emotions
Neurotic delinquency

Excludes   *compulsive conduct disorder (312.3)*

● **312.8 Other specified disturbances of conduct, not else-where classified**

312.81 Conduct disorder, childhood onset type

312.82 Conduct disorder, adolescent onset type

❏ **312.89 Other conduct disorder**
Conduct disorder of unspecified onset   ◀

❏ **312.9 Unspecified disturbance of conduct**
Delinquency (juvenile)
Disruptive behavior disorder NOS   ◀

● **313 Disturbance of emotions specific to childhood and ado-lescence**

Excludes   *adjustment reaction (309.0–309.9)*
emotional disorder of neurotic type (300.0–300.9)
masturbation, nail-biting, thumb-sucking, and other isolated symptoms (307.0–307.9)

313.0 Overanxious disorder
Anxiety and fearfulness of childhood and adoles-cence
Overanxious disorder of childhood and adoles-cence

Excludes   *abnormal separation anxiety (309.21)*
anxiety states (300.00–300.09)
hospitalism in children (309.83)
phobic state (300.20–300.29)

313.1 Misery and unhappiness disorder

Excludes   *depressive neurosis (300.4)*

● **313.2 Sensitivity, shyness, and social withdrawal disor-der**

Excludes   *infantile autism (299.0)*
schizoid personality (301.20–301.22)
schizophrenia (295.0–295.9)

313.21 Shyness disorder of childhood
Sensitivity reaction of childhood or adoles-cence

313.22 Introverted disorder of childhood
Social withdrawal of childhood or adoles-cence
Withdrawal reaction of childhood or ado-lescence

313.23 Selective mutism   ◀▥

Excludes   *elective mutism as adjustment reaction (309.83)*

313.3 Relationship problems
Sibling jealousy

Excludes   *relationship problems associated with aggression, destruction, or other forms of conduct dis-turbance (312.0–312.9)*

● **313.8 Other or mixed emotional disturbances of child-hood or adolescence**

313.81 Oppositional defiant disorder   ◀▥

313.82 Identity disorder
Identity problem   ◀

313.83 Academic underachievement disorder

❏ **313.89 Other**
Reactive attachment disorder of infancy or early childhood   ◀

❏ **313.9 Unspecified emotional disturbance of childhood or adolescence**   ◀▥
Mental disorder of infancy, childhood or adoles-cence NOS   ◀

● **314 Hyperkinetic syndrome of childhood**

Excludes   *hyperkinesis as symptom of underlying disorder-code the underlying disorder*

● **314.0 Attention deficit disorder**
Adult
Child

314.00 Without mention of hyperactivity
Predominantly inattentive type

314.01 With hyperactivity
Combined type
Overactivity NOS
Predominantly hyperactive/impulsive type
Simple disturbance of attention with over-activity

314.1 Hyperkinesis with developmental delay
Developmental disorder of hyperkinesis

Use additional code to identify any associated neu-rological disorder

314.2 Hyperkinetic conduct disorder
Hyperkinetic conduct disorder without develop-mental delay

Excludes   *hyperkinesis with significant delays in specific skills (314.1)*

❏ **314.8 Other specified manifestations of hyperkinetic syn-drome**

❏ **314.9 Unspecified hyperkinetic syndrome**
Hyperkinetic reaction of childhood or adolescence NOS
Hyperkinetic syndrome NOS

● **315 Specific delays in development**

Excludes   *that due to a neurological disorder (320.0–389.9)*

● **315.0 Specific reading disorder**

❏ **315.00 Reading disorder, unspecified**

315.01 Alexia

315.02 Developmental dyslexia

❏ **315.09 Other**
Specific spelling difficulty

315.1 Mathematics disorder   ◀▥
Dyscalculia

ICD-9-CM

300-399

Vol. 1

❑ 315.2 **Other specific learning difficulties**
Disorder of written expression   ◀

    | **Excludes** | *specific arithmetical disorder (315.1)* |
    | | *specific reading disorder (315.00–315.09)* |

● 315.3 **Developmental speech or language disorder**

    315.31 **Expressive language disorder**   ◀▦
        Developmental aphasia
        Word deafness

    | **Excludes** | *acquired aphasia (784.3)* |
    | | *elective mutism (309.83, 313.0, 313.23)* |

    315.32 **Mixed receptive-expressive language disorder**   ◀▦

    ❑ 315.39 **Other**
        Developmental articulation disorder
        Dyslalia
        Phonological disorder   ◀

    | **Excludes** | *lisping and lalling (307.9)* |
    | | *stammering and stuttering (307.0)* |

315.4 **Developmental coordination disorder**   ◀▦
    Clumsiness syndrome
    Dyspraxia syndrome
    Specific motor development disorder

315.5 **Mixed development disorder**

❑ 315.8 **Other specified delays in development**

❑ 315.9 **Unspecified delay in development**
    Developmental disorder NOS
    Learning disorder NOS   ◀

316 **Psychic factors associated with diseases classified elsewhere**
    Psychologic factors in physical conditions classified elsewhere

Use additional code to identify the associated physical condition, as:
    psychogenic:
        asthma (493.9)
        dermatitis (692.9)
        duodenal ulcer (532.0–532.9)
        eczema (691.8, 692.9)
        gastric ulcer (531.0–531.9)
        mucous colitis (564.9)
        paroxysmal tachycardia (427.2)
        ulcerative colitis (556)
        urticaria (708.0–708.9)
    psychosocial dwarfism (259.4)

    | **Excludes** | *physical symptoms and physiological malfunctions, not involving tissue damage, of mental origin (306.0–306.9)* |

MENTAL RETARDATION (317–319)

Use additional code (s) to identify any associated psychiatric or physical condition(s)

317 **Mild mental retardation**
    High-grade defect
    IQ 50–70
    Mild mental subnormality

● 318 **Other specified mental retardation**

    318.0 **Moderate mental retardation**
        IQ 35–49
        Moderate mental subnormality

    318.1 **Severe mental retardation**
        IQ 20–34
        Severe mental subnormality

    318.2 **Profound mental retardation**
        IQ under 20
        Profound mental subnormality

❑ 319 **Unspecified mental retardation**
    Mental deficiency NOS
    Mental subnormality NOS

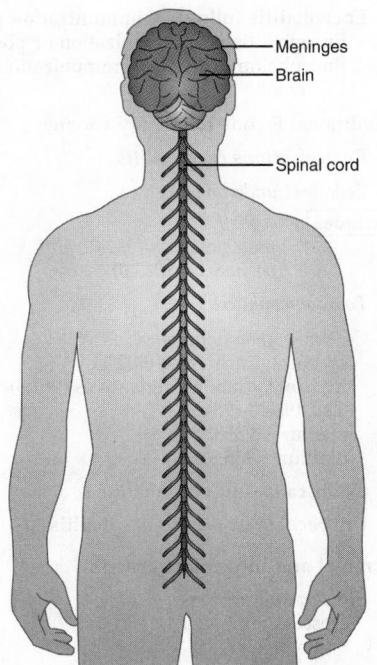

Figure 6-1   The brain and spinal cord make up the central nervous system.

Item 6-1   The two major classifications of the nervous system are the peripheral nervous system and the central nervous system (CNS). The central nervous system contains the brain and the spinal cord. **Encephalitis** is the swelling of the brain. **Meningitis** is swelling of the covering of the brain, the meninges. Types and causes of brain infections are:

Type	Cause
purulent	bacterial
aseptic/abacterial	viral
chronic meningitis	mycobacterial and fungal

6.   DISEASES OF THE NERVOUS SYSTEM AND SENSE ORGANS (320–389)

INFLAMMATORY DISEASES OF THE CENTRAL NERVOUS SYSTEM (320–326)

● **320   Bacterial meningitis**

Includes: arachnoiditis bacterial
leptomeningitis bacterial
meningitis bacterial
meningoencephalitis bacterial
meningomyelitis bacterial
pachymeningitis bacterial

320.0   Haemophilus meningitis
Meningitis due to Haemophilus influenzae [H. influenzae]

320.1   Pneumococcal meningitis

320.2   Streptococcal meningitis

320.3   Staphylococcal meningitis

● **320.7   Meningitis in other bacterial diseases classified elsewhere**

Code first underlying disease as:
actinomycosis (039.8)
listeriosis (027.0)
typhoid fever (002.0)
whooping cough (033.0–033.9)

Excludes   *meningitis (in):*
epidemic (036.0)
gonococcal (098.82)
meningococcal (036.0)
salmonellosis (003.21)
syphilis:
NOS (094.2)
congenital (090.42)
meningovascular (094.2)
secondary (091.81)
tuberculosis (013.0)

● **320.8   Meningitis due to other specified bacteria**

320.81   Anaerobic meningitis
Bacteroides (fragilis)
Gram-negative anaerobes

320.82   Meningitis due to gram-negative bacteria, not elsewhere classified
Aerobacter aerogenes
Escherichia coli [E. coli]
Friedlander bacillus
Klebsiella pneumoniae
Proteus morganii
Pseudomonas

Excludes   *gram-negative anaerobes (320.81)*

❑ **320.89   Meningitis due to other specified bacteria**
Bacillus pyocyaneus

❑ **320.9   Meningitis due to unspecified bacterium**
Meningitis:

bacterial NOS	pyogenic NOS
purulent NOS	suppurative NOS

● **321   Meningitis due to other organisms**

Includes: arachnoiditis due to organisms other than bacteria
leptomeningitis due to organisms other than bacteria
meningitis due to organisms other than bacteria
pachymeningitis due to organisms other than bacteria

● **321.0   Cryptococcal meningitis**

Code first underlying disease (117.5)

●❑ **321.1   Meningitis in other fungal diseases**

Code first underlying disease (110.0–118)

Excludes   *meningitis in:*
candidiasis (112.83)
coccidioidomycosis (114.2)
histoplasmosis (115.01, 115.11, 115.91)

● **321.2   Meningitis due to viruses not elsewhere classified**

Code first underlying disease, as:
meningitis due to arbovirus (060.0–066.9)

Excludes   *meningitis (due to):*
abacterial (047.0–047.9)
adenovirus (049.1)
aseptic NOS (047.9)
Coxsackie (virus) (047.0)
ECHO virus (047.1)
enterovirus (047.0–047.9)
herpes simplex virus (054.72)
herpes zoster virus (053.0)
lymphocytic choriomeningitis virus (049.0)
mumps (072.1)
viral NOS (047.9)
meningo-eruptive syndrome (047.1)

ICD-9-CM

300-399

Vol. 1

● *321.3* *Meningitis due to trypanosomiasis*

     Code first underlying disease (086.0–086.9)

● *321.4* *Meningitis in sarcoidosis*

     Code first underlying disease (135)

●❑ *321.8* *Meningitis due to other nonbacterial organisms classified elsewhere*

     Code first underlying disease

     Excludes *leptospiral meningitis (100.81)*

● **322** **Meningitis of unspecified cause**

     Includes: arachnoiditis with no organism specified as cause

               leptomeningitis with no organism specified as cause

               meningitis with no organism specified as cause

               pachymeningitis with no organism specified as cause

     322.0 **Nonpyogenic meningitis**

          Meningitis with clear cerebrospinal fluid

     322.1 **Eosinophilic meningitis**

     322.2 **Chronic meningitis**

     ❑ **322.9** **Meningitis, unspecified**

● **323** **Encephalitis, myelitis, and encephalomyelitis**

     Includes: acute disseminated encephalomyelitis

               meningoencephalitis, except bacterial

               meningomyelitis, except bacterial

               myelitis (acute):

                  ascending

                  transverse

     Excludes *bacterial:*

            meningoencephalitis (320.0–320.9)

            meningomyelitis (320.0–320.9)

  ● *323.0* *Encephalitis in viral diseases classified elsewhere*

       Code first underlying disease, as:

          cat-scratch disease (078.3)

          infectious mononucleosis (075)

          ornithosis (073.7)

       Excludes *encephalitis (in):*

            arthropod-borne viral (062.0–064)

            herpes simplex (054.3)

            mumps (072.2)

            poliomyelitis (045.0–045.9)

            rubella (056.01)

            slow virus infections of central nervous system (046.0–046.9)

            other viral diseases of central nervous system (049.8–049.9)

            viral NOS (049.9)

  ● *323.1* *Encephalitis in rickettsial diseases classified elsewhere*

       Code first underlying disease (080–083.9)

  ● *323.2* *Encephalitis in protozoal diseases classified elsewhere*

       Code first underlying disease, as:

          malaria (084.0–084.9)

          trypanosomiasis (086.0–086.9)

  ●❑ *323.4* *Other encephalitis due to infection classified elsewhere*

       Code first underlying disease

       Excludes *encephalitis (in):*

            meningococcal (036.1)

            syphilis:

               NOS (094.81)

               congenital (090.41)

            toxoplasmosis (130.0)

            tuberculosis (013.6)

          meningoencephalitis due to free-living ameba [Naegleria] (136.2)

● *323.5* **Encephalitis following immunization procedures**

     Encephalitis postimmunization or postvaccinal

     Encephalomyelitis postimmunization or postvaccinal

Use additional E code to identify vaccine

● *323.6* *Postinfectious encephalitis*

     Code first underlying disease

     Excludes *encephalitis:*

          postchickenpox (052.0)

          postmeasles (055.0)

● *323.7* *Toxic encephalitis*

     Code first underlying cause, as:

        carbon tetrachloride (982.1)

        hydroxyquinoline derivatives (961.3)

        lead (984.0–984.9)

        mercury (985.0)

        thallium (985.8)

❑ **323.8** **Other causes of encephalitis**

❑ **323.9** **Unspecified cause of encephalitis**

● **324** **Intracranial and intraspinal abscess**

     324.0 **Intracranial abscess**

          Abscess (embolic):

            cerebellar

            cerebral

          Abscess (embolic) of brain [any part]:

            epidural

            extradural

            otogenic

            subdural

       Excludes *tuberculous (013.3)*

     324.1 **Intraspinal abscess**

          Abscess (embolic) of spinal cord [any part]:

            epidural

            extradural

            subdural

       Excludes *tuberculous (013.5)*

     ❑ **324.9** **Of unspecified site**

          Extradural or subdural abscess NOS

325 **Phlebitis and thrombophlebitis of intracranial venous sinuses**

     Embolism of cavernous, lateral, or other intracranial or unspecified intracranial venous sinus

     Endophlebitis of cavernous, lateral, or other intracranial or unspecified intracranial venous sinus

     Phlebitis, septic or suppurative of cavernous, lateral, or other intracranial or unspecified intracranial venous sinus

     Thrombophlebitis of cavernous, lateral, or other intracranial or unspecified intracranial venous sinus

     Thrombosis of cavernous, lateral, or other intracranial or unspecified intracranial venous sinus

     Excludes *that specified as:*

          complicating pregnancy, childbirth, or the puerperium (671.5)

          of nonpyogenic origin (437.6)

❑ **326** **Late effects of intracranial abscess or pyogenic infection**

     Note: This category is to be used to indicate conditions whose primary classification is to 320–325 [excluding 320.7, 321.0–321.8, 323.0–323.4, 323.6–323.7] as the cause of late effects, themselves classifiable elsewhere. The "late effects" include conditions specified as such, or as sequelae, which may occur at any time after the resolution of the causal condition.

Use additional code to identify condition, as:

     hydrocephalus (331.4)

     paralysis (342.0–342.9, 344.0–344.9)

Item 6-2   Leukodystrophy is characterized by degeneration and/or failure of the myelin formation of the central nervous system and sometimes of the peripheral nervous system. The disease is inherited and progressive.

HEREDITARY AND DEGENERATIVE DISEASES OF THE CENTRAL NERVOUS SYSTEM (330–337)

> **Excludes**   *hepatolenticular degeneration (275.1)*
> *multiple sclerosis (340)*
> *other demyelinating diseases of central nervous system (341.0–341.9)*

● **330   Cerebral degenerations usually manifest in childhood**

Use additional code to identify associated mental retardation

330.0   Leukodystrophy
Krabbe's disease
Leukodystrophy:
   NOS
   globoid cell
   metachromatic
   sudanophilic
Pelizaeus-Merzbacher disease
Sulfatide lipidosis

330.1   Cerebral lipidoses
Amaurotic (familial) idiocy
Disease:
   Batten
   Jansky-Bielschowsky
   Kufs'
   Spielmeyer-Vogt
   Tay-Sachs
Gangliosidosis

● *330.2   Cerebral degeneration in generalized lipidoses*

Code first underlying disease, as:
   Fabry's disease (272.7)
   Gaucher's disease (272.7)
   Niemann-Pick disease (272.7)
   sphingolipidosis (272.7)

●❑ *330.3   Cerebral degeneration of childhood in other diseases classified elsewhere*

Code first underlying disease, as:
   Hunter's disease (277.5)
   mucopolysaccharidosis (277.5)

❑ **330.8   Other specified cerebral degenerations in childhood**
Alpers' disease or gray-matter degeneration
Infantile necrotizing encephalomyelopathy
Leigh's disease
Subacute necrotizing encephalopathy or encephalomyelopathy

❑ **330.9   Unspecified cerebral degeneration in childhood**

Item 6-3   Pick's disease is the atrophy of the frontal and temporal lobes, causing dementia; **Alzheimer's** is characterized by a more diffuse cerebral atrophy.

● **331   Other cerebral degenerations**

331.0   Alzheimer's disease

● **331.1   Frontotemporal dementia**
Use additional code for associated behavioral disturbance (294.10–294.11)

331.11   Pick's disease

331.19   Other frontotemporal dementia
Frontal dementia

331.2   Senile degeneration of brain
> **Excludes**   *senility NOS (797)*

331.3   Communicating hydrocephalus
> **Excludes**   *congenital hydrocephalus (741.0, 742.3)*

331.4   Obstructive hydrocephalus
Acquired hydrocephalus NOS
> **Excludes**   *congenital hydrocephalus (741.0, 742.3)*

● *331.7   Cerebral degeneration in diseases classified elsewhere*

Code first underlying disease, as:
   alcoholism (303.0–303.9)
   beriberi (265.0)
   cerebrovascular disease (430–438)
   congenital hydrocephalus (741.0, 742.3)
   neoplastic disease (140.0–239.9)
   myxedema (244.0–244.9)
   vitamin B_{12} deficiency (266.2)

> **Excludes**   *cerebral degeneration in:*
> *Jakob-Creutzfeldt disease (046.1)*
> *progressive multifocal leukoencephalopathy (046.3)*
> *subacute spongiform encephalopathy (046.1)*

● **331.8   Other cerebral degeneration**

331.81   Reye's syndrome

331.82   Dementia with Lewy bodies
Dementia with Parkinsonism
Lewy body dementia
Lewy body disease

Use additional code for associated behavioral disturbance (294.10–294.11)

❑ **331.89   Other**
Cerebral ataxia

❑ **331.9   Cerebral degeneration, unspecified**

● **332   Parkinson's disease**
> **Excludes**   *dementia with Parkinsonism (331.82)*

332.0   Paralysis agitans
Parkinsonism or Parkinson's disease:
   NOS
   idiopathic
   primary

332.1   Secondary Parkinsonism
Parkinsonism due to drugs

Use additional E code to identify drug, if drug-induced

> **Excludes**   *Parkinsonism (in):*
> *Huntington's disease (333.4)*
> *progressive supranuclear palsy (333.0)*
> *Shy-Drager syndrome (333.0)*
> *syphilitic (094.82)*

● **333   Other extrapyramidal disease and abnormal movement disorders**

Includes: other forms of extrapyramidal, basal ganglia, or striatopallidal disease

> **Excludes**   *abnormal movements of head NOS (781.0)*

❑ **333.0   Other degenerative diseases of the basal ganglia**
Atrophy or degeneration:
   olivopontocerebellar [Déjérine-Thomas syndrome]
   pigmentary pallidal [Hallervorden-Spatz disease] striatonigral
Parkinsonian syndrome associated with:
   idiopathic orthostatic hypotension
   symptomatic orthostatic hypotension
Progressive supranuclear ophthalmoplegia
Shy-Drager syndrome

❑ **333.1   Essential and other specified forms of tremor**
Benign essential tremor
Familial tremor

Use additional E code to identify drug, if drug-induced

> **Excludes**   *tremor NOS (781.0)*

ICD-9-CM

300-
Vol.

333.2 Myoclonus
　　Familial essential myoclonus
　　Progressive myoclonic epilepsy
　　Unverricht-Lundborg disease

　　Use additional E code to identify drug, if drug-induced

333.3 Tics of organic origin

　　Excludes | *Gilles de la Tourette's syndrome (307.23)*
　　　　　　　habit spasm (307.22)
　　　　　　　tic NOS (307.20)

　　Use additional E code to identify drug, if drug-induced

Item 6-4 Huntington's disease is characterized by ceaseless, jerky movements and progressive cognitive and behavioral deterioration.

333.4 Huntington's chorea

☐ **333.5 Other choreas**
　　Hemiballism(us)
　　Paroxysmal choreo-athetosis

　　Excludes | *Sydenham's or rheumatic chorea (392.0–392.9)*

　　Use additional E code to identify drug, if drug-induced

333.6 Idiopathic torsion dystonia
　　Dystonia:
　　　deformans progressiva
　　　musculorum deformans
　　(Schwalbe-) Ziehen-Oppenheim disease

333.7 Symptomatic torsion dystonia
　　Athetoid cerebral palsy [Vogt's disease]
　　Double athetosis (syndrome)

　　Use additional E code to identify drug, if drug-induced

● **333.8 Fragments of torsion dystonia**

　　Use additional E code to identify drug, if drug-induced

　　333.81 Blepharospasm

　　333.82 Orofacial dyskinesia

　　333.83 Spasmodic torticollis
　　Excludes | *torticollis:*
　　　　　　　NOS (723.5)
　　　　　　　hysterical (300.11)
　　　　　　　psychogenic (306.0)

　　333.84 Organic writers' cramp
　　Excludes | *psychogenic (300.89)*

　　☐ **333.89 Other**

● **333.9 Other and unspecified extrapyramidal diseases and abnormal movement disorders**

　　☐ **333.90 Unspecified extrapyramidal disease and abnormal movement disorder**

　　333.91 Stiff-man syndrome

　　333.92 Neuroleptic malignant syndrome

　　　Use additional E to identify drug

　　333.93 Benign shuddering attacks

　　☐ **333.99 Other**
　　　Restless legs

● **334 Spinocerebellar disease**
　　Excludes | *olivopontocerebellar degeneration (333.0)*
　　　　　　　peroneal muscular atrophy (356.1)

334.0 Friedreich's ataxia

334.1 Hereditary spastic paraplegia

334.2 Primary cerebellar degeneration
　　Cerebellar ataxia:
　　　Marie's
　　　Sanger-Brown
　　Dyssynergia cerebellaris myoclonica
　　Primary cerebellar degeneration:
　　　NOS
　　　hereditary
　　　sporadic

☐ **334.3 Other cerebellar ataxia**
　　Cerebellar ataxia NOS

　　Use additional E code to identify drug, if drug-induced

● **334.4 Cerebellar ataxia in diseases classified elsewhere**

　　Code first underlying disease, as:
　　　alcoholism (303.0–303.9)
　　　myxedema (244.0–244.9)
　　　neoplastic disease (140.0–239.9)

☐ **334.8 Other spinocerebellar diseases**
　　Ataxia-telangiectasia [Louis-Bar syndrome]
　　Corticostriatal-spinal degeneration

☐ **334.9 Spinocerebellar disease, unspecified**

● **335 Anterior horn cell disease**

　　335.0 Werdnig-Hoffmann disease
　　　Infantile spinal muscular atrophy
　　　Progressive muscular atrophy of infancy

● **335.1 Spinal muscular atrophy**

　　☐ **335.10 Spinal muscular atrophy, unspecified**

　　335.11 Kugelberg-Welander disease
　　　Spinal muscular atrophy:
　　　　familial
　　　　juvenile

　　☐ **335.19 Other**
　　　Adult spinal muscular atrophy

● **335.2 Motor neuron disease**

　　335.20 Amyotrophic lateral sclerosis
　　　Motor neuron disease (bulbar) (mixed type)

　　335.21 Progressive muscular atrophy
　　　Duchenne-Aran muscular atrophy
　　　Progressive muscular atrophy (pure)

　　335.22 Progressive bulbar palsy

　　335.23 Pseudobulbar palsy

　　335.24 Primary lateral sclerosis

　　☐ **335.29 Other**

☐ **335.8 Other anterior horn cell diseases**

☐ **335.9 Anterior horn cell disease, unspecified**

● **336 Other diseases of spinal cord**

　　336.0 Syringomyelia and syringobulbia

　　336.1 Vascular myelopathies
　　　Acute infarction of spinal cord (embolic) (nonembolic)
　　　Arterial thrombosis of spinal cord
　　　Edema of spinal cord
　　　Hematomyelia
　　　Subacute necrotic myelopathy

● **336.2 Subacute combined degeneration of spinal cord in diseases classified elsewhere**

　　Code first underlying disease, as:
　　　pernicious anemia (281.0)
　　　other vitamin B_{12} deficiency anemia (281.1)
　　　vitamin B_{12} deficiency (266.2)

● **336.3** *Myelopathy in other diseases classified elsewhere*

    Code first underlying disease, as:
        myelopathy in neoplastic disease (140.0–239.9)

    Excludes   *myelopathy in:*
        intervertebral disc disorder (722.70–722.73)
        spondylosis (721.1, 721.41–721.42, 721.91)

❑ **336.8   Other myelopathy**
    Myelopathy:
        drug-induced   radiation-induced

    Use additional E code to identify cause

❑ **336.9   Unspecified disease of spinal cord**
    Cord compression NOS
    Myelopathy NOS

    Excludes   *myelitis (323.0–323.9)*
        spinal (canal) stenosis (723.0, 724.00–724.09)

● **337   Disorders of the autonomic nervous system**

    Includes: disorders of peripheral autonomic, sympathetic, parasympathetic, or vegetative system

    Excludes   *familial dysautonomia [Riley-Day syndrome] (742.8)*

    337.0   Idiopathic peripheral autonomic neuropathy
        Carotid sinus syncope or syndrome
        Cervical sympathetic dystrophy or paralysis

● **337.1   *Peripheral autonomic neuropathy in disorders classified elsewhere***

    Code first underlying disease, as:
        amyloidosis (277.3)
        diabetes (250.6)

● **337.2   Reflex sympathetic dystrophy**

    ❑ **337.20   Reflex sympathetic dystrophy, unspecified**

    337.21   Reflex sympathetic dystrophy of the upper limb

    337.22   Reflex sympathetic dystrophy of the lower limb

    ❑ **337.29   Reflex sympathetic dystrophy of other specified site**

    337.3   Autonomic dysreflexia

    Use additional code to identify the cause, such as:
        decubitus ulcer (707.00–707.09)   ◀▥
        fecal impaction (560.39)
        urinary tract infection (599.0)

❑ **337.9   Unspecified disorder of autonomic nervous system**

OTHER DISORDERS OF THE CENTRAL NERVOUS SYSTEM (340–349)

340   Multiple sclerosis
    Disseminated or multiple sclerosis:
        NOS   cord
        brain stem   generalized

● **341   Other demyelinating diseases of central nervous system**

    341.0   Neuromyelitis optica

    341.1   Schilder's disease
        Balo's concentric sclerosis
        Encephalitis periaxialis:
            concentrica [Balo's]
            diffusa [Schilder's]

    ❑ **341.8   Other demyelinating diseases of central nervous system**
        Central demyelination of corpus callosum
        Central pontine myelinosis
        Marchiafava (-Bignami) disease

    ❑ **341.9   Demyelinating disease of central nervous system, unspecified**

● **342   Hemiplegia and hemiparesis**

    Note: This category is to be used when hemiplegia (complete) (incomplete) is reported without further specification, or is stated to be old or long-standing but of unspecified cause. The category is also for use in multiple coding to identify these types of hemiplegia resulting from any cause.

    Excludes   *congenital (343.1)*
        hemiplegia due to late effect of cerebrovascular accident (438.20–438.22)
        infantile NOS (343.4)

    The following fifth digits are for use with codes 342.0–342.9
    ❑ **0   affecting unspecified side**
      1   affecting dominant side
      2   affecting nondominant side

● **342.0   Flaccid hemiplegia**

● **342.1   Spastic hemiplegia**

● ❑ **342.8   Other specified hemiplegia**

● ❑ **342.9   Hemiplegia, unspecified**

● **343   Infantile cerebral palsy**

    Includes: cerebral:
        palsy NOS
        spastic infantile paralysis
        congenital spastic paralysis (cerebral)
        Little's disease
        paralysis (spastic) due to birth injury:
            intracranial
            spinal

    Excludes   *hereditary cerebral paralysis, such as:*
        hereditary spastic paraplegia (334.1)
        Vogt's disease (333.7)
        spastic paralysis specified as noncongenital or noninfantile (344.0–344.9)

    343.0   Diplegic
        Congenital diplegia
        Congenital paraplegia

    343.1   Hemiplegic
        Congenital hemiplegia

    Excludes   *infantile hemiplegia NOS (343.4)*

    343.2   Quadriplegic
        Tetraplegic

    343.3   Monoplegic

    343.4   Infantile hemiplegia
        Infantile hemiplegia (postnatal) NOS

    ❑ **343.8   Other specified infantile cerebral palsy**

    ❑ **343.9   Infantile cerebral palsy, unspecified**
        Cerebral palsy NOS

ICD-9-CM

300-
3??

Vol. 1

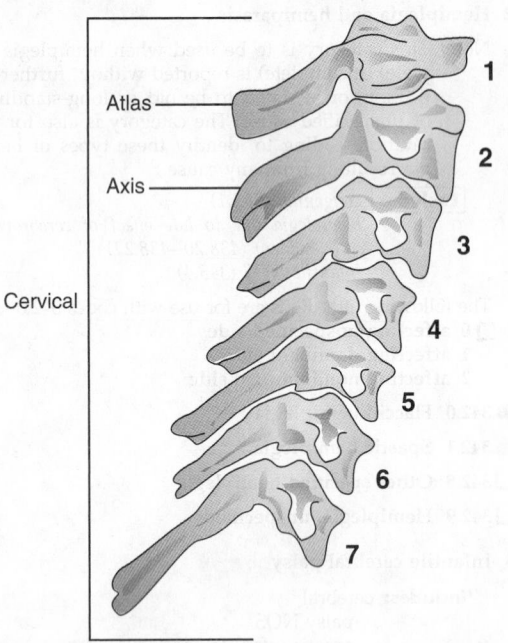

Figure 6-2 Cervical vertebrae.

Item 6-5 Quadriplegia, also called tetraplegia, is the paralysis of all four limbs. **Quadriparesis** is the incomplete paralysis of all four limbs. Nerve damage in C1–C4 is associated with lower limb paralysis and C5–C7 damage is associated with upper limb paralysis. **Diplegia** is the paralysis of the upper limbs. **Monoplegia** is the paralysis of the lower limbs.
Cauda equina syndrome is due to pressure on the roots of the spinal nerves and causes paresthesia (abnormal sensations).

● 344   **Other paralytic syndromes**

   Note: This category is to be used when the listed conditions are reported without further specification or are stated to be old or long-standing but of unspecified cause. The category is also for use in multiple coding to identify these conditions resulting from any cause.

   Includes: paralysis (complete) (incomplete), except as classifiable to 342 and 343

   Excludes   *congenital or infantile cerebral palsy (343.0–343.9)*
   hemiplegia (342.0–342.9)
   congenital or infantile (343.1, 343.4)

● 344.0   **Quadriplegia and quadriparesis**

   ❏ 344.00   **Quadriplegia, unspecified**

   344.01 C_1-C_4, complete

   344.02 C_1-C_4, incomplete

   344.03 C_5-C_7, complete

   344.04 C_5-C_7, incomplete

   ❏ 344.09   **Other**

   344.1   **Paraplegia**
   Paralysis of both lower limbs
   Paraplegia (lower)

   344.2   **Diplegia of upper limbs**
   Diplegia (upper)
   Paralysis of both upper limbs

● 344.3   **Monoplegia of lower limb**
   Paralysis of lower limb

   Excludes   *Monoplegia of lower limb due to late effect of cerebrovascular accident (438.40–438.42)*

   ❏ 344.30   **Affecting unspecified side**

   344.31   **Affecting dominant side**

   344.32   **Affecting nondominant side**

● 344.4   **Monoplegia of upper limb**
   Paralysis of upper limb

   Excludes   *monoplegia of upper limb due to late effect of cerebrovascular accident (438.30–438.32)*

   ❏ 344.40   **Affecting unspecified side**

   344.41   **Affecting dominant side**

   344.42   **Affecting nondominant side**

❏ 344.5   **Unspecified monoplegia**

● 344.6   **Cauda equina syndrome**

   344.60   **Without mention of neurogenic bladder**

   344.61   **With neurogenic bladder**
   Acontractile bladder
   Autonomic hyperreflexia of bladder
   Cord bladder
   Detrusor hyperreflexia

● 344.8   **Other specified paralytic syndromes**

   344.81   **Locked-in state**

   ❏ 344.89   **Other specified paralytic syndrome**

❏ 344.9   **Paralysis, unspecified**

● 345   **Epilepsy**
   The following fifth-digit subclassification is for use with categories 345.0, .1, .4–.9:
   0 without mention of intractable epilepsy
   1 with intractable epilepsy

   Excludes   *progressive myoclonic epilepsy (333.2)*

● 345.0   **Generalized nonconvulsive epilepsy**
   Absences: Petit mal
   atonic   Pykno-epilepsy
   typical   Seizures:
   Minor epilepsy   akinetic
                             atonic
● 345.1   **Generalized convulsive epilepsy**
   Epileptic seizures: Epileptic seizures:
   clonic   tonic-clonic
   myoclonic   Grand mal
   tonic   Major epilepsy

   Excludes   *convulsions:*
   NOS (780.3)
   infantile (780.3)
   newborn (779.0)
   infantile spasms (345.6)

   345.2   **Petit mal status**
   Epileptic absence status

   345.3   **Grand mal status**
   Status epilepticus NOS

   Excludes   *epilepsia partialis continua (345.7) status:*
   psychomotor (345.7)
   temporal lobe (345.7)

● 345.4   **Partial epilepsy, with impairment of consciousness**
   Epilepsy:
   limbic system
   partial:
   secondarily generalized
   with memory and ideational disturbances
   psychomotor
   psychosensory
   temporal lobe
   Epileptic automatism

●345.5 **Partial epilepsy, without mention of impairment of consciousness**
Epilepsy:
  Bravais-Jacksonian NOS
  focal (motor) NOS
  Jacksonian NOS
  motor partial
  partial NOS
Epilepsy:
  sensory-induced
  somatomotor
  somatosensory
  visceral
  visual

●345.6 **Infantile spasms**
Hypsarrhythmia   Salaam attacks
Lightning spasms
Excludes salaam tic (781.0)

●345.7 **Epilepsia partialis continua**
Kojevnikov's epilepsy

● □345.8 **Other forms of epilepsy**
Epilepsy: Epilepsy:
  cursive [running]   gelastic

● □345.9 **Epilepsy, unspecified**
Epileptic convulsions, fits, or seizures NOS
Excludes convulsive seizure or fit NOS (780.3)

●346 **Migraine**
The following fifth-digit subclassification is for use with category 346:
  0 without mention of intractable migraine
  1 with intractable migraine, so stated

●346.0 **Classical migraine**
Migraine preceded or accompanied by transient focal neurological phenomena
Migraine with aura

●346.1 **Common migraine**
Atypical migraine   Sick headache

●346.2 **Variants of migraine**
Cluster headache
Histamine cephalgia
Horton's neuralgia
Migraine:
  abdominal
  basilar
Migraine:
  lower half
  retinal
Neuralgia:
  ciliary
  migrainous

● □346.8 **Other forms of migraine**
Migraine: Migraine:
  hemiplegic   ophthalmoplegic

● □346.9 **Migraine, unspecified**

●347 **Cataplexy and narcolepsy**
●347.0 **Narcolepsy** ◀
  347.00 **Without category** ◀
    Narcolepsy NOS ◀
  347.01 **With cataplexy** ◀
●347.1 **Narcolepsy in conditions classified elsewhere** ◀
  Code first underlying condition ◀
  347.10 **Without cataplexy** ◀
  347.11 **With cataplexy** ◀

●348 **Other conditions of brain**
348.0 **Cerebral cysts**
Arachnoid cyst   Porencephaly, acquired
Porencephalic cyst   Pseudoporencephaly
Excludes porencephaly (congenital) (724.4)

348.1 **Anoxic brain damage**
Excludes that occurring in:
  abortion (634–638 with .7, 639.8)
  ectopic or molar pregnancy (639.8)
  labor or delivery (668.2, 669.4)
  that of newborn (767.0, 768.0–768.9, 772.1–772.2)
Use additional E code to identify cause

348.2 **Benign intracranial hypertension**
Pseudotumor cerebri
Excludes hypertensive encephalopathy (437.2)

●348.3 **Encephalopathy, not elsewhere classified**
□348.30 **Encephalopathy, unspecified**
348.31 **Metabolic encephalopathy**
Septic encephalopathy
□348.39 **Other encephalopathy**
Excludes alcoholic (291.2)
  hepatic encephalopathy (572.2)
  hypertensive (437.2)
  toxic encephalopathy (349.82)

348.4 **Compression of brain**
Compression brain (stem)
Herniation brain (stem)
Posterior fossa compression syndrome

348.5 **Cerebral edema**

□348.8 **Other conditions of brain**
Cerebral: Cerebral:
  calcification   fungus

□348.9 **Unspecified condition of brain**

●349 **Other and unspecified disorders of the nervous system**
349.0 **Reaction to spinal or lumbar puncture**
Headache following lumbar puncture

349.1 **Nervous system complications from surgically implanted device**
Excludes immediate postoperative complications (997.00–997.09)
  mechanical complications of nervous system device (996.2)

□349.2 **Disorders of meninges, not elsewhere classified**
Adhesions, meningeal (cerebral) (spinal)
Cyst, spinal meninges
Meningocele, acquired
Pseudomeningocele, acquired

●349.8 **Other specified disorders of nervous system**
349.81 **Cerebrospinal fluid rhinorrhea**
Excludes cerebrospinal fluid otorrhea (388.61)
349.82 **Toxic encephalopathy**
Use additional E code to identify cause
□349.89 **Other**

□349.9 **Unspecified disorders of nervous system**
Disorder of nervous system (central) NOS

ICD-9-CM
300-399
Vol. 1

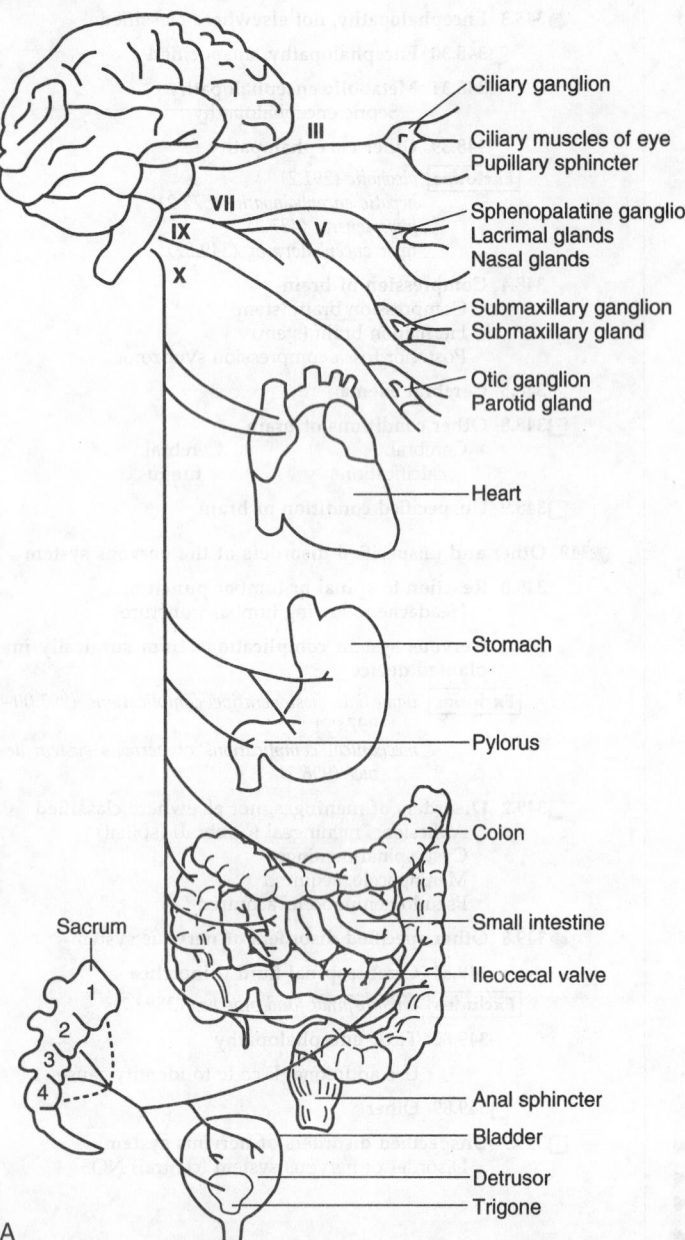

Ciliary ganglion

Ciliary muscles of eye
Pupillary sphincter

Sphenopalatine ganglion
Lacrimal glands
Nasal glands

Submaxillary ganglion
Submaxillary gland

Otic ganglion
Parotid gland

Heart

Stomach

Pylorus

Colon

Small intestine

Ileocecal valve

Sacrum

Anal sphincter
Bladder
Detrusor
Trigone

A

Item 6-6 The peripheral nervous system consists of 31 pairs of spinal nerves, 12 pairs of cranial nerves, and the autonomic nerves, which are divided into the parasympathetic and sympathetic nerves. The cranial nerves are: olfactory (I), optic (II), oculomotor (III), trochlear (IV), trigeminal (V), abducens (VI), facial (VII), vestibulocochlear (VIII), glossopharyngeal (IX), vagus (X), accessory (XI), and hypoglossal (XII).

DISORDERS OF THE PERIPHERAL NERVOUS SYSTEM (350–359)

Excludes *diseases of:*
  acoustic [8th] nerve (388.5)
  oculomotor [3rd, 4th, 6th] nerves (378.0–378.9)
  optic [2nd] nerve (377.0–377.9)
  peripheral autonomic nerves (337.0–337.9)
  neuralgia NOS or "rheumatic" (729.2)
  neuritis NOS or "rheumatic" (729.2)
  radiculitis NOS or "rheumatic" (729.2)
  peripheral neuritis in pregnancy (646.4)

Figure 6-3 A. Parasympathetic nervous system.

● 350 Trigeminal nerve disorders

  Includes: disorders of 5th cranial nerve

  350.1 **Trigeminal neuralgia**
      Tic douloureux
      Trifacial neuralgia
      Trigeminal neuralgia NOS
      Excludes *postherpetic (053.12)*

  350.2 **Atypical face pain**

  ❏ 350.8 **Other specified trigeminal nerve disorders**

  ❏ 350.9 **Trigeminal nerve disorder, unspecified**

● 351 Facial nerve disorders

  Includes: disorders of 7th cranial nerve
  Excludes *that in newborn (767.5)*

  351.0 **Bell's palsy**
      Facial palsy

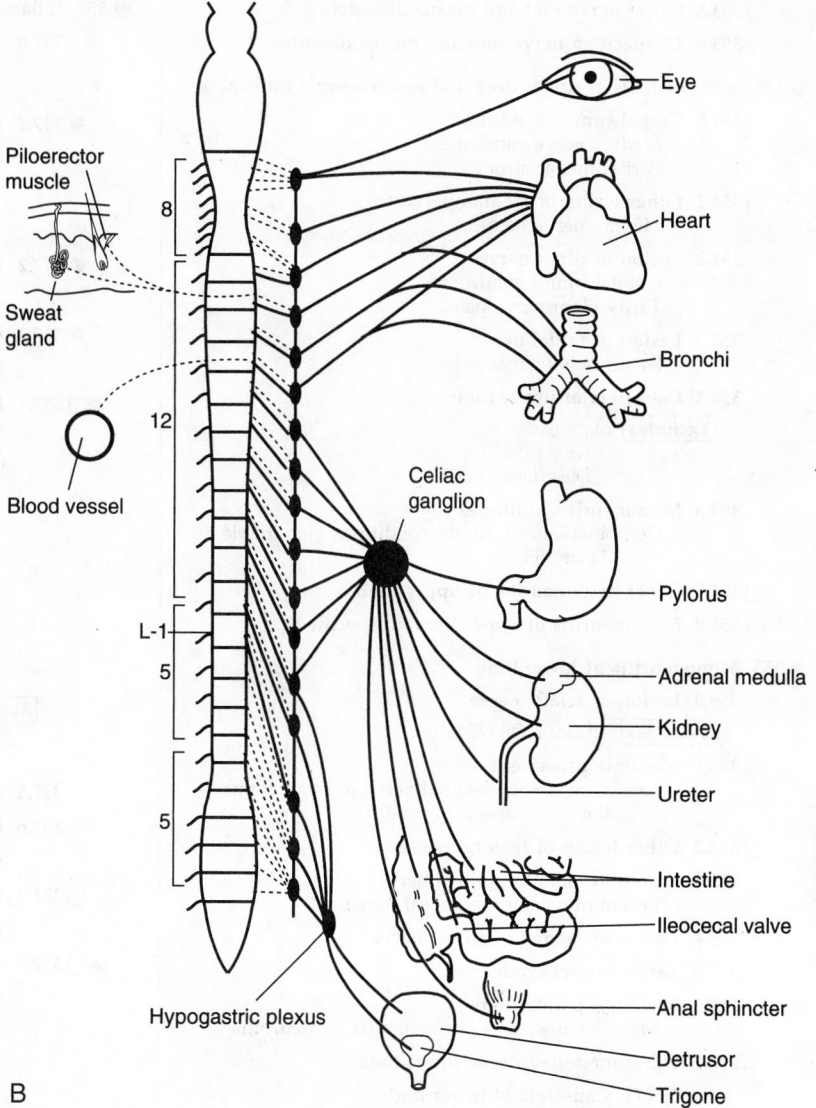

Figure 6–3 B. Sympathetic nervous system. (From Buck CJ: Step-by-Step Medical Coding, 2nd ed. Philadelphia, WB Saunders, 1998, pp 186 and 187.)

B

351.1 **Geniculate ganglionitis**
    Geniculate ganglionitis NOS
    Excludes *herpetic (053.11)*

☐ 351.8 **Other facial nerve disorders**
    Facial myokymia
    Melkersson's syndrome

☐ 351.9 **Facial nerve disorder, unspecified**

● 352 **Disorders of other cranial nerves**

352.0 **Disorders of olfactory [1st] nerve**

352.1 **Glossopharyngeal neuralgia**

☐ 352.2 **Other disorders of glossopharyngeal [9th] nerve**

352.3 **Disorders of pneumogastric [10th] nerve**
    Disorders of vagal nerve
    Excludes *paralysis of vocal cords or larynx (478.30–478.34)*

352.4 **Disorders of accessory [11th] nerve**

352.5 **Disorders of hypoglossal [12th] nerve**

352.6 **Multiple cranial nerve palsies**
    Collet-Sicard syndrome
    Polyneuritis cranialis

☐ 352.9 **Unspecified disorder of cranial nerves**

● 353 **Nerve root and plexus disorders**
    Excludes *conditions due to:*
      intervertebral disc disorders (722.0–722.9)
      spondylosis (720.0–721.9)
      vertebrogenic disorders (723.0–724.9)

353.0 **Brachial plexus lesions**
    Cervical rib syndrome
    Costoclavicular syndrome
    Scalenus anticus syndrome
    Thoracic outlet syndrome
    Excludes *brachial neuritis or radiculitis NOS (723.4)*
      that in newborn (767.6)

353.1 **Lumbosacral plexus lesions**

353.2 **Cervical root lesions, not elsewhere classified**

353.3 **Thoracic root lesions, not elsewhere classified**

353.4 **Lumbosacral root lesions, not elsewhere classified**

353.5 **Neuralgic amyotrophy**
    Parsonage-Aldren-Turner syndrome

353.6 **Phantom limb (syndrome)**

ICD-9-CM

300-399

Vol. 1

☐ **353.8 Other nerve root and plexus disorders**

☐ **353.9 Unspecified nerve root and plexus disorder**

● **354 Mononeuritis of upper limb and mononeuritis multiplex**

    354.0 Carpal tunnel syndrome
        Median nerve entrapment
        Partial thenar atrophy

  ☐ **354.1 Other lesion of median nerve**
        Median nerve neuritis

    354.2 Lesion of ulnar nerve
        Cubital tunnel syndrome
        Tardy ulnar nerve palsy

    354.3 Lesion of radial nerve
        Acute radial nerve palsy

    354.4 Causalgia of upper limb

        | **Excludes** | *causalgia:* |
                NOS (355.9)
                lower limb (355.71)

    354.5 Mononeuritis multiplex
        Combinations of single conditions classifiable to
        354 or 355

  ☐ **354.8 Other mononeuritis of upper limb**

  ☐ **354.9 Mononeuritis of upper limb, unspecified**

● **355 Mononeuritis of lower limb**

    355.0 Lesion of sciatic nerve

        | **Excludes** | *sciatica NOS (724.3)* |

    355.1 Meralgia paresthetica
        Lateral cutaneous femoral nerve of thigh compres-
        sion or syndrome

  ☐ **355.2 Other lesion of femoral nerve**

    355.3 Lesion of lateral popliteal nerve
        Lesion of common peroneal nerve

    355.4 Lesion of medial popliteal nerve

    355.5 Tarsal tunnel syndrome

    355.6 Lesion of plantar nerve
        Morton's metatarsalgia, neuralgia, or neuroma

  ● **355.7 Other mononeuritis of lower limb**

      355.71 Causalgia of lower limb

        | **Excludes** | *causalgia:* |
                NOS (355.9)
                upper limb (354.4)

      ☐ **355.79 Other mononeuritis of lower limb**

  ☐ **355.8 Mononeuritis of lower limb, unspecified**

  ☐ **355.9 Mononeuritis of unspecified site**
        Causalgia NOS

        | **Excludes** | *causalgia:* |
                lower limb (355.71)
                upper limb (354.4)

● **356 Hereditary and idiopathic peripheral neuropathy**

    356.0 Hereditary peripheral neuropathy
        Déjérine-Sottas disease

    356.1 Peroneal muscular atrophy
        Charcot-Marie-Tooth disease
        Neuropathic muscular atrophy

    356.2 Hereditary sensory neuropathy

    356.3 Refsum's disease
        Heredopathia atactica polyneuritiformis

    356.4 Idiopathic progressive polyneuropathy

  ☐ **356.8 Other specified idiopathic peripheral neuropathy**
        Supranuclear paralysis

  ☐ **356.9 Unspecified**

● **357 Inflammatory and toxic neuropathy**

    357.0 Acute infective polyneuritis
        Guillain-Barre syndrome
        Postinfectious polyneuritis

  ● **357.1 *Polyneuropathy in collagen vascular disease***

    Code first underlying disease, as:
        disseminated lupus erythematosus (710.0)
        polyarteritis nodosa (446.0)
        rheumatoid arthritis (714.0)

  ● **357.2 *Polyneuropathy in diabetes***

    Code first underlying disease (250.6)

  ● **357.3 *Polyneuropathy in malignant disease***

    Code first underlying disease (140.0–208.9)

  ●☐ **357.4 *Polyneuropathy in other diseases classified else-
        where***

    Code first underlying disease, as:
        amyloidosis (277.3)
        beriberi (265.0)
        deficiency of B vitamins (266.0–266.9)
        diphtheria (032.0–032.9)
        hypoglycemia (251.2)
        pellagra (265.2)
        porphyria (277.1)
        sarcoidosis (135)
        uremia (585)

        | **Excludes** | *polyneuropathy in:* |
                herpes zoster (053.13)
                mumps (072.72)

    357.5 Alcoholic polyneuropathy

    357.6 Polyneuropathy due to drugs

    Use additional E code to identify drug

  ☐ **357.7 Polyneuropathy due to other toxic agents**

    Use additional E code to identify toxic agent

  ●☐ **357.8 Other**

      **357.81 Chronic inflammatory demyelinating
             polyneuritis**

      357.82 Critical illness polyneuropathy
             Acute motor neuropathy

      ☐ **357.89 Other inflammatory and toxic neuropathy**

  ☐ **357.9 Unspecified**

● **358 Myoneural disorders**

  ● **358.0 Myasthenia gravis**

      **358.00 Myasthenia gravis without (acute) exacerba-
             tion**
             Myasthenia gravis NOS

      358.01 Myasthenia gravis with acute exacerbation
             Myasthenia gravis in crisis

  ● **358.1 *Myasthenic syndromes in diseases classified else-
        where***
        Amyotrophy from stated cause classified else-
        where
        Eaton-Lambert syndrome from stated cause classi-
        fied elsewhere

    Code first underlying disease, as:
        botulism (005.1)
        diabetes mellitus (250.6)
        hypothyroidism (244.0–244.9)
        malignant neoplasm (140.0–208.9)
        pernicious anemia (281.0)
        thyrotoxicosis (242.0–242.9)

    358.2 Toxic myoneural disorders

    Use additional E code to identify toxic agent

❏ 358.8 **Other specified myoneural disorders**

❏ 358.9 **Myoneural disorders, unspecified**

● 359 **Muscular dystrophies and other myopathies**

> Excludes | *idiopathic polymyositis (710.4)*

359.0 **Congenital hereditary muscular dystrophy**
  Benign congenital myopathy
  Central core disease
  Centronuclear myopathy
  Myotubular myopathy
  Nemaline body disease

> Excludes | *arthrogryposis multiplex congenita (754.89)*

359.1 **Hereditary progressive muscular dystrophy**
  Muscular dystrophy:
    NOS
    distal
    Duchenne
    Erb's
    fascioscapulohumeral
    Gower's
    Landouzy-Déjérine
    limb-girdle
    ocular
    oculopharyngeal

359.2 **Myotonic disorders**
  Dystrophia myotonica   Paramyotonia congenita
  Eulenburg's disease   Steinert's disease
  Myotonia congenita   Thomsen's disease

359.3 **Familial periodic paralysis**
  Hypokalemic familial periodic paralysis

359.4 **Toxic myopathy**
  Use additional E code to identify toxic agent

● 359.5 *Myopathy in endocrine diseases classified elsewhere*
  Code first underlying disease, as:
    Addison's disease (255.4)
    Cushing's syndrome (255.0)
    hypopituitarism (253.2)
    myxedema (244.0–244.9)
    thyrotoxicosis (242.0–242.9)

● 359.6 *Symptomatic inflammatory myopathy in diseases classified elsewhere*
  Code first underlying disease, as:
    amyloidosis (277.3)
    disseminated lupus erythematosus (710.0)
    malignant neoplasm (140.0–208.9)
    polyarteritis nodosa (446.0)
    rheumatoid arthritis (714.0)
    sarcoidosis (135)
    scleroderma (710.1)
    Sjögren's disease (710.2)

● ❏ 359.8 **Other myopathies**

359.81 **Critical illness myopathy**
  Acute necrotizing myopathy
  Acute quadriplegic myopathy
  Intensive care (ICU) myopathy
  Myopathy of critical illness

❏ 359.89 **Other myopathies**

❏ 359.9 **Myopathy, unspecified**

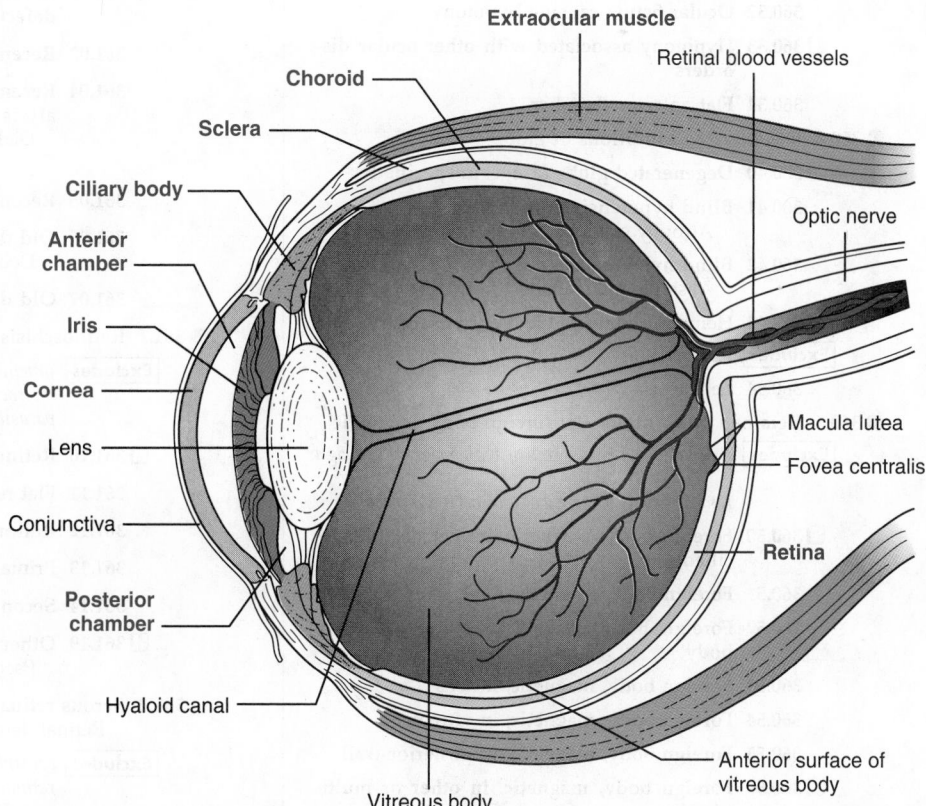

Figure 6–4 Eye and ocular adnexa. (From Buck CJ: Step-by-Step Medical Coding, 2005 ed. Philadelphia, WBS, 2005.)

◀ **New**   ⬅ **Revised**   ● **Not a Principal Diagnosis**   ● **Use Additional Digit(s)**   ❏ **Nonspecific Code**

DISORDERS OF THE EYE AND ADNEXA (360–379)

● **360   Disorders of the globe**

    Includes: disorders affecting multiple structures of eye

  ● **360.0   Purulent endophthalmitis**

    ❏ **360.00   Purulent endophthalmitis, unspecified**

    360.01   Acute endophthalmitis

    360.02   Panophthalmitis

    360.03   Chronic endophthalmitis

    360.04   Vitreous abscess

  ● **360.1   Other endophthalmitis**

    360.11   Sympathetic uveitis

    360.12   Panuveitis

    360.13   Parasitic endophthalmitis NOS

    360.14   Ophthalmia nodosa

    ❏ **360.19   Other**
              Phacoanaphylactic endophthalmitis

  ● **360.2   Degenerative disorders of globe**

    ❏ **360.20   Degenerative disorder of globe, unspecified**

    360.21   Progressive high (degenerative) myopia
              Malignant myopia

    360.23   Siderosis

    ❏ **360.24   Other metallosis**
              Chalcosis

    ❏ **360.29   Other**

    Excludes   *xerophthalmia (264.7)*

  ● **360.3   Hypotony of eye**

    ❏ **360.30   Hypotony, unspecified**

    360.31   Primary hypotony

    360.32   Ocular fistula causing hypotony

    ❏ **360.33   Hypotony associated with other ocular disorders**

    360.34   Flat anterior chamber

  ● **360.4   Degenerated conditions of globe**

    ❏ **360.40   Degenerated globe or eye, unspecified**

    360.41   Blind hypotensive eye
              Atrophy of globe   Phthisis bulbi

    360.42   Blind hypertensive eye
              Absolute glaucoma

    360.43   Hemophthalmos, except current injury

    Excludes   *traumatic (871.0–871.9, 921.0–921.9)*

    360.44   Leucocoria

  ● **360.5   Retained (old) intraocular foreign body, magnetic**

    Excludes   *current penetrating injury with magnetic foreign body (871.5)*
              retained (old) foreign body of orbit (376.6)

    ❏ **360.50   Foreign body, magnetic, intraocular, unspecified**

    360.51   Foreign body, magnetic, in anterior chamber

    360.52   Foreign body, magnetic, in iris or ciliary body

    360.53   Foreign body, magnetic, in lens

    360.54   Foreign body, magnetic, in vitreous

    360.55   Foreign body, magnetic, in posterior wall

    ❏ **360.59   Foreign body, magnetic, in other or multiple sites**

● **360.6   Retained (old) intraocular foreign body, nonmagnetic**
     Retained (old) foreign body:
       NOS
       nonmagnetic

    Excludes   *current penetrating injury with (nonmagnetic) foreign body (871.6)*
              retained (old) foreign body in orbit (376.6)

    ❏ **360.60   Foreign body, intraocular, unspecified**

    360.61   Foreign body in anterior chamber

    360.62   Foreign body in iris or ciliary body

    360.63   Foreign body in lens

    360.64   Foreign body in vitreous

    360.65   Foreign body in posterior wall

    ❏ **360.69   Foreign body in other or multiple sites**

  ● **360.8   Other disorders of globe**

    360.81   Luxation of globe

    ❏ **360.89   Other**

  ❏ **360.9   Unspecified disorder of globe**

● **361   Retinal detachments and defects**

  ● **361.0   Retinal detachment with retinal defect**
     Rhegmatogenous retinal detachment

    Excludes   *detachment of retinal pigment epithelium (362.42–362.43)*
              retinal detachment (serous) (without defect) (361.2)

    ❏ **361.00   Retinal detachment with retinal defect, unspecified**

    361.01   Recent detachment, partial, with single defect

    361.02   Recent detachment, partial, with multiple defects

    361.03   Recent detachment, partial, with giant tear

    361.04   Recent detachment, partial, with retinal dialysis
              Dialysis (juvenile) of retina (with detachment)

    361.05   Recent detachment, total or subtotal

    361.06   Old detachment, partial
              Delimited old retinal detachment

    361.07   Old detachment, total or subtotal

  ● **361.1   Retinoschisis and retinal cysts**

    Excludes   *juvenile retinoschisis (362.73)*
              microcystoid degeneration of retina (362.62)
              parasitic cyst of retina (360.13)

    ❏ **361.10   Retinoschisis, unspecified**

    361.11   Flat retinoschisis

    361.12   Bullous retinoschisis

    361.13   Primary retinal cysts

    361.14   Secondary retinal cysts

    ❏ **361.19   Other**
              Pseudocyst of retina

  ● **361.2   Serous retinal detachment**
     Retinal detachment without retinal defect

    Excludes   *central serous retinopathy (362.41)*
              retinal pigment epithelium detachment (362.42–362.43)

● **361.3　Retinal defects without detachment**

> | **Excludes** | *chorioretinal scars after surgery for detachment (363.30–363.35)* |
> | | *peripheral retinal degeneration without defect (362.60–362.66)* |

❑ **361.30　Retinal defect, unspecified**
　　　　　　Retinal break(s) NOS

361.31　Round hole of retina without detachment

361.32　Horseshoe tear of retina without detachment
　　　　　　Operculum of retina without mention of detachment

❑ **361.33　Multiple defects of retina without detachment**

● **361.8　Other forms of retinal detachment**

361.81　Traction detachment of retina
　　　　　　Traction detachment with vitreoretinal organization

❑ **361.89　Other**

❑ **361.9　Unspecified retinal detachment**

● **362　Other retinal disorders**

> | **Excludes** | *chorioretinal scars (363.30–363.35)* |
> | | *chorioretinitis (363.0–363.2)* |

● **362.0　Diabetic retinopathy**

　　Code first diabetes (250.5)

● **362.01　Background diabetic retinopathy**
　　　　　　Diabetic macular edema
　　　　　　Diabetic retinal edema
　　　　　　Diabetic retinal microaneurysms
　　　　　　Diabetic retinopathy NOS

● **362.02　Proliferative diabetic retinopathy**

● **362.1　Other background retinopathy and retinal vascular changes**

❑ **362.10　Background retinopathy, unspecified**

362.11　Hypertensive retinopathy

362.12　Exudative retinopathy
　　　　　　Coats'syndrome

362.13　Changes in vascular appearance
　　　　　　Vascular sheathing of retina

　　　　　　Use additional code for any associated atherosclerosis (440.8)

362.14　Retinal microaneurysms NOS

362.15　Retinal telangiectasia

362.16　Retinal neovascularization NOS
　　　　　　Neovascularization:
　　　　　　　　choroidal
　　　　　　　　subretinal

❑ **362.17　Other intraretinal microvascular abnormalities**
　　　　　　Retinal varices

362.18　Retinal vasculitis
　　　　　　Eales' disease　　　Retinal:
　　　　　　Retinal:　　　　　　　perivasculitis
　　　　　　　arteritis　　　　　　phlebitis
　　　　　　　endarteritis

● **362.2　Other proliferative retinopathy**

362.21　Retrolental fibroplasia

❑ **362.29　Other nondiabetic proliferative retinopathy**

● **362.3　Retinal vascular occlusion**

❑ **362.30　Retinal vascular occlusion, unspecified**

362.31　Central retinal artery occlusion

362.32　Arterial branch occlusion

362.33　Partial arterial occlusion
　　　　　　Hollenhorst plaque
　　　　　　Retinal microembolism

362.34　Transient arterial occlusion
　　　　　　Amaurosis fugax

362.35　Central retinal vein occlusion

362.36　Venous tributary (branch) occlusion

362.37　Venous engorgement
　　　　　　Occlusion:
　　　　　　　of retinal vein
　　　　　　　incipient of retinal vein
　　　　　　　partial of retinal vein

● **362.4　Separation of retinal layers**

> | **Excludes** | *retinal detachment (serous) (361.2)* |
> | | *rhegmatogenous (361.00–361.07)* |

❑ **362.40　Retinal layer separation, unspecified**

362.41　Central serous retinopathy

362.42　Serous detachment of retinal pigment epithelium
　　　　　　Exudative detachment of retinal pigment epithelium

362.43　Hemorrhagic detachment of retinal pigment epithelium

● **362.5　Degeneration of macula and posterior pole**

> | **Excludes** | *degeneration of optic disc (377.21–377.24)* |
> | | *hereditary retinal degeneration [dystrophy] (362.70–362.77)* |

❑ **362.50　Macular degeneration (senile), unspecified**

362.51　Nonexudative senile macular degeneration
　　　　　　Senile macular degeneration:
　　　　　　　atrophic
　　　　　　　dry

362.52　Exudative senile macular degeneration
　　　　　　Kuhnt-Junius degeneration
　　　　　　Senile macular degeneration:
　　　　　　　disciform
　　　　　　　wet

362.53　Cystoid macular degeneration
　　　　　　Cystoid macular edema

362.54　Macular cyst, hole, or pseudohole

362.55　Toxic maculopathy

　　　　　　Use additional E code to identify drug, if drug induced

362.56　Macular puckering
　　　　　　Preretinal fibrosis

362.57　Drusen (degenerative)

● **362.6　Peripheral retinal degenerations**

> | **Excludes** | *hereditary retinal degeneration [dystrophy] (362.70–362.77)* |
> | | *retinal degeneration with retinal defect (361.00–361.07)* |

❑ **362.60　Peripheral retinal degeneration, unspecified**

362.61　Paving stone degeneration

362.62　Microcystoid degeneration
　　　　　　Blessig's cysts
　　　　　　Iwanoff's cysts

362.63　Lattice degeneration
　　　　　　Palisade degeneration of retina

362.64　Senile reticular degeneration

362.65　Secondary pigmentary degeneration
　　　　　　Pseudoretinitis pigmentosa

362.66　Secondary vitreoretinal degenerations

● **362.7　Hereditary retinal dystrophies**

❑ **362.70　Hereditary retinal dystrophy, unspecified**

ICD-9-CM

300-399

Vol. 1

● 362.71 *Retinal dystrophy in systemic or cerebro-retinal lipidoses*

Code first underlying disease, as:
cerebroretinal lipidoses (330.1)
systemic lipidoses (272.7)

●❑ 362.72 *Retinal dystrophy in other systemic disorders and syndromes*

Code first underlying disease, as:
Bassen-Kornzweig syndrome (272.5)
Refsum's disease (356.3)

362.73 **Vitreoretinal dystrophies**
Juvenile retinoschisis

362.74 **Pigmentary retinal dystrophy**
Retinal dystrophy, albipunctate
Retinitis pigmentosa

❑ 362.75 **Other dystrophies primarily involving the sensory retina**
Progressive cone (-rod) dystrophy
Stargardt's disease

362.76 **Dystrophies primarily involving the retinal pigment epithelium**
Fundus flavimaculatus
Vitelliform dystrophy

362.77 **Dystrophies primarily involving Bruch's membrane**
Dystrophy:
hyaline
pseudoinflammatory foveal
Hereditary drusen

● 362.8 **Other retinal disorders**

Excludes *chorioretinal inflammations (363.0–363.2)*
chorioretinal scars (363.30–363.35)

362.81 **Retinal hemorrhage**
Hemorrhage:
preretinal
retinal (deep) (superficial)
subretinal

362.82 **Retinal exudates and deposits**

362.83 **Retinal edema**
Retinal:
cotton wool spots
edema (localized) (macular) (peripheral)

362.84 **Retinal ischemia**

362.85 **Retinal nerve fiber bundle defects**

❑ 362.89 **Other retinal disorders**

❑ 362.9 **Unspecified retinal disorder**

● 363 **Chorioretinal inflammations, scars, and other disorders of choroid**

● 363.0 **Focal chorioretinitis and focal retinochoroiditis**

Excludes *focal chorioretinitis or retinochoroiditis in:*
histoplasmosis (115.02, 115.12, 115.92)
toxoplasmosis (130.2)
congenital infection (771.2)

❑ 363.00 **Focal chorioretinitis, unspecified**
Focal:
choroiditis or chorioretinitis NOS
retinitis or retinochoroiditis NOS

363.01 **Focal choroiditis and chorioretinitis, juxtapapillary**

❑ 363.03 **Focal choroiditis and chorioretinitis of other posterior pole**

363.04 **Focal choroiditis and chorioretinitis, peripheral**

363.05 **Focal retinitis and retinochoroiditis, juxtapapillary**
Neuroretinitis

363.06 **Focal retinitis and retinochoroiditis, macular or paramacular**

❑ 363.07 **Focal retinitis and retinochoroiditis of other posterior pole**

❑ 363.08 **Focal retinitis and retinochoroiditis, peripheral**

● 363.1 **Disseminated chorioretinitis and disseminated retinochoroiditis**

Excludes *disseminated choroiditis or chorioretinitis in secondary syphilis (091.51)*
neurosyphilitic disseminated retinitis or retinochoroiditis (094.83)
retinal (peri)vasculitis (362.18)

❑ 363.10 **Disseminated chorioretinitis, unspecified**
Disseminated:
choroiditis or chorioretinitis NOS
retinitis or retinochoroiditis NOS

363.11 **Disseminated choroiditis and chorioretinitis, posterior pole**

363.12 **Disseminated choroiditis and chorioretinitis, peripheral**

363.13 **Disseminated choroiditis and chorioretinitis, generalized**

Code first any underlying disease, as:
tuberculosis (017.3)

363.14 **Disseminated retinitis and retinochoroiditis, metastatic**

363.15 **Disseminated retinitis and retinochoroiditis, pigment epitheliopathy**
Acute posterior multifocal placoid pigment epitheliopathy

● 363.2 **Other and unspecified forms of chorioretinitis and retinochoroiditis**

Excludes *panophthalmitis (360.02)*
sympathetic uveitis (360.11)
uveitis NOS (364.3)

❑ 363.20 **Chorioretinitis, unspecified**
Choroiditis NOS
Retinitis NOS
Uveitis, posterior NOS

363.21 **Pars planitis**
Posterior cyclitis

363.22 **Harada's disease**

● 363.3 **Chorioretinal scars**
Scar (postinflammatory) (postsurgical) (posttraumatic):
choroid
retina

❑ 363.30 **Chorioretinal scar, unspecified**

363.31 **Solar retinopathy**

❑ 363.32 **Other macular scars**

❑ 363.33 **Other scars of posterior pole**

363.34 **Peripheral scars**

363.35 **Disseminated scars**

● 363.4 **Choroidal degenerations**

❑ 363.40 **Choroidal degeneration, unspecified**
Choroidal sclerosis NOS

363.41 **Senile atrophy of choroid**

363.42 **Diffuse secondary atrophy of choroid**

363.43 **Angioid streaks of choroid**

● **363.5 Hereditary choroidal dystrophies**
Hereditary choroidal atrophy:
    partial [choriocapillaris]
    total [all vessels]

❑ **363.50 Hereditary choroidal dystrophy or atrophy, unspecified**

363.51 Circumpapillary dystrophy of choroid, partial

363.52 Circumpapillary dystrophy of choroid, total
    Helicoid dystrophy of choroid

363.53 Central dystrophy of choroid, partial
    Dystrophy, choroidal:
        central areolar
        circinate

363.54 Central choroidal atrophy, total
    Dystrophy, choroidal:
        central gyrate
        serpiginous

363.55 Choroideremia

❑ **363.56 Other diffuse or generalized dystrophy, partial**
    Diffuse choroidal sclerosis

❑ **363.57 Other diffuse or generalized dystrophy, total**
    Generalized gyrate atrophy, choroid

● **363.6 Choroidal hemorrhage and rupture**

❑ **363.61 Choroidal hemorrhage, unspecified**

363.62 Expulsive choroidal hemorrhage

363.63 Choroidal rupture

● **363.7 Choroidal detachment**

❑ **363.70 Choroidal detachment, unspecified**

363.71 Serous choroidal detachment

363.72 Hemorrhagic choroidal detachment

❑ **363.8 Other disorders of choroid**

❑ **363.9 Unspecified disorder of choroid**

● **364 Disorders of iris and ciliary body**

● **364.0 Acute and subacute iridocyclitis**
    Anterior uveitis, acute, subacute
    Cyclitis, acute, subacute
    Iridocyclitis, acute, subacute
    Iritis, acute, subacute

Excludes	*gonococcal (098.41)*
	herpes simplex (054.44)
	herpes zoster (053.22)

❑ **364.00 Acute and subacute iridocyclitis, unspecified**

364.01 Primary iridocyclitis

364.02 Recurrent iridocyclitis

364.03 Secondary iridocyclitis, infectious

364.04 Secondary iridocyclitis, noninfectious
    Aqueous:
        cells
        fibrin
        flare

364.05 Hypopyon

● **364.1 Chronic iridocyclitis**

Excludes	*posterior cyclitis (363.21)*

❑ **364.10 Chronic iridocyclitis, unspecified**

● *364.11 Chronic iridocyclitis in diseases classified elsewhere*

    Code first underlying disease, as:
        sarcoidosis (135)
        tuberculosis (017.3)

Excludes	*syphilitic iridocyclitis (091.52)*

● **364.2 Certain types of iridocyclitis**

Excludes	*posterior cyclitis (363.21)*
	sympathetic uveitis (360.11)

364.21 Fuchs' heterochromic cyclitis

364.22 Glaucomatocyclitic crises

364.23 Lens-induced iridocyclitis

364.24 Vogt-Koyanagi syndrome

❑ **364.3 Unspecified iridocyclitis**
    Uveitis NOS

● **364.4 Vascular disorders of iris and ciliary body**

364.41 Hyphema
    Hemorrhage of iris or ciliary body

364.42 Rubeosis iridis
    Neovascularization of iris or ciliary body

● **364.5 Degenerations of iris and ciliary body**

364.51 Essential or progressive iris atrophy

364.52 Iridoschisis

364.53 Pigmentary iris degeneration
    Acquired heterochromia of iris
    Pigment dispersion syndrome of iris
    Translucency of iris

364.54 Degeneration of pupillary margin
    Atrophy of sphincter of iris
    Ectropion of pigment epithelium of iris

364.55 Miotic cysts of pupillary margin

364.56 Degenerative changes of chamber angle

364.57 Degenerative changes of ciliary body

❑ **364.59 Other iris atrophy**
    Iris atrophy (generalized) (sector shaped)

● **364.6 Cysts of iris, ciliary body, and anterior chamber**

Excludes	*miotic pupillary cyst (364.55)*
	parasitic cyst (360.13)

364.60 Idiopathic cysts

364.61 Implantation cysts
    Epithelial down-growth, anterior chamber
    Implantation cysts (surgical) (traumatic)

364.62 Exudative cysts of iris or anterior chamber

364.63 Primary cyst of pars plana

364.64 Exudative cyst of pars plana

● **364.7 Adhesions and disruptions of iris and ciliary body**

Excludes	*flat anterior chamber (360.34)*

❑ **364.70 Adhesions of iris, unspecified**
    Synechiae (iris) NOS

364.71 Posterior synechiae

364.72 Anterior synechiae

364.73 Goniosynechiae
    Peripheral anterior synechiae

364.74 Pupillary membranes
    Iris bombé
    Pupillary:
        occlusion
        seclusion

364.75 Pupillary abnormalities
    Deformed pupil
    Ectopic pupil
    Rupture of sphincter, pupil

364.76 Iridodialysis

364.77 Recession of chamber angle

ICD-9-CM

300-
~~399~~

Vol.

☐ **364.8 Other disorders of iris and ciliary body**
Prolapse of iris NOS

> **Excludes** *prolapse of iris in recent wound (871.1)*

☐ **364.9 Unspecified disorder of iris and ciliary body**

● **365 Glaucoma**

> **Excludes** *hypertensive eye [absolute glaucoma] (360.42)*
> *congenital glaucoma (743.20–743.22)*

● **365.0 Borderline glaucoma [glaucoma suspect]**

☐ **365.00 Preglaucoma, unspecified**

365.01 Open angle with borderline findings
Open angle with:
borderline intraocular pressure
cupping of optic discs

365.02 Anatomical narrow angle

365.03 Steroid responders

☐ **365.04 Ocular hypertension**

● **365.1 Open-angle glaucoma**

☐ **365.10 Open-angle glaucoma, unspecified**
Wide-angle glaucoma NOS

365.11 Primary open angle glaucoma
Chronic simple glaucoma

365.12 Low tension glaucoma

365.13 Pigmentary glaucoma

365.14 Glaucoma of childhood
Infantile or juvenile glaucoma

365.15 Residual stage of open angle glaucoma

● **365.2 Primary angle-closure glaucoma**

☐ **365.20 Primary angle-closure glaucoma, unspecified**

365.21 Intermittent angle-closure glaucoma
Angle-closure glaucoma:
interval
subacute

365.22 Acute angle-closure glaucoma

365.23 Chronic angle-closure glaucoma

365.24 Residual stage of angle-closure glaucoma

● **365.3 Corticosteroid-induced glaucoma**

365.31 Glaucomatous stage

365.32 Residual stage

● **365.4 Glaucoma associated with congenital anomalies, dystrophies, and systemic syndromes**

● ☐ **365.41 *Glaucoma associated with chamber angle anomalies***
Code first associated disorder, as:
Axenfeld's anomaly (743.44)
Rieger's anomaly or syndrome (743.44)

● **365.42 *Glaucoma associated with anomalies of iris***
Code first associated disorder, as:
aniridia (743.45)
essential iris atrophy (364.51)

● ☐ **365.43 *Glaucoma associated with other anterior segment anomalies***
Code first associated disorder, as:
microcornea (743.41)

● **365.44 *Glaucoma associated with systemic syndromes***
Code first associated disease, as:
neurofibromatosis (237.7)
Sturge-Weber (-Dimitri) syndrome (759.6)

● **365.5 Glaucoma associated with disorders of the lens**

365.51 Phacolytic glaucoma
Use additional code for associated hypermature cataract (366.18)

365.52 Pseudoexfoliation glaucoma
Use additional code for associated pseudoexfoliation of capsule (366.11)

☐ **365.59 Glaucoma associated with other lens disorders**
Use additional code for associated disorder, as:
dislocation of lens (379.33–379.34)
spherophakia (743.36)

● **365.6 Glaucoma associated with other ocular disorders**

☐ **365.60 Glaucoma associated with unspecified ocular disorder**

365.61 Glaucoma associated with pupillary block
Use additional code for associated disorder, as:
seclusion of pupil [iris bombé] (364.74)

365.62 Glaucoma associated with ocular inflammations
Use additional code for associated disorder, as:
glaucomatocyclitic crises (364.22)
iridocyclitis (364.0–364.3)

365.63 Glaucoma associated with vascular disorders
Use additional code for associated disorder, as:
central retinal vein occlusion (362.35)
hyphema (364.41)

365.64 Glaucoma associated with tumors or cysts
Use additional code for associated disorder, as:
benign neoplasm (224.0–224.9)
epithelial down-growth (364.61)
malignant neoplasm (190.0–190.9)

365.65 Glaucoma associated with ocular trauma
Use additional code for associated condition, as:
contusion of globe (921.3)
recession of chamber angle (364.77)

● **365.8 Other specified forms of glaucoma**

365.81 Hypersecretion glaucoma

365.82 Glaucoma with increased episcleral venous pressure

365.83 Aqueous misdirection
Malignant glaucoma

☐ **365.89 Other specified glaucoma**

☐ **365.9 Unspecified glaucoma**

● **366 Cataract**

> **Excludes** *congenital cataract (743.30–743.34)*

● **366.0 Infantile, juvenile, and presenile cataract**

☐ **366.00 Nonsenile cataract, unspecified**

366.01 Anterior subcapsular polar cataract

366.02 Posterior subcapsular polar cataract

366.03 Cortical, lamellar, or zonular cataract

366.04 Nuclear cataract

☐ **366.09 Other and combined forms of nonsenile cataract**

Figure 6–5 Mature cataract with gray fissures. (From Pau H: Differential Diagnosis of Eye Diseases. Philadelphia, WB Saunders, 1978, p 240.)

Item 6–7 Senile cataracts are linked to the aging process. The most common area for the formation of a cataract is the cortical area of the lens. **Polar cataracts** can be either anterior or posterior. **Anterior polar cataracts** are more common and are small, white, capsular cataracts located on the anterior portion of the lens.
Total cataracts, also called **complete** or **mature**, cause an opacity of all fibers of the lens.
Hypermature describes a mature cataract with a swollen, milky cortex that covers the entire lens.
Immature, also called **incipient**, cataracts have a clear cortex and are only slightly opaque.

● 366.1 Senile cataract

   ❑ 366.10 Senile cataract, unspecified

   366.11 Pseudoexfoliation of lens capsule

   366.12 Incipient cataract
            Cataract:
               coronary
               immature NOS
               punctate
            Water clefts

   366.13 Anterior subcapsular polar senile cataract

   366.14 Posterior subcapsular polar senile cataract

   366.15 Cortical senile cataract

   366.16 Nuclear sclerosis
            Cataracta brunescens
            Nuclear cataract

   366.17 Total or mature cataract

   366.18 Hypermature cataract
            Morgagni cataract

   ❑ 366.19 Other and combined forms of senile cataract

● 366.2 Traumatic cataract

   ❑ 366.20 Traumatic cataract, unspecified

   366.21 Localized traumatic opacities
            Vossius' ring

   366.22 Total traumatic cataract

   366.23 Partially resolved traumatic cataract

Figure 6–6 Perforation rosette of the lens; feathery opacities along suture lines beneath the posterior capsule. (From Pau H: Differential Diagnosis of Eye Diseases. Philadelphia, WB Saunders, 1978, p 250.)

Item 6–8 Vossius' ring is the result of contusion-type traumatic injury and results in a ring of iris pigment pressed onto the anterior lens capsule.

● 366.3 Cataract secondary to ocular disorders

   ❑ 366.30 Cataracta complicata, unspecified

   366.31 Glaucomatous flecks (subcapsular)
            Code first underlying glaucoma (365.0–365.9)

   366.32 Cataract in inflammatory disorders
            Code first underlying condition, as:
               chronic choroiditis (363.0–363.2)

   366.33 Cataract with neovascularization
            Code first underlying condition, as:
               chronic iridocyclitis (364.10)

   366.34 Cataract in degenerative disorders
            Sunflower cataract

            Code first underlying condition, as:
               chalcosis (360.24)
               degenerative myopia (360.21)
               pigmentary retinal dystrophy (362.74)

● 366.4 Cataract associated with other disorders

   ● 366.41 *Diabetic cataract*
            Code first diabetes (250.5)

   ● 366.42 *Tetanic cataract*
            Code first underlying disease, as:
               calcinosis (275.4)
               hypoparathyroidism (252.1)

   ● 366.43 *Myotonic cataract*
            Code first underlying disorder (359.2)

   ●❑ 366.44 *Cataract associated with other syndromes*
            Code first underlying condition, as:
               craniofacial dysostosis (756.0)
               galactosemia (271.1)

   366.45 Toxic cataract
            Drug-induced cataract

            Use additional E code to identify drug or other toxic substance

   ❑ 366.46 Cataract associated with radiation and other physical influences

            Use additional E code to identify cause

ICD-9-CM

300-
399

Vol. 1

● **366.5 After-cataract**

  □ **366.50 After-cataract, unspecified**
         Secondary cataract NOS

     366.51 Soemmering's ring

  □ **366.52 Other after-cataract, not obscuring vision**

     366.53 After-cataract, obscuring vision

□ **366.8 Other cataract**
     Calcification of lens

□ **366.9 Unspecified cataract**

● **367 Disorders of refraction and accommodation**

  367.0 Hypermetropia
     Far-sightedness
     Hyperopia

  367.1 Myopia
     Near-sightedness

● **367.2 Astigmatism**

  □ **367.20 Astigmatism, unspecified**

     367.21 Regular astigmatism

     367.22 Irregular astigmatism

● **367.3 Anisometropia and aniseikonia**

     367.31 Anisometropia

     367.32 Aniseikonia

  367.4 Presbyopia

● **367.5 Disorders of accommodation**

     367.51 Paresis of accommodation
         Cycloplegia

     367.52 Total or complete internal ophthalmoplegia

     367.53 Spasm of accommodation

● **367.8 Other disorders of refraction and accommodation**

     367.81 Transient refractive change

  □ **367.89 Other**
         Drug-induced disorders of refraction and
           accommodation
         Toxic disorders of refraction and accom-
           modation

□ **367.9 Unspecified disorder of refraction and accommodation**

● **368 Visual disturbances**

  | **Excludes** | *electrophysiological disturbances (794.11–794.14)* |

● **368.0 Amblyopia ex anopsia**

  □ **368.00 Amblyopia, unspecified**

     368.01 Strabismic amblyopia
         Suppression amblyopia

     368.02 Deprivation amblyopia

     368.03 Refractive amblyopia

● **368.1 Subjective visual disturbances**

  □ **368.10 Subjective visual disturbance, unspecified**

     368.11 Sudden visual loss

     368.12 Transient visual loss
         Concentric fading
         Scintillating scotoma

     368.13 Visual discomfort
         Asthenopia
         Eye strain
         Photophobia

     368.14 Visual distortions of shape and size
         Macropsia
         Metamorphopsia
         Micropsia

□ **368.15 Other visual distortions and entoptic phenomena**
     Photopsia
     Refractive:
       diplopia
       polyopia
     Visual halos

     368.16 Psychophysical visual disturbances
         Visual:
           agnosia
           disorientation syndrome
           hallucinations

  368.2 Diplopia
     Double vision

● **368.3 Other disorders of binocular vision**

  □ **368.30 Binocular vision disorder, unspecified**

     368.31 Suppression of binocular vision

     **368.32 Simultaneous visual perception without fu-
sion**

     368.33 Fusion with defective stereopsis

     368.34 Abnormal retinal correspondence

● **368.4 Visual field defects**

  □ **368.40 Visual field defect, unspecified**

     368.41 Scotoma involving central area
         Scotoma:
           central
           centrocecal
           paracentral

     368.42 Scotoma of blind spot area
         Enlarged:
           angioscotoma
           blind spot
         Paracecal scotoma

     368.43 Sector or arcuate defects
         Scotoma:
           arcuate
           Bjerrum
           Seidel

  □ **368.44 Other localized visual field defect**
         Scotoma:
           NOS
           ring
         Visual field defect:
           nasal step
           peripheral

     368.45 Generalized contraction or constriction

     368.46 Homonymous bilateral field defects
         Hemianopsia (altitudinal) (homonymous)
         Quadrant anopia

     368.47 Heteronymous bilateral field defects
         Hemianopsia:
           binasal
           bitemporal

● **368.5 Color vision deficiencies**
     Color blindness

     368.51 Protan defect
         Protanomaly
         Protanopia

     368.52 Deutan defect
         Deuteranomaly
         Deuteranopia

     368.53 Tritan defect
         Tritanomaly
         Tritanopia

368.54 Achromatopsia
Monochromatism (cone) (rod)

368.55 Acquired color vision deficiencies

☐ **368.59 Other color vision deficiencies**

● **368.6 Night blindness**
Nyctalopia

☐ **368.60 Night blindness, unspecified**

368.61 Congenital night blindness
Hereditary night blindness
Oguchi's disease

368.62 Acquired night blindness

Excludes *that due to vitamin A deficiency (264.5)*

368.63 Abnormal dark adaptation curve
Abnormal threshold of cones or rods
Delayed adaptation of cones or rods

☐ **368.69 Other night blindness**

☐ **368.8 Other specified visual disturbances**
Blurred vision NOS

☐ **368.9 Unspecified visual disturbance**

Classification		Levels of Visual Impairment	Additional Descriptors Which May Be Encountered
"Legal"	WHO	Visual Acuity and/or Visual Field Limitation (Whichever Is Worse)	
	(Near-)normal vision	Range of Normal Vision 20/10 20/13 20/16 20/20 20/25 2.0 1.6 1.25 1.0 0.8	
		Near-Normal Vision 20/30 20/40 20/50 20/60 0.7 0.6 0.5 0.4 0.3	
	Low vision	Moderate Visual Impairment 20/70 20/80 20/100 20/125 20/160 0.25 0.20 0.16 0.12	Moderate low vision
Legal Blindness (U.S.A.) both eyes		Severe Visual Impairment 20/200 20/250 20/320 20/400 0.10 0.08 0.06 0.05 Visual field: 20 degrees or less	Severe low vision, "Legal" blindness
	Blindness (WHO) one or both eyes	Profound Visual Impairment 20/500 20/630 20/800 20/1000 0.04 0.03 0.025 0.02 Count fingers at: less than 3 m (10 ft) Visual field: 10 degrees or less	Profound low vision, Moderate blindness
		Near-Total Visual Impairment Visual acuity: less than 0.02 (20/1000) Count fingers: 1 m (3 ft) or less Hand movements: 5 m (15 ft) or less Light projection, light perception Visual field: 5 degrees or less	Severe blindness, Near-total blindness
		Total Visual Impairment No light perception (NLP)	Total blindness

Visual acuity refers to best achievable acuity with correction.
Non-listed Snellen fractions may be classified by converting to the nearest decimal equivalent, e.g., 10/200 = 0.05, 6/30 = 0.20.
CF (count fingers) without designation of distance, may be classified to profound impairment.
HM (hand motion) without designation of distance, may be classified to near-total impairment.
Visual field measurements refer to the largest field diameter for a 1/100 white test object.

● **369 Blindness and low vision**

Excludes *correctable impaired vision due to refractive errors (367.0–367.9)*

Note: Visual impairment refers to a functional limitation of the eye (e.g., limited visual acuity or visual field). It should be distinguished from visual disability, indicating a limitation of the abilities of the individual (e.g., limited reading skills, vocational skills), and from visual handicap, indicating a limitation of personal and socioeconomic independence (e.g., limited mobility, limited employability).

The levels of impairment defined in the table after 369.9 are based on the recommendations of the WHO Study Group on Prevention of Blindness (Geneva, November 6–10, 1972; WHO Technical Report Series 518), and of the International Council of Ophthalmology (1976).

Note that definitions of blindness vary in different settings.

For international reporting, WHO defines blindness as profound impairment. This definition can be applied to blindness of one eye (369.1, 369.6) and to blindness of the individual (369.0).

For determination of benefits in the U.S.A., the definition of legal blindness as severe impairment is often used. This definition applies to blindness of the individual only.

● **369.0 Profound impairment, both eyes**

☐ **369.00 Impairment level not further specified**
Blindness:
NOS according to WHO definition
both eyes

☐ **369.01 Better eye: total impairment; lesser eye: total impairment**

☐ **369.02 Better eye: near-total impairment; lesser eye: not further specified**

☐ **369.03 Better eye: near-total impairment; lesser eye: total impairment**

☐ **369.04 Better eye: near-total impairment; lesser eye: near-total impairment**

☐ **369.05 Better eye: profound impairment; lesser eye: not further specified**

☐ **369.06 Better eye: profound impairment; lesser eye: total impairment**

☐ **369.07 Better eye: profound impairment; lesser eye: near-total impairment**

☐ **369.08 Better eye: profound impairment; lesser eye: profound impairment**

● **369.1 Moderate or severe impairment, better eye, profound impairment, lesser eye**

☐ **369.10 Impairment level not further specified**
Blindness, one eye, low vision, other eye

☐ **369.11 Better eye: severe impairment; lesser eye: blind, not further specified**

369.12 Better eye: severe impairment; lesser eye: total impairment

369.13 Better eye: severe impairment; lesser eye: near-total impairment

369.14 Better eye: severe impairment; lesser eye: profound impairment

☐ **369.15 Better eye: moderate impairment; lesser eye: blind, not further specified**

369.16 Better eye: moderate impairment; lesser eye: total impairment

369.17 Better eye: moderate impairment; lesser eye: near-total impairment

369.18 Better eye: moderate impairment; lesser eye: profound impairment

ICD-9-CM

300-399

Vol. 1

● 369.2 **Moderate or severe impairment, both eyes**

    ❑ 369.20 **Impairment level not further specified**
          Low vision, both eyes NOS

    ❑ 369.21 **Better eye: severe impairment; lesser eye: not further specified**

    369.22 **Better eye: severe impairment; lesser eye: severe impairment**

    ❑ 369.23 **Better eye: moderate impairment; lesser eye: not further specified**

    369.24 **Better eye: moderate impairment; lesser eye: severe impairment**

    369.25 **Better eye: moderate impairment; lesser eye: moderate impairment**

369.3 **Unqualified visual loss, both eyes**

    Excludes   *blindness NOS:*
          legal [U.S.A. definition] (369.4)
          WHO definition (369.00)

369.4 **Legal blindness, as defined in U.S.A.**
    Blindness NOS according to U.S.A. definition

    Excludes   *legal blindness with specification of impairment*
          level   (369.01–369.08,   369.11–369.14,
          369.21–369.22)

● 369.6 **Profound impairment, one eye**

    ❑ 369.60 **Impairment level not further specified**
          Blindness, one eye

    ❑ 369.61 **One eye: total impairment; other eye: not specified**

    369.62 **One eye: total impairment; other eye: near-normal vision**

    369.63 **One eye: total impairment; other eye: normal vision**

    ❑ 369.64 **One eye: near-total impairment; other eye: not specified**

    369.65 **One eye: near-total impairment; other eye: near-normal vision**

    369.66 **One eye: near-total impairment; other eye: normal vision**

    ❑ 369.67 **One eye: profound impairment; other eye: not specified**

    369.68 **One eye: profound impairment; other eye: near-normal vision**

    369.69 **One eye: profound impairment; other eye: normal vision**

● 369.7 **Moderate or severe impairment, one eye**

    ❑ 369.70 **Impairment level not further specified**
          Low vision, one eye

    ❑ 369.71 **One eye: severe impairment; other eye: not specified**

    369.72 **One eye: severe impairment; other eye: near-normal vision**

    369.73 **One eye: severe impairment; other eye: normal vision**

    ❑ 369.74 **One eye: moderate impairment; other eye: not specified**

    369.75 **One eye: moderate impairment; other eye: near-normal vision**

    369.76 **One eye: moderate impairment; other eye: normal vision**

369.8 **Unqualified visual loss, one eye**

❑ 369.9 **Unspecified visual loss**

● 370.0 **Corneal ulcer**

    Excludes   *that due to vitamin A deficiency (264.3)*

    ❑ 370.00 **Corneal ulcer, unspecified**

    370.01 **Marginal corneal ulcer**

    370.02 **Ring corneal ulcer**

    370.03 **Central corneal ulcer**

    370.04 **Hypopyon ulcer**
          Serpiginous ulcer

    370.05 **Mycotic corneal ulcer**

    370.06 **Perforated corneal ulcer**

    370.07 **Mooren's ulcer**

● 370.2 **Superficial keratitis without conjunctivitis**

    Excludes   *dendritic [herpes simplex] keratitis (054.42)*

    ❑ 370.20 **Superficial keratitis, unspecified**

    370.21 **Punctate keratitis**
          Thygeson's superficial punctate keratitis

Item 6-9 An infected ulcer is usually called a **serpiginous** or **hypopyon** ulcer which is a pus sac in the anterior chamber of the eye.
Marginal ulcers are usually asymptomatic, not primary, and are often superficial and simple. More severe marginal ulcers spread to form a ring ulcer. **Ring** ulcers can extend around the entire corneal periphery.
Central corneal ulcers develop when there is an abrasion to the epithelium and an infection develops in the eroded area.
The **pyocyaneal** ulcer is the most serious corneal infection, which, if left untreated, can lead to loss of the eye.

Marginal (catarrhal) ulcer   Ring ulcer   Central corneal ulcer   Rosacea ulcer   Mooren's (rodent) ulcer

Figure 6-7   Corneal ulcers: marginal, ring, central corneal, rosacea, and Mooren's.

370.22 Macular keratitis
Keratitis:
areolar
nummular
stellate
striate

370.23 Filamentary keratitis

370.24 Photokeratitis
Snow blindness
Welders' keratitis

● **370.3 Certain types of keratoconjunctivitis**

370.31 Phlyctenular keratoconjunctivitis
Phlyctenulosis

Use additional code for any associated tuberculosis (017.3)

370.32 Limbal and corneal involvement in vernal conjunctivitis

Use additional code for vernal conjunctivitis (372.13)

❏ **370.33 Keratoconjunctivitis sicca, not specified as Sjögren's**
Excludes   *Sjögren's syndrome (710.2)*

370.34 Exposure keratoconjunctivitis

370.35 Neurotrophic keratoconjunctivitis

● **370.4 Other and unspecified keratoconjunctivitis**

❏ **370.40 Keratoconjunctivitis, unspecified**
Superficial keratitis with conjunctivitis NOS

● **370.44 *Keratitis or keratoconjunctivitis in exanthema***

Code first underlying condition (050.0–052.9)
Excludes   *herpes simplex (054.43)*
herpes zoster (053.21)
measles (055.71)

❏ **370.49 Other**
Excludes   *epidemic keratoconjunctivitis (077.1)*

● **370.5 Interstitial and deep keratitis**

❏ **370.50 Interstitial keratitis, unspecified**

370.52 Diffuse interstitial keratitis
Cogan's syndrome

370.54 Sclerosing keratitis

370.55 Corneal abscess

❏ **370.59 Other**
Excludes   *disciform herpes simplex keratitis (054.43)*
syphilitic keratitis (090.3)

● **370.6 Corneal neovascularization**

❏ **370.60 Corneal neovascularization, unspecified**

370.61 Localized vascularization of cornea

370.62 Pannus (corneal)

370.63 Deep vascularization of cornea

370.64 Ghost vessels (corneal)

❏ **370.8 Other forms of keratitis**

❏ **370.9 Unspecified keratitis**

● **371 Corneal opacity and other disorders of cornea**

● **371.0 Corneal scars and opacities**
Excludes   *that due to vitamin A deficiency (264.6)*

❏ **371.00 Corneal opacity, unspecified**
Corneal scar NOS

371.01 Minor opacity of cornea
Corneal nebula

371.02 Peripheral opacity of cornea
Corneal macula not interfering with central vision

371.03 Central opacity of cornea
Corneal:
leucoma interfering with central vision
macula interfering with central vision

371.04 Adherent leucoma

● **371.05 *Phthisical cornea***

Code first underlying tuberculosis (017.3)

● **371.1 Corneal pigmentations and deposits**

❏ **371.10 Corneal deposit, unspecified**

371.11 Anterior pigmentations
Stähli's lines

371.12 Stromal pigmentations
Hematocornea

371.13 Posterior pigmentations
Krukenberg spindle

371.14 Kayser-Fleischer ring

❏ **371.15 Other deposits associated with metabolic disorders**

371.16 Argentous deposits

● **371.2 Corneal edema**

❏ **371.20 Corneal edema, unspecified**

371.21 Idiopathic corneal edema

371.22 Secondary corneal edema

371.23 Bullous keratopathy

371.24 Corneal edema due to wearing of contact lenses

● **371.3 Changes of corneal membranes**

❏ **371.30 Corneal membrane change, unspecified**

371.31 Folds and rupture of Bowman's membrane

371.32 Folds in Descemet's membrane

371.33 Rupture in Descemet's membrane

● **371.4 Corneal degenerations**

❏ **371.40 Corneal degeneration, unspecified**

371.41 Senile corneal changes
Arcus senilis   Hassall-Henle bodies

371.42 Recurrent erosion of cornea
Excludes   *Mooren's ulcer (370.07)*

371.43 Band-shaped keratopathy

❏ **371.44 Other calcerous degenerations of cornea**

371.45 Keratomalacia NOS
Excludes   *that due to vitamin A deficiency (264.4)*

371.46 Nodular degeneration of cornea
Salzmann's nodular dystrophy

371.48 Peripheral degenerations of cornea
Marginal degeneration of cornea [Terrien's]

❏ **371.49 Other**
Discrete colliquative keratopathy

● **371.5 Hereditary corneal dystrophies**

❏ **371.50 Corneal dystrophy, unspecified**

371.51 Juvenile epithelial corneal dystrophy

❏ **371.52 Other anterior corneal dystrophies**
Corneal dystrophy:
microscopic cystic
ring-like

371.53 Granular corneal dystrophy

371.54 Lattice corneal dystrophy

ICD-9-CM

300-399

Vol. 1

Figure 6–8   Keratoconus. (From Adler FH: Textbook of Ophthalmology, 7th ed. Philadelphia, WB Saunders, 1962, p 223.)

Item 6-10 Keratoconus is corneal degeneration that begins in childhood and gradually forms a cone at the apex of the eye even though the intraocular pressure is normal. The apex of the cornea becomes increasingly thin and can rupture, resulting in scarring.

    371.55   Macular corneal dystrophy

    371.56   Other stromal corneal dystrophies
               Crystalline corneal dystrophy

    371.57   Endothelial corneal dystrophy
               Combined corneal dystrophy
               Cornea guttata
               Fuchs' endothelial dystrophy

    371.58   Other posterior corneal dystrophies
               Polymorphous corneal dystrophy

● 371.6   Keratoconus

    371.60   Keratoconus, unspecified

    371.61   Keratoconus, stable condition

    371.62   Keratoconus, acute hydrops

● 371.7   Other corneal deformities

    371.70   Corneal deformity, unspecified

    371.71   Corneal ectasia

    371.72   Descemetocele

    371.73   Corneal staphyloma

● 371.8   Other corneal disorders

    371.81   Corneal anesthesia and hypoesthesia

    371.82   Corneal disorder due to contact lens

      Excludes *corneal edema due to contact lens (371.24)*

    371.89   Other

  371.9   Unspecified corneal disorder

● 372   Disorders of conjunctiva
      Excludes *keratoconjunctivitis (370.3–370.4)*

● 372.0   Acute conjunctivitis

    372.00   Acute conjunctivitis, unspecified

    372.01   Serous conjunctivitis, except viral

      Excludes *viral conjunctivitis NOS (077.9)*

    372.02   Acute follicular conjunctivitis
               Conjunctival folliculosis NOS

      Excludes *conjunctivitis:*
           adenoviral (acute follicular) (077.3)
           epidemic hemorrhagic (077.4)
           inclusion (077.0)
           Newcastle (077.8)
        epidemic keratoconjunctivitis (077.1)
        pharyngoconjunctival fever (077.2)

    372.03   Other mucopurulent conjunctivitis
               Catarrhal conjunctivitis

      Excludes *blennorrhea neonatorum (gonococcal) (098.40)*
          neonatal conjunctivitis (771.6)
          ophthalmia neonatorum NOS (771.6)

    372.04   Pseudomembranous conjunctivitis
               Membranous conjunctivitis

      Excludes *diphtheritic conjunctivitis (032.81)*

    372.05   Acute atopic conjunctivitis

● 372.1   Chronic conjunctivitis

    372.10   Chronic conjunctivitis, unspecified

    372.11   Simple chronic conjunctivitis

    372.12   Chronic follicular conjunctivitis

    372.13   Vernal conjunctivitis

    372.14   Other chronic allergic conjunctivitis

  ● 372.15   *Parasitic conjunctivitis*

      Code first underlying disease, as:
        filariasis (125.0–125.9)
        mucocutaneous leishmaniasis (085.5)

● 372.2   Blepharoconjunctivitis

    372.20   Blepharoconjunctivitis, unspecified

    372.21   Angular blepharoconjunctivitis

    372.22   Contact blepharoconjunctivitis

● 372.3   Other and unspecified conjunctivitis

    372.30   Conjunctivitis, unspecified

  ● 372.31   *Rosacea conjunctivitis*

      Code first underlying rosacea dermatitis (695.3)

  ● 372.33   *Conjunctivitis in mucocutaneous disease*

      Code first underlying disease, as:
        erythema multiforme (695.1)
        Reiter's disease (099.3)

      Excludes *ocular pemphigoid (694.61)*

    372.39   Other

Figure 6–9   Pterygium. (From Adler FH: Textbook of Ophthalmology, 7th ed. Philadelphia, WB Saunders, 1962, p 194.)

Item 6-11 Pterygium is Greek for batlike. The condition is characterized by a membrane that extends from the limbus to the center of the cornea and resembles a wing.

● 372.4   Pterygium

    | Excludes | *pseudopterygium (372.52)*

    ❑ 372.40   Pterygium, unspecified

       372.41   Peripheral pterygium, stationary

       372.42   Peripheral pterygium, progressive

       372.43   Central pterygium

       372.44   Double pterygium

       372.45   Recurrent pterygium

● 372.5   Conjunctival degenerations and deposits

    ❑ 372.50   Conjunctival degeneration, unspecified

       372.51   Pinguecula

       372.52   Pseudopterygium

       372.53   Conjunctival xerosis

    | Excludes | *conjunctival xerosis due to vitamin A deficiency (264.0, 264.1, 264.7)*

       372.54   Conjunctival concretions

       372.55   Conjunctival pigmentations
            Conjunctival argyrosis

       372.56   Conjunctival deposits

● 372.6   Conjunctival scars

       372.61   Granuloma of conjunctiva

       372.62   Localized adhesions and strands of conjunctiva

       372.63   Symblepharon
            Extensive adhesions of conjunctiva

       372.64   Scarring of conjunctiva
            Contraction of eye socket (after enucleation)

● 372.7   Conjunctival vascular disorders and cysts

       372.71   Hyperemia of conjunctiva

       372.72   Conjunctival hemorrhage
            Hyposphagma
            Subconjunctival hemorrhage

       372.73   Conjunctival edema
            Chemosis of conjunctiva
            Subconjunctival edema

       372.74   Vascular abnormalities of conjunctiva
            Aneurysm(ata) of conjunctiva

       372.75   Conjunctival cysts

●❑ 372.8   Other disorders of conjunctiva

       372.81   Conjunctivochalasis

    ❑ 372.89   Other disorders of conjunctiva

❑ 372.9   Unspecified disorder of conjunctiva

Figure 6-10   Ulcerating blepharitis caused by a staphylococcal infection. (From Pau H: Differential Diagnosis of Eye Diseases. Philadelphia, WB Saunders, 1978, p 106.)

Item 6-12 Blepharitis is a common condition in which the lid is swollen and yellow scaling and conjunctivitis develop. Usually the hair on the scalp and brow is involved.

Item 6-13 Hordeolum is the inflammation of the sebaceous gland of the eyelid.

● 373   Inflammation of eyelids

    ● 373.0   Blepharitis

       | Excludes | *blepharoconjunctivitis (372.20–372.22)*

       ❑ 373.00   Blepharitis, unspecified

          373.01   Ulcerative blepharitis

          373.02   Squamous blepharitis

    ● 373.1   Hordeolum and other deep inflammation of eyelid

          373.11   Hordeolum externum
               Hordeolum NOS
               Stye

          373.12   Hordeolum internum
               Infection of meibomian gland

          373.13   Abscess of eyelid
               Furuncle of eyelid

      373.2   Chalazion
          Meibomian (gland) cyst

      | Excludes | *infected meibomian gland (373.12)*

    ● 373.3   Noninfectious dermatoses of eyelid

          373.31   Eczematous dermatitis of eyelid

          373.32   Contact and allergic dermatitis of eyelid

          373.33   Xeroderma of eyelid

          373.34   Discoid lupus erythematosus of eyelid

    ● 373.4   *Infective dermatitis of eyelid of types resulting in deformity*

       Code first underlying disease, as:
          leprosy (030.0–030.9)
          lupus vulgaris (tuberculous) (017.0)
          yaws (102.0–102.9)

    ●❑ 373.5   *Other infective dermatitis of eyelid*

       Code first underlying disease, as:
          actinomycosis (039.3)
          impetigo (684)
          mycotic dermatitis (110.0–111.9)
          vaccinia (051.0)
             postvaccination (999.0)

      | Excludes | *herpes:*
               simplex (054.41)
               zoster (053.20)

    ● 373.6   *Parasitic infestation of eyelid*

       Code first underlying disease, as:
          leishmaniasis (085.0–085.9)
          loiasis (125.2)
          onchocerciasis (125.3)
          pediculosis (132.0)

❑ 373.8   Other inflammations of eyelids

❑ 373.9   Unspecified inflammation of eyelid

ICD-9-CM

300-399

Vol. 1

Figure 6-11 **A.** A 72-year-old male with senile ectropion on the left and postsurgical correction on the right. **B.** Entropion in a 6-month-old male infant. (From Pau H: Differential Diagnosis of Eye Diseases. Philadelphia, WB Saunders, 1978, p 90.)

● **374 Other disorders of eyelids**

  ● **374.0 Entropion and trichiasis of eyelid**

     □ **374.00 Entropion, unspecified**

     374.01 Senile entropion

     374.02 Mechanical entropion

     374.03 Spastic entropion

     374.04 Cicatricial entropion

     374.05 Trichiasis without entropion

  ● **374.1 Ectropion**

     □ **374.10 Ectropion, unspecified**

     374.11 Senile ectropion

     374.12 Mechanical ectropion

     374.13 Spastic ectropion

     374.14 Cicatricial ectropion

  ● **374.2 Lagophthalmos**

     □ **374.20 Lagophthalmos, unspecified**

     374.21 Paralytic lagophthalmos

     374.22 Mechanical lagophthalmos

     374.23 Cicatricial lagophthalmos

  ● **374.3 Ptosis of eyelid**

     □ **374.30 Ptosis of eyelid, unspecified**

     374.31 Paralytic ptosis

     374.32 Myogenic ptosis

     374.33 Mechanical ptosis

     374.34 Blepharochalasis
           Pseudoptosis

● **374.4 Other disorders affecting eyelid function**

    | Excludes | blepharoclonus (333.81) |

        blepharospasm (333.81)
        facial nerve palsy (351.0)
        third nerve palsy or paralysis (378.51–378.52)
        tic (psychogenic) (307.20–307.23)
          organic (333.3)

     374.41 Lid retraction or lag

     374.43 Abnormal innervation syndrome
         Jaw-blinking
         Paradoxical facial movements

     374.44 Sensory disorders

     □ **374.45 Other sensorimotor disorders**
         Deficient blink reflex

     374.46 Blepharophimosis
         Ankyloblepharon

● **374.5 Degenerative disorders of eyelid and periocular area**

     □ **374.50 Degenerative disorder of eyelid, unspecified**

     374.51 *Xanthelasma*
         Xanthoma (planum) (tuberosum) of eyelid

       Code first underlying condition (272.0–272.9)

     374.52 Hyperpigmentation of eyelid
         Chloasma
         Dyspigmentation

     374.53 Hypopigmentation of eyelid
         Vitiligo of eyelid

     374.54 Hypertrichosis of eyelid

     374.55 Hypotrichosis of eyelid
         Madarosis of eyelid

     □ **374.56 Other degenerative disorders of skin affecting eyelid**

● **374.8 Other disorders of eyelid**

     374.81 Hemorrhage of eyelid

    | Excludes | *black eye (921.0)* |

     374.82 Edema of eyelid
         Hyperemia of eyelid

     374.83 Elephantiasis of eyelid

     374.84 Cysts of eyelids
         Sebaceous cyst of eyelid

     374.85 Vascular anomalies of eyelid

     374.86 Retained foreign body of eyelid

     374.87 Dermatochalasis

     □ **374.89 Other disorders of eyelid**

□ **374.9 Unspecified disorder of eyelid**

Figure 6-12 Lacrimal apparatus. (From Buck CJ: Step-by-Step Medical Coding, 3rd ed. Philadelphia, WB Saunders, 2000, p. 205.)

   ◀ **New**   ◀▥ **Revised**   ● **Not a Principal Diagnosis**   ● **Use Additional Digit(s)**   □ **Nonspecific Code**

● 375 Disorders of lacrimal system

  ● 375.0 Dacryoadenitis

    ❏ 375.00 Dacryoadenitis, unspecified

    375.01 Acute dacryoadenitis

    375.02 Chronic dacryoadenitis

    375.03 Chronic enlargement of lacrimal gland

  ● 375.1 Other disorders of lacrimal gland

    ❏ 375.11 Dacryops

    ❏ 375.12 Other lacrimal cysts and cystic degeneration

    375.13 Primary lacrimal atrophy

    375.14 Secondary lacrimal atrophy

    ❏ 375.15 Tear film insufficiency, unspecified
              Dry eye syndrome

    375.16 Dislocation of lacrimal gland

  ● 375.2 Epiphora

    ❏ 375.20 Epiphora, unspecified as to cause

    375.21 Epiphora due to excess lacrimation

    375.22 Epiphora due to insufficient drainage

  ● 375.3 Acute and unspecified inflammation of lacrimal passages

    Excludes *neonatal dacryocystitis (771.6)*

    ❏ 375.30 Dacryocystitis, unspecified

    375.31 Acute canaliculitis, lacrimal

    375.32 Acute dacryocystitis
              Acute peridacryocystitis

    375.33 Phlegmonous dacryocystitis

  ● 375.4 Chronic inflammation of lacrimal passages

    375.41 Chronic canaliculitis

    375.42 Chronic dacryocystitis

    375.43 Lacrimal mucocele

  ● 375.5 Stenosis and insufficiency of lacrimal passages

    375.51 Eversion of lacrimal punctum

    375.52 Stenosis of lacrimal punctum

    375.53 Stenosis of lacrimal canaliculi

    375.54 Stenosis of lacrimal sac

    375.55 Obstruction of nasolacrimal duct, neonatal

    Excludes *congenital anomaly of nasolacrimal duct (743.65)*

    375.56 Stenosis of nasolacrimal duct, acquired

    375.57 Dacryolith

  ● 375.6 Other changes of lacrimal passages

    375.61 Lacrimal fistula

    ❏ 375.69 Other

  ● 375.8 Other disorders of lacrimal system

    375.81 Granuloma of lacrimal passages

    ❏ 375.89 Other

  ❏ 375.9 Unspecified disorder of lacrimal system

● 376 Disorders of the orbit

  ● 376.0 Acute inflammation of orbit

    ❏ 376.00 Acute inflammation of orbit, unspecified

    376.01 Orbital cellulitis
              Abscess of orbit

    376.02 Orbital periostitis

    376.03 Orbital osteomyelitis

    376.04 Tenonitis

  ● 376.1 Chronic inflammatory disorders of orbit

    ❏ 376.10 Chronic inflammation of orbit, unspecified

    376.11 Orbital granuloma
              Pseudotumor (inflammatory) of orbit

    376.12 Orbital myositis

    ● 376.13 *Parasitic infestation of orbit*

          Code first underlying disease, as:
              hydatid infestation of orbit (122.3, 122.6, 122.9)
              myiasis of orbit (134.0)

  ● 376.2 *Endocrine exophthalmos*

    Code first underlying thyroid disorder (242.0–242.9)

    ● 376.21 *Thyrotoxic exophthalmos*

    ● 376.22 *Exophthalmic ophthalmoplegia*

  ● 376.3 Other exophthalmic conditions

    ❏ 376.30 Exophthalmos, unspecified

    376.31 Constant exophthalmos

    376.32 Orbital hemorrhage

    376.33 Orbital edema or congestion

    376.34 Intermittent exophthalmos

    376.35 Pulsating exophthalmos

    376.36 Lateral displacement of globe

  ● 376.4 Deformity of orbit

    ❏ 376.40 Deformity of orbit, unspecified

    376.41 Hypertelorism of orbit

    376.42 Exostosis of orbit

    376.43 Local deformities due to bone disease

    376.44 Orbital deformities associated with craniofacial deformities

    376.45 Atrophy of orbit

    376.46 Enlargement of orbit

    376.47 Deformity due to trauma or surgery

  ● 376.5 Enophthalmos

    ❏ 376.50 Enophthalmos, unspecified as to cause

    376.51 Enophthalmos due to atrophy of orbital tissue

    376.52 Enophthalmos due to trauma or surgery

  376.6 Retained (old) foreign body following penetrating wound of orbit
          Retrobulbar foreign body

  ● 376.8 Other orbital disorders

    376.81 Orbital cysts
          Encephalocele of orbit

    376.82 Myopathy of extraocular muscles

    ❏ 376.89 Other

  ❏ 376.9 Unspecified disorder of orbit

● 377 Disorders of optic nerve and visual pathways

  ● 377.0 Papilledema

    ❏ 377.00 Papilledema, unspecified

    377.01 Papilledema associated with increased intracranial pressure

    377.02 Papilledema associated with decreased ocular pressure

    377.03 Papilledema associated with retinal disorder

    377.04 Foster-Kennedy syndrome

ICD-9-CM

300-399

Vol. 1

● **377.1 Optic atrophy**

❑ **377.10** Optic atrophy, unspecified

377.11 Primary optic atrophy

　Excludes　*neurosyphilitic optic atrophy (094.84)*

377.12 Postinflammatory optic atrophy

377.13 Optic atrophy associated with retinal dystrophies

377.14 Glaucomatous atrophy [cupping] of optic disc

377.15 Partial optic atrophy
　　Temporal pallor of optic disc

377.16 Hereditary optic atrophy
　　Optic atrophy:
　　　dominant hereditary
　　　Leber's

● **377.2 Other disorders of optic disc**

377.21 Drusen of optic disc

377.22 Crater-like holes of optic disc

377.23 Coloboma of optic disc

377.24 Pseudopapilledema

● **377.3 Optic neuritis**

　Excludes　*meningococcal optic neuritis (036.81)*

❑ **377.30** Optic neuritis, unspecified

377.31 Optic papillitis

377.32 Retrobulbar neuritis (acute)

　Excludes　*syphilitic retrobulbar neuritis (094.85)*

377.33 Nutritional optic neuropathy

377.34 Toxic optic neuropathy
　　Toxic amblyopia

❑ **377.39** Other

　Excludes　*ischemic optic neuropathy (377.41)*

● **377.4 Other disorders of optic nerve**

377.41 Ischemic optic neuropathy

377.42 Hemorrhage in optic nerve sheaths

❑ **377.49** Other
　　Compression of optic nerve

● **377.5 Disorders of optic chiasm**

377.51 Associated with pituitary neoplasms and disorders

❑ **377.52** Associated with other neoplasms

377.53 Associated with vascular disorders

377.54 Associated with inflammatory disorders

● **377.6 Disorders of other visual pathways**

377.61 Associated with neoplasms

377.62 Associated with vascular disorders

377.63 Associated with inflammatory disorders

● **377.7 Disorders of visual cortex**

　Excludes　*visual:*
　　agnosia (368.16)
　　hallucinations (368.16)
　　halos (368.15)

377.71 Associated with neoplasms

377.72 Associated with vascular disorders

377.73 Associated with inflammatory disorders

377.75 Cortical blindness

❑ **377.9** Unspecified disorder of optic nerve and visual pathways

● **378 Strabismus and other disorders of binocular eye movements**

　Excludes　*nystagmus and other irregular eye movements (379.50–379.59)*

● **378.0 Esotropia**
　Convergent concomitant strabismus

　Excludes　*intermittent esotropia (378.20–378.22)*

❑ **378.00** Esotropia, unspecified

378.01 Monocular esotropia

378.02 Monocular esotropia with A pattern

378.03 Monocular esotropia with V pattern

❑ **378.04** Monocular esotropia with other noncomitancies
　　Monocular esotropia with X or Y pattern

378.05 Alternating esotropia

378.06 Alternating esotropia with A pattern

378.07 Alternating esotropia with V pattern

❑ **378.08** Alternating esotropia with other noncomitancies
　　Alternating esotropia with X or Y pattern

● **378.1 Exotropia**
　Divergent concomitant strabismus

　Excludes　*intermittent exotropia (378.20, 378.23–378.24)*

❑ **378.10** Exotropia, unspecified

378.11 Monocular exotropia

378.12 Monocular exotropia with A pattern

378.13 Monocular exotropia with V pattern

❑ **378.14** Monocular exotropia with other noncomitancies
　　Monocular exotropia with X or Y pattern

378.15 Alternating exotropia

378.16 Alternating exotropia with A pattern

378.17 Alternating exotropia with V pattern

❑ **378.18** Alternating exotropia with other noncomitancies
　　Alternating exotropia with X or Y pattern

● **378.2 Intermittent heterotropia**

　Excludes　*vertical heterotropia (intermittent) (378.31)*

❑ **378.20** Intermittent heterotropia, unspecified
　　Intermittent:
　　　esotropia NOS
　　　exotropia NOS

378.21 Intermittent esotropia, monocular

378.22 Intermittent esotropia, alternating

378.23 Intermittent exotropia, monocular

378.24 Intermittent exotropia, alternating

● **378.3 Other and unspecified heterotropia**

❑ **378.30** Heterotropia, unspecified

378.31 Hypertropia
　　Vertical heterotropia (constant) (intermittent)

378.32 Hypotropia

378.33 Cyclotropia

378.34 Monofixation syndrome
　　Microtropia

378.35 Accommodative component in esotropia

● **378.4 Heterophoria**

❑ **378.40** Heterophoria, unspecified

378.41 Esophoria

378.42 Exophoria

378.43 Vertical heterophoria

378.44 Cyclophoria

378.45 Alternating hyperphoria

● 378.5 Paralytic strabismus

❑ 378.50 Paralytic strabismus, unspecified

378.51 Third or oculomotor nerve palsy, partial

378.52 Third or oculomotor nerve palsy, total

378.53 Fourth or trochlear nerve palsy

378.54 Sixth or abducens nerve palsy

378.55 External ophthalmoplegia

378.56 Total ophthalmoplegia

● 378.6 Mechanical strabismus

❑ 378.60 Mechanical strabismus, unspecified

378.61 Brown's (tendon) sheath syndrome

❑ 378.62 Mechanical strabismus from other musculo-fascial disorders

❑ 378.63 Limited duction associated with other conditions

● 378.7 Other specified strabismus

378.71 Duane's syndrome

378.72 Progressive external ophthalmoplegia

❑ 378.73 Strabismus in other neuromuscular disorders

● 378.8 Other disorders of binocular eye movements

| Excludes | nystagmus (379.50–379.56) |

378.81 Palsy of conjugate gaze

378.82 Spasm of conjugate gaze

378.83 Convergence insufficiency or palsy

378.84 Convergence excess or spasm

378.85 Anomalies of divergence

378.86 Internuclear ophthalmoplegia

❑ 378.87 Other dissociated deviation of eye movements
Skew deviation

❑ 378.9 Unspecified disorder of eye movements
Ophthalmoplegia NOS
Strabismus NOS

● 379 Other disorders of eye

● 379.0 Scleritis and episcleritis

| Excludes | syphilitic episcleritis (095.0) |

❑ 379.00 Scleritis, unspecified
Episcleritis NOS

379.01 Episcleritis periodica fugax

379.02 Nodular episcleritis

379.03 Anterior scleritis

379.04 Scleromalacia perforans

379.05 Scleritis with corneal involvement
Scleroperikeratitis

379.06 Brawny scleritis

379.07 Posterior scleritis
Sclerotenonitis

❑ 379.09 Other
Scleral abscess

● 379.1 Other disorders of sclera

| Excludes | blue sclera (743.47) |

379.11 Scleral ectasia
Scleral staphyloma NOS

379.12 Staphyloma posticum

379.13 Equatorial staphyloma

379.14 Anterior staphyloma, localized

379.15 Ring staphyloma

❑ 379.16 Other degenerative disorders of sclera

❑ 379.19 Other

● 379.2 Disorders of vitreous body

379.21 Vitreous degeneration
Vitreous:
cavitation
detachment
liquefaction

379.22 Crystalline deposits in vitreous
Asteroid hyalitis
Synchysis scintillans

379.23 Vitreous hemorrhage

❑ 379.24 Other vitreous opacities
Vitreous floaters

379.25 Vitreous membranes and strands

379.26 Vitreous prolapse

❑ 379.29 Other disorders of vitreous

| Excludes | vitreous abscess (360.04) |

● 379.3 Aphakia and other disorders of lens

| Excludes | after-cataract (366.50–366.53) |

379.31 Aphakia

| Excludes | cataract extraction status (V45.61) |

379.32 Subluxation of lens

379.33 Anterior dislocation of lens

379.34 Posterior dislocation of lens

❑ 379.39 Other disorders of lens

● 379.4 Anomalies of pupillary function

❑ 379.40 Abnormal pupillary function, unspecified

379.41 Anisocoria

379.42 Miosis (persistent), not due to miotics

379.43 Mydriasis (persistent), not due to mydriatics

379.45 Argyll Robertson pupil, atypical
Argyll Robertson phenomenon or pupil, nonsyphilitic

| Excludes | Argyll Robertson pupil (syphilitic) (094.89) |

379.46 Tonic pupillary reaction
Adie's pupil or syndrome

❑ 379.49 Other
Hippus
Pupillary paralysis

● 379.5 Nystagmus and other irregular eye movements

❑ 379.50 Nystagmus, unspecified

379.51 Congenital nystagmus

379.52 Latent nystagmus

379.53 Visual deprivation nystagmus

379.54 Nystagmus associated with disorders of the vestibular system

379.55 Dissociated nystagmus

❑ 379.56 Other forms of nystagmus

379.57 Deficiencies of saccadic eye movements
Abnormal optokinetic response

ICD-9-CM

300-399

Vol. 1

379.58   Deficiencies of smooth pursuit movements

❏379.59   Other irregularities of eye movements
Opsoclonus

❏379.8   **Other specified disorders of eye and adnexa**

●379.9   **Unspecified disorder of eye and adnexa**

❏379.90   Disorder of eye, unspecified

379.91   Pain in or around eye

379.92   Swelling or mass of eye

379.93   Redness or discharge of eye

❏379.99   Other ill-defined disorders of eye

Excludes   *blurred vision NOS (368.8)*

DISEASES OF THE EAR AND MASTOID PROCESS (380–389)

●380   **Disorders of external ear**

●380.0   **Perichondritis and chondritis of pinna**   ◀▥
Chondritis of auricle   ◀
Perichondritis of auricle

❏380.00   Perichondritis of pinna, unspecified

380.01   Acute perichondritis of pinna

380.02   Chronic perichondritis of pinna

380.03   Chondritis of pinna   ◀

●380.1   **Infective otitis externa**

❏380.10   Infective otitis externa, unspecified
Otitis externa (acute):
NOS
circumscribed
diffuse
hemorrhagica
infective NOS

380.11   Acute infection of pinna

Excludes   *furuncular otitis externa (680.0)*

380.12   Acute swimmers' ear
Beach ear
Tank ear

●❏380.13   *Other acute infections of external ear*

Code first underlying disease, as:
erysipelas (035)
impetigo (684)
seborrheic dermatitis (690.10–690.18)

Excludes   *herpes simplex (054.73)*
herpes zoster (053.71)

380.14   Malignant otitis externa

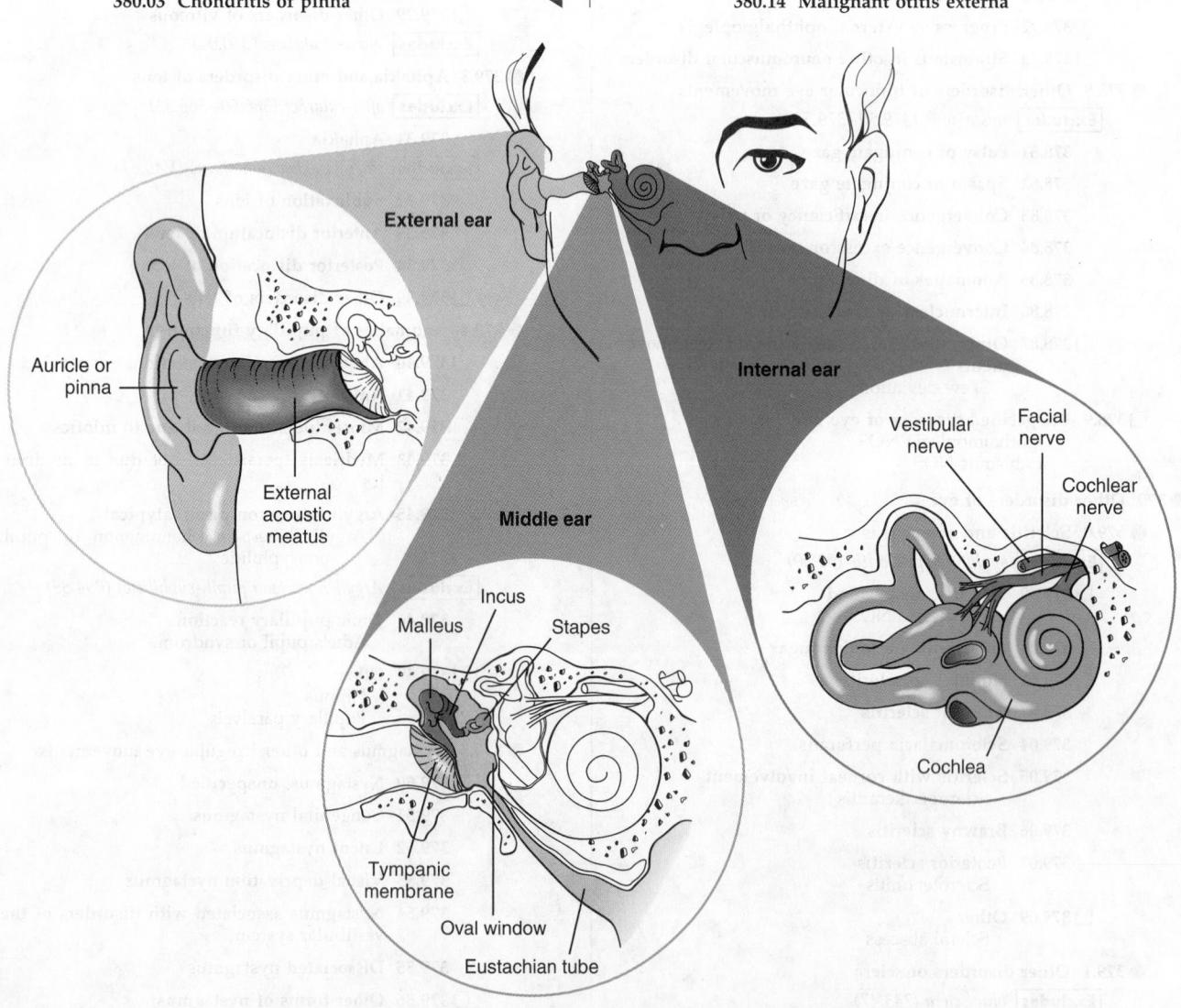

Figure 6-13   Auditory system. (From Buck CJ: Step-by-Step Medical Coding, 2005 ed. Philadelphia, WBS, 2005.)

● **380.15   Chronic mycotic otitis externa**

     Code first underlying disease, as:
        aspergillosis (117.3)
        otomycosis NOS (111.9)

   Excludes *candidal otitis externa (112.82)*

❑ **380.16 Other chronic infective otitis externa**
     Chronic infective otitis externa NOS

● **380.2 Other otitis externa**

  380.21 Cholesteatoma of external ear
     Keratosis obturans of external ear (canal)

  Excludes *cholesteatoma NOS (385.30–385.35)*
         postmastoidectomy (383.32)

❑ **380.22 Other acute otitis externa**
     Acute otitis externa:
       actinic
       chemical
       contact
       eczematoid
       reactive

❑ **380.23 Other chronic otitis externa**
     Chronic otitis externa NOS

● **380.3 Noninfectious disorders of pinna**

❑ **380.30 Disorder of pinna, unspecified**

  380.31 Hematoma of auricle or pinna

  380.32 Acquired deformities of auricle or pinna

  Excludes *cauliflower ear (738.7)*

❑ **380.39 Other**

  Excludes *gouty tophi of ear (274.81)*

  380.4 Impacted cerumen
     Wax in ear

● **380.5 Acquired stenosis of external ear canal**
     Collapse of external ear canal

❑ **380.50 Acquired stenosis of external ear canal, unspecified as to cause**

  380.51 Secondary to trauma

  380.52 Secondary to surgery

  380.53 Secondary to inflammation

● **380.8 Other disorders of external ear**

  380.81 Exostosis of external ear canal

❑ **380.89 Other**

❑ **380.9 Unspecified disorder of external ear**

● **381 Nonsuppurative otitis media and Eustachian tube disorders**

● **381.0 Acute nonsuppurative otitis media**
     Acute tubotympanic catarrh
     Otitis media, acute or subacute:
       catarrhal
       exudative
       transudative
       with effusion

  Excludes *otitic barotrauma (993.0)*

❑ **381.00 Acute nonsuppurative otitis media, unspecified**

  381.01 Acute serous otitis media
     Acute or subacute secretory otitis media

  381.02 Acute mucoid otitis media
     Acute or subacute seromucinous otitis media
     Blue drum syndrome

  381.03 Acute sanguinous otitis media

  381.04 Acute allergic serous otitis media

  381.05 Acute allergic mucoid otitis media

  381.06 Acute allergic sanguinous otitis media

● **381.1 Chronic serous otitis media**
     Chronic tubotympanic catarrh

  381.10 Chronic serous otitis media, simple or unspecified

❑ **381.19 Other**
     Serosanguinous chronic otitis media

● **381.2 Chronic mucoid otitis media**
     Glue ear

  Excludes *adhesive middle ear disease (385.10–385.19)*

  381.20 Chronic mucoid otitis media, simple or unspecified

❑ **381.29 Other**
     Mucosanguinous chronic otitis media

❑ **381.3 Other and unspecified chronic nonsuppurative otitis media**

    Otitis media, chronic: Otitis media, chronic:
      allergic   seromucinous
      exudative   transudative
      secretory   with effusion

❑ **381.4 Nonsuppurative otitis media, not specified as acute or chronic**

    Otitis media: Otitis media:
      allergic   seromucinous
      catarrhal   serous
      exudative   transudative
      mucoid   with effusion
      secretory

● **381.5 Eustachian salpingitis**

❑ **381.50 Eustachian salpingitis, unspecified**

  381.51 Acute Eustachian salpingitis

  381.52 Chronic Eustachian salpingitis

● **381.6 Obstruction of Eustachian tube**
     Stenosis of Eustachian tube
     Stricture of Eustachian tube

❑ **381.60 Obstruction of Eustachian tube, unspecified**

  381.61 Osseous obstruction of Eustachian tube
     Obstruction of Eustachian tube from cholesteatoma, polyp, or other osseous lesion

  381.62 Intrinsic cartilaginous obstruction of Eustachian tube

  381.63 Extrinsic cartilaginous obstruction of Eustachian tube
     Compression of Eustachian tube

  381.7 Patulous Eustachian tube

● **381.8 Other disorders of Eustachian tube**

  381.81 Dysfunction of Eustachian tube

❑ **381.89 Other**

❑ **381.9 Unspecified Eustachian tube disorder**

● **382 Suppurative and unspecified otitis media**

● **382.0 Acute suppurative otitis media**
     Otitis media, acute:
       necrotizing NOS
       purulent

  382.00 Acute suppurative otitis media without spontaneous rupture of ear drum

  382.01 Acute suppurative otitis media with spontaneous rupture of ear drum

ICD-9-CM

**300-
399**

Vol. 1

●❑ 382.02 *Acute suppurative otitis media in diseases classified elsewhere*

> *Code first underlying disease, as:*
> influenza (487.8)
> scarlet fever (034.1)

> **Excludes** *postmeasles otitis (055.2)*

382.1 **Chronic tubotympanic suppurative otitis media**
> Benign chronic suppurative otitis media (with anterior perforation of ear drum)
> Chronic tubotympanic disease (with anterior perforation of ear drum)

382.2 **Chronic atticoantral suppurative otitis media**
> Chronic atticoantral disease (with posterior or superior marginal perforation of ear drum)
> Persistent mucosal disease (with posterior or superior marginal perforation of ear drum)

❑382.3 **Unspecified chronic suppurative otitis media**
> Chronic purulent otitis media

> **Excludes** *tuberculous otitis media (017.4)*

❑382.4 **Unspecified suppurative otitis media**
> Purulent otitis media NOS

❑382.9 **Unspecified otitis media**
> Otitis media:
> NOS
> acute NOS
> chronic NOS

● 383 **Mastoiditis and related conditions**

● 383.0 **Acute mastoiditis**
> Abscess of mastoid
> Empyema of mastoid

383.00 **Acute mastoiditis without complications**

383.01 **Subperiosteal abscess of mastoid**

❑383.02 **Acute mastoiditis with other complications**
> Gradenigo's syndrome

383.1 **Chronic mastoiditis**
> Caries of mastoid
> Fistula of mastoid

> **Excludes** *tuberculous mastoiditis (015.6)*

● 383.2 **Petrositis**
> Coalescing osteitis of petrous bone
> Inflammation of petrous bone
> Osteomyelitis of petrous bone

❑383.20 **Petrositis, unspecified**

383.21 **Acute petrositis**

383.22 **Chronic petrositis**

● 383.3 **Complications following mastoidectomy**

❑383.30 **Postmastoidectomy complication, unspecified**

383.31 **Mucosal cyst of postmastoidectomy cavity**

383.32 **Recurrent cholesteatoma of postmastoidectomy cavity**

383.33 **Granulations of postmastoidectomy cavity**
> Chronic inflammation of postmastoidectomy cavity

● 383.8 **Other disorders of mastoid**

383.81 **Postauricular fistula**

❑383.89 **Other**

❑383.9 **Unspecified mastoiditis**

● 384 **Other disorders of tympanic membrane**

● 384.0 **Acute myringitis without mention of otitis media**

❑384.00 **Acute myringitis, unspecified**
> Acute tympanitis NOS

384.01 **Bullous myringitis**
> Myringitis bullosa hemorrhagica

❑384.09 **Other**

384.1 **Chronic myringitis without mention of otitis media**
> Chronic tympanitis

● 384.2 **Perforation of tympanic membrane**
> Perforation of ear drum:
> NOS
> persistent posttraumatic
> postinflammatory

> **Excludes** *otitis media with perforation of tympanic membrane (382.00–382.9)*
> *traumatic perforation [current injury] (872.61)*

❑384.20 **Perforation of tympanic membrane, unspecified**

384.21 **Central perforation of tympanic membrane**

384.22 **Attic perforation of tympanic membrane**
> Pars flaccida

❑384.23 **Other marginal perforation of tympanic membrane**

384.24 **Multiple perforations of tympanic membrane**

384.25 **Total perforation of tympanic membrane**

● 384.8 **Other specified disorders of tympanic membrane**

384.81 **Atrophic flaccid tympanic membrane**
> Healed perforation of ear drum

384.82 **Atrophic nonflaccid tympanic membrane**

❑384.9 **Unspecified disorder of tympanic membrane**

● 385 **Other disorders of middle ear and mastoid**

> **Excludes** *mastoiditis (383.0–383.9)*

● 385.0 **Tympanosclerosis**

❑385.00 **Tympanosclerosis, unspecified as to involvement**

385.01 **Tympanosclerosis involving tympanic membrane only**

385.02 **Tympanosclerosis involving tympanic membrane and ear ossicles**

385.03 **Tympanosclerosis involving tympanic membrane, ear ossicles, and middle ear**

❑385.09 **Tympanosclerosis involving other combination of structures**

● 385.1 **Adhesive middle ear disease**
> Adhesive otitis
> Otitis media:
> chronic adhesive
> fibrotic

> **Excludes** *glue ear (381.20–381.29)*

❑385.10 **Adhesive middle ear disease, unspecified as to involvement**

385.11 **Adhesions of drum head to incus**

385.12 **Adhesions of drum head to stapes**

385.13 **Adhesions of drum head to promontorium**

❑385.19 **Other adhesions and combinations**

● 385.2 **Other acquired abnormality of ear ossicles**

385.21 **Impaired mobility of malleus**
> Ankylosis of malleus

❑385.22   **Impaired mobility of other ear ossicles**
Ankylosis of ear ossicles, except malleus

385.23   **Discontinuity or dislocation of ear ossicles**

385.24   **Partial loss or necrosis of ear ossicles**

● 385.3   **Cholesteatoma of middle ear and mastoid**
Cholesterosis of (middle) ear
Epidermosis of (middle) ear
Keratosis of (middle) ear
Polyp of (middle) ear

   | **Excludes** | *cholesteatoma:*
external ear canal (380.21)
recurrent of postmastoidectomy cavity (383.32)

❑385.30   **Cholesteatoma, unspecified**

385.31   **Cholesteatoma of attic**

385.32   **Cholesteatoma of middle ear**

385.33   **Cholesteatoma of middle ear and mastoid**

385.35   **Diffuse cholesteatosis**

● 385.8   **Other disorders of middle ear and mastoid**

385.82   **Cholesterin granuloma**

385.83   **Retained foreign body of middle ear**

❑385.89   **Other**

❑385.9   **Unspecified disorder of middle ear and mastoid**

● 386   **Vertiginous syndromes and other disorders of vestibular system**

   | **Excludes** | *vertigo NOS (780.4)*

● 386.0   **Ménière's disease**
Endolymphatic hydrops
Lermoyez's syndrome
Ménière's syndrome or vertigo

❑386.00   **Ménière's disease, unspecified**
Ménière's disease (active)

386.01   **Active Ménière's disease, cochleovestibular**

386.02   **Active Ménière's disease, cochlear**

386.03   **Active Ménière's disease, vestibular**

386.04   **Inactive Ménière's disease**
Ménière's disease in remission

● 386.1   **Other and unspecified peripheral vertigo**

   | **Excludes** | *epidemic vertigo (078.81)*

❑386.10   **Peripheral vertigo, unspecified**

386.11   **Benign paroxysmal positional vertigo**
Benign paroxysmal positional nystagmus

386.12   **Vestibular neuronitis**
Acute (and recurrent) peripheral vestibulopathy

❑386.19   **Other**
Aural vertigo
Otogenic vertigo

386.2   **Vertigo of central origin**
Central positional nystagmus
Malignant positional vertigo

● 386.3   **Labyrinthitis**

❑386.30   **Labyrinthitis, unspecified**

386.31   **Serous labyrinthitis**
Diffuse labyrinthitis

386.32   **Circumscribed labyrinthitis**
Focal labyrinthitis

386.33   **Suppurative labyrinthitis**
Purulent labyrinthitis

386.34   **Toxic labyrinthitis**

386.35   **Viral labyrinthitis**

● 386.4   **Labyrinthine fistula**

❑386.40   **Labyrinthine fistula, unspecified**

386.41   **Round window fistula**

386.42   **Oval window fistula**

386.43   **Semicircular canal fistula**

386.48   **Labyrinthine fistula of combined sites**

● 386.5   **Labyrinthine dysfunction**

❑386.50   **Labyrinthine dysfunction, unspecified**

386.51   **Hyperactive labyrinth, unilateral**

386.52   **Hyperactive labyrinth, bilateral**

386.53   **Hypoactive labyrinth, unilateral**

386.54   **Hypoactive labyrinth, bilateral**

386.55   **Loss of labyrinthine reactivity, unilateral**

386.56   **Loss of labyrinthine reactivity, bilateral**

❑386.58   **Other forms and combinations**

❑386.8   **Other disorders of labyrinth**

❑386.9   **Unspecified vertiginous syndromes and labyrinthine disorders**

● 387   **Otosclerosis**

   Includes: otospongiosis

387.0   **Otosclerosis involving oval window, nonobliterative**

387.1   **Otosclerosis involving oval window, obliterative**

387.2   **Cochlear otosclerosis**
Otosclerosis involving:
otic capsule
round window

❑387.8   **Other otosclerosis**

❑387.9   **Otosclerosis, unspecified**

● 388   **Other disorders of ear**

● 388.0   **Degenerative and vascular disorders of ear**

❑388.00   **Degenerative and vascular disorders, unspecified**

388.01   **Presbyacusis**

388.02   **Transient ischemic deafness**

● 388.1   **Noise effects on inner ear**

❑388.10   **Noise effects on inner ear, unspecified**

388.11   **Acoustic trauma (explosive) to ear**
Otitic blast injury

388.12   **Noise-induced hearing loss**

❑388.2   **Sudden hearing loss, unspecified**

● 388.3   **Tinnitus**

❑388.30   **Tinnitus, unspecified**

388.31   **Subjective tinnitus**

388.32   **Objective tinnitus**

● 388.4   **Other abnormal auditory perception**

❑388.40   **Abnormal auditory perception, unspecified**

388.41   **Diplacusis**

388.42   **Hyperacusis**

388.43   **Impairment of auditory discrimination**

388.44   **Recruitment**

ICD-9-CM

300-399

Vol. 1

388.5 **Disorders of acoustic nerve**
Acoustic neuritis
Degeneration of acoustic or eighth nerve
Disorder of acoustic or eighth nerve

> **Excludes** *acoustic neuroma (225.1)*
> *syphilitic acoustic neuritis (094.86)*

● 388.6 **Otorrhea**

❏ 388.60 **Otorrhea, unspecified**
Discharging ear NOS

388.61 **Cerebrospinal fluid otorrhea**

> **Excludes** *cerebrospinal fluid rhinorrhea (349.81)*

❏ 388.69 **Other**
Otorrhagia

● 388.7 **Otalgia**

❏ 388.70 **Otalgia, unspecified**
Earache NOS

388.71 **Otogenic pain**

388.72 **Referred pain**

❏ 388.8 **Other disorders of ear**

❏ 388.9 **Unspecified disorder of ear**

● 389 **Hearing loss**

● 389.0 **Conductive hearing loss**
Conductive deafness

❏ 389.00 **Conductive hearing loss, unspecified**

389.01 **Conductive hearing loss, external ear**

389.02 **Conductive hearing loss, tympanic membrane**

389.03 **Conductive hearing loss, middle ear**

389.04 **Conductive hearing loss, inner ear**

389.08 **Conductive hearing loss of combined types**

● 389.1 **Sensorineural hearing loss**
Perceptive hearing loss or deafness

> **Excludes** *abnormal auditory perception (388.40–388.44)*
> *psychogenic deafness (306.7)*

❏ 389.10 **Sensorineural hearing loss, unspecified**

389.11 **Sensory hearing loss**

389.12 **Neural hearing loss**

389.14 **Central hearing loss**

389.18 **Sensorineural hearing loss of combined types**

389.2 **Mixed conductive and sensorineural hearing loss**
Deafness or hearing loss of type classifiable to 389.0 with type classifiable to 389.1

389.7 **Deaf mutism, not elsewhere classifiable**
Deaf, nonspeaking

❏ 389.8 **Other specified forms of hearing loss**

❏ 389.9 **Unspecified hearing loss**
Deafness NOS

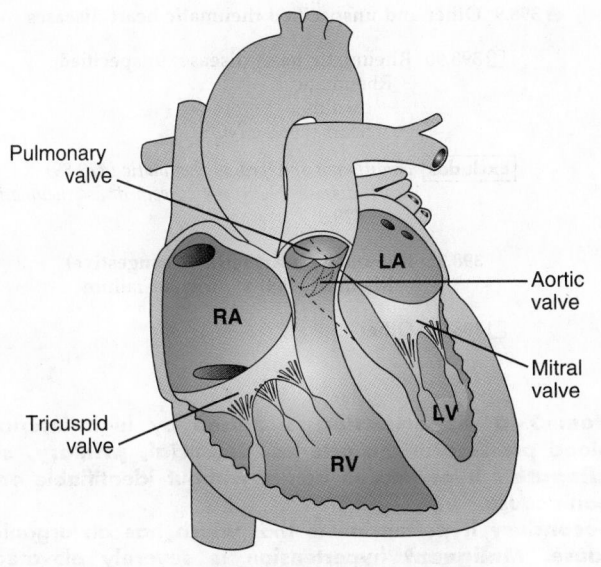

Figure 7-1 Cardiovascular valves.

Item 7-1 Rheumatic fever is the inflammation of the valve(s) of the heart, usually the mitral or aortic, which leads to valve damage. Rheumatic heart inflammations are usually **pericarditis** (heart), **endocarditis** (heart cavity), or **myocarditis** (heart muscle).

Item 7-2 Rheumatic chorea, also called Sydenham's, juvenile, minor, simple, or St. Vitus' dance, is a condition linked with rheumatic fever and is characterized by ceaseless, jerky movements.

7. DISEASES OF THE CIRCULATORY SYSTEM (390–459)

ACUTE RHEUMATIC FEVER (390–392)

390 **Rheumatic fever without mention of heart involvement**
 Arthritis, rheumatic, acute or subacute
 Rheumatic fever (active) (acute)
 Rheumatism, articular, acute or subacute
 Excludes *that with heart involvement (391.0–391.9)*

● 391 **Rheumatic fever with heart involvement**
 Excludes *chronic heart diseases of rheumatic origin (393.0–398.9) unless rheumatic fever is also present or there is evidence of recrudescence or activity of the rheumatic process*

391.0 **Acute rheumatic pericarditis**
 Rheumatic:
  fever (active) (acute) with pericarditis
  pericarditis (acute)
 Any condition classifiable to 390 with pericarditis
 Excludes *that not specified as rheumatic (420.0–420.9)*

391.1 **Acute rheumatic endocarditis**
 Rheumatic:
  endocarditis, acute
  fever (active) (acute) with endocarditis or valvulitis
  valvulitis, acute
 Any condition classifiable to 390 with endocarditis or valvulitis

391.2 **Acute rheumatic myocarditis**
 Rheumatic fever (active) (acute) with myocarditis
 Any condition classifiable to 390 with myocarditis

❏391.8 **Other acute rheumatic heart disease**
 Rheumatic:
  fever (active) (acute) with other or multiple types of heart involvement
  pancarditis, acute
 Any condition classifiable to 390 with other or multiple types of heart involvement

❏391.9 **Acute rheumatic heart disease, unspecified**
 Rheumatic:
  carditis, acute
  fever (active) (acute) with unspecified type of heart involvement
  heart disease, active or acute
 Any condition classifiable to 390 with unspecified type of heart involvement

● 392 **Rheumatic chorea**
 Includes: Sydenham's chorea
 Excludes *chorea:*
  NOS (333.5)
  Huntington's (333.4)

392.0 **With heart involvement**
 Rheumatic chorea with heart involvement of any type classifiable to 391

392.9 **Without mention of heart involvement**

CHRONIC RHEUMATIC HEART DISEASE (393–398)

393 **Chronic rheumatic pericarditis**
 Adherent pericardium, rheumatic
 Chronic rheumatic:
  mediastinopericarditis
  myopericarditis
 Excludes *pericarditis NOS or not specified as rheumatic (423.0–423.9)*

Item 7-3 Mitral stenosis is the narrowing of the mitral valve. **Mitral insufficiency** is the improper closure of the mitral valve. These conditions lead to enlargement (hypertrophy) of the left atrium.

● 394 **Diseases of mitral valve**
 Excludes *that with aortic valve involvement (396.0–396.9)*

394.0 **Mitral stenosis**
 Mitral (valve):
  obstruction (rheumatic)
  stenosis NOS

394.1 **Rheumatic mitral insufficiency**
 Rheumatic mitral:
  incompetence
  regurgitation
 Excludes *that not specified as rheumatic (424.0)*

394.2 **Mitral stenosis with insufficiency**
 Mitral stenosis with incompetence or regurgitation

❏394.9 **Other and unspecified mitral valve diseases**
 Mitral (valve):
  disease (chronic)
  failure

Item 7-4 Aortic stenosis is the narrowing of the aortic valve. **Aortic insufficiency** is the improper closure of the aortic valve. These conditions lead to enlargement (hypertrophy) of the left ventricle.

ICD-9-CM
300-399
Vol. 1

● 395 Diseases of aortic valve

> **Excludes** *that not specified as rheumatic (424.1)*
> *that with mitral valve involvement (396.0–*
> *396.9)*

395.0 **Rheumatic aortic stenosis**
Rheumatic aortic (valve) obstruction

395.1 **Rheumatic aortic insufficiency**
Rheumatic aortic:
incompetence
regurgitation

395.2 **Rheumatic aortic stenosis with insufficiency**
Rheumatic aortic stenosis with incompetence or
regurgitation

☐ 395.9 **Other and unspecified rheumatic aortic diseases**
Rheumatic aortic (valve) disease

Item 7–5 Mitral and aortic valve stenosis is the narrowing of these valves, which leads to enlargement (hypertrophy) of the left atrium and left ventricle.
Mitral and aortic insufficiency is the improper closure of the mitral and aortic valves, which leads to enlargement (hypertrophy) of the left atrium and left ventricle.

● 396 Diseases of mitral and aortic valves

> **Includes:** involvement of both mitral and aortic valves, whether specified as rheumatic or not

396.0 **Mitral valve stenosis and aortic valve stenosis**
Atypical aortic (valve) stenosis
Mitral and aortic (valve) obstruction (rheumatic)

396.1 **Mitral valve stenosis and aortic valve insufficiency**

396.2 **Mitral valve insufficiency and aortic valve stenosis**

396.3 **Mitral valve insufficiency and aortic valve insufficiency**
Mitral and aortic (valve):
incompetence
regurgitation

396.8 **Multiple involvement of mitral and aortic valves**
Stenosis and insufficiency of mitral or aortic valve
with stenosis or insufficiency, or both, of the
other valve

☐ 396.9 **Mitral and aortic valve diseases, unspecified**

● 397 Diseases of other endocardial structures

397.0 **Diseases of tricuspid valve**
Tricuspid (valve) (rheumatic):
disease
insufficiency
obstruction
regurgitation
stenosis

397.1 **Rheumatic diseases of pulmonary valve**
> **Excludes** *that not specified as rheumatic (424.3)*

☐ 397.9 **Rheumatic diseases of endocardium, valve unspecified**
Rheumatic:
endocarditis (chronic)
valvulitis (chronic)
> **Excludes** *that not specified as rheumatic (424.90–424.99)*

● 398 Other rheumatic heart disease

398.0 **Rheumatic myocarditis**
Rheumatic degeneration of myocardium
> **Excludes** *myocarditis not specified as rheumatic (429.0)*

● 398.9 **Other and unspecified rheumatic heart diseases**

☐ 398.90 **Rheumatic heart disease, unspecified**
Rheumatic:
carditis
heart disease NOS

> **Excludes** *carditis not specified as rheumatic (429.89)*
> *heart disease NOS not specified as rheumatic*
> *(429.9)*

398.91 **Rheumatic heart failure (congestive)**
Rheumatic left ventricular failure

☐ 398.99 **Other**

Item 7–6 Hypertension is caused by high arterial blood pressure in the arteries. **Essential, primary,** or **idiopathic** hypertension occurs without identifiable organic cause.
Secondary hypertension is that which has an organic cause. **Malignant** hypertension is severely elevated blood pressure. **Benign** hypertension is mildly elevated blood pressure.

HYPERTENSIVE DISEASE (401–405)

> **Excludes** *that complicating pregnancy, childbirth, or the*
> *puerperium (642.0–642.9)*
> *that involving coronary vessels (410.00–414.9)*

● 401 Essential hypertension

> **Includes:** high blood pressure
> hyperpiesia
> hyperpiesis
> hypertension (arterial) (essential) (primary)
> (systemic)
> hypertensive vascular:
> degeneration
> disease

> **Excludes** *elevated blood pressure without diagnosis of hypertension (796.2)*
> *pulmonary hypertension (416.0–416.9)*
> *that involving vessels of:*
> *brain (430–438)*
> *eye (362.11)*

401.0 **Malignant**

401.1 **Benign**

☐ 401.9 **Unspecified**

● 402 Hypertensive heart disease

> **Includes:** hypertensive:
> cardiomegaly
> cardiopathy
> cardiovascular disease
> heart (disease) (failure)
> any condition classifiable to 429.0–429.3, 429.8, 429.9 due to hypertension ◀⏴⏴

Use additional code to specify type of heart failure (428.0, 428.20–428.23, 428.30–428.33, 428.40–428.43)

● 402.0 **Malignant**

402.00 **Without heart failure**

☐ 402.01 **With heart failure**

● 402.1 **Benign**

    402.10 **Without heart failure**

    402.11 **With heart failure**

● 402.9 **Unspecified**

    ❏ 402.90 **Without heart failure**

    ❏ 402.91 **With heart failure**

● 403 **Hypertensive renal disease**

    Includes: arteriolar nephritis
              arteriosclerosis of:
                kidney
                renal arterioles
              arteriosclerotic nephritis (chronic) (interstitial)
              hypertensive:
                nephropathy
                renal failure
                uremia (chronic)
              nephrosclerosis
              renal sclerosis with hypertension
              any condition classifiable to 585, 586, or 587
                with any condition classifiable to 401

    Excludes *acute renal failure (584.5–584.9)*
              renal disease stated as not due to hypertension
              renovascular hypertension (405.0–405.9 with
                fifth-digit 1)

    The following fifth-digit subclassification is for use with
    category 403:
      0 without mention of renal failure
      1 with renal failure

    ● 403.0 **Malignant**

    ● 403.1 **Benign**

    ● ❏ 403.9 **Unspecified**

● 404 **Hypertensive heart and renal disease**

    Includes: disease:
              cardiorenal
              cardiovascular renal
              any condition classifiable to 402 with any con-
                dition classifiable to 403

    Use additional code to specify type of heart failure (428.0,
    428.20–428.23, 428.30–428.33, 428.40–428.43)
    The following fifth-digit subclassification is for use with cate-
    gory 404:
      0 without mention of heart failure or renal failure
      1 with heart failure
      2 with renal failure
      3 with heart failure and renal failure

    ● 404.0 **Malignant**

    ● 404.1 **Benign**

    ● ❏ 404.9 **Unspecified**

● 405 **Secondary hypertension**

    ● 405.0 **Malignant**

        405.01 **Renovascular**

        ❏ 405.09 **Other**

    ● 405.1 **Benign**

        405.11 **Renovascular**

        ❏ 405.19 **Other**

    ● 405.9 **Unspecified**

        ❏ 405.91 **Renovascular**

        ❏ 405.99 **Other**

Figure 7-2 Myocardial infarction.

Item 7-7 Myocardial infarction is a sudden decrease in the coronary artery blood flow that results in death of the heart muscle. Classifications are based on the affected heart tissue.

ISCHEMIC HEART DISEASE (410–414)

    Includes: that with mention of hypertension

Use additional code to identify presence of hypertension
(401.0–405.9)

● 410 **Acute myocardial infarction**

    Includes: cardiac infarction
              coronary (artery):
                embolism
                occlusion
                rupture
                thrombosis
              infarction of heart, myocardium, or ventricle
              rupture of heart, myocardium, or ventricle
              any condition classifiable to 414.1–414.9 speci-
                fied as acute or with a stated duration of
                8 weeks or less

    The following fifth-digit subclassification is for use with
    category 410:
    ❏ **0 episode of care unspecified**
        Use when the source document does not contain
        sufficient information for the assignment of fifth-
        digit 1 or 2.
    1 initial episode of care
        Use fifth-digit 1 to designate the first episode of
        care (regardless of facility site) for a newly diag-
        nosed myocardial infarction. The fifth-digit 1 is
        assigned regardless of the number of times a pa-
        tient may be transferred during the initial episode
        of care.
    2 subsequent episode of care
        Use fifth-digit 2 to designate an episode of care
        following the initial episode when the patient is
        admitted for further observation, evaluation or
        treatment for a myocardial infarction that has re-
        ceived initial treatment, but is still less than 8
        weeks old.

    ● 410.0 **Of anterolateral wall**

    ● ❏ 410.1 **Of other anterior wall**
        Infarction:
            anterior (wall) NOS (with contiguous portion of
                intraventricular septum)
            anteroapical (with contiguous portion of intra-
                ventricular septum)
            anteroseptal (with contiguous portion of intra-
                ventricular septum)

Zone of injury
Zone of infarction
Zone of ischemia

ICD-9-CM

400-409
Vol. 1

● 410.2   Of inferolateral wall

● 410.3   Of inferoposterior wall

● ☐ 410.4   Of other inferior wall
     Infarction:
         diaphragmatic wall NOS (with contiguous por-
             tion of intraventricular septum)
         inferior (wall) NOS (with contiguous portion of
             intraventricular septum)

● ☐ 410.5   Of other lateral wall
     Infarction:
         apical-lateral
         basal-lateral
         high lateral
         posterolateral

● 410.6   True posterior wall infarction
     Infarction:
         posterobasal
         strictly posterior

● 410.7   Subendocardial infarction
     Nontransmural infarction

● ☐ 410.8   Of other specified sites
     Infarction of:
         atrium
         papillary muscle
         septum alone

● ☐ 410.9   Unspecified site
     Acute myocardial infarction NOS
     Coronary occlusion NOS

● **411   Other acute and subacute forms of ischemic heart disease**

     411.0   Postmyocardial infarction syndrome
         Dressler's syndrome

     411.1   Intermediate coronary syndrome
         Impending infarction
         Preinfarction angina
         Preinfarction syndrome
         Unstable angina

         Excludes   *angina (pectoris) (413.9)*
                          decubitus (413.0)

     411.8   Other

         411.81   Acute coronary occlusion without myocar-
                 dial infarction
             Acute coronary (artery):
                 embolism without or not resulting in
                     myocardial infarction
                 obstruction without or not resulting in
                     myocardial infarction
                 occlusion without or not resulting in
                     myocardial infarction
                 thrombosis without or not resulting in
                     myocardial infarction

         Excludes   *obstruction without infarction due to atheroscle-*
                        rosis (414.00–414.07)
                         occlusion without infarction due to atherosclero-
                        sis (414.00–414.07)

         ☐ 411.89   Other
             Coronary insufficiency (acute)
             Subendocardial ischemia

     412   Old myocardial infarction
         Healed myocardial infarction
         Past myocardial infarction diagnosed on ECG [EKG] or
             other special investigation, but currently presenting
             no symptoms

● **413   Angina pectoris**

     413.0   Angina decubitus
         Nocturnal angina

     413.1   Prinzmetal angina
         Variant angina pectoris

☐ 413.9   Other and unspecified angina pectoris
     Angina:
         NOS
         cardiac
         of effort
     Anginal syndrome
     Status anginosus
     Stenocardia
     Syncope anginosa

     Excludes   *preinfarction angina (411.1)*

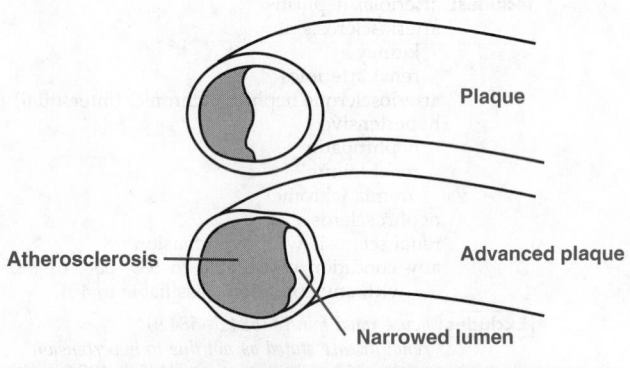

Figure 7–3   Atherosclerosis. (From Buck CJ: Step-by-Step Medical Coding, 2005 ed. Philadelphia, WBS, 2005.)

Item 7–8   Classification is based on the location of the atherosclerosis. "Of native coronary artery" indicates the atherosclerosis is within an original heart artery. "Of autologous vein bypass graft" indicates that the atherosclerosis is within a vein graft that was taken from within the patient. "Of nonautologous biological by-pass graft" indicates the atherosclerosis is within a ves-sel grafted from other than the patient. "Of artery by-pass graft" indicates the atherosclerosis is within an artery that was grafted from within the patient.

● **414   Other forms of chronic ischemic heart disease**

     Excludes   *arteriosclerotic cardiovascular disease [ASCVD]*
                     (429.2)
                 cardiovascular:
                     arteriosclerosis or sclerosis (429.2)
                     degeneration or disease (429.2)

● 414.0   Coronary atherosclerosis
     Arteriosclerotic heart disease [ASHD]
     Atherosclerotic heart disease
     Coronary (artery):
         arteriosclerosis
         arteritis or endarteritis
         atheroma
         sclerosis
         stricture

     Excludes   *embolism of graft (996.72)*
                 occlusion NOS of graft (996.72)
                 thrombus of graft (996.72)

☐ 414.00   Of unspecified type of vessel, native or graft

     414.01   Of native coronary artery

     414.02   Of autologous biological bypass graft

     414.03   Of nonautologous biological bypass graft

     414.04   Of artery bypass graft
         Internal mammary artery

     414.05   Of unspecified type of bypass graft
         Bypass graft NOS

414.06 Of native coronary artery of transplanted heart

414.07 Of bypass graft (artery) (vein) of transplanted heart

● **414.1 Aneurysm and dissection of heart**

414.10 Aneurysm of heart (wall)
Aneurysm (arteriovenous):
mural
ventricular

414.11 Aneurysm of coronary vessels
Aneurysm (arteriovenous) of coronary vessels

414.12 Dissection of coronary artery

❏ **414.19 Other aneurysm of heart**
Arteriovenous fistula, acquired, of heart

❏ **414.8 Other specified forms of chronic ischemic heart disease**
Chronic coronary insufficiency
Ischemia, myocardial (chronic)
Any condition classifiable to 410 specified as chronic, or presenting with symptoms after 8 weeks from date of infarction

Excludes *coronary insufficiency (acute) (411.89)*

❏ **414.9 Chronic ischemic heart disease, unspecified**
Ischemic heart disease NOS

DISEASES OF PULMONARY CIRCULATION (415–417)

● **415 Acute pulmonary heart disease**

415.0 Acute cor pulmonale

Excludes *cor pulmonale NOS (416.9)*

● **415.1 Pulmonary embolism and infarction**
Pulmonary (artery) (vein):
apoplexy
embolism
infarction (hemorrhagic)
thrombosis

Excludes *that complicating:*
abortion (634–638 with .6, 639.6)
ectopic or molar pregnancy (639.6)
pregnancy, childbirth, or the puerperium (673.0–673.8)

415.11 Iatrogenic pulmonary embolism and infarction

❏ **415.19 Other**

● **416 Chronic pulmonary heart disease**

416.0 Primary pulmonary hypertension
Idiopathic pulmonary arteriosclerosis
Pulmonary hypertension (essential) (idiopathic) (primary)

416.1 Kyphoscoliotic heart disease

❏ **416.8 Other chronic pulmonary heart diseases**
Pulmonary hypertension, secondary

❏ **416.9 Chronic pulmonary heart disease, unspecified**
Chronic cardiopulmonary disease
Cor pulmonale (chronic) NOS

● **417 Other diseases of pulmonary circulation**

417.0 Arteriovenous fistula of pulmonary vessels

Excludes *congenital arteriovenous fistula (747.3)*

417.1 Aneurysm of pulmonary artery

Excludes *congenital aneurysm (747.3)*

❏ **417.8 Other specified diseases of pulmonary circulation**
Pulmonary:
arteritis
endarteritis
Rupture of pulmonary vessel
Stricture of pulmonary vessel

❏ **417.9 Unspecified disease of pulmonary circulation**

OTHER FORMS OF HEART DISEASE (420–429)

● **420 Acute pericarditis**

Includes: acute:
mediastinopericarditis
myopericarditis
pericardial effusion
pleuropericarditis
pneumopericarditis

Excludes *acute rheumatic pericarditis (391.0)*
postmyocardial infarction syndrome [Dressler's] (411.0)

● ❏ **420.0 Acute pericarditis in diseases classified elsewhere**

Code first underlying disease, as:
actinomycosis (039.8)
amebiasis (006.8)
nocardiosis (039.8)
tuberculosis (017.9)
uremia (585)

Excludes *pericarditis (acute) (in):*
Coxsackie (virus) (074.21)
gonococcal (098.83)
histoplasmosis (115.0–115.9 with fifth-digit 3)
meningococcal infection (036.41)
syphilitic (093.81)

● **420.9 Other and unspecified acute pericarditis**

❏ **420.90 Acute pericarditis, unspecified**
Pericarditis (acute):
NOS
infective NOS
sicca

420.91 Acute idiopathic pericarditis
Pericarditis, acute:
benign   viral
nonspecific

❏ **420.99 Other**
Pericarditis (acute):
pneumococcal
purulent
staphylococcal
streptococcal
suppurative
Pneumopyopericardium
Pyopericardium

Excludes *pericarditis in diseases classified elsewhere (420.0)*

● **421 Acute and subacute endocarditis**

421.0 Acute and subacute bacterial endocarditis
Endocarditis (acute) (chronic) (subacute):
bacterial
infective NOS
lenta
malignant
purulent
septic
ulcerative
vegetative
Infective aneurysm
Subacute bacterial endocarditis [SBE]

Use additional code, if desired, to identify infectious organism [e.g., Streptococcus 041.0, Staphylococcus 041.1]

ICD-9-CM

400-
...

Vol. 1

●❏ **421.1 Acute and subacute infective endocarditis in diseases classified elsewhere**

Code first underlying disease, as:
blastomycosis (116.0)
Q fever (083.0)
typhoid (fever) (002.0)

Excludes *endocarditis (in):*
Coxsackie (virus) (074.22)
gonococcal (098.84)
histoplasmosis (115.0–115.9 with fifth-digit 4)
meningococcal infection (036.42)
monilial (112.81)

❏ **421.9 Acute endocarditis, unspecified**
Endocarditis, acute or subacute
Myoendocarditis, acute or subacute
Periendocarditis, acute or subacute

Excludes *acute rheumatic endocarditis (391.1)*

● **422 Acute myocarditis**

Excludes *acute rheumatic myocarditis (391.2)*

●❏ **422.0 Acute myocarditis in diseases classified elsewhere**

Code first underlying disease, as:
myocarditis (acute):
influenzal (487.8)
tuberculous (017.9)

Excludes *myocarditis (acute) (due to):*
aseptic, of newborn (074.23)
Coxsackie (virus) (074.23)
diphtheritic (032.82)
meningococcal infection (036.43)
syphilitic (093.82)
toxoplasmosis (130.3)

● **422.9 Other and unspecified acute myocarditis**

❏ **422.90 Acute myocarditis, unspecified**
Acute or subacute (interstitial) myocarditis

422.91 Idiopathic myocarditis
Myocarditis (acute or subacute):
Fiedler's
giant cell
isolated (diffuse) (granulomatous)
nonspecific granulomatous

422.92 Septic myocarditis
Myocarditis, acute or subacute:
pneumococcal
staphylococcal

Use additional code to identify infectious organism [e.g., Staphylococcus 041.1]

Excludes *myocarditis, acute or subacute:*
in bacterial diseases classified elsewhere (422.0)
streptococcal (391.2)

422.93 Toxic myocarditis

❏ **422.99 Other**

● **423 Other diseases of pericardium**

Excludes *that specified as rheumatic (393)*

423.0 Hemopericardium

423.1 Adhesive pericarditis
Adherent pericardium
Fibrosis of pericardium
Milk spots
Pericarditis:
adhesive
obliterative
Soldiers' patches

423.2 Constrictive pericarditis
Concato's disease
Pick's disease of heart (and liver)

❏ **423.8 Other specified diseases of pericardium**
Calcification of pericardium
Fistula of pericardium

❏ **423.9 Unspecified disease of pericardium**

● **424 Other diseases of endocardium**

Excludes *bacterial endocarditis (421.0–421.9)*
rheumatic endocarditis (391.1, 394.0–397.9)
syphilitic endocarditis (093.20–093.24)

424.0 Mitral valve disorders
Mitral (valve):
incompetence NOS of specified cause, except rheumatic
insufficiency NOS of specified cause, except rheumatic
regurgitation NOS of specified cause, except rheumatic

Excludes *mitral (valve):*
disease (394.9)
failure (394.9)
stenosis (394.0)
the listed conditions:
specified as rheumatic (394.1)
unspecified as to cause but with mention of:
diseases of aortic valve (396.0–396.9)
mitral stenosis or obstruction (394.2)

424.1 Aortic valve disorders
Aortic (valve):
incompetence NOS of specified cause, except rheumatic
insufficiency NOS of specified cause, except rheumatic
regurgitation NOS of specified cause, except rheumatic
stenosis NOS of specified cause, except rheumatic

Excludes *hypertrophic subaortic stenosis (425.1)*
that specified as rheumatic (395.0–395.9)
that of unspecified cause but with mention of diseases of mitral valve (396.0–396.9)

424.2 Tricuspid valve disorders, specified as nonrheumatic
Tricuspid valve:
incompetence of specified cause, except rheumatic
insufficiency of specified cause, except rheumatic
regurgitation of specified cause, except rheumatic
stenosis of specified cause, except rheumatic

Excludes *rheumatic or of unspecified cause (397.0)*

424.3 Pulmonary valve disorders
Pulmonic:
incompetence NOS
insufficiency NOS
regurgitation NOS
stenosis NOS

Excludes *that specified as rheumatic (397.1)*

● **424.9 Endocarditis, valve unspecified**

❏ **424.90 Endocarditis, valve unspecified, unspecified cause**
Endocarditis (chronic):
NOS
nonbacterial thrombotic
Valvular:
incompetence of unspecified valve, unspecified cause
insufficiency of unspecified valve, unspecified cause
regurgitation of unspecified valve, unspecified cause
stenosis of unspecified valve, unspecified cause
Valvulitis (chronic)

● ❑ **424.91 Endocarditis in diseases classified elsewhere**

Code first underlying disease, as:
       atypical verrucous endocarditis [Libman-Sacks] (710.0)
       disseminated lupus erythematosus (710.0)
       tuberculosis (017.9)

Excludes	syphilitic (093.20–093.24)

❑ **424.99 Other**

Any condition classifiable to 424.90 with specified cause, except rheumatic

Excludes	endocardial fibroelastosis (425.3)
	that specified as rheumatic (397.9)

● **425 Cardiomyopathy**

Includes: myocardiopathy

425.0 Endomyocardial fibrosis

425.1 Hypertrophic obstructive cardiomyopathy
Hypertrophic subaortic stenosis (idiopathic)

425.2 Obscure cardiomyopathy of Africa
Becker's disease
Idiopathic mural endomyocardial disease

425.3 Endocardial fibroelastosis
Elastomyofibrosis

❑ **425.4 Other primary cardiomyopathies**
Cardiomyopathy:
   NOS
   congestive
   constrictive
   familial
   hypertrophic
   idiopathic
   nonobstructive
   obstructive
   restrictive
Cardiovascular collagenosis

425.5 Alcoholic cardiomyopathy

● **425.7 Nutritional and metabolic cardiomyopathy**

Code first underlying disease, as:
   amyloidosis (277.3)
   beriberi (265.0)
   cardiac glycogenosis (271.0)
   mucopolysaccharidosis (277.5)
   thyrotoxicosis (242.0–242.9)

Excludes	gouty tophi of heart (274.82)

● ❑ **425.8 Cardiomyopathy in other diseases classified elsewhere**

Code first underlying disease, as:
   Friedreich's ataxia (334.0)
   myotonia atrophica (359.2)
   progressive muscular dystrophy (359.1)
   sarcoidosis (135)

Excludes	cardiomyopathy in Chagas' disease (086.0)

❑ **425.9 Secondary cardiomyopathy, unspecified**

● **426 Conduction disorders**

426.0 Atrioventricular block, complete
Third degree atrioventricular block

● **426.1 Atrioventricular block, other and unspecified**

❑ **426.10 Atrioventricular block, unspecified**
Atrioventricular [AV] block (incomplete) (partial)

426.11 First degree atrioventricular block
Incomplete atrioventricular block, first degree
Prolonged P-R interval NOS

426.12 Mobitz (type) II atrioventricular block
Incomplete atrioventricular block:
   Mobitz (type) II
   second degree, Mobitz (type) II

❑ **426.13 Other second degree atrioventricular block**
Incomplete atrioventricular block:
   Mobitz (type) I [Wenckebach's]
   second degree:
     NOS
     Mobitz (type) I
     with 2:1 atrioventricular response [block]
Wenckebach's phenomenon

426.2 Left bundle branch hemiblock
Block:
   left anterior fascicular
   left posterior fascicular

❑ **426.3 Other left bundle branch block**
Left bundle branch block:
   NOS
   anterior fascicular with posterior fascicular
   complete
   main stem

426.4 Right bundle branch block

● **426.5 Bundle branch block, other and unspecified**

❑ **426.50 Bundle branch block, unspecified**

426.51 Right bundle branch block and left posterior fascicular block

426.52 Right bundle branch block and left anterior fascicular block

❑ **426.53 Other bilateral bundle branch block**
Bifascicular block NOS
Bilateral bundle branch block NOS
Right bundle branch with left bundle branch block (incomplete) (main stem)

426.54 Trifascicular block

❑ **426.6 Other heart block**
Intraventricular block:
   NOS
   diffuse
   myofibrillar
Sinoatrial block
Sinoauricular block

426.7 Anomalous atrioventricular excitation
Atrioventricular conduction:
   accelerated
   accessory
   pre-excitation
Ventricular pre-excitation
Wolff-Parkinson-White syndrome

● **426.8 Other specified conduction disorders**

426.81 Lown-Ganong-Levine syndrome
Syndrome of short P-R interval, normal QRS complexes, and supraventricular tachycardias

❑ **426.89 Other**
Dissociation:
   atrioventricular [AV]
   interference
   isorhythmic
Nonparoxysmal AV nodal tachycardia

❑ **426.9 Conduction disorder, unspecified**
Heart block NOS
Stokes-Adams syndrome

ICD-9-CM

400-
Vol.

● 427 **Cardiac dysrhythmias**

> **Excludes** *that complicating:*
> *abortion (634–638 with .7, 639.8)*
> *ectopic or molar pregnancy (639.8)*
> *labor or delivery (668.1, 669.4)*

427.0 **Paroxysmal supraventricular tachycardia**
Paroxysmal tachycardia:
  atrial [PAT]   junctional
  atrioventricular [AV] nodal

427.1 **Paroxysmal ventricular tachycardia**
Ventricular tachycardia (paroxysmal)

❑427.2 **Paroxysmal tachycardia, unspecified**
Bouveret-Hoffmann syndrome
Paroxysmal tachycardia:
  NOS   essential

● 427.3 **Atrial fibrillation and flutter**
427.31 **Atrial fibrillation**
427.32 **Atrial flutter**

● 427.4 **Ventricular fibrillation and flutter**
427.41 **Ventricular fibrillation**
427.42 **Ventricular flutter**

❑427.5 **Cardiac arrest**
Cardiorespiratory arrest

● 427.6 **Premature beats**
❑427.60 **Premature beats, unspecified**
Ectopic beats
Extrasystoles
Extrasystolic arrhythmia
Premature contractions or systoles NOS

427.61 **Supraventricular premature beats**
Atrial premature beats, contractions, or systoles

❑427.69 **Other**
Ventricular premature beats, contractions, or systoles

● 427.8 **Other specified cardiac dysrhythmias**
427.81 **Sinoatrial node dysfunction**
Sinus bradycardia: Syndrome:
  persistent   sick sinus
  severe   tachycardia-
                        bradycardia

> **Excludes** *sinus bradycardia NOS (427.89)*

❑427.89 **Other**
Rhythm disorder: Wandering
  coronary sinus   (atrial)
  ectopic   pacemaker
  nodal

> **Excludes** *carotid sinus syncope (337.0)*
> *neonatal bradycardia (779.81)*
> *neonatal tachycardia (779.82)*
> *reflex bradycardia (337.0)*
> *tachycardia NOS (785.0)*

❑427.9 **Cardiac dysrhythmia, unspecified**
Arrhythmia (cardiac) NOS

● 428 **Heart failure**

> **Excludes** *rheumatic (398.91)*
> *that complicating:*
> *abortion (634–638 with .7, 639.8)*
> *ectopic or molar pregnancy (639.8)*
> *labor or delivery (668.1, 669.4)*

Code, if applicable, heart failure due to hypertension first (402.0–402.9, with fifth-digit 1 or 404.0–404.9 with fifth-digit 1 or 3)

❑428.0 **Congestive heart failure, unspecified**
Congestive heart disease
Right heart failure (secondary to left heart failure)

> **Excludes** *fluid overload NOS (276.6)*

428.1 **Left heart failure**
Acute edema of lung with heart disease NOS or heart failure
Acute pulmonary edema with heart disease NOS or heart failure
Cardiac asthma
Left ventricular failure

● 428.2 **Systolic heart failure**

> **Excludes** *combined systolic and diastolic heart failure (428.40–428.43)*

❑428.20 **Unspecified**
428.21 **Acute**
428.22 **Chronic**
428.23 **Acute on chronic**

● 428.3 **Diastolic heart failure**

> **Excludes** *combined systolic and diastolic heart failure (428.40–428.43)*

❑428.30 **Unspecified**
428.31 **Acute**
428.32 **Chronic**
428.33 **Acute on chronic**

● 428.4 **Combined systolic and diastolic heart failure**
❑428.40 **Unspecified**
428.41 **Acute**
428.42 **Chronic**
428.43 **Acute on chronic**

❑428.9 **Heart failure, unspecified**
Cardiac failure NOS
Heart failure NOS
Myocardial failure NOS
Weak heart

● 429 **Ill-defined descriptions and complications of heart disease**
❑429.0 **Myocarditis, unspecified**
Myocarditis (with mention of arteriosclerosis):
  NOS (with mention of arteriosclerosis)
  chronic (interstitial) (with mention of arteriosclerosis)
  fibroid (with mention of arteriosclerosis)
  senile (with mention of arteriosclerosis)

Use additional code to identify presence of arteriosclerosis

> **Excludes** *acute or subacute (422.0–422.9)*
> *rheumatic (398.0)*
> *acute (391.2)*
> *that due to hypertension (402.0–402.9)*

429.1 **Myocardial degeneration**
Degeneration of heart or myocardium (with mention of arteriosclerosis):
  fatty (with mention of arteriosclerosis)
  mural (with mention of arteriosclerosis)
  muscular (with mention of arteriosclerosis)
Myocardial (with mention of arteriosclerosis):
  degeneration (with mention of arteriosclerosis)
  disease (with mention of arteriosclerosis)

Use additional code to identify presence of arteriosclerosis

> **Excludes** *that due to hypertension (402.0–402.9)*

❑429.2 **Cardiovascular disease, unspecified**
Arteriosclerotic cardiovascular disease [ASCVD]
Cardiovascular arteriosclerosis
Cardiovascular:
  degeneration (with mention of arteriosclerosis)
  disease (with mention of arteriosclerosis)
  sclerosis (with mention of arteriosclerosis)

Use additional code to identify presence of arteriosclerosis

> **Excludes** *that due to hypertension (402.0–402.9)*

429.3 Cardiomegaly
  Cardiac:
    dilatation
    hypertrophy
  Ventricular dilatation

> **Excludes** *that due to hypertension (402.0–402.9)*

429.4 Functional disturbances following cardiac surgery
  Cardiac insufficiency following cardiac surgery or
    due to prosthesis
  Heart failure following cardiac surgery or due to
    prosthesis
  Postcardiotomy syndrome
  Postvalvulotomy syndrome

> **Excludes** *cardiac failure in the immediate postoperative period (997.1)*

429.5 Rupture of chordae tendineae

429.6 Rupture of papillary muscle

● **429.7 Certain sequelae of myocardial infarction, not elsewhere classified**

  Use additional code to identify the associated myocardial infarction:
    with onset of 8 weeks or less (410.00–410.92)
    with onset of more than 8 weeks (414.8)

> **Excludes** *congenital defects of heart (745, 746)*
> *coronary aneurysm (414.11)*
> *disorders of papillary muscle (429.6, 429.81)*
> *postmyocardial infarction syndrome (411.0)*
> *rupture of chordae tendineae (429.5)*

  429.71 Acquired cardiac septal defect

> **Excludes** *acute septal infarction (410.00–410.92)*

  ❏**429.79 Other**
    Mural thrombus (atrial) (ventricular) acquired, following myocardial infarction

● **429.8 Other ill-defined heart diseases**

  ❏**429.81 Other disorders of papillary muscle**
    Papillary muscle: Papillary muscle:
     atrophy   incompetence
     degeneration   incoordination
     dysfunction   scarring

  429.82 Hyperkinetic heart disease

  ❏**429.89 Other**
    Carditis

> **Excludes** *that due to hypertension (402.0–402.9)*

❏**429.9 Heart disease, unspecified**
  Heart disease (organic) NOS
  Morbus cordis NOS

> **Excludes** *that due to hypertension (402.0–402.9)*

CEREBROVASCULAR DISEASE (430–438)

Includes: with mention of hypertension (conditions classifiable to 401–405)

Use additional code to identify presence of hypertension

> **Excludes** *any condition classifiable to 430–434, 436, 437 occurring during pregnancy, childbirth, or the puerperium, or specified as puerperal (674.0)*
> *iatrogenic cerebrovascular infarction or hemorrhage (997.02)*

430 Subarachnoid hemorrhage
  Meningeal hemorrhage
  Ruptured:
    berry aneurysm
    (congenital) cerebral aneurysm NOS

> **Excludes** *syphilitic ruptured cerebral aneurysm (094.87)*

431 Intracerebral hemorrhage
  Hemorrhage (of):   Hemorrhage (of):
    basilar   internal capsule
    bulbar   intrapontine
    cerebellar   pontine
    cerebral   subcortical
    cerebromeningeal   ventricular
    cortical
  Rupture of blood vessel in brain

● **432 Other and unspecified intracranial hemorrhage**

  432.0 Nontraumatic extradural hemorrhage
    Nontraumatic epidural hemorrhage

  432.1 Subdural hemorrhage
    Subdural hematoma, nontraumatic

  ❏**432.9 Unspecified intracranial hemorrhage**
    Intracranial hemorrhage NOS

● **433 Occlusion and stenosis of precerebral arteries**

  The following fifth-digit subclassification is for use with category 433:
  0 without mention of cerebral infarction
  1 with cerebral infarction

  Includes: embolism of basilar, carotid, and vertebral arteries
    narrowing of basilar, carotid, and vertebral arteries
    obstruction of basilar, carotid, and vertebral arteries
    thrombosis of basilar, carotid, and vertebral arteries

> **Excludes** *insufficiency NOS of precerebral arteries (435.0–435.9)*

● **433.0 Basilar artery**

● **433.1 Carotid artery**

● **433.2 Vertebral artery**

● **433.3 Multiple and bilateral**

● ❏**433.8 Other specified precerebral artery**

● ❏**433.9 Unspecified precerebral artery**
  Precerebral artery NOS

● **434 Occlusion of cerebral arteries**

  The following fifth-digit subclassification is for use with category 434:
  0 without mention of cerebral infarction
  1 with cerebral infarction

● **434.0 Cerebral thrombosis**
  Thrombosis of cerebral arteries

● **434.1 Cerebral embolism**

● ❏**434.9 Cerebral artery occlusion, unspecified**

● **435 Transient cerebral ischemia**

  Includes: cerebrovascular insufficiency (acute) with transient focal neurological signs and symptoms
    insufficiency of basilar, carotid, and vertebral arteries
    spasm of cerebral arteries

> **Excludes** *acute cerebrovascular insufficiency NOS (437.1)*
> *that due to any condition classifiable to 433 (433.0–433.9)*

435.0 Basilar artery syndrome

435.1 Vertebral artery syndrome

435.2 Subclavian steal syndrome

435.3 **Vertebrobasilar artery syndrome**

❏ 435.8 **Other specified transient cerebral ischemias**

❏ 435.9 **Unspecified transient cerebral ischemia**
        Impending cerebrovascular accident
        Intermittent cerebral ischemia
        Transient ischemic attack [TIA]

436 **Acute, but ill-defined, cerebrovascular disease**
      Apoplexy, apoplectic:
        NOS
        attack
        cerebral
        seizure
      Cerebral seizure

> **Excludes** *any condition classifiable to categories 430–435*
>   *cerebrovascular accident (434.91)* ◀
>   *CVA (ischemic) (434.91)* ◀
>   *embolic (434.11)* ◀
>   *hemorrhagic (430, 431, 432.0–432.9)* ◀
>   *thrombotic (434.01)* ◀
>   *postoperative cerebrovascular accident (997.02)*
>   *stroke (ischemic) (434.91)* ◀
>   *embolic (434.11)* ◀
>   *hemorrhagic (430, 431, 432.0–432.9)* ◀
>   *thrombotic (434.01)* ◀

● 437 **Other and ill-defined cerebrovascular disease**

437.0 **Cerebral atherosclerosis**
      Atheroma of cerebral arteries
      Cerebral arteriosclerosis

❏ 437.1 **Other generalized ischemic cerebrovascular disease**
      Acute cerebrovascular insufficiency NOS
      Cerebral ischemia (chronic)

437.2 **Hypertensive encephalopathy**

437.3 **Cerebral aneurysm, nonruptured**
      Internal carotid artery, intracranial portion
      Internal carotid artery NOS

> **Excludes** *congenital cerebral aneurysm, nonruptured*
>   *(747.81)*
>   *internal carotid artery, extracranial portion*
>   *(442.81)*

437.4 **Cerebral arteritis**

437.5 **Moyamoya disease**

437.6 **Nonpyogenic thrombosis of intracranial venous sinus**

> **Excludes** *pyogenic (325)*

437.7 **Transient global amnesia**

❏ 437.8 **Other**

❏ 437.9 **Unspecified**
      Cerebrovascular disease or lesion NOS

● 438 **Late effects of cerebrovascular disease**

Note: This category is to be used to indicate conditions in 430–437 as the cause of late effects. The "late effects" include conditions specified as such, or as sequelae, which may occur at any time after the onset of the causal condition.

438.0 **Cognitive deficits**

● 438.1 **Speech and language deficits**

❏ 438.10 **Speech and language deficit, unspecified**

438.11 **Aphasia**

438.12 **Dysphasia**

❏ 438.19 **Other speech and language deficits**

● 438.2 **Hemiplegia/hemiparesis**

❏ 438.20 **Hemiplegia affecting unspecified side**

438.21 **Hemiplegia affecting dominant side**

438.22 **Hemiplegia affecting nondominant side**

● 438.3 **Monoplegia of upper limb**

❏ 438.30 **Monoplegia of upper limb affecting unspecified side**

438.31 **Monoplegia of upper limb affecting dominant side**

438.32 **Monoplegia of upper limb affecting nondominant side**

● 438.4 **Monoplegia of lower limb**

❏ 438.40 **Monoplegia of lower limb affecting unspecified side**

438.41 **Monoplegia of lower limb affecting dominant side**

438.42 **Monoplegia of lower limb affecting nondominant side**

● 438.5 **Other paralytic syndrome**

Use additional code to identify type of paralytic syndrome, such as:
    locked-in state (344.81)
    quadriplegia (344.00–344.09)

438.6 **Alterations of sensations**

Use additional code to identify the altered sensation

438.7 **Disturbances of vision**

Use additional code to identify the visual disturbance

> **Excludes** *late effects of cerebrovascular accident with:*
>   *hemiplegia/hemiparesis (438.20–438.22)*
>   *monoplegia of lower limb (438.40–438.42)*
>   *monoplegia of upper limb (438.30–438.32)*

❏ 438.50 **Other paralytic syndrome affecting unspecified side**

438.51 **Other paralytic syndrome affecting dominant side**

438.52 **Other paralytic syndrome affecting nondominant side**

438.53 **Other paralytic syndrome, bilateral**

● 438.8 **Other late effects of cerebrovascular disease**

438.81 **Apraxia**

438.82 **Dysphagia**

438.83 **Facial weakness**
      Facial droop

438.84 **Ataxia**

438.85 **Vertigo**

❏ 438.89 **Other late effects of cerebrovascular disease**

❏ 438.9 **Unspecified late effects of cerebrovascular disease**
      Use additional code to identify the late effect

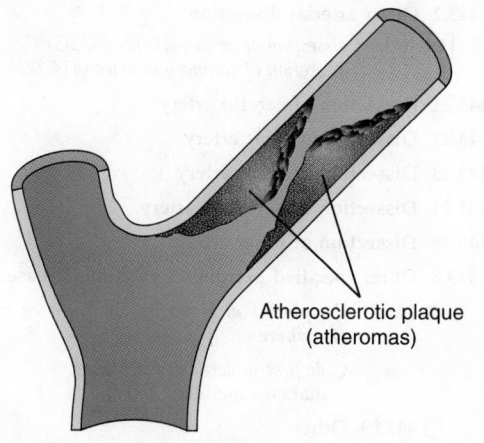

Figure 7-4   Atherosclerotic plaque.

Item 7-9   Classification is based on the location of the atherosclerosis.

DISEASES OF ARTERIES, ARTERIOLES, AND CAPILLARIES (440–448)

● **440   Atherosclerosis**

    Includes: arteriolosclerosis
                arteriosclerosis (obliterans) (senile)
                arteriosclerotic vascular disease
                atheroma
                degeneration:
                    arterial
                    arteriovascular
                    vascular
                endarteritis deformans or obliterans
                senile:
                    arteritis
                    endarteritis

      Excludes   *atheroembolism (445.01–445.89)*
                     atherosclerosis of bypass graft of the extremities
                     (440.30–440.32)

    440.0   Of aorta

    440.1   Of renal artery

      Excludes   *atherosclerosis of renal arterioles (403.00–403.91)*

● **440.2   Of native arteries of the extremities**

      Excludes   *atherosclerosis of bypass graft of the extremities*
                     (440.30–440.32)

       ❑ **440.20   Atherosclerosis of the extremities, unspecified**

       440.21   Atherosclerosis of the extremities with intermittent claudication

       440.22   Atherosclerosis of the extremities with rest pain
             Includes any condition classifiable to 440.21

       440.23   Atherosclerosis of the extremities with ulceration
             Includes any condition classifiable to 440.21–440.22
             Use additional code for any associated ulceration (707.10–707.9)

       440.24   Atherosclerosis of the extremities with gangrene
             Includes any condition classifiable to 440.21, 440.22, and 440.23 with ischemic gangrene 785.4

      Excludes   *gas gangrene (040.0)*

       ❑ **440.29   Other**

● **440.3   Of bypass graft of the extremities**

      Excludes   *atherosclerosis of native artery of the extremity*
                     (440.21–440.24)
                     embolism [occlusion NOS] [thrombus] of graft
                     (996.74)

       ❑ **440.30   Of unspecified graft**

       440.31   Of autologous vein bypass graft

       440.32   Of nonautologous vein bypass graft

❑ **440.8   Of other specified arteries**

      Excludes   *basilar (433.0)*
                     carotid (433.1)
                     cerebral (437.0)
                     coronary (414.00–414.07)
                     mesenteric (557.1)
                     precerebral (433.0–433.9)
                     pulmonary (416.0)
                     vertebral (433.2)

❑ **440.9   Generalized and unspecified atherosclerosis**
        Arteriosclerotic vascular disease NOS

      Excludes   *arteriosclerotic cardiovascular disease [ASCVD]*
                     (429.2)

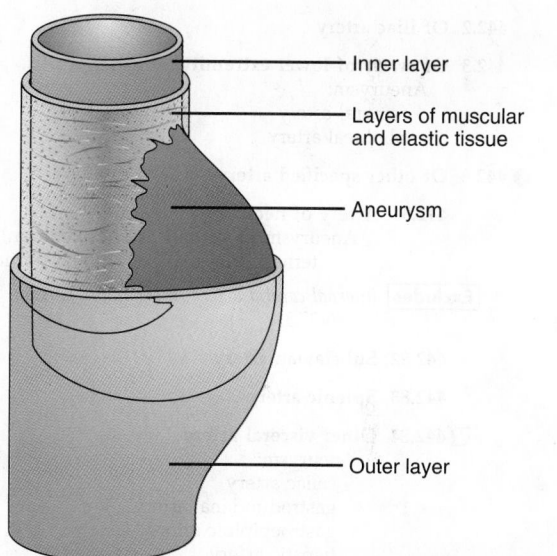

Figure 7-5   An aneurysm is an enclosed swelling on the wall of the vessel.

Item 7-10   Rupture is the tearing of the aneurysm.

● **441   Aortic aneurysm and dissection**

      Excludes   *syphilitic aortic aneurysm (093.0)*
                     traumatic aortic aneurysm (901.0, 902.0)

● **441.0   Dissection of aorta**

       ❑ **441.00   Unspecified site**

       441.01   Thoracic

       441.02   Abdominal

       441.03   Thoracoabdominal

    441.1   Thoracic aneurysm, ruptured

    441.2   Thoracic aneurysm without mention of rupture

    441.3   Abdominal aneurysm, ruptured

    441.4   Abdominal aneurysm without mention of rupture

ICD-9-CM

400-
449

Vol. 1

❏ **441.5 Aortic aneurysm of unspecified site, ruptured**
Rupture of aorta NOS

441.6 Thoracoabdominal aneurysm, ruptured

441.7 Thoracoabdominal aneurysm, without mention of rupture

❏ **441.9 Aortic aneurysm of unspecified site without mention of rupture**
Aneurysm
Dilatation of aorta
Hyaline necrosis of aorta

● **442 Other aneurysm**

Includes: aneurysm (ruptured) (cirsoid) (false) (varicose)
         aneurysmal varix

Excludes	*arteriovenous aneurysm or fistula:*
	acquired (447.0)
	congenital (747.60–747.69)
	traumatic (900.0–904.9)

442.0 Of artery of upper extremity

442.1 Of renal artery

442.2 Of iliac artery

442.3 Of artery of lower extremity
Aneurysm:
     femoral artery
     popliteal artery

● **442.8 Of other specified artery**

442.81 Artery of neck
Aneurysm of carotid artery (common) (external) (internal, extracranial portion)

Excludes	*internal carotid artery, intracranial portion (437.3)*

442.82 Subclavian artery

442.83 Splenic artery

❏ **442.84 Other visceral artery**
Aneurysm:
     celiac artery
     gastroduodenal artery
     gastroepiploic artery
     hepatic artery
     pancreaticoduodenal artery
     superior mesenteric artery

❏ **442.89 Other**
Aneurysm:
     mediastinal artery
     spinal artery

Excludes	*cerebral (nonruptured) (437.3)*
	congenital (747.81)
	ruptured (430)
	coronary (414.11)
	heart (414.10)
	pulmonary (417.1)

❏ **442.9 Of unspecified site**

● **443 Other peripheral vascular disease**

443.0 Raynaud's syndrome
Raynaud's:
     disease
     phenomenon (secondary)

Use additional code to identify gangrene (785.4)

443.1 Thromboangiitis obliterans [Buerger's disease]
Presenile gangrene

● **443.2 Other arterial dissection**

Excludes	*dissection of aorta (441.00–441.03)*
	dissection of coronary arteries (414.12)

443.21 Dissection of carotid artery

443.22 Dissection of iliac artery

443.23 Dissection of renal artery

443.24 Dissection of vertebral artery

❏ **443.29 Dissection of other artery**

● **443.8 Other specified peripheral vascular diseases**

● *443.81 Peripheral angiopathy in diseases classified elsewhere*

     Code first underlying disease, as:
         diabetes mellitus (250.7)

❏ **443.89 Other**
Acrocyanosis
Acroparesthesia:
     simple [Schultze's type]
     vasomotor [Nothnagel's type]
Erythrocyanosis
Erythromelalgia

Excludes	*chilblains (991.5)*
	frostbite (991.0–991.3)
	immersion foot (991.4)

❏ **443.9 Peripheral vascular disease, unspecified**
Intermittent claudication NOS
Peripheral:
     angiopathy NOS
     vascular disease NOS
Spasm of artery

Excludes	*atherosclerosis of the arteries of the extremities (440.20–440.22)*
	spasm of cerebral artery (435.0–435.9)

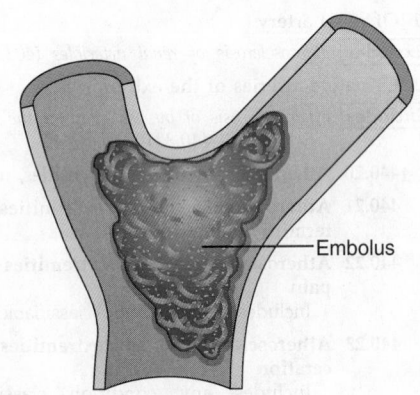

Figure 7–6 An arterial embolism.

Item 7-11 An embolus is a mass of undissolved matter present in the blood that is transported by the blood current. A **thrombus** is a blood clot that occludes or shuts off a vessel. When a thrombus is dislodged, it becomes an embolus.

● **444 Arterial embolism and thrombosis**

Includes: infarction:
embolic
thrombotic
occlusion

Excludes   *that complicating:*
abortion (634–638 with .6, 639.6)
atheroembolism (445.01–445.89)
ectopic or molar pregnancy (639.6)
pregnancy, childbirth, or the puerperium (673.0–673.8)

444.0 Of abdominal aorta
Aortic bifurcation syndrome
Aortoiliac obstruction
Leriche's syndrome
Saddle embolus

444.1 Of thoracic aorta
Embolism or thrombosis of aorta (thoracic)

● **444.2 Of arteries of the extremities**

444.21 Upper extremity

444.22 Lower extremity
Arterial embolism or thrombosis:
femoral
peripheral NOS
popliteal

Excludes   *iliofemoral (444.81)*

● **444.8 Of other specified artery**

444.81 Iliac artery

❏ **444.89 Other**

Excludes   *basilar (433.0)*
carotid (433.1)
cerebral (434.0–434.9)
coronary (410.00–410.92)
mesenteric (557.0)
ophthalmic (362.30–362.34)
precerebral (433.0–433.9)
pulmonary (415.19)
renal (593.81)
retinal (362.30–362.34)
vertebral (433.2)

❏ **444.9 Of unspecified artery**

● **445 Atheroembolism**

Includes: atherothrombotic microembolism
cholesterol embolism

● **445.0 Of extremities**

445.01 Upper extremity

445.02 Lower extremity

● **445.8 Of other sites**

445.81 Kidney
Use additional code for any associated kidney failure
(584, 585)

❏ **445.89 Other site**

● **446 Polyarteritis nodosa and allied conditions**

446.0 Polyarteritis nodosa
Disseminated necrotizing periarteritis
Necrotizing angiitis
Panarteritis (nodosa)
Periarteritis (nodosa)

446.1 Acute febrile mucocutaneous lymph node syndrome [MCLS]
Kawasaki disease

● **446.2 Hypersensitivity angiitis**

Excludes   *antiglomerular basement membrane disease without pulmonary hemorrhage (583.89)*

❏ **446.20 Hypersensitivity angiitis, unspecified**

446.21 Goodpasture's syndrome
Antiglomerular basement membrane antibody-mediated nephritis with pulmonary hemorrhage

Use additional code to identify renal disease
(583.81)

❏ **446.29 Other specified hypersensitivity angiitis**

446.3 Lethal midline granuloma
Malignant granuloma of face

446.4 Wegener's granulomatosis
Necrotizing respiratory granulomatosis
Wegener's syndrome

446.5 Giant cell arteritis
Cranial arteritis
Horton's disease
Temporal arteritis

446.6 Thrombotic microangiopathy
Moschcowitz's syndrome
Thrombotic thrombocytopenic purpura

446.7 Takayasu's disease
Aortic arch arteritis
Pulseless disease

● **447 Other disorders of arteries and arterioles**

447.0 Arteriovenous fistula, acquired
Arteriovenous aneurysm, acquired

Excludes   *cerebrovascular (437.3)*
coronary (414.19)
pulmonary (417.0)
surgically created arteriovenous shunt or fistula:
complication (996.1, 996.61–996.62)
status or presence (V45.1)
traumatic (900.0–904.9)

447.1 Stricture of artery

447.2 Rupture of artery
Erosion of artery
Fistula, except arteriovenous, of artery
Ulcer of artery

Excludes   *traumatic rupture of artery (900.0–904.9)*

447.3 Hyperplasia of renal artery
Fibromuscular hyperplasia of renal artery

447.4 Celiac artery compression syndrome
Celiac axis syndrome
Marable's syndrome

447.5 Necrosis of artery

❏ **447.6 Arteritis, unspecified**
Aortitis NOS
Endarteritis NOS

Excludes   *arteritis, endarteritis:*
aortic arch (446.7)
cerebral (437.4)
coronary (414.00–414.07)
deformans (440.0–440.9)
obliterans (440.0–440.9)
pulmonary (417.8)
senile (440.0–440.9)
polyarteritis NOS (446.0)
syphilitic aortitis (093.1)

ICD-9-CM

400-
499

Vol. 1

❏ **447.8 Other specified disorders of arteries and arterioles**
Fibromuscular hyperplasia of arteries, except renal

❏ **447.9 Unspecified disorders of arteries and arterioles**

● **448 Disease of capillaries**

448.0 Hereditary hemorrhagic telangiectasia
Rendu-Osler-Weber disease

448.1 Nevus, non-neoplastic
Nevus: Nevus:
  araneus   spider
  senile   stellar

Excludes *neoplastic (216.0–216.9)*
port wine (757.32)
strawberry (757.32)

❏ **448.9 Other and unspecified capillary diseases**
Capillary:
  hemorrhage
  hyperpermeability
  thrombosis

Excludes *capillary fragility (hereditary) (287.8)*

**DISEASES OF VEINS AND LYMPHATICS, AND OTHER DISEASES
OF CIRCULATORY SYSTEM (451–459)**

● **451 Phlebitis and thrombophlebitis**

Includes: endophlebitis
          inflammation, vein
          periphlebitis
          suppurative phlebitis

Use additional E code to identify drug, if drug-induced

Excludes *that complicating:*
abortion (634–638 with .7, 639.8)
ectopic or molar pregnancy (639.8)
*pregnancy, childbirth, or the puerperium
(671.0–671.9)*
that due to or following:
implant or catheter device (996.61–996.62)
infusion, perfusion, or transfusion (999.2)

451.0 Of superficial vessels of lower extremities
Saphenous vein (greater) (lesser)

● **451.1 Of deep vessels of lower extremities**

451.11 Femoral vein (deep) (superficial)

❏ **451.19 Other**
Femoropopliteal vein
Popliteal vein
Tibial vein

❏ **451.2 Of lower extremities, unspecified**

● **451.8 Of other sites**

Excludes *intracranial venous sinus (325)*
nonpyogenic (437.6)
portal (vein) (572.1)

451.81 Iliac vein

451.82 Of superficial veins of upper extremities
Antecubital vein   Cephalic vein
Basilic vein

451.83 Of deep veins of upper extremities
Brachial vein   Ulnar vein
Radial vein

❏ **451.84 Of upper extremities, unspecified**

❏ **451.89 Other**
Axillary vein
Jugular vein
Subclavian vein
Thrombophlebitis of breast (Mondor's disease)

❏ **451.9 Of unspecified site**

452 Portal vein thrombosis
Portal (vein) obstruction

Excludes *hepatic vein thrombosis (453.0)*
phlebitis of portal vein (572.1)

● **453 Other venous embolism and thrombosis**

Excludes *that complicating:*
abortion (634–638 with .7, 639.8)
ectopic or molar pregnancy (639.8)
*pregnancy, childbirth, or the puerperium
(671.0–671.9)*
*that with inflammation, phlebitis, and thrombo-
phlebitis (451.0–451.9)*

453.0 Budd-Chiari syndrome
Hepatic vein thrombosis

453.1 Thrombophlebitis migrans

453.2 Of vena cava

453.3 Of renal vein

● **453.4 Venous embolism and thrombosis of deep vessels
of lower extremity** ◀

❏ **453.40 Venous embolism and thrombosis of un-
specified deep vessels of lower extremity** ◀
Deep vein thrombosis NOS ◀
DVT NOS ◀

**453.41 Venous embolism and thrombosis of deep
vessels of proximal lower extremity** ◀
Femoral ◀
Iliac ◀
Popliteal ◀
Thigh ◀
Upper leg NOS ◀

**453.42 Venous embolism and thrombosis of deep
vessels of distal lower extremity** ◀
Calf ◀
Lower leg NOS ◀
Peroneal ◀
Tibial ◀

❏ **453.8 Of other specified veins**

Excludes *cerebral (434.0–434.9)*
coronary (410.00–410.92)
intracranial venous sinus (325)
nonpyogenic (437.6)
mesenteric (557.0)
portal (452)
precerebral (433.0–433.9)
pulmonary (415.19)

❏ **453.9 Of unspecified site**
Embolism of vein   Thrombosis (vein)

● **454 Varicose veins of lower extremities**

Excludes *that complicating pregnancy, childbirth, or the
puerperium (671.0)*

454.0 With ulcer
Varicose ulcer (lower extremity, any part)
Varicose veins with ulcer of lower extremity [any
part] or of unspecified site
Any condition classifiable to 454.9 with ulcer or
specified as ulcerated

454.1 With inflammation
Stasis dermatitis
Varicose veins with inflammation of lower ex-
tremity [any part] or of unspecified site
Any condition classifiable to 454.9 with inflamma-
tion or specified as inflamed

454.2 With ulcer and inflammation
Varicose veins with ulcer and inflammation of lower
extremity [any part] or of unspecified site
Any condition classifiable to 454.9 with ulcer and
inflammation

❏ **454.8 With other complications**
Edema
Pain
Swelling

454.9 Asymptomatic varicose veins
Phlebectasia of lower extremity [any part] or of
unspecified site
Varicose veins NOS
Varicose veins of lower extremity [any part] or of
unspecified site
Varix of lower extremity [any part] or of unspeci-
fied site

● **455 Hemorrhoids**

Includes: hemorrhoids (anus) (rectum)
piles
varicose veins, anus or rectum

Excludes *that complicating pregnancy, childbirth, or the*
puerperium (671.8)

455.0 Internal hemorrhoids without mention of compli-
cation

455.1 Internal thrombosed hemorrhoids

❏ **455.2 Internal hemorrhoids with other complication**
Internal hemorrhoids: Internal hemorrhoids:
   bleeding   strangulated
   prolapsed   ulcerated

455.3 External hemorrhoids without mention of compli-
cation

455.4 External thrombosed hemorrhoids

❏ **455.5 External hemorrhoids with other complication**
External hemorrhoids:
   bleeding
   prolapsed
   strangulated
   ulcerated

❏ **455.6 Unspecified hemorrhoids without mention of com-**
plication
Hemorrhoids NOS

❏ **455.7 Unspecified thrombosed hemorrhoids**
Thrombosed hemorrhoids, unspecified whether
internal or external

❏ **455.8 Unspecified hemorrhoids with other complication**
Hemorrhoids, unspecified whether internal or external:
   bleeding
   prolapsed
   strangulated
   ulcerated

455.9 Residual hemorrhoidal skin tags
Skin tags, anus or rectum

● **456 Varicose veins of other sites**

456.0 Esophageal varices with bleeding

456.1 Esophageal varices without mention of bleeding

● *456.2 Esophageal varices in diseases classified elsewhere*

   Code first underlying disease, as:
     cirrhosis of liver (571.0–571.9)
     portal hypertension (572.3)

   ● *456.20 With bleeding*

   ● *456.21 Without mention of bleeding*

456.3 Sublingual varices

456.4 Scrotal varices
Varicocele

456.5 Pelvic varices
Varices of broad ligament

456.6 Vulval varices
Varices of perineum

Excludes *that complicating pregnancy, childbirth, or the*
puerperium (671.1)

❏ **456.8 Varices of other sites**
Varicose veins of nasal septum (with ulcer)

Excludes *placental varices (656.7)*
retinal varices (362.17)
varicose ulcer of unspecified site (454.0)
varicose veins of unspecified site (454.9)

● **457 Noninfectious disorders of lymphatic channels**

457.0 Postmastectomy lymphedema syndrome
Elephantiasis due to mastectomy
Obliteration of lymphatic vessel due to mastectomy

❏ **457.1 Other lymphedema**
Elephantiasis (nonfilarial) NOS
Lymphangiectasis
Lymphedema: Lymphedema:
   acquired (chronic)   secondary
   praecox
Obliteration, lymphatic vessel

Excludes *elephantiasis (nonfilarial):*
   congenital (757.0)
   eyelid (374.83)
   vulva (624.8)

457.2 Lymphangitis
Lymphangitis:
   NOS
   chronic
   subacute

Excludes *acute lymphangitis (682.0–682.9)*

❏ **457.8 Other noninfectious disorders of lymphatic channels**
Chylocele (nonfilarial)
Chylous:
   ascites
   cyst
Lymph node or vessel:
   fistula
   infarction
   rupture

Excludes *chylocele:*
   filarial (125.0–125.9)
   tunica vaginalis (nonfilarial) (608.84)

❏ **457.9 Unspecified noninfectious disorder of lymphatic**
channels

● **458 Hypotension**

Includes: hypopiesis

Excludes *cardiovascular collapse (785.50)*
maternal hypotension syndrome (669.2)
shock (785.50–785.59)
Shy-Drager syndrome (333.0)

458.0 Orthostatic hypotension
Hypotension:
   orthostatic (chronic)
   postural

458.1 Chronic hypotension
Permanent idiopathic hypotension

458.2 Iatrogenic hypotension

   458.21 Hypotension of hemodialysis
Intra-dialytic hypotension

   458.29 Other iatrogenic hypodialysis
Postoperative hypotension

❏ **458.8 Other specified hypotension**

❏ **458.9 Hypotension, unspecified**
Hypotension (arterial) NOS

ICD-9-CM

400-
499

Vol. 1

● **459 Other disorders of circulatory system**

❏ **459.0 Hemorrhage, unspecified**
Rupture of blood vessel NOS
Spontaneous hemorrhage NEC

Excludes *hemorrhage:*
gastrointestinal NOS (578.9)
in newborn NOS (772.9)
*secondary or recurrent following trauma
(958.2)*
*traumatic rupture of blood vessel (900.0–
904.9)*

● **459.1 Postphlebitic syndrome**
Chronic venous hypertension due to deep vein
thrombosis

Excludes *chronic venous hypertension without deep vein
thrombosis (459.30–459.39)*

459.10 Postphlebetic syndrome without complications
Asymptomatic postphlebetic syndrome
Postphlebetic syndrome NOS

459.11 Postphlebetic syndrome with ulcer

459.12 Postphlebetic syndrome with inflammation

**459.13 Postphlebetic syndrome with ulcer and
inflammation**

❏ **459.19 Postphlebetic syndrome with other complication**

459.2 Compression of vein
Stricture of vein
Vena cava syndrome (inferior) (superior)

● **459.3 Chronic venous hypertension (idiopathic)**
Stasis edema

Excludes *chronic venous hypertension due to deep vein
thrombosis (459.10–459.19)*
varicose veins (454.0–454.9)

**459.30 Chronic venous hypertension without
complications**
Asymptomatic chronic venous hypertension
Chronic venous hypertension NOS

459.31 Chronic venous hypertension with ulcer

**459.32 Chronic venous hypertension with inflam-
mation**

**459.33 Chronic venous hypertension with ulcer
and inflammation**

❏ **459.39 Chronic venous hypertension with other
complication**

● **459.8 Other specified disorders of circulatory system**

❏ **459.81 Venous (peripheral) insufficiency, unspecified**
Chronic venous insufficiency NOS

Use additional code for any associated ulceration (707.10–707.9)

❏ **459.89 Other**
Collateral circulation (venous), any site
Phlebosclerosis
Venofibrosis

❏ **459.9 Unspecified circulatory system disorder**

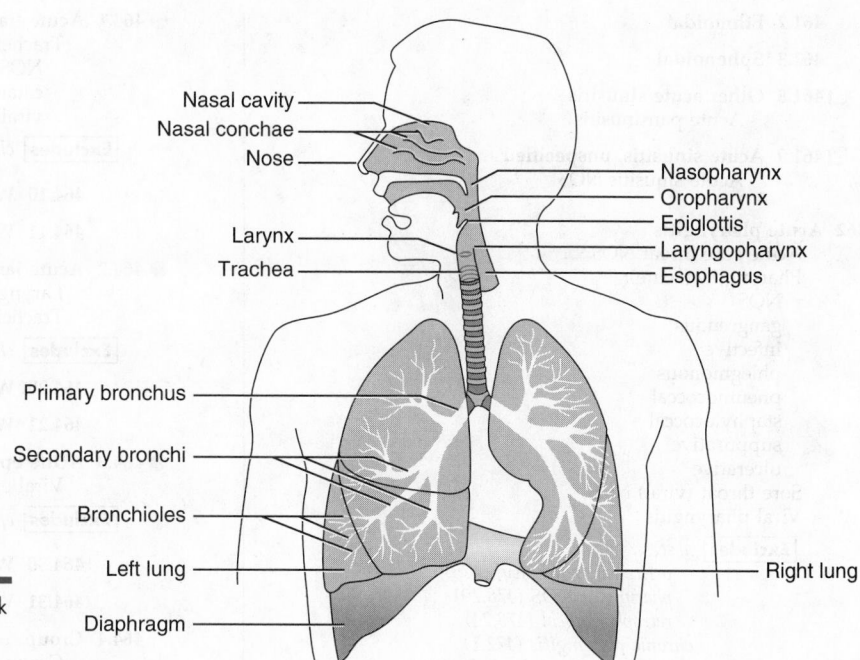

Figure 8-1 Respiratory system. (From Buck CJ: Step-by-Step Medical Coding, 2005 ed. Philadelphia, WBS, 2005.)

8. DISEASES OF THE RESPIRATORY SYSTEM (460-519)

Use additional code to identify infectious organism

ACUTE RESPIRATORY INFECTIONS (460-466)

| Excludes | *pneumonia and influenza (480.0-487.8)* |

460 Acute nasopharyngitis [common cold]
Coryza (acute)
Nasal catarrh, acute
Nasopharyngitis:
    NOS
    acute
    infective NOS
Rhinitis:
    acute
    infective

| Excludes | *nasopharyngitis, chronic (472.2)*
pharyngitis:
    acute or unspecified (462)
    chronic (472.1)
rhinitis:
    allergic (477.0-477.9)
    chronic or unspecified (472.0)
sore throat:
    acute or unspecified (462)
    chronic (472.1) |

Figure 8-2 Paranasal sinuses. (From Buck CJ: Step-by-Step Medical Coding, 2005 ed. Philadelphia, WBS, 2005.)

● **461 Acute sinusitis**

Includes: abscess, acute, of sinus (accessory) (nasal)
empyema, acute, of sinus (accessory) (nasal)
infection, acute, of sinus (accessory) (nasal)
inflammation, acute, of sinus (accessory) (nasal)
suppuration, acute, of sinus (accessory) (nasal)

| Excludes | *chronic or unspecified sinusitis (473.0-473.9)* |

461.0 Maxillary
Acute antritis

461.1 Frontal

461.2   Ethmoidal

461.3   Sphenoidal

☐ **461.8   Other acute sinusitis**
     Acute pansinusitis

☐ **461.9   Acute sinusitis, unspecified**
     Acute sinusitis NOS

462   Acute pharyngitis
     Acute sore throat NOS
     Pharyngitis (acute):
         NOS
         gangrenous
         infective
         phlegmonous
         pneumococcal
         staphylococcal
         suppurative
         ulcerative
     Sore throat (viral) NOS
     Viral pharyngitis

> **Excludes**   *abscess:*
>   *peritonsillar [quinsy] (475)*
>   *pharyngeal NOS (478.29)*
>   *retropharyngeal (478.24)*
>   *chronic pharyngitis (472.1)*
>   *infectious mononucleosis (075)*
>   *that specified as (due to):*
>   *Coxsackie (virus) (074.0)*
>   *gonococcus (098.6)*
>   *herpes simplex (054.79)*
>   *influenza (487.1)*
>   *septic (034.0)*
>   *streptococcal (034.0)*

463   Acute tonsillitis
     Tonsillitis (acute):
         NOS
         follicular
         gangrenous
         infective
         pneumococcal
         septic
         staphylococcal
         suppurative
         ulcerative
         viral

> **Excludes**   *chronic tonsillitis (474.0)*
>   *hypertrophy of tonsils (474.1)*
>   *peritonsillar abscess [quinsy] (475)*
>   *sore throat:*
>   *acute or NOS (462)*
>   *septic (034.0)*
>   *streptococcal tonsillitis (034.0)*

● **464   Acute laryngitis and tracheitis**

> **Excludes**   *that associated with influenza (487.1)*
>   *that due to Streptococcus (034.0)*

● **464.0   Acute laryngitis**
     Laryngitis (acute):
         NOS
         edematous
         Hemophilus influenzae [H. influenzae]
         pneumococcal
         septic
         suppurative
         ulcerative

> **Excludes**   *chronic laryngitis (476.0–476.1)*
>   *influenzal laryngitis (487.1)*

     464.00   Without mention of obstruction

     464.01   With obstruction

● **464.1   Acute tracheitis**
     Tracheitis (acute):
         NOS
         catarrhal
         viral

> **Excludes**   *chronic tracheitis (491.8)*

     464.10   Without mention of obstruction

     464.11   With obstruction

● **464.2   Acute laryngotracheitis**
     Laryngotracheitis (acute)
     Tracheitis (acute) with laryngitis (acute)

> **Excludes**   *chronic laryngotracheitis (476.1)*

     464.20   Without mention of obstruction

     464.21   With obstruction

● **464.3   Acute epiglottitis**
     Viral epiglottitis

> **Excludes**   *epiglottitis, chronic (476.1)*

     464.30   Without mention of obstruction

     464.31   With obstruction

     464.4   Croup
         Croup syndrome

● **464.5   Supraglottitis, unspecified**

     464.50   Without mention of obstruction

     464.51   With obstruction

● **465   Acute upper respiratory infections of multiple or unspecified sites**

> **Excludes**   *upper respiratory infection due to:*
>   *influenza (487.1)*
>   *Streptococcus (034.0)*

     465.0   Acute laryngopharyngitis

☐ **465.8   Other multiple sites**
     Multiple URI

☐ **465.9   Unspecified site**
     Acute URI NOS
     Upper respiratory infection (acute)

● **466   Acute bronchitis and bronchiolitis**

> **Includes:**   that with:
>   bronchospasm
>   obstruction

     466.0   Acute bronchitis

Bronchitis, acute or subacute:	Bronchitis, acute or subacute:
fibrinous	septic
membranous	viral
pneumococcal	with tracheitis
purulent	
Croupous bronchitis	
Tracheobronchitis, acute	

> **Excludes**   *acute bronchitis with chronic obstructive pulmonary disease (491.22)* ◀

● **466.1   Acute bronchiolitis**
     Bronchiolitis (acute)
     Capillary pneumonia

     466.11   Acute bronchiolitis due to respiratory syncytial virus (RSV)

☐ **466.19   Acute bronchiolitis due to other infectious organisms**

     Use additional code to identify organism

Figure 8-3 Deviated nasal septum.

Item 8-1 **A deviated nasal septum is the displacement of the septal cartilage.**

OTHER DISEASES OF THE UPPER RESPIRATORY TRACT (470–478)

470   Deviated nasal septum
Deflected septum (nasal) (acquired)

    Excludes   *congenital (754.0)*

● 471   Nasal polyps

    Excludes   *adenomatous polyps (212.0)*

471.0   Polyp of nasal cavity
Polyp:
    choanal
    nasopharyngeal

471.1   Polypoid sinus degeneration
Woakes' syndrome or ethmoiditis

❑ 471.8   Other polyp of sinus
Polyp of sinus:
    accessory
    ethmoidal
    maxillary
    sphenoidal

❑ 471.9   Unspecified nasal polyp
Nasal polyp NOS

● 472   Chronic pharyngitis and nasopharyngitis

472.0   Chronic rhinitis
Ozena
Rhinitis: Rhinitis:
    NOS   obstructive
    atrophic   purulent
    granulomatous   ulcerative
    hypertrophic

    Excludes   *allergic rhinitis (477.0–477.9)*

472.1   Chronic pharyngitis
Chronic sore throat
Pharyngitis:
    atrophic
    granular (chronic)
    hypertrophic

472.2   Chronic nasopharyngitis

    Excludes   *acute or unspecified nasopharyngitis (460)*

● 473   Chronic sinusitis

    Includes: abscess (chronic) of sinus (accessory) (nasal)
              empyema (chronic) of sinus (accessory) (nasal)
              infection (chronic) of sinus (accessory) (nasal)
              suppuration (chronic) of sinus (accessory) (nasal)

    Excludes   *acute sinusitis (461.0–461.9)*

473.0   Maxillary
Antritis (chronic)

473.1   Frontal

473.2   Ethmoidal

    Excludes   *Woakes' ethmoiditis (471.1)*

473.3   Sphenoidal

❑ 473.8   Other chronic sinusitis
Pansinusitis (chronic)

❑ 473.9   Unspecified sinusitis (chronic)
Sinusitis (chronic) NOS

● 474   Chronic disease of tonsils and adenoids

● 474.0   Chronic tonsillitis and adenoiditis

    Excludes   *acute or unspecified tonsillitis (463)*

    474.00   Chronic tonsillitis

    474.01   Chronic adenoiditis

    474.02   Chronic tonsillitis and adenoiditis

● 474.1   Hypertrophy of tonsils and adenoids
Enlargement of tonsils or adenoids
Hyperplasia of tonsils or adenoids
Hypertrophy of tonsils or adenoids

    Excludes   *that with:*
           adenoiditis (474.01)
           adenoiditis and tonsillitis (474.02)
           tonsillitis (474.00)

    474.10   Tonsils with adenoids

    474.11   Tonsils alone

    474.12   Adenoids alone

474.2   Adenoid vegetations

❑ 474.8   Other chronic disease of tonsils and adenoids
Amygdalolith
Calculus, tonsil
Cicatrix of tonsil (and adenoid)
Tonsillar tag
Ulcer, tonsil

❑ 474.9   Unspecified chronic disease of tonsils and adenoids
Disease (chronic) of tonsils (and adenoids)

475   Peritonsillar abscess
Abscess of tonsil
Peritonsillar cellulitis
Quinsy

    Excludes   *tonsillitis:*
           acute or NOS (463)
           chronic (474.0)

● 476   Chronic laryngitis and laryngotracheitis

476.0   Chronic laryngitis
Laryngitis:
    catarrhal
    hypertrophic
    sicca

ICD-9-CM

400-499

Vol. 1

476.1 Chronic laryngotracheitis
  Laryngitis, chronic, with tracheitis (chronic)
  Tracheitis, chronic, with laryngitis
  | Excludes | *chronic tracheitis (491.8)*
  laryngitis and tracheitis, acute or unspecified
  (464.00–464.51)

● **477 Allergic rhinitis**
  Includes: allergic rhinitis (nonseasonal) (seasonal)
  hay fever
  spasmodic rhinorrhea
  | Excludes | *allergic rhinitis with asthma (bronchial) (493.0)*

  477.0 Due to pollen
    Pollinosis

  477.1 Due to food

  477.2 Due to animal (cat) (dog) hair and dander ◀

  ❑ **477.8 Due to other allergen**

  ❑ **477.9 Cause unspecified**

● **478 Other diseases of upper respiratory tract**

  478.0 Hypertrophy of nasal turbinates

  ❑ **478.1 Other diseases of nasal cavity and sinuses**
    Abscess of nose (septum)
    Necrosis of nose (septum)
    Ulcer of nose (septum)
    Cyst or mucocele of sinus (nasal)
    Rhinolith
    | Excludes | *varicose ulcer of nasal septum (456.8)*

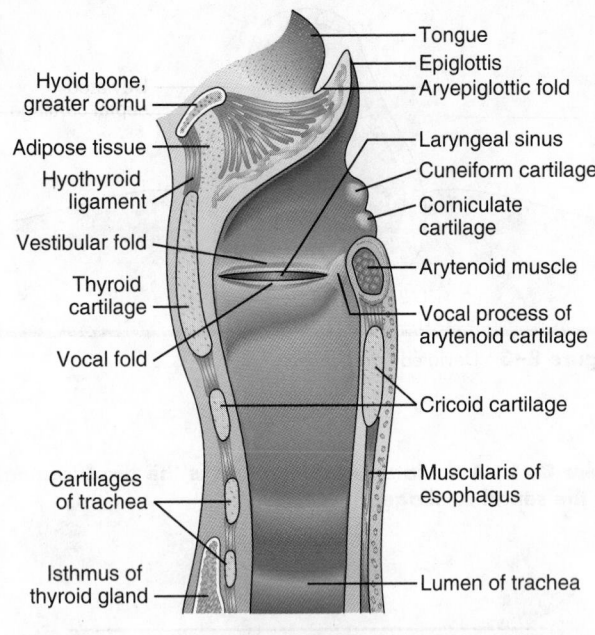

Figure 8–5 Coronal section of the larynx.

Item 8–3 The larynx extends from the tongue to the trachea and is divided into an upper and lower portion separated by folds. The framework of the larynx is cartilage composed of the single cricoid, thyroid, and epiglottic cartilages, and the paired arytenoid, cuneiform, and corniculate cartilages.

● **478.3 Paralysis of vocal cords or larynx**

  ❑ **478.30 Paralysis, unspecified**
    Laryngoplegia   Paralysis of glottis

  478.31 Unilateral, partial

  478.32 Unilateral, complete

  478.33 Bilateral, partial

  478.34 Bilateral, complete

  478.4 Polyp of vocal cord or larynx
    | Excludes | *adenomatous polyps (212.1)*

  ❑ **478.5 Other diseases of vocal cords**
    Abscess of vocal cords
    Cellulitis of vocal cords
    Granuloma of vocal cords
    Leukoplakia of vocal cords
    Chorditis (fibrinous) (nodosa) (tuberosa)
    Singers' nodes

  478.6 Edema of larynx
    Edema (of):   Edema (of):
     glottis   supraglottic
     subglottic

● **478.7 Other diseases of larynx, not elsewhere classified**

  ❑ **478.70 Unspecified disease of larynx**

  478.71 Cellulitis and perichondritis of larynx

  478.74 Stenosis of larynx

  478.75 Laryngeal spasm
    Laryngismus (stridulus)

  ❑ **478.79 Other**
    Abscess of larynx
    Necrosis of larynx
    Obstruction of larynx
    Pachyderma of larynx
    Ulcer of larynx
    | Excludes | *ulcerative laryngitis (464.00–464.01)*

Figure 8–4 The pharynx.

Item 8–2 The pharynx is the passage for both food and air between the mouth and the esophagus and is divided into three areas: nasopharynx, oropharynx, and hypopharynx. The hypopharynx branches into the esophagus and the voice box.

● **478.2 Other diseases of pharynx, not elsewhere classified**

  ❑ **478.20 Unspecified disease of pharynx**

  478.21 Cellulitis of pharynx or nasopharynx

  478.22 Parapharyngeal abscess

  478.24 Retropharyngeal abscess

  478.25 Edema of pharynx or nasopharynx

  478.26 Cyst of pharynx or nasopharynx

  ❑ **478.29 Other**
    Abscess of pharynx or nasopharynx
    | Excludes | *ulcerative pharyngitis (462)*

☐ **478.8   Upper respiratory tract hypersensitivity reaction, site unspecified**

> **Excludes**   *hypersensitivity reaction of lower respiratory tract, as:*
> > *extrinsic allergic alveolitis (495.0–495.9)*
> > *pneumoconiosis (500–505)*

☐ **478.9   Other and unspecified diseases of upper respiratory tract**

> Abscess of trachea   Cicatrix of trachea

PNEUMONIA AND INFLUENZA (480–487)

> **Excludes**   *pneumonia:*
> > *allergic or eosinophilic (518.3)*
> > *aspiration:*
> > > *NOS (507.0)*
> > > *newborn (770.1)*
> > > *solids and liquids (507.0–507.8)*
> > *congenital (770.0)*
> > *lipoid (507.1)*
> > *passive (514)*
> > *rheumatic (390)*

● **480   Viral pneumonia**

    480.0   Pneumonia due to adenovirus

    480.1   Pneumonia due to respiratory syncytial virus

    480.2   Pneumonia due to parainfluenza virus

    480.3   Pneumonia due to SARS-associated coronavirus

    ☐ **480.8   Pneumonia due to other virus not elsewhere classified**

> **Excludes**   *congenital rubella pneumonitis (771.0)*
> > *influenza with pneumonia, any form (487.0)*
> > *pneumonia complicating viral diseases classified elsewhere (484.1–484.8)*

    ☐ **480.9   Viral pneumonia, unspecified**

481   Pneumococcal pneumonia [Streptococcus pneumoniae pneumonia]

> Lobar pneumonia, organism unspecified

● **482   Other bacterial pneumonia**

    482.0   Pneumonia due to Klebsiella pneumoniae

    482.1   Pneumonia due to Pseudomonas

    482.2   Pneumonia due to Haemophilus influenzae [H. influenzae]

●   **482.3   Pneumonia due to Streptococcus**

> **Excludes**   *Streptococcus pneumoniae pneumonia (481)*

    ☐ **482.30   Streptococcus, unspecified**

    482.31   Group A

    482.32   Group B

    ☐ **482.39   Other Streptococcus**

●   **482.4   Pneumonia due to Staphylococcus**

    ☐ **482.40   Pneumonia due to *Staphylococcus*, unspecified**

    482.41   Pneumonia due to *Staphylococcus aureus*

    ☐ **482.49   Other *Staphylococcus* pneumonia**

● **482.8   Pneumonia due to other specified bacteria**

> **Excludes**   *pneumonia complicating infectious disease classified elsewhere (484.1–484.8)*

    482.81   Anaerobes

> Bacteroides (melaninogenicus)
> Gram-negative anaerobes

    482.82   Escherichia coli [E. coli]

    ☐ **482.83   Other gram-negative bacteria**

> Gram-negative pneumonia NOS
> Proteus
> Serratia marcescens

> **Excludes**   *gram-negative anaerobes (482.81)*
> > *Legionnaires' disease (482.84)*

    482.84   Legionnaires' disease

    ☐ **482.89   Other specified bacteria**

☐ **482.9   Bacterial pneumonia unspecified**

● **483   Pneumonia due to other specified organism**

    483.0   Mycoplasma pneumoniae

> Eaton's agent
> Pleuropneumonia-like organisms [PPLO]

    483.1   Chlamydia

    ☐ **483.8   Other specified organism**

● **484   Pneumonia in infectious diseases classified elsewhere**

> **Excludes**   *influenza with pneumonia, any form (487.0)*

●   **484.1   *Pneumonia in cytomegalic inclusion disease***

> *Code first underlying disease, as: (078.5)*

●   **484.3   *Pneumonia in whooping cough***

> *Code first underlying disease, as: (033.0–033.9)*

●   **484.5   *Pneumonia in anthrax***

> *Code first underlying disease (022.1)*

●   **484.6   *Pneumonia in aspergillosis***

> *Code first underlying disease (117.3)*

●☐   **484.7   *Pneumonia in other systemic mycoses***

> *Code first underlying disease*

> **Excludes**   *pneumonia in:*
> > *candidiasis (112.4)*
> > *coccidioidomycosis (114.0)*
> > *histoplasmosis (115.0–115.9 with fifth-digit 5)*

●☐   **484.8   *Pneumonia in other infectious diseases classified elsewhere***

> *Code first underlying disease, as:*
> Q fever (083.0)
> typhoid fever (002.0)

> **Excludes**   *pneumonia in:*
> > *actinomycosis (039.1)*
> > *measles (055.1)*
> > *nocardiosis (039.1)*
> > *ornithosis (073.0)*
> > *Pneumocystis carinii (136.3)*
> > *salmonellosis (003.22)*
> > *toxoplasmosis (130.4)*
> > *tuberculosis (011.6)*
> > *tularemia (021.2)*
> > *varicella (052.1)*

☐ **485   Bronchopneumonia, organism unspecified**

Bronchopneumonia:	Pneumonia:
hemorrhagic	lobular
terminal	segmental

> Pleurobronchopneumonia

> **Excludes**   *bronchiolitis (acute) (466.11– 466.19)*
> > *chronic (491.8)*
> > *lipoid pneumonia (507.1)*

ICD-9-CM

400- 499

Vol. 1

☐ **486 Pneumonia, organism unspecified**

> | Excludes | *hypostatic or passive pneumonia (514)* |
> |---|---|
> | | *influenza with pneumonia, any form (487.0)* |
> | | *inhalation or aspiration pneumonia due to for-* |
> | | *eign materials (507.0–507.8)* |
> | | *pneumonitis due to fumes and vapors (506.0)* |

● **487 Influenza**

> | Excludes | *Hemophilus influenzae [H. influenzae]:* |
> |---|---|
> | | *infection NOS (041.5)* |
> | | *laryngitis (464.00–464.01)* |
> | | *meningitis (320.0)* |
> | | *pneumonia (482.2)* |

487.0 With pneumonia
Influenza with pneumonia, any form
Influenzal:
bronchopneumonia
pneumonia

☐ **487.1 With other respiratory manifestations**
Influenza NOS
Influenzal:
laryngitis
pharyngitis
respiratory infection (upper) (acute)

☐ **487.8 With other manifestations**
Encephalopathy due to influenza
Influenza with involvement of gastrointestinal tract

> | Excludes | *"intestinal flu" [viral gastroenteritis] (008.8)* |
> |---|---|

CHRONIC OBSTRUCTIVE PULMONARY DISEASE AND ALLIED CONDITIONS (490–496)

Item 8-4 Chronic bronchitis is usually defined as being present in any patient who has persistent cough with sputum production for at least three months in at least two consecutive years. **Simple chronic bronchitis** is marked by a productive cough but no pathological airflow obstruction. **Chronic obstructive pulmonary disease (COPD)** is a group of conditions—bronchitis, emphysema, asthma, bronchiectasis, allergic alveolitis—marked by dyspnea. **Catarrhal** bronchitis is an acute form of bronchitis marked by profuse mucus and pus production (**mucopurulent** discharge). **Croupous** bronchitis, also known as pseudomembranous, fibrinous, plastic, exudative, or membranous, is marked by a violent cough and dyspnea.

☐ **490 Bronchitis, not specified as acute or chronic**
Bronchitis NOS:
catarrhal
with tracheitis NOS
Tracheobronchitis NOS

> | Excludes | *bronchitis:* |
> |---|---|
> | | *allergic NOS (493.9)* |
> | | *asthmatic NOS (493.9)* |
> | | *due to fumes and vapors (506.0)* |

● **491 Chronic bronchitis**

> | Excludes | *chronic obstructive asthma (493.2)* |
> |---|---|

491.0 Simple chronic bronchitis
Catarrhal bronchitis, chronic
Smokers' cough

491.1 Mucopurulent chronic bronchitis
Bronchitis (chronic) (recurrent):
fetid
mucopurulent
purulent

● **491.2 Obstructive chronic bronchitis**
Bronchitis:
emphysematous
obstructive (chronic) (diffuse)
Bronchitis with:
chronic airway obstruction
emphysema

> | Excludes | *asthmatic bronchitis (acute) (NOS) 493.9* |
> |---|---|
> | | *chronic obstructive asthma 493.2* |

491.20 Without exacerbation
Emphysema with chronic bronchitis

491.21 With (acute) exacerbation
Decompensated chronic obstructive pulmonary disease [COPD]
Decompensated chronic obstructive pulmonary disease [COPD] with exacerbation

> | Excludes | *chronic obstructive asthma with acute exacerbation (493.22)* |
> |---|---|

491.22 With acute bronchitis ◀

☐ **491.8 Other chronic bronchitis**
Chronic:
tracheitis
tracheobronchitis

☐ **491.9 Unspecified chronic bronchitis**

● **492 Emphysema**

492.0 Emphysematous bleb
Giant bullous emphysema
Ruptured emphysematous bleb
Tension pneumatocele
Vanishing lung

☐ **492.8 Other emphysema**

Emphysema (lung or pulmonary):	Emphysema (lung or pulmonary):
NOS	panacinar
centriacinar	panlobular
centrilobular	unilateral
obstructive	vesicular

MacLeod's syndrome
Swyer-James syndrome
Unilateral hyperlucent lung

> | Excludes | *emphysema:* |
> |---|---|
> | | *with chronic bronchitis (491.20–491.22)* ◀ |
> | | *compensatory (518.2)* |
> | | *due to fumes and vapors (506.4)* |
> | | *interstitial (518.1)* |
> | | *newborn (770.2)* |
> | | *mediastinal (518.1)* |
> | | *surgical (subcutaneous) (998.81)* |
> | | *traumatic (958.7)* |
> | | *with chronic bronchitis (491.20)* |

Item 8-5 Asthma is a bronchial condition marked by airway obstruction, hyper-responsiveness, and inflammation. **Extrinsic** asthma, also known as allergic asthma, is characterized by the same symptoms that occur with exposure to allergens and is divided into the following types: **atopic, occupational, and allergic bronchopulmonary aspergillosis. Intrinsic** asthma occurs in patients who have no history of allergy or sensitivities to allergens and is divided into the following types: **nonreaginic and pharmacologic. Status asthmaticus** is the most severe form of asthma attack and can last for days or weeks.

● 493 **Asthma**

The following fifth-digit subclassification is for use with codes 493.0–493.2, 493.9:

  0 unspecified
  1 with status asthmaticus
  2 with (acute) exacerbation

  | **Excludes** | *wheezing NOS (786.07)* |

● 493.0 **Extrinsic asthma**
  Asthma:
    allergic with stated cause
    atopic
    childhood
    hay
    platinum
  Hay fever with asthma

Excludes	*asthma:*
	allergic NOS (493.9)
	detergent (507.8)
	miners' (500)
	wood (495.8)

● 493.1 **Intrinsic asthma**
  Late-onset asthma

● 493.2 **Chronic obstructive asthma**
  Asthma with chronic obstructive pulmonary disease (COPD)
  Chronic asthmatic bronchitis

  | **Excludes** | *acute bronchitis (466.0)* |
  | | *chronic obstructive bronchitis (491.20–491.22)* ◀▥ |

● 493.8 **Other forms of asthma**

  493.81 **Exercise induced bronchospasm**

  493.82 **Cough variant asthma**

● ❑ 493.9 **Asthma, unspecified**
  Asthma (bronchial) (allergic NOS)
  Bronchitis:
    allergic
    asthmatic

● 494 **Bronchiectasis**
  Bronchiectasis (fusiform) (postinfectious) (recurrent)
  Bronchiolectasis

  | **Excludes** | *congenital (748.61)* |
  | | *tuberculous bronchiectasis (current disease) (011.5)* |

  494.0 **Bronchiectasis without acute exacerbation**

  494.1 **Bronchiectasis with acute exacerbation**

● 495 **Extrinsic allergic alveolitis**

  Includes: allergic alveolitis and pneumonitis due to inhaled organic dust particles of fungal, thermophilic actinomycete, or other origin

  495.0 **Farmers' lung**

  495.1 **Bagassosis**

  495.2 **Bird-fanciers' lung**
    Budgerigar-fanciers' disease or lung
    Pigeon-fanciers' disease or lung

  495.3 **Suberosis**
    Cork-handlers' disease or lung

  495.4 **Malt workers' lung**
    Alveolitis due to Aspergillus clavatus

  495.5 **Mushroom workers' lung**

  495.6 **Maple bark-strippers' lung**
    Alveolitis due to Cryptostroma corticale

  495.7 **"Ventilation" pneumonitis**
    Allergic alveolitis due to fungal, thermophilic actinomycete, and other organisms growing in ventilation [air conditioning] systems

❑ 495.8 **Other specified allergic alveolitis and pneumonitis**
    Cheese-washers' lung
    Coffee workers' lung
    Fish-meal workers' lung
    Furriers' lung
    Grain-handlers' disease or lung
    Pituitary snuff-takers' disease
    Sequoiosis or red-cedar asthma
    Wood asthma

❑ 495.9 **Unspecified allergic alveolitis and pneumonitis**
    Alveolitis, allergic (extrinsic)
    Hypersensitivity pneumonitis

❑ 496 **Chronic airway obstruction, not elsewhere classified**
  Chronic:
    nonspecific lung disease
    obstructive lung disease
    obstructive pulmonary disease [COPD] NOS

  Note: This code is not to be used with any code from categories 491–493

Excludes	*chronic obstructive lung disease [COPD] specified (as) (with):*
	allergic alveolitis (495.0–495.9)
	asthma (493.2)
	bronchiectasis (494.0–494.1)
	bronchitis (491.20–491.22) ◀▥
	with emphysema (491.20–491.22) ◀▥
emphysema (492.0–492.8)

ICD-9-CM

400-499

Vol. 1

Figure 8-6 Progressive massive fibrosis superimposed on coalworkers' pneumoconiosis. The large, blackened scars are located principally in the upper lobe. Note extensions of scars into surrounding parenchyma and retraction of adjacent pleura. (From Cotran R, Kumar V, Collins T: Robbins Pathologic Basis of Disease, 6/e. Philadelphia, WBS, 1999, pg. 730. Courtesy of Dr. Warner Laquer, Dr. Jerome Kleinerman, and the National Institute of Occupational Safety and Health, Morgantown, WV.)

Item 8-6 Pneumoconiosis refers to a lung condition resulting from exposure to inorganic or organic airborne particles, such as coal dust or moldy hay, as well as chemical fumes and vapors, such as insecticides. In this condition, the lungs retain the airborne particles.

PNEUMOCONIOSES AND OTHER LUNG DISEASES DUE TO EXTERNAL AGENTS (500–508)

500   Coal workers' pneumoconiosis
Anthracosilicosis
Anthracosis
Black lung disease
Coal workers' lung
Miners' asthma

501   Asbestosis

☐ **502   Pneumoconiosis due to other silica or silicates**
Pneumoconiosis due to talc
Silicotic fibrosis (massive) of lung
Silicosis (simple) (complicated)

☐ **503   Pneumoconiosis due to other inorganic dust**
Aluminosis (of lung)
Bauxite fibrosis (of lung)
Berylliosis
Graphite fibrosis (of lung)
Siderosis
Stannosis

☐ **504   Pneumonopathy due to inhalation of other dust**
Byssinosis
Cannabinosis
Flax-dressers' disease

> **Excludes**   allergic alveolitis (495.0–495.9)
> asbestosis (501)
> bagassosis (495.1)
> farmers' lung (495.0)

☐ **505   Pneumoconiosis, unspecified**

● **506   Respiratory conditions due to chemical fumes and vapors**
Use additional E code to identify cause

506.0   Bronchitis and pneumonitis due to fumes and vapors
Chemical bronchitis (acute)

506.1   Acute pulmonary edema due to fumes and vapors
Chemical pulmonary edema (acute)

> **Excludes**   acute pulmonary edema NOS (518.4)
> chronic or unspecified pulmonary edema (514)

506.2   Upper respiratory inflammation due to fumes and vapors

☐ **506.3   Other acute and subacute respiratory conditions due to fumes and vapors**

506.4   Chronic respiratory conditions due to fumes and vapors
Emphysema (diffuse) (chronic) due to inhalation of chemical fumes and vapors
Obliterative bronchiolitis (chronic) (subacute) due to inhalation of chemical fumes and vapors
Pulmonary fibrosis (chronic) due to inhalation of chemical fumes and vapors

☐ **506.9   Unspecified respiratory conditions due to fumes and vapors**
Silo-fillers' disease

● **507   Pneumonitis due to solids and liquids**

> **Excludes**   fetal aspiration pneumonitis (770.1)

507.0   Due to inhalation of food or vomitus
Aspiration pneumonia (due to):
NOS   milk
food (regurgitated)   saliva
gastric secretions   vomitus

507.1   Due to inhalation of oils and essences
Lipoid pneumonia (exogenous)

> **Excludes**   endogenous lipoid pneumonia (516.8)

☐ **507.8   Due to other solids and liquids**
Detergent asthma

● **508   Respiratory conditions due to other and unspecified external agents**
Use additional E code to identify cause

508.0   Acute pulmonary manifestations due to radiation
Radiation pneumonitis

508.1   Chronic and other pulmonary manifestations due to radiation
Fibrosis of lung following radiation

☐ **508.8   Respiratory conditions due to other specified external agents**

☐ **508.9   Respiratory conditions due to unspecified external agent**

Figure 8–7   The apex of a lung (to the right) in a heavy cigarette smoker with severe emphysema (enlargement and distortion of the airspaces). (From Cotran R, Kumar V, Robbins S: Robbins Pathologic Basis of Disease. Philadelphia, WB Saunders, 1994, p 381.)

Item 8–7   Empyema is a condition in which pus accumulates in a body cavity. **Empyema with fistula** occurs when the pus passes from one cavity to another organ or structure.

OTHER DISEASES OF RESPIRATORY SYSTEM (510–519)

● 510 **Empyema**

Use additional code to identify infectious organism (041.0–041.9)

> **Excludes** *abscess of lung (513.0)*

510.0 **With fistula**

Fistula:	Fistula:
bronchocutaneous	mediastinal
bronchopleural	pleural
hepatopleural	thoracic

Any condition classifiable to 510.9 with fistula

510.9 **Without mention of fistula**
Abscess:
pleura
thorax
Empyema (chest) (lung) (pleura)
Fibrinopurulent pleurisy
Pleurisy:
purulent
septic
seropurulent
suppurative
Pyopneumothorax
Pyothorax

● 511 **Pleurisy**

> **Excludes** *malignant pleural effusion (197.2)*
> *pleurisy with mention of tuberculosis, current disease (012.0)*

511.0 **Without mention of effusion or current tuberculosis**
Adhesion, lung or pleura
Calcification of pleura
Pleurisy (acute) (sterile):
diaphragmatic
fibrinous
interlobar
Pleurisy:
NOS
pneumococcal
staphylococcal
streptococcal
Thickening of pleura

❑ 511.1 **With effusion, with mention of a bacterial cause other than tuberculosis**
Pleurisy with effusion (exudative) (serous):
pneumococcal
staphylococcal
streptococcal
other specified nontuberculous bacterial cause

❑ 511.8 **Other specified forms of effusion, except tuberculous**
Encysted pleurisy
Hemopneumothorax
Hemothorax
Hydropneumothorax
Hydrothorax

> **Excludes** *traumatic (860.2–860.5, 862.29, 862.39)*

❑ 511.9 **Unspecified pleural effusion**
Pleural effusion NOS
Pleurisy:
exudative
serofibrinous
serous
with effusion NOS

● 512 **Pneumothorax**

512.0 **Spontaneous tension pneumothorax**

512.1 **Iatrogenic pneumothorax**
Postoperative pneumothorax

❑ 512.8 **Other spontaneous pneumothorax**
Pneumothorax:
NOS
acute
chronic

> **Excludes** *pneumothorax:*
> *congenital (770.2)*
> *traumatic (860.0–860.1, 860.4–860.5)*
> *tuberculous, current disease (011.7)*

● 513 **Abscess of lung and mediastinum**

513.0 **Abscess of lung**
Abscess (multiple) of lung
Gangrenous or necrotic pneumonia
Pulmonary gangrene or necrosis

513.1 **Abscess of mediastinum**

514 **Pulmonary congestion and hypostasis**
Hypostatic:
bronchopneumonia
pneumonia
Passive pneumonia
Pulmonary congestion (chronic) (passive)
Pulmonary edema:
NOS
chronic

> **Excludes** *acute pulmonary edema:*
> *NOS (518.4)*
> *with mention of heart disease or failure (428.1)*

515 **Postinflammatory pulmonary fibrosis**
Cirrhosis of lung chronic or unspecified
Fibrosis of lung (atrophic) (confluent) (massive) (perialveolar) (peribronchial) chronic or unspecified
Induration of lung chronic or unspecified

● 516 **Other alveolar and parietoalveolar pneumonopathy**

516.0 **Pulmonary alveolar proteinosis**

● 516.1 *Idiopathic pulmonary hemosiderosis*
Essential brown induration of lung

Code first underlying disease (275.0)

516.2 **Pulmonary alveolar microlithiasis**

516.3 **Idiopathic fibrosing alveolitis**
Alveolar capillary block
Diffuse (idiopathic) (interstitial) pulmonary fibrosis
Hamman-Rich syndrome

❑ 516.8 **Other specified alveolar and parietoalveolar pneumonopathies**
Endogenous lipoid pneumonia
Interstitial pneumonia (desquamative) (lymphoid)

> **Excludes** *lipoid pneumonia, exogenous or unspecified (507.1)*

❑ 516.9 **Unspecified alveolar and parietoalveolar pneumonopathy**

● 517 **Lung involvement in conditions classified elsewhere**

> **Excludes** *rheumatoid lung (714.81)*

● 517.1 *Rheumatic pneumonia*

Code first underlying disease (390)

● 517.2 *Lung involvement in systemic sclerosis*

Code first underlying disease (710.1)

517.3 *Acute chest syndrome*

Code first sickle-cell disease in crisis (282.42, 282.62, 282.64, 282.69)

ICD-9-CM

500-599

Vol. 1

●❑ **517.8** *Lung involvement in other diseases classified else-where*

        Code first underlying disease, as:
           amyloidosis (277.3)
           polymyositis (710.4)
           sarcoidosis (135)
           Sjögren's disease (710.2)
           systemic lupus erythematosus (710.0)

        | **Excludes** | *syphilis (095.1)*

● **518   Other diseases of lung**

    518.0   Pulmonary collapse
        Atelectasis
        Collapse of lung
        Middle lobe syndrome

      | **Excludes** | *atelectasis:*
           congenital (partial) (770.5)
           primary (770.4)
           tuberculous, current disease (011.8)

    518.1   Interstitial emphysema
        Mediastinal emphysema

      | **Excludes** | *surgical (subcutaneous) emphysema (998.81)*
           that in fetus or newborn (770.2)
           traumatic emphysema (958.7)

    518.2   Compensatory emphysema

    518.3   Pulmonary eosinophilia
        Eosinophilic asthma
        Löffler's syndrome
        Pneumonia:
           allergic
           eosinophilic
        Tropical eosinophilia

 ❑ **518.4   Acute edema of lung, unspecified**
        Acute pulmonary edema NOS
        Pulmonary edema, postoperative

      | **Excludes** | *pulmonary edema:*
           acute, with mention of heart disease or failure (428.1)
           chronic or unspecified (514)
           due to external agents (506.0–508.9)

    518.5   Pulmonary insufficiency following trauma and sur-gery
        Adult respiratory distress syndrome
        Pulmonary insufficiency following:
           shock
           surgery
           trauma
        Shock lung

      | **Excludes** | *adult respiratory distress syndrome associated with other conditions (518.82)*
           pneumonia:
           aspiration (507.0)
           hypostatic (514)
           respiratory failure in other conditions (518.81, 518.83–518.84)

    518.6   Allergic bronchopulmonary aspergillosis

 ● **518.8   Other diseases of lung**

       518.81   Acute respiratory failure
           Respiratory failure NOS

     | **Excludes** | *acute and chronic respiratory failure (518.84)*
          acute respiratory distress (518.82)
          chronic respiratory failure (518.83)
          respiratory arrest (799.1)
          respiratory failure, newborn (770.84)

❑ **518.82   Other pulmonary insufficiency, not else-where classified**
        Acute respiratory distress
        Acute respiratory insufficiency
        Adult respiratory distress syndrome NEC

      | **Excludes** | *adult respiratory distress syndrome associated with trauma or surgery (518.5)*
           pulmonary insufficiency following trauma or surgery (518.5)
           respiratory distress:
           NOS (786.09)
           newborn (770.89)
           syndrome, newborn (769)
           shock lung (518.5)

    518.83   Chronic respiratory failure

    518.84   Acute and chronic respiratory failure
        Acute on chronic respiratory failure

❑ **518.89   Other diseases of lung, not elsewhere classified**
        Broncholithiasis   Lung disease NOS
        Calcification of lung   Pulmolithiasis

● **519   Other diseases of respiratory system**

 ● **519.0   Tracheostomy complications**

  ❑ **519.00   Tracheostomy complication, unspecified**

    519.01   Infection of tracheostomy

    Use additional code to identify type of infection, such as:
        abscess or cellulitis of neck (682.1)
        septicemia (038.0–038.9)

    Use additional code to identify organism (041.00–041.9)

    519.02   Mechanical complication of tracheostomy
        Tracheal stenosis due to tracheostomy

    519.09   Other tracheostomy complications
        Hemorrhage due to tracheostomy
        Tracheoesophageal fistula due to tracheostomy

 ❑ **519.1   Other diseases of trachea and bronchus, not else-where classified**
        Calcification of bronchus or trachea
        Stenosis of bronchus or trachea
        Ulcer of bronchus or trachea

    519.2   Mediastinitis

 ❑ **519.3   Other diseases of mediastinum, not elsewhere classified**
        Fibrosis of mediastinum
        Hernia of mediastinum
        Retraction of mediastinum

    519.4   Disorders of diaphragm
        Diaphragmitis
        Paralysis of diaphragm
        Relaxation of diaphragm

      | **Excludes** | *congenital defect of diaphragm (756.6)*
           diaphragmatic hernia (551–553 with .3)
           congenital (756.6)

 ❑ **519.8   Other diseases of respiratory system, not else-where classified**

 ❑ **519.9   Unspecified disease of respiratory system**
        Respiratory disease (chronic) NOS

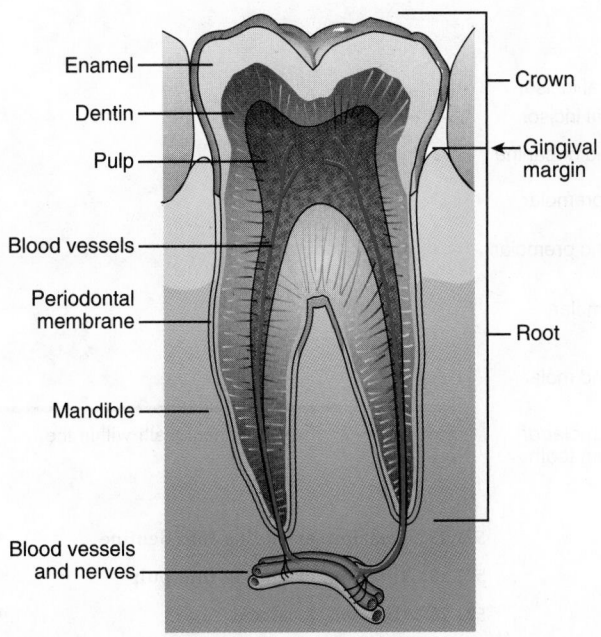

Figure 9-1   Anatomy of a tooth.

Item 9-1 Anodontia is the congenital absence of teeth. **Hypodontia** is partial anodontia. **Oligodontia** is the congenital absence of some teeth, whereas **supernumerary** is having more teeth than the normal number. **Mesiodens** are small extra teeth that often appear in pairs, although single small teeth are not uncommon.

9.   DISEASES OF THE DIGESTIVE SYSTEM (520–579)

DISEASES OF ORAL CAVITY, SALIVARY GLANDS, AND JAWS (520–529)

● **520   Disorders of tooth development and eruption**

    520.0   Anodontia
         Absence of teeth (complete) (congenital) (partial)
         Hypodontia
         Oligodontia
         Excludes   *acquired absence of teeth (525.10–525.19)*

    520.1   Supernumerary teeth
         Distomolar
         Fourth molar
         Mesiodens
         Paramolar
         Supplemental teeth
         Excludes   *supernumerary roots (520.2)*

520.2   Abnormalities of size and form
     Concrescence of teeth
     Fusion of teeth
     Gemination of teeth
     Dens evaginatus
     Dens in dente
     Dens invaginatus
     Enamel pearls
     Macrodontia
     Microdontia
     Peg-shaped [conical] teeth
     Supernumerary roots
     Taurodontism
     Tuberculum paramolare
     Excludes   *that due to congenital syphilis (090.5)*
                 tuberculum Carabelli, which is regarded as a normal variation

520.3   Mottled teeth
     Dental fluorosis
     Mottling of enamel
     Nonfluoride enamel opacities

520.4   Disturbances of tooth formation
     Aplasia and hypoplasia of cementum
     Dilaceration of tooth
     Enamel hypoplasia (neonatal) (postnatal) (prenatal)
     Horner's teeth
     Hypocalcification of teeth
     Regional odontodysplasia
     Turner's tooth
     Excludes   *Hutchinson's teeth and mulberry molars in congenital syphilis (090.5)*
                 mottled teeth (520.3)

520.5   Hereditary disturbances in tooth structure, not elsewhere classified
     Amelogenesis imperfecta
     Dentinogenesis imperfecta
     Odontogenesis imperfecta
     Dentinal dysplasia
     Shell teeth

520.6   Disturbances in tooth eruption
     Teeth:
         embedded
         impacted
         natal
         neonatal
         primary [deciduous]:
             persistent
             shedding, premature
     Tooth eruption:
         late
         obstructed
         premature
     Excludes   *exfoliation of teeth (attributable to disease of surrounding tissues) (525.0–525.19)*

520.7   Teething syndrome

☐ **520.8   Other specified disorders of tooth development and eruption**
     Color changes during tooth formation
     Pre-eruptive color changes
     Excludes   *posteruptive color changes (521.7)*

☐ **520.9   Unspecified disorder of tooth development and eruption**

ICD-9-CM

500-599

Vol. 1

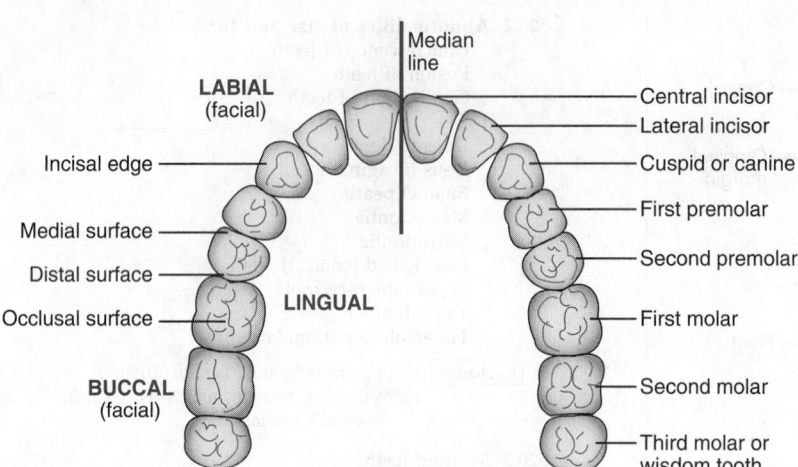

Figure 9-2 The permanent teeth within the dental arch.

Item 9-2 Each dental arch (jaw) normally contains 16 teeth. Tooth decay or **dental caries** is a disease of the enamel, dentin, and cementum of the tooth and can result in a cavity.

● 521 **Diseases of hard tissues of teeth**

  ● 521.0 **Dental caries**

    ❑ 521.00 **Dental caries, unspecified**

    521.01 **Dental caries limited to enamel**
       Initial caries
       White spot lesion

    521.02 **Dental caries extending into dentin**

    521.03 **Dental caries extending into pulp**

    521.04 **Arrested dental caries**

    521.05 **Odontoclasia**
       Infantile melanodontia
       Melanodontoclasia

    ⎣Excludes⎦ *internal and external resorption of teeth (521.40–521.49)* ◀┅

    521.06 **Dental caries pit and fissure** ◀

    521.07 **Dental caries of smooth surface** ◀

    521.08 **Dental caries of root surface** ◀

    ❑ 521.09 **Other dental caries**

  ● 521.1 **Excessive attrition (approximal wear) (occlusal wear)** ◀┅

    ❑ 521.10 **Excessive attrition, unspecified** ◀

    521.11 **Excessive attrition, limited to enamel** ◀

    521.12 **Excessive attrition, extending into dentine** ◀

    521.13 **Excessive attrition, extending into pulp** ◀

    521.14 **Excessive attrition, localized** ◀

    521.15 **Excessive attrition, generalized** ◀

  ● 521.2 **Abrasion**
    Abrasion of teeth: Abrasion of teeth:
      dentifrice   ritual
      habitual   traditional
      occupational
    Wedge defect NOS of teeth

    ❑ 521.20 **Abrasion, unspecified** ◀

    521.21 **Abrasion, limited to enamel** ◀

    521.22 **Abrasion, extending into dentine** ◀

    521.23 **Abrasion, extending into pulp** ◀

    521.24 **Abrasion, localized** ◀

    521.25 **Abrasion, generalized** ◀

  ● 521.3 **Erosion**
    Erosion of teeth:
      NOS
      due to:
        medicine
          persistent vomiting
      idiopathic
      occupational

    ❑ 521.30 **Erosion, unspecified** ◀

    521.31 **Erosion, limited to enamel** ◀

    521.32 **Erosion, extending into dentine** ◀

    521.33 **Erosion, extending into pulp** ◀

    521.34 **Erosion, localized** ◀

    521.35 **Erosion, generalized** ◀

  ● 521.4 **Pathological resorption**

    ❑ 521.40 **Pathological resorption, unspecified** ◀

    521.41 **Pathological resorption, internal** ◀

    521.42 **Pathological resorption, external** ◀

    ❑ 521.49 **Other pathological resorption** ◀
       Internal granuloma of pulp

  521.5 **Hypercementosis**
    Cementation hyperplasia

  521.6 **Ankylosis of teeth**

  521.7 **Intrinsic posteruptive color changes** ◀┅
    Staining [discoloration] of teeth:
      NOS
      due to:
        drugs
        metals
      pulpal bleeding

    ⎣Excludes⎦ *accretions [deposits] on teeth (523.6)*
            extrinsic color changes (523.6) ◀
            pre-eruptive color changes (520.8)

  ❑ 521.8 **Other specified diseases of hard tissues of teeth**
    Irradiated enamel   Sensitive dentin

  ❑ 521.9 **Unspecified disease of hard tissues of teeth**

● **522   Diseases of pulp and periapical tissues**

     522.0   Pulpitis
         Pulpal:
            abscess
            polyp
         Pulpitis:
            acute
            chronic (hyperplastic) (ulcerative)
            suppurative

     522.1   Necrosis of the pulp
         Pulp gangrene

     522.2   Pulp degeneration
         Denticles
         Pulp stones
         Pulp calcifications

     522.3   Abnormal hard tissue formation in pulp
         Secondary or irregular dentin

     522.4   Acute apical periodontitis of pulpal origin

     522.5   Periapical abscess without sinus
         Abscess:
            dental
            dentoalveolar

         Excludes   *periapical abscess with sinus (522.7)*

     522.6   Chronic apical periodontitis
         Apical or periapical granuloma
         Apical periodontitis NOS

     522.7   Periapical abscess with sinus
         Fistula:
            alveolar process
            dental

     522.8   Radicular cyst
         Cyst:
            apical (periodontal)
            periapical
            radiculodental
            residual radicular

         Excludes   *lateral developmental or lateral periodontal cyst (526.0)*

     ❑ **522.9   Other and unspecified diseases of pulp and periapical tissues**

Item 9-3   Acute gingivitis, also known as orilitis or ulitis, is the short-term, severe inflammation of the gums (gingiva) caused by bacteria. **Chronic gingivitis** is persistent inflammation of the gums. When the gingivitis moves into the periodontium it is called periodontitis, also known as paradentitis.

● **523   Gingival and periodontal diseases**

     523.0   Acute gingivitis

         Excludes   *acute necrotizing ulcerative gingivitis (101)*
                        herpetic gingivostomatitis (054.2)

     523.1   Chronic gingivitis
         Gingivitis (chronic):
            NOS
            desquamative
            hyperplastic
            simple marginal
            ulcerative
         Gingivostomatitis

         Excludes   *herpetic gingivostomatitis (054.2)*

❑ **523.2   Gingival recession**
         Gingival recession (postinfective) (postoperative) ◀━

     ❑ **523.20   Gingival recession, unspecified**   ◀

     523.21   Gingival recession, minimal   ◀

     523.22   Gingival recession, moderate   ◀

     523.23   Gingival recession, severe   ◀

     523.24   Gingival recession, localized   ◀

     523.25   Gingival recession, generalized   ◀

     523.3   Acute periodontitis
         Acute:
            pericementitis
            pericoronitis
         Paradontal abscess
         Periodontal abscess

         Excludes   *acute apical periodontitis (522.4)*
                        periapical abscess (522.5, 522.7)

     523.4   Chronic periodontitis
         Alveolar pyorrhea
         Chronic pericoronitis
         Pericementitis (chronic)
         Periodontitis:
            NOS
            complex
            simplex

         Excludes   *chronic apical periodontitis (522.6)*

     523.5   Periodontosis

     523.6   Accretions on teeth
         Dental calculus:
            subgingival
            supragingival
         Deposits on teeth:
            betel
            materia alba
            soft
            tartar
            tobacco
         Extrinsic discoloration of teeth   ◀

         Excludes   *intrinsic discoloration of teeth (521.7)*   ◀

❑ **523.8   Other specified periodontal diseases**
         Giant cell:
            epulis
            peripheral granuloma
         Gingival:
            cysts
            enlargement NOS
            fibromatosis
         Gingival polyp
         Periodontal lesions due to traumatic occlusion
         Peripheral giant cell granuloma

         Excludes   *leukoplakia of gingiva (528.6)*

❑ **523.9   Unspecified gingival and periodontal disease**

ICD-9-CM

500-599

Vol. 1

Figure 9-3 Dentofacial malocclusion.

Item 9-4 Hyperplasia is a condition of overdevelopment, whereas hypoplasia is a condition of underdevelopment. Macrogenia is overdevelopment of the chin, whereas microgenia is underdevelopment of the chin.

● 524 Dentofacial anomalies, including malocclusion

  ● 524.0 Major anomalies of jaw size

    Excludes *hemifacial atrophy or hypertrophy (754.0)*
    unilateral condylar hyperplasia or hypoplasia of
    mandible

    ❑ 524.00 Unspecified anomaly

    524.01 Maxillary hyperplasia

    524.02 Mandibular hyperplasia

    524.03 Maxillary hypoplasia

    524.04 Mandibular hypoplasia

    524.05 Macrogenia

    524.06 Microgenia

    524.07 Excessive tuberosity of jaw ◄

    ❑ 524.09 Other specified anomaly

  ● 524.1 Anomalies of relationship of jaw to cranial base

    ❑ 524.10 Unspecified anomaly
    Prognathism
    Retrognathism

    524.11 Maxillary asymmetry

    ❑ 524.12 Other jaw asymmetry

    ❑ 524.19 Other specified anomaly

  ● 524.2 Anomalies of dental arch relationship

    Excludes *hemifacial atrophy or hypertrophy (754.0)*
    soft tissue impingement (524.81–524.82) ◄
    unilateral condylar hyperplasia or hypoplasia of
    mandible (526.89)

    ❑ 524.20 Unspecified anomaly of dental arch relationship ◄

    524.21 Angle's class I ◄
    Neutro-occlusion ◄

    524.22 Angle's class II ◄
    Disto-occlusion Division I ◄
    Disto-occlusion Division II ◄

    524.23 Angle's class III ◄
    Mesio-occlusion ◄

    524.24 Open anterior occlusal relationship ◄

    524.25 Open posterior occlusal relationship ◄

    524.26 Excessive horizontal overlap ◄

    524.27 Reverse articulation ◄
    Anterior articulation ◄
    Posterior articulation ◄

    524.28 Anomalies of interarch distance ◄
    Excessive interarch distance ◄
    Inadequate interarch distance ◄

    524.29 Other anomalies of dental arch relationship ◄

  ● 524.3 Anomalies of tooth position of fully erupted teeth ◄▥

    Excludes *impacted or embedded teeth with abnormal position of such teeth or adjacent teeth (520.6)* ◄

    ❑ 524.30 Unspecified anomaly of tooth position ◄
    Diastema of teeth NOS ◄
    Displacement of teeth NOS ◄
    Transposition of teeth NOS ◄

    524.31 Crowding of teeth ◄

    524.32 Excessive spacing of teeth ◄

    524.33 Horizontal displacement of teeth ◄
    Tipping of teeth ◄

    524.34 Vertical displacement of teeth ◄
    Infraeruption of teeth ◄
    Supraeruption of teeth ◄

    524.35 Rotation of teeth ◄

    524.36 Insufficient interocclusal distance of teeth (ridge) ◄

    524.37 Excessive interocclusal distance of teeth ◄
    Loss of occlusal vertical dimension ◄

    524.39 Other anomalies of tooth position ◄

  ❑ 524.4 Malocclusion, unspecified

  ● 524.5 Dentofacial functional abnormalities

    ❑ 524.50 Dentofacial functional abnormality, unspecified ◄

    524.51 Abnormal jaw closure ◄
    Dyskinesia ◄

    524.52 Limited mandibular range of motion ◄

    524.53 Deviation in opening and closing of the mandible ◄

    524.54 Insufficient anterior guidance ◄

    524.55 Centric occlusion maximum intercuspation discrepancy ◄

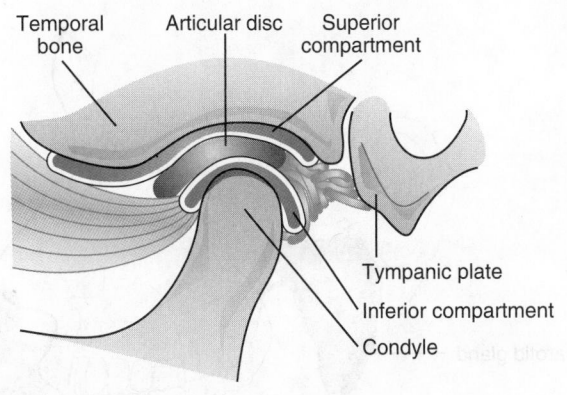

Figure 9–4   Temporomandibular joint.

Item 9–5   **Dysfunction of the temporomandibular joint is termed temporomandibular joint (TMJ) syndrome and is characterized by pain and tenderness/spasm of the muscles of mastication, joint noise, and in the later stages, limited mandibular movement.**

524.56   Non-working side interference ◄

524.57   Lack of posterior occlusal support ◄

524.59   Other dentofacial functional abnormalities ◄
     Abnormal swallowing ◄
     Mouth breathing ◄
     Sleep postures ◄
     Tongue, lip, or finger habits ◄

● 524.6   Temporomandibular joint disorders

     Excludes   *current temporomandibular joint:*
     dislocation (830.0–830.1)
     strain (848.1)

524.60   Temporomandibular joint disorders, unspecified
     Temporomandibular joint-pain-dysfunction syndrome [TMJ]

524.61   Adhesions and ankylosis (bony or fibrous)

524.62   Arthralgia of temporomandibular joint

524.63   Articular disc disorder (reducing or nonreducing)

524.64   Temporomandibular joint sounds on opening and/or closing the jaw ◄

524.69   Other specified temporomandibular joint disorders

● 524.7   Dental alveolar anomalies

524.70   Unspecified alveolar anomaly

524.71   Alveolar maxillary hyperplasia

524.72   Alveolar mandibular hyperplasia

524.73   Alveolar maxillary hypoplasia

524.74   Alveolar mandibular hypoplasia

524.75   Vertical displacement of alveolus and teeth ◄
     Extrusion of alveolus and teeth ◄

524.76   Occlusal plane deviation ◄

524.79   Other specified alveolar anomaly

● 524.8   Other specified dentofacial anomalies

524.81   Anterior soft tissue impingement ◄

524.82   Posterior soft tissue impingement ◄

524.89   Other specified dentofacial anomalies ◄

524.9   Unspecified dentofacial anomalies

● 525   Other diseases and conditions of the teeth and supporting structures

525.0   Exfoliation of teeth due to systemic causes

● 525.1   Loss of teeth due to trauma, extraction, or periodontal disease

525.10   Acquired absence of teeth, unspecified
     Edentulism
     Tooth extraction status, NOS

525.11   Loss of teeth due to trauma

525.12   Loss of teeth due to periodontal disease

525.13   Loss of teeth due to caries

525.19   Other loss of teeth

● 525.2   Atrophy of edentulous alveolar ridge

525.20   Unspecified atrophy of edentulous alveolar ridge ◄
     Atrophy of the mandible NOS ◄
     Atrophy of the maxilla NOS ◄

525.21   Minimal atrophy of the mandible ◄

525.22   Moderate atrophy of the mandible ◄

525.23   Severe atrophy of the mandible ◄

525.24   Minimal atrophy of the maxilla ◄

525.25   Moderate atrophy of the maxilla ◄

525.26   Severe atrophy of the maxilla ◄

525.3   Retained dental root

525.8   Other specified disorders of the teeth and supporting structures
     Enlargement of alveolar ridge NOS
     Irregular alveolar process

525.9   Unspecified disorder of the teeth and supporting structures

ICD-9-CM

500-599

Vol. 1

● 526   Diseases of the jaws

526.0   **Developmental odontogenic cysts**
Cyst:
    dentigerous
    eruption
    follicular
    lateral developmental
    lateral periodontal
    primordial
Keratocyst

| Excludes | radicular cyst (522.8) |

526.1   **Fissural cysts of jaw**
Cyst:
    globulomaxillary
    incisor canal
    median anterior maxillary
    median palatal
    nasopalatine
    palatine of papilla

| Excludes | cysts of oral soft tissues (528.4) |

❏ 526.2   **Other cysts of jaws**
Cyst of jaw:
    NOS
    aneurysmal
    hemorrhagic
    traumatic

526.3   **Central giant cell (reparative) granuloma**

| Excludes | peripheral giant cell granuloma (523.8) |

526.4   **Inflammatory conditions**
Abscess of jaw (acute) (chronic) (suppurative)
Osteitis of jaw (acute) (chronic) (suppurative)
Osteomyelitis (neonatal) of jaw (acute) (chronic)
    (suppurative)
Periostitis of jaw (acute) (chronic) (suppurative)
Sequestrum of jaw bone

| Excludes | alveolar osteitis (526.5) |

526.5   **Alveolitis of jaw**
Alveolar osteitis
Dry socket

● 526.8   **Other specified diseases of the jaws**

526.81   **Exostosis of jaw**
Torus mandibularis
Torus palatinus

❏ 526.89   **Other**
Cherubism
Fibrous dysplasia of jaw(s)
Latent bone cyst of jaw(s)
Osteoradionecrosis of jaw(s)
Unilateral condylar hyperplasia or hypo-
    plasia of mandible

❏ 526.9   **Unspecified disease of the jaws**

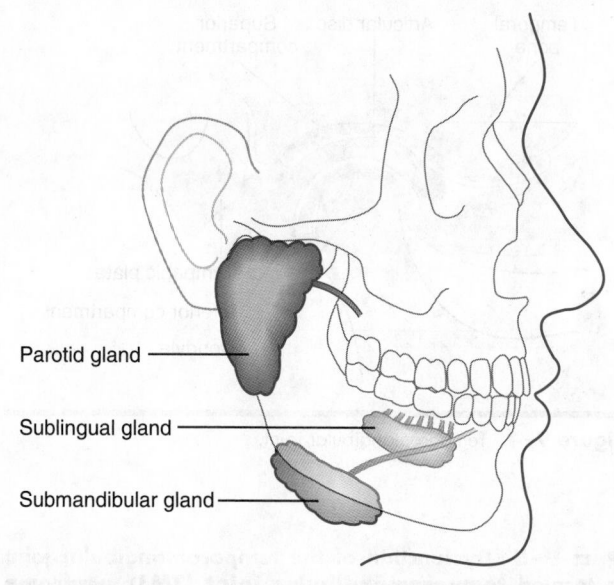

Figure 9–5   Major salivary glands.

Parotid gland
Sublingual gland
Submandibular gland

Item 9–6   **Atrophy** is wasting away of a tissue or organ, whereas **hypertrophy** is overdevelopment or enlargement of a tissue or organ. **Sialoadenitis** is salivary
gland inflammation. **Parotitis** is the inflammation of the
parotid gland. In the epidemic form, parotitis is also
known as mumps.
Sialolithiasis is the formation of calculus within a salivary gland. **Mucocele** is a polyp composed of mucus.

● 527   Diseases of the salivary glands

527.0   **Atrophy**

527.1   **Hypertrophy**

527.2   **Sialoadenitis**
Parotitis:
    NOS
    allergic
    toxic
Sialoangitis
Sialodochitis

| Excludes | epidemic or infectious parotitis (072.0–072.9) |
| | uveoparotid fever (135) |

527.3   **Abscess**

527.4   **Fistula**

| Excludes | congenital fistula of salivary gland (750.24) |

527.5   **Sialolithiasis**
Calculus of salivary gland or duct
Stone of salivary gland or duct
Sialodocholithiasis

527.6 Mucocele
Mucous:
extravasation cyst of salivary gland
retention cyst of salivary gland
Ranula

527.7 Disturbance of salivary secretion
Hyposecretion
Ptyalism
Sialorrhea
Xerostomia

❑ **527.8 Other specified diseases of the salivary glands**
Benign lymphoepithelial lesion of salivary gland
Sialectasia
Sialosis
Stenosis of salivary duct
Stricture of salivary duct

❑ **527.9 Unspecified disease of the salivary glands**

Item 9-7 Stomatitis is the inflammation of the oral mucosa. **Cancrum oris,** also known as **noma** or **gangrenous stomatitis,** begins as an ulcer of the gingiva and results in a progressive gangrenous process.

● **528 Diseases of the oral soft tissues, excluding lesions specific for gingiva and tongue**

528.0 Stomatitis
Stomatitis:
NOS
ulcerative
Vesicular stomatitis

Excludes   *stomatitis:*
acute necrotizing ulcerative (101)
aphthous (528.2)
gangrenous (528.1)
herpetic (054.2)
Vincent's (101)

528.1 Cancrum oris
Gangrenous stomatitis
Noma

528.2 Oral aphthae
Aphthous stomatitis
Canker sore
Periadenitis mucosa necrotica recurrens
Recurrent aphthous ulcer
Stomatitis herpetiformis

Excludes   *herpetic stomatitis (054.2)*

528.3 Cellulitis and abscess
Cellulitis of mouth (floor)
Ludwig's angina
Oral fistula

Excludes   *abscess of tongue (529.0)*
cellulitis or abscess of lip (528.5)
fistula (of):
dental (522.7)
lip (528.5)
gingivitis (523.0–523.1)

528.4 Cysts
Dermoid cyst of mouth
Epidermoid cyst of mouth
Epstein's pearl of mouth
Lymphoepithelial cyst of mouth
Nasoalveolar cyst of mouth
Nasolabial cyst of mouth

Excludes   *cyst:*
gingiva (523.8)
tongue (529.8)

528.5 Diseases of lips
Abscess of lip(s)
Cellulitis of lip(s)
Fistula of lip(s)
Hypertrophy of lip(s)
Cheilitis:
NOS
angular
Cheilodynia
Cheilosis

Excludes   *actinic cheilitis (692.79)*
congenital fistula of lip (750.25)
leukoplakia of lips (528.6)

528.6 Leukoplakia of oral mucosa, including tongue
Leukokeratosis of oral mucosa
Leukoplakia of:
gingiva
lips
tongue

Excludes   *carcinoma in situ (230.0, 232.0)* ◀━━ ICD-9-CM
leukokeratosis nicotina palati (528.79)

500-
599

Vol. 1

Figure 9–6 A. Lingual leukoplakia. **B.** Buccal leukoplakia. (From Pindborg JJ: In Jones JH, Mason DK (eds): Oral Manifestations of Systemic Disease. Philadelphia, WB Saunders, 1980, p 322.)

● 528.7 **Other disturbances of oral epithelium, including tongue**

> **Excludes** *carcinoma in situ (230.0, 232.0)*
> *leukokeratosis NOS (702)*

528.71 **Mimimal keratinized residual ridge mucosa** ◀

528.72 **Excessive keratinized residual ridge mucosa** ◀

☐528.79 **Other disturbances of oral epithelium, including tongue** ◀
  Erythroplakia of mouth or tongue ◀
  Focal epithelial hyperplasia of mouth or tongue ◀
  Leukoedema of mouth or tongue ◀
  Leukokeratosis nicotina palate ◀

528.8 **Oral submucosal fibrosis, including of tongue**

☐528.9 **Other and unspecified diseases of the oral soft tissues**
  Cheek and lip biting
  Denture sore mouth
  Denture stomatitis
  Melanoplakia
  Papillary hyperplasia of palate
  Eosinophilic granuloma of oral mucosa
  Irritative hyperplasia of oral mucosa
  Pyogenic granuloma of oral mucosa
  Ulcer (traumatic) of oral mucosa

● 529 **Diseases and other conditions of the tongue**

529.0 **Glossitis**
  Abscess of tongue
  Ulceration (traumatic) of tongue

> **Excludes** *glossitis:*
> *benign migratory (529.1)*
> *Hunter's (529.4)*
> *median rhomboid (529.2)*
> *Moeller's (529.4)*

529.1 **Geographic tongue**
  Benign migratory glossitis
  Glossitis areata exfoliativa

529.2 **Median rhomboid glossitis**

529.3 **Hypertrophy of tongue papillae**
  Black hairy tongue
  Coated tongue
  Hypertrophy of foliate papillae
  Lingua villosa nigra

529.4 **Atrophy of tongue papillae**
  Bald tongue
  Glazed tongue
  Glossitis:
    Hunter's
    Moeller's
  Glossodynia exfoliativa
  Smooth atrophic tongue

529.5 **Plicated tongue**
  Fissured tongue
  Furrowed tongue
  Scrotal tongue

> **Excludes** *fissure of tongue, congenital (750.13)*

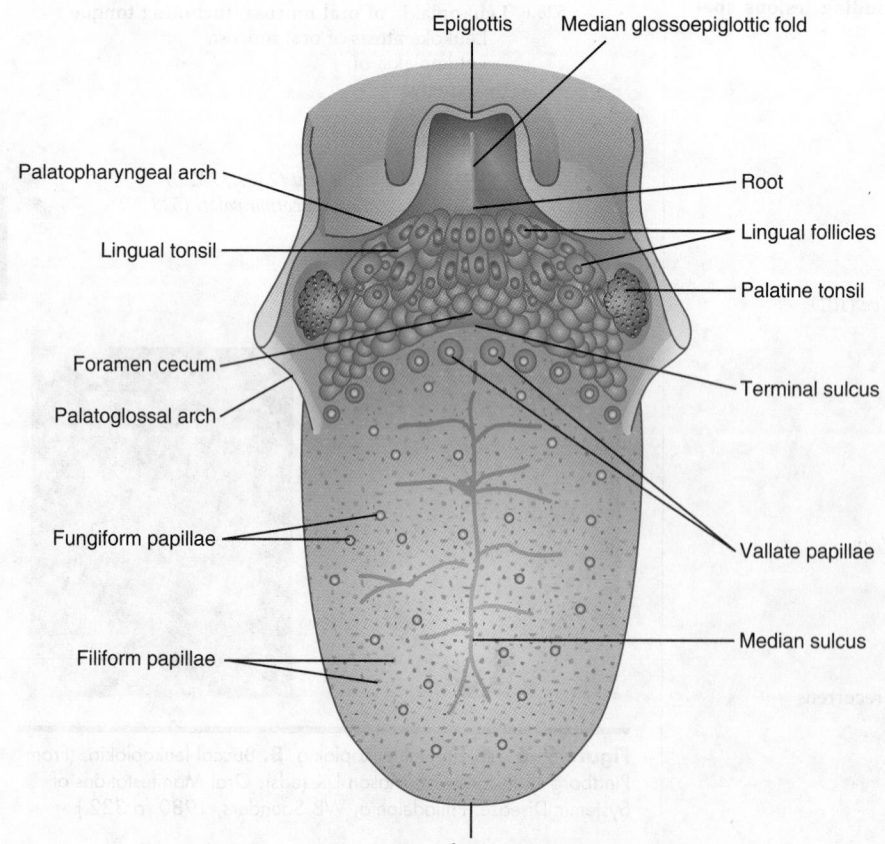

Epiglottis
Median glossoepiglottic fold
Palatopharyngeal arch
Lingual tonsil
Foramen cecum
Palatoglossal arch
Fungiform papillae
Filiform papillae
Root
Lingual follicles
Palatine tonsil
Terminal sulcus
Vallate papillae
Median sulcus
Apex

Figure 9–7 Structure of the tongue.

◀ **New**   ◀▦ **Revised**   ● **Not a Principal Diagnosis**   ● **Use Additional Digit(s)**   ☐ **Nonspecific Code**

529.6 Glossodynia
Glossopyrosis
Painful tongue

| Excludes | *glossodynia exfoliativa (529.4)* |

□ 529.8 Other specified conditions of the tongue
Atrophy (of) tongue
Crenated (of) tongue
Enlargement (of) tongue
Hypertrophy (of) tongue
Glossocele
Glossoptosis

Excludes	*erythroplasia of tongue (528.79)*
	leukoplakia of tongue (528.6)
	macroglossia (congenital) (750.15)
	microglossia (congenital) (750.16)
	oral submucosal fibrosis (528.8)

□ 529.9 Unspecified condition of the tongue

CERVICAL ESOPHAGUS
First rib
Left subclavian artery
Arch of aorta
THORACIC ESOPHAGUS
Diaphragm
ABDOMINAL ESOPHAGUS
Stomach

Figure 9–8 The esophagus is the muscular tube that connects the pharynx and the stomach. The 10 inch (25 cm) long esophagus is divided into three parts: **cervical, thoracic,** and **abdominal.**

Item 9–8 Achalasia is a condition in which the smooth muscle fibers of the esophagus do not relax. Most frequently, this condition occurs at the esophagogastric sphincter. **Cardiospasm,** also known as **megaesophagus,** is achalasia of the thoracic esophagus.

Item 9–9 Dyskinesia is difficulty in moving, and **diverticulum** is a sac or pouch.

DISEASES OF ESOPHAGUS, STOMACH, AND DUODENUM (530–537)

● **530 Diseases of esophagus**

| Excludes | *esophageal varices (456.0–456.2)* |

530.0 Achalasia and cardiospasm
Achalasia (of cardia)
Aperistalsis of esophagus
Megaesophagus

| Excludes | *congenital cardiospasm (750.7)* |

● ### 530.1 Esophagitis
Abscess of esophagus
Esophagitis:	Esophagitis:
NOS	postoperative
chemical	regurgitant
peptic	

Use additional E code to identify cause, if induced by chemical

| Excludes | *tuberculous esophagitis (017.8)* |

□ 530.10 Esophagitis, unspecified

530.11 Reflux esophagitis

530.12 Acute esophagitis

□ 530.19 Other esophagitis

● ### 530.2 Ulcer of esophagus
| Ulcer of esophagus | |
| fungal | peptic |
Ulcer of esophagus due to ingestion of:
| aspirin | chemicals |
| medicines | |

Use additional E code to identify cause, if induced by chemical or drug

530.20 Ulcer of esophagus without bleeding
Ulcer of esophagus NOS

530.21 Ulcer of esophagus with bleeding

| Excludes | *bleeding esophageal varices (456.0, 456.20)* |

530.3 Stricture and stenosis of esophagus
Compression of esophagus
Obstruction of esophagus

| Excludes | *congenital stricture of esophagus (750.3)* |

530.4 Perforation of esophagus
Rupture of esophagus

| Excludes | *traumatic perforation of esophagus (862.22, 862.32, 874.4–874.5)* |

530.5 Dyskinesia of esophagus
Corkscrew esophagus
Curling esophagus
Esophagospasm
Spasm of esophagus

| Excludes | *cardiospasm (530.0)* |

ICD-9-CM

500-599

Vol. 1

530.6 Diverticulum of esophagus, acquired
   Diverticulum, acquired:
      epiphrenic
      pharyngoesophageal
      pulsion
      subdiaphragmatic
      traction
      Zenker's (hypopharyngeal)
   Esophageal pouch, acquired
   Esophagocele, acquired

   | Excludes | *congenital diverticulum of esophagus (750.4)*

530.7 Gastroesophageal laceration-hemorrhage syndrome
   Mallory-Weiss syndrome

● **530.8 Other specified disorders of esophagus**

   530.81 Esophageal reflux
      Gastroesophageal reflux

   | Excludes | *reflux esophagitis (530.11)*

   530.82 Esophageal hemorrhage

   | Excludes | *hemorrhage due to esophageal varices (456.0–456.2)*

   530.83 Esophageal leukoplakia

   530.84 Tracheoesophageal fistula

   | Excludes | *congenital tracheoesophageal fistula (750.3)*

   530.85 Barrett's esophagus

   530.86 Infection of esophagostomy ◄

      Use additional code to specify infection ◄

   530.87 Mechanical complication of esophagostomy ◄
      Malfunction of esophagostomy ◄

   ☐ **530.89 Other**

   | Excludes | *Paterson-Kelly syndrome (280.8)*

☐ **530.9 Unspecified disorder of esophagus**

Item 9–10 Esophageal reflux is the return flow of the contents of the stomach to the esophagus. **Gastroesophageal reflux** is the return flow of the contents of the stomach and duodenum to the esophagus. **Esophageal leukoplakia** are white areas on the mucous membrane of the esophagus for which no specific cause can be identified.

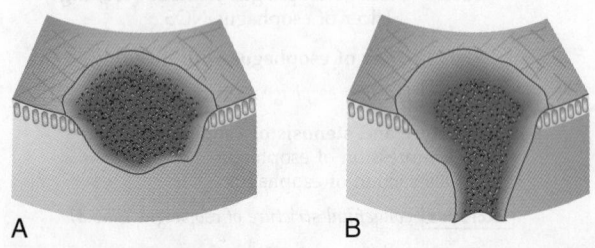

Figure 9–9   A. Ulcer. **B.** Perforated ulcer.

Item 9–11   Gastric ulcers are lesions of the stomach that result in the death of the tissue and a defect of the surface. **Perforated ulcers** are those in which the lesion penetrates the gastric wall, leaving a hole. **Peptic ulcers** are lesions of the stomach or the duodenum. **Peptic** refers to the gastric juice, pepsin.

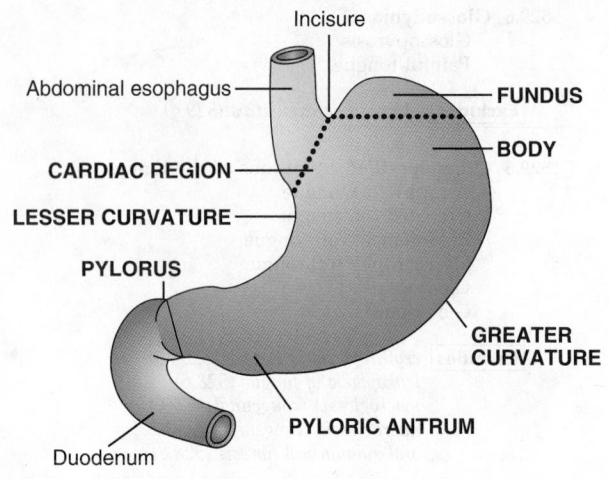

Figure 9–10   Parts of the stomach.

● 531 **Gastric ulcer**

   Includes: ulcer (peptic):
      prepyloric
      pylorus
      stomach

   Use additional E code to identify drug, if drug-induced
   | Excludes | *peptic ulcer NOS (533.0–533.9)*

   The following fifth-digit subclassification is for use with category 531:
      0 **without mention of obstruction**
      1 **with obstruction**

● **531.0 Acute with hemorrhage**

● **531.1 Acute with perforation**

● **531.2 Acute with hemorrhage and perforation**

● **531.3 Acute without mention of hemorrhage or perforation**

● **531.4 Chronic or unspecified with hemorrhage**

● **531.5 Chronic or unspecified with perforation**

● **531.6 Chronic or unspecified with hemorrhage and perforation**

● **531.7 Chronic without mention of hemorrhage or perforation**

● ☐ **531.9 Unspecified as acute or chronic, without mention of hemorrhage or perforation**

● 532 **Duodenal ulcer**

   Includes: erosion (acute) of duodenum
      ulcer (peptic):
         duodenum
         postpyloric

   Use additional E code to identify drug, if drug-induced
   | Excludes | *peptic ulcer NOS (533.0–533.9)*

   The following fifth-digit subclassification is for use with category 532:
      0 **without mention of obstruction**
      1 **with obstruction**

● **532.0 Acute with hemorrhage**

● **532.1 Acute with perforation**

● **532.2 Acute with hemorrhage and perforation**

● **532.3 Acute without mention of hemorrhage or perforation**

● 532.4   Chronic or unspecified with hemorrhage

● 532.5   Chronic or unspecified with perforation

● 532.6   Chronic or unspecified with hemorrhage and perforation

● 532.7   Chronic without mention of hemorrhage or perforation

● ❑ 532.9   Unspecified as acute or chronic, without mention of hemorrhage or perforation

● 533   Peptic ulcer, site unspecified

     Includes: gastroduodenal ulcer NOS
                     peptic ulcer NOS
                     stress ulcer NOS

     Use additional E code to identify drug, if drug-induced

     | **Excludes** | *peptic ulcer:*
                    duodenal (532.0–532.9)
                    gastric (531.0–531.9)

     The following fifth-digit subclassification is for use with category 533:
       0 **without mention of obstruction**
       1 **with obstruction**

● 533.0   Acute with hemorrhage

● 533.1   Acute with perforation

● 533.2   Acute with hemorrhage and perforation

● 533.3   Acute without mention of hemorrhage and perforation

● 533.4   Chronic or unspecified with hemorrhage

● 533.5   Chronic or unspecified with perforation

● 533.6   Chronic or unspecified with hemorrhage and perforation

● 533.7   Chronic without mention of hemorrhage or perforation

● ❑ 533.9   Unspecified as acute or chronic, without mention of hemorrhage or perforation

● 534   Gastrojejunal ulcer

     Includes: ulcer (peptic) or erosion:
                     anastomotic
                     gastrocolic
                     gastrointestinal
                     gastrojejunal
                     jejunal
                     marginal
                     stomal

     | **Excludes** | *primary ulcer of small intestine (569.82)*

     The following fifth-digit subclassification is for use with category 534:
       0 **without mention of obstruction**
       1 **with obstruction**

● 534.0   Acute with hemorrhage

● 534.1   Acute with perforation

● 534.2   Acute with hemorrhage and perforation

● 534.3   Acute without mention of hemorrhage or perforation

● 534.4   Chronic or unspecified with hemorrhage

● 534.5   Chronic or unspecified with perforation

● 534.6   Chronic or unspecified with hemorrhage and perforation

● 534.7   Chronic without mention of hemorrhage or perforation

● ❑ 534.9   Unspecified as acute or chronic, without mention of hemorrhage or perforation

Item 9-12 Gastritis is a severe inflammation of the stomach. **Atrophic gastritis** is a chronic inflammation of the stomach that results in destruction of the cells of the mucosa of the stomach.

● 535   Gastritis and duodenitis

     The following fifth-digit subclassification is for use with category 535:
       0 **without mention of hemorrhage**
       1 **with hemorrhage**

● 535.0   Acute gastritis

● 535.1   Atrophic gastritis
       Gastritis:
          atrophic-hyperplastic   chronic (atrophic)

● 535.2   Gastric mucosal hypertrophy
       Hypertrophic gastritis

● 535.3   Alcoholic gastritis

● ❑ 535.4   Other specified gastritis

     Gastritis: Gastritis:
       allergic   superficial
       bile induced   toxic
       irritant

● ❑ 535.5   Unspecified gastritis and gastroduodenitis

● 535.6   Duodenitis

Item 9-13 Achlorhydria, also known as gastric anacidity, is the absence of gastric acid. **Gastroparesis** is paralysis of the stomach.

● 536   Disorders of function of stomach

     | **Excludes** | *functional disorders of stomach specified as psychogenic (306.4)*

   536.0   Achlorhydria

   536.1   Acute dilatation of stomach
       Acute distention of stomach

   536.2   Persistent vomiting
       Habit vomiting
       Persistent vomiting [not of pregnancy]
       Uncontrollable vomiting

     | **Excludes** | *excessive vomiting in pregnancy (643.0–643.9)*
                   vomiting NOS (787.0)

   536.3   Gastroparesis
       Gastroparalysis

● 536.4   Gastrostomy complications

     ❑ 536.40   Gastrostomy complication, unspecified

     536.41   Infection of gastrostomy

     Use additional code to specify type of infection, such as:
       abscess or cellulitis of abdomen (682.2)
       septicemia (038.0–038.9)

     Use additional code to identify organism (041.00–041.9)

     536.42   Mechanical complication of gastrostomy

     ❑ 536.49   Other gastrostomy complications

   ❑ 536.8   Dyspepsia and other specified disorders of function of stomach
       Achylia gastrica   Hyperchlorhydria
       Hourglass contraction   Hypochlorhydria
         of stomach   Indigestion
       Hyperacidity

     | **Excludes** | *achlorhydria (536.0)*
                   heartburn (787.1)

ICD-9-CM

**500-
599**

Vol. 1

☐ **536.9 Unspecified functional disorder of stomach**
Functional gastrointestinal:
    disorder
    disturbance
    irritation

● **537 Other disorders of stomach and duodenum**

  537.0 Acquired hypertrophic pyloric stenosis
    Constriction of pylorus, acquired or adult
    Obstruction of pylorus, acquired or adult
    Stricture of pylorus, acquired or adult

    Excludes   *congenital or infantile pyloric stenosis (750.5)*

  537.1 Gastric diverticulum

    Excludes   *congenital diverticulum of stomach (750.7)*

  537.2 Chronic duodenal ileus

  ☐ **537.3 Other obstruction of duodenum**
    Cicatrix of duodenum
    Stenosis of duodenum
    Stricture of duodenum
    Volvulus of duodenum

    Excludes   *congenital obstruction of duodenum (751.1)*

  537.4 Fistula of stomach or duodenum
    Gastrocolic fistula
    Gastrojejunocolic fistula

  537.5 Gastroptosis

  537.6 Hourglass stricture or stenosis of stomach
    Cascade stomach

    Excludes   *congenital hourglass stomach (750.7)*
                   hourglass contraction of stomach (536.8)

● **537.8 Other specified disorders of stomach and duodenum**

    537.81 Pylorospasm

    Excludes   *congenital pylorospasm (750.5)*

    **537.82 Angiodysplasia of stomach and duodenum
            without mention of hemorrhage**

    **537.83 Angiodysplasia of stomach and duodenum
            with hemorrhage**

    **537.84 Dieulafoy lesion (hemorrhagic) of stomach
            and duodenum**

    ☐ **537.89 Other**
        Gastric or duodenal:
          prolapse   rupture
        Intestinal metaplasia of gastric mucosa
        Passive congestion of stomach

    Excludes   *diverticula of duodenum (562.00–562.01)*
                    gastrointestinal hemorrhage (578.0–578.9)

☐ **537.9 Unspecified disorder of stomach and duodenum**

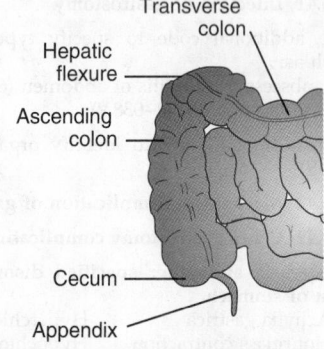

Figure 9-11 Acute appendicitis is the inflammation of the appendix, usually associated with obstruction. Most often this is a disease of adolescents and young adults.

APPENDICITIS (540–543)

● **540 Acute appendicitis**

  540.0 With generalized peritonitis
    Appendicitis (acute) with: perforation, peritonitis
      (generalized), rupture:
      fulminating
      gangrenous
      obstructive
    Cecitis (acute) with: perforation, peritonitis (gener-
      alized), rupture
    Rupture of appendix

    Excludes   *acute appendicitis with peritoneal abscess (540.1)*

  540.1 With peritoneal abscess
    Abscess of appendix
      With generalized peritonitis

  540.9 Without mention of peritonitis
    Acute:
      appendicitis without mention of perforation,
        peritonitis, or rupture:
        fulminating
        gangrenous
        inflamed
        obstructive
      cecitis without mention of perforation, peritoni-
        tis, or rupture

☐ **541 Appendicitis, unqualified**

☐ **542 Other appendicitis**
  Appendicitis: Appendicitis:
    chronic   relapsing
    recurrent   subacute

    Excludes   *hyperplasia (lymphoid) of appendix (543.0)*

● **543 Other diseases of appendix**

  543.0 Hyperplasia of appendix (lymphoid)

  ☐ **543.9 Other and unspecified diseases of appendix**
    Appendicular or appendiceal:
      colic
      concretion
      fistula
    Diverticulum of appendix
    Fecalith of appendix
    Intussusception of appendix
    Mucocele of appendix
    Stercolith of appendix

Figure 9-12 Inguinal hernias are those that are located in the inguinal or iliac areas of the abdomen.

Item 9-14 Hernias of the groin are the most common type, accounting for 80 percent of all hernias. There are two major types of inguinal hernias: indirect (oblique) and direct. **Indirect inguinal hernias** result when the intestines emerge through the abdominal wall in an indirect fashion through the inguinal canal. **Direct inguinal hernias** penetrate through the abdominal wall in a direct fashion.

Femoral hernias occur at the femoral ring where the femoral vessels enter the thigh.

Classification is based on location of the hernia and whether there is obstruction or gangrene.

HERNIA OF ABDOMINAL CAVITY (550–553)

Includes: hernia:
    acquired
    congenital, except diaphragmatic or hiatal

● **550 Inguinal hernia**

    Includes: bubonocele
        inguinal hernia (direct) (double) (indirect) (oblique) (sliding)
        scrotal hernia

    The following fifth-digit subclassification is for use with category 550:
    ❏ 0 **unilateral or unspecified (not specified as recurrent)**
        Unilateral NOS
      1 **unilateral or unspecified, recurrent**
      2 **bilateral (not specified as recurrent)**
        Bilateral NOS
      3 **bilateral, recurrent**

  ● **550.0 Inguinal hernia, with gangrene**
    Inguinal hernia with gangrene (and obstruction)

  ● **550.1 Inguinal hernia, with obstruction, without mention of gangrene**
    Inguinal hernia with mention of incarceration, irreducibility, or strangulation

  ● **550.9 Inguinal hernia, without mention of obstruction or gangrene**
    Inguinal hernia NOS

● **551 Other hernia of abdominal cavity, with gangrene**

    Includes: that with gangrene (and obstruction)

  ● **551.0 Femoral hernia with gangrene**

    ❏ **551.00 Unilateral or unspecified (not specified as recurrent)**
        Femoral hernia NOS with gangrene

    551.01 Unilateral or unspecified, recurrent

    551.02 Bilateral (not specified as recurrent)

    551.03 Bilateral, recurrent

  551.1 Umbilical hernia with gangrene
    Parumbilical hernia specified as gangrenous

  ● **551.2 Ventral hernia with gangrene**

    ❏ **551.20 Ventral, unspecified, with gangrene**

    551.21 Incisional, with gangrene
        Hernia:
          postoperative specified as gangrenous
          recurrent, ventral specified as gangrenous

    ❏ **551.29 Other**
        Epigastric hernia specified as gangrenous

551.3 Diaphragmatic hernia with gangrene
    Hernia:
        hiatal (esophageal) (sliding) specified as gangrenous
        paraesophageal specified as gangrenous
    Thoracic stomach specified as gangrenous

Excludes	congenital diaphragmatic hernia (756.6)

❏ **551.8 Hernia of other specified sites, with gangrene**
    Any condition classifiable to 553.8 if specified as gangrenous

❏ **551.9 Hernia of unspecified site, with gangrene**
    Any condition classifiable to 553.9 if specified as gangrenous

● **552 Other hernia of abdominal cavity, with obstruction, but without mention of gangrene**

Excludes	that with mention of gangrene (551.0–551.9)

● **552.0 Femoral hernia with obstruction**
    Femoral hernia specified as incarcerated, irreducible, strangulated, or causing obstruction

    ❏ **552.00 Unilateral or unspecified (not specified as recurrent)**

    552.01 Unilateral or unspecified, recurrent

    552.02 Bilateral (not specified as recurrent)

    552.03 Bilateral, recurrent

  552.1 Umbilical hernia with obstruction
    Parumbilical hernia specified as incarcerated, irreducible, strangulated, or causing obstruction

● **552.2 Ventral hernia with obstruction**
    Ventral hernia specified as incarcerated, irreducible, strangulated, or causing obstruction

    ❏ **552.20 Ventral, unspecified, with obstruction**

    552.21 Incisional, with obstruction
        Hernia:
          postoperative specified as incarcerated, irreducible, strangulated, or causing obstruction
          recurrent, ventral specified as incarcerated, irreducible, strangulated, or causing obstruction

    ❏ **552.29 Other**
        Epigastric hernia specified as incarcerated, irreducible, strangulated, or causing obstruction

  552.3 Diaphragmatic hernia with obstruction
    Hernia:
        hiatal (esophageal) (sliding) specified as incarcerated, irreducible, strangulated, or causing obstruction
        paraesophageal specified as incarcerated, irreducible, strangulated, or causing obstruction
    Thoracic stomach specified as incarcerated, irreducible, strangulated, or causing obstruction

Excludes	congenital diaphragmatic hernia (756.6)

❏ **552.8 Hernia of other specified sites, with obstruction**
    Any condition classifiable to 553.8 if specified as incarcerated, irreducible, strangulated, or causing obstruction

❏ **552.9 Hernia of unspecified site, with obstruction**
    Any condition classifiable to 553.9 if specified as incarcerated, irreducible, strangulated, or causing obstruction

ICD-9-CM

500-
Vol.

● 553 **Other hernia of abdominal cavity without mention of obstruction or gangrene**

> **Excludes** *the listed conditions with mention of:*
> *gangrene (and obstruction) (551.0–551.9)*
> *obstruction (552.0–552.9)*

● 553.0 **Femoral hernia**

❑ 553.00 **Unilateral or unspecified (not specified as recurrent)**
Femoral hernia NOS

553.01 **Unilateral or unspecified, recurrent**

553.02 **Bilateral (not specified as recurrent)**

553.03 **Bilateral, recurrent**

553.1 **Umbilical hernia**
Parumbilical hernia

● 553.2 **Ventral hernia**

❑ 553.20 **Ventral, unspecified**

553.21 **Incisional**
Hernia:
postoperative
recurrent, ventral

❑ 553.29 **Other**
Hernia:
epigastric
spigelian

553.3 **Diaphragmatic hernia**
Hernia:
hiatal (esophageal) (sliding)
paraesophageal
Thoracic stomach

> **Excludes** *congenital:*
> *diaphragmatic hernia (756.6)*
> *hiatal hernia (750.6)*
> *esophagocele (530.6)*

❑ 553.8 **Hernia of other specified sites**
Hernia:
ischiatic
ischiorectal
lumbar
obturator
pudendal
retroperitoneal
sciatic
Other abdominal hernia of specified site

> **Excludes** *vaginal enterocele (618.6)*

❑ 553.9 **Hernia of unspecified site**
Enterocele
Epiplocele
Hernia:
NOS
interstitial
intestinal
intra-abdominal
Rupture (nontraumatic)
Sarcoepiplocele

NONINFECTIOUS ENTERITIS AND COLITIS (555–558)

● 555 **Regional enteritis**

> **Includes:** Crohn's disease
> Granulomatous enteritis

> **Excludes** *ulcerative colitis (556)*

555.0 **Small intestine**
Ileitis:
regional
segmental
terminal
Regional enteritis or Crohn's disease of:
duodenum
ileum
jejunum

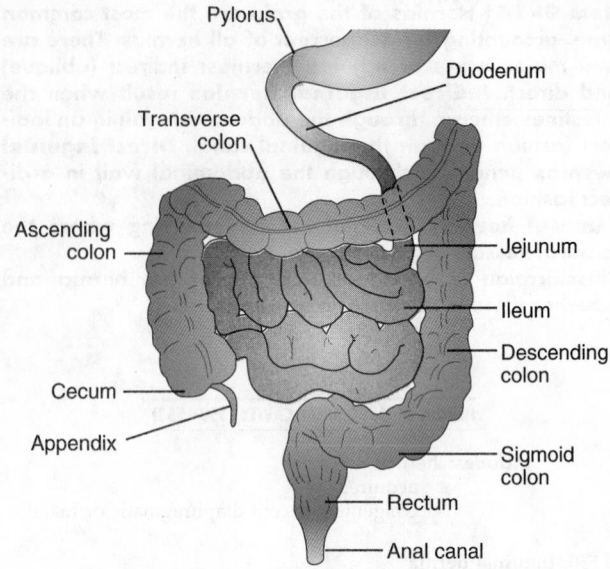

Figure 9–13 Small and large intestines.

Item 9–15 Crohn's disease, also known as regional enteritis, is a chronic inflammatory disease of the intestines. Classification is based on location in the small (duodenum, ileum, jejunum) or large (cecum, colon, rectum, anal canal) intestine.

555.1 **Large intestine**
Colitis:
granulomatous
regional
transmural
Regional enteritis or Crohn's disease of:
colon
large bowel
rectum

555.2 **Small intestine with large intestine**
Regional ileocolitis

❑ 555.9 **Unspecified site**
Crohn's disease NOS
Regional enteritis NOS

● 556 **Ulcerative colitis**

556.0 **Ulcerative (chronic) enterocolitis**

556.1 **Ulcerative (chronic) ileocolitis**

556.2 **Ulcerative (chronic) proctitis**

Item 9–16 Ulcerative colitis attacks the colonic mucosa and forms abscesses. The disease involves the intestines.
Classification is based on the location:
enterocolitis: large and small intestine
ileocolitis: ileum and colon
proctitis: rectum
proctosigmoiditis: sigmoid colon and rectum

556.3 Ulcerative (chronic) proctosigmoiditis

556.4 Pseudopolyposis of colon

556.5 Left-sided ulcerative (chronic) colitis

556.6 Universal ulcerative (chronic) colitis
Pancolitis

☐ **556.8 Other ulcerative colitis**

☐ **556.9 Ulcerative colitis, unspecified**
Ulcerative enteritis NOS

● **557 Vascular insufficiency of intestine**

> **Excludes** *necrotizing enterocolitis of the newborn (777.5)*

557.0 Acute vascular insufficiency of intestine
Acute:
hemorrhagic enterocolitis
ischemic colitis, enteritis, or enterocolitis
massive necrosis of intestine
Bowel infarction
Embolism of mesenteric artery
Fulminant enterocolitis
Hemorrhagic necrosis of intestine
Infarction of appendices epiploicae
Intestinal gangrene
Intestinal infarction (acute) (agnogenic) (hemor-
rhagic) (nonocclusive)
Mesenteric infarction (embolic) (thrombotic)
Necrosis of intestine
Terminal hemorrhagic enteropathy
Thrombosis of mesenteric artery

557.1 Chronic vascular insufficiency of intestine
Angina, abdominal
Chronic ischemic colitis, enteritis, or enterocolitis
Ischemic stricture of intestine
Mesenteric:
angina
artery syndrome (superior)
vascular insufficiency

☐ **557.9 Unspecified vascular insufficiency of intestine**
Alimentary pain due to vascular insufficiency
Ischemic colitis, enteritis, or enterocolitis NOS

● **558 Other and unspecified noninfectious gastroenteritis and colitis**

> **Excludes** *infectious:*
> *colitis, enteritis, or gastroenteritis (009.0–009.1)*
> *diarrhea (009.2–009.3)*

558.1 Gastroenteritis and colitis due to radiation
Radiation enterocolitis

558.2 Toxic gastroenteritis and colitis
Use additional E code to identify cause

558.3 Allergic gastroenteritis and colitis
Use additional code to identify type of food allergy
(V15.01–V15.05)

☐ **558.9 Other and unspecified noninfectious gastroenteritis and colitis**
Colitis, NOS, dietetic, or noninfectious
Enteritis, NOS, dietetic, or noninfectious
Gastroenteritis, NOS, dietetic, or noninfectious
Ileitis, NOS, dietetic, or noninfectious
Jejunitis, NOS, dietetic, or noninfectious
Sigmoiditis, NOS, dietetic, or noninfectious

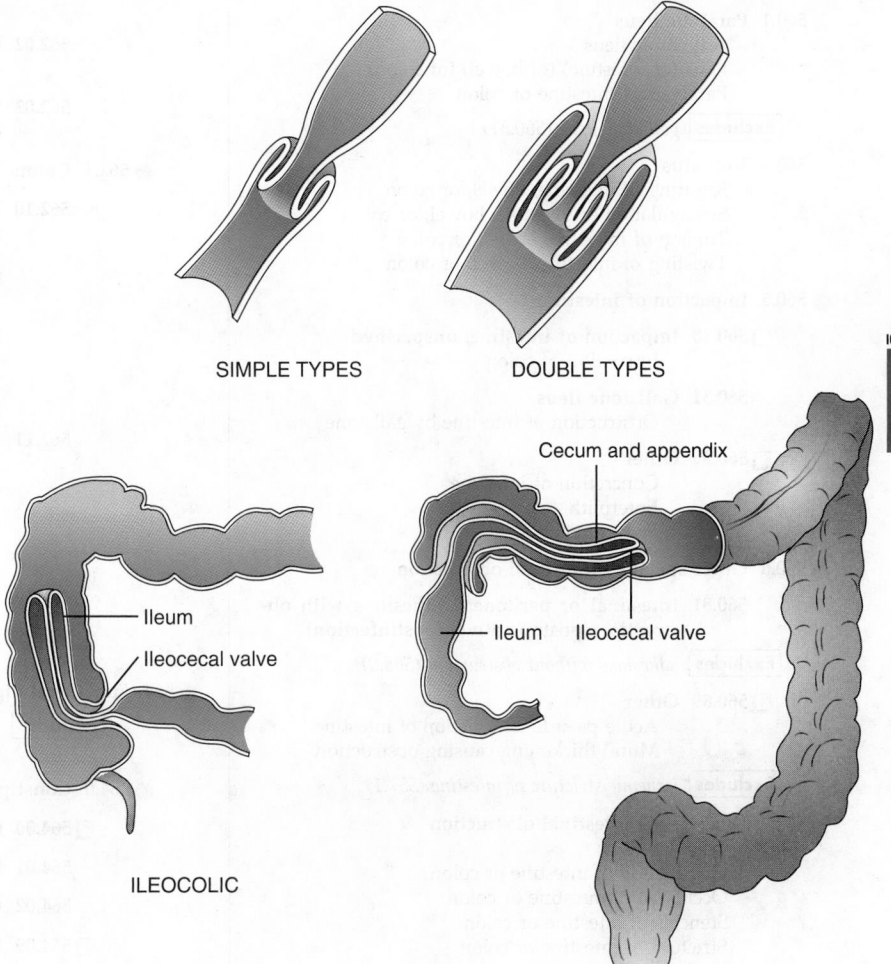

SIMPLE TYPES   DOUBLE TYPES

Cecum and appendix

Ileum

Ileocecal valve

Ileum   Ileocecal valve

ILEOCOLIC   ILEOCECAL

ICD-9-CM

**500-
599**

Vol. 1

Figure 9–14 Types of intussusception.

Item 9-17 Intussusception is the prolapse of a part of the intestine into another adjacent part of the intestine. Intussusception may be enteric (ileoileal, jejunoileal, jejunojejunal), colic (colocolic), or intracolic (ileocecal, ileocolic).

Item 9-18 Volvulus is the twisting of a segment of the intestine, resulting in obstruction.

OTHER DISEASES OF INTESTINES AND PERITONEUM (560–569)

● 560   Intestinal obstruction without mention of hernia

> | Excludes | duodenum (537.2–537.3)
> inguinal hernia with obstruction (550.1)
> intestinal obstruction complicating hernia (552.0–552.9)
> mesenteric:
>   embolism (557.0)
>   infarction (557.0)
>   thrombosis (557.0)
> neonatal intestinal obstruction (277.01, 777.1–777.2, 777.4)

    560.0   **Intussusception**
        Intussusception (colon) (intestine) (rectum)
        Invagination of intestine or colon

> | Excludes | intussusception of appendix (543.9)

    560.1   **Paralytic ileus**
        Adynamic ileus
        Ileus (of intestine) (of bowel) (of colon)
        Paralysis of intestine or colon

> | Excludes | gallstone ileus (560.31)

    560.2   **Volvulus**
        Knotting of intestine, bowel, or colon
        Strangulation of intestine, bowel, or colon
        Torsion of intestine, bowel, or colon
        Twisting of intestine, bowel, or colon

● 560.3   **Impaction of intestine**

    ☐ 560.30   **Impaction of intestine, unspecified**
           Impaction of colon

    560.31   **Gallstone ileus**
           Obstruction of intestine by gallstone

    ☐ 560.39   **Other**
           Concretion of intestine
           Enterolith
           Fecal impaction

● 560.8   **Other specified intestinal obstruction**

    560.81   **Intestinal or peritoneal adhesions with obstruction (postoperative) (postinfection)**

> | Excludes | adhesions without obstruction (568.0)

    ☐ 560.89   **Other**
           Acute pseudo-obstruction of intestine ◄
           Mural thickening causing obstruction

> | Excludes | ischemic stricture of intestine (557.1)

☐ 560.9   **Unspecified intestinal obstruction**
        Enterostenosis
        Obstruction of intestine or colon
        Occlusion of intestine or colon
        Stenosis of intestine or colon
        Stricture of intestine or colon

> | Excludes | congenital stricture or stenosis of intestine (751.1–751.2)

Item 9-19 Diverticula of the intestines are acquired herniations of the mucosa.
Classification is based on location (small intestine or colon) and whether it occurs with or without hemorrhage.

● 562   Diverticula of intestine
        Use additional code to identify any associated:
        peritonitis (567.0–567.9)

> | Excludes | congenital diverticulum of colon (751.5)
> diverticulum of appendix (543.9)
> Meckel's diverticulum (751.0)

● 562.0   **Small intestine**

    562.00   **Diverticulosis of small intestine (without mention of hemorrhage)**
           Diverticulosis:
              duodenum without mention of diverticulitis
              ileum without mention of diverticulitis
              jejunum without mention of diverticulitis

    562.01   **Diverticulitis of small intestine (without mention of hemorrhage)**
           Diverticulitis (with diverticulosis):
              duodenum
              ileum
              jejunum
              small intestine

    562.02   **Diverticulosis of small intestine with hemorrhage**

    562.03   **Diverticulitis of small intestine with hemorrhage**

● 562.1   **Colon**

    562.10   **Diverticulosis of colon (without mention of hemorrhage)**
           Diverticulosis without mention of diverticulitis:
              NOS
              intestine (large) without mention of diverticulitis
           Diverticular disease (colon) without mention of diverticulitis

    562.11   **Diverticulitis of colon without mention of hemorrhage**
           Diverticulitis (with diverticulosis):
              NOS
              colon
              intestine (large)

    562.12   **Diverticulosis of colon with hemorrhage**

    562.13   **Diverticulitis of colon with hemorrhage**

● 564   **Functional digestive disorders, not elsewhere classified**

> | Excludes | functional disorders of stomach (536.0–536.9)
> those specified as psychogenic (306.4)

● 564.0   **Constipation**

    ☐ 564.00   **Constipation, unspecified**

    564.01   **Slow transit constipation**

    564.02   **Outlet dysfunction constipation**

    ☐ 564.09   **Other constipation**

564.1   **Irritable bowel syndrome**
        Irritable colon

564.2 Postgastric surgery syndromes
Dumping syndrome
Jejunal syndrome
Postgastrectomy syndrome
Postvagotomy syndrome

Excludes *malnutrition following gastrointestinal surgery (579.3)*
postgastrojejunostomy ulcer (534.0–534.9)

564.3 Vomiting following gastrointestinal surgery
Vomiting (bilious) following gastrointestinal surgery

❑**564.4 Other postoperative functional disorders**
Diarrhea following gastrointestinal surgery

Excludes *colostomy and enterostomy complications (569.60–569.69)*

564.5 Functional diarrhea

Excludes *diarrhea:*
NOS (787.91)
psychogenic (306.4)

564.6 Anal spasm
Proctalgia fugax

564.7 Megacolon, other than Hirschsprung's
Dilatation of colon

Excludes *megacolon:*
congenital [Hirschsprung's] (751.3)
toxic (556)

●**564.8 Other specified functional disorders of intestine**

Excludes *malabsorption (579.0–579.9)*

    564.81 Neurogenic bowel

    ❑**564.89 Other functional disorders of intestine**
Atony of colon

❑**564.9 Unspecified functional disorder of intestine**

Item 9-20 A **fissure** is a groove in the surface, whereas a **fistula** is an abnormal passage.

●**565 Anal fissure and fistula**

565.0 Anal fissure
Tear of anus, nontraumatic

Excludes *traumatic (863.89, 863.99)*

565.1 Anal fistula
Fistula:
anorectal
rectal
rectum to skin

Excludes *fistula of rectum to internal organs - see Alphabetic Index*
ischiorectal fistula (566)
rectovaginal fistula (619.1)

566 Abscess of anal and rectal regions
Abscess:
ischiorectal
perianal
perirectal
Cellulitis:
anal
perirectal
rectal
Ischiorectal fistula

●**567 Peritonitis**

Excludes *peritonitis:*
benign paroxysmal (277.3)
pelvic, female (614.5, 614.7)
periodic familial (277.3)
puerperal (670)
with or following:
abortion (634–638 with .0, 639.0)
appendicitis (540.0–540.1)
ectopic or molar pregnancy (639.0)

●**567.0 Peritonitis in infectious diseases classified elsewhere**

Code first underlying disease

Excludes *peritonitis:*
gonococcal (098.86)
syphilitic (095.2)
tuberculous (014.0)

567.1 Pneumococcal peritonitis

❑**567.2 Other suppurative peritonitis**
Abscess (of):   Abscess (of):
abdominopelvic   retroperitoneal
mesenteric   subdiaphragmatic
omentum   subhepatic
peritoneum   subphrenic
retrocecal
Peritonitis (acute):   Peritonitis (acute):
general   subphrenic
pelvic, male   suppurative

❑**567.8 Other specified peritonitis**
Chronic proliferative peritonitis
Fat necrosis of peritoneum
Mesenteric saponification
Peritonitis due to:
bile   urine

❑**567.9 Unspecified peritonitis**
Peritonitis: Peritonitis:
NOS   of unspecified cause

●**568 Other disorders of peritoneum**

568.0 Peritoneal adhesions (postoperative) (postinfection)
Adhesions (of):   Adhesions (of):
abdominal (wall)   mesenteric
diaphragm   omentum
intestine   stomach
male pelvis
Adhesive bands

Excludes *adhesions:*
pelvic, female (614.6)
with obstruction:
duodenum (537.3)
intestine (560.81)

●**568.8 Other specified disorders of peritoneum**

    568.81 Hemoperitoneum (nontraumatic)

    568.82 Peritoneal effusion (chronic)

Excludes *ascites NOS (789.5)*

    ❑**568.89 Other**
Peritoneal:
cyst   granuloma

❑**568.9 Unspecified disorder of peritoneum**

●**569 Other disorders of intestine**

569.0 Anal and rectal polyp
Anal and rectal polyp NOS

Excludes *adenomatous anal and rectal polyp (211.4)*

569.1 Rectal prolapse
Procidentia: Prolapse:
anus (sphincter)   anal canal
rectum (sphincter)   rectal mucosa
Proctoptosis

Excludes *prolapsed hemorrhoids (455.2, 455.5)*

569.2 Stenosis of rectum and anus
Stricture of anus (sphincter)

ICD-9-CM

500-599

Vol. 1

569.3   Hemorrhage of rectum and anus

> **Excludes**   *gastrointestinal bleeding NOS (578.9)*
> *melena (578.1)*

● **569.4   Other specified disorders of rectum and anus**

     569.41   Ulcer of anus and rectum
          Solitary ulcer of anus (sphincter) or rectum (sphincter)
          Stercoral ulcer of anus (sphincter) or rectum (sphincter)

     569.42   Anal or rectal pain

     ☐ **569.49   Other**
          Granuloma of rectum (sphincter)
          Rupture of rectum (sphincter)
          Hypertrophy of anal papillae
          Proctitis NOS

> **Excludes**   *fistula of rectum to:*
> *internal organs - see Alphabetic Index*
> *skin (565.1)*
> *hemorrhoids (455.0–455.9)*
> *incontinence of sphincter ani (787.6)*

569.5   Abscess of intestine

> **Excludes**   *appendiceal abscess (540.1)*

● **569.6   Colostomy and enterostomy complications**

     ☐ **569.60   Colostomy and enterostomy complication, unspecified**

     569.61   Infection of colostomy or enterostomy

          Use additional code to identify organism (041.00–041.9)

          Use additional code to specify type of infection, such as:
          abscess or cellulitis of abdomen (682.2)
          septicemia (038.0–038.9)

     569.62   Mechanical complication of colostomy and enterostomy
          Malfunction of colostomy and enterostomy

     ☐ **569.69   Other complication**
          Fistula
          Hernia
          Prolapse

● **569.8   Other specified disorders of intestine**

     569.81   Fistula of intestine, excluding rectum and anus
          Fistula:
          abdominal wall
          enterocolic
          enteroenteric
          ileorectal

> **Excludes**   *fistula of intestine to internal organs-see Alphabetic Index*
> *persistent postoperative fistula (998.6)*

     569.82   Ulceration of intestine
          Primary ulcer of intestine
          Ulceration of colon

> **Excludes**   *that with perforation (569.83)*

     569.83   Perforation of intestine

     569.84   Angiodysplasia of intestine (without mention of hemorrhage)

     569.85   Angiodysplasia of intestine with hemorrhage

     569.86   Dieulafoy lesion (hemorrhagic) of intestine

☐ **569.89   Other**
     Enteroptosis
     Granuloma of intestine
     Prolapse of intestine
     Pericolitis
     Perisigmoiditis
     Visceroptosis

> **Excludes**   *gangrene of intestine, mesentery, or omentum (557.0)*
> *hemorrhage of intestine NOS (578.9)*
> *obstruction of intestine (560.0–560.9)*

☐ **569.9   Unspecified disorder of intestine**

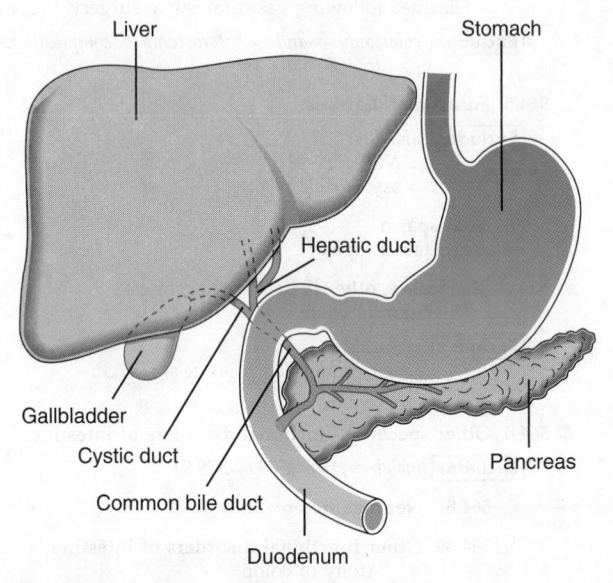

Figure 9–15   Liver and bile ducts.

Item 9–21   Cirrhosis is the progressive fibrosis of the liver resulting in loss of liver function. The main causes of cirrhosis of the liver are alcohol abuse, chronic hepatitis (inflammation of the liver), biliary disease, and excessive amounts of iron. **Alcoholic cirrhosis of the liver** is also called portal, Laënnec's, or fatty nutritional cirrhosis.

OTHER DISEASES OF DIGESTIVE SYSTEM (570–579)

570   Acute and subacute necrosis of liver
     Acute hepatic failure
     Acute or subacute hepatitis, not specified as infective
     Necrosis of liver (acute) (diffuse) (massive) (subacute)
     Parenchymatous degeneration of liver
     Yellow atrophy (liver) (acute) (subacute)

> **Excludes**   *icterus gravis of newborn (773.0–773.2)*
> *serum hepatitis (070.2–070.3)*
> *that with:*
> *abortion (634–638 with .7, 639.8)*
> *ectopic or molar pregnancy (639.8)*
> *pregnancy, childbirth, or the puerperium (646.7)*
> *viral hepatitis (070.0–070.9)*

● **571   Chronic liver disease and cirrhosis**

     571.0   Alcoholic fatty liver

     571.1   Acute alcoholic hepatitis
          Acute alcoholic liver disease

571.2 Alcoholic cirrhosis of liver
Florid cirrhosis
Laënnec's cirrhosis (alcoholic)

☐**571.3 Alcoholic liver damage, unspecified**

●**571.4 Chronic hepatitis**

| **Excludes** | viral hepatitis (acute) (chronic) (070.0–070.9) |

☐**571.40 Chronic hepatitis, unspecified**

571.41 Chronic persistent hepatitis

☐**571.49 Other**
Chronic hepatitis:
active
aggressive
Recurrent hepatitis

571.5 Cirrhosis of liver without mention of alcohol
Cirrhosis of liver:
NOS
cryptogenic
macronodular
micronodular
posthepatitic
postnecrotic
Healed yellow atrophy (liver)
Portal cirrhosis

571.6 Biliary cirrhosis
Chronic nonsuppurative destructive cholangitis
Cirrhosis:
cholangitic
cholestatic

☐**571.8 Other chronic nonalcoholic liver disease**
Chronic yellow atrophy (liver)
Fatty liver, without mention of alcohol

☐**571.9 Unspecified chronic liver disease without mention of alcohol**

●**572 Liver abscess and sequelae of chronic liver disease**

572.0 Abscess of liver

| **Excludes** | amebic liver abscess (006.3) |

572.1 Portal pyemia
Phlebitis of portal vein
Portal thrombophlebitis
Pylephlebitis
Pylethrombophlebitis

572.2 Hepatic coma
Hepatic encephalopathy
Hepatocerebral intoxication
Portal-systemic encephalopathy

572.3 Portal hypertension

572.4 Hepatorenal syndrome

| **Excludes** | that following delivery (674.8) |

☐**572.8 Other sequelae of chronic liver disease**

●**573 Other disorders of liver**

| **Excludes** | amyloid or lardaceous degeneration of liver (277.3)
congenital cystic disease of liver (751.62)
glycogen infiltration of liver (271.0)
hepatomegaly NOS (789.1)
portal vein obstruction (452) |

573.0 Chronic passive congestion of liver

●**573.1 Hepatitis in viral diseases classified elsewhere**

Code first underlying disease, as:
Coxsackie virus disease (074.8)
cytomegalic inclusion virus disease (078.5)
infectious mononucleosis (075)

| **Excludes** | hepatitis (in):
mumps (072.71)
viral (070.0–070.9)
yellow fever (060.0–060.9) |

●☐**573.2 Hepatitis in other infectious diseases classified elsewhere**

Code first underlying disease, as:
malaria (084.9)

| **Excludes** | hepatitis in:
late syphilis (095.3)
secondary syphilis (091.62)
toxoplasmosis (130.5) |

☐**573.3 Hepatitis, unspecified**
Toxic (noninfectious) hepatitis

Use additional E code to identify cause

573.4 Hepatic infarction

☐**573.8 Other specified disorders of liver**
Hepatoptosis

☐**573.9 Unspecified disorder of liver**

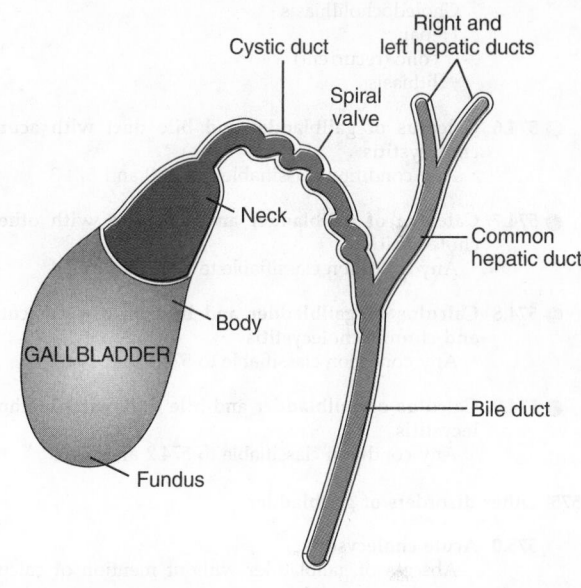

Figure 9-16 Gallbladder and bile ducts.

●**574 Cholelithiasis**

The following fifth-digit subclassification is for use with category 574:
0 **without mention of obstruction**
1 **with obstruction**

●**574.0 Calculus of gallbladder with acute cholecystitis**
Biliary calculus with acute cholecystitis
Calculus of cystic duct with acute cholecystitis
Cholelithiasis with acute cholecystitis
Any condition classifiable to 574.2 with acute cholecystitis

●☐**574.1 Calculus of gallbladder with other cholecystitis**
Biliary calculus with cholecystitis
Calculus of cystic duct with cholecystitis
Cholelithiasis with cholecystitis
Cholecystitis with cholelithiasis NOS
Any condition classifiable to 574.2 with cholecystitis (chronic)

●**574.2 Calculus of gallbladder without mention of cholecystitis**
Biliary:
calculus NOS
colic NOS
Calculus of cystic duct
Cholelithiasis NOS
Colic (recurrent) of gallbladder
Gallstone (impacted)

● **574.3 Calculus of bile duct with acute cholecystitis**
Calculus of bile duct [any] with acute cholecystitis
Choledocholithiasis with acute cholecystitis
Any condition classifiable to 574.5 with acute cholecystitis

● ❑ **574.4 Calculus of bile duct with other cholecystitis**
Calculus of bile duct [any] with cholecystitis (chronic)
Choledocholithiasis with cholecystitis (chronic)
Any condition classifiable to 574.5 with cholecystitis (chronic)

● **574.5 Calculus of bile duct without mention of cholecystitis**
Calculus of:
   bile duct [any]
   common duct
   hepatic duct
Choledocholithiasis
Hepatic:
   colic (recurrent)
   lithiasis

● **574.6 Calculus of gallbladder and bile duct with acute cholecystitis**
Any condition classifiable to 574.0 and 574.3

● **574.7 Calculus of gallbladder and bile duct with other cholecystitis**
Any condition classifiable to 574.1 and 574.4

● **574.8 Calculus of gallbladder and bile duct with acute and chronic cholecystitis**
Any condition classifiable to 574.6 and 574.7

● **574.9 Calculus of gallbladder and bile duct without cholecystitis**
Any condition classifiable to 574.2 and 574.5

● **575 Other disorders of gallbladder**

575.0 Acute cholecystitis
Abscess of gallbladder without mention of calculus
Angiocholecystitis without mention of calculus
Cholecystitis without mention of calculus:
   emphysematous (acute)
   gangrenous
   suppurative
Empyema of gallbladder without mention of calculus
Gangrene of gallbladder without mention of calculus

   | Excludes | *that with:*
   acute and chronic cholecystitis (575.12)
   choledocholithiasis (574.3)
   choledocholithiasis and cholelithiasis (574.6)
   cholelithiasis (574.0)

● **575.1 Other cholecystitis**
Cholecystitis without mention of calculus:
   NOS without mention of calculus
   chronic without mention of calculus

   | Excludes | *that with:*
   choledocholithiasis (574.4)
   choledocholithiasis and cholelithiasis (574.8)
   cholelithiasis (574.1)

❑ **575.10 Cholecystitis, unspecified**
Cholecystitis NOS

575.11 Chronic cholecystitis

575.12 Acute and chronic cholecystitis

575.2 Obstruction of gallbladder
Occlusion of cystic duct or gallbladder without mention of calculus
Stenosis of cystic duct or gallbladder without mention of calculus
Stricture of cystic duct or gallbladder without mention of calculus

   | Excludes | *that with calculus (574.0–574.2 with fifth digit 1)*

575.3 Hydrops of gallbladder
Mucocele of gallbladder

575.4 Perforation of gallbladder
Rupture of cystic duct or gallbladder

575.5 Fistula of gallbladder
Fistula:
   cholecystoduodenal
   cholecystoenteric

575.6 Cholesterolosis of gallbladder
Strawberry gallbladder

❑ **575.8 Other specified disorders of gallbladder**
Adhesions (of) cystic duct gallbladder
Atrophy (of) cystic duct gallbladder
Cyst (of) cystic duct gallbladder
Hypertrophy (of) cystic duct gallbladder
Nonfunctioning (of) cystic duct gallbladder
Ulcer (of) cystic duct gallbladder
Biliary dyskinesia

   | Excludes | *Hartmann's pouch of intestine (V44.3)*
   nonvisualization of gallbladder (793.3)

❑ **575.9 Unspecified disorder of gallbladder**

● **576 Other disorders of biliary tract**

   | Excludes | *that involving the:*
   cystic duct (575.0–575.9)
   gallbladder (575.0–575.9)

576.0 Postcholecystectomy syndrome

576.1 Cholangitis
Cholangitis: Cholangitis:
   NOS   recurrent
   acute   sclerosing
   ascending   secondary
   chronic   stenosing
   primary   suppurative

576.2 Obstruction of bile duct
Occlusion of bile duct, except cystic duct, without mention of calculus
Stenosis of bile duct, except cystic duct, without mention of calculus
Stricture of bile duct, except cystic duct, without mention of calculus

   | Excludes | *congenital (751.61)*
   that with calculus (574.3–574.5 with fifth-digit 1)

576.3 Perforation of bile duct
Rupture of bile duct, except cystic duct

576.4 Fistula of bile duct
Choledochoduodenal fistula

576.5 Spasm of sphincter of Oddi

❑ **576.8 Other specified disorders of biliary tract**
Adhesions of bile duct [any]
Atrophy of bile duct [any]
Cyst of bile duct [any]
Hypertrophy of bile duct [any]
Stasis of bile duct [any]
Ulcer of bile duct [any]

   | Excludes | *congenital choledochal cyst (751.69)*

❑ **576.9 Unspecified disorder of biliary tract**

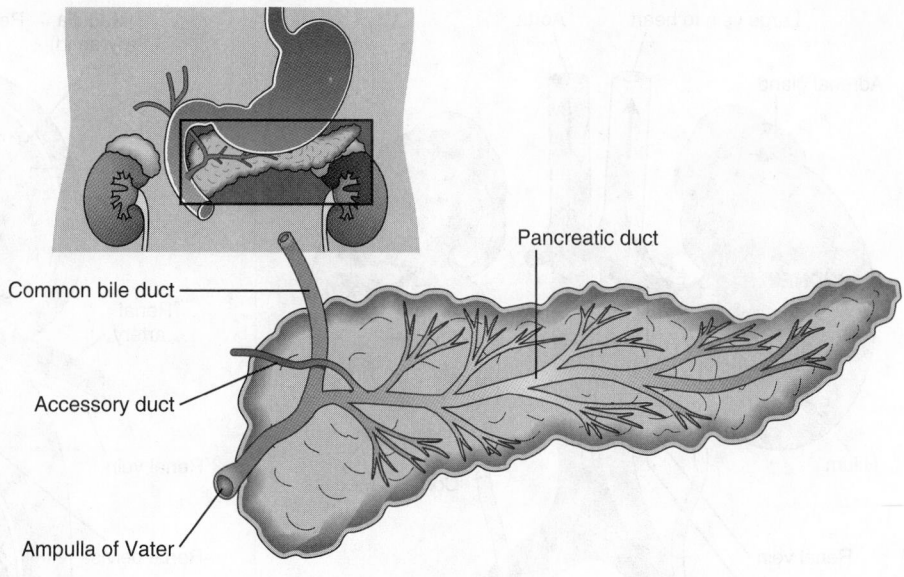

Figure 9–17 Pancreas.

Common bile duct

Accessory duct

Ampulla of Vater

Pancreatic duct

● 577 **Diseases of pancreas**

577.0 **Acute pancreatitis**
Abscess of pancreas
Necrosis of pancreas:
  acute   infective
Pancreatitis: Pancreatitis:
  NOS   hemorrhagic
  acute (recurrent)   subacute
  apoplectic   suppurative
Excludes *mumps pancreatitis (072.3)*

577.1 **Chronic pancreatitis**
Chronic pancreatitis: Pancreatitis:
  NOS   painless
  infectious   recurrent
  interstitial   relapsing

577.2 **Cyst and pseudocyst of pancreas**

☐577.8 **Other specified diseases of pancreas**
Atrophy of pancreas
Calculus of pancreas
Cirrhosis of pancreas
Fibrosis of pancreas
Pancreatic:
  infantilism
  necrosis:
    NOS   fat
    aseptic
Pancreatolithiasis
Excludes *fibrocystic disease of pancreas (277.00–277.09)*
islet cell tumor of pancreas (211.7)
pancreatic steatorrhea (579.4)

☐577.9 **Unspecified disease of pancreas**

● 578 **Gastrointestinal hemorrhage**
Excludes *that with mention of:*
angiodysplasia of stomach and duodenum (537.83)
angiodysplasia of intestine (569.85)
diverticulitis, intestine:
  large (562.13)
  small (562.03)
diverticulosis, intestine:
  large (562.12)
  small (562.02)
gastritis and duodenitis (535.0–535.6)
ulcer:
  duodenal, gastric, gastrojejunal, or peptic (531.00–534.91)

578.0 **Hematemesis**
Vomiting of blood

578.1 **Blood in stool**
Melena
Excludes *melena of the newborn (772.4, 777.3)*
occult blood (792.1)

☐578.9 **Hemorrhage of gastrointestinal tract, unspecified**
Gastric hemorrhage   Intestinal hemorrhage

● 579 **Intestinal malabsorption**

579.0 **Celiac disease**
Celiac: Gee (-Herter) disease
  crisis   Gluten enteropathy
  infantilism   Idiopathic steatorrhea
  rickets   Nontropical sprue

579.1 **Tropical sprue**
Sprue:
  NOS
  tropical
Tropical steatorrhea

579.2 **Blind loop syndrome**
Postoperative blind loop syndrome

☐579.3 **Other and unspecified postsurgical nonabsorption**
Hypoglycemia following gastrointestinal surgery
Malnutrition following gastrointestinal surgery

579.4 **Pancreatic steatorrhea**

☐579.8 **Other specified intestinal malabsorption**
Enteropathy:
  exudative
  protein-losing
Steatorrhea (chronic)

☐579.9 **Unspecified intestinal malabsorption**
Malabsorption syndrome NOS

ICD-9-CM

500-
599

Vol. 1

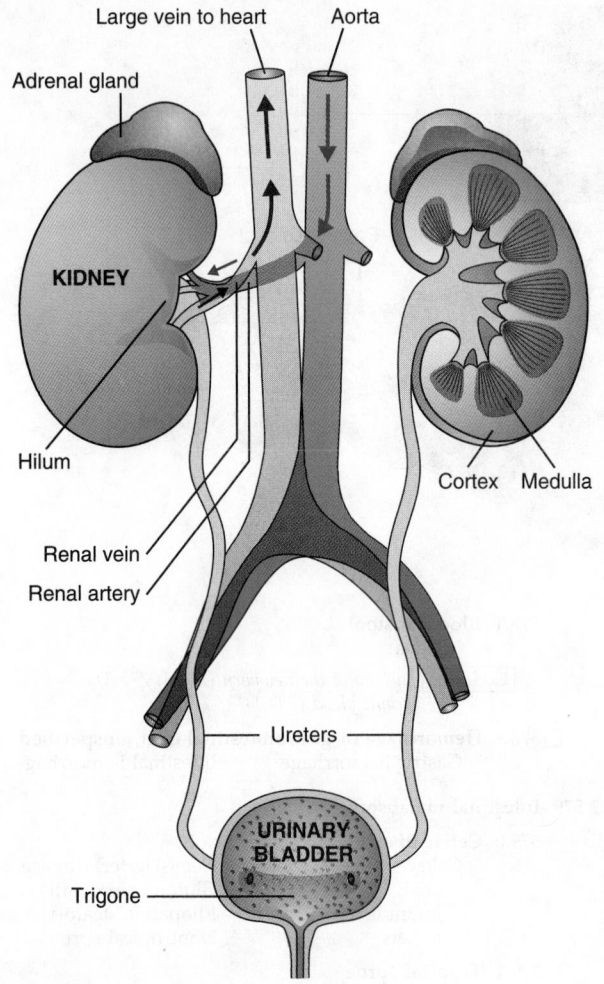

Figure 10-1   Kidneys within the urinary system.

Item 10-1 Glomerulonephritis is nephritis accompanied by inflammation of the glomeruli of the kidney, resulting in the degeneration of the glomeruli and the nephrons.
Acute glomerulonephritis primarily affects children and young adults and is usually a result of a streptococcal infection.
Proliferative glomerulonephritis is the acute form of the disease resulting from a streptococcal infection.
Rapidly progressive glomerulonephritis, also known as **crescentic** or **malignant glomerulonephritis,** is the acute form of the disease, which leads quickly to rapid and progressive decline in renal function.

10.   DISEASES OF THE GENITOURINARY SYSTEM (580–629)

NEPHRITIS, NEPHROTIC SYNDROME, AND NEPHROSIS (580–589)

> **Excludes** *hypertensive renal disease (403.00–403.91)*

● 580 Acute glomerulonephritis

  Includes: acute nephritis

  580.0 **With lesion of proliferative glomerulonephritis**
    Acute (diffuse) proliferative glomerulonephritis
    Acute poststreptococcal glomerulonephritis

Figure 10-2   Kidney.

580.4 **With lesion of rapidly progressive glomerulonephritis**
    Acute nephritis with lesion of necrotizing glomerulitis

● 580.8 **With other specified pathological lesion in kidney**

  ● 580.81 *Acute glomerulonephritis in diseases classified elsewhere*

    Code first underlying disease, as:
      infectious hepatitis (070.0–070.9)
      mumps (072.79)
      subacute bacterial endocarditis (421.0)
      typhoid fever (002.0)

  ☐ 580.89 **Other**
      Glomerulonephritis, acute, with lesion of:
        exudative nephritis
        interstitial (diffuse) (focal) nephritis

☐ 580.9 **Acute glomerulonephritis with unspecified pathological lesion in kidney**
      Glomerulonephritis: specified as acute
        NOS specified as acute
        hemorrhagic specified as acute
      Nephritis specified as acute
      Nephropathy specified as acute

Item 10-2 Nephrotic syndrome (NS) is marked by massive proteinuria (protein in the urine) and water retention. Patients with NS are particularly vulnerable to staphylococcal and pneumococcal infections.
NS with lesion of proliferative glomerulonephritis results from a streptococcal infection.
NS with lesion of membranous glomerulonephritis results in thickening of the capillary walls.
NS with lesion of minimal change glomerulonephritis is usually a benign disorder that occurs mostly in children and requires electron microscopy to verify changes in the glomeruli.

Item 10-3 Chronic glomerulonephritis (GN) persists over a period of years, with remissions and exacerbation.
Chronic GN with lesion of proliferative glomerulonephritis results from a streptococcal infection.
Chronic GN with lesion of membranous glomerulonephritis, also known as membranous nephropathy, is characterized by deposits along the epithelial side of the basement membrane.
Chronic GN with lesion of membranoproliferative glomerulonephritis (MPGN) is a group of disorders characterized by alterations in the basement membranes of the kidney and the glomerular cells.
Chronic GN with lesion of rapidly progressive glomerulonephritis is characterized by necrosis, endothelial proliferation, and mesangial proliferation. The condition is marked by rapid and progressive decline in renal function.

● 581 Nephrotic syndrome

    581.0 **With lesion of proliferative glomerulonephritis**

    581.1 **With lesion of membranous glomerulonephritis**
        Epimembranous nephritis
        Idiopathic membranous glomerular disease
        Nephrotic syndrome with lesion of:
            focal glomerulosclerosis
            sclerosing membranous glomerulonephritis
            segmental hyalinosis

    581.2 **With lesion of membranoproliferative glomerulonephritis**
        Nephrotic syndrome with lesion (of):
            endothelial glomerulonephritis
            hypocomplementemic glomerulonephritis
                persistent glomerulonephritis
            lobular glomerulonephritis
            mesangiocapillary glomerulonephritis
            mixed membranous and proliferative glomerulonephritis

    581.3 **With lesion of minimal change glomerulonephritis**
        Foot process disease
        Lipoid nephrosis
        Minimal change:
            glomerular disease
            glomerulitis
            nephrotic syndrome

● 581.8 **With other specified pathological lesion in kidney**

    ● 581.81 *Nephrotic syndrome in diseases classified elsewhere*

        Code first underlying disease, as:
            amyloidosis (277.3)
            diabetes mellitus (250.4)
            malaria (084.9)
            polyarteritis (446.0)
            systemic lupus erythematosus (710.0)

    | Excludes | nephrosis in epidemic hemorrhagic fever (078.6)

    ❑ 581.89 **Other**
        Glomerulonephritis with edema and lesion of:
            exudative nephritis
            interstitial (diffuse) (focal) nephritis

    ❑ 581.9 **Nephrotic syndrome with unspecified pathological lesion in kidney**
        Glomerulonephritis with edema NOS
        Nephritis:
            nephrotic NOS
            with edema NOS
        Nephrosis NOS
        Renal disease with edema NOS

● 582 Chronic glomerulonephritis

    Includes: chronic nephritis

    582.0 **With lesion of proliferative glomerulonephritis**
        Chronic (diffuse) proliferative glomerulonephritis

    582.1 **With lesion of membranous glomerulonephritis**
        Chronic glomerulonephritis:
            membranous
            sclerosing
        Focal glomerulosclerosis
        Segmental hyalinosis

    582.2 **With lesion of membranoproliferative glomerulonephritis**
        Chronic glomerulonephritis:
            endothelial
            hypocomplementemic persistent
            lobular
            membranoproliferative
            mesangiocapillary
            mixed membranous and proliferative

    582.4 **With lesion of rapidly progressive glomerulonephritis**
        Chronic nephritis with lesion of necrotizing glomerulitis

● 582.8 **With other specified pathological lesion in kidney**

    ● 582.81 *Chronic glomerulonephritis in diseases classified elsewhere*

        Code first underlying disease, as:
            amyloidosis (277.3)
            systemic lupus erythematosus (710.0)

    ❑ 582.89 **Other**
        Chronic glomerulonephritis with lesion of:
            exudative nephritis
            interstitial (diffuse) (focal) nephritis

    ❑ 582.9 **Chronic glomerulonephritis with unspecified pathological lesion in kidney**
        Glomerulonephritis: specified as chronic
            NOS specified as chronic
            hemorrhagic specified as chronic
        Nephritis specified as chronic
        Nephropathy specified as chronic

ICD-9-CM

500-599

Vol.

Item 10-4 Nephritis (inflammation) or nephropathy (disease) with lesion of proliferative glomerulonephritis results from a streptococcal infection.
Nephritis (inflammation) or nephropathy (disease) with lesion of membranous glomerulonephritis is characterized by deposits along the epithelial side of the basement membrane.
Nephritis (inflammation) or nephropathy (disease) with lesion of membranoproliferative glomerulonephritis is characterized by alterations in the basement membranes of the kidney and the glomerular cells.
Nephritis (inflammation) or nephropathy (disease) with lesion of rapidly progressive glomerulonephritis is characterized by rapid and progressive decline in renal function.
Nephritis (inflammation) or nephropathy (disease) with lesion of renal cortical necrosis is characterized by death of the cortical tissues.
Nephritis (inflammation) or nephropathy (disease) with lesion of renal medullary necrosis is characterized by death of the tissues that collect urine.

● 583 Nephritis and nephropathy, not specified as acute or chronic

> **Includes:** "renal disease" so stated, not specified as acute or chronic but with stated pathology or cause

583.0 **With lesion of proliferative glomerulonephritis**
Proliferative:
glomerulonephritis (diffuse) NOS
nephritis NOS
nephropathy NOS

583.1 **With lesion of membranous glomerulonephritis**
Membranous:
glomerulonephritis NOS
nephritis NOS
Membranous nephropathy NOS

583.2 **With lesion of membranoproliferative glomerulonephritis**
Membranoproliferative:
glomerulonephritis NOS
nephritis NOS
nephropathy NOS
Nephritis NOS, with lesion of:
hypocomplementemic persistent glomerulonephritis
lobular glomerulonephritis
mesangiocapillary glomerulonephritis
mixed membranous and proliferative glomerulonephritis

583.4 **With lesion of rapidly progressive glomerulonephritis**
Necrotizing or rapidly progressive:
glomerulitis NOS
glomerulonephritis NOS
nephritis NOS
nephropathy NOS
Nephritis, unspecified, with lesion of necrotizing glomerulitis

583.6 **With lesion of renal cortical necrosis**
Nephritis NOS with (renal) cortical necrosis
Nephropathy NOS with (renal) cortical necrosis
Renal cortical necrosis NOS

583.7 **With lesion of renal medullary necrosis**
Nephritis NOS with (renal) medullary [papillary] necrosis
Nephropathy NOS with (renal) medullary [papillary] necrosis

● 583.8 **With other specified pathological lesion in kidney**

> ● 583.81 *Nephritis and nephropathy, not specified as acute or chronic, in diseases classified elsewhere*
>
> *Code first underlying disease, as:*
> amyloidosis (277.3)
> diabetes mellitus (250.4)
> gonococcal infection (098.19)
> Goodpasture's syndrome (446.21)
> systemic lupus erythematosus (710.0)
> tuberculosis (016.0)

Excludes	*gouty nephropathy (274.10)*
	syphilitic nephritis (095.4)

☐ 583.89 **Other**
Glomerulitis with lesion of:
exudative nephritis
interstitial nephritis
Glomerulonephritis with lesion of:
exudative nephritis
interstitial nephritis
Nephritis with lesion of:
exudative nephritis
interstitial nephritis
Nephropathy with lesion of:
exudative nephritis
interstitial nephritis
Renal disease with lesion of:
exudative nephritis
interstitial nephritis

☐ 583.9 **With unspecified pathological lesion in kidney**
Glomerulitis NOS   Nephritis NOS
Glomerulonephritis NOS   Nephropathy NOS

Excludes	*nephropathy complicating pregnancy, labor, or the puerperium (642.0–642.9, 646.2)*
	renal disease NOS with no stated cause (593.9)

Item 10-5 Decreased blood flow is the usual cause of acute renal failure that offers a good prognosis for recovery. Chronic renal failure is usually the result of long-standing kidney disease and is a very serious condition that generally results in death.

● 584 Acute renal failure

Excludes	*following labor and delivery (669.3)*
	posttraumatic (958.5)
	that complicating:
	abortion (634–638 with .3, 639.3)
	ectopic or molar pregnancy (639.3)

584.5 **With lesion of tubular necrosis**
Lower nephron nephrosis
Renal failure with (acute) tubular necrosis
Tubular necrosis:
NOS
acute

584.6 **With lesion of renal cortical necrosis**

584.7 **With lesion of renal medullary [papillary] necrosis**
Necrotizing renal papillitis

☐ 584.8 **With other specified pathological lesion in kidney**

☐ 584.9 **Acute renal failure, unspecified**

585 Chronic renal failure
Chronic uremia

Use additional code to identify manifestation as:
uremic:
neuropathy (357.4)
pericarditis (420.0)

Excludes	*that with any condition classifiable to 401 (403.0–403.9 with fifth-digit 1)*

□ **586 Renal failure, unspecified**
Uremia NOS

| Excludes | *following labor and delivery (669.3)*
posttraumatic renal failure (958.5)
that complicating:
  abortion (634–638 with .3, 639.3)
  ectopic or molar pregnancy (639.3)
uremia:
  extrarenal (788.9)
  prerenal (788.9)
with any condition classifiable to 401 (403.0–403.9 with fifth-digit 1)

□ **587 Renal sclerosis, unspecified**
Atrophy of kidney
Contracted kidney
Renal:
  cirrhosis
  fibrosis

| Excludes | *nephrosclerosis (arteriolar) (arteriosclerotic)
(403.00–403.92)*
with hypertension (403.00–403.92)

● **588 Disorders resulting from impaired renal function**

588.0 Renal osteodystrophy
Azotemic osteodystrophy
Phosphate-losing tubular disorders
Renal:
  dwarfism
  infantilism
  rickets

588.1 Nephrogenic diabetes insipidus

| Excludes | *diabetes insipidus NOS (253.5)*

● **588.8 Other specified disorders resulting from impaired renal function**

| Excludes | *secondary hypertension (405.0–405.9)*

588.81 Secondary hyperparathyroidism (of renal origin) ◀
Secondary hyperparathyroidism NOS ◀

588.89 Other specified disorders resulting from impaired renal function ◀
Hypokalemic nephropathy ◀

□ **588.9 Unspecified disorder resulting from impaired renal function**

● **589 Small kidney of unknown cause**

589.0 Unilateral small kidney

589.1 Bilateral small kidneys

□ **589.9 Small kidney, unspecified**

Figure 10–3 Acute pyelonephritis. Cortical surface is dotted with abscesses. (From Cotran R, Kumar V, Robbins S: Robbins Pathologic Basis of Disease. Philadelphia, WB Saunders, 1994, p 969.)

OTHER DISEASES OF URINARY SYSTEM (590–599)

● **590 Infections of kidney**
Use additional code to identify organism, such as Escherichia coli [E. coli] (041.4)

● **590.0 Chronic pyelonephritis**
Chronic pyelitis
Chronic pyonephrosis

Code, if applicable, any causal condition first

590.00 Without lesion of renal medullary necrosis

590.01 With lesion of renal medullary necrosis

● **590.1 Acute pyelonephritis**
Acute pyelitis
Acute pyonephrosis

590.10 Without lesion of renal medullary necrosis

590.11 With lesion of renal medullary necrosis

590.2 Renal and perinephric abscess
Abscess:
  kidney
  nephritic
  perirenal
Carbuncle of kidney

590.3 Pyeloureteritis cystica
Infection of renal pelvis and ureter
Ureteritis cystica

ICD-9-CM

500–599

Vol. 1

● **590.8 Other pyelonephritis or pyonephrosis, not specified as acute or chronic**

   ❑ **590.80 Pyelonephritis, unspecified**
      Pyelitis NOS
      Pyelonephritis NOS

   ● *590.81 Pyelitis or pyelonephritis in diseases classified elsewhere*

      Code first underlying disease, as:
      tuberculosis (016.0)

❑ **590.9 Infection of kidney, unspecified**

   | **Excludes** | *urinary tract infection NOS (599.0)*

591 Hydronephrosis
   Hydrocalycosis
   Hydronephrosis
   Hydroureteronephrosis

   | **Excludes** | *congenital hydronephrosis (753.29)*
      hydroureter (593.5)

Multiple calculi

Figure 10–5 Multiple urinary calculi.

● **592 Calculus of kidney and ureter**

   | **Excludes** | *nephrocalcinosis (275.4)*

   592.0 Calculus of kidney
      Nephrolithiasis NOS
      Renal calculus or stone
      Staghorn calculus
      Stone in kidney

     | **Excludes** | *uric acid nephrolithiasis (274.11)*

   592.1 Calculus of ureter
      Ureteric stone
      Ureterolithiasis

   ❑ **592.9 Urinary calculus, unspecified**

● **593 Other disorders of kidney and ureter**

   593.0 Nephroptosis
      Floating kidney   Mobile kidney

   593.1 Hypertrophy of kidney

   593.2 Cyst of kidney, acquired
      Cyst (multiple) (solitary) of kidney, not congenital
      Peripelvic (lymphatic) cyst

     | **Excludes** | *calyceal or pyelogenic cyst of kidney (591)*
      congenital cyst of kidney (753.1)
      polycystic (disease of) kidney (753.1)

   593.3 Stricture or kinking of ureter
      Angulation of ureter (postoperative)
      Constriction of ureter (postoperative)
      Stricture of pelviureteric junction

   ❑ **593.4 Other ureteric obstruction**
      Idiopathic retroperitoneal fibrosis
      Occlusion NOS of ureter

     | **Excludes** | *that due to calculus (592.1)*

   593.5 Hydroureter

     | **Excludes** | *congenital hydroureter (753.22)*
      hydroureteronephrosis (591)

   593.6 Postural proteinuria
      Benign postural proteinuria
      Orthostatic proteinuria

     | **Excludes** | *proteinuria NOS (791.0)*

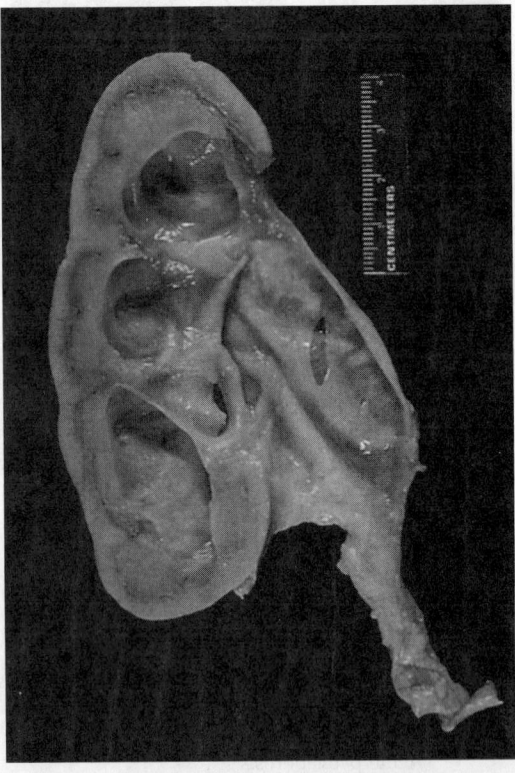

Figure 10–4 Hydronephrosis of the kidney, with marked dilatation of pelvis and calyces and thinning of renal parenchyma. (From Cotran R, Kumar V, Collins T: Robbins Pathologic Basis of Disease, 6/e. Philadelphia, WBS 1999, pg. 989.)

Item 10-6 Vesicoureteral reflux occurs when urine flows from the bladder back into the ureters, often resulting in urinary tract infection.

● **593.7 Vesicoureteral reflux**

    ❑ **593.70 Unspecified or without reflux nephropathy**

    593.71 With reflux nephropathy, unilateral

    593.72 With reflux nephropathy, bilateral

    ❑ **593.73 With reflux nephropathy NOS**

● **593.8 Other specified disorders of kidney and ureter**

    593.81 Vascular disorders of kidney
        Renal (artery):
           embolism
           hemorrhage
           thrombosis
        Renal infarction

    593.82 Ureteral fistula
        Intestinoureteral fistula

    | Excludes | fistula between ureter and female genital tract (619.0) |

    ❑ **593.89 Other**
        Adhesions, kidney or ureter
        Periureteritis
        Polyp of ureter
        Pyelectasia
        Ureterocele

    | Excludes | tuberculosis of ureter (016.2) |
    | | ureteritis cystica (590.3) |

❑ **593.9 Unspecified disorder of kidney and ureter**
    Renal disease (chronic) NOS
    Renal insufficiency (acute) (chronic)
    Salt-losing nephritis or syndrome

    | Excludes | cystic kidney disease (753.1) |
    | | nephropathy, so stated (583.0–583.9) |
    | | renal disease: |
    | | acute (580.0–580.9) |
    | | arising in pregnancy or the puerperium (642.1–642.2, 642.4–642.7, 646.2) |
    | | chronic (582.0–582.9) |
    | | not specified as acute or chronic, but with stated pathology or cause (583.0–583.9) |

● **594 Calculus of lower urinary tract**

    594.0 Calculus in diverticulum of bladder

    ❑ **594.1 Other calculus in bladder**
        Urinary bladder stone

    | Excludes | staghorn calculus (592.0) |

    594.2 Calculus in urethra

    ❑ **594.8 Other lower urinary tract calculus**

    ❑ **594.9 Calculus of lower urinary tract, unspecified**
    | Excludes | calculus of urinary tract NOS (592.9) |

● **595 Cystitis**

    | Excludes | prostatocystitis (601.3) |

    Use additional code to identify organism, such as Escherichia coli [E. coli] (041.4)

    595.0 Acute cystitis

    | Excludes | trigonitis (595.3) |

    595.1 Chronic interstitial cystitis
        Hunner's ulcer
        Panmural fibrosis of bladder
        Submucous cystitis

❑ **595.2 Other chronic cystitis**
    Chronic cystitis NOS
    Subacute cystitis

    | Excludes | trigonitis (595.3) |

    595.3 Trigonitis
        Follicular cystitis
        Trigonitis (acute) (chronic)
        Urethrotrigonitis

● **595.4 *Cystitis in diseases classified elsewhere***
    Code first underlying disease, as:
        actinomycosis (039.8)
        amebiasis (006.8)
        bilharziasis (120.0–120.9)
        Echinococcus infestation (122.3, 122.6)

    | Excludes | cystitis: |
    | | diphtheritic (032.84) |
    | | gonococcal (098.11, 098.31) |
    | | monilial (112.2) |
    | | trichomonal (131.09) |
    | | tuberculous (016.1) |

● **595.8 Other specified types of cystitis**

    595.81 Cystitis cystica

    595.82 Irradiation cystitis
        Use additional E code to identify cause

    ❑ **595.89 Other**
        Abscess of bladder
        Cystitis:
           bullous
           emphysematous
           glandularis

❑ **595.9 Cystitis, unspecified**

Item 10-7 Intestinovesical fistula is a passage between the bladder and the intestine. **Diverticulum of the bladder** is the formation of a sac from a herniation of the wall of the bladder through a deviation. **Atony of the bladder** is diminished tone of the bladder muscle.

● **596 Other disorders of bladder**
    Use additional code to identify urinary incontinence (625.6, 788.30–788.39)

    596.0 Bladder neck obstruction
        Contracture (acquired) of bladder neck or vesicourethral orifice
        Obstruction (acquired) of bladder neck or vesicourethral orifice
        Stenosis (acquired) of bladder neck or vesicourethral orifice

    | Excludes | congenital (753.6) |

    596.1 Intestinovesical fistula

Fistula:	Fistula:
enterovesical	vesicoenteric
vesicocolic	vesicorectal

    596.2 Vesical fistula, not elsewhere classified

Fistula:	Fistula:
bladder NOS	vesicocutaneous
urethrovesical	vesicoperineal

    | Excludes | fistula between bladder and female genital tract (619.0) |

    596.3 Diverticulum of bladder
        Diverticulitis of bladder
        Diverticulum (acquired) (false) of bladder

    | Excludes | that with calculus in diverticulum of bladder (594.0) |

ICD-9-CM

500-599

Vol. 1

◀ **New**   ◀||| **Revised**   ● **Not a Principal Diagnosis**   ● **Use Additional Digit(s)**   ❑ **Nonspecific Code**

596.4 Atony of bladder
High compliance bladder
Hypotonicity of bladder
Inertia of bladder

Excludes *neurogenic bladder (596.54)*

● **596.5 Other functional disorders of bladder**

Excludes *cauda equina syndrome with neurogenic bladder (344.61)*

596.51 Hypertonicity of bladder
Hyperactivity
Overactive bladder

596.52 Low bladder compliance

596.53 Paralysis of bladder

596.54 Neurogenic bladder NOS

596.55 Detrusor sphincter dyssynergia

❑ **596.59 Other functional disorder of bladder**
Detrusor instability

596.6 Rupture of bladder, nontraumatic

596.7 Hemorrhage into bladder wall
Hyperemia of bladder

Excludes *acute hemorrhagic cystitis (595.0)*

❑ **596.8 Other specified disorders of bladder**
Calcified
Contracted
Hemorrhage
Hypertrophy

Excludes *cystocele, female (618.01–618.02, 618.09, 618.2– 618.4)* ◀▥
hernia or prolapse of bladder, female (618.01– 618.02, 618.09, 618.2–618.4) ◀▥

❑ **596.9 Unspecified disorder of bladder**

● **597 Urethritis, not sexually transmitted, and urethral syndrome**

Excludes *nonspecific urethritis, so stated (099.4)*

597.0 Urethral abscess
Abscess of:
bulbourethral gland
Cowper's gland
Littré's gland
Abscess:
periurethral
urethral (gland)
Periurethral cellulitis

Excludes *urethral caruncle (599.3)*

● **597.8 Other urethritis**

❑ **597.80 Urethritis, unspecified**

597.81 Urethral syndrome NOS

❑ **597.89 Other**
Adenitis, Skene's glands
Cowperitis
Meatitis, urethral
Ulcer, urethra (meatus)
Verumontanitis

Excludes *trichomonal (131.02)*

● **598 Urethral stricture**

Includes: pinhole meatus
stricture of urinary meatus

Use additional code to identify urinary incontinence (625.6, 788.30–788.39)

Excludes *congenital stricture of urethra and urinary meatus (753.6)*

● **598.0 Urethral stricture due to infection**

❑ **598.00 Due to unspecified infection**

● **598.01 Due to infective diseases classified elsewhere**

Code first underlying disease, as:
gonococcal infection (098.2)
schistosomiasis (120.0–120.9)
syphilis (095.8)

598.1 Traumatic urethral stricture
Stricture of urethra:
late effect of injury
postobstetric

Excludes *postoperative following surgery on genitourinary tract (598.2)*

598.2 Postoperative urethral stricture
Postcatheterization stricture of urethra

❑ **598.8 Other specified causes of urethral stricture**

❑ **598.9 Urethral stricture, unspecified**

● **599 Other disorders of urethra and urinary tract**

❑ **599.0 Urinary tract infection, site not specified**

Excludes *Candidiasis of urinary tract (112.2)*
urinary tract infection of newborn (771.82)

Use additional code to identify organism, such as Escherichia coli [E. coli] (041.4)

599.1 Urethral fistula
Fistula:
urethroperineal
urethrorectal
Urinary fistula NOS

Excludes *fistula:*
urethroscrotal (608.89)
urethrovaginal (619.0)
urethrovesicovaginal (619.0)

599.2 Urethral diverticulum

599.3 Urethral caruncle
Polyp of urethra

599.4 Urethral false passage

599.5 Prolapsed urethral mucosa
Prolapse of urethra
Urethrocele

Excludes *urethrocele, female (618.03, 618.09, 618.2– 618.4)* ◀▥

❑ **599.6 Urinary obstruction, unspecified**
Obstructive uropathy NOS
Urinary (tract) obstruction NOS

Use additional code to identify urinary incontinence (625.6, 788.30–788.39)

Excludes *obstructive nephropathy NOS (593.89)*

599.7 Hematuria
Hematuria (benign) (essential)

Excludes *hemoglobinuria (791.2)*

● **599.8 Other specified disorders of urethra and urinary tract**

Use additional code to identify urinary incontinence (625.6, 788.30–788.39)

Excludes *symptoms and other conditions classifiable to 788.0–788.2, 788.4–788.9, 791.0–791.9*

599.81 Urethral hypermobility

599.82 Intrinsic (urethral) sphincter deficiency [ISD]

599.83 Urethral instability

❑ **599.84 Other specified disorders of urethra**
Rupture of urethra (nontraumatic)
Urethral:
cyst
granuloma

❑ **599.89 Other specified disorders of urinary tract**

❑ **599.9 Unspecified disorder of urethra and urinary tract**

Figure 10-6 **A.** Male genital system. **B.** Testis.

DISEASES OF MALE GENITAL ORGANS (600–608)

● **600 Hyperplasia of prostate**

Use additional code to identify urinary incontinence (788.30–788.39)

● **600.0 Hypertrophy (benign) of prostate**
Benign prostatic hypertrophy
Enlargement of prostate
Smooth enlarged prostate
Soft enlarged prostate

600.00 Hypertropy (benign) of prostate without urinary obstruction
Hypertrophy (benign) of prostate NOS

600.01 Hypertrophy (benign) of prostate with urinary obstruction
Hypertrophy (benign) of prostate with urinary retention

● **600.1 Nodular prostate**
Hard, firm prostate
Multinodular prostate

Excludes malignant neoplasm of prostate (185)

600.10 Nodular prostate without urinary obstruction
Nodular prostate NOS

600.11 Nodular prostate with urinary obstruction
Nodular prostate with urinary retention

● **600.2 Benign localized hyperplasia of prostate**
Adenofibromatous hypertrophy of prostate
Adenoma of prostate
Fibroadenoma of prostate
Fibroma of prostate
Myoma of prostate
Polyp of prostate

Excludes benign neoplasms of prostate (222.2)
hypertrophy of prostate (600.00–600.01)
malignant neoplasm of prostate (185)

600.20 Benign localized hyperplasia of prostate without urinary obstruction
Benign localized hyperplasia of prostate NOS

600.21 Benign localized hyperplasia of prostate with urinary obstruction
Benign localized hyperplasia of prostate with urinary retention

600.3 Cyst of prostate

● **600.9 Hyperplasia of prostate, unspecified**
Median bar
Prostatic obstruction NOS

❑ **600.90 Hyperplasia of prostate, unspecified, without urinary obstruction**
Hyperplasia of prostate NOS

❑ **600.91 Hyperplasia of prostate, unspecified, with urinary obstruction**
Hyperplasia of prostate, unspecified, with urinary retention

● **601 Inflammatory diseases of prostate**

Use additional code to identify organism, such as Staphylococcus (041.1), or Streptococcus (041.0)

601.0 Acute prostatitis

601.1 Chronic prostatitis

601.2 Abscess of prostate

601.3 Prostatocystitis

● **601.4 Prostatitis in diseases classified elsewhere**

Code first underlying disease, as:
actinomycosis (039.8)
blastomycosis (116.0)
syphilis (095.8)
tuberculosis (016.5)

Excludes prostatitis:
gonococcal (098.12, 098.32)
monilial (112.2)
trichomonal (131.03)

❑ **601.8 Other specified inflammatory diseases of prostate**
Prostatitis:
cavitary   granulomatous
diverticular

❑ **601.9 Prostatitis, unspecified**
Prostatitis NOS

● **602 Other disorders of prostate**

602.0 Calculus of prostate
Prostatic stone

602.1 Congestion or hemorrhage of prostate

602.2 Atrophy of prostate

602.3 Dysplasia of prostate
Prostatic intraepithelial neoplasia I (PIN I)
Prostatic intraepithelial neoplasia II (PIN II)

Excludes Prostatic intraepithelial neoplasia III (PIN III) (233.4)

❑ **602.8 Other specified disorders of prostate**
Fistula of prostate
Infarction of prostate
Stricture of prostate
Periprostatic adhesions

❑ **602.9 Unspecified disorder of prostate**

ICD-9-CM

600-699

Vol. 1

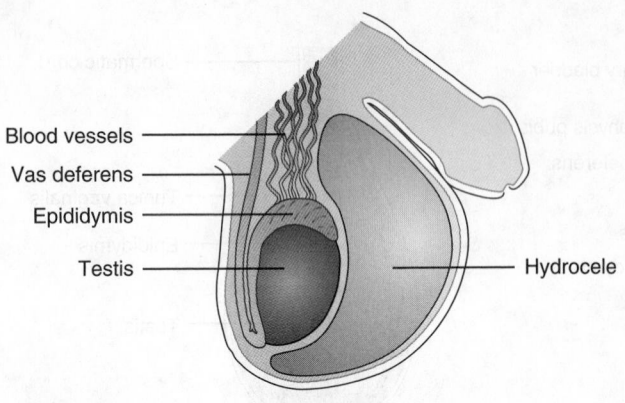

Figure 10-7   Hydrocele.

Item 10-8 Hydrocele is a sac of fluid in the testes membrane.

● **603 Hydrocele**

> **Includes:** hydrocele of spermatic cord, testis, or tunica vaginalis
>
> Excludes   *congenital (778.6)*

    603.0 Encysted hydrocele

    603.1 Infected hydrocele

> Use additional code to identify organism

    ❑**603.8 Other specified types of hydrocele**

    ❑**603.9 Hydrocele, unspecified**

● **604 Orchitis and epididymitis**

> Use additional code to identify organism, such as Escherichia coli [E. coli] (041.4), Staphylococcus (041.1), or Streptococcus (041.0)

    604.0 Orchitis, epididymitis, and epididymo-orchitis, with abscess

> Abscess of epididymis or testis

●   **604.9 Other orchitis, epididymitis, and epididymo-orchitis, without mention of abscess**

      ❑**604.90 Orchitis and epididymitis, unspecified**

●   **604.91 *Orchitis and epididymitis in diseases classified elsewhere***

> *Code first underlying disease, as:*
> diphtheria (032.89)
> filariasis (125.0–125.9)
> syphilis (095.8)
>
> Excludes   *orchitis:*
> *gonococcal (098.13, 098.33)*
> *mumps (072.0)*
> *tuberculous (016.5)*
> *tuberculous epididymitis (016.4)*

      ❑**604.99 Other**

605 Redundant prepuce and phimosis
> Adherent prepuce
> Paraphimosis
> Phimosis (congenital)
> Tight foreskin

● **606 Infertility, male**

    606.0 Azoospermia
> Absolute infertility
> Infertility due to:
> germinal (cell) aplasia
> spermatogenic arrest (complete)

    606.1 Oligospermia
> Infertility due to:
> germinal cell desquamation
> hypospermatogenesis
> incomplete spermatogenic arrest

    606.8 Infertility due to extratesticular causes
> Infertility due to:
> drug therapy
> infection
> obstruction of efferent ducts
> radiation
> systemic disease

    ❑**606.9 Male infertility, unspecified**

● **607 Disorders of penis**
> Excludes   *phimosis (605)*

    607.0 Leukoplakia of penis
> Kraurosis of penis
>
> Excludes   *carcinoma in situ of penis (233.5)*
> *erythroplasia of Queyrat (233.5)*

    607.1 Balanoposthitis
> Balanitis
>
> Use additional code to identify organism

    ❑**607.2 Other inflammatory disorders of penis**
> Abscess of corpus cavernosum or penis
> Boil of corpus cavernosum or penis
> Carbuncle of corpus cavernosum or penis
> Cellulitis of corpus cavernosum or penis
> Cavernitis (penis)
>
> Use additional code to identify organism
>
> Excludes   *herpetic infection (054.13)*

    607.3 Priapism
> Painful erection

● **607.8 Other specified disorders of penis**

    607.81 Balanitis xerotica obliterans
> Induratio penis plastica

    607.82 Vascular disorders of penis
> Embolism of corpus cavernosum or penis
> Hematoma (nontraumatic) of corpus cavernosum or penis
> Hemorrhage of corpus cavernosum or penis
> Thrombosis of corpus cavernosum or penis

    607.83 Edema of penis

    607.84 Impotence of organic origin
> Excludes   *nonorganic or unspecified (302.72)*

    607.85 Peyronie's disease

    ❑**607.89 Other**
> Atrophy of corpus cavernosum or penis
> Fibrosis of corpus cavernosum or penis
> Hypertrophy of corpus cavernosum or penis
> Ulcer (chronic) of corpus cavernosum or penis

❑**607.9 Unspecified disorder of penis**

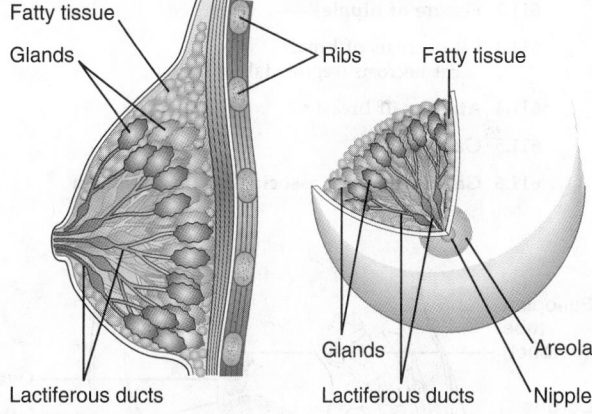

Figure 10-8 Torsion of testis.

Item 10-9 **Rotation of the spermatic cord causes strangulation and infarction of the testis.**

● **608 Other disorders of male genital organs**

608.0 Seminal vesiculitis
Abscess of seminal vesicle
Cellulitis of seminal vesicle
Vesiculitis (seminal)

Use additional code to identify organism

| Excludes | gonococcal infection (098.14, 098.34) |

608.1 Spermatocele

608.2 Torsion of testis
Torsion of:
epididymis
spermatic cord
testicle

608.3 Atrophy of testis

❑ **608.4 Other inflammatory disorders of male organs**
Abscess of scrotum, spermatic cord, testis [except abscess], tunica vaginalis, or vas deferens
Boil of scrotum, spermatic cord, testis [except abscess], tunica vaginalis, or vas deferens
Carbuncle of scrotum, spermatic cord, testis [except abscess], tunica vaginalis, or vas deferens
Cellulitis of scrotum, spermatic cord, testis [except abscess], tunica vaginalis, or vas deferens
Vasitis

Use additional code to identify organism

| Excludes | abscess of testis (604.0) |

● **608.8 Other specified disorders of male genital organs**

● *608.81 Disorders of male genital organs in diseases classified elsewhere*

Code first underlying disease, as:
filariasis (125.0–125.9)
tuberculosis (016.5)

608.82 Hematospermia

608.83 Vascular disorders
Hematoma (nontraumatic) of seminal vesicle, spermatic cord, testis, scrotum, tunica vaginalis, or vas deferens
Hemorrhage of seminal vesicle, spermatic cord, testis, scrotum, tunica vaginalis, or vas deferens
Thrombosis of seminal vesicle, spermatic cord, testis, scrotum, tunica vaginalis, or vas deferens
Hematocele NOS, male

608.84 Chylocele of tunica vaginalis

608.85 Stricture
Stricture of:
spermatic cord
tunica vaginalis
vas deferens

608.86 Edema

608.87 Retrograde ejaculation

❑ **608.89 Other**
Atrophy of seminal vesicle, spermatic cord, testis, scrotum, tunica vaginalis, or vas deferens
Fibrosis of seminal vesicle, spermatic cord, testis, scrotum, tunica vaginalis, or vas deferens
Hypertrophy of seminal vesicle, spermatic cord, testis, scrotum, tunica vaginalis, or vas deferens
Ulcer of seminal vesicle, spermatic cord, testis, scrotum, tunica vaginalis, or vas deferens

| Excludes | atrophy of testis (608.3) |

❑ **608.9 Unspecified disorder of male genital organs**

Fatty tissue
Glands
Ribs
Fatty tissue
Glands
Areola
Lactiferous ducts
Lactiferous ducts
Nipple

ICD-9-CM
608-699
Vol. 1

Figure 10-9 Breast.

DISORDERS OF BREAST (610–611)

● **610 Benign mammary dysplasias**

610.0 Solitary cyst of breast
Cyst (solitary) of breast

610.1 Diffuse cystic mastopathy
Chronic cystic mastitis
Cystic breast
Fibrocystic disease of breast

610.2 Fibroadenosis of breast

Fibroadenosis of breast:	Fibroadenosis of breast:
NOS	diffuse
chronic	periodic
cystic	segmental

610.3 Fibrosclerosis of breast

610.4 Mammary duct ectasia
Comedomastitis
Duct ectasia
Mastitis:
periductal
plasma cell

☐ **610.8 Other specified benign mammary dysplasias**
Mazoplasia
Sebaceous cyst of breast

☐ **610.9 Benign mammary dysplasia, unspecified**

● **611 Other disorders of breast**

> **Excludes** *that associated with lactation or the puerperium (675.0–676.9)*

611.0 Inflammatory disease of breast
Abscess (acute) (chronic) (nonpuerperal) of:
areola
breast
Mammillary fistula
Mastitis (acute) (subacute) (nonpuerperal):
NOS   retromammary
infective   submammary

> **Excludes** *carbuncle of breast (680.2)*
> *chronic cystic mastitis (610.1)*
> *neonatal infective mastitis (771.5)*
> *thrombophlebitis of breast [Mondor's disease] (451.89)*

611.1 Hypertrophy of breast
Gynecomastia
Hypertrophy of breast:
NOS
massive pubertal

611.2 Fissure of nipple

611.3 Fat necrosis of breast
Fat necrosis (segmental) of breast

611.4 Atrophy of breast

611.5 Galactocele

611.6 Galactorrhea not associated with childbirth

● **611.7 Signs and symptoms in breast**

611.71 Mastodynia
Pain in breast

611.72 Lump or mass in breast

☐ **611.79 Other**
Induration of breast
Inversion of nipple
Nipple discharge
Retraction of nipple

☐ **611.8 Other specified disorders of breast**
Hematoma (nontraumatic) of breast
Infarction of breast
Occlusion of breast duct
Subinvolution of breast (postlactational) (postpartum)

☐ **611.9 Unspecified breast disorder**

INFLAMMATORY DISEASE OF FEMALE PELVIC ORGANS (614–616)

Use additional code to identify organism, such as Staphylococcus (041.1), or Streptococcus (041.0)

> **Excludes** *that associated with pregnancy, abortion, childbirth, or the puerperium (630–676.9)*

● **614 Inflammatory disease of ovary, fallopian tube, pelvic cellular tissue, and peritoneum**

> **Excludes** *endometritis (615.0–615.9)*
> *major infection following delivery (670)*
> *that complicating:*
> *abortion (634–638 with .0, 639.0)*
> *ectopic or molar pregnancy (639.0)*
> *pregnancy or labor (646.6)*

614.0 Acute salpingitis and oophoritis
Any condition classifiable to 614.2, specified as acute or subacute

614.1 Chronic salpingitis and oophoritis
Hydrosalpinx
Salpingitis:
follicularis
isthmica nodosa
Any condition classifiable to 614.2, specified as chronic

A

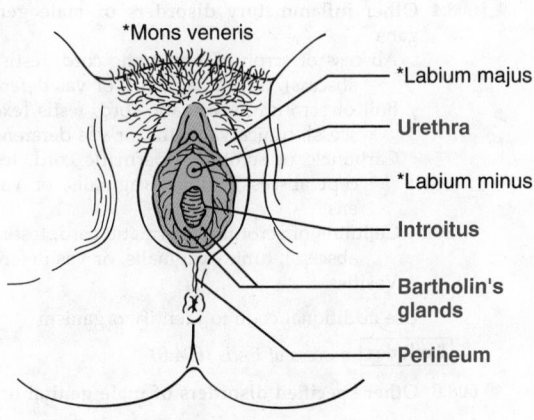

B   *The three parts of the vulva

Figure 10–10 A. Female genital system. **B.** External female genital system. (From Buck CJ: Step-by-Step Medical Coding, 2005 ed. Philadelphia, WBS, 2005.)

❑614.2 **Salpingitis and oophoritis not specified as acute, subacute, or chronic**

    Abscess (of):
        fallopian tube
        ovary
        tubo-ovarian
    Oophoritis
    Tubo-ovarian inflammatory disease

    Perioophoritis
    Perisalpingitis
    Pyosalpinx
    Salpingitis
    Salpingo-oophoritis

Excludes	*gonococcal infection (chronic) (098.37)*
	acute (098.17)
	tuberculous (016.6)

614.3 **Acute parametritis and pelvic cellulitis**

    Acute inflammatory pelvic disease
    Any condition classifiable to 614.4, specified as acute

614.4 **Chronic or unspecified parametritis and pelvic cellulitis**

    Abscess (of):
        broad ligament chronic or NOS
        parametrium chronic or NOS
        pelvis, female chronic or NOS
        pouch of Douglas chronic or NOS
    Chronic inflammatory pelvic disease
    Pelvic cellulitis, female

Excludes	*tuberculous (016.7)*

614.5 **Acute or unspecified pelvic peritonitis, female**

614.6 **Pelvic peritoneal adhesions, female (postoperative) (postinfection)**

    Adhesions:
        peritubal
        tubo-ovarian

    Use additional code to identify any associated infertility (628.2)

❑614.7 **Other chronic pelvic peritonitis, female**

Excludes	*tuberculous (016.7)*

❑614.8 **Other specified inflammatory disease of female pelvic organs and tissues**

❑614.9 **Unspecified inflammatory disease of female pelvic organs and tissues**

    Pelvic infection or inflammation, female NOS
    Pelvic inflammatory disease [PID]

●615 **Inflammatory diseases of uterus, except cervix**

Excludes	*following delivery (670)*
	hyperplastic endometritis (621.30–621.33) ◀▥
	that complicating:
	abortion (634–638 with .0, 639.0)
	ectopic or molar pregnancy (639.0)
	pregnancy or labor (646.6)

615.0 **Acute**

    Any condition classifiable to 615.9, specified as acute or subacute

615.1 **Chronic**

    Any condition classifiable to 615.9, specified as chronic

❑615.9 **Unspecified inflammatory disease of uterus**

    Endometritis
    Endomyometritis
    Metritis
    Myometritis

    Perimetritis
    Pyometra
    Uterine abscess

●616 **Inflammatory disease of cervix, vagina, and vulva**

Excludes	*that complicating:*
	abortion (634–638 with .0, 639.0)
	ectopic or molar pregnancy (639.0)
	pregnancy, childbirth, or the puerperium (646.6)

616.0 **Cervicitis and endocervicitis**

    Cervicitis with or without mention of erosion or ectropion
    Endocervicitis with or without mention of erosion or ectropion
    Nabothian (gland) cyst or follicle

Excludes	*erosion or ectropion without mention of cervicitis (622.0)*

●616.1 **Vaginitis and vulvovaginitis**

❑616.10 **Vaginitis and vulvovaginitis, unspecified**

    Vaginitis:
        NOS
        postirradiation
    Vulvitis NOS
    Vulvovaginitis NOS

    Use additional code to identify organism, such as Escherichia coli [E. coli] (041.4), Staphylococcus (041.1), or Streptococcus (041.0)

Excludes	*noninfective leukorrhea (623.5)*
	postmenopausal or senile vaginitis (627.3)

●616.11 *Vaginitis and vulvovaginitis in diseases classified elsewhere*

    Code first underlying disease, as:
        pinworm vaginitis (127.4)

Excludes	*herpetic vulvovaginitis (054.11)*
	monilial vulvovaginitis (112.1)
	trichomonal vaginitis or vulvovaginitis (131.01)

616.2 **Cyst of Bartholin's gland**

    Bartholin's duct cyst

616.3 **Abscess of Bartholin's gland**

    Vulvovaginal gland abscess

❑616.4 **Other abscess of vulva**

    Abscess of vulva   Furuncle of vulva
    Carbuncle of vulva

●616.5 **Ulceration of vulva**

❑616.50 **Ulceration of vulva, unspecified**

    Ulcer NOS of vulva

●616.51 *Ulceration of vulva in diseases classified elsewhere*

    Code first underlying disease, as:
        Behçet's syndrome (136.1)
        tuberculosis (016.7)

Excludes	*vulvar ulcer (in):*
	gonococcal (098.0)
	herpes simplex (054.12)
	syphilitic (091.0)

❑616.8 **Other specified inflammatory diseases of cervix, vagina, and vulva**

    Caruncle, vagina or labium
    Ulcer, vagina

Excludes	*noninflammatory disorders of:*
	cervix (622.0–622.9)
	vagina (623.0–623.9)
	vulva (624.0–624.9)

❑616.9 **Unspecified inflammatory disease of cervix, vagina, and vulva**

ICD-9-CM

600-600

Vol.

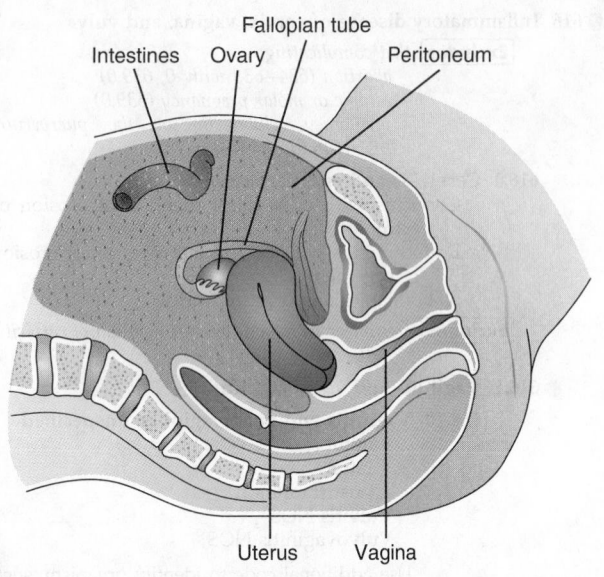

Fallopian tube
Intestines   Ovary   Peritoneum

Uterus   Vagina

Figure 10–11 Sites of potential endometrial implants.

Item 10-10 Endometriosis is a condition for which no clear cause has been identified. Endometrial tissue is expelled from the uterus into the body and can implant onto a variety of organs. Classification is based on the site of implant of the endometrial tissue.

OTHER DISORDERS OF FEMALE GENITAL TRACT (617–629)

● 617 **Endometriosis**

  617.0 **Endometriosis of uterus**
      Adenomyosis
      Endometriosis: Endometriosis:
        cervix   myometrium
        internal

      Excludes *stromal endometriosis (236.0)*

  617.1 **Endometriosis of ovary**
      Chocolate cyst of ovary
      Endometrial cystoma of ovary

  617.2 **Endometriosis of fallopian tube**

  617.3 **Endometriosis of pelvic peritoneum**
      Endometriosis:
        broad ligament   parametrium
        cul-de-sac (Douglas')   round ligament

  617.4 **Endometriosis of rectovaginal septum and vagina**
  617.5 **Endometriosis of intestine**
      Endometriosis:
        appendix
        colon
        rectum

  617.6 **Endometriosis in scar of skin**
☐ 617.8 **Endometriosis of other specified sites**
      Endometriosis:
        bladder
        lung
        umbilicus
        vulva

☐ 617.9 **Endometriosis, site unspecified**

● 618 **Genital prolapse**

  Use additional code to identify urinary incontinence (625.6, 788.31, 788.33–788.39)
      Excludes *that complicating pregnancy, labor, or delivery (654.4)*

● 618.0 **Prolapse of vaginal walls without mention of uterine prolapse**
      Excludes *that with uterine prolapse (618.2–618.4)*
                enterocele (618.6)
                vaginal vault prolapse following hysterectomy (618.5)

  ☐ 618.00 **Unspecified prolapse of vaginal walls** ◄
        Vaginal prolapse NOS ◄
    618.01 **Cystocele, midline** ◄
        Cystocele NOS ◄
    618.02 **Cystocele, lateral** ◄
        Paravaginal ◄
    618.03 **Urethrocele** ◄
    618.04 **Rectocele** ◄
        Proctocele ◄
    618.05 **Perineocele** ◄
  ☐ 618.09 **Other prolapse of vaginal walls without mention of uterine prolapse** ◄
        Cystourethrocele ◄

  618.1 **Uterine prolapse without mention of vaginal wall prolapse**
      Descensus uteri
      Uterine prolapse:
        NOS
        complete
        first degree
        second degree
        third degree
      Excludes *that with mention of cystocele, urethrocele, or rectocele (618.2–618.4)*

  618.2 **Uterovaginal prolapse, incomplete**
  618.3 **Uterovaginal prolapse, complete**

A

B

C

Figure 10–12 Three stages of uterine prolapse. **A.** Uterus is prolapsed. **B.** Vagina and uterus are prolapsed (incomplete uterovaginal prolapse). **C.** Vagina and uterus are completely prolapsed and are exposed through the external genitalia (complete uterovaginal prolapse).

❏ **618.4 Uterovaginal prolapse, unspecified**

618.5 Prolapse of vaginal vault after hysterectomy

618.6 Vaginal enterocele, congenital or acquired
    Pelvic enterocele, congenital or acquired

618.7 Old laceration of muscles of pelvic floor

● **618.8 Other specified genital prolapse**

    618.81 Incompetence or weakening of pubocervical tissue ◀

    618.82 Incompetence or weakening of rectovaginal tissue ◀

    618.83 Pelvic muscle wasting ◀
        Disuse atrophy of pelvic muscles and anal sphincter ◀

    ❏ **618.89 Other specified genital prolapse** ◀

❏ **618.9 Unspecified genital prolapse**

● **619 Fistula involving female genital tract**

    Excludes *vesicorectal and intestinovesical fistula (596.1)*

619.0 Urinary-genital tract fistula, female
    Fistula:
      cervicovesical   uteroureteric
      ureterovaginal   uterovesical
      urethrovaginal   vesicocervicovaginal
      urethrovesicovaginal   vesicovaginal

619.1 Digestive-genital tract fistula, female
    Fistula: Fistula:
      intestinouterine   rectovulval
      intestinovaginal   sigmoidovaginal
      rectovaginal   uterorectal

619.2 Genital tract-skin fistula, female
    Fistula:
      uterus to abdominal wall
      vaginoperineal

❏ **619.8 Other specified fistulas involving female genital tract**
    Fistula:
      cervix   uterus
      cul-de-sac (Douglas')   vagina

❏ **619.9 Unspecified fistula involving female genital tract**

● **620 Noninflammatory disorders of ovary, fallopian tube, and broad ligament**

    Excludes *hydrosalpinx (614.1)*

620.0 Follicular cyst of ovary
    Cyst of graafian follicle

620.1 Corpus luteum cyst or hematoma
    Corpus luteum hemorrhage or rupture
    Lutein cyst

❏ **620.2 Other and unspecified ovarian cyst**
    Cyst of ovary: Cyst of ovary:
      NOS   serous
      corpus albicans   theca-lutein
      retention NOS
    Simple cystoma of ovary

    Excludes *cystadenoma (benign) (serous) (220)*
      developmental cysts (752.0)
      neoplastic cysts (220)
      polycystic ovaries (256.4)
      Stein-Leventhal syndrome (256.4)

620.3 Acquired atrophy of ovary and fallopian tube
    Senile involution of ovary

620.4 Prolapse or hernia of ovary and fallopian tube
    Displacement of ovary and fallopian tube
    Salpingocele

620.5 Torsion of ovary, ovarian pedicle, or fallopian tube
    Torsion:
      accessory tube
      hydatid of Morgagni

620.6 Broad ligament laceration syndrome
    Masters-Allen syndrome

620.7 Hematoma of broad ligament
    Hematocele, broad ligament

❏ **620.8 Other noninflammatory disorders of ovary, fallopian tube, and broad ligament**
    Cyst of broad ligament or fallopian tube
    Polyp of broad ligament or fallopian tube
    Infarction of ovary or fallopian tube
    Rupture of ovary or fallopian tube
    Hematosalpinx of ovary or fallopian tube

    Excludes *hematosalpinx in ectopic pregnancy (639.2)*
      peritubal adhesions (614.6)
      torsion of ovary, ovarian pedicle, or fallopian tube (620.5)

❏ **620.9 Unspecified noninflammatory disorder of ovary, fallopian tube, and broad ligament**

● **621 Disorders of uterus, not elsewhere classified**

621.0 Polyp of corpus uteri
    Polyp:
      endometrium
      uterus NOS

    Excludes *cervical polyp NOS (622.7)*

621.1 Chronic subinvolution of uterus
    Excludes *puerperal (674.8)*

621.2 Hypertrophy of uterus
    Bulky or enlarged uterus
    Excludes *puerperal (674.8)*

● **621.3 Endometrial hyperplasia** ◀▥
    Hyperplasia (adenomatous) (cystic) (glandular) of endometrium
    Hyperplastic endometritis

    ❏ **621.30 Endometrial hyperplasia, unspecified** ◀
      Endometrial hyperplasia NOS ◀

    621.31 Simple endometrial hyperplasia without atypia ◀

    621.32 Complex endometrial hyperplasia without atypia ◀

    621.33 Endometrial hyperplasia with atypia ◀

621.4 Hematometra
    Hemometra
    Excludes *that in congenital anomaly (752.2–752.3)*

621.5 Intrauterine synechiae
    Adhesions of uterus   Band(s) of uterus

621.6 Malposition of uterus
    Anteversion of uterus   Retroversion of uterus
    Retroflexion of uterus

    Excludes *malposition complicating pregnancy, labor, or delivery (654.3–654.4)*
      prolapse of uterus (618.1–618.4)

621.7 Chronic inversion of uterus
    Excludes *current obstetrical trauma (665.2)*
      prolapse of uterus (618.1–618.4)

❏ **621.8 Other specified disorders of uterus, not elsewhere classified**
    Atrophy, acquired of uterus
    Cyst of uterus
    Fibrosis NOS of uterus
    Old laceration (postpartum) of uterus
    Ulcer of uterus

    Excludes *bilharzial fibrosis (120.0–120.9)*
      endometriosis (617.0)
      fistulas (619.0–619.8)
      inflammatory diseases (615.0–615.9)

❏ **621.9 Unspecified disorder of uterus**

● **622 Noninflammatory disorders of cervix**

    Excludes *abnormality of cervix complicating pregnancy, labor, or delivery (654.5–654.6)*
      fistula (619.0–619.8)

622.0 Erosion and ectropion of cervix
    Eversion of cervix
    Ulcer of cervix
    Excludes *that in chronic cervicitis (616.0)*

ICD-9-CM

600-699

Vol. 1

622.1 Dysplasia of cervix (uteri)

Excludes	*abnormal results from cervical cytologic examination* ◄

carcinoma in situ of cervix (233.1)
cervical intraepithelial neoplasia III [CIN III] (233.1)
without histologic confirmation (795.00–795.09) ◄

☐ **622.10 Dysplasia of cervix, unspecified** ◄
Anaplasia of cervix ◄
Cervical atypism ◄
Cervical dysplasia NOS ◄

622.11 Mild dysplasia of cervix ◄
Cervical intraepithelial neoplasia I [CIN I] ◄

622.12 Moderate dysplasia of cervix ◄
Cervical intraepithelial neoplasia II [CIN II] ◄

Excludes	*carcinoma in situ of cervix (233.1)* ◄

cervical intraepithelial neoplasia III [CIN III] (233.1)
severe dysplasia (233.1) ◄

622.2 Leukoplakia of cervix (uteri)

Excludes	*carcinoma in situ of cervix (233.1)*

622.3 Old laceration of cervix
Adhesions of cervix
Band(s) of cervix
Cicatrix (postpartum) of cervix

Excludes	*current obstetrical trauma (665.3)*

622.4 Stricture and stenosis of cervix
Atresia (acquired) of cervix   Occlusion of cervix
Contracture of cervix   Pinpoint os uteri

Excludes	*congenital (752.49)*

that complicating labor (654.6)

622.5 Incompetence of cervix

Excludes	*complicating pregnancy (654.5)*

that affecting fetus or newborn (761.0)

622.6 Hypertrophic elongation of cervix

622.7 Mucous polyp of cervix
Polyp NOS of cervix

Excludes	*adenomatous polyp of cervix (219.0)*

☐ **622.8 Other specified noninflammatory disorders of cervix**
Atrophy (senile) of cervix   Fibrosis of cervix
Cyst of cervix   Hemorrhage of cervix

Excludes	*endometriosis (617.0)*

fistula (619.0–619.8)
inflammatory diseases (616.0)

☐ **622.9 Unspecified noninflammatory disorder of cervix**

● **623 Noninflammatory disorders of vagina**

Excludes	*abnormality of vagina complicating pregnancy, labor, or delivery (654.7)*

congenital absence of vagina (752.49)
congenital diaphragm or bands (752.49)
fistulas involving vagina (619.0–619.8)

623.0 Dysplasia of vagina

Excludes	*carcinoma in situ of vagina (233.3)*

623.1 Leukoplakia of vagina

623.2 Stricture or atresia of vagina
Adhesions (postoperative) (postradiation) of vagina
Occlusion of vagina
Stenosis, vagina

Use additional E code to identify any external cause

Excludes	*congenital atresia or stricture (752.49)*

623.3 Tight hymenal ring
Rigid hymen acquired or congenital
Tight hymenal ring acquired or congenital
Tight introitus acquired or congenital

Excludes	*imperforate hymen (752.42)*

623.4 Old vaginal laceration

Excludes	*old laceration involving muscles of pelvic floor (618.7)*

623.5 Leukorrhea, not specified as infective
Leukorrhea NOS of vagina
Vaginal discharge NOS

Excludes	*trichomonal (131.00)*

623.6 Vaginal hematoma

Excludes	*current obstetrical trauma (665.7)*

623.7 Polyp of vagina

☐ **623.8 Other specified noninflammatory disorders of vagina**
Cyst of vagina
Hemorrhage of vagina

☐ **623.9 Unspecified noninflammatory disorder of vagina**

● **624 Noninflammatory disorders of vulva and perineum**

Excludes	*abnormality of vulva and perineum complicating pregnancy, labor, or delivery (654.8)*

condyloma acuminatum (078.1)
fistulas involving:
perineum-see Alphabetic Index
vulva (619.0–619.8)
vulval varices (456.6)
vulvar involvement in skin conditions (690–709.9)

624.0 Dystrophy of vulva
Kraurosis of vulva
Leukoplakia of vulva

Excludes	*carcinoma in situ of vulva (233.3)*

624.1 Atrophy of vulva

624.2 Hypertrophy of clitoris

Excludes	*that in endocrine disorders (255.2, 256.1)*

624.3 Hypertrophy of labia
Hypertrophy of vulva NOS

624.4 Old laceration or scarring of vulva

624.5 Hematoma of vulva

Excludes	*that complicating delivery (664.5)*

624.6 Polyp of labia and vulva

☐ **624.8 Other specified noninflammatory disorders of vulva and perineum**
Cyst of vulva
Edema of vulva
Stricture of vulva

☐ **624.9 Unspecified noninflammatory disorder of vulva and perineum**

● **625 Pain and other symptoms associated with female genital organs**

625.0 Dyspareunia

Excludes	*psychogenic dyspareunia (302.76)*

625.1 Vaginismus
Colpospasm
Vulvismus

Excludes	*psychogenic vaginismus (306.51)*

625.2 Mittelschmerz
Intermenstrual pain
Ovulation pain

625.3 Dysmenorrhea
Painful menstruation

Excludes	*psychogenic dysmenorrhea (306.52)*

625.4 Premenstrual tension syndrome
Menstrual:
migraine
molimen
Premenstrual dysphoric disorder
Premenstrual syndrome
Premenstrual tension NOS

625.5 **Pelvic congestion syndrome**
    Congestion-fibrosis syndrome
    Taylor's syndrome

625.6 **Stress incontinence, female**
    Excludes *mixed incontinence (788.33)*
          stress incontinence, male (788.32)

❑ 625.8 **Other specified symptoms associated with female genital organs**

❑ 625.9 **Unspecified symptoms associated with female genital organs**

● 626 **Disorders of menstruation and other abnormal bleeding from female genital tract**
    Excludes *menopausal and premenopausal bleeding (627.0)*
          pain and other symptoms associated with menstrual cycle (625.2–625.4)
          postmenopausal bleeding (627.1)

626.0 **Absence of menstruation**
    Amenorrhea (primary) (secondary)

626.1 **Scanty or infrequent menstruation**
    Hypomenorrhea   Oligomenorrhea

626.2 **Excessive or frequent menstruation**
    Heavy periods   Menorrhagia
    Menometrorrhagia   Polymenorrhea
    Excludes *premenopausal (627.0)*
          that in puberty (626.3)

626.3 **Puberty bleeding**
    Excessive bleeding associated with onset of menstrual periods
    Pubertal menorrhagia

626.4 **Irregular menstrual cycle**
    Irregular:
        bleeding NOS   periods
        menstruation

626.5 **Ovulation bleeding**
    Regular intermenstrual bleeding

626.6 **Metrorrhagia**
    Bleeding unrelated to menstrual cycle
    Irregular intermenstrual bleeding

626.7 **Postcoital bleeding**

❑ 626.8 **Other**
    Dysfunctional or functional uterine hemorrhage NOS
    Menstruation:
        retained   suppression of

❑ 626.9 **Unspecified**

● 627 **Menopausal and postmenopausal disorders**
    Excludes *asymptomatic age-related (natural) postmenopausal status (V49.81)*

627.0 **Premenopausal menorrhagia**
    Excessive bleeding associated with onset of menopause
    Menorrhagia:
        climacteric   preclimacteric
        menopausal

627.1 **Postmenopausal bleeding**

627.2 **Symptomatic or female climacteric states**
    Symptoms, such as flushing, sleeplessness, headache, lack of concentration, associated with the menopause

627.3 **Postmenopausal atrophic vaginitis**
    Senile (atrophic) vaginitis

627.4 **Symptomatic states associated with artificial menopause**
    Postartificial menopause syndromes
    Any condition classifiable to 627.1, 627.2, or 627.3 which follows induced menopause

❑ 627.8 **Other specified menopausal and postmenopausal disorders**
    Excludes *premature menopause NOS (256.31)*

❑ 627.9 **Unspecified menopausal and postmenopausal disorder**

● 628 **Infertility, female**
    Includes: primary and secondary sterility

628.0 **Associated with anovulation**
    Anovulatory cycle
    Use additional code for any associated Stein-Leventhal syndrome (256.4)

● 628.1 *Of pituitary-hypothalamic origin*
    Code first underlying disease, as:
        adiposogenital dystrophy (253.8)
        anterior pituitary disorder (253.0–253.4)

628.2 **Of tubal origin**
    Infertility associated with congenital anomaly of tube
    Tubal:
        block   stenosis
        occlusion
    Use additional code for any associated peritubal adhesions (614.6)

628.3 **Of uterine origin**
    Infertility associated with congenital anomaly of uterus
    Nonimplantation
    Use additional code for any associated tuberculous endometritis (016.7)

628.4 **Of cervical or vaginal origin**
    Infertility associated with:
        anomaly or cervical mucus
        congenital structural anomaly
        dysmucorrhea

❑ 628.8 **Of other specified origin**

❑ 628.9 **Of unspecified origin**

● 629 **Other disorders of female genital organs**

629.0 **Hematocele, female, not elsewhere classified**
    Excludes *hematocele or hematoma:*
        broad ligament (620.7)
        fallopian tube (620.8)
        that associated with ectopic pregnancy (633.00–633.91)
        uterus (621.4)
        vagina (623.6)
        vulva (624.5)

629.1 **Hydrocele, canal of Nuck**
    Cyst of canal of Nuck (acquired)
    Excludes *congenital (752.41)*

● 629.2 **Female genital multilation status** ◄
    Female circumcision status ◄

❑ 629.20 **Female genital mutilation status, unspecified** ◄
    Female genital mutilation status NOS ◄

629.21 **Female genital mutilation Type I status** ◄
    Clitorectomy status ◄

629.22 **Female genital mutilation Type II status** ◄
    Clitorectomy with excision of labia minora status ◄

629.23 **Female genital mutilation Type III status** ◄
    Infibulation status ◄

❑ 629.8 **Other specified disorders of female genital organs**

❑ 629.9 **Unspecified disorder of female genital organs**
    Habitual aborter without current pregnancy

ICD-9-CM
600–609
Vol. 1

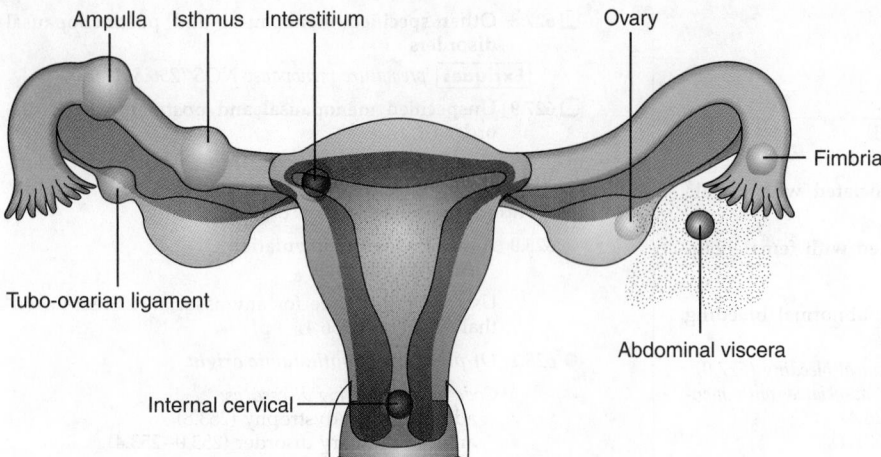

Ampulla   Isthmus   Interstitium   Ovary

Fimbria

Tubo-ovarian ligament

Abdominal viscera

Internal cervical

Figure 11–1 Implantation sites of ectopic pregnancy.

Item 11–1 A hydatidiform mole is a benign tumor of the placenta. The tumor secretes a hormone, chorionic gonadotropic hormone (CGH), that indicates a positive pregnancy test.

Item 11–2 Ectopic pregnancy most often occurs in the fallopian tube. Pregnancy outside the uterus may end in a life-threatening rupture.

11. COMPLICATIONS OF PREGNANCY, CHILDBIRTH, AND THE PUERPERIUM (630–677)

ECTOPIC AND MOLAR PREGNANCY (630–633)

Use additional code from category 639 to identify any complications

630 Hydatidiform mole
    Trophoblastic disease NOS
    Vesicular mole

    Excludes   *chorioadenoma (destruens) (236.1)*
                  chorioepithelioma (181)
                  malignant hydatidiform mole (236.1)

☐ **631 Other abnormal product of conception**
    Blighted ovum
    Mole: Mole:
      NOS   fleshy
      carneous   stone

632 Missed abortion
    Early fetal death before completion of 22 weeks' gestation with retention of dead fetus
    Retained products of conception, not following spontaneous or induced abortion or delivery

    Excludes   *failed induced abortion (638.0–638.9)*
                  fetal death (intrauterine) (late) (656.4)
                  missed delivery (656.4)
                  that with abnormal product of conception (630, 631)

● **633 Ectopic pregnancy**

    Includes: ruptured ectopic pregnancy

  ● **633.0 Abdominal pregnancy**
      Intraperitoneal pregnancy

      633.00 Abdominal pregnancy without intrauterine pregnancy

      633.01 Abdominal pregnancy with intrauterine pregnancy

● **633.1 Tubal pregnancy**
    Fallopian pregnancy
    Rupture of (fallopian) tube due to pregnancy
    Tubal abortion

    633.10 Tubal pregnancy without intrauterine pregnancy

    633.11 Tubal pregnancy with intrauterine pregnancy

● **633.2 Ovarian pregnancy**

    633.20 Ovarian pregnancy without intrauterine pregnancy

    633.21 Ovarian pregnancy with intrauterine pregnancy

● ☐ **633.8 Other ectopic pregnancy**
    Pregnancy: Pregnancy:
      cervical   intraligamentous
      combined   mesometric
      cornual   mural

    633.80 Other ectopic pregnancy without intrauterine pregnancy

    633.81 Other ectopic pregnancy with intrauterine pregnancy

● ☐ **633.9 Unspecified ectopic pregnancy**

    633.90 Unspecified ectopic pregnancy without intrauterine pregnancy

    633.91 Unspecified ectopic pregnancy with intrauterine pregnancy

OTHER PREGNANCY WITH ABORTIVE OUTCOME (634–639)

The following fourth digit subdivisions are for use with categories 634–638:

.0 Complicated by genital tract and pelvic infection
    Endometritis   Sepsis NOS
    Salpingo-oophoritis   Septicemia NOS
    Any condition classifiable to 639.0, with condition classifiable to 634–638

    Excludes   *urinary tract infection (634–638 with .7)*

.1 Complicated by delayed or excessive hemorrhage
    Afibrinogenemia   Intravascular hemolysis
    Defibrination syndrome
    Any condition classifiable to 639.1, with condition classifiable to 634–638

.2 Complicated by damage to pelvic organs and tissues
    Laceration, perforation, or tear of:
      bladder   uterus
    Any condition classifiable to 639.2, with condition classifiable to 634–638

.3 Complicated by renal failure
    Oliguria   Uremia
    Any condition classifiable to 639.3, with condition classifiable to 634–638

.4 **Complicated by metabolic disorder**
    Electrolyte imbalance with conditions classifia-
    ble to 634–638

.5 **Complicated by shock**
    Circulatory collapse
    Shock (postoperative) (septic)
    Any condition classifiable to 639.5, with condi-
      tion classifiable to 634–638

.6 **Complicated by embolism**
    Embolism: Embolism:
      NOS   pulmonary
      amniotic fluid
Any condition classifiable to 639.6, with condi   tion
classifiable to 634–638

☐ .7 **With other specified complications**
    Cardiac arrest or failure
    Urinary tract infection
    Any condition classifiable to 639.8, with condi-
      tion classifiable to 634–638

☐ .8 **With unspecified complications**

.9 **Without mention of complication**

● 634 **Spontaneous abortion**

Requires fifth digit to identify stage:
☐ 0 **unspecified**
  1 **incomplete**
  2 **complete**

Includes: miscarriage
            spontaneous abortion

● 634.0 **Complicated by genital tract and pelvic infection**

● 634.1 **Complicated by delayed or excessive hemorrhage**

● 634.2 **Complicated by damage to pelvic organs or tissues**

● 634.3 **Complicated by renal failure**

● 634.4 **Complicated by metabolic disorder**

● 634.5 **Complicated by shock**

● 634.6 **Complicated by embolism**

● ☐ 634.7 **With other specified complications**

● ☐ 634.8 **With unspecified complication**

● 634.9 **Without mention of complication**

● 635 **Legally induced abortion**

Requires fifth digit to identify stage:
☐ 0 **unspecified**
  1 **incomplete**
  2 **complete**

Includes: abortion or termination of pregnancy:
            elective
            legal
            therapeutic

Excludes *menstrual extraction or regulation (V25.3)*

● 635.0 **Complicated by genital tract and pelvic infection**

● 635.1 **Complicated by delayed or excessive hemorrhage**

● 635.2 **Complicated by damage to pelvic organs or tissues**

● 635.3 **Complicated by renal failure**

● 635.4 **Complicated by metabolic disorder**

● 635.5 **Complicated by shock**

● 635.6 **Complicated by embolism**

● ☐ 635.7 **With other specified complications**

● ☐ 635.8 **With unspecified complication**

● 635.9 **Without mention of complication**

● 636 **Illegally induced abortion**

Requires fifth digit to identify stage:
☐ 0 **unspecified**
  1 **incomplete**
  2 **complete**

Includes: abortion:
         criminal
         illegal
         self-induced

● 636.0 **Complicated by genital tract and pelvic infection**

● 636.1 **Complicated by delayed or excessive hemorrhage**

● 636.2 **Complicated by damage to pelvic organs or tissues**

● 636.3 **Complicated by renal failure**

● 636.4 **Complicated by metabolic disorder**

● 636.5 **Complicated by shock**

● 636.6 **Complicated by embolism**

● ☐ 636.7 **With other specified complications**

● ☐ 636.8 **With unspecified complication**

● 636.9 **Without mention of complication**

● 637 **Unspecified abortion**

Requires following fifth digit to identify stage:
☐ 0 **unspecified**
  1 **incomplete**
  2 **complete**

Includes: abortion NOS
           retained products of conception following
           abortion, not classifiable elsewhere

● ☐ 637.0 **Complicated by genital tract and pelvic infection**

● ☐ 637.1 **Complicated by delayed or excessive hemorrhage**

● ☐ 637.2 **Complicated by damage to pelvic organs or tissues**

● ☐ 637.3 **Complicated by renal failure**

● ☐ 637.4 **Complicated by metabolic disorder**

● ☐ 637.5 **Complicated by shock**

● ☐ 637.6 **Complicated by embolism**

● ☐ 637.7 **With other specified complications**

● ☐ 637.8 **With unspecified complication**

● ☐ 637.9 **Without mention of complication**

● 638 **Failed attempted abortion**

Includes: failure of attempted induction of (legal) abortion
Excludes *incomplete abortion (634.0–637.9)*

638.0 **Complicated by genital tract and pelvic infection**

638.1 **Complicated by delayed or excessive hemorrhage**

638.2 **Complicated by damage to pelvic organs or tissues**

638.3 **Complicated by renal failure**

638.4 **Complicated by metabolic disorder**

638.5 **Complicated by shock**

638.6 **Complicated by embolism**

☐ 638.7 **With other specified complications**

☐ 638.8 **With unspecified complication**

638.9 **Without mention of complication**

● 639 **Complications following abortion and ectopic and molar pregnancies**

Note: This category is provided for use when it is required
    to classify separately the complications classifiable to
    the fourth digit level in categories 634–638; for ex-
    ample:
    a) when the complication itself was responsible for
       an episode of medical care, the abortion, ectopic
       or molar pregnancy itself having been dealt with
       at a previous episode
    b) when these conditions are immediate complica-
       tions of ectopic or molar pregnancies classifiable
       to 630–633 where they cannot be identified at
       fourth digit level.

ICD-9-CM

600-609

Vol. 1

639.0   Genital tract and pelvic infection

Endometritis following conditions classifiable to 630–638

Parametritis following conditions classifiable to 630–638

Pelvic peritonitis following conditions classifiable to 630–638

Salpingitis following conditions classifiable to 630–638

Salpingo-oophoritis following conditions classifiable to 630–638

Sepsis NOS following conditions classifiable to 630–638

Septicemia NOS following conditions classifiable to 630–638

Excludes   *urinary tract infection (639.8)*

639.1   Delayed or excessive hemorrhage

Afibrinogenemia following conditions classifiable to 630–638

Defibrination syndrome following conditions classifiable to 630–638

Intravascular hemolysis following conditions classifiable to 630–638

639.2   Damage to pelvic organs and tissues

Laceration, perforation, or tear of:

bladder following conditions classifiable to 630–638

bowel following conditions classifiable to 630–638

broad ligament following conditions classifiable to 630–638

cervix following conditions classifiable to 630–638

periurethral tissue following conditions classifiable to 630–638

uterus following conditions classifiable to 630–638

vagina following conditions classifiable to 630–638

639.3   Renal failure

Oliguria following conditions classifiable to 630–638

Renal:

failure (acute) following conditions classifiable to 630–638

shutdown following conditions classifiable to 630–638

tubular necrosis following conditions classifiable to 630–638

Uremia following conditions classifiable to 630–638

639.4   Metabolic disorders

Electrolyte imbalance following conditions classifiable to 630–638

639.5   Shock

Circulatory collapse following conditions classifiable to 630–638

Shock (postoperative) (septic) following conditions classifiable to 630–638

639.6   Embolism

Embolism:

NOS following conditions classifiable to 630–638

air following conditions classifiable to 630–638

amniotic fluid following conditions classifiable to 630–638

blood-clot following conditions classifiable to 630–638

fat following conditions classifiable to 630–638

pulmonary following conditions classifiable to 630–638

pyemic following conditions classifiable to 630–638

septic following conditions classifiable to 630–638

septic following conditions classifiable to 630–638

soap following conditions classifiable to 630–638

☐ 639.8   Other specified complications following abortion or ectopic and molar pregnancy

Acute yellow atrophy or necrosis of liver following conditions classifiable to 630–638

Cardiac arrest or failure following conditions classifiable to 630–638

Cerebral anoxia following conditions classifiable to 630–638

Urinary tract infection following conditions classifiable to 630–638

☐ 639.9   Unspecified complication following abortion or ectopic and molar pregnancy

Complication(s) not further specified following conditions classifiable to 630–638

COMPLICATIONS MAINLY RELATED TO PREGNANCY (640–648)

Includes: the listed conditions even if they arose or were present during labor, delivery, or the puerperium

A   B   C

Figure 11–2   **A.** Marginal placenta previa. **B.** Partial placenta previa. **C.** Total placenta previa.

Figure 11-3 Abruptio placentae is classified according to the grade of separation of the placenta from the uterine wall. **A.** Mild separation in which hemorrhage is internal. **B.** Moderate separation in which there is external hemorrhage. **C.** Severe separation in which there is external hemorrhage and extreme separation.

A   B   C

Item 11-3 Placenta previa is a condition in which the opening of the cervix is obstructed by the displaced placenta. The three types, marginal, partial, and total, are varying degrees of placenta displacement.

The following fifth-digit subclassification is for use with categories 640–648 to denote the current episode of care:

☐ **0** unspecified as to episode of care or not applicable

1 delivered, with or without mention of antepartum condition

Antepartum condition with delivery

Delivery NOS (with mention of antepartum complication during current episode of care)

Intrapartum

obstetric condition (with mention of antepartum complication during current episode of care)

Pregnancy, delivered (with mention of antepartum complication during current episode of care)

2 delivered, with mention of postpartum complication

Delivery with mention of puerperal complication during current episode of care

3 antepartum condition or complication

Antepartum obstetric condition, not delivered during the current episode of care

4 postpartum condition or complication

Postpartum or puerperal obstetric condition or complication following delivery that occurred:

during previous episode of care

outside hospital, with subsequent admission for observation or care

● **640 Hemorrhage in early pregnancy**

Requires fifth digit; valid digits are in [brackets] under each code. See beginning of section 640–648 for definitions.

Includes: hemorrhage before completion of 22 weeks' gestation

● **640.0 Threatened abortion**
[0,1,3]

● ☐**640.8 Other specified hemorrhage in early pregnancy**
[0,1,3]

● ☐**640.9 Unspecified hemorrhage in early pregnancy**
[0,1,3]

● **641 Antepartum hemorrhage, abruptio placentae, and placenta previa**

Requires fifth digit; valid digits are in [brackets] under each code. See beginning of section 640–648 for definitions.

● **641.0 Placenta previa without hemorrhage**
[0,1,3]   Low implantation of placenta without hemorrhage
Placenta previa noted:
during pregnancy without hemorrhage
before labor (and delivered by cesarean delivery) without hemorrhage

● **641.1 Hemorrhage from placenta previa**
[0,1,3]   Low-lying placenta NOS or with hemorrhage (intrapartum)
Placenta previa:
incomplete NOS or with hemorrhage (intrapartum)
marginal NOS or with hemorrhage (intrapartum)
partial NOS or with hemorrhage (intrapartum)
total NOS or with hemorrhage (intrapartum)

Excludes hemorrhage from vasa previa (663.5)

● **641.2 Premature separation of placenta**
[0,1,3]   Ablatio placentae
Abruptio placentae
Accidental antepartum hemorrhage
Couvelaire uterus
Detachment of placenta (premature)
Premature separation of normally implanted placenta

● **641.3 Antepartum hemorrhage associated with coagula-**
[0,1,3] **tion defects**
Antepartum or intrapartum hemorrhage associated with:
afibrinogenemia
hyperfibrinolysis
hypofibrinogenemia

● ☐**641.8 Other antepartum hemorrhage**
[0,1,3]   Antepartum or intrapartum hemorrhage associated with:
trauma
uterine leiomyoma

● ☐**641.9 Unspecified antepartum hemorrhage**
[0,1,3]   Hemorrhage:
antepartum NOS
intrapartum NOS
of pregnancy NOS

● **642 Hypertension complicating pregnancy, childbirth, and the puerperium**

Requires fifth digit; valid digits are in [brackets] under each code. See beginning of section 640–648 for definitions.

ICD-9-CM

600-

Vol.

● **642.0** **Benign essential hypertension complicating preg-**
[0–4] **nancy, childbirth, and the puerperium**
    Hypertension:
       benign essential specified as complicating, or as
         a reason for obstetric care during preg-
         nancy, childbirth, or the puerperium
       chronic NOS specified as complicating, or as a
         reason for obstetric care during pregnancy,
         childbirth, or the puerperium
       essential specified as complicating, or as a rea-
         son for obstetric care during pregnancy,
         childbirth, or the puerperium
       pre-existing NOS specified as complicating, or
         as a reason for obstetric care during preg-
         nancy, childbirth, or the puerperium

● **642.1** **Hypertension secondary to renal disease, compli-**
[0–4] **cating pregnancy, childbirth, and the puerperium**
    Hypertension secondary to renal disease, specified
       as complicating, or as a reason for obstetric
       care during pregnancy, childbirth, or the pu-
       erperium

● ❑ **642.2** **Other pre-existing hypertension complicating preg-**
[0–4] **nancy, childbirth, and the puerperium**
    Hypertensive:
       heart and renal disease specified as complicat-
         ing, or as a reason for obstetric care during
         pregnancy, childbirth, or the puerperium
       heart disease specified as complicating, or as a
         reason for obstetric care during pregnancy,
         childbirth, or the puerperium
       renal disease specified as complicating, or as a
         reason for obstetric care during pregnancy,
         childbirth, or the puerperium
    Malignant hypertension specified as complicating,
       or as a reason for obstetric care during preg-
       nancy, childbirth, or the puerperium

● **642.3** **Transient hypertension of pregnancy**
[0–4]   Gestational hypertension
    Transient hypertension, so described, in preg-
       nancy, childbirth, or the puerperium

● **642.4** **Mild or unspecified pre-eclampsia**
[0–4]   Hypertension in pregnancy, childbirth, or the pu-
       erperium, not specified as pre-existing, with
       either albuminuria or edema, or both; mild or
       unspecified

    Pre-eclampsia: Toxemia (pre-eclamptic):
    NOS   NOS
    mild   mild

    Excludes   *albuminuria in pregnancy, without mention of*
               hypertension (646.2)
            edema in pregnancy, without mention of hyper-
               tension (646.1)

● **642.5** **Severe pre-eclampsia**
[0–4]   Hypertension in pregnancy, childbirth, or the pu-
       erperium, not specified as pre-existing, with
       either albuminuria or edema, or both; speci-
       fied as severe
    Pre-eclampsia, severe
    Toxemia (pre-eclamptic), severe

● **642.6** **Eclampsia**
[0–4]   Toxemia: Toxemia:
       eclamptic   with convulsions

● **642.7** **Pre-eclampsia or eclampsia superimposed on pre-**
[0–4] **existing hypertension**
    Conditions classifiable to 642.4–642.6, with condi-
       tions classifiable to 642.0–642.2

● ❑ **642.9** **Unspecified hypertension complicating pregnancy,**
[0–4] **childbirth, or the puerperium**
    Hypertension NOS, without mention of albumin-
       uria or edema, complicating pregnancy, child-
       birth, or the puerperium

● **643** **Excessive vomiting in pregnancy**

    Requires fifth digit; valid digits are in [brackets] under each
    code. See beginning of section 640–648 for definitions.

    Includes: hyperemesis arising during pregnancy
               hyperemesis gravidarum
               vomiting:
                  persistent arising during pregnancy
                  vicious arising during pregnancy

● **643.0** **Mild hyperemesis gravidarum**
[0,1,3]   Hyperemesis gravidarum, mild or unspecified,
       starting before the end of the 22nd week of
       gestation

● **643.1** **Hyperemesis gravidarum with metabolic distur-**
[0,1,3] **bance**
    Hyperemesis gravidarum, starting before the end
       of the 22nd week of gestation, with metabolic
       disturbance, such as:
    carbohydrate depletion
    dehydration
    electrolyte imbalance

● **643.2** **Late vomiting of pregnancy**
[0,1,3]   Excessive vomiting starting after 22 completed
       weeks of gestation

● ❑ **643.8** **Other vomiting complicating pregnancy**
[0,1,3]   Vomiting due to organic disease or other cause,
       specified as complicating pregnancy, or as a
       reason for obstetric care during pregnancy

    Use additional code to specify cause

● ❑ **643.9** **Unspecified vomiting of pregnancy**
[0,1,3]   Vomiting as a reason for care during pregnancy,
       length of gestation unspecified

● **644** **Early or threatened labor**

    Requires fifth digit; valid digits are in [brackets] under
    each code. See beginning of section 640–648 for defini-
    tions.

● **644.0** **Threatened premature labor**
[0,3]   Premature labor after 22 weeks, but before 37 com-
       pleted weeks of gestation without delivery

    Excludes   *that occurring before 22 completed weeks of ges-*
               tation (640.0)

● ❑ **644.1** **Other threatened labor**
[0,3]   False labor:
       NOS without delivery
       after 37 completed weeks of gestation without
         delivery
    Threatened labor NOS without delivery

● **644.2** **Early onset of delivery**
[0–1]   Onset (spontaneous) of delivery before 37 com-
       pleted weeks of gestation
    Premature labor with onset of delivery before 37
       completed weeks of gestation

● **645** **Late pregnancy**

    Requires fifth digit; valid digits are in [brackets] under
    each code. See beginning of section 640–648 for defini-
    tions.

    645.1 **Post term pregnancy**
[0,1,3]   Pregnancy over 40 completed weeks to 42 com-
       pleted weeks gestation

    645.2 **Prolonged pregnancy**
[0,1,3]   Pregnancy which has advanced beyond 42 com-
       pleted weeks of gestation

● **646** **Other complications of pregnancy, not elsewhere classi-**
fied

    Use additional code(s) to further specify complication

    Requires fifth digit; valid digits are in [brackets] under each
    code. See beginning of section 640–648 for definitions.

● **646.0 Papyraceous fetus**
[0,1,3]

● **646.1 Edema or excessive weight gain in pregnancy,**
[0–4] **without mention of hypertension**
　　　Gestational edema
　　　Maternal obesity syndrome
　　Excludes *that with mention of hypertension (642.0–642.9)*

● ❑ **646.2 Unspecified renal disease in pregnancy, without**
[0–4] **mention of hypertension**
　　　Albuminuria in pregnancy or the puerperium, without mention of hypertension
　　　Nephropathy NOS in pregnancy or the puerperium, without mention of hypertension
　　　Renal disease NOS in pregnancy or the puerperium, without mention of hypertension
　　　Uremia in pregnancy or the puerperium, without mention of hypertension
　　　Gestational proteinuria in pregnancy or the puerperium, without mention of hypertension
　　Excludes *that with mention of hypertension (642.0–642.9)*

● **646.3 Habitual aborter**
[0–1,3]
　　Excludes *with current abortion (634.0–634.9)*
　　　　　　without current pregnancy (629.9)

● **646.4 Peripheral neuritis in pregnancy**
[0–4]

● **646.5 Asymptomatic bacteriuria in pregnancy**
[0–4]

● **646.6 Infections of genitourinary tract in pregnancy**
[0–4] Conditions classifiable to 590, 595, 597, 599.0, 616 complicating pregnancy, childbirth, or the puerperium
　　　Conditions classifiable to 614.0–614.5, 614.7–614.9, 615
　　Excludes *major puerperal infection (670)*

● **646.7 Liver disorders in pregnancy**
[0,1,3] Acute yellow atrophy of liver (obstetric) (true) of pregnancy
　　　Icterus gravis of pregnancy
　　　Necrosis of liver of pregnancy
　　Excludes *hepatorenal syndrome following delivery (674.8)*
　　　　　　viral hepatitis (647.6)

● ❑ **646.8 Other specified complications of pregnancy**
[0–4] Fatigue during pregnancy
　　　Herpes gestationis
　　　Insufficient weight gain of pregnancy
　　　Uterine size-date discrepancy

● ❑ **646.9 Unspecified complication of pregnancy**
[0,1,3]

● **647 Infectious and parasitic conditions in the mother classifiable elsewhere, but complicating pregnancy, childbirth, or the puerperium**

Use additional code(s) to further specify complication

Requires fifth digit; valid digits are in [brackets] under each code. See beginning of section 640–648 for definitions.

Includes: the listed conditions when complicating the pregnant state, aggravated by the pregnancy, or when a main reason for obstetric care

Excludes *those conditions in the mother known or suspected to have affected the fetus (655.0–655.9)*

● **647.0 Syphilis**
[0–4] Conditions classifiable to 090–097

● **647.1 Gonorrhea**
[0–4] Conditions classifiable to 098

● ❑ **647.2 Other venereal diseases**
[0–4] Conditions classifiable to 099

● **647.3 Tuberculosis**
[0–4] Conditions classifiable to 010–018

● **647.4 Malaria**
[0–4] Conditions classifiable to 084

● **647.5 Rubella**
[0–4] Conditions classifiable to 056

● ❑ **647.6 Other viral diseases**
[0–4] Conditions classifiable to 042 and 050–079, except 056

● ❑ **647.8 Other specified infectious and parasitic diseases**
[0–4]

● ❑ **647.9 Unspecified infection or infestation**
[0–4]

● **648 Other current conditions in the mother classifiable elsewhere, but complicating pregnancy, childbirth, or the puerperium**

Use additional code(s) to identify the condition

Requires fifth digit; valid digits are in [brackets] under each code. See beginning of section 640–648 for definitions.

Includes: the listed conditions when complicating the pregnant state, aggravated by the pregnancy, or when a main reason for obstetric care

Excludes *those conditions in the mother known or suspected to have affected the fetus (655.0–665.9)*

● **648.0 Diabetes mellitus**
[0–4] Conditions classifiable to 250
　　Excludes *gestational diabetes (648.8)*

● **648.1 Thyroid dysfunction**
[0–4] Conditions classifiable to 240–246

● **648.2 Anemia**
[0–4] Conditions classifiable to 280–285

● **648.3 Drug dependence**
[0–4] Conditions classifiable to 304

● **648.4 Mental disorders**
[0–4] Conditions classifiable to 290–303, 305–316, 317–319

● **648.5 Congenital cardiovascular disorders**
[0–4] Conditions classifiable to 745–747

● ❑ **648.6 Other cardiovascular diseases**
[0–4] Conditions classifiable to 390–398, 410–429
　　Excludes *cerebrovascular disorders in the puerperium (674.0)*
　　　　　　peripartum cardiomyopathy (674.5)
　　　　　　venous complications (671.0–671.9)

● **648.7 Bone and joint disorders of back, pelvis, and**
[0–4] **lower limbs**
　　　Conditions classifiable to 720–724, and those classifiable to 711–719 or 725–738, specified as affecting the lower limbs

● **648.8 Abnormal glucose tolerance**
[0–4] Conditions classifiable to 790.2
　　　Gestational diabetes

● ❑ **648.9 Other current conditions classifiable elsewhere**
[0–4] Conditions classifiable to 440–459
　　　Nutritional deficiencies [conditions classifiable to 260–269]

ICD-9-CM
600-
679
Vol. 1

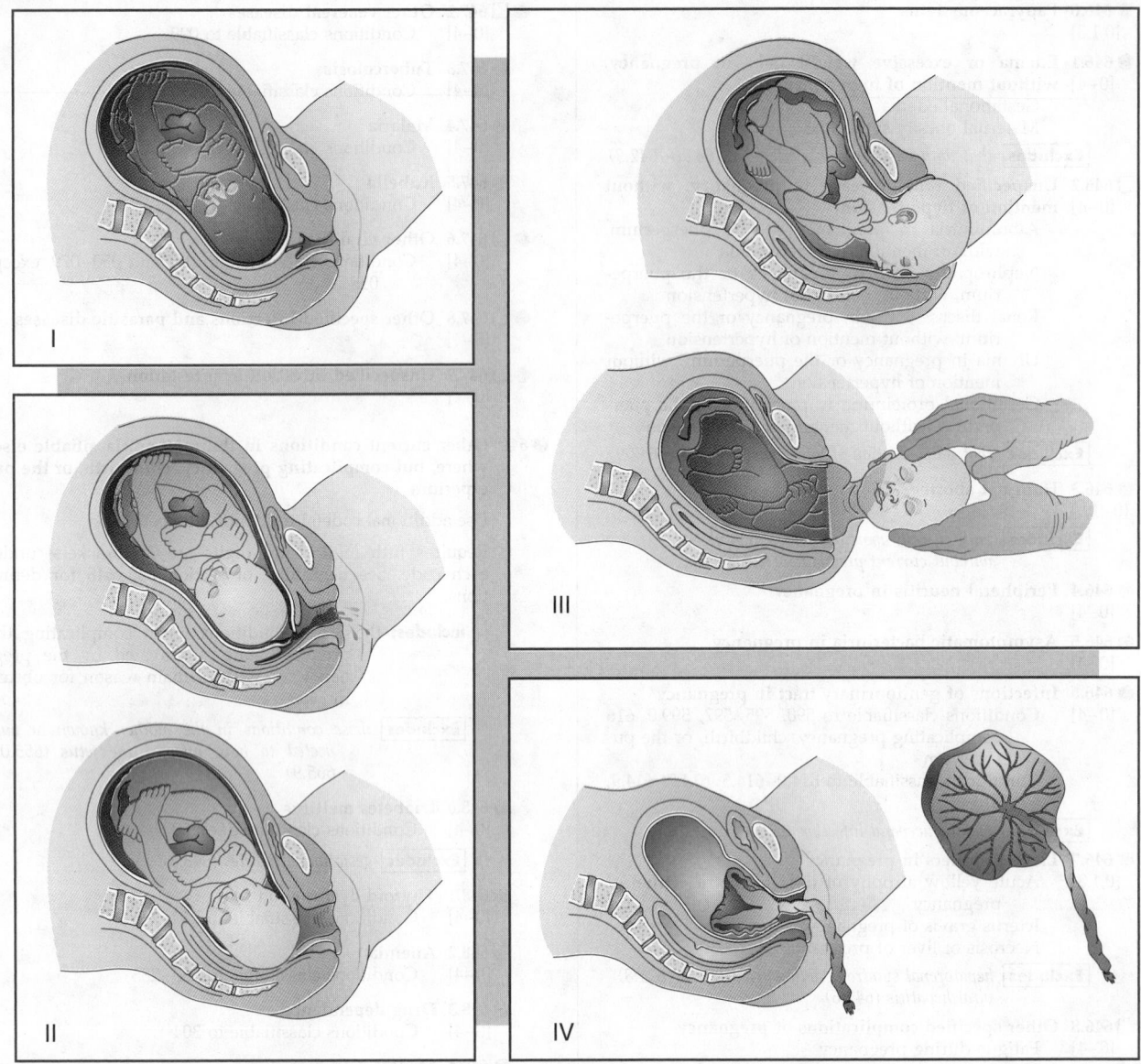

Figure 11-4 The four stages of normal delivery: **I.** Lightening, which occurs 2 to 4 weeks before birth, at which time the fetus turns with head toward the vagina. **II.** Regular contractions begin, the amniotic sac ruptures, and dilation is complete. **III.** Delivery of the head and rotation. **IV.** Recovery of the mother to full homeostasis.

NORMAL DELIVERY, AND OTHER INDICATIONS FOR CARE IN PREGNANCY, LABOR, AND DELIVERY (650-659)

The following fifth-digit subclassification is for use with categories 651-659 to denote the current episode of care:

☐ 0 unspecified as to episode of care or not applicable
  1 delivered, with or without mention of antepartum condition
  2 delivered, with mention of postpartum complication
  3 antepartum condition or complication
  4 postpartum condition or complication

650 Normal delivery

Delivery requiring minimal or no assistance, with or without episiotomy, without fetal manipulation [e.g., rotation version] or instrumentation [forceps] of a spontaneous, cephalic, vaginal, full-term, single, live-born infant. This code is for use as a single diagnosis code and is not to be used with any other code in the range 630-676.

Use additional code to indicate outcome of delivery (V27.0)

Excludes *breech delivery (assisted) (spontaneous) NOS (652.2)*

delivery by vacuum extractor, forceps, cesarean section, or breech extraction, without specified complication (669.5-669.7)

◀ **New** ◀▥▥ **Revised** ● **Not a Principal Diagnosis** ● **Use Additional Digit(s)** ☐ **Nonspecific Code**

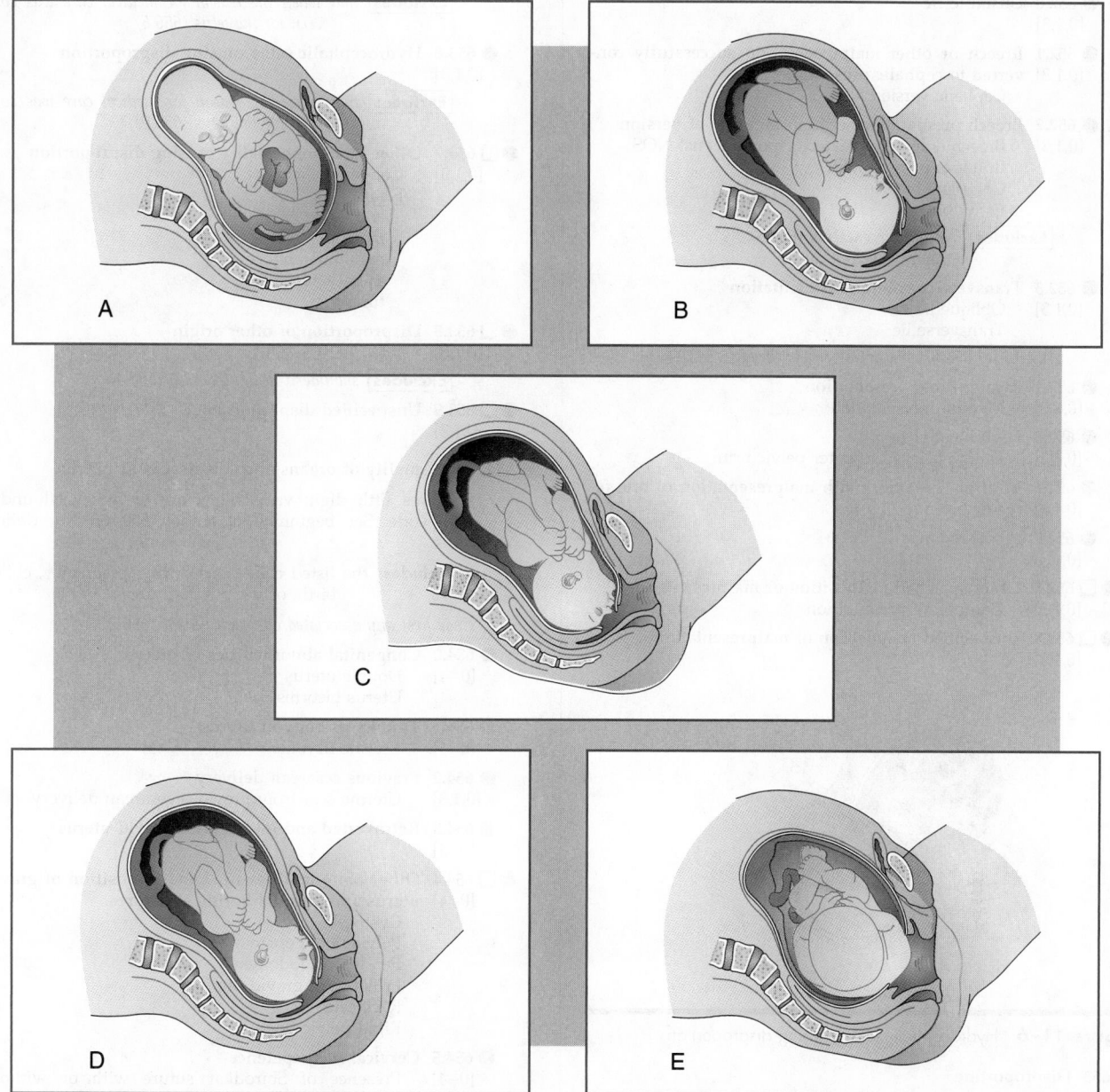

Figure 11–5 Five types of malposition and malpresentation of the fetus: **A.** Breech. **B.** Vertex. **C.** Face. **D.** Brow. **E.** Shoulder.

ICD-9-CM

600-
699

Vol. 1

● **651 Multiple gestation**

Requires fifth digit; valid digits are in [brackets] under each code. See beginning of section 650–659 for definitions.

● **651.0 Twin pregnancy**
[0,1,3]

● **651.1 Triplet pregnancy**
[0,1,3]

● **651.2 Quadruplet pregnancy**
[0,1,3]

● **651.3 Twin pregnancy with fetal loss and retention of**
[0,1,3] **one fetus**

● **651.4 Triplet pregnancy with fetal loss and retention of**
[0,1,3] **one or more fetus(es)**

● **651.5 Quadruplet pregnancy with fetal loss and reten-**
[0,1,3] **tion of one or more fetus(es)**

● ❑**651.6 Other multiple pregnancy with fetal loss and re-**
[0,1,3] **tention of one or more fetus(es)**

● ❑**651.8 Other specified multiple gestation**
[0,1,3]

● ❑**651.9 Unspecified multiple gestation**
[0,1,3]

● **652 Malposition and malpresentation of fetus**

Requires fifth digit; valid digits are in [brackets] under each code. See beginning of section 650–659 for definitions.

Code first any associated obstructed labor (660.0)

● 652.0 Unstable lie
[0,1,3]

● 652.1 Breech or other malpresentation successfully con-
[0,1,3] verted to cephalic presentation
       Cephalic version NOS

● 652.2 Breech presentation without mention of version
[0,1,3]   Breech delivery (assisted) (spontaneous) NOS
       Buttocks presentation
       Complete breech
       Frank breech

   Excludes *footling presentation (652.8)*
                 incomplete breech (652.8)

● 652.3 Transverse or oblique presentation
[0,1,3]   Oblique lie
       Transverse lie

   Excludes *transverse arrest of fetal head (660.3)*

● 652.4 Face or brow presentation
[0,1,3]   Mentum presentation

● 652.5 High head at term
[0,1,3]   Failure of head to enter pelvic brim

● 652.6 Multiple gestation with malpresentation of one fe-
[0,1,3] tus or more

● 652.7 Prolapsed arm
[0,1,3]

● ❑ 652.8 Other specified malposition or malpresentation
[0,1,3]   Compound presentation

● ❑ 652.9 Unspecified malposition or malpresentation
[0,1,3]

Figure 11–6 Hydrocephalic fetus causing disproportion.

● 653 Disproportion

Requires fifth digit; valid digits are in [brackets] under each code. See beginning of section 650–659 for definitions.

Code first any associated obstructed labor (660.1)

● 653.0 Major abnormality of bony pelvis, not further
[0,1,3] specified
       Pelvic deformity NOS

● 653.1 Generally contracted pelvis
[0,1,3]   Contracted pelvis NOS

● 653.2 Inlet contraction of pelvis
[0,1,3]   Inlet contraction (pelvis)

● 653.3 Outlet contraction of pelvis
[0,1,3]   Outlet contraction (pelvis)

● 653.4 Fetopelvic disproportion
[0,1,3]   Cephalopelvic disproportion NOS
       Disproportion of mixed maternal and fetal origin,
          with normally formed fetus

● 653.5 Unusually large fetus causing disproportion
[0,1,3]   Disproportion of fetal origin with normally
          formed fetus
       Fetal disproportion NOS

   Excludes *that when the reason for medical care was con-*
             cern for the fetus (656.6)

● 653.6 Hydrocephalic fetus causing disproportion
[0,1,3]

   Excludes *that when the reason for medical care was con-*
             cern for the fetus (655.0)

● ❑ 653.7 Other fetal abnormality causing disproportion
[0,1,3]   Conjoined twins
       Fetal:
          ascites
          hydrops
          myelomeningocele
          sacral teratoma
          tumor

● ❑ 653.8 Disproportion of other origin
[0,1,3]

   Excludes *shoulder (girdle) dystocia (660.4)*

● ❑ 653.9 Unspecified disproportion
[0,1,3]

● 654 Abnormality of organs and soft tissues of pelvis

Requires fifth digit; valid digits are in [brackets] under each code. See beginning of section 650–659 for defini-tions.

Includes: the listed conditions during pregnancy, child-birth, or the puerperium

Code first any associated obstructed labor (660.2)

● 654.0 Congenital abnormalities of uterus
[0–4]   Double uterus
       Uterus bicornis

● 654.1 Tumors of body of uterus
[0–4]   Uterine fibroids

● 654.2 Previous cesarean delivery
[0,1,3]   Uterine scar from previous cesarean delivery

● 654.3 Retroverted and incarcerated gravid uterus
[0–4]

● ❑ 654.4 Other abnormalities in shape or position of gravid
[0–4] uterus and of neighboring structures
       Cystocele
       Pelvic floor repair
       Pendulous abdomen
       Prolapse of gravid uterus
       Rectocele
       Rigid pelvic floor

● 654.5 Cervical incompetence
[0–4]   Presence of Shirodkar suture with or without
          mention of cervical incompetence

● ❑ 654.6 Other congenital or acquired abnormality of cervix
[0–4]   Cicatricial cervix
       Polyp of cervix
       Previous surgery to cervix
       Rigid cervix (uteri)
       Stenosis or stricture of cervix
       Tumor of cervix

● 654.7 Congenital or acquired abnormality of vagina
[0–4]   Previous surgery to vagina
       Septate vagina
       Stenosis of vagina (acquired) (congenital)
       Stricture of vagina
       Tumor of vagina

● 654.8 Congenital or acquired abnormality of vulva
[0–4]   Fibrosis of perineum
       Persistent hymen
       Previous surgery to perineum or vulva
       Rigid perineum
       Tumor of vulva

   Excludes *varicose veins of vulva (671.1)*

● ❑ **654.9 Other and unspecified**
[0–4]   Uterine scar NEC

● **655 Known or suspected fetal abnormality affecting management of mother**

Requires fifth digit; valid digits are in [brackets] under each code. See beginning of section 650–659 for definitions.

Includes: the listed conditions in the fetus as a reason for observation or obstetrical care of the mother, or for termination of pregnancy

● **655.0 Central nervous system malformation in fetus**
[0,1,3]   Fetal or suspected fetal:
     anencephaly
     hydrocephalus
     spina bifida (with myelomeningocele)

● **655.1 Chromosomal abnormality in fetus**
[0,1,3]

● **655.2 Hereditary disease in family possibly affecting fetus**
[0,1,3]

● **655.3 Suspected damage to fetus from viral disease in the mother**
[0,1,3]   Suspected damage to fetus from maternal rubella

● ❑ **655.4 Suspected damage to fetus from other disease in the mother**
[0,1,3]   Suspected damage to fetus from maternal:
     alcohol addiction
     listeriosis
     toxoplasmosis

● **655.5 Suspected damage to fetus from drugs**
[0,1,3]

● **655.6 Suspected damage to fetus from radiation**
[0,1,3]

● **655.7 Decreased fetal movements**
[0,1,3]

● ❑ **655.8 Other known or suspected fetal abnormality, not elsewhere classified**
[0,1,3]   Suspected damage to fetus from:
     environmental toxins
     intrauterine contraceptive device

● ❑ **655.9 Unspecified**
[0,1,3]

● **656 Other fetal and placental problems affecting management of mother**

Requires fifth digit; valid digits are in [brackets] under each code. See beginning of section 650–659 for definitions.

● **656.0 Fetal-maternal hemorrhage**
[0,1,3]   Leakage (microscopic) of fetal blood into maternal circulation

● **656.1 Rhesus isoimmunization**
[0,1,3]   Anti-D [Rh] antibodies
     Rh incompatibility

● ❑ **656.2 Isoimmunization from other and unspecified blood-group incompatibility**
[0,1,3]   ABO isoimmunization

● **656.3 Fetal distress**
[0,1,3]   Fetal metabolic acidemia

Excludes abnormal fetal acid-base balance (656.8)
abnormality in fetal heart rate or rhythm (659.7)
fetal bradycardia (659.7)
fetal tachycardia (659.7)
meconium in liquor (656.8)

● **656.4 Intrauterine death**
[0,1,3]   Fetal death:
     NOS
     after completion of 22 weeks' gestation
     late
   Missed delivery

Excludes missed abortion (632)

● **656.5 Poor fetal growth**
[0,1,3]   "Light-for-dates"
     "Placental insufficiency"
     "Small-for-dates"

● **656.6 Excessive fetal growth**
[0,1,3]   "Large-for-dates"

● ❑ **656.7 Other placental conditions**
[0,1,3]   Abnormal placenta
     Placental infarct

Excludes placental polyp (674.4)
placentitis (658.4)

● ❑ **656.8 Other specified fetal and placental problems**
[0,1,3]   Abnormal acid-base balance
     Intrauterine acidosis
     Lithopedian
     Meconium in liquor

● ❑ **656.9 Unspecified fetal and placental problem**
[0,1,3]

● **657 Polyhydramnios**
[0,1,3]   Hydramnios

Requires fifth digit; valid digits are in [brackets] under each code. See beginning of section 650–659 for definitions.

Use 0 as fourth digit for category 657

● **658 Other problems associated with amniotic cavity and membranes**

Requires fifth digit; valid digits are in [brackets] under each code. See beginning of section 650–659 for definitions.

Excludes amniotic fluid embolism (673.1)

● **658.0 Oligohydramnios**
[0,1,3]   Oligohydramnios without mention of rupture of membranes

● **658.1 Premature rupture of membranes**
[0,1,3]   Rupture of amniotic sac less than 24 hours prior to the onset of labor

● **658.2 Delayed delivery after spontaneous or unspecified rupture of membranes**
[0,1,3]   Prolonged rupture of membranes NOS
     Rupture of amniotic sac 24 hours or more prior to the onset of labor

● **658.3 Delayed delivery after artificial rupture of membranes**
[0,1,3]

● **658.4 Infection of amniotic cavity**
[0,1,3]   Amnionitis
     Chorioamnionitis
     Membranitis
     Placentitis

● ❑ **658.8 Other**
[0,1,3]   Amnion nodosum
     Amniotic cyst

● ❑ **658.9 Unspecified**
[0,1,3]

● **659 Other indications for care or intervention related to labor and delivery, not elsewhere classified**

Requires fifth digit; valid digits are in [brackets] under each code. See beginning of section 650–659 for definitions.

● **659.0 Failed mechanical induction**
[0,1,3]   Failure of induction of labor by surgical or other instrumental methods

ICD-9-CM

600-
609

Vol. 1

● **659.1 Failed medical or unspecified induction**
[0,1,3]   Failed induction NOS
          Failure of induction of labor by medical methods,
             such as oxytocic drugs

● ❑ **659.2 Maternal pyrexia during labor, unspecified**
[0,1,3]

● **659.3 Generalized infection during labor**
[0,1,3]   Septicemia during labor

● **659.4 Grand multiparity**
[0,1,3]

    Excludes   *supervision only, in pregnancy (V23.3)*
                   without current pregnancy (V61.5)

● **659.5 Elderly primigravida**
[0,1,3]   First pregnancy in a woman who will be 35 years
            of age or older at expected date of delivery

    Excludes   *supervision only, in pregnancy (V23.81)*

● ❑ **659.6 Elderly multigravida**
[0,1,3]   Second or more pregnancy in a woman who will
            be 35 years of age or older at expected date
            of delivery

    Excludes   *elderly primigravida (659.5)*

● ❑ **659.7 Abnormality in fetal heart rate or rhythm**
[0,1,3]   Depressed fetal heart tones
          Fetal:
            bradycardia
            tachycardia
          Fetal heart rate decelerations
          Non-reassuring fetal heart rate or rhythm

● ❑ **659.8 Other specified indications for care or intervention**
[0,1,3] **related to labor and delivery**
          Pregnancy in a female less than 16 years old at
            expected date of delivery
          Very young maternal age

● ❑ **659.9 Unspecified indication for care or intervention re-**
[0,1,3] **lated to labor and delivery**

COMPLICATIONS OCCURRING MAINLY IN THE COURSE OF LABOR AND DELIVERY (660–669)

The following fifth-digit subclassification is for use with
categories 660–669 to denote the current episode of care:
❑ 0   **unspecified as to episode of care or not applicable**
   1   **delivered, with or without mention of antepartum**
       condition
   2   **delivered, with mention of postpartum complication**
   3   **antepartum condition or complication**
   4   **postpartum condition or complication**

● **660 Obstructed labor**

    Requires fifth digit; valid digits are in [brackets] under each
    code. See beginning of section 660–669 for definitions.

● **660.0 Obstruction caused by malposition of fetus at on-**
[0,1,3] **set of labor**
          Any condition classifiable to 652, causing obstruc-
            tion during labor

          Use additional code from 652.0–652.9 to identify
            condition

● **660.1 Obstruction by bony pelvis**
[0,1,3]   Any condition classifiable to 653, causing obstruc-
            tion during labor

          Use additional code from 653.0–653.9 to identify
            condition

● **660.2 Obstruction by abnormal pelvic soft tissues**
[0,1,3]   Prolapse of anterior lip of cervix
          Any condition classifiable to 654, causing obstruc-
            tion during labor

          Use additional code from 654.0–654.9 to identify
            condition

● **660.3 Deep transverse arrest and persistent occipitopos-**
[0,1,3] **terior position**

● **660.4 Shoulder (girdle) dystocia**
[0,1,3]   Impacted shoulders

● **660.5 Locked twins**
[0,1,3]

● ❑ **660.6 Failed trial of labor, unspecified**
[0,1,3]   Failed trial of labor, without mention of condition
            or suspected condition

● ❑ **660.7 Failed forceps or vacuum extractor, unspecified**
[0,1,3]   Application of ventouse or forceps, without men-
            tion of condition

● ❑ **660.8 Other causes of obstructed labor**
[0,1,3]

● ❑ **660.9 Unspecified obstructed labor**
[0,1,3]   Dystocia:
            NOS
            fetal NOS
            maternal NOS

● **661 Abnormality of forces of labor**

    Requires fifth digit; valid digits are in [brackets] under each
    code. See beginning of section 660–669 for definitions.

● **661.0 Primary uterine inertia**
[0,1,3]   Failure of cervical dilation
          Hypotonic uterine dysfunction, primary
          Prolonged latent phase of labor

● **661.1 Secondary uterine inertia**
[0,1,3]   Arrested active phase of labor
          Hypotonic uterine dysfunction, secondary

● ❑ **661.2 Other and unspecified uterine inertia**
[0,1,3]   Desultory labor
          Irregular labor
          Poor contractions
          Slow slope active phase of labor

● **661.3 Precipitate labor**
[0,1,3]

● ❑ **661.4 Hypertonic, incoordinate, or prolonged uterine**
[0,1,3] **contractions**
          Cervical spasm
          Contraction ring (dystocia)
          Dyscoordinate labor
          Hourglass contraction of uterus
          Hypertonic uterine dysfunction
          Incoordinate uterine action
          Retraction ring (Bandl's) (pathological)
          Tetanic contractions
          Uterine dystocia NOS
          Uterine spasm

● ❑ **661.9 Unspecified abnormality of labor**
[0,1,3]

● **662 Long labor**

    Requires fifth digit; valid digits are in [brackets] under each
    code. See beginning of section 660–669 for definitions.

● **662.0 Prolonged first stage**
[0,1,3]

● ❑ **662.1 Prolonged labor, unspecified**
[0,1,3]

● **662.2 Prolonged second stage**
[0,1,3]

● **662.3 Delayed delivery of second twin, triplet, etc.**
[0,1,3]

● **663 Umbilical cord complications**

    Requires fifth digit; valid digits are in [brackets] under each
    code. See beginning of section 660–669 for definitions.

● **663.0 Prolapse of cord**
[0,1,3]   Presentation of cord

Vaginal opening   Urethral opening

A
B
C
D

Anus

Figure 11-7   Perineal lacerations: **A.** First-degree is laceration of superficial tissues. **B.** Second-degree is limited to the pelvic floor and may involve the perineal or vaginal muscles. **C.** Third-degree involves the anal sphincter. **D.** Fourth-degree involves anal or rectal mucosa.

● **663.1** **Cord around neck, with compression**
[0,1,3]   Cord tightly around neck

● ❑ **663.2** **Other and unspecified cord entanglement, with**
[0,1,3]   **compression**
    Entanglement of cords of twins in mono-amniotic sac
    Knot in cord (with compression)

● ❑ **663.3** **Other and unspecified cord entanglement, without**
[0,1,3]   **mention of compression**

● **663.4** **Short cord**
[0,1,3]

● **663.5** **Vasa previa**
[0,1,3]

● **663.6** **Vascular lesions of cord**
[0,1,3]   Bruising of cord
    Hematoma of cord
    Thrombosis of vessels of cord

● ❑ **663.8** **Other umbilical cord complications**
[0,1,3]   Velamentous insertion of umbilical cord

● ❑ **663.9** **Unspecified umbilical cord complication**
[0,1,3]

● **664** **Trauma to perineum and vulva during delivery**

    Requires fifth digit; valid digits are in [brackets] under each code. See beginning of section 660–669 for definitions.

    Includes: damage from instruments
        that from extension of episiotomy

● **664.0** **First-degree perineal laceration**
[0,1,4]   Perineal laceration, rupture, or tear involving:
        fourchette   skin
        hymen   vagina
        labia   vulva

● **664.1** **Second-degree perineal laceration**
[0,1,4]   Perineal laceration, rupture, or tear (following episiotomy) involving:
            pelvic floor
            perineal muscles
            vaginal muscles

    Excludes *that involving anal sphincter (664.2)*

● **664.2** **Third-degree perineal laceration**
[0,1,4]   Perineal laceration, rupture, or tear (following episiotomy) involving:
        anal sphincter
        rectovaginal septum
        sphincter NOS

    Excludes *that with anal or rectal mucosal laceration (664.3)*

● **664.3** **Fourth-degree perineal laceration**
[0,1,4]   Perineal laceration, rupture, or tear as classifiable to 664.2 and involving also:
        anal mucosa
        rectal mucosa

● ❑ **664.4** **Unspecified perineal laceration**
[0,1,4]   Central laceration

● **664.5** **Vulval and perineal hematoma**
[0,1,4]

● ❑ **664.8** **Other specified trauma to perineum and vulva**
[0,1,4]

● ❑ **664.9** **Unspecified trauma to perineum and vulva**
[0,1,4]

● **665** **Other obstetrical trauma**

    Requires fifth digit; valid digits are in [brackets] under each code. See beginning of section 660–669 for definitions.

    Includes: damage from instruments

● **665.0** **Rupture of uterus before onset of labor**
[0,1,3]

● **665.1** **Rupture of uterus during labor**
[0,1]   Rupture of uterus NOS

● **665.2** **Inversion of uterus**
[0,2,4]

● **665.3** **Laceration of cervix**
[0,1,4]

● **665.4** **High vaginal laceration**
[0,1,4]   Laceration of vaginal wall or sulcus without mention of perineal laceration

ICD-9-CM

660-
669

Vol. 1

◀ **New**   ◀▥ **Revised**   ● **Not a Principal Diagnosis**   ● **Use Additional Digit(s)**   ❑ **Nonspecific Code**

● ❑ **665.5 Other injury to pelvic organs**
[0,1,4]   Injury to:
               bladder
               urethra

● **665.6 Damage to pelvic joints and ligaments**
[0,1,4]   Avulsion of inner symphyseal cartilage
           Damage to coccyx
           Separation of symphysis (pubis)

● **665.7 Pelvic hematoma**
[0–2,4]   Hematoma of vagina

● ❑ **665.8 Other specified obstetrical trauma**
[0–4]

● ❑ **665.9 Unspecified obstetrical trauma**
[0–4]

● **666 Postpartum hemorrhage**

    Requires fifth digit; valid digits are in [brackets] under each code. See beginning of section 660–669 for definitions.

● **666.0 Third-stage hemorrhage**
[0,2,4]   Hemorrhage associated with retained, trapped, or
           adherent placenta
           Retained placenta NOS

● ❑ **666.1 Other immediate postpartum hemorrhage**
[0,2,4]   Atony of uterus
           Hemorrhage within the first 24 hours following
             delivery of placenta
           Postpartum hemorrhage (atonic) NOS

● **666.2 Delayed and secondary postpartum hemorrhage**
[0,2,4]   Hemorrhage:
             after the first 24 hours following delivery
             associated with retained portions of placenta or
               membranes
           Postpartum hemorrhage specified as delayed or
             secondary
           Retained products of conception NOS, following
             delivery

● **666.3 Postpartum coagulation defects**
[0,2,4]   Postpartum:
           afibrinogenemia
           fibrinolysis

● **667 Retained placenta without hemorrhage**

    Requires fifth digit; valid digits are in [brackets] under each code. See beginning of section 660–669 for definitions.

● **667.0 Retained placenta without hemorrhage**
[0,2,4]   Placenta accreta without hemorrhage
           Retained placenta:
             NOS without hemorrhage
             total without hemorrhage

● **667.1 Retained portions of placenta or membranes, with-**
[0,2,4] **out hemorrhage**
           Retained products of conception following deliv-
             ery, without hemorrhage

● **668 Complications of the administration of anesthetic or other sedation in labor and delivery**

    Use additional code(s) to further specify complication

    Requires fifth digit; valid digits are in [brackets] under each code. See beginning of section 660–669 for definitions.

    Includes: complications arising from the administration
                   of a general or local anesthetic, analgesic,
                   or other sedation in labor and delivery

    | **Excludes** | *reaction to spinal or lumbar puncture (349.0)*
                 spinal headache (349.0)

● **668.0 Pulmonary complications**
[0–4]   Inhalation [aspiration] of stomach contents or se-
           cretions following anesthesia or other seda-
             tion in labor or delivery
           Mendelson's syndrome following anesthesia or
             other sedation in labor or delivery
           Pressure collapse of lung following anesthesia or
             other sedation in labor or delivery

● **668.1 Cardiac complications**
[0–4]   Cardiac arrest or failure following anesthesia or
           other sedation in labor and delivery

● **668.2 Central nervous system complications**
[0–4]   Cerebral anoxia following anesthesia or other se-
           dation in labor and delivery

● ❑ **668.8 Other complications of anesthesia or other seda-**
[0–4] **tion in labor and delivery**

● ❑ **668.9 Unspecified complication of anesthesia and other**
[0–4] **sedation**

● **669 Other complications of labor and delivery, not elsewhere classified**

    Requires fifth digit; valid digits are in [brackets] under each code. See beginning of section 660–669 for definitions.

● **669.0 Maternal distress**
[0–4]   Metabolic disturbance in labor and delivery

● **669.1 Shock during or following labor and delivery**
[0–4]   Obstetric shock

● **669.2 Maternal hypotension syndrome**
[0–4]

● **669.3 Acute renal failure following labor and delivery**
[0,2,4]

● ❑ **669.4 Other complications of obstetrical surgery and pro-**
[0–4] **cedures**
           Cardiac:
             arrest following cesarean or other obstetrical
               surgery or procedure, including delivery
               NOS
             failure following cesarean or other obstetrical
               surgery or procedure, including delivery
               NOS
           Cerebral anoxia following cesarean or other ob-
             stetrical surgery or procedure, including de-
             livery NOS

    | **Excludes** | *complications of obstetrical surgical wounds*
                (674.1–674.3)

● **669.5 Forceps or vacuum extractor delivery without men-**
[0,1] **tion of indication**
           Delivery by ventouse, without mention of indica-
             tion

● **669.6 Breech extraction, without mention of indication**
[0,1]

    | **Excludes** | *breech delivery NOS (652.2)*

● **669.7 Cesarean delivery, without mention of indication**
[0,1]

● ❑ **669.8 Other complications of labor and delivery**
[0–4]

● ❑ **669.9 Unspecified complication of labor and delivery**
[0–4]

COMPLICATIONS OF THE PUERPERIUM (670–677)

Note: Categories 671 and 673–676 include the listed conditions even if they occur during pregnancy or childbirth.

The following fifth-digit subclassification is for use with categories 670–676 to denote the current episode of care:
☐ 0 unspecified as to episode of care or not applicable
1 delivered, with or without mention of antepartum condition
2 delivered, with mention of postpartum complication
3 antepartum condition or complication
4 postpartum condition or complication

● 670 Major puerperal infection
[0,2,4]
Requires fifth digit; valid digits are in [brackets] under each code. See beginning of section 670–676 for definitions.

Use 0 as fourth digit for category 670
Puerperal:
  endometritis
  fever (septic)
  pelvic:
    cellulitis
    sepsis
  peritonitis
  pyemia
  salpingitis
  septicemia

Excludes infection following abortion (639.0)
          minor genital tract infection following delivery (646.6)
          puerperal fever NOS (672)
          puerperal pyrexia NOS (672)
          puerperal pyrexia of unknown origin (672)
          urinary tract infection following delivery (646.6)

● 671 Venous complications in pregnancy and the puerperium

Requires fifth digit; valid digits are in [brackets] under each code. See beginning of section 670–676 for definitions.

● 671.0 Varicose veins of legs
[0–4]   Varicose veins NOS

● 671.1 Varicose veins of vulva and perineum
[0–4]

● 671.2 Superficial thrombophlebitis
[0–4]   Thrombophlebitis (superficial)

● 671.3 Deep phlebothrombosis, antepartum
[0,1,3] Deep-vein thrombosis, antepartum

● 671.4 Deep phlebothrombosis, postpartum
[0,2,4] Deep-vein thrombosis, postpartum
         Pelvic thrombophlebitis, postpartum
         Phlegmasia alba dolens (puerperal)

● ☐ 671.5 Other phlebitis and thrombosis
[0–4]   Cerebral venous thrombosis
         Thrombosis of intracranial venous sinus

● ☐ 671.8 Other venous complications
[0–4]   Hemorrhoids

● ☐ 671.9 Unspecified venous complication
[0–4]   Phlebitis NOS
         Thrombosis NOS

● 672 Pyrexia of unknown origin during the puerperium
[0,2,4]   Postpartum fever NOS
              Puerperal fever NOS
              Puerperal pyrexia NOS

Requires fifth digit; valid digits are in [brackets] under each code. See beginning of section 670–676 for definitions.

Use 0 as fourth digit for category 672

● 673 Obstetrical pulmonary embolism

Requires fifth digit; valid digits are in [brackets] under each code. See beginning of section 670–676 for definitions.

Includes: pulmonary emboli in pregnancy, childbirth, or the puerperium, or specified as puerperal

Excludes embolism following abortion (639.6)

● 673.0 Obstetrical air embolism
[0–4]

● 673.1 Amniotic fluid embolism
[0–4]

● 673.2 Obstetrical blood-clot embolism
[0–4]   Puerperal pulmonary embolism NOS

● 673.3 Obstetrical pyemic and septic embolism
[0–4]

● ☐ 673.8 Other pulmonary embolism
[0–4]   Fat embolism

● 674 Other and unspecified complications of the puerperium, not elsewhere classified

Requires fifth digit; valid digits are in [brackets] under each code. See beginning of section 670–676 for definitions.

● 674.0 Cerebrovascular disorders in the puerperium
[0–4]   Any condition classifiable to 430–434, 436–437 occurring during pregnancy, childbirth, or the puerperium, or specified as puerperal

Excludes intracranial venous sinus thrombosis (671.5)

● 674.1 Disruption of cesarean wound
[0,2,4] Dehiscence or disruption of uterine wound

Excludes uterine rupture before onset of labor (665.0)
          uterine rupture during labor (665.1)

● 674.2 Disruption of perineal wound
[0,2,4] Breakdown of perineum
         Disruption of wound of:
           episiotomy
           perineal laceration
         Secondary perineal tear

● ☐ 674.3 Other complications of obstetrical surgical wounds
[0,2,4] Hematoma of cesarean section or perineal wound
         Hemorrhage of cesarean section or perineal wound
         Infection of cesarean section or perineal wound

Excludes damage from instruments in delivery (664.0–665.9)

● 674.4 Placental polyp
[0,2,4]

674.5 Peripartum cardiomyopathy
[0–4]   Postpartum cardiomyopathy

● ☐ 674.8 Other
[0,2,4] Hepatorenal syndrome, following delivery
         Postpartum:
           subinvolution of uterus
           uterine hypertrophy

● ☐ 674.9 Unspecified
[0,2,4] Sudden death of unknown cause during the puerperium

● 675 Infections of the breast and nipple associated with childbirth

Requires fifth digit; valid digits are in [brackets] under each code. See beginning of section 670–676 for definitions.

Includes: the listed conditions during pregnancy, childbirth, or the puerperium

● 675.0 Infections of nipple
[0–4]   Abscess of nipple

ICD-9-CM

675-699

Vol. 1

● **675.1 Abscess of breast**
[0–4]   Abscess:
          mammary
          subareolar
          submammary
        Mastitis:
          purulent
          retromammary
          submammary

● **675.2 Nonpurulent mastitis**
[0–4]   Lymphangitis of breast
        Mastitis:
          NOS
          interstitial
          parenchymatous

● ❑ **675.8 Other specified infections of the breast and nipple**
[0–4]

● ❑ **675.9 Unspecified infection of the breast and nipple**
[0–4]

● **676 Other disorders of the breast associated with childbirth and disorders of lactation**

Requires fifth digit; valid digits are in [brackets] under each code. See beginning of section 670–676 for definitions.

Includes: the listed conditions during pregnancy, the puerperium, or lactation

● **676.0 Retracted nipple**
[0–4]

● **676.1 Cracked nipple**
[0–4]   Fissure of nipple

● **676.2 Engorgement of breasts**
[0–4]

● ❑ **676.3 Other and unspecified disorder of breast**
[0–4]

● **676.4 Failure of lactation**
[0–4]   Agalactia

● **676.5 Suppressed lactation**
[0–4]

● **676.6 Galactorrhea**
[0–4]

     Excludes *galactorrhea not associated with childbirth (611.6)*

● ❑ **676.8 Other disorders of lactation**
[0–4]   Galactocele

● ❑ **676.9 Unspecified disorder of lactation**
[0–4]

❑ **677 Late effect of complication of pregnancy, childbirth, and the puerperium**

Note: This category is to be used to indicate conditions in 632–648.9 and 651–676.9 as the cause of the late effect, themselves classifiable elsewhere. The "late effects" include conditions specified as such, or as sequelae, which may occur at any time after the puerperium.

Code first any sequelae

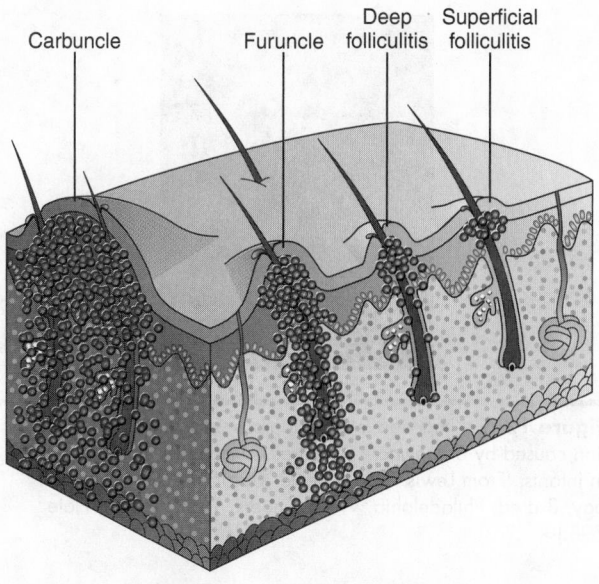

Carbuncle   Furuncle   Deep folliculitis   Superficial folliculitis

Figure 12–1 Furuncle, also known as a boil, is a staphylococcal infection. The organism enters the body through a hair follicle and so furuncles usually appear in hairy areas of the body. A cluster of furuncles is known as a carbuncle and involves infection into the deep subcutaneous fascia. These usually appear on the back and neck.

12. DISEASES OF THE SKIN AND SUBCUTANEOUS TISSUE (680–709)

INFECTIONS OF SKIN AND SUBCUTANEOUS TISSUE (680–686)

> **Excludes** *certain infections of skin classified under "Infectious and Parasitic Diseases," such as:*
> *erysipelas (035)*
> *erysipeloid of Rosenbach (027.1)*
> *herpes:*
> *simplex (054.0–054.9)*
> *zoster (053.0–053.9)*
> *molluscum contagiosum (078.0)*
> *viral warts (078.1)*

● **680 Carbuncle and furuncle**

> **Includes:** boil
> furunculosis

680.0 Face
Ear [any part]   Nose (septum)
Face [any part, except eye]   Temple (region)

> **Excludes** *eyelid (373.13)*
> *lacrimal apparatus (375.31)*
> *orbit (376.01)*

680.1 Neck

680.2 Trunk
Abdominal wall
Back [any part, except buttocks]
Breast
Chest wall
Flank
Groin
Pectoral region
Perineum
Umbilicus

> **Excludes** *buttocks (680.5)*
> *external genital organs:*
> *female (616.4)*
> *male (607.2, 608.4)*

680.3 Upper arm and forearm
Arm [any part, except hand]
Axilla
Shoulder

680.4 Hand
Finger [any]   Wrist
Thumb

680.5 Buttock
Anus   Gluteal region

680.6 Leg, except foot
Ankle   Knee
Hip   Thigh

680.7 Foot
Heel   Toe

☐ **680.8 Other specified sites**
Head [any part, except face]
Scalp

> **Excludes** *external genital organs:*
> *female (616.4)*
> *male (607.2, 608.4)*

☐ **680.9 Unspecified site**
Boil NOS   Furuncle NOS
Carbuncle NOS

● **681 Cellulitis and abscess of finger and toe**

> **Includes:** that with lymphangitis

Use additional code to identify organism, such as Staphylococcus (041.1)

● **681.0 Finger**

681.00 Cellulitis and abscess, unspecified

681.01 Felon
Pulp abscess   Whitlow

> **Excludes** *herpetic whitlow (054.6)*

681.02 Onychia and paronychia of finger
Panaritium of finger
Perionychia of finger

● **681.1 Toe**

☐ **681.10 Cellulitis and abscess, unspecified**

681.11 Onychia and paronychia of toe
Panaritium of toe
Perionychia of toe

☐ **681.9 Cellulitis and abscess of unspecified digit**
Infection of nail NOS

● **682 Other cellulitis and abscess**

> **Includes:** abscess (acute) (with lymphangitis) except of finger or toe
> cellulitis (diffuse) (with lymphangitis) except of finger or toe
> lymphangitis, acute (with lymphangitis) except of finger or toe

Use additional code to identify organism, such as Staphylococcus (041.1)

> **Excludes** *lymphangitis (chronic) (subacute) (457.2)*

682.0 Face
Cheek, external   Nose, external
Chin   Submandibular
Forehead   Temple (region)

> **Excludes** *ear [any part] (380.10–380.16)*
> *eyelid (373.13)*
> *lacrimal apparatus (375.31)*
> *lip (528.5)*
> *mouth (528.3)*
> *nose (internal) (478.1)*
> *orbit (376.01)*

ICD-9-CM

680–699

Vol. 1

682.1 Neck

682.2 Trunk
        Abdominal wall
        Back [any part, except buttocks]
        Chest wall
        Flank
        Groin
        Pectoral region
        Perineum
        Umbilicus, except newborn

> **Excludes**   *anal and rectal regions (566)*
>   *breast:*
>   *NOS (611.0)*
>   *puerperal (675.1)*
>   *external genital organs:*
>   *female (616.3–616.4)*
>   *male (604.0, 607.2, 608.4)*
>   *umbilicus, newborn (771.4)*

682.3 Upper arm and forearm
        Arm [any part, except hand]
        Axilla
        Shoulder

> **Excludes**   *hand (682.4)*

682.4 Hand, except fingers and thumb
        Wrist

> **Excludes**   *fingers and thumb (681.00–681.02)*

682.5 Buttocks
        Gluteal region

> **Excludes**   *anal and rectal regions (566)*

682.6 Leg, except foot
        Ankle
        Hip
        Knee
        Thigh

682.7 Foot, except toes
        Heel

> **Excludes**   *toe (681.10–681.11)*

☐ 682.8 Other specified sites
        Head [except face]
        Scalp

> **Excludes**   *face (682.0)*

☐ 682.9 Unspecified site
        Abscess NOS
        Cellulitis NOS
        Lymphangitis, acute NOS

> **Excludes**   *lymphangitis NOS (457.2)*

683 Acute lymphadenitis
        Abscess (acute) lymph gland or node, except mesenteric
        Adenitis, acute lymph gland or node, except mesenteric
        Lymphadenitis, acute lymph gland or node, except mesenteric

Use additional code to identify organism such as Staphylococcus (041.1)

> **Excludes**   *enlarged glands NOS (785.6)*
>   *lymphadenitis:*
>   *chronic or subacute, except mesenteric (289.1)*
>   *mesenteric (acute) (chronic) (subacute) (289.2)*
>   *unspecified (289.3)*

684 Impetigo
        Impetiginization of other dermatoses
        Impetigo (contagiosa) [any site] [any organism]:
          bullous   neonatorum
          circinate   simplex
        Pemphigus neonatorum

> **Excludes**   *impetigo herpetiformis (694.3)l*

Figure 12–2   Impetigo is a contagious, superficial skin infection caused by *Staphylococcus aureus*. It appears most frequently in infants. (From Lewis GM, Wheeler CE, Jr: Practical Dermatology, 3rd ed. Philadelphia, WB Saunders, 1967, p 234, Plate 79B.)

Item 12–1 Pilonidal cyst, also called a coccygeal cyst, is the result of a disorder called pilonidal disease. The cyst usually contains hair and pus.

● 685 Pilonidal cyst

> **Includes:** fistula, coccygeal or pilonidal
>   sinus, coccygeal or pilonidal

  685.0 With abscess

  685.1 Without mention of abscess

● 686 Other local infections of skin and subcutaneous tissue

Use additional code to identify any infectious organism (041.0–041.8)

● 686.0 Pyoderma
        Dermatitis:
          purulent
          septic
          suppurative

  ☐ 686.00 Pyoderma, unspecified

  686.01 Pyoderma gangrenosum

  ☐ 686.09 Other pyoderma

686.1 Pyogenic granuloma
        Granuloma:
          septic
          suppurative
          telangiectaticum

> **Excludes**   *pyogenic granuloma of oral mucosa (528.9)*

☐ 686.8 Other specified local infections of skin and subcutaneous tissue
        Bacterid (pustular)   Ecthyma
        Dermatitis vegetans   Perlèche

> **Excludes**   *dermatitis infectiosa eczematoides (690.8)*
>   *panniculitis (729.30–729.39)*

☐ 686.9 Unspecified local infection of skin and subcutaneous tissue
        Fistula of skin NOS
        Skin infection NOS

> **Excludes**   *fistula to skin from internal organs—see Alphabetic Index*

Figure 12-3 Severe seborrheic dermatitis. (From Arnold HL, Odom RB, James WD: Andrews' Diseases of the Skin, Clinical Dermatology, 8th ed. Philadelphia, WB Saunders, 1990, p 195.)

Item 12-2 Seborrheic dermatitis is characterized by greasy, scaly, red patches and is associated with oily skin and scalp.

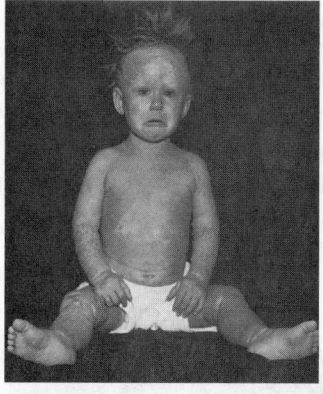

Figure 12-4 Atopic dermatitis. (From Moschella SL, Hurley HJ: Dermatology, 2nd ed. Philadelphia, WB Saunders, 1985, p 336.)

Item 12-3 Atopic dermatitis, also known as atopic eczema, infantile eczema, disseminated neurodermatitis, flexural eczema, and *prurigo diathesique* (Besnier), is characterized by intense itching and is often hereditary.

OTHER INFLAMMATORY CONDITIONS OF SKIN AND SUBCUTANEOUS TISSUE (690–698)

Excludes *panniculitis (729.30–729.39)*

● **690 Erythematosquamous dermatosis**

Excludes *eczematous dermatitis of eyelid (373.31)*
parakeratosis variegata (696.2)
psoriasis (696.0–696.1)
seborrheic keratosis (702.11–702.19)

● **690.1 Seborrheic dermatitis**

❑ **690.10 Seborrheic dermatitis, unspecified**
Seborrheic dermatitis NOS

690.11 Seborrhea capitis
Cradle cap

690.12 Seborrheic infantile dermatitis

❑ **690.18 Other seborrheic dermatitis**

❑ **690.8 Other erythematosquamous dermatosis**

● **691 Atopic dermatitis and related conditions**

691.0 Diaper or napkin rash
Ammonia dermatitis
Diaper or napkin:
dermatitis
erythema
rash
Psoriasiform napkin eruption

❑ **691.8 Other atopic dermatitis and related conditions**
Atopic dermatitis
Besnier's prurigo
Eczema:
atopic
flexural
intrinsic (allergic)
Neurodermatitis:
atopic
diffuse (of Brocq)

● **692 Contact dermatitis and other eczema**

Includes: dermatitis:
NOS
contact
occupational
venenata
eczema (acute) (chronic):
NOS
allergic
erythematous
occupational

Excludes *allergy NOS (995.3)*
contact dermatitis of eyelids (373.32)
dermatitis due to substances taken internally (693.0–693.9)
eczema of external ear (380.22)
perioral dermatitis (695.3)
urticarial reactions (708.0–708.9, 995.1)

692.0 Due to detergents

692.1 Due to oils and greases

692.2 Due to solvents
Dermatitis due to solvents of:
chlorocompound group
cyclohexane group
ester group
glycol group
hydrocarbon group
ketone group

692.3 Due to drugs and medicines in contact with skin
Dermatitis (allergic) (contact) due to:
arnica
fungicides
iodine
keratolytics
mercurials
neomycin
pediculocides
phenols
scabicides
any drug applied to skin
Dermatitis medicamentosa due to drug applied to skin

Use additional E code to identify drug

Excludes *allergy NOS due to drugs (995.2)*
dermatitis due to ingested drugs (693.0)
dermatitis medicamentosa NOS (693.0)

❑ **692.4 Due to other chemical products**

Dermatitis due to:	Dermatitis due to:
acids	insecticide
adhesive plaster	nylon
alkalis	plastic
caustics	rubber
dichromate	

ICD-9-CM

600-699

Vol.

692.5 Due to food in contact with skin
  Dermatitis, contact, due to:
    cereals
    fish
    flour
    fruit
    meat
    milk

  | Excludes | *dermatitis due to:*
              dyes (692.89)
              ingested foods (693.1)
              preservatives (692.89)

692.6 Due to plants [except food]
  Dermatitis due to:
    lacquer tree [Rhus verniciflua]
    poison:
      ivy [Rhus toxicodendron]
      oak [Rhus diversiloba]
      sumac [Rhus venenata]
      vine [Rhus radicans]
    primrose [Primula]
    ragweed [Senecio jacobae]
    other plants in contact with the skin

  | Excludes | *allergy NOS due to pollen (477.0)*
              nettle rash (708.8)

● **692.7 Due to solar radiation**

  | Excludes | *sunburn due to other ultraviolet radiation expo-*
              sure (692.82)

  ❏ **692.70 Unspecified dermatitis due to sun**

  692.71 Sunburn
    First degree sunburn
    Sunburn NOS

  692.72 Acute dermatitis due to solar radiation
    Berloque dermatitis
    Photoallergic response
    Phototoxic response
    Polymorphous light eruption
    Acute solar skin damage NOS

  | Excludes | *sunburn (692.71, 692.76–692.77)*

    Use additional E code to identify drug, if
    drug induced

  692.73 Actinic reticuloid and actinic granuloma

  ❏ **692.74 Other chronic dermatitis due to solar radia-**
             tion
    Chronic solar skin damage NOS
    Solar elastosis

  | Excludes | *actinic [solar] keratosis (702.0)*

  692.75 Disseminated superficial actinic porokerato-
           sis (DSAP)

  692.76 Sunburn of second degree

  692.77 Sunburn of third degree

  ❏ **692.79 Other dermatitis due to solar radiation**
    Hydroa aestivale
    Photodermatitis (due to sun)
    Photosensitiveness (due to sun)
    Solar skin damage NOS

● **692.8 Due to other specified agents**

  692.81 Dermatitis due to cosmetics

  ❏ **692.82 Dermatitis due to other radiation**
    Infrared rays
    Light, except from sun
    Radiation NOS
    Tanning bed
    Ultraviolet rays, except from sun
    X-rays

  | Excludes | *that due to solar radiation (692.70–692.79)*

692.83 Dermatitis due to metals
    Jewelry

692.84 Due to animal (cat) (dog) dander ◄
    Due to animal (cat) (dog) hair ◄

❏ **692.89 Other**
    Dermatitis due to:
      cold weather   hot weather
      dyes   preservatives

  | Excludes | *allergy (NOS) (rhinitis) due to animal hair or*
              dander (477.2) ◄
              allergy to dust (477.8)
              sunburn (692.71, 692.76–692.77)

❏ **692.9 Unspecified cause**
    Dermatitis:
      NOS
      contact NOS
      venenata NOS
    Eczema NOS

● **693 Dermatitis due to substances taken internally**

  | Excludes | *adverse effect NOS of drugs and medicines (995.2)*
              allergy NOS (995.3)
              contact dermatitis (692.0–692.9)
              urticarial reactions (708.0–708.9, 995.1)

  693.0 Due to drugs and medicines
    Dermatitis medicamentosa NOS

    Use additional E code to identify drug

  | Excludes | *that due to drugs in contact with skin (692.3)*

  693.1 Due to food

  ❏ **693.8 Due to other specified substances taken internally**

  ❏ **693.9 Due to unspecified substance taken internally**

  | Excludes | *dermatitis NOS (692.9)*

Figure 12–5 Dermatitis herpetiformis. (From Arnold HL, Odom
RB, James WD: Andrews' Diseases of the Skin, Clinical
Dermatology, 8th ed. Philadelphia, WB Saunders, 1990, p 553.)

Item 12–4 Dermatitis herpetiformis, also known as
Duhring's disease, is a systemic disease characterized by
small blisters (3 to 5 mm) and occasionally large bullae
(+5 mm).

● 694 **Bullous dermatoses**

694.0 **Dermatitis herpetiformis**
Dermatosis herpetiformis
Duhring's disease
Hydroa herpetiformis

Excludes *herpes gestationis (646.8)*
dermatitis herpetiformis:
juvenile (694.2)
senile (694.5)

694.1 **Subcorneal pustular dermatosis**
Sneddon-Wilkinson disease or syndrome

694.2 **Juvenile dermatitis herpetiformis**
Juvenile pemphigoid

694.3 **Impetigo herpetiformis**

694.4 **Pemphigus**
Pemphigus:
NOS
erythematosus
foliaceus
malignant
vegetans
vulgaris

Excludes *pemphigus neonatorum (684)*

694.5 **Pemphigoid**
Benign pemphigus NOS
Bullous pemphigoid
Herpes circinatus bullosus
Senile dermatitis herpetiformis

● 694.6 **Benign mucous membrane pemphigoid**
Cicatricial pemphigoid
Mucosynechial atrophic bullous dermatitis

694.60 **Without mention of ocular involvement**

694.61 **With ocular involvement**
Ocular pemphigus

❏ 694.8 **Other specified bullous dermatoses**
Excludes *herpes gestationis (646.8)*

❏ 694.9 **Unspecified bullous dermatoses**

● 695 **Erythematous conditions**

695.0 **Toxic erythema**
Erythema venenatum

695.1 **Erythema multiforme**
Erythema iris
Herpes iris
Lyell's syndrome
Scalded skin syndrome
Stevens-Johnson syndrome
Toxic epidermal necrolysis

695.2 **Erythema nodosum**
Excludes *tuberculous erythema nodosum (017.1)*

695.3 **Rosacea**
Acne: Perioral dermatitis
erythematosa   Rhinophyma
rosacea

695.4 **Lupus erythematosus**
Lupus:
erythematodes (discoid)
erythematosus (discoid), not disseminated

Excludes *lupus (vulgaris) NOS (017.0)*
systemic [disseminated] lupus erythematosus
(710.0)

● 695.8 **Other specified erythematous conditions**

695.81 **Ritter's disease**
Dermatitis exfoliativa neonatorum

Figure 12-6 Psoriasis. (From Moschella SL, Hurley HJ: Dermatology, 2nd ed. Philadelphia, WB Saunders, 1985, p 512.)

Item 12-5 Psoriasis is a chronic, recurrent inflammatory skin disease characterized by small patches covered with thick silvery scales. **Parapsoriasis** is a treatment-resistant erythroderma. **Pityriasis rosea** is characterized by a herald patch that is a single large lesion and that usually appears on the trunk and is followed by scattered, smaller lesions.

❏695.89 **Other**
Erythema intertrigo
Intertrigo
Pityriasis rubra (Hebra)

Excludes *mycotic intertrigo (111.0–111.9)*

❏695.9 **Unspecified erythematous condition**
Erythema NOS
Erythroderma (secondary)

● 696 **Psoriasis and similar disorders**

696.0 **Psoriatic arthropathy**

❏696.1 **Other psoriasis**
Acrodermatitis continua
Dermatitis repens
Psoriasis:
NOS
any type, except arthropathic

Excludes *psoriatic arthropathy (696.0)*

696.2 **Parapsoriasis**
Parakeratosis variegata
Parapsoriasis lichenoides chronica
Pityriasis lichenoides et varioliformis

696.3 **Pityriasis rosea**
Pityriasis circinata (et maculata)

696.4 **Pityriasis rubra pilaris**
Devergie's disease
Lichen ruber acuminatus

Excludes *pityriasis rubra (Hebra) (695.89)*

❏696.5 **Other and unspecified pityriasis**
Pityriasis:
NOS
alba
streptogenes

ICD-9-CM

699-709

Vol. 1

Excludes | pityriasis:
simplex (690.18)
versicolor (111.0)

☐ **696.8 Other**

● **697 Lichen**

Excludes | lichen:
obtusus corneus (698.3)
pilaris (congenital) (757.39)
ruber acuminatus (696.4)
sclerosus et atrophicus (701.0)
scrofulosus (017.0)
simplex chronicus (698.3)
spinulosus (congenital) (757.39)
urticatus (698.2)

697.0 Lichen planus
Lichen:
planopilaris
ruber planus

697.1 Lichen nitidus
Pinkus' disease

☐ **697.8 Other lichen, not elsewhere classified**
Lichen:
ruber moniliforme
striata

☐ **697.9 Lichen, unspecified**

● **698 Pruritus and related conditions**

Excludes | pruritus specified as psychogenic (306.3)

698.0 Pruritus ani
Perianal itch

698.1 Pruritus of genital organs

698.2 Prurigo
Lichen urticatus
Prurigo:
NOS
Hebra's
mitis
simplex
Urticaria papulosa (Hebra)

Excludes | prurigo nodularis (698.3)

698.3 Lichenification and lichen simplex chronicus
Hyde's disease
Neurodermatitis (circumscripta) (local)
Prurigo nodularis

Excludes | neurodermatitis, diffuse (of Brocq) (691.8)

698.4 Dermatitis factitia [artefacta]
Dermatitis ficta
Neurotic excoriation

Use additional code to identify any associated mental disorder

☐ **698.8 Other specified pruritic conditions**
Pruritus:
hiemalis
senilis
Winter itch

☐ **698.9 Unspecified pruritic disorder**
Itch NOS
Pruritus NOS

Item 12-6 **Keratoderma** is characterized by firm horny papules that have a cobblestone appearance. **Keratoderma climactericum,** also known as endocrine keratoderma, is hyperkeratosis located on the palms and soles.

OTHER DISEASES OF SKIN AND SUBCUTANEOUS TISSUE (700–709)

Excludes | conditions confined to eyelids (373.0–374.9)
congenital conditions of skin, hair, and nails (757.0–757.9)

700 Corns and callosities
Callus
Clavus

● **701 Other hypertrophic and atrophic conditions of skin**

Excludes | dermatomyositis (710.3)
hereditary edema of legs (757.0)
scleroderma (generalized) (710.1)

701.0 Circumscribed scleroderma
Addison's keloid
Dermatosclerosis, localized
Lichen sclerosus et atrophicus
Morphea
Scleroderma, circumscribed or localized

701.1 Keratoderma, acquired
Acquired:
ichthyosis
keratoderma palmaris et plantaris
Elastosis perforans serpiginosa
Hyperkeratosis:
NOS
follicularis in cutem penetrans
palmoplantaris climacterica
Keratoderma:
climactericum
tylodes, progressive
Keratosis (blennorrhagica)

Excludes | Darier's disease [keratosis follicularis] (congenital) (757.39)
keratosis:
arsenical (692.4)
gonococcal (098.81)

701.2 Acquired acanthosis nigricans
Keratosis nigricans

701.3 Striae atrophicae
Atrophic spots of skin
Atrophoderma maculatum
Atrophy blanche (of Milian)
Degenerative colloid atrophy
Senile degenerative atrophy
Striae distensae

701.4 Keloid scar
Cheloid
Hypertrophic scar
Keloid

☐ **701.5 Other abnormal granulation tissue**
Excessive granulation

☐ **701.8 Other specified hypertrophic and atrophic conditions of skin**
Acrodermatitis atrophicans chronica
Atrophia cutis senilis
Atrophoderma neuriticum
Confluent and reticulate papillomatosis
Cutis laxa senilis
Elastosis senilis
Folliculitis ulerythematosa reticulata
Gougerot-Carteaud syndrome or disease

☐ **701.9 Unspecified hypertrophic and atrophic conditions of skin**
Atrophoderma

● **702 Other dermatoses**

Excludes | carcinoma in situ (232.0–232.9)

702.0 Actinic keratosis

● **702.1 Seborrheic keratosis**

     702.11 Inflamed seborrheic keratosis

❑ **702.19 Other seborrheic keratosis**
     Seborrheic keratosis NOS

❑ **702.8 Other specified dermatoses**

● **703 Diseases of nail**
    Excludes *congenital anomalies (757.5)*
             onychia and paronychia (681.02, 681.11)

   703.0 Ingrowing nail
     Ingrowing nail with infection
     Unguis incarnatus
    Excludes *infection, nail NOS (681.9)*

❑ **703.8 Other specified diseases of nail**
     Dystrophia unguium
     Hypertrophy of nail
     Koilonychia
     Leukonychia (punctata) (striata)
     Onychauxis
     Onychogryposis
     Onycholysis

❑ **703.9 Unspecified disease of nail**

Figure 12-7 Male pattern alopecia.

Item 12-7 Alopecia is lack of hair and takes many forms. The most common is male pattern alopecia, also known as **androgenetic alopecia. Telogen effluvium** is early and excessive loss of hair resulting from a trauma to the hair (fever, drugs, surgery, etc.).

● **704 Diseases of hair and hair follicles**
    Excludes *congenital anomalies (757.4)*

● **704.0 Alopecia**
    Excludes *madarosis (374.55)*
             syphilitic alopecia (091.82)

❑ **704.00 Alopecia, unspecified**
     Baldness   Loss of hair

     704.01 Alopecia areata
        Ophiasis

     704.02 Telogen effluvium

❑ **704.09 Other**
     Folliculitis decalvans
     Hypotrichosis:
       NOS
       postinfectional NOS
     Pseudopelade

Item 12-8 Hirsutism is excessive growth of hair.

     704.1 Hirsutism
       Hypertrichosis: Polytrichia
       NOS
       lanuginosa, acquired
    Excludes *hypertrichosis of eyelid (374.54)*

     704.2 Abnormalities of the hair
       Atrophic hair   Trichiasis:
       Clastothrix   NOS
       Fragilitas crinium   cicatrical
                      Trichorrhexis (nodosa)
    Excludes *trichiasis of eyelid (374.05)*

     704.3 Variations in hair color
       Canities (premature)
       Grayness, hair (premature)
       Heterochromia of hair
       Poliosis:
         NOS
         circumscripta, acquired

❑ **704.8 Other specified diseases of hair and hair follicles**
     Folliculitis:
       NOS
       abscedens et suffodiens
       pustular
     Perifolliculitis:
       NOS
       capitis abscedens et suffodiens
       scalp
     Sycosis:
       NOS
       barbae [not parasitic]
       lupoid
       vulgaris

❑ **704.9 Unspecified disease of hair and hair follicles**

● **705 Disorders of sweat glands**

     705.0 Anhidrosis
       Hypohidrosis   Oligohidrosis

     705.1 Prickly heat
       Heat rash   Sudamina
       Miliaria rubra (tropicalis)

     705.2 Focal hyperhidrosis ◄
    Excludes *generalized (secondary) hyperhidrosis (780.8)* ◄

       705.21 Primary focal hyperhidrosis ◄
         Focal hyperhidrosis NOS ◄
         Hyperhidrosis NOS ◄
         Hyperhidrosis of: ◄
           axilla ◄
           face ◄
           palms ◄
           soles ◄
       705.22 Secondary focal hyperhidrosis ◄
         Frey's syndrome ◄

ICD-9-CM
700-
799
Vol. 1

● **705.8 Other specified disorders of sweat glands**

    705.81 Dyshidrosis
        Cheiropompholyx
        Pompholyx

    705.82 Fox-Fordyce disease

    705.83 Hidradenitis
        Hidradenitis suppurativa

    ❑ **705.89 Other**
        Bromhidrosis   Granulosis rubra nasi
        Chromhidrosis   Urhidrosis

        | **Excludes** | *hidrocystoma (216.0–216.9)* |
                    generalized hyperhidrosis (780.8) ◀▥

❑ **705.9 Unspecified disorder of sweat glands**
    Disorder of sweat glands NOS

● **706 Diseases of sebaceous glands**

    706.0 Acne varioliformis
        Acne: Acne:
          frontalis   necrotica

    ❑ **706.1 Other acne**
        Acne:
          NOS
          conglobata
          cystic
          pustular
          vulgaris
        Blackhead
        Comedo

        | **Excludes** | *acne rosacea (695.3)* |

    706.2 Sebaceous cyst
        Atheroma, skin   Wen
        Keratin cyst

    706.3 Seborrhea

        | **Excludes** | *seborrhea:* |
                capitis (690.11)
                sicca (690.18)
           seborrheic:
                dermatitis (690.10)
                keratosis (702.11–702.19)

    ❑ **706.8 Other specified diseases of sebaceous glands**
        Asteatosis (cutis)
        Xerosis cutis

    ❑ **706.9 Unspecified disease of sebaceous glands**

● **707 Chronic ulcer of skin**

    Includes: non-infected sinus of skin
               non-healing ulcer

    | **Excludes** | *specific infections classified under "Infectious and Parasitic Diseases" (001.0–136.9)* |
                    varicose ulcer (454.0, 454.2)

● **707.0 Decubitus ulcer**
    Bed sore   Plaster ulcer
    Decubitus ulcer [any site] Pressure ulcer

    ❑ **707.00 Unspecified site** ◀

    707.01 Elbow ◀

    707.02 Upper back ◀
        Shoulder blades

    707.03 Lower back ◀
        Sacrum

    707.04 Hip ◀

    707.05 Buttock ◀

    707.06 Ankle ◀

    707.07 Heel ◀

    707.09 Other site ◀
        Head

707.1 Ulcer of lower limbs, except decubitus
    Ulcer, chronic, of lower limb:
        neurogenic of lower limb
        trophic of lower limb

    Code if applicable, any causal condition first:
        atherosclerosis of the extremities with ulceration
          (440.23)
        chronic venous hypertension with ulcer (459.31)
        chronic venous hypertension with ulcer and in-
          flammation (459.33)
        diabetes mellitus (250.80–250.83)
        postphlebetic syndrome with ulcer (459.11)
        postphlebetic syndrome with ulcer and inflamma-
          tion (459.13)

    707.10 Ulcer of lower limb, unspecified

    707.11 Ulcer of thigh

    707.12 Ulcer of calf

    707.13 Ulcer of ankle

    707.14 Ulcer of heel and midfoot
        Plantar surface of midfoot

    707.15 Ulcer of other part of foot
        Toes

    707.19 Ulcer of other part of lower limb

❑ **707.8 Chronic ulcer of other specified sites**
    Ulcer, chronic, of other specified sites:
        neurogenic of other specified sites
        trophic of other specified sites

❑ **707.9 Chronic ulcer of unspecified site**
    Chronic ulcer NOS   Tropical ulcer NOS
    Trophic ulcer NOS   Ulcer of skin NOS

● **708 Urticaria**

    | **Excludes** | *edema:* |
                angioneurotic (995.1)
                Quincke's (995.1)
          hereditary angioedema (277.6)
          urticaria:
                giant (995.1)
                papulosa (Hebra) (698.2)
                pigmentosa (juvenile) (congenital) (757.33)

708.0 Allergic urticaria

708.1 Idiopathic urticaria

Figure 12–8   Urticaria, or hives. (From Arnold HL, Odom RB, James WD: Andrews' Diseases of the Skin, Clinical Dermatology, 8th ed. Philadelphia, WB Saunders, 1990, p 148.)

Item 12-9   Urticaria is a vascular reaction in which wheals surrounded by a red halo appear and cause severe itching. The causes of urticaria or hives are extensive and varied (e.g., food, heat, cold, drugs, stress, infections).

708.2 Urticaria due to cold and heat
Thermal urticaria

708.3 Dermatographic urticaria
Dermatographia
Factitial urticaria

708.4 Vibratory urticaria

708.5 Cholinergic urticaria

❑ **708.8 Other specified urticaria**
Nettle rash
Urticaria:
  chronic
  recurrent periodic

❑ **708.9 Urticaria, unspecified**
Hives NOS

● **709 Other disorders of skin and subcutaneous tissue**

  ● **709.0 Dyschromia**

  Excludes   albinism (270.2)
      pigmented nevus (216.0–216.9)
      that of eyelid (374.52–374.53)

   ❑ **709.00 Dyschromia, unspecified**

   709.01 Vitiligo

   ❑ **709.09 Other**

  709.1 Vascular disorders of skin
  Angioma serpiginosum
  Purpura (primary) annularis telangiectodes

709.2 Scar conditions and fibrosis of skin
Adherent scar (skin)
Cicatrix
Disfigurement (due to scar)
Fibrosis, skin NOS
Scar NOS

Excludes   keloid scar (701.4)

709.3 Degenerative skin disorders
Calcinosis:
  circumscripta
  cutis
Colloid milium
Degeneration, skin
Deposits, skin
Senile dermatosis NOS
Subcutaneous calcification

709.4 Foreign body granuloma of skin and subcutaneous tissue

Excludes   residual foreign body without granuloma of skin
      and subcutaneous tissue (729.6)
      that of muscle (728.82)

❑ **709.8 Other specified disorders of skin**
Epithelial hyperplasia
Menstrual dermatosis
Vesicular eruption

❑ **709.9 Unspecified disorder of skin and subcutaneous tissue**
Dermatosis NOS

ICD-9-CM

700-799

Vol. 1

13. DISEASES OF THE MUSCULOSKELETAL SYSTEM AND CONNECTIVE TISSUE (710–739)

The following fifth-digit subclassification is for use with categories 711–712, 715–716, 718–719, and 730:

☐ 0 site unspecified
   1 shoulder region
      Acromioclavicular joint(s)
      Clavicle
      Glenohumeral joint(s)
      Scapula
      Sternoclavicular joint(s)
   2 upper arm
      Elbow joint
      Humerus
   3 forearm
      Radius
      Ulna
      Wrist joint
   4 hand
      Carpus
      Metacarpus
      Phalanges [fingers]
   5 pelvic region and thigh
      Buttock
      Femur
      Hip (joint)
   6 lower leg
      Fibula
      Knee joint
      Patella
      Tibia
   7 ankle and foot
      Ankle joint
      Digits [toes]
      Metatarsus
      Phalanges, foot
      Tarsus
      Other joints in foot
☐ 8 other specified sites
      Head
      Neck
      Ribs
      Skull
      Trunk
      Vertebral column
☐ 9 multiple sites

ARTHROPATHIES AND RELATED DISORDERS (710–719)

| Excludes | *disorders of spine (720.0–724.9)* |

● **710 Diffuse diseases of connective tissue**

   Includes: all collagen diseases whose effects are not mainly confined to a single system

   | Excludes | *those affecting mainly the cardiovascular system, i.e., polyarteritis nodosa and allied conditions (446.0–446.7)* |

   710.0 Systemic lupus erythematosus
      Disseminated lupus erythematosus
      Libman-Sacks disease

      Use additional code to identify manifestation, as:
         endocarditis (424.91)
         nephritis (583.81)
            chronic (582.81)
         nephrotic syndrome (581.81)

   | Excludes | *lupus erythematosus (discoid) NOS (695.4)* |

   710.1 Systemic sclerosis
      Acrosclerosis
      CRST syndrome
      Progressive systemic sclerosis
      Scleroderma

      Use additional code to identify manifestations, as:
         lung involvement (517.2)
         myopathy (359.6)

   | Excludes | *circumscribed scleroderma (701.0)* |

   710.2 Sicca syndrome
      Keratoconjunctivitis sicca
      Sjögren's disease

   710.3 Dermatomyositis
      Poikilodermatomyositis
      Polymyositis with skin involvement

   710.4 Polymyositis

   710.5 Eosinophilia myalgia syndrome
      Toxic oil syndrome

      Use additional E code to identify drug, if drug induced

☐ **710.8 Other specified diffuse diseases of connective tissue**
      Multifocal fibrosclerosis (idiopathic) NEC
      Systemic fibrosclerosing syndrome

☐ **710.9 Unspecified diffuse connective tissue disease**
      Collagen disease NOS

● **711 Arthropathy associated with infections**

   Includes: arthritis associated with conditions classifiable below
   arthropathy associated with conditions classifiable below
   polyarthritis associated with conditions classifiable below
   polyarthropathy associated with conditions classifiable below

   | Excludes | *rheumatic fever (390)* |

   The following fifth-digit subclassification is for use with category 711; valid digits are in [brackets] under each code. See list at beginning of chapter for definitions:

☐ 0 site unspecified
   1 shoulder region
   2 upper arm
   3 forearm
   4 hand
   5 pelvic region and thigh
   6 lower leg
   7 ankle and foot
☐ 8 other specified sites
☐ 9 multiple sites

● **711.0 Pyogenic arthritis**
   [0–9]   Arthritis or polyarthritis (due to):
             coliform [Escherichia coli]
             Hemophilus influenzae [H. influenzae]
             pneumococcal
             Pseudomonas
             staphylococcal
             streptococcal
             Pyarthrosis

      Use additional code to identify infectious organism (041.0–041.8)

●● ***711.1 Arthropathy associated with Reiter's disease and***
   [0–9] ***nonspecific urethritis***

      Code first underlying disease, as:
         nonspecific urethritis (099.4)
         Reiter's disease (099.3)

●● ***711.2 Arthropathy in Behçet's syndrome***
   [0–9] *Code first underlying disease (136.1)*

●● **711.3** *Postdysentericarthropathy*
[0–9]
    Code first underlying disease, as:
        dysentery (009.0)
        enteritis, infectious (008.0–009.3)
        paratyphoid fever (002.1–002.9)
        typhoid fever (002.0)
    Excludes *salmonella arthritis (003.23)*

●●❑ **711.4** *Arthropathy associated with other bacterial diseases*
[0–9]
    Code first underlying disease, as:
        diseases classifiable to 010–040, 090–099, except as in 711.1, 711.3, and 713.5
        leprosy (030.0–030.9)
        tuberculosis (015.0–015.9)
    Excludes *gonococcal arthritis (098.50)*
                 meningococcal arthritis (036.82)

●●❑ **711.5** *Arthropathy associated with other viral diseases*
[0–9]
    Code first underlying disease, as:
        diseases classifiable to 045–049, 050–079, 480, 487
        O'nyong-nyong (066.3)
    Excludes *that due to rubella (056.71)*

●● **711.6** *Arthropathy associated with mycoses*
[0–9]
    Code first underlying disease (110.0–118)

●● **711.7** *Arthropathy associated with helminthiasis*
[0–9]
    Code first underlying disease, as:
        filariasis (125.0–125.9)

●●❑ **711.8** *Arthropathy associated with other infectious and parasitic diseases*
[0–9]
    Code first underlying disease, as:
        diseases classifiable to 080–088, 100–104, 130–136
    Excludes *arthropathy associated with sarcoidosis (713.7)*

●❑ **711.9** **Unspecified infective arthritis**
[0–9]
    Infective arthritis or polyarthritis (acute) (chronic) (subacute) NOS

● **712** **Crystal arthropathies**

    Includes: crystal-induced arthritis and synovitis
    Excludes *gouty arthropathy (274.0)*

The following fifth-digit subclassification is for use with category 712; valid digits are in [brackets] under each code. See list at beginning of chapter for definitions:
❑ 0 site unspecified
   1 shoulder region
   2 upper arm
   3 forearm
   4 hand
   5 pelvic region and thigh
   6 lower leg
   7 ankle and foot
❑ 8 other specified sites
❑ 9 multiple sites

●● **712.1** *Chondrocalcinosis due to dicalcium phosphate crystals*
[0–9]
    Chondrocalcinosis due to dicalcium phosphate crystals (with other crystals)
    Code first underlying disease (275.4)

●● **712.2** *Chondrocalcinosis due to pyrophosphate crystals*
[0–9]
    Code first underlying disease (275.4)

●●❑ **712.3** *Chondrocalcinosis, unspecified*
[0–9]
    Code first underlying disease (275.4)

●❑ **712.8** *Other specified crystal arthropathies*
[0–9]

●❑ **712.9** **Unspecified crystal arthropathy**
[0–9]

● **713** **Arthropathy associated with other disorders classified elsewhere**

    Includes: arthritis associated with conditions classifiable below
              arthropathy associated with conditions classifiable below
              polyarthritis associated with conditions classifiable below
              polyarthropathy associated with conditions classifiable below

●❑ **713.0** *Arthropathy associated with other endocrine and metabolic disorders*

    Code first underlying disease, as:
        acromegaly (253.0)
        hemochromatosis (275.0)
        hyperparathyroidism (252.00–252.08)   ◀━━
        hypogammaglobulinemia (279.00–279.09)
        hypothyroidism (243–244.9)
        lipoid metabolism disorder (272.0–272.9)
        ochronosis (270.2)
    Excludes *arthropathy associated with:*
           amyloidosis (713.7)
           crystal deposition disorders, except gout (712.1–712.9)
           diabetic neuropathy (713.5)
           gouty arthropathy (274.0)

● **713.1** *Arthropathy associated with gastrointestinal conditions other than infections*

    Code first underlying disease, as:
        regional enteritis (555.0–555.9)
        ulcerative colitis (556)

● **713.2** *Arthropathy associated with hematological disorders*

    Code first underlying disease, as:
        hemoglobinopathy (282.4–282.7)
        hemophilia (286.0–286.2)
        leukemia (204.0–208.9)
        malignant reticulosis (202.3)
        multiple myelomatosis (203.0)
    Excludes *arthropathy associated with Henoch-Schönlein purpura (713.6)*

● **713.3** *Arthropathy associated with dermatological disorders*

    Code first underlying disease, as:
        erythema multiforme (695.1)
        erythema nodosum (695.2)
    Excludes *psoriatic arthropathy (696.0)*

● **713.4** *Arthropathy associated with respiratory disorders*

    Code first underlying disease, as:
        diseases classifiable to 490–519
    Excludes *arthropathy associated with respiratory infections (711.0, 711.4–711.8)*

● **713.5** *Arthropathy associated with neurological disorders*
    Charcot's arthropathy associated with diseases classifiable elsewhere
    Neuropathic arthritis associated with diseases classifiable elsewhere

    Code first underlying disease, as:
        neuropathic joint disease [Charcot's joints]:
          NOS (094.0)
          diabetic (250.6)
          syringomyelic (336.0)
          tabetic [syphilitic] (094.0)

ICD-9-CM

**700-
799**

Vol. 1

● **713.6** *Arthropathy associated with hypersensitivity reaction*

Code first underlying disease, as:
    Henoch (-Schönlein) purpura (287.0)
    serum sickness (999.5)

Excludes *allergic arthritis NOS (716.2)*

●❑ **713.7** *Other general diseases with articular involvement*

Code first underlying disease, as:
    amyloidosis (277.3)
    familial Mediterranean fever (277.3)
    sarcoidosis (135)

●❑ **713.8** *Arthropathy associated with other conditions classifiable elsewhere*

Code first underlying disease, as:
    conditions classifiable elsewhere except as in 711.1–711.8, 712, and 713.0–713.7

● **714** Rheumatoid arthritis and other inflammatory polyarthropathies

Excludes *rheumatic fever (390)*
    rheumatoid arthritis of spine NOS (720.0)

714.0 **Rheumatoid arthritis**
Arthritis or polyarthritis:
    atrophic
    rheumatic (chronic)

Use additional code to identify manifestation, as:
    myopathy (359.6)
    polyneuropathy (357.1)

Excludes *juvenile rheumatoid arthritis NOS (714.30)*

714.1 **Felty's syndrome**
Rheumatoid arthritis with splenoadenomegaly and leukopenia

❑ **714.2** **Other rheumatoid arthritis with visceral or systemic involvement**
Rheumatoid carditis

● **714.3** **Juvenile chronic polyarthritis**

❑ **714.30** **Polyarticular juvenile rheumatoid arthritis, chronic or unspecified**
Juvenile rheumatoid arthritis NOS
Still's disease

714.31 **Polyarticular juvenile rheumatoid arthritis, acute**

714.32 **Pauciarticular juvenile rheumatoid arthritis**

714.33 **Monoarticular juvenile rheumatoid arthritis**

714.4 **Chronic postrheumatic arthropathy**
Chronic rheumatoid nodular fibrositis
Jaccoud's syndrome

● **714.8** **Other specified inflammatory polyarthropathies**

714.81 **Rheumatoid lung**
Caplan's syndrome
Diffuse interstitial rheumatoid disease of lung
Fibrosing alveolitis, rheumatoid

❑ **714.89** **Other**

❑ **714.9** **Unspecified inflammatory polyarthropathy**
Inflammatory polyarthropathy or polyarthritis NOS

Excludes *polyarthropathy NOS (716.5)*

● **715** Osteoarthrosis and allied disorders

Note: Localized, in the subcategories below, includes bilateral involvement of the same site.

Includes: arthritis or polyarthritis:
    degenerative
    hypertrophic
    degenerative joint disease
    osteoarthritis

Excludes *Marie-Strümpell spondylitis (720.0)*
    osteoarthrosis [osteoarthritis] of spine (721.0–721.9)

The following fifth-digit subclassification is for use with category 715; valid digits are in [brackets] under each code. See list at beginning of chapter for definitions:
❑ 0 site unspecified
  1 shoulder region
  2 upper arm
  3 forearm
  4 hand
  5 pelvic region and thigh
  6 lower leg
  7 ankle and foot
❑ 8 other specified sites
❑ 9 multiple sites

● **715.0** **Osteoarthrosis, generalized**
[0,4,9]   Degenerative joint disease, involving multiple joints
    Primary generalized hypertrophic osteoarthrosis

● **715.1** **Osteoarthrosis, localized, primary**
[0–8]   Localized osteoarthropathy, idiopathic

● **715.2** **Osteoarthrosis, localized, secondary**
[0–8]   Coxae malum senilis

●❑ **715.3** **Osteoarthrosis, localized, not specified whether**
[0–8] **primary or secondary**
    Otto's pelvis

●❑ **715.8** **Osteoarthrosis involving, or with mention of more**
[0,9] **than one site, but not specified as generalized**

●❑ **715.9** **Osteoarthrosis, unspecified whether generalized or**
[0–8] **localized**

● **716** Other and unspecified arthropathies

Excludes *cricoarytenoid arthropathy (478.79)*

The following fifth-digit subclassification is for use with category 716; valid digits are in [brackets] under each code. See list at beginning of chapter for definitions:
❑ 0 site unspecified
  1 shoulder region
  2 upper arm
  3 forearm
  4 hand
  5 pelvic region and thigh
  6 lower leg
  7 ankle and foot
❑ 8 other specified sites
❑ 9 multiple sites

● **716.0** **Kaschin-Beck disease**
[0–9]   Endemic polyarthritis

● **716.1** **Traumatic arthropathy**
[0–9]

● **716.2** **Allergic arthritis**
[0–9]

Excludes *arthritis associated with Henoch-Schönlein purpura or serum sickness (713.6)*

● **716.3** **Climacteric arthritis**
[0–9]   Menopausal arthritis

● **716.4** **Transient arthropathy**
[0–9]

Excludes *palindromic rheumatism (719.3)*

● ❑ **716.5 Unspecified polyarthropathy or polyarthritis**
[0–9]

● ❑ **716.6 Unspecified monoarthritis**
[0–8]   Coxitis

● ❑ **716.8 Other specified arthropathy**
[0–9]

● ❑ **716.9 Arthropathy, unspecified**
[0–9]   Arthritis (acute) (chronic) (subacute)
        Arthropathy (acute) (chronic) (subacute)
        Articular rheumatism (chronic)
        Inflammation of joint NOS

● **717 Internal derangement of knee**

    Includes: degeneration of articular cartilage or meniscus
            of knee
          rupture, old of articular cartilage or meniscus
            of knee
          tear, old of articular cartilage or meniscus of
            knee

    | **Excludes** | *acute derangement of knee (836.0–836.6)*
                ankylosis (718.5)
                contracture (718.4)
                current injury (836.0–836.6)
                deformity (736.4–736.6)
                recurrent dislocation (718.3)

    717.0 Old bucket handle tear of medial meniscus
        Old bucket handle tear of unspecified cartilage

    717.1 Derangement of anterior horn of medial meniscus

    717.2 Derangement of posterior horn of medial meniscus

    ❑ **717.3 Other and unspecified derangement of medial meniscus**
        Degeneration of internal semilunar cartilage

●   **717.4 Derangement of lateral meniscus**

      ❑ **717.40 Derangement of lateral meniscus, unspecified**

      717.41 Bucket handle tear of lateral meniscus

      717.42 Derangement of anterior horn of lateral meniscus

      717.43 Derangement of posterior horn of lateral meniscus

      ❑ **717.49 Other**

    717.5 Derangement of meniscus, not elsewhere classified
        Congenital discoid meniscus
        Cyst of semilunar cartilage
        Derangement of semilunar cartilage NOS

    717.6 Loose body in knee
        Joint mice, knee
        Rice bodies, knee (joint)

    717.7 Chondromalacia of patella
        Chondromalacia patellae
        Degeneration [softening] of articular cartilage of
        patella

●   **717.8 Other internal derangement of knee**

      717.81 Old disruption of lateral collateral ligament

      717.82 Old disruption of medial collateral ligament

      717.83 Old disruption of anterior cruciate ligament

      717.84 Old disruption of posterior cruciate ligament

      ❑ **717.85 Old disruption of other ligaments of knee**
          Capsular ligament of knee

      ❑ **717.89 Other**
          Old disruption of ligaments of knee NOS

    ❑ **717.9 Unspecified internal derangement of knee**
        Derangement NOS of knee

● **718 Other derangement of joint**

    | **Excludes** | *current injury (830.0–848.9)*
                jaw (524.60–524.69) ◀▥

    The following fifth-digit subclassification is for use with
    category 718; valid digits are in [brackets] under each
    code. See list at beginning of chapter for definitions:
    ❑ **0 site unspecified**
      1 shoulder region
      2 upper arm
      3 forearm
      4 hand
      5 pelvic region and thigh
      6 lower leg
      7 ankle and foot
    ❑ **8 other specified sites**
    ❑ **9 multiple sites**

●   **718.0 Articular cartilage disorder**
[0–5,7–9]   Meniscus:
            disorder
            rupture, old
            tear, old
         Old rupture of ligament(s) of joint NOS

    | **Excludes** | *articular cartilage disorder:*
                in ochronosis (270.2)
                knee (717.0–717.9)
                chondrocalcinosis (275.4)
                metastatic calcification (275.4)

●   **718.1 Loose body in joint**
[0–5,7–9]   Joint mice

    | **Excludes** | *knee (717.6)*

●   **718.2 Pathological dislocation**
[0–9]   Dislocation or displacement of joint, not recurrent
            and not current

●   **718.3 Recurrent dislocation of joint**
[0–9]

●   **718.4 Contracture of joint**
[0–9]

●   **718.5 Ankylosis of joint**
[0–9]   Ankylosis of joint (fibrous) (osseous)

    | **Excludes** | *spine (724.9)*
                stiffness of joint without mention of ankylosis
                (719.5)

● ❑ **718.6 Unspecified intrapelvic protrusion of acetabulum**
    [0,5]   Protrusio acetabuli, unspecified

●   **718.7 Developmental dislocation of joint**
[0–9]

    | **Excludes** | *congenital dislocation of joint (754.0–755.8)*
                traumatic dislocation of joint (830–839)

● ❑ **718.8 Other joint derangement, not elsewhere classified**
    [0–9]   Flail joint (paralytic)
            Instability of joint

    | **Excludes** | *deformities classifiable to 736 (736.0–736.9)*

● ❑ **718.9 Unspecified derangement of joint**
[0–5,7–9]

    | **Excludes** | *knee (717.9)*

ICD-9-CM

700–799

Vol. 1

● 719 **Other and unspecified disorders of joint**

    Excludes *jaw (524.60–524.69)*   ◀▥

The following fifth-digit subclassification is for use with codes 719.0–719.6, 719.8–719.9; valid digits are in [brackets] under each code. See list at beginning of chapter for definitions:

❑ 0 site unspecified
   1 shoulder region
   2 upper arm
   3 forearm
   4 hand
   5 pelvic region and thigh
   6 lower leg
   7 ankle and foot
❑ 8 other specified sites
❑ 9 multiple sites

● **719.0 Effusion of joint**
   [0–9]   Hydrarthrosis
           Swelling of joint, with or without pain
     Excludes *intermittent hydrarthrosis (719.3)*

● **719.1 Hemarthrosis**
   [0–9]
     Excludes *current injury (840.0–848.9)*

● **719.2 Villonodular synovitis**
   [0–9]

● **719.3 Palindromic rheumatism**
   [0–9]   Hench-Rosenberg syndrome
           Intermittent hydrarthrosis

● **719.4 Pain in joint**
   [0–9]   Arthralgia

● **719.5 Stiffness of joint, not elsewhere classified**
   [0–9]

● ❑ **719.6 Other symptoms referable to joint**
   [0–9]   Joint crepitus   Snapping hip

  719.7 Difficulty in walking
     Excludes *abnormality of gait (781.2)*

● ❑ **719.8 Other specified disorders of joint**
   [0–9]   Calcification of joint   Fistula of joint
     Excludes *temporomandibular joint-pain-dysfunction syndrome [Costen's syndrome] (524.60)* ◀▥

● ❑ **719.9 Unspecified disorder of joint**
   [0–9]

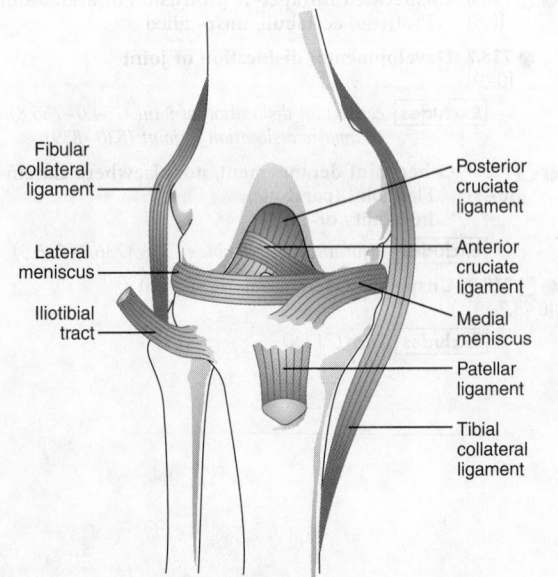

Figure 13–1   Anterior aspect of the right knee joint.

Fibular collateral ligament
Lateral meniscus
Iliotibial tract
Posterior cruciate ligament
Anterior cruciate ligament
Medial meniscus
Patellar ligament
Tibial collateral ligament

    Excludes *curvature of spine (737.0–737.9)*
                 osteochondrosis of spine (juvenile) (732.0) adult (732.8)

● 720 **Ankylosing spondylitis and other inflammatory spondylopathies**

  720.0 Ankylosing spondylitis
      Rheumatoid arthritis of spine NOS
      Spondylitis: Spondylitis:
        Marie-Strümpell   rheumatoid

  720.1 Spinal enthesopathy
      Disorder of peripheral ligamentous or muscular attachments of spine
      Romanus lesion

  720.2 Sacroiliitis, not elsewhere classified
      Inflammation of sacroiliac joint NOS

● **720.8 Other inflammatory spondylopathies**

   ● **720.81 Inflammatory spondylopathies in diseases classified elsewhere**
        Code first underlying disease, as:
          tuberculosis (015.0)

   ❑ **720.89 Other**

  ❑ **720.9 Unspecified inflammatory spondylopathy**
      Spondylitis NOS

● 721 **Spondylosis and allied disorders**

  721.0 Cervical spondylosis without myelopathy
      Cervical or cervicodorsal:
        arthritis   spondylarthritis
        osteoarthritis

  721.1 Cervical spondylosis with myelopathy
      Anterior spinal artery compression syndrome
      Spondylogenic compression of cervical spinal cord
      Vertebral artery compression syndrome

  721.2 Thoracic spondylosis without myelopathy
      Thoracic:
        arthritis   spondylarthritis
        osteoarthritis

  721.3 Lumbosacral spondylosis without myelopathy
      Lumbar or lumbosacral:
        arthritis   spondylarthritis
        osteoarthritis

● **721.4 Thoracic or lumbar spondylosis with myelopathy**

   721.41 Thoracic region
        Spondylogenic compression of thoracic spinal cord

   721.42 Lumbar region
        Spondylogenic compression of lumbar spinal cord

  721.5 Kissing spine
      Baastrup's syndrome

  721.6 Ankylosing vertebral hyperostosis

  721.7 Traumatic spondylopathy
      Kümmell's disease or spondylitis

 ❑ **721.8 Other allied disorders of spine**

● **721.9 Spondylosis of unspecified site**

   721.90 Without mention of myelopathy
        Spinal:
          arthritis (deformans) (degenerative) (hypertrophic)
          osteoarthritis NOS
        Spondylarthrosis NOS

   721.91 With myelopathy
        Spondylogenic compression of spinal cord NOS

● **722 Intervertebral disc disorders**

  722.0 Displacement of cervical intervertebral disc without myelopathy

    Neuritis (brachial) or radiculitis due to displacement or rupture of cervical intervertebral disc

    Any condition classifiable to 722.2 of the cervical or cervicothoracic intervertebral disc

● **722.1 Displacement of thoracic or lumbar intervertebral disc without myelopathy**

    722.10 Lumbar intervertebral disc without myelopathy

      Lumbago or sciatica due to displacement of intervertebral disc

      Neuritis or radiculitis due to displacement or rupture of lumbar intervertebral disc

      Any condition classifiable to 722.2 of the lumbar or lumbosacral intervertebral disc

    722.11 Thoracic intervertebral disc without myelopathy

      Any condition classifiable to 722.2 of thoracic intervertebral disc

☐ **722.2 Displacement of intervertebral disc, site unspecified, without myelopathy**

    Discogenic syndrome NOS

    Herniation of nucleus pulposus NOS

    Intervertebral disc NOS:

      extrusion

      prolapse

      protrusion

      rupture

    Neuritis or radiculitis due to displacement or rupture of intervertebral disc

● **722.3 Schmorl's nodes**

  ☐ **722.30 Unspecified region**

    722.31 Thoracic region

    722.32 Lumbar region

  ☐ **722.39 Other**

  722.4 Degeneration of cervical intervertebral disc

    Degeneration of cervicothoracic intervertebral disc

● **722.5 Degeneration of thoracic or lumbar intervertebral disc**

    722.51 Thoracic or thoracolumbar intervertebral disc

    722.52 Lumbar or lumbosacral intervertebral disc

☐ **722.6 Degeneration of intervertebral disc, site unspecified**

    Degenerative disc disease NOS

    Narrowing of intervertebral disc or space NOS

● **722.7 Intervertebral disc disorder with myelopathy**

  ☐ **722.70 Unspecified region**

    722.71 Cervical region

    722.72 Thoracic region

    722.73 Lumbar region

● **722.8 Postlaminectomy syndrome**

  ☐ **722.80 Unspecified region**

    722.81 Cervical region

    722.82 Thoracic region

    722.83 Lumbar region

● **722.9 Other and unspecified disc disorder**

    Calcification of intervertebral cartilage or disc Discitis

  ☐ **722.90 Unspecified region**

    722.91 Cervical region

    722.92 Thoracic region

    722.93 Lumbar region

● **723 Other disorders of cervical region**

    | Excludes | conditions due to: |
    intervertebral disc disorders (722.0–722.9)
    spondylosis (721.0–721.9)

  723.0 Spinal stenosis of cervical region

  723.1 Cervicalgia

    Pain in neck

  723.2 Cervicocranial syndrome

    Barré-Liéou syndrome

    Posterior cervical sympathetic syndrome

  723.3 Cervicobrachial syndrome (diffuse)

  723.4 Brachia neuritis or radiculitis NOS

    Cervical radiculitis

    Radicular syndrome of upper limbs

☐ **723.5 Torticollis, unspecified**

    Contracture of neck

    Excludes *congenital (754.1)*
    due to birth injury (767.8)
    hysterical (300.11)
    ocular torticollis (781.93)
    psychogenic (306.0)
    spasmodic (333.83)
    traumatic, current (847.0)

  723.6 Panniculitis specified as affecting neck

  723.7 Ossification of posterior longitudinal ligament in cervical region

☐ **723.8 Other syndromes affecting cervical region**

    Cervical syndrome NEC

    Klippel's disease

    Occipital neuralgia

☐ **723.9 Unspecified musculoskeletal disorders and symptoms referable to neck**

    Cervical (region) disorder NOS

● **724 Other and unspecified disorders of back**

    Excludes *collapsed vertebra (code to cause, e.g., osteoporosis, 733.00–733.09)*
    conditions due to:
    intervertebral disc disorders (722.0–722.9)
    spondylosis (721.0–721.9)

● **724.0 Spinal stenosis, other than cervical**

  ☐ **724.00 Spinal stenosis, unspecified region**

    724.01 Thoracic region

    724.02 Lumbar region

  ☐ **724.09 Other**

  724.1 Pain in thoracic spine

  724.2 Lumbago

    Low back pain

    Low back syndrome

    Lumbalgia

  724.3 Sciatica

    Neuralgia or neuritis of sciatic nerve

    Excludes *specified lesion of sciatic nerve (355.0)*

☐ **724.4 Thoracic or lumbosacral neuritis or radiculitis, unspecified**

    Radicular syndrome of lower limbs

ICD-9-CM

700-799

Vol.

❏ **724.5 Backache, unspecified**
Vertebrogenic (pain) syndrome NOS

724.6 Disorders of sacrum
Ankylosis, lumbosacral or sacroiliac (joint)
Instability, lumbosacral or sacroiliac (joint)

● **724.7 Disorders of coccyx**

❏ **724.70 Unspecified disorder of coccyx**

724.71 Hypermobility of coccyx

❏ **724.79 Other**
Coccygodynia

❏ **724.8 Other symptoms referable to back**
Ossification of posterior longitudinal ligament NOS
Panniculitis specified as sacral or affecting back

❏ **724.9 Other unspecified back disorders**
Ankylosis of spine NOS
Compression of spinal nerve root NEC
Spinal disorder NOS

Excludes *sacroiliitis (720.2)*

Item 13-1 Polymyalgia rheumatica is a syndrome characterized by aching and morning stiffness and is related to aging and hereditary predisposition.

RHEUMATISM, EXCLUDING THE BACK (725–729)

Includes: disorders of muscles and tendons and their attachments, and of other soft tissues

725 Polymyalgia rheumatica

● **726 Peripheral enthesopathies and allied syndromes**

Note: Enthesopathies are disorders of peripheral ligamentous or muscular attachments.

Excludes *spinal enthesopathy (720.1)*

726.0 Adhesive capsulitis of shoulder

● **726.1 Rotator cuff syndrome of shoulder and allied disorders**

❏ **726.10 Disorders of bursae and tendons in shoulder region, unspecified**
Rotator cuff syndrome NOS
Supraspinatus syndrome NOS

726.11 Calcifying tendinitis of shoulder

726.12 Bicipital tenosynovitis

❏ **726.19 Other specified disorders**
Excludes *complete rupture of rotator cuff, nontraumatic (727.61)*

❏ **726.2 Other affections of shoulder region, not elsewhere classified**
Periarthritis of shoulder
Scapulohumeral fibrositis

● **726.3 Enthesopathy of elbow region**

❏ **726.30 Enthesopathy of elbow, unspecified**

726.31 Medial epicondylitis

726.32 Lateral epicondylitis
Epicondylitis NOS   Tennis elbow
Golfers' elbow

726.33 Olecranon bursitis
Bursitis of elbow

❏ **726.39 Other**

726.4 Enthesopathy of wrist and carpus
Bursitis of hand or wrist
Periarthritis of wrist

726.5 Enthesopathy of hip region
Bursitis of hip
Gluteal tendinitis
Iliac crest spur
Psoas tendinitis
Trochanteric tendinitis

● **726.6 Enthesopathy of knee**

❏ **726.60 Enthesopathy of knee, unspecified**
Bursitis of knee NOS

726.61 Pes anserinus tendinitis or bursitis

726.62 Tibial collateral ligament bursitis
Pellegrini-Stieda syndrome

726.63 Fibular collateral ligament bursitis

726.64 Patellar tendinitis

726.65 Prepatellar bursitis

❏ **726.69 Other**
Bursitis:
infrapatellar
subpatellar

● **726.7 Enthesopathy of ankle and tarsus**

❏ **726.70 Enthesopathy of ankle and tarsus, unspecified**
Metatarsalgia NOS
Excludes *Morton's metatarsalgia (355.6)*

726.71 Achilles bursitis or tendinitis

726.72 Tibialis tendinitis
Tibialis (anterior) (posterior) tendinitis

726.73 Calcaneal spur

❏ **726.79 Other**
Peroneal tendinitis

❏ **726.8 Other peripheral enthesopathies**

● **726.9 Unspecified enthesopathy**

❏ **726.90 Enthesopathy of unspecified site**
Capsulitis NOS
Periarthritis NOS
Tendinitis NOS

❏ **726.91 Exostosis of unspecified site**
Bone spur NOS

● **727 Other disorders of synovium, tendon, and bursa**

● **727.0 Synovitis and tenosynovitis**

❏ **727.00 Synovitis and tenosynovitis, unspecified**
Synovitis NOS
Tenosynovitis NOS

● **727.01 *Synovitis and tenosynovitis in diseases classified elsewhere***

Code first underlying disease, as:
tuberculosis (015.0–015.9)

Excludes *crystal-induced (275.4)*
gonococcal (098.51)
gouty (274.0)
syphilitic (095.7)

727.02 Giant cell tumor of tendon sheath

727.03 Trigger finger (acquired)

727.04 Radial styloid tenosynovitis
de Quervain's disease

❏ **727.05 Other tenosynovitis of hand and wrist**

727.06 Tenosynovitis of foot and ankle

❏ **727.09 Other**

727.1 Bunion

Figure 13–2   Hallux valgus or bunion.

Item 13-2   Hallux valgus, or bunion, is a bursa usually found along the medial aspect of the big toe. It is most often attributed to heredity or poorly fitted shoes.

❑ **727.2   Specific bursitides often of occupational origin**
Beat:
    elbow
    hand
    knee
Chronic crepitant synovitis of wrist
Miners':
    elbow
    knee

❑ **727.3   Other bursitis**
Bursitis NOS

Excludes	*bursitis:*
	gonococcal (098.52)
	subacromial (726.19)
	subcoracoid (726.19)
	subdeltoid (726.19)
	syphilitic (095.7)
	"frozen shoulder" (726.0)

● **727.4   Ganglion and cyst of synovium, tendon, and bursa**

  ❑ **727.40   Synovial cyst, unspecified**

Excludes	*that of popliteal space (727.51)*

  727.41   Ganglion of joint

  727.42   Ganglion of tendon sheath

  ❑ **727.43   Ganglion, unspecified**

  ❑ **727.49   Other**
      Cyst of bursa

● **727.5   Rupture of synovium**

  ❑ **727.50   Rupture of synovium, unspecified**

  727.51   Synovial cyst of popliteal space

Baker's cyst (knee)

  ❑ **727.59   Other**

● **727.6   Rupture of tendon, nontraumatic**

  ❑ **727.60   Nontraumatic rupture of unspecified tendon**

  727.61   Complete rupture of rotator cuff

  727.62   Tendons of biceps (long head)

  727.63   Extensor tendons of hand and wrist

  727.64   Flexor tendons of hand and wrist

  727.65   Quadriceps tendon

  727.66   Patellar tendon

  727.67   Achilles tendon

  ❑ **727.68   Other tendons of foot and ankle**

  ❑ **727.69   Other**

● **727.8   Other disorders of synovium, tendon, and bursa**

  727.81   Contracture of tendon (sheath)
      Short Achilles tendon (acquired)

  727.82   Calcium deposits in tendon and bursa
      Calcification of tendon NOS
      Calcific tendinitis NOS

Excludes	*peripheral ligamentous or muscular attachments (726.0–726.9)*

  727.83   Plica syndrome
      Plica knee

  ❑ **727.89   Other**
      Abscess of bursa or tendon

Excludes	*xanthomatosis localized to tendons (272.7)*

❑ **727.9   Unspecified disorder of synovium, tendon, and bursa**

● **728   Disorders of muscle, ligament, and fascia**

Excludes	*enthesopathies (726.0–726.9)*
	muscular dystrophies (359.0–359.1)
	myoneural disorders (358.00–358.9)
	myopathies (359.2–359.9)
	old disruption of ligaments of knee (717.81–717.89)

  728.0   Infective myositis
    Myositis:
      purulent
      suppurative

Excludes	*myositis:*
	epidemic (074.1)
	interstitial (728.81)
	syphilitic (095.6)
	tropical (040.81)

● **728.1   Muscular calcification and ossification**

  ❑ **728.10   Calcification and ossification, unspecified**
      Massive calcification (paraplegic)

  728.11   Progressive myositis ossificans

  728.12   Traumatic myositis ossificans
      Myositis ossificans (circumscripta)

  728.13   Postoperative heterotopic calcification

  ❑ **728.19   Other**
      Polymyositis ossificans

  728.2   Muscular wasting and disuse atrophy, not elsewhere classified
    Amyotrophia NOS
    Myofibrosis

Excludes	*neuralgic amyotrophy (353.5)*
	pelvic muscle wasting and disuse atrophy (618.83)
	progressive muscular atrophy (335.0–335.9)

ICD-9-CM

700-799

Vol. 1

❑ **728.3 Other specific muscle disorders**
Arthrogryposis
Immobility syndrome (paraplegic)
Excludes	*arthrogryposis multiplex congenita (754.89)*
	stiff-man syndrome (333.91)

728.4 Laxity of ligament

728.5 Hypermobility syndrome

728.6 Contracture of palmar fascia
Dupuytren's contracture

● **728.7 Other fibromatoses**

     728.71 Plantar fascial fibromatosis
         Contracture of plantar fascia
         Plantar fasciitis (traumatic)

     ❑ **728.79 Other**
         Garrod's or knuckle pads
         Nodular fasciitis
         Pseudosarcomatous fibromatosis (prolifera-
         tive) (subcutaneous)

● **728.8 Other disorders of muscle, ligament, and fascia**

     728.81 Interstitial myositis

     728.82 Foreign body granuloma of muscle
         Talc granuloma of muscle

     728.83 Rupture of muscle, nontraumatic

     728.84 Diastasis of muscle
         Diastasis recti (abdomen)

Excludes	*diastasis recti complicating pregnancy, labor, and*
	delivery (665.8)

     728.85 Spasm of muscle

     728.86 Necrotizing fasciitis

         Use additional code to identify:
         infectious organism (041.00–041.89)
         gangrene (785.4), if applicable

     728.87 Muscle weakness

Excludes	*generalized weakness (780.79)*

     728.88 Rhabdomyolysis

     ❑ **728.89 Other**
         Eosinophilic fasciitis

         Use additional E code to identify drug, if
         drug induced

❑ **728.9 Unspecified disorder of muscle, ligament, and fascia**

● **729 Other disorders of soft tissues**

Excludes	*acroparesthesia (443.89)*
	carpal tunnel syndrome (354.0)
	disorders of the back (720.0–724.9)
	entrapment syndromes (354.0–355.9)
	palindromic rheumatism (719.3)
	periarthritis (726.0–726.9)
	psychogenic rheumatism (306.0)

❑ **729.0 Rheumatism, unspecified, and fibrositis**

❑ **729.1 Myalgia and myositis, unspecified**
Fibromyositis NOS

❑ **729.2 Neuralgia, neuritis, and radiculitis, unspecified**

Excludes	*brachia radiculitis (723.4)*
	cervical radiculitis (723.4)
	lumbosacral radiculitis (724.4)
	mononeuritis (354.0–355.9)
	radiculitis due to intervertebral disc involvement
	(722.0–722.2,722.7)
	sciatica (724.3)

Item 13–3 Panniculitis is an inflammation of the adipose tissue of the heel pad.

● **729.3 Panniculitis, unspecified**

     ❑ **729.30 Panniculitis, unspecified site**
         Weber-Christian disease

     729.31 Hypertrophy of fat pad, knee
         Hypertrophy of infrapatellar fat pad

     ❑ **729.39 Other site**

Excludes	*panniculitis specified as (affecting):*
	back (724.8)
	neck (723.6)
	sacral (724.8)

Figure 13–3 Suppurative osteomyelitis. The initial radiograph **(A)** shows only minimal periosteal reaction along the lateral aspect of the proximal femur *(arrow)*. Eight months after onset **(B)** there is gross destruction of the joint and the proximal femur. (From Aegerter E, Kirkpatrick J Jr: Orthopedic Diseases, 4th ed. Philadelphia, WB Saunders, 1975, p 257.)

□ **729.4 Fasciitis, unspecified**

> | Excludes | *necrotizing fasciitis (728.86)*
> *nodular fasciitis (728.79)*

729.5 Pain in limb

729.6 Residual foreign body in soft tissue

> | Excludes | *foreign body granuloma:*
> *muscle (728.82)*
> *skin and subcutaneous tissue (709.4)*

● **729.8 Other musculoskeletal symptoms referable to limbs**

729.81 Swelling of limb

729.82 Cramp

□ **729.89 Other**

> | Excludes | *abnormality of gait (781.2)*
> *tetany (781.7)*
> *transient paralysis of limb (781.4)*

□ **729.9 Other and unspecified disorders of soft tissue**
Polyalgia

Item 13-4 Osteomyelitis is an inflammation of the bone. Acute osteomyelitis is a rapidly destructive, pus-producing infection capable of causing severe bone destruction. Chronic osteomyelitis can remain long after the initial acute episode has passed and may lead to a recurrence of the acute phase. Brodie's abscess is an encapsulated focal abscess that must be surgically drained.

OSTEOPATHIES, CHONDROPATHIES, AND ACQUIRED MUSCULOSKELETAL DEFORMITIES (730–739)

● **730 Osteomyelitis, periostitis, and other infections involving bone**

> | Excludes | *jaw (526.4–526.5)*
> *petrous bone (383.2)*

Use additional code to identify organism, such as Staphylococcus (041.1)

The following fifth-digit subclassification is for use with category 730; valid digits are in [brackets] under each code. See list at beginning of chapter for definitions:

□ 0 site unspecified
1 shoulder region
2 upper arm
3 forearm
4 hand
5 pelvic region and thigh
6 lower leg
7 ankle and foot
□ 8 other specified sites
□ 9 multiple sites

● **730.0 Acute osteomyelitis**
[0–9] Abscess of any bone except accessory sinus, jaw, or mastoid
Acute or subacute osteomyelitis, with or without mention of periostitis

● **730.1 Chronic osteomyelitis**
[0–9] Brodie's abscess
Chronic or old osteomyelitis, with or without mention of periostitis
Sequestrum
Sclerosing osteomyelitis of Garré

> | Excludes | *aseptic necrosis of bone (733.40–733.49)*

● □ **730.2 Unspecified osteomyelitis**
[0–9] Osteitis or osteomyelitis NOS, with or without mention of periostitis

● **730.3 Periostitis without mention of osteomyelitis**
[0–9] Abscess of periosteum, without mention of osteomyelitis
Periostosis, without mention of osteomyelitis

> | Excludes | *that in secondary syphilis (091.61)*

●● **730.7 Osteopathy resulting from poliomyelitis**
[0–9] *Code first underlying disease (045.0–045.9)*

●●□ **730.8 Other infections involving bone in disease classified elsewhere**
[0–9]
> *Code first underlying disease, as:*
> *tuberculosis (015.0–015.9)*
> *typhoid fever (002.0)*

> | Excludes | *syphilitis of bone NOS (095.5)*

●□ **730.9 Unspecified infection of bone**
[0–9]

● **731 Osteitis deformans and osteopathies associated with other disorders classified elsewhere**

731.0 Osteitis deformans without mention of bone tumor
Paget's disease of bone

● **731.1 Osteitis deformans in diseases classified elsewhere**

> *Code first underlying disease, as:*
> *malignant neoplasm of bone (170.0–170.9)*

731.2 Hypertrophic pulmonary osteoarthropathy
Bamberger-Marie disease

●□ **731.8 Other bone involvement in diseases classified elsewhere**

> *Code first underlying disease, as:*
> *diabetes mellitus (250.8)*

> Use additional code to specify bone condition, such as: acute osteomyelitis (730.00–730.09)

● **732 Osteochondropathies**

732.0 Juvenile osteochondrosis of spine
Juvenile osteochondrosis (of):
marginal or vertebral ephiphysis (of Scheuermann) spine NOS
Vertebral epiphysitis

> | Excludes | *adolescent postural kyphosis (737.0)*

732.1 Juvenile osteochondrosis of hip and pelvis
Coxa plana
Ischiopubic synchondrosis (of van Neck)
Osteochondrosis (juvenile) of:
acetabulum
head of femur (of Legg-Calvé-Perthes)
iliac crest (of Buchanan)
symphysis pubis (of Pierson)
Pseudocoxalgia

732.2 Nontraumatic slipped upper femoral epiphysis
Slipped upper femoral epiphysis NOS

732.3 Juvenile osteochondrosis of upper extremity
Osteochondrosis (juvenile) of:
capitulum of humerus (of Panner)
carpal lunate (of Kienbock)
hand NOS
head of humerus (of Haas)
heads of metacarpals (of Mauclaire)
lower ulna (of Burns)
radial head (of Brailsford)
upper extremity NOS

732.4 Juvenile osteochondrosis of lower extremity, excluding foot
Osteochondrosis (juvenile) of:
lower extremity NOS
primary patellar center (of Köhler)
proximal tibia (of Blount)
secondary patellar center (of Sinding-Larsen)
tibial tubercle (of Osgood-Schlatter)
Tibia vara

ICD-9-CM

700-
Vol.

732.5 Juvenile osteochondrosis of foot
Calcaneal apophysitis
Epiphysitis, os calcis
Osteochondrosis (juvenile) of:
astragalus (of Diaz)
calcaneum (of Sever)
foot NOS
metatarsal:
second (of Freiberg)
fifth (of Iselin)
os tibiale externum (of Haglund)
tarsal navicular (of Köhler)

☐ **732.6 Other juvenile osteochondrosis**
Apophysitis specified as juvenile, of other site, or site NOS
Epiphysitis specified as juvenile, of other site, or site NOS
Osteochondritis specified as juvenile, of other site, or site NOS
Osteochondrosis specified as juvenile, of other site, or site NOS

732.7 Osteochondritis dissecans

☐ **732.8 Other specified forms of osteochondropathy**
Adult osteochondrosis of spine

☐ **732.9 Unspecified osteochondropathy**
Apophysitis
NOS
not specified as adult or juvenile, of unspecified site
Epiphysitis
NOS
not specified as adult or juvenile, of unspecified site
Osteochondritis
NOS
not specified as adult or juvenile, of unspecified site
Osteochondrosis
NOS
not specified as adult or juvenile, of unspecified site

● **733 Other disorders of bone and cartilage**
Excludes   bone spur (726.91)
cartilage of, or loose body in, joint (717.0–717.9, 718.0–718.9)
giant cell granuloma of jaw (526.3)
osteitis fibrosa cystica generalisata (252.01) ◄
osteomalacia (268.2)
polyostotic fibrous dysplasia of bone (756.54)
prognathism, retrognathism (524.1)
xanthomatosis localized to bone (272.7)

● **733.0 Osteoporosis**
☐ **733.00 Osteoporosis, unspecified**
Wedging of vertebra NOS

733.01 Senile osteoporosis
Postmenopausal osteoporosis

733.02 Idiopathic osteoporosis

733.03 Disuse osteoporosis

☐ **733.09 Other**
Drug-induced osteoporosis
Use additional E code to identify drug

● **733.1 Pathologic fracture**
Spontaneous fracture
Excludes   stress fracture (733.93–733.95)
traumatic fractures (800–829)

☐ **733.10 Pathologic fracture, unspecified site**

733.11 Pathologic fracture of humerus

733.12 Pathologic fracture of distal radius and ulna
Wrist NOS

733.13 Pathologic fracture of vertebrae
Collapse of vertebra NOS

733.14 Pathologic fracture of neck of femur
Femur NOS
Hip NOS

☐ **733.15 Pathologic fracture of other specified part of femur**

733.16 Pathologic fracture of tibia and fibula
Ankle NOS

☐ **733.19 Pathologic fracture of other specified site**

● **733.2 Cyst of bone**
☐ **733.20 Cyst of bone (localized), unspecified**

733.21 Solitary bone cyst
Unicameral bone cyst

733.22 Aneurysmal bone cyst

☐ **733.29 Other**
Fibrous dysplasia (monostotic)
Excludes   cyst of jaw (526.0–526.2, 526.89)
osteitis fibrosa cystica (252.01) ◄
polyostotic fibrous dysplasia of bone (756.54)

733.3 Hyperostosis of skull
Hyperostosis interna frontalis
Leontiasis ossium

● **733.4 Aseptic necrosis of bone**
Excludes   osteochondropathies (732.0–732.9)
☐ **733.40 Aseptic necrosis of bone, site unspecified**

733.41 Head of humerus

733.42 Head and neck of femur
Femur NOS
Excludes   Legg-Calvé-Perthes disease (732.1)

733.43 Medial femoral condyle

733.44 Talus

☐ **733.49 Other**

733.5 Osteitis condensans
Piriform sclerosis of ilium

733.6 Tietze's disease
Costochondral junction syndrome
Costochondritis

733.7 Algoneurodystrophy
Disuse atrophy of bone
Sudeck's atrophy

● **733.8 Malunion and nonunion of fracture**
733.81 Malunion of fracture

733.82 Nonunion of fracture
Pseudoarthrosis (bone)

● **733.9 Other and unspecified disorders of bone and cartilage**
☐ **733.90 Disorder of bone and cartilage, unspecified**

733.91 Arrest of bone development or growth
Epiphyseal arrest

733.92 Chondromalacia
Chondromalacia:
NOS
localized, except patella
systemic
tibial plateau
Excludes   chondromalacia of patella (717.7)

733.93 **Stress fracture of tibia or fibula**
Stress reaction of tibia or fibula

733.94 **Stress fracture of the metatarsals**
Stress reaction of metatarsals

☐ 733.95 **Stress fracture of other bone**
Stress reaction of other bone

☐ 733.99 **Other**
Diaphysitis
Hypertrophy of bone
Relapsing polychondritis

734 **Flat foot**
Pes planus (acquired)
Talipes planus (acquired)

Excludes	congenital (754.61)
	rigid flat foot (754.61)
	spastic (everted) flat foot (754.61)

Figure 13-4   Claw toe.

Item 13-5   **Claw toe** is caused by a contraction of the flexor tendon producing a flexion deformity characterized by hyperextension of the big toe.

● 735 **Acquired deformities of toe**

Excludes	congenital (754.60–754.69, 755.65–755.66)

735.0 **Hallux valgus (acquired)**

735.1 **Hallux varus (acquired)**

735.2 **Hallux rigidus**

735.3 **Hallux malleus**

☐ 735.4 **Other hammer toe (acquired)**

735.5 **Claw toe (acquired)**

☐ 735.8 **Other acquired deformities of toe**

☐ 735.9 **Unspecified acquired deformity of toe**

● 736 **Other acquired deformities of limbs**

Excludes	congenital (754.3–755.9)

● 736.0 **Acquired deformities of forearm, excluding fingers**

☐ 736.00 **Unspecified deformity**
Deformity of elbow, forearm, hand, or wrist (acquired) NOS

736.01 **Cubitus valgus (acquired)**

736.02 **Cubitus varus (acquired)**

736.03 **Valgus deformity of wrist (acquired)**

736.04 **Varus deformity of wrist (acquired)**

736.05 **Wrist drop (acquired)**

736.06 **Claw hand (acquired)**

736.07 **Club hand (acquired)**

☐ 736.09 **Other**

736.1 **Mallet finger**

● 736.2 **Other acquired deformities of finger**

☐ 736.20 **Unspecified deformity**
Deformity of finger (acquired) NOS

736.21 **Boutonniere deformity**

736.22 **Swan-neck deformity**

☐ 736.29 **Other**

Excludes	trigger finger (727.03)

● 736.3 **Acquired deformities of hip**

☐ 736.30 **Unspecified deformity**
Deformity of hip (acquired) NOS

736.31 **Coxa valga (acquired)**

736.32 **Coxa vara (acquired)**

☐ 736.39 **Other**

● 736.4 **Genu valgum or varum (acquired)**

736.41 **Genu valgum (acquired)**

736.42 **Genu varum (acquired)**

736.5 **Genu recurvatum (acquired)**

☐ 736.6 **Other acquired deformities of knee**
Deformity of knee (acquired) NOS

Figure 13-5   Pes cavovarus, meaning "foot with high arch."

Item 13-6   **Equinus foot** is a term referring to the hoof of a horse. The deformity is usually congenital or spastic.

● 736.7 **Other acquired deformities of ankle and foot**

Excludes	deformities of toe (acquired) (735.0–735.9)
	pes planus (acquired) (734)

☐ 736.70 **Unspecified deformity of ankle and foot, acquired**

736.71 **Acquired equinovarus deformity**
Clubfoot, acquired

Excludes	clubfoot not specified as acquired (754.5–754.7)

736.72 **Equinus deformity of foot, acquired**

736.73 **Cavus deformity of foot**

Excludes	that with claw foot (736.74)

736.74 **Claw foot, acquired**

736.75 **Cavovarus deformity of foot, acquired**

☐ 736.76 **Other calcaneus deformity**

☐ 736.79 **Other**
Acquired:
    pes not elsewhere classified
    talipes not elsewhere classified

ICD-9-CM

700-799

Vol. 1

● **736.8   Acquired deformities of other parts of limbs**

     736.81   Unequal leg length (acquired)

☐ **736.89   Other**
         Deformity (acquired):
            arm or leg, not elsewhere classified
            shoulder

☐ **736.9   Acquired deformity of limb, site unspecified**

Item 13-7   Kyphosis is an abnormal curvature of the spine. **Senile kyphosis** is a result of disc degeneration causing ossification (turning to bone). **Adolescent** or **juvenile kyphosis** is also known as **Scheuermann's disease**, a condition in which the discs of the lower thoracic spine herniate, causing the disc space to narrow and the spine to tilt forward. This condition is attributed to poor posture.

Item 13-8   Spondylolisthesis is a condition caused by the slipping forward of one disc over another.

● **737   Curvature of spine**
     Excludes   *congenital (754.2)*

     737.0   Adolescent postural kyphosis
         Excludes   *osteochondrosis of spine (juvenile) (732.0)*
                     adult (732.8)

☐ **737.1   Kyphosis (acquired)**
     737.10   Kyphosis (acquired) (postural)
     737.11   Kyphosis due to radiation
     737.12   Kyphosis, postlaminectomy
     ☐ **737.19   Other**
     Excludes   *that associated with conditions classifiable elsewhere (737.41)*

● **737.2   Lordosis (acquired)**
     737.20   Lordosis (acquired) (postural)
     737.21   Lordosis, postlaminectomy
     737.22   Other postsurgical lordosis
     ☐ **737.29   Other**
     Excludes   *that associated with conditions classifiable elsewhere (737.42)*

● **737.3   Kyphoscoliosis and scoliosis**

     737.30   Scoliosis [and kyphoscoliosis], idiopathic
     737.31   Resolving infantile idiopathic scoliosis
     737.32   Progressive infantile idiopathic scoliosis
     737.33   Scoliosis due to radiation
     737.34   Thoracogenic scoliosis
     ☐ **737.39   Other**
     Excludes   *that associated with conditions classifiable elsewhere (737.43)*
                   that in kyphoscoliotic heart disease (416.1)

●● **737.4   *Curvature of spine associated with other conditions***

     Code first associated condition, as:
         Charcot-Marie-Tooth disease (356.1)
         mucopolysaccharidosis (277.5)
         neurofibromatosis (237.7)
         osteitis deformans (731.0)
         osteitis fibrosa cystica (252.01)   ⬅
         osteoporosis (733.00–733.09)
         poliomyelitis (138)
         tuberculosis [Pott's curvature] (015.0)

     ●● ☐ **737.40   *Curvature of spine, unspecified***
     ● **737.41   *Kyphosis***
     ● **737.42   *Lordosis***
     ● **737.43   *Scoliosis***

☐ **737.8   Other curvatures of spine**

☐ **737.9   Unspecified curvature of spine**
         Curvature of spine (acquired) (idiopathic) NOS
         Hunchback, acquired
     Excludes   *deformity of spine NOS (738.5)*

● **738   Other acquired deformity**
     Excludes   *congenital (754.0–756.9, 758.0–759.9)*
                 dentofacial anomalies (524.0–524.9)

     738.0   Acquired deformity of nose
         Deformity of nose (acquired)
         Overdevelopment of nasal bones
     Excludes   *deflected or deviated nasal septum (470)*

● **738.1   Other acquired deformity of head**
     ☐ **738.10   Unspecified deformity**
     738.11   Zygomatic hyperplasia
     738.12   Zygomatic hypoplasia
     ☐ **738.19   Other specified deformity**

     738.2   Acquired deformity of neck

     738.3   Acquired deformity of chest and rib
         Deformity:
            chest (acquired)
            rib (acquired)
         Pectus:
            carinatum, acquired
            excavatum, acquired

     738.4   Acquired spondylolisthesis
         Degenerative spondylolisthesis
         Spondylolysis, acquired
     Excludes   *congenital (756.12)*

☐ **738.5   Other acquired deformity of back or spine**
         Deformity of spine NOS
     Excludes   *curvature of spine (737.0–737.9)*

     738.6   Acquired deformity of pelvis
         Pelvic obliquity
     Excludes   *intrapelvic protrusion of acetabulum (718.6)*
                   that in relation to labor and delivery (653.0–
                   653.4, 653.8–653.9)

Figure 13-6   Scoliosis is a lateral curvature of the spine.

738.7 **Cauliflower ear**

☐ 738.8 **Acquired deformity of other specified site**
Deformity of clavicle

☐ 738.9 **Acquired deformity of unspecified site**

● 739 **Nonallopathic lesions, not elsewhere classified**

Includes: segmental dysfunction
somatic dysfunction

739.0 **Head region**
Occipitocervical region

739.1 **Cervical region**
Cervicothoracic region

739.2 **Thoracic region**
Thoracolumbar region

739.3 **Lumbar region**
Lumbosacral region

739.4 **Sacral region**
Sacrococcygeal region
Sacroiliac region

739.5 **Pelvic region**
Hip region
Pubic region

739.6 **Lower extremities**

739.7 **Upper extremities**
Acromioclavicular region
Sternoclavicular region

739.8 **Rib cage**
Costochondral region
Costovertebral region
Sternochondral region

739.9 **Abdomen and other**

Figure 14-1 Generalized craniosynostosis in a 4-year-old girl without symptoms or signs of increased intracranial pressure. The child was referred for medical evaluation because of abnormal facial characteristics, features similar to those of her mother and aunt. Her fronto-occipital head circumference was found to be 47 cm. (From Bell WE, McCormick WF: Increased Intracranial Pressure in Children, 2nd ed. Philadelphia, WB Saunders, 1978, p 116.)

Item 14-1 Anencephalus is a congenital deformity of the cranial vault. **Craniosynostosis,** also known as craniostenosis and stenocephaly, signifies any form of congenital deformity of the skull that results from the premature closing of the sutures of the skull. **Iniencephaly** is a deformity in which the head and neck are flexed backward to a great extent and the head is very large in comparison to the shortened body.

14. CONGENITAL ANOMALIES (740-759)

● 740 **Anencephalus and similar anomalies**

   740.0 **Anencephalus**
       Acrania
       Amyelencephalus
       Hemianencephaly
       Hemicephaly

   740.1 **Craniorachischisis**

   740.2 **Iniencephaly**

Item 14-2 Spina bifida is a midline spinal defect in which one or more vertebrae fail to fuse, leaving an opening in the vertebral canal. When the defect is not visible, it is called spina bifida occulta, and when it is visible, it is called spina bifida cystica.

● 741 **Spina bifida**

   Excludes *spina bifida occulta (756.17)*

   The following fifth-digit subclassification is for use with category 741:
   ❏ 0 unspecified region
       1 cervical region
       2 dorsal (thoracic) region
       3 lumbar region

● 741.0 **With hydrocephalus**
       Arnold-Chiari syndrome, type II
       Any condition classifiable to 741.9 with any condition classifiable to 742.3
       Chiari malformation, type II

● 741.9 **Without mention of hydrocephalus**
       Hydromeningocele (spinal)
       Hydromyelocele
       Meningocele (spinal)
       Meningomyelocele
       Myelocele
       Myelocystocele
       Rachischisis
       Spina bifida (aperta)
       Syringomyelocele

Spina bifida occulta

A

Dura

B

C

Central canal

Hydromyelia

D

Figure 14–2 **A.** Spina bifida occulta. **B.** Meningocele. **C.** Myelomeningocele. **D.** Myelocystocele (syringomyelocele) or hydromyelia.

Figure 14-3 Encephalocele is a protrusion of the brain through an opening in the skull.

- **742 Other congenital anomalies of nervous system**

  742.0 Encephalocele
  Encephalocystocele
  Encephalomyelocele
  Hydroencephalocele
  Hydromeningocele, cranial
  Meningocele, cerebral
  Meningoencephalocele

  742.1 Microcephalus
  Hydromicrocephaly   Micrencephaly

  742.2 Reduction deformities of brain
  Absence of part of brain
  Agenesis of part of brain
  Agyria
  Aplasia of part of brain
  Arhinencephaly
  Holoprosencephaly
  Hypoplasia of part of brain
  Microgyria

  742.3 Congenital hydrocephalus
  Aqueduct of Sylvius:
      anomaly
      obstruction, congenital
      stenosis
  Atresia of foramina of Magendie and Luschka
  Hydrocephalus in newborn
  Excludes *hydrocephalus:*
      acquired (331.3–331.4)
      due to congenital toxoplasmosis (771.2)
      with any condition classifiable to 741.9 (741.0)

  ☐ **742.4 Other specified anomalies of brain**
  Congenital cerebral cyst
  Macroencephaly
  Macrogyria
  Megalencephaly
  Multiple anomalies of brain NOS
  Porencephaly
  Ulegyria

- **742.5 Other specified anomalies of spinal cord**

  742.51 Diastematomyelia

  742.53 Hydromyelia
  Hydrorhachis

  ☐ **742.59 Other**
  Amyelia
  Atelomyelia
  Congenital anomaly of spinal meninges
  Defective development of cauda equina
  Hypoplasia of spinal cord
  Myelatelia
  Myelodysplasia

☐ **742.8 Other specified anomalies of nervous system**
Agenesis of nerve
Displacement of brachial plexus
Familial dysautonomia
Jaw-winking syndrome
Marcus-Gunn syndrome
Riley-Day syndrome
Excludes *neurofibromatosis (237.7)*

☐ **742.9 Unspecified anomaly of brain, spinal cord, and nervous system**
Anomaly of brain, nervous system, and spinal cord
Congenital, of brain, nervous system, and spinal cord:
    disease of brain, nervous system, and spinal cord
    lesion of brain, nervous system, and spinal cord
Deformity of brain, nervous system, and spinal cord

Item 14-3 Anophthalmia is the absence of the eye and the optic pit. **Microphthalmia** is the partial absence of the eye and optic pit.

- **743 Congenital anomalies of eye**

  - **743.0 Anophthalmos**

    ☐ **743.00 Clinical anophthalmos, unspecified**
    Agenesis
    Congenital absence of eye
    Anophthalmos NOS

    743.03 Cystic eyeball, congenital

    743.06 Cryptophthalmos

  - **743.1 Microphthalmos**
    Dysplasia of eye
    Hypoplasia of eye
    Rudimentary eye

    ☐ **743.10 Microphthalmos, unspecified**

    743.11 Simple microphthalmos

    ☐ **743.12 Microphthalmos associated with other anomalies of eye and adnexa**

Figure 14-4 Bilateral congenital hydrophthalmia, in which the eyes are very large in comparison to the other facial features.

● **743.2 Buphthalmos**
       Glaucoma:
          congenital
          newborn
       Hydrophthalmos

> **Excludes**   *glaucoma of childhood (365.14)*
> *traumatic glaucoma due to birth injury (767.8)*

❑ **743.20 Buphthalmos, unspecified**

   743.21 Simple buphthalmos

❑ **743.22 Buphthalmos associated with other ocular anomalies**
       Keratoglobus, congenital, associated with buphthalmos
       Megalocornea associated with buphthalmos

● **743.3 Congenital cataract and lens anomalies**

> **Excludes**   *infantile cataract (366.00–366.09)*

❑ **743.30 Congenital cataract, unspecified**

   743.31 Capsular and subcapsular cataract

   743.32 Cortical and zonular cataract

   743.33 Nuclear cataract

   743.34 Total and subtotal cataract, congenital

   743.35 Congenital aphakia
       Congenital absence of lens

   743.36 Anomalies of lens shape
       Microphakia
       Spherophakia

   743.37 Congenital ectopic lens

❑ **743.39 Other**

● **743.4 Coloboma and other anomalies of anterior segment**

   743.41 Anomalies of corneal size and shape
       Microcornea

> **Excludes**   *that associated with buphthalmos (743.22)*

❑ **743.42 Corneal opacities, interfering with vision, congenital**

❑ **743.43 Other corneal opacities, congenital**

❑ **743.44 Specified anomalies of anterior chamber, chamber angle, and related structures**
       Anomaly:
          Axenfeld's
          Peters'
          Rieger's

   743.45 Aniridia

❑ **743.46 Other specified anomalies of iris and ciliary body**
       Anisocoria, congenital
       Atresia of pupil
       Coloboma of iris
       Corectopia

❑ **743.47 Specified anomalies of sclera**

❑ **743.48 Multiple and combined anomalies of anterior segment**

❑ **743.49 Other**

● **743.5 Congenital anomalies of posterior segment**

   743.51 Vitreous anomalies
       Congenital vitreous opacity

   743.52 Fundus coloboma

   743.53 Chorioretinal degeneration, congenital

   743.54 Congenital folds and cysts of posterior segment

   743.55 Congenital macular changes

❑ **743.56 Other retinal changes, congenital**

❑ **743.57 Specified anomalies of optic disc**
       Coloboma of optic disc (congenital)

   743.58 Vascular anomalies
       Congenital retinal aneurysm

❑ **743.59 Other**

● **743.6 Congenital anomalies of eyelids, lacrimal system, and orbit**

   743.61 Congenital ptosis

   743.62 Congenital deformities of eyelids
       Ablepharon
       Absence of eyelid
       Accessory eyelid
       Congenital:
          ectropion
          entropion

❑ **743.63 Other specified congenital anomalies of eyelid**
       Absence, agenesis, of cilia

❑ **743.64 Specified congenital anomalies of lacrimal gland**

❑ **743.65 Specified congenital anomalies of lacrimal passages**
       Absence, agenesis, of:
          lacrimal apparatus
          punctum lacrimale
       Accessory lacrimal canal

❑ **743.66 Specified congenital anomalies of orbit**

❑ **743.69 Other**
       Accessory eye muscles

❑ **743.8 Other specified anomalies of eye**

> **Excludes**   *congenital nystagmus (379.51)*
> *ocular albinism (270.2)*
> *retinitis pigmentosa (362.74)*

❑ **743.9 Unspecified anomaly of eye**
       Congenital:
          anomaly NOS of eye [any part]
          deformity NOS of eye [any part]

● **744 Congenital anomalies of ear, face, and neck**

> **Excludes**   *anomaly of:*
> *cervical spine (754.2, 756.10–756.19)*
> *larynx (748.2–748.3)*
> *nose (748.0–748.1)*
> *parathyroid gland (759.2)*
> *thyroid gland (759.2)*
> *cleft lip (749.10–749.25)*

● ❑ **744.0 Anomalies of ear causing impairment of hearing**

> **Excludes**   *congenital deafness without mention of cause (380.0–389.9)*

❑ **744.00 Unspecified anomaly of ear with impairment of hearing**

   744.01 Absence of external ear
       Absence of:
          auditory canal (external)
          auricle (ear) (with stenosis or atresia of auditory canal)

❑ **744.02 Other anomalies of external ear with impairment of hearing**
       Atresia or stricture of auditory canal (external)

   744.03 Anomaly of middle ear, except ossicles
       Atresia or stricture of osseous meatus (ear)

   744.04 Anomalies of ear ossicles
       Fusion of ear ossicles

ICD-9-CM

700-799

Vol. 1

Figure 14–5   Multiple auricular appendage.

Figure 14–6   Webbing of the neck.

      744.05 Anomalies of inner ear
            Congenital anomaly of:
                membranous labyrinth
                organ of Corti

    ❑ **744.09 Other**
            Absence of ear, congenital

  744.1 Accessory auricle
        Accessory tragus
        Polyotia
        Preauricular appendage
        Supernumerary:
          ear
          lobule

● **744.2 Other specified anomalies of ear**
      Excludes *that with impairment of hearing (744.00–744.09)*

      744.21 Absence of ear lobe, congenital

      744.22 Macrotia

      744.23 Microtia

    ❑ **744.24 Specified anomalies of Eustachian tube**
            Absence of Eustachian tube

    ❑ **744.29 Other**
            Bat ear   Prominence of auricle
            Darwin's tubercle   Ridge ear
            Pointed ear
      Excludes *preauricular sinus (744.46)*

  ❑ **744.3 Unspecified anomaly of ear**
        Congenital:
          anomaly NOS of ear, NEC
          deformity NOS of ear, NEC

● **744.4 Branchial cleft cyst or fistula; preauricular sinus**

      744.41 Branchial cleft sinus or fistula
            Branchial:
              sinus (external) (internal)
              vestige

      744.42 Branchial cleft cyst

      744.43 Cervical auricle

      744.46 Preauricular sinus or fistula

      744.47 Preauricular cyst

    ❑ **744.49 Other**
            Fistula (of):
              auricle, congenital
              cervicoaural

  744.5 Webbing of neck
        Pterygium colli

● **744.8 Other specified anomalies of face and neck**

      744.81 Macrocheilia
            Hypertrophy of lip, congenital

      744.82 Microcheilia

      744.83 Macrostomia

      744.84 Microstomia

    ❑ **744.89 Other**
      Excludes *congenital fistula of lip (750.25)*
                 musculoskeletal anomalies (754.0–754.1, 756.0)

  ❑ **744.9 Unspecified anomalies of face and neck**
        Congenital:
          anomaly NOS of face [any part] or neck [any
            part]
          deformity NOS of face [any part] or neck [any
            part]

● **745 Bulbus cordis anomalies and anomalies of cardiac septal closure**

  745.0 Common truncus
        Absent septum between aorta and pulmonary artery
        Communication (abnormal) between aorta and
          pulmonary artery
        Aortic septal defect
        Common aortopulmonary trunk
        Persistent truncus arteriosus

● **745.1 Transposition of great vessels**

      745.10 Complete transposition of great vessels
            Transposition of great vessels:
              NOS
              classical

      745.11 Double outlet right ventricle
            Dextrotransposition of aorta
            Incomplete transposition of great vessels
            Origin of both great vessels from right
              ventricle
            Taussig-Bing syndrome or defect

      745.12 Corrected transposition of great vessels

    ❑ **745.19 Other**

745.2 Tetralogy of Fallot
    Fallot's pentalogy
    Ventricular septal defect with pulmonary stenosis
      or atresia, dextroposition of aorta, and hyper-
      trophy of right ventricle

    Excludes *Fallot's triad (746.09)*

745.3 Common ventricle
    Cor triloculare biatriatum
    Single ventricle

745.4 Ventricular septal defect
    Eisenmenger's defect or complex
    Gerbode defect
    Interventricular septal defect
    Left ventricular-right atrial communication
    Roger's disease

    Excludes *common atrioventricular canal type (745.69)*
                  single ventricle (745.3)

745.5 Ostium secundum type atrial septal defect
    Defect:
      atrium secundum
      fossa ovalis
    Lutembacher's syndrome
    Patent or persistent:
      foramen ovale
      ostium secundum

● **745.6 Endocardial cushion defects**

   ❏ **745.60 Endocardial cushion defect, unspecified type**

   745.61 Ostium primum defect
      Persistent ostium primum

   ❏ **745.69 Other**
      Absence of atrial septum
      Atrioventricular canal type ventricular
        septal defect
      Common atrioventricular canal
      Common atrium

745.7 Cor biloculare
    Absence of atrial and ventricular septa

❏ **745.8 Other**

❏ **745.9 Unspecified defect of septal closure**
    Septal defect NOS

● **746 Other congenital anomalies of heart**

    Excludes *endocardial fibroelastosis (425.3)*

● **746.0 Anomalies of pulmonary valve**

    Excludes *infundibular or subvalvular pulmonic stenosis*
                (746.83)
          tetralogy of Fallot (745.2)

   ❏ **746.00 Pulmonary valve anomaly, unspecified**

   746.01 Atresia, congenital
      Congenital absence of pulmonary valve

   746.02 Stenosis, congenital

   ❏ **746.09 Other**
      Congenital insufficiency of pulmonary
        valve
      Fallot's triad or trilogy

746.1 Tricuspid atresia and stenosis, congenital
    Absence of tricuspid valve

746.2 Ebstein's anomaly

746.3 Congenital stenosis of aortic valve
    Congenital aortic stenosis

    Excludes *congenital:*
        subaortic stenosis (746.81)
        supravalvular aortic stenosis (747.22)

746.4 Congenital insufficiency of aortic valve
    Bicuspid aortic valve
    Congenital aortic insufficiency

746.5 Congenital mitral stenosis
    Fused commissure of mitral valve
    Parachute deformity of mitral valve
    Supernumerary cusps of mitral valve

746.6 Congenital mitral insufficiency

746.7 Hypoplastic left heart syndrome
    Atresia, or marked hypoplasia, of aortic orifice or
      valve, with hypoplasia of ascending aorta
      and defective development of left ventricle
      (with mitral valve atresia)

● **746.8 Other specified anomalies of heart**

   746.81 Subaortic stenosis

   746.82 Cor triatriatum

   746.83 Infundibular pulmonic stenosis
      Subvalvular pulmonic stenosis

   746.84 Obstructive anomalies of heart, NEC
      Uhl's disease

   746.85 Coronary artery anomaly
      Anomalous origin or communication of
        coronary artery
      Arteriovenous malformation of coronary
        artery
      Coronary artery:
        absence
        arising from aorta or pulmonary trunk
        single

   746.86 Congenital heart block
      Complete or incomplete atrioventricular
        [AV] block

   746.87 Malposition of heart and cardiac apex
      Abdominal heart
      Dextrocardia
      Ectopia cordis
      Levocardia (isolated)
      Mesocardia

    Excludes *dextrocardia with complete transposition of vis-*
        cera (759.3)

   ❏ **746.89 Other**
      Atresia of cardiac vein
      Hypoplasia of cardiac vein
      Congenital:
        cardiomegaly
        diverticulum, left ventricle
        pericardial defect

❏ **746.9 Unspecified anomaly of heart**
    Congenital:
      anomaly of heart NOS
      heart disease NOS

● **747 Other congenital anomalies of circulatory system**

   747.0 Patent ductus arteriosus
      Patent ductus Botalli
      Persistent ductus arteriosus

● **747.1 Coarctation of aorta**

   747.10 Coarctation of aorta (preductal) (postductal)
      Hypoplasia of aortic arch

   747.11 Interruption of aortic arch

● **747.2 Other anomalies of aorta**

   ❏ **747.20 Anomaly of aorta, unspecified**

ICD-9-CM

700-
799

Vol. 1

747.21 Anomalies of aortic arch
   Anomalous origin, right subclavian artery
   Dextroposition of aorta
   Double aortic arch
   Kommerell's diverticulum
   Overriding aorta
   Persistent:
      convolutions, aortic arch
      right aortic arch
   Vascular ring

   Excludes *hypoplasia of aortic arch (747.10)*

747.22 Atresia and stenosis of aorta
   Absence of aorta
   Aplasia of aorta
   Hypoplasia of aorta
   Stricture of aorta
   Supra (valvular)-aortic stenosis

   Excludes *congenital aortic (valvular) stenosis or stricture, so stated (746.3)*
   hypoplasia of aorta in hypoplastic left heart syndrome (746.7)

☐ **747.29 Other**
   Aneurysm of sinus of Valsalva
   Congenital:
      aneurysm of aorta
      dilation of aorta

747.3 Anomalies of pulmonary artery
   Agenesis of pulmonary artery
   Anomaly of pulmonary artery
   Atresia of pulmonary artery
   Coarctation of pulmonary artery
   Hypoplasia of pulmonary artery
   Stenosis of pulmonary artery
   Pulmonary arteriovenous aneurysm

● **747.4 Anomalies of great veins**

   ☐ **747.40 Anomaly of great veins, unspecified**
      Anomaly NOS of:
         pulmonary veins
         vena cava

   747.41 Total anomalous pulmonary venous connection
      Total anomalous pulmonary venous return [TAPVR]:
         subdiaphragmatic
         supradiaphragmatic

   747.42 Partial anomalous pulmonary venous connection
      Partial anomalous pulmonary venous return

   ☐ **747.49 Other anomalies of great veins**
      Absence of vena cava (inferior) (superior)
      Congenital stenosis of vena cava (inferior) (superior)
      Persistent:
         left posterior cardinal vein
         left superior vena cava
      Scimitar syndrome
      Transposition of pulmonary veins NOS

747.5 Absence or hypoplasia of umbilical artery
   Single umbilical artery

● **747.6 Other anomalies of peripheral vascular system**
   Absence of artery or vein, NEC
   Anomaly of artery or vein, NEC
   Atresia of artery or vein, NEC
   Arteriovenous aneurysm (peripheral)
   Arteriovenous malformation of the peripheral vascular system
   Congenital:
      aneurysm (peripheral)
      phlebectasia
      stricture, artery
      varix
   Multiple renal arteries

   Excludes *anomalies of:*
      cerebral vessels (747.81)
      pulmonary artery (747.3)
   congenital retinal aneurysm (743.58)
   hemangioma (228.00–228.09)
   lymphangioma (228.1)

   ☐ **747.60 Anomaly of the peripheral vascular system, unspecified site**

   747.61 Gastrointestinal vessel anomaly

   747.62 Renal vessel anomaly

   747.63 Upper limb vessel anomaly

   747.64 Lower limb vessel anomaly

   ☐ **747.69 Anomalies of other specified sites of peripheral vascular system**

● **747.8 Other specified anomalies of circulatory system**

   747.81 Anomalies of cerebrovascular system
      Arteriovenous malformation of brain
      Cerebral arteriovenous aneurysm, congenital
      Congenital anomalies of cerebral vessels

   Excludes *ruptured cerebral (arteriovenous) aneurysm (430)*

   747.82 Spinal vessel anomaly
      Arteriovenous malformation of spinal vessel

   747.83 Persistent fetal circulation
      Persistent pulmonary hypertension
      Primary pulmonary hypertension of newborn

   ☐ **747.89 Other**
      Aneurysm, congenital, specified site not elsewhere classified

   Excludes *congenital aneurysm:*
      coronary (746.85)
      peripheral (747.6)
      pulmonary (747.3)
      retinal (743.58)

   ☐ **747.9 Unspecified anomaly of circulatory system**

● **748 Congenital anomalies of respiratory system**
   Excludes *congenital defect of diaphragm (756.6)*

   748.0 Choanal atresia
      Atresia of nares (anterior) (posterior)
      Congenital stenosis of nares (anterior) (posterior)

   ☐ **748.1 Other anomalies of nose**
      Absent nose
      Accessory nose
      Cleft nose
      Deformity of wall of nasal sinus
      Congenital:
         deformity of nose
         notching of tip of nose
         perforation of wall of nasal sinus

   Excludes *congenital deviation of nasal septum (754.0)*

748.2 Web of larynx
    Web of larynx:
      NOS
      glottic
      subglottic

❑**748.3 Other anomalies of larynx, trachea, and bronchus**
    Absence or agenesis of:
      bronchus
      larynx
      trachea
    Anomaly (of):
      cricoid cartilage
      epiglottis
      thyroid cartilage
      tracheal cartilage
    Atresia (of):
      epiglottis
      glottis
      larynx
      trachea
    Cleft thyroid, cartilage, congenital
    Congenital:
      dilation, trachea
      stenosis:
        larynx
        trachea
      tracheocele
    Diverticulum:
      bronchus
      trachea
    Fissure of epiglottis
    Laryngocele
    Posterior cleft of cricoid cartilage (congenital)
    Rudimentary tracheal bronchus
    Stridor, laryngeal, congenital

748.4 Congenital cystic lung
    Disease, lung:
      cystic, congenital
      polycystic, congenital
    Honeycomb lung, congenital
    Excludes *acquired or unspecified cystic lung (518.89)*

748.5 Agenesis, hypoplasia, and dysplasia of lung
    Absence of lung (fissures) (lobe)
    Aplasia of lung
    Hypoplasia of lung (lobe)
    Sequestration of lung

●**748.6 Other anomalies of lung**

  ❑**748.60 Anomaly of lung, unspecified**

  748.61 Congenital bronchiectasis

  ❑**748.69 Other**
      Accessory lung (lobe)
      Azygos lobe (fissure), lung

❑**748.8 Other specified anomalies of respiratory system**
    Abnormal communication between pericardial and pleural sacs
    Anomaly, pleural folds
    Atresia of nasopharynx
    Congenital cyst of mediastinum

❑**748.9 Unspecified anomaly of respiratory system**
    Anomaly of respiratory system NOS

Figure 14–7 Cleft palate.

●**749 Cleft palate and cleft lip**

  ●**749.0 Cleft palate**

    ❑**749.00 Cleft palate, unspecified**

    749.01 Unilateral, complete

    749.02 Unilateral, incomplete
      Cleft uvula

    749.03 Bilateral, complete

    749.04 Bilateral, incomplete

  ●**749.1 Cleft lip**
    Cheiloschisis
    Congenital fissure of lip
    Harelip
    Labium leporinum

    ❑**749.10 Cleft lip, unspecified**

    749.11 Unilateral, complete

    749.12 Unilateral, incomplete

    749.13 Bilateral, complete

    749.14 Bilateral, incomplete

  ●**749.2 Cleft palate with cleft lip**
    Cheilopalatoschisis

    ❑**749.20 Cleft palate with cleft lip, unspecified**

    749.21 Unilateral, complete

    749.22 Unilateral, incomplete

    749.23 Bilateral, complete

    749.24 Bilateral, incomplete

    ❑**749.25 Other combinations**

●**750 Other congenital anomalies of upper alimentary tract**
    Excludes *dentofacial anomalies (524.0–524.9)*

  750.0 Tongue tie
    Ankyloglossia

  ●**750.1 Other anomalies of tongue**

    ❑**750.10 Anomaly of tongue, unspecified**

    750.11 Aglossia

    750.12 Congenital adhesions of tongue

    750.13 Fissure of tongue
      Bifid tongue
      Double tongue

ICD-9-CM
700-799
Vol. 1

750.15   **Macroglossia**
> Congenital hypertrophy of tongue

750.16   **Microglossia**
> Hypoplasia of tongue

❑ 750.19   **Other**

● 750.2   **Other specified anomalies of mouth and pharynx**

750.21   **Absence of salivary gland**

750.22   **Accessory salivary gland**

750.23   **Atresia, salivary gland**
> Imperforate salivary duct

750.24   **Congenital fistula of salivary gland**

750.25   **Congenital fistula of lip**
> Congenital (mucus) lip pits

❑ 750.26   **Other specified anomalies of mouth**
> Absence of uvula

750.27   **Diverticulum of pharynx**
> Pharyngeal pouch

❑ 750.29   **Other specified anomalies of pharynx**
> Imperforate pharynx

750.3   **Tracheoesophageal fistula, esophageal atresia and stenosis**
> Absent esophagus
> Atresia of esophagus
> Congenital:
>> esophageal ring
>> stenosis of esophagus
>> stricture of esophagus
> Congenital fistula:
>> esophagobronchial
>> esophagotracheal
> Imperforate esophagus
> Webbed esophagus

❑ 750.4   **Other specified anomalies of esophagus**
> Dilatation, congenital, of esophagus
> Displacement, congenital, of esophagus
> Diverticulum of esophagus
> Duplication of esophagus
> Esophageal pouch
> Giant esophagus

> **Excludes**   *congenital hiatus hernia (750.6)*

750.5   **Congenital hypertrophic pyloric stenosis**
> Congenital or infantile:
>> constriction of pylorus
>> hypertrophy of pylorus
>> spasm of pylorus
>> stenosis of pylorus
>> stricture of pylorus

750.6   **Congenital hiatus hernia**
> Displacement of cardia through esophageal hiatus

> **Excludes**   *congenital diaphragmatic hernia (756.6)*

❑ 750.7   **Other specified anomalies of stomach**
> Congenital:
>> cardiospasm
>> hourglass stomach
> Displacement of stomach
> Diverticulum of stomach, congenital
> Duplication of stomach
> Megalogastria
> Microgastria
> Transposition of stomach

❑ 750.8   **Other specified anomalies of upper alimentary tract**

❑ 750.9   **Unspecified anomaly of upper alimentary tract**
> Congenital:
>> anomaly NOS of upper alimentary tract [any part, except tongue]
>> deformity NOS of upper alimentary tract [any part, except tongue]

● 751   **Other congenital anomalies of digestive system**

751.0   **Meckel's diverticulum**
> Meckel's diverticulum (displaced) (hypertrophic)
> Persistent:
>> omphalomesenteric duct
>> vitelline duct

751.1   **Atresia and stenosis of small intestine**
> Atresia of: Atresia of:
>> duodenum   intestine NOS
>> ileum
> Congenital:
>> absence of small intestine or intestine NOS
>> obstruction of small intestine or intestine NOS
>> stenosis of small intestine or intestine NOS
>> stricture of small intestine or intestine NOS
> Imperforate jejunum

751.2   **Atresia and stenosis of large intestine, rectum, and anal canal**
> Absence:
>> anus (congenital)
>> appendix, congenital
>> large instestine, congenital
>> rectum
> Atresia of: Atresia of:
>> anus   rectum
>> colon
> Congenital or infantile:
>> obstruction of large intestine
>> occlusion of anus
>> stricture of anus
> Imperforate:
>> anus
>> rectum
> Stricture of rectum, congenital

❑ 751.3   **Hirschsprung's disease and other congenital functional disorders of colon**
> Aganglionosis
> Congenital dilation of colon
> Congenital megacolon
> Macrocolon

751.4   **Anomalies of intestinal fixation**
> Congenital adhesions:
>> omental, anomalous
>> peritoneal
> Jackson's membrane
> Malrotation of colon
> Rotation of cecum or colon:
>> failure of
>> incomplete
>> insufficient
> Universal mesentery

❑ 751.5   **Other anomalies of intestine**
> Congenital diverticulum,   Megaloappendix
>> colon   Megaloduodenum
> Dolichocolon   Microcolon
> Duplication of: Persistent cloaca
>> anus   Transposition of:
>> appendix   appendix
>> cecum   colon
>> intestine   intestine
> Ectopic anus

● 751.6   **Anomalies of gallbladder, bile ducts, and liver**

❑ 751.60   **Unspecified anomaly of gallbladder, bile ducts, and liver**

751.61   **Biliary atresia**
> Congenital:
>> absence of bile duct (common) or passage
>> hypoplasia of bile duct (common) or passage
>> obstruction of bile duct (common) or passage
>> stricture of bile duct (common) or passage

751.62 Congenital cystic disease of liver
Congenital polycystic disease of liver
Fibrocystic disease of liver

☐ **751.69 Other anomalies of gallbladder, bile ducts, and liver**

Absence of:
    gallbladder, congenital
Accessory:
    hepatic ducts
Congenital:
    choledochal cyst
Duplication of:
    biliary duct
    cystic duct
Floating:
    gallbladder
Intrahepatic gallbladder

Absence of:
    liver (lobe)
Accessory:
    liver
Congenital:
    hepatomegaly
Duplication of:
    gallbladder
    liver
Floating:
    liver

751.7 Anomalies of pancreas
Absence of pancreas
Accessory pancreas
Agenesis of pancreas
Annular pancreas
Ectopic pancreatic tissue
Hypoplasia of pancreas
Pancreatic heterotopia

Excludes *diabetes mellitus:*
    congenital (250.0–250.9)
    neonatal (775.1)
    fibrocystic disease of pancreas (277.00–277.09)

☐ **751.8 Other specified anomalies of digestive system**
Absence (complete) (partial) of alimentary tract NOS
Duplication of digestive organs NOS
Malposition, congenital, of digestive organs NOS

Excludes *congenital diaphragmatic hernia (756.6)*
    congenital hiatus hernia (750.6)

☐ **751.9 Unspecified anomaly of digestive system**
Congenital:
    anomaly NOS of digestive system NOS
    deformity NOS of digestive system NOS

● **752 Congenital anomalies of genital organs**

Excludes *syndromes associated with anomalies in the number and form of chromosomes (758.0–758.9)*
    testicular feminization syndrome (257.8)

752.0 Anomalies of ovaries
Absence, congenital, of ovary   Ectopic ovary
Accessory ovary   Streak of ovary

● **752.1 Anomalies of fallopian tubes and broad ligaments**

☐ **752.10 Unspecified anomaly of fallopian tubes and broad ligaments**

752.11 Embryonic cyst of fallopian tubes and broad ligaments
Cyst:
    epoöphoron   Gartner's duct
    fimbrial   parovarian

☐ **752.19 Other**
Absence of fallopian tube or broad ligament
Accessory fallopian tube or broad ligament
Atresia of fallopian tube or broad ligament

752.2 Doubling of uterus
Didelphic uterus
Doubling of uterus [any degree] (associated with doubling of cervix and vagina)

☐ **752.3 Other anomalies of uterus**
Absence, congenital, of uterus
Agenesis of uterus
Aplasia of uterus
Bicornuate uterus
Uterus unicornis
Uterus with only one functioning horn

● **752.4 Anomalies of cervix, vagina, and external female genitalia**

☐ **752.40 Unspecified anomaly of cervix, vagina, and external female genitalia**

752.41 Embryonic cyst of cervix, vagina, and external female genitalia
Cyst of:
    canal of Nuck, congenital
    vagina, embryonal
    vulva, congenital

752.42 Imperforate hymen

ECTOPIC TESTES
Penile
Superficial inguinal (most common)
Femoral

CRYPTORCHID TESTES
Abdominal
Inguinal
Prepubic (most common)

Penile
Internal inguinal ring
Superficial inguinal (most common)
Femoral

Abdominal
Inguinal
External inguinal ring
Prepubic (most common)

Figure 14–8 Undescended testes and the positions of the testes in various types of cryptorchidism or abnormal paths of descent.

ICD-9-CM

700-799

Vol.

☐ **752.49 Other anomalies of cervix, vagina, and external female genitalia**
    Absence of cervix, clitoris, vagina, or vulva
    Agenesis of cervix, clitoris, vagina, or vulva
    Congenital stenosis or stricture of:
      cervical canal
      vagina
    Excludes *double vagina associated with total duplication (752.2)*

● **752.5 Undescended and retractile testicle**
    752.51 Undescended testis
      Cryptorchism
      Ectopic testis
    752.52 Retractile testis

● **752.6 Hypospadias and epispadias and other penile anomalies**
    752.61 Hypospadias
    752.62 Epispadias
      Anaspadias
    752.63 Congenital chordee
    752.64 Micropenis
    752.65 Hidden penis
    ☐ **752.69 Other penile anomalies**

752.7 Indeterminate sex and pseudohermaphroditism
    Gynandrism
    Hermaphroditism
    Ovotestis
    Pseudohermaphroditism (male) (female)
    Pure gonadal dysgenesis
    Excludes *pseudohermaphroditism:*
      female, with adrenocortical disorder (255.2)
      male, with gonadal disorder (257.8)
      with specified chromosomal anomaly (758.0–758.9)
      testicular feminization syndrome (257.8)

● **752.8 Other specified anomalies of genital organs**
    Excludes *congenital hydrocele (778.6)*
      penile anomalies (752.61–752.69)
      phimosis or paraphimosis (605)
    752.81 Scrotal transposition
    ☐ **752.89 Other specified anomalies of genital organs**
      Absence of:
        prostate
        spermatic cord
        vas deferens
      Anorchism
      Aplasia (congenital) of:
        prostate
        round ligament
        testicle:
      Atresia of:
        ejaculatory duct
        vas deferens
      Fusion of testes
      Hypoplasia of testis
      Monorchism
      Polyorchism

☐ **752.9 Unspecified anomaly of genital organs**
    Congenital:
      anomaly NOS of genital organ, NEC
      deformity NOS of genital organ, NEC

● **753 Congenital anomalies of urinary system**
    753.0 Renal agenesis and dysgenesis
      Atrophy of kidney:
        congenital
        infantile
      Congenital absence of kidney(s)
      Hypoplasia of kidney(s)

● **753.1 Cystic kidney disease**
    Excludes *acquired cyst of kidney (593.2)*
    ☐ **753.10 Cystic kidney disease, unspecified**
    753.11 Congenital single renal cyst
    ☐ **753.12 Polycystic kidney, unspecified type**
    753.13 Polycystic kidney, autosomal dominant
    753.14 Polycystic kidney, autosomal recessive
    753.15 Renal dysplasia
    753.16 Medullary cystic kidney
      Nephronophthisis
    753.17 Medullary sponge kidney
    ☐ **753.19 Other specified cystic kidney disease**
      Multicystic kidney

● **753.2 Obstructive defects of renal pelvis and ureter**
    ☐ **753.20 Unspecified obstructive defect of renal pelvis and ureter**
    753.21 Congenital obstruction of ureteropelvic junction
    753.22 Congenital obstruction of ureterovesical junction
      Adynamic ureter
      Congenital hydroureter
    753.23 Congenital ureterocele
    ☐ **753.29 Other**

☐ **753.3 Other specified anomalies of kidney**
    Accessory kidney
    Congenital:
      calculus of kidney
      displaced kidney
    Discoid kidney
    Double kidney with double pelvis
    Ectopic kidney
    Fusion of kidneys
    Giant kidney
    Horseshoe kidney
    Hyperplasia of kidney
    Lobulation of kidney
    Malrotation of kidney
    Trifid kidney (pelvis)

☐ **753.4 Other specified anomalies of ureter**
    Absent ureter
    Accessory ureter
    Deviaton of ureter
    Displaced ureteric orifice
    Double ureter
    Ectopic ureter
    Implantation, anomalous, of ureter

753.5 Exstrophy of urinary bladder
    Ectopia vesicae
    Extroversion of bladder

753.6 Atresia and stenosis of urethra and bladder neck
    Congenital obstruction:
      bladder neck
      urethra
    Congenital stricture of:
      urethra (valvular)
      urinary meatus
      vesicourethral orifice
    Imperforate urinary meatus
    Impervious urethra
    Urethral valve formation

753.7 Anomalies of urachus
    Cyst (of) urachus
    Fistula (of) urachus
    Patent (of) urachus
    Persistent umbilical sinus

❑ **753.8 Other specified anomalies of bladder and urethra**

Absence, congenital, of:
    bladder
    urethra
Accessory:
    bladder
    urethra
Congenital:
    diverticulum of bladder
    hernia of bladder
Congenital urethrorectal fistula
Congenital prolapse of:
    bladder (mucosa)
    urethra
Double:
    urethra
    urinary meatus

❑ **753.9 Unspecified anomaly of urinary system**

Congenital:
    anomaly NOS of urinary system [any part, except urachus]
    deformity NOS of urinary system [any part, except urachus]

● **754 Certain congenital musculoskeletal deformities**

Includes: nonteratogenic deformities which are considered to be due to intrauterine malposition and pressure

754.0 Of skull, face, and jaw

Asymmetry of face
Compression facies
Depressions in skull
Deviation of nasal septum, congenital
Dolichocephaly
Plagiocephaly
Potter's facies
Squashed or bent nose, congenital

Excludes	dentofacial anomalies (524.0–524.9)
	syphilitic saddle nose (090.5)

754.1 Of sternocleidomastoid muscle

Congenital sternomastoid torticollis
Congenital wryneck
Contracture of sternocleidomastoid (muscle)
Sternomastoid tumor

754.2 Of spine

Congenital postural:
    lordosis
    scoliosis

Figure 14–9 Mild to moderate inbowing of the lower leg. (From Jones KL: Smith's Recognizable Patterns of Human Malformation, 4th ed. Philadelphia, WB Saunders, 1988, p 671.)

● **754.3 Congenital dislocation of hip**

754.30 Congenital dislocation of hip, unilateral
Congenital dislocation of hip NOS

754.31 Congenital dislocation of hip, bilateral

754.32 Congenital subluxation of hip, unilateral
Congenital flexion deformity, hip or thigh
Predislocation status of hip at birth
Preluxation of hip, congenital

754.33 Congenital subluxation of hip, bilateral

754.35 Congenital dislocation of one hip with subluxation of other hip

● **754.4 Congenital genu recurvatum and bowing of long bones of leg**

754.40 Genu recurvatum

754.41 Congenital dislocation of knee (with genu recurvatum)

754.42 Congenital bowing of femur

754.43 Congenital bowing of tibia and fibula

❑ **754.44 Congenital bowing of unspecified long bones of leg**

● **754.5 Varus deformities of feet**

Excludes	acquired (736.71, 736.75, 736.79)

754.50 Talipes varus
Congenital varus deformity of foot, unspecified
Pes varus

754.51 Talipes equinovarus
Equinovarus (congenital)

754.52 Metatarsus primus varus

754.53 Metatarsus varus

❑ **754.59 Other**
Talipes calcaneovarus

● **754.6 Valgus deformities of feet**

Excludes	valgus deformity of foot (acquired) (736.79)

754.60 Talipes valgus
Congenital valgus deformity of foot, unspecified

754.61 Congenital pes planus
Congenital rocker bottom flat foot
Flat foot, congenital

Excludes	pes planus (acquired) (734)

754.62 Talipes calcaneovalgus

❑ **754.69 Other**
Talipes:
    equinovalgus   planovalgus

● **754.7 Other deformities of feet**

Excludes	acquired (736.70–736.79)

❑ **754.70 Talipes, unspecified**
Congenital deformity of foot NOS

754.71 Talipes cavus
Cavus foot (congenital)

❑ **754.79 Other**
Asymmetric talipes
Talipes:
    calcaneus   equinus

● **754.8 Other specified nonteratogenic anomalies**

754.81 Pectus excavatum
Congenital funnel chest

754.82 Pectus carinatum
Congenital pigeon chest [breast]

❑ **754.89 Other**
Club hand (congenital)
Congenital:
    deformity of chest wall
    dislocation of elbow
Generalized flexion contractures of lower limb joints, congenital
Spade-like hand (congenital)

ICD-9-CM

700-799

Vol. 1

Figure 14-10 Polydactyly. (From Tachdjian MO: Pediatric Orthopedics, 2nd ed, Vol 4. Philadelphia, WB Saunders, 1990, p 2644.)

● **755 Other congenital anomalies of limbs**
    Excludes *those deformities classifiable to 754.0–754.8*

● **755.0 Polydactyly**

❑ **755.00 Polydactyly, unspecified digits**
    Supernumerary digits

755.01 Of fingers
    Accessory fingers

755.02 Of toes
    Accessory toes

● **755.1 Syndactyly**
    Symphalangy
    Webbing of digits

❑ **755.10 Of multiple and unspecified sites**

755.11 Of fingers without fusion of bone

755.12 Of fingers with fusion of bone

755.13 Of toes without fusion of bone

755.14 Of toes with fusion of bone

● **755.2 Reduction deformities of upper limb**

❑ **755.20 Unspecified reduction deformity of upper limb**
    Ectromelia NOS of upper limb
    Hemimelia NOS of upper limb
    Shortening of arm, congenital

755.21 Transverse deficiency of upper limb
    Amelia of upper limb
    Congenital absence of:
        fingers, all (complete or partial)
        forearm, including hand and fingers
        upper limb, complete
    Congenital amputation of upper limb
    Transverse hemimelia of upper limb

755.22 Longitudinal deficiency of upper limb, NEC
    Phocomelia NOS of upper limb
    Rudimentary arm

755.23 Longitudinal deficiency, combined, involving humerus, radius, and ulna (complete or incomplete)
    Congenital absence of arm and forearm (complete or incomplete) with or without metacarpal deficiency and/or phalangeal deficiency, incomplete
    Phocomelia, complete, of upper limb

755.24 Longitudinal deficiency, humeral, complete or partial (with or without distal deficiencies, incomplete)
    Congenital absence of humerus (with or without absence of some [but not all] distal elements)
    Proximal phocomelia of upper limb

755.25 Longitudinal deficiency, radioulnar, complete or partial (with or without distal deficiencies, incomplete)
    Congenital absence of radius and ulna (with or without absence of some [but not all] distal elements)
    Distal phocomelia of upper limb

755.26 Longitudinal deficiency, radial, complete or partial (with or without distal deficiencies, incomplete)
    Agenesis of radius
    Congenital absence of radius (with or without absence of some [but not all] distal elements)

755.27 Longitudinal deficiency, ulnar, complete or partial (with or without distal deficiencies, incomplete)
    Agenesis of ulna
    Congenital absence of ulna (with or without absence of some [but not all] distal elements)

755.28 Longitudinal deficiency, carpals or metacarpals, complete or partial (with or without incomplete phalangeal deficiency)

755.29 Longitudinal deficiency, phalanges, complete or partial
    Absence of finger, congenital
    Aphalangia of upper limb, terminal, complete or partial
    Excludes *terminal deficiency of all five digits (755.21)*
    transverse deficiency of phalanges (755.21)

● **755.3 Reduction deformities of lower limb**

❑ **755.30 Unspecified reduction deformity of lower limb**
    Ectromelia NOS of lower limb
    Hemimelia NOS of lower limb
    Shortening of leg, congenital

755.31 Transverse deficiency of lower limb
    Amelia of lower limb
    Congenital absence of:
        foot
        leg, including foot and toes
        lower limb, complete
        toes, all, complete
    Transverse hemimelia of lower limb

755.32 Longitudinal deficiency of lower limb, NEC
    Phocomelia NOS of lower limb

755.33 Longitudinal deficiency, combined, involving femur, tibia, and fibula (complete or incomplete)
    Congenital absence of thigh and (lower) leg (complete or incomplete) with or without metacarpal deficiency and/or phalangeal deficiency, incomplete
    Phocomelia, complete, of lower limb

755.34 Longitudinal deficiency, femoral, complete or partial (with or without distal deficiencies, incomplete)
     Congenital absence of femur (with or without absence of some [but not all] distal elements)
     Proximal phocomelia of lower limb

755.35 Longitudinal deficiency, tibiofibular, complete or partial (with or without distal deficiencies, incomplete)
     Congenital absence of tibia and fibula (with or without absence of some [but not all] distal elements)
     Distal phocomelia of lower limb

755.36 Longitudinal deficiency, tibia, complete or partial (with or without distal deficiencies, incomplete)
     Agenesis of tibia
     Congenital absence of tibia (with or without absence of some [but not all] distal elements)

755.37 Longitudinal deficiency, fibular, complete or partial (with or without distal deficiencies, incomplete)
     Agenesis of fibula
     Congenital absence of fibula (with or without absence of some [but not all] distal elements)

755.38 Longitudinal deficiency, tarsals or metatarsals, complete or partial (with or without incomplete phalangeal deficiency)

755.39 Longitudinal deficiency, phalanges, complete or partial
     Absence of toe, congenital
     Aphalangia of lower limb, terminal, complete or partial

Excludes	terminal deficiency of all five digits (755.31)
	transverse deficiency of phalanges (755.31)

❏ **755.4 Reduction deformities, unspecified limb**
     Absence, congenital (complete or partial) of limb NOS
     Amelia of unspecified limb
     Ectromelia of unspecified limb
     Hemimelia of unspecified limb
     Phocomelia of unspecified limb

● **755.5 Other anomalies of upper limb, including shoulder girdle**

  ❏ **755.50 Unspecified anomaly of upper limb**

  755.51 Congenital deformity of clavicle

  755.52 Congenital elevation of scapula
     Sprengel's deformity

  755.53 Radioulnar synostosis

  755.54 Madelung's deformity

  755.55 Acrocephalosyndactyly
     Apert's syndrome

  755.56 Accessory carpal bones

  755.57 Macrodactylia (fingers)

  755.58 Cleft hand, congenital
     Lobster-claw hand

  ❏ **755.59 Other**
     Cleidocranial dysostosis
     Cubitus:
       valgus, congenital
       varus, congenital

Excludes	club hand (congenital) (754.89)
	congenital dislocation of elbow (754.89)

● **755.6 Other anomalies of lower limb, including pelvic girdle**

  ❏ **755.60 Unspecified anomaly of lower limb**

  755.61 Coxa valga, congenital

  755.62 Coxa vara, congenital

  ❏ **755.63 Other congenital deformity of hip (joint)**
     Congenital anteversion of femur (neck)

Excludes	congenital dislocation of hip (754.30–754.35)

  755.64 Congenital deformity of knee (joint)
     Congenital:
       absence of patella
       genu valgum [knock-knee]
       genu varum [bowleg]
       Rudimentary patella

  755.65 Macrodactylia of toes

  ❏ **755.66 Other anomalies of toes**
     Congenital:
       hallux valgus
       hallux varus
       hammer toe

  755.67 Anomalies of foot, NEC
     Astragaloscaphoid synostosis
     Calcaneonavicular bar
     Coalition of calcaneus
     Talonavicular synostosis
     Tarsal coalitions

  ❏ **755.69 Other**
     Congenital:
       angulation of tibia
       deformity (of):
         ankle (joint)
         sacroiliac (joint)
       fusion of sacroiliac joint

❏ **755.8 Other specified anomalies of unspecified limb**

❏ **755.9 Unspecified anomaly of unspecified limb**
     Congenital:
       anomaly NOS of unspecified limb
       deformity NOS of unspecified limb

Excludes	reduction deformity of unspecified limb (755.4)

● **756 Other congenital musculoskeletal anomalies**

Excludes	those deformities classifiable to 754.0–754.8

756.0 Anomalies of skull and face bones
     Absence of skull bones
     Acrocephaly
     Congenital deformity of forehead
     Craniosynostosis
     Crouzon's disease
     Hypertelorism
     Imperfect fusion of skull
     Oxycephaly
     Platybasia
     Premature closure of cranial sutures
     Tower skull
     Trigonocephaly

Excludes	acrocephalosyndactyly [Apert's syndrome] (755.55)
	dentofacial anomalies (524.0–524.9)
	skull defects associated with brain anomalies, such as:
	anencephalus (740.0)
	encephalocele (742.0)
	hydrocephalus (742.3)
	microcephalus (742.1)

ICD-9-CM

700-799

Vol. 1

● 756.1 **Anomalies of spine**

❑ 756.10 **Anomaly of spine, unspecified**

756.11 **Spondylolysis, lumbosacral region**
Prespondylolisthesis (lumbosacral)

756.12 **Spondylolisthesis**

756.13 **Absence of vertebra, congenital**

756.14 **Hemivertebra**

756.15 **Fusion of spine [vertebra], congenital**

756.16 **Klippel-Feil syndrome**

756.17 **Spina bifida occulta**

Excludes *spina bifida (aperta) (741.0–741.9)*

❑ 756.19 **Other**
Platyspondylia
Supernumerary vertebra

756.2 **Cervical rib**
Supernumerary rib in the cervical region

❑ 756.3 **Other anomalies of ribs and sternum**
Congenital absence of:
   rib
   sternum
Congenital:
   fissure of sternum
   fusion of ribs
Sternum bifidum

Excludes *nonteratogenic deformity of chest wall (754.81–754.89)*

756.4 **Chondrodystrophy**
Achondroplasia   Enchondromatosis
Chondrodystrophia (fetalis)   Ollier's disease
Dyschondroplasia

Excludes *lipochondrodystrophy [Hurler's syndrome] (277.5)*
Morquio's disease (277.5)

● 756.5 **Osteodystrophies**

❑ 756.50 **Osteodystrophy, unspecified**

756.51 **Osteogenesis imperfecta**
Fragilitas ossium
Osteopsathyrosis

756.52 **Osteopetrosis**

756.53 **Osteopoikilosis**

756.54 **Polyostotic fibrous dysplasia of bone**

756.55 **Chondroectodermal dysplasia**
Ellis-van Creveld syndrome

756.56 **Multiple epiphyseal dysplasia**

❑ 756.59 **Other**
Albright (-McCune)-Sternberg syndrome

756.6 **Anomalies of diaphragm**
Absence of diaphragm
Congenital hernia:
   diaphragmatic
   foramen of Morgagni
Eventration of diaphragm

Excludes *congenital hiatus hernia (750.6)*

● 756.7 **Anomalies of abdominal wall**

❑ 756.70 **Anomaly of abdominal wall, unspecified**

756.71 **Prune belly syndrome**
Eagle-Barrett syndrome
Prolapse of bladder mucosa

❑ 756.79 **Other congenital anomalies of abdominal wall**
Exomphalos   Omphalocele
Gastroschisis

Excludes *umbilical hernia (551–553 with .1)*

● 756.8 **Other specified anomalies of muscle, tendon, fascia, and connective tissue**

756.81 **Absence of muscle and tendon**
Absence of muscle (pectoral)

756.82 **Accessory muscle**

756.83 **Ehlers-Danlos syndrome**

❑ 756.89 **Other**
Amyotrophia congenita
Congenital shortening of tendon

❑ 756.9 **Other and unspecified anomalies of musculoskeletal system**
Congenital:
   anomaly NOS of musculoskeletal system, NEC
   deformity NOS of musculoskeletal system, NEC

● 757 **Congenital anomalies of the integument**

Includes: anomalies of skin, subcutaneous tissue, hair, nails, and breast

Excludes *hemangioma (228.00–228.09)*
pigmented nevus (216.0–216.9)

757.0 **Hereditary edema of legs**
Congenital lymphedema
Hereditary trophedema
Milroy's disease

757.1 **Ichthyosis congenita**
Congenital ichthyosis
Harlequin fetus
Ichthyosiform erythroderma

757.2 **Dermatoglyphic anomalies**
Abnormal palmar creases

● 757.3 **Other specified anomalies of skin**

757.31 **Congenital ectodermal dysplasia**

757.32 **Vascular hamartomas**
Birthmarks
Port-wine stain
Strawberry nevus

757.33 **Congenital pigmentary anomalies of skin**
Congenital poikiloderma
Urticaria pigmentosa
Xeroderma pigmentosum

Excludes *albinism (270.2)*

❑ 757.39 **Other**
Accessory skin tags, congenital
Congenital scar
Epidermolysis bullosa
Keratoderma (congenital)

Excludes *pilonidal cyst (685.0–685.1)*

❑ 757.4 **Specified anomalies of hair**
Congenital:
   alopecia
   atrichosis
   beaded hair
   hypertrichosis
   monilethrix
Persistent lanugo

❑ 757.5 **Specified anomalies of nails**
Anonychia
Congenital:
   clubnail
   koilonychia
   leukonychia
   onychauxis
   pachyonychia

❑ **757.6 Specified anomalies of breast**
Absent breast or nipple
Accessory breast or nipple
Supernumerary breast or nipple
Hypoplasia of breast

    Excludes *absence of pectoral muscle (756.81)*

❑ **757.8 Other specified anomalies of the integument**

❑ **757.9 Unspecified anomaly of the integument**
Congenital:
   anomaly NOS of integument
   deformity NOS of integument

● **758 Chromosomal anomalies**

Use additional codes for conditions associated with the
chromosomal anomalies   ◀

   Includes: syndromes associated with anomalies in the
           number and form of chromosomes

758.0 Down's syndrome
Mongolism
Translocation Down's syndrome
Trisomy:
  21 or 22
  G

758.1 Patau's syndrome
Trisomy:
  13
  D_1

758.2 Edwards's syndrome
Trisomy:
  18
  E_3

● **758.3 Autosomal deletion syndromes**

   758.31 Cri-du-chat syndrome   ◀
      Deletion 5p   ◀

   758.32 Velo-cardio-facial syndrome   ◀
      Deletion 22q 11.2   ◀

   ❑ **758.33 Other microdeletions**   ◀
      Miller-Dieker syndrome   ◀
      Smith-Magenis syndrome   ◀

   ❑ **758.39 Other autosomal deletions**   ◀

758.4 Balanced autosomal translocation in normal individual

❑ **758.5 Other conditions due to autosomal anomalies**
Accessory autosomes, NEC

758.6 Gonadal dysgenesis
Ovarian dysgenesis
Turner's syndrome
XO syndrome

    Excludes *pure gonadal dysgenesis (752.7)*

758.7 Klinefelter's syndrome
XXY syndrome

● **758.8 Other conditions due to chromosome anomalies**

   ❑ **758.81 Other conditions due to sex chromosome anomalies**

   ❑ **758.89 Other**

❑ **758.9 Conditions due to anomaly of unspecified chromosome**

● **759 Other and unspecified congenital anomalies**

759.0 Anomalies of spleen
Aberrant spleen   Congenital splenomegaly
Absent spleen   Ectopic spleen
Accessory spleen   Lobulation of spleen

759.1 Anomalies of adrenal gland
Aberrant adrenal gland
Absent adrenal gland
Accessory adrenal gland

    Excludes *adrenogenital disorders (255.2)*
                congenital disorders of steroid metabolism (255.2)

❑ **759.2 Anomalies of other endocrine glands**
Absent parathyroid gland
Accessory thyroid gland
Persistent thyroglossal or thyrolingual duct
Thyroglossal (duct) cyst

    Excludes *congenital:*
         goiter (246.1)
         hypothyroidism (243)

759.3 Situs inversus
Situs inversus or transversus:
  abdominalis
  thoracis
Transposition of viscera:
  abdominal
  thoracic

    Excludes *dextrocardia without mention of complete transposition (746.87)*

759.4 Conjoined twins
Craniopagus   Thoracopagus
Dicephalus   Xiphopagus
Pygopagus

759.5 Tuberous sclerosis
Bourneville's disease
Epiloia

❑ **759.6 Other hamartoses, NEC**
Syndrome:
  Peutz-Jeghers
  Sturge-Weber (-Dimitri)
  von Hippel-Lindau

    Excludes *neurofibromatosis (237.7)*

759.7 Multiple congenital anomalies, so described
Congenital:
  anomaly, multiple NOS
  deformity, multiple NOS

● **759.8 Other specified anomalies**

   759.81 Prader-Willi syndrome

   759.82 Marfan syndrome

   759.83 Fragile X syndrome

   ❑ **759.89 Other**
      Congenital malformation syndromes affecting multiple systems, NEC
      Laurence-Moon-Biedl syndrome

❑ **759.9 Congenital anomaly, unspecified**

15. CERTAIN CONDITIONS ORIGINATING IN THE PERINATAL PERIOD (760–779)

Includes: conditions which have their origin in the perinatal period even though death or morbidity occurs later

Use additional code(s) to further specify condition

MATERNAL CAUSES OF PERINATAL MORBIDITY AND MORTALITY (760–763)

● **760 Fetus or newborn affected by maternal conditions which may be unrelated to present pregnancy**

Includes: the listed maternal conditions only when specified as a cause of mortality or morbidity of the fetus or newborn

Excludes maternal endocrine and metabolic disorders affecting fetus or newborn (775.0–775.9)

760.0 Maternal hypertensive disorders
Fetus or newborn affected by maternal conditions classifiable to 642

760.1 Maternal renal and urinary tract diseases
Fetus or newborn affected by maternal conditions classifiable to 580–599

760.2 Maternal infections
Fetus or newborn affected by maternal infectious disease classifiable to 001–136 and 487, but fetus or newborn not manifesting that disease

Excludes congenital infectious diseases (771.0–771.8)
maternal genital tract and other localized infections (760.8)

☐ **760.3 Other chronic maternal circulatory and respiratory diseases**
Fetus or newborn affected by chronic maternal conditions classifiable to 390–459, 490–519, 745–748

760.4 Maternal nutritional disorders
Fetus or newborn affected by:
maternal disorders classifiable to 260–269
maternal malnutrition NOS

Excludes fetal malnutrition (764.10–764.29)

760.5 Maternal injury
Fetus or newborn affected by maternal conditions classifiable to 800–995

760.6 Surgical operation on mother

Excludes cesarean section for present delivery (763.4)
damage to placenta from amniocentesis, cesarean section, or surgical induction (762.1)
previous surgery to uterus or pelvic organs (763.89)

● **760.7 Noxious influences affecting fetus or newborn via placenta or breast milk** ◀▥
Fetus or newborn affected by noxious substance transmitted via placenta or breast milk

Excludes anesthetic and analgesic drugs administered during labor and delivery (763.5)
drug withdrawal syndrome in newborn (779.5)

☐ **760.70 Unspecified noxious substance**
Fetus or newborn affected by:
Drug, NEC

760.71 Alcohol
Fetal alcohol syndrome

760.72 Narcotics

760.73 Hallucinogenic agents

760.74 Anti-infectives
Antibiotics

760.75 Cocaine

760.76 Diethylstilbestrol [DES]

☐ **760.79 Other**
Fetus or newborn affected by:
immune sera transmitted via placenta or breast milk
medicinal agents, NEC, transmitted via placenta or breast milk
toxic substance, NEC, transmitted via placenta or breast milk

☐ **760.8 Other specified maternal conditions affecting fetus or newborn**
Maternal genital tract and other localized infection affecting fetus or newborn, but fetus or newborn not manifesting that disease

Excludes maternal urinary tract infection affecting fetus or newborn (760.1)

☐ **760.9 Unspecified maternal condition affecting fetus or newborn**

● **761 Fetus or newborn affected by maternal complications of pregnancy**

Includes: the listed maternal conditions only when specified as a cause of mortality or morbidity of the fetus or newborn

761.0 Incompetent cervix

761.1 Premature rupture of membranes

761.2 Oligohydramnios

Excludes that due to premature rupture of membranes (761.1)

761.3 Polyhydramnios
Hydramnios (acute) (chronic)

761.4 Ectopic pregnancy
Pregnancy:
abdominal
intraperitoneal
tubal

761.5 Multiple pregnancy
Triplet (pregnancy)
Twin (pregnancy)

761.6 Maternal death

761.7 Malpresentation before labor
Breech presentation before labor
External version before labor
Oblique lie before labor
Transverse lie before labor
Unstable lie before labor

☐ **761.8 Other specified maternal complications of pregnancy affecting fetus or newborn**
Spontaneous abortion, fetus

☐ **761.9 Unspecified maternal complication of pregnancy affecting fetus or newborn**

● **762 Fetus or newborn affected by complications of placenta, cord, and membranes**

Includes: the listed maternal conditions only when specified as a cause of mortality or morbidity in the fetus or newborn

762.0 Placenta previa

☐ **762.1 Other forms of placental separation and hemorrhage**
Abruptio placentae
Antepartum hemorrhage
Damage to placenta from amniocentesis, cesarean section, or surgical induction
Maternal blood loss
Premature separation of placenta
Rupture of marginal sinus

☐ **762.2 Other and unspecified morphological and functional abnormalities of placenta**
Placental:
dysfunction
infarction
insufficiency

762.3 Placental transfusion syndromes
Placental and cord abnormality resulting in twin-to-twin or other transplacental transfusion

Use additional code to indicate resultant condition in fetus or newborn:
fetal blood loss (772.0)
polycythemia neonatorum (776.4)

762.4 Prolapsed cord
Cord presentation

☐ **762.5 Other compression of umbilical cord**
Cord around neck
Entanglement of cord
Knot in cord
Torsion of cord

☐ **762.6 Other and unspecified conditions of umbilical cord**
Short cord
Thrombosis of umbilical cord
Varices of umbilical cord
Velamentous insertion of umbilical cord
Vasa previa

> **Excludes** *infection of umbilical cord (771.4)*
> *single umbilical artery (747.5)*

762.7 Chorioamnionitis
Amnionitis
Membranitis
Placentitis

☐ **762.8 Other specified abnormalities of chorion and amnion**

☐ **762.9 Unspecified abnormality of chorion and amnion**

● **763 Fetus or newborn affected by other complications of labor and delivery**

> **Includes:** the listed conditions only when specified as a cause of mortality or morbidity in the fetus or newborn

763.0 Breech delivery and extraction

☐ **763.1 Other malpresentation, malposition, and disproportion during labor and delivery**
Fetus or newborn affected by:
abnormality of bony pelvis
contracted pelvis
persistent occipitoposterior position
shoulder presentation
transverse lie
conditions classifiable to 652, 653, and 660

763.2 Forceps delivery
Fetus or newborn affected by forceps extraction

763.3 Delivery by vacuum extractor

763.4 Cesarean delivery

> **Excludes** *placental separation or hemorrhage from cesarean section (762.1)*

763.5 Maternal anesthesia and analgesia
Reactions and intoxications from maternal opiates and tranquilizers during labor and delivery

> **Excludes** *drug withdrawal syndrome in newborn (779.5)*

763.6 Precipitate delivery
Rapid second stage

763.7 Abnormal uterine contractions
Fetus or newborn affected by:
contraction ring
hypertonic labor
hypotonic uterine dysfunction
uterine inertia or dysfunction
conditions classifiable to 661, except 661.3

● **763.8 Other specified complications of labor and delivery affecting fetus or newborn**

     763.81 Abnormality in fetal heart rate or rhythm before the onset of labor

     763.82 Abnormality in fetal heart rate or rhythm during labor

     ☐ **763.83 Abnormality in fetal heart rate or rhythm, unspecified as to time of onset**

     ☐ **763.89 Other specified complications of labor and delivery affecting fetus or newborn**
Fetus or newborn affected by:
abnormality of maternal soft tissues
destructive operation on live fetus to facilitate delivery
induction of labor (medical)
previous surgery to uterus or pelvic organs
other conditions classifiable to 650–669
other procedures used in labor and delivery

☐ **763.9 Unspecified complication of labor and delivery affecting fetus or newborn**

OTHER CONDITIONS ORIGINATING IN THE PERINATAL PERIOD (764–779)

The following fifth-digit subclassification is for use with category 764 and codes 765.0 and 765.1 to denote birthweight:

☐ 0 unspecified [weight]
1 less than 500 grams
2 500–749 grams
3 750–999 grams
4 1,000–1,249 grams
5 1,250–1,499 grams
6 1,500–1,749 grams
7 1,750–1,999 grams
8 2,000–2,499 grams
9 2,500 grams and over

● **764 Slow fetal growth and fetal malnutrition**

Requires fifth digit. See beginning of section 764–779 for codes and definitions.

● **764.0 "Light-for-dates" without mention of fetal malnutrition**
Infants underweight for gestational age
"Small-for-dates"

● **764.1 "Light-for-dates" with signs of fetal malnutrition**
Infants "light-for-dates" classifiable to 764.0, who in addition show signs of fetal malnutrition, such as dry peeling skin and loss of subcutaneous tissue

● **764.2 Fetal malnutrition without mention of "light-for-dates"**
Infants, not underweight for gestational age, showing signs of fetal malnutrition, such as dry peeling skin and loss of subcutaneous tissue
Intrauterine malnutrition

● ☐ **764.9 Fetal growth retardation, unspecified**
Intrauterine growth retardation

ICD-9-CM

700–799

Vol. 1

● 765 **Disorders relating to short gestation and low birthweight**

Requires fifth digit. See beginning of section 764–779 for codes and definitions.

Includes: the listed conditions, without further specification, as causes of mortality, morbidity, or additional care, in fetus or newborn

● 765.0 **Extreme immaturity**

Note: Usually implies a birthweight of less than 1,000 grams

Use additional code for weeks of gestation (765.20–765.29)

● ☐ 765.1 **Other preterm infants**

Note: Usually implies birthweight of 1,000–2,499 grams

Prematurity NOS

Prematurity or small size, not classifiable to 765.0 or as "light-for-dates" in 764

Use additional code for weeks of gestation (765.20–765.29)

● 765.2 **Weeks of gestation**

☐ 765.20 Unspecified weeks of gestation

765.21 Less than 24 completed weeks of gestation

765.22 24 completed weeks of gestation

765.23 25–26 completed weeks of gestation

765.24 27–28 completed weeks of gestation

765.25 29–30 completed weeks of gestation

765.26 31–32 completed weeks of gestation

765.27 33–34 completed weeks of gestation

765.28 35–36 completed weeks of gestation

765.29 37 or more completed weeks of gestation

● 766 **Disorders relating to long gestation and high birthweight**

Includes: the listed conditions, without further specification, as causes of mortality, morbidity, or additional care, in fetus or newborn

766.0 **Exceptionally large baby**

Note: Usually implies a birthweight of 4,500 grams or more.

☐ 766.1 **Other "heavy-for-dates" infants**

Other fetus or infant "heavy-" or "large-for-dates" regardless of period of gestation

● 766.2 **Late infant, not "heavy-for-dates"**

766.21 **Post-term infant**

Infant with gestation period over 40 completed weeks to 42 completed weeks

766.22 **Prolonged gestation of infant**

Infant with gestation period over 42 completed weeks

Postmaturity NOS

● 767 **Birth trauma**

767.0 **Subdural and cerebral hemorrhage**

Subdural and cerebral hemorrhage, whether described as due to birth trauma or to intrapartum anoxia or hypoxia

Subdural hematoma (localized)

Tentorial tear

Use additional code to identify cause

Excludes *intraventricular hemorrhage (772.10–772.14) subarachnoid hemorrhage (772.2)*

● 767.1 **Injuries to scalp**

767.11 **Epicranial subaponeurotic hemorrhage (massive)**

Subgaleal hemorrhage

☐ 767.19 **Other injuries to scalp**

Caput succedaneum

Cephalhematoma

Chignon (from vacuum extraction)

767.2 **Fracture of clavicle**

☐ 767.3 **Other injuries to skeleton**

Fracture of:

long bones

skull

Excludes *congenital dislocation of hip (754.30–754.35) fracture of spine, congenital (767.4)*

767.4 **Injury to spine and spinal cord**

Dislocation of spine or spinal cord due to birth trauma

Fracture of spine or spinal cord due to birth trauma

Laceration of spine or spinal cord due to birth trauma

Rupture of spine or spinal cord due to birth trauma

767.5 **Facial nerve injury**

Facial palsy

767.6 **Injury to brachial plexus**

Palsy or paralysis:

brachial

Erb (-Duchenne)

Klumpke (-Déjérine)

☐ 767.7 **Other cranial and peripheral nerve injuries**

Phrenic nerve paralysis

☐ 767.8 **Other specified birth trauma**

Eye damage

Hematoma of:

liver (subcapsular)

testes

vulva

Rupture of:

liver

spleen

Scalpel wound

Traumatic glaucoma

Excludes *hemorrhage classifiable to 772.0–772.9*

☐ 767.9 **Birth trauma, unspecified**

Birth injury NOS

● 768 **Intrauterine hypoxia and birth asphyxia**

Use only when associated with newborn morbidity classifiable elsewhere

☐ 768.0 **Fetal death from asphyxia or anoxia before onset of labor or at unspecified time**

768.1 **Fetal death from asphyxia or anoxia during labor**

768.2 **Fetal distress before onset of labor, in liveborn infant**

Fetal metabolic acidemia before onset of labor, in liveborn infant

768.3 **Fetal distress first noted during labor, in liveborn infant**

Fetal metabolic acidemia first noted during labor, in liveborn infant

☐ 768.4 **Fetal distress, unspecified as to time of onset, in liveborn infant**

Fetal metabolic acidemia unspecified as to time of onset, in liveborn infant

768.5 Severe birth asphyxia
Birth asphyxia with neurologic involvement

768.6 Mild or moderate birth asphyxia
Other specified birth asphyxia (without mention of neurologic involvement)

❑ **768.9 Unspecified birth asphyxia in liveborn infant**
Anoxia NOS, in liveborn infant
Asphyxia NOS, in liveborn infant
Hypoxia NOS, in liveborn infant

769 Respiratory distress syndrome
Cardiorespiratory distress syndrome of newborn
Hyaline membrane disease (pulmonary)
Idiopathic respiratory distress syndrome [IRDS or RDS] of newborn
Pulmonary hypoperfusion syndrome
Excludes *transient tachypnea of newborn (770.6)*

● **770 Other respiratory conditions of fetus and newborn**

770.0 Congenital pneumonia
Infective pneumonia acquired prenatally
Excludes *pneumonia from infection acquired after birth (480.0–486)*

770.1 Meconium aspiration syndrome
Aspiration of contents of birth canal NOS
Meconium aspiration below vocal cords
Pneumonitis:
fetal aspiration
meconium

770.2 Interstitial emphysema and related conditions
Pneumomediastinum originating in the perinatal period
Pneumopericardium originating in the perinatal period
Pneumothorax originating in the perinatal period

770.3 Pulmonary hemorrhage
Hemorrhage:
alveolar (lung) originating in the perinatal period
intra-alveolar (lung) originating in the perinatal period
massive pulmonary originating in the perinatal period

770.4 Primary atelectasis
Pulmonary immaturity NOS

❑ **770.5 Other and unspecified atelectasis**
Atelectasis:
NOS originating in the perinatal period
partial originating in the perinatal period
secondary originating in the perinatal period
Pulmonary collapse originating in the perinatal period

770.6 Transitory tachypnea of newborn
Idiopathic tachypnea of newborn
Wet lung syndrome
Excludes *respiratory distress syndrome (769)*

770.7 Chronic respiratory disease arising in the perinatal period
Bronchopulmonary dysplasia
Interstitial pulmonary fibrosis of prematurity
Wilson-Mikity syndrome

● ❑ **770.8 Other respiratory problems after birth**

770.81 Primary apnea of newborn
Apneic spells of newborn NOS
Essential apnea of newborn
Sleep apnea of newborn

770.82 Other apnea of newborn
Obstructive apnea of newborn

770.83 Cyanotic attacks of newborn

770.84 Respiratory failure of newborn
Excludes *respiratory distress syndrome (769)*

❑ **770.89 Other respiratory problems after birth**

❑ **770.9 Unspecified respiratory condition of fetus and newborn**

● **771 Infections specific to the perinatal period**
Includes: infections acquired before or during birth or via the umbilicus
Excludes *congenital pneumonia (770.0)*
congenital syphilis (090.0–090.9)
maternal infectious disease as a cause of mortality or morbidity in fetus or newborn, but fetus or newborn not manifesting the disease (760.2)
ophthalmia neonatorum due to gonococcus (098.40)
other infections not specifically classified to this category

771.0 Congenital rubella
Congenital rubella pneumonitis

771.1 Congenital cytomegalovirus infection
Congenital cytomegalic inclusion disease

❑ **771.2 Other congenital infections**
Congenital: Congenital:
herpes simplex   toxoplasmosis
listeriosis   tuberculosis
malaria

771.3 Tetanus neonatorum
Tetanus omphalitis
Excludes *hypocalcemic tetany (775.4)*

771.4 Omphalitis of the newborn
Infection: Infection:
navel cord   umbilical stump
Excludes *tetanus omphalitis (771.3)*

771.5 Neonatal infective mastitis
Excludes *noninfective neonatal mastitis (778.7)*

771.6 Neonatal conjunctivitis and dacryocystitis
Ophthalmia neonatorum NOS
Excludes *ophthalmia neonatorum due to gonococcus (098.40)*

771.7 Neonatal Candida infection
Neonatal moniliasis
Thrush in newborn

● ❑ **771.8 Other infections specific to the perinatal period**
Use additional code to identify organism (041.00–041.9) ◄▥

771.81 Septicemia [sepsis] of newborn

771.82 Urinary tract infection of newborn

771.83 Bacteremia of newborn

❑ **771.89 Other infections specific to the perinatal period**
Intra-amniotic infection of fetus NOS
Infection of newborn NOS

● **772 Fetal and neonatal hemorrhage**
Excludes *hematological disorders of fetus and newborn (776.0–776.9)*

772.0 Fetal blood loss
Fetal blood loss from:
cut end of co-twin's cord
placenta
ruptured cord
vasa previa
Fetal exsanguination
Fetal hemorrhage into:
co-twin
mother's circulation

ICD-9-CM

700-799

Vol. 1

● **772.1 Intraventricular hemorrhage**
Intraventricular hemorrhage from any perinatal cause

❑ **772.10 Unspecified grade**

772.11 Grade I
Bleeding into germinal matrix

772.12 Grade II
Bleeding into ventricle

772.13 Grade III
Bleeding with enlargement of ventricle

772.14 Grade IV
Bleeding into cerebral cortex

772.2 Subarachnoid hemorrhage
Subarachnoid hemorrhage from any perinatal cause
| **Excludes** | *subdural and cerebral hemorrhage (767.0)* |

772.3 Umbilical hemorrhage after birth
Slipped umbilical ligature

772.4 Gastrointestinal hemorrhage
| **Excludes** | *swallowed maternal blood (777.3)* |

772.5 Adrenal hemorrhage

772.6 Cutaneous hemorrhage
Bruising in fetus or newborn
Ecchymoses in fetus or newborn
Petechiae in fetus or newborn
Superficial hematoma in fetus or newborn

❑ **772.8 Other specified hemorrhage of fetus or newborn**
| **Excludes** | *hemorrhagic disease of newborn (776.0)* |
| | *pulmonary hemorrhage (770.3)* |

❑ **772.9 Unspecified hemorrhage of newborn**

● **773 Hemolytic disease of fetus or newborn, due to isoimmunization**

773.0 Hemolytic disease due to Rh isoimmunization
Anemia due to RH:
  antibodies
  isoimmunization
  maternal/fetal incompatibility
Erythroblastosis (fetalis) due to RH:
  antibodies
  isoimmunization
  maternal/fetal incompatibility
Hemolytic disease (fetus) (newborn) due to RH:
  antibodies
  isoimmunization
  maternal/fetal incompatibility
Jaundice due to RH:
  antibodies
  isoimmunization
  maternal/fetal incompatibility
Rh hemolytic disease
Rh isoimmunization

773.1 Hemolytic disease due to ABO isoimmunization
ABO hemolytic disease
ABO isoimmunization
Anemia due to ABO:
  antibodies
  isoimmunization
  maternal/fetal incompatibility
Erythroblastosis (fetalis) due to ABO:
  antibodies
  isoimmunization
  maternal/fetal incompatibility
Hemolytic disease (fetus) (newborn) due to ABO:
  antibodies
  isoimmunization
  maternal/fetal incompatibility
Jaundice due to ABO:
  antibodies
  isoimmunization
  maternal/fetal incompatibility

❑ **773.2 Hemolytic disease due to other and unspecified isoimmunization**
Erythroblastosis (fetalis) (neonatorum) NOS
Hemolytic disease (fetus) (newborn) NOS
Jaundice or anemia due to other and unspecified blood-group incompatibility

773.3 Hydrops fetalis due to isoimmunization
Use additional code , if desired, to identify type of isoimmunization (773.0–773.2)

773.4 Kernicterus due to isoimmunization
Use additional code , if desired, to identify type of isoimmunization (773.0–773.2)

773.5 Late anemia due to isoimmunization

● **774 Other perinatal jaundice**

● **774.0 *Perinatal jaundice from hereditary hemolytic anemias***
Code first underlying disease (282.0–282.9)

❑ **774.1 Perinatal jaundice from other excessive hemolysis**
Fetal or neonatal jaundice from:
  bruising
  drugs or toxins transmitted from mother
  infection
  polycythemia
  swallowed maternal blood
Use additional code to identify cause
| **Excludes** | *jaundice due to isoimmunization (773.0–773.2)* |

774.2 Neonatal jaundice associated with preterm delivery
Hyperbilirubinemia of prematurity
Jaundice due to delayed conjugation associated with preterm delivery

● **774.3 Neonatal jaundice due to delayed conjugation from other causes**

❑ **774.30 Neonatal jaundice due to delayed conjugation, cause unspecified**

● **774.31 *Neonatal jaundice due to delayed conjugation in diseases classified elsewhere***
Code first underlying diseases, as:
  congenital hypothyroidism (243)
  Crigler-Najjar syndrome (277.4)
  Gilbert's syndrome (277.4)

❑ **774.39 Other**
Jaundice due to delayed conjugation from causes, such as:
  breast milk inhibitors
  delayed development of conjugating system

774.4 Perinatal jaundice due to hepatocellular damage
Fetal or neonatal hepatitis
Giant cell hepatitis
Inspissated bile syndrome

● ❑ **774.5 *Perinatal jaundice from other causes***
Code first underlying cause, as:
  congenital obstruction of bile duct (751.61)
  galactosemia (271.1)
  mucoviscidosis (277.00–277.09)

❑ **774.6 Unspecified fetal and neonatal jaundice**
Icterus neonatorum
Neonatal hyperbilirubinemia (transient)
Physiologic jaundice NOS in newborn
| **Excludes** | *that in preterm infants (774.2)* |

774.7 Kernicterus not due to isoimmunization
Bilirubin encephalopathy
Kernicterus of newborn NOS

Excludes *kernicterus due to isoimmunization (773.4)*

● **775 Endocrine and metabolic disturbances specific to the fetus and newborn**

Includes: transitory endocrine and metabolic disturbances caused by the infant's response to maternal endocrine and metabolic factors, its removal from them, or its adjustment to extrauterine existence

775.0 Syndrome of "infant of a diabetic mother"
Maternal diabetes mellitus affecting fetus or newborn (with hypoglycemia)

775.1 Neonatal diabetes mellitus
Diabetes mellitus syndrome in newborn infant

775.2 Neonatal myasthenia gravis

775.3 Neonatal thyrotoxicosis
Neonatal hyperthyroidism (transient)

775.4 Hypocalcemia and hypomagnesemia of newborn
Cow's milk hypocalcemia
Hypocalcemic tetany, neonatal
Neonatal hypoparathyroidism
Phosphate-loading hypocalcemia

☐ 775.5 Other transitory neonatal electrolyte disturbances
Dehydration, neonatal

775.6 Neonatal hypoglycemia

Excludes *infant of mother with diabetes mellitus (775.0)*

775.7 Late metabolic acidosis of newborn

☐ 775.8 Other transitory neonatal endocrine and metabolic disturbances
Amino-acid metabolic disorders described as transitory

☐ 775.9 Unspecified endocrine and metabolic disturbances specific to the fetus and newborn

● **776 Hematological disorders of fetus and newborn**

Includes: disorders specific to the fetus or newborn

776.0 Hemorrhagic disease of newborn
Hemorrhagic diathesis of newborn
Vitamin K deficiency of newborn

Excludes *fetal or neonatal hemorrhage (772.0–772.9)*

776.1 Transient neonatal thrombocytopenia
Neonatal thrombocytopenia due to:
exchange transfusion
idiopathic maternal thrombocytopenia
isoimmunization

776.2 Disseminated intravascular coagulation in newborn

☐ 776.3 Other transient neonatal disorders of coagulation
Transient coagulation defect, newborn

776.4 Polycythemia neonatorum
Plethora of newborn
Polycythemia due to:
donor twin transfusion
maternal-fetal transfusion

776.5 Congenital anemia
Anemia following fetal blood loss

Excludes *anemia due to isoimmunization (773.0–773.2, 773.5)*
hereditary hemolytic anemias (282.0–282.9)

776.6 Anemia of prematurity

776.7 Transient neonatal neutropenia
Isoimmune neutropenia
Maternal transfer neutropenia

Excludes *congenital neutropenia (nontransient) (288.0)*

☐ 776.8 Other specified transient hematological disorders

☐ 776.9 Unspecified hematological disorder specific to fetus or newborn

● **777 Perinatal disorders of digestive system**

Includes: disorders specific to the fetus and newborn

Excludes *intestinal obstruction classifiable to 560.0–560.9*

777.1 Meconium obstruction
Congenital fecaliths
Delayed passage of meconium
Meconium ileus NOS
Meconium plug syndrome

Excludes *meconium ileus in cystic fibrosis (277.01)*

777.2 Intestinal obstruction due to inspissated milk

777.3 Hematemesis and melena due to swallowed maternal blood
Swallowed blood syndrome in newborn

Excludes *that not due to swallowed maternal blood (772.4)*

777.4 Transitory ileus of newborn

Excludes *Hirschsprung's disease (751.3)*

777.5 Necrotizing enterocolitis in fetus or newborn
Pseudomembranous enterocolitis in newborn

777.6 Perinatal intestinal perforation
Meconium peritonitis

☐ 777.8 Other specified perinatal disorders of digestive system

☐ 777.9 Unspecified perinatal disorder of digestive system

● **778 Conditions involving the integument and temperature regulation of fetus and newborn**

778.0 Hydrops fetalis not due to isoimmunization
Idiopathic hydrops

Excludes *hydrops fetalis due to isoimmunization (773.3)*

778.1 Sclerema neonatorum

778.2 Cold injury syndrome of newborn

☐ 778.3 Other hypothermia of newborn

☐ 778.4 Other disturbances of temperature regulation of newborn
Dehydration fever in newborn
Environmentally induced pyrexia
Hyperthermia in newborn
Transitory fever of newborn

☐ 778.5 Other and unspecified edema of newborn
Edema neonatorum

778.6 Congenital hydrocele
Congenital hydrocele of tunica vaginalis

778.7 Breast engorgement in newborn
Noninfective mastitis of newborn

Excludes *infective mastitis of newborn (771.5)*

☐ 778.8 Other specified conditions involving the integument of fetus and newborn
Urticaria neonatorum

Excludes *impetigo neonatorum (684)*
pemphigus neonatorum (684)

☐ 778.9 Unspecified condition involving the integument and temperature regulation of fetus and newborn

ICD-9-CM

700-799

Vol. 1

● **779 Other and ill-defined conditions originating in the perinatal period**

    779.0 Convulsions in newborn
        Fits in newborn
        Seizures in newborn

    ❑ **779.1 Other and unspecified cerebral irritability in newborn**

    779.2 Cerebral depression, coma, and other abnormal cerebral signs
        CNS dysfunction in newborn NOS

    779.3 Feeding problems in newborn
        Regurgitation of food in newborn
        Slow feeding in newborn
        Vomiting in newborn

    779.4 Drug reactions and intoxications specific to newborn
        Gray syndrome from chloramphenicol administration in newborn

      | **Excludes** | *fetal alcohol syndrome (760.71)* |
                reactions and intoxications from maternal opiates and tranquilizers (763.5)

    779.5 Drug withdrawal syndrome in newborn
        Drug withdrawal syndrome in infant of dependent mother

      | **Excludes** | *fetal alcohol syndrome (760.71)* |

    779.6 Termination of pregnancy (fetus)
        Fetal death due to:
          induced abortion
          termination of pregnancy

      | **Excludes** | *spontaneous abortion (fetus) (761.8)* |

    779.7 Periventricular leukomalacia

● ❑ **779.8 Other specified conditions originating in the perinatal period**

    779.81 Neonatal bradycardia

      | **Excludes** | *abnormality in fetal heart rate or rhythm complicating labor and delivery (763.81–763.83)* |
                bradycardia due to birth asphyxia (768.5–768.9)

    779.82 Neonatal tachycardia

      | **Excludes** | *abnormality in fetal heart rate or rhythm complicating labor and delivery (763.81–763.83)* |

    779.83 Delayed separation of umbilical cord

    ❑ **779.89 Other specified conditions originating in the perinatal period**

    ❑ **779.9 Unspecified condition originating in the perinatal period**
        Congenital debility NOS
        Stillbirth, NEC

16. SYMPTOMS, SIGNS, AND ILL-DEFINED CONDITIONS (780–799)

This section includes symptoms, signs, abnormal results of laboratory or other investigative procedures, and ill-defined conditions regarding which no diagnosis classifiable elsewhere is recorded.

Signs and symptoms that point rather definitely to a given diagnosis are assigned to some category in the preceding part of the classification. In general, categories 780–796 include the more ill-defined conditions and symptoms that point with perhaps equal suspicion to two or more diseases or to two or more systems of the body, and without the necessary study of the case to make a final diagnosis. Practically all categories in this group could be designated as "not otherwise specified," or as "unknown etiology," or as "transient." The Alphabetic Index should be consulted to determine which symptoms and signs are to be allocated here and which to more specific sections of the classification; the residual subcategories numbered .9 are provided for other relevant symptoms which cannot be allocated elsewhere in the classification.

The conditions and signs or symptoms included in categories 780–796 consist of: (a) cases for which no more specific diagnosis can be made even after all facts bearing on the case have been investigated; (b) signs or symptoms existing at the time of initial encounter that proved to be transient and whose causes could not be determined; (c) provisional diagnoses in a patient who failed to return for further investigation or care; (d) cases referred elsewhere for investigation or treatment before the diagnosis was made; (e) cases in which a more precise diagnosis was not available for any other reason; (f) certain symptoms which represent important problems in medical care and which it might be desired to classify in addition to a known cause.

SYMPTOMS (780–789)

● **780 General symptoms**

  ● **780.0 Alteration of consciousness**

    | Excludes | coma:
        diabetic (250.2–250.3)
        hepatic (572.2)
        originating in the perinatal period (779.2)

    780.01 Coma

    780.02 Transient alteration of awareness

    780.03 Persistent vegetative state

    ☐ **780.09 Other**
        Drowsiness
        Semicoma
        Somnolence
        Stupor
        Unconsciousness

  780.1 Hallucinations
    Hallucinations:
      NOS
      auditory
      gustatory
      olfactory
      tactile

    | Excludes | those associated with mental disorders, as functional psychoses (295.0–298.9)
        organic brain syndromes (290.0–294.9, 310.0–310.9)
        visual hallucinations (368.16)

780.2 Syncope and collapse
    Blackout   (Near) (Pre)syncope
    Fainting   Vasovagal attack

    | Excludes | carotid sinus syncope (337.0)
        heat syncope (992.1)
        neurocirculatory asthenia (306.2)
        orthostatic hypotension (458.0)
        shock NOS (785.50)

● **780.3 Convulsions**

    | Excludes | convulsions:
        epileptic (345.10–345.91)
        in newborn (779.0)

    780.31 Febrile convulsions
        Febrile seizures

    ☐ **780.39 Other convulsions**
        Convulsive disorder NOS
        Fits NOS
        Seizures NOS

  780.4 Dizziness and giddiness
    Light-headedness
    Vertigo NOS

    | Excludes | Ménière's disease and other specified vertiginous syndromes (386.0–386.9)

● **780.5 Sleep disturbances**

    | Excludes | that of nonorganic origin (307.40–307.49)

    ☐ **780.50 Sleep disturbance, unspecified**

    780.51 Insomnia with sleep apnea

    ☐ **780.52 Other insomnia**
        Insomnia NOS

    780.53 Hypersomnia with sleep apnea

    ☐ **780.54 Other hypersomnia**
        Hypersomnia NOS

    780.55 Disruptions of 24-hour sleep-wake cycle
        Inversion of sleep rhythm
        Irregular sleep-wake rhythm NOS
        Non-24-hour sleep-wake rhythm

    780.56 Dysfunctions associated with sleep stages or arousal from sleep

    ☐ **780.57 Other and unspecified sleep apnea**

    ☐ **780.58 Sleep related movement disorder** ◀
        Periodic limb movement disorder ◀

    | Excludes | restless leg syndrome (333.99) ◀

    ☐ **780.59 Other**

780.6 Fever
    Chills with fever   Hyperpyrexia NOS
    Fever NOS   Pyrexia NOS
    Fever of unknown   Pyrexia of unknown
      origin (FUO)   origin

    | Excludes | pyrexia of unknown origin (during):
        in newborn (778.4)
        labor (659.2)
        the puerperium (672)

● **780.7 Malaise and fatigue**

    | Excludes | debility, unspecified (799.3)
        fatigue (during):
        combat (308.0–308.9)
        heat (992.6)
        pregnancy (646.8)
        neurasthenia (300.5)
        senile asthenia (797)

    780.71 Chronic fatigue syndrome

    ☐ **780.79 Other malaise and fatigue**
        Asthenia NOS
        Lethargy
        Postviral (asthenic) syndrome
        Tiredness

ICD-9-CM

700-799

Vol. 1

780.8 Generalized hyperhidrosis ◀▥▥▥
Diaphoresis
Excessive sweating
Secondary hyperhidrosis ◀

Excludes *focal (localized) (primary) (secondary) hyperhidrosis (705.21–705.22)* ◀
Frey's syndrome (705.22) ◀

● **780.9 Other general symptoms**

Excludes *hypothermia:*
NOS (accidental) (991.6)
due to anesthesia (995.89)
memory disturbance as part of a pattern of mental disorder
of newborn (778.2–778.3)

780.91 Fussy infant (baby)

780.92 Excessive crying of infant (baby)

780.93 Memory loss
Amnesia (retrograde)
Memory loss NOS

Excludes *mild memory disturbance due to organic brain damage (310.1)*
transient global amnesia (437.7)

780.94 Early satiety

780.99 Other general symptoms
Chill(s) NOS
Generalized pain
Hypothermia, not associated with low environmental temperature

● **781 Symptoms involving nervous and musculoskeletal systems**

Excludes *depression NOS (311)*
disorders specifically relating to:
back (724.0–724.9)
hearing (388.0–389.9)
joint (718.0–719.9)
limb (729.0–729.9)
neck (723.0–723.9)
vision (368.0–369.9)
pain in limb (729.5)

781.0 Abnormal involuntary movements
Abnormal head movements   Spasms NOS
Fasciculation   Tremor NOS

Excludes *abnormal reflex (796.1)*
chorea NOS (333.5)
infantile spasms (345.60–345.61)
spastic paralysis (342.1, 343.0–344.9)
specified movement disorders classifiable to 333 (333.0–333.9)
that of nonorganic origin (307.2–307.3)

781.1 Disturbances of sensation of smell and taste
Anosmia   Parosmia
Parageusia

781.2 Abnormality of gait
Gait:
ataxic   spastic
paralytic   staggering

Excludes *ataxia:*
NOS (781.3)
locomotor (progressive) (094.0)
difficulty in walking (719.7)

781.3 Lack of coordination
Ataxia NOS
Muscular incoordination

Excludes *ataxic gait (781.2)*
cerebellar ataxia (334.0–334.9)
difficulty in walking (719.7)
vertigo NOS (780.4)

781.4 Transient paralysis of limb
Monoplegia, transient NOS

Excludes *paralysis (342.0–344.9)*

781.5 Clubbing of fingers

781.6 Meningismus
Dupré's syndrome
Meningism

781.7 Tetany
Carpopedal spasm

Excludes *tetanus neonatorum (771.3)*
tetany:
hysterical (300.11)
newborn (hypocalcemic) (775.4)
parathyroid (252.1)
psychogenic (306.0)

781.8 Neurologic neglect syndrome
Asomatognosia   Left-sided neglect
Hemi-akinesia   Sensory extinction
Hemi-inattention   Sensory neglect
Hemispatial neglect   Visuospatial neglect

● **781.9 Other symptoms involving nervous and musculoskeletal systems**

781.91 Loss of height

Excludes *osteoporosis (733.00–733.09)*

781.92 Abnormal posture

781.93 Ocular torticollis

781.94 Facial weakness
Facial droop

Excludes *facial weakness due to late effect of cerebrovascular accident (438.83)*

781.99 Other symptoms involving nervous and musculoskeletal system

● **782 Symptoms involving skin and other integumentary tissue**

Excludes *symptoms relating to breast (611.71–611.79)*

782.0 Disturbance of skin sensation
Anesthesia of skin
Burning or prickling sensation
Hyperesthesia
Hypoesthesia
Numbness
Paresthesia
Tingling

☐ **782.1 Rash and other nonspecific skin eruption**
Exanthem

Excludes *vesicular eruption (709.8)*

782.2 Localized superficial swelling, mass, or lump
Subcutaneous nodules

Excludes *localized adiposity (278.1)*

782.3 Edema
Anasarca
Dropsy
Localized edema NOS

Excludes *ascites (789.5)*
edema of:
newborn NOS (778.5)
pregnancy (642.0–642.9, 646.1)
fluid retention (276.6)
hydrops fetalis (773.3, 778.0)
hydrothorax (511.8)
nutritional edema (260, 262)

❑ **782.4 Jaundice, unspecified, not of newborn**
     Cholemia NOS
     Icterus NOS

     Excludes *due to isoimmunization (773.0–773.2, 773.4)*
                 jaundice in newborn (774.0–774.7)

782.5 Cyanosis

     Excludes *newborn (770.83)*

● **782.6 Pallor and flushing**

     ❑ **782.61 Pallor**

     ❑ **782.62 Flushing**
            Excessive blushing

782.7 Spontaneous ecchymoses
     Petechiae

     Excludes *ecchymosis in fetus or newborn (772.6)*
                  purpura (287.0–287.9)

782.8 Changes in skin texture
     Induration of skin
     Thickening of skin

❑ **782.9 Other symptoms involving skin and integumentary tissues**

● **783 Symptoms concerning nutrition, metabolism, and development**

     783.0 Anorexia
         Loss of appetite

         Excludes *anorexia nervosa (307.1)*
                     loss of appetite of nonorganic origin (307.59)

     783.1 Abnormal weight gain

         Excludes *excessive weight gain in pregnancy (646.1)*
                     obesity (278.00)
                         morbid (278.01)

● **783.2 Abnormal loss of weight and underweight**

         783.21 Loss of weight

         783.22 Underweight

     783.3 Feeding difficulties and mismanagement
         Feeding problem (elderly) (infant)

         Excludes *feeding disturbance or problems:*
                     in newborn (779.3)
                     of nonorganic origin (307.50–307.59)

● **783.4 Lack of expected normal physiological development in childhood**

         Excludes *delay in sexual development and puberty (259.0)*
                     gonadal dysgenesis (758.6)
                     pituitary dwarfism (253.3)
                     slow fetal growth and fetal malnutrition (764.00–764.99)
                     specific delays in mental development (315.0–315.9)

         ❑ **783.40 Lack of normal physiological development, unspecified**
             Inadequate development
             Lack of development

         783.41 Failure to thrive
             Failure to gain weight

         783.42 Delayed milestones
             Late talker
             Late walker

         783.43 Short stature
             Growth failure
             Growth retardation
             Lack of growth
             Physical retardation

     783.5 Polydipsia
         Excessive thirst

783.6 Polyphagia
     Excessive eating
     Hyperalimentation NOS

     Excludes *disorders of eating of nonorganic origin (307.50–307.59)*

783.7 Adult failure to thrive

❑ **783.9 Other symptoms concerning nutrition, metabolism, and development**
     Hypometabolism

     Excludes *abnormal basal metabolic rate (794.7)*
                  dehydration (276.5)
                  other disorders of fluid, electrolyte, and acid-base balance (276.0–276.9)

● **784 Symptoms involving head and neck**

     Excludes *encephalopathy NOS (348.30)*
                  specific symptoms involving neck classifiable to 723 (723.0–723.9)

     784.0 Headache
         Facial pain
         Pain in head NOS

         Excludes *atypical face pain (350.2)*
                     migraine (346.0–346.9)
                     tension headache (307.81)

     784.1 Throat pain

         Excludes *dysphagia (787.2)*
                     neck pain (723.1)
                     sore throat (462)
                     chronic (472.1)

     784.2 Swelling, mass, or lump in head and neck
         Space-occupying lesion, intracranial NOS

     784.3 Aphasia

         Excludes *developmental aphasia (315.31)*

● **784.4 Voice disturbance**

     ❑ **784.40 Voice disturbance, unspecified**

         784.41 Aphonia
             Loss of voice

     ❑ **784.49 Other**
             Change in voice
             Dysphonia
             Hoarseness
             Hypernasality
             Hyponasality

❑ **784.5 Other speech disturbance**
     Dysarthria
     Dysphasia
     Slurred speech

     Excludes *stammering and stuttering (307.0)*
                  that of nonorganic origin (307.0, 307.9)

● **784.6 Other symbolic dysfunction**

     Excludes *developmental learning delays (315.0–315.9)*

     ❑ **784.60 Symbolic dysfunction, unspecified**

         784.61 Alexia and dyslexia
             Alexia (with agraphia)

     ❑ **784.69 Other**
             Acalculia
             Agnosia
             Agraphia NOS
             Apraxia

     784.7 Epistaxis
         Hemorrhage from nose
         Nosebleed

     784.8 Hemorrhage from throat

         Excludes *hemoptysis (786.3)*

ICD-9-CM

700-799

Vol. 1

❑784.9 **Other symptoms involving head and neck**
Choking sensation
Halitosis
Mouth breathing
Sneezing

●785 **Symptoms involving cardiovascular system**
Excludes *heart failure NOS (428.9)*

❑785.0 **Tachycardia, unspecified**
Rapid heart beat
Excludes *neonatal tachycardia (779.82)*
paroxysmal tachycardia (427.0–427.2)

785.1 **Palpitations**
Awareness of heart beat
Excludes *specified dysrhythmias (427.0–427.9)*

785.2 **Undiagnosed cardiac murmurs**
Heart murmur NOS

❑785.3 **Other abnormal heart sounds**
Cardiac dullness, increased or decreased
Friction fremitus, cardiac
Precordial friction

785.4 **Gangrene**
Gangrene:
NOS
spreading cutaneous
Gangrenous cellulitis
Phagedena

Code first any associated underlying condition
diabetes
Raynaud's syndrome (443.0)
Excludes *gangrene of certain sites—see Alphabetic Index*
gangrene with atherosclerosis of the extremities (440.24)
gas gangrene (040.0)

●785.5 **Shock without mention of trauma**

❑785.50 **Shock, unspecified**
Failure of peripheral circulation

785.51 **Cardiogenic shock**

785.52 **Septic shock**
Endotoxic ◀
Gram-negative ◀
Code first: ◀▥
systemic inflammatory response syndrome
due to infectious process with organ
dysfunction (995.92) ◀▥
systemic inflammatory response syndrome
due to non-infectious process with organ dysfuction (995.94) ◀

❑785.59 **Other**
Shock:
hypovolemic
Excludes *shock (due to):*
anesthetic (995.4)
anaphylactic (995.0)
due to serum (999.4)
electric (994.8)
following abortion (639.5)
lightning (994.0)
obstetrical (669.1)
postoperative (998.0)
traumatic (958.4)

785.6 **Enlargement of lymph nodes**
Lymphadenopathy
"Swollen glands"
Excludes *lymphadenitis (chronic) (289.1–289.3)*
acute (683)

❑785.9 **Other symptoms involving cardiovascular system**
Bruit (arterial)   Weak pulse

●786 **Symptoms involving respiratory system and other chest symptoms**

●786.0 **Dyspnea and respiratory abnormalities**

❑786.00 **Respiratory abnormality, unspecified**

786.01 **Hyperventilation**
Excludes *hyperventilation, psychogenic (306.1)*

786.02 **Orthopnea**

786.03 **Apnea**
Excludes *apnea of newborn (770.81, 770.82)*
sleep apnea (780.51, 780.53, 780.57)

786.04 **Cheyne-Stokes respiration**

786.05 **Shortness of breath**

786.06 **Tachypnea**
Excludes *transitory tachypnea of newborn (770.6)*

786.07 **Wheezing**
Excludes *asthma (493.00–493.92)*

❑786.09 **Other**
Respiratory:
distress
insufficiency
Excludes *respiratory distress:*
following trauma and surgery (518.5)
newborn (770.89)
respiratory failure (518.81, 518.83–518.84)
newborn (770.84)
syndrome (newborn) (769)
adult (518.5)

786.1 **Stridor**
Excludes *congenital laryngeal stridor (748.3)*

786.2 **Cough**
Excludes *cough:*
psychogenic (306.1)
smokers' (491.0)
with hemorrhage (786.3)

786.3 **Hemoptysis**
Cough with hemorrhage
Pulmonary hemorrhage NOS
Excludes *pulmonary hemorrhage of newborn (770.3)*

786.4 **Abnormal sputum**
Abnormal:
amount of sputum
color of sputum
odor of sputum
Excessive sputum

●786.5 **Chest pain**

❑786.50 **Chest pain, unspecified**

786.51 **Precordial pain**

786.52 **Painful respiration**
Pain:
anterior chest wall
pleuritic
pleurodynia
Excludes *epidemic pleurodynia (074.1)*

❑786.59 **Other**
Discomfort in chest
Pressure in chest
Tightness in chest
Excludes *pain in breast (611.71)*

786.6 **Swelling, mass, or lump in chest**
Excludes *lump in breast (611.72)*

◀ **New** ◀▥ **Revised** ● **Not a Principal Diagnosis** ● **Use Additional Digit(s)** ❑ **Nonspecific Code**

786.7 Abnormal chest sounds
    Abnormal percussion, chest   Rales
    Friction sounds, chest   Tympany, chest
    Excludes *wheezing (786.07)*

786.8 Hiccough
    Excludes *psychogenic hiccough (306.1)*

☐**786.9 Other symptoms involving respiratory system and chest**
    Breath-holding spell

● **787 Symptoms involving digestive system**
    Excludes *constipation (564.00–564.09)*
           pylorospasm (537.81)
              congenital (750.5)

● **787.0 Nausea and vomiting**
    Emesis
    Excludes *hematemesis NOS (578.0)*
           vomiting:
              bilious, following gastrointestinal surgery (564.3)
              cyclical (536.2)
                psychogenic (306.4)
              excessive, in pregnancy (643.0–643.9)
              habit (536.2)
              of newborn (779.3)
              psychogenic NOS (307.54)

    787.01 Nausea with vomiting

    787.02 Nausea alone

    787.03 Vomiting alone

787.1 Heartburn
    Pyrosis
    Waterbrash
    Excludes *dyspepsia or indigestion (536.8)*

787.2 Dysphagia
    Difficulty in swallowing

787.3 Flatulence, eructation, and gas pain
    Abdominal distention (gaseous)
    Bloating
    Tympanites (abdominal) (intestinal)
    Excludes *aerophagy (306.4)*

787.4 Visible peristalsis
    Hyperperistalsis

787.5 Abnormal bowel sounds
    Absent bowel sounds
    Hyperactive bowel sounds

787.6 Incontinence of feces
    Encopresis NOS
    Incontinence of sphincter ani
    Excludes *that of nonorganic origin (307.7)*

787.7 Abnormal feces
    Bulky stools
    Excludes *abnormal stool content (792.1)*
           melena:
              NOS (578.1)
              newborn (772.4, 777.3)

● **787.9 Other symptoms involving digestive system**
    Excludes *gastrointestinal hemorrhage (578.0–578.9)*
           intestinal obstruction (560.0–560.9)
           specific functional digestive disorders:
              esophagus (530.0–530.9)
              stomach and duodenum (536.0–536.9)
              those not elsewhere classified (564.00–564.9)

    787.91 Diarrhea
        Diarrhea NOS

    787.99 Other
        Change in bowel habits
        Tenesmus (rectal)

● **788 Symptoms involving urinary system**
    Excludes *hematuria (599.7)*
           nonspecific findings on examination of the urine (791.0–791.9)
           small kidney of unknown cause (589.0–589.9)
           uremia NOS (586)

788.0 Renal colic
    Colic (recurrent) of:
        kidney
        ureter

788.1 Dysuria
    Painful urination
    Strangury

● **788.2 Retention of urine**

    ☐**788.20 Retention of urine, unspecified**

    788.21 Incomplete bladder emptying

    ☐**788.29 Other specified retention of urine**

● **788.3 Urinary incontinence** ◀▥
    Excludes *that of nonorganic origin (307.6)*
    Code, if applicable, any causal condition first, such as:
        congenital ureterocele (753.23)
        genital prolapse (618.00–618.9) ◀▥

    ☐**788.30 Urinary incontinence, unspecified**
        Enuresis NOS

    788.31 Urge incontinence

    788.32 Stress incontinence, male
    Excludes *stress incontinence, female (625.6)*

    788.33 Mixed incontinence (female) (male)
        Urge and stress

    788.34 Incontinence without sensory awareness

    788.35 Post-void dribbling

    788.36 Nocturnal enuresis

    788.37 Continuous leakage

    788.38 Overflow incontinence ◀

    ☐**788.39 Other urinary incontinence**

● **788.4 Frequency of urination and polyuria**

    788.41 Urinary frequency
        Frequency of micturition

    788.42 Polyuria

    788.43 Nocturia

788.5 Oliguria and anuria
    Deficient secretion of urine
    Suppression of urinary secretion
    Excludes *that complicating:*
           abortion (634–638 with .3, 639.3)
           ectopic or molar pregnancy (639.3)
           pregnancy, childbirth, or the puerperium (642.0–642.9, 646.2)

● **788.6 Other abnormality of urination**

    788.61 Splitting of urinary stream
        Intermittent urinary stream

    788.62 Slowing of urinary stream
        Weak stream

    788.63 Urgency of urination
    Excludes *urge incontinence (788.31, 788.33)*

    ☐**788.69 Other**

ICD-9-CM

700-799

Vol. 1

788.7 Urethral discharge
    Penile discharge   Urethrorrhea

788.8 Extravasation of urine

☐ **788.9 Other symptoms involving urinary system**
    Extrarenal uremia
    Vesical:
        pain
        tenesmus

● **789 Other symptoms involving abdomen and pelvis**

The following fifth-digit subclassification is to be used for
codes 789.0, 789.3, 789.4, 789.6

☐ **0 unspecified site**
  1 right upper quadrant
  2 left upper quadrant
  3 right lower quadrant
  4 left lower quadrant
  5 periumbilic
  6 epigastric
☐ **7 generalized**
☐ **9 other specified site**
    multiple sites

    | Excludes | symptoms referable to genital organs:
                  female (625.0–625.9)
                  male (607.0–608.9)
                  psychogenic (302.70–302.79)

● **789.0 Abdominal pain**
    Colic:
        NOS
        infantile
    Cramps, abdominal

    | Excludes | renal colic (788.0)

789.1 Hepatomegaly
    Enlargement of liver

789.2 Splenomegaly
    Enlargement of spleen

● **789.3 Abdominal or pelvic swelling, mass, or lump**
    Diffuse or generalized swelling or mass:
        abdominal NOS
        umbilical

    | Excludes | abdominal distention (gaseous) (787.3)
                ascites (789.5)

● **789.4 Abdominal rigidity**

789.5 Ascites
    Fluid in peritoneal cavity

● **789.6 Abdominal tenderness**
    Rebound tenderness

☐ **789.9 Other symptoms involving abdomen and pelvis**
    Umbilical:
        bleeding
        discharge

NONSPECIFIC ABNORMAL FINDINGS (790–796)

● **790 Nonspecific findings on examination of blood**

    | Excludes | abnormality of:
              platelets (287.0–287.9)
              thrombocytes (287.0–287.9)
              white blood cells (288.0–288.9)

● **790.0 Abnormality of red blood cells**

    | Excludes | anemia:
              congenital (776.5)
              newborn, due to isoimmunization (773.0–
                  773.2, 773.5)
              of premature infant (776.6)
              other specified types (280.0–285.9)
        hemoglobin disorders (282.5–282.7)
        polycythemia:
              familial (289.6)
              neonatorum (776.4)
              secondary (289.0)
              vera (238.4)

  790.01 Precipitous drop in hematocrit
      Drop in hematocrit

☐ **790.09 Other abnormality of red blood cells**
      Abnormal red cell morphology NOS
      Abnormal red cell volume NOS
      Anisocytosis
      Poikilocytosis

☐ **790.1 Elevated sedimentation rate**

● **790.2 Abnormal glucose**

    | Excludes | diabetes mellitus (250.00–250.93)
              dysmetabolic syndrome X (277.7)
              gestational diabetes (648.8)
              glycosuria (791.5)
              hypoglycemia (251.2)
              that complicating pregnancy, childbirth or the
                  puerperium (648.8)

  790.21 Impaired fasting glucose
      Elevated fasting glucose

  790.22 Impaired glucose tolerance test (oral)
      Elevated glucose tolerance test

  790.29 Other abnormal glucose
      Abnormal glucose NOS
      Abnormal non-fasting glucose
      Pre-diabetes NOS

  790.3 Excessive blood level of alcohol
      Elevated blood-alcohol

☐ **790.4 Nonspecific elevation of levels of transaminase or
lactic acid dehydrogenase [LDH]**

☐ **790.5 Other nonspecific abnormal serum enzyme levels**
      Abnormal serum level of:
        acid phosphatase
        alkaline phosphatase
        amylase
        lipase

    | Excludes | deficiency of circulating enzymes (277.6)

❑ **790.6 Other abnormal blood chemistry**
    Abnormal blood levels of:
      cobalt
      copper
      iron
      lithium
      magnesium
      mineral
      zinc

    | Excludes | *abnormality of electrolyte or acid-base balance (276.0–276.9)*
                hypoglycemia NOS (251.2)
                specific finding indicating abnormality of:
                    amino-acid transport and metabolism (270.0–270.9)
                    carbohydrate transport and metabolism (271.0–271.9)
                    lipid metabolism (272.0–272.9)
                uremia NOS (586)

   790.7 Bacteremia

    | Excludes | *bacteremia of newborn (771.83)*
                septicemia (038)

    Use additional code to identify organism (041)

❑ **790.8 Viremia, unspecified**

● ❑ **790.9 Other nonspecific findings on examination of blood**

    ❑ **790.91 Abnormal arterial blood gases**

    ❑ **790.92 Abnormal coagulation profile**
        Abnormal or prolonged:
          bleeding time
          coagulation time
          partial thromboplastin time [PTT]
          prothrombin time [PT]

    | Excludes | *coagulation (hemorrhagic) disorders (286.0–286.9)*

    790.93 Elevated prostate specific antigen [PSA]

    790.94 Euthyroid sick syndrome

    790.95 Elevated C-reactive protein (CRP) ◄

    ❑ **790.99 Other**

● **791 Nonspecific findings on examination of urine**

    | Excludes | *hematuria NOS (599.7)*
                specific findings indicating abnormality of:
                    amino-acid transport and metabolism (270.0–270.9)
                    carbohydrate transport and metabolism (271.0–271.9)

   791.0 Proteinuria
      Albuminuria
      Bence-Jones proteinuria

    | Excludes | *postural proteinuria (593.6)*
                that arising during pregnancy or the puerperium (642.0–642.9, 646.2)

   791.1 Chyluria

    | Excludes | *filarial (125.0–125.9)*

   791.2 Hemoglobinuria

   791.3 Myoglobinuria

   791.4 Biliuria

   791.5 Glycosuria

    | Excludes | *renal glycosuria (271.4)*

   791.6 Acetonuria
      Ketonuria

❑ **791.7 Other cells and casts in urine**

● ❑ **791.9 Other nonspecific findings on examination of urine**
    Crystalluria
    Elevated urine levels of:
      17-ketosteroids
      catecholamines
      indolacetic acid
      vanillylmandelic acid [VMA]
    Melanuria

● **792 Nonspecific abnormal findings in other body substances**

    | Excludes | *that in chromosomal analysis (795.2)*

   792.0 Cerebrospinal fluid

   792.1 Stool contents
      Abnormal stool color
      Fat in stool
      Mucus in stool
      Occult blood
      Pus in stool

    | Excludes | *blood in stool [melena] (578.1)*
                newborn (772.4, 777.3)

   792.2 Semen
      Abnormal spermatozoa

    | Excludes | *azoospermia (606.0)*
                oligospermia (606.1)

   792.3 Amniotic fluid

   792.4 Saliva

    | Excludes | *that in chromosomal analysis (795.2)*

   792.5 Cloudy (hemodialysis) (peritoneal) dialysis effluent

   ❑ **792.9 Other nonspecific abnormal findings in body substances**
      Peritoneal fluid
      Pleural fluid
      Synovial fluid
      Vaginal fluids

● **793 Nonspecific abnormal findings on radiological and other examination of body structure**

    Includes: nonspecific abnormal findings of:
        thermography
        ultrasound examination [echogram]
        x-ray examination

    | Excludes | *abnormal results of function studies and radioisotope scans (794.0–794.9)*

   793.0 Skull and head

    | Excludes | *nonspecific abnormal echoencephalogram (794.01)*

   793.1 Lung field
      Coin lesion lung
      Shadow, lung

   ❑ **793.2 Other intrathoracic organ**
      Abnormal:
        echocardiogram
        heart shadow
        ultrasound cardiogram
      Mediastinal shift

   793.3 Biliary tract
      Nonvisualization of gallbladder

   793.4 Gastrointestinal tract

   793.5 Genitourinary organs
      Filling defect:
        bladder
        kidney
        ureter

   793.6 Abdominal area, including retroperitoneum

   793.7 Musculoskeletal system

ICD-9-CM

700-799

Vol. 1

● **793.8 Breast**

❑ **793.80 Abnormal mammogram, unspecified**

793.81 Mammographic microcalcification

❑ **793.89 Other abnormal findings on radiological examination of breast**

❑ **793.9 Other**
Abnormal:
placental finding by x-ray or ultrasound method
radiological findings in skin and subcutaneous tissue
| **Excludes** | *abnormal finding by radioisotope localization of placenta (794.9)* |

● **794 Nonspecific abnormal results of function studies**

Includes: radioisotope:
scans
uptake studies
scintiphotography

● **794.0 Brain and central nervous system**

❑ **794.00 Abnormal function study, unspecified**

794.01 Abnormal echoencephalogram

794.02 Abnormal electroencephalogram [EEG]

❑ **794.09 Other**
Abnormal brain scan

● **794.1 Peripheral nervous system and special senses**

❑ **794.10 Abnormal response to nerve stimulation, unspecified**

794.11 Abnormal retinal function studies
Abnormal electroretinogram [ERG]

794.12 Abnormal electro-oculogram [EOG]

794.13 Abnormal visually evoked potential

794.14 Abnormal oculomotor studies

794.15 Abnormal auditory function studies

794.16 Abnormal vestibular function studies

794.17 Abnormal electromyogram [EMG]
| **Excludes** | *that of eye (794.14)* |

❑ **794.19 Other**

794.2 Pulmonary
Abnormal lung scan
Reduced:
ventilatory capacity
vital capacity

● **794.3 Cardiovascular**

❑ **794.30 Abnormal function study, unspecified**

794.31 Abnormal electrocardiogram [ECG] [EKG]

❑ **794.39 Other**
Abnormal:
ballistocardiogram
phonocardiogram
vectorcardiogram

794.4 Kidney
Abnormal renal function test

794.5 Thyroid
Abnormal thyroid:
scan   uptake

❑ **794.6 Other endocrine function study**

794.7 Basal metabolism
Abnormal basal metabolic rate [BMR]

794.8 Liver
Abnormal liver scan

❑ **794.9 Other**
Bladder   Placenta
Pancreas   Spleen

● **795 Other and nonspecific abnormal cytological, histological, immunological and DNA test findings**
| **Excludes** | *nonspecific abnormalities of red blood cells (790.01–790.09)* |

● ❑ **795.0 Abnormal Papanicolaou smear of cervix and cervical HPV**
Abnormal thin preparation smear of cervice
Abnormal cervical cytology
Excludes	*carcinoma in-situ of cervix (233.1)*
	cervical intraepithelial neoplasia I (CIN I) (622.11)
	cervical intraepithelial neoplasia II (CIN II) (622.12)
	cervical intraepithelial neoplasia III (CIN III) (233.1)
	dysplasia (histologically confirmed) of cervix (uteri) NOS (622.10)
	mild dysplasia (histologically confirmed) (622.11)
	moderate dysplasia (histologically confirmed) (622.12)
	severe dysplasia (histological confirmed) (233.1)

❑ **795.00 Abnormal glandular Papanicolaou smear of cervix**
Atypical endocervical cells NOS
Atypical endometrial cells NOS
Atypical glandular cells NOS

795.01 Papanicolaou smear of cervix with atypical squamous cells of undetermined significance (ASC-US)

795.02 Papanicolaou smear of cervix with atypical squamous cells cannot exclude high grade squamous intraepithelial lesion (ASC-H)

795.03 Papanicolaou smear of cervix with low grade sqaumous intraepithelial lesion (LGSIL)

795.04 Papanicolaou smear of cervix with high grade squamous intraepithelial lesion (HGSIL)
Cytologic evidence of carcinoma

795.05 Cervical high risk human papillomavirus (HPV) DNA test positive

795.08 Unsatisfactory smear
Inadequate sample

❑ **795.09 Other abnormal Papanicolaou smear of cervix and cervical HVP**
Papanicolaou smear of cervix with low risk human papillomavirus (HPV) DNA test positive

Use additional code for associated human papillomavirus (079.4)
| **Excludes** | *encounter for Papanicolaou cervical smear to confirm findings of recent normal smear following initial abnormal smear (V72.32)* |

❑ **795.1 Nonspecific abnormal Papanicolaou smear of other site**

❑ **795.2 Nonspecific abnormal findings on chromosomal analysis**
Abnormal karyotype

● ❑ **795.3 Nonspecific positive culture findings**
Positive culture findings in:
nose   throat
sputum   wound
Excludes	*that of:*
	blood (790.7–790.8)
	urine (791.9)

795.31 Nonspecific positive findings for anthrax
Positive findings by nasal swab

❑ **795.39 Other nonspecific positive culture findings**

❑ **795.4 Other nonspecific abnormal histological findings**

☐ **795.5 Nonspecific reaction to tuberculin skin test without active tuberculosis**
Abnormal result of Mantoux test
PPD positive
Tuberculin (skin test):
   positive
   reactor

795.6 False positive serological test for syphilis
False positive Wassermann reaction

● **795.7 Other nonspecific immunological findings**

Excludes	isoimmunization, in pregnancy (656.1–656.2)
	affecting fetus or newborn (773.0–773.2)

☐ **795.71 Nonspecific serologic evidence of human immunodeficiency virus [HIV]**
Inconclusive human immunodeficiency virus [HIV] test (adult) (infant)

Note: This code is ONLY to be used when a test finding is reported as nonspecific. Asymptomatic positive findings are coded to V08. If any HIV infection symptom or condition is present, see code 042. Negative findings are not coded.

Excludes	acquired immunodeficiency syndrome [AIDS] (042)
	asymptomatic human immunodeficiency virus [HIV] infection status (V08)
	HIV infection, symptomatic (042)
	human immunodeficiency virus [HIV] disease (042)
	positive (status) NOS (V08)

☐ **795.79 Other and unspecified nonspecific immunological findings**
Raised antibody titer
Raised level of immunoglobulins

● **796 Other nonspecific abnormal findings**

☐ **796.0 Nonspecific abnormal toxicological findings**
Abnormal levels of heavy metals or drugs in blood, urine, or other tissue

Excludes	excessive blood level of alcohol (790.3)

796.1 Abnormal reflex

796.2 Elevated blood pressure reading without diagnosis of hypertension

Note: This category is to be used to record an episode of elevated blood pressure in a patient in whom no formal diagnosis of hypertension has been made, or as an incidental finding.

☐ **796.3 Nonspecific low blood pressure reading**

☐ **796.4 Other abnormal clinical findings**

☐ **796.5 Abnormal finding on antenatal screening**

☐ **796.6 Abnormal findings on neonatal screening** ◀

Excludes	nonspecific serologic evidence of human immunodeficiency virus [HIV] (795.71) ◀

☐ **796.9 Other**

ILL-DEFINED AND UNKNOWN CAUSES OF MORBIDITY AND MORTALITY (797–799)

797 Senility without mention of psychosis
Old age   Senile:
Senescence   debility
Senile asthenia   exhaustion

Excludes	senile psychoses (290.0–290.9)

● **798 Sudden death, cause unknown**

798.0 Sudden infant death syndrome
Cot death
Crib death
Sudden death of nonspecific cause in infancy

● **798.1 Instantaneous death**

● **798.2 Death occurring in less than 24 hours from onset of symptoms, not otherwise explained**
Death known not to be violent or instantaneous, for which no cause could be discovered
Died without sign of disease

● **798.9 Unattended death**
Death in circumstances where the body of the deceased was found and no cause could be discovered
Found dead

● **799 Other ill-defined and unknown causes of morbidity and mortality**

799.0 Asphyxia

Excludes	asphyxia (due to):
	carbon monoxide (986)
	inhalation of food or foreign body (932–934.9)
	newborn (768.0–768.9)
	traumatic (994.7)

799.1 Respiratory arrest
Cardiorespiratory failure

Excludes	cardiac arrest (427.5)
	failure of peripheral circulation (785.50)
	respiratory distress:
	NOS (786.09)
	acute (518.82)
	following trauma or surgery (518.5)
	newborn (770.89)
	syndrome (newborn) (769)
	adult (following trauma or surgery) (518.5)
	other (518.82)
	respiratory failure (518.81, 518.83–518.84)
	newborn (770.84)
	respiratory insufficiency (786.09)
	acute (518.82)

799.2 Nervousness
"Nerves"

☐ **799.3 Debility, unspecified**

Excludes	asthenia (780.79)
	nervous debility (300.5)
	neurasthenia (300.5)
	senile asthenia (797)

799.4 Cachexia
Wasting disease

Excludes	nutritional marasmus (261)

● **799.8 Other ill-defined conditions**

799.81 Decreased libido
Decreased sexual desire

Excludes	psychosexual dysfunction with inhibited sexual desire (302.71)

☐ **799.89 Other ill-defined conditions**

☐ **799.9 Other unknown and unspecified cause**
Undiagnosed disease, not specified as to site or system involved
Unknown cause of morbidity or mortality

ICD-9-CM

700-799

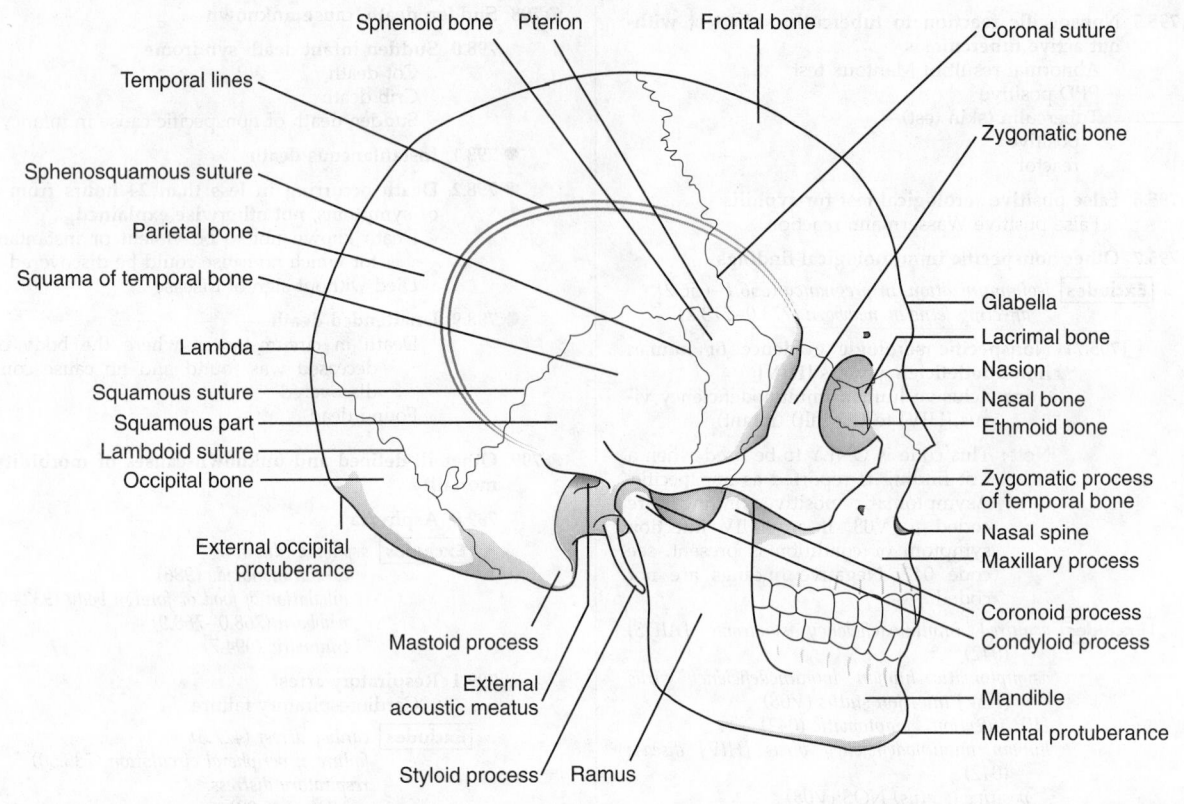

Figure 17-1 Lateral view of skull.

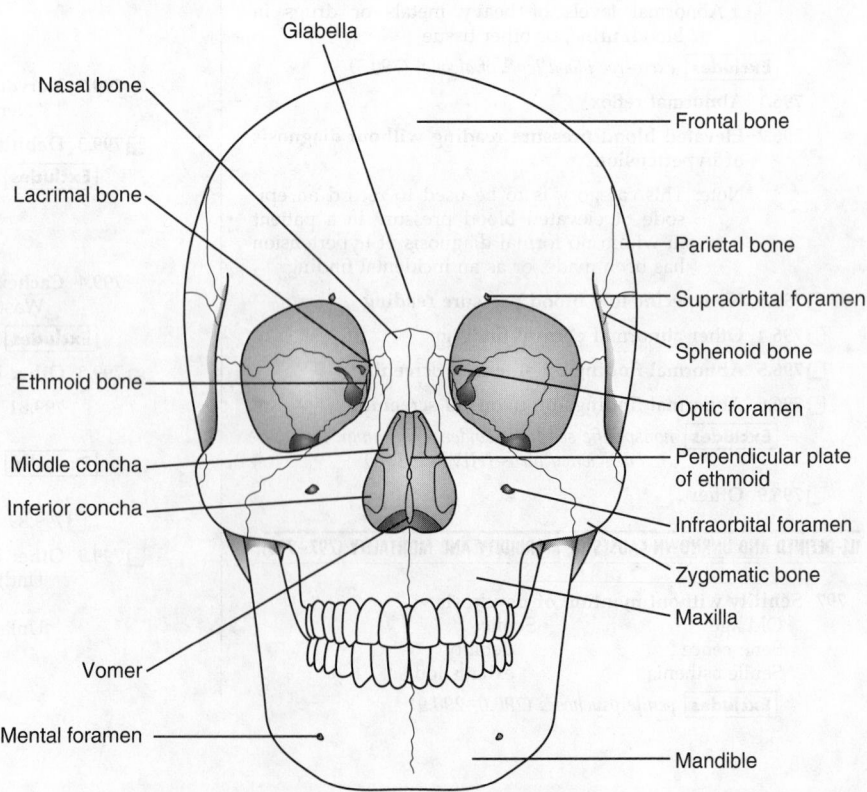

Figure 17-2 Frontal view of skull.

Figure 17-3 Anterior view of vertebral column.

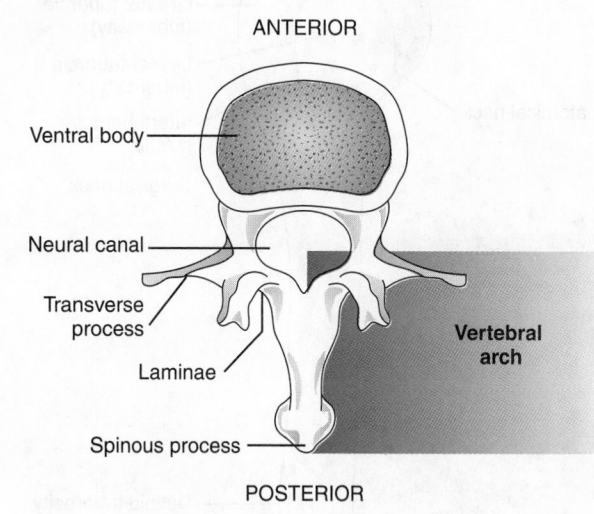

Figure 17-4 Vertebra viewed from above.

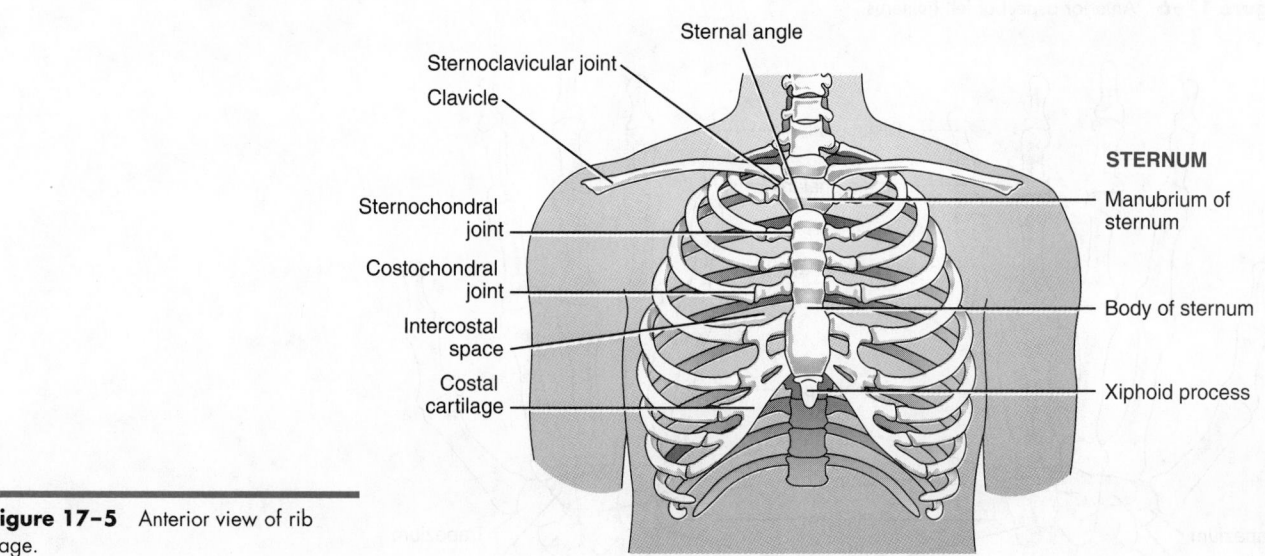

Figure 17-5 Anterior view of rib cage.

ICD-9-CM

800-999

Vol. 1

Head

Greater tubercle
(tuberosity)

Lesser tubercle
(tuberosity)

Intertubercular
sulcus

Surgical neck

Anatomical neck

Deltoid tuberosity

Medial
supracondylar
ridge

Lateral
supracondylar
ridge

Coronoid fossa

Radial fossa

Medial
epicondyle

Lateral
epicondyle

Trochlea

Capitulum

Figure 17-6   Anterior aspect of left humerus.

Olecranon

Trochlear notch

Radial notch

Coronoid process

Head

Neck

Radial tuberosity

Head

Styloid process

Styloid process

ULNA   RADIUS

Figure 17-7   Anterior aspect of left radius and ulna.

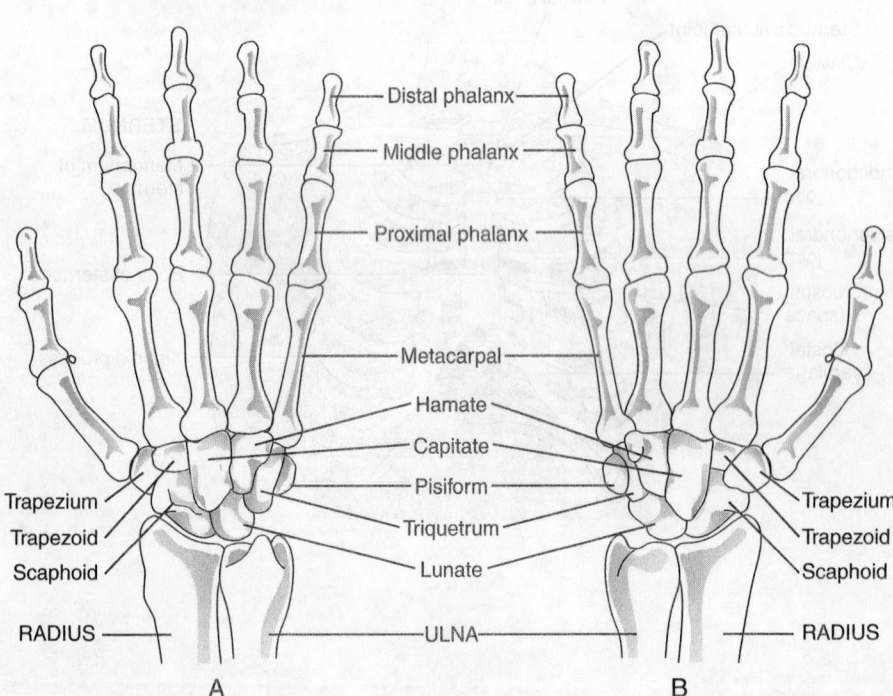

Distal phalanx

Middle phalanx

Proximal phalanx

Metacarpal

Hamate

Capitate

Pisiform

Triquetrum

Lunate

Trapezium

Trapezoid

Scaphoid

Trapezium

Trapezoid

Scaphoid

RADIUS

ULNA

RADIUS

A   B

Figure 17-8   Right hand and wrist:
A. Dorsal surface. **B.** Palmar surface.

◄ **New**   ◄▥ **Revised**   ● **Not a Principal Diagnosis**   ● **Use Additional Digit(s)**   ❑ **Nonspecific Code**

Greater trochanter

Fovea on head

Head

Neck

Intertrochanteric line

Lesser trochanter

Shaft

Abductor tubercle

Lateral epicondyle

Medial epicondyle

Lateral condyle

Medial condyle

Patellar surface

Figure 17-9 Anterior aspect of right femur.

Tubercles of intercondyle eminence

Medial condyle of tibia

Lateral condyle of tibia

Apex

Head of tibia

Tuberosity of tibia

Anterior border

Interosseous border

Interosseous border

Medial crest

Anterior border

Anterior surface

Medial surface

Medial part of posterior surface

Lateral surface

Triangular subcutaneous area

Medial malleolus

Lateral malleolus

Figure 17-10 Anterior aspect of left tibia and fibula.

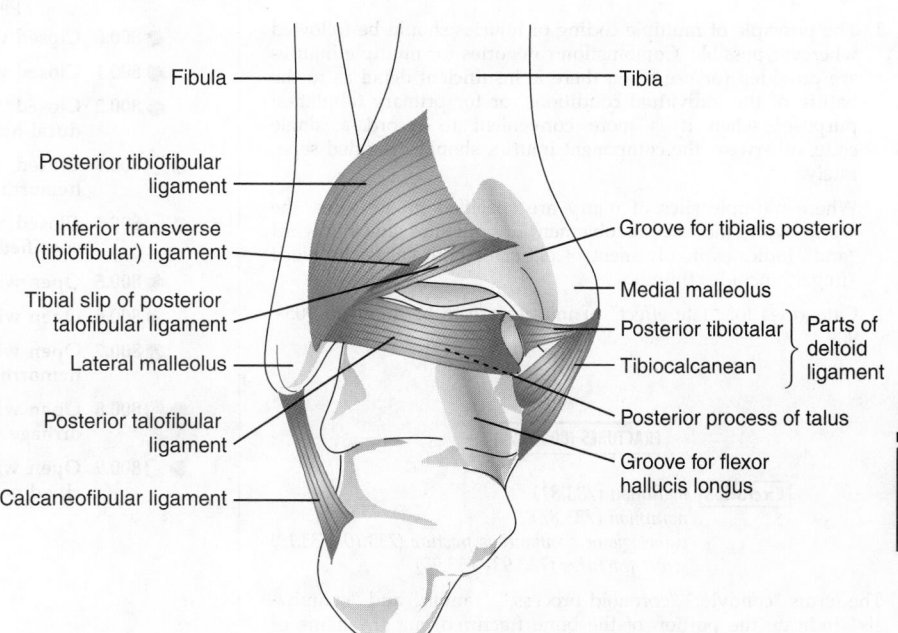

Fibula

Tibia

Posterior tibiofibular ligament

Groove for tibialis posterior

Inferior transverse (tibiofibular) ligament

Medial malleolus

Tibial slip of posterior talofibular ligament

Posterior tibiotalar

Parts of deltoid ligament

Lateral malleolus

Tibiocalcanean

Posterior process of talus

Posterior talofibular ligament

Groove for flexor hallucis longus

Calcaneofibular ligament

Figure 17-11 Posterior aspect of the left ankle joint.

ICD-9-CM

800-999

Vol. 1

Row of distal phalanges
Row of middle phalanges
Row of proximal phalanges

Metatarsals

Cuneiforms

Navicular

Cuboid

Talus

Calcaneus

Figure 17-12 Right foot viewed from above.

17. INJURY AND POISONING (800–999)

Use E code(s) to identify the cause and intent of the injury or poisoning (E800-E999)

Note:

1. The principle of multiple coding of injuries should be followed wherever possible. Combination categories for multiple injuries are provided for use when there is insufficient detail as to the nature of the individual conditions, or for primary tabulation purposes when it is more convenient to record a single code; otherwise, the component injuries should be coded separately.

   Where multiple sites of injury are specified in the titles, the word "with" indicates involvement of both sites, and the word "and" indicates involvement of either or both sites. The word "finger" includes thumb.

2. Categories for "late effect" of injuries are to be found at 905–909.

FRACTURES (800–829)

Excludes *malunion (733.81)*
nonunion (733.82)
pathologic or spontaneous fracture (733.10–733.19)
stress fractures (733.93–733.95)

The terms "condyle," "coronoid process," "ramus," and "symphysis" indicate the portion of the bone fractured, not the name of the bone involved.

The descriptions "closed" and "open" used in the fourth-digit subdivisions include the following terms:
    closed (with or without delayed healing):
        comminuted
        depressed
        elevated
        fissured
        fracture NOS
        greenstick
        impacted
        linear
        simple
        slipped epiphysis
        spiral
    open (with or without delayed healing):
        compound
        infected
        missile
        puncture
        with foreign body

Note: A fracture not indicated as closed or open should be classified as closed.

FRACTURE OF SKULL (800–804)

The following fifth-digit subclassification is for use with the appropriate codes in categories 800, 801, 803, and 804:
☐ 0 unspecified state of consciousness
  1 with no loss of consciousness
  2 with brief [less than one hour] loss of consciousness
  3 with moderate [1–24 hours] loss of consciousness
  4 with prolonged [more than 24 hours] loss of consciousness and return to pre-existing conscious level
  5 with prolonged [more than 24 hours] loss of consciousness, without return to pre-existing conscious level

      Use fifth-digit 5 to designate when a patient is unconscious and dies before regaining consciousness, regardless of the duration of the loss of consciousness
☐ 6 with loss of consciousness of unspecified duration
☐ 9 with concussion, unspecified

● 800 **Fracture of vault of skull**

    Requires fifth digit. See beginning of section 800–804 for codes and definitions.

    Includes: frontal bone
            parietal bone

    ● 800.0 **Closed without mention of intracranial injury**

    ● 800.1 **Closed with cerebral laceration and contusion**

    ● 800.2 **Closed with subarachnoid, subdural, and extradural hemorrhage**

    ●☐ 800.3 **Closed with other and unspecified intracranial hemorrhage**

    ●☐ 800.4 **Closed with intracranial injury of other and unspecified nature**

    ● 800.5 **Open without mention of intracranial injury**

    ● 800.6 **Open with cerebral laceration and contusion**

    ● 800.7 **Open with subarachnoid, subdural, and extradural hemorrhage**

    ●☐ 800.8 **Open with other and unspecified intracranial hemorrhage**

    ●☐ 800.9 **Open with intracranial injury of other and unspecified nature**

● **801 Fracture of base of skull**

Requires fifth digit. See beginning of section 800–804 for codes and definitions.

Includes: fossa:
　　　　anterior
　　　　middle
　　　　posterior
　　　　occiput bone
　　　　orbital roof
　　　　sinus:
　　　　　　ethmoid
　　　　　　frontal
　　　　sphenoid bone
　　　　temporal bone

● **801.0 Closed without mention of intracranial injury**

● **801.1 Closed with cerebral laceration and contusion**

● **801.2 Closed with subarachnoid, subdural, and extradural hemorrhage**

● ❑ **801.3 Closed with other and unspecified intracranial hemorrhage**

● ❑ **801.4 Closed with intracranial injury of other and unspecified nature**

● **801.5 Open without mention of intracranial injury**

● **801.6 Open with cerebral laceration and contusion**

● **801.7 Open with subarachnoid, subdural, and extradural hemorrhage**

● ❑ **801.8 Open with other and unspecified intracranial hemorrhage**

● ❑ **801.9 Open with intracranial injury of other and unspecified nature**

● **802 Fracture of face bones**

　802.0 Nasal bones, closed

　802.1 Nasal bones, open

● **802.2 Mandible, closed**
　　　Inferior maxilla
　　　Lower jaw (bone)

　❑ **802.20 Unspecified site**

　802.21 Condylar process

　802.22 Subcondylar

　802.23 Coronoid process

　❑ **802.24 Ramus, unspecified**

　802.25 Angle of jaw

　802.26 Symphysis of body

　802.27 Alveolar border of body

　❑ **802.28 Body, other and unspecified**

　❑ **802.29 Multiple sites**

● **802.3 Mandible, open**

　❑ **802.30 Unspecified site**

　802.31 Condylar process

　802.32 Subcondylar

　802.33 Coronoid process

　❑ **802.34 Ramus, unspecified**

　802.35 Angle of jaw

　802.36 Symphysis of body

　802.37 Alveolar border of body

　❑ **802.38 Body, other and unspecified**

　❑ **802.39 Multiple sites**

　802.4 Malar and maxillary bones, closed
　　　Superior maxilla
　　　Upper jaw (bone)
　　　Zygoma
　　　Zygomatic arch

　802.5 Malar and maxillary bones, open

　802.6 Orbital floor (blow-out), closed

　802.7 Orbital floor (blow-out), open

❑ **802.8 Other facial bones, closed**
　　　Alveolus
　　　Orbit:
　　　　NOS
　　　　part other than roof or floor
　　　Palate

　| **Excludes** | orbital:
　　　　floor (802.6)
　　　　roof (801.0–801.9)

❑ **802.9 Other facial bones, open**

● **803 Other and unqualified skull fractures**

Requires fifth digit. See beginning of section 800–804 for codes and definitions.

Includes: skull NOS
　　　　skull multiple NOS

● **803.0 Closed without mention of intracranial injury**

● **803.1 Closed with cerebral laceration and contusion**

● **803.2 Closed with subarachnoid, subdural, and extradural hemorrhage**

● ❑ **803.3 Closed with other and unspecified intracranial hemorrhage**

● ❑ **803.4 Closed with intracranial injury of other and unspecified nature**

● **803.5 Open without mention of intracranial injury**

● **803.6 Open with cerebral laceration and contusion**

● **803.7 Open with subarachnoid, subdural, and extradural hemorrhage**

● ❑ **803.8 Open with other and unspecified intracranial hemorrhage**

● ❑ **803.9 Open with intracranial injury of other and unspecified nature**

● **804 Multiple fractures involving skull or face with other bones**

Requires fifth digit. See beginning of section 800–804 for codes and definitions.

● **804.0 Closed without mention of intracranial injury**

● **804.1 Closed with cerebral laceration and contusion**

● **804.2 Closed with subarachnoid, subdural, and extradural hemorrhage**

● ❑ **804.3 Closed with other and unspecified intracranial hemorrhage**

● ❑ **804.4 Closed with intracranial injury of other and unspecified nature**

● **804.5 Open without mention of intracranial injury**

● **804.6 Open with cerebral laceration and contusion**

● **804.7 Open with subarachnoid, subdural, and extradural hemorrhage**

● ❑ **804.8 Open with other and unspecified intracranial hemorrhage**

● ❑ **804.9 Open with intracranial injury of other and unspecified nature**

ICD-9-CM

800–899

Vol. 1

FRACTURE OF NECK AND TRUNK (805–809)

● 805 **Fracture of vertebral column without mention of spinal cord injury**

Includes: neural arch
spine
spinous process
transverse process
vertebra

The following fifth-digit subclassification is for use with codes 805.0–805.1:

❑ 0 cervical vertebra, unspecified level
1 first cervical vertebra
2 second cervical vertebra
3 third cervical vertebra
4 fourth cervical vertebra
5 fifth cervical vertebra
6 sixth cervical vertebra
7 seventh cervical vertebra
❑ 8 multiple cervical vertebrae

● 805.0 **Cervical, closed**
Atlas
Axis

● 805.1 **Cervical, open**

805.2 **Dorsal [thoracic], closed**

805.3 **Dorsal [thoracic], open**

805.4 **Lumbar, closed**

805.5 **Lumbar, open**

805.6 **Sacrum and coccyx, closed**

805.7 **Sacrum and coccyx, open**

❑ 805.8 **Unspecified, closed**

❑ 805.9 **Unspecified, open**

● 806 **Fracture of vertebral column with spinal cord injury**

Includes: any condition classifiable to 805 with:
complete or incomplete transverse lesion (of cord)
hematomyelia
injury to:
cauda equina
nerve
paralysis
paraplegia
quadriplegia
spinal concussion

● 806.0 **Cervical, closed**

❑ 806.00 C_1-C_4 level with unspecified spinal cord injury
Cervical region NOS with spinal cord injury NOS

806.01 C_1-C_4 level with complete lesion of cord

806.02 C_1-C_4 level with anterior cord syndrome

806.03 C_1-C_4 level with central cord syndrome

❑ 806.04 C_1-C_4 level with other specified spinal cord injury
C_1-C_4 level with:
incomplete spinal cord lesion NOS
posterior cord syndrome

❑ 806.05 C_5-C_7 level with unspecified spinal cord injury

806.06 C_5-C_7 level with complete lesion of cord

806.07 C_5-C_7 level with anterior cord syndrome

806.08 C_5-C_7 level with central cord syndrome

❑ 806.09 C_5-C_7 level with other specified spinal cord injury
C_5-C_7 level with:
incomplete spinal cord lesion NOS
posterior cord syndrome

● 806.1 **Cervical, open**

❑ 806.10 C_1-C_4 level with unspecified spinal cord injury

806.11 C_1-C_4 level with complete lesion of cord

806.12 C_1-C_4 level with anterior cord syndrome

806.13 C_1-C_4 level with central cord syndrome

❑ 806.14 C_1-C_4 level with other specified spinal cord injury
C_1-C_4 level with:
incomplete spinal cord lesion NOS
posterior cord syndrome

❑ 806.15 C_5-C_7 level with unspecified spinal cord injury

806.16 C_5-C_7 level with complete lesion of cord

806.17 C_5-C_7 level with anterior cord syndrome

806.18 C_5-C_7 level with central cord syndrome

❑ 806.19 C_5-C_7 level with other specified spinal cord injury
C_5-C_7 level with:
incomplete spinal cord lesion NOS
posterior cord syndrome

● 806.2 **Dorsal [thoracic], closed**

❑ 806.20 T_1-T_6 level with unspecified spinal cord injury
Thoracic region NOS with spinal cord injury NOS

806.21 T_1-T_6 level with complete lesion of cord

806.22 T_1-T_6 level with anterior cord syndrome

806.23 T_1-T_6 level with central cord syndrome

❑ 806.24 T_1-T_6 level with other specified spinal cord injury
T_1-T_6 level with:
incomplete spinal cord lesion NOS
posterior cord syndrome

❑ 806.25 T_7-T_{12} level with unspecified spinal cord injury

806.26 T_7-T_{12} level with complete lesion of cord

806.27 T_7-T_{12} level with anterior cord syndrome

806.28 T_7-T_{12} level with central cord syndrome

❑ 806.29 T_7-T_{12} level with other specified spinal cord injury
T_7-T_{12} level with:
incomplete spinal cord lesion NOS
posterior cord syndrome

● 806.3 **Dorsal [thoracic], open**

❑ 806.30 T_1-T_6 level with unspecified spinal cord injury

806.31 T_1-T_6 level with complete lesion of cord

806.32 T_1-T_6 level with anterior cord syndrome

806.33 T_1-T_6 level with central cord syndrome

❑ 806.34 T_1-T_6 level with other specified spinal cord injury
T_1-T_6 level with:
incomplete spinal cord lesion NOS
posterior cord syndrome

❑ 806.35 T_7-T_{12} level with unspecified spinal cord injury

806.36   T$_7$-T$_{12}$ level with complete lesion of cord

806.37   T$_7$-T$_{12}$ level with anterior cord syndrome

806.38   T$_7$-T$_{12}$ level with central cord syndrome

☐ 806.39   T$_7$-T$_{12}$ level with other specified spinal cord injury
> T$_7$-T$_{12}$ level with:
>   incomplete spinal cord lesion NOS
>   posterior cord syndrome

806.4   Lumbar, closed

806.5   Lumbar, open

● 806.6   Sacrum and coccyx, closed

☐ 806.60   With unspecified spinal cord injury

806.61   With complete cauda equina lesion

☐ 806.62   With other cauda equina injury

☐ 806.69   With other spinal cord injury

● 806.7   Sacrum and coccyx, open

☐ 806.70   With unspecified spinal cord injury

806.71   With complete cauda equina lesion

☐ 806.72   With other cauda equina injury

☐ 806.79   With other spinal cord injury

☐ 806.8   Unspecified, closed

☐ 806.9   Unspecified, open

● 807   Fracture of rib(s), sternum, larynx, and trachea

The following fifth-digit subclassification is for use with codes 807.0–807.1:

☐ 0   rib(s), unspecified
1   one rib
2   two ribs
3   three ribs
4   four ribs
5   five ribs
6   six ribs
7   seven ribs
8   eight or more ribs
☐ 9   multiple ribs, unspecified

● 807.0   Rib(s), closed

● 807.1   Rib(s), open

807.2   Sternum, closed

807.3   Sternum, open

807.4   Flail chest

807.5   Larynx and trachea, closed
> Hyoid bone   Trachea
> Thyroid cartilage

807.6   Larynx and trachea, open

● 808   Fracture of pelvis

808.0   Acetabulum, closed

808.1   Acetabulum, open

808.2   Pubis, closed

808.3   Pubis, open

● 808.4   Other specified part, closed

808.41   Ilium

808.42   Ischium

☐ 808.43   Multiple pelvic fractures with disruption of pelvic circle

☐ 808.49   Other
> Innominate bone   Pelvic rim

● 808.5   Other specified part, open

808.51   Ilium

808.52   Ischium

☐ 808.53   Multiple pelvic fractures with disruption of pelvic circle

☐ 808.59   Other

☐ 808.8   Unspecified, closed

☐ 808.9   Unspecified, open

● 809   Ill-defined fractures of bones of trunk

Includes: bones of trunk with other bones except those of skull and face
multiple bones of trunk

Excludes	*multiple fractures of:*

> *multiple fractures of:*
>   *pelvic bones alone (808.0–808.9)*
>   *ribs alone (807.0–807.1, 807.4)*
>   *ribs or sternum with limb bones (819.0–819.1,*
>   *828.0–828.1)*
>   *skull or face with other bones (804.0–804.9)*

809.0   Fracture of bones of trunk, closed

809.1   Fracture of bones of trunk, open

FRACTURE OF UPPER LIMB (810–819)

● 810   Fracture of clavicle

Includes: collar bone
interligamentous part of clavicle

The following fifth-digit subclassification is for use with category 810:

☐ 0   unspecified part
> clavicle NOS
1   sternal end of clavicle
2   shaft of clavicle
3   acromial end of clavicle

● 810.0   Closed

● 810.1   Open

● 811   Fracture of scapula

Includes: shoulder blade

The following fifth-digit subclassification is for use with category 811:

☐ 0   unspecified part
1   acromial process
> acromion (process)
2   coracoid process
3   glenoid cavity and neck of scapula
☐ 9   other

● 811.0   Closed

● 811.1   Open

● 812   Fracture of humerus

● 812.0   Upper end, closed

☐ 812.00   Upper end, unspecified part
> Proximal end
> Shoulder

812.01   Surgical neck
> Neck of humerus NOS

812.02   Anatomical neck

812.03   Greater tuberosity

☐ 812.09   Other
> Head
> Upper epiphysis

● 812.1   Upper end, open

☐ 812.10   Upper end, unspecified part

ICD-9-CM

**800-
899**

Vol. 1

812.11   Surgical neck

812.12   Anatomical neck

812.13   Greater tuberosity

❏ 812.19   Other

● 812.2   Shaft or unspecified part, closed

❏ 812.20   Unspecified part of humerus
     Humerus NOS
     Upper arm NOS

812.21   Shaft of humerus

● 812.3   Shaft or unspecified part, open

❏ 812.30   Unspecified part of humerus

812.31   Shaft of humerus

● 812.4   Lower end, closed
     Distal end of humerus
     Elbow

❏ 812.40   Lower end, unspecified part

812.41   Supracondylar fracture of humerus

812.42   Lateral condyle
     External condyle

812.43   Medial condyle
     Internal epicondyle

❏ 812.44   Condyle(s), unspecified
     Articular process NOS
     Lower epiphysis

❏ 812.49   Other
     Multiple fractures of lower end
     Trochlea

● 812.5   Lower end, open

❏ 812.50   Lower end, unspecified part

812.51   Supracondylar fracture of humerus

812.52   Lateral condyle

812.53   Medial condyle

❏ 812.54   Condyle(s), unspecified

❏ 812.59   Other

● 813   Fracture of radius and ulna

● 813.0   Upper end, closed
     Proximal end

❏ 813.00   Upper end of forearm, unspecified

813.01   Olecranon process of ulna

813.02   Coronoid process of ulna

813.03   Monteggia's fracture

❏ 813.04   Other and unspecified fractures of proximal
     end of ulna (alone)
     Multiple fractures of ulna, upper end

813.05   Head of radius

813.06   Neck of radius

❏ 813.07   Other and unspecified fractures of proximal
     end of radius (alone)
     Multiple fractures of radius, upper end

813.08   Radius with ulna, upper end [any part]

● 813.1   Upper end, open

❏ 813.10   Upper end of forearm, unspecified

813.11   Olecranon process of ulna

813.12   Coronoid process of ulna

813.13   Monteggia's fracture

❏ 813.14   Other and unspecified fractures of proximal
     end of ulna (alone)

813.15   Head of radius

813.16   Neck of radius

❏ 813.17   Other and unspecified fractures of proximal
     end of radius (alone)

813.18   Radius with ulna, upper end [any part]

● 813.2   Shaft, closed

❏ 813.20   Shaft, unspecified

813.21   Radius (alone)

813.22   Ulna (alone)

813.23   Radius with ulna

● 813.3   Shaft, open

❏ 813.30   Shaft, unspecified

813.31   Radius (alone)

813.32   Ulna (alone)

813.33   Radius with ulna

● 813.4   Lower end, closed
     Distal end

❏ 813.40   Lower end of forearm, unspecified

813.41   Colles' fracture
     Smith's fracture

❏ 813.42   Other fractures of distal end of radius
     (alone)
     Dupuytren's fracture, radius
     Radius, lower end

813.43   Distal end of ulna (alone)
     Ulna:
       head
       lower end
       lower epiphysis
       styloid process

813.44   Radius with ulna, lower end

813.45   Torus fracture of radius

● 813.5   Lower end, open

❏ 813.50   Lower end of forearm, unspecified

813.51   Colles' fracture

❏ 813.52   Other fractures of distal end of radius
     (alone)

813.53   Distal end of ulna (alone)

813.54   Radius with ulna, lower end

● 813.8   Unspecified part, closed

❏ 813.80   Forearm, unspecified

❏ 813.81   Radius (alone)

❏ 813.82   Ulna (alone)

❏ 813.83   Radius with ulna

● 813.9   Unspecified part, open

❏ 813.90   Forearm, unspecified

❏ 813.91   Radius (alone)

❏ 813.92   Ulna (alone)

❏ 813.93   Radius with ulna

● 814   Fracture of carpal bone(s)

The following fifth-digit subclassification is for use with category 814:

☐ 0   carpal bone, unspecified
     Wrist NOS
   1   navicular [scaphoid] of wrist
   2   lunate [semilunar] bone of wrist
   3   triquetral [cuneiform] bone of wrist
   4   pisiform
   5   trapezium bone [larger multangular]
   6   trapezoid bone [smaller multangular]
   7   capitate bone [os magnum]
   8   hamate [unciform] bone
☐ 9   other

● 814.0   Closed

● 814.1   Open

● 815   Fracture of metacarpal bone(s)

Includes: hand [except finger]
          metacarpus

The following fifth-digit subclassification is for use with category 815:

☐ 0   metacarpal bone(s), site unspecified
   1   base of thumb [first] metacarpal
     Bennett's fracture
   2   base of other metacarpal bone(s)
   3   shaft of metacarpal bone(s)
   4   neck of metacarpal bone(s)
☐ 9   multiple sites of metacarpus

● 815.0   Closed

● 815.1   Open

● 816   Fracture of one or more phalanges of hand

Includes: finger(s)
          thumb

The following fifth-digit subclassification is for use with category 816:

☐ 0   phalanx or phalanges, unspecified
   1   middle or proximal phalanx or phalanges
   2   distal phalanx or phalanges
☐ 3   multiple sites

● 816.0   Closed

● 816.1   Open

● 817   Multiple fractures of hand bones

Includes: metacarpal bone(s) with phalanx or phalanges
          of same hand

817.0   Closed

817.1   Open

● 818   Ill-defined fractures of upper limb

Includes: arm NOS
          multiple bones of same upper limb

Excludes   *multiple fractures of:*
      metacarpal bone(s) with phalanx or phalanges
         (817.0–817.1)
      phalanges of hand alone (816.0–816.1)
      radius with ulna (813.0–813.9)

☐ 818.0   Closed

☐ 818.1   Open

● 819   Multiple fractures involving both upper limbs, and upper limb with rib(s) and sternum

Includes: arm(s) with rib(s) or sternum
          both arms [any bones]

819.0   Closed

819.1   Open

FRACTURE OF LOWER LIMB (820–829)

● 820   Fracture of neck of femur

● 820.0   Transcervical fracture, closed

☐ 820.00   Intracapsular section, unspecified

820.01   Epiphysis (separation) (upper)
       Transepiphyseal

820.02   Midcervical section
       Transcervical NOS

820.03   Base of neck
       Cervicotrochanteric section

☐ 820.09   Other
       Head of femur
       Subcapital

● 820.1   Transcervical fracture, open

☐ 820.10   Intracapsular section, unspecified

820.11   Epiphysis (separation) (upper)

820.12   Midcervical section

820.13   Base of neck

☐ 820.19   Other

● 820.2   Pertrochanteric fracture, closed

☐ 820.20   Trochanteric section, unspecified
       Trochanter:
         NOS
         greater
         lesser

820.21   Intertrochanteric section

820.22   Subtrochanteric section

● 820.3   Pertrochanteric fracture, open

☐ 820.30   Trochanteric section, unspecified

820.31   Intertrochanteric section

820.32   Subtrochanteric section

☐ 820.8   Unspecified part of neck of femur, closed
       Hip NOS
       Neck of femur NOS

☐ 820.9   Unspecified part of neck of femur, open

● 821   Fracture of other and unspecified parts of femur

● 821.0   Shaft or unspecified part, closed

☐ 821.00   Unspecified part of femur
       Thigh
       Upper leg

Excludes   *hip NOS (820.8)*

821.01   Shaft

● 821.1   Shaft or unspecified part, open

☐ 821.10   Unspecified part of femur

821.11   Shaft

● 821.2   Lower end, closed
       Distal end

☐ 821.20   Lower end, unspecified part

821.21   Condyle, femoral

821.22   Epiphysis, lower (separation)

821.23   Supracondylar fracture of femur

☐ 821.29   Other
       Multiple fractures of lower end

ICD-9-CM

808-
849

Vol. 1

● **821.3 Lower end, open**

❑ 821.30 Lower end, unspecified part

821.31 Condyle, femoral

821.32 Epiphysis, lower (separation)

821.33 Supracondylar fracture of femur

❑ 821.39 Other

● **822 Fracture of patella**

822.0 Closed

822.1 Open

● **823 Fracture of tibia and fibula**

Excludes *Dupuytren's fracture (824.4–824.5)*
ankle (824.4–824.5)
radius (813.42, 813.52)
Pott's fracture (824.4–824.5)
that involving ankle (824.0–824.9)

The following fifth-digit subclassification is for use with category 823:
0 tibia alone
1 fibula alone
2 fibula with tibia

● 823.0 Upper end, closed
Head
Proximal end
Tibia:
condyles
tuberosity

● 823.1 Upper end, open

● 823.2 Shaft, closed

● 823.3 Shaft, open

● 823.4 Torus fracture

● ❑ 823.8 Unspecified part, closed
Lower leg NOS

● ❑ 823.9 Unspecified part, open

● **824 Fracture of ankle**

824.0 Medial malleolus, closed
Tibia involving:
ankle
malleolus

824.1 Medial malleolus, open

824.2 Lateral malleolus, closed
Fibula involving:
ankle
malleolus

824.3 Lateral malleolus, open

824.4 Bimalleolar, closed
Dupuytren's fracture, fibula
Pott's fracture

824.5 Bimalleolar, open

824.6 Trimalleolar, closed
Lateral and medial malleolus with anterior or posterior lip of tibia

824.7 Trimalleolar, open

❑ 824.8 Unspecified, closed
Ankle NOS

❑ 824.9 Unspecified, open

● **825 Fracture of one or more tarsal and metatarsal bones**

❑ 825.0 Fracture of calcaneus, closed
Heel bone
Os calcis

825.1 Fracture of calcaneus, open

● 825.2 Fracture of other tarsal and metatarsal bones, closed

❑ 825.20 Unspecified bone(s) of foot [except toes]
Instep

825.21 Astragalus
Talus

825.22 Navicular [scaphoid], foot

825.23 Cuboid

825.24 Cuneiform, foot

825.25 Metatarsal bone(s)

❑ 825.29 Other
Tarsal with metatarsal bone(s) only

Excludes *calcaneus (825.0)*

● 825.3 Fracture of other tarsal and metatarsal bones, open

❑ 825.30 Unspecified bone(s) of foot [except toes]

825.31 Astragalus

825.32 Navicular [scaphoid], foot

825.33 Cuboid

825.34 Cuneiform, foot

825.35 Metatarsal bone(s)

❑ 825.39 Other

● **826 Fracture of one or more phalanges of foot**

Includes: toe(s)

826.0 Closed

826.1 Open

● **827 Other, multiple, and ill-defined fractures of lower limb**

Includes: leg NOS
multiple bones of same lower limb

Excludes *multiple fractures of:*
ankle bones alone (824.4–824.9)
phalanges of foot alone (826.0–826.1)
tarsal with metatarsal bones (825.29, 825.39)
tibia with fibula (823.0–823.9 with fifth-digit 2)

827.0 Closed

827.1 Open

● **828 Multiple fractures involving both lower limbs, lower with upper limb, and lower limb(s) with rib(s) and sternum**

Includes: arm(s) with leg(s) [any bones]
both legs [any bones]
leg(s) with rib(s) or sternum

828.0 Closed

828.1 Open

● **829 Fracture of unspecified bones**

❑ 829.0 Unspecified bone, closed

❑ 829.1 Unspecified bone, open

DISLOCATION (830–839)

Includes: displacement
subluxation

Excludes *congenital dislocation (754.0–755.8)*
pathological dislocation (718.2)
recurrent dislocation (718.3)

The descriptions "closed" and "open," used in the fourth-digit subdivisions, include the following terms:

closed:
  complete   simple
  dislocation NOS   uncomplicated
  partial
open:
  compound   with foreign body
  infected

Note: A dislocation not indicated as closed or open should be classified as closed.

● 830   Dislocation of jaw

  Includes: jaw (cartilage) (meniscus)
          mandible
          maxilla (inferior)
          temporomandibular (joint)

  830.0   Closed dislocation

  830.1   Open dislocation

● 831   Dislocation of shoulder

  Excludes *sternoclavicular joint (839.61, 839.71)*
          sternum (839.61, 839.71)

  The following fifth-digit subclassification is for use with category 831:
  ❏ 0   shoulder, unspecified
       humerus NOS
     1   anterior dislocation of humerus
     2   posterior dislocation of humerus
     3   inferior dislocation of humerus
     4   acromioclavicular (joint)
       clavicle
  ❏ 9   other
       Scapula

  ● 831.0   Closed dislocation

  ● 831.1   Open dislocation

● 832   Dislocation of elbow

  The following fifth-digit subclassification is for use with category 832:
  ❏ 0   elbow unspecified
     1   anterior dislocation of elbow
     2   posterior dislocation of elbow
     3   medial dislocation of elbow
     4   lateral dislocation of elbow
  ❏ 9   other

  ● 832.0   Closed dislocation

  ● 832.1   Open dislocation

● 833   Dislocation of wrist

  The following fifth-digit subclassification is for use with category 833:
  ❏ 0   wrist, unspecified part
       carpal (bone)
       radius, distal end
     1   radioulnar (joint), distal
     2   radiocarpal (joint)
     3   midcarpal (joint)
     4   carpometacarpal (joint)
     5   metacarpal (bone), proximal end
  ❏ 9   other
       ulna, distal end

  ● 833.0   Closed dislocation

  ● 833.1   Open dislocation

● 834   Dislocation of finger

  Includes: finger(s)
          phalanx of hand
          thumb

  The following fifth-digit subclassification is for use with category 834:
  ❏ 0   finger, unspecified part
     1   metacarpophalangeal (joint)
       metacarpal (bone), distal end
     2   interphalangeal (joint), hand

  ● 834.0   Closed dislocation

  ● 834.1   Open dislocation

● 835   Dislocation of hip

  The following fifth-digit subclassification is for use with category 835:
  ❏ 0   dislocation of hip, unspecified
     1   posterior dislocation
     2   obturator dislocation
  ❏ 3   other anterior dislocation

  ● 835.0   Closed dislocation

  ● 835.1   Open dislocation

● 836   Dislocation of knee

  Excludes *dislocation of knee:*
       old or pathological (718.2)
       recurrent (718.3)
       internal derangement of knee joint (717.0–717.5, 717.8–717.9)
       old tear of cartilage or meniscus of knee (717.0–717.5, 717.8–717.9)

  836.0   Tear of medial cartilage or meniscus of knee, current
       Bucket handle tear:
         NOS current injury
         medial meniscus current injury

  836.1   Tear of lateral cartilage or meniscus of knee, current

  ❏ 836.2   Other tear of cartilage or meniscus of knee, current
       Tear of:
         cartilage (semilunar) current injury, not specified as medial or lateral
         meniscus current injury, not specified as medial or lateral

  836.3   Dislocation of patella, closed

  836.4   Dislocation of patella, open

  ● 836.5   Other dislocation of knee, closed

    ❏ 836.50   Dislocation of knee, unspecified

       836.51   Anterior dislocation of tibia, proximal end
         Posterior dislocation of femur, distal end

       836.52   Posterior dislocation of tibia, proximal end
         Anterior dislocation of femur, distal end

       836.53   Medial dislocation of tibia, proximal end

       836.54   Lateral dislocation of tibia, proximal end

    ❏ 836.59   Other

  ● 836.6   Other dislocation of knee, open

    ❏ 836.60   Dislocation of knee, unspecified

       836.61   Anterior dislocation of tibia, proximal end

       836.62   Posterior dislocation of tibia, proximal end

       836.63   Medial dislocation of tibia, proximal end

       836.64   Lateral dislocation of tibia, proximal end

    ❏ 836.69   Other

ICD-9-CM
830-839
Vol. 1

● 837 **Dislocation of ankle**

Includes: astragalus
fibula, distal end   scaphoid, foot
navicular, foot   tibia, distal end

837.0 **Closed dislocation**

837.1 **Open dislocation**

● 838 **Dislocation of foot**

The following fifth-digit subclassification is for use with category 838:
❑ 0 **foot, unspecified**
1 **tarsal (bone), joint unspecified**
2 **midtarsal (joint)**
3 **tarsometatarsal (joint)**
4 **metatarsal (bone), joint unspecified**
5 **metatarsophalangeal (joint)**
6 **interphalangeal (joint), foot**
❑ 9 **other**
phalanx of foot
toe(s)

● 838.0 **Closed dislocation**

● 838.1 **Open dislocation**

● 839 **Other, multiple, and ill-defined dislocations**

● 839.0 **Cervical vertebra, closed**
Cervical spine
Neck

❑ 839.00 **Cervical vertebra, unspecified**

839.01 **First cervical vertebra**

839.02 **Second cervical vertebra**

839.03 **Third cervical vertebra**

839.04 **Fourth cervical vertebra**

839.05 **Fifth cervical vertebra**

839.06 **Sixth cervical vertebra**

839.07 **Seventh cervical vertebra**

❑ 839.08 **Multiple cervical vertebrae**

● 839.1 **Cervical vertebra, open**

❑ 839.10 **Cervical vertebra, unspecified**

839.11 **First cervical vertebra**

839.12 **Second cervical vertebra**

839.13 **Third cervical vertebra**

839.14 **Fourth cervical vertebra**

839.15 **Fifth cervical vertebra**

839.16 **Sixth cervical vertebra**

839.17 **Seventh cervical vertebra**

❑ 839.18 **Multiple cervical vertebrae**

● 839.2 **Thoracic and lumbar vertebra, closed**

839.20 **Lumbar vertebra**

839.21 **Thoracic vertebra**
Dorsal [thoracic] vertebra

● 839.3 **Thoracic and lumbar vertebra, open**

839.30 **Lumbar vertebra**

839.31 **Thoracic vertebra**

● 839.4 **Other vertebra, closed**

❑ 839.40 **Vertebra, unspecified site**
Spine NOS

839.41 **Coccyx**

839.42 **Sacrum**
Sacroiliac (joint)

❑ 839.49 **Other**

● 839.5 **Other vertebra, open**

❑ 839.50 **Vertebra, unspecified site**

839.51 **Coccyx**

839.52 **Sacrum**

❑ 839.59 **Other**

● 839.6 **Other location, closed**

839.61 **Sternum**
Sternoclavicular joint

❑ 839.69 **Other**
Pelvis

● 839.7 **Other location, open**

839.71 **Sternum**

❑ 839.79 **Other**

❑ 839.8 **Multiple and ill-defined, closed**
Arm
Back
Hand
Multiple locations, except fingers or toes alone
Other ill-defined locations
Unspecified location

❑ 839.9 **Multiple and ill-defined, open**

SPRAINS AND STRAINS OF JOINTS AND ADJACENT MUSCLES (840–848)

Includes: avulsion of joint capsule, ligament, muscle, tendon
hemarthrosis of joint capsule, ligament, muscle, tendon
laceration of joint capsule, ligament, muscle, tendon
rupture of joint capsule, ligament, muscle, tendon
sprain of joint capsule, ligament, muscle, tendon
strain of joint capsule, ligament, muscle, tendon
tear of joint capsule, ligament, muscle, tendon

Excludes *laceration of tendon in open wounds (880–884 and 890–894 with .2)*

● 840 **Sprains and strains of shoulder and upper arm**

840.0 **Acromioclavicular (joint) (ligament)**

840.1 **Coracoclavicular (ligament)**

840.2 **Coracohumeral (ligament)**

840.3 **Infraspinatus (muscle) (tendon)**

840.4 **Rotator cuff (capsule)**

Excludes *complete rupture of rotator cuff, nontraumatic (727.61)*

840.5 **Subscapularis (muscle)**

840.6 **Supraspinatus (muscle) (tendon)**

840.7 **Superior glenoid labrum lesion**
SLAP lesion

❑ 840.8 **Other specified sites of shoulder and upper arm**

❑ 840.9 **Unspecified site of shoulder and upper arm**
Arm NOS
Shoulder NOS

● 841 **Sprains and strains of elbow and forearm**

841.0 **Radial collateral ligament**

841.1 **Ulnar collateral ligament**

841.2 **Radiohumeral (joint)**

841.3 **Ulnohumeral (joint)**

❑ 841.8 **Other specified sites of elbow and forearm**

❑ 841.9 **Unspecified site of elbow and forearm**
Elbow NOS

● **842 Sprains and strains of wrist and hand**

  ● **842.0 Wrist**

    ❑ **842.00 Unspecified site**

      842.01 **Carpal (joint)**

      842.02 **Radiocarpal (joint) (ligament)**

    ❑ **842.09 Other**
        Radioulnar joint, distal

  ● **842.1 Hand**

    ❑ **842.10 Unspecified site**

      842.11 **Carpometacarpal (joint)**

      842.12 **Metacarpophalangeal (joint)**

      842.13 **Interphalangeal (joint)**

    ❑ **842.19 Other**
        Midcarpal (joint)

● **843 Sprains and strains of hip and thigh**

  843.0 **Iliofemoral (ligament)**

  843.1 **Ischiocapsular (ligament)**

  ❑ **843.8 Other specified sites of hip and thigh**

  ❑ **843.9 Unspecified site of hip and thigh**
     Hip NOS
     Thigh NOS

● **844 Sprains and strains of knee and leg**

  844.0 **Lateral collateral ligament of knee**

  844.1 **Medial collateral ligament of knee**

  844.2 **Cruciate ligament of knee**

  844.3 **Tibiofibular (joint) (ligament), superior**

  ❑ **844.8 Other specified sites of knee and leg**

  ❑ **844.9 Unspecified site of knee and leg**
     Knee NOS
     Leg NOS

● **845 Sprains and strains of ankle and foot**

  ● **845.0 Ankle**

    ❑ **845.00 Unspecified site**

      845.01 **Deltoid (ligament), ankle**
        Internal collateral (ligament), ankle

      845.02 **Calcaneofibular (ligament)**

      845.03 **Tibiofibular (ligament), distal**

    ❑ **845.09 Other**
        Achilles tendon

  ● **845.1 Foot**

    ❑ **845.10 Unspecified site**

      845.11 **Tarsometatarsal (joint) (ligament)**

      845.12 **Metatarsophalangeal (joint)**

      845.13 **Interphalangeal (joint), toe**

    ❑ **845.19 Other**

● **846 Sprains and strains of sacroiliac region**

  846.0 **Lumbosacral (joint) (ligament)**

  846.1 **Sacroiliac ligament**

  846.2 **Sacrospinatus (ligament)**

  846.3 **Sacrotuberous (ligament)**

  ❑ **846.8 Other specified sites of sacroiliac region**

  ❑ **846.9 Unspecified site of sacroiliac region**

● **847 Sprains and strains of other and unspecified parts of back**

  Excludes *lumbosacral (846.0)*

  847.0 **Neck**
     Anterior longitudinal (ligament), cervical
     Atlanto-axial (joints)
     Atlanto-occipital (joints)
     Whiplash injury

    Excludes *neck injury NOS (959.09)*
           thyroid region (848.2)

  847.1 **Thoracic**

  847.2 **Lumbar**

  847.3 **Sacrum**
     Sacrococcygeal (ligament)

  847.4 **Coccyx**

  ❑ **847.9 Unspecified site of back**
     Back NOS

● **848 Other and ill-defined sprains and strains**

  848.0 **Septal cartilage of nose**

  848.1 **Jaw**
     Temporomandibular (joint) (ligament)

  848.2 **Thyroid region**
     Cricoarytenoid (joint) (ligament)
     Cricothyroid (joint) (ligament)
     Thyroid cartilage

  848.3 **Ribs**
     Chondrocostal (joint) without mention of injury to sternum
     Costal cartilage without mention of injury to sternum

  ● **848.4 Sternum**

    ❑ **848.40 Unspecified site**

      848.41 **Sternoclavicular (joint) (ligament)**

      848.42 **Chondrosternal (joint)**

    ❑ **848.49 Other**
        Xiphoid cartilage

  848.5 **Pelvis**
     Symphysis pubis

  Excludes *that in childbirth (665.6)*

  ❑ **848.8 Other specified sites of sprains and strains**

  ❑ **848.9 Unspecified site of sprain and strain**

ICD-9-CM

800-
999

Vol. 1

INTRACRANIAL INJURY, EXCLUDING THOSE WITH SKULL FRACTURE (850–854)

> **Excludes** *intracranial injury with skull fracture (800–801 and 803–804, except .0 and .5)*
> *open wound of head without intracranial injury (870.0–873.9)*
> *skull fracture alone (800–801 and 803–804 with .0, .5)*

Note: The description "with open intracranial wound," used in the fourth-digit subdivisions, includes those specified as open or with mention of infection or foreign body.

The following fifth-digit subclassification is for use with categories 851–854:

❑ 0 unspecified state of consciousness
1 with no loss of consciousness
2 with brief [less than one hour] loss of consciousness
3 with moderate [1–24 hours] loss of consciousness
4 with prolonged [more than 24 hours] loss of consciousness and return to pre-existing conscious level
5 with prolonged [more than 24 hours] loss of consciousness without return to pre-existing conscious level

> Use fifth-digit 5 to designate when a patient is unconscious and dies before regaining consciousness, regardless of the duration of the loss of consciousness

❑ 6 with loss of consciousness of unspecified duration
❑ 9 with concussion, unspecified

● 850 Concussion

Includes: commotio cerebri

> **Excludes** *concussion with:*
> *cerebral laceration or contusion (851.0–851.9)*
> *cerebral hemorrhage (852–853)*
> *head injury NOS (959.01)*

850.0 With no loss of consciousness
Concussion with mental confusion or disorientation, without loss of consciousness

● 850.1 With brief loss of consciousness
Loss of consciousness for less than one hour

850.11 with loss of consciousness less than 30 minutes

850.12 with loss of consciousness from 31 to 59 minutes

850.2 With moderate loss of consciousness
Loss of consciousness for 1–24 hours

850.3 With prolonged loss of consciousness and return to pre-existing conscious level
Loss of consciousness for more than 24 hours with complete recovery

850.4 With prolonged loss of consciousness, without return to pre-existing conscious level

❑ 850.5 With loss of consciousness of unspecified duration

❑ 850.9 Concussion, unspecified

● 851 Cerebral laceration and contusion

Requires fifth digit. See beginning of section 850–854 for codes and definitions.

● 851.0 Cortex (cerebral) contusion without mention of open intracranial wound

● 851.1 Cortex (cerebral) contusion with open intracranial wound

● 851.2 Cortex (cerebral) laceration without mention of open intracranial wound

● 851.3 Cortex (cerebral) laceration with open intracranial wound

● 851.4 Cerebellar or brain stem contusion without mention of open intracranial wound

● 851.5 Cerebellar or brain stem contusion with open intracranial wound

● 851.6 Cerebellar or brain stem laceration without mention of open intracranial wound

● 851.7 Cerebellar or brain stem laceration with open intracranial wound

● ❑ 851.8 Other and unspecified cerebral laceration and contusion, without mention of open intracranial wound
Brain (membrane) NOS

● ❑ 851.9 Other and unspecified cerebral laceration and contusion, with open intracranial wound

● 852 Subarachnoid, subdural, and extradural hemorrhage, following injury

Requires fifth digit. See beginning of section 850–854 for codes and definitions.

> **Excludes** *cerebral contusion or laceration (with hemorrhage) (851.0–851.9)*

● 852.0 Subarachnoid hemorrhage following injury without mention of open intracranial wound
Middle meningeal hemorrhage following injury

● 852.1 Subarachnoid hemorrhage following injury with open intracranial wound

● 852.2 Subdural hemorrhage following injury without mention of open intracranial wound

● 852.3 Subdural hemorrhage following injury with open intracranial wound

● 852.4 Extradural hemorrhage following injury without mention of open intracranial wound
Epidural hematoma following injury

● 852.5 Extradural hemorrhage following injury with open intracranial wound

● 853 Other and unspecified intracranial hemorrhage following injury

Requires fifth digit. See beginning of section 850–854 for codes and definitions.

● ❑ 853.0 Without mention of open intracranial wound
Cerebral compression due to injury
Intracranial hematoma following injury
Traumatic cerebral hemorrhage

● ❑ 853.1 With open intracranial wound

● 854 Intracranial injury of other and unspecified nature

Includes: injury:
brain NOS
cavernous sinus
intracranial

> **Excludes** *any condition classifiable to 850–853*
> *head injury NOS (959.01)*

● ❑ 854.0 Without mention of open intracranial wound

● ❑ 854.1 With open intracranial wound

INTERNAL INJURY OF THORAX, ABDOMEN, AND PELVIS (860–869)

Includes: blast injuries of internal organs
blunt trauma of internal organs
bruise of internal organs
concussion injuries (except cerebral) of internal organs
crushing of internal organs
hematoma of internal organs
laceration of internal organs
puncture of internal organs
tear of internal organs
traumatic rupture of internal organs

Excludes concussion NOS (850.0–850.9)
flail chest (807.4)
foreign body entering through orifice (930.0–939.9)
injury to blood vessels (901.0–902.9)

Note: The description "with open wound," used in the fourth-digit subdivisions, includes those with mention of infection or foreign body.

● **860   Traumatic pneumothorax and hemothorax**

860.0   Pneumothorax without mention of open wound into thorax

860.1   Pneumothorax with open wound into thorax

860.2   Hemothorax without mention of open wound into thorax

860.3   Hemothorax with open wound into thorax

860.4   Pneumohemothorax without mention of open wound into thorax

860.5   Pneumohemothorax with open wound into thorax

● **861   Injury to heart and lung**

Excludes injury to blood vessels of thorax (901.0–901.9)

● **861.0   Heart, without mention of open wound into thorax**

☐ **861.00   Unspecified injury**

861.01   Contusion
Cardiac contusion
Myocardial contusion

861.02   Laceration without penetration of heart chambers

861.03   Laceration with penetration of heart chambers

● **861.1   Heart, with open wound into thorax**

☐ **861.10   Unspecified injury**

861.11   Contusion

861.12   Laceration without penetration of heart chambers

861.13   Laceration with penetration of heart chambers

● **861.2   Lung, without mention of open wound into thorax**

☐ **861.20   Unspecified injury**

861.21   Contusion

861.22   Laceration

● **861.3   Lung, with open wound into thorax**

☐ **861.30   Unspecified injury**

861.31   Contusion

861.32   Laceration

● **862   Injury to other and unspecified intrathoracic organs**

Excludes injury to blood vessels of thorax (901.0–901.9)

862.0   Diaphragm, without mention of open wound into cavity

862.1   Diaphragm, with open wound into cavity

● **862.2   Other specified intrathoracic organs, without mention of open wound into cavity**

862.21   Bronchus

862.22   Esophagus

☐ **862.29   Other**
Pleura
Thymus gland

● **862.3   Other specified intrathoracic organs, with open wound into cavity**

862.31   Bronchus

862.32   Esophagus

☐ **862.39   Other**

☐ **862.8   Multiple and unspecified intrathoracic organs, without mention of open wound into cavity**
Crushed chest
Multiple intrathoracic organs

☐ **862.9   Multiple and unspecified intrathoracic organs, with open wound into cavity**

● **863   Injury to gastrointestinal tract**

Excludes anal sphincter laceration during delivery (664.2)
bile duct (868.0–868.1 with fifth-digit 2)
gallbladder (868.0–868.1 with fifth-digit 2)

863.0   Stomach, without mention of open wound into cavity

863.1   Stomach, with open wound into cavity

● **863.2   Small intestine, without mention of open wound into cavity**

☐ **863.20   Small intestine, unspecified site**

863.21   Duodenum

☐ **863.29   Other**

● **863.3   Small intestine, with open wound into cavity**

☐ **863.30   Small intestine, unspecified site**

863.31   Duodenum

☐ **863.39   Other**

● **863.4   Colon or rectum, without mention of open wound into cavity**

☐ **863.40   Colon, unspecified site**

863.41   Ascending [right] colon

863.42   Transverse colon

863.43   Descending [left] colon

863.44   Sigmoid colon

863.45   Rectum

☐ **863.46   Multiple sites in colon and rectum**

☐ **863.49   Other**

● **863.5   Colon or rectum, with open wound into cavity**

☐ **863.50   Colon, unspecified site**

863.51   Ascending [right] colon

863.52   Transverse colon

863.53   Descending [left] colon

863.54   Sigmoid colon

863.55   Rectum

☐ **863.56   Multiple sites in colon and rectum**

☐ **863.59   Other**

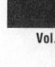

ICD-9-CM

860-869

Vol. 1

● 863.8 Other and unspecified gastrointestinal sites, without mention of open wound into cavity

  ☐ 863.80 Gastrointestinal tract, unspecified site

  863.81 Pancreas, head

  863.82 Pancreas, body

  863.83 Pancreas, tail

  ☐ 863.84 Pancreas, multiple and unspecified sites

  863.85 Appendix

  ☐ 863.89 Other
  Intestine NOS

● 863.9 Other and unspecified gastrointestinal sites, with open wound into cavity

  ☐ 863.90 Gastrointestinal tract, unspecified site

  863.91 Pancreas, head

  863.92 Pancreas, body

  863.93 Pancreas, tail

  ☐ 863.94 Pancreas, multiple and unspecified sites

  863.95 Appendix

  ☐ 863.99 Other

● 864 Injury to liver

The following fifth-digit subclassification is for use with category 864:

☐ 0 unspecified injury
  1 hematoma and contusion
  2 laceration, minor
  Laceration involving capsule only, or without significant involvement of hepatic parenchyma [i.e., less than 1 cm deep]
  3 laceration, moderate
  Laceration involving parenchyma but without major disruption of parenchyma [i.e., less than 10 cm long and less than 3 cm deep]
  4 laceration, major
  Laceration with significant disruption of hepatic parenchyma [i.e., 10 cm long and 3 cm deep]
  Multiple moderate lacerations, with or without hematoma
  Stellate lacerations of liver
☐ 5 laceration, unspecified
☐ 9 other

  ● 864.0 Without mention of open wound into cavity

  ● 864.1 With open wound into cavity

● 865 Injury to spleen

The following fifth-digit subclassification is for use with category 865:

☐ 0 unspecified injury
  1 hematoma without rupture of capsule
  2 capsular tears, without major disruption of parenchyma
  3 laceration extending into parenchyma
  4 massive parenchymal disruption
☐ 9 other

  ● 865.0 Without mention of open wound into cavity

  ● 865.1 With open wound into cavity

● 866 Injury to kidney

The following fifth-digit subclassification is for use with category 866:

☐ 0 unspecified injury
  1 hematoma without rupture of capsule
  2 laceration
  3 complete disruption of kidney parenchyma

  ● 866.0 Without mention of open wound into cavity

  ● 866.1 With open wound into cavity

● 867 Injury to pelvic organs

  Excludes injury during delivery (664.0–665.9)

  867.0 Bladder and urethra, without mention of open wound into cavity

  867.1 Bladder and urethra, with open wound into cavity

  867.2 Ureter, without mention of open wound into cavity

  867.3 Ureter, with open wound into cavity

  867.4 Uterus, without mention of open wound into cavity

  867.5 Uterus, with open wound into cavity

  ☐ 867.6 Other specified pelvic organs, without mention of open wound into cavity
  Fallopian tube
  Ovary
  Prostate
  Seminal vesicle
  Vas deferens

  ☐ 867.7 Other specified pelvic organs, with open wound into cavity

  ☐ 867.8 Unspecified pelvic organ, without mention of open wound into cavity

  ☐ 867.9 Unspecified pelvic organ, with open wound into cavity

● 868 Injury to other intra-abdominal organs

The following fifth-digit subclassification is for use with category 868:

☐ 0 unspecified intra-abdominal organ
  1 adrenal gland
  2 bile duct and gallbladder
  3 peritoneum
  4 retroperitoneum
☐ 9 other and multiple intra-abdominal organs

  ● 868.0 Without mention of open wound into cavity

  ● 868.1 With open wound into cavity

● 869 Internal injury to unspecified or ill-defined organs

  Includes: internal injury NOS
  multiple internal injury NOS

  ☐ 869.0 Without mention of open wound into cavity

  ☐ 869.1 With open wound into cavity

OPEN WOUNDS (870–897)

Note: The description "complicated" used in the fourth-digit subdivisions includes those with mention of delayed healing, delayed treatment, foreign body, or infection.

Includes: animal bite
avulsion
cut
laceration
puncture wound
traumatic amputation

Excludes *burn (940.0–949.5)*
crushing (925–929.9)
puncture of internal organs (860.0–869.1)
superficial injury (910.0–919.9)
that incidental to:
   dislocation (830.0–839.9)
   fracture (800.0–829.1)
   internal injury (860.0–869.1)
   intracranial injury (851.0–854.1)

Use additional code to identify infection

OPEN WOUND OF HEAD, NECK, AND TRUNK (870–879)

● 870   Open wound of ocular adnexa

    870.0   Laceration of skin of eyelid and periocular area

    870.1   Laceration of eyelid, full-thickness, not involving lacrimal passages

    870.2   Laceration of eyelid involving lacrimal passages

    870.3   Penetrating wound of orbit, without mention of foreign body

    870.4   Penetrating wound of orbit with foreign body
      Excludes *retained (old) foreign body in orbit (376.6)*

    ❏ 870.8   Other specified open wounds of ocular adnexa

    ❏ 870.9   Unspecified open wound of ocular adnexa

● 871   Open wound of eyeball
      Excludes *2nd cranial nerve [optic] injury (950.0–950.9)*
        3rd cranial nerve [oculomotor] injury (951.0)

    871.0   Ocular laceration without prolapse of intraocular tissue

    871.1   Ocular laceration with prolapse or exposure of intraocular tissue

    871.2   Rupture of eye with partial loss of intraocular tissue

    871.3   Avulsion of eye
      Traumatic enucleation

    ❏ 871.4   Unspecified laceration of eye

    871.5   Penetration of eyeball with magnetic foreign body
      Excludes *retained (old) magnetic foreign body in globe (360.50–360.59)*

    871.6   Penetration of eyeball with (nonmagnetic) foreign body
      Excludes *retained (old) (nonmagnetic) foreign body in globe (360.60–360.69)*

    ❏ 871.7   Unspecified ocular penetration

    ❏ 871.9   Unspecified open wound of eyeball

● 872   Open wound of ear

    ● 872.0   External ear, without mention of complication

      ❏ 872.00   External ear, unspecified site

      872.01   Auricle, ear
        Pinna

      872.02   Auditory canal

    ● 872.1   External ear, complicated

      ❏ 872.10   External ear, unspecified site

      872.11   Auricle, ear

      872.12   Auditory canal

    ● 872.6   Other specified parts of ear, without mention of complication

      872.61   Ear drum
        Drumhead
        Tympanic membrane

      872.62   Ossicles

      872.63   Eustachian tube

      872.64   Cochlea

      ❏ 872.69   Other and multiple sites

    ● 872.7   Other specified parts of ear, complicated

      872.71   Ear drum

      872.72   Ossicles

      872.73   Eustachian tube

      872.74   Cochlea

      ❏ 872.79   Other and multiple sites

    ❏ 872.8   Ear, part unspecified, without mention of complication
      Ear NOS

    ❏ 872.9   Ear, part unspecified, complicated

● 873   Other open wound of head

    873.0   Scalp, without mention of complication

    873.1   Scalp, complicated

    ● 873.2   Nose, without mention of complication

      ❏ 873.20   Nose, unspecified site

      873.21   Nasal septum

      873.22   Nasal cavity

      873.23   Nasal sinus

      ❏ 873.29   Multiple sites

    ● 873.3   Nose, complicated

      ❏ 873.30   Nose, unspecified site

      873.31   Nasal septum

      873.32   Nasal cavity

      873.33   Nasal sinus

      ❏ 873.39   Multiple sites

    ● 873.4   Face, without mention of complication

      ❏ 873.40   Face, unspecified site

      873.41   Cheek

      873.42   Forehead
        Eyebrow

      873.43   Lip

      873.44   Jaw

      ❏ 873.49   Other and multiple sites

    ● 873.5   Face, complicated

      ❏ 873.50   Face, unspecified site

      873.51   Cheek

      873.52   Forehead

      873.53   Lip

      873.54   Jaw

      ❏ 873.59   Other and multiple sites

ICD-9-CM

868–999

Vol. 1

● 873.6 **Internal structures of mouth, without mention of complication**

   ❏ 873.60 Mouth, unspecified site

   873.61 Buccal mucosa

   873.62 Gum (alveolar process)

   873.63 Tooth (broken)

   873.64 Tongue and floor of mouth

   873.65 Palate

   ❏ 873.69 Other and multiple sites

● 873.7 **Internal structures of mouth, complicated**

   ❏ 873.70 Mouth, unspecified site

   873.71 Buccal mucosa

   873.72 Gum (alveolar process)

   873.73 Tooth (broken)

   873.74 Tongue and floor of mouth

   873.75 Palate

   ❏ 873.79 Other and multiple sites

❏ 873.8 **Other and unspecified open wound of head without mention of complication**
   Head NOS

❏ 873.9 **Other and unspecified open wound of head, complicated**

● 874 **Open wound of neck**

  ● 874.0 **Larynx and trachea, without mention of complication**

    874.00 Larynx with trachea

    874.01 Larynx

    874.02 Trachea

  ● 874.1 **Larynx and trachea, complicated**

    874.10 Larynx with trachea

    874.11 Larynx

    874.12 Trachea

  874.2 **Thyroid gland, without mention of complication**

  874.3 **Thyroid gland, complicated**

  874.4 **Pharynx, without mention of complication**
    Cervical esophagus

  874.5 **Pharynx, complicated**

  ❏ 874.8 **Other and unspecified parts, without mention of complication**
    Nape of neck   Throat NOS
    Supraclavicular region

  ❏ 874.9 **Other and unspecified parts, complicated**

● 875 **Open wound of chest (wall)**

   Excludes *open wound into thoracic cavity (860.0–862.9)*
   traumatic pneumothorax and hemothorax (860.1, 860.3, 860.5)

  875.0 **Without mention of complication**

  875.1 **Complicated**

● 876 **Open wound of back**

   Includes: loin
    lumbar region

   Excludes *open wound into thoracic cavity (860.0–862.9)*
   traumatic pneumothorax and hemothorax (860.1, 860.3, 860.5)

  876.0 **Without mention of complication**

  876.1 **Complicated**

● 877 **Open wound of buttock**

   Includes: sacroiliac region

  877.0 **Without mention of complication**

  877.1 **Complicated**

● 878 **Open wound of genital organs (external), including traumatic amputation**

   Excludes *injury during delivery (664.0–665.9)*
   internal genital organs (867.0–867.9)

  878.0 **Penis, without mention of complication**

  878.1 **Penis, complicated**

  878.2 **Scrotum and testes, without mention of complication**

  878.3 **Scrotum and testes, complicated**

  878.4 **Vulva, without mention of complication**
    Labium (majus) (minus)

  878.5 **Vulva, complicated**

  878.6 **Vagina, without mention of complication**

  878.7 **Vagina, complicated**

  ❏ 878.8 **Other and unspecified parts, without mention of complication**

  ❏ 878.9 **Other and unspecified parts, complicated**

● 879 **Open wound of other and unspecified sites, except limbs**

  879.0 **Breast, without mention of complication**

  879.1 **Breast, complicated**

  879.2 **Abdominal wall, anterior, without mention of complication**
    Abdominal wall NOS   Pubic region
    Epigastric region   Umbilical region
    Hypogastric region

  879.3 **Abdominal wall, anterior, complicated**

  879.4 **Abdominal wall, lateral, without mention of complication**
    Flank   Iliac (region)
    Groin   Inguinal region
    Hypochondrium

  879.5 **Abdominal wall, lateral, complicated**

  ❏ 879.6 **Other and unspecified parts of trunk, without mention of complication**
    Pelvic region   Trunk NOS
    Perineum

  ❏ 879.7 **Other and unspecified parts of trunk, complicated**

  ❏ 879.8 **Open wound(s) (multiple) of unspecified site(s), without mention of complication**
    Multiple open wounds NOS
    Open wound NOS

  ❏ 879.9 **Open wound(s) (multiple) of unspecified site(s), complicated**

OPEN WOUND OF UPPER LIMB (880–887)

● 880 **Open wound of shoulder and upper arm**

  The following fifth-digit subclassification is for use with category 880:
   0 shoulder region
   1 scapular region
   2 axillary region
   3 upper arm
  ❏ 9 multiple sites

● 880.0 **Without mention of complication**

● 880.1 **Complicated**

● 880.2 **With tendon involvement**

● **881 Open wound of elbow, forearm, and wrist**

The following fifth-digit subclassification is for use with category 881:
0 forearm
1 elbow
2 wrist

● 881.0 Without mention of complication
● 881.1 Complicated
● 881.2 With tendon involvement

● **882 Open wound of hand except finger(s) alone**

882.0 Without mention of complication
882.1 Complicated
882.2 With tendon involvement

● **883 Open wound of finger(s)**

Includes: fingernail
thumb (nail)

883.0 Without mention of complication
883.1 Complicated
883.2 With tendon involvement

● **884 Multiple and unspecified open wound of upper limb**

Includes: arm NOS
multiple sites of one upper limb
upper limb NOS

❏ 884.0 Without mention of complication
❏ 884.1 Complicated
❏ 884.2 With tendon involvement

● **885 Traumatic amputation of thumb (complete) (partial)**

Includes: thumb(s) (with finger(s) of either hand)

885.0 Without mention of complication
885.1 Complicated

● **886 Traumatic amputation of other finger(s) (complete) (partial)**

Includes: finger(s) of one or both hands, without mention of thumb(s)

886.0 Without mention of complication
886.1 Complicated

● **887 Traumatic amputation of arm and hand (complete) (partial)**

887.0 Unilateral, below elbow, without mention of complication
887.1 Unilateral, below elbow, complicated
887.2 Unilateral, at or above elbow, without mention of complication
887.3 Unilateral, at or above elbow, complicated
❏ 887.4 Unilateral, level not specified, without mention of complication
❏ 887.5 Unilateral, level not specified, complicated
887.6 Bilateral [any level], without mention of complication
One hand and other arm
887.7 Bilateral [any level], complicated

OPEN WOUND OF LOWER LIMB (890–897)

● **890 Open wound of hip and thigh**

890.0 Without mention of complication
890.1 Complicated
890.2 With tendon involvement

● **891 Open wound of knee, leg [except thigh], and ankle**

Includes: leg NOS
multiple sites of leg, except thigh
Excludes *that of thigh (890.0–890.2)*
with multiple sites of lower limb (894.0–894.2)

891.0 Without mention of complication
891.1 Complicated
891.2 With tendon involvement

● **892 Open wound of foot except toe(s) alone**

Includes: heel

892.0 Without mention of complication
892.1 Complicated
892.2 With tendon involvement

● **893 Open wound of toe(s)**

Includes: toenail

893.0 Without mention of complication
893.1 Complicated
893.2 With tendon involvement

● **894 Multiple and unspecified open wound of lower limb**

Includes: lower limb NOS
multiple sites of one lower limb, with thigh

❏ 894.0 Without mention of complication
❏ 894.1 Complicated
❏ 894.2 With tendon involvement

● **895 Traumatic amputation of toe(s) (complete) (partial)**

Includes: toe(s) of one or both feet

895.0 Without mention of complication
895.1 Complicated

● **896 Traumatic amputation of foot (complete) (partial)**

896.0 Unilateral, without mention of complication
896.1 Unilateral, complicated
896.2 Bilateral, without mention of complication
Excludes *one foot and other leg (897.6–897.7)*
896.3 Bilateral, complicated

● **897 Traumatic amputation of leg(s) (complete) (partial)**

897.0 Unilateral, below knee, without mention of complication
897.1 Unilateral, below knee, complicated
897.2 Unilateral, at or above knee, without mention of complication
897.3 Unilateral, at or above knee, complicated
❏ 897.4 Unilateral, level not specified, without mention of complication
❏ 897.5 Unilateral, level not specified, complicated
897.6 Bilateral [any level], without mention of complication
One foot and other leg
897.7 Bilateral [any level], complicated

ICD-9-CM
898-900

Vol. 1

INJURY TO BLOOD VESSELS (900–904)

Includes: arterial hematoma of blood vessel, secondary to other injuries, e.g., fracture or open wound

avulsion of blood vessel, secondary to other injuries, e.g., fracture or open wound

cut of blood vessel, secondary to other injuries, e.g., fracture or open wound

laceration of blood vessel, secondary to other injuries, e.g., fracture or open wound

rupture of blood vessel, secondary to other injuries, e.g., fracture or open wound

traumatic aneurysm or fistula (arteriovenous) of blood vessel, secondary to other injuries, e.g., fracture or open wound

Excludes accidental puncture or laceration during medical procedure (998.2)

intracranial hemorrhage following injury (851.0–854.1)

● 900   **Injury to blood vessels of head and neck**

   ● 900.0   **Carotid artery**

     ❑ 900.00   Carotid artery, unspecified

     900.01   Common carotid artery

     900.02   External carotid artery

     900.03   Internal carotid artery

   900.1   **Internal jugular vein**

   ● 900.8   **Other specified blood vessels of head and neck**

     900.81   External jugular vein
       Jugular vein NOS

     ❑ 900.82   Multiple blood vessels of head and neck

     ❑ 900.89   Other

   ❑ 900.9   **Unspecified blood vessel of head and neck**

● 901   **Injury to blood vessels of thorax**

   Excludes traumatic hemothorax (860.2–860.5)

   901.0   **Thoracic aorta**

   901.1   **Innominate and subclavian arteries**

   901.2   **Superior vena cava**

   901.3   **Innominate and subclavian veins**

   ● 901.4   **Pulmonary blood vessels**

     ❑ 901.40   Pulmonary vessel(s), unspecified

     901.41   Pulmonary artery

     901.42   Pulmonary vein

   ● 901.8   **Other specified blood vessels of thorax**

     901.81   Intercostal artery or vein

     901.82   Internal mammary artery or vein

     901.83   Multiple blood vessels of thorax

     ❑ 901.89   Other
       Azygos vein
       Hemiazygos vein

   ❑ 901.9   **Unspecified blood vessel of thorax**

● 902   **Injury to blood vessels of abdomen and pelvis**

   902.0   **Abdominal aorta**

   ● 902.1   **Inferior vena cava**

     ❑ 902.10   Inferior vena cava, unspecified

     902.11   Hepatic veins

     ❑ 902.19   Other

● 902.2   **Celiac and mesenteric arteries**

   ❑ 902.20   Celiac and mesenteric arteries, unspecified

   902.21   Gastric artery

   902.22   Hepatic artery

   902.23   Splenic artery

   ❑ 902.24   Other specified branches of celiac axis

   902.25   Superior mesenteric artery (trunk)

   902.26   Primary branches of superior mesenteric artery
     Ileo-colic artery

   902.27   Inferior mesenteric artery

   ❑ 902.29   Other

● 902.3   **Portal and splenic veins**

   902.31   Superior mesenteric vein and primary subdivisions
     Ileo-colic vein

   902.32   Inferior mesenteric vein

   902.33   Portal vein

   902.34   Splenic vein

   ❑ 902.39   Other
     Cystic vein
     Gastric vein

● 902.4   **Renal blood vessels**

   ❑ 902.40   Renal vessel(s), unspecified

   902.41   Renal artery

   902.42   Renal vein

   ❑ 902.49   Other
     Suprarenal arteries

● 902.5   **Iliac blood vessels**

   ❑ 902.50   Iliac vessel(s), unspecified

   902.51   Hypogastric artery

   902.52   Hypogastric vein

   902.53   Iliac artery

   902.54   Iliac vein

   902.55   Uterine artery

   902.56   Uterine vein

   ❑ 902.59   Other

● 902.8   **Other specified blood vessels of abdomen and pelvis**

   902.81   Ovarian artery

   902.82   Ovarian vein

   ❑ 902.87   Multiple blood vessels of abdomen and pelvis

   ❑ 902.89   Other

❑ 902.9   **Unspecified blood vessel of abdomen and pelvis**

● 903   **Injury to blood vessels of upper extremity**

   ● 903.0   **Axillary blood vessels**

     ❑ 903.00   Axillary vessel(s), unspecified

     903.01   Axillary artery

     903.02   Axillary vein

   903.1   **Brachial blood vessels**

   903.2   **Radial blood vessels**

   903.3   **Ulnar blood vessels**

   903.4   **Palmar artery**

   903.5   **Digital blood vessels**

   ❑ 903.8   **Other specified blood vessels of upper extremity**
     Multiple blood vessels of upper extremity

   ❑ 903.9   **Unspecified blood vessel of upper extremity**

● 904 **Injury to blood vessels of lower extremity and unspecified sites**

  904.0 **Common femoral artery**
     Femoral artery above profunda origin

  904.1 **Superficial femoral artery**

  904.2 **Femoral veins**

  904.3 **Saphenous veins**
     Saphenous vein (greater) (lesser)

  ● 904.4 **Popliteal blood vessels**

    ❏ 904.40 **Popliteal vessel(s), unspecified**

    904.41 **Popliteal artery**

    904.42 **Popliteal vein**

  ● 904.5 **Tibial blood vessels**

    ❏ 904.50 **Tibial vessel(s), unspecified**

    904.51 **Anterior tibial artery**

    904.52 **Anterior tibial vein**

    904.53 **Posterior tibial artery**

    904.54 **Posterior tibial vein**

  904.6 **Deep plantar blood vessels**

  ❏ 904.7 **Other specified blood vessels of lower extremity**
     Multiple blood vessels of lower extremity

  ❏ 904.8 **Unspecified blood vessel of lower extremity**

  ❏ 904.9 **Unspecified site**
     Injury to blood vessel NOS

LATE EFFECTS OF INJURIES, POISONINGS, TOXIC EFFECTS, AND OTHER EXTERNAL CAUSES (905–909)

Note: These categories are to be used to indicate conditions classifiable to 800–999 as the cause of late effects, which are themselves classified elsewhere. The "late effects" include those specified as such, or as sequelae, which may occur at any time after the acute injury.

● 905 **Late effects of musculoskeletal and connective tissue injuries**

  ❏ 905.0 **Late effect of fracture of skull and face bones**
     Late effect of injury classifiable to 800–804

  ❏ 905.1 **Late effect of fracture of spine and trunk without mention of spinal cord lesion**
     Late effect of injury classifiable to 805, 807–809

  ❏ 905.2 **Late effect of fracture of upper extremities**
     Late effect of injury classifiable to 810–819

  ❏ 905.3 **Late effect of fracture of neck of femur**
     Late effect of injury classifiable to 820

  ❏ 905.4 **Late effect of fracture of lower extremities**
     Late effect of injury classifiable to 821–827

  ❏ 905.5 **Late effect of fracture of multiple and unspecified bones**
     Late effect of injury classifiable to 828–829

  ❏ 905.6 **Late effect of dislocation**
     Late effect of injury classifiable to 830–839

  ❏ 905.7 **Late effect of sprain and strain without mention of tendon injury**
     Late effect of injury classifiable to 840–848, except tendon injury

  ❏ 905.8 **Late effect of tendon injury**
     Late effect of tendon injury due to:
       open wound [injury classifiable to 880–884 with .2, 890–894 with .2]
       sprain and strain [injury classifiable to 840–848]

  ❏ 905.9 **Late effect of traumatic amputation**
     Late effect of injury classifiable to 885–887, 895–897

    Excludes *late amputation stump complication (997.60–997.69)*

● 906 **Late effects of injuries to skin and subcutaneous tissues**

  ❏ 906.0 **Late effect of open wound of head, neck, and trunk**
     Late effect of injury classifiable to 870–879

  ❏ 906.1 **Late effect of open wound of extremities without mention of tendon injury**
     Late effect of injury classifiable to 880–884, 890–894 except .2

  ❏ 906.2 **Late effect of superficial injury**
     Late effect of injury classifiable to 910–919

  ❏ 906.3 **Late effect of contusion**
     Late effect of injury classifiable to 920–924

  ❏ 906.4 **Late effect of crushing**
     Late effect of injury classifiable to 925–929

  ❏ 906.5 **Late effect of burn of eye, face, head, and neck**
     Late effect of injury classifiable to 940–941

  ❏ 906.6 **Late effect of burn of wrist and hand**
     Late effect of injury classifiable to 944

  ❏ 906.7 **Late effect of burn of other extremities**
     Late effect of injury classifiable to 943 or 945

  ❏ 906.8 **Late effect of burns of other specified sites**
     Late effect of injury classifiable to 942, 946–947

  ❏ 906.9 **Late effect of burn of unspecified site**
     Late effect of injury classifiable to 948–949

● 907 **Late effects of injuries to the nervous system**

  ❏ 907.0 **Late effect of intracranial injury without mention of skull fracture**
     Late effect of injury classifiable to 850–854

  ❏ 907.1 **Late effect of injury to cranial nerve**
     Late effect of injury classifiable to 950–951

  ❏ 907.2 **Late effect of spinal cord injury**
     Late effect of injury classifiable to 806, 952

  ❏ 907.3 **Late effect of injury to nerve root(s), spinal plexus(es), and other nerves of trunk**
     Late effect of injury classifiable to 953–954

  ❏ 907.4 **Late effect of injury to peripheral nerve of shoulder girdle and upper limb**
     Late effect of injury classifiable to 955

  ❏ 907.5 **Late effect of injury to peripheral nerve of pelvic girdle and lower limb**
     Late effect of injury classifiable to 956

  ❏ 907.9 **Late effect of injury to other and unspecified nerve**
     Late effect of injury classifiable to 957

● 908 **Late effects of other and unspecified injuries**

  ❏ 908.0 **Late effect of internal injury to chest**
     Late effect of injury classifiable to 860–862

  ❏ 908.1 **Late effect of internal injury to intra-abdominal organs**
     Late effect of injury classifiable to 863–866, 868

  ❏ 908.2 **Late effect of internal injury to other internal organs**
     Late effect of injury classifiable to 867 or 869

  ❏ 908.3 **Late effect of injury to blood vessel of head, neck, and extremities**
     Late effect of injury classifiable to 900, 903–904

  ❏ 908.4 **Late effect of injury to blood vessel of thorax, abdomen, and pelvis**
     Late effect of injury classifiable to 901–902

  ❏ 908.5 **Late effect of foreign body in orifice**
     Late effect of injury classifiable to 930–939

  ❏ 908.6 **Late effect of certain complications of trauma**
     Late effect of complications classifiable to 958

  ❏ 908.9 **Late effect of unspecified injury**
     Late effect of injury classifiable to 959

● **909 Late effects of other and unspecified external causes**

❏ **909.0 Late effect of poisoning due to drug, medicinal or biological substance**
Late effect of conditions classifiable to 960–979

> **Excludes** *Late effect of adverse effect of drug, medicinal or biological substance (909.5)*

❏ **909.1 Late effect of toxic effects of nonmedical substances**
Late effect of conditions classifiable to 980–989

❏ **909.2 Late effect of radiation**
Late effect of conditions classifiable to 990

❏ **909.3 Late effect of complications of surgical and medical care**
Late effect of conditions classifiable to 996–999

❏ **909.4 Late effect of certain other external causes**
Late effect of conditions classifiable to 991–994

❏ **909.5 Late effect of adverse effect of drug, medicinal or biological substance**

> **Excludes** *late effect of poisoning due to drug, medicinal or biological substances (909.0)*

❏ **909.9 Late effect of other and unspecified external causes**

SUPERFICIAL INJURY (910–919)

> **Excludes** *burn (blisters) (940.0–949.5)*
> *contusion (920–924.9)*
> *foreign body:*
>   *granuloma (728.82)*
>   *inadvertently left in operative wound (998.4)*
>   *residual, in soft tissue (729.6)*
> *insect bite, venomous (989.5)*
> *open wound with incidental foreign body (870.0–897.7)*

● **910 Superficial injury of face, neck, and scalp except eye**

Includes: cheek   lip
          ear   nose
          gum   throat

> **Excludes** *eye and adnexa (918.0–918.9)*

910.0 Abrasion or friction burn without mention of infection

910.1 Abrasion or friction burn, infected

910.2 Blister without mention of infection

910.3 Blister, infected

910.4 Insect bite, nonvenomous, without mention of infection

910.5 Insect bite, nonvenomous, infected

910.6 Superficial foreign body (splinter) without major open wound and without mention of infection

910.7 Superficial foreign body (splinter) without major open wound, infected

❏ **910.8 Other and unspecified superficial injury of face, neck, and scalp without mention of infection**

❏ **910.9 Other and unspecified superficial injury of face, neck, and scalp, infected**

● **911 Superficial injury of trunk**

Includes: abdominal wall   interscapular region
          anus   labium (majus) (minus)
          back   penis
          breast   perineum
          buttock   scrotum
          chest wall   testis
          flank   vagina
          groin   vulva

> **Excludes** *hip (916.0–916.9)*
> *scapular region (912.0–912.9)*

911.0 Abrasion or friction burn without mention of infection

911.1 Abrasion or friction burn, infected

911.2 Blister without mention of infection

911.3 Blister, infected

911.4 Insect bite, nonvenomous, without mention of infection

911.5 Insect bite, nonvenomous, infected

911.6 Superficial foreign body (splinter) without major open wound and without mention of infection

911.7 Superficial foreign body (splinter) without major open wound, infected

❏ **911.8 Other and unspecified superficial injury of trunk without mention of infection**

❏ **911.9 Other and unspecified superficial injury of trunk, infected**

● **912 Superficial injury of shoulder and upper arm**

Includes: axilla
          scapular region

912.0 Abrasion or friction burn without mention of infection

912.1 Abrasion or friction burn, infected

912.2 Blister without mention of infection

912.3 Blister, infected

912.4 Insect bite, nonvenomous, without mention of infection

912.5 Insect bite, nonvenomous, infected

912.6 Superficial foreign body (splinter) without major open wound and without mention of infection

912.7 Superficial foreign body (splinter) without major open wound, infected

❏ **912.8 Other and unspecified superficial injury of shoulder and upper arm without mention of infection**

❏ **912.9 Other and unspecified superficial injury of shoulder and upper arm, infected**

● **913 Superficial injury of elbow, forearm, and wrist**

913.0 Abrasion or friction burn without mention of infection

913.1 Abrasion or friction burn, infected

913.2 Blister without mention of infection

913.3 Blister, infected

913.4 Insect bite, nonvenomous, without mention of infection

913.5 Insect bite, nonvenomous, infected

913.6 Superficial foreign body (splinter) without major open wound and without mention of infection

913.7 Superficial foreign body (splinter) without major open wound, infected

◀ **New**   ◀▥ **Revised**   ● **Not a Principal Diagnosis**   ● **Use Additional Digit(s)**   ❏ **Nonspecific Code**

❑ **913.8** Other and unspecified superficial injury of elbow, forearm, and wrist without mention of infection

❑ **913.9** Other and unspecified superficial injury of elbow, forearm, and wrist, infected

● **914 Superficial injury of hand(s) except finger(s) alone**

914.0 Abrasion or friction burn without mention of infection

914.1 Abrasion or friction burn, infected

914.2 Blister without mention of infection

914.3 Blister, infected

914.4 Insect bite, nonvenomous, without mention of infection

914.5 Insect bite, nonvenomous, infected

914.6 Superficial foreign body (splinter) without major open wound and without mention of infection

914.7 Superficial foreign body (splinter) without major open wound, infected

❑ **914.8** Other and unspecified superficial injury of hand without mention of infection

❑ **914.9** Other and unspecified superficial injury of hand, infected

● **915 Superficial injury of finger(s)**

Includes: fingernail
thumb (nail)

915.0 Abrasion or friction burn without mention of infection

915.1 Abrasion or friction burn, infected

915.2 Blister without mention of infection

915.3 Blister, infected

915.4 Insect bite, nonvenomous, without mention of infection

915.5 Insect bite, nonvenomous, infected

915.6 Superficial foreign body (splinter) without major open wound and without mention of infection

915.7 Superficial foreign body (splinter) without major open wound, infected

❑ **915.8** Other and unspecified superficial injury of fingers without mention of infection

❑ **915.9** Other and unspecified superficial injury of fingers, infected

● **916 Superficial injury of hip, thigh, leg, and ankle**

916.0 Abrasion or friction burn without mention of infection

916.1 Abrasion or friction burn, infected

916.2 Blister without mention of infection

916.3 Blister, infected

916.4 Insect bite, nonvenomous, without mention of infection

916.5 Insect bite, nonvenomous, infected

916.6 Superficial foreign body (splinter) without major open wound and without mention of infection

916.7 Superficial foreign body (splinter) without major open wound, infected

❑ **916.8** Other and unspecified superficial injury of hip, thigh, leg, and ankle without mention of infection

❑ **916.9** Other and unspecified superficial injury of hip, thigh, leg, and ankle, infected

● **917 Superficial injury of foot and toe(s)**

Includes: heel
toenail

917.0 Abrasion or friction burn without mention of infection

917.1 Abrasion or friction burn, infected

917.2 Blister without mention of infection

917.3 Blister, infected

917.4 Insect bite, nonvenomous, without mention of infection

917.5 Insect bite, nonvenomous, infected

917.6 Superficial foreign body (splinter) without major open wound and without mention of infection

917.7 Superficial foreign body (splinter) without major open wound, infected

❑ **917.8** Other and unspecified superficial injury of foot and toes without mention of infection

❑ **917.9** Other and unspecified superficial injury of foot and toes, infected

● **918 Superficial injury of eye and adnexa**

Excludes *burn (940.0–940.9)*
foreign body on external eye (930.0–930.9)

918.0 Eyelids and periocular area
Abrasion
Insect bite
Superficial foreign body (splinter)

918.1 Cornea
Corneal abrasion
Superficial laceration

Excludes *corneal injury due to contact lens (371.82)*

918.2 Conjunctiva

❑ **918.9** Other and unspecified superficial injuries of eye
Eye (ball) NOS

● **919 Superficial injury of other, multiple, and unspecified sites**

Excludes *multiple sites classifiable to the same three-digit category (910.0–918.9)*

❑ **919.0** Abrasion or friction burn without mention of infection

❑ **919.1** Abrasion or friction burn, infected

❑ **919.2** Blister without mention of infection

❑ **919.3** Blister, infected

❑ **919.4** Insect bite, nonvenomous, without mention of infection

❑ **919.5** Insect bite, nonvenomous, infected

❑ **919.6** Superficial foreign body (splinter) without major open wound and without mention of infection

❑ **919.7** Superficial foreign body (splinter) without major open wound, infected

❑ **919.8** Other and unspecified superficial injury without mention of infection

❑ **919.9** Other and unspecified superficial injury, infected

CONTUSION WITH INTACT SKIN SURFACE (920–924)

Includes: bruise without fracture or open wound
hematoma without fracture or open wound

Excludes	concussion (850.0–850.9)
	hemarthrosis (840.0–848.9)
	internal organs (860.0–869.1)
	that incidental to:
	crushing injury (925–929.9)
	dislocation (830.0–839.9)
	fracture (800.0–829.1)
	internal injury (860.0–869.1)
	intracranial injury (850.0–854.1)
	nerve injury (950.0–957.9)
	open wound (870.0–897.7)

920   Contusion of face, scalp, and neck except eye(s)

Cheek	Mandibular joint area
Ear (auricle)	Nose
Gum	Throat
Lip	

● **921   Contusion of eye and adnexa**

❑ **921.0   Black eye, NOS**

921.1   Contusion of eyelids and periocular area

921.2   Contusion of orbital tissues

921.3   Contusion of eyeball

❑ **921.9   Unspecified contusion of eye**
Injury of eye NOS

● **922   Contusion of trunk**

922.0   Breast

922.1   Chest wall

922.2   Abdominal wall
Flank
Groin

● **922.3   Back**

922.31   Back

Excludes	interscapular region (922.33)

922.32   Buttock

922.33   Interscapular region

Excludes	scapular region (923.01)

922.4   Genital organs
Labium (majus) (minus)
Penis
Perineum
Scrotum
Testis
Vagina
Vulva

❑ **922.8   Multiple sites of trunk**

❑ **922.9   Unspecified part**
Trunk NOS

● **923   Contusion of upper limb**

● **923.0   Shoulder and upper arm**

923.00   Shoulder region

923.01   Scapular region

923.02   Axillary region

923.03   Upper arm

❑ **923.09   Multiple sites**

● **923.1   Elbow and forearm**

923.10   Forearm

923.11   Elbow

● **923.2   Wrist and hand(s), except finger(s) alone**

923.20   Hand(s)

923.21   Wrist

923.3   Finger
Fingernail
Thumb (nail)

❑ **923.8   Multiple sites of upper limb**

❑ **923.9   Unspecified part of upper limb**
Arm NOS

● **924   Contusion of lower limb and of other and unspecified sites**

● **924.0   Hip and thigh**

924.00   Thigh

924.01   Hip

● **924.1   Knee and lower leg**

924.10   Lower leg

924.11   Knee

● **924.2   Ankle and foot, excluding toe(s)**

924.20   Foot
Heel

924.21   Ankle

924.3   Toe
Toenail

❑ **924.4   Multiple sites of lower limb**

❑ **924.5   Unspecified part of lower limb**
Leg NOS

❑ **924.8   Multiple sites, not elsewhere classified**

❑ **924.9   Unspecified site**

CRUSHING INJURY (925–929)

Use additional code to identify any associated injuries, such as:
fractures (800–829)
internal organs (860.0–869.1)
intracranial injury (850.0–854.1)

● **925   Crushing injury of face, scalp, and neck**

Cheek	Pharynx
Ear	Throat
Larynx	

925.1   Crushing injury of face and scalp
Cheek
Ear

925.2   Crushing injury of neck
Larynx
Throat
Pharynx

● **926   Crushing injury of trunk**

926.0   External genitalia

Labium (majus) (minus)	Testis
Penis	Vulva
Scrotum	

● **926.1   Other specified sites**

926.11   Back

926.12   Buttock

❑ **926.19   Other**
Breast

❑ **926.8   Multiple sites of trunk**

❑ **926.9   Unspecified site**
Trunk NOS

● 927 **Crushing injury of upper limb**

  ● 927.0 **Shoulder and upper arm**

    927.00 **Shoulder region**

    927.01 **Scapular region**

    927.02 **Axillary region**

    927.03 **Upper arm**

    ❏ 927.09 **Multiple sites**

  ● 927.1 **Elbow and forearm**

    927.10 **Forearm**

    927.11 **Elbow**

  ● 927.2 **Wrist and hand(s), except finger(s) alone**

    927.20 **Hand(s)**

    927.21 **Wrist**

  927.3 **Finger(s)**

  ❏ 927.8 **Multiple sites of upper limb**

  ❏ 927.9 **Unspecified site**
    Arm NOS

● 928 **Crushing injury of lower limb**

  ● 928.0 **Hip and thigh**

    928.00 **Thigh**

    928.01 **Hip**

  ● 928.1 **Knee and lower leg**

    928.10 **Lower leg**

    928.11 **Knee**

  ● 928.2 **Ankle and foot, excluding toe(s) alone**

    928.20 **Foot**
      Heel

    928.21 **Ankle**

  928.3 **Toe(s)**

  ❏ 928.8 **Multiple sites of lower limb**

  ❏ 928.9 **Unspecified site**
    Leg NOS

● 929 **Crushing injury of multiple and unspecified sites**

  ❏ 929.0 **Multiple sites, not elsewhere classified**

  ❏ 929.9 **Unspecified site**

EFFECTS OF FOREIGN BODY ENTERING THROUGH ORIFICE (930–939)

  Excludes *foreign body:*
    granuloma (728.82)
    inadvertently left in operative wound (998.4, 998.7)
    in open wound (800–839, 851–897)
    residual, in soft tissues (729.6)
    superficial without major open wound (910– 919 with .6 or .7)

● 930 **Foreign body on external eye**

  Excludes *foreign body in penetrating wound of:*
    eyeball (871.5–871.6)
    retained (old) (360.5–360.6)
    ocular adnexa (870.4)
    retained (old) (376.6)

  930.0 **Corneal foreign body**

  930.1 **Foreign body in conjunctival sac**

  930.2 **Foreign body in lacrimal punctum**

  ❏ 930.8 **Other and combined sites**

  ❏ 930.9 **Unspecified site**
    External eye NOS

● 931 **Foreign body in ear**
  Auditory canal
  Auricle

● 932 **Foreign body in nose**
  Nasal sinus
  Nostril

● 933 **Foreign body in pharynx and larynx**

  933.0 **Pharynx**
    Nasopharynx
    Throat NOS

  933.1 **Larynx**
    Asphyxia due to foreign body
    Choking due to:
      food (regurgitated)
      phlegm

● 934 **Foreign body in trachea, bronchus, and lung**

  934.0 **Trachea**

  934.1 **Main bronchus**

  ❏ 934.8 **Other specified parts**
    Bronchioles
    Lung

  ❏ 934.9 **Respiratory tree, unspecified**
    Inhalation of liquid or vomitus, lower respiratory tract NOS

● 935 **Foreign body in mouth, esophagus, and stomach**

  935.0 **Mouth**

  935.1 **Esophagus**

  935.2 **Stomach**

  936 **Foreign body in intestine and colon**

  937 **Foreign body in anus and rectum**
    Rectosigmoid (junction)

❏ 938 **Foreign body in digestive system, unspecified**
  Alimentary tract NOS
  Swallowed foreign body

● 939 **Foreign body in genitourinary tract**

  939.0 **Bladder and urethra**

  939.1 **Uterus, any part**

    Excludes *intrauterine contraceptive device:*
    complications from (996.32, 996.65)
    presence of (V45.51)

  939.2 **Vulva and vagina**

  939.3 **Penis**

  ❏ 939.9 **Unspecified site**

BURNS (940–949)

Includes: burns from:
  electrical heating appliance
  electricity
  flame
  hot object
  lightning
  radiation
  chemical burns (external) (internal)
  scalds

  Excludes *friction burns (910–919 with .0, .1)*
  sunburn (692.71, 692.76–692.77)

● **940   Burn confined to eye and adnexa**

    940.0   Chemical burn of eyelids and periocular area

☐ 940.1   Other burns of eyelids and periocular area

    940.2   Alkaline chemical burn of cornea and conjunctival sac

    940.3   Acid chemical burn of cornea and conjunctival sac

☐ 940.4   Other burn of cornea and conjunctival sac

    940.5   Burn with resulting rupture and destruction of eyeball

☐ 940.9   Unspecified burn of eye and adnexa

● **941   Burn of face, head, and neck**

    | Excludes | *mouth (947.0)*

    The following fifth-digit subclassification is for use with category 941:
    ☐ 0   face and head, unspecified site
       1   ear [any part]
       2   eye (with other parts of face, head, and neck)
       3   lip(s)
       4   chin
       5   nose (septum)
       6   scalp [any part]
           temple (region)
       7   forehead and cheek
       8   neck
    ☐ 9   multiple sites [except with eye] of face, head, and neck

● ☐ 941.0   Unspecified degree

● 941.1   Erythema [first degree]

● 941.2   Blisters, epidermal loss [second degree]

● 941.3   Full-thickness skin loss [third degree NOS]

● 941.4   Deep necrosis of underlying tissues [deep third degree] without mention of loss of a body part

● 941.5   Deep necrosis of underlying tissues [deep third degree] with loss of a body part

● **942   Burn of trunk**

    | Excludes | *scapular region (943.0–943.5 with fifth-digit 6)*

    The following fifth-digit subclassification is for use with category 942:
    ☐ 0   trunk, unspecified site
       1   breast
       2   chest wall, excluding breast and nipple
       3   abdominal wall
           flank
           groin
       4   back [any part]
           buttock
           interscapular region
       5   genitalia
           labium (majus) (minus)
           penis
           perineum
           scrotum
           testis
           vulva
    ☐ 9   other and multiple sites of trunk

● ☐ 942.0   Unspecified degree

● 942.1   Erythema [first degree]

● 942.2   Blisters, epidermal loss [second degree]

● 942.3   Full-thickness skin loss [third degree NOS]

● 942.4   Deep necrosis of underlying tissues [deep third degree] without mention of loss of a body part

● 942.5   Deep necrosis of underlying tissues [deep third degree] with loss of a body part

● **943   Burn of upper limb, except wrist and hand**

    The following fifth-digit subclassification is for use with category 943:
    ☐ 0   upper limb, unspecified site
       1   forearm
       2   elbow
       3   upper arm
       4   axilla
       5   shoulder
       6   scapular region
    ☐ 9   multiple sites of upper limb, except wrist and hand

● ☐ 943.0   Unspecified degree

● 943.1   Erythema [first degree]

● 943.2   Blisters, epidermal loss [second degree]

● 943.3   Full-thickness skin loss [third degree NOS]

● 943.4   Deep necrosis of underlying tissues [deep third degree] without mention of loss of a body part

● 943.5   Deep necrosis of underlying tissues [deep third degree] with loss of a body part

● **944   Burn of wrist(s) and hand(s)**

    The following fifth-digit subclassification is for use with category 944:
    ☐ 0   hand, unspecified site
       1   single digit [finger (nail)] other than thumb
       2   thumb (nail)
       3   two or more digits, not including thumb
       4   two or more digits including thumb
       5   palm
       6   back of hand
       7   wrist
    ☐ 8   multiple sites of wrist(s) and hand(s)

● ☐ 944.0   Unspecified degree

● 944.1   Erythema [first degree]

● 944.2   Blisters, epidermal loss [second degree]

● 944.3   Full-thickness skin loss [third degree NOS]

● 944.4   Deep necrosis of underlying tissues [deep third degree] without mention of loss of a body part

● 944.5   Deep necrosis of underlying tissues [deep third degree] with loss of a body part

● **945   Burn of lower limb(s)**

    The following fifth-digit subclassification is for use with category 945:
    ☐ 0   lower limb [leg], unspecified site
       1   toe(s) (nail)
       2   foot
       3   ankle
       4   lower leg
       5   knee
       6   thigh [any part]
    ☐ 9   multiple sites of lower limb(s)

● ☐ 945.0   Unspecified degree

● 945.1   Erythema [first degree]

● 945.2   Blisters, epidermal loss [second degree]

● 945.3   Full-thickness skin loss [third degree NOS]

● 945.4   Deep necrosis of underlying tissues [deep third degree] without mention of loss of a body part

● 945.5   Deep necrosis of underlying tissues [deep third degree] with loss of a body part

● **946 Burns of multiple specified sites**

 Includes: burns of sites classifiable to more than one three-digit category in 940–945

  Excludes *multiple burns NOS (949.0–949.5)*

❏ **946.0 Unspecified degree**

946.1 Erythema [first degree]

946.2 Blisters, epidermal loss [second degree]

946.3 Full-thickness skin loss [third degree NOS]

946.4 Deep necrosis of underlying tissues [deep third degree] without mention of loss of a body part

946.5 Deep necrosis of underlying tissues [deep third degree] with loss of a body part

● **947 Burn of internal organs**

 Includes: burns from chemical agents (ingested)

947.0 Mouth and pharynx
 Gum   Tongue

947.1 Larynx, trachea, and lung

947.2 Esophagus

947.3 Gastrointestinal tract
 Colon   Small intestine
 Rectum   Stomach

947.4 Vagina and uterus

❏ **947.8 Other specified sites**

❏ **947.9 Unspecified site**

● **948 Burns classified according to extent of body surface involved**

 Note: This category is to be used when the site of the burn is unspecified, or with categories 940–947 when the site is specified.

  Excludes *sunburn (692.71, 692.76–692.77)*

 The following fifth-digit subclassification is for use with category 948 to indicate the percent of body surface with third degree burn; valid digits are in [brackets] under each code:

 0 less than 10 percent or unspecified
 1 10–19%
 2 20–29%
 3 30–39%
 4 40–49%
 5 50–59%
 6 60–69%
 7 70–79%
 8 80–89%
 9 90% or more of body surface

● **948.0 Burn [any degree] involving less than 10 percent**
[0] **of body surface**

● **948.1 10–19 percent of body surface**
[0–1]

● **948.2 20–29 percent of body surface**
[0–2]

● **948.3 30–39 percent of body surface**
[0–3]

● **948.4 40–49 percent of body surface**
[0–4]

● **948.5 50–59 percent of body surface**
[0–5]

● **948.6 60–69 percent of body surface**
[0–6]

● **948.7 70–79 percent of body surface**
[0–7]

● **948.8 80–89 percent of body surface**
[0–8]

● **948.9 90 percent or more of body surface**
[0–9]

● **949 Burn, unspecified**

 Includes: burn NOS
     multiple burns NOS

  Excludes *burn of unspecified site but with statement of the extent of body surface involved (948.0–948.9)*

❏ **949.0 Unspecified degree**

❏ **949.1 Erythema [first degree]**

❏ **949.2 Blisters, epidermal loss [second degree]**

❏ **949.3 Full-thickness skin loss [third degree NOS]**

❏ **949.4 Deep necrosis of underlying tissues [deep third degree] without mention of loss of a body part**

❏ **949.5 Deep necrosis of underlying tissues [deep third degree] with loss of a body part**

INJURY TO NERVES AND SPINAL CORD (950–957)

 Includes: division of nerve
     lesion in continuity (with open wound)
     traumatic neuroma (with open wound)
     traumatic transient paralysis (with open wound)

  Excludes *accidental puncture or laceration during medical procedure (998.2)*

● **950 Injury to optic nerve and pathways**

950.0 Optic nerve injury
 Second cranial nerve

950.1 Injury to optic chiasm

950.2 Injury to optic pathways

950.3 Injury to visual cortex

❏ **950.9 Unspecified**
 Traumatic blindness NOS

● **951 Injury to other cranial nerve(s)**

951.0 Injury to oculomotor nerve
 Third cranial nerve

951.1 Injury to trochlear nerve
 Fourth cranial nerve

951.2 Injury to trigeminal nerve
 Fifth cranial nerve

951.3 Injury to abducens nerve
 Sixth cranial nerve

951.4 Injury to facial nerve
 Seventh cranial nerve

951.5 Injury to acoustic nerve
 Auditory nerve
 Eighth cranial nerve
 Traumatic deafness NOS

951.6 Injury to accessory nerve
 Eleventh cranial nerve

951.7 Injury to hypoglossal nerve
 Twelfth cranial nerve

❏ **951.8 Injury to other specified cranial nerves**
 Glossopharyngeal [9th cranial] nerve
 Olfactory [1st cranial] nerve
 Pneumogastric [10th cranial] nerve
 Traumatic anosmia NOS
 Vagus [10th cranial] nerve

❏ **951.9 Injury to unspecified cranial nerve**

● **952 Spinal cord injury without evidence of spinal bone injury**

  ● **952.0 Cervical**

    ❑ **952.00** C_1-C_4 level with unspecified spinal cord injury
        Spinal cord injury, cervical region NOS

    952.01 C_1-C_4 level with complete lesion of spinal cord

    952.02 C_1-C_4 level with anterior cord syndrome

    952.03 C_1-C_4 level with central cord syndrome

    ❑ **952.04** C_1-C_4 level with other specified spinal cord injury
        Incomplete spinal cord lesion at C_1-C_4 level:
          NOS
        with posterior cord syndrome

    ❑ **952.05** C_5-C_7 level with unspecified spinal cord injury

    952.06 C_5-C_7 level with complete lesion of spinal cord

    952.07 C_5-C_7 level with anterior cord syndrome

    952.08 C_5-C_7 level with central cord syndrome

    ❑ **952.09** C_5-C_7 level with other specified spinal cord injury
        Incomplete spinal cord lesion at C_5-C_7 level:
          NOS
        with posterior cord syndrome

  ● **952.1 Dorsal [thoracic]**

    ❑ **952.10** T_1-T_6 level with unspecified spinal cord injury
        Spinal cord injury, thoracic region NOS

    952.11 T_1-T_6 level with complete lesion of spinal cord

    952.12 T_1-T_6 level with anterior cord syndrome

    952.13 T_1-T_6 level with central cord syndrome

    ❑ **952.14** T_1-T_6 level with other specified spinal cord injury
        Incomplete spinal cord lesion at T_1-T_6 level:
          NOS
        with posterior cord syndrome

    ❑ **952.15** T_7-T_{12} level with unspecified spinal cord injury

    952.16 T_7-T_{12} level with complete lesion of spinal cord

    952.17 T_7-T_{12} level with anterior cord syndrome

    952.18 T_7-T_{12} level with central cord syndrome

    ❑ **952.19** T_7-T_{12} level with other specified spinal cord injury
        Incomplete spinal cord lesion at T_7-T_{12} level:
          NOS
        with posterior cord syndrome

    952.2 Lumbar

    952.3 Sacral

    952.4 Cauda equina

    ❑ **952.8 Multiple sites of spinal cord**

    ❑ **952.9 Unspecified site of spinal cord**

● **953 Injury to nerve roots and spinal plexus**

    953.0 Cervical root

    953.1 Dorsal root

    953.2 Lumbar root

    953.3 Sacral root

    953.4 Brachial plexus

    953.5 Lumbosacral plexus

    ❑ **953.8 Multiple sites**

    ❑ **953.9 Unspecified site**

● **954 Injury to other nerve(s) of trunk, excluding shoulder and pelvic girdles**

    954.0 Cervical sympathetic

    ❑ **954.1 Other sympathetic**
      Celiac ganglion or plexus   Splanchnic nerve(s)
      Inferior mesenteric plexus   Stellate ganglion

    ❑ **954.8 Other specified nerve(s) of trunk**

    ❑ **954.9 Unspecified nerve of trunk**

● **955 Injury to peripheral nerve(s) of shoulder girdle and upper limb**

    955.0 Axillary nerve

    955.1 Median nerve

    955.2 Ulnar nerve

    955.3 Radial nerve

    955.4 Musculocutaneous nerve

    955.5 Cutaneous sensory nerve, upper limb

    955.6 Digital nerve

    ❑ **955.7 Other specified nerve(s) of shoulder girdle and upper limb**

    ❑ **955.8 Multiple nerves of shoulder girdle and upper limb**

    ❑ **955.9 Unspecified nerve of shoulder girdle and upper limb**

● **956 Injury to peripheral nerve(s) of pelvic girdle and lower limb**

    956.0 Sciatic nerve

    956.1 Femoral nerve

    956.2 Posterior tibial nerve

    956.3 Peroneal nerve

    956.4 Cutaneous sensory nerve, lower limb

    ❑ **956.5 Other specified nerve(s) of pelvic girdle and lower limb**

    ❑ **956.8 Multiple nerves of pelvic girdle and lower limb**

    ❑ **956.9 Unspecified nerve of pelvic girdle and lower limb**

● **957 Injury to other and unspecified nerves**

    957.0 Superficial nerves of head and neck

    ❑ **957.1 Other specified nerve(s)**

    ❑ **957.8 Multiple nerves in several parts**
      Multiple nerve injury NOS

    ❑ **957.9 Unspecified site**
      Nerve injury NOS

CERTAIN TRAUMATIC COMPLICATIONS AND UNSPECIFIED INJURIES (958–959)

● **958 Certain early complications of trauma**

Excludes	adult respiratory distress syndrome (518.5)

                flail chest (807.4)
                shock lung (518.5)
                that occurring during or following medical pro-
                   cedures (996.0–999.9)

    958.0 Air embolism
        Pneumathemia

    Excludes *that complicating:*
          abortion (634–638 with .6, 639.6)
          ectopic or molar pregnancy (639.6)
          pregnancy, childbirth, or the puerperium
            (673.0)

    958.1 Fat embolism

    Excludes *that complicating:*
          abortion (634–638 with .6, 639.6)
          pregnancy, childbirth, or the puerperium
            (673.8)

    958.2 Secondary and recurrent hemorrhage

    958.3 Posttraumatic wound infection, not elsewhere classified

    Excludes *infected open wounds—code to complicated open wound of site*

    958.4 Traumatic shock
        Shock (immediate) (delayed) following injury

    Excludes *shock:*
          anaphylactic (995.0)
            due to serum (999.4)
          anesthetic (995.4)
          electric (994.8)
          following abortion (639.5)
          lightning (994.0)
          nontraumatic NOS (785.50)
          obstetric (669.1)
          postoperative (998.0)

    958.5 Traumatic anuria
        Crush syndrome
        Renal failure following crushing

    Excludes *that due to a medical procedure (997.5)*

    958.6 Volkmann's ischemic contracture
        Posttraumatic muscle contracture

    958.7 Traumatic subcutaneous emphysema

    Excludes *subcutaneous emphysema resulting from a procedure (998.81)*

    ❏ **958.8 Other early complications of trauma**

● **959 Injury, other and unspecified**

    Includes: injury NOS

    Excludes *injury NOS of:*
          blood vessels (900.0–904.9)
          eye (921.0–921.9)
          internal organs (860.0–869.1)
          intracranial sites (854.0–854.1)
          nerves (950.0–951.9, 953.0–957.9)
          spinal cord (952.0–952.9)

    ● **959.0 Head, face and neck**

        ❏ **959.01 Head injury, unspecified**

        Excludes *concussion (850.1–850.9)*
             with head injury NOS (850.1–850.5)
          head injury NOS with loss of consciousness
             (850.1–850.5)
          specified intracranial injuries (850.0–854.1)

        959.09 Injury of face and neck

● **959.1 Trunk**

    Excludes *scapular region (959.2)*

    ❏ **959.11 Other injury of chest wall**

    ❏ **959.12 Other injury of abdomen**

    959.13 Fracture of corpus cavernosum penis

    959.14 Other injury of external genitals

    ❏ **959.19 Other injury of other sites of trunk**
        Injury of trunk NOS

    959.2 Shoulder and upper arm
        Axilla
        Scapular region

    959.3 Elbow, forearm, and wrist

    959.4 Hand, except finger

    959.5 Finger
        Fingernail
        Thumb (nail)

    959.6 Hip and thigh
        Upper leg

    959.7 Knee, leg, ankle, and foot

    ❏ **959.8 Other specified sites, including multiple**

    Excludes *multiple sites classifiable to the same four-digit category (959.0–959.7)*

    ❏ **959.9 Unspecified site**

POISONING BY DRUGS, MEDICINAL AND BIOLOGICAL SUBSTANCES (960–979)

    Includes: overdose of these substances
               wrong substance given or taken in error

    Excludes *adverse effects ["hypersensitivity," "reaction," etc.] of correct substance properly administered. Such cases are to be classified according to the nature of the adverse effect, such as:*
          adverse effect NOS (995.2)
          allergic lymphadenitis (289.3)
          aspirin gastritis (535.4)
          blood disorders (280.0–289.9)
          dermatitis:
            contact (692.0–692.9)
            due to ingestion (693.0–693.9)
          nephropathy (583.9)
          [The drug giving rise to the adverse effect may be identified by use of categories E930–E949.]
          drug dependence (304.0–304.9)
          drug reaction and poisoning affecting the newborn (760.0–779.9)
          nondependent abuse of drugs (305.0–305.9)
          pathological drug intoxication (292.2)

    Use additional code to specify the effects of the poisoning

● **960 Poisoning by antibiotics**

    Excludes *antibiotics:*
          ear, nose, and throat (976.6)
          eye (976.5)
          local (976.0)

    960.0 Penicillins

Ampicillin	Cloxacillin
Carbenicillin	Penicillin G

    960.1 Antifungal antibiotics

Amphotericin B	Nystatin
Griseofulvin	Trichomycin

    Excludes *preparations intended for topical use (976.0–976.9)*

960.2 Chloramphenicol group
Chloramphenicol   Thiamphenicol

960.3 Erythromycin and other macrolides
Oleandomycin   Spiramycin

960.4 Tetracycline group
Doxycycline   Oxytetracycline
Minocycline

960.5 Cephalosporin group
Cephalexin   Cephaloridine
Cephaloglycin   Cephalothin

960.6 Antimycobacterial antibiotics
Cycloserine   Rifampin
Kanamycin   Streptomycin

960.7 Antineoplastic antibiotics
Actinomycin such as: Dactinomycin
   Bleomycin   Daunorubicin
   Cactinomycin   Mitomycin

☐ **960.8 Other specified antibiotics**

☐ **960.9 Unspecified antibiotic**

● **961 Poisoning by other anti-infectives**

   Excludes *anti-infectives:*
      ear, nose, and throat (976.6)
      eye (976.5)
      local (976.0)

961.0 Sulfonamides
Sulfadiazine
Sulfafurazole
Sulfamethoxazole

961.1 Arsenical anti-infectives

961.2 Heavy metal anti-infectives
Compounds of: Compounds of:
   antimony   lead
   bismuth   mercury

   Excludes *mercurial diuretics (974.0)*

961.3 Quinoline and hydroxyquinoline derivatives
Chiniofon
Diiodohydroxyquin

   Excludes *antimalarial drugs (961.4)*

961.4 Antimalarials and drugs acting on other blood protozoa
Chloroquine
Cycloguanil
Primaquine
Proguanil [chloroguanide]
Pyrimethamine
Quinine

☐ **961.5 Other antiprotozoal drugs**
Emetine

961.6 Anthelmintics
Hexylresorcinol   Thiabendazole
Piperazine

961.7 Antiviral drugs
Methisazone

   Excludes *amantadine (966.4)*
      cytarabine (963.1)
      idoxuridine (976.5)

☐ **961.8 Other antimycobacterial drugs**
Ethambutol
Ethionamide
Isoniazid
Para-aminosalicylic acid derivatives
Sulfones

☐ **961.9 Other and unspecified anti-infectives**
Flucytosine
Nitrofuran derivatives

● **962 Poisoning by hormones and synthetic substitutes**

   Excludes *oxytocic hormones (975.0)*

962.0 Adrenal cortical steroids
Cortisone derivatives
Desoxycorticosterone derivatives
Fluorinated corticosteroids

962.1 Androgens and anabolic congeners
Methandriol
Nandrolone
Oxymetholone
Testosterone

962.2 Ovarian hormones and synthetic substitutes
Contraceptives, oral
Estrogens
Estrogens and progestogens, combined
Progestogens

962.3 Insulins and antidiabetic agents
Acetohexamide
Biguanide derivatives, oral
Chlorpropamide
Glucagon
Insulin
Phenformin
Sulfonylurea derivatives, oral
Tolbutamide

962.4 Anterior pituitary hormones
Corticotropin
Gonadotropin
Somatotropin [growth hormone]

962.5 Posterior pituitary hormones
Vasopressin

   Excludes *oxytocic hormones (975.0)*

962.6 Parathyroid and parathyroid derivatives

962.7 Thyroid and thyroid derivatives
Dextrothyroxin
Levothyroxine sodium
Liothyronine
Thyroglobulin

962.8 Antithyroid agents
Iodides
Thiouracil
Thiourea

☐ **962.9 Other and unspecified hormones and synthetic substitutes**

● **963 Poisoning by primarily systemic agents**

963.0 Antiallergic and antiemetic drugs
Antihistamines   Diphenylpyraline
Chlorpheniramine   Thonzylamine
Diphenhydramine   Tripelennamine

   Excludes *phenothiazine-based tranquilizers (969.1)*

963.1 Antineoplastic and immunosuppressive drugs
Azathioprine
Busulfan
Chlorambucil
Cyclophosphamide
Cytarabine
Fluorouracil
Mercaptopurine
thio-TEPA

   Excludes *antineoplastic antibiotics (960.7)*

963.2 Acidifying agents

963.3 Alkalizing agents

963.4 **Enzymes, not elsewhere classified**
Penicillinase

963.5 **Vitamins, not elsewhere classified**
Vitamin A
Vitamin D

Excludes   *nicotinic acid (972.2)*
vitamin K (964.3)

☐963.8 **Other specified systemic agents**
Heavy metal antagonists

☐963.9 **Unspecified systemic agent**

● 964 **Poisoning by agents primarily affecting blood constituents**

964.0 **Iron and its compounds**
Ferric salts
Ferrous sulfate and other ferrous salts

964.1 **Liver preparations and other antianemic agents**
Folic acid

964.2 **Anticoagulants**
Coumarin
Heparin
Phenindione
Warfarin sodium

964.3 **Vitamin K [phytonadione]**

964.4 **Fibrinolysis-affecting drugs**
Aminocaproic acid
Streptodornase
Streptokinase
Urokinase

964.5 **Anticoagulant antagonists and other coagulants**
Hexadimethrine
Protamine sulfate

964.6 **Gamma globulin**

964.7 **Natural blood and blood products**
Blood plasma   Packed red cells
Human fibrinogen   Whole blood

Excludes   *transfusion reactions (999.4–999.8)*

☐964.8 **Other specified agents affecting blood constituents**
Macromolecular blood substitutes
Plasma expanders

☐964.9 **Unspecified agents affecting blood constituents**

● 965 **Poisoning by analgesics, antipyretics, and antirheumatics**

Excludes   *drug dependence (304.0–304.9)*
nondependent abuse (305.0–305.9)

● 965.0 **Opiates and related narcotics**

☐965.00 **Opium (alkaloids), unspecified**

965.01 **Heroin**
Diacetylmorphine

965.02 **Methadone**

☐965.09 **Other**
Codeine [methylmorphine]
Meperidine [pethidine]
Morphine

965.1 **Salicylates**
Acetylsalicylic acid [aspirin]
Salicylic acid salts

965.4 **Aromatic analgesics, not elsewhere classified**
Acetanilid
Paracetamol [acetaminophen]
Phenacetin [acetophenetidin]

965.5 **Pyrazole derivatives**
Aminophenazone [aminopyrine]
Phenylbutazone

● 965.6 **Antirheumatics [antiphlogistics]**

Excludes   *salicylates (965.1)*
steroids (962.0–962.9)

965.61 **Propionic acid derivatives**
Fenoprofen
Flurbiprofen
Ibuprofen
Ketoprofen
Naproxen
Oxaprozin

☐965.69 **Other antirheumatics**
Gold salts
Indomethacin

☐965.7 **Other non-narcotic analgesics**
Pyrabital

☐965.8 **Other specified analgesics and antipyretics**
Pentazocine

☐965.9 **Unspecified analgesic and antipyretic**

● 966 **Poisoning by anticonvulsants and anti-Parkinsonism drugs**

966.0 **Oxazolidine derivatives**
Paramethadione
Trimethadione

966.1 **Hydantoin derivatives**
Phenytoin

966.2 **Succinimides**
Ethosuximide
Phensuximide

☐966.3 **Other and unspecified anticonvulsants**
Primidone

Excludes   *barbiturates (967.0)*
sulfonamides (961.0)

966.4 **Anti-Parkinsonism drugs**
Amantadine
Ethopropazine [profenamine]
Levodopa [L-dopa]

● 967 **Poisoning by sedatives and hypnotics**

Excludes   *drug dependence (304.0–304.9)*
nondependent abuse (305.0–305.9)

967.0 **Barbiturates**
Amobarbital [amylobarbitone]
Barbital [barbitone]
Butabarbital [butabarbitone]
Pentobarbital [pentobarbitone]
Phenobarbital [phenobarbitone]
Secobarbital [quinalbarbitone]

Excludes   *thiobarbiturate anesthetics (968.3)*

967.1 **Chloral hydrate group**

967.2 **Paraldehyde**

967.3 **Bromine compounds**
Bromide
Carbromal (derivatives)

967.4 **Methaqualone compounds**

967.5 **Glutethimide group**

967.6 **Mixed sedatives, not elsewhere classified**

☐967.8 **Other sedatives and hypnotics**

☐967.9 **Unspecified sedative or hypnotic**
Sleeping:
drug NOS
pill NOS
tablet NOS

● 968 Poisoning by other central nervous system depressants and anesthetics

Excludes drug dependence (304.0–304.9)
          nondependent abuse (305.0–305.9)

968.0 Central nervous system muscle-tone depressants
       Chlorphenesin (carbamate)
       Mephenesin
       Methocarbamol

968.1 Halothane

❑ 968.2 Other gaseous anesthetics
       Ether
       Halogenated hydrocarbon derivatives, except halothane
       Nitrous oxide

968.3 Intravenous anesthetics
       Ketamine
       Methohexital [methohexitone]
       Thiobarbiturates, such as thiopental sodium

❑ 968.4 Other and unspecified general anesthetics

968.5 Surface [topical] and infiltration anesthetics
       Cocaine
       Lidocaine [lignocaine]
       Procaine
       Tetracaine

968.6 Peripheral nerve- and plexus-blocking anesthetics

968.7 Spinal anesthetics

❑ 968.9 Other and unspecified local anesthetics

● 969 Poisoning by psychotropic agents

Excludes drug dependence (304.0–304.9)
          nondependent abuse (305.0–305.9)

969.0 Antidepressants
       Amitriptyline
       Imipramine
       Monoamine oxidase [MAO] inhibitors

969.1 Phenothiazine-based tranquilizers
       Chlorpromazine
       Fluphenazine
       Prochlorperazine
       Promazine

969.2 Butyrophenone-based tranquilizers
       Haloperidol   Trifluperidol
       Spiperone

❑ 969.3 Other antipsychotics, neuroleptics, and major tranquilizers

969.4 Benzodiazepine-based tranquilizers
       Chlordiazepoxide   Lorazepam
       Diazepam   Medazepam
       Flurazepam   Nitrazepam

❑ 969.5 Other tranquilizers
       Hydroxyzine
       Meprobamate

969.6 Psychodysleptics [hallucinogens]
       Cannabis (derivatives)
       Lysergide [LSD]
       Marijuana (derivatives)
       Mescaline
       Psilocin
       Psilocybin

969.7 Psychostimulants
       Amphetamine
       Caffeine

Excludes central appetite depressants (977.0)

❑ 969.8 Other specified psychotropic agents

❑ 969.9 Unspecified psychotropic agent

● 970 Poisoning by central nervous system stimulants

970.0 Analeptics
       Lobeline
       Nikethamide

970.1 Opiate antagonists
       Levallorphan
       Nalorphine
       Naloxone

❑ 970.8 Other specified central nervous system stimulants

❑ 970.9 Unspecified central nervous system stimulant

● 971 Poisoning by drugs primarily affecting the autonomic nervous system

971.0 Parasympathomimetics [cholinergics]
       Acetylcholine
       Anticholinesterase:
         organophosphorus
         reversible
       Pilocarpine

971.1 Parasympatholytics [anticholinergics and antimuscarinics] and spasmolytics
       Atropine
       Homatropine
       Hyoscine [scopolamine]
       Quaternary ammonium derivatives

Excludes papaverine (972.5)

971.2 Sympathomimetics [adrenergics]
       Epinephrine [adrenalin]
       Levarterenol [noradrenalin]

971.3 Sympatholytics [antiadrenergics]
       Phenoxybenzamine
       Tolazoline hydrochloride

❑ 971.9 Unspecified drug primarily affecting autonomic nervous system

● 972 Poisoning by agents primarily affecting the cardiovascular system

972.0 Cardiac rhythm regulators
       Practolol
       Procainamide
       Propranolol
       Quinidine

Excludes lidocaine (968.5)

972.1 Cardiotonic glycosides and drugs of similar action
       Digitalis glycosides
       Digoxin
       Strophanthins

972.2 Antilipemic and antiarteriosclerotic drugs
       Clofibrate
       Nicotinic acid derivatives

972.3 Ganglion-blocking agents
       Pentamethonium bromide

972.4 Coronary vasodilators
       Dipyridamole
       Nitrates [nitroglycerin]
       Nitrites

❑ 972.5 Other vasodilators
       Cyclandelate
       Diazoxide
       Papaverine

Excludes nicotinic acid (972.2)

❑ 972.6 Other antihypertensive agents
       Clonidine
       Guanethidine
       Rauwolfia alkaloids
       Reserpine

972.7 Antivaricose drugs, including sclerosing agents
Sodium morrhuate
Zinc salts

972.8 Capillary-active drugs
Adrenochrome derivatives
Metaraminol

❑**972.9 Other and unspecified agents primarily affecting the cardiovascular system**

● **973 Poisoning by agents primarily affecting the gastrointestinal system**

973.0 Antacids and antigastric secretion drugs
Aluminum hydroxide
Magnesium trisilicate

973.1 Irritant cathartics
Bisacodyl
Castor oil
Phenolphthalein

973.2 Emollient cathartics
Dioctyl sulfosuccinates

❑**973.3 Other cathartics, including intestinal atonia drugs**
Magnesium sulfate

973.4 Digestants
Pancreatin
Papain
Pepsin

973.5 Antidiarrheal drugs
Kaolin
Pectin
| **Excludes** | *anti-infectives (960.0–961.9)* |

973.6 Emetics

❑**973.8 Other specified agents primarily affecting the gastrointestinal system**

❑**973.9 Unspecified agent primarily affecting the gastrointestinal system**

● **974 Poisoning by water, mineral, and uric acid metabolism drugs**

974.0 Mercurial diuretics
Chlormerodrin
Mercaptomerin
Mersalyl

974.1 Purine derivative diuretics
Theobromine
Theophylline
| **Excludes** | *aminophylline [theophylline ethylenediamine] (975.7)* |
| | *caffeine (969.7)* |

974.2 Carbonic acid anhydrase inhibitors
Acetazolamide

974.3 Saluretics
Benzothiadiazides
Chlorothiazide group

❑**974.4 Other diuretics**
Ethacrynic acid
Furosemide

974.5 Electrolytic, caloric, and water-balance agents

❑**974.6 Other mineral salts, not elsewhere classified**

974.7 Uric acid metabolism drugs
Allopurinol
Colchicine
Probenecid

● **975 Poisoning by agents primarily acting on the smooth and skeletal muscles and respiratory system**

975.0 Oxytocic agents
Ergot alkaloids
Oxytocin
Prostaglandins

975.1 Smooth muscle relaxants
Adiphenine
Metaproterenol [orciprenaline]
| **Excludes** | *papaverine (972.5)* |

975.2 Skeletal muscle relaxants

❑**975.3 Other and unspecified drugs acting on muscles**

975.4 Antitussives
Dextromethorphan
Pipazethate

975.5 Expectorants
Acetylcysteine
Guaifenesin
Terpin hydrate

975.6 Anti-common cold drugs

975.7 Antiasthmatics
Aminophylline [theophylline ethylenediamine]

❑**975.8 Other and unspecified respiratory drugs**

● **976 Poisoning by agents primarily affecting skin and mucous membrane, ophthalmological, otorhinolaryngological, and dental drugs**

976.0 Local anti-infectives and anti-inflammatory drugs

976.1 Antipruritics

976.2 Local astringents and local detergents

976.3 Emollients, demulcents, and protectants

976.4 Keratolytics, keratoplastics, other hair treatment drugs and preparations

976.5 Eye anti-infectives and other eye drugs
Idoxuridine

976.6 Anti-infectives and other drugs and preparations for ear, nose, and throat

976.7 Dental drugs topically applied
| **Excludes** | *anti-infectives (976.0)* |
| | *local anesthetics (968.5)* |

❑**976.8 Other agents primarily affecting skin and mucous membrane**
Spermicides [vaginal contraceptives]

❑**976.9 Unspecified agent primarily affecting skin and mucous membrane**

● **977 Poisoning by other and unspecified drugs and medicinal substances**

977.0 Dietetics
Central appetite depressants

977.1 Lipotropic drugs

977.2 Antidotes and chelating agents, not elsewhere classified

977.3 Alcohol deterrents

977.4 Pharmaceutical excipients
Pharmaceutical adjuncts

❑**977.8 Other specified drugs and medicinal substances**
Contrast media used for diagnostic x-ray procedures
Diagnostic agents and kits

❑**977.9 Unspecified drug or medicinal substance**

● **978 Poisoning by bacterial vaccines**

   978.0 BCG

   978.1 Typhoid and paratyphoid

   978.2 Cholera

   978.3 Plague

   978.4 Tetanus

   978.5 Diphtheria

   978.6 Pertussis vaccine, including combinations with a pertussis component

   ☐978.8 Other and unspecified bacterial vaccines

   978.9 Mixed bacterial vaccines, except combinations with a pertussis component

● **979 Poisoning by other vaccines and biological substances**

   Excludes *gamma globulin (964.6)*

   979.0 Smallpox vaccine

   979.1 Rabies vaccine

   979.2 Typhus vaccine

   979.3 Yellow fever vaccine

   979.4 Measles vaccine

   979.5 Poliomyelitis vaccine

   ☐979.6 Other and unspecified viral and rickettsial vaccines
      Mumps vaccine

   979.7 Mixed viral-rickettsial and bacterial vaccines, except combinations with a pertussis component

   Excludes *combinations with a pertussis component (978.6)*

   ☐979.9 Other and unspecified vaccines and biological substances

TOXIC EFFECTS OF SUBSTANCES CHIEFLY NONMEDICINAL AS TO SOURCE (980–989)

   Excludes *burns from chemical agents (ingested) (947.0–947.9)*
localized toxic effects indexed elsewhere (001.0–799.9)
respiratory conditions due to external agents (506.0–508.9)

Use additional code to specify the nature of the toxic effect

● **980 Toxic effect of alcohol**

   980.0 Ethyl alcohol
      Denatured alcohol
      Ethanol
      Grain alcohol

   Use additional code to identify any associated:
   acute alcohol intoxication (305.0)
     in alcoholism (303.0)
   drunkenness (simple) (305.0)
     pathological (291.4)

   980.1 Methyl alcohol
      Methanol
      Wood alcohol

   980.2 Isopropyl alcohol
      Dimethyl carbinol
      Isopropanol
      Rubbing alcohol

   980.3 Fusel oil
      Alcohol:
       amyl
       butyl
       propyl

   ☐980.8 Other specified alcohols

   ☐980.9 Unspecified alcohol

● **981 Toxic effect of petroleum products**
   Benzine   Petroleum:
   Gasoline   ether
   Kerosene   naphtha
   Paraffin wax   spirit

● **982 Toxic effect of solvents other than petroleum based**

   982.0 Benzene and homologues

   982.1 Carbon tetrachloride

   982.2 Carbon disulfide
      Carbon bisulfide

   ☐982.3 Other chlorinated hydrocarbon solvents
      Tetrachloroethylene
      Trichloroethylene

   Excludes *chlorinated hydrocarbon preparations other than solvents (989.2)*

   982.4 Nitroglycol

   ☐982.8 Other nonpetroleum-based solvents
      Acetone

● **983 Toxic effect of corrosive aromatics, acids, and caustic alkalis**

   983.0 Corrosive aromatics
      Carbolic acid or phenol   Cresol

   983.1 Acids
      Acid:
       hydrochloric
       nitric
       sulfuric

   983.2 Caustic alkalis
      Lye
      Potassium hydroxide
      Sodium hydroxide

   ☐983.9 Caustic, unspecified

● **984 Toxic effect of lead and its compounds (including fumes)**

   Includes: that from all sources except medicinal substances

   984.0 Inorganic lead compounds
      Lead dioxide
      Lead salts

   984.1 Organic lead compounds
      Lead acetate
      Tetraethyl lead

   ☐984.8 Other lead compounds

   ☐984.9 Unspecified lead compound

● **985 Toxic effect of other metals**

   Includes: that from all sources except medicinal substances

   985.0 Mercury and its compounds
      Minamata disease

   985.1 Arsenic and its compounds

   985.2 Manganese and its compounds

   985.3 Beryllium and its compounds

   985.4 Antimony and its compounds

   985.5 Cadmium and its compounds

   985.6 Chromium

   ☐985.8 Other specified metals
      Brass fumes
      Copper salts
      Iron compounds
      Nickel compounds

   ☐985.9 Unspecified metal

986   Toxic effect of carbon monoxide

● 987   Toxic effect of other gases, fumes, or vapors

     987.0   Liquefied petroleum gases
         Butane
         Propane

     ❏987.1   Other hydrocarbon gas

     987.2   Nitrogen oxides
         Nitrogen dioxide
         Nitrous fumes

     987.3   Sulfur dioxide

     987.4   Freon
         Dichloromonofluoromethane

     987.5   Lacrimogenic gas
         Bromobenzyl cyanide
         Chloroacetophenone
         Ethyliodoacetate

     987.6   Chlorine gas

     987.7   Hydrocyanic acid gas

     ❏987.8   Other specified gases, fumes, or vapors
         Phosgene
         Polyester fumes

     ❏987.9   Unspecified gas, fume, or vapor

● 988   Toxic effect of noxious substances eaten as food

     | Excludes | *allergic reaction to food, such as:*
         gastroenteritis (558.3)
         rash (692.5, 693.1)
       food poisoning (bacterial) (005.0–005.9)
       toxic effects of food contaminants, such as:
         aflatoxin and other mycotoxin (989.7)
         mercury (985.0)

     988.0   Fish and shellfish

     988.1   Mushrooms

     988.2   Berries and other plants

     ❏988.8   Other specified noxious substances eaten as food

     ❏988.9   Unspecified noxious substance eaten as food

● 989   Toxic effect of other substances, chiefly nonmedicinal as to source

     989.0   Hydrocyanic acid and cyanides
         Potassium cyanide
         Sodium cyanide

     | Excludes | *gas and fumes (987.7)*

     989.1   Strychnine and salts

     989.2   Chlorinated hydrocarbons
         Aldrin
         Chlordane
         DDT
         Dieldrin

     | Excludes | *chlorinated hydrocarbon solvents (982.0–982.3)*

     989.3   Organophosphate and carbamate

Carbaryl	Parathion
Dichlorvos	Phorate
Malathion	Phosdrin

     ❏989.4   Other pesticides, not elsewhere classified
         Mixtures of insecticides

     989.5   Venom
         Bites of venomous snakes, lizards, and spiders
         Tick paralysis

     989.6   Soaps and detergents

     989.7   Aflatoxin and other mycotoxin [food contaminants]

● 989.8   Other substances, chiefly nonmedicinal as to source

     989.81   Asbestos

     | Excludes | *asbestosis (501)*
         exposure to asbestos (V15.84)

     989.82   Latex

     989.83   Silicone

     | Excludes | *silicone used in medical devices, implants and grafts (996.00–996.79)*

     989.84   Tobacco

     ❏989.89   Other

     ❏989.9   Unspecified substance, chiefly nonmedicinal as to source

OTHER AND UNSPECIFIED EFFECTS OF EXTERNAL CAUSES (990–995)

❏990   Effects of radiation, unspecified
     Complication of:
         phototherapy
         radiation therapy
     Radiation sickness

     | Excludes | *specified adverse effects of radiation. Such conditions are to be classified according to the nature of the adverse effect, as:*
       burns (940.0–949.5)
       dermatitis (692.7–692.8)
       leukemia (204.0–208.9)
       pneumonia (508.0)
       sunburn (692.71, 692.76–692.77)
     [The type of radiation giving rise to the adverse effect may be identified by use of the E codes.]

● 991   Effects of reduced temperature

     991.0   Frostbite of face

     991.1   Frostbite of hand

     991.2   Frostbite of foot

     ❏991.3   Frostbite of other and unspecified sites

     991.4   Immersion foot
         Trench foot

     991.5   Chilblains
         Erythema pernio
         Perniosis

     991.6   Hypothermia
         Hypothermia (accidental)

     | Excludes | *hypothermia following anesthesia (995.89)*
       hypothermia not associated with low environmental temperature (780.99)

     ❏991.8   Other specified effects of reduced temperature

     ❏991.9   Unspecified effect of reduced temperature
         Effects of freezing or excessive cold NOS

● 992   Effects of heat and light

     | Excludes | *burns (940.0–949.5)*
       diseases of sweat glands due to heat (705.0–705.9)
       malignant hyperpyrexia following anesthesia (995.86)
       sunburn (692.71, 692.76–692.77)

     992.0   Heat stroke and sunstroke

Heat apoplexy	Siriasis
Heat pyrexia	Thermoplegia
Ictus solaris	

     992.1   Heat syncope
         Heat collapse

992.2 Heat cramps

992.3 Heat exhaustion, anhydrotic
Heat prostration due to water depletion
> **Excludes** *that associated with salt depletion (992.4)*

992.4 Heat exhaustion due to salt depletion
Heat prostration due to salt (and water) depletion

☐ **992.5 Heat exhaustion, unspecified**
Heat prostration NOS

992.6 Heat fatigue, transient

992.7 Heat edema

☐ **992.8 Other specified heat effects**

☐ **992.9 Unspecified**

● **993 Effects of air pressure**

993.0 Barotrauma, otitic
Aero-otitis media
Effects of high altitude on ears

993.1 Barotrauma, sinus
Aerosinusitis
Effects of high altitude on sinuses

☐ **993.2 Other and unspecified effects of high altitude**
Alpine sickness
Andes disease
Anoxia due to high altitude
Hypobaropathy
Mountain sickness

993.3 Caisson disease
Bends
Compressed-air disease
Decompression sickness
Divers' palsy or paralysis

993.4 Effects of air pressure caused by explosion

☐ **993.8 Other specified effects of air pressure**

☐ **993.9 Unspecified effect of air pressure**

● **994 Effects of other external causes**
> **Excludes** *certain adverse effects not elsewhere classified (995.0–995.8)*

994.0 Effects of lightning
Shock from lightning
Struck by lightning NOS
> **Excludes** *burns (940.0–949.5)*

994.1 Drowning and nonfatal submersion
Bathing cramp   Immersion

994.2 Effects of hunger
Deprivation of food   Starvation

994.3 Effects of thirst
Deprivation of water

994.4 Exhaustion due to exposure

994.5 Exhaustion due to excessive exertion
Overexertion

994.6 Motion sickness
Air sickness   Travel sickness
Seasickness

994.7 Asphyxiation and strangulation
Suffocation (by):   Suffocation (by):
  bedclothes   plastic bag
  cave-in   pressure
  constriction   strangulation
  mechanical
> **Excludes** *asphyxia from:*
>   *carbon monoxide (986)*
>   *inhalation of food or foreign body (932–934.9)*
>   *other gases, fumes, and vapors (987.0–987.9)*

994.8 Electrocution and nonfatal effects of electric current
Shock from electric current
> **Excludes** *electric burns (940.0–949.5)*

☐ **994.9 Other effects of external causes**
Effects of:
  abnormal gravitational [G] forces or states
  weightlessness

● **995 Certain adverse effects not elsewhere classified**
> **Excludes** *complications of surgical and medical care (996.0–999.9)*

☐ **995.0 Other anaphylactic shock**
Allergic shock NOS or due to adverse effect of correct medicinal substance properly administered
Anaphylactic reaction NOS or due to adverse effect of correct medicinal substance properly administered
Anaphylaxis NOS or due to adverse effect of correct medicinal substance properly administered
> **Excludes** *anaphylactic reaction to serum (999.4)*
>   *anaphylactic shock due to adverse food reaction (995.60–995.69)*

Use additional E code to identify external cause, such as:
  adverse effects of correct medicinal substance properly administered [E930–E949]

995.1 Angioneurotic edema
Giant urticaria
> **Excludes** *urticaria:*
>   *due to serum (999.5)*
>   *other specified (698.2, 708.0–708.9, 757.33)*

☐ **995.2 Unspecified adverse effect of drug, medicinal and biological substance (due) to correct medicinal substance properly administered**
Adverse effect to correct medicinal substance properly administered
Allergic reaction to correct medicinal substance properly administered
Hypersensitivity to correct medicinal substance properly administered
Idiosyncrasy due to correct medicinal substance properly administered
Drug:
  hypersensitivity NOS
  reaction NOS
> **Excludes** *pathological drug intoxication (292.2)*

☐ **995.3 Allergy, unspecified**
Allergic reaction NOS
Hypersensitivity NOS
Idiosyncrasy NOS
> **Excludes** *allergic reaction NOS to correct medicinal substance properly administered (995.2)*
>   *specific types of allergic reaction, such as:*
>   *allergic diarrhea (558.3)*
>   *dermatitis (691.0–693.9)*
>   *hayfever (477.0–477.9)*

995.4 Shock due to anesthesia
Shock due to anesthesia in which the correct substance was properly administered
> **Excludes** *complications of anesthesia in labor or delivery (668.0–668.9)*
>   *overdose or wrong substance given (968.0–969.9)*
>   *postoperative shock NOS (998.0)*
>   *specified adverse effects of anesthesia classified elsewhere, such as:*
>   *anoxic brain damage (348.1)*
>   *hepatitis (070.0–070.9), etc.*
>   *unspecified adverse effect of anesthesia (995.2)*

- **995.5   Child maltreatment syndrome**

  Use additional code(s), if applicable, to identify any associated injuries

  Use additional E code to identify:
  nature of abuse (E960-E968)
  perpetrator (E967.0-E967.9)

  ☐ **995.50   Child abuse, unspecified**

  995.51   Child emotional/psychological abuse

  995.52   Child neglect (nutritional)

  995.53   Child sexual abuse

  995.54   Child physical abuse
  Battered baby or child syndrome

  | **Excludes** | *Shaken infant syndrome (995.55)* |

  995.55   Shaken infant syndrome

  Use additional code(s) to identify any associated injuries

  ☐ **995.59   Other child abuse and neglect**
  Multiple forms of abuse

- **995.6   Anaphylactic shock due to adverse food reaction**
  Anaphylactic shock due to nonpoisonous foods

  ☐ **995.60   Due to unspecified food**

  995.61   Due to peanuts

  995.62   Due to crustaceans

  995.63   Due to fruits and vegetables

  995.64   Due to tree nuts and seeds

  995.65   Due to fish

  995.66   Due to food additives

  995.67   Due to milk products

  995.68   Due to eggs

  ☐ **995.69   Due to other specified food**

  995.7   Other adverse food reactions, not elsewhere classified

  Use additional code to identify the type of reaction, such as:
  hives (708.0)
  wheezing (786.07)

Excludes	*anaphylactic shock due to adverse food reaction (995.60–995.69)*
	asthma (493.0, 493.9)
	dermatitis due to food (693.1)
	in contact with the skin (692.5)
	gastroenteritis and colitis due to food (558.3)
	rhinitis due to food (477.1)

- **995.8   Other specified adverse effects, not elsewhere classified**

  ☐ **995.80   Adult maltreatment, unspecified**
  Abused person NOS

  Use additional code to identify:
  any associated injury
  perpetrator (E967.0-E967.9)

  995.81   Adult physical abuse
  Battered:
  person syndrome, NEC
  man
  spouse
  woman

  Use additional code to identify:
  any associated injury
  nature of abuse (E960-E968)
  perpetrator (E967.0-E967.9)

  995.82   Adult emotional/psychological abuse

  Use additional E code to identify perpetrator (E967.0-E967.9)

  995.83   Adult sexual abuse

  Use additional code to identify:
  any associated injury
  perpetrator (E967.0-E967.9)

  995.84   Adult neglect (nutritional)

  Use additional code to identify:
  intent of neglect (E904.0-E968.4)
  perpetrator (E967.0-E967.9)

  ☐ **995.85   Other adult abuse and neglect**
  Multiple forms of abuse and neglect

  Use additional code to identify any associated injury
  intent of neglect (E904.0, E968.4)
  nature of abuse (E960-E968)
  perpetrator (E967.0-E967.9)

  995.86   Malignant hyperthermia
  Malignant hyperpyrexia due to anesthesia

  ☐ **995.89   Other**
  Hypothermia due to anesthesia

- **995.9   Systemic inflammatory response syndrome (SIRS)**
  Code first underlying systemic infection   ◄▦

  ☐ **995.90   Systemic inflammatory response syndrome, unspecified SIRS NOS**

  995.91   Systemic inflammatory response syndrome due to infectious process without organ dysfunction
  Sepsis

  995.92   Systemic inflammatory response syndrome due to infectious process with organ dysfunction
  Severe sepsis

  Use additional code to specify organ dysfunction, such as:
  acute renal failure (584.5–584.9)
  acute respiratory failure (518.81)
  critical illness myopathy (359.81)
  critical illness polyneuropathy (357.82)
  encephalopathy (348.31)
  hepatic failure (570)
  septic shock (785.52)

  995.93   Systemic inflammatory response syndrome due to noninfectious process without organ dysfunction

  995.94   Systemic inflammatory response syndrome due to noninfectious process with organ dysfunction

  Use additional code to specify organ dysfunction, such as:
  acute renal failure (584.5–584.9)
  acute respiratory failure (518.81)
  critical illness myopathy (359.81)
  critical illness polyneuropathy (357.82)
  encephalopathy (348.31)
  hepatic failure (570)
  septic shock (785.52)

COMPLICATIONS OF SURGICAL AND MEDICAL CARE, NOT ELSEWHERE CLASSIFIED (996–999)

| Excludes | adverse effects of medicinal agents (001.0–799.9, 995.0–995.8) |

burns from local applications and irradiation (940.0–949.5)

complications of:
    conditions for which the procedure was performed
    surgical procedures during abortion, labor, and delivery (630–676.9)

poisoning and toxic effects of drugs and chemicals (960.0–989.9)

postoperative conditions in which no complications are present, such as:
    artificial opening status (V44.0–V44.9)
    closure of external stoma (V55.0–V55.9)
    fitting of prosthetic device (V52.0–V52.9)

specified complications classified elsewhere:
    anesthetic shock (995.4)
    electrolyte imbalance (276.0–276.9)
    postlaminectomy syndrome (722.80–722.83)
    postmastectomy lymphedema syndrome (457.0)
    postoperative psychosis (293.0–293.9)
    any other condition classified elsewhere in the Alphabetic Index when described as due to a procedure

● **996   Complications peculiar to certain specified procedures**

Includes: complications, not elsewhere classified, in the use of artificial substitutes [e.g., Dacron, metal, Silastic, Teflon] or natural sources [e.g., bone] involving:
    anastomosis (internal)
    graft (bypass) (patch)
    implant
    internal device:
        catheter
        electronic
        fixation
        prosthetic
    reimplant
    transplant

| Excludes | accidental puncture or laceration during procedure (998.2) |

complications of internal anastomosis of:
    gastrointestinal tract (997.4)
    urinary tract (997.5)

other specified complications classified elsewhere, such as:
    hemolytic anemia (283.1)
    functional cardiac disturbances (429.4)
    serum hepatitis (070.2–070.3)

● **996.0   Mechanical complication of cardiac device, implant, and graft**
    Breakdown (mechanical)
    Displacement
    Leakage
    Obstruction, mechanical
    Perforation
    Protrusion

❏ **996.00   Unspecified device, implant, and graft**

996.01   Due to cardiac pacemaker (electrode)

996.02   Due to heart valve prosthesis

996.03   Due to coronary bypass graft

| Excludes | atherosclerosis of graft (414.02, 414.03) |

embolism [occlusion NOS] [thrombus] of graft (996.72)

996.04   Due to automatic implantable cardiac defibrillator

❏ **996.09   Other**

❏ **996.1   Mechanical complication of other vascular device, implant, and graft**
    Mechanical complications involving:
    aortic (bifurcation) graft (replacement)
    arteriovenous:
        dialysis catheter
        fistula surgically created
        shunt surgically created
    balloon (counterpulsation) device, intra-aortic
    carotid artery bypass graft
    femoral-popliteal bypass graft
    umbrella device, vena cava

| Excludes | atherosclerosis of biological graft (440.30–440.32) |

embolism [occlusion NOS] [thrombus] of (biological) (synthetic) graft (996.74)

peritoneal dialysis catheter (996.56)

996.2   Mechanical complication of nervous system device, implant, and graft
    Mechanical complications involving:
    dorsal column stimulator
    electrodes implanted in brain [brain "pacemaker"]
    peripheral nerve graft
    ventricular (communicating) shunt

● **996.3   Mechanical complication of genitourinary device, implant, and graft**

❏ **996.30   Unspecified device, implant, and graft**

996.31   Due to urethral [indwelling] catheter

996.32   Due to intrauterine contraceptive device

❏ **996.39   Other**
    Cystostomy catheter
    Prosthetic reconstruction of vas deferens
    Repair (graft) of ureter without mention of resection

| Excludes | complications due to: |

external stoma of urinary tract (997.5)
internal anastomosis of urinary tract (997.5)

996.4   Mechanical complication of internal orthopedic device, implant, and graft
    Mechanical complications involving:
    external (fixation) device utilizing internal screw(s), pin(s) or other methods of fixation
    grafts of bone, cartilage, muscle, or tendon
    internal (fixation) device such as nail, plate, rod, etc.

| Excludes | complications of external orthopedic device, such as: |

pressure ulcer due to cast (707.00–707.09) ◀▥

● **996.5   Mechanical complication of other specified prosthetic device, implant, and graft**
    Mechanical complications involving:
    prosthetic implant in:
        bile duct
        breast
        chin
        orbit of eye
    nonabsorbable surgical material NOS
    other graft, implant, and internal device, not elsewhere classified

996.51   Due to corneal graft

❏ **996.52   Due to graft of other tissue, not elsewhere classified**
    Skin graft failure or rejection

| Excludes | failure of artificial skin graft (996.55) |

failure of decellularized allodermis (996.55)
sloughing of temporary skin allografts or xenografts (pigskin)-omit code

996.53 Due to ocular lens prosthesis
> **Excludes** contact lenses—code to condition

996.54 Due to breast prosthesis
Breast capsule (prosthesis)
Mammary implant

996.55 Due to artificial skin graft and decellularized allodermis
Dislodgement　　　Non-adherence
Displacement　　　Poor incorporation
Failure　　　　　　Shearing

996.56 Due to peritoneal dialysis catheter
> **Excludes** mechanical complication of arteriovenous dialysis catheter (996.1)

996.57 Due to insulin pump

❑ **996.59 Due to other implant and internal device, not elsewhere classified**
Nonabsorbable surgical material NOS
Prosthetic implant in:
　bile duct　　　　orbit of eye
　chin

● **996.6 Infection and inflammatory reaction due to internal prosthetic device, implant, and graft**
Infection (causing obstruction) due to (presence of) any device, implant, and graft classifiable to 996.0–996.5
Inflammation due to (presence of) any device, implant, and graft classifiable to 996.0–996.5

Use additional code to identify specified infections

❑ **996.60 Due to unspecified device, implant and graft**

996.61 Due to cardiac device, implant and graft
Cardiac pacemaker or defibrillator:
　electrode(s), lead(s)
　pulse generator
　subcutaneous pocket
Coronary artery bypass graft
Heart valve prosthesis

❑ **996.62 Due to vascular device, implant and graft**
Arterial graft
Arteriovenous fistula or shunt
Infusion pump
Vascular catheter (arterial) (dialysis) (venous)

996.63 Due to nervous system device, implant and graft
Electrodes implanted in brain
Peripheral nerve graft
Spinal canal catheter
Ventricular (communicating) shunt (catheter)

996.64 Due to indwelling urinary catheter
Use additional code to identify specified infections, such as:
Cystitis (595.0–595.9)
Sepsis (038.0–038.9)

❑ **996.65 Due to other genitourinary device, implant and graft**
Intrauterine contraceptive device

996.66 Due to internal joint prosthesis

❑ **996.67 Due to other internal orthopedic device, implant and graft**
Bone growth stimulator (electrode)
Internal fixation device (pin) (rod) (screw)

996.68 Due to peritoneal dialysis catheter
Exit-site infection or inflammation

❑ **996.69 Due to other internal prosthetic device, implant, and graft**
Breast prosthesis
Ocular lens prosthesis
Prosthetic orbital implant

● **996.7 Other complications of internal (biological) (synthetic) prosthetic device, implant, and graft**
Complication NOS due to (presence of) any device, implant, and graft classifiable to 996.0–996.5
occlusion NOS
Embolism due to (presence of) any device, implant, and graft classifiable to 996.0–996.5
Fibrosis due to (presence of) any device, implant, and graft classifiable to 996.0–996.5
Hemorrhage due to (presence of) any device, implant, and graft classifiable to 996.0–996.5
Pain due to (presence of) any device, implant, and graft classifiable to 996.0–996.5
Stenosis due to (presence of) any device, implant, and graft classifiable to 996.0–996.5
Thrombus due to (presence of) any device, implant, and graft classifiable to 996.0–996.5
> **Excludes** transplant rejection (996.8)

❑ **996.70 Due to unspecified device, implant, and graft**

996.71 Due to heart valve prosthesis

996.72 Due to other cardiac device, implant, and graft
Cardiac pacemaker or defibrillator:
　electrode(s), lead(s)
　subcutaneous pocket
Coronary artery bypass (graft)
> **Excludes** occlusion due to atherosclerosis (414.00–414.06)

996.73 Due to renal dialysis device, implant, and graft

❑ **996.74 Due to vascular device, implant, and graft**
> **Excludes** occlusion of biological graft due to atherosclerosis (440.30–440.32)

996.75 Due to nervous system device, implant, and graft

996.76 Due to genitourinary device, implant, and graft

996.77 Due to internal joint prosthesis

❑ **996.78 Due to other internal orthopedic device, implant, and graft**

❑ **996.79 Due to other internal prosthetic device, implant, and graft**

● **996.8 Complications of transplanted organ**
Transplant failure or rejection

Use additional code to identify nature of complication, such as:
Cytomegalovirus [CMV] infection (078.5)

❑ **996.80 Transplanted organ, unspecified**

996.81 Kidney

996.82 Liver

996.83 Heart

996.84 Lung

996.85 Bone marrow
Graft-versus-host disease (acute) (chronic)

996.86 Pancreas

996.87 Intestine

❑ **996.89 Other specified transplanted organ**

● **996.9 Complications of reattached extremity or body part**

   ❑ **996.90 Unspecified extremity**

   996.91 Forearm

   996.92 Hand

   996.93 Finger(s)

   ❑ **996.94 Upper extremity, other and unspecified**

   996.95 Foot and toe(s)

   ❑ **996.96 Lower extremity, other and unspecified**

   ❑ **996.99 Other specified body part**

● **997 Complications affecting specified body systems, not elsewhere classified**

   Use additional code to identify complication

    | **Excludes** | *the listed conditions when specified as:*
          causing shock (998.0)
          complications of:
            anesthesia:
              adverse effect (001.0–799.9, 995.0–995.8)
              in labor or delivery (668.0–668.9)
              poisoning (968.0–969.9)
            implanted device or graft (996.0–996.9)
            obstetrical procedures (669.0–669.4)
            reattached extremity (996.90–996.96)
            transplanted organ (996.80–996.89)

● **997.0 Nervous system complications**

   ❑ **997.00 Nervous system complication, unspecified**

   997.01 Central nervous system complication
       Anoxic brain damage
       Cerebral hypoxia

    | **Excludes** | *Cerebrovascular hemorrhage or infarction (997.02)*

   997.02 Iatrogenic cerebrovascular infarction or hemorrhage
       Postoperative stroke

   ❑ **997.09 Other nervous system complications**

997.1 Cardiac complications
    Cardiac:
       arrest during or resulting from a procedure
       insufficiency during or resulting from a procedure
    Cardiorespiratory failure during or resulting from a procedure
    Heart failure during or resulting from a procedure

    | **Excludes** | *the listed conditions as long-term effects of cardiac surgery or due to the presence of cardiac prosthetic device (429.4)*

997.2 Peripheral vascular complications
    Phlebitis or thrombophlebitis during or resulting from a procedure

    | **Excludes** | *the listed conditions due to:*
          implant or catheter device (996.62)
          infusion, perfusion, or transfusion (999.2)
          complications affecting blood vessels (997.71–997.79)

997.3 Respiratory complications
    Mendelson's syndrome resulting from a procedure
    Pneumonia (aspiration) resulting from a procedure

    | **Excludes** | *iatrogenic [postoperative] pneumothorax (512.1)*
          iatrogenic pulmonary embolism (415.11)
          Mendelson's syndrome in labor and delivery (668.0)
          specified complications classified elsewhere, such as:
            adult respiratory distress syndrome (518.5)
            pulmonary edema, postoperative (518.4)
            respiratory insufficiency, acute, postoperative (518.5)
            shock lung (518.5)
            tracheostomy complication (519.00–519.09)

997.4 Digestive system complications
    Complications of:
       Intestinal (internal) anastomosis and bypass, not elsewhere classified, except that involving urinary tract
       Hepatic failure specified as due to a procedure
       Hepatorenal syndrome specified as due to a procedure
       Intestinal obstruction NOS specified as due to a procedure

    | **Excludes** | *specified gastrointestinal complications classified elsewhere, such as:*
          blind loop syndrome (579.2)
          colostomy or enterostomy complications (569.60–569.69)
          gastrojejunal ulcer (534.0–534.9)
          gastrostomy complications (536.40–536.49)
          infection of esophagostomy (530.86) ◄
          infection of external stoma (569.61)
          mechanical complication of esophagostomy (530.87) ◄
          pelvic peritoneal adhesions, female (614.6)
          peritoneal adhesions (568.0)
          peritoneal adhesions with obstruction (560.81)
          postcholecystectomy syndrome (576.0)
          postgastric surgery syndromes (564.2)
          vomiting following gastrointestinal surgery (564.3)

997.5 Urinary complications
    Complications of:
       external stoma of urinary tract
       internal anastomosis and bypass of urinary tract, including that involving intestinal tract
       Oliguria or anuria specified as due to procedure
       Renal:
          failure (acute) specified as due to procedure
          insufficiency (acute) specified as due to procedure
       Tubular necrosis (acute) specified as due to procedure

    | **Excludes** | *specified complications classified elsewhere, such as:*
          postoperative stricture of:
            ureter (593.3)
            urethra (598.2)

● **997.6 Amputation stump complication**

    | **Excludes** | *admission for treatment for a current traumatic amputation—code to complicated traumatic amputation*
         phantom limb (syndrome) (353.6)

   ❑ **997.60 Unspecified complication**

   997.61 Neuroma of amputation stump

   997.62 Infection (chronic)
       Use additional code to identify the organism

   ❑ **997.69 Other**

● **997.7 Vascular complications of other vessels**

    | **Excludes** | *peripheral vascular complications (997.2)*

   997.71 Vascular complications of mesenteric artery

   997.72 Vascular complications of renal artery

   ❑ **997.79 Vascular complications of other vessels**

● **997.9 Complications affecting other specified body systems, not elsewhere classified**

Excludes specified complications classified elsewhere, such as:
broad ligament laceration syndrome (620.6)
postartificial menopause syndrome (627.4)
postoperative stricture of vagina (623.2)

997.91 Hypertension

Excludes Essential hypertension (401.0–401.9)

❑ **997.99 Other**
Vitreous touch syndrome

● **998 Other complications of procedures, NEC**

998.0 Postoperative shock
Collapse NOS during or resulting from a surgical procedure
Shock (endotoxic) (hypovolemic) (septic) during or resulting from a surgical procedure

Excludes shock:
anaphylactic due to serum (999.4)
anesthetic (995.4)
electric (994.8)
following abortion (639.5)
obstetric (669.1)
traumatic (958.4)

● **998.1 Hemorrhage or hematoma or seroma complicating a procedure**

Excludes hemorrhage, hematoma or seroma:
complicating cesarean section or puerperal perineal wound (674.3)

998.11 Hemorrhage complicating a procedure

998.12 Hematoma complicating a procedure

998.13 Seroma complicating a procedure

998.2 Accidental puncture or laceration during a procedure
Accidental perforation by catheter or other instrument during a procedure on:
blood vessel
nerve
organ

Excludes iatrogenic [postoperative] pneumothorax (512.1)
puncture or laceration caused by implanted device intentionally left in operation wound (996.0–996.5)
specified complications classified elsewhere, such as:
broad ligament laceration syndrome (620.6)
trauma from instruments during delivery (664.0–665.9)

● **998.3 Disruption of operation wound**
Dehiscence of operation wound
Rupture of operation wound

Excludes disruption of:
cesarean wound (674.1)
perineal wound, puerperal (674.2)

998.31 Disruption of internal operation wound

998.32 Disruption of external operation wound
Disruption of operation wound NOS

998.4 Foreign body accidentally left during a procedure
Adhesions due to foreign body accidentally left in operative wound or body cavity during a procedure
Obstruction due to foreign body accidentally left in operative wound or body cavity during a procedure
Perforation due to foreign body accidentally left in operative wound or body cavity during a procedure

Excludes obstruction or perforation caused by implanted device intentionally left in body (996.0–996.5)

● **998.5 Postoperative infection**

Excludes infection due to:
implanted device (996.60–996.69)
infusion, perfusion, or transfusion (999.3)
postoperative obstetrical wound infection (674.3)

998.51 Infected postoperative seroma
Use additional code to identify organism

❑ **998.59 Other postoperative infection**
Abscess: postoperative
intra-abdominal postoperative
stitch postoperative
subphrenic postoperative
wound postoperative
Septicemia postoperative

Use additional code to identify infection

998.6 Persistent postoperative fistula

998.7 Acute reaction to foreign substance accidentally left during a procedure
Peritonitis:
aseptic
chemical

● **998.8 Other specified complications of procedures, not elsewhere classified**

998.81 Emphysema (subcutaneous) (surgical) resulting from a procedure

998.82 Cataract fragments in eye following cataract surgery

998.83 Non-healing surgical wound

❑ **998.89 Other specified complications**

❑ **998.9 Unspecified complication of procedure, not elsewhere classified**
Postoperative complication NOS

Excludes complication NOS of obstetrical surgery or procedure (669.4)

● **999 Complications of medical care, not elsewhere classified**

Includes: complications, not elsewhere classified, of:
dialysis (hemodialysis) (peritoneal) (renal)
extracorporeal circulation
hyperalimentation therapy
immunization
infusion
inhalation therapy
injection
inoculation
perfusion
transfusion
vaccination
ventilation therapy

Excludes specified complications classified elsewhere such as:
complications of implanted device (996.0–996.9)
contact dermatitis due to drugs (692.3)
dementia dialysis (294.8)
transient (293.9)
dialysis disequilibrium syndrome (276.0–276.9)
poisoning and toxic effects of drugs and chemicals (960.0–989.9)
postvaccinal encephalitis (323.5)
water and electrolyte imbalance (276.0–276.9)

999.0 Generalized vaccinia

999.1 Air embolism
> Air embolism to any site following infusion, perfusion, or transfusion
>
> **Excludes** *embolism specified as:*
> > *complicating:*
> > > *abortion (634–638 with .6, 639.6)*
> > > *ectopic or molar pregnancy (639.6)*
> > > *pregnancy, childbirth, or the puerperium (673.0)*
> > *due to implanted device (996.7)*
> > *traumatic (958.0)*

❑ **999.2 Other vascular complications**
> Phlebitis following infusion, perfusion, or transfusion
> Thromboembolism following infusion, perfusion, or transfusion
> Thrombophlebitis following infusion, perfusion, or transfusion
>
> **Excludes** *the listed conditions when specified as:*
> > *due to implanted device (996.61–996.62, 996.72–996.74)*
> > *postoperative NOS (997.2, 997.71–997.79)*

❑ **999.3 Other infection**
> Infection following infusion, injection, transfusion, or vaccination
> Sepsis following infusion, injection, transfusion, or vaccination
> Septicemia following infusion, injection, transfusion, or vaccination
>
> **Excludes** *the listed conditions when specified as:*
> > *due to implanted device (996.60–996.69)*
> > *postoperative NOS (998.51–998.59)*

999.4 Anaphylactic shock due to serum
> **Excludes** *shock:*
> > *allergic NOS (995.0)*
> > *anaphylactic:*
> > > *NOS (995.0)*
> > > *due to drugs and chemicals (995.0)*

❑ **999.5 Other serum reaction**
> Intoxication by serum   Serum sickness
> Protein sickness   Urticaria due to serum
> Serum rash
>
> **Excludes** *serum hepatitis (070.2–070.3)*

999.6 ABO incompatibility reaction
> Incompatible blood transfusion
> Reaction to blood group incompatibility in infusion or transfusion

999.7 Rh incompatibility reaction
> Reactions due to Rh factor in infusion or transfusion

❑ **999.8 Other transfusion reaction**
> Septic shock due to transfusion
> Transfusion reaction NOS
>
> **Excludes** *postoperative shock (998.0)*

❑ **999.9 Other and unspecified complications of medical care, not elsewhere classified**
> Complications, not elsewhere classified, of:
> > electroshock therapy
> > inhalation therapy
> > ultrasound therapy
> > ventilation therapy
> Unspecified misadventure of medical care
>
> **Excludes** *unspecified complication of:*
> > *phototherapy (990)*
> > *radiation therapy (990)*

V-Codes—SUPPLEMENTARY CLASSIFICATION OF FACTORS INFLUENCING HEALTH STATUS AND CONTACT WITH HEALTH SERVICES (V01–V84) ◀▥

This classification is provided to deal with occasions when circumstances other than a disease or injury classifiable to categories 001–999 (the main part of ICD) are recorded as "diagnoses" or "problems." This can arise mainly in three ways:

a) When a person who is not currently sick encounters the health services for some specific purpose, such as to act as a donor of an organ or tissue, to receive prophylactic vaccination, or to discuss a problem which is in itself not a disease or injury. This will be a fairly rare occurrence among hospital inpatients, but will be relatively more common among hospital outpatients and patients of family practitioners, health clinics, etc.

b) When a person with a known disease or injury, whether it is current or resolving, encounters the health care system for a specific treatment of that disease or injury (e.g., dialysis for renal disease; chemotherapy for malignancy; cast change).

c) When some circumstance or problem is present which influences the person's health status but is not in itself a current illness or injury. Such factors may be elicited during population surveys, when the person may or may not be currently sick, or be recorded as an additional factor to be borne in mind when the person is receiving care for some current illness or injury classifiable to categories 001–999.

In the latter circumstances the V code should be used only as a supplementary code and should not be the one selected for use in primary, single cause tabulations. Examples of these circumstances are a personal history of certain diseases, or a person with an artificial heart valve in situ.

PERSONS WITH POTENTIAL HEALTH HAZARDS RELATED TO COMMUNICABLE DISEASES (V01–V06)

> **Excludes** *family history of infectious and parasitic diseases (V18.8)*
> *personal history of infectious and parasitic diseases (V12.0)*

● **V01   Contact with or exposure to communicable diseases**

   ● **V01.0   Cholera**
       Conditions classifiable to 001

   ● **V01.1   Tuberculosis**
       Conditions classifiable to 010–018

   ● **V01.2   Poliomyelitis**
       Conditions classifiable to 045

   ● **V01.3   Smallpox**
       Conditions classifiable to 050

   ● **V01.4   Rubella**
       Conditions classifiable to 056

   ● **V01.5   Rabies**
       Conditions classifiable to 071

   ● **V01.6   Venereal diseases**
       Conditions classifiable to 090–099

   ● **V01.7   Other viral diseases**
       Conditions classifiable to 042–078, and V08, except as above

     ● **V01.71   Varicella** ◀

     ●□ **V01.79   Other viral diseases** ◀

● **V01.8   Other communicable diseases**
       Conditions classifiable to 001–136, except as above

   ● **V01.81   Anthrax**

   V01.82   Exposure to SARS-associated coronavirus

   V01.83   Escherichia coli (E. coli) ◀

   V01.84   Meningococcus ◀

   ●□ **V01.89   Other communicable diseases**

●□ **V01.9   Unspecified communicable disease**

● **V02   Carrier or suspected carrier of infectious diseases**

   ● **V02.0   Cholera**

   ● **V02.1   Typhoid**

   ● **V02.2   Amebiasis**

   ●□ **V02.3   Other gastrointestinal pathogens**

   ● **V02.4   Diphtheria**

   ● **V02.5   Other specified bacterial diseases**

     V02.51   Group B streptococcus

     ●□ **V02.52   Other streptococcus**

     ●□ **V02.59   Other specified bacterial diseases**
         Meningococcal
         Staphylococcal

   ● **V02.6   Viral hepatitis**

     ●□ **V02.60   Viral hepatitis carrier, unspecified**

     ● **V02.61   Hepatitis B carrier**

     ● **V02.62   Hepatitis C carrier**

     ●□ **V02.69   Other viral hepatitis carrier**

   ● **V02.7   Gonorrhea**

   ●□ **V02.8   Other venereal diseases**

   ●□ **V02.9   Other specified infectious organism**

● **V03   Need for prophylactic vaccination and inoculation against bacterial diseases**

> **Excludes** *vaccination not carried out because of contraindication (V64.0)*
> *vaccines against combinations of diseases (V06.0–V06.9)*

   ● **V03.0   Cholera alone**

   ● **V03.1   Typhoid-paratyphoid alone [TAB]**

   ● **V03.2   Tuberculosis [BCG]**

   ● **V03.3   Plague**

   ● **V03.4   Tularemia**

   ● **V03.5   Diphtheria alone**

   ● **V03.6   Pertussis alone**

   ● **V03.7   Tetanus toxoid alone**

   ● **V03.8   Other specified vaccinations against single bacterial diseases**

     ● **V03.81   Haemophilus influenzae, type B [Hib]**

     ● **V03.82   Streptococcus pneumoniae [pneumococcus]**

     ●□ **V03.89   Other specified vaccination**

   ●□ **V03.9   Unspecified single bacterial disease**

ICD-9-CM

V01–V09

Vol. 1

● **V04 Need for prophylactic vaccination and inoculation against certain diseases**

Excludes *vaccines against combinations of diseases(V06.0– V06.9)*

- ● V04.0 Poliomyelitis
- ● V04.1 Smallpox
- ● V04.2 Measles alone
- ● V04.3 Rubella alone
- ● V04.4 Yellow fever
- ● V04.5 Rabies
- ● V04.6 Mumps alone
- ● V04.7 Common cold
- ● V04.8 Other viral diseases
  - ● V04.81 Influenza
  - ● V04.82 Respiratory syncytial virus (RSV)
  - ●☐ V04.89 Other viral disease

● **V05 Need for prophylactic vaccination and inoculation against single diseases**

Excludes *vaccines against combinations of diseases (V06.0–V06.9)*

- ● V05.0 Arthropod-borne viral encephalitis
- ●☐ V05.1 Other arthropod-borne viral diseases
- ● V05.2 Leishmaniasis
- ● V05.3 Viral hepatitis
- ● V05.4 Varicella
  - Chicken pox
- ●☐ V05.8 Other specified disease
- ●☐ V05.9 Unspecified single disease

● **V06 Need for prophylactic vaccination and inoculation against combinations of diseases**

Note: Use additional single vaccination codes from categories V03–V05 to identify any vaccinations not included in a combination code.

- ● V06.0 Cholera with typhoid-paratyphoid [cholera TAB]
- ● V06.1 Diphtheria-tetanus-pertussis, combined [DTP] [DTaP]
- ● V06.2 Diphtheria-tetanus-pertussis with typhoid-paratyphoid [DTP TAB]
- ● V06.3 Diphtheria-tetanus-pertussis with poliomyelitis [DTP+polio]
- ● V06.4 Measles-mumps-rubella [MMR]
- ● V06.5 Tetanus-diphtheria [Td] [DT]
- ● V06.6 Streptococcus pneumoniae [pneumococcus] and influenza
- ●☐ V06.8 Other combinations

Excludes *multiple single vaccination codes (V03.0–V05.9)*

- ●☐ V06.9 Unspecified combined vaccine

PERSONS WITH NEED FOR ISOLATION, OTHER POTENTIAL HEALTH HAZARDS AND PROPHYLACTIC MEASURES (V07–V09)

● **V07 Need for isolation and other prophylactic measures**

Excludes *prophylactic organ removal (V50.41–V50.49)*

- V07.0 Isolation
  - Admission to protect the individual from his surroundings or for isolation of individual after contact with infectious diseases
- ● V07.1 Desensitization to allergens
- ● V07.2 Prophylactic immunotherapy
  - Administration of:
    - antivenin
    - immune sera [gamma globulin]
    - RhoGAM
    - tetanus antitoxin
- ● V07.3 Other prophylactic chemotherapy
  - ● V07.31 Prophylactic fluoride administration
  - ☐ V07.39 Other prophylactic chemotherapy

Excludes *maintenance chemotherapy following disease (V58.1)*

- ● V07.4 Hormone replacement therapy (post-menopausal) ◀▥
- ☐ V07.8 Other specified prophylactic measure
- ●☐ V07.9 Unspecified prophylactic measure

● **V08 Asymptomatic human immunodeficiency virus [HIV] infection status**

HIV positive NOS

Note: This code is ONLY to be used when NO HIV infection symptoms or conditions are present. If any HIV infection symptoms or conditions are present, see code 042.

Excludes *AIDS (042)*
human immunodeficiency virus [HIV] disease (042)
exposure to HIV (V01.79) ◀▥
nonspecific serologic evidence of HIV (795.71)
symptomatic human immunodeficiency virus [HIV] infection (042)

● **V09 Infection with drug-resistant microorganisms**

Note: This category is intended for use as an additional code for infectious conditions classified elsewhere to indicate the presence of drug-resistance of the infectious organism.

- ● V09.0 Infection with microorganisms resistant to penicillins
  - Methicillin-resistant staphylococcus aureus (MRSA) ◀
- ● V09.1 Infection with microorganisms resistant to cephalosporins and other B-lactam antibiotics
- ● V09.2 Infection with microorganisms resistant to macrolides
- ● V09.3 Infection with microorganisms resistant to tetracyclines
- ● V09.4 Infection with microorganisms resistant to aminoglycosides

● **V09.5 Infection with microorganisms resistant to quinolones and fluoroquinolones**

  ● **V09.50 Without mention of resistance to multiple quinolones and fluoroquinols**

  ● **V09.51 With resistance to multiple quinolones and fluoroquinols**

● **V09.6 Infection with microorganisms resistant to sulfonamides**

● **V09.7 Infection with microorganisms resistant to other specified antimycobacterial agents**

  Excludes *amikacin (V09.4)*
              kanamycin (V09.4)
              streptomycin [SM] (V09.4)

  ●❑ **V09.70 Without mention of resistance to multiple antimycobacterial agents**

  ●❑ **V09.71 With resistance to multiple antimycobacterial agents**

● **V09.8 Infection with microorganisms resistant to other specified drugs**
  Vancomycin (glycopeptide) intermediate staphylococcus aureus (VISA/GISA) ◀
  Vancomycin (glycopeptide) resistant enterococcus (VRE) ◀
  Vancomycin (glycopeptide) resistant staphylococcus aureus (VRSA/GRSA) ◀

  ●❑ **V09.80 Without mention of resistance to multiple drugs**

  ●❑ **V09.81 With resistance to multiple drugs**

● **V09.9 Infection with drug-resistant microorganisms, unspecified**
  Drug resistance NOS

  ●❑ **V09.90 Without mention of multiple drug resistance**

  ●❑ **V09.91 With multiple drug resistance**
    Multiple drug resistance NOS

PERSONS WITH POTENTIAL HEALTH HAZARDS RELATED TO PERSONAL AND FAMILY HISTORY (V10–V19)

  Excludes *obstetric patients where the possibility that the fetus might be affected is the reason for observation or management during pregnancy (655.0–655.9)*

● **V10 Personal history of malignant neoplasm**

  ● **V10.0 Gastrointestinal tract**
    History of conditions classifiable to 140–159

    ●❑ **V10.00 Gastrointestinal tract, unspecified**

    ● **V10.01 Tongue**

    ●❑ **V10.02 Other and unspecified oral cavity and pharynx**

    ● **V10.03 Esophagus**

    ● **V10.04 Stomach**

    ● **V10.05 Large intestine**

    ● **V10.06 Rectum, rectosigmoid junction, and anus**

    ● **V10.07 Liver**

    ●❑ **V10.09 Other**

● **V10.1 Trachea, bronchus, and lung**
  History of conditions classifiable to 162

  ● **V10.11 Bronchus and lung**

  ● **V10.12 Trachea**

● **V10.2 Other respiratory and intrathoracic organs**
  History of conditions classifiable to 160, 161, 163–165

  ●❑ **V10.20 Respiratory organ, unspecified**

  ● **V10.21 Larynx**

  ● **V10.22 Nasal cavities, middle ear, and accessory sinuses**

  ●❑ **V10.29 Other**

● **V10.3 Breast**
  History of conditions classifiable to 174 and 175

● **V10.4 Genital organs**
  History of conditions classifiable to 179–187

  ●❑ **V10.40 Female genital organ, unspecified**

  ● **V10.41 Cervix uteri**

  ●❑ **V10.42 Other parts of uterus**

  ● **V10.43 Ovary**

  ●❑ **V10.44 Other female genital organs**

  ●❑ **V10.45 Male genital organ, unspecified**

  ● **V10.46 Prostate**

  ● **V10.47 Testis**

  ● **V10.48 Epididymis**

  ●❑ **V10.49 Other male genital organs**

● **V10.5 Urinary organs**
  History of conditions classifiable to 188 and 189

  ●❑ **V10.50 Urinary organ, unspecified**

  ● **V10.51 Bladder**

  ● **V10.52 Kidney**

  Excludes *renal pelvis (V10.53)*

  ● **V10.53 Renal pelvis**

  ●❑ **V10.59 Other**

● **V10.6 Leukemia**
  Conditions classifiable to 204–208

  Excludes *leukemia in remission (204–208)*

  ●❑ **V10.60 Leukemia, unspecified**

  ● **V10.61 Lymphoid leukemia**

  ● **V10.62 Myeloid leukemia**

  ● **V10.63 Monocytic leukemia**

  ●❑ **V10.69 Other**

● **V10.7 Other lymphatic and hematopoietic neoplasms**
  Conditions classifiable to 200–203

  Excludes *listed conditions in 200–203 in remission*

  ● **V10.71 Lymphosarcoma and reticulosarcoma**

  ● **V10.72 Hodgkin's disease**

  ●❑ **V10.79 Other**

● **V10.8 Personal history of malignant neoplasm of other sites**
    History of conditions classifiable to 170–173, 190–195

   ● **V10.81 Bone**

   ● **V10.82 Malignant melanoma of skin**

   ●❑ **V10.83 Other malignant neoplasm of skin**

   ● **V10.84 Eye**

   ● **V10.85 Brain**

   ●❑ **V10.86 Other parts of nervous system**

   Excludes *peripheral, sympathetic, and parasympathetic nerves (V10.89)*

   ● **V10.87 Thyroid**

   ●❑ **V10.88 Other endocrine glands and related structures**

   ●❑ **V10.89 Other**

●❑ **V10.9 Unspecified personal history of malignant neoplasm**

● **V11 Personal history of mental disorder**

   ● **V11.0 Schizophrenia**

   Excludes *that in remission (295.0–295.9 with fifth-digit 5)*

   ● **V11.1 Affective disorders**
      Personal history of manic-depressive psychosis

   Excludes *that in remission (296.0–296.6 with fifth-digit 5, 6)*

   ● **V11.2 Neurosis**

   ● **V11.3 Alcoholism**

   ●❑ **V11.8 Other mental disorders**

   ●❑ **V11.9 Unspecified mental disorder**

● **V12 Personal history of certain other diseases**

   ● **V12.0 Infectious and parasitic diseases**

     ●❑ **V12.00 Unspecified infectious and parasitic disease**

     ● **V12.01 Tuberculosis**

     ● **V12.02 Poliomyelitis**

     ● **V12.03 Malaria**

     ●❑ **V12.09 Other**

   ● **V12.1 Nutritional deficiency**

   ● **V12.2 Endocrine, metabolic, and immunity disorders**

   Excludes *history of allergy (V14.0–V14.9, V15.01–V15.09)*

   ● **V12.3 Diseases of blood and blood-forming organs**

   ● **V12.4 Disorders of nervous system and sense organs**

     ●❑ **V12.40 Unspecified disorder of nervous system and sense organs**

     ● **V12.41 Benign neoplasm of the brain**

     ●❑ **V12.49 Other disorders of nervous system and sense organs**

● **V12.5 Diseases of circulatory system**

   Excludes *old myocardial infarction (412)*
      postmyocardial infarction syndrome (411.0)

   ●❑ **V12.50 Unspecified circulatory disease**

   ● **V12.51 Venous thrombosis and embolism**
      Pulmonary embolism

   ● **V12.52 Thrombophlebitis**

   ●❑ **V12.59 Other**

● **V12.6 Diseases of respiratory system**

● **V12.7 Diseases of digestive system**

   ●❑ **V12.70 Unspecified digestive disease**

   ● **V12.71 Peptic ulcer disease**

   ● **V12.72 Colonic polyps**

   ●❑ **V12.79 Other**

● **V13 Personal history of other diseases**

   ● **V13.0 Disorders of urinary system**

     ●❑ **V13.00 Unspecified urinary disorder**

     ● **V13.01 Urinary calculi**

     ●❑ **V13.09 Other**

   ● **V13.1 Trophoblastic disease**

   Excludes *supervision during a current pregnancy (V23.1)*

   ●❑ **V13.2 Other genital system and obstetric disorders**

   Excludes *supervision during a current pregnancy of a woman with poor obstetric history (V23.0–V23.9)*
      habitual aborter (646.3)
        without current pregnancy (629.9)

     ● **V13.21 Personal history of pre-term labor**

   Excludes *current pregnancy with history of pre-term labor (V23.41)*

     ●❑ **V13.29 Other genital system and obstetric disorders**

   ● **V13.3 Diseases of skin and subcutaneous tissue**

   ● **V13.4 Arthritis**

   ●❑ **V13.5 Other musculoskeletal disorders**

   ● **V13.6 Congenital malformations**

     ● **V13.61 Hypospadias**

     ●❑ **V13.69 Other congenital malformations**

   ● **V13.7 Perinatal problems**

   Excludes *low birth weight status (V21.30–V21.35)*

   ●❑ **V13.8 Other specified diseases**

   ●❑ **V13.9 Unspecified disease**

● **V14 Personal history of allergy to medicinal agents**

   ● **V14.0 Penicillin**

   ●❑ **V14.1 Other antibiotic agent**

   ● **V14.2 Sulfonamides**

   ●❑ **V14.3 Other anti-infective agent**

   ● **V14.4 Anesthetic agent**

   ● **V14.5 Narcotic agent**

- V14.6 **Analgesic agent**
- V14.7 **Serum or vaccine**
- ☐ V14.8 **Other specified medicinal agents**
- ☐ V14.9 **Unspecified medicinal agent**
- V15 **Other personal history presenting hazards to health**
- ☐ V15.0 **Allergy, other than to medicinal agents**

  Excludes *allergy to food substance used as base for medicinal agent (V14.0–V14.9)*

  - V15.01 **Allergy to peanuts**
  - V15.02 **Allergy to milk products**

    Excludes *lactose intolerance (271.3)*

  - V15.03 **Allergy to eggs**
  - V15.04 **Allergy to seafood**
    Seafood (octopus) (squid) ink
    Shellfish
  - V15.05 **Allergy to other foods**
    Food additives
    Nuts other than peanuts
  - V15.06 **Allergy to insects**
    Bugs
    Insect bites and stings
    Spiders
  - V15.07 **Allergy to latex**
    Latex sensitivity
  - V15.08 **Allergy to radiographic dye**
    Contrast media used for diagnostic x-ray procedures
  - V15.09 **Other allergy, other than to medicinal agents**

- V15.1 **Surgery to heart and great vessels**

  Excludes *replacement by transplant or other means (V42.1–V42.2, V43.2–V43.4)*

- ☐ V15.2 **Surgery to other major organs**

  Excludes *replacement by transplant or other means (V42.0–V43.8)*

- V15.3 **Irradiation**
  Previous exposure to therapeutic or other ionizing radiation
- V15.4 **Psychological trauma**

  Excludes *history of condition classifiable to 290–316 (V11.0–V11.9)*

  - V15.41 **History of physical abuse**
    Rape
  - V15.42 **History of emotional abuse**
    Neglect
  - ☐ V15.49 **Other**

- V15.5 **Injury**
- V15.6 **Poisoning**
- V15.7 **Contraception**

  Excludes *current contraceptive management (V25.0–V25.4)*
  presence of intrauterine contraceptive device as incidental finding (V45.5)

- V15.8 **Other specified personal history presenting hazards to health**

  - V15.81 **Noncompliance with medical treatment**
  - V15.82 **History of tobacco use**

    Excludes *tobacco dependence (305.1)*

- V15.84 **Exposure to asbestos**
- V15.85 **Exposure to potentially hazardous body fluids**
- V15.86 **Exposure to lead**
- V15.87 **History of Extracorporeal Membrane Oxygenation [ECMO]**
- ☐ V15.89 **Other**
- ☐ V15.9 **Unspecified personal history presenting hazards to health**

- V16 **Family history of malignant neoplasm**
  - V16.0 **Gastrointestinal tract**
    Family history of condition classifiable to 140–159
  - V16.1 **Trachea, bronchus, and lung**
    Family history of condition classifiable to 162
  - ☐ V16.2 **Other respiratory and intrathoracic organs**
    Family history of condition classifiable to 160–161, 163–165
  - V16.3 **Breast**
    Family history of condition classifiable to 174
  - V16.4 **Genital organs**
    Family history of condition classifiable to 179–187

    - ☐ V16.40 **Genital organ, unspecified**
    - V16.41 **Ovary**
    - V16.42 **Prostate**
    - V16.43 **Testis**
    - ☐ V16.49 **Other**

  - V16.5 **Urinary organs**
    Family history of condition classifiable to 189

    - V16.51 **Kidney**
    - ☐ V16.59 **Other**

  - V16.6 **Leukemia**
    Family history of condition classifiable to 204–208
  - ☐ V16.7 **Other lymphatic and hematopoietic neoplasms**
    Family history of condition classifiable to 200–203
  - ☐ V16.8 **Other specified malignant neoplasm**
    Family history of other condition classifiable to 140–199
  - ☐ V16.9 **Unspecified malignant neoplasm**

- V17 **Family history of certain chronic disabling diseases**
  - V17.0 **Psychiatric condition**

    Excludes *family history of mental retardation (V18.4)*

  - V17.1 **Stroke (cerebrovascular)**
  - ☐ V17.2 **Other neurological diseases**
    Epilepsy
    Huntington's chorea
  - V17.3 **Ischemic heart disease**
  - ☐ V17.4 **Other cardiovascular diseases**
  - V17.5 **Asthma**

ICD-9-CM
V01-V99
Vol. 1

●❏V17.6 Other chronic respiratory conditions

● V17.7 Arthritis

●❏V17.8 Other musculoskeletal diseases

● V18 Family history of certain other specific conditions

● V18.0 Diabetes mellitus

●❏V18.1 Other endocrine and metabolic diseases

● V18.2 Anemia

●❏V18.3 Other blood disorders

● V18.4 Mental retardation

● V18.5 Digestive disorders

● V18.6 Kidney diseases

● V18.61 Polycystic kidney

●❏V18.69 Other kidney diseases

●❏V18.7 Other genitourinary diseases

● V18.8 Infectious and parasitic diseases

● V19 Family history of other conditions

● V19.0 Blindness or visual loss

●❏V19.1 Other eye disorders

● V19.2 Deafness or hearing loss

●❏V19.3 Other ear disorders

● V19.4 Skin conditions

● V19.5 Congenital anomalies

● V19.6 Allergic disorders

● V19.7 Consanguinity

●❏V19.8 Other condition

PERSONS ENCOUNTERING HEALTH SERVICES IN CIRCUMSTANCES RELATED TO REPRODUCTION AND DEVELOPMENT (V20–V29)

● V20 Health supervision of infant or child

  V20.0 Foundling

●❏V20.1 Other healthy infant or child receiving care
    Medical or nursing care supervision of
      healthy infant in cases of:
    maternal illness, physical or psychiatric
    socioeconomic adverse condition at home
    too many children at home preventing or
      interfering with normal care

● V20.2 Routine infant or child health check
    Developmental testing of infant or child
    Immunizations appropriate for age
    Routine vision and hearing testing

Excludes special screening for developmental handicaps
          (V79.3)

    Use additional code(s) to identify:
    Special screening examination(s) performed
      (V73.0–V82.9)

● V21 Constitutional states in development

● V21.0 Period of rapid growth in childhood

● V21.1 Puberty

●❏V21.2 Other adolescence

● V21.3 Low birth weight status

Excludes history of perinatal problems (V13.7)

●❏V21.30 Low birth weight status,
          unspecified

●❏V21.31 Low birth weight status, less than
          500 grams

●❏V21.32 Low birth weight status, 500–999
          grams

●❏V21.33 Low birth weight status, 1000–1499
          grams

●❏V21.34 Low birth weight status, 1500–1999
          grams

●❏V21.35 Low birth weight status, 2000–2500
          grams

●❏V21.8 Other specified constitutional states in devel-
         opment

●❏V21.9 Unspecified constitutional state in develop-
         ment

● V22 Normal pregnancy

Excludes pregnancy examination or test, pregnancy un-
          confirmed (V72.40)   ◀▬

● V22.0 Supervision of normal first pregnancy

● V22.1 Supervision of other normal pregnancy

● V22.2 Pregnant state, incidental
          Pregnant state NOS

● V23 Supervision of high-risk pregnancy

● V23.0 Pregnancy with history of infertility

● V23.1 Pregnancy with history of trophoblastic disease
          Pregnancy with history of:
            hydatidiform mole
            vesicular mole

Excludes that without current pregnancy (V13.1)

● V23.2 Pregnancy with history of abortion
          Pregnancy with history of conditions classi-
            fiable to 634–638

Excludes habitual aborter:
            care during pregnancy (646.3)
            that without current pregnancy (629.9)

● V23.3 Grand multiparity

Excludes care in relation to labor and delivery (659.4)
            that without current pregnancy (V61.5)

●❏V23.4 Pregnancy with other poor obstetric history
          Pregnancy with history of other conditions
            classifiable to 630–676

● V23.41 Pregnancy with history of pre-term
           labor

●❏V23.49 Pregnancy with other poor obstetric
          history

●❏V23.5 Pregnancy with other poor reproductive his-
         tory
          Pregnancy with history of stillbirth or neo-
            natal death

● V23.7 Insufficient prenatal care
          History of little or no prenatal care

● V23.8 Other high-risk pregnancy

● V23.81 Elderly primigravida
           First pregnancy in a woman who
             will be 35 years of age or older
             at expected date of delivery

Excludes elderly primigravida complcating pregnancy
          (659.5)

● **V23.82 Elderly multigravida**
　　Second or more pregnancy in a woman who will be 35 years of age or older at expected date of delivery

Excludes *elderly multigravida complicating pregnancy (659.6)*

● **V23.83 Young primigravida**
　　First pregnancy in a female less than 16 years old at expected date of delivery

Excludes *young primigravida complicating pregnancy (659.8)*

● **V23.84 Young multigravida**
　　Second or more pregnancy in a female less than 16 years old at expected date of delivery

Excludes *young multigravida complicating pregnancy (659.8)*

●▢ **V23.89 Other high-risk pregnancy**

●▢ **V23.9 Unspecified high-risk pregnancy**

● **V24 Postpartum care and examination**

V24.0 Immediately after delivery
　　Care and observation in uncomplicated cases

● **V24.1 Lactating mother**
　　Supervision of lactation

● **V24.2 Routine postpartum follow-up**

● **V25 Encounter for contraceptive management**

● **V25.0 General counseling and advice**

● **V25.01 Prescription of oral contraceptives**

●▢ **V25.02 Initiation of other contraceptive measures**
　　Fitting of diaphragm
　　Prescription of foams, creams, or other agents

● **V25.03 Encounter for emergency contraceptive counseling and prescription**
　　Encounter for postcoital contraceptive counseling and prescription

●▢ **V25.09 Other**
　　Family planning advice

● **V25.1 Insertion of intrauterine contraceptive device**

V25.2 Sterilization
　　Admission for interruption of fallopian tubes or vas deferens

V25.3 Menstrual extraction
　　Menstrual regulation

● **V25.4 Surveillance of previously prescribed contraceptive methods**
　　Checking, reinsertion, or removal of contraceptive device
　　Repeat prescription for contraceptive method
　　Routine examination in connection with contraceptive maintenance

Excludes *presence of intrauterine contraceptive device as incidental finding (V45.5)*

●▢ **V25.40 Contraceptive surveillance, unspecified**

● **V25.41 Contraceptive pill**

● **V25.42 Intrauterine contraceptive device**
　　Checking, reinsertion, or removal of intrauterine device

● **V25.43 Implantable subdermal contraceptive**

●▢ **V25.49 Other contraceptive method**

● **V25.5 Insertion of implantable subdermal contraceptive**

●▢ **V25.8 Other specified contraceptive management**
　　Postvasectomy sperm count

Excludes *sperm count following sterilization reversal (V26.22)*
　　sperm count for fertility testing (V26.21)

●▢ **V25.9 Unspecified contraceptive management**

● **V26 Procreative management**

V26.0 Tuboplasty or vasoplasty after previous sterilization

● **V26.1 Artificial insemination**

● **V26.2 Investigation and testing**

Excludes *postvasectomy sperm count (V25.8)*

● **V26.21 Fertility testing**
　　Fallopian insufflation
　　Sperm count for fertility testing

Excludes *Genetic counseling and testing (V26.3)*

● **V26.22 Aftercare following sterilization reversal**
　　Fallopian insufflation following sterilization reversal
　　Sperm count following sterilization reversal

● **V26.29 Other investigation and testing**

● **V26.3 Genetic counseling and testing**

Excludes *fertility testing (V26.21)*

● **V26.4 General counseling and advice**

● **V26.5 Sterilization status**

V26.51 Tubal ligation status

Excludes *infertility not due to previous tubal ligation (628.0–628.9)*

V26.52 Vasectomy status

●▢ **V26.8 Other specified procreative management**

●▢ **V26.9 Unspecified procreative management**

● **V27 Outcome of delivery**
　　Note: This category is intended for the coding of the outcome of delivery on the mother's record.

● **V27.0 Single liveborn**

● **V27.1 Single stillborn**

● **V27.2 Twins, both liveborn**

● **V27.3 Twins, one liveborn and one stillborn**

● **V27.4 Twins, both stillborn**

●▢ **V27.5 Other multiple birth, all liveborn**

ICD-9-CM

V01-
V09

● ◻ **V27.6** Other multiple birth, some liveborn

● ◻ **V27.7** Other multiple birth, all stillborn

● ◻ **V27.9** Unspecified outcome of delivery
     Single birth, outcome to infant unspecified
     Multiple birth, outcome to infant unspecified

● **V28** Antenatal screening

    Excludes *abnormal findings on screening—code to findings*
          routine prenatal care (V22.0–V23.9)

  ● **V28.0** Screening for chromosomal anomalies by amniocentesis

  ● **V28.1** Screening for raised alpha-fetoprotein levels in amniotic fluid

  ● ◻ **V28.2** Other screening based on amniocentesis

  ● **V28.3** Screening for malformation using ultrasonics

  ● **V28.4** Screening for fetal growth retardation using ultrasonics

  ● **V28.5** Screening for isoimmunization

  ● **V28.6** Screening for Streptococcus B

  ● ◻ **V28.8** Other specified antenatal screening

  ● ◻ **V28.9** Unspecified antenatal screening

● **V29** Observation and evaluation of newborns for suspected condition not found

    Note: This category is to be used for newborns, within the neonatal period (the first 28 days of life), who are suspected of having an abnormal condition resulting from exposure from the mother or the birth process, but without signs or symptoms, and which, after examination and observation, is found not to exist.

    V29.0 Observation for suspected infectious condition

    V29.1 Observation for suspected neurological condition

    V29.2 Observation for suspected respiratory condition

  ● **V29.3** Observation for suspected genetic or metabolic condition

  ◻ **V29.8** Observation for other specified suspected condition

  ● ◻ **V29.9** Observation for unspecified suspected condition

LIVEBORN INFANTS ACCORDING TO TYPE OF BIRTH (V30–V39)

    Note: These categories are intended for the coding of liveborn infants who are consuming health care [e.g., crib or bassinet occupancy].

    The following fourth-digit subdivisions are for use with categories V30–V39:
    .0 **Born in hospital**
    .1 **Born before admission to hospital**
  ● .2 **Born outside hospital and not hospitalized**

    The following two fifth-digits are for use with the fourth-digit .0, born in hospital:
    0 **delivered without mention of cesarean delivery**
    1 **delivered by cesarean delivery**

● **V30** Single liveborn

● **V31** Twin, mate liveborn

● **V32** Twin, mate stillborn

● ◻ **V33** Twin, unspecified

● ◻ **V34** Other multiple, mates all liveborn

● ◻ **V35** Other multiple, mates all stillborn

● ◻ **V36** Other multiple, mates live- and stillborn

● ◻ **V37** Other multiple, unspecified

● ◻ **V39** Unspecified

PERSONS WITH A CONDITION INFLUENCING THEIR HEALTH STATUS (V40–V49)

    Note: These categories are intended for use when these conditions are recorded as "diagnoses" or "problems."

● **V40** Mental and behavioral problems

  ● **V40.0** Problems with learning

  ● **V40.1** Problems with communication [including speech]

  ● ◻ **V40.2** Other mental problems

  ● ◻ **V40.3** Other behavioral problems

  ● ◻ **V40.9** Unspecified mental or behavioral problem

● **V41** Problems with special senses and other special functions

  ● **V41.0** Problems with sight

  ● ◻ **V41.1** Other eye problems

  ● **V41.2** Problems with hearing

  ● ◻ **V41.3** Other ear problems

  ● **V41.4** Problems with voice production

  ● **V41.5** Problems with smell and taste

  ● **V41.6** Problems with swallowing and mastication

  ● **V41.7** Problems with sexual function

    Excludes *marital problems (V61.10)*
          psychosexual disorders (302.0–302.9)

  ● **V41.8** Other problems with special functions

  ● **V41.9** Unspecified problem with special functions

● **V42** Organ or tissue replaced by transplant

    Includes: homologous or heterologous (animal) (human) transplant organ status

  ● **V42.0** Kidney

  ● **V42.1** Heart

  ● **V42.2** Heart valve

  ● **V42.3** Skin

  ● **V42.4** Bone

  ● **V42.5** Cornea

  ● **V42.6** Lung

  ● **V42.7** Liver

  ● **V42.8** Other specified organ or tissue

    ● **V42.81** Bone marrow

    ● **V42.82** Peripheral stem cells

    ● **V42.83** Pancreas

    ● **V42.84** Intestines

    ● ◻ **V42.89** Other

  ● ◻ **V42.9** Unspecified organ or tissue

● **V43　Organ or tissue replaced by other means**

Includes: organ or tissue assisted by other means
　　　　　replacement of organ by:
　　　　　　　artificial device
　　　　　　　mechanical device
　　　　　　　prosthesis

Excludes cardiac pacemaker in situ (V45.01)
　　　　　fitting and adjustment of prosthetic device
　　　　　　(V52.0–V52.9)
　　　　　renal dialysis status (V45.1)

● **V43.0　Eye globe**

● **V43.1　Lens**
　　　　Pseudophakos

●● **V43.2　Heart**

　　　V43.21　Heart assist device

　　　V43.22　Fully implantable artificial heart

● **V43.3　Heart valve**

● **V43.4　Blood vessel**

● **V43.5　Bladder**

● **V43.6　Joint**

　●❑ **V43.60　Unspecified joint**

　● **V43.61　Shoulder**

　● **V43.62　Elbow**

　● **V43.63　Wrist**

　● **V43.64　Hip**

　● **V43.65　Knee**

　● **V43.66　Ankle**

　●❑ **V43.69　Other**

● **V43.7　Limb**

● **V43.8　Other organ or tissue**

　● **V43.81　Larynx**

　● **V43.82　Breast**

　● **V43.83　Artificial skin**

　●❑ **V43.89　Other**

● **V44　Artificial opening status**

Excludes artificial openings requiring attention or manage-
　　　　　ment (V55.0–V55.9)

● **V44.0　Tracheostomy**

● **V44.1　Gastrostomy**

● **V44.2　Ileostomy**

● **V44.3　Colostomy**

●❑ **V44.4　Other artificial opening of gastrointestinal
　　　　　tract**

● **V44.5　Cystostomy**

　●❑ **V44.50　Cystostomy, unspecified**

　● **V44.51　Cutaneous-vesicostomy**

　● **V44.52　Appendico-vesicostomy**

　●❑ **V44.59　Other cystostomy**

●❑ **V44.6　Other artificial opening of urinary tract**
　　　　Nephrostomy
　　　　Ureterostomy
　　　　Urethrostomy

● **V44.7　Artificial vagina**

●❑ **V44.8　Other artificial opening status**

●❑ **V44.9　Unspecified artificial opening status**

● **V45　Other postprocedural states**

Excludes aftercare management (V51–V58.9)
　　　　　malfunction or other complication—code to con-
　　　　　　dition

● **V45.0　Cardiac device in situ**

Excludes artificial heart (V43.22)
　　　　　heart assist device (V43.21)

　●❑ **V45.00　Unspecified cardiac device**

　● **V45.01　Cardiac pacemaker**

　● **V45.02　Automatic implantable cardiac defib-
　　　　　rillator**

　●❑ **V45.09　Other specified cardiac device**
　　　　　Carotid sinus pacemaker in situ

● **V45.1　Renal dialysis status**
　　　　Patient requiring intermittent renal dialysis
　　　　Presence of arterial-venous shunt (for dialy-
　　　　　sis)

Excludes admission for dialysis treatment or session
　　　　　(V56.0)

● **V45.2　Presence of cerebrospinal fluid drainage device**
　　　　Cerebral ventricle (communicating) shunt,
　　　　　valve, or device in situ

Excludes malfunction (996.2)

● **V45.3　Intestinal bypass or anastomosis status**

● **V45.4　Arthrodesis status**

● **V45.5　Presence of contraceptive device**

Excludes checking, reinsertion, or removal of device
　　　　　(V25.42)
　　　　　complication from device (996.32)
　　　　　insertion of device (V25.1)

　● **V45.51　Intrauterine contraceptive device**

　● **V45.52　Subdermal contraceptive implant**

　●❑ **V45.59　Other**

● **V45.6　States following surgery of eye and adnexa**

Excludes aphakia (379.31)
　　　　　artificial:
　　　　　　eye globe (V43.0)

　● **V45.61　Cataract extraction status**

　　　　Use additional code for associated ar-
　　　　　tificial lens status (V43.1)

　●❑ **V45.69　Other states following surgery of eye
　　　　　and adnexa**

● **V45.7　Acquired absence of organ**

　● **V45.71　Acquired absence of breast**

　● **V45.72　Acquired absence of intestine (large)
　　　　　(small)**

　● **V45.73　Acquired absence of kidney**

　● **V45.74　Other parts of urinary tract**
　　　　Bladder

　● **V45.75　Stomach**

　● **V45.76　Lung**

　● **V45.77　Genital organs**

Excludes female genital mutilation status
　　　　　(629.20–629.23)　　　　　　　　　　◄

　● **V45.78　Eye**

　● **V45.79　Other acquired absence of organ**

◄ **New**　　◄▬ **Revised**　　● **Not a Principal Diagnosis**　　● **Use Additional Digit(s)**　　❑ **Nonspecific Code**　　871

● **V45.8 Other postprocedural status**

  ● **V45.81 Aortocoronary bypass status**

  ● **V45.82 Percutaneous transluminal coronary angioplasty status**

  ● **V45.83 Breast implant removal status**

  ● **V45.84 Dental restoration status**
       Dental crowns status
       Dental fillings status

  ● **V45.85 Insulin pump status**

  ●❑ **V45.89 Other**
       Presence of neuropacemaker or other electronic device

  Excludes *artificial heart valve in situ (V43.3)*
       vascular prosthesis in situ (V43.4)

● **V46 Other dependence on machines**

  ● **V46.0 Aspirator**

  ● **V46.1 Respirator**
      Iron lung

    ● **V46.11 Dependence on respirator, status** ◀

    ● **V46.12 Encounter for respirator dependence during power failure** ◀

  ● **V46.2 Supplemental oxygen**
      Long-term oxygen therapy

  ●❑ **V46.8 Other enabling machines**
      Hyperbaric chamber
      Possum [Patient-Operated-Selector-Mechanism]

  Excludes *cardiac pacemaker (V45.0)*
       kidney dialysis machine (V45.1)

  ●❑ **V46.9 Unspecified machine dependence**

● **V47 Other problems with internal organs**

  ● **V47.0 Deficiencies of internal organs**

  ● **V47.1 Mechanical and motor problems with internal organs**

  ●❑ **V47.2 Other cardiorespiratory problems**
      Cardiovascular exercise intolerance with pain (with):
       at rest
       less than ordinary activity
       ordinary activity

  ●❑ **V47.3 Other digestive problems**

  ●❑ **V47.4 Other urinary problems**

  ●❑ **V47.5 Other genital problems**

  ●❑ **V47.9 Unspecified**

● **V48 Problems with head, neck, and trunk**

  ● **V48.0 Deficiencies of head**

  Excludes *deficiencies of ears, eyelids, and nose (V48.8)*

  ● **V48.1 Deficiencies of neck and trunk**

  ● **V48.2 Mechanical and motor problems with head**

  ● **V48.3 Mechanical and motor problems with neck and trunk**

  ● **V48.4 Sensory problem with head**

● **V48.5 Sensory problem with neck and trunk**

● **V48.6 Disfigurements of head**

● **V48.7 Disfigurements of neck and trunk**

●❑ **V48.8 Other problems with head, neck, and trunk**

●❑ **V48.9 Unspecified problem with head, neck, or trunk**

● **V49 Other conditions influencing health status**

  ● **V49.0 Deficiencies of limbs**

  ● **V49.1 Mechanical problems with limbs**

  ● **V49.2 Motor problems with limbs**

  ● **V49.3 Sensory problems with limbs**

  ● **V49.4 Disfigurements of limbs**

  ●❑ **V49.5 Other problems of limbs**

  ● **V49.6 Upper limb amputation status**

    ●❑ **V49.60 Unspecified level**

    ● **V49.61 Thumb**

    ●❑ **V49.62 Other finger(s)**

    ● **V49.63 Hand**

    ● **V49.64 Wrist**
       Disarticulation of wrist

    ● **V49.65 Below elbow**

    ● **V49.66 Above elbow**
       Disarticulation of elbow

    ● **V49.67 Shoulder**
       Disarticulation of shoulder

  ● **V49.7 Lower limb amputation status**

    ●❑ **V49.70 Unspecified level**

    ● **V49.71 Great toe**

    ●❑ **V49.72 Other toe(s)**

    ● **V49.73 Foot**

    ● **V49.74 Ankle**
       Disarticulation of ankle

    ● **V49.75 Below knee**

    ● **V49.76 Above knee**
       Disarticulation of knee

    ● **V49.77 Hip**
       Disarticulation of hip

  ● **V49.8 Other specified conditions influencing health status**

    ● **V49.81 Asymptomatic postmenopausal status (age-related) (natural)**

  Excludes *menopausal and premenopausal disorders (627.0–627.9)*
       postsurgical menopause (256.2)
       premature menopause (256.31)
       symptomatic menopause (627.0–627.9)

    ● **V49.82 Dental sealant status**

    V49.83 Awaiting organ transplant status ◀

    ● **V49.89 Other specified conditions influencing health status**

  ●❑ **V49.9 Unspecified**

PERSONS ENCOUNTERING HEALTH SERVICES FOR SPECIFIC PROCEDURES AND AFTERCARE (V50–V59)

Note: Categories V51–V58 are intended for use to indicate a reason for care in patients who may have already been treated for some disease or injury not now present, or who are receiving care to consolidate the treatment, to deal with residual states, or to prevent recurrence.

Excludes *follow-up examination for medical surveillance following treatment (V67.0–V67.9)*

● **V50 Elective surgery for purposes other than remedying health states**

    V50.0 Hair transplant

☐ **V50.1 Other plastic surgery for unacceptable cosmetic appearance**
    Breast augmentation or reduction
    Face-lift

Excludes *plastic surgery following healed injury or operation (V51)*

    V50.2 Routine or ritual circumcision
        Circumcision in the absence of significant medical indication

● **V50.3 Ear piercing**

● **V50.4 Prophylactic organ removal**

Excludes *organ donations (V59.0–V59.9)*
    therapeutic organ removal—code to condition

    V50.41 Breast

    V50.42 Ovary

☐ **V50.49 Other**

●☐ **V50.8 Other**

●☐ **V50.9 Unspecified**

V51 Aftercare involving the use of plastic surgery
    Plastic surgery following healed injury or operation

Excludes *cosmetic plastic surgery (V50.1)*
    plastic surgery as treatment for current injury—code to condition
    repair of scar tissue—code to scar

● **V52 Fitting and adjustment of prosthetic device and implant**

Includes: removal of device

Excludes *malfunction or complication of prosthetic device (996.0–996.7)*
    status only, without need for care (V43.0–V43.8)

    V52.0 Artificial arm (complete) (partial)

    V52.1 Artificial leg (complete) (partial)

    V52.2 Artificial eye

    V52.3 Dental prosthetic device

    V52.4 Breast prosthesis and implant

Excludes *admission for breast implant insertion (V50.1)*

☐ **V52.8 Other specified prosthetic device**

☐ **V52.9 Unspecified prosthetic device**

● **V53 Fitting and adjustment of other device**

Includes: removal of device
    replacement of device

Excludes *status only, without need for care (V45.0–V45.8)*

● **V53.0 Devices related to nervous system and special senses**

    V53.01 Fitting and adjustment of cerebral ventricle (communicating) shunt

    V53.02 Neuropacemaker (brain) (peripheral nerve) (spinal cord)

    V53.09 Fitting and adjustment of other devices related to nervous system and special senses
        Auditory substitution device
        Visual substitution device

    V53.1 Spectacles and contact lenses

    V53.2 Hearing aid

● **V53.3 Cardiac device**
    Reprogramming

    V53.31 Cardiac pacemaker

Excludes *mechanical complication of cardiac pacemaker (996.01)*

    V53.32 Automatic implantable cardiac defibrillator

☐ **V53.39 Other cardiac device**

    V53.4 Orthodontic devices

    V53.5 Other intestinal appliance

Excludes *colostomy (V55.3)*
    ileostomy (V55.2)
    other artifical opening of digestive tract (V55.4)

    V53.6 Urinary devices
    Urinary catheter

Excludes *cystostomy (V55.5)*
    nephrostomy (V55.6)
    ureterostomy (V55.6)
    urethrostomy (V55.6)

    V53.7 Orthopedic devices
    Orthopedic:
        brace
        cast
        corset
        shoes

Excludes *other orthopedic aftercare (V54)*

    V53.8 Wheelchair

● **V53.9 Other and unspecified device**

☐ **V53.90 Unspecified device**

    V53.91 Fitting and adjustment of insulin pump
        Insulin pump titration

☐ **V53.99 Other device**

● **V54 Other orthopedic aftercare**

Excludes *fitting and adjustment of orthopedic devices (V53.7)*
    malfunction of internal orthopedic device (996.4)
    other complication of nonmechanical nature (996.60–996.79)

● **V54.0 Aftercare involving internal fixation device**

Excludes *removal of external fixation device (V54.89)*

    V54.01 Encounter for removal of internal fixation device

    V54.02 Encounter for lengthening/adjustment of growth rod

☐ **V54.09 Other aftercare involving internal fixation device**

● V54.1 Aftercare for healing traumatic fracture

❑ V54.10 Aftercare for healing traumatic fracture of arm, unspecified

V54.11 Aftercare for healing traumatic fracture of upper arm

V54.12 Aftercare for healing traumatic fracture of lower arm

V54.13 Aftercare for healing traumatic fracture of hip

❑ V54.14 Aftercare for healing traumatic fracture of leg, unspecified

V54.15 Aftercare for healing traumatic fracture of upper leg

| Excludes | *aftercare for healing traumatic fracture of hip (V54.13)* |

V54.16 Aftercare for healing traumatic fracture of lower leg

V54.17 Aftercare for healing traumatic fracture of vertebrae

❑ V54.19 Aftercare for healing traumatic fracture of other bone

● V54.2 Aftercare for healing pathologic fracture

❑ V54.20 Aftercare for healing pathologic fracture of arm, unspecified

V54.21 Aftercare for healing pathologic fracture of upper arm

V54.22 Aftercare for healing pathologic fracture of lower arm

V54.23 Aftercare for healing pathologic fracture of hip

❑ V54.24 Aftercare for healing pathologic fracture of leg, unspecified

V54.25 Aftercare for healing pathologic fracture of upper leg

| Excludes | *aftercare for healing pathologic fracture of hip (V54.23)* |

V54.26 Aftercare for healing pathologic fracture of lower leg

V54.27 Aftercare for healing pathologic fracture of vertebrae

❑ V54.29 Aftercare for healing pathologic fracture of other bone

● ❑ V54.8 Other orthopedic aftercare

V54.81 Aftercare following joint replacement
Use additional code to identify joint replacement site (V43.60–V43.69)

❑ V54.89 Other orthopedic aftercare
Aftercare for healing fracture NOS

❑ V54.9 Unspecified orthopedic aftercare

● V55 Attention to artificial openings

Includes: adjustment or repositioning of catheter
closure
passage of sounds or bougies
reforming
removal or replacement of catheter
toilet or cleansing

| Excludes | *complications of external stoma (519.00–519.09, 569.60–569.69, 997.4, 997.5)* |
| | *status only, without need for care (V44.0–V44.9)* |

V55.0 Tracheostomy

V55.1 Gastrostomy

V55.2 Ileostomy

V55.3 Colostomy

❑ V55.4 Other artificial opening of digestive tract

V55.5 Cystostomy

❑ V55.6 Other artificial opening of urinary tract
Nephrostomy
Ureterostomy
Urethrostomy

V55.7 Artificial vagina

❑ V55.8 Other specified artificial opening

❑ V55.9 Unspecified artificial opening

● V56 Encounter for dialysis and dialysis catheter care
Use additional code to identify the associated condition

| Excludes | *dialysis preparation—code to condition* |

V56.0 Extracorporeal dialysis
Dialysis (renal) NOS

| Excludes | *dialysis status (V45.1)* |

V56.1 Fitting and adjustment of extracoporeal dialysis catheter
Removal or replacement of catheter
Toilet or cleansing

Use additional code for any concurrent extra-corporeal dialysis (V56.0)

V56.2 Fitting and adjustment of peritoneal dialysis catheter

Use additional code for any concurrent peritoneal dialysis (V56.8)

● V56.3 Encounter for adequacy testing for dialysis

● V56.31 Encounter for adequacy testing for hemodialysis

● V56.32 Encounter for adequacy testing for peritoneal dialysis
Peritoneal equilibration test

❑ V56.8 Other dialysis
Peritoneal dialysis

● V57 Care involving use of rehabilitation procedures
Use additional code to identify underlying condition

V57.0 Breathing exercises

❑ V57.1 Other physical therapy
Therapeutic and remedial exercises, except breathing

● V57.2 Occupational therapy and vocational rehabilitation

V57.21 Encounter for occupational therapy

V57.22 Encounter for vocational therapy

V57.3 Speech therapy

V57.4 Orthoptic training

● V57.8 Other specified rehabilitation procedure

V57.81 Orthotic training
Gait training in the use of artificial limbs

❑ V57.89 Other
Multiple training or therapy

❑ V57.9 Unspecified rehabilitation procedure

● **V58   Encounter for other and unspecified procedures and aftercare**

> **Excludes**   *convalescence and palliative care (V66.0–V66.9)*

V58.0   Radiotherapy
> Encounter or admission for radiotherapy

> **Excludes**   *encounter for radioactive implant—code to condition*
> *radioactive iodine therapy—code to condition*

V58.1   Chemotherapy
> Encounter or admission for chemotherapy

> **Excludes**   *prophylactic chemotherapy against disease which has never been present (V03.0–V07.9)*

V58.2   Blood transfusion, without reported diagnosis

V58.3   Attention to surgical dressings and sutures
> Change of dressings
> Removal of sutures

● **V58.4   Other aftercare following surgery**

> Note: Codes from this subcategory should be used in conjunction with other after care codes to fully identify the reason for the aftercare encounter.

> **Excludes**   *aftercare following sterilization reversal surgery (V26.22)*
> *attention to artificial openings (V55.0–V55.9)*
> *orthopedic aftercare (V54.0–V54.9)*

V58.41   Encounter for planned post-operative wound closure

> **Excludes**   *disruption of operative wound (998.3)*

V58.42   Aftercare following surgery for neoplasm
> Conditions classifiable to 140–239

V58.43   Aftercare following surgery for injury and trauma
> Conditions classifiable to 800–999

> **Excludes**   *aftercare for healing traumatic fracture (V54.10–V54.19)*

V58.44   Aftercare following organ transplant ◄
> Use additional code to identify the organ transplanted (V42.0–V42.9) ◄

❑ **V58.49   Other specified aftercare following surgery**

V58.5   Orthodontics

> **Excludes**   *fitting and adjustment of orthodontic device (V53.4)*

● **V58.6   Long-term (current) drug use**

> **Excludes**   *drug abuse (305.00–305.93)*
> *drug dependence (304.00–304.93)*
> *hormone replacement therapy (postmenopausal) (V07.4)* ◄

V58.61   Long-term (current) use of anticoagulants

> **Excludes**   *long-term (current) use of aspirin (V58.66)* ◄

V58.62   Long-term (current) use of antibiotics

V58.63   Long-term (current) use of antiplatelet/antithrombotic

> **Excludes**   *long-term (current) use of aspirin (V58.66)* ◄

V58.64   Long-term (current) use of non-steroidal anti-inflammatories (NSAID)

> **Excludes**   *long-term (current) use of aspirin (V58.66)* ◄

V58.65   Long-term (current) use of steroids

V58.66   Long-term (current) use of aspirin ◄

V58.67   Long-term (current) use of insulin ◄

❑ **V58.69   Long-term (current) use of other medications**
> High-risk medications

● **V58.7   Aftercare following surgery to specified body systems, not elsewhere classified**

> Note: Codes from this subcategory should be used in conjunction with other aftercare codes to fully identify the reason for the aftercare encounter

> **Excludes**   *aftercare following organ transplant (V58.44)* ◄
> *aftercare following surgery for neoplasm (V58.42)* ◄

V58.71   Aftercare following surgery of the sense organs, NEC
> Conditions classifiable to 360–379, 380–389

V58.72   Aftercare following surgery of the nervous system, NEC
> Conditions classifiable to 320–359

> **Excludes**   *aftercare following surgery of the sense organs, NEC (V58.71)*

V58.73   Aftercare following surgery of the circulatory system, NEC
> Conditions classifiable to 390–459

V58.74   Aftercare following surgery of the respiratory system, NEC
> Conditions classifiable to 460–519

V58.75   Aftercare following surgery of the teeth, oral cavity and digestive system, NEC
> Conditions classifiable to 520–579

V58.76   Aftercare following surgery of the genitourinary system, NEC
> Conditions classifiable to 580–629

> **Excludes**   *aftercare following sterilization reversal (V26.22)*

V58.77   Aftercare following surgery of the skin and subcutaneous tissue, NEC
> Conditions classifiable to 680–709

V58.78   Aftercare following surgery of the musculoskeletal system, NEC
> Conditions classifiable to 710–739

● **V58.8   Other specified procedures and aftercare**

V58.81   Fitting and adjustment of vascular catheter
> Removal or replacement of catheter
> Toilet or cleansing

> **Excludes**   *complications of renal dialysis (996.73)*
> *complications of vascular catheter (996.74)*
> *dialysis preparation—code to condition*
> *encounter for dialysis (V56.0–V56.8)*
> *fitting and adjustment of dialysis catheter (V56.2)*

V58.82   Fitting and adjustment of non-vascular catheter, NEC
> Removal or replacement of catheter
> Toilet or cleansing

> **Excludes**   *fitting and adjustment of peritoneal dialysis catheter (V56.2)*
> *fitting and adjustment of urinary catheter (V53.6)*

V01–V99   Vol. 1   ICD-9-CM

V58.83 Encounter for therapeutic drug monitoring

> Use additional code for any associated long-term (current) drug use (V58.61–V58.69)

> Excludes | *blood-drug testing for medicolegal reasons (V70.4)*

❏ **V58.89 Other specified aftercare**

❏ **V58.9 Unspecified aftercare**

● **V59 Donors**

> Excludes | *examination of potential donor (V70.8)*
> *self-donation of organ or tissue—code to condition*

● **V59.0 Blood**

V59.01 Whole blood

V59.02 Stem cells

❏ **V59.09 Other**

V59.1 Skin

V59.2 Bone

V59.3 Bone marrow

V59.4 Kidney

V59.5 Cornea

V59.6 Liver

V59.8 Other specified organ or tissue

V59.9 Unspecified organ or tissue

PERSONS ENCOUNTERING HEALTH SERVICES IN OTHER CIRCUMSTANCES (V60–V68)

● **V60 Housing, household, and economic circumstances**

V60.0 Lack of housing
> Hobos
> Social migrants
> Tramps
> Transients
> Vagabonds

● **V60.1 Inadequate housing**
> Lack of heating
> Restriction of space
> Technical defects in home preventing adequate care

● **V60.2 Inadequate material resources**
> Economic problem
> Poverty NOS

● **V60.3 Person living alone**

● **V60.4 No other household member able to render care**
> Person requiring care (has) (is):
> family member too handicapped, ill, or otherwise unsuited to render care
> partner temporarily away from home
> temporarily away from usual place of abode

> Excludes | *holiday relief care (V60.5)*

● **V60.5 Holiday relief care**
> Provision of health care facilities to a person normally cared for at home, to enable relatives to take a vacation

● **V60.6 Person living in residential institution**
> Boarding school resident

●❏ **V60.8 Other specified housing or economic circumstances**

●❏ **V60.9 Unspecified housing or economic circumstance**

● **V61 Other family circumstances**

Includes: when these circumstances or fear of them, affecting the person directly involved or others, are mentioned as the reason, justified or not, for seeking or receiving medical advice or care

● **V61.0 Family disruption**
> Divorce
> Estrangement

● **V61.1 Counseling for marital and partner problems**

> Excludes | *problems related to:*
> *psychosexual disorders (302.0–302.9)*
> *sexual function (V41.7)*

● **V61.10 Counseling for marital and partner problems, unspecified**
> Marital conflict
> Partner conflict

● **V61.11 Counseling for victim of spousal and partner abuse**

> Excludes | *encounter for treatment of current injuries due to abuse (995.80–995.85)*

● **V61.12 Counseling for perpetrator of spousal and partner abuse**

● **V61.2 Parent-child problems**

●❏ **V61.20 Counseling for parent-child problem, unspecified**
> Concern about behavior of child
> Parent-child conflict

● **V61.21 Counseling for victim of child abuse**
> Child battering
> Child neglect

> Excludes | *current injuries due to abuse (995.50–995.59)*

● **V61.22 Counseling for perpetrator of parental child abuse**

> Excludes | *counseling for non-parental abuser (V62.83)*

●❏ **V61.29 Other**
> Problem concerning adopted or foster child

● **V61.3 Problems with aged parents or in-laws**

● **V61.4 Health problems within family**

● **V61.41 Alcoholism in family**

●❏ **V61.49 Other**
> Care of sick or handicapped person in family or household
> Presence of sick or handicapped person in family or household

● **V61.5 Multiparity**

● **V61.6 Illegitimacy or illegitimate pregnancy**

●❏ **V61.7 Other unwanted pregnancy**

●❏ **V61.8 Other specified family circumstances**
> Problems with family members, NEC

●❏ **V61.9 Unspecified family circumstance**

● **V62 Other psychosocial circumstances**

Includes: those circumstances or fear of them, affecting the person directly involved or others, mentioned as the reason, justified or not, for seeking or receiving medical advice or care

> Excludes | *previous psychological trauma (V15.41–V15.49)*

● **V62.0 Unemployment**

Excludes *circumstances when main problem is economic inadequacy or poverty (V60.2)*

● **V62.1 Adverse effects of work environment**

●❑ **V62.2 Other occupational circumstances or maladjustment**
    Career choice problem
    Dissatisfaction with employment

● **V62.3 Educational circumstances**
    Dissatisfaction with school environment
    Educational handicap

● **V62.4 Social maladjustment**
    Cultural deprivation
    Political, religious, or sex discrimination
    Social:
        isolation
        persecution

● **V62.5 Legal circumstances**
    Imprisonment
    Legal investigation
    Litigation
    Prosecution

● **V62.6 Refusal of treatment for reasons of religion or conscience**

● **V62.8 Other psychological or physical stress, not elsewhere classified**

  ● **V62.81 Interpersonal problems, not elsewhere classified**

  ● **V62.82 Bereavement, uncomplicated**

Excludes *bereavement as adjustment reaction (309.0)*

  ● **V62.83 Counseling for perpetrator of physical/sexual abuse**

Excludes *counseling for perpetrator of parental child abuse (V61.22)*
counseling for perpetrator of spousal and partner abuse (V61.12)

  ●❑ **V62.89 Other**
        Life circumstance problems
        Phase of life problems

●❑ **V62.9 Unspecified psychosocial circumstance**

● **V63 Unavailability of other medical facilities for care**

  ● **V63.0 Residence remote from hospital or other health care facility**

  ● **V63.1 Medical services in home not available**

Excludes *no other household member able to render care (V60.4)*

  ● **V63.2 Person awaiting admission to adequate facility elsewhere**

  ●❑ **V63.8 Other specified reasons for unavailability of medical facilities**
        Person on waiting list undergoing social agency investigation

  ●❑ **V63.9 Unspecified reason for unavailability of medical facilities**

● **V64 Persons encountering health services for specific procedures, not carried out**

  ● **V64.0 Vaccination not carried out because of contraindication**

  ● **V64.1 Surgical or other procedure not carried out because of contraindication**

  ● **V64.2 Surgical or other procedure not carried out because of patient's decision**

  ●❑ **V64.3 Procedure not carried out for other reasons**

  ● **V64.4 Closed surgical procedure converted to open procedure**

    ● **V64.41 Laparoscopic surgical procedure converted to open procedure**

    ● **V64.42 Thoracoscopic surgical procedure converted to open procedure**

    ● **V64.43 Arthroscopic surgical procedure converted to open procedure**

● **V65 Other persons seeking consultation**

  V65.0 Healthy person accompanying sick person
    Boarder

  ● **V65.1 Person consulting on behalf of another person**
    Advice or treatment for nonattending third party

Excludes *concern (normal) about sick person in family (V61.41–V61.49)*

    ● **V65.11 Pediatric pre-birth visit for expectant mother**

    ● **V65.19 Other person consulting on behalf of another person**

  V65.2 Person feigning illness
    Malingerer
    Peregrinating patient

  ● **V65.3 Dietary surveillance and counseling**
    Dietary surveillance and counseling (in):
        NOS
        colitis
        diabetes mellitus
        food allergies or intolerance
        gastritis
        hypercholesterolemia
        hypoglycemia
        obesity

  ● **V65.4 Other counseling, not elsewhere classified**
    Health:
        advice
        education
        instruction

Excludes *counseling (for):*
contraception (V25.40–V25.49)
genetic (V26.3)
on behalf of third party (V65.11–V65.19)
procreative management (V26.4)

    ● **V65.40 Counseling NOS**

    ● **V65.41 Exercise counseling**

    ● **V65.42 Counseling on substance use and abuse**

    ● **V65.43 Counseling on injury prevention**

    ● **V65.44 Human immunodeficiency virus [HIV] counseling**

    ●❑ **V65.45 Counseling on other sexually transmitted diseases**

    ● **V65.46 Encounter for insulin pump training**

    ●❑ **V65.49 Other specified counseling**

● **V65.5 Person with feared complaint in whom no diagnosis was made**
    Feared condition not demonstrated
    Problem was normal state
    "Worried well"

●☐ **V65.8 Other reasons for seeking consultation**
    Excludes *specified symptoms*

●☐ **V65.9 Unspecified reason for consultation**

● **V66 Convalescence and palliative care**

    V66.0 Following surgery

    V66.1 Following radiotherapy

    V66.2 Following chemotherapy

    V66.3 Following psychotherapy and other treatment for mental disorder

    V66.4 Following treatment of fracture

    ●☐ **V66.5 Following other treatment**

    ☐ **V66.6 Following combined treatment**

    ● **V66.7 Encounter for palliative care**
        End-of-life care
        Hospice care
        Terminal care

        Code first underlying disease

    ●☐ **V66.9 Unspecified convalescence**

● **V67 Follow-up examination**

    Includes: surveillance only following completed treatment
    Excludes *surveillance of contraception (V25.40–V25.49)*

    ● **V67.0 Following surgery**

        V67.00 Following surgery, unspecified

        V67.01 Follow-up vaginal pap smear
            Vaginal pap smear, status-post hysterectomy for malignant condition

            Use additional code to identify:
            acquired absence of uterus (V45.77)
            personal history of malignant neoplasm (V10.40–V10.44)

        Excludes *vaginal pap smear status-post hysterectomy for non-malignant condition (V76.47)*

        V67.09 Following other surgery

        Excludes *sperm count following sterilization reversal (V26.22)*
        sperm count for fertility testing (V26.21)

    V67.1 Following radiotherapy

    V67.2 Following chemotherapy
        Cancer chemotherapy follow-up

    V67.3 Following psychotherapy and other treatment for mental disorder

    V67.4 Following treatment of healed fracture
    Excludes *current (healing) fracture aftercare (V54.0–V54.9)*

    ● **V67.5 Following other treatment**

        V67.51 Following completed treatment with high-risk medication, not elsewhere classified
        Excludes *Long-term (current) drug use (V58.61–V58.69)*

        ☐ **V67.59 Other**

☐ **V67.6 Following combined treatment**

●☐ **V67.9 Unspecified follow-up examination**

● **V68 Encounters for administrative purposes**

    ● **V68.0 Issue of medical certificates**
        Issue of medical certificate of:
        cause of death
        fitness
        incapacity

    Excludes *encounter for general medical examination (V70.0–V70.9)*

    ● **V68.1 Issue of repeat prescriptions**
        Issue of repeat prescription for:
        appliance
        glasses
        medications

    Excludes *repeat prescription for contraceptives (V25.41–V25.49)*

    ● **V68.2 Request for expert evidence**

    ● **V68.8 Other specified administrative purpose**

        ● **V68.81 Referral of patient without examination or treatment**

        ●☐ **V68.89 Other**

    ●☐ **V68.9 Unspecified administrative purpose**

● **V69 Problems related to lifestyle**

    ● **V69.0 Lack of physical exercise**

    ● **V69.1 Inappropriate diet and eating habits**

    Excludes *anorexia nervosa (307.1)*
    bulimia (783.6)
    malnutrition and other nutritional deficiencies (260–269.9)
    other and unspecified eating disorders (307.50–307.59)

    ● **V69.2 High-risk sexual behavior**

    ● **V69.3 Gambling and betting**
    Excludes *pathological gambling (312.31)*

    ● **V69.4 Lack of adequate sleep** ◀
        Sleep deprivation ◀
    Excludes *insomnia (780.52)* ◀

    ●☐ **V69.8 Other problems related to lifestyle**
        Self-damaging behavior

    ●☐ **V69.9 Problem related to lifestyle, unspecified**

PERSONS WITHOUT REPORTED DIAGNOSIS ENCOUNTERED DURING EXAMINATION AND INVESTIGATION OF INDIVIDUALS AND POPULATIONS (V70–V84) ◀▥

Note: Nonspecific abnormal findings disclosed at the time of these examinations are classifiable to categories 790–796.

● **V70 General medical examination**

    Use additional code(s) to identify any special screening examination(s) performed (V73.0–V82.9)

    ● **V70.0 Routine general medical examination at a health care facility**
        Health checkup

    Excludes *health checkup of infant or child (V20.2)*

    V70.1 General psychiatric examination, requested by the authority

●❑ **V70.2 General psychiatric examination, other and unspecified**

●❑ **V70.3 Other medical examination for administrative purposes**
General medical examination for:
admission to old age home
adoption
camp
driving license
immigration and naturalization
insurance certification
marriage
prison
school admission
sports competition

Excludes *attendance for issue of medical certificates (V68.0)*
pre-employment screening (V70.5)

V70.4 Examination for medicolegal reasons
Blood-alcohol tests
Blood-drug tests
Paternity testing

Excludes *examination and observation following:*
accidents (V71.3, V71.4)
assault (V71.6)
rape (V71.5)

V70.5 Health examination of defined subpopulations
Armed forces personnel
Inhabitants of institutions
Occupational health examinations
Pre-employment screening
Preschool children
Prisoners
Prostitutes
Refugees
School children
Students

● **V70.6 Health examination in population surveys**

Excludes *special screening (V73.0–V82.9)*

V70.7 Examination of participant in clinical trial
Examination of participant or control in clinical research

●❑ **V70.8 Other specified general medical examinations**
Examination of potential donor of organ or tissue

●❑ **V70.9 Unspecified general medical examination**

● **V71 Observation and evaluation for suspected conditions not found**

Note: This category is to be used when persons without a diagnosis are suspected of having an abnormal condition, without signs or symptoms, which requires study, but after examination and observation, is found not to exist. This category is also for use for administrative and legal observation status.

● **V71.0 Observation for suspected mental condition**

V71.01 Adult antisocial behavior
Dyssocial behavior or gang activity in adult without manifest psychiatric disorder

V71.02 Childhood or adolescent antisocial behavior
Dyssocial behavior or gang activity in child or adolescent without manifest psychiatric disorder

❑ **V71.09 Other suspected mental condition**

V71.1 Observation for suspected malignant neoplasm

V71.2 Observation for suspected tuberculosis

V71.3 Observation following accident at work

❑ **V71.4 Observation following other accident**
Examination of individual involved in motor vehicle traffic accident

V71.5 Observation following alleged rape or seduction
Examination of victim or culprit

❑ **V71.6 Observation following other inflicted injury**
Examination of victim or culprit

V71.7 Observation for suspected cardiovascular disease

●❑ **V71.8 Observation and evaluation for other specified suspected conditions**

V71.81 Abuse and neglect

V71.82 Observation and evaluation for suspected exposure to anthrax

❑ **V71.83 Observation and evaluation for suspected exposure to other biological agent**

Excludes *adult abuse and neglect (995.80–995.85)*
child abuse and neglect (995.50–995.59)

V71.89 Other specified suspected conditions

●❑ **V71.9 Observation for unspecified suspected condition**

● **V72 Special investigations and examinations**

Includes: routine examination of specific system

Excludes *general medical examination (V70.0–70.4)*
general screening examination of defined population groups (V70.5, V70.6, V70.7)
routine examination of infant or child (V20.2)

Use additional code(s) to identify any special screening examination(s) performed (V73.0–V82.9)

V72.0 Examination of eyes and vision

● **V72.1 Examination of ears and hearing**

● **V72.2 Dental examination**

● **V72.3 Gynecological examination** ◄▥

Excludes *cervical Papanicolaou smear without general gynecological examination (V76.2)*
routine examination in contraceptive management (V25.40–V25.49)

● **V72.31 Routine gynecological examination** ◄
General gynecological examination with or without Papanicolaou cervical smear
Pelvic examination (annual) (periodic) ◄
Use additional code to identify routine vaginal Papanicolaou smear (V76.47) ◄

● **V72.32 Encounter for Papanicolaou cervical smear to confirm findings of recent normal smear following initial abnormal smear** ◄

● **V72.4 Pregnancy examination or test**   ◄▥

Excludes   *pregnancy examination with immediate confirma-*
           tion (V22.0–V22.1)

   ● **V72.40 Pregnancy examination or test, preg-**
       nancy unconfirmed   ◄
         Possible   pregnancy,   not   (yet)
          confirmed   ◄

   ● **V72.41 Pregnancy examination or test, nega-**
       tive result   ◄

● **V72.5 Radiological   examination,   not   elsewhere**
   classified
     Routine chest x-ray

Excludes   *examination for suspected tuberculosis (V71.2)*

● **V72.6 Laboratory examination**

Excludes   *that for suspected disorder (V71.0–V71.9)*

● **V72.7 Diagnostic skin and sensitization tests**
     Allergy tests
     Skin tests for hypersensitivity

Excludes   *diagnostic skin tests for bacterial diseases*
           (V74.0–V74.9)

● **V72.8 Other specified examinations**

   V72.81 Preoperative cardiovascular examina-
       tion

   V72.82 Preoperative respiratory examination

   ☐ **V72.83 Other specified preoperative exami-**
       nation

   ●☐ **V72.84 Preoperative examination, unspeci-**
       fied

   ●☐ **V72.85 Other specified examination**

●☐ **V72.9 Unspecified examination**

● **V73 Special screening examination for viral and chla-**
   mydial diseases

   ● **V73.0 Poliomyelitis**

   ● **V73.1 Smallpox**

   ● **V73.2 Measles**

   ● **V73.3 Rubella**

   ● **V73.4 Yellow fever**

   ●☐ **V73.5 Other arthropod-borne viral diseases**
      Dengue fever
      Hemorrhagic fever
      Viral encephalitis:
        mosquito-borne
        tick-borne

   ● **V73.6 Trachoma**

   ● **V73.8 Other specified viral and chlamydial dis-**
     eases

     ●☐ **V73.88 Other specified chlamydial diseases**

     ●☐ **V73.89 Other specified viral diseases**

   ● **V73.9 Unspecified viral and chlamydial disease**

     ●☐ **V73.98 Unspecified chlamydial disease**

     ●☐ **V73.99 Unspecified viral disease**

● **V74 Special screening examination for bacterial and spi-**
   rochetal diseases

Includes: diagnostic skin tests for these diseases

   ● **V74.0 Cholera**

   ● **V74.1 Pulmonary tuberculosis**

   ● **V74.2 Leprosy [Hansen's disease]**

   ● **V74.3 Diphtheria**

   ● **V74.4 Bacterial conjunctivitis**

   ● **V74.5 Venereal disease**

   ● **V74.6 Yaws**

   ●☐ **V74.8 Other specified bacterial and spirochetal dis-**
     eases
      Brucellosis
      Leptospirosis
      Plague
      Tetanus
      Whooping cough

   ●☐ **V74.9 Unspecified bacterial and spirochetal disease**

● **V75 Special screening examination for other infectious**
   diseases

   ● **V75.0 Rickettsial diseases**

   ● **V75.1 Malaria**

   ● **V75.2 Leishmaniasis**

   ● **V75.3 Trypanosomiasis**
      Chagas' disease
      Sleeping sickness

   ● **V75.4 Mycotic infections**

   ● **V75.5 Schistosomiasis**

   ● **V75.6 Filariasis**

   ● **V75.7 Intestinal helminthiasis**

   ●☐ **V75.8 Other specified parasitic infections**

   ●☐ **V75.9 Unspecified infectious disease**

● **V76 Special screening for malignant neoplasms**

   ● **V76.0 Respiratory organs**

   ● **V76.1 Breast**

     ●☐ **V76.10 Breast screening, unspecified**

     ● **V76.11 Screening mammogram for high-risk**
       patient

     ● **V76.12 Other screening mammogram**

     ●☐ **V76.19 Other screening breast examination**

   ● **V76.2 Cervix**
     Routine cervical Papanicolaou smear

Excludes   *that as part of a general gynecological examina-*
           tion (V72.31)   ◄▥

   ● **V76.3 Bladder**

   ● **V76.4 Other sites**

     ● **V76.41 Rectum**

     ● **V76.42 Oral cavity**

     ● **V76.43 Skin**

     V76.44 Prostate

     ● **V76.45 Testis**

     ● **V76.46 Ovary**

     ● **V76.47 Vagina**
       Vaginal   pap   smear   status-post
       hysterectomy   for   nonmalignant
       condition

       Use additional code to identify ac-
       quired absence of uterus (V45.77)

Excludes   *vaginal pap smear status-post hysterectomy for*
           malignant condition (V67.01)

     ●☐ **V76.49 Other sites**

● V76.5   Intestine
- ● V76.50   Intestine, unspecified
- ● V76.51   Colon

Excludes   *rectum (V76.41)*

- ● V76.52   Small intestine

●☐ V76.8   Other neoplasm
- ● V76.81   Nervous system
- ● V76.89   Other neoplasm

☐ V76.9   Unspecified

● V77   Special screening for endocrine, nutritional, metabolic, and immunity disorders
- ● V77.0   Thyroid disorders
- ● V77.1   Diabetes mellitus
- ● V77.2   Malnutrition
- ● V77.3   Phenylketonuria [PKU]
- ● V77.4   Galactosemia
- ● V77.5   Gout
- ● V77.6   Cystic fibrosis
  Screening for mucoviscidosis
- ●☐ V77.7   Other inborn errors of metabolism
- ● V77.8   Obesity
- ● V77.9   Other and unspecified endocrine, nutritional, metabolic, and immunity disorders
  - ● V77.91   Screening for lipoid disorders
    Screening cholesterol level
    Screening for hypercholesterolemia
    Screening for hyperlipidemia
  - ● V77.99   Other and unspecified endocrine, nutritional, metabolic, and immunity disorders

● V78   Special screening for disorders of blood and blood-forming organs
- ● V78.0   Iron deficiency anemia
- ●☐ V78.1   Other and unspecified deficiency anemia
- ● V78.2   Sickle-cell disease or trait
- ●☐ V78.3   Other hemoglobinopathies
- ●☐ V78.8   Other disorders of blood and blood-forming organs
- ●☐ V78.9   Unspecified disorder of blood and blood-forming organs

● V79   Special screening for mental disorders and developmental handicaps
- ● V79.0   Depression
- ● V79.1   Alcoholism
- ● V79.2   Mental retardation
- ● V79.3   Developmental handicaps in early childhood
- ●☐ V79.8   Other specified mental disorders and developmental handicaps
- ●☐ V79.9   Unspecified mental disorder and developmental handicap

● V80   Special screening for neurological, eye, and ear diseases
- ● V80.0   Neurological conditions
- ● V80.1   Glaucoma

●☐ V80.2   Other eye conditions
  Screening for:
  cataract
  congenital anomaly of eye
  senile macular lesions

Excludes   *general vision examination (V72.0)*

- ● V80.3   Ear diseases

Excludes   *general hearing examination (V72.1)*

● V81   Special screening for cardiovascular, respiratory, and genitourinary diseases
- ● V81.0   Ischemic heart disease
- ● V81.1   Hypertension
- ●☐ V81.2   Other and unspecified cardiovascular conditions
- ● V81.3   Chronic bronchitis and emphysema
- ●☐ V81.4   Other and unspecified respiratory conditions

Excludes   *screening for:*
lung neoplasm (V76.0)
pulmonary tuberculosis (V74.1)

- ● V81.5   Nephropathy
  Screening for asymptomatic bacteriuria
- ●☐ V81.6   Other and unspecified genitourinary conditions

● V82   Special screening for other conditions
- ● V82.0   Skin conditions
- ● V82.1   Rheumatoid arthritis
- ●☐ V82.2   Other rheumatic disorders
- ● V82.3   Congenital dislocation of hip
- ● V82.4   Maternal screening for chromosomal anomalies

Excludes   *antenatal screening by amniocentesis (V28.0)*

- ● V82.5   Chemical poisoning and other contamination
  Screening for:
  heavy metal poisoning
  ingestion of radioactive substance
  poisoning from contaminated water supply
  radiation exposure
- ● V82.6   Multiphasic screening
- ● V82.8   Other specified conditions
  - ● V82.81   Osteoporosis
    Use additional code to identify:
    hormone replacement therapy (postmenopausal) status (V07.4)
    postmenopausal (natural) status (V49.81)
  - ● V82.89   Other specified conditions
- ●☐ V82.9   Unspecified condition

● V83   Generic carrier status
- ● V83.0   Hemophilia A carrier
  - ● V83.01   Asymptomatic hemophilia A carrier
  - ● V83.02   Symptomatic hemophilia A carrier
- ●☐ V83.8   Other genetic carrier status
  - ● V83.81   Cystic fibrosis gene carrier
  - ●☐ V83.89   Other genetic carrier status

ICD-9-CM
V01-V99
Vol. 1

● **V84 Genetic susceptibility to disease** ◄

Includes: Confirmed abnormal gene ◄

Use additional code, if applicable, for any associated family history of the disease (V16–V19) ◄

● **V84.0 Genetic susceptibility to malignant neoplasm**

Code first, if applicable, any current malignant neoplasms (140.0–195.8, 200.0–208.9, 230.0–234.9) ◄

Use additional code, if applicable, for any personal history of malignant neoplasm (V10.0–V10.9) ◄

● **V84.01 Genetic susceptibility to malignant neoplasm of breast** ◄

● **V84.02 Genetic susceptibility to malignant neoplasm of ovary** ◄

● **V84.03 Genetic susceptibility to malignant neoplasm of prostate** ◄

● **V84.04 Genetic susceptibility to malignant neoplasm of endometrium** ◄

● **V84.09 Genetic susceptibility to other malignant neoplasm** ◄

● **V84.8 Genetic susceptibility to other disease** ◄

E-Codes—SUPPLEMENTARY CLASSIFICATION OF EXTERNAL CAUSES OF INJURY AND POISONING (E800-E999)

This section is provided to permit the classification of environmental events, circumstances, and conditions as the cause of injury, poisoning, and other adverse effects. Where a code from this section is applicable, it is intended that it shall be used in addition to a code from one of the main chapters of ICD-9-CM, indicating the nature of the condition. Certain other conditions which may be stated to be due to external causes are classified in Chapters 1 to 16 of ICD-9-CM. For these, the "E" code classification should be used as an additional code for more detailed analysis.

Machinery accidents [other than those connected with transport] are classifiable to category E919, in which the fourth digit allows a broad classification of the type of machinery involved. If a more detailed classification of type of machinery is required, it is suggested that the "Classification of Industrial Accidents according to Agency," prepared by the International Labor Office, be used in addition; it is included in this publication.

Categories for "late effects" of accidents and other external causes are to be found at E929, E959, E969, E977, E989, and E999.

Definitions and examples related to transport accidents:

(a) A transport accident (E800-E848) is any accident involving a device designed primarily for, or being used at the time primarily for, conveying persons or goods from one place to another.

> **Includes:** accidents involving:
> aircraft and spacecraft (E840-E845)
> watercraft (E830-E838)
> motor vehicle (E810-E825)
> railway (E800-E807)
> other road vehicles (E826-E829)

In classifying accidents which involve more than one kind of transport, the above order of precedence of transport accidents should be used.

Accidents involving agricultural and construction machines, such as tractors, cranes, and bulldozers, are regarded as transport accidents only when these vehicles are under their own power on a highway [otherwise the vehicles are regarded as machinery]. Vehicles which can travel on land or water, such as hovercraft and other amphibious vehicles, are regarded as watercraft when on the water, as motor vehicles when on the highway, and as off-road motor vehicles when on land, but off the highway.

> **Excludes** *accidents:*
> *in sports which involve the use of transport but where the transport vehicle itself was not involved in the accident*
> *involving vehicles which are part of industrial equipment used entirely on industrial premises*
> *occurring during transportation but unrelated to the hazards associated with the means of transportation [e.g., injuries received in a fight on board ship; transport vehicle involved in a cataclysm such as an earthquake]*
> *to persons engaged in the maintenance or repair of transport equipment or vehicle not in motion, unless injured by another vehicle in motion*

(b) A railway accident is a transport accident involving a railway train or other railway vehicle operated on rails, whether in motion or not.

> **Excludes** *accidents:*
> *in repair shops*
> *in roundhouse or on turntable*
> *on railway premises but not involving a train or other railway vehicle*

(c) A railway train or railway vehicle is any device with or without cars coupled to it, designed for traffic on a railway.

> **Includes:** interurban:
> electric car (operated chiefly on its own right-of-way, not open to other traffic)
> streetcar (operated chiefly on its own right-of-way, not open to other traffic)
> railway train, any power [diesel] [electric] [steam]
> funicular
> monorail or two-rail
> subterranean or elevated
> other vehicle designed to run on a railway track

> **Excludes** *interurban electric cars [streetcars] specified to be operating on a right-of-way that forms part of the public street or highway [definition (n)]*

(d) A railway or railroad is a right-of-way designed for traffic on rails, which is used by carriages or wagons transporting passengers or freight, and by other rolling stock, and which is not open to other public vehicular traffic

(e) A motor vehicle accident is a transport accident involving a motor vehicle. It is defined as a motor vehicle traffic accident or as a motor vehicle nontraffic accident according to whether the accident occurs on a public highway or elsewhere.

> **Excludes** *injury or damage due to cataclysm*
> *injury or damage while a motor vehicle, not under its own power, is being loaded on, or unloaded from, another conveyance*

(f) A motor vehicle traffic accident is any motor vehicle accident occurring on a public highway [i.e., originating, terminating, or involving a vehicle partially on the highway]. A motor vehicle accident is assumed to have occurred on the highway unless another place is specified, except in the case of accidents involving only off-road motor vehicles which are classified as nontraffic accidents unless the contrary is stated.

(g) A motor vehicle nontraffic accident is any motor vehicle accident which occurs entirely in any place other than a public highway.

(h) A public highway [trafficway] or street is the entire width between property lines [or other boundary lines] of every way or place, of which any part is open to the use of the public for purposes of vehicular traffic as a matter of right or custom. A roadway is that part of the public highway designed, improved, and ordinarily used, for vehicular travel.

> **Includes:** approaches (public) to:
> docks
> public building
> station

> **Excludes** *driveway (private)*
> *parking lot*
> *ramp*
> *roads in:*
> *airfield*
> *farm*
> *industrial premises*
> *mine*
> *private grounds*
> *quarry*

(i) A motor vehicle is any mechanically or electrically powered device, not operated on rails, upon which any person or property may be transported or drawn upon a highway. Any object such as a trailer, coaster, sled, or wagon being towed by a motor vehicle is considered a part of the motor vehicle.

> **Includes:** automobile [any type]
> bus
> construction machinery, farm and industrial machinery, steam roller, tractor, army tank, highway grader, or similar vehicle on wheels or treads, while in transport under own power
> fire engine (motorized)
> motorcycle
> motorized bicycle [moped] or scooter
> trolley bus not operating on rails
> truck
> van

> **Excludes** *devices used solely to move persons or materials within the confines of a building and its premises, such as:*
> *building elevator*
> *coal car in mine*
> *electric baggage or mail truck used solely within a railroad station*
> *electric truck used solely within an industrial plant*
> *moving overhead crane*

(j) A motorcycle is a two-wheeled motor vehicle having one or two riding saddles and sometimes having a third wheel for the support of a sidecar. The sidecar is considered part of the motorcycle.

> **Includes:** motorized:
> bicycle [moped]
> scooter
> tricycle

(k) An off-road motor vehicle is a motor vehicle of special design, to enable it to negotiate rough or soft terrain or snow. Examples of special design are high construction, special wheels and tires, driven by treads, or support on a cushion of air.

> **Includes:** all terrain vehicle [ATV]
> army tank
> hovercraft, on land or swamp
> snowmobile

(l) A driver of a motor vehicle is the occupant of the motor vehicle operating it or intending to operate it. A motorcyclist is the driver of a motorcycle. Other authorized occupants of a motor vehicle are passengers.

(m) An other road vehicle is any device, except a motor vehicle, in, on, or by which any person or property may be transported on a highway.

> **Includes:** animal carrying a person or goods
> animal-drawn vehicle
> animal harnessed to conveyance
> bicycle [pedal cycle]
> streetcar
> tricycle (pedal)

> **Excludes** *pedestrian conveyance [definition (q)]*

(n) A streetcar is a device designed and used primarily for transporting persons within a municipality, running on rails, usually subject to normal traffic control signals, and operated principally on a right-of-way that forms part of the traffic way. A trailer being towed by a streetcar is considered a part of the streetcar.

> **Includes:** interurban or intraurban electric or streetcar, when specified to be operating on a street or public highway
> tram (car)
> trolley (car)

(o) A pedal cycle is any road transport vehicle operated solely by pedals.

> **Includes:** bicycle
> pedal cycle
> tricycle

> **Excludes** *motorized bicycle [definition (i)]*

(p) A pedal cyclist is any person riding on a pedal cycle or in a sidecar attached to such a vehicle.

(q) A pedestrian conveyance is any human powered device by which a pedestrian may move other than by walking or by which a walking person may move another pedestrian.

> **Includes:** baby carriage
> coaster wagon
> ice skates
> perambulator
> pushcart
> pushchair
> roller skates
> scooter
> skateboard
> skis
> sled
> wheelchair

(r) A pedestrian is any person involved in an accident who was not at the time of the accident riding in or on a motor vehicle, railroad train, streetcar, animal-drawn or other vehicle, or on a bicycle or animal.

> **Includes:** person:
> changing tire of vehicle
> in or operating a pedestrian conveyance
> making adjustment to motor of vehicle
> on foot

(s) A watercraft is any device for transporting passengers or goods on the water.

(t) A small boat is any watercraft propelled by paddle, oars, or small motor, with a passenger capacity of less than ten.

> **Includes:** boat NOS
> canoe
> coble
> dinghy
> punt
> raft
> rowboat
> rowing shell
> scull
> skiff
> small motorboat

> **Excludes** *barge*
> *lifeboat (used after abandoning ship)*
> *raft (anchored) being used as a diving platform*
> *yacht*

(u) An aircraft is any device for transporting passengers or goods in the air.

> **Includes:** airplane [any type]
> balloon
> bomber
> dirigible
> glider (hang)
> military aircraft
> parachute

(v) A commercial transport aircraft is any device for collective passenger or freight transportation by air, whether run on commercial lines for profit or by government authorities, with the exception of military craft.

RAILWAY ACCIDENTS (E800-E807)

Note: For definitions of railway accident and related terms see definitions (a) to (d).

Excludes *accidents involving railway train and:*
    aircraft (E840.0-E845.9)
    motor vehicle (E810.0-E825.9)
    watercraft (E830.0-E838.9)

The following fourth-digit subdivisions are for use with categories E800-E807 to identify the injured person:

.0 Railway employee
Any person who by virtue of his employment in connection with a railway, whether by the railway company or not, is at increased risk of involvement in a railway accident, such as:
    catering staff of train
    driver
    guard
    porter
    postal staff on train
    railway fireman
    shunter
    sleeping car attendant

.1 Passenger on railway
Any authorized person traveling on a train, except a railway employee.

Excludes *intending passenger waiting at station (8)*
    unauthorized rider on railway vehicle (8)

.2 Pedestrian
See definition (r)

.3 Pedal cyclist
See definition (p)

.8 Other specified person
Intending passenger or bystander waiting at station
Unauthorized rider on railway vehicle

.9 Unspecified person

● **E800 Railway accident involving collision with rolling stock**

Requires fourth digit. See beginning of section E800-E845 for codes and definitions.

Includes: collision between railway trains or railway vehicles, any kind
collision NOS on railway
derailment with antecedent collision with rolling stock or NOS

● **E801 Railway accident involving collision with other object**

Requires fourth digit. See beginning of section E800-E845 for codes and definitions.

Includes: collision of railway train with:
    buffers
    fallen tree on railway
    gates
    platform
    rock on railway
    streetcar
    other nonmotor vehicle
    other object

Excludes *collision with:*
    aircraft (E840.0-E842.9)
    motor vehicle (E810.0-E810.9, E820.0-E822.9)

● **E802 Railway accident involving derailment without antecedent collision**

Requires fourth digit. See beginning of section E800-E845 for codes and definitions.

● **E803 Railway accident involving explosion, fire, or burning**

Requires fourth digit. See beginning of section E800-E845 for codes and definitions.

Excludes *explosion or fire, with antecedent derailment (E802.0-E802.9)*
explosion or fire, with mention of antecedent collision (E800.0-E801.9)

● **E804 Fall in, on, or from railway train**

Requires fourth digit. See beginning of section E800-E845 for codes and definitions.

Includes: fall while alighting from or boarding railway train

Excludes *fall related to collision, derailment, or explosion of railway train (E800.0-E803.9)*

● **E805 Hit by rolling stock**

Requires fourth digit. See beginning of section E800-E845 for codes and definitions.

Includes: crushed by railway train or part
injured by railway train or part
killed by railway train or part
knocked down by railway train or part
run over by railway train or part

Excludes *pedestrian hit by object set in motion by railway train (E806.0-E806.9)*

● **E806 Other specified railway accident**

Requires fourth digit. See beginning of section E800-E845 for codes and definitions.

Includes: hit by object falling in railway train
injured by door or window on railway train
nonmotor road vehicle or pedestrian hit by object set in motion by railway train
railway train hit by falling:
    earth NOS
    rock
    tree
    other object

Excludes *railway accident due to cataclysm (E908-E909)*

● **E807 Railway accident of unspecified nature**

Requires fourth digit. See beginning of section E800-E845 for codes and definitions.

Includes: found dead on railway right-of-way NOS
injured on railway right-of-way NOS
railway accident NOS

MOTOR VEHICLE TRAFFIC ACCIDENTS (E810-E819)

Note: For definitions of motor vehicle traffic accident, and related terms, see definitions (e) to (k).

| Excludes | *accidents involving motor vehicle and aircraft (E840.0-E845.9)* |

The following fourth-digit subdivisions are for use with categories E810-E819 to identify the injured person:

.0 Driver of motor vehicle other than motorcycle
    See definition (l)
.1 Passenger in motor vehicle other than motorcycle
    See definition (l)
.2 Motorcyclist
    See definition (l)
.3 Passenger on motorcycle
    See definition (l)
.4 Occupant of streetcar
.5 Rider of animal; occupant of animal-drawn vehicle
.6 Pedal cyclist
    See definition (p)
.7 Pedestrian
    See definition (r)
☐ .8 Other specified person
    Occupant of vehicle other than above
    Person in railway train involved in accident
    Unauthorized rider of motor vehicle
☐ .9 Unspecified person

● E810 Motor vehicle traffic accident involving collision with train

Requires fourth digit. See beginning of section E800-E845 for codes and definitions.

| Excludes | *motor vehicle collision with object set in motion by railway train (E815.0-E815.9)* |
| | *railway train hit by object set in motion by motor vehicle (E818.0-E818.9)* |

● E811 Motor vehicle traffic accident involving re-entrant collision with another motor vehicle

Requires fourth digit. See beginning of section E800-E845 for codes and definitions.

Includes: collision between motor vehicle which accidentally leaves the roadway then re-enters the same roadway, or the opposite roadway on a divided highway, and another motor vehicle

| Excludes | *collision on the same roadway when none of the motor vehicles involved have left and re-entered the roadway (E812.0-E812.9)* |

● ☐ E812 Other motor vehicle traffic accident involving collision with motor vehicle

Requires fourth digit. See beginning of section E800-E845 for codes and definitions.

Includes: collision with another motor vehicle parked, stopped, stalled, disabled, or abandoned on the highway
    motor vehicle collision NOS

| Excludes | *collision with object set in motion by another motor vehicle (E815.0-E815.9)* |
| | *re-entrant collision with another motor vehicle (E811.0-E811.9)* |

● ☐ E813 Motor vehicle traffic accident involving collision with other vehicle

Requires fourth digit. See beginning of section E800-E845 for codes and definitions.

Includes: collision between motor vehicle, any kind, and:
    other road (nonmotor transport) vehicle, such as:
Includes: animal carrying a person
Includes: animal-drawn vehicle
Includes: pedal cycle
Includes: streetcar

Excludes	*collision with:*
	object set in motion by nonmotor road vehicle (E815.0-E815.9)
	pedestrian (E814.0-E814.9)
	nonmotor road vehicle hit by object set in motion by motor vehicle (E818.0-E818.9)

● E814 Motor vehicle traffic accident involving collision with pedestrian

Requires fourth digit. See beginning of section E800-E845 for codes and definitions.

Includes: collision between motor vehicle, any kind, and pedestrian
    pedestrian dragged, hit, or run over by motor vehicle, any kind

| Excludes | *pedestrian hit by object set in motion by motor vehicle (E818.0-E818.9)* |

● ☐ E815 Other motor vehicle traffic accident involving collision on the highway

Requires fourth digit. See beginning of section E800-E845 for codes and definitions.

Includes: collision (due to loss of control) (on highway)
    between motor vehicle, any kind, and:
    abutment (bridge) (overpass)
    animal (herded) (unattended)
    fallen stone, traffic sign, tree, utility pole
    guard rail or boundary fence
    interhighway divider
    landslide (not moving)
    object set in motion by railway train or road vehicle (motor) (nonmotor)
    object thrown in front of motor vehicle
    safety island
    temporary traffic sign or marker
    wall of cut made for road
    other object, fixed, movable, or moving

Excludes	*collision with:*
	any object off the highway (resulting from loss of control) (E816.0-E816.9)
	any object which normally would have been off the highway and is not stated to have been on it (E816.0-E816.9)
	motor vehicle parked, stopped, stalled, disabled, or abandoned on highway (E812.0-E812.9)
	moving landslide (E909.2)
	motor vehicle hit by object:
	set in motion by railway train or road vehicle (motor) (nonmotor) (E818.0-E818.9)
	thrown into or on vehicle (E818.0-E818.9)

     ◀ **New**   ◀▥ **Revised**   ● **Not a Principal Diagnosis**   ● **Use Additional Digit(s)**   ☐ **Nonspecific Code**

● **E816 Motor vehicle traffic accident due to loss of control, without collision on the highway**

Requires fourth digit. See beginning of section E800-E845 for codes and definitions.

Includes: motor vehicle:
         failing to make curve and:
Includes: colliding with object off the highway
Includes: overturning
Includes: stopping abruptly off the highway
         going out of control (due to)
Includes: blowout and:
         colliding with object off the highway
         overturning
         stopping abruptly off the highway
         burst tire and:
           colliding with object off the highway
           overturning
           stopping abruptly off the highway
         driver falling asleep and:
           colliding with object off the highway
           overturning
           stopping abruptly off the highway
         driver inattention and:
           colliding with object off the highway
           overturning
           stopping abruptly off the highway
         excessive speed and:
           colliding with object off the highway
           overturning
           stopping abruptly off the highway
         failure of mechanical part and:
           colliding with object off the highway
           overturning
           stopping abruptly off the highway

Excludes *collision on highway following loss of control (E810.0-E815.9)*
loss of control of motor vehicle following collision on the highway (E810.0-E815.9)

● **E817 Noncollision motor vehicle traffic accident while boarding or alighting**

Requires fourth digit. See beginning of section E800-E845 for codes and definitions.

Includes: fall down stairs of motor bus while boarding or alighting
fall from car in street while boarding or alighting
injured by moving part of the vehicle while boarding or alighting
trapped by door of motor bus while boarding or alighting

● ☐ **E818 Other noncollision motor vehicle traffic accident**

Requires fourth digit. See beginning of section E800-E845 for codes and definitions.

Includes: accidental poisoning from exhaust gas generated by motor vehicle while in motion
breakage of any part of motor vehicle while in motion
explosion of any part of motor vehicle while in motion
fall, jump, or being accidentally pushed from motor vehicle while in motion
fire starting in motor vehicle while in motion
hit by object thrown into or on motor vehicle while in motion
injured by being thrown against some part of, or object in, motor vehicle while in motion
injury from moving part of motor vehicle while in motion
object falling in or on motor vehicle while in motion
object thrown on motor vehicle while in motion
collision of railway train or road vehicle except motor vehicle, with object set in motion by motor vehicle
motor vehicle hit by object set in motion by railway train or road vehicle (motor) (nonmotor)
pedestrian, railway train, or road vehicle (motor) (nonmotor) hit by object set in motion by motor vehicle

Excludes *collision between motor vehicle and:*
object set in motion by railway train or road vehicle (motor) (nonmotor) (E815.0-E815.9)
object thrown towards the motor vehicle (E815.0-E815.9)
person overcome by carbon monoxide generated by stationary motor vehicle off the roadway with motor running (E868.2)

● ☐ **E819 Motor vehicle traffic accident of unspecified nature**

Requires fourth digit. See beginning of section E800-E845 for codes and definitions.

Includes: motor vehicle traffic accident NOS
traffic accident NOS

ICD-9-CM

E800-E999

Vol.

MOTOR VEHICLE NONTRAFFIC ACCIDENTS (E820-E825)

Note: For definitions of motor vehicle nontraffic accident and related terms see definitions (a) to (k).

Includes: accidents involving motor vehicles being used in recreational or sporting activities off the highway

collision and noncollision motor vehicle accidents occurring entirely off the highway

> **Excludes** *accidents involving motor vehicle and:*
> *aircraft (E840.0-E845.9)*
> *watercraft (E830.0-E838.9)*
> *accidents, not on the public highway, involving agricultural and construction machinery but not involving another motor vehicle (E919.0, E919.2, E919.7)*

The following fourth-digit subdivisions are for use with categories E820-E825 to identify the injured person:

.0 **Driver of motor vehicle other than motorcycle**
See definition (l)
.1 **Passenger in motor vehicle other than motorcycle**
See definition (l)
.2 **Motorcyclist**
See definition (l)
.3 **Passenger on motorcycle**
See definition (l)
.4 **Occupant of streetcar**
.5 **Rider of animal; occupant of animal-drawn vehicle**
.6 **Pedal cyclist**
See definition (p)
.7 **Pedestrian**
See definition (r)
☐ .8 **Other specified person**
Occupant of vehicle other than above
Person on railway train involved in accident
Unauthorized rider of motor vehicle
☐ .9 **Unspecified person**

● E820 **Nontraffic accident involving motor-driven snow vehicle**

Requires fourth digit. See beginning of section E800-E845 for codes and definitions.

Includes: breakage of part of motor-driven snow vehicle (not on public highway)
fall from motor-driven snow vehicle (not on public highway)
hit by motor-driven snow vehicle (not on public highway)
overturning of motor-driven snow vehicle (not on public highway)
run over or dragged by motor-driven snow vehicle (not on public highway)
collision of motor-driven snow vehicle with:
animal (being ridden) (-drawn vehicle)
another off-road motor vehicle
other motor vehicle, not on public highway
railway train
other object, fixed or movable
injury caused by rough landing of motor-driven snow vehicle (after leaving ground on rough terrain)

> **Excludes** *accident on the public highway involving motor driven snow vehicle (E810.0-E819.9)*

● ☐ E821 **Nontraffic accident involving other off-road motor vehicle**

Requires fourth digit. See beginning of section E800-E845 for codes and definitions.

Includes: breakage of part of off-road motor vehicle, except snow vehicle (not on public highway)
fall from off-road motor vehicle, except snow vehicle (not on public highway)
hit by off-road motor vehicle, except snow vehicle (not on public highway)
overturning of off-road motor vehicle, except snow vehicle (not on public highway)
run over or dragged by off-road motor vehicle, except snow vehicle (not on public highway)
thrown against some part of or object in off-road motor vehicle, except snow vehicle (not on public highway)
collision with:
animal (being ridden) (-drawn vehicle)
another off-road motor vehicle, except snow vehicle
other motor vehicle, not on public highway
other object, fixed or movable

> **Excludes** *accident on public highway involving off-road motor vehicle (E810.0-E819.9)*
> *collision between motor driven snow vehicle and other off-road motor vehicle (E820.0-E820.9)*
> *hovercraft accident on water (E830.0-E838.9)*

● ☐ E822 **Other motor vehicle nontraffic accident involving collision with moving object**

Requires fourth digit. See beginning of section E800-E845 for codes and definitions.

Includes: collision, not on public highway, between motor vehicle, except off-road motor vehicle and:
animal
nonmotor vehicle
other motor vehicle, except off-road motor vehicle
pedestrian
railway train
other moving object

> **Excludes** *collision with:*
> *motor-driven snow vehicle (E820.0-E820.9)*
> *other off-road motor vehicle (E821.0-E821.9)*

● ☐ E823 **Other motor vehicle nontraffic accident involving collision with stationary object**

Requires fourth digit. See beginning of section E800-E845 for codes and definitions.

Includes: collision, not on public highway, between motor vehicle, except off-road motor vehicle, and any object, fixed or movable, but not in motion

● ☐ E824 **Other motor vehicle nontraffic accident while boarding and alighting**

Requires fourth digit. See beginning of section E800-E845 for codes and definitions.

Includes: fall while boarding or alighting from motor vehicle except off-road motor vehicle, not on public highway
injury from moving part of motor vehicle while boarding or alighting from motor vehicle except off-road motor vehicle, not on public highway
trapped by door of motor vehicle while boarding or alighting from motor vehicle except off-road motor vehicle, not on public highway

● ❏**E825 Other motor vehicle nontraffic accident of other and unspecified nature**

Requires fourth digit. See beginning of section E800-E845 for codes and definitions.

Includes: accidental poisoning from carbon monoxide generated by motor vehicle while in motion, not on public highway

breakage of any part of motor vehicle while in motion, not on public highway

explosion of any part of motor vehicle while in motion, not on public highway

fall, jump, or being accidentally pushed from motor vehicle while in motion, not on public highway

fire starting in motor vehicle while in motion, not on public highway

hit by object thrown into, towards, or on motor vehicle while in motion, not on public highway

injured by being thrown against some part of, or object in, motor vehicle while in motion, not on public highway

injury from moving part of motor vehicle while in motion, not on public highway

object falling in or on motor vehicle while in motion, not on public highway

motor vehicle nontraffic accident NOS

Excludes *fall from or in stationary motor vehicle (E884.9, E885.9)*

overcome by carbon monoxide or exhaust gas generated by stationary motor vehicle off the roadway with motor running (E868.2)

struck by falling object from or in stationary motor vehicle (E916)

OTHER ROAD VEHICLE ACCIDENTS (E826-E829)

Note: Other road vehicle accidents are transport accidents involving road vehicles other than motor vehicles. For definitions of other road vehicle and related terms see definitions (m) to (o).

Includes: accidents involving other road vehicles being used in recreational or sporting activities

Excludes *collision of other road vehicle [any] with:*
aircraft (E840.0-E845.9)
motor vehicle (E813.0-E813.9, E820.0-E822.9)
railway train (E801.0-E801.9)

ICD-9-CM

E800-E999

Vol. 1

The following fourth-digit subdivisions are for use with categories E826-E829 to identify the injured person:

.0 **Pedestrian**
See definition (r)

.1 **Pedal cyclist**
See definition (p)

.2 **Rider of animal**

.3 **Occupant of animal-drawn vehicle**

.4 **Occupant of streetcar**

❏ .8 **Other specified person**

❏ .9 **Unspecified person**

● **E826 Pedal cycle accident**

[0–9]   Requires fourth digit. See beginning of section E800-E845 for codes and definitions.

Includes: breakage of any part of pedal cycle

collision between pedal cycle and:
animal (being ridden) (herded) (unattended)
another pedal cycle
nonmotor road vehicle, any
pedestrian
other object, fixed, movable, or moving, not set in motion by motor vehicle, railway train, or aircraft

entanglement in wheel of pedal cycle

fall from pedal cycle

hit by object falling or thrown on the pedal cycle

pedal cycle accident NOS

pedal cycle overturned

● **E827 Animal-drawn vehicle accident**

[0,2–4,8,9]   Requires fourth digit. See beginning of section E800-E845 for codes and definitions.

Includes: breakage of any part of vehicle

collision between animal-drawn vehicle and:
animal (being ridden) (herded) (unattended)
nonmotor road vehicle, except pedal cycle
pedestrian, pedestrian conveyance, or pedestrian vehicle
other object, fixed, movable, or moving, not set in motion by motor vehicle, railway train, or aircraft

fall from animal-drawn vehicle

knocked down by animal-drawn vehicle

overturning of animal-drawn vehicle

run over by animal-drawn vehicle

thrown from animal-drawn vehicle

Excludes *collision of animal-drawn vehicle with pedal cycle (E826.0-E826.9)*

● **E828   Accident involving animal being ridden**

[0,2,4,8,9]

Requires fourth digit. See beginning of section E800-E845 for codes and definitions.

Includes: collision between animal being ridden and:
    another animal
    nonmotor road vehicle, except pedal cycle, and animal-drawn vehicle
    pedestrian, pedestrian conveyance, or pedestrian vehicle
    other object, fixed, movable, or moving, not set in motion by motor vehicle, railway train, or aircraft
  fall from animal being ridden
  knocked down by animal being ridden
  thrown from animal being ridden
  trampled by animal being ridden
  ridden animal stumbled and fell

Excludes *collision of animal being ridden with:*
    animal-drawn vehicle (E827.0-E827.9)
    pedal cycle (E826.0-E826.9)

● ❑ **E829   Other road vehicle accidents**

[0,4,8,9]

Requires fourth digit. See beginning of section E800-E845 for codes and definitions.

Includes: accident while boarding or alighting from
    streetcar
    nonmotor road vehicle not classifiable to E826-E828
  blow from object in
    streetcar
    nonmotor road vehicle not classifiable to E826-E828
  breakage of any part of
    streetcar
    nonmotor road vehicle not classifiable to E826-E828
  caught in door of
    streetcar
    nonmotor road vehicle not classifiable to E826-E828
  derailment of
    streetcar
    nonmotor road vehicle not classifiable to E826-E828
  fall in, on, or from
    streetcar
    nonmotor road vehicle not classifiable to E826-E828
  fire in
    streetcar
    nonmotor road vehicle not classifiable to E826-E828
  collision between streetcar or nonmotor road vehicle, except as in E826-E828, and:
    animal (not being ridden)
    another nonmotor road vehicle not classifiable to E826-E828
    pedestrian
    other object, fixed, movable, or moving, not set in motion by motor vehicle, railway train, or aircraft
  nonmotor road vehicle accident NOS
  streetcar accident NOS

Excludes *collision with:*
    animal being ridden (E828.0-E828.9)
    animal-drawn vehicle (E827.0-E827.9)
    pedal cycle (E826.0-E826.9)

WATER TRANSPORT ACCIDENTS (E830-E838)

Note: For definitions of water transport accident and related terms see definitions (a), (s), and (t).

Includes: watercraft accidents in the course of recreational activities

Excludes *accidents involving both aircraft, including objects set in motion by aircraft, and watercraft (E840.0-E845.9)*

The following fourth-digit subdivisions are for use with categories E830-E838 to identify the injured person:

  .0 Occupant of small boat, unpowered
  .1 Occupant of small boat, powered
    See definition (t)

Excludes *water skier (4)*

❑ **.2 Occupant of other watercraft-crew**
    Persons:
      engaged in operation of watercraft
      providing passenger services [cabin attendants, ship's physician, catering personnel]
      working on ship during voyage in other capacity [musician in band, operators of shops and beauty parlors]

❑ **.3 Occupant of other watercraft -- other than crew**
    Passenger
      Occupant of lifeboat, other than crew, after abandoning ship

  .4 Water skier
  .5 Swimmer
  .6 Dockers, stevedores
    Longshoreman employed on the dock in loading and unloading ships

❑ **.8 Other specified person**
    Immigration and customs officials on board ship
    Person:
      accompanying passenger or member of crew visiting boat
    Pilot (guiding ship into port)

❑ **.9 Unspecified person**

● **E830   Accident to watercraft causing submersion**

Requires fourth digit. See beginning of section E800-E845 for codes and definitions.

Includes: submersion and drowning due to:
    boat overturning
    boat submerging
    falling or jumping from burning ship
    falling or jumping from crushed watercraft
    ship sinking
    other accident to watercraft

● ❑ **E831   Accident to watercraft causing other injury**

Requires fourth digit. See beginning of section E800-E845 for codes and definitions.

Includes: any injury, except submersion and drowning, as a result of an accident to watercraft
    burned while ship on fire
    crushed between ships in collision
    crushed by lifeboat after abandoning ship
    fall due to collision or other accident to watercraft
    hit by falling object due to accident to watercraft
    injured in watercraft accident involving collision
    struck by boat or part thereof after fall or jump from damaged boat

Excludes *burns from localized fire or explosion on board ship (E837.0-E837.9)*

● ☐ **E832 Other accidental submersion or drowning in water transport accident**

Requires fourth digit. See beginning of section E800-E845 for codes and definitions.

Includes: submersion or drowning as a result of an accident other than accident to the watercraft, such as:
     fall:
Includes: from gangplank
Includes: from ship
Includes: overboard
     thrown overboard by motion of ship
     washed overboard

Excludes *submersion or drowning of swimmer or diver who voluntarily jumps from boat not involved in an accident (E910.0-E910.9)*

● **E833 Fall on stairs or ladders in water transport**

Requires fourth digit. See beginning of section E800-E845 for codes and definitions.

Excludes *fall due to accident to watercraft (E831.0-E831.9)*

● ☐ **E834 Other fall from one level to another in water transport**

Requires fourth digit. See beginning of section E800-E845 for codes and definitions.

Excludes *fall due to accident to watercraft (E831.0-E831.9)*

● ☐ **E835 Other and unspecified fall in water transport**

Requires fourth digit. See beginning of section E800-E845 for codes and definitions.

Excludes *fall due to accident to watercraft (E831.0-E831.9)*

● **E836 Machinery accident in water transport**

Requires fourth digit. See beginning of section E800-E845 for codes and definitions.

Includes: injuries in water transport caused by:
     deck machinery
     engine room machinery
     galley machinery
     laundry machinery
     loading machinery

● **E837 Explosion, fire, or burning in watercraft**

Requires fourth digit. See beginning of section E800-E845 for codes and definitions.

Includes: explosion of boiler on steamship
     localized fire on ship

Excludes *burning ship (due to collision or explosion) resulting in:*
     submersion or drowning (E830.0-E830.9)
     other injury (E831.0-E831.9)

● ☐ **E838 Other and unspecified water transport accident**

Requires fourth digit. See beginning of section E800-E845 for codes and definitions.

Includes: accidental poisoning by gases or fumes on ship
     atomic power plant malfunction in watercraft
     crushed between ship and stationary object [wharf]
     crushed between ships without accident to watercraft
     crushed by falling object on ship or while loading or unloading
     hit by boat while water skiing
     struck by boat or part thereof (after fall from boat)
     watercraft accident NOS

AIR AND SPACE TRANSPORT ACCIDENTS (E840-E845)

Note: For definition of aircraft and related terms see definitions (u) and (v).

The following fourth-digit subdivisions are for use with categories E840-E845 to identify the injured person:

.0 Occupant of spacecraft

.1 Occupant of military aircraft, any
     Crew in military aircraft [air force] [army] [national guard] [navy]
     Passenger (civilian) (military) in military aircraft [air force] [army] [national guard] [navy]
     Troops in military aircraft [air force] [army] [national guard] [navy]

Excludes *occupants of aircraft operated under jurisdiction of police departments (5)*
     parachutist (7)

.2 Crew of commercial aircraft (powered) in surface-to-surface transport

☐ **.3 Other occupant of commercial aircraft (powered) in surface-to-surface transport**
     Flight personnel:
         not part of crew
         on familiarization flight
     Passenger on aircraft (powered) NOS

.4 Occupant of commercial aircraft (powered) in surface-to-air transport
     Occupant [crew] [passenger] of aircraft (powered) engaged in activities, such as:
         aerial spraying (crops) (fire retardants)
         air drops of emergency supplies
         air drops of parachutists, except from military craft
         crop dusting
         lowering of construction material [bridge or telephone pole]
         sky writing

☐ **.5 Occupant of other powered aircraft**
     Occupant [crew] [passenger] of aircraft [powered] engaged in activities, such as:
         aerobatic flying
         aircraft racing
         rescue operation
         storm surveillance
         traffic surveillance
     Occupant of private plane NOS

.6 Occupant of unpowered aircraft, except parachutist
     Occupant of aircraft classifiable to E842

.7 Parachutist (military) (other)
     Person making voluntary descent

Excludes *person making descent after accident to aircraft (.1-.6)*

.8 Ground crew, airline employee
     Persons employed at airfields (civil) (military) or launching pads, not occupants of aircraft

☐ **.9 Other person**

● **E840 Accident to powered aircraft at takeoff or landing**

Requires fourth digit. See beginning of section E800-E845 for codes and definitions.

Includes: collision of aircraft with any object, fixed, movable, or moving while taking off or landing
     crash while taking off or landing
     explosion on aircraft while taking off or landing
     fire on aircraft while taking off or landing
     forced landing

ICD-9-CM

E800-E999

Vol. 1

● ☐ **E841 Accident to powered aircraft, other and unspecified**

> Requires fourth digit. See beginning of section E800-E845 for codes and definitions.

Includes: aircraft accident NOS
> aircraft crash or wreck NOS
> any accident to powered aircraft while in transit or when not specified whether in transit, taking off, or landing
> collision of aircraft with another aircraft, bird, or any object, while in transit
> explosion on aircraft while in transit
> fire on aircraft while in transit

● **E842 Accident to unpowered aircraft**
[6–9]

> Requires fourth digit. See beginning of section E800-E845 for codes and definitions.

Includes: any accident, except collision with powered aircraft, to:
> balloon
> glider
> hang glider
> kite carrying a person
> hit by object falling from unpowered aircraft

● **E843 Fall in, on, or from aircraft**
[0–9]

> Requires fourth digit. See beginning of section E800-E845 for codes and definitions.

Includes: accident in boarding or alighting from aircraft, any kind
> fall in, on, or from aircraft [any kind], while in transit, taking off, or landing, except when as a result of an accident to aircraft

● ☐ **E844 Other specified air transport accidents**
[0–9]

> Requires fourth digit. See beginning of section E800-E845 for codes and definitions.

Includes: hit by aircraft without accident to aircraft
> hit by object falling from aircraft without accident to aircraft
> injury by or from machinery on aircraft without accident to aircraft
> injury by or from rotating propeller without accident to aircraft
> injury by or from voluntary parachute descent without accident to aircraft
> poisoning by carbon monoxide from aircraft while in transit without accident to aircraft
> sucked into jet without accident to aircraft
> any accident involving other transport vehicle (motor) (nonmotor) due to being hit by object set in motion by aircraft (powered)

> **Excludes** *air sickness (E903)*
> *effects of:*
>   *high altitude (E902.0-E902.1)*
>   *pressure change (E902.0-E902.1)*
> *injury in parachute descent due to accident to aircraft (E840.0-E842.9)*

● **E845 Accident involving spacecraft**
[0,8,9]

> Requires fourth digit. See beginning of section E800-E845 for codes and definitions.

Includes: launching pad accident

> **Excludes** *effects of weightlessness in spacecraft (E928.0)*

VEHICLE ACCIDENTS NOT ELSEWHERE CLASSIFIABLE (E846-E848)

E846 Accidents involving powered vehicles used solely within the buildings and premises of industrial or commercial establishment

> Accident to, on, or involving:
>   battery-powered airport passenger vehicle
>   battery-powered trucks (baggage) (mail)
>   coal car in mine
>   logging car
>   self-propelled truck, industrial
>   station baggage truck (powered)
>   tram, truck, or tub (powered) in mine or quarry
> Breakage of any part of vehicle
> Collision with:
>   pedestrian
>   other vehicle or object within premises
> Explosion of powered vehicle, industrial or commercial
> Fall from powered vehicle, industrial or commercial
> Overturning of powered vehicle, industrial or commercial
> Struck by powered vehicle, industrial or commercial

> **Excludes** *accidental poisoning by exhaust gas from vehicle not elsewhere classifiable (E868.2)*
> *injury by crane, lift (fork), or elevator (E919.2)*

E847 Accidents involving cable cars not running on rails

> Accident to, on, or involving:
>   cable car, not on rails
>   ski chair-lift
>   ski-lift with gondola
>   teleferique
> Breakage of cable
>   Caught or dragged by cable car, not on rails
>   Fall or jump from cable car, not on rails
>   Object thrown from or in cable car not on rails

☐ **E848 Accidents involving other vehicles, not elsewhere classifiable**

> Accident to, on, or involving:
>   ice yacht
>   land yacht
>   nonmotor, nonroad vehicle NOS

● *E849 Place of occurrence*

> *Note: The following category is for use to denote the place where the injury or poisoning occurred.*

E849.0 Home
> *Apartment*
> *Boarding house*
> *Farm house*
> *Home premises*
> *House (residential)*
> *Noninstitutional place of residence*
> *Private:*
>   *driveway*
>   *garage*
>   *garden*
>   *home*
>   *walk*
> *Swimming pool in private house or garden*
> *Yard of home*

> **Excludes** *home under construction but not yet occupied (E849.3)*
> *institutional place of residence (E849.7)*

E849.1 Farm
> *buildings*
> *land under cultivation*

> **Excludes** *farm house and home premises of farm (E849.0)*

E849.2   Mine and quarry
Gravel pit
Sand pit
Tunnel under construction

E849.3   Industrial place and premises
Building under construction
Dockyard
Dry dock
Factory
    building
    premises
Garage (place of work)
Industrial yard
Loading platform (factory) (store)
Plant, industrial
Railway yard
Shop (place of work)
Warehouse
Workhouse

E849.4   Place for recreation and sport
Amusement park	Playground, including
Baseball field	school playground
Basketball court	Public park
Beach resort	Racecourse
Cricket ground	Resort NOS
Fives court	Riding school
Football field	Rifle range
Golf course	Seashore resort
Gymnasium	Skating rink
Hockey field	Sports palace
Holiday camp	Stadium
Ice palace	Swimming pool, public
Lake resort	Tennis court
Mountain resort	Vacation resort

Excludes   that in private house or garden (E849.0)

E849.5   Street and highway

E849.6   Public building
Building (including adjacent grounds) used by
    the general public or by a particular group
    of the public, such as:
airport
bank
cafe
casino
church
cinema
clubhouse
courthouse
dance hall
garage building (for car storage)
hotel
market (grocery or other commodity)
movie house
music hall
nightclub
office
office building
opera house
post office
public hall
radio broadcasting station
restaurant
school (state) (public) (private)
shop, commercial
station (bus) (railway)
store
theater

Excludes   home garage (E849.0)
           industrial building or workplace (E849.3)

E849.7   Residential institution
Children's home
Dormitory
Hospital
Jail
Old people's home
Orphanage
Prison
Reform school

☐E849.8   Other specified places
Beach NOS
Canal
Caravan site NOS
Derelict house
Desert
Dock
Forest
Harbor
Hill
Lake NOS
Mountain
Parking lot
Parking place
Pond or pool (natural)
Prairie
Public place NOS
Railway line
Reservoir
River
Sea
Seashore NOS
Stream
Swamp
Trailer court
Woods

☐E849.9   Unspecified place

ACCIDENTAL POISONING BY DRUGS, MEDICINAL SUBSTANCES, AND BIOLOGICALS (E850-E858)

Includes: accidental overdose of drug, wrong drug
         given or taken in error, and drug taken
         inadvertently
         accidents in the use of drugs and biologicals
         in medical and surgical procedures

Excludes   administration with suicidal or homicidal intent
       or intent to harm, or in circumstances clas-
       sifiable to E980-E989 (E950.0-E950.5,
       E962.0, E980.0-E980.5)
       correct drug properly administered in therapeutic
       or prophylactic dosage, as the cause of ad-
       verse effect (E930.0-E949.9)

Note: See Alphabetic Index for more complete list of
       specific drugs to be classified under the fourth-
       digit subdivisions. The American Hospital For-
       mulary numbers can be used to classify new
       drugs listed by the American Hospital Formu-
       lary Service (AHFS). See appendix C.

●E850   Accidental poisoning by analgesics, antipyretics, and antirheumatics

E850.0   Heroin
Diacetylmorphine

E850.1   Methadone

☐E850.2   Other opiates and related narcotics
Codeine [methylmorphine]
Meperidine [pethidine]
Morphine
Opium (alkaloids)

E850.3 **Salicylates**
Acetylsalicylic acid [aspirin]
Amino derivatives of salicylic acid
Salicylic acid salts

E850.4 **Aromatic analgesics, not elsewhere classified**
Acetanilid
Paracetamol [acetaminophen]
Phenacetin [acetophenetidin]

E850.5 **Pyrazole derivatives**
Aminophenazone [amidopyrine]
Phenylbutazone

E850.6 **Antirheumatics [antiphlogistics]**
Gold salts
Indomethacin
Excludes *salicylates (E850.3)*
steroids (E858.0)

☐ E850.7 **Other non-narcotic analgesics**
Pyrabital

☐ E850.8 **Other specified analgesics and antipyretics**
Pentazocine

☐ E850.9 **Unspecified analgesic or antipyretic**

E851 **Accidental poisoning by barbiturates**
Amobarbital [amylobarbitone]
Barbital [barbitone]
Butabarbital [butabarbitone]
Pentobarbital [pentobarbitone]
Phenobarbital [phenobarbitone]
Secobarbital [quinalbarbitone]
Excludes *thiobarbiturates (E855.1)*

● E852 **Accidental poisoning by other sedatives and hypnotics**

E852.0 **Chloral hydrate group**

E852.1 **Paraldehyde**

E852.2 **Bromine compounds**
Bromides
Carbromal (derivatives)

E852.3 **Methaqualone compounds**

E852.4 **Glutethimide group**

E852.5 **Mixed sedatives, not elsewhere classified**

☐ E852.8 **Other specified sedatives and hypnotics**

☐ E852.9 **Unspecified sedative or hypnotic**
Sleeping:
drug NOS
pill NOS
tablet NOS

● E853 **Accidental poisoning by tranquilizers**

E853.0 **Phenothiazine-based tranquilizers**
Chlorpromazine
Fluphenazine
Prochlorperazine
Promazine

E853.1 **Butyrophenone-based tranquilizers**
Haloperidol
Spiperone
Trifluperidol

E853.2 **Benzodiazepine-based tranquilizers**
Chlordiazepoxide   Lorazepam
Diazepam   Medazepam
Flurazepam   Nitrazepam

☐ E853.8 **Other specified tranquilizers**
Hydroxyzine
Meprobamate

☐ E853.9 **Unspecified tranquilizer**

● E854 **Accidental poisoning by other psychotropic agents**

E854.0 **Antidepressants**
Amitriptyline
Imipramine
Monoamine oxidase [MAO] inhibitors

E854.1 **Psychodysleptics [hallucinogens]**
Cannabis derivatives
Lysergide [LSD]
Marihuana (derivatives)
Mescaline
Psilocin
Psilocybin

E854.2 **Psychostimulants**
Amphetamine
Caffeine
Excludes *central appetite depressants (E858.8)*

E854.3 **Central nervous system stimulants**
Analeptics
Opiate antagonists

E854.8 **Other psychotropic agents**

● E855 **Accidental poisoning by other drugs acting on central and autonomic nervous system**

E855.0 **Anticonvulsant and anti-Parkinsonism drugs**
Amantadine
Hydantoin derivatives
Levodopa [L-dopa]
Oxazolidine derivatives [paramethadione] [trimethadione]
Succinimides

☐ E855.1 **Other central nervous system depressants**
Ether
Gaseous anesthetics
Halogenated hydrocarbon derivatives
Intravenous anesthetics
Thiobarbiturates, such as thiopental sodium

E855.2 **Local anesthetics**
Cocaine
Lidocaine [lignocaine]
Procaine
Tetracaine

E855.3 **Parasympathomimetics [cholinergics]**
Acetylcholine
Anticholinesterase:
organophosphorus
reversible
Pilocarpine

E855.4 **Parasympatholytics [anticholinergics and antimuscarinics] and spasmolytics**
Atropine
Homatropine
Hyoscine [scopolamine]
Quaternary ammonium derivatives

E855.5 **Sympathomimetics [adrenergics]**
Epinephrine [adrenalin]
Levarterenol [noradrenalin]

E855.6 **Sympatholytics [antiadrenergics]**
Phenoxybenzamine
Tolazoline hydrochloride

☐ E855.8 **Other specified drugs acting on central and autonomic nervous systems**

☐ E855.9 **Unspecified drug acting on central and autonomic nervous systems**

E856 **Accidental poisoning by antibiotics**

☐ E857 **Accidental poisoning by other anti-infectives**

● **E858 Accidental poisoning by other drugs**

E858.0 Hormones and synthetic substitutes

E858.1 Primarily systemic agents

E858.2 Agents primarily affecting blood constituents

E858.3 Agents primarily affecting cardiovascular system

E858.4 Agents primarily affecting gastrointestinal system

E858.5 Water, mineral, and uric acid metabolism drugs

E858.6 Agents primarily acting on the smooth and skeletal muscles and respiratory system

E858.7 Agents primarily affecting skin and mucous membrane, ophthalmological, otorhinolaryngological, and dental drugs

☐ **E858.8 Other specified drugs**
Central appetite depressants

☐ **E858.9 Unspecified drug**

ACCIDENTAL POISONING BY OTHER SOLID AND LIQUID SUBSTANCES, GASES, AND VAPORS (E860-E869)

Note: Categories in this section are intended primarily to indicate the external cause of poisoning states classifiable to 980–989. They may also be used to indicate external causes of localized effects classifiable to 001–799.

● **E860 Accidental poisoning by alcohol, not elsewhere classified**

E860.0 Alcoholic beverages
Alcohol in preparations intended for consumption

☐ **E860.1 Other and unspecified ethyl alcohol and its products**
Denatured alcohol
Ethanol NOS
Grain alcohol NOS
Methylated spirit

E860.2 Methyl alcohol
Methanol
Wood alcohol

E860.3 Isopropyl alcohol
Dimethyl carbinol
Isopropanol
Rubbing alcohol substitute
Secondary propyl alcohol

E860.4 Fusel oil
Alcohol:
amyl
butyl
propyl

☐ **E860.8 Other specified alcohols**

☐ **E860.9 Unspecified alcohol**

● **E861 Accidental poisoning by cleansing and polishing agents, disinfectants, paints, and varnishes**

E861.0 Synthetic detergents and shampoos

E861.1 Soap products

E861.2 Polishes

☐ **E861.3 Other cleansing and polishing agents**
Scouring powders

E861.4 Disinfectants
Household and other disinfectants not ordinarily used on the person

Excludes	carbolic acid or phenol (E864.0)

E861.5 Lead paints

☐ **E861.6 Other paints and varnishes**
Lacquers
Oil colors
Paints, other than lead
Whitewashes

☐ **E861.9 Unspecified**

● **E862 Accidental poisoning by petroleum products, other solvents and their vapors, not elsewhere classified**

E862.0 Petroleum solvents
Petroleum:
ether
benzine
naphtha

E862.1 Petroleum fuels and cleaners
Antiknock additives to petroleum fuels
Gas oils
Gasoline or petrol
Kerosene

Excludes	kerosene insecticides (E863.4)

E862.2 Lubricating oils

E862.3 Petroleum solids
Paraffin wax

☐ **E862.4 Other specified solvents**
Benzene

☐ **E862.9 Unspecified solvent**

● **E863 Accidental poisoning by agricultural and horticultural chemical and pharmaceutical preparations other than plant foods and fertilizers**

Excludes	plant foods and fertilizers (E866.5)

E863.0 Insecticides of organochlorine compounds

Benzene hexachloride	Dieldrin
Chlordane	Endrine
DDT	Toxaphene

E863.1 Insecticides of organophosphorus compounds

Demeton	Parathion
Diazinon	Phenylsulphthion
Dichlorvos	Phorate
Malathion	Phosdrin
Methyl parathion	

E863.2 Carbamates
Aldicarb
Carbaryl
Propoxur

E863.3 Mixtures of insecticides

☐ **E863.4 Other and unspecified insecticides**
Kerosene insecticides

E863.5 Herbicides
2,4-Dichlorophenoxyacetic acid [2, 4-D]
2,4,5-Trichlorophenoxyacetic acid [2, 4, 5-T]
Chlorates
Diquat
Mixtures of plant foods and fertilizers with herbicides
Paraquat

E863.6 Fungicides
Organic mercurials (used in seed dressing)
Pentachlorophenols

E863.7 **Rodenticides**
Fluoroacetates Warfarin
Squill and derivatives Zinc phosphide
Thallium

E863.8 **Fumigants**
Cyanides Phosphine
Methyl bromide

☐E863.9 **Other and unspecified**

●E864 **Accidental poisoning by corrosives and caustics, not elsewhere classified**

Excludes *those as components of disinfectants (E861.4)*

E864.0 **Corrosive aromatics**
Carbolic acid or phenol

E864.1 **Acids**
Acid:
hydrochloric
nitric
sulfuric

E864.2 **Caustic alkalis**
Lye

☐E864.3 **Other specified corrosives and caustics**

☐E864.4 **Unspecified corrosives and caustics**

●E865 **Accidental poisoning from poisonous foodstuffs and poisonous plants**

Includes: any meat, fish, or shellfish
plants, berries, and fungi eaten as, or in mistake for food, or by a child

Excludes *anaphlyactic shock due to adverse food reaction (995.60–995.69)*
food poisoning (bacterial) (005.0–005.9)
poisoning and toxic reactions to venomous plants (E905.6-E905.7)

E865.0 **Meat**

E865.1 **Shellfish**

☐E865.2 **Other fish**

E865.3 **Berries and seeds**

☐E865.4 **Other specified plants**

E865.5 **Mushrooms and other fungi**

☐E865.8 **Other specified foods**

☐E865.9 **Unspecified foodstuff or poisonous plant**

●E866 **Accidental poisoning by other and unspecified solid and liquid substances**

Excludes *these substances as a component of:*
medicines (E850.0-E858.9)
paints (E861.5-E861.6)
pesticides (E863.0-E863.9)
petroleum fuels (E862.1)

E866.0 **Lead and its compounds and fumes**

E866.1 **Mercury and its compounds and fumes**

E866.2 **Antimony and its compounds and fumes**

E866.3 **Arsenic and its compounds and fumes**

☐E866.4 **Other metals and their compounds and fumes**
Beryllium (compounds)
Brass fumes
Cadmium (compounds)
Copper salts
Iron (compounds)
Manganese (compounds)
Nickel (compounds)
Thallium (compounds)

E866.5 **Plant foods and fertilizers**

Excludes *mixtures with herbicides (E863.5)*

E866.6 **Glues and adhesives**

E866.7 **Cosmetics**

☐E866.8 **Other specified solid or liquid substances**

☐E866.9 **Unspecified solid or liquid substance**

E867 **Accidental poisoning by gas distributed by pipeline**
Carbon monoxide from incomplete combustion of piped gas
Coal gas NOS
Liquefied petroleum gas distributed through pipes (pure or mixed with air)
Piped gas (natural) (manufactured)

●E868 **Accidental poisoning by other utility gas and other carbon monoxide**

E868.0 **Liquefied petroleum gas distributed in mobile containers**
Butane or carbon monoxide from incomplete combustion of these gases
Liquefied hydrocarbon gas NOS or carbon monoxide from incomplete combustion of these gases
Propane or carbon monoxide from incomplete combustion of these gases

☐E868.1 **Other and unspecified utility gas**
Acetylene or carbon monoxide from incomplete combustion of these gases
Gas NOS used for lighting, heating, or cooking or carbon monoxide from incomplete combustion of these gases
Water gas or carbon monoxide from incomplete combustion of these gases

E868.2 **Motor vehicle exhaust gas**
Exhaust gas from:
farm tractor, not in transit
gas engine
motor pump
motor vehicle, not in transit
any type of combustion engine not in watercraft

Excludes *poisoning by carbon monoxide from:*
aircraft while in transit (E844.0-E844.9)
motor vehicle while in transit (E818.0-E818.9)
watercraft whether or not in transit (E838.0-E838.9)

☐E868.3 **Carbon monoxide from incomplete combustion of other domestic fuels**
Carbon monoxide from incomplete combustion of:
coal in domestic stove or fireplace
coke in domestic stove or fireplace
kerosene in domestic stove or fireplace
wood in domestic stove or fireplace

Excludes *carbon monoxide from smoke and fumes due to conflagration (E890.0-E893.9)*

☐E868.8 **Carbon monoxide from other sources**
Carbon monoxide from:
blast furnace gas
incomplete combustion of fuels in industrial use
kiln vapor

☐E868.9 **Unspecified carbon monoxide**

● **E869 Accidental poisoning by other gases and vapors**

> **Excludes** *effects of gases used as anesthetics (E855.1, E938.2)*
> *fumes from heavy metals (E866.0-E866.4)*
> *smoke and fumes due to conflagration or explosion (E890.0-E899)*

   E869.0 Nitrogen oxides

   E869.1 Sulfur dioxide

   E869.2 Freon

   E869.3 Lacrimogenic gas [tear gas]
      Bromobenzyl cyanide
      Chloroacetophenone
      Ethyliodoacetate

   E869.4 Second-hand tobacco smoke

   ❏ **E869.8 Other specified gases and vapors**
      Chlorine
      Hydrocyanic acid gas

   ❏ **E869.9 Unspecified gases and vapors**

MISADVENTURES TO PATIENTS DURING SURGICAL AND MEDICAL CARE (E870-E876)

> **Excludes** *accidental overdose of drug and wrong drug given in error (E850.0-E858.9)*
> *surgical and medical procedures as the cause of abnormal reaction by the patient, without mention of misadventure at the time of procedure (E878.0-E879.9)*

● **E870 Accidental cut, puncture, perforation, or hemorrhage during medical care**

   E870.0 Surgical operation

   E870.1 Infusion or transfusion

   E870.2 Kidney dialysis or other perfusion

   E870.3 Injection or vaccination

   E870.4 Endoscopic examination

   E870.5 Aspiration of fluid or tissue, puncture, and catheterization
      Abdominal paracentesis
      Aspirating needle biopsy
      Blood sampling
      Lumbar puncture
      Thoracentesis

> **Excludes** *heart catheterization (E870.6)*

   E870.6 Heart catheterization

   E870.7 Administration of enema

   ❏ **E870.8 Other specified medical care**

   ❏ **E870.9 Unspecified medical care**

● **E871 Foreign object left in body during procedure**

   E871.0 Surgical operation

   E871.1 Infusion or transfusion

   E871.2 Kidney dialysis or other perfusion

   E871.3 Injection or vaccination

   E871.4 Endoscopic examination

   E871.5 Aspiration of fluid or tissue, puncture, and catheterization
      Abdominal paracentesis
      Aspiration needle biopsy
      Blood sampling
      Lumbar puncture
      Thoracentesis

> **Excludes** *heart catheterization (E871.6)*

   E871.6 Heart catheterization

   E871.7 Removal of catheter or packing

   ❏ **E871.8 Other specified procedures**

   ❏ **E871.9 Unspecified procedure**

● **E872 Failure of sterile precautions during procedure**

   E872.0 Surgical operation

   E872.1 Infusion or transfusion

   E872.2 Kidney dialysis and other perfusion

   E872.3 Injection or vaccination

   E872.4 Endoscopic examination

   E872.5 Aspiration of fluid or tissue, puncture, and catheterization
      Abdominal paracentesis
      Aspirating needle biopsy
      Blood sampling
      Lumbar puncture
      Thoracentesis

> **Excludes** *heart catheterization (E872.6)*

   E872.6 Heart catheterization

   ❏ **E872.8 Other specified procedures**

   ❏ **E872.9 Unspecified procedure**

● **E873 Failure in dosage**

> **Excludes** *accidental overdose of drug, medicinal or biological substance (E850.0-E858.9)*

   ❏ **E873.0 Excessive amount of blood or other fluid during transfusion or infusion**

   E873.1 Incorrect dilution of fluid during infusion

   E873.2 Overdose of radiation in therapy

   E873.3 Inadvertent exposure of patient to radiation during medical care

   E873.4 Failure in dosage in electroshock or insulin-shock therapy

   E873.5 Inappropriate [too hot or too cold] temperature in local application and packing

   E873.6 Nonadministration of necessary drug or medicinal substance

   ❏ **E873.8 Other specified failure in dosage**

   ❏ **E873.9 Unspecified failure in dosage**

● **E874 Mechanical failure of instrument or apparatus during procedure**

   E874.0 Surgical operation

   E874.1 Infusion and transfusion
      Air in system

   E874.2 Kidney dialysis and other perfusion

   E874.3 Endoscopic examination

   E874.4 Aspiration of fluid or tissue, puncture, and catheterization
      Abdominal paracentesis
      Aspirating needle biopsy
      Blood sampling
      Lumbar puncture
      Thoracentesis

> **Excludes** *heart catheterization (E874.5)*

   E874.5 Heart catheterization

   ❏ **E874.8 Other specified procedures**

   ❏ **E874.9 Unspecified procedure**

ICD-9-CM

E800–E899

Vol. 1

● E875 **Contaminated or infected blood, other fluid, drug, or biological substance**

Includes: presence of:
    bacterial pyrogens
    endotoxin-producing bacteria
    serum hepatitis-producing agent

    E875.0 **Contaminated substance transfused or infused**

    E875.1 **Contaminated substance injected or used for vaccination**

    ☐ E875.2 **Contaminated drug or biological substance administered by other means**

    ☐ E875.8 **Other**

    ☐ E875.9 **Unspecified**

● E876 **Other and unspecified misadventures during medical care**

    E876.0 **Mismatched blood in transfusion**

    E876.1 **Wrong fluid in infusion**

    E876.2 **Failure in suture and ligature during surgical operation**

    E876.3 **Endotracheal tube wrongly placed during anesthetic procedure**

    ☐ E876.4 **Failure to introduce or to remove other tube or instrument**

       | **Excludes** | *foreign object left in body during procedure (E871.0-E871.9)* |

    E876.5 **Performance of inappropriate operation**

    ☐ E876.8 **Other specified misadventures during medical care**
        Performance of inappropriate treatment, NEC

    ☐ E876.9 **Unspecified misadventure during medical care**

SURGICAL AND MEDICAL PROCEDURES AS THE CAUSE OF ABNORMAL REACTION OF PATIENT OR LATER COMPLICATION, WITHOUT MENTION OF MISADVENTURE AT THE TIME OF PROCEDURE (E878-E879)

Includes: procedures as the cause of abnormal reaction, such as:
    displacement or malfunction of prosthetic device
    hepatorenal failure, postoperative
    malfunction of external stoma
    postoperative intestinal obstruction
    rejection of transplanted organ

| **Excludes** | *anesthetic management properly carried out as the cause of adverse effect (E937.0-E938.9)* |
| | *infusion and transfusion, without mention of misadventure in the technique of procedure (E930.0-E949.9)* |

● E878 **Surgical operation and other surgical procedures as the cause of abnormal reaction of patient, or of later complication, without mention of misadventure at the time of operation**

    E878.0 **Surgical operation with transplant of whole organ**
        Transplantation of:
          heart
          kidney
          liver

    E878.1 **Surgical operation with implant of artificial internal device**
        Cardiac pacemaker
        Electrodes implanted in brain
        Heart valve prosthesis
        Internal orthopedic device

    E878.2 **Surgical operation with anastomosis, bypass, or graft, with natural or artificial tissues used as implant**
        Anastomosis:
          arteriovenous
          gastrojejunal
        Graft of blood vessel, tendon, or skin

    | **Excludes** | *external stoma (E878.3)* |

    E878.3 **Surgical operation with formation of external stoma**
        Colostomy
        Cystostomy
        Duodenostomy
        Gastrostomy
        Ureterostomy

    ☐ E878.4 **Other restorative surgery**

    E878.5 **Amputation of limb(s)**

    ☐ E878.6 **Removal of other organ (partial) (total)**

    ☐ E878.8 **Other specified surgical operations and procedures**

    ☐ E878.9 **Unspecified surgical operations and procedures**

● E879 **Other procedures, without mention of misadventure at the time of procedure, as the cause of abnormal reaction of patient, or of later complication**

    E879.0 **Cardiac catheterization**

    E879.1 **Kidney dialysis**

    E879.2 **Radiological procedure and radiotherapy**

    | **Excludes** | *radio-opaque dyes for diagnostic x-ray procedures (E947.8)* |

    E879.3 **Shock therapy**
        Electroshock therapy
        Insulin-shock therapy

    E879.4 **Aspiration of fluid**
        Lumbar puncture   Thoracentesis

    E879.5 **Insertion of gastric or duodenal sound**

    E879.6 **Urinary catheterization**

    E879.7 **Blood sampling**

    ☐ E879.8 **Other specified procedures**
        Blood transfusion

    ☐ E879.9 **Unspecified procedure**

ACCIDENTAL FALLS (E880-E888)

Excludes	*falls (in or from):*
	burning building (E890.8, E891.8)
	into fire (E890.0-E899)
	into water (with submersion or drowning) (E910.0-E910.9)
	machinery (in operation) (E919.0-E919.9)
	on edged, pointed, or sharp object (E920.0-E920.9)
	transport vehicle (E800.0-E845.9)
	vehicle not elsewhere classifiable (E846-E848)

● E880 **Fall on or from stairs or steps**

    E880.0 **Escalator**

    E880.1 **Fall on or from sidewalk curb**

    | **Excludes** | *fall from moving sidewalk (E885.9)* |

    ☐ E880.9 **Other stairs or steps**

● E881 **Fall on or from ladders or scaffolding**

    E881.0 **Fall from ladder**

    E881.1 **Fall from scaffolding**

☐ **E882 Fall from or out of building or other structure**
Fall from:
    balcony
    bridge
    building
    flagpole
    tower
    turret
    viaduct
    wall
    window
Fall through roof

Excludes	collapse of a building or structure (E916)
	fall or jump from burning building (E890.8, E891.8)

● **E883 Fall into hole or other opening in surface**

Includes: fall into:
    cavity
    dock
    hole
    pit
    quarry
    shaft
    swimming pool
    tank
    well

Excludes	fall into water NOS (E910.9)
	that resulting in drowning or submersion without mention of injury (E910.0-E910.9)

E883.0 Accident from diving or jumping into water [swimming pool]
Strike or hit:
    against bottom when jumping or diving into water
    wall or board of swimming pool
    water surface

Excludes	diving with insufficient air supply (E913.2)
	effects of air pressure from diving (E902.2)

E883.1 Accidental fall into well

E883.2 Accidental fall into storm drain or manhole

☐ **E883.9 Fall into other hole or other opening in surface**

● **E884 Other fall from one level to another**

E884.0 Fall from playground equipment

Excludes	recreational machinery (E919.8)

E884.1 Fall from cliff

E884.2 Fall from chair

E884.3 Fall from wheelchair

E884.4 Fall from bed

E884.5 Fall from other furniture

E884.6 Fall from commode
Toilet

☐ **E884.9 Other fall from one level to another**
Fall from:
    embankment
    haystack
    stationary vehicle
    tree

● **E885 Fall on same level from slipping, tripping, or stumbling**

E885.0 Fall from (nonmotorized) scooter

E885.1 Fall from roller skates
In-line skates

E885.2 Fall from skateboard

E885.3 Fall from skis

E885.4 Fall from snowboard

E885.9 Fall from other slipping, tripping, or stumbling
Fall on moving sidewalk

● **E886 Fall on same level from collision, pushing, or shoving, by or with other person**

Excludes	crushed or pushed by a crowd or human stampede (E917.1, E917.6)

E886.0 In sports
Tackles in sports

Excludes	kicked, stepped on, struck by object, in sports (E917.0, E917.5)

☐ **E886.9 Other and unspecified**
Fall from collision of pedestrian (conveyance) with another pedestrian (conveyance)

☐ **E887 Fracture, cause unspecified**

● **E888 Other and unspecified fall**
Accidental fall NOS

E888.0 Fall resulting in striking against sharp object
Use additional external cause code to identify object (E920)

E888.1 Fall resulting in striking against other object

E888.8 Other fall

E888.9 Unspecified fall
Fall NOS

ACCIDENTS CAUSED BY FIRE AND FLAMES (E890-E899)

Includes: asphyxia or poisoning due to conflagration or ignition
    burning by fire
    secondary fires resulting from explosion

Excludes	arson (E968.0)
	fire in or on:
	machinery (in operation) (E919.0-E919.9)
	transport vehicle other than stationary vehicle (E800.0-E845.9)
	vehicle not elsewhere classifiable (E846-E848)

● **E890 Conflagration in private dwelling**

Includes: conflagration in:
    apartment
    boarding house
    camping place
    caravan
    farmhouse
    house
    lodging house
    mobile home
    private garage
    rooming house
    tenement
conflagration originating from sources classifiable to E893-E898 in the above buildings

E890.0 Explosion caused by conflagration

E890.1 Fumes from combustion of polyvinylchloride [PVC] and similar material in conflagration

☐ **E890.2 Other smoke and fumes from conflagration**
Carbon monoxide from conflagration in private building
Fumes NOS from conflagration in private building
Smoke NOS from conflagration in private building

E890.3 Burning caused by conflagration

☐ **E890.8 Other accident resulting from conflagration**
   Collapse of burning private building
   Fall from burning private building
   Hit by object falling from burning private
      building
   Jump from burning private building

☐ **E890.9 Unspecified accident resulting from conflagration in private dwelling**

● **E891 Conflagration in other and unspecified building or
   structure**
   Conflagration in:
      barn
      church
      convalescent and other residential home
      dormitory of educational institution
      factory
      farm outbuildings
      hospital
      hotel
      school
      store
      theater
   Conflagration originating from sources classifiable
      to E893-E898, in the above buildings

E891.0 Explosion caused by conflagration

**E891.1 Fumes from combustion of polyvinylchlor-
   ide [PVC] and similar material in conflagration**

☐ **E891.2 Other smoke and fumes from conflagration**
   Carbon monoxide from conflagration in
      building or structure
   Fumes NOS from conflagration in building
      or structure
   Smoke NOS from conflagration in building
      or structure

E891.3 Burning caused by conflagration

☐ **E891.8 Other accident resulting from conflagration**
   Collapse of burning building or structure
   Fall from burning building or structure
   Hit by object falling from burning building
      or structure
   Jump from burning building or structure

☐ **E891.9 Unspecified accident resulting from conflagration of other and unspecified building or
   structure**

E892 Conflagration not in building or structure
   Fire (uncontrolled) (in) (of):
      forest
      grass
      hay
      lumber
      mine
      prairie
      transport vehicle [any], except while in transit
      tunnel

● **E893 Accident caused by ignition of clothing**
   | **Excludes** | *ignition of clothing:
      from highly inflammable material (E894)
      with conflagration (E890.0-E892)* |

E893.0 From controlled fire in private dwelling
   Ignition of clothing from:
      normal fire (charcoal) (coal) (electric)
         (gas) (wood) in:
      brazier in private dwelling (as listed in
         E890)
      fireplace in private dwelling (as listed
         in E890)

   furnace in private dwelling (as listed in
      E890)
   stove in private dwelling (as listed in
      E890)

☐ **E893.1 From controlled fire in other building or
   structure**
   Ignition of clothing from:
      normal fire (charcoal) (coal) (electric)
         (gas) (wood) in:
      brazier in other building or structure
         (as listed in E891)
      fireplace in other building or structure
         (as listed in E891)
      furnace in other building or structure
         (as listed in E891)
      stove in other building or structure (as
         listed in E891)

**E893.2 From controlled fire not in building or struc-
   ture**
   Ignition of clothing from:
      bonfire (controlled)
      brazier fire (controlled), not in building
         or structure
      trash fire (controlled)

| **Excludes** | *conflagration not in building (E892)
   trash fire out of control (E892)* |

☐ **E893.8 From other specified sources**
   Ignition of clothing from:
      blowlamp
      blowtorch
      burning bedspread
      candle
      cigar
      cigarette
      lighter
      matches
      pipe
      welding torch

☐ **E893.9 Unspecified source**
   Ignition of clothing (from controlled fire
      NOS) (in building NOS) NOS

E894 Ignition of highly inflammable material
   Ignition of:
      benzine (with ignition of clothing)
      gasoline (with ignition of clothing)
      fat (with ignition of clothing)
      kerosene (with ignition of clothing)
      paraffin (with ignition of clothing)
      petrol (with ignition of clothing)

| **Excludes** | *ignition of highly inflammable material with:
   conflagration (E890.0-E892)
   explosion (E923.0-E923.9)* |

**E895 Accident caused by controlled fire in private dwell-
   ing**
   Burning by (flame of) normal fire (charcoal) (coal)
      (electric) (gas) (wood) in:
   brazier in private dwelling (as listed in E890)
   fireplace in private dwelling (as listed in E890)
   furnace in private dwelling (as listed in E890)
   stove in private dwelling (as listed in E890)

| **Excludes** | *burning by hot objects not producing fire or
   flames (E924.0-E924.9)
   ignition of clothing from these sources (E893.0)
   poisoning by carbon monoxide from incomplete
   combustion of fuel (E867-E868.9)
   that with conflagration (E890.0-E890.9)* |

☐ **E896 Accident caused by controlled fire in other and un-specified building or structure**

> Burning by (flame of) normal fire (charcoal) (coal) (electric) (gas) (wood) in:
> > brazier in other building or structure (as listed in E891)
> > fireplace in other building or structure (as listed in E891)
> > furnace in other building or structure (as listed in E891)
> > stove in other building or structure (as listed in E891)

> **Excludes** *burning by hot objects not producing fire or flames (E924.0-E924.9)*
> > *ignition of clothing from these sources (E893.1)*
> > *poisoning by carbon monoxide from incomplete combustion of fuel (E867-E868.9)*
> > *that with conflagration (E891.0-E891.9)*

E897 Accident caused by controlled fire not in building or structure

> Burns from flame of:
> > bonfire (controlled)
> > brazier fire (controlled), not in building or structure
> > trash fire (controlled)

> **Excludes** *ignition of clothing from these sources (E893.2)*
> > *trash fire out of control (E892)*
> > *that with conflagration (E892)*

● **E898 Accident caused by other specified fire and flames**

> **Excludes** *conflagration (E890.0-E892)*
> > *that with ignition of:*
> > > *clothing (E893.0-E893.9)*
> > > *highly inflammable material (E894)*

E898.0 Burning bedclothes
> Bed set on fire NOS

☐ **E898.1 Other**

Burning by:	Burning by:
blowlamp	lamp
blowtorch	lighter
candle	matches
cigar	pipe
cigarette	welding torch
fire in room NOS	

☐ **E899 Accident caused by unspecified fire**
> Burning NOS

ACCIDENTS DUE TO NATURAL AND ENVIRONMENTAL FACTORS (E900-E909)

● **E900 Excessive heat**

E900.0 Due to weather conditions
> Excessive heat as the external cause of:
> > ictus solaris
> > siriasis
> > sunstroke

E900.1 Of man-made origin
> Heat (in):
> > boiler room
> > drying room
> > factory
> > furnace room
> > generated in transport vehicle
> > kitchen

☐ **E900.9 Of unspecified origin**

● **E901 Excessive cold**

E901.0 Due to weather conditions
> Excessive cold as the cause of:
> > chilblains NOS
> > immersion foot

E901.1 Of man-made origin
> Contact with or inhalation of:
> > dry ice
> > liquid air
> > liquid hydrogen
> > liquid nitrogen
> Prolonged exposure in:
> > deep freeze unit
> > refrigerator

☐ **E901.8 Other specified origin**

☐ **E901.9 Of unspecified origin**

● **E902 High and low air pressure and changes in air pressure**

E902.0 Residence or prolonged visit at high altitude
> Residence or prolonged visit at high altitude as the cause of:
> > Acosta syndrome
> > Alpine sickness
> > altitude sickness
> > Andes disease
> > anoxia, hypoxia
> > barotitis, barodontalgia, barosinusitis, otitic barotrauma
> > hypobarism, hypobaropathy
> > mountain sickness
> > range disease

E902.1 In aircraft
> Sudden change in air pressure in aircraft during ascent or descent as the cause of:
> > aeroneurosis
> > aviators' disease

E902.2 Due to diving
> High air pressure from rapid descent in water as the cause of:
> > caisson disease
> > divers' disease
> > divers' palsy or paralysis
> Reduction in atmospheric pressure while surfacing from deep water diving as the cause of:
> > caisson disease
> > divers' disease
> > divers' palsy or paralysis

☐ **E902.8 Due to other specified causes**
> Reduction in atmospheric pressure while surfacing from under ground

☐ **E902.9 Unspecified cause**

E903 Travel and motion

● **E904 Hunger, thirst, exposure, and neglect**

> **Excludes** *any condition resulting from homicidal intent (E968.0-E968.9)*
> > *hunger, thirst, and exposure resulting from accidents connected with transport (E800.0-E848)*

E904.0 Abandonment or neglect of infants and helpless persons
> Exposure to weather conditions resulting from abandonment or neglect
> Hunger or thirst resulting from abandonment or neglect
> Desertion of newborn
> Inattention at or after birth
> Lack of care (helpless person) (infant)

> **Excludes** *criminal [purposeful] neglect (E968.4)*

ICD-9-CM

E800-E999

Vol. 1

E904.1 Lack of food
Lack of food as the cause of:
   inanition
   insufficient nourishment
   starvation

| Excludes | *hunger resulting from abandonment or neglect (E904.0)* |

E904.2 Lack of water
Lack of water as the cause of:
   dehydration
   inanition

| Excludes | *dehydration due to acute fluid loss (276.5)* |

E904.3 Exposure (to weather conditions), not elsewhere classifiable
   Exposure NOS
   Humidity
   Struck by hailstones

| Excludes | *struck by lightning (E907)* |

E904.9 Privation, unqualified
   Destitution

● **E905 Venomous animals and plants as the cause of poisoning and toxic reactions**

Includes: chemical released by animal
            insects
            release of venom through fangs, hairs, spines, tentacles, and other venom apparatus

| Excludes | *eating of poisonous animals or plants (E865.0-E865.9)* |

E905.0 Venomous snakes and lizards

Cobra	Mamba
Copperhead snake	Rattlesnake
Coral snake	Sea snake
Fer de lance	Snake (venomous)
Gila monster	Viper
Krait	Water moccasin

| Excludes | *bites of snakes and lizards known to be nonvenomous (E906.2)* |

E905.1 Venomous spiders
   Black widow spider
   Brown recluse spider
   Tarantula (venomous)

E905.2 Scorpion

E905.3 Hornets, wasps, and bees
   Yellow jacket

E905.4 Centipede and venomous millipede (tropical)

☐ **E905.5 Other venomous arthropods**
   Sting of:
      ant
      caterpillar

E905.6 Venomous marine animals and plants
   Puncture by sea urchin spine
   Sting of:
      coral
      jelly fish
      nematocysts
      sea anemone
      sea cucumber
      other marine animal or plant

| Excludes | *bites and other injuries caused by nonvenomous marine animal (E906.2-E906.8)*
 bite of sea snake (venomous) (E905.0) |

☐ **E905.7 Poisoning and toxic reactions caused by other plants**
   Injection of poisons or toxins into or through skin by plant thorns, spines, or other mechanisms

| Excludes | *puncture wound NOS by plant thorns or spines (E920.8)* |

☐ **E905.8 Other specified**

☐ **E905.9 Unspecified**
   Sting NOS
   Venomous bite NOS

● **E906 Other injury caused by animals**

| Excludes | *poisoning and toxic reactions caused by venomous animals and insects (E905.0-E905.9)*
 road vehicle accident involving animals (E827.0-E828.9)
 tripping or falling over an animal (E885.9) |

E906.0 Dog bite

E906.1 Rat bite

E906.2 Bite of nonvenomous snakes and lizards

☐ **E906.3 Bite of other animal except arthropod**

Cats	Rodents, except rats
Moray eel	Shark

E906.4 Bite of nonvenomous arthropod
   Insect bite NOS

E906.5 Bite by unspecified animal
   Animal bite NOS

☐ **E906.8 Other specified injury caused by animal**
   Butted by animal
   Fallen on by horse or other animal, not being ridden
   Gored by animal
   Implantation of quills of porcupine
   Pecked by bird
   Run over by animal, not being ridden
   Stepped on by animal, not being ridden

| Excludes | *injury by animal being ridden (E828.0-E828.9)* |

☐ **E906.9 Unspecified injury caused by animal**

E907 Lightning

| Excludes | *injury from:*
    fall of tree or other object caused by lightning (E916)
    fire caused by lightning (E890.0-E892) |

● **E908 Cataclysmic storms, and floods resulting from storms**

| Excludes | *collapse of dam or man-made structure causing flood (E909.3)* |

E908.0 Hurricane
   Storm surge
   "Tidal wave" caused by storm action
   Typhoon

E908.1 Tornado
   Cyclone
   Twisters

E908.2 Floods
   Torrential rainfall
   Flash flood

| Excludes | *collapse of dam or man-made structure causing flood (E909.3)* |

E908.3 Blizzard (snow) (ice)

E908.4 Dust storm

E908.8 Other cataclysmic storms

E908.9 Unspecified cataclysmic storms, and floods resulting from storms
Storm NOS

E909 Cataclysmic earth surface movements and eruptions

E909.0 Earthquakes

E909.1 Volcanic eruptions
Burns from lava   Ash inhalation

E909.2 Avalanche, landslide, or mudslide

E909.3 Collapse of dam or man-made structure

E909.4 Tidal wave caused by earthquake
Tidal wave NOS   Tsunami

Excludes *tidal wave caused by tropical storm (E908.0)*

E909.8 Other cataclysmic earth surface movements and eruptions

E909.9 Unspecified cataclysmic earth surface movements and eruptions

ACCIDENTS CAUSED BY SUBMERSION, SUFFOCATION, AND FOREIGN BODIES (E910-E915)

● **E910 Accidental drowning and submersion**

Includes: immersion
swimmers' cramp

Excludes *diving accident (NOS) (resulting in injury except drowning) (E883.0)*
diving with insufficient air supply (E913.2)
drowning and submersion due to:
    cataclysm (E908-E909)
    machinery accident (E919.0-E919.9)
    transport accident (E800.0-E845.9)
effect of high and low air pressure (E902.2)
injury from striking against objects while in running water (E917.2)

E910.0 While water-skiing
Fall from water skis with submersion or drowning

Excludes *accident to water-skier involving a watercraft and resulting in submersion or other injury (E830.4, E831.4)*

☐ **E910.1 While engaged in other sport or recreational activity with diving equipment**
Scuba diving NOS
Skin diving NOS
Underwater spear fishing NOS

☐ **E910.2 While engaged in other sport or recreational activity without diving equipment**
Fishing or hunting, except from boat or with diving equipment
Ice skating
Playing in water
Surfboarding
Swimming NOS
Voluntarily jumping from boat, not involved in accident, for swim NOS
Wading in water

Excludes *jumping into water to rescue another person (E910.3)*

E910.3 While swimming or diving for purposes other than recreation or sport
Marine salvage (with diving equipment)
Pearl diving (with diving equipment)
Placement of fishing nets (with diving equipment)
Rescue (attempt) of another person (with diving equipment)
Underwater construction or repairs (with diving equipment)

E910.4 In bathtub

☐ **E910.8 Other accidental drowning or submersion**
Drowning in:
    quenching tank
    swimming pool

☐ **E910.9 Unspecified accidental drowning or submersion**
Accidental fall into water NOS
Drowning NOS

E911 Inhalation and ingestion of food causing obstruction of respiratory tract or suffocation
Aspiration and inhalation of food [any] (into respiratory tract) NOS
Asphyxia by food [including bone, seed in food, regurgitated food]
Choked on food [including bone, seed in food, regurgitated food]
Suffocation by food [including bone, seed in food, regurgitated food]
Compression of trachea by food lodged in esophagus
Interruption of respiration by food lodged in esophagus
Obstruction of respiration by food lodged in esophagus
Obstruction of pharynx by food (bolus)

Excludes *injury, except asphyxia and obstruction of respiratory passage, caused by food (E915)*
obstruction of esophagus by food without mention of asphyxia or obstruction of respiratory passage (E915)

☐ **E912 Inhalation and ingestion of other object causing obstruction of respiratory tract or suffocation**
Aspiration and inhalation of foreign body except food (into respiratory tract) NOS
Foreign object [bean] [marble] in nose
Obstruction of pharynx by foreign body
Compression by foreign body in esophagus
Interruption of respiration by foreign body in esophagus
Obstruction of respiration by foreign body in esophagus

Excludes *injury, except asphyxia and obstruction of respiratory passage, caused by foreign body (E915)*
obstruction of esophagus by foreign body without mention of asphyxia or obstruction in respiratory passage (E915)

● **E913 Accidental mechanical suffocation**

Excludes *mechanical suffocation from or by:*
    accidental inhalation or ingestion of:
      food (E911)
      foreign object (E912)
    cataclysm (E908-E909)
    explosion (E921.0-E921.9, E923.0-E923.9)
    machinery accident (E919.0-E919.9)

E913.0 In bed or cradle
Excludes *suffocation by plastic bag (E913.1)*

E913.1 By plastic bag

E913.2 Due to lack of air (in closed place)
Accidentally closed up in refrigerator or other airtight enclosed space
Diving with insufficient air supply
Excludes *suffocation by plastic bag (E913.1)*

E913.3 By falling earth or other substance
Cave-in NOS

Excludes *cave-in caused by cataclysmic earth surface movements and eruptions (E909.8)*
struck by cave-in without asphyxiation or suffocation (E916)

☐ **E913.8 Other specified means**
Accidental hanging, except in bed or cradle

☐ **E913.9 Unspecified means**
Asphyxia, mechanical NOS
Strangulation NOS
Suffocation NOS

E914 Foreign body accidentally entering eye and adnexa
Excludes *corrosive liquid (E924.1)*

☐ **E915 Foreign body accidentally entering other orifice**
Excludes *aspiration and inhalation of foreign body, any, (into respiratory tract) NOS (E911-E912)*

OTHER ACCIDENTS (E916-E928)

E916 Struck accidentally by falling object
Collapse of building, except on fire
Falling: Falling:
    rock   stone
    snowslide NOS   tree
Object falling from:
    machine, not in operation
    stationary vehicle

Code first: collapse of building on fire (E890.0-E891.9)
    falling object in:
       cataclysm (E908-E909)
       machinery accidents (E919.0-E919.9)
       transport accidents (E800.0-E845.9)
       vehicle accidents not elsewhere classifiable (E846-E848)
    object set in motion by:
       explosion (E921.0-E921.9, E923.0-E923.9)
       firearm (E922.0-E922.9)
       projected object (E917.0-E917.9)

● **E917 Striking against or struck accidentally by objects or persons**
Includes: bumping into or against
       object (moving) (projected) (stationary)
       pedestrian conveyance
       person
    colliding with
       object (moving) (projected) (stationary)
       pedestrian conveyance
       person
    kicking against
       object (moving) (projected) (stationary)
       pedestrian conveyance
       person
    stepping on
       object (moving) (projected) (stationary)
       pedestrian conveyance
       person
    struck by
       object (moving) (projected) (stationary)
       pedestrian conveyance
       person

Excludes *fall from:*
       collision with another person, except when caused by a crowd (E886.0-E886.9)
       stumbling over object (E885.9)
    fall resulting in striking against object (E888.0, E888.1)
    injury caused by:
       assault (E960.0-E960.1, E967.0-E967.9)
       cutting or piercing instrument (E920.0-E920.9)
       explosion (E921.0-E921.9, E923.0-E923.9)
       firearm (E922.0-E922.9)
       machinery (E919.0-E919.9)
       transport vehicle (E800.0-E845.9)
       vehicle not elsewhere classifiable (E846-E848)

E917.0 In sports without subsequent fall
Kicked or stepped on during game (football) (rugby)

Struck by hit or thrown ball
Struck by hockey stick or puck

E917.1 Caused by a crowd, by collective fear or panic without subsequent fall
Crushed by crowd or human stampede
Pushed by crowd or human stampede
Stepped on by crowd or human stampede

E917.2 In running water without subsequent fall
Excludes *drowning or submersion (E910.0-E910.9) that in sports (E917.0, E917.5)*

E917.3 Furniture without subsequent fall
Excludes *fall from furniture (E884.2, E884.4-E884.5)*

E917.4 Other stationary object without subsequent fall
Bath tub
Fence
Lamp-post

E917.5 Object in sports with subsequent fall
Knocked down while boxing

E917.6 Caused by a crowd, by collective fear or panic with subsequent fall

E917.7 Furniture with subsequent fall
Excludes *fall from furniture (E884.2, E884.4-E884.5)*

☐ **E917.8 Other stationary object with subsequent fall**
Bath tub
Fence
Lamp-post

☐ **E917.9 Other striking against with or without subsequent fall**

E918 Caught accidentally in or between objects
Caught, crushed, jammed, or pinched in or between moving or stationary objects, such as:
escalator
folding object
hand tools, appliances, or implements
sliding door and door frame
under packing crate
washing machine wringer

Excludes *injury caused by:*
       cutting or piercing instrument (E920.0-E920.9)
       machinery (E919.0-E919.9)
       transport vehicle (E800.0-E845.9)
       vehicle not elsewhere classifiable (E846-E848)
    struck accidentally by:
       falling object (E916)
       object (moving) (projected) (E917.0-E917.9)

● **E919 Accidents caused by machinery**
Includes: burned by machinery (accident)
    caught in (moving parts of) machinery (accident)
    collapse of machinery (accident)
    crushed by machinery (accident)
    cut or pierced by machinery (accident)
    drowning or submersion caused by machinery (accident)
    explosion of, on, in machinery (accident)
    fall from or into moving part of machinery (accident)
    fire starting in or on machinery (accident)
    mechanical suffocation caused by machinery (accident)
    object falling from, on, in motion by machinery (accident)
    overturning of machinery (accident)
    pinned under machinery (accident)
    run over by machinery (accident)
    struck by machinery (accident)
    thrown from machinery (accident)
    caught between machinery and other object
    machinery accident NOS

Excludes *accidents involving machinery, not in operation (E884.9, E916-E918)*

injury caused by:
    electric current in connection with machinery (E925.0-E925.9)
    escalator (E880.0, E918)
    explosion of pressure vessel in connection with machinery (E921.0-E921.9)
    moving sidewalk (E885.9)
    powered hand tools, appliances, and implements (E916-E918, E920.0-E921.9, E923.0-E926.9)
    transport vehicle accidents involving machinery (E800.0-E848.9)
    poisoning by carbon monoxide generated by machine (E868.8)

E919.0 Agricultural machines
    Animal-powered agricultural machine
    Combine
    Derrick, hay
    Farm machinery NOS
    Farm tractor
    Harvester
    Hay mower or rake
    Reaper
    Thresher

Excludes *that in transport under own power on the highway (E810.0-E819.9)*
that being towed by another vehicle on the highway (E810.0-E819.9, E827.0-E827.9, E829.0-E829.9)
that involved in accident classifiable to E820-E829 (E820.0-E829.9)

E919.1 Mining and earth-drilling machinery
    Bore or drill (land) (seabed)
    Shaft hoist
    Shaft lift
    Under-cutter

Excludes *coal car, tram, truck, and tub in mine (E846)*

E919.2 Lifting machines and appliances
    Chain hoist except in agricultural or mining operations
    Crane except in agricultural or mining operations
    Derrick except in agricultural or mining operations
    Elevator (building) (grain) except in agricultural or mining operations
    Forklift truck except in agricultural or mining operations
    Lift except in agricultural or mining operations
    Pulley block except in agricultural or mining operations
    Winch except in agricultural or mining operations

Excludes *that being towed by another vehicle on the highway (E810.0-E819.9, E827.0-E827.9, E829.0-E829.9)*
that in transport under own power on the highway (E810.0-E819.9)
that involved in accident classifiable to E820-E829 (E820.0-E829.9)

E919.3 Metalworking machines
    Abrasive wheel
    Forging machine
    Lathe
    Mechanical shears
    Metal:
        drilling machine
    Metal:
        milling machine
        power press
        rolling-mill
        sawing machine

E919.4 Woodworking and forming machines
    Band saw
    Bench saw
    Circular saw
    Molding machine
    Overhead plane
    Powered saw
    Radial saw
    Sander

Excludes *hand saw (E920.1)*

E919.5 Prime movers, except electrical motors
    Gas turbine
    Internal combustion engine
    Steam engine
    Water driven turbine

Excludes *that being towed by other vehicle on the highway (E810.0-E819.9, E827.0-E827.9, E829.0-E829.9)*
that in transport under own power on the highway (E810.0-E819.9)

E919.6 Transmission machinery
Transmission:	Transmission:
belt	pinion
cable	pulley
chain	shaft
gear	

E919.7 Earth moving, scraping, and other excavating machines
Bulldozer	Steam shovel
Road scraper	

Excludes *that being towed by other vehicle on the highway (E810.0-E819.9)*
that in transport under own power on the highway (E810.0-E819.9)

☐**E919.8 Other specified machinery**
    Machines for manufacture of:
        clothing
        foodstuffs and beverages
        paper
    Printing machine
    Recreational machinery
    Spinning, weaving, and textile machines

☐**E919.9 Unspecified machinery**

●**E920 Accidents caused by cutting and piercing instruments or objects**

Includes: accidental injury (by) object:
    edged
    pointed
    sharp

E920.0 Powered lawn mower

☐**E920.1 Other powered hand tools**
    Any powered hand tool [compressed air] [electric] [explosive cartridge] [hydraulic power], such as:
        drill
        hand saw
        hedge clipper
        rivet gun
        snow blower
        staple gun

Excludes *band saw (E919.4)*
bench saw (E919.4)

E920.2 Powered household appliances and implements
    Blender
    Electric:
        beater or mixer
        can opener
        fan
        knife
        sewing machine
    Garbage disposal appliance

E920.3 Knives, swords, and daggers

☐**E920.4 Other hand tools and implements**
    Axe
    Can opener NOS
    Chisel
    Fork
    Hand saw

ICD-9-CM

E900-F999

Vol. 1

Hoe
Ice pick
Needle (sewing)
Paper cutter
Pitchfork
Rake
Scissors
Screwdriver
Sewing machine, not powered
Shovel

E920.5 Hypodermic needle
Contaminated needle
Needle stick

☐ **E920.8 Other specified cutting and piercing instruments or objects**

Arrow	Nail
Broken glass	Plant thorn
Dart	Splinter
Edge of stiff paper	Tin can lid
Lathe turnings	

Excludes *animal spines or quills (E906.8)*
flying glass due to explosion (E921.0-E923.9)

☐ **E920.9 Unspecified cutting and piercing instrument or object**

● **E921 Accident caused by explosion of pressure vessel**

Includes: accidental explosion of pressure vessels, whether or not part of machinery

Excludes *explosion of pressure vessel on transport vehicle (E800.0-E845.9)*

E921.0 Boilers

E921.1 Gas cylinders
Air tank   Pressure gas tank

☐ **E921.8 Other specified pressure vessels**
Aerosol can
Automobile tire
Pressure cooker

☐ **E921.9 Unspecified pressure vessel**

● **E922 Accident caused by firearm and air gun missile**

E922.0 Handgun
Pistol
Revolver

Excludes *Very pistol (E922.8)*

E922.1 Shotgun (automatic)

E922.2 Hunting rifle

E922.3 Military firearms
Army rifle
Machine gun

E922.4 Air gun
BB gun
Pellet gun

E922.5 Paintball gun

☐ **E922.8 Other specified firearm missile**
Very pistol [flare]

☐ **E922.9 Unspecified firearm missile**
Gunshot wound NOS
Shot NOS

● **E923 Accident caused by explosive material**

Includes: flash burns and other injuries resulting from explosion of explosive material
ignition of highly explosive material with explosion

Excludes *explosion:*
in or on machinery (E919.0-E919.9)
on any transport vehicle, except stationary motor vehicle (E800.0-E848)
with conflagration (E890.0, E891.0, E892)
secondary fires resulting from explosion (E890.0-E899)

E923.0 Fireworks

E923.1 Blasting materials
Blasting cap
Detonator
Dynamite
Explosive [any] used in blasting operations

E923.2 Explosive gases
Acetylene
Butane
Coal gas
Explosion in mine NOS
Fire damp
Gasoline fumes
Methane
Propane

☐ **E923.8 Other explosive materials**
Bomb
Explosive missile
Grenade
Mine
Shell
Torpedo
Explosion in munitions:
dump
factory

☐ **E923.9 Unspecified explosive material**
Explosion NOS

● **E924 Accident caused by hot substance or object, caustic or corrosive material, and steam**

Excludes *burning NOS (E899)*
chemical burn resulting from swallowing a corrosive substance (E860.0-E864.4)
fire caused by these substances and objects (E890.0-E894)
radiation burns (E926.0-E926.9)
therapeutic misadventures (E870.0-E876.9)

E924.0 Hot liquids and vapors, including steam
Burning or scalding by:
boiling water
hot or boiling liquids not primarily caustic or corrosive
liquid metal
steam
other hot vapor

Excludes *hot (boiling) tap water (E924.2)*

E924.1 Caustic and corrosive substances
Burning by:
acid [any kind]
ammonia
caustic oven cleaner or other substance
corrosive substance
lye
vitriol

E924.2 Hot (boiling) tap water

☐ **E924.8 Other**
Burning by:
heat from electric heating appliance
hot object NOS
light bulb
steam pipe

☐ **E924.9 Unspecified**

● **E925 Accident caused by electric current**

Includes: electric current from exposed wire, faulty appliance, high voltage cable, live rail, or open electric socket as the cause of:
burn
cardiac fibrillation
convulsion
electric shock
electrocution
puncture wound
respiratory paralysis

Excludes *burn by heat from electrical appliance (E924.8)*
lightning (E907)

E925.0 Domestic wiring and appliances

E925.1 Electric power generating plants, distribution stations, transmission lines
> Broken power line

E925.2 Industrial wiring, appliances, and electrical machinery
> Conductors
> Control apparatus
> Electrical equipment and machinery
> Transformers

☐ **E925.8 Other electric current**
> Wiring and appliances in or on:
>> farm [not farmhouse]
>> outdoors
>> public building
>> residential institutions
>> schools

☐ **E925.9 Unspecified electric current**
> Burns or other injury from electric current NOS
> Electric shock NOS
> Electrocution NOS

● **E926 Exposure to radiation**

Excludes *abnormal reaction to or complication of treatment without mention of misadventure (E879.2)*
atomic power plant malfunction in water transport (E838.0-E838.9)
misadventure to patient in surgical and medical procedures (E873.2-E873.3)
use of radiation in war operations (E996-E997.9)

E926.0 Radiofrequency radiation
> Overexposure to:
>> microwave radiation from:
>>> high-powered radio and television transmitters
>>> industrial radiofrequency induction heaters
>>> radar installations
>> radar radiation from:
>>> high-powered radio and television transmitters
>>> industrial radiofrequency induction heaters
>>> radar installations
>> radiofrequency from:
>>> high-powered radio and television transmitters
>>> industrial radiofrequency induction heaters
>>> radar installations
>> radiofrequency radiation [any] from:
>>> high-powered radio and television transmitters
>>> industrial radiofrequency induction heaters
>>> radar installations

E926.1 Infra-red heaters and lamps
> Exposure to infra-red radiation from heaters and lamps as the cause of:
>> blistering
>> burning
>> charring
>> inflammatory change

Excludes *physical contact with heater or lamp (E924.8)*

E926.2 Visible and ultraviolet light sources
> Arc lamps
> Black light sources
> Electrical welding arc
> Oxygas welding torch
> Sun rays
> Tanning bed

Excludes *excessive heat from these sources (E900.1-E900.9)*

E926.3 X-rays and other electromagnetic ionizing radiation
> Gamma rays
> X-rays (hard) (soft)

E926.4 Lasers

E926.5 Radioactive isotopes
> Radiobiologicals
> Radiopharmaceuticals

☐ **E926.8 Other specified radiation**
> Artificially accelerated beams of ionized particles generated by:
>> betatrons
>> synchrotrons

☐ **E926.9 Unspecified radiation**
> Radiation NOS

E927 Overexertion and strenuous movements
> Excessive physical exercise
> Overexertion (from):
>> lifting
>> pulling
>> pushing
> Strenuous movements in:
>> recreational activities
>> other activities

● **E928 Other and unspecified environmental and accidental causes**

E928.0 Prolonged stay in weightless environment
> Weightlessness in spacecraft (simulator)

E928.1 Exposure to noise
> Noise (pollution)
> Sound waves
> Supersonic waves

E928.2 Vibration

E928.3 Human bite

E928.4 External constriction caused by hair

E928.5 External constriction caused by other object

☐ **E928.8 Other**

☐ **E928.9 Unspecified accident**
> Accident NOS stated as accidentally inflicted
> Blow NOS stated as accidentally inflicted
> Casualty (not due to war) stated as accidentally inflicted
> Decapitation stated as accidentally inflicted
> Injury [any part of body, or unspecified] stated as accidentally inflicted, but not otherwise specified
> Killed stated as accidentally inflicted, but not otherwise specified
> Knocked down stated as accidentally inflicted, but not otherwise specified
> Mangled stated as accidentally inflicted, but not otherwise specified
> Wound stated as accidentally inflicted, but not otherwise specified

Excludes *fracture, cause unspecified (E887)*
injuries undetermined whether accidentally or purposely inflicted (E980.0-E989)

ICD-9-CM

E900-E999

Vol. 1

LATE EFFECTS OF ACCIDENTAL INJURY (E929)

Note: This category is to be used to indicate accidental injury as the cause of death or disability from late effects, which are themselves classifiable elsewhere. The "late effects" include conditions reported as such or as sequelae, which may occur at any time after the acute accidental injury.

● E929 Late effects of accidental injury

Excludes *late effects of:*
surgical and medical procedures (E870.0-E879.9)
therapeutic use of drugs and medicines (E930.0-E949.9)

E929.0 Late effects of motor vehicle accident
Late effects of accidents classifiable to E810-E825

☐ E929.1 Late effects of other transport accident
Late effects of accidents classifiable to E800-E807, E826-E838, E840-E848

E929.2 Late effects of accidental poisoning
Late effects of accidents classifiable to E850-E858, E860-E869

E929.3 Late effects of accidental fall
Late effects of accidents classifiable to E880-E888

E929.4 Late effects of accident caused by fire
Late effects of accidents classifiable to E890-E899

E929.5 Late effects of accident due to natural and environmental factors
Late effects of accidents classifiable to E900-E909

☐ E929.8 Late effects of other accidents
Late effects of accidents classifiable to E910-E928.8

☐ E929.9 Late effects of unspecified accident
Late effects of accidents classifiable to E928.9

DRUGS, MEDICINAL AND BIOLOGICAL SUBSTANCES CAUSING ADVERSE EFFECTS IN THERAPEUTIC USE (E930-E949)

Includes: correct drug properly administered in therapeutic or prophylactic dosage, as the cause of any adverse effect including allergic or hypersensitivity reactions

Excludes *accidental overdose of drug and wrong drug given or taken in error (E850.0-E858.9)*
accidents in the technique of administration of drug or biological substance such as accidental puncture during injection, or contamination of drug (E870.0-E876.9)
administration with suicidal or homicidal intent or intent to harm, or in circumstances classifiable to E980-E989 (E950.0-E950.5, E962.0, E980.0-E980.5)
See Alphabetic Index for more complete list of specific drugs to be classified under the fourth-digit subdivisions. The American Hospital Formulary numbers can be used to classify new drugs listed by the American Hospital Formulary Service (AHFS). See appendix C.

● E930 Antibiotics

Excludes *that used as eye, ear, nose, and throat [ENT], and local anti-infectives (E946.0-E946.9)*

E930.0 Penicillins
Natural
Synthetic
Semisynthetic, such as:
ampicillin
cloxacillin
nafcillin
oxacillin

E930.1 Antifungal antibiotics
Amphotericin B
Griseofulvin
Hachimycin [trichomycin]
Nystatin

E930.2 Chloramphenicol group
Chloramphenicol   Thiamphenicol

E930.3 Erythromycin and other macrolides
Oleandomycin   Spiramycin

E930.4 Tetracycline group
Doxycycline   Oxytetracycline
Minocycline

E930.5 Cephalosporin group
Cephalexin
Cephaloglycin
Cephaloridine
Cephalothin

E930.6 Antimycobacterial antibiotics
Cycloserine
Kanamycin
Rifampin
Streptomycin

E930.7 Antineoplastic antibiotics
Actinomycins, such as:
Bleomycin
Cactinomycin
Dactinomycin
Daunorubicin
Mitomycin

Excludes *other antineoplastic drugs (E933.1)*

❑ **E930.8 Other specified antibiotics**

❑ **E930.9 Unspecified antibiotic**

● **E931 Other anti-infectives**

> **Excludes** *ENT, and local anti-infectives (E946.0-E946.9)*

E931.0 Sulfonamides
> Sulfadiazine
> Sulfafurazole
> Sulfamethoxazole

E931.1 Arsenical anti-infectives

E931.2 Heavy metal anti-infectives
> Compounds of:
>> antimony
>> bismuth
>> lead
>> mercury

> **Excludes** *mercurial diuretics (E944.0)*

E931.3 Quinoline and hydroxyquinoline derivatives
> Chiniofon
> Diiodohydroxyquin

> **Excludes** *antimalarial drugs (E931.4)*

E931.4 Antimalarials and drugs acting on other blood protozoa
> Chloroquine phosphate
> Cycloguanil
> Primaquine
> Proguanil [chloroguanide]
> Pyrimethamine
> Quinine (sulphate)

❑ **E931.5 Other antiprotozoal drugs**
> Emetine

E931.6 Anthelmintics
> Hexylresorcinol
> Male fern oleoresin
> Piperazine
> Thiabendazole

E931.7 Antiviral drugs
> Methisazone

> **Excludes** *amantadine (E936.4)*
> *cytarabine (E933.1)*
> *idoxuridine (E946.5)*

❑ **E931.8 Other antimycobacterial drugs**
> Ethambutol
> Ethionamide
> Isoniazid
> Para-aminosalicylic acid derivatives
> Sulfones

❑ **E931.9 Other and unspecified anti-infectives**
> Flucytosine
> Nitrofuran derivatives

● **E932 Hormones and synthetic substitutes**

E932.0 Adrenal cortical steroids
> Cortisone derivatives
> Desoxycorticosterone derivatives
> Fluorinated corticosteroids

E932.1 Androgens and anabolic congeners
> Nandrolone phenpropionate
> Oxymetholone
> Testosterone and preparations

E932.2 Ovarian hormones and synthetic substitutes
> Contraceptives, oral
> Estrogens
> Estrogens and progestogens combined
> Progestogens

E932.3 Insulins and antidiabetic agents
> Acetohexamide
> Biguanide derivatives, oral
> Chlorpropamide
> Glucagon
> Insulin
> Phenformin
> Sulfonylurea derivatives, oral
> Tolbutamide

> **Excludes** *adverse effect of insulin administered for shock therapy (E879.3)*

E932.4 Anterior pituitary hormones
> Corticotropin
> Gonadotropin
> Somatotropin [growth hormone]

E932.5 Posterior pituitary hormones
> Vasopressin

> **Excludes** *oxytocic agents (E945.0)*

E932.6 Parathyroid and parathyroid derivatives

E932.7 Thyroid and thyroid derivatives
> Dextrothyroxine
> Levothyroxine sodium
> Liothyronine
> Thyroglobulin

E932.8 Antithyroid agents
> Iodides
> Thiouracil
> Thiourea

❑ **E932.9 Other and unspecified hormones and synthetic substitutes**

● **E933 Primarily systemic agents**

E933.0 Antiallergic and antiemetic drugs
> Antihistamines
> Chlorpheniramine
> Diphenhydramine
> Diphenylpyraline
> Thonzylamine
> Tripelennamine

> **Excludes** *phenothiazine-based tranquilizers (E939.1)*

E933.1 Antineoplastic and immunosuppressive drugs
> Azathioprine
> Busulfan
> Chlorambucil
> Cyclophosphamide
> Cytarabine
> Fluorouracil
> Mechlorethamine hydrochloride
> Mercaptopurine
> Triethylenethiophosphoramide [thio-TEPA]

> **Excludes** *antineoplastic antibiotics (E930.7)*

E933.2 Acidifying agents

E933.3 Alkalizing agents

E933.4 Enzymes, not elsewhere classified
> Penicillinase

E933.5 Vitamins, not elsewhere classified
> Vitamin A
> Vitamin D

> **Excludes** *nicotinic acid (E942.2)*
> *vitamin K (E934.3)*

❑ **E933.8 Other systemic agents, not elsewhere classified**
> Heavy metal antagonists

❑ **E933.9 Unspecified systemic agent**

ICD-9-CM

E900-
E999

Vol. 1

● **E934**   **Agents primarily affecting blood constituents**

E934.0   **Iron and its compounds**
Ferric salts
Ferrous sulphate and other ferrous salts

❑ **E934.1**   **Liver preparations and other antianemic agents**
Folic acid

E934.2   **Anticoagulants**
Coumarin
Heparin
Phenindione
Prothrombin synthesis inhibitor
Warfarin sodium

E934.3   **Vitamin K [phytonadione]**

E934.4   **Fibrinolysis-affecting drugs**
Aminocaproic acid
Streptodornase
Streptokinase
Urokinase

❑ **E934.5**   **Anticoagulant antagonists and other coagulants**
Hexadimethrine bromide
Protamine sulfate

E934.6   **Gamma globulin**

E934.7   **Natural blood and blood products**
Blood plasma
Human fibrinogen
Packed red cells
Whole blood

❑ **E934.8**   **Other agents affecting blood constituents**
Macromolecular blood substitutes

❑ **E934.9**   **Unspecified agent affecting blood constituents**

● **E935**   **Analgesics, antipyretics, and antirheumatics**

E935.0   **Heroin**
Diacetylmorphine

E935.1   **Methadone**

❑ **E935.2**   **Other opiates and related narcotics**
Codeine [methylmorphine]
Morphine
Opium (alkaloids)
Meperidine [pethidine]

E935.3   **Salicylates**
Acetylsalicylic acid [aspirin]
Amino derivatives of salicylic acid
Salicylic acid salts

E935.4   **Aromatic analgesics, not elsewhere classified**
Acetanilid
Paracetamol [acetaminophen]
Phenacetin [acetophenetidin]

E935.5   **Pyrazole derivatives**
Aminophenazone [aminopyrine]
Phenylbutazone

E935.6   **Antirheumatics [antiphlogistics]**
Gold salts
Indomethacin

Excludes	*salicylates (E935.3)*
	steroids (E932.0)

❑ **E935.7**   **Other non-narcotic analgesics**
Pyrabital

❑ **E935.8**   **Other specified analgesics and antipyretics**
Pentazocine

❑ **E935.9**   **Unspecified analgesic and antipyretic**

● **E936**   **Anticonvulsants and anti-Parkinsonism drugs**

E936.0   **Oxazolidine derivatives**
Paramethadione
Trimethadione

E936.1   **Hydantoin derivatives**
Phenytoin

E936.2   **Succinimides**
Ethosuximide
Phensuximide

❑ **E936.3**   **Other and unspecified anticonvulsants**
Beclamide
Primidone

E936.4   **Anti-Parkinsonism drugs**
Amantadine
Ethopropazine [profenamine]
Levodopa [L-dopa]

● **E937**   **Sedatives and hypnotics**

E937.0   **Barbiturates**
Amobarbital [amylobarbitone]
Barbital [barbitone]
Butabarbital [butabarbitone]
Pentobarbital [pentobarbitone]
Phenobarbital [phenobarbitone]
Secobarbital [quinalbarbitone]

Excludes	*thiobarbiturates (E938.3)*

E937.1   **Chloral hydrate group**

E937.2   **Paraldehyde**

E937.3   **Bromine compounds**
Bromide
Carbromal (derivatives)

E937.4   **Methaqualone compounds**

E937.5   **Glutethimide group**

E937.6   **Mixed sedatives, not elsewhere classified**

❑ **E937.8**   **Other sedatives and hypnotics**

❑ **E937.9**   **Unspecified**
Sleeping:
drug NOS
pill NOS
tablet NOS

● **E938**   **Other central nervous system depressants and anesthetics**

E938.0   **Central nervous system muscle-tone depressants**
Chlorphenesin (carbamate)
Mephenesin
Methocarbamol

E938.1   **Halothane**

❑ **E938.2**   **Other gaseous anesthetics**
Ether
Halogenated hydrocarbon derivatives, except halothane
Nitrous oxide

E938.3   **Intravenous anesthetics**
Ketamine
Methohexital [methohexitone]
Thiobarbiturates, such as thiopental sodium

☐ **E938.4 Other and unspecified general anesthetics**

E938.5 Surface and infiltration anesthetics
    Cocaine
    Lidocaine [lignocaine]
    Procaine
    Tetracaine

E938.6 Peripheral nerve- and plexus-blocking anesthetics

E938.7 Spinal anesthetics

☐ **E938.9 Other and unspecified local anesthetics**

● **E939 Psychotropic agents**

E939.0 Antidepressants
    Amitriptyline
    Imipramine
    Monoamine oxidase [MAO] inhibitors

E939.1 Phenothiazine-based tranquilizers
    Chlorpromazine
    Fluphenazine
    Phenothiazine
    Prochlorperazine
    Promazine

E939.2 Butyrophenone-based tranquilizers
    Haloperidol
    Spiperone
    Trifluperidol

☐ **E939.3 Other antipsychotics, neuroleptics, and major tranquilizers**

E939.4 Benzodiazepine-based tranquilizers
    Chlordiazepoxide
    Diazepam
    Flurazepam
    Lorazepam
    Medazepam
    Nitrazepam

☐ **E939.5 Other tranquilizers**
    Hydroxyzine
    Meprobamate

E939.6 Psychodysleptics [hallucinogens]
    Cannabis (derivatives)
    Lysergide [LSD]
    Marihuana (derivatives)
    Mescaline
    Psilocin
    Psilocybin

E939.7 Psychostimulants
    Amphetamine
    Caffeine

| Excludes | central appetite depressants (E947.0) |

☐ **E939.8 Other psychotropic agents**

☐ **E939.9 Unspecified psychotropic agent**

● **E940 Central nervous system stimulants**

E940.0 Analeptics
    Lobeline
    Nikethamide

E940.1 Opiate antagonists
    Levallorphan
    Nalorphine
    Naloxone

☐ **E940.8 Other specified central nervous system stimulants**

☐ **E940.9 Unspecified central nervous system stimulant**

● **E941 Drugs primarily affecting the autonomic nervous system**

E941.0 Parasympathomimetics [cholinergics]
    Acetylcholine
    Anticholinesterase:
      organophosphorus
      reversible
    Pilocarpine

E941.1 Parasympatholytics [anticholinergics and antimuscarinics] and spasmolytics
    Atropine
    Homatropine
    Hyoscine [scopolamine]
    Quaternary ammonium derivatives

| Excludes | papaverine (E942.5) |

E941.2 Sympathomimetics [adrenergics]
    Epinephrine [adrenalin]
    Levarterenol [noradrenalin]

E941.3 Sympatholytics [antiadrenergics]
    Phenoxybenzamine
    Tolazoline hydrochloride

☐ **E941.9 Unspecified drug primarily affecting the autonomic nervous system**

● **E942 Agents primarily affecting the cardiovascular system**

E942.0 Cardiac rhythm regulators
    Practolol
    Procainamide
    Propranolol
    Quinidine

E942.1 Cardiotonic glycosides and drugs of similar action
    Digitalis glycosides
    Digoxin
    Strophanthins

E942.2 Antilipemic and antiarteriosclerotic drugs
    Cholestyramine
    Clofibrate
    Nicotinic acid derivatives
    Sitosterols

| Excludes | dextrothyroxine (E932.7) |

E942.3 Ganglion-blocking agents
    Pentamethonium bromide

E942.4 Coronary vasodilators
    Dipyridamole
    Nitrates [nitroglycerin]
    Nitrites
    Prenylamine

☐ **E942.5 Other vasodilators**
    Cyclandelate
    Diazoxide
    Hydralazine
    Papaverine

☐ **E942.6 Other antihypertensive agents**
    Clonidine
    Guanethidine
    Rauwolfia alkaloids
    Reserpine

E942.7 Antivaricose drugs, including sclerosing agents
    Monoethanolamine
    Zinc salts

ICD-9-CM

E900-F000

Vol.

E942.8 Capillary-active drugs
Adrenochrome derivatives
Bioflavonoids
Metaraminol

☐ **E942.9 Other and unspecified agents primarily affecting the cardiovascular system**

● **E943 Agents primarily affecting gastrointestinal system**

E943.0 Antacids and antigastric secretion drugs
Aluminum hydroxide
Magnesium trisilicate

E943.1 Irritant cathartics
Bisacodyl
Castor oil
Phenolphthalein

E943.2 Emollient cathartics
Sodium dioctyl sulfosuccinate

☐ **E943.3 Other cathartics, including intestinal atonia drugs**
Magnesium sulfate

E943.4 Digestants
Pancreatin
Papain
Pepsin

E943.5 Antidiarrheal drugs
Bismuth subcarbonate
Kaolin
Pectin

Excludes *anti-infectives (E930.0-E931.9)*

E943.6 Emetics

☐ **E943.8 Other specified agents primarily affecting the gastrointestinal system**

☐ **E943.9 Unspecified agent primarily affecting the gastrointestinal system**

● **E944 Water, mineral, and uric acid metabolism drugs**

E944.0 Mercurial diuretics
Chlormerodrin
Mercaptomerin
Mercurophylline
Mersalyl

E944.1 Purine derivative diuretics
Theobromine
Theophylline

Excludes *aminophylline [theophylline ethylenediamine] (E945.7)*

E944.2 Carbonic acid anhydrase inhibitors
Acetazolamide

E944.3 Saluretics
Benzothiadiazides
Chlorothiazide group

☐ **E944.4 Other diuretics**
Ethacrynic acid
Furosemide

E944.5 Electrolytic, caloric, and water-balance agents

☐ **E944.6 Other mineral salts, not elsewhere classified**

E944.7 Uric acid metabolism drugs
Cinchophen and congeners
Colchicine
Phenoquin
Probenecid

● **E945 Agents primarily acting on the smooth and skeletal muscles and respiratory system**

E945.0 Oxytocic agents
Ergot alkaloids
Prostaglandins

E945.1 Smooth muscle relaxants
Adiphenine
Metaproterenol [orciprenaline]

Excludes *papaverine (E942.5)*

E945.2 Skeletal muscle relaxants
Alcuronium chloride
Suxamethonium chloride

☐ **E945.3 Other and unspecified drugs acting on muscles**

E945.4 Antitussives
Dextromethorphan
Pipazethate hydrochloride

E945.5 Expectorants
Acetylcysteine
Cocillana
Guaifenesin [glyceryl guaiacolate]
Ipecacuanha
Terpin hydrate

E945.6 Anti-common cold drugs

E945.7 Antiasthmatics
Aminophylline [theophylline ethylenediamine]

☐ **E945.8 Other and unspecified respiratory drugs**

● **E946 Agents primarily affecting skin and mucous membrane, ophthalmological, otorhinolaryngological, and dental drugs**

E946.0 Local anti-infectives and anti-inflammatory drugs

E946.1 Antipruritics

E946.2 Local astringents and local detergents

E946.3 Emollients, demulcents, and protectants

E946.4 Keratolytics, keratoplastics, other hair treatment drugs and preparations

E946.5 Eye anti-infectives and other eye drugs
Idoxuridine

E946.6 Anti-infectives and other drugs and preparations for ear, nose, and throat

E946.7 Dental drugs topically applied

☐ **E946.8 Other agents primarily affecting skin and mucous membrane**
Spermicides

☐ **E946.9 Unspecified agent primarily affecting skin and mucous membrane**

● **E947 Other and unspecified drugs and medicinal substances**

E947.0 Dietetics

E947.1 Lipotropic drugs

E947.2 Antidotes and chelating agents, not elsewhere classified

E947.3 Alcohol deterrents

E947.4 Pharmaceutical excipients

☐ **E947.8 Other drugs and medicinal substances**
Contrast media used for diagnostic x-ray procedures
Diagnostic agents and kits

☐ **E947.9 Unspecified drug or medicinal substance**

● **E948 Bacterial vaccines**

E948.0 BCG vaccine

E948.1 Typhoid and paratyphoid

E948.2 Cholera

E948.3 Plague

E948.4 Tetanus

E948.5 Diphtheria

E948.6 Pertussis vaccine, including combinations with a pertussis component

☐ **E948.8 Other and unspecified bacterial vaccines**

E948.9 Mixed bacterial vaccines, except combinations with a pertussis component

● **E949 Other vaccines and biological substances**

Excludes *gamma globulin (E934.6)*

E949.0 Smallpox vaccine

E949.1 Rabies vaccine

E949.2 Typhus vaccine

E949.3 Yellow fever vaccine

E949.4 Measles vaccine

E949.5 Poliomyelitis vaccine

☐ **E949.6 Other and unspecified viral and rickettsial vaccines**
Mumps vaccine

E949.7 Mixed viral-rickettsial and bacterial vaccines, except combinations with a pertussis component

Excludes *combinations with a pertussis component (E948.6)*

☐ **E949.9 Other and unspecified vaccines and biological substances**

SUICIDE AND SELF-INFLICTED INJURY (E950-E959)

Includes: injuries in suicide and attempted suicide
self-inflicted injuries specified as intentional

● **E950 Suicide and self-inflicted poisoning by solid or liquid substances**

E950.0 Analgesics, antipyretics, and antirheumatics

E950.1 Barbiturates

☐ **E950.2 Other sedatives and hypnotics**

E950.3 Tranquilizers and other psychotropic agents

☐ **E950.4 Other specified drugs and medicinal substances**

☐ **E950.5 Unspecified drug or medicinal substance**

E950.6 Agricultural and horticultural chemical and pharmaceutical preparations other than plant foods and fertilizers

E950.7 Corrosive and caustic substances
Suicide and self-inflicted poisoning by substances classifiable to E864

E950.8 Arsenic and its compounds

☐ **E950.9 Other and unspecified solid and liquid substances**

● **E951 Suicide and self-inflicted poisoning by gases in domestic use**

E951.0 Gas distributed by pipeline

E951.1 Liquefied petroleum gas distributed in mobile containers

☐ **E951.8 Other utility gas**

● **E952 Suicide and self-inflicted poisoning by other gases and vapors**

E952.0 Motor vehicle exhaust gas

☐ **E952.1 Other carbon monoxide**

☐ **E952.8 Other specified gases and vapors**

☐ **E952.9 Unspecified gases and vapors**

● **E953 Suicide and self-inflicted injury by hanging, strangulation, and suffocation**

E953.0 Hanging

E953.1 Suffocation by plastic bag

☐ **E953.8 Other specified means**

☐ **E953.9 Unspecified means**

E954 Suicide and self-inflicted injury by submersion [drowning]

● **E955 Suicide and self-inflicted injury by firearms, air guns and explosives**

E955.0 Handgun

E955.1 Shotgun

E955.2 Hunting rifle

E955.3 Military firearms

☐ **E955.4 Other and unspecified firearm**
Gunshot NOS
Shot NOS

E955.5 Explosives

E955.6 Air gun
BB gun
Pellet gun

E955.7 Paintball gun

☐ **E955.9 Unspecified**

E956 Suicide and self-inflicted injury by cutting and piercing instrument

● **E957 Suicide and self-inflicted injuries by jumping from high place**

E957.0 Residential premises

☐ **E957.1 Other man-made structures**

E957.2 Natural sites

☐ **E957.9 Unspecified**

● **E958 Suicide and self-inflicted injury by other and unspecified means**

E958.0 Jumping or lying before moving object

E958.1 Burns, fire

E958.2 Scald

E958.3 Extremes of cold

E958.4 Electrocution

ICD-9-CM

E900-
E999

Vol.

E958.5   Crashing of motor vehicle

E958.6   Crashing of aircraft

E958.7   Caustic substances, except poisoning

> Excludes   *poisoning by caustic substance (E950.7)*

☐ **E958.8   Other specified means**

☐ **E958.9   Unspecified means**

E959   Late effects of self-inflicted injury

> Note: This category is to be used to indicate circum-
> stances classifiable to E950-E958 as the cause of
> death or disability from late effects, which are
> themselves classifiable elsewhere. The "late ef-
> fects" include conditions reported as such or as
> sequelae which may occur at any time after the
> attempted suicide or self-inflicted injury.

HOMICIDE AND INJURY PURPOSELY INFLICTED BY OTHER PERSONS (E960-E969)

> **Includes:** injuries inflicted by another person with in-
> tent to injure or kill, by any means

> Excludes   *injuries due to:*
> *legal intervention (E970-E978)*
> *operations of war (E990-E999)*
> *terrorism (E979)*

● **E960   Fight, brawl, rape**

E960.0   Unarmed fight or brawl
     Beatings NOS
     Brawl or fight with hands, fists, feet
     Injured or killed in fight NOS

> Excludes   *homicidal:*
> *injury by weapons (E965.0-E966, E969)*
> *strangulation (E963)*
> *submersion (E964)*

E960.1   Rape

**E961   Assault by corrosive or caustic substance, except
poisoning**
     Injury or death purposely caused by corrosive or
     caustic substance, such as:
     acid [any]
     corrosive substance
     vitriol

> Excludes   *burns from hot liquid (E968.3)*
> *chemical burns from swallowing a corrosive sub-
> stance (E962.0-E962.9)*

● **E962   Assault by poisoning**

E962.0   Drugs and medicinal substances
     Homicidal poisoning by any drug or medic-
     inal substance

☐ **E962.1   Other solid and liquid substances**

☐ **E962.2   Other gases and vapors**

☐ **E962.9   Unspecified poisoning**

E963   Assault by hanging and strangulation
     Homicidal (attempt):
     garrotting or ligature
     hanging
     strangulation
     suffocation

E964   Assault by submersion [drowning]

● **E965   Assault by firearms and explosives**

E965.0   Handgun
     Pistol
     Revolver

E965.1   Shotgun

E965.2   Hunting rifle

E965.3   Military firearms

☐ **E965.4   Other and unspecified firearm**

E965.5   Antipersonnel bomb

E965.6   Gasoline bomb

E965.7   Letter bomb

☐ **E965.8   Other specified explosive**
     Bomb NOS (placed in):
        car
        house
     Dynamite

☐ **E965.9   Unspecified explosive**

E966   Assault by cutting and piercing instrument
     Assassination (attempt), homicide (attempt) by any
       instrument classifiable under E920
     Homicidal:
       cut any part of body
       puncture any part of body
       stab any part of body
     Stabbed any part of body

● **E967   Perpetrator of child and adult abuse**

> Note: selection of the correct perpetrator code is
> based on the relationship between the perpe-
> trator and the victim

E967.0   By father, stepfather, or boyfriend
     Male partner of child's parent or
     guardian

☐ **E967.1   By other specified person**

E967.2   By mother, stepmother, or girlfriend
     Female partner of child's parent or
     guardian

E967.3   By spouse or partner
     Abuse of spouse or partner by ex-spouse or
     ex-partner

E967.4   By child

E967.5   By sibling

E967.6   By grandparent

☐ **E967.7   By other relative**

☐ **E967.8   By non-related caregiver**

☐ **E967.9   By unspecified person**

● **E968   Assault by other and unspecified means**

E968.0   Fire
     Arson
     Homicidal burns NOS

> Excludes   *burns from hot liquid (E968.3)*

E968.1   Pushing from a high place

E968.2   Striking by blunt or thrown object

E968.3   Hot liquid
     Homicidal burns by scalding

E968.4   Criminal neglect
     Abandonment of child, infant, or other
     helpless person with intent to injure or
     kill

E968.5   Transport vehicle
     Being struck by other vehicle or run down
     with intent to injure
     Pushed in front of, thrown from, or
     dragged by moving vehicle with intent
     to injure

E968.6   Air gun
     BB gun
     Pellet gun

E968.7   Human bite

☐ **E968.8   Other specified means**

❏**E968.9 Unspecified means**
    Assassination (attempt) NOS
    Homicidal (attempt):
      injury NOS
      wound NOS
    Manslaughter (nonaccidental)
    Murder (attempt) NOS
    Violence, non-accidental

E969 Late effects of injury purposely inflicted by other person

Note: This category is to be used to indicate circumstances classifiable to E960-E968 as the cause of death or disability from late effects, which are themselves classifiable elsewhere. The "late effects" include conditions reported as such, or as sequelae which may occur at any time after the injury purposely inflicted by another person.

LEGAL INTERVENTION (E970-E978)

Includes: injuries inflicted by the police or other law-enforcing agents, including military on duty, in the course of arresting or attempting to arrest lawbreakers, suppressing disturbances, maintaining order, and other legal action
    legal execution

Excludes *injuries caused by civil insurrections (E990.0-E999)*

E970 Injury due to legal intervention by firearms
    Gunshot wound
    Injury by:
      machine gun
      revolver
      rifle pellet or rubber bullet
      shot NOS

E971 Injury due to legal intervention by explosives
    Injury by:
      dynamite
      explosive shell
      grenade
      motor bomb

E972 Injury due to legal intervention by gas
    Asphyxiation by gas
    Injury by tear gas
    Poisoning by gas

E973 Injury due to legal intervention by blunt object
    Hit, struck by:
      baton (nightstick)
      blunt object
      stave

E974 Injury due to legal intervention by cutting and piercing instrument
    Cut
    Incised wound
    Injured by bayonet
    Stab wound

❏**E975 Injury due to legal intervention by other specified means**
    Blow
    Manhandling

❏**E976 Injury due to legal intervention by unspecified means**

E977 Late effects of injuries due to legal intervention

Note: This category is to be used to indicate circumstances classifiable to E970-E976 as the cause of death or disability from late effects, which are themselves classifiable elsewhere. The "late effects" include conditions reported as such, or as sequelae which may occur at any time after the injury due to legal intervention.

E978 Legal execution
    All executions performed at the behest of the judiciary or ruling authority [whether permanent or temporary] as:
    asphyxiation by gas
    beheading, decapitation (by guillotine)
    capital punishment
    electrocution
    hanging
    poisoning
    shooting
    other specified means

TERRORISM (E979)

●**E979 Terrorism**
Includes: injuries resulting from the unlawful use of force or violence against persons or property to intimidate or coerce a Government, the civilian population, or any segment thereof, in furtherance of political or social objective

E979.0 Terrorism involving explosion of marine weapons
    Depth-charge
    Marine mine
    mine NOS, at sea or in harbour
    Sea-based artillery shell
    Torpedo
    Underwater blast

E979.1 Terrorism involving destruction of aircraft
    Aircraft used as a weapon
    Aircraft:
      burned
      exploded
      shot down
    Crushed by falling aircraft

❏**E979.2 Terrorism involving other explosions and fragments**
    Antipersonnel bomb (fragments)
    Blast NOS
    Explosion (of):
      artillery shell
      breech-block
      cannon block
      mortar bomb
      munitions being used in terrorism
      NOS
    Fragments from:
      artillery shell
      bomb
      grenade
      guided missile
      land-mine
      rocket
      shell
      shrapnel
    Mine NOS

E979.3 Terrorism involving fires, conflagration and hot substances
    Burning building or structure
      collapse of
      fall from
      hit by falling object in
      jump from
    Conflagration NOS
    Fire (causing)
      Asphyxia
      Burns
      NOS
      Other injury
    Melting of fittings and furniture in burning
    Petrol bomb
    Smouldering building or structure

ICD-9-CM
E900-E999
Vol. 1

E979.4 **Terrorism involving firearms**
Bullet:
carbine
machine gun
pistol
rifle
rubber (rifle)
Pellets (shotgun)

E979.5 **Terrorism involving nuclear weapons**
Blast effects
Exposure to ionizing radiation from nuclear
weapon
Fireball effects
Heat from nuclear weapon
Other direct and secondary effects of nu-
clear weapons

E979.6 **Terrorism involving biological weapons**
Anthrax
Cholera
Smallpox

E979.7 **Terrorism involving chemical weapons**
Gases, fumes, chemicals
Hydrogen cyanide
Phosgene
Sarin

☐ E979.8 **Terrorism involving other means**
Drowning and submersion
Lasers
Piercing or stabbing instruments
Terrorism NOS

☐ E979.9 **Terrorism secondary effects**

Note: This code is for use to identify conditions occurring subsequent to a terrorist attack not
those that are due to the initial terrorist act.

Excludes *late effect of terrorist attack (E999.1)*

INJURY UNDETERMINED WHETHER ACCIDENTALLY OR PURPOSELY INFLICTED (E980-E989)

Note: Categories E980-E989 are for use when it is
unspecified or it cannot be determined
whether the injuries are accidental (unintentional), suicide (attempted), or assault.

● E980 **Poisoning by solid or liquid substances, under-
mined whether accidentally or purposely inflicted**

E980.0 **Analgesics, antipyretics, and antirheumatics**

E980.1 **Barbiturates**

☐ E980.2 **Other sedatives and hypnotics**

E980.3 **Tranquilizers and other psychotropic agents**

☐ E980.4 **Other specified drugs and medicinal substances**

☐ E980.5 **Unspecified drug or medicinal substance**

E980.6 **Corrosive and caustic substances**
Poisoning, undetermined whether accidental or purposeful, by substances classifiable to E864

E980.7 **Agricultural and horticultural chemical and
pharmaceutical preparations other than plant
foods and fertilizers**

E980.8 **Arsenic and its compounds**

☐ E980.9 **Other and unspecified solid and liquid substances**

● E981 **Poisoning by gases in domestic use, undetermined
whether accidentally or purposely inflicted**

E981.0 **Gas distributed by pipeline**

E981.1 **Liquefied petroleum gas distributed in mobile containers**

☐ E981.8 **Other utility gas**

● E982 **Poisoning by other gases, undetermined whether accidentally or purposely inflicted**

E982.0 **Motor vehicle exhaust gas**

☐ E982.1 **Other carbon monoxide**

☐ E982.8 **Other specified gases and vapors**

☐ E982.9 **Unspecified gases and vapors**

● E983 **Hanging, strangulation, or suffocation, undetermined whether accidentally or purposely inflicted**

E983.0 **Hanging**

E983.1 **Suffocation by plastic bag**

☐ E983.8 **Other specified means**

☐ E983.9 **Unspecified means**

E984 **Submersion [drowning], undetermined whether accidentally or purposely inflicted**

● E985 **Injury by firearms, air guns and explosives, undetermined whether accidentally or purposely inflicted**

E985.0 **Handgun**

E985.1 **Shotgun**

E985.2 **Hunting rifle**

E985.3 **Military firearms**

☐ E985.4 **Other and unspecified firearm**

E985.5 **Explosives**

E985.6 **Air gun**
BB gun
Pellet gun

E985.7 **Paintball gun**

E986 **Injury by cutting and piercing instruments, undetermined whether accidentally or purposely inflicted**

● E987 **Falling from high place, undetermined whether accidentally or purposely inflicted**

E987.0 **Residential premises**

☐ E987.1 **Other man-made structures**

E987.2 **Natural sites**

☐ E987.9 **Unspecified site**

● E988 **Injury by other and unspecified means, undetermined whether accidentally or purposely inflicted**

E988.0 **Jumping or lying before moving object**

E988.1 **Burns, fire**

E988.2 **Scald**

E988.3 **Extremes of cold**

E988.4 **Electrocution**

E988.5 **Crashing of motor vehicle**

E988.6 **Crashing of aircraft**

E988.7 **Caustic substances, except poisoning**

☐ E988.8 **Other specified means**

☐ E988.9 **Unspecified means**

E989 **Late effects of injury, undetermined whether accidentally or purposely inflicted**

Note: This category is to be used to indicate circumstances classifiable to E980-E988 as the cause of
death or disability from late effects, which are
themselves classifiable elsewhere. The "late effects" include conditions reported as such or as
sequelae which may occur at any time after
injury, undetermined whether accidentally or
purposely inflicted.

INJURY RESULTING FROM OPERATIONS OF WAR (E990-E999)

Includes: injuries to military personnel and civilians caused by war and civil insurrections and occurring during the time of war and insurrection

Excludes *accidents during training of military personnel, manufacture of war material and transport, unless attributable to enemy action*

● **E990 Injury due to war operations by fires and conflagrations**

Includes: asphyxia, burns, or other injury originating from fire caused by a fire-producing device or indirectly by any conventional weapon

    E990.0 From gasoline bomb

    ❏ **E990.9 From other and unspecified source**

● **E991 Injury due to war operations by bullets and fragments**

    E991.0 Rubber bullets (rifle)

    E991.1 Pellets (rifle)

    ❏ **E991.2 Other bullets**
        Bullet [any, except rubber bullets and pellets]
        carbine
        machine gun
        pistol
        rifle
        shotgun

    E991.3 Antipersonnel bomb (fragments)

    ❏ **E991.9 Other and unspecified fragments**
        Fragments from:
        artillery shell
        bombs, except antipersonnel
        grenade
        guided missile
        land mine
        rockets
        shell
        Shrapnel

E992 Injury due to war operations by explosion of marine weapons
    Depth charge
    Marine mines
    Mine NOS, at sea or in harbor
    Sea-based artillery shell
    Torpedo
    Underwater blast

❏ **E993 Injury due to war operations by other explosion**
    Accidental explosion of munitions being used in war
    Accidental explosion of own weapons
    Air blast NOS
    Blast NOS
    Explosion NOS
    Explosion of:
        artillery shell
        breech block
        cannon block
        mortar bomb
    Injury by weapon burst

E994 Injury due to war operations by destruction of aircraft
    Airplane:
        burned
        exploded
        shot down
    Crushed by falling airplane

❏ **E995 Injury due to war operations by other and unspecified forms of conventional warfare**
    Battle wounds
    Bayonet injury
    Drowned in war operations

E996 Injury due to war operations by nuclear weapons
    Blast effects
    Exposure to ionizing radiation from nuclear weapons
    Fireball effects
    Heat
    Other direct and secondary effects of nuclear weapons

● **E997 Injury due to war operations by other forms of unconventional warfare**

    E997.0 Lasers

    E997.1 Biological warfare

    E997.2 Gases, fumes, and chemicals

    ❏ **E997.8 Other specified forms of unconventional warfare**

    ❏ **E997.9 Unspecified form of unconventional warfare**

E998 Injury due to war operations but occurring after cessation of hostilities
    Injuries due to operations of war but occurring after cessation of hostilities by any means classifiable under E990-E997
    Injuries by explosion of bombs or mines placed in the course of operations of war, if the explosion occurred after cessation of hostilities

● **E999 Late effect of injury due to war operations and terrorism**

    Note: This category is to be used to indicate circumstances classifiable to E979, E990-E998 as the cause of death or disability from late effects, which are themselves classifiable elsewhere. The "late effects" include conditions reported as such or as sequelae which may occur at any time after injury resulting from operations of war or terrorism.

    E999.0 Late effect of injury due to war operations

    E999.1 Late effect of injury due to terrorism

ICD-9-CM

E900-E999

Vol. 1

APPENDIX A
MORPHOLOGY OF NEOPLASMS

The World Health Organization has published an adaptation of the International Classification of Diseases for Oncology (ICD-O). It contains a coded nomenclature for the morphology of neoplasms, which is reproduced here for those who wish to use it in conjunction with Chapter 2 of the International Classification of Diseases, 9th Revision, Clinical Modification.

The morphology code numbers consist of five digits; the first four identify the histological type of the neoplasm and the fifth indicates its behavior. The one-digit behavior code is as follows:

/0 Benign
/1 Uncertain whether benign or malignant
    Borderline malignancy
/2 Carcinoma in situ
    Intraepithelial
    Noninfiltrating
    Noninvasive
/3 Malignant, primary site
/6 Malignant, metastatic site
    Secondary site
/9 Malignant, uncertain whether primary or metastatic site

In the nomenclature below, the morphology code numbers include the behavior code appropriate to the histological type of neoplasm, but this behavior code should be changed if other reported information makes this necessary. For example, "chordoma (M9370/3)" is assumed to be malignant; the term "benign chordoma" should be coded M9370/0. Similarly, "superficial spreading adenocarcinoma (M8143/3)" described as "noninvasive" should be coded M8143/2 and "melanoma (M8720/3)" described as "secondary" should be coded M8720/6.

The following table shows the correspondence between the morphology code and the different sections of Chapter 2:

Morphology Code Histology/Behavior		ICD-9-CM Chapter 2	
Any	0	210-229	Benign neoplasms
M800-M8004	1	239	Neoplasms of unspecified nature
M8010+	1	235-238	Neoplasms of uncertain behavior
Any	2	230-234	Carcinoma in situ
Any	3	140-195 200-208	Malignant neoplasms, stated or presumed to be primary
Any	6	196-198	Malignant neoplasms, stated or presumed to be secondary

The ICD-O behavior digit/9 is inapplicable in an ICD context, since all malignant neoplasms are presumed to be primary (/3) or secondary (/6) according to other information on the medical record.

Only the first-listed term of the full ICD-O morphology nomenclature appears against each code number in the list below. The ICD-9-CM Alphabetical Index (Volume 2), however, includes all the ICD-O synonyms as well as a number of other morphological names still likely to be encountered on medical records but omitted from ICD-O as outdated or otherwise undesirable.

A coding difficulty sometimes arises where a morphological diagnosis contains two qualifying adjectives that have different code numbers. An example is "transitional cell epidermoid carcinomas." "Transitional cell carcinoma NOS" is M8120/3 and "epidermoid carcinoma NOS" is M8070/3. In such circumstances, the higher number (M8120/3 in this example) should be used, as it is usually more specific.

CODED NOMENCLATURE FOR MORPHOLOGY OF NEOPLASMS

M800	Neoplasms NOS
M8000/0	Neoplasm, benign
M8000/1	Neoplasm, uncertain whether benign or malignant
M8000/3	Neoplasm, malignant
M8000/6	Neoplasm, metastatic

M8000/9	Neoplasm, malignant, uncertain whether primary or metastatic
M8001/0	Tumor cells, benign
M8001/1	Tumor cells, uncertain whether benign or malignant
M8001/3	Tumor cells, malignant
M8002/3	Malignant tumor, small cell type
M8003/3	Malignant tumor, giant cell type
M8004/3	Malignant tumor, fusiform cell type

M801-M804	Epithelial neoplasms NOS
M8010/0	Epithelial tumor, benign
M8010/2	Carcinoma in situ NOS
M8010/3	Carcinoma NOS
M8010/6	Carcinoma, metastatic NOS
M8010/9	Carcinomatosis
M8011/0	Epithelioma, benign
M8011/3	Epithelioma, malignant
M8012/3	Large cell carcinoma NOS
M8020/3	Carcinoma, undifferentiated type NOS
M8021/3	Carcinoma, anaplastic type NOS
M8022/3	Pleomorphic carcinoma
M8030/3	Giant cell and spindle cell carcinoma
M8031/3	Giant cell carcinoma
M8032/3	Spindle cell carcinoma
M8033/3	Pseudosarcomatous carcinoma
M8034/3	Polygonal cell carcinoma
M8035/3	Spheroidal cell carcinoma
M8040/1	Tumorlet
M8041/3	Small cell carcinoma NOS
M8042/3	Oat cell carcinoma
M8043/3	Small cell carcinoma, fusiform cell type

M805-M808	Papillary and squamous cell neoplasms
M8050/0	Papilloma NOS (except Papilloma of urinary bladder M8120/1)
M8050/2	Papillary carcinoma in situ
M8050/3	Papillary carcinoma NOS
M8051/0	Verrucous papilloma
M8051/3	Verrucous carcinoma NOS
M8052/0	Squamous cell papilloma
M8052/3	Papillary squamous cell carcinoma
M8053/0	Inverted papilloma
M8060/0	Papillomatosis NOS
M8070/2	Squamous cell carcinoma in situ NOS
M8070/3	Squamous cell carcinoma NOS
M8070/6	Squamous cell carcinoma, metastatic NOS
M8071/3	Squamous cell carcinoma, keratinizing type NOS
M8072/3	Squamous cell carcinoma, large cell, nonkeratinizing type
M8073/3	Squamous cell carcinoma, small cell, nonkeratinizing type
M8074/3	Squamous cell carcinoma, spindle cell type
M8075/3	Adenoid squamous cell carcinoma
M8076/2	Squamous cell carcinoma in situ with questionable stromal invasion
M8076/3	Squamous cell carcinoma, microinvasive
M8080/2	Queyrat's erythroplasia
M8081/2	Bowen's disease
M8082/3	Lymphoepithelial carcinoma

M809-M811	Basal cell neoplasms
M8090/1	Basal cell tumor
M8090/3	Basal cell carcinoma NOS
M8091/3	Multicentric basal cell carcinoma
M8092/3	Basal cell carcinoma, morphea type
M8093/3	Basal cell carcinoma, fibroepithelial type
M8094/3	Basosquamous carcinoma
M8095/3	Metatypical carcinoma
M8096/0	Intraepidermal epithelioma of Jadassohn
M8100/0	Trichoepithelioma
M8101/0	Trichofolliculoma
M8102/0	Tricholemmoma

M8110/0	*Pilomatrixoma*

M812-M813   **Transitional cell papillomas and carcinomas**

M8120/0	*Transitional cell papilloma NOS*
M8120/1	*Urothelial papilloma*
M8120/2	*Transitional cell carcinoma in situ*
M8120/3	*Transitional cell carcinoma NOS*
M8121/0	*Schneiderian papilloma*
M8121/1	*Transitional cell papilloma, inverted type*
M8121/3	*Schneiderian carcinoma*
M8122/3	*Transitional cell carcinoma, spindle cell type*
M8123/3	*Basaloid carcinoma*
M8124/3	*Cloacogenic carcinoma*
M8130/3	*Papillary transitional cell carcinoma*

M814-M838   **Adenomas and adenocarcinomas**

M8140/0	*Adenoma NOS*
M8140/1	*Bronchial adenoma NOS*
M8140/2	*Adenocarcinoma in situ*
M8140/3	*Adenocarcinoma NOS*
M8140/6	*Adenocarcinoma, metastatic NOS*
M8141/3	*Scirrhous adenocarcinoma*
M8142/3	*Linitis plastica*
M8143/3	*Superficial spreading adenocarcinoma*
M8144/3	*Adenocarcinoma, intestinal type*
M8145/3	*Carcinoma, diffuse type*
M8146/0	*Monomorphic adenoma*
M8147/0	*Basal cell adenoma*
M8150/0	*Islet cell adenoma*
M8150/3	*Islet cell carcinoma*
M8151/0	*Insulinoma NOS*
M8151/3	*Insulinoma, malignant*
M8152/0	*Glucagonoma NOS*
M8152/3	*Glucagonoma, malignant*
M8153/1	*Gastrinoma NOS*
M8153/3	*Gastrinoma, malignant*
M8154/3	*Mixed islet cell and exocrine adenocarcinoma*
M8160/0	*Bile duct adenoma*
M8160/3	*Cholangiocarcinoma*
M8161/0	*Bile duct cystadenoma*
M8161/3	*Bile duct cystadenocarcinoma*
M8170/0	*Liver cell adenoma*
M8170/3	*Hepatocellular carcinoma NOS*
M8180/0	*Hepatocholangioma, benign*
M8180/3	*Combined hepatocellular carcinoma and cholangiocarcinoma*
M8190/0	*Trabecular adenoma*
M8190/3	*Trabecular adenocarcinoma*
M8191/0	*Embryonal adenoma*
M8200/0	*Eccrine dermal cylindroma*
M8200/3	*Adenoid cystic carcinoma*
M8201/3	*Cribriform carcinoma*
M8210/0	*Adenomatous polyp NOS*
M8210/3	*Adenocarcinoma in adenomatous polyp*
M8211/0	*Tubular adenoma NOS*
M8211/3	*Tubular adenocarcinoma*
M8220/0	*Adenomatous polyposis coli*
M8220/3	*Adenocarcinoma in adenomatous polyposis coli*
M8221/0	*Multiple adenomatous polyps*
M8230/3	*Solid carcinoma NOS*
M8231/3	*Carcinoma simplex*
M8240/1	*Carcinoid tumor NOS*
M8240/3	*Carcinoid tumor, malignant*
M8241/1	*Carcinoid tumor, argentaffin NOS*
M8241/3	*Carcinoid tumor, argentaffin, malignant*
M8242/1	*Carcinoid tumor, nonargentaffin NOS*
M8242/3	*Carcinoid tumor, nonargentaffin, malignant*
M8243/3	*Mucocarcinoid tumor, malignant*
M8244/3	*Composite carcinoid*
M8250/1	*Pulmonary adenomatosis*
M8250/3	*Bronchiolo-alveolar adenocarcinoma*
M8251/0	*Alveolar adenoma*
M8251/3	*Alveolar adenocarcinoma*
M8260/0	*Papillary adenoma NOS*
M8260/3	*Papillary adenocarcinoma NOS*

M8261/1	*Villous adenoma NOS*
M8261/3	*Adenocarcinoma in villous adenoma*
M8262/3	*Villous adenocarcinoma*
M8263/0	*Tubulovillous adenoma*
M8270/0	*Chromophobe adenoma*
M8270/3	*Chromophobe carcinoma*
M8280/0	*Acidophil adenoma*
M8280/3	*Acidophil carcinoma*
M8281/0	*Mixed acidophil-basophil adenoma*
M8281/3	*Mixed acidophil-basophil carcinoma*
M8290/0	*Oxyphilic adenoma*
M8290/3	*Oxyphilic adenocarcinoma*
M8300/0	*Basophil adenoma*
M8300/3	*Basophil carcinoma*
M8310/0	*Clear cell adenoma*
M8310/3	*Clear cell adenocarcinoma NOS*
M8311/1	*Hypernephroid tumor*
M8312/3	*Renal cell carcinoma*
M8313/0	*Clear cell adenofibroma*
M8320/3	*Granular cell carcinoma*
M8321/0	*Chief cell adenoma*
M8322/0	*Water-clear cell adenoma*
M8322/3	*Water-clear cell adenocarcinoma*
M8323/0	*Mixed cell adenoma*
M8323/3	*Mixed cell adenocarcinoma*
M8324/0	*Lipoadenoma*
M8330/0	*Follicular adenoma*
M8330/3	*Follicular adenocarcinoma NOS*
M8331/3	*Follicular adenocarcinoma, well differentiated type*
M8332/3	*Follicular adenocarcinoma, trabecular type*
M8333/0	*Microfollicular adenoma*
M8334/0	*Macrofollicular adenoma*
M8340/3	*Papillary and follicular adenocarcinoma*
M8350/3	*Nonencapsulated sclerosing carcinoma*
M8360/1	*Multiple endocrine adenomas*
M8361/1	*Juxtaglomerular tumor*
M8370/0	*Adrenal cortical adenoma NOS*
M8370/3	*Adrenal cortical carcinoma*
M8371/0	*Adrenal cortical adenoma, compact cell type*
M8372/0	*Adrenal cortical adenoma, heavily pigmented variant*
M8373/0	*Adrenal cortical adenoma, clear cell type*
M8374/0	*Adrenal cortical adenoma, glomerulosa cell type*
M8375/0	*Adrenal cortical adenoma, mixed cell type*
M8380/0	*Endometrioid adenoma NOS*
M8380/1	*Endometrioid adenoma, borderline malignancy*
M8380/3	*Endometrioid carcinoma*
M8381/0	*Endometrioid adenofibroma NOS*
M8381/1	*Endometrioid adenofibroma, borderline malignancy*
M8381/3	*Endometrioid adenofibroma, malignant*

M839-M842   **Adnexal and skin appendage neoplasms**

M8390/0	*Skin appendage adenoma*
M8390/3	*Skin appendage carcinoma*
M8400/0	*Sweat gland adenoma*
M8400/1	*Sweat gland tumor NOS*
M8400/3	*Sweat gland adenocarcinoma*
M8401/0	*Apocrine adenoma*
M8401/3	*Apocrine adenocarcinoma*
M8402/0	*Eccrine acrospiroma*
M8403/0	*Eccrine spiradenoma*
M8404/0	*Hidrocystoma*
M8405/0	*Papillary hydradenoma*
M8406/0	*Papillary syringadenoma*
M8407/0	*Syringoma NOS*
M8410/0	*Sebaceous adenoma*
M8410/3	*Sebaceous adenocarcinoma*
M8420/0	*Ceruminous adenoma*
M8420/3	*Ceruminous adenocarcinoma*

M843   **Mucoepidermoid neoplasms**

M8430/1	*Mucoepidermoid tumor*
M8430/3	*Mucoepidermoid carcinoma*

M844-M849   **Cystic, mucinous, and serous neoplasms**

M8440/0	*Cystadenoma NOS*
M8440/3	*Cystadenocarcinoma NOS*

M8441/0	Serous cystadenoma NOS
M8441/1	Serous cystadenoma, borderline malignancy
M8441/3	Serous cystadenocarcinoma NOS
M8450/0	Papillary cystadenoma NOS
M8450/1	Papillary cystadenoma, borderline malignancy
M8450/3	Papillary cystadenocarcinoma NOS
M8460/0	Papillary serous cystadenoma NOS
M8460/1	Papillary serous cystadenoma, borderline malignancy
M8460/3	Papillary serous cystadenocarcinoma
M8461/0	Serous surface papilloma NOS
M8461/1	Serous surface papilloma, borderline malignancy
M8461/3	Serous surface papillary carcinoma
M8470/0	Mucinous cystadenoma NOS
M8470/1	Mucinous cystadenoma, borderline malignancy
M8470/3	Mucinous cystadenocarcinoma NOS
M8471/0	Papillary mucinous cystadenoma NOS
M8471/1	Papillary mucinous cystadenoma, borderline malignancy
M8471/3	Papillary mucinous cystadenocarcinoma
M8480/0	Mucinous adenoma
M8480/3	Mucinous adenocarcinoma
M8480/6	Pseudomyxoma peritonei
M8481/3	Mucin-producing adenocarcinoma
M8490/3	Signet ring cell carcinoma
M8490/6	Metastatic signet ring cell carcinoma

M850-M854 Ductal, lobular, and medullary neoplasms

M8500/2	Intraductal carcinoma, noninfiltrating NOS
M8500/3	Infiltrating duct carcinoma
M8501/2	Comedocarcinoma, noninfiltrating
M8501/3	Comedocarcinoma NOS
M8502/3	Juvenile carcinoma of the breast
M8503/0	Intraductal papilloma
M8503/2	Noninfiltrating intraductal papillary adenocarcinoma
M8504/0	Intracystic papillary adenoma
M8504/2	Noninfiltrating intracystic carcinoma
M8505/0	Intraductal papillomatosis NOS
M8506/0	Subareolar duct papillomatosis
M8510/3	Medullary carcinoma NOS
M8511/3	Medullary carcinoma with amyloid stroma
M8512/3	Medullary carcinoma with lymphoid stroma
M8520/2	Lobular carcinoma in situ
M8520/3	Lobular carcinoma NOS
M8521/3	Infiltrating ductular carcinoma
M8530/3	Inflammatory carcinoma
M8540/3	Paget's disease, mammary
M8541/3	Paget's disease and infiltrating duct carcinoma of breast
M8542/3	Paget's disease, extramammary (except Paget's disease of bone)

M855 Acinar cell neoplasms

M8550/0	Acinar cell adenoma
M8550/1	Acinar cell tumor
M8550/3	Acinar cell carcinoma

M856-M858 Complex epithelial neoplasms

M8560/3	Adenosquamous carcinoma
M8561/0	Adenolymphoma
M8570/3	Adenocarcinoma with squamous metaplasia
M8571/3	Adenocarcinoma with cartilaginous and osseous metaplasia
M8572/3	Adenocarcinoma with spindle cell metaplasia
M8573/3	Adenocarcinoma with apocrine metaplasia
M8580/0	Thymoma, benign
M8580/3	Thymoma, malignant

M859-M867 Specialized gonadal neoplasms

M8590/1	Sex cord-stromal tumor
M8600/0	Thecoma NOS
M8600/3	Theca cell carcinoma
M8610/0	Luteoma NOS
M8620/1	Granulosa cell tumor NOS
M8620/3	Granulosa cell tumor, malignant
M8621/1	Granulosa cell-theca cell tumor
M8630/0	Androblastoma, benign
M8630/1	Androblastoma NOS
M8630/3	Androblastoma, malignant
M8631/0	Sertoli-Leydig cell tumor
M8632/1	Gynandroblastoma
M8640/0	Tubular androblastoma NOS
M8640/3	Sertoli cell carcinoma
M8641/0	Tubular androblastoma with lipid storage
M8650/0	Leydig cell tumor, benign
M8650/1	Leydig cell tumor NOS
M8650/3	Leydig cell tumor, malignant
M8660/0	Hilar cell tumor
M8670/0	Lipid cell tumor of ovary
M8671/0	Adrenal rest tumor

M868-M871 Paragangliomas and glomus tumors

M8680/1	Paraganglioma NOS
M8680/3	Paraganglioma, malignant
M8681/1	Sympathetic paraganglioma
M8682/1	Parasympathetic paraganglioma
M8690/1	Glomus jugulare tumor
M8691/1	Aortic body tumor
M8692/1	Carotid body tumor
M8693/1	Extra-adrenal paraganglioma NOS
M8693/3	Extra-adrenal paraganglioma, malignant
M8700/0	Pheochromocytoma NOS
M8700/3	Pheochromocytoma, malignant
M8710/3	Glomangiosarcoma
M8711/0	Glomus tumor
M8712/0	Glomangioma

M872-M879 Nevi and melanomas

M8720/0	Pigmented nevus NOS
M8720/3	Malignant melanoma NOS
M8721/3	Nodular melanoma
M8722/0	Balloon cell nevus
M8722/3	Balloon cell melanoma
M8723/0	Halo nevus
M8724/0	Fibrous papule of the nose
M8725/0	Neuronevus
M8726/0	Magnocellular nevus
M8730/0	Nonpigmented nevus
M8730/3	Amelanotic melanoma
M8740/0	Junctional nevus
M8740/3	Malignant melanoma in junctional nevus
M8741/2	Precancerous melanosis NOS
M8741/3	Malignant melanoma in precancerous melanosis
M8742/2	Hutchinson's melanotic freckle
M8742/3	Malignant melanoma in Hutchinson's melanotic freckle
M8743/3	Superficial spreading melanoma
M8750/0	Intradermal nevus
M8760/0	Compound nevus
M8761/1	Giant pigmented nevus
M8761/3	Malignant melanoma in giant pigmented nevus
M8770/0	Epithelioid and spindle cell nevus
M8771/3	Epithelioid cell melanoma
M8772/3	Spindle cell melanoma NOS
M8773/3	Spindle cell melanoma, type A
M8774/3	Spindle cell melanoma, type B
M8775/3	Mixed epithelioid and spindle cell melanoma
M8780/0	Blue nevus NOS
M8780/3	Blue nevus, malignant
M8790/0	Cellular blue nevus

M880 Soft tissue tumors and sarcomas NOS

M8800/0	Soft tissue tumor, benign
M8800/3	Sarcoma NOS
M8800/9	Sarcomatosis NOS
M8801/3	Spindle cell sarcoma
M8802/3	Giant cell sarcoma (except of bone M9250/3)
M8803/3	Small cell sarcoma
M8804/3	Epithelioid cell sarcoma

M881-M883 Fibromatous neoplasms

M8810/0	Fibroma NOS
M8810/3	Fibrosarcoma NOS
M8811/0	Fibromyxoma
M8811/3	Fibromyxosarcoma

M8812/0	*Periosteal fibroma*
M8812/3	*Periosteal fibrosarcoma*
M8813/0	*Fascial fibroma*
M8813/3	*Fascial fibrosarcoma*
M8814/3	*Infantile fibrosarcoma*
M8820/0	*Elastofibroma*
M8821/1	*Aggressive fibromatosis*
M8822/1	*Abdominal fibromatosis*
M8823/1	*Desmoplastic fibroma*
M8830/0	*Fibrous histiocytoma NOS*
M8830/1	*Atypical fibrous histiocytoma*
M8830/3	*Fibrous histiocytoma, malignant*
M8831/0	*Fibroxanthoma NOS*
M8831/1	*Atypical fibroxanthoma*
M8831/3	*Fibroxanthoma, malignant*
M8832/0	*Dermatofibroma NOS*
M8832/1	*Dermatofibroma protuberans*
M8832/3	*Dermatofibrosarcoma NOS*
M884	**Myxomatous neoplasms**
M8840/0	*Myxoma NOS*
M8840/3	*Myxosarcoma*
M885-M888	**Lipomatous neoplasms**
M8850/0	*Lipoma NOS*
M8850/3	*Liposarcoma NOS*
M8851/0	*Fibrolipoma*
M8851/3	*Liposarcoma, well differentiated type*
M8852/0	*Fibromyxolipoma*
M8852/3	*Myxoid liposarcoma*
M8853/3	*Round cell liposarcoma*
M8854/3	*Pleomorphic liposarcoma*
M8855/3	*Mixed type liposarcoma*
M8856/0	*Intramuscular lipoma*
M8857/0	*Spindle cell lipoma*
M8860/0	*Angiomyolipoma*
M8860/3	*Angiomyoliposarcoma*
M8861/0	*Angiolipoma NOS*
M8861/1	*Angiolipoma, infiltrating*
M8870/0	*Myelolipoma*
M8880/0	*Hibernoma*
M8881/0	*Lipoblastomatosis*
M889-M892	**Myomatous neoplasms**
M8890/0	*Leiomyoma NOS*
M8890/1	*Intravascular leiomyomatosis*
M8890/3	*Leiomyosarcoma NOS*
M8891/1	*Epithelioid leiomyoma*
M8891/3	*Epithelioid leiomyosarcoma*
M8892/1	*Cellular leiomyoma*
M8893/0	*Bizarre leiomyoma*
M8894/0	*Angiomyoma*
M8894/3	*Angiomyosarcoma*
M8895/0	*Myoma*
M8895/3	*Myosarcoma*
M8900/0	*Rhabdomyoma NOS*
M8900/3	*Rhabdomyosarcoma NOS*
M8901/3	*Pleomorphic rhabdomyosarcoma*
M8902/3	*Mixed type rhabdomyosarcoma*
M8903/0	*Fetal rhabdomyoma*
M8904/0	*Adult rhabdomyoma*
M8910/3	*Embryonal rhabdomyosarcoma*
M8920/3	*Alveolar rhabdomyosarcoma*
M893-M899	**Complex mixed and stromal neoplasms**
M8930/3	*Endometrial stromal sarcoma*
M8931/1	*Endolymphatic stromal myosis*
M8932/0	*Adenomyoma*
M8940/0	*Pleomorphic adenoma*
M8940/3	*Mixed tumor, malignant NOS*
M8950/3	*Mullerian mixed tumor*
M8951/3	*Mesodermal mixed tumor*
M8960/1	*Mesoblastic nephroma*
M8960/3	*Nephroblastoma NOS*
M8961/3	*Epithelial nephroblastoma*
M8962/3	*Mesenchymal nephroblastoma*

M8970/3	*Hepatoblastoma*
M8980/3	*Carcinosarcoma NOS*
M8981/3	*Carcinosarcoma, embryonal type*
M8982/0	*Myoepithelioma*
M8990/0	*Mesenchymoma, benign*
M8990/1	*Mesenchymoma NOS*
M8990/3	*Mesenchymoma, malignant*
M8991/3	*Embryonal sarcoma*
M900-M903	**Fibroepithelial neoplasms**
M9000/0	*Brenner tumor NOS*
M9000/1	*Brenner tumor, borderline malignancy*
M9000/3	*Brenner tumor, malignant*
M9010/0	*Fibroadenoma NOS*
M9011/0	*Intracanalicular fibroadenoma NOS*
M9012/0	*Pericanalicular fibroadenoma*
M9013/0	*Adenofibroma NOS*
M9014/0	*Serous adenofibroma*
M9015/0	*Mucinous adenofibroma*
M9020/0	*Cellular intracanalicular fibroadenoma*
M9020/1	*Cystosarcoma phyllodes NOS*
M9020/3	*Cystosarcoma phyllodes, malignant*
M9030/0	*Juvenile fibroadenoma*
M904	**Synovial neoplasms**
M9040/0	*Synovioma, benign*
M9040/3	*Synovial sarcoma NOS*
M9041/3	*Synovial sarcoma, spindle cell type*
M9042/3	*Synovial sarcoma, epithelioid cell type*
M9043/3	*Synovial sarcoma, biphasic type*
M9044/3	*Clear cell sarcoma of tendons and aponeuroses*
M905	**Mesothelial neoplasms**
M9050/0	*Mesothelioma, benign*
M9050/3	*Mesothelioma, malignant*
M9051/0	*Fibrous mesothelioma, benign*
M9051/3	*Fibrous mesothelioma, malignant*
M9052/0	*Epithelioid mesothelioma, benign*
M9052/3	*Epithelioid mesothelioma, malignant*
M9053/0	*Mesothelioma, biphasic type, benign*
M9053/3	*Mesothelioma, biphasic type, malignant*
M9054/0	*Adenomatoid tumor NOS*
M906-M909	**Germ cell neoplasms**
M9060/3	*Dysgerminoma*
M9061/3	*Seminoma NOS*
M9062/3	*Seminoma, anaplastic type*
M9063/3	*Spermatocytic seminoma*
M9064/3	*Germinoma*
M9070/3	*Embryonal carcinoma NOS*
M9071/3	*Endodermal sinus tumor*
M9072/3	*Polyembryoma*
M9073/1	*Gonadoblastoma*
M9080/0	*Teratoma, benign*
M9080/1	*Teratoma NOS*
M9080/3	*Teratoma, malignant NOS*
M9081/3	*Teratocarcinoma*
M9082/3	*Malignant teratoma, undifferentiated type*
M9083/3	*Malignant teratoma, intermediate type*
M9084/0	*Dermoid cyst*
M9084/3	*Dermoid cyst with malignant transformation*
M9090/0	*Struma ovarii NOS*
M9090/3	*Struma ovarii, malignant*
M9091/1	*Strumal carcinoid*
M910	**Trophoblastic neoplasms**
M9100/0	*Hydatidiform mole NOS*
M9100/1	*Invasive hydatidiform mole*
M9100/3	*Choriocarcinoma*
M9101/3	*Choriocarcinoma combined with teratoma*
M9102/3	*Malignant teratoma, trophoblastic*
M911	**Mesonephromas**
M9110/0	*Mesonephroma, benign*
M9110/1	*Mesonephric tumor*
M9110/3	*Mesonephroma, malignant*
M9111/1	*Endosalpingioma*

M912-M916	**Blood vessel tumors**		M9282/0	Complex odontoma
M9120/0	Hemangioma NOS		M9290/0	Ameloblastic fibro-odontoma
M9120/3	Hemangiosarcoma		M9290/3	Ameloblastic odontosarcoma
M9121/0	Cavernous hemangioma		M9300/0	Adenomatoid odontogenic tumor
M9122/0	Venous hemangioma		M9301/0	Calcifying odontogenic cyst
M9123/0	Racemose hemangioma		M9310/0	Ameloblastoma NOS
M9124/3	Kupffer cell sarcoma		M9310/3	Ameloblastoma, malignant
M9130/0	Hemangioendothelioma, benign		M9311/0	Odontoameloblastoma
M9130/1	Hemangioendothelioma NOS		M9312/0	Squamous odontogenic tumor
M9130/3	Hemangioendothelioma, malignant		M9320/0	Odontogenic myxoma
M9131/0	Capillary hemangioma		M9321/0	Odontogenic fibroma NOS
M9132/0	Intramuscular hemangioma		M9330/0	Ameloblastic fibroma
M9140/3	Kaposi's sarcoma		M9330/3	Ameloblastic fibrosarcoma
M9141/0	Angiokeratoma		M9340/0	Calcifying epithelial odontogenic tumor
M9142/0	Verrucous keratotic hemangioma			
M9150/0	Hemangiopericytoma, benign		**M935-M937**	**Miscellaneous tumors**
M9150/1	Hemangiopericytoma NOS		M9350/1	Craniopharyngioma
M9150/3	Hemangiopericytoma, malignant		M9360/1	Pinealoma
M9160/0	Angiofibroma NOS		M9361/1	Pineocytoma
M9161/1	Hemangioblastoma		M9362/3	Pineoblastoma
			M9363/0	Melanotic neuroectodermal tumor
M917	**Lymphatic vessel tumors**		M9370/3	Chordoma
M9170/0	Lymphangioma NOS			
M9170/3	Lymphangiosarcoma		**M938-M948**	**Gliomas**
M9171/0	Capillary lymphangioma		M9380/3	Glioma, malignant
M9172/0	Cavernous lymphangioma		M9381/3	Gliomatosis cerebri
M9173/0	Cystic lymphangioma		M9382/3	Mixed glioma
M9174/0	Lymphangiomyoma		M9383/1	Subependymal glioma
M9174/1	Lymphangiomyomatosis		M9384/1	Subependymal giant cell astrocytoma
M9175/0	Hemolymphangioma		M9390/0	Choroid plexus papilloma NOS
			M9390/3	Choroid plexus papilloma, malignant
M918-M920	**Osteomas and osteosarcomas**		M9391/3	Ependymoma NOS
M9180/0	Osteoma NOS		M9392/3	Ependymoma, anaplastic type
M9180/3	Osteosarcoma NOS		M9393/1	Papillary ependymoma
M9181/3	Chondroblastic osteosarcoma		M9394/1	Myxopapillary ependymoma
M9182/3	Fibroblastic osteosarcoma		M9400/3	Astrocytoma NOS
M9183/3	Telangiectatic osteosarcoma		M9401/3	Astrocytoma, anaplastic type
M9184/3	Osteosarcoma in Paget's disease of bone		M9410/3	Protoplasmic astrocytoma
M9190/3	Juxtacortical osteosarcoma		M9411/3	Gemistocytic astrocytoma
M9191/0	Osteoid osteoma NOS		M9420/3	Fibrillary astrocytoma
M9200/0	Osteoblastoma		M9421/3	Pilocytic astrocytoma
			M9422/3	Spongioblastoma NOS
M921-M924	**Chondromatous neoplasms**		M9423/3	Spongioblastoma polare
M9210/0	Osteochondroma		M9430/3	Astroblastoma
M9210/1	Osteochondromatosis NOS		M9440/3	Glioblastoma NOS
M9220/0	Chondroma NOS		M9441/3	Giant cell glioblastoma
M9220/1	Chondromatosis NOS		M9442/3	Glioblastoma with sarcomatous component
M9220/3	Chondrosarcoma NOS		M9443/3	Primitive polar spongioblastoma
M9221/0	Juxtacortical chondroma		M9450/3	Oligodendroglioma NOS
M9221/3	Juxtacortical chondrosarcoma		M9451/3	Oligodendroglioma, anaplastic type
M9230/0	Chondroblastoma NOS		M9460/3	Oligodendroblastoma
M9230/3	Chondroblastoma, malignant		M9470/3	Medulloblastoma NOS
M9240/3	Mesenchymal chondrosarcoma		M9471/3	Desmoplastic medulloblastoma
M9241/0	Chondromyxoid fibroma		M9472/3	Medullomyoblastoma
			M9480/3	Cerebellar sarcoma NOS
M925	**Giant cell tumors**		M9481/3	Monstrocellular sarcoma
M9250/1	Giant cell tumor of bone NOS			
M9250/3	Giant cell tumor of bone, malignant		**M949-M952**	**Neuroepitheliomatous neoplasms**
M9251/1	Giant cell tumor of soft parts NOS		M9490/0	Ganglioneuroma
M9251/3	Malignant giant cell tumor of soft parts		M9490/3	Ganglioneuroblastoma
			M9491/0	Ganglioneuromatosis
M926	**Miscellaneous bone tumors**		M9500/3	Neuroblastoma NOS
M9260/3	Ewing's sarcoma		M9501/3	Medulloepithelioma NOS
M9261/3	Adamantinoma of long bones		M9502/3	Teratoid medulloepithelioma
M9262/0	Ossifying fibroma		M9503/3	Neuroepithelioma NOS
			M9504/3	Spongioneuroblastoma
M927-M934	**Odontogenic tumors**		M9505/1	Ganglioglioma
M9270/0	Odontogenic tumor, benign		M9506/0	Neurocytoma
M9270/1	Odontogenic tumor NOS		M9507/0	Pacinian tumor
M9270/3	Odontogenic tumor, malignant		M9510/3	Retinoblastoma NOS
M9271/0	Dentinoma		M9511/3	Retinoblastoma, differentiated type
M9272/0	Cementoma NOS		M9512/3	Retinoblastoma, undifferentiated type
M9273/0	Cementoblastoma, benign		M9520/3	Olfactory neurogenic tumor
M9274/0	Cementifying fibroma		M9521/3	Esthesioneurocytoma
M9275/0	Gigantiform cementoma		M9522/3	Esthesioneuroblastoma
M9280/0	Odontoma NOS		M9523/3	Esthesioneuroepithelioma
M9281/0	Compound odontoma			

M953   **Meningiomas**
M9530/0   *Meningioma NOS*
M9530/1   *Meningiomatosis NOS*
M9530/3   *Meningioma, malignant*
M9531/0   *Meningotheliomatous meningioma*
M9532/0   *Fibrous meningioma*
M9533/0   *Psammomatous meningioma*
M9534/0   *Angiomatous meningioma*
M9535/0   *Hemangioblastic meningioma*
M9536/0   *Hemangiopericytic meningioma*
M9537/0   *Transitional meningioma*
M9538/1   *Papillary meningioma*
M9539/3   *Meningeal sarcomatosis*

M954-M957   **Nerve sheath tumor**
M9540/0   *Neurofibroma NOS*
M9540/1   *Neurofibromatosis NOS*
M9540/3   *Neurofibrosarcoma*
M9541/0   *Melanotic neurofibroma*
M9550/0   *Plexiform neurofibroma*
M9560/0   *Neurilemmoma NOS*
M9560/1   *Neurinomatosis*
M9560/3   *Neurilemmoma, malignant*
M9570/0   *Neuroma NOS*

M958   **Granular cell tumors and alveolar soft part sarcoma**
M9580/0   *Granular cell tumor NOS*
M9580/3   *Granular cell tumor, malignant*
M9581/3   *Alveolar soft part sarcoma*

M959-M963   **Lymphomas, NOS or diffuse**
M9590/0   *Lymphomatous tumor, benign*
M9590/3   *Malignant lymphoma NOS*
M9591/3   *Malignant lymphoma, non Hodgkin's type*
M9600/3   *Malignant lymphoma, undifferentiated cell type NOS*
M9601/3   *Malignant lymphoma, stem cell type*
M9602/3   *Malignant lymphoma, convoluted cell type NOS*
M9610/3   *Lymphosarcoma NOS*
M9611/3   *Malignant lymphoma, lymphoplasmacytoid type*
M9612/3   *Malignant lymphoma, immunoblastic type*
M9613/3   *Malignant lymphoma, mixed lymphocytic-histiocytic NOS*
M9614/3   *Malignant lymphoma, centroblastic-centrocytic, diffuse*
M9615/3   *Malignant lymphoma, follicular center cell NOS*
M9620/3   *Malignant lymphoma, lymphocytic, well differentiated NOS*
M9621/3   *Malignant lymphoma, lymphocytic, intermediate differentiation NOS*
M9622/3   *Malignant lymphoma, centrocytic*
M9623/3   *Malignant lymphoma, follicular center cell, cleaved NOS*
M9630/3   *Malignant lymphoma, lymphocytic, poorly differentiated NOS*
M9631/3   *Prolymphocytic lymphosarcoma*
M9632/3   *Malignant lymphoma, centroblastic type NOS*
M9633/3   *Malignant lymphoma, follicular center cell, noncleaved NOS*

M964   **Reticulosarcomas**
M9640/3   *Reticulosarcoma NOS*
M9641/3   *Reticulosarcoma, pleomorphic cell type*
M9642/3   *Reticulosarcoma, nodular*

M965-M966   **Hodgkin's disease**
M9650/3   *Hodgkin's disease NOS*
M9651/3   *Hodgkin's disease, lymphocytic predominance*
M9652/3   *Hodgkin's disease, mixed cellularity*
M9653/3   *Hodgkin's disease, lymphocytic depletion NOS*
M9654/3   *Hodgkin's disease, lymphocytic depletion, diffuse fibrosis*
M9655/3   *Hodgkin's disease, lymphocytic depletion, reticular type*
M9656/3   *Hodgkin's disease, nodular sclerosis NOS*
M9657/3   *Hodgkin's disease, nodular sclerosis, cellular phase*
M9660/3   *Hodgkin's paragranuloma*
M9661/3   *Hodgkin's granuloma*

M9662/3   *Hodgkin's sarcoma*

M969   **Lymphomas, nodular or follicular**
M9690/3   *Malignant lymphoma, nodular NOS*
M9691/3   *Malignant lymphoma, mixed lymphocytic-histiocytic, nodular*
M9692/3   *Malignant lymphoma, centroblastic-centrocytic, follicular*
M9693/3   *Malignant lymphoma, lymphocytic, well differentiated, nodular*
M9694/3   *Malignant lymphoma, lymphocytic, intermediate differentiation, nodular*
M9695/3   *Malignant lymphoma, follicular center cell, cleaved, follicular*
M9696/3   *Malignant lymphoma, lymphocytic, poorly differentiated, nodular*
M9697/3   *Malignant lymphoma, centroblastic type, follicular*
M9698/3   *Malignant lymphoma, follicular center cell, noncleaved, follicular*

M970   **Mycosis fungoides**
M9700/3   *Mycosis fungoides*
M9701/3   *Sezary's disease*

M971-M972   **Miscellaneous reticuloendothelial neoplasms**
M9710/3   *Microglioma*
M9720/3   *Malignant histiocytosis*
M9721/3   *Histiocytic medullary reticulosis*
M9722/3   *Letterer-Siwe's disease*

M973   **Plasma cell tumors**
M9730/3   *Plasma cell myeloma*
M9731/0   *Plasma cell tumor, benign*
M9731/1   *Plasmacytoma NOS*
M9731/3   *Plasma cell tumor, malignant*

M974   **Mast cell tumors**
M9740/1   *Mastocytoma NOS*
M9740/3   *Mast cell sarcoma*
M9741/3   *Malignant mastocytosis*

M975   **Burkitt's tumor**
M9750/3   *Burkitt's tumor*

M980-M994   **Leukemias**

M980   **Leukemias NOS**
M9800/3   *Leukemia NOS*
M9801/3   *Acute leukemia NOS*
M9802/3   *Subacute leukemia NOS*
M9803/3   *Chronic leukemia NOS*
M9804/3   *Aleukemic leukemia NOS*

M981   **Compound leukemias**
M9810/3   *Compound leukemia*

M982   **Lymphoid leukemias**
M9820/3   *Lymphoid leukemia NOS*
M9821/3   *Acute lymphoid leukemia*
M9822/3   *Subacute lymphoid leukemia*
M9823/3   *Chronic lymphoid leukemia*
M9824/3   *Aleukemic lymphoid leukemia*
M9825/3   *Prolymphocytic leukemia*

M983   **Plasma cell leukemias**
M9830/3   *Plasma cell leukemia*

M984   **Erythroleukemias**
M9840/3   *Erythroleukemia*
M9841/3   *Acute erythremia*
M9842/3   *Chronic erythremia*

M985   **Lymphosarcoma cell leukemias**
M9850/3   *Lymphosarcoma cell leukemia*

M986   **Myeloid leukemias**
M9860/3   *Myeloid leukemia NOS*
M9861/3   *Acute myeloid leukemia*
M9862/3   *Subacute myeloid leukemia*

M9863/3	*Chronic myeloid leukemia*
M9864/3	*Aleukemic myeloid leukemia*
M9865/3	*Neutrophilic leukemia*
M9866/3	*Acute promyelocytic leukemia*

M987   **Basophilic leukemias**
M9870/3	*Basophilic leukemia*

M988   **Eosinophilic leukemias**
M9880/3	*Eosinophilic leukemia*

M989   **Monocytic leukemias**
M9890/3	*Monocytic leukemia NOS*
M9891/3	*Acute monocytic leukemia*
M9892/3	*Subacute monocytic leukemia*
M9893/3	*Chronic monocytic leukemia*
M9894/3	*Aleukemic monocytic leukemia*

M990-M994   **Miscellaneous leukemias**
M9900/3	*Mast cell leukemia*
M9910/3	*Megakaryocytic leukemia*
M9920/3	*Megakaryocytic myelosis*
M9930/3	*Myeloid sarcoma*
M9940/3	*Hairy cell leukemia*

M995-M997   **Miscellaneous myeloproliferative and lympho-proliferative disorders**
M9950/1	*Polycythemia vera*
M9951/1	*Acute panmyelosis*
M9960/1	*Chronic myeloproliferative disease*
M9961/1	*Myelosclerosis with myeloid metaplasia*
M9962/1	*Idiopathic thrombocythemia*
M9970/1	*Chronic lymphoproliferative disease*

APPENDIX B

GLOSSARY OF MENTAL DISORDERS

Deleted as of October 1, 2004

APPENDIX C

CLASSIFICATION OF DRUGS BY AMERICAN HOSPITAL FORMULARY SERVICES LIST NUMBER AND THEIR ICD-9-CM EQUIVALENTS

The coding of adverse effects of drugs is keyed to the continually revised Hospital Formulary of the American Hospital Formulary Service (AHFS) published under the direction of the American Society of Hospital Pharmacists.

The following section gives the ICD-9-CM diagnosis code for each AHFS list.

AHFS List		ICD-9-CM Diagnosis Code
4:00	**ANTIHISTAMINE DRUGS**	**963.0**
8:00	**ANTI-INFECTIVE AGENTS**	
8:04	Amebicides	961.5
	hydroxyquinoline derivatives	961.3
	arsenical anti-infectives	961.1
8:08	Anthelmintics	961.6
	quinoline derivatives	961.3
8:12.04	Antifungal Antibiotics	960.1
	nonantibiotics	961.9
8:12.06	Cephalosporins	960.5
8:12.08	Chloramphenicol	960.2
8:12.12	The Erythromycins	960.3
8:12.16	The Penicillins	960.0
8:12.20	The Streptomycins	960.6
8:12.24	The Tetracyclines	960.4
8:12.28	Other Antibiotics	960.8
	antimycobacterial antibiotics	960.6
	macrolides	960.3
8:16	Antituberculars	961.8
	antibiotics	960.6
8:18	Antivirals	961.7
8:20	Plasmodicides (antimalarials)	961.4
8:24	Sulfonamides	961.0
8:26	The Sulfones	961.8
8:28	Treponemicides	961.2
8:32	Trichomonacides	961.5
	hydroxyquinoline derivatives	961.3
	nitrofuran derivatives	961.9
8:36	Urinary Germicides	961.9
	quinoline derivatives	961.3
8:40	Other Anti-Infectives	961.9
10:00	**ANTINEOPLASTIC AGENTS**	**963.1**
	antibiotics	960.7
	progestogens	962.2
12:00	**AUTONOMIC DRUGS**	
12:04	Parasympathomimetic (Cholinergic) Agents	971.0
12:08	Parasympatholytic (Cholinergic Blocking) Agents	971.1
12:12	Sympathomimetic (Adrenergic) Agents	971.2
12:16	Sympatholytic (Adrenergic Blocking) Agents	971.3
12:20	Skeletal Muscle Relaxants	975.2
	central nervous system muscle-tone depressants	968.0
16:00	**BLOOD DERIVATIVES**	**964.7**
20:00	**BLOOD FORMATION AND COAGULATION**	
20:04	Antianemia Drugs	964.1
20:04.04	Iron Preparations	964.0
20:04.08	Liver and Stomach Preparations	964.1
20:12.04	Anticoagulants	964.2
20:12.08	Antiheparin agents	964.5
20:12.12	Coagulants	964.5
20.12.16	Hemostatics	964.5
	capillary-active drugs	972.8
	fibrinolysis-affecting agents	964.4
	natural products	964.7

24:00	**CARDIOVASCULAR DRUGS**	
24:04	Cardiac Drugs	972.9
	cardiotonic agents	972.1
	rhythm regulators	972.0
24:06	Antilipemic Agents	972.2
	thyroid derivatives	962.7
24:08	Hypotensive Agents	972.6
	adrenergic blocking agents	971.3
	ganglion-blocking agents	972.3
	vasodilators	972.5
24:12	Vasodilating Agents	972.5
	coronary	972.4
	nicotinic acid derivatives	972.2
24:16	Sclerosing Agents	972.7
28:00	**CENTRAL NERVOUS SYSTEM DRUGS**	
28:04	General Anesthetics	968.4
	gaseous anesthetics	968.2
	halothane	968.1
	intravenous anesthetics	968.3
28:08	Analgesics and Antipyretics	965.9
	antirheumatics	965.6
	aromatic analgesics	965.4
	non-narcotics NEC	965.7
	opium alkaloids	965.00
	heroin	965.01
	methadone	965.02
	specified type NEC	965.09
	pyrazole derivatives	965.5
	salicylates	965.1
	specified type NEC	965.8
28:10	Narcotic Antagonists	970.1
28:12	Anticonvulsants	966.3
	barbiturates	967.0
	benzodiazepine-based tranquilizers	969.4
	bromides	967.3
	hydantoin derivatives	966.1
	oxazolidone derivative	966.0
	succinamides	966.2
28:16.04	Antidepressants	969.0
28:16.08	Tranquilizers	969.5
	benzodiazepine-based	969.4
	butyrophenone-based	969.2
	major NEC	969.3
	phenothiazine-based	969.1
28:16.12	Other Psychotherapeutic Agents	969.8
28:20	Respiratory and Cerebral Stimulants	970.9
	analeptics	970.0
	anorexigenic agents	977.0
	psychostimulants	969.7
	specified type NEC	970.8
28:24	Sedatives and Hypnotics	967.9
	barbiturates	967.0
	benzodiazepine-based tranquilizers	969.4
	chloral hydrate group	967.1
	glutethimide group	967.5
	intravenous anesthetics	968.3
	methaqualone	967.4
	paraldehyde	967.2
	phenothiazine-based tranquilizers	969.1
	specified type NEC	967.8
	thiobarbiturates	968.3
	tranquilizer NEC	969.5
36:00	**DIAGNOSTIC AGENTS**	**977.8**
40:00	**ELECTROLYTE, CALORIC, AND WATER BALANCE AGENTS NEC**	**974.5**

ICD-9-CM

Appx C

Vol.

APPENDIX D

CLASSIFICATION OF INDUSTRIAL ACCIDENTS ACCORDING TO AGENCY

Annex B to the Resolution concerning Statistics of Employment Injuries adopted by the Tenth International Conference of Labor Statisticians on 12 October 1962

1 MACHINES

11 Prime-Movers, except Electrical Motors
111 *Steam engines*
112 *Internal combustion engines*
119 *Others*

12 Transmission Machinery
121 *Transmission shafts*
122 *Transmission belts, cables, pulleys, pinions, chains, gears*
129 *Others*

13 Metalworking Machines
131 *Power presses*
132 *Lathes*
133 *Milling machines*
134 *Abrasive wheels*
135 *Mechanical shears*
136 *Forging machines*
137 *Rolling-mills*
139 *Others*

14 Wood and Assimilated Machines
141 *Circular saws*
142 *Other saws*
143 *Molding machines*
144 *Overhand planes*
149 *Others*

15 Agricultural Machines
151 *Reapers (including combine reapers)*
152 *Threshers*
159 *Others*

16 Mining Machinery
161 *Under-cutters*
169 *Others*

19 Other Machines Not Elsewhere Classified
191 *Earth-moving machines, excavating and scraping machines, except means of transport*
192 *Spinning, weaving and other textile machines*
193 *Machines for the manufacture of foodstuffs and beverages*
194 *Machines for the manufacture of paper*
195 *Printing machines*
199 *Others*

2 MEANS OF TRANSPORT AND LIFTING EQUIPMENT

21 Lifting Machines and Appliances
211 *Cranes*
212 *Lifts and elevators*
213 *Winches*
214 *Pulley blocks*
219 *Others*

22 Means of Rail Transport
221 *Inter-urban railways*
222 *Rail transport in mines, tunnels, quarries, industrial establishments, docks, etc.*
229 *Others*

23 Other Wheeled Means of Transport, Excluding Rail Transport
231 *Tractors*
232 *Lorries*
233 *Trucks*
234 *Motor vehicles, not elsewhere classified*
235 *Animal-drawn vehicles*
236 *Hand-drawn vehicles*
239 *Others*

24 Means of Air Transport

25 Means of Water Transport
251 *Motorized means of water transport*
252 *Non-motorized means of water transport*

26 Other Means of Transport
261 *Cable-cars*
262 *Mechanical conveyors, except cable-cars*
269 *Others*

3 OTHER EQUIPMENT

31 Pressure Vessels
311 *Boilers*
312 *Pressurized containers*
313 *Pressurized piping and accessories*
314 *Gas cylinders*
315 *Caissons, diving equipment*
319 *Others*

32 Furnaces, Ovens, Kilns
321 *Blast furnaces*
322 *Refining furnaces*
323 *Other furnaces*
324 *Kilns*
325 *Ovens*

33 Refrigerating Plants

34 Electrical Installations, Including Electric Motors, but Excluding Electric Hand Tools
341 *Rotating machines*
342 *Conductors*
343 *Transformers*
344 *Control apparatus*
349 *Others*

35 Electric Hand Tools

36 Tools, Implements, and Appliances, Except Electric Hand Tools
361 *Power-driven hand tools, except electric hand tools*
362 *Hand tools, not power-driven*
369 *Others*

37 Ladders, Mobile Ramps

38 Scaffolding

39 Other Equipment, Not Elsewhere Classified

4 MATERIALS, SUBSTANCES, AND RADIATIONS

41 Explosives

42 Dusts, Gases, Liquids and Chemicals, Excluding Explosives
421 *Dusts*
422 *Gases, vapors, fumes*
423 *Liquids, not elsewhere classified*
424 *Chemicals, not elsewhere classified*

43 Flying Fragments

44 Radiations
441 *Ionizing radiations*
449 *Others*

49   Other Materials and Substances Not Elsewhere
      Classified

5 WORKING ENVIRONMENT

51   **Outdoor**
      511 *Weather*
      512 *Traffic and working surfaces*
      513 *Water*
      519 *Others*

52   **Indoor**
      521 *Floors*
      522 *Confined quarters*
      523 *Stairs*
      524 *Other traffic and working surfaces*
      525 *Floor openings and wall openings*
      526 *Environmental factors (lighting, ventilation, temperature, noise, etc.)*
      529 *Others*

53   **Underground**
      531 *Roofs and faces of mine roads and tunnels, etc.*
      532 *Floors of mine roads and tunnels, etc.*
      533 *Working-faces of mines, tunnels, etc.*
      534 *Mine shafts*
      535 *Fire*
      536 *Water*
      539 *Others*

6 OTHER AGENCIES, NOT ELSEWHERE CLASSIFIED

61   **Animals**
      611 *Live animals*
      612 *Animals products*

69   **Other Agencies, Not Elsewhere Classified**

7 AGENCIES NOT CLASSIFIED FOR LACK OF SUFFICIENT DATA

APPENDIX E
LIST OF THREE-DIGIT CATEGORIES

1. INFECTIOUS AND PARASITIC DISEASES

Intestinal infectious diseases (001–009)
001 Cholera
002 Typhoid and paratyphoid fevers
003 Other salmonella infections
004 Shigellosis
005 Other food poisoning (bacterial)
006 Amebiasis
007 Other protozoal intestinal diseases
008 Intestinal infections due to other organisms
009 Ill-defined intestinal infections

Tuberculosis (010–018)
010 Primary tuberculous infection
011 Pulmonary tuberculosis
012 Other respiratory tuberculosis
013 Tuberculosis of meninges and central nervous system
014 Tuberculosis of intestines, peritoneum, and mesenteric glands
015 Tuberculosis of bones and joints
016 Tuberculosis of genitourinary system
017 Tuberculosis of other organs
018 Miliary tuberculosis

Zoonotic bacterial diseases (020–027)
020 Plague
021 Tularemia
022 Anthrax
023 Brucellosis
024 Glanders
025 Melioidosis
026 Rat-bite fever
027 Other zoonotic bacterial diseases

Other bacterial diseases (030–041)
030 Leprosy
031 Diseases due to other mycobacteria
032 Diphtheria
033 Whooping cough
034 Streptococcal sore throat and scarlet fever
035 Erysipelas
036 Meningococcal infection
037 Tetanus
038 Septicemia
039 Actinomycotic infections
040 Other bacterial diseases
041 Bacterial infection in conditions classified elsewhere and of unspecified site

Human immunodeficiency virus (042)
042 Human immunodeficiency virus [HIV] disease

Poliomyelitis and other non-arthropod-borne viral diseases of central nervous system (045–049)
045 Acute poliomyelitis
046 Slow virus infection of central nervous system
047 Meningitis due to enterovirus
048 Other enterovirus diseases of central nervous system
049 Other non-arthropod-borne viral diseases of central nervous system

Viral diseases accompanied by exanthem (050–057)
050 Smallpox
051 Cowpox and paravaccinia
052 Chickenpox
053 Herpes zoster
054 Herpes simplex
055 Measles
056 Rubella
057 Other viral exanthemata

Arthropod-borne viral diseases (060–066)
060 Yellow fever
061 Dengue
062 Mosquito-borne viral encephalitis
063 Tick-borne viral encephalitis
064 Viral encephalitis transmitted by other and unspecified arthropods
065 Arthropod-borne hemorrhagic fever
066 Other arthropod-borne viral diseases

Other diseases due to viruses and Chlamydiae (070–079)
070 Viral hepatitis
071 Rabies
072 Mumps
073 Ornithosis
074 Specific diseases due to Coxsackie virus
075 Infectious mononucleosis
076 Trachoma
077 Other diseases of conjunctiva due to viruses and Chlamydiae
078 Other diseases due to viruses and Chlamydiae
079 Viral infection in conditions classified elsewhere and of unspecified site

Rickettsioses and other arthropod-borne diseases (080–088)
080 Louse-borne [epidemic] typhus
081 Other typhus
082 Tick-borne rickettsioses
083 Other rickettsioses
084 Malaria
085 Leishmaniasis
086 Trypanosomiasis
087 Relapsing fever
088 Other arthropod-borne diseases

Syphilis and other venereal diseases (090–099)
090 Congenital syphilis
091 Early syphilis, symptomatic
092 Early syphilis, latent
093 Cardiovascular syphilis
094 Neurosyphilis
095 Other forms of late syphilis, with symptoms
096 Late syphilis, latent
097 Other and unspecified syphilis
098 Gonococcal infections
099 Other venereal diseases

Other spirochetal diseases (100–104)
100 Leptospirosis
101 Vincent's angina
102 Yaws
103 Pinta
104 Other spirochetal infection

Mycoses (110–118)
110 Dermatophytosis
111 Dermatomycosis, other and unspecified
112 Candidiasis
114 Coccidioidomycosis
115 Histoplasmosis
116 Blastomycotic infection
117 Other mycoses
118 Opportunistic mycoses

Helminthiases (120–129)
120 Schistosomiasis [bilharziasis]
121 Other trematode infections
122 Echinococcosis
123 Other cestode infection
124 Trichinosis
125 Filarial infection and dracontiasis
126 Ancylostomiasis and necatoriasis
127 Other intestinal helminthiases
128 Other and unspecified helminthiases
129 Intestinal parasitism, unspecified

Other infectious and parasitic diseases (130–136)
130 Toxoplasmosis
131 Trichomoniasis
132 Pediculosis and phthirus infestation
133 Acariasis
134 Other infestation
135 Sarcoidosis
136 Other and unspecified infectious and parasitic diseases

Late effects of infectious and parasitic diseases (137–139)
137 Late effects of tuberculosis
138 Late effects of acute poliomyelitis
139 Late effects of other infectious and parasitic diseases

2. NEOPLASMS

Malignant neoplasm of lip, oral cavity, and pharynx (140–149)
140 Malignant neoplasm of lip
141 Malignant neoplasm of tongue
142 Malignant neoplasm of major salivary glands
143 Malignant neoplasm of gum
144 Malignant neoplasm of floor of mouth
145 Malignant neoplasm of other and unspecified parts of mouth
146 Malignant neoplasm of oropharynx
147 Malignant neoplasm of nasopharynx
148 Malignant neoplasm of hypopharynx
149 Malignant neoplasm of other and ill-defined sites within the lip, oral cavity, and pharynx

Malignant neoplasm of digestive organs and peritoneum (150–159)
150 Malignant neoplasm of esophagus
151 Malignant neoplasm of stomach
152 Malignant neoplasm of small intestine, including duodenum
153 Malignant neoplasm of colon
154 Malignant neoplasm of rectum, rectosigmoid junction, and anus
155 Malignant neoplasm of liver and intrahepatic bile ducts
156 Malignant neoplasm of gallbladder and extrahepatic bile ducts
157 Malignant neoplasm of pancreas
158 Malignant neoplasm of retroperitoneum and peritoneum
159 Malignant neoplasm of other and ill-defined sites within the digestive organs and peritoneum

Malignant neoplasm of respiratory and intrathoracic organs (160–165)
160 Malignant neoplasm of nasal cavities, middle ear, and accessory sinuses
161 Malignant neoplasm of larynx
162 Malignant neoplasm of trachea, bronchus, and lung
163 Malignant neoplasm of pleura
164 Malignant neoplasm of thymus, heart, and mediastinum
165 Malignant neoplasm of other and ill-defined sites within the respiratory system and intrathoracic organs

Malignant neoplasm of bone, connective tissue, skin, and breast (170–176)
170 Malignant neoplasm of bone and articular cartilage
171 Malignant neoplasm of connective and other soft tissue
172 Malignant melanoma of skin
173 Other malignant neoplasm of skin
174 Malignant neoplasm of female breast
175 Malignant neoplasm of male breast

Kaposi's sarcoma (176)
176 Kaposi's sarcoma

Malignant neoplasm of genitourinary organs (179–189)
179 Malignant neoplasm of uterus, part unspecified
180 Malignant neoplasm of cervix uteri
181 Malignant neoplasm of placenta
182 Malignant neoplasm of body of uterus
183 Malignant neoplasm of ovary and other uterine adnexa
184 Malignant neoplasm of other and unspecified female genital organs
185 Malignant neoplasm of prostate
186 Malignant neoplasm of testis
187 Malignant neoplasm of penis and other male genital organs
188 Malignant neoplasm of bladder
189 Malignant neoplasm of kidney and other and unspecified urinary organs

Malignant neoplasm of other and unspecified sites (190–199)
190 Malignant neoplasm of eye
191 Malignant neoplasm of brain
192 Malignant neoplasm of other and unspecified parts of nervous system
193 Malignant neoplasm of thyroid gland
194 Malignant neoplasm of other endocrine glands and related structures
195 Malignant neoplasm of other and ill-defined sites
196 Secondary and unspecified malignant neoplasm of lymph nodes
197 Secondary malignant neoplasm of respiratory and digestive systems
198 Secondary malignant neoplasm of other specified sites
199 Malignant neoplasm without specification of site

Malignant neoplasm of lymphatic and hematopoietic tissue (200–208)
200 Lymphosarcoma and reticulosarcoma
201 Hodgkin's disease
202 Other malignant neoplasm of lymphoid and histiocytic tissue
203 Multiple myeloma and immunoproliferative neoplasms
204 Lymphoid leukemia
205 Myeloid leukemia
206 Monocytic leukemia
207 Other specified leukemia
208 Leukemia of unspecified cell type

Benign neoplasms (210–229)
210 Benign neoplasm of lip, oral cavity, and pharynx
211 Benign neoplasm of other parts of digestive system
212 Benign neoplasm of respiratory and intrathoracic organs
213 Benign neoplasm of bone and articular cartilage
214 Lipoma
215 Other benign neoplasm of connective and other soft tissue
216 Benign neoplasm of skin
217 Benign neoplasm of breast
218 Uterine leiomyoma
219 Other benign neoplasm of uterus
220 Benign neoplasm of ovary
221 Benign neoplasm of other female genital organs
222 Benign neoplasm of male genital organs
223 Benign neoplasm of kidney and other urinary organs
224 Benign neoplasm of eye
225 Benign neoplasm of brain and other parts of nervous system
226 Benign neoplasm of thyroid gland
227 Benign neoplasm of other endocrine glands and related structures
228 Hemangioma and lymphangioma, any site
229 Benign neoplasm of other and unspecified sites

Carcinoma in situ (230–234)
230 Carcinoma in situ of digestive organs
231 Carcinoma in situ of respiratory system
232 Carcinoma in situ of skin
233 Carcinoma in situ of breast and genitourinary system
234 Carcinoma in situ of other and unspecified sites

Neoplasms of uncertain behavior (235–238)
235 Neoplasm of uncertain behavior of digestive and respiratory systems
236 Neoplasm of uncertain behavior of genitourinary organs
237 Neoplasm of uncertain behavior of endocrine glands and nervous system
238 Neoplasm of uncertain behavior of other and unspecified sites and tissues

Neoplasms of unspecified nature (239)
239   Neoplasm of unspecified nature

3. ENDOCRINE, NUTRITIONAL AND METABOLIC DISEASES, AND IMMUNITY DISORDERS

Disorders of thyroid gland (240–246)
240   Simple and unspecified goiter
241   Nontoxic nodular goiter
242   Thyrotoxicosis with or without goiter
243   Congenital hypothyroidism
244   Acquired hypothyroidism
245   Thyroiditis
246   Other disorders of thyroid

Diseases of other endocrine glands (250–259)
250   Diabetes mellitus
251   Other disorders of pancreatic internal secretion
252   Disorders of parathyroid gland
253   Disorders of the pituitary gland and its hypothalamic control
254   Diseases of thymus gland
255   Disorders of adrenal glands
256   Ovarian dysfunction
257   Testicular dysfunction
258   Polyglandular dysfunction and related disorders
259   Other endocrine disorders

Nutritional deficiencies (260–269)
260   Kwashiorkor
261   Nutritional marasmus
262   Other severe protein-calorie malnutrition
263   Other and unspecified protein-calorie malnutrition
264   Vitamin A deficiency
265   Thiamine and niacin deficiency states
266   Deficiency of B-complex components
267   Ascorbic acid deficiency
268   Vitamin D deficiency
269   Other nutritional deficiencies

Other metabolic disorders and immunity disorders (270–279)
270   Disorders of amino-acid transport and metabolism
271   Disorders of carbohydrate transport and metabolism
272   Disorders of lipid metabolism
273   Disorders of plasma protein metabolism
274   Gout
275   Disorders of mineral metabolism
276   Disorders of fluid, electrolyte, and acid-base balance
277   Other and unspecified disorders of metabolism
278   Obesity and other hyperalimentation
279   Disorders involving the immune mechanism

4. DISEASES OF BLOOD AND BLOOD-FORMING ORGANS

Diseases of the blood and blood-forming organs (280–289)
280   Iron deficiency anemias
281   Other deficiency anemias
282   Hereditary hemolytic anemias
283   Acquired hemolytic anemias
284   Aplastic anemia
285   Other and unspecified anemias
286   Coagulation defects
287   Purpura and other hemorrhagic conditions
288   Diseases of white blood cells
289   Other diseases of blood and blood-forming organs

5. MENTAL DISORDERS

Organic psychotic conditions (290–294)
290   Senile and presenile organic psychotic conditions
291   Alcoholic psychoses
292   Drug psychoses
293   Transient organic psychotic conditions
294   Other organic psychotic conditions (chronic)

Other psychoses (295–299)
295   Schizophrenic psychoses

296   Affective psychoses
297   Paranoid states
298   Other nonorganic psychoses
299   Psychoses with origin specific to childhood

Neurotic disorders, personality disorders, and other nonpsychotic mental disorders (300–316)
300   Neurotic disorders
301   Personality disorders
302   Sexual deviations and disorders
303   Alcohol dependence syndrome
304   Drug dependence
305   Nondependent abuse of drugs
306   Physiological malfunction arising from mental factors
307   Special symptoms or syndromes, not elsewhere classified
308   Acute reaction to stress
309   Adjustment reaction
310   Specific nonpsychotic mental disorders following organic brain damage
311   Depressive disorder, not elsewhere classified
312   Disturbance of conduct, not elsewhere classified
313   Disturbance of emotions specific to childhood and adolescence
314   Hyperkinetic syndrome of childhood
315   Specific delays in development
316   Psychic factors associated with diseases classified elsewhere

Mental retardation (317–319)
317   Mild mental retardation
318   Other specified mental retardation
319   Unspecified mental retardation

6. DISEASES OF THE NERVOUS SYSTEM AND SENSE ORGANS

Inflammatory diseases of the central nervous system (320–326)
320   Bacterial meningitis
321   Meningitis due to other organisms
322   Meningitis of unspecified cause
323   Encephalitis, myelitis, and encephalomyelitis
324   Intracranial and intraspinal abscess
325   Phlebitis and thrombophlebitis of intracranial venous sinuses
326   Late effects of intracranial abscess or pyogenic infection

Hereditary and degenerative diseases of the central nervous system (330–337)
330   Cerebral degenerations usually manifest in childhood
331   Other cerebral degenerations
332   Parkinson's disease
333   Other extrapyramidal disease and abnormal movement disorders
334   Spinocerebellar disease
335   Anterior horn cell disease
336   Other diseases of spinal cord
337   Disorders of the autonomic nervous system

Other disorders of the central nervous system (340–349)
340   Multiple sclerosis
341   Other demyelinating diseases of central nervous system
342   Hemiplegia and hemiparesis
343   Infantile cerebral palsy
344   Other paralytic syndromes
345   Epilepsy
346   Migraine
347   Cataplexy and narcolepsy
348   Other conditions of brain
349   Other and unspecified disorders of the nervous system

Disorders of the peripheral nervous system (350–359)
350   Trigeminal nerve disorders
351   Facial nerve disorders
352   Disorders of other cranial nerves
353   Nerve root and plexus disorders
354   Mononeuritis of upper limb and mononeuritis multiplex
355   Mononeuritis of lower limb

356 Hereditary and idiopathic peripheral neuropathy
357 Inflammatory and toxic neuropathy
358 Myoneural disorders
359 Muscular dystrophies and other myopathies

Disorders of the eye and adnexa (360–379)
360 Disorders of the globe
361 Retinal detachments and defects
362 Other retinal disorders
363 Chorioretinal inflammations and scars and other disorders of choroid
364 Disorders of iris and ciliary body
365 Glaucoma
366 Cataract
367 Disorders of refraction and accommodation
368 Visual disturbances
369 Blindness and low vision
370 Keratitis
371 Corneal opacity and other disorders of cornea
372 Disorders of conjunctiva
373 Inflammation of eyelids
374 Other disorders of eyelids
375 Disorders of lacrimal system
376 Disorders of the orbit
377 Disorders of optic nerve and visual pathways
378 Strabismus and other disorders of binocular eye movements
379 Other disorders of eye

Diseases of the ear and mastoid process (380–389)
380 Disorders of external ear
381 Nonsuppurative otitis media and eustachian tube disorders
382 Suppurative and unspecified otitis media
383 Mastoiditis and related conditions
384 Other disorders of tympanic membrane
385 Other disorders of middle ear and mastoid
386 Vertiginous syndromes and other disorders of vestibular system
387 Otosclerosis
388 Other disorders of ear
389 Hearing loss

7. DISEASES OF THE CIRCULATORY SYSTEM

Acute rheumatic fever (390–392)
390 Rheumatic fever without mention of heart involvement
391 Rheumatic fever with heart involvement
392 Rheumatic chorea

Chronic rheumatic heart disease (393–398)
393 Chronic rheumatic pericarditis
394 Diseases of mitral valve
395 Diseases of aortic valve
396 Diseases of mitral and aortic valves
397 Diseases of other endocardial structures
398 Other rheumatic heart disease

Hypertensive disease (401–405)
401 Essential hypertension
402 Hypertensive heart disease
403 Hypertensive renal disease
404 Hypertensive heart and renal disease
405 Secondary hypertension

Ischemic heart disease (410–414)
410 Acute myocardial infarction
411 Other acute and subacute form of ischemic heart disease
412 Old myocardial infarction
413 Angina pectoris
414 Other forms of chronic ischemic heart disease

Diseases of pulmonary circulation (415–417)
415 Acute pulmonary heart disease
416 Chronic pulmonary heart disease
417 Other diseases of pulmonary circulation

Other forms of heart disease (420–429)
420 Acute pericarditis
421 Acute and subacute endocarditis
422 Acute myocarditis
423 Other diseases of pericardium
424 Other diseases of endocardium
425 Cardiomyopathy
426 Conduction disorders
427 Cardiac dysrhythmias
428 Heart failure
429 Ill-defined descriptions and complications of heart disease

Cerebrovascular disease (430–438)
430 Subarachnoid hemorrhage
431 Intracerebral hemorrhage
432 Other and unspecified intracranial hemorrhage
433 Occlusion and stenosis of precerebral arteries
434 Occlusion of cerebral arteries
435 Transcient cerebral ischemia
436 Acute but ill-defined cerebrovascular disease
437 Other and ill-defined cerebrovascular disease
438 Late effects of cerebrovascular disease

Diseases of arteries, arterioles, and capillaries (440–448)
440 Atherosclerosis
441 Aortic aneurysm and dissection
442 Other aneurysm
443 Other peripheral vascular disease
444 Arterial embolism and thrombosis
446 Polyarteritis nodosa and allied conditions
447 Other disorders of arteries and arterioles
448 Diseases of capillaries

Diseases of veins and lymphatics, and other diseases of circulatory system (451–459)
451 Phlebitis and thrombophlebitis
452 Portal vein thrombosis
453 Other venous embolism and thrombosis
454 Varicose veins of lower extremities
455 Hemorrhoids
456 Varicose veins of other sites
457 Noninfective disorders of lymphatic channels
458 Hypotension
459 Other disorders of circulatory system

8. DISEASES OF THE RESPIRATORY SYSTEM

Acute respiratory infections (460–466)
460 Acute nasopharyngitis [common cold]
461 Acute sinusitis
462 Acute pharyngitis
463 Acute tonsillitis
464 Acute laryngitis and tracheitis
465 Acute upper respiratory infections of multiple or unspecified sites
466 Acute bronchitis and bronchiolitis

Other diseases of upper respiratory tract (470–478)
470 Deviated nasal septum
471 Nasal polyps
472 Chronic pharyngitis and nasopharyngitis
473 Chronic sinusitis
474 Chronic disease of tonsils and adenoids
475 Peritonsillar abscess
476 Chronic laryngitis and laryngotracheitis
477 Allergic rhinitis
478 Other diseases of upper respiratory tract

Pneumonia and influenza (480–487)
480 Viral pneumonia
481 Pneumococcal pneumonia [*Streptococcus pneumoniae* pneumonia]
482 Other bacterial pneumonia
483 Pneumonia due to other specified organism
484 Pneumonia in infectious diseases classified elsewhere
485 Bronchopneumonia, organism unspecified

486 Pneumonia, organism unspecified
487 Influenza

Chronic obstructive pulmonary disease and allied conditions (490–496)
490 Bronchitis, not specified as acute or chronic
491 Chronic bronchitis
492 Emphysema
493 Asthma
494 Bronchiectasis
495 Extrinsic allergic alveolitis
496 Chronic airways obstruction, not elsewhere classified

Pneumoconioses and other lung diseases due to external agents (500–508)
500 Coalworkers' pneumoconiosis
501 Asbestosis
502 Pneumoconiosis due to other silica or silicates
503 Pneumoconiosis due to other inorganic dust
504 Pneumopathy due to inhalation of other dust
505 Pneumoconiosis, unspecified
506 Respiratory conditions due to chemical fumes and vapors
507 Pneumonitis due to solids and liquids
508 Respiratory conditions due to other and unspecified external agents

Other diseases of respiratory system (510–519)
510 Empyema
511 Pleurisy
512 Pneumothorax
513 Abscess of lung and mediastinum
514 Pulmonary congestion and hypostasis
515 Postinflammatory pulmonary fibrosis
516 Other alveolar and parietoalveolar pneumopathy
517 Lung involvement in conditions classified elsewhere
518 Other diseases of lung
519 Other diseases of respiratory system

9. DISEASES OF THE DIGESTIVE SYSTEM

Diseases of oral cavity, salivary glands, and jaws (520–529)
520 Disorders of tooth development and eruption
521 Diseases of hard tissues of teeth
522 Diseases of pulp and periapical tissues
523 Gingival and periodontal diseases
524 Dentofacial anomalies, including malocclusion
525 Other diseases and conditions of the teeth and supporting structures
526 Diseases of the jaws
527 Diseases of the salivary glands
528 Diseases of the oral soft tissues, excluding lesions specific for gingiva and tongue
529 Diseases and other conditions of the tongue

Diseases of esophagus, stomach, and duodenum (530–537)
530 Diseases of esophagus
531 Gastric ulcer
532 Duodenal ulcer
533 Peptic ulcer, site unspecified
534 Gastrojejunal ulcer
535 Gastritis and duodenitis
536 Disorders of function of stomach
537 Other disorders of stomach and duodenum

Appendicitis (540–543)
540 Acute appendicitis
541 Appendicitis, unqualified
542 Other appendicitis
543 Other diseases of appendix

Hernia of abdominal cavity (550–553)
550 Inguinal hernia
551 Other hernia of abdominal cavity, with gangrene
552 Other hernia of abdominal cavity, with obstruction, but without mention of gangrene
553 Other hernia of abdominal cavity without mention of obstruction or gangrene

Noninfective enteritis and colitis (555–558)
555 Regional enteritis
556 Ulcerative colitis
557 Vascular insufficiency of intestine
558 Other noninfective gastroenteritis and colitis

Other diseases of intestines and peritoneum (560–569)
560 Intestinal obstruction without mention of hernia
562 Diverticula of intestine
564 Functional digestive disorders, not elsewhere classified
565 Anal fissure and fistula
566 Abscess of anal and rectal regions
567 Peritonitis
568 Other disorders of peritoneum
569 Other disorders of intestine

Other diseases of digestive system (570–579)
570 Acute and subacute necrosis of liver
571 Chronic liver disease and cirrhosis
572 Liver abscess and sequelae of chronic liver disease
573 Other disorders of liver
574 Cholelithiasis
575 Other disorders of gallbladder
576 Other disorders of biliary tract
577 Diseases of pancreas
578 Gastrointestinal hemorrhage
579 Intestinal malabsorption

10. DISEASES OF THE GENITOURINARY SYSTEM

Nephritis, nephrotic syndrome, and nephrosis (580–589)
580 Acute glomerulonephritis
581 Nephrotic syndrome
582 Chronic glomerulonephritis
583 Nephritis and nephropathy, not specified as acute or chronic
584 Acute renal failure
585 Chronic renal failure
586 Renal failure, unspecified
587 Renal sclerosis, unspecified
588 Disorders resulting from impaired renal function
589 Small kidney of unknown cause

Other diseases of urinary system (590–599)
590 Infections of kidney
591 Hydronephrosis
592 Calculus of kidney and ureter
593 Other disorders of kidney and ureter
594 Calculus of lower urinary tract
595 Cystitis
596 Other disorders of bladder
597 Urethritis, not sexually transmitted, and urethral syndrome
598 Urethral stricture
599 Other disorders of urethra and urinary tract

Diseases of male genital organs (600–608)
600 Hyperplasia of prostate
601 Inflammatory diseases of prostate
602 Other disorders of prostate
603 Hydrocele
604 Orchitis and epididymitis
605 Redundant prepuce and phimosis
606 Infertility, male
607 Disorders of penis
608 Other disorders of male genital organs

Disorders of breast (610–611)
610 Benign mammary dysplasias
611 Other disorders of breast

Inflammatory disease of female pelvic organs (614–616)
614 Inflammatory disease of ovary, fallopian tube, pelvic cellular tissue, and peritoneum
615 Inflammatory diseases of uterus, except cervix
616 Inflammatory disease of cervix, vagina, and vulva

ICD-9-CM
Appx E
Vol. 1

Other disorders of female genital tract (617–629)

617	Endometriosis
618	Genital prolapse
619	Fistula involving female genital tract
620	Noninflammatory disorders of ovary, fallopian tube, and broad ligament
621	Disorders of uterus, not elsewhere classified
622	Noninflammatory disorders of cervix
623	Noninflammatory disorders of vagina
624	Noninflammatory disorders of vulva and perineum
625	Pain and other symptoms associated with female genital organs
626	Disorders of menstruation and other abnormal bleeding from female genital tract
627	Menopausal and postmenopausal disorders
628	Infertility, female
629	Other disorders of female genital organs

11. COMPLICATIONS OF PREGNANCY, CHILDBIRTH, AND THE PUERPERIUM

Ectopic and molar pregnancy and other pregnancy with abortive outcome (630–639)

630	Hydatidiform mole
631	Other abnormal product of conception
632	Missed abortion
633	Ectopic pregnancy
634	Spontaneous abortion
635	Legally induced abortion
636	Illegally induced abortion
637	Unspecified abortion
638	Failed attempted abortion
639	Complications following abortion and ectopic and molar pregnancies

Complications mainly related to pregnancy (640–648)

640	Hemorrhage in early pregnancy
641	Antepartum hemorrhage, abruptio placentae, and placenta previa
642	Hypertension complicating pregnancy, childbirth, and the puerperium
643	Excessive vomiting in pregnancy
644	Early or threatened labor
645	Prolonged pregnancy
646	Other complications of pregnancy, not elsewhere classified
647	Infective and parasitic conditions in the mother classifiable elsewhere but complicating pregnancy, childbirth, and the puerperium
648	Other current conditions in the mother classifiable elsewhere but complicating pregnancy, childbirth, and the puerperium

Normal delivery, and other indications for care in pregnancy, labor, and delivery (650–659)

650	Normal delivery
651	Multiple gestation
652	Malposition and malpresentation of fetus
653	Disproportion
654	Abnormality of organs and soft tissues of pelvis
655	Known or suspected fetal abnormality affecting management of mother
656	Other fetal and placental problems affecting management of mother
657	Polyhydramnios
658	Other problems associated with amniotic cavity and membranes
659	Other indications for care or intervention related to labor and delivery and not elsewhere classified

Complications occurring mainly in the course of labor and delivery (660–669)

660	Obstructed labor
661	Abnormality of forces of labor
662	Long labor
663	Umbilical cord complications
664	Trauma to perineum and vulva during delivery
665	Other obstetrical trauma
666	Postpartum hemorrhage
667	Retained placenta or membranes, without hemorrhage
668	Complications of the administration of anesthetic or other sedation in labor and delivery
669	Other complications of labor and delivery, not elsewhere classified

Complications of the puerperium (670–677)

670	Major puerperal infection
671	Venous complications in pregnancy and the puerperium
672	Pyrexia of unknown origin during the puerperium
673	Obstetrical pulmonary embolism
674	Other and unspecified complications of the puerperium, not elsewhere classified
675	Infections of the breast and nipple associated with childbirth
676	Other disorders of the breast associated with childbirth, and disorders of lactation
677	Late effect of complication of pregnancy, childbirth, and the puerperium

12. DISEASES OF THE SKIN AND SUBCUTANEOUS TISSUE

Infections of skin and subcutaneous tissue (680–686)

680	Carbuncle and furuncle
681	Cellulitis and abscess of finger and toe
682	Other cellulitis and abscess
683	Acute lymphadenitis
684	Impetigo
685	Pilonidal cyst
686	Other local infections of skin and subcutaneous tissue

Other inflammatory conditions of skin and subcutaneous tissue (690–698)

690	Erythematosquamous dermatosis
691	Atopic dermatitis and related conditions
692	Contact dermatitis and other eczema
693	Dermatitis due to substances taken internally
694	Bullous dermatoses
695	Erythematous conditions
696	Psoriasis and similar disorders
697	Lichen
698	Pruritus and related conditions

Other diseases of skin and subcutaneous tissue (700–709)

700	Corns and callosities
701	Other hypertrophic and atrophic conditions of skin
702	Other dermatoses
703	Diseases of nail
704	Diseases of hair and hair follicles
705	Disorders of sweat glands
706	Diseases of sebaceous glands
707	Chronic ulcer of skin
708	Urticaria
709	Other disorders of skin and subcutaneous tissue

13. DISEASES OF THE MUSCULOSKELETAL SYSTEM AND CONNECTIVE TISSUE

Arthropathies and related disorders (710–719)

710	Diffuse diseases of connective tissue
711	Arthropathy associated with infections
712	Crystal arthropathies
713	Arthropathy associated with other disorders classified elsewhere
714	Rheumatoid arthritis and other inflammatory polyarthropathies
715	Osteoarthrosis and allied disorders
716	Other and unspecified arthropathies
717	Internal derangement of knee
718	Other derangement of joint
719	Other and unspecified disorder of joint

Dorsopathies (720–724)
720 Ankylosing spondylitis and other inflammatory spondylopathies
721 Spondylosis and allied disorders
722 Intervertebral disc disorders
723 Other disorders of cervical region
724 Other and unspecified disorders of back

Rheumatism, excluding the back (725–729)
725 Polymyalgia rheumatica
726 Peripheral enthesopathies and allied syndromes
727 Other disorders of synovium, tendon, and bursa
728 Disorders of muscle, ligament, and fascia
729 Other disorders of soft tissues

Osteopathies, chondropathies, and acquired musculoskeletal deformities (730–739)
730 Osteomyelitis, periostitis, and other infections involving bone
731 Osteitis deformans and osteopathies associated with other disorders classified elsewhere
732 Osteochondropathies
733 Other disorders of bone and cartilage
734 Flat foot
735 Acquired deformities of toe
736 Other acquired deformities of limbs
737 Curvature of spine
738 Other acquired deformity
739 Nonallopathic lesions, not elsewhere classified

14. CONGENITAL ANOMALIES

Congential anomalies (740–759)
740 Anencephalus and similar anomalies
741 Spina bifida
742 Other congenital anomalies of nervous system
743 Congenital anomalies of eye
744 Congenital anomalies of ear, face, and neck
745 Bulbus cordis anomalies and anomalies of cardiac septal closure
746 Other congenital anomalies of heart
747 Other congenital anomalies of circulatory system
748 Congenital anomalies of respiratory system
749 Cleft palate and cleft lip
750 Other congenital anomalies of upper alimentary tract
751 Other congenital anomalies of digestive system
752 Congenital anomalies of genital organs
753 Congenital anomalies of urinary system
754 Certain congenital musculoskeletal deformities
755 Other congenital anomalies of limbs
756 Other congenital musculoskeletal anomalies
757 Congenital anomalies of the integument
758 Chromosomal anomalies
759 Other and unspecified congenital anomalies

15. CERTAIN CONDITIONS ORIGINATING IN THE PERINATAL PERIOD

Maternal causes of perinatal morbidity and mortality (760–763)
760 Fetus or newborn affected by maternal conditions which may be unrelated to present pregnancy
761 Fetus or newborn affected by maternal complications of pregnancy
762 Fetus or newborn affected by complications of placenta, cord, and membranes
763 Fetus or newborn affected by other complications of labor and delivery

Other conditions originating in the perinatal period (764–779)
764 Slow fetal growth and fetal malnutrition
765 Disorders relating to short gestation and unspecified low birthweight
766 Disorders relating to long gestation and high birthweight
767 Birth trauma
768 Intrauterine hypoxia and birth asphyxia
769 Respiratory distress syndrome
770 Other respiratory conditions of fetus and newborn
771 Infections specific to the perinatal period
772 Fetal and neonatal hemorrhage
773 Hemolytic disease of fetus or newborn, due to isoimmunization
774 Other perinatal jaundice
775 Endocrine and metabolic disturbances specific to the fetus and newborn
776 Hematological disorders of fetus and newborn
777 Perinatal disorders of digestive system
778 Conditions involving the integument and temperature regulation of fetus and newborn
779 Other and ill-defined conditions originating in the perinatal period

16. SYMPTOMS, SIGNS, AND ILL-DEFINED CONDITIONS

Symptoms (780–789)
780 General symptoms
781 Symptoms involving nervous and musculoskeletal systems
782 Symptoms involving skin and other integumentary tissue
783 Symptoms concerning nutrition, metabolism, and development
784 Symptoms involving head and neck
785 Symptoms involving cardiovascular system
786 Symptoms involving respiratory system and other chest symptoms
787 Symptoms involving digestive system
788 Symptoms involving urinary system
789 Other symptoms involving abdomen and pelvis

Nonspecific abnormal findings (790–796)
790 Nonspecific findings on examination of blood
791 Nonspecific findings on examination of urine
792 Nonspecific abnormal findings in other body substances
793 Nonspecific abnormal findings on radiological and other examination of body structure
794 Nonspecific abnormal results of function studies
795 Nonspecific abnormal histological and immunological findings
796 Other nonspecific abnormal findings

Ill-defined and unknown causes of morbidity and mortality (797–799)
797 Senility without mention of psychosis
798 Sudden death, cause unknown
799 Other ill-defined and unknown causes of morbidity and mortality

17. INJURY AND POISONING

Fracture of skull (800–804)
800 Fracture of vault of skull
801 Fracture of base of skull
802 Fracture of face bones
803 Other and unqualified skull fractures
804 Multiple fractures involving skull or face with other bones

Fracture of spine and trunk (805–809)
805 Fracture of vertebral column without mention of spinal cord lesion
806 Fracture of vertebral column with spinal cord lesion
807 Fracture of rib(s), sternum, larynx, and trachea
808 Fracture of pelvis
809 Ill-defined fractures of bones of trunk

Fracture of upper limb (810–819)
810 Fracture of clavicle
811 Fracture of scapula
812 Fracture of humerus
813 Fracture of radius and ulna
814 Fracture of carpal bone(s)
815 Fracture of metacarpal bone(s)
816 Fracture of one or more phalanges of hand
817 Multiple fractures of hand bones

ICD-9-CM

Appx E

Vol. 1

818	Ill-defined fractures of upper limb
819	Multiple fractures involving both upper limbs, and upper limb with rib(s) and sternum

Fracture of lower limb (820–829)

820	Fracture of neck of femur
821	Fracture of other and unspecified parts of femur
822	Fracture of patella
823	Fracture of tibia and fibula
824	Fracture of ankle
825	Fracture of one or more tarsal and metatarsal bones
826	Fracture of one or more phalanges of foot
827	Other, multiple, and ill-defined fractures of lower limb
828	Multiple fractures involving both lower limbs, lower with upper limb, and lower limb(s) with rib(s) and sternum
829	Fracture of unspecified bones

Dislocation (830–839)

830	Dislocation of jaw
831	Dislocation of shoulder
832	Dislocation of elbow
833	Dislocation of wrist
834	Dislocation of finger
835	Dislocation of hip
836	Dislocation of knee
837	Dislocation of ankle
838	Dislocation of foot
839	Other, multiple, and ill-defined dislocations

Sprains and strains of joints and adjacent muscles (840–848)

840	Sprains and strains of shoulder and upper arm
841	Sprains and strains of elbow and forearm
842	Sprains and strains of wrist and hand
843	Sprains and strains of hip and thigh
844	Sprains and strains of knee and leg
845	Sprains and strains of ankle and foot
846	Sprains and strains of sacroiliac region
847	Sprains and strains of other and unspecified parts of back
848	Other and ill-defined sprains and strains

Intracranial injury, excluding those with skull fracture (850–854)

850	Concussion
851	Cerebral laceration and contusion
852	Subarachnoid, subdural, and extradural hemorrhage, following injury
853	Other and unspecified intracranial hemorrhage following injury
854	Intracranial injury of other and unspecified nature

Internal injury of chest, abdomen, and pelvis (860–869)

860	Traumatic pneumothorax and hemothorax
861	Injury to heart and lung
862	Injury to other and unspecified intrathoracic organs
863	Injury to gastrointestinal tract
864	Injury to liver
865	Injury to spleen
866	Injury to kidney
867	Injury to pelvic organs
868	Injury to other intra-abdominal organs
869	Internal injury to unspecified or ill-defined organs

Open wound of head, neck, and trunk (870–879)

870	Open wound of ocular adnexa
871	Open wound of eyeball
872	Open wound of ear
873	Other open wound of head
874	Open wound of neck
875	Open wound of chest (wall)
876	Open wound of back
877	Open wound of buttock
878	Open wound of genital organs (external), including traumatic amputation
879	Open wound of other and unspecified sites, except limbs

Open wound of upper limb (880–887)

880	Open wound of shoulder and upper arm
881	Open wound of elbow, forearm, and wrist
882	Open wound of hand except finger(s) alone
883	Open wound of finger(s)
884	Multiple and unspecified open wound of upper limb
885	Traumatic amputation of thumb (complete) (partial)
886	Traumatic amputation of other finger(s) (complete) (partial)
887	Traumatic amputation of arm and hand (complete) (partial)

Open wound of lower limb (890–897)

890	Open wound of hip and thigh
891	Open wound of knee, leg [except thigh], and ankle
892	Open wound of foot except toe(s) alone
893	Open wound of toe(s)
894	Multiple and unspecified open wound of lower limb
895	Traumatic amputation of toe(s) (complete) (partial)
896	Traumatic amputation of foot (complete) (partial)
897	Traumatic amputation of leg(s) (complete) (partial)

Injury to blood vessels (900–904)

900	Injury to blood vessels of head and neck
901	Injury to blood vessels of thorax
902	Injury to blood vessels of abdomen and pelvis
903	Injury to blood vessels of upper extremity
904	Injury to blood vessels of lower extremity and unspecified sites

Late effects of injuries, poisonings, toxic effects, and other external causes (905–909)

905	Late effects of musculoskeletal and connective tissue injuries
906	Late effects of injuries to skin and subcutaneous tissues
907	Late effects of injuries to the nervous system
908	Late effects of other and unspecified injuries
909	Late effects of other and unspecified external causes

Superficial injury (910–919)

910	Superficial injury of face, neck, and scalp except eye
911	Superficial injury of trunk
912	Superficial injury of shoulder and upper arm
913	Superficial injury of elbow, forearm, and wrist
914	Superficial injury of hand(s) except finger(s) alone
915	Superficial injury of finger(s)
916	Superficial injury of hip, thigh, leg, and ankle
917	Superficial injury of foot and toe(s)
918	Superficial injury of eye and adnexa
919	Superficial injury of other, multiple, and unspecified sites

Contusion with intact skin surface (920–924)

920	Contusion of face, scalp, and neck except eye(s)
921	Contusion of eye and adnexa
922	Contusion of trunk
923	Contusion of upper limb
924	Contusion of lower limb and of other and unspecified sites

Crushing injury (925–929)

925	Crushing injury of face, scalp, and neck
926	Crushing injury of trunk
927	Crushing injury of upper limb
928	Crushing injury of lower limb
929	Crushing injury of multiple and unspecified sites

Effects of foreign body entering through orifice (930–939)

930	Foreign body on external eye
931	Foreign body in ear
932	Foreign body in nose
933	Foreign body in pharynx and larynx
934	Foreign body in trachea, bronchus, and lung
935	Foreign body in mouth, esophagus, and stomach
936	Foreign body in intestine and colon
937	Foreign body in anus and rectum
938	Foreign body in digestive system, unspecified
939	Foreign body in genitourinary tract

Burns (940–949)

940	Burn confined to eye and adnexa
941	Burn of face, head, and neck

942 Burn of trunk
943 Burn of upper limb, except wrist and hand
944 Burn of wrist(s) and hand(s)
945 Burn of lower limb(s)
946 Burns of multiple specified sites
947 Burn of internal organs
948 Burns classified according to extent of body surface involved
949 Burn, unspecified

Injury to nerves and spinal cord (950–957)
950 Injury to optic nerve and pathways
951 Injury to other cranial nerve(s)
952 Spinal cord injury without evidence of spinal bone injury
953 Injury to nerve roots and spinal plexus
954 Injury to other nerve(s) of trunk excluding shoulder and pelvic girdles
955 Injury to peripheral nerve(s) of shoulder girdle and upper limb
956 Injury to peripheral nerve(s) of pelvic girdle and lower limb
957 Injury to other and unspecified nerves

Certain traumatic complications and unspecified injuries (958–959)
958 Certain early complications of trauma
959 Injury, other and unspecified

Poisoning by drugs, medicinals and biological substances (960–979)
960 Poisoning by antibiotics
961 Poisoning by other anti-infectives
962 Poisoning by hormones and synthetic substitutes
963 Poisoning by primarily systemic agents
964 Poisoning by agents primarily affecting blood constituents
965 Poisoning by analgesics, antipyretics, and antirheumatics
966 Poisoning by anticonvulsants and anti-parkinsonism drugs
967 Poisoning by sedatives and hypnotics
968 Poisoning by other central nervous system depressants and anesthetics
969 Poisoning by psychotropic agents
970 Poisoning by central nervous system stimulants
971 Poisoning by drugs primarily affecting the autonomic nervous system
972 Poisoning by agents primarily affecting the cardiovascular system
973 Poisoning by agents primarily affecting the gastrointestinal system
974 Poisoning by water, mineral, and uric acid metabolism drugs
975 Poisoning by agents primarily acting on the smooth and skeletal muscles and respiratory system
976 Poisoning by agents primarily affecting skin and mucous membrane, ophthalmological, otorhinolaryngological, and dental drugs
977 Poisoning by other and unspecified drugs and medicinals
978 Poisoning by bacterial vaccines
979 Poisoning by other vaccines and biological substances

Toxic effects of substances chiefly nonmedicinal as to source (980–989)
980 Toxic effect of alcohol
981 Toxic effect of petroleum products
982 Toxic effect of solvents other than petroleum-based
983 Toxic effect of corrosive aromatics, acids, and caustic alkalis
984 Toxic effect of lead and its compounds (including fumes)
985 Toxic effect of other metals
986 Toxic effect of carbon monoxide
987 Toxic effect of other gases, fumes, or vapors
988 Toxic effect of noxious substances eaten as food
989 Toxic effect of other substances, chiefly nonmedicinal as to source

Other and unspecified effects of external causes (990–995)
990 Effects of radiation, unspecified
991 Effects of reduced temperature
992 Effects of heat and light
993 Effects of air pressure
994 Effects of other external causes
995 Certain adverse effects, not elsewhere classified

Complications of surgical and medical care, not elsewhere classified (996–999)
996 Complications peculiar to certain specified procedures
997 Complications affecting specified body systems, not elsewhere classified
998 Other complications of procedures, not elsewhere classified
999 Complications of medical care, not elsewhere classified

SUPPLEMENTARY CLASSIFICATION OF FACTORS INFLUENCING HEALTH STATUS AND CONTACT WITH HEALTH SERVICES

Persons with potential health hazards related to communicable diseases (V01–V09)
V01 Contact with or exposure to communicable diseases
V02 Carrier or suspected carrier of infectious diseases
V03 Need for prophylactic vaccination and inoculation against bacterial diseases
V04 Need for prophylactic vaccination and inoculation against certain viral diseases
V05 Need for other prophylactic vaccination and inoculation against single diseases
V06 Need for prophylactic vaccination and inoculation against combinations of diseases
V07 Need for isolation and other prophylactic measures
V08 Asymptomatic human immunodeficiency virus [HIV] infection status
V09 Infection with drug-resistant microorganisms

Persons with potential health hazards related to personal and family history (V10–V19)
V10 Personal history of malignant neoplasm
V11 Personal history of mental disorder
V12 Personal history of certain other diseases
V13 Personal history of other diseases
V14 Personal history of allergy to medicinal agents
V15 Other personal history presenting hazards to health
V16 Family history of malignant neoplasm
V17 Family history of certain chronic disabling diseases
V18 Family history of certain other specific conditions
V19 Family history of other conditions

Persons encountering health services in circumstances related to reproduction and development (V20–V29)
V20 Health supervision of infant or child
V21 Constitutional states in development
V22 Normal pregnancy
V23 Supervision of high-risk pregnancy
V24 Postpartum care and examination
V25 Encounter for contraceptive management
V26 Procreative management
V27 Outcome of delivery
V28 Antenatal screening
V29 Observation and evaluation of newborns and infants for suspected condition not found

Liveborn infants according to type of birth (V30–V39)
V30 Single liveborn
V31 Twin, mate liveborn
V32 Twin, mate stillborn
V33 Twin, unspecified
V34 Other multiple, mates all liveborn
V35 Other multiple, mates all stillborn
V36 Other multiple, mates live- and stillborn
V37 Other multiple, unspecified
V39 Unspecified

Persons with a condition influencing their health status (V40–V49)
V40 Mental and behavioral problems

ICD-9-CM

Appx E

Vol. 1

V41 Problems with special senses and other special functions
V42 Organ or tissue replaced by transplant
V43 Organ or tissue replaced by other means
V44 Artificial opening status
V45 Other postsurgical states
V46 Other dependence on machines
V47 Other problems with internal organs
V48 Problems with head, neck, and trunk
V49 Problems with limbs and other problems

Persons encountering health services for specific procedures and aftercare (V50–V59)

V50 Elective surgery for purposes other than remedying health states
V51 Aftercare involving the use of plastic surgery
V52 Fitting and adjustment of prosthetic device
V53 Fitting and adjustment of other device
V54 Other orthopedic aftercare
V55 Attention to artificial openings
V56 Encounter for dialysis and dialysis catheter care
V57 Care involving use of rehabilitation procedures
V58 Other and unspecified aftercare
V59 Donors

Persons encountering health services in other circumstances (V60–V69)

V60 Housing, household, and economic circumstances
V61 Other family circumstances
V62 Other psychosocial circumstances
V63 Unavailability of other medical facilities for care
V64 Persons encountering health services for specific procedures, not carried out
V65 Other persons seeking consultation without complaint or sickness
V66 Convalescence and palliative care
V67 Follow-up examination
V68 Encounters for administrative purposes
V69 Problems related to lifestyle

Persons without reported diagnosis encountered during examination and investigation of individuals and populations (V70–V82)

V70 General medical examination
V71 Observation and evaluation for suspected conditions
V72 Special investigations and examinations
V73 Special screening examination for viral and chlamydial diseases
V74 Special screening examination for bacterial and spirochetal diseases
V75 Special screening examination for other infectious diseases
V76 Special screening for malignant neoplasms
V77 Special screening for endocrine, nutritional, metabolic, and immunity disorders
V78 Special screening for disorders of blood and blood-forming organs
V79 Special screening for mental disorders and developmental handicaps
V80 Special screening for neurological, eye, and ear diseases
V81 Special screening for cardiovascular, respiratory, and genitourinary diseases
V82 Special screening for other conditions

SUPPLEMENTARY CLASSIFICATION OF EXTERNAL CAUSES OF INJURY AND POISONING

Railway accidents (E800–E807)

E800 Railway accident involving collision with rolling stock
E801 Railway accident involving collision with other object
E802 Railway accident involving derailment without antecedent collision
E803 Railway accident involving explosion, fire, or burning
E804 Fall in, on, or from railway train
E805 Hit by rolling stock
E806 Other specified railway accident
E807 Railway accident of unspecified nature

Motor vehicle traffic accidents (E810–E819)

E810 Motor vehicle traffic accident involving collision with train
E811 Motor vehicle traffic accident involving re-entrant collision with another motor vehicle
E812 Other motor vehicle traffic accident involving collision with another motor vehicle
E813 Motor vehicle traffic accident involving collision with other vehicle
E814 Motor vehicle traffic accident involving collision with pedestrian
E815 Other motor vehicle traffic accident involving collision on the highway
E816 Motor vehicle traffic accident due to loss of control, without collision on the highway
E817 Noncollision motor vehicle traffic accident while boarding or alighting
E818 Other noncollision motor vehicle traffic accident
E819 Motor vehicle traffic accident of unspecified nature

Motor vehicle nontraffic accidents (E820–E825)

E820 Nontraffic accident involving motor-driven snow vehicle
E821 Nontraffic accident involving other off-road motor vehicle
E822 Other motor vehicle nontraffic accident involving collision with moving object
E823 Other motor vehicle nontraffic accident involving collision with stationary object
E824 Other motor vehicle nontraffic accident while boarding and alighting
E825 Other motor vehicle nontraffic accident of other and unspecified nature

Other road vehicle accidents (E826–E829)

E826 Pedal cycle accident
E827 Animal-drawn vehicle accident
E828 Accident involving animal being ridden
E829 Other road vehicle accidents

Water transport accidents (E830–E838)

E830 Accident to watercraft causing submersion
E831 Accident to watercraft causing other injury
E832 Other accidental submersion or drowning in water transport accident
E833 Fall on stairs or ladders in water transport
E834 Other fall from one level to another in water transport
E835 Other and unspecified fall in water transport
E836 Machinery accident in water transport
E837 Explosion, fire, or burning in watercraft
E838 Other and unspecified water transport accident

Air and space transport accidents (E840–E845)

E840 Accident to powered aircraft at takeoff or landing
E841 Accident to powered aircraft, other and unspecified
E842 Accident to unpowered aircraft
E843 Fall in, on, or from aircraft
E844 Other specified air transport accidents
E845 Accident involving spacecraft

Vehicle accidents, not elsewhere classifiable (E846–E849)

E846 Accidents involving powered vehicles used solely within the buildings and premises of an industrial or commercial establishment
E847 Accidents involving cable cars not running on rails
E848 Accidents involving other vehicles, not elsewhere classifiable
E849 Place of occurrence

Accidental poisoning by drugs, medicinal substances, and biologicals (E850–E858)

E850 Accidental poisoning by analgesics, antipyretics, and antirheumatics
E851 Accidental poisoning by barbiturates
E852 Accidental poisoning by other sedatives and hypnotics
E853 Accidental poisoning by tranquilizers
E854 Accidental poisoning by other psychotropic agents

E855 Accidental poisoning by other drugs acting on central and autonomic nervous systems
E856 Accidental poisoning by antibiotics
E857 Accidental poisoning by anti-infectives
E858 Accidental poisoning by other drugs

Accidental poisoning by other solid and liquid substances, gases, and vapors (E860–E869)
E860 Accidental poisoning by alcohol, not elsewhere classified
E861 Accidental poisoning by cleansing and polishing agents, disinfectants, paints, and varnishes
E862 Accidental poisoning by petroleum products, other solvents and their vapors, not elsewhere classified
E863 Accidental poisoning by agricultural and horticultural chemical and pharmaceutical preparations other than plant foods and fertilizers
E864 Accidental poisoning by corrosives and caustics, not elsewhere classified
E865 Accidental poisoning from poisonous foodstuffs and poisonous plants
E866 Accidental poisoning by other and unspecified solid and liquid substances
E867 Accidental poisoning by gas distributed by pipeline
E868 Accidental poisoning by other utility gas and other carbon monoxide
E869 Accidental poisoning by other gases and vapors

Misadventures to patients during surgical and medical care (E870–E876)
E870 Accidental cut, puncture, perforation, or hemorrhage during medical care
E871 Foreign object left in body during procedure
E872 Failure of sterile precautions during procedure
E873 Failure in dosage
E874 Mechanical failure of instrument or apparatus during procedure
E875 Contaminated or infected blood, other fluid, drug, or biological substance
E876 Other and unspecified misadventures during medical care

Surgical and medical procedures as the cause of abnormal reaction of patient or later complication, without mention of misadventure at the time of procedure (E878–E879)
E878 Surgical operation and other surgical procedures as the cause of abnormal reaction of patient, or of later complication, without mention of misadventure at the time of operation
E879 Other procedures, without mention of misadventure at the time of procedure, as the cause of abnormal reaction of patient, or of later complication

Accidental falls (E880–E888)
E880 Fall on or from stairs or steps
E881 Fall on or from ladders or scaffolding
E882 Fall from or out of building or other structure
E883 Fall into hole or other opening in surface
E884 Other fall from one level to another
E885 Fall on same level from slipping, tripping, or stumbling
E886 Fall on same level from collision, pushing or shoving, by or with other person
E887 Fracture, cause unspecified
E888 Other and unspecified fall

Accidents caused by fire and flames (E890–E899)
E890 Conflagration in private dwelling
E891 Conflagration in other and unspecified building or structure
E892 Conflagration not in building or structure
E893 Accident caused by ignition of clothing
E894 Ignition of highly inflammable material
E895 Accident caused by controlled fire in private dwelling
E896 Accident caused by controlled fire in other and unspecified building or structure
E897 Accident caused by controlled fire not in building or structure

E898 Accident caused by other specified fire and flames
E899 Accident caused by unspecified fire

Accidents due to natural and environmental factors (E900–E909)
E900 Excessive heat
E901 Excessive cold
E902 High and low air pressure and changes in air pressure
E903 Travel and motion
E904 Hunger, thirst, exposure, and neglect
E905 Venomous animals and plants as the cause of poisoning and toxic reactions
E906 Other injury caused by animals
E907 Lightning
E908 Cataclysmic storms, and floods resulting from storms
E909 Cataclysmic earth surface movements and eruptions

Accidents caused by submersion, suffocation, and foreign bodies (E910–E915)
E910 Accidental drowning and submersion
E911 Inhalation and ingestion of food causing obstruction of respiratory tract or suffocation
E912 Inhalation and ingestion of other object causing obstruction of respiratory tract or suffocation
E913 Accidental mechanical suffocation
E914 Foreign body accidentally entering eye and adnexa
E915 Foreign body accidentally entering other orifice

Other accidents (E916–E928)
E916 Struck accidentally by falling object
E917 Striking against or struck accidentally by objects or persons
E918 Caught accidentally in or between objects
E919 Accidents caused by machinery
E920 Accidents caused by cutting and piercing instruments or objects
E921 Accident caused by explosion of pressure vessel
E922 Accident caused by firearm missile
E923 Accident caused by explosive material
E924 Accident caused by hot substance or object, caustic or corrosive material, and steam
E925 Accident caused by electric current
E926 Exposure to radiation
E927 Overexertion and strenuous movements
E928 Other and unspecified environmental and accidental causes

Late effects of accidental injury (E929)
E929 Late effects of accidental injury

Drugs, medicinal and biological substances causing adverse effects in therapeutic use (E930–E949)
E930 Antibiotics
E931 Other anti-infectives
E932 Hormones and synthetic substitutes
E933 Primarily systemic agents
E934 Agents primarily affecting blood constituents
E935 Analgesics, antipyretics, and antirheumatics
E936 Anticonvulsants and anti-parkinsonism drugs
E937 Sedatives and hypnotics
E938 Other central nervous system depressants and anesthetics
E939 Psychotropic agents
E940 Central nervous system stimulants
E941 Drugs primarily affecting the autonomic nervous system
E942 Agents primarily affecting the cardiovascular system
E943 Agents primarily affecting gastrointestinal system
E944 Water, mineral, and uric acid metabolism drugs
E945 Agents primarily acting on the smooth and skeletal muscles and respiratory system
E946 Agents primarily affecting skin and mucous membrane, ophthalmological, otorhinolaryngological, and dental drugs
E947 Other and unspecified drugs and medicinal substances
E948 Bacterial vaccines
E949 Other vaccines and biological substances

Suicide and self-inflicted injury (E950–E959)

E950 Suicide and self-inflicted poisoning by solid or liquid substances
E951 Suicide and self-inflicted poisoning by gases in domestic use
E952 Suicide and self-inflicted poisoning by other gases and vapors
E953 Suicide and self-inflicted injury by hanging, strangulation, and suffocation
E954 Suicide and self-inflicted injury by submersion [drowning]
E955 Suicide and self-inflicted injury by firearms and explosives
E956 Suicide and self-inflicted injury by cutting and piercing instruments
E957 Suicide and self-inflicted injuries by jumping from high place
E958 Suicide and self-inflicted injury by other and unspecified means
E959 Late effects of self-inflicted injury

Homicide and injury purposely inflicted by other persons (E960–E969)

E960 Fight, brawl, and rape
E961 Assault by corrosive or caustic substance, except poisoning
E962 Assault by poisoning
E963 Assault by hanging and strangulation
E964 Assault by submersion [drowning]
E965 Assault by firearms and explosives
E966 Assault by cutting and piercing instrument
E967 Child and adult battering and other maltreatment
E968 Assault by other and unspecified means
E969 Late effects of injury purposely inflicted by other person

Legal intervention (E970–E978)

E970 Injury due to legal intervention by firearms
E971 Injury due to legal intervention by explosives
E972 Injury due to legal intervention by gas
E973 Injury due to legal intervention by blunt object
E974 Injury due to legal intervention by cutting and piercing instruments
E975 Injury due to legal intervention by other specified means

E976 Injury due to legal intervention by unspecified means
E977 Late effects of injuries due to legal intervention
E978 Legal execution

Injury undetermined whether accidentally or purposely inflicted (E980–E989)

E980 Poisoning by solid or liquid substances, undetermined whether accidentally or purposely inflicted
E981 Poisoning by gases in domestic use, undetermined whether accidentally or purposely inflicted
E982 Poisoning by other gases, undetermined whether accidentally or purposely inflicted
E983 Hanging, strangulation, or suffocation, undetermined whether accidentally or purposely inflicted
E984 Submersion [drowning], undetermined whether accidentally or purposely inflicted
E985 Injury by firearms and explosives, undetermined whether accidentally or purposely inflicted
E986 Injury by cutting and piercing instruments, undetermined whether accidentally or purposely inflicted
E987 Falling from high place, undetermined whether accidentally or purposely inflicted
E988 Injury by other and unspecified means, undetermined whether accidentally or purposely inflicted
E989 Late effects of injury, undetermined whether accidentally or purposely inflicted

Injury resulting from operations of war (E990–E999)

E990 Injury due to war operations by fires and conflagrations
E991 Injury due to war operations by bullets and fragments
E992 Injury due to war operations by explosion of marine weapons
E993 Injury due to war operations by other explosion
E994 Injury due to war operations by destruction of aircraft
E995 Injury due to war operations by other and unspecified forms of conventional warfare
E996 Injury due to war operations by nuclear weapons
E997 Injury due to war operations by other forms of unconventional warfare
E998 Injury due to war operations but occurring after cessation of hostilities
E999 Late effects of injury due to war operations

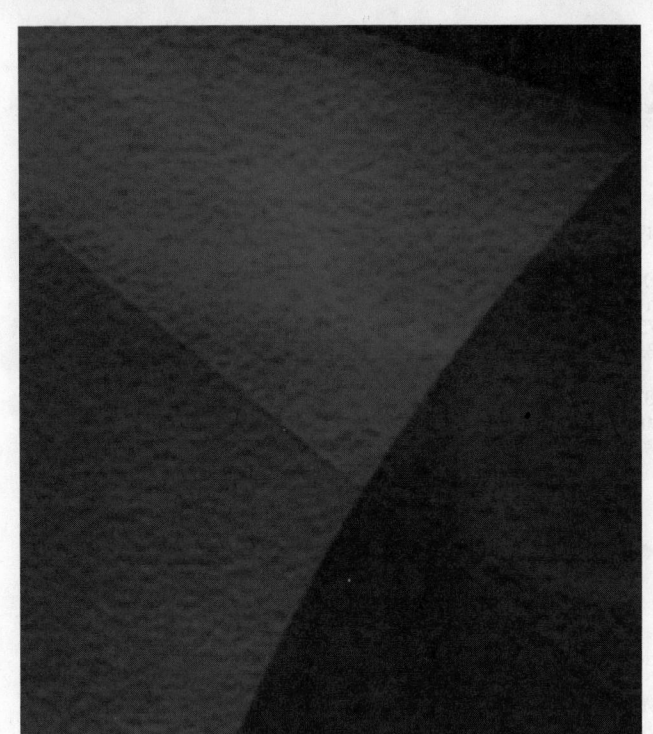

PART IV

Procedures
Volume 3

◄ New   ◄▥ Revised

Alveolectomy (interradicular) (intraseptal) (radical) (simple) (with graft) (with implant) 24.5
Alveoloplasty (with graft or implant) 24.5
Alveolotomy (apical) 24.0
Ambulatory cardiac monitoring (ACM) 89.50
Ammon operation (dacryocystotomy) 09.53
Amniocentesis (transuterine) (diagnostic) 75.1
   with intra-amniotic injection of saline 75.0
Amniography 87.81
Amnioinfusion 75.37
Amnioscopy, internal 75.31
Amniotomy 73.09
   to induce labor 73.01
Amputation (cineplastic) (closed flap) (guillotine) (kineplastic) (open) 84.91
   abdominopelvic 84.19
   above-elbow 84.07
   above-knee (AK) 84.17
   ankle (disarticulation) 84.13
      through malleoli of tibia and fibula 84.14
   arm NEC 84.00
      through
         carpals 84.03
         elbow (disarticulation) 84.06
         forearm 84.05
         humerus 84.07
         shoulder (disarticulation) 84.08
         wrist (disarticulation) 84.04
      upper 84.07
   Batch-Spittler-McFaddin (knee disarticulation) 84.16
   below-knee (BK) NEC 84.15
      conversion into above-knee amputation 84.17
   Boyd (hip disarticulation) 84.18
   Callander's (knee disarticulation) 84.16
   carpals 84.03
   cervix 67.4
   Chopart's (midtarsal) 84.12
   clitoris 71.4
   Dieffenbach (hip disarticulation) 84.18
   Dupuytren's (shoulder disarticulation) 84.08
   ear, external 18.39
   elbow (disarticulation) 84.06
   finger, except thumb 84.01
      thumb 84.02
   foot (middle) 84.12
   forearm 84.05
   forefoot 84.12
   forequarter 84.09
   Gordon-Taylor (hindquarter) 84.19
   Gritti-Stokes (knee disarticulation) 84.16
   Guyon (ankle) 84.13
   hallux 84.11
   hand 84.03
   Hey's (foot) 84.12
   hindquarter 84.19
   hip (disarticulation) 84.18
   humerus 84.07
   interscapulothoracic 84.09
   interthoracoscapular 84.09
   King-Steelquist (hindquarter) 84.19
   Kirk (thigh) 84.17
   knee (disarticulation) 84.16
   Kutler (revision of current traumatic amputation of finger) 84.01
   Larry (shoulder disarticulation) 84.08

Amputation (Continued)
   leg NEC 84.10
      above knee (AK) 84.17
      below knee (BK) 84.15
      through
         ankle (disarticulation) 84.13
         femur (AK) 84.17
         foot 84.12
         hip (disarticulation) 84.18
         tibia and fibula (BK) 84.15
   Lisfranc
      foot 84.12
      shoulder (disarticulation) 84.08
   Littlewood (forequarter) 84.09
   lower limb NEC (see also Amputation, leg) 84.10
   Mazet (knee disarticulation) 84.16
   metacarpal 84.03
   metatarsal 84.11
      head (bunionectomy) 77.59
   metatarsophalangeal (joint) 84.11
   midtarsal 84.12
   nose 21.4
   penis (circle) (complete) (flap) (partial) (radical) 64.3
   Pirogoff's (ankle amputation through malleoli of tibia and fibula) 84.14
   ray
      finger 84.01
      foot 84.11
      toe (metatarsal head) 84.11
   root (tooth) (apex) 23.73
      with root canal therapy 23.72
   shoulder (disarticulation) 84.08
   Sorondo-Ferre (hindquarter) 84.19
   S. P. Rogers (knee disarticulation) 84.16
   supracondylar, above-knee 84.17
   supramalleolar, foot 84.14
   Syme's (ankle amputation through malleoli of tibia and fibula) 84.14
   thigh 84.17
   thumb 84.02
   toe (through metatarsophalangeal joint) 84.11
   transcarpal 84.03
   transmetatarsal 84.12
   upper limb NEC (see also Amputation, arm) 84.00
   wrist (disarticulation) 84.04
Amygdalohippocampotomy 01.39
Amygdalotomy 01.39
Analysis
   cardiac rhythm device (CRT-D) (CRT-P) (AICD) (pacemaker) - see Interrogation ◀
   character 94.03
   gastric 89.39
   psychologic 94.31
   transactional
      group 94.44
      individual 94.39
Anastomosis
   abdominal artery to coronary artery 36.17
   accessory-facial nerve 04.72
   accessory-hypoglossal nerve 04.73
   anus (with formation of endorectal ileal pouch) 45.95
   aorta (descending)-pulmonary (artery) 39.0
   aorta-renal artery 39.24
   aorta-subclavian artery 39.22
   aortoceliac 39.26

Anastomosis (Continued)
   aorto(ilio)femoral 39.25
   aortomesenteric 39.26
   appendix 47.99
   arteriovenous NEC 39.29
      for renal dialysis 39.27
   artery (suture of distal to proximal end) 39.31
      with
         bypass graft 39.29
            extracranial-intracranial [EC-IC] 39.28
         excision or resection of vessel - see Arteriectomy, with anastomosis, by site
         revision 39.49
   bile ducts 51.39
   bladder NEC 57.88
      with
         isolated segment of intestine 57.87 [45.50]
            colon (sigmoid) 57.87 [45.52]
            ileum 57.87 [45.51]
            open loop of ileum 57.87 [45.51]
         to intestine 57.88
            ileum 57.87 [45.51]
   bowel - see also Anastomosis, intestine 45.90
   bronchotracheal 33.48
   bronchus 33.48
   carotid-subclavian artery 39.22
   caval-mesenteric vein 39.1
   caval-pulmonary artery 39.21
   cervicoesophageal 42.59
   colohypopharyngeal (intrathoracic) 42.55
      antesternal or antethoracic 42.65
   common bile duct 51.39
   common pulmonary trunk and left atrium (posterior wall) 35.82
   cystic bile duct 51.39
   cystocolic 57.88
   epididymis to vas deferens 63.83
   esophagocolic (intrathoracic) NEC 42.56
      with interposition 42.55
      antesternal or antethoracic NEC 42.66
         with interposition 42.65
   esophagocologastric (intrathoracic) 42.55
      antesternal or antethoracic 42.65
   esophagoduodenal (intrathoracic) NEC 42.54
      with interposition 42.53
   esophagoenteric (intrathoracic) NEC - see also Anastomosis, esophagus, to intestinal segment 42.54
      antesternal or antethoracic NEC - see also Anastomosis, esophagus, antesternal, to intestinal segment 42.64
   esophagoesophageal (intrathoracic) 42.51
      antesternal or antethoracic 42.61
   esophagogastric (intrathoracic) 42.52
      antesternal or antethoracic 42.62
   esophagus (intrapleural) (intrathoracic) (retrosternal) NEC 42.59
      with
         gastrectomy (partial) 43.5
            complete or total 43.99
         interposition (of) NEC 42.58
            colon 42.55
            jejunum 42.53
            small bowel 42.53

Anastomosis (*Continued*)
  esophagus (*Continued*)
    antesternal or antethoracic NEC
      42.69
      with
        interposition (of) NEC 42.68
          colon 42.65
          jejunal loop 42.63
          small bowel 42.63
          rubber tube 42.68
      to intestinal segment NEC 42.64
        with interposition 42.68
        colon NEC 42.66
          with interposition 42.65
        small bowel NEC 42.64
          with interposition 42.63
    to intestinal segment (intrathoracic)
      NEC 42.54
      with interposition 42.58
      antesternal or antethoracic NEC
        42.64
        with interposition 42.68
      colon (intrathoracic) NEC 42.56
        with interposition 42.55
        antesternal or antethoracic 42.66
          with interposition 42.65
      small bowel NEC 42.54
        with interposition 42.53
        antesternal or antethoracic 42.64
          with interposition 42.63
  facial-accessory nerve 04.72
  facial-hypoglossal nerve 04.71
  fallopian tube 66.73
    by reanastomosis 66.79
  gallbladder 51.35
    to
      hepatic ducts 51.31
      intestine 51.32
      pancreas 51.33
      stomach 51.34
  gastroepiploic artery to coronary artery
    36.17
  hepatic duct 51.39
  hypoglossal-accessory nerve 04.73
  hypoglossal-facial nerve 04.71
  ileal loop to bladder 57.87 [45.51]
  ileoanal 45.95
  ileorectal 45.93
  inferior vena cava and portal vein 39.1
  internal mammary artery (to)
    coronary artery (single vessel) 36.15
      double vessel 36.16
    myocardium 36.2
  intestine 45.90
    large-to-anus 45.95
    large-to-large 45.94
    large-to-rectum 45.94
    large-to-small 45.93
    small-to-anus 45.95
    small-to-large 45.93
    small-to-rectal stump 45.92
    small-to-small 45.91
  intrahepatic 51.79
  intrathoracic vessel NEC 39.23
  kidney (pelvis) 55.86
  lacrimal sac to conjunctiva 09.82
  left-to-right (systemic-pulmonary ar-
    tery) 39.0
  lymphatic (channel) (peripheral) 40.9
  mesenteric-caval 39.1
  mesocaval 39.1
  nasolacrimal 09.81
  nerve (cranial) (peripheral) NEC
    04.74

Anastomosis (*Continued*)
  nerve (*Continued*)
    accessory-facial 04.72
    accessory-hypoglossal 04.73
    hypoglossal-facial 04.71
  pancreas (duct) (to) 52.96
    bile duct 51.39
    gall bladder 51.33
    intestine 52.96
    jejunum 52.96
    stomach 52.96
  pleurothecal (with valve) 03.79
  portacaval 39.1
  portal vein to inferior vena cava 39.1
  pulmonary-aortic (Pott's) 39.0
  pulmonary artery and superior vena
    cava 39.21
  pulmonary-innominate artery (Blalock)
    39.0
  pulmonary-subclavian artery (Blalock-
    Taussig) 39.0
  pulmonary vein and azygos vein
    39.23
  pyeloileocutaneous 56.51
  pyeloureterovesical 55.86
  radial artery 36.19
  rectum, rectal NEC 48.74
    stump to small intestine 45.92
  renal (pelvis) 55.86
    vein and splenic vein 39.1
  renoportal 39.1
  salpingothecal (with valve) 03.79
  splenic to renal veins 39.1
  splenorenal (venous) 39.1
    arterial 39.26
  subarachnoid-peritoneal (with valve)
    03.71
  subarachnoid-ureteral (with valve)
    03.72
  subclavian-aortic 39.22
  superior vena cava to pulmonary ar-
    tery 39.21
  systemic-pulmonary artery 39.0
  thoracic artery (to)
    coronary artery (single) 36.15
      double 36.16
    myocardium 36.2
  ureter (to) NEC 56.79
    bladder 56.74
    colon 56.71
    ileal pouch (bladder) 56.51
    ileum 56.71
    intestine 56.71
    skin 56.61
  ureterocalyceal 55.86
  ureterocolic 56.71
  ureterovesical 56.74
  urethra (end-to-end) 58.44
  vas deferens 63.82
  veins (suture of proximal to distal end)
    (with bypass graft) 39.29
    with excision or resection of vessel -
      see Phlebectomy, with anasto-
      mosis, by site
    mesenteric to vena cava 39.1
    portal to inferior vena cava 39.1
    revision 39.49
    splenic and renal 39.1
  ventricle, ventricular (intracerebral)
    (with valve) (*see also* Shunt, ven-
    tricular) 02.2
  ventriculoatrial (with valve) 02.32
  ventriculocaval (with valve) 02.32
  ventriculomastoid (with valve) 02.31

Anastomosis (*Continued*)
  ventriculopleural (with valve) 02.33
  vesicle - *see* Anastomosis, bladder
Anderson operation (tibial lengthening)
  78.37
Anel operation (dilation of lacrimal
  duct) 09.42
Anesthesia
  acupuncture for 99.91
  cryoanalgesia nerve (cranial) (periph-
    eral) 04.2
  spinal - *omit code*
Aneurysmectomy 38.60
  with
    anastomosis 38.30
      abdominal
        artery 38.36
        vein 38.37
      aorta (arch) (ascending) (descend-
        ing) 38.34
      head and neck NEC 38.32
      intracranial NEC 38.31
      lower limb
        artery 38.38
        vein 38.39
      thoracic NEC 38.35
      upper limb (artery) (vein) 38.33
    graft replacement (interposition) 38.40
      abdominal
        aorta 38.44
        artery 38.46
        vein 38.47
      aorta (arch) (ascending) (descend-
        ing thoracic)
        abdominal 38.44
        thoracic 38.45
        thoracoabdominal 38.45
          [38.44]
      head and neck NEC 38.42
      intracranial NEC 38.41
      lower limb
        artery 38.48
        vein 38.49
      thoracic NEC 38.45
      upper limb (artery) (vein) 38.43
    abdominal
      artery 38.66
      vein 38.67
    aorta (arch) (ascending) (descending)
      38.64
    atrial, auricular 37.32
    head and neck NEC 38.62
    heart 37.32
    intracranial NEC 38.61
    lower limb
      artery 38.68
      vein 38.69
    sinus of Valsalva 35.39
    thoracic NEC 38.65
    upper limb (artery) (vein) 38.63
    ventricle (myocardium) 37.32
Aneurysmoplasty - *see* Aneurysmorrhaphy
Aneurysmorrhaphy NEC 39.52
  by or with
    anastomosis - *see* Aneurysmectomy,
      with anastomosis, by site
    clipping 39.51
    coagulation 39.52
    electrocoagulation 39.52
    endovascular graft
      abdominal aorta 39.71
      lower extremity artery(ies) 39.79
      thoracic aorta 39.79

◄ **New**   ⫷ **Revised**

Aneurysmorrhaphy NEC *(Continued)*
  by or with *(Continued)*
    endovascular graft *(Continued)*
      upper extremity artery(ies) 39.79
    excision or resection - *see also* Aneu-
      rysmectomy, by site
      with
        anastomosis - *see* Aneurysmec-
          tomy, with anastomosis, by
          site
        graft replacement - *see* Aneurys-
          mectomy, with graft re-
          placement, by site
    filipuncture 39.52
    graft replacement - *see* Aneurysmec-
      tomy, with graft replacement,
      by site
    methyl methacrylate 39.52
    suture 39.52
    wiring 39.52
    wrapping 39.52
    Matas' 39.52
Aneurysmotomy - *see* Aneurysmectomy
Angiectomy
  with
    anastomosis 38.30
      abdominal
        artery 38.36
        vein 38.37
      aorta (arch) (ascending) (descend-
        ing) 38.34
      head and neck NEC 38.32
      intracranial NEC 38.31
      lower limb
        artery 38.38
        vein 38.39
      thoracic vessel NEC 38.35
      upper limb (artery) (vein) 38.33
    graft replacement (interposition)
      38.40
      abdominal
        aorta 38.44
        artery 38.46
        vein 38.47
      aorta (arch) (ascending) (descend-
        ing thoracic)
        abdominal 38.44
        thoracic 38.45
        thoracoabdominal 38.45 *[38.44]*
      head and neck NEC 38.42
      intracranial NEC 38.41
      lower limb
        artery 38.48
        vein 38.49
      thoracic vessel NEC 38.45
      upper limb (artery) (vein) 38.43
Angiocardiography (selective) 88.50
  carbon dioxide (negative contrast)
    88.58
  combined right and left heart 88.54
  left heart (aortic valve) (atrium) (ven-
    tricle) (ventricular outflow tract)
    88.53
    combined with right heart 88.54
  right heart (atrium) (pulmonary valve)
    (ventricle) (ventricular outflow
    tract) 88.52
    combined with left heart 88.54
  vena cava (inferior) (superior) 88.51
Angiography (arterial) - *see also* Arteriography 88.40
  by radioisotope - *see* Scan, radioiso-
    tope, by site
  by ultrasound - *see* Ultrasonography,
    by site

Angiography *(Continued)*
  basilar 88.41
  brachial 88.49
  carotid (internal) 88.41
  celiac 88.47
  cerebral (posterior circulation) 88.41
  coronary NEC 88.57
  eye (fluorescein) 95.12
  femoral 88.48
  heart 88.50
  intra-abdominal NEC 88.47
  intracranial 88.41
  intrathoracic vessels NEC 88.44
  lower extremity NEC 88.48
  neck 88.41
  placenta 88.46
  pulmonary 88.43
  renal 88.45
  specified artery NEC 88.49
  transfemoral 88.48
  upper extremity NEC 88.49
  veins - *see* Phlebography
  vertebral 88.41
Angioplasty (laser) - *see also* Repair,
  blood vessel
  balloon (percutaneous transluminal)
    NEC 39.50
    coronary artery (single vessel)
      36.01
      with thrombolytic agent infusion
        36.02
      multiple vessels 36.05
  coronary 36.09
    open chest approach 36.03
    percutaneous transluminal (balloon)
      (single vessel) 36.01
      with thrombolytic agent infusion
        36.02
    multiple vessels 36.05
  percutaneous transluminal (balloon)
    (single vessel) ◄▥
    basilar 00.61 ◄▥
    carotid 00.61 ◄▥
    cerebral (intracranial) 00.62 ◄
    cerebrovascular ◄
      cerebral (intracranial) 00.62 ◄
      precerebral (extracranial) 00.61 ◄
        carotid 00.61 ◄
    coronary (balloon) (single vessel)
      36.01
      with thrombolytic agent infusion
        36.02
      multiple vessels 36.05
    femoropopliteal 39.50
    iliac 39.50
    lower extremity NOS 39.50
    mesenteric 39.50
    peripheral NEC 39.50 ◄
    precerebral (extracranial) 00.61 ◄
      carotid 00.61 ◄
    renal 39.50
    subclavian 39.50
    upper extremity NOS 39.50 ◄
    vertebral 00.61 ◄▥
  specified site NEC 39.50
    cerebrovascular ◄
      cerebral (intracranial) 00.62 ◄
      precerebral (extracranial) 00.61 ◄
    peripheral 39.50 ◄
Angiorrhaphy 39.30
  artery 39.31
  vein 39.32
Angioscopy, percutaneous 38.22
  eye (fluorescein) 95.12

Angiotomy 38.00
  abdominal
    artery 38.06
    vein 38.07
  aorta (arch) (ascending) (descending)
    38.04
  head and neck NEC 38.02
  intracranial NEC 38.01
  lower limb
    artery 38.08
    vein 38.09
  thoracic NEC 38.05
  upper limb (artery) (vein) 38.03
Angiotripsy 39.98
Ankylosis, production of - *see* Arthrodesis
Annuloplasty (heart) (posteromedial)
  35.33
Anoplasty 49.79
  with hemorrhoidectomy 49.46
Anoscopy 49.21
Antibiogram - *see* Examination, microscopic
Antiembolic filter, vena cava 38.7
Antiphobic treatment 94.39
Antrectomy
  mastoid 20.49
  maxillary 22.39
    radical 22.31
  pyloric 43.6
Antrostomy - *see* Antrotomy
Antrotomy (exploratory) (nasal sinus)
  22.2
  Caldwell-Luc (maxillary sinus) 22.39
    with removal of membrane lining
      22.31
  intranasal 22.2
    with external approach (Caldwell-
      Luc) 22.39
      radical 22.31
  maxillary (simple) 22.2
    with Caldwell-Luc approach 22.39
      with removal of membrane lining
        22.31
    external (Caldwell-Luc approach)
      22.39
      with removal of membrane lining
        22.31
    radical (with removal of membrane
      lining) 22.31
Antrum window operation - *see* Antrotomy, maxillary
Aorticopulmonary window operation
  39.59
Aortogram, aortography (abdominal)
  (retrograde) (selective) (translumbar)
  88.42
Aortoplasty (aortic valve) (gusset type)
  35.11
Aortotomy 38.04
Apexcardiogram (with ECG lead)
  89.57
Apheresis, therapeutic - *see* category
  99.7
Apicectomy
  lung 32.3
  petrous pyramid 20.59
  tooth (root) 23.73
    with root canal therapy 23.72
Apicoectomy 23.73
  with root canal therapy 23.72
Apicolysis (lung) 33.39
Apicostomy, alveolar 24.0
Aponeurectomy 83.42
  hand 82.33

Aponeurorrhaphy - *see also* Suture, tendon 83.64
  hand - *see also* Suture, tendon, hand 82.45
Aponeurotomy 83.13
  hand 82.11
Appendectomy (with drainage) 47.09
  incidental 47.19
    laparoscopic 47.11
  laparoscopic 47.01
Appendicectomy (with drainage) 47.09
  incidental 47.19
    laparoscopic 47.11
  laparoscopic 47.01
Appendicocecostomy 47.91
Appendicoenterostomy 47.91
Appendicolysis 54.59
  with appendectomy 47.09
    laparoscopic 47.01
    other 47.09
  laparoscopic 54.51
Appendicostomy 47.91
  closure 47.92
Appendicotomy 47.2
Application
  adhesion barrier substance 99.77
  anti-shock trousers 93.58
  arch bars (orthodontic) 24.7
    for immobilization (fracture) 93.55
  barrier substance, adhesion 99.77
  Barton's tongs (skull) (with synchronous skeletal traction) 02.94
  bone growth stimulator (surface) (transcutaneous) 99.86
  bone morphogenetic protein (recombinant) (rhBMP) 84.52
  Bryant's traction 93.44
    with reduction of fracture or dislocation - *see* Reduction, fracture *and* Reduction, dislocation
  Buck's traction 93.46
  caliper tongs (skull) (with synchronous skeletal traction) 02.94
  cast (fiberglass) (plaster) (plastic) NEC 93.53
    with reduction of fracture or dislocation - *see* Reduction, fracture *and* Reduction, dislocation
    spica 93.51
  cervical collar 93.52
    with reduction of fracture or dislocation - *see* Reduction, fracture *and* Reduction, dislocation
  clamp, cerebral aneurysm (Crutchfield) (Silverstone) 39.51
  croupette, croup tent 93.94
  crown (artificial) 23.41
  Crutchfield tongs (skull) (with synchronous skeletal traction) 02.94
  Dunlop's traction 93.44
    with reduction of fracture or dislocation - *see* Reduction, fracture *and* Reduction, dislocation
  elastic stockings 93.59
  electronic gaiter 93.59
  external fixation device (bone) 78.10
    carpal, metacarpal 78.14
    clavicle 78.11
    femur 78.15
    fibula 78.17
    humerus 78.12
    patella 78.16
    pelvic 78.19
    phalanges (foot) (hand) 78.19

Application (*Continued*)
  external fixation device (*Continued*)
    radius 78.13
    scapula 78.11
    specified site NEC 78.19
    tarsal, metatarsal 78.18
    thorax (ribs) (sternum) 78.11
    tibia 78.17
    ulna 78.13
    vertebrae 78.19
  forceps, with delivery - *see* Delivery, forceps
  graft - *see* Graft
  gravity (G-) suit 93.59
  intermittent pressure device 93.59
  Jewett extension brace 93.59
  Jobst pumping unit (reduction of edema) 93.59
  Lyman Smith traction 93.44
    with reduction of fracture or dislocation - *see* Reduction, fracture *and* Reduction, dislocation
  MAST (military anti-shock trousers) 93.58
  Minerva jacket 93.52
  minifixator device (bone) - *see* category 78.1
  neck support (molded) 93.52
  obturator (orthodontic) 24.7
  orthodontic appliance (obturator) (wiring) 24.7
  pelvic sling 93.44
    with reduction of fracture or dislocation - *see* Reduction, fracture *and* Reduction, dislocation
  peridontal splint (orthodontic) 24.7
  plaster jacket 93.51
    Minerva 93.52
  pressure
    dressing (bandage) (Gibney) (Robert Jones') (Shanz) 93.56
    trousers (anti-shock) (MAST) 93.58
  prosthesis for missing ear 18.71
  Russell's traction 93.44
    with reduction of fracture or dislocation - *see* Reduction, fracture *and* Reduction, dislocation
  splint, for immobilization (plaster) (pneumatic) (tray) 93.54
    with fracture reduction - *see* Reduction, fracture
  stereotactic head frame 93.59
  substance, adhesion barrier 99.77
  Thomas' collar 93.52
    with reduction of fracture or dislocation - *see* Reduction, fracture *and* Reduction, dislocation
  traction
    with reduction of fracture or dislocation - *see* Reduction, fracture *and* Reduction, dislocation
    adhesive tape (skin) 93.46
    boot 93.46
    Bryant's 93.44
    Buck's 93.46
    Cotrel's 93.42
    Dunlop's 93.44
    gallows 93.46
    Lyman Smith 93.44
    Russell's 93.44
    skeletal NEC 93.44
      intermittent 93.43
    skin, limbs NEC 93.46

Application (*Continued*)
  traction (*Continued*)
    spinal NEC 93.42
      with skull device (halo) (caliper) (Crutchfield) (Gardner-Wells) (Vinke) (tongs) 93.41
        with synchronous insertion 02.94
    Thomas' splint 93.45
  Unna's paste boot 93.53
  vasopneumatic device 93.58
  Velpeau dressing 93.59
  Vinke tongs (skull) (with synchronous skeletal traction) 02.94
  wound dressing NEC 93.57
Aquapheresis 99.78 ◀
Arc lamp - *see* Photocoagulation
Arrest
  bone growth (epiphyseal) 78.20
    by stapling - *see* Stapling, epiphyseal plate
    femur 78.25
    fibula 78.27
    humerus 78.22
    radius 78.23
    tibia 78.27
    ulna 78.23
  cardiac, induced (anoxic) (circulatory) 39.63
  circulatory, induced (anoxic) 39.63
  hemorrhage - *see* Control, hemorrhage
Arslan operation (fenestration of inner ear) 20.61
Arteriectomy 38.60
  with
    anastomosis 38.30
      abdominal 38.36
      aorta (arch) (ascending) (descending) 38.34
      head and neck NEC 38.32
      intracranial NEC 38.31
      lower limb 38.38
      thoracic NEC 38.35
      upper limb 38.33
    graft replacement (interposition) 38.40
      abdominal 38.36
        aorta 38.44
      aorta (arch) (ascending) (descending thoracic)
        abdominal 38.44
        thoracic 38.45
        thoracoabdominal 38.45 [38.44]
      head and neck NEC 38.42
      intracranial NEC 38.41
      lower limb 38.48
      thoracic NEC 38.45
      upper limb 38.43
  abdominal 38.66
  aorta (arch) (ascending) (descending) 38.64
  head and neck NEC 38.62
  intracranial NEC 38.61
  lower-limb 38.68
  thoracic NEC 38.65
  upper limb 38.63
Arteriography (contrast) (fluoroscopic) (retrograde) 88.40
  by
    radioisotope - *see* Scan, radioisotope
    ultrasound (Doppler) - *see* Ultrasonography, by site
  aorta (arch) (ascending) (descending) 88.42
  basilar 88.41
  brachial 88.49

Arteriography *(Continued)*
  carotid (internal) 88.41
  cerebral (posterior circulation) 88.41
  coronary (direct) (selective) NEC 88.57
    double catheter technique (Judkins)
      (Ricketts and Abrams) 88.56
    single catheter technique (Sones)
      88.55
  Doppler (ultrasonic) - *see* Ultrasonography, by site
  femoral 88.48
  head and neck 88.41
  intra-abdominal NEC 88.47
  intrathoracic NEC 88.44
  lower extremity 88.48
  placenta 88.46
  pulmonary 88.43
  radioisotope - *see* Scan, radioisotope
  renal 88.45
  specified site NEC 88.49
  superior mesenteric artery 88.47
  transfemoral 88.48
  ultrasound - *see* Ultrasonography, by site
  upper extremity 88.49
Arterioplasty - *see* Repair, artery
Arteriorrhaphy 39.31
Arteriotomy 38.00
  abdominal 38.06
  aorta (arch) (ascending) (descending)
    38.04
  head and neck NEC 38.02
  intracranial NEC 38.01
  lower limb 38.08
  thoracic NEC 38.05
  upper limb 38.03
Arteriovenostomy 39.29
  for renal dialysis 39.27
Arthrectomy 80.90
  ankle 80.97
  elbow 80.92
  foot and toe 80.98
  hand and finger 80.94
  hip 80.95
  intervertebral disc - *see* category 80.5
  knee 80.96
  semilunar cartilage 80.6
  shoulder 80.91
  specified site NEC 80.99
  spine NEC 80.99
  wrist 80.93
Arthrocentesis 81.91
  for arthrography - *see* Arthrogram
Arthrodesis (compression) (extra-articular) (intra-articular) (with bone graft)
    (with fixation device) 81.20
  ankle 81.11
  carporadial 81.25
  cricoarytenoid 31.69
  elbow 81.24
  finger 81.28
  foot NEC 81.17
  hip 81.21
  interphalangeal
    finger 81.28
    toe NEC 77.58
      claw toe repair 77.57
      hammer toe repair 77.56
  ischiofemoral 81.21
  knee 81.22
  lumbosacral, lumbar NEC 81.08
    anterior (interbody), anterolateral
      technique 81.06
    lateral transverse process technique
      81.07

Arthrodesis *(Continued)*
  lumbosacral, lumbar NEC *(Continued)*
    posterior (interbody), posterolateral
      technique 81.08
  McKeever (metatarsophalangeal) 81.16
  metacarpocarpal 81.26
  metacarpophalangeal 81.27
  metatarsophalangeal 81.16
  midtarsal 81.14
  plantar 81.11
  sacroiliac 81.08
  shoulder 81.23
  specified joint NEC 81.29
  spinal - *see also* Fusion, spinal 81.00
  subtalar 81.13
  tarsometatarsal 81.15
  tibiotalar 81.11
  toe NEC 77.58
    claw toe repair 77.57
    hammer toe repair 77.56
  triple 81.12
  wrist 81.26
Arthroendoscopy - *see* Arthroscopy
Arthrogram, arthrography 88.32
  temporomandibular 87.13
Arthrolysis 93.26
Arthroplasty (with fixation device) (with
    traction) 81.96
  ankle 81.49
  carpals 81.75
    with prosthetic implant 81.74
  carpocarpal, carpometacarpal 81.75
    with prosthetic implant 81.74
  Carroll and Taber (proximal interphalangeal joint) 81.72
  cup (partial hip) 81.52
  Curtis (interphalangeal joint) 81.72
  elbow 81.85
    with prosthetic replacement (total)
      81.84
  femoral head NEC 81.40
    with prosthetic implant 81.52
  finger(s) 81.72
    with prosthetic implant 81.71
  foot (metatarsal) with joint replacement 81.57
  Fowler (metacarpophalangeal joint)
    81.72
  hand (metacarpophalangeal) (interphalangeal) 81.72
    with prosthetic implant 81.71
  hip (with bone graft) 81.40
    cup (partial hip) 81.52
    femoral head NEC 81.40
      with prosthetic implant 81.52
        with total replacement 81.51
    partial replacement 81.52
    total replacement 81.51
  interphalangeal joint 81.72
    with prosthetic implant 81.71
  Kessler (carpometacarpal joint) 81.74
  knee (*see also* Repair, knee) 81.47
    prosthetic replacement (bicompartmental) (hemijoint) (partial) (total) (tricompartmental) (unicompartmental) 81.54
    revision 81.55
  metacarpophalangeal joint 81.72
    with prosthetic implant 81.71
  shoulder 81.83
    prosthetic replacement (partial) 81.81
      total 81.80
    for recurrent dislocation 81.82
  temporomandibular 76.5

Arthroplasty *(Continued)*
  toe NEC 77.58
    with prosthetic replacement 81.57
    for hallux valgus repair 77.59
  wrist 81.75
    with prosthetic implant 81.74
      total replacement 81.73
Arthroscopy 80.20
  ankle 80.27
  elbow 80.22
  finger 80.24
  foot 80.28
  hand 80.24
  hip 80.25
  knee 80.26
  shoulder 80.21
  specified site NEC 80.29
  toe 80.28
  wrist 80.23
Arthrostomy - *see also* Arthrotomy 80.10
Arthrotomy 80.10
  as operative approach - *omit code*
  with
    arthrography - *see* Arthrogram
    arthroscopy - *see* Arthroscopy
    injection of drug 81.92
    removal of prosthesis (*see also* Removal, prosthesis, joint structures) 80.00
  ankle 80.17
  elbow 80.12
  foot and toe 80.18
  hand and finger 80.14
  hip 80.15
  knee 80.16
  shoulder 80.11
  specified site NEC 80.19
  spine 80.19
  wrist 80.13
Artificial
  insemination 69.92
  kidney 39.95
  rupture of membranes 73.09
Arytenoidectomy 30.29
Arytenoidopexy 31.69
Asai operation (larynx) 31.75
Aspiration
  abscess - *see* Aspiration, by site
  anterior chamber, eye (therapeutic) 12.91
    diagnostic 12.21
  aqueous (eye) (humor) (therapeutic)
    12.91
    diagnostic 12.21
  ascites 54.91
  Bartholin's gland (cyst) (percutaneous)
    71.21
  biopsy - *see* Biopsy, by site
  bladder (catheter) 57.0
    percutaneous (needle) 57.11
  bone marrow (for biopsy) 41.31
    from donor for transplant 41.91
    stem cell 99.79
  branchial cleft cyst 29.0
  breast 85.91
  bronchus 96.05
    with lavage 96.56
  bursa (percutaneous) 83.94
    hand 82.92
  calculus, bladder 57.0
  cataract 13.3
    with
      phacoemulsification 13.41
      phacofragmentation 13.43
        posterior route 13.42

Aspiration *(Continued)*
chest 34.91
cisternal 01.01
cranial (puncture) 01.09
craniobuccal pouch 07.72
craniopharyngioma 07.72
cul-de-sac (abscess) 70.0
curettage, uterus 69.59
after abortion or delivery 69.52
diagnostic 69.59
to terminate pregnancy 69.51
cyst - *see* Aspiration, by site
diverticulum, pharynx 29.0
endotracheal 96.04
with lavage 96.56
extradural 01.09
eye (anterior chamber) (therapeutic) 12.91
diagnostic 12.21
fallopian tube 66.91
fascia 83.95
hand 82.93
gallbladder (percutaneous) 51.01
hematoma - *see also* Aspiration, by site
obstetrical 75.92
incisional 75.91
hydrocele, tunica vaginalis 61.91
hygroma - *see* Aspiration, by site
hyphema 12.91
hypophysis 07.72
intracranial space (epidural) (extra-dural) (subarachnoid) (subdural) (ventricular) 01.09
through previously implanted catheter or reservoir (Ommaya) (Rickham) 01.02
joint 81.91
for arthrography - *see* Arthrogram
kidney (cyst) (pelvis) (percutaneous) (therapeutic) 55.92
diagnostic 55.23
liver (percutaneous) 50.91
lung (percutaneous) (puncture) (needle) (trocar) 33.93
middle ear 20.09
with intubation 20.01
muscle 83.95
hand 82.93
nail 86.01
nasal sinus 22.00
by puncture 22.01
through natural ostium 22.02
nasotracheal 96.04
with lavage 96.56
orbit, diagnostic 16.22
ovary 65.91
percutaneous - *see* Aspiration, by site
pericardium (wound) 37.0
pituitary gland 07.72
pleural cavity 34.91
prostate (percutaneous) 60.91
Rathke's pouch 07.72

Aspiration *(Continued)*
seminal vesicles 60.71
seroma - *see* Aspiration, by site
skin 86.01
soft tissue NEC 83.95
hand 82.93
spermatocele 63.91
spinal (puncture) 03.31
spleen (cyst) 41.1
stem cell 99.79
subarachnoid space (cerebral) 01.09
subcutaneous tissue 86.01
subdural space (cerebral) 01.09
tendon 83.95
hand 82.93
testis 62.91
thymus 07.92
thyroid (field) (gland) 06.01
postoperative 06.02
trachea 96.04
with lavage 96.56
percutaneous 31.99
tunica vaginalis (hydrocele) (percutaneous) 61.91
vitreous (and replacement) 14.72
diagnostic 14.11
Assessment
fitness to testify 94.11
mental status 94.11
nutritional status 89.39
personality 94.03
temperament 94.02
vocational 93.85
Assistance
cardiac - *see also* Resuscitation, cardiac
extracorporeal circulation 39.61
endotracheal respiratory - *see* category 96.7
hepatic, extracorporeal 50.92
respiratory (endotracheal) (mechanical) - *see* Ventilation, mechanical
Astragalectomy 77.98
Asymmetrogammagram - *see* Scan, radioisotope
Atherectomy
cerebrovascular - *see* angioplasty ◀
coronary - *see* Angioplasty
peripheral 39.50
Atriocommissuropexy (mitral valve) 35.12
Atrioplasty NEC 37.99
combined with repair of valvular and ventricular septal defects - *see* Repair, endocardial cushion defect
septum (heart) NEC 35.71
Atrioseptopexy - *see also* Repair, atrial septal defect 35.71
Atrioseptoplasty - *see also* Repair, atrial septal defect 35.71
Atrioseptostomy (balloon) 35.41
Atriotomy 37.11

Atrioventriculostomy (cerebral-heart) 02.32
Attachment
eye muscle
orbicularis oculi to eyebrow 08.36
rectus to frontalis 15.9
pedicle (flap) graft 86.74
hand 86.73
lip 27.57
mouth 27.57
pharyngeal flap (for cleft palate repair) 27.62
secondary or subsequent 27.63
retina - *see* Reattachment, retina
Atticoantrostomy (ear) 20.49
Atticoantrotomy (ear) 20.49
Atticotomy (ear) 20.23
Audiometry (Bekesy 5-tone) (impedance) (stapedial reflex response) (subjective) 95.41
Augmentation
bladder 57.87
breast - *see* Mammoplasty, augmentation
buttock ("fanny-lift") 86.89
chin 76.68
genioplasty 76.68
mammoplasty - *see* Mammoplasty, augmentation
outflow tract (pulmonary valve) (gusset type) 35.26
in total repair of tetralogy of Fallot 35.81
vocal cord(s) 31.0
Auriculectomy 18.39
Autograft - *see* Graft
Autologous - *see* Blood, transfusion
Autopsy 89.8
Autotransfusion (whole blood) 99.02 - *see* Blood, transfusion
Autotransplant, autotransplantation - *see also* Reimplantation
adrenal tissue (heterotopic) (orthotopic) 07.45
kidney 55.61
lung - *see* Transplant, transplantation, lung
ovary 65.72
laparoscopic 65.75
pancreatic tissue 52.81
parathyroid tissue (heterotopic) (orthotopic) 06.95
thyroid tissue (heterotopic) (orthotopic) 06.94
tooth 23.5
Avulsion, nerve (cranial) (peripheral) NEC 04.07
acoustic 04.01
phrenic 33.31
sympathetic 05.29
Azygography 88.63

◀ New ◀▬ Revised

B

Bacterial smear - *see* Examination, microscopic
Baffes operation (interatrial transposition of venous return) 35.91
Baffle, atrial or interatrial 35.91
Balanoplasty 64.69
Baldy-Webster operation (uterine suspension) 69.22
Ballistocardiography 89.59
Balloon
   angioplasty - *see* Angioplasty, balloon
   pump, intra-aortic 37.61
   systostomy (atrial) 35.41
Ball operation
   herniorrhaphy - *see* Repair, hernia, inguinal
   undercutting 49.02
Bandage 93.37
   elastic 93.56
Banding
   gastric 44.68
      vertical 44.68
   pulmonary artery 38.85
Bankhart operation (capsular repair into glenoid, for shoulder dislocation) 81.82
Bardenheurer operation (ligation of innominate artery) 38.85
Barium swallow 87.61
Barkan operation (goniotomy) 12.52
   with goniopuncture 12.53
Barr operation (transfer of tibialis posterior tendon) 83.75
Barsky operation (closure of cleft hand) 82.82
Basal metabolic rate 89.39
Basiotripsy 73.8
Bassett operation (vulvectomy with inguinal lymph node dissection) 71.5 *[40.3]*
Bassini operation - *see* Repair, hernia, inguinal
Batch-Spittler-McFaddin operation (knee disarticulation) 84.16
Batista operation (partial ventriculectomy) (ventricular reduction) (ventricular remodeling) 37.35
Beck operation
   aorta-coronary sinus shunt 36.39
   epicardial poudrage 36.39
Beck-Jianu operation (permanent gastrostomy) 43.19
Behavior modification 94.33
Bell-Beuttner operation (subtotal abdominal hysterectomy) 68.39
   laparoscopic 68.31
Belsey operation (esophagogastric sphincter) 44.65
Benenenti operation (rotation of bulbous urethra) 58.49
Berke operation (levator resection of eyelid) 08.33
Bicuspidization of heart valve 35.10
   aortic 35.11
   mitral 35.12
Bicycle dynamometer 93.01
Biesenberger operation (size reduction of breast, bilateral) 85.32
   unilateral 85.31
Bifurcation, bone - *see also* Osteotomy 77.30
Bigelow operation (litholapaxy) 57.0
Bililite therapy (ultraviolet) 99.82

Billroth I operation (partial gastrectomy with gastroduodenostomy) 43.6
Billroth II operation (partial gastrectomy with gastrojejunostomy) 43.7
Binnie operation (hepatopexy) 50.69
Biofeedback, psychotherapy 94.39
Biopsy
   abdominal wall 54.22
   adenoid 28.11
   adrenal gland NEC 07.11
      closed 07.11
      open 07.12
      percutaneous (aspiration) (needle) 07.11
   alveolus 24.12
   anus 49.23
   appendix 45.26
   artery (any site) 38.21
   aspiration - *see* Biopsy, by site
   bile ducts 51.14
      closed (endoscopic) 51.14
      open 51.13
      percutaneous (needle) 51.12
   bladder 57.33
      closed 57.33
      open 57.34
      transurethral 57.33
   blood vessel (any site) 38.21
   bone 77.40
      carpal, metacarpal 77.44
      clavicle 77.41
      facial 76.11
      femur 77.45
      fibula 77.47
      humerus 77.42
      marrow 41.31
      patella 77.46
      pelvic 77.49
      phalanges (foot) (hand) 77.49
      radius 77.43
      scapula 77.41
      specified site NEC 77.49
      tarsal, metatarsal 77.48
      thorax (ribs) (sternum) 77.41
      tibia 77.47
      ulna 77.43
      vertebrae 77.49
   bowel - *see* Biopsy, intestine
   brain NEC 01.13
      closed 01.13
      open 01.14
      percutaneous (needle) 01.13
   breast 85.11
      blind 85.11
      closed 85.11
      open 85.12
      percutaneous (needle) (Vimm-Silverman) 85.11
   bronchus NEC 33.24
      brush 33.24
      closed (endoscopic) 33.24
      open 33.25
      washings 33.24
   bursa 83.21
   cardioesophageal (junction) 44.14
      closed (endoscopic) 44.14
      open 44.14
   cecum 45.25
      brush 45.25
      closed (endoscopic) 45.25
      open 45.26
   cerebral meninges NEC 01.11
      closed 01.11
      open 01.12
      percutaneous (needle) 01.11
   cervix (punch) 67.12

Biopsy *(Continued)*
   cervix *(Continued)*
      conization (sharp) 67.2
   chest wall 34.23
   clitoris 71.11
   colon 45.25
      brush 45.25
      closed (endoscopic) 45.25
      open 45.26
   conjunctiva 10.21
   cornea 11.22
   cul-de-sac 70.23
   diaphragm 34.27
   duodenum 45.14
      brush 45.14
      closed (endoscopic) 45.14
      open 45.15
   ear (external) 18.12
      middle or inner 20.32
   endocervix 67.11
   endometrium NEC 68.16
      by
         aspiration curettage 69.59
         dilation and curettage 69.09
      closed (endoscopic) 68.16
      open 68.13
   epididymis 63.01
   esophagus 42.24
      closed (endoscopic) 42.24
      open 42.25
   extraocular muscle or tendon 15.01
   eye 16.23
      muscle (oblique) (rectus) 15.01
   eyelid 08.11
   fallopian tube 66.11
   fascia 83.21
   fetus 75.33
   gallbladder 51.12
      closed (endoscopic) 51.14
      open 51.13
      percutaneous (needle) 51.12
   ganglion (cranial) (peripheral) NEC 04.11
      closed 04.11
      open 04.12
      percutaneous (needle) 04.11
      sympathetic nerve 05.11
   gum 24.11
   heart 37.25
   hypophysis - *see also* Biopsy, pituitary gland 07.15
   ileum 45.14
      brush 45.14
      closed (endoscopic) 45.14
      open 45.15
   intestine NEC 45.27
      large 45.25
         brush 45.25
         closed (endoscopic) 45.25
         open 45.26
      small 45.14
         brush 45.14
         closed (endoscopic) 45.14
         open 45.15
   intra-abdominal mass 54.24
      closed 54.24
      percutaneous (needle) 54.24
   iris 12.22
   jejunum 45.14
      brush 45.14
      closed (endoscopic) 45.14
      open 45.15
   joint structure (aspiration) 80.30
      ankle 80.37

Biopsy *(Continued)*
  joint structure *(Continued)*
    elbow 80.32
    foot and toe 80.38
    hand and finger 80.34
    hip 80.35
    knee 80.36
    shoulder 80.31
    specified site NEC 80.39
    spine 80.39
    wrist 80.33
  kidney 55.23
    closed 55.23
    open 55.24
    percutaneous (aspiration) (needle) 55.23
  labia 71.11
  lacrimal
    gland 09.11
    sac 09.12
  larynx 31.43
    brush 31.43
    closed (endoscopic) 31.43
    open 31.45
  lip 27.23
  liver 50.11
    closed 50.11
    laparoscopic 50.19
    open 50.12
    percutaneous (aspiration) (needle) 50.11
  lung NEC 33.27
    brush 33.24
    closed (percutaneous) (needle) 33.26
      brush 33.24
      endoscopic 33.27
        brush 33.24
    endoscopic 33.27
      brush 33.24
    open 33.28
    transbronchial 33.27
  lymphatic structure (channel) (node) (vessel) 40.11
  mediastinum NEC 34.25
    closed 34.25
    open 34.26
    percutaneous (needle) 34.25
  meninges (cerebral) NEC 01.11
    closed 01.11
    open 01.12
    percutaneous (needle) 01.11
    spinal 03.32
  mesentery 54.23
  mouth NEC 27.24
  muscle 83.21
    extraocular 15.01
    ocular 15.01
  nasopharynx 29.12
  nerve (cranial) (peripheral) NEC 04.11
    closed 04.11
    open 04.12
    percutaneous (needle) 04.11
    sympathetic 05.11
  nose, nasal 21.22
    sinus 22.11
      closed (endoscopic) (needle) 22.11
      open 22.12
  ocular muscle or tendon 15.01
  omentum
    closed 54.24
    open 54.23
    percutaneous (needle) 54.24
  orbit 16.23
    by aspiration 16.22
  ovary 65.12

Biopsy *(Continued)*
  ovary *(Continued)*
    by aspiration 65.11
    laparoscopic 65.13
  palate (bony) 27.21
    soft 27.22
  pancreas 52.11
    closed (endoscopic) 52.11
    open 52.12
    percutaneous (aspiration) (needle) 52.11
  pancreatic duct 52.14
    closed (endoscopic) 52.14
  parathyroid gland 06.13
  penis 64.11
  perianal tissue 49.22
  pericardium 37.24
  periprostatic 60.15
  perirectal tissue 48.26
  perirenal tissue 59.21
  peritoneal implant
    closed 54.24
    open 54.23
    percutaneous (needle) 54.24
  peritoneum
    closed 54.24
    open 54.23
    percutaneous (needle) 54.24
  periurethral tissue 58.24
  perivesical tissue 59.21
  pharynx, pharyngeal 29.12
  pineal gland 07.17
  pituitary gland 07.15
    transfrontal approach 07.13
    transsphenoidal approach 07.14
  pleura, pleural 34.24
  prostate NEC 60.11
    closed (transurethral) 60.11
    open 60.12
    percutaneous (needle) 60.11
    transrectal 60.11
  rectum 48.24
    brush 48.24
    closed (endoscopic) 48.24
    open 48.25
  retroperitoneal tissue 54.24
  salivary gland or duct 26.11
    closed (needle) 26.11
    open 26.12
  scrotum 61.11
  seminal vesicle NEC 60.13
    closed 60.13
    open 60.14
    percutaneous (needle) 60.13
  sigmoid colon 45.25
    brush 45.25
    closed (endoscopic) 45.25
    open 45.26
  sinus, nasal 22.11
    closed (endoscopic) (needle) 22.11
    open 22.12
  skin (punch) 86.11
  skull 01.15
  soft palate 27.22
  soft tissue NEC 83.21
  spermatic cord 63.01
  sphincter of Oddi 51.14
    closed (endoscopic) 51.14
    open 51.13
  spinal cord (meninges) 03.32
  spleen 41.32
    closed 41.32
    open 41.33

Biopsy *(Continued)*
  spleen *(Continued)*
    percutaneous (aspiration) (needle) 41.32
  stomach 44.14
    brush 44.14
    closed (endoscopic) 44.14
    open 44.15
  subcutaneous tissue (punch) 86.11
  supraglottic mass 29.12
  sympathetic nerve 05.11
  tendon 83.21
    extraocular 15.01
    ocular 15.01
  testis NEC 62.11
    closed 62.11
    open 62.12
    percutaneous (needle) 62.11
  thymus 07.16
  thyroid gland NEC 06.11
    closed 06.11
    open 06.12
    percutaneous (aspiration) (needle) 06.11
      tongue 25.01
      closed (needle) 25.01
      open 25.02
  tonsil 28.11
  trachea 31.44
    brush 31.44
    closed (endoscopic) 31.44
    open 31.45
  tunica vaginalis 61.11
  umbilicus 54.22
  ureter 56.33
    closed (percutaneous) 56.32
      endoscopic 56.33
    open 56.34
    transurethral 56.33
  urethra 58.23
  uterus, uterine (endometrial) 68.16
    by
      aspiration curettage 69.59
      dilation and curettage 69.09
    closed (endoscopic) 68.16
    ligaments 68.15
      closed (endoscopic) 68.15
      open 68.14
    open 68.13
  uvula 27.22
  vagina 70.24
  vas deferens 63.01
  vein (any site) 38.21
  vulva 71.11
Bischoff operation (ureteroneocystostomy) 56.74
Bisection - *see also* Excision
  hysterectomy 68.39
    laparoscopic 68.31
  ovary 65.29
    laparoscopic 65.25
  stapes foot plate 19.19
    with incus replacement 19.11
Bischoff operation (spinal myelotomy) 03.29
Blalock operation (systemic-pulmonary anastomosis) 39.0
Blalock-Hanlon operation (creation of atrial septal defect) 35.42
Blalock-Taussig operation (subclavian-pulmonary anastomosis) 39.0
Blascovic operation (resection and advancement of levator palpebrae superioris) 08.33
Blepharectomy 08.20

◀ **New**   ◀◁◁ **Revised**

ICD-9-CM

Vol. 3

Bypass (*Continued*)
vascular NEC (*Continued*)
aortic-superior mesenteric 39.26
aortocarotid 39.22
aortoceliac 39.26
aortocoronary - *see also* Bypass,
aortocoronary 36.10
aortofemoral 39.25
aortofemoral-popliteal 39.25
aortoiliac 39.25
to popliteal 39.25
aortoiliofemoral 39.25
aortomesenteric 39.26
aortopopliteal 39.25
aortorenal 39.24
aortosubclavian 39.22
axillary-brachial 39.29
axillary-femoral (superficial) 39.29
axillofemoral (superficial) 39.29

Bypass (*Continued*)
vascular NEC (*Continued*)
carotid-cerebral 39.28
carotid-vertebral 39.28
carotid to subclavian artery
39.22
common hepatic-common iliac-renal
39.26
coronary - *see also* Bypass, aortocoronary 36.10
extracranial-intracranial [EC-IC]
39.28
femoral-femoral 39.29
femoroperoneal 39.29
femoropopliteal (reversed saphenous
vein) (saphenous) 39.29
femorotibial (anterior) (posterior)
39.29
iliofemoral 39.25

Bypass (*Continued*)
vascular NEC (*Continued*)
ilioiliac 39.26
internal mammary-coronary
artery (single) 36.15
double vessel 36.16
intra-abdominal (arterial) NEC
39.26
venous NEC 39.1
intrathoracic NEC 39.23
peripheral artery NEC 39.29
popliteal-tibial 39.29
renal artery 39.24
splenorenal (venous) 39.1
arterial 39.26
subclavian-axillary 39.29
subclavian-carotid 39.22
subclavian-subclavian 39.22
Y graft to renal arteries 39.24

◀ **New**   ◀**▮** **Revised**

C

Caldwell operation (sulcus extension) 24.91
Caldwell-Luc operation (maxillary sinusotomy) 22.39
with removal of membrane lining 22.31
Calibration, urethra 89.29
Calicectomy (renal) 55.4
Callander operation (knee disarticulation) 84.16
Caloric test, vestibular function 95.44
Calycectomy (renal) 55.4
Calyco-ileoneocystostomy 55.86
Calycotomy (renal) 55.11
Campbell operation
bone block, ankle 81.11
fasciotomy (iliac crest) 83.14
reconstruction of anterior cruciate ligament 81.45
Campimetry 95.05
Canaliculodacryocystorhinostomy 09.81
Canaliculoplasty 09.73
Canaliculorhinostomy 09.81
Canaloplasty, external auditory meatus 18.6
Cannulation - *see also* Insertion, catheter
ampulla of Vater 51.99
antrum 22.01
arteriovenous 39.93
artery 38.91
caval-mesenteric vein 39.1
cisterna chyli 40.61
Eustachian tube 20.8
lacrimal apparatus 09.42
lymphatic duct, left (thoracic) 40.61
nasal sinus (by puncture) 22.01
through natural ostium 22.02
pancreatic duct 52.92
by retrograde endoscopy (ERP) 52.93
renoportal 39.1
sinus (nasal) (by puncture) 22.01
through natural ostium 22.02
splenorenal (venous) 39.1
arterial 39.26
thoracic duct (cervical approach) (thoracic approach) 40.61
Cannulization - *see* Cannulation
Canthocystostomy 09.82
Canthoplasty 08.59
Canthorrhaphy 08.52
division or severing 08.02
Canthotomy 08.51
Capsulectomy
joint - *see also* Arthrectomy 80.90
kidney 55.91
lens 13.65
with extraction of lens 13.51
ovary 65.29
laparoscopic 65.25
Capsulo-iridectomy 13.65
Capsuloplasty - *see* Arthroplasty
Capsulorrhaphy 81.96
with arthroplasty - *see* Arthroplasty
ankle 81.94
foot 81.94
lower extremity NEC 81.95
upper extremity 81.93
Capsulotomy
joint - *see also* Division, joint capsule 80.40
for claw toe repair 77.57
lens 13.64

Capsulotomy (*Continued*)
lens (*Continued*)
with
discission of lens 13.2
removal of foreign body 13.02
by magnet extraction 13.01
Cardiac
mapping 37.27
massage (external) (closed chest) 99.63
open chest 37.91
retraining 93.36
Cardiectomy (stomach) 43.5
Cardiocentesis 37.0
Cardiography - *see also* Angiocardiography 88.50
Cardiolysis 37.10
Cardiomyopexy 36.39
Cardiomyotomy 42.7
Cardio-omentopexy 36.39
Cardiopericardiopexy 36.39
Cardioplasty (stomach and esophagus) 44.65
stomach alone 44.66
laparoscopic 44.67 ◄
Cardioplegia 39.63
Cardiopneumopexy 36.39
Cardiorrhaphy 37.4
Cardioschisis 37.12
Cardiosplenopexy 36.39
Cardiotomy (exploratory) 37.11
Cardiovalvulotomy - *see* Valvulotomy, heart
Cardioversion (external) 99.62
atrial 99.61
Carotid pulse tracing with ECG lead 89.56
Carpectomy (partial) 77.84
total 77.94
Carroll and Taber arthroplasty (proximal interphalangeal joint) 81.72
Casting (for immobilization) NEC 93.53
with fracture-reduction - *see* Reduction, fracture
Castration
female (oophorectomy, bilateral) 65.51
laparoscopic 65.53
male 62.41
C.A.T. (computerized axial tomography) - *see also* Scan, C.A.T. 88.38
Catheterization - *see also* Insertion, catheter
arteriovenous 39.93
artery 38.91
bladder, indwelling 57.94
percutaneous (cystostomy) 57.17
suprapubic NEC 57.18
bronchus 96.05
with lavage 96.56
cardiac (right) 37.21
combined left and right 37.23
left 37.22
combined with right heart 37.23
right 37.21
combined with left heart 37.23
central venous NEC 38.93
peripherally inserted central catheter (PICC) 38.93
chest 34.04
revision (with lysis of adhesions) 34.04
Eustachian tube 20.8
heart (right) 37.21
combined left and right 37.23
left 37.22
combined with right heart 37.23
right 37.21
combined with left heart 37.23

Catheterization (*Continued*)
hepatic vein 38.93
inferior vena cava 38.93
intercostal space (with water seal), for drainage 34.04
revision (with lysis of adhesions) 34.04
lacrimonasal duct 09.44
laryngeal 96.05
nasolacrimal duct 09.44
pancreatic cyst 52.01
renal vein 38.93
Swan-Ganz (pulmonary) 89.64
transtracheal for oxygenation 31.99
umbilical vein 38.92
ureter (to kidney) 59.8
for retrograde pyelogram 87.74
urethra, indwelling 57.94
vein NEC 38.93
for renal dialysis 38.95
Cattell operation (herniorrhaphy) 53.51
Cauterization - *see also* Destruction, lesion, by site
anus NEC 49.39
endoscopic 49.31
Bartholin's gland 71.24
broad ligament 69.19
bronchus 32.09
endoscopic 32.01
canaliculi 09.73
cervix 67.32
chalazion 08.25
choroid plexus 02.14
conjunctiva 10.33
lesion 10.32
cornea (fistula) (ulcer) 11.42
ear, external 18.29
endometrial implant - *see* Excision, lesion, by site
entropion 08.41
esophagus 42.39
endoscopic 42.33
eyelid 08.25
for entropion or ectropion 08.41
fallopian tube 66.61
by endoscopy (hysteroscopy) (laparoscopy) 66.29
hemorrhoids 49.43
iris 12.41
lacrimal
gland 09.21
punctum 09.72
for eversion 09.71
sac 09.6
larynx 30.09
liver 50.29
lung 32.29
endoscopic 32.28
meibomian gland 08.25
nose, for epistaxis (with packing) 21.03
ovary 65.29
laparoscopic 65.25
palate (bony) 27.31
pannus (superficial) 11.42
pharynx 29.39
punctum, lacrimal 09.72
for eversion 09.71
rectum 48.32
radical 48.31
round ligament 69.19
sclera 12.84
with iridectomy 12.62
skin 86.3
subcutaneous tissue 86.3
tonsillar fossa 28.7

◄ New ◄≋ Revised

Chondrectomy (Continued)
  hand and finger 80.94
  hip 80.95
  intervertebral cartilage - see category 80.5
  knee (semilunar cartilage) 80.6
  nasal (submucous) 21.5
  semilunar cartilage (knee) 80.6
  shoulder 80.91
  specified site NEC 80.99
  spine - see category 80.5
  wrist 80.93
Chondroplasty - see Arthroplasty
Chondrosternoplasty (for pectus excavatum repair) 34.74
Chondrotomy - see also Division, cartilage 80.40
  nasal 21.1
Chopart operation (midtarsal amputation) 84.12
Chordectomy, vocal 30.22
Chordotomy (spinothalamic) (anterior) (posterior) NEC 03.29
  percutaneous 03.21
  stereotactic 03.21
Ciliarotomy 12.55
Ciliectomy (ciliary body) 12.44
  eyelid margin 08.20
Cinch, cinching
  for scleral buckling - see also Buckling, scleral 14.49
  ocular muscle (oblique) (rectus) 15.22
    multiple (two or more muscles) 15.4
Cineangiocardiography - see also Angiocardiography 88.50
Cineplasty, cineplastic prosthesis
  amputation - see Amputation
  arm 84.44
  biceps 84.44
  extremity 84.40
    lower 84.48
    upper 84.44
  leg 84.48
Cineradiograph - see Radiography
Cingulumotomy (brain) (percutaneous radiofrequency) 01.32
Circumcision (male) 64.0
  female 71.4
CISH [classic infrafascial SEMM hysterectomy] 68.31
Clagett operation (closure of chest wall following open flap drainage) 34.72
Clamp and cautery, hemorrhoids 49.43
Clamping
  aneurysm (cerebral) 39.51
  blood vessel - see Ligation, blood vessel
  ventricular shunt 02.43
Clavicotomy 77.31
  fetal 73.8
Claviculectomy (partial) 77.81
  total 77.91
Clayton operation (resection of metatarsal heads and bases of phalanges) 77.88
Cleaning, wound 96.59
Clearance
  bladder (transurethral) 57.0
  pelvic
    female 68.8
    male 57.71
  prescalene fat pad 40.21
  renal pelvis (transurethral) 56.0
  ureter (transurethral) 56.0
Cleidotomy 77.31
  fetal 73.8

Clipping
  aneurysm (basilar) (carotid) (cerebellar) (cerebellopontine) (communicating artery) (vertebral) 39.51
  arteriovenous fistula 39.53
  frenulum, frenum
    labia (lips) 27.91
    lingual (tongue) 25.91
  tip of uvula 27.72
Clitoridectomy 71.4
Clitoridotomy 71.4
Clivogram 87.02
Closure - see also Repair
  abdominal wall 54.63
    delayed (granulating wound) 54.62
    secondary 54.61
    tertiary 54.62
  amputation stump, secondary 84.3
  aorticopulmonary fenestration (fistula) 39.59
  appendicostomy 47.92
  artificial opening
    bile duct 51.79
    bladder 57.82
    bronchus 33.42
    common duct 51.72
    esophagus 42.83
    gallbladder 51.92
    hepatic duct 51.79
    intestine 46.50
      large 46.52
      small 46.51
    kidney 55.82
    larynx 31.62
    rectum 48.72
    stomach 44.62
    thorax 34.72
    trachea 31.72
    ureter 56.83
    urethra 58.42
  atrial septal defect - see also Repair, atrial septal defect 35.71
    with umbrella device (King-Mills type) 35.52
    combined with repair of valvular and ventricular septal defects - see Repair, endocardial cushion defect
  bronchostomy 33.42
  cecostomy 46.52
  cholecystostomy 51.92
  cleft hand 82.82
  colostomy 46.52
  cystostomy 57.82
  diastema (alveolar) (dental) 24.8
  disrupted abdominal wall (postoperative) 54.61
  duodenostomy 46.51
  encephalocele 02.12
  endocardial cushion defect - see also Repair, endocardial cushion defect 35.73
  enterostomy 46.50
  esophagostomy 42.83
  fenestration
    aorticopulmonary 39.59
    septal, heart - see also Repair, heart, septum 35.70
  filtering bleb, corneoscleral (postglaucoma) 12.66
  fistula
    abdominothoracic 34.83
    anorectal 48.73
    anovaginal 70.73
    antrobuccal 22.71
    anus 49.73
    aorticopulmonary (fenestration) 39.59

Closure (Continued)
  fistula (Continued)
    aortoduodenal 39.59
    appendix 47.92
    biliary tract 51.79
    bladder NEC 57.84
    branchial cleft 29.52
    bronchocutaneous 33.42
    bronchoesophageal 33.42
    bronchomediastinal 34.73
    bronchopleural 34.73
    bronchopleurocutaneous 34.73
    bronchopleuromediastinal 34.73
    bronchovisceral 33.42
    bronchus 33.42
    cecosigmoidal 46.76
    cerebrospinal fluid 02.12
    cervicoaural 18.79
    cervicosigmoidal 67.62
    cervicovesical 57.84
    cervix 67.62
    cholecystocolic 51.93
    cholecystoduodenal 51.93
    cholecystoenteric 51.93
    cholecystogastric 51.93
    cholecystojejunal 51.93
    cisterna chyli 40.63
    colon 46.76
    colovaginal 70.72
    common duct 51.72
    cornea 11.49
      with lamellar graft (homograft) 11.62
        autograft 11.61
    diaphragm 34.83
    duodenum 46.72
    ear, middle 19.9
    ear drum 19.4
    enterocolic 46.74
    enterocutaneous 46.74
    enterouterine 69.42
    enterovaginal 70.74
    enterovesical 57.83
    esophagobronchial 33.42
    esophagocutaneous 42.84
    esophagopleurocutaneous 34.73
    esophagotracheal 31.73
    esophagus NEC 42.84
    fecal 46.79
    gallbladder 51.93
    gastric NEC 44.63
    gastrocolic 44.63
    gastroenterocolic 44.63
    gastroesophageal 42.84
    gastrojejunal 44.63
    gastrojejunocolic 44.63
    heart valve - see Repair, heart, valve
    hepatic duct 51.79
    hepatopleural 34.73
    hepatopulmonary 34.73
    ileorectal 46.74
    ileosigmoidal 46.74
    ileovesical 57.83
    ileum 46.74
    in ano 49.73
    intestine 46.79
      large 46.76
      small NEC 46.74
    intestinocolonic 46.74
    intestinoureteral 56.84
    intestinouterine 69.42
    intestinovaginal 70.74
    intestinovesical 57.83
    jejunum 46.74
    kidney 55.83

Closure *(Continued)*
fistula *(Continued)*
lacrimal 09.99
laryngotracheal 31.62
larynx 31.62
lymphatic duct, left (thoracic) 40.63
mastoid (antrum) 19.9
mediastinobronchial 34.73
mediastinocutaneous 34.73
mouth (external) 27.53
nasal 21.82
sinus 22.71
nasolabial 21.82
nasopharyngeal 21.82
oroantral 22.71
oronasal 21.82
oval window (ear) 20.93
pancreaticoduodenal 52.95
perilymph 20.93
perineorectal 48.73
perineosigmoidal 46.76
perineourethroscrotal 58.43
perineum 71.72
perirectal 48.93
pharyngoesophageal 29.53
pharynx NEC 29.53
pleura, pleural NEC 34.93
pleurocutaneous 34.73
pleuropericardial 37.4
pleuroperitoneal 34.83
pulmonoperitoneal 34.83
rectolabial 48.73
rectoureteral 56.84
rectourethral 58.43
rectovaginal 70.73
rectovesical 57.83
rectovesicovaginal 57.83
rectovulvar 48.73
rectum NEC 48.73
renal 55.83
reno-intestinal 55.83
round window 20.93
salivary (gland) (duct) 26.42
scrotum 61.42
sigmoidovaginal 70.74
sigmoidovesical 57.83
splenocolic 41.95
stomach NEC 44.63
thoracic duct 40.63
thoracoabdominal 34.83
thoracogastric 34.83
thoracointestinal 34.83
thorax NEC 34.73
trachea NEC 31.73
tracheoesophageal 31.73
tympanic membrane - *see also* Tympanoplasty 19.4
umbilicourinary 57.51
ureter 56.84
ureterocervical 56.84
ureterorectal 56.84
ureterosigmoidal 56.84
ureterovaginal 56.84
ureterovesical 56.84
urethra 58.43
urethroperineal 58.43
urethroperineovesical 57.84
urethrorectal 58.43
urethroscrotal 58.43
urethrovaginal 58.43
uteroenteric 69.42
uterointestinal 69.42
uterorectal 69.42
uteroureteric 56.84

Closure *(Continued)*
fistula *(Continued)*
uterovaginal 69.42
uterovesical 57.84
vagina 70.75
vaginocutaneous 70.75
vaginoenteric 70.74
vaginoperineal 70.75
vaginovesical 57.84
vesicocervicovaginal 57.84
vesicocolic 57.83
vesicocutaneous 57.84
vesicoenteric 57.83
vesicometrorectal 57.83
vesicoperineal 57.84
vesicorectal 57.83
vesicosigmoidal 57.83
vesicosigmoidovaginal 57.83
vesicoureteral 56.84
vesicoureterovaginal 56.84
vesicourethral 57.84
vesicourethrorectal 57.83
vesicouterine 57.84
vesicovaginal 57.84
vulva 71.72
vulvorectal 48.73
foramen ovale (patent) 35.71
with
prosthesis (open heart technique) 35.51
closed heart technique 35.52
tissue graft 35.61
gastroduodenostomy 44.5
gastrojejunostomy 44.5
gastrostomy 44.62
ileostomy 46.51
jejunostomy 46.51
laceration - *see also* Suture, by site
liver 50.61
laparotomy, delayed 54.62
meningocele (spinal) 03.51
cerebral 02.12
myelomeningocele 03.52
nephrostomy 55.82
palmar cleft 82.82
patent ductus arteriosus 38.85
pelviostomy 55.82
peptic ulcer (bleeding) (perforated) 44.40
perforation
ear drum - *see also* Tympanoplasty 19.4
esophagus 42.82
nasal septum 21.88
tympanic membrane - *see also* Tympanoplasty 19.4
proctostomy 48.72
punctum, lacrimal (papilla) 09.91
pyelostomy 55.82
rectostomy 48.72
septum defect (heart) - *see also* Repair, heart, septum 35.70
sigmoidostomy 46.52
skin (V-Y type) 86.59
stoma
bile duct 51.79
bladder 57.82
bronchus 33.42
common duct 51.72
esophagus 42.83
gallbladder 51.92
hepatic duct 51.79
intestine 46.50
large 46.52
small 46.51

Closure *(Continued)*
stoma *(Continued)*
kidney 55.82
larynx 31.62
rectum 48.72
stomach 44.62
thorax 34.72
trachea 31.72
ureter 56.83
urethra 58.42
thoracostomy 34.72
tracheostomy 31.72
ulcer (bleeding) (peptic) (perforated) 44.40
duodenum 44.42
gastric 44.41
intestine (perforated) 46.79
skin 86.59
stomach 44.41
ureterostomy 56.83
urethrostomy 58.42
vagina 70.8
vascular
percutaneous puncture - *omit code*
vesicostomy 57.22
wound - *see also* Suture, by site
with graft - *see* Graft
with tissue adhesive 86.59
Coagulation, electrocoagulation - *see also* Destruction, lesion, by site
aneurysm (cerebral) (peripheral vessel) 39.52
arteriovenous fistula 39.53
brain tissue (incremental) (radiofrequency) 01.59
broad ligament 69.19
cervix 67.32
ear
external 18.29
inner 20.79
middle 20.51
fallopian tube 66.61
gasserian ganglion 04.05
nose, for epistaxis (with packing) 21.03
ovary 65.29
laparoscopic 65.25
pharynx (by diathermy) 29.39
prostatic bed 60.94
rectum (polyp) 48.32
radical 48.31
retina (for)
destruction of lesion 14.21
reattachment 14.51
repair for tear 14.31
round ligament 69.19
semicircular canals 20.79
spinal cord (lesion) 03.4
urethrovesical junction, transurethral 57.49
uterosacral ligament 69.19
uterus 68.29
vagina 70.33
vulva 71.3
Coating, aneurysm of brain 39.52
Cobalt-60 therapy (treatment) 92.23
Coccygectomy (partial) 77.89
total 77.99
Coccygotomy 77.39
"Cocked hat" procedure (metacarpal lengthening and transfer of local flap) 82.69
Cockett operation (varicose vein)
lower limb 38.59
upper limb 38.53

ICD-9-CM

c

Vol.

Cooling, gastric 96.31
Cordectomy, vocal 30.22
Cordopexy, vocal 31.69
Cordotomy
  spinal (bilateral) NEC 03.29
    percutaneous 03.21
  vocal 31.3
Corectomy 12.12
Corelysis 12.35
Coreoplasty 12.35
Corneoconjunctivoplasty 11.53
Correction - *see also* Repair
  atresia
    esophageal 42.85
      by magnetic forces 42.99
    external meatus (ear) 18.6
    nasopharynx, nasopharyngeal 29.4
    rectum 48.0
    tricuspid 35.94
  atrial septal defect - *see also* Repair,
    atrial septal defect 35.71
    combined with repair of valvular
      and ventricular septal defects -
      see Repair, endocardial cushion
      defect
  blepharoptosis - *see also* Repair, ble-
    pharoptosis 08.36
  bunionette (with osteotomy) 77.54
  chordee 64.42
  claw toe 77.57
  cleft
    lip 27.54
    palate 27.62
  clubfoot NEC 83.84
  coarctation of aorta
    with
      anastomosis 38.34
      graft replacement 38.44
  cornea NEC 11.59
    refractive NEC 11.79
      epikeratophakia 11.76
      keratomileusis 11.71
      keratophakia 11.72
      radial keratotomy 11.75
  esophageal atresia 42.85
    by magnetic forces 42.99
  everted lacrimal punctum 09.71
  eyelid
    ptosis - *see also* Repair, blepharopto-
      sis 08.36
    retraction 08.38
  fetal defect 75.36
  forcible, of musculoskeletal deformity
    NEC 93.29
  hammer toe 77.56
  hydraulic pressure, open surgery for
    penile inflatable prosthesis 64.99
    urinary artificial sphincter 58.99
  intestinal malrotation 46.80
    large 46.82
    small 46.81
  inverted uterus - *see* Repair, inverted
    uterus
  lymphedema (of limb) 40.9
    excision with graft 40.9
    obliteration of lymphatics 40.9
    transplantation of autogenous lym-
      phatics 40.9
  nasopharyngeal atresia 29.4
  overlapping toes 77.58
  palate (cleft) 27.62
  prognathism NEC 76.64
  prominent ear 18.5
  punctum (everted) 09.71

Correction *(Continued)*
  spinal pseudarthrosis - *see* Refusion,
    spinal
  syndactyly 86.85
  tetralogy of Fallot
    one-stage 35.81
    partial - *see* specific procedure
    total 35.81
  total anomalous pulmonary venous
    connection
    one-stage 35.82
    partial - *see* specific procedure
    total 35.82
  transposition, great arteries, total 35.84
  tricuspid atresia 35.94
  truncus arteriosus
    one-stage 35.83
    partial - *see* specific procedure
    total 35.83
  ureteropelvic junction 55.87
  ventricular septal defect - *see also* Re-
    pair, ventricular septal defect
    35.72
    combined with repair of valvular
      and atrial septal defects - *see* Re-
      pair, endocardial cushion defect
Costectomy 77.91
  with lung excision - *see* Excision, lung
  associated with thoracic operation -
    omit code
Costochondrectomy 77.91
  associated with thoracic operation -
    omit code
Costosternoplasty (pectus excavatum repair) 34.74
Costotomy 77.31
Costotransversectomy 77.91
  associated with thoracic operation -
    omit code
Counseling (for) NEC 94.49
  alcoholism 94.46
  drug addiction 94.45
  employers 94.49
  family (medical) (social) 94.49
  marriage 94.49
  ophthalmologic (with instruction) 95.36
  pastoral 94.49
Countershock, cardiac NEC 99.62
Coventry operation (tibial wedge osteotomy) 77.27
CPAP (continuous positive airway pressure) 93.90
Craniectomy 01.25
  linear (opening of cranial suture) 02.01
  reopening of site 01.23
  strip (opening of cranial suture) 02.01
Cranioclasis, fetal 73.8
Cranioplasty 02.06
  with synchronous repair of encephalo-
    cele 02.12
Craniotomy 01.24
  as operative approach - *omit code*
  fetal 73.8
  for decompression of fracture 02.02
  reopening of site 01.23
Craterization, bone - *see also* Excision, lesion, bone 77.60
Crawford operation (tarso-frontalis sling
  of eyelid) 08.32
Creation - *see also* Formation
  cardiac pacemaker pocket
    with initial insertion of pacemaker -
      omit code
    new site (skin) (subcutaneous) 37.79

Creation *(Continued)*
  conduit
    ileal (urinary) 56.51
    left ventricle and aorta 35.93
    right atrium and pulmonary artery
      35.94
    right ventricle and pulmonary (dis-
      tal) artery 35.92
    in repair of
      pulmonary artery atresia 35.92
      transposition of great vessels
        35.92
      truncus arteriosus 35.83
  endorectal ileal pouch (H-pouch) (J-
    pouch) (S-pouch) (with anastomo-
    sis to anus) 45.95
  esophagogastric sphincteric compe-
    tence NEC 44.66
    laparoscopic 44.67 ◄
  Hartmann pouch - *see* Colectomy, by
    site
  interatrial fistula 35.42
  pericardial window 37.12
  pleural window, for drainage 34.09
  pocket
    cardiac pacemaker
      with initial insertion of pacemaker
        - *omit code*
      new site (skin) (subcutaneous)
        37.79
    loop recorder 86.09
    thalamic stimulator pulse generator
      with initial insertion of battery
        package - *omit code*
      new site (skin) (subcutaneous)
        86.09
  shunt - *see also* Shunt
    arteriovenous fistula, for dialysis
      39.93
    left-to-right (systemic to pulmonary
      circulation) 39.0
  subcutaneous tunnel for esophageal
    anastomosis 42.86
    with anastomosis - *see* Anastomosis,
      esophagus, antesternal
  syndactyly (finger) (toe) 86.89
  thalamic stimulator pulse generator
    with initial insertion of battery pack-
      age - *omit code*
    new site (skin) (subcutaneous) 86.09
  tracheoesophageal fistula 31.95
  window
    pericardial 37.12
    pleura, for drainage 34.09
Credé maneuver 73.59
Cricoidectomy 30.29
Cricothyreotomy (for assistance in
  breathing) 31.1
Cricothyroidectomy 30.29
Cricothyrostomy 31.1
Cricothyrotomy (for assistance in
  breathing) 31.1
Cricotomy (for assistance in breathing)
  31.1
Cricotracheotomy (for assistance in
  breathing) 31.1
Crisis intervention 94.35
Croupette, croup tent 93.94
Crown, dental (ceramic) (gold) 23.41
Crushing
  bone - *see* category 78.4
  calculus
    bile (hepatic) passage 51.49
      endoscopic 51.88

ICD-9-CM

C

Vol. 3

Crushing (Continued)
  calculus (Continued)
    bladder (urinary) 57.0
    pancreatic duct 52.09
      endoscopic 52.94
    fallopian tube - see also Ligation, fallo-
      pian tube 66.39
    ganglion - see Crushing, nerve
    hemorrhoids 49.45
    nasal septum 21.88
    nerve (cranial) (peripheral) NEC 04.03
      acoustic 04.01
      auditory 04.01
      phrenic 04.03
        for collapse of lung 33.31
      sympathetic 05.0
      trigeminal 04.02
      vestibular 04.01
    vas deferens 63.71
Cryoablation - see Ablation
Cryoanalgesia, nerve (cranial) (periph-
  eral) 04.2
Cryoconization, cervix 67.33
Cryodestruction - see Destruction, lesion,
  by site
Cryoextraction, lens - see also Extraction,
  cataract, intracapsular 13.19
Cryohypophysectomy (complete) (total) -
  see also Hypophysectomy 07.69
Cryoleucotomy 01.32
Cryopexy, retinal - see Cryotherapy, retina
Cryoprostatectomy 60.62
Cryoretinopexy (for)
  reattachment 14.52
  repair of tear or defect 14.32
Cryosurgery - see Cryotherapy
Cryothalamectomy 01.41
Cryotherapy - see also Destruction, lesion,
  by site
  bladder 57.59
  brain 01.59
  cataract 13.19
  cervix 67.33
  choroid - see Cryotherapy, retina
  ciliary body 12.72
  corneal lesion (ulcer) 11.43
    to reshape cornea 11.79
  ear
    external 18.29
    inner 20.79
  esophagus 42.39
    endoscopic 42.33
  eyelid 08.25
  hemorrhoids 49.44
  iris 12.41
  nasal turbinates 21.61
  palate (bony) 27.31
  prostate 60.62
  retina (for)
    destruction of lesion 14.22
    reattachment 14.52
    repair of tear 14.32
  skin 86.3
  stomach 43.49
    endoscopic 43.41
  subcutaneous tissue 86.3
  turbinates (nasal) 21.61
  warts 86.3
    genital 71.3
Cryptectomy (anus) 49.39
  endoscopic 49.31

Cryptorchidectomy (unilateral) 62.3
  bilateral 62.41
Cryptotomy (anus) 49.39
  endoscopic 49.31
Cuirass 93.99
Culdocentesis 70.0
Culdoplasty 70.92
Culdoscopy (exploration) (removal of
  foreign body or lesion) 70.22
Culdotomy 70.12
Culp-Deweerd operation (spiral flap
  pyeloplasty) 55.87
Culp-Scardino operation (ureteral flap
  pyeloplasty) 55.87
Culture (and sensitivity) - see Examination, microscopic
Curettage (with packing) (with secondary closure) - see also Dilation and
  curettage
  adenoids 28.6
  anus 49.39
    endoscopic 49.31
  bladder 57.59
    transurethral 57.49
  bone - see also Excision, lesion, bone
    77.60
  brain 01.59
  bursa 83.39
    hand 82.29
  cartilage - see also Excision, lesion, joint
    80.80
  cerebral meninges 01.51
  chalazion 08.25
  conjunctiva (trachoma follicles) 10.33
  corneal epithelium 11.41
    for smear or culture 11.21
  ear, external 18.29
  eyelid 08.25
  joint - see also Excision, lesion, joint
    80.80
  meninges (cerebral) 01.51
    spinal 03.4
  muscle 83.32
    hand 82.22
  nerve (peripheral) 04.07
    sympathetic 05.29
  sclera 12.84
  skin 86.3
  spinal cord (meninges) 03.4
  subgingival 24.31
  tendon 83.39
    sheath 83.31
      hand 82.21
  uterus (with dilation) 69.09
    aspiration (diagnostic) NEC 69.59
      after abortion or delivery 69.52
      to terminate pregnancy 69.51
    following delivery or abortion
      69.02
Curette evacuation, lens 13.2
Curtis operation (interphalangeal joint
  arthroplasty) 81.72
Cutaneolipectomy 86.83
Cutdown, venous 38.94
Cutting
  nerve (cranial) (peripheral) NEC 04.03
    acoustic 04.01
    auditory 04.01
    root, spinal 03.1
    sympathetic 05.0
    trigeminal 04.02
    vestibular 04.01

Cutting (Continued)
  pedicle (flap) graft 86.71
  pylorus (with wedge resection) 43.3
  spinal nerve root 03.1
  ureterovesical orifice 56.1
  urethral sphincter 58.5
CVP (central venous pressure monitoring) 89.62
Cyclectomy (ciliary body) 12.44
  eyelid margin 08.20
Cyclicotomy 12.55
Cycloanemization 12.74
Cyclocryotherapy 12.72
Cyclodialysis (initial) (subsequent)
  12.55
Cyclodiathermy (penetrating) (surface)
  12.71
Cycloelectrolysis 12.71
Cyclophotocoagulation 12.73
Cyclotomy 12.55
Cystectomy - see also Excision, lesion, by
  site
  gallbladder - see Cholecystectomy
  urinary (partial) (subtotal) 57.6
    complete (with urethrectomy) 57.79
    radical 57.71
      with pelvic exenteration (female)
        68.8
    total (with urethrectomy) 57.79
Cystocolostomy 57.88
Cystogram, cystography NEC 87.77
Cystolitholapaxy 57.0
Cystolithotomy 57.19
Cystometrogram 89.22
Cystopexy NEC 57.89
Cystoplasty NEC 57.89
Cystoproctostomy 57.88
Cystoprostatectomy, radical 57.71
Cystopyelography 87.74
Cystorrhaphy 57.81
Cystoscopy (transurethral) 57.32
  with biopsy 57.33
  for
    control of hemorrhage
      bladder 57.93
      prostate 60.94
    retrograde pyelography 87.74
  ileal conduit 56.35
  through stoma (artificial) 57.31
Cystostomy
  closed (suprapubic) (percutaneous)
    57.17
  open (suprapubic) 57.18
  percutaneous (closed) (suprapubic)
    57.17
  suprapubic
    closed 57.17
    open 57.18
Cystotomy (open) (for removal of calculi) 57.19
Cystourethrogram (retrograde) (voiding)
  87.76
Cystourethropexy (by) 59.79
  levator muscle sling 59.71
  retropubic suspension 59.5
  suprapubic suspension 59.4
Cystourethroplasty 57.85
Cystourethroscopy 57.32
  with biopsy
    bladder 57.33
    ureter 56.33
Cytology - see Examination, microscopic

D

Dacryoadenectomy 09.20
  partial 09.22
  total 09.23
Dacryoadenotomy 09.0
Dacryocystectomy (complete) (partial) 09.6
Dacryocystogram 87.05
Dacryocystorhinostomy (DCR) (by intubation) (external) (intranasal) 09.81
Dacryocystostomy 09.53
Dacryocystosyringotomy 09.53
Dacryocystotomy 09.53
Dahlman operation (excision of esophageal diverticulum) 42.31
Dana operation (posterior rhizotomy) 03.1
Danforth operation (fetal) 73.8
Darrach operation (ulnar resection) 77.83
Davis operation (intubated ureterotomy) 56.2
Deaf training 95.49
Debridement
  abdominal wall 54.3
  bone - *see also* Excision, lesion, bone 77.60
    fracture - *see* Debridement, open fracture
  brain 01.59
  burn (skin) 86.28
    excisional 86.22
    nonexcisional 86.28
  cerebral meninges 01.51
  dental 96.54
  flap graft 86.75
  graft (flap) (pedicle) 86.75
  heart valve (calcified) - *see* Valvuloplasty, heart
  infection (skin) 86.28
    excisional 86.22
    nail (bed) (fold) 86.27
    nonexcisional 86.28
  joint - *see* Excision, lesion, joint
  meninges (cerebral) 01.51
    spinal 03.4
  muscle 83.45
    hand 82.36
  nail (bed) (fold) 86.27
  nerve (peripheral) 04.07
  open fracture (compound) 79.60
    arm NEC 79.62
    carpal, metacarpal 79.63
    facial bone 76.2
    femur 79.65
    fibula 79.66
    foot NEC 79.67
    hand NEC 79.63
    humerus 79.61
    leg NEC 79.66
    phalanges
      foot 79.68
      hand 79.64
    radius 79.62
    specified site NEC 79.69
    tarsal, metatarsal 79.67
    tibia 79.66
    ulna 79.62
  patella 77.66
  pedicle graft 86.75
  skin or subcutaneous tissue (burn) (infection) (wound) 86.28

Debridement *(Continued)*
  skin or subcutaneous tissue *(Continued)*
    cardioverter/defibrillator (automatic) pocket 37.99
    excisional 86.22
    graft 86.75
    nail, nail bed, or nail fold 86.27
    nonexcisional 86.28
    pacemaker pocket 37.79
    pocket
      cardiac pacemaker 37.79
      cardioverter/defibrillator (automatic) 37.99
  skull 01.25
    compound fracture 02.02
  spinal cord (meninges) 03.4
  wound (skin) 86.28
    excisional 86.22
    nonexcisional 86.28
Decapitation, fetal 73.8
Decapsulation, kidney 55.91
Declotting - *see also* Removal, thrombus
  arteriovenous cannula or shunt 39.49
Decompression
  anus (imperforate) 48.0
  biliary tract 51.49
    by intubation 51.43
      endoscopic 51.87
      percutaneous 51.98
  brain 01.24
  carpal tunnel 04.43
  cauda equina 03.09
  chamber 93.97
  colon 96.08
    by incision 45.03
    endoscopic (balloon) 46.85
  common bile duct 51.42
    by intubation 51.43
      endoscopic 51.87
      percutaneous 51.98
  cranial 01.24
    for skull fracture 02.02
  endolymphatic sac 20.79
  ganglion (peripheral) NEC 04.49
    cranial NEC 04.42
  gastric 96.07
  heart 37.0
  intestine 96.08
    by incision 45.00
    endoscopic (balloon) 46.85
  intracranial 01.24
  labyrinth 20.79
  laminectomy 03.09
  laminotomy 03.09
  median nerve 04.43
  muscle 83.02
    hand 82.02
  nerve (peripheral) NEC 04.49
    auditory 04.42
    cranial NEC 04.42
    median 04.43
    trigeminal (root) 04.41
  orbit - *see also* Orbitotomy 16.09
  pancreatic duct 52.92
    endoscopic 52.93
  pericardium 37.0
  rectum 48.0
  skull fracture 02.02
  spinal cord (canal) 03.09
  tarsal tunnel 04.44
  tendon (sheath) 83.01
    hand 82.01

Decompression *(Continued)*
  thoracic outlet
    by
      myotomy (division of scalenus anticus muscle) 83.19
      tenotomy 83.13
  trigeminal (nerve root) 04.41
Decortication
  arterial 05.25
  brain 01.51
  cerebral meninges 01.51
  heart 37.31
  kidney 55.91
  lung (partial) (total) 34.51
  nasal turbinates - *see* Turbinectomy
  nose 21.89
  ovary 65.29
    laparoscopic 65.25
  periarterial 05.25
  pericardium 37.31
  ventricle, heart (complete) 37.31
Decoy, E2F 00.16 ◀
Deepening
  alveolar ridge 24.5
  buccolabial sulcus 24.91
  lingual sulcus 24.91
Defatting, flap or pedicle graft 86.75
Defibrillation, electric (external) (internal) 99.62
  automatic cardioverter/defibrillator - *see* category 37.9
de Grandmont operation (tarsectomy) 08.35
Delaying of pedicle graft 86.71
Delivery (with)
  assisted spontaneous 73.59
  breech extraction (assisted) 72.52
    partial 72.52
      with forceps to aftercoming head 72.51
    total 72.54
      with forceps to aftercoming head 72.53
    unassisted (spontaneous delivery) - *omit code*
  cesarean section - *see* Cesarean section
  Credé maneuver 73.59
  De Lee maneuver 72.4
  forceps 72.9
    application to aftercoming head (Piper) 72.6
      with breech extraction
        partial 72.51
        total 72.53
    Barton's 72.4
    failed 73.3
    high 72.39
      with episiotomy 72.31
    low (outlet) 72.0
      with episiotomy 72.1
    mid- 72.29
      with episiotomy 72.21
    outlet (low) 72.0
      with episiotomy 72.1
    rotation of fetal head 72.4
    trial 73.3
    instrumental NEC 72.9
      specified NEC 72.8
  key-in-lock rotation 72.4
  Kielland rotation 72.4
  Malstrom's extraction 72.79
    with episiotomy 72.71
  manually assisted (spontaneous) 73.59
  spontaneous (unassisted) 73.59
    assisted 73.59

◀ **New**　　　◀■ **Revised**

Delivery (Continued)
  vacuum extraction 72.79
    with episiotomy 72.71
Delorme operation
  pericardiectomy 37.31
  proctopexy 48.76
  repair of prolapsed rectum 48.76
  thoracoplasty 33.34
Denervation
  aortic body 39.8
  carotid body 39.8
  facet, percutaneous (radiofrequency) 03.96
  ovarian 65.94
  paracervical uterine 69.3
  uterosacral 69.3
Denker operation (radical maxillary antrotomy) 22.31
Dennis-Barco operation - see Repair, hernia, femoral
Denonvilliers operation (limited rhinoplasty) 21.86
Densitometry, bone (serial) (radiographic) 88.98
Depilation, skin 86.92
Derlacki operation (tympanoplasty) 19.4
Dermabond 86.59
Dermabrasion (laser) 86.25
  for wound debridement 86.28
Derotation - see Reduction, torsion
Desensitization
  allergy 99.12
  psychologic 94.33
Desmotomy - see also Division, ligament 80.40
Destruction
  breast 85.20
  chorioretinopathy - see also Destruction, lesion, choroid 14.29
  ciliary body 12.74
  epithelial downgrowth, anterior chamber 12.93
  fallopian tube 66.39
    with
      crushing (and ligation) 66.31
        by endoscopy (laparoscopy) 66.21
      division (and ligation) 66.32
        by endoscopy (culdoscopy) (hysteroscopy) (laparoscopy) (peritoneoscopy) 66.22
      ligation 66.39
        with
          crushing 66.31
            by endoscopy (laparoscopy) 66.21
          division 66.32
            by endoscopy (culdoscopy) (hysteroscopy) (laparoscopy) (peritoneoscopy) 66.22
  fetus 73.8
  hemorrhoids 49.49
    by
      cryotherapy 49.44
      sclerotherapy 49.42
  inner ear NEC 20.79
    by injection 20.72
  intervertebral disc (NOS) 80.50
    by injection 80.52
    by other specified method 80.59
    herniated (nucleus pulposus) 80.51
  lacrimal sac 09.6
  lesion (local)
    anus 49.39
      endoscopic 49.31

Destruction (Continued)
  lesion (Continued)
    Bartholin's gland 71.24
      by
        aspiration 71.21
        excision 71.24
        incision 71.22
        marsupialization 71.23
    biliary ducts 51.69
      endoscopic 51.64
    bladder 57.59
      transurethral 57.49
    bone - see Excision, lesion, bone
    bowel - see Destruction, lesion, intestine
    brain (transtemporal approach) NEC 01.59
      by stereotactic radiosurgery 92.30
        cobalt 60 92.32
        linear accelerator (LINAC) 92.31
        multi-source 92.32
        particle beam 92.33
        particulate 92.33
        radiosurgery NEC 92.39
        single source photon 92.31
    breast NEC 85.20
    bronchus NEC 32.09
      endoscopic 32.01
    cerebral NEC 01.59
      meninges 01.51
    cervix 67.39
      by
        cauterization 67.32
        cryosurgery, cryoconization 67.33
        electroconization 67.32
    choroid 14.29
      by
        cryotherapy 14.22
        diathermy 14.21
        implantation of radiation source 14.27
        photocoagulation 14.25
          laser 14.24
          xenon arc 14.23
        radiation therapy 14.26
    ciliary body (nonexcisional) 12.43
      by excision 12.44
    conjunctiva 10.32
      by excision 10.31
    cornea NEC 11.49
      by
        cryotherapy 11.43
        electrocauterization 11.42
        thermocauterization 11.42
    cul-de-sac 70.32
    duodenum NEC 45.32
      by excision 45.31
        endoscopic 45.30
      endoscopic 45.30
    esophagus (chemosurgery) (cryosurgery) (electroresection) (fulguration) NEC 42.39
      by excision 42.32
        endoscopic 42.33
      endoscopic 42.33
    eye NEC 16.93
    eyebrow 08.25
    eyelid 08.25
      excisional - see Excision, lesion, eyelid
    heart 37.33
      by catheter ablation 37.34

Destruction (Continued)
  lesion (Continued)
    intestine (large) 45.49
      by excision 45.41
        endoscopic 45.43
          polypectomy 45.42
      endoscopic 45.43
        polypectomy 45.42
      small 45.34
        by excision 45.33
    intranasal 21.31
    iris (nonexcisional) NEC 12.41
      by excision 12.42
    kidney 55.39
      by marsupialization 55.31
    lacrimal sac 09.6
    larynx 30.09
    liver 50.29
    lung 32.29
      endoscopic 32.28
    meninges (cerebral) 01.51
      spinal 03.4
    nerve (peripheral) 04.07
      sympathetic 05.29
    nose 21.30
      intranasal 21.31
      specified NEC 21.32
    ovary
      by
        aspiration 65.91
        excision 65.29
          laparoscopic 65.25
      cyst by rupture (manual) 65.93
    palate (bony) (local) 27.31
      wide 27.32
    pancreas 52.22
      by marsupialization 52.3
      endoscopic 52.21
    pancreatic duct 52.22
      endoscopic 52.21
    penis 64.2
    pharynx (excisional) 29.39
    pituitary gland
      by stereotactic radiosurgery 92.30
        cobalt 60 92.32
        linear accelerator (LINAC) 92.31
        multi-source 92.32
        particle beam 92.33
        particulate 92.33
        radiosurgery NEC 92.39
        single source photon 92.31
    rectum (local) 48.32
      by
        cryosurgery 48.34
        electrocoagulation 48.32
        excision 48.35
        fulguration 48.32
        laser (Argon) 48.33
      polyp 48.36
      radical 48.31
    retina 14.29
      by
        cryotherapy 14.22
        diathermy 14.21
        implantation of radiation source 14.27
        photocoagulation 14.25
          laser 14.24
          xenon arc 14.23
        radiation therapy 14.26
    salivary gland NEC 26.29
      by marsupialization 26.21
    sclera 12.84
    scrotum 61.3

ICD-9-CM

Vol. 3

Destruction *(Continued)*
  lesion *(Continued)*
    skin NEC 86.3
    sphincter of Oddi 51.69
      endoscopic 51.64
    spinal cord (meninges) 03.4
    spleen 41.42
      by marsupialization 41.41
    stomach NEC 43.49
      by excision 43.42
        endoscopic 43.41
      endoscopic 43.41
    subcutaneous tissue NEC 86.3
    testis 62.2
    tongue 25.1
    urethra (excisional) 58.39
      endoscopic 58.31
    uterus 68.29
  nerve (cranial) (peripheral) (by cryon-
      algesia) (by radiofrequency) 04.2
    sympathetic, by injection of neuro-
        lytic agent 05.32
  neuroma
    acoustic 04.01
      by craniotomy 04.01
      by stereotactic radiosurgery 92.30
        cobalt 60 92.32
        linear accelerator (LINAC)
            92.31
        multi-source 92.32
        particle beam 92.33
        particulate 92.33
        radiosurgery NEC 92.39
        single source photon 92.31
    cranial 04.07
    Morton's 04.07
    peripheral
      Morton's 04.07
  prostate (prostatic tissue)
    by
      cryotherapy 60.62
      microwave 60.96
      radiofrequency 60.97
    transurethral microwave thermother-
        apy (TUMT) 60.96
    transurethral needle ablation
        (TUNA) 60.97
    TULIP (transurethral (ultrasound)
        guided laser induced prostatec-
        tomy) 60.21
    TUMT (transurethral microwave
        thermotherapy) 60.96
    TUNA (transurethral needle abla-
        tion) 60.97
  semicircular canals, by injection 20.72
  vestibule, by injection 20.72
Detachment, uterosacral ligaments 69.3
Determination
  mental status (clinical) (medicolegal)
      (psychiatric) NEC 94.11
    psychologic NEC 94.09
  vital capacity (pulmonary) 89.37
Detorsion
  intestine (twisted) (volvulus) 46.80
    large 46.82
      endoscopic (balloon) 46.85
    small 46.81
  kidney 55.84
  ovary 65.95
  spermatic cord 63.52
    with orchiopexy 62.5
  testis 63.52
    with orchiopexy 62.5
  volvulus 46.80
    endoscopic (balloon) 46.85

Detoxification therapy 94.25
  alcohol 94.62
    with rehabilitation 94.63
    combined alcohol and drug 94.68
      with rehabilitation 94.69
  drug 94.65
    with rehabilitation 94.66
    combined alcohol and drug 94.68
      with rehabilitation 94.69
Devascularization, stomach 44.99
Dewebbing
  esophagus 42.01
  syndactyly (fingers) (toes) 86.85
Dextrorotation - *see* Reduction, torsion
Dialysis
  hemodiafiltration, hemofiltration (ex-
      tracorporeal) 39.95
  kidney (extracorporeal) 39.95
  liver 50.92
  peritoneal 54.98
  renal (extracorporeal) 39.95
Diaphanoscopy
  nasal sinuses 89.35
  skull (newborn) 89.16
Diaphysectomy - *see* category 77.8
Diathermy 93.34
  choroid - *see* Diathermy, retina
  nasal turbinates 21.61
  retina
    for
      destruction of lesion 14.21
      reattachment 14.51
      repair of tear 14.31
    surgical - *see* Destruction, lesion, by site
  turbinates (nasal) 21.61
Dickson operation (fascial transplant)
    83.82
Dickson-Diveley operation (tendon
    transfer and arthrodesis to correct
    claw toe) 77.57
Dieffenbach operation (hip disarticula-
    tion) 84.18
Dilation
  achalasia 42.92
  ampulla of Vater 51.81
    endoscopic 51.84
  anus, anal (sphincter) 96.23
  biliary duct
    endoscopic 51.84
    pancreatic duct 52.99
      endoscopic 52.98
    percutaneous (endoscopy) 51.98
    sphincter
      of Oddi 51.81
        endoscopic 51.84
      pancreatic 51.82
        endoscopic 51.85
  bladder 96.25
    neck 57.92
  bronchus 33.91
  cervix (canal) 67.0
    obstetrical 73.1
    to assist delivery 73.1
  choanae (nasopharynx) 29.91
  colon (endoscopic) (balloon) 46.85
  colostomy stoma 96.24
  duodenum (endoscopic) (balloon) 46.85
  endoscopic - *see* Dilation, by site
  enterostomy stoma 96.24
  esophagus (by bougie) (by sound) 42.92
  fallopian tube 66.96
  foreskin (newborn) 99.95
  frontonasal duct 96.21
  gastrojejunostomy site, endoscopic 44.22
  heart valve - *see* Valvulotomy, heart

Dilation *(Continued)*
  ileostomy stoma 96.24
  ileum (endoscopic) (balloon) 46.85
  intestinal stoma (artificial) 96.24
  intestine (endoscopic) (balloon) 46.85
  jejunum (endoscopic) (balloon) 46.85
  lacrimal
    duct 09.42
    punctum 09.41
  larynx 31.98
  lymphatic structure(s) (peripheral) 40.9
  nares 21.99
  nasolacrimal duct (retrograde) 09.43
    with insertion of tube or stent 09.44
  nasopharynx 29.91
  pancreatic duct 52.99
    endoscopic 52.98
  pharynx 29.91
  prostatic urethra (transurethral) (bal-
      loon) 60.95
  punctum, lacrimal papilla 09.41
  pylorus
    by incision 44.21
    endoscopic 44.22
  rectum 96.22
  salivary duct 26.91
  sphenoid ostia 22.52
  sphincter
    anal 96.23
    cardiac 42.92
    of Oddi 51.81
      endoscopic 51.84
    pancreatic 51.82
      endoscopic 51.85
    pylorus, endoscopic 44.22
      by incision 44.21
  Stenson's duct 26.91
  trachea 31.99
  ureter 59.8
    meatus 56.91
  ureterovesical orifice 59.8
  urethra 58.6
    prostatic (transurethral) (balloon) 60.95
  urethrovesical junction 58.6
  vagina (instrumental) (manual) NEC
      96.16
  vesical neck 57.92
  Wharton's duct 26.91
  Wirsung's duct 52.99
    endoscopic 52.98
Dilation and curettage, uterus (diagnos-
    tic) 69.09
  after
    abortion 69.02
    delivery 69.02
  to terminate pregnancy 69.01
Diminution, ciliary body 12.74
Disarticulation 84.91
  ankle 84.13
  elbow 84.06
  finger, except thumb 84.01
    thumb 84.02
  hip 84.18
  knee 84.16
  shoulder 84.08
  thumb 84.02
  toe 84.11
  wrist 84.04
Discectomy - *see* Diskectomy   ◄
Discission
  capsular membrane 13.64
  cataract (Wheeler knife) (Ziegler knife)
      13.2
    congenital 13.69
    secondary membrane 13.64

Discission (Continued)
iris 12.12
lens (capsule) (Wheeler knife) (Ziegler knife) (with capsulotomy) 13.2
orbitomaxillary, radical 16.51
pupillary 13.2
secondary membrane (after cataract) 13.64
vitreous strands (posterior approach) 14.74
anterior approach 14.73
Discogram, diskogram 87.21
Discolysis (by injection) 80.52
Diskectomy, (discectomy) intervertebral 80.51 ◀▥
herniated (nucleus pulposus) 80.51
percutaneous 80.59
Dispensing (with fitting)
contact lens 95.32
low vision aids NEC 95.33
spectacles 95.31
Dissection - see also Excision
aneurysm 38.60
artery-vein-nerve bundle 39.91
branchial cleft fistula or sinus 29.52
bronchus 32.1
femoral hernia 53.29
groin, radical 40.54
larynx block (en bloc) 30.3
mediastinum with pneumonectomy 32.5
neck, radical 40.40
with laryngectomy 30.4
bilateral 40.42
unilateral 40.41
orbital fibrous bands 16.92
pterygium (with reposition) 11.31
radical neck - see Dissection, neck, radical
retroperitoneal NEC 59.00
thoracic structures (block) (brachial plexus, bronchus, lobe of lung, ribs, and sympathetic nerves) (en bloc) (radical) 32.6
vascular bundle 39.91
Distention, bladder (therapeutic) (intermittent) 96.25
Diversion
biliopancreatic (BPD) 43.7 [45.51] [45.91]
with duodenal switch 43.89 [45.51] [45.91]
urinary
cutaneous 56.61
ileal conduit 56.51
internal NEC 56.71
ureter to
intestine 56.71
skin 56.61
uretero-ileostomy 56.51
Diversional therapy 93.81
Diverticulectomy
bladder (suprapubic) 57.59
transurethral approach 57.49
duodenum 45.31
endoscopic 45.30
esophagus 42.31
endoscopic 42.33
esophagomyotomy 42.7
hypopharyngeal (by cricopharyngeal myotomy) 29.32
intestine
large 45.41
endoscopic 45.43
small 45.33

Diverticulectomy (Continued)
kidney 55.39
Meckel's 45.33
pharyngeal (by cricopharyngeal myotomy) 29.32
pharyngoesophageal (by cricopharyngeal myotomy) 29.32
stomach 43.42
endoscopic 43.41
urethra 58.39
endoscopic 58.31
Division
Achilles tendon 83.11
adductor tendon (hip) 83.12
adhesions - see Lysis, adhesions
angle of mandible (open) 76.62
closed 76.61
anterior synechiae 12.32
aponeurosis 83.13
arcuate ligament (spine) - omit code
arteriovenous fistula (with ligation) 39.53
artery (with ligation) 38.80
abdominal 38.86
aorta (arch) (ascending) (descending) 38.84
head and neck NEC 38.82
intracranial NEC 38.81
lower limb 38.88
thoracic NEC 38.85
upper limb 38.83
bladder neck 57.91
blepharorrhaphy 08.02
blood vessels, cornea 10.1
bone - see also Osteotomy 77.30
brain tissue 01.32
cortical adhesions 02.91
canaliculus 09.52
canthorrhaphy 08.02
cartilage 80.40
ankle 80.47
elbow 80.42
foot and toe 80.48
hand and finger 80.44
hip 80.45
knee 80.46
shoulder 80.41
specified site NEC 80.49
spine 80.49
wrist 80.43
cerebral tracts 01.32
chordae tendineae 35.32
common wall between posterior left atrium and coronary sinus (with roofing of resultant defect with patch graft) 35.82
congenital web
larynx 31.98
pharynx 29.54
endometrial synechiae 68.21
fallopian tube - see Ligation, fallopian tube
fascia 83.14
hand 82.12
frenulum, frenum
labial 27.91
lingual 25.91
tongue 25.91
ganglion, sympathetic 05.0
glossopharyngeal nerve 29.92
goniosynechiae 12.31
hypophyseal stalk - see also Hypophysectomy, partial 07.63
iliotibial band 83.14

Division (Continued)
isthmus
horseshoe kidney 55.85
thyroid 06.91
joint capsule 80.40
ankle 80.47
elbow 80.42
foot and toe 80.48
hand and finger 80.44
hip 80.45
knee 80.46
shoulder 80.41
specified site NEC 80.49
wrist 80.43
labial frenum 27.91
lacrimal ductules 09.0
laryngeal nerve (external) (recurrent) (superior) 31.91
ligament 80.40
ankle 80.47
arcuate (spine) - omit code
canthal 08.36
elbow 80.42
foot and toe 80.48
hand and finger 80.44
hip 80.45
knee 80.46
palpebrae 08.36
shoulder 80.41
specified site NEC 80.49
spine 80.49
arcuate - omit code
flavum - omit code
uterosacral 69.3
wrist 80.43
ligamentum flavum (spine) - omit code
meninges (cerebral) 01.31
muscle 83.19
hand 82.19
nasolacrimal duct stricture (with drainage) 09.59
nerve (cranial) (peripheral) NEC 04.03
acoustic 04.01
adrenal gland 07.42
auditory 04.01
glossopharyngeal 29.92
lacrimal branch 05.0
laryngeal (external) (recurrent) (superior) 31.91
phrenic 04.03
for collapse of lung 33.31
root, spinal or intraspinal 03.1
sympathetic 05.0
tracts
cerebral 01.32
spinal cord 03.29
percutaneous 03.21
trigeminal 04.02
vagus - see also Vagotomy 44.00
vestibular 04.01
otosclerotic process or material, middle ear 19.0
papillary muscle (heart) 35.31
patent ductus arteriosus 38.85
penile adhesions 64.93
posterior synechiae 12.33
pylorus (with wedge resection) 43.3
rectum (stricture) 48.91
scalenus anticus muscle 83.19
Skene's gland 71.3
soft tissue NEC 83.19
hand 82.19

ICD-9-CM
Vol. 3

Division (*Continued*)
sphincter
anal (external) (internal) 49.59
left lateral 49.51
posterior 49.52
cardiac 42.7
of Oddi 51.82
endoscopic 51.85
pancreatic 51.82
endoscopic 51.85
spinal
cord tracts 03.29
percutaneous 03.21
nerve root 03.1
symblepharon (with insertion of conformer) 10.5
synechiae
endometrial 68.21
iris (posterior) 12.33
anterior 12.32
tarsorrhaphy 08.02
tendon 83.13
Achilles 83.11
adductor (hip) 83.12
hand 82.11
trabeculae carneae cordis (heart)
35.35
tympanum 20.23
uterosacral ligaments 69.3
vaginal septum 70.14
vas deferens 63.71
vein (with ligation) 38.80
abdominal 38.87
head and neck NEC 38.82
intracranial NEC 38.81
lower limb 38.89
varicose 38.59
thoracic NEC 38.85
upper limb 38.83
varicose 38.50
abdominal 38.57
head and neck NEC 38.52
intracranial NEC 38.51
lower limb 38.59
thoracic NEC 38.55
upper limb 38.53
vitreous, cicatricial bands (posterior
approach) 14.74
anterior approach 14.73
Doleris operation (shortening of round
ligaments) 69.22
D'Ombrain operation (excision of pterygium with corneal graft) 11.32
Domestic tasks therapy 93.83
Dopplergram, Doppler flow mapping -
see also Ultrasonography
aortic arch 88.73
head and neck 88.71
heart 88.72
thorax NEC 88.73
Dorrance operation (push-back operation for cleft palate) 27.62
Dotter operation (transluminal angioplasty) 39.59
Douche, vagina 96.44
Douglas' operation (suture of tongue to
lip for micrognathia) 25.59
Doyle operation (paracervical uterine
denervation) 69.3
Drainage
by
anastomosis - *see* Anastomosis
aspiration - *see* Aspiration
incision - *see* Incision

Drainage (*Continued*)
abdomen 54.19
percutaneous 54.91
abscess - *see also* Drainage, by site and
Incision, by site
appendix 47.2
with appendectomy 47.09
laparoscopic 47.01
parapharyngeal (oral) (transcervical)
28.0
peritonsillar (oral) (transcervical)
28.0
retropharyngeal (oral) (transcervical)
28.0
thyroid (field) (gland) 06.09
percutaneous (needle) 06.01
postoperative 06.02
tonsil, tonsillar (oral) (transcervical)
28.0
antecubital fossa 86.04
appendix 47.91
with appendectomy 47.09
laparoscopic 47.01
abscess 47.2
with appendectomy 47.09
laparoscopic 47.01
axilla 86.04
bladder (without incision) 57.0
by indwelling catheter 57.94
percutaneous suprapubic (closed)
57.17
suprapubic NEC 57.18
buccal space 27.0
bursa 83.03
by aspiration 83.94
hand 82.92
hand 82.03
by aspiration 82.92
radial 82.03
ulnar 82.03
cerebrum, cerebral (meninges) (ventricle) (incision) (trephination)
01.39
by
anastomosis - *see* Shunt, ventricular
aspiration 01.09
through previously implanted
catheter 01.02
chest (closed) 34.04
open (by incision) 34.09
cranial sinus (incision) (trephination)
01.21
by aspiration 01.09
cul-de-sac 70.12
by aspiration 70.0
cyst - *see also* Drainage, by site and
Incision, by site
pancreas (by catheter) 52.01
by marsupialization 52.3
internal (anastomosis) 52.4
pilonidal 86.03
spleen, splenic (by marsupialization)
41.41
duodenum (tube) 46.39
by incision 45.01
ear
external 18.09
inner 20.79
middle (by myringotomy) 20.09
with intubation 20.01
epidural space, cerebral (incision)
(trephination) 01.24
by aspiration 01.09

Drainage (*Continued*)
extradural space, cerebral (incision)
(trephination) 01.24
by aspiration 01.09
extraperitoneal 54.0
facial region 27.0
fascial compartments, head and neck
27.0
fetal hydrocephalic head (needling)
(trocar) 73.8
gallbladder 51.04
by
anastomosis 51.35
aspiration 51.01
incision 51.04
groin region (abdominal wall) (inguinal) 54.0
skin 86.04
subcutaneous tissue 86.04
hematoma - *see* Drainage, by site and
Incision, by site
hydrocephalic head (needling) (trocar)
73.8
hypochondrium 54.0
intra-abdominal 54.19
iliac fossa 54.0
infratemporal fossa 27.0
intracranial space (epidural) (extradural) (incision) (trephination)
01.24
by aspiration 01.09
subarachnoid or subdural (incision)
(trephination) 01.31
by aspiration 01.09
intraperitoneal 54.19
percutaneous 54.91
kidney (by incision) 55.01
by
anastomosis 55.86
catheter 59.8
pelvis (by incision) 55.11
liver 50.0
by aspiration 50.91
Ludwig's angina 27.0
lung (by incision) 33.1
by punch (needle) (trocar) 33.93
midpalmar space 82.04
mouth floor 27.0
mucocele, nasal sinus 22.00
by puncture 22.01
through natural ostium 22.02
omentum 54.19
percutaneous 54.91
ovary (aspiration) 65.91
by incision 65.09
laparoscopic 65.01
palmar space (middle) 82.04
pancreas (by catheter) 52.01
by anastomosis 52.96
parapharyngeal 28.0
paronychia 86.04
parotid space 27.0
pelvic peritoneum (female) 70.12
male 54.19
pericardium 37.0
perigastric 54.19
percutaneous 54.91
perineum
female 71.09
male 86.04
perisplenic tissue 54.19
percutaneous 54.91
peritoneum 54.19
pelvic (female) 70.12
percutaneous 54.91

◀ **New**   ◀▦ **Revised**

Drainage *(Continued)*
peritonsillar 28.0
pharyngeal space, lateral 27.0
pilonidal cyst or sinus 86.03
pleura (closed) 34.04
open (by incision) 34.09
popliteal space 86.04
postural 93.99
postzygomatic space 27.0
pseudocyst, pancreas 52.3
by anastomosis 52.4
pterygopalatine fossa 27.0
retropharyngeal 28.0
scrotum 61.0
skin 86.04
spinal (canal) (cord) 03.09
by anastomosis - *see* Shunt, spinal
diagnostic 03.31
spleen 41.2
cyst (by marsupialization) 41.41
subarachnoid space, cerebral (incision)
(trephination) 01.31
by aspiration 01.09
subcutaneous tissue 86.04
subdiaphragmatic 54.19
percutaneous 54.91
subdural space, cerebral (incision)
(trephination) 01.31
by aspiration 01.09
subhepatic space 54.19
percutaneous 54.91
sublingual space 27.0
submental space 27.0
subphrenic space 54.19
percutaneous 54.91
supraclavicular fossa 86.04
temporal pouches 27.0
tendon (sheath) 83.01
hand 82.01

Drainage *(Continued)*
thenar space 82.04
thorax (closed) 34.04
open (by incision) 34.09
thyroglossal tract (by incision) 06.09
by aspiration 06.01
thyroid (field) (gland) (by incision)
06.09
by aspiration 06.01
postoperative 06.02
tonsil 28.0
tunica vaginalis 61.0
ureter (by catheter) 59.8
by
anastomosis NEC - *see also* Anastomosis, ureter 56.79
incision 56.2
ventricle (cerebral) (incision) NEC
02.39
by
anastomosis - *see* Shunt, ventricular
aspiration 01.09
through previously implanted
catheter 01.02
vertebral column 03.09
Drawing test 94.08
Dressing
burn 93.57
ulcer 93.56
wound 93.57
Drilling ◀▥
bone - *see also* Incision, bone 77.10 ◀
ovary 65.99 ◀
Drotrecogin alfa (activated) infusion
00.11
Ductogram, mammary 87.35
Duhamel operation (abdominoperineal
pull-through) 48.65

Duhrssen's
incisions (cervix, to assist delivery)
73.93
operation (vaginofixation of uterus)
69.22
Dunn operation (triple arthrodesis)
81.12
Duodenectomy 45.62
with
gastrectomy - *see* Gastrectomy
pancreatectomy - *see* Pancreatectomy
Duodenocholedochotomy 51.51
Duodenoduodenostomy 45.91
proximal to distal segment 45.62
Duodenoileostomy 45.91
Duodenojejunostomy 45.91
Duodenoplasty 46.79
Duodenorrhaphy 46.71
Duodenoscopy 45.13
through stoma (artificial) 45.12
transabdominal (operative) 45.11
Duodenostomy 46.39
Duodenotomy 45.01
Dupuytren operation
fasciectomy 82.35
fasciotomy 82.12
with excision 82.35
shoulder disarticulation 84.08
Durabond 86.59
Duraplasty 02.12
Durham (-Caldwell) operation (transfer
of biceps femoris tendon) 83.75
DuToit and Roux operation (staple cap-
sulorrhaphy of shoulder) 81.82
DuVries operation (tenoplasty) 83.88
Dwyer operation
fasciotomy 83.14
soft tissue release NEC 83.84
wedge osteotomy, calcaneus 77.28

ICD-9-CM

▯

Vol. 3

E

E2F decoy 00.16 ◄
Eagleton operation (extrapetrosal drainage) 20.22
ECG - *see* Electrocardiogram
Echocardiography 88.72
  intracardiac (heart chambers) (ICE) 37.28 ◄
  intravascular (coronary vessels) 00.24 ◄
  transesophageal 88.72
    monitoring (Doppler) (ultrasound) 89.68
Echoencephalography 88.71
Echography - *see* Ultrasonography
Echogynography 88.79
Echoplacentogram 88.78
ECMO (extracorporeal membrane oxygenation) 39.65
Eden-Hybinette operation (glenoid bone block) 78.01
Educational therapy (bed-bound children) (handicapped) 93.82
EEG (electroencephalogram) 89.14
  monitoring (radiographic) (video) 89.19
Effler operation (heart) 36.2
Effleurage 93.39
EGD (esophagogastroduodenoscopy) 45.13
  with closed biopsy 45.16
Eggers operation
  tendon release (patellar retinacula) 83.13
  tendon transfer (biceps femoris tendon) (hamstring tendon) 83.75
EKG - *see also* Electrocardiogram 89.52
Elastic hosiery 93.59
Electrocardiogram (with 12 or more leads) 89.52
  with vectorcardiogram 89.53
  fetal (scalp), intrauterine 75.32
  rhythm (with one to three leads) 89.51
Electrocautery - *see also* Cauterization
  cervix 67.32
  corneal lesion (ulcer) 11.42
  esophagus 42.39
    endoscopic 42.33
Electrocoagulation - *see also* Destruction, lesion, by site
  aneurysm (cerebral) (peripheral vessels) 39.52
  cervix 67.32
  cystoscopic 57.49
  ear
    external 18.29
    inner 20.79
    middle 20.51
  fallopian tube (lesion) 66.61
    for tubal ligation - *see* Ligation, fallopian tube
  gasserian ganglion 04.02
  nasal turbinates 21.61
  nose, for epistaxis (with packing) 21.03
  ovary 65.29
    laparoscopic 65.25
  prostatic bed 60.94
  rectum (polyp) 48.32
    radical 48.31
  retina (for)
    destruction of lesion 14.21
    reattachment 14.51
    repair of tear 14.31

Electrocoagulation *(Continued)*
  round ligament 69.19
  semicircular canals 20.79
  urethrovesical junction, transurethral 57.49
  uterine ligament 69.19
  uterosacral ligament 69.19
  uterus 68.29
  vagina 70.33
  vulva 71.3
Electrocochleography 20.31
Electroconization, cervix 67.32
Electroconvulsive therapy (ECT) 94.27
Electroencephalogram (EEG) 89.14
  monitoring (radiographic) (video) 89.19
Electrogastrogram 44.19
Electrokeratotomy 11.49
Electrolysis
  ciliary body 12.71
  hair follicle 86.92
  retina (for)
    destruction of lesion 14.21
    reattachment 14.51
    repair of tear 14.31
  skin 86.92
  subcutaneous tissue 86.92
Electromyogram, electromyography (EMG) (muscle) 93.08
  eye 95.25
  urethral sphincter 89.23
Electronarcosis 94.29
Electronic gaiter 93.59
Electronystagmogram (ENG) 95.24
Electro-oculogram (EOG) 95.22
Electroresection - *see also* Destruction, lesion, by site
  bladder neck (transurethral) 57.49
  esophagus 42.39
    endoscopic 42.33
  prostate (transurethral) 60.29
  stomach 43.49
    endoscopic 43.41
Electroretinogram (ERG) 95.21
Electroshock therapy (EST) 94.27
  subconvulsive 94.26
Elevation
  bone fragments (fractured)
    orbit 76.79
    sinus (nasal)
      frontal 22.79
      maxillary 22.79
    skull (with debridement) 02.02
    spinal 03.53
  pedicle graft 86.71
Elliot operation (scleral trephination with iridectomy) 12.61
Ellis Jones operation (repair of peroneal tendon) 83.88
Ellison operation (reinforcement of collateral ligament) 81.44
Elmslie-Cholmeley operation (tarsal wedge osteotomy) 77.28
Eloesser operation
  thoracoplasty 33.34
  thoracostomy 34.09
Elongation - *see* Lengthening
Embolectomy 38.00
  with endarterectomy - *see* Endarterectomy
  abdominal
    artery 38.06
    vein 38.07
  aorta (arch) (ascending) (descending) 38.04

Embolectomy *(Continued)*
  head and neck NEC 38.02
  intracranial NEC 38.01
  lower limb
    artery 38.08
    vein 38.09
  thoracic NEC 38.05
  upper limb (artery) (vein) 38.03
Embolization (transcatheter)
  adhesive (glue) 39.79
    head and neck 39.72
  arteriovenous fistula 39.53
    endovascular 39.72
  artery (selective) 38.80
    by
      endovascular approach 39.79
        head and neck vessels 39.72
      percutaneous transcatheter infusion 99.29
    abdominal NEC 38.86
      duodenal (transcatheter) 44.44
      gastric (transcatheter) 44.44
      renal (transcatheter) 38.86
    aorta (arch) (ascending) (descending) 38.84
    duodenal (transcatheter) 44.44
    gastric (transcatheter) 44.44
    head and neck NEC 38.82
    intracranial NEC 38.81
    lower limb 38.88
    renal (transcatheter) 38.86
    thoracic NEC 38.85
    upper limb 38.83
  AVM intracranial, endovascular approach 39.72
  carotid cavernous fistula 39.53
  chemoembolization 99.25
  coil, endovascular 39.79
    head and neck 39.72
  vein (selective) 38.80
    by
      endovascular approach 39.79
        head and neck 39.72
    abdominal NEC 38.87
      duodenal (transcatheter) 44.44
      gastric (transcatheter) 44.44
    duodenal (transcatheter) 44.44
    gastric (transcatheter) 44.44
Embryotomy 73.8
EMG - *see* Electromyogram
Emmet operation (cervix) 67.61
Encephalocentesis - *see also* Puncture 01.09
  fetal head, transabdominal 73.8
Encephalography (cisternal puncture) (fractional) (lumbar) (pneumoencephalogram) 87.01
Encephalopuncture 01.09
Encircling procedure - *see also* Cerclage
  sclera, for buckling 14.49
    with implant 14.41
Endarterectomy (gas) (with patch graft) 38.10
  abdominal 38.16
  aorta (arch) (ascending) (descending) 38.14
  coronary artery - *see* category 36.0
    open chest approach 36.03
  head and neck (open) NEC 38.12 ◄
    percutaneous approach, intracranial vessel(s) 00.62 ◄
    percutaneous approach, precerebral (extracranial) vessel(s) 00.61 ◄

◄ **New** ◄▥ **Revised**

Endarterectomy (Continued)
  intracranial (open) NEC 38.11 ◄▦
    percutaneous approach, intracranial vessel(s) 00.62 ◄
    percutaneous approach, precerebral (extracranial) vessel(s) 00.61 ◄
  lower limb 38.18
  thoracic NEC 38.15
  upper limb 38.13
Endoaneurysmorrhaphy - see also Aneurysmorrhaphy 39.52
  by or with
    endovascular graft
      abdominal aorta 39.71
      lower extremity artery(ies) 39.79
      thoracic aorta 39.79
      upper extremity artery(ies) 39.79
Endolymphatic (-subarachnoid) shunt 20.71
Endometrectomy (uterine) (internal) 68.29
  bladder 57.59
  cul-de-sac 70.32
Endoprosthesis
  bile duct 51.87
  femoral head (bipolar) 81.52
Endoscopy
  with biopsy - see Biopsy, by site, closed
  anus 49.21
  biliary tract (operative) 51.11
    by retrograde cholangiography (ERC) 51.11
    by retrograde cholangiopancreatography (ERCP) 51.10
    intraoperative 51.11
    percutaneous (via T-tube or other tract) 51.98
      with removal of common duct stones 51.96
  bladder 57.32
    through stoma (artificial) 57.31
  bronchus NEC 33.23
    with biopsy 33.24
    fiberoptic 33.22
    through stoma (artificial) 33.21
  colon 45.23
    through stoma (artificial) 45.22
    transabdominal (operative) 45.21
  cul-de-sac 70.22
  ear 18.11
  esophagus NEC 42.23
    through stoma (artificial) 42.22
    transabdominal (operative) 42.21
  ileum 45.13
    through stoma (artificial) 45.12
    transabdominal (operative) 45.11
  intestine NEC 45.24
    large 45.24
      fiberoptic (flexible) 45.23
      through stoma (artificial) 45.22
      transabdominal (intraoperative) 45.21
    small 45.13
      esophagogastroduodenoscopy (EGD) 45.13
        with closed biopsy 45.16
      through stoma (artificial) 45.12
      transabdominal (operative) 45.11
  jejunum 45.13
    through stoma (artificial) 45.12
    transabdominal (operative) 45.11
  kidney 55.21
  larynx 31.42
    through stoma (artificial) 31.41

Endoscopy (Continued)
  lung - see Bronchoscopy
  mediastinum (transpleural) 34.22
  nasal sinus 22.19
  nose 21.21
  pancreatic duct 52.13
  pelvis 55.22
  peritoneum 54.21
  pharynx 29.11
  rectum 48.23
    through stoma (artificial) 48.22
    transabdominal (operative) 48.21
  sinus, nasal 22.19
  stomach NEC 44.13
    through stoma (artificial) 44.12
    transabdominal (operative) 44.11
  thorax (transpleural) 34.21
  trachea NEC 31.42
    through stoma (artificial) 31.41
  transpleural
    mediastinum 34.22
    thorax 34.21
  ureter 56.31
  urethra 58.22
  uterus 68.12
  vagina 70.21
Enema (transanal) NEC 96.39
  for removal of impacted feces 96.38
ENG (electronystagmogram) 95.24
Enlargement
  aortic lumen, thoracic 38.14
  atrial septal defect (pre-existing) 35.41
    in repair of total anomalous pulmonary venous connection 35.82
  eye socket 16.64
  foramen ovale (pre-existing) 35.41
    in repair of total anomalous pulmonary venous connection 35.82
  intestinal stoma 46.40
    large intestine 46.43
    small intestine 46.41
  introitus 96.16
  orbit (eye) 16.64
  palpebral fissure 08.51
  punctum 09.41
  sinus tract (skin) 86.89
Enterectomy NEC 45.63
Enteroanastomosis
  large-to-large intestine 45.94
  small-to-large intestine 45.93
  small-to-small intestine 45.91
Enterocelectomy 53.9
  female 70.92
  vaginal 70.92
Enterocentesis 45.00
  duodenum 45.01
  large intestine 45.03
  small intestine NEC 45.02
Enterocholecystostomy 51.32
Enteroclysis (small bowel) 96.43
Enterocolectomy NEC 45.79
Enterocolostomy 45.93
Enteroentectropy 46.99
Enteroenterostomy 45.90
  small-to-large intestine 45.93
  small-to-small intestine 45.91
Enterogastrostomy 44.39
  laparoscopic 44.38 ◄
Enterolithotomy 45.00
Enterolysis 54.59
  laparoscopic 54.51
Enteropancreatostomy 52.96
Enterorrhaphy 46.79
  large intestine 46.75
  small intestine 46.73

Enterostomy NEC 46.39
  cecum - see also Colostomy 46.10
  colon (transverse) - see also Colostomy 46.10
    loop 46.03
  delayed opening 46.31
  duodenum 46.39
    loop 46.01
  feeding NEC 46.39
    percutaneous (endoscopic) 46.32
  ileum (Brooke) (Dragstedt) 46.20
    loop 46.01
  jejunum (feeding) 46.39
    loop 46.01
    percutaneous (endoscopic) 46.32
  sigmoid colon - see also Colostomy 46.10
    loop 46.03
  transverse colon - see also Colostomy 46.10
    loop 46.03
Enterotomy 45.00
  large intestine 45.03
  small intestine 45.02
Enucleation - see also Excision, lesion, by site
  cyst
    broad ligament 69.19
    dental 24.4
    liver 50.29
    ovarian 65.29
      laparoscopic 65.25
    parotid gland 26.29
    salivary gland 26.29
    skin 86.3
    subcutaneous tissue 86.3
  eyeball 16.49
    with implant (into Tenon's capsule) 16.42
    with attachment of muscles 16.41
EOG (electro-oculogram) 95.22
Epicardiectomy 36.39
Epididymectomy 63.4
  with orchidectomy (unilateral) 62.3
    bilateral 62.41
Epididymogram 87.93
Epididymoplasty 63.59
Epididymorrhaphy 63.81
Epididymotomy 63.92
Epididymovasostomy 63.83
Epiglottidectomy 30.21
Epikeratophakia 11.76
Epilation
  eyebrow (forceps) 08.93
    cryosurgical 08.92
    electrosurgical 08.91
  eyelid (forceps) NEC 08.93
    cryosurgical 08.92
    electrosurgical 08.91
  skin 86.92
Epiphysiodesis - see also Arrest, bone growth - see category 78.2
Epiphysiolysis - see also Arrest, bone growth - see category 78.2
Epiploectomy 54.4
Epiplopexy 54.74
Epiplorrhaphy 54.74
Episioperineoplasty 71.79
Episioperineorrhaphy 71.71
  obstetrical 75.69
Episioplasty 71.79
Episioproctotomy 73.6

ICD-9-CM

▣

Vol. 3

> Note   Use the following fourth-digit subclassification with categories 90-91 to identify type of examination:
>
> 1 bacterial smear
> 2 culture
> 3 culture and sensitivity
> 4 parasitology
> 5 toxicology
> 6 cell block and Papanicolaou smear
> 9 other microscopic examination

◄ New   ◄█ Revised

Examination (*Continued*)
microscopic (*Continued*)
chorion 91.4
colon 90.9
cul-de-sac 91.1
dental 90.8
diaphragm 90.4
duodenum 90.8
ear 90.3
endocrine gland NEC 90.1
esophagus 90.8
eye 90.2
fallopian tube 91.4
fascia 91.5
female genital tract 91.4
fetus 91.4
gallbladder 91.0
hair 91.6
ileum 90.9
jejunum 90.9
joint fluid 91.5
kidney 91.2
large intestine 90.9
larynx 90.3
ligament 91.5
liver 91.0
lung 90.4
lymph (node) 90.7
meninges 90.0
mesentery 91.1
mouth 90.8
muscle 91.5
musculoskeletal system 91.5
nails 91.6
nerve 90.0
nervous system 90.0
nose 90.3
omentum 91.1
operative wound 91.7
ovary 91.4
pancreas 91.0
parathyroid gland 90.1
penis 91.3
perirenal tissue 91.2
peritoneum (fluid) 91.1
periureteral tissue 91.2
perivesical (tissue) 91.3
pharynx 90.3
pineal gland 90.1
pituitary gland 90.1
placenta 91.4
pleura (fluid) 90.4
prostate 91.3
rectum 90.9
retroperitoneum 91.1
semen 91.3
seminal vesicle 91.3
sigmoid 90.9
skin 91.6
small intestine 90.9
specified site NEC 91.8
spinal fluid 90.0
spleen 90.6
sputum 90.4
stomach 90.8
stool 90.9
synovial membrane 91.5
tendon 91.5
thorax NEC 90.4
throat 90.3
thymus 90.1
thyroid gland 90.1
tonsil 90.3
trachea 90.4

Examination (*Continued*)
microscopic (*Continued*)
ureter 91.2
urethra 91.3
urine 91.3
uterus 91.4
vagina 91.4
vas deferens 91.3
vomitus 90.8
vulva 91.4
neurologic 89.13
neuro-ophthalmology 95.03
ophthalmoscopic 16.21
panorex, mandible 87.12
pelvic (manual) 89.26
instrumental (by pelvimeter) 88.25
pelvimetric 88.25
physical, general 89.7
postmortem 89.8
rectum (digital) 89.34
endoscopic 48.23
through stoma (artificial) 48.22
transabdominal 48.21
retinal disease 95.03
specified type (manual) NEC 89.39
thyroid field, postoperative 06.02
uterus (digital) 68.11
endoscopic 68.12
vagina 89.26
endoscopic 70.21
visual field 95.05
Exchange transfusion 99.01
intrauterine 75.2
Excision
aberrant tissue - *see* Excision, lesion, by site of tissue origin
abscess - *see* Excision, lesion, by site
accessory tissue - *see also* Excision, lesion, by site of tissue origin
lung 32.29
endoscopic 32.28
spleen 41.93
adenoids (tag) 28.6
with tonsillectomy 28.3
adenoma - *see* Excision, lesion, by site
adrenal gland - *see also* Adrenalectomy 07.22
ampulla of Vater (with reimplantation of common duct) 51.62
anal papilla 49.39
endoscopic 49.31
aneurysm (arteriovenous) - *see also* Aneurysmectomy 38.60
coronary artery 36.91
heart 37.32
myocardium 37.32
sinus of Valsalva 35.39
ventricle (heart) 37.32
anus (complete) (partial) 49.6
aortic subvalvular ring 35.35
apocrine gland 86.3
aponeurosis 83.42
hand 82.33
appendiceal stump 47.09
laparoscopic 47.01
appendices epiploicae 54.4
appendix - *see also* Appendectomy
epididymis 63.3
testis 62.2
arcuate ligament (spine) - *omit code*
arteriovenous fistula - *see also* Aneurysmectomy 38.60
artery - *see also* Arteriectomy 38.60
Baker's cyst, knee 83.39

Excision (*Continued*)
Bartholin's gland 71.24
basal ganglion 01.59
bile duct 51.69
endoscopic 51.64
bladder - *see also* Cystectomy
bleb (emphysematous), lung 32.29
endoscopic 32.28
blood vessel - *see also* Angiectomy 38.60
bone (ends) (partial), except facial - *see* category 77.8
facial NEC 76.39
total 76.45
with reconstruction 76.44
for graft (autograft) (homograft) - *see* category 77.7
fragments (chips) - *see also* Incision, bone 77.10
joint - *see also* Arthrotomy 80.10
necrotic - *see also* Sequestrectomy, bone 77.00
heterotopic, from
muscle 83.32
hand 82.22
skin 86.3
tendon 83.31
hand 82.21
mandible 76.31
with arthrodesis - *see* Arthrodesis
total 76.42
with reconstruction 76.41
spur - *see* Excision, lesion, bone
total, except facial - *see* category 77.9
facial NEC 76.45
with reconstruction 76.44
mandible 76.42
with reconstruction 76.41
brain 01.59
hemisphere 01.52
lobe 01.53
branchial cleft cyst or vestige 29.2
breast - *see also* Mastectomy 85.41
aberrant tissue 85.24
accessory 85.24
ectopic 85.24
nipple 85.25
accessory 85.24
segmental 85.23
supernumerary 85.24
wedge 85.21
broad ligament 69.19
bronchogenic cyst 32.09
endoscopic 32.01
bronchus (wide sleeve) NEC 32.1
buccal mucosa 27.49
bulbourethral gland 58.92
bulbous tuberosities (mandible) (maxilla) (fibrous) (osseous) 24.31
bunion - *see also* Bunionectomy 77.59
bunionette (with osteotomy) 77.54
bursa 83.5
hand 82.31
canal of Nuck 69.19
cardioma 37.33
carotid body (lesion) (partial) (total) 39.8
cartilage - *see also* Chondrectomy 80.90
intervertebral - *see* category 80.5
knee (semilunar) 80.6
larynx 30.29
nasal (submucous) 21.5
caruncle, urethra 58.39
endoscopic 58.31
cataract - *see also* Extraction, cataract 13.19

ICD-9-CM Vol. 3

Excision *(Continued)*
  cataract *(Continued)*
    secondary membrane (after cataract) 13.65
  cervical
    rib 77.91
    stump 67.4
  cervix (stump) NEC 67.4
    cold (knife) 67.2
    conization 67.2
    cryoconization 67.33
    electroconization 67.32
  chalazion (multiple) (single) 08.21
  cholesteatoma - *see* Excision, lesion, by site
  choroid plexus 02.14
  cicatrix (skin) 86.3
  cilia base 08.20
  ciliary body, prolapsed 12.98
  clavicle (head) (partial) 77.81
    total (complete) 77.91
  clitoris 71.4
  coarctation of aorta (end-to-end anastomosis) 38.64
    with
      graft replacement (interposition)
        abdominal 38.44
        thoracic 38.45
        thoracoabdominal 38.45 *[38.44]*
  common
    duct 51.63
    wall between posterior and coronary sinus (with roofing or resultant defect with patch graft) 35.82
  condyle - *see* category 77.8
    mandible 76.5
  conjunctival ring 10.31
  cornea 11.49
    epithelium (with chemocauterization) 11.41
      for smear or culture 11.21
  costal cartilage 80.99
  cul-de-sac (Douglas') 70.92
  cusp, heart valve 35.10
    aortic 35.11
    mitral 35.12
    tricuspid 35.14
  cyst - *see also* Excision, lesion, by site
    apical (tooth) 23.73
      with root canal therapy 23.72
    Baker's (popliteal) 83.39
    breast 85.21
    broad ligament 69.19
    bronchogenic 32.09
      endoscopic 32.01
    cervix 67.39
    dental 24.4
    dentigerous 24.4
    epididymis 63.2
    fallopian tube 66.61
    Gartner's duct 70.33
    hand 82.29
    labia 71.3
    lung 32.29
      endoscopic 32.28
    mesonephric duct 69.19
    Morgagni
      female 66.61
      male 62.2
    mullerian duct 60.73
    nasolabial 27.49
    nasopalatine 27.31
      by wide excision 27.32
    ovary 65.29
      laparoscopic 65.25

Excision *(Continued)*
  cyst *(Continued)*
    parovarian 69.19
    pericardium 37.31
    periodontal (apical) (lateral) 24.4
    popliteal (Baker's), knee 83.39
    radicular 24.4
    spleen 41.42
    synovial (membrane) 83.39
    thyroglossal (with resection of hyoid bone) 06.7
    urachal (bladder) 57.51
      abdominal wall 54.3
    vagina (Gartner's duct) 70.33
  cystic
    duct remnant 51.61
    hygroma 40.29
  dentinoma 24.4
  diaphragm 34.81
  disc, intervertebral NOS 80.50
    herniated (nucleus pulposus) 80.51
    other specified (diskectomy) 80.51
  diverticulum
    ampulla of Vater 51.62
    anus 49.39
      endoscopic 49.31
    bladder 57.59
      transurethral 57.49
    duodenum 45.31
      endoscopic 45.30
    esophagus (local) 42.31
      endoscopic 42.33
    hypopharyngeal (by cricopharyngeal myotomy) 29.32
    intestine
      large 45.41
        endoscopic 45.43
      small NEC 45.33
    Meckel's 45.33
    pharyngeal (by cricopharyngeal myotomy) 29.32
    pharyngoesophageal (by cricopharyngeal myotomy) 29.32
    stomach 43.42
      endoscopic 43.41
    urethra 58.39
      endoscopic 58.31
    ventricle, heart 37.33
  duct
    mullerian 69.19
    paramesonephric 69.19
    thyroglossal (with resection of hyoid bone) 06.7
  ear, external (complete) NEC 18.39
    partial 18.29
      radical 18.31
  ectopic
    abdominal fetus 74.3
    tissue - *see also* Excision, lesion, by site of tissue origin
      bone, from muscle 83.32
      breast 85.24
      lung 32.29
        endoscopic 32.28
      spleen 41.93
  empyema pocket, lung 34.09
  epididymis 63.4
  epiglottis 30.21
  epithelial downgrowth, anterior chamber (eye) 12.93
  epulis (gingiva) 24.31
  esophagus - *see also* Esophagectomy 42.40
  exostosis - *see also* Excision, lesion, bone 77.60

Excision *(Continued)*
  exostosis *(Continued)*
    auditory canal, external 18.29
    facial bone 76.2
    first metatarsal (hallux valgus repair) - *see* Bunionectomy
  eye 16.49
    with implant (into Tenon's capsule) 16.42
    with attachment of muscles 16.41
  eyelid 08.20
    redundant skin 08.86
  falciform ligament 54.4
  fallopian tube - *see* Salpingectomy
  fascia 83.44
    for graft 83.43
      hand 82.34
    hand 82.35
      for graft 82.34
  fat pad NEC 86.3
    knee (infrapatellar) (prepatellar) 86.3
    scalene 40.21
  fibroadenoma, breast 85.21
  fissure, anus 49.39
    endoscopic 49.31
  fistula - *see also* Fistulectomy
    anal 49.12
    arteriovenous - *see also* Aneurysmectomy 38.60
    ileorectal 46.74
    lacrimal
      gland 09.21
      sac 09.6
    rectal 48.73
    vesicovaginal 57.84
  frenulum, frenum
    labial (lip) 27.41
    lingual (tongue) 25.92
  ganglion (hand) (tendon sheath) (wrist) 82.21
    gasserian 04.05
    site other than hand or nerve 83.31
    sympathetic nerve 05.29
    trigeminal nerve 04.05
  gastrocolic ligament 54.4
  gingiva 24.31
  glomus jugulare tumor 20.51
  goiter - *see* Thyroidectomy
  gum 24.31
  hallux valgus - *see also* Bunionectomy
    with prosthetic implant 77.59
  hamartoma, mammary 85.21
  heart assist system - *see* Removal ◄
  hematocele, tunica vaginalis 61.92
  hematoma - *see* Drainage, by site
  hemorrhoids (external) (internal) (tag) 49.46
  heterotopic bone, from
    muscle 83.32
      hand 82.22
    skin 86.3
    tendon 83.31
      hand 82.21
  hydatid of Morgagni
    female 66.61
    male 62.2
  hydatid cyst, liver 50.29
  hydrocele
    canal of Nuck (female) 69.19
    male 63.1
    round ligament 69.19
    spermatic cord 63.1
    tunica vaginalis 61.2
  hygroma, cystic 40.29

◄ New   ◄⊪ Revised

Excision (*Continued*)
  hymen (tag) 70.31
  hymeno-urethral fusion 70.31
  intervertebral disc - *see* Excision, disc,
      intervertebral (NOS) 80.50
  intestine - *see also* Resection, intestine
      45.8
    for interposition 45.50
      large 45.52
      small 45.51
    large (total) 45.8
      for interposition 45.52
      local 45.41
        endoscopic 45.43
      segmental 45.79
        multiple 45.71
    small (total) 45.63
      for interposition 45.51
      local 45.33
      partial 45.62
      segmental 45.62
        multiple 45.61
  intraductal papilloma 85.21
  iris prolapse 12.13
  joint - *see also* Arthrectomy 80.90
  keloid (scar), skin 86.3
  labia - *see* Vulvectomy
  lacrimal
    gland 09.20
      partial 09.22
      total 09.23
    passage 09.6
    sac 09.6
  lesion (local)
    abdominal wall 54.3
    accessory sinus - *see* Excision, lesion,
        nasal sinus
    adenoids 28.92
    adrenal gland(s) 07.21
    alveolus 24.4
    ampulla of Vater 51.62
    anterior chamber (eye) NEC 12.40
    anus 49.39
      endoscopic 49.31
    apocrine gland 86.3
    artery 38.60
      abdominal 38.66
      aorta (arch) (ascending) (descend-
          ing thoracic) 38.64
        with end-to-end anastomosis
            38.45
          abdominal 38.44
          thoracic 38.45
          thoracoabdominal 38.45
              [38.44]
        with graft interposition graft re-
            placement 38.45
          abdominal 38.44
          thoracic 38.45
          thoracoabdominal 38.45
              [38.44]
      head and neck NEC 38.62
      intracranial NEC 38.61
      lower limb 38.68
      thoracic NEC 38.65
      upper limb 38.63
    atrium 37.33
    auditory canal or meatus, external
        18.29
      radical 18.31
    auricle, ear 18.29
      radical 18.31
    biliary ducts 51.69
      endoscopic 51.64

Excision (*Continued*)
  lesion (*Continued*)
    bladder (transurethral) 57.49
      open 57.59
      suprapubic 57.59
    blood vessel 38.60
      abdominal
        artery 38.66
        vein 38.67
      aorta (arch) (ascending) (descend-
          ing) 38.64
      head and neck NEC 38.62
      intracranial NEC 38.61
      lower limb
        artery 38.68
        vein 38.69
      thoracic NEC 38.65
      upper limb (artery) (vein) 38.63
    bone 77.60
      carpal, metacarpal 77.64
      clavicle 77.61
      facial 76.2
      femur 77.65
      fibula 77.67
      humerus 77.62
      jaw 76.2
        dental 24.4
      patella 77.66
      pelvic 77.69
      phalanges (foot) (hand) 77.69
      radius 77.63
      scapula 77.61
      skull 01.6
      specified site NEC 77.69
      tarsal, metatarsal 77.68
      thorax (ribs) (sternum) 77.61
      tibia 77.67
      ulna 77.63
      vertebrae 77.69
    brain (transtemporal approach) NEC
        01.59
      by stereotactic radiosurgery 92.30
        cobalt 60 92.32
        linear accelerator (LINAC) 92.31
        multi-source 92.32
        particle beam 92.33
        particulate 92.33
        radiosurgery NEC 92.39
        single source photon 92.31
    breast (segmental) (wedge) 85.21
    broad ligament 69.19
    bronchus NEC 32.09
      endoscopic 32.01
    cerebral (cortex) NEC 01.59
      meninges 01.51
    cervix (myoma) 67.39
    chest wall 34.4
    choroid plexus 02.14
    ciliary body 12.44
    colon 45.41
      endoscopic NEC 45.43
        polypectomy 45.42
    conjunctiva 10.31
    cornea 11.49
    cranium 01.6
    cul-de-sac (Douglas') 70.32
    dental (jaw) 24.4
    diaphragm 34.81
    duodenum (local) 45.31
      endoscopic 45.30
    ear, external 18.29
      radical 18.31
    endometrium 68.29
    epicardium 37.31

Excision (*Continued*)
  lesion (*Continued*)
    epididymis 63.3
    epiglottis 30.09
    esophagus NEC 42.32
      endoscopic 42.33
    eye, eyeball 16.93
      anterior segment NEC 12.40
    eyebrow (skin) 08.20
    eyelid 08.20
      by
        halving procedure 08.24
        wedge resection 08.24
      major
        full-thickness 08.24
        partial-thickness 08.23
      minor 08.22
    fallopian tube 66.61
    fascia 83.39
      hand 82.29
    groin region (abdominal wall) (in-
        guinal) 54.3
      skin 86.3
      subcutaneous tissue 86.3
    gum 24.31
    heart 37.33
    hepatic duct 51.69
    inguinal canal 54.3
    intestine
      large 45.41
        endoscopic NEC 45.43
          polypectomy 45.42
      small NEC 45.33
    intracranial NEC 01.59
    intranasal 21.31
    intraspinal 03.4
    iris 12.42
    jaw 76.2
      dental 24.4
    joint 80.80
      ankle 80.87
      elbow 80.82
      foot and toe 80.88
      hand and finger 80.84
      hip 80.85
      knee 80.86
      shoulder 80.81
      specified site NEC 80.89
      spine 80.89
      wrist 80.83
    kidney 55.39
      with partial nephrectomy 55.4
    labia 71.3
    lacrimal
      gland (frontal approach) 09.21
      passage 09.6
      sac 09.6
    larynx 30.09
    ligament (joint) - *see also* Excision, le-
        sion, joint 80.80
      broad 69.19
      round 69.19
      uterosacral 69.19
    lip 27.43
      by wide excision 27.42
    liver 50.29
    lung NEC 32.29
      by lung volume reduction surgery
          32.22
      by wide excision 32.3
      endoscopic 32.28
    lymph structure(s) (channel) (vessel)
        NEC 40.29
      node - *see* Excision, lymph, node

ICD-9-CM

Vol. 3

Excision *(Continued)*
lesion *(Continued)*
mammary duct 85.21
mastoid (bone) 20.49
mediastinum 34.3
meninges (cerebral) 01.51
spinal 03.4
mesentery 54.4
middle ear 20.51
mouth NEC 27.49
muscle 83.32
hand 82.22
ocular 15.13
myocardium 37.33
nail 86.23
nasal sinus 22.60
antrum 22.62
with Caldwell-Luc approach 22.61
specified approach NEC 22.62
ethmoid 22.63
frontal 22.42
maxillary 22.62
with Caldwell-Luc approach 22.61
specified approach NEC 22.62
sphenoid 22.64
nasopharynx 29.3
nerve (cranial) (peripheral) 04.07
sympathetic 05.29
nonodontogenic 24.31
nose 21.30
intranasal 21.31
polyp 21.31
skin 21.32
specified site NEC 21.32
odontogenic 24.4
omentum 54.4
orbit 16.92
ovary 65.29
by wedge resection 65.22
laparoscopic 65.24
that by laparoscope 65.25
palate (bony) 27.31
by wide excision 27.32
soft 27.49
pancreas (local) 52.22
endoscopic 52.21
parathyroid 06.89
parotid gland or duct NEC 26.29
pelvic wall 54.3
pelvirectal tissue 48.82
penis 64.2
pericardium 37.31
perineum (female) 71.3
male 86.3
periprostatic tissue 60.82
perirectal tissue 48.82
perirenal tissue 59.91
peritoneum 54.4
perivesical tissue 59.91
pharynx 29.3
diverticulum 29.32
pineal gland 07.53
pinna 18.29
radical 18.31
pituitary (gland) - *see also* Hypophysectomy, partial 07.63
by stereotactic radiosurgery 92.30
cobalt 60 92.32
linear accelerator (LINAC) 92.31

Excision *(Continued)*
lesion *(Continued)*
pituitary *(Continued)*
by stereotactic radiosurgery *(Continued)*
multi-source 92.32
particle beam 92.33
particulate 92.33
radiosurgery NEC 92.39
single source photon 92.31
pleura 34.59
pouch of Douglas 70.32
preauricular (ear) 18.21
presacral 54.4
prostate (transurethral) 60.61
pulmonary (fibrosis) 32.29
endoscopic 32.28
rectovaginal septum 48.82
rectum 48.35
polyp (endoscopic) 48.36
retroperitoneum 54.4
salivary gland or duct NEC 26.29
en bloc 26.32
sclera 12.84
scrotum 61.3
sinus (nasal) - *see* Excision, lesion, nasal sinus
Skene's gland 71.3
skin 86.3
breast 85.21
nose 21.32
radical (wide) (involving underlying or adjacent structure)
(with flap closure) 86.4
scrotum 61.3
skull 01.6
soft tissue NEC 83.39
hand 82.29
spermatic cord 63.3
sphincter of Oddi 51.62
endoscopic 51.64
spinal cord (meninges) 03.4
spleen (cyst) 41.42
stomach NEC 43.42
endoscopic 43.41
polyp 43.41
polyp (endoscopic) 43.41
subcutaneous tissue 86.3
breast 85.21
subgingival 24.31
sweat gland 86.3
tendon 83.39
hand 82.29
ocular 15.13
sheath 83.31
hand 82.21
testis 62.2
thorax 34.4
thymus 07.81
thyroid 06.31
substernal or transsternal route 06.51
tongue 25.1
tonsil 28.92
trachea 31.5
tunica vaginalis 61.92
ureter 56.41
urethra 58.39
endoscopic 58.31
uterine ligament 69.19
uterosacral ligament 69.19
uterus 68.29
vagina 70.33
vein 38.60

Excision *(Continued)*
leision *(Continued)*
vein *(Continued)*
abdominal 38.67
head and neck NEC 38.62
intracranial NEC 38.61
lower limb 38.69
thoracic NEC 38.65
upper limb 38.63
ventricle (heart) 37.33
vocal cords 30.09
vulva 71.3
ligament - *see also* Arthrectomy 80.90
broad 69.19
round 69.19
uterine 69.19
uterosacral 69.19
ligamentum flavum (spine) - *omit code*
lingual tonsil 28.5
lip 27.43
liver (partial) 50.22
loose body
bone - *see* Sequestrectomy, bone
joint 80.10
lung (complete) (with mediastinal dissection) 32.5
accessory or ectopic tissue 32.29
endoscopic 32.28
segmental 32.3
specified type NEC 32.29
endoscopic 32.28
volume reduction surgery 32.22
wedge 32.29
lymph, lymphatic
drainage area 40.29
radical - *see* Excision, lymph, node, radical
regional (with lymph node, skin, subcutaneous tissue, and fat) 40.3
node (simple) NEC 40.29
with
lymphatic drainage area (including skin, subcutaneous tissue, and fat) 40.3
mastectomy - *see* Mastectomy, radical
muscle and deep fascia - *see* Excision, lymph, node, radical
axillary 40.23
radical 40.51
regional (extended) 40.3
cervical (deep) (with excision of
scalene fat pad) 40.21
with laryngectomy 30.4
radical (including muscle and deep fascia) 40.40
bilateral 40.42
unilateral 40.41
regional (extended) 40.3
superficial 40.29
groin 40.24
radical 40.54
regional (extended) 40.3
iliac 40.29
radical 40.53
regional (extended) 40.3
inguinal (deep) (superficial) 40.24
radical 40.54
regional (extended) 40.3
jugular - *see* Excision, lymph, node, cervical
mammary (internal) 40.22

Excision (*Continued*)
 lymph, lymphatic (*Continued*)
  node (*Continued*)
   mammary (*Continued*)
    external 40.29
     radical 40.59
      regional (extended) 40.3
    radical 40.59
     regional (extended) 40.3
    paratracheal - *see* Excision, lymph, node, cervical
    periaortic 40.29
     radical 40.52
      regional (extended) 40.3
    radical 40.50
     with mastectomy - *see* Mastectomy, radical
     specified site NEC 40.59
    regional (extended) 40.3
    sternal - *see* Excision, lymph, node, mammary
   structure(s) (simple) NEC 40.29
    radical 40.59
    regional (extended) 40.3
 lymphangioma (simple) - *see also* Excision, lymph, lymphatic, node, 40.29
 lymphocele 40.29
 mastoid - *see also* Mastoidectomy 20.49
 median bar, transurethral approach 60.29
 meibomian gland 08.20
 meniscus (knee) 80.6
  acromioclavicular 80.91
  jaw 76.5
  sternoclavicular 80.91
  temporomandibular (joint) 76.5
  wrist 80.93
 mullerian duct cyst 60.73
 muscle 83.45
  for graft 83.43
   hand 82.34
  hand 82.36
   for graft 82.34
 myositis ossificans 83.32
  hand 82.22
 nail (bed) (fold) 86.23
 nasolabial cyst 27.49
 nasopalatine cyst 27.31
  by wide excision 27.32
 neoplasm - *see* Excision, lesion, by site
 nerve (cranial) (peripheral) NEC 04.07
  sympathetic 05.29
 neuroma (Morton's) (peripheral nerve) 04.07
  acoustic
   by craniotomy 04.01
   by stereotactic radiosurgery 92.30
    cobalt 60 92.32
    linear accelerator (LINAC) 92.31
    multi-source 92.32
    particle beam 92.33
    particulate 92.33
    radiosurgery NEC 92.39
    single source photon 92.31
  sympathetic nerve 05.29
 nipple 85.25
  accessory 85.24
 odontoma 24.4
 orbital contents - *see also* Exenteration, orbit 16.59
 osteochondritis dissecans - *see also* Excision, lesion, joint 80.80

Excision (*Continued*)
 ovary - *see also* Oophorectomy
  partial 65.29
   by wedge resection 65.22
    laparoscopic 65.24
   that by laparoscope 65.25
 Pancoast tumor (lung) 32.6
 pancreas (total) (with synchronous duodenectomy) 52.6
  partial NEC 52.59
   distal (tail) (with part of body) 52.52
   proximal (head) (with part of body) (with synchronous duodenectomy) 52.51
   radical subtotal 52.53
  radical (one-stage) (two-stage) 52.7
  subtotal 52.53
 paramesonephric duct 69.19
 parathyroid gland (partial) (subtotal) NEC - *see also* Parathyroidectomy 06.89
 parotid gland - *see also* Excision, salivary gland 26.30
 parovarian cyst 69.19
 patella (complete) 77.96
  partial 77.86
 pelvirectal tissue 48.82
 perianal tissue 49.04
  skin tags 49.03
 pericardial adhesions 37.31
 periprostatic tissue 60.82
 perirectal tissue 48.82
 perirenal tissue 59.91
 periurethral tissue 58.92
 perivesical tissue 59.91
 petrous apex cells 20.59
 pharyngeal bands 29.54
 pharynx (partial) 29.33
 pilonidal cyst or sinus (open) (with partial closure) 86.21
 pineal gland (complete) (total) 07.54
  partial 07.53
 pituitary gland (complete) (total) - *see also* Hypophysectomy 07.69
 pleura NEC 34.59
 polyp - *see also* Excision, lesion, by site
  esophagus 42.32
   endoscopic 42.33
  large intestine 45.41
   endoscopic 45.42
  nose 21.31
  rectum (endoscopic) 48.36
  stomach (endoscopic) 43.41
 preauricular
  appendage (remnant) 18.29
  cyst, fistula, or sinus (congenital) 18.21
  remnant 18.29
 prolapsed iris (in wound) 12.13
 prostate - *see* Prostatectomy
 pterygium (simple) 11.39
  with corneal graft 11.32
 radius (head) (partial) 77.83
  total 77.93
 ranula, salivary gland NEC 26.29
 rectal mucosa 48.35
 rectum - *see* Resection, rectum
 redundant mucosa
  colostomy 45.41
   endoscopic 45.43
  duodenostomy 45.31
   endoscopic 45.30
  ileostomy 45.33
  jejunostomy 45.33

Excision (*Continued*)
 redundant mucosa (*Continued*)
  perineum 71.3
  rectum 48.35
  vulva 71.3
 renal vessel, aberrant 38.66
 rib (cervical) 77.91
 ring of conjunctiva around cornea 10.31
 round ligament 69.19
 salivary gland 26.30
  complete 26.32
  partial 26.31
  radical 26.32
 scalene fat pad 40.21
 scar - *see also* Excision, lesion, by site
  epicardium 37.31
  mastoid 20.92
  pericardium 37.31
  pleura 34.59
  skin 86.3
  thorax 34.4
 secondary membrane, lens 13.65
 seminal vesicle 60.73
  with radical prostatectomy 60.5
 septum - *see also* Excision, by site
  uterus (congenital) 68.22
  vagina 70.33
 sinus - *see also* Excision, lesion, by site
  nasal - *see* Sinusectomy
  pilonidal 86.21
  preauricular (ear) (radical) 18.21
  tarsi 80.88
  thyroglossal (with resection of hyoid bone) 06.7
  urachal (bladder) 57.51
   abdominal wall 54.3
 Skene's gland 71.3
 skin (local) 86.3
  for graft (with closure of donor site) 86.91
  radical (wide) (involving underlying or adjacent structure) (with flap closure) 86.4
  tags
   perianal 49.03
   periauricular 18.29
 soft tissue NEC 83.49
  hand 82.39
 spermatocele 63.2
 spinous process 77.89
 spleen (total) 41.5
  accessory 41.93
  partial 41.43
 stomach - *see* Gastrectomy
 sublingual gland (salivary) - *see also* Excision, salivary gland 26.30
 submaxillary gland - *see also* Excision, salivary gland 26.30
 supernumerary
  breast 85.24
  digits 86.26
 sweat gland 86.3
 synechiae - *see also* Lysis, synechiae
  endometrial 68.21
 tarsal plate (eyelid) 08.20
  by wedge resection 08.24
 tattoo 86.3
  by dermabrasion 86.25
 tendon (sheath) 83.42
  for graft 83.41
   hand 82.32
  hand 82.33
   for graft 82.32

ICD-9-CM

E

Vol.

Excision *(Continued)*
  thymus - *see also* Thymectomy 07.80
  thyroglossal duct or tract (with resection of hyoid bone) 06.7
  thyroid NEC - *see also* Thyroidectomy 06.39
  tongue (complete) (total) 25.3
    partial or subtotal 25.2
    radical 25.4
  tonsil 28.2
    with adenoidectomy 28.3
    lingual 28.5
    tag 28.4
  tooth NEC - *see also* Removal, tooth, surgical 23.19
    from nasal sinus 22.60
  torus
    lingual 76.2
    mandible, mandibularis 76.2
    palate, palatinus 27.31
      by wide excision 27.32
  trabeculae carneae cordis (heart) 35.35
  trochanteric lipomatosis 86.83
  tumor - *see* Excision, lesion, by site
  ulcer - *see also* Excision, lesion, by site
    duodenum 45.31
      endoscopic 45.30
    stomach 43.42
      endoscopic 43.41
  umbilicus 54.3
  urachus, urachal (cyst) (bladder) 57.51
    abdominal wall 54.3
  ureter, ureteral 56.40
    with nephrectomy - *see* Nephrectomy
    partial 56.41
    stricture 56.41
    total 56.42
  ureterocele 56.41
  urethra, urethral 58.39
    with complete cystectomy 57.79
    endoscopic 58.31
    septum 58.0
    stricture 58.39
      endoscopic 58.31
    valve (congenital) 58.39
      endoscopic (transurethral) (transvesical) 58.31
  urethrovaginal septum 70.33
  uterus (corpus) - *see also* Hysterectomy 68.9
    cervix 67.4
      lesion 67.39
    lesion 68.29
    septum 68.22
  uvula 27.72
  vagina (total) 70.4
  varicocele, spermatic cord 63.1
  vein - *see also* Phlebectomy 38.60
    varicose 38.50
      abdominal 38.57
      head and neck NEC 38.52
      intracranial NEC 38.51
      lower limb 38.59
      ovarian 38.67
      thoracic NEC 38.55
      upper limb 38.53
  verucca - *see also* Excision, lesion, by site
    eyelid 08.22
  vesicovaginal septum 70.33
  vitreous opacity 14.74
    anterior approach 14.73

Excision *(Continued)*
  vocal cord(s) (submucous) 30.22
  vulva (bilateral) (simple) - *see also* Vulvectomy 71.62
  wart - *see also* Excision, lesion, by site
    eyelid 08.22
  wolffian duct 69.19
  xanthoma (tendon sheath, hand) 82.21
    site other than hand 83.31
Excisional biopsy - *see* Biopsy
Exclusion, pyloric 44.39
  laparoscopic 44.38 ◄
Exenteration
  ethmoid air cells 22.63
  orbit 16.59
    with
      removal of adjacent structures 16.51
      temporalis muscle transplant 16.59
      therapeutic removal of bone 16.52
  pelvic (organs) (female) 68.8
    male 57.71
  petrous pyramid air cells 20.59
Exercise (physical therapy) NEC 93.19
  active musculoskeletal NEC 93.12
  assisting 93.11
    in pool 93.31
  breathing 93.18
  musculoskeletal
    active NEC 93.12
    passive NEC 93.17
  neurologic 89.13
  passive musculoskeletal NEC 93.17
  resistive 93.13
Exfoliation, skin, by chemical 86.24
Exostectomy - *see also* Excision, lesion, bone 77.60
  first metatarsal (hallux valgus repair) - *see* Bunionectomy
  hallux valgus repair (with wedge osteotomy) - *see* Bunionectomy
Expiratory flow rate 89.38
Explant, explanation - *see* Removal ◄
Exploration - *see also* Incision
  abdomen 54.11
  abdominal wall 54.0
  adrenal (gland) 07.41
    field 07.00
      bilateral 07.02
      unilateral 07.01
  artery 38.00
    abdominal 38.06
    aorta (arch) (ascending) (descending) 38.04
    head and neck NEC 38.02
    intracranial NEC 38.01
    lower limb 38.08
    thoracic NEC 38.05
    upper limb 38.03
  auditory canal, external 18.02
  axilla 86.09
  bile duct(s) 51.59
    common duct 51.51
      endoscopic 51.11
      for
        relief of obstruction 51.42
          endoscopic 51.84
        removal of calculus 51.41
          endoscopic 51.88
      laparoscopic 51.11
    for relief of obstruction 51.49
      endoscopic 51.84
  bladder (by incision) 57.19
    endoscopic 57.32
      through stoma (artificial) 57.31

Exploration *(Continued)*
  bone - *see also* Incision, bone 77.10
  brain (tissue) 01.39
  breast 85.0
  bronchus 33.0
    endoscopic - *see* Bronchoscopy
  bursa 83.03
    hand 82.03
  carotid body 39.8
  carpal tunnel 04.43
  choroid 14.9
  ciliary body 12.44
  colon 45.03
  common bile duct 51.51
    endoscopic 51.11
    for
      relief of obstruction 51.42
        endoscopic 51.84
      removal of calculus 51.41
        endoscopic 51.88
  coronary artery 36.99
  cranium 01.24
  cul-de-sac 70.12
    endoscopic 70.22
  disc space 03.09
  duodenum 45.01
  endoscopic - *see* Endoscopy, by site
  epididymis 63.92
  esophagus (by incision) NEC 42.09
    endoscopic - *see* Esophagoscopy
  ethmoid sinus 22.51
  eyelid 08.09
  fallopian tube 66.01
  fascia 83.09
    hand 82.09
  flank 54.0
  fossa (superficial) NEC 86.09
    pituitary 07.71
  frontal sinus 22.41
  frontonasal duct 96.21
  gallbladder 51.04
  groin (region) (abdominal wall) (inguinal) 54.0
    skin and subcutaneous tissue 86.09
  heart 37.11
  hepatic duct 51.59
  hypophysis 07.72
  ileum 45.02
  inguinal canal (groin) 54.0
  intestine (by incision) NEC 45.00
    large 45.03
    small 45.02
  intrathoracic 34.02
  jejunum 45.02
  joint structures - *see also* Arthrotomy 80.10
  kidney 55.01
    pelvis 55.11
  labia 71.09
  lacrimal
    gland 09.0
    sac 09.53
  laparotomy site 54.12
  larynx (by incision) 31.3
    endoscopic 31.42
  liver 50.0
  lung (by incision) 33.1
  lymphatic structure(s) (channel) (node) (vessel) 40.0
  mastoid 20.21
  maxillary antrum or sinus (Caldwell-Luc approach) 22.39
  mediastinum 34.1
    endoscopic 34.22

◄ **New**   ◄═ **Revised**

ICD-9-CM

Vol. 3

Extraction *(Continued)*
  cataract *(Continued)*
    intracapsular *(Continued)*
      by temporal inferior route (in presence of fistulization bleb) 13.11
      linear extraction (extracapsular approach) 13.2
      phacoemulsification (and aspiration) 13.41
      phacofragmentation (mechanical)
        with aspiration by
          posterior route 13.42
          specified route NEC 13.43
        ultrasonic 13.41
      rotoextraction (mechanical)
        with aspiration by
          posterior route 13.42
          specified route NEC 13.43

Extraction *(Continued)*
  cataract *(Continued)*
    secondary membranous (after cataract) (by)
      capsulectomy 13.65
      capsulotomy 13.64
      discission 13.64
      excision 13.65
      iridocapsulectomy 13.65
      mechanical fragmentation 13.66
      needling 13.64
      phacofragmentation (mechanical) 13.66
  common duct stones (percutaneous) (through sinus tract) (with basket) 51.96
  foreign body - *see* Removal, foreign body
  kidney stone(s), percutaneous 55.03
    with fragmentation procedure 55.04

Extraction *(Continued)*
  lens (eye) - *see also* Extraction, cataract 13.19
  Malstrom's 72.79
    with episiotomy 72.71
  menstrual, menses 69.6
  milk from lactating breast (manual) (pump) 99.98
  tooth (by forceps) (multiple) (single) NEC 23.09
    with mucoperiosteal flap elevation 23.19
    deciduous 23.01
    surgical NEC - *see also* Removal, tooth, surgical 23.19
  vacuum, fetus 72.79
    with episiotomy 72.71
  vitreous - *see also* Removal, vitreous 14.72

F

Face lift 86.82
Facetectomy 77.89
Facilitation, intraocular circulation NEC 12.59
Failed (trial) forceps 73.3
Family
    counselling (medical) (social) 94.49
    therapy 94.42
Farabeuf operation (ischiopubiotomy) 77.39
Fasanella-Servatt operation (blepharoptosis repair) 08.35
Fasciaplasty - see Fascioplasty
Fascia sling operation - see Operation, sling
Fasciectomy 83.44
    for graft 83.43
        hand 82.34
    hand 82.35
        for graft 82.34
    palmar (release of Dupuytren's contracture) 82.35
Fasciodesis 83.89
    hand 82.89
Fascioplasty - see also Repair, fascia 83.89
    hand - see also Repair, fascia, hand 82.89
Fasciorrhaphy - see Suture, fascia
Fasciotomy 83.14
    Dupuytren's 82.12
        with excision 82.35
    Dwyer 83.14
    hand 82.12
    Ober-Yount 83.14
    orbital - see also Orbitotomy 16.09
    palmar (release of Dupuytren's contracture) 82.12
        with excision 82.35
Fenestration
    aneurysm (dissecting), thoracic aorta 39.54
    aortic aneurysm 39.54
    cardiac valve 35.10
    chest wall 34.01
    ear
        inner (with graft) 20.61
            revision 20.62
        tympanic 19.55
    labyrinth (with graft) 20.61
    Lempert's (endaural) 19.9
    operation (aorta) 39.54
    oval window, ear canal 19.55
    palate 27.1
    pericardium 37.12
    semicircular canals (with graft) 20.61
    stapes foot plate (with vein graft) 19.19
        with incus replacement 19.11
    tympanic membrane 19.55
    vestibule (with graft) 20.61
Ferguson operation (hernia repair) 53.00
Fetography 87.81
Fetoscopy 75.31
Fiberoscopy - see Endoscopy, by site
Fibroidectomy, uterine 68.29
Fick operation (perforation of foot plate) 19.0
Filipuncture (aneurysm) (cerebral) 39.52
Filleting
    hammer toe 77.56
    pancreas 52.3

Filling, tooth (amalgam) (plastic) (silicate) 23.2
    root canal - see also Therapy, root canal 23.70
Fimbriectomy - see also Salpingectomy, partial 66.69
    Uchida (with tubal ligation) 66.32
Finney operation (pyloroplasty) 44.29
Fissurectomy, anal 49.39
    endoscopic 49.31
    skin (subcutaneous tissue) 49.04
Fistulectomy - see also Closure, fistula, by site
    abdominothoracic 34.83
    abdominouterine 69.42
    anus 49.12
    appendix 47.92
    bile duct 51.79
    biliary tract NEC 51.79
    bladder (transurethral approach) 57.84
    bone - see also Excision, lesion, bone 77.60
    branchial cleft 29.52
    bronchocutaneous 33.42
    bronchoesophageal 33.42
    bronchomediastinal 34.73
    bronchopleural 34.73
    bronchopleurocutaneous 34.73
    bronchopleuromediastinal 34.73
    bronchovisceral 33.42
    cervicosigmoidal 67.62
    cholecystogastroenteric 51.93
    cornea 11.49
    diaphragm 34.83
    enterouterine 69.42
    esophagopleurocutaneous 34.73
    esophagus NEC 42.84
    fallopian tube 66.73
    gallbladder 51.93
    gastric NEC 44.63
    hepatic duct 51.79
    hepatopleural 34.73
    hepatopulmonary 34.73
    intestine
        large 46.76
        small 46.74
    intestinouterine 69.42
    joint - see also Excision, lesion, joint 80.80
    lacrimal
        gland 09.21
        sac 09.6
    laryngotracheal 31.62
    larynx 31.62
    mediastinocutaneous 34.73
    mouth NEC 27.53
    nasal 21.82
        sinus 22.71
    nasolabial 21.82
    nasopharyngeal 21.82
    oroantral 22.71
    oronasal 21.82
    pancreas 52.95
    perineorectal 71.72
    perineosigmoidal 71.72
    perirectal, not opening into rectum 48.93
    pharyngoesophageal 29.53
    pharynx NEC 29.53
    pleura 34.73
    rectolabial 71.72
    rectourethral 58.43
    rectouterine 69.42
    rectovaginal 70.73

Fistulectomy (Continued)
    rectovesical 57.83
    rectovulvar 71.72
    rectum 48.73
    salivary (duct) (gland) 26.42
    scrotum 61.42
    skin 86.3
    stomach NEC 44.63
    subcutaneous tissue 86.3
    thoracoabdominal 34.83
    thoracogastric 34.83
    thoracointestinal 34.83
    thorax NEC 34.73
    trachea NEC 31.73
    tracheoesophageal 31.73
    ureter 56.84
    urethra 58.43
    uteroenteric 69.42
    uterointestinal 69.42
    uterorectal 69.42
    uterovaginal 69.42
    vagina 70.75
    vesicosigmoidovaginal 57.83
    vocal cords 31.62
    vulvorectal 71.72
Fistulization
    appendix 47.91
    arteriovenous 39.27
    cisterna chyli 40.62
    endolymphatic sac (for decompression) 20.79
    esophagus, external 42.10
        cervical 42.11
        specified technique NEC 42.19
    interatrial 35.41
    labyrinth (for decompression) 20.79
    lacrimal sac into nasal cavity 09.81
    larynx 31.29
    lymphatic duct, left (thoracic) 40.62
    orbit 16.09
    peritoneal 54.93
    salivary gland 26.49
    sclera 12.69
        by trephination 12.61
        with iridectomy 12.65
    sinus, nasal NEC 22.9
    subarachnoid space 02.2
    thoracic duct 40.62
    trachea 31.29
    tracheoesophageal 31.95
    urethrovaginal 58.0
    ventricle, cerebral - see also Shunt, ventricular 02.2
Fistulogram
    abdominal wall 88.03
    chest wall 87.38
    retroperitoneum 88.14
Fistulotomy, anal 49.11
Fitting
    arch bars (orthodontic) 24.7
        for immobilization (fracture) 93.55
    artificial limb 84.40
    contact lens 95.32
    denture (total) 99.97
        bridge (fixed) 23.42
            removable 23.43
        partial (fixed) 23.42
            removable 23.43
    hearing aid 95.48
    obturator (orthodontic) 24.7
    ocular prosthetics 95.34
    orthodontic
        appliance 24.7
        obturator 24.7

ICD-9-CM

F

Vol. 3

Fitting *(Continued)*
orthodontic *(Continued)*
wiring 24.7
orthotic device 93.23
periodontal splint (orthodontic) 24.7
prosthesis, prosthetic device
above knee 84.45
arm 84.43
lower (and hand) 84.42
upper (and shoulder) 84.41
below knee 84.46
hand (and lower arm) 84.42
leg 84.47
above knee 84.45
below knee 84.46
limb NEC 84.40
ocular 95.34
penis (external) 64.94
shoulder (and upper arm) 84.41
spectacles 95.31
Five-in-one repair, knee 81.42
Fixation
bone
external, without reduction 93.59
with fracture reduction - *see* Reduction, fracture
cast immobilization NEC 93.53
splint 93.54
traction (skeletal) NEC 93.44
intermittent 93.43
internal (without fracture reduction) 78.50
with fracture reduction - *see* Reduction, fracture
carpal, metacarpal 78.54
clavicle 78.51
femur 78.55
fibula 78.57
humerus 78.52
patella 78.56
pelvic 78.59
phalanges (foot) (hand) 78.59
radius 78.53
scapula 78.51
specified site NEC 78.59
tarsal, metatarsal 78.58
thorax (ribs) (sternum) 78.51
tibia 78.57
ulna 78.53
vertebrae 78.59
breast (pendulous) 85.6
cardinal ligaments 69.22
duodenum 46.62
to abdominal wall 46.61
external (without manipulation for reduction) 93.59
with fracture reduction - *see* Reduction, fracture
cast immobilization NEC 93.53
pressure dressing 93.56
splint 93.54
traction (skeletal) NEC 93.44
intermittent 93.43
hip 81.40
ileum 46.62
to abdominal wall 46.61
internal
with fracture reduction - *see* Reduction, fracture
without fracture reduction - *see* Fixation, bone, internal
intestine 46.60

Fixation *(Continued)*
intestine *(Continued)*
large 46.64
to abdominal wall 46.63
small 46.62
to abdominal wall 46.61
to abdominal wall 46.60
iris (bombé) 12.11
jejunum 46.62
to abdominal wall 46.61
joint - *see* Arthroplasty
kidney 55.7
ligament
cardinal 69.22
palpebrae 08.36
omentum 54.74
parametrial 69.22
rectum (sling) 48.76
spine, with fusion - *see also* Fusion, spinal 81.00
spleen 41.95
tendon 83.88
hand 82.85
testis in scrotum 62.5
tongue 25.59
urethrovaginal (to Cooper's ligament) 70.77
uterus (abdominal) (vaginal) (ventrofixation) 69.22
vagina 70.77
Flooding (psychologic desensitization) 94.33
Flowmetry, Doppler (ultrasonic) - *see also* Ultrasonography
aortic arch 88.73
head and neck 88.71
heart 88.72
thorax NEC 88.73
Fluoroscopy - *see* Radiography
Fog therapy (respiratory) 93.94
Folding, eye muscle 15.22
multiple (two or more muscles) 15.4
Foley operation (pyeloplasty) 55.87
Fontan operation (creation of conduit between right atrium and pulmonary artery) 35.94
Foraminotomy 03.09
Forced extension, limb 93.25
Forceps delivery - *see* Delivery, forceps
Formation
adhesions
pericardium 36.39
pleura 34.6
anus, artificial - *see also* Colostomy 46.13
duodenostomy 46.39
ileostomy - *see also* Ileostomy 46.23
jejunostomy 46.39
percutaneous (endoscopic) (PEJ) 46.32
arteriovenous fistula (for kidney dialysis) (peripheral) (shunt) 39.27
external cannula 39.93
bone flap, cranial 02.03
cardiac pacemaker pocket
with initial insertion of pacemaker - *omit code*
new site (skin) (subcutaneous) 37.79
colostomy - *see also* Colostomy 46.13
conduit
ileal (urinary) 56.51

Formation *(Continued)*
conduit *(Continued)*
left ventricle and aorta 35.93
right atrium and pulmonary artery 35.94
right ventricle and pulmonary (distal) artery 35.92
in repair of
pulmonary artery atresia 35.92
transposition of great vessels 35.92
truncus arteriosus 35.83
endorectal ileal pouch (H-pouch) (J-pouch) (S-pouch) (with anastomosis to anus) 45.95
fistula
arteriovenous (for kidney dialysis) (peripheral shunt) 39.27
external cannula 39.93
bladder to skin NEC 57.18
with bladder flap 57.21
percutaneous 57.17
cutaneoperitoneal 54.93
gastric 43.19
percutaneous (endoscopic) (transabdominal) 43.11
mucous - *see also* Colostomy 46.13
rectovaginal 48.99
tracheoesophageal 31.95
tubulovalvular (Beck-Jianu) (Frank's) (Janeway) (Spivack's) (Ssabanejew-Frank) 43.19
urethrovaginal 58.0
ileal
bladder
closed 57.87 [45.51]
open 56.51
conduit 56.51
interatrial fistula 35.42
mucous fistula - *see also* Colostomy 46.13
pericardial
baffle, interatrial 35.91
window 37.12
pleural window (for drainage) 34.09
pocket
cardiac pacemaker
with initail insertion of pacemaker - *omit code*
new site (skin) (subcutaneous) 37.79
thalamic stimulator pulse generator
with initial insertion of battery package - *omit code*
new site (skin) (subcutaneous) 86.09
pupil 12.39
by iridectomy 12.14
rectovaginal fistula 48.99
reversed gastric tube (intrathoracic) (retrosternal) 42.58
antesternal or antethoracic 42.68
septal defect, interatrial 35.42
shunt
abdominovenous 54.94
arteriovenous 39.93
peritoneojugular 54.94
peritoneo-vascular 54.94
pleuroperitoneal 34.05
transjugular intrahepatic portosystemic (TIPS) 39.1
subcutaneous tunnel

ICD-9-CM

Vol. 3

Fusion (*Continued*)
  spinal (*Continued*)
    dorsal (*Continued*)
      posterior (interbody), posterolateral technique 81.05
        for pseudarthrosis 81.35
    lumbar, lumbosacral NEC 81.08
      anterior (interbody), anterolateral technique 81.06
        for pseudarthrosis 81.36
      for pseudarthrosis 81.38

Fusion (*Continued*)
  spinal (*Continued*)
    lumbar (*Continued*)
      lateral transverse process technique 81.07
        for pseudarthrosis 81.37
      posterior (interbody), posterolateral technique 81.08
        for pseudarthrosis 81.38
      number of vertebrae - *see* codes 81.62-81.64

Fusion (*Continued*)
  spinal (*Continued*)
    occiput-C2 (anterior transoral) (posterior) 81.01
      for pseudarthrosis 81.31

> Note   Also use either 81.62, 81.63, or 81.64 as an additional code to show the total number of vertebrae fused

  tongue (to lip) 25.59

◀ **New**   ◀▦ **Revised**

G

Gait training 93.22
Galeaplasty 86.89
Galvanoionization 99.27
Games
    competitive 94.39
    organized 93.89
Gamma irradiation, stereotactic 92.32
Ganglionectomy
    gasserian 04.05
    lumbar sympathetic 05.23
    nerve (cranial) (peripheral) NEC 04.06
        sympathetic 05.29
    sphenopalatine (Meckel's) 05.21
    tendon sheath (wrist) 82.21
        site other than hand 83.31
    trigeminal 04.05
Ganglionotomy, trigeminal (radiofrequency) 04.02
Gant operation (wedge osteotomy of trochanter) 77.25
Garceau operation (tibial tendon transfer) 83.75
Gardner operation (spinal meningocele repair) 03.51
Gas endarterectomy 38.10
    abdominal 38.16
    aorta (arch) (ascending) (descending) 38.14
    coronary artery 36.09
    head and neck NEC 38.12
    intracranial NEC 38.11
    lower limb 38.18
    thoracic NEC 38.15
    upper limb 38.13
Gastrectomy (partial) (subtotal) NEC 43.89
    with
        anastomosis (to) NEC 43.89
            duodenum 43.6
            esophagus 43.5
            gastrogastric 43.89
            jejunum 43.7
        esophagogastrostomy 43.5
        gastroduodenostomy (bypass) 43.6
        gastroenterostomy (bypass) 43.7
        gastrogastrostomy (bypass) 43.89
        gastrojejunostomy (bypass) 43.7
        jejunal transposition 43.81
    complete NEC 43.99
        with intestinal interposition 43.91
    distal 43.6
    Hofmeister 43.7
    Polya 43.7
    proximal 43.5
    radical NEC 43.99
        with intestinal interposition 43.91
    total NEC 43.99
        with intestinal interposition 43.91
Gastrocamera 44.19
Gastroduodenectomy - *see* Gastrectomy
Gastroduodenoscopy 45.13
    through stoma (artificial) 45.12
    transabdominal (operative) 45.11
Gastroduodenostomy (bypass) (Jaboulay's) 44.39
    with partial gastrectomy 43.6
    laparoscopic 44.38 ◄
Gastroenterostomy (bypass) NEC 44.39
    with partial gastrectomy 43.7
    laparoscopic 44.38 ◄
Gastrogastrostomy (bypass) 44.39
    with partial gastrectomy 43.89
    laparoscopic 44.38 ◄
Gastrojejunostomy (bypass) 44.39
    with partial gastrectomy 43.7
    laparoscopic 44.38 ◄
    percutaneous (endoscopic) 44.32

Gastrolysis 54.59
    laparoscopic 54.51
Gastropexy 44.64
Gastroplasty NEC 44.69
    laparoscopic 44.68 ◄
    vertical banded gastroplasty (VBG) 44.68 ◄
Gastroplication 44.69
    laparoscopic 44.68 ◄
Gastropylorectomy 43.6
Gastrorrhaphy 44.61
Gastroscopy NEC 44.13
    through stoma (artificial) 44.12
    transabdominal (operative) 44.11
Gastrostomy (Brunschwig's) (decompression) (fine caliber tube) (Kader) (permanent) (Stamm) (Stamm-Kader) (temporary) (tube) (Witzel) 43.19
    Beck-Jianu 43.19
    Frank's 43.19
    Janeway 43.19
    percutaneous (endoscopic) (PEG) 43.11
    Spivack's 43.19
    Ssabanejew-Frank 43.19
Gastrotomy 43.0
    for control of hemorrhage 44.49
Gavage, gastric 96.35
Gelman operation (release of clubfoot) 83.84
Genioplasty (augmentation) (with graft) (with implant) 76.68
    reduction 76.67
Ghormley operation (hip fusion) 81.21
Gifford operation
    destruction of lacrimal sac 09.6
    keratotomy (delimiting) 11.1
        radial (refractive) 11.75
Gill operation
    arthrodesis of shoulder 81.23
    laminectomy 03.09
Gill-Stein operation (carporadial arthrodesis) 81.25
Gilliam operation (uterine suspension) 69.22
Gingivectomy 24.31
Gingivoplasty (with bone graft) (with soft tissue graft) 24.2
Girdlestone operation
    laminectomy with spinal fusion 81.00
    muscle transfer for claw toe repair 77.57
    resection of femoral head and neck 77.85
Girdlestone-Taylor operation (muscle transfer for claw toe repair) 77.57
Glenn operation (anastomosis of superior vena cava to right pulmonary artery) 39.21
Glenoplasty, shoulder 81.83
    with
        partial replacement 81.81
        total replacement 81.80
    for recurrent dislocation 81.82
Glomectomy
    carotid 39.8
    jugulare 20.51
Glossectomy (complete) (total) 25.3
    partial or subtotal 25.2
    radical 25.4
Glossopexy 25.59
Glossoplasty NEC 25.59
Glossorrhaphy 25.51
Glossotomy NEC 25.94
    for tongue tie 25.91
Glycoprotein IIB/IIIa inhibitor 99.20
Goebel-Frangenheim-Stoeckel operation (urethrovesical suspension) 59.4

Goldner operation (clubfoot release) 80.48
Goldthwaite operation
    ankle stabilization 81.11
    patellar stabilization 81.44
    tendon transfer for stabilization of patella 81.44
Gonadectomy
    ovary
        bilateral 65.51
            laparoscopic 65.53
        unilateral 65.39
            laparoscopic 65.31
    testis
        bilateral 62.41
        unilateral 62.3
Goniopuncture 12.51
    with goniotomy 12.53
Gonioscopy 12.29
Goniospasis 12.59
Goniotomy (Barkan's) 12.52
    with goniopuncture 12.53
Goodal-Power operation (vagina) 70.8
Gordon-Taylor operation (hindquarter amputation) 84.19
GP IIB/IIIa inhibitor, infusion 99.20
Graber-Duvernay operation (drilling of femoral head) 77.15
Graft, grafting
    aneurysm 39.52
        endovascular
            abdominal aorta 39.71
            lower extremity artery(ies) 39.79
            thoracic aorta 39.79
            upper extremity artery(ies) 39.79
    artery, arterial (patch) 39.58
        with
            excision or resection of vessel - *see* Arteriectomy, with graft replacement
            synthetic patch (Dacron) (Teflon) 39.57
            tissue patch (vein) (autogenous) (homograft) 39.56
    blood vessel (patch) 39.58
        with
            excision or resection of vessel - *see* Angiectomy, with graft replacement
            synthetic patch (Dacron) (Teflon) 39.57
            tissue patch (vein) (autogenous) (homograft) 39.56
    bone (autogenous) (bone bank) (dual onlay) (heterogeneous) (inlay) (massive onlay) (multiple) (osteoperiosteal) (peg) (subperiosteal) (with metallic fixation) 78.00
        with
            arthrodesis - *see* Arthrodesis
            arthroplasty - *see* Arthroplasty
            gingivoplasty 24.2
            lengthening - *see* Lengthening, bone
        carpals, metacarpals 78.04
        clavicle 78.01
        facial NEC 76.91
            with total ostectomy 76.44
        femur 78.05
        fibula 78.07
        humerus 78.02
        joint - *see* Arthroplasty
        mandible 76.91
            with total mandibulectomy 76.41
        marrow - *see* Transplant, bone, marrow
        nose - *see* Graft, nose

ICD-9-CM

G

Vol. 3

Graft, grafting (*Continued*)
  bone (*Continued*)
    patella 78.06
    pelvic 78.09
    pericranial 02.04
    phalanges (foot) (hand) 78.09
    radius 78.03
    scapula 78.01
    skull 02.04
    specified site NEC 78.09
    spine 78.09
      with fusion - *see* Fusion, spinal
    tarsal, metatarsal 78.08
    thorax (ribs) (sternum) 78.01
    thumb (with transfer of skin flap)
        82.69
    tibia 78.07
    ulna 78.03
    vertebrae 78.09
      with fusion - *see* Fusion, spinal
  breast - *see also* Mammoplasty 85.89
  buccal sulcus 27.99
  cartilage (joint) - *see also* Arthroplasty
    nose - *see* Graft, nose
  chest wall (mesh) (silastic) 34.79
  conjunctiva (free) (mucosa) 10.44
    for symblepharon repair 10.41
  cornea - *see also* Keratoplasty 11.60
  dermal-fat 86.69
  dermal regenerative 86.67
  dura 02.12
  ear
    auricle 18.79
    external auditory meatus 18.6
    inner 20.61
    pedicle preparation 86.71
  esophagus NEC 42.87
    with interposition (intrathoracic)
        NEC 42.58
      antesternal or antethoracic NEC
          42.68
      colon (intrathoracic) 42.55
        antesternal or antethoracic 42.65
      small bowel (intrathoracic) 42.53
        antesternal or antethoracic 42.63
  eyebrow - *see also* Reconstruction, eye-
      lid, with graft 08.69
  eyelid - *see also* Reconstruction, eyelid,
      with graft 08.69
    free mucous membrane 08.62
  eye socket (bone) (cartilage) (skin)
      16.63
  fallopian tube 66.79
  fascia 83.82
    with hernia repair - *see* Repair, her-
        nia
    eyelid 08.32
    hand 82.72
    tarsal cartilage 08.69
  fat pad NEC 86.89
    with skin graft - *see* Graft, skin, full-
        thickness
  flap (advanced) (rotating) (sliding) - *see*
      also Graft, skin, pedicle
    tarsoconjunctival 08.64
  hair-bearing skin 86.64
  hand
    fascia 82.72
    free skin 86.62
    muscle 82.72
    pedicle (flap) 86.73
    tendon 82.79
  heart, for revascularization, *see*
      category 36.3

Graft, grafting (*Continued*)
  joint - *see* Arthroplasty
  larynx 31.69
  lip 27.56
    full-thickness 27.55
  lymphatic structure(s) (channel) (node)
      (vessel) 40.9
  mediastinal fat to myocardium 36.39
  meninges (cerebral) 02.12
  mouth, except palate 27.56
    full-thickness 27.55
  muscle 83.82
    hand 82.72
  myocardium, for revascularization 36.39
  nasolabial flaps 21.86
  nerve (cranial) (peripheral) 04.5
  nipple 85.86
  nose 21.89
    with
      augmentation 21.85
      rhinoplasty - *see* Rhinoplasty
      total reconstruction 21.83
    septum 21.88
    tip 21.86
  omentum 54.74
    to myocardium 36.39
  orbit (bone) (cartilage) (skin) 16.63
  outflow tract (patch) (pulmonary
      valve) 35.26
    in total repair of tetralogy of Fallot
        35.81
  ovary 65.92
  palate 27.69
    for cleft palate repair 27.62
  pedicle - *see* Graft, skin, pedicle
  penis (rib) (skin) 64.49
  pigskin 86.65
  pinch - *see* Graft, skin, free
  pocket - *see* Graft, skin, pedicle
  porcine 86.65
  postauricular (Wolff) 18.79
  razor - *see* Graft, skin, free
  rope - *see* Graft, skin, pedicle
  saphenous vein in aortocoronary by-
      pass - *see* Bypass, aorto-coronary
  scrotum 61.49
  skin (partial-thickness) (split-thickness)
      86.69
    amnionic membrane 86.66
    auditory meatus (ear) 18.6
    dermal-fat 86.69
      for breast augmentation 85.50
    dermal regenerative 86.67
    ear
      auditory meatus 18.6
      postauricular 18.79
    eyelid 08.61
    flap - *see* Graft, skin, pedicle
    free (autogenous) NEC 86.60
      lip 27.56
      thumb 86.62
        for
          pollicization 82.61
          reconstruction 82.69
      full-thickness 86.63
        breast 85.83
        hand 86.61
      hair-bearing 86.64
        eyelid or eyebrow 08.63
      hand 86.62
        full-thickness 86.61
      heterograft 86.65
      homograft 86.66
      island flap 86.70

Graft, grafting (*Continued*)
  skin (*Continued*)
    mucous membrane 86.69
      eyelid 08.62
    nose - *see* Graft, nose
    pedicle (flap) (tube) 86.70
      advancement 86.72
      attachment to site (advanced)
          (double) (rotating) (sliding)
          86.74
        hand (cross finger) (pocket)
            86.73
        lip 27.57
        mouth 27.57
        thumb 86.73
          for
            pollicization 82.61
            reconstruction NEC 82.69
      breast 85.84
        transverse rectus abdominis
            musculocutaneous (TRAM)
            85.7
      defatting 86.75
      delayed 86.71
      design and raising 86.71
      elevation 86.71
      preparation of (cutting) 86.71
      revision 86.75
      sculpturing 86.71
      transection 86.71
      transfer 86.74
      trimming 86.71
    postauricular 18.79
    rotation flap 86.70
    specified site NEC 86.69
      full-thickness 86.63
  tarsal cartilage 08.69
  temporalis muscle to orbit 16.63
    with exenteration of orbit 16.59
  tendon 83.81
    for joint repair - *see* Arthroplasty
    hand 82.79
  testicle 62.69
  thumb (for reconstruction) NEC 82.69
  tongue (mucosal) (skin) 25.59
  trachea 31.79
  tubular (tube) - *see* Graft, skin, pedicle
  tunnel - *see* Graft, skin, pedicle
  tympanum - *see also* Tympanoplasty
      19.4
  ureter 56.89
  vein (patch) 39.58
    with
      excision or resection of vessel - *see*
          Phlebectomy, with graft re-
          placement
      synthetic patch (Dacron) (Teflon)
          39.57
      tissue patch (vein) (autogenous)
          (homograft) 39.56
  vermilion border (lip) 27.56
Grattage, conjunctiva 10.31
Green operation (scapulopexy) 78.41
Grice operation (subtalar arthrodesis)
    81.13
Grip, strength 93.04
Gritti-Stokes operation (knee disarticula-
    tion) 84.16
Gross operation (herniorrhaphy) 53.49
Group therapy 94.44
Guttering, bone - *see also* Excision, le-
    sion, bone 77.60
Guyon operation (amputation of ankle)
    84.13

◀ New   ◀▥ Revised

H

Hagner operation (epididymotomy) 63.92
Halsted operation - *see* Repair, hernia, inguinal
Hampton operation (anastomosis small intestine to rectal stump) 45.92
Hanging hip operation (muscle release) 83.19
Harelip operation 27.54
Harrison-Richardson operation (vaginal suspension) 70.77
Hartmann resection (of intestine) (with pouch) - *see* Colectomy, by site
Harvesting
  bone marrow 41.91
  stem cells 99.79
Hauser operation
  achillotenotomy 83.11
  bunionectomy with adductor tendon transfer 77.53
  stabilization of patella 81.44
Heaney operation (vaginal hysterectomy) 68.59
  laparoscopically assisted (LAVH) 68.51
Hearing aid (with battery replacement) 95.49
Hearing test 95.47
Hegar operation (perineorrhaphy) 71.79
Heine operation (cyclodialysis) 12.55
Heineke-Mikulicz operation (pyloroplasty) 44.29
Heller operation (esophagomyotomy) 42.7
Hellström operation (transplantation of aberrant renal vessel) 39.55
Hemicolectomy
  left 45.75
  right (extended) 45.73
Hemicystectomy 57.6
Hemigastrectomy - *see* Gastrectomy
Hemiglossectomy 25.2
Hemilaminectomy (decompression) (exploration) 03.09
Hemilaryngectomy (anterior) (lateral) (vertical) 30.1
Hemimandibulectomy 76.31
Hemimastectomy (radical) 85.23
Hemimaxillectomy (with bone graft) (with prosthesis) 76.39
Heminephrectomy 55.4
Hemipelvectomy 84.19
Hemispherectomy (cerebral) 01.52
Hemithyroidectomy (with removal of isthmus) (with removal of portion of remaining lobe) 06.2
Hemodiafiltration (extracorporeal) 39.95
Hemodialysis (extracorporeal) 39.95
Hemodilution 99.03
Hemofiltration (extracorporeal) 39.95
Hemorrhage control - *see* Control, hemorrhage
Hemorrhoidectomy 49.46
  by
    cautery, cauterization 49.43
    crushing 49.45
    cryotherapy, cryosurgery 49.44
    excision 49.46
    injection 49.42
    ligation 49.45
Hemostasis - *see* Control, hemorrhage
Henley operation (jejunal transposition) 43.81
Hepatectomy (complete) (total) 50.4
  partial or subtotal 50.22
Hepatic assistance, extracorporeal 50.92

Hepaticocholangiojejunostomy 51.37
Hepaticocystoduodenostomy 51.37
Hepaticodochotomy 51.59
Hepaticoduodenostomy 51.37
Hepaticojejunostomy 51.37
Hepaticolithectomy 51.49
  endoscopic 51.88
Hepaticolithotomy 51.49
  endoscopic 51.88
Hepaticostomy 51.59
Hepaticotomy 51.59
Hepatocholangiocystoduodenostomy 51.37
Hepatocholedochostomy 51.43
  endoscopic 51.87
Hepatoduodenostomy 50.69
Hepatogastrostomy 50.69
Hepatojejunostomy 50.69
Hepatolithotomy
  hepatic duct 51.49
  liver 50.0
Hepatopexy 50.69
Hepatorrhaphy 50.61
Hepatostomy (external) (internal) 50.69
Hepatotomy (with packing) 50.0
Hernioplasty - *see* Repair, hernia
Herniorrhaphy - *see* Repair, hernia
Herniotomy - *see* Repair, hernia
Heterograft - *see* Graft
Heterotransplant, heterotransplantation - *see* Transplant
Hey operation (amputation of foot) 84.12
Hey-Groves operation (reconstruction of anterior cruciate ligament) 81.45
Heyman operation (soft tissue release for clubfoot) 83.84
Heyman-Herndon (-Strong) operation (correction of metatarsus varus) 80.48
Hibbs operation (lumbar spinal fusion) - *see* Fusion, lumbar
Higgins operation - *see* Repair, hernia, femoral
High forceps delivery 72.39
  with episiotomy 72.31
Hill-Allison operation (hiatal hernia repair, transpleural approach) 53.80
Hinging, mitral valve 35.12
His bundle recording 37.29
Hitchcock operation (anchoring tendon of biceps) 83.88
Hofmeister operation (gastrectomy) 43.7
Hoke operation
  midtarsal fusion 81.14
  triple arthrodesis 81.12
Holth operation
  iridencleisis 12.63
  sclerectomy 12.65
Homans operation (correction of lymphedema) 40.9
Homograft - *see* Graft
Homotransplant, homotransplantation - *see* Transplant
Hosiery, elastic 93.59
Hutch operation (ureteroneocystostomy) 56.74
Hybinette-Eden operation (glenoid bone block) 78.01
Hydrocelectomy
  canal of Nuck (female) 69.19
    male 63.1
  round ligament 69.19
  spermatic cord 63.1
  tunica vaginalis 61.2
Hydrotherapy 93.33
  assisted exercise in pool 93.31
  whirlpool 93.32

Hymenectomy 70.31
Hymenoplasty 70.76
Hymenorrhaphy 70.76
Hymenotomy 70.11
Hyperalimentation (parenteral) 99.15
Hyperbaric oxygenation 93.95
  wound 93.59
Hyperextension, joint 93.25
Hyperthermia NEC 93.35
  for cancer treatment (interstitial) (local) (radiofrequency) (regional) (ultrasound) (whole-body) 99.85
Hypnodrama, psychiatric 94.32
Hypnosis (psychotherapeutic) 94.32
  for anesthesia - *omit code*
Hypnotherapy 94.32
Hypophysectomy (complete) (total) 07.69
  partial or subtotal 07.63
    transfrontal approach 07.61
    transsphenoidal approach 07.62
  specified approach NEC 07.68
  transfrontal approach (complete) (total) 07.64
    partial 07.61
  transsphenoidal approach (complete) (total) 07.65
    partial 07.62
Hypothermia (central) (local) 99.81
  gastric (cooling) 96.31
    freezing 96.32
  systemic (in open heart surgery) 39.62
Hypotympanotomy 20.23
Hysterectomy 68.9
  abdominal 68.4
    partial or subtotal (supracervical) (supravaginal) 68.39
    radical (modified) (Wertheim's) 68.6
    supracervical 68.39
      classic infrafasical SEMM hysterectomy [CISH] 68.31
      laparoscopically assisted [LASH] 68.31
  vaginal (complete) (partial) (subtotal) (total) 68.59
    laparoscopically assisted (LAVH) 68.51
    radical (Schauta) 68.7
Hysterocolpectomy (radical) (vaginal) 68.7
  abdominal 68.6
Hysterogram NEC 87.85
  percutaneous 87.84
Hysterolysis 54.59
  laparoscopic 54.51
Hysteromyomectomy 68.29
Hysteropexy 69.22
Hysteroplasty 69.49
Hysterorrhaphy 69.41
Hysterosalpingography gas (contrast) 87.82
  opaque dye (contrast) 87.83
Hysterosalpingostomy 66.74
Hysteroscopy 68.12
  with
    ablation
      endometrial 68.23
    biopsy 68.16
Hysterotomy (with removal of foreign body) (with removal of hydatidiform mole) 68.0
  for intrauterine transfusion 75.2
  obstetrical 74.99
    for termination of pregnancy 74.91
Hysterotrachelectomy 67.4
Hysterotracheloplasty 69.49
Hysterotrachelorrhaphy 69.41
Hysterotrachelotomy 69.95

ICD-9-CM
H
Vol. 3

I

◄ **New**   ◄▥ **Revised**

Implant, implantation (*Continued*)
CRT-P (cardiac resynchronization
pacemaker) 00.50
left ventricular coronary venous lead
only 00.52
pulse generator only 00.53
custodis eye 14.41
dental (endosseous) (prosthetic) 23.6
device ◀▥
adjustable gastric band and port
44.95 ◀
Lap-Band™ 44.95 ◀
left atrial appendage 37.90 ◀
left atrial filter 37.90 ◀
left atrial occluder 37.90 ◀
vascular access 86.07 ◀
diaphragmatic pacemaker 34.85
electrode(s)
brain 02.93
depth 02.93
foramen ovale 02.93
sphenoidal 02.96
cardiac (initial) (transvenous)
37.70
atrium (initial) 37.73
replacement 37.76
atrium and ventricle (initial)
37.72
replacement 37.76
epicardium (sternotomy or thoracotomy approach) 37.74
left ventricular coronary venous
system 00.52
temporary transvenous pacemaker
system 37.78
during and immediately following cardiac surgery
39.64
ventricle (initial) 37.71
replacement 37.76
depth 02.93
foramen ovale 02.93
heart - *see also* Implant, electrode(s),
cardiac 37.70
intracranial 02.93
osteogenic (invasive) for bone
growth stimulation - *see* category 78.9
peripheral nerve 04.92
sacral nerve 04.92 ◀
sphenoidal 02.96
spine 03.93
electroencephalographic receiver
brain 02.93
intracranial 02.93
electronic stimulator
anus (subcutaneous) 49.92
bladder 57.96
bone growth (invasive) (percutaneous) (semi-invasive) 78.9
brain - *see* Implant, neurostimulator,
brain ◀▥
carotid sinus 39.8
cochlear 20.96
channel (single) 20.97
multiple 20.98
intracranial - *see* Implant, neurostimulator, intracranial ◀▥
peripheral nerve - *see* Implant, neurostimulator, peripheral nerve ◀▥
phrenic nerve 34.85
skeletal muscle 83.92
spine - *see* Implant, neurostimulator,
spine ◀▥
ureter 56.92

Implant, implantation (*Continued*)
electrostimulator - *see* Implant, electronic stimulator, by site
endoprosthesis
bile duct 51.87
femoral head (bipolar) 81.52
pancreatic duct 52.93
endosseous (dental) 23.6
epidural pegs 02.93
epikeratoprosthesis 11.73
estradiol (pellet) 99.23
eye (Iowa type) 16.61
integrated 16.41
facial bone, synthetic (alloplastic)
76.92
fallopian tube (Mulligan hood) (silastic
tube) (stent) 66.93
into uterus 66.74
gastroepiploic artery to coronary artery
36.17
half-heart 37.62
hearing device, electromagnetic
20.95
heart
artificial 37.52
total replacement system 37.52
assist system NEC 37.62
external 37.65 ◀▥
extrinsic 37.68 ◀
implantable 37.66 ◀▥
non-implantable 37.62 ◀
percutaneous external 37.68 ◀
pVAD 37.68 ◀
auxiliary ventricle 37.62
circulatory assist system - *see* Implant, heart, assist system ◀
pacemaker - *see also* Implant, pacemaker, cardiac 37.80
valve(s)
prosthesis or synthetic device
(partial) (synthetic) (total)
35.20
aortic 35.22
mitral 35.24
pulmonary 35.26
tricuspid 35.28
tissue graft 35.20
aortic 35.21
mitral 35.23
pulmonary 35.25
tricuspid 35.27
total replacement system 37.52
inert material
breast (for augmentation) (bilateral)
85.54
unilateral 85.53
larynx 31.0
nose 21.85
orbit (eye socket) 16.69
reinsertion 16.62
scleral shell (cup) (with evisceration
of eyeball) 16.31
reinsertion 16.62
Tenon's capsule (with enucleation of
eyeball) 16.42
with attachment of muscles
16.41
reinsertion 16.62
urethra 59.79
vocal cord(s) 31.0
interbody spinal fusion device
84.51 ◀
infusion pump 86.06

Implant, implantation (*Continued*)
joint (prosthesis) (silastic) (Swanson
type) NEC 81.96
ankle (total) 81.56
revision 81.59
carpocarpal, carpometacarpal
81.74
elbow (total) 81.84
revision 81.97
extremity (bioelectric) (cineplastic)
(kineplastic) 84.40
lower 84.48
revision 81.59
upper 84.44
revision 81.97
femoral (bipolar endoprosthesis)
81.52
finger 81.71
hand (metacarpophalangeal) (interphalangeal) 81.71
revision 81.97
hip (partial) 81.52
revision 81.53
total 81.51
revision 81.53
interphalangeal 81.71
revision 81.97
knee (partial) (total) 81.54
revision 81.55
metacarpophalangeal 81.71
revision 81.97
shoulder (partial) 81.81
revision 81.97
total replacement 81.80
toe 81.57
for hallux valgus repair 77.59
revision 81.59
wrist (partial) 81.74
revision 81.97
total replacement 81.73
kidney, mechanical 55.97
Lap-Band™ 44.95 ◀
larynx 31.0
leads (cardiac) - *see* Implant, elec-
trode(s), cardiac
limb lengthening device, internal
(NOS) 84.54 ◀
with kinetic distraction 84.53 ◀
mammary artery
in ventricle (Vineberg) 36.2
to coronary artery (single vessel)
36.15
double vessel 36.16
Mulligan hood, fallopian tube 66.93
nerve (peripheral) 04.79
neuropacemaker - *see* Implant, neurostimulator, by site ◀▥
neurostimulator
electrodes ◀
brain 02.93 ◀▥
intracranial 02.93 ◀▥
peripheral nerve 04.92 ◀▥
sacral nerve 04.92 ◀
spine 03.93 ◀▥
pulse generator 86.96 ◀
dual array 86.95 ◀
single array 86.94 ◀
nose 21.85
Ommaya reservoir 02.2
orbit 16.69
reinsertion 16.62
outflow tract prosthesis (heart) (gusset
type)

ICD-9-CM
—
Vol. 3

Implant, implantation (*Continued*)
  outflow tract prosthesis (*Continued*)
    in
      pulmonary valvuloplasty 35.26
      total repair of tetralogy of Fallot
        35.81
  ovary into uterine cavity 65.72
    laparoscopic 65.75
  pacemaker
    brain - *see* Implant, neurostimulator,
      brain
    cardiac (device) (initial) (permanent)
      (replacement) 37.80
      dual-chamber device (initial)
        37.83
        replacement 37.87
      resynchronization device (CRT-P)
        device only (initial) (replace-
          ment) 00.53
        total system 00.50
        transvenous lead into left ven-
          tricular coronary
      single-chamber device (initial)
        37.81
        rate responsive 37.82
        replacement 37.85
          rate responsive 37.86
      temporary transvenous pacemaker
        system 37.78
        during and immediately follow-
          ing cardiac surgery
          39.64
      venous system 00.52
    carotid sinus 39.8
    diaphragm 34.85
    intracranial - *see* Implant, neuro-
      stimulator, intracranial
    neural - *see* Implant, neurostimula-
      tor, by site
    peripheral nerve - *see* Implant, neu-
      rostimulator, peripheral nerve
    spine - *see* Implant, neurostimulator,
      spine
  pancreas (duct) 52.96
  penis, prosthesis (internal)
    inflatable 64.97
    non-inflatable 64.95
  port, vascular access device 86.07
  premaxilla 76.68
  progesterone (subdermal) 99.23
  prosthesis, prosthetic device
    acetabulum (Aufranc-Turner)
      81.52
    ankle (total) 81.56
    arm (bioelectric) (cineplastic) (kine-
      plastic) 84.44
    breast (bilateral) (Cronin) (Dow-
      Corning) (Perras-Pappillon)
      85.54
      unilateral 85.53
    cochlear 20.96
      channel (single) 20.97
        multiple 20.98
    extremity (bioelectric) (cineplastic)
      (kineplastic) 84.40
      lower 84.48
      upper 84.44
    fallopian tube (Mulligan hood)
      (stent) 66.93
    femoral head (Austin-Moore) (bipo-
      lar) (Eicher) (Thompson)
      81.52
    joint (Swanson type) NEC 81.96
      ankle (total) 81.56

Implant, implantation (*Continued*)
  prosthesis (*Continued*)
    carpocarpal, carpometacarpal
      81.74
    elbow (total) 81.84
    finger 81.71
    hand (metacarpophalangeal) (in-
      terphalangeal) 81.71
    hip (partial) 81.52
      total 81.51
    interphalangeal 81.71
    knee (partial) (total) 81.54
      revision 81.55
    metacarpophalangeal 81.71
    shoulder (partial) 81.81
      total 81.80
    toe 81.57
      for hallux valgus repair 77.59
    wrist (partial) 81.74
      total 81.73
    leg (bioelectric) (cineplastic) (kine-
      plastic) 84.48
    outflow tract (heart) (gusset type)
      in
        pulmonary valvuloplasty
          35.26
        total repair of tetralogy of Fallot
          35.81
    penis (internal) (non-inflatable)
      64.95
      inflatable (internal) 64.97
    skin (dermal regenerative) (matrix)
      86.67
    testicular (bilateral) (unilateral)
      62.7
  pulsation balloon (phase-shift)
    37.61
  pump, infusion 86.06
  radial artery 36.19
  radioactive isotope 92.27
  radium (radon) 92.27
  retinal attachment 14.41
    with buckling 14.41
  Rickham reservoir 02.2
  silicone
    breast (bilateral) 85.54
      unilateral 85.53
    skin (for filling of defect) 86.02
      for augmentation NEC 86.89
  skin (dermal regenerative) (matrix)
    86.67
  stimoceiver - *see* Implant, neurostimu-
    lator, by site
  sudural
    grids 02.93
    strips 02.93
  Swanson prosthesis (joint) (silastic)
    NEC 81.96
    carpocarpal, carpometacarpal
      81.74
    finger 81.71
    hand (interphalangeal) (metacarpo-
      phalangeal) 81.71
    interphalangeal 81.71
    knee (partial) (total) 81.54
      revision 81.55
    metacarpophalangeal 81.71
    toe 81.57
      for hallux valgus repair 77.59
    wrist (partial) 81.74
      total 81.73
  systemic arteries into myocardium
    (Vineberg type operation)
    36.2

Implant, implantation (*Continued*)
  Tandem™ heart 37.68 ◄
  testicular prosthesis (bilateral) (unilat-
    eral) 62.7
  tissue expander (skin) NEC 86.93
    breast 85.95
  tissue mandril (for vascular graft)
    39.99
    with
      blood vessel repair 39.56
      vascular bypass or shunt - *see* By-
        pass, vascular
  tooth (bud) (germ) 23.5
    prosthetic 23.6
  umbrella, vena cava 38.7
  ureters into
    bladder 56.74
    intestine 56.71
      external diversion 56.51
    skin 56.61
  urethra
    for repair of urinary stress inconti-
      nence
      collagen 59.72
      fat 59.72
      polytef 59.72
  urethral sphincter, artificial (inflatable)
    58.93
  urinary sphincter, artificial (inflatable)
    58.93
  vascular access device 86.07
  vitreous (silicone) 14.75
    for retinal reattachment 14.41
      with buckling 14.41
  vocal cord(s) (paraglottic) 31.98
Implosion (psychologic desensitization)
  94.33
Incision (and drainage)
  with
    exploration - *see* Exploration
    removal of foreign body - *see* Re-
      moval, foreign body
  abdominal wall 54.0
    as operative approach - *omit code*
  abscess - *see also* Incision, by site
    appendix 47.2
      with appendectomy 47.09
        laparoscopic 47.01
    extraperitoneal 54.0
    ischiorectal 49.01
    lip 27.0
    omental 54.19
    perianal 49.01
    perigastric 54.19
    perisplenic 54.19
    peritoneal NEC 54.19
      pelvic (female) 70.12
    retroperitoneal 54.0
    sclera 12.89
    skin 86.04
    subcutaneous tissue 86.04
    subdiaphragmatic 54.19
    subhepatic 54.19
    subphrenic 54.19
    vas deferens 63.6
  adrenal gland 07.41
  alveolus, alveolar bone 24.0
  antecubital fossa 86.09
  anus NEC 49.93
    fistula 49.11
    septum 49.91
  appendix 47.2
  artery 38.00
    abdominal 38.06

Incision *(Continued)*
  artery *(Continued)*
    abdominal *(Continued)*
      aorta (arch) (ascending) (descending) 38.04
      head and neck NEC 38.02
      intracranial NEC 38.01
      lower limb 38.08
      thoracic NEC 38.05
      upper limb 38.03
  atrium (heart) 37.11
  auditory canal or meatus, external 18.02
  auricle 18.09
  axilla 86.09
  Bartholin's gland or cyst 71.22
  bile duct (with T or Y tube insertion) NEC 51.59
    common (exploratory) 51.51
      for
        relief of obstruction NEC 51.42
        removal of calculus 51.41
    for
      exploration 51.59
      relief of obstruction 51.49
  bladder 57.19
    neck (transurethral) 57.91
    percutaneous suprapubic (closed) 57.17
    suprapubic NEC 57.18
  blood vessel - *see also* Angiotomy 38.00
  bone 77.10
    alveolus, alveolar 24.0
    carpals, metacarpals 77.14
    clavicle 77.11
    facial 76.09
    femur 77.15
    fibula 77.17
    humerus 77.12
    patella 77.16
    pelvic 77.19
    phalanges (foot) (hand) 77.19
    radius 77.13
    scapula 77.11
    skull 01.24
    specified site NEC 77.19
    tarsals, metatarsals 77.18
    thorax (ribs) (sternum) 77.11
    tibia 77.17
    ulna 77.13
    vertebrae 77.19
  brain 01.39
    cortical adhesions 02.91
  breast (skin) 85.0
    with removal of tissue expander 85.96
  bronchus 33.0
  buccal space 27.0
  bulbourethral gland 58.91
  bursa 83.03
    hand 82.03
    pharynx 29.0
  carotid body 39.8
  cerebral (meninges) 01.39
    epidural or extradural space 01.24
    subarachnoid or subdural space 01.31
  cerebrum 01.39
  cervix 69.95
    to
      assist delivery 73.93

Incision *(Continued)*
  cervix *(Continued)*
    to *(Continued)*
      replace inverted uterus 75.93
  chalazion 08.09
    with removal of capsule 08.21
  cheek 86.09
  chest wall (for extrapleural drainage) (for removal of foreign body) 34.01
    as operative approach - *omit code*
  common bile duct (for exploration) 51.51
    for
      relief of obstruction 51.42
      removal of calculus 51.41
  common wall between posterior left atrium and coronary sinus (with roofing of resultant defect with patch graft) 35.82
  conjunctiva 10.1
  cornea 11.1
    radial (refractive) 11.75
  cranial sinus 01.21
  craniobuccal pouch 07.72
  cul-de-sac 70.12
  cyst
    dentigerous 24.0
    radicular (apical) (periapical) 24.0
  Duhrssen's (cervix, to assist delivery) 73.93
  duodenum 45.01
  ear
    external 18.09
    inner 20.79
    middle 20.23
  endocardium 37.11
  endolymphatic sac 20.79
  epididymis 63.92
  epidural space, cerebral 01.24
  epigastric region 54.0
    intra-abdominal 54.19
  esophagus, esophageal NEC 42.09
    web 42.01
  exploratory - *see* Exploration
  extradural space (cerebral) 01.24
  extrapleural 34.01
  eyebrow 08.09
  eyelid 08.09
    margin (trichiasis) 08.01
  face 86.09
  fallopian tube 66.01
  fascia 83.09
    with division 83.14
      hand 82.12
    hand 82.09
      with division 82.12
  fascial compartments, head and neck 27.0
  fistula, anal 49.11
  flank 54.0
  furuncle - *see* Incision, by site
  gallbladder 51.04
  gingiva 24.0
  gluteal 86.09
  groin region (abdominal wall) (inguinal) 54.0
    skin 86.09
    subcutaneous tissue 86.09
  gum 24.0
  hair follicles 86.09
  heart 37.10
    valve - *see* Valvulotomy
  hematoma - *see also* Incision, by site

Incision *(Continued)*
  hematoma *(Continued)*
    axilla 86.04
    broad ligament 69.98
    ear 18.09
    episiotomy site 75.91
    fossa (superficial) NEC 86.04
    groin region (abdominal wall) (inguinal) 54.0
      skin 86.04
      subcutaneous tissue 86.04
    laparotomy site 54.12
    mediastinum 34.1
    perineum (female) 71.09
      male 86.04
    popliteal space 86.04
    scrotum 61.0
    skin 86.04
    space of Retzius 59.19
    subcutaneous tissue 86.04
    vagina (cuff) 70.14
      episiotomy site 75.91
      obstetrical NEC 75.92
  hepatic ducts 51.59
  hordeolum 08.09
  hygroma - *see also* Incision, by site
    cystic 40.0
  hymen 70.11
  hypochondrium 54.0
    intra-abdominal 54.19
  hypophysis 07.72
  iliac fossa 54.0
  infratemporal fossa 27.0
  ingrown nail 86.09
  intestine 45.00
    large 45.03
    small 45.02
  intracerebral 01.39
  intracranial (epidural space) (extradural space) 01.24
    subarachnoid or subdural space 01.31
  intraperitoneal 54.19
  ischiorectal tissue 49.02
    abscess 49.01
  joint structures - *see also* Arthrotomy 80.10
  kidney 55.01
    pelvis 55.11
  labia 71.09
  lacrimal
    canaliculus 09.52
    gland 09.0
    passage NEC 09.59
    punctum 09.51
    sac 09.53
  larynx NEC 31.3
  ligamentum flavum (spine) - *omit code*
  liver 50.0
  lung 33.1
  lymphangioma 40.0
  lymphatic structure (channel) (node) (vessel) 40.0
  mastoid 20.21
  mediastinum 34.1
  meibomian gland 08.09
  meninges (cerebral) 01.31
    spinal 03.09
  midpalmar space 82.04
  mouth NEC 27.92
    floor 27.0
  muscle 83.02
    with division 83.19
      hand 82.19

ICD-9-CM
Vol. 3

Incision (*Continued*)
muscle (*Continued*)
  hand 82.02
    with division 82.19
myocardium 37.11
nailbed or nailfold 86.09
nasolacrimal duct (stricture) 09.59
neck 86.09
nerve (cranial) (peripheral) NEC 04.04
  root (spinal) 03.1
nose 21.1
omentum 54.19
orbit - *see also* Orbitotomy 16.09
ovary 65.09
  laparoscopic 65.01
palate 27.1
palmar space (middle) 82.04
pancreas 52.09
pancreatic sphincter 51.82
  endoscopic 51.85
parapharyngeal (oral) (transcervical)
  28.0
paronychia 86.09
parotid
  gland or duct 26.0
  space 27.0
pelvirectal tissue 48.81
penis 64.92
perianal (skin) (tissue) 49.02
  abscess 49.01
perigastric 54.19
perineum (female) 71.09
  male 86.09
peripheral vessels
  lower limb
    artery 38.08
    vein 38.09
  upper limb (artery) (vein) 38.03
periprostatic tissue 60.81
perirectal tissue 48.81
perirenal tissue 59.09
perisplenic 54.19
peritoneum 54.95
  by laparotomy 54.19
  pelvic (female) 70.12
    male 54.19
periureteral tissue 59.09
periurethral tissue 58.91
perivesical tissue 59.19
petrous pyramid (air cells) (apex)
  (mastoid) 20.22
pharynx, pharyngeal (bursa) 29.0
  space, lateral 27.0
pilonidal sinus (cyst) 86.03
pineal gland 07.52
pituitary (gland) 07.72
pleura NEC 34.09
popliteal space 86.09
postzygomatic space 27.0
pouch of Douglas 70.12
prostate (perineal approach) (transurethral approach) 60.0
pterygopalatine fossa 27.0
pulp canal (tooth) 24.0
Rathke's pouch 07.72
rectovaginal septum 48.81
rectum 48.0
  stricture 48.91
renal pelvis 55.11
retroperitoneum 54.0
retropharyngeal (oral) (transcervical)
  28.0
salivary gland or duct 26.0
sclera 12.89

Incision (*Continued*)
scrotum 61.0
sebaceous cyst 86.04
seminal vesicle 60.72
sinus - *see* Sinusotomy
Skene's duct or gland 71.09
skin 86.09
  with drainage 86.04
  breast 85.0
  cardiac pacemaker pocket, new site
    37.79
  ear 18.09
  nose 21.1
  subcutaneous tunnel for pulse gen-
    erator lead wire 86.99
    with initial procedure - *omitcode*
  thalamic stimulator pulse generator
    pocket, new site 86.09
    with initial insertion of battery
      package - *omit code*
  tunnel, subcutaneous, for pulse gen-
    erator lead wire 86.99
    with initial procedure - *omit code*
skull (bone) 01.24
soft tissue NEC 83.09
  with division 83.19
    hand 82.19
  hand 82.09
    with division 82.19
space of Retzius 59.19
spermatic cord 63.93
sphincter of Oddi 51.82
  endoscopic 51.85
spinal
  cord 03.09
  nerve root 03.1
spleen 41.2
stomach 43.0
stye 08.09
subarachnoid space, cerebral 01.31
subcutaneous tissue 86.09
  with drainage 86.04
  tunnel
    esophageal 42.86
      with anastomosis - *see* Anasto-
        mosis, esophagus, antester-
        nal
    pulse generator lead wire 86.99
      with initial procedure - *omit
      code*
subdiaphragmatic space 54.19
subdural space, cerebral 01.31
sublingual space 27.0
submandibular space 27.0
submaxillary 86.09
  with drainage 86.04
submental space 27.0
subphrenic space 54.19
supraclavicular fossa 86.09
  with drainage 86.04
sweat glands, skin 86.04
temporal pouches 27.0
tendon (sheath) 83.01
  with division 83.13
    hand 82.11
  hand 82.01
    with division 82.11
testis 62.0
thenar space 82.04
thymus 07.92
thyroid (field) (gland) NEC 06.09
  postoperative 06.02
tongue NEC 25.94
  for tongue tie 25.91

Incision (*Continued*)
tonsil 28.0
trachea NEC 31.3
tunica vaginalis 61.0
umbilicus 54.0
urachal cyst 54.0
ureter 56.2
urethra 58.0
uterus (corpus) 68.0
  cervix 69.95
  for termination of pregnancy 74.91
  septum (congenital) 68.22
uvula 27.71
vagina (cuff) (septum) (stenosis) 70.14
  for
    incisional hematoma (episiotomy)
      75.91
    obstetrical hematoma NEC 75.92
    pelvic abscess 70.12
vas deferens 63.6
vein 38.00
  abdominal 38.07
  head and neck NEC 38.02
  intracranial NEC 38.01
  lower limb 38.09
  thoracic NEC 38.05
  upper limb 38.03
vertebral column 03.09
vulva 71.09
  obstetrical 75.92
web, esophageal 42.01
Incudectomy NEC 19.3
with
  stapedectomy - *see also* Stapedec-
    tomy 19.19
  tympanoplasty - *see* Tympanoplasty
Incudopexy 19.19
Incudostapediopexy 19.19
  with incus replacement 19.11
Indentation, sclera, for buckling - *see
  also* Buckling, scleral 14.49
Indicator dilution flow measurement
  89.68
Induction
abortion
  by
    D and C 69.01
    insertion of prostaglandin suppos-
      itory 96.49
    intra-amniotic injection (prosta-
      glandin) (saline) 75.0
labor
  medical 73.4
  surgical 73.01
    intra- and extra-amniotic injection
      73.1
    stripping of membranes 73.1
Inflation
belt wrap 93.99
Eustachian tube 20.8
fallopian tube 66.8
  with injection of therapeutic agent
    66.95
Infolding, sclera, for buckling - *see also*
  Buckling, scleral 14.49
Infraction, turbinates (nasal) 21.62
Infundibulectomy
hypophyseal - *see also* Hypophysectomy, partial 07.63
ventricle (heart) (right) 35.34
  in total repair of tetralogy of Fallot
    35.81
Infusion (intra-arterial) (intravenous)
Abciximab 99.20

◀ **New**   ⬅▥ **Revised**

Infusion (*Continued*)
antibiotic
  oxazolidinone class 00.14
antineoplastic agent (chemotherapeutic) 99.25
  biological response modifier [BRM] 99.28
    high-dose interleukin-2 00.15
    low-dose interleukin-2 99.28
biological response modifier [BRM], antineoplastic agent 99.28
  high-dose interleukin-2 00.15
  low-dose interleukin-2 99.28
cancer chemotherapy agent NEC 99.25
drotrecogin alfa (activated) 00.11
electrolytes 99.18
enzymes, thrombolytic (streptokinase) (tissue plasminogen activator) (TPA) (urokinase)
  direct coronary artery 36.04
  intravenous 99.10
Eptifibatide 99.20
GP IIB/IIIa inhibitor 99.20
hormone substance NEC 99.24
human B-type natriuretic peptide (hBNP) 00.13
nesiritide 00.13
neuroprotective agent 99.75
nimodipine 99.75
nutritional substance - *see* Nutrition
platelet inhibitor
  direct coronary artery 36.04
  intravenous 99.20
Proleukin (low-dose) 99.28
  high-dose 00.15
prophylactic substance NEC 99.29
radioimmunoconjugate 92.28
radioimmunotherapy 92.28
recombinant protein 00.11
reteplase 99.10
therapeutic substance NEC 99.29
thrombolytic agent (enzyme) (streptokinase) 99.10
  with percutaneous transluminal angioplasty
    coronary (single vessel) 36.02
      multiple vessels 36.05
    non-coronary vessel(s) 39.50
      specified site NEC 39.50
    direct intracoronary artery 36.04
tirofiban (HCl) 99.20
vaccine
  tumor 99.28
vasopressor 00.17 ◄

Injection (into) (hypodermically) (intramuscularly) (intravenously) (acting locally or systemically)
Actinomycin D, for cancer chemotherapy 99.25
adhesion barrier substance 99.77
alcohol
  nerve - *see* Injection, nerve
  spinal 03.8
anterior chamber, eye (air) (liquid) (medication) 12.92
antibiotic 99.21
  oxazolidinone class 00.14
anticoagulant 99.19
anti-D (Rhesus) globulin 99.11
antidote NEC 99.16
anti-infective NEC 99.22
antineoplastic agent (chemotherapeutic) NEC 99.25

Injection (*Continued*)
antineoplastic agent (*Continued*)
  biological response modifier [BRM] 99.28
    high-dose interleukin-2 00.15
    low-dose interleukin-2 99.28
antivenin 99.16
barrier substance, adhesion 99.77
BCG
  for chemotherapy 99.25
  vaccine 99.33
biological response modifier [BRM], antineoplastic agent 99.28
  high-dose interleukin-2 00.15
  low-dose interleukin-2 99.28
bone marrow 41.92
  transplant - *see* Transplant, bone, marrow
breast (therapeutic agent) 85.92
  inert material (silicone) (bilateral) 85.52
    unilateral 85.51
bursa (therapeutic agent) 83.96
  hand 82.94
cancer chemotherapeutic agent 99.25
caudal - *see* Injection, spinal
cortisone 99.23
costochondral junction 81.92
dinoprost-tromethine, intra-amniotic 75.0
disc, intervertebral (herniated) 80.52
ear, with alcohol 20.72
electrolytes 99.18
enzymes, thrombolytic (streptokinase) (tissue plasminogen activator) (TPA) (urokinase)
  direct coronary artery 36.04
  intravenous 99.10
epidural, spinal - *see* Injection, spinal
esophageal varices or blood vessel (endoscopic) (sclerosing agent) 42.33
Eustachian tube (inert material) 20.8
eye (orbit) (retrobulbar) 16.91
  anterior chamber 12.92
  subconjunctival 10.91
fascia 83.98
  hand 82.96
gamma globulin 99.14
ganglion, sympathetic 05.39
  ciliary 12.79
  paravertebral stellate 05.39
gel, adhesion barrier - *see* Injection, adhesion barrier substances
globulin
  anti-D (Rhesus) 99.11
  gamma 99.14
  Rh immune 99.11
heart 37.92
heavy metal antagonist 99.16
hemorrhoids (sclerosing agent) 49.42
hormone NEC 99.24
human B-type natriuretic peptide (hBNP) 00.13
immune sera 99.14
inert material - *see* Implant, inert material
inner ear, for destruction 20.72
insulin 99.17
intervertebral space for herniated disc 80.52
intra-amniotic
  for induction of
    abortion 75.0
    labor 73.1

Injection (*Continued*)
intrathecal - *see* Injection, spinal
joint (therapeutic agent) 81.92
  temporomandibular 76.96
kidney (cyst) (therapeutic substance) NEC 55.96
larynx 31.0
ligament (joint) (therapeutic substance) 81.92
liver 50.94
lung, for surgical collapse 33.32
Methotrexate, for cancer chemotherapy 99.25
nerve (cranial) (peripheral) 04.80
  agent NEC 04.89
    alcohol 04.2
    anesthetic for analgesia 04.81
      for operative anesthesia - *omit code*
    neurolytic 04.2
    phenol 04.2
  laryngeal (external) (recurrent) (superior) 31.91
  optic 16.91
  sympathetic 05.39
    alcohol 05.32
    anesthetic for analgesia 05.31
    neurolytic agent 05.32
    phenol 05.32
nesiritide 00.13
neuroprotective agent 99.75
nimodipine 99.75
orbit 16.91
pericardium 37.93
peritoneal cavity
  air 54.96
  locally-acting therapeutic substance 54.97
platelet inhibitor
  direct coronary artery 36.04
  intravenous 99.20
prophylactic substance NEC 99.29
prostate 60.92
radioimmunoconjugate 92.28
radioimmunotherapy 92.28
radioisotopes (intracavitary) (intravenous) 92.28
renal pelvis (cyst) 55.96
retrobulbar (therapeutic substance) 16.91
  for anesthesia - *omit code*
Rh immune globulin 99.11
RhoGAM 99.11
sclerosing agent NEC 99.29
  esophageal varices (endoscopic) 42.33
  hemorrhoids 49.42
  pleura 34.92
    treatment of malignancy (cytotoxic agent) 34.92 [99.25]
      with tetracycline 34.92 [99.21]
  varicose vein 39.92
  vein NEC 39.92
semicircular canals, for destruction 20.72
silicone - *see* Implant, inert material
skin (sclerosing agent) (filling material) 86.02
soft tissue 83.98
  hand 82.96
spinal (canal) NEC 03.92
  alcohol 03.8
  anesthetic agent for analgesia 03.91
    for operative anesthesia - *omit code*

ICD-9-CM
Vol. 3

Injection *(Continued)*
spinal *(Continued)*
contrast material (for myelogram) 87.21
destructive agent NEC 03.8
neurolytic agent NEC 03.8
phenol 03.8
proteolytic enzyme (chymodiactin) (chymopapain) 80.52
saline (hypothermic) 03.92
steroid NEC 03.92
spinal nerve root (intrathecal) - *see* Injection, spinal
steroid NEC 99.23
subarachnoid, spinal - *see* Injection, spinal
subconjunctival 10.91
tendon 83.97
hand 82.95
testis 62.92
therapeutic agent NEC 99.29
thoracic cavity 34.92
thrombolytic agent (enzyme) (streptokinase) 99.10
with percutaneous transluminal angioplasty
coronary (single vessel) 36.02
multiple vessels 36.05
non-coronary vessels 39.50
specified site NEC 39.50
direct intracoronary artery 36.04
trachea 31.94
tranquilizer 99.26
tunica vaginalis (with aspiration) 61.91
tympanum 20.94
urethra (inert material)
for repair of urinary stress incontinence
collagen implant 59.72
endoscopic injection of implant 59.72
fat implant 59.72
polytef implant 59.72
vaccine
tumor 99.28
varices, esophagus (endoscopic) (sclerosing agent) 42.33
varicose vein (sclerosing agent) 39.92
esophagus (endoscopic) 42.33
vestibule, for destruction 20.72
vitreous substitute (silicone) 14.75
for reattachment of retina 14.59
vocal cords 31.0
Inlay, tooth 23.3
Inoculation
antitoxins - *see* Administration, antitoxins
toxoids - *see* Administration, toxoids
vaccine - *see* Administration, vaccine
Insemination, artificial 69.92
Insertion
airway
esophageal obturator 96.03
nasopharynx 96.01
oropharynx 96.02
Allen-Brown cannula 39.93
arch bars (orthodontic) 24.7
for immobilization (fracture) 93.55
atrial septal umbrella 35.52
Austin-Moore prosthesis 81.52
baffle, heart (atrial) (interatrial) (intraatrial) 35.91
bag, cervix (nonobstetrical) 67.0
after delivery or abortion 75.8

Insertion *(Continued)*
bag, cervix *(Continued)*
to assist delivery or induce labor 73.1
Baker's (tube) (for stenting) 46.85
balloon
gastric 44.93
heart (pulsation-type) (Kantrowitz) 37.61
intestine (for decompression) (for dilation) 46.85
band (adjustable) ◄
gastric, laparoscopic 44.95 ◄
Lap-Band™ 44.95 ◄
Barton's tongs (skull) (with synchronous skeletal traction) 02.94
bipolar endoprosthesis (femoral head) 81.52
Blakemore-Sengstaken tube 96.06
bone growth stimulator (invasive) (percutaneous) (semi-invasive) - *see* category 78.9
bone morphogenetic protein (recombinant) (rhBMP) 84.52
bone void filler 84.55 ◄
that with kyphoplasty 81.66 ◄
that with vertebroplasty 81.65 ◄
bougie, cervix, nonobstetrical 67.0
to assist delivery or induce labor 73.1
breast implant (for augmentation) (bilateral) 85.54
unilateral 85.53
bridge (dental) (fixed) 23.42
removable 23.43
bubble (balloon), stomach 44.93
caliper tongs (skull) (with synchronous skeletal traction) 02.94
cannula
Allen-Brown 39.93
for extracorporeal membrane oxygenation (ECMO) - *omit code*
nasal sinus (by puncture) 22.01
through natural ostium 22.02
pancreatic duct 52.92
endoscopic 52.93
vessel to vessel 39.93
cardiac resynchronization device
defibrillator (CRT-D) (total system) 00.51
left ventricular coronary venous lead only 00.52
pulse generator only 00.54
pacemaker (CRT-P) (total system) 00.50
left ventricular coronary venous lead only 00.52
pulse generator only 00.53
carotid artery stent(s) (stent graft) (00.63) ◄
catheter
abdomen of fetus, for intrauterine transfusion 75.2
anterior chamber (eye), for permanent drainage (glaucoma) 12.79
artery 38.91
bile duct(s) 51.59
common 51.51
endoscopic 51.87
endoscopic 51.87
bladder, indwelling 57.94
suprapubic 57.18
percutaneous (closed) 57.17

Insertion *(Continued)*
catheter *(Continued)*
bronchus 96.05
with lavage 96.56
central venous NEC 38.93
for
hemodialysis 38.95
pressure monitoring 89.62
peripherally inserted central catheter (PICC) 38.93
chest 34.04
revision (with lysis of adhesions) 34.04
esophagus (nonoperative) 96.06
permanent tube 42.81
intercostal (with water seal), for drainage 34.04
revision (with lysis of adhesions) 34.04
spinal canal space (epidural) (subarachnoid) (subdural) for infusion of therapeutic or palliative substances 03.90
Swan-Ganz (pulmonary) 89.64
transtracheal for oxygenation 31.99
vein NEC 38.93
for renal dialysis 38.95
chest tube 34.04
choledochohepatic tube (for decompression) 51.43
endoscopic 51.87
cochlear prosthetic device - *see* Implant, cochlear prosthetic device
contraceptive device (intrauterine) 69.7
cordis cannula 54.98
coronary (artery)
stent, drug-eluting 36.07 ◄
stent, non-drug-eluting 36.06 ◄
Crosby-Cooney button 54.98
CRT-D (cardiac resynchronization defibrillator) 00.51
left ventricular coronary venous lead only 00.52
pulse generator only 00.54
CRT-P (cardiac resynchronization pacemaker) 00.50
left ventricular coronary venous lead only 00.52
pulse generator only 00.53
Crutchfield tongs (skull) (with synchronous skeletal traction) 02.94
Davidson button 54.98
denture (total) 99.97
device ◄
adjustable gastric band and port 44.95 ◄
Lap-Band™ 44.95 ◄
left atrial appendage 37.90 ◄
left atrial filter 37.90 ◄
left atrial occluder 37.90 ◄
vascular access 86.07 ◄
diaphragm, vagina 96.17
drainage tube
kidney 55.02
pelvis 55.12
renal pelvis 55.12
elbow prosthesis (total) 81.84
revision 81.97
electrode(s)
bone growth stimulator (invasive) (percutaneous) (semi-invasive) - *see* category 78.9
brain 02.93
depth 02.93

Insertion (*Continued*)
electrode(s) (*Continued*)
brain (*Continued*)
foramen ovale 02.93
sphenoidal 02.96
depth 02.93
foramen ovale 02.93
sacral nerve 04.92 ◄
sphenoidal 02.96
heart (initial) (transvenous) 37.70
atrium (initial) 37.73
replacement 37.76
atrium and ventricle (initial) 37.72
replacement 37.76
epicardium (sternotomy or thoracotomy approach) 37.74
left ventricular coronary venous system 00.52
temporary transvenous pacemaker system 37.78
during and immediately following cardiac surgery 39.64
ventricle (initial) 37.71
replacement 37.76
intracranial 02.93
osteogenic (for bone growth stimulation) - *see* category 78.9
peripheral nerve 04.92
sphenoidal 02.96
spine 03.93
electroencephalographic receiver - *see* Implant, electroencephalographic receiver, by site
electronic stimulator - *see* Implant, electronic stimulator, by site
electrostimulator - *see* Implant, electronic stimulator, by site
endograft(s), endovascular graft(s)
endovascular, head and neck vessels 39.72
endovascular, other vessels (for aneurysm) 39.79
endoprosthesis
bile duct 51.87
femoral head (bipolar) 81.52
pancreatic duct 52.93
epidural pegs 02.93
external fixation device (bone) - *see* category 78.1
facial bone implant (alloplastic) (synthetic) 76.92
filling material, skin (filling of defect) 86.02
filter
vena cava (inferior) (superior) (transvenous) 38.7
fixator, mini device (bone) - *see* category 78.1
frame (stereotactic)
for radiosurgery 93.59
Gardner Wells tongs (skull) (with synchronous skeletal traction) 02.94
gastric bubble (balloon) 44.93
globe, into eye socket 16.69
Greenfield filter 38.7
halo device (skull) (with synchronous skeletal traction) 02.94
Harrington rod - *see also* Fusion, spinal, by level
with dorsal, dorsolumbar fusion 81.05
Harris pin 79.15

Insertion (*Continued*)
heart
assist system - *see* Implant, heart assist system ◄
circulatory assist system - *see* Implant, heart assist system ◄
pacemaker - *see* Insertion, pacemaker, cardiac
pump (Kantrowitz) 37.62
valve - *see* Replacement, heart valve
hip prosthesis (partial) 81.52
revision 81.53
total 81.51
revision 81.53
Holter valve 02.2
Hufnagel valve - *see* Replacement, heart valve
implant - *see* Insertion, prosthesis
infusion pump 86.06
interbody spinal fusion device 84.51 ◄
intercostal catheter (with water seal) for drainage 34.04
intra-arterial blood gas monitoring system 89.60
intrauterine
contraceptive device 69.7
radium (intracavitary) 69.91
tamponade (nonobstetric) 69.91
Kantrowitz
heart pump 37.62
pulsation balloon (phase-shift) 37.61
keratoprosthesis 11.73
King-Mills umbrella device (heart) 35.52
Kirschner wire 93.44
with reduction of fracture or dislocation - *see* Reduction, fracture *and* Reduction, dislocation
laminaria, cervix 69.93
Lap-Band™ 44.95 ◄
larynx, valved tube 31.75
leads - *see* Insertion, electrode(s) ◄
lens, prosthetic (intraocular) 13.70
with cataract extraction, one-stage 13.71
limb lengthening device, internal, NOS 84.54 ◄
with kinetic distraction 84.53 ◄
secondary (subsequent to cataract extraction) 13.72
loop recorder 86.09
metal staples into epiphyseal plate - *see also* Stapling, epiphyseal plate 78.20
minifixator device (bone) - *see* category 78.1
Mobitz-Uddin umbrella, vena cava 38.7
mold, vagina 96.15
Moore (cup) 81.52
myringotomy device (button) (tube) 20.01
with intubation 20.01
nasobiliary drainage tube (endoscopic) 51.86
nasogastric tube
for
decompression, intestinal 96.07
feeding 96.6
naso-intestinal tube 96.08
nasolacrimal tube or stent 09.44

Insertion (*Continued*)
nasopancreatic drainage tube (endoscopic) 52.97
neuropacemaker - *see* Implant, neurostimulator, by site ◄
neurostimulator - *see* Implant, neurostimulator, by site
non-coronary vessel
stent(s) (stent graft) ◄
basilar 00.64 ◄
carotid 00.63 ◄
extracranial 00.64 ◄
intracranial 00.65 ◄
peripheral 39.90 ◄
bare, drug-coated 39.90 ◄
drug-eluting 00.55 ◄
vertebral 00.64 ◄
with angioplasty or atherectomy 39.50
with bypass - *omit code*
non-invasive (surface) (transcutaneous) stimulator 99.86
obturator (orthodontic) 24.7
ocular implant
with synchronous
enucleation 16.42
with muscle attachment to implant 16.41
evisceration 16.31
following or secondary to
enucleation 16.61
evisceration 16.61
Ommaya reservoir 02.2
orbital implant (stent) (outside muscle cone) 16.69
with orbitotomy 16.02
orthodontic appliance (obturator) (wiring) 24.7
outflow tract prosthesis (heart) (gusset type)
in
pulmonary valvuloplasty 35.26
total repair of tetralogy of Fallot 35.81
pacemaker
brain - *see* Implant, neurostimulator, brain ◄
cardiac (device) (initial) (permanent) (replacement) 37.80
dual-chamber device (initial) 37.83
replacement 37.87
during and immediately following cardiac surgery 39.64
resynchronization (CRT-P) (device)
device only (initial) (replacement) 00.53
total system 00.50
transvenous lead into left ventricular coronary
single-chamber device (initial) 37.81
rate responsive 37.82
replacement 37.85
rate responsive 37.86
temporary transvenous pacemaker system 37.78
during and immediately following cardiac surgery 39.64
venous system 00.52
carotid 39.8

ICD-9-CM

—

Vol. 3

Insertion (*Continued*)
  pacemaker (*Continued*)
    heart - *see* Insertion, pacemaker, cardiac
    intracranial - *see* Implant, neurostimulator, intracranial ◄▥
    neural - *see* Implant, neurostimulator, by site ◄▥
    peripheral nerve - *see* Implant, neurostimulator, peripheral nerve ◄▥
    spine - *see* Implant, neurostimulator, spine ◄▥
  pacing catheter - *see* Insertion, pacemaker, cardiac
  pack
    auditory canal, external 96.11
    cervix (nonobstetrical) 67.0
      after delivery or abortion 75.8
      to assist delivery or induce labor 73.1
    rectum 96.19
    sella turcica 07.79
    vagina (nonobstetrical) 96.14
      after delivery or abortion 75.8
  palatal implant 27.64 ◄
  penile prosthesis (internal) (non-inflatable) 64.95
    inflatable (internal) 64.97
  periodontal splint (orthodontic) 24.7
  peripheral blood vessel - *see* non-coronary
  pessary
    cervix 96.18
      to assist delivery or induce labor 73.1
    vagina 96.18
  pharyngeal valve, artificial 31.75
  port, vascular access 86.07
  prostaglandin suppository (for abortion) 96.49
  prosthesis, prosthetic device
    acetabulum (partial) 81.52
      revision 81.53
    ankle (total) 81.56
    arm (bioelectric) (cineplastic) (kineplastic) 84.44
    biliary tract 51.99
    breast (bilateral) 85.54
      unilateral 85.53
    chin (polyethylene) (silastic) 76.68
    elbow (total) 81.84
      revision 81.97
    extremity (bioelectric) (cineplastic) (kineplastic) 84.40
      lower 84.48
      upper 84.44
    fallopian tube 66.93
    femoral head (Austin-Moore) (bipolar) (Eicher) (Thompson) 81.52
    hip (partial) 81.52
      revision 81.53
      total 81.51
        revision 81.53
    joint - *see* Arthroplasty
    knee (partial) (total) 81.54
      revision 81.55
    leg (bioelectric) (cineplastic) (kineplastic) 84.48

Insertion (*Continued*)
  prosthesis (*Continued*)
    ocular (secondary) 16.61
      with orbital exenteration 16.42
    outflow tract (heart) (gusset type)
      in
        pulmonary valvuloplasty 35.26
        total repair of tetralogy of Fallot 35.81
    penis (internal) (noninflatable) 64.95
      with
        construction 64.43
        reconstruction 64.44
      inflatable (internal) 64.97
    Rosen (for urinary incontinence) 59.79
    shoulder
      partial 81.81
      revision 81.97
      total 81.80
    spine ◄
      artificial, NOS 84.60 ◄
        cervical 84.62 ◄
          nucleus 84.61 ◄
          partial 84.61 ◄
          total 84.62 ◄
        lumbar, lumbosacral 84.65 ◄
          nucleus 84.64 ◄
          partial 84.64 ◄
          total 84.65 ◄
        thoracic (partial) (total) 84.63 ◄
      other device 84.59 ◄
    testicular (bilateral) (unilateral) 62.7
    toe 81.57
      hallux valgus repair 77.59
  pseudophakos - *see also* Insertion, lens 13.70
  pump, infusion 86.06
  radioactive isotope 92.27
  radium 92.27
  radon seeds 92.27
  Reuter bobbin (with intubation) 20.01
  Rickham reservoir 02.2
  Rosen prosthesis (for urinary incontinence) 59.79
  Scribner shunt 39.93
  Sengstaken-Blakemore tube 96.06
  sensor
    intra-arterial, for continuous blood gas monitoring 89.60
  sieve, vena cava 38.7
  skeletal muscle stimulator 83.92
  skull
    plate 02.05
    stereotactic frame 93.59
    tongs (Barton) (caliper) (Gardner Wells) (Vinke) (with synchronous skeletal traction) 02.94
  spacer (cement) in joint 80.00
    spine 84.51
  sphenoidal electrodes 02.96
  spine
    bone void filler ◄
      that with kyphoplasty 81.66 ◄
      that with vertebroplasty 81.65 ◄
    cage (BAK) 84.51
    interbody spinal fusion device 84.51 ◄
    spacer 84.51

Insertion (*Continued*)
  Spitz-Holter valve 02.2
  Steinmann pin 93.44
    with reduction of fracture or dislocation - *see* Reduction, fracture *and* Reduction, dislocation
  stent(s) (stent graft)
    artery (bare) (bonded) (drug coated) (non-drug-eluting) ◄▥
      basilar 00.64 ◄
      carotid 00.63 ◄
      cerebrovascular ◄
        cerebral (intracranial) 00.65 ◄
        precerebral (extracranial) 00.64◄
          carotid 00.63 ◄
        extracranial 00.64 ◄
          carotid 00.63 ◄
        intracranial 00.65 ◄
      coronary (bare) (bonded) (drug coated) (non-drug-eluting) 36.06
      non-coronary vessel ◄▥
        basilar 00.64 ◄
        carotid 00.63 ◄
        extracranial 00.64 ◄
        intracranial 00.65 ◄
        peripheral 39.90 ◄
          bare, drug-coated 39.90 ◄
          drug-eluting 00.55 ◄
        vertebral 00.64 ◄
    bile duct 51.43
      endoscopic 51.87
      percutaneous transhepatic 51.98
    coronary (artery) (bare) (bonded) (drug-coated) (non-drug-eluting) 36.06 ◄▥
      drug-eluting 36.07 ◄
    esophagus (endoscopic) (fluoroscopic) 42.81
    non-coronary vessel ◄▥
      with angioplasty or atherectomy 39.50
      with bypass - *omit code*
      basilar 00.64 ◄
      carotid 00.63 ◄
      extracranial 00.64 ◄
      intracranial 00.65 ◄
      peripheral 39.90 ◄
        bare, drug-coated 39.90 ◄
        drug-eluting 00.55 ◄
      vertebral 00.64 ◄
    pancreatic duct 52.92
      endoscopic 52.93
    peripheral 39.90 ◄▥
      bare, drug-coated 39.90 ◄
      drug-eluting 00.55 ◄
    precerebral 00.64 ◄
    subclavian 39.90 ◄
      bare, drug-coated 39.90 ◄
      drug-eluting 00.55 ◄
    tracheobronchial 96.05
    vertebral 00.64 ◄
  stimoceiver - *see* Implant, neurostimulator, by site ◄▥
  stimulator for bone growth - *see* category 78.9
  subdural
    grids 02.93
    strips 02.93
  suppository
    prostaglandin (for abortion) 96.49
    vagina 96.49
  Swan-Ganz catheter (pulmonary) 89.64

◄ **New**   ◄▥ **Revised**

Insertion (*Continued*)
tampon
esophagus 96.06
uterus 69.91
vagina 96.14
after delivery or abortion 75.8
Tandem™ heart 37.68 ◄
testicular prosthesis (bilateral) (unilateral) 62.7
tissue expander (skin) NEC 86.93
breast 85.95
tissue mandril (peripheral vessel) (Dacron) (Spark's type) 39.99
with
blood vessel repair 39.56
vascular bypass or shunt - *see* Bypass, vascular
tongs, skull (with synchronous skeletal traction) 02.94
totally implanted device for bone growth (invasive) - *see* category 78.9
tube - *see also* Catheterization and Intubation
bile duct 51.43
endoscopic 51.87
chest 34.04
revision (with lysis of adhesions) 34.04
endotracheal 96.04
esophagus (nonoperative) (Sengstaken) 96.06
permanent (silicone) (Souttar) 42.81
feeding
esophageal 42.81
gastric 96.6
nasogastric 96.6
gastric
by gastrostomy - *see* category 43.1
for
decompression, intestinal 96.07
feeding 96.6
intercostal (with water seal), for drainage 34.04
revision (with lysis of adhesions) 34.04
Miller-Abbott (for intestinal decompression) 96.08
nasobiliary (drainage) 51.86
nasogastric (for intestinal decompression) NEC 96.07
naso-intestinal 96.08
nasopancreatic drainage (endoscopic) 52.97
pancreatic duct 52.92
endoscopic 52.93
rectum 96.09
stomach (nasogastric) (for intestinal decompression) NEC 96.07
for feeding 96.6
tracheobronchial 96.05
umbrella device
atrial septum (King-Mills) 35.52
vena cava (Mobitz-Uddin) 38.7
ureteral stent (transurethral) 59.8
with ureterotomy 59.8 [56.2]
urinary sphincter, artificial (AUS) (inflatable) 58.93
vaginal mold 96.15
valve
Holter 02.2

Insertion (*Continued*)
valve (*Continued*)
Hufnagel - *see* Replacement, heart valve
pharyngeal (artificial) 31.75
Spitz-Holter 02.2
vas deferens 63.95
vascular access device, totally implantable 86.07
vena cava sieve or umbrella 38.7
Vinke tongs (skull) (with synchronous skeletal traction) 02.94
Instillation
bladder 96.49
digestive tract, except gastric gavage 96.43
genitourinary NEC 96.49
radioisotope (intracavitary) (intravenous) 92.28
Insufflation
Eustachian tube 20.8
fallopian tube (air) (dye) (gas) (saline) 66.8
for radiography - *see* Hysterosalpingography
therapeutic substance 66.95
lumbar retroperitoneal, bilateral 88.15
Intercricothyroidotomy (for assistance in breathing) 31.1
Intermittent positive pressure breathing (IPPB) 93.91
Interposition operation
esophageal reconstruction (intrathoracic) (retrosternal) NEC - *see also* Anastomosis, esophagus, with, interposition 42.58
antesternal or antethoracic NEC - *see also* Anastomosis, esophagus, antesternal, with, interposition 42.68
uterine suspension 69.21
Interrogation ◄
cardioverter-defibrillator, automatic (AICD) ◄
with NIPS (arrhythmia induction) 37.26 ◄
interrogation only (bedside device check) 89.49 ◄
CRT-D (cardiac resynchronization defibrillator) ◄
with NIPS (arrhythmia induction) 37.26 ◄
interrogation only (bedside device check) 89.49 ◄
CRT-P (cardiac resynchronization pacemaker) ◄
with NIPS (arrhythmia induction) 37.26 ◄
interrogation only (bedside device check) 89.45 ◄
pacemaker ◄
with NIPS (arrhythmia induction) 37.26 ◄
interrogation only (bedside device check) 89.45 ◄
Interruption
vena cava (inferior) (superior) 38.7
Interview (evaluation) (diagnostic)
medical, except psychiatric 89.05
brief (abbreviated history) 89.01
comprehensive (history and evaluation of new problem) 89.03

Interview (*Continued*)
medical, except psychiatric (*Continued*)
limited (interval history) 89.02
specified type NEC 89.04
psychiatric NEC 94.19
follow-up 94.19
initial 94.19
pre-commitment 94.13
Intimectomy 38.10
abdominal 38.16
aorta (arch) (ascending) (descending) 38.14
head and neck NEC 38.12
intracranial NEC 38.11
lower limb 38.18
thoracic NEC 38.15
upper limb 38.13
Introduction
orthodontic appliance 24.7
therapeutic substance (acting locally or systemically) NEC 99.29
bursa 83.96
hand 82.94
fascia 83.98
hand 82.96
heart 37.92
joint 81.92
temporomandibular 76.96
ligament (joint) 81.92
pericardium 37.93
soft tissue NEC 83.98
hand 82.96
tendon 83.97
hand 82.95
vein 39.92
Intubation - *see also* Catheterization and Insertion
bile duct(s) 51.59
common 51.51
endoscopic 51.87
endoscopic 51.87
esophagus (nonoperative) (Sengstaken) 96.06
permanent tube (silicone) (Souttar) 42.81
Eustachian tube 20.8
intestine (for decompression) 96.08
lacrimal for
dilation 09.42
tear drainage, intranasal 09.81
larynx 96.05
nasobiliary (drainage) 51.86
nasogastric
for
decompression, intestinal 96.07
feeding 96.6
naso-intestinal 96.08
nasolacrimal (duct) (with irrigation) 09.44
nasopancreatic drainage (endoscopic) 52.97
respiratory tract NEC 96.05
small intestine (Miller-Abbott) 96.08
stomach (nasogastric) (for intestinal decompression) NEC 96.07
for feeding 96.6
trachea 96.04
ventriculocisternal 02.2
Invagination, diverticulum
gastric 44.69
laparoscopic 44.68 ◄
pharynx 29.59

ICD-9-CM

–

Vol. 3

Invagination, diverticulum *(Continued)*
  stomach 44.69
    laparoscopic 44.68 ◀
Inversion
  appendix 47.99
  diverticulum
    gastric 44.69
      laparoscopic 44.68 ◀
    intestine
      large 45.49
        endoscopic 45.43
      small 45.34
    stomach 44.69
      laparoscopic 44.68 ◀
  tunica vaginalis 61.49
Ionization, medical 99.27
Iontherapy 99.27
Iontophoresis 99.27
Iridectomy (basal) (buttonhole) (optical)
    (peripheral) (total) 12.14
  with
    capsulectomy 13.65
    cataract extraction - *see* Extraction,
      cataract
    filtering operation (for glaucoma)
      NEC 12.65
    scleral
      fistulization 12.65
      thermocauterization 12.62
      trephination 12.61
Iridencleisis 12.63
Iridesis 12.63
Irido-capsulectomy 13.65
Iridocyclectomy 12.44
Iridocystectomy 12.42
Iridodesis 12.63
Iridoplasty NEC 12.39
Iridosclerectomy 12.65
Iridosclerotomy 12.69
Iridotasis 12.63
Iridotomy 12.12
  by photocoagulation 12.12
  with transfixion 12.11
  for iris bombé 12.11
  specified type NEC 12.12
Iron lung 93.99
Irradiation
  gamma, stereotactic 92.32
Irrigation
  anterior chamber (eye) 12.91
  bronchus NEC 96.56
  canaliculus 09.42
  catheter
    ureter 96.46
    urinary, indwelling NEC 96.48
    vascular 96.57
    ventricular 02.41
    wound 96.58
  cholecystostomy 96.41
  cornea 96.51
    with removal of foreign body
      98.21
  corpus cavernosum 64.98
  cystostomy 96.47
  ear (removal of cerumen) 96.52
  enterostomy 96.36
  eye 96.51
    with removal of foreign body 98.21
  gastrostomy 96.36
  lacrimal
    canaliculi 09.42
    punctum 09.41
  muscle 83.02
    hand 82.02

Irrigation *(Continued)*
  nasal
    passages 96.53
    sinus 22.00
  nasolacrimal duct 09.43
    with insertion of tube or stent
      09.44
  nephrostomy 96.45
  peritoneal 54.25
  pyelostomy 96.45
  rectal 96.39
  stomach 96.33
  tendon (sheath) 83.01
    hand 82.01
  trachea NEC 96.56
  traumatic cataract 13.3
  tube
    biliary NEC 96.41
    nasogastric NEC 96.34
    pancreatic 96.42
  ureterostomy 96.46
  ventricular shunt 02.41
  wound (cleaning) NEC 96.59
Irving operation (tubal ligation) 66.32
Irwin operation - *see also* Osteotomy
    77.30
Ischiectomy (partial) 77.89
  total 77.99
Ischiopubiotomy 77.39
Isolation
  after contact with infectious disease
    99.84
  ileal loop 45.51
  intestinal segment or pedicle flap
    large 45.52
    small 45.51
Isthmectomy, thyroid - *see also* Thyroid-
    ectomy, partial 06.39

J

Jaboulay operation (gastroduodenos-
    tomy) 44.39
  laparoscopic 44.38 ◀
Janeway operation (permanent gastros-
    tomy) 43.19
Jatene operation (arterial switch)
    35.84
Jejunectomy 45.62
Jejunocecostomy 45.93
Jejunocholecystostomy 51.32
Jejunocolostomy 45.93
Jejunoileostomy 45.91
Jejunojejunostomy 45.91
Jejunopexy 46.61
Jejunorrhaphy 46.73
Jejunostomy (feeding) 46.39
  delayed opening 46.31
  loop 46.01
  percutaneous (endoscopic) (PEJ)
    46.32
  revision 46.41
Jejunotomy 45.02
Johanson operation (urethral reconstruc-
    tion) 58.46
Jones operation
  claw toe (transfer of extensor hallucis
    longus tendon) 77.57
  modified (with arthrodesis)
    77.57
  dacryocystorhinostomy 09.81

Jones operation *(Continued)*
  hammer toe (interphalangeal fusion)
    77.56
  modified (tendon transfer with ar-
    throdesis) 77.57
  repair of peroneal tendon 83.88
Joplin operation (exostectomy with ten-
    don transfer) 77.53

K

Kader operation (temporary gastros-
    tomy) 43.19
Kasai portoenterostomy 51.37
Kaufman operation (for urinary stress
    incontinence) 59.79
Kazanjian operation (buccal vestibular
    sulcus extension) 24.91
Kehr operation (hepatopexy) 50.69
Keller operation (bunionectomy)
    77.59
Kelly (-Kennedy) **operation** (urethrovesi-
    cal plication) 59.3
Kelly-Stoeckel operation (urethrovesical
    plication) 59.3
Kelotomy 53.9
Keratectomy (complete) (partial) (super-
    ficial) 11.49
  for pterygium 11.39
    with corneal graft 11.32
Keratocentesis (for hyphema) 12.91
Keratomileusis 11.71
Keratophakia 11.72
Keratoplasty (tectonic) (with autograft)
    (with homograft) 11.60
  lamellar (nonpenetrating) (with homo-
    graft) 11.62
    with autograft 11.61
  penetrating (full-thickness) (with ho-
    mograft) 11.64
    with autograft 11.63
  perforating - *see* Keratoplasty, pene-
    trating
  refractive 11.71
  specified type NEC 11.69
Keratoprosthesis 11.73
Keratotomy (delimiting) (posterior)
    11.1
  radial (refractive) 11.75
Kerr operation (low cervical cesarean
    section) 74.1
Kessler operation (arthroplasty, carpo-
    metacarpal joint) 81.74
Kidner operation (excision of accessory
    navicular bone) (with tendon trans-
    fer) 77.98
Killian operation (frontal sinusotomy)
    22.41
Kineplasty - *see* Cineplasty
King-Steelquist operation (hindquarter
    amputation) 84.19
Kirk operation (amputation through
    thigh) 84.17
Kock pouch
  bowel anastomosis - *omit code*
  continent ileostomy 46.22
  cutaneous uretero-ileostomy 56.51
  ESWL (electrocorporeal shock wave
    lithotripsy) 98.51
  removal, calculus 57.19
  revision, cutaneous uretero-ileostomy
    56.52
  urinary diversion procedure 56.51

Kockogram (ileal conduitogram) 87.78

Kockoscopy 45.12

Kondoleon operation (correction of lymphedema) 40.9

Krause operation (sympathetic denervation) 05.29

Kroener operation (partial salpingectomy) 66.69

Kroenlein operation (lateral orbitotomy) 16.01

Krönig operation (low cervical cesarean section) 74.1

Krunkenberg operation (reconstruction of below-elbow amputation) 82.89

Kuhnt-Szymanowski operation (ectropion repair with lid reconstruction) 08.44

Kyphoplasty 81.66   ◀▦

ICD-9-CM

Vol. 3

L

Labbe operation (gastrotomy) 43.0
Labiectomy (bilateral) 71.62
  unilateral 71.61
Labyrinthectomy (transtympanic) 20.79
Labyrinthotomy (transtympanic) 20.79
Ladd operation (mobilization of intestine) 54.95
Lagrange operation (iridosclerectomy) 12.65
Lambrinudi operation (triple arthrodesis) 81.12
Laminectomy (decompression) (for exploration) 03.09
  as operative approach - *omit code*
  with
    excision of herniated intervertebral disc (nucleus pulposus) 80.51
    excision of other intraspinal lesion (tumor) 03.4
  reopening of site 03.02
Laminography - *see* Radiography
Laminoplasty, expansile 03.09
Laminotomy (decompression) (for exploration) 03.09
  as operative approach - *omit code*
  reopening of site 03.02
Langenbeck operation (cleft palate repair) 27.62
Laparoamnioscopy 75.31
Lapararrhaphy 54.63
Laparoscopy 54.21
  with
    biopsy (intra-abdominal) 54.24
      uterine ligaments 68.15
      uterus 68.16
    destruction of fallopian tubes - *see* Destruction, fallopian tube
Laparotomy NEC 54.19
  as operative approach - *omit code*
  exploratory (pelvic) 54.11
  reopening of recent operative site (for control of hemorrhage) (for exploration) (for incision of hematoma) 54.12
Laparotrachelotomy 74.1
Lapidus operation (bunionectomy with metatarsal osteotomy) 77.51
Larry operation (shoulder disarticulation) 84.08
Laryngectomy
  with radical neck dissection (with synchronous thyroidectomy) (with synchronous tracheostomy) 30.4
  complete (with partial laryngectomy) (with synchronous tracheostomy) 30.3
    with radical neck dissection (with synchronous thyroidectomy) (with synchronous tracheostomy) 30.4
  frontolateral partial (extended) 30.29
  glottosupraglottic partial 30.29
  lateral partial 30.29
  partial (frontolateral) (glottosupraglottic) (lateral) (submucous) (supraglottic) (vertical) 30.29
  radical (with synchronous thyroidectomy) (with synchronous tracheostomy) 30.4
  submucous (partial) 30.29
  supraglottic partial 30.29
  total (with partial pharyngectomy) (with synchronous tracheostomy) 30.3

Laryngectomy *(Continued)*
  total *(Continued)*
    with radical neck dissection (with synchronous thyroidectomy) (with synchronous tracheostomy) 30.4
  vertical partial 30.29
  wide field 30.3
Laryngocentesis 31.3
Laryngoesophagectomy 30.4
Laryngofissure 30.29
Laryngogram 87.09
  contrast 87.07
Laryngopharyngectomy (with synchronous tracheostomy) 30.3
  radical (with synchronous thyroidectomy) 30.4
Laryngopharyngoesophagectomy (with synchronous tracheostomy) 30.3
  with radical neck dissection (with synchronous thyroidectomy) 30.4
Laryngoplasty 31.69
Laryngorrhaphy 31.61
Laryngoscopy (suspension) (through artificial stoma) 31.42
Laryngostomy (permanent) 31.29
  revision 31.63
  temporary (emergency) 31.1
Laryngotomy 31.3
Laryngotracheobronchoscopy 33.23
  with biopsy 33.24
Laryngotracheoscopy 31.42
Laryngotracheostomy (permanent) 31.29
  temporary (emergency) 31.1
Laryngotracheotomy (temporary) 31.1
  permanent 31.29
Laser - *see also* Coagulation, Destruction, *and* Photocoagulation, by site
  angioplasty, percutaneous transluminal 39.59
    coronary - *see* Angioplasty, coronary
Lash operation
  internal cervical os repair 67.59
  laparoscopic supracervical hysterectomy 68.31
LASIK (Laser-assisted in situ keratomileusis) 11.71
Latzko operation
  cesarean section 74.2
  colpocleisis 70.4
Lavage
  antral 22.00
  bronchus NEC 96.56
    diagnostic (endoscopic) bronchoalveolar lavage (BAL) 33.24
  endotracheal 96.56
  gastric 96.33
  lung (total) (whole) 33.99
    diagnostic (endoscopic) bronchoalveolar lavage (BAL) 33.24
  nasal sinus(es) 22.00
    by puncture 22.01
    through natural ostium 22.02
  peritoneal (diagnostic) 54.25
  trachea NEC 96.56
Leadbetter operation (urethral reconstruction) 58.46
Leadbetter-Politano operation (ureteroneocystostomy) 56.74
LEEP (loop electrosurgical excision procedure) of cervix 67.32
Le Fort operation (colpocleisis) 70.8
LeMesurier operation (cleft lip repair) 27.54
Lengthening
  bone (with bone graft) 78.30
    femur 78.35

Lengthening *(Continued)*
  bone *(Continued)*
    for reconstruction of thumb 82.69
    specified site NEC - *see also* category 78.3, 78.39
    tibia 78.37
    ulna 78.33
  extraocular muscle NEC 15.21
    multiple (two or more muscles) 15.4
  fascia 83.89
    hand 82.89
  hamstring NEC 83.85
  heel cord 83.85
  leg
    femur 78.35
    tibia 78.37
  levator palpebrae muscle 08.38
  muscle 83.85
    extraocular 15.21
      multiple (two or more muscles) 15.4
    hand 82.55
  palate 27.62
    secondary or subsequent 27.63
  tendon 83.85
    for claw toe repair 77.57
    hand 82.55
Leriche operation (periarterial sympathectomy) 05.25
Leucotomy, leukotomy 01.32
Leukopheresis, therapeutic 99.72
Lid suture operation (blepharoptosis) 08.31
Ligation
  adrenal vessel (artery) (vein) 07.43
  aneurysm 39.52
  appendages, dermal 86.26
  arteriovenous fistula 39.53
    coronary artery 36.99
  artery 38.80
    abdominal 38.86
    adrenal 07.43
    aorta (arch) (ascending) (descending) 38.84
    coronary (anomalous) 36.99
    ethmoidal 21.04
    external carotid 21.06
    for control of epistaxis - *see* Control, epistaxis
    head and neck NEC 38.82
    intracranial NEC 38.81
    lower limb 38.88
    maxillary (transantral) 21.05
    middle meningeal 02.13
    thoracic NEC 38.85
    thyroid 06.92
    upper limb 38.83
  atrium, heart 37.99
  auricle, heart 37.99
  bleeding vessel - *see* Control, hemorrhage
  blood vessel 38.80
    abdominal
      artery 38.86
      vein 38.87
    adrenal 07.43
    aorta (arch) (ascending) (descending) 38.84
    esophagus 42.91
      endoscopic 42.33
    head and neck 38.82
    intracranial NEC 38.81
    lower limb
      artery 38.88
      vein 38.89

ICD-9-CM

Vol. 3

Lymphangiogram (Continued)
  lower limb 88.36
  pelvic 88.04
  upper limb 88.34
Lymphangioplasty 40.9
Lymphangiorrhaphy 40.9
Lymphangiotomy 40.0
Lymphaticostomy 40.9
  thoracic duct 40.62
Lysis

> Note blunt - *omit code*
>   digital - *omit code*
>   manual - *omit code*
>   mechanical - *omit code*
>   without instrumentation - *omit code*

  adhesions
    abdominal 54.59
      laparoscopic 54.51
    appendiceal 54.59
      laparoscopic 54.51
    artery-vein-nerve bundle 39.91
    biliary tract 54.59
      laparoscopic 54.51
    bladder (neck) (intraluminal) 57.12
      external 59.11
        laparoscopic 59.12
      transurethral 57.41
    blood vessels 39.91
    bone - *see* category 78.4
    bursa 83.91
      by stretching or manipulation 93.28
      hand 82.91
    cartilage of joint 93.26
    chest wall 33.99
    choanae (nasopharynx) 29.54
    conjunctiva 10.5
    corneovitreal 12.34
    cortical (brain) 02.91
    ear, middle 20.23
    Eustachian tube 20.8
    extraocular muscle 15.7
    extrauterine 54.59
      laparoscopic 54.51
    eyelid 08.09
      and conjunctiva 10.5
    eye muscle 15.7
    fallopian tube 65.89
      laparoscopic 65.81

Lysis (Continued)
  adhesions (Continued)
    fascia 83.91
      hand 82.91
        by stretching or manipulation 93.26
    gallbladder 54.59
      laparoscopic 54.51
    ganglion (peripheral) NEC 04.49
      cranial NEC 04.42
    hand 82.91
      by stretching or manipulation 93.26
    heart 37.10
    intestines 54.59
      laparoscopic 54.51
    iris (posterior) 12.33
      anterior 12.32
    joint (capsule) (structure) - *see also* Division, joint capsule 80.40
    kidney 59.02
      laparoscopic 59.03
    labia (vulva) 71.01
    larynx 31.92
    liver 54.59
      laparoscopic 54.51
    lung (for collapse of lung) 33.39
    mediastinum 34.99
    meninges (spinal) 03.6
      cortical 02.91
    middle ear 20.23
    muscle 83.91
      by stretching or manipulation 93.27
      extraocular 15.7
      hand 82.91
        by stretching or manipulation 93.26
    nasopharynx 29.54
    nerve (peripheral) NEC 04.49
      cranial NEC 04.42
      roots, spinal 03.6
      trigeminal 04.41
    nose, nasal 21.91
    ocular muscle 15.7
    ovary 65.89
      laparoscopic 65.81
    pelvic 54.59
      laparoscopic 54.51
    penile 64.93
    pericardium 37.12

Lysis (Continued)
  adhesions (Continued)
    perineal (female) 71.01
    peripheral vessels 39.91
    perirectal 48.81
    perirenal 59.02
      laparoscopic 59.03
    peritoneum (pelvic) 54.59
      laparoscopic 54.51
    periureteral 59.02
      laparoscopic 59.03
    perivesical 59.11
      laparoscopic 59.12
    pharynx 29.54
    pleura (for collapse of lung) 33.39
    spermatic cord 63.94
    spinal (cord) (meninges) (nerve roots) 03.6
    spleen 54.59
      laparoscopic 54.51
    tendon 83.91
      by stretching or manipulation 93.27
      hand 82.91
        by stretching or manipulation 93.26
    thorax 34.99
    tongue 25.93
    trachea 31.92
    tubo-ovarian 65.89
      laparoscopic 65.81
    ureter 59.02
      with freeing or repositioning of ureter 59.02
      intraluminal 56.81
      laparoscopic 59.03
    urethra (intraluminal) 58.5
    uterus 54.59
      intraluminal 68.21
      laparoscopic 54.51
      peritoneal 54.59
        laparoscopic 54.51
    vagina (intraluminal) 70.13
    vitreous (posterior approach) 14.74
      anterior approach 14.73
    vulva 71.01
  goniosynechiae (with injection of air or liquid) 12.31
  synechiae (posterior) 12.33
    anterior (with injection of air or liquid) 12.32

M

Madlener operation (tubal ligation) 66.31
Magnet extraction
 foreign body
  anterior chamber, eye 12.01
  choroid 14.01
  ciliary body 12.01
  conjunctiva 98.22
  cornea 11.0
  eye, eyeball NEC 98.21
   anterior segment 12.01
   posterior segment 14.01
  intraocular (anterior segment) 12.01
  iris 12.01
  lens 13.01
  orbit 98.21
  retina 14.01
  sclera 12.01
  vitreous 14.01
Magnetic resonance imaging (nuclear) -
  see Imaging, magnetic resonance
Magnuson (-Stack) operation (arthroplasty for recurrent shoulder dislocation) 81.82
Malleostapediopexy 19.19
 with incus replacement 19.11
Malström's vacuum extraction 72.79
 with episiotomy 72.71
Mammaplasty - see Mammoplasty
Mammectomy - see also Mastectomy
 subcutaneous (unilateral) 85.34
  with synchronous implant 85.33
   bilateral 85.36
    with synchronous implant 85.35
Mammilliplasty 85.87
Mammography NEC 87.37
Mammoplasty 85.89
 with
  full-thickness graft 85.83
  muscle flap 85.85
  pedicle graft 85.84
  split-thickness graft 85.82
 amputative (reduction) (bilateral) 85.32
  unilateral 85.31
 augmentation 85.50
  with
   breast implant (bilateral) 85.54
    unilateral 85.53
   injection into breast (bilateral)
    85.52
    unilateral 85.51
 reduction (bilateral) 85.32
  unilateral 85.31
 revision 85.89
 size reduction (gynecomastia) (bilateral) 85.32
  unilateral 85.31
Mammotomy 85.0
Manchester (-Donald) (-Fothergill) operation (uterine suspension) 69.22
Mandibulectomy (partial) 76.31
 total 76.42
  with reconstruction 76.41
Maneuver (method)
 Bracht 72.52
 Credé 73.59
 De Lee (key-in-lock) 72.4
 Kristeller 72.54
 Loveset's (extraction of arms in breech
  birth) 72.52
 Mauriceau (-Smellie-Veit) 72.52
 Pinard (total breech extraction) 72.54

Maneuver (Continued)
 Prague 72.52
 Ritgen 73.59
 Scanzoni (rotation) 72.4
 Van Hoorn 72.52
 Wigand-Martin 72.52
Manipulation
 with reduction of fracture or dislocation - see Reduction, fracture and
  Reduction, dislocation
 enterostomy stoma (with dilation)
  96.24
 intestine (intra-abdominal) 46.80
  large 46.82
  small 46.81
 joint
  adhesions 93.26
   temporomandibular 76.95
  dislocation - see Reduction, dislocation
 lacrimal passage (tract) NEC 09.49
 muscle structures 93.27
 musculoskeletal (physical therapy)
  NEC 93.29
 nasal septum, displaced 21.88
 osteopathic NEC 93.67
  for general mobilization (general articulation) 93.61
  high-velocity, low-amplitude forces
   (thrusting) 93.62
  indirect forces 93.65
  isotonic, isometric forces 93.64
  low-velocity, high-amplitude forces
   (springing) 93.63
  to move tissue fluids 93.66
 rectum 96.22
 salivary duct 26.91
 stomach, intraoperative 44.92
 temporomandibular joint NEC 76.95
 ureteral calculus by catheter
  with removal 56.0
  without removal 59.8
 uterus NEC 69.98
  gravid 75.99
  inverted
   manual replacement (following
    delivery) 75.94
  surgical - see Repair, inverted uterus
Manometry
 esophageal 89.32
 spinal fluid 89.15
 urinary 89.21
Manual arts therapy 93.81
Mapping
 cardiac (electrophysiologic) 37.27
  doppler (flow) 88.72
 electrocardiogram only 89.52
Marckwald operation (cervical os repair)
  67.59
Marshall-Marchetti (-Krantz) operation
  (retropubic urethral suspension) 59.5
Marsupialization - see also Destruction,
  lesion, by site
 cyst
  Bartholin's 71.23
  brain 01.59
  cervical (nabothian) 67.31
  dental 24.4
  dentigerous 24.4
  kidney 55.31
  larynx 30.01
  liver 50.21
  ovary 65.21
   laparoscopic 65.23

Marsupialization (Continued)
 cyst (Continued)
  pancreas 52.3
  pilonidal (open excision) (with partial closure) 86.21
  salivary gland 26.21
  spinal (intraspinal) (meninges) 03.4
  spleen, splenic 41.41
 lesion
  brain 01.59
  cerebral 01.59
  liver 50.21
 pilonidal cyst or sinus (open excision)
  (with partial closure) 86.21
 pseudocyst, pancreas 52.3
 ranula, salivary gland 26.21
Massage
 cardiac (external) (manual) (closed)
  99.63
  open 37.91
 prostatic 99.94
 rectal (for levator spasm) 99.93
MAST (military anti-shock trousers)
  93.58
Mastectomy (complete) (prophylactic)
  (simple) (unilateral) 85.41
 with
  excision of regional lymph nodes
   85.43
   bilateral 85.44
  preservation of skin and nipple
   85.34
   with synchronous implant 85.33
   bilateral 85.36
    with synchronous implant
     85.35
 bilateral 85.42
 extended
  radical (Urban) (unilateral) 85.47
   bilateral 85.48
  simple (with regional lymphadenectomy) (unilateral) 85.43
   bilateral 85.44
 modified radical (unilateral) 85.43
  bilateral 85.44
 partial 85.23
 radical (Halsted) (Meyer) (unilateral)
  85.45
  bilateral 85.46
  extended (Urban) (unilateral) 85.47
   bilateral 85.48
  modified (unilateral) 85.43
   bilateral 85.44
 subcutaneous 85.34
  with synchronous implant 85.33
   bilateral 85.36
    with synchronous implant 85.35
 subtotal 85.23
Masters' stress test (two-step) 89.42
Mastoidectomy (cortical) (conservative)
  20.49
 complete (simple) 20.41
 modified radical 20.49
 radical 20.42
  modified 20.49
 simple (complete) 20.41
Mastoidotomy 20.21
Mastoidotympanectomy 20.42
Mastopexy 85.6
Mastoplasty - see Mammoplasty
Mastorrhaphy 85.81
Mastotomy 85.0
Matas operation (aneurysmorrhaphy)
  39.52

ICD-9-CM

M

Vol. 3

Mayo operation
bunionectomy 77.59
herniorrhaphy 53.49
vaginal hysterectomy 68.59
laparoscopically assisted (LAVH) 68.51
Mazet operation (knee disarticulation) 84.16
McBride operation (bunionectomy with soft tissue correction) 77.53
McBurney operation - *see* Repair, hernia, inguinal
McCall operation (enterocele repair) 70.92
McCauley operation (release of clubfoot) 83.84
McDonald operation (encirclement suture, cervix) 67.59
McIndoe operation (vaginal construction) 70.61
McKeever operation (fusion of first metatarsophalangeal joint for hallux valgus repair) 77.52
McKissock operation (breast reduction) 85.33
McReynolds operation (transposition of pterygium) 11.31
McVay operation
femoral hernia - *see* Repair, hernia, femoral
inguinal hernia - *see* Repair, hernia, inguinal
Measurement
airway resistance 89.38
anatomic NEC 89.39
arterial blood gases 89.65
basal metabolic rate (BMR) 89.39
blood gases
arterial 89.65
continuous intra-arterial 89.60
venous 89.66
body 93.07
cardiac output (by)
Fick method 89.67
indicator dilution technique 89.68
oxygen consumption technique 89.67
thermodilution indicator 89.68
cardiovascular NEC 89.59
central venous pressure 89.62
coronary blood flow 89.69
gastric function NEC 89.39
girth 93.07
intelligence 94.01
intracranial pressure 01.18
intraocular tension or pressure 89.11
as part of extended ophthalmologic work-up 95.03
intrauterine pressure 89.62
limb length 93.06
lung volume 89.37
mixed venous blood gases 89.66
physiologic NEC 89.39
portovenous pressure 89.62
range of motion 93.05
renal clearance 89.29
respiratory NEC 89.38
skin fold thickness 93.07
skull circumference 93.07
sphincter of Oddi pressure 51.15
systemic arterial
blood gases 89.65
continuous intra-arterial 89.60
pressure 89.61
urine (bioassay) (chemistry) 89.29
vascular 89.59

Measurement (*Continued*)
venous blood gases 89.66
vital capacity (pulmonary) 89.37
Meatoplasty
ear 18.6
urethra 58.47
Meatotomy
ureter 56.1
urethra 58.1
internal 58.5
Mechanical ventilation - *see* Ventilation
Mediastinectomy 34.3
Mediastinoscopy (transpleural) 34.22
Mediastinotomy 34.1
with pneumonectomy 32.5
Meloplasty, facial 86.82
Meningeorrhaphy (cerebral) 02.12
spinal NEC 03.59
for
meningocele 03.51
myelomeningocele 03.52
Meniscectomy (knee) NEC 80.6
acromioclavicular 80.91
sternoclavicular 80.91
temporomandibular (joint) 76.5
wrist 80.93
Menstrual extraction or regulation 69.6
Mentoplasty (augmentation) (with graft) (with implant) 76.68
reduction 76.67
Mesenterectomy 54.4
Mesenteriopexy 54.75
Mesenteriplication 54.75
Mesocoloplication 54.75
Mesopexy 54.75
Metatarsectomy 77.98
Metroplasty 69.49
Mid-forceps delivery 72.29
Mikulicz operation (exteriorization of intestine) (first stage) 46.03
second stage 46.04
Miles operation (proctectomy) 48.5
Military anti-shock trousers (MAST) 93.58
Millard operation (cheiloplasty) 27.54
Miller operation
midtarsal arthrodesis 81.14
urethrovesical suspension 59.4
Millin-Read operation (urethrovesical suspension) 59.4
Mist therapy 93.94
Mitchell operation (hallux valgus repair) 77.51
Mobilization
joint NEC 93.16
mandible 76.95
neostrophingic (mitral valve) 35.12
spine 93.15
stapes (transcrural) 19.0
testis in scrotum 62.5
Mohs operation (chemosurgical excision of skin) 86.24
Molegraphy 87.81
Monitoring
cardiac output (by)
ambulatory (ACM) 89.50
electrographic 89.54
during surgery - *omit code*
Fick method 89.67
Holter-type device 89.50
indicator dilution technique 89.68
oxygen consumption technique 89.67
specified technique NEC 89.68
telemetry (cardiac) 89.54
thermodilution indicator 89.68

Monitoring (*Continued*)
cardiac output (*Continued*)
transesophageal (Doppler) (ultrasound) 89.68
central venous pressure 89.62
circulatory NEC 89.69
continuous intra-arterial blood gas 89.60
coronary blood flow (coincidence counting technique) 89.69
electroencephalographic 89.19
radio-telemetered 89.19
video 89.19
fetus (fetal heart)
antepartum
nonstress (fetal activity acceleration determinations) 75.34 ◀━
oxytocin challenge (contraction stress test) 75.35
ultrasonography (early pregnancy) (Doppler) 88.78
intrapartum (during labor) (extrauterine) (external) 75.34
auscultatory (stethoscopy) - *omit code*
internal (with contraction measurements) (ECG) 75.32
intrauterine (direct) (ECG) 75.32
phonocardiographic (extrauterine) 75.34
pulsed ultrasound (Doppler) 88.78
transcervical fetal oxygen saturation monitoring 75.38
transcervical fetal SpO$_2$ monitoring 75.38
Holter-type device (cardiac) 89.50
intracranial pressure 01.18
pulmonary artery
pressure 89.63
wedge 89.64
sleep (recording) - *see* categories 89.17-89.18
systemic arterial pressure 89.61
telemetry (cardiac) 89.54
transesophageal cardiac output (Doppler) 89.68
ventricular pressure (cardiac) 89.62
Moore operation (arthroplasty) 81.52
Moschowitz
enterocele repair 70.92
herniorrhaphy - *see* Repair, hernia, femoral
sigmoidopexy 46.63
Mountain resort sanitarium 93.98
Mouth-to-mouth resuscitation 93.93
Moxibustion 93.35
MRI - *see* Imaging, magnetic resonance
Muller operation (banding of pulmonary artery) 38.85
Multiple sleep latency test (MSLT) 89.18
Mumford operation (partial claviculectomy) 77.81
Musculoplasty - *see also* Repair, muscle 83.87
hand - *see also* Repair, muscle, hand 82.89
Music therapy 93.84
Mustard operation (interatrial transposition of venous return) 35.91
Myectomy 83.45
anorectal 48.92
eye muscle 15.13
multiple 15.3
for graft 83.43
hand 82.34

Myectomy (Continued)
  hand 82.36
    for graft 82.34
  levator palpebrae 08.33
  rectal 48.92
Myelogram, myelography (air) (gas)
  87.21
  posterior fossa 87.02
Myelotomy
  spine, spinal (cord) (tract) (one-stage)
    (two-stage) 03.29
    percutaneous 03.21
Myocardiectomy (infarcted area) 37.33
Myocardiotomy 37.11
Myoclasis 83.99
  hand 82.99
Myomectomy (uterine) 68.29
  broad ligament 69.19
Myoplasty - see also Repair, muscle 83.87
  hand - see also Repair, muscle, hand
    82.89
  mastoid 19.9
Myorrhaphy 83.65
  hand 82.46
Myosuture 83.65
  hand 82.46
Myotasis 93.27
Myotenontoplasty - see also Repair, tendon 83.88
  hand 82.86
Myotenoplasty - see also Repair, tendon
  83.88
  hand 82.86
Myotenotomy 83.13
  hand 82.11
Myotomy 83.02
  with division 83.19
    hand 82.19
  colon NEC 46.92
    sigmoid 46.91
  cricopharyngeal 29.31
    that for pharyngeal (pharyngoesoph-
      ageal) diverticulectomy 29.32
  esophagus 42.7
  eye (oblique) (rectus) 15.21
    multiple (two or more muscles) 15.4
  hand 82.02
    with division 82.19
  levator palpebrae 08.38
  sigmoid (colon) 46.91
Myringectomy 20.59
Myringodectomy 20.59
Myringomalleolabyrinthopexy 19.52
Myringoplasty (epitympanic, type I) (by
  cauterization) (by graft) 19.4
  revision 19.6
Myringostapediopexy 19.53
Myringostomy 20.01
Myringotomy (with aspiration) (with
  drainage) 20.09
  with insertion of tube or drainage de-
    vice (button) (grommet) 20.01

N

Nailing, intramedullary - see Reduction,
  fracture with internal fixation
Narcoanalysis 94.21
Narcosynthesis 94.21
Narrowing, palpebral fissure 08.51
Nasopharyngogram 87.09
  contrast 87.06
Necropsy 89.8
Needleoscopy (fetus) 75.31
Needling
  Bartholin's gland (cyst) 71.21
  cataract (secondary) 13.64
  fallopian tube 66.91
  hydrocephalic head 73.8
  lens (capsule) 13.2
  pupillary membrane (iris) 12.35
Nephrectomy (complete) (total) (unilat-
  eral) 55.51
  bilateral 55.54
  partial (wedge) 55.4
  remaining or solitary kidney 55.52
  removal, transplanted kidney 55.53
Nephrocolopexy 55.7
Nephrocystanastomosis NEC 56.73
Nephrolithotomy 55.01
Nephrolysis 59.02
  laparoscopic 59.03
Nephropexy 55.7
Nephroplasty 55.89
Nephropyeloplasty 55.87
Nephropyeloureterostomy 55.86
Nephrorrhaphy 55.81
Nephroscopy 55.21
Nephrostolithotomy, percutaneous
  55.03
Nephrostomy (with drainage tube)
  55.02
  closure 55.82
  percutaneous 55.03
    with fragmentation (ultrasound)
      55.04
Nephrotomogram, nephrotomography
  NEC 87.72
Nephrotomy 55.01
Nephroureterectomy (with bladder cuff)
  55.51
Nephroureterocystectomy 55.51 [57.79]
Nerve block (cranial) (peripheral) NEC -
  see also Block, by site 04.81
Neurectasis (cranial) (peripheral) 04.91
Neurectomy (cranial) (infraorbital) (occipital) (peripheral) (spinal) NEC
  04.07
  gastric (vagus) - see also Vagotomy
    44.00
  opticociliary 12.79

Neurectomy NEC (Continued)
  paracervical 05.22
  presacral 05.24
  retrogasserian 04.07
  sympathetic - see Sympathectomy
  trigeminal 04.07
  tympanic 20.91
Neurexeresis NEC 04.07
Neuroablation
  radiofrequency 04.2
Neuroanastomosis (cranial) (peripheral)
  NEC 04.74
  accessory-facial 04.72
  accessory-hypoglossal 04.73
  hypoglossal-facial 04.71
Neurolysis (peripheral nerve) NEC
  04.49
  carpal tunnel 04.43
  cranial nerve NEC 04.42
  spinal (cord) (nerve roots) 03.6
  tarsal tunnel 04.44
  trigeminal nerve 04.41
Neuroplasty (cranial) (peripheral) NEC
  04.79
  of old injury (delayed repair) 04.76
  revision 04.75
Neurorrhaphy (cranial) (peripheral)
  04.3
Neurotomy (cranial) (peripheral) (spinal)
  NEC 04.04
  acoustic 04.01
  glossopharyngeal 29.92
  lacrimal branch 05.0
  retrogasserian 04.02
  sympathetic 05.0
  vestibular 04.01
Neurotripsy (peripheral) NEC 04.03
  trigeminal 04.02
Nicola operation (tenodesis for recurrent
  dislocation of shoulder) 81.82
Nimodipine, infusion 99.75
NIPS (non-invasive programmed electrical stimulation) 37.26
Nissen operation (fundoplication of
  stomach) 44.66
  laparoscopic 44.67 ◀
Noble operation (plication of small intestine) 46.62
Norman Miller operation (vaginopexy)
  70.77
Norton operation (extraperitoneal cesarean section) 74.2
Nuclear magnetic resonance imaging -
  see Imaging, magnetic resonance
Nutrition, concentrated substances
  enteral infusion (of) 96.6
  parenteral (total) 99.15
  peripheral parenteral 99.15

O

Ober (-Yount) operation (gluteal-iliotibial fasciotomy) 83.14

Obliteration
bone cavity - *see also* Osteoplasty 78.40
calyceal diverticulum 55.39
canaliculi 09.6
cerebrospinal fistula 02.12
cul-de-sac 70.92
frontal sinus (with fat) 22.42
lacrimal punctum 09.91
lumbar pseudomeningocele 03.51
lymphatic structure(s) (peripheral) 40.9
maxillary sinus 22.31
meningocele (sacral) 03.51
pelvic 68.8
pleural cavity 34.6
sacral meningocele 03.51
Skene's gland 71.3
tympanomastoid cavity 19.9
vagina, vaginal (partial) (total) 70.4
vault 70.8

Occlusal molds (dental) 89.31

Occlusion
artery
by embolization - *see* Embolization, artery
by endovascular approach - *see* Embolization, artery
by ligation - *see* Ligation, artery
fallopian tube - *see* Ligation, fallopian tube
patent ductus arteriosus (PDA) 38.85
vein
by embolization - *see* Embolization, vein
by endovascular approach - *see* Embolization, vein
by ligation - *see* Ligation, vein
vena cava (surgical) 38.7

Occupational therapy 93.83

O'Donoghue operation (triad knee repair) 81.43

Odontectomy NEC - *see also* Removal, tooth, surgical 23.19

Oleothorax 33.39

Olshausen operation (uterine suspension) 69.22

Omentectomy 54.4
Omentofixation 54.74
Omentopexy 54.74
Omentoplasty 54.74
Omentorrhaphy 54.74
Omentotomy 54.19
Omphalectomy 54.3
Onychectomy 86.23
Onychoplasty 86.86
Onychotomy 86.09
with drainage 86.04

Oophorectomy (unilateral) 65.39
with salpingectomy 65.49
laparoscopic 65.41
bilateral (same operative episode) 65.51
laparoscopic 65.53
with salpingectomy 65.61
laparoscopic 65.63
laparoscopic 65.31
partial 65.29
laparoscopic 65.25
wedge 65.22
that by laparoscope 65.24
remaining ovary 65.52
laparoscopic 65.54
with tube 65.62
laparoscopic 65.64

Oophorocystectomy 65.29
laparoscopic 65.25
Oophoropexy 65.79
Oophoroplasty 65.79
Oophororrhaphy 65.71
laparoscopic 65.74
Oophorostomy 65.09
laparoscopic 65.01
Oophorotomy 65.09
laparoscopic 65.01

Opening
bony labyrinth (ear) 20.79
cranial suture 02.01
heart valve
closed heart technique - *see* Valvulotomy, by site
open heart technique - *see* Valvuloplasty, by site
spinal dura 03.09

Operation
Abbe
construction of vagina 70.61
intestinal anastomosis - *see* Anastomosis, intestine
abdominal (region) NEC 54.99
abdominoperineal NEC 48.5
Aburel (intra-amniotic injection for abortion) 75.0
Adams
advancement of round ligament 69.22
crushing of nasal septum 21.88
excision of palmar fascia 82.35
adenoids NEC 28.99
adrenal (gland) (nerve) (vessel) NEC 07.49
Albee
bone peg, femoral neck 78.05
graft for slipping patella 78.06
sliding inlay graft, tibia 78.07
Albert (arthrodesis, knee) 81.22
Aldridge (-Studdiford) (urethral sling) 59.5
Alexander
prostatectomy
perineal 60.62
suprapubic 60.3
shortening of round ligaments of uterus 69.22
Alexander-Adams (shortening of round ligaments of uterus) 69.22
Almoor (extrapetrosal drainage) 20.22
Altemeier (perineal rectal pull-through) 48.49
Ammon (dacryocystotomy) 09.53
Anderson (tibial lengthening) 78.37
Anel (dilation of lacrimal duct) 09.42
anterior chamber (eye) NEC 12.99
anti-incontinence NEC 59.79
antrum window (nasal sinus) 22.2
with Caldwell-Luc approach 22.39
anus NEC 49.99
aortic body NEC 39.8
aorticopulmonary window 39.59
appendix NEC 47.99
Arslan (fenestration of inner ear) 20.61
artery NEC 39.99
Asai (larynx) 31.75
Baffes (interatrial transposition of venous return) 35.91
Baldy-Webster (uterine suspension) 69.22
Ball
herniorrhaphy - *see* Repair, hernia, inguinal
undercutting 49.02

Operation (*Continued*)
Bankhart (capsular repair into glenoid, for shoulder dislocation) 81.82
Bardenheurer (ligation of innominate artery) 38.85
Barkan (goniotomy) 12.52
with goniopuncture 12.53
Barr (transfer of tibialis posterior tendon) 83.75
Barsky (closure of cleft hand) 82.82
Bassett (vulvectomy with inguinal lymph node dissection) 71.5 [40.3]
Bassini (herniorrhaphy) - *see* Repair, hernia, inguinal
Batch-Spittler-McFaddin (knee disarticulation) 84.16
Batista (partial ventriculectomy) (ventricular reduction) (ventricular remodeling) 37.35
Beck I (epicardial poudrage) 36.39
Beck II (aorta-coronary sinus shunt) 36.39
Beck-Jianu (permanent gastrostomy) 43.19
Bell-Beuttner (subtotal abdominal hysterectomy) 68.39
Belsey (esophagogastric sphincter) 44.65
Benenenti (rotation of bulbous urethra) 58.49
Berke (levator resection, eyelid) 08.33
Biesenberger (size reduction of breast, bilateral) 85.32
unilateral 85.31
Bigelow (litholapaxy) 57.0
biliary (duct) (tract) NEC 51.99
Billroth I (partial gastrectomy with gastroduodenostomy) 43.6
Billroth II (partial gastrectomy with gastrojejunostomy) 43.7
Binnie (hepatopexy) 50.69
Bischoff (ureteroneocystostomy) 56.74
bisection hysterectomy 68.39
laparoscopic 68.31
Bishoff (spinal myelotomy) 03.29
bladder NEC 57.99
flap 56.74
Blalock (systemic-pulmonary anastomosis) 39.0
Blalock-Hanlon (creation of atrial septal defect) 35.42
Blalock-Taussig (subclavian-pulmonary anastomosis) 39.0
Blascovic (resection and advancement of levator palpebrae superioris) 08.33
blood vessel NEC 39.99
Blount
femoral shortening (with blade plate) 78.25
by epiphyseal stapling 78.25
Boari (bladder flap) 56.74
Bobb (cholelithotomy) 51.04
bone NEC - *see* category 78.4
facial 76.99
injury NEC - *see* category 79.9
marrow NEC 41.98
skull NEC 02.99
Bonney (abdominal hysterectomy) 68.4
Borthen (iridotasis) 12.63
Bost
plantar dissection 80.48
radiocarpal fusion 81.26
Bosworth
arthroplasty for acromioclavicular separation 81.83

Operation *(Continued)*

Bosworth *(Continued)*

fusion of posterior lumbar spine 81.08
for pseudarthrosis 81.38
resection of radial head ligaments
(for tennis elbow) 80.92
shelf procedure, hip 81.40

Bottle (repair of hydrocele of tunica
vaginalis) 61.2

Boyd (hip disarticulation) 84.18

brain NEC 02.99

Brauer (cardiolysis) 37.10

breast NEC 85.99

Bricker (ileoureterostomy) 56.51

Bristow (repair of shoulder dislocation)
81.82

Brock (pulmonary valvulotomy) 35.03

Brockman (soft tissue release for clubfoot) 83.84

bronchus NEC 33.98

Browne (-Denis) (hypospadias repair)
58.45

Brunschwig (temporary gastrostomy)
43.19

buccal cavity NEC 27.99

Bunnell (tendon transfer) 82.56

Burch procedure (retropubic urethral
suspension for urinary stress incontinence) 59.5

Burgess (amputation of ankle) 84.14

bursa NEC 83.99
hand 82.99

bypass - *see* Bypass

Caldwell (sulcus extension) 24.91

Caldwell-Luc (maxillary sinusotomy)
22.39
with removal of membrane lining
22.31

Callander (knee disarticulation) 84.16

Campbell
bone block, ankle 81.11
fasciotomy (iliac crest) 83.14
reconstruction of anterior cruciate
ligaments 81.45

canthus NEC 08.99

cardiac NEC 37.99
septum NEC 35.98
valve NEC 35.99

carotid body or gland NEC 39.8

Carroll and Taber (arthroplasty, proximal interphalangeal joint) 81.72

Cattell (herniorrhaphy) 53.51

Cecil (urethral reconstruction) 58.46

cecum NEC 46.99

cerebral (meninges) NEC 02.99

cervix NEC 69.99

Chandler (hip fusion) 81.21

Charles (correction of lymphedema) 40.9

Charnley (compression arthrodesis)
ankle 81.11
hip 81.21
knee 81.22

Cheatle-Henry - *see* Repair, hernia,
femoral

chest cavity NEC 34.99

Chevalier-Jackson (partial laryngectomy) 30.29

Child (radical subtotal pancreatectomy) 52.53

Chopart (midtarsal amputation) 84.12

chordae tendineae NEC 35.32

choroid NEC 14.9

ciliary body NEC 12.98

cisterna chyli NEC 40.69

Operation *(Continued)*

Clagett (closure of chest wall following
open flap drainage) 34.72

Clayton (resection of metatarsal heads
and bases of phalanges) 77.88

clitoris NEC 71.4

cocked hat (metacarpal lengthening
and transfer of local flap) 82.69

Cockett (varicose vein)
lower limb 38.59
upper limb 38.53

Cody tack (perforation of footplate) 19.0

Coffey (uterine suspension) (Meig's
modification) 69.22

Cole (anterior tarsal wedge osteotomy)
77.28

Collis-Nissen (hiatal hernia repair) 53.80

colon NEC 46.99

Colonna
adductor tenotomy (first stage) 83.12
hip arthroplasty (second stage) 81.40
reconstruction of hip (second stage)
81.40

commando (radical glossectomy) 25.4

conjunctiva NEC 10.99
destructive NEC 10.33

Cox-maze procedure (ablation or destruction of heart tissue) - *see*
maze procedure

cornea NEC 11.99

Coventry (tibial wedge osteotomy) 77.27

Crawford (tarso-frontalis sling of eyelid) 08.32

cul-de-sac NEC 70.92

Culp-Deweerd (spiral flap pyeloplasty)
55.87

Culp-Scardino (ureteral flap pyeloplasty) 55.87

Curtis (interphalangeal joint arthroplasty) 81.72

cystocele NEC 70.51

Dahlman (excision of esophageal diverticulum) 42.31

Dana (posterior rhizotomy) 03.1

Danforth (fetal) 73.8

Darrach (ulnar resection) 77.83

Davis (intubated ureterotomy) 56.2

de Grandmont (tarsectomy) 08.35

Delorme
pericardiectomy 37.31
proctopexy 48.76
repair of prolapsed rectum 48.76
thoracoplasty 33.34

Denker (radical maxillary antrotomy)
22.31

Dennis-Varco (herniorrhaphy) - *see* Repair, hernia, femoral

Denonvilliers (limited rhinoplasty)
21.86

dental NEC 24.99
orthodontic NEC 24.8

Derlacki (tympanoplasty) 19.4

diaphragm NEC 34.89

Dickson (fascial transplant) 83.82

Dickson-Diveley (tendon transfer and
arthrodesis to correct claw toe)
77.57

Dieffenbach (hip disarticulation) 84.18

digestive tract NEC 46.99

Doléris (shortening of round ligaments) 69.22

D'Ombrain (excision of pterygium
with corneal graft) 11.32

Dorrance (push-back operation for
cleft palate) 27.62

Operation *(Continued)*

Dotter (transluminal angioplasty)
39.59

Douglas (suture of tongue to lip for
micrognathia) 25.59

Doyle (paracervical uterine denervation) 69.3

Dühamel (abdominoperineal pull-
through) 48.65

Duhrssen's (vaginofixation of uterus)
69.22

Dunn (triple arthrodesis) 81.12

duodenum NEC 46.99

Dupuytren
fasciectomy 82.35
fasciotomy 82.12
with excision 82.35
shoulder disarticulation 84.08

Durham (-Caldwell) (transfer of biceps
femoris tendon) 83.75

DuToit and Roux (staple capsulorrhaphy of shoulder) 81.82

DuVries (tenoplasty) 83.88

Dwyer
fasciotomy 83.14
soft tissue release NEC 83.84
wedge osteotomy, calcaneus 77.28

Eagleton (extrapetrosal drainage)
20.22

ear (external) NEC 18.9
middle or inner NEC 20.99

Eden-Hybinette (glenoid bone block)
78.01

Effler (heart) 36.2

Eggers
tendon release (patellar retinacula)
83.13
tendon transfer (biceps femoris tendon) (hamstring tendon) 83.75

Elliot (scleral trephination with iridectomy) 12.61

Ellis Jones (repair of peroneal tendon)
83.88

Ellison (reinforcement of collateral ligament) 81.44

Elmslie-Cholmeley (tarsal wedge osteotomy) 77.28

Eloesser
thoracoplasty 33.34
thoracostomy 34.09

Emmet (cervix) 67.61

endorectal pull-through 48.41

epididymis NEC 63.99

esophagus NEC 42.99

Estes (ovary) 65.72
laparoscopic 65.75

Estlander (thoracoplasty) 33.34

Evans (release of clubfoot) 83.84

extraocular muscle NEC 15.9
multiple (two or more muscles) 15.4
with temporary detachment from
globe 15.3
revision 15.6
single 15.29
with temporary detachment from
globe 15.19

eyeball NEC 16.99

eyelid(s) NEC 08.99

face NEC 27.99

facial bone or joint NEC 76.99

fallopian tube NEC 66.99

Farabeuf (ischiopubiotomy) 77.39

Fasanella-Servatt (blepharoptosis repair) 08.35

Operation *(Continued)*
fascia NEC 83.99
  hand 82.99
female (genital organs) NEC 71.9
  hysterectomy NEC 68.9
fenestration (aorta) 39.54
Ferguson (hernia repair) 53.00
Fick (perforation of footplate) 19.0
filtering (for glaucoma) 12.79
  with iridectomy 12.65
Finney (pyloroplasty) 44.2
fistulizing, sclera NEC 12.69
Foley (pyeloplasty) 55.87
Fontan (creation of conduit between
  right atrium and pulmonary artery) 35.94
Fothergill (-Donald) (uterine suspension) 69.22
Fowler
  arthroplasty of metacarpophalangeal
    joint 81.72
    release (mallet finger repair) 82.84
    tenodesis (hand) 82.85
    thoracoplasty 33.34
Fox (entropion repair with wedge resection) 08.43
Franco (suprapubic cystotomy) 57.19
Frank (permanent gastrostomy)
  43.19
Frazier (-Spiller) (subtemporal trigeminal rhizotomy) 04.02
Fredet-Ramstedt (pyloromyotomy)
  (with wedge resection) 43.3
Frenckner (intrapetrosal drainage)
  20.22
Frickman (abdominal proctopexy)
  48.75
Frommel (shortening of uterosacral ligaments) 69.22
Gabriel (abdominoperineal resection of
  rectum) 48.5
gallbladder NEC 51.99
ganglia NEC 04.99
  sympathetic 05.89
Gant (wedge osteotomy of trochanter)
  77.25
Garceau (tibial tendon transfer)
  83.75
Gardner (spinal meningocele repair)
  03.51
gastric NEC 44.99
Gelman (release of clubfoot) 83.84
genital organ NEC
  female 71.9
  male 64.99
Ghormley (hip fusion) 81.21
Giffod
  destruction of lacrimal sac 09.6
  keratotomy (delimiting) 11.1
Gill
  arthrodesis of shoulder 81.23
  laminectomy 03.09
Gill-Stein (carporadial arthrodesis)
  81.25
Gilliam (uterine suspension) 69.22
Girdlestone
  laminectomy with spinal fusion
    81.00
  muscle transfer for claw toe 77.57
  resection of femoral head and neck
    77.85
Girdlestone-Taylor (muscle transfer for
  claw toe repair) 77.57
glaucoma NEC 12.79

Operation *(Continued)*
Glenn (anastomosis of superior vena
  cava to right pulmonary artery)
  39.21
globus pallidus NEC 01.42
Goebel-Frangenheim-Stoeckel (urethro-
  vesical suspension) 59.4
Goldner (clubfoot release) 80.48
Goldthwaite
  ankle stabilization 81.11
  patella stabilization 81.44
  tendon transfer for patella disloca-
    tion 81.44
Goodall-Power (vagina) 70.4
Gordon-Taylor (hindquarter amputa-
  tion) 84.19
Graber-Duvernay (drilling femoral
  head) 77.15
Green (scapulopexy) 78.41
Grice (subtalar arthrodesis) 81.13
Gritti-Stokes (knee disarticulation)
  84.16
Gross (herniorrhaphy) 53.49
gum NEC 24.39
Guyon (amputation of ankle) 84.13
Hagner (epididymotomy) 63.92
Halsted - see Repair, hernia, inguinal
Hampton (anastomosis, small intestine
  to rectal stump) 45.92
hanging hip (muscle release) 83.19
harelip 27.54
Harrison-Richardson (vaginal suspen-
  sion) 70.77
Hartmann - see Colectomy, by site
Hauser
  achillotenotomy 83.11
  bunionectomy with adductor tendon
    transfer 77.53
  stabilization of patella 81.44
Heaney (vaginal hysterectomy) 68.59
  laparoscopically assisted (LAVH)
    68.51
heart NEC 37.99
  valve NEC 35.99
    adjacent structure NEC 35.39
Hegar (perineorrhaphy) 71.79
Heine (cyclodialysis) 12.55
Heineke-Mikulicz (pyloroplasty) - see
  category 44.2
Heller (esophagomyotomy) 42.7
Hellström (transplantation of aberrant
  renal vessel) 39.55
hemorrhoids NEC 49.49
Henley (jejunal transposition) 43.81
hepatic NEC 50.99
hernia - see Repair, hernia
Hey (amputation of foot) 84.12
Hey-Groves (reconstruction of anterior
  cruciate ligament) 81.45
Heyman (soft tissue release for club-
  foot) 83.84
Heyman-Herndon (-Strong) (correction
  of metatarsus varus) 80.48
Hibbs (lumbar spinal fusion) - see Fusion, lumbar
Higgins - see Repair, hernia, femoral
Hill-Allison (hiatal hernia repair, transpleural approach) 53.80
Hitchcock (anchoring tendon of biceps)
  83.88
Hofmeister (gastrectomy) 43.7
Hoke
  midtarsal fusion 81.14
  triple arthrodesis 81.12

Operation *(Continued)*
Holth
  iridencleisis 12.63
  sclerectomy 12.65
Homans (correction of lymphedema)
  40.9
Hutch (ureteroneocystostomy) 56.74
Hybinette-Eden (glenoid bone block)
  78.01
hymen NEC 70.91
hypopharynx NEC 29.99
hypophysis NEC 07.79
ileal loop 56.51
ileum NEC 46.99
intestine NEC 46.99
iris NEC 12.97
  inclusion 12.63
Irving (tubal ligation) 66.32
Irwin - see also Osteotomy 77.30
Jaboulay (gastroduodenostomy) 44.39 ◀
  laparoscopic 44.38
Janeway (permanent gastrostomy) 43.19
Jatene (arterial switch) 35.84
jejunum NEC 46.99
Johanson (urethral reconstruction)
  58.46
joint (capsule) (ligament) (structure)
  NEC 81.99
  facial NEC 76.99
Jones
  claw toe (transfer of extensor hallu-
    cis longus tendon) 77.57
    modified (with arthrodesis) 77.57
  dacryocystorhinostomy 09.81
  hammer toe (interphalangeal fusion)
    77.56
  modified (tendon transfer with ar-
    throdesis) 77.57
  repair of peroneal tendon 83.88
Joplin (exostectomy with tendon transfer) 77.53
Kader (temporary gastrostomy) 43.19
Kaufman (for urinary stress incontinence) 59.79
Kazanjian (buccal vestibular sulcus ex-
  tension) 24.91
Kehr (hepatopexy) 50.69
Keller (bunionectomy) 77.59
Kelly (-Kennedy) (urethrovesical plication) 59.3
Kelly-Stoeckel (urethrovesical plication) 59.3
Kerr (cesarean section) 74.1
Kessler (arthroplasty, carpometacarpal
  joint) 81.74
Kidner (excision of accessory navicular
  bone) (with tendon transfer) 77.98
kidney NEC 55.99
Killian (frontal sinusotomy) 22.41
King-Steelquist (hindquarter amputation) 84.19
Kirk (amputation through thigh) 84.17
Kock pouch
  bowel anastomosis - *omit code*
  continent ileostomy 46.22
  cutaneous uretero-ileostomy 56.51
  ESWL (electrocorporeal shock wave
    lithotripsy) 98.51
  removal, calculus 57.19
  revision, cutaneous uretero-ileos-
    tomy 56.52
  urinary diversion procedure 56.51
Kondoleon (correction of lymphedema)
  40.9

Operation (Continued)

Krause (sympathetic denervation) 05.29
Kroener (partial salpingectomy) 66.69
Kroenlein (lateral orbitotomy) 16.01
Krönig (low cervical cesarean section) 74.1
Krukenberg (reconstruction of below-elbow amputation) 82.89
Kuhnt-Szymanowski (ectropion repair with lid reconstruction) 08.44
Labbe (gastrotomy) 43.0
labia NEC 71.8
lacrimal
    gland 09.3
    system NEC 09.99
Ladd (mobilization of intestine) 54.95
Lagrange (iridosclerectomy) 12.65
Lambrinudi (triple arthrodesis) 81.12
Langenbeck (cleft palate repair) 27.62
Lapidus (bunionectomy with metatarsal osteotomy) 77.51
Larry (shoulder disarticulation) 84.08
larynx NEC 31.98
Lash
    internal cervical os repair 67.59
    laparoscopic supracervical hysterectomy 68.31
Latzko
    cesarean section, extraperitoneal 74.2
    colpocleisis 70.8
Leadbetter (urethral reconstruction) 58.46
Leadbetter-Politano (ureteroneocystostomy) 56.74
Le Fort (colpocleisis) 70.8
LeMesurier (cleft lip repair) 27.54
lens NEC 13.9
Leriche (periarterial sympathectomy) 05.25
levator muscle sling
    eyelid ptosis repair 08.33
    urethrovesical suspension 59.71
    urinary stress incontinence 59.71
lid suture (blepharoptosis) 08.31
ligament NEC 81.99
    broad NEC 69.98
    round NEC 69.98
    uterine NEC 69.98
Lindholm (repair of ruptured tendon) 83.88
Linton (varicose vein) 38.59
lip NEC 27.99
Lisfranc
    foot amputation 84.12
    shoulder disarticulation 84.08
Littlewood (forequarter amputation) 84.09
liver NEC 50.99
Lloyd-Davies (abdominoperineal resection) 48.5
Longmire (bile duct anastomosis) 51.39
Lord
    dilation of anal canal for hemorrhoids 49.49
    hemorrhoidectomy 49.49
    orchidopexy 62.5
Lucas and Murray (knee arthrodesis with plate) 81.22
lung NEC 33.99
lung volume reduction 32.22
lymphatic structure(s) NEC 40.9
    duct, left (thoracic) NEC 40.69
Madlener (tubal ligation) 66.31
Magnuson (-Stack) (arthroplasty for recurrent shoulder dislocation) 81.82

Operation (Continued)

male genital organs NEC 64.99
Manchester (-Donald) (-Fothergill) (uterine suspension) 69.22
mandible NEC 76.99
    orthognathic 76.64
Marckwald (cervical os repair) 67.59
Marshall-Marchetti (-Krantz) (retropubic urethral suspension) 59.5
Matas (aneurysmorrhaphy) 39.52
Mayo
    bunionectomy 77.59
    herniorrhaphy 53.49
    vaginal hysterectomy 68.59
        laparoscopically assisted (LAVH) 68.51
Maze procedure (ablation or destruction of heart tissue)
    by incision (open) 37.33
    by peripherally inserted catheter 37.34
    endovascular approach 37.34
    trans-thoracic approach 37.33
Mazet (knee disarticulation) 84.16
McBride (bunionectomy with soft tissue correction) 77.53
McBurney - see Repair, hernia, inguinal
McCall (enterocele repair) 70.92
McCauley (release of clubfoot) 83.84
McDonald (encirclement suture, cervix) 67.59
McIndoe (vaginal construction) 70.61
McKeever (fusion of first metatarsophalangeal joint for hallux valgus repair) 77.52
McKissock (breast reduction) 85.33
McReynolds (transposition of pterygium) 11.31
McVay
    femoral hernia - see Repair, hernia, femoral
    inguinal hernia - see Repair, hernia, inguinal
meninges (spinal) NEC 03.99
    cerebral NEC 02.99
mesentery NEC 54.99
Mikulicz (exteriorization of intestine) (first stage) 46.03
    second stage 46.04
Miles (complete proctectomy) 48.5
Millard (cheiloplasty) 27.54
Miller
    midtarsal arthrodesis 81.14
    urethrovesical suspension 59.4
Millin-Read (urethrovesical suspension) 59.4
Mitchell (hallux valgus repair) 77.51
Mohs (chemosurgical excision of skin) 86.24
Moore (arthroplasty) 81.52
Moschowitz
    enterocele repair 70.92
    herniorrhaphy - see Repair, hernia, femoral
    sigmoidopexy 46.63
mouth NEC 27.99
Muller (banding of pulmonary artery) 38.85
Mumford (partial claviculectomy) 77.81
muscle NEC 83.99
    extraocular - see Operation, extraocular
    hand NEC 82.99
    papillary heart NEC 35.31
musculoskeletal system NEC 84.99
Mustard (interatrial transposition of venous return) 35.91

Operation (Continued)

nail (finger) (toe) NEC 86.99
nasal sinus NEC 22.9
nasopharynx NEC 29.99
nerve (cranial) (peripheral) NEC 04.99
    adrenal NEC 07.49
    sympathetic NEC 05.89
nervous system NEC 05.9
Nicola (tenodesis for recurrent dislocation of shoulder) 81.82
nipple NEC 85.99
Nissen (fundoplication of stomach) 44.66
    laparoscopic 44.67 ◀
Noble (plication of small intestine) 46.62
node (lymph) NEC 40.9
Norman Miller (vaginopexy) 70.77
Norton (extraperitoneal cesarean operation) 74.2
nose, nasal NEC 21.99
    sinus NEC 22.9
Ober (-Yount) (gluteal-iliotibial fasciotomy) 83.14
obstetric NEC 75.99
ocular NEC 16.99
    muscle - see Operation, extraocular muscle
O'Donoghue (triad knee repair) 81.43
Olshausen (uterine suspension) 69.22
omentum NEC 54.99
ophthalmologic NEC 16.99
oral cavity NEC 27.99
orbicularis muscle sling 08.36
orbit NEC 16.98
oropharynx NEC 29.99
orthodontic NEC 24.8
orthognathic NEC 76.69
Oscar Miller (midtarsal arthrodesis) 81.14
Osmond-Clark (soft tissue release with peroneus brevis tendon transfer) 83.75
ovary NEC 65.99
Oxford (for urinary incontinence) 59.4
palate NEC 27.99
palpebral ligament sling 08.36
Panas (linear proctotomy) 48.0
Pancoast (division of trigeminal nerve at foramen ovale) 04.02
pancreas NEC 52.99
pantaloon (revision of gastric anastomosis) 44.5
papillary muscle (heart) NEC 35.31
Paquin (ureteroneocystostomy) 56.74
parathyroid gland(s) NEC 06.99
parotid gland or duct NEC 26.99
Partsch (marsupialization of dental cyst) 24.4
Pattee (auditory canal) 18.6
Peet (splanchnic resection) 05.29
Pemberton
    osteotomy of ilium 77.39
    rectum (mobilization and fixation for prolapse repair) 48.76
penis NEC 64.98
Pereyra (paraurethral suspension) 59.6
pericardium NEC 37.99
perineum (female) NEC 71.8
    male NEC 86.99
perirectal tissue NEC 48.99
perirenal tissue NEC 59.92
peritoneum NEC 54.99
periurethral tissue NEC 58.99
perivesical tissue NEC 59.92

Operation (Continued)

pharyngeal flap (cleft palate repair) 27.62
  secondary or subsequent 27.63
pharynx, pharyngeal (pouch) NEC 29.99
pineal gland NEC 07.59
Pinsker (obliteration of nasoseptal telangiectasia) 21.07
Piper (forceps) 72.6
Pirogoff (ankle amputation through malleoli of tibia and fibula) 84.14
pituitary gland NEC 07.79
plastic - *see* Repair, by site
pleural cavity NEC 34.99
Politano-Leadbetter (ureteroneocystostomy) 56.74
pollicization (with nerves and blood supply) 82.61
Polya (gastrectomy) 43.7
Pomeroy (ligation and division of fallopian tubes) 66.32
Poncet
  lengthening of Achilles tendon 83.85
  urethrostomy, perineal 58.0
Porro (cesarean section) 74.99
posterior chamber (eye) NEC 14.9
Potts-Smith (descending aorta-left pulmonary artery anastomosis) 39.0
Printen and Mason (high gastric bypass) 44.31
prostate NEC - *see also* Prostatectomy 60.69
  specified type 60.99
pterygium 11.39
  with corneal graft 11.32
Puestow (pancreaticojejunostomy) 52.96
pull-through NEC 48.49
pulmonary NEC 33.99
push-back (cleft palate repair) 27.62
Putti-Platt (capsulorrhaphy of shoulder for recurrent dislocation) 81.82
pyloric exclusion 44.39
  laparoscopic 44.38 ◄
pyriform sinus NEC 29.99
"rabbit ear" (anterior urethropexy) (Tudor) 59.79
Ramadier (intrapetrosal drainage) 20.22
Ramstedt (pyloromyotomy) (with wedge resection) 43.3
Rankin
  exteriorization of intestine 46.03
  proctectomy (complete) 48.5
Rashkind (balloon septostomy) 35.41
Rastelli (creation of conduit between right ventricle and pulmonary artery) 35.92
  in repair of
    pulmonary artery atresia 35.92
    transposition of great vessels 35.92
    truncus arteriosus 35.83
Raz-Pereyra procedure (bladder neck suspension) 59.79
rectal NEC 48.99
rectocele NEC 70.52
re-entry (aorta) 39.54
renal NEC 55.99
respiratory (tract) NEC 33.99
retina NEC 14.9
Ripstein (repair of rectal prolapse) 48.75

Operation (Continued)

Rodney Smith (radical subtotal pancreatectomy) 52.53
Roux-en-Y
  bile duct 51.36
  cholecystojejunostomy 51.32
  esophagus (intrathoracic) 42.54
  gastroenterostomy 44.39
    laparoscopic 44.38 ◄
  gastrojejunostomy 44.39
    laparoscopic 44.38 ◄
  pancreaticojejunostomy 52.96
Roux-Goldthwait (repair of patellar dislocation) 81.44
Roux-Herzen-Judine (jejunal loop interposition) 42.63
Ruiz-Mora (proximal phalangectomy for hammer toe) 77.99
Russe (bone graft of scaphoid) 78.04
Saemisch (corneal section) 11.1
salivary gland or duct NEC 26.99
Salter (innominate osteotomy) 77.39
Sauer-Bacon (abdominoperineal resection) 48.5
Schanz (femoral osteotomy) 77.35
Schauta (-Amreich) (radical vaginal hysterectomy) 68.7
Schede (thoracoplasty) 33.34
Scheie
  cautery of sclera 12.62
  sclerostomy 12.62
Schlatter (total gastrectomy) 43.99
Schroeder (endocervical excision) 67.39
Schuchardt (nonobstetrical episiotomy) 71.09
Schwartze (simple mastoidectomy) 20.41
sclera NEC 12.89
Scott
  intestinal bypass for obesity 45.93
  jejunocolostomy (bypass) 45.93
scrotum NEC 61.99
Seddon-Brooks (transfer of pectoralis major tendon) 83.75
Semb (apicolysis of lung) 33.39
seminal vesicle NEC 60.79
Senning (correction of transposition of great vessels) 35.91
Sever (division of soft tissue of arm) 83.19
Sewell (heart) 36.2
sex transformation NEC 64.5
Sharrard (iliopsoas muscle transfer) 83.77
shelf (hip arthroplasty) 81.40
Shirodkar (encirclement suture, cervix) 67.59
sigmoid NEC 46.99
Silver (bunionectomy) 77.59
Sistrunk (excision of thyroglossal cyst) 06.7
Skene's gland NEC 71.8
skin NEC 86.99
skull NEC 02.99
sling
  eyelid
    fascia lata, palpebral 08.36
    frontalis fascial 08.32
    levator muscle 08.33
    orbicularis muscle 08.36
    palpebrae ligament, fascia lata 08.36
    tarsus muscle 08.35
  fascial (fascia lata)
    eye 08.32

Operation (Continued)

sling (Continued)
  fascial (Continued)
    for facial weakness (trigeminal nerve paralysis) 86.81
    palpebral ligament 08.36
    tongue 25.59
  tongue (fascial) 25.59
  urethra (suprapubic) 59.4
    retropubic 59.5
  urethrovesical 59.5
Slocum (pes anserinus transfer) 81.47
Sluder (tonsillectomy) 28.2
Smith (open osteotomy of mandible) 76.62
Smith-Peterson (radiocarpal arthrodesis) 81.25
Smithwick (sympathectomy) 05.29
Soave (endorectal pull-through) 48.41
soft tissue NEC 83.99
  hand 82.99
Sonneberg (inferior maxillary neurectomy) 04.07
Sorondo-Ferré (hindquarter amputation) 84.19
Soutter (iliac crest fasciotomy) 83.14
Spalding-Richardson (uterine suspension) 69.22
spermatic cord NEC 63.99
sphincter of Oddi NEC 51.89
spinal (canal) (cord) (structures) NEC 03.99
Spinelli (correction of inverted uterus) 75.93
Spivack (permanent gastrostomy) 43.19
spleen NEC 41.99
S.P. Rogers (knee disarticulation) 84.16
Ssabanejew-Frank (permanent gastrostomy) 43.19
Stacke (simple mastoidectomy) 20.41
Stallard (conjunctivocystorhinostomy) 09.82
  with insertion of tube or stent 09.83
Stamm (-Kader) (temporary gastrostomy) 43.19
Steinberg 44.5
Steindler
  fascia stripping (for cavus deformity) 83.14
  flexorplasty (elbow) 83.77
  muscle transfer 83.77
sterilization NEC
  female - *see also* specific operation 66.39
  male - *see also* Ligation, vas deferens 63.70
Stewart (renal plication with pyeloplasty) 55.87
stomach NEC 44.99
Stone (anoplasty) 49.79
Strassman (metroplasty) 69.49
  metroplasty (Jones modification) 69.49
  uterus 68.22
Strayer (gastrocnemius recession) 83.72
stress incontinence - *see* Repair, stress incontinence
Stromeyer-Little (hepatotomy) 50.0
Strong (unbridling of celiac artery axis) 39.91
Sturmdorf (conization of cervix) 67.2
subcutaneous tissue NEC 86.99
sublingual gland or duct NEC 26.99
submaxillary gland or duct NEC 26.99

Operation (*Continued*)
Summerskill (dacryocystorhinostomy by intubation) 09.81
Surmay (jejunostomy) 46.39
Swenson
  bladder reconstruction 57.87
  proctectomy 48.49
Swinney (urethral reconstruction) 58.46
Syme
  ankle amputation through malleoli of tibia and fibula 84.14
  urethrotomy, external 58.0
sympathetic nerve NEC 05.89
Taarnhoj (trigeminal nerve root decompression) 04.41
Tack (sacculotomy) 20.79
Talma-Morison (omentopexy) 54.74
Tanner (devascularization of stomach) 44.99
TAPVC NEC 35.82
tarsus NEC 08.99
  muscle sling 08.35
tendon NEC 83.99
  extraocular NEC 15.9
  hand NEC 82.99
testis NEC 62.99
tetralogy of Fallot
  partial repair - *see* specific procedure
  total (one-stage) 35.81
Thal (repair of esophageal stricture) 42.85
thalamus 01.41
  by stereotactic radiosurgery 92.32
    cobalt 60 92.32
    linear accelerator (LINAC) 92.31
    multi-source 92.32
    particle beam 92.33
    particulate 92.33
    radiosurgery NEC 92.39
    single source photon 92.31
Thiersch
  anus 49.79
  skin graft 86.69
    hand 86.62
Thompson
  cleft lip repair 27.54
  correction of lymphedema 40.9
  quadricepsplasty 83.86
  thumb apposition with bone graft 82.69
thoracic duct NEC 40.69
thorax NEC 34.99
Thorek (partial cholecystectomy) 51.21
three-snip, punctum 09.51
thymus NEC 07.99
thyroid gland NEC 06.98
TKP (thermokeratoplasty) 11.74
Tomkins (metroplasty) 69.49
tongue NEC 25.99
  flap, palate 27.62
  tie 25.91
tonsil NEC 28.99
Torek (-Bevan) (orchidopexy) (first stage) (second stage) 62.5
Torkildsen (ventriculocisternal shunt) 02.2
Torpin (cul-de-sac resection) 70.92
Toti (dacryocystorhinostomy) 09.81
Touchas 86.83
Touroff (ligation of subclavian artery) 38.85
trabeculae corneae cordis (heart) NEC 35.35
trachea NEC 31.99

Operation (*Continued*)
Trauner (lingual sulcus extension) 24.91
truncus arteriosus NEC 35.83
Tsuge (macrodactyly repair) 82.83
Tudor "rabbit ear" (anterior urethropexy) 59.79
Tuffier
  apicolysis of lung 33.39
  vaginal hysterectomy 68.59
    laparoscopically assisted (LAVH) 68.51
tunica vaginalis NEC 61.99
Turco (release of joint capsules in clubfoot) 80.48
Uchida (tubal ligation with or without fimbriectomy) 66.32
umbilicus NEC 54.99
urachus NEC 57.51
Urban (mastectomy) (unilateral) 85.47
  bilateral 85.48
ureter NEC 56.99
urethra NEC 58.99
urinary system NEC 59.99
uterus NEC 69.99
  supporting structures NEC 69.98
uvula NEC 27.79
vagina NEC 70.91
vascular NEC 39.99
vas deferens NEC 63.99
  ligation NEC 63.71
vein NEC 39.99
vena cava sieve 38.7
vertebra NEC 78.49
vesical (bladder) NEC 57.99
vessel NEC 39.99
  cardiac NEC 36.99
Vicq d'Azyr (larynx) 31.1
Vidal (varicocele ligation) 63.1
Vineberg (implantation of mammary artery into ventricle) 36.2
vitreous NEC 14.79
vocal cord NEC 31.98
von Kraske (proctectomy) 48.64
Voss (hanging hip operation) 83.19
Vulpius (-Compere) (lengthening of gastrocnemius muscle) 83.85
vulva NEC 71.8
Ward-Mayo (vaginal hysterectomy) 68.59
  laparoscopically assisted (LAVH) 68.51
Wardill (cleft palate) 27.62
Waters (extraperitoneal cesarean section) 74.2
Waterston (aorta-right pulmonary artery anastomosis) 39.0
Watkins (-Wertheim) (uterus interposition) 69.21
Watson-Jones
  hip arthrodesis 81.21
  reconstruction of lateral ligaments, ankle 81.49
  shoulder arthrodesis (extra-articular) 81.23
  tenoplasty 83.88
Weir
  appendicostomy 47.91
  correction of nostrils 21.86
Wertheim (radical hysterectomy) 68.6
West (dacryocystorhinostomy) 09.81
Wheeler
  entropion repair 08.44
  halving procedure (eyelid) 08.24
Whipple (radical pancreaticoduodenec-

Operation (*Continued*)
  tomy) 52.7
  Child modification (radical subtotal pancreatectomy) 52.53
  Rodney Smith modification (radical subtotal pancreatectomy) 52.53
White (lengthening of tendo calcaneus by incomplete tenotomy) 83.11
Whitehead
  glossectomy, radical 25.4
  hemorrhoidectomy 49.46
Whitman
  foot stabilization (talectomy) 77.98
  hip reconstruction 81.40
  repair of serratus anterior muscle 83.87
  talectomy 77.98
  trochanter wedge osteotomy 77.25
Wier (entropion repair) 08.44
Williams-Richardson (vaginal construction) 70.61
Wilms (thoracoplasty) 33.34
Wilson (angulation osteotomy for hallux valgus) 77.51
window
  antrum (nasal sinus) - *see* Antrotomy, maxillary
  aorticopulmonary 39.59
  bone cortex - *see also* Incision, bone 77.10
    facial 76.09
  nasoantral - *see* Antrotomy, maxillary
  pericardium 37.12
  pleural 34.09
Winiwarter (cholecystoenterostomy) 51.32
Witzel (temporary gastrostomy) 43.19
Woodward (release of high riding scapula) 81.83
Young
  epispadias repair 58.45
  tendon transfer (anterior tibialis) (repair of flat foot) 83.75
Yount (division of iliotibial band) 83.14
Zancolli
  capsuloplasty 81.72
  tendon transfer (biceps) 82.56
Ziegler (iridectomy) 12.14
Operculectomy 24.6
Ophthalmectomy 16.49
  with implant (into Tenon's capsule) 16.42
  with attachment of muscles 16.41
Ophthalmoscopy 16.21
Opponensplasty (hand) 82.56
Orbitomaxillectomy, radical 16.51
Orbitotomy (anterior) (frontal) (temporofrontal) (transfrontal) NEC 16.09
  with
    bone flap 16.01
    insertion of implant 16.02
  Kroenlein (lateral) 16.01
  lateral 16.01
Orchidectomy (with epididymectomy) (unilateral) 62.3
  bilateral (radical) 62.41
  remaining or solitary testis 62.42
Orchidopexy 62.5
Orchidoplasty 62.69
Orchidorrhaphy 62.61
Orchidotomy 62.0
Orchiectomy (with epididymectomy) (unilateral) 62.3
  bilateral (radical) 62.41
  remaining or solitary testis 62.42

ICD-9-CM

P

Vol. 3

P

Pacemaker
cardiac - *see also* Insertion, pacemaker, cardiac
intraoperative (temporary) 39.64
temporary (during and immediately following cardiac surgery) 39.64
Packing - *see also* Insertion, pack
auditory canal 96.11
nose, for epistaxis (anterior) 21.01
posterior (and anterior) 21.02
rectal 96.19
sella turcica 07.79
vaginal 96.14
Palatoplasty 27.69
for cleft palate 27.62
secondary or subsequent 27.63
Palatorrhaphy 27.61
for cleft palate 27.62
Pallidectomy 01.42
Pallidoansotomy 01.42
Pallidotomy 01.42
by stereotactic radiosurgery 92.32
cobalt 60 92.32
linear accelerator (LINAC) 92.31
multi-source 92.32
particle beam 92.33
particulate 92.33
radiosurgery NEC 92.39
single source photon 92.31
Panas operation (linear proctotomy) 48.0
Pancoast operation (division of trigeminal nerve at foramen ovale) 04.02
Pancreatectomy (total) (with synchronous duodenectomy) 52.6
partial NEC 52.59
distal (tail) (with part of body) 52.52
proximal (head) (with part of body) (with synchronous duodenectomy) 52.51
radical 52.53
subtotal 52.53
radical 52.7
subtotal 52.53
Pancreaticocystoduodenostomy 52.4
Pancreaticocystoenterostomy 52.4
Pancreaticocystogastrostomy 52.4
Pancreaticocystojejunostomy 52.4
Pancreaticoduodenectomy (total) 52.6
partial NEC 52.59
proximal 52.51
radical subtotal 52.53
radical (one-stage) (two-stage) 52.7
subtotal 52.53
Pancreaticoduodenostomy 52.96
Pancreaticoenterostomy 52.96
Pancreaticogastrostomy 52.96
Pancreaticoileostomy 52.96
Pancreaticojejunostomy 52.96
Pancreatoduodenectomy (total) 52.6
partial NEC 52.59
radical (one-stage) (two-stage) 52.7
subtotal 52.53
Pancreatogram 87.66
endoscopic retrograde (ERP) 52.13
Pancreatolithotomy 52.09
endoscopic 52.94
Pancreatotomy 52.09
Pancreolithotomy 52.09
endoscopic 52.94
Panendoscopy 57.32
specified site, other than bladder - *see* Endoscopy, by site

Panendoscopy (*Continued*)
through artificial stoma 57.31
Panhysterectomy (abdominal) 68.4
vaginal 68.59
laparoscopically assisted (LAVH) 68.51
Panniculectomy 86.83
Panniculotomy 86.83
Pantaloon operation (revision of gastric anastomosis) 44.5
Papillectomy, anal 49.39
endoscopic 49.31
Papillotomy (pancreas) 51.82
endoscopic 51.85
Paquin operation (ureteroneocystostomy) 56.74
Paracentesis
abdominal (percutaneous) 54.91
anterior chamber, eye 12.91
bladder 57.11
cornea 12.91
eye (anterior chamber) 12.91
thoracic, thoracis 34.91
tympanum 20.09
with intubation 20.01
Parasitology - *see* Examination, microscopic
Parathyroidectomy (partial) (subtotal) NEC 06.89
complete 06.81
ectopic 06.89
global removal 06.81
mediastinal 06.89
total 06.81
Parenteral nutrition, total 99.15
peripheral 99.15
Parotidectomy 26.30
complete 26.32
partial 26.31
radical 26.32
Partsch operation (marsupialization of dental cyst) 24.4
Passage - *see* Insertion and Intubation
Passage of sounds, urethra 58.6
Patch
blood, spinal (epidural) 03.95
graft - *see* Graft
spinal, blood (epidural) 03.95
subdural, brain 02.12
Patellapexy 78.46
Patellaplasty NEC 78.46
Patellectomy 77.96
partial 77.86
Pattee operation (auditory canal) 18.6
Pectenotomy - *see also* Sphincterotomy, anal 49.59
Pedicle flap - *see* Graft, skin, pedicle
Peet operation (splanchnic resection) 05.29
PEG (percutaneous endoscopic gastrostomy) 43.11
PEJ (percutaneous endoscopic jejunostomy) 46.32
Pelvectomy, kidney (partial) 55.4
Pelvimetry 88.25
gynecological 89.26
Pelviolithotomy 55.11
Pelvioplasty, kidney 55.87
Pelviostomy 55.12
closure 55.82
Pelviotomy 77.39
to assist delivery 73.94
Pelvi-ureteroplasty 55.87

Pemberton operation
osteotomy of ilium 77.39
rectum (mobilization and fixation for prolapse repair) 48.76
Penectomy 64.3
Pereyra operation (paraurethral suspension) 59.6
Perforation
stapes footplate 19.0
Perfusion NEC 39.97
carotid artery 39.97
coronary artery 39.97
for
chemotherapy NEC 99.25
hormone therapy NEC 99.24
head 39.97
hyperthermic (lymphatic), localized region or site 93.35
intestine (large) (local) 46.96
small 46.95
kidney, local 55.95
limb (lower) (upper) 39.97
liver, localized 50.93
neck 39.97
subarachnoid (spinal cord) (refrigerated saline) 03.92
total body 39.96
Pericardiectomy 37.31
Pericardiocentesis 37.0
Pericardiolysis 37.12
Pericardioplasty 37.4
Pericardiorrhaphy 37.4
Pericardiostomy (tube) 37.12
Pericardiotomy 37.12
Peridectomy 10.31
Perilimbal suction 89.11
Perimetry 95.05
Perineoplasty 71.79
Perineorrhaphy 71.71
obstetrical laceration (current) 75.69
Perineotomy (nonobstetrical) 71.09
to assist delivery - *see* Episiotomy
Periosteotomy - *see also* Incision, bone 77.10
facial bone 76.09
Perirectofistulectomy 48.93
Peritectomy 10.31
Peritomy 10.1
Peritoneocentesis 54.91
Peritoneoscopy 54.21
Peritoneotomy 54.19
Peritoneumectomy 54.4
Phacoemulsification (ultrasonic) (with aspiration) 13.41
Phacofragmentation (mechanical) (with aspiration) 13.43
posterior route 13.42
ultrasonic 13.41
Phalangectomy (partial) 77.89
claw toe 77.57
cockup toe 77.58
hammer toe 77.56
overlapping toe 77.58
total 77.99
Phalangization (fifth metacarpal) 82.81
Pharyngeal flap operation (cleft palate repair) 27.62
secondary or subsequent 27.63
Pharyngectomy (partial) 29.33
with laryngectomy 30.3
Pharyngogram 87.09
contrast 87.06
Pharyngolaryngectomy 30.3

Pharyngoplasty (with silastic implant) 29.4
for cleft palate 27.62
secondary or subsequent 27.63
Pharyngorrhaphy 29.51
for cleft palate 27.62
Pharyngoscopy 29.11
Pharyngotomy 29.0
Phenopeel (skin) 86.24
Phlebectomy 38.60
with
anastomosis 38.30
abdominal 38.37
head and neck NEC 38.32
intracranial NEC 38.31
lower limb 38.39
thoracic NEC 38.35
upper limb 38.33
graft replacement 38.40
abdominal 38.47
head and neck NEC 38.42
intracranial NEC 38.41
lower limb 38.49
thoracic NEC 38.45
upper limb 38.43
abdominal 38.67
head and neck NEC 38.62
intracranial NEC 38.61
lower limb 38.69
thoracic NEC 38.65
upper limb 38.63
varicose 38.50
abdominal 38.57
head and neck NEC 38.52
intracranial NEC 38.51
lower limb 38.59
thoracic NEC 38.55
upper limb 38.53
Phlebogoniostomy 12.52
Phlebography (contrast) (retrograde) 88.60
by radioisotope - *see* Scan, radioisotope, by site
adrenal 88.65
femoral 88.66
head 88.61
hepatic 88.64
impedance 88.68
intra-abdominal NEC 88.65
intrathoracic NEC 88.63
lower extremity NEC 88.66
neck 88.61
portal system 88.64
pulmonary 88.62
specified site NEC 88.67
vena cava (inferior) (superior) 88.51
Phleborrhaphy 39.32
Phlebotomy 38.99
Phonocardiogram, with ECG lead 89.55
Photochemotherapy NEC 99.83
extracorporeal 99.88
Photocoagulation
ciliary body 12.73
eye, eyeball 16.99
iris 12.41
macular hole - *see* Photocoagulation, retina
orbital lesion 16.92
retina
for
destruction of lesion 14.25
reattachment 14.55
repair of tear or defect 14.35

Photocoagulation *(Continued)*
retina *(Continued)*
laser (beam)
for
destruction of lesion 14.24
reattachment 14.54
repair of tear or defect 14.34
xenon arc
for
destruction of lesion 14.23
reattachment 14.53
repair of tear or defect 14.33
Photography 89.39
fundus 95.11
Photopheresis, therapeutic 99.88
Phototherapy NEC 99.83
newborn 99.83
ultraviolet 99.82
Phrenemphraxis 04.03
for collapse of lung 33.31
Phrenicectomy 04.03
for collapse of lung 33.31
Phrenicoexeresis 04.03
for collapse of lung 33.31
Phrenicotomy 04.03
for collapse of lung 33.31
Phrenicotripsy 04.03
for collapse of lung 33.31
Phrenoplasty 34.84
Physical medicine - *see* Therapy, physical
Physical therapy - *see* Therapy, physical
Physiotherapy, chest 93.99
PICC (peripherally inserted central catheter) 38.93
Piercing ear, external (pinna) 18.01
Pigmenting, skin 86.02
Pilojection (aneurysm) (Gallagher) 39.52
Pinealectomy (complete) (total) 07.54
partial 07.53
Pinealotomy (with drainage) 07.52
Pinning
bone - *see* Fixation, bone, internal
ear 18.5
Pinsker operation (obliteration of nasoseptal telangiectasia) 21.07
Piper operation (forceps) 72.6
Pirogoff operation (ankle amputation through malleoli of tibia and fibula) 84.14
Pituitectomy (complete) (total) - *see also* Hypophysectomy 07.69
Placentogram, placentography 88.46
with radioisotope (RISA) 92.17
Planing, skin 86.25
Plantation, tooth (bud) (germ) 23.5
prosthetic 23.6
Plasma exchange 99.07
Plasmapheresis, therapeutic 99.71
Plastic repair - *see* Repair, by site
Plasty - *see also* Repair, by site
bladder neck (V-Y) 57.85
skin (without graft) 86.89
subcutaneous tissue 86.89
Platelet inhibitor (GP IIB/IIIa inhibitor only), infusion 99.20
Plateletpheresis, therapeutic 99.74
Play
psychotherapy 94.36
therapy 93.81
Pleating
eye muscle 15.22
multiple (two or more muscles) 15.4

Pleating *(Continued)*
sclera, for buckling - *see also* Buckling, scleral 14.49
Plethysmogram (carotid) 89.58
air-filled (pneumatic) 89.58
capacitance 89.58
cerebral 89.58
differential 89.58
oculoplethysmogram 89.58
penile 89.58
photoelectric 89.58
regional 89.58
respiratory function measurement (body) 89.38
segmental 89.58
strain-gauge 89.58
thoracic impedance 89.38
venous occlusion 89.58
water-filled 89.58
Plethysmography
penile 89.58
Pleurectomy NEC 34.59
Pleurocentesis 34.91
Pleurodesis 34.6
chemical 34.92
with cancer chemotherapy substance 34.92 [99.25]
tetracycline 34.92 [99.21]
Pleurolysis (for collapse of lung) 33.39
Pleuropexy 34.99
Pleurosclerosis 34.6
chemical 34.92
with cancer chemotherapy substance 34.92 [99.25]
tetracycline 34.92 [99.21]
Pleurotomy 34.09
Plexectomy
choroid 02.14
hypogastric 05.24
Plication
aneurysm
heart 37.32
annulus, heart valve 35.33
bleb (emphysematous), lung 32.21
broad ligament 69.22
diaphragm (for hernia repair) (thoracic approach) (thoracoabdominal approach) 53.81
eye muscle (oblique) (rectus) 15.22
multiple (two or more muscles) 15.4
fascia 83.89
hand 82.89
inferior vena cava 38.7
intestine (jejunum) (Noble) 46.62
Kelly (-Stoeckel) (urethrovesical junction) 59.3
levator, for blepharoptosis 08.34
ligament - *see also* Arthroplasty 81.96
broad 69.22
round 69.22
uterosacral 69.22
mesentery 54.75
round ligament 69.22
sphincter, urinary bladder 57.85
stomach 44.69
laparoscopic 44.68 ◄
superior vena cava 38.7
tendon 83.85
hand 82.55
tricuspid valve (with repositioning) 35.14
ureter 56.89
urethra 58.49
urethrovesical junction 59.3
vein (peripheral) 39.59

◄ **New**   ◀▥ **Revised**

Plication (Continued)
vena cava (inferior) (superior) 38.7
ventricle (heart)
aneurysm 37.32
Plicotomy, tympanum 20.23
Plombage, lung 33.39
Pneumocentesis 33.93
Pneumocisternogram 87.02
Pneumoencephalogram 87.01
Pneumogram, pneumography
extraperitoneal 88.15
mediastinal 87.33
orbit 87.14
pelvic 88.13
peritoneum NEC 88.13
presacral 88.15
retroperitoneum 88.15
Pneumogynecography 87.82
Pneumomediastinography 87.33
Pneumonectomy (complete) (extended)
(radical) (standard) (total) (with mediastinal dissection) 32.5
partial
complete excision, one lobe 32.4
resection (wedge), one lobe 32.3
Pneumonolysis (for collapse of lung)
33.39
Pneumonotomy (with exploration) 33.1
Pneumoperitoneum (surgically-induced)
54.96
for collapse of lung 33.33
pelvic 88.12
Pneumothorax (artificial) (surgical) 33.32
intrapleural 33.32
Pneumoventriculogram 87.02
Politano-Leadbetter operation (ureteroneocystostomy) 56.74
Politzerization, eustachian tube 20.8
Pollicization (with carry over of nerves
and blood supply) 82.61
Polya operation (gastrectomy) 43.7
Polypectomy - see also Excision, lesion,
by site
esophageal 42.32
endoscopic 42.33
gastric (endoscopic) 43.41
large intestine (colon) 45.42
nasal 21.31
rectum (endoscopic) 48.36
Polysomnogram 89.17
Pomeroy operation (ligation and division
of fallopian tubes) 66.32
Poncet operation
lengthening of Achilles tendon 83.85
urethrostomy, perineal 58.0
Porro operation (cesarean section) 74.99
Portoenterostomy (Kasai) 51.37
Positrocephalogram 92.11
Positron emission tomography (PET) -
see Scan, radioisotope
Postmortem examination 89.8
Potts-Smith operation (descending aorta-
left pulmonary artery anastomosis)
39.0
Poudrage
intrapericardial 36.39
pleural 34.6
PPN (peripheral parenteral nutrition) 99.15
Preparation (cutting), pedicle (flap) graft
86.71
Preputiotomy 64.91
Prescription for glasses 95.31 ◀
Pressurized
graft treatment 00.16 ◀
Pressure support
ventilation [PSV] - see category 96.7

Printen and Mason operation (high gastric bypass) 44.31
Probing
canaliculus, lacrimal (with irrigation)
09.42
lacrimal
canaliculi 09.42
punctum (with irrigation) 09.41
nasolacrimal duct (with irrigation)
09.43
with insertion of tube or stent 09.44
salivary duct (for dilation of duct) (for
removal of calculus) 26.91
with incision 26.0
Procedure - see also specific procedure
diagnostic NEC
abdomen (region) 54.29
adenoid 28.19
adrenal gland 07.19
alveolus 24.19
amnion 75.35
anterior chamber, eye 12.29
anus 49.29
appendix 45.28
biliary tract 51.19
bladder 57.39
blood vessel (any site) 38.29
bone 78.80
carpal, metacarpal 78.84
clavicle 78.81
facial 76.19
femur 78.85
fibula 78.87
humerus 78.82
marrow 41.38
patella 78.86
pelvic 78.89
phalanges (foot) (hand) 78.89
radius 78.83
scapula 78.81
specified site NEC 78.89
tarsal, metatarsal 78.88
thorax (ribs) (sternum) 78.81
tibia 78.87
ulna 78.83
vertebrae 78.89
brain 01.18
breast 85.19
bronchus 33.29
buccal 27.24
bursa 83.29
canthus 08.19
cecum 45.28
cerebral meninges 01.18
cervix 67.19
chest wall 34.28
choroid 14.19
ciliary body 12.29
clitoris 71.19
colon 45.28
conjunctiva 10.29
cornea 11.29
cul-de-sac 70.29
dental 24.19
diaphragm 34.28
duodenum 45.19
ear
external 18.19
inner and middle 20.39
epididymis 63.09
esophagus 42.29
eustachian tube 20.39
extraocular muscle or tendon 15.09
eye 16.29

Procedure (Continued)
diagnostic NEC (Continued)
eye (Continued)
anterior chamber 12.29
posterior chamber 14.19
eyeball 16.29
eyelid 08.19
fallopian tube 66.19
fascia (any site) 83.29
fetus 75.35
gallbladder 51.19
ganglion (cranial) (peripheral)
04.19
sympathetic 05.19
gastric 44.19
globus pallidus 01.18
gum 24.19
heart 37.29
hepatic 50.19
hypophysis 07.19
ileum 45.19
intestine 45.29
large 45.28
small 45.19
iris 12.29
jejunum 45.19
joint (capsule) (ligament) (structure)
NEC 81.98
facial 76.19
kidney 55.29
labia 71.19
lacrimal (system) 09.19
large intestine 45.28
larynx 31.48
ligament 81.98
uterine 68.19
liver 50.19
lung 33.29
lymphatic structure (channel)
(gland) (node) (vessel) 40.19
mediastinum 34.29
meninges (cerebral) 01.18
spinal 03.39
mouth 27.29
muscle 83.29
extraocular (oblique) (rectus)
15.09
papillary (heart) 37.29
nail 86.19
nasopharynx 29.19
nerve (cranial) (peripheral) NEC
04.19
sympathetic 05.19
nipple 85.19
nose, nasal 21.29
sinus 22.19
ocular 16.29
muscle 15.09
omentum 54.29
ophthalmologic 16.29
oral (cavity) 27.29
orbit 16.29
orthodontic 24.19
ovary 65.19
laparoscopic 65.14
palate 27.29
pancreas 52.19
papillary muscle (heart) 37.29
parathyroid gland 06.19
penis 64.19
perianal tissue 49.29
pericardium 37.29
periprostatic tissue 60.18
perirectal tissue 48.29

ICD-9-CM

Vol. 3

Procedure *(Continued)*
  diagnostic NEC *(Continued)*
    perirenal tissue 59.29
    peritoneum 54.29
    periurethral tissue 58.29
    perivesical tissue 59.29
    pharynx 29.19
    pineal gland 07.19
    pituitary gland 07.19
    pleura 34.28
    posterior chamber, eye 14.19
    prostate 60.18
    pulmonary 33.29
    rectosigmoid 48.29
    rectum 48.29
    renal 55.29
    respiratory 33.29
    retina 14.19
    retroperitoneum 59.29
    salivary gland or duct 26.19
    sclera 12.29
    scrotum 61.19
    seminal vesicle 60.19
    sigmoid 45.28
    sinus, nasal 22.19
    skin 86.19
    skull 01.19
    soft tissue 83.29
    spermatic cord 63.09
    sphincter of Oddi 51.19
    spine, spinal (canal) (cord) (menin-
      ges) (structure) 03.39
    spleen 41.39
    stomach 44.19
    subcutaneous tissue 86.19
    sympathetic nerve 05.19
    tarsus 09.19
    tendon NEC 83.29
      extraocular 15.09
    testicle 62.19
    thalamus 01.18
    thoracic duct 40.19
    thorax 34.28
    thymus 07.19
    thyroid gland 06.19
    tongue 25.09
    tonsils 28.19
    tooth 24.19
    trachea 31.49
    tunica vaginalis 61.19
    ureter 56.39
    urethra 58.29
    uterus and supporting structures
      68.19
    uvula 27.29
    vagina 70.29
    vas deferens 63.09
    vesical 57.39
    vessel (blood) (any site) 38.2
    vitreous 14.19
    vulva 71.19
  fistulizing, sclera NEC 12.69
  miscellaneous (nonoperative) NEC
    99.99
  respiratory (nonoperative) NEC 93.99
  surgical - *see* Operation
Proctectasis 96.22
Proctectomy (partial) - *see also* Resection,
  rectum 48.69
  abdominoperineal 48.5
  complete (Miles) (Rankin) 48.5
  pull-through 48.49
Proctoclysis 96.37
Proctolysis 48.99

Proctopexy (Delorme) 48.76
  abdominal (Ripstein) 48.75
Proctoplasty 48.79
Proctorrhaphy 48.71
Proctoscopy 48.23
  with biopsy 48.24
  through stoma (artificial) 48.22
  transabdominal approach 48.21
Proctosigmoidectomy - *see also* Resection,
  rectum 48.69
Proctosigmoidopexy 48.76
Proctosigmoidoscopy (rigid) 48.23
  with biopsy 48.24
  flexible 45.24
  through stoma (artificial) 48.22
  transabdominal approach 48.21
Proctostomy 48.1
Proctotomy (decompression) (linear)
  48.0
Production - *see also* Formation *and* Creation
  atrial septal defect 35.42
  subcutaneous tunnel for esophageal
    anastomosis 42.86
    with anastomosis - *see* Anastomosis,
      esophagus, antesternal
Prognathic recession 76.64
Prophylaxis, dental (scaling) (polishing)
  96.54
Prostatectomy (complete) (partial) NEC
  60.69
  loop 60.29
  perineal 60.62
  radical (any approach) 60.5
  retropubic (punch) (transcapsular) 60.4
  suprapubic (punch) (transvesical) 60.3
  transcapsular NEC 60.69
    retropubic 60.4
  transperineal 60.62
  transurethral 60.29
    ablation (contact) (noncontact) by la-
      ser 60.21
    electrovaporization 60.29
    enucleative 60.29
    resection of prostate (TURP) 60.29
    ultrasound guided, laser induced
      (TULIP) 60.21
  transvesical punch (suprapubic) 60.3
Prostatocystotomy 60.0
Prostatolithotomy 60.0
Prostatotomy (perineal) 60.0
Prostatovesiculectomy 60.5
Protection (of)
  individual from his surroundings 99.84
  surroundings from individual 99.84
Psychoanalysis 94.31
Psychodrama 94.43
Psychotherapy NEC 94.39
  biofeedback 94.39
  exploratory verbal 94.37
  group 94.44
    for psychosexual dysfunctions 94.41
  play 94.36
  psychosexual dysfunctions 94.34
  supportive verbal 94.38
PTCA (percutaneous transluminal coro-
  nary angioplasty) - *see* Angioplasty,
  balloon, coronary
Ptyalectasis 26.91
Ptyalithotomy 26.0
Ptyalolithotomy 26.0
Pubiotomy 77.39
  assisting delivery 73.94
Pubococcygeoplasty 59.71

Puestow operation (pancreaticojejunostomy) 52.96
Pull-through
  abdomino-anal 48.49
  abdominoperineal 48.49
    Duhamel type 48.65
  endorectal 48.41
Pulmowrap 93.99
Pulpectomy - *see also* Therapy, root canal
  23.70
Pulpotomy - *see also* Therapy, root canal
  23.70
**Pump-oxygenator, for extracorporeal cir-
  culation** 39.61
  percutaneous 39.66
Punch
  operation
    bladder neck, transurethral 57.49
    prostate - *see* Prostatectomy
  resection, vocal cords 30.22
Puncture
  antrum (nasal) (bilateral) (unilateral)
    22.01
  artery NEC 38.98
    for
      arteriography - *see also* Arteriogra-
        phy 88.40
    for
      coronary arteriography - *see also*
        Arteriography, coronary
        88.57
    percutaneous vascular closure - *omit
      code*
  bladder, suprapubic (for drainage)
    NEC 57.18
    needle 57.11
    percutaneous (suprapubic) 57.17
  bursa 83.94
    hand 82.92
  cisternal 01.01
    with contrast media 87.02
  cranial 01.09
    with contrast media 87.02
  craniobuccal pouch 07.72
  craniopharyngioma 07.72
  fallopian tube 66.91
  fontanel, anterior 01.09
  heart 37.0
    for intracardiac injection 37.92
  hypophysis 07.72
  iris 12.12
  joint 81.91
  kidney (percutaneous) 55.92
  larynx 31.98
  lumbar (diagnostic) (removal of dye)
    03.31
  lung (for aspiration) 33.93
  nasal sinus 22.01
  pericardium 37.0
  pituitary gland 07.72
  pleural cavity 34.91
  Rathke's pouch 07.72
  spinal 03.31
  spleen 41.1
    for biopsy 41.32
  sternal (for bone marrow biopsy) 41.31
    donor for bone marrow transplant
      41.91
  vein NEC 38.99
    for
      phlebography - *see also* Phlebogra-
        phy 88.60
      transfusion - *see* Transfusion
  ventricular shunt tubing 01.02

Pupillotomy 12.35
Push-back operation (cleft palate repair) 27.62
Putti-Platt operation (capsulorrhaphy of shoulder for recurrent dislocation) 81.82
pVAD (percutaneous ventricular assist device) 37.68 ◄
Pyelogram (intravenous) 87.73
  infusion (continuous) (diuretic) 87.73
  percutaneous 87.75
  retrograde 87.74
Pyeloileostomy 56.71
Pyelolithotomy 55.11
Pyeloplasty 55.87
Pyelorrhaphy 55.81
Pyeloscopy 55.22

Pyelostolithotomy, percutaneous 55.03
Pyelostomy 55.12
  closure 55.82
Pyelotomy 55.11
Pyeloureteroplasty 55.87
Pylorectomy 43.6
Pyloroduodenotomy - *see* category 44.2
Pyloromyotomy (Ramstedt) (with wedge resection) 43.3
Pyloroplasty (Finney) (Heineke-Mikulicz) 44.29
  dilation, endoscopic 44.22
    by incision 44.21
  not elsewhere classified 44.29
  revision 44.29
Pylorostomy - *see* Gastrostomy

Q

Quadrant resection of breast 85.22
Quadricepsplasty (Thompson) 83.86
Quarantine 99.84
Quenuthoracoplasty 77.31
Quotient, respiratory 89.38

R

Rachicentesis 03.31
Rachitomy 03.09
Radiation therapy - *see also* Therapy, radiation
  teleradiotherapy - *see* Teleradiotherapy
Radical neck dissection - *see* Dissection, neck
Radicotomy 03.1
Radiculectomy 03.1
Radiculotomy 03.1
Radiography (diagnostic) NEC 88.39
  abdomen, abdominal (flat plate) NEC 88.19
    wall (soft tissue) NEC 88.09
  adenoid 87.09
  ankle (skeletal) 88.28
    soft tissue 88.37
  bone survey 88.31
  bronchus 87.49
  chest (routine) 87.44
    wall NEC 87.39
  clavicle 87.43
  computer assisted surgery (CAS) with fluoroscopy 00.33 ◄
  contrast (air) (gas) (radio-opaque substance) NEC
    abdominal wall 88.03
    arteries (by fluoroscopy) - *see* Arteriography
    bile ducts NEC 87.54
    bladder NEC 87.77
    brain 87.02
    breast 87.35
    bronchus NEC (transcricoid) 87.32
      endotracheal 87.31
    epididymis 87.93
    esophagus 87.61
    fallopian tubes
      gas 87.82
      opaque dye 87.83
    fistula (sinus tract) - *see also* Radiography, contrast, by site
      abdominal wall 88.03
      chest wall 87.38
    gallbladder NEC 87.59
    intervertebral disc(s) 87.21
    joints 88.32
    larynx 87.07
    lymph - *see* Lymphangiogram
    mammary ducts 87.35
    mediastinum 87.33
    nasal sinuses 87.15
    nasolacrimal ducts 87.05
    nasopharynx 87.06
    orbit 87.14
    pancreas 87.66
    pelvis
      gas 88.12
      opaque dye 88.11
    peritoneum NEC 88.13
    retroperitoneum NEC 88.15
    seminal vesicles 87.91
    sinus tract - *see also* Radiography, contrast, by site
      abdominal wall 88.03
      chest wall 87.38
      nose 87.15
    skull 87.02
    spinal disc(s) 87.21
    trachea 87.32
    uterus
      gas 87.82
      opaque dye 87.83

Radiography NEC *(Continued)*
  contrast *(Continued)*
    vas deferens 87.94
    veins (by fluoroscopy) - *see* Phlebography
    vena cava (inferior) (superior) 88.51
  dental NEC 87.12
  diaphragm 87.49
  digestive tract NEC 87.69
    barium swallow 87.61
    lower GI series 87.64
    small bowel series 87.63
    upper GI series 87.62
  elbow (skeletal) 88.22
    soft tissue 88.35
  epididymis NEC 87.95
  esophagus 87.69
    barium-swallow 87.61
  eye 95.14
  face, head, and neck 87.09
  facial bones 87.16
  fallopian tubes 87.85
  foot 88.28
  forearm (skeletal) 88.22
    soft tissue 88.35
  frontal area, facial 87.16
  genital organs
    female NEC 87.89
    male NEC 87.99
  hand (skeletal) 88.23
    soft tissue 88.35
  head NEC 87.09
  heart 87.49
  hip (skeletal) 88.26
    soft tissue 88.37
  intestine NEC 87.65
  kidney-ureter-bladder (KUB) 87.79
  knee (skeletal) 88.27
    soft tissue 88.37
  KUB (kidney-ureter-bladder) 87.79
  larynx 87.09
  lower leg (skeletal) 88.27
    soft tissue 88.37
  lower limb (skeletal) NEC 88.29
    soft tissue NEC 88.37
  lung 87.49
  mandible 87.16
  maxilla 87.16
  mediastinum 87.49
  nasal sinuses 87.16
  nasolacrimal duct 87.09
  nasopharynx 87.09
  neck NEC 87.09
  nose 87.16
  orbit 87.16
  pelvis (skeletal) 88.26
    pelvimetry 88.25
    soft tissue 88.19
  prostate NEC 87.92
  retroperitoneum NEC 88.16
  ribs 87.43
  root canal 87.12
  salivary gland 87.09
  seminal vesicles NEC 87.92
  shoulder (skeletal) 88.21
    soft tissue 88.35
  skeletal NEC 88.33
    series (whole or complete) 88.31
  skull (lateral, sagittal or tangential projection) NEC 87.17
  spine NEC 87.29
    cervical 87.22
    lumbosacral 87.24
    sacrococcygeal 87.24
    thoracic 87.23

Radiography NEC *(Continued)*
  sternum 87.43
  supraorbital area 87.16
  symphysis menti 87.16
  teeth NEC 87.12
    full-mouth 87.11
  thigh (skeletal) 88.27
    soft tissue 88.37
  thyroid region 87.09
  tonsils and adenoids 87.09
  trachea 87.49
  ultrasonic - *see* Ultrasonography
  upper arm (skeletal) 88.21
    soft tissue 88.35
  upper limb (skeletal) NEC 88.24
    soft tissue NEC 88.35
  urinary system NEC 87.79
  uterus NEC 87.85
    gravid 87.81
  uvula 87.09
  vas deferens NEC 87.95
  wrist 88.23
  zygomaticomaxillary complex 87.16
Radioimmunotherapy 92.28
Radioisotope
  scanning - *see* Scan, radioisotope
  therapy - *see* Therapy, radioisotope
Radiology
  diagnostic - *see* Radiography
  therapeutic - *see* Therapy, radiation
Radiosurgery, stereotactic 92.30
  cobalt 60 92.32
  linear accelerator (LINAC) 92.31
  multi-source 92.32
  particle beam 92.33
  particulate 92.33
  radiosurgery NEC 92.39
  single source photon 92.31
Raising, pedicle graft 86.71
Ramadier operation (intrapetrosal drainage) 20.22
Ramisection (sympathetic) 05.0
Ramstedt operation (pyloromyotomy) (with wedge resection) 43.3
Range of motion testing 93.05
Rankin operation
  exteriorization of intestine 46.03
  proctectomy (complete) 48.5
Rashkind operation (balloon septostomy) 35.41
Rastelli operation (creation of conduit between right ventricle and pulmonary artery) 35.92
  in repair of
    pulmonary artery atresia 35.92
    transposition of great vessels 35.92
    truncus arteriosus 35.83
Raz-Pereyra procedure (bladder neck suspension) 59.79
RCSA (radical cryosurgical ablation) of prostate 60.62
Readjustment - *see* Adjustment
Reamputation, stump 84.3
Reanastomosis - *see* Anastomosis
Reattachment
  amputated ear 18.72
  ankle 84.27
  arm (upper) NEC 84.24
  choroid and retina NEC 14.59
    by
      cryotherapy 14.52
      diathermy 14.51
      electrocoagulation 14.51
      photocoagulation 14.55
        laser 14.54
        xenon arc 14.53

ICD-9-CM

R

Vol.

Reattachment (Continued)
ear (amputated) 18.72
extremity 84.29
ankle 84.27
arm (upper) NEC 84.24
fingers, except thumb 84.22
thumb 84.21
foot 84.26
forearm 84.23
hand 84.23
leg (lower) NEC 84.27
thigh 84.28
thumb 84.21
toe 84.25
wrist 84.23
finger 84.22
thumb 84.21
foot 84.26
forearm 84.23
hand 84.23
joint capsule - see also Arthroplasty 81.96
leg (lower) NEC 84.27
ligament - see also Arthroplasty
uterosacral 69.22
muscle 83.74
hand 82.54
papillary (heart) 35.31
nerve (peripheral) 04.79
nose (amputated) 21.89
papillary muscle (heart) 35.31
penis (amputated) 64.45
retina (and choroid) NEC 14.59
by
cryotherapy 14.52
diathermy 14.51
electrocoagulation 14.51
photocoagulation 14.55
laser 14.54
xenon arc 14.53
tendon (to tendon) 83.73
hand 82.53
to skeletal attachment 83.88
hand 82.85
thigh 84.28
thumb 84.21
toe 84.25
tooth 23.5
uterosacral ligament(s) 69.22
vessels (peripheral) 39.59
renal, aberrant 39.55
wrist 84.23
Recession
extraocular muscle 15.11
multiple (two or more muscles)
(with advancement or resection)
15.3
gastrocnemius tendon (Strayer operation) 83.72
levator palpebrae (superioris) muscle
08.38
prognathic jaw 76.64
tendon 83.72
hand 82.52
Reclosure - see also Closure
disrupted abdominal wall (postoperative) 54.61
Reconstruction (plastic) - see also Construction and Repair, by site
alveolus, alveolar (process) (ridge)
(with graft or implant) 24.5
artery (graft) - see Graft, artery
artificial stoma, intestine 46.40
auditory canal (external) 18.6
auricle (ear) 18.71

Reconstruction (Continued)
bladder 57.87
with
ileum 57.87 [45.51]
sigmoid 57.87 [45.52]
bone, except facial - see also Osteoplasty 78.40
facial NEC 76.46
with total ostectomy 76.44
mandible 76.43
with total mandibulectomy 76.41
breast, total 85.7
bronchus 33.48
canthus (lateral) 08.59
cardiac annulus 35.33
chest wall (mesh) (silastic) 34.79
cleft lip 27.54
conjunctival cul-de-sac 10.43
with graft (buccal mucous membrane) (free) 10.42
cornea NEC 11.79
diaphragm 34.84
ear (external) (auricle) 18.71
external auditory canal 18.6
meatus (new) (osseous skin-lined)
18.6
ossicles 19.3
prominent or protruding 18.5
eyebrow 08.70
eyelid 08.70
with graft or flap 08.69
hair follicle 08.63
mucous membrane 08.62
skin 08.61
tarsoconjunctival (one-stage) (two-stage) 08.64
full-thickness 08.74
involving lid margin 08.73
partial-thickness 08.72
involving lid margin 08.71
eye socket 16.64
with graft 16.63
fallopian tube 66.79
foot and toes (with fixation device)
81.57
with prosthetic implant 81.57
frontonasal duct 22.79
hip (total) (with prosthesis) 81.51
intraoral 27.59
joint - see Arthroplasty
lymphatic (by transplantation) 40.9
mandible 76.43
with total mandibulectomy 76.41
mastoid cavity 19.9
mouth 27.59
nipple NEC 85.87
nose (total) (with arm flap) (with forehead flap) 21.83
ossicles (graft) (prosthesis) NEC 19.3
with
stapedectomy 19.19
tympanoplasty 19.53
pelvic floor 71.79
penis (rib graft) (skin graft) (myocutaneous flap) 64.44
pharynx 29.4
scrotum (with pedicle flap) (with rotational flap) 61.49
skin (plastic) (without graft) NEC
86.89
with graft - see Graft, skin
subcutaneous tissue (plastic) (without
skin graft) NEC 86.89
with graft - see Graft, skin

Reconstruction (Continued)
tendon pulley (with graft) (with local
tissue) 83.83
for opponensplasty 82.71
hand 82.71
thumb (osteoplastic) (with bone graft)
(with skin graft) 82.69
trachea (with graft) 31.75
umbilicus 53.49
ureteropelvic junction 55.87
urethra 58.46
vagina 70.62
vas deferens, surgically divided 63.82
Recontour, gingiva 24.2
Recreational therapy 93.81
Rectectomy - see also Resection, rectum
48.69
Rectopexy (Delorme) 48.76
abdominal (Ripstein) 48.75
Rectoplasty 48.79
Rectorectostomy 48.74
Rectorrhaphy 48.71
Rectosigmoidectomy - see also Resection,
rectum 48.69
transsacral 48.61
Rectosigmoidostomy 45.94
Rectostomy 48.1
closure 48.72
Red cell survival studies 92.05
Reduction
adipose tissue 86.83
batwing arms 86.83
breast (bilateral) 85.32
unilateral 85.31
bulbous tuberosities (mandible) (maxilla) (fibrous) (osseous) 24.31
buttocks 86.83
diastasis, ankle mortise (closed) 79.77
open 79.87
dislocation (of joint) (manipulation)
(with cast) (with splint) (with
traction device) (closed) 79.70
with fracture - see Reduction, fracture, by site
ankle (closed) 79.77
open 79.87
elbow (closed) 79.72
open 79.82
finger (closed) 79.74
open 79.84
foot (closed) 79.78
open 79.88
hand (closed) 79.74
open 79.84
hip (closed) 79.75
open 79.85
knee (closed) 79.76
open 79.86
open (with external fixation) (with
internal fixation) 79.80
specified site NEC 79.89
shoulder (closed) 79.71
open 79.81
specified site (closed) NEC 79.79
open 79.89
temporomandibular (closed) 76.93
open 76.94
toe (closed) 79.78
open 79.88
wrist (closed) 79.73
open 79.83
elephantiasis, scrotum 61.3
epistaxis - see also Control, epistaxis
21.00

Reduction *(Continued)*
  fracture (bone) (with cast) (with splint)
      (with traction device) (closed)
      79.00
    with internal fixation 79.10
    alveolar process (with stabilization
        of teeth)
      mandible (closed) 76.75
        open 76.77
      maxilla (closed) 76.73
        open 76.77
        open 76.77
    ankle - *see* Reduction, fracture, leg
    arm (closed) NEC 79.02
      with internal fixation 79.12
      open 79.22
        with internal fixation 79.32
    blow-out - *see* Reduction, fracture,
        orbit
    carpal, metacarpal (closed) 79.03
      with internal fixation 79.13
      open 79.23
        with internal fixation 79.33
    epiphysis - *see* Reduction, separation
    facial (bone) NEC 76.70
      closed 76.78
      open 76.79
    femur (closed) 79.05
      with internal fixation 79.15
      open 79.25
        with internal fixation 79.35
    fibula (closed) 79.06
      with internal fixation 79.16
      open 79.26
        with internal fixation 79.36
    foot (closed) NEC 79.07
      with internal fixation 79.17
      open 79.27
        with internal fixation 79.37
    hand (closed) NEC 79.03
      with internal fixation 79.13
      open 79.23
        with internal fixation 79.33
    humerus (closed) 79.01
      with internal fixation 79.11
      open 79.21
        with internal fixation 79.31
    jaw (lower) - *see also* Reduction, frac-
        ture, mandible
      upper - *see* Reduction, fracture,
          maxilla
    larynx 31.64
    leg (closed) NEC 79.06
      with internal fixation 79.16
      open 79.26
        with internal fixation 79.36
    malar (closed) 76.71
      open 76.72
    mandible (with dental wiring)
        (closed) 76.75
      open 76.76
    maxilla (with dental wiring) (closed)
        76.73
      open 76.74
    nasal (closed) 21.71
      open 21.72
    open 79.20
      with internal fixation 79.30
      specified site NEC 79.29
        with internal fixation 79.39
    orbit (rim) (wall) (closed) 76.78
      open 76.79
    patella (open) (with internal fixation)
        79.36

Reduction *(Continued)*
  fracture *(Continued)*
    phalanges
      foot (closed) 79.08
        with internal fixation 79.18
        open 79.28
          with internal fixation 79.38
      hand (closed) 79.04
        with internal fixation 79.14
        open 79.24
          with internal fixation 79.34
    radius (closed) 79.02
      with internal fixation 79.12
      open 79.22
        with internal fixation 79.32
    skull 02.02
    specified site (closed) NEC 79.09
      with internal fixation 79.19
      open 79.29
        with internal fixation 79.39
    spine 03.53
    tarsal, metatarsal (closed) 79.07
      with internal fixation 79.17
      open 79.27
        with internal fixation 79.37
    tibia (closed) 79.06
      with internal fixation 79.16
      open 79.26
        with internal fixation 79.36
    ulna (closed) 79.02
      with internal fixation 79.12
      open 79.22
        with internal fixation 79.32
    vertebra 03.53
    zygoma, zygomatic arch (closed) 76.71
      open 76.72
  fracture dislocation - *see* Reduction,
      fracture
  heart volume 37.35
  hemorrhoids (manual) 49.41
  hernia - *see also* Repair, hernia
    manual 96.27
  intussusception (open) 46.80
    with
      fluoroscopy 96.29
      ionizing radiation enema 96.29
      ultrasonography guidance 96.29
    hydrostatic 96.29
    large intestine 46.82
      endoscopic (balloon) 46.85
    pneumatic 96.29
    small intestine 46.81
  lung volume 32.22
  malrotation, intestine (manual) (surgi-
      cal) 46.80
    large 46.82
      endoscopic (balloon) 46.85
    small 46.81
  mammoplasty (bilateral) 85.32
    unilateral 85.31
  prolapse
    anus (operative) 49.94
    colostomy (manual) 96.28
    enterostomy (manual) 96.28
    ileostomy (manual) 96.28
    rectum (manual) 96.26
    uterus
      by pessary 96.18
      surgical 69.22
  ptosis overcorrection 08.37
  retroversion, uterus by pessary 96.18
  separation, epiphysis (with internal
      fixation) (closed)
      79.40

Reduction *(Continued)*
  separation, epiphysis *(Continued)*
    femur (closed) 79.45
      open 79.55
    fibula (closed) 79.46
      open 79.56
    humerus (closed) 79.41
      open 79.51
    open 79.50
    specified site (closed) NEC - *see also*
        category 79.4
      open - *see* category 79.5
    tibia (closed) 79.46
      open 79.56
  size
    abdominal wall (adipose) (pendu-
        lous) 86.83
    arms (adipose) (batwing) 86.83
    breast (bilateral) 85.32
      unilateral 85.31
    buttocks (adipose) 86.83
    finger (macrodactyly repair) 82.83
    skin 86.83
    subcutaneous tissue 86.83
    thighs (adipose) 86.83
  torsion
    intestine (manual) (surgical)
        46.80
      large 46.82
        endoscopic (balloon) 46.85
      small 46.81
    kidney pedicle 55.84
    omentum 54.74
    spermatic cord 63.52
      with orchiopexy 62.5
    testis 63.52
      with orchiopexy 62.5
    uterus NEC 69.98
      gravid 75.99
  ventricular 37.35
  volvulus
    intestine 46.80
      large 46.82
        endoscopic (balloon) 46.85
      small 46.81
    stomach 44.92
Reefing, joint capsule - *see also* Arthro-
    plasty 81.96
Re-entry operation (aorta) 39.54
Re-establishment, continuity - *see also*
    Anastomosis
  bowel 46.50
  fallopian tube 66.79
  vas deferens 63.82
Referral (for)
  psychiatric aftercare (halfway house)
      (outpatient clinic) 94.52
  psychotherapy 94.51
  rehabilitation
    alcoholism 94.53
    drug addiction 94.54
    psychologic NEC 94.59
    vocational 94.55
Reformation
  cardiac pacemaker pocket, new site
      (skin) (subcutaneous) 37.79
  cardioverter/defibrillator (automatic)
      pocket, new site (skin) (subcutane-
      ous) 37.99
  chamber of eye 12.99
Refracture
  bone (for faulty union) - *see also* Oste-
      oclasis 78.70
  nasal bones 21.88

ICD-9-CM

R

Vol. 3

Refusion
spinal, NOS 81.30
  atlas-axis (anterior) (transoral) (posterior) 81.31
  cervical (C2 level or below) NEC 81.32
    anterior (interbody), anterolateral technique 81.32
    C1-C2 level (anterior) (posterior) 81.31
    posterior (interbody), posterolateral technique 81.33
  craniocervical (anterior) (transoral) (posterior) 81.31
  dorsal, dorsolumbar NEC 81.35
    anterior (interbody), anterolateral technique 81.34
    posterior (interbody), posterolateral technique 81.35
  lumbar, lumbosacral NEC 81.38
    anterior (interbody), anterolateral technique 81.36
    lateral transverse process technique 81.37
    posterior (interbody), posterolateral technique 81.38
  number of vertebrae - see codes 81.62–81.64.
  occiput–C2 (anterior) (transoral) (posterior) 81.31
  refusion NEC 81.39

Note Also use either 81.62, 81.63, or 81.64 as an additional code to show the total number of vertebrae fused

Regional blood flow study 92.05
Regulation, menstrual 69.6
Rehabilitation programs NEC 93.89
alcohol 94.61
  with detoxification 94.63
  combined alcohol and drug 94.67
    with detoxification 94.69
drug 94.64
  with detoxification 94.66
  combined drug and alcohol 94.67
    with detoxification 94.69
sheltered employment 93.85
vocational 93.85
Reimplantation
adrenal tissue (heterotopic) (orthotopic) 07.45
artery 39.59
  renal, aberrant 39.55
bile ducts following excision of ampulla of Vater 51.62
extremity - see Reattachment, extremity
fallopian tube into uterus 66.74
kidney 55.61
lung 33.5
ovary 65.72
  laparoscopic 65.75
pancreatic tissue 52.81
parathyroid tissue (heterotopic) (orthotopic) 06.95
pulmonary artery for hemitruncus repair 35.83
renal vessel, aberrant 39.55
testis in scrotum 62.5
thyroid tissue (heterotopic) (orthotopic) 06.94
tooth 23.5
ureter into bladder 56.74
Reinforcement - see also Repair, by site
sclera NEC 12.88
  with graft 12.87

Reinsertion - see also Insertion or Revision
cystostomy tube 59.94
fixation device (internal) - see also Fixation, bone, internal 78.50
heart valve (prosthetic) 35.95
Holter (-Spitz) valve 02.42
implant (expelled) (extruded)
  eyeball (with conjunctival graft) 16.62
  orbital 16.62
nephrostomy tube 55.93
pyelostomy tube 55.94
ureteral stent (transurethral) 59.8
  with ureterotomy 59.8 [56.2]
ureterostomy tube 59.93
valve
  heart (prosthetic) 35.95
  ventricular (cerebral) 02.42
Relaxation - see also Release training 94.33
Release
carpal tunnel (for nerve decompression) 04.43
celiac artery axis 39.91
central slip, extensor tendon, hand (mallet finger repair) 82.84
chordee 64.42
clubfoot NEC 83.84
de Quervain's tenosynovitis 82.01
Dupuytren's contracture (by palmar fasciectomy) 82.35
  by fasciotomy (subcutaneous) 82.12
  with excision 82.35
Fowler (mallet finger repair) 82.84
joint (capsule) (adherent) (constrictive) - see also Division, joint capsule 80.40
laryngeal 31.92
ligament - see also Division, ligament 80.40
  median arcuate 39.91
median arcuate ligament 39.91
muscle (division) 83.19
  hand 82.19
nerve (peripheral) NEC 04.49
  cranial NEC 04.42
  trigeminal 04.41
pressure, intraocular 12.79
scar tissue
  skin 86.84
  stoma - see Revision, stoma
tarsal tunnel 04.44
tendon 83.13
  hand 82.11
    extensor, central slip (mallet finger repair) 82.84
  sheath 83.01
    hand 82.01
tenosynovitis 83.01
  abductor pollicis longus 82.01
  de Quervain's 82.01
  external pollicis brevis 82.01
  hand 82.01
torsion
  intestine 46.80
    large 46.82
      endoscopic (balloon) 46.85
    small 46.81
  kidney pedicle 55.84
  ovary 65.95
  testes 63.52
transverse carpal ligament (for nerve decompression) 04.43
trigger finger or thumb 82.01
urethral stricture 58.5

Release (Continued)
Volkmann's contracture
  excision of scar, muscle 83.32
  fasciotomy 83.14
  muscle transplantation 83.77
web contracture (skin) 86.84
Relief - see Release
Relocation - see also Revision
cardiac pacemaker pocket, new site (skin) (subcutaneous) 37.79
CRT-D pocket 37.99
CRT-P pocket 37.79
subcutaneous device pocket NEC 86.09
Remobilization
joint 93.16
stapes 19.0
Remodel
ventricle 37.35
Removal - see also Excision
Abrams bar (chest wall) 34.01
abscess - see Incision, by site
adenoid tag(s) 28.6
anal sphincter
  with revision 49.75
  without revision 49.76
arch bars (orthodontic) 24.8
  immobilization device 97.33
arterial graft or prosthesis 39.49
arteriovenous shunt (device) 39.43
  with creation of new shunt 39.42
Barton's tongs (skull) 02.95
  with synchronous replacement 02.94
bladder sphincter, artificial 58.99
  with replacement 58.93
blood clot - see also Incision, by site
  bladder (by incision) 57.19
    without incision 57.0
  kidney (without incision) 56.0
    by incision 55.01
  ureter
    by incision 56.2
bone fragment (chip) - see also Incision, bone 77.10
  joint - see also Arthrotomy 80.10
  necrotic - see also Sequestrectomy, bone 77.00
    joint - see also Arthrotomy 80.10
  skull 01.25
    with debridement of compound fracture 02.02
bone growth stimulator - see category 78.6
bony spicules, spinal canal 03.53
brace 97.88
breast implant 85.94
  tissue expander 85.96
calcareous deposit
  bursa 83.03
    hand 82.03
  tendon, intratendinous 83.39
    hand 82.29
calcification, heart valve leaflets - see Valvuloplasty, heart
calculus
  bile duct (by incision) 51.49
    endoscopic 51.88
    laparoscopic 51.88
    percutaneous 51.98
  bladder (by incision) 57.19
    without incision 57.0
  common duct (by incision) 51.41
    endoscopic 51.88
    laparoscopic 51.88
    percutaneous 51.96

Removal *(Continued)*
calculus *(Continued)*
gallbladder 51.04
endoscopic 51.88
laparoscopic 51.88
kidney (by incision) 55.01
without incision (transurethral) 56.0
percutaneous 55.03
with fragmentation (ultrasound) 55.04
renal pelvis (by incision) 55.11
percutaneous nephrostomy 55.03
with fragmentation 55.04
transurethral 56.0
lacrimal
canaliculi 09.42
by incision 09.52
gland 09.3
by incision 09.0
passage(s) 09.49
by incision 09.59
punctum 09.41
by incision 09.51
sac 09.49
by incision 09.53
pancreatic duct (by incision) 52.09
endoscopic 52.94
perirenal tissue 59.09
pharynx 29.39
prostate 60.0
salivary gland (by incision) 26.0
by probe 26.91
ureter (by incision) 56.2
without incision 56.0
urethra (by incision) 58.0
without incision 58.6
caliper tongs (skull) 02.95
cannula
for extracorporeal membrane oxygenation (ECMO) - *omit code*
cardiac pacemaker (device) (initial) (permanent) (cardiac resynchronization device, CRT-P) 37.89
with replacement (by)
cardiac resynchronization pacemaker (CRT-P)
device only 00.53
total system 00.50
dual chamber device 37.87
single-chamber device 37.85
rate responsive 37.86
cardioverter/defibrillator pulse generator without replacement (cardiac resynchronization defibrillator device (CRT-D) 37.99
cast 97.88
with reapplication 97.13
lower limb 97.12
upper limb 97.11
catheter (indwelling) - *see also* Removal, tube
bladder 97.64
middle ear (tympanum) 20.1
ureter 97.62
urinary 97.64
ventricular (cerebral) 02.43
with synchronous replacement 02.42
cerclage material, cervix 69.96
cerumen, ear 96.52
corneal epithelium 11.41
for smear or culture 11.21

Removal *(Continued)*
coronary artery obstruction (thrombus) 36.09
direct intracoronary artery infusion 36.04
open chest approach 36.03
percutaneous transluminal (balloon) (single vessel) 36.01
with thrombolytic agent infusion 36.02
multiple vessels 36.05
Crutchfield tongs (skull) 02.95
with synchronous replacement 02.94
cyst - *see also* Excision, lesion, by site
dental 24.4
lung 32.29
endoscopic 32.28
cystic duct remnant 51.61
decidua (by)
aspiration curettage 69.52
curettage (D and C) 69.02
manual 75.4
dental wiring (immobilization device) 97.33
orthodontic 24.8
device (therapeutic) NEC 97.89
abdomen NEC 97.86
digestive system NEC 97.59
drainage - *see* Removal, tube
external fixation device 97.88
mandibular NEC 97.36
minifixator (bone) - *see category* 78.6
for musculoskeletal immobilization NEC 97.88
genital tract NEC 97.79
head and neck NEC 97.39
intrauterine contraceptive 97.71
thorax NEC 97.49
trunk NEC 97.87
urinary system NEC 97.69
diaphragm, vagina 97.73
drainage device - *see* Removal, tube
dye, spinal canal 03.31
ectopic fetus (from) 66.02
abdominal cavity 74.3
extraperitoneal (intraligamentous) 74.3
fallopian tube (by salpingostomy) 66.02
by salpingotomy 66.01
with salpingectomy 66.62
intraligamentous 74.3
ovarian 74.3
peritoneal (following uterine or tubal rupture) 74.3
site NEC 74.3
tubal (by salpingostomy) 66.02
by salpingotomy 66.01
with salpingectomy 66.62
electrodes
bone growth stimulator - *see* category 78.6
brain 01.22
depth 01.22
with synchronous replacement 02.93
foramen ovale 01.22
with synchronous replacement 02.93
sphenoidal - *omit code*
with synchronous replacement 02.96
cardiac pacemaker (atrial) (transvenous) (ventricular) 37.77
with replacement 37.76

Removal *(Continued)*
electrodes *(Continued)*
depth 01.22
with synchronous replacement 02.93
epicardial (myocardial) 37.77
with replacement (by)
atrial and/or ventricular lead(s) (electrode) 37.76
epicardial lead 37.74
epidural pegs 01.22
with synchronous replacement 02.93
foramen ovale 01.22
with synchronous replacement 02.93
intracranial 01.22
with synchronous replacement 02.93
peripheral nerve 04.93
with synchronous replacement 04.92
sacral nerve 04.93 ◄
sphenoidal - *omit code*
with synchronous replacement 02.96
spinal 03.94
with synchronous replacement 03.93
temporary transvenous pacemaker system - *omit code*
electroencephalographic receiver (brain) (intracranial) 01.22
with synchronous replacement 02.93
electronic
stimulator - *see* Removal, neurostimulator, by site ◄⦙⦙
bladder 57.98
bone 78.6
skeletal muscle 83.93
with synchronous replacement 83.92
ureter 56.94
electrostimulator - *see* Removal, electronic, stimulator, by site
embolus 38.00
with endarterectomy - *see* Endarterectomy
abdominal
artery 38.06
vein 38.07
aorta (arch) (ascending) (descending) 38.04
arteriovenous shunt or cannula 39.49
bovine graft 39.49
head and neck vessel NEC 38.02
intracranial vessel NEC 38.01
lower limb
artery 38.08
vein 38.09
pulmonary (artery) (vein) 38.05
thoracic vessel NEC 38.05
upper limb (artery) (vein) 38.03
embryo - *see* Removal, ectopic fetus
encircling tube, eye (episcleral) 14.6
epithelial downgrowth, anterior chamber 12.93
external fixation device 97.88
mandibular NEC 97.36
minifixator (bone) - *see* category 78.6
extrauterine embryo - *see* Removal, ectopic fetus
eyeball 16.49
with implant 16.42
with attachment of muscles 16.41

Removal (*Continued*)
fallopian tube - *see* Salpingectomy
feces (impacted) (by flushing) (manual) 96.38
fetus, ectopic - *see* Removal, ectopic fetus
fingers, supernumerary 86.26
fixation device
  external 97.88
    mandibular NEC 97.36
    minifixator (bone) - *see* category 78.6
  internal 78.60
    carpal, metacarpal 78.64
    clavicle 78.61
    facial (bone) 76.97
    femur 78.65
    fibula 78.67
    humerus 78.62
    patella 78.66
    pelvic 78.69
    phalanges (foot) (hand) 78.69
    radius 78.63
    scapula 78.61
    specified site NEC 78.69
    tarsal, metatarsal 78.68
    thorax (ribs) (sternum) 78.61
    tibia 78.67
    ulna 78.63
    vertebrae 78.69
foreign body NEC - *see also* Incision, by site 98.20
  abdominal (cavity) 54.92
    wall 54.0
  adenoid 98.13
    by incision 28.91
  alveolus, alveolar bone 98.22
    by incision 24.0
  antecubital fossa 98.27
    by incision 86.05
  anterior chamber 12.00
    by incision 12.02
      with use of magnet 12.01
  anus (intraluminal) 98.05
    by incision 49.93
  artificial stoma (intraluminal) 98.18
  auditory canal, external 18.02
  axilla 98.27
    by incision 86.05
  bladder (without incision) 57.0
    by incision 57.19
  bone, except fixation device - *see also* Incision, bone 77.10
    alveolus, alveolar 98.22
      by incision 24.0
  brain 01.39
    without incision into brain 01.24
  breast 85.0
  bronchus (intraluminal) 98.15
    by incision 33.0
  bursa 83.03
    hand 82.03
  canthus 98.22
    by incision 08.51
  cerebral meninges 01.31
  cervix (intraluminal) NEC 98.16
    penetrating 69.97
  choroid (by incision) 14.00
    with use of magnet 14.01
    without use of magnet 14.02
  ciliary body (by incision) 12.00
    with use of magnet 12.01
    without use of magnet 12.02
  conjunctiva (by magnet) 98.22
    by incision 10.0

Removal (*Continued*)
foreign body NEC (*Continued*)
  cornea 98.21
    by
      incision 11.1
      magnet 11.0
  duodenum 98.03
    by incision 45.01
  ear (intraluminal) 98.11
    with incision 18.09
  epididymis 63.92
  esophagus (intraluminal) 98.02
    by incision 42.09
  extrapleural (by incision) 34.01
  eye, eyeball (by magnet) 98.21
    anterior segment (by incision) 12.00
      with use of magnet 12.01
      without use of magnet 12.02
    posterior segment (by incision) 14.00
      with use of magnet 14.01
      without use of magnet 14.02
    superficial 98.21
  eyelid 98.22
    by incision 08.09
  fallopian tube
    by salpingostomy 66.02
    by salpingotomy 66.01
  fascia 83.09
    hand 82.09
  foot 98.28
  gallbladder 51.04
  groin region (abdominal wall) (inguinal) 54.0
  gum 98.22
    by incision 24.0
  hand 98.26
  head and neck NEC 98.22
  heart 37.11
  internal fixation device - *see* Removal, fixation device, internal
  intestine
    by incision 45.00
    large (intraluminal) 98.04
      by incision 45.03
    small (intraluminal) 98.03
      by incision 45.02
  intraocular (by incision) 12.00
    with use of magnet 12.01
    without use of magnet 12.02
  iris (by incision) 12.00
    with use of magnet 12.01
    without use of magnet 12.02
  joint structures - *see also* Arthrotomy 80.10
  kidney (transurethral) (by endoscopy) 56.0
    by incision 55.01
    pelvis (transurethral) 56.0
      by incision 55.11
  labia 98.23
    by incision 71.09
  lacrimal
    canaliculi 09.42
      by incision 09.52
    gland 09.3
      by incision 09.0
    passage(s) 09.49
      by incision 09.59
    punctum 09.41
      by incision 09.51
    sac 09.49
      by incision 09.53
  large intestine (intraluminal) 98.04
    by incision 45.03

Removal (*Continued*)
foreign body NEC (*Continued*)
  larynx (intraluminal) 98.14
    by incision 31.3
  lens 13.00
    by incision 13.02
      with use of magnet 13.01
  liver 50.0
  lower limb, except foot 98.29
    foot 98.28
  lung 33.1
  mediastinum 34.1
  meninges (cerebral) 01.31
    spinal 03.01
  mouth (intraluminal) 98.01
    by incision 27.92
  muscle 83.02
    hand 82.02
  nasal sinus 22.50
    antrum 22.2
      with Caldwell-Luc approach 22.39
    ethmoid 22.51
    frontal 22.41
    maxillary 22.2
      with Caldwell-Luc approach 22.39
    sphenoid 22.52
  nerve (cranial) (peripheral) NEC 04.04
    root 03.01
  nose (intraluminal) 98.12
    by incision 21.1
  oral cavity (intraluminal) 98.01
    by incision 27.92
  orbit (by magnet) 98.21
    by incision 16.1
  palate (penetrating) 98.22
    by incision 27.1
  pancreas 52.09
  penis 98.24
    by incision 64.92
  pericardium 37.12
  perineum (female) 98.23
    by incision 71.09
    male 98.25
      by incision 86.05
  perirenal tissue 59.09
  peritoneal cavity 54.92
  perivesical tissue 59.19
  pharynx (intraluminal) 98.13
    by pharyngotomy 29.0
  pleura (by incision) 34.09
  popliteal space 98.29
    by incision 86.05
  rectum (intraluminal) 98.05
    by incision 48.0
  renal pelvis (transurethral) 56.0
    by incision 56.1
  retina (by incision) 14.00
    with use of magnet 14.01
    without use of magnet 14.02
  retroperitoneum 54.92
  sclera (by incision) 12.00
    with use of magnet 12.01
    without use of magnet 12.02
  scrotum 98.24
    by incision 61.0
  sinus (nasal) 22.50
    antrum 22.2
      with Caldwell-Luc approach 22.39
    ethmoid 22.51
    frontal 22.41
    maxillary 22.2
      with Caldwell-Luc approach 22.39
    sphenoid 22.52

ICD-9-CM

R

Vol. 3

Removal *(Continued)*
  foreign body NEC *(Continued)*
    skin NEC 98.20
      by incision 86.05
    skull 01.24
      with incision into brain 01.39
    small intestine (intraluminal) 98.03
      by incision 45.02
    soft tissue NEC 83.09
      hand 82.09
    spermatic cord 63.93
    spinal (canal) (cord) (meninges) 03.01
    stomach (intraluminal) 98.03
      bubble (balloon) 44.94
      by incision 43.0
    subconjunctival (by magnet) 98.22
      by incision 10.0
    subcutaneous tissue NEC 98.20
      by incision 86.05
    supraclavicular fossa 98.27
      by incision 86.05
    tendon (sheath) 83.01
      hand 82.01
    testis 62.0
    thorax (by incision) 34.09
    thyroid (field) (gland) (by incision) 06.09
    tonsil 98.13
      by incision 28.91
    trachea (intraluminal) 98.15
      by incision 31.3
    trunk NEC 98.25
    tunica vaginalis 98.24
    upper limb, except hand 98.27
      hand 98.26
    ureter (transurethral) 56.0
      by incision 56.2
    urethra (intraluminal) 98.19
      by incision 58.0
    uterus (intraluminal) 98.16
    vagina (intraluminal) 98.17
      by incision 70.14
    vas deferens 63.6
    vitreous (by incision) 14.00
      with use of magnet 14.01
      without use of magnet 14.02
    vulva 98.23
      by incision 71.09
  gallstones
    bile duct (by incision) NEC 51.49
      endoscopic 51.88
    common duct (by incision) 51.41
      endoscopic 51.88
      percutaneous 51.96
    duodenum 45.01
    gallbladder 51.04
      endoscopic 51.88
      laparoscopic 51.88
    hepatic ducts 51.49
      endoscopic 51.88
    intestine 45.00
      large 45.03
      small NEC 45.02
    liver 50.0
  Gardner Wells tongs (skull) 02.95
    with synchronous replacement 02.94
  gastric band (adjustable), laparoscopic 44.97
  gastric bubble (balloon) 44.94
  granulation tissue - *see also* Excision, lesion, by site
    with repair - *see* Repair, by site
    cranial 01.6
    skull 01.6

Removal *(Continued)*
  halo traction device (skull) 02.95
    with synchronous replacement 02.94
  heart assist system
    with replacement 37.63
    intra-aortic balloon pump (IABP) 97.44
    nonoperative 97.44
    open removal 37.64
    percutaneous external device 97.44
  hematoma - *see* Drainage, by site
  Hoffman minifixator device (bone) - *see* category 78.6
  hydatidiform mole 68.0
  impacted
    feces (rectum) (by flushing) (manual) 96.38
    tooth 23.19
    from nasal sinus (maxillary) 22.61
  implant
    breast 85.94
    cochlear prosthetic device 20.99
    cornea 11.92
    lens (prosthetic) 13.8
    middle ear NEC 20.99
    ocular 16.71
      posterior segment 14.6
    orbit 16.72
    retina 14.6
    tympanum 20.1
  internal fixation device - *see* Removal, fixation device, internal
  intra-aortic balloon pump (IABP) 97.44
  intrauterine contraceptive device (IUD) 97.71
  joint (structure) NOS 80.90
    ankle 80.97
    elbow 80.92
    foot and toe 80.98
    hand and finger 80.94
    hip 80.95
    knee 80.96
    other specified sites 80.99
    shoulder 80.91
    spine 80.99
    toe 80.98
    wrist 80.93
  Kantrowitz heart pump 37.64
    nonoperative 97.44
  keel (tantalum plate), larynx 31.98
  kidney - *see also* Nephrectomy
    mechanical 55.98
    transplanted or rejected 55.53
  laminaria (tent), uterus 97.79
  leads (cardiac) - *see* Removal, electrodes, cardiac pacemaker
  lesion - *see* Excision, lesion, by site
  ligamentum flavum (spine) - *omit code*
  ligature
    fallopian tube 66.79
    ureter 56.86
    vas deferens 63.84
  limb lengthening device, internal - *see* category 78.6
  loop recorder 86.05
  loose body
    bone - *see* Sequestrectomy, bone
    joint 80.10
    mesh (surgical) - *see* Removal, foreign body, by site
  lymph node - *see* Excision, lymph, node
  minifixator device (bone) - *see* category 78.6
    external fixation device 97.88
  Mulligan hood, fallopian tube 66.94
    with synchronous replacement 66.93

Removal *(Continued)*
  muscle stimulator (skeletal) 83.93
    with replacement 83.92
  myringotomy device or tube 20.1
  nail (bed) (fold) 86.23
    internal fixation device - *see* Removal, fixation device, internal
  necrosis
    skin 86.28
      excisional 86.22
  neuropacemaker - *see* Removal, neurostimulator, by site
  neurostimulator
    brain 01.22
      with synchronous replacement 02.93
    electrodes
      brain 01.22
        with synchronous replacement 02.93
      intracranial 01.22
        with synchronous replacement 02.93
      peripheral nerve 04.93
        with synchronous replacement 04.92
      sacral nerve 04.93
        with synchronous replacement 04.92
      spinal 03.94
        with synchronous replacement 03.93
    pulse generator (single array, dual array) 86.05
      with synchronous replacement 86.96
      dual array 86.95
      single array 86.94
  nonabsorbable surgical material NEC - *see* Removal, foreign body, by site
  odontoma (tooth) 24.4
  orbital implant 16.72
  osteocartilaginous loose body, joint structures - *see also* Arthrotomy 80.10
  outer attic wall (middle ear) 20.59
  ovo-testis (unilateral) 62.3
    bilateral 62.41
  pacemaker
    brain (intracranial) - *see* Removal, neurostimulator
    cardiac (device) (initial) (permanent) 37.89
      with replacement
        dual-chamber device 37.87
        single-chamber device 37.85
          rate responsive 37.86
      electrodes (atrial) (transvenous) (ventricular) 37.77
        with replacement 37.76
      epicardium (myocardium) 37.77
        with replacement (by)
          atrial and/or ventricular lead(s) (electrode) 37.76
          epicardial lead 37.74
      temporary transvenous pacemaker system - *omit code*
    intracranial - *see* Removal, neurostimulator
    neural - *see* Removal, neurostimulator
    peripheral nerve - *see* Removal, neurostimulator
    spinal - *see* Removal, neurostimulator

◄ **New**   ◄⦀ **Revised**

Removal (*Continued*)
pack, packing
  dental 97.34
  intrauterine 97.72
  nasal 97.32
  rectum 97.59
  trunk NEC 97.85
  vagina 97.75
  vulva 97.75
pantopaque dye, spinal canal 03.31
patella (complete) 77.96
  partial 77.86
pectus deformity implant device 34.01
pelvic viscera, en masse (female) 68.8
  male 57.71
pessary, vagina NEC 97.74
pharynx (partial) 29.33
phlebolith - *see* Removal, embolus
placenta (by)
  aspiration curettage 69.52
  D and C 69.02
  manual 75.4
plaque, dental 96.54
plate, skull 02.07
  with synchronous replacement 02.05
polyp - *see also* Excision, lesion, by site
  esophageal 42.32
    endoscopic 42.33
  gastric (endoscopic) 43.41
  intestine 45.41
    endoscopic 45.42
  nasal 21.31
prosthesis
  bile duct 51.95
    nonoperative 97.55
  cochlear prosthetic device 20.99
  dental 97.35
  eye 97.31
  facial bone 76.99
  fallopian tube 66.94
    with synchronous replacement 66.93
  joint structures 80.00
    ankle 80.07
    elbow 80.02
    foot and toe 80.08
    hand and finger 80.04
    hip 80.05
    knee 80.06
    shoulder 80.01
    specified site NEC 80.09
    spine 80.09
    wrist 80.03
  lens 13.8
  penis (internal), without replacement 64.96
  Rosen (urethra) 59.99
  testicular, by incision 62.0
  urinary sphincter, artificial 58.99
    with replacement 58.93
pseudophakos 13.8
pterygium 11.39
  with corneal graft 11.32
pulse generator
  cardiac pacemaker 37.86
  cardioverter/defibrillator 37.99
  neurostimulator - *see* Removal, neurostimulator, pulse generator ◄
pump assist device, heart 37.64
  with replacement 37.63
  nonoperative 97.44
radioactive material - *see* Removal, foreign body, by site
redundant skin, eyelid 08.86

Removal (*Continued*)
rejected organ
  kidney 55.53
  testis 62.42
reservoir, ventricular (Ommaya) (Rickham) 02.43
  with synchronous replacement 02.42
retained placenta (by)
  aspiration curettage 69.52
  D and C 69.02
  manual 75.4
retinal implant 14.6
rhinolith 21.31
rice bodies, tendon sheaths 83.01
  hand 82.01
Roger-Anderson minifixator device (bone) - *see* category 78.6
root, residual (tooth) (buried) (retained) 23.11
Rosen prosthesis (urethra) 59.99
scleral buckle or implant 14.6
Scribner shunt 39.43
secondary membranous cataract (with iridectomy) 13.65
secundines (by)
  aspiration curettage 69.52
  D and C 69.02
  manual 75.4
sequestrum - *see* Sequestrectomy
seton, anus 49.93
Shepard's tube (ear) 20.1
Shirodkar suture, cervix 69.96
shunt
  arteriovenous 39.43
    with creation of new shunt 39.42
  lumbar-subarachnoid NEC 03.98
  pleurothecal 03.98
  salpingothecal 03.98
  spinal (thecal) NEC 03.98
  subarachnoid-peritoneal 03.98
  subarachnoid-ureteral 03.98
silastic tubes
  ear 20.1
  fallopian tubes 66.94
    with synchronous replacement 66.93
skin
  necrosis or slough 86.28
    excisional 86.22
    superficial layer (by dermabrasion) 86.25
skull tongs 02.95
  with synchronous replacement 02.94
splint 97.88
stent
  bile duct 97.55
  larynx 31.98
  ureteral 97.62
  urethral 97.65
stimoceiver - *see* Removal, neurostimulator ◄▥
subdural
  grids 01.22
  strips 01.22
supernumerary digit(s) 86.26
suture(s) NEC 97.89
  abdominal wall 97.83
  by incision - *see* Incision, by site
  genital tract 97.79
  head and neck 97.38
  thorax 97.43
  trunk NEC 97.84
symblepharon - *see* Repair, symblepharon

Removal (*Continued*)
temporary transvenous pacemaker system - *omit code*
testis (unilateral) 62.3
  bilateral 62.41
  remaining or solitary 62.42
thrombus 36.09
  with endarterectomy - *see* Endarterectomy
  abdominal
    artery 38.06
    vein 38.07
  aorta (arch) (ascending) (descending) 38.04
  arteriovenous shunt or cannula 39.49
  bovine graft 39.49
  coronary artery 36.09
  head and neck vessel NEC 38.02
  intracranial vessel NEC 38.01
  lower limb
    artery 38.08
    vein 38.09
  pulmonary (artery) (vein) 38.05
  thoracic vessel NEC 38.05
  upper limb (artery) (vein) 38.03
tissue expander (skin) NEC 86.05
  breast 85.96
toes, supernumerary 86.26
tongs, skull 02.95
  with synchronous replacement 02.94
tonsil tag 28.4
tooth (by forceps) (multiple) (single) NEC 23.09
  deciduous 23.01
  surgical NEC 23.19
    impacted 23.19
    residual root 23.11
    root apex 23.73
      with root canal therapy 23.72
trachoma follicles 10.33
T-tube (bile duct) 97.55
tube
  appendix 97.53
  bile duct (T-tube) NEC 97.55
  cholecystostomy 97.54
  cystostomy 97.63
  ear (button) 20.1
  gastrostomy 97.51
  large intestine 97.53
  liver 97.55
  mediastinum 97.42
  nephrostomy 97.61
  pancreas 97.56
  peritoneum 97.82
  pleural cavity 97.41
  pyelostomy 97.61
  retroperitoneum 97.81
  small intestine 97.52
  thoracotomy 97.41
  tracheostomy 97.37
  tympanostomy 20.1
  tympanum 20.1
  ureterostomy 97.62
ureteral splint (stent) 97.62
urethral sphincter, artificial 58.99
  with replacement 58.93
urinary sphincter, artificial 58.99
  with replacement 58.93
utricle 20.79
valve
  vas deferens 63.85
  ventricular (cerebral) 02.43
vascular graft or prosthesis 39.49
ventricular shunt or reservoir 02.43
  with synchronous replacement 02.42

ICD-9-CM
R
Vol. 3

Removal *(Continued)*
  Vinke tongs (skull) 02.95
    with synchronous replacement 02.94
  vitreous (with replacement) 14.72
    anterior approach (partial) 14.71
    open sky technique 14.71
  Wagner-Brooker minifixator device
    (bone) - *see* category 78.6
  wiring, dental (immobilization device)
    97.33
    orthodontic 24.8

Renipuncture (percutaneous) 55.92
Renogram 92.03
Renotransplantation NEC 55.69

Note: To report donor source: ◀
    cadaver 00.93 ◀
    live non-related donor
      00.92 ◀
    live related donor 00.91 ◀
    live unrelated donor 00.92 ◀

Reopening - *see also* Incision, by site
  blepharorrhaphy 08.02
  canthorrhaphy 08.02
  cilia base 08.71
  craniotomy or craniectomy site 01.23
  fallopian tube (divided) 66.79
  iris in anterior chambers 12.97
  laminectomy or laminotomy site 03.02
  laparotomy site 54.12
  osteotomy site - *see also* Incision, bone
    77.10
    facial bone 76.09
  tarsorrhaphy 08.02
  thoracotomy site (for control of hemor-
    rhage) (for examination) (for ex-
    ploration) 34.03
  thyroid field wound (for control of
    hemorrhage) (for examination)
    (for exploration) (for removal of
    hematoma) 06.02

Repacking - *see* Replacement, pack, by
  site
Repair
  abdominal wall 54.72
  adrenal gland 07.44
  alveolus, alveolar (process) (ridge)
    (with graft) (with implant) 24.5
  anal sphincter 49.79
    artificial sphincter
      implantation 49.75
      revision 49.75
    laceration (by suture) 49.71
    obstetric (current) 75.62
      old 49.79
  aneurysm (false) (true) 39.52
    by or with
      clipping 39.51
      coagulation 39.52
      coil (endovascular approach)
        39.79
        head and neck 39.72
      electrocoagulation 39.52
      excision or resection of vessel -
        see also Aneurysmectomy,
        by site
      with
        anastomosis - *see* Aneurys-
          mectomy, with anastomo-
          sis, by site
        graft replacement - *see* Aneu-
          rysmectomy, with graft
          replacement, by site

Repair *(Continued)*
  aneurysm *(Continued)*
    by or with *(Continued)*
      endovascular graft 39.79
        abdominal aorta 39.71
        head and neck 39.72
        lower extremity artery(ies)
          39.79
        thoracic aorta 39.79
        upper extremity artery(ies)
          39.79
      filipuncture 39.52
      graft replacement - *see* Aneurys-
        mectomy, with graft
        replacement, by site
      ligation 39.52
      liquid tissue adhesive (glue) 39.79
        endovascular approach 39.79
        head and neck 39.72
      methyl methacrylate 39.52
        endovascular approach 39.79
        head and neck 39.72
      occlusion 39.52
        endovascular approach 39.79
        head and neck 39.72
      suture 39.52
      trapping 39.52
      wiring 39.52
      wrapping (gauze) (methyl methac-
        rylate) (plastic) 39.52
    coronary artery 36.91
    heart 37.4
      total replacement system 37.52
        implantable battery 37.54
        implantable controller 37.54
        thoracic unit 37.53
        transcutaneous energy transfer
          [TET] device 37.54
    sinus of Valsalva 35.39
    thoracic aorta (dissecting), by fenes-
      tration 39.54
  anomalous pulmonary venous connec-
    tion (total)
    one-stage 35.82
    partial - *see* specific procedure
    total 35.82
  anus 49.79
    laceration (by suture) 49.71
      obstetric (current) 75.62
      old 49.79
  aorta 39.31
  aorticopulmonary window 39.59
  arteriovenous fistula 39.53
    by or with
      clipping 39.53
      coagulation 39.53
      coil (endovascular approach) 39.79
        head and neck vessels 39.72
      division 39.53
      excision or resection - *see also*
        Aneurysmectomy, by site
      with
        anastomosis - *see* Aneurys-
          mectomy, with anastomo-
          sis, by site
        graft replacement - *see* Aneu-
          rysmectomy, with graft
          replacement, by site
      ligation 39.53
        coronary artery 36.99
      occlusion 39.53
        endovascular approach 39.79
        head and neck 39.72
      suture 39.53

Repair *(Continued)*
  artery NEC 39.59
    by
      endovascular approach ⬅
        head and neck (embolization or
          occlusion) 39.72 ⬅
        other repair (of aneurysms)
          39.79 ◀
        percutaneous repair of intracra-
          nial vessel(s) (for stent in-
          sertion) 00.62 ◀
        percutaneous repair of precere-
          bral (extracranial) vessel(s)
          (for stent insertion) 00.61 ◀
      non-coronary percutaneous trans-
        luminal angioplasty or ather-
        ectomy
        basilar 00.61 ⬅
        carotid 00.61 ⬅
        femoropopliteal 39.50
        iliac 39.50
        lower extremity NOS 39.50
        mesenteric 39.50
        renal 39.50
        upper extremity NOS 39.50
        vertebral 00.61 ⬅
    with
      patch graft 39.58
        with excision or resection of ves-
          sel - *see* Arteriectomy, with
          graft replacement, by site
        synthetic (Dacron) (Teflon) 39.57
        tissue (vein) (autogenous) (ho-
          mograft) 39.56
      suture 39.31
  coronary NEC 36.99
    by angioplasty - *see* Angioplasty,
      coronary
    by atherectomy - *see* Angioplasty,
      coronary
  artificial opening - *see* Repair, stoma
  atrial septal defect 35.71
    with
      prosthesis (open heart technique)
        35.51
        closed heart technique 35.52
      tissue graft 35.61
    combined with repair of valvular and
      ventricular septal defects - *see* Re-
      pair, endocardial cushion defect
    in total repair of total anomalous pul-
      monary venous connection 35.82
  atrioventricular canal defect (any type)
    35.73
    with
      prosthesis 35.54
      tissue graft 35.63
  bifid digit (finger) 82.89
  bile duct NEC 51.79
    laceration (by suture) NEC 51.79
      common bile duct 51.71
  bladder NEC 57.89
    exstrophy 57.86
    for stress incontinence - *see* Repair,
      stress incontinence
    laceration (by suture) 57.81
      obstetric (current) 75.61
      old 57.89
    neck 57.85
  blepharophimosis 08.59
  blepharoptosis 08.36
    by
      frontalis muscle technique (with)
        fascial sling 08.32
        suture 08.31

◀ **New**　　⬅ **Revised**

ICD-9-CM

R

Vol. 3

Repair *(Continued)*
  blepharoptosis *(Continued)*
    levator muscle technique 08.34
      with resection or advancement 08.33
    orbicularis oculi muscle sling 08.36
    tarsal technique 08.35
  blood vessel NEC 39.59
    patch graft 39.58
      with excision or resection - *see*
        Angiectomy, with graft re-
        placement
        synthetic (Dacron) (Teflon) 39.57
        tissue (vein) (autogenous) (ho-
        mograft) 39.56
    resection - *see* Angiectomy
    suture 39.30
  coronary artery NEC 36.99
    by angioplasty - *see* Angioplasty,
      coronary
    by atherectomy - *see* Angioplasty,
      coronary
  peripheral vessel NEC 39.59
    by angioplasty 39.50
    by atherectomy 39.50
    by endovascular approach 39.79
  bone NEC - *see also* Osteoplasty - *see*
    category 78.4
    by synostosis technique - *see* Ar-
      throdesis
    accessory sinus 22.79
    cranium NEC 02.06
      with
        flap (bone) 02.03
        graft (bone) 02.04
    for malunion, nonunion, or delayed
      union of fracture - *see* Repair,
      fracture, malunion or nonunion
    nasal 21.89
    skull NEC 02.06
      with
        flap (bone) 02.03
        graft (bone) 02.04
  bottle, hydrocele of tunica vaginalis 61.2
  brain (trauma) NEC 02.92
  breast (plastic) - *see also* Mammoplasty
    85.89
  broad ligament 69.29
  bronchus NEC 33.48
    laceration (by suture) 33.41
  bunionette (with osteotomy) 77.54
  canaliculus, lacrimal 09.73
  canthus (lateral) 08.59
  cardiac pacemaker NEC 37.89
    electrode(s) (lead) NEC 37.75
  cardioverter/defibrillator (automatic)
    pocket (skin) (subcutaneous) 37.99
  cerebral meninges 02.12
  cervix 67.69
    internal os 67.59
      transabdominal 67.51
      transvaginal 67.59
    laceration (by suture) 67.61
      obstetric (current) 75.51
      old 67.69
  chest wall (mesh) (silastic) NEC 34.79
  chordae tendineae 35.32
  choroid NEC 14.9
    with retinal repair - *see* Repair, ret-
      ina
  cisterna chyli 40.69
  claw toe 77.57
  cleft
    hand 82.82
    laryngotracheal 31.69

Repair *(Continued)*
  cleft *(Continued)*
    lip 27.54
    palate 27.62
      secondary or subsequent 27.63
  coarctation of aorta - *see* Excision, co-
    arctation of aorta
  cochlear prosthetic device 20.99
    external components only 95.49
  cockup toe 77.58
  colostomy 46.43
  conjunctiva NEC 10.49
    with scleral repair 12.81
    laceration 10.6
      with repair of sclera 12.81
    late effect of trachoma 10.49
  cornea NEC 11.59
    with
      conjunctival flap 11.53
      transplant - *see* Keratoplasty
    postoperative dehiscence 11.52
  coronary artery NEC 36.99
    by angioplasty - *see* Angioplasty,
      coronary
    by atherectomy - *see* Angioplasty,
      coronary
  cranium NEC 02.06
    with
      flap (bone) 02.03
      graft (bone) 02.04
  cusp, valve - *see* Repair, heart, valve
  cystocele 70.51
    and rectocele 70.50
  dental arch 24.8
  diaphragm NEC 34.84
  diastasis recti 83.65
  diastematomyelia 03.59
  ear (external) 18.79
    auditory canal or meatus 18.6
    auricle NEC 18.79
    cartilage NEC 18.79
    laceration (by suture) 18.4
    lop ear 18.79
    middle NEC 19.9
    prominent or protruding 18.5
  ectropion 08.49
    by or with
      lid reconstruction 08.44
      suture (technique) 08.42
      thermocauterization 08.41
      wedge resection 08.43
  encephalocele (cerebral) 02.12
  endocardial cushion defect 35.73
    with
      prosthesis (grafted to septa) 35.54
      tissue graft 35.63
  enterocele (female) 70.92
    male 53.9
  enterostomy 46.40
  entropion 08.49
    by or with
      lid reconstruction 08.44
      suture (technique) 08.42
      thermocauterization 08.41
      wedge resection 08.43
  epicanthus (fold) 08.59
  epididymis (and spermatic cord) NEC
    63.59
    with vas deferens 63.89
  epiglottis 31.69
  episiotomy
    routine following delivery - *see* Epis-
      iotomy
    secondary 75.69

Repair *(Continued)*
  epispadias 58.45
  esophagus, esophageal NEC 42.89
    fistula NEC 42.84
    stricture 42.85
  exstrophy of bladder 57.86
  eye, eyeball 16.89
    multiple structures 16.82
    rupture 16.82
    socket 16.64
      with graft 16.63
  eyebrow 08.89
    linear 08.81
  eyelid 08.89
    full-thickness 08.85
      involving lid margin 08.84
    laceration 08.81
      full-thickness 08.85
        involving lid margin 08.84
      partial-thickness 08.83
        involving lid margin 08.82
    linear 08.81
    partial-thickness 08.83
      involving lid margin 08.82
    retraction 08.38
  fallopian tube (with prosthesis) 66.79
    by
      anastomosis 66.73
      reanastomosis 66.79
      reimplantation into
        ovary 66.72
        uterus 66.74
      suture 66.71
  false aneurysm - *see* Repair, aneurysm
  fascia 83.89
    by or with
      arthroplasty - *see* Arthroplasty
      graft (fascial) (muscle) 83.82
        hand 82.72
        tendon 83.81
          hand 82.79
      suture (direct) 83.65
        hand 82.46
    hand 82.89
      by
        graft NEC 82.79
          fascial 82.72
          muscle 82.72
        suture (direct) 82.46
  joint - *see* Arthroplasty
  filtering bleb (corneal) (scleral) (by ex-
    cision) 12.82
    by
      corneal graft - *see also* Kerato-
        plasty 11.60
      scleroplasty 12.82
      suture 11.51
        with conjunctival flap 11.53
  fistula - *see also* Closure, fistula
    anovaginal 70.73
    arteriovenous 39.53
      clipping 39.53
      coagulation 39.53
        endovascular approach 39.79
          head and neck 39.72
      division 39.53
      excision or resection - *see also*
        Aneurysmectomy, by site
        with
          anastomosis - *see* Aneurys-
            mectomy, with anastomo-
            sis, by site
          graft replacement - *see* Aneu-
            rysmectomy, with graft
            replacement, by site

Repair *(Continued)*
  fistula *(Continued)*
    arteriovenous *(Continued)*
      ligation 39.53
        coronary artery 36.99
      occlusion 39.53
        endovascular approach 39.79
          head and neck 39.72
      suture 39.53
    cervicovesical 57.84
    cervix 67.62
    choledochoduodenal 51.72
    colovaginal 70.72
    enterovaginal 70.74
    enterovesical 57.83
    esophagocutaneous 42.84
    ileovesical 57.83
    intestinovaginal 70.74
    intestinovesical 57.83
    oroantral 22.71
    perirectal 48.93
    pleuropericardial 37.4
    rectovaginal 70.73
    rectovesical 57.83
    rectovesicovaginal 57.83
    scrotum 61.42
    sigmoidovaginal 70.74
    sinus
      nasal 22.71
      of Valsalva 35.39
    splenocolic 41.95
    urethroperineovesical 57.84
    urethrovesical 57.84
    urethrovesicovaginal 57.84
    uterovesical 57.84
    vagina NEC 70.75
    vaginocutaneous 70.75
    vaginoenteric NEC 70.74
    vaginoileal 70.74
    vaginoperineal 70.75
    vaginovesical 57.84
    vesicocervicovaginal 57.84
    vesicocolic 57.83
    vesicocutaneous 57.84
    vesicoenteric 57.83
    vesicointestinal 57.83
    vesicometrorectal 57.83
    vesicoperineal 57.84
    vesicorectal 57.83
    vesicosigmoidal 57.83
    vesicosigmoidovaginal 57.83
    vesicourethral 57.84
    vesicourethrorectal 57.83
    vesicouterine 57.84
    vesicovaginal 57.84
    vulva 71.72
    vulvorectal 48.73
  foramen ovale (patent) 35.71
    with
      prosthesis (open heart technique) 35.51
        closed heart technique 35.52
      tissue graft 35.61
  fracture - *see also* Reduction, fracture
    larynx 31.64
    malunion or nonunion (delayed)
      NEC - *see* category 78.4
      with
        graft - *see* Graft, bone
        insertion (of)
          bone growth stimulator (invasive) - *see* category 78.9
          internal fixation device 78.5

Repair *(Continued)*
  fracture *(Continued)*
    malunion or nonunion *(Continued)*
      with *(Continued)*
        manipulation for realignment - *see* Reduction, fracture, by site, closed
        osteotomy
          with
            correction of alignment - *see* category 77.3
            with internal fixation device - *see* categories 77.3 [78.5]
            with intramedullary rod - *see* categories 77.3 [78.5]
        replacement arthroplasty - *see* Arthroplasty
        sequestrectomy - *see* category 77.0
        Sofield type procedure - *see* categories 77.3 [78.5]
        synostosis technique - *see* Arthrodesis
    vertebra 03.53
  funnel chest (with implant) 34.74
  gallbladder 51.91
  gastroschisis 54.71
  great vessels NEC 39.59
    laceration (by suture) 39.30
      artery 39.31
      vein 39.32
  hallux valgus NEC 77.59
    resection of joint with prosthetic implant 77.59
  hammer toe 77.56
  hand 82.89
    with graft or implant 82.79
      fascia 82.72
      muscle 82.72
      tendon 82.79
  heart 37.4
    assist system 37.63
    septum 35.70
      with
        prosthesis 35.50
        tissue graft 35.60
      atrial 35.71
        with
          prosthesis (open heart technique) 35.51
          closed heart technique 35.52
          tissue graft 35.61
        combined with repair of valvular and ventricular septal defects - *see* Repair, endocardial cushion defect
        in total repair of
          tetralogy of Fallot 35.81
          total anomalous pulmonary venous connection 35.82
          truncus arteriosus 35.83
        combined with repair of valvular defect - *see* Repair, endocardial cushion defect
      ventricular 35.72
        with
          prosthesis 35.53
          tissue graft 35.62
        combined with repair of valvular and atrial septal defects - *see* Repair, endocardial cushion defect

Repair *(Continued)*
  heart *(Continued)*
    septum *(Continued)*
      ventricular *(Continued)*
        in total repair of
          tetralogy of Fallot 35.81
          total anomalous pulmonary venous connection 35.82
          truncus arteriosus 35.83
    total replacement system 37.52
      implantable battery 37.54
      implantable controller 37.54
      thoracic unit 37.53
      transcutaneous energy transfer [TET] device 37.54
    valve (cusps) (open heart technique) 35.10
      with prosthesis or tissue graft 35.20
      aortic (without replacement) 35.11
        with
          prosthesis 35.22
          tissue graft 35.21
        combined with repair of atrial and ventricular septal defects - *see* Repair, endocardial cushion defect
      mitral (without replacement) 35.12
        with
          prosthesis 35.24
          tissue graft 35.23
      pulmonary (without replacement) 35.13
        with
          prosthesis 35.26
            in total repair of tetralogy of Fallot 35.81
          tissue graft 35.25
      tricuspid (without replacement) 35.14
        with
          prosthesis 35.28
          tissue graft 35.27
  hepatic duct 51.79
  hernia NEC 53.9
    anterior abdominal wall NEC 53.59
      with prosthesis or graft 53.69
    colostomy 46.42
    crural 53.29
    cul-de-sac (Douglas') 70.92
    diaphragmatic
      abdominal approach 53.7
      thoracic, thoracoabdominal approach 53.80
    epigastric 53.59
      with prosthesis or graft 53.69
    esophageal hiatus
      abdominal approach 53.7
      thoracic, thoracoabdominal approach 53.80
    fascia 83.89
      hand 82.89
    femoral (unilateral) 53.29
      with prosthesis or graft 53.21
      bilateral 53.39
        with prosthesis or graft 53.31
    Ferguson 53.00
    Halsted 53.00
    Hill-Allison (hiatal hernia repair, transpleural approach) 53.80
    hypogastric 53.59
      with prosthesis or graft 53.69
    incisional 53.51
      with prosthesis or graft 53.61
    inguinal (unilateral) 53.00

◀ **New**   ◀▦ **Revised**

Repair *(Continued)*
  hernia NEC *(Continued)*
    inguinal *(Continued)*
      with prosthesis or graft 53.05
      bilateral 53.10
        with prosthesis or graft 53.17
        direct 53.11
          with prosthesis or graft 53.14
        direct and indirect 53.13
          with prosthesis or graft 53.16
        indirect 53.12
          with prosthesis or graft 53.15
      direct (unilateral) 53.01
        with prosthesis or graft 53.03
        and indirect (unilateral) 53.01
          with prosthesis or graft 53.03
          bilateral 53.13
            with prosthesis or graft 53.16
        bilateral 53.11
          with prosthesis or graft 53.14
      indirect (unilateral) 53.02
        with prosthesis or graft 53.04
        and direct (unilateral) 53.01
          with prosthesis or graft 53.03
          bilateral 53.13
            with prosthesis or graft 53.16
        bilateral 53.12
          with prosthesis or graft 53.15
    internal 53.9
    ischiatic 53.9
    ischiorectal 53.9
    lumbar 53.9
    manual 96.27
    obturator 53.9
    omental 53.9
    paraesophageal 53.7
    parahiatal 53.7
    paraileostomy 46.41
    parasternal 53.82
    paraumbilical 53.49
      with prosthesis 53.41
    pericolostomy 46.42
    perineal (enterocele) 53.9
    preperitoneal 53.29
    pudendal 53.9
    retroperitoneal 53.9
    sciatic 53.9
    scrotal - *see* Repair, hernia, inguinal
    spigelian 53.59
      with prosthesis or graft 53.69
    umbilical 53.49
      with prosthesis 53.41
    uveal 12.39
    ventral 53.59
      incisional 53.51
        with prosthesis or graft 53.61
  hydrocele
    round ligament 69.19
    spermatic cord 63.1
    tunica vaginalis 61.2
  hymen 70.76
  hypospadias 58.45
  ileostomy 46.41
  ingrown toenail 86.23
  intestine, intestinal NEC 46.79
    fistula - *see* Closure, fistula, intestine
    laceration
      large intestine 46.75
      small intestine NEC 46.73
    stoma - *see* Repair, stoma
  inverted uterus NEC 69.29
    manual
      nonobstetric 69.94
      obstetric 75.94

Repair *(Continued)*
  inverted uterus NEC *(Continued)*
    obstetrical
      manual 75.94
      surgical 75.93
    vaginal approach 69.23
  iris (rupture) NEC 12.39
  jejunostomy 46.41
  joint (capsule) (cartilage) NEC - *see also* Arthroplasty 81.96
  kidney NEC 55.89
  knee (joint) NEC 81.47
    collateral ligaments 81.46
    cruciate ligaments 81.45
    five-in-one 81.42
    triad 81.43
  labia - *see* Repair, vulva
  laceration - *see* Suture, by site
  lacrimal system NEC 09.99
    canaliculus 09.73
    punctum 09.72
      for eversion 09.71
  laryngostomy 31.62
  laryngotracheal cleft 31.69
  larynx 31.69
    fracture 31.64
    laceration 31.61
  leads (cardiac) NEC 37.75
  ligament - *see also* Arthroplasty 81.96
    broad 69.29
    collateral, knee NEC 81.46
    cruciate, knee NEC 81.45
    round 69.29
    uterine 69.29
  lip NEC 27.59
    cleft 27.54
    laceration (by suture) 27.51
  liver NEC 50.69
    laceration 50.61
  lop ear 18.79
  lung NEC 33.49
  lymphatic (channel) (peripheral) NEC 40.9
    duct, left (thoracic) NEC 40.69
  macrodactyly 82.83
  mallet finger 82.84
  mandibular ridge 76.64
  mastoid (antrum) (cavity) 19.9
  meninges (cerebral) NEC 02.12
    spinal NEC 03.59
      meningocele 03.51
      myelomeningocele 03.52
  meningocele (spinal) 03.51
    cranial 02.12
  mesentery 54.75
  mouth NEC 27.59
    laceration NEC 27.52
  muscle NEC 83.87
    by
      graft or implant (fascia) (muscle) 83.82
      hand 82.72
      tendon 83.81
        hand 82.79
      suture (direct) 83.65
        hand 82.46
      transfer or transplantation (muscle) 83.77
        hand 82.58
    hand 82.89
      by
        graft or implant NEC 82.79
          fascia 82.72
        suture (direct) 82.46
        transfer or transplantation (muscle) 82.58

Repair *(Continued)*
  musculotendinous cuff, shoulder 83.63
  myelomeningocele 03.52
  nasal
    septum (perforation) NEC 21.88
    sinus NEC 22.79
      fistula 22.71
  nasolabial flaps (plastic) 21.86
  nasopharyngeal atresia 29.4
  nerve (cranial) (peripheral) NEC 04.79
    old injury 04.76
    revision 04.75
    sympathetic 05.81
  nipple NEC 85.87
  nose (external) (internal) (plastic) NEC - *see also* Rhinoplasty 21.89
    laceration (by suture) 21.81
  notched lip 27.59
  omentum 54.74
  omphalocele 53.49
    with prosthesis 53.41
  orbit 16.89
    wound 16.81
  ostium
    primum defect 35.73
      with
        prosthesis 35.54
        tissue graft 35.63
    secundum defect 35.71
      with
        prosthesis (open heart technique) 35.51
          closed heart technique 35.52
        tissue graft 35.61
  ovary 65.79
    with tube 65.73
      laparoscopic 65.76
  overlapping toe 77.58
  pacemaker
    cardiac
      device (permanent) 37.89
      electrodes (leads) NEC 37.75
      pocket (skin) (subcutaneous) 37.79
  palate NEC 27.69
    cleft 27.62
      secondary or subsequent 27.63
    laceration (by suture) 27.61
  pancreas NEC 52.95
    Wirsung's duct 52.99
  papillary muscle (heart) 35.31
  patent ductus arteriosus 38.85
  pectus deformity (chest) (carinatum) (excavatum) 34.74
  pelvic floor NEC 70.79
    obstetric laceration (current) 75.69
      old 70.79
  penis NEC 64.49
    for epispadias or hypospadias 58.45
    inflatable prosthesis 64.99
    laceration 64.41
  pericardium 37.4
  perineum (female) 71.79
    laceration (by suture) 71.71
      obstetric (current) 75.69
        old 71.79
    male NEC 86.89
      laceration (by suture) 86.59
  peritoneum NEC 54.73
    by suture 54.64
  pharynx NEC 29.59
    laceration (by suture) 29.51
    plastic 29.4
  pleura NEC 34.93
  postcataract wound dehiscence 11.52
    with conjunctival flap 11.53

ICD-9-CM

Vol. 3

Repair (Continued)
pouch of Douglas 70.52
primum ostium defect 35.73
  with
      prosthesis 35.54
      tissue graft 35.63
prostate 60.93
ptosis, eyelid - *see* Repair, blepharoptosis
punctum, lacrimal NEC 09.72
  for correction of eversion 09.71
quadriceps (mechanism) 83.86
rectocele (posterior colporrhaphy) 70.52
  and cystocele 70.50
rectum NEC 48.79
  laceration (by suture) 48.71
  prolapse NEC 48.76
      abdominal approach 48.75
retina, retinal
  detachment 14.59
      by
          cryotherapy 14.52
          diathermy 14.51
          photocoagulation 14.55
              laser 14.54
              xenon arc 14.53
          scleral buckling - *see also* Buckling, scleral 14.49
  tear or defect 14.39
      by
          cryotherapy 14.32
          diathermy 14.31
          photocoagulation 14.35
              laser 14.34
              xenon arc 14.33
retroperitoneal tissue 54.73
rotator cuff (suture) 83.63
round ligament 69.29
ruptured tendon NEC 83.88
  hand 82.86
salivary gland or duct NEC 26.49
sclera, scleral 12.89
  fistula 12.82
  staphyloma NEC 12.86
      with graft 12.85
scrotum 61.49
sinus
  nasal NEC 22.79
  of Valsalva (aneurysm) 35.39
skin (plastic) (without graft) 86.89
  laceration (by suture) 86.59
skull NEC 02.06
  with
      flap (bone) 02.03
      graft (bone) 02.04
spermatic cord NEC 63.59
  laceration (by suture) 63.51
sphincter ani 49.79
  laceration (by suture) 49.71
      obstetric (current) 75.62
      old 49.79
spina bifida NEC 03.59
  meningocele 03.51
  myelomeningocele 03.52
spinal (cord) (meninges) (structures) NEC 03.59
  meningocele 03.51
  myelomeningocele 03.52
spleen 41.95
sternal defect 78.41
stoma
  bile duct 51.79
  bladder 57.22
  bronchus 33.42

Repair (Continued)
stoma (Continued)
  common duct 51.72
  esophagus 42.89
  gallbladder 51.99
  hepatic duct 51.79
  intestine 46.40
      large 46.43
      small 46.41
  kidney 55.89
  larynx 31.63
  rectum 48.79
  stomach 44.69
      laparoscopic 44.68   ◀
  thorax 34.79
  trachea 31.74
  ureter 56.62
  urethra 58.49
stomach NEC 44.69
  laceration (by suture) 44.61
  laparoscopic 44.68   ◀
stress incontinence (urinary) NEC 59.79
  by
      anterior urethropexy 59.79
      Burch 59.5
      cystourethropexy (with levator muscle sling) 59.71
      injection of implant (fat) (collagen) (polytef) 59.72
      paraurethral suspension (Pereyra) 59.6
      periurethral suspension 59.6
      plication of urethrovesical junction 59.3
      pubococcygeal sling 59.71
      retropubic urethral suspension 59.5
      suprapubic sling 59.4
      tension free vaginal tape 59.79
      urethrovesical suspension 59.4
          gracilis muscle transplant 59.71
          levator muscle sling 59.71
subcutaneous tissue (plastic) (without skin graft) 86.89
  laceration (by suture) 86.59
supracristal defect (heart) 35.72
  with
      prosthesis 35.53
      tissue graft 35.62
symblepharon NEC 10.49
  by division (with insertion of conformer) 10.5
  with free graft 10.41
syndactyly 86.85
synovial membrane, joint - *see* Arthroplasty
telecanthus 08.59
tendon 83.88
  by or with
      arthroplasty - *see* Arthroplasty
      graft or implant (tendon) 83.81
          fascia 83.82
              hand 82.72
          hand 82.79
          muscle 83.82
              hand 82.72
      suture (direct) (immediate) (primary) - *see also* Suture, tendon 83.64
          hand 82.45
      transfer for transplantation (tendon) 83.75
          hand 82.56

Repair (Continued)
tendon (Continued)
  hand 82.86
      by
          graft or implant (tendon) 82.79
          suture (direct) (immediate) (primary) - *see also* Suture, tendon, hand 82.45
          transfer or transplantation (tendon) 82.56
  rotator cuff (direct suture) 83.63
  ruptured NEC 83.88
      hand 82.86
  sheath (direct suture) 83.61
      hand 82.41
testis NEC 62.69
tetralogy of Fallot
  partial - *see* specific procedure
  total (one-stage) 35.81
thoracic duct NEC 40.69
thoracostomy 34.72
thymus (gland) 07.93
tongue NEC 25.59
tooth NEC 23.2
  by
      crown (artificial) 23.41
      filling (amalgam) (plastic) (silicate) 23.2
      inlay 23.3
total anomalous pulmonary venous connection
  partial - *see* specific procedure
  total (one-stage) 35.82
trachea NEC 31.79
  laceration (by suture) 31.71
tricuspid atresia 35.94
truncus arteriosus
  partial - *see* specific procedure
  total (one-stage) 35.83
tunica vaginalis 61.49
  laceration (by suture) 61.41
tympanum - *see* Tympanoplasty
ureter NEC 56.89
  laceration (by suture) 56.82
ureterocele 56.89
urethra NEC 58.49
  laceration (by suture) 58.41
      obstetric (current) 75.61
      old 58.49
  meatus 58.47
urethrocele (anterior colporrhaphy) (female) 70.51
  and rectocele 70.50
urinary sphincter, artificial (component) 58.99
urinary stress incontinence - *see* Repair, stress incontinence
uterus, uterine 69.49
  inversion - *see* Repair, inverted uterus
  laceration (by suture) 69.41
      obstetric (current) 75.50
      old 69.49
  ligaments 69.29
      by
          interposition 69.21
          plication 69.22
uvula 27.73
  with synchronous cleft palate repair 27.62
vagina, vaginal (cuff) (wall) NEC 70.79
  anterior 70.51
      with posterior repair 70.50
  cystocele 70.51
      and rectocele 70.50

◀ **New**   ◀▥ **Revised**

ICD-9-CM
Vol. 3

Replacement *(Continued)*
  mechanical kidney 55.97
  mitral valve (with prosthesis) 35.24
    with tissue graft 35.23
  Mulligan hood, fallopian tube 66.93
  muscle stimulator (skeletal) 83.92
  nephrostomy tube 55.93
  neuropacemaker - *see* Implant, neuro-
    stimulator by site ◀▥
  neurostimulator - *see* Implant, neuro-
    stimulator, by site ◀▥
  skeletal muscle 83.92
  pacemaker
    brain - *see* Implant, neurostimulator,
      brain ◀▥
    cardiac device (initial) (permanent)
      resynchronization - *see* Replace-
        ment, CRT-P
      dual-chamber device 37.87
      single-chamber device 37.85
        rate responsive 37.86
    electrode(s), cardiac (atrial) (trans-
      venous) (ventricular) 37.76
      epicardium (myocardium) 37.74
      left ventricular coronary venous
        system 00.52
    intracranial - *see* Implant, neurosti-
      mulator, intracranial ◀▥
    neural - *see* Implant, neurostimula-
      tor, by site ◀▥
    peripheral nerve - *see* Implant, neu-
      rostimulator, peripheral nerve ◀
    sacral nerve - *see* Implant, neurosti-
      mulator, sacral nerve ◀
    spine - *see* Implant, neurostimulator,
      spine ◀▥
    temporary transvenous pacemaker
      system 37.78
  pack or bag
    nose 97.21
    teeth, tooth 97.22
    vagina 97.26
    vulva 97.26
    wound 97.16
  pessary, vagina NEC 97.25
  prosthesis
    acetabulum 81.53
    arm (bioelectric) (cineplastic) (kine-
      plastic) 84.44
    biliary tract 51.99
    cochlear 20.96
    channel (single) 20.97
      multiple 20.98
    elbow 81.97
    extremity (bioelectric) (cineplastic)
      (kineplastic) 84.40
      lower 84.48
      upper 84.44
    fallopian tube (Mulligan hood)
      (stent) 66.93
    femur 81.53
    knee 81.55
    leg (bioelectric) (cineplastic) (kine-
      plastic) 84.48
    penis (internal) (non-inflatable) 64.95
      inflatable (internal) 64.97
    pulmonary valve (with prosthesis) 35.26
      with tissue graft 35.25
      in total repair of tetralogy of Fallot
        35.81
    pyelostomy tube 55.94
    rectal tube 96.09
    shoulder NEC 81.83
      partial 81.81
      total 81.80

Replacement *(Continued)*
  skull
    plate 02.05
    tongs 02.94
  specified appliance or device NEC 97.29
  stent
    bile duct 97.05
    fallopian tube 66.93
    larynx 31.93
    pancreatic duct 97.05
    trachea 31.93
  stimoceiver - *see* Implant, stimoceiver,
    by site
  subdural
    grids 02.93
    strips 02.93
  testis in scrotum 62.5
  tongs, skull 02.94
  tracheal stent 31.93
  tricuspid valve (with prosthesis) 35.28
    with tissue graft 35.27
  tube
    bile duct 97.05
    bladder 57.95
    cystostomy 59.94
    esophagostomy 97.01
    gastrostomy 97.02
    large intestine 97.04
    nasogastric 97.01
    nephrostomy 55.93
    pancreatic duct 97.05
    pyelostomy 55.94
    rectal 96.09
    small intestine 97.03
    tracheostomy 97.23
    ureterostomy 59.93
    ventricular (cerebral) 02.42
  umbilical cord, prolapsed 73.92
  ureter (with)
    bladder flap 56.74
    ileal segment implanted into bladder
      56.89 [45.51]
  ureterostomy tube 59.93
  urethral sphincter, artificial 58.93
  urinary sphincter, artificial 58.93
  valve
    heart - *see also* Replacement, heart
      valve, poppet (prosthetic) 35.95
    ventricular (cerebral) 02.42
  ventricular shunt (catheter) (valve) 02.42
  Vinke tongs (skull) 02.94
  vitreous (silicone) 14.75
    for retinal reattachment 14.59
Replant, replantation - *see also* Reattachment
  extremity - *see* Reattachment, extremity
  penis 64.45
  scalp 86.51
  tooth 23.5
Reposition
  cardiac pacemaker
    electrode(s) (atrial) (transvenous)
      (ventricular) 37.75
    pocket 37.79
  cardioverter/defibrillator (automatic)
    lead(s) (sensing) (pacing) (epicardial
      patch) 37.99
    pocket 37.99
    pulse generator 37.99
  cilia base 08.71
  iris 12.39
  neurostimulator ◀
    leads ◀
      subcutaneous, without device re-
        placement 86.09 ◀

Reposition *(Continued)*
  neurostimulator *(Continued)*
    leads *(Continued)*
      within brain 02.93 ◀
      within or over peripheral nerve
        04.92 ◀
      within or over sacral nerve 04.92◀
      within spine 03.93 ◀
    pulse generator ◀
      subcutaneous, without device re-
        placement 86.09 ◀
  renal vessel, aberrant 39.55
  subcutaneous device pocket NEC
    86.09 ◀
  thyroid tissue 06.94
  tricuspid valve (with plication) 35.14
Resection - *see also* Excision, by site
  abdominoendorectal (combined) 48.5
  abdominoperineal (rectum) 48.5
    pull-through (Altemeier) (Swenson)
      NEC 48.49
      Duhamel type 48.65
  alveolar process and palate (en bloc) 27.32
  aneurysm - *see* Aneurysmectomy
  aortic valve (for subvalvular stenosis)
    35.11
  artery - *see* Arteriectomy
  bile duct NEC 51.69
    common duct NEC 51.63
  bladder (partial) (segmental) (transves-
    ical) (wedge) 57.6
    complete or total 57.79
    lesion NEC 57.59
      transurethral approach 57.49
    neck 57.59
      transurethral approach 57.49
  blood vessel - *see* Angiectomy
  brain 01.59
    by
      stereotactic radiosurgery 92.30
        cobalt 60 92.32
        linear accelerator (LINAC) 92.31
        multi-source 92.32
        particle beam 92.33
        particulate 92.33
        radiosurgery NEC 92.39
        single source photon 92.31
    hemisphere 01.52
    lobe 01.53
  breast - *see also* Mastectomy
    quadrant 85.22
    segmental 85.23
  broad ligament 69.19
  bronchus (sleeve) (wide sleeve) 32.1
    block (en bloc) (with radical dissec-
      tion of brachial plexus, bron-
      chus, lobe of lung, ribs, and
      sympathetic nerves) 32.6
  bursa 83.5
    hand 82.31
  cecum (and terminal ileum) 45.72
  cerebral meninges 01.51
  chest wall 34.4
  clavicle 77.81
  clitoris 71.4
  colon (partial) (segmental) 45.79
    ascending (cecum and terminal il-
      eum) 45.72
    cecum (and terminal ileum) 45.72
    complete 45.8
    descending (sigmoid) 45.76
    for interposition 45.52
    Hartmann 45.75
    hepatic flexure 45.73
    left radical (hemicolon) 45.75

◀ **New**   ◀▥ **Revised**

Resection *(Continued)*
  colon *(Continued)*
    multiple segmental 45.71
    right radical (hemicolon) (ileocolectomy) 45.73
    segmental NEC 45.79
      multiple 45.71
    sigmoid 45.76
    splenic flexure 45.75
    total 45.8
    transverse 45.74
  conjunctiva, for pterygium 11.39
    corneal graft 11.32
  cornual (fallopian tube) (unilateral) 66.69
    bilateral 66.63
  diaphragm 34.81
  endaural 20.79
  endorectal (pull-through) (Soave) 48.41
    combined abdominal 48.5
  esophagus (partial) (subtotal) - *see also* Esophagectomy 42.41
    total 42.42
  exteriorized intestine - *see* Resection, intestine, exteriorized
  fascia 83.44
    for graft 83.43
      hand 82.34
    hand 82.35
      for graft 82.34
  gallbladder (total) 51.22
  gastric (partial) (sleeve) (subtotal) NEC - *see also* Gastrectomy 43.89
    with anastomosis NEC 43.89
      esophagogastric 43.5
      gastroduodenal 43.6
      gastrogastric 43.89
      gastrojejunal 43.7
    complete or total NEC 43.99
      with intestinal interposition 43.91
    radical NEC 43.99
      with intestinal interposition 43.91
    wedge 43.42
      endoscopic 43.41
  hallux valgus (joint) - *see also* Bunionectomy with prosthetic implant 77.59
  hepatic
    duct 51.69
    flexure (colon) 45.73
  infundibula, heart (right) 35.34
  intestine (partial) NEC 45.79
    cecum (with terminal ileum) 45.72
    exteriorized (large intestine) 46.04
      small intestine 46.02
    for interposition 45.50
      large intestine 45.52
      small intestine 45.51
    hepatic flexure 45.73
    ileum 45.62
      with cecum 45.72
    large (partial) (segmental) NEC 45.79
      for interposition 45.52
      multiple segmental 45.71
      total 45.8
    left hemicolon 45.75
    multiple segmental (large intestine) 45.71
      small intestine 45.61
    right hemicolon 45.73
    segmental (large intestine) 45.79
      multiple 45.71
      small intestine 45.62
        multiple 45.61
    sigmoid 45.76

Resection *(Continued)*
  intestine (partial) NEC *(Continued)*
    small (partial) (segmental) NEC 45.62
      for interposition 45.51
      multiple segmental 45.61
      total 45.63
    total
      large intestine 45.8
      small intestine 45.63
  joint structure NEC - *see also* Arthrectomy 80.90
  kidney (segmental) (wedge) 55.4
  larynx - *see also* Laryngectomy
    submucous 30.29
  lesion - *see* Excision, lesion, by site
  levator palpebrae muscle 08.33
  ligament - *see also* Arthrectomy 80.90
    broad 69.19
    round 69.19
    uterine 69.19
  lip (wedge) 27.43
  liver (partial) (wedge) 50.22
    lobe (total) 50.3
    total 50.4
  lung (wedge) NEC 32.29
    endoscopic 32.28
    segmental (any part) 32.3
    volume reduction 32.22
  meninges (cerebral) 01.51
    spinal 03.4
  mesentery 54.4
  muscle 83.45
    extraocular 15.13
      with
        advancement or recession of other eye muscle 15.3
        suture of original insertion 15.13
      levator palpebrae 08.33
      Muller's, for blepharoptosis 08.35
      orbicularis oculi 08.20
      tarsal, for blepharoptosis 08.35
    for graft 83.43
      hand 82.34
    hand 82.36
      for graft 82.34
    ocular - *see* Resection, muscle, extraocular
  myocardium 37.33
  nasal septum (submucous) 21.5
  nerve (cranial) (peripheral) NEC 04.07
    phrenic 04.03
      for collapse of lung 33.31
    sympathetic 05.29
    vagus - *see* Vagotomy
  nose (complete) (extended) (partial) (radical) 21.4
  omentum 54.4
  orbitomaxillary, radical 16.51
  ovary - *see also* Oophorectomy
    wedge 65.22
      laparoscopic 65.24
  palate (bony) (local) 27.31
    by wide excision 27.32
    soft 27.49
  pancreas (total) (with synchronous duodenectomy) 52.6
    partial NEC 52.59
      distal (tail) (with part of body) 52.52
      proximal (head) (with part of body) (with synchronous duodenectomy) 52.51
      radical subtotal 52.53
    radical (one-stage) (two-stage) 52.7
      subtotal 52.53

Resection *(Continued)*
  pancreaticoduodenal - *see also* Pancreatectomy 52.6
  pelvic viscera (en masse) (female) 68.8
    male 57.71
  penis 64.3
  pericardium (partial) (for)
    chronic constrictive pericarditis 37.31
    drainage 37.12
    removal of adhesions 37.31
  peritoneum 54.4
  pharynx (partial) 29.33
  phrenic nerve 04.03
    for collapse of lung 33.31
  prostate - *see also* Prostatectomy
    transurethral (punch) 60.29
  pterygium 11.39
  radial head 77.83
  rectosigmoid - *see also* Resection, rectum 48.69
  rectum (partial) NEC 48.69
    with
      pelvic exenteration 68.8
      transsacral sigmoidectomy 48.61
    abdominoendorectal (combined) 48.5
    abdominoperineal 48.5
      pull-through NEC 48.49
        Duhamel type 48.65
    anterior 48.63
      with colostomy (synchronous) 48.62
    Duhamel 48.65
    endorectal 48.41
      combined abdominal 48.5
    posterior 48.64
    pull-through NEC 48.49
      endorectal 48.41
    submucosal (Soave) 48.41
      combined abdominal 48.5
  rib (transaxillary) 77.91
    as operative approach - *omit code*
    incidental to thoracic operation - *omit code*
  right ventricle (heart), for infundibular stenosis 35.34
  root (tooth) (apex) 23.73
    with root canal therapy 23.72
    residual or retained 23.11
  round ligament 69.19
  sclera 12.65
    with scleral buckling - *see also* Buckling, scleral 14.49
    lamellar (for retinal reattachment) 14.49
      with implant 14.41
  scrotum 61.3
  soft tissue NEC 83.49
    hand 82.39
  sphincter of Oddi 51.89
  spinal cord (meninges) 03.4
  splanchnic 05.29
  splenic flexure (colon) 45.75
  sternum 77.81
  stomach (partial) (sleeve) (subtotal) NEC - *see also* Gastrectomy 43.89
    with anastomosis NEC 43.89
      esophagogastric 43.5
      gastroduodenal 43.6
      gastrogastric 43.89
      gastrojejunal 43.7
    complete or total NEC 43.99
      with intestinal interposition 43.91
    fundus 43.89
    radical NEC 43.99
      with intestinal interposition 43.91
    wedge 43.42
      endoscopic 43.41

ICD-9-CM

Vol. 3

Resection (*Continued*)
submucous
  larynx 30.29
  nasal septum 21.5
  vocal cords 30.22
synovial membrane (complete) (partial) - *see also* Synovectomy 80.70
tarsoelevator 08.33
tendon 83.42
  hand 82.33
thoracic structures (block) (en bloc) (radical) (brachial plexus, bronchus, lobes of lung, ribs, and sympathetic nerves) 32.6
thorax 34.4
tongue 25.2
  wedge 25.1
tooth root 23.73
  with root canal therapy 23.72
  apex (abscess) 23.73
    with root canal therapy 23.72
  residual or retained 23.11
trachea 31.5
transurethral
  bladder NEC 57.49
  prostate 60.29
transverse colon 45.74
turbinates - *see* Turbinectomy
ureter (partial) 56.41
  total 56.42
uterus - *see* Hysterectomy
vein - *see* Phlebectomy
ventricle (heart) 37.35
  infundibula 35.34
vesical neck 57.59
  transurethral 57.49
vocal cords (punch) 30.22
Respirator, volume-controlled (Bennett) (Byrd) - *see* Ventilation
Restoration
cardioesophageal angle 44.66
  laparoscopic 44.67 ◀
dental NEC 23.49
  by
    application of crown (artificial) 23.41
    insertion of bridge (fixed) 23.42
      removable 23.43
extremity - *see* Reattachment, extremity
eyebrow 08.70
  with graft 08.63
eye socket 16.64
  with graft 16.63
tooth NEC 23.2
  by
    crown (artificial) 23.41
    filling (amalgam) (plastic) (silicate) 23.2
    inlay 23.3
Restrictive ◀
gastric band, laparoscopic 44.95 ◀
Resuscitation
artificial respiration 93.93
cardiac 99.60
  cardioversion 99.62
    atrial 99.61
  defibrillation 99.62
  external massage 99.63
    open chest 37.91
  intracardiac injection 37.92
cardiopulmonary 99.60
endotracheal intubation 96.04
manual 93.93
mouth-to-mouth 93.93
pulmonary 93.93

Resuture
abdominal wall 54.61
cardiac septum prosthesis 35.95
chest wall 34.71
heart valve prosthesis (poppet) 35.95
wound (skin and subcutaneous tissue) (without graft) NEC 86.59
Retavase, infusion 99.10
Reteplase, infusion 99.10
Retinaculotomy NEC - *see also* Division, ligament 80.40
carpal tunnel (flexor) 04.43
Retraining
cardiac 93.36
vocational 93.85
Retrogasserian neurotomy 04.02
Revascularization
cardiac (heart muscle) (myocardium) (direct) 36.10
  with
    bypass anastomosis
      abdominal artery to coronary artery 36.17
      aortocoronary (catheter stent) (homograft) (prosthesis) (saphenous vein graft) 36.10
      one coronary vessel 36.11
      two coronary vessels 36.12
      three coronary vessels 36.13
      four coronary vessels 36.14
      gastroepiploic artery to coronary artery 36.17
      internal mammary-coronary artery (single vessel) 36.15
      double vessel 36.16
      specified type NEC 36.19
      thoracic artery-coronary artery (single vessel) 36.15
      double vessel 36.16
    implantation of artery into heart (muscle) (myocardium) (ventricle) 36.2
  indirect 36.2
  specified type NEC 36.39
  transmyocardial
    open chest 36.31
    percutaneous 36.32
    specified type NEC 36.32
    thoracoscopic 36.32
Reversal, intestinal segment 45.50
large 45.52
small 45.51
Revision
amputation stump 84.3
  current traumatic - *see* Amputation
anastomosis
  biliary tract 51.94
  blood vessel 39.49
  gastric, gastrointestinal (with jejunal interposition) 44.5
  intestine (large) 46.94
    small 46.93
  pleurothecal 03.97
  pyelointestinal 56.72
  salpingothecal 03.97
  subarachnoid-peritoneal 03.97
  subarachnoid-ureteral 03.97
  ureterointestinal 56.72
ankle replacement (prosthesis) 81.59
anterior segment (eye) wound (operative) NEC 12.83
arteriovenous shunt (cannula) (for dialysis) 39.42
arthroplasty - *see* Arthroplasty

Revision (*Continued*)
bone flap, skull 02.06
breast implant 85.93
bronchostomy 33.42
bypass graft (vascular) 39.49
  abdominal - coronary artery 36.17
  aortocoronary (catheter stent) (with prosthesis) (with saphenous vein graft) (with vein graft) 36.10
  one coronary vessel 36.11
  two coronary vessels 36.12
  three coronary vessels 36.13
  four coronary vessels 36.14
  CABG - *see* Revision, aortocoronary bypass graft
  chest tube - *see* intercostal catheter
  coronary artery bypass graft (CABG) see Revision, aortocoronary bypass graft, abdominal - coronary artery bypass, and internal mammary - coronary artery bypass
  intercostal catheter (with lysis of adhesions) 34.04
  internal mammary - coronary artery (single) 36.15
  double vessel 36.16
cannula, vessel-to-vessel (arteriovenous) 39.94
canthus, lateral 08.59
cardiac pacemaker
  device (permanent) 37.89
  electrode(s) (atrial) (transvenous) (ventricular) 37.75
  pocket 37.79
cardiac resynchronization defibrillator (CRT-D) 37.99
cardiac resynchronization pacemaker (CRT-P)
  device (permanent) 37.89
  electrode(s) (atrial) (transvenous) (ventricular) 37.75
  pocket 37.79
cardioverter/defibrillator (automatic) pocket 37.99
cholecystostomy 51.99
cleft palate repair 27.63
colostomy 46.43
conduit, urinary 56.52
cystostomy (stoma) 57.22
disc - *see* Revision, intervertebral disc ◀
elbow replacement (prosthesis) 81.97
enterostomy (stoma) 46.40
  large intestine 46.43
  small intestine 46.41
enucleation socket 16.64
  with graft 16.63
esophagostomy 42.83
exenteration cavity 16.66
  with secondary graft 16.65
extraocular muscle surgery 15.6
fenestration, inner ear 20.62
filtering bleb 12.66
fixation device (broken) (displaced) - *see also* Fixation, bone, internal 78.50
flap or pedicle graft (skin) 86.75
foot replacement (prosthesis) 81.59
gastric anastomosis (with jejunal interposition) 44.5
gastric band, laparoscopic 44.96 ◀
gastric port device ◀
  laparoscopic 44.96 ◀
gastroduodenostomy (with jejunal interposition) 44.5

Revision *(Continued)*
  gastrointestinal anastomosis (with je-
    junal interposition) 44.5
  gastrojejunostomy 44.5
  gastrostomy 44.69
    laparoscopic 44.68 ◄
  hand replacement (prosthesis) 81.97
  heart procedure NEC 35.95
  hip replacement (acetabulum) (femoral
    head) (partial) (total) 81.53
  Holter (-Spitz) valve 02.42
  ileal conduit 56.52
  ileostomy 46.41
  intervertebral disc, artificial (partial)
    (total) NOS 84.69 ◄
    cervical 84.66 ◄
    lumbar, lumbosacral 84.68 ◄
    thoracic 84.67 ◄
  jejunoileal bypass 46.93
  jejunostomy 46.41
  joint replacement
    acetabulum 81.53
    ankle 81.59
    elbow 81.97
    femoral head 81.53
    foot 81.59
    hand 81.97
    hip (partial) (total) 81.53
    knee 81.55
    lower extremity NEC 81.59
    toe 81.59
    upper extremity 81.97
    wrist 81.97
  knee replacement (prosthesis) 81.55
  laryngostomy 31.63
  lateral canthus 08.59
  mallet finger 82.84
  mastoid antrum 19.9
  mastoidectomy 20.92
  nephrostomy 55.89
  neuroplasty 04.75
  ocular implant 16.62
  orbital implant 16.62
  pocket
    cardiac pacemaker
      with initial insertion of pacemaker
        - omit code
      new site (skin) (subcutaneous) 37.79
    subcutaneous device pocket NEC ◄
      with initial insertion of generator
        or device *- omit code* ◄
      new site 86.09 ◄
    thalamic stimulator pulse generator
      with initial insertion of battery
        package *- omit code*
      new site (skin) (subcutaneous)
        86.09
  previous mastectomy site *- see* catego-
    ries 85.0-85.99
  proctostomy 48.79
  prosthesis
    acetabulum
      hip 81.53
    ankle 81.59
    breast 85.93
    elbow 81.97
    femoral head 81.53
    foot 81.59
    hand 81.97
    heart valve (poppet) 35.95
    hip (partial) (total) 81.53
    knee 81.55
    lower extremity NEC 81.59

Revision *(Continued)*
  prosthesis *(Continued)*
    shoulder 81.97
    toe 81.59
    upper extremity 81.97
    wrist 81.97
  ptosis overcorrection 08.37
  pyelostomy 55.12
  pyloroplasty 44.29
  rhinoplasty 21.84
    scar
      skin 86.84
        with excision 86.3
  scleral fistulization 12.66
  shoulder replacement (prosthesis)
    81.97
  shunt
    arteriovenous (cannula) (for dialysis)
      39.42
    lumbar-subarachnoid NEC 03.97
    peritoneojugular 54.99
    peritoneovascular 54.99
    pleurothecal 03.97
    salpingothecal 03.97
    spinal (thecal) NEC 03.97
    subarachnoid-peritoneal 03.97
    subarachnoid-ureteral 03.97
    ventricular (cerebral) 02.42
    ventriculoperitoneal
      at peritoneal site 54.95
      at ventricular site 02.42
  stapedectomy NEC 19.29
    with incus replacement (homograft)
      (prosthesis) 19.21
  stoma
    bile duct 51.79
    bladder (vesicostomy) 57.22
    bronchus 33.42
    common duct 51.72
    esophagus 42.89
    gallbladder 51.99
    hepatic duct 51.79
    intestine 46.40
      large 46.43
      small 46.41
    kidney 55.89
    larynx 31.63
    rectum 48.79
    stomach 44.69
      laparoscopic 44.68 ◄
    thorax 34.79
    trachea 31.74
    ureter 56.62
    urethra 58.49
  tack operation 20.79
  toe replacement (prosthesis) 81.59
  tracheostomy 31.74
  tunnel
    pulse generator lead wire 86.99
      with initial procedure *- omit code*
  tympanoplasty 19.6
  uretero-ileostomy, cutaneous 56.52
  ureterostomy (cutaneous) (stoma) NEC
    56.62
    ileal 56.52
  urethrostomy 58.49
  urinary conduit 56.52
  vascular procedure (previous) NEC
    39.49
  ventricular shunt (cerebral) 02.42
  vesicostomy stoma 57.22
  wrist replacement (prosthesis) 81.97
Rhinectomy 21.4

Rhinocheiloplasty 27.59
  cleft lip 27.54
Rhinomanometry 89.12
Rhinoplasty (external) (internal) NEC
  21.87
  augmentation (with graft) (with syn-
    thetic implant) 21.85
  limited 21.86
  revision 21.84
  tip 21.86
  twisted nose 21.84
Rhinorrhaphy (external) (internal) 21.81
  for epistaxis 21.09
Rhinoscopy 21.21
Rhinoseptoplasty 21.84
Rhinotomy 21.1
Rhizotomy (radiofrequency) (spinal)
  03.1
  acoustic 04.01
  trigeminal 04.02
Rhytidectomy (facial) 86.82
  eyelid
    lower 08.86
    upper 08.87
Rhytidoplasty (facial) 86.82
Ripstein operation (repair of prolapsed
  rectum) 48.75
Rodney Smith operation (radical subtotal pancreatectomy) 52.53
Roentgenography - *see also* Radiography
  cardiac, negative contrast 88.58
Rolling of conjunctiva 10.33
Root
  canal (tooth) (therapy) 23.70
    with
      apicoectomy 23.72
      irrigation 23.71
  resection (tooth) (apex) 23.73
    with root canal therapy 23.72
    residual or retained 23.11
Rotation of fetal head
  forceps (instrumental) (Kielland) (Scan-
    zoni) (key-in-lock) 72.4
  manual 73.51
Routine
  chest x-ray 87.44
  psychiatric visit 94.12
Roux-en-Y operation
  bile duct 51.36
  cholecystojejunostomy 51.32
  esophagus (intrathoracic) 42.54
  gastroenterostomy 44.39
    laparoscopic 44.38 ◄
  gastrojejunostomy 44.39
    laparoscopic 44.38 ◄
  pancreaticojejunostomy 52.96
Roux-Goldthwait operation (repair of
  recurrent patellar dislocation)
  81.44
Roux-Herzen-Judine operation (jejunal
  loop interposition) 42.63
Rubin test (insufflation of fallopian tube)
  66.8
Ruiz-Mora operation (proximal phalangectomy for hammer toe) 77.99
Rupture
  esophageal web 42.01
  joint adhesions, manual 93.26
  membranes, artificial 73.09
    for surgical induction of labor 73.01
  ovarian cyst, manual 65.93
Russe operation (bone graft of scaphoid)
  78.04

ICD-9-CM

R

Vol. 3

S

Sacculotomy (tack) 20.79
Sacrectomy (partial) 77.89
  total 77.99
Saemisch operation (corneal section) 11.1
Salpingectomy (bilateral) (total) (transvaginal) 66.51
  with oophorectomy 65.61
    laparoscopic 65.63
  partial (unilateral) 66.69
    with removal of tubal pregnancy 66.62
    bilateral 66.63
      for sterilization 66.39
        by endoscopy 66.29
  remaining or solitary tube 66.52
    with ovary 65.62
      laparoscopic 65.64
  unilateral (total) 66.4
    with
      oophorectomy 65.49
        laparoscopic 65.41
      removal of tubal pregnancy 66.62
    partial 66.69
Salpingography 87.85
Salpingohysterostomy 66.74
Salpingo-oophorectomy (unilateral) 65.49
  that by laparoscope 65.41
  bilateral (same operative episode) 65.61
    laparoscopic 65.63
  remaining or solitary tube and ovary 65.62
    laparoscopic 65.64
Salpingo-oophoroplasty 65.73
  laparoscopic 65.76
Salpingo-oophororrhaphy 65.79
Salpingo-oophorostomy 66.72
Salpingo-oophorotomy 65.09
  laparoscopic 65.01
Salpingoplasty 66.79
Salpingorrhaphy 66.71
Salpingosalpingostomy 66.73
Salpingostomy (for removal of non-ruptured ectopic pregnancy) 66.02
Salpingotomy 66.01
Salpingo-uterostomy 66.74
Salter operation (innominate osteotomy) 77.39
Salvage (autologous blood) (intraoperative) (perioperative) (postoperative) 99.00
Sampling, blood for genetic determination of fetus 75.33
Sandpapering (skin) 86.25
Saucerization
  bone - see also Excision, lesion, bone 77.60
  rectum 48.99
Sauer-Bacon operation (abdominoperineal resection) 48.5
Scalenectomy 83.45
Scalenotomy 83.19
Scaling and polishing, dental 96.54
Scan, scanning
  C.A.T. (computerized axial tomography) 88.38
    with computer assisted surgery (CAS) 00.31
    abdomen 88.01

Scan, scanning (Continued)
  computerized axial tomography (C.A.T.) (Continued)
    bone 88.38
      mineral density 88.98
    brain 87.03
    head 87.03
    kidney 87.71
    skeletal 88.38
      mineral density 88.98
    thorax 87.41
  computerized axial tomography (C.A.T.) - see also Scan, C.A.T. 88.38
  C.T. - see Scan, C.A.T.
  gallium - see Scan, radioisotope
  liver 92.02
  MUGA (multiple gated acquisition) - see Scan, radioiostope
  positron emission tomography (PET) - see Scan, radioisotope
  radioisotope
    adrenal 92.09
    bone 92.14
      marrow 92.05
    bowel 92.04
    cardiac output 92.05
    cardiovascular 92.05
    cerebral 92.11
    circulation time 92.05
    eye 95.16
    gastrointestinal 92.04
    head NEC 92.12
    hematopoietic 92.05
    intestine 92.04
    iodine-131 92.01
    kidney 92.03
    liver 92.02
    lung 92.15
    lymphatic system 92.16
    myocardial infarction 92.05
    pancreatic 92.04
    parathyroid 92.13
    pituitary 92.11
    placenta 92.17
    protein-bound iodine 92.01
    pulmonary 92.15
    radio-iodine uptake 92.01
    renal 92.03
    specified site NEC 92.19
    spleen 92.05
    thyroid 92.01
    total body 92.18
    uterus 92.19
  renal 92.03
  thermal - see Thermography
Scapulectomy (partial) 77.81
  total 77.91
Scapulopexy 78.41
Scarification
  conjunctiva 10.33
  nasal veins (with packing) 21.03
  pericardium 36.39
  pleura 34.6
    chemical 34.92
      with cancer chemotherapy substance 34.92 [99.25]
      tetracycline 34.92 [99.21]
Schanz operation (femoral osteotomy) 77.35
Schauta (-Amreich) operation (radical vaginal hysterectomy) 68.7
Schede operation (thoracoplasty) 33.34
Scheie operation
  cautery of sclera 12.62
  sclerostomy 12.62

Schlatter operation (total gastrectomy) 43.99
Schroeder operation (endocervical excision) 67.39
Schuchardt operation (nonobstetrical episiotomy) 71.09
Schwartze operation (simple mastoidectomy) 20.41
Scintiphotography - see Scan, radioisotope
Scintiscan - see Scan, radioisotope
Sclerectomy (punch) (scissors) 12.65
  for retinal reattachment 14.49
  Holth's 12.65
  trephine 12.61
    with implant 14.41
Scleroplasty 12.89
Sclerosis - see Sclerotherapy
Sclerostomy (Scheie's) 12.62
Sclerotherapy
  esophageal varices (endoscopic) 42.33
  hemorrhoids 49.42
  pleura 34.92
    treatment of malignancy (cytotoxic agent) 34.92 [99.25]
      with tetracycline 34.92 [99.21]
  varicose vein 39.92
  vein NEC 39.92
Sclerotomy (exploratory) 12.89
  anterior 12.89
    with
      iridectomy 12.65
      removal of vitreous 14.71
  posterior 12.89
    with
      iridectomy 12.65
      removal of vitreous 14.72
Scott operation
  intestinal bypass for obesity 45.93
  jejunocolostomy (bypass) 45.93
Scraping
  corneal epithelium 11.41
    for smear or culture 11.21
  trachoma follicles 10.33
Scrotectomy (partial) 61.3
Scrotoplasty 61.49
Scrotorrhaphy 61.41
Scrototomy 61.0
Scrub, posterior nasal (adhesions) 21.91
Sculpturing, heart valve - see Valvuloplasty, heart
Section - see also Division and Incision
  cesarean - see Cesarean section
  ganglion, sympathetic 05.0
  hypophyseal stalk - see also Hypophysectomy, partial 07.63
  ligamentum flavum (spine) - omit code
  nerve (cranial) (peripheral) NEC 04.03
    acoustic 04.01
    spinal root (posterior) 03.1
    sympathetic 05.0
    trigeminal tract 04.02
  Saemisch (corneal) 11.1
  spinal ligament 80.49
    arcuate - omit code
    flavum - omit code
  tooth (impacted) 23.19
Seddon-Brooks operation (transfer of pectoralis major tendon) 83.75
Semb operation (apicolysis of lung) 33.39
Senning operation (correction of transposition of great vessels) 35.91
Separation
  twins (attached) (conjoined) (Siamese) 84.93
    asymmetrical (unequal) 84.93
    symmetrical (equal) 84.92

Septectomy
 atrial (closed) 35.41
  open 35.42
  transvenous method (balloon) 35.41
 submucous (nasal) 21.5
Septoplasty NEC 21.88
 with submucous resection of septum
  21.5
Septorhinoplasty 21.84
Septostomy (atrial) (balloon) 35.41
Septotomy, nasal 21.1
Sequestrectomy
 bone 77.00
  carpals, metacarpals 77.04
  clavicle 77.01
  facial 76.01
  femur 77.05
  fibula 77.07
  humerus 77.02
  nose 21.32
  patella 77.06
  pelvic 77.09
  phalanges (foot) (hand) 77.09
  radius 77.03
  scapula 77.01
  skull 01.25
  specified site NEC 77.09
  tarsals, metatarsals 77.08
  thorax (ribs) (sternum) 77.01
  tibia 77.07
  ulna 77.03
  vertebrae 77.09
 nose 21.32
 skull 01.25
Sesamoidectomy 77.98
Setback, ear 18.5
Sever operation (division of soft tissue
  of arm) 83.19
Severing of blepharorrhaphy 08.02
Sewell operation (heart) 36.2
Sharrard operation (iliopsoas muscle
  transfer) 83.77
Shaving
 bone - *see also* Excision, lesion, bone
  77.60
 cornea (epithelium) 11.41
  for smear or culture 11.21
 patella 77.66
Shelf operation (hip arthroplasty) 81.40
Shirodkar operation (encirclement suture, cervix) 67.59
Shock therapy
 chemical 94.24
 electroconvulsive 94.27
 electrotonic 94.27
 insulin 94.24
 subconvulsive 94.26
Shortening
 bone (fusion) 78.20
  femur 78.25
  specified site NEC - *see* category 78.2
  tibia 78.27
  ulna 78.23
 endopelvic fascia 69.22
 extraocular muscle NEC 15.22
  multiple (two or more muscles) 15.4
 eyelid margin 08.71
 eye muscle NEC 15.22
  multiple (two or more muscles)
   (with lengthening) 15.4
 finger (macrodactyly repair) 82.83
 heel cord 83.85
 levator palpebrae muscle 08.33
 ligament - *see also* Arthroplasty

Shortening (Continued)
 ligament (Continued)
  round 69.22
  uterosacral 69.22
 muscle 83.85
  extraocular 15.22
   multiple (two or more muscles)
    15.4
  hand 82.55
 sclera (for repair of retinal detachment) 14.59
  by scleral buckling - *see also* Buckling, scleral 14.49
 tendon 83.85
  hand 82.55
 ureter (with reimplantation) 56.41
Shunt - *see also* Anastomosis and Bypass,
  vascular
 abdominovenous 54.94
 aorta-coronary sinus 36.39
 aorta (descending)-pulmonary (artery)
  39.0
 aortocarotid 39.22
 aortoceliac 39.26
 aortofemoral 39.25
 aortoiliac 39.25
 aortoiliofemoral 39.25
 aortomesenteric 39.26
 aorto-myocardial (graft) 36.2
 aortorenal 39.24
 aortosubclavian 39.22
 apicoaortic 35.93
 arteriovenous NEC 39.29
  for renal dialysis (by)
   anastomosis 39.27
   external cannula 39.93
 ascending aorta to pulmonary artery
  (Waterston) 39.0
 axillary-femoral 39.29
 carotid-carotid 39.22
 carotid-subclavian 39.22
 caval-mesenteric 39.1
 corpora cavernosa-corpus spongiosum
  64.98
 corpora-saphenous 64.98
 descending aorta to pulmonary artery
  (Potts-Smith) 39.0
 endolymphatic (-subarachnoid) 20.71
 endolymph-perilymph 20.71
 extracranial-intracranial (EC-IC) 39.28
 femoroperoneal 39.29
 femoropopliteal 39.29
 iliofemoral 39.25
 ilioiliac 39.25
 intestinal
  large-to-large 45.94
  small-to-large 45.93
  small-to-small 45.91
 left subclavian to descending aorta
  (Blalock-Park) 39.0
 left-to-right (systemic-pulmonary artery) 39.0
 left ventricle (heart) (apex) and aorta
  35.93
 lienorenal 39.1
 lumbar-subarachnoid (with valve)
  NEC 03.79
 mesocaval 39.1
 peritoneal-jugular 54.94
 peritoneo-vascular 54.94
 peritoneovenous 54.94
 pleuroperitoneal 34.05
 pleurothecal (with valve) 03.79
 portacaval (double) 39.1

Shunt (Continued)
 portal-systemic 39.1
 portal vein to vena cava 39.1
 pulmonary-innominate 39.0
 pulmonary vein to atrium 35.82
 renoportal 39.1
 right atrium and pulmonary artery
  35.94
 right ventricle and pulmonary artery
  (distal) 35.92
  in repair of
   pulmonary artery atresia 35.92
   transposition of great vessels 35.92
   truncus arteriosus 35.83
 salpingothecal (with valve) 03.79
 semicircular subarachnoid 20.71
 spinal (thecal) (with valve) NEC 03.79
  subarachnoid-peritoneal 03.71
  subarachnoid-ureteral 03.72
 splenorenal (venous) 39.1
  arterial 39.26
 subarachnoid-peritoneal (with valve)
  03.71
 subarachnoid-ureteral (with valve) 03.72
 subclavian-pulmonary 39.0
 subdural-peritoneal (with valve) 02.34
 superior mesenteric-caval 39.1
 systemic-pulmonary artery 39.0
 transjugular intrahepatic portosystemic
  [TIPS] 39.1
 vena cava to pulmonary artery (Green)
  39.21
 ventricular (cerebral) (with valve) 02.2
  to
   abdominal cavity or organ 02.34
   bone marrow 02.39
   cervical subarachnoid space 02.2
   circulatory system 02.32
   cisterna magna 02.2
   extracranial site NEC 02.39
   gallbladder 02.34
   head or neck structure 02.31
   intracerebral site NEC 02.2
   lumbar site 02.39
   mastoid 02.31
   nasopharynx 02.31
   thoracic cavity 02.33
   ureter 02.35
   urinary system 02.35
   venous system 02.32
 ventriculoatrial (with valve) 02.32
 ventriculocaval (with valve) 02.32
 ventriculocisternal (with valve) 02.2
 ventriculolumbar (with valve) 02.39
 ventriculomastoid (with valve) 02.31
 ventriculonasopharyngeal 02.31
 ventriculopleural (with valve) 02.33
Sialoadenectomy (parotid) (sublingual)
  (submaxillary) 26.30
 complete 26.32
 partial 26.31
 radical 26.32
Sialoadenolithotomy 26.0
Sialoadenotomy 26.0
Sialodochoplasty NEC 26.49
Sialogram 87.09
Sialolithotomy 26.0
Sieve, vena cava 38.7
Sigmoid bladder 57.87 [45.52]
Sigmoidectomy 45.76
Sigmoidomyotomy 46.91
Sigmoidopexy (Moschowitz) 46.63
Sigmoidoproctectomy - *see also* Resec-
  tion, rectum 48.69

ICD-9-CM

S

Vol. 3

Sigmoidoproctostomy 45.94
Sigmoidorectostomy 45.94
Sigmoidorrhaphy 46.75
Sigmoidoscopy (rigid) 48.23
    with biopsy 45.25
    flexible 45.24
    through stoma (artificial) 45.22
    transabdominal 45.21
Sigmoidosigmoidostomy 45.94
    proximal to distal segment 45.76
Sigmoidostomy - see also Colostomy 46.10
Sigmoidotomy 45.03
Sign language 93.75
Silver operation (bunionectomy) 77.59
Sinogram
    abdominal wall 88.03
    chest wall 87.38
    retroperitoneum 88.14
Sinusectomy (nasal) (complete) (partial)
        (with turbinectomy) 22.60
    antrum 22.62
        with Caldwell-Luc approach 22.61
    ethmoid 22.63
    frontal 22.42
    maxillary 22.62
        with Caldwell-Luc approach 22.61
    sphenoid 22.64
Sinusotomy (nasal) 22.50
    antrum (intranasal) 22.2
        with external approach (Caldwell-
            Luc) 22.39
            radical (with removal of mem-
                brane lining) 22.31
    ethmoid 22.51
    frontal 22.41
    maxillary (intranasal) 22.2
        external approach (Caldwell-Luc)
            22.39
            radical (with removal of mem-
                brane lining) 22.31
    multiple 22.53
    perinasal 22.50
    sphenoid 22.52
Sistrunk operation (excision of thyro-
        glossal cyst) 06.7
Size reduction
    abdominal wall (adipose) (pendulous)
        86.83
    arms (adipose) (batwing) 86.83
    breast (bilateral) 85.32
        unilateral 85.31
    buttocks (adipose) 86.83
    skin 86.83
    subcutaneous tissue 86.83
    thighs (adipose) 86.83
Skeletal series (x-ray) 88.31
Sling - see also Operation, sling
    fascial (fascia lata)
        for facial weakness (trigeminal nerve
            paralysis) 86.81
        mouth 86.81
        orbicularis (mouth) 86.81
        tongue 25.59
    levator muscle (urethrocystopexy)
        59.71
    pubococcygeal 59.71
    rectum (puborectalis) 48.76
    tongue (fascial) 25.59
Slitting
    canaliculus for
        passage of tube 09.42
        removal of streptothrix 09.42
    lens 13.2
    prepuce (dorsal) (lateral) 64.91

Slocum operation (pes anserinus trans-
    fer) 81.47
Sluder operation (tonsillectomy) 28.2
Small bowel series (x-ray) 87.63
Smith operation (open osteotomy of
    mandible) 76.62
Smith-Peterson operation (radiocarpal
    arthrodesis) 81.25
Smithwick operation (sympathectomy)
    05.29
Snaring, polyp, colon (endoscopic) 45.42
Snip, punctum (with dilation) 09.51
Soave operation (endorectal pull-
    through) 48.41
Somatotherapy, psychiatric NEC 94.29
Sonneberg operation (inferior maxillary
    neurectomy) 04.07
Sorondo-Ferré operation (hindquarter
    amputation) 84.19
Soutter operation (iliac crest fasciotomy)
    83.14
Spaulding-Richardson operation (uter-
    ine suspension) 69.22
Spectrophotometry NEC 89.39
    blood 89.39
    placenta 89.29
    urine 89.29
Speech therapy NEC 93.75
Spermatocelectomy 63.2
Spermatocystectomy 60.73
Spermatocystotomy 60.72
Sphenoidectomy 22.64
Sphenoidotomy 22.52
Sphincterectomy, anal 49.6
Sphincteroplasty
    anal 49.79
        obstetrical laceration (current) 75.62
        old 49.79
    bladder neck 57.85
    pancreas 51.83
    sphincter of Oddi 51.83
Sphincterorrhaphy, anal 49.71
    obstetrical laceration (current) 75.62
    old 49.79
Sphincterotomy
    anal (external) (internal) 49.59
        left lateral 49.51
        posterior 49.52
    bladder (neck) (transurethral) 57.91
    choledochal 51.82
        endoscopic 51.85
    iris 12.12
    pancreatic 51.82
        endoscopic 51.85
    sphincter of Oddi 51.82
        endoscopic 51.85
    transduodenal ampullary 51.82
        endoscopic 51.85
Spinal anesthesia - omit code
Spinelli operation (correction of inverted
    uterus) 75.93
Spirometry (incentive) (respiratory) 89.37
Spivack operation (permanent gastros-
    tomy) 43.19
Splanchnicectomy 05.29
Splanchnicotomy 05.0
Splenectomy (complete) (total) 41.5
    partial 41.43
Splenogram 88.64
    radioisotope 92.05
Splenolysis 54.59
    laparoscopic 54.51
Splenopexy 41.95
Splenoplasty 41.95

Splenoportogram (by splenic arteriogra-
    phy) 88.64
Splenorrhaphy 41.95
Splenotomy 41.2
Splinting
    dental (for immobilization) 93.55
        orthodontic 24.7
    musculoskeletal 93.54
    ureteral 56.2
Splitting - see also Division
    canaliculus 09.52
    lacrimal papilla 09.51
    spinal cord tracts 03.29
        percutaneous 03.21
    tendon sheath 83.01
        hand 82.01
Spondylosyndesis - see also Fusion, spi-
    nal 81.00
S.P. Rogers operation (knee disarticula-
    tion) 84.16
Ssabanejew-Frank operation (permanent
    gastrostomy) 43.19
Stab, intercostal 34.09
Stabilization, joint - see also Arthrodesis
    patella (for recurrent dislocation) 81.44
Stacke operation (simple mastoidec-
    tomy) 20.41
Stallard operation (conjunctivocystorhi-
    nostomy) 09.82
    with insertion of tube or stent 09.83
Stamm (-Kader) operation (temporary
    gastrostomy) 43.19
Stapedectomy 19.19
    with incus replacement (homograft)
        (prosthesis) 19.11
    revision 19.29
        with incus replacement 19.21
Stapediolysis 19.0
Stapling
    artery 39.31
    blebs, lung (emphysematous) 32.21
    diaphysis - see also Stapling, epiphyseal
        plate 78.20
    epiphyseal plate 78.20
        femur 78.25
        fibula 78.27
        humerus 78.22
        radius 78.23
        specified site NEC 78.29
        tibia 78.27
        ulna 78.23
    gastric varices 44.91
    graft - see Graft
    vein 39.32
Steinberg operation 44.5
Steindler operation
    fascia stripping (for cavus deformity)
        83.14
    flexorplasty (elbow) 83.77
    muscle transfer 83.77
Stereotactic head frame application
    93.59
Stereotactic radiosurgery 92.30
    cobalt 60 92.32
    linear accelerator (LINAC) 92.31
    multi-source 92.32
    particle beam 92.33
    particulate 92.33
    radiosurgery NEC 92.39
    single source photon 92.31
Sterilization
    female - see also specific operation 66.39
    male NEC - see also Ligation, vas def-
        erens 63.70

Sternotomy 77.31
    as operative approach - *omit code*
    for bone marrow biopsy 41.31
Stewart operation (renal plication with
    pyeloplasty) 55.87
Stimulation (electronic) - *see also* Implant, electronic stimulator
    bone growth (percutaneous) - see category 78.9
        transcutaneous (surface) 99.86
    cardiac (external) 99.62
        internal 37.91
    carotid sinus 99.64
    defibrillator
        non-invasive programmed electrical
            stimulation (NIPS) 37.26
    electrophysiologic, cardiac 37.26
    nerve, peripheral or spinal cord, transcutaneous 93.39
Stitch, Kelly-Stoeckel (urethra) 59.3
Stomatoplasty 27.59
Stomatorrhaphy 27.52
Stone operation (anoplasty) 49.79
Strassman operation (metroplasty) 69.49
Strayer operation (gastrocnemius recession) 83.72
Stretching
    eyelid (with elongation) 08.71
    fascia 93.28
    foreskin 99.95
    iris 12.63
    muscle 93.27
    nerve (cranial) (peripheral) 04.91
    tendon 93.27
Stripping
    bone - *see also* Incision, bone 77.10
    carotid sinus 39.8
    cranial suture 02.01
    fascia 83.14
        hand 82.12
    membranes for surgical induction of
        labor 73.1
    meninges (cerebral) 01.51
        spinal 03.4
    saphenous vein, varicose 38.59
    subdural membrane (cerebral) 01.51
        spinal 03.4
    varicose veins (lower limb) 38.59
        upper limb 38.53
    vocal cords 30.09
Stromeyer-Little operation (hepatotomy)
    50.0
Strong operation (unbridling of celiac artery axis) 39.91
Stryker frame 93.59
Study
    bone mineral density 88.98
    bundle of His 37.29
    color vision 95.06
    conduction, nerve (median) 89.15
    dark adaptation, eye 95.07
    electrophysiologic stimulation and recording, cardiac 37.26
    function - *see also* Function, study
        radioisotope - see Scan, radioisotope
    lacrimal flow (radiographic) 87.05
    ocular motility 95.15
    pulmonary function - see categories
        89.37-89.38
    radiographic - see Radiography
    radio-iodinated triolein 92.04
    renal clearance 92.03
    spirometer 89.37
    tracer - *see also* Scan, radioisotope, eye
        (P32) 95.16

Study (Continued)
    ultrasonic - see Ultrasonography
    visual field 95.05
    xenon flow NEC 92.19
        cardiovascular 92.05
        pulmonary 92.15
Sturmdorf operation (conization of cervix) 67.2
Submucous resection
    larynx 30.29
    nasal septum 21.5
Summerskill operation (dacryocystorhinostomy by intubation) 09.81
Surgery ◀
    computer assisted (CAS) 00.39 ◀
        CAS with CT/CTA 00.31 ◀
        CAS with fluoroscopy 00.33 ◀
        CAS with MR/MRA 00.32 ◀
        CAS with multiple datasets 00.35 ◀
            imageless 00.34 ◀
        other CAS 00.39 ◀
    IGS - *see* Surgery, computer
        assisted ◀
    image guided - *see* Surgery, computer assisted ◀
    navigation (CT-free, IGN image
        guided, imageless) - *see* Surgery,
        computer assisted ◀
Surmay operation (jejunostomy) 46.39
Suspension
    balanced, for traction 93.45
    bladder NEC 57.89
    diverticulum, pharynx 29.59
    kidney 55.7
    Olshausen (uterus) 69.22
    ovary 65.79
    paraurethral (Pereyra) 59.6
    periurethral 59.6
    urethra (retropubic) (sling) 59.5
    urethrovesical
        Goebel-Frangenheim-Stoeckel 59.4
        gracilis muscle transplant 59.71
        levator muscle sling 59.71
        Marshall-Marchetti (-Krantz) 59.5
        Millin-Read 59.4
        suprapubic 59.4
    uterus (abdominal or vaginal approach) 69.22
    vagina 70.77
Suture (laceration)
    abdominal wall 54.63
        secondary 54.61
    adenoid fossa 28.7
    adrenal (gland) 07.44
    aneurysm (cerebral) (peripheral) 39.52
    anus 49.71
        obstetric laceration (current) 75.62
        old 49.79
    aorta 39.31
    aponeurosis - *see also* Suture, tendon
        83.64
    arteriovenous fistula 39.53
    artery 39.31
        percutaneous puncture closure - *omit code*
    bile duct 51.79
    bladder 57.81
        obstetric laceration (current) 75.61
    blood vessel NEC 39.30
        artery 39.31
            percutaneous puncture closure -
                omit code
        vein 39.32
    breast (skin) 85.81
    bronchus 33.41

Suture (Continued)
    bursa 83.99
        hand 82.99
    canaliculus 09.73
    cecum 46.75
    cerebral meninges 02.11
    cervix (traumatic laceration) 67.61
        internal os, encirclement 67.59
        obstetric laceration (current) 75.51
            old 67.69
    chest wall 34.71
    cleft palate 27.62
    clitoris 71.4
    colon 46.75
    common duct 51.71
    conjunctiva 10.6
    cornea 11.51
        with conjunctival flap 11.53
    corneoscleral 11.51
        with conjunctival flap 11.53
    diaphragm 34.82
    duodenum 46.71
        ulcer (bleeding) (perforated) 44.42
            endoscopic 44.43
    dura mater (cerebral) 02.11
        spinal 03.59
    ear, external 18.4
    enterocele 70.92
    entropion 08.42
    epididymis (and)
        spermatic cord 63.51
        vas deferens 63.81
    episiotomy - see Episiotomy
    esophagus 42.82
    eyeball 16.89
    eyebrow 08.81
    eyelid 08.81
        with entropion or ectropion repair
            08.42
    fallopian tube 66.71
    fascia 83.65
        hand 82.46
        to skeletal attachment 83.89
            hand 82.89
    gallbladder 51.91
    ganglion, sympathetic 05.81
    gingiva 24.32
    great vessel 39.30
        artery 39.31
        vein 39.32
    gum 24.32
    heart 37.4
    hepatic duct 51.79
    hymen 70.76
    ileum 46.73
    intestine 46.79
        large 46.75
        small 46.73
    jejunum 46.73
    joint capsule 81.96
        with arthroplasty - see Arthroplasty
            ankle 81.94
            foot 81.94
            lower extremity NEC 81.95
            upper extremity 81.93
    kidney 55.81
    labia 71.71
    laceration - see Suture, by site
    larynx 31.61
    ligament 81.96
        with arthroplasty - see Arthroplasty
            ankle 81.94
            broad 69.29
            Cooper's 54.64
            foot and toes 81.94

ICD-9-CM

S

Vol.

Suture *(Continued)*
  ligament *(Continued)*
    gastrocolic 54.73
    knee 81.95
    lower extremity NEC 81.95
    sacrouterine 69.29
    upper extremity 81.93
    uterine 69.29
  ligation - see Ligation
  lip 27.51
  liver 50.61
  lung 33.43
  meninges (cerebral) 02.11
    spinal 03.59
  mesentery 54.75
  mouth 27.52
  muscle 83.65
    hand 82.46
    ocular (oblique) (rectus) 15.7
  nerve (cranial) (peripheral) 04.3
    sympathetic 05.81
  nose (external) (internal) 21.81
    for epistaxis 21.09
  obstetric laceration NEC 75.69
    bladder 75.61
    cervix 75.51
    corpus uteri 75.52
    pelvic floor 75.69
    perineum 75.69
    rectum 75.62
    sphincter ani 75.62
    urethra 75.61
    uterus 75.50
    vagina 75.69
    vulva 75.69
  omentum 54.64
  ovary 65.71
    laparoscopic 65.74
  palate 27.61
    cleft 27.62
  palpebral fissure 08.59
  pancreas 52.95
  pelvic floor 71.71
    obstetric laceration (current) 75.69
  penis 64.41
  peptic ulcer (bleeding) (perforated) 44.40
  pericardium 37.4
  perineum (female) 71.71
    after delivery 75.69
      episiotomy repair - see Episiotomy
    male 86.59
  periosteum 78.20
    carpal, metacarpal 78.24
    femur 78.25
    fibula 78.27
    humerus 78.22
    pelvic 78.29
    phalanges (foot) (hand) 78.29
    radius 78.23
    specified site NEC 78.29
    tarsal, metatarsal 78.28
    tibia 78.27
    ulna 78.23
    vertebrae 78.29
  peritoneum 54.64
  periurethral tissue to symphysis pubis 59.5
  pharynx 29.51
  pleura 34.93
  rectum 48.71
    obstetric laceration (current) 75.62
  retina (for reattachment) 14.59
  sacrouterine ligament 69.29

Suture *(Continued)*
  salivary gland 26.41
  scalp 86.59
    replantation 86.51
  sclera (with repair of conjunctiva) 12.81
  scrotum (skin) 61.41
  secondary
    abdominal wall 54.61
    episiotomy 75.69
    peritoneum 54.64
  sigmoid 46.75
  skin (mucous membrane) (without graft) 86.59
    with graft - see Graft, skin
    breast 85.81
    ear 18.4
    eyebrow 08.81
    eyelid 08.81
    nose 21.81
    penis 64.41
    scalp 86.59
      replantation 86.51
    scrotum 61.41
    vulva 71.71
  specified site NEC - see Repair, by site
  spermatic cord 63.51
  sphincter ani 49.71
    obstetric laceration (current) 75.62
    old 49.79
  spinal meninges 03.59
  spleen 41.95
  stomach 44.61
    ulcer (bleeding) (perforated) 44.41
      endoscopic 44.43
  subcutaneous tissue (without skin graft) 86.59
    with graft - see Graft, skin
  tendon (direct) (immediate) (primary) 83.64
    delayed (secondary) 83.62
      hand NEC 82.43
        flexors 82.42
    hand NEC 82.45
      delayed (secondary) 82.43
      flexors 82.44
        delayed (secondary) 82.42
    ocular 15.7
    rotator cuff 83.63
    sheath 83.61
      hand 82.41
    supraspinatus (rotator cuff repair) 83.63
    to skeletal attachment 83.88
      hand 82.85
  Tenon's capsule 15.7
  testis 62.61
  thymus 07.93
  thyroid gland 06.93
  tongue 25.51
  tonsillar fossa 28.7
  trachea 31.71
  tunica vaginalis 61.41
  ulcer (bleeding) (perforated) (peptic) 44.40
    duodenum 44.42
      endoscopic 44.43
    gastric 44.41
      endoscopic 44.43
    intestine 46.79
    skin 86.59
    stomach 44.41
      endoscopic 44.43
  ureter 56.82

Suture *(Continued)*
  urethra 58.41
    obstetric laceration (current) 75.61
  uterosacral ligament 69.29
  uterus 69.41
    obstetric laceration (current) 75.50
    old 69.49
  uvula 27.73
  vagina 70.71
    obstetric laceration (current) 75.69
    old 70.79
  vas deferens 63.81
  vein 39.32
  vulva 71.71
    obstetric laceration (current) 75.69
    old 71.79
Suture-ligation - *see also* Ligation
  blood vessel - see Ligation, blood vessel
Sweep, anterior iris 12.97
Swenson operation
  bladder reconstruction 57.87
  proctectomy 48.49
Swinney operation (urethral reconstruction) 58.46
Switch, switching
  coronary arteries 35.84
  great arteries, total 35.84
Syme operation
  ankle amputation through malleoli of tibia and fibula 84.14
  urethrotomy, external 58.0
Sympathectomy NEC 05.29
  cervical 05.22
  cervicothoracic 05.22
  lumbar 05.23
  periarterial 05.25
  presacral 05.24
  renal 05.29
  thoracolumbar 05.23
  tympanum 20.91
Sympatheticotripsy 05.0
Symphysiotomy 77.39
  assisting delivery (obstetrical) 73.94
  kidney (horseshoe) 55.85
Symphysis, pleural 34.6
Synchondrotomy - *see also* Division, cartilage 80.40
Syndactylization 86.89
Syndesmotomy - *see also* Division, ligament 80.40
Synechiotomy
  endometrium 68.21
  iris (posterior) 12.33
    anterior 12.32
Synovectomy (joint) (complete) (partial) 80.70
  ankle 80.77
  elbow 80.72
  foot and toe 80.78
  hand and finger 80.74
  hip 80.75
  knee 80.76
  shoulder 80.71
  specified site NEC 80.79
  spine 80.79
  tendon sheath 83.42
    hand 82.33
  wrist 80.73
Syringing
  lacrimal duct or sac 09.43
  nasolacrimal duct 09.43
    with
      dilation 09.43
      insertion of tube or stent 09.44

T

Taarnhoj operation (trigeminal nerve root decompression) 04.41
Tack operation (sacculotomy) 20.79
Take-down
  anastomosis
    arterial 39.49
    blood vessel 39.49
    gastric, gastrointestinal 44.5
    intestine 46.93
    stomach 44.5
    vascular 39.49
    ventricular 02.43
  arterial bypass 39.49
  arteriovenous shunt 39.43
    with creation of new shunt 39.42
  cecostomy 46.52
  colostomy 46.52
  duodenostomy 46.51
  enterostomy 46.50
  esophagostomy 42.83
  gastroduodenostomy 44.5
  gastrojejunostomy 44.5
  ileostomy 46.51
  intestinal stoma 46.50
    large 46.52
    small 46.51
  jejunoileal bypass 46.93
  jejunostomy 46.51
  laryngostomy 31.62
  sigmoidostomy 46.52
  stoma
    bile duct 51.79
    bladder 57.82
    bronchus 33.42
    common duct 51.72
    esophagus 42.83
    gallbladder 51.92
    hepatic duct 51.79
    intestine 46.50
      large 46.52
      small 46.51
    kidney 55.82
    larynx 31.62
    rectum 48.72
    stomach 44.62
    thorax 34.72
    trachea 31.72
    ureter 56.83
    urethra 58.42
  systemic-pulmonary artery anastomosis 39.49
    in total repair of tetralogy of Fallot 35.81
  tracheostomy 31.72
  vascular anastomosis or bypass 39.49
  ventricular shunt (cerebral) 02.43
Talectomy 77.98
Talma-Morison operation (omentopexy) 54.74
Tamponade
  esophageal 96.06
  intrauterine (nonobstetric) 69.91
    after delivery or abortion 75.8
    antepartum 73.1
  vagina 96.14
    after delivery or abortion 75.8
    antepartum 73.1
Tanner operation (devascularization of stomach) 44.99
Tap
  abdomen 54.91

Tap (Continued)
  chest 34.91
  cisternal 01.01
  cranial 01.09
  joint 81.91
  lumbar (diagnostic) (removal of dye) 03.31
  perilymphatic 20.79
  spinal (diagnostic) 03.31
  subdural (through fontanel) 01.09
  thorax 34.91
Tarsectomy 08.20
  de Grandmont 08.35
Tarsoplasty - see also Reconstruction, eyelid 08.70
Tarsorrhaphy (lateral) 08.52
  division or severing 08.02
Tattooing
  cornea 11.91
  skin 86.02
Tautening, eyelid for entropion 08.42
Telemetry (cardiac) 89.54
Teleradiotherapy
  beta particles 92.25
  Betatron 92.24
  cobalt-60 92.23
  electrons 92.25
  iodine-125 92.23
  linear accelerator 92.24
  neutrons 92.26
  particulate radiation NEC 92.26
  photons 92.24
  protons 92.26
  radioactive cesium 92.23
  radioisotopes NEC 92.23
Temperament assessment 94.02
Temperature gradient study - see also Thermography 88.89
Tendinoplasty - see Repair, tendon
Tendinosuture (immediate) (primary) - see also Suture, tendon 83.64
  hand - see also Suture, tendon, hand 82.45
Tendolysis 83.91
  hand 82.91
Tendoplasty - see Repair, tendon
Tenectomy 83.39
  eye 15.13
    levator palpebrae 08.33
    multiple (two or more tendons) 15.3
  hand 82.29
  levator palpebrae 08.33
  tendon sheath 83.31
    hand 82.21
Tenodesis (tendon fixation to skeletal attachment) 83.88
  Fowler 82.85
  hand 82.85
Tenolysis 83.91
  hand 82.91
Tenomyoplasty - see also Repair, tendon 83.88
  hand - see also Repair, tendon, hand 82.86
Tenomyotomy - see Tenonectomy
Tenonectomy 83.42
  for graft 83.41
    hand 82.32
  hand 82.33
    for graft 82.32
Tenontomyoplasty - see Repair, tendon
Tenontoplasty - see Repair, tendon
Tenoplasty - see also Repair, tendon 83.88

Tenoplasty (Continued)
  hand - see also Repair, tendon, hand 82.86
Tenorrhaphy - see also Suture, tendon 83.64
  hand - see also Suture, tendon, hand 82.45
  to skeletal attachment 83.88
    hand 82.85
Tenosuspension 83.88
  hand 82.86
Tenosuture - see also Suture, tendon 83.64
  hand - see also Suture, tendon, hand 82.45
  to skeletal attachment 83.88
    hand 82.85
Tenosynovectomy 83.42
  hand 82.33
Tenotomy 83.13
  Achilles tendon 83.11
  adductor (hip) (subcutaneous) 83.12
  eye 15.12
    levator palpebrae 08.38
    multiple (two or more tendons) 15.4
  hand 82.11
  levator palpebrae 08.38
  pectoralis minor tendon (decompression, thoracic outlet) 83.13
  stapedius 19.0
  tensor tympani 19.0
Tenovaginotomy - see Tenotomy
Tensing, orbicularis oculi 08.59
Termination of pregnancy
  by
    aspiration curettage 69.51
    dilation and curettage 69.01
    hysterectomy - see Hysterectomy
    hysterotomy 74.91
    intra-amniotic injection (saline) 75.0
Test, testing (for)
  14 C-Urea breath 89.39
  auditory function NEC 95.46
  Bender Visual-Motor Gestalt 94.02
  Benton Visual Retention 94.02
  cardiac (vascular)
    function NEC 89.59
    stress 89.44
      bicycle ergometer 89.43
      Masters' two-step 89.42
      treadmill 89.41
  Denver developmental (screening) 94.02
  fetus, fetal
    nonstress (fetal activity acceleration determinations) 75.35
    oxytocin challenge (contraction stress) 75.35
    sensitivity (to oxytocin) - omit code
  function
    cardiac NEC 89.59
    hearing NEC 95.46
    muscle (by)
      electromyography 93.08
      manual 93.04
    neurologic NEC 89.15
    vestibular 95.46
      clinical 95.44
  glaucoma NEC 95.26
  hearing 95.47
    clinical NEC 95.42
  intelligence 94.01
  internal jugular-subclavian venous reflux 89.62

ICD-9-CM

T

Vol.

Test, testing *(Continued)*
  intracarotid amobarbital (Wada) 89.10
  Masters' two-step stress (cardiac) 89.42
  muscle function (by)
    electromyography 93.08
    manual 93.04
  neurologic function NEC 89.15
  nocturnal penile tumescence 89.29
  provocative, for glaucoma 95.26
  psychologic NEC 94.08
  psychometric 94.01
  radio-cobalt B12 Schilling 92.04
  range of motion 93.05
  rotation (Bárány chair) (hearing) 95.45
  sleep disorder function - *see* categories
    89.17-89.18
  Stanford-Binet 94.01
  Thallium stress (transesophageal pacing) 89.44
  tuning fork (hearing) 95.42
  urea breath (14 C) 89.39
  vestibular function NEC 95.46
    thermal 95.44
  Wada (hemispheric function) 89.10
  whispered speech (hearing) 95.42
TEVAP (transurethral electrovaporization of prostate) 60.29
Thalamectomy 01.41
Thalamotomy 01.41
  by stereotactic radiosurgery 92.32
    cobalt 60 92.32
    linear accelerator (LINAC) 92.31
    multi-source 92.32
    particle beam 92.33
    particulate 92.33
    radiosurgery NEC 92.39
    single source photon 92.31
Thal operation (repair of esophageal stricture) 42.85
Theleplasty 85.87
Therapy
  Antabuse 94.25
  art 93.89
  aversion 94.33
  behavior 94.33
  Bennett respirator - *see* category 96.7
  blind rehabilitation NEC 93.78
  Byrd respirator - *see* category 96.7
  carbon dioxide 94.25
  cobalt-60 92.23
  conditioning, psychiatric 94.33
  continuous positive airway pressure (CPAP) 93.90
  croupette, croup tent 93.94
  daily living activities 93.83
    for the blind 93.78
  dance 93.89
  desensitization 94.33
  detoxification 94.25
  diversional 93.81
  domestic tasks 93.83
    for the blind 93.78
  educational (bed-bound children) (handicapped) 93.82
  electroconvulsive (ECT) 94.27
  electroshock (EST) 94.27
    subconvulsive 94.26
  electrotonic (ETT) 94.27
  encounter group 94.44
  extinction 94.33
  family 94.42
  fog (inhalation) 93.94
  gamma ray 92.23
  group NEC 94.44

Therapy *(Continued)*
  group NEC *(Continued)*
    for psychosexual dysfunctions 94.41
  hearing NEC 95.49
  heat NEC 93.35
    for cancer treatment 99.85
  helium 93.98
  hot pack(s) 93.35
  hyperbaric oxygen 93.95
    wound 93.59
  hyperthermia NEC 93.35
    for cancer treatment 99.85
  individual, psychiatric NEC 94.39
    for psychosexual dysfunction 94.34
  industrial 93.89
  infrared irradiation 93.35
  inhalation NEC 93.96
    nitric oxide 00.12
  insulin shock 94.24
  intermittent positive pressure breathing (IPPB) 93.91
  IPPB (intermittent positive pressure breathing) 93.91
  leech 99.99
  lithium 94.22
  maggot 86.28
  manipulative, osteopathic - *see also* Manipulation, osteopathic 93.67
  manual arts 93.81
  methadone 94.25
  mist (inhalation) 93.94
  music 93.84
  nebulizer 93.94
  neuroleptic 94.23
  nitric oxide 00.12
  occupational 93.83
  oxygen 93.96
    catalytic 93.96
    hyperbaric 93.95
      wound 93.59
    wound (hyperbaric) 93.59
  paraffin bath 93.35
  physical NEC 93.39
    combined (without mention of components) 93.38
    diagnostic NEC 93.09
  play 93.81
    psychotherapeutic 94.36
  positive and expiratory pressure - *see* category 96.7
  psychiatric NEC 94.39
    drug NEC 94.25
    lithium 94.22
  radiation 92.29
    contact (150 KVP or less) 92.21
    deep (200-300 KVP) 92.22
    high voltage (200-300 KVP) 92.22
    low voltage (150 KVP or less) 92.21
    megavoltage 92.24
    orthovoltage 92.22
    particle source NEC 92.26
    photon 92.24
    radioisotope (teleradiotherapy) 92.23
    retinal lesion 14.26
    superficial (150 KVP or less) 92.21
    supervoltage 92.24
  radioisotope, radioisotopic NEC 92.29
    implantation or insertion 92.27
    injection or instillation 92.28
    teleradiotherapy 92.23
  radium (radon) 92.23
  recreational 93.81
  rehabilitation NEC 93.89
  respiratory NEC 93.99
    bi-level airway pressure 93.90
    continuous positive airway pressure [CPAP] 93.90

Therapy *(Continued)*
  respiratory NEC *(Continued)*
    endotracheal respiratory assistance - *see* category 96.7
    intermittent mandatory ventilation [IMV] - *see* category 96.7
    intermittent positive pressure breathing [IPPB] 93.91
    negative pressure (continuous) [CNP] 93.99
    nitric oxide 00.12
    non-invasive positive pressure (NIPPV) 93.90 ◄
    other continuous (unspecified duration) 96.70
      for less than 96 consecutive hours 96.71
      for 96 consecutive hours or more 96.72
    positive end-expiratory pressure [PEEP] - *see* category 96.7
    pressure support ventilation [PSV] - *see* category 96.7
  root canal 23.70
    with
      apicoectomy 23.72
      irrigation 23.71
  shock
    chemical 94.24
    electric 94.27
      subconvulsive 94.26
    insulin 94.24
  speech 93.75
    for correction of defect 93.74
  ultrasound
    heat therapy 93.35
    hyperthermia for cancer treatment 99.85
    physical therapy 93.35
    therapeutic - *see* Ultrasound
  ultraviolet light 99.82
Thermocautery - *see* Cauterization
Thermography 88.89
  blood vessel 88.86
  bone 88.83
  breast 88.85
  cerebral 88.81
  eye 88.82
  lymph gland 88.89
  muscle 88.84
  ocular 88.82
  osteoarticular 88.83
  specified site NEC 88.89
  vein, deep 88.86
Thermokeratoplasty 11.74
Thermosclerectomy 12.62
Thermotherapy (hot packs) (paraffin bath) NEC 93.35
  prostate
    by
      microwave 60.96
      radiofrequency 60.97
      transurethral microwave thermotherapy (TUMT) 60.96
      transurethral needle ablation (TUNA) 60.97
    TUMT (transurethral microwave thermotherapy) 60.96
    TUNA (transurethral needle ablation 60.97
Thiersch operation
  anus 49.79
  skin graft 86.69
    hand 86.62
Thompson operation
  cleft lip repair 27.54
  correction of lymphedema 40.9

Thompson operation (Continued)
  quadricepsplasty 83.86
  thumb apposition with bone graft 82.69
Thoracectomy 34.09
  for lung collapse 33.34
Thoracentesis 34.91
Thoracocentesis 34.91
Thoracolysis (for collapse of lung) 33.39
Thoracoplasty (anterior) (extrapleural)
    (paravertebral) (posterolateral) (com-
    plete) (partial) 33.34
Thoracoscopy, transpleural (for explora-
    tion) 34.21
Thoracostomy 34.09
  for lung collapse 33.32
Thoracotomy (with drainage) 34.09
  as operative approach - omit code
  exploratory 34.02
Three-snip operation, punctum 09.51
Thrombectomy 38.00
  with endarterectomy - see Endarterec-
    tomy
  abdominal
    artery 38.06
    vein 38.07
  aorta (arch) (ascending) (descending)
    38.04
  bovine graft 39.49
  coronary artery 36.09
  head and neck vessel NEC 38.02
  intracranial vessel NEC 38.01
  lower limb
    artery 38.08
    vein 38.09
  pulmonary vessel 38.05
  thoracic vessel NEC 38.05
  upper limb (artery) (vein) 38.03
Thromboendarterectomy 38.10
  abdominal 38.16
  aorta (arch) (ascending) (descending)
    38.14
  coronary artery 36.09
    open chest approach 36.03
  head and neck NEC 38.12
  intracranial NEC 38.11
  lower limb 38.18
  thoracic NEC 38.15
  upper limb 38.13
Thymectomy 07.80
  partial 07.81
  total 07.82
Thymopexy 07.99
Thyrochondrotomy 31.3
Thyrocricoidectomy 30.29
Thyrocricotomy (for assistance in
    breathing) 31.1
Thyroidectomy NEC 06.39
  by mediastinotomy - see also Thyroid-
    ectomy, substernal 06.50
  with laryngectomy - see Laryngectomy
  complete or total 06.4
    substernal (by mediastinotomy)
      (transsternal route) 06.52
    transoral route (lingual) 06.6
  lingual (complete) (partial) (subtotal)
    (total) 06.6
  partial or subtotal NEC 06.39
    with complete removal of remaining
      lobe 06.2
    submental route (lingual) 06.6
    substernal (by mediastinotomy)
      (transsternal route) 06.51
  remaining tissue 06.4
  submental route (lingual) 06.6

Thyroidectomy NEC (Continued)
  substernal (by mediastinotomy)
      (transsternal route) 06.50
    complete or total 06.52
    partial or subtotal 06.51
  transoral route (lingual) 06.6
  transsternal route - see also Thyroidec-
    tomy, substernal 06.50
  unilateral (with removal of isthmus)
      (with removal of portion of other
      lobe) 06.2
Thyroidorrhaphy 06.93
Thyroidotomy (field) (gland) NEC 06.09
  postoperative 06.02
Thyrotomy 31.3
  with tantalum plate 31.69
Tirofiban (HCl), infusion 99.20
Toilette
  skin - see Debridement, skin or subcu-
    taneous tissue
  tracheostomy 96.55
Token economy (behavior therapy) 94.33
Tomkins operation (metroplasty) 69.49
Tomography - see also Radiography
  abdomen NEC 88.02
  cardiac 87.42
  computerized axial NEC 88.38
    abdomen 88.01
    bone 88.38
      quantitative 88.98
    brain 87.03
    head 87.03
    kidney 87.71
    skeletal 88.38
      quantitative 88.98
    thorax 87.41
  head NEC 87.04
  kidney NEC 87.72
  lung 87.42
  thorax NEC 87.42
Tongue tie operation 25.91
Tonography 95.26
Tonometry 89.11
Tonsillectomy 28.2
  with adenoidectomy 28.3
Tonsillotomy 28.0
Topectomy 01.32
Torek (-Bevan) operation (orchidopexy)
    (first stage) (second stage) 62.5
Torkildsen operation (ventriculocisternal
    shunt) 02.2
Torpin operation (cul-de-sac resection)
    70.92
Toti operation (dacryocystorhinostomy)
    09.81
Touchas operation 86.83
Touroff operation (ligation of subclavian
    artery) 38.85
Toxicology - see Examination, microscopic
TPN (total parenteral nutrition) 99.15
Trabeculectomy ab externo 12.64
Trabeculodialysis 12.59
Trabeculotomy ab externo 12.54
Trachelectomy 67.4
Trachelopexy 69.22
Tracheloplasty 67.69
Trachelorrhaphy (Emmet) (suture) 67.61
  obstetrical 75.51
Trachelotomy 69.95
  obstetrical 73.93
Tracheocricotomy (for assistance in
    breathing) 31.1
Tracheofissure 31.1
Tracheography 87.32
Tracheolaryngotomy (emergency) 31.1
  permanent opening 31.29

Tracheoplasty 31.79
  with artificial larynx 31.75
Tracheorrhaphy 31.71
Tracheoscopy NEC 31.42
  through tracheotomy (stoma) 31.41
Tracheostomy (emergency) (temporary)
    (for assistance in breathing) 31.1
  mediastinal 31.21
  permanent NEC 31.29
  revision 31.74
Tracheotomy (emergency) (temporary)
    (for assistance in breathing) 31.1
  permanent 31.29
Tracing, carotid pulse with ECG lead
    89.56
Traction
  with reduction of fracture or disloca-
    tion - see Reduction, fracture, and
    Reduction, dislocation
  adhesive tape (skin) 93.46
  boot 93.46
  Bryant's (skeletal) 93.44
  Buck's 93.46
  caliper tongs 93.41
    with synchronous insertion of device
      02.94
  Cortel's (spinal) 93.42
  Crutchfield tongs 93.41
    with synchronous insertion of device
      02.94
  Dunlop's (skeletal) 93.44
  gallows 93.46
  Gardner Wells 93.41
    with synchronous insertion of device
      02.94
  halo device, skull 93.41
    with synchronous insertion of device
      02.94
  Lyman Smith (skeletal) 93.44
  manual, intermittent 93.21
  mechanical, intermittent 93.21
  Russell's (skeletal) 93.44
  skeletal NEC 93.44
    intermittent 93.43
  skin, limbs NEC 93.46
  spinal NEC 93.42
    with skull device (halo) (caliper)
      (Crutchfield) (Gardner Wells)
      (Vinke) (tongs) 93.41
    with synchronous insertion of de-
      vice 02.94
  Thomas' splint 93.45
  Vinke tongs 93.41
    with synchronous insertion of device
      02.94
Tractotomy
  brain 01.32
  medulla oblongata 01.32
  mesencephalon 01.32
  percutaneous 03.21
  spinal cord (one-stage) (two-stage)
    03.29
  trigeminal (percutaneous) (radiofre-
    quency) 04.02
Training (for) (in)
  ADL (activities of daily living) 93.83
    for the blind 93.78
  ambulation 93.22
  braille 93.77
  crutch walking 93.24
  dyslexia 93.71
  dysphasia 93.72
  esophageal speech (postlaryngectomy)
    93.73

ICD-9-CM

T

Vol. 3

Training *(Continued)*
  gait 93.22
  joint movements 93.14
  lip reading 93.75
  Moon (blind reading) 93.77
  orthoptic 95.35
  prenatal (natural childbirth) 93.37
  prosthetic or orthotic device usage
    93.24
  relaxation 94.33
  speech NEC 93.75
    esophageal type 93.73
    for correction of defect 93.74
  use of lead dog for the blind 93.76
  vocational 93.85
TRAM (transverse rectus abdominis musculocutaneous) flap of breast 85.7
Transactional analysis
  group 94.44
  individual 94.39
Transection - *see also* Division
  artery (with ligation) - *see also* Divi-
    sion, artery 38.80
    renal, aberrant (with reimplantation)
      39.55
  bone - *see also* Osteotomy 77.30
  fallopian tube (bilateral) (remaining)
    (solitary) 66.39
    by endoscopy 66.22
    unilateral 66.92
  isthmus, thyroid 06.91
  muscle 83.19
    eye 15.13
      multiple (two or more muscles) 15.3
    hand 82.19
  nerve (cranial) (peripheral) NEC 04.03
    acoustic 04.01
    root (spinal) 03.1
    sympathetic 05.0
    tracts in spinal cord 03.29
    trigeminal 04.02
    vagus (transabdominal) - *see also* Va-
      gotomy 44.00
  pylorus (with wedge resection) 43.3
  renal vessel, aberrant (with reimplan-
    tation) 39.55
  spinal
    cord tracts 03.29
    nerve root 03.1
  tendon 83.13
    hand 82.11
  uvula 27.71
  vas deferens 63.71
  vein (with ligation) - *see also* Division,
    vein 38.80
    renal, aberrant (with reimplantation)
      39.55
    varicose (lower limb) 38.59
Transfer, transference
  bone shaft, fibula into tibia 78.47
  digital (to replace absent thumb) 82.69
    finger (to thumb) (same hand) 82.61
    to
      finger, except thumb 82.81
      opposite hand (with amputa-
        tion) 82.69 *[84.01]*
    toe (to thumb) (with amputation)
      82.69 *[84.11]*
      to finger, except thumb 82.81 *[84.11]*
  fat pad NEC 86.89
    with skin graft - *see* Graft, skin, full-
      thickness
  finger (to replace absent thumb) (same
    hand) 82.61

Transfer, transference *(Continued)*
  finger *(Continued)*
    to
      finger, except thumb 82.81
      opposite hand (with amputation)
        82.69 *[84.01]*
  muscle origin 83.77
    hand 82.58
  nerve (cranial) (peripheral) (radial an-
    terior) (ulnar) 04.6
  pedicle graft 86.74
  pes anserinus (tendon) (repair of knee)
    81.47
  tarsoconjunctival flap, from opposing
    lid 08.64
  tendon 83.75
    hand 82.56
    pes anserinus (repair of knee)
      81.47
  toe-to-thumb (free) (pedicle) (with am-
    putation) 82.69 *[84.11]*
Transfixion - *see also* Fixation
  iris (bombé) 12.11
Transfusion (of) 99.03
  antihemophilic factor 99.06
  antivenin 99.16
  autologous blood
    collected prior to surgery 99.02
    intraoperative 99.00
    perioperative 99.00
    postoperative 99.00
    previously collected 99.02
    salvage 99.00
  blood (whole) NOS 99.03
    expander 99.08
    surrogate 99.09
  bone marrow 41.00
    allogeneic 41.03
      with purging 41.02
    allograft 41.03
      with purging 41.02
    autograft 41.01
      with purging 41.09
    autologous 41.01
      with purging 41.09
  coagulation factors 99.06
  Dextran 99.08
  exchange 99.01
    intraperitoneal 75.2
    in utero (with hysterotomy) 75.2
  exsanguination 99.01
  gamma globulin 99.14
  granulocytes 99.09
  hemodilution 99.03
  intrauterine 75.2
  packed cells 99.04
  plasma 99.07
  platelets 99.05
  replacement, total 99.01
  serum NEC 99.07
  substitution 99.01
  thrombocytes 99.05
Transillumination
  nasal sinuses 89.35
  skull (newborn) 89.16
Translumbar aortogram 88.42
Transplant, transplantation

Note:	To report donor source: ◀
	cadaver 00.93 ◀
	live non-related donor
	00.92 ◀
	live related donor 00.91 ◀
	live unrelated donor 00.92◀

Transplant, transplantation *(Continued)*
  artery 39.59
    renal, aberrant 39.55
  autotransplant - *see* Reimplantation
  blood vessel 39.59
    renal, aberrant 39.55
  bone - *see also* Graft, bone 78.00
    marrow 41.00
      allogeneic 41.03
        with purging 41.02
      allograft 41.03
        with purging 41.02
      autograft 41.01
        with purging 41.09
      autologous 41.01
        with purging 41.09
      stem cell
        allogeneic (hematopoietic) 41.05
          with purging 41.08
        autologous (hematopoietic) 41.04
          with purging 41.07
        cord blood 41.06
    stem cell
      allogeneic (hematopoietic) 41.05
        with purging 41.08
      autologous (hematopoietic) 41.04
        with purging 41.07
      cord blood 41.06
  combined heart-lung 33.6
  conjunctiva, for pterygium 11.39
  corneal - *see also* Keratoplasty 11.60
  dura 02.12
  fascia 83.82
    hand 82.72
  finger (replacing absent thumb) (same
    hand) 82.61
    to
      finger, except thumb 82.81
      opposite hand (with amputation)
        82.69 *[84.01]*
  gracilis muscle (for) 83.77
    anal incontinence 49.74
    urethrovesical suspension 59.71
  hair follicles
    eyebrow 08.63
    eyelid 08.63
    scalp 86.64
  heart (orthotopic) 37.51
    combined with lung 33.6
  ileal stoma to new site 46.23
  intestine 46.97
  Islets of Langerhans (cells) 52.86
    allotransplantation of cells 52.85
    autotransplantation of cells 52.84
    heterotransplantation 52.85
    homotransplantation 52.84
  kidney NEC 55.69
  liver 50.59
    auxiliary (permanent) (temporary)
      (recipient's liver in situ) 50.51
    cells into spleen via percutaneous
      catheterization 38.91
  lung 33.50
    bilateral 33.52
    combined with heart 33.6
    double 33.52
    single 33.51
    unilateral 33.51
  lymphatic structure(s) (peripheral) 40.9
  mammary artery to myocardium or
    ventricular wall 36.2
  muscle 83.77
    gracilis (for) 83.77
      anal incontinence 49.74
      urethrovesical suspension 59.71

Transplant, transplantation (*Continued*)
  muscle (*Continued*)
    hand 82.58
    temporalis 83.77
      with orbital exenteration 16.59
  nerve (cranial) (peripheral) 04.6
  ovary 65.92
  pancreas 52.80
    heterotransplant 52.83
    homotransplant 52.82
    Islets of Langerhans (cells) 52.86
      allotransplantation of cells 52.85
      autotransplantation of cells 52.84
      heterotransplantation 52.85
      homotransplantation 52.84
      reimplantation 52.81
  pes anserinus (tendon) (repair of knee)
    81.47
  renal NEC 55.69
    vessel, aberrant 39.55
  salivary duct opening 26.49
  skin - *see* Graft, skin
  spermatic cord 63.53
  spleen 41.94
  stem cell(s)
    allogeneic (hematopoietic) 41.05
      with purging 41.08
    autologous (hematopoietic) 41.04
      with purging 41.07
    cord blood 41.06
  tendon 83.75
    hand 82.56
    pes anserinus (repair of knee) 81.47
    superior rectus (blepharoptosis)
      08.36
  testis to scrotum 62.5
  thymus 07.94
  thyroid tissue 06.94
  toe (replacing absent thumb) (with am-
    putation) 82.69 *[84.11]*
    to finger, except thumb 82.81 *[84.11]*
  tooth 23.5
  ureter to
    bladder 56.74
    ileum (external diversion) 56.51
      internal diversion only 56.71
    intestine 56.71
    skin 56.61
  vein (peripheral) 39.59
    renal, aberrant 39.55
  vitreous 14.72
    anterior approach 14.71
Transposition
  extraocular muscles 15.5

Transposition (*Continued*)
  eyelash flaps 08.63
  eye muscle (oblique) (rectus) 15.5
  finger (replacing absent thumb) (same
    hand) 82.61
    to
      finger, except thumb 82.81
      opposite hand (with amputation)
        82.69 *[84.01]*
  interatrial venous return 35.91
  jejunal (Henley) 43.81
  joint capsule - *see also* Arthroplasty
    81.96
  muscle NEC 83.79
    extraocular 15.5
    hand 82.59
  nerve (cranial) (peripheral) (radial an-
    terior) (ulnar) 04.6
  nipple 85.86
  pterygium 11.31
  tendon NEC 83.76
    hand 82.57
  vocal cords 31.69
Transureteroureterostomy 56.75
Transversostomy - *see also* Colostomy
  46.10
Trapping, aneurysm (cerebral) 39.52
Trauner operation (lingual sulcus extension) 24.91
Trephination, trephining
  accessory sinus - *see* Sinusotomy
  corneoscleral 12.89
  cranium 01.24
  nasal sinus - *see* Sinusotomy
  sclera (with iridectomy) 12.61
Trial (failed) forceps 73.3
Trigonectomy 57.6
Trimming, amputation stump 84.3
Triple arthrodesis 81.12
Trochanterplasty 81.40
Tsuge operation (macrodactyly repair)
  82.83
Tuck, tucking - *see also* Plication
  eye muscle 15.22
    multiple (two or more muscles)
      15.4
    levator palpebrae, for blepharoptosis
      08.34
Tudor "rabbit ear" operation (anterior
  urethropexy) 59.79
Tuffier operation
  apicolysis of lung 33.39
  vaginal hysterectomy 68.59
    laparoscopically assisted (LAVH)
      68.51

TULIP (transurethral ultrasound guided
  laser induced prostatectomy)
  60.21
TUMT (transurethral microwave thermotherapy) of prostate 60.96
TUNA (transurethral needle ablation) of
  prostate 60.97
Tunnel, subcutaneous (antethoracic)
  42.86
  esophageal 42.68
    with anastomosis - *see* Anastomosis,
      esophagus, antesternal
  pulse generator lead wire 86.99
    with initial procedure - *omit code*
Turbinectomy (complete) (partial) NEC
  21.69
  by
    cryosurgery 21.61
    diathermy 21.61
  with sinusectomy - *see* Sinusectomy
Turco operation (release of joint capsules
  in clubfoot) 80.48
TURP (transurethral resection of prostate) 60.29
Tylectomy (breast) (partial) 85.21
Tympanectomy 20.59
  with tympanoplasty - *see* Tympano-
    plasty
Tympanogram 95.41
Tympanomastoidectomy 20.42
Tympanoplasty (type I) (with graft)
  19.4
  with
    air pocket over round window
      19.54
    fenestra in semicircular canal
      19.55
    graft against
      incus or malleus 19.52
      mobile and intact stapes 19.53
    incudostapediopexy 19.52
  epitympanic, type I 19.4
  revision 19.6
  type
    II (graft against incus or malleus)
      19.52
    III (graft against mobile and intact
      stapes) 19.53
    IV (air pocket over round window)
      19.54
    V (fenestra in semicircular canal)
      19.55
Tympanosympathectomy 20.91
Tympanotomy 20.09
  with intubation 20.01

ICD-9-CM

T

Vol. 3

U

Uchida operation (tubal ligation with or without fimbriectomy) 66.32
UFR (uroflowmetry) 89.24
Ultrafiltration 99.78 ◀
  hemodiafiltration 39.95 ◀
  hemodialysis (kidney) 39.95 ◀
  removal, plasma water 99.78 ◀
  therapeutic plasmapheresis 99.71 ◀
Ultrasonography
  abdomen 88.76
  aortic arch 88.73
  biliary tract 88.74
  breast 88.73
  deep vein thrombosis 88.77
  digestive system 88.74
  eye 95.13
  head and neck 88.71
  heart 88.72 ◀
  intestine 88.74
  intravascular - *see* Ultrasound, intra-
    vascular (IVUS) ◀
  lung 88.73
  midline shift, brain 88.71
  multiple sites 88.79
  peripheral vascular system 88.77
  retroperitoneum 88.76
  therapeutic - *see* Ultrasound
  thorax NEC 88.73
  total body 88.79
  urinary system 88.75
  uterus 88.79
    gravid 88.78
Ultrasound
  diagnostic - *see* Ultrasonography
  fragmentation (of)
    cataract (with aspiration) 13.41
    urinary calculus, stones (Kock pouch) 59.95
  heart ◀
    intracardiac (heart chambers) (ICE) 37.28 ◀
    intravascular (coronary vessels) (IVUS) 00.24 ◀
    non-invasive 88.72 ◀
  inner ear 20.79
  intravascular (IVUS) 00.29 ◀
    aorta 00.22 ◀
    aortic arch 00.22 ◀
    cerebral vessel, extracranial 00.21 ◀
    coronary vessel 00.24 ◀
    intrathoracic vessel 00.22 ◀
    other specified vessel 00.28 ◀
    peripheral vessel 00.23 ◀
    renal vessel 00.25 ◀
    vena cava (inferior) (superior) 00.22 ◀
  therapeutic
    head 00.01
    heart 00.02

Ultrasound *(Continued)*
  therapeutic *(Continued)*
    neck 00.01
    other therapeutic ultrasound 00.09
    peripheral vascular vessels 00.03
    vessels of head and neck 00.01
    therapy 93.35
Umbilectomy 54.3
Unbridling
  blood vessel, peripheral 39.91
  celiac artery axis 39.91
Uncovering - *see* Incision, by site
Undercutting
  hair follicle 86.09
  perianal tissue 49.02
Unroofing - *see also* Incision, by site
  external
    auditory canal 18.02
    ear NEC 18.09
  kidney cyst 55.39
UPP (urethral pressure profile) 89.25
Upper GI series (x-ray) 87.62
UPPP (uvulopalatopharyngoplasty) 27.69 *[29.4]*
Uranoplasty (for cleft palate repair) 27.62
Uranorrhaphy (for cleft palate repair) 27.62
Uranostaphylorrhaphy 27.62
Urban operation (mastectomy) (unilateral) 85.47
  bilateral 85.48
Ureterectomy 56.40
  with nephrectomy 55.51
  partial 56.41
  total 56.42
Ureterocecostomy 56.71
Ureterocelectomy 56.41
Ureterocolostomy 56.71
Ureterocystostomy 56.74
Ureteroenterostomy 56.71
Ureteroileostomy (internal diversion) 56.71
  external diversion 56.51
Ureterolithotomy 56.2
Ureterolysis 59.02
  with freeing or repositioning of ureter 59.02
  laparoscopic 59.03
Ureteroneocystostomy 56.74
Ureteropexy 56.85
Ureteroplasty 56.89
Ureteroplication 56.89
Ureteroproctostomy 56.71
Ureteropyelography (intravenous) (diuretic infusion) 87.73
  percutaneous 87.75
  retrograde 87.74
Ureteropyeloplasty 55.87
Ureteropyelostomy 55.86

Ureterorrhaphy 56.82
Ureteroscopy 56.31
  with biopsy 56.33
Ureterosigmoidostomy 56.71
Ureterostomy (cutaneous) (external) (tube) 56.61
  closure 56.83
  ileal 56.51
Ureterotomy 56.2
Ureteroureterostomy (crossed) 56.75
  lumbar 56.41
  resection with end-to-end anastomosis 56.41
  spatulated 56.41
Urethral catheterization, indwelling 57.94
Urethral pressure profile (UPP) 89.25
Urethrectomy (complete) (partial) (radical) 58.39
  with
    complete cystectomy 57.79
    pelvic exenteration 68.8
    radical cystectomy 57.71
Urethrocystography (retrograde) (voiding) 87.76
Urethrocystopexy (by) 59.79
  levator muscle sling 59.71
  retropubic suspension 59.5
  suprapubic suspension 59.4
Urethrolithotomy 58.0
Urethrolysis 58.5
Urethropexy 58.49
  anterior 59.79
Urethroplasty 58.49
  augmentation 59.79
    collagen implant 59.72
    fat implant 59.72
    injection (endoscopic) of implant into urethra 59.72
    polytef implant 59.72
Urethrorrhaphy 58.41
Urethroscopy 58.22
  for control of hemorrhage of prostate 60.94
  perineal 58.21
Urethrostomy (perineal) 58.0
Urethrotomy (external) 58.0
  internal (endoscopic) 58.5
Uroflowmetry (UFR) 89.24
Urography (antegrade) (excretory) (intravenous) 87.73
  retrograde 87.74
Uteropexy (abdominal approach) (vaginal approach) 69.22
UVP (uvulopalatopharyngoplasty) 27.69 *[29.4]*
Uvulectomy 27.72
Uvulopalatopharyngoplasty (UPPP) 27.69 *[29.4]*
Uvulotomy 27.71

V

Vaccination (prophylactic) (against) 99.59
  anthrax 99.55
  brucellosis 99.55
  cholera 99.31
  common cold 99.51
  disease NEC 99.55
    arthropod-borne viral NEC 99.54
  encephalitis, arthropod-borne viral 99.53
  German measles 99.47
  hydrophobia 99.44
  infectious parotitis 99.46
  influenza 99.52
  measles 99.45
  mumps 99.46
  paratyphoid fever 99.32
  pertussis 99.37
  plague 99.34
  poliomyelitis 99.41
  rabies 99.44
  Rocky Mountain spotted fever 99.55
  rubella 99.47
  rubeola 99.45
  smallpox 99.42
  Staphylococcus 99.55
  Streptococcus 99.55
  tuberculosis 99.33
  tularemia 99.35
  tumor 99.28
  typhoid 99.32
  typhus 99.55
  undulant fever 99.55
  yellow fever 99.43
Vacuum extraction, fetal head 72.79
  with episiotomy 72.71
VAD (vascular access device) - *see* Implant, heart assist system
Vagectomy (subdiaphragmatic) - *see also* Vagotomy 44.00
Vaginal douche 96.44
Vaginectomy 70.4
Vaginofixation 70.77
Vaginoperineotomy 70.14
Vaginoplasty 70.79
Vaginorrhaphy 70.71
  obstetrical 75.69
Vaginoscopy 70.21
Vaginotomy 70.14
  for
    culdocentesis 70.0
    pelvic abscess 70.12
Vagotomy (gastric) 44.00
  parietal cell 44.02
  selective NEC 44.03
    highly 44.02
    Holle's 44.02
    proximal 44.02
  truncal 44.01
Valvotomy - *see* Valvulotomy
Valvulectomy, heart - *see* Valvuloplasty, heart
Valvuloplasty
  heart (open heart technique) (without valve replacement) 35.10
    with prosthesis or tissue graft - *see* Replacement, heart, valve, by site
    aortic valve 35.11
      percutaneous (balloon) 35.96
    combined with repair of atrial and ventricular septal defects - *see* Repair, endocardial cushion defect

Valvuloplasty (*Continued*)
  heart (*Continued*)
    mitral valve 35.12
    percutaneous (balloon) 35.96
    pulmonary valve 35.13
      in total repair of tetralogy of Fallot 35.81
      percutaneous (balloon) 35.96
    tricuspid valve 35.14
Valvulotomy
  heart (closed heart technique) (transatrial) (transventricular) 35.00
    aortic valve 35.01
    mitral valve 35.02
    open heart technique - *see* Valvuloplasty, heart
    pulmonary valve 35.03
      in total repair of tetralogy of Fallot 35.81
    tricuspid valve 35.04
Varicocelectomy, spermatic cord 63.1
Varicotomy, peripheral vessels (lower limb) 38.59
  upper limb 38.53
Vascular closure, percutaneous puncture - *omit code*
Vascularization - *see* Revascularization
Vasectomy (complete) (partial) 63.73
Vasogram 87.94
Vasoligation 63.71
  gastric 38.86
Vasorrhaphy 63.81
Vasostomy 63.6
Vasotomy 63.6
Vasotripsy 63.71
Vasovasostomy 63.82
Vectorcardiogram (VCG) (with ECG) 89.53
Venectomy - *see* Phlebectomy
Venipuncture NEC 38.99
  for injection of contrast material - *see* Phlebography
Venography - *see* Phlebography
Venorrhaphy 39.32
Venotomy 38.00
  abdominal 38.07
  head and neck NEC 38.02
  intracranial NEC 38.01
  lower limb 38.09
  thoracic NEC 38.05
  upper limb 38.03
Venotripsy 39.98
Venovenostomy 39.29
Ventilation
  bi-level airway pressure 93.90
  continuous positive airway pressure [CPAP] 93.90
  endotracheal respiratory assistance - *see* category 96.7
  intermittent mandatory ventilation [IMV] - *see* category 96.7
  intermittent positive pressure breathing [IPPB] 93.91
  mechanical
    endotracheal respiratory assistance - *see* category 96.7
    intermittent mandatory ventilation [IMV] - *see* category 96.7
    other continuous (unspecified duration) 96.70
      for less than 96 consecutive hours 96.71
      for 96 consecutive hours or more 96.72
    positive end-expiratory pressure [PEEP] - *see* category 96.7

Ventilation (*Continued*)
  mechanical (*Continued*)
    pressure support ventilation [PSV] - *see* category 96.7
  negative pressure (continuous) [CNP] 93.99
  non-invasive positive pressure (NIPPV) 93.90 ◄
Ventriculectomy, heart
  partial 37.35
Ventriculocholecystostomy 02.34
Ventriculocisternostomy 02.2
Ventriculocordectomy 30.29
Ventriculogram, ventriculography (cerebral) 87.02
  cardiac
    left ventricle (outflow tract) 88.53
      combined with right heart 88.54
    right ventricle (outflow tract) 88.52
      combined with left heart 88.54
  radionuclide cardiac 92.05
Ventriculomyocardiotomy 37.11
Ventriculoperitoneostomy 02.34
Ventriculopuncture 01.09
  through previously implanted catheter or reservoir (Ommaya) (Rickham) 01.02
Ventriculoseptopexy - *see also* Repair, ventricular septal defect 35.72
Ventriculoseptoplasty - *see also* Repair, ventricular septal defect 35.72
Ventriculostomy 02.2
Ventriculotomy
  cerebral 02.2
  heart 37.11
Ventriculoureterostomy 02.35
Ventriculovenostomy 02.32
Ventrofixation, uterus 69.22
Ventrohysteropexy 69.22
Ventrosuspension, uterus 69.22
VEP (visual evoked potential) 95.23
Version, obstetrical (bimanual) (cephalic) (combined) (internal) (podalic) 73.21
  with extraction 73.22
  Braxton Hicks 73.21
    with extraction 73.22
  external (bipolar) 73.91
  Potter's (podalic) 73.21
    with extraction 73.22
  Wigand's (external) 73.91
  Wright's (cephalic) 73.21
    with extraction 73.22
Vesicolithotomy (suprapubic) 57.19
Vesicostomy 57.21
Vesicourethroplasty 57.85
Vesiculectomy 60.73
  with radical prostatectomy 60.5
Vesiculogram, seminal 87.92
  contrast 87.91
Vesiculotomy 60.72
Vestibuloplasty (buccolabial) (lingual) 24.91
Vestibulotomy 20.79
Vertebroplasty (percutaneous) 81.65 ◄▥
Vicq D'Azyr operation (larynx) 31.1
Vidal operation (varicocele ligation) 63.1
Vidianectomy 05.21
Villusectomy - *see also* Synovectomy 80.70
Vision check 95.09
Visual evoked potential (VEP) 95.23

ICD-9-CM

V–Z

Vol. 3

Vitrectomy (mechanical) (posterior approach) 14.74
   with scleral buckling 14.49
   anterior approach 14.73
Vocational
   assessment 93.85
   retraining 93.85
   schooling 93.82
Voice training (postlaryngectomy) 93.73
von Kraske operation (proctectomy) 48.64
Voss operation (hanging hip operation) 83.19
Vulpius (-Compere) operation (lengthening of gastrocnemius muscle) 83.85
Vulvectomy (bilateral) (simple) 71.62
   partial (unilateral) 71.61
   radical (complete) 71.5
   unilateral 71.61
V-Y operation (repair)
   bladder 57.89
      neck 57.85
   ectropion 08.44
   lip 27.59
   skin (without graft) 86.89
   subcutaneous tissue (without skin graft) 86.89
   tongue 25.59

W

Wada test (hemispheric function) 89.10
Ward-Mayo operation (vaginal hysterectomy) 68.59
   laparoscopically assisted (LAVH) 68.51
Washing - see Lavage and Irrigation
Waterston operation (aorta-right pulmonary artery anastomosis) 39.0
Watkins (-Wertheim) operation (uterus interposition) 69.21
Watson-Jones operation
   hip arthrodesis 81.21
   reconstruction of lateral ligaments, ankle 81.49
   shoulder arthrodesis (extra-articular) 81.23
   tenoplasty 83.88
Webbing (syndactylization) 86.89
Weir operation
   appendicostomy 47.91
   correction of nostrils 21.86

Wertheim operation (radical hysterectomy) 68.6
West operation (dacryocystorhinostomy) 09.81
Wheeler operation
   entropion repair 08.44
   halving procedure (eyelid) 08.24
Whipple operation (radical pancreaticoduodenectomy) 52.7
   Child modification (radical subtotal pancreatectomy) 52.53
   Rodney Smith modification (radical subtotal pancreatectomy) 52.53
White operation (lengthening of tendo calcaneus by incomplete tenotomy) 83.11
Whitehead operation
   glossectomy, radical 25.4
   hemorrhoidectomy 49.46
Whitman operation
   foot stabilization (talectomy) 77.98
   hip reconstruction 81.40
   repair of serratus anterior muscle 83.87
   talectomy 77.98
   trochanter wedge osteotomy 77.25
Wier operation (entropion repair) 08.44
Williams-Richardson operation (vaginal construction) 70.61
Wilms operation (thoracoplasty) 33.34
Wilson operation (angulation osteotomy for hallux valgus) 77.51
Window operation
   antrum (nasal sinus) - see Antrotomy, maxillary
   aorticopulmonary 39.59
   bone cortex - see also Incision, bone 77.10
      facial 76.09
   nasoantral - see Antrotomy, maxillary
   pericardium 37.12
   pleura 34.09
Winiwarter operation (cholecystoenterostomy) 51.32
Wiring
   aneurysm 39.52
   dental (for immobilization) 93.55
      with fracture-reduction - see Reduction, fracture
      orthodontic 24.7
Wirsungojejunostomy 52.96

Witzel operation (temporary gastrostomy) 43.19
Woodward operation (release of high riding scapula) 81.83
Wrapping, aneurysm (gauze) (methyl methacrylate) (plastic) 39.52

X

Xenograft 86.65
Xerography, breast 87.36
Xeromammography 87.36
Xiphoidectomy 77.81
X-ray
   chest (routine) 87.44
      wall NEC 87.39
   contrast - see Radiography, contrast
   diagnostic - see Radiography
   injection of radio-opaque substance - see Radiography, contrast
   skeletal series, whole or complete 88.31
   therapeutic - see Therapy, radiation

Y

Young operation
   epispadias repair 58.45
   tendon transfer (anterior tibialis) (repair of flat foot) 83.75
Yount operation (division of iliotibial band) 83.14

Z

Zancolli operation
   capsuloplasty 81.72
   tendon transfer (biceps) 82.56
Ziegler operation (iridectomy) 12.14
Zonulolysis (with lens extraction) - see also Extraction, cataract, intracapsular 13.19
Z-plasty
   epicanthus 08.59
   eyelid - see also Reconstruction, eyelid 08.70
   hypopharynx 29.4
   skin (scar) (web contracture) 86.84
      with excision of lesion 86.3

◀ New   ◀▦ Revised

TABULAR LIST OF PROCEDURES

00   PROCEDURES AND INTERVENTIONS, NOT ELSEWHERE CLASSIFIED (00)

● **00.0   Therapeutic ultrasound**

> **Excludes**   *diagnostic ultrasound (non-invasive) (88.71–88.79)* ◀
> *intracardiac echocardiography [ICE] (heart chambers(s)) (37.28)* ◀
> *intravascular imaging (adjunctive) (00.21–00.29)* ◀

00.01   Therapeutic ultrasound of vessels of head and neck
> Anti-restenotic ultrasound
> Intravascular non-ablative ultrasound

> **Excludes**   *diagnostic ultrasound of:*
> *eye (95.13)*
> *head and neck (88.71)*
> *that of inner ear (20.79)*
> *ultrasonic:*
> *angioplasty of non-coronary vessel (39.50)*
> *embolectomy (38.01, 38.02)*
> *endarterectomy (38.11, 38.12)*
> *thrombectomy (38.01, 38.02)*

00.02   Therapeutic ultrasound of heart
> Anti-restenotic ultrasound
> Intravascular non-ablative ultrasound

> **Excludes**   *diagnostic ultrasound of heart (88.72)*
> *ultrasonic ablation of heart lesion (37.34)*
> *ultrasonic angioplasty of coronary vessels (36.01, 36.02, 36.05, 36.09)*

00.03   Therapeutic ultrasound of peripheral vascular vessels
> Anti-restenotic ultrasound
> Intravascular non-ablative ultrasound

> **Excludes**   *diagnostic ultrasound of peripheral vascular system (88.77)*
> *ultrasonic angioplasty of:*
> *non-coronary vessel (39.50)*

00.09   Other therapeutic ultrasound
> **Excludes**   *ultrasonic:*
> *fragmentation of urinary stones (59.95)*
> *percutaneous nephrostomy with fragmentation (55.04)*
> *physical therapy (93.35)*
> *transurethral guided laster induced prostatectomy (TULIP) (60.21)*

● **00.1   Pharmaceuticals**

00.10   Implantation of chemotherapeutic agent
> Brain wafer chemotherapy
> Interstitial/intracavitary

> **Excludes**   *injection or infusion of cancer chemotherapeutic substance (99.25)*

00.11   Infusion of drotrecogin alfa (activated)
> Infusion of recombinant protein

00.12   Administration of inhaled nitric oxide
> Nitric oxide therapy

00.13   Injection or infusion of nesiritide
> Human B-type natriuretic peptide (hBNP)

00.14   Injection or infusion of oxazolidinone class of antibiotics
> Linezolid injection

00.15   High-dose infusion interleukin-2 (IL-2)
> Infusion (IV bolus, CIV) interleukin
> Infusion aldesleukin

> **Excludes**   *low-dose infusion interleukin-2 (99.28)*

00.16   Pressurized treatment of venous bypass graft [conduit] with pharmaceutical substance ◀
> Ex-vivo treatment of vessel ◀
> Hyperbaric pressurized graft [conduit] ◀

00.17   Infusion of vasopressor agent ◀

● **00.2   Intravascular imaging of blood vessels** ◀
> Endovascular ultrasonography ◀
> Intravascular ultrasound (IVUS) ◀

> Code also any synchronous diagnostic or therapeutic procedures ◀

> **Excludes**   *therapeutic ultrasound (00.01–00.09)* ◀

00.21   Intravascular imaging of extracranial cerebral vessels ◀
> Common carotid arteries and branches ◀
> Intravascular ultrasound (IVUS), extracranial cerebral vessels ◀

> **Excludes**   *diagnostic ultrasound (non-invasive) of head and neck (88.71)* ◀

00.22   Intravascular imaging of intrathoracic vessels ◀
> Aorta and aortic arch ◀
> Intravascular ultrasound (IVUS), intrathoracic vessels ◀
> Vena cava (superior) (inferior) ◀

> **Excludes**   *diagnostic ultrasound (non-invasive) of other sites of thorax (88.73)* ◀

00.23   Intravascular imaging of peripheral vessels ◀
> Imaging of: ◀
> vessels of arm(s) ◀
> vessels of leg(s) ◀
> Intravascular ultrasound (IVUS), peripheral vessels ◀

> **Excludes**   *diagnostic ultrasound (non-invasive) of peripheral vascular system (88.77)* ◀

00.24   Intravascular imaging of coronary vessels ◀
> Intravascular ultrasound (IVUS), coronary vessels ◀

> **Excludes**   *diagnostic ultrasound (non-invasive) of heart (88.72)* ◀
> *intracardiac echocardiography [ICE] (ultrasound of heart chamber(s) (37.28)* ◀

00.25   Intravascular imaging, renal vessel(s) ◀
> Intravascular ultrasound (IVUS), renal vessels ◀
> Renal artery ◀

> **Excludes**   *diagnostic ultrasound (non-invasive) of urinary system (88.75)* ◀

00.28   Intravascular imaging, other specified vessel(s) ◀

☐ **00.29   Intravascular imaging, unspecified vessels** ◀

● **00.3   Computer assisted surgery [CAS]** ◀
> CT-free navigation ◀
> Image guided navigation (IGN) ◀
> Image guided surgery (IGS) ◀
> Imageless navigation ◀

> Code also diagnostic or therapeutic procedure ◀

> **Excludes**   *sterotactic frame application only (93.59)* ◀

00.31   Computer assisted surgery with CT/CTA ◀

00.32   Computer assisted surgery with MR/MRA ◀

● **Use Additional Digit(s)**   ✖ **Valid O.R. Procedure**   ◀ **New**   ◀▥ **Revised**

00.33 Computer assisted surgery with fluoroscopy ◄

00.34 Imageless computer assisted surgery ◄

00.35 Computer assisted surgery with multiple datasets ◄

00.39 Other computer assisted surgery ◄
Computer assisted surgery NOS ◄

● 00.5 Other cardiovascular procedures

✖ 00.50 Implantation of cardiac resynchronization pacemaker without mention of defibrillation, total system [CRT-P]
Biventricular pacing without internal cardiac defibrillator
Implantation of cardiac resynchronization (biventricular) pulse generator pacing device, formation of pocket, transvenous leads including placement of lead into left ventricular coronary venous system, and intraoperative procedures for evaluation of lead signals.

Excludes *implantation of cardiac resynchronization defibrillator, total system [CRT-D] (00.51)*
insertion or replacement of any type pacemaker device (37.80–37.87)
replacement of cardiac resynchronization defibrillator pulse generator only [CRT-D] (00.54)
replacement of cardiac resynchronization pacemaker pulse generator only [CRT-P] (00.53)

✖ 00.51 Implantation of cardiac resynchronization defibrillator, total system [CRT-D]
Biventricular pacing with internal cardiac defibrillator
Implantation of a cardiac resynchronization (biventricular) pulse generator with defibrillator [AICD], formation of pocket, transvenous leads, including placement of lead into left ventricular coronary venous system, intraoperative procedures for evaluation of lead signals, and obtaining defibrillator threshold measurements.

Excludes *implantation of cardiac resynchronization pacemaker, total system [CRT-P] (00.50)*
implantation or replacement of automatic cardioverter/defibrillator, total system [AICD] (37.94)
replacement of cardiac resynchronization defibrillator pulse generator, only [CRT-D] (00.54)

✖ 00.52 Implantation or replacement of transvenous lead [electrode] into left ventricular coronary venous system

Excludes *implantation of cardiac resynchronization defibrillator, total system [CRT-D] (00.51)*
implantation of cardiac resynchronization pacemaker, total system [CRT-P] (00.50)
initial insertion of transvenous lead [electrode] (37.70–37.72)
replacement of transvenous atrial and/or ventricular lead(s) [electrodes] (37.76)

✖ 00.53 Implantation or replacement of cardiac resynchronization pacemaker pulse generator only [CRT-P]
Implantation of CRT-P device with removal of any existing CRT-P or other pacemaker device

Excludes *implantation of cardiac resynchronization pacemaker, total system [CRT-P] (00.50)*
implantation or replacement of cardiac resynchronization defibrillator pulse generator only [CRT-D] (00.54)
insertion or replacement of any type pacemaker device (37.80–37.87)

✖ 00.54 Implantation or replacement of cardiac resynchronization defibrillator pulse generator device only [CRT-D]
Implantation of CRT-D device with removal of any existing CRT-D, CRT-P, pacemaker, or defibrillator device

Excludes *implantation of automatic cardioverter/defibrillator pulse generator only (37.96)*
implantation of cardiac resynchronization defibrillator, total system [CRT-D] (00.51)
implantation or replacement of cardiac resynchronization pacemaker pulse generator only [CRT-P] (00.53)

00.55 Insertion of drug-eluting peripheral vessel stent(s) ◄▥
Endograft(s)
Endovascular graft(s)
Stent grafts

Code also any angioplasty or atherectomy of other non-coronary vessel(s) (39.50) ◄▥

Excludes *drug-coated peripheral stents, e.g., heparin coated (39.90)*
insertion of cerebrovascular stent(s) (00.63–00.65) ◄
insertion of drug-eluting coronary artery stent (36.07)
insertion of non-drug-eluting stent(s):
coronary artery (36.06)
peripheral vessel (39.90) ◄▥
that for aneurysm repair (39.71–39.79)

● 00.6 Procedures on blood vessels ◄

Excludes *angioplasty or atherectomy of other non-coronary vessel(s) (39.50)* ◄
insertion of coronary artery stent(s) (36.06–36.07)
insertion of drug-eluting peripheral vessel stent(s) (00.55)
insertion of non-drug-eluting peripheral vessel stent(s) (39.90) ◄

00.61 Percutaneous angioplasty or atherectomy of precerebral (extracranial) vessel(s) ◄
Basilar ◄
Carotid ◄
Vertebral ◄

Code also any: ◄
injection or infusion of thrombolytic agent (99.10) ◄
percutaneous insertion of carotid artery stent(s) (00.63) ◄
percutaneous insertion of other precerebral artery stent(s) (00.64) ◄

Excludes *angioplasty or atherectomy of other non-coronary vessel(s) (39.50)* ◄
removal of cerebrovascular obstruction of vessel(s) by open approach (38.01–38.02, 38.11–38.12, 38.31–38.32, 38.41–38.42) ◄

00.62 Percutaneous angioplasty or atherectomy of intracranial vessel(s) ◄

Code also any: ◄
injection or infusion of thrombolytic agent (99.10) ◄
percutaneous insertion of intracranial stent(s) (00.65) ◄

Excludes *angioplasty or atherectomy of other non-coronary vessel(s) (39.50)* ◄
removal of cerebrovascular obstruction of vessel(s) by open approach (38.01–38.02, 38.11–38.12, 38.31–38.32, 38.41–38.42) ◄

00.63 Percutaneous insertion of carotid artery stent(s) ◀

    Includes the use of any embolic protection device, distal protection device, filter device, or stent delivery system ◀

    Non-drug-eluting stents ◀

    Code also percutaneous angioplasty or atherectomy of precerebral vessel(s) (00.61) ◀

00.64 Percutaneous insertion of other precerebral (extracranial) artery stent(s) ◀

    Includes the use of any embolic protection device, distal protection device, filter device, or stent delivery system ◀

    Basilar stent ◀
    Vertebral stent ◀

    Code also percutaneous angioplasty or atherectomy of precerebral vessel(s) (00.61) ◀

00.65 Percutaneous insertion of intracranial vascular stent(s) ◀

    Includes the use of any embolic protection device, distal protection device, filter device, or stent delivery system ◀

    Code also percutaneous angioplasty or atherectomy of intracranial vessel(s) (00.62) ◀

● **00.9 Other procedures and interventions** ◀

00.91 Transplant from live related donor ◀

    Code also organ transplant procedure ◀

00.92 Transplant from live non-related donor ◀

    Code also organ transplant procedure ◀

00.93 Transplant from cadaver ◀

    Code also organ transplant procedure ◀

1. OPERATIONS ON THE NERVOUS SYSTEM (01–05)

● 01 Incision and excision of skull, brain, and cerebral meninges

● 01.0 Cranial puncture

01.01 Cisternal puncture
Cisternal tap

Excludes *pneumocisternogram (87.02)*

01.02 Ventriculopuncture through previously implanted catheter
Puncture of ventricular shunt tubing

01.09 Other cranial puncture
Aspiration of:
subarachnoid space
subdural space
Cranial aspiration NOS
Puncture of anterior fontanel
Subdural tap (through fontanel)

● 01.1 Diagnostic procedures on skull, brain, and cerebral meninges

01.11 Closed [percutaneous] [needle] biopsy of cerebral meninges
Burr hole approach

✖ 01.12 Open biopsy of cerebral meninges

01.13 Closed [percutaneous] [needle] biopsy of brain
Burr hole approach
Stereotactic method

✖ 01.14 Open biopsy of brain

✖ 01.15 Biopsy of skull

✖ 01.18 Other diagnostic procedures on brain and cerebral meninges

Excludes *cerebral:*
arteriography (88.41)
thermography (88.81)
contrast radiogram of brain (87.01–87.02)
echoencephalogram (88.71)
electroencephalogram (89.14)
microscopic examination of specimen from nervous system and of spinal fluid (90.01–90.09)
neurologic examination (89.13)
phlebography of head and neck (88.61)
pneumoencephalogram (87.01)
radioisotope scan:
cerebral (92.11)
head NEC (92.12)
tomography of head:
C.A.T. scan (87.03)
other (87.04)

✖ 01.19 Other diagnostic procedures on skull

Excludes *transillumination of skull (89.16)*
x-ray of skull (87.17)

● 01.2 Craniotomy and craniectomy

Excludes *decompression of skull fracture (02.02)*
exploration of orbit (16.01–16.09)
that as operative approach—omit code

✖ 01.21 Incision and drainage of cranial sinus

✖ 01.22 Removal of intracranial neurostimulator lead(s) ◀▦

Code also any removal of neurostimulator pulse generator (86.05) ◀

Excludes *removal with synchronous replacement (02.93)*

✖ 01.23 Reopening of craniotomy site

✖ 01.24 Other craniotomy
Cranial:
decompression
exploration
trephination
Craniotomy NOS
Craniotomy with removal of:
epidural abscess
extradural hematoma
foreign body of skull

Excludes *removal of foreign body with incision into brain (01.39)*

✖ 01.25 Other craniectomy
Debridement of skull NOS
Sequestrectomy of skull

Excludes *debridement of compound fracture of skull (02.02)*
strip craniectomy (02.01)

● 01.3 Incision of brain and cerebral meninges

✖ 01.31 Incision of cerebral meninges
Drainage of:
intracranial hygroma
subarachnoid abscess (cerebral)
subdural empyema

✖ 01.32 Lobotomy and tractotomy
Division of:
brain tissue
cerebral tracts
Percutaneous (radiofrequency) cingulotomy

✖ 01.39 Other incision of brain
Amygdalohippocampotomy
Drainage of intracerebral hematoma
Incision of brain NOS

Excludes *division of cortical adhesions (02.91)*

● 01.4 Operations on thalamus and globus pallidus

✖ 01.41 Operations on thalamus
Chemothalamectomy
Thalamotomy

Excludes *that by stereotactic radiosurgery (92.30–92.39)*

✖ 01.42 Operations on globus pallidus
Pallidoansectomy
Pallidotomy

Excludes *that by stereotactic radiosurgery (92.30–92.39)*

● 01.5 Other excision or destruction of brain and meninges

✖ 01.51 Excision of lesion or tissue of cerebral meninges
Decortication of (cerebral) meninges
Resection of (cerebral) meninges
Stripping of subdural membrane of (cerebral) meninges

Excludes *biopsy of cerebral meninges (01.11–01.12)*

✖ 01.52 Hemispherectomy

✖ 01.53 Lobectomy of brain

✖ 01.59 Other excision or destruction of lesion or tissue of brain
Curettage of brain
Debridement of brain
Marsupialization of brain cyst
Transtemporal (mastoid) excision of brain tumor

Excludes *biopsy of brain (01.13–01.14)*
that by stereotactic radiosurgery (92.30–92.39)

�ख़ **01.6 Excision of lesion of skull**
Removal of granulation tissue of cranium

> Excludes   *biopsy of skull (01.15)*
> *sequestrectomy (01.25)*

● **02 Other operations on skull, brain, and cerebral meninges**

   ● **02.0 Cranioplasty**

> Excludes   *that with synchronous repair of encephalocele*
> *(02.12)*

     ✗ **02.01 Opening of cranial suture**
Linear craniectomy
Strip craniectomy

     ✗ **02.02 Elevation of skull fracture fragments**
Debridement of compound fracture of skull
Decompression of skull fracture
Reduction of skull fracture

Code also any synchronous debridement of brain (01.59)

> Excludes   *debridement of skull NOS (01.25)*
> *removal of granulation tissue of cranium (01.6)*

     ✗ **02.03 Formation of cranial bone flap**
Repair of skull with flap

     ✗ **02.04 Bone graft to skull**
Pericranial graft (autogenous) (heterogenous)

     ✗ **02.05 Insertion of skull plate**
Replacement of skull plate

     ✗ **02.06 Other cranial osteoplasty**
Repair of skull NOS
Revision of bone flap of skull

     ✗ **02.07 Removal of skull plate**

> Excludes   *removal with synchronous replacement (02.05)*

   ● **02.1 Repair of cerebral meninges**

> Excludes   *marsupialization of cerebral lesion (01.59)*

     ✗ **02.11 Simple suture of dura mater of brain**

     ✗ **02.12 Other repair of cerebral meninges**
Closure of fistula of cerebrospinal fluid
Dural graft
Repair of encephalocele including synchronous cranioplasty
Repair of meninges NOS
Subdural patch

     ✗ **02.13 Ligation of meningeal vessel**
Ligation of:
longitudinal sinus
middle meningeal artery

     ✗ **02.14 Choroid plexectomy**
Cauterization of choroid plexus

   ✗ **02.2 Ventriculostomy**
Anastomosis of ventricle to:
cervical subarachnoid space
cisterna magna
Insertion of Holter valve
Ventriculocisternal intubation

   ● **02.3 Extracranial ventricular shunt**

   Includes: that with insertion of valve

     ✗ **02.31 Ventricular shunt to structure in head and neck**
Ventricle to nasopharynx shunt
Ventriculomastoid anastomosis

     ✗ **02.32 Ventricular shunt to circulatory system**
Ventriculoatrial anastomosis
Ventriculocaval shunt

     ✗ **02.33 Ventricular shunt to thoracic cavity**
Ventriculopleural anastomosis

     ✗ **02.34 Ventricular shunt to abdominal cavity and organs**
Ventriculocholecystostomy
Ventriculoperitoneostomy

     ✗ **02.35 Ventricular shunt to urinary system**
Ventricle to ureter shunt

     ✗ **02.39 Other operations to establish drainage of ventricle**
Ventricle to bone marrow shunt
Ventricular shunt to extracranial site NEC

   ● **02.4 Revision, removal, and irrigation of ventricular shunt**

> Excludes   *revision of distal catheter of ventricular shunt (54.95)*

     02.41 Irrigation and exploration of ventricular shunt
Exploration of ventriculoperitoneal shunt at ventricular site
Re-programming of ventriculoperitoneal shunt

     ✗ **02.42 Replacement of ventricular shunt**
Reinsertion of Holter valve
Replacement of ventricular catheter
Revision of ventriculoperitoneal shunt at ventricular site

     ✗ **02.43 Removal of ventricular shunt**

   ● **02.9 Other operations on skull, brain, and cerebral meninges**

> Excludes   *operations on:*
> *pineal gland (07.17, 07.51–07.59)*
> *pituitary gland [hypophysis] (07.13–07.15,*
> *07.61–07.79)*

     ✗ **02.91 Lysis of cortical adhesions**

     ✗ **02.92 Repair of brain**

     ✗ **02.93 Implantation or replacement of intracranial neurostimulator lead(s)** ◀▥
Implantation, insertion, placement, or replacement of intracranial:
brain pacemaker [neuropacemaker]
depth electrodes
epidural pegs
electroencephalographic receiver
foramen ovale electrodes
intracranial electrostimulator
subdural grids
subdural strips

Code also any insertion of neurostimulator pulse generator (86.94–86.96) ◀

     ✗ **02.94 Insertion or replacement of skull tongs or halo traction device**

     02.95 Removal of skull tongs or halo traction device

     02.96 Insertion of sphenoidal electrodes

     ✗ **02.99 Other**

> Excludes   *chemical shock therapy (94.24)*
> *electroshock therapy:*
> *subconvulsive (94.26)*
> *other (94.27)*

● **03 Operations on spinal cord and spinal canal structures**
Code also any application or administration of an adhesion barrier substance (99.77)

   ● **03.0 Exploration and decompression of spinal canal structures**

     ✗ **03.01 Removal of foreign body from spinal canal**

     ✗ **03.02 Reopening of laminectomy site**

✖ 03.09 Other exploration and decompression of spinal canal
Decompression:
  laminectomy
  laminotomy
Expansile laminoplasty
Exploration of spinal nerve root
Foraminotomy
> **Excludes** *drainage of spinal fluid by anastomosis (03.71–03.79)*
> *laminectomy with excision of intervertebral disc (80.51)*
> *spinal tap (03.31)*
> *that as operative approach—omit code*

✖ 03.1 Division of intraspinal nerve root
Rhizotomy

● 03.2 Chordotomy

✖ 03.21 Percutaneous chordotomy
Stereotactic chordotomy

✖ 03.29 Other chordotomy
Chordotomy NOS
Tractotomy (one-stage) (two-stage) of spinal cord
Transection of spinal cord tracts

● 03.3 Diagnostic procedures on spinal cord and spinal canal structures

03.31 Spinal tap
Lumbar puncture for removal of dye
> **Excludes** *lumbar puncture for injection of dye [myelogram] (87.21)*

✖ 03.32 Biopsy of spinal cord or spinal meninges

✖ 03.39 Other diagnostic procedures on spinal cord and spinal canal structures
> **Excludes** *microscopic examination of specimen from nervous system or of spinal fluid (90.01–90.09)*
> *x-ray of spine (87.21–87.29)*

✖ 03.4 Excision or destruction of lesion of spinal cord or spinal meninges
Curettage of spinal cord or spinal meninges
Debridement of spinal cord or spinal meninges
Marsupialization of cyst of spinal cord or spinal meninges
Resection of spinal cord or spinal meninges
> **Excludes** *biopsy of spinal cord or meninges (03.32)*

● 03.5 Plastic operations on spinal cord structures

✖ 03.51 Repair of spinal meningocele
Repair of meningocele NOS

✖ 03.52 Repair of spinal myelomeningocele

✖ 03.53 Repair of vertebral fracture
Elevation of spinal bone fragments
Reduction of fracture of vertebrae
Removal of bony spicules from spinal canal
> **Excludes** *kyphoplasty (78.49)*
> *vertebroplasty (78.49)*

✖ 03.59 Other repair and plastic operations on spinal cord structures
Repair of:
  diastematomyelia
  spina bifida NOS
  spinal cord NOS
  spinal meninges NOS
  vertebral arch defect

✖ 03.6 Lysis of adhesions of spinal cord and nerve roots

● 03.7 Shunt of spinal theca
Includes: that with valve

✖ 03.71 Spinal subarachnoid-peritoneal shunt

✖ 03.72 Spinal subarachnoid-ureteral shunt

✖ 03.79 Other shunt of spinal theca
Lumbar-subarachnoid shunt NOS
Pleurothecal anastomosis
Salpingothecal anastomosis

03.8 Injection of destructive agent into spinal canal

● 03.9 Other operations on spinal cord and spinal canal structures

03.90 Insertion of catheter into spinal canal for infusion of therapeutic or palliative substances
Insertion of catheter into epidural, subarachnoid, or subdural space of spine with intermittent or continuous infusion of drug (with creation of any reservoir)
Code also any implantation of infusion pump (86.06)

03.91 Injection of anesthetic into spinal canal for analgesia
> **Excludes** *that for operative anesthesia—omit code*

03.92 Injection of other agent into spinal canal
Intrathecal injection of steroid
Subarachnoid perfusion of refrigerated saline
> **Excludes** *injection of:*
> *contrast material for myelogram (87.21)*
> *destructive agent into spinal canal (03.8)*

✖ 03.93 Implantation or replacement of spinal neurostimulator lead(s) ◀━
Code also any insertion of neurostimulator pulse generator (86.94–86.96) ◀

✖ 03.94 Removal of spinal neurostimulator lead(s) ◀━
Code also any removal of neurostimulator pulse generator (86.05) ◀

03.95 Spinal blood patch

03.96 Percutaneous denervation of facet

✖ 03.97 Revision of spinal thecal shunt

✖ 03.98 Removal of spinal thecal shunt

✖ 03.99 Other

● 04 Operations on cranial and peripheral nerves

● 04.0 Incision, division, and excision of cranial and peripheral nerves
> **Excludes** *opticociliary neurectomy (12.79)*
> *sympathetic ganglionectomy (05.21–05.29)*

✖ 04.01 Excision of acoustic neuroma
That by craniotomy
> **Excludes** *that by stereotactic radiosurgery (92.3)*

✖ 04.02 Division of trigeminal nerve
Retrogasserian neurotomy

✖ 04.03 Division or crushing of other cranial and peripheral nerves
> **Excludes** *that of:*
> *glossopharyngeal nerve (29.92)*
> *laryngeal nerve (31.91)*
> *nerves to adrenal glands (07.42)*
> *phrenic nerve for collapse of lung (33.31)*
> *vagus nerve (44.00–44.03)*

✖ 04.04 Other incision of cranial and peripheral nerves

✖ 04.05 Gasserian ganglionectomy

✖ 04.06 Other cranial or peripheral ganglionectomy
> **Excludes** *sympathetic ganglionectomy (05.21–05.29)*

✖ 04.07　Other excision or avulsion of cranial and peripheral nerves
> Curettage of peripheral nerve
> Debridement of peripheral nerve
> Resection of peripheral nerve
> Excision of peripheral neuroma [Morton's]

> | Excludes | biopsy of cranial or peripheral nerve (04.11–04.12) |

● 04.1　Diagnostic procedures on peripheral nervous system

04.11　Closed [percutaneous] [needle] biopsy of cranial or peripheral nerve or ganglion

✖ 04.12　Open biopsy of cranial or peripheral nerve or ganglion

✖ 04.19　Other diagnostic procedures on cranial and peripheral nerves and ganglia

> | Excludes | microscopic examination of specimen from nervous system (90.01–90.09) |
> | | neurologic examination (89.13) |

04.2　Destruction of cranial and peripheral nerves
> Destruction of cranial or peripheral nerves by:
> cryoanalgesia
> injection of neurolytic agent
> radiofrequency
> Radiofrequency ablation

✖ 04.3　Suture of cranial and peripheral nerves

● 04.4　Lysis of adhesions and decompression of cranial and peripheral nerves

✖ 04.41　Decompression of trigeminal nerve root

✖ 04.42　Other cranial nerve decompression

✖ 04.43　Release of carpal tunnel

✖ 04.44　Release of tarsal tunnel

✖ 04.49　Other peripheral nerve or ganglion decompression or lysis of adhesions
> Peripheral nerve neurolysis NOS

✖ 04.5　Cranial or peripheral nerve graft

✖ 04.6　Transposition of cranial and peripheral nerves
> Nerve transplantation

● 04.7　Other cranial or peripheral neuroplasty

✖ 04.71　Hypoglossal-facial anastomosis

✖ 04.72　Accessory-facial anastomosis

✖ 04.73　Accessory-hypoglossal anastomosis

✖ 04.74　Other anastomosis of cranial or peripheral nerve

✖ 04.75　Revision of previous repair of cranial and peripheral nerves

✖ 04.76　Repair of old traumatic injury of cranial and peripheral nerves

✖ 04.79　Other neuroplasty

● 04.8　Injection into peripheral nerve

> | Excludes | destruction of nerve (by injection of neurolytic agent) (04.2) |

04.80　Peripheral nerve injection, not otherwise specified

04.81　Injection of anesthetic into peripheral nerve for analgesia

> | Excludes | that for operative anesthesia—omit code |

04.89　Injection of other agent, except neurolytic

> | Excludes | injection of neurolytic agent (04.2) |

● 04.9　Other operations on cranial and peripheral nerves

✖ 04.91　Neurectasis

✖ 04.92　Implantation or replacement of peripheral neurostimulator lead(s)　◀▥

> Code also any insertion of neurostimulator pulse generator (86.94–86.96)　◀

✖ 04.93　Removal of peripheral neurostimulator lead(s)　◀▥

> Code also any removal of neurostimulator pulse generator (86.05)　◀

✖ 04.99　Other

● 05　Operations on sympathetic nerves or ganglia

> | Excludes | paracervical uterine denervation (69.3) |

✖ 05.0　Division of sympathetic nerve or ganglion

> | Excludes | that of nerves to adrenal glands (07.42) |

● 05.1　Diagnostic procedures on sympathetic nerves or ganglia

✖ 05.11　Biopsy of sympathetic nerve or ganglion

✖ 05.19　Other diagnostic procedures on sympathetic nerves or ganglia

● 05.2　Sympathectomy

✖ 05.21　Sphenopalatine ganglionectomy

✖ 05.22　Cervical sympathectomy

✖ 05.23　Lumbar sympathectomy

✖ 05.24　Presacral sympathectomy

✖ 05.25　Periarterial sympathectomy

✖ 05.29　Other sympathectomy and ganglionectomy
> Excision or avulsion of sympathetic nerve NOS
> Sympathetic ganglionectomy NOS

> | Excludes | biopsy of sympathetic nerve or ganglion (05.11) |
> | | opticociliary neurectomy (12.79) |
> | | periarterial sympathectomy (05.25) |
> | | tympanosympathectomy (20.91) |

● 05.3　Injection into sympathetic nerve or ganglion

> | Excludes | injection of ciliary sympathetic ganglion (12.79) |

05.31　Injection of anesthetic into sympathetic nerve for analgesia

05.32　Injection of neurolytic agent into sympathetic nerve

05.39　Other injection into sympathetic nerve or ganglion

● 05.8　Other operations on sympathetic nerves or ganglia

✖ 05.81　Repair of sympathetic nerve or ganglion

✖ 05.89　Other

✖ 05.9　Other operations on nervous system

---

2.   OPERATIONS ON THE ENDOCRINE SYSTEM (06–07)

● **06**   **Operations on thyroid and parathyroid glands**

> **Includes:** incidental resection of hyoid bone

06.0   **Incision of thyroid field**

> **Excludes**   *division of isthmus (06.91)*

06.01   **Aspiration of thyroid field**
> Percutaneous or needle drainage of thyroid field

> **Excludes**   *aspiration biopsy of thyroid (06.11)*
> *drainage by incision (06.09)*
> *postoperative aspiration of field (06.02)*

✖ **06.02**   **Reopening of wound of thyroid field**
> Reopening of wound of thyroid field for:
> control of (postoperative) hemorrhage
> examination
> exploration
> removal of hematoma

✖ **06.09**   **Other incision of thyroid field**
> Drainage of hematoma by incision
> Drainage of thyroglossal tract by incision
> Exploration:
> neck by incision
> thyroid (field) by incision
> Removal of foreign body by incision
> Thyroidotomy NOS by incision

> **Excludes**   *postoperative exploration (06.02)*
> *removal of hematoma by aspiration (06.01)*

● **06.1**   **Diagnostic procedures on thyroid and parathyroid glands**

06.11   **Closed [percutaneous] [needle] biopsy of thyroid gland**
> Aspiration biopsy of thyroid

✖ **06.12**   **Open biopsy of thyroid gland**

✖ **06.13**   **Biopsy of parathyroid gland**

✖ **06.19**   **Other diagnostic procedures on thyroid and parathyroid glands**

> **Excludes**   *radioisotope scan of:*
> *parathyroid (92.13)*
> *thyroid (92.01)*
> *soft tissue x-ray of thyroid field (87.09)*

✖ **06.2**   **Unilateral thyroid lobectomy**
> Complete removal of one lobe of thyroid (with removal of isthmus or portion of other lobe)
> Hemithyroidectomy

> **Excludes**   *partial substernal thyroidectomy (06.51)*

● **06.3**   **Other partial thyroidectomy**

✖ **06.31**   **Excision of lesion of thyroid**
> **Excludes**   *biopsy of thyroid (06.11–06.12)*

✖ **06.39**   **Other**
> Isthmectomy
> Partial thyroidectomy NOS
> **Excludes**   *partial substernal thyroidectomy (06.51)*

✖ **06.4**   **Complete thyroidectomy**
> **Excludes**   *complete substernal thyroidectomy (06.52)*
> *that with laryngectomy (30.3–30.4)*

● **06.5**   **Substernal thyroidectomy**

✖ **06.50**   **Substernal thyroidectomy, not otherwise specified**

✖ **06.51**   **Partial substernal thyroidectomy**

✖ **06.52**   **Complete substernal thyroidectomy**

✖ **06.6**   **Excision of lingual thyroid**
> Excision of thyroid by:
> submental route
> transoral route

✖ **06.7**   **Excision of thyroglossal duct or tract**

● **06.8**   **Parathyroidectomy**

✖ **06.81**   **Complete parathyroidectomy**

✖ **06.89**   **Other parathyroidectomy**
> Parathyroidectomy NOS
> Partial parathyroidectomy

> **Excludes**   *biopsy of parathyroid (06.13)*

● **06.9**   **Other operations on thyroid (region) and parathyroid**

✖ **06.91**   **Division of thyroid isthmus**
> Transection of thyroid isthmus

✖ **06.92**   **Ligation of thyroid vessels**

✖ **06.93**   **Suture of thyroid gland**

✖ **06.94**   **Thyroid tissue reimplantation**
> Autotransplantation of thyroid tissue

✖ **06.95**   **Parathyroid tissue reimplantation**
> Autotransplantation of parathyroid tissue

✖ **06.98**   **Other operations on thyroid glands**

✖ **06.99**   **Other operations on parathyroid glands**

● **07**   **Operations on other endocrine glands**

> **Includes:** operations on:
> adrenal glands
> pineal gland
> pituitary gland
> thymus

> **Excludes**   *operations on:*
> *aortic and carotid bodies (39.8)*
> *ovaries (65.0–65.99)*
> *pancreas (52.01–52.99)*
> *testes (62.0–62.99)*

● **07.0**   **Exploration of adrenal field**
> **Excludes**   *incision of adrenal (gland) (07.41)*

✖ **07.00**   **Exploration of adrenal field, not otherwise specified**

✖ **07.01**   **Unilateral exploration of adrenal field**

✖ **07.02**   **Bilateral exploration of adrenal field**

● **07.1**   **Diagnostic procedures on adrenal glands, pituitary gland, pineal gland, and thymus**

07.11   **Closed [percutaneous] [needle] biopsy of adrenal gland**

✖ **07.12**   **Open biopsy of adrenal gland**

✖ **07.13**   **Biopsy of pituitary gland, transfrontal approach**

✖ **07.14**   **Biopsy of pituitary gland, transsphenoidal approach**

✖ **07.15**   **Biopsy of pituitary gland, unspecified approach**

✖ **07.16**   **Biopsy of thymus**

✖ **07.17**   **Biopsy of pineal gland**

✖ **07.19**   **Other diagnostic procedures on adrenal glands, pituitary gland, pineal gland, and thymus**

> **Excludes**   *microscopic examination of specimen from endocrine gland (90.11–90.19)*
> *radioisotope scan of pituitary gland (92.11)*

● **07.2**   **Partial adrenalectomy**

✖ **07.21**   **Excision of lesion of adrenal gland**
> **Excludes**   *biopsy of adrenal gland (07.11–07.12)*

✖ **07.22 Unilateral adrenalectomy**
Adrenalectomy NOS

Excludes *excision of remaining adrenal gland (07.3)*

✖ **07.29 Other partial adrenalectomy**
Partial adrenalectomy NOS

✖ **07.3 Bilateral adrenalectomy**
Excision of remaining adrenal gland

Excludes *bilateral partial adrenalectomy (07.29)*

● **07.4 Other operations on adrenal glands, nerves, and vessels**

✖ **07.41 Incision of adrenal gland**
Adrenalotomy (with drainage)

✖ **07.42 Division of nerves to adrenal glands**

✖ **07.43 Ligation of adrenal vessels**

✖ **07.44 Repair of adrenal gland**

✖ **07.45 Reimplantation of adrenal tissue**
Autotransplantation of adrenal tissue

✖ **07.49 Other**

● **07.5 Operations on pineal gland**

✖ **07.51 Exploration of pineal field**

Excludes *that with incision of pineal gland (07.52)*

✖ **07.52 Incision of pineal gland**

✖ **07.53 Partial excision of pineal gland**

Excludes *biopsy of pineal gland (07.17)*

✖ **07.54 Total excision of pineal gland**
Pinealectomy (complete) (total)

✖ **07.59 Other operations on pineal gland**

● **07.6 Hypophysectomy**

✖ **07.61 Partial excision of pituitary gland, transfrontal approach**
Cryohypophysectomy, partial transfrontal approach
Division of hypophyseal stalk transfrontal approach
Excision of lesion of pituitary [hypophysis] transfrontal approach
Hypophysectomy, subtotal transfrontal approach
Infundibulectomy, hypophyseal transfrontal approach

Excludes *biopsy of pituitary gland, transfrontal approach (07.13)*

✖ **07.62 Partial excision of pituitary gland, transsphenoidal approach**

Excludes *biopsy of pituitary gland, transsphenoidal approach (07.14)*

✖ **07.63 Partial excision of pituitary gland, unspecified approach**

Excludes *biopsy of pituitary gland NOS (07.15)*

✖ **07.64 Total excision of pituitary gland, transfrontal approach**
Ablation of pituitary by implantation (strontium-yttrium) (Y) transfrontal approach
Cryohypophysectomy, complete transfrontal approach

✖ **07.65 Total excision of pituitary gland, transsphenoidal approach**

✖ **07.68 Total excision of pituitary gland, other specified approach**

✖ **07.69 Total excision of pituitary gland, unspecified approach**
Hypophysectomy NOS
Pituitectomy NOS

● **07.7 Other operations on hypophysis**

✖ **07.71 Exploration of pituitary fossa**

Excludes *exploration with incision of pituitary gland (07.72)*

✖ **07.72 Incision of pituitary gland**
Aspiration of:
craniobuccal pouch
craniopharyngioma
hypophysis
pituitary gland
Rathke's pouch

✖ **07.79 Other**
Insertion of pack into sella turcica

● **07.8 Thymectomy**

✖ **07.80 Thymectomy, not otherwise specified**

✖ **07.81 Partial excision of thymus**

Excludes *biopsy of thymus (07.16)*

✖ **07.82 Total excision of thymus**

● **07.9 Other operations on thymus**

✖ **07.91 Exploration of thymus field**

Excludes *exploration with incision of thymus (07.92)*

✖ **07.92 Incision of thymus**

✖ **07.93 Repair of thymus**

✖ **07.94 Transplantation of thymus**

✖ **07.99 Other**
Thymopexy

3.   OPERATIONS ON THE EYE (08–16)

● 08 Operations on eyelids

    Includes: operations on the eyebrow

  ● 08.0 Incision of eyelid

    08.01 Incision of lid margin

    08.02 Severing of blepharorrhaphy

    08.09 Other incision of eyelid

  ● 08.1 Diagnostic procedures on eyelid

    ✖ 08.11 Biopsy of eyelid

    08.19 Other diagnostic procedures on eyelid

  ● 08.2 Excision or destruction of lesion or tissue of eyelid

    Code also any synchronous reconstruction (08.61–08.74)

    Excludes *biopsy of eyelid (08.11)*

    ✖ 08.20 Removal of lesion of eyelid, not otherwise specified

      Removal of meibomian gland NOS

    ✖ 08.21 Excision of chalazion

    ✖ 08.22 Excision of other minor lesion of eyelid

      Excision of:

        verucca

        wart

    ✖ 08.23 Excision of major lesion of eyelid, partial-thickness

      Excision involving one-fourth or more of lid margin, partial-thickness

    ✖ 08.24 Excision of major lesion of eyelid, full-thickness

      Excision involving one-fourth or more of lid margin, full-thickness

      Wedge resection of eyelid

    ✖ 08.25 Destruction of lesion of eyelid

  ● 08.3 Repair of blepharoptosis and lid retraction

    ✖ 08.31 Repair of blepharoptosis by frontalis muscle technique with suture

    ✖ 08.32 Repair of blepharoptosis by frontalis muscle technique with fascial sling

    ✖ 08.33 Repair of blepharoptosis by resection or advancement of levator muscle or aponeurosis

    ✖ 08.34 Repair of blepharoptosis by other levator muscle techniques

    ✖ 08.35 Repair of blepharoptosis by tarsal technique

    ✖ 08.36 Repair of blepharoptosis by other techniques

      Correction of eyelid ptosis NOS

      Orbicularis oculi muscle sling for correction of blepharoptosis

    ✖ 08.37 Reduction of overcorrection of ptosis

    ✖ 08.38 Correction of lid retraction

  ● 08.4 Repair of entropion or ectropion

    ✖ 08.41 Repair of entropion or ectropion by thermocauterization

    ✖ 08.42 Repair of entropion or ectropion by suture technique

    ✖ 08.43 Repair of entropion or ectropion with wedge resection

    ✖ 08.44 Repair of entropion or ectropion with lid reconstruction

    ✖ 08.49 Other repair of entropion or ectropion

  ● 08.5 Other adjustment of lid position

    ✖ 08.51 Canthotomy

      Enlargement of palpebral fissure

    ✖ 08.52 Blepharorrhaphy

      Canthorrhaphy

      Tarsorrhaphy

    ✖ 08.59 Other

      Canthoplasty NOS

      Repair of epicanthal fold

  ● 08.6 Reconstruction of eyelid with flaps or grafts

    Excludes *that associated with repair of entropion and ectropion (08.44)*

    ✖ 08.61 Reconstruction of eyelid with skin flap or graft

    ✖ 08.62 Reconstruction of eyelid with mucous membrane flap or graft

    ✖ 08.63 Reconstruction of eyelid with hair follicle graft

    ✖ 08.64 Reconstruction of eyelid with tarsoconjunctival flap

      Transfer of tarsoconjunctival flap from opposing lid

    ✖ 08.69 Other reconstruction of eyelid with flaps or grafts

  ● 08.7 Other reconstruction of eyelid

    Excludes *that associated with repair of entropion and ectropion (08.44)*

    ✖ 08.70 Reconstruction of eyelid, not otherwise specified

    ✖ 08.71 Reconstruction of eyelid involving lid margin, partial-thickness

    ✖ 08.72 Other reconstruction of eyelid, partial-thickness

    ✖ 08.73 Reconstruction of eyelid involving lid margin, full-thickness

    ✖ 08.74 Other reconstruction of eyelid, full-thickness

  ● 08.8 Other repair of eyelid

    08.81 Linear repair of laceration of eyelid or eyebrow

    08.82 Repair of laceration involving lid margin, partial-thickness

    08.83 Other repair of laceration of eyelid, partial-thickness

    08.84 Repair of laceration involving lid margin, full-thickness

    08.85 Other repair of laceration of eyelid, full-thickness

    08.86 Lower eyelid rhytidectomy

    08.87 Upper eyelid rhytidectomy

    08.89 Other eyelid repair

  ● 08.9 Other operations on eyelids

    ✖ 08.91 Electrosurgical epilation of eyelid

    ✖ 08.92 Cryosurgical epilation of eyelid

    ✖ 08.93 Other epilation of eyelid

    ✖ 08.99 Other

● 09 Operations on lacrimal system

  ✖ 09.0 Incision of lacrimal gland

    Incision of lacrimal cyst (with drainage)

  ● 09.1 Diagnostic procedures on lacrimal system

    ✖ 09.11 Biopsy of lacrimal gland

    ✖ 09.12 Biopsy of lacrimal sac

    ✖ 09.19 Other diagnostic procedures on lacrimal system

    Excludes *contrast dacryocystogram (87.05)*

      soft tissue x-ray of nasolacrimal duct (87.09)

● **09.2 Excision of lesion or tissue of lacrimal gland**

✳ **09.20 Excision of lacrimal gland, not otherwise specified**

✳ **09.21 Excision of lesion of lacrimal gland**

Excludes *biopsy of lacrimal gland (09.11)*

✳ **09.22 Other partial dacryoadenectomy**

Excludes *biopsy of lacrimal gland (09.11)*

✳ **09.23 Total dacryoadenectomy**

✳ **09.3 Other operations on lacrimal gland**

● **09.4 Manipulation of lacrimal passage**

Includes: removal of calculus
that with dilation

Excludes *contrast dacryocystogram (87.05)*

✳ **09.41 Probing of lacrimal punctum**

✳ **09.42 Probing of lacrimal canaliculi**

✳ **09.43 Probing of nasolacrimal duct**

Excludes *that with insertion of tube or stent (09.44)*

✳ **09.44 Intubation of nasolacrimal duct**
Insertion of stent into nasolacrimal duct

✳ **09.49 Other manipulation of lacrimal passage**

● **09.5 Incision of lacrimal sac and passages**

✳ **09.51 Incision of lacrimal punctum**

✳ **09.52 Incision of lacrimal canaliculi**

✳ **09.53 Incision of lacrimal sac**

✳ **09.59 Other incision of lacrimal passages**
Incision (and drainage) of nasolacrimal duct
NOS

✳ **09.6 Excision of lacrimal sac and passage**

Excludes *biopsy of lacrimal sac (09.12)*

● **09.7 Repair of canaliculus and punctum**

Excludes *repair of eyelid (08.81–08.89)*

✳ **09.71 Correction of everted punctum**

✳ **09.72 Other repair of punctum**

✳ **09.73 Repair of canaliculus**

● **09.8 Fistulization of lacrimal tract to nasal cavity**

✳ **09.81 Dacryocystorhinostomy [DCR]**

✳ **09.82 Conjunctivocystorhinostomy**
Conjunctivodacryocystorhinostomy [CDCR]

Excludes *that with insertion of tube or stent (09.83)*

✳ **09.83 Conjunctivorhinostomy with insertion of tube or stent**

● **09.9 Other operations on lacrimal system**

✳ **09.91 Obliteration of lacrimal punctum**

✳ **09.99 Other**

● **10 Operations on conjunctiva**

✳ **10.0 Removal of embedded foreign body from conjunctiva by incision**

Excludes *removal of:*
embedded foreign body without incision (98.22)
superficial foreign body (98.21)

✳ **10.1 Other incision of conjunctiva**

● **10.2 Diagnostic procedures on conjunctiva**

✳ **10.21 Biopsy of conjunctiva**

✳ **10.29 Other diagnostic procedures on conjunctiva**

● **10.3 Excision or destruction of lesion or tissue of conjunctiva**

✳ **10.31 Excision of lesion or tissue of conjunctiva**
Excision of ring of conjunctiva around cornea

Excludes *biopsy of conjunctiva (10.21)*

✳ **10.32 Destruction of lesion of conjunctiva**

Excludes *excision of lesion (10.31)*
thermocauterization for entropion (08.41)

✳ **10.33 Other destructive procedures on conjunctiva**
Removal of trachoma follicles

● **10.4 Conjunctivoplasty**

✳ **10.41 Repair of symblepharon with free graft**

✳ **10.42 Reconstruction of conjunctival cul-de-sac with free graft**

Excludes *revision of enucleation socket with graft (16.63)*

✳ **10.43 Other reconstruction of conjunctival cul-de-sac**

Excludes *revision of enucleation socket (16.64)*

✳ **10.44 Other free graft to conjunctiva**

✳ **10.49 Other conjunctivoplasty**

Excludes *repair of cornea with conjunctival flap (11.53)*

✳ **10.5 Lysis of adhesions of conjunctiva and eyelid**
Division of symblepharon (with insertion of conformer)

✳ **10.6 Repair of laceration of conjunctiva**

Excludes *that with repair of sclera (12.81)*

● **10.9 Other operations on conjunctiva**

✳ **10.91 Subconjunctival injection**

✳ **10.99 Other**

● **11 Operations on cornea**

✳ **11.0 Magnetic removal of embedded foreign body from cornea**

Excludes *that with incision (11.1)*

✳ **11.1 Incision of cornea**
Incision of cornea for removal of foreign body

● **11.2 Diagnostic procedures on cornea**

✳ **11.21 Scraping of cornea for smear or culture**

✳ **11.22 Biopsy of cornea**

✳ **11.29 Other diagnostic procedures on cornea**

● **11.3 Excision of pterygium**

✳ **11.31 Transposition of pterygium**

✳ **11.32 Excision of pterygium with corneal graft**

✳ **11.39 Other excision of pterygium**

● **11.4 Excision or destruction of tissue or other lesion of cornea**

✳ **11.41 Mechanical removal of corneal epithelium**
That by chemocauterization

Excludes *that for smear or culture (11.21)*

✳ **11.42 Thermocauterization of corneal lesion**

✳ **11.43 Cryotherapy of corneal lesion**

✳ **11.49 Other removal or destruction of corneal lesion**
Excision of cornea NOS

Excludes *biopsy of cornea (11.22)*

● **11.5 Repair of cornea**

✳ **11.51 Suture of corneal laceration**

✳ **11.52 Repair of postoperative wound dehiscence of cornea**

✳ **11.53 Repair of corneal laceration or wound with conjunctival flap**

✳ **11.59 Other repair of cornea**

● **11.6 Corneal transplant**

> **Excludes** *excision of pterygium with corneal graft (11.32)*

> ✖ **11.60 Corneal transplant, not otherwise specified**
> Keratoplasty NOS

> > **Note: To report donor source -** *see* codes 00.91–
> > 00.93) ◀

> ✖ **11.61 Lamellar keratoplasty with autograft**

> ✖ **11.62 Other lamellar keratoplasty**

> ✖ **11.63 Penetrating keratoplasty with autograft**
> Perforating keratoplasty with autograft

> ✖ **11.64 Other penetrating keratoplasty**
> Perforating keratoplasty (with homograft)

> ✖ **11.69 Other corneal transplant**

● **11.7 Other reconstructive and refractive surgery on cornea**

> ✖ **11.71 Keratomileusis**

> ✖ **11.72 Keratophakia**

> ✖ **11.73 Keratoprosthesis**

> ✖ **11.74 Thermokeratoplasty**

> ✖ **11.75 Radial keratotomy**

> ✖ **11.76 Epikeratophakia**

> ✖ **11.79 Other**

● **11.9 Other operations on cornea**

> ✖ **11.91 Tattooing of cornea**

> ✖ **11.92 Removal of artificial implant from cornea**

> ✖ **11.99 Other**

● **12 Operations on iris, ciliary body, sclera, and anterior chamber**

> **Excludes** *operations on cornea (11.0–11.99)*

● **12.0 Removal of intraocular foreign body from anterior segment of eye**

> ✖ **12.00 Removal of intraocular foreign body from anterior segment of eye, not otherwise specified**

> ✖ **12.01 Removal of intraocular foreign body from anterior segment of eye with use of magnet**

> ✖ **12.02 Removal of intraocular foreign body from anterior segment of eye without use of magnet**

● **12.1 Iridotomy and simple iridectomy**

> **Excludes** *iridectomy associated with:*
> *cataract extraction (13.11–13.69)*
> *removal of lesion (12.41–12.42)*
> *scleral fistulization (12.61–12.69)*

> ✖ **12.11 Iridotomy with transfixion**

> ✖ **12.12 Other iridotomy**
> Corectomy
> Discission of iris
> Iridotomy NOS

> ✖ **12.13 Excision of prolapsed iris**

> ✖ **12.14 Other iridectomy**
> Iridectomy (basal) (peripheral) (total)

● **12.2 Diagnostic procedures on iris, ciliary body, sclera, and anterior chamber**

> ✖ **12.21 Diagnostic aspiration of anterior chamber of eye**

> ✖ **12.22 Biopsy of iris**

> ✖ **12.29 Other diagnostic procedures on iris, ciliary body, sclera, and anterior chamber**

● **12.3 Iridoplasty and coreoplasty**

> ✖ **12.31 Lysis of goniosynechiae**
> Lysis of goniosynechiae by injection of air or liquid

> ✖ **12.32 Lysis of other anterior synechiae**
> Lysis of anterior synechiae:
> NOS
> by injection of air or liquid

> ✖ **12.33 Lysis of posterior synechiae**
> Lysis of iris adhesions NOS

> ✖ **12.34 Lysis of corneovitreal adhesions**

> ✖ **12.35 Coreoplasty**
> Needling of pupillary membrane

> ✖ **12.39 Other iridoplasty**

● **12.4 Excision or destruction of lesion of iris and ciliary body**

> ✖ **12.40 Removal of lesion of anterior segment of eye, not otherwise specified**

> ✖ **12.41 Destruction of lesion of iris, nonexcisional**
> Destruction of lesion of iris by:
> cauterization
> cryotherapy
> photocoagulation

> ✖ **12.42 Excision of lesion of iris**

> **Excludes** *biopsy of iris (12.22)*

> ✖ **12.43 Destruction of lesion of ciliary body, nonexcisional**

> ✖ **12.44 Excision of lesion of ciliary body**

● **12.5 Facilitation of intraocular circulation**

> ✖ **12.51 Goniopuncture without goniotomy**

> ✖ **12.52 Goniotomy without goniopuncture**

> ✖ **12.53 Goniotomy with goniopuncture**

> ✖ **12.54 Trabeculotomy ab externo**

> ✖ **12.55 Cyclodialysis**

> ✖ **12.59 Other facilitation of intraocular circulation**

● **12.6 Scleral fistulization**

> **Excludes** *exploratory sclerotomy (12.89)*

> ✖ **12.61 Trephination of sclera with iridectomy**

> ✖ **12.62 Thermocauterization of sclera with iridectomy**

> ✖ **12.63 Iridencleisis and iridotasis**

> ✖ **12.64 Trabeculectomy ab externo**

> ✖ **12.65 Other scleral fistulization with iridectomy**

> ✖ **12.66 Postoperative revision of scleral fistulization procedure**
> Revision of filtering bleb

> **Excludes** *repair of fistula (12.82)*

> ✖ **12.69 Other fistulizing procedure**

● **12.7 Other procedures for relief of elevated intraocular pressure**

> ✖ **12.71 Cyclodiathermy**

> ✖ **12.72 Cyclocryotherapy**

> ✖ **12.73 Cyclophotocoagulation**

> ✖ **12.74 Diminution of ciliary body, not otherwise specified**

> ✖ **12.79 Other glaucoma procedures**

● **12.8 Operations on sclera**

> **Excludes** *those associated with:*
> *retinal reattachment (14.41–14.59)*
> *scleral fistulization (12.61–12.69)*

> ✖ **12.81 Suture of laceration of sclera**
> Suture of sclera with synchronous repair of conjunctiva

✖ **12.82   Repair of scleral fistula**

> **Excludes**   *postoperative revision of scleral fistulization procedure (12.66)*

✖ **12.83   Revision of operative wound of anterior segment, not elsewhere classified**

> **Excludes**   *postoperative revision of scleral fistulization procedure (12.66)*

✖ **12.84   Excision or destruction of lesion of sclera**

✖ **12.85   Repair of scleral staphyloma with graft**

✖ **12.86   Other repair of scleral staphyloma**

✖ **12.87   Scleral reinforcement with graft**

✖ **12.88   Other scleral reinforcement**

✖ **12.89   Other operations on sclera**
> Exploratory sclerotomy

● **12.9   Other operations on iris, ciliary body, and anterior chamber**

✖ **12.91   Therapeutic evacuation of anterior chamber**
> Paracentesis of anterior chamber

> **Excludes**   *diagnostic aspiration (12.21)*

✖ **12.92   Injection into anterior chamber**
> Injection of:
>> air into anterior chamber
>> liquid into anterior chamber
>> medication into anterior chamber

✖ **12.93   Removal or destruction of epithelial downgrowth from anterior chamber**

> **Excludes**   *that with iridectomy (12.41–12.42)*

✖ **12.97   Other operations on iris**

✖ **12.98   Other operations on ciliary body**

✖ **12.99   Other operations on anterior chamber**

● **13   Operations on lens**

● **13.0   Removal of foreign body from lens**

> **Excludes**   *removal of pseudophakos (13.8)*

✖ **13.00   Removal of foreign body from lens, not otherwise specified**

✖ **13.01   Removal of foreign body from lens with use of magnet**

✖ **13.02   Removal of foreign body from lens without use of magnet**

● **13.1   Intracapsular extraction of lens**

> Code also any synchronous insertion of pseudophakos (13.71)

✖ **13.11   Intracapsular extraction of lens by temporal inferior route**

✖ **13.19   Other intracapsular extraction of lens**
> Cataract extraction NOS
> Cryoextraction of lens
> Erysiphake extraction of cataract
> Extraction of lens NOS

✖ **13.2   Extracapsular extraction of lens by linear extraction technique**

✖ **13.3   Extracapsular extraction of lens by simple aspiration (and irrigation) technique**
> Irrigation of traumatic cataract

● **13.4   Extracapsular extraction of lens by fragmentation and aspiration technique**

✖ **13.41   Phacoemulsification and aspiration of cataract**

✖ **13.42   Mechanical phacofragmentation and aspiration of cataract by posterior route**

> Code also any synchronous vitrectomy (14.74)

✖ **13.43   Mechanical phacofragmentation and other aspiration of cataract**

● **13.5   Other extracapsular extraction of lens**

> Code also any synchronous insertion of pseudophakos (13.71)

✖ **13.51   Extracapsular extraction of lens by temporal inferior route**

✖ **13.59   Other extracapsular extraction of lens**

● **13.6   Other cataract extraction**

> Code also any synchronous insertion of pseudophakos (13.71)

✖ **13.64   Discission of secondary membrane [after cataract]**

✖ **13.65   Excision of secondary membrane [after cataract]**
> Capsulectomy

✖ **13.66   Mechanical fragmentation of secondary membrane [after cataract]**

✖ **13.69   Other cataract extraction**

● **13.7   Insertion of prosthetic lens [pseudophakos]**

✖ **13.70   Insertion of pseudophakos, not otherwise specified**

✖ **13.71   Insertion of intraocular lens prosthesis at time of cataract extraction, one-stage**

> Code also synchronous extraction of cataract (13.11–13.69)

✖ **13.72   Secondary insertion of intraocular lens prosthesis**

✖ **13.8   Removal of implanted lens**
> Removal of pseudophakos

✖ **13.9   Other operations on lens**

● **14   Operations on retina, choroid, vitreous, and posterior chamber**

● **14.0   Removal of foreign body from posterior segment of eye**

> **Excludes**   *removal of surgically implanted material (14.6)*

✖ **14.00   Removal of foreign body from posterior segment of eye, not otherwise specified**

✖ **14.01   Removal of foreign body from posterior segment of eye with use of magnet**

✖ **14.02   Removal of foreign body from posterior segment of eye without use of magnet**

● **14.1   Diagnostic procedures on retina, choroid, vitreous, and posterior chamber**

✖ **14.11   Diagnostic aspiration of vitreous**

✖ **14.19   Other diagnostic procedures on retina, choroid, vitreous, and posterior chamber**

● **14.2   Destruction of lesion of retina and choroid**

> **Includes:** destruction of chorioretinopathy or isolated chorioretinal lesion

> **Excludes**   *that for repair of retina (14.31–14.59)*

✖ **14.21   Destruction of chorioretinal lesion by diathermy**

✖ **14.22   Destruction of chorioretinal lesion by cryotherapy**

14.23   Destruction of chorioretinal lesion by xenon arc photocoagulation

14.24   Destruction of chorioretinal lesion by laser photocoagulation

---

14.25 Destruction of chorioretinal lesion by photocoagulation of unspecified type

✖ **14.26** Destruction of chorioretinal lesion by radiation therapy

✖ **14.27** Destruction of chorioretinal lesion by implantation of radiation source

✖ **14.29** Other destruction of chorioretinal lesion
Destruction of lesion of retina and choroid NOS

● **14.3** Repair of retinal tear

Includes: repair of retinal defect

Excludes *repair of retinal detachment (14.41–14.59)*

✖ **14.31** Repair of retinal tear by diathermy

✖ **14.32** Repair of retinal tear by cryotherapy

14.33 Repair of retinal tear by xenon arc photocoagulation

14.34 Repair of retinal tear by laser photocoagulation

14.35 Repair of retinal tear by photocoagulation of unspecified type

✖ **14.39** Other repair of retinal tear

● **14.4** Repair of retinal detachment with scleral buckling and implant

✖ **14.41** Scleral buckling with implant

✖ **14.49** Other scleral buckling
Scleral buckling with:
air tamponade
resection of sclera
vitrectomy

● **14.5** Other repair of retinal detachment

Includes: that with drainage

✖ **14.51** Repair of retinal detachment with diathermy

✖ **14.52** Repair of retinal detachment with cryotherapy

✖ **14.53** Repair of retinal detachment with xenon arc photocoagulation

✖ **14.54** Repair of retinal detachment with laser photocoagulation

✖ **14.55** Repair of retinal detachment with photocoagulation of unspecified type

✖ **14.59** Other

✖ **14.6** Removal of surgically implanted material from posterior segment of eye

● **14.7** Operations on vitreous

✖ **14.71** Removal of vitreous, anterior approach
Open sky technique
Removal of vitreous, anterior approach (with replacement)

✖ **14.72** Other removal of vitreous
Aspiration of vitreous by posterior sclerotomy

✖ **14.73** Mechanical vitrectomy by anterior approach

✖ **14.74** Other mechanical vitrectomy

✖ **14.75** Injection of vitreous substitute

Excludes *that associated with removal (14.71–14.72)*

✖ **14.79** Other operations on vitreous

✖ **14.9** Other operations on retina, choroid, and posterior chamber

● **15** Operations on extraocular muscles

● **15.0** Diagnostic procedures on extraocular muscles or tendons

✖ **15.01** Biopsy of extraocular muscle or tendon

✖ **15.09** Other diagnostic procedures on extraocular muscles and tendons

● **15.1** Operations on one extraocular muscle involving temporary detachment from globe

✖ **15.11** Recession of one extraocular muscle

✖ **15.12** Advancement of one extraocular muscle

✖ **15.13** Resection of one extraocular muscle

✖ **15.19** Other operations on one extraocular muscle involving temporary detachment from globe

Excludes *transposition of muscle (15.5)*

● **15.2** Other operations on one extraocular muscle

✖ **15.21** Lengthening procedure on one extraocular muscle

✖ **15.22** Shortening procedure on one extraocular muscle

✖ **15.29** Other

✖ **15.3** Operations on two or more extraocular muscles involving temporary detachment from globe, one or both eyes

✖ **15.4** Other operations on two or more extraocular muscles, one or both eyes

✖ **15.5** Transposition of extraocular muscles

Excludes *that for correction of ptosis (08.31–08.36)*

✖ **15.6** Revision of extraocular muscle surgery

✖ **15.7** Repair of injury of extraocular muscle
Freeing of entrapped extraocular muscle
Lysis of adhesions of extraocular muscle
Repair of laceration of extraocular muscle, tendon, or Tenon's capsule

✖ **15.9** Other operations on extraocular muscles and tendons

● **16** Operations on orbit and eyeball

Excludes *reduction of fracture of orbit (76.78–76.79)*

● **16.0** Orbitotomy

✖ **16.01** Orbitotomy with bone flap
Orbitotomy with lateral approach

✖ **16.02** Orbitotomy with insertion of orbital implant

Excludes *that with bone flap (16.01)*

✖ **16.09** Other orbitotomy

✖ **16.1** Removal of penetrating foreign body from eye, not otherwise specified

Excludes *removal of nonpenetrating foreign body (98.21)*

● **16.2** Diagnostic procedures on orbit and eyeball

16.21 Ophthalmoscopy

✖ **16.22** Diagnostic aspiration of orbit

✖ **16.23** Biopsy of eyeball and orbit

✖ **16.29** Other diagnostic procedures on orbit and eyeball

Excludes *examination of form and structure of eye (95.11–95.16)*
general and subjective eye examination (95.01–95.09)
microscopic examination of specimen from eye (90.21–90.29)
objective functional tests of eye (95.21–95.26)
ocular thermography (88.82)
tonometry (89.11)
x-ray of orbit (87.14, 87.16)

● **16.3 Evisceration of eyeball**

✖ **16.31 Removal of ocular contents with synchronous implant into scleral shell**

✖ **16.39 Other evisceration of eyeball**

● **16.4 Enucleation of eyeball**

✖ **16.41 Enucleation of eyeball with synchronous implant into Tenon's capsule with attachment of muscles**
Integrated implant of eyeball

✖ **16.42 Enucleation of eyeball with other synchronous implant**

✖ **16.49 Other enucleation of eyeball**
Removal of eyeball NOS

● **16.5 Exenteration of orbital contents**

✖ **16.51 Exenteration of orbit with removal of adjacent structures**
Radical orbitomaxillectomy

✖ **16.52 Exenteration of orbit with therapeutic removal of orbital bone**

✖ **16.59 Other exenteration of orbit**
Evisceration of orbit NOS
Exenteration of orbit with temporalis muscle transplant

● **16.6 Secondary procedures after removal of eyeball**

Excludes   *that with synchronous:*
     enucleation of eyeball (16.41–16.42)
     evisceration of eyeball (16.31)

✖ **16.61 Secondary insertion of ocular implant**

✖ **16.62 Revision and reinsertion of ocular implant**

✖ **16.63 Revision of enucleation socket with graft**

✖ **16.64 Other revision of enucleation socket**

✖ **16.65 Secondary graft to exenteration cavity**

✖ **16.66 Other revision of exenteration cavity**

✖ **16.69 Other secondary procedures after removal of eyeball**

● **16.7 Removal of ocular or orbital implant**

✖ **16.71 Removal of ocular implant**

✖ **16.72 Removal of orbital implant**

● **16.8 Repair of injury of eyeball and orbit**

✖ **16.81 Repair of wound of orbit**

Excludes   *reduction of orbital fracture (76.78–76.79)*
     repair of extraocular muscles (15.7)

✖ **16.82 Repair of rupture of eyeball**
Repair of multiple structures of eye

Excludes   *repair of laceration of:*
     cornea (11.51–11.59)
     sclera (12.81)

✖ **16.89 Other repair of injury of eyeball or orbit**

● **16.9 Other operations on orbit and eyeball**

Excludes   *irrigation of eye (96.51)*
     prescription and fitting of low vision aids
       (95.31–95.33)
     removal of:
       eye prosthesis NEC (97.31)
       nonpenetrating foreign body from eye without
         incision (98.21)

16.91 Retrobulbar injection of therapeutic agent

Excludes   *injection of radiographic contrast material (87.14)*
     opticociliary injection (12.79)

✖ **16.92 Excision of lesion of orbit**

Excludes   *biopsy of orbit (16.23)*

✖ **16.93 Excision of lesion of eye, unspecified structure**

Excludes   *biopsy of eye NOS (16.23)*

✖ **16.98 Other operations on orbit**

✖ **16.99 Other operations on eyeball**

4. OPERATIONS ON THE EAR (18-20)

● **18 Operations on external ear**

Includes: operations on:
external auditory canal
skin and cartilage of:
auricle
meatus

● **18.0 Incision of external ear**

   Excludes *removal of intraluminal foreign body (98.11)*

   18.01 Piercing of ear lobe
   Piercing of pinna

   18.02 Incision of external auditory canal

   18.09 Other incision of external ear

● **18.1 Diagnostic procedures on external ear**

   18.11 Otoscopy

   18.12 Biopsy of external ear

   18.19 Other diagnostic procedures on external ear

   Excludes *microscopic examination of specimen from ear (90.31–90.39)*

● **18.2 Excision or destruction of lesion of external ear**

   ✖ **18.21 Excision of preauricular sinus**
   Radical excision of preauricular sinus or cyst

   Excludes *excision of preauricular remnant [appendage] (18.29)*

   18.29 Excision or destruction of other lesion of external ear
   Cauterization of external ear
   Coagulation of external ear
   Cryosurgery of external ear
   Curettage of external ear
   Electrocoagulation of external ear
   Enucleation of external ear
   Excision of:
   exostosis of external auditory canal
   preauricular remnant [appendage]
   Partial excision of ear

   Excludes *biopsy of external ear (18.12)*
   radical excision of lesion (18.31)
   removal of cerumen (96.52)

● **18.3 Other excision of external ear**

   Excludes *biopsy of external ear (18.12)*

   ✖ **18.31 Radical excision of lesion of external ear**
   Excludes *radical excision of preauricular sinus (18.21)*

   ✖ **18.39 Other**
   Amputation of external ear
   Excludes *excision of lesion (18.21–18.29, 18.31)*

   18.4 Suture of laceration of external ear

   ✖ **18.5 Surgical correction of prominent ear**
   Ear:
   pinning
   setback

   ✖ **18.6 Reconstruction of external auditory canal**
   Canaloplasty of external auditory meatus
   Construction [reconstruction] of external meatus
   of ear:
   osseous portion
   skin-lined portion (with skin graft)

● **18.7 Other plastic repair of external ear**

   ✖ **18.71 Construction of auricle of ear**
   Prosthetic appliance for absent ear
   Reconstruction:
   auricle
   ear

   ✖ **18.72 Reattachment of amputated ear**

   ✖ **18.79 Other plastic repair of external ear**
   Otoplasty NOS
   Postauricular skin graft
   Repair of lop ear

   ✖ **18.9 Other operations on external ear**
   Excludes *irrigation of ear (96.52)*
   packing of external auditory canal (96.11)
   removal of:
   cerumen (96.52)
   foreign body (without incision) (98.11)

● **19 Reconstructive operations on middle ear**

   ✖ **19.0 Stapes mobilization**
   Division, otosclerotic:
   material
   process
   Remobilization of stapes
   Stapediolysis
   Transcrural stapes mobilization
   Excludes *that with synchronous stapedectomy (19.11–19.19)*

● **19.1 Stapedectomy**
   Excludes *revision of previous stapedectomy (19.21–19.29)*
   stapes mobilization only (19.0)

   ✖ **19.11 Stapedectomy with incus replacement**
   Stapedectomy with incus:
   homograft
   prosthesis

   ✖ **19.19 Other stapedectomy**

● **19.2 Revision of stapedectomy**

   ✖ **19.21 Revision of stapedectomy with incus replacement**

   ✖ **19.29 Other revision of stapedectomy**

   ✖ **19.3 Other operations on ossicular chain**
   Incudectomy NOS
   Ossiculectomy NOS
   Reconstruction of ossicles, second stage

   ✖ **19.4 Myringoplasty**
   Epitympanic, type I
   Myringoplasty by:
   cauterization
   graft
   Tympanoplasty (type I)

● **19.5 Other tympanoplasty**

   ✖ **19.52 Type II tympanoplasty**
   Closure of perforation with graft against incus
   or malleus

   ✖ **19.53 Type III tympanoplasty**
   Graft placed in contact with mobile and intact
   stapes

   ✖ **19.54 Type IV tympanoplasty**
   Mobile footplate left exposed with air pocket
   between round window and graft

   ✖ **19.55 Type V tympanoplasty**
   Fenestra in horizontal semicircular canal covered by graft

   ✖ **19.6 Revision of tympanoplasty**

   ✖ **19.9 Other repair of middle ear**
   Closure of mastoid fistula
   Mastoid myoplasty
   Obliteration of tympanomastoid cavity

● **20 Other operations on middle and inner ear**

   ● **20.0 Myringotomy**

✖ **20.01 Myringotomy with insertion of tube**
Myringostomy

✖ **20.09 Other myringotomy**
Aspiration of middle ear NOS

20.1 Removal of tympanostomy tube

● **20.2 Incision of mastoid and middle ear**

✖ **20.21 Incision of mastoid**

✖ **20.22 Incision of petrous pyramid air cells**

✖ **20.23 Incision of middle ear**
Atticotomy
Division of tympanum
Lysis of adhesions of middle ear

> **Excludes** *division of otosclerotic process (19.0)*
> *stapediolysis (19.0)*
> *that with stapedectomy (19.11–19.19)*

● **20.3 Diagnostic procedures on middle and inner ear**

20.31 Electrocochleography

✖ **20.32 Biopsy of middle and inner ear**

✖ **20.39 Other diagnostic procedures on middle and inner ear**

> **Excludes** *auditory and vestibular function tests (89.13, 95.41–95.49)*
> *microscopic examination of specimen from ear (90.31–90.39)*

● **20.4 Mastoidectomy**
Code also any:
skin graft (18.79)
tympanoplasty (19.4–19.55)

> **Excludes** *that with implantation of cochlear prosthetic device (20.96–20.98)*

✖ **20.41 Simple mastoidectomy**

✖ **20.42 Radical mastoidectomy**

✖ **20.49 Other mastoidectomy**
Atticoantrostomy
Mastoidectomy:
NOS
modified radical

● **20.5 Other excision of middle ear**

> **Excludes** *that with synchronous mastoidectomy (20.41–20.49)*

✖ **20.51 Excision of lesion of middle ear**

> **Excludes** *biopsy of middle ear (20.32)*

✖ **20.59 Other**
Apicectomy of petrous pyramid
Tympanectomy

● **20.6 Fenestration of inner ear**

✖ **20.61 Fenestration of inner ear (initial)**
Fenestration of:
labyrinth with graft (skin) (vein)
semicircular canals with graft (skin) (vein)
vestibule with graft (skin) (vein)

> **Excludes** *that with tympanoplasty, type V (19.55)*

✖ **20.62 Revision of fenestration of inner ear**

● **20.7 Incision, excision, and destruction of inner ear**

✖ **20.71 Endolymphatic shunt**

✖ **20.72 Injection into inner ear**
Destruction by injection (alcohol):
inner ear
semicircular canals
vestibule

✖ **20.79 Other incision, excision, and destruction of inner ear**
Decompression of labyrinth
Drainage of inner ear
Fistulization:
endolymphatic sac
labyrinth
Incision of endolymphatic sac
Labyrinthectomy (transtympanic)
Opening of bony labyrinth
Perilymphatic tap

> **Excludes** *biopsy of inner ear (20.32)*

20.8 Operations on Eustachian tube
Catheterization of eustachian tube
Inflation of eustachian tube
Injection (Teflon paste) of eustachian tube
Insufflation (boric acid-salicylic acid)
Intubation of eustachian tube
Politzerization of eustachian tube

● **20.9 Other operations on inner and middle ear**

✖ **20.91 Tympanosympathectomy**

✖ **20.92 Revision of mastoidectomy**

✖ **20.93 Repair of oval and round windows**
Closure of fistula:
oval window
perilymph
round window

20.94 Injection of tympanum

✖ **20.95 Implantation of electromagnetic hearing device**
Bone conduction hearing device

> **Excludes** *cochlear prosthetic device (20.96–20.98)*

✖ **20.96 Implantation or replacement of cochlear prosthetic device, not otherwise specified**
Implantation of receiver (within skull) and insertion of electrode(s) in the cochlea

Includes: mastoidectomy

> **Excludes** *electromagnetic hearing device (20.95)*

✖ **20.97 Implantation or replacement of cochlear prosthetic device, single channel**
Implantation of receiver (within skull) and insertion of electrode in the cochlea

Includes: mastoidectomy

> **Excludes** *electromagnetic hearing device (20.95)*

✖ **20.98 Implantation or replacement of cochlear prosthetic device, multiple channel**
Implantation of receiver (within skull) and insertion of electrodes in the cochlea

Includes: mastoidectomy

> **Excludes** *electromagnetic hearing device (20.95)*

✖ **20.99 Other operations on middle and inner ear**
Repair or removal of cochlear prosthetic device (receiver) (electrode)

> **Excludes** *adjustment (external components) of cochlear prosthetic device (95.49)*
> *fitting of hearing aid (95.48)*

5. OPERATIONS ON THE NOSE, MOUTH, AND PHARYNX (21–29)

● 21 Operations on nose

>   **Includes:** operations on:
>   bone of nose
>   skin of nose

● 21.0 Control of epistaxis

21.00 Control of epistaxis, not otherwise specified

21.01 Control of epistaxis by anterior nasal packing

21.02 Control of epistaxis by posterior (and anterior) packing

21.03 Control of epistaxis by cauterization (and packing)

✖ 21.04 Control of epistaxis by ligation of ethmoidal arteries

✖ 21.05 Control of epistaxis by (transantral) ligation of the maxillary artery

✖ 21.06 Control of epistaxis by ligation of the external carotid artery

✖ 21.07 Control of epistaxis by excision of nasal mucosa and skin grafting of septum and lateral nasal wall

✖ 21.09 Control of epistaxis by other means

21.1 Incision of nose
>   Chondrotomy
>   Incision of skin of nose
>   Nasal septotomy

● 21.2 Diagnostic procedures on nose

21.21 Rhinoscopy

21.22 Biopsy of nose

21.29 Other diagnostic procedures on nose

> **Excludes** microscopic examination of specimen from nose (90.31–90.39)
>   nasal:
>   function study (89.12)
>   x-ray (87.16)
>   rhinomanometry (89.12)

● 21.3 Local excision or destruction of lesion of nose

> **Excludes** biopsy of nose (21.22)
>   nasal fistulectomy (21.82)

21.30 Excision or destruction of lesion of nose, not otherwise specified

21.31 Local excision or destruction of intranasal lesion
>   Nasal polypectomy

21.32 Local excision or destruction of other lesion of nose

✖ 21.4 Resection of nose
>   Amputation of nose

✖ 21.5 Submucous resection of nasal septum

● 21.6 Turbinectomy

✖ 21.61 Turbinectomy by diathermy or cryosurgery

✖ 21.62 Fracture of the turbinates

✖ 21.69 Other turbinectomy

> **Excludes** turbinectomy associated with sinusectomy (22.31–22.39, 22.42, 22.60–22.64)

● 21.7 Reduction of nasal fracture

21.71 Closed reduction of nasal fracture

✖ 21.72 Open reduction of nasal fracture

● 21.8 Repair and plastic operations on the nose

21.81 Suture of laceration of nose

✖ 21.82 Closure of nasal fistula
>   Nasolabial fistulectomy
>   Nasopharyngeal fistulectomy
>   Oronasal fistulectomy

✖ 21.83 Total nasal reconstruction
>   Reconstruction of nose with:
>   arm flap
>   forehead flap

✖ 21.84 Revision rhinoplasty
>   Rhinoseptoplasty
>   Twisted nose rhinoplasty

✖ 21.85 Augmentation rhinoplasty
>   Augmentation rhinoplasty with:
>   graft
>   synthetic implant

✖ 21.86 Limited rhinoplasty
>   Plastic repair of nasolabial flaps
>   Tip rhinoplasty

✖ 21.87 Other rhinoplasty
>   Rhinoplasty NOS

✖ 21.88 Other septoplasty
>   Crushing of nasal septum
>   Repair of septal perforation

> **Excludes** septoplasty associated with submucous resection of septum (21.5)

✖ 21.89 Other repair and plastic operations on nose
>   Reattachment of amputated nose

● 21.9 Other operations on nose

21.91 Lysis of adhesions of nose
>   Posterior nasal scrub

✖ 21.99 Other

> **Excludes** dilation of frontonasal duct (96.21)
>   irrigation of nasal passages (96.53)
>   removal of:
>   intraluminal foreign body without incision (98.12)
>   nasal packing (97.32)
>   replacement of nasal packing (97.21)

● 22 Operations on nasal sinuses

● 22.0 Aspiration and lavage of nasal sinus

22.00 Aspiration and lavage of nasal sinus, not otherwise specified

22.01 Puncture of nasal sinus for aspiration or lavage

22.02 Aspiration or lavage of nasal sinus through natural ostium

● 22.1 Diagnostic procedures on nasal sinus

22.11 Closed [endoscopic] [needle] biopsy of nasal sinus

✖ 22.12 Open biopsy of nasal sinus

22.19 Other diagnostic procedures on nasal sinuses
>   Endoscopy without biopsy

> **Excludes** transillumination of sinus (89.35)
>   x-ray of sinus (87.15–87.16)

22.2 Intranasal antrotomy

> **Excludes** antrotomy with external approach (22.31–22.39)

● 22.3 External maxillary antrotomy

✖ 22.31 Radical maxillary antrotomy
>   Removal of lining membrane of maxillary sinus using Caldwell-Luc approach

✖ **22.39 Other external maxillary antrotomy**
Exploration of maxillary antrum with Caldwell-Luc approach

● **22.4 Frontal sinusotomy and sinusectomy**

✖ **22.41 Frontal sinusotomy**

✖ **22.42 Frontal sinusectomy**
Excision of lesion of frontal sinus
Obliteration of frontal sinus (with fat)

Excludes *biopsy of nasal sinus (22.11–22.12)*

● **22.5 Other nasal sinusotomy**

✖ **22.50 Sinusotomy, not otherwise specified**

✖ **22.51 Ethmoidotomy**

✖ **22.52 Sphenoidotomy**

✖ **22.53 Incision of multiple nasal sinuses**

● **22.6 Other nasal sinusectomy**

Includes: that with incidental turbinectomy

Excludes *biopsy of nasal sinus (22.11–22.12)*

✖ **22.60 Sinusectomy, not otherwise specified**

✖ **22.61 Excision of lesion of maxillary sinus with Caldwell-Luc approach**

✖ **22.62 Excision of lesion of maxillary sinus with other approach**

✖ **22.63 Ethmoidectomy**

✖ **22.64 Sphenoidectomy**

● **22.7 Repair of nasal sinus**

✖ **22.71 Closure of nasal sinus fistula**
Repair of oro-antral fistula

✖ **22.79 Other repair of nasal sinus**
Reconstruction of frontonasal duct
Repair of bone of accessory sinus

✖ **22.9 Other operations on nasal sinuses**
Exteriorization of maxillary sinus
Fistulization of sinus

Excludes *dilation of frontonasal duct (96.21)*

● **23 Removal and restoration of teeth**

● **23.0 Forceps extraction of tooth**

23.01 Extraction of deciduous tooth

23.09 Extraction of other tooth
Extraction of tooth NOS

● **23.1 Surgical removal of tooth**

23.11 Removal of residual root

23.19 Other surgical extraction of tooth
Odontectomy NOS
Removal of impacted tooth
Tooth extraction with elevation of mucoperiosteal flap

23.2 Restoration of tooth by filling

23.3 Restoration of tooth by inlay

● **23.4 Other dental restoration**

23.41 Application of crown

23.42 Insertion of fixed bridge

23.43 Insertion of removable bridge

23.49 Other

23.5 Implantation of tooth

23.6 Prosthetic dental implant
Endosseous dental implant

● **23.7 Apicoectomy and root canal therapy**

23.70 Root canal, not otherwise specified

23.71 Root canal therapy with irrigation

23.72 Root canal therapy with apicoectomy

23.73 Apicoectomy

● **24 Other operations on teeth, gums, and alveoli**

24.0 Incision of gum or alveolar bone
Apical alveolotomy

● **24.1 Diagnostic procedures on teeth, gums, and alveoli**

24.11 Biopsy of gum

24.12 Biopsy of alveolus

24.19 Other diagnostic procedures on teeth, gums, and alveoli

Excludes *dental:*
        examination (89.31)
        x-ray:
            full-mouth (87.11)
            other (87.12)
        microscopic examination of dental specimen (90.81–90.89)

✖ **24.2 Gingivoplasty**
Gingivoplasty with bone or soft tissue graft

● **24.3 Other operations on gum**

24.31 Excision of lesion or tissue of gum

Excludes *biopsy of gum (24.11)*
        excision of odontogenic lesion (24.4)

24.32 Suture of laceration of gum

24.39 Other

✖ **24.4 Excision of dental lesion of jaw**
Excision of odontogenic lesion

✖ **24.5 Alveoloplasty**
Alveolectomy (interradicular) (intraseptal) (radical) (simple) (with graft or implant)

Excludes *biopsy of alveolus (24.12)*
        en bloc resection of alveolar process and palate (27.32)

24.6 Exposure of tooth

24.7 Application of orthodontic appliance
Application, insertion, or fitting of:
    arch bars
    orthodontic obturator
    orthodontic wiring
    periodontal splint

Excludes *nonorthodontic dental wiring (93.55)*

24.8 Other orthodontic operation
Closure of diastema (alveolar) (dental)
Occlusal adjustment
Removal of arch bars
Repair of dental arch

Excludes *removal of nonorthodontic wiring (97.33)*

● **24.9 Other dental operations**

24.91 Extension or deepening of buccolabial or lingual sulcus

24.99 Other

> **Excludes** *dental:*
> *debridement (96.54)*
> *examination (89.31)*
> *prophylaxis (96.54)*
> *scaling and polishing (96.54)*
> *wiring (93.55)*
> *fitting of dental appliance [denture] (99.97)*
> *microscopic examination of dental specimen (90.81–90.89)*
> *removal of dental:*
> *packing (97.34)*
> *prosthesis (97.35)*
> *wiring (97.33)*
> *replacement of dental packing (97.22)*

● **25   Operations on tongue**

● **25.0   Diagnostic procedures on tongue**

  25.01   Closed [needle] biopsy of tongue

✖ **25.02   Open biopsy of tongue**
     Wedge biopsy

  25.09   Other diagnostic procedures on tongue

✖ **25.1   Excision or destruction of lesion or tissue of tongue**

> **Excludes** *biopsy of tongue (25.01–25.02)*
> *frenumectomy:*
> *labial (27.41)*
> *lingual (25.92)*

✖ **25.2   Partial glossectomy**

✖ **25.3   Complete glossectomy**
     Glossectomy NOS

  Code also any neck dissection (40.40–40.42)

✖ **25.4   Radical glossectomy**

  Code also any:
     neck dissection (40.40–40.42)
     tracheostomy (31.1–31.29)

● **25.5   Repair of tongue and glossoplasty**

  25.51   Suture of laceration of tongue

✖ **25.59   Other repair and plastic operations on tongue**
     Fascial sling of tongue
     Fusion of tongue (to lip)
     Graft of mucosa or skin to tongue

> **Excludes** *lysis of adhesions of tongue (25.93)*

● **25.9   Other operations on tongue**

  25.91   Lingual frenotomy
> **Excludes** *labial frenotomy (27.91)*

  25.92   Lingual frenectomy
> **Excludes** *labial frenectomy (27.41)*

  25.93   Lysis of adhesions of tongue

✖ **25.94   Other glossotomy**

✖ **25.99   Other**

● **26   Operations on salivary glands and ducts**

> **Includes:** operations on:
> lesser salivary gland and duct
> parotid gland and duct
> sublingual gland and duct
> submaxillary gland and duct

Code also any neck dissection (40.40–40.42)

  26.0   Incision of salivary gland or duct

● **26.1   Diagnostic procedures on salivary glands and ducts**

  26.11   Closed [needle] biopsy of salivary gland or duct

✖ **26.12   Open biopsy of salivary gland or duct**

  26.19   Other diagnostic procedures on salivary glands and ducts

> **Excludes** *x-ray of salivary gland (87.09)*

● **26.2   Excision of lesion of salivary gland**

✖ **26.21   Marsupialization of salivary gland cyst**

✖ **26.29   Other excision of salivary gland lesion**

> **Excludes** *biopsy of salivary gland (26.11–26.12)*
> *salivary fistulectomy (26.42)*

● **26.3   Sialoadenectomy**

✖ **26.30   Sialoadenectomy, not otherwise specified**

✖ **26.31   Partial sialoadenectomy**

✖ **26.32   Complete sialoadenectomy**
     En bloc excision of salivary gland lesion
     Radical sialoadenectomy

● **26.4   Repair of salivary gland or duct**

✖ **26.41   Suture of laceration of salivary gland**

✖ **26.42   Closure of salivary fistula**

✖ **26.49   Other repair and plastic operations on salivary gland or duct**
     Fistulization of salivary gland
     Plastic repair of salivary gland or duct NOS
     Transplantation of salivary duct opening

● **26.9   Other operations on salivary gland or duct**

  26.91   Probing of salivary duct

✖ **26.99   Other**

● **27   Other operations on mouth and face**

> **Includes:** operations on:
> lips
> palate
> soft tissue of face and mouth, except tongue and gingiva

> **Excludes** *operations on:*
> *gingiva (24.0–24.99)*
> *tongue (25.01–25.99)*

✖ **27.0   Drainage of face and floor of mouth**
     Drainage of:
     facial region (abscess)
     fascial compartment of face
     Ludwig's angina

> **Excludes** *drainage of thyroglossal tract (06.09)*

✖ **27.1   Incision of palate**

● **27.2   Diagnostic procedures on oral cavity**

✖ **27.21   Biopsy of bony palate**

✖ **27.22   Biopsy of uvula and soft palate**

  27.23   Biopsy of lip

  27.24   Biopsy of mouth, unspecified structure

  27.29   Other diagnostic procedures on oral cavity
> **Excludes** *soft tissue x-ray (87.09)*

● **27.3   Excision of lesion or tissue of bony palate**

✖ **27.31   Local excision or destruction of lesion or tissue of bony palate**
     Local excision or destruction of palate by:
     cautery
     chemotherapy
     cryotherapy

> **Excludes** *biopsy of bony palate (27.21)*

✖ **27.32   Wide excision or destruction of lesion or tissue of bony palate**
     En bloc resection of alveolar process and palate

● **27.4 Excision of other parts of mouth**

  27.41 Labial frenectomy

  Excludes | *division of labial frenum (27.91)*

  ✖ **27.42 Wide excision of lesion of lip**

  ✖ **27.43 Other excision of lesion or tissue of lip**

  ✖ **27.49 Other excision of mouth**

  Excludes | *biopsy of mouth NOS (27.24)*
    excision of lesion of:
      palate (27.31–27.32)
      tongue (25.1)
      uvula (27.72)
    fistulectomy of mouth (27.53)
    frenectomy of:
      lip (27.41)
      tongue (25.92)

● **27.5 Plastic repair of mouth**

  Excludes | *palatoplasty (27.61–27.69)*

  27.51 Suture of laceration of lip

  27.52 Suture of laceration of other part of mouth

  ✖ **27.53 Closure of fistula of mouth**

  Excludes | *fistulectomy:*
    nasolabial (21.82)
    oro-antral (22.71)
    oronasal (21.82)

  ✖ **27.54 Repair of cleft lip**

  ✖ **27.55 Full-thickness skin graft to lip and mouth**

  ✖ **27.56 Other skin graft to lip and mouth**

  ✖ **27.57 Attachment of pedicle or flap graft to lip and mouth**

  ✖ **27.59 Other plastic repair of mouth**

● **27.6 Palatoplasty**

  ✖ **27.61 Suture of laceration of palate**

  ✖ **27.62 Correction of cleft palate**
    Correction of cleft palate by push-back operation

  Excludes | *revision of cleft palate repair (27.63)*

  ✖ **27.63 Revision of cleft palate repair**
    Secondary:
      attachment of pharyngeal flap
      lengthening of palate

  ✖ **27.64 Insertion of palatal implant** ◀

  ✖ **27.69 Other plastic repair of palate**
    Code also any insertion of palatal implant (27.64) ◀

  Excludes | *fistulectomy of mouth (27.53)*

● **27.7 Operations on uvula**

  ✖ **27.71 Incision of uvula**

  ✖ **27.72 Excision of uvula**

  Excludes | *biopsy of uvula (27.22)*

  ✖ **27.73 Repair of uvula**

  Excludes | *that with synchronous cleft palate repair (27.62)*
    uranostaphylorrhaphy (27.62)

  ✖ **27.79 Other operations on uvula**

● **27.9 Other operations on mouth and face**

  27.91 Labial frenotomy
    Division of labial frenum

  Excludes | *lingual frenotomy (25.91)*

  ✖ **27.92 Incision of mouth, unspecified structure**

  Excludes | *incision of:*
    gum (24.0)
    palate (27.1)
    salivary gland or duct (26.0)
    tongue (25.94)
    uvula (27.71)

  ✖ **27.99 Other operations on oral cavity**
    Graft of buccal sulcus

  Excludes | *removal of:*
    intraluminal foreign body (98.01)
    penetrating foreign body from mouth without incision (98.22)

● **28 Operations on tonsils and adenoids**

  28.0 Incision and drainage of tonsil and peritonsillar structures
    Drainage (oral) (transcervical) of:
      parapharyngeal abscess
      peritonsillar abscess
      retropharyngeal abscess
      tonsillar abscess

● **28.1 Diagnostic procedures on tonsils and adenoids**

  ✖ **28.11 Biopsy of tonsils and adenoids**

  ✖ **28.19 Other diagnostic procedures on tonsils and adenoids**

  Excludes | *soft tissue x-ray (87.09)*

✖ **28.2 Tonsillectomy without adenoidectomy**

✖ **28.3 Tonsillectomy with adenoidectomy**

✖ **28.4 Excision of tonsil tag**

✖ **28.5 Excision of lingual tonsil**

✖ **28.6 Adenoidectomy without tonsillectomy**
  Excision of adenoid tag

✖ **28.7 Control of hemorrhage after tonsillectomy and adenoidectomy**

● **28.9 Other operations on tonsils and adenoids**

  ✖ **28.91 Removal of foreign body from tonsil and adenoid by incision**

  Excludes | *that without incision (98.13)*

  ✖ **28.92 Excision of lesion of tonsil and adenoid**

  Excludes | *biopsy of tonsil and adenoid (28.11)*

  ✖ **28.99 Other**

● **29 Operations on pharynx**

  Includes: operations on:
    hypopharynx
    nasopharynx
    oropharynx
    pharyngeal pouch
    pyriform sinus

✖ **29.0 Pharyngotomy**
  Drainage of pharyngeal bursa

  Excludes | *incision and drainage of retropharyngeal abscess (28.0)*
    removal of foreign body (without incision) (98.13)

● 29.1   Diagnostic procedures on pharynx

     29.11   Pharyngoscopy

     29.12   Pharyngeal biopsy
          Biopsy of supraglottic mass

     29.19   Other diagnostic procedures on pharynx

     | Excludes | *x-ray of nasopharynx:*
                contrast (87.06)
                other (87.09)

✖ 29.2   Excision of branchial cleft cyst or vestige

     | Excludes | *branchial cleft fistulectomy (29.52)*

● 29.3   Excision or destruction of lesion or tissue of pharynx

     ✖ 29.31   Cricopharyngeal myotomy

     | Excludes | *that with pharyngeal diverticulectomy (29.32)*

     ✖ 29.32   Pharyngeal diverticulectomy

     ✖ 29.33   Pharyngectomy (partial)

     | Excludes | *laryngopharyngectomy (30.3)*

     ✖ 29.39   Other excision or destruction of lesion or tissue of pharynx

✖ 29.4   Plastic operation on pharynx
          Correction of nasopharyngeal atresia

     | Excludes | *pharyngoplasty associated with cleft palate repair (27.62–27.63)*

● 29.5   Other repair of pharynx

     ✖ 29.51   Suture of laceration of pharynx

     ✖ 29.52   Closure of branchial cleft fistula

     ✖ 29.53   Closure of other fistula of pharynx
            Pharyngoesophageal fistulectomy

     ✖ 29.54   Lysis of pharyngeal adhesions

     ✖ 29.59   Other

● 29.9   Other operations on pharynx

     29.91   Dilation of pharynx
          Dilation of nasopharynx

     ✖ 29.92   Division of glossopharyngeal nerve

     ✖ 29.99   Other

     | Excludes | *insertion of radium into pharynx and nasopharynx (92.27)*
                removal of intraluminal foreign body (98.13)

6. OPERATIONS ON THE RESPIRATORY SYSTEM (30–34)

● 30 Excision of larynx

  ● 30.0 Excision or destruction of lesion or tissue of larynx

    ✖ 30.01 Marsupialization of laryngeal cyst

    ✖ 30.09 Other excision or destruction of lesion or tissue of larynx
        Stripping of vocal cords

    Excludes *biopsy of larynx (31.43)*
          laryngeal fistulectomy (31.62)
          laryngotracheal fistulectomy (31.62)

  ✖ 30.1 Hemilaryngectomy

  ● 30.2 Other partial laryngectomy

    ✖ 30.21 Epiglottidectomy

    ✖ 30.22 Vocal cordectomy
        Excision of vocal cords

    ✖ 30.29 Other partial laryngectomy
        Excision of laryngeal cartilage

  ✖ 30.3 Complete laryngectomy
    Block dissection of larynx (with thyroidectomy) (with synchronous tracheostomy)
    Laryngopharyngectomy

    Excludes *that with radical neck dissection (30.4)*

  ✖ 30.4 Radical laryngectomy
    Complete [total] laryngectomy with radical neck dissection (with thyroidectomy) (with synchronous tracheostomy)

● 31 Other operations on larynx and trachea

  31.0 Injection of larynx
    Injection of inert material into larynx or vocal cords

  31.1 Temporary tracheostomy
    Tracheotomy for assistance in breathing

  ● 31.2 Permanent tracheostomy

    ✖ 31.21 Mediastinal tracheostomy

    ✖ 31.29 Other permanent tracheostomy
    Excludes *that with laryngectomy (30.3–30.4)*

  ✖ 31.3 Other incision of larynx or trachea
    Excludes *that for assistance in breathing (31.1–31.29)*

  ● 31.4 Diagnostic procedures on larynx and trachea

    31.41 Tracheoscopy through artificial stoma
    Excludes *that with biopsy (31.43–31.44)*

    31.42 Laryngoscopy and other tracheoscopy
    Excludes *that with biopsy (31.43–31.44)*

    31.43 Closed [endoscopic] biopsy of larynx

    31.44 Closed [endoscopic] biopsy of trachea

    ✖ 31.45 Open biopsy of larynx or trachea

    31.48 Other diagnostic procedures on larynx
    Excludes *contrast laryngogram (87.07)*
          microscopic examination of specimen from larynx (90.31–90.39)
          soft tissue x-ray of larynx NEC (87.09)

    31.49 Other diagnostic procedures on trachea
    Excludes *microscopic examination of specimen from trachea (90.41–90.49)*
          x-ray of trachea (87.49)

  ✖ 31.5 Local excision or destruction of lesion or tissue of trachea
    Excludes *biopsy of trachea (31.44–31.45)*
          laryngotracheal fistulectomy (31.62)
          tracheoesophageal fistulectomy (31.73)

  ● 31.6 Repair of larynx

    ✖ 31.61 Suture of laceration of larynx

    ✖ 31.62 Closure of fistula of larynx
        Laryngotracheal fistulectomy
        Take-down of laryngostomy

    ✖ 31.63 Revision of laryngostomy

    ✖ 31.64 Repair of laryngeal fracture

    ✖ 31.69 Other repair of larynx
        Arytenoidopexy
        Graft of larynx
        Transposition of vocal cords
    Excludes *construction of artificial larynx (31.75)*

  ● 31.7 Repair and plastic operations on trachea

    ✖ 31.71 Suture of laceration of trachea

    ✖ 31.72 Closure of external fistula of trachea
        Closure of tracheotomy

    ✖ 31.73 Closure of other fistula of trachea
        Tracheoesophageal fistulectomy
    Excludes *laryngotracheal fistulectomy (31.62)*

    ✖ 31.74 Revision of tracheostomy

    ✖ 31.75 Reconstruction of trachea and construction of artificial larynx
        Tracheoplasty with artificial larynx

    ✖ 31.79 Other repair and plastic operations on trachea

  ● 31.9 Other operations on larynx and trachea

    ✖ 31.91 Division of laryngeal nerve

    ✖ 31.92 Lysis of adhesions of trachea or larynx

    31.93 Replacement of laryngeal or tracheal stent

    31.94 Injection of locally-acting therapeutic substance into trachea

    31.95 Tracheoesophageal fistulization

    ✖ 31.98 Other operations on larynx
        Dilation of larynx
        Division of congenital web of larynx
        Removal of keel or stent of larynx
    Excludes *removal of intraluminal foreign body from larynx without incision (98.14)*

    ✖ 31.99 Other operations on trachea
    Excludes *removal of:*
          intraluminal foreign body from trachea without incision (98.15)
          tracheostomy tube (97.37)
          replacement of tracheostomy tube (97.23)
          tracheostomy toilette (96.55)

● 32 Excision of lung and bronchus

  Includes: rib resection as operative approach
           sternotomy as operative approach
           sternum-splitting incision as operative approach
           thoracotomy as operative approach

  Code also any synchronous bronchoplasty (33.48)

● **32.0 Local excision or destruction of lesion or tissue of bronchus**

> **Excludes** *biopsy of bronchus (33.24–33.25)*
> *bronchial fistulectomy (33.42)*

    32.01 Endoscopic excision or destruction of lesion or tissue of bronchus

✖ **32.09 Other local excision or destruction of lesion or tissue of bronchus**

> **Excludes** *that by endoscopic approach (32.01)*

✖ **32.1 Other excision of bronchus**
      Resection (wide sleeve) of bronchus

> **Excludes** *radical dissection [excision] of bronchus (32.6)*

● **32.2 Local excision or destruction of lesion or tissue of lung**

✖ **32.21 Plication of emphysematous bleb**

✖ **32.22 Lung volume reduction surgery**

    32.28 Endoscopic excision or destruction of lesion or tissue of lung

> **Excludes** *biopsy of lung (33.26–33.27)*

✖ **32.29 Other local excision or destruction of lesion or tissue of lung**
      Resection of lung:
        NOS
        wedge

> **Excludes** *biopsy of lung (33.26–33.27)*
> *that by endoscopic approach (32.28)*
> *wide excision of lesion of lung (32.3)*

✖ **32.3 Segmental resection of lung**
      Partial lobectomy

✖ **32.4 Lobectomy of lung**
      Lobectomy with segmental resection of adjacent lobes of lung

> **Excludes** *that with radical dissection [excision] of thoracic structures (32.6)*

✖ **32.5 Complete pneumonectomy**
      Excision of lung NOS
      Pneumonectomy (with mediastinal dissection)

✖ **32.6 Radical dissection of thoracic structures**
      Block [en bloc] dissection of bronchus, lobe of lung, brachial plexus, intercostal structure, ribs (transverse process), and sympathetic nerves

✖ **32.9 Other excision of lung**

> **Excludes** *biopsy of lung and bronchus (33.24–33.27)*
> *pulmonary decortication (34.51)*

● **33 Other operations on lung and bronchus**

    Includes: rib resection as operative approach
             sternotomy as operative approach
             sternum-splitting incision as operative approach
             thoracotomy as operative approach

✖ **33.0 Incision of bronchus**

✖ **33.1 Incision of lung**

> **Excludes** *puncture of lung (33.93)*

● **33.2 Diagnostic procedures on lung and bronchus**

    33.21 Bronchoscopy through artificial stoma

> **Excludes** *that with biopsy (33.24, 33.27)*

    33.22 Fiber-optic bronchoscopy

> **Excludes** *that with biopsy (33.24, 33.27)*

    33.23 Other bronchoscopy

> **Excludes** *that for:*
> *aspiration (96.05)*
> *biopsy (33.24, 33.27)*

✖ **33.24 Closed [endoscopic] biopsy of bronchus**
      Bronchoscopy (fiberoptic) (rigid) with:
        brush biopsy of "lung"
        brushing or washing for specimen collection
        excision (bite) biopsy
      Diagnostic bronchoalveolar lavage (BAL)

> **Excludes** *closed biopsy of lung, other than brush biopsy of "lung" (33.26, 33.27)*
> *whole lung lavage (33.99)*

✖ **33.25 Open biopsy of bronchus**

> **Excludes** *open biopsy of lung (33.28)*

    33.26 Closed [percutaneous] [needle] biopsy of lung

> **Excludes** *endoscopic biopsy of lung (33.27)*

✖ **33.27 Closed endoscopic biopsy of lung**
      Fiber-optic (flexible) bronchoscopy with fluoroscopic guidance with biopsy
      Transbronchial lung biopsy

> **Excludes** *brush biopsy of "lung" (33.24)*
> *percutaneous biopsy of lung (33.26)*

✖ **33.28 Open biopsy of lung**

✖ **33.29 Other diagnostic procedures on lung and bronchus**

> **Excludes** *contrast bronchogram:*
> *endotracheal (87.31)*
> *other (87.32)*
> *lung scan (92.15)*
> *magnetic resonance imaging (88.92)*
> *microscopic examination of specimen from bronchus or lung (90.41–90.49)*
> *routine chest x-ray (87.44)*
> *ultrasonography of lung (88.73)*
> *vital capacity determination (89.37)*
> *x-ray of bronchus or lung NOS (87.49)*

● **33.3 Surgical collapse of lung**

    33.31 Destruction of phrenic nerve for collapse of lung

    33.32 Artificial pneumothorax for collapse of lung
      Thoracotomy for collapse of lung

    33.33 Pneumoperitoneum for collapse of lung

✖ **33.34 Thoracoplasty**

✖ **33.39 Other surgical collapse of lung**
      Collapse of lung NOS

● **33.4 Repair and plastic operation on lung and bronchus**

✖ **33.41 Suture of laceration of bronchus**

✖ **33.42 Closure of bronchial fistula**
      Closure of bronchostomy
      Fistulectomy:
        bronchocutaneous
        bronchoesophageal
        bronchovisceral

> **Excludes** *closure of fistula:*
> *bronchomediastinal (34.73)*
> *bronchopleural (34.73)*
> *bronchopleuromediastinal (34.73)*

✖ **33.43 Closure of laceration of lung**

✖ **33.48 Other repair and plastic operations on bronchus**

✖ **33.49 Other repair and plastic operations on lung**

> **Excludes** *closure of pleural fistula (34.73)*

✖ **33.5 Lung transplant**

    Note: **To report donor source** - *see* codes 00.91–00.93 ◄

> **Excludes** *combined heart-lung transplantation (33.6)*

    Code also cardiopulmonary bypass [extracorporeal circulation] [heart-lung machine] (39.61)

✖ **33.50 Lung transplantation, not otherwise specified**

✖ **33.51 Unilateral lung transplantation**

✖ **33.52 Bilateral lung transplantation**
Double-lung transplantation
En bloc transplantation

Code also cardiopulmonary bypass [extracorporeal circulation] [heart-lung machine] (39.61)

✖ **33.6 Combined heart-lung transplantation**

Note: To report donor source - *see* codes 00.91–00.93 ◄

Code also cardiopulmonary bypass [extracorporeal circulation] [heart-lung machine] (39.61)

● **33.9 Other operations on lung and bronchus**

33.91 Bronchial dilation

✖ **33.92 Ligation of bronchus**

✖ **33.93 Puncture of lung**

Excludes | *needle biopsy (33.26)*

✖ **33.98 Other operations on bronchus**

Excludes | *bronchial lavage (96.56)*
removal of intraluminal foreign body from bronchus without incision (98.15)

✖ **33.99 Other operations on lung**
Whole lung lavage

Excludes | *other continuous mechanical ventilation (96.70–96.72)*
respiratory therapy (93.90–93.99)

● **34 Operations on chest wall, pleura, mediastinum, and diaphragm**

Excludes | *operations on breast (85.0–85.99)*

● **34.0 Incision of chest wall and pleura**

Excludes | *that as operative approach—omit code*

34.01 Incision of chest wall
Extrapleural drainage

Excludes | *incision of pleura (34.09)*

✖ **34.02 Exploratory thoracotomy**

✖ **34.03 Reopening of recent thoracotomy site**

34.04 Insertion of intercostal catheter for drainage
Chest tube
Closed chest drainage
Revision of intercostal catheter (chest tube) (with lysis of adhesions)

34.05 Creation of pleuroperitoneal shunt

34.09 Other incision of pleura
Creation of pleural window for drainage
Intercostal stab
Open chest drainage

Excludes | *thoracoscopy (34.21)*
thoracotomy for collapse of lung (33.32)

✖ **34.1 Incision of mediastinum**

Excludes | *mediastinoscopy (34.22)*
mediastinotomy associated with pneumonectomy (32.5)

● **34.2 Diagnostic procedures on chest wall, pleura, mediastinum, and diaphragm**

✖ **34.21 Transpleural thoracoscopy**

✖ **34.22 Mediastinoscopy**

Code also any lymph node biopsy (40.11)

34.23 Biopsy of chest wall

34.24 Pleural biopsy

34.25 Closed [percutaneous] [needle] biopsy of mediastinum

✖ **34.26 Open mediastinal biopsy**

✖ **34.27 Biopsy of diaphragm**

✖ **34.28 Other diagnostic procedures on chest wall, pleura, and diaphragm**

Excludes | *angiocardiography (88.50–88.58)*
aortography (88.42)
arteriography of:
intrathoracic vessels NEC (88.44)
pulmonary arteries (88.43)
microscopic examination of specimen from chest wall, pleura, and diaphragm (90.41–90.49)
phlebography of:
intrathoracic vessels NEC (88.63)
pulmonary veins (88.62)
radiological examinations of thorax:
C.A.T. scan (87.41)
diaphragmatic x-ray (87.49)
intrathoracic lymphangiogram (87.34)
routine chest x-ray (87.44)
sinogram of chest wall (87.38)
soft tissue x-ray of chest wall NEC (87.39)
tomogram of thorax NEC (87.42)
ultrasonography of thorax 88.73)

✖ **34.29 Other diagnostic procedures on mediastinum**

Excludes | *mediastinal:*
pneumogram (87.33)
x-ray NEC (87.49)

✖ **34.3 Excision or destruction of lesion or tissue of mediastinum**

Excludes | *biopsy of mediastinum (34.25–34.26)*
mediastinal fistulectomy (34.73)

✖ **34.4 Excision or destruction of lesion of chest wall**
Excision of lesion of chest wall NOS (with excision of ribs)

Excludes | *biopsy of chest wall (34.23)*
costectomy not incidental to thoracic procedure (77.91)
excision of lesion of:
breast (85.20–85.25)
cartilage (80.89)
skin (86.2–86.3)
fistulectomy (34.73)

● **34.5 Pleurectomy**

✖ **34.51 Decortication of lung**

✖ **34.59 Other excision of pleura**
Excision of pleural lesion

Excludes | *biopsy of pleura (34.24)*
pleural fistulectomy (34.73)

✖ **34.6 Scarification of pleura**
Pleurosclerosis

Excludes | *injection of sclerosing agent (34.92)*

● **34.7 Repair of chest wall**

34.71 Suture of laceration of chest wall

Excludes | *suture of skin and subcutaneous tissue alone (86.59)*

34.72 Closure of thoracostomy

✖ **34.73 Closure of other fistula of thorax**
Closure of:
bronchopleural fistula
bronchopleurocutaneous fistula
bronchopleuromediastinal fistula

✖ **34.74 Repair of pectus deformity**
Repair of:
pectus carinatum (with implant)
pectus excavatum (with implant)

✖ **34.79 Other repair of chest wall**
Repair of chest wall NOS

● **Use Additional Digit(s)**   ✖ **Valid O.R. Procedure**   ◄ **New**   ◄▦ **Revised**

● 34.8 **Operations on diaphragm**

✖ 34.81 **Excision of lesion or tissue of diaphragm**
   Excludes | *biopsy of diaphragm (34.27)*

✖ 34.82 **Suture of laceration of diaphragm**

✖ 34.83 **Closure of fistula of diaphragm**
   Thoracicoabdominal fistulectomy
   Thoracicogastric fistulectomy
   Thoracicointestinal fistulectomy

✖ 34.84 **Other repair of diaphragm**
   Excludes | *repair of diaphragmatic hernia (53.7–53.82)*

✖ 34.85 **Implantation of diaphragmatic pacemaker**

✖ 34.89 **Other operations on diaphragm**

● 34.9 **Other operations on thorax**

34.91 **Thoracentesis**

34.92 **Injection into thoracic cavity**
   Chemical pleurodesis
   Injection of cytotoxic agent or tetracycline
   Requires additional code for any cancer
      chemotherapeutic substance (99.25)
   Excludes | *that for collapse of lung (33.32)*

✖ 34.93 **Repair of pleura**

✖ 34.99 **Other**
   Excludes | *removal of:*
      mediastinal drain (97.42)
      sutures (97.43)
      thoracotomy tube (97.41)

7. OPERATIONS ON THE CARDIOVASCULAR SYSTEM (35–39)

● **35   Operations on valves and septa of heart**

Includes: sternotomy (median) (transverse) as operative approach
thoracotomy as operative approach

Code also cardiopulmonary bypass [extracorporeal circulation] [heart-lung machine] (39.61)

● **35.0   Closed heart valvotomy**

Excludes percutaneous (balloon) valvuloplasty (35.96)

✖ **35.00   Closed heart valvotomy, unspecified valve**

✖ **35.01   Closed heart valvotomy, aortic valve**

✖ **35.02   Closed heart valvotomy, mitral valve**

✖ **35.03   Closed heart valvotomy, pulmonary valve**

✖ **35.04   Closed heart valvotomy, tricuspid valve**

● **35.1   Open heart valvuloplasty without replacement**

Includes: open heart valvotomy

Excludes that associated with repair of:
endocardial cushion defect (35.54, 35.63, 35.73)
percutaneous (balloon) valvuloplasty (35.96)
valvular defect associated with atrial and ventricular septal defects (35.54, 35.63, 35.73)

Code also cardiopulmonary bypass if performed [extracorporeal circulation] [heart-lung machine] (39.61)

✖ **35.10   Open heart valvuloplasty without replacement, unspecified valve**

✖ **35.11   Open heart valvuloplasty of aortic valve without replacement**

✖ **35.12   Open heart valvuloplasty of mitral valve without replacement**

✖ **35.13   Open heart valvuloplasty of pulmonary valve without replacement**

✖ **35.14   Open heart valvuloplasty of tricuspid valve without replacement**

● **35.2   Replacement of heart valve**

Includes: excision of heart valve with replacement

Code also cardiopulmonary bypass [extracorporeal circulation] [heart-lung machine] (39.61)

Excludes that associated with repair of:
endocardial cushion defect (35.54, 35.63, 35.73)
valvular defect associated with atrial and ventricular septal defects (35.54, 35.63, 35.73)

✖ **35.20   Replacement of unspecified heart valve**
Repair of unspecified heart valve with tissue graft or prosthetic implant

✖ **35.21   Replacement of aortic valve with tissue graft**
Repair of aortic valve with tissue graft (autograft) (heterograft) (homograft)

✖ **35.22   Other replacement of aortic valve**
Repair of aortic valve with replacement:
NOS
prosthetic (partial) (synthetic) (total)

✖ **35.23   Replacement of mitral valve with tissue graft**
Repair of mitral valve with tissue graft (autograft) (heterograft) (homograft)

✖ **35.24   Other replacement of mitral valve**
Repair of mitral valve with replacement:
NOS
prosthetic (partial) (synthetic) (total)

✖ **35.25   Replacement of pulmonary valve with tissue graft**
Repair of pulmonary valve with tissue graft (autograft) (heterograft) (homograft)

✖ **35.26   Other replacement of pulmonary valve**
Repair of pulmonary valve with replacement:
NOS
prosthetic (partial) (synthetic) (total)

✖ **35.27   Replacement of tricuspid valve with tissue graft**
Repair of tricuspid valve with tissue graft (autograft) (heterograft) (homograft)

✖ **35.28   Other replacement of tricuspid valve**
Repair of tricuspid valve with replacement:
NOS
prosthetic (partial) (synthetic) (total)

● **35.3   Operations on structures adjacent to heart valves**

Code also cardiopulmonary bypass [extracorporeal circulation] [heart-lung machine] (39.61)

✖ **35.31   Operations on papillary muscle**
Division of papillary muscle
Reattachment of papillary muscle
Repair of papillary muscle

✖ **35.32   Operations on chordae tendineae**
Division of chordae tendineae
Repair of chordae tendineae

✖ **35.33   Annuloplasty**
Plication of annulus

✖ **35.34   Infundibulectomy**
Right ventricular infundibulectomy

✖ **35.35   Operations on trabeculae carneae cordis**
Division of trabeculae carneae cordis
Excision of trabeculae carneae cordis
Excision of aortic subvalvular ring

✖ **35.39   Operations on other structures adjacent to valves of heart**
Repair of sinus of Valsalva (aneurysm)

● **35.4   Production of septal defect in heart**

35.41   Enlargement of existing atrial septal defect
Rashkind procedure
Septostomy (atrial) (balloon)

✖ **35.42   Creation of septal defect in heart**
Blalock-Hanlon operation

● **35.5   Repair of atrial and ventricular septa with prosthesis**

Includes: repair of septa with synthetic implant or patch

Code also cardiopulmonary bypass [extracorporeal circulation] [heart-lung machine] (39.61)

✖ **35.50   Repair of unspecified septal defect of heart with prosthesis**

Excludes that associated with repair of:
endocardial cushion defect (35.54)
septal defect associated with valvular defect (35.54)

✖ **35.51   Repair of atrial septal defect with prosthesis, open technique**
Atrioseptoplasty with prosthesis
Correction of atrial septal defect with prosthesis
Repair:
foramen ovale (patent)
with prosthesis ostium secundum defect with prosthesis

Excludes that associated with repair of:
atrial septal defect associated with valvular and ventricular septal defects (35.54)
endocardial cushion defect (35.54)

✖ **35.52 Repair of atrial septal defect with prosthesis, closed technique**
> Insertion of atrial septal umbrella [King-Mills]

✖ **35.53 Repair of ventricular septal defect with prosthesis**
> Correction of ventricular septal defect with prosthesis
> Repair of supracristal defect with prosthesis

> **Excludes** *that associated with repair of:*
> *endocardial cushion defect (35.54)*
> *ventricular defect associated with valvular and atrial septal defects (35.54)*

✖ **35.54 Repair of endocardial cushion defect with prosthesis**
> Repair:
> atrioventricular canal with prosthesis (grafted to septa)
> ostium primum defect with prosthesis (grafted to septa)
> valvular defect associated with atrial and ventricular septal defects with prosthesis (grafted to septa)

> **Excludes** *repair of isolated:*
> *atrial septal defect (35.51–35.52)*
> *valvular defect (35.20, 35.22, 35.24, 35.26, 35.28)*
> *ventricular septal defect (35.53)*

● **35.6 Repair of atrial and ventricular septa with tissue graft**

> Code also cardiopulmonary bypass [extracorporeal circulation] [heart-lung machine] (39.61)

✖ **35.60 Repair of unspecified septal defect of heart with tissue graft**

> **Excludes** *that associated with repair of:*
> *endocardial cushion defect (35.63)*
> *septal defect associated withvalvular defect (35.63)*

✖ **35.61 Repair of atrial septal defect with tissue graft**
> Atrioseptoplasty with tissue graft
> Correction of atrial septal defect with tissue graft
> Repair:
> foramen ovale (patent) with tissue graft
> ostium secundum defect with tissue graft

> **Excludes** *that associated with repair of:*
> *atrial septal defect associated with valvular and ventricular septal defects (35.63)*
> *endocardial cushion defect (35.63)*

✖ **35.62 Repair of ventricular septal defect with tissue graft**
> Correction of ventricular septal defect with tissue graft
> Repair of supracristal defect with tissue graft

> **Excludes** *that associated with repair of:*
> *endocardial cushion defect(35.63)*
> *ventricular defect associate with valvular and atrial septal defects (35.63)*

✖ **35.63 Repair of endocardial cushion defect with tissue graft**
> Repair of:
> atrioventricular canal with tissue graft
> ostium primum defect with tissue graft
> valvular defect associated with atrial and ventricular septal defects with tissue graft

> **Excludes** *repair of isolated:*
> *atrial septal defect (35.61)*
> *valvular defect (35.20–35.21, 35.23, 35.25, 35.27)*
> *ventricular septal defect (35.62)*

● **35.7 Other and unspecified repair of atrial and ventricular septa**

> Code also cardiopulmonary bypass [extracorporeal circulation] [heart-lung machine] (39.61)

✖ **35.70 Other and unspecified repair of unspecified septal defect of heart**
> Repair of septal defect NOS

> **Excludes** *that associated with repair of:*
> *endocardial cushion defect (35.73)*
> *septal defect associated with valvular defect (35.73)*

✖ **35.71 Other and unspecified repair of atrial septal defect**
> Repair NOS:
> atrial septum
> foramen ovale (patent)
> ostium secundum defect

> **Excludes** *that associated with repair of:*
> *atrial septal defect associated with valvular ventricular septal defects (35.73)*
> *endocardial cushion defect (35.73)*

✖ **35.72 Other and unspecified repair of ventricular septal defect**
> Repair NOS:
> supracristal defect
> ventricular septum

> **Excludes** *that associated with repair of:*
> *endocardial cushion defect (35.73)*
> *ventricular septal defect associated with valvular and atrial septal defects (35.73)*

✖ **35.73 Other and unspecified repair of endocardial cushion defect**
> Repair NOS:
> atrioventricular canal
> ostium primum defect
> valvular defect associated with atrial and ventricular septal defects

> **Excludes** *repair of isolated:*
> *atrial septal defect (35.71)*
> *valvular defect (35.20, 35.22, 35.24, 35.26, 35.28)*
> *ventricular septal defect (35.72)*

● **35.8 Total repair of certain congenital cardiac anomalies**

> Note: For partial repair of defect [e.g. repair of atrial septal defect in tetralogy of Fallot]—code to specific procedure

✖ **35.81 Total repair of tetralogy of Fallot**
> One-stage total correction of tetralogy of Fallot with or without:
> commissurotomy of pulmonary valve
> infundibulectomy
> outflow tract prosthesis
> patch graft of outflow tract
> prosthetic tube for pulmonary artery
> repair of ventricular septal defect (with prosthesis)
> take-down of previous systemic-pulmonary artery anastomosis

�ത **35.82 Total repair of total anomalous venous connection**

One-stage total correction of total anomalous pulmonary venous connection with or without:

anastomosis between (horizontal) common pulmonary trunk and posterior wall of left atrium (side-to-side)

enlargement of foramen ovale

incision [excision] of common wall between posterior left atrium and coronary sinus and roofing of resultant defect with patch graft (synthetic)

ligation of venous connection (descending anomalous vein) (to left innominate vein) (to superior vena cava)

repair of atrial septal defect (with prosthesis)

�ത **35.83 Total repair of truncus arteriosus**

One-stage total correction of truncus arteriosus with or without:

construction (with aortic homograft) (with prosthesis) of a pulmonary artery placed from right ventricle to arteries supplying the lung

ligation of connections between aorta and pulmonary artery

repair of ventricular septal defect (with prosthesis)

✯ **35.84 Total correction of transposition of great vessels, not elsewhere classified**

Arterial switch operation [Jatene]

Total correction of transposition of great arteries at the arterial level by switching the great arteries, including the left or both coronary arteries, implanted in the wall of the pulmonary artery

Excludes | baffle operation [Mustard] [Senning] (35.91)
creation of shunt between right ventricle and pulmonary artery [Rastelli] (35.92)

● **35.9 Other operations on valves and septa of heart**

Code also cardiopulmonary bypass, if performed [extracorporeal circulation] [heart-lung machine] (39.61)

✯ **35.91 Interatrial transposition of venous return**

Baffle:
atrial
interatrial

Mustard's operation

Resection of atrial septum and insertion of patch to direct systemic venous return to tricuspid valve and pulmonary venous return to mitral valve

✯ **35.92 Creation of conduit between right ventricle and pulmonary artery**

Creation of shunt between right ventricle and (distal) pulmonary artery

Excludes | that associated with total repair of truncus arteriosus (35.83)

✯ **35.93 Creation of conduit between left ventricle and aorta**

Creation of apicoaortic shunt

Shunt between apex of left ventricle and aorta

✯ **35.94 Creation of conduit between atrium and pulmonary artery**

Fontan procedure

✯ **35.95 Revision of corrective procedure on heart**

Replacement of prosthetic heart valve poppet

Resuture of prosthesis of:
septum
valve

Excludes | complete revision—code to specific procedure replacement of prosthesis or graft of:
septum (35.50–35.63)
valve (35.20–35.28)

✯ **35.96 Percutaneous valvuloplasty**

Percutaneous balloon valvuloplasty

✯ **35.98 Other operations on septa of heart**

✯ **35.99 Other operations on valves of heart**

● **36 Operations on vessels of heart**

Includes: sternotomy (median) (transverse) as operative approach
thoracotomy as operative approach

Code also cardiopulmonary bypass, if performed [extracorporeal circulation] [heart-lung machine] (39.61)

Code also any injection or infusion of platelet inhibitor (99.20)

● **36.0 Removal of coronary artery obstruction and insertion of stent(s)**

✯ **36.01 Single vessel percutaneous transluminal coronary angioplasty [PTCA] or coronary atherectomy without mention of thrombolytic agent**

Balloon angioplasty of coronary artery

Coronary atherectomy

Percutaneous coronary angioplasty NOS

PTCA NOS

Excludes | multiple vessel percutaneous transluminal coronary angioplasty [PTCA] or coronary atherectomy performed during the same operation (36.05)

Code also any insertion of coronary stent(s)(36.06)

✯ **36.02 Single vessel percutaneous transluminal coronary angioplasty [PTCA] or coronary atherectomy with mention of thrombolytic agent**

Balloon angioplasty of coronary artery with infusion of thrombolytic agent [streptokinase]

Coronary atherectomy

Excludes | multiple vessel percutaneous transluminal coronary angioplasty [PTCA] or coronary atherectomy performed during the same operation (36.05)
single vessel PTCA or coronary atherectomy without mention of thrombolytic agent (36.01)

Code also any insertion of coronary stent(s) (36.06)

✯ **36.03 Open chest coronary artery angioplasty**

Coronary (artery):
endarterectomy (with patch graft)
thromboendarterectomy (with patch graft)

Open surgery for direct relief of coronary artery obstruction

Excludes | that with coronary artery bypass graft (36.10–36.19)

Code also any insertion of coronary stent(s) (36.06)

36.04 Intracoronary artery thrombolytic infusion

That by direct coronary artery injection, infusion, or catheterization
enzyme infusion
platelet inhibitor

Excludes | infusion of platelet inhibitor (99.20)
infusion of thrombolytic agent (99.10)

✖ **36.05 Multiple vessel percutaneous transluminal coronary angioplasty [PTCA] or coronary atherectomy performed during the same operation, with or without mention of thrombolytic agent**
     Balloon angioplasty of multiple coronary arteries
     Coronary atherectomy

     Code also any:
         intracoronary artery thrombolytic infusion (36.04)
         insertion of coronary stent(s) (36.06)

     Excludes   *single vessel PTCA or coronary atherectomy*
         without mention of thrombolytic agent (36.01)
         with mention of thrombolytic agent (36.02)

✖ **36.06 Insertion of non-drug-eluting coronary artery stent(s)**
     Bare stent(s)
     Bonded stent(s)
     Drug-coated stent(s), i.e., heparin coated
     Endograft(s)
     Endovascular graft(s)
     Stent graft(s)

     Code also any:
         open chest coronary artery angioplasty (36.03)
         percutaneous transluminal coronary angioplasty [PTCA] or coronary atherectomy (36.01, 36.02, 36.05)

     Excludes   *insertion of drug-eluting coronary artery stent(s) (36.07)*

36.07 Insertion of drug-eluting coronary artery stent(s)
     Endograft(s)
     Endovascular graft(s)
     Stent graft(s)

     Code also any:
         open chest coronary artery angioplasty (36.03)
         percutaneous transluminal coronary angioplasty [PCTA] or coronary atherectomy (36.01, 36.02, 36.05)

     Excludes   *drug-coated stents, e.g., heparin coated (36.06)*
         insertion of non-drug-eluting coronary artery stent(s) (36.06)

✖ **36.09 Other removal of coronary artery obstruction**
     Coronary angioplasty NOS

     Excludes   *that by open angioplasty (36.03)*
         that by percutaneous transluminal coronary angioplasty [PTCA] or coronary atherectomy (36.01–36.02, 36.05)

● **36.1 Bypass anastomosis for heart revascularization**

     Code also cardiopulmonary bypass [extracorporeal circulation] [heart-lung machine] (39.61)

     Code also pressurized treatment of venous bypass graft [conduit] with pharmaceutical substance, if performed (00.16) ◄

✖ **36.10 Aortocoronary bypass for heart revascularization, not otherwise specified**
     Direct revascularization:
         cardiac with catheter stent, prosthesis, or vein graft
         coronary with catheter stent, prosthesis, or vein graft
         heart muscle with catheter stent, prosthesis, or vein graft
         myocardial with catheter stent, prosthesis, or vein graft
     Heart revascularization NOS

✖ **36.11 (Aorto)coronary bypass of one coronary artery** ⬅

✖ **36.12 (Aorto)coronary bypass of two coronary arteries** ⬅

✖ **36.13 (Aorto)coronary bypass of three coronary arteries** ⬅

✖ **36.14 (Aorto)coronary bypass of four or more coronary arteries** ⬅

✖ **36.15 Single internal mammary-coronary artery bypass**
     Anastomosis (single):
         mammary artery to coronary artery
         thoracic artery to coronary artery

✖ **36.16 Double internal mammary-coronary artery bypass**
     Anastomosis, double:
         mammary artery to coronary artery
         thoracic artery to coronary artery

✖ **36.17 Abdominal-coronary artery bypass**
     Anastomosis:
         Gastroepiploic-coronary artery

✖ **36.19 Other bypass anastomosis for heart revascularization**

✖ **36.2 Heart revascularization by arterial implant**
     Implantation of:
         aortic branches [ascending aortic branches] into heart muscle
         blood vessels into myocardium
         internal mammary artery [internal thoracic artery] into:
            heart muscle
            myocardium
            ventricle
            ventricular wall
         indirect heart revascularization NOS

● **36.3 Other heart revascularization**

✖ **36.31 Open chest transmyocardial revascularization**

✖ **36.32 Other transmyocardial revascularization**
     Percutaneous transmyocardial revascularization
     Thoracoscopic transmyocardial revascularization

✖ **36.39 Other heart revascularization**
     Abrasion of epicardium
     Cardio-omentopexy
     Intrapericardial poudrage
     Myocardial graft:
         mediastinal fat
         omentum
         pectoral muscles

● **36.9 Other operations on vessels of heart**

     Code also cardiopulmonary bypass [extracorporeal circulation] [heart-lung machine] (39.61)

✖ **36.91 Repair of aneurysm of coronary vessel**

✖ **36.99 Other operations on vessels of heart**
     Exploration of coronary artery
     Incision of coronary artery
     Ligation of coronary artery
     Repair of arteriovenous fistula

● **37 Other operations on heart and pericardium**

     Code also any injection or infusion of platelet inhibitor (99.20)

37.0 Pericardiocentesis

● **37.1 Cardiotomy and pericardiotomy**

     Code also cardiopulmonary bypass [extracorporeal circulation] [heart-lung machine] (39.61)

✖ **37.10 Incision of heart, not otherwise specified**
     Cardiolysis NOS

✷ **37.11 Cardiotomy**
Incision of:
    atrium
    endocardium
    myocardium
    ventricle

✷ **37.12 Pericardiotomy**
Pericardial window operation
Pericardiolysis
Pericardiotomy

● **37.2 Diagnostic procedures on heart and pericardium**

37.21 Right heart cardiac catheterization
Cardiac catheterization NOS

> Excludes | *that with catheterization of left heart (37.23)*

37.22 Left heart cardiac catheterization

> Excludes | *that with catheterization of right heart (37.23)*

37.23 Combined right and left heart cardiac catheterization

✷ **37.24 Biopsy of pericardium**

37.25 Biopsy of heart

37.26 Cardiac electrophysiologic stimulation and recording studies
Electrophysiologic studies [EPS]
Non-invasive programmed electrical stimulation (NIPS)
Programmed electrical stimulation

Code also any concomitant procedure

> Excludes | *device interrogation only without arrhythmia induction (bedside check) (89.45–89.49)* ◀
> *His bundle recording (37.29)*

37.27 Cardiac mapping

Code also any concomitant procedure

> Excludes | *electrocardiogram (89.52)*
> *His bundle recording (37.29)*

37.28 Intracardiac echocardiography
Echocardiography of heart chambers ◀
ICE

Code also any synchronous Doppler flow mapping (88.72)

> Excludes | *intravascular imagining of coronary vessels (intravascular ultrasound) (IVUS) (00.24)* ◀

37.29 Other diagnostic procedures on heart and pericardium

> Excludes | *angiocardiography (88.50–88.58)*
> *cardiac function tests (89.41–89.69)*
> *cardiovascular radioisotopic scan and function study (92.05)*
> *coronary arteriography (88.55–88.57)*
> *diagnostic pericardiocentesis (37.0)*
> *diagnostic ultrasound of heart (88.72)*
> *x-ray of heart (87.49)*

● **37.3 Pericardiectomy and excision of lesion of heart**

Code also cardiopulmonary bypass [extracorporeal circulation] [heart-lung machine] (39.61)

✷ **37.31 Pericardiectomy**
Excision of:
    adhesions of pericardium
    constricting scar of:
        epicardium
        pericardium

✷ **37.32 Excision of aneurysm of heart**

Repair of aneurysm of heart

✷ **37.33 Excision or destruction of other lesion or tissue of heart, open approach**
Ablation of heart tissue (cryoablation) (electrocurrent) (laser) (microwave) (radiofrequency) (resection), open chest approach
Cox-maze procedure
Maze procedure
Modified maze procedure, trans-thoracic approach

> Excludes | *ablation, excision or destruction of lesion or tissue of heart, endovascular approach (37.34)*

✷ **37.34 Excision or destruction of other lesion or tissue of heart, other approach**
Ablation of heart tissue (cryoablation) (electrocurrent) (laser) (microwave) (radiofrequency) (resection), via peripherally inserted catheter
Modified maze procedure, endovascular approach

✷ **37.35 Partial ventriculectomy**
Ventricular reduction surgery
Ventricular remodeling
Code also any synchronous:
    mitral valve repair (35.02, 35.12)
    mitral valve replacement (35.23–35.24)

✷ **37.4 Repair of heart and pericardium**

● **37.5 Heart replacement procedures**

> Excludes | *combined heart-lung transplantation (33.6)*

✷ **37.51 Heart transplantation**

> Excludes | *combined heart-lung transplantation (33.6)*

✷ **37.52 Implantation of total replacement heart system**
Artificial heart
Implantation of fully implantable total replacement heart system, including ventriculectomy

> Excludes | *implantation of heart assist system [VAD] (37.62, 37.65, 37.66)* ◀▥

✷ **37.53 Replacement or repair of thoracic unit of total replacement heart system**

> Excludes | *replacement and repair of heart assist system [VAD] (37.63)* ◀▥

✷ **37.54 Replacement or repair of other implantable component of total replacement heart system**
Implantable battery
Implantable controller
Transcutaneous energy transfer (TET) device

> Excludes | *replacement and repair of heart assist system [VAD] (37.63)*
> *replacement or repair of thoracic unit of total replacement heart system (37.53)*

● **37.6 Implantation of heart circulatory assist system** ◀▥

✷ **37.61 Implant of pulsation balloon**

✷ **37.62 Insertion of non-implantable heart assist system** ◀▥
Insertion of heart assist system, NOS
Insertion of heart pump

> Excludes | *implantation of total replacement heart system (37.52)*
> *insertion of percutaneous external heart assist device (37.68)* ◀

✷ **37.63 Repair of heart assist system** ◀▥
Replacement of parts of an existing ventricular assist device (VAD) ◀

> Excludes | *replacement or repair of other implantable component of total replacement heart system [artificial heart] (37.54)* ◀▥
> *replacement or repair of thoracic unit of total replacement heart system [artificial heart] (37.53)* ◀▥

✖**37.64 Removal of heart assist system**

Excludes *explanation [removal] of percutaneous external heart assist device (97.44)* ◄
that with replacement of implant (37.63)

✖**37.65 Implant of external heart assist system** ◄▥

Note: Device (outside the body but connected to heart) with external circulation and pump. Includes open chest (sternotomy) procedure for cannulae attachments ◄▥

Excludes *implant of pulsation balloon (37.61)*
implantation of total replacement heart system (37.52)
insertion of percutaneous external heart assist device (37.68) ◄

✖**37.66 Insertion of implantable, heart assist system** ◄▥
Axial flow heart assist system ◄
Diagonal pump heart assist system ◄
Left ventricular assist device (LVAD) ◄
Pulsatile heart assist system ◄
Right ventricular assist device (RVAD) ◄
Rotary pump heart assist system ◄
Transportable, implantable heart assist system
Ventricular assist device (VAD) not otherwise specified ◄

Note: Device directly connected to the heart and implanted in the upper left quadrant of peritoneal cavity.

Excludes *implant of pulsation balloon (37.61)*
implantation of total replacement heart system [artificial heart] (37.52) ◄▥
insertion of percutaneous external heart assist device (37.68) ◄

✖**37.67 Implantation of cardiomyostimulation system**

Note: Two-step open procedure consisting of transfer of one end of the latissimus dorsi muscle; wrapping it around the heart; rib resection; implantation of epicardial cardiac pacing leads into the right ventricle; tunneling and pocket creation for the cardiomyostimulator.

✖**37.68 Insertion of percutaneous external heart assist device** ◄
Includes percutaneous [femoral] insertion of cannulae attachments ◄
Circulatory assist device ◄
Extrinsic heart assist device ◄
pVAD ◄
Percutaneous heart assist device ◄

●**37.7 Insertion, revision, replacement, and removal of pacemaker leads; insertion of temporary pacemaker system; or revision of pocket**

Code also any insertion and replacement of pacemaker device (37.80–37.87)

Excludes *implantation or replacement of transvenous lead [electrode] into left ventricular cardiac venous system (00.52)*

37.70 Initial insertion of lead [electrode], not otherwise specified

Excludes *insertion of temporary transvenous pacemaker system (37.78)*
replacement of atrial and/or ventricular lead(s) (37.76)

37.71 Initial insertion of transvenous lead [electrode] into ventricle

Excludes *insertion of temporary transvenous pacemaker system (37.78)*
replacement of atrial and/or ventricular lead(s) (37.76)

37.72 Initial insertion of transvenous leads [electrodes] into atrium and ventricle

Excludes *insertion of temporary transvenous pacemaker system (37.78)*
replacement of atrial and/or ventricular lead(s) (37.76)

37.73 Initial insertion of transvenous lead [electrode] into atrium

Excludes *insertion of temporary transvenous pacemaker system (37.78)*
replacement of atrial and/or ventricular lead(s) (37.76)

✖**37.74 Insertion or replacement of epicardial lead [electrode] into epicardium**
Insertion or replacement of epicardial by:
sternotomy
thoracotomy

Excludes *replacement of atrial and/or ventricular lead(s) (37.76)*

✖**37.75 Revision of lead [electrode]**
Repair of electrode [removal with re-insertion]
Repositioning of lead [electrode]
Revision of lead NOS

Excludes *repositioning of temporary transvenous pacemaker system—omit code*

✖**37.76 Replacement of transvenous atrial and/or ventricular lead(s) [electrode]**
Removal or abandonment of existing transvenous or epicardial lead(s) with transvenous lead(s) replacement

Excludes *replacement of epicardial lead [electrode] (37.74)*

✖**37.77 Removal of lead(s) [electrode] without replacement**
Removal:
epicardial lead (transthoracic approach)
transvenous lead(s)

Excludes *removal of temporary transvenous pacemaker system—omit code*
that with replacement of:
atrial and/or ventricular lead(s) [electrode] (37.76)
epicardial lead [electrode] (37.74)

37.78 Insertion of temporary transvenous pacemaker system

Excludes *intraoperative cardiac pacemaker (39.64)*

✖**37.79 Revision or relocation of pacemaker pocket**
Debridement and reforming pocket (skin and subcutaneous tissue)
Relocation of pocket [creation of new pocket] pacemaker or CRT-P

●**37.8 Insertion, replacement, removal, and revision of pacemaker device**

Code also any lead insertion, lead replacement, lead removal and/or lead revision (37.70–37.77)

Excludes *implantation of cardiac resynchronization pacemaker [CRT-P] (00.50)*
implantation or replacement of cardiac resynchronization pacemaker pulse generator only [CRT-P] (00.53)

✖**37.80 Insertion of permanent pacemaker, initial or replacement, type of device not specified**

37.81 Initial insertion of single-chamber device, not specified as rate responsive

Excludes *replacement of existing pacemaker device (37.85–37.87)*

37.82 Initial insertion of single-chamber device, rate responsive
Rate responsive to physiologic stimuli other than atrial rate

> **Excludes** *replacement of existing pacemaker device (37.85–37.87)*

37.83 Initial insertion of dual-chamber device
Atrial ventricular sequential device

> **Excludes** *replacement of existing pacemaker device (37.85–37.87)*

�ö **37.85 Replacement of any type pacemaker device with single-chamber device, not specified as rate responsive**

✖ **37.86 Replacement of any type of pacemaker device with single-chamber device, rate responsive**
Rate responsive to physiologic stimuli other than atrial rate

✖ **37.87 Replacement of any type pacemaker device with dual-chamber device**
Atrial ventricular sequential device

✖ **37.89 Revision or removal of pacemaker device**
Removal without replacement of cardiac resynchronization pacemaker device [CRT-P]
Repair of pacemaker device

> **Excludes** *removal of temporary transvenous pacemaker system—omit code*
> *replacement of existing pacemaker device (37.85–37.87)*
> *replacement of existing pacemaker device with CRT-P pacemaker device (00.53)*

● **37.9 Other operations on heart and pericardium**

✖ **37.90 Insertion of left atrial appendage device** ◀
Left atrial filter ◀
Left atrial occluder ◀
Transeptal catheter technique ◀

✖ **37.91 Open chest cardiac massage**

> **Excludes** *closed chest cardiac massage (99.63)*

37.92 Injection of therapeutic substance into heart

37.93 Injection of therapeutic substance into pericardium

✖ **37.94 Implantation or replacement of automatic cardioverter/defibrillator, total system [AICD]**
Implantation of defibrillator with leads (epicardial patches), formation of pocket (abdominal fascia) (subcutaneous), any transvenous leads, intraoperative procedures for evaluation of lead signals, and obtaining defibrillator threshold measurements (electrophysiologic studies [EPS])
Techniques:
lateral thoracotomy
medial sternotomy
subxiphoid procedure

Code also extracorporeal circulation, if performed (39.61)

Code also any concomitant procedure [e.g., coronary bypass] (36.00–36.19)

> **Excludes** *implantation of cardiac resynchronization defibrillator, total system [CRT-D] (00.51)*

✖ **37.95 Implantation of automatic cardioverter/defibrillator lead(s) only**

✖ **37.96 Implantation of automatic cardioverter/defibrillator pulse generator only**

> **Excludes** *implantation or replacement of cardiac resynchronization defibrillator, pulse generator device only [CRT-D] (00.54)*

✖ **37.97 Replacement of automatic cardioverter/defibrillator lead(s) only**

✖ **37.98 Replacement of automatic cardioverter/defibrillator pulse generator only**

> **Excludes** *replacement of cardiac resynchronization defibrillator, pulse generator device only [CRT-D] (00.54)*

✖ **37.99 Other**
Removal of cardioverter/defibrillator pulse generator only without replacement
Removal without replacement of cardiac resynchronization defibrillator device [CRT-D]
Repositioning of lead(s) (sensing) (pacing) [electrode]
Repositioning of pulse generator
Revision of cardioverter/defibrillator (automatic) pocket
Revision or relocation of CRT-D pocket

> **Excludes** *cardiac retraining (93.36)*
> *conversion of cardiac rhythm (99.60–99.69)*
> *insertion of left atrial appendage device (37.90)* ◀
> *maze procedure (Cox-maze), open (37.33)*
> *maze procedure, endovascular approach (37.34)*

● **38 Incision, excision, and occlusion of vessels**

Code also any application or administration of an adhesion barrier substance (99.77)

Code also cardiopulmonary bypass [extracorporeal circulation] [heart-lung machine] (39.61)

> **Excludes** *that of coronary vessels (36.01–36.99)*

The following fourth-digit subclassification is for use with appropriate categories in section 38.0, 38.1, 38.3, 38.5, 38.6, 38.8, and 38.9 according to site. Valid fourth-digits are in [brackets] at the end of each code/description.

0 unspecified site
1 intracranial vessels
Cerebral (anterior) (middle)
Circle of Willis
Posterior communicating artery
2 other vessels of head and neck
Carotid artery (common) (external) (internal)
Jugular vein (external) (internal)
3 upper limb vessels
Axillary
Brachial
Radial
Ulnar
4 aorta
5 other thoracic vessels
Innominate
Pulmonary (artery) (vein)
Subclavian
Vena cava, superior
6 abdominal arteries
Celiac
Gastric
Hepatic
Iliac
Mesenteric
Renal
Splenic
Umbilical

> **Excludes** *abdominal aorta (4)*

● **Use Additional Digit(s)**   ✖ **Valid O.R. Procedure**   ◀ **New**   ◀▌ **Revised**

7 abdominal veins
    Iliac
    Portal
    Renal
    Splenic
    Vena cava (inferior)
8 lower limb arteries
    Femoral (common) (superficial)
    Popliteal
    Tibial
9 lower limb veins
    Femoral
    Popliteal
    Saphenous
    Tibial

✖ ● 38.0 Incision of vessel
[0–9] Embolectomy
    Thrombectomy

   Excludes *puncture or catheterization of any:*
      artery (38.91, 38.98)
      vein (38.92–38.95, 38.99)

✖ ● 38.1 Endarterectomy
[0–6, 8] Endarterectomy with:
    embolectomy
    patch graft
    temporary bypass during procedure
    thrombectomy

● 38.2 Diagnostic procedures on blood vessels

  ✖ 38.21 Biopsy of blood vessel

  38.22 Percutaneous angioscopy

   Excludes *angioscopy of eye (95.12)*

  ✖ 38.29 Other diagnostic procedures on blood vessels

   Excludes *blood vessel thermography (88.86)*
    circulatory monitoring (89.61–89.69)
    contrast:
     angiocardiography (88.50–88.58)
     arteriography (88.40–88.49)
     phlebography (88.60–88.67)
    impedance phlebography (88.68)
    peripheral vascular ultrasonography (88.77)
    plethysmogram (89.58)

✖ ● 38.3 Resection of vessel with anastomosis
[0–9] Angiectomy
    Excision of:
     aneurysm (arteriovenous) with anastomosis
     blood vessel (lesion) with anastomosis

✖ ● 38.4 Resection of vessel with replacement
[0–9] Angiectomy
    Excision of:
     aneurysm (arteriovenous) or blood vessel (lesion)
     with replacement

   Excludes *endovascular repair of aneurysm (39.71–39.79)*

Requires the use of one of the following fourth-digit subclassifications to identify site:
0 unspecified site
1 intracranial vessels
    Cerebral (anterior) (middle)
    Circle of Willis
    Posterior communicating artery
2 other vessels of head and neck
    Carotid artery (common) (external) (internal)
    Jugular vein (external) (internal)
3 upper limb vessels
    Axillary
    Brachial
    Radial
    Ulnar
4 aorta, abdominal
    Code also any thoracic vessel involvement (thoracoabdominal procedure) (38.45)

5 thoracic vessels
    Aorta (thoracic)
    Innominate
    Pulmonary (artery) (vein)
    Subclavian
    Vena cava, superior
     Code also any abdominal aorta involvement (thoracoabdominal procedure) (38.44)
6 abdominal arteries
    Celiac
    Gastric
    Hepatic
    Iliac
    Mesenteric
    Renal
    Splenic
    Umbilical

   Excludes *abdominal aorta (4)*

7 abdominal veins
    Iliac
    Portal
    Renal
    Splenic
    Vena cava (inferior)
8 lower limb arteries
    Femoral (common) (superficial)
    Popliteal
    Tibial
9 lower limb veins
    Femoral
    Popliteal
    Saphenous
    Tibial

✖ ● 38.5 Ligation and stripping of varicose veins
[0–3, 5, 7, 9]

   Excludes *ligation of varices:*
    esophageal (42.91)
    gastric (44.91)

✖ ● 38.6 Other excision of vessel
[0–9] Excision of blood vessel (lesion) NOS

   Excludes *excision of vessel for aortocoronary bypass (36.10–36.14)*
    excision with:
    anastomosis (38.30–38.39)
    graft replacement (38.40–38.49)
    implant (38.40–38.49)

38.7 Interruption of the vena cava
    Insertion of implant or sieve in vena cava
    Ligation of vena cava (inferior) (superior)
    Plication of vena cava

✖ ● 38.8 Other surgical occlusion of vessels
[0–9] Clamping of blood vessel
    Division of blood vessel
    Ligation of blood vessel
    Occlusion of blood vessel

   Excludes *adrenal vessels (07.43)*
    esophageal varices (42.91)
    gastric or duodenal vessel for ulcer (44.40–44.49)
    gastric varices (44.91)
    meningeal vessel (02.13)
    percutaneous transcatheter infusion embolization (99.29)
    spermatic vein for varicocele (63.1)
    surgical occlusion of vena cava (38.7)
    that for chemoembolization (99.25)
    that for control of (postoperative) hemorrhage:
     anus (49.95)
     bladder (57.93)
     following vascular procedure (39.41)
     nose (21.00–21.09)
     prostate (60.94)
     tonsil (28.7)
     thyroid vessel (06.92)
    transcatheter (infusion) (99.29)

● **38.9 Puncture of vessel**

> Excludes   *that for circulatory monitoring (89.60–89.69)*

38.91 Arterial catheterization

38.92 Umbilical vein catheterization

38.93 Venous catheterization, not elsewhere classified

> Excludes   *that for cardiac catheterization (37.21–37.23)*
> *that for renal dialysis (38.95)*

38.94 Venous cutdown

38.95 Venous catheterization for renal dialysis

> Excludes   *insertion of totally implantable vascular access device [VAD] (86.07)*

38.98 Other puncture of artery

> Excludes   *that for:*
> *arteriography (88.40–88.49)*
> *coronary arteriography (88.55–88.57)*

38.99 Other puncture of vein
Phlebotomy

> Excludes   *that for:*
> *angiography (88.60–88.69)*
> *extracorporeal circulation (39.61, 50.92)*
> *injection or infusion of:*
> *sclerosing solution (39.92)*
> *therapeutic or prophylactic substance (99.11–99.29)*
> *perfusion (39.96–39.97)*
> *phlebography (88.60–88.69)*
> *transfusion (99.01–99.09)*

● **39 Other operations on vessels**

> Excludes   *those on coronary vessels (36.00–36.99)*

✖ **39.0 Systemic to pulmonary artery shunt**
Descending aorta-pulmonary artery anastomosis (graft)
Left to right anastomosis (graft)
Subclavian-pulmonary anastomosis (graft)

Code also cardiopulmonary bypass [extracorporeal circulation] [heart-lung machine] (39.61)

✖ **39.1 Intra-abdominal venous shunt**
Anastomosis:
mesocaval
portacaval
portal vein to inferior vena cava
splenic and renal veins
transjugular intrahepatic portosystemic shunt (TIPS)

> Excludes   *peritoneovenous shunt (54.94)*

● **39.2 Other shunt or vascular bypass**

Code also pressurized treatment of venous bypass graft [conduit] with pharmaceutical substance, if performed (00.16) ◄

✖ **39.21 Caval-pulmonary artery anastomosis**

Code also cardiopulmonary bypass (39.61)

✖ **39.22 Aorta-subclavian-carotid bypass**
Bypass (arterial):
aorta to carotid and brachial
aorta to subclavian and carotid
carotid to subclavian

✖ **39.23 Other intrathoracic vascular shunt or bypass**
Intrathoracic (arterial) bypass graft NOS

> Excludes   *coronary artery bypass (36.10–36.19)*

✖ **39.24 Aorta-renal bypass**

✖ **39.25 Aorta-iliac-femoral bypass**
Bypass:
aortofemoral
aortoiliac
aortoiliac to popliteal
aortopopliteal
iliofemoral [iliac-femoral]

✖ **39.26 Other intra-abdominal vascular shunt or bypass**
Bypass:
aortoceliac
aortic-superior mesenteric
common hepatic-common iliac-renal
Intra-abdominal arterial bypass graft NOS

> Excludes   *peritoneovenous shunt (54.94)*

✖ **39.27 Arteriovenostomy for renal dialysis**
Anastomosis for renal dialysis
Formation of (peripheral) arteriovenous
fistula for renal [kidney] dialysis

Code also any renal dialysis (39.95)

✖ **39.28 Extracranial-intracranial (EC-IC) vascular bypass**

✖ **39.29 Other (peripheral) vascular shunt or bypass**
Bypass (graft):
axillary-brachial
axillary-femoral [axillofemoral] (superficial)
brachial
femoral-femoral
femoroperoneal
femoropopliteal (arteries)
femorotibial (anterior) (posterior)
popliteal
vascular NOS

> Excludes   *peritoneovenous shunt (54.94)*

● **39.3 Suture of vessel**
Repair of laceration of blood vessel

> Excludes   *any other vascular puncture closure device-omit code*
> *suture of aneurysm (39.52)*
> *that for control of hemorrhage (postoperative):*
> *anus (49.95)*
> *bladder (57.93)*
> *following vascular procedure (39.41)*
> *nose (21.00–21.09)*
> *prostate (60.94)*
> *tonsil (28.7)*

✖ **39.30 Suture of unspecified blood vessel**

✖ **39.31 Suture of artery**

✖ **39.32 Suture of vein**

● **39.4 Revision of vascular procedure**

✖ **39.41 Control of hemorrhage following vascular surgery**

> Excludes   *that for control of hemorrhage (post operative):*
> *anus (49.95)*
> *bladder (57.93)*
> *nose (21.00–21.09)*
> *prostate (60.94)*
> *tonsil (28.7)*

✖ **39.42 Revision of arteriovenous shunt for renal dialysis**
Conversion of renal dialysis:
end-to-end anastomosis to end-to-side
end-to-side anastomosis to end-to-end
vessel-to-vessel cannula to arteriovenous shunt
Removal of old arteriovenous shunt and creation of new shunt

> Excludes   *replacement of vessel-to-vessel cannula (39.94)*

✖ **39.43 Removal of arteriovenous shunt for renal dialysis**

> **Excludes**   *that with replacement [revision] of shunt (39.42)*

✖ **39.49 Other revision of vascular procedure**
Declotting (graft)
Revision of:
    anastomosis of blood vessel
    vascular procedure (previous)

● **39.5   Other repair of vessels**

✖ **39.50 Angioplasty or atherectomy of other non-coronary vessel(s)** ◀▥
Percutaneous transluminal angioplasty (PTA)
    of non-coronary vessels:
    Lower extremity vessels
    Mesenteric artery
    Renal artery
    Upper extremity vessels

Code also any:
    injection or infusion of thrombolytic agent
      (99.10)
    insertion of non-coronary stent(s) or stent
      grafts(s) (39.90)
    percutaneous insertion of carotid artery
      stent(s) (00.63) ◀

> **Excludes**   *percutaneous angioplasty or atherectomy of precerebral or cerebral vessel(s) (00.61–00.62)* ◀

✖ **39.51 Clipping of aneurysm**

> **Excludes**   *clipping of arteriovenous fistula (39.53)*

✖ **39.52 Other repair of aneurysm**
Repair of aneurysm by:
    coagulation
    electrocoagulation
    filipuncture
    methyl methacrylate
    suture
    wiring
    wrapping

> **Excludes**   *endovascular repair of aneurysm (39.71–39.79)*
> *re-entry operation (aorta) (39.54)*
> *that with:*
>   *graft replacement (38.40–38.49)*
>   *resection (38.30–38.49, 38.60–38.69)*

✖ **39.53 Repair of arteriovenous fistula**
Embolization of carotid cavernous fistula
Repair of arteriovenous fistula by:
    clipping
    coagulation
    ligation and division

> **Excludes**   *repair of:*
>   *arteriovenous shunt for renal dialysis*
>   *(39.42)*
>   *head and neck vessels, endovascular approach*
>   *(39.72)*
>   *that with:*
>   *graft replacement (38.40–38.49)*
>   *resection (38.30–38.49, 38.60–38.69)*

✖ **39.54 Re-entry operation (aorta)**
Fenestration of dissecting aneurysm of thoracic aorta

Code also cardiopulmonary bypass [extracorporeal circulation] [heart-lung machine] (39.61)

✖ **39.55 Reimplantation of aberrant renal vessel**

✖ **39.56 Repair of blood vessel with tissue patch graft**

> **Excludes**   *that with resection (38.40–38.49)*

✖ **39.57 Repair of blood vessel with synthetic patch graft**

> **Excludes**   *that with resection (38.40–38.49)*

✖ **39.58 Repair of blood vessel with unspecified type of patch graft**

> **Excludes**   *that with resection (38.40–38.49)*

✖ **39.59 Other repair of vessel**
Aorticopulmonary window operation
Arterioplasty NOS
Construction of venous valves (peripheral)
Plication of vein (peripheral)
Reimplantation of artery

Code also cardiopulmonary bypass [extracorporeal circulation] [heart-lung machine] (39.61)

> **Excludes**   *interruption of the vena cava (38.7)*
> *reimplantation of renal artery (39.55)*
> *that with:*
>   *graft (39.56–39.58)*
>   *resection (38.30–38.49, 38.60–38.69)*

● **39.6   Extracorporeal circulation and procedures auxiliary to heart surgery**

39.61 Extracorporeal circulation auxiliary to open heart surgery
Artificial heart and lung
Cardiopulmonary bypass
Pump oxygenator

> **Excludes**   *extracorporeal hepatic assistance (50.92)*
> *extracorporeal membrane oxygenation [ECMO]*
>   *(39.65)*
> *hemodialysis (39.95)*
> *percutaneous cardiopulmonary bypass (39.66)*

39.62 Hypothermia (systemic) incidental to open heart surgery

39.63 Cardioplegia
Arrest:
    anoxic
    circulatory

39.64 Intraoperative cardiac pacemaker
Temporary pacemaker used during and immediately following cardiac surgery

39.65 Extracorporeal membrane oxygenation [ECMO]

> **Excludes**   *extracorporeal circulation auxiliary to open heart*
>   *surgery (39.61)*
> *percutaneous cardiopulmonary bypass (39.66)*

39.66 Percutaneous cardiopulmonary bypass
Closed chest

> **Excludes**   *extracorporeal circulation auxiliary to open heart*
>   *surgery (39.61)*
> *extracorporeal hepatic assistance (50.92)*
> *extracorporeal membrane oxygenation [ECMO]*
>   *(39.65)*
> *hemodialysis (39.95)*

660-100

Vol.

● **39.7 Endovascular repair of vessel**
Endoluminal repair

> **Excludes** angioplasty or atherectomy of other non-coronary vessel (39.50) ◀▥
>
> insertion of non-drug-eluting peripheral vessel stent(s) (39.90) ◀▥
>
> other repair of aneurysm (39.52)
>
> percutaneous insertion of carotid artery stent(s) (00.63) ◀
>
> percutaneous insertion of intracranial stent(s) (00.65) ◀
>
> percutaneous insertion of other precerebral artery stent(s) (00.64) ◀
>
> resection of abdominal aorta with replacement (38.44)
>
> resection of lower limb arteries with replacement (38.48)
>
> resection of thoracic aorta with replacement (38.45)
>
> resection of upper limb vessels with replacement (38.43)

✖ **39.71 Endovascular implantation of graft in abdominal aorta**
Endovascular repair of abdominal aortic aneurysm with graft
Stent graft(s)

✖ **39.72 Endovascular repair or occlusion of head and neck vessels**
Coil embolization or occlusion
Endograft(s)
Endovascular graft(s)
Liquid tissue adhesive (glue) embolization or occlusion
Other implant or substance for repair, embolization or occlusion
That for repair of aneurysm, arteriovenous malformation [AVM] or fistula

✖ **39.79 Other endovascular repair (of aneurysm) of other vessels**
Coil embolization or occlusion
Endograft(s)
Endovascular graft(s)
Liquid tissue adhesive (glue) embolization or occlusion
Other implant or substance for repair, embolization or occlusion

> **Excludes** endovascular repair or occlusion of head and neck vessels (39.72)
>
> insertion of drug-eluting peripheral vessel stent(s) (00.55) ◀▥
>
> insertion of non-drug-eluting peripheral vessel stent(s) (for other than aneurysm repair) (39.90) ◀▥
>
> non-endovascular repair of arteriovenous fistula (39.53)
>
> other surgical occlusion of vessels - see category 38.8
>
> percutaneous transcatheter infusion (99.29)
>
> transcatheter embolization for gastric or duodenal bleeding (44.44)

✖ **39.8 Operations on carotid body and other vascular bodies**
Chemodectomy
Denervation of:
  aortic body
  carotid body
Glomectomy, carotid
Implantation into carotid body:
  electronic stimulator
  pacemaker

> **Excludes** excision of glomus jugulare (20.51)

● **39.9 Other operations on vessels**

39.90 Insertion of non-drug-eluting, peripheral vessel stent(s) ◀▥
Bare stent(s)
Bonded stent(s)
Drug-coated stent(s), i.e., heparin coated
Endograft(s)
Endovascular graft(s)

> **Excludes** insertion of drug-eluting, peripheral vessel stent(s) (00.55) ◀▥
>
> percutaneous insertion of carotid artery stent(s) (00.63) ◀
>
> percutaneous insertion of intracranial stent(s) (00.65) ◀
>
> percutaneous insertion of other precerebral artery stent(s) (00.64) ◀
>
> that for aneurysm repair (39.71–39.79)
>   Endovascular recanalization techniques
>   Stent graft(s)

Code also any non-coronary angioplasty or atherectomy (39.50)

✖ **39.91 Freeing of vessel**
Dissection and freeing of adherent tissue:
  artery-vein-nerve bundle
  vascular bundle

✖ **39.92 Injection of sclerosing agent into vein**

> **Excludes** injection:
>   esophageal varices (42.33)
>   hemorrhoids (49.42)

✖ **39.93 Insertion of vessel-to-vessel cannula**
Formation of:
  arteriovenous:
    fistula by external cannula
    shunt by external cannula

Code also any renal dialysis (39.95)

✖ **39.94 Replacement of vessel-to-vessel cannula**
Revision of vessel-to-vessel cannula

39.95 Hemodialysis
Artificial kidney
Hemodiafiltration
Hemofiltration
Renal dialysis

> **Excludes** peritoneal dialysis (54.98)

39.96 Total body perfusion
Code also substance perfused (99.21–99.29)

● **Use Additional Digit(s)**   ✖ **Valid O.R. Procedure**   ◀ **New**   ◀▥ **Revised**

39.97 Other perfusion
     Perfusion NOS
     Perfusion, local [regional] of:
         carotid artery
         coronary artery
         head
         lower limb
         neck
         upper limb

     Code also substance perfused (99.21–99.29)

     | Excludes | *perfusion of:*
         kidney (55.95)
         large intestine (46.96)
         liver (50.93)
         small intestine (46.95)

�х 39.98 Control of hemorrhage, not otherwise specified
     Angiotripsy
     Control of postoperative hemorrhage NOS
     Venotripsy

     | Excludes | *control of hemorrhage (postoperative):*
         anus (49.95)
         bladder (57.93)
         following vascular procedure (39.41)
         nose (21.00–21.09)
         prostate (60.94)
         tonsil (28.7)
     that by:
         ligation (38.80–38.89)
         suture (39.30–39.32)

✖ 39.99 Other operations on vessels

     | Excludes | *injection or infusion of therapeutic or prophylac-*
         tic substance (99.11–99.29)
     transfusion of blood and blood components
         (99.01–99.09)

8. OPERATIONS ON THE HEMIC AND LYMPHATIC SYSTEM (40–41)

● **40 Operations on lymphatic system**

✖ **40.0 Incision of lymphatic structures**

● **40.1 Diagnostic procedures on lymphatic structures**

✖ **40.11 Biopsy of lymphatic structure**

✖ **40.19 Other diagnostic procedures on lymphatic structures**

> Excludes | *lymphangiogram:*
> *abdominal (88.04)*
> *cervical (87.08)*
> *intrathoracic (87.34)*
> *lower limb (88.36)*
> *upper limb (88.34)*
> *microscopic examination of specimen (90.71–90.79)*
> *radioisotope scan (92.16)*
> *thermography (88.89)*

● **40.2 Simple excision of lymphatic structure**

> Excludes | *biopsy of lymphatic structure (40.11)*

✖ **40.21 Excision of deep cervical lymph node**

✖ **40.22 Excision of internal mammary lymph node**

✖ **40.23 Excision of axillary lymph node**

✖ **40.24 Excision of inguinal lymph node**

✖ **40.29 Simple excision of other lymphatic structure**
Excision of:
cystic hygroma
lymphangioma
Simple lymphadenectomy

✖ **40.3 Regional lymph node excision**
Extended regional lymph node excision
Regional lymph node excision with excision of lymphatic drainage area including skin, subcutaneous tissue, and fat

● **40.4 Radical excision of cervical lymph nodes**
Resection of cervical lymph nodes down to muscle and deep fascia

> Excludes | *that associated with radical laryngectomy (30.4)*

✖ **40.40 Radical neck dissection, not otherwise specified**

✖ **40.41 Radical neck dissection, unilateral**

✖ **40.42 Radical neck dissection, bilateral**

● **40.5 Radical excision of other lymph nodes**

> Excludes | *that associated with radical mastectomy (85.45–85.48)*

✖ **40.50 Radical excision of lymph nodes, not otherwise specified**
Radical (lymph) node dissection NOS

✖ **40.51 Radical excision of axillary lymph nodes**

✖ **40.52 Radical excision of periaortic lymph nodes**

✖ **40.53 Radical excision of iliac lymph nodes**

✖ **40.54 Radical groin dissection**

✖ **40.59 Radical excision of other lymph nodes**

> Excludes | *radical neck dissection (40.40–40.42)*

● **40.6 Operations on thoracic duct**

✖ **40.61 Cannulation of thoracic duct**

✖ **40.62 Fistulization of thoracic duct**

✖ **40.63 Closure of fistula of thoracic duct**

✖ **40.64 Ligation of thoracic duct**

✖ **40.69 Other operations on thoracic duct**

✖ **40.9 Other operations on lymphatic structures**
Anastomosis of peripheral lymphatics
Dilation of peripheral lymphatics
Ligation of peripheral lymphatics
Obliteration of peripheral lymphatics
Reconstruction of peripheral lymphatics
Repair of peripheral lymphatics
Transplantation of peripheral lymphatics
Correction of lymphedema of limb, NOS

> Excludes | *reduction of elephantiasis of scrotum (61.3)*

● **41 Operations on bone marrow and spleen**

● **41.0 Bone marrow or hematopoietic stem cell transplant**

Note: To report donor source - *see* codes 00.91–00.93 ◀

> Excludes | *aspiration of bone marrow from donor (41.91)*

✖ **41.00 Bone marrow transplant, not otherwise specified**

✖ **41.01 Autologous bone marrow transplant without purging**

> Excludes | *that with purging (41.09)*

✖ **41.02 Allogeneic bone marrow transplant with purging**
Allograft of bone marrow with in vitro removal (purging) of T-cells

✖ **41.03 Allogeneic bone marrow transplant without purging**
Allograft of bone marrow NOS

✖ **41.04 Autologous hematopoietic stem cell transplant without purging**

> Excludes | *that with purging (41.07)*

✖ **41.05 Allogeneic hematopoietic stem cell transplant without purging**

> Excludes | *that with purging (41.08)*

✖ **41.06 Cord blood stem cell transplant**

✖ **41.07 Autologous hematopoietic stem cell transplant with purging**
Cell depletion

✖ **41.08 Allogeneic hematopoietic stem cell transplant with purging**
Cell depletion

✖ **41.09 Autologous bone marrow transplant with purging**
with extracorporeal purging of malignant cells from marrow
Cell depletion

41.1 Puncture of spleen

> Excludes | *aspiration biopsy of spleen (41.32)*

✖ **41.2 Splenotomy**

● **41.3 Diagnostic procedures on bone marrow and spleen**

41.31 Biopsy of bone marrow

41.32 Closed [aspiration] [percutaneous] biopsy of spleen

✖ **41.33 Open biopsy of spleen**

41.38 Other diagnostic procedures on bone marrow

> Excludes | *microscopic examination of specimen from bone marrow (90.61–90.69)*
> *radioisotope scan (92.05)*

● Use Additional Digit(s)   ✖ Valid O.R. Procedure   ◀ New   ◀▥ Revised

41.39 Other diagnostic procedures on spleen

Excludes *microscopic examination of specimen from spleen (90.61–90.69)*
radioisotope scan (92.05)

● **41.4 Excision or destruction of lesion or tissue of spleen**

Excludes *excision of accessory spleen (41.93)*

Code also any application or administration of an adhesion barrier substance (99.77)

✖ **41.41 Marsupialization of splenic cyst**

✖ **41.42 Excision of lesion or tissue of spleen**

Excludes *biopsy of spleen (41.32–41.33)*

✖ **41.43 Partial splenectomy**

✖ **41.5 Total splenectomy**
Splenectomy NOS

Code also any application or administration of an adhesion barrier substance (99.77)

● **41.9 Other operations on spleen and bone marrow**

Code also any application or administration of an adhesion barrier substance (99.77)

41.91 Aspiration of bone marrow from donor for transplant

Excludes *biopsy of bone marrow (41.31)*

41.92 Injection into bone marrow

Excludes *bone marrow transplant (41.00–41.03)*

✖ **41.93 Excision of accessory spleen**

✖ **41.94 Transplantation of spleen**

✖ **41.95 Repair and plastic operations on spleen**

41.98 Other operations on bone marrow

✖ **41.99 Other operations on spleen**

9.   OPERATIONS ON THE DIGESTIVE SYSTEM (42–54)

● **42   Operations on esophagus**

  ● **42.0   Esophagotomy**

    �za **42.01   Incision of esophageal web**

    �za **42.09   Other incision of esophagus**
         Esophagotomy NOS

       Excludes   *esophagomyotomy (42.7)*
                 esophagostomy (42.10–42.19)

  ● **42.1   Esophagostomy**

    �za **42.10   Esophagostomy, not otherwise specified**

    �za **42.11   Cervical esophagostomy**

    �za **42.12   Exteriorization of esophageal pouch**

    �za **42.19   Other external fistulization of esophagus**
         Thoracic esophagostomy

         Code also any resection (42.40–42.42)

  ● **42.2   Diagnostic procedures on esophagus**

    �za **42.21   Operative esophagoscopy by incision**

    42.22   Esophagoscopy through artificial stoma

     Excludes   *that with biopsy (42.24)*

    42.23   Other esophagoscopy

     Excludes   *that with biopsy (42.24)*

    42.24   Closed [endoscopic] biopsy of esophagus
         Brushing or washing for specimen collection
         Esophagoscopy with biopsy
         Suction biopsy of the esophagus

     Excludes   *esophagogastroduodenoscopy [EGD] with closed biopsy (45.16)*

    �za **42.25   Open biopsy of esophagus**

    42.29   Other diagnostic procedures on esophagus

     Excludes   *barium swallow (87.61)*
                 esophageal manometry (89.32)
                 microscopic examination of specimen from esophagus (90.81–90.89)

  ● **42.3   Local excision or destruction of lesion or tissue of esophagus**

    �za **42.31   Local excision of esophageal diverticulum**

    �za **42.32   Local excision of other lesion or tissue of esophagus**

     Excludes   *biopsy of esophagus (42.24–42.25)*
                 esophageal fistulectomy (42.84)

    42.33   Endoscopic excision or destruction of lesion or tissue of esophagus
         Ablation of esophageal neoplasm by endoscopic approach
         Control of esophageal bleeding by endoscopic approach
         Esophageal polypectomy by endoscopic approach
         Esophageal varices by endoscopic approach
         Injection of esophageal varices by endoscopic approach

     Excludes   *biopsy of esophagus (42.24–42.25)*
                 fistulectomy (42.84)
                 open ligation of esophageal varices (42.91)

    �za **42.39   Other destruction of lesion or tissue of esophagus**

     Excludes   *that by endoscopic approach (42.33)*

  ● **42.4   Excision of esophagus**

     Excludes   *esophagogastrectomy NOS (43.99)*

    �za **42.40   Esophagectomy, not otherwise specified**

    �za **42.41   Partial esophagectomy**
         Code also any synchronous:
            anastomosis other than end-to-end (42.51–42.69)
            esophagostomy (42.10–42.19)
            gastrostomy (43.11–43.19)

    �za **42.42   Total esophagectomy**
         Code also any synchronous:
            gastrostomy (43.11–43.19)
            interposition or anastomosis other than end-to-end (42.51–42.69)

     Excludes   *esophagogastrectomy (43.99)*

  ● **42.5   Intrathoracic anastomosis of esophagus**

     Code also any synchronous:
       esophagectomy (42.40–42.42)
       gastrostomy (43.1)

    �za **42.51   Intrathoracic esophagoesophagostomy**

    �za **42.52   Intrathoracic esophagogastrostomy**

    �za **42.53   Intrathoracic esophageal anastomosis with interposition of small bowel**

    �za **42.54   Other intrathoracic esophagoenterostomy**
         Anastomosis of esophagus to intestinal segment NOS

    �za **42.55   Intrathoracic esophageal anastomosis with interposition of colon**

    �za **42.56   Other intrathoracic esophagocolostomy**
         Esophagocolostomy NOS

    �za **42.58   Intrathoracic esophageal anastomosis with other interposition**
         Construction of artificial esophagus
         Retrosternal formation of reversed gastric tube

    �za **42.59   Other intrathoracic anastomosis of esophagus**

  ● **42.6   Antesternal anastomosis of esophagus**

     Code also any synchronous:
       esophagectomy (42.40–42.42)
       gastrostomy (43.1)

    �za **42.61   Antesternal esophagoesophagostomy**

    �za **42.62   Antesternal esophagogastrostomy**

    �za **42.63   Antesternal esophageal anastomosis with interposition of small bowel**

    �za **42.64   Other antesternal esophagoenterostomy**
         Antethoracic:
            esophagoenterostomy
            esophagoileostomy
            esophagojejunostomy

    �za **42.65   Antesternal esophageal anastomosis with interposition of colon**

    �za **42.66   Other antesternal esophagocolostomy**
         Antethoracic esophagocolostomy

    �za **42.68   Other antesternal esophageal anastomosis with interposition**

    �za **42.69   Other antesternal anastomosis of esophagus**

  �za **42.7   Esophagomyotomy**

  ● **42.8   Other repair of esophagus**

    42.81   Insertion of permanent tube into esophagus

    ✚ **42.82   Suture of laceration of esophagus**

    ✚ **42.83   Closure of esophagostomy**

✖ **42.84 Repair of esophageal fistula, not elsewhere classified**

> **Excludes**   *repair of fistula:*
> *bronchoesophageal (33.42)*
> *esophagopleurocutaneous (34.73)*
> *pharyngoesophageal (29.53)*
> *tracheoesophageal (31.73)*

✖ **42.85 Repair of esophageal stricture**

✖ **42.86 Production of subcutaneous tunnel without esophageal anastomosis**

✖ **42.87 Other graft of esophagus**

> **Excludes**   *antesternal esophageal anastomosis with interposition of:*
> *colon (42.65)*
> *small bowel (42.63)*
> *antesternal esophageal anastomosis with other interposition (42.68)*
> *intrathoracic esophageal anastomosis with interposition of:*
> *colon (42.55)*
> *small bowel (42.53)*
> *intrathoracic esophageal anastomosis with other interposition (42.58)*

✖ **42.89 Other repair of esophagus**

● **42.9 Other operations on esophagus**

✖ **42.91 Ligation of esophageal varices**

> **Excludes**   *that by endoscopic approach (42.33)*

42.92 Dilation of esophagus
Dilation of cardiac sphincter

> **Excludes**   *intubation of esophagus (96.03, 96.06–96.08)*

42.99 Other

> **Excludes**   *insertion of Sengstaken tube (96.06)*
> *intubation of esophagus (96.03, 96.06–96.08)*
> *removal of intraluminal foreign body from esophagus without incision (98.02)*
> *tamponade of esophagus (96.06)*

● **43 Incision and excision of stomach**

Code also any application or administration of an adhesion barrier substance (99.77)

✖ **43.0 Gastrotomy**

> **Excludes**   *gastrostomy (43.11–43.19)*
> *that for control of hemorrhage (44.49)*

● **43.1 Gastrostomy**

43.11 Percutaneous [endoscopic] gastrostomy [PEG]
Percutaneous transabdominal gastrostomy

43.19 Other gastrostomy

> **Excludes**   *percutaneous [endoscopic] gastrostomy [PEG] (43.11)*

✖ **43.3 Pyloromyotomy**

● **43.4 Local excision or destruction of lesion or tissue of stomach**

43.41 Endoscopic excision or destruction of lesion or tissue of stomach
Gastric polypectomy by endoscopic approach
Gastric varices by endoscopic approach

> **Excludes**   *biopsy of stomach (44.14–44.15)*
> *control of hemorrhage (44.43)*
> *open ligation of gastric varices (44.91)*

✖ **43.42 Local excision of other lesion or tissue of stomach**

> **Excludes**   *biopsy of stomach (44.14–44.15)*
> *gastric fistulectomy (44.62–44.63)*
> *partial gastrectomy (43.5–43.89)*

✖ **43.49 Other destruction of lesion or tissue of stomach**

> **Excludes**   *that by endoscopic approach (43.41)*

✖ **43.5 Partial gastrectomy with anastomosis to esophagus**
Proximal gastrectomy

✖ **43.6 Partial gastrectomy with anastomosis to duodenum**
Billroth I operation
Distal gastrectomy
Gastropylorectomy

✖ **43.7 Partial gastrectomy with anastomosis to jejunum**
Billroth II operation

● **43.8 Other partial gastrectomy**

✖ **43.81 Partial gastrectomy with jejunal transposition**
Henley jejunal transposition operation

Code also any synchronous intestinal resection (45.51)

✖ **43.89 Other**
Partial gastrectomy with bypass gastrogastrostomy
Sleeve resection of stomach

● **43.9 Total gastrectomy**

✖ **43.91 Total gastrectomy with intestinal interposition**

✖ **43.99 Other total gastrectomy**
Complete gastroduodenectomy
Esophagoduodenostomy with complete gastrectomy
Esophagogastrectomy NOS
Esophagojejunostomy with complete gastrectomy
Radical gastrectomy

● **44 Other operations on stomach**

Code also any application or administration of an adhesion barrier substance (99.77)

● **44.0 Vagotomy**

✖ **44.00 Vagotomy, not otherwise specified**
Division of vagus nerve NOS

✖ **44.01 Truncal vagotomy**

✖ **44.02 Highly selective vagotomy**
Parietal cell vagotomy
Selective proximal vagotomy

✖ **44.03 Other selective vagotomy**

● **44.1 Diagnostic procedures on stomach**

✖ **44.11 Transabdominal gastroscopy**
Intraoperative gastroscopy

> **Excludes**   *that with biopsy (44.14)*

44.12 Gastroscopy through artificial stoma

> **Excludes**   *that with biopsy (44.14)*

44.13 Other gastroscopy

> **Excludes**   *that with biopsy (44.14)*

44.14 Closed [endoscopic] biopsy of stomach
Brushing or washing for specimen collection

> **Excludes**   *esophagogastroduodenoscopy [EGD] with closed biopsy (45.16)*

✖ **44.15 Open biopsy of stomach**

44.19 Other diagnostic procedures on stomach

> **Excludes**   *gastric lavage (96.33)*
> *microscopic examination of specimen from stomach (90.81–90.89)*
> *upper GI series (87.62)*

● **44.2 Pyloroplasty**

✖ **44.21 Dilation of pylorus by incision**

44.22 Endoscopic dilation of pylorus
Dilation with balloon endoscope
Endoscopic dilation of gastrojejunostomy site

✖ **44.29 Other pyloroplasty**
Pyloroplasty NOS
Revision of pylorus

● **44.3 Gastroenterostomy without gastrectomy**

✖ **44.31 High gastric bypass**
Printen and Mason gastric bypass

✖ **44.32 Percutaneous [endoscopic] gastrojejunostomy**
Endoscopic conversion of gastrostomy or jejunostomy

44.38 Laparoscopic gastroenterostomy ◄
Bypass: ◄
    gastroduodenostomy ◄
    gastroenterostomy ◄
    gastrogastrostomy ◄
Laparoscopic gastrojejunostomy without gastrectomy NEC ◄

Excludes gastroenterostomy, open approach (44.39) ◄

✖ **44.39 Other gastroenterostomy**
Bypass:
    gastroduodenostomy
    gastroenterostomy
    gastrogastrostomy
Gastrojejunostomy without gastrectomy NOS

● **44.4 Control of hemorrhage and suture of ulcer of stomach or duodenum**

✖ **44.40 Suture of peptic ulcer, not otherwise specified**

✖ **44.41 Suture of gastric ulcer site**

Excludes ligation of gastric varices (44.91)

✖ **44.42 Suture of duodenal ulcer site**

44.43 Endoscopic control of gastric or duodenal bleeding

44.44 Transcatheter embolization for gastric or duodenal bleeding

Excludes surgical occlusion of abdominal vessels (38.86–38.87)

44.49 Other control of hemorrhage of stomach or duodenum
That with gastrotomy

✖ **44.5 Revision of gastric anastomosis**
Closure of:
    gastric anastomosis
    gastroduodenostomy
    gastrojejunostomy
Pantaloon operation

● **44.6 Other repair of stomach**

✖ **44.61 Suture of laceration of stomach**

Excludes that of ulcer site (44.41)

44.62 Closure of gastrostomy

✖ **44.63 Closure of other gastric fistula**
Closure of:
    gastrocolic fistula
    gastrojejunocolic fistula

✖ **44.64 Gastropexy**

✖ **44.65 Esophagogastroplasty**
Belsey operation
Esophagus and stomach cardioplasty

✖ **44.66 Other procedures for creation of esophagogastric sphincteric competence**
Fundoplication
Gastric cardioplasty
Nissen's fundoplication
Restoration of cardio-esophageal angle

Excludes that by laparoscopy (44.67) ◄

44.67 Laparoscopic procedures for creation of esophagogastric sphincteric competence ◄
Fundoplication ◄
Gastric cardioplasty ◄
Nissen's fundoplication ◄
Restoration of cardio-esophageal angle ◄

44.68 Laparoscopic gastroplasty ◄
Banding ◄
Silastic vertical banding ◄
Vertical banded gastroplasty (VBG) ◄

Code also any syndhronous laparoscopic gastroenterostomy (44.38) ◄

Excludes insertion, laparoscopic adjustable gastric band (restrictive procedure) (44.95) ◄
other repair of stomach, open approach (44.61–44.65, 44.69) ◄

✖ **44.69 Other**
Inversion of gastric diverticulum
Repair of stomach NOS

● **44.9 Other operations on stomach**

✖ **44.91 Ligation of gastric varices**

Excludes that by endoscopic approach (43.41)

✖ **44.92 Intraoperative manipulation of stomach**
Reduction of gastric volvulus

44.93 Insertion of gastric bubble (balloon)

44.94 Removal of gastric bubble (balloon)

✖ **44.95 Laparoscopic gastric restrictive procedure** ◄
Adjustable gastric band and port insertion ◄

Excludes laparoscopic gastroplasty (44.68) ◄
other repair of stomach (44.69) ◄

✖ **44.96 Laparoscopic revision of gastric restrictive procedure** ◄
Revision or replacement of: ◄
    adjustable gastric band ◄
    subcutaneous port device ◄

✖ **44.97 Laparoscopic removal of gastric restrictive device(s)** ◄
Removal of either or both: ◄
    adjustable gastric band ◄
    subcutaneous port device ◄

Excludes nonoperative removal of gastric restrictive device(s) (97.86) ◄
open removal of gastric restrictive device(s) (44.99) ◄

✖ **44.98 (Laparoscopic) adjustment of size of adjustable gastric restrictive device** ◄
Infusion of saline for device tightening ◄
Widthdrawal of saline for device loosening ◄

Code also any: ◄
    abdominal ultrasound (88.76) ◄
    abdominal wall fluoroscopy (88.09) ◄
    barium swallow (87.61) ◄

✖ **44.99 Other**

> **Excludes**   *change of gastrostomy tube (97.02)*
> *dilation of cardiac sphincter (42.92)*
> *gastric:*
>   *cooling (96.31)*
>   *freezing (96.32)*
>   *gavage (96.35)*
>   *hypothermia (96.31)*
>   *lavage (96.33)*
> *insertion of nasogastric tube (96.07)*
> *irrigation of gastrostomy (96.36)*
> *irrigation of nasogastric tube (96.34)*
> *removal of:*
>   *gastrostomy tube (97.51)*
>   *intraluminal foreign body from stomach with-*
>   *out incision (98.03)*
> *replacement of:*
>   *gastrostomy tube (97.02)*
>   *(naso-)gastric tube (97.01)*

● **45   Incision, excision, and anastomosis of intestine**

Code also any application or administration of an adhesion barrier substance (99.77)

● **45.0   Enterotomy**

> **Excludes**   *duodenocholedochotomy (51.41–51.42, 51.51)*
> *that for destruction of lesion (45.30–45.34)*
> *that of exteriorized intestine (46.14, 46.24, 46.31)*

✖ **45.00   Incision of intestine, not otherwise specified**

✖ **45.01   Incision of duodenum**

✖ **45.02   Other incision of small intestine**

✖ **45.03   Incision of large intestine**

> **Excludes**   *proctotomy (48.0)*

● **45.1   Diagnostic procedures on small intestine**

Code also any laparotomy (54.11–54.19)

✖ **45.11   Transabdominal endoscopy of small intestine**
Intraoperative endoscopy of small intestine

> **Excludes**   *that with biopsy (45.14)*

45.12   Endoscopy of small intestine through artificial stoma

> **Excludes**   *that with biopsy (45.14)*

45.13   Other endoscopy of small intestine
Esophagogastroduodenoscopy [EGD]

> **Excludes**   *that with biopsy (45.14, 45.16)*

45.14   Closed [endoscopic] biopsy of small intestine
Brushing or washing for specimen collection

> **Excludes**   *esophagogastroduodenoscopy [EGD] with closed biopsy (45.16)*

✖ **45.15   Open biopsy of small intestine**

45.16   Esophagogastroduodenoscopy [EGD] with closed biopsy
Biopsy of one or more sites involving esophagus, stomach, and/or duodenum

45.19   Other diagnostic procedures on small intestine

> **Excludes**   *microscopic examination of specimen from small intestine (90.91–90.99)*
> *radioisotope scan (92.04)*
> *ultrasonography (88.74)*
> *x-ray (87.61–87.69)*

● **45.2   Diagnostic procedures on large intestine**

Code also any laparotomy (54.11–54.19)

✖ **45.21   Transabdominal endoscopy of large intestine**
Intraoperative endoscopy of large intestine

> **Excludes**   *that with biopsy (45.25)*

45.22   Endoscopy of large intestine through artificial stoma

> **Excludes**   *that with biopsy (45.25)*

45.23   Colonoscopy
Flexible fiberoptic colonoscopy

> **Excludes**   *endoscopy of large intestine through artificial stoma (45.22)*
> *flexible sigmoidoscopy (45.24)*
> *rigid proctosigmoidoscopy (48.23)*
> *transabdominal endoscopy of large intestine (45.21)*

45.24   Flexible sigmoidoscopy
Endoscopy of descending colon

> **Excludes**   *rigid proctosigmoidoscopy (48.23)*

45.25   Closed [endoscopic] biopsy of large intestine
Biopsy, closed, of unspecified intestinal site
Brushing or washing for specimen collection
Colonoscopy with biopsy

> **Excludes**   *proctosigmoidoscopy with biopsy (48.24)*

✖ **45.26   Open biopsy of large intestine**

45.27   Intestinal biopsy, site unspecified

45.28   Other diagnostic procedures on large intestine

45.29   Other diagnostic procedures on intestine, site unspecified

> **Excludes**   *microscopic examination of specimen (90.91–90.99)*
> *scan and radioisotope function study (92.04)*
> *ultrasonography (88.74)*
> *x-ray (87.61–87.69)*

● **45.3   Local excision or destruction of lesion or tissue of small intestine**

45.30   Endoscopic excision or destruction of lesion of duodenum

> **Excludes**   *biopsy of duodenum (45.14–45.15)*
> *control of hemorrhage (44.43)*
> *fistulectomy (46.72)*

✖ **45.31   Other local excision of lesion of duodenum**

> **Excludes**   *biopsy of duodenum (45.14–45.15)*
> *fistulectomy (46.72)*
> *multiple segmental resection (45.61)*
> *that by endoscopic approach (45.30)*

✖ **45.32   Other destruction of lesion of duodenum**

> **Excludes**   *that by endoscopic approach (45.30)*

✖ **45.33   Local excision of lesion or tissue of small intestine, except duodenum**
Excision of redundant mucosa of ileostomy

> **Excludes**   *biopsy of small intestine (45.14–45.15)*
> *fistulectomy (46.74)*
> *multiple segmental resection (45.61)*

✖ **45.34   Other destruction of lesion of small intestine, except duodenum**

● **45.4   Local excision or destruction of lesion or tissue of large intestine**

✖ **45.41   Excision of lesion or tissue of large intestine**
Excision of redundant mucosa of colostomy

> **Excludes**   *biopsy of large intestine (45.25–45.27)*
> *endoscopic polypectomy of large intestine (45.42)*
> *fistulectomy (46.76)*
> *multiple segmental resection (45.71)*
> *that by endoscopic approach (45.42–45.43)*

45.42   Endoscopic polypectomy of large intestine

> **Excludes**   *that by open approach (45.41)*

45.43 Endoscopic destruction of other lesion or tissue of large intestine
Endoscopic ablation of tumor of large intestine
Endoscopic control of colonic bleeding

Excludes *endoscopic polypectomy of large intestine (45.42)*

✖ **45.49 Other destruction of lesion of large intestine**

Excludes *that by endoscopic approach (45.43)*

● **45.5 Isolation of intestinal segment**
Code also any synchronous:
anastomosis other than end-to-end (45.90–45.94)
enterostomy (46.10–46.39)

✖ **45.50 Isolation of intestinal segment, not otherwise specified**
Isolation of intestinal pedicle flap
Reversal of intestinal segment

✖ **45.51 Isolation of segment of small intestine**
Isolation of ileal loop
Resection of small intestine for interposition

✖ **45.52 Isolation of segment of large intestine**
Resection of colon for interposition

● **45.6 Other excision of small intestine**
Code also any synchronous:
anastomosis other than end-to-end (45.90–45.93, 45.95)
colostomy (46.10–46.13)
enterostomy (46.10–46.39)

Excludes *cecectomy (45.72)*
enterocolectomy (45.79)
gastroduodenectomy (43.6–43.99)
ileocolectomy (45.73)
pancreatoduodenectomy (52.51–52.7)

✖ **45.61 Multiple segmental resection of small intestine**
Segmental resection for multiple traumatic lesions of small intestine

✖ **45.62 Other partial resection of small intestine**
Duodenectomy
Ileectomy
Jejunectomy

Excludes *duodenectomy with synchronous pancreatectomy (52.51–52.7)*
resection of cecum and terminal ileum (45.72)

✖ **45.63 Total removal of small intestine**

● **45.7 Partial excision of large intestine**
Code also any synchronous:
anastomosis other than end-to-end (45.92–45.94)
enterostomy (46.10–46.39)

✖ **45.71 Multiple segmental resection of large intestine**
Segmental resection for multiple traumatic lesions of large intestine

✖ **45.72 Cecectomy**
Resection of cecum and terminal ileum

✖ **45.73 Right hemicolectomy**
Ileocolectomy
Right radical colectomy

✖ **45.74 Resection of transverse colon**

✖ **45.75 Left hemicolectomy**

Excludes *proctosigmoidectomy (48.41–48.69)*
second stage Mikulicz operation (46.04)

✖ **45.76 Sigmoidectomy**

✖ **45.79 Other partial excision of large intestine**
Enterocolectomy NEC

✖ **45.8 Total intra-abdominal colectomy**
Excision of cecum, colon, and sigmoid

Excludes *coloproctectomy (48.41–48.69)*

● **45.9 Intestinal anastomosis**
Code also any synchronous resection (45.31–45.8, 48.41–48.69)

Excludes *end-to-end anastomosis—omit code*

✖ **45.90 Intestinal anastomosis, not otherwise specified**

✖ **45.91 Small-to-small intestinal anastomosis**

✖ **45.92 Anastomosis of small intestine to rectal stump**
Hampton procedure

✖ **45.93 Other small-to-large intestinal anastomosis**

✖ **45.94 Large-to-large intestinal anastomosis**

Excludes *rectorectostomy (48.74)*

✖ **45.95 Anastomosis to anus**
Formation of endorectal ileal pouch (H-pouch) (J-pouch) (S-pouch) with anastomosis of small intestine to anus

● **46 Other operations on intestine**
Code also any application or administration of an adhesion barrier substance (99.77)

● **46.0 Exteriorization of intestine**

Includes: loop enterostomy
multiple stage resection of intestine

✖ **46.01 Exteriorization of small intestine**
Loop ileostomy

✖ **46.02 Resection of exteriorized segment of small intestine**

✖ **46.03 Exteriorization of large intestine**
Exteriorization of intestine NOS
First stage Mikulicz exteriorization of intestine
Loop colostomy

✖ **46.04 Resection of exteriorized segment of large intestine**
Resection of exteriorized segment of intestine NOS
Second stage Mikulicz operation

● **46.1 Colostomy**
Code also any synchronous resection (45.49, 45.71–45.79, 45.8)

Excludes *loop colostomy (46.03)*
that with abdominoperineal resection of rectum (48.5)
that with synchronous anterior rectal resection (48.62)

✖ **46.10 Colostomy, not otherwise specified**

✖ **46.11 Temporary colostomy**

✖ **46.13 Permanent colostomy**

46.14 Delayed opening of colostomy

● **46.2 Ileostomy**
Code also any synchronous resection (45.34, 45.61–45.63)

Excludes *loop ileostomy (46.01)*

✖ **46.20 Ileostomy, not otherwise specified**

✖ **46.21 Temporary ileostomy**

✖ **46.22 Continent ileostomy**

✖ **46.23 Other permanent ileostomy**

46.24 Delayed opening of ileostomy

● **Use Additional Digit(s)**　　　　✖ **Valid O.R. Procedure**　　　　◀ **New**　　　　◀◀ **Revised**

● **46.3 Other enterostomy**

Code also any synchronous resection (45.61–45.8)

46.31 Delayed opening of other enterostomy

46.32 Percutaneous (endoscopic) jejunostomy [PEJ]

46.39 Other
Duodenostomy
Feeding enterostomy

● **46.4 Revision of intestinal stoma**

✖ **46.40 Revision of intestinal stoma, not otherwise specified**
Plastic enlargement of intestinal stoma
Reconstruction of stoma of intestine
Release of scar tissue of intestinal stoma

Excludes │ *excision of redundant mucosa (45.41)*

✖ **46.41 Revision of stoma of small intestine**

Excludes │ *excision of redundant mucosa (45.33)*

✖ **46.42 Repair of pericolostomy hernia**

✖ **46.43 Other revision of stoma of large intestine**

Excludes │ *excision of redundant mucosa (45.41)*

● **46.5 Closure of intestinal stoma**

Code also any synchronous resection (45.34, 45.49, 45.61–45.8)

✖ **46.50 Closure of intestinal stoma, not otherwise specified**

✖ **46.51 Closure of stoma of small intestine**

✖ **46.52 Closure of stoma of large intestine**
Closure or take-down of:
cecostomy
colostomy
sigmoidostomy

● **46.6 Fixation of intestine**

✖ **46.60 Fixation of intestine, not otherwise specified**
Fixation of intestine to abdominal wall

✖ **46.61 Fixation of small intestine to abdominal wall**
Ileopexy

✖ **46.62 Other fixation of small intestine**
Noble plication of small intestine
Plication of jejunum

✖ **46.63 Fixation of large intestine to abdominal wall**
Cecocoloplicopexy
Sigmoidopexy (Moschowitz)

✖ **46.64 Other fixation of large intestine**
Cecofixation
Colofixation

● **46.7 Other repair of intestine**

Excludes │ *closure of:*
ulcer of duodenum (44.42)
vesicoenteric fistula (57.83)

✖ **46.71 Suture of laceration of duodenum**

✖ **46.72 Closure of fistula of duodenum**

✖ **46.73 Suture of laceration of small intestine, except duodenum**

✖ **46.74 Closure of fistula of small intestine, except duodenum**

Excludes │ *closure of:*
artificial stoma (46.51)
vaginal fistula (70.74)
repair of gastrojejunocolic fistula (44.63)

✖ **46.75 Suture of laceration of large intestine**

✖ **46.76 Closure of fistula of large intestine**

Excludes │ *closure of:*
gastrocolic fistula (44.63)
rectal fistula (48.73)
sigmoidovesical fistula (57.83)
stoma (46.52)
vaginal fistula (70.72–70.73)
vesicocolic fistula (57.83)
vesicosigmoidovaginal fistula (57.83)

✖ **46.79 Other repair of intestine**
Duodenoplasty

● **46.8 Dilation and manipulation of intestine**

✖ **46.80 Intra-abdominal manipulation of intestine, not otherwise specified**
Correction of intestinal malrotation
Reduction of:
intestinal torsion
intestinal volvulus
intussusception

Excludes │ *reduction of intussusception with:*
fluoroscopy (96.29)
ionizing radiation enema (96.29)
ultrasonography guidance (96.29)

✖ **46.81 Intra-abdominal manipulation of small intestine**

✖ **46.82 Intra-abdominal manipulation of large intestine**

46.85 Dilation of intestine
Dilation (balloon) of duodenum
Dilation (balloon) of jejunum
Endoscopic dilation (balloon) of large intestine
That through rectum or colostomy

● **46.9 Other operations on intestines**

✖ **46.91 Myotomy of sigmoid colon**

✖ **46.92 Myotomy of other parts of colon**

✖ **46.93 Revision of anastomosis of small intestine**

✖ **46.94 Revision of anastomosis of large intestine**

46.95 Local perfusion of small intestine

Code also substance perfused (99.21–99.29)

46.96 Local perfusion of large intestine

Code also substance perfused (99.21–99.29)

46.97 Transplant of intestine

Note: To report donor source - *see* codes 00.91–00.93 ◄

✖ **46.99 Other**
Ileoentectropy

Excludes │ *diagnostic procedures on intestine (45.11–45.29)*
dilation of enterostomy stoma (96.24)
intestinal intubation (96.08)
removal of:
intraluminal foreign body from large intestine
without incision (98.04)
intraluminal foreign body from small intestine
without incision (98.03)
tube from large intestine (97.53)
tube from small intestine (97.52)
replacement of:
large intestine tube or enterostomy device
(97.04)
small intestine tube or enterostomy device
(97.03)

● 47   **Operations on appendix**

Code also any application or administration of an adhesion barrier substance (99.77)

    Includes: appendiceal stump

✖ **47.0   Appendectomy**

    Excludes   incidental appendectomy, so described
                   laparoscopic (47.11)
                   other (47.19)

    ✖ **47.01   Laparoscopic appendectomy**

    ✖ **47.09   Other appendectomy**

● **47.1   Incidental appendectomy**

    ✖ **47.11   Laparoscopic incidental appendectomy**

    ✖ **47.19   Other incidental appendectomy**

✖ **47.2   Drainage of appendiceal abscess**

    Excludes   that with appendectomy (47.0)

● **47.9   Other operations on appendix**

    ✖ **47.91   Appendicostomy**

    ✖ **47.92   Closure of appendiceal fistula**

    ✖ **47.99   Other**
            Anastomosis of appendix
        Excludes   diagnostic procedures on appendix (45.21–45.29)

● 48   **Operations on rectum, rectosigmoid and perirectal tissue**

Code also any application or administration of an adhesion barrier substance (99.77)

✖ **48.0   Proctotomy**
         Decompression of imperforate anus
         Panas' operation [linear proctotomy]
    Excludes   incision of perirectal tissue (48.81)

✖ **48.1   Proctostomy**

● **48.2   Diagnostic procedures on rectum, rectosigmoid and perirectal tissue**

    ✖ **48.21   Transabdominal proctosigmoidoscopy**
            Intraoperative proctosigmoidoscopy
        Excludes   that with biopsy (48.24)

    48.22   Proctosigmoidoscopy through artificial stoma
        Excludes   that with biopsy (48.24)

    48.23   Rigid proctosigmoidoscopy
        Excludes   flexible sigmoidoscopy (45.24)

    48.24   Closed [endoscopic] biopsy of rectum
            Brushing or washing for specimen collection
            Proctosigmoidoscopy with biopsy

    ✖ **48.25   Open biopsy of rectum**

    48.26   Biopsy of perirectal tissue

    48.29   Other diagnostic procedures on rectum, rectosigmoid and perirectal tissue
        Excludes   digital examination of rectum (89.34)
                    lower GI series (87.64)
                    microscopic examination of specimen from rectum (90.91–90.99)

● **48.3   Local excision or destruction of lesion or tissue of rectum**

    48.31   Radical electrocoagulation of rectal lesion or tissue

    48.32   Other electrocoagulation of rectal lesion or tissue

    48.33   Destruction of rectal lesion or tissue by laser

    48.34   Destruction of rectal lesion or tissue by cryosurgery

✖ **48.35   Local excision of rectal lesion or tissue**
    Excludes   biopsy of rectum (48.24–48.25)
                excision of perirectal tissue (48.82)
                hemorrhoidectomy (49.46)
                [endoscopic] polypectomy of rectum (48.36)
                rectal fistulectomy (48.73)

    48.36   [Endoscopic] polypectomy of rectum

● **48.4   Pull-through resection of rectum**

Code also any synchronous anastomosis other than end-to-end (45.90, 45.92–45.95)

    ✖ **48.41   Save submucosal resection of rectum**
            Endorectal pull-through operation

    ✖ **48.49   Other pull-through resection of rectum**
            Abdominoperineal pull-through
            Altemeier operation
            Swenson proctectomy
        Excludes   Duhamel abdominoperineal pull-through (48.65)

✖ **48.5   Abdominoperineal resection of rectum**

    Includes: with synchronous colostomy
    Combined abdominoendorectal resection
    Complete proctectomy

Code also any synchronous anastomosis other than end-to-end (45.90, 45.92–45.95)

    Excludes   Duhamel abdominoperineal pull-through (48.65)
                that as part of pelvic exenteration (68.8)

● **48.6   Other resection of rectum**

Code also any synchronous anastomosis other than end-to-end (45.90, 45.92–45.95)

    ✖ **48.61   Transsacral rectosigmoidectomy**

    ✖ **48.62   Anterior resection of rectum with synchronous colostomy**

    ✖ **48.63   Other anterior resection of rectum**
        Excludes   that with synchronous colostomy (48.62)

    ✖ **48.64   Posterior resection of rectum**

    ✖ **48.65   Duhamel resection of rectum**
            Duhamel abdominoperineal pull-through

    ✖ **48.69   Other**
            Partial proctectomy
            Rectal resection NOS

● **48.7   Repair of rectum**
    Excludes   repair of:
                current obstetric laceration (75.62)
                vaginal rectocele (70.50, 70.52)

    ✖ **48.71   Suture of laceration of rectum**

    ✖ **48.72   Closure of proctostomy**

    ✖ **48.73   Closure of other rectal fistula**
    Excludes   fistulectomy:
                perirectal (48.93)
                rectourethral (58.43)
                rectovaginal (70.73)
                rectovesical (57.83)
                rectovesicovaginal (57.83)

    ✖ **48.74   Rectorectostomy**
            Rectal anastomosis NOS

    ✖ **48.75   Abdominal proctopexy**
            Frickman procedure
            Ripstein repair of rectal prolapse

    ✖ **48.76   Other proctopexy**
            Delorme repair of prolapsed rectum
            Proctosigmoidopexy
            Puborectalis sling operation
    Excludes   manual reduction of rectal prolapse (96.26)

✖ **48.79 Other repair of rectum**
Repair of old obstetric laceration of rectum

| **Excludes** | *anastomosis to:*
large intestine (45.94)
small intestine (45.92–45.93)
repair of:
current obstetric laceration (75.62)
vaginal rectocele (70.50, 70.52)

● **48.8 Incision or excision of perirectal tissue or lesion**

Includes: pelvirectal tissue
rectovaginal septum

✖ **48.81 Incision of perirectal tissue**
Incision of rectovaginal septum

✖ **48.82 Excision of perirectal tissue**

| **Excludes** | *perirectal biopsy (48.26)*
perirectofistulectomy (48.93)
rectal fistulectomy (48.73)

● **48.9 Other operations on rectum and perirectal tissue**

✖ **48.91 Incision of rectal stricture**

✖ **48.92 Anorectal myectomy**

✖ **48.93 Repair of perirectal fistula**

| **Excludes** | *that opening into rectum (48.73)*

✖ **48.99 Other**

| **Excludes** | *digital examination of rectum (89.34)*
dilation of rectum (96.22)
insertion of rectal tube (96.09)
irrigation of rectum (96.38–96.39)
manual reduction of rectal prolapse (96.26)
proctoclysis (96.37)
rectal massage (99.93)
rectal packing (96.19)
removal of:
impacted feces (96.38)
intraluminal foreign body from rectum without incision (98.05)
rectal packing (97.59)
transanal enema (96.39)

● **49 Operations on anus**

Code also any application or administration of an adhesion barrier substance (99.77)

● **49.0 Incision or excision of perianal tissue**

✖ **49.01 Incision of perianal abscess**

✖ **49.02 Other incision of perianal tissue**
Undercutting of perianal tissue

| **Excludes** | *anal fistulotomy (49.11)*

49.03 Excision of perianal skin tags

✖ **49.04 Other excision of perianal tissue**

| **Excludes** | *anal fistulectomy (49.12)*
biopsy of perianal tissue (49.22)

● **49.1 Incision or excision of anal fistula**

| **Excludes** | *closure of anal fistula (49.73)*

✖ **49.11 Anal fistulotomy**

✖ **49.12 Anal fistulectomy**

● **49.2 Diagnostic procedures on anus and perianal tissue**

49.21 Anoscopy

49.22 Biopsy of perianal tissue

49.23 Biopsy of anus

49.29 Other diagnostic procedures on anus and perianal tissue

| **Excludes** | *microscopic examination of specimen from anus (90.91–90.99)*

● **49.3 Local excision or destruction of other lesion or tissue of anus**
Anal cryptotomy
Cauterization of lesion of anus

| **Excludes** | *biopsy of anus (49.23)*
control of (postoperative) hemorrhage of anus (49.95)
hemorrhoidectomy (49.46)

49.31 Endoscopic excision or destruction of lesion or tissue of anus

✖ **49.39 Other local excision or destruction of lesion or tissue of anus**

| **Excludes** | *that by endoscopic approach (49.31)*

● **49.4 Procedures on hemorrhoids**

49.41 Reduction of hemorrhoids

49.42 Injection of hemorrhoids

49.43 Cauterization of hemorrhoids
Clamp and cautery of hemorrhoids

✖ **49.44 Destruction of hemorrhoids by cryotherapy**

✖ **49.45 Ligation of hemorrhoids**

✖ **49.46 Excision of hemorrhoids**
Hemorrhoidectomy NOS

49.47 Evacuation of thrombosed hemorrhoids

✖ **49.49 Other procedures on hemorrhoids**
Lord procedure

● **49.5 Division of anal sphincter**

✖ **49.51 Left lateral anal sphincterotomy**

✖ **49.52 Posterior anal sphincterotomy**

✖ **49.59 Other anal sphincterotomy**
Division of sphincter NOS

✖ **49.6 Excision of anus**

● **49.7 Repair of anus**

| **Excludes** | *repair of current obstetric laceration (75.62)*

✖ **49.71 Suture of laceration of anus**

✖ **49.72 Anal cerclage**

✖ **49.73 Closure of anal fistula**

| **Excludes** | *excision of anal fistula (49.12)*

✖ **49.74 Gracilis muscle transplant for anal incontinence**

✖ **49.75 Implantation or revision of artificial anal sphincter**
Removal with subsequent replacement
Replacement during same or subsequent operative episode

✖ **49.76 Removal of artificial anal sphincter**
Explanation or removal without replacement

| **Excludes** | *revision with implantation during same operative episode (49.75)*

✖ **49.79 Other repair of anal sphincter**
Repair of old obstetric laceration of anus

| **Excludes** | *anoplasty with synchronous hemorrhoidectomy (49.46)*
repair of current obstetric laceration (75.62)

● **49.9 Other operations on anus**

| **Excludes** | *dilation of anus (sphincter) (96.23)*

✖ **49.91 Incision of anal septum**

✖ **49.92 Insertion of subcutaneous electrical anal stimulator**

✖ **49.93   Other incision of anus**
Removal of:
    foreign body from anus with incision
    seton from anus

> **Excludes**   *anal fistulotomy (49.11)*
> *removal of intraluminal foreign body without in-
> cision (98.05)*

✖ **49.94   Reduction of anal prolapse**

> **Excludes**   *manual reduction of rectal prolapse (96.26)*

✖ **49.95   Control of (postoperative) hemorrhage of anus**

✖ **49.99   Other**

● **50   Operations on liver**

Code also any application or administration of an adhesion
barrier substance (99.77)

✖ **50.0   Hepatotomy**
Incision of abscess of liver
Removal of gallstones from liver
Stromeyer-Little operation

● **50.1   Diagnostic procedures on liver**

    50.11   Closed (percutaneous) [needle] biopsy of liver
       Diagnostic aspiration of liver

✖ **50.12   Open biopsy of liver**
       Wedge biopsy

✖ **50.19   Other diagnostic procedures on liver**
       Laparoscopic liver biopsy ◀

> **Excludes**   *liver scan and radioisotope function study*
> *(92.02)*
> *microscopic examination of specimen from liver*
> *(91.01–91.09)*

● **50.2   Local excision or destruction of liver tissue or lesion**

✖ **50.21   Marsupialization of lesion of liver**

✖ **50.22   Partial hepatectomy**
       Wedge resection of liver

> **Excludes**   *biopsy of liver (50.11–50.12)*
> *hepatic lobectomy (50.3)*

✖ **50.29   Other destruction of lesion of liver**
       Cauterization of hepatic lesion
       Enucleation of hepatic lesion
       Evacuation of hepatic lesion

> **Excludes**   *percutaneous aspiration of lesion (50.91)*

✖ **50.3   Lobectomy of liver**
Total hepatic lobectomy with partial excision of
    other lobe

✖ **50.4   Total hepatectomy**

● **50.5   Liver transplant**

Note: To report donor source - *see* codes 00.91–00.93 ◀

✖ **50.51   Auxiliary liver transplant**
       Auxiliary hepatic transplantation leaving pa-
       tient's own liver in situ

✖ **50.59   Other transplant of liver**

● **50.6   Repair of liver**

✖ **50.61   Closure of laceration of liver**

✖ **50.69   Other repair of liver**
       Hepatopexy

● **50.9   Other operations on liver**

> **Excludes**   *lysis of adhesions (54.5)*

    50.91   Percutaneous aspiration of liver

> **Excludes**   *percutaneous biopsy (50.11)*

    50.92   Extracorporeal hepatic assistance

Includes: Liver dialysis

    50.93   Localized perfusion of liver

    50.94   Other injection of therapeutic substance into liver

    50.99   Other

● **51   Operations on gallbladder and biliary tract**

Code also any application or administration of an adhesion
barrier substance (99.77)

Includes: operations on:
       ampulla of Vater
       common bile duct
       cystic duct
       hepatic duct
       intrahepatic bile duct
       sphincter of Oddi

● **51.0   Cholecystotomy and cholecystostomy**

    51.01   Percutaneous aspiration of gallbladder
       Percutaneous cholecystotomy for drainage
       That by: needle or catheter

> **Excludes**   *needle biopsy (51.12)*

✖ **51.02   Trocar cholecystostomy**

✖ **51.03   Other cholecystostomy**

✖ **51.04   Other cholecystotomy**
       Cholelithotomy NOS

● **51.1   Diagnostic procedures on biliary tract**

> **Excludes**   *that for endoscopic procedures classifiable to*
> *51.64, 51.84–51.88, 52.14, 52.21, 52.93–*
> *52.94, 52.97–52.98*

    51.10   Endoscopic retrograde cholangiopancreatography [ERCP]

> **Excludes**   *endoscopic retrograde:*
> *cholangiography [ERC] (51.11)*
> *pancreatography [ERP] (52.13)*

    51.11   Endoscopic retrograde cholangiography [ERC]

Includes: Laparoscopic exploration of common
            bile duct

> **Excludes**   *endoscopic retrograde:*
> *cholangiopancreatography [ERCP] (51.10)*
> *pancreatography [ERP] (52.13)*

    51.12   Percutaneous biopsy of gallbladder or bile ducts
       Needle biopsy of gallbladder

✖ **51.13   Open biopsy of gallbladder or bile ducts**

    51.14   Other closed [endoscopic] biopsy of biliary duct or sphincter of Oddi
       Brushing or washing for specimen collection
       Closed biopsy of biliary duct or sphincter of
       Oddi by procedures classifiable to 51.10–
       51.11, 52.13

    51.15   Pressure measurement of sphincter of Oddi
       Pressure measurement of sphincter by proce-
       dures classifiable to 51.10–51.11, 52.13

✖ **51.19   Other diagnostic procedures on biliary tract**

> **Excludes**   *biliary tract x-ray (87.51–87.59)*
> *microscopic examination of specimen from biliary*
> *tract (91.01–91.09)*

● **51.2   Cholecystectomy**

✖ **51.21   Other partial cholecystectomy**
       Revision of prior cholecystectomy

> **Excludes**   *that by laparoscope (51.24)*

✖ **51.22 Cholecystectomy**
> Excludes *laparoscopic cholecystectomy (51.23)*

✖ **51.23 Laparoscopic cholecystectomy**
That by laser

✖ **51.24 Laparoscopic partial cholecystectomy**

● **51.3 Anastomosis of gallbladder or bile duct**
> Excludes *resection with end-to-end anastomosis (51.61–51.69)*

✖ **51.31 Anastomosis of gallbladder to hepatic ducts**

✖ **51.32 Anastomosis of gallbladder to intestine**

✖ **51.33 Anastomosis of gallbladder to pancreas**

✖ **51.34 Anastomosis of gallbladder to stomach**

✖ **51.35 Other gallbladder anastomosis**
Gallbladder anastomosis NOS

✖ **51.36 Choledochoenterostomy**

✖ **51.37 Anastomosis of hepatic duct to gastrointestinal tract**
Kasai portoenterostomy

✖ **51.39 Other bile duct anastomosis**
Anastomosis of bile duct NOS
Anastomosis of unspecified bile duct to:
    intestine
    liver
    pancreas
    stomach

● **51.4 Incision of bile duct for relief of obstruction**

✖ **51.41 Common duct exploration for removal of calculus**
> Excludes *percutaneous extraction (51.96)*

✖ **51.42 Common duct exploration for relief of other obstruction**

✖ **51.43 Insertion of choledochohepatic tube for decompression**
Hepatocholedochostomy

✖ **51.49 Incision of other bile ducts for relief of obstruction**

● **51.5 Other incision of bile duct**
> Excludes *that for relief of obstruction (51.41–51.49)*

✖ **51.51 Exploration of common duct**
Incision of common bile duct

✖ **51.59 Incision of other bile duct**

● **51.6 Local excision or destruction of lesion or tissue of biliary ducts and sphincter of Oddi**
Code also anastomosis other than end-to-end (51.31, 51.36–51.39)
> Excludes *biopsy of bile duct (51.12–51.13)*

✖ **51.61 Excision of cystic duct remnant**

✖ **51.62 Excision of ampulla of Vater (with reimplantation of common duct)**

✖ **51.63 Other excision of common duct**
Choledochectomy
> Excludes *fistulectomy (51.72)*

51.64 Endoscopic excision or destruction of lesion of biliary ducts or sphincter of Oddi
Excision or destruction of lesion of biliary duct by procedures classifiable to 51.10–51.11, 52.13

✖ **51.69 Excision of other bile duct**
Excision of lesion of bile duct NOS
> Excludes *fistulectomy (51.79)*

● **51.7 Repair of bile ducts**

✖ **51.71 Simple suture of common bile duct**

✖ **51.72 Choledochoplasty**
Repair of fistula of common bile duct

✖ **51.79 Repair of other bile ducts**
Closure of artificial opening of bile duct NOS
Suture of bile duct NOS
> Excludes *operative removal of prosthetic device (51.95)*

● **51.8 Other operations on biliary ducts and sphincter of Oddi**

✖ **51.81 Dilation of sphincter of Oddi**
Dilation of ampulla of Vater
> Excludes *that by endoscopic approach (51.84)*

✖ **51.82 Pancreatic sphincterotomy**
Incision of pancreatic sphincter
Transduodenal ampullary sphincterotomy
> Excludes *that by endoscopic approach (51.85)*

✖ **51.83 Pancreatic sphincteroplasty**

51.84 Endoscopic dilation of ampulla and biliary duct
Dilation of ampulla and biliary duct by procedures classifiable to 51.10–51.11, 52.13

51.85 Endoscopic sphincterotomy and papillotomy
Sphincterotomy and papillotomy by procedures classifiable to 51.10–51.11, 52.13

51.86 Endoscopic insertion of nasobiliary drainage tube
Insertion of nasobiliary tube by procedures classifiable to 51.10–51.11, 52.13

51.87 Endoscopic insertion of stent (tube) into bile duct
Endoprosthesis of bile duct
Insertion of stent into bile duct by procedures classifiable to 51.10–51.11, 52.13
> Excludes *nasobiliary drainage tube (51.86)*
> *replacement of stent (tube) (97.05)*

51.88 Endoscopic removal of stone(s) from biliary tract
Laparoscopic removal of stone(s) from biliary tract
Removal of biliary tract stone(s) by procedures classifiable to 51.10–51.11, 52.13
> Excludes *percutaneous extraction of common duct stones (51.96)*

✖ **51.89 Other operations on sphincter of Oddi**

● **51.9 Other operations on biliary tract**

✖ **51.91 Repair of laceration of gallbladder**

✖ **51.92 Closure of cholecystostomy**

✖ **51.93 Closure of other biliary fistula**
Cholecystogastroenteric fistulectomy

✖ **51.94 Revision of anastomosis of biliary tract**

✖ **51.95 Removal of prosthetic device from bile duct**
> Excludes *nonoperative removal (97.55)*

51.96 Percutaneous extraction of common duct stones

51.98   Other percutaneous procedures on biliary tract
Percutaneous biliary endoscopy via existing T-tube or other tract for:
dilation of biliary duct stricture
removal of stone(s) except common duct stone
exploration (postoperative)
Percutaneous transhepatic biliary drainage

> **Excludes**   *percutaneous aspiration of gallbladder (51.01)*
> *percutaneous biopsy and/or collection of specimen by brushing or washing (51.12)*
> *percutaneous removal of common duct stone(s) (51.96)*

✖ **51.99   Other**
Insertion or replacement of biliary tract prosthesis

> **Excludes**   *biopsy of gallbladder (51.12–51.13)*
> *irrigation of cholecystostomy and other biliary tube (96.41)*
> *lysis of peritoneal adhesions (54.5)*
> *nonoperative removal of:*
>   *cholecystostomy tube (97.54)*
>   *tube from biliary tract or liver (97.55)*

● **52   Operations on pancreas**

Code also any application or administration of an adhesion barrier substance (99.77)

    Includes: operations on pancreatic duct

● **52.0   Pancreatotomy**

    ✖ **52.01   Drainage of pancreatic cyst by catheter**

    ✖ **52.09   Other pancreatotomy**
      Pancreatolithotomy

> **Excludes**   *drainage by anastomosis (52.4, 52.96)*
> *incision of pancreatic sphincter (51.82)*
> *marsupialization of cyst (52.3)*

● **52.1   Diagnostic procedures on pancreas**

    52.11   Closed [aspiration] [needle] [percutaneous] biopsy of pancreas

    ✖ **52.12   Open biopsy of pancreas**

    52.13   Endoscopic retrograde pancreatography [ERP]

> **Excludes**   *endoscopic retrograde:*
>   *cholangiography [ERC] (51.11)*
>   *cholangiopancreatography [ERCP] (51.10)*
> *that for procedures classifiable to 51.14–51.15, 51.64, 51.84–51.88, 52.14, 52.21, 52.92–52.94, 52.97–52.98*

    52.14   Closed [endoscopic] biopsy of pancreatic duct
      Closed biopsy of pancreatic duct by procedures classifiable to 51.10–51.11, 52.13

    ✖ **52.19   Other diagnostic procedures on pancreas**

> **Excludes**   *contrast pancreatogram (87.66)*
> *endoscopic retrograde pancreatography [ERP] (52.13)*
> *microscopic examination of specimen from pancreas (91.01–91.09)*

● **52.2   Local excision or destruction of pancreas and pancreatic duct**

> **Excludes**   *biopsy of pancreas (52.11–52.12, 52.14)*
> *pancreatic fistulectomy (52.95)*

    52.21   Endoscopic excision or destruction of lesion or tissue of pancreatic duct
      Excision or destruction of lesion or tissue of pancreatic duct by procedures classifiable to 51.10–51.11, 52.13

    ✖ **52.22   Other excision or destruction of lesion or tissue of pancreas or pancreatic duct**

✖ **52.3   Marsupialization of pancreatic cyst**

> **Excludes**   *drainage of cyst by catheter (52.01)*

✖ **52.4   Internal drainage of pancreatic cyst**
Pancreaticocystoduodenostomy
Pancreaticocystogastrostomy
Pancreaticocystojejunostomy

● **52.5   Partial pancreatectomy**

> **Excludes**   *pancreatic fistulectomy (52.95)*

    ✖ **52.51   Proximal pancreatectomy**
      Excision of head of pancreas (with part of body)
      Proximal pancreatectomy with synchronous duodenectomy

    ✖ **52.52   Distal pancreatectomy**
      Excision of tail of pancreas (with part of body)

    ✖ **52.53   Radical subtotal pancreatectomy**

    ✖ **52.59   Other partial pancreatectomy**

✖ **52.6   Total pancreatectomy**
Pancreatectomy with synchronous duodenectomy

✖ **52.7   Radical pancreaticoduodenectomy**
One-stage pancreaticoduodenal resection with choledochojejunal anastomosis, pancreaticojejunal anastomosis, and gastrojejunostomy
Two-stage pancreaticoduodenal resection (first stage) (second stage)
Radical resection of the pancreas
Whipple procedure

> **Excludes**   *radical subtotal pancreatectomy (52.53)*

● **52.8   Transplant of pancreas**

    Note: To report donor source - *see* codes 00.91–00.93 ◄

    ✖ **52.80   Pancreatic transplant, not otherwise specified**

    ✖ **52.81   Reimplantation of pancreatic tissue**

    ✖ **52.82   Homotransplant of pancreas**

    ✖ **52.83   Heterotransplant of pancreas**

    52.84   Autotransplantation of cells of Islets of Langerhans
      Homotransplantation of islet cells of pancreas

    52.85   Allotransplantation of cells of Islets of Langerhans
      Heterotransplantation of islet cells of pancreas

    ✖ **52.86   Transplantation of cells of Islets of Langerhans, not otherwise specified**

● **52.9   Other operations on pancreas**

    ✖ **52.92   Cannulation of pancreatic duct**

> **Excludes**   *that by endoscopic approach (52.93)*

    52.93   Endoscopic insertion of stent (tube) into pancreatic duct
      Insertion of cannula or stent into pancreatic duct by procedures classifiable to 51.10–51.11, 52.13

> **Excludes**   *endoscopic insertion of nasopancreatic drainage tube (52.97)*
> *replacement of stent (tube) (97.05)*

    52.94   Endoscopic removal of stone(s) from pancreatic duct
      Removal of stone(s) from pancreatic duct by procedures classifiable to 51.10–51.11, 52.13

    ✖ **52.95   Other repair of pancreas**
      Fistulectomy of pancreas
      Simple suture of pancreas

✖**52.96 Anastomosis of pancreas**
Anastomosis of pancreas (duct) to:
     intestine
     jejunum
     stomach

     Excludes   *anastomosis to:*
         bile duct (51.39)
         gallbladder (51.33)

52.97 Endoscopic insertion of nasopancreatic drainage tube
Insertion of nasopancreatic drainage tube by procedures classifiable to 51.10–51.11, 52.13

     Excludes   *drainage of pancreatic cyst by catheter (52.01)*
         replacement of stent (tube) (97.05)

52.98 Endoscopic dilation of pancreatic duct
Dilation of Wirsung's duct by procedures classifiable to 51.10–51.11, 52.13

✖**52.99 Other**
Dilation of pancreatic [Wirsung's] duct by open approach
Repair of pancreatic [Wirsung's] duct by open approach

     Excludes   *irrigation of pancreatic tube (96.42)*
         removal of pancreatic tube (97.56)

●**53   Repair of hernia**

Code also any application or administration of an adhesion barrier substance (99.77)

     Includes: hernioplasty
           herniorrhaphy

     Excludes   *manual reduction of hernia (96.27)*

●**53.0   Unilateral repair of inguinal hernia**

✖**53.00 Unilateral repair of inguinal hernia, not otherwise specified**
Inguinal herniorrhaphy NOS

✖**53.01 Repair of direct inguinal hernia**

✖**53.02 Repair of indirect inguinal hernia**

✖**53.03 Repair of direct inguinal hernia with graft or prosthesis**

✖**53.04 Repair of indirect inguinal hernia with graft or prosthesis**

✖**53.05 Repair of inguinal hernia with graft or prosthesis, not otherwise specified**

●**53.1   Bilateral repair of inguinal hernia**

✖**53.10 Bilateral repair of inguinal hernia, not otherwise specified**

✖**53.11 Bilateral repair of direct inguinal hernia**

✖**53.12 Bilateral repair of indirect inguinal hernia**

✖**53.13 Bilateral repair of inguinal hernia, one direct and one indirect**

✖**53.14 Bilateral repair of direct inguinal hernia with graft or prosthesis**

✖**53.15 Bilateral repair of indirect inguinal hernia with graft or prosthesis**

✖**53.16 Bilateral repair of inguinal hernia, one direct and one indirect, with graft or prosthesis**

✖**53.17 Bilateral inguinal hernia repair with graft or prosthesis, not otherwise specified**

●**53.2   Unilateral repair of femoral hernia**

✖**53.21 Unilateral repair of femoral hernia with graft or prosthesis**

✖**53.29 Other unilateral femoral herniorrhaphy**

●**53.3   Bilateral repair of femoral hernia**

✖**53.31 Bilateral repair of femoral hernia with graft or prosthesis**

✖**53.39 Other bilateral femoral herniorrhaphy**

●**53.4   Repair of umbilical hernia**

     Excludes   *repair of gastroschisis (54.71)*

✖**53.41 Repair of umbilical hernia with prosthesis**

✖**53.49 Other umbilical herniorrhaphy**

●**53.5   Repair of other hernia of anterior abdominal wall (without graft or prosthesis)**

✖**53.51 Incisional hernia repair**

✖**53.59 Repair of other hernia of anterior abdominal wall**
Repair of hernia:
     epigastric
     hypogastric
     spigelian
     ventral

●**53.6   Repair of other hernia of anterior abdominal wall with graft or prosthesis**

✖**53.61 Incisional hernia repair with prosthesis**

✖**53.69 Repair of other hernia of anterior abdominal wall with prosthesis**

✖**53.7   Repair of diaphragmatic hernia, abdominal approach**

●**53.8   Repair of diaphragmatic hernia, thoracic approach**

✖**53.80 Repair of diaphragmatic hernia with thoracic approach, not otherwise specified**
Thoracoabdominal repair of diaphragmatic hernia

✖**53.81 Plication of the diaphragm**

✖**53.82 Repair of parasternal hernia**

✖**53.9   Other hernia repair**
Repair of hernia:
     ischiatic
     ischiorectal
     lumbar
     obturator
     omental
     retroperitoneal
     sciatic

     Excludes   *relief of strangulated hernia with exteriorization of intestine (46.01, 46.03)*
         repair of pericolostomy hernia (46.42)
         repair of vaginal enterocele (70.92)

●**54   Other operations on abdominal region**

Code also any application or administration of an adhesion barrier substance (99.77)

     Includes: operations on:
           epigastric region
           flank
           groin region
           hypochondrium
           inguinal region
           loin region
           male pelvic cavity
           mesentery
           omentum
           peritoneum
           retroperitoneal tissue space

     Excludes   *female pelvic cavity (69.01–70.92)*
         hernia repair (53.00–53.9)
         obliteration of cul-de-sac (70.92)
         retroperitoneal tissue dissection (59.00–59.09)
         skin and subcutaneous tissue of abdominal wall (86.01–86.99)

✖ **54.0   Incision of abdominal wall**
Drainage of:
abdominal wall
extraperitoneal abscess
retroperitoneal abscess

> **Excludes**   incision of peritoneum (54.95)
> laparotomy (54.11–54.19)

● **54.1   Laparotomy**

✖ **54.11   Exploratory laparotomy**

> **Excludes**   exploration incidental to intra- abdominal sur-
> gery—omit code

✖ **54.12   Reopening of recent laparotomy site**
Reopening of recent laparotomy site for:
control of hemorrhage
exploration
incision of hematoma

✖ **54.19   Other laparotomy**
Drainage of intraperitoneal abscess or hematoma

> **Excludes**   culdocentesis (70.0)
> drainage of appendiceal abscess (47.2)
> exploration incidental to intra-abdominal sur-
> gery—omit code
> Ladd operation (54.95)
> percutaneous drainage of abdomen (54.91)
> removal of foreign body (54.92)

● **54.2   Diagnostic procedures of abdominal region**

✖ **54.21   Laparoscopy**
Peritoneoscopy

> **Excludes**   laparoscopic cholecystectomy (51.23)
> that incidental to destruction of fallopian tubes
> (66.21–66.29)

✖ **54.22   Biopsy of abdominal wall or umbilicus**

✖ **54.23   Biopsy of peritoneum**
Biopsy of:
mesentery
omentum
peritoneal implant

> **Excludes**   closed biopsy of:
> omentum (54.24)
> peritoneum (54.24)

**54.24   Closed [percutaneous] [needle] biopsy of intra-
abdominal mass**
Closed biopsy of:
omentum
peritoneal implant
peritoneum

> **Excludes**   that of:
> fallopian tube (66.11)
> ovary (65.11)
> uterine ligaments (68.15)
> uterus (68.16)

54.25   Peritoneal lavage
Diagnostic peritoneal lavage

> **Excludes**   peritoneal dialysis (54.98)

✖ **54.29   Other diagnostic procedures on abdominal region**

> **Excludes**   abdominal lymphangiogram (88.04)
> abdominal x-ray NEC (88.19)
> angiocardiography of venae cava (88.51)
> C.A.T. scan of abdomen (88.01)
> contrast x-ray of abdominal cavity (88.11–88.15)
> intra-abdominal arteriography NEC (88.47)
> microscopic examination of peritoneal and retro-
> peritoneal specimen (91.11–91.19)
> phlebography of:
> intra-abdominal vessels NEC (88.65)
> portal venous system (88.64)
> sinogram of abdominal wall (88.03)
> soft tissue x-ray of abdominal wall NEC (88.09)
> tomography of abdomen NEC (88.02)
> ultrasonography of abdomen and retroperitoneum
> (88.76)

✖ **54.3   Excision or destruction of lesion or tissue of abdomi-
nal wall or umbilicus**
Debridement of abdominal wall
Omphalectomy

> **Excludes**   biopsy of abdominal wall or umbilicus (54.22)
> size reduction operation (86.83)
> that of skin of abdominal wall (86.22, 86.26, 86.3)

✖ **54.4   Excision or destruction of peritoneal tissue**
Excision of:
appendices epiploicae
falciform ligament
gastrocolic ligament
lesion of:
mesentery
omentum
peritoneum
presacral lesion NOS
retroperitoneal lesion NOS

> **Excludes**   biopsy of peritoneum (54.23)
> endometrectomy of cul-de-sac (70.32)

54.5   Lysis of peritoneal adhesions
Freeing of adhesions of:
biliary tract
intestines
liver
pelvic peritoneum
peritoneum
spleen
uterus

> **Excludes**   lysis of adhesions of:
> bladder (59.11)
> fallopian tube and ovary
> laparoscopic (65.81)
> other (65.89)
> kidney (59.02)
> ureter (59.02)

✖ **54.51   Laparoscopic lysis of peritoneal adhesions**

✖ **54.59   Other lysis of peritoneal adhesions**

● **54.6   Suture of abdominal wall and peritoneum**

✖ **54.61   Reclosure of postoperative disruption of abdominal wall**

✖ **54.62   Delayed closure of granulating abdominal
wound**
Tertiary subcutaneous wound closure

✖ **54.63   Other suture of abdominal wall**
Suture of laceration of abdominal wall

> **Excludes**   closure of operative wound—omit code

✖ **54.64   Suture of peritoneum**
Secondary suture of peritoneum

> **Excludes**   closure of operative wound—omit code

- ● **54.7 Other repair of abdominal wall and peritoneum**
  - ✖ **54.71 Repair of gastroschisis**
  - ✖ **54.72 Other repair of abdominal wall**
  - ✖ **54.73 Other repair of peritoneum**
    Suture of gastrocolic ligament
  - ✖ **54.74 Other repair of omentum**
    Epiplorrhaphy
    Graft of omentum
    Omentopexy
    Reduction of torsion of omentum
    Excludes *cardio-omentopexy (36.39)*
  - ✖ **54.75 Other repair of mesentery**
    Mesenteric plication
    Mesenteropexy
- ● **54.9 Other operations of abdominal region**
  Excludes *removal of ectopic pregnancy (74.3)*
  - **54.91 Percutaneous abdominal drainage**
    Paracentesis
    Excludes *creation of cutaneoperitoneal fistula (54.93)*
  - ✖ **54.92 Removal of foreign body from peritoneal cavity**
  - ✖ **54.93 Creation of cutaneoperitoneal fistula**
  - ✖ **54.94 Creation of peritoneovascular shunt**
    Peritoneovenous shunt

- ✖ **54.95 Incision of peritoneum**
  Exploration of ventriculoperitoneal shunt at peritoneal site
  Ladd operation
  Revision of distal catheter of ventricular shunt
  Revision of ventriculoperitoneal shunt at peritoneal site
  Excludes *that incidental to laparotomy (54.11–54.19)*
- **54.96 Injection of air into peritoneal cavity**
  Pneumoperitoneum
  Excludes *that for:*
  collapse of lung (33.33)
  radiography (88.12–88.13, 88.15)
- **54.97 Injection of locally-acting therapeutic substance into peritoneal cavity**
  Excludes *peritoneal dialysis (54.98)*
- **54.98 Peritoneal dialysis**
  Excludes *peritoneal lavage (diagnostic) (54.25)*
- **54.99 Other**
  Excludes *removal of:*
  abdominal wall suture (97.83)
  peritoneal drainage device (97.82)
  retroperitoneal drainage device (97.81)

10. OPERATIONS ON THE URINARY SYSTEM (55–59)

● **55 Operations on kidney**

Code also any application or administration of an adhesion barrier substance (99.77)

> **Includes:** operations on renal pelvis
>
> **Excludes** *perirenal tissue (59.00–59.09, 59.21–59.29, 59.91–59.92)*

● **55.0 Nephrotomy and nephrostomy**

> **Excludes** *drainage by:*
> *anastomosis (55.86)*
> *aspiration (55.92)*
> *incision of kidney pelvis (55.11–55.12)*

✖ **55.01 Nephrotomy**
Evacuation of renal cyst
Exploration of kidney
Nephrolithotomy

✖ **55.02 Nephrostomy**

✖ **55.03 Percutaneous nephrostomy without fragmentation**
Nephrostolithotomy, percutaneous (nephroscopic)
Percutaneous removal of kidney stone(s) by:
basket extraction
forceps extraction (nephroscopic)
Pyelostolithotomy, percutaneous (nephroscopic)
With placement of catheter down ureter

> **Excludes** *percutaneous removal by fragmentation (55.04)*
> *repeat nephroscopic removal during current episode (55.92)*

✖ **55.04 Percutaneous nephrostomy with fragmentation**
Percutaneous nephrostomy with disruption of kidney stone by ultrasonic energy and extraction (suction) through endoscope
With placement of catheter down ureter
With fluoroscopic guidance

> **Excludes** *repeat fragmentation during current episode (59.95)*

● **55.1 Pyelotomy and pyelostomy**

> **Excludes** *drainage by anastomosis (55.86)*
> *percutaneous pyelostolithotomy (55.03)*
> *removal of calculus without incision (56.0)*

✖ **55.11 Pyelotomy**
Exploration of renal pelvis
Pyelolithotomy

✖ **55.12 Pyelostomy**
Insertion of drainage tube into renal pelvis

● **55.2 Diagnostic procedures on kidney**

55.21 Nephroscopy

55.22 Pyeloscopy

55.23 Closed [percutaneous] [needle] biopsy of kidney
Endoscopic biopsy via existing nephrostomy, nephrotomy, pyelostomy, or pyelotomy

✖ **55.24 Open biopsy of kidney**

✖ **55.29 Other diagnostic procedures on kidney**

> **Excludes** *microscopic examination of specimen from kidney (91.21–91.29)*
> *pyelogram:*
> *intravenous (87.73)*
> *percutaneous (87.75)*
> *retrograde (87.74)*
> *radioisotope scan (92.03)*
> *renal arteriography (88.45)*
> *tomography:*
> *C.A.T. scan (87.71)*
> *other (87.72)*

● **55.3 Local excision or destruction of lesion or tissue of kidney**

✖ **55.31 Marsupialization of kidney lesion**

✖ **55.39 Other local destruction or excision of renal lesion or tissue**
Obliteration of calyceal diverticulum

> **Excludes** *biopsy of kidney (55.23–55.24)*
> *partial nephrectomy (55.4)*
> *percutaneous aspiration of kidney (55.92)*
> *wedge resection of kidney (55.4)*

✖ **55.4 Partial nephrectomy**
Calycectomy
Wedge resection of kidney

Code also any synchronous resection of ureter (56.40–56.42)

● **55.5 Complete nephrectomy**

Code also any synchronous excision of:
adrenal gland (07.21–07.3) ◄
bladder segment (57.6)
lymph nodes (40.3, 40.52–40.59)

✖ **55.51 Nephroureterectomy**
Nephroureterectomy with bladder cuff
Total nephrectomy (unilateral)

> **Excludes** *removal of transplanted kidney (55.53)*

✖ **55.52 Nephrectomy of remaining kidney**
Removal of solitary kidney

> **Excludes** *removal of transplanted kidney (55.53)*

✖ **55.53 Removal of transplanted or rejected kidney**

✖ **55.54 Bilateral nephrectomy**

> **Excludes** *complete nephrectomy NOS (55.51)*

● **55.6 Transplant of kidney**

Note: To report donor source - *see* codes 00.91–00.93) ◄

✖ **55.61 Renal autotransplantation**

✖ **55.69 Other kidney transplantation**

✖ **55.7 Nephropexy**
Fixation or suspension of movable [floating] kidney

● **55.8 Other repair of kidney**

✖ **55.81 Suture of laceration of kidney**

✖ **55.82 Closure of nephrostomy and pyelostomy**

✖ **55.83 Closure of other fistula of kidney**

✖ **55.84 Reduction of torsion of renal pedicle**

✖ **55.85 Symphysiotomy for horseshoe kidney**

✖ **55.86 Anastomosis of kidney**
Nephropyeloureterostomy
Pyeloureterovesical anastomosis
Ureterocalyceal anastomosis

> **Excludes** *nephrocystanastomosis NOS (56.73)*

✖ **55.87 Correction of ureteropelvic junction**

✖ **55.89 Other**

● **55.9 Other operations on kidney**

> **Excludes** *lysis of perirenal adhesions (59.02)*

✖ **55.91 Decapsulation of kidney**
Capsulectomy of kidney
Decortication of kidney

55.92 Percutaneous aspiration of kidney (pelvis)
Aspiration of renal cyst
Renipuncture

> **Excludes** *percutaneous biopsy of kidney (55.23)*

55.93 Replacement of nephrostomy tube

55.94 Replacement of pyelostomy tube

● **Use Additional Digit(s)**   ✖ **Valid O.R. Procedure**   ◄ **New**   ◄|||| **Revised**

55.95   Local perfusion of kidney

55.96   Other injection of therapeutic substance into kidney
> Injection into renal cyst

✖ 55.97   Implantation or replacement of mechanical kidney

✖ 55.98   Removal of mechanical kidney

✖ 55.99   Other

> **Excludes**   *removal of pyelostomy or nephrostomy tube (97.61)*

● 56   **Operations on ureter**

Code also any application or administration of an adhesion barrier substance (99.77)

✖ 56.0   **Transurethral removal of obstruction from ureter and renal pelvis**
> Removal of:
>> blood clot from ureter or renal pelvis without incision
>> calculus from ureter or renal pelvis without incision
>> foreign body from ureter or renal pelvis without incision

> **Excludes**   *manipulation without removal of obstruction (59.8)*
> *that by incision (55.11, 56.2)*
> *transurethral insertion of ureteral stent for passage of calculus (59.8)*

✖ 56.1   **Ureteral meatotomy**

✖ 56.2   **Ureterotomy**
> Incision of ureter for:
>> drainage
>> exploration
>> removal of calculus

> **Excludes**   *cutting of ureterovesical orifice (56.1)*
> *removal of calculus without incision (56.0)*
> *transurethral insertion of ureteral stent for passage of calculus (59.8)*
> *urinary diversion (56.51–56.79)*

● 56.3   **Diagnostic procedures on ureter**

56.31   Ureteroscopy

56.32   Closed percutaneous biopsy of ureter

> **Excludes**   *endoscopic biopsy of ureter (56.33)*

56.33   Closed endoscopic biopsy of ureter
> Cystourethroscopy with ureteral biopsy
> Transurethral biopsy of ureter
> Ureteral endoscopy with biopsy through ureterotomy
> Ureteroscopy with biopsy

> **Excludes**   *percutaneous biopsy of ureter (56.32)*

✖ 56.34   Open biopsy of ureter

56.35   Endoscopy (cystoscopy) (looposcopy) of ileal conduit

✖ 56.39   Other diagnostic procedures on ureter

> **Excludes**   *microscopic examination of specimen from ureter (91.21–91.29)*

● 56.4   **Ureterectomy**

Code also anastomosis other than end-to-end (56.51–56.79)

> **Excludes**   *fistulectomy (56.84)*
> *nephroureterectomy (55.51–55.54)*

✖ 56.40   Ureterectomy, not otherwise specified

✖ 56.41   Partial ureterectomy
> Excision of lesion of ureter
> Shortening of ureter with reimplantation

> **Excludes**   *biopsy of ureter (56.32–56.34)*

✖ 56.42   Total ureterectomy

● 56.5   **Cutaneous uretero-ileostomy**

✖ 56.51   Formation of cutaneous uretero-ileostomy
> Construction of ileal conduit
> External ureteral ileostomy
> Formation of open ileal bladder
> Ileal loop operation
> Ileoureterostomy (Bricker's) (ileal bladder)
> Transplantation of ureter into ileum with external diversion

> **Excludes**   *closed ileal bladder (57.87)*
> *replacement of ureteral defect by ileal segment (56.89)*

✖ 56.52   Revision of cutaneous uretero-ileostomy

● 56.6   **Other external urinary diversion**

✖ 56.61   Formation of other cutaneous ureterostomy
> Anastomosis of ureter to skin
> Ureterostomy NOS

✖ 56.62   Revision of other cutaneous ureterostomy
> Revision of ureterostomy stoma

> **Excludes**   *nonoperative removal of ureterostomy tube (97.62)*

● 56.7   **Other anastomosis or bypass of ureter**

> **Excludes**   *ureteropyelostomy (55.86)*

✖ 56.71   Urinary diversion to intestine
> Anastomosis of ureter to intestine
> Internal urinary diversion NOS

> Code also any synchronous colostomy (46.10–46.13)

> **Excludes**   *external ureteral ileostomy (56.51)*

✖ 56.72   Revision of ureterointestinal anastomosis

> **Excludes**   *revision of external ureteral ileostomy (56.52)*

✖ 56.73   Nephrocystanastomosis, not otherwise specified

✖ 56.74   Ureteroneocystostomy
> Replacement of ureter with bladder flap
> Ureterovesical anastomosis

✖ 56.75   Transureteroureterostomy

> **Excludes**   *ureteroureterostomy associated with partial resection (56.41)*

✖ 56.79   Other

● 56.8   **Repair of ureter**

✖ 56.81   Lysis of intraluminal adhesions of ureter

> **Excludes**   *lysis of periureteral adhesions (59.01–59.02)*
> *ureterolysis (59.01–59.02)*

✖ 56.82   Suture of laceration of ureter

✖ 56.83   Closure of ureterostomy

✖ 56.84   Closure of other fistula of ureter

✖ 56.85   Ureteropexy

✖ 56.86   Removal of ligature from ureter

✖ 56.89   Other repair of ureter
> Graft of ureter
> Replacement of ureter with ileal segment implanted into bladder
> Ureteroplication

● **56.9 Other operations on ureter**

     56.91 Dilation of ureteral meatus

     ✖ **56.92 Implantation of electronic ureteral stimulator**

     ✖ **56.93 Replacement of electronic ureteral stimulator**

     ✖ **56.94 Removal of electronic ureteral stimulator**

     Excludes *that with synchronous replacement (56.93)*

     ✖ **56.95 Ligation of ureter**

     ✖ **56.99 Other**

     Excludes *removal of ureterostomy tube and ureteral catheter (97.62)*
ureteral catheterization (59.8)

● **57 Operations on urinary bladder**

Code also any application or administration of an adhesion barrier substance (99.77)

     Excludes *perivesical tissue (59.11–59.29, 59.91–59.92)*
ureterovesical orifice (56.0–56.99)

     57.0 Transurethral clearance of bladder
Drainage of bladder without incision
Removal of:
     blood clots from bladder without incision
     calculus from bladder without incision
     foreign body from bladder without incision

     Excludes *that by incision (57.19)*

● **57.1 Cystotomy and cystostomy**

     Excludes *cystotomy and cystostomy as operative approach—omit code*

     57.11 Percutaneous aspiration of bladder

     ✖ **57.12 Lysis of intraluminal adhesions with incision into bladder**

     Excludes *transurethral lysis of intraluminal adhesions (57.41)*

     57.17 Percutaneous cystostomy
Closed cystostomy
Percutaneous suprapubic cystostomy

     Excludes *removal of cystostomy tube (97.63)*
replacement of cystostomy tube (59.94)

     ✖ **57.18 Other suprapubic cystostomy**

     Excludes *percutaneous cystostomy (57.17)*
removal of cystostomy tube (97.63)
replacement of cystostomy tube (59.94)

     ✖ **57.19 Other cystotomy**
Cystolithotomy

     Excludes *percutaneous cystostomy (57.17)*
suprapubic cystostomy (57.18)

● **57.2 Vesicostomy**

     Excludes *percutaneous cystostomy (57.17)*
suprapubic cystostomy (57.18)

     ✖ **57.21 Vesicostomy**
Creation of permanent opening from bladder to skin using a bladder flap

     ✖ **57.22 Revision or closure of vesicostomy**

     Excludes *closure of cystostomy (57.82)*

● **57.3 Diagnostic procedures on bladder**

     57.31 Cystoscopy through artificial stoma

     57.32 Other cystoscopy
Transurethral cystoscopy

     Excludes *cystourethroscopy with ureteral biopsy (56.33)*
retrograde pyelogram (87.74)
that for control of hemorrhage (postoperative):
     bladder (57.93)
     prostate (60.94)

✖ **57.33 Closed [transurethral] biopsy of bladder**

✖ **57.34 Open biopsy of bladder**

✖ **57.39 Other diagnostic procedures on bladder**

     Excludes *cystogram NEC (87.77)*
microscopic examination of specimen from bladder (91.31–91.39)
retrograde cystourethrogram (87.76)
therapeutic distention of bladder (96.25)

● **57.4 Transurethral excision or destruction of bladder tissue**

     ✖ **57.41 Transurethral lysis of intraluminal adhesions**

     ✖ **57.49 Other transurethral excision or destruction of lesion or tissue of bladder**
Endoscopic resection of bladder lesion

     Excludes *transurethral biopsy of bladder (57.33)*
transurethral fistulectomy (57.83–57.84)

● **57.5 Other excision or destruction of bladder tissue**

     Excludes *that with transurethral approach (57.41–57.49)*

     ✖ **57.51 Excision of urachus**
Excision of urachal sinus of bladder

     Excludes *excision of urachal cyst of abdominal wall (54.3)*

     ✖ **57.59 Open excision or destruction of other lesion or tissue of bladder**
Endometrectomy of bladder
Suprapubic excision of bladder lesion

     Excludes *biopsy of bladder (57.33–57.34)*
fistulectomy of bladder (57.83–57.84)

✖ **57.6 Partial cystectomy**
Excision of bladder dome
Trigonectomy
Wedge resection of bladder

● **57.7 Total cystectomy**

     Includes: total cystectomy with urethrectomy

     ✖ **57.71 Radical cystectomy**
Pelvic exenteration in male
Removal of bladder, prostate, seminal vesicles, and fat
Removal of bladder, urethra, and fat in a female

     Code also any:
lymph node dissection (40.3, 40.5)
urinary diversion (56.51–56.79)

     Excludes *that as part of pelvic exenteration in female (68.8)*

     ✖ **57.79 Other total cystectomy**

● **57.8 Other repair of urinary bladder**

     Excludes *repair of:*
     current obstetric laceration (75.61)
     cystocele (70.50–70.51)
     that for stress incontinence (59.3–59.79)

     ✖ **57.81 Suture of laceration of bladder**

     ✖ **57.82 Closure of cystostomy**

     ✖ **57.83 Repair of fistula involving bladder and intestine**
Rectovesicovaginal fistulectomy
Vesicosigmoidovaginal fistulectomy

     ✖ **57.84 Repair of other fistula of bladder**
Cervicovesical fistulectomy
Urethroperineovesical fistulectomy
Uterovesical fistulectomy
Vaginovesical fistulectomy

     Excludes *vesicoureterovaginal fistulectomy (56.84)*

● **Use Additional Digit(s)**   ✖ **Valid O.R. Procedure**   ◀ **New**   ◀■ **Revised**

✖ **57.85 Cystourethroplasty and plastic repair of bladder neck**
Plication of sphincter of urinary bladder
V-Y plasty of bladder neck

✖ **57.86 Repair of bladder exstrophy**

✖ **57.87 Reconstruction of urinary bladder**
Anastomosis of bladder with isolated segment of ileum
Augmentation of bladder
Replacement of bladder with ileum or sigmoid [closed ileal bladder]
Code also resection of intestine (45.50–45.52)

✖ **57.88 Other anastomosis of bladder**
Anastomosis of bladder to intestine NOS
Cystocolic anastomosis
Excludes *formation of closed ileal bladder (57.87)*

✖ **57.89 Other repair of bladder**
Bladder suspension, not elsewhere classified
Cystopexy NOS
Repair of old obstetric laceration of bladder
Excludes *repair of current obstetric laceration (75.61)*

● **57.9 Other operations on bladder**

✖ **57.91 Sphincterotomy of bladder**
Division of bladder neck

57.92 Dilation of bladder neck

✖ **57.93 Control of (postoperative) hemorrhage of bladder**

57.94 Insertion of indwelling urinary catheter

57.95 Replacement of indwelling urinary catheter

✖ **57.96 Implantation of electronic bladder stimulator**

✖ **57.97 Replacement of electronic bladder stimulator**

✖ **57.98 Removal of electronic bladder stimulator**
Excludes *that with synchronous replacement (57.97)*

✖ **57.99 Other**
Excludes *irrigation of:*
cystostomy (96.47)
other indwelling urinary catheter (96.48)
lysis of external adhesions (59.11)
removal of:
cystostomy tube (97.63)
other urinary drainage device (97.64)
therapeutic distention of bladder (96.25)

● **58 Operations on urethra**
Code also any application or administration of an adhesion barrier substance (99.77)
Includes: operations on:
bulbourethral gland [Cowper's gland]
periurethral tissue

✖ **58.0 Urethrotomy**
Excision of urethral septum
Formation of urethrovaginal fistula
Perineal urethrostomy
Removal of calculus from urethra by incision
Excludes *drainage of bulbourethral gland or periurethral tissue (58.91)*
internal urethral meatotomy (58.5)
removal of urethral calculus without incision (58.6)

✖ **58.1 Urethral meatotomy**
Excludes *internal urethral meatotomy (58.5)*

● **58.2 Diagnostic procedures on urethra**

58.21 Perineal urethroscopy

58.22 Other urethroscopy

58.23 Biopsy of urethra

58.24 Biopsy of periurethral tissue

58.29 Other diagnostic procedures on urethra and periurethral tissue
Excludes *microscopic examination of specimen from urethra (91.31–91.39)*
retrograde cystourethrogram (87.76)
urethral pressure profile (89.25)
urethral sphincter electromyogram (89.23)

● **58.3 Excision or destruction of lesion or tissue of urethra**
Excludes *biopsy of urethra (58.23)*
excision of bulbourethral gland (58.92)
fistulectomy (58.43)
urethrectomy as part of:
complete cystectomy (57.79)
pelvic evisceration (68.8)
radical cystectomy (57.71)

58.31 Endoscopic excision or destruction of lesion or tissue of urethra
Fulguration of urethral lesion

58.39 Other local excision or destruction of lesion or tissue of urethra
Excision of:
congenital valve of urethra
lesion of urethra
stricture of urethra
Urethrectomy
Excludes *that by endoscopic approach (58.31)*

● **58.4 Repair of urethra**
Excludes *repair of current obstetric laceration (75.61)*

✖ **58.41 Suture of laceration of urethra**

✖ **58.42 Closure of urethrostomy**

✖ **58.43 Closure of other fistula of urethra**
Excludes *repair of urethroperineovesical fistula (57.84)*

✖ **58.44 Reanastomosis of urethra**
Anastomosis of urethra

✖ **58.45 Repair of hypospadias or epispadias**

✖ **58.46 Other reconstruction of urethra**
Urethral construction

✖ **58.47 Urethral meatoplasty**

✖ **58.49 Other repair of urethra**
Benenenti rotation of bulbous urethra
Repair of old obstetric laceration of urethra
Urethral plication
Excludes *repair of:*
current obstetric laceration (75.61)
urethrocele (70.50–70.51)

✖ **58.5 Release of urethral stricture**
Cutting of urethral sphincter
Internal urethral meatotomy
Urethrolysis

58.6 Dilation of urethra
Dilation of urethrovesical junction
Passage of sounds through urethra
Removal of calculus from urethra without incision
Excludes *urethral calibration (89.29)*

● **58.9 Other operations on urethra and periurethral tissue**

✖ **58.91 Incision of periurethral tissue**
Drainage of bulbourethral gland

✖ **58.92   Excision of periurethral tissue**

    Excludes   *biopsy of periurethral tissue (58.24)*
             lysis of periurethral adhesions
                laparoscopic (59.12)
                other (59.11)

✖ **58.93   Implantation of artificial urinary sphincter [AUS]**

    Placement of inflatable:
       bladder sphincter
       urethral sphincter
    Removal with replacement of sphincter device [AUS]
    With pump and/or reservoir

✖ **58.99   Other**

    Removal of inflatable urinary sphincter without replacement
    Repair of inflatable sphincter pump and/or reservoir
    Surgical correction of hydraulic pressure of inflatable sphincter device

    Excludes   *removal of:*
             intraluminal foreign body from urethra without incision (98.19)
             urethral stent (97.65)

● **59   Other operations on urinary tract**

Code also any application or administration of an adhesion barrier substance (99.77)

● **59.0   Dissection of retroperitoneal tissue**

✖ **59.00   Retroperitoneal dissection, not otherwise specified**

✖ **59.02   Other lysis of perirenal or periureteral adhesions**

    Excludes   *that by laparoscope (59.03)*

✖ **59.03   Laparoscopic lysis of perirenal or periureteral adhesions**

✖ **59.09   Other incision of perirenal or periureteral tissue**

    Exploration of perinephric area
    Incision of perirenal abscess

● **59.1   Incision of perivesical tissue**

✖ **59.11   Other lysis of perivesical adhesions**

✖ **59.12   Laparoscopic lysis of perivesical adhesions**

✖ **59.19   Other incision of perivesical tissue**

    Exploration of perivesical tissue
    Incision of hematoma of space of Retzius
    Retropubic exploration

● **59.2   Diagnostic procedures on perirenal and perivesical tissue**

✖ **59.21   Biopsy of perirenal or perivesical tissue**

✖ **59.29   Other diagnostic procedures on perirenal tissue, perivesical tissue, and retroperitoneum**

    Excludes   *microscopic examination of specimen from:*
             perirenal tissue (91.21–91.29)
             perivesical tissue (91.31–91.39)
             retroperitoneum NEC (91.11–91.19)
             retroperitoneal x-ray (88.14–88.16)

✖ **59.3   Plication of urethrovesical junction**

    Kelly-Kennedy operation on urethra
    Kelly-Stoeckel urethral plication

✖ **59.4   Suprapubic sling operation**

    Goebel-Frangenheim-Stoeckel urethrovesical suspension
    Millin-Read urethrovesical suspension
    Oxford operation for urinary incontinence
    Urethrocystopexy by suprapubic suspension

✖ **59.5   Retropubic urethral suspension**

    Burch procedure
    Marshall-Marchetti-Krantz operation
    Suture of periurethral tissue to symphysis pubis
    Urethral suspension NOS

✖ **59.6   Paraurethral suspension**

    Pereyra paraurethral suspension
    Periurethral suspension

● **59.7   Other repair of urinary stress incontinence**

✖ **59.71   Levator muscle operation for urethrovesical suspension**

    Cystourethropexy with levator muscle sling
    Gracilis muscle transplant for urethrovesical suspension
    Pubococcygeal sling

59.72   Injection of implant into urethra and/or bladder neck

    Collagen implant
    Endoscopic injection of implant
    Fat implant
    Polytef implant

✖ **59.79   Other**

    Anterior urethropexy
    Repair of stress incontinence NOS
    Tudor "rabbit ear" urethropexy

59.8   Ureteral catheterization

    Drainage of kidney by catheter
    Insertion of ureteral stent
    Ureterovesical orifice dilation

    Code also any ureterotomy (56.2)

    Excludes   *that for:*
             retrograde pyelogram (87.74)
             transurethral removal of calculus or clot from ureter and renal pelvis (56.0)

● **59.9   Other operations on urinary system**

    Excludes   *nonoperative removal of therapeutic device (97.61–97.69)*

✖ **59.91   Excision of perirenal or perivesical tissue**

    Excludes   *biopsy of perirenal or perivesical tissue (59.21)*

✖ **59.92   Other operations on perirenal or perivesical tissue**

59.93   Replacement of ureterostomy tube

    Change of ureterostomy tube
    Reinsertion of ureterostomy tube

    Excludes   *nonoperative removal of ureterostomy tube (97.62)*

59.94   Replacement of cystostomy tube

    Excludes   *nonoperative removal of cystostomy tube (97.63)*

59.95   Ultrasonic fragmentation of urinary stones

    Shattered urinary stones

    Excludes   *percutaneous nephrostomy with fragmentation (55.04)*
             shock-wave disintegration (98.51)

59.99   Other

    Excludes   *instillation of medication into urinary tract (96.49)*
             irrigation of urinary tract (96.45–96.48)

11. OPERATIONS ON THE MALE GENITAL ORGANS (60–64)

● **60 Operations on prostate and seminal vesicles**

Code also any application or administration of an adhesion barrier substance (99.77)

Includes: operations on periprostatic tissue

Excludes | *that associated with radical cystectomy (57.71)*

✖ **60.0 Incision of prostate**
Drainage of prostatic abscess
Prostatolithotomy

Excludes | *drainage of periprostatic tissue only (60.81)*

● **60.1 Diagnostic procedures on prostate and seminal vesicles**

60.11 Closed [percutaneous] [needle] biopsy of prostate
Approach:
transrectal
transurethral
Punch biopsy

✖ **60.12 Open biopsy of prostate**

60.13 Closed [percutaneous] biopsy of seminal vesicles
Needle biopsy of seminal vesicles

✖ **60.14 Open biopsy of seminal vesicles**

✖ **60.15 Biopsy of periprostatic tissue**

✖ **60.18 Other diagnostic procedures on prostate and periprostatic tissue**

Excludes | *microscopic examination of specimen from prostate (91.31–91.39)*
x-ray of prostate (87.92)

✖ **60.19 Other diagnostic procedures on seminal vesicles**

Excludes | *microscopic examination of specimen from seminal vesicles (91.31–91.39)*
x-ray:
contrast seminal vesiculogram (87.91)
other (87.92)

● **60.2 Transurethral prostatectomy**

Excludes | *local excision of lesion of prostate (60.61)*

✖ **60.21 Transurethral (ultrasound) guided laser induced prostatectomy (TULIP)**
Ablation (contact) (noncontact) by laser

✖ **60.29 Other transurethral prostatectomy**
Excision of median bar by transurethral approach
Transurethral electrovaporization of prostrate (TEVAP)
Transurethral enucleative procedure
Transurethral prostatectomy NOS
Transurethral resection of prostate (TURP)

✖ **60.3 Suprapubic prostatectomy**
Transvesical prostatectomy

Excludes | *local excision of lesion of prostate (60.61)*
radical prostatectomy (60.5)

✖ **60.4 Retropubic prostatectomy**

Excludes | *local excision of lesion of prostate (60.61)*
radical prostatectomy (60.5)

✖ **60.5 Radical prostatectomy**
Prostatovesiculectomy
Radical prostatectomy by any approach

Excludes | *cystoprostatectomy (57.71)*

● **60.6 Other prostatectomy**

✖ **60.61 Local excision of lesion of prostate**
Excision of prostatic lesion by any approach

Excludes | *biopsy of prostate (60.11–60.12)*

✖ **60.62 Perineal prostatectomy**
Cryoablation of prostate
Cryoprostatectomy
Cryosurgery of prostate
Radical cryosurgical ablation of prostate (RCSA)

Excludes | *local excision of lesion of prostate (60.61)*

✖ **60.69 Other**

● **60.7 Operations on seminal vesicles**

60.71 Percutaneous aspiration of seminal vesicle

Excludes | *needle biopsy of seminal vesicle (60.13)*

✖ **60.72 Incision of seminal vesicle**

✖ **60.73 Excision of seminal vesicle**
Excision of Müllerian duct cyst
Spermatocystectomy

Excludes | *biopsy of seminal vesicle (60.13–60.14)*
prostatovesiculectomy (60.5)

✖ **60.79 Other operations on seminal vesicles**

● **60.8 Incision or excision of periprostatic tissue**

✖ **60.81 Incision of periprostatic tissue**
Drainage of periprostatic abscess

✖ **60.82 Excision of periprostatic tissue**
Excision of lesion of periprostatic tissue

Excludes | *biopsy of periprostatic tissue (60.15)*

● **60.9 Other operations on prostate**

60.91 Percutaneous aspiration of prostate

Excludes | *needle biopsy of prostate (60.11)*

60.92 Injection into prostate

✖ **60.93 Repair of prostate**

✖ **60.94 Control of (postoperative) hemorrhage of prostate**
Coagulation of prostatic bed
Cystoscopy for control of prostatic hemorrhage

✖ **60.95 Transurethral balloon dilation of the prostatic urethra**

60.96 Transurethral destruction of prostate tissue by microwave thermotherapy
Transurethral microwave thermotherapy (TUMT) of prostate

Excludes | *prostatectomy:*
other (60.61–60.69)
radical (60.5)
retropubic (60.4)
suprapubic (60.3)
transurethral (60.21–60.29)

60.97 Other transurethral destruction of prostate tissue by other thermotherapy
Radiofrequency thermotherapy
Transurethral needle ablation (TUNA) of prostate

Excludes | *prostatectomy:*
other (60.61–60.69)
radical (60.5)
retropubic (60.4)
suprapubic (60.3)
transurethral (60.21–60.29)

✖ **60.99 Other**

Excludes | *prostatic massage (99.94)*

● 61 **Operations on scrotum and tunica vaginalis**

   61.0 **Incision and drainage of scrotum and tunica vaginalis**

   Excludes *percutaneous aspiration of hydrocele (61.91)*

● 61.1 **Diagnostic procedures on scrotum and tunica vaginalis**

   61.11 **Biopsy of scrotum or tunica vaginalis**

   61.19 **Other diagnostic procedures on scrotum and tunica vaginalis**

✖ 61.2 **Excision of hydrocele (of tunica vaginalis)**
   Bottle repair of hydrocele of tunica vaginalis

   Excludes *percutaneous aspiration of hydrocele (61.91)*

   61.3 **Excision or destruction of lesion or tissue of scrotum**
   Fulguration of lesion of scrotum
   Reduction of elephantiasis of scrotum
   Partial scrotectomy of scrotum

   Excludes *biopsy of scrotum (61.11)*
   scrotal fistulectomy (61.42)

● 61.4 **Repair of scrotum and tunica vaginalis**

   61.41 **Suture of laceration of scrotum and tunica vaginalis**

✖ 61.42 **Repair of scrotal fistula**

✖ 61.49 **Other repair of scrotum and tunica vaginalis**
   Reconstruction with rotational or pedicle flaps

● 61.9 **Other operations on scrotum and tunica vaginalis**

   61.91 **Percutaneous aspiration of tunica vaginalis**
   Aspiration of hydrocele of tunica vaginalis

✖ 61.92 **Excision of lesion of tunica vaginalis other than hydrocele**
   Excision of hematocele of tunica vaginalis

✖ 61.99 **Other**

   Excludes *removal of foreign body from scrotum without incision (98.24)*

● 62 **Operations on testes**

✖ 62.0 **Incision of testis**

● 62.1 **Diagnostic procedures on testes**

   62.11 **Closed [percutaneous] [needle] biopsy of testis**

✖ 62.12 **Open biopsy of testis**

✖ 62.19 **Other diagnostic procedures on testes**

✖ 62.2 **Excision or destruction of testicular lesion**
   Excision of appendix testis
   Excision of cyst of Morgagni in the male

   Excludes *biopsy of testis (62.11–62.12)*

✖ 62.3 **Unilateral orchiectomy**
   Orchidectomy (with epididymectomy) NOS

● 62.4 **Bilateral orchiectomy**
   Male castration
   Radical bilateral orchiectomy (with epididymectomy)

   Code also any synchronous lymph node dissection (40.3, 40.5)

✖ 62.41 **Removal of both testes at same operative episode**
   Bilateral orchidectomy NOS

✖ 62.42 **Removal of remaining testis**
   Removal of solitary testis

✖ 62.5 **Orchiopexy**
   Mobilization and replacement of testis in scrotum
   Orchiopexy with detorsion of testis
   Torek (-Bevan) operation (orchidopexy) (first stage) (second stage)
   Transplantation to and fixation of testis in scrotum

● 62.6 **Repair of testes**

   Excludes *reduction of torsion (63.52)*

✖ 62.61 **Suture of laceration of testis**

✖ 62.69 **Other repair of testis**
   Testicular graft

✖ 62.7 **Insertion of testicular prosthesis**

● 62.9 **Other operations on testes**

   62.91 **Aspiration of testis**

   Excludes *percutaneous biopsy of testis (62.11)*

   62.92 **Injection of therapeutic substance into testis**

✖ 62.99 **Other**

● 63 **Operations on spermatic cord, epididymis, and vas deferens**

● 63.0 **Diagnostic procedures on spermatic cord, epididymis, and vas deferens**

   63.01 **Biopsy of spermatic cord, epididymis, or vas deferens**

✖ 63.09 **Other diagnostic procedures on spermatic cord, epididymis, and vas deferens**

   Excludes *contrast epididymogram (87.93)*
   contrast vasogram (87.94)
   other x-ray of epididymis and vas deferens (87.95)

✖ 63.1 **Excision of varicocele and hydrocele of spermatic cord**
   High ligation of spermatic vein
   Hydrocelectomy of canal of Nuck

✖ 63.2 **Excision of cyst of epididymis**
   Spermatocelectomy

✖ 63.3 **Excision of other lesion or tissue of spermatic cord and epididymis**
   Excision of appendix epididymis

   Excludes *biopsy of spermatic cord or epididymis (63.01)*

✖ 63.4 **Epididymectomy**

   Excludes *that synchronous with orchiectomy (62.3–62.42)*

● 63.5 **Repair of spermatic cord and epididymis**

✖ 63.51 **Suture of laceration of spermatic cord and epididymis**

   63.52 **Reduction of torsion of testis or spermatic cord**

   Excludes *that associated with orchiopexy (62.5)*

✖ 63.53 **Transplantation of spermatic cord**

✖ 63.59 **Other repair of spermatic cord and epididymis**

   63.6 **Vasotomy**
   Vasostomy

● 63.7 **Vasectomy and ligation of vas deferens**

   63.70 **Male sterilization procedure, not otherwise specified**

   63.71 **Ligation of vas deferens**
   Crushing of vas deferens
   Division of vas deferens

   63.72 **Ligation of spermatic cord**

   63.73 **Vasectomy**

● **63.8 Repair of vas deferens and epididymis**

✖ **63.81 Suture of laceration of vas deferens and epididymis**

✖ **63.82 Reconstruction of surgically divided vas deferens**

✖ **63.83 Epididymovasostomy**

    63.84 Removal of ligature from vas deferens

✖ **63.85 Removal of valve from vas deferens**

✖ **63.89 Other repair of vas deferens and epididymis**

● **63.9 Other operations on spermatic cord, epididymis, and vas deferens**

    63.91 Aspiration of spermatocele

✖ **63.92 Epididymotomy**

✖ **63.93 Incision of spermatic cord**

✖ **63.94 Lysis of adhesions of spermatic cord**

✖ **63.95 Insertion of valve in vas deferens**

✖ **63.99 Other**

● **64 Operations on penis**

    Includes: operations on:
           corpora cavernosa
           glans penis
           prepuce

✖ **64.0 Circumcision**

● **64.1 Diagnostic procedures on the penis**

✖ **64.11 Biopsy of penis**

    64.19 Other diagnostic procedures on penis

✖ **64.2 Local excision or destruction of lesion of penis**

    | **Excludes** | *biopsy of penis (64.11)* |

✖ **64.3 Amputation of penis**

● **64.4 Repair and plastic operation on penis**

✖ **64.41 Suture of laceration of penis**

✖ **64.42 Release of chordee**

✖ **64.43 Construction of penis**

✖ **64.44 Reconstruction of penis**

✖ **64.45 Replantation of penis**
        Reattachment of amputated penis

✖ **64.49 Other repair of penis**

    | **Excludes** | *repair of epispadias and hypospadias (58.45)* |

✖ **64.5 Operations for sex transformation, not elsewhere classified**

● **64.9 Other operations on male genital organs**

    64.91 Dorsal or lateral slit of prepuce

✖ **64.92 Incision of penis**

✖ **64.93 Division of penile adhesions**

    64.94 Fitting of external prosthesis of penis
        Penile prosthesis NOS

✖ **64.95 Insertion or replacement of non-inflatable penile prosthesis**
        Insertion of semi-rigid rod prosthesis into shaft of penis

    | **Excludes** | *external penile prosthesis (64.94)* |
        inflatable penile prosthesis (64.97)
        plastic repair, penis (64.43–64.49)
        that associated with:
            construction (64.43)
            reconstruction (64.44)

✖ **64.96 Removal of internal prosthesis of penis**
        Removal without replacement of non-inflatable or inflatable penile prosthesis

✖ **64.97 Insertion or replacement of inflatable penile prosthesis**
        Insertion of cylinders into shaft of penis and placement of pump and reservoir

    | **Excludes** | *external penile prosthesis (64.94)* |
        non-inflatable penile prosthesis (64.95)
        plastic repair, penis (64.43–64.49)

✖ **64.98 Other operations on penis**
        Corpora cavernosa-corpus spongiosum shunt
        Corpora-saphenous shunt
        Irrigation of corpus cavernosum

    | **Excludes** | *removal of foreign body:* |
        intraluminal (98.19)
        without incision (98.24)
        stretching of foreskin (99.95)

✖ **64.99 Other**

    | **Excludes** | *collection of sperm for artificial insemination (99.96)* |

12. OPERATIONS ON THE FEMALE GENITAL ORGANS (65–71)

● 65 Operations on ovary

Code also any application or administration of an adhesion barrier substance (99.77)

● 65.0 Oophorotomy
Salpingo-oophorotomy

✖ 65.01 Laparoscopic oophorotomy

✖ 65.09 Other oophorotomy

● 65.1 Diagnostic procedures on ovaries

✖ 65.11 Aspiration biopsy of ovary

✖ 65.12 Other biopsy of ovary

✖ 65.13 Laparoscopic biopsy of ovary

✖ 65.14 Other laparoscopic diagnostic procedures on ovaries

✖ 65.19 Other diagnostic procedures on ovaries

Excludes microscopic examination of specimen from ovary (91.41–91.49)

● 65.2 Local excision or destruction of ovarian lesion or tissue

✖ 65.21 Marsupialization of ovarian cyst

Excludes that by laparoscope (65.23)

✖ 65.22 Wedge resection of ovary

Excludes that by laparoscope (65.24)

✖ 65.23 Laparoscopic marsupialization of ovarian cyst

✖ 65.24 Laparoscopic wedge resection of ovary

✖ 65.25 Other laparoscopic local excision or destruction of ovary

✖ 65.29 Other local excision or destruction of ovary
Bisection of ovary
Cauterization of ovary
Partial excision of ovary

Excludes biopsy of ovary (65.11–65.13)
that by laparoscope (65.25)

● 65.3 Unilateral oophorectomy

✖ 65.31 Laparoscopic unilateral oophorectomy

✖ 65.39 Other unilateral oophorectomy

Excludes that by laparoscope (65.31)

● 65.4 Unilateral salpingo-oophorectomy

✖ 65.41 Laparoscopic unilateral salpingo-oophorectomy

✖ 65.49 Other unilateral salpingo-oophorectomy

● 65.5 Bilateral oophorectomy

✖ 65.51 Other removal of both ovaries at same operative episode
Female castration

Excludes that by laparoscope (65.53)

✖ 65.52 Other removal of remaining ovary
Removal of solitary ovary

Excludes that by laparoscope (65.54)

✖ 65.53 Laparoscopic removal of both ovaries at same operative episode

✖ 65.54 Laparoscopic removal of remaining ovary

● 65.6 Bilateral salpingo-oophorectomy

✖ 65.61 Other removal of both ovaries and tubes at same operative episode

Excludes that by laparoscope (65.63)

✖ 65.62 Other removal of remaining ovary and tube
Removal of solitary ovary and tube

Excludes that by laparoscope (65.64)

✖ 65.63 Laparoscopic removal of both ovaries and tubes at same operative episode

✖ 65.64 Laparoscopic removal of remaining ovary and tube

● 65.7 Repair of ovary

Excludes salpingo-oophorostomy (66.72)

✖ 65.71 Other simple suture of ovary

Excludes that by laparoscope (65.74)

✖ 65.72 Other reimplantation of ovary

Excludes that by laparoscope (65.75)

✖ 65.73 Other salpingo-oophoroplasty

Excludes that by laparoscope (65.76)

✖ 65.74 Laparoscopic simple suture of ovary

✖ 65.75 Laparoscopic reimplantation of ovary

✖ 65.76 Laparoscopic salpingo-oophoroplasty

✖ 65.79 Other repair of ovary
Oophoropexy

● 65.8 Lysis of adhesions of ovary and fallopian tube

✖ 65.81 Laparoscopic lysis of adhesions of ovary and fallopian tube

✖ 65.89 Other lysis of adhesions of ovary and fallopian tube

Excludes that by laparoscope (65.81)

● 65.9 Other operations on ovary

✖ 65.91 Aspiration of ovary

Excludes aspiration biopsy of ovary (65.11)

✖ 65.92 Transplantation of ovary

Excludes reimplantation of ovary
laparoscopic (65.75))
other (65.72)

✖ 65.93 Manual rupture of ovarian cyst

✖ 65.94 Ovarian denervation

✖ 65.95 Release of torsion of ovary

✖ 65.99 Other
Ovarian drilling ◄

● 66 Operations on fallopian tubes

Code also any application or administration of an adhesion barrier substance (99.77)

● 66.0 Salpingotomy and salpingostomy

✖ 66.01 Salpingotomy

✖ 66.02 Salpingostomy

● 66.1 Diagnostic procedures on fallopian tubes

✖ 66.11 Biopsy of fallopian tube

✖ 66.19 Other diagnostic procedures on fallopian tubes

Excludes microscopic examination of specimen from fallopian tubes (91.41–91.49)
radiography of fallopian tubes (87.82–87.83, 87.85)
Rubin's test (66.8)

● **66.2 Bilateral endoscopic destruction or occlusion of fallopian tubes**

> **Includes:** bilateral endoscopic destruction or occlusion of fallopian tubes by:
> culdoscopy
> endoscopy
> hysteroscopy
> laparoscopy
> peritoneoscopy
> endoscopic destruction of solitary fallopian tube

✖ **66.21 Bilateral endoscopic ligation and crushing of fallopian tubes**

✖ **66.22 Bilateral endoscopic ligation and division of fallopian tubes**

✖ **66.29 Other bilateral endoscopic destruction or occlusion of fallopian tubes**

● **66.3 Other bilateral destruction or occlusion of fallopian tubes**

> **Includes:** destruction of solitary fallopian tube
> **Excludes** *endoscopic destruction or occlusion of fallopian tubes (66.21–66.29)*

✖ **66.31 Other bilateral ligation and crushing of fallopian tubes**

✖ **66.32 Other bilateral ligation and division of fallopian tubes**
> Pomeroy operation

✖ **66.39 Other bilateral destruction or occlusion of fallopian tubes**
> Female sterilization operation NOS

✖ **66.4 Total unilateral salpingectomy**

● **66.5 Total bilateral salpingectomy**

> **Excludes** *bilateral partial salpingectomy for sterilization (66.39)*
> *that with oophorectomy (65.61–65.64)*

✖ **66.51 Removal of both fallopian tubes at same operative episode**

✖ **66.52 Removal of remaining fallopian tube**
> Removal of solitary fallopian tube

● **66.6 Other salpingectomy**

> **Includes:** salpingectomy by:
> cauterization
> coagulation
> electrocoagulation
> excision
> **Excludes** *fistulectomy (66.73)*

✖ **66.61 Excision or destruction of lesion of fallopian tube**
> **Excludes** *biopsy of fallopian tube (66.11)*

✖ **66.62 Salpingectomy with removal of tubal pregnancy**
> Code also any synchronous oophorectomy (65.31, 65.39)

✖ **66.63 Bilateral partial salpingectomy, not otherwise specified**

✖ **66.69 Other partial salpingectomy**

● **66.7 Repair of fallopian tube**

✖ **66.71 Simple suture of fallopian tube**

✖ **66.72 Salpingo-oophorostomy**

✖ **66.73 Salpingo-salpingostomy**

✖ **66.74 Salpingo-uterostomy**

✖ **66.79 Other repair of fallopian tube**
> Graft of fallopian tube
> Reopening of divided fallopian tube
> Salpingoplasty

● **66.8 Insufflation of fallopian tube**

> Insufflation of fallopian tube with:
> air
> dye
> gas
> saline
> Rubin's test
> **Excludes** *insufflation of therapeutic agent (66.95)*
> *that for hysterosalpingography (87.82–87.83)*

● **66.9 Other operations on fallopian tubes**

66.91 Aspiration of fallopian tube

✖ **66.92 Unilateral destruction or occlusion of fallopian tube**
> **Excludes** *that of solitary tube (66.21–66.39)*

✖ **66.93 Implantation or replacement of prosthesis of fallopian tube**

✖ **66.94 Removal of prosthesis of fallopian tube**

✖ **66.95 Insufflation of therapeutic agent into fallopian tubes**

✖ **66.96 Dilation of fallopian tube**

✖ **66.97 Burying of fimbriae in uterine wall**

✖ **66.99 Other**
> **Excludes** *lysis of adhesions of ovary and tube*
> *laparoscopic (65.81)*
> *other (65.89)*

● **67 Operations on cervix**

Code also any application or administration of an adhesion barrier substance (99.77)

67.0 Dilation of cervical canal
> **Excludes** *dilation and curettage (69.01–69.09)*
> *that for induction of labor (73.1)*

● **67.1 Diagnostic procedures on cervix**

✖ **67.11 Endocervical biopsy**
> **Excludes** *conization of cervix (67.2)*

✖ **67.12 Other cervical biopsy**
> Punch biopsy of cervix NOS
> **Excludes** *conization of cervix (67.2)*

✖ **67.19 Other diagnostic procedures on cervix**
> **Excludes** *microscopic examination of specimen from cervix (91.41–91.49)*

✖ **67.2 Conization of cervix**
> **Excludes** *that by:*
> *cryosurgery (67.33)*
> *electrosurgery (67.32)*

● **67.3 Other excision or destruction of lesion or tissue of cervix**

✖ **67.31 Marsupialization of cervical cyst**

✖ **67.32 Destruction of lesion of cervix by cauterization**
> Electroconization of cervix
> LEEP (loop electrosurgical excision procedure)
> LLETZ (large loop excision of the transformation zone)

✖ **67.33 Destruction of lesion of cervix by cryosurgery**
> Cryoconization of cervix

✖ **67.39 Other excision or destruction of lesion or tissue of cervix**
> **Excludes** *biopsy of cervix (67.11–67.12)*
> *cervical fistulectomy (67.62)*
> *conization of cervix (67.2)*

✖ **67.4 Amputation of cervix**
> Cervicectomy with synchronous colporrhaphy

● **67.5 Repair of internal cervical os**

✖ **67.51 Transabdominal cerclage of cervix**

✖ **67.59 Other repair of internal cervical os**
Cerclage of isthmus uteri
McDonald operation
Shirodkar operation
Transvaginal cerclage

Excludes *transabdominal cerclage of cervix (67.51)*
laparoscopically assisted supracervical hysterec-
tomy [LASH] (68.31)

● **67.6 Other repair of cervix**

Excludes *repair of current obstetric laceration (75.51)*

✖ **67.61 Suture of laceration of cervix**

✖ **67.62 Repair of fistula of cervix**
Cervicosigmoidal fistulectomy

Excludes *fistulectomy:*
cervicovesical (57.84)
ureterocervical (56.84)
vesicocervicovaginal (57.84)

✖ **67.69 Other repair of cervix**
Repair of old obstetric laceration of cervix

● **68 Other incision and excision of uterus**

Code also any application or administration of an adhesion barrier substance (99.77)

✖ **68.0 Hysterotomy**
Hysterotomy with removal of hydatidiform mole

Excludes *hysterotomy for termination of pregnancy (74.91)*

● **68.1 Diagnostic procedures on uterus and supporting**
structures

68.11 Digital examination of uterus

Excludes *pelvic examination, so described (89.26)*
postpartal manual exploration of uterine cavity
(75.7)

68.12 Hysteroscopy

Excludes *that with biopsy (68.16)*

✖ **68.13 Open biopsy of uterus**

Excludes *closed biopsy of uterus(68.16)*

✖ **68.14 Open biopsy of uterine ligaments**

Excludes *closed biopsy of uterine ligaments (68.15)*

✖ **68.15 Closed biopsy of uterine ligaments**
Endoscopic (laparoscopy) biopsy of uterine
adnexa, except ovary and fallopian tube

✖ **68.16 Closed biopsy of uterus**
Endoscopic (laparoscopy) (hysteroscopy) biopsy of uterus

Excludes *open biopsy of uterus (68.13)*

✖ **68.19 Other diagnostic procedures on uterus and**
supporting structures

Excludes *diagnostic:*
aspiration curettage (69.59)
dilation and curettage (69.09)
microscopic examination of specimen from uterus
(91.41–91.49)
pelvic examination (89.26)
radioisotope scan of:
placenta (92.17)
uterus (92.19)
ultrasonography of uterus (88.78–88.79)
x-ray of uterus (87.81–87.89)

● **68.2 Excision or destruction of lesion or tissue of uterus**

✖ **68.21 Division of endometrial synechiae**
Lysis of intraluminal uterine adhesions

✖ **68.22 Incision or excision of congenital septum of**
uterus

✖ **68.23 Endometrial ablation**
Dilation and curettage
Hysteroscopic endometrial ablation

✖ **68.29 Other excision or destruction of lesion of**
uterus
Uterine myomectomy

Excludes *biopsy of uterus (68.13)*
uterine fistulectomy (69.42)

● **68.3 Subtotal abdominal hysterectomy**

✖ **68.31 Laparoscopic supracervical hysterectomy**
[LSH]
Classic infrafascial SEMM hysterectomy
[CISH]
Laparoscopically assisted supracervical hys-
terectomy [LASH]

✖ **68.39 Other subtotal abdominal hysterectomy,**
NOS
Supracervical hysterectomy

Excludes *classic infrafascial SEMM hysterectomy [CISH]*
(68.31)
laparoscopic supracervical hysterectomy [LSH]
(68.31)

✖ **68.4 Total abdominal hysterectomy**
Hysterectomy:
extended

Code also any synchronous removal of tubes and
ovaries (65.3–65.6)

● **68.5 Vaginal hysterectomy**

Code also any synchronous:
removal of tubes and ovaries (65.31–65.64)
repair of cystocele or rectocele (70.50–70.52)
repair of pelvic floor (70.79)

✖ **68.51 Laparoscopically assisted vaginal hysterec-**
tomy (LAVH)

✖ **68.59 Other vaginal hysterectomy**

Excludes *laparoscopically assisted vaginal hysterectomy*
(LAVH) (68.51)
radical vaginal hysterectomy (68.7)

✖ **68.6 Radical abdominal hysterectomy**
Modified radical hysterectomy
Wertheim's operation

Code also any synchronous:
lymph gland dissection (40.3, 40.5)
removal of tubes and ovaries (65.61–65.64)

Excludes *pelvic evisceration (68.8)*

✖ **68.7 Radical vaginal hysterectomy**
Schauta operation

Code also any synchronous:
lymph gland dissection (40.3, 40.5)
removal of tubes and ovaries (65.61–65.64)

✖ **68.8 Pelvic evisceration**
Removal of ovaries, tubes, uterus, vagina, bladder,
and urethra (with removal of sigmoid colon
and rectum)

Code also any synchronous:
colostomy (46.12–46.13)
lymph gland dissection (40.3, 40.5)
urinary diversion (56.51–56.79)

✖ **68.9 Other and unspecified hysterectomy**
Hysterectomy NOS

Excludes *abdominal hysterectomy, any approach (68.31–*
68.39, 68.4, 68.6)
vaginal hysterectomy, any approach (68.51,
68.59, 68.7)

● 69 Other operations on uterus and supporting structures

Code also any application or administration of an adhesion barrier substance (99.77)

● 69.0 Dilation and curettage of uterus

> **Excludes** *aspiration curettage of uterus (69.51–69.59)*

✖ 69.01 Dilation and curettage for termination of pregnancy

✖ 69.02 Dilation and curettage following delivery or abortion

✖ 69.09 Other dilation and curettage
Diagnostic D and C

● 69.1 Excision or destruction of lesion or tissue of uterus and supporting structures

✖ 69.19 Other excision or destruction of uterus and supporting structures

> **Excludes** *biopsy of uterine ligament (68.14)*

● 69.2 Repair of uterine supporting structures

✖ 69.21 Interposition operation
Watkins procedure

✖ 69.22 Other uterine suspension
Hysteropexy
Manchester operation
Plication of uterine ligament

✖ 69.23 Vaginal repair of chronic inversion of uterus

✖ 69.29 Other repair of uterus and supporting structures

✖ 69.3 Paracervical uterine denervation

● 69.4 Uterine repair

> **Excludes** *repair of current obstetric laceration (75.50–75.52)*

✖ 69.41 Suture of laceration of uterus

✖ 69.42 Closure of fistula of uterus

> **Excludes** *uterovesical fistulectomy (57.84)*

✖ 69.49 Other repair of uterus
Repair of old obstetric laceration of uterus

● 69.5 Aspiration curettage of uterus

> **Excludes** *menstrual extraction (69.6)*

✖ 69.51 Aspiration curettage of uterus for termination of pregnancy
Therapeutic abortion NOS

✖ 69.52 Aspiration curettage following delivery or abortion

69.59 Other aspiration curettage of uterus

69.6 Menstrual extraction or regulation

69.7 Insertion of intrauterine contraceptive device

● 69.9 Other operations on uterus, cervix, and supporting structures

> **Excludes** *obstetric dilation or incision of cervix (73.1, 73.93)*

69.91 Insertion of therapeutic device into uterus

> **Excludes** *insertion of:*
> *intrauterine contraceptive device (69.7)*
> *laminaria (69.93)*
> *obstetric insertion of bag, bougie, or pack (73.1)*

69.92 Artificial insemination

69.93 Insertion of laminaria

69.94 Manual replacement of inverted uterus

> **Excludes** *that in immediate postpartal period (75.94)*

✖ 69.95 Incision of cervix

> **Excludes** *that to assist delivery (73.93)*

69.96 Removal of cerclage material from cervix

✖ 69.97 Removal of other penetrating foreign body from cervix

> **Excludes** *removal of intraluminal foreign body from cervix (98.16)*

✖ 69.98 Other operations on supporting structures of uterus

> **Excludes** *biopsy of uterine ligament (68.14)*

✖ 69.99 Other operations on cervix and uterus

> **Excludes** *removal of:*
> *foreign body (98.16)*
> *intrauterine contraceptive device (97.71)*
> *obstetric bag, bougie, or pack (97.72)*
> *packing (97.72)*

● 70 Operations on vagina and cul-de-sac

Code also any application or administration of an adhesion barrier substance (99.77)

70.0 Culdocentesis

● 70.1 Incision of vagina and cul-de-sac

70.11 Hymenotomy

✖ 70.12 Culdotomy

✖ 70.13 Lysis of intraluminal adhesions of vagina

✖ 70.14 Other vaginotomy
Division of vaginal septum
Drainage of hematoma of vaginal cuff

● 70.2 Diagnostic procedures on vagina and cul-de-sac

70.21 Vaginoscopy

70.22 Culdoscopy

✖ 70.23 Biopsy of cul-de-sac

✖ 70.24 Vaginal biopsy

✖ 70.29 Other diagnostic procedures on vagina and cul-de-sac

● 70.3 Local excision or destruction of vagina and cul-de-sac

✖ 70.31 Hymenectomy

✖ 70.32 Excision or destruction of lesion of cul-de-sac
Endometrectomy of cul-de-sac

> **Excludes** *biopsy of cul-de-sac (70.23)*

✖ 70.33 Excision or destruction of lesion of vagina

> **Excludes** *biopsy of vagina (70.24)*
> *vaginal fistulectomy (70.72–70.75)*

✖ 70.4 Obliteration and total excision of vagina
Vaginectomy

> **Excludes** *obliteration of vaginal vault (70.8)*

● 70.5 Repair of cystocele and rectocele

✖ 70.50 Repair of cystocele and rectocele

✖ 70.51 Repair of cystocele
Anterior colporrhaphy (with urethrocele repair)

✖ 70.52 Repair of rectocele
Posterior colporrhaphy

● 70.6 Vaginal construction and reconstruction

✖ 70.61 Vaginal construction

✖ 70.62 Vaginal reconstruction

- **70.7 Other repair of vagina**

  Excludes *lysis of intraluminal adhesions (70.13)*
  repair of current obstetric laceration (75.69)
  that associated with cervical amputation (67.4)

  - ✖ **70.71 Suture of laceration of vagina**

  - ✖ **70.72 Repair of colovaginal fistula**

  - ✖ **70.73 Repair of rectovaginal fistula**

  - ✖ **70.74 Repair of other vaginoenteric fistula**

  - ✖ **70.75 Repair of other fistula of vagina**

    Excludes *repair of fistula:*
    rectovesicovaginal (57.83)
    ureterovaginal (56.84)
    urethrovaginal (58.43)
    uterovaginal (69.42)
    vesicocervicovaginal (57.84)
    vesicosigmoidovaginal (57.83)
    vesicoureterovaginal (56.84)
    vesicovaginal (57.84)

  - ✖ **70.76 Hymenorrhaphy**

  - ✖ **70.77 Vaginal suspension and fixation**

  - ✖ **70.79 Other repair of vagina**
    Colpoperineoplasty
    Repair of old obstetric laceration of vagina

- ✖ **70.8 Obliteration of vaginal vault**
  LeFort operation

- **70.9 Other operations on vagina and cul-de-sac**

  - ✖ **70.91 Other operations on vagina**

    Excludes *insertion of:*
    diaphragm (96.17)
    mold (96.15)
    pack (96.14)
    pessary (96.18)
    suppository (96.49)
    removal of:
    diaphragm (97.73)
    foreign body (98.17)
    pack (97.75)
    pessary (97.74)
    replacement of:
    diaphragm (97.24)
    pack (97.26)
    pessary (97.25)
    vaginal dilation (96.16)
    vaginal douche (96.44)

  - ✖ **70.92 Other operations on cul-de-sac**
    Obliteration of cul-de-sac
    Repair of vaginal enterocele

- ● **71 Operations on vulva and perineum**

  Code also any application or administration of an adhesion
  barrier substance (99.77)

  - **71.0 Incision of vulva and perineum**

    - ✖ **71.01 Lysis of vulvar adhesions**

    - ✖ **71.09 Other incision of vulva and perineum**
      Enlargement of introitus NOS

      Excludes *removal of foreign body without incision (98.23)*

- **71.1 Diagnostic procedures on vulva**

  - ✖ **71.11 Biopsy of vulva**

  - ✖ **71.19 Other diagnostic procedures on vulva**

- **71.2 Operations on Bartholin's gland**

  - **71.21 Percutaneous aspiration of Bartholin's gland (cyst)**

  - ✖ **71.22 Incision of Bartholin's gland (cyst)**

  - ✖ **71.23 Marsupialization of Bartholin's gland (cyst)**

  - ✖ **71.24 Excision or other destruction of Bartholin's gland (cyst)**

  - ✖ **71.29 Other operations on Bartholin's gland**

- ✖ **71.3 Other local excision or destruction of vulva and perineum**
  Division of Skene's gland

  Excludes *biopsy of vulva (71.11)*
  vulvar fistulectomy (71.72)

- ✖ **71.4 Operations on clitoris**
  Amputation of clitoris
  Clitoridotomy
  Female circumcision

- ✖ **71.5 Radical vulvectomy**

  Code also any synchronous lymph gland dissection
  (40.3, 40.5)

- **71.6 Other vulvectomy**

  - ✖ **71.61 Unilateral vulvectomy**

  - ✖ **71.62 Bilateral vulvectomy**
    Vulvectomy NOS

- **71.7 Repair of vulva and perineum**

  Excludes *repair of current obstetric laceration (75.69)*

  - ✖ **71.71 Suture of laceration of vulva or perineum**

  - ✖ **71.72 Repair of fistula of vulva or perineum**

    Excludes *repair of fistula:*
    urethroperineal (58.43)
    urethroperineovesical (57.84)
    vaginoperineal (70.75)

  - ✖ **71.79 Other repair of vulva and perineum**
    Repair of old obstetric laceration of vulva or
    perineum

- ✖ **71.8 Other operations on vulva**

  Excludes *removal of:*
  foreign body without incision (98.23)
  packing (97.75)
  replacement of packing (97.26)

- ✖ **71.9 Other operations on female genital organs**

13. OBSTETRICAL PROCEDURES (72–75)

- **72 Forceps, vacuum, and breech delivery**

  72.0 Low forceps operation
  Outlet forceps operation

  72.1 Low forceps operation with episiotomy
  Outlet forceps operation with episiotomy

  - **72.2 Mid forceps operation**

    72.21 Mid forceps operation with episiotomy

    72.29 Other mid forceps operation

  - **72.3 High forceps operation**

    72.31 High forceps operation with episiotomy

    72.39 Other high forceps operation

  72.4 Forceps rotation of fetal head
  De Lee maneuver
  Key-in-lock rotation
  Kielland rotation
  Scanzoni's maneuver

  Code also any associated forceps extraction (72.0–72.39)

  - **72.5 Breech extraction**

    72.51 Partial breech extraction with forceps to after-coming head

    72.52 Other partial breech extraction

    72.53 Total breech extraction with forceps to after-coming head

    72.54 Other total breech extraction

  72.6 Forceps application to aftercoming head
  Piper forceps operation

  | Excludes | partial breech extraction with forceps to after-coming head (72.51)
  total breech extraction with forceps to aftercoming head (72.53)

  - **72.7 Vacuum extraction**

    Includes: Malström's extraction

    72.71 Vacuum extraction with episiotomy

    72.79 Other vacuum extraction

  72.8 Other specified instrumental delivery

  72.9 Unspecified instrumental delivery

- **73 Other procedures inducing or assisting delivery**

  - **73.0 Artificial rupture of membranes**

    73.01 Induction of labor by artificial rupture of membranes
    Surgical induction NOS

    | Excludes | artificial rupture of membranes after onset of labor (73.09)

    73.09 Other artificial rupture of membranes
    Artificial rupture of membranes at time of delivery

  73.1 Other surgical induction of labor
  Induction by cervical dilation

  | Excludes | injection for abortion (75.0)
  insertion of suppository for abortion (96.49)

  - **73.2 Internal and combined version and extraction**

    73.21 Internal and combined version without extraction
    Version NOS

    73.22 Internal and combined version with extraction

  73.3 Failed forceps
  Application of forceps without delivery
  Trial forceps

  73.4 Medical induction of labor

  | Excludes | medication to augment active labor— omit code

  - **73.5 Manually assisted delivery**

    73.51 Manual rotation of fetal head

    73.59 Other manually assisted delivery
    Assisted spontaneous delivery
    Credé maneuver

  73.6 Episiotomy
  Episioproctotomy
  Episiotomy with subsequent episiorrhaphy

  | Excludes | that with:
  high forceps (72.31)
  low forceps (72.1)
  mid forceps (72.21)
  outlet forceps (72.1)
  vacuum extraction (72.71)

  73.8 Operations on fetus to facilitate delivery
  Clavicotomy on fetus
  Destruction of fetus
  Needling of hydrocephalic head

  - **73.9 Other operations assisting delivery**

    73.91 External version

    73.92 Replacement of prolapsed umbilical cord

    73.93 Incision of cervix to assist delivery
    Dührssen's incisions

    ✖ **73.94 Pubiotomy to assist delivery**
    Obstetric symphysiotomy

    ✖ **73.99 Other**

    | Excludes | dilation of cervix, obstetrical to induce labor (73.1)
    insertion of bag or bougie to induce labor (73.1)
    removal of cerclage material (69.96)

- **74 Cesarean section and removal of fetus**

  Code also any synchronous:
  hysterectomy (68.3–68.4, 68.6, 68.8)
  myomectomy (68.29)
  sterilization (66.31–66.39, 66.63)

  ✖ **74.0 Classical cesarean section**
  Transperitoneal classical cesarean section

  ✖ **74.1 Low cervical cesarean section**
  Lower uterine segment cesarean section

  ✖ **74.2 Extraperitoneal cesarean section**
  Supravesical cesarean section

  ✖ **74.3 Removal of extratubal ectopic pregnancy**
  Removal of:
  ectopic abdominal pregnancy
  fetus from peritoneal or extraperitoneal cavity following uterine or tubal rupture

  | Excludes | that by salpingostomy (66.02)
  that by salpingotomy (66.01)
  that with synchronous salpingectomy (66.62)

  ✖ **74.4 Cesarean section of other specified type**
  Peritoneal exclusion cesarean section
  Transperitoneal cesarean section NOS
  Vaginal cesarean section

  - **74.9 Cesarean section of unspecified type**

    ✖ **74.91 Hysterotomy to terminate pregnancy**
    Therapeutic abortion by hysterotomy

    ✖ **74.99 Other cesarean section of unspecified type**
    Cesarean section NOS
    Obstetrical abdominouterotomy
    Obstetrical hysterotomy

● 75 Other obstetric operations

75.0 Intra-amniotic injection for abortion
Injection of:
prostaglandin for induction of abortion
saline for induction of abortion
Termination of pregnancy by intrauterine injection

Excludes insertion of prostaglandin suppository for abortion (96.49)

75.1 Diagnostic amniocentesis

75.2 Intrauterine transfusion
Exchange transfusion in utero
Insertion of catheter into abdomen of fetus for transfusion

Code also any hysterotomy approach (68.0)

● 75.3 Other intrauterine operations on fetus and amnion
Code also any hysterotomy approach (68.0)

75.31 Amnioscopy
Fetoscopy
Laparoamnioscopy

75.32 Fetal EKG (scalp)

75.33 Fetal blood sampling and biopsy

75.34 Other fetal monitoring
Antepartum fetal nonstress test   ◀

Includes: Fetal monitoring, not otherwise specified

Excludes fetal pulse oximetry (75.38)

75.35 Other diagnostic procedures on fetus and amnion
Intrauterine pressure determination

Excludes amniocentesis (75.1)
diagnostic procedures on gravid uterus and placenta (87.81, 88.46, 88.78, 92.17)

�excludes 75.36 Correction of fetal defect

75.37 Amnioinfusion
Code also injection of antibiotic (99.21)

75.38 Fetal pulse oximetry
Transcervical fetal oxygen saturation monitoring
Transcervical fetal SpO₂ monitoring

75.4 Manual removal of retained placenta

Excludes aspiration curettage (69.52)
dilation and curettage (69.02)

● 75.5 Repair of current obstetric laceration of uterus

✖ 75.50 Repair of current obstetric laceration of uterus, not otherwise specified

✖ 75.51 Repair of current obstetric laceration of cervix

✖ 75.52 Repair of current obstetric laceration of corpus uteri

● 75.6 Repair of other current obstetric laceration

✖ 75.61 Repair of current obstetric laceration of bladder and urethra

75.62 Repair of current obstetric laceration of rectum and sphincter ani

75.69 Repair of other current obstetric laceration
Episioperineorrhaphy
Repair of:
pelvic floor
perineum
vagina
vulva
Secondary repair of episiotomy

Excludes repair of routine episiotomy (73.6)

75.7 Manual exploration of uterine cavity, postpartum

75.8 Obstetric tamponade of uterus or vagina

Excludes antepartum tamponade (73.1)

● 75.9 Other obstetric operations

75.91 Evacuation of obstetric incisional hematoma of perineum
Evacuation of hematoma of:
episiotomy
perineorrhaphy

75.92 Evacuation of other hematoma of vulva or vagina

✖ 75.93 Surgical correction of inverted uterus
Spinelli operation

Excludes vaginal repair of chronic inversion of uterus (69.23)

75.94 Manual replacement of inverted uterus

✖ 75.99 Other

14. OPERATIONS ON THE MUSCULOSKELETAL SYSTEM (76–84)

● **76 Operations on facial bones and joints**

> **Excludes** *accessory sinuses (22.00–22.9)*
> *nasal bones (21.00–21.99)*
> *skull (01.01–02.99)*

● **76.0 Incision of facial bone without division**

✖ **76.01 Sequestrectomy of facial bone**
Removal of necrotic bone chip from facial bone

✖ **76.09 Other incision of facial bone**
Reopening of osteotomy site of facial bone

> **Excludes** *osteotomy associated with orthognathic surgery (76.61–76.69)*
> *removal of internal fixation device (76.97)*

● **76.1 Diagnostic procedures on facial bones and joints**

✖ **76.11 Biopsy of facial bone**

✖ **76.19 Other diagnostic procedures on facial bones and joints**

> **Excludes** *contrast arthrogram of temporomandibular joint (87.13)*
> *other x-ray (87.11–87.12, 87.14–87.16)*

✖ **76.2 Local excision or destruction of lesion of facial bone**

> **Excludes** *biopsy of facial bone (76.11)*
> *excision of odontogenic lesion (24.4)*

● **76.3 Partial ostectomy of facial bone**

✖ **76.31 Partial mandibulectomy**
Hemimandibulectomy

> **Excludes** *that associated with temporomandibular arthroplasty (76.5)*

✖ **76.39 Partial ostectomy of other facial bone**
Hemimaxillectomy (with bone graft or prosthesis)

● **76.4 Excision and reconstruction of facial bones**

✖ **76.41 Total mandibulectomy with synchronous reconstruction**

✖ **76.42 Other total mandibulectomy**

✖ **76.43 Other reconstruction of mandible**

> **Excludes** *genioplasty (76.67–76.68)*
> *that with synchronous total mandibulectomy (76.41)*

✖ **76.44 Total ostectomy of other facial bone with synchronous reconstruction**

✖ **76.45 Other total ostectomy of other facial bone**

✖ **76.46 Other reconstruction of other facial bone**

> **Excludes** *that with synchronous total ostectomy (76.44)*

✖ **76.5 Temporomandibular arthroplasty**

● **76.6 Other facial bone repair and orthognathic surgery**

> Code also any synchronous:
> bone graft (76.91)
> synthetic implant (76.92)

> **Excludes** *reconstruction of facial bones (76.41–76.46)*

✖ **76.61 Closed osteoplasty [osteotomy] of mandibular ramus**
Gigli saw osteotomy

✖ **76.62 Open osteoplasty [osteotomy] of mandibular ramus**

✖ **76.63 Osteoplasty [osteotomy] of body of mandible**

✖ **76.64 Other orthognathic surgery on mandible**
Mandibular osteoplasty NOS
Segmental or subapical osteotomy

✖ **76.65 Segmental osteoplasty [osteotomy] of maxilla**
Maxillary osteoplasty NOS

✖ **76.66 Total osteoplasty [osteotomy] of maxilla**

✖ **76.67 Reduction genioplasty**
Reduction mentoplasty

✖ **76.68 Augmentation genioplasty**
Mentoplasty:
NOS
with graft or implant

✖ **76.69 Other facial bone repair**
Osteoplasty of facial bone NOS

● **76.7 Reduction of facial fracture**

> **Includes:** internal fixation
> Code also any synchronous:
> bone graft (76.91)
> synthetic implant (76.92)

> **Excludes** *that of nasal bones (21.71–21.72)*

✖ **76.70 Reduction of facial fracture, not otherwise specified**

76.71 Closed reduction of malar and zygomatic fracture

✖ **76.72 Open reduction of malar and zygomatic fracture**

76.73 Closed reduction of maxillary fracture

✖ **76.74 Open reduction of maxillary fracture**

76.75 Closed reduction of mandibular fracture

✖ **76.76 Open reduction of mandibular fracture**

✖ **76.77 Open reduction of alveolar fracture**
Reduction of alveolar fracture with stabilization of teeth

76.78 Other closed reduction of facial fracture
Closed reduction of orbital fracture

> **Excludes** *nasal bone (21.71)*

✖ **76.79 Other open reduction of facial fracture**
Open reduction of orbit rim or wall

> **Excludes** *nasal bone (21.72)*

● **76.9 Other operations on facial bones and joints**

✖ **76.91 Bone graft to facial bone**
Autogenous graft to facial bone
Bone bank graft to facial bone
Heterogenous graft to facial bone

✖ **76.92 Insertion of synthetic implant in facial bone**
Alloplastic implant to facial bone

76.93 Closed reduction of temporomandibular dislocation

✖ **76.94 Open reduction of temporomandibular dislocation**

76.95 Other manipulation of temporomandibular joint

76.96 Injection of therapeutic substance into temporomandibular joint

✖ **76.97 Removal of internal fixation device from facial bone**

> **Excludes** *removal of:*
> *dental wiring (97.33)*
> *external mandibular fixation device NEC (97.36)*

✖ **76.99 Other**

● **Use Additional Digit(s)** ✖ **Valid O.R. Procedure** ◀ **New** ◀▦ **Revised**

● **77 Incision, excision, and division of other bones**

> **Excludes** *laminectomy for decompression (03.09)*
> *operations on:*
> *accessory sinuses (22.00–22.9)*
> *ear ossicles (19.0–19.55)*
> *facial bones (76.01–76.99)*
> *joint structures (80.00–81.99)*
> *mastoid (19.9–20.99)*
> *nasal bones (21.00–21.99)*
> *skull (01.01–02.99)*

The following fourth-digit subclassification is for use with appropriate categories in section 77 to identify the site. Valid fourth-digit categories are in brackets under each code.

  0 unspecified site
  1 scapula, clavicle, and thorax [ribs and sternum]
  2 humerus
  3 radius and ulna
  4 carpals and metacarpals
  5 femur
  6 patella
  7 tibia and fibula
  8 tarsals and metatarsals
  9 other
    Pelvic bones
    Phalanges (of foot) (of hand)
    Vertebrae

✖ ● **77.0 Sequestrectomy**
  [0–9]

✖ ● **77.1 Other incision of bone without division**
  [0–9]   Reopening of osteotomy site

> **Excludes** *aspiration of bone marrow (41.31, 41.91)*
> *removal of internal fixation device (78.60–78.69)*

✖ ● **77.2 Wedge osteotomy**
  [0–9]

> **Excludes** *that for hallux valgus (77.51)*

✖ ● **77.3 Other division of bone**
  [0–9]   Osteoarthrotomy

> **Excludes** *clavicotomy of fetus (73.8)*
> *laminotomy or incision of vertebra (03.01–03.09)*
> *pubiotomy to assist delivery (73.94)*
> *sternotomy incidental to thoracic operation—omit code*

✖ ● **77.4 Biopsy of bone**
  [0–9]

● **77.5 Excision and repair of bunion and other toe deformities**

✖ **77.51 Bunionectomy with soft tissue correction and osteotomy of the first metatarsal**

✖ **77.52 Bunionectomy with soft tissue correction and arthrodesis**

✖ **77.53 Other bunionectomy with soft tissue correction**

✖ **77.54 Excision or correction of bunionette**
    That with osteotomy

✖ **77.56 Repair of hammer toe**
    Filleting of hammer toe
    Fusion of hammer toe
    Phalangectomy (partial) of hammer toe

✖ **77.57 Repair of claw toe**
    Capsulotomy of claw toe
    Fusion of claw toe
    Phalangectomy (partial) of claw toe
    Tendon lengthening of claw toe

✖ **77.58 Other excision, fusion and repair of toes**
    Cockup toe repair
    Overlapping toe repair
    That with use of prosthetic materials

✖ **77.59 Other bunionectomy**
    Resection of hallux valgus joint with insertion of prosthesis

✖ ● **77.6 Local excision of lesion or tissue of bone**
  [0–9]

> **Excludes** *biopsy of bone (77.40–77.49)*
> *debridement of compound fracture (79.60–79.69)*

✖ ● **77.7 Excision of bone for graft**
  [0–9]

✖ ● **77.8 Other partial ostectomy**
  [0–9]   Condylectomy

> **Excludes** *amputation (84.00–84.19, 84.91)*
> *arthrectomy (80.90–80.99)*
> *excision of bone ends associated with:*
> *arthrodesis (81.00–81.29)*
> *arthroplasty (81.31–81.87)*
> *excision of cartilage (80.5–80.6, 80.80–80.99)*
> *excision of head of femur with synchronous replacement (81.51–81.53)*
> *hemilaminectomy (03.01–03.09)*
> *laminectomy (03.01–03.09)*
> *ostectomy for hallux valgus (77.51–77.59)*
> *partial amputation:*
> *finger (84.01)*
> *thumb (84.02)*
> *toe (84.11)*
> *resection of ribs incidental to thoracic operation—omit code*
> *that incidental to other operation—omit code*

✖ ● **77.9 Total ostectomy**
  [0–9]

> **Excludes** *amputation of limb (84.00–84.19, 84.91)*
> *that incidental to other operation—omit code*

● **78 Other operations on bones, except facial bones**

> **Excludes** *operations on:*
> *accessory sinuses (22.00–22.9)*
> *facial bones (76.01–76.99)*
> *joint structures (80.00–81.99)*
> *nasal bones (21.00–21.99)*
> *skull (01.01–02.99)*

The following fourth-digit subclassification is for use with categories in section 78 to identify the site. Valid fourth-digit categories are in [brackets] under each code.

  0 unspecified site
  1 scapula, clavicle, and thorax [ribs and sternum]
  2 humerus
  3 radius and ulna
  4 carpals and metacarpals
  5 femur
  6 patella
  7 tibia and fibula
  8 tarsals and metatarsals
  9 other
    Pelvic bones
    Phalanges (of foot) (of hand)
    Vertebrae

✖ ● **78.0 Bone graft**
  [0–9]   Bone:
    bank graft
    graft (autogenous) (heterogenous)
    That with debridement of bone graft site (removal of sclerosed, fibrous or necrotic bone or tissue)
    Transplantation of bone

Code also any excision of bone for graft (77.70–77.79)

> **Excludes** *that for bone lengthening (78.30–78.39)*

✖ ● **78.1 Application of external fixation device**
  [0–9]   Minifixator with insertion of pins/wires/screws into
           bone

  | Excludes | *other immobilization, pressure, and attention to wound (93.51–93.59)* |

✖ ● **78.2 Limb shortening procedures**
  [0, 2–5, 7–9] Epiphyseal stapling
           Open epiphysiodesis
           Percutaneous epiphysiodesis
           Resection/osteotomy

✖ ● **78.3 Limb lengthening procedures**
  [0, 2–5, 7–9] Bone graft with or without internal fixation devices
           or osteotomy
           Distraction technique with or without corticotomy/
           osteotomy

  Code also any application of an external fixation device (78.10–78.19)

✖ ● **78.4 Other repair or plastic operations on bone**
  [0–9]   Other operation on bone NEC
           Repair of malunion or nonunion fracture NEC

Excludes	*application of external fixation device (78.10–78.19)*
	limb lengthening procedures (78.30–78.39)
	limb shortening procedures (78.20–78.29)
	osteotomy (77.3)
	reconstruction of thumb (82.61–82.69)
	repair of pectus deformity (34.74)
	repair with bone graft (78.00–78.09)

✖ ● **78.5 Internal fixation of bone without fracture reduction**
  [0–9]   Internal fixation of bone (prophylactic)
           Reinsertion of internal fixation device
           Revision of displaced or broken fixation device

Excludes	*arthroplasty and arthrodesis (81.00–81.85)*
	bone graft (78.00–78.09)
	limb shortening procedures (78.20–78.29)
	that for fracture reduction (79.10–79.19, 79.30–79.59)

✖ ● **78.6 Removal of implanted devices from bone**
  [0–9]   External fixator device (invasive)
           Internal fixation device
           Removal of bone growth stimulator (invasive)
           Removal of internal limb lengthening device   ◄

  | Excludes | *removal of cast, splint, and traction device (Kirschner wire) (Steinmann pin) (97.88)* |
  | | *removal of skull tongs or halo traction device (02.95)* |

✖ ● **78.7 Osteoclasis**
  [0–9]

✖ ● **78.8 Diagnostic procedures on bone, not elsewhere classi-
       fied**
  [0–9]

Excludes	*biopsy of bone (77.40–77.49)*
	magnetic resonance imaging (88.94)
	microscopic examination of specimen from bone (91.51–91.59)
	radioisotope scan (92.14)
	skeletal x-ray (87.21–87.29, 87.43, 88.21–88.33)
	thermography (88.83)

✖ ● **78.9 Insertion of bone growth stimulator**
  [0–9]   Insertion of:
           bone stimulator (electrical) to aid bone healing
           osteogenic electrodes for bone growth stimulation
           totally implanted device (invasive)

  | Excludes | *non-invasive (transcutaneous) (surface) stimulator (99.86)* |

● **79 Reduction of fracture and dislocation**

  Includes: application of cast or splint
           Reduction with insertion of traction device
           (Kirschner wire) (Steinmann pin)

  Code also any application of external fixation device (78.10–
  78.19)

Excludes	*external fixation alone for immobilization of fracture (93.51–93.56, 93.59)*
	internal fixation without reduction of fracture (78.50–78.59)
	operations on:
	facial bones (76.70–76.79)
	nasal bones (21.71–21.72)
	orbit (76.78–76.79)
	skull (02.02)
	vertebrae (03.53)
	removal of cast or splint (97.88)
	replacement of cast or splint (97.11–97.14)
	traction alone for reduction of fracture (93.41–93.46)

  The following fourth-digit subclassification is for use with
  appropriate categories in section 79 to identify the site. Valid
  fourth-digit categories are in [brackets] under each code.
   0 unspecified site
   1 humerus
   2 radius and ulna
        Arm NOS
   3 carpals and metacarpals
        Hand NOS
   4 phalanges of hand
   5 femur
   6 tibia and fibula
        Leg NOS
   7 tarsals and metatarsals
        Foot NOS
   8 phalanges of foot
   9 other specified bone

● **79.0 Closed reduction of fracture without internal fixation**
  | Excludes | *that for separation of epiphysis (79.40–79.49)* |

✖ ● **79.1 Closed reduction of fracture with internal fixation**
  | Excludes | *that for separation of epiphysis (79.40–79.49)* |

✖ ● **79.2 Open reduction of fracture without internal fixation**
  [0–9]
  | Excludes | *that for separation of epiphysis (79.50–79.59)* |

✖ ● **79.3 Open reduction of fracture with internal fixation**
  [0–9]
  | Excludes | *that for separation of epiphysis (79.50–79.59)* |

✖ ● **79.4 Closed reduction of separated epiphysis**
  [0–2, 5, 6, 9] Reduction with or without internal fixation

✖ ● **79.5 Open reduction of separated epiphysis**
  [0–2, 5, 6, 9] Reduction with or without internal fixation

✖ ● **79.6 Debridement of open fracture site**
  [0–9]   Debridement of compound fracture

● **79.7 Closed reduction of dislocation**

  Includes: closed reduction (with external traction de-
           vice)

  | Excludes | *closed reduction of dislocation of temporomandibular joint (76.93)* |

  **79.70 Closed reduction of dislocation of unspecified
       site**

  79.71 Closed reduction of dislocation of shoulder

  79.72 Closed reduction of dislocation of elbow

  79.73 Closed reduction of dislocation of wrist

  **79.74 Closed reduction of dislocation of hand and
       finger**

79.75　Closed reduction of dislocation of hip

79.76　Closed reduction of dislocation of knee

79.77　Closed reduction of dislocation of ankle

79.78　Closed reduction of dislocation of foot and toe

79.79　Closed reduction of dislocation of other specified sites

● 79.8　Open reduction of dislocation

Includes: open reduction (with internal and external fixation devices)

Excludes open reduction of dislocation of temporomandibular joint (76.94)

✖ 79.80　Open reduction of dislocation of unspecified site

✖ 79.81　Open reduction of dislocation of shoulder

✖ 79.82　Open reduction of dislocation of elbow

✖ 79.83　Open reduction of dislocation of wrist

✖ 79.84　Open reduction of dislocation of hand and finger

✖ 79.85　Open reduction of dislocation of hip

✖ 79.86　Open reduction of dislocation of knee

✖ 79.87　Open reduction of dislocation of ankle

✖ 79.88　Open reduction of dislocation of foot and toe

✖ 79.89　Open reduction of dislocation of other specified sites

✖ ● 79.9　Unspecified operation on bone injury
[0–9]

● 80　Incision and excision of joint structures

Includes: operations on:
　　capsule of joint
　　cartilage
　　condyle
　　ligament
　　meniscus
　　synovial membrane

Excludes cartilage of:
　　ear (18.01–18.9)
　　nose (21.00–21.99)
　　temporomandibular joint (76.01–76.99)

The following fourth-digit subclassification is for use with appropriate categories in section 80 to identify the site:
0 unspecified site
1 shoulder
2 elbow
3 wrist
4 hand and finger
5 hip
6 knee
7 ankle
8 foot and toe
9 other specified sites
　Spine

✖ ● 80.0　Arthrotomy for removal of prosthesis
Cement spacer

✖ ● 80.1　Other arthrotomy
Arthrostomy

Excludes that for:
　　arthrography (88.32)
　　arthroscopy (80.20–80.29)
　　injection of drug (81.92)
　　operative approach—omit code

✖ ● 80.2　Arthroscopy

● 80.3　Biopsy of joint structure
Aspiration biopsy

✖ ● 80.4　Division of joint capsule, ligament, or cartilage
Goldner clubfoot release
Heyman-Herndon(-Strong) correction of metatarsus varus
Release of:
　adherent or constrictive joint capsule
　joint
　ligament

Excludes symphysiotomy to assist delivery (73.94)
　　that for:
　　　carpal tunnel syndrome (04.43)
　　　tarsal tunnel syndrome (04.44)

● 80.5　Excision or destruction of intervertebral disc

✖ 80.50　Excision or destruction of intervertebral disc, unspecified
Unspecified as to excision or destruction

✖ 80.51　Excision of intervertebral disc
Diskectomy
Removal of herniated nucleus pulposus
Level:
　cervical
　thoracic
　lumbar (lumbosacral)
That by laminotomy or hemilaminectomy
That with decompression of spinal nerve root at same level
Requires additional code for any concomitant decompression of spinal nerve root at different level from excision site

Code also any concurrent spinal fusion (81.00–81.09)

Excludes intervertebral chemonucleolysis (80.52)
　laminectomy for exploration of intraspinal canal (03.09)
　laminotomy for decompression of spinal nerve root only (03.09)
　that for insertion of (non-fusion) spinal disc replacement device (84.60–84.69)　◀

80.52　Intervertebral chemonucleolysis
With aspiration of disc fragments
With diskography
Injection of proteolytic enzyme into intervertebral space (chymopapain)

Excludes injection of anesthetic substance (03.91)
　injection of other substances (03.92)

✖ 80.59　Other destruction of intervertebral disc
Destruction NEC
That by laser

✖ 80.6　Excision of semilunar cartilage of knee
Excision of meniscus of knee

✖ ● 80.7　Synovectomy
Complete or partial resection of synovial membrane

Excludes excision of Baker's cyst (83.39)

✖ ● 80.8　Other local excision or destruction of lesion of joint

✖ ● 80.9　Other excision of joint

Excludes cheilectomy of joint (77.80–77.89)
　excision of bone ends (77.80–77.89)

● **81 Repair and plastic operations on joint structures**

  ● **81.0 Spinal fusion**

      Code also the total number of vertebrae fused (81.62–81.64)

      Code also any 360 degree spinal fusion by a single incision (81.61)

      Code also any insertion of interbody spinal fusion device (84.51)

      Code also any insertion of recombinant bone morphogenetic protein (84.52)

      Includes: arthrodesis of spine with:
          bone graft
          internal fixation

      Excludes *correction of pseudarthrosis of spine (81.30–81.39)*
          refusion of spine (81.30–81.39)

    �֍ **81.00 Spinal fusion, not otherwise specified**

    ✖ **81.01 Atlas-axis spinal fusion**
        Craniocervical fusion by anterior, transoral, or posterior technique
        C1-C2 fusion by anterior, transoral, or posterior technique
        Occiput C2 fusion by anterior, transoral, or posterior technique

    ✖ **81.02 Other cervical fusion, anterior technique**
        Arthrodesis of C2 level or below:
          anterior (interbody) technique
          anterolateral technique

    ✖ **81.03 Other cervical fusion, posterior technique**
        Arthrodesis of C2 level or below:
          posterior (interbody) technique
          posterolateral technique

    ✖ **81.04 Dorsal and dorsolumbar fusion, anterior technique**
        Arthrodesis of thoracic or thoracolumbar region:
          anterior (interbody) technique
          anterolateral technique

    ✖ **81.05 Dorsal and dorsolumbar fusion, posterior technique**
        Arthrodesis of thoracic or thoracolumbar region:
          posterior (interbody) technique
          posterolateral technique

    ✖ **81.06 Lumbar and lumbosacral fusion, anterior technique**
        Arthrodesis of lumbar or lumbosacral region:
          anterior (interbody) technique
          anterolateral technique

    ✖ **81.07 Lumbar and lumbosacral fusion, lateral transverse process technique**

    ✖ **81.08 Lumbar and lumbosacral fusion, posterior technique**
        Arthrodesis of lumbar or lumbosacral region:
          posterior (interbody) technique
          posterolateral technique

  ● **81.1 Arthrodesis of foot and ankle**

      Includes: arthrodesis of foot and ankle with:
          bone graft
          external fixation device

    ✖ **81.11 Ankle fusion**
        Tibiotalar fusion

    ✖ **81.12 Triple arthrodesis**
        Talus to calcaneus and calcaneus to cuboid and navicular

    ✖ **81.13 Subtalar fusion**

    ✖ **81.14 Midtarsal fusion**

    ✖ **81.15 Tarsometatarsal fusion**

    ✖ **81.16 Metatarsophalangeal fusion**

    ✖ **81.17 Other fusion of foot**

● **81.2 Arthrodesis of other joint**

      Includes: arthrodesis with:
          bone graft
          external fixation device
          excision of bone ends and compression

    ✖ **81.20 Arthrodesis of unspecified joint**

    ✖ **81.21 Arthrodesis of hip**

    ✖ **81.22 Arthrodesis of knee**

    ✖ **81.23 Arthrodesis of shoulder**

    ✖ **81.24 Arthrodesis of elbow**

    ✖ **81.25 Carporadial fusion**

    ✖ **81.26 Metacarpocarpal fusion**

    ✖ **81.27 Metacarpophalangeal fusion**

    ✖ **81.28 Interphalangeal fusion**

    ✖ **81.29 Arthrodesis of other specified joints**

● **81.3 Refusion of spine**

      Includes: arthrodesis of spine with:
          bone graft
          internal fixation
          correction of pseudarthrosis of spine

      Code also any 360 degree spinal fusion by a single incision (81.61)

      Code also any insertion of interbody spinal fusion device (84.51)

      Code also any insertion of recombinant bone morphogenetic protein (84.52)

      Code also the total number of vertebra fused (81.62–81.64)

    ✖ **81.30 Refusion of spine, not otherwise specified**

    ✖ **81.31 Refusion of atlas-axis spine**
        Craniocervical fusion by anterior, transoral or posterior technique
        C1-C2 fusion by anterior, transoral or posterior technique
        Occiput C2 fusion by anterior, transoral or posterior technique

    ✖ **81.32 Refusion of other cervical spine, anterior technique**
        Arthrodesis of C2 level or below:
          anterior (interbody) technique
          anterolateral technique

    ✖ **81.33 Refusion of other cervical spine, posterior technique**
        Arthrodesis of C2 level or below:
          posterior (interbody) technique
          posterolateral technique

    ✖ **81.34 Refusion of dorsal and dorsolumbar spine, anterior technique**
        Arthrodesis of thoracic or thoracolumbar region:
          anterior (interbody) technique
          anterolateral technique

    ✖ **81.35 Refusion of dorsal and dorsolumbar spine, posterior technique**
        Arthrodesis of thoracic or thoracolumbar region:
          posterior (interbody) technique
          posterolateral technique

    ✖ **81.36 Refusion of lumbar and lumbosacral spine, anterior technique**
        Arthrodesis of lumbar or lumbosacral region:
          anterior (interbody) technique
          anterolateral technique

    ✖ **81.37 Refusion of lumbar and lumbosacral spine, lateral transverse process technique**

    ✖ **81.38 Refusion of lumbar and lumbosacral spine, posterior technique**
        Arthrodesis of lumbar or lumbosacral region:
          posterior (interbody) technique
          posterolateral technique

    ✖ **81.39 Refusion of spine, not elsewhere classified**

● **81.4   Other repair of joint of lower extremity**

> **Includes:** arthroplasty of lower extremity with:
> external traction or fixation
> graft of bone (chips) or cartilage
> internal fixation device

✖ **81.40   Repair of hip, not elsewhere classified**

✖ **81.42   Five-in-one repair of knee**
> Medial meniscectomy, medial collateral ligament repair, vastus medialis advancement, semitendinosus advancement, and pes anserinus transfer

✖ **81.43   Triad knee repair**
> Medial meniscectomy with repair of the anterior cruciate ligament and the medial collateral ligament
> O'Donoghue procedure

✖ **81.44   Patellar stabilization**
> Roux-Goldthwait operation for recurrent dislocation of patella

✖ **81.45   Other repair of the cruciate ligaments**

✖ **81.46   Other repair of the collateral ligaments**

✖ **81.47   Other repair of knee**

✖ **81.49   Other repair of ankle**

● **81.5   Joint replacement of lower extremity**

> **Includes:** arthroplasty of lower extremity with:
> external traction or fixation
> graft of bone (chips) or cartilage
> internal fixation device or prosthesis
> removal of cement spacer

✖ **81.51   Total hip replacement**
> Replacement of both femoral head and acetabulum by prosthesis
> Total reconstruction of hip

✖ **81.52   Partial hip replacement**
> Bipolar endoprosthesis

✖ **81.53   Revision of hip replacement**
> Partial
> Total

✖ **81.54   Total knee replacement**
> Bicompartmental
> Tricompartmental
> Unicompartmental (hemijoint)

✖ **81.55   Revision of knee replacement**
> **Excludes**   *arthrodesis of knee (81.22)*

✖ **81.56   Total ankle replacement**

✖ **81.57   Replacement of joint of foot and toe**

✖ **81.59   Revision of joint replacement of lower extremity, not elsewhere classified**

● **81.6   Other procedures on spine**
Note: Number of vertebrae
The vertebral spine consists of 25 vertebrae in the following order and number:
> Cervical: C1 (atlas), C2 (axis), C3, C4, C5, C6, C7
> Thoracic or Dorsal: T1, T2, T3, T4, T5, T6, T7, T8, T9, T10, T11. T12
> Lumbar and Sacral: L1, L2, L3, L4, L5, S1

Coders should report only one code from the series 81.62 or 81.63 or 81.64 to show the total number of vertebrae fused on the patient.

Code also the level and approach of the fusion or refusion (81.00–81.08, 81.30–81.39)

● **81.61   360 degree spinal fusion, single incision approach**
> That by a single incision but fusing or refusion both anterior and posterior spine

Code also refusion of spine (81.30–81.39)

Code also spinal fusion (81.00–81.08)

Code also the total number of vertebrae fused (81.62–81.64)

✖ **81.62   Fusion or refusion of 2–3 vertebrae**

✖ **81.63   Fusion or refusion of 4–8 vertebrae**

✖ **81.64   Fusion or refusion of 9 or more vertebrae**

✖ **81.65   Vertebroplasty** ◄
> Injection of bone void filler (cement) (polymethylmethacrylate) (PMMA) into the diseased or fractured vertebral body ◄
> **Excludes**   *kyphoplasty (81.66)* ◄

✖ **81.66   Kyphoplasty** ◄
> Insertion of an inflatable balloon, bone tamp, or other device to create a cavity for a partial restoration of height of diseased or fractured vertebral body prior to injection of bone void filler (cement) (polymethylmethacrylate) (PMMA) ◄
> **Excludes**   *vertebroplasty (81.65)* ◄

● **81.7   Arthroplasty and repair of hand, fingers and wrist**

> **Includes:** arthroplasty of hand and finger with:
> external traction or fixation
> graft of bone (chips) or cartilage
> internal fixation device or prosthesis

> **Excludes**   *operations on muscle, tendon and fascia of hand (82.01–82.99)*

✖ **81.71   Arthroplasty of metacarpophalangeal and interphalangeal joint with implant**

✖ **81.72   Arthroplasty of metacarpophalangeal and interphalangeal joint without implant**

✖ **81.73   Total wrist replacement**

✖ **81.74   Arthroplasty of carpocarpal or carpometacarpal joint with implant**

✖ **81.75   Arthroplasty of carpocarpal or carpometacarpal joint without implant**

✖ **81.79   Other repair of hand, fingers and wrist**

● **81.8   Arthroplasty and repair of shoulder and elbow**

> **Includes:** arthroplasty of upper limb NEC with:
> external traction or fixation
> graft of bone (chips) or cartilage
> internal fixation device or prosthesis

✖ **81.80   Total shoulder replacement**

✖ **81.81   Partial shoulder replacement**

✖ **81.82   Repair of recurrent dislocation of shoulder**

✖ **81.83   Other repair of shoulder**
Revision of arthroplasty of shoulder

✖ **81.84   Total elbow replacement**

✖ **81.85   Other repair of elbow**

● **81.9   Other operations on joint structures**

81.91   Arthrocentesis
Joint aspiration

Excludes   *that for:*
    arthrography (88.32)
    biopsy of joint structure (80.30–80.39)
    injection of drug (81.92)

81.92   Injection of therapeutic substance into joint or ligament

✖ **81.93   Suture of capsule or ligament of upper extremity**

Excludes   *that associated with arthroplasty (81.71–81.75, 81.80–81.81, 81.84)*

✖ **81.94   Suture of capsule or ligament of ankle and foot**

Excludes   *that associated with arthroplasty (81.56–81.59)*

✖ **81.95   Suture of capsule or ligament of other lower extremity**

Excludes   *that associated with arthroplasty (81.51–81.55, 81.59)*

✖ **81.96   Other repair of joint**

✖ **81.97   Revision of joint replacement of upper extremity**
Partial
Removal of cement spacer
Total

✖ **81.98   Other diagnostic procedures on joint structures**

Excludes   *arthroscopy (80.20–80.29)*
    biopsy of joint structure (80.30–80.39)
    microscopic examination of specimen from joint (91.51–91.59)
    thermography (88.83)
    x-ray (87.21–87.29, 88.21–88.33)

✖ **81.99   Other**

● **82   Operations on muscle, tendon, and fascia of hand**

Includes: operations on:
    aponeurosis
    synovial membrane (tendon sheath)
    tendon sheath

● **82.0   Incision of muscle, tendon, fascia, and bursa of hand**

✖ **82.01   Exploration of tendon sheath of hand**
Incision of tendon sheath of hand
Removal of rice bodies in tendon sheath of hand

Excludes   *division of tendon (82.11)*

✖ **82.02   Myotomy of hand**

Excludes   *myotomy for division (82.19)*

✖ **82.03   Bursotomy of hand**

82.04   Incision and drainage of palmar or thenar space

✖ **82.09   Other incision of soft tissue of hand**

Excludes   *incision of skin and subcutaneous tissue alone (86.01–86.09)*

● **82.1   Division of muscle, tendon, and fascia of hand**

✖ **82.11   Tenotomy of hand**
Division of tendon of hand

✖ **82.12   Fasciotomy of hand**
Division of fascia of hand

✖ **82.19   Other division of soft tissue of hand**
Division of muscle of hand

● **82.2   Excision of lesion of muscle, tendon, and fascia of hand**

✖ **82.21   Excision of lesion of tendon sheath of hand**
Ganglionectomy of tendon sheath (wrist)

✖ **82.22   Excision of lesion of muscle of hand**

✖ **82.29   Excision of other lesion of soft tissue of hand**

Excludes   *excision of lesion of skin and subcutaneous tissue (86.21–86.3)*

● **82.3   Other excision of soft tissue of hand**

Code also any skin graft (86.61–86.62, 86.73)

Excludes   *excision of skin and subcutaneous tissue (86.21–86.3)*

✖ **82.31   Bursectomy of hand**

✖ **82.32   Excision of tendon of hand for graft**

✖ **82.33   Other tenonectomy of hand**
Tenosynovectomy of hand

Excludes   *excision of lesion of:*
    tendon (82.29)
    sheath (82.21)

✖ **82.34   Excision of muscle or fascia of hand for graft**

✖ **82.35   Other fasciectomy of hand**
Release of Dupuytren's contracture

Excludes   *excision of lesion of fascia (82.29)*

✖ **82.36   Other myectomy of hand**

Excludes   *excision of lesion of muscle (82.22)*

✖ **82.39   Other excision of soft tissue of hand**

Excludes   *excision of skin (86.21–86.3)*
    excision of soft tissue lesion (82.29)

● **82.4   Suture of muscle, tendon, and fascia of hand**

✖ **82.41   Suture of tendon sheath of hand**

✖ **82.42   Delayed suture of flexor tendon of hand**

✖ **82.43   Delayed suture of other tendon of hand**

✖ **82.44   Other suture of flexor tendon of hand**

Excludes   *delayed suture of flexor tendon of hand (82.42)*

✖ **82.45   Other suture of other tendon of hand**

Excludes   *delayed suture of other tendon of hand (82.43)*

✖ **82.46   Suture of muscle or fascia of hand**

● **82.5   Transplantation of muscle and tendon of hand**

✖ **82.51   Advancement of tendon of hand**

✖ **82.52   Recession of tendon of hand**

✖ **82.53   Reattachment of tendon of hand**

✖ **82.54   Reattachment of muscle of hand**

✖ **82.55   Other change in hand muscle or tendon length**

✖ **82.56   Other hand tendon transfer or transplantation**

Excludes   *pollicization of thumb (82.61)*
    transfer of finger, except thumb (82.81)

✖ **82.57   Other hand tendon transposition**

✖ **82.58   Other hand muscle transfer or transplantation**

✖ **82.59   Other hand muscle transposition**

● **82.6   Reconstruction of thumb**

Includes: digital transfer to act as thumb

Code also any amputation for digital transfer (84.01, 84.11)

✖ **82.61   Pollicization operation carrying over nerves and blood supply**

✖ **82.69   Other reconstruction of thumb**
"Cocked-hat" procedure [skin flap and bone]
Grafts:
    bone to thumb skin (pedicle) to thumb

● **82.7 Plastic operation on hand with graft or implant**

✖ **82.71 Tendon pulley reconstruction**
Reconstruction for opponensplasty

✖ **82.72 Plastic operation on hand with graft of muscle or fascia**

✖ **82.79 Plastic operation on hand with other graft or implant**
Tendon graft to hand

● **82.8 Other plastic operations on hand**

✖ **82.81 Transfer of finger, except thumb**

<u>Excludes</u> *pollicization of thumb (82.61)*

✖ **82.82 Repair of cleft hand**

✖ **82.83 Repair of macrodactyly**

✖ **82.84 Repair of mallet finger**

✖ **82.85 Other tenodesis of hand**
Tendon fixation of hand NOS

✖ **82.86 Other tenoplasty of hand**
Myotenoplasty of hand

✖ **82.89 Other plastic operations on hand**
Plication of fascia
Repair of fascial hernia

<u>Excludes</u> *that with graft or implant (82.71–82.79)*

● **82.9 Other operations on muscle, tendon, and fascia of hand**

<u>Excludes</u> *diagnostic procedures on soft tissue of hand (83.21–83.29)*

✖ **82.91 Lysis of adhesions of hand**
Freeing of adhesions of fascia, muscle, and tendon of hand

<u>Excludes</u> *decompression of carpal tunnel (04.43)*
that by stretching or manipulation only (93.26)

82.92 Aspiration of bursa of hand

82.93 Aspiration of other soft tissue of hand

<u>Excludes</u> *skin and subcutaneous tissue (86.01)*

82.94 Injection of therapeutic substance into bursa of hand

82.95 Injection of therapeutic substance into tendon of hand

82.96 Other injection of locally-acting therapeutic substance into soft tissue of hand

<u>Excludes</u> *subcutaneous or intramuscular injection (99.11–99.29)*

✖ **82.99 Other operations on muscle, tendon, and fascia of hand**

● **83 Operations on muscle, tendon, fascia, and bursa, except hand**

Includes: operations on:
    aponeurosis
    synovial membrane of bursa and tendon sheaths
    tendon sheaths

<u>Excludes</u> *diaphragm (34.81–34.89)*
hand (82.01–82.99)
muscles of eye (15.01–15.9)

● **83.0 Incision of muscle, tendon, fascia, and bursa**

✖ **83.01 Exploration of tendon sheath**
Incision of tendon sheath
Removal of rice bodies from tendon sheath

✖ **83.02 Myotomy**

<u>Excludes</u> *cricopharyngeal myotomy (29.31)*

✖ **83.03 Bursotomy**
Removal of calcareous deposit of bursa

<u>Excludes</u> *aspiration of bursa (percutaneous) (83.94)*

✖ **83.09 Other incision of soft tissue**
Incision of fascia

<u>Excludes</u> *incision of skin and subcutaneous tissue alone (86.01–86.09)*

● **83.1 Division of muscle, tendon, and fascia**

✖ **83.11 Achillotenotomy**

✖ **83.12 Adductor tenotomy of hip**

✖ **83.13 Other tenotomy**
Aponeurotomy
Division of tendon
Tendon release
Tendon transection
Tenotomy for thoracic outlet decompression

✖ **83.14 Fasciotomy**
Division of fascia
Division of iliotibial band
Fascia stripping
Release of Volkmann's contracture by fasciotomy

✖ **83.19 Other division of soft tissue**
Division of muscle
Muscle release
Myotomy for thoracic outlet decompression
Myotomy with division
Scalenotomy
Transection of muscle

● **83.2 Diagnostic procedures on muscle, tendon, fascia, and bursa, including that of hand**

✖ **83.21 Biopsy of soft tissue**

<u>Excludes</u> *biopsy of chest wall (34.23)*
biopsy of skin and subcutaneous tissue (86.11)

✖ **83.29 Other diagnostic procedures on muscle, tendon, fascia, and bursa, including that of hand**

<u>Excludes</u> *microscopic examination of specimen (91.51–91.59)*
soft tissue x-ray (87.09, 87.38–87.39, 88.09, 88.35, 88.37)
thermography of muscle (88.84)

● **83.3 Excision of lesion of muscle, tendon, fascia, and bursa**

<u>Excludes</u> *biopsy of soft tissue (83.21)*

✖ **83.31 Excision of lesion of tendon sheath**
Excision of ganglion of tendon sheath, except of hand

✖ **83.32 Excision of lesion of muscle**
Excision of:
    heterotopic bone
    muscle scar for release of Volkmann's contracture
    myositis ossificans

✖ **83.39 Excision of lesion of other soft tissue**
Excision of Baker's cyst

<u>Excludes</u> *bursectomy (83.5)*
excision of lesion of skin and subcutaneous tissue (86.3)
synovectomy (80.70–80.79)

● 83.4 **Other excision of muscle, tendon, and fascia**

✖ 83.41 **Excision of tendon for graft**

✖ 83.42 **Other tenonectomy**
Excision of:
aponeurosis
tendon sheath
Tenosynovectomy

✖ 83.43 **Excision of muscle or fascia for graft**

✖ 83.44 **Other fasciectomy**

✖ 83.45 **Other myectomy**
Debridement of muscle NOS
Scalenectomy

✖ 83.49 **Other excision of soft tissue**

✖ 83.5 **Bursectomy**

● 83.6 **Suture of muscle, tendon, and fascia**

✖ 83.61 **Suture of tendon sheath**

✖ 83.62 **Delayed suture of tendon**

✖ 83.63 **Rotator cuff repair**

✖ 83.64 **Other suture of tendon**
Achillorrhaphy
Aponeurorrhaphy
| **Excludes** | delayed suture of tendon (83.62) |

✖ 83.65 **Other suture of muscle or fascia**
Repair of diastasis recti

● 83.7 **Reconstruction of muscle and tendon**
| **Excludes** | reconstruction of muscle and tendon associated with arthroplasty |

✖ 83.71 **Advancement of tendon**

✖ 83.72 **Recession of tendon**

✖ 83.73 **Reattachment of tendon**

✖ 83.74 **Reattachment of muscle**

✖ 83.75 **Tendon transfer or transplantation**

✖ 83.76 **Other tendon transposition**

✖ 83.77 **Muscle transfer or transplantation**
Release of Volkmann's contracture by muscle transplantation

✖ 83.79 **Other muscle transposition**

● 83.8 **Other plastic operations on muscle, tendon, and fascia**
| **Excludes** | plastic operations on muscle, tendon, and fascia associated with arthroplasty |

✖ 83.81 **Tendon graft**

✖ 83.82 **Graft of muscle or fascia**

✖ 83.83 **Tendon pulley reconstruction**

✖ 83.84 **Release of clubfoot, not elsewhere classified**
Evans operation on clubfoot

✖ 83.85 **Other change in muscle or tendon length**
Hamstring lengthening
Heel cord shortening
Plastic achillotenotomy
Tendon plication

✖ 83.86 **Quadricepsplasty**

✖ 83.87 **Other plastic operations on muscle**
Musculoplasty
Myoplasty

✖ 83.88 **Other plastic operations on tendon**
Myotenoplasty
Tendon fixation
Tenodesis
Tenoplasty

✖ 83.89 **Other plastic operations on fascia**
Fascia lengthening
Fascioplasty
Plication of fascia

● 83.9 **Other operations on muscle, tendon, fascia, and bursa**
| **Excludes** | nonoperative: manipulation (93.25–93.29) stretching (93.27–93.29) |

✖ 83.91 **Lysis of adhesions of muscle, tendon, fascia, and bursa**
| **Excludes** | that for tarsal tunnel syndrome (04.44) |

✖ 83.92 **Insertion or replacement of skeletal muscle stimulator**
Implantation, insertion, placement, or replacement of skeletal muscle:
electrodes
stimulator

✖ 83.93 **Removal of skeletal muscle stimulator**

83.94 **Aspiration of bursa**

83.95 **Aspiration of other soft tissue**
| **Excludes** | that of skin and subcutaneous tissue (86.01) |

83.96 **Injection of therapeutic substance into bursa**

83.97 **Injection of therapeutic substance into tendon**

83.98 **Injection of locally-acting therapeutic substance into other soft tissue**
| **Excludes** | subcutaneous or intramuscular injection (99.11–99.29) |

✖ 83.99 **Other operations on muscle, tendon, fascia, and bursa**
Suture of bursa

● 84 **Other procedures on musculoskeletal system**

● 84.0 **Amputation of upper limb**
| **Excludes** | revision of amputation stump (84.3) |

✖ 84.00 **Upper limb amputation, not otherwise specified**
Closed flap amputation of upper limb NOS
Kineplastic amputation of upper limb NOS
Open or guillotine amputation of upper limb NOS
Revision of current traumatic amputation of upper limb NOS

✖ 84.01 **Amputation and disarticulation of finger**
| **Excludes** | ligation of supernumerary finger (86.26) |

✖ 84.02 **Amputation and disarticulation of thumb**

✖ 84.03 **Amputation through hand**
Amputation through carpals

✖ 84.04 **Disarticulation of wrist**

✖ 84.05 **Amputation through forearm**
Forearm amputation

✖ 84.06 **Disarticulation of elbow**

✖ 84.07 **Amputation through humerus**
Upper arm amputation

✖ 84.08 **Disarticulation of shoulder**

✖ 84.09 **Interthoracoscapular amputation**
Forequarter amputation

● **Use Additional Digit(s)** ✖ **Valid O.R. Procedure** ◄ **New** ◄▬ **Revised**

● 84.1　**Amputation of lower limb**

> Excludes　*revision of amputation stump (84.3)*

✖ 84.10　**Lower limb amputation, not otherwise specified**
> Closed flap amputation of lower limb NOS
> Kineplastic amputation of lower limb NOS
> Open or guillotine amputation of lower limb NOS
> Revision of current traumatic amputation of lower limb NOS

✖ 84.11　**Amputation of toe**
> Amputation through metatarsophalangeal joint
> Disarticulation of toe
> Metatarsal head amputation
> Ray amputation of foot (disarticulation of the metatarsal head of the toe extending across the forefoot just proximal to the metatarsophalangeal crease)

> Excludes　*ligation of supernumerary toe (86.26)*

✖ 84.12　**Amputation through foot**
> Amputation of forefoot
> Amputation through middle of foot
> Chopart's amputation
> Midtarsal amputation
> Transmetatarsal amputation (amputation of the forefoot, including all the toes)

> Excludes　*ray amputation of foot (84.11)*

✖ 84.13　**Disarticulation of ankle**

✖ 84.14　**Amputation of ankle through malleoli of tibia and fibula**

✖ 84.15　**Other amputation below knee**
> Amputation of leg through tibia and fibula NOS

✖ 84.16　**Disarticulation of knee**
> Batch, Spitler, and McFaddin amputation
> Mazet amputation
> S.P. Roger's amputation

✖ 84.17　**Amputation above knee**
> Amputation of leg through femur
> Amputation of thigh
> Conversion of below-knee amputation into above-knee amputation
> Supracondylar above-knee amputation

✖ 84.18　**Disarticulation of hip**

✖ 84.19　**Abdominopelvic amputation**
> Hemipelvectomy
> Hindquarter amputation

● 84.2　**Reattachment of extremity**

✖ 84.21　**Thumb reattachment**

✖ 84.22　**Finger reattachment**

✖ 84.23　**Forearm, wrist, or hand reattachment**

✖ 84.24　**Upper arm reattachment**
> Reattachment of arm NOS

✖ 84.25　**Toe reattachment**

✖ 84.26　**Foot reattachment**

✖ 84.27　**Lower leg or ankle reattachment**
> Reattachment of leg NOS

✖ 84.28　**Thigh reattachment**

✖ 84.29　**Other reattachment**

✖ 84.3　**Revision of amputation stump**
> Reamputation of stump
> Secondary closure of stump
> Trimming of stump

> Excludes　*revision of current traumatic amputation [revision by further amputation of current injury] (84.00–84.19, 84.91)*

● 84.4　**Implantation or fitting of prosthetic limb device**

✖ 84.40　**Implantation or fitting of prosthetic limb device, not otherwise specified**

84.41　**Fitting of prosthesis of upper arm and shoulder**

84.42　**Fitting of prosthesis of lower arm and hand**

84.43　**Fitting of prosthesis of arm, not otherwise specified**

✖ 84.44　**Implantation of prosthetic device of arm**

84.45　**Fitting of prosthesis above knee**

84.46　**Fitting of prosthesis below knee**

84.47　**Fitting of prosthesis of leg, not otherwise specified**

✖ 84.48　**Implantation of prosthetic device of leg**

● 84.5　**Implantation of other musculoskeletal devices an substances**

84.51　**Insertion of interbody spinal fusion device**
> Insertion of: cages (carbon, ceramic, metal, plastic or titanium)
>   interbody fusion cage
>   synthetic cages or spacers
>   threaded bone dowels

> Code also refusion of spine (81.30–81.39)

> Code also spinal fusion (81.00–81.08)

> Excludes　*insertion of (non-fusion) spinal disc replacement device (84.60–84.69)*　◀

84.52　**Insertion of recombinant bone morphogenetic protein rhBMP**
> That via collagen sponge, coral, ceramic, and other carriers

> Code also primary procedure performed:
>   fracture repair (79.00–79.99)
>   spinal fusion (81.00–81.08)
>   spinal refusion (81.30–81.39)

84.53　**Implantation of internal limb lengthening device with kinetic distraction**　◀

> Code also limb lengthening procedure (78.30–78.39)　◀

84.54　**Implantation of other internal limb lengthening device**　◀
> Implantation of internal limb lengthening device Not Otherwise Specified (NOS)　◀

> Code also limb lengthening procedure (78.30–78.39)　◀

84.55　**Insertion of bone void filler**　◀
> Insertion of:　◀
>   acrylic cement (PMMA)　◀
>   bone void cement　◀
>   calcium based bone void filler　◀
>   polymethylmethacrylate (PMMA)　◀

> Excludes　*that with kyphoplasty (81.66)*　◀
>   *that with vertebroplasty (81.65)*　◀

84.59　**Insertion of other spinal devices**　◀

● **Use Additional Digit(s)**　　　✖ **Valid O.R. Procedure**　　　◀ **New**　　　◀▥ **Revised**

84.6   Replacement of spinal disc ◄

Includes: non-fusion arthroplasty of the spine with insertion of artificial disc prosthesis ◄

84.60   Insertion of spinal disc prosthesis, not otherwise specified ◄
Replacement of spinal disc, NOS ◄

Includes: diskectomy (discectomy) ◄

84.61   Insertion of partial spinal disc prosthesis, cervical ◄
Nuclear replacement device, cervical ◄
Partial artificial disc prosthesis (flexible), cervical ◄
Replacement of nuclear disc (nucleus pulposus), cervical ◄

Includes: diskectomy (discectomy) ◄

84.62   Insertion of total spinal disc prosthesis, cervical ◄
Replacement of cervical spinal disc, NOS ◄
Replacement of total spinal disc, cervical ◄
Total artificial disc prosthesis (flexible), cervical ◄

Includes: diskectomy (discectomy) ◄

84.63   Insertion of spinal disc prosthesis, thoracic ◄
Artificial disc prosthesis (flexible), thoracic ◄
Replacement of thoracic spinal disc, partial or total ◄

Includes: diskectomy (discectomy) ◄

84.64   Insertion of partial spinal disc prosthesis, lumbosacral ◄
Nuclear replacement device, lumbar ◄
Partial artificial disc prosthesis (flexible), lumbar ◄
Replacement of nuclear disc (nucleus pulposus), lumbar ◄

Includes: diskectomy (discectomy) ◄

84.65   Insertion of total spinal disc prosthesis, lumbosacral ◄
Replacement of lumbar spinal disc, NOS ◄
Replacement of total spinal disc, lumbar ◄
Total artificial disc prosthesis (flexible), lumbar ◄

Includes: diskectomy (discectomy) ◄

84.66   Revision or replacement of artificial spinal disc prosthesis, cervical ◄
Removal of (partial) (total) spinal disc prosthesis with synchronous insertion of new (partial) (total) spinal disc prosthesis, cervical ◄
Repair of previously inserted spinal disc prosthesis, cervical ◄

84.67   Revision or replacement of artificial spinal disc prosthesis, thoracic ◄
Removal of (partial) (total) spinal disc prosthesis with synchronous insertion of new (partial) (total) spinal disc prosthesis, thoracic
Repair of previously inserted spinal disc prosthesis, thoracic ◄

84.68   Revision or replacement of artificial spinal disc prosthesis, lumbosacral ◄
Removal of (partial) (total) spinal disc prosthesis with synchronous insertion of new (partial) (total) spinal disc prosthesis, lumbosacral
Repair of previously inserted spinal disc prosthesis, lumbosacral

☐**84.69   Revision or replacement of artificial spinal disc prosthesis, not otherwise specified** ◄
Removal of (partial) (total) spinal disc prosthesis with synchronous insertion of new (partial) (total) spinal disc prosthesis ◄
Repair of previously inserted spinal disc prosthesis ◄

● **84.9   Other operations on musculoskeletal system**
    Excludes   *nonoperative manipulation (93.25–93.29)*

✖ **84.91   Amputation, not otherwise specified**

✖ **84.92   Separation of equal conjoined twins**

✖ **84.93   Separation of unequal conjoined twins**
Separation of conjoined twins NOS

✖ **84.99   Other**

---

15. OPERATIONS ON THE INTEGUMENTARY SYSTEM (85–86)

● 85 Operations on the breast

Includes: operations on the skin and subcutaneous tissue of:
    breast female or male
    previous mastectomy site female or male
    revision of previous mastectomy site

85.0 **Mastotomy**
    Incision of breast (skin)
    Mammotomy

    Excludes | *aspiration of breast (85.91)*
    removal of implant (85.94)

● 85.1 **Diagnostic procedures on breast**

    85.11 **Closed [percutaneous] [needle] biopsy of breast**

  ✱ 85.12 **Open biopsy of breast**

    85.19 **Other diagnostic procedures on breast**

    Excludes | *mammary ductogram (87.35)*
    mammography NEC (87.37)
    manual examination (89.36)
    microscopic examination of specimen (91.61–91.69)
    thermography (88.85)
    ultrasonography (88.73)
    xerography (87.36)

● 85.2 **Excision or destruction of breast tissue**

    Excludes | *mastectomy (85.41–85.48)*
    reduction mammoplasty (85.31–85.32)

  ✱ 85.20 **Excision or destruction of breast tissue, not otherwise specified**

  ✱ 85.21 **Local excision of lesion of breast**
    Lumpectomy
    Removal of area of fibrosis from breast

    Excludes | *biopsy of breast (85.11–85.12)*

  ✱ 85.22 **Resection of quadrant of breast**

  ✱ 85.23 **Subtotal mastectomy**

    Excludes | *quadrant resection (85.22)*

  ✱ 85.24 **Excision of ectopic breast tissue**
    Excision of accessory nipple

  ✱ 85.25 **Excision of nipple**

    Excludes | *excision of accessory nipple (85.24)*

● 85.3 **Reduction mammoplasty and subcutaneous mammectomy**

  ✱ 85.31 **Unilateral reduction mammoplasty**
    Unilateral:
      amputative mammoplasty
      size reduction mammoplasty

  ✱ 85.32 **Bilateral reduction mammoplasty**
    Amputative mammoplasty
    Reduction mammoplasty (for gynecomastia)

  ✱ 85.33 **Unilateral subcutaneous mammectomy with synchronous implant**

    Excludes | *that without synchronous implant (85.34)*

  ✱ 85.34 **Other unilateral subcutaneous mammectomy**
    Removal of breast tissue with preservation of skin and nipple
    Subcutaneous mammectomy NOS

  ✱ 85.35 **Bilateral subcutaneous mammectomy with synchronous implant**

    Excludes | *that without synchronous implant (85.36)*

  ✱ 85.36 **Other bilateral subcutaneous mammectomy**

● 85.4 **Mastectomy**

  ✱ 85.41 **Unilateral simple mastectomy**
    Mastectomy:
      NOS
      complete

  ✱ 85.42 **Bilateral simple mastectomy**
    Bilateral complete mastectomy

  ✱ 85.43 **Unilateral extended simple mastectomy**
    Extended simple mastectomy NOS
    Modified radical mastectomy
    Simple mastectomy with excision of regional lymph nodes

  ✱ 85.44 **Bilateral extended simple mastectomy**

  ✱ 85.45 **Unilateral radical mastectomy**
    Excision of breast, pectoral muscles, and regional lymph nodes [axillary, clavicular, supraclavicular]
    Radical mastectomy NOS

  ✱ 85.46 **Bilateral radical mastectomy**

  ✱ 85.47 **Unilateral extended radical mastectomy**
    Excision of breast, muscles, and lymph nodes [axillary, clavicular, supraclavicular, internal mammary, and mediastinal]
    Extended radical mastectomy NOS

  ✱ 85.48 **Bilateral extended radical mastectomy**

● 85.5 **Augmentation mammoplasty**

    Excludes | *that associated with subcutaneous mammectomy (85.33, 85.35)*

  ✱ 85.50 **Augmentation mammoplasty, not otherwise specified**

    85.51 **Unilateral injection into breast for augmentation**

    85.52 **Bilateral injection into breast for augmentation**
    Injection into breast for augmentation NOS

  ✱ 85.53 **Unilateral breast implant**

  ✱ 85.54 **Bilateral breast implant**
    Breast implant NOS

✱ 85.6 **Mastopexy**

✱ 85.7 **Total reconstruction of breast**

● 85.8 **Other repair and plastic operations on breast**

    Excludes | *that for:*
    augmentation (85.50–85.54)
    reconstruction (85.7)
    reduction (85.31–85.32)

    85.81 **Suture of laceration of breast**

  ✱ 85.82 **Split-thickness graft to breast**

  ✱ 85.83 **Full-thickness graft to breast**

  ✱ 85.84 **Pedicle graft to breast**

  ✱ 85.85 **Muscle flap graft to breast**

  ✱ 85.86 **Transposition of nipple**

  ✱ 85.87 **Other repair or reconstruction of nipple**

  ✱ 85.89 **Other mammoplasty**

● 85.9 **Other operations on the breast**

    85.91 **Aspiration of breast**

    Excludes | *percutaneous biopsy of breast (85.11)*

    85.92 **Injection of therapeutic agent into breast**

    Excludes | *that for augmentation of breast (85.51–85.52)*

  ✱ 85.93 **Revision of implant of breast**

  ✱ 85.94 **Removal of implant of breast**

  ✱ 85.95 **Insertion of breast tissue expander**
    Insertion (soft tissue) of tissue expander (one or more) under muscle or platysma to develop skin flaps for donor use

---

● **Use Additional Digit(s)**   ✱ **Valid O.R. Procedure**   ◄ **New**   ◄◀▥ **Revised**   1127

✖ **85.96   Removal of breast tissue expander(s)**

✖ **85.99   Other**

● **86   Operations on skin and subcutaneous tissue**

> **Includes:**   operations on:
> hair follicles
> male perineum
> nails
> sebaceous glands
> subcutaneous fat pads
> sudoriferous glands
> superficial fossae

> | Excludes | *those on skin of:*
>   *anus (49.01–49.99)*
>   *breast (mastectomy site) (85.0–85.99)*
>   *ear (18.01–18.9)*
>   *eyebrow (08.01–08.99)*
>   *eyelid (08.01–08.99)*
>   *female perineum (71.01–71.9)*
>   *lips (27.0–27.99)*
>   *nose (21.00–21.99)*
>   *penis (64.0–64.99)*
>   *scrotum (61.0–61.99)*
>   *vulva (71.01–71.9)*

● **86.0   Incision of skin and subcutaneous tissue**

86.01   Aspiration of skin and subcutaneous tissue
Aspiration of:
    abscess of nail, skin, or subcutaneous tissue
    hematoma of nail, skin, or subcutaneous tissue
    seroma of nail, skin, or subcutaneous tissue

86.02   Injection or tattooing of skin lesion or defect
Injection of filling material
Insertion of filling material
Pigmenting of skin of filling material

86.03   Incision of pilonidal sinus or cyst

> | Excludes | *marsupialization (86.21)*

86.04   Other incision with drainage of skin and subcutaneous tissue

> | Excludes | *drainage of:*
>   *fascial compartments of face and mouth (27.0)*
>   *palmar or thenar space 82.04*
>   *pilonidal sinus or cyst 86.03*

86.05   Incision with removal of foreign body or device from skin and subcutaneous tissue ◀▥
Removal of loop recorder
Removal of neurostimulator pulse generator (single array, dual array) ◀
Removal of tissue expander(s) from skin or soft tissue other than breast tissue

> | Excludes | *removal of foreign body without incision (98.20–98.29)*

✖ **86.06   Insertion of totally implantable infusion pump**

Code also any associated catheterization

> | Excludes | *insertion of totally implantable vascular access device (86.07)*

86.07   Insertion of totally implantable vascular access device [VAD]
Totally implanted port

> | Excludes | *insertion of totally implantable infusion pump (86.06)*

86.09   Other incision of skin and subcutaneous tissue
Creation of loop recorder pocket, new site and insertion/relocation of device
Creation of pocket for implantable, patient-activated cardiac event recorder and insertion/relocation of device
Creation of thalamic stimulator pulse generator pocket, new site
Escharotomy
Exploration:
    sinus tract, skin
    superficial fossa
Relocation of subcutaneous device pocket NEC ◀
Reopening subcutaneous pocket for device revision without replacement ◀
Undercutting of hair follicle

> | Excludes | *that of:*
>   *cardiac pacemaker pocket, new site (37.79)*
>   *fascial compartments of face and mouth (27.0)*

● **86.1   Diagnostic procedures on skin and subcutaneous tissue**

86.11   Biopsy of skin and subcutaneous tissue

86.19   Other diagnostic procedures on skin and subcutaneous tissue

> | Excludes | *microscopic examination of specimen from skin and subcutaneous tissue (91.61–91.79)*

● **86.2   Excision or destruction of lesion or tissue of skin and subcutaneous tissue**

✖ **86.21   Excision of pilonidal cyst or sinus**
Marsupialization of cyst

> | Excludes | *incision of pilonidal cyst or sinus (86.03)*

✖ **86.22   Excisional debridement of wound, infection, or burn**
Removal by excision of:
    devitalized tissue
    necrosis
    slough

> | Excludes | *debridement of:*
>   *abdominal wall (wound) (54.3)*
>   *bone (77.60–77.69)*
>   *muscle (83.45)*
>   *of hand (82.36)*
>   *nail (bed) (fold) (86.27)*
>   *nonexcisional debridement of wound, infection, or burn (86.28)*
>   *open fracture site (79.60–79.69)*
>   *pedicle or flap graft (86.75)*

86.23   Removal of nail, nail bed, or nail fold

86.24   Chemosurgery of skin
Chemical peel of skin

✖ **86.25   Dermabrasion**
That with laser

> | Excludes | *dermabrasion of wound to remove embedded debris (86.28)*

86.26   Ligation of dermal appendage

> | Excludes | *excision of preauricular appendage (18.29)*

86.27   Debridement of nail, nail bed, or nail fold
Removal of:
    necrosis
    slough

> | Excludes | *removal of nail, nail bed, or nail fold (86.23)*

86.28 Nonexcisional debridement of wound, infection or burn
   Debridement NOS
   Maggot therapy
   Removal of devitalized tissue, necrosis and slough by such methods as:
      brushing
      irrigation (under pressure)
      scrubbing
      washing

86.3 Other local excision or destruction of lesion or tissue of skin and subcutaneous tissue
   Destruction of skin by:
      cauterization cryosurgery
      fulguration
      laser beam
   That with Z-plasty

   Excludes | adipectomy (86.83)
              biopsy of skin (86.11)
              wide or radical excision of skin (86.4)
              Z-plasty without excision (86.84)

�303 86.4 Radical excision of skin lesion
   Wide excision of skin lesion involving underlying or adjacent structure

   Code also any lymph node dissection (40.3–40.5)

● 86.5 Suture or other closure of skin and subcutaneous tissue

   86.51 Replantation of scalp

   86.59 Closure of skin and subcutaneous tissue of other sites
      Adhesives (surgical) (tissue)
      Staples
      Sutures

   Excludes | application of adhesive strips (butterfly)—omit code

● 86.6 Free skin graft

   Includes: excision of skin for autogenous graft

   Excludes | construction or reconstruction of:
              penis (64.43–64.44)
              trachea (31.75)
              vagina (70.61–70.62)

   �303 86.60 Free skin graft, not otherwise specified

   �303 86.61 Full-thickness skin graft to hand

   Excludes | heterograft (86.65)
              homograft (86.66)

   �303 86.62 Other skin graft to hand

   Excludes | heterograft (86.65)
              homograft (86.66)

   �303 86.63 Full-thickness skin graft to other sites

   Excludes | heterograft (86.65)
              homograft (86.66)

   86.64 Hair transplant

   Excludes | hair follicle transplant to eyebrow or eyelash (08.63)

   �303 86.65 Heterograft to skin
      Pigskin graft
      Porcine graft

   Excludes | application of dressing only (93.57)

   �303 86.66 Homograft to skin
      Graft to skin of:
         amnionic membrane from donor skin from donor

86.67 Dermal regenerative graft
   Artificial skin, NOS
   Creation of "neodermis"
   Decellularized allodermis
   Integumentary matrix implants
   Prosthetic implant of dermal layer of skin
   Regenerate dermal layer of skin

   Excludes | heterograft to skin (86.65)
              homograft to skin (86.66)

✖ 86.69 Other skin graft to other sites

   Excludes | heterograft (86.65)
              homograft (86.66)

● 86.7 Pedicle grafts or flaps

   Excludes | construction or reconstruction of:
              penis (64.43–64.44)
              trachea (31.75)
              vagina (70.61–70.62)

✖ 86.70 Pedicle or flap graft, not otherwise specified

✖ 86.71 Cutting and preparation of pedicle grafts or flaps
   Elevation of pedicle from its bed
   Flap design and raising
   Partial cutting of pedicle or tube
   Pedicle delay

   Excludes | pollicization or digital transfer (82.61, 82.81)
              revision of pedicle (86.75)

✖ 86.72 Advancement of pedicle graft

✖ 86.73 Attachment of pedicle or flap graft to hand

   Excludes | pollicization or digital transfer (82.61, 82.81)

✖ 86.74 Attachment of pedicle or flap graft to other sites
   Attachment by:
      advanced flap
      double pedicled flap
      pedicle graft
      rotating flap
      sliding flap
      tube graft

✖ 86.75 Revision of pedicle or flap graft
   Debridement of pedicle or flap graft
   Defatting of pedicle or flap graft

● 86.8 Other repair and reconstruction of skin and subcutaneous tissue

   ✖ 86.81 Repair for facial weakness

   ✖ 86.82 Facial rhytidectomy
      Face lift

   Excludes | rhytidectomy of eyelid (08.86–08.87)

   ✖ 86.83 Size reduction plastic operation
      Reduction of adipose tissue of:
         abdominal wall (pendulous)
         arms (batwing)
         buttock
         liposuction
         thighs (trochanteric lipomatosis)

   Excludes | breast (85.31–85.32)

   ✖ 86.84 Relaxation of scar or web contracture of skin
      Z-plasty of skin

   Excludes | Z-plasty with excision of lesion (86.3)

   ✖ 86.85 Correction of syndactyly

   ✖ 86.86 Onychoplasty

   ✖ 86.89 Other repair and reconstruction of skin and subcutaneous tissue

   Excludes | mentoplasty (76.67–76.68)

● 86.9 Other operations on skin and subcutaneous tissue

✖ 86.91 **Excision of skin for graft**
Excision of skin with closure of donor site

   Excludes *that with graft at same operative episode (86.60–86.69)*

86.92 **Electrolysis and other epilation of skin**

   Excludes *epilation of eyelid (08.91–08.93)*

✖ 86.93 **Insertion of tissue expander**
Insertion (subcutaneous) (soft tissue) of expander (one or more) in scalp (subgaleal space), face, neck, trunk except breast, and upper and lower extremities for development of skin flaps for donor use

   Excludes *flap graft preparation (86.71)*
tissue expander, breast (85.95)

86.94 **Insertion or replacement of single array neurostimulator pulse generator** ◄
Pulse generator (single array, single channel) for intracranial, spinal, or peripheral neurostimulator ◄

Code also any associated lead implantation (02.93, 03.93, 04.92) ◄

86.95 **Insertion or replacement of dual array neurostimulator pulse generator** ◄
Pulse generator (dual array, dual channel) for intracranial, spinal, or peripheral neurostimulator ◄

Code also any associated lead implantation (02.93, 03.93, 04.92) ◄

86.96 **Insertion or replacement of other neurostimulator pulse generator** ◄
Code also any associated lead implantation (02.93, 03.93, 04.92) ◄

   Excludes *insertion of dual array neurostimulator pulse generator (86.95)* ◄
insertion of single array neurostimulator pulse generator (86.94) ◄

   Excludes *insertion of dual array neurostimulator pulse generator (86.95)* ◄
insertion of single array neurostimulator pulse generator (86.94) ◄

86.99 **Other**

   Excludes *removal of sutures from:*
abdomen (97.83)
head and neck (97.38)
thorax (97.43)
trunk NEC (97.84)
wound catheter:
irrigation (96.58)
replacement (97.15)

16. MISCELLANEOUS DIAGNOSTIC AND THERAPEUTIC PROCEDURES (87–99)

● **87 Diagnostic Radiology**

● **87.0 Soft tissue x-ray of face, head, and neck**

Excludes | *angiography (88.40–88.68)*

87.01 Pneumoencephalogram

87.02 Other contrast radiogram of brain and skull
Pneumocisternogram
Pneumoventriculogram
Posterior fossa myelogram

87.03 Computerized axial tomography of head
C.A.T. scan of head

87.04 Other tomography of head

87.05 Contrast dacryocystogram

87.06 Contrast radiogram of nasopharynx

87.07 Contrast laryngogram

87.08 Cervical lymphangiogram

87.09 Other soft tissue x-ray of face, head, and neck
Noncontrast x-ray of:
adenoid
larynx
nasolacrimal duct
nasopharynx
salivary gland
thyroid region
uvula

Excludes | *x-ray study of eye (95.14)*

● **87.1 Other x-ray of face, head, and neck**

Excludes | *angiography (88.40–88.68)*

87.11 Full-mouth x-ray of teeth

87.12 Other dental x-ray
Orthodontic cephalogram or cephalometrics
Panorex examination of mandible
Root canal x-ray

87.13 Temporomandibular contrast arthrogram

87.14 Contrast radiogram of orbit

87.15 Contrast radiogram of sinus

87.16 Other x-ray of facial bones
X-ray of:
frontal area
mandible
maxilla
nasal sinuses
nose
orbit
supraorbital area
symphysis menti
zygomaticomaxillary complex

87.17 Other x-ray of skull
Lateral projection of skull
Sagittal projection of skull
Tangential projection of skull

● **87.2 X-ray of spine**

87.21 Contrast myelogram

87.22 Other x-ray of cervical spine

87.23 Other x-ray of thoracic spine

87.24 Other x-ray of lumbosacral spine
Sacrococcygeal x-ray

87.29 Other x-ray of spine
Spinal x-ray NOS

● **87.3 Soft tissue x-ray of thorax**

Excludes | *angiocardiography (88.50–88.58)*
angiography (88.40–88.68)

87.31 Endotracheal bronchogram

87.32 Other contrast bronchogram
Transcricoid bronchogram

87.33 Mediastinal pneumogram

87.34 Intrathoracic lymphangiogram

87.35 Contrast radiogram of mammary ducts

87.36 Xerography of breast

87.37 Other mammography

87.38 Sinogram of chest wall
Fistulogram of chest wall

87.39 Other soft tissue x-ray of chest wall

● **87.4 Other x-ray of thorax**

Excludes | *angiocardiography (88.50–88.58)*
angiography (88.40–88.68)

87.41 Computerized axial tomography of thorax
C.A.T. scan of thorax
Crystal linear scan of x-ray beam of thorax
Electronic subtraction of thorax
Photoelectric response of thorax
Tomography with use of computer, x-rays, and camera of thorax

87.42 Other tomography of thorax
Cardiac tomogram

87.43 X-ray of ribs, sternum, and clavicle
Examination for:
cervical rib
fracture

87.44 Routine chest x-ray, so described
X-ray of chest NOS

87.49 Other chest x-ray
X-ray of:
bronchus NOS
diaphragm NOS
heart NOS
lung NOS
mediastinum NOS
trachea NOS

● **87.5 Biliary tract x-ray**

87.51 Percutaneous hepatic cholangiogram

87.52 Intravenous cholangiogram

✖ **87.53 Intraoperative cholangiogram**

87.54 Other cholangiogram

87.59 Other biliary tract x-ray
Cholecystogram

● **87.6 Other x-ray of digestive system**

87.61 Barium swallow

87.62 Upper GI series

87.63 Small bowel series

87.64 Lower GI series

87.65 Other x-ray of intestine

87.66 Contrast pancreatogram

87.69 Other digestive tract x-ray

● 87.7　X-ray of urinary system

> **Excludes** *angiography of renal vessels (88.45, 88.65)*

　87.71　Computerized axial tomography of kidney
　　　　　C.A.T. scan of kidney

　87.72　Other nephrotomogram

　87.73　Intravenous pyelogram
　　　　　Diuretic infusion pyelogram

　87.74　Retrograde pyelogram

　87.75　Percutaneous pyelogram

　87.76　Retrograde cystourethrogram

　87.77　Other cystogram

　87.78　Ileal conduitogram

　87.79　Other x-ray of the urinary system
　　　　　KUB x-ray

● 87.8　X-ray of female genital organs

　87.81　X-ray of gravid uterus
　　　　　Intrauterine cephalometry by x-ray

　87.82　Gas contrast hysterosalpingogram

　87.83　Opaque dye contrast hysterosalpingogram

　87.84　Percutaneous hysterogram

　87.85　Other x-ray of fallopian tubes and uterus

　87.89　Other x-ray of female genital organs

● 87.9　X-ray of male genital organs

　87.91　Contrast seminal vesiculogram

　87.92　Other x-ray of prostate and seminal vesicles

　87.93　Contrast epididymogram

　87.94　Contrast vasogram

　87.95　Other x-ray of epididymis and vas deferens

　87.99　Other x-ray of male genital organs

● 88　Other diagnostic radiology and related techniques

● 88.0　Soft tissue x-ray of abdomen

> **Excludes** *angiography (88.40–88.68)*

　88.01　Computerized axial tomography of abdomen
　　　　　C.A.T. scan of abdomen

> **Excludes** *C.A.T. scan of kidney (87.71)*

　88.02　Other abdomen tomography

> **Excludes** *nephrotomogram (87.72)*

　88.03　Sinogram of abdominal wall
　　　　　Fistulogram of abdominal wall

　88.04　Abdominal lymphangiogram

　88.09　Other soft tissue x-ray of abdominal wall

● 88.1　Other x-ray of abdomen

　88.11　Pelvic opaque dye contrast radiography

　88.12　Pelvic gas contrast radiography
　　　　　Pelvic pneumoperitoneum

　88.13　Other peritoneal pneumogram

　88.14　Retroperitoneal fistulogram

　88.15　Retroperitoneal pneumogram

　88.16　Other retroperitoneal x-ray

　88.19　Other x-ray of abdomen
　　　　　Flat plate of abdomen

● 88.2　Skeletal x-ray of extremities and pelvis

> **Excludes** *contrast radiogram of joint (88.32)*

　88.21　Skeletal x-ray of shoulder and upper arm

　88.22　Skeletal x-ray of elbow and forearm

　88.23　Skeletal x-ray of wrist and hand

　88.24　Skeletal x-ray of upper limb, not otherwise specified

　88.25　Pelvimetry

　88.26　Other skeletal x-ray of pelvis and hip

　88.27　Skeletal x-ray of thigh, knee, and lower leg

　88.28　Skeletal x-ray of ankle and foot

　88.29　Skeletal x-ray of lower limb, not otherwise specified

● 88.3　Other x-ray

　88.31　Skeletal series
　　　　　X-ray of whole skeleton

　88.32　Contrast arthrogram

> **Excludes** *that of temporomandibular joint (87.13)*

　88.33　Other skeletal x-ray

> **Excludes** *skeletal x-ray of:*
> *extremities and pelvis 88.21–88.29)*
> *face, head, and neck (87.11–87.17)*
> *spine (87.21–87.29)*
> *thorax (87.43)*

　88.34　Lymphangiogram of upper limb

　88.35　Other soft tissue x-ray of upper limb

　88.36　Lymphangiogram of lower limb

　88.37　Other soft tissue x-ray of lower limb

> **Excludes** *femoral angiography (88.48, 88.66)*

　88.38　Other computerized axial tomography
　　　　　C.A.T. scan NOS

> **Excludes** *C.A.T. scan of:*
> *abdomen (88.01)*
> *head (87.03)*
> *kidney (87.71)*
> *thorax (87.41)*

　88.39　X-ray, other and unspecified

● 88.4　Arteriography using contrast material

Includes: angiography of arteries
　　　　arterial puncture for injection of contrast material
　　　　radiography of arteries (by fluoroscopy)
　　　　retrograde arteriography

Note: The fourth-digit subclassification identifies the site to be viewed, not the site of injection.

> **Excludes** *arteriography using:*
> *radioisotopes or radionuclides (92.01–92.19)*
> *ultrasound (88.71–88.79)*
> *fluorescein angiography of eye (95.12)*

　88.40　Arteriography using contrast material, unspecified site

　88.41　Arteriography of cerebral arteries
　　　　　Angiography of:
　　　　　　basilar artery
　　　　　　carotid (internal)
　　　　　　posterior cerebral circulation
　　　　　　vertebral artery

　88.42　Aortography
　　　　　Arteriography of aorta and aortic arch

　88.43　Arteriography of pulmonary arteries

　88.44　Arteriography of other intrathoracic vessels

> **Excludes** *angiocardiography (88.50–88.58)*
> *arteriography of coronary arteries (88.55–88.57)*

　88.45　Arteriography of renal arteries

88.46 Arteriography of placenta
Placentogram using contrast material

88.47 Arteriography of other intra-abdominal arteries

88.48 Arteriography of femoral and other lower extremity arteries

88.49 Arteriography of other specified sites

● **88.5 Angiocardiography using contrast material**

Includes: arterial puncture and insertion of arterial catheter for injection of contrast material
cineangiocardiography
selective angiocardiography

Code also synchronous cardiac catheterization (37.21–37.23)

| **Excludes** | *angiography of pulmonary vessels (88.43, 88.62)* |

88.50 Angiocardiography, not otherwise specified

88.51 Angiocardiography of venae cavae
Inferior vena cavography
Phlebography of vena cava (inferior) (superior)

88.52 Angiocardiography of right heart structures
Angiocardiography of:
pulmonary valve
right atrium
right ventricle (outflow tract)

| **Excludes** | *that combined with left heart angiocardiography (88.54)* |

88.53 Angiocardiography of left heart structures
Angiocardiography of:
aortic valve
left atrium
left ventricle (outflow tract)

| **Excludes** | *that combined with right heart angiocardiography (88.54)* |

88.54 Combined right and left heart angiocardiography

88.55 Coronary arteriography using a single catheter
Coronary arteriography by Sones technique
Direct selective coronary arteriography using a single catheter

88.56 Coronary arteriography using two catheters
Coronary arteriography by:
Judkins technique
Ricketts and Abrams technique
Direct selective coronary arteriography using two catheters

88.57 Other and unspecified coronary arteriography
Coronary arteriography NOS

88.58 Negative-contrast cardiac roentgenography
Cardiac roentgenography with injection of carbon dioxide

● **88.6 Phlebography**

Includes: angiography of veins
radiography of veins (by fluoroscopy)
retrograde phlebography
venipuncture for injection of contrast material
venography using contrast material

Note: The fourth-digit subclassification (88.60–88.67) identifies the site to be viewed, not the site of injection.

Excludes	*angiography using:*
	radioisotopes or radionuclides (92.01–92.19)
	ultrasound (88.71–88.79)
	fluorescein angiography of eye (95.12)

88.60 Phlebography using contrast material, unspecified site

88.61 Phlebography of veins of head and neck using contrast material

88.62 Phlebography of pulmonary veins using contrast material

88.63 Phlebography of other intrathoracic veins using contrast material

88.64 Phlebography of the portal venous system using contrast material
Splenoportogram (by splenic arteriography)

88.65 Phlebography of other intra-abdominal veins using contrast material

88.66 Phlebography of femoral and other lower extremity veins using contrast material

88.67 Phlebography of other specified sites using contrast material

88.68 Impedance phlebography

● **88.7 Diagnostic ultrasound**　　　　　　　　　　◀
Non-invasive ultrasound

Includes: echography
ultrasonic angiography
ultrasonography

Excludes	*intravascular imaging (adjunctive) (IVUS)* ◀
	(00.21–00.29)
	therapeutic ultrasound (00.01–00.09)

88.71 Diagnostic ultrasound of head and neck
Determination of midline shift of brain
Echoencephalography

| **Excludes** | *eye (95.13)* |

88.72 Diagnostic ultrasound of heart
Echocardiography
Transesophageal echocardiography　　　◀

Excludes	*echocardiography of heart chambers (37.28)* ◀
	intracardiac echocardiography (ICE) (37.28) ◀
	intravascular (IVUS) imaging of coronary vessels (00.24) ◀

88.73 Diagnostic ultrasound of other sites of thorax
Aortic arch ultrasonography
Breast ultrasonography
Lung ultrasonography

88.74 Diagnostic ultrasound of digestive system

88.75 Diagnostic ultrasound of urinary system

88.76 Diagnostic ultrasound of abdomen and retroperitoneum

88.77 Diagnostic ultrasound of peripheral vascular system
Deep vein thrombosis ultrasonic scanning

88.78 Diagnostic ultrasound of gravid uterus
Intrauterine cephalometry:
echo
ultrasonic
Placental localization by ultrasound

88.79 Other diagnostic ultrasound
Ultrasonography of:
multiple sites
nongravid uterus
total body

● **88.8 Thermography**

    88.81 Cerebral thermography

    88.82 Ocular thermography

    88.83 Bone thermography
         Osteoarticular thermography

    88.84 Muscle thermography

    88.85 Breast thermography

    88.86 Blood vessel thermography
         Deep vein thermography

    88.89 Thermography of other sites
         Lymph gland thermography
         Thermography NOS

● **88.9 Other diagnostic imaging**

    88.90 Diagnostic imaging, not elsewhere classified

    88.91 Magnetic resonance imaging of brain and brain stem

         | Excludes | *intraoperative magnetic resonance imaging (88.96)*
                   real-time magnetic resonance imaging (88.96)

    88.92 Magnetic resonance imaging of chest and myocardium
         For evaluation of hilar and mediastinal lymphadenopathy

    88.93 Magnetic resonance imaging of spinal canal
         Spinal cord levels:
            cervical
            thoracic
            lumbar (lumbosacral)
         Spinal cord
         Spine

    88.94 Magnetic resonance imaging of musculoskeletal
         Bone marrow blood supply
         Extremities (upper) (lower)

    88.95 Magnetic resonance imaging of pelvis, prostate, and bladder

    88.96 Other intraoperative magnetic resonance imaging
         iMRI
         Real-time magnetic resonance imaging

    88.97 Magnetic resonance imaging of other and unspecified sites
         Abdomen
         Eye orbit
         Face
         Neck

    88.98 Bone mineral density studies
         Dual photon absorptiometry
         Quantitative computed tomography (CT) studies
         Radiographic densitometry
         Single photon absorptiometry

● **89 Interview, evaluation, consultation, and examination**

 ● **89.0 Diagnostic interview, consultation, and evaluation**

         | Excludes | *psychiatric diagnostic interview (94.11–94.19)*

    89.01 Interview and evaluation, described as brief
         Abbreviated history and evaluation

    89.02 Interview and evaluation, described as limited
         Interval history and evaluation

    89.03 Interview and evaluation, described as comprehensive
         History and evaluation of new problem

    89.04 Other interview and evaluation

    89.05 Diagnostic interview and evaluation, not otherwise specified

    89.06 Consultation, described as limited
         Consultation on a single organ system

    89.07 Consultation, described as comprehensive

    89.08 Other consultation

    89.09 Consultation, not otherwise specified

● **89.1 Anatomic and physiologic measurements and manual examinations—nervous system and sense organs**

         | Excludes | *ear examination (95.41–95.49)*
                   eye examination (95.01–95.26)
                   the listed procedures when done as part of a general physical examination (89.7)

    89.10 Intracarotid amobarbital test
         Wada test

    89.11 Tonometry

    89.12 Nasal function study
         Rhinomanometry

    89.13 Neurologic examination

    89.14 Electroencephalogram

         | Excludes | *that with polysomnogram (89.17)*

    89.15 Other nonoperative neurologic function tests

    89.16 Transillumination of newborn skull

    89.17 Polysomnogram
         Sleep recording

    89.18 Other sleep disorder function tests
         Multiple sleep latency test [MSLT]

    89.19 Video and radio-telemetered electroencephalographic monitoring
         Radiographic EEG monitoring
         Video EEG monitoring

● **89.2 Anatomic and physiologic measurements and manual examinations—genitourinary system**

         | Excludes | *the listed procedures when done as part of a general physical examination (89.7)*

    89.21 Urinary manometry
         Manometry through:
            indwelling ureteral catheter
            nephrostomy
            pyelostomy
            ureterostomy

    89.22 Cystometrogram

    89.23 Urethral sphincter electromyogram

    89.24 Uroflowmetry [UFR]

    89.25 Urethral pressure profile [UPP]

    89.26 Gynecological examination
         Pelvic examination

    89.29 Other nonoperative genitourinary system measurements
         Bioassay of urine
         Renal clearance
         Urine chemistry

● **89.3 Other anatomic and physiologic measurements and manual examinations**

         | Excludes | *the listed procedures when done as part of a general physical examination (89.7)*

    89.31 Dental examination
         Oral mucosal survey
         Periodontal survey

    89.32 Esophageal manometry

    89.33 Digital examination of enterostomy stoma
         Digital examination of colostomy stoma

89.34   Digital examination of rectum

89.35   Transillumination of nasal sinuses

89.36   Manual examination of breast

89.37   Vital capacity determination

89.38   Other nonoperative respiratory measurements
     Plethysmography for measurement of respiratory function
     Thoracic impedance plethysmography

89.39   Other nonoperative measurements and examinations
     14 C-Urea breath test
     Basal metabolic rate [BMR]
     Gastric:
         analysis
         function NEC

> **Excludes**   *body measurement (93.07)*
> *cardiac tests (89.41–89.69)*
> *fundus photography (95.11)*
> *limb length measurement (93.06)*

● 89.4   Cardiac stress tests, pacemaker and defibrillator checks ◂▥

89.41   Cardiovascular stress test using treadmill

89.42   Masters' two-step stress test

89.43   Cardiovascular stress test using bicycle ergometer

89.44   Other cardiovascular stress test
     Thallium stress test with or without transesophageal pacing

89.45   Artificial pacemaker rate check
     Artificial pacemaker function check NOS
     Bedside device check of pacemaker or cardiac resynchronization pacemaker [CRT-P] ◂
     Interrogation only without arrhythmia induction ◂

> **Excludes**   *electrophysiologic studies [EPS] (37.26)* ◂
> *non-invasive programmed electrical stimulation [NIPS] (arrhythmia induction) (37.26)* ◂

89.46   Artificial pacemaker artifact wave form check

89.47   Artificial pacemaker electrode impedance check

89.48   Artificial pacemaker voltage or amperage threshold check

89.49   Automatic implantable cardioverter/defibrillator (AICD) check ◂
     Bedside check of an AICD or cardiac resynchronization defibrillator [CRT-D] ◂
     Checking pacing thresholds of device ◂
     Interrogation only without arrhythmia induction ◂

> **Excludes**   *electrophysiologic studies [EPS] (37.26)* ◂
> *non-invasive programmed electrical stimulation [NIPS] (arrhythmia induction) (37.26)* ◂

● 89.5   Other nonoperative cardiac and vascular diagnostic procedures

> **Excludes**   *fetal EKG (75.32)*

89.50   Ambulatory cardiac monitoring
     Analog devices [Holter-type]

89.51   Rhythm electrocardiogram
     Rhythm EKG (with one to three leads)

89.52   Electrocardiogram
     ECG NOS
     EKG (with 12 or more leads)

89.53   Vectorcardiogram (with ECG)

89.54   Electrographic monitoring
     Telemetry

> **Excludes**   *ambulatory cardiac monitoring (89.50)*
> *electrographic monitoring during surgery—omit code*

89.55   Phonocardiogram with ECG lead

89.56   Carotid pulse tracing with ECG lead

> **Excludes**   *oculoplethysmography (89.58)*

89.57   Apexcardiogram (with ECG lead)

89.58   Plethysmogram

> **Includes:** Penile plethysmography with nerve stimulation

> **Excludes**   *plethysmography (for):*
> *measurement of respiratory function (89.38)*
> *thoracic impedance (89.38)*

89.59   Other nonoperative cardiac and vascular measurements

89.60   Continuous intra-arterial blood gas monitoring
     Insertion of blood gas monitoring system and continuous monitoring of blood gases through an intra-arterial sensor

● 89.6   Circulatory monitoring

> **Excludes**   *electrocardiographic monitoring during surgery—omit code*

89.61   Systemic arterial pressure monitoring

89.62   Central venous pressure monitoring

89.63   Pulmonary artery pressure monitoring

> **Excludes**   *pulmonary artery wedge monitoring (89.64)*

89.64   Pulmonary artery wedge monitoring
     Pulmonary capillary wedge [PCW] monitoring
     Swan-Ganz catheterization

89.65   Measurement of systemic arterial blood gases

> **Excludes**   *continuous intra-arterial blood gas monitoring (89.60)*

89.66   Measurement of mixed venous blood gases

89.67   Monitoring of cardiac output by oxygen consumption technique
     Fick method

89.68   Monitoring of cardiac output by other technique
     Cardiac output monitor by thermodilution indicator

89.69   Monitoring of coronary blood flow
     Coronary blood flow monitoring by coincidence counting technique

89.7   General physical examination

89.8   Autopsy

● 90   Microscopic examination-I

The following fourth-digit subclassification is for use with categories in section 90 to identify type of examination:
     1 bacterial smear
     2 culture
     3 culture and sensitivity
     4 parasitology
     5 toxicology
     6 cell block and Papanicolaou smear
     9 other microscopic examination

● 90.0   Microscopic examination of specimen from nervous system and of spinal fluid

- **90.1** Microscopic examination of specimen from endocrine gland, not elsewhere classified
- **90.2** Microscopic examination of specimen from eye
- **90.3** Microscopic examination of specimen from ear, nose, throat, and larynx
- **90.4** Microscopic examination of specimen from trachea, bronchus, pleura, lung, and other thoracic specimen, and of sputum
- **90.5** Microscopic examination of blood
- **90.6** Microscopic examination of specimen from spleen and of bone marrow
- **90.7** Microscopic examination of specimen from lymph node and of lymph
- **90.8** Microscopic examination of specimen from upper gastrointestinal tract and of vomitus
- **90.9** Microscopic examination of specimen from lower gastrointestinal tract and of stool

● **91 Microscopic examination-II**

The following fourth-digit subclassification is for use with categories in section 91 to identify type of examination
- 1 bacterial smear
- 2 culture
- 3 culture and sensitivity
- 4 parasitology
- 5 toxicology
- 6 cell block and Papanicolaou smear
- 9 other microscopic examination

- **91.0** Microscopic examination of specimen from liver, biliary tract, and pancreas
- **91.1** Microscopic examination of peritoneal and retroperitoneal specimen
- **91.2** Microscopic examination of specimen from kidney, ureter, perirenal and periureteral tissue
- **91.3** Microscopic examination of specimen from bladder, urethra, prostate, seminal vesicle, perivesical tissue, and of urine and semen
- **91.4** Microscopic examination of specimen from female genital tract
  - Amnionic sac
  - Fetus
- **91.5** Microscopic examination of specimen from musculoskeletal system and of joint fluid
  - Microscopic examination of:
    - bone
    - bursa
    - cartilage
    - fascia
    - ligament
    - muscle
    - synovial membrane
    - tendon
- **91.6** Microscopic examination of specimen from skin and other integument
  - Microscopic examination of:
    - hair
    - nails
    - skin

  Excludes *mucous membrane—code to organ site that of operative wound (91.70–91.79)*

- **91.7** Microscopic examination of specimen from operative wound
- **91.8** Microscopic examination of specimen from other site
- **91.9** Microscopic examination of specimen from unspecified site

● **92 Nuclear medicine**
- ● **92.0** Radioisotope scan and function study
  - **92.01** Thyroid scan and radioisotope function studies
    - Iodine-131 uptake
    - Protein-bound iodine
    - Radio-iodine uptake
  - **92.02** Liver scan and radioisotope function study
  - **92.03** Renal scan and radioisotope function study
    - Renal clearance study
  - **92.04** Gastrointestinal scan and radioisotope function study
    - Radio-cobalt B12 Schilling test
    - Radio-iodinated triolein study
  - **92.05** Cardiovascular and hematopoietic scan and radioisotope function study
    - Bone marrow scan or function study
    - Cardiac output scan or function study
    - Circulation time scan or function study
    - Radionuclide cardiac ventriculogram scan or function study
    - Spleen scan or function study
  - **92.09** Other radioisotope function studies
- ● **92.1** Other radioisotope scan
  - **92.11** Cerebral scan
    - Pituitary
  - **92.12** Scan of other sites of head
    - **Excludes** *eye (95.16)*
  - **92.13** Parathyroid scan
  - **92.14** Bone scan
  - **92.15** Pulmonary scan
  - **92.16** Scan of lymphatic system
  - **92.17** Placental scan
  - **92.18** Total body scan
  - **92.19** Scan of other sites
- ● **92.2** Therapeutic radiology and nuclear medicine
  - **Excludes** *that for:*
    - *ablation of pituitary gland (07.64–07.69)*
    - *destruction of chorioretinal lesion (14.26–14.27)*
  - **92.21** Superficial radiation
    - Contact radiation [up to 150 KVP]
  - **92.22** Orthovoltage radiation
    - Deep radiation [200–300 KVP]
  - **92.23** Radioisotopic teleradiotherapy
    - Teleradiotherapy using:
      - Cobalt-60
      - Iodine-125
      - radioactive cesium
  - **92.24** Teleradiotherapy using photons
    - Megavoltage NOS
    - Supervoltage NOS
    - Use of:
      - Betatron
      - linear accelerator
  - **92.25** Teleradiotherapy using electrons
    - Beta particles
  - **92.26** Teleradiotherapy of other particulate radiation
    - Neutrons
    - Protons NOS
- ✖ **92.27** Implantation or insertion of radioactive elements
  - Code also incision of site
  - **Includes:** Intravascular brachytherapy

92.28 Injection or instillation of radioisotopes
Injection or infusion of radioimmunocon-
jugate
Intracavitary injection or instillation
Intravenous injection or instillation
Iodine-131 [I-131] tositumomab
Radioimmunotherapy
Ytrium-90 [Y-90] ibritumomab tiuxetan

92.29 Other radiotherapeutic procedure

● **92.3 Stereotactic radiosurgery**

| Excludes | *stereotactic biopsy*

Code also stereotactic head frame application (93.59)

**92.30 Stereotactic radiosurgery, not otherwise speci-
fied**

92.31 Single source photon radiosurgery
High energy x-rays
Linear accelerator (LINAC)

92.32 Multi-source photon radiosurgery
Cobalt 60 radiation
Gamma irradiation

92.33 Particulate radiosurgery
Particle beam radiation (cyclotron)
Proton accelerator

**92.39 Stereotactic radiosurgery, not elsewhere classi-
fied**

● **93 Physical therapy, respiratory therapy, rehabilitation, and
related procedures**

● **93.0 Diagnostic physical therapy**

93.01 Functional evaluation

93.02 Orthotic evaluation

93.03 Prosthetic evaluation

93.04 Manual testing of muscle function

93.05 Range of motion testing

93.06 Measurement of limb length

93.07 Body measurement
Girth measurement
Measurement of skull circumference

93.08 Electromyography

| Excludes | *eye EMG (95.25)*
that with polysomnogram (89.17)
urethral sphincter EMG (89.23)

93.09 Other diagnostic physical therapy procedure

● **93.1 Physical therapy exercises**

93.11 Assisting exercise

| Excludes | *assisted exercise in pool (93.31)*

93.12 Other active musculoskeletal exercise

93.13 Resistive exercise

93.14 Training in joint movements

93.15 Mobilization of spine

93.16 Mobilization of other joints

| Excludes | *manipulation of temporomandibular joint (76.95)*

93.17 Other passive musculoskeletal exercise

93.18 Breathing exercise

93.19 Exercise, not elsewhere classified

● **93.2 Other physical therapy musculoskeletal manipulation**

93.21 Manual and mechanical traction

| Excludes | *skeletal traction (93.43–93.44)*
skin traction (93.45–93.46)
spinal traction (93.41–93.42)

93.22 Ambulation and gait training

93.23 Fitting of orthotic device

93.24 Training in use of prosthetic or orthotic device
Training in crutch walking

93.25 Forced extension of limb

93.26 Manual rupture of joint adhesions

93.27 Stretching of muscle or tendon

93.28 Stretching of fascia

93.29 Other forcible correction of deformity

● **93.3 Other physical therapy therapeutic procedures**

93.31 Assisted exercise in pool

93.32 Whirlpool treatment

93.33 Other hydrotherapy

93.34 Diathermy

93.35 Other heat therapy
Acupuncture with smoldering moxa
Hot packs
Hyperthermia NEC
Infrared irradiation
Moxibustion
Paraffin bath

| Excludes | *hyperthermia for treatment of cancer (99.85)*

93.36 Cardiac retraining

93.37 Prenatal training
Training for natural childbirth

**93.38 Combined physical therapy without mention
of the components**

93.39 Other physical therapy

● **93.4 Skeletal traction and other traction**

93.41 Spinal traction using skull device
Traction using:
caliper tongs
Crutchfield tongs
halo device
Vinke tongs

| Excludes | *insertion of tongs or halo traction device (02.94)*

93.42 Other spinal traction
Cotrel's traction

| Excludes | *cervical collar (93.52)*

93.43 Intermittent skeletal traction

93.44 Other skeletal traction
Bryant's traction
Dunlop's traction
Lyman Smith traction
Russell's traction

93.45 Thomas' splint traction

93.46 Other skin traction of limbs
Adhesive tape traction
Boot traction
Buck's traction
Gallows traction

● **93.5** **Other immobilization, pressure, and attention to wound**

> **Excludes** *wound cleansing (96.58–96.59)*

93.51 Application of plaster jacket

> **Excludes** *Minerva jacket (93.52)*

93.52 Application of neck support
Application of:
    cervical collar
    Minerva jacket
    molded neck support

93.53 Application of other cast

93.54 Application of splint
Plaster splint
Tray splint

> **Excludes** *periodontal splint (24.7)*

93.55 Dental wiring

> **Excludes** *that for orthodontia (24.7)*

93.56 Application of pressure dressing
Application of:
    Gibney bandage
    Robert Jones' bandage
    Shanz dressing

93.57 Application of other wound dressing
Porcine wound dressing

93.58 Application of pressure trousers
Application of:
    anti-shock trousers
    MAST trousers
    vasopneumatic device

93.59 Other immobilization, pressure, and attention to wound
Elastic stockings
Electronic gaiter
Intermittent pressure device
Oxygenation of wound (hyperbaric)
Stereotactic head frame application
Velpeau dressing

● **93.6** **Osteopathic manipulative treatment**

93.61 Osteopathic manipulative treatment for general mobilization
General articulatory treatment

93.62 Osteopathic manipulative treatment using high- velocity, low-amplitude forces
Thrusting forces

93.63 Osteopathic manipulative treatment using low-velocity, high-amplitude forces
Springing forces

93.64 Osteopathic manipulative treatment using isotonic, isometric forces

93.65 Osteopathic manipulative treatment using indirect forces

93.66 Osteopathic manipulative treatment to move tissue fluids
Lymphatic pump

93.67 Other specified osteopathic manipulative treatment

● **93.7** **Speech and reading rehabilitation and rehabilitation of the blind**

93.71 Dyslexia training

93.72 Dysphasia training

93.73 Esophageal speech training

93.74 Speech defect training

93.75 Other speech training and therapy

93.76 Training in use of lead dog for the blind

93.77 Training in braille or Moon

93.78 Other rehabilitation for the blind

● **93.8** **Other rehabilitation therapy**

93.81 Recreation therapy
Diversional therapy
Play therapy

> **Excludes** *play psychotherapy (94.36)*

93.82 Educational therapy
Education of bed-bound children
Special schooling for the handicapped

93.83 Occupational therapy
Daily living activities therapy

> **Excludes** *training in activities of daily living for the blind (93.78)*

93.84 Music therapy

93.85 Vocational rehabilitation
Sheltered employment
Vocational:
    assessment
    retraining
    training

93.89 Rehabilitation, not elsewhere classified

● **93.9** **Respiratory therapy**

> **Excludes** *insertion of airway (96.01–96.05)*
> *other continuous mechanical ventilation (96.70–96.72)*

93.90 Continuous positive airway pressure [CPAP]
Bi-level airway pressure ◀
Non-invasive positive pressure (NIPPV) ◀

93.91 Intermittent positive pressure breathing [IPPB]

93.93 Nonmechanical methods of resuscitation
Artificial respiration
Manual resuscitation
Mouth-to-mouth resuscitation

93.94 Respiratory medication administered by nebulizer
Mist therapy

93.95 Hyperbaric oxygenation

> **Excludes** *oxygenation of wound (93.59)*

93.96 Other oxygen enrichment
Catalytic oxygen therapy
Cytoreductive effect
Oxygenators
Oxygen therapy

> **Excludes** *oxygenation of wound (93.59)*

93.97 Decompression chamber

93.98 Other control of atmospheric pressure and composition
Antigen-free air conditioning
Helium therapy

> **Excludes** *inhaled nitric oxide therapy (INO) (00.12)*

93.99 Other respiratory procedures
Continuous negative pressure ventilation [CNP]
Postural drainage

● 94 Procedures related to the psyche
  ● 94.0 Psychologic evaluation and testing
    94.01 Administration of intelligence test
           Administration of:
             Stanford-Binet
             Wechsler Adult Intelligence Scale
             Wechsler Intelligence Scale for Children
    94.02 Administration of psychologic test
           Administration of:
             Bender Visual-Motor Gestalt Test
             Benton Visual Retention Test
             Minnesota Multiphasic Personality Inventory
             Wechsler Memory Scale
    94.03 Character analysis
    94.08 Other psychologic evaluation and testing
    94.09 Psychologic mental status determination, not
           otherwise specified
  ● 94.1 Psychiatric interviews, consultations, and evaluations
    94.11 Psychiatric mental status determination
           Clinical psychiatric mental status determina-
             tion
           Evaluation for criminal responsibility
           Evaluation for testimentary capacity
           Medicolegal mental status determination
           Mental status determination NOS
    94.12 Routine psychiatric visit, not otherwise speci-
           fied
    94.13 Psychiatric commitment evaluation
           Pre-commitment interview
    94.19 Other psychiatric interview and evaluation
           Follow-up psychiatric interview NOS
  ● 94.2 Psychiatric somatotherapy
    94.21 Narcoanalysis
           Narcosynthesis
    94.22 Lithium therapy
    94.23 Neuroleptic therapy
    94.24 Chemical shock therapy
    94.25 Other psychiatric drug therapy
    94.26 Subconvulsive electroshock therapy
    94.27 Other electroshock therapy
           Electroconvulsive therapy (ECT)
           EST
    94.29 Other psychiatric somatotherapy
  ● 94.3 Individual psychotherapy
    94.31 Psychoanalysis
    94.32 Hypnotherapy
           Hypnodrome
           Hypnosis
    94.33 Behavior therapy
           Aversion therapy
           Behavior modification
           Desensitization therapy
           Extinction therapy
           Relaxation training
           Token economy
    94.34 Individual therapy for psychosexual dysfunction
           Excludes that performed in group setting (94.41)
    94.35 Crisis intervention
    94.36 Play psychotherapy
    94.37 Exploratory verbal psychotherapy
    94.38 Supportive verbal psychotherapy
    94.39 Other individual psychotherapy
           Biofeedback

  ● 94.4 Other psychotherapy and counselling
    94.41 Group therapy for psychosexual dysfunction
    94.42 Family therapy
    94.43 Psychodrama
    94.44 Other group therapy
    94.45 Drug addiction counselling
    94.46 Alcoholism counselling
    94.49 Other counselling
  ● 94.5 Referral for psychologic rehabilitation
    94.51 Referral for psychotherapy
    94.52 Referral for psychiatric aftercare:
           That in:
             halfway house
             outpatient (clinic) facility
    94.53 Referral for alcoholism rehabilitation
    94.54 Referral for drug addiction rehabilitation
    94.55 Referral for vocational rehabilitation
    94.59 Referral for other psychologic rehabilitation
  ● 94.6 Alcohol and drug rehabilitation and detoxification
    94.61 Alcohol rehabilitation
    94.62 Alcohol detoxification
    94.63 Alcohol rehabilitation and detoxification
    94.64 Drug rehabilitation
    94.65 Drug detoxification
    94.66 Drug rehabilitation and detoxification
    94.67 Combined alcohol and drug rehabilitation
    94.68 Combined alcohol and drug detoxification
    94.69 Combined alcohol and drug rehabilitation and
           detoxification
● 95 Ophthalmologic and otologic diagnosis and treatment
  ● 95.0 General and subjective eye examination
    95.01 Limited eye examination
           Eye examination with prescription of spectacles
    95.02 Comprehensive eye examination
           Eye examination covering all aspects of the
             visual system
    95.03 Extended ophthalmologic work-up
           Examination (for):
             glaucoma
             neuro-ophthalmology
             retinal disease
  ✖ 95.04 Eye examination under anesthesia
           Code also type of examination
    95.05 Visual field study
    95.06 Color vision study
    95.07 Dark adaptation study
    95.09 Eye examination, not otherwise specified
           Vision check NOS
  ● 95.1 Examinations of form and structure of eye
    95.11 Fundus photography
    95.12 Fluorescein angiography or angioscopy of eye
    95.13 Ultrasound study of eye
    95.14 X-ray study of eye
    95.15 Ocular motility study
    95.16 P32 and other tracer studies of eye

● **95.2   Objective functional tests of eye**

> **Excludes**   *that with polysomnogram (89.17)*

>> **95.21   Electroretinogram [ERG]**

>> **95.22   Electro-oculogram [EOG]**

>> **95.23   Visual evoked potential [VEP]**

>> **95.24   Electronystagmogram [ENG]**

>> **95.25   Electromyogram of eye [EMG]**

>> **95.26   Tonography, provocative tests, and other glaucoma testing**

● **95.3   Special vision services**

>> **95.31   Fitting and dispensing of spectacles**

>> **95.32   Prescription, fitting, and dispensing of contact lens**

>> **95.33   Dispensing of other low vision aids**

>> **95.34   Ocular prosthetics**

>> **95.35   Orthoptic training**

>> **95.36   Ophthalmologic counselling and instruction**
>> Counselling in:
>> adaptation to visual loss
>> use of low vision aids

● **95.4   Nonoperative procedures related to hearing**

>> **95.41   Audiometry**
>> Békésy 5-tone audiometry
>> Impedance audiometry
>> Stapedial reflex response
>> Subjective audiometry
>> Tympanogram

>> **95.42   Clinical test of hearing**
>> Tuning fork test
>> Whispered speech test

>> **95.43   Audiological evaluation**
>> Audiological evaluation by:
>> Bárány noise machine
>> blindfold test
>> delayed feedback
>> masking
>> Weber lateralization

>> **95.44   Clinical vestibular function tests**
>> Thermal test of vestibular function

>> **95.45   Rotation tests**
>> Bárány chair

>> **95.46   Other auditory and vestibular function tests**

>> **95.47   Hearing examination, not otherwise specified**

>> **95.48   Fitting of hearing aid**

> **Excludes**   *implantation of electromagnetic hearing device (20.95)*

>> **95.49   Other nonoperative procedures related to hearing**
>> Adjustment (external components) of cochlear prosthetic device

● **96   Nonoperative intubation and irrigation**

● **96.0   Nonoperative intubation of gastrointestinal and respiratory tracts**

>> **96.01   Insertion of nasopharyngeal airway**

>> **96.02   Insertion of oropharyngeal airway**

>> **96.03   Insertion of esophageal obturator airway**

>> **96.04   Insertion of endotracheal tube**

>> **96.05   Other intubation of respiratory tract**

>> **96.06   Insertion of Sengstaken tube**
>> Esophageal tamponade

>> **96.07   Insertion of other (naso-)gastric tube**
>> Intubation for decompression

> **Excludes**   *that for enteral infusion of nutritional substance (96.6)*

>> **96.08   Insertion of (naso-)intestinal tube**
>> Miller-Abbott tube (for decompression)

>> **96.09   Insertion of rectal tube**
>> Replacement of rectal tube

● **96.1   Other nonoperative insertion**

> **Excludes**   *nasolacrimal intubation (09.44)*

>> **96.11   Packing of external auditory canal**

>> **96.14   Vaginal packing**

>> **96.15   Insertion of vaginal mold**

>> **96.16   Other vaginal dilation**

>> **96.17   Insertion of vaginal diaphragm**

>> **96.18   Insertion of other vaginal pessary**

>> **96.19   Rectal packing**

● **96.2   Nonoperative dilation and manipulation**

>> **96.21   Dilation of frontonasal duct**

>> **96.22   Dilation of rectum**

>> **96.23   Dilation of anal sphincter**

>> **96.24   Dilation and manipulation of enterostomy stoma**

>> **96.25   Therapeutic distention of bladder**
>> Intermittent distention of bladder

>> **96.26   Manual reduction of rectal prolapse**

>> **96.27   Manual reduction of hernia**

>> **96.28   Manual reduction of enterostomy prolapse**

>> **96.29   Reduction of intussusception of alimentary tract**
>> With:
>> Fluoroscopy
>> Ionizing radiation enema
>> Ultrasonography guidance
>> Hydrostatic reduction
>> Pneumatic reduction

> **Excludes**   *intra-abdominal manipulation of intestine, not otherwise specified (46.80)*

● **96.3   Nonoperative alimentary tract irrigation, cleaning, and local instillation**

>> **96.31   Gastric cooling**
>> Gastric hypothermia

>> **96.32   Gastric freezing**

>> **96.33   Gastric lavage**

>> **96.34   Other irrigation of (naso-)gastric tube**

>> **96.35   Gastric gavage**

>> **96.36   Irrigation of gastrostomy or enterostomy**

>> **96.37   Proctoclysis**

>> **96.38   Removal of impacted feces**
>> Removal of impaction:
>> by flushing
>> manually

>> **96.39   Other transanal enema**
>> Rectal irrigation

> **Excludes**   *reduction of intussusception of alimentary tract by ionizing radiation enema (96.29)*

● 96.4 Nonoperative irrigation, cleaning, and local instillation of other digestive and genitourinary organs

     96.41   Irrigation of cholecystostomy and other biliary
tube

     96.42   Irrigation of pancreatic tube

     96.43   Digestive tract instillation, except gastric gavage

     96.44   Vaginal douche

     96.45   Irrigation of nephrostomy and pyelostomy

     96.46   Irrigation of ureterostomy and ureteral catheter

     96.47   Irrigation of cystostomy

     96.48   Irrigation of other indwelling urinary catheter

     96.49   Other genitourinary instillation
               Insertion of prostaglandin suppository

● 96.5 Other nonoperative irrigation and cleaning

     96.51   Irrigation of eye
               Irrigation of cornea

        Excludes   *irrigation with removal of foreign body (98.21)*

     96.52   Irrigation of ear
               Irrigation with removal of cerumen

     96.53   Irrigation of nasal passages

     96.54   Dental scaling, polishing, and debridement
               Dental prophylaxis
               Plaque removal

     96.55   Tracheostomy toilette

     96.56   Other lavage of bronchus and trachea

        Excludes   *diagnostic bronchoalveolar lavage (BAL)*
                      (33.24)
                 whole lung lavage (33.99)

     96.57   Irrigation of vascular catheter

     96.58   Irrigation of wound catheter

     96.59   Other irrigation of wound
               Wound cleaning NOS

        Excludes   *debridement (86.22, 86.27–86.28)*

● 96.6 Enteral infusion of concentrated nutritional substances

● 96.7 Other continuous mechanical ventilation

   Includes: Endotracheal respiratory assistance
               Intermittent mandatory ventilation [IMV]
               Positive end expiratory pressure [PEEP]
               Pressure support ventilation [PSV]
               That by tracheostomy
               Weaning of an intubated (endotracheal tube)
               patient

     Excludes   *bi-level airway pressure (93.90)*
                 continuous negative pressure ventilation [CNP]
                    (iron lung) (cuirass) (93.99)
                 continuous positive airway pressure [CPAP]
                    (93.90)
                 intermittent positive pressure breathing [IPPB]
                    (93.91)
                 non-invasive positive pressure (NIPPV) (93.90) ◄
                    that by face mask (93.90–93.99)
                 that by nasal cannula (93.90–93.99)
                 that by nasal catheter (93.90–93.99)

   Code also any associated:
      endotracheal tube insertion (96.04)
      tracheostomy (31.1–31.29)

   Note: Endotracheal Intubation

                To calculate the number of hours (dura-
tion) of continuous mechanical ventila-
tion during a hospitalization, begin the
count from the start of the (endotracheal)
intubation. The duration ends with (endotracheal) extubation.

                If a patient is intubated prior to admis-
sion, begin counting the duration from
the time of the admission. If a patient is
transferred (discharged) while intubated,
the duration would end at the time of
transfer (discharge).

                For patients who begin on (endotracheal)
intubation and subsequently have a
tracheostomy performed for mechanical
ventilation, the duration begins with the
(endotracheal) intubation and ends when
the mechanical ventilation is turned off
(after the weaning period).

                Tracheostomy

                To calculate the number of hours of con-
tinuous mechanical ventilation during a
hospitalization, begin counting the duration when mechanical ventilation is
started. The duration ends when the mechanical ventilator is turned off (after the
weaning period).

                If a patient has received a tracheostomy
prior to admission and is on mechanical
ventilation at the time of admission, begin counting the duration from the time
of admission. If a patient is transferred
(discharged) while still on mechanical
ventilation via tracheostomy, the duration would end at the time of the transfer (discharge).

     96.70   Continuous mechanical ventilation of unspeci-
fied duration
               Mechanical ventilation NOS

     96.71   Continuous mechanical ventilation for less
than 96 consecutive hours

     96.72   Continuous mechanical ventilation for 96 con-
secutive hours or more

●   **Use Additional Digit(s)**   ✖   **Valid O.R. Procedure**   ◄   **New**   ◀═   **Revised**

● **97 Replacement and removal of therapeutic appliances**

  ● **97.0 Nonoperative replacement of gastrointestinal appliance**

    97.01 Replacement of (naso-)gastric or esophagostomy tube

    97.02 Replacement of gastrostomy tube

    97.03 Replacement of tube or enterostomy device of small intestine

    97.04 Replacement of tube or enterostomy device of large intestine

    97.05 Replacement of stent (tube) in biliary or pancreatic duct

  ● **97.1 Nonoperative replacement of musculoskeletal and integumentary system appliance**

    97.11 Replacement of cast on upper limb

    97.12 Replacement of cast on lower limb

    97.13 Replacement of other cast

    97.14 Replacement of other device for musculoskeletal immobilization

    97.15 Replacement of wound catheter

    97.16 Replacement of wound packing or drain

      | **Excludes** | *repacking of:* |

        dental wound (97.22)
        vulvar wound (97.26)

  ● **97.2 Other nonoperative replacement**

    97.21 Replacement of nasal packing

    97.22 Replacement of dental packing

    97.23 Replacement of tracheostomy tube

    97.24 Replacement and refitting of vaginal diaphragm

    97.25 Replacement of other vaginal pessary

    97.26 Replacement of vaginal or vulvar packing or drain

    97.29 Other nonoperative replacements

  ● **97.3 Nonoperative removal of therapeutic device from head and neck**

    97.31 Removal of eye prosthesis

      | **Excludes** | *removal of ocular implant (16.71)* |

        removal of orbital implant (16.72)

    97.32 Removal of nasal packing

    97.33 Removal of dental wiring

    97.34 Removal of dental packing

    97.35 Removal of dental prosthesis

    97.36 Removal of other external mandibular fixation device

    97.37 Removal of tracheostomy tube

    97.38 Removal of sutures from head and neck

    97.39 Removal of other therapeutic device from head and neck

      | **Excludes** | *removal of skull tongs (02.94)* |

  ● **97.4 Nonoperative removal of therapeutic device from thorax**

    97.41 Removal of thoracotomy tube or pleural cavity drain

    97.42 Removal of mediastinal drain

    97.43 Removal of sutures from thorax

    97.44 Nonoperative removal of heart assist system

      Explantation [removal] of circulatory assist device ◄

      Explantation [removal] of percutaneous external heart assist device ◄

      Intra-aortic balloon pump [IABP]

      Removal of extrinsic heart assist device ◄

      Removal of pVAD ◄

      Removal of percutaneous heart assist device ◄

    97.49 Removal of other device from thorax

  ● **97.5 Nonoperative removal of therapeutic device from digestive system**

    97.51 Removal of gastrostomy tube

    97.52 Removal of tube from small intestine

    97.53 Removal of tube from large intestine or appendix

    97.54 Removal of cholecystostomy tube

    97.55 Removal of T-tube, other bile duct tube, or liver tube

      Includes: Removal of bile duct stent

    97.56 Removal of pancreatic tube or drain

    97.59 Removal of other device from digestive system
      Removal of rectal packing

  ● **97.6 Nonoperative removal of therapeutic device from urinary system**

    97.61 Removal of pyelostomy and nephrostomy tube

    97.62 Removal of ureterostomy tube and ureteral catheter

    97.63 Removal of cystostomy tube

    97.64 Removal of other urinary drainage device
      Removal of indwelling urinary catheter

    97.65 Removal of urethral stent

    97.69 Removal of other device from urinary system

  ● **97.7 Nonoperative removal of therapeutic device from genital system**

    97.71 Removal of intrauterine contraceptive device

    97.72 Removal of intrauterine pack

    97.73 Removal of vaginal diaphragm

    97.74 Removal of other vaginal pessary

    97.75 Removal of vaginal or vulvar packing

    97.79 Removal of other device from genital tract
      Removal of sutures

  ● **97.8 Other nonoperative removal of therapeutic device**

    97.81 Removal of retroperitoneal drainage device

    97.82 Removal of peritoneal drainage device

    97.83 Removal of abdominal wall sutures

    97.84 Removal of sutures from trunk, not elsewhere classified

    97.85 Removal of packing from trunk, not elsewhere classified

    97.86 Removal of other device from abdomen

    97.87 Removal of other device from trunk

    97.88 Removal of external immobilization device
      Removal of:
        brace
        cast
        splint

    97.89 Removal of other therapeutic device

● **98   Nonoperative removal of foreign body or calculus**

  ● **98.0   Removal of intraluminal foreign body from digestive system without incision**

    | **Excludes** | *removal of therapeutic device (97.51–97.59)* |

    98.01   Removal of intraluminal foreign body from mouth without incision

    98.02   Removal of intraluminal foreign body from esophagus without incision

    98.03   Removal of intraluminal foreign body from stomach and small intestine without incision

    98.04   Removal of intraluminal foreign body from large intestine without incision

    98.05   Removal of intraluminal foreign body from rectum and anus without incision

  ● **98.1   Removal of intraluminal foreign body from other sites without incision**

    | **Excludes** | *removal of therapeutic device (97.31–97.49, 97.61–97.89)* |

    98.11   Removal of intraluminal foreign body from ear without incision

    98.12   Removal of intraluminal foreign body from nose without incision

    98.13   Removal of intraluminal foreign body from pharynx without incision

    98.14   Removal of intraluminal foreign body from larynx without incision

    98.15   Removal of intraluminal foreign body from trachea and bronchus without incision

    98.16   Removal of intraluminal foreign body from uterus without incision

    | **Excludes** | *removal of intrauterine contraceptive device (97.71)* |

    98.17   Removal of intraluminal foreign body from vagina without incision

    98.18   Removal of intraluminal foreign body from artificial stoma without incision

    98.19   Removal of intraluminal foreign body from urethra without incision

  ● **98.2   Removal of other foreign body without incision**

    | **Excludes** | *removal of intraluminal foreign body (98.01–98.19)* |

    98.20   Removal of foreign body, not otherwise specified

    98.21   Removal of superficial foreign body from eye without incision

    98.22   Removal of other foreign body without incision from head and neck
        Removal of embedded foreign body from eyelid or conjunctiva without incision

    98.23   Removal of foreign body from vulva without incision

    98.24   Removal of foreign body from scrotum or penis without incision

    98.25   Removal of other foreign body without incision from trunk except scrotum, penis, or vulva

    98.26   Removal of foreign body from hand without incision

    98.27   Removal of foreign body without incision from upper limb, except hand

    98.28   Removal of foreign body from foot without incision

    98.29   Removal of foreign body without incision from lower limb, except foot

  ● **98.5   Extracorporeal shockwave lithotripsy [ESWL]**
      Lithotriptor tank procedure
      Disintegration of stones by extracorporeal induced shockwaves
      That with insertion of stent

    98.51   Extracorporeal shockwave lithotripsy [ESWL] of the kidney, ureter and/or bladder

    98.52   Extracorporeal shockwave lithotripsy [ESWL] of the gallbladder and/or bile duct

    98.59   Extracorporeal shockwave lithotripsy of other sites

● **99   Other nonoperative procedures**

  ● **99.0   Transfusion of blood and blood components**
      Use additional code for that done via catheter or cutdown (38.92–38.94)

    99.00   Perioperative autologous transfusion of whole blood or blood components
        Intraoperative blood collection
        Postoperative blood collection
        Salvage

    99.01   Exchange transfusion
        Transfusion:
          exsanguination
          replacement

    99.02   Transfusion of previously collected autologous blood
        Blood component

    99.03   Other transfusion of whole blood
        Transfusion:
          blood NOS
          hemodilution
          NOS

    99.04   Transfusion of packed cells

    99.05   Transfusion of platelets
        Transfusion of thrombocytes

    99.06   Transfusion of coagulation factors
        Transfusion of antihemophilic factor

    99.07   Transfusion of other serum
        Transfusion of plasma

    | **Excludes** | *injection [transfusion] of:* |
        antivenin (99.16)
        gamma globulin (99.14)

    99.08   Transfusion of blood expander
        Transfusion of Dextran

    99.09   Transfusion of other substance
        Transfusion of:
          blood surrogate
          granulocytes

    | **Excludes** | *transplantation [transfusion] of bone marrow (41.0)* |

  ● **99.1   Injection or infusion of therapeutic or prophylactic substance**

    Includes: injection or infusion given:
        hypodermically acting locally or systemically
        intramuscularly acting locally or systemically
        intravenously acting locally or systemically

99.10 Injection or infusion of thrombolytic agent
Streptokinase
Tissue plasminogen activator (TPA)
Urokinase
Excludes *aspirin—omit code*
GP IIB/IIIa platelet inhibitors (99.20)
heparin (99.19)
single vessel percutaneous transluminal coronary angioplasty [PTCA] or coronary atherectomy with mention of thrombolytic agent (36.02)
warfarin—omit code

99.11 Injection of Rh immune globulin
Injection of:
Anti-D (Rhesus) globulin
RhoGAM

99.12 Immunization for allergy
Desensitization

99.13 Immunization for autoimmune disease

99.14 Injection of gamma globulin
Injection of immune sera

99.15 Parenteral infusion of concentrated nutritional substances
Hyperalimentation
Total parenteral nutrition [TPN]
Peripheral parenteral nutrition [PPN]

99.16 Injection of antidote
Injection of:
antivenin
heavy metal antagonist

99.17 Injection of insulin

99.18 Injection or infusion of electrolytes

99.19 Injection of anticoagulant
Excludes *infusion of drotrecogin alfa (activated) (00.11)*

● **99.2 Injection or infusion of other therapeutic or prophylactic substance**
Includes: injection or infusion given:
hypodermically acting locally or systemically
intramuscularly acting locally or systemically
intravenously acting locally or systemically

Use additional code for:
injection (into):
breast (85.92)
bursa (82.94, 83.96)
intraperitoneal (cavity) (54.97)
intrathecal (03.92)
joint (76.96, 81.92)
kidney (55.96)
liver (50.94)
orbit (16.91)
other sites—see Alphabetic Index
perfusion:
NOS (39.97)
intestine (46.95, 46.96)
kidney (55.95)
liver (50.93)
total body (39.96)

99.20 Injection or infusion of platelet inhibitor
Glycoprotein IIB/IIIa inhibitor
GP IIB/IIIa inhibitor
GP IIB/IIa inhibitor
Excludes *infusion of heparin (99.19)*
injection or infusion of thrombolytic agent (99.10)

99.21 Injection of antibiotic
Excludes *injection or infusion of oxazolidinones class of antibiotics (00.14)*

99.22 Injection of other anti-infective
Excludes *injection or infusion of oxazolidinones class of antibiotics (00.14)*

99.23 Injection of steroid
Injection of cortisone
Subdermal implantation of progesterone

99.24 Injection of other hormone

99.25 Injection or infusion of cancer chemotherapeutic substance
Chemoembolization
Injection or infusion of antineoplastic agent
Excludes *immunotherapy, antineoplastic (00.15, 99.28)*
implantation of chemotherapeutic agent (00.10)
injection of radioisotope (92.28)
injection or infusion of biological response modifier [BRM] as an antineoplastic agent (99.28)

99.26 Injection of tranquilizer

99.27 Iontophoresis

99.28 Injection or infusion of biological response modifier [BRM] as an antineoplastic agent
Low-dose interleukin-2 (IL-2) therapy
Immunotherapy, antineoplastic
Interleukin therapy
Tumor vaccine
Excludes *high-dose infusion interleukin-2 [IL-2] (00.15)*

99.29 Injection or infusion of other therapeutic or prophylactic substance
Excludes *administration of neuroprotective agent (99.75)*
immunization (99.31–99.59)
injection of sclerosing agent into:
esophageal varices (42.33)
hemorrhoids (49.42)
veins (39.92)
injection or infusion of human B-type natriuretic peptide (hBNP) (00.13)
injection or infusion of nesiritide (00.13)
injection or infusion of platelet inhibitor (99.20)
injection or infusion of thrombolytic agent (99.10)

● **99.3 Prophylactic vaccination and inoculation against certain bacterial diseases**

99.31 Vaccination against cholera

99.32 Vaccination against typhoid and paratyphoid fever
Administration of TAB vaccine

99.33 Vaccination against tuberculosis
Administration of BCG vaccine

99.34 Vaccination against plague

99.35 Vaccination against tularemia

99.36 Administration of diphtheria toxoid
Excludes *administration of:*
diphtheria antitoxin (99.58)
diphtheria-tetanus-pertussis, combined (99.39)

99.37 Vaccination against pertussis
Excludes *administration of diphtheria-tetanus-pertussis, combined (99.39)*

99.38 Administration of tetanus toxoid
Excludes *administration of:*
diphtheria-tetanus-pertussis, combined (99.39)
tetanus antitoxin (99.56)

99.39 Administration of diphtheria-tetanus-pertussis, combined

● **99.4 Prophylactic vaccination and inoculation against certain viral diseases**

99.41 Administration of poliomyelitis vaccine

99.42 Vaccination against smallpox

99.43 Vaccination against yellow fever

99.44 Vaccination against rabies

99.45 Vaccination against measles

> Excludes   *administration of measles-mumps-rubella vaccine (99.48)*

99.46 Vaccination against mumps

> Excludes   *administration of measles-mumps-rubella vaccine (99.48)*

99.47 Vaccination against rubella

> Excludes   *administration of measles-mumps-rubella vaccine (99.48)*

99.48 Administration of measles-mumps-rubella vaccine

● **99.5 Other vaccination and inoculation**

99.51 Prophylactic vaccination against the common cold

99.52 Prophylactic vaccination against influenza

99.53 Prophylactic vaccination against arthropod-borne viral encephalitis

99.54 Prophylactic vaccination against other arthropod-borne viral diseases

99.55 Prophylactic administration of vaccine against other diseases
> Vaccination against:
> anthrax
> brucellosis
> Rocky Mountain spotted fever
> Staphylococcus
> Streptococcus
> typhus

99.56 Administration of tetanus antitoxin

99.57 Administration of botulism antitoxin

99.58 Administration of other antitoxins
> Administration of:
> diphtheria antitoxin
> gas gangrene antitoxin
> scarlet fever antitoxin

99.59 Other vaccination and inoculation
> Vaccination NOS

> Excludes   *injection of:*
> *gamma globulin (99.14)*
> *Rh immune globulin (99.11)*
> *immunization for:*
> *allergy (99.12)*
> *autoimmune disease (99.13)*

● **99.6 Conversion of cardiac rhythm**

> Excludes   *open chest cardiac:*
> *electric stimulation (37.91)*
> *massage (37.91)*

99.60 Cardiopulmonary resuscitation, not otherwise specified

99.61 Atrial cardioversion

99.62 Other electric countershock of heart
> Cardioversion:
> NOS
> external
> Conversion to sinus rhythm
> Defibrillation
> External electrode stimulation

99.63 Closed chest cardiac massage
> Cardiac massage NOS
> Manual external cardiac massage

99.64 Carotid sinus stimulation

99.69 Other conversion of cardiac rhythm

● **99.7 Therapeutic apheresis or other injection, administration, or infusion of other therapeutic or prophylactic substance**

99.71 Therapeutic plasmapheresis

> Excludes   *extracorporeal immunoadsorption [ECI] 99.76*

99.72 Therapeutic leukopheresis
> Therapeutic leukocytapheresis

99.73 Therapeutic erythrocytapheresis
> Therapeutic erythropheresis

99.74 Therapeutic plateletpheresis

99.75 Administration of neuroprotective agent

99.76 Extracorporeal immunoadsorption
> Removal of antibodies from plasma with protein A columns

99.77 Application or administration of adhesion barrier substance

99.78 Aquapheresis ◀
> Plasma water removal ◀
> Ultrafiltration [for water removal] ◀

> Excludes   *hemodiafiltration (39.95)* ◀
> *hemodialysis (39.95)* ◀
> *therapeutic plasmapheresis (99.71)* ◀

99.79 Other
> Apheresis (harvest) of stem cells

● **99.8 Miscellaneous physical procedures**

99.81 Hypothermia (central) (local)

> Excludes   *gastric cooling (96.31)*
> *gastric freezing (96.32)*
> *that incidental to open heart surgery (39.62)*

99.82 Ultraviolet light therapy
> Actinotherapy

99.83 Other phototherapy
> Phototherapy of the newborn

> Excludes   *extracorporeal photochemotherapy (99.88)*
> *photocoagulation of retinal lesion (14.23–14.25, 14.33–14.35, 14.53–14.55)*

99.84 Isolation
> Isolation after contact with infectious disease
> Protection of individual from his surroundings
> Protection of surroundings from individual

99.85 Hyperthermia for treatment of cancer
> Hyperthermia (adjunct therapy) induced by microwave, ultrasound, low energy radio frequency, probes (interstitial), or other means in the treatment of cancer
>
> Code also any concurrent chemotherapy or radiation therapy

99.86 Non-invasive placement of bone growth stimulator
> Transcutaneous (surface) placement of pads or patches for stimulation to aid bone healing

> Excludes   *insertion of invasive or semi-invasive bone growth stimulators (device) (percutaneous electrodes) (78.90–78.99)*

99.88 Therapeutic photopheresis
    Extracorporeal photochemotherapy
    Extracorporeal photopheresis
    Excludes *other phototherapy (99.83)*
        ultraviolet light therapy (99.82)

● **99.9 Other miscellaneous procedures**

99.91 Acupuncture for anesthesia

99.92 Other acupuncture
    Excludes *that with smoldering moxa (93.35)*

99.93 Rectal massage (for levator spasm)

99.94 Prostatic massage

99.95 Stretching of foreskin

99.96 Collection of sperm for artificial insemination

99.97 Fitting of denture

99.98 Extraction of milk from lactating breast

99.99 Other
    Leech therapy

UNIT TWO

HCPCS 2004: LEVEL II NATIONAL CODES

2005 HCPCS Updates available on the companion website at:
http://evolve.elsevier.com/Buck/icd

DISCLAIMER

Every effort has been made to make this text complete and accurate, but no guarantee, warranty, or representation is made for its accuracy or completeness. It is based on the Centers for Medicare and Medicaid Services Healthcare Common Procedure Coding System (HCPCS).

Contains the March 31, 2004, quarterly updates.

PART I

Introduction

2005 HCPCS Updates available on the companion website at: http://evolve.elsevier.com/Buck/icd

The Centers for Medicare and Medicaid Services (CMS) (formerly Health Care Financing Administration [HCFA]) Healthcare Common Procedure Coding System (HCPCS) is a collection of codes and descriptors that represent procedures, supplies, products, and services that may be provided to Medicare beneficiaries and to individuals enrolled in private health insurance programs. The codes are divided as follows:

Level I: Codes and descriptors copyrighted by the American Medical Association's (AMA's) Current Procedural Terminology, ed. 4 (CPT-4). Five-position numeric codes primarily represent physician services.

Level II: Five-position alpha-numeric codes representing primarily items and nonphysician services that are not represented in the Level I codes. Codes and descriptors copyrighted by the American Dental Association's (ADA's) Current Dental Terminology, ed. 2 (CDT-2), are five-position alpha-numeric codes comprising the D series. **This book does not contain codes D0100 through D9999.** They can be purchased from the ADA. All other Level II codes and descriptors are approved and maintained jointly by the Alpha-Numeric Editorial Panel.

Level III: The CMS has eliminated Level III local codes. See Program Memorandum AB-02-113.

Headings are provided as a means of grouping similar or closely related items. The placement of a code under a heading does not indicate additional means of classification, nor does it relate to any health insurance coverage categories.

HCPCS also contains modifiers, which are two-position codes and descriptors used to indicate that a service or procedure that has been performed has been altered by some specific circumstance but not changed in its definition or code. Modifiers are grouped by the three levels. Level I modifiers and descriptors are copyrighted by the AMA. Modifiers in the D series are copyrighted by the ADA. **This book does not contain D series modifiers.** They are available directly from the ADA.

HCPCS is designed to promote uniform reporting and statistical data collection of medical procedures, supplies, products, and services.

HCPCS Disclaimer

Inclusion or exclusion of a procedure, supply, product, or service does not imply any health insurance coverage or reimbursement policy.

HCPCS makes as much use as possible of generic descriptions, but the inclusion of brand names to describe devices or drugs is intended only for indexing purposes; it is not meant to convey endorsement of any particular product or drug.

Updating HCPCS

The primary updates are made annually.

Legend
⊙ Special coverage instructions
◆ Not covered by or valid for Medicare
✳ Carrier discretion
◀▶ New
◀▥▥▶ Revised

The revised symbol is placed in front of items with data, payment, or miscellaneous changes.

LEVEL II NATIONAL MODIFIERS

✳ A1   Dressing for one wound

✳ A2   Dressing for two wounds

✳ A3   Dressing for three wounds

✳ A4   Dressing for four wounds

✳ A5   Dressing for five wounds

✳ A6   Dressing for six wounds

✳ A7   Dressing for seven wounds

✳ A8   Dressing for eight wounds

✳ A9   Dressing for nine or more wounds

❂ AA   Anesthesia services performed personally by anesthesiologist

❂ AD   Medical supervision by a physician: more than four concurrent anesthesia procedures MCM 3350.5

❂ AH   Clinical psychologist MCM 2150, MCM 5112

❂ AJ   Clinical social worker MCM 2152, MCM 5113

❂ AM   Physician, team member service MCM 4105.7, Cross Reference QM

✳ AP   Determination of refractive state was not performed in the course of diagnostic ophthalmological examination

✳ AS   Physician assistant, nurse practitioner, or clinical nurse specialist services for assistant at surgery

✳ AT   Acute treatment (this modifier should be used when reporting service 98940, 98941, 98942✳)

✳ AU   Item furnished in conjunction with a urological, ostomy, or tracheostomy supply

✳ AV   Item furnished in conjunction with a prosthetic device, prosthetic or orthotic

✳ AW   Item furnished in conjunction with a surgical dressing

✳ AX   Item furnished in conjunction with dialysis services

✳ BA   Item furnished in conjunction with parenteral enteral nutrition (PEN) services

✳ BO   Orally administered nutrition, not by feeding tube

✳ BP   The beneficiary has been informed of the purchase and rental options and has elected to purchase the item.

✳ BR   The beneficiary has been informed of the purchase and rental options and has elected to rent the item.

✳ BU   The beneficiary has been informed of the purchase and rental options and after 30 days has not informed the supplier of his/her decision.

✳ CA   Procedure payable only in inpatient setting when performed emergently on an outpatient who expires prior to admission

➡✳ CB   Service ordered by a renal dialysis facility (RDF) physician as part of the ESRD beneficiary's dialysis benefit, is not part of the composite rate, and is separately reimbursable

✳ CC   Procedure code change. (Use CC when the procedure code submitted was changed either for administrative reasons or because an incorrect code was filed.)

▶ CD   AMCC test has been ordered by an ESRD facility or MCP physician that is part of the composite rate and is not separately billable

▶ CE   AMCC test has been ordered by an ESRD facility or MCP physician that is a composite rate test but is beyond the normal frequency covered under the rate and is separately reimbursable based on medical necessity

▶ CF   AMCC test has been ordered by an ESRD facility or MCP physician that is not part of the composite rate and is separately billable

✳ E1   Upper left eyelid

✳ E2   Lower left eyelid

✳ E3   Upper right eyelid

✳ E4   Lower right eyelid

❂ EJ   Subsequent claim for a defined course of therapy (e.g., EPO, sodium hyaluronate, infliximab

❂ EM   Emergency reserve supply (for end state renal disease [ESRD] benefit only)

✳ EP   Service provided as part of Medicaid early periodic screening diagnosis and treatment (EPSDT) program

✳ ET   Emergency services

✳ EY   No physician or other licensed health care provider order for this item or service

✳ F1   Left hand, second digit

✳ F2   Left hand, third digit

✳ F3   Left hand, fourth digit

✳ F4   Left hand, fifth digit

✳ F5   Right hand, thumb

✳ F6   Right hand, second digit

✳ F7   Right hand, third digit

✳ F8   Right hand, fourth digit

✳ F9   Right hand, fifth digit

✳ FA   Left hand, thumb

✳ FP   Service provided as part of Medicaid Family Planning Program

✳ G1   Most recent URR reading of less than 60

✳ G2   Most recent URR reading of 60 to 64.9

✳ G3   Most recent URR reading of 65 to 69.9

✳ G4   Most recent URR reading of 70 to 74.9

✳ G5	Most recent URR reading of 75 or greater		GX	Deleted 01/01/02
✳ G6	ESRD patient for whom less than six dialysis sessions have been provided in a month	◆ GY	Item or service statutorily excluded or does not meet the definition of any Medicare benefit
☺ G7	Pregnancy resulting from rape or incest or pregnancy certified by physician as life threatening MCM 2005.1, CIM 35-99	◆ GZ	Item or service expected to be denied as not reasonable or necessary MCM 2000

✳ G5 — Most recent URR reading of 75 or greater

✳ G6 — ESRD patient for whom less than six dialysis sessions have been provided in a month

☺ G7 — Pregnancy resulting from rape or incest or pregnancy certified by physician as life threatening
MCM 2005.1, CIM 35-99

✳ G8 — Monitored anesthesia care (MAC) for deep complex, complicated, or markedly invasive surgical procedure

✳ G9 — Monitored anesthesia care patient who has history of severe cardio-pulmonary condition

✳ GA — Waiver of liability statement on file

✳ GB — Claims being resubmitted for payment because it is no longer covered under a global payment demonstration

☺ GC — This service has been performed in part by a resident under the direction of a teaching physician.
MCM 3350.5, MCM 4116

☺ GE — This service has been performed by a resident without the presence of a teaching physician under the primary care exception.
MCM 4116

✳ GG — Performance and payment of a screening mammogram and diagnostic mammogram on the same patient, same day

✳ GH — Diagnostic mammogram converted from screening mammogram on same day

✳ GJ — "Opt out" physician or practitioner emergency or urgent service

✳ GK — Actual item/service ordered by physician, item associated with GA or GZ modifier

✳ GL — Medically unnecessary upgrade provided instead of standard item, no charge, no Advance Beneficiary Notice (ABN)

✳ GM — Multiple patients on one ambulance trip

✳ GN — Services delivered under an outpatient speech-language pathology plan of care

✳ GO — Services delivered under an outpatient occupational therapy plan of care

✳ GP — Services delivered under an outpatient physical therapy plan of care

✳ GQ — Via asynchronous telecommunications system

☺ GT — Via interactive audio and video telecommunication systems

GU — Deleted 01/01/02

☺ GV — Attending physician not employed or paid under arrangement by the patient's hospice provider
MCM 4175-5

☺ GW — Service not related to the hospice patient's terminal condition
MCM 4175-5

GX — Deleted 01/01/02

◆ GY — Item or service statutorily excluded or does not meet the definition of any Medicare benefit

◆ GZ — Item or service expected to be denied as not reasonable or necessary
MCM 2000

◆ H9 — Court-ordered

◆ HA — Child/adolescent program

◆ HB — Adult program, non geriatric

◆ HC — Adult program, geriatric

◆ HD — Pregnant/parenting women's program

◆ HE — Mental health program

◆ HF — Substance abuse program

◆ HG — Opioid addiction treatment program

◆ HH — Integrated mental health/substance abuse program

◆ HI — Integrated mental health and mental retardation/developmental disabilities program

◆ HJ — Employee assistance program

◆ HK — Specialized mental health programs for high-risk populations

◆ HL — Intern

◆ HM — Less than bachelor degree level

◆ HN — Bachelor's degree level

◆ HO — Master's degree level

◆ HP — Doctoral level

◆ HQ — Group setting

◆ HR — Family/couple with client present

◆ HS — Family/couple without client present

◆ HT — Multi-disciplinary team

◆ HU — Funded by child welfare agency

◆ HV — Funded state addictions agency

◆ HW — Funded by state mental health agency

◆ HX — Funded by county/local agency

◆ HY — Funded by juvenile justice agency

◆ HZ — Funded by criminal justice agency

✳ JW — Drug amount discarded/not administered to any patient

✳ K0 — Lower extremity prosthesis functional Level 0 does not have the ability or potential to ambulate or transfer safely with or without assistance and a prosthesis does not enhance their quality of life or mobility

✳ K1 — Lower extremity prosthesis functional Level 1 has the ability or potential to use a prosthesis for transfers or ambulation on level surfaces at fixed cadence. Typical of the limited and unlimited household ambulator.

✳ K2 — Lower extremity prosthesis functional Level 2 has the ability or potential for ambulation with the ability to traverse low level environmental barriers such as curbs, stairs or uneven surfaces. Typical of the limited community ambulator.

* K3   Lower extremity prosthesis functional Level 3 has the ability or potential for ambulation with variable cadence. Typical of the community ambulator who has the ability to traverse most environmental barriers and may have vocational, therapeutic, or exercise activity that demands prosthetic utilization beyond simple locomotion.

* K4   Lower extremity prosthesis functional Level 4 has the ability or potential for prosthetic ambulation that exceeds the basic ambulation skills, exhibiting high impact, stress, or energy levels, typical of the prosthetic demands of the child, active adult, or athlete.

* KA   Add on option/accessory for wheelchair

* KB   Beneficiary requested upgrade for ABN, more than 4 modifiers identified on claim

▶ KD   Drug or biological infused through DME

▶ KF   Item designated by FDA as Class III device

* KH   Durable medical equipment prosthetics and orthotics supplies (DMEPOS) item, initial claim, purchase or first month rental

* KI   DMEPOS item, second or third month rental

* KJ   DMEPOS item, parenteral enteral nutrition (PEN) pump or capped rental, months four to fifteen

* KM   Replacement of facial prosthesis including new impression/moulage

* KN   Replacement of facial prosthesis using previous master model

* KO   Single drug unit dose formulation

* KP   First drug of a multiple drug unit dose formulation

* KQ   Second or subsequent drug of a multiple drug unit dose formulation

* KR   Rental item, billing for partial month

◎ KS   Glucose monitor supply for diabetic beneficiary not treated with insulin

* KX   Specific required documentation on file

▶* KZ   New coverage not implemented by managed care

* LC   Left circumflex coronary artery

* LD   Left anterior descending coronary artery

* LL   Lease/rental (use the LL modifier when durable medical equipment [DME] rental is to be applied against the purchase price)

* LR   Laboratory round trip
        CIM 65-7

◎ LS   Food and Drug Administration (FDA)–monitored intraocular lens implant

* LT   Left side (used to identify procedures performed on the left side of the body)

* MS   Six-month maintenance and servicing fee for reasonable and necessary parts and labor, which are not covered under any manufacturer or supplier warranty

* NR   New when rented (use the NR modifier when DME which was new at the time of rental is subsequently purchased)

* NU   New equipment

* PL   Progressive addition lenses

* Q2   HCFA/ORD demonstration project procedure/service

* Q3   Live kidney donor surgery and related services

* Q4   Service for ordering/referring physician qualifies as a service exemption

◎ Q5   Service furnished by a substitute physician under a reciprocal billing arrangement
        MCM 3060.6

◎ Q6   Service furnished by a locum tenens physician
        MCM 3060.7

* Q7   One Class A finding

* Q8   Two Class B findings

* Q9   One Class B and two Class C findings

* QA   FDA investigational device exemption

◎ QB   Physician providing service in a rural health professional shortage area (HPSA)
        MCM 3050.3

* QC   Single channel monitoring

* QD   Recording and storage in solid state memory by a digital recorder

* QE   Prescribed amount of oxygen is less than 1 liter per minute (LPM)

* QF   Prescribed amount of oxygen exceeds 4 LPM and portable oxygen is prescribed

* QG   Prescribed amount of oxygen is greater than 4 LPM

* QH   Oxygen-conserving device is being used with an oxygen delivery system

◎ QJ   Services/items provided to a prisoner or patient in state or local custody, however the state or local government, as applicable, meets the requirements in 42 CFR 411.4 (B)

◎ QK   Medical direction of two, three, or four concurrent anesthesia procedures involving qualified individuals
        MCM 3350.5

* QL   Patient pronounced dead after ambulance called

* QM   Ambulance service provided under arrangement by a provider of services

* QN   Ambulance service furnished directly by a provider of services

⊚ QP Documentation is on file showing that the laboratory test(s) was ordered individually or ordered as a CPT-recognized panel other than automated profile codes 80002 to 80019,* G0058, G0059, and G0060
MCM 7517.1

∗ QQ Claim submitted with a written statement of intent

⊚ QS Monitored anesthesia care service
MCM 150181

∗ QT Recording and storage on tape by an analog tape recorder

⊚ QU Physician providing service in an urban HPSA
MCM 3350.3

⊚ QV Item or service provided as routine care in a Medicare qualifying clinical trial
CIM 30-1

∗ QW CLIA-waived test

∗ QX Certified registered nurse anesthetist (CRNA) service: with medical direction by a physician

⊚ QY Medical direction of one CRNA by an anesthesiologist
MCM 3350.5

∗ QZ CRNA service: without medical direction by a physician

∗ RC Right coronary artery

∗ RP Replacement and repair (RP may be used to indicate replacement of DME or orthotic and prosthetic devices that have been in use for sometime.) The claim shows the code for the part, followed by the *RP* modifier and the charge for the part.

∗ RR Rental (use the RR modifier when DME is to be rented)

∗ RT Right side (used to identify procedures performed on the right side of the body

◆ SA Nurse practitioner rendering service in collaboration with a physician

◆ SB Nurse midwife

◆ SC Medically necessary service or supply

◆ SD Services provided by registered nurse with specialized, highly technical home infusion training

◆ SE State and/or federally funded programs/services

∗ SF Second opinion ordered by a professional review organization (PRO) per Section 9401, P.L. 99-272 (100% reimbursement/no Medicare deductible or coinsurance)

∗ SG Ambulatory surgical center (ASC) facility service

◆ SH Second concurrently administered infusion therapy

◆ SJ Third or more concurrently administered infusion therapy

◆ SK Member of high risk population (use only with codes for immunization)

◆ SL State supplied vaccine

▶◆ SM Second surgical opinion

▶◆ SN Third surgical opinion

▶◆ SQ Item ordered by home health

◆ ST Related to trauma or injury

◆ SU Procedure performed in physician's office (to denote use of facility and equipment)

◆ SV Pharmaceuticals delivered to patient's home but not utilized

▶ SW Services provided by a certified diabetic educator

∗ T1 Left foot, second digit

∗ T2 Left foot, third digit

∗ T3 Left foot, fourth digit

∗ T4 Left foot, fifth digit

∗ T5 Right foot, great toe

∗ T6 Right foot, second digit

∗ T7 Right foot, third digit

∗ T8 Right foot, fourth digit

∗ T9 Right foot, fifth digit

∗ TA Left foot, great toe

∗ TC Technical component (Under certain circumstances, a charge may be made for the technical component alone. Under those circumstances the technical component charge is identified by adding modifier TC to the usual procedure number. Technical component charges are institutional charges and not billed separately by physicians. However, portable x-ray suppliers only bill for technical component and should utilize modifier TC. The charge data from portable x-ray suppliers will then be used to build customary and prevailing profiles.)

◆ TD RN

◆ TE LPN/LVN

◆ TF Intermediate level of care

◆ TG Complex/high-tech level of care

◆ TH Obstetrical treatment/services, prenatal or postpartum

◆ TJ Program group, child, and/or adolescent

◆ TK Extra patient or passenger, non-ambulance

◆ TL Early intervention/individualized family services plan (IFSP)

◆ TM Individualized education program (IEP)

◆ TN Rural/outside providers customary service area

◆ TP Medical transport, unloaded vehicle

◆ TQ Basic life support (BLS) transport by a volunteer ambulance provider

◆ TR School-based IEP services provided outside the public school district responsible for the student

◆ TS Follow-up service

- ◆ TT   Individualized service provided to more than one patient in same setting
- ◆ TU   Special payment rate, overtime
- ◆ TV   Special payment rates, holidays/weekends
- ◆ TW   Back-up equipment
- ◆ U1   Medicaid Level of Care 1, as defined by each State
- ◆ U2   Medicaid Level of Care 2, as defined by each State
- ◆ U3   Medicaid Level of Care 3, as defined by each State
- ◆ U4   Medicaid Level of Care 4, as defined by each State
- ◆ U5   Medicaid Level of Care 5, as defined by each State
- ◆ U6   Medicaid Level of Care 6, as defined by each State
- ◆ U7   Medicaid Level of Care 7, as defined by each State
- ◆ U8   Medicaid Level of Care 8, as defined by each State
- ◆ U9   Medicaid Level of Care 9, as defined by each State
- ◆ UA   Medicaid Level of Care 10, as defined by each State
- ◆ UB   Medicaid Level of Care 11, as defined by each State
- ◆ UC   Medicaid Level of Care 12, as defined by each State
- ◆ UD   Medicaid Level of Care 13, as defined by each State
- ✳ UE   Used DME
- ▶◆ UF   Services provided in the morning
- ▶◆ UG   Services provided in the afternoon
- ▶◆ UH   Services provided in the evening
- ▶◆ UJ   Services provided at night
- ▶◆ UK   Services provided on behalf of the client to someone other than the client (collateral relationship)
- ▶✳ UN   Two patients served
- ▶✳ UP   Three patients served
- ▶✳ UQ   Four patients served
- ▶✳ UR   Five patients served
- ▶✳ US   Six or more patients served
- ✳ VP   Aphakic patient

Ambulance Modifiers

Modifiers that are used on claims for ambulance services are created by combining two alpha characters. Each alpha character, with the exception of X, represents an origin (source) code or a destination code. The pair of alpha codes creates one modifier. The first position alpha-code = origin; the second position alpha-code = destination. On form HCFA-1491, used to report ambulance services, Item 12 should contain the origin code and Item 13 should contain the destination code. Origin and destination codes and their descriptions are as follows:

- D   Diagnostic or therapeutic site other than *P* or *H* when these are used as origin codes
- E   Residential, domiciliary, custodial facility (other than an 1819 facility)
- G   Hospital-based dialysis facility (hospital or hospital related)
- H   Hospital
- I   Site of transfer (e.g., airport or helicopter pad) between modes of ambulance transport
- J   Non–hospital-based dialysis facility
- N   Skilled nursing facility (SNF) (1819 facility)
- P   Physician's office (includes HMO non-hospital facility, clinic, etc.)
- R   Residence
- S   Scene of accident or acute event
- X   Destination code only. Intermediate stop at physician's office en route to the hospital (includes non-hospital facility, clinic, etc.)

TRANSPORT SERVICES INCLUDING AMBULANCE (A0000-A0999)

- ◆ A0021   Ambulance service, outside state per mile, transport (Medicaid only) Cross Reference A0030
- ◆ A0080   Non-emergency transportation: per mile—vehicle provided by volunteer (individual or organization), with no vested interest
- ◆ A0090   Non-emergency transportation, per mile—vehicle provided by volunteer (individual or organization), with no vested interest
- ◆ A0100   Non-emergency transportation: taxi
- ◆ A0110   Non-emergency transportation and bus, intra or inter state carrier
- ◆ A0120   Non-emergency transportation: minibus, mountain area transports, or other transportation systems
- ◆ A0130   Non-emergency transportation: wheelchair van
- ◆ A0140   Non-emergency transportation and air travel (private or commercial), intra or inter state
- ◆ A0160   Non-emergency transportation: per mile—caseworker or social worker
- ◆ A0170   Transportation: ancillary: parking fees, tolls, other
- ◆ A0180   Non-emergency transportation: ancillary: lodging—recipient
- ◆ A0190   Non-emergency transportation: ancillary: meals—recipient
- ◆ A0200   Non-emergency transportation: ancillary: lodging—escort
- ◆ A0210   Non-emergency transportation: ancillary: meals—escort
- ⟱✳ A0225   Ambulance service, neonatal transport, base rate, emergency transport, one way

* A0380 BLS mileage (per mile)
         Cross Reference A0425
* A0382 BLS routine disposable supplies
* A0384 BLS specialized service disposable sup-
         plies; defibrillation (used by advanced
         life support [ALS] ambulances and BLS
         ambulances in jurisdictions where de-
         fibrillation is permitted in BLS ambu-
         lances)
* A0390 ALS mileage (per mile)
         Cross Reference A0425
* A0392 ALS specialized service disposable sup-
         plies; defibrillation (to be used only in
         jurisdictions where defibrillation cannot
         be performed in BLS ambulances)
* A0394 ALS specialized service disposable sup-
         plies; intravenous (IV) drug therapy
* A0396 ALS specialized service disposable sup-
         plies; esophageal intubation
* A0398 ALS routine disposable supplies
* A0420 Ambulance waiting time (ALS or BLS),
         one half (½) hour increments

Waiting Time Table

Units	Time	Units	Time
1	½ to 1 hrs.	6	3 to 3½ hrs.
2	1 to 1½ hrs.	7	3½ to 4 hrs.
3	1½ to 2 hrs	8	4 to 4½ hrs.
4	2 to 2½ hrs.	9	4½ to 5 hrs.
5	2½ to 3 hrs.	10	5 to 5½ hrs.

* A0422 Ambulance (ALS or BLS) oxygen and
         oxygen supplies, life-sustaining situa-
         tion
* A0424 Extra ambulance attendant, ALS or BLS
         or air (fixed or rotary winged); (re-
         quires medical review)
* A0425 Ground mileage, per statute mile
* A0426 Ambulance service, advanced life sup-
         port, non-emergency transport, Level 1
         (ALS1)
* A0427 Ambulance service, advanced life sup-
         port, emergency transport, Level 1
         (ALS1-Emergency)
* A0428 Ambulance service, BLS, non-emer-
         gency transport
* A0429 Ambulance service, basic life support,
         emergency transport (BLS-Emergency)
* A0430 Ambulance service, conventional air
         services, transport, one way (fixed
         wing)
* A0431 Ambulance service, conventional air
         services, transport, one way (rotary
         wing)
* A0432 Paramedic intercept (PI), rural area,
         transport furnished by a volunteer am-
         bulance company, which is prohibited
         by state law from billing third-party
         payers
* A0433 Advanced life support, Level 2 (ALS2)
* A0434 Specialty care transport (SCT)

* A0435 Fixed wing air mileage, per statute
         mile
* A0436 Rotary wing air mileage, per statute
         mile
▶* A0800 Ambulance transport provided between
         the hours of 7 pm and 7 am
◆ A0888 Noncovered ambulance mileage, per
         mile (e.g., for miles traveled beyond
         closest appropriate facility)
         MCM 2125
☺ A0999 Unlisted ambulance service
         MCM 2120.1, MCM 2125

MEDICAL AND SURGICAL SUPPLIES (A4000-A8999)

◆ A4206 Syringe with needle, sterile 1 cc, each
◆ A4207 Syringe with needle, sterile 2 cc, each
◆ A4208 Syringe with needle, sterile 3 cc, each
◆ A4209 Syringe with needle, sterile 5 cc or
         greater, each
◆ A4210 Needle-free injection device, each
         CIM 60-9
☺ A4211 Supplies for self-administered injections
         MCM 2049
* A4212 Non-coring needle or stylet with or
         without catheter
◆ A4213 Syringe, sterile, 20 cc or greater, each
  A4214 Deleted 10/01/03
◆ A4215 Needles only, sterile, any size, each
▶☺ A4216 Sterile water/saline, 10 ml
         MCM 2049
▶☺ A4217 Sterile water/saline, 500 ml
         MCM 2049
☺ A4220 Refill kit for implantable infusion pump
         CIM 60-14
* A4221 Supplies for maintenance of drug infu-
         sion catheter, per week (list drug sepa-
         rately)
* A4222 Supplies for external drug infusion
         pump, per cassette or bag (list drug
         separately)
☺ A4230 Infusion set for external insulin pump,
         non-needle cannula type
         CIM 60-14
☺ A4231 Infusion set for external insulin pump,
         needle type
         CIM 60-14
⇒◆ A4232 Syringe with needle for external insulin
         pump, sterile, 3 cc
         CIM 60-14
◆ A4244 Alcohol or peroxide, per pint
◆ A4245 Alcohol wipes, per box
◆ A4246 Betadine or pHisoHex solution, per pint
◆ A4247 Betadine or iodine swabs/wipes, per
         box
▶* A4248 Chlorhexidine containing antiseptic,
         1 ml

◆ A4250   Urine test or reagent strips or tablets (100 tablets or strips)
MCM 2100

� A4253   Blood glucose test or reagent strips for home blood glucose monitor, per 50 strips
CIM 60-11

☼ A4254   Replacement battery, any type, for use with medically necessary home blood glucose monitor owned by patient, each
CIM 60-11

☼ A4255   Platforms for home blood glucose monitor, 50 per box
CIM 60-11

☼ A4256   Normal, low and high calibrator solution/chips
CIM 60-11

∗ A4257   Replacement lens shield cartridge for use with laser skin piercing device, each

☼ A4258   Spring-powered device for lancet, each
CIM 60-11

☼ A4259   Lancets, per box of 100
CIM 60-11

◆ A4260   Levonorgestrel (contraceptive) implants system, including implants and supplies
Medicare Statute 1862a1A

◆ A4261   Cervical cap for contraceptive use
Medicare Statute 1862a1

☼ A4262   Temporary, absorbable lacrimal duct implant, each

☼ A4263   Permanent, long-term, non-dissolvable lacrimal duct implant, each
MCM 15030

☼ A4265   Paraffin, per pound
CIM 60-9

◆ A4266   Diaphragm for contraceptive use

◆ A4267   Contraceptive supply, condom, male, each

◆ A4268   Contraceptive supply, condom, female, each

◆ A4269   Contraceptive supply, spermicide (e.g., foam, gel), each

∗ A4270   Disposable endoscope sheath, each

∗ A4280   Adhesive skin support attachment for use with external breast prosthesis, each

◆ A4281   Tubing for breast pump, replacement

◆ A4282   Adapter for breast pump, replacement

◆ A4283   Cap for breast pump bottle, replacement

◆ A4284   Breast shield and splash protector for use with breast pump, replacement

◆ A4285   Polycarbonate bottle for use with breast pump, replacement

◆ A4286   Locking ring for breast pump, replacement

∗ A4290   Sacral nerve stimulation test lead, each

Vascular Catheters

☼ A4300   Implantable access catheter, (e.g., venous, arterial, epidural subarachnoid, or peritoneal, etc.) external access
MCM 2130

∗ A4301   Implantable access total; catheter, port/reservoir (e.g., venous, arterial, epidural, or subarachnoid, peritoneal etc.)

∗ A4305   Disposable drug delivery system, flow rate of 50 ml or greater per hour

∗ A4306   Disposable drug delivery system, flow rate of 5 ml or less per hour

Incontinence Appliances and Care Supplies

☼ A4310   Insertion tray without drainage bag and without catheter (accessories only)
MCM 2130

☼ A4311   Insertion tray without drainage bag with indwelling catheter, Foley type, two-way latex with coating (Teflon, silicone, silicone elastomer or hydrophilic, etc.)
MCM 2130

☼ A4312   Insertion tray without drainage bag with indwelling catheter, Foley type, two-way, all silicone
MCM 2130

☼ A4313   Insertion tray without drainage bag with indwelling catheter, Foley type, three-way, for continuous irrigation
MCM 2130

☼ A4314   Insertion tray with drainage bag with indwelling catheter, Foley type, two-way latex with coating (Teflon, silicone, silicone elastomer or hydrophilic, etc.)
MCM 2130

☼ A4315   Insertion tray with drainage bag with indwelling catheter, Foley type, two-way, all silicone
MCM 2130

☼ A4316   Insertion tray with drainage bag with indwelling catheter, Foley type, three-way, for continuous irrigation
MCM 2130

A4319   Deleted 12/31/03

☼ A4320   Irrigation tray with bulb or piston syringe, any purpose
MCM 2130

∗ A4321   Therapeutic agent for urinary catheter irrigation

☼ A4322   Irrigation syringe, bulb or piston, each
MCM 2130

A4323   Deleted 12/31/03

∗ A4324   Male external catheter, with adhesive coating, each

∗ A4325   Male external catheter, with adhesive strip, each

☼ **Special coverage instructions**   ◆ **Not covered by or valid for Medicare**   ∗ **Carrier discretion**   ◀▶ **New**   ⬅▦▦➡ **Revised**

➠ ⊘ A4326 Male external catheter specialty type with integral collection chamber, each
MCM 2130

⊘ A4327 Female external urinary collection device; metal cup, each
MCM 2130

⊘ A4328 Female external urinary collection device; pouch, each
MCM 2130

A4329 Deleted 01/01/02

⊘ A4330 Perianal fecal collection pouch with adhesive, each
MCM 2130

✳ A4331 Extension drainage tubing, any type, any length, with connector/adaptor, for use with urinary leg bag or urostomy pouch, each

✳ A4332 Lubricant, individual sterile packet, for insertion of urinary catheter, each

✳ A4333 Urinary catheter anchoring device, adhesive skin attachment, each

✳ A4334 Urinary catheter anchoring device, leg strap, each

⊘ A4335 Incontinence supply; miscellaneous
MCM 2130

⊘ A4338 Indwelling catheter; Foley type, two-way latex with coating (Teflon, silicone, silicone elastomer, or hydrophilic, etc.), each
MCM 2130

⊘ A4340 Indwelling catheter; specialty type (e.g., coudé, mushroom, wing, etc.), each
MCM 2130

⊘ A4344 Indwelling catheter, Foley type, two-way, all silicone, each
MCM 2130A

⊘ A4346 Indwelling catheter; Foley type, three-way for continuous irrigation, each
MCM 2130

⊘ A4347 Male external catheter with or without adhesive, with or without anti-reflux device; per dozen
MCM 2130

✳ A4348 Male external catheter with integral collection compartment, extended wear, (e.g., two per month)

⊘ A4351 Intermittent urinary catheter; straight tip, with or without coating (Teflon, silicone, silicone elastomer, or hydrophilic, etc.), each
MCM 2130

⊘ A4352 Intermittent urinary catheter; coudé (curved) tip, with or without coating (Teflon, silicone, silicone elastomeric, or hydrophilic, etc.), each
MCM 2130

✳ A4353 Intermittent urinary catheter, with insertion supplies

⊘ A4354 Insertion tray with drainage bag but without catheter
MCM 2130

⊘ A4355 Irrigation tubing set for continuous bladder irrigation through a three-way indwelling Foley catheter, each
MCM 2130

External Urinary Supplies

⊘ A4356 External urethral clamp or compression device (not to be used for catheter clamp), each
MCM 2130

⊘ A4357 Bedside drainage bag, day or night, with or without anti-reflux device, with or without tube, each
MCM 2130

⊘ A4358 Urinary drainage bag, leg or abdomen, vinyl, with or without tube, with straps, each
MCM 2130

⊘ A4359 Urinary suspensory without leg bag, each
MCM 2130

A4360 Deleted 12/31/02

Ostomy Supplies

⊘ A4361 Ostomy faceplate, each
MCM 2130A

⊘ A4362 Skin barrier; solid, 4 × 4 or equivalent; each
MCM 2130

A4363 Deleted 01/01/00; Cross Reference A4369, A4370, A4371

✳ A4364 Adhesive, liquid or equal, any type, per ounce (oz)

✳ A4365 Adhesive remover wipes, any type, per 50

▶✳ A4366 Ostomy vent, any type, each

⊘ A4367 Ostomy belt, each
MCM 2130A

✳ A4368 Ostomy filter, any type, each

✳ A4369 Ostomy skin barrier, liquid (spray, brush, etc.), per oz

A4370 Deleted 12/31/02

✳ A4371 Ostomy skin barrier, powder, per oz

✳ A4372 Ostomy skin barrier, solid 4 × 4 or with built-in convexity, each
MCM 2130

✳ A4373 Ostomy skin barrier, with flange (solid, flexible, or accordion), with built-in convexity, any size, each
MCM 2130

A4374 Deleted 12/31/02

✳ A4375 Ostomy pouch, drainable, with faceplate attached, plastic, each

✻ A4376 Ostomy pouch, drainable, with face-plate attached, rubber, each

✻ A4377 Ostomy pouch, drainable, for use on faceplate, plastic, each

✻ A4378 Ostomy pouch, drainable, for use on faceplate, rubber, each

✻ A4379 Ostomy pouch, urinary, with faceplate attached, plastic, each

✻ A4380 Ostomy pouch, urinary, with faceplate attached, rubber, each

✻ A4381 Ostomy pouch, urinary, with faceplate attached, plastic, each

✻ A4382 Ostomy pouch, urinary, for use on faceplate, heavy plastic, each

✻ A4383 Ostomy pouch, urinary, for use on faceplate, rubber, each

✻ A4384 Ostomy faceplate equivalent, silicone ring, each

✻ A4385 Ostomy skin barrier, solid 4 × 4 or equivalent, extended wear, without built-in convexity, each

A4386 Deleted 12/31/02

✻ A4387 Ostomy pouch closed, with barrier attached, with built-in convexity (1 piece), each
MCM 2130

✻ A4388 Ostomy pouch, drainable, with extended wear barrier attached (1 piece), each
MCM 2130

✻ A4389 Ostomy pouch, drainable, with barrier attached, with built-in convexity (1 piece), each
MCM 2130

✻ A4390 Ostomy pouch, drainable, with extended wear barrier attached, with built-in convexity (1 piece), each

✻ A4391 Ostomy pouch, urinary, with extended wear barrier attached (1 piece), each
MCM 2130

✻ A4392 Ostomy pouch, urinary, with standard wear barrier attached, with built-in convexity (1 piece), each

✻ A4393 Ostomy pouch, urinary, with extended wear barrier attached, with built-in convexity (1 piece), each

✻ A4394 Ostomy deodorant for use in ostomy pouch, liquid, per fluid ounce

✻ A4395 Ostomy deodorant for use in ostomy pouch, solid, per tablet

✻ A4396 Ostomy belt with peristomal hernia support

⊘ A4397 Irrigation supply; sleeve, each
MCM 2130

⊘ A4398 Ostomy irrigation supply; bag, each
MCM 2130A

⊘ A4399 Ostomy irrigation supply; cone/catheter, including brush
MCM 2130A

⊘ A4400 Ostomy irrigation set
MCM 2130

⊘ A4402 Lubricant, per ounce
MCM 2130

⊘ A4404 Ostomy ring, each
MCM 2130

⊘ A4405 Ostomy skin barrier, non-pectin based, paste, per ounce
MCM 2130

⊘ A4406 Ostomy skin barrier, pectin-based, paste, per ounce
MCM 2130

⊘ A4407 Ostomy skin barrier, with flange (solid, flexible, or accordion), extended wear, with built-in convexity, 4 x 4 inches or smaller, each
MCM 2130

⊘ A4408 Ostomy skin barrier, with flange (solid, flexible or accordion), extended wear, with built-in convexity, larger than 4 x 4 inches, each
MCM 2130

⊘ A4409 Ostomy skin barrier, with flange (solid, flexible or accordion), extended wear, without built-in convexity, 4 x 4 inches or smaller, each
MCM 2130

⊘ A4410 Ostomy skin barrier, with flange (solid, flexible or accordion), extended wear, without built-in convexity, larger than 4 × 4 inches, each
MCM 2130

⊘ A4413 Ostomy pouch, drainable, high output, for use on a barrier with flange (2 piece system), with filter, each
MCM 2130

⊘ A4414 Ostomy skin barrier, with flange (solid, flexible or accordion), without built-in convexity, 4 × 4 inches or smaller, each
MCM 2130

⊘ A4415 Ostomy skin barrier, with flange (solid, flexible or accordion), without built-in convexity, larger than 4 × 4 inches, each
MCM 2130

▶✻ A4416 Ostomy pouch, closed, with barrier attached, with filter (1 piece), each

▶✻ A4417 Ostomy pouch, closed, with barrier attached, with built-in convexity, with filter (1 piece), each

▶✻ A4418 Ostomy pouch, closed; without barrier attached, with filter (1 piece), each

▶✻ A4419 Ostomy pouch, closed; for use on barrier with non-locking flange, with filter (2 piece), each

▶✻ A4420 Ostomy pouch, closed; for use on barrier with locking flange (2 piece), each

⟼ ◆ A4421 Ostomy supply; miscellaneous
MCM 2130

⊘ A4422 Ostomy absorbent material (sheet/pad/crystal packet) for use in ostomy pouch to thicken liquid stomal output, each
MCM 2130

▶* A4423 Ostomy pouch, closed; for use on barrier with locking flange, with filter (2 piece), each

▶* A4424 Ostomy pouch, drainable, with barrier attached, with filter (1 piece), each

▶* A4425 Ostomy pouch, drainable; for use on barrier with non-locking flange, with filter (2 piece system), each

▶* A4426 Ostomy pouch, drainable; for use on barrier with locking flange (2 piece system), each

▶* A4427 Ostomy pouch, drainable; for use on barrier with locking flange, with filter (2 piece system), each

▶* A4428 Ostomy pouch, urinary, with extended wear barrier attached, with faucet-type tap with valve (1 piece), each

▶* A4429 Ostomy pouch, urinary, with barrier attached, with built-in convexity, with faucet-type tap with valve (1 piece), each

▶* A4430 Ostomy pouch, urinary, with extended wear barrier attached, with built-in convexity, with faucet-type tap with valve (1 piece), each

▶* A4431 Ostomy pouch, urinary; with barrier attached, with faucet-type tap with valve (1 piece), each

▶* A4432 Ostomy pouch, urinary; for use on barrier with non-locking flange, with faucet-type tap with valve (2 piece), each

▶* A4433 Ostomy pouch, urinary; for use on barrier with locking flange (2 piece), each

▶* A4434 Ostomy pouch, urinary; for use on barrier with locking flange, with faucet-type tap with valve (2 piece), each

Miscellaneous Supplies

⊙ A4450 Tape, non-waterproof, per 18 square inches
MCM 2130

⊙ A4452 Tape, waterproof, per 18 square inches
MCM 2130

A4454 Deleted 12/31/02

⊙ A4455 Adhesive remover or solvent (for tape, cement or other adhesive), per ounce
MCM 2130

◆ A4458 Enema bag with tubing, reusable

A4460 Deleted 12/31/02

* A4462 Abdominal dressing holder, each
MCM 2130

A4464 Deleted 12/31/02

* A4465 Non-elastic binder for extremity

⊙ A4470 Gravlee jet washer
MCM 2320, CIM 50-4

⊙ A4480 VABRA aspirator
MCM 2320, CIM 50-4

* A4481 Tracheostoma filter, any type, any size, each

* A4483 Moisture exchanger, disposable, for use with invasive mechanical ventilation

◆ A4490 Surgical stockings above knee length, each
MCM 2079, MCM 2133, CIM 60-9

◆ A4495 Surgical stockings thigh length, each
MCM 2079, MCM 2133, CIM 60-9

◆ A4500 Surgical stockings below knee length, each
MCM 2079, MCM 2133, CIM 60-9

◆ A4510 Surgical stockings full length, each
MCM 2079, MCM 2133, CIM 60-9

◆ A4521 Adult-sized incontinence product, diaper, small size, each
CIM 60-9

◆ A4522 Adult-sized incontinence product, diaper, medium size, each
CIM 60-9

◆ A4523 Adult-sized incontinence product, diaper, large size, each
CIM 60-9

◆ A4524 Adult-sized incontinence product, diaper, extra large size, each
CIM 60-9

◆ A4525 Adult-sized incontinence product, brief, small size, each
CIM 60-9

◆ A4526 Adult-sized incontinence product, brief, medium size, each
CIM 60-9

◆ A4527 Adult-sized incontinence product, brief, large size, each
CIM 60-9

◆ A4528 Adult-sized incontinence product, brief, extra-large size, each
CIM 60-9

◆ A4529 Child-sized incontinence product, diaper, small/medium size, each
CIM 60-9

◆ A4530 Child-sized incontinence product, diaper, large size, each
CIM 60-9

◆ A4531 Child-sized incontinence product, brief, small/medium size, each
CIM 60-9

◆ A4532 Child-sized incontinence product, brief, large size, each
CIM 60-9

◆ A4533 Youth-sized incontinence product, diaper, each
CIM 60-9

◆ A4534 Youth-sized incontinence product, brief, each
CIM 60-9

◆ A4535 Disposable liner/shield for incontinence, each
CIM 60-9

◆ A4536   Protective underwear, washable, any
          size, each
          CIM 60-9

◆ A4537   Under pad, reusable/washable, any
          size, each
          CIM 60-9

➠◆ A4538 Diaper, reusable, provided by a diaper
          service, each diaper
          CIM 60-9

⊘ A4550   Surgical trays
          MCM 15030

◆ A4554   Disposable underpads, all sizes, (e.g.,
          Chux's)
          MCM 2130, CIM 60-9

✳ A4556   Electrodes, (e.g., apnea monitor), per
          pair

✳ A4557   Lead wires, (e.g., apnea monitor), per
          pair

✳ A4558   Conductive paste or gel

✳ A4561   Pessary, rubber, any type

✳ A4562   Pessary, non-rubber, any type

✳ A4565   Slings

◆ A4570   Splint
          MCM 2079

  A4572   Deleted 12/31/02, Cross Reference
          L0210

◆ A4575   Topical hyperbaric oxygen chamber,
          disposable
          CIM 35-10

◆ A4580   Cast supplies (e.g., plaster)
          MCM 2079

◆ A4590   Special casting material (e.g., fiberglass)

✳ A4595   Electrical stimulators supplies, 2-lead,
          per month (e.g. tens, NMES)
          CIM 45-25

Supplies for Respiratory and Oxygen Equipment

✳ A4606   Oxygen probe for use with oximeter
          device, replacement

✳ A4608   Transtracheal oxygen catheter, each

✳ A4609   Tracheal suction catheter, closed sys-
          tem, for less than 72 hours of use, each

✳ A4610   Tracheal suction catheter, closed sys-
          tem, for 72 or more hours of use, each

✳ A4611   Battery, heavy duty; replacement for
          patient-owned ventilator

✳ A4612   Battery cables; replacement for patient-
          owned ventilator

✳ A4613   Battery charger; replacement for pa-
          tient-owned ventilator

✳ A4614   Peak expiratory flow rate meter, hand-
          held

⊘ A4615   Cannula, nasal
          MCM 3312, CIM 60-4

⊘ A4616   Tubing (oxygen), per foot
          MCM 3312, CIM 60-4

⊘ A4617   Mouth piece
          MCM 3312, CIM 60-4

⊘ A4618   Breathing circuits
          MCM 3312, CIM 60-4

⊘ A4619   Face tent
          MCM 3312, CIM 60-4

⊘ A4620   Variable concentration mask
          MCM 3312, CIM 60-4

  A4621   Deleted 12/31/03

  A4622   Deleted 12/31/03

➠◆ A4623 Tracheostomy, inner cannula
          MCM 2130, CIM 65-16

✳ A4624   Tracheal suction catheter, any type,
          other than closed system, each

✳ A4625   Tracheostomy care kit for new trach-
          eostomy

✳ A4626   Tracheostomy cleaning brush, each

◆ A4627   Spacer, bag or reservoir, with or with-
          out mask, for use with metered dose
          inhaler
          MCM 2100

✳ A4628   Oropharyngeal suction catheter, each

✳ A4629   Tracheostomy care kit for established
          tracheostomy

Supplies for Other Durable Medical Equipment

⊘ A4630   Replacement batteries; medically neces-
          sary TENS owned by patient
          CIM 65-8

  A4631   Deleted 12/31/03

◆ A4632   Replacement battery for external infu-
          sion pump, any type, each

✳ A4633   Replacement bulb/lamp for ultraviolet
          light therapy system, each

✳ A4634   Replacement bulb for therapeutic light
          box, tabletop model

⊘ A4635   Underarm pad, crutch, replacement, each
          CIM 60-9

⊘ A4636   Replacement, handgrip, cane, crutch, or
          walker, each
          CIM 60-9

⊘ A4637   Replacement, tip, cane, crutch, walker,
          each
          CIM 60-9

▶✳ A4638 Replacement battery for patient-owned
          ear pulse generator, each

✳ A4639   Replacement pad for infrared heating
          pad system, each

⊘ A4640   Replacement pad for use with medi-
          cally necessary alternating pressure pad
          owned by patient
          MCM 4107.6, CIM 60-9

Supplies for Radiological Procedures

✳ A4641   Supply of radiopharmaceutical diagnos-
          tic imaging agent, not otherwise classi-
          fied
          MCM 15030

* A4642 Supply of satumomab pendetide, radiopharmaceutical diagnostic imaging agent, per dose
MCM 15030

* A4643 Supply of additional high dose contrast material(s) during magnetic resonance imaging (e.g., gadoteridol injection)
MCM 15030

▶ ☺ A4644 Supply of low osmolar contrast material (100 to 199 milligram [mg] of iodine)
MCM 15022, MCM 15030

▶ ☺ A4645 Supply of low osmolar contrast material (200 to 299 mg of iodine)
MCM 15022, MCM 15030

▶ ☺ A4646 Supply of low osmolar contrast material (300 to 399 mg of iodine)
MCM 15022, MCM 15030

☺ A4647 Supply of paramagnetic contrast material (e.g., gadolinium)
MCM 15022, MCM 15030

* A4649 Surgical supply, miscellaneous

Supplies for End State Renal Disease

NOTE: For DME items for ESRD see procedures codes E1550 to E1699.

A4650 Deleted 01/01/02

☺ A4651 Calibrated microcapillary tube, each
MCM 4270

☺ A4652 Microcapillary tube sealant
MCM 4270

* A4653 Peritoneal dialysis catheter anchoring device, belt, each

A4655 Deleted 01/01/02

☺ A4656 Needle, any size, each
MCM 4270

☺ A4657 Syringe, with or without needle, each
MCM 4270

☺ A4660 Sphygmomanometer/blood pressure apparatus with cuff and stethoscope
MCM 4270

☺ A4663 Blood pressure cuff only
MCM 4270

◆ A4670 Automatic blood pressure monitor
MCM 4270, CIM 50-42

▶ ☺ A4671 Disposable cycler set used with cycler dialysis machine, each
MCM 4270

▶ ☺ A4672 Drainage extension line, sterile, for dialysis, each
MCM 4270

▶ ☺ A4673 Extension line with easy lock connectors, used with dialysis
MCM 4270

▶ ☺ A4674 Chemicals/antiseptics solution used to clean/sterilize dialysis equipment, per 8 oz
MCM 4270

☺ A4680 Activated carbon filters for hemodialysis, each
MCM 4270, CIM 55-1

☺ A4690 Dialyzers (artificial kidneys) all types, all sizes, for hemodialysis, each
MCM 4270

A4700 Deleted 01/01/02

A4705 Deleted 01/01/02

☺ A4706 Bicarbonate concentrate, solution, for hemodialysis, per gallon
MCM 4270

☺ A4707 Bicarbonate concentrate, powder, for hemodialysis, per packet
MCM 4270

☺ A4708 Acetate concentrate solution, for hemodialysis, per gallon
MCM 4270

☺ A4709 Acid concentrate, solution, for hemodialysis, per gallon
MCM 4270

A4712 Deleted 12/31/03

☺ A4714 Treated water (deionized, distilled, reverse osmosis) for peritoneal dialysis, per gallon
MCM 4270, CIM 55-1

☺ A4719 "Y set" tubing for peritoneal dialysis
MCM 4270

☺ A4720 Dialysate solution, any concentrate of dextrose, fluid volume greater than 249 cc, but less than or equal to 999 cc, for peritoneal dialysis
MCM 4270

☺ A4721 Dialysate solution, any concentrate of dextrose, fluid volume greater than 999 cc, but less than or equal to 1999 cc, for peritoneal dialysis
MCM 4270

☺ A4722 Dialysate solution, any concentrate of dextrose, fluid volume greater than 1999 cc, but less than or equal to 2999 cc, for peritoneal dialysis
MCM 4270

☺ A4723 Dialysate solution, any concentrate of dextrose, fluid volume greater than 2999 cc, but less than or equal to 3999 cc, for peritoneal dialysis
MCM 4270

☺ A4724 Dialysate solution, any concentrate of dextrose, fluid volume greater than 3999 cc, but less than or equal to 4999 cc, for peritoneal dialysis
MCM 4270

☺ A4725 Dialysate solution, any concentrate of dextrose, fluid volume greater than 4999 cc, but less than or equal to 5999 cc, for peritoneal dialysis
MCM 4270

☺ A4726 Dialysate solution, any concentrate of dextrose, fluid volume greater than 5999 cc, for peritoneal dialysis
MCM 4270

▶* A4728　Dialysate solution, non-dextrose containing, 500 ml

⊛ A4730　Fistula cannulation set for hemodialysis, each
MCM 4270

　A4735　Deleted 01/01/02

⊛ A4736　Topical anesthetic, for dialysis, per gram
MCM 4270

⊛ A4737　Injectable anesthetic, for dialysis, per 10 ml
MCM 4270

⊛ A4740　Shunt accessories for hemodialysis, any type, each
MCM 4270

⊛ A4750　Blood tubing, arterial or venous for hemodialysis, each
MCM 4270

⊛ A4755　Blood tubing, arterial and venous combined, for hemodialysis, each
MCM 4270

⊛ A4760　Dialysate solution test kit, for peritoneal dialysis, any type, each
MCM 4270

⊛ A4765　Dialysate concentrate, powder, additive for peritoneal dialysis, per packet
MCM 4270

⊛ A4766　Dialysate concentrate, solution, additive for peritoneal dialysis, per 10 ml
MCM 4270

⊛ A4770　Blood collection tube, vacuum, for dialysis, per 50
MCM 4270

⊛ A4771　Serum clotting time tube, for dialysis, per 50
MCM 4270

⊛ A4772　Blood glucose test strips, for dialysis, per 50
MCM 4270

⊛* A4773　Occult blood test strips, for dialysis, per 50
MCM 4270

⊛ A4774　Ammonia test strips, for dialysis, per 50
MCM 4270

　A4780　Deleted 01/01/02

　A4790　Deleted 01/01/02

　A4800　Deleted 01/01/02, Cross Reference A4801

　A4801　Deleted 12/31/02, Cross Reference J1644

⊛ A4802　Protamine sulfate, for hemodialysis, per 50 mg
MCM 4270

　A4820　Deleted 01/01/02

　A4850　Deleted 01/01/02, Cross Reference E1637

⊛ A4860　Disposable catheter tips for peritoneal dialysis, per 10

⊛ A4870　Plumbing and/or electrical work for home dialysis equipment

　A4880　Deleted 12/31/01

⊛ A4890　Contracts, repair and maintenance, for hemodialysis equipment
MCM 2100.4

　A4900　Deleted 01/01/02

　A4901　Deleted 01/01/02

　A4905　Deleted 01/01/02

　A4910　Deleted 01/01/02

⊛ A4911　Drain bag/bottle, for dialysis, each

　A4912　Deleted 01/01/02, Cross Reference A4911

⊛ A4913　Miscellaneous dialysis supplies, not otherwise specified

　A4914　Deleted 01/01/02

⊛ A4918　Venous pressure clamp, for hemodialysis, each

　A4919　Deleted 01/01/02

　A4920　Deleted 01/01/02

　A4921　Deleted 01/01/02

⊛ A4927　Gloves, non-sterile, per 100

⊛ A4928　Surgical mask, per 20

⊛ A4929　Tourniquet for dialysis, each

⊛ A4930　Gloves, sterile, per pair

* A4931　Oral thermometer, reusable, any type, each

♦ A4932　Rectal thermometer, reusable, any type, each

Additional Ostomy Supplies

⊛ A5051　Ostomy pouch, closed; with barrier attached (1 piece), each
MCM 2130

⊛ A5052　Ostomy pouch, closed; without barrier attached (1 piece), each
MCM 2130

⊛ A5053　Ostomy pouch, closed; for use on faceplate, each
MCM 2130

⊛ A5054　Ostomy pouch, closed; for use on barrier with flange (2 piece), each
MCM 2130

⊛ A5055　Stoma cap
MCM 2130

⊛ A5061　Ostomy pouch, drainable; with barrier attached (1 piece), each
MCM 2130

⊛ A5062　Ostomy pouch, drainable; without barrier attached (1 piece), each
MCM 2130

⊛ A5063　Ostomy pouch, drainable; for use on barrier with flange (2 piece), each
MCM 2130

　A5064　Deleted 01/01/02

⊛ A5071　Ostomy pouch, urinary; with barrier attached (1 piece), each
MCM 2130

⊛ A5072　Ostomy pouch, urinary; without barrier attached (1 piece), each
MCM 2130

⊛ A5073 Ostomy pouch, urinary; for use on barrier with flange (2 piece), each
MCM 2130
A5074 Deleted 01/01/02
A5075 Deleted 01/01/02
⊛ A5081 Continent device; plug for continent stoma
MCM 2130
⊛ A5082 Continent device; catheter for continent stoma
MCM 2130
⊛ A5093 Ostomy accessory; convex insert
MCM 2130

Additional Incontinence Appliances/Supplies

⊛ A5102 Bedside drainage bottle with or without tubing, rigid or expandable, each
MCM 2130
⊛ A5105 Urinary suspensory; with leg bag, with or without tube
MCM 2130
⊛ A5112 Urinary leg bag; latex
MCM 2130
⊛ A5113 Leg strap; latex, replacement only, per set
MCM 2130
⊛ A5114 Leg strap; foam or fabric, replacement only, per set
MCM 2130

Supplies for Either Incontinence or Ostomy Appliances

⊛ A5119 Skin barrier; wipes, box per 50
MCM 2130
⊛ A5121 Skin barrier; solid, 6 × 6 or equivalent, each
MCM 2130
⊛ A5122 Skin barrier; solid, 8 × 8 or equivalent, each
MCM 2130
A5123 Deleted 12/31/02
⊛ A5126 Adhesive or non-adhesive; disc or foam pad
MCM 2130
⊛ A5131 Appliance cleaner, incontinence and ostomy appliances, per 16 oz
MCM 2130
✳ A5200 Percutaneous catheter/tube anchoring device, adhesive skin attachment

Diabetic Shoes, Fitting and Modifications

⊛ A5500 For diabetics only, fitting (including follow-up), custom preparation and supply of off-the-shelf depth-inlay shoe manufactured to accommodate multi-density insert(s), per shoe
MCM 2134
⊛ A5501 For diabetics only, fitting (including follow-up), custom preparation and supply of shoe molded from cast(s) of patient's foot (custom molded shoe), per shoe
MCM 2134
A5502 Deleted 01/01/02
⊛ A5503 For diabetics only, modification (including fitting) of off-the-shelf depth-inlay shoe or custommolded shoe with roller or rigid rocker bottom, per shoe
MCM 2134
⊛ A5504 For diabetics only, modification (including fitting) of off-the-shelf depth-inlay shoe or custom-molded shoe with wedge(s), per shoe
MCM 2134
⊛ A5505 For diabetics only, modification (including fitting) of off-the-shelf depth-inlay shoe or custom-molded shoe with metatarsal bar, per shoe
MCM 2134
⊛ A5506 For diabetics only, modification (including fitting) of off-the-shelf depth-inlay shoe or custom-molded shoe with offset heel(s), per shoe
MCM 2134
⊛ A5507 For diabetics only, not otherwise specified modification (including fitting) of off-the-shelf depth-inlay shoe or custom-molded shoe, per shoe
MCM 2134
✳ A5508 For diabetics only, deluxe feature of off-the-shelf depth-inlay shoe or custom-molded shoe, per shoe
⊛ A5509 For diabetics only, direct formed, molded to foot with external heat source (e.g., heat gun) multiple density insert(s), prefabricated, per shoe
MCM 2134
⊛ A5510 For diabetics only, direct formed, compression molded to patient's foot without external heat source, multiple-density insert(s) prefabricated, per shoe
MCM 2134
⊛ A5511 For diabetics only, custom-molded from model of patient's foot, multiple density insert(s), custom-fabricated, per shoe
MCM 2134

Dressings

* A6000   Non-contact wound warming wound cover for use with the non-contact wound warming device and warming card

* A6010   Collagen based wound filler, dry form, per gram of collagen

⊙ A6011   Collagen based wound filler, gel/paste, per gram of collagen
     MCM 2079

* A6021   Collagen dressing, pad size 16 square inch (in²) or less, each

* A6022   Collagen dressing, pad size more than 16 in² but less than or equal to 48 in², each

* A6023   Collagen dressing, pad size more than 48 in², each

* A6024   Collagen dressing wound filler, per 6 in

➠ ◆ A6025   Gel sheet for dermal or epidermal application, (e.g., silicon, hydrogel, other), each

* A6154   Wound pouch, each

* A6196   Alginate or other fiber gelling dressing, wound cover, pad size 16 in² or less, each dressing

* A6197   Alginate or other fiber gelling dressing, wound cover, pad size more than 16 in², but less than or equal to 48 in², each dressing

* A6198   Alginate or other fiber gelling dressing, wound cover, pad size more than 48 in², each dressing

* A6199   Alginate or other fiber gelling dressing, wound filler, per 6 in

* A6200   Composite dressing, pad size 16 in² or less, without adhesive border, each dressing

* A6201   Composite dressing, pad size more than 16 in² but less than or equal to 48 in², without adhesive border, each dressing

* A6202   Composite dressing, pad size more than 48 in², without adhesive border, each dressing

* A6203   Composite dressing, pad size 16 in² or less, with any size adhesive border, each dressing

* A6204   Composite dressing, pad size more than 16 in² but less than or equal to 48 in, with any size adhesive border, each dressing

* A6205   Composite dressing, pad size more than 48 in², with any size adhesive, each dressing

* A6206   Contact layer, 16 in² or less, each dressing

* A6207   Contact layer, more than 16 in² but less than or equal to 48 in², each dressing

* A6208   Contact layer, more than 48 in², each dressing

* A6209   Foam dressing, wound cover, pad size 16 in² or less, without adhesive border, each dressing

* A6210   Foam dressing, wound cover, pad size more than 16 in² but less than or equal to 48 in², without adhesive border, each dressing

* A6211   Foam dressing, wound cover, pad size more than 48 in², without adhesive border, each dressing

* A6212   Foam dressing, wound cover, pad size 16 in² or less, with any size adhesive border, each dressing

* A6213   Foam dressing, wound cover, pad size more than 16 in² but less than or equal to 48 in², with any size adhesive border, each dressing

* A6214   Foam dressing, wound cover, pad size more than 48 in², with any size adhesive border, each dressing

* A6215   Foam dressing, wound filler, per gram

* A6216   Gauze, non-impregnated, non-sterile, pad size 16 in² or less, without adhesive border, each dressing

* A6217   Gauze, non-impregnated, non-sterile, pad size more than 16 in² but less than or equal to 48 in², without adhesive border, each dressing

* A6218   Gauze, non-impregnated, non-sterile, pad size more than 48 in², without adhesive border, each dressing

* A6219   Gauze, non-impregnated, pad size 16 in² or less, with any size adhesive border, each dressing

* A6220   Gauze, non-impregnated, pad size more than 16 in² but less than or equal to 48 in², with any size adhesive border, each dressing

* A6221   Gauze, non-impregnated, pad size more than 48 in², with any size adhesive border, each dressing

* A6222   Gauze, impregnated, other than water, normal saline or hydrogel, pad size 16 in² or less, without adhesive border, each dressing

* A6223   Gauze, impregnated, with other than water, normal saline or hydrogel, pad size more than 16 in² but less than or equal to 48 in², without adhesive border, each dressing

* A6224   Gauze, impregnated, other than water or normal saline or hydrogel, pad size more than 48 in², without adhesive border, each dressing

* A6228   Gauze, impregnated, water or normal saline, pad size 16 in² or less, without adhesive border, each dressing

* A6229 Gauze, impregnated, water or normal saline, pad size more than 16 in² but less than or equal to 48 in², without adhesive border, each dressing

* A6230 Gauze, impregnated, water or normal saline, pad size more than 48 in², without adhesive border, each dressing

* A6231 Gauze, impregnated, hydrogel, for direct wound contact, pad size 16 in² or less, each dressing

* A6232 Gauze, impregnated, hydrogel, for direct wound contact, pad size greater than 16 in², but less than or equal to 48 in², each dressing

* A6233 Gauze, impregnated, hydrogel, for direct wound contact, pad size more than 48 in², each dressing

* A6234 Hydrocolloid dressing, wound cover, pad size 16 in² or less, without adhesive border, each dressing

* A6235 Hydrocolloid dressing, wound cover, pad size more than 16 in² but less than or equal to 48 in², without adhesive border, each dressing

* A6236 Hydrocolloid dressing, wound cover, pad size more than 48 in², without adhesive border, each dressing

* A6237 Hydrocolloid dressing, wound cover, pad size 16 in² or less, with any size adhesive border, each dressing

* A6238 Hydrocolloid dressing, wound cover, pad size more than 16 in² but less than or equal to 48 in², with any size adhesive border, each dressing

* A6239 Hydrocolloid dressing, wound cover, pad size more than 48 in², with any size adhesive border, each dressing

* A6240 Hydrocolloid dressing, wound filler, paste, per fluid ounce

* A6241 Hydrocolloid dressing, wound filler, dry form, per gram

* A6242 Hydrogel dressing, wound cover, pad size 16 in² or less, without adhesive border, each dressing

* A6243 Hydrogel dressing, wound cover, pad size more than 16 in² but less than or equal to 48 in², without adhesive border, each dressing

* A6244 Hydrogel dressing, wound cover, pad size more than 48 in², without adhesive border, each dressing

* A6245 Hydrogel dressing, wound cover, pad size 16 in² or less, with any size adhesive border, each dressing

* A6246 Hydrogel dressing, wound cover, pad size more than 16 in² but less than or equal to 48 in², with any size adhesive border, each dressing

* A6247 Hydrogel dressing, wound cover, pad size more than 48 in², with any size adhesive border, each dressing

* A6248 Hydrogel dressing, wound filler, gel, per fluid ounce

* A6250 Skin sealants, protectants, moisturizers, ointments, any type, any size

* A6251 Specialty absorptive dressing, wound cover, pad size 16 in² or less, without adhesive border, each dressing

* A6252 Specialty absorptive dressing, wound cover, pad size more than 16 in² but less than or equal to 48 in², without adhesive border, each dressing

* A6253 Specialty absorptive dressing, wound cover, pad size more than 48 in², without adhesive border, each dressing

* A6254 Specialty absorptive dressing, wound cover, pad size 16 in² or less, with any size adhesive border, each dressing

* A6255 Specialty absorptive dressing, wound cover, pad size more than 16 in² but less than or equal to 48 in², with any size adhesive border, each dressing

* A6256 Specialty absorptive dressing, wound cover, pad size more than 48 in², with any size adhesive border, each dressing

* A6257 Transparent film, 16 in² or less, each dressing

* A6258 Transparent film, more than 16 in² but less than or equal to 48 in², each dressing

* A6259 Transparent film, more than 48 in², each dressing

* A6260 Wound cleansers, any type, any size

* A6261 Wound filler, not elsewhere classified, gel/paste, per fluid ounce

* A6262 Wound filler, not elsewhere classified, dry form, per gram

A6263 Deleted 12/31/02

A6264 Deleted 12/31/02

A6265 Deleted 12/31/02

* A6266 Gauze, impregnated, other than water normal saline, or zinc paste, any width, per linear yard
MCM 2079

* A6402 Gauze, non-impregnated, sterile, pad size 16 in² or less, without adhesive border, each dressing

* A6403 Gauze, non-impregnated, sterile, pad size more than 16 in², less than or equal to 48 in², without adhesive border, each dressing

* A6404 Gauze, non-impregnated, sterile, pad size more than 48 in², without adhesive border, each dressing

A6405 Deleted 12/31/02

A6406 Deleted 12/31/02

▶* A6407 Packing strips, non-impregnated, up to 2 inches in width, per linear yard

⊚ A6410 Eye pad, sterile, each
MCM 2079

⊚ A6411 Eye pad, non-sterile, each
MCM 2079

◆ A6412   Eye patch, occlusive, each
A6421   Deleted 12/31/03
A6422   Deleted 12/31/03
A6424   Deleted 12/31/03
A6426   Deleted 12/31/03
A6428   Deleted 12/31/03
A6430   Deleted 12/31/03
A6432   Deleted 12/31/03
A6434   Deleted 12/31/03
A6436   Deleted 12/31/03
A6438   Deleted 12/31/03
A6440   Deleted 12/31/03

▶✳ A6441   Padding bandage, non-elastic, non-woven/non-knitted, width greater than or equal to three inches and less than five inches, per yard

▶✳ A6442   Conforming bandage, non-elastic, knitted/woven, non-sterile, width less than three inches, per yard

▶✳ A6443   Conforming bandage, non-elastic, knitted/woven, non-sterile, width greater than or equal to three inches and less than five inches, per yard

▶✳ A6444   Conforming bandage, non-elastic, knitted/woven, non-sterile, width greater than or equal to 5 inches, per yard

▶✳ A6445   Conforming bandage, non-elastic, knitted/woven, sterile, width less than three inches, per yard

▶✳ A6446   Conforming bandage, non-elastic, knitted/woven, sterile, width greater than or equal to three inches and less than five inches, per yard

▶✳ A6447   Conforming bandage, non-elastic, knitted/woven, sterile, width greater than or equal to five inches, per yard

▶✳ A6448   Light compression bandage, elastic, knitted/woven, width less than three inches, per yard

▶✳ A6449   Light compression bandage, elastic, knitted/woven, width greater than or equal to three inches and less than five inches, per yard

▶✳ A6450   Light compression bandage, elastic, knitted/woven, width greater than or equal to five inches, per yard

▶✳ A6451   Moderate compression bandage, elastic, knitted/woven, load resistance of 1.25 to 1.34 foot pounds at 50% maximum stretch, width greater than or equal to three inches and less than five inches, per yard

▶✳ A6452   High compression bandage, elastic, knitted/woven, load resistance greater than or equal to 1.35 foot pounds at 50% maximum stretch, width greater than or equal to three inches and less than five inches, per yard

▶✳ A6453   Self-adherent bandage, elastic, non-knitted/non-woven, width less than three inches, per yard

▶✳ A6454   Self-adherent bandage, elastic, non-knitted/non-woven, width greater than or equal to three inches and less than five inches, per yard

▶✳ A6455   Self-adherent bandage, elastic, non-knitted/non-woven, width greater than or equal to five inches, per yard

▶✳ A6456   Zinc paste impregnated bandage, non-elastic, knitted/woven, width greater than or equal to three inches and less than five inches, per yard

☉ A6501   Compression burn garment, bodysuit (head to foot), custom fabricated
MCM 2079

☉ A6502   Compression burn garment, chin strap, custom fabricated
MCM 2079

☉ A6503   Compression burn garment, facial hood, custom fabricated
MCM 2079

☉ A6504   Compression burn garment, glove to wrist, custom fabricated
MCM 2079

☉ A6505   Compression burn garment, glove to elbow, custom fabricated
MCM 2079

☉ A6506   Compression burn garment, glove to axilla, custom fabricated
MCM 2079

☉ A6507   Compression burn garment, foot to knee length, custom fabricated
MCM 2079

☉ A6508   Compression burn garment, foot to thigh length, custom fabricated
MCM 2079

☉ A6509   Compression burn garment, upper trunk to waist including arm openings (vest), custom fabricated
MCM 2079

☉ A6510   Compression burn garment, trunk, including arms down to leg openings (leotard), custom fabricated
MCM 2079

☉ A6511   Compression burn garment, lower trunk including leg openings (panty), custom fabricated
MCM 2079

☉ A6512   Compression burn garment, not otherwise classified
MCM 2079

▶✳ A6550   Dressing set for negative pressure wound therapy electrical pump, stationary or portable, each

▶✳ A6551   Canister set for negative pressure wound therapy electrical pump, stationary or portable, each

RESPIRATORY DURABLE MEDICAL EQUIPMENT, INEXPENSIVE AND ROUTINELY PURCHASED (A7700-A7509)

* A7700 Canister, disposable, used with suction pump, each
* A7001 Canister, non-disposable, used with suction pump, each
* A7002 Tubing, used with suction pump, each
* A7003 Administration set, with small volume nonfiltered pneumatic nebulizer, disposable
* A7004 Small volume nonfiltered pneumatic nebulizer, disposable
* A7005 Administration set, with small volume nonfiltered pneumatic nebulizer, non-disposable
* A7006 Administration set, with small volume filtered pneumatic nebulizer
* A7007 Large volume nebulizer, disposable, unfilled, used with aerosol compressor
* A7008 Large volume nebulizer, disposable, prefilled, used with aerosol compressor
* A7009 Reservoir bottle, nondisposable, used with large volume ultrasonic nebulizer
* A7010 Corrugated tubing, disposable, used with large volume nebulizer, 100 feet
* A7011 Corrugated tubing, non-disposable, used with large volume nebulizer, 10 feet
* A7012 Water collection device, used with large volume nebulizer
* A7013 Filter, disposable, used with aerosol compressor
* A7014 Filter, non-disposable, used with aerosol compressor or ultrasonic generator
* A7015 Aerosol mask, used with DME nebulizer
* A7016 Dome and mouthpiece, used with small volume ultrasonic nebulizer
⊙ A7017 Nebulizer, durable, glass or autoclavable plastic, bottle type, not used with oxygen
CIM 60-9
* A7018 Water, distilled, used with large volume nebulizer, 1000 ml
  A7019 Deleted 12/31/03
  A7020 Deleted 12/31/03
* A7025 High frequency chest wall oscillation system vest, replacement for use with patient-owned equipment, each
* A7026 High frequency chest wall oscillation system hose, replacement for use with patient-owned equipment, each
* A7030 Full face mask used with positive airway pressure device, each
* A7031 Face mask interface, replacement for full-face mask, each

* A7032 Replacement cushion for nasal application device, each
* A7033 Replacement pillows for nasal application device, pair
* A7034 Nasal interface (mask or cannula type) used with positive airway pressure device, with or without head strap
* A7035 Headgear used with positive airway pressure device
* A7036 Chinstrap used with positive airway pressure device
* A7037 Tubing used with positive airway pressure device
* A7038 Filter, disposable, used with positive airway pressure device
* A7039 Filter, non disposable, used with positive airway pressure device
* A7042 Implanted pleural catheter, each
* A7043 Vacuum drainage bottle and tubing for use with implanted catheter
* A7044 Oral interface used with positive airway pressure device, each
▶⊙ A7046 Water chamber for humidifier, used with positive airway pressure device, replacement, each
CIM 60-17
⊙ A7501 Tracheostoma valve, including diaphragm, each
MCM 2130
⊙ A7502 Replacement diaphragm/faceplate for tracheostoma valve, each
MCM 2130
⊙ A7503 Filter holder or filter cap, reusable, for use in a tracheostoma heat and moisture exchange system, each
MCM 2130
⊙ A7504 Filter for use in a tracheostoma heat and moisture exchange system, each
MCM 2130
⊙ A7505 Housing, reusable without adhesive, for use in a heat and moisture exchange system and/or with a tracheostoma valve, each
MCM 2130
⊙ A7506 Adhesive disc for use in a heat and moisture exchange system and/or with tracheostoma valve, any type, each
MCM 2130
⊙ A7507 Filter holder and integrated filter without adhesive, for use in a tracheostoma heat and moisture exchange system, each
MCM 2130
⊙ A7508 Housing and integrated adhesive, for use in a tracheostoma heat and moisture exchange system and/or with a tracheostoma valve, each
MCM 2130

⊘ A7509   Filter holder and integrated filter housing, and adhesive, for use as a tracheostoma heat and moisture exchange system, each
MCM 2130

▶∗ A7520   Tracheostomy/laryngectomy tube, noncuffed, polyvinylchloride (PVC), silicone or equal, each

▶∗ A7521   Tracheostomy/laryngectomy tube, cuffed, polyvinylchloride (PVC), silicone or equal, each

▶∗ A7522   Tracheostomy/laryngectomy tube, stainless steel or equal (sterilizable and reusable), each

▶∗ A7523   Tracheostomy shower protector, each

▶∗ A7524   Tracheostoma stent/stud/button, each

▶∗ A7525   Tracheostomy mask, each

▶∗ A7526   Tracheostomy tube collar/holder, each

ADMINISTRATIVE, MISCELLANEOUS AND INVESTIGATIONAL (A9000-A9999)

NOTE: The following codes do not imply that codes in other sections are necessarily covered.

⊘ A9150   Non-prescription drugs
MCM 2050.5

A9160   Deleted 01/01/02

A9170   Deleted 12/31/01

A9190   Deleted 12/31/01

◆ A9270   Non-covered item or service
MCM 2303

▶◆ A9280   Alert or alarm device, not otherwise classified
Medicare Statute 1861

◆ A9300   Exercise equipment
MCM 2100.1, CIM 60-9

Supplies for Radiology Procedures

⊘ A9500   Supply of radiopharmaceutical diagnostic imaging agent, technetium Tc99m sestamibi, per dose
MCM 15022

⊘ A9502   Supply of radiopharmaceutical diagnostic imaging agent, technetium Tc99m tetrofosmin, per unit dose
MCM 15022

⊘ A9503   Supply of radiopharmaceutical diagnostic imaging agent, technetium Tc99m, medronate, up to 30 mCi
MCM 15022

∗ A9504   Supply of radiopharmaceutical diagnostic imaging agent, technetium Tc99m apcitide
MCM 15022

⊘ A9505   Supply of radiopharmaceutical diagnostic imaging agent, thallous chloride Tl-201, per mCi
MCM 15022

∗ A9507   Supply of radiopharmaceutical diagnostic imaging agent, indium In 111-capromab pendetide, per dose
MCM 15022

⊘ A9508   Supply of radiopharmaceutical diagnostic imaging agent, iobenguane sulfate I-131, per 0.5 mCi
MCM 15030

⊘ A9510   Supply of radiopharmaceutical diagnostic imaging agent, technetium Tc99m disofenin, per vial
MCM 15030

∗ A9511   Supply of radiopharmaceutical diagnostic imaging agent, technetium Tc99m, depreotide, per mCi

∗ A9512   Supply of radiopharmaceutical diagnostic imaging agent, technetium Tc-99m pertechnetate, per mCi

∗ A9513   Supply of radiopharmaceutical diagnostic imaging agent, technetium Tc-99m mebrofenin, per mCi

∗ A9514   Supply of radiopharmaceutical diagnostic imaging agent, technetium Tc-99m pyrophosphate, per mCi

∗ A9515   Supply of radiopharmaceutical diagnostic imaging agent, technetium Tc-99m pentetate, per mCi

∗ A9516   Supply of radiopharmaceutical diagnostic imaging agent, i-123 sodium iodide capsule, per 100 uCi

∗ A9517   Supply of radiopharmaceutical therapeutic imaging agent, I-131 sodium iodide capsule, per mCi

A9518   Deleted 12/31/03, Cross Reference A9530

∗ A9519   Supply of radiopharmaceutical diagnostic imaging agent, technetium Tc-99m macroaggregated albumin, per mCi

∗ A9520   Supply of radiopharmaceutical diagnostic imaging agent, technetium Tc-99m sulfur colloid, per mCi

∗ A9521   Supply of radiopharmaceutical diagnostic imaging agent, technetium Tc-99m exametazime, per dose

⊘ A9522   Supply of radiopharmaceutical diagnostic imaging agent, indium-111 ibritumomab tiuxetan, per mCi
MCM 15022

⊘ A9523   Supply of radiopharmaceutical therapeutic imaging agent, yttrium 90 ibritumomab tiuxetan, per mCi
MCM 15022

⊘ A9524   Supply of radiopharmaceutical diagnostic imaging agent, iodinated I-131 serum albumin, 5 uCi
MCM 15022

▶ ⊕ **A9525** Supply of low or ISO-osmolar contrast material, 10 mg of iodine
MCM 15022, MCM 15030

▶ ⊕ **A9526** Supply of radiopharmaceutical diagnostic imaging agent, ammonia N-13, per dose
CIM 50-36

▶ ✳ **A9528** Supply of radiopharmaceutical diagnostic agent, I-131 sodium iodide capsule, per millicurie

▶ ✳ **A9529** Supply of radiopharmaceutical diagnostic agent, I-131 sodium iodide solution, per millicurie

▶ ✳ **A9530** Supply of radiopharmaceutical therapeutic agent, I-131 sodium iodide solution, per millicurie

▶ ✳ **A9531** Supply of radiopharmaceutical diagnostic agent, I-131 sodium iodide, per microcurie (up to 100 microcuries)

▶ ✳ **A9532** Supply of radiopharmaceutical therapeutic agent, iodinated I-125, serum albumin, 5 microcuries

▶ ✳ **A9533** Supply of radiopharmaceutical diagnostic imaging agent, I-131 tositumomab, per millicurie

▶ ✳ **A9534** Supply of radiopharmaceutical therapeutic imaging agent, I-131 tositumomab, per millicurie

✳ **A9600** Supply of therapeutic radiopharmaceutical, strontium-89 chloride, per mCi

✳ **A9605** Supply of therapeutic radiopharmaceutical, samarium Sm-153 lexidronamm, 50 mCi

✳ **A9699** Supply of radiopharmaceutical therapeutic imaging agent, not otherwise classified

⊕ **A9700** Supply of injectable contrast material for use in echocardiography, per study
MCM 15360

Miscellaneous Service Component

✳ **A9900** Miscellaneous DME supply, accessory, and/or service component of another HCPCS code

✳ **A9901** DME delivery, set up, and/or dispensing service component of another HCPCS code

▶ ✳ **A9999** Miscellaneous DME supply or accessory, not otherwise specified

ENTERAL AND PARENTERAL THERAPY (B4000-B9999)

Enteral Formulae and Enteral Medical Supplies

⊕ **B4034** Enteral feeding supply kit; syringe, per day
MCM 2130, MCM 4450, CIM 65-10

⊕ **B4035** Enteral feeding supply kit; pump fed, per day
MCM 2130, MCM 4450, CIM 65-10

⊕ **B4036** Enteral feeding supply kit; gravity fed, per day
MCM 2130, MCM 4450, CIM 65-10

⊕ **B4081** Nasogastric tubing with stylet
MCM 2130, MCM 4450, CIM 65-10

⊕ **B4082** Nasogastric tubing without stylet
MCM 2130, MCM 4450, CIM 65-10

⊕ **B4083** Stomach tube, Levine type
MCM 2130, MCM 4450, CIM

B4084 Deleted 01/01/02

B4085 Deleted 01/01/02

✳ **B4086** Gastrostomy/jejunostomy tube, any material, any type, (standard or low profile), each

◆ **B4100** Food thickener, administered orally, per ounce

⊕ **B4150** Enteral formulae; category I; semi-synthetic intact protein/protein isolates, administered through an enteral feeding tube at 100 calories = 1 unit
MCM 2130, MCM 4450, CIM 65-10

⊕ **B4151** Enteral formulae; category I: natural intact protein/protein isolates, administered through an enteral feeding tube at 100 calories = 1 unit
MCM 2130, MCM 4450, CIM 65-10

⊕ **B4152** Enteral formulae; category II: intact protein/protein isolates (calorically dense), administered through an enteral feeding tube at 100 calories = 1 unit
MCM 2130, MCM 4450, CIM 65-10

⊕ **B4153** Enteral formulae; category III: hydrolized protein/amino acids, administered through an enteral feeding tube at 100 calories = 1 unit
MCM 2130, MCM 4450, CIM 65-10

⊕ **B4154** Enteral formulae; category IV: defined formula for special metabolic need, administered through an enteral feeding tube at 100 calories = 1 unit
MCM 2130, MCM 4450, CIM 65-10

⊕ **B4155** Enteral formulae; category V: modular components, administered through an enteral feeding tube at 100 calories = 1 unit
MCM 2130, MCM 4450, CIM 65-10

◎ B4156   Enteral formulae; category VI: standardized nutrients, administered through an enteral feeding tube at 100 calories = 1 unit
MCM 2130, MCM 4450, CIM 65-10

Parenteral Nutritional Solutions and Supplies

◎ B4164   Parenteral nutrition solution: carbohydrates (dextrose), 50% or less (500 cc = 1 unit)—home mix
MCM 2130, MCM 4450, CIM 65-10

◎ B4168   Parenteral nutrition solution; amino acid, 3.5% (500 cc = 1 unit)—home mix
MCM 2130, MCM 4450, CIM 65-10

◎ B4172   Parenteral nutrition solution; amino acid, 5.5% through 7% (500 cc = 1 unit)—home mix
MCM 2130, MCM 4450, CIM 65-10

◎ B4176   Parenteral nutrition solution; amino acid, 7% through 8.5% (500 cc = 1 unit)—home mix
MCM 2130, MCM 4450, CIM 65-10

◎ B4178   Parenteral nutrition solution: amino acid, greater than 8.5% (500 cc = 1 unit)—home mix
MCM 2130, MCM 4450, CIM 65-10

◎ B4180   Parenteral nutrition solution; carbohydrates (dextrose), greater than 50% (500 cc = 1 unit)—home mix
MCM 2130, MCM 4450, CIM 65-10

◎ B4184   Parenteral nutrition solution; lipids, 10% with administration set (500 cc = 1 unit)
MCM 2130, MCM 4450, CIM 65-10

◎ B4186   Parenteral nutrition solution, lipids, 20% with administration set (500 cc = 1 unit)
MCM 2130, MCM 4450, CIM 65-10

◎ B4189   Parenteral nutrition solution; compounded amino acid and carbohydrates with electrolytes, trace elements, and vitamins, including preparation, any strength, 10 to 51 gram (gm) of protein—premix
MCM 2130, MCM 4450, CIM 65-10

◎ B4193   Parenteral nutrition solution; compounded amino acid and carbohydrates with electrolytes, trace elements, and vitamins, including preparation, any strength, 52 to 73 gm of protein—premix
MCM 2130, MCM 4450, CIM 65-10

◎ B4197   Parenteral nutrition solution; compounded amino acid and carbohydrates with electrolytes, trace elements and vitamins, including preparation, any strength, 74 to 100 gm of protein—premix
MCM 2130, MCM 4450, CIM 65-10

◎ B4199   Parenteral nutrition solution; compounded amino acid and carbohydrates with electrolytes, trace elements and vitamins, including preparation, any strength, over 100 gm of protein—premix

◎ B4216   Parenteral nutrition additives (vitamins, trace elements, heparin, electrolytes) home mix, per day
MCM 2130, MCM 4450, CIM 65-10

◎ B4220   Parenteral nutrition supply kit; premix, per day
MCM 2130, MCM 4450, CIM 65-10

◎ B4222   Parenteral nutrition supply kit; home mix, per day
MCM 2130, MCM 4450, CIM 65-10

◎ B4224   Parenteral nutrition administration kit, per day
MCM 2130, MCM 4450, CIM 65-10

◎ B5000   Parenteral nutrition solution; compounded amino acid and carbohydrates with electrolytes, trace elements, and vitamins, including preparation, any strength, renal—Amirosyn-RF, NephrAmine, RenAmine—premix
MCM 2130, MCM 4450, CIM 65-10

◎ B5100   Parenteral nutrition solution; compounded amino acid and carbohydrates with electrolytes, trace elements, and vitamins, including preparation, any strength, hepatic—FreAmine HBC, HepatAmine—premix
MCM 2130, MCM 4450, CIM 65-10

◎ B5200   Parenteral nutrition solution; compounded amino acid and carbohydrates with electrolytes, trace elements, and vitamins, including preparation, any strength, stress—branch chain amino acids—premix
MCM 2130, MCM 4450, CIM 65-10

Enteral and Parenteral Pumps

◎ B9000   Enteral nutrition infusion pump, without alarm
MCM 2130, MCM 4450, CIM 65-10

◎ B9002   Enteral nutrition infusion pump, with alarm
MCM 2130, MCM 4450, CIM 65-10

◎ B9004   Parenteral nutrition infusion pump, portable
MCM 2130, MCM 4450, CIM 65-10

◎ B9006   Parenteral nutrition infusion pump, stationary
MCM 2130, MCM 4450, CIM 65-10

◎ B9998   NOC for enteral supplies
MCM 2130, MCM 4450, CIM 65-10

◎ B9999   NOC for parenteral supplies
MCM 2130, MCM 4450, CIM 65-10

C CODES FOR USE ONLY UNDER THE HOSPITAL OUTPATIENT PROSPECTIVE PAYMENT SYSTEM (C1000-C9999)

Note: C-codes are used ONLY as a part of Hospital Outpatient Prospective Payment System (OPPS) and are not to be used to report other services. C-codes are updated quarterly by the Centers for Medicare and Medicaid Services.

C1010   Deleted 12/31/03
C1011   Deleted 12/31/03
C1012   Deleted 12/31/02, Cross Reference P9003
C1013   Deleted 12/31/02, Cross Reference P9031
C1014   Deleted 12/31/02, Cross Reference P9035
C1015-C1018 Deleted 12/31/03
C1019   Deleted 01/01/02
C1020-C1022 Deleted 12/31/03
C1058   Deleted 12/31/02, Cross Reference Q3009
C1064   Deleted 12/31/02
C1065   Deleted 12/31/02
C1066   Deleted 12/31/02, Cross Reference A4642
⊗ C1079   Supply of radiopharmaceutical diagnostic imaging agent, cyanocobalamin Co-58/57, per 0.5 mCi
Medicare Statute 1833(t)
▶⊗ C1080   Supply of radiopharmaceutical diagnostic imaging agent, I-131 tositumomab, per dose
▶⊗ C1081   Supply of radiopharmaceutical therapeutic imaging agent, I-131 tositumomab, per dose
▶⊗ C1082   Supply of radiopharmaceutical diagnostic imaging agent, indium-111 ibritumomab tiuxetan, per dose
▶⊗ C1083   Supply of radiopharmaceutical therapeutic imaging agent, Yttrium 90 ibritumomab tiuxetan, per dose
C1087   Deleted 12/31/02
⊗ C1088   Laser optic treatment system, Indigo LaserOptic Treatment System
Medicare Statute 1833(t)
C1090   Deleted 01/01/02
⊗ C1091   Supply of radiopharmaceutical diagnostic imaging agent, indium-111 oxyquinoline, per 0.5 mCi
Medicare Statute 1833(t)
⊗ C1092   Supply of radiopharmaceutical diagnostic imaging agent, indium-111 pentetate, per 0.5 mCi
Medicare Statute 1833(t)
C1094   Deleted 12/31/02
C1095   Deleted 01/01/02
C1096   Deleted 12/31/02

C1097   Deleted 12/31/02
C1098   Deleted 12/31/02
C1099   Deleted 12/31/02
⊗ C1122   Supply of radiopharmaceutical diagnostic imaging agent, technetium Tc99m arcitumomab, per vial
Medicare Statute 1833(t)
C1166   Deleted 12/31/03
C1167   Deleted 12/31/03
⊗ C1178   Injection, bisulfan, per 6 mg
Medicare Statute 1833(t)
C1188   Deleted 12/31/02
⊗ C1200   Supply of radiopharmaceutical diagnostic imaging agent, technetium Tc99m sodium glucoheptonate, per vial
Medicare Statute 1833(t)
⊗ C1201   Supply of radiopharmaceutical diagnostic imaging agent, technetium Tc99m succimer, per vial
Medicare Statute 1833(t)
C1202   Deleted 12/31/02
C1207   Deleted 06/30/03
⊗ C1300   Hyperbaric oxygen under pressure, full body chamber, per 30-minute, TVL SQ01
Medicare Statute 1833(t)
⊗ C1305   Apligraf, per 44 sqare centimeter (cm²)
Medicare Statute 1833(t)
C1348   Deleted 12/31/02
▶⊗ C1713   Anchor/Screw for opposing bone-to-bone or soft tissue-to-bone (implantable)
Medicare Statute 1833(t)
▶⊗ C1714   Catheter, transluminal atherectomy, directional
Medicare Statute 1833(t)
▶⊗ C1715   Brachytherapy needle
Medicare Statute 1833(t)
➡⊗ C1716   Brachytherapy seed source, gold-198
Medicare Statute 1833(t)
▶⊗ C1717   Brachytherapy seed, high dose rate iridium 192
Medicare Statute 1833(t)
➡⊗ C1718   Brachytherapy source, iodine 125
Medicare Statute 1833(t)
➡⊗ C1719   Brachytherapy source, non-high dose rate iridium-192
Medicare Statute 1833(t)
➡⊗ C1720   Brachytherapy source, palladium 103
Medicare Statute 1833(t)
▶⊗ C1721   Cardioverter-defibrillator, dual chamber (implantable)
Medicare Statute 1833(t)
▶⊗ C1722   Cardioverter-defibrillator, single chamber (implantable)
Medicare Statute 1833(t)
▶⊗ C1724   Catheter, transluminal atherectomy, rotational
Medicare Statute 1833(t)

▶ ✪ C1725 Catheter, transluminal angioplasty, non-laser (may include guidance, infusion/perfusion capability)
Medicare Statute 1833(t)

▶ ✪ C1726 Catheter, balloon dilatation, non-vascular
Medicare Statute 1833(t)

▶ ✪ C1727 Catheter, balloon tissue dissector, non-vascular (insertable)
Medicare Statute 1833(t)

▶ ✪ C1728 Catheter, brachytherapy seed administration
Medicare Statute 1833(t)

▶ ✪ C1729 Catheter, drainage
Medicare Statute 1833(t)

▶ ✪ C1730 Catheter, electrophysiology, diagnostic, other than 3D mapping (19 or fewer electrodes)
Medicare Statute 1833(t)

▶ ✪ C1731 Catheter, electrophysiology, diagnostic, other than 3D mapping (20 or more electrodes)
Medicare Statute 1833(t)

▶ ✪ C1732 Catheter, electrophysiology, diagnostic/ablation, 3D or vector mapping
Medicare Statute 1833(t)

▶ ✪ C1733 Catheter, electrophysiology, diagnostic/ablation, orther than 3D or vector mapping, other than cool-tip
Medicare Statute 1833(t)

▶ ✪ C1750 Catheter, hemodialysis, long term
Medicare Statute 1833(t)

▶ ✪ C1751 Catheter, infusion, inserted peripherally, centrally or midline (other than hemodialysis)
Medicare Statute 1833(t)

▶ ✪ C1752 Catheter, hemodialysis, short term
Medicare Statute 1833(t)

▶ ✪ C1753 Catheter, intravascular ultrasound
Medicare Statute 1833(t)

▶ ✪ C1754 Catheter, intradiscal
Medicare Statute 1833(t)

▶ ✪ C1755 Catheter, instraspinal
Medicare Statute 1833(t)

▶ ✪ C1756 Catheter, pacing transesophageal
Medicare Statute 1833(t)

▶ ✪ C1757 Catheter, thrombectomy/embolectomy
Medicare Statute 1833(t)

▶ ✪ C1758 Catheter, ureteral
Medicare Statute 1833(t)

▶ ✪ C1759 Catheter, intracardiac echocardiography
Medicare Statute 1833(t)

▶ ✪ C1760 Closure device, vascular (implantable/insertable)
Medicare Statute 1833(t)

▶ ✪ C1762 Connective tissue, human (includes fascia lata)
Medicare Statute 1833(t)

▶ ✪ C1763 Connective tissue, non-human (includes synthetic)
Medicare Statute 1833(t)

▶ ✪ C1764 Event recorder, cardiac (implantable)
Medicare Statute 1833(t)

✪ C1765 Adhesion barrier
Medicare Statute 1833 (t)

▶ ✪ C1766 Introduction/sheath, guiding, intracardiac electrophysiological steerable, other than peel-away
Medicare Statute 1833(t)

▶ ✪ C1767 Generator, neurostimulator (implantable)
Medicare Statute 1833(t)

▶ ✪ C1768 Graft, vascular
Medicare Statute 1833(t)

▶ ✪ C1769 Guidewire
Medicare Statute 1833(t)

▶ ✪ C1770 Imaging coil, magnetic reasonance (insertable)
Medicare Statute 1833(t)

▶ ✪ C1771 Repair device, urinary, incontinence, with sling graft
Medicare Statute 1833(t)

▶ ✪ C1772 Infusion pump, programmable (implantable)
Medicare Statute 1833(t)

▶ ✪ C1773 Retrieval device, insertable (used to retrieve fractured medical devices)
Medicare Statute 1833(t)

C1774 Deleted 12/31/03

✪ C1775 Supply of radiopharmaceutical diagnostic imaging agent, fluorodeoxyglucose f18 (2-deoxy-2-[18f] fluoro-d-glucose), per dose (4-40 mCi/ml)
Medicare Statute 1833(t)

▶ ✪ C1776 Joint device (implantable)
Medicare Statute 1833(t)

▶ ✪ C1777 Lead, cardioverter-defibrillator, endocardial single coil (implantable)
Medicare Statute 1833(t)

▶ ✪ C1778 Lead, neurostimulator (implantable)
Medicare Statute 1833(t)

▶ ✪ C1779 Lead, pacemaker, trasvenous VDD single pass
Medicare Statute 1833(t)

▶ ✪ C1780 Lens, intraocular (new technology)
Medicare Statute 1833(t)

▶ ✪ C1781 Mesh (implantable)
Medicare Statute 1833(t)

▶ ✪ C1782 Morcellator
Medicare Statute 1833(t)

▶ ✪ C1783 Ocular implant, aqueous drainage assist device
Medicare Statute 1833(t)

▶ ✪ C1784 Ocular device, intraoperative, detached retina
Medicare Statute 1833(t)

▶ ✪ C1785 Pacemaker, dual chamber, rate-responsive (implantable)
Medicare Statute 1833(t)

▶ ✪ C1786 Pacemaker, single chamber, rate-responsive (implantable)
Medicare Statute 1833(t)

▶ ⊙ C1787 Patient programmer, neurostimulator
Medicare Statute 1833(t)

▶ ⊙ C1788 Port, indwelling (implantable)
Medicare Statute 1833(t)

▶ ⊙ C1789 Prosthesis, breast (implantable)
Medicare Statute 1833(t)

▶ ⊙ C1813 Prosthesis, penile, inflatable
Medicare Statute 1833(t)

▶ ⊙ C1814 Retinal tamponade device, silicone oil
Medicare Statute 1833(t)

▶ ⊙ C1815 Prosthesis, urinary sphincter (implantable)
Medicare Statute 1833(t)

▶ ⊙ C1816 Receiver and/or transmitter, neurostimulator (implantable)
Medicare Statute 1833(t)

▶ ⊙ C1817 Septal defect implant system, intracardiac
Medicare Statute 1833(t)

▶ ⊙ C1818 Integrated keratoprosthesic
Medicare Statute 1833(t)

▶ ⊙ C1819 Surgical tissue localization and excision device (implantable)
Medicare Statute 1833(t)

▶ ⊙ C1874 Stent, coated/covered, with delivery system
Medicare Statute 1833(t)

▶ ⊙ C1875 Stent, coated/covered, without delivery system
Medicare Statute 1833(t)

▶ ⊙ C1876 Stent, non-coated/non-covered, with delivery system
Medicare Statute 1833(t)

▶ ⊙ C1877 Stent, non-coated/non-covered, without delivery system
Medicare Statute 1833(t)

▶ ⊙ C1878 Material for vocal cord medialization, synthetic (implantable)
Medicare Statute 1833(t)

▶ ⊙ C1879 Tissue marker (implantable)
Medicare Statute 1833(t)

▶ ⊙ C1880 Vena cava filter
Medicare Statute 1833(t)

▶ ⊙ C1881 Dialysis access system (implantable)
Medicare Statute 1833(t)

▶ ⊙ C1882 Cardioverter-defibrillator, other than single or dual chamber (implantable)
Medicare Statute 1833(t)

▶ ⊙ C1883 Adaptor/Extension, pacing lead or neurostimulator lead (implantable)
Medicare Statute 1833(t)

▶ ⊙ C1884 Embolization protection system
Medicare Statute 1833(t)

▶ ⊙ C1885 Catheter, transluminal angioplasty, laser
Medicare Statute 1833(t)

▶ ⊙ C1887 Catheter, guiding (may include infusion/perfusion capability)
Medicare Statute 1833(t)

⊙ C1888 Catheter, ablation, non-cardiac, endovascular (implantable)
Medicare Statute 1833(t)

▶ ⊙ C1891 Infusion pump, on-programmable, permanent (implantable)
Medicare Statute 1833(t)

▶ ⊙ C1892 Introducer/sheath, guiding, intracardiac electrophysiological, fixed-curve, peel-away
Medicare Statute 1833(t)

▶ ⊙ C1893 Introducer/Sheath, guiding, intracardiac electrophysiological, fixed-curve, other than peel-away
Medicare Statute 1833(t)

▶ ⊙ C1894 Introducer/Sheath, other than guiding, intracardiac electrophysiological, non-laser
Medicare Statute 1833(t)

▶ ⊙ C1895 Lead, cardioverter-defibrillator, endocardial dual coil (implantable)
Medicare Statute 1833(t)

▶ ⊙ C1896 Lead, cardioverter-defibrillator, other than endocardial single or dual coil (implantable)
Medicare Statute 1833(t)

▶ ⊙ C1897 Lead, neurostimulator test kit (implantable)
Medicare Statute 1833(t)

▶ ⊙ C1898 Lead, pacemaker, other than transvenous VDD single pass
Medicare Statute 1833(t)

▶ ⊙ C1899 Lead, pacemaker/cardioverter-defibrillator combination (implantable)
Medicare Statute 1833(t)

⊙ C1900 Lead, left ventricular coronary venous system
Medicare Statute 1833(t)

⊙ C2614 Probe, percutaneous lumbar disectomy
Medicare Statute 1833(t)

▶ ⊙ C2615 Sealant, pulmonary, liquid
Medicare Statute 1833(t)

➠ ⊙ C2616 Brachytherapy source, yttrium-90
Medicare Statute 1833(T)

▶ ⊙ C2617 Stent, non-coronary, temporary, without delivery system
Medicare Statute 1833(t)

⊙ C2618 Probe, cryoablation
Medicare Statute 1833(t)

▶ ⊙ C2619 Pacemaker, dual chamber, non-rate-responsiveness (implantable)
Medicare Statute 1833(t)

▶ ⊙ C2620 Pacemaker, single chamber, non-rate-responsiveness (implantable)
Medicare Statute 1833(t)

▶ ⊙ C2621 Pacemaker, other than single or dual chamber (implantable)
Medicare Statute 1833(t)

▶ ⊙ C2622 Prosthesis, penile, non-inflatable
Medicare Statute 1833(t)

▶ ⊙ C2625 Stent, non-coronary, temporary, with delivery system
Medicare Statute 1833(t)

▶ ⊙ C2626 Infusion pump, non-programmable, temporary (implantable)
Medicare Statute 1833(t)

▶ ✪ C2627 Catheter, suprapubic/cystoscopic
Medicare Statute 1833(t)

▶ ✪ C2628 Catheter, occlusion
Medicare Statute 1833(t)

▶ ✪ C2629 Introducer/Sheath, other than guiding, intracaradiac electrophysiological, laser
Medicare Statute 1833(t)

▶ ✪ C2630 Catheter, electrophysiology, diagnostic/ablation, other than 3D or vector mapping, cool-tip
Medicare Statute 1833(t)

▶ ✪ C2631 Repair device, urinary, incontinence, without sling graft
Medicare Statute 1833(t)

✪ C2632 Brachytherapy solution, iodine-125, per mCi
Medicare Statute 1833(t)

▶ ✪ C2633 Brachytherapy source, Cesium-131
Medicare Statute 1833(t)

✪ C8900 Magnetic resonance angiography (MRA) with contrast, abdomen
Medicare Statute 1833(t)(2)

✪ C8901 MRA without contrast, abdomen
Medicare Statute 1833(t)(2)

✪ C8902 MRA without contrast followed by with contrast, abdomen
Medicare Statute 1833(t)(2)

✪ C8903 Magnetic resonance imaging (MRI) with contrast, breast; unilateral
Medicare Statute 1833(t)(2)

✪ C8904 MRI without contrast, breast; unilateral
Medicare Statute 1833(t)(2)

✪ C8905 MRI without contrast followed by with contrast, breast; unilateral
Medicare Statute 1833(t)(2)

✪ C8906 MRI with contrast, breast; bilateral
Medicare Statute 1833(t)(2)

✪ C8907 MRI without contrast, breast; bilateral
Medicare Statute 1833(t)(2)

✪ C8908 MRI without contrast followed by with contrast, breast; bilateral
Medicare Statute 1833(t)(2)

✪ C8909 MRA with contrast, chest (excluding myocardium)
Medicare Statute 1833(t)(2)

✪ C8910 MRA without contrast, chest (excluding myocardium)
Medicare Statute 1833(t)(2)

✪ C8911 MRA without contrast followed by with contrast, chest (excluding myocardium)
Medicare Statute 1833(t)(2)

✪ C8912 MRA with contrast, lower extremity
Medicare Statute 1833(t)(2)

✪ C8913 MRA without contrast, lower extremity
Medicare Statute 1833(t)(2)

✪ C8914 MRA without contrast followed by with contrast, lower extremity
Medicare Statute 1833(t)(2)

▶ ✪ C8918 Magnetic resonance angiography with contrast, pelvis
Medicare Statute 430 BIPA

▶ ✪ C8919 Magnetic resonance angiography without contrast, pelvis
Medicare Statute 430 BIPA

▶ ✪ C8920 Magnetic resonance angiography without contrast followed by with contrast, pelvis
Medicare Statute 430 BIPA

✪ C9000 Injection, sodium chromate Cr51, per 0.25 mCi
Medicare Statute 1833(t)

✪ C9003 Palivizumab-RSV-IGM, per 50 mg
Medicare Statute 1833(t)

✪ C9007 Baclofen intrathecal screening kit (1 amp)
Medicare Statute 1833(t)

✪ C9008 Baclofen intrathecal refill kit, per 500 micrograms (mcg)
Medicare Statute 1833(t)

✪ C9009 Baclofen intrathecal refill kit, per 2000 mcg
Medicare Statute 1833(t)

C9010 Deleted 12/31/03

✪ C9013 Supply of cobaltous chloride Co 57, radiopharmaceutical diagnostic imaging agent
Medicare Statute 1833(t)(2)

C9018 Deleted 01/01/02

C9019 Deleted 12/31/02, Cross Reference J0637

C9020 Deleted 01/01/02, Cross Reference J7520

C9100 Deleted 12/31/02

✪ C9102 Supply of radiopharmaceutical diagnostic imaging agent, 51-sodium chromate, per 50 mCi
Medicare Statute 1833(t)

✪ C9103 Supply of radiopharmaceutical diagnostic imaging agent, sodium iothalamate I-125 injection, per 10 mCi
Medicare Statute 1833(t)

C9104 Deleted 01/01/02

✪ C9105 Injection, hepatitis B immune globulin, per 1 ml
Medicare Statute 1833(t)

C9108 Deleted 12/31/02, Cross Reference J3240

✪ C9109 Injection, tirofiban HCl, 6.25 mg
Medicare Statute 1833(t)

C9110 Deleted 12/31/02, Cross Reference J9010

C9111 Deleted 12/31/03

✪ C9112 Injection, perflutren lipid microsphere, per 2 ml vial
Medicare Statute 1833(t)

✪ C9113 Injection, pantoprazole sodium, per vial
Medicare Statute 1833(t)

C9114 Deleted 12/31/02, Cross Reference J2324

C9115 Deleted 12/31/02 Cross Reference J3487

C9116 Deleted 12/31/03

C9117 Deleted 12/31/02, Cross Reference A9523

C9118 Deleted 12/31/02, Cross Reference A9522

C9119 Deleted 6/30/03

C9120 Deleted 12/31/03

⊛ C9121 Injection, argatroban, per 5 mg Medicare Statute 1833(t)

▶⊛ C9123 Transcyte, per 247 square centimeters Medicare Statute 1833(t)

⊛ C9200 Orcel, per 36 cm² Medicare Statute 1833(t)

⊛ C9201 Dermagraft, per 37.5 cm² Medicare Statute 1833(t)

▶⊛ C9202 Injection, suspension of microspheres of human serum albumin with octafluoropropane, per 3 ml Medicare Statute 1833(t)

▶⊛ C9203 Injection, perflexane lipid microspheres, per 10 ml vial Medicare Statute 1833(t)

C9204 Deleted 12/31/03

▶⊛ C9205 Injection, oxaliplatin, per 5 mg Medicare Statute 1833(t)

▶⊛ C9207 Injection, bortezomib, per 3.5 mg Medicare Statute 1833(t)

▶⊛ C9208 Injection, agalsidase beta, per 1 mg Medicare Statute 1833(t)

▶⊛ C9209 Injection, laronidase, per 2.9 mg Medicare Statute 1833(t)

▶⊛ C9210 Injection, palonesetron hydrochloride, per 250 mcg Medicare Statute 1833(t)

▶⊛ C9211 Injection, alefacept, for intravenous use, per 7.5 mg Medicare Statute 1833(t)

▶⊛ C9212 Injection, alefacept, for intramuscular use, per 7.5 mg Medicare Statute 1833(t)

C9503 Deleted 12/31/03

⊛ C9701 STRETTA system Medicare Statute 1833(t)

⊛ C9703 Bard endoscopic suturing system Medicare Statute 1833(t)

▶⊛ C9704 Injection or insertion of inert substance for submucosal/intramuscular injection(s) into the upper gastrointestinal tract, under fluoroscopic guidance Medicare Statute 1833(t)

C9708 Deleted 12/31/02

C9711 Deleted 12/31/03

DENTAL PROCEDURES (D0000-D9999)

Codes D0100-D9999 are dental codes copyrighted to the ADA. A copy of the Current Dental Terminology (CDT), which contains all of the dental codes, can be purchased from the ADA.

DURABLE MEDICAL EQUIPMENT (E0100-E9999)

Canes

⊛ E0100 Cane, includes canes of all materials, adjustable or fixed, with tip MCM 2100.1, CIM 60-3, CIM 60-9

⊛ E0105 Cane, quad or three prong, includes canes of all materials, adjustable or fixed, with tips MCM 2100.1, CIM 60-9, CIM 60-15

Crutches

⊛ E0110 Crutches, forearm, includes crutches of various materials, adjustable or fixed, pair, complete with tips and handgrips MCM 2100.1, CIM 60-9

⊛ E0111 Crutches, forearm, includes crutches of various materials, adjustable or fixed, each, with tips and handgrips MCM 2100.1, CIM 60-9

⊛ E0112 Crutches, underarm, wood, adjustable or fixed, pair, with pads, tips and handgrips MCM 2100.1, CIM 60-9

⊛ E0113 Crutches, underarm, wood, adjustable or fixed, each, with pads, tips and handgrip MCM 2100.1, CIM 60-9

⊛ E0114 Crutches, underarm, other than wood, adjustable or fixed, pair, with pads, tips and handgrips MCM 2100.1, CIM 60-9

⊛ E0116 Crutches, underarm, other than wood, adjustable or fixed, each, with pads, tips and handgrips MCM 2100.1, CIM 60-9

⊛ E0117 Crutch, underarm, articulating, spring assisted, each MCM 2100.1

▶✱ E0118 Crutch substitute, lower leg platform, with or without wheels, each

Walkers

⊛ E0130 Walker, rigid (pickup), adjustable or fixed height MCM 2100.1, CIM 60-9

⊛ E0135 Walker, folding (pickup), adjustable or fixed height MCM 2100.1, CIM 60-9

▶⊛ E0140 Walker, with trunk support, adjustable or fixed height, any type MCM 2100.1, CIM 60-9

⇒⊛ E0141 Walker, rigid, wheeled, adjustable or fixed height MCM 2100.1, CIM 60-9

E0142   Deleted 12/31/02

➡ ✪ E0143   Walker, folding, wheeled, adjustable or fixed height
      MCM 2100.1, CIM 60-9

➡ ✪ E0144   Walker, enclosed, four-sided framed, rigid or folding, wheeled, with posterior seat
      MCM 2100.1, CIM 60-9

E0145   Deleted 12/31/03

E0146   Deleted 12/31/03

➡ ✪ E0147   Walker, heavy duty, multiple braking system, variable wheel resistance
      MCM 2100.1, CIM 60-9

✳ E0148   Walker, heavy duty, without wheels, rigid or folding, any type, each

➡ ✳ E0149   Walker, heavy duty, wheeled, rigid or folding, any type

✳ E0153   Platform attachment, forearm crutch, each

✳ E0154   Platform attachment, walker, each

✳ E0155   Wheel attachment, rigid pick-up walker, per pair

Attachments

✳ E0156   Seat attachment, walker

✳ E0157   Crutch attachment, walker, each

✳ E0158   Leg extensions for a walker, per set of four (4)

✳ E0159   Brake attachment for wheeled walker, replacement, each

Commodes

✪ E0160   Sitz type bath or equipment, portable, used with or without commode
      CIM 60-9

✪ E0161   Sitz type bath or equipment, portable, used with or without commode, with faucet attachment/s
      CIM 60-9

✪ E0162   Sitz bath chair
      CIM 60-9

✪ E0163   Commode chair, stationary, with fixed arms
      MCM 2100.1, CIM 60-9

✪ E0164   Commode chair, mobile, with fixed arms
      MCM 2100.1, CIM 60-9

E0165   Deleted 12/31/03

✪ E0166   Commode chair, mobile, with detachable arms
      MCM 2100.1, CIM 60-9

✪ E0167   Pail or pan for use with commode chair
      CIM 60-9

✳ E0168   Commode chair, extra wide and/or heavy duty, stationary or mobile, with or without arms, any type, each

✳ E0169   Commode chair with seat lift mechanism

✳ E0175   Foot rest, for use with commode chair, each

Decubitus Care Equipment

✪ E0176   Air pressure pad or cushion, nonpositioning
      CIM 60-9

✪ E0177   Water pressure pad or cushion, nonpositioning
      CIM 60-9

✪ E0178   Gel or gel-like pressure pad or cushion, nonpositioning
      CIM 60-9

✪ E0179   Dry pressure pad or cushion, nonpositioning
      CIM 60-9

✪ E0180   Pressure pad, alternating with pump
      MCM 4107.6, CIM 60-9

✪ E0181   Pressure pad, alternating with pump, heavy duty
      MCM 4107.6, CIM 60-9

✪ E0182   Pump for alternating pressure pad
      MCM 4107.6, CIM 60-9

✪ E0184   Dry pressure mattress
      MCM 4107.6, CIM 60-9

✪ E0185   Gel or gel-like pressure pad for mattress, standard mattress length and width
      MCM 4107.6, CIM 60-9

✪ E0186   Air pressure mattress
      CIM 60-9

✪ E0187   Water pressure mattress
      CIM 60-9

✪ E0188   Synthetic sheepskin pad
      MCM 4107.6, CIM 60-9

✪ E0189   Lambswool sheepskin pad, any size
      MCM 4107.6, CIM 60-9

▶ ✪ E0190   Positioning cushion/pillow/wedge, any shape or size

✳ E0191   Heel or elbow protector, each

✪ E0192   Low pressure and positioning equalization pad, for wheelchair
      MCM 4107.6, CIM 60-9

✳ E0193   Powered air flotation bed (low air loss therapy)

✪ E0194   Air fluidized bed
      CIM 60-19, Cross Reference Q0049

✪ E0196   Gel pressure mattress
      CIM 60-9

✪ E0197   Air pressure pad for mattress, standard mattress length and width
      CIM 60-9

⊗ E0198   Water pressure pad for mattress, standard mattress length and width
CIM 60-9

⊗ E0199   Dry pressure pad for mattress, standard mattress length and width
CIM 60-9

Heat/Cold Application

⊗ E0200   Heat lamp, without stand (table model), includes bulb, or infrared element
MCM 2100.1, CIM 60-9

✳ E0202   Phototherapy (bilirubin) light with photometer

◆ E0203   Therapeutic lightbox, minimum 10,000 lux, table top model

⊗ E0205   Heat lamp, with stand, includes bulb, or infrared element
MCM 2100.1, CIM 60-9

⊗ E0210   Electric heat pad, standard
CIM 60-9

⊗ E0215   Electric heat pad, moist
CIM 60-9

⊗ E0217   Water circulating heat pad with pump
CIM 60-9

⊗ E0218   Water circulating cold pad with pump
CIM 60-9

✳ E0220   Hot water bottle

✳ E0221   Infrared heating pad system

⊗ E0225   Hydrocollator unit, includes pads
MCM 2210.3, CIM 60-9

✳ E0230   Ice cap or collar

✳ E0231   Non-contact wound warming device (temperature control unit, AC adapter and power cord) for use with warming card and wound cover

✳ E0232   Warming card for use with the non-contact wound warming device and non-contact wound warming wound cover

⊗ E0235   Paraffin bath unit, portable (see medical supply code A4265 for paraffin)
MCM 2210.3, CIM 60-9

⊗ E0236   Pump for water circulating pad
CIM 60-9

⊗ E0238   Non-electric heat pad, moist
CIM 60-9

⊗ E0239   Hydrocollator unit, portable
MCM 2210.3, CIM 60-9

▶⊗ E0240   Bath/shower chair, with or without wheels, any size
CIM 60-9

Bath and Toilet Aids

◆ E0241   Bath tub wall rail, each
MCM 2100.1, CIM 60-9

◆ E0242   Bath tub rail, floor base
MCM 2100.1, CIM 60-9

◆ E0243   Toilet rail, each
MCM 2100.1, CIM 60-9

◆ E0244   Raised toilet seat
CIM 60-9

◆ E0245   Tub stool or bench
CIM 60-9

✳ E0246   Transfer tub rail attachment

▶⊗ E0247   Transfer bench for tub or toilet with or without commode opening
CIM 60-9

▶⊗ E0248   Transfer bench, heavy duty, for tub or toilet with or without commode opening
CIM 60-9

⊗ E0249   Pad for water circulating heat unit
CIM 60-9

Hospital Beds and Accessories

⊗ E0250   Hospital bed, fixed height, with any type side rails, with mattress
MCM 2100.1, CIM 60-18

⊗ E0251   Hospital bed, fixed height, with any type side rails, without mattress
MCM 2100.1, CIM 60-18

⊗ E0255   Hospital bed, variable height, high-low (hi-lo), with any type side rails, with mattress
MCM 2100.1, CIM 60-18

⊗ E0256   Hospital bed, variable height, hi-lo, with any type side rails, without mattress
MCM 2100.1, CIM 60-18

⊗ E0260   Hospital bed, semi-electric (head and foot adjustment), with any type side rails, with mattress
MCM 2100.1, CIM 60-18

⊗ E0261   Hospital bed, semi-electric (head and foot adjustment), with any type side rails, without mattress
MCM 2100.1, CIM 60-18

⊗ E0265   Hospital bed, total electric (head, foot and height adjustments), with any type side rails, with mattress
MCM 2100.1, CIM 60-18

⊗ E0266   Hospital bed, total electric (head, foot and height adjustments), with any type side rails, without mattress
MCM 2100.1, CIM 60-18

◆ E0270   Hospital bed, institutional type includes: oscillating, circulating and Stryker frame, with mattress
CIM 60-9

⊗ E0271   Mattress, innerspring
CIM 60-9, CIM 60-18

⊗ E0272   Mattress, foam rubber
CIM 60-9, CIM 60-18

◆ E0273　Bed board
　　　　　CIM 60-9
◆ E0274　Over-bed table
　　　　　CIM 60-9
☺ E0275　Bed pan, standard, metal or plastic
　　　　　CIM 60-9
☺ E0276　Bed pan, fracture, metal or plastic
　　　　　CIM 60-9
☺ E0277　Powered pressure-reducing air mattress
　　　　　CIM 60-9
✻ E0280　Bed cradle, any type
☺ E0290　Hospital bed, fixed height, without side
　　　　　rails, with mattress
　　　　　MCM 2100.1, CIM 60-18
☺ E0291　Hospital bed, fixed height, without side
　　　　　rails, without mattress
　　　　　MCM 2100.1, CIM 60-18
☺ E0292　Hospital bed, variable height, hi-lo,
　　　　　without side rails, with mattress
　　　　　MCM 2100.1, CIM 60-18
☺ E0293　Hospital bed, variable height, hi-lo,
　　　　　without side rails, without mattress
　　　　　MCM 2100.1, CIM 60-18
☺ E0294　Hospital bed, semi-electric (head and
　　　　　foot adjustment), without side rails,
　　　　　with mattress
　　　　　MCM 2100.1, CIM 60-18
☺ E0295　Hospital bed, semi-electric (head and
　　　　　foot adjustment), without side rails,
　　　　　without mattress
　　　　　MCM 2100.1, CIM 60-18
☺ E0296　Hospital bed, total electric (head, foot
　　　　　and height adjustments), without side
　　　　　rails, with mattress
　　　　　MCM 2100.1, CIM 60-18
☺ E0297　Hospital bed, total electric (head, foot
　　　　　and height adjustments), without side
　　　　　rails, without mattress
　　　　　MCM 2100.1, CIM 60-18
　 E0298　Deleted 01/01/02, Cross Reference
　　　　　K0549
▶✻ E0300　Pediatric crib, hospital grade, fully en-
　　　　　closed
▶☺ E0301　Hospital bed, heavy duty, extra wide,
　　　　　with weight capacity greater than 350
　　　　　pounds, but less than or equal to 600
　　　　　pounds, with any type side rails, with-
　　　　　out mattress
　　　　　CIM 60-18
▶☺ E0302　Hospital bed, extra heavy duty, extra
　　　　　wide, with weight capacity greater than
　　　　　600 pounds, with any type side rails,
　　　　　without mattress
　　　　　CIM 60-18
▶☺ E0303　Hospital bed, heavy duty, extra wide,
　　　　　with weight capacity greater than 350
　　　　　pounds, but less than or equal to 600
　　　　　pounds, with any type side rails, with
　　　　　mattress
　　　　　CIM 60-18

▶☺ E0304　Hospital bed, extra heavy duty, extra
　　　　　wide, with weight capacity greater than
　　　　　600 pounds, with any type side rails,
　　　　　with mattress
　　　　　CIM 60-18

Bed Accessories

☺ E0305　Bed side rails, half length
　　　　　CIM 60-18
☺ E0310　Bed side rails, full length
　　　　　CIM 60-18
◆ E0315　Bed accessory: board, table, or support
　　　　　device, any type
　　　　　CIM 60-9
✻ E0316　Safety enclosure frame/canopy for use
　　　　　with hospital bed, any type
☺ E0325　Urinal; male, jug-type, any material
　　　　　CIM 60-9
☺ E0326　Urinal; female, jug-type, any material
　　　　　CIM 60-9
✻ E0350　Control unit for electronic bowel irriga-
　　　　　tion/evacuation system
✻ E0352　Disposable pack (water reservoir bag,
　　　　　speculum, valving mechanism and col-
　　　　　lection bag/box) for use with the elec-
　　　　　tronic bowel irrigation/evacuation sys-
　　　　　tem
✻ E0370　Air pressure elevator for heel
✻ E0371　Non-powered advanced pressure-re-
　　　　　ducing overlay for mattress, standard
　　　　　mattress length and width
✻ E0372　Powered air overlay for mattress, stan-
　　　　　dard mattress length and width
✻ E0373　Non-powered advanced pressure-re-
　　　　　ducing mattress

Oxygen and Related Respiratory Equipment

☺ E0424　Stationary compressed gaseous oxygen
　　　　　system, rental; includes container, con-
　　　　　tents, regulator, flowmeter, humidifier,
　　　　　nebulizer, cannula or mask, and tubing
　　　　　MCM 4107.9, CIM 60-4
☺ E0425　Stationary compressed gas system, pur-
　　　　　chase; includes regulator, flowmeter,
　　　　　humidifier, nebulizer, cannula or mask,
　　　　　and tubing
　　　　　MCM 4107.9, CIM 60-4
☺ E0430　Portable gaseous oxygen system, pur-
　　　　　chase; includes regulator, flowmeter, hu-
　　　　　midifier, cannula or mask, and tubing
　　　　　MCM 4107.9, CIM 60-4
☺ E0431　Portable gaseous oxygen system, rental;
　　　　　includes portable container, regulator,
　　　　　flowmeter, humidifier, cannula or
　　　　　mask, and tubing
　　　　　MCM 4107.9, CIM 60-4

⊛ E0434 Portable liquid oxygen system, rental; includes portable container, supply reservoir, humidifier, flowmeter, refill adaptor, contents gauge, cannula or mask, and tubing
MCM 4107.9, CIM 60-4

⊛ E0435 Portable liquid oxygen system, purchase; includes portable container, supply reservoir, flowmeter, humidifier, contents gauge, cannula or mask, tubing and refill adaptor
MCM 4107.9, CIM 60-4

⊛ E0439 Stationary liquid oxygen system, rental; includes container, contents, regulator, flowmeter, humidifier, nebulizer, cannula or mask, and tubing
MCM 4107.9, CIM 60-4

⊛ E0440 Stationary liquid oxygen system, purchase; includes use of reservoir, contents indicator, regulator, flowmeter, humidifier, nebulizer, cannula or mask, and tubing
MCM 4107.9, CIM 60-4

⊛ E0441 Oxygen contents, gaseous (for use with owned gaseous stationary systems or when both a stationary and portable gaseous system are owned), 1 month's supply = 1 unit
MCM 4107.9, CIM 60-4

⊛ E0442 Oxygen contents, liquid, (for use with owned liquid stationary systems or when both a stationary and portable liquid system are owned), 1 month's supply = 1 unit
MCM 4107.9, CIM 60-4

⊛ E0443 Portable oxygen contents, gaseous, (for use only with portable gaseous systems when no stationary gas or liquid system is used), 1 month's supply = 1 unit
MCM 4107.9, CIM 60-4

⊛ E0444 Portable oxygen contents, liquid (for use only with portable liquid systems when no stationary gas or liquid system is used), 1 month's supply = 1 unit
MCM 4107.9, CIM 60-4

✳ E0445 Oximeter device for measuring blood oxygen levels non-invasively

⊛ E0450 Volume ventilator, stationary or portable, with backup rate feature, used with invasive interface (e.g., tracheostomy tube)
CIM 60-9

⊛ E0454 Pressure ventilator with pressure control, pressure support and flow triggering features
CIM 60-9

⊛ E0455 Oxygen tent, excluding croup or pediatric tents
MCM 4107.9, CIM 60-4

✳ E0457 Chest shell (cuirass)

✳ E0459 Chest wrap

⊛ E0460 Negative pressure ventilator, portable or stationary
CIM 60-9

⊛ E0461 Volume ventilator, stationary or portable, with backup rate feature, used with non-invasive interface
CIM 60-9

✳ E0462 Rocking bed, with or without side rails
CIM 60-9

▶⊛ E0470 Respiratory assist device, bi-level pressure capability, without backup rate feature, used with noninvasive interface, e.g., nasal or facial mask (intermittent assist device with continuous positive airway pressure device)
CIM 60-9

▶⊛ E0471 Respiratory assist device, bi-level pressure capability, with back-up rate feature, used with noninvasive interface, e.g., nasal or facial mask (intermittent assist device with continuous positive airway pressure device)
CIM 60-9

▶⊛ E0472 Respiratory assist device, bi-level pressure capability, with backup rate feature, used with invasive interface, e.g., tracheostomy tube (intermittent assist device with continuous positive airway pressure device)
CIM 60-9

⊛ E0480 Percussor, electric or pneumatic, home model
CIM 60-9

◆ E0481 Intrapulmonary percussive ventilation system and related accessories
CIM 60-21

✳ E0482 Cough stimulating device, alternating positive and negative airway pressure

✳ E0483 High frequency chest wall oscillation air-pulse generator system, (includes hoses and vest), each

✳ E0484 Oscillatory positive expiratory pressure device, non-electric, any type, each

IPPB Machines

⊛ E0500 IPPB machine, all types, with built-in nebulization; manual or automatic valves; internal or external power source
CIM 60-9

Humidifiers/Nebulizers/Compressors for Use with Oxygen IPPB Equipment

☼ E0550   Humidifier, durable for extensive supplemental humidification during IPPB treatments or oxygen delivery
CIM 60-9

☼ E0555   Humidifier, durable, glass or autoclavable plastic bottle type, for use with regulator or flowmeter
MCM 4107.9, CIM 60-9

☼ E0560   Humidifier, durable for supplemental humidification during IPPB treatment or oxygen delivery
CIM 60-9

▶* E0561   Humidifier, non-heated, used with positive airway pressure device

▶* E0562   Humidifier, heated, used with positive airway pressure device

* E0565   Compressor, air power source for equipment which is not self-contained or cylinder driven

☼ E0570   Nebulizer, with compressor
MCM 4107.9, CIM 60-9

☼ E0571   Aerosol compressor, battery powered, for use with small volume nebulizer
CIM 60-9

* E0572   Aerosol compressor, adjustable pressure, light duty for intermittent use

* E0574   Ultrasonic electronic aerosol generator with small volume nebulizer

☼ E0575   Nebulizer, ultrasonic, large volume
CIM 60-9

☼ E0580   Nebulizer, durable, glass or autoclavable plastic, bottle type, for use with regulator or flowmeter
MCM 4107.9, CIM 60-9

☼ E0585   Nebulizer, with compressor and heater
MCM 4107.9, CIM 60-9

* E0590   Dispensing fee for covered drug administered through DME nebulizer

Suction Pump/Room Vaporizers

☼ E0600   Respiratory such pump, home model, portable or stationary, electric
CIM 60-9

☼ E0601   Continuous airway pressure (CPAP) device
CIM 60-17

* E0602   Breast pump, manual, any type

* E0603   Breast pump, electric (AC and/or DC), any type

* E0604   Breast pump, heavy duty, hospital grade, piston operated, pulsatile, vacuum suction/release cycles, vacuum regulator, supplies, transformer, electric (AC and/or DC)

☼ E0605   Vaporizer, room type
CIM 60-9

☼ E0606   Postural drainage board
CIM 60-9

Monitoring Equipment

☼ E0607   Home blood glucose monitor
CIM 60-11

E0608   Deleted 12/31/02, Cross Reference E0618

E0609   Deleted 01/01/02

Pacemaker Monitor

☼ E0610   Pacemaker monitor, self-contained (checks battery depletion, includes audible and visible check systems)
CIM 50-1, CIM 60-7

☼ E0615   Pacemaker monitor, self-contained (checks battery depletion and other pacemaker components, includes digital/visible check systems)
CIM 50-1, CIM 60-7

* E0616   Implantable cardiac event recorder with memory, activator, and programmer

* E0617   External defibrillator with integrated electrocardiogram analysis

* E0618   Apnea monitor, without recording feature

* E0619   Apnea monitor, with recording feature

* E0620   Skin piercing device for collection of capillary blood, laser, each

Patient Lifts

☼ E0621   Sling or seat, patient lift, canvas or nylon
CIM 60-9

◆ E0625   Patient lift, Kartop, bathroom or toilet
CIM 60-9

☼ E0627   Seat lift mechanism incorporated into a combination lift-chair mechanism
MCM 4107.8, CIM 60-8, Cross Reference Q0080

☼ E0628   Separate seat lift mechanism for use with patient owned furniture—electric
MCM 4107.8, CIM 60-8, Cross Reference Q0078

☼ E0629   Separate seat lift mechanism for use with patient owned furniture—nonelectric
MCM 4107.8, Cross Reference Q0079

☼ E0630   Patient lift, hydraulic, with seat or sling
CIM 60-9

⊘ E0635 Patient lift, electric, with seat or sling
CIM 60-9

✻ E0636 Multipositional patient support system, with integrated lift, patient accessible controls

▶⊘ E0637 Combination sit to stand system, any size, with seat lift feature, with or without wheels

▶⊘ E0638 Standing frame system, any size, with or without wheels

Pneumatic Compressor and Appliances

⊘ E0650 Pneumatic compressor, non-segmental home model
CIM 60-16

⊘ E0651 Pneumatic compressor, segmental home model without calibrated gradient pressure
CIM 60-16

⊘ E0652 Pneumatic compressor, segmental home model with calibrated gradient pressure
CIM 60-16

⊘ E0655 Non-segmental pneumatic appliance for use with pneumatic compressor, half arm
CIM 60-16

⊘ E0660 Non-segmental pneumatic appliance for use with pneumatic compressor, full leg
CIM 60-16

⊘ E0665 Non-segmental pneumatic appliance for use with pneumatic compressor, full arm
CIM 60-16

⊘ E0666 Non-segmental pneumatic appliance for use with pneumatic compressor, half leg
CIM 60-16

⊘ E0667 Segmental pneumatic appliance for use with pneumatic compressor, full leg
CIM 60-16

⊘ E0668 Segmental pneumatic appliance for use with pneumatic compressor, full arm
CIM 60-16

⊘ E0669 Segmental pneumatic appliance for use with pneumatic compressor, half leg
CIM 60-16

⊘ E0671 Segmental gradient pressure pneumatic appliance, full leg
CIM 60-16

⊘ E0672 Segmental gradient pressure pneumatic appliance, full arm
CIM 60-16

⊘ E0673 Segmental gradient pressure pneumatic appliance, half leg
CIM 60-16

▶✻ E0675 Pneumatic compression device, high pressure, rapid inflation/deflation cycle, for arterial insufficiency (unilateral or bilateral system)

Ultraviolet Cabinet

E0690 Deleted 12/31/02

✻ E0691 Ultraviolet light therapy system panel, includes bulbs/lamps, timer and eye protection; treatment area 2 square feet or less

✻ E0692 Ultraviolet light therapy system panel, includes bulbs/lamps, timer and eye protection, 4 foot panel

✻ E0693 Ultraviolet light therapy system panel, includes bulbs/lamps, timer and eye protection, 6 foot panel

✻ E0694 Ultraviolet multidirectional light therapy system in 6 foot cabinet, includes bulbs/lamps, timer and eye protection

Safety Equipment

✻ E0700 Safety equipment (e.g., belt, harness or vest)

✻ E0701 Helmet with face guard and soft interface material, prefabricated

Restraints

✻ E0710 Restraints, any type (body, chest, wrist or ankle)

Transcutaneous and/or Neuromuscular Electrical Nerve Stimulators

⊘ E0720 TENS, two lead, localized stimulation
MCM 4107.6, CIM 35-20, CIM 35-46

⊘ E0730 Transcutaneous electrical nerve stimulation device, four or more leads, for multiple nerve stimulation
MCM 4107.6, CIM 35-20, CIM 35-46

⊘ E0731 Form fitting conductive garment for delivery of TENS or NMES (with conductive fibers separated from the patient's skin by layers of fabric)
CIM 45-25

⊘ E0740 Incontinence treatment system, pelvic floor stimulator, monitor, sensor and/or trainer
CIM 65-24

✻ E0744 Neuromuscular stimulator for scoliosis

☼ E0745   Neuromuscular stimulator, electronic shock unit
CIM 35-77

☼ E0746   Electromyography (EMG), biofeedback device
CIM 35-27

☼ E0747   Osteogenesis stimulator, electrical, non-invasive, other than spinal applications
CIM 35-48

☼ E0748   Osteogenesis stimulator, electrical, non-invasive, spinal applications
CIM 35-48

☼ E0749   Osteogenesis stimulator, electrical, surgically implanted
CIM 35-48

☼ E0752   Implantable neurostimulator electrode, each
CIM 65-8

E0753   Deleted 01/01/02

☼ E0754   Patient programmer (external) for use with implantable programmable neurostimulator pulse generator
CIM 65-8

∗ E0755   Electronic salivary reflex stimulator (intra-oral/non-invasive)

☼ E0756   Implantable neurostimulator pulse generator
CIM 65-8

☼ E0757   Implantable neurostimulator radiofrequency receiver
CIM 65-8

☼ E0758   Radiofrequency transmitter (external) for use with implantable neurostimulator radiofrequency receiver
CIM 65-8

∗ E0759   Radiofrequency transmitter (external) for use with implantable sacral root neurostimulator receiver for bowel and bladder management, replacement
CIM 65-8

☼ E0760   Osteogenesis stimulator, low intensity ultrasound, non-invasive
CIM 35-48

◆ E0761   Non-thermal pulsed high frequency radio waves, high peak power electromagnetic energy treatment device

∗ E0765   FDA-approved nerve stimulator, with replaceable batteries, for treatment of nausea and vomiting

Infusion Supplies

∗ E0776   IV pole

∗ E0779   Ambulatory infusion pump, mechanical, reusable, for infusion 8 hours or greater

∗ E0780   Ambulatory infusion pump, mechanical, reusable, for infusion less than 8 hours

☼ E0781   Ambulatory infusion pump, single or multiple channels, electric or battery operated with administrative equipment, worn by patient
CIM 60-14

☼ E0782   Infusion pump, implantable, non-programmable (includes all components, e.g., pump, cathether, connectors, etc.)
CIM 60-14

☼ E0783   Infusion pump system, implantable, programmable (includes all components, e.g., pump, catheter, connectors, etc.)
CIM 60-14

☼ E0784   External ambulatory infusion pump, insulin
CIM 60-14

☼ E0785   Implantable intraspinal (epidural/intrathecal) catheter used with implantable infusion pump, replacement
CIM 60-14

☼ E0786   Implantable programmable infusion pump, replacement (excludes implantable intraspinal catheter
CIM 60-14

☼ E0791   Parenteral infusion pump, stationary, single or multi-channel
MCM 2130, MCM 4450, CIM 65-10

Traction Equipment: All Types and Cervical

☼ E0830   Ambulatory tract device, all types, each
CIM 60-9

☼ E0840   Traction frame, attached to headboard, cervical traction
CIM 60-9

☼ E0850   Traction stand, free-standing, cervical traction
CIM 60-9

∗ E0855   Cervical traction equipment not requiring additional stand or frame

Traction: Overdoor

☼ E0860   Traction equipment, overdoor, cervical
CIM 60-9

Traction: Extremity

☼ E0870   Traction frame, attached to footboard, extremity traction (e.g., Buck's)
CIM 60-9

☼ E0880   Traction stand, free-standing, extremity traction (e.g., Buck's)
CIM 60-9

Traction: Pelvic

- ✪ E0890 Traction frame, attached to footboard, pelvic traction
CIM 60-9
- ✪ E0900 Traction stand, free-standing, pelvic traction (e.g., Buck's)
CIM 60-9

Trapeze Equipment, Fracture Frame and Other Orthopedic Devices

- ✪ E0910 Trapeze bars, also known as patient helper, attached to bed, with grab bar
CIM 60-9
- ✪ E0920 Fracture frame, attached to bed, includes weights
CIM 60-9
- ✪ E0930 Fracture frame, free-standing, includes weights
CIM 60-9
- ✪ E0935 Passive motion exercise device
CIM 60-9
- ✪ E0940 Trapeze bar, free-standing, complete with grab bar
CIM 60-9
- ✪ E0941 Gravity assisted traction device, any type
CIM 60-9
- ✱ E0942 Cervical head harness/halter
- E0943 Deleted 12/31/03
- ✱ E0944 Pelvic belt/harness/boot
- ✱ E0945 Extremity belt/harness
- ✪ E0946 Fracture, frame, dual with cross bars, attached to bed, (e.g., Balken, Four Poster)
CIM 60-9
- ✪ E0947 Fracture frame, attachments for complex pelvic traction
CIM 60-9
- ✪ E0948 Fracture frame, attachments for complex cervical traction
CIM 60-9

Wheelchairs

- ➡ ✪ E0950 Wheelchair accessory, tray, each
CIM 60-9
- ➡ ✱ E0951 Heel loop/holder, with or without ankle strap, each
CIM 60-9
- ➡ ✪ E0952 Toe loop/holder, each
CIM 60-9
- ◆ E0953 Pneumatic tire, each
CIM 60-9, Cross Reference K0067
- ◆ E0954 Semi-pneumatic caster, each
CIM 60-9, Cross Reference K0075
- ▶✱ E0955 Wheelchair accessory, headrest, cushioned, prefabricated, including fixed mounting hardware, each
- ▶✱ E0956 Wheelchair accessory, lateral trunk or hip support, prefabricated, including fixed mounting hardware, each
- ▶✱ E0957 Wheelchair accessory, medial thigh support, prefabricated, including fixed mounting hardware, each

Wheelchair Accessories

- ➡ ✪ E0958 Manual wheelchair accessory, one-arm drive attachment, each
CIM 60-9
- ➡ ✱ E0959 Manual wheelchair accessory, adapter for amputee, each
CIM 60-9
- ▶✱ E0960 Wheelchair accessory, shoulder harness/straps or chest strap, including any type mounting hardware
- ➡ ✱ E0961 Manual wheelchair accessory, wheel lock brake extension (handle), each
CIM 60-9
- ✪ E0962 1" cushion, for wheelchair
CIM 60-9
- ✪ E0963 2" cushion, for wheelchair
CIM 60-9
- ✪ E0964 3" cushion, for wheelchair
CIM 60-9
- ✪ E0965 4" cushion, for wheelchair
CIM 60-9
- ➡ ✱ E0966 Manual wheelchair accessory, headrest extension, each
CIM 60-9
- ➡ ✪ E0967 Manual wheelchair accessory, hand rim with projections, each
CIM 60-9
- ✪ E0968 Commode seat, wheelchair
CIM 60-9
- ✪ E0969 Narrowing device, wheelchair
CIM 60-9
- ◆ E0970 No. 2 footplates, except for elevating leg rest
CIM 60-9; Cross Reference K0037, K0042
- ◆ E0971 Anti-tipping device wheelchair
CIM 60-9, Cross Reference K0021
- ➡ ✱ E0972 Wheelchair accessory, transfer board or device, each
- ➡ ✪ E0973 Wheelchair accessory, adjustable height, detachable armrest, complete assembly, each
CIM 60-9

➡ ⊘ E0974 Manual wheelchair accessory, anti-roll-back device, each
CIM 60-9

E0975 Deleted 12/31/03

E0976 Deleted 12/31/03

✻ E0977 Wedge cushion, wheelchair

➡✻ E0978 Wheelchair accessory, safety belt/pelvic strap, each

E0979 Deleted 12/31/03

✻ E0980 Safety vest, wheelchair

▶✻ E0981 Wheelchair accessory, seat upholstery, replacement only, each

▶✻ E0982 Wheelchair accessory, back upholstery, replacement only, each

▶✻ E0983 Manual wheelchair accessory, power add-on to convert manual wheelchair to motorized wheelchair, joystick control

▶✻ E0984 Manual wheelchair accessory, power add-on to convert manual wheelchair to motorized wheelchair, tiller control

▶✻ E0985 Wheelchair accessory, seat lift mechanism

▶✻ E0986 Manual wheelchair accessory, push-rim activated power assist, each

➡✻ E0990 Wheelchair accessory, elevating leg rest, complete assembly, each
CIM 60-9

E0991 Deleted 12/31/03

➡✻ E0992 Manual wheelchair accessory, solid seat insert

E0993 Deleted 12/31/03

⊘ E0994 Arm rest, each
CIM 60-9

➡✻ E0995 Wheelchair accessory, calf rest/pad, each

◆ E0996 Tire, solid, each
CIM 60-9, Cross Reference K0066

⊘ E0997 Caster with a fork
CIM 60-9

⊘ E0998 Caster without fork
CIM 60-9

⊘ E0999 Pneumatic tire with wheel
CIM 60-9

◆ E1000 Tire, pneumatic caster
CIM 60-9, Cross Reference K0074

⊘ E1001 Wheel, single
CIM 60-9

▶✻ E1002 Wheelchair accessory, power seating system, tilt only

▶✻ E1003 Wheelchair accessory, power seating system, recline only, without shear reduction

▶✻ E1004 Wheelchair accessory, power seating system, recline only, with mechanical shear reduction

▶✻ E1005 Wheelchair accessory, power seating system, recline only, with power shear reduction

▶✻ E1006 Wheelchair accessory, power seating system, combination tilt and recline, without shear reduction

▶✻ E1007 Wheelchair accessory, power seating system, combination tilt and recline, with mechanical shear reduction

▶✻ E1008 Wheelchair accessory, power seating system, combination tilt and recline, with power shear reduction

▶✻ E1009 Wheelchair accessory, addition to power seating system, mechanically linked leg elevation system, including pushrod and leg rest, each

▶✻ E1010 Wheelchair accessory, addition to power seating system, power leg elevation system, including leg rest, each

⊘ E1011 Modification to pediatric wheelchair, width adjustment package (not to be dispensed with initial chair)
CIM 60-9

⊘ E1012 Integrated seating system, planar, for pediatric wheelchair
CIM 60-9

⊘ E1013 Integrated seating system, contoured, for pediatric wheelchair
CIM 60-9

⊘ E1014 Reclining back, addition to pediatric wheelchair
CIM 60-9

⊘ E1015 Shock absorber for manual wheelchair, each
CIM 60-9

⊘ E1016 Shock absorber for power wheelchair, each
CIM 60-9

⊘ E1017 Heavy duty shock absorber for heavy duty or extra heavy duty manual wheelchair, each
CIM 60-9

⊘ E1018 Heavy duty shock absorber for heavy duty or extra heavy duty power wheelchair, each
CIM 60-9

▶◆ E1019 Wheelchair accessory, power seating system, heavy duty feature, patient weight capacity greater than 250 pounds and less than or equal to 400 pounds

⊘ E1020 Residual limb support system for wheelchair
CIM 60-6

▶◆ E1021 Wheelchair accessory, power seating system, extra heavy duty feature, weight capacity greater than 400 pounds

Introduction

© E1025 Lateral thoracic support, non-contoured, for pediatric wheelchair, each (includes hardware)
CIM 60-9

© E1026 Lateral thoracic support, contoured, for pediatric wheelchair, each (includes hardware)
CIM 60-9

© E1027 Lateral/anterior support, for pediatric wheelchair, each (includes hardware)
CIM 60-9

▶✱ E1028 Wheelchair accessory, manual swing away, retractable or removable mounting hardware for joystick, other control interface or positioning accessory

▶✱ E1029 Wheelchair accessory, ventilator tray, fixed

▶✱ E1030 Wheelchair accessory, ventilator tray, gimbaled

Rollabout Chair and Transfer System

© E1031 Rollabout chair, any and all types with castors 5 inches or greater
CIM 60-9

© E1035 Multi-positional patient transfer system, with integrated seat, operated by care giver
MCM 2100

© E1037 Transport chair, pediatric size
CIM 60-9

© E1038 Transport chair, adult size
CIM 60-9

Wheelchair: Fully Reclining

© E1050 Fully reclining wheelchair, fixed full-length arms, swing-away detachable elevating leg rests
CIM 60-9

© E1060 Fully reclining wheelchair, detachable arms, desk or full-length, swing-away detachable elevating leg rests
CIM 60-9

E1065 Deleted 12/31/03
E1066 Deleted 12/31/03
E1069 Deleted 12/31/03

© E1070 Fully reclining wheelchair, detachable arms (desk or full-length), swing-away detachable foot rests
CIM 60-9

© E1083 Hemi-wheelchair, fixed full-length arms, swing-away detachable elevating leg rests
CIM 60-9

© E1084 Hemi-wheelchair, detachable arms (desk or full-length) arms, swing-away detachable elevating leg rests
CIM 60-9

◆ E1085 Hemi-wheelchair, fixed full-length arms, swing-away detachable foot rests
CIM 60-9, Cross Reference K0002

◆ E1086 Hemi-wheelchair, detachable arms (desk or full-length), swing-away detachable foot rests
CIM 60-9, Cross Reference K0002

© E1087 High-strength lightweight wheelchair, fixed full-length arms, swing-away detachable elevating leg rests
CIM 60-9

© E1088 High-strength lightweight wheelchair, detachable arms (desk or full-length), swing-away detachable elevating leg rests
CIM 60-9

◆ E1089 High-strength lightweight wheelchair, fixed-length arms, swing-away detachable foot rests
CIM 60-9, Cross Reference K0004

◆ E1090 High-strength lightweight wheelchair, detachable arms (desk or full-length), swing-away detachable foot rests
CIM 60-9, Cross Reference K0004

E1091 Deleted 12/31/02

© E1092 Wide, heavy duty wheelchair, detachable arms (desk or full-length), swing-away detachable elevating leg rests
CIM 60-9

© E1093 Wide, heavy duty wheelchair, detachable arms (desk or full-length) swing-away detachable foot rests
CIM 60-9

Wheelchair: Semi-reclining

© E1100 Semi-reclining wheelchair, fixed full-length arms, swing-away detachable elevating leg rests
CIM 60-9

© E1110 Semi-reclining wheelchair, detachable arms (desk or full-length), elevating leg rests
CIM 60-9

Wheelchair: Standard

◆ E1130 Standard wheelchair, fixed full-length arms, fixed or swing-away detachable foot rests
CIM 60-9, Cross Reference K0001

◆ E1140   Wheelchair, detachable arms (desk or full-length), swing-away detachable foot rests
CIM 60-9, Cross Reference K0001

✿ E1150   Wheelchair, detachable arms (desk or full-length), swing-away detachable elevating leg rests
CIM 60-9

✿ E1160   Wheelchair, fixed full-length arms, swing-away detachable elevating leg rests
CIM 60-9

✱ E1161   Manual adult size wheelchair, includes tilt in space

Wheelchair: Amputee

✿ E1170   Amputee wheelchair, fixed full-length arms, swing-away detachable elevating leg rests
CIM 60-9

✿ E1171   Amputee wheelchair, fixed full-length arms, without foot rests or leg rests
CIM 60-9

✿ E1172   Amputee wheelchair, detachable arms (desk or full-length), without foot rests or leg rests
CIM 60-9

✿ E1180   Amputee wheelchair, detachable arms (desk or full-length) swing-away detachable foot rests
CIM 60-9

✿ E1190   Amputee wheelchair, detachable arms (desk or full-length), swing-away detachable elevating leg rests
CIM 60-9

✿ E1195   Heavy duty wheelchair, fixed full-length arms, swing-away detachable elevating leg rests
CIM 60-9

✿ E1200   Amputee wheelchair, fixed full-length arms, swing-away detachable foot rests
CIM 60-9

Wheelchair: Power

✿ E1210   Motorized wheelchair, fixed full-length arms, swing-away detachable elevating leg rests
CIM 60-5, CIM 60-9

✿ E1211   Motorized wheelchair, detachable arms (desk or full-length) swing-away, detachable elevating leg rests
CIM 60-5, CIM 60-9

◆ E1212   Motorized wheelchair, fixed full-length arms, swing-away detachable foot rests
CIM 60-5, CIM 60-9, Cross Reference K0010

◆ E1213   Motorized wheelchair, detachable arms (desk or full-length), swing-away detachable foot rests
CIM 60-5, CIM 60-9, Cross Reference K0010

Wheelchair: Special Size

✿ E1220   Wheelchair; specially sized or constructed (indicate brand name, model number, if any) and justification
CIM 60-6

✿ E1221   Wheelchair with fixed arm, foot rests
CIM 60-6

✿ E1222   Wheelchair with fixed arm, elevating leg rests
CIM 60-6

✿ E1223   Wheelchair with detachable arms, foot rests
CIM 60-6

✿ E1224   Wheelchair with detachable arms, elevating leg rests
CIM 60-6

➠ ✿ E1225   Manual wheelchair accessory, semi-reclining back (recline greater than 15 degrees, but less than 80 degrees), each
CIM 60-6

➠ ✿ E1226   Manual wheelchair accessory, fully reclining back, each
CIM 60-6

✿ E1227   Special height arms for wheelchair
CIM 60-6

✿ E1228   Special back height for wheelchair
CIM 60-6

✿ E1230   Power operated vehicle (three- or four-wheel non-highway); specify brand name and model number
MCM 4107.6, CIM 60-5

✿ E1231   Wheelchair, pediatric size, tilt-in-space, rigid, adjustable, with seating system
CIM 60-9

✿ E1232   Wheelchair, pediatric size, tilt-in-space, folding, adjustable, with seating system
CIM 60-9

✿ E1233   Wheelchair, pediatric size, tilt-in-space, rigid, adjustable, without seating system
CIM 60-9

✿ E1234   Wheelchair, pediatric size, tilt-in-space, folding, adjustable, without seating system
CIM 60-9

✿ E1235   Wheelchair, pediatric size, rigid, adjustable, with seating system
CIM 60-9

⊕ E1236 Wheelchair, pediatric size, folding, adjustable, with seating system
CIM 60-9

⊕ E1237 Wheelchair, pediatric size, rigid, adjustable, without seating system
CIM 60-9

⊕ E1238 Wheelchair, pediatric size, folding, adjustable, without seating system
CIM 60-9

Wheelchair: Lightweight

⊕ E1240 Lightweight wheelchair, detachable arms (desk or full-length), swing-away detachable, elevating leg rests
CIM 60-9

◆ E1250 Lightweight wheelchair, fixed full-length arms, swing-away detachable foot rests
CIM 60-9, Cross Reference K0003

◆ E1260 Lightweight wheelchair, detachable arms (desk or full-length), swing-away detachable foot rests
CIM 60-9, Cross Reference K0003

⊕ E1270 Lightweight wheelchair, fixed full-length arms, swing-away detachable elevating leg rests
CIM 60-9

Wheelchair: Heavy Duty

⊕ E1280 Heavy duty wheelchair, detachable arms (desk or full-length), elevating leg rests
CIM 60-9

◆ E1285 Heavy duty wheelchair, fixed full-length arms, swing-away detachable foot rests
CIM 60-9, Cross Reference K0006

◆ E1290 Heavy duty wheelchair, detachable arms (desk or full-length), swing-away detachable foot rests
CIM 60-9, Cross Reference K0006

⊕ E1295 Heavy duty wheelchair, fixed full-length arms, elevating leg rests
CIM 60-9

⊕ E1296 Special wheelchair seat, height from floor
CIM 60-6

⊕ E1297 Special wheelchair seat depth, by upholstery
CIM 60-6

⊕ E1298 Special wheelchair seat depth and/or width, by construction
CIM 60-6

Whirlpool Equipment

◆ E1300 Whirlpool, portable (overtub type)
CIM 60-9

⊕ E1310 Whirlpool, non-portable (built-in type)
CIM 60-9

Repairs and Replacement Parts

⊕ E1340 Repair or nonroutine service for durable medical equipment requiring the skill of a technician, labor component, per 15 minutes
MCM 2100.4

Additional Oxygen Related Equipment

⊕ E1353 Regulator
MCM 4107.9, CIM 60-4

⊕ E1355 Stand/rack
CIM 60-4

⊕ E1372 Immersion external heater for nebulizer
CIM 60-4

⇒ ⊕ E1390 Oxygen concentrator, single delivery port, capable of delivering 85 percent or greater oxygen concentration at the prescribed flow rate
CIM 60-4

▶ ⊕ E1391 Oxygen concentrator, dual delivery port, capable of delivering 85 percent or greater oxygen concentration at the prescribed flow rate, each
CIM 60-4

✳ E1399 Durable medical equipment, miscellaneous

⊕ E1405 Oxygen and water vapor enriching system with heated delivery
MCM 4107, CIM 60-4

⊕ E1406 Oxygen and water vapor enriching system without heated delivery
MCM 4107, CIM 60-4

⊕ E1500 Centrifuge, for dialysis

Artificial Kidney Machines and Accessories

⊕ E1510 Kidney, dialysate delivery system, kidney machine, pump recirculating, air removal system, flow rate meter, power off, heater and temperature control with alarm, IV poles, pressure gauge, concentrate container

⊕ E1520 Heparin infusion pump for hemodialysis

⊕ E1530 Air bubble detector for hemodialysis, each, replacement

✪ E1540 Pressure alarm for hemodialysis, each
✪ E1550 Bath conductivity meter for hemodialysis, each
✪ E1560 Blood leak detector for hemodialysis, each, replacement
✪ E1570 Adjustable chair, for ESRD patients
✪ E1575 Transducer protectors/fluid barriers for hemohemodialysis, any size, per 10
✪ E1580 Unipuncture control system for hemodialysis
✪ E1590 Hemodialysis machine
✪ E1592 Automatic intermittent peritoneal dialysis system
✪ E1594 Cycler dialysis machine for peritoneal dialysis
✪ E1600 Delivery and/or installation charges for hemodialysis equipment
✪ E1610 Reverse osmosis water purification system, for hemodialysis
CIM 55-1A
✪ E1615 Deionizer water purification system, for hemodialysis
CIM 55-1A
✪ E1620 Blood pump for hemodialysis replacement
✪ E1625 Water softening system, for hemodialysis
CIM 55-1B
✳ E1630 Reciprocating peritoneal dialysis system
✪ E1632 Wearable artificial kidney, each
▶✪ E1634 Peritoneal dialysis clamps, each
MCM 4270
✪ E1635 Compact (portable) travel hemodialyzer system
✪ E1636 Sorbent cartridges, per case, for hemodialysis, per 10
✪ E1637 Hemostats, each
E1638 Deleted 12/31/02, Cross Reference E0210
✪ E1639 Scale, each
E1640 Deleted 01/01/02
✪ E1699 Dialysis equipment, not otherwise specified

Jaw Motion Rehabilitation System and Accessories

✳ E1700 Jaw motion rehabilitation system
✳ E1701 Replacement cushions for jaw motion rehabilitation system, package of 6
✳ E1702 Replacement measuring scales for jaw motion rehabilitation system, package of 200

Other Orthopedic Devices

✳ E1800 Dynamic adjustable elbow extension/flexion device, includes soft interface material

✳ E1801 Bi-directional static progressive stretch elbow device with range of motion adjustment, includes cuffs
✳ E1802 Dynamic adjustable forearm pronation/supination device, includes soft interface material
✳ E1805 Dynamic adjustable wrist extension/flexion device, includes soft interface material
✳ E1806 Bi-directional static progressive stretch wrist device with range of motion adjustment, includes cuffs
✳ E1810 Dynamic adjustable knee extension/flexion device, includes soft interface material
✳ E1811 Bi-directional static progressive stretch knee device with range of motion adjustment, includes cuffs
✳ E1815 Dynamic adjustable ankle extension/flexion device, includes soft interface material
✳ E1816 Bi-directional static progressive stretch ankle device with range of motion adjustment, includes cuffs
✳ E1818 Bi-directional static progressive stretch forearm pronation/supination device with range of motion adjustment, includes cuffs
✳ E1820 Replacement of soft interface material, dynamic adjustable extension/flexion device
✳ E1821 Replacement of soft interface material/cuffs for bi-directional static progressive stretch device
✳ E1825 Dynamic adjustable finger extension/flexion device, includes soft interface material
✳ E1830 Dynamic adjustable toe extension/flexion device, includes soft interface material
✳ E1840 Dynamic adjustable shoulder flexion/abduction/rotation device, includes soft interface material
E1900 Deleted 01/01/02
✳ E1902 Communication board, non-electronic augmentative or alternative communication device
✳ E2000 Gastric suction pump, home model, portable or stationary, electric
✪ E2100 Blood glucose monitor with integrated voice synthesizer
CIM 60-11
✪ E2101 Blood glucose monitor with integrated lancing/blood sample
CIM 60-11
▶✳ E2120 Pulse generator system for tympanic treatment of inner ear endolymphatic fluid

▶✳ E2201   Manual wheelchair accessory, nonstandard seat frame, width greater than or equal to 20 inches and less than 24 inches

▶✳ E2202   Manual wheelchair accessory, nonstandard seat frame width, 24-27 inches

▶✳ E2203   Manual wheelchair accessory, nonstandard seat frame depth, 20 to less than 22 inches

▶✳ E2204   Manual wheelchair accessory, nonstandard seat frame depth, 22 to 25 inches

▶✳ E2300   Power wheelchair accessory, power seat elevation system

▶✳ E2301   Power wheelchair accessory, power standing system

▶✳ E2310   Power wheelchair accessory, electronic connection between wheelchair controller and one power seating system motor, including all related electronics, indicator feature, mechanical function selection switch, and fixed mounting hardware

▶✳ E2311   Power wheelchair accessory, electronic connection between wheelchair controller and two or more power seating system motors, including all related electronics, indicator feature, mechanical function selection switch, and fixed mounting hardware

▶✳ E2320   Power wheelchair accessory, hand or chin control interface, remote joystick or touchpad, proportional, including all related electronics, and fixed mounting hardware

▶✳ E2321   Power wheelchair accessory, hand control interface, remote joystick, nonproportional, including all related electronics, mechanical stop switch, and fixed mounting hardware

▶✳ E2322   Power wheelchair accessory, hand control interface, multiple mechanical switches, nonproportional, including all related electronics, mechanical stop switch, and fixed mounting hardware

▶✳ E2323   Power wheelchair accessory, specialty joystick handle for hand control interface, prefabricated

▶✳ E2324   Power wheelchair accessory, chin cup for chin control interface

▶✳ E2325   Power wheelchair accessory, sip and puff interface, nonproportional, including all related electronics, mechanical stop switch, and manual swingaway mounting hardware

▶✳ E2326   Power wheelchair accessory, breath tube kit for sip and puff interface

▶✳ E2327   Power wheelchair accessory, head control interface, mechanical, proportional, including all related electronics, mechanical direction change switch, and fixed mounting hardware

▶✳ E2328   Power wheelchair accessory, head control or extremity control interface, electronic, proportional, including all related electronics and fixed mounting hardware

▶✳ E2329   Power wheelchair accessory, head control interface, contact switch mechanism, nonproportional, including all related electronics, mechanical stop switch, mechanical direction change switch, head array, and fixed mounting hardware

▶✳ E2330   Power wheelchair accessory, head control interface, proximity switch mechanism, nonproportional, including all related electronics, mechanical stop switch, mechanical direction change switch, head array, and fixed mounting hardware

▶✳ E2331   Power wheelchair accessory, attendant control, proportional, including all related electronics and fixed mounting hardware

▶✳ E2340   Power wheelchair accessory, nonstandard seat frame width, 20-23 inches

▶✳ E2341   Power wheelchair accessory, nonstandard seat frame width, 24-27 inches

▶✳ E2342   Power wheelchair accessory, nonstandard seat frame depth, 20 or 21 inches

▶✳ E2343   Power wheelchair accessory, nonstandard seat frame depth, 22-25 inches

▶✳ E2351   Power wheelchair accessory, electronic interface to operate speech generating device using power wheelchair control interface

▶✳ E2360   Power wheelchair accessory, 22 NF non-sealed lead acid battery, each

▶✳ E2361   Power wheelchair accessory, 22 NF sealed lead acid battery, each, (e.g., gel cell, absorbed glassmat)

▶✳ E2362   Power wheelchair accessory, group 24 non-sealed lead acid battery, each

▶✳ E2363   Power wheelchair accessory, group 24 sealed lead acid battery, each (e.g., gel cell, absorbed glassmat)

▶✳ E2364   Power wheelchair accessory, U-1 non-sealed lead acid battery, each

▶✳ E2365   Power wheelchair accessory, U-1 sealed lead acid battery, each (e.g., gel cell, absorbed glassmat)

▶✳ E2366   Power wheelchair accessory, battery charger, single mode, for use with only one battery type, sealed or non-sealed, each

▶✳ E2367   Power wheelchair accessory, battery charger, dual mode, for use with either battery type, sealed or non-sealed, each

▶✳ E2399   Power wheelchair accessory, not otherwise classified interface, including all related electronics and any type mounting hardware

▶* E2402   Negative pressure wound therapy electrical pump, stationary or portable

▶⊙ E2500   Speech generating device, digitized speech, using pre-recorded messages, less than or equal to 8 minutes recording time
CIM 60-23

▶⊙ E2502   Speech generating device, digitized speech, using pre-recorded messages, greater than 8 minutes but less than or equal to 20 minutes recording time
CIM 60-23

▶⊙ E2504   Speech generating device, digitized speech, using pre-recorded messages, greater than 20 minutes but less than or equal to 40 minutes recording time
CIM 60-23

▶⊙ E2506   Speech generating device, digitized speech, using pre-recorded messages, greater than 40 minutes recording time
CIM 60-23

▶⊙ E2508   Speech generating device, synthesized speech, requiring message formulation by spelling and access by physical contact with the device
CIM 60-23

▶⊙ E2510   Speech generating device, synthesized speech, permitting multiple methods of message formulation and multiple methods of device access
CIM 60-23

▶⊙ E2511   Speech generating software program, for personal computer or personal digital assistant
CIM 60-23

▶⊙ E2512   Accessory for speech generating device, mounting system
CIM 60-23

▶⊙ E2599   Accessory for speech generating device, not otherwise classified
CIM 60-23

PROCEDURES/PROFESSIONAL SERVICES (TEMPORARY) (G0000-G9999)

NOTE: This section contains national codes assigned by CMS on a temporary basis to identify procedures/professional services.

Positron Emission Tomography Scan Code Modifiers

Modifiers that are used on claims for positron emission tomography (PET) myocardial perfusion imaging are created by combining two alpha characters. Each alpha character represents the results of the PET scan and the previous test, with the first letter indicating the results of the PET scan, while the second letter indicates the test done prior to the PET scan. The test result codes and their descriptions are listed below:

Code
N   Negative
E   Equivocal
P   Positive, but not suggestive of extensive ischemia
S   Positive and suggestive of extensive ischemia (greater than 20% of the left ventricle)

* G0001   Routine venipuncture for collection of specimen(s)

G0002   Deleted 12/31/02, Cross Reference 51702*, 51703*

G0004   Deleted 12/31/02, Cross Reference 93268

G0005   Deleted 12/31/02, Cross Reference 93270

G0006   Deleted 12/31/02, Cross Reference 93271

G0007   Deleted 12/31/02, Cross Reference 93272

* G0008   Administration of influenza virus vaccine

* G0009   Administration of pneumococcal vaccine

* G0010   Administration of hepatitis B vaccine

G0015   Deleted 12/31/02, Cross Reference 93012

G0016   Deleted 01/01/02

G0025   Deleted 04/01/03, Cross Reference Q3031

G0026   Deleted 12/31/02

▶* G0027   Semen analysis; presence and/or motility of sperm excluding Huhner

⊙ G0030   PET myocardial perfusion imaging (following previous PET, G0030-G0047); single study, rest or stress (exercise and/or pharmacologic)
CIM 50-36

⊙ G0031   PET myocardial perfusion imaging (following previous PET, G0030-G0047); multiple studies, rest or stress (exercise and/or pharmacologic)
CIM 50-36

⊙ G0032   PET myocardial perfusion imaging (following rest SPECT, 78464); single study, rest or stress (exercise and/or pharmacologic)
CIM 50-36

⊙ G0033   PET myocardial perfusion imaging (following rest SPECT, 78464*); multiple studies, rest or stress (exercise and/or pharmacologic)
CIM 50-36

⊙ G0034 PET myocardial perfusion imaging (following stress SPECT, 78465*); single study, rest or stress (exercise and/or pharmacologic)
CIM 50-36

⊙ G0035 PET myocardial perfusion imaging (following stress SPECT, 78465*); multiple studies, rest or stress (exercise and/or pharmacologic)
CIM 50-36

⊙ G0036 PET myocardial perfusion imaging (following coronary angiography, 93510-93529*); single study, rest or stress (exercise and/or pharmacologic)
CIM 50-36

⊙ G0037 PET myocardial perfusion imaging (following coronary angiography, 93510-93529*); multiple studies, rest or stress (exercise and/or pharmacologic)
CIM 50-36

⊙ G0038 PET myocardial perfusion imaging, (following stress planar myocardial perfusion, 78460*); single study, rest or stress (exercise and/or pharmacologic)
CIM 50-36

⊙ G0039 PET myocardial perfusion imaging (following stress planar myocardial perfusion, 78460*); multiple studies, rest or stress (exercise and/or pharmacologic)
CIM 50-36

⊙ G0040 PET myocardial perfusion imaging (following stress echocardiogram, 93350*); single study, rest or stress (exercise and/or pharmacologic)
CIM 50-36

⊙ G0041 PET myocardial perfusion imaging (following stress echocardiogram, 93350*); multiple studies, rest or stress (exercise and/or pharmacologic)
CIM 50-36

⊙ G0042 PET myocardial perfusion imaging (following stress nuclear ventriculogram, 78481 or 78483*); single study, rest or stress (exercise and/or pharmacologic)
CIM 50-36

⊙ G0043 PET myocardial perfusion imaging, (following stress nuclear ventriculogram, 78488 or 78483*); multiple studies, rest or stress (exercise and/or pharmacologic)
CIM 50-36

⊙ G0044 PET myocardial perfusion imaging (following rest electrocardiogram [ECG], 93000*); single study, rest or stress (exercise and/or pharmacologic)
CIM 50-36

⊙ G0045 PET myocardial perfusion imaging (following rest ECG, 93000*); multiple studies, rest or stress (exercise and/or pharmacologic)
CIM 50-36

⊙ G0046 PET myocardial perfusion imaging (following stress ECG, 93015*); single study, rest or stress (exercise and/or pharmacologic)
CIM 50-36

⊙ G0047 PET myocardial perfusion imaging, (following stress ECG, 93015*); multiple studies, rest or stress (exercise and/or pharmacologic)
CIM 50-36

G0050 Deleted 12/31/02, Cross Reference 51798*

⊙ G0101 Cervical or vaginal cancer screening; pelvic and clinical breast examination

⊙ G0102 Prostate cancer screening; digital rectal examination
MCM 4182, CIM 50-55

⊙ G0103 Prostate cancer screening; prostate specific antigen test (PSA), total
MCM 4182, CIM 50-55

⊙ G0104 Colorectal cancer screening; flexible sigmoidoscopy

⊙ G0105 Colorectal cancer screening; colonoscopy on individual at high risk

⊙ G0106 Colorectal cancer screening; alternative to G0104, screening sigmoidoscopy, barium enema

⊙ G0107 Colorectal cancer screening; fecal-occult blood test, 1-3 simultaneous determinations

✳ G0108 Diabetes outpatient self-management training services, individual, per 30 minute

✳ G0109 Diabetes outpatient self-management training services, group session, two or more, per 30 minutes

G0110 Deleted 12/31/03, Cross Reference Q3031

G0111-G0116 Deleted 12/31/03

✳ G0117 Glaucoma screening for high risk patients furnished by optometrist or ophthalmologist

✳ G0118 Glaucoma screening for high risk patient furnished under direct supervision by optometrist or ophthalmologist

⊙ G0120 Colorectal cancer screening; alternative to G0105, screening colonoscopy, barium enema

⊙ G0121 Colorectal cancer screening; colonoscopy on individual not meeting criteria for high risk

◆ G0122 Colorectal cancer screening; barium enema

*CPT only © 2003. *Current Procedural Terminology, 2004, Professional Edition,* American Medical Association. All Rights Reserved.

⊙ **Special coverage instructions**   ◆ **Not covered by or valid for Medicare**   ✳ **Carrier discretion**   ◀▶ **New**   ◀▦▦▶ **Revised**   1191

⊙ G0123 Screening cytopathology, cervical or vaginal (any reporting system); collected in preservative fluid, automated thin layer preparation, screening by cytotechnologist under physician supervision
CIM 50-20, Laboratory Certification: cytology

⊙ G0124 Screening cytopathology, cervical or vaginal (any reporting system); collected in preservative fluid, automated thin layer preparation, requiring interpretation by physician
CIM 50-20, Laboratory Certification: cytology

⊙ G0125 PET imaging regional or whole body; single pulmonary nodule
MCM 4173, CIM 50-36

⊙ G0127 Trimming of dystrophic nails, any number
MCM 2323, MCM 4120

⊙ G0128 Direct (face-to-face with patient) skilled nursing services of a registered nurse provided in a comprehensive outpatient rehabilitation facility, each 10 minutes beyond the first 5 minutes
Medicare Statute 1833a

G0129 Occupational therapy requiring the skills of a qualified occupational therapist, furnished as a component of a partial hospitalization treatment program, per day

⊙ G0130 Single energy x-ray absorptiometry (SEXA) bone density study, one or more sites; appendicular skeleton (peripheral) (e.g., radius, wrist, heel)
CIM 50-44

G0131 Deleted 12/31/02, Cross Reference 76070*

G0132 Deleted 12/31/02, Cross Reference 76071*

✳ G0141 Screening cytopathology smears, cervical or vaginal, performed by automated system, with manual rescreening requiring interpretation by physician;
Laboratory Certification: cytology

✳ G0143 Screening cytopathology, cervical or vaginal (any reporting system); collected in preservative fluid, automated thin layer preparation, with manual screening and rescreening by cytotechnologist under physician supervision;
Laboratory Certification: cytology

✳ G0144 Screening cytopathology, cervical or vaginal (any reporting system); collected in preservative fluid, automated thin layer preparation, with screening by automated system, under physician supervision; Laboratory Certification: cytology

✳ G0145 Screening cytopathology, cervical or vaginal (any reporting system); collected in preservative fluid, automated thin layer preparation, with screening by automated system and manual rescreening under physician supervision; Laboratory Certification: cytology

✳ G0147 Screening cytopathology smears, cervical or vaginal; performed by automated system under physician supervision; Laboratory Certification: cytology

✳ G0148 Screening cytopathology smears, cervical or vaginal; performed by automated system with manual rescreening; Laboratory Certification: cytology

✳ G0151 Services of physical therapist in home health setting, each 15 minutes

✳ G0152 Services of occupational therapist in home health setting, each 15 minutes

✳ G0153 Services of speech and language pathologist in home health setting, each 15 minutes

✳ G0154 Services of skilled nurse in home health setting, each 15 minutes

✳ G0155 Services of clinical social worker in home health setting, each 15 minutes

✳ G0156 Services of home health aide in home health setting, each 15 minutes

⊙ G0166 External counterpulsation, per treatment session
CIM 35-74

G0167 Deleted 12/31/03

✳ G0168 Wound closure utilizing tissue adhesive(s) only

⊙ G0173 Stereotactic radiosurgery, complete course of therapy in one session

⊙ G0174 Deleted 01/01/02

✳ G0175 Scheduled interdisciplinary team conference (minimum of three exclusive of patient care nursing staff) with patient present

⊙ G0176 Activity therapy, such as music, dance, art or play therapies not for recreation, related to the care and treatment of patient's disabling mental health problems, per session (45 minutes or more)

⊙ G0177 Training and educational services related to the care and treatment of patient's disabling mental health problems per session (45 minutes or more)

G0178 Deleted 01/01/02

* G0179 Physician re-certification for Medicare-covered home health services under a home health plan of care (patient not present), including contacts with home health agency and review of reports of patient status required by physicians to affirm the initial implementation of the plan of care that meets patient's needs, per re-certification period

* G0180 Physician certification for Medicare-covered home health services under a home health plan of care (patient not present), including contacts with home health agency and review of reports of patient status required by physicians to affirm the initial implementation of the plan of care that meets patient's needs, per certification period

* G0181 Physician supervision of a patient receiving Medicare-covered services provided by a participating home health agency (patient not present) requiring complex and multidisciplinary care modalities involving regular physician development and/or revision of care plans, review of subsequent reports of patient status, review of laboratory and other studies, communication (including telephone calls) with other health care professionals involved in the patient's care, integration of new information into the medical treatment plan, and/or adjustment of medical therapy, within a calendar month, 30 minutes or more

* G0182 Physician supervision of a patient under a Medicare-approved hospice (patient not present) requiring complex and multidisciplinary care modalities involving regular physician development and/or revision of care plans, review of subsequent reports of patient status, review of laboratory and other studies, communication (including telephone calls) with other health care professionals involved in the patient's care, integration of new information into the medical treatment plan, and/or adjustment of medical therapy, within a calendar month, 30 minutes or more

G0184 Deleted 01/01/02

G0185 Deleted 12/31/02, Cross Reference 0016T*

* G0186 Destruction of localized lesion of choroid (for example, choroidal neovascularization); photocoagulation, feeder vessel technique (one or more sessions)

G0187 Deleted 12/31/02

G0188 Deleted 01/01/02

G0190 Deleted 01/01/02
G0191 Deleted 01/01/02
G0192 Deleted 12/31/02
G0193 Deleted 12/31/02, Cross Reference 92612*
G0194 Deleted 12/31/02, Cross Reference 92614*
G0195 Deleted 12/31/02, Cross Reference 92610*
G0196 Deleted 12/31/02, Cross Reference 92611*
G0197 Deleted 12/31/02, Cross Reference 92607*
G0198 Deleted 12/31/02, Cross Reference 92609*
G0199 Deleted 12/31/02, Cross Reference 92607 and 92608*
G0200 Deleted 12/31/02, Cross Reference 92506*
G0201 Deleted 12/31/02, Cross Reference 92507*
* G0202 Screening mammography, producing direct digital image, bilateral, all views
G0203 Deleted 01/01/02
* G0204 Diagnostic mammography, producing direct digital image, bilateral, all views
G0205 Deleted 01/01/02
* G0206 Diagnostic mammography, producing direct digital image, unilateral, all views
G0207 Deleted 01/01/02
G0210 PET imaging whole body; diagnosis; lung cancer, non-small cell MCM 4173 CIM 50-36
G0211 PET imaging whole body; initial staging; lung cancer; non-small cell (replaces G0126) MCM 4173 CIM 50-36
G0212 PET imaging whole body; restaging; lung cancer; non-small cell MCM 4173 CIM 50-36
G0213 PET imaging whole body; diagnosis; colorectal cancer MCM 4173 CIM 50-36
G0214 PET imaging whole body; initial staging; colorectal cancer MCM 4173 CIM 50-36
G0215 PET imaging whole body; restaging; colorectal cancer (replaces G0163) MCM 4173 CIM 50-36
G0216 PET imaging whole body; diagnosis; melanoma MCM 4173 CIM 50-36
G0217 PET imaging whole body; initial staging; melanoma MCM 4173 CIM 50-36
G0218 PET imaging whole body; restaging; melanoma (replaces G0165) MCM 4173 CIM 50-36
G0219 PET imaging whole body melanoma; for non-covered indications MCM 4173 CIM 50-36

⊛ G0220 PET imaging whole body; diagnosis; lymphoma
MCM 4173 CIM 50-36

⊛ G0221 PET imaging whole body; initial staging; lymphoma (replaces G0164)
MCM 4173 CIM 50-36

⊛ G0222 PET imaging whole body; restaging; lymphoma (replaces G0164)
MCM 4173 CIM 50-36

⊛ G0223 PET imaging whole body or regional; diagnosis; head and neck cancer; excluding thyroid and CNS cancers
MCM 4173 CIM 50-36

⊛ G0224 PET imaging whole body or regional; initial staging; head and neck cancer; excluding thyroid and CNS cancers
MCM 4173 CIM 50-36

⊛ G0225 PET imaging whole body or regional; restaging; head and neck cancer, excluding thyroid and CNS cancers
MCM 4173 CIM 50-36

⊛ G0226 PET imaging whole body; diagnosis; esophageal cancer
MCM 4173 CIM 50-36

⊛ G0227 PET imaging whole body; initial staging; esophageal cancer
MCM 4173 CIM 50-36

⊛ G0228 PET imaging whole body; restaging; esophageal cancer
MCM 4173 CIM 50-36

⊛ G0229 PET imaging; metabolic brain imaging for pre-surgical evaluation of refractory seizures
MCM 4173 CIM 50-36

⊛ G0230 PET imaging; metabolic assessment for myocardial viability following inconclusive SPECT study
MCM 4173 CIM 50-36

⊛ G0231 PET, whole body, for recurrence of colorectal or colorectal metastatic cancer; gamma cameras only
CIM 50-36

⊛ G0232 PET, whole body, staging and characterization of lymphoma; gamma cameras only
CIM 50-36

⊛ G0233 PET, whole body, for recurrence of melanoma or melanoma metastatic cancer; gamma cameras only
CIM 50-36

⊛ G0234 PET, regional or whole body, for solitary pulmonary nodule following CT or for initial staging of pathologically diagnosed non-small cell lung cancer; gamma cameras only
CIM 50-36

G0236 Deleted 12/31/03

∗ G0237 Therapeutic procedures to increase strength or endurance of respiratory muscles, face to face, one on one, each 15 minutes

∗ G0238 Therapeutic procedures to improve respiratory function, other than described by G0237, one on one, face to face, per 15 minutes

∗ G0239 Therapeutic procedures to improve respiratory function or increase strength or endurance of respiratory muscles, two or more individuals (includes monitoring)

G0240 Deleted 12/31/02
G0241 Deleted 12/31/02

⊛ G0242 Multi-source photon stereotactic radiosurgery (cobalt-60 multi-source converging beams) plan, including dose volume histograms for target and critical structure tolerances, plan optimization performed for highly conformal distributions, plan positional accuracy and dose verification, all lesions treated, per course of treatment

⊛ G0243 Multi-source photon stereotactic radiosurgery, delivery including collimator changes and custom plugging, complete course of treatment, all lesions

⊛ G0244 Observation care provided by a facility to a patient with congestive heart failure, chest pain, or asthma, minimum 8 hours, maximum 48 hours

LOSS OF PROTECTIVE SENSATION (LOPS)

⊛ G0245 Initial physician evaluation of a diabetic patient with diabetic sensory neuropathy resulting in a loss of protective sensation (LOPS) which must include (1) the diagnosis of LOPS; (2) a patient history; (3) a physical examination that consist of *at least* the following elements:
   a. Visual inspection of the forefoot, hindfoot and toeweb spaces
   b. Evaluation of a protective sensation
   c. Evaluation of foot structure and biomechanics
   d. Evaluation of vascular status and skin integrity
   e. Evaluation and recommendation of footwear
   4. Patient education
   CIM 50-81

⊛ G0246 Follow-up physician evaluation and management of a diabetic patient with diabetic sensory neuropathy resulting in a loss of protective sensation (LOPS) to include at least the following, (1) a patient history (2) a physical examination that includes:

a. Visual inspection of the forefoot, hindfoot and toe web spaces
b. Evaluation of protective sensation
c. Evaluation of foot structure and biomechanics
d. Evaluation of vascular status and skin integrity
e. Evaluation and recommendation of footwear
3. Patient education

➟ ✪ **G0247** Routine foot care by a physician of a diabetic patient with diabetic sensory neuropathy resulting in a loss of protective sensation (LOPS) to include the local care of superficial wounds (i.e. superficial to muscle and fascia) and at least the following if present: (1) local care of superficial wounds, (2) debridement of corns and calluses, and (3) trimming and debridement of nails
CIM 50-81

"G" Codes for International Normalized Ratio Monitoring

Codes established for CIM 50.55 effective for services furnished on or after July 1, 2002. Use of the International Normalized Ratio (INR) allows physician to determine the level of anti-coagulation in a patient independent of the laboratory reagents used. Home prothrombin monitoring with the use of INR devices is only covered for patients with mechanical heart valves.

CIM reference 50-36 details coverage indications. FDG Positron Emission Tomography is a minimally invasive diagnostic procedure using positron camera (tomograph) to measure the decay of radioisotopes such as FDG, CMS determined that the benefit category for the requested indications fell under 1861(s)(3) of the Social Security Act diagnostic service.

✪ **G0248** Demonstration, at initial use, of home INR monitoring for patient with mechanical heart valve(s) who meets Medicare coverage criteria, under the direction of a physician; includes: demonstrating use and care of the INR monitor, obtaining at least one blood sample, provision of instructions for reporting home INR test results, and documentation of patient ability to perform testing.
CIM 50-55

✪ **G0249** Provision of test materials and equipment for home INR monitoring to patient with mechanical heart valve(s) who meets Medicare coverage criteria; includes provision of materials for use in the home and reporting of test results to physician; per 4 tests.
CIM 50-55

✪ **G0250** Physician review, interpretation and patient management of home INR testing for a patient with mechanical heart valve(s) who meets other coverage criteria; per 4 tests (does not require face-to-face service)
CIM 50-55

✪ **G0251** Linear accelerator based stereotactic radiosurgery, delivery including collimator changes and custom plugging, fractionated treatment, all lesions, per session, maximum five sessions per course of treatment

✪ **G0252** PET imaging, full and partial-ring PET scanners only, for initial diagnosis of breast cancer and/or surgical planning for breast cancer (e.g. initial staging of axillary lymph nodes)
CIM 50-36

✱ **G0253** PET imaging for breast cancer, full and partial-ring PET scanners only, staging/restaging of local regional recurrence or distant metastases (i.e., staging/restaging after or prior to course of treatment)
CIM 50-36

✱ **G0254** PET imaging for breast cancer, full and partial ring PET scanners only, evaluation of response to treatment, performed during course of treatment
CIM 50-36

◆ **G0255** Current perception threshold/sensory nerve conduction test, (SNCT) per limb, any nerve
CIM 50-57

G0256 Deleted 12/31/03

✪ **G0257** Unscheduled or emergency dialysis treatment for an ESRD patient in a hospital outpatient department that is not certified as an ESRD facility

✪ **G0258** Intravenous infusion during separately payable observation stay, per observation stay (must be reported with G0244)

✪ **G0259** Injection procedure for sacroiliac joint; arthrography

✪ **G0260** Injection procedure for sacroiliac joint; provision of anesthetic, steroid and/or other therapeutic agent and arthrography

G0261 Deleted 12/31/03
G0262 Deleted 12/31/03

✪ **G0263** Direct admission of patient with diagnosis of congestive heart failure, chest pain or asthma for observation services that meet all criteria from G0244

✪ G0264   Initial nursing assessment of patient directly admitted to observation with diagnosis other than congestive heart failure, chest pain or asthma or patient directly admitted to observation with diagnosis of CHF, chest pain or asthma when the observation stay does not qualify for G0244

∗ G0265   Cryopreservation, freezing and storage of cells for therapeutic use, each cell line

∗ G0266   Thawing and expansion of frozen cells for therapeutic use, each aliquot

∗ G0267   Bone marrow or peripheral stem cell harvest, modification or treatment to eliminate cell type(s) (e.g. t-cells, metastatic carcinoma)

∗ G0268   Removal of impacted cerumen (one or both ears) by physician on same date of service as audiologic function testing

✪ G0269   Placement of occlusive device into either a venous or arterial access site, post surgical or interventional procedure (e.g. angioseal plug, vascular plug)

∗ G0270   Medical nutrition therapy; reassessment and subsequent intervention(s) following second referral in same year for change in diagnosis, medical condition or treatment regimen (including additional hours needed for renal disease), individual, face to face with the patient, each 15 minutes

∗ G0271   Medical nutrition therapy, reassessment and subsequent intervention(s) following second referral in same year for change in diagnosis, medical condition, or treatment regimen (including additional hours needed for renal disease), group (2 or more individuals), each 30 minutes

G0272-G0274 Deleted 12/31/03

∗ G0275   Renal artery angiography (unilateral or bilateral) performed at the time of cardiac catheterization, includes catheter placement, injection of dye, flush aortogram and radiologic supervision and interpretation and production of images (list separately in addition to primary procedure)

∗ G0278   Iliac artery angiography performed at the same time of cardiac catheterization, includes catheter placement, injection of dye, radiologic supervision and interpretation and production of images (list separately in addition to primary procedure)

∗ G0279   Extracorporeal shock wave therapy; involving elbow epicondylitis

∗ G0280   Extracorporeal shock wave therapy; involving other than elbow epicondylitis or plantar fascitis

∗ G0281   Electrical stimulation, (unattended), to one or more areas, for chronic stage iii and stage iv pressure ulcers, arterial ulcers, diabetic ulcers, and venous stasis ulcers not demonstrating measurable signs of healing after 30 days of conventional care, as part of a therapy plan of care

∗ G0282   Electrical stimulation, (unattended), to one or more areas, for wound care other than described in G0281
CIM 35-98

∗ G0283   Electrical stimulation (unattended), to one or more areas for indication(s) other than wound care, as part of a therapy plan of care

∗ G0288   Reconstruction, computed tomographic angiography of aorta for surgical planning for vascular surgery

∗ G0289   Arthroscopy, knee, surgical, for removal of loose body, foreign body, debridement/shaving of articular cartilage (chondroplasty) at the time of other surgical knee arthroscopy in a different compartment of the same knee

✪ G0290   Transcatheter placement of a drug eluting intracoronary stent(s), percutaneous, with or without other therapeutic intervention, any method; single vessel

✪ G0291   Transcatheter placement of a drug eluting intracoronary stent(s), percutaneous, with or without other therapeutic intervention, any method; each additional vessel

✪ G0292   Administration(s) of experimental drug(s) only in a Medicare qualifying clinical trial (includes administration for chemotherapy and other types of therapy via infusion and/or other than infusion), per day

✪ G0293   Noncovered surgical procedure(s) using conscious sedation, regional, general or spinal anesthesia in a Medicare qualifying clinical trial, per day

✪ G0294   Noncovered procedure(s) using either no anesthesia or local anesthesia only, in a Medicare qualifying clinical trial, per day

◆ G0295   Electromagnetic stimulation, to one or more areas
CIM 35-98

▶∗ G0296   PET imaging, full and partial ring PET scanner only, for restaging of previously treated thyroid cancer of follicular cell origin following negative I-131 whole body scan

▶∗ G0297   Insertion of single chamber pacing cardioverter defibrillator pulse generator

▶✳ G0298   Insertion of dual chamber pacing cardioverter defibrillator pulse generator

▶✳ G0299   Insertion or repositioning of electrode lead for single chamber pacing cardioverter defibrillator and insertion of pulse generator

▶✳ G0300   Insertion or repositioning of electrode lead(s) for dual chamber pacing cardioverter defibrillator and insertion of pulse generator

▶✳ G0302   Pre-operative pulmonary surgery services for preparation for LVRS, complete course of services, to include a minimum of 16 days of services

▶✳ G0303   Pre-operative pulmonary surgery services for preparation for LVRS, 10 to 15 days of services

▶✳ G0304   Pre-operative pulmonary surgery services for preparation for LVRS, 1 to 9 days of services

▶✳ G0305   Post-discharge pulmonary surgery services after LVRS, minimum of 6 days of services

▶✳ G0306   Complete CBC, automated (HgB, HCT, RBC, WBC, without platelet count) and automated WBC differential count
Laboratory Certification 400

▶✳ G0307   Complete CBC, automated (HgB, HCT, RBC, WBC; without platelet count)

▶✿ G0308   End Stage Renal Disease (ESRD) related services during the course of treatment, for patients under 2 years of age to include monitoring for the adequacy of nutrition, assessment of growth and development, and counseling of parents; with 4 or more face-to-face physician visits per month
MCM 2230

▶✿ G0309   End Stage Renal Disease (ESRD) related services during the course of treatment, for patients under 2 years of age to include monitoring for the adequacy of nutrition, assessment of growth and development, and counseling of parents; with 2 or 3 face-to-face physician visits per month
MCM 2230

▶✿ G0310   End Stage Renal Disease (ESRD) related services during the course of treatment, for patients under 2 years of age to include monitoring for the adequacy of nutrition, assessment of growth and development, and counseling of parents; with 1 face-to-face physician visit per month
MCM 2230

▶✿ G0311   End Stage Renal Disease (ESRD) related services during the course of treatment, for patients between 2 and 11 years of age to include monitoring for the adequacy of nutrition, assessment of growth and development, and counseling of parents; with 4 or more face-to-face physician visits per month
MCM 2230

▶✿ G0312   End Stage Renal Disease (ESRD) related services during the course of treatment, for patients between 2 and 11 years of age to include monitoring for the adequacy of nutrition, assessment of growth and development, and counseling of parents; with 2 or 3 face-to-face physician visits per month
MCM 2230

▶✿ G0313   End Stage Renal Disease (ESRD) related services during the course of treatment, for patients between 2 and 11 years of age to include monitoring for the adequacy of nutrition, assessment of growth and development, and counseling of parents; with 1 face-to-face physician visits per month
MCM 2230

▶✿ G0314   End Stage Renal Disease (ESRD) related services during the course of treatment, for patients between 12 and 19 years of age to include monitoring for the adequacy of nutrition, assessment of growth and development, and counseling of parents; with 4 or more face-to-face physician visits per month
MCM 2230

▶✿ G0315   End Stage Renal Disease (ESRD) related services during the course of treatment, for patients between 12 and 19 years of age to include monitoring for the adequacy of nutrition, assessment of growth and development, and counseling of parents; with 2 or 3 face-to-face physician visits per month
MCM 2230

▶✿ G0316   End Stage Renal Disease (ESRD) related services during the course of treatment, for patients between 12 and 19 years of age to include monitoring for the adequacy of nutrition, assessment of growth and development, and counseling of parents; with 1 face-to-face physician visits per month
MCM 2230

▶✿ G0317   End Stage Renal Disease (ESRD) related services during the course of treatment, for patients 20 years of age and over; with 4 or more face-to-face physician visits per month
MCM 2230

▶ ✪ G0318   End Stage Renal Disease (ESRD) related services during the course of treatment, for patients 20 years of age and over; with 2 or 3 face-to-face physician visits per month
MCM 2230

▶ ✪ G0319   End Stage Renal Disease (ESRD) related services during the course of treatment, for patients 20 years of age and over; with 1 face-to-face physician visit per month
MCM 2230

▶ ✪ G0320   End stage renal disease (ESRD) related services for home dialysis patients per full month; for patients under two years of age to include monitoring for adequacy of nutrition, assessment of growth and development, and counseling of parents
MCM 2230

▶ ✪ G0321   End stage renal disease (ESRD) related services for home dialysis patients per full month; for patients two to eleven years of age to include monitoring for adequacy of nutrition, assessment of growth and development, and counseling of parents
MCM 2230

▶ ✪ G0322   End stage renal disease (ESRD) related services for home dialysis patients per full month; for patients twelve to nineteen years of age to include monitoring for adequacy of nutrition, assessment of growth and development, and counseling of parents
MCM 2230

▶ ✪ G0323   End stage renal disease (ESRD) related services for home dialysis patients per full month; for patients twenty years of age and older
MCM 2230

▶ ✪ G0324   End stage renal disease (ESRD) related services for home dialysis (less than full month), per day; for patients under two years of age
MCM 2230

▶ ✪ G0325   End stage renal disease (ESRD) related services for home dialysis (less than full month), per day; for patients between two and eleven years of age
MCM 2230

▶ ✪ G0326   End stage renal disease (ESRD) related services for home dialysis (less than full month), per day; for patients between twelve and nineteen years of age
MCM 2230

▶ ✪ G0327   End stage renal disease (ESRD) related services for home dialysis (less than full month), per day; for patients twenty years of age and over
MCM 2230

▶ ✪ G0328   Colorectal cancer screening; fecal occult blood test, immunoassay, 1-3 simultaneous
Laboratory Certification 310, 400

▶ ✱ G0338   Linear-accelerator-based stereotactic radiosurgery plan, including dose volume histograms for target and critical structure tolerances, plan optimization performed for highly conformal distributions, plan positional accuracy and dose verification, all lesions treated, per course of treatment

▶ ✱ G0339   Image-guided robotic linear accelerator-based stereotactic radiosurgery, complete course of therapy in one session or first session or fractionated treatment

▶ ✱ G0340   Image-guided robotic linear accelerator-based stereotactic radiosurgery, delivery including collimator changes and custom plugging, fractionated treatment, all lesions, per session, second through fifth sessions, maximum five sessions per course of treatment

▶ ✱ G3001   Administration and supply of tositumomab, 450 mg

✪ G9001   Coordination fee, initial rate

✪ G9002   Coordinated care fee, maintenance rate

✪ G9003   Coordinated care fee, risk adjusted high, initial

✪ G9004   Coordinated care fee, risk adjusted low, initial

✪ G9005   Coordinated care fee, risk adjusted maintenance

✪ G9006   Coordinated care fee, home monitoring

✪ G9007   Coordinated care fee, scheduled team conference

✪ G9008   Coordinated care fee, physician coordinated care oversight services

✪ G9009   Coordination care fee, risk adjustment maintenance, level 3

✪ G9010   Coordination care fee, risk adjustment maintenance, level 4

✪ G9011   Coordination care fee, risk adjustment maintenance, level 5

✪ G9012   Other specified care management services not elsewhere classified

◆ G9016   Smoking cessation counseling, individual, in the absence of or in addition to any other evaluation and management service, per session (6-10 minutes) (demo project code only)

ALCOHOL AND/OR DRUG SERVICES (H0001-H1005)

◆ H0001   Alcohol and/or drug assessment

◆ H0002   Behavioral health screening to determine eligibility for admission to treatment program

- H0003 Alcohol and/or drug screening; laboratory analysis of specimens for presence of alcohol and/or drugs
- H0004 Behavioral health counseling and therapy, per 15 minutes
- H0005 Alcohol and/or drug services; group counseling by a clinician
- H0006 Alcohol and/or drug services; case management
- H0007 Alcohol and/or drug services; crisis intervention (outpatient)
- H0008 Alcohol and/or drug services; subacute detoxification (hospital inpatient)
- H0009 Alcohol and/or drug services; acute detoxification (hospital inpatient)
- H0010 Alcohol and/or drug services; subacute detoxification (residential addiction program inpatient)
- H0011 Alcohol and/or drug services; acute detoxification (residential addiction program inpatient)
- H0012 Alcohol and/or drug services; subacute detoxification (residential addiction program outpatient)
- H0013 Alcohol and/or drug services; acute detoxification (residential addiction program outpatient)
- H0014 Alcohol and/or drug services; ambulatory detoxification
- H0015 Alcohol and/or drug services; intensive outpatient (treatment program that operates at least 3 hours per day and at least 3 days per week and is based on an individualized treatment plan), including assessment, counseling; crisis intervention, and activity therapies or education
- H0016 Alcohol and/or drug services; medical/somatic (medical intervention in ambulatory setting)
- H0017 Behavioral health; residential (hospital residential treatment program), without room and board, per diem
- H0018 Behavioral health; short-term residential (non-hospital residential treatment program), without room and board, per diem
- H0019 Behavioral health; long-term residential (non-medial, non-acute care in a residential treatment program where stay is typically longer than 30 days), without room and board, per diem
- H0020 Alcohol and/or drug services; methadone administration and/or service (provision of the drug by a licensed program)
- H0021 Alcohol and/or drug training service (for staff and personnel not employed by providers)
- H0022 Alcohol and/or drug intervention service (planned facilitation)
- H0023 Behavioral health outreach service (planned approach to reach a target population)
- H0024 Behavioral health prevention information dissemination service (one-way direct or non-direct contact with service audiences to affect knowledge or attitude)
- H0025 Behavioral health prevention education service (delivery of services with target population to affect knowledge, attitude, and/or behavior)
- H0026 Alcohol and/or drug prevention process service, community-based (delivery of services to develop skills of impactors)
- H0027 Alcohol and/or drug prevention environmental service (broad range of external activities geared toward modifying systems in order to mainstream prevention through policy and law)
- H0028 Alcohol and/or drug prevention problem identification and referral service (e.g., student assistance and employee assistance programs), does not include assessment
- H0029 Alcohol and/or drug prevention alternatives service (services for populations that exclude alcohol and other drug use [e.g., alcohol-free social events])
- H0030 Behavioral health hotline service
- H0031 Mental health assessment, by non-physician
- H0032 Mental health service plan development by non-physician
- H0033 Oral medication administration, direct observation
- H0034 Medication training and support, per 15 minutes
- H0035 Mental health partial hospitalization, treatment, less than 24 hours
- H0036 Community psychiatric supportive treatment, face-to-face, per 15 minutes
- H0037 Community psychiatric supportive treatment program, per diem
- H0038 Self-help/peer services, per 15 minutes
- H0039 Assertive community treatment, face-to-face, per 15 minutes
- H0040 Assertive community treatment program, per diem
- H0041 Foster care, child, non-therapeutic, per diem
- H0042 Foster care, child, non-therapeutic, per month?
- H0043 Supported housing, per diem
- H0044 Supported housing, per month
- H0045 Respite care services, not in the home, per diem
- H0046 Mental health services, not otherwise specified

◆ H0047 Alcohol and/or other drug abuse services, not otherwise specified

◆ H0048 Alcohol and/or other drug testing: collection and handling only, specimens other than blood

◆ H1000 Prenatal care, at-risk assessment

◆ H1001 Prenatal care, at-risk enhanced service; antepartum management

◆ H1002 Prenatal care, at-risk enhanced service; care coordination

◆ H1003 Prenatal care, at-risk enhanced service; education

◆ H1004 Prenatal care, at-risk enhanced service; follow-up home visit

◆ H1005 Prenatal care, at-risk enhanced service package (includes H1001-H1004)

◆ H1010 Non-medical family planning education, per session

◆ H1011 Family assessment by licensed behavioral health professional for state defined purposes

◆ H2000 Comprehensive multidisciplinary evaluation

◆ H2001 Rehabilitation program, per 1/2 day

▶◆ H2010 Comprehensive medication services, per 15 minutes

▶◆ H2011 Crisis intervention service, per 15 minutes

▶◆ H2012 Behavioral health day treatment, per hour

▶◆ H2013 Psychiatric health facility service, per diem

▶◆ H2014 Skills training and development, per 15 minutes

▶◆ H2015 Comprehensive community support services, per 15 minutes

▶◆ H2016 Comprehensive community support services, per diem

▶◆ H2017 Psychosocial rehabilitation services, per 15 minutes

▶◆ H2018 Psychosocial rehabilitation services, per diem

▶◆ H2019 Therapeutic behavioral services, per 15 minutes

▶◆ H2020 Therapeutic behavioral services, per diem

▶◆ H2021 Community-based wrap-around services, per 15 minutes

▶◆ H2022 Community-based wrap-around services, per diem

▶◆ H2023 Supported employment, per 15 minutes

▶◆ H2024 Supported employment, per diem

▶◆ H2025 Ongoing support to maintain employment, per 15 minutes

▶◆ H2026 Ongoing support to maintain employment, per diem

▶◆ H2027 Psychoeducational service, per 15 minutes

▶◆ H2028 Sexual offender treatment service, per 15 minutes

▶◆ H2029 Sexual offender treatment service, per diem

▶◆ H2030 Mental health clubhouse services, per 15 minutes

▶◆ H2031 Mental health clubhouse services, per diem

▶◆ H2032 Activity therapy, per 15 minutes

▶◆ H2033 Multisystemic therapy for juveniles, per 15 minutes

▶◆ H2034 Alcohol and/or drug abuse halfway house services, per diem

▶◆ H2035 Alcohol and/or other drug treatment program, per hour

▶◆ H2036 Alcohol and/or other drug treatment program, per diem

▶◆ H2037 Developmental delay prevention activities, dependent child of client, per 15 minutes

DRUGS OTHER THAN CHEMOTHERAPY (J0100-J8999)

☺ J0120 Injection, tetracycline, up to 250 mg
MCM 2049

☺ J0130 Injection abciximab, 10 mg
MCM 2049

☺ J0150 Injection, adenosine, 6 mg (not to be used to report any adenosine phosphate compounds; instead use A9270)
MCM 2049

J0151 Deleted 12/31/03, Cross Reference J0152

▶✳ J0152 Injection, adenosine, 30 mg (not to be used to report any adenosine phosphate compounds; instead use A9270)

☺ J0170 Injection, adrenalin, epinephrine, up to 1 ml ampule
MCM 2049

☺ J0190 Injection, biperiden lactate, per 5 mg
MCM 2049

☺ J0200 Injection, alatrofloxacin mesylate, 100 mg
MCM 2049.5

☺ J0205 Injection, alglucerase, per 10 units
MCM 2049

☺ J0207 Injection, amifostine, 500 mg
MCM 2049

☺ J0210 Injection, methyldopate HCl, up to 250 mg
MCM 2049

▶✳ J0215 Injection, alefacept, 0.5 mg

☺ J0256 Injection, alpha-1-proteinase inhibitor (human), 10 mg
MCM 2049

☺ J0270 Injection, alprostadil, per 1.25 mcg (Code may be used for Medicare when drug administered under the direct supervision of a physician, not for use when drug is self-administered.)
MCM 2049

⊗ J0275 Alprostadil urethral suppository (Code may be used for Medicare when drug administered under the direct supervision of a physician, not for use when drug is self-administered.)
MCM 2049

⊗ J0280 Injection, aminophylline, up to 250 mg
MCM 2049

⊗ J0282 Injection, amiodarone HCl, 30 mg
MCM 2049

⊗ J0285 Injection, amphotericin B, 50 mg
MCM 2049

   J0286 Deleted 12/31/02

⊗ J0287 Injection, amphotericin B lipid complex, 10 mg
MCM 2049

⊗ J0288 Injection, amphotericin B cholesteryl sulfate complex, 10 mg
MCM 2049

⊗ J0289 Injection, amphotericin B liposome, 10 mg
MCM 2049

⊗ J0290 Injection, ampicillin sodium, 500 mg
MCM 2049

⊗ J0295 Injection, ampicillin sodium/sulbactam sodium, per 1.5 gm
MCM 2049

⊗ J0300 Injection, amobarbital, up to 125 mg
MCM 2049

⊗ J0330 Injection, succinylcholine chloride, up to 20 mg
MCM 2049

   J0340 Deleted 01/01/02

⊗ J0350 Injection, anistreplase, per 30 units
MCM 2049

⊗ J0360 Injection, hydralazine HCl, up to 20 mg
MCM 2049

⊗ J0380 Injection, metaraminol bitartrate, per 10 mg
MCM 2049

⊗ J0390 Injection, chloroquine HCl, up to 250 mg
MCM 2049

⊗ J0395 Injection, arbutamine HCl, 1 mg
MCM 2049

   J0400 Deleted 01/01/02

⊗ J0456 Injection, azithromycin, 500 mg
MCM 2049.5

⊗ J0460 Injection, atropine sulfate, up to 0.3 mg
MCM 2049

⊗ J0470 Injection, dimercaprol, per 100 mg
MCM 2049

⊗ J0475 Injection, baclofen, 10 mg
MCM 2049

⊗ J0476 Injection, baclofen 50 mcg for intrathecal trial
MCM 2049

⊗ J0500 Injection, dicyclomine HCl, up to 20 mg
MCM 2049

   J0510 Deleted 01/01/02

⊗ J0515 Injection, benztropine mesylate, per 1 mg
MCM 2049

⊗ J0520 Injection, bethanechol chloride, myotonachol or urecholine, up to 5 mg
MCM 2049

⊗ J0530 Injection, penicillin G benzathine and penicillin G procaine, up to 600,000 units
MCM 2049

⊗ J0540 Injection, penicillin G benzathine and penicillin G procaine, up to 1,200,000 units
MCM 2049

⊗ J0550 Injection, penicillin G benzathine and penicillin G procaine, up to 2,400,000 units
MCM 2049

⊗ J0560 Injection, penicillin G benzathine, up to 600,000 units
MCM 2049

⊗ J0570 Injection, penicillin G benzathine, up to 1,200,000 units
MCM 2049

⊗ J0580 Injection, penicillin G benzathine, up to 2,400,000 units
MCM 2049

▶* J0583 Injection, bivalirudin, 1 mg

⊗ J0585 Botulinum toxin type A, per unit
MCM 2049

⊗ J0587 Botulinum toxin type B, per 100 units

   J0590 Deleted 01/01/02

⊗ J0592 Injection, buprenorphine hydrochloride, 0.1 mg
MCM 2049

▶* J0595 Injection, butorphanol tartrate, 1 mg

⊗ J0600 Injection, edetate calcium disodium, up to 1000 mg
MCM 2049

⊗ J0610 Injection, calcium gluconate, per 10 ml
MCM 2049

⊗ J0620 Injection, calcium glycerophosphate and calcium lactate, per 10 ml
MCM 2049

⊗ J0630 Injection, calcitonin (salmon), up to 400 units
MCM 2049

   J0635 Deleted 12/31/02

⊗ J0636 Injection, calcitriol, 0.1 mcg
MCM 2049

* J0637 Injection, caspofungin acetate, 5 mg

⊗ J0640 Injection, leucovorin calcium, per 50 mg
MCM 2049

⊗ J0670 Injection, mepivacaine HCl, per 10 ml
MCM 2049

⊗ J0690 Injection, cefazolin sodium, 500 mg
MCM 2049

   J0690 Injection, cefepime HCl, 500 mg

* J0692 Injection, cefepime HCl, 500 mg

⊗ J0694 Injection, cefoxitin sodium, 1 gm
MCM 2049, Cross Reference Q0090

J0695   Deleted 01/01/02

⊘ J0696   Injection, ceftriaxone sodium, per 250 mg
MCM 2049

⊘ J0697   Injection, sterile cefuroxime sodium, per 750 mg
MCM 2049

⊘ J0698   Injection, cefotaxime sodium, per gm
MCM 2049

⊘ J0702   Injection, betamethasone acetate and betamethasone sodium phosphate, per 3 mg
MCM 2049

⊘ J0704   Injection, betamethasone sodium phosphate, per 4 mg
MCM 2049

✳ J0706   Injection, caffeine citrate, 5 mg

⊘ J0710   Injection, cephapirin sodium, up to 1 gm
MCM 2049

⊘ J0713   Injection, ceftazidime, per 500 mg
MCM 2049

⊘ J0715   Injection, ceftizoxime sodium, per 500 mg
MCM 2049

⊘ J0720   Injection, chloramphenicol sodium succinate, up to 1 gm
MCM 2049

⊘ J0725   Injection, chorionic gonadotropin, per 1,000 USP units
MCM 2049

J0730   Deleted 01/01/02

⊘ J0735   Injection, clonidine HCl, 1 mg
MCM 2049

⊘ J0740   Injection, cidofovir, 375 mg
MCM 2049

⊘ J0743   Injection, cilastatin sodium; imipenem, per 250 mg
MCM 2049

✳ J0744   Injection, ciprofloxacin for IV infusion, 200 mg

⊘ J0745   Injection, codeine phosphate, per 30 mg
MCM 2049

⊘ J0760   Injection, colchicine, per 1 mg
MCM 2049

⊘ J0770   Injection, colistimethate sodium, up to 150 mg
MCM 2049

⊘ J0780   Injection, prochlorperazine, up to 10 mg
MCM 2049

⊘ J0800   Injection, corticotropin, up to 40 units
MCM 2049

J0810   Deleted 01/01/02

⊘ J0835   Injection, cosyntropin, per 0.25 mg
MCM 2049

⊘ J0850   Injection, cytomegalovirus immune globulin IV (human), per vial
MCM 2049

➡✳ J0880   Injection, darbepoetin alfa, 5 mcg

⊘ J0895   Injection, deferoxamine mesylate, 500 mg
MCM 2049, Cross Reference Q0087

⊘ J0900   Injection, testosterone enanthate and estradiol valerate, up to 1 cc
MCM 2049

⊘ J0945   Injection, brompheniramine maleate, per 10 mg
MCM 2049

⊘ J0970   Injection, estradiol valerate, up to 40 mg
MCM 2049

⊘ J1000   Injection, depo-estradiol cypionate, up to 5 mg
MCM 2049

⊘ J1020   Injection, methylprednisolone acetate, 20 mg
MCM 2049

⊘ J1030   Injection, methylprednisolone acetate, 40 mg
MCM 2049

⊘ J1040   Injection, methylprednisolone acetate, 80 mg
MCM 2049

J1050   Deleted 12/31/02

⊘ J1051   Injection, medroxyprogesterone acetate, 50 mg
MCM 2049

◆ J1055   Injection, medroxyprogesterone acetate for contraceptive use, 150 mg
Medicare Statute 1862A1

✳ J1056   Injection, medroxyprogesterone acetate/ estradiol cypionate, 5 mg/ 25 mg

⊘ J1060   Injection, testosterone cypionate and estradiol cypionate, up to 1 ml
MCM 2049

⊘ J1070   Injection, testosterone cypionate, up to 100 mg
MCM 2049

⊘ J1080   Injection, testosterone cypionate, 1 cc, 200 mg
MCM 2049

J1090   Deleted 01/01/02

⊘ J1094   Injection, dexamethasone acetate, 1 mg
MCM 2049

J1095   Deleted 12/31/02

⊘ J1100   Injection, dexamethasone sodium phosphate, 1 mg
MCM 2049

⊘ J1110   Injection, dihydroergotamine mesylate, per 1 mg
MCM 2049

⊘ J1120   Injection, acetazolamide sodium, up to 500 mg
MCM 2049

⊘ J1160   Injection, digoxin, up to 0.5 mg
MCM 2049

⊘ J1165   Injection, phenytoin sodium, per 50 mg
MCM 2049

⊘ J1170   Injection, hydromorphone, up to 4 mg
MCM 2049

✪ J1180	Injection, dyphylline, up to 500 mg MCM 2049
✪ J1190	Injection, dexrazoxane HCl, per 250 mg MCM 2049
✪ J1200	Injection, diphenhydramine HCl, up to 50 mg MCM 2049
✪ J1205	Injection, chlorothiazide sodium, per 500 mg MCM 2049
✪ J1212	Injection, dimethyl sulfoxide, DMSO, 50%, 50 ml MCM 2049, CIM 45-23
✪ J1230	Injection, methadone HCl, up to 10 mg MCM 2049
✪ J1240	Injection, dimenhydrinate, up to 50 mg MCM 2049
✪ J1245	Injection, dipyridamole, per 10 mg MCM 2049, MCM 15030
✪ J1250	Injection, dobutamine HCl, per 250 mg MCM 2049
✪ J1260	Injection, dolasetron mesylate, 10 mg MCM 2049
✱ J1270	Injection, doxercalciferol, 1 mcg
✪ J1320	Injection, amitriptyline HCl, up to 20 mg MCM 2049
✪ J1325	Injection, epoprostenol, 0.5 mg MCM 2049
✪ J1327	Injection, eptifibatide, 5 mg MCM 2049
✪ J1330	Injection, ergonovine maleate, up to 0.2 mg MCM 2049
▶✱ J1335	Injection, ertapenem sodium, 500 mg
J1362	Deleted 01/01/02
✪ J1364	Injection, erythromycin lactobionate, per 500 mg MCM 2049
✪ J1380	Injection, estradiol valerate, up to 10 mg MCM 2049
✪ J1390	Injection, estradiol valerate, up to 20 mg MCM 2049
✪ J1410	Injection, estrogen conjugated, per 25 mg MCM 2049
✪ J1435	Injection, estrone, per 1 mg MCM 2049
✪ J1436	Injection, etidronate disodium, per 300 mg MCM 2049
✪ J1438	Injection, etanercept, 25 mg (Code may be used for Medicare when drug administered under the direct supervision of a physician, not for use when drug is self-administered.)
✪ J1440	Injection, filgrastim (G-CSF), 300 mcg MCM 2049
✪ J1441	Injection, filgrastim (G-CSF), 480 mcg MCM 2049
✪ J1450	Injection, fluconazole, 200 mg MCM 2049.5
✪ J1452	Injection, fomivirsen sodium, intraocular, 1.65 mg MCM 2049.3
✪ J1455	Injection, foscarnet sodium, per 1000 mg MCM 2049
✪ J1460	Injection, gamma globulin, intramuscular, 1 cc MCM 2049
✪ J1470	Injection, gamma globulin, intramuscular, 2 cc MCM 2049
✪ J1480	Injection, gamma globulin, intramuscular, 3 cc MCM 2049
✪ J1490	Injection, gamma globulin, intramuscular, 4 cc MCM 2049
✪ J1500	Injection, gamma globulin, intramuscular, 5 cc MCM 2049
✪ J1510	Injection, gamma globulin, intramuscular, 6 cc MCM 2049
✪ J1520	Injection, gamma globulin, intramuscular, 7 cc MCM 2049
✪ J1530	Injection, gamma globulin, intramuscular, 8 cc MCM 2049
✪ J1540	Injection, gamma globulin, intramuscular, 9 cc MCM 2049
✪ J1550	Injection, gamma globulin, intramuscular, 10 cc MCM 2049
✪ J1560	Injection, gamma globulin, intramuscular, over 10 cc MCM 2049
J1561	Deleted 12/31/02
J1562	Deleted 01/01/01
✪ J1563	Injection, immune globulin, IV, 1 gm MCM 2049
✪ J1564	Injection, immune globulin, 10 mg MCM 2049
✪ J1565	Injection, respiratory syncytial virus immune globulin, IV, 50 mg MCM 2049
✪ J1570	Injection, ganciclovir sodium, 500 mg MCM 2049
✪ J1580	Injection, Garamycin, gentamicin, up to 80 mg MCM 2049
✱ J1590	Injection, gatifloxacin, 10 mg
▶✪ J1595	Injection, glatiramer acetate, 20 mg MCM 2049

✿	J1600	Injection, gold sodium thiomalate, up to 50 mg MCM 2049
✿	J1610	Injection, glucagon HCl, per 1 mg MCM 2049
✿	J1620	Injection, gonadorelin HCl, per 100 mcg MCM 2049
✿	J1626	Injection, granisetron HCl, 100 mcg MCM 2049
✿	J1630	Injection, haloperidol, up to 5 mg MCM 2049
✿	J1631	Injection, haloperidol decanoate, per 50 mg MCM 2049
✿	J1642	Injection, heparin sodium, (heparin lock flush), per 10 units MCM 2049
✿	J1644	Injection, heparin sodium, per 1000 units MCM 2049
✿	J1645	Injection, dalteparin sodium, per 2500 IU MCM 2049
➡ ✳	J1650	Injection, enoxaparin sodium, 10 mg
✿	J1652	Injection, fondaparinux sodium, 0.5 mg MCM 2049
✳	J1655	Injection, tinzaparin sodium 1000 IU
✿	J1670	Injection, tetanus immune globulin (human), up to 250 units MCM 2049
	J1690	Deleted 01/01/02
✿	J1700	Injection, hydrocortisone acetate, up to 25 mg MCM 2049
✿	J1710	Injection, hydrocortisone sodium phosphate, up to 50 mg MCM 2049
✿	J1720	Injection, hydrocortisone sodium succinate, up to 100 mg MCM 2049
✿	J1730	Injection, diazoxide, up to 300 mg MCM 2049
	J1739	Deleted 01/01/02
	J1741	Deleted 01/01/02
✿	J1742	Injection, ibutilide fumarate, 1 mg MCM 2049
✿	J1745	Injection, infliximab, 10 mg MCM 2049
✿	J1750	Injection, iron dextran, 50 mg MCM 2049.5
	J1755	Deleted 12/31/02
✳	J1756	Injection, iron sucrose, 1 mg
✿	J1785	Injection, imiglucerase, per unit MCM 2049
✿	J1790	Injection, droperidol, up to 5 mg MCM 2049
✿	J1800	Injection, propranolol HCl, up to 1 mg MCM 2049
✿	J1810	Injection, droperidol and fentanyl citrate, up to 2 ml ampule MCM 2049
✿	J1815	Injection, insulin, per 5 units MCM 2049, CIM 60-14
✳	J1817	Insulin for administration through DME (i.e., insulin pump) per 50 units
	J1820	Deleted 12/31/02, Cross Reference J1815
✿	J1825	Injection, interferon beta-1a, 33 mcg MCM 2049
✿	J1830	Injection interferon beta-1b, per 0.25 mg (Code may be used for Medicare when drug administered under the direct supervision of a physician, not for use when drug is self-administered.) MCM 2049
✳	J1835	Injection, itraconazole, 50 mg
✿	J1840	Injection, kanamycin sulfate, up to 500 mg MCM 2049
✿	J1850	Injection, kanamycin sulfate, up to 75 mg MCM 2049
✿	J1885	Injection, ketorolac tromethamine, per 15 mg MCM 2049
✿	J1890	Injection, cephalothin sodium, up to 1 gm MCM 2049
	J1910	Deleted 12/31/03
	J1930	Deleted 01/01/02
✿	J1940	Injection, furosemide, up to 20 mg MCM 2049
✿	J1950	Injection, leuprolide acetate (for depot suspension), per 3.75 mg MCM 2049
✿	J1955	Injection, levocarnitine, per 1 gm MCM 2049
✿	J1956	Injection, levofloxacin, 250 mg MCM 2049
✿	J1960	Injection, levorphanol tartrate, up to 2 mg MCM 2049
	J1970	Deleted 01/01/02
✿	J1980	Injection, hyoscyamine sulfate, up to 0.25 mg MCM 2049
✿	J1990	Injection, chlordiazepoxide HCl, up to 100 mg MCM 2049
	J2000	Deleted 12/31/03
▶ ✿	J2001	Injection, lidocaine HCL for intravenous infusion, 10 mg MCM 2049
✿	J2010	Injection, lincomycin HCl, up to 300 mg MCM 2049
✳	J2020	Injection, linezolid, 200 mg
✿	J2060	Injection, lorazepam, 2 mg MCM 2049
✿	J2150	Injection, mannitol, 25% in 50 ml MCM 2049
✿	J2175	Injection, meperidine HCl, per 100 mg MCM 2049

✪	J2180	Injection, meperidine and promethazine HCl, up to 50 mg MCM 2049
▶✳	J2185	Injection, meropenem, 100 mg
✪	J2210	Injection, methylergonovine maleate, up to 0.2 mg MCM 2049
	J2240	Deleted 01/01/02
✪	J2250	Injection, midazolam HCl, per 1 mg MCM 2049
✪	J2260	Injection milrinone lactate, 5 mg MCM 2049
✪	J2270	Injection, morphine sulfate, up to 10 mg MCM 2049
✪	J2271	Injection, morphine sulfate, 100 mg MCM 2049, CIM 60-14a
✪	J2275	Injection, morphine sulfate (preservative-free sterile solution), per 10 mg MCM 2049, CIM 60-14b
▶✳	J2280	Injection, moxifloxacin, 100 mg
✪	J2300	Injection, nalbuphine HCl, per 10 mg MCM 2049
✪	J2310	Injection, naloxone HCl, per 1 mg MCM 2049
✪	J2320	Injection, nandrolone decanoate, up to 50 mg MCM 2049
✪	J2321	Injection, nandrolone decanoate, up to 100 mg MCM 2049
✪	J2322	Injection, nandrolone decanoate, up to 200 mg MCM 2049
✪	J2324	Injection, nesiritide, 0.5 mg MCM 2049
	J2330	Deleted 01/01/02
	J2350	Deleted 01/01/02
	J2352	Deleted 12/31/03
▶✳	J2353	Injection, octreotide, depot form for intramuscular injection, 1 mg
▶✳	J2354	Injection, octreotide, non-depot form for subcutaneous or intravenous injection, 25 mcg
✪	J2355	Injection, oprelvekin, 5 mg MCM 2049
✪	J2360	Injection, orphenadrine citrate, up to 60 mg MCM 2049
✪	J2370	Injection, phenylephrine HCl, up to 1 ml MCM 2049
✪	J2400	Injection, chloroprocaine HCl, per 30 ml MCM 2049
✪	J2405	Injection, ondansetron HCl, per 1 mg MCM 2049
✪	J2410	Injection, oxymorphone HCl, up to 1 mg MCM 2049
✪	J2430	Injection, pamidronate disodium, per 30 mg MCM 2049

✪	J2440	Injection, papaverine HCl, up to 60 mg MCM 2049
✪	J2460	Injection, oxytetracycline HCl, up to 50 mg MCM 2049
	J2480	Deleted 01/01/02
	J2500	Deleted 12/31/02
✪	J2501	Injection, paricalcitol, 1 mcg MCM 2049
▶✳	J2505	Injection, pegfilgrastim, 6 mg
✪	J2510	Injection, penicillin G procaine, aqueous, up to 600,000 units MCM 2049
	J2512	Deleted 01/01/02
✪	J2515	Injection, pentobarbital sodium, per 50 mg MCM 2049
✪	J2540	Injection, penicillin G potassium, up to 600,000 units MCM 2049
✪	J2543	Injection, piperacillin sodium/tazobactam sodium, 1/0.125 gm (1.125 gm) MCM 2049
✪	J2545	Pentamidine isethionate, inhalation solution, per 300 mg, administered through a DME MCM 2049, Cross Reference Q0077
✪	J2550	Injection, promethazine HCl, up to 50 mg MCM 2049
✪	J2560	Injection, phenobarbital sodium, up to 120 mg MCM 2049
✪	J2590	Injection, oxytocin, up to 10 units MCM 2049
✪	J2597	Injection, desmopressin acetate, per 1 mcg MCM 2049
	J2640	Deleted 01/01/02
✪	J2650	Injection, prednisolone acetate, up to 1 ml MCM 2049
✪	J2670	Injection, tolazoline HCl, up to 25 mg MCM 2049
✪	J2675	Injection, progesterone, per 50 mg MCM 2049
✪	J2680	Injection, fluphenazine decanoate, up to 25 mg MCM 2049
✪	J2690	Injection, procainamide HCl, up to 1 gm MCM 2049
✪	J2700	Injection, oxacillin sodium, up to 250 mg MCM 2049
✪	J2710	Injection, neostigmine methylsulfate, up to 0.5 mg MCM 2049
✪	J2720	Injection, protamine sulfate, per 10 mg MCM 2049

✪	J2725	Injection, protirelin, per 250 mcg MCM 2049
✪	J2730	Injection, pralidoxime chloride, up to 1 gm MCM 2049
✪	J2760	Injection, phentolamine mesylate, up to 5 mg MCM 2049
✪	J2765	Injection, metoclopramide HCl, up to 10 mg MCM 2049
	J2770	Injection quinupristin/dalfopristin, 500 mg (150/350) MCM 2049
✪	J2780	Injection, ranitidine HCl, 25 mg MCM 2049
▶✱	J2783	Injection, rasburicase, 0.5 mg
✪	J2788	Injection, Rho (d) immune globulin, human, minidose, 50 mcg MCM 2049
✪	J2790	Injection, Rho (D) immune globulin, human, full dose, 300 mcg MCM 2049
✪	J2792	Injection, Rho (D) immune globulin (human), IV, solvent detergent, 100 IU MDC 2049
✱	J2795	Injection, ropivacaine HCl, 1 mg
✪	J2800	Injection, methocarbamol, up to 10 ml MCM 2049
✪	J2810	Injection, theophylline, per 40 mg MCM 2049
✪	J2820	Injection, sargramostim (GM-CSF), 50 mcg MCM 2049
	J2860	Deleted 01/01/02
✪	J2910	Injection, aurothioglucose, up to 50 mg MCM 2049
✪	J2912	Injection, sodium chloride, 0.9%, per 2 ml MCM 2049
	J2915	Deleted 12/31/02
✪	J2916	Injection, sodium ferric gluconate complex in sucrose injection, 12.5 mg MCM 2049.2, MCM 2049.4
✪	J2920	Injection, methylprednisolone sodium succinate, up to 40 mg MCM 2049
✪	J2930	Injection, methylprednisolone sodium succinate, up to 125 mg MCM 2049
✪	J2940	Injection, somatrem, 1 mg MCM 2049, Medicare Statute 1861s2b
✪	J2941	Injection, somatropin, 1 mg MCM 2049, Medicare Statute 1861s2b
✪	J2950	Injection, promazine HCl, up to 25 mg MCM 2049
	J2970	Deleted 01/01/02
✪	J2993	Injection, reteplase, 18.1 mg MCM 2049
✪	J2995	Injection, streptokinase, per 250,000 IU MCM 2049

✪	J2997	Injection, alteplase recombinant, 1 mg MCM 2049
✪	J3000	Injection, streptomycin, up to 1 gm MCM 2049
✪	J3010	Injection, fentanyl citrate, 0.1 mg MCM 2049
✪	J3030	Injection, sumatriptan succinate, 6 mg (Code may be used for Medicare when drug administered under the direct supervision of a physician, not for use when drug is self-administered.) MCM 2049
✪	J3070	Injection, pentazocine 30 mg MCM 2049
	J3080	Deleted 01/01/02
✱	J3100	Injection, tenecteplase, 50 mg
✪	J3105	Injection, terbutaline sulfate, up to 1 mg MCM 2049
✪	J3120	Injection, testosterone enanthate, up to 100 mg MCM 2049
✪	J3130	Injection, testosterone enanthate, up to 200 mg MCM 2049
✪	J3140	Injection, testosterone suspension, up to 50 mg provided in 1.1 mg vial MCM 2049
✪	J3150	Injection, testosterone propionate, up to 100 mg MCM 2049
✪	J3230	Injection, chlorpromazine HCl, up to 50 mg MCM 2049
✪	J3240	Injection, thyrotropin alfa, 0.9 mg provided in 1.1 mg vial MCM 2049
✪	J3245	Injection, tirofiban HCl, 12.5 mg MCM 2049
✪	J3250	Injection, trimethobenzamide HCl, up to 200 mg MCM 2049
✪	J3260	Injection, tobramycin sulfate, up to 80 mg MCM 2049
✪	J3265	Injection, torsemide, 10 mg/cc MCM 2049
	J3270	Deleted 01/01/02
✪	J3280	Injection, thiethylperazine maleate, up to 10 mg MCM 2049
✪	J3301	Injection triamcinolone acetonide, per 10 mg MCM 2049
✪	J3302	Injection triamcinolone diacetate, per 5 mg MCM 2049
✪	J3303	Injection triamcinolone hexacetonide, per 5 mg MCM 2049

⊘ J3305   Injection, trimetrexate glucuronate, per 25 mg
MCM 2049

⊘ J3310   Injection, perphenazine, up to 5 mg
MCM 2049

⊘ J3315   Injection, triptorelin pamoate, 3.75 mg
MCM 2049

⊘ J3320   Injection, spectinomycin dihydrochloride, up to 2 gm
MCM 2049

⊘ J3350   Injection, urea, up to 40 gm
MCM 2049

⊘ J3360   Injection, diazepam, up to 5 mg
MCM 2049

⊘ J3364   Injection, urokinase, 5000 IU vial
MCM 2049

⊘ J3365   Injection, IV, urokinase, 250,000 IU vial
MCM 2049, Cross Reference Q0089

⊘ J3370   Injection, vancomycin HCl, 500 mg
MCM 2049, CIM 60-14

J3390   Deleted 01/01/02

⊘ J3395   Injection, verteporfin, 15 mg
CIM 35-100, CIM 45-30

⊘ J3400   Injection, triflupromazine HCl, up to 20 mg
MCM 2049

⊘ J3410   Injection, hydroxyzine HCl, up to 25 mg
MCM 2049

▶✳ J3411   Injection, thiamine HCL, 100 mg

▶✳ J3415   Injection, pyridoxine HCL, 100 mg

⊘ J3420   Injection, vitamin B-12 cyanocobalamin, up to 1000 mcg
MCM 2049, CIM 45-4

⊘ J3430   Injection, phytonadione (vitamin K), per 1 mg
MCM 2049

⊘ J3450   Deleted 01/01/02

▶⊘ J3465   Injection, voriconazole, 10 mg
MCM 2049

⊘ J3470   Injection, hyaluronidase, up to 150 units
MCM 2049

⊘ J3475   Injection, magnesium sulfate, per 500 mg
MCM 2049

⊘ J3480   Injection, potassium chloride, per 2 milliequivalents (mEq)
MCM 2049

⊘ J3485   Injection, zidovudine, 10 mg
MCM 2049

▶✳ J3486   Injection, ziprasidone mesylate, 10 mg

✳ J3487   Injection, zoledronic acid, 1 mg

⊘ J3490   Unclassified drugs
MCM 2049

◆ J3520   Edetate disodium, per 150 mg
CIM 35-64, CIM 45-20

⊘ J3530   Nasal vaccine inhalation
MCM 2049

◆ J3535   Drug administered through a metered dose inhaler
MCM 2050.5

◆ J3570   Laetrile, amygdalin, vitamin B-17
CIM 45-10

✳ J3590   Unclassified biologics

Miscellaneous Drugs and Solutions

⊘ J7030   Infusion, normal saline solution, 1000 cc
MCM 2049

⊘ J7040   Infusion, normal saline solution, sterile (500 ml = 1 unit)
MCM 2049

⊘ J7042   5% dextrose/normal saline (500 ml = 1 unit)
MCM 2049

⊘ J7050   Infusion, normal saline solution, 250 cc
MCM 2049

⊘ J7051   Sterile saline or water, up to 5 cc
MCM 2049

⊘ J7060   5% dextrose/water (500 ml = 1 unit)
MCM 2049

⊘ J7070   Infusion, D-5-W, 1000 cc
MCM 2049

⊘ J7100   Infusion, dextran 40, 500 ml
MCM 2049

⊘ J7110   Infusion, dextran 75, 500 ml
MCM 2049

⊘ J7120   Ringer's lactate infusion, up to 1000 cc
MCM 2049

⊘ J7130   Hypertonic saline solution, 50 or 100 mEq, 20 cc vial
MCM 2049

⊘ J7190   Factor VIII, anti-hemophilic factor (human), per IU
MCM 2049

⊘ J7191   Factor VIII, anti-hemophilic factor (porcine), per IU
MCM 2049

⊘ J7192   Factor VIII (anti-hemophilic factor recombinant), per IU
MCM 2049

⊘ J7193   Factor IX (anti-hemophilic factor, purified, non-recombinant) per IU
MCM 2049

⊘ J7194   Factor IX, complex, per IU
MCM 2049

⊘ J7195   Factor IX (anti-hemophilic factor, recombinant) per IU
MCM 2049

J7196   Deleted 01/01/00

⊘ J7197   Anti-thrombin III (human), per IU
MCM 2049

⊘ J7198   Anti-inhibitor, per IU
MCM 2049, CIM 45-24

⊘ J7199   Hemophilia clotting factor, not otherwise classified
MCM 2049, CIM 45-24

◆ J7300   Intrauterine copper contraceptive
Medicare Statute 1862A1

◆ J7302   Levonorgestrel-releasing intrauterine
contraceptive system, 52 mg
Medicare Statute 1862a1

▶◆ J7303   Contraceptive supply, hormone containing vaginal ring, each
Medicare Statute 1862.1

⇒ ✳ J7308   Aminolevulinic acid HCl for topical administration, 20%, single unit dosage
form (354 mg)

۞ J7310   Ganciclovir, 4.5 mg, long-acting implant
MCM 2049

    J7315   Deleted 01/01/02

    J7316   Deleted 12/31/02, Cross Reference
J7317

✳ J7317   Sodium hyaluronate, per 20 to 25 mg
dose for intra-articular injection

✳ J7320   Hylan G-F 20, 16 mg, for intra-articular
injection

✳ J7330   Autologous cultured chondrocytes, implant

✳   J7340   Dermal and epidermal, tissue of human
origin, with or without bioengineered
of processed elements, with metabolically active elements, per square centimeter

✳ J7342   Dermal tissue, of human origin, with or
without other bioengineered or processed elements, with metabolically active elements, per square centimeter

✳ J7350   Dermal tissue of human origin, injectable, with or without other bioengineered or processed elements, but without metabolized active elements, per
10 mg

Immunosuppressive Drugs (Includes Non-injectibles)

۞ J7500   Azathioprine, oral, 50 mg
MCM 2049.5

۞ J7501   Azathioprine, parenteral, 100 mg
MCM 2049

۞ J7502   Cyclosporine, oral, 100 mg
MCM 2049.5

۞ J7504   Lymphocyte immune globulin, anti-thymocyte globulin, equine, parenteral 250
mg
MCM 2049, CIM 45-22

۞ J7505   Muromonab-CD3, parenteral, 5 mg
MCM 2049

۞ J7506   Prednisone, oral, per 5 mg
MCM 2049.5

۞ J7507   Tacrolimus, oral, per 1 mg
MCM 2049.5

    J7508   Deleted 12/31/03

۞ J7509   Methylprednisolone oral, per 4 mg
MCM 2049.5

۞ J7510   Prednisolone oral, per 5 mg
MCM 2049.5

✳ J7511   Lymphocyte immune globulin, anti-thymocyte globulin, rabbit, parenteral, 25
mg

۞ J7513   Daclizumab, parenteral, 25 mg
MCM 2049.5

✳ J7515   Cyclosporine, oral, 25 mg

✳ J7516   Cyclosporin, parenteral, 250 mg

✳ J7517   Mycophenolate mofetil, oral, 250 mg

۞ J7520   Sirolimus, oral, 1 mg
MCM 2049.5

۞ J7525   Tacrolimus, parenteral, 5 mg
MCM 2049.5

۞ J7599   Immunosuppressive drug, not otherwise classified
MCM 2049.5

Inhalation Solutions

۞ J7608   Acetylcysteine, inhalation solution administered through DME, unit dose
form, per gm
MCM 2100.5

۞ J7618   Albuterol, all formulations including
separated isomers, inhalation solution
administered through DME, concentrated form, per 1 mg (albuterol) or per
0.5 mg (levalbuterol)
MCM 2100.5

۞ J7619   Albuterol, all formulations including
separated isomers, inhalation solution
administered through DME, unit dose
form, per 1 mg (albuterol) or per 0.5
mg (levalbuterol)
MCM 2100.5

▶✳ J7621   Albuterol, all formulations, including
separated isomers, up to 5 mg (albuterol) or 2.5 mg (levoalbuterol), and
ipratropium bromide, up to 1 mg,
compounded inhalation solution, administered through DME

✳ J7622   Beclomethasone, inhalation solution administered through DME, unit dose
form, per mg

✳ J7624   Betamethasone, inhalation solution administered through DME, unit dose
form, per mg

✳ J7626   Budesonide inhalation solution, administered through DME, unit dose form,
0.25 to 0.50 mg

۞ J7628   Bitolterol mesylate, inhalation solution
administered through DME, concentrated form, per mg
MCM 2100.5

۞ J7629   Bitolterol mesylate, inhalation solution
administered through DME, unit dose
form, per mg
MCM 2100.5

⊛ J7631   Cromolyn sodium, inhalation solution administered through DME, unit dose form, per 10 mg
MCM 2100.5

✱ J7633   Budesonide, inhalation solution administered through DME, concentrated form, per 0.25 milligram

⊛ J7635   Atropine, inhalation solution administered through DME, concentrated form, per mg
MCM 2100.5

⊛ J7636   Atropine, inhalation solution administered through DME, unit dose form, per mg
MCM 2100.5

⊛ J7637   Dexamethasone, inhalation solution administered through DME, concentrated form, per mg
MCM 2100.5

⊛ J7638   Dexamethasone, inhalation solution administered through DME, unit dose form, per mg
MCM 2100.5

⊛ J7639   Dornase alpha, inhalation solution administered through DME, unit dose form, per mg
MCM 2100.5

✱ J7641   Flunisolide, inhalation solution administered through DME, unit dose, per mg

⊛ J7642   Glycopyrrolate, inhalation solution administered through DME, concentrated form, per mg
MCM 2100.5

⊛ J7643   Glycopyrrolate, inhalation solution administered through DME, unit dose form, per mg
MCM 2100.5

⊛ J7644   Ipratropium bromide, inhalation solution administered through DME, unit dose form, per mg
MCM 2100.5

⊛ J7648   Isoetharine HCl, inhalation solution administered through DME, concentrated form, per mg
MCM 2100.5

⊛ J7649   Isoetharine HCl, inhalation solution administered through DME, unit dose form, per mg
MCM 2100.5

⊛ J7658   Isoproterenol HCl, inhalation solution administered through DME, concentrated form, per mg
MCM 2100.5

⊛ J7659   Isoproterenol HCl, inhalation solution administered through DME, unit dose form, per mg
MCM 2100.5

⊛ J7668   Metaproterenol sulfate, inhalation solution administered through DME, concentrated form, per 10 mg
MCM 2100.5

⊛ J7669   Metaproterenol sulfate, inhalation solution administered through DME, unit dose form, per 10 mg
MCM 2100.5

⊛ J7680   Terbutaline sulfate, inhalation solution administered through DME, concentrated form, per mg
MCM 2100.5

⊛ J7681   Terbutaline sulfate, inhalation solution administered through DME, unit dose form, per mg
MCM 2100.5

⊛ J7682   Tobramycin, unit dose form, 300 mg, inhalation solution, administered through DME
MCM 2100.5

⊛ J7683   Triamcinolone, inhalation solution administered through DME, concentrated form, per mg
MCM 2100.5

⊛ J7684   Triamcinolone, inhalation solution administered through DME, unit dose form, per mg
MCM 2100.5

⊛ J7699   NOC drugs, inhalation solution administered through DME
MCM 2100.5

⊛ J7799   NOC drugs, other than inhalation drugs, administered through DME
MCM 2100.5

◆ J8499   Prescription drug, oral, non-chemotherapeutic, NOS
MCM 2049

⊛ J8510   Busulfan; oral, 2 mg
MCM 2049.5

⊛ J8520   Capecitabine, oral, 150 mg
MCM 2049.5

⊛ J8521   Capecitabine, oral, 500 mg
MCM 2049.5

⊛ J8530   Cyclophosphamide, oral, 25 mg
MCM 2049.5

⊛ J8560   Etoposide, oral, 50 mg
MCM 2049.5

⊛ J8600   Melphalan, oral, 2 mg
MCM 2049.5

⊛ J8610   Methotrexate, oral, 2.5 mg
MCM 2049.5

⊛ J8700   Temozolomide, oral, 5 mg
MCM 2049.5c

⊛ J8999   Prescription drug, oral, chemotherapeutic, NOS
MCM 2049.5

CHEMOTHERAPY DRUGS (J9000-J9999)

NOTE: These codes cover the cost of the chemotherapy drug only, not to include the administration

⊛ J9000   Doxorubicin HCl, 10 mg
MCM 2049

⊘ J9001   Doxorubicin HCl, all lipid formulations, 10 mg
MCM 2049

⊘ J9010   Alemtuzumab, 10 mg
Medicare Statute 1833(t)

⊘ J9015   Aldesleukin, per single use vial
MCM 2049

✳ J9017   Arsenic trioxide, 1 mg

⊘ J9020   Asparaginase, 10,000 units
MCM 2049

⊘ J9031   BCG (intravesical), per instillation
MCM 2049

⊘ J9040   Bleomycin sulfate, 15 units
MCM 2049

⊘ J9045   Carboplatin, 50 mg
MCM 2049

⊘ J9050   Carmustine, 100 mg
MCM 2049

⊘ J9060   Cisplatin, powder or solution, per 10 mg
MCM 2049

⊘ J9062   Cisplatin, 50 mg
MCM 2049

⊘ J9065   Injection, cladribine, per 1 mg
MCM 2049

⊘ J9070   Cyclophosphamide, 100 mg
MCM 2049

⊘ J9080   Cyclophosphamide, 200 mg
MCM 2049

⊘ J9090   Cyclophosphamide, 500 mg
MCM 2049

⊘ J9091   Cyclophosphamide, 1 gm
MCM 2049

⊘ J9092   Cyclophosphamide, 2 gm
MCM 2049

⊘ J9093   Cyclophosphamide, lyophilized, 100 mg
MCM 2049

⊘ J9094   Cyclophosphamide, lyophilized, 200 mg
MCM 2049

⊘ J9095   Cyclophosphamide, lyophilized, 500 mg
MCM 2049

⊘ J9096   Cyclophosphamide, lyophilized, 1 gm
MCM 2049

⊘ J9097   Cyclophosphamide, lyophilized, 2 gm
MCM 2049

▶✳ J9098   Cytarabine liposome, 10 mg

⊘ J9100   Cytarabine 100 mg
MCM 2049

⊘ J9110   Cytarabine, 500 mg
MCM 2049

⊘ J9120   Dactinomycin, 0.5 mg
MCM 2049

⊘ J9130   Dacarbazine, 100 mg
MCM 2049

⊘ J9140   Dacarbazine, 200 mg
MCM 2049

⊘ J9150   Daunorubicin, HCl, 10 mg
MCM 2049

⊘ J9151   Daunorubicin citrate liposomal formulation, 10 mg
MCM 2049

✳ J9160   Denileukin diftitox, 300 mcg

⊘ J9165   Diethylstilbestrol diphosphate, 250 mg
MCM 2049

⊘ J9170   Docetaxel, 20 mg
MCM 2049

▶✳ J9178   Injection, epirubicin HCl, 2 mg

J9180   Deleted 12/31/03

⊘ J9181   Etoposide, 10 mg
MCM 2049

⊘ J9182   Etoposide, 100 mg
MCM 2049

⊘ J9185   Fludarabine phosphate, 50 mg
MCM 2049

⊘ J9190   Fluorouracil, 500 mg
MCM 2049

⊘ J9200   Floxuridine, 500 mg
MCM 2049

⊘ J9201   Gemcitabine HCl, 200 mg
MCM 2049

⊘ J9202   Goserelin acetate implant, per 3.6 mg
MCM 2049

⊘ J9206   Irinotecan, 20 mg
MCM 2049

⊘ J9208   Ifosfamide, 1 gm
MCM 2049

⊘ J9209   Mesna, 200 mg
MCM 2049

⊘ J9211   Idarubicin HCl, 5 mg
MCM 2049

⊘ J9212   Injection, interferon alfacon-1, recombinant, 1 mcg
MCM 2049

⊘ J9213   Interferon, alfa-2a, recombinant, 3 million units
MCM 2049

⊘ J9214   Interferon, alfa-2b, recombinant, 1 million units
MCM 2049

⊘ J9215   Interferon, alfa-n3 (human leukocyte derived), 250,000 IU
MCM 2049

⊘ J9216   Interferon, gamma-1B, 3 million units
MCM 2049

⊘ J9217   Leuprolide acetate (for depot suspension), 7.5 mg
MCM 2049

⊘ J9218   Leuprolide acetate, per 1 mg
MCM 2049

⊘ J9219   Leuprolide acetate implant, 65 mg
MCM 2049

⊘ J9230   Mechlorethamine HCl (nitrogen mustard), 10 mg
MCM 2049

⊘ J9245   Injection, melphalan HCl, 50 mg
MCM 2049

⊘ J9250   Methotrexate sodium, 5 mg
MCM 2049

⊘ J9260   Methotrexate sodium, 50 mg
MCM 2049

▶✳ J9263   Injection, oxaliplatin, 0.5 mg

✪	J9265	Paclitaxel, 30 mg MCM 2049
✪	J9266	Pegaspargase, per single dose vial MCM 2049
✪	J9268	Pentostatin, per 10 mg MCM 2049
✪	J9270	Plicamycin, 2.5 mg MCM 2049
✪	J9280	Mitomycin, 5 mg MCM 2049
✪	J9290	Mitomycin, 20 mg MCM 2049
✪	J9291	Mitomycin, 40 mg MCM 2049
✪	J9293	Injection, mitoxantrone HCl, per 5 mg MCM 2049
✳	J9300	Gemtuzumab ozogamicin, 5 mg, not for use for Gemzer
✪	J9310	Rituximab, 100 mg MCM 2049
✪	J9320	Streptozocin, 1 gm MCM 2049
✪	J9340	Thiotepa, 15 mg MCM 2049
✪	J9350	Topotecan, 4 mg MCM 2049
✳	J9355	Trastuzumab, 10 mg
✪	J9357	Valrubicin, intravesical, 200 mg MCM 2049
✪	J9360	Vinblastine sulfate, 1 mg MCM 2049
✪	J9370	Vincristine sulfate, 1 mg MCM 2049
✪	J9375	Vincristine sulfate, 2 mg MCM 2049
✪	J9380	Vincristine sulfate, 5 mg MCM 2049
✪	J9390	Vinorelbine tartrate, per 10 mg MCM 2049
▶✳	J9395	Injection, fulvestrant, 25 mg
✪	J9600	Porfimer sodium, 75 mg MCM 2049
✪	J9999	Not otherwise classified, anti-neoplastic drugs MCM 2049, CIM 45-16

K CODES FOR DURABLE MEDICAL EQUIPMENT: TEMPORARY CODES (K0000-K9999)

Wheelchairs

NOTE: This section contains national codes assigned by CMS on a temporary basis and for the exclusive use of the durable medical equipment regional carriers (DMERC).

✳	K0001	Standard wheelchair
✳	K0002	Standard hemi (low seat) wheelchair
✳	K0003	Lightweight wheelchair

✳	K0004	High-strength, lightweight wheelchair
✳	K0005	Ultra lightweight wheelchair
✳	K0006	Heavy-duty wheelchair
✳	K0007	Extra heavy-duty wheelchair
✳	K0009	Other manual wheelchair/base
✳	K0010	Standard-weight frame motorized/power wheelchair
✳	K0011	Standard-weight frame motorized/power wheelchair, with programmable control parameters for speed adjustment, tremor dampening, acceleration control and braking
✳	K0012	Lightweight portable motorized/power wheelchair
✳	K0014	Other motorized/power wheelchair base
✳	K0015	Detachable, non-adjustable height arm rest, each
	K0016	Deleted 12/31/03, Cross Reference E0973
✳	K0017	Detachable, adjustable height arm rest, base, each
✳	K0018	Detachable, adjustable height arm rest, upper portion, each
✳	K0019	Arm pad, each
✳	K0020	Fixed, adjustable height arm rest, pair
	K0021	Deleted 12/31/02, Cross Reference E0971
	K0022	Deleted 12/31/03, Cross Reference E0982
✳	K0023	Solid back insert, planar back, single density foam, attached with straps
✳	K0024	Solid back insert, planar back, single density form, with adjustable hook-on hardware
	K0025	Deleted 12/31/03, Cross Reference E0966
	K0026	Deleted 12/31/03
	K0027	Deleted 12/31/03
	K0028	Deleted 12/31/03, Cross Reference E1226
	K0029	Deleted 12/31/03
	K0030	Deleted 12/31/03, Cross Reference E0992
	K0031	Deleted 12/31/03
	K0032	Deleted 12/31/03
	K0033	Deleted 12/31/03
	K0034	Deleted 12/31/02, Cross Reference E0951
	K0035	Deleted 12/31/03, Cross Reference E0951
	K0036	Deleted 12/31/03, Cross Reference E0952
✳	K0037	High mount flip-up footrest, each
✳	K0038	Leg strap, each
✳	K0039	Leg strap, H-style, each
✳	K0040	Adjustable angle footplate, each
✳	K0041	Large size footplate, each
✳	K0042	Standard size footplate, each
✳	K0043	Foot rest, lower extension tube, each

* K0044   Foot rest, upper hanger bracket, each
* K0045   Foot rest, complete assembly
* K0046   Elevating leg rests, lower extension tube, each
* K0047   Elevating leg rests, upper hanger bracket, each
  K0048   Deleted 12/31/03, Cross Reference E0990
  K0049   Deleted 12/31/03, Cross Reference E0995
* K0050   Ratchet assembly
* K0051   Cam release assembly, footrest or leg rests, each
* K0052   Swing-away, detachable foot rests, each
* K0053   Elevating foot rests, articulating (telescoping), each
  K0054   Deleted 12/31/03
  K0055   Deleted 12/31/03
* K0056   Seat height less than 17″ or equal to or greater than 21″ for a high-strength, lightweight, or ultra lightweight wheelchair
  K0057   Deleted 12/31/03
  K0058   Deleted 12/31/03
* K0059   Plastic coated hand rim, each
* K0060   Steel hand rim, each
* K0061   Aluminum hand rim, each
  K0062   Deleted 12/31/03, Cross Reference E0967
  K0063   Deleted 12/31/03, Cross Reference E0967
* K0064   Zero pressure tube (flat-free inserts), any size, each
* K0065   Spoke protectors, each
* K0066   Solid tire, any size, each
* K0067   Pneumatic tire, any size, each
* K0068   Pneumatic tire tube, each
* K0069   Rear wheel assembly, complete, with solid tire, spokes or molded, each
* K0070   Rear wheel assembly, complete, with pneumatic tire, spokes or molded, each
* K0071   Front caster assembly, complete, with pneumatic tire, each
* K0072   Front caster assembly, complete, with semi-pneumatic tire, each
* K0073   Caster pin lock, each
* K0074   Pneumatic caster tire, any size, each
* K0075   Semi-pneumatic caster tire, any size, each
* K0076   Solid caster tire, any size, each
* K0077   Front caster assembly, complete, with solid tire, each
* K0078   Pneumatic caster tire tube, each
  K0079   Deleted 12/31/03, Cross Reference E0961
  K0080   Deleted 12/31/03, Cross Reference E0974
* K0081   Wheel lock assembly, complete each
  K0082   Deleted 12/31/03, Cross Reference E2360

  K0083   Deleted 12/31/03, Cross Reference E2361
  K0084   Deleted 12/31/03, Cross Reference E2362
  K0085   Deleted 12/31/03, Cross Reference E2363
  K0086   Deleted 12/31/03, Cross Reference E2364
  K0087   Deleted 12/31/03, Cross Reference E2365
  K0088   Deleted 12/31/03, Cross Reference E2366
  K0089   Deleted 12/31/03, Cross Reference E2367
* K0090   Rear wheel tire for power wheelchair, any size, each
* K0091   Rear wheel tire tube other than zero pressure for power wheelchair, any size, each
* K0092   Rear wheel assembly for power wheelchair, complete each
* K0093   Rear wheel, zero pressure tire tube (flat-free insert) for power wheelchair, any size, each
* K0094   Wheel tire for power base, any size, each
* K0095   Wheel tire tube other than zero pressure for each base, any size, each
* K0096   Wheel assembly for power base, complete, each
* K0097   Wheel zero pressure tire tube (flat-free insert) for power base, any size, each
* K0098   Drive belt for power wheelchair
* K0099   Front caster for power wheelchair, each
  K0100   Deleted 12/31/03, Cross Reference E0959
  K0101   Deleted 12/31/02, Cross Reference E0958
* K0102   Crutch and cane holder, each
  K0103   Deleted 12/31/03, Cross Reference E0972
* K0104   Cylinder tank carrier, each
* K0105   IV hanger, each
* K0106   Arm trough, each
  K0107   Deleted 12/31/03, Cross Reference E0950
* K0108   Wheelchair component or accessory, not otherwise specified

Spinal Orthotics

  K0112   Deleted 12/31/03
  K0113   Deleted 12/31/03
* K0114   Back support system for use with a wheelchair, with inner frame, prefabricated
* K0115   Seating system, back module, posterior-lateral control, with or without lateral supports, custom fabricated for attachment to wheelchair base

✳ K0116 Seating system, combined back and seat module, custom fabricated for attachment to wheelchair base

Other

K0183 Deleted 12/31/02, Cross Reference A7034

K0184 Deleted 12/31/02, Cross Reference A7032, A7033

K0185 Deleted 12/31/02, Cross Reference A7035

K0186 Deleted 12/31/02, Cross Reference A7036

K0187 Deleted 12/31/02, Cross Reference A7037

K0188 Deleted 12/31/02, Cross Reference A7038

K0189 Deleted 12/31/02, Cross Reference A7039

⊘ K0195 Elevating leg rests, pair (for use with capped rental wheelchair base)
CIM 60-9

K0268 Deleted 12/31/03, Cross Reference E0561

⊘ K0415 Prescription antiemetic drug, oral, per 1 mg, for use in conjunction with oral anti-cancer drug, not otherwise specified
MCM 2049.5C

⊘ K0416 Prescription antiemetic drug, rectal, per 1 mg, for use in conjunction with oral anti-cancer drug, not otherwise specified
MCM 2049.5C

✳ K0452 Wheelchair bearings, any type

➠⊘ K0455 Infusion pump used for uninterrupted parenteral administration of medication (e.g., epoprostenol or treprostinol)
CIM 60-14

K0460 Deleted 12/31/03, Cross Reference E0983

K0461 Deleted 12/31/03, Cross Reference E0984

⊘ K0462 Temporary replacement for patient owned equipment being repaired, any type
MCM 5102.3

K0531 Deleted 12/31/03, Cross Reference E0562

K0532 Deleted 12/31/03, Cross Reference E0470

K0533 Deleted 12/31/03, Cross Reference E0471

K0534 Deleted 12/31/03, Cross Reference E0472

K0538 Deleted 12/31/03, Cross Reference E2402

K0539 Deleted 12/31/03, Cross Reference A6550

K0540 Deleted 12/31/03, Cross Reference A6551

K0541 Deleted 12/31/03, Cross Reference E2500

K0542 Deleted 12/31/03

K0543 Deleted 12/31/03, Cross Reference E2508

K0544 Deleted 12/31/03, Cross Reference E2510

K0545 Deleted 12/31/03, Cross Reference E2511

K0546 Deleted 12/31/03, Cross Reference E2512

K0547 Deleted 12/31/03, Cross Reference E2599

✳ K0548 Deleted 12/31/02, Cross Reference J1817

K0549 Deleted 12/31/03, Cross Reference E0303

K0550 Deleted 12/31/03, Cross Reference E0304

K0551 Deleted 12/31/02, Cross Reference E1020

▶⊘ K0552 Supplies for external drug infusion pump, syringe type cartridge, sterile, each
CIM 60-14

K0556 Deleted 12/31/03, Cross Reference L5673

K0557 Deleted 12/31/03, Cross Reference L5679

K0558 Deleted 12/31/03, Cross Reference L5681

K0559 Deleted 12/31/03, Cross Reference L5683

K0560 Deleted 12/31/03, Cross Reference L8631

Ostomy Supplies

K0561 Deleted 12/31/02, Cross Reference A4405

K0562 Deleted 12/31/02, Cross Reference A4406

K0563 Deleted 12/31/02, Cross Reference A4407

K0564 Deleted 12/31/02, Cross Reference A4408

K0565 Deleted 12/31/02, Cross Reference A4409

K0566 Deleted 12/31/02, Cross Reference A4410

K0567 Deleted 12/31/02

K0568 Deleted 12/31/02

K0569 Deleted 12/31/02, Cross Reference A4413

K0570 Deleted 12/31/02, Cross Reference A4414

K0571 Deleted 12/31/02, Cross Reference A4415

K0572 Deleted 12/31/02, Cross Reference A4450

K0573 Deleted 12/31/02, Cross Reference A4452

K0574-K0578 Deleted 12/31/02

K0579 Deleted 12/31/02, Cross Reference A4422

K0580 Deleted 12/31/02

K0581 Deleted 12/31/03, Cross Reference A4416

K0582 Deleted 12/31/03, Cross Reference A4417

K0583 Deleted 12/31/03, Cross Reference A4418

K0584 Deleted 12/31/03, Cross Reference A4419

K0585 Deleted 12/31/03, Cross Reference A4420

K0586 Deleted 12/31/03, Cross Reference A4423

K0587 Deleted 12/31/03, Cross Reference A4424

K0588 Deleted 12/31/03, Cross Reference A4425

K0589 Deleted 12/31/03, Cross Reference A4426

K0590 Deleted 12/31/03, Cross Reference A4427

K0591 Deleted 12/31/03, Cross Reference A4428

K0592 Deleted 12/31/03, Cross Reference A4429

K0593 Deleted 12/31/03, Cross Reference A4430

K0594 Deleted 12/31/03, Cross Reference A4431

K0595 Deleted 12/31/03, Cross Reference A4432

K0596 Deleted 12/31/03, Cross Reference A4433

K0597 Deleted 12/31/03, Cross Reference A4434

▶ ✪ K0600 Functional neuromuscular stimulator transcutaneous stimulation of muscles of ambulation with computer control, used for walking by spinal cord injured, entire system, after completion of training program
CIM 35-77

▶✳ K0601 Replacement battery for external infusion pump owned by patient, silver oxide, 1.5 volt, each

▶✳ K0602 Replacement battery for external infusion pump owned by patient, silver oxide, 3 volt, each

▶✳ K0603 Replacement battery for external infusion pump owned by patient, alkaline, 1.5 volt, each

▶✳ K0604 Replacement battery for external infusion pump owned by patient, lithium, 3.6 volt, each

▶✳ K0605 Replacement battery for external infusion pump owned by patient, lithium, 4.5 volt, each

▶✳ K0606 Automatic external defibrillator, with integrated electrocardiogram analysis, garment type

▶✳ K0607 Replacement battery for automated external defibrillator, garment type only, each

▶✳ K0608 Replacement garment for use with automated external defibrillator, each

▶✳ K0609 Replacement electrodes for use with automated external defibrillator, garment type only, each

K0610 Deleted 12/31/03, Cross Reference E1634

K0611 Deleted 12/31/03, Cross Reference A4671

K0612 Deleted 12/31/03, Cross Reference A4672

K0613 Deleted 12/31/03, Cross Reference A4673

K0614 Deleted 12/31/03, Cross Reference A4674

K0615 Deleted 12/31/03, Cross Reference E2502

K0616 Deleted 12/31/03, Cross Reference E2504

K0617 Deleted 12/31/03, Cross Reference E2506

▶✳ K0618 TLSO, sagittal-coronal control, modular segmented spinal system, two rigid plastic shells, posterior extends from the sacrococcygeal junction and terminates just inferior to the scapular spine, anterior extends from the symphysis pubis to the xiphoid, soft liner, restricts gross trunk motion in the sagittal and coronal planes, lateral strength is provided by overlapping plastic and stabilizing closures, includes straps and closures, prefabricated, includes fitting and adjustment

▶✳ K0619 TLSO, sagittal-coronal control, modular segmented spinal system, three rigid plastic shells, posterior extends from the sacrococcygeal junction and terminates just inferior to the scapular spine, anterior extends from the symphysis pubis to the xiphoid, soft liner, restricts gross trunk motion in the sagittal and coronal planes, lateral strength is provided by overlapping plastic and stabilizing closures, includes straps and closures, prefabricated, includes fitting and adjustment

▶✳ K0620 Tubular elastic dressing, any width, per linear yard

K0621   Deleted 12/31/03
K0622   Deleted 12/31/03
K0623   Deleted 12/31/03
K0624   Deleted 12/31/03
K0625   Deleted 12/31/03
K0626   Deleted 12/31/03

▶✳ K0627   Traction equipment, cervical, free-standing, pneumatic, applying traction force to other than mandible

▶⊙ K0628   For diabetics only, multiple density insert, direct formed, molded to foot after external heat source of 230 degrees Fahrenheit or higher, total contact with patient's foot, including arch, base layer minimum of 1/4 inch material of shore a 35 durometer or 3/16 inch material of shore a 40 (or higher), prefabricated, each

▶⊙ K0629   For diabetics only, multiple density insert, custom molded from model of patient's foot, total contact with patient's foot, including arch, base layer minimum of 3/16 inch material of shore a 35 durometer or higher, includes arch filler and other shaping material, custom fabricated, each

▶✳ K0630   Sacroiliac orthosis, flexible, provides pelvic-sacral support, reduces motion about the sacroiliac joint, includes straps, closures, may include pendulous abdomen design, prefabricated, includes fitting and adjustment

▶✳ K0631   Sacroiliac orthosis, flexible, provides pelvic-sacral support, reduces motion about the sacroiliac joint, includes straps, closures, may include pendulous abdomen design, custom fabricated

▶✳ K0632   Sacroiliac orthosis, provides pelvic-sacral support, with rigid or semi-rigid panels over the sacrum and abdomen, reduces motion about the sacroiliac joint, includes straps, closures, may include pendulous abdomen design, prefabricated, includes fitting and adjustment

▶✳ K0633   Sacroiliac orthosis, provides pelvic-sacral support, with rigid or semi-rigid panels placed over the sacrum and abdomen, reduces motion about the sacroiliac joint, includes straps, closures, may include pendulous abdomen design, custom fabricated

▶✳ K0634   Lumbar orthosis, flexible, provides lumbar support, posterior extends from L-1 to below L-5 vertebra, produces intracavitary pressure to reduce load on the intervertebral discs, includes straps, closures, may include pendulous abdomen design, shoulder straps, stays, prefabricated, includes fitting and adjustment

▶✳ K0635   Lumbar orthosis, sagittal control, with rigid posterior panel(s), posterior extends from L-1 to below L-5 vertebra, produces intracavitary pressure to reduce load on the intervertebral discs, includes straps, closures, may include padding, stays, shoulder straps, pendulous abdomen design, prefabricated, includes fitting and adjustment

▶✳ K0636   Lumbar orthosis, sagittal control, with rigid anterior and posterior panels, posterior extends from L-1 to below L-5 vertebra, produces intracavitary pressure to reduce load on the intervertebral discs, includes straps, closures, may include padding, shoulder straps, pendulous abdomen design, prefabricated, includes fitting and adjustment

▶✳ K0637   Lumbar-sacral orthosis, flexible, provides lumbo-sacral support, posterior extends from sacrococcygeal junction to T-9 vertebra, produces intracavitary pressure to reduce load on the intervertebral discs, includes straps, closures, may include stays, shoulder straps, pendulous abdomen design, prefabricated, includes fitting and adjustment

▶✳ K0638   Lumbar-sacral orthosis, flexible, provides lumbo-sacral support, posterior extends from sacrococcygeal junction to T-9 vertebra, produces intracavitary pressure to reduce load on the intervertebral discs, includes straps, closures, may include stays, shoulder straps, pendulous abdomen design, custom fabricated

▶✳ K0639   Lumbar-sacral orthosis, sagittal control, with rigid posterior panel(s), posterior extends from sacrococcygeal junction to T-9 vertebra, produces intracavitary pressure to reduce load on the intervertebral discs, includes straps, closures, may include padding, stays, shoulder straps, pendulous abdomen design, prefabricated, includes fitting and adjustment

▶✳ K0640   Lumbar-sacral orthosis, sagittal-coronal control, with rigid anterior and posterior panels, posterior extends from sacrococcygeal junction to T-9 vertebra, produces intracavitary pressure to reduce load on the intervertebral discs, includes straps, closures, may include padding, shoulder straps, pendulous abdomen design, prefabricated, includes fitting and adjustment

▶ ✳ K0641 Lumbar-sacral orthosis, sagittal-coronal control, with rigid anterior and posterior panels, posterior extends from sacrococcygeal junction to T-9 vertebra, produces intracavitary pressure to reduce load on the intervertebral discs, includes straps, closures, may include padding, shoulder straps, pendulous abdomen design, custom fabricated

▶ ✳ K0642 Lumbar-sacral orthosis, sagittal-coronal control, with rigid posterior frame/panel(s), posterior extends from sacrococcygeal junction to T-9 vertebra, lateral strength provided by rigid lateral frame/panels, produces intracavitary pressure to reduce load on intervertebral discs, includes straps, closures, may include padding, stays, shoulder straps, pendulous abdomen design, prefabricated, includes fitting and adjustment

▶ ✳ K0643 Lumbar-sacral orthosis, sagittal-coronal control, with rigid posterior frame/panel(s), posterior extends from sacrococcygeal junction to T-9 vertebra, lateral strength provided by rigid lateral frame/panels, produces intracavitary pressure to reduce load on intervertebral discs, includes straps, closures, may include padding, stays, shoulder straps, pendulous abdomen design, custom fabricated

▶ ✳ K0644 Lumbar-sacral orthosis, sagittal-coronal control, lumbar flexion, rigid posterior frame/panels, lateral articulating design to flex the lumbar spine, posterior extends from sacrococcygeal junction to T-9 vertebra, lateral strength provided by rigid lateral frame/panels, produces intracavitary pressure to reduce load on intervertebral discs, includes straps, closures, may include padding, anterior panel, pendulous abdomen design, prefabricated, includes fitting and adjustment

▶ ✳ K0645 Lumbar sacral orthosis, sagittal-coronal control, lumbar flexion, rigid posterior frame/panels, lateral articulating design to flex the lumbar spine, posterior extends from sacrococcygeal junction to T-9 vertebra, lateral strength provided by rigid lateral frame/panels, produces intracavitary pressure to reduce load on intervertebral discs, includes straps, closures, may include padding, anterior panel, pendulous abdomen design, custom fabricated

▶ ✳ K0646 Lumbar-sacral orthosis, sagittal-coronal control, with rigid anterior and posterior frame/panels, posterior extends from sacrococcygeal junction to T-9 vertebra, lateral strength provided by rigid lateral frame/panels, produces intracavitary pressure to reduce load on intervertebral discs, includes straps, closures, may include padding, shoulder straps, pendulous abdomen design, prefabricated, includes fitting and adjustment

▶ ✳ K0647 Lumbar-sacral orthosis, sagittal-coronal control, with rigid anterior and posterior frame/panels, posterior extends from sacrococcygeal junction to T-9 vertebra, lateral strength provided by rigid lateral frame/panels, produces intracavitary pressure to reduce load on intervertebral discs, includes straps, closures, may include padding, shoulder straps, pendulous abdomen design, custom fabricated

▶ ✳ K0648 Lumbar-sacral orthosis, sagittal-coronal control, rigid shell(s)/panel(s), posterior extends from sacrococcygeal junction to T-9 vertebra, anterior extends from symphysis pubis to xiphoid, produces intracavitary pressure to reduce load on the intervertebral discs, overall strength is provided by overlapping rigid material and stabilizing closures, includes straps, closures, may include soft interface, pendulous abdomen design, prefabricated, includes fitting and adjustment

▶ ✳ K0649 Lumbar-sacral orthosis, sagittal-coronal control, rigid shell(s)/panel(s), posterior extends from sacrococcygeal junction to T-9 vertebra, anterior extends from symphysis pubis to xiphoid, produces intracavitary pressure to reduce load on the intervertebral discs, overall strength is provided by overlapping rigid material and stabilizing closures, includes straps, closures, may include soft interface, pendulous abdomen design, custom fabricated

▶ ✳ K0650 General use wheelchair seat cushion, width less than 22 inches, any depth

▶ ✳ K0651 General use wheelchair seat cushion, width 22 inches or greater, any depth

▶ ✳ K0652 Skin protection wheelchair seat cushion, width less than 22 inches, any depth

▶ ✳ K0653 Skin protection wheelchair seat cushion, width 22 inches or greater, any depth

▶ ✳ K0654 Positioning wheelchair seat cushion, width less than 22 inches, any depth

▶ ✳ K0655 Positioning wheelchair seat cushion, width 22 inches or greater, any depth

▶※ K0656   Skin protection and positioning wheelchair seat cushion, width less than 22 inches, any depth

▶※ K0657   Skin protection and positioning wheelchair seat cushion, width 22 inches or greater, any depth

▶※ K0658   Custom fabricated wheelchair seat cushion, any size

▶※ K0659   Wheelchair seat cushion, powered

▶※ K0660   General use wheelchair back cushion, width less than 22 inches, any height, including any type mounting hardware

▶※ K0661   General use wheelchair back cushion, width 22 inches or greater, any height, including any type mounting hardware

▶※ K0662   Positioning wheelchair back cushion, posterior, width less than 22 inches, any height, including any type mounting hardware

▶※ K0663   Positioning wheelchair back cushion, posterior, width 22 inches or greater, any height, including any type mounting hardware

▶※ K0664   Positioning wheelchair back cushion, posterior-lateral, width less than 22 inches, any height, including any type mounting hardware

▶※ K0665   Positioning wheelchair back cushion, posterior-lateral, width 22 inches or greater, any height, including any type mounting hardware

▶※ K0666   Custom fabricated wheelchair back cushion, any size, including any type mounting hardware

▶※ K0667   Mounting hardware, any type, for seat cushion or seat support base attached to a manual wheelchair or lightweight power wheelchair, per cushion/base

▶※ K0668   Replacement cover for wheelchair seat cushion or back cushion, each

▶※ K0669   Wheelchair seat or back cushion, no written coding verifcation from SADMERC (Statistical Analysis Durable Medical Equipment Regional Carrier)

ORTHOTIC PROCEDURES (L0100-L4999)

Orthotic Devices: Spinal

Cervical

※ L0100   Cranial orthosis (helmet,), with or without soft interface, molded to patient model

※ L0110   Cranial orthosis (helmet), with or without soft-interface, non-molded

▶※ L0112   Cranial cervical orthosis, congenital torticollis type, with or without soft interface material, adjustable range of motion joint, custom fabricated

※ L0120   Cervical, flexible, non-adjustable (foam collar)

※ L0130   Cervical, flexible, thermoplastic collar, molded to patient

※ L0140   Cervical, semi-rigid, adjustable (plastic collar)

※ L0150   Cervical, semi-rigid, adjustable molded chin cup (plastic collar with mandibular/occipital piece)

※ L0160   Cervical, semi-rigid, wire frame occipital/mandibular support

※ L0170   Cervical, collar, molded to patient model

※ L0172   Cervical, collar, semi-rigid thermoplastic foam, two piece

※ L0174   Cervical, collar, semi-rigid, thermoplastic foam, two piece with thoracic extension

Multiple Post Collar

※ L0180   Cervical, multiple post collar, occipital/mandibular supports, adjustable

※ L0190   Cervical, multiple post collar, occipital/mandibular supports, adjustable cervical bars (SOMI, Guilford, Taylor types)

※ L0200   Cervical, multiple post collar, occipital/mandibular supports, adjustable cervical bars, and thoracic extension

Thoracic

※ L0210   Thoracic, rib belt

※ L0220   Thoracic, rib belt, custom fabricated

Thoracic-Lumbar-Sacral

Flexible

L0300	Deleted 12/31/02
L0310	Deleted 12/31/02
L0315	Deleted 12/31/02
L0317	Deleted 12/31/02

Anterior-Posterior Control

L0320	Deleted 12/31/02
L0321	Deleted 12/31/02
L0330	Deleted 12/31/02
L0331	Deleted 12/31/02

Anterior-Posterior-Lateral Rotary-Control

	L0340	Deleted 12/31/02
	L0350	Deleted 12/31/02
	L0360	Deleted 12/31/02
	L0370	Deleted 12/31/02
	L0380	Deleted 12/31/02
	L0390	Deleted 12/31/02
	L0391	Deleted 12/31/02
	L0400	Deleted 12/31/02
	L0410	Deleted 12/31/02
	L0420	Deleted 12/31/02
	L0430	Deleted 12/31/02
	L0440	Deleted 12/31/02

✳ L0450   TLSO, flexible, provides trunk support, upper thoracic region, produces intracavitary pressure to reduce load on the intevertebral disks with rigid stays or panel(s), includes shoulder straps and closures, prefabricated, includes fitting and adjustment

✳ L0452   TLSO TLSO, flexible, provides trunk support, upper thoracic region, produces intracavitary pressure to reduce load on the intervertebral disks with rigid stays or panel(s), includes shoulder straps and closures, custom fabricated

✳ L0454   TLSO flexible, provides trunk support, extends from sacrococcygeal junction to above t-9 vertebra, restricts gross trunk motion in the sagittal plane, produces intracavitary pressure to reduce load on the intervertebral disks with rigid stays or panel(s), includes shoulder straps and closures, prefabricated, includes fitting and adjustment

✳ L0456   TLSO, flexible, provides trunk support, thoracic region, rigid posterior panel and soft anterior apron, extends from the sacrococcygeal junction and terminates just inferior to the scapular spine, restricts gross trunk motion in the sagittal plane, produces intracavitary pressure to reduce load on the intervertebral disks, includes straps and closures, prefabricated, includes fitting and adjustment

✳ L0458   TLSO, triplanar control, modular segmented spinal system, two rigid plastic shells, posterior extends from the sacrococcygeal junction and terminates just inferior to the scapular spine, anterior extends from the symphysis pubis to the xiphoid, soft liner, restricts gross trunk motion in the sagittal, coronal, and transverse planes, lateral strength is provided by overlapping plastic and stabilizing closures, includes straps and closures, prefabricated, includes fitting and adjustment

✳ L0460   TLSO, triplanar control, modular segmented spinal system, two rigid plastic shells, posterior extends from the sacrococcygeal junction and terminates just inferior to the scapular spine, anterior extends from the symphysis pubis to the sternal notch, soft liner, restricts gross trunk motion in the sagittal, coronal, and transverse planes, lateral strength is provided by overlapping plastic and stabilizing closures, includes straps and closures, prefabricated, includes fitting and adjustment

✳ L0462   TLSO, triplanar control, modular segmented spinal system, three rigid plastic shells, posterior extends from the sacrococcygeal junction and terminates just inferior to the scapular spine, anterior extends from the symphysis pubis to the sternal notch, soft liner, restricts gross trunk motion in the sagittal, coronal, and transverse planes, lateral strength is provided by overlapping plastic and stabilizing closures, includes straps and closures, prefabricated, includes fitting and adjustment

✳ L0464   TLSO, triplanar control, modular segmented spinal system, four rigid plastic shells, posterior extends from sacrococcygeal junction and terminates just inferior to scapular spine, anterior extends from symphysis pubis to the sternal notch, soft liner, restricts gross trunk motion in sagittal, coronal, and transverse planes, lateral strength is provided by overlapping plastic and stabilizing closures, includes straps and closures, prefabricated, includes fitting and adjustment

✳ L0466   TLSO, sagittal control, rigid posterior frame and flexible soft anterior apron with straps, closures and padding, restricts gross trunk motion in sagittal plane, produces intracavitary pressure to reduce load on intervertebral disks, includes fitting and shaping the frame, prefabricated, includes fitting and adjustment

✳ L0468   TLSO, sagittal-coronal control, rigid posterior frame and flexible soft anterior apron with straps, closures and padding, extends from sacrococcygeal junction over scapulae, lateral strength provided by pelvic, thoracic, and lateral frame pieces, restricts gross trunk motion in sagittal, and coronal planes, produces intracavitary pressure to reduce load on intervertebral disks, includes fitting and shaping the frame, prefabricated, includes fitting and adjustment

❋ L0470   TLSO, triplanar control, rigid posterior frame and flexible soft anterior apron with straps, closures and padding, extends from sacrococcygeal junction to scapula, lateral strength provided by pelvic, thoracic, and lateral frame pieces, rotational strength provided by subclavicular extensions, restricts gross trunk motion in sagittal, coronal, and transverse planes, produces intracavitary pressure to reduce load on the intervertebral disks, includes fitting and shaping the frame, prefabricated, includes fitting and adjustment

❋ L0472   TLSO, triplanar control, hyperextension, rigid anterior and lateral frame extends from symphysis pubis to sternal notch with two anterior components (one pubic and one sternal), posterior and lateral pads with straps and closures, limits spinal flexion, restricts gross trunk motion in sagittal, coronal, and transverse planes, includes fitting and shaping the frame, prefabricated, includes fitting and adjustment

❋ L0476   TLSO, sagittal-coronal control, flexion compression jacket, two rigid plastic shells with soft liner, posterior extends from sacrococcygeal junction and terminates at or before the T-9 vertebra, anterior extends from symphysis pubis to xiphoid, usually laced together on one side, restricts gross trunk motion in sagittal and coronal planes, allows free flexion and compression of the LS region, includes straps and closures, prefabricated, includes fitting and adjustment

❋ L0478   TLSO, sagittal-coronal control, flexion compression jacket, two rigid plastic shells with soft liner, posterior extends from sacrococcygeal junction and terminates at or before the T-9 vertebra, anterior extends from symphysis pubis to xiphoid, usually laced together on one side, restricts gross trunk motion in sagittal and coronal planes, allows free flexion and compression of LS region, includes straps and closures, custom fabricated

❋ L0480   TLSO, triplanar control, one piece rigid plastic shell without interface liner, with multiple straps and closures, posterior extends from sacrococcygeal junction and terminates just inferior to scapular spine, anterior extends from symphysis pubis to sternal notch, anterior or posterior opening, restricts gross trunk motion in sagittal, coronal, and transverse planes, includes a carved plaster or CAD-CAM model, custom fabricated

❋ L0482   TLSO, triplanar control, one piece rigid plastic shell with interface liner, multiple straps and closures, posterior extends from sacrococcygeal junction and terminates just inferior to scapular spine, anterior extends from symphysis pubis to sternal notch, anterior or posterior opening, restricts gross trunk motion in sagittal, coronal, and transverse planes, includes a carved plaster or CAD-CAM model, custom fabricated

❋ L0484   TLSO, triplanar control, two piece rigid plastic shell without interface liner, with multiple straps and closures, posterior extends from sacrococcygeal junction and terminates just inferior to scapular spine, anterior extends from symphysis pubis to sternal notch, lateral strength is enhanced by overlapping plastic, restricts gross trunk motion in the sagittal, coronal, and transverse planes, includes a carved plaster or CAD-CAM model, custom fabricated

❋ L0486   TLSO, triplanar control, two piece rigid plastic shell with interface liner, multiple straps and closures, posterior extends from sacrococcygeal junction and terminates just inferior to scapular spine, anterior extends from symphysis pubis to sternal notch, lateral strength is enhanced by overlapping plastic, restricts gross trunk motion in the sagittal, coronal, and transverse planes, includes a carved plaster or CAD-CAM model, custom fabricated

❋ L0488   TLSO, triplanar control, one piece rigid plastic shell with interface liner, multiple straps and closures, posterior extends from sacrococcygeal junction and terminates just inferior to scapular spine, anterior extends from symphysis pubis to sternal notch, anterior or posterior opening, restricts gross trunk motion in sagittal, coronal, and transverse planes, prefabricated, includes fitting and adjustment

❋ L0490   TLSO, sagittal-coronal control, one piece rigid plastic shell, with overlapping reinforced anterior, with multiple straps and closures, posterior extends from sacrococcygeal junction and terminates at or before the T-9 vertebra, anterior extends from symphysis pubis to xiphoid, anterior opening, restricts gross trunk motion in sagittal and coronal planes, prefabricated, includes fitting and adjustment

Lumbar-Sacral

Flexible

* L0500 Lumbar-sacral orthosis (LSO), flexible, (lumbar-sacral support)
* L0510 LSO, flexible (lumbar-sacral support), custom fabricated
* L0515 LSO, anterior-posterior control, with rigid or semi-rigid posterior panel, prefabricated

Anterior-Posterior-Lateral Control

* L0520 LSO, anterior-posterior-lateral control (Knight, Wilcox types), with apron front

Anterior-Posterior Control

* L0530 LSO, anterior-posterior control (Macausland type), with apron front

Lumbar-Flexion

* L0540 LSO, lumbar flexion (Williams flexion type)

Anterior-Posterior-Lateral Control (Body Jacket)

* L0550 LSO, anterior-posterior-lateral control, molded to patient model
* L0560 LSO, anterior-posterior lateral control, molded to patient model, with interface material
* L0561 LSO, anterior-posterior-lateral control, with rigid or semi-rigid posterior panel, prefabricated
* L0565 LSO, anterior-posterior-lateral control, custom fitted

Sacroiliac

Flexible

* L0600 Sacroiliac, flexible (sacroiliac surgical support)
* L0610 Sacroiliac, flexible (sacroiliac surgical support), custom fabricated

Semi-rigid

* L0620 Sacroiliac, semi-rigid (Goldthwaite, Osgood types), with apron front

Cervical-Thoracic-Lumbar-Sacral

Anterior-Posterior-Lateral Control

* L0700 Cervical-thoracic-lumbar-sacral orthosis (CTLSO), anterior-posterior-lateral control, molded to patient model (Minerva type)
* L0710 CTLSO, anterior-posterior-lateral control, molded to patient model, with interface material (Minerva type)

HALO Procedure

* L0810 HALO procedure, cervical halo incorporated into jacket vest
* L0820 HALO procedure, cervical halo incorporated into plaster body jacket
* L0830 HALO procedure, cervical halo incorporated into Milwaukee type orthosis
* L0860 Addition to HALO procedures, magnetic resonance image compatible system
▶* L0861 Addition to halo procedure, replacement liner/interface material

Torso Supports

L0900 Deleted 12/31/02, Cross Reference L0500
L0910 Deleted 12/31/02, Cross Reference L0510
L0920 Deleted 12/31/02, Cross Reference L0500
L0930 Deleted 12/31/02, Cross Reference L0510
L0940 Deleted 12/31/02, Cross Reference L0500
L0950 Deleted 12/31/02, Cross Reference L0510
* L0960 Torso support, postsurgical support, pads for postsurgical support

Additions to Spinal Orthoses

* L0970 TLSO, corset front
* L0972 LSO, corset front
* L0974 TLSO, full corset
* L0976 LSO, full corset
* L0978 Axillary crutch extension
* L0980 Peroneal straps, pair
* L0982 Stocking supporter grips, set of four (4)
* L0984 Protective body sock, each
L0986 Deleted 12/31/02
* L0999 Addition to spinal orthosis, not otherwise specified

Orthotic Devices: Scoliosis Procedures (L1000-L1499)

NOTE: Orthotic care of scoliosis differs from other orthotic care in that the treatment is more dynamic in nature and uses ongoing continual modification of the orthosis to the patient's changing condition. This coding structure uses the proper names, or eponyms, of the procedures because they have historic and universal acceptance in the profession. It should be recognized that variations to the basic procedures described by the founders/developers are accepted in various medical and orthotic practices throughout the country. All procedures include a model of patient when indicated.

Scoliosis: Cervical-Thoracic-Lumbar-Sacral (CTLSO) (Milwaukee)

* L1000 CTLSO (Milwaukee), inclusive of furnishing initial orthosis, including model
* L1005 Tension-based scoliosis orthosis and accessory pads, includes fitting and adjustment
* L1010 Addition to CTLSO or scoliosis orthosis, axilla sling

Correction Pads

* L1020 Addition to CTLSO or scoliosis orthosis, kyphosis pad
* L1025 Addition to CTLSO or scoliosis orthosis, kyphosis pad, floating
* L1030 Addition to CTLSO or scoliosis orthosis, lumbar bolster pad
* L1040 Addition to CTLSO or scoliosis orthosis, lumbar or lumbar rib pad
* L1050 Addition to CTLSO or scoliosis orthosis, sternal pad
* L1060 Addition to CTLSO or scoliosis orthosis, thoracic pad
* L1070 Addition to CTLSO or scoliosis orthosis, trapezius sling
* L1080 Addition to CTLSO or scoliosis orthosis, outrigger
* L1085 Addition to CTLSO or scoliosis orthosis, outrigger, bilateral with vertical extensions
* L1090 Addition to CTLSO or scoliosis orthosis, lumbar sling
* L1100 Addition to CTLSO or scoliosis orthosis, ring flange, plastic or leather
* L1110 Addition to CTLSO or scoliosis orthosis, ring flange, plastic or leather, molded to patient model
* L1120 Addition to CTLSO, scoliosis orthosis, cover for upright, each

Scoliosis: Cervical-Thoracic-Lumbar-Sacral (Low Profile)

* L1200 TLSO, inclusive of furnishing initial orthosis only
* L1210 Addition to TLSO, (low profile), lateral thoracic extension
* L1220 Addition to TLSO (low profile), anterior thoracic extension
* L1230 Addition to TLSO (low profile), Milwaukee type superstructure
* L1240 Addition to TLSO (low profile), lumbar derotation pad
* L1250 Addition to TLSO (low profile), anterior ASIS pad
* L1260 Addition to TLSO (low profile), anterior thoracic derotation pad
* L1270 Addition to TLSO (low profile), abdominal pad
* L1280 Addition to TLSO (low profile), rib gusset (elastic), each
* L1290 Addition to TLSO (low profile), lateral trochanteric pad

Other Scoliosis Procedures

* L1300 Other scoliosis procedure, body jacket molded to patient model
* L1310 Other scoliosis procedure, postoperative body jacket
* L1499 Spinal orthosis, NOS

Scoliosis: Thoracic-Hip-Knee-Ankle (THKA)

* L1500 Thoracic-hip-knee-ankle orthosis (THKAO), mobility frame (Newington, Parapodium types)
* L1510 THKAO, standing frame, with or without tray and accessories
* L1520 THKAO, swivel walker

Orthotic Devices: Lower Limb

NOTE: the procedures in L1600-L2999 are considered as *base* or *basic procedures* and may be modified by listing procedure from the Additions Sections and adding them to the base procedure.

Hip: Flexible

* L1600 Hip orthosis (HO), abduction control of hip joints, flexible, Frejka type with cover, prefabricated, includes fitting and adjustment
* L1610 HO, abduction control of hip joints, flexible, Frejka cover only, prefabricated, includes fitting and adjustment

* L1620   HO, abduction control of hip joints, flexible, Pavlik harness, prefabricated, includes fitting and adjustment

* L1630   HO, abduction control of hip joints, semi-flexible (Von Rosen type), custom fabrication

* L1640   HO, abduction control of hip joints, static, pelvic band or spreader bar, thigh cuffs, custom fabrication

* L1650   HO, abduction control of hip joints, static, adjustable, (Ilfeld type), prefabricated, includes fitting and adjustment

* L1652   Hip orthosis, bilateral thigh cuffs with adjustable abductor spreader bar, adult size, prefabricated, includes fitting and adjustment, any type

* L1660   HO, abduction control of hip joints, static, plastic, prefabricated, includes fitting and adjustment

* L1680   HO, abduction control of hip joints, dynamic, pelvic control, adjustable hip motion control, thigh cuffs (Rancho hip action type), custom fabrication

* L1685   HO, abduction control of hip joint, postoperative hip abduction type, custom fabricated

* L1686   HO, abduction control of hip joint, postoperative hip abduction type, prefabricated, includes fitting and adjustment

* L1690   Combination, bilateral, lumbar sacral, hip, femur orthosis providing adduction and internal rotation control, prefabricated, includes fitting and adjustment

Legg-Perthes

* L1700   Legg-Perthes orthosis (Toronto type), custom fabrication

* L1710   Legg-Perthes orthosis (Newington type), custom fabrication

* L1720   Legg-Perthes orthosis, trilateral (Tachdjian type), custom fabrication

* L1730   Legg-Perthes orthosis (Scottish Rite type), custom fabrication

* L1750   Legg-Perthes orthosis, Legg Perthes sling (Sam Browne type), prefabricated, includes fitting and adjustment

* L1755   Legg-Perthes orthosis (Patten bottom type), custom fabrication

Knee (KO)

* L1800   Knee orthosis (KO), elastic with stays, prefabricated, includes fitting and adjustment

* L1810   KO, elastic with joints, prefabricated, includes fitting and adjustment

* L1815   KO, elastic or other elastic type material with condylar pads, prefabricated, includes fitting and adjustment

* L1820   KO, elastic with condylar pads and joints, prefabricated, includes fitting and adjustment

* L1825   KO, elastic kneecap, prefabricated, includes fitting and adjustment

* L1830   KO, immobilizer, canvas longitudinal, prefabricated, includes fitting and adjustment

▶* L1831   Knee orthosis, locking knee joint(s), positional orthosis, prefabricated, includes fitting and adjustment

* L1832   KO, adjustable knee joints, positional orthosis, rigid support, prefabricated, includes fitting and adjustment

* L1834   KO, without knee joint, rigid, custom fabrication

* L1836   Knee orthosis, rigid, without joint(s), includes soft interface material, prefabricated, includes fitting and adjustment

* L1840   KO, derotation, medial-lateral, anterior cruciate ligament, custom fabricated

⇒* L1843   Knee orthosis, single upright, thigh and calf, with adjustable flexion and extension joint, medial-lateral and rotation control, with or without varus/valgus adjustment; prefabricated, includes fitting and adjustment

⇒* L1844   Knee orthosis, single upright, thigh and calf, with adjustable flexion and extension joint, medial-lateral and rotation control, with or without varus/valgus adjustment, custom fabricated

* L1845   KO, double upright, thigh and calf, with adjustable flexion and extension joint, medial-lateral and rotation control; prefabricated, includes fitting and adjustment

* L1846   KO, double upright, thigh and calf, with adjustable flexion and extension joint, medial-lateral and rotation control, custom fabrication

* L1847   Knee orthosis, double upright with adjustable joint, with inflatable air support chambers, prefabricated, includes fitting and adjustment

* L1850   KO, Swedish type, prefabricated, includes fitting and adjustment

* L1855   KO, molded plastic, thigh and calf sections, with double upright knee joints, custom fabrication

* L1858   KO, molded plastic, polycentric knee joints, pneumatic knee pads (CTI), custom fabrication

* L1860   KO, modification of supracondylar prosthetic socket, custom fabrication (SK)

* L1870   KO, double upright, thigh and calf lacers, with knee joints, custom fabrication
* L1880   KO, double upright, non-molded thigh and calf cuffs/lacers with knee joints, custom fabrication
L1885   Deleted 12/31/03, Cross Reference E1810

Ankle-Foot (AFO)

* L1900   Ankle-foot orthosis (AFO), spring wire, dorsiflexion assist calf band, custom fabrication
* L1901   Ankle orthosis, elastic, prefabricated, includes fitting and adjustment (e.g. neoprene, Lycra)
* L1902   AFO, ankle gauntlet, prefabricated, includes fitting and adjustment
* L1904   AFO, molded ankle gauntlet, custom fabrication
* L1906   AFO, multiligamentus ankle support, prefabricated, includes fitting and adjustment
▶* L1907   AFO (ankle foot orthosis), supramalleolar with straps, with or without interface/pads, custom fabricated
* L1910   AFO, posterior, single bar, clasp attachment to shoe counter, prefabricated, includes fitting and adjustment
* L1920   AFO, single upright with static or adjustable stop (Phelps or Perlstein type), custom fabrication
* L1930   AFO, plastic or other material, prefabricated, includes fitting and adjustment
* L1940   AFO, plastic or other material, custom fabrication
* L1945   AFO, plastic, rigid anterior tibial section (floor reaction), custom fabrication
⇒* L1950   Ankle foot orthosis, spiral, (Institute of Rehabilitation Medicine type), plastic, custom-fabrication
▶* L1951   Ankle foot orthosis, spiral, (Institute of Rehabilitative Medicine type), plastic or other material, prefabricated, includes fitting and adjustment
* L1960   AFO, posterior solid ankle, plastic, custom fabrication
* L1970   AFO, plastic, with ankle joint, custom fabrication
▶* L1971   Ankle foot orthosis, plastic or other material with ankle joint, prefabricated, includes fitting and adjustment
* L1980   AFO, single upright free plantar dorsiflexion, solid stirrup, calf band/cuff (single bar BK orthosis), custom fabrication
* L1990   AFO, double upright free plantar dorsiflexion, solid stirrup, calf band/cuff (double bar BK orthosis), custom fabrication

Hip-Knee-Ankle-Foot (or Any Combination)

NOTE: L2000, L2020, and L2036 are base procedures to be used with any knee joint. L2010 and L2030 are to be used only with no knee joint.

* L2000   Knee-ankle-foot orthosis (KAFO), single upright, free knee, free ankle, solid stirrup, thigh and calf bands/cuffs (single bar 'AK' orthosis), custom fabrication
* L2010   KAFO, single upright, free ankle, solid stirrup, thigh and calf bands/cuffs (single bar AK orthosis), without knee joint, custom fabrication
* L2020   KAFO, double upright, free knee, free ankle, solid stirrup, thigh and calf bands/cuffs (double bar AK orthosis), custom fabrication
* L2030   KAFO, double upright, free ankle, solid stirrup, thigh and calf bands/cuffs (double bar AK orthosis), without knee joint, custom fabrication
* L2035   KAFO, full plastic, static, prefabricated (pediatric size), prefabricated, includes fitting and adjustment
* L2036   KAFO, full plastic, double upright, free knee, custom fabrication
* L2037   KAFO, full plastic, single upright, free knee, custom fabrication
* L2038   KAFO, full plastic, without knee joint, multi-axis ankle, (lively orthosis or equal), custom fabrication
* L2039   KAFO, full plastic, single upright, polyaxial hinge, medial-lateral rotation control, custom fabrication

Torsion Control

* L2040   Hip-knee-ankle-foot orthosis (HKAFO), torsion control, bilateral rotation straps, pelvic band/belt, custom fabrication
* L2050   HKAFO, torsion control, bilateral torsion cables, hip joint, pelvic band/belt, custom fabrication
* L2060   HKAFO, torsion control, bilateral torsion cables, ball bearing hip joint, pelvic band/belt, custom fabrication
* L2070   HKAFO, torsion control, unilateral rotation straps, pelvic band/belt, custom fabrication
* L2080   HKAFO, torsion control, unilateral torsion cable, hip joint, pelvic band/belt, custom fabrication
* L2090   HKAFO, torsion control, unilateral torsion cable, ball bearing hip joint, pelvic band/belt, custom fabrication

Fracture Orthoses

L2102   Deleted 12/31/03
L2104   Deleted 12/31/03

* L2106 AFO, fracture orthosis, tibial fracture cast orthosis, thermoplastic type casting material, custom fabrication

* L2108 AFO, fracture orthosis, tibial fracture cast orthosis, custom fabrication

* L2112 AFO, fracture orthosis, tibial fracture orthosis, soft, prefabricated, includes fitting and adjustment

* L2114 AFO, fracture orthosis, tibial fracture orthosis, semi-rigid, prefabricated, includes fitting and adjustment

* L2116 AFO, fracture orthosis, tibial fracture orthosis, rigid, prefabricated, includes fitting and adjustment

L2122 Deleted 12/31/03

L2124 Deleted 12/31/03

* L2126 KAFO, fracture orthosis, femoral fracture cast orthosis, thermoplastic type casting material, custom fabrication

* L2128 KAFO, fracture orthosis, femoral fracture cast orthosis, custom fabrication

* L2132 KAFO, fracture orthosis, femoral fracture cast orthosis, soft, prefabricated, includes fitting and adjustment

* L2134 KAFO, fracture orthosis, femoral fracture cast orthosis, semi-rigid, prefabricated, includes fitting and adjustment

* L2136 KAFO, fracture orthosis, femoral fracture cast orthosis, rigid, prefabricated, includes fitting and adjustment

Additions to Fracture Orthosis

* L2180 Addition to lower extremity fracture orthosis, plastic shoe insert with ankle joints

* L2182 Addition to lower extremity fracture orthosis, drop lock knee joint

* L2184 Addition to lower extremity fracture orthosis, limited motion knee joint

* L2186 Addition to lower extremity fracture orthosis, adjustable motion knee joint (Lerman type)

* L2188 Addition to lower extremity fracture orthosis, quadrilateral brim

* L2190 Addition to lower extremity fracture orthosis, waist belt

* L2192 Addition to lower extremity fracture orthosis, hip joint, pelvic band, thigh flange, and pelvic belt

Additions to Lower Extremity Orthosis

Shoe-Ankle-Shin-Knee

* L2200 Addition to lower extremity, limited ankle motion, each joint

* L2210 Addition to lower extremity, dorsiflexion assist (plantar flexion resist), each joint

* L2220 Addition to lower extremity, dorsiflexion and plantar flexion assist/resist, each joint

* L2230 Addition to lower extremity, split flat caliper stirrups and plate attachment

* L2240 Addition to lower extremity, round caliper and plate attachment

* L2250 Addition to lower extremity, footplate, molded to patient model, stirrup attachment

* L2260 Addition to lower extremity, reinforced solid stirrup (Scott-Craig type)

* L2265 Addition to lower extremity, long tongue stirrup

* L2270 Addition to lower extremity, varus/valgus correction (T) strap, padded/lined or malleolus pad

* L2275 Addition to lower extremity, varus/valgus correction, plastic modification, padded/lined

* L2280 Addition to lower extremity, molded inner boot

* L2300 Addition to lower extremity, abduction bar (bilateral hip involvement), jointed, adjustable

* L2310 Addition to lower extremity, abduction bar, straight

* L2320 Addition to lower extremity, non-molded lacer

* L2330 Addition to lower extremity, lacer molded to patient model

* L2335 Addition to lower extremity, anterior swing band

* L2340 Addition to lower extremity, pre-tibial shell, molded to patient model

* L2350 Addition to lower extremity, prosthetic type, (BK) socket, molded to patient model, (used for PTB and AFO orthoses)

* L2360 Addition to lower extremity, extended steel shank

* L2370 Addition to lower extremity, Patten bottom

* L2375 Addition to lower extremity, torsion control, ankle joint and half solid stirrup

* L2380 Addition to lower extremity, torsion control, straight knee joint, each joint

* L2385 Addition to lower extremity, straight knee joint, heavy duty, each joint

* L2390 Addition to lower extremity, offset knee joint, each joint

* L2395 Addition to lower extremity, offset knee joint, heavy duty, each joint

* L2397 Addition to lower extremity orthosis, suspension sleeve

Additions to Straight Knee or Offset Knee Joints

➡ * L2405 Addition to knee joint, lock, drop, stance or swing phase, each joint

⊙ **Special coverage instructions** ◆ **Not covered by or valid for Medicare** * **Carrier discretion** ◀ ▶ **New** ⬤➡ **Revised**

* L2415 Addition to knee lock with integrated release mechanism (bail, cable, or equal), any material, each joint
* L2425 Addition to knee joint, disc or dial lock for adjustable knee flexion, each joint
* L2430 Addition to knee joint, ratchet lock for active and progressive knee extension, each joint
* L2435 Addition to knee joint, polycentric joint, each joint
* L2492 Addition to knee joint, lift loop for drop lock ring

Additions to Thigh/Weight Bearing

Gluteal/Ischial Weight Bearing

* L2500 Addition to lower extremity, thigh/weight bearing, gluteal/ischial weight bearing, ring
* L2510 Addition to lower extremity, thigh/weight bearing, quadri-lateral brim, molded to patient model
* L2520 Addition to lower extremity, thigh/weight bearing, quadri-lateral brim, custom fitted
* L2525 Addition to lower extremity, thigh/weight bearing, ischial containment/narrow M-L brim molded to patient model
* L2526 Addition to lower extremity, thigh/weight bearing, ischial containment/narrow M-L brim, custom fitted
* L2530 Addition to lower extremity, thigh-weight bearing, lacer, non-molded
* L2540 Addition to lower extremity, thigh/weight bearing, lacer, molded to patient model
* L2550 Addition to lower extremity, thigh/weight bearing, high roll cuff

Additions to Pelvic and Thoracic Control

* L2570 Addition to lower extremity, pelvic control, hip joint, Clevis type two position joint, each
* L2580 Addition to lower extremity, pelvic control, pelvic sling
* L2600 Addition to lower extremity, pelvic control, hip joint, Clevis type, or thrust bearing, free, each
* L2610 Addition to lower extremity, pelvic control, hip joint, Clevis or thrust bearing, lock, each
* L2620 Addition to lower extremity, pelvic control, hip joint, heavy duty, each
* L2622 Addition to lower extremity, pelvic control, hip joint, adjustable flexion, each

* L2624 Addition to lower extremity, pelvic control, hip joint, adjustable flexion, extension, abduction control, each
* L2627 Addition to lower extremity, pelvic control, plastic, molded to patient model, reciprocating hip joint and cables
* L2628 Addition to lower extremity, pelvic control, metal frame, reciprocating hip joint and cables
* L2630 Addition to lower extremity, pelvic control, band and belt, unilateral
* L2640 Addition to lower extremity, pelvic control, band and belt, bilateral
* L2650 Addition to lower extremity, pelvic and thoracic control, gluteal pad, each
* L2660 Addition to lower extremity, thoracic control, thoracic band
* L2670 Addition to lower extremity, thoracic control, paraspinal uprights
* L2680 Addition to lower extremity, thoracic control, lateral support uprights

General Additions

* L2750 Addition to lower extremity orthosis, plating chrome or nickel, per bar
* L2755 Addition to lower extremity orthosis, high strength, lightweight material, all hybrid lamination/prepreg composite, per segment
* L2760 Addition to lower extremity orthosis, extension, per extension, per bar (for lineal adjustment for growth)
* L2768 Orthotic side bar disconnect device, per bar
* L2770 Addition to lower extremity orthosis, any material—per bar or joint
* L2780 Addition to lower extremity orthosis, non-corrosive finish, per bar
* L2785 Addition to lower extremity orthosis, drop lock retainer, each
* L2795 Addition to lower extremity orthosis, knee control, full kneecap
* L2800 Addition to lower extremity orthosis, knee control, knee cap, medial or lateral pull
* L2810 Addition to lower extremity orthosis, knee control, condylar pad
* L2820 Addition to lower extremity orthosis, soft interface for molded plastic, below knee section
* L2830 Addition to lower extremity orthosis, soft interface for molded plastic, above knee section
* L2840 Addition to lower extremity orthosis, tibial length sock, fracture or equal, each
* L2850 Addition to lower extremity orthosis, femoral length sock, fracture or equal, each

* L2860   Addition to lower extremity joint, knee or ankle, concentric adjustable torsion style mechanism, each

* L2999   Lower extremity orthoses, not otherwise specified

Foot (Orthopedic Shoes)

Insert, Removable, Molded to Patient Model

⊗ L3000   Foot, insert, removable, molded to patient model, UCB type, Berkeley shell, each
MCM 2323

⊗ L3001   Foot, insert, removable, molded to patient model, Spenco, each
MCM 2323

⊗ L3002   Foot, insert, removable, molded to patient model, Plastazote or equal, each
MCM 2323

⊗ L3003   Foot, insert, removable, molded to patient model, silicone gel, each
MCM 2323

⊗ L3010   Foot, insert, removable, molded to patient model, longitudinal arch support, each
MCM 2323

⊗ L3020   Foot, insert, removable, molded to patient model, longitudinal/metatarsal support, each
MCM 2323

⊗ L3030   Foot, insert, removable, formed to patient foot, each
MCM 2323

▶◆ L3031   Foot, insert/plate, removable, addition to lower extremity orthosis, high strength, lightweight material, all hybrid lamination/prepreg composite, each

Arch Support, Removable, Premolded

⊗ L3040   Foot, arch support, removable, premolded, longitudinal, each
MCM 2323

⊗ L3050   Foot, arch support, removable, premolded, metatarsal, each
MCM 2323

⊗ L3060   Foot, arch support, removable, premolded, longitudinal/metatarsal, each
MCM 2323

Arch Support, Non-removable, Attached to Shoe

⊗ L3070   Foot, arch support, non-removable attached to shoe, longitudinal, each
MCM 2323

⊗ L3080   Foot, arch support, non-removable attached to shoe, metatarsal, each
MCM 2323

⊗ L3090   Foot, arch support, non-removable attached to shoe, longitudinal/metatarsal, each
MCM 2323

⊗ L3100   Hallus-valgus night dynamic splint
MCM 2323

Abduction and Rotation Bars

⊗ L3140   Foot, abduction rotation bar, including shoes
MCM 2323

⊗ L3150   Foot, abduction rotation bar, without shoes
MCM 2323

* L3160   Foot, adjustable shoe-styled positioning device

⊗ L3170   Foot, plastic heel stabilizer
MCM 2323

Orthopedic Footwear

⊗ L3201   Orthopedic shoe, oxford with supinator or pronator, infant
MCM 2323

⊗ L3202   Orthopedic shoe, oxford with supinator or pronator, child
MCM 2323

⊗ L3203   Orthopedic shoe, oxford with supinator or pronator, junior
MCM 2323

⊗ L3204   Orthopedic shoe, hightop with supinator or pronator, infant
MCM 2323

⊗ L3206   Orthopedic shoe, hightop with supinator or pronator, child
MCM 2323

⊗ L3207   Orthopedic shoe, hightop with supinator or pronator, junior
MCM 2323

⊗ L3208   Surgical boot, infant, each
MCM 2079

⊗ L3209   Surgical boot, each, child
MCM 2079

⊗ L3211   Surgical boot, each, junior
MCM 2079

⊗ L3212   Benesch boot, pair, infant
MCM 2079

⊗ L3213   Benesch boot, pair, child
MCM 2079

⊗ L3214   Benesch boot, pair, junior
MCM 2079

◆ L3215   Orthopedic footwear, ladies' shoes, oxford
Medicare Statute 1862A8

◆ L3216 Orthopedic footwear, ladies' shoes, depth inlay
Medicare Statute 1862A8

◆ L3217 Orthopedic footwear, ladies' shoes, hightop, depth inlay
Medicare Statute 1862A8

L3218 Deleted 12/31/02, Cross Reference L3260

◆ L3219 Orthopedic footwear, men's shoes, oxford
Medicare Statute 1862A8

◆ L3221 Orthopedic footwear, men's shoes, depth inlay
Medicare Statute 1862A8

◆ L3222 Orthopedic footwear, men's shoes, high-top, depth inlay
Medicare Statute 1862A8

L3223 Deleted 12/31/02, Cross Reference L3260

✪ L3224 Orthopedic footwear, ladies' shoe, oxford, used as an integral part of a brace (orthosis)
MCM 2323D

✪ L3225 Orthopedic footwear, men's shoe, oxford, used as an integral part of a brace (orthosis)
MCM 2323D

✪ L3230 Orthopedic footwear, custom shoes, depth inlay
MCM 2323

✪ L3250 Orthopedic footwear, custom molded shoe, removable inner mold, prosthetic shoe, each
MCM 2323

✪ L3251 Foot, shoe molded to patient model, silicone shoe, each
MCM 2323

✪ L3252 Foot, shoe molded to patient model, Plastazote (or similar), custom fabricated, each
MCM 2323

✪ L3253 Foot, molded shoe Plastazote (or similar), custom fitted, each
MCM 2323

✪ L3254 Non-standard size or width
MCM 2323

✪ L3255 Non-standard size or length
MCM 2323

✪ L3257 Orthopedic footwear, additional charge for split size
MCM 2323

✪ L3260 Surgical boot/shoe, each
MCM 2079

∗ L3265 Plastazote sandal, each

Shoe Modifications

Lifts

✪ L3300 Lift, elevation, heel, tapered to metatarsals, per inch
MCM 2323

✪ L3310 Lift, elevation, heel and sole, Neoprene, per inch
MCM 2323

✪ L3320 Lift, elevation, heel and sole, cork, per inch
MCM 2323

✪ L3330 Lift, elevation, metal extension (skate)
MCM 2323

✪ L3332 Lift, elevation, inside shoe, tapered, up to 0.5 in
MCM 2323

✪ L3334 Lift, elevation, heel, per inch
MCM 2323

Wedges

✪ L3340 Heel wedge, SACH
MCM 2323

✪ L3350 Heel wedge
MCM 2323

✪ L3360 Sole wedge, outside sole
MCM 2323

✪ L3370 Sole wedge, between sole
MCM 2323

✪ L3380 Clubfoot wedge
MCM 2323

✪ L3390 Outflare wedge
MCM 2323

✪ L3400 Metatarsal bar wedge, rocker
MCM 2323

✪ L3410 Metatarsal bar wedge, between sole
MCM 2323

✪ L3420 Full sole and heel wedge, between sole
MCM 2323

Heels

✪ L3430 Heel, counter, plastic reinforced
MCM 2323

✪ L3440 Heel, counter, leather reinforced
MCM 2323

✪ L3450 Heel, SACH cushion type
MCM 2323

✪ L3455 Heel, new leather, standard
MCM 2323

✪ L3460 Heel, new rubber, standard
MCM 2323

✪ L3465 Heel, Thomas with wedge
MCM 2323

✪ L3470 Heel, Thomas extended to ball
MCM 2323

✪ L3480 Heel, pad and depression for spur
MCM 2323

⊘ L3485   Heel, pad, removable for spur
MCM 2323

Additions to Orthopedic Shoes

⊘ L3500   shoe addition, insole, leather
MCM 2323

⊘ L3510   Orthopedic shoe addition, insole,
rubber
MCM 2323

⊘ L3520   Orthopedic shoe addition, insole, felt
covered with leather
MCM 2323

⊘ L3530   Orthopedic shoe addition, sole, half
MCM 2323

⊘ L3540   Orthopedic shoe addition, sole, full
MCM 2323

⊘ L3550   Orthopedic shoe addition, toe tap, standard
MCM 2323

⊘ L3560   Orthopedic shoe addition, toe tap,
horseshoe
MCM 2323

⊘ L3570   Orthopedic shoe addition, special extension to instep (leather with eyelets)
MCM 2323

⊘ L3580   Orthopedic shoe addition, convert instep to Velcro closure
MCM 2323

⊘ L3590   Orthopedic shoe addition, convert firm
shoe counter to soft counter
MCM 2323

⊘ L3595   Orthopedic shoe addition, March bar
MCM 2323

Transfer or Replacement

⊘ L3600   Transfer of an orthosis from one shoe
to another, caliper plate, existing
MCM 2323

⊘ L3610   Transfer of an orthosis from one shoe
to another, caliper plate, new
MCM 2323

⊘ L3620   Transfer of an orthosis from one shoe
to another, solid stirrup, existing
MCM 2323

⊘ L3630   Transfer of an orthosis from one shoe
to another, solid stirrup, new
MCM 2323

⊘ L3640   Transfer of an orthosis from one shoe
to another, Dennis Browne splint (Rive-
ton), both shoes
MCM 2323

⊘ L3649   Orthopedic shoe, modification, addition
or transfer, not otherwise specified
MCM 2323

Orthotic Devices: Upper Limb

NOTE: The procedures in this section are considered as *base* or *basic procedures* and may be modified by listing procedures from the Additions section and adding them to the base procedure.

Shoulder

∗ L3650   Shoulder orthosis, (SO), figure of eight
(8) design abduction restrainer, prefabricated, includes fitting and adjustment

∗ L3651   Shoulder orthosis, single shoulder, elastic, prefabricated, includes fitting and
adjustment (e.g. neoprene, Lycra)

∗ L3652   Shoulder orthosis, double shoulder,
elastic, prefabricated, includes fitting
and adjustment (e.g. neoprene, Lycra)

∗ L3660   SO, figure of eight (8) design abduction
restrainer, canvas and webbing, prefabricated, includes fitting and adjustment

∗ L3670   SO, acromio/clavicular (canvas and
webbing type), prefabricated, includes
fitting and adjustment

∗ L3675   SO, vest type abduction restrainer, canvas webbing type, or equal, prefabricated, includes fitting and adjustment

⊘ L3677   SO, hard plastic, shoulder stabilizer,
pre-fabricated, includes fitting and adjustment
MCM 2130

Elbow

∗ L3700   Elbow orthosis (EO), elastic with stays,
prefabricated, includes fitting and adjustment

∗ L3701   Elbow orthosis, elastic, prefabricated,
includes fitting and adjustment (e.g. neoprene, Lycra)

∗ L3710   EO, elastic with metal joints, prefabricated, includes fitting and adjustment

∗ L3720   EO, double upright with forearm/arm
cuffs, free motion, custom fabrication

∗ L3730   EO, double upright with forearm/arm
cuffs, extension/flexion assist, custom
fabrication

∗ L3740   EO, double upright with forearm/arm
cuffs, adjustable position lock with active control, custom fabrication

∗ L3760   Elbow orthosis, with adjustable position
locking joint(s), prefabricated, includes
fitting and adjustments, any type

∗ L3762   Elbow orthosis, rigid, without joints, includes soft interface material, prefabricated, includes fitting and adjustment

Wrist-Hand-Finger Orthosis (WHFO)

∗ L3800   Wrist-hand-finger orthosis (WHFO), short opponens, no attachments, custom fabrication

∗ L3805   Wrist-hand-finger orthosis (WHFO), long opponens, no attachment, custom fabrication

∗ L3807   Wrist-hand-finger orthosis (WHFO), without joint(s), prefabricated, includes fitting and adjustments, any type

Additions and Extensions

∗ L3810   Wrist-hand-finger orthosis (WHFO), addition to short and long opponens, thumb abduction (C) bar

∗ L3815   Wrist-hand-finger orthosis (WHFO), addition to short and long opponens, second MP abduction assist

∗ L3820   Wrist-hand-finger orthosis (WHFO), addition to short and long opponens, IP extension assist, with MP extension stop

∗ L3825   Wrist-hand-finger orthosis (WHFO), addition to short and long opponens, MP extension stop

∗ L3830   Wrist-hand-finger orthosis (WHFO), addition to short and long opponens, MP extension assist

∗ L3835   Wrist-hand-finger orthosis (WHFO), addition to short and long opponens, MP spring extension assist

∗ L3840   Wrist-hand-finger orthosis (WHFO), addition to short and long opponens, spring swivel thumb

∗ L3845   Wrist-hand-finger orthosis (WHFO), addition to short and long opponens, thumb IP extension assist, with MP stop

∗ L3850   WHO, addition to short and long opponens, action wrist, with dorsiflexion assist

∗ L3855   Wrist-hand-finger orthosis (WHFO), addition to short and long opponens, adjustable MP flexion control

∗ L3860   Wrist-hand-finger orthosis (WHFO), addition to short and long opponens, adjustable MP flexion control and IP

∗ L3890   Addition to upper extremity joint, wrist or elbow, concentric adjustable torsion style mechanism, each

∗ L3900   Wrist-hand-finger orthosis (WHFO), dynamic flexor hinge, reciprocal wrist extension/flexion, finger flexion/extension, wrist or finger driven, custom fabrication

∗ L3901   Wrist-hand-finger orthosis (WHFO), dynamic flexor hinge, reciprocal wrist extension/flexion, finger flexion/extension, cable driven, custom fabrication

External Power

⇥ ◆ L3902   Wrist-hand-finger orthosis (WHFO), external powered, compressed gas, custom fabrication

∗ L3904   Wrist-hand-finger orthosis (WHFO), external powered, electric, custom fabrication

Other Wrist-Hand-Finger Orthoses: Custom Fitted

∗ L3906   WHO, wrist gauntlet, molded to patient model, custom fabrication

∗ L3907   Wrist-hand-finger orthosis (WHFO), wrist gauntlet with thumb spica, molded to patient model, custom fabrication

∗ L3908   WHO, wrist extension control cock-up, non-molded, prefabricated, includes fitting and adjustment

∗ L3909   Wrist orthosis, elastic, prefabricated, includes fitting and adjustment (e.g. neoprene, Lycra)

∗ L3910   Wrist-hand-finger orthosis (WHFO), Swanson design, prefabricated, includes fitting and adjustment

∗ L3911   Wrist hand finger orthosis, elastic, prefabricated, includes fitting and adjustment (e.g. neoprene, Lycra)

∗ L3912   HFO, flexion glove with elastic finger control, prefabricated, includes fitting and adjustment

∗ L3914   WHO, wrist extension cock-up, prefabricated, includes fitting and adjustment

∗ L3916   Wrist-hand-finger orthosis (WHFO), wrist extension cock-up, with outrigger, prefabricated, includes fitting and adjustment

▶ ∗ L3917   Hand orthosis, metacarpal fracture orthosis, prefabricated, includes fitting and adjustment

∗ L3918   HFO, knuckle bender, prefabricated, includes fitting and adjustment

∗ L3920   HFO, knuckle bender, with outrigger, prefabricated, includes fitting and adjustment

∗ L3922   HFO, knuckle bender, two segment to flex joints, prefabricated, includes fitting and adjustment

∗ L3923   HFO, without joint(s), prefabricated, includes fitting and adjustments, any type

∗ L3924   Wrist-hand-finger orthosis (WHFO), Oppenheimer, prefabricated, includes fitting and adjustment

∗ L3926   Wrist-hand-finger orthosis (WHFO), Thomas suspension, prefabricated, includes fitting and adjustment

∗ L3928   HFO, finger extension, with clock spring, prefabricated, includes fitting and adjustment

* L3930 Wrist-hand-finger orthosis (WHFO), finger extension, with wrist support, prefabricated, includes fitting and adjustment

* L3932 FO, safety pin, spring wire, prefabricated, includes fitting and adjustment

* L3934 FO, safety pin, modified, prefabricated, includes fitting and adjustment

* L3936 Wrist-hand-finger orthosis (WHFO), palmar, prefabricated, includes fitting and adjustment

* L3938 Wrist-hand-finger orthosis (WHFO), dorsal wrist, prefabricated, includes fitting and adjustment

* L3940 Wrist-hand-finger orthosis (WHFO), dorsal wrist, with outrigger attachment, prefabricated, includes fitting and adjustment

* L3942 HFO, reverse knuckle bender, prefabricated, includes fitting and adjustment

* L3944 HFO, reverse knuckle bender, with outrigger, prefabricated, includes fitting and adjustment

* L3946 HFO, composite elastic, prefabricated, includes fitting and adjustment

* L3948 FO, finger knuckle bender, prefabricated, includes fitting and adjustment

* L3950 Wrist-hand-finger orthosis (WHFO), combination Oppenheimer, with knuckle bender and two attachments, prefabricated, includes fitting and adjustment

* L3952 Wrist-hand-finger orthosis (WHFO), combination Oppenheimer, with reverse knuckle and two attachments, prefabricated, includes fitting and adjustment

* L3954 HFO, spreading hand, prefabricated, includes fitting and adjustment

* L3956 Addition of joint to upper extremity orthosis, any material, per joint

Shoulder-Elbow-Wrist-Hand Orthosis (SEWHO)

Abduction Positioning: Custom Fitted

* L3960 Shoulder-elbow-wrist-hand orthosis, (SEWHO), abduction positioning, airplane design, prefabricated, includes fitting and adjustment

* L3962 SEWHO, abduction positioning, Erb's palsy design, prefabricated, includes fitting and adjustment

* L3963 SEWHO, molded shoulder, arm, forearm, and wrist, with articulating elbow joint, custom fabrication

* L3964 SEO, mobile arm support attached to wheelchair, balanced, adjustable, prefabricated, includes fitting and adjustment

* L3965 SEO, mobile arm support attached to wheelchair, balanced, adjustable Rancho type, prefabricated, includes fitting and adjustment

* L3966 SEO, mobile arm support attached to wheelchair, balanced, reclining, prefabricated, includes fitting and adjustment

* L3968 SEO, mobile arm support attached to wheelchair, balanced, friction arm support (friction dampening to proximal and distal joints), prefabricated, includes fitting and adjustment

* L3969 SEO, mobile arm support, monosuspension arm and hand support, overhead elbow forearm hand sling support, yoke type arm suspension support, prefabricated, includes fitting and adjustment

Additions to Mobile Arm Supports

* L3970 SEO, addition to mobile arm support, elevating proximal arm

* L3972 SEO, addition to mobile arm support, offset or lateral rocker arm with elastic balance control

* L3974 SEO, addition to mobile arm support, supinator

Fracture Orthoses

* L3980 Upper extremity fracture orthosis, humeral, prefabricated, includes fitting and adjustment

* L3982 Upper extremity fracture orthosis, radius/ulnar, prefabricated, includes fitting and adjustment

* L3984 Upper extremity fracture orthosis, wrist, prefabricated, includes fitting and adjustment

* L3985 Upper extremity fracture orthosis, forearm, hand with wrist hinge, custom fabrication

* L3986 Upper extremity fracture orthosis, combination of humeral, radius/ulnar, wrist, (e.g., Colles' fracture), custom fabrication

* L3995 Addition to upper extremity orthosis, sock, fracture or equal, each

* L3999 Upper limb orthosis, not otherwise specified

Specific Repair

* L4000 Replace girdle for spinal orthosis (CTLSO or SO)

* L4010 Replace trilateral socket brim

* L4020 Replace quadrilateral socket brim, molded to patient model

* L4030 Replace quadrilateral socket brim, custom fitted
* L4040 Replace molded thigh lacer
* L4045 Replace non-molded thigh lacer
* L4050 Replace molded calf lacer
* L4055 Replace non-molded calf lacer
* L4060 Replace high roll cuff
* L4070 Replace proximal and distal upright for KAFO
* L4080 Replace metal bands, KAFO, proximal thigh
* L4090 Replace metal bands, KAFO-AFO, calf or distal thigh
* L4100 Replace leather cuff, KAFO, proximal thigh
* L4110 Replace leather cuff, KAFO-AFO, calf or distal thigh
* L4130 Replace pretibial shell

Repairs

⊘ L4205 Repair of orthotic device, labor component, per 15 minutes
MCM 2100.4
⊘ L4210 Repair of orthotic device, repair or replace minor parts
MCM 2100.4, MCM 2130D, MCM 2133

Ancillary Orthotic Services

➡ * L4350 Ankle control orthosis, stirrup style, rigid, includes any type interface (e.g., pneumatic, gel), prefabricated, includes fitting and adjustment
➡ * L4360 Walking boot, pneumatic, with or without joints, with or without interface material, prefabricated, includes fitting and adjustment
* L4370 Pneumatic full leg splint, prefabricated, includes fitting and adjustment
* L4380 Pneumatic knee splint, prefabricated, includes fitting and adjustment
➡ * L4386 Walking boot, non-pneumatic, with or without joints, with or without interface material, prefabricated, includes fitting and adjustment
* L4392 Replace soft interface material, static AFO
* L4394 Replace soft interface material, foot drop splint
* L4396 Static AFO, including soft interface material, adjustable for fit, for positioning, pressure reduction, may be used for minimal ambulation, prefabricated, includes fitting and adjustment
* L4398 Foot drop splint, recumbent positioning device, prefabricated, includes fitting and adjustment

PROSTHETIC PROCEDURES (L5000-L9999)

Lower Limb (L5000-L5999)

NOTE: The procedures in this sections are considered as *base* or *basic procedures* and may be modified by listing items/procedures or special materials from the Additions section and adding them to the base procedure.

Partial Foot

⊘ L5000 Partial foot, shoe insert with longitudinal arch, toe filler
MCM 2323
⊘ L5010 Partial foot, molded socket, ankle height, with toe filler
MCM 2323
⊘ L5020 Partial foot, molded socket, tibial tubercle height, with toe filler
MCM 2323

Ankle

* L5050 Ankle, Symes, molded socket, SACH (solid ankle cushion heel) foot
* L5060 Ankle, Symes, metal frame, molded leather socket, articulated ankle/foot

Below Knee

* L5100 Below knee, molded socket, shin, SACH (solid ankle cushion heel) foot
* L5105 Below knee, plastic socket, joints and thigh lacer, SACH (solid ankle cushion heel) foot

Knee Disarticulation

* L5150 Knee disarticulation (or through knee), molded socket, external knee joints, shin, SACH (solid ankle cushion heel) foot
* L5160 Knee disarticulation (or through knee), molded socket, bent knee configuration, external knee joints, shin, SACH (solid ankle cushion heel) foot

Above Knee

* L5200 Above knee, molded socket, single axis constant friction knee, shin, SACH (solid ankle cushion heel) foot
* L5210 Above knee, short prosthesis, no knee joint ('stubbies'), with foot blocks, no ankle joints, each
* L5220 Above knee, short prosthesis, no knee joint ('stubbies'), with articulated ankle/foot, dynamically aligned, each

* L5230   Above knee, for proximal femoral focal deficiency, constant friction knee, shin, SACH (solid ankle cushion heel) foot

Hip Disarticulation

* L5250   Hip disarticulation, Canadian type; molded socket, hip joint, single axis constant friction knee, shin, SACH (solid ankle cushion heel) foot

* L5270   Hip disarticulation, tilt table type; molded socket, locking hip joint, single axis constant friction knee, shin, SACH (solid ankle cushion heel) foot

Hemipelvectomy

* L5280   Hemipelvectomy, Canadian type; molded socket, hip joint, single axis constant friction knee, shin, SACH (solid ankle cushion heel) foot

Endoskeleton: Below Knee

* L5301   Below knee, molded socket, shin, SACH (solid ankle cushion heel) foot, endoskeletal system

Endoskeletal: Knee Disarticulation

* L5311   Knee disarticulation (or through knee), molded socket, external knee joints, shin, SACH (solid ankle cushion heel) foot, endoskeletal system

Endoskeletal: Above Knee

* L5321   Above knee, molded socket, open end, SACH (solid ankle cushion heel) foot, endoskeletal system, single axis knee

Endoskeletal: Hip Disarticulation

* L5331   Hip disarticulation, Canadian type, molded socket, endoskeletal system, hip joint, single axis knee, SACH (solid ankle cushion heel) foot

Endoskeletal: Hemipelvectomy

L5340   Deleted 01/01/02, Cross Reference L5341

* L5341   Hemipelvectomy, Canadian type, molded socket, endoskeletal system, hip joint, single axis knee, SACH (solid ankle cushion heel) foot

Immediate Postsurgical or Early Fitting Procedures

* L5400   Immediate postsurgical or early fitting, application of initial rigid dressing, including fitting, alignment, suspension, and one cast change, below knee

* L5410   Immediate post surgical or early fitting, application of initial rigid dressing, including fitting, alignment and suspension, below knee, each additional cast change and realignment

* L5420   Immediate postsurgical or early fitting, application of initial rigid dressing, including fitting, alignment and suspension and one cast change AK or knee disarticulation

* L5430   Immediate postsurgical or early fitting, application of initial rigid dressing, including fitting, alignment and suspension, AK or knee disarticulation, each additional cast change and realignment

* L5450   Immediate postsurgical or early fitting, application of non-weight bearing rigid dressing, below knee

* L5460   Immediate postsurgical or early fitting, application of non-weight bearing rigid dressing, above knee

Initial Prosthesis

* L5500   Initial, below knee PTB type socket, non-alignable system, pylon, no cover, SACH (solid ankle cushion heel) foot, plaster socket, direct formed

* L5505   Initial, above knee–knee disarticulation, ischial level socket, non-alignable system, pylon, no cover, SACH (solid ankle cushion heel) foot, plaster socket, direct formed

Preparatory Prosthesis

* L5510   Preparatory, below knee PTB type socket, non-alignable system, pylon, no cover, SACH (solid ankle cushion heel) foot, plaster socket, molded to model

* L5520   Preparatory, below knee PTB type socket, non-alignable system, pylon, no cover, SACH (solid ankle cushion heel) foot, thermoplastic or equal, direct formed

* L5530   Preparatory, below knee PTB type socket, non-alignable system, pylon, no cover, SACH (solid ankle cushion heel) foot, thermoplastic or equal, molded to model

* L5535   Preparatory, below knee PTB type socket, non-alignable system, no cover, SACH (solid ankle cushion heel) foot, prefabricated, adjustable open end socket

* L5540 Preparatory, below knee PTB type socket, non-alignable system, pylon, no cover, SACH (solid ankle cushion heel) foot, laminated socket, molded to model

* L5560 Preparatory, above knee-knee disarticulation, ischial level socket, non-alignable system, pylon, no cover, SACH (solid ankle cushion heel) foot, plaster socket, molded to model

* L5570 Preparatory, above knee-knee disarticulation, ischial level socket, non-alignable system, pylon, no cover, SACH (solid ankle cushion heel) foot, thermoplastic or equal, direct formed

* L5580 Preparatory, above knee-knee disarticulation, ischial level socket, non-alignable system, pylon, no cover, SACH (solid ankle cushion heel) foot, thermoplastic or equal, molded to model

* L5585 Preparatory, above knee-knee disarticulation, ischial level socket, non-alignable system, pylon, no cover, SACH (solid ankle cushion heel) foot, prefabricated adjustable open end socket

* L5590 Preparatory, above knee-knee disarticulation, ischial level socket, non-alignable system, pylon, no cover, SACH (solid ankle cushion heel) foot, laminated socket, molded to model

* L5595 Preparatory, hip disarticulation-hemipelvectomy, pylon, no cover, SACH (solid ankle cushion heel) foot, thermoplastic or equal, molded to patient model

* L5600 Preparatory, hip disarticulation-hemipelvectomy, pylon, no cover, SACH (solid ankle cushion heel) foot, laminated socket, molded to patient model

Additions to Lower Extremity

* L5610 Addition to lower extremity, endoskeletal system, above knee, hydracadence system

* L5611 Addition to lower extremity, endoskeletal system, above knee-knee disarticulation, 4-bar link-age, with friction wing phase control

* L5613 Addition to lower extremity, endoskeletal system, above knee-knee disarticulation, 4-bar linkage, with hydraulic swing phase control

* L5614 Addition to lower extremity, exoskeletal system, above knee-knee disarticulation, 4-bar linkage, with pneumatic swing phase control

* L5616 Addition to lower extremity, endoskeletal system, above knee, universal multiplex system, friction swing phase control

* L5617 Addition to lower extremity, quick change self-aligning unit, above knee or below knee, each

Additions to Test Sockets

* L5618 Addition to lower extremity, test socket, Symes

* L5620 Addition to lower extremity, test socket, below knee

* L5622 Addition to lower extremity, test socket, knee disarticulation

* L5624 Addition to lower extremity, test socket, above knee

* L5626 Addition to lower extremity, test socket, hip disarticulation

* L5628 Addition to lower extremity, test socket, hemipelvectomy

* L5629 Addition to lower extremity, below knee, acrylic socket

Additions to Socket Variations

* L5630 Addition to lower extremity, Symes type, expandable wall socket

* L5631 Addition to lower extremity, above knee or knee disarticulation, acrylic socket

* L5632 Addition to lower extremity, Symes type, PTB brim design socket

* L5634 Addition to lower extremity, Symes type, posterior opening (Canadian) socket

* L5636 Addition to lower extremity, Symes type, medial opening socket

* L5637 Addition to lower extremity, below knee, total contact

* L5638 Addition to lower extremity, below knee, leather socket

* L5639 Addition to lower extremity, below knee, wood socket

* L5640 Addition to lower extremity, knee disarticulation, leather socket

* L5642 Addition to lower extremity, above knee, leather socket

* L5643 Addition to lower extremity, hip disarticulation, flexible inner socket, external frame

* L5644 Addition to lower extremity, above knee, wood socket

* L5645 Addition to lower extremity, below knee, flexible inner socket, external frame

➡ * L5646 Addition to lower extremity, below knee, air, fluid, gel or equal, cushion socket

* L5647 Addition to lower extremity, below knee, suction socket

➠∗ L5648　Addition to lower extremity, above knee, air, fluid, gel or equal, cushion socket

∗ L5649　Addition to lower extremity, ischial containment/narrow M-L socket

∗ L5650　Additions to lower extremity, total contact, above knee or knee disarticulation socket

∗ L5651　Addition to lower extremity, above knee, flexible inner socket, external frame

∗ L5652　Addition to lower extremity, suction suspension, above knee or knee disarticulation socket

∗ L5653　Addition to lower extremity, knee disarticulation, expandable wall socket

Additions to Socket Insert and Suspension

∗ L5654　Addition to lower extremity, socket insert, Symes, (Kemblo, Pelite, Aliplast, Plastazote or equal)

∗ L5655　Addition to lower extremity, socket insert, below knee (Kemblo, Pelite, Aliplast, Plastazote or equal)

∗ L5656　Addition to lower extremity, socket insert, knee disarticulation (Kemblo, Pelite, Aliplast, Plastazote or equal)

∗ L5658　Addition to lower extremity, socket insert, above knee (Kemblo, Pelite, Aliplast, Plastazote or equal)

L5660　Deleted 12/31/02

∗ L5661　Addition to lower extremity, socket insert, multi-durometer Symes

L5662　Deleted 12/31/02

L5663　Deleted 12/31/02

L5664　Deleted 12/31/02

∗ L5665　Addition to lower extremity, socket insert, multi-durometer, below knee

∗ L5666　Addition to lower extremity, below knee, cuff suspension

L5667　Deleted 01/01/02

∗ L5668　Addition to lower extremity, below knee, molded distal cushion

L5669　Deleted 01/01/02; Cross Reference L5660, L5662, L5663, L5664

∗ L5670　Addition to lower extremity, below knee, molded supracondylar suspension (PTS or similar)

∗ L5671　Addition to lower extremity, below knee/above knee suspension locking mechanism (shuttle, lanyard or equal), excludes socket insert

∗ L5672　Addition to lower extremity, below knee, removable medial brim suspension

▶∗ L5673　Addition to lower extremity, below knee/above knee, custom fabricated from existing mold or prefabricated, socket insert, silicone gel, elastomeric or equal, for use with locking mechanism

∗ L5674　Addition to lower extremity, below knee, suspension sleeve, any material, each

∗ L5675　Addition to lower extremity, below knee, suspension sleeve, heavy duty, any material, each

∗ L5676　Addition to lower extremity, below knee, knee joints, single axis, pair

∗ L5677　Addition to lower extremity, below knee, knee joints, polycentric, pair

∗ L5678　Addition to lower extremity, below knee, joint covers, pair

▶∗ L5679　Addition to lower extremity, below knee/above knee, custom fabricated from existing mold or prefabricated, socket insert, silicone gel, elastomeric or equal, not for use with locking mechanism

∗ L5680　Addition to lower extremity, below knee, thigh lacer, non-molded

▶∗ L5681　Addition to lower extremity, below knee/above knee, custom fabricated socket insert for congenital or atypical traumatic amputee, silicone gel, elastomeric or equal, for use with or without locking mechanism, initial only (for other than initial, use code L5673 or L5679)

∗ L5682　Addition to lower extremity, below knee, thigh lacer, gluteal/ischial, molded

▶∗ L5683　Addition to lower extremity, below knee/above knee, custom fabricated socket insert for other than congenital or atypical traumatic amputee, silicone gel, elastomeric or equal, for use with or without locking mechanism, initial only (for other than initial, use code L5673 or L5679)

∗ L5684　Addition to lower extremity, below knee, fork strap

∗ L5686　Addition to lower extremity, below knee, back check (extension control)

∗ L5688　Addition to lower extremity, below knee, waist belt, webbing

∗ L5690　Addition to lower extremity, below knee, waist belt, padded and lined

∗ L5692　Addition to lower extremity, above knee, pelvic control belt, light

∗ L5694　Addition to lower extremity, above knee, pelvic control belt, padded and lined

∗ L5695　Addition to lower extremity, above knee, pelvic control, sleeve suspension, neoprene or equal, each

* L5696 Addition to lower extremity, above knee or knee disarticulation, pelvic joint
* L5697 Addition to lower extremity, above knee or knee disarticulation, pelvic band
* L5698 Addition to lower extremity, above knee or knee disarticulation, Silesian bandage
* L5699 All lower extremity prostheses, shoulder harness

Additions to Feet-Ankle Units

* L5700 Replacement, socket, below knee, molded to patient model
* L5701 Replacement, socket, above knee-knee disarticulation, including attachment plate, molded to patient model
* L5702 Replacement, socket, hip disarticulation, including hip joint, molded to patient model
* L5704 Custom shaped protective cover, below knee
* L5705 Custom shaped protective cover, above knee
* L5706 Custom shaped protective cover, knee disarticulation
* L5707 Custom shaped protective cover, hip disarticulation

Additions to Exoskeletal–Knee-Shin System

* L5710 Addition, exoskeletal knee-shin system, single axis, manual lock
* L5711 Addition, exoskeletal knee-shin system, single axis, manual lock, ultralight material
* L5712 Addition, exoskeletal knee-shin system, single axis, friction swing and stance phase control (safety knee)
* L5714 Addition, exoskeletal knee-shin system, single axis, variable friction swing phase control
* L5716 Addition, exoskeletal knee-shin system, polycentric, mechanical stance phase lock
* L5718 Addition, exoskeletal knee-shin system, polycentric, friction swing and stance phase control
* L5722 Addition, exoskeletal knee-shin system, single axis, pneumatic swing, friction stance phase control
* L5724 Addition, exoskeletal knee-shin system, single axis, fluid swing phase control
* L5726 Addition, exoskeletal knee-shin system, single axis, external joints, fluid swing phase control
* L5728 Addition, exoskeletal knee-shin system, single axis, fluid swing and stance phase control

* L5780 Addition, exoskeletal knee-shin system, single axis, pneumatic/hydra pneumatic swing phase control
* L5781 Addition to lower limb prosthesis, vacuum pump, residual limb volume management and moisture evacuation system
* L5782 Addition to lower limb prosthesis, vacuum pump, residual limb volume management and moisture evacuation system, heavy duty

Component Modification

* L5785 Addition, exoskeletal system, below knee, ultra-light material (titanium, carbon fiber or equal)
* L5790 Addition, exoskeletal system, above knee, ultra-light material (titanium, carbon fiber or equal)
* L5795 Addition, exoskeletal system, hip disarticulation, ultra-light material (titanium, carbon fiber or equal)

Endoskeletal

* L5810 Addition, endoskeletal knee-shin system, single axis, manual lock
* L5811 Addition, endoskeletal knee-shin system, single axis, manual lock, ultra light material
* L5812 Addition, endoskeletal knee-shin system, single axis, friction swing and stance phase control (safety knee)
* L5814 Addition, endoskeletal knee-shin system, polycentric, hydraulic swing phase control, mechanical stance phase lock
* L5816 Addition, endoskeletal knee-shin system, polycentric, mechanical stance phase lock
* L5818 Addition, endoskeletal knee-shin system, polycentric, friction swing, and stance phase control
* L5822 Addition, endoskeletal knee-shin system, single axis, pneumatic swing, friction stance phase control
* L5824 Addition, endoskeletal knee-shin system, single axis, fluid swing phase control
* L5826 Addition, endoskeletal knee-shin system, single axis, hydraulic swing phase control, with miniature high activity frame
* L5828 Addition, endoskeletal knee-shin system, single axis, fluid swing and stance phase control
* L5830 Addition, endoskeletal knee-shin system, single axis, pneumatic/ swing phase control

＊ L5840 Addition, endoskeletal knee-shin system, four-bar linkage or multiaxial, pneumatic swing phase control

＊ L5845 Addition, endoskeletal, knee-shin system, stance flexion feature, adjustable

＊ L5846 Addition, endoskeletal, knee-shin system, microprocessor control feature, swing phase only

＊ L5847 Addition, endoskeletal knee-shin system, microprocessor control feature, stance phase

➡ ＊ L5848 Addition to endoskeletal, knee-shin system, hydraulic stance extension, dampening feature, with or without adjustability

＊ L5850 Addition, endoskeletal system, above knee or hip disarticulation, knee extension assist

＊ L5855 Addition, endoskeletal system, hip disarticulation, mechanical hip extension assist

＊ L5910 Addition, endoskeletal system, below knee, alignable system

＊ L5920 Addition, endoskeletal system, above knee or hip disarticulation, alignable system

＊ L5925 Addition, endoskeletal system, above knee, knee disarticulation or hip disarticulation, manual lock

＊ L5930 Addition, endoskeletal system, high activity knee control frame

＊ L5940 Addition, endoskeletal system, below knee, ultra light material (titanium, carbon fiber or equal)

＊ L5950 Addition, endoskeletal system, above knee, ultra light material (titanium, carbon fiber or equal)

＊ L5960 Addition, endoskeletal system, hip disarticulation, ultra light material (titanium, carbon fiber or equal)

＊ L5962 Addition, endoskeletal system, below knee, flexible protective outer surface covering system

＊ L5964 Addition, endoskeletal system, above knee, flexible protective outer surface covering system

＊ L5966 Addition, endoskeletal system, hip disarticulation, flexible protective outer surface covering system

＊ L5968 Addition to lower limb prosthesis, multiaxial ankle with swing phase active dorsiflexion feature

＊ L5970 All lower extremity prostheses, foot, external heel, SACH foot

＊ L5972 All lower extremity prostheses, flexible heel foot (Safe, Sten, Bock Dynamic or equal)

＊ L5974 All lower extremity prostheses, foot, single axis ankle/foot

＊ L5975 All lower extremity prostheses, combination single axis ankle and flexible heel foot

＊ L5976 All lower extremity prostheses, energy storing foot (Seattle Carbon Copy II or equal)

＊ L5978 All lower extremity prostheses, foot, multiaxial ankle/foot

＊ L5979 All lower extremity prostheses, multiaxial ankle, dynamic response foot, one piece system

＊ L5980 All lower extremity prostheses, flex foot system

＊ L5981 All lower extremity prostheses, flex-walk system or equal

＊ L5982 All exoskeletal lower extremity prostheses, axial rotation unit

➡ ＊ L5984 All endoskeletal lower extremity prostheses, axial rotation unit, with or without adjustability

＊ L5985 All endoskeletal lower extremity prostheses, dynamic prosthetic pylon

＊ L5986 All lower extremity prostheses, multiaxial rotation unit (MCP or equal)

＊ L5987 All lower extremity prostheses, shank foot system with vertical loading pylon

＊ L5988 Addition to lower limb prosthesis, vertical shock reducing pylon feature

＊ L5989 Addition to lower extremity prosthesis, endoskeletal system, pylon with integrated electronic force sensors

＊ L5990 Addition to lower extremity prosthesis, user adjustable heel height

＊ L5995 Addition to lower extremity prosthesis, heavy duty feature (for patient weight > 300 lbs)

＊ L5999 Lower extremity prosthesis, not otherwise specified

Upper Limb

NOTE: The procedures in L6000-L6599 are considered as base or basic procedures and may be modified by listing procedures from the additions sections. The base procedures include only standard friction wrist and control cable system unless otherwise specified.

Partial Hand

＊ L6000 Partial hand, Robin-Aids, thumb remaining (or equal)

＊ L6010 Partial hand, Robin-Aids, little and/or ring finger remaining (or equal)

＊ L6020 Partial hand, Robin-Aids, no finger remaining (or equal)

* L6025 Transcarpal/metacarpal or partial hand disarticulation prosthesis, external power, self-suspended, inner socket with removable forearm section, electrodes and cables, two batteries, charger, myoelectric control of terminal device

Wrist Disarticulation

* L6050 Wrist disarticulation, molded socket, flexible elbow hinges, triceps pad
* L6055 Wrist disarticulation, molded socket with expandable interface, flexible elbow hinges, triceps pad

Below Elbow

* L6100 Below elbow, molded socket, flexible elbow hinge, triceps pad
* L6110 Below elbow, molded socket, (Muenster or Northwestern suspension types)
* L6120 Below elbow, molded double wall split socket, step-up hinges, half cuff
* L6130 Below elbow, molded double wall split socket, stump activated locking hinge, half cuff

Elbow Disarticulation

* L6200 Elbow disarticulation, molded socket, outside locking hinge, forearm
* L6205 Elbow disarticulation, molded socket with expandable interface, outside locking hinges, forearm

Above Elbow

* L6250 Above elbow, molded double wall socket, internal locking elbow, forearm

Shoulder Disarticulation

* L6300 Shoulder disarticulation, molded socket, shoulder bulkhead, humeral section, internal locking elbow, forearm
* L6310 Shoulder disarticulation, passive restoration (complete prosthesis)
* L6320 Shoulder disarticulation, passive restoration (shoulder cap only)

Interscapular Thoracic

* L6350 Interscapular thoracic, molded socket, shoulder bulkhead, humeral section, internal locking elbow, forearm

* L6360 Interscapular thoracic, passive restoration (complete prosthesis)
* L6370 Interscapular thoracic, passive restoration (shoulder cap only)

Immediate and Early Postsurgical Procedures

* L6380 Immediate postsurgical or early fitting, application of initial rigid dressing, including fitting alignment and suspension of components, and one cast change, wrist disarticulation or below elbow
* L6382 Immediate postsurgical or early fitting, application of initial rigid dressing including fitting alignment and suspension of components, and one cast change, elbow disarticulation or above elbow
* L6384 Immediate postsurgical or early fitting, application of initial rigid dressing including fitting alignment and suspension of components, and one cast change, shoulder disarticulation or interscapular thoracic
* L6386 Immediate postsurgical or early fitting, each additional cast change and re-alignment
* L6388 Immediate postsurgical or early fitting, application of rigid dressing only

Endoskeletal: Below Elbow

* L6400 Below elbow, molded socket, endoskeletal system, including soft prosthetic tissue shaping

Endoskeletal: Elbow Disarticulation

* L6450 Elbow disarticulation, molded socket, endoskeletal system, including soft prosthetic tissue shaping

Endoskeletal: Above Elbow

* L6500 Above elbow, molded socket, endoskeletal system, including soft prosthetic tissue shaping

Endoskeletal: Shoulder Disarticulation

* L6550 Shoulder disarticulation, molded socket, endoskeletal system, including soft prosthetic tissue shaping

Endoskeletal: Interscapular Thoracic

* L6570 Interscapular thoracic, molded socket, endoskeletal system, including soft prosthetic tissue shaping

* L6580 Preparatory, wrist disarticulation or below elbow, single wall plastic socket, friction wrist, flexible elbow hinges, figure of eight harness, humeral cuff, Bowden cable control, USMC or equal pylon, no cover, molded to patient model

* L6582 Preparatory, wrist disarticulation or below elbow, single wall socket, friction wrist, flexible elbow hinges, figure of eight harness, humeral cuff, Bowden cable control, USMC or equal pylon, no cover, direct formed

* L6584 Preparatory, elbow disarticulation or above elbow, single wall plastic socket, friction wrist, locking elbow, figure of eight harness, fair lead cable control, USMC or equal pylon, no cover, molded to patient model

* L6586 Preparatory, elbow disarticulation or above elbow, single wall socket, friction wrist, locking elbow, figure of eight harness, fair lead cable control, USMC or equal pylon, no cover, direct formed

* L6588 Preparatory, shoulder disarticulation or interscapular thoracic, single wall plastic socket, shoulder joint, locking elbow, friction wrist, chest strap, fair lead cable control, USMC or equal pylon, no cover, molded to patient model

* L6590 Preparatory, shoulder disarticulation or interscapular thoracic, single wall socket, shoulder joint, locking elbow, friction wrist, chest strap, fair lead cable control, USMC or equal pylon, no cover, direct formed

Additions to Upper Limb

NOTE: The following procedures/modifications/components may be added to other base procedures. The items in this section should reflect the additional complexity of each modification procedure, in addition to base procedure, at the time of the original order.

* L6600 Upper extremity addition, polycentric hinge, pair

* L6605 Upper extremity addition, single pivot hinge, pair

* L6610 Upper extremity addition, flexible metal hinge, pair

* L6615 Upper extremity addition, disconnect locking wrist unit

* L6616 Upper extremity addition, additional disconnect insert for locking wrist unit, each

➡ * L6620 Upper extremity addition, flexion-friction wrist unit, with or without friction

* L6623 Upper extremity addition, spring assisted rotational wrist unit with latch release

* L6625 Upper extremity addition, rotation wrist unit with cable lock

* L6628 Upper extremity addition, quick disconnect hook adapter, Otto Bock or equal

* L6629 Upper extremity addition, quick disconnect lamination collar with coupling piece, Otto Bock or equal

* L6630 Upper extremity addition, stainless steel, any wrist

* L6632 Upper extremity addition, latex suspension sleeve, each

* L6635 Upper extremity addition, lift assist for elbow

* L6637 Upper extremity addition, nudge control elbow lock

* L6638 Upper extremity addition to prosthesis, electric locking feature, only for use with manually powered elbow

* L6640 Upper extremity additions, shoulder abduction joint, pair

* L6641 Upper extremity addition, excursion amplifier, pulley type

* L6642 Upper extremity addition, excursion amplifier, lever type

* L6645 Upper extremity addition, shoulder flexion-abduction joint, each

* L6646 Upper extremity addition, shoulder joint, multipositional locking, flexion, adjustable abduction friction control, for use with body powered or external powered system

* L6647 Upper extremity addition, shoulder lock mechanism, body powered actuator

* L6648 Upper extremity addition, shoulder lock mechanism, external powered actuator

* L6650 Upper extremity addition, shoulder universal joint, each

* L6655 Upper extremity addition, standard control cable, extra

* L6660 Upper extremity addition, heavy duty control cable

* L6665 Upper extremity addition, Teflon, or equal, cable lining

* L6670 Upper extremity addition, hook to hand, cable adapter

* L6672 Upper extremity addition, harness, chest or shoulder, saddle type

➡ * L6675 Upper extremity addition, harness, (e.g. figure of eight type), single cable design

➡ * L6676 Upper extremity addition, harness, (e.g. figure of eight type), dual cable design

* L6680 Upper extremity addition, test socket, wrist disarticulation or below elbow

* L6682 Upper extremity addition, test socket, elbow disarticulation or above elbow

* L6684 Upper extremity addition, test socket, shoulder disarticulation or interscapular thoracic

* L6686 Upper extremity addition, suction socket

* L6687 Upper extremity addition, frame type socket, below elbow or wrist disarticulation

* L6688 Upper extremity addition, frame type socket, above elbow or elbow disarticulation

* L6689 Upper extremity addition, frame type socket, shoulder disarticulation

* L6690 Upper extremity addition, frame type socket, interscapular-thoracic

* L6691 Upper extremity addition, removable insert, each

* L6692 Upper extremity addition, silicone gel insert or equal, each

* L6693 Upper extremity addition, locking elbow, forearm counterbalance

Terminal Devices

Hooks

⊛ L6700 Terminal device, hook, Dorrance, or equal, model #3
MCM 2133

⊛ L6705 Terminal device, hook, Dorrance, or equal, model #5
MCM 2133

⊛ L6710 Terminal device, hook, Dorrance, or equal, model #5X
MCM 2133

⊛ L6715 Terminal device, hook, Dorrance, or equal, model #5XA
MCM 2133

⊛ L6720 Terminal device, hook, Dorrance, or equal, model #6
MCM 2133

⊛ L6725 Terminal device, hook, Dorrance, or equal, model #7
MCM 2133

⊛ L6730 Terminal device, hook, Dorrance, or equal, model #7LO
MCM 2133

⊛ L6735 Terminal device, hook, Dorrance, or equal, model #8
MCM 2133

⊛ L6740 Terminal device, hook, Dorrance, or equal, model #8X
MCM 2133

⊛ L6745 Terminal device, hook, Dorrance, or equal, model #88X
MCM 2133

⊛ L6750 Terminal device, hook, Dorrance, or equal, model #10P
MCM 2133

⊛ L6755 Terminal device, hook, Dorrance, or equal, model #10X
MCM 2133

⊛ L6765 Terminal device, hook, Dorrance, or equal, model #12P
MCM 2133

⊛ L6770 Terminal device, hook, Dorrance, or equal, model #99X
MCM 2133

⊛ L6775 Terminal device, hook, Dorrance, or equal, model #555
MCM 2133

⊛ L6780 Terminal device, hook, Dorrance, or equal, model #SS555
MCM 2133

⊛ L6790 Terminal device, hook, Accu hook, or equal
MCM 2133

⊛ L6795 Terminal device, hook, 2 load, or equal
MCM 2133

⊛ L6800 Terminal device, hook, APRL VC, or equal
MCM 2133

⊛ L6805 Terminal device, modifier wrist flexion unit
MCM 2133

⊛ L6806 Terminal device, hook, TRS Grip, Grip III, VC, or equal
MCM 2133

⊛ L6807 Terminal device, hook, Grip I, Grip II, VC, or equal
MCM 2133

⊛ L6808 Terminal device, hook, TRS Adept, infant or child, VC, or equal
MCM 2133

⊛ L6809 Terminal device, hook, TRS Super Sport, passive
MCM 2133

⊛ L6810 Terminal device, pincher tool, Otto Bock or equal
MCM 2133

Hands

⊛ L6825 Terminal device, hand, Dorrance, VO
MCM 2133

⊛ L6830 Terminal device, hand, APRL, VC
MCM 2133

⊛ L6835 Terminal device, hand, Sierra, VO
MCM 2133

⊛ L6840 Terminal device, hand, Becker Imperial
MCM 2133

⊘ L6845 Terminal device, hand, Becker Lock
Grip
MCM 2133

⊘ L6850 Terminal device, hand, Becker Plylite
MCM 2133

⊘ L6855 Terminal device, hand, Robin-Aids, VO
MCM 2133

⊘ L6860 Terminal device, hand, Robin-Aids, VO
soft
MCM 2133

⊘ L6865 Terminal device, hand, passive hand
MCM 2133

⊘ L6867 Terminal device, hand, Detroit infant
hand (mechanical)
MCM 2133

⊘ L6868 Terminal device, hand, passive infant
hand, (Steeper, Hosmer or equal)
MCM 2133

⊘ L6870 Terminal device, hand, child MITT
MCM 2133

⊘ L6872 Terminal device, hand, NYU child hand
MCM 2133

⊘ L6873 Terminal device, hand, mechanical infant hand, Steeper or equal
MCM 2133

⊘ L6875 Terminal device, hand, Bock, VC
MCM 2133

⊘ L6880 Terminal device, hand, Bock, VO
MCM 2133

✳ L6881 Automatic grasp feature, addition to
upper limb prosthetic terminal device

⊘ L6882 Microprocessor control feature, addition
to upper limb prosthetic terminal device
MCM 2133

Gloves for Above Hands

✳ L6890 Terminal device, glove for above hands,
production glove

✳ L6895 Terminal device, glove for above hands,
custom glove

Hand Restoration

✳ L6900 Hand restoration (casts, shading and
measurements included), partial hand,
with glove, thumb or one finger remaining

✳ L6905 Hand restoration (casts, shading and
measurements included), partial hand,
with glove, multiple fingers remaining

✳ L6910 Hand restoration (casts, shading and
measurements included), partial hand,
with glove, no fingers remaining

✳ L6915 Hand restoration (shading, and measurements included), replacement glove
for above

External Power

Base Devices

✳ L6920 Wrist disarticulation, external power,
self-suspended inner socket, removable
forearm shell, Otto Bock or equal,
switch, cables, two batteries and one
charger, switch control of terminal device

✳ L6925 Wrist disarticulation, external power,
self-suspended inner socket, removable
forearm shell, Otto Bock or equal, electrodes, cables, two batteries and one
charger, myoelectronic control of terminal device

✳ L6930 Below elbow, external power, self-suspended inner socket, removable forearm shell, Otto Bock or equal, switch,
cables, two batteries and one charger,
switch control of terminal device

✳ L6935 Below elbow, external power, self-suspended inner socket, removable forearm shell, Otto Bock or equal, electrodes, cables, two batteries and one
charger, myoelectronic control of terminal device

✳ L6940 Elbow disarticulation, external power,
molded inner socket, removable humeral shell, outside locking hinges,
forearm, Otto Bock or equal, switch, cables, two batteries and one charger,
switch control of terminal device

✳ L6945 Elbow disarticulation, external power,
molded inner socket, removable humeral shell, outside locking hinges,
forearm, Otto Bock or equal, electrodes,
cables, two batteries and one charger,
myoelectronic control of terminal device

✳ L6950 Above elbow, external power, molded
inner socket, removable humeral shell,
internal locking elbow, forearm, Otto
Bock or equal, switch, cables, two batteries and one charger, switch control
of terminal device

✳ L6955 Above elbow, external power, molded
inner socket, removable humeral shell,
internal locking elbow, forearm, Otto
Bock or equal, electrodes, cables, two
batteries and one charger, myoelectronic control of terminal device

✳ L6960 Shoulder disarticulation, external
power, molded inner socket, removable
shoulder shell, shoulder bulkhead, humeral section, mechanical elbow, forearm, Otto Bock or equal, switch, cables,
two batteries and one charger, switch
control of terminal device

* L6965 Shoulder disarticulation, external power, molded inner socket, removable shoulder shell, shoulder bulkhead, humeral section, mechanical elbow, forearm, Otto Bock or equal, electrodes, cables, two batteries and one charger, myoelectronic control of terminal device
* L6970 Interscapular-thoracic, external power, molded inner socket, removable shoulder shell, shoulder bulkhead, humeral section, mechanical elbow, forearm, Otto Bock or equal, switch, cables, two batteries and one charger, switch control of terminal device
* L6975 Interscapular-thoracic, external power, molded inner socket, removable shoulder shell, shoulder bulkhead, humeral section, mechanical elbow, forearm, Otto Bock or equal, electrodes, cables, two batteries and one charger, myoelectronic control of terminal device

Terminal Devices

* L7010 Electronic hand, Otto Bock, Steeper or equal, switch controlled
* L7015 Electronic hand, System Teknik, Variety Village or equal, switch controlled
* L7020 Electronic greifer, Otto Bock or equal, switch controlled
* L7025 Electronic hand, Otto Bock or equal, myoelectronically controlled
* L7030 Electronic hand, System Teknik, Variety Village or equal, myoelectronically controlled
* L7035 Electronic greifer, Otto Bock or equal, myoelectronically controlled
* L7040 Prehensile actuator, Hosmer or equal, switch controlled
* L7045 Electronic hook, child, Michigan or equal, switch controlled

Elbow

* L7170 Electronic elbow, Hosmer or equal, switch controlled
* L7180 Electronic elbow, Boston, Utah or equal, myoelectronically controlled
* L7185 Electronic elbow, adolescent, Variety Village or equal, switch controlled
* L7186 Electronic elbow, child, Variety Village or equal, switch controlled
* L7190 Electronic elbow, adolescent, Variety Village or equal, myoelectronically controlled
* L7191 Electronic elbow, child, Variety Village or equal, myoelectronically controlled
* L7260 Electronic wrist rotator, Otto Bock or equal
* L7261 Electronic wrist rotator, for Utah arm

* L7266 Servo control, Steeper or equal
* L7272 Analogue control, UNB or equal
* L7274 Proportional control, 6-12 volt, Liberty, Utah or equal

Battery Components

* L7360 Six-volt battery, Otto Bock or equal, each
* L7362 Battery charger, 6 volt, Otto Bock or equal
* L7364 Twelve volt battery, Utah or equal, each
* L7366 Battery charger, 12 volt, Utah or equal
* L7367 Lithium ion battery, replacement
* L7368 Lithium ion battery charger
* L7499 Upper extremity prosthesis, not otherwise specified

Repairs

☺ L7500 Repair of prosthetic device, hourly rate (excludes V5335 repair of oral or laryngeal prosthesis or artificial larynx) MCM 2100.4, MCM 2130D, MCM 2133
☺ L7510 Repair of prosthetic device, repair or replace minor parts MCM 2100.4, MCM 2130D, MCM 2133
* L7520 Repair prosthetic device, labor component, per 15 minutes

General

* L7900 Male vacuum erection system

Breast Prostheses

☺ L8000 Breast prosthesis, mastectomy bra MCM 2130A
☺ L8001 Breast prosthesis, mastectomy bra, with integrated breast prosthesis form, unilateral MCM 2130A
☺ L8002 Breast prosthesis, mastectomy bra, with integrated breast prosthesis form, bilateral MCM 2130A
☺ L8010 Breast prosthesis, mastectomy sleeve MCM 2130A
☺ L8015 External breast prosthesis garment, with mastectomy form, post mastectomy MCM 2130
☺ L8020 Breast prosthesis, mastectomy form MCM 2130A
☺ L8030 Breast prosthesis, silicone or equal MCM 2130A
☺ L8035 Custom breast prosthesis, post mastectomy, molded to patient mode lMCM 2130

* L8039   Breast prosthesis, not otherwise specified

Nasal, Orbital, Auricular Prosthesis

* L8040   Nasal prosthesis, provided by a non-physician

* L8041   Midfacial prosthesis, provided by a non-physician

* L8042   Orbital prosthesis, provided by a non-physician

* L8043   Upper facial prosthesis, provided by a non-physician

* L8044   Hemi-facial prosthesis, provided by a non-physician

* L8045   Auricular prosthesis, provided by a non-physician

* L8046   Partial facial prosthesis, provided by a non-physician

* L8047   Nasal septal prosthesis, provided by a non-physician

* L8048   Unspecified maxillofacial prosthesis, by report, provided by a non-physician

* L8049   Repair or modification of maxillofacial prosthesis, labor component, 15-minute increments, provided by a non-physician

Elastic Supports

◆ L8100   Gradient compression stocking, below knee, 18-30 mm Hg, each
MCM 2133, CIM 60-9

➡ ◎ L8110   Gradient compression stocking, below knee, 30-40 mm Hg, each
MCM 2133, CIM 60-9

➡ ◎ L8120   Gradient compression stocking, below knee, 40-50 mm Hg, each
MCM 2133, CIM 60-9

◆ L8130   Gradient compression stocking, thigh length, 18-30 mm Hg, each
MCM 2133, CIM 60-9

◆ L8140   Gradient compression stocking, thigh length, 30-40 mm Hg, each
MCM 2133, CIM 60-9

◆ L8150   Gradient compression stocking, thigh length, 40-50 mm Hg, each
MCM 2133, CIM 60-9

◆ L8160   Gradient compression stocking, full length/chap style, 18-30 mm Hg, each
MCM 2133, CIM 60-9

◆ L8170   Gradient compression stocking, full length/chap style, 30-40 mm Hg, each
MCM 2133, CIM 60-9

◆ L8180   Gradient compression stocking, full length/chap style, 40-50 mm Hg, each
MCM 2133, CIM 60-9

◆ L8190   Gradient compression stocking, waist length, 18-30 mm Hg, each
MCM 2133, CIM 60-9

◆ L8195   Gradient compression stocking, waist length, 30-40 mm Hg, each
MCM 2133, CIM 60-9

◆ L8200   Gradient compression stocking, waist length, 40-50 mm Hg, each
MCM 2133, CIM 60-9

◆ L8210   Gradient compression stocking, custom made
MCM 2133, CIM 60-9

◆ L8220   Gradient compression stocking, lymphedema
MCM 2133, CIM 60-9

◆ L8230   Gradient compression stocking, garter belt
MCM 2133, CIM 60-9

* L8239   Gradient compression stocking, not otherwise specified

Trusses

◎ L8300   Truss, single with standard pad
MCM 2133, CIM 70-1, CIM 70-2

◎ L8310   Truss, double with standard pads
MCM 2133, CIM 70-1, CIM 70-2

◎ L8320   Truss, addition to standard pad, water pad
MCM 2133, CIM 70-1, CIM 70-2

◎ L8330   Truss, addition to standard pad, scrotal pad
MCM 2133, CIM 70-1, CIM 70-2

Prosthetic Socks

◎ L8400   Prosthetic sheath, below knee, each
MCM 2133

◎ L8410   Prosthetic sheath, above knee, each
MCM 2133

◎ L8415   Prosthetic sheath, upper limb, each
MCM 2133

* L8417   Prosthetic sheath/sock, including a gel cushion layer, below knee or above knee, each

◎ L8420   Prosthetic sock, multiple ply, below knee, each
MCM 2133

◎ L8430   Prosthetic sock, multiple ply, above knee, each
MCM 2133

◎ L8435   Prosthetic sock, multiple ply, upper limb, each
MCM 2133

◎ L8440   Prosthetic shrinker, below knee, each
MCM 2133

◎ L8460   Prosthetic shrinker, above knee, each
MCM 2133

◎ L8465   Prosthetic shrinker, upper limb, each
MCM 2133

◎ L8470   Prosthetic sock, single ply, fitting, below knee, each
MCM 2133

⊛ L8480   Prosthetic sock, single ply, fitting, above knee, each
MCM 2133
⊛ L8485   Prosthetic sock, single ply, fitting, upper limb, each
MCM 2133
✻ L8490   Addition to prosthetic sheath/sock, air seal suction retention system
✻ L8499   Unlisted procedure for miscellaneous prosthetic services

Prosthetic Implants

Integumentary System

⊛ L8500   Artificial larynx, any type
MCM 2130, CIM 65-5
⊛ L8501   Tracheostomy speaking valve
CIM 65-16
✻ L8505   Artificial larynx replacement battery/accessory, any type
✻ L8507   Tracheo-esophageal voice prosthesis, patient inserted, any type, each
✻ L8509   Tracheo-esophageal voice prosthesis, inserted by licensed health car provider, any type
⊛ L8510   Voice amplifier
CIM 65-5
▶✻ L8511   Insert for indwelling tracheoesophageal prosthesis, with or without valve, replacement only, each
▶✻ L8512   Gelatin capsules or equivalent, for use with tracheoesophageal voice prosthesis, replacement only, per 10
▶✻ L8513   Cleaning device used with tracheoesophageal voice prosthesis, pipet, brush, or equal, replacement only, each
▶✻ L8514   Tracheoesophageal puncture dilator, replacement only, each
⊛ L8600   Implantable breast prosthesis, silicone or equal
MCM 2130, CIM 35-47

Urinary System

⊛ L8603   Injectable bulking agent, collagen implant, urinary tract, per 2.5 cc syringe, includes shipping and necessary supplies
CIM 65-9
⊛ L8606   Injectable bulking agent, synthetic implant, urinary tract, 1 cc syringe, includes shipping and necessary supplies
CIM 65.9

Head (Skull, Facial Bones, and Temporomandibular Joint)

⊛ L8610   Ocular implant
MCM 2130

⊛ L8612   Aqueous shunt
MCM 2130, Cross Reference Q0074
⊛ L8613   Ossicula implant
MCM 2130
⊛ L8614   Cochlear device/system
MCM 2130, CIM 65-14
⊛ L8619   Cochlear implant external speech processor, replacement
CIM 65-14

Upper Extremity

⊛ L8630   Metacarpophalangeal joint implant
MCM 2130
▶⊛ L8631   Metacarpal phalangeal joint replacement, two or more pieces, metal (e.g., stainless steel or cobalt chrome), ceramic-like material (e.g., pyrocarbon), for surgical implantation (all sizes, includes entire system)
MCM 2130

Lower Extremity (Joint: Knee, Ankle, Toe)

⊛ L8641   Metatarsal joint implant
MCM 2130
⊛ L8642   Hallux implant
MCM 2130, Cross Reference Q0073

Miscellaneous Muscular-Skeletal

➡⊛ L8658   Interphalangeal joint spacer, silicone or equal, each
MCM 2130
▶⊛ L8659   Interphalangeal finger joint replacement, 2 or more pieces, metal (e.g., stainless steel or cobalt chrome), ceramic-like material (e.g., pyrocarbon) for surgical implantation, any size
MCM 2130

Cardiovascular System

⊛ L8670   Vascular graft material, synthetic, implant
MCM 2130

Genital

✻ L8699   Prosthetic implant, not otherwise specified
✻ L9900   Orthotic and prosthetic supply, accessory, and/or service component of another HCPCS L code

MEDICAL SERVICES (M0000-M0399)

Other Medical Services

✪ M0064   Brief office visit for the sole purpose of monitoring or changing drug prescriptions used in the treatment of mental psychoneurotic and personality disorders
MCM 2476.3

◆ M0075   Cellular therapy
CIM 35-5

◆ M0076   Prolotherapy
CIM 35-13

⇒◆ M0100   Intragastric hypothermia using gastric freezing
CIM 35-65

◆ M0300   IV chelation therapy (chemical endarterectomy)
CIM 35-64

⇒◆ M0301   Fabric wrapping of abdominal aneurysm
CIM 35-34

M0302   Deleted 01/01/02, Cross Reference CPT

PATHOLOGY AND LABORATORY TESTS (P0000-P2999)

Chemistry and Toxicology Tests

✪ P2028   Cephalin flocculation, blood
CIM 50-34

✪ P2029   Congo red, blood
CIM 50-34

◆ P2031   Hair analysis (excluding arsenic)
CIM 50-24

✪ P2033   Thymol turbidity, blood
CIM 50-34

✪ P2038   Mucoprotein, blood (seromucoid) (medical necessity procedure)
CIM 50-34

Pathology Screening Tests

✪ P3000   Screening Papanicolaou smear, cervical or vaginal, up to three smears, by technician under physician supervision
CIM 50-20, Laboratory Certification: cytology

✪ P3001   Screening Papanicolaou smear, cervical or vaginal, up to three smears, requiring interpretation by physician
CIM 50-20, Laboratory Certification: cytology

Microbiology Tests

◆ P7001   Culture, bacterial, urine; quantitative, sensitivity study
Cross Reference CPT, Laboratory Certification: bacteriology

Miscellaneous Pathology

✪ P9010   Blood (whole), for transfusion, per unit
MCM 2455A

✪ P9011   Blood (split unit), specify amount
MCM 2455A

✪ P9012   Cryoprecipitate, each unit
MCM 2455B

✪ P9016   Red blood cells, leukocytes reduced, each unit
MCM 2455B

⇒✪ P9017   Fresh frozen plasma (single donor), frozen within 8 hours of collection, each unit
MCM 2455B

P9018   Deleted 01/01/01

✪ P9019   Platelets, each unit
MCM 2455B

✪ P9020   Platelet rich plasma, each unit
MCM 2455B

✪ P9021   Red blood cells, each unit
MCM 2455A

✪ P9022   Red blood cells, washed, each unit
MCM 2455A

✪ P9023   Plasma, pooled multiple donor, solvent/detergent treated, frozen, each unit
MCM 2455B

✪ P9031   Platelets, leukocytes reduced, each unit
MCM 2455

✪ P9032   Platelets, irradiated, each unit
MCM 2455

✪ P9033   Platelets, leukocytes reduced, irradiated, each unit
MCM 2455

✪ P9034   Platelets, pheresis, each unit
MCM 2455

✪ P9035   Platelets, pheresis, leukocytes reduced, each unit
MCM 2455

✪ P9036   Platelets, pheresis, irradiated, each unit
MCM 2455

✪ P9037   Platelets, pheresis, leukocytes reduced, irradiated, each unit
MCM 2455

✪ P9038   Red blood cells, irradiated, each unit
MCM 2455

✪ P9039   Red blood cells, deglycerolized, each unit
MCM 2455

⊕ P9040 Red blood cells, leukocytes reduced, irradiated, each unit
MCM 2455

∗ P9041 Infusion, albumin (human), 5%, 50 ml

P9042 Deleted 01/01/02, Cross Reference
P9046

⊕ P9043 Infusion, plasma protein fraction (human), 5%, 50 ml
MCM 2455B

⊕ P9044 Plasma, cryoprecipitate reduced, each
unit
MCM 2455B

∗ P9045 Infusion, albumin (human), 5%, 250 ml

∗ P9046 Infusion, albumin (human), 25%, 20 ml

∗ P9047 Infusion, albumin (human), 25%, 50 ml

∗ P9048 Infusion, plasma protein fraction (human), 5%, 250 ml

∗ P9050 Granulocytes, pheresis, each unit

▶⊕ P9051 Whole blood or red blood cells, leukocytes reduced, CMV-negative, each unit
Medicare Statute 1833(t)

▶⊕ P9052 Platelets, HLA-matched leukocytes reduced, apheresis/pheresis, each unit
Medicare Statute 1833(t)

▶⊕ P9053 Platelets, pheresis, leukocytes reduced,
CMV-negative, irradiated, each unit
Medicare Statute 1833(t)

▶⊕ P9054 Whole blood or red blood cells, leukocytes reduced, frozen, deglycerol,
washed, each unit
Medicare Statute 1833(t)

▶⊕ P9055 Platelets, leukocytes reduced, CMV-
negative, apheresis/pheresis, each unit
Medicare Statute 1833(t)

▶⊕ P9056 Whole blood, leukocytes reduced, irradiated, each unit
Medicare Statute 1833(t)

▶⊕ P9057 Red blood cells, frozen/deglycerolized/
washed, leukocytes reduced, irradiated,
each unit
Medicare Statute 1833(t)

▶⊕ P9058 Red blood cells, leukocytes reduced,
CMV-negative, irradiated, each unit
Medicare Statute 1833(t)

▶⊕ P9059 Fresh frozen plasma between 8-24
hours of collection, each unit
Medicare Statute 1833(t)

▶⊕ P9060 Fresh frozen plasma, donor retested,
each unit
Medicare Statute 1833(t)

⊕ P9603 Travel allowance one way in connection with medically necessary laboratory specimen collection drawn from
home bound or nursing home bound
patient; prorated miles actually traveled.
MCM 5114.1K

⊕ P9604 Travel allowance one way in connection with medically necessary laboratory specimen collection drawn from
home bound or nursing home bound
patient; prorated trip charge
MCM 5114.1K

⊕ P9612 Catheterization for collection of specimen, single patient, all places of service
MCM 5114.1D

⊕ P9615 Catheterization for collection of speci-
men(s) (multiple patients)
MCM 5114.1D

Q CODES: TEMPORARY CODES (Q0000-Q9999)

⊕ Q0035 Cardiokymography
CIM 50-50

⊕ Q0081 Infusion therapy, using other than
chemotherapy drugs, per visit
CIM 60-14

∗ Q0083 Chemotherapy administration by other
than infusion technique only (e.g., subcutaneous, intramuscular, push), per
visit

⊕ Q0084 Chemotherapy administration by infusion technique only, per visit
CIM 60-14

∗ Q0085 Chemotherapy administration by both
infusion technique and other tech-
nique(s) (e.g., subcutaneous, intramuscular, push), per visit

Q0086 Deleted 12/31/03

⊕ Q0091 Screening Papanicolaou smear; obtaining, preparing and conveyance of cervical or vaginal smear to laboratory
CIM 50-20

⊕ Q0092 Setup portable x-ray equipment
MCM 2070.4

∗ Q0111 Wet mounts, including preparations of
vaginal, cervical or skin specimens;
Laboratory Certification: bacteriology,
mycology, parasitology

∗ Q0112 All potassium hydroxide (KOH) preparations; Laboratory Certification: mycology

∗ Q0113 Pinworm examinations; Laboratory Certification: parasitology

∗ Q0114 Fern test; Laboratory certification: routine chemistry

∗ Q0115 Post-coital direct, qualitative examinations of vaginal or cervical mucus; Laboratory Certification: hematology

⊕ Q0136 Injection, epoetin alfa, (for non-ESRD
use), per 1000 units
MCM 2049

▶⊕ Q0137 Injection, darbepoetin alfa, 1 mcg (non-
ESRD use)
MCM 4273.1

◆ Q0144 Azithromycin dihydrate, oral, capsules/
powder, 1 gm

Q0160 Deleted 01/01/02, Cross Reference J7193

Q0161 Deleted 01/01/02, Cross Reference J7195

⊛ Q0163 Diphenhydramine HCl, 50 mg, oral, FDA-approved prescription antiemetic, for use as a complete therapeutic substitute for an IV antiemetic at time of chemotherapy treatment not to exceed a 48-hour dosage regimen
Medicare Statute 4557

⊛ Q0164 Prochlorperazine maleate, 5 mg, oral, FDA-approved prescription antiemetic, for use as a complete therapeutic substitute for an IV antiemetic at the time of chemotherapy treatment, not to exceed a 48-hour dosage regimen
Medicare Statute 4557

⊛ Q0165 Prochlorperazine maleate, 10 mg, oral, FDA-approved prescription antiemetic, for use as a complete therapeutic substitute for an IV antiemetic at the time of chemotherapy treatment, not to exceed a 48-hour dosage regimen
Medicare Statute 4557

⊛ Q0166 Granisetron HCl, 1 mg, oral, FDA-approved prescription antiemetic, for use as a complete therapeutic substitute for an IV antiemetic at the time of chemotherapy treatment, not to exceed a 24-hour dosage regimen
Medicare Statute 4557

⊛ Q0167 Dronabinol, 2.5 mg, oral, FDA-approved prescription antiemetic, for use as a complete therapeutic substitute for an IV antiemetic at the time of chemotherapy treatment, not to exceed a 48-hour dosage regimen
Medicare Statute 4557

⊛ Q0168 Dronabinol, 5 mg, oral, FDA-approved prescription antiemetic, for use as a complete therapeutic substitute for an IV antiemetic at the time of chemotherapy treatment, not to exceed a 48-hour dosage regimen
Medicare Statute 4557

⊛ Q0169 Promethazine HCl, 12.5 mg, oral, FDA-approved prescription antiemetic, for use as a complete therapeutic substitute for an IV antiemetic at the time of chemotherapy treatment, not to exceed a 48-hour dosage regimen
Medicare Statute 4557

⊛ Q0170 Promethazine HCl, 25 mg, oral, FDA-approved prescription antiemetic, for use as a complete therapeutic substitute for an IV antiemetic at the time of chemotherapy treatment, not to exceed a 48-hour dosage regimen
Medicare Statute 4557

⊛ Q0171 Chlorpromazine HCl, 10 mg, oral, FDA-approved prescription antiemetic, for use as a complete therapeutic substitute for an IV antiemetic at the time of chemotherapy treatment, not to exceed a 48-hour dosage regimen
Medicare Statute 4557

⊛ Q0172 Chlorpromazine HCl, 25 mg, oral, FDA-approved prescription antiemetic, for use as a complete therapeutic substitute for an IV antiemetic at the time of chemotherapy treatment, not to exceed a 48-hour dosage regimen
Medicare Statute 4557

⊛ Q0173 Trimethobenzamide HCl, 250 mg, oral, FDA-approved prescription antiemetic, for use as a complete therapeutic substitute for an IV antiemetic at the time of chemotherapy treatment, not to exceed a 48-hour dosage regimen
Medicare Statute 4557

⊛ Q0174 Thiethylperazine maleate, 10 mg, oral, FDA-approved prescription antiemetic, for use as a complete therapeutic substitute for an IV antiemetic at the time of chemotherapy treatment, not to exceed a 48-hour dosage regimen
Medicare Statute 4557

⊛ Q0175 Perphenazine, 4 mg, oral, FDA-approved prescription antiemetic, for use as a complete therapeutic substitute for an IV antiemetic at the time of chemotherapy treatment, not to exceed a 48-hour dosage regimen
Medicare Statute 4557

⊛ Q0176 Perphenazine, 8 mg, oral, FDA-approved prescription antiemetic, for use as a complete therapeutic substitute for an IV antiemetic at the time of chemotherapy treatment, not to exceed a 48-hour dosage regimen
Medicare Statute 4557

⊛ Q0177 Hydroxyzine pamoate, 25 mg, oral, FDA-approved prescription antiemetic, for use as a complete therapeutic substitute for an IV antiemetic at the time of chemotherapy treatment, not to exceed a 48-hour dosage regimen
Medicare Statute 4557

⊛ Q0178 Hydroxyzine pamoate, 50 mg, oral, FDA-approved prescription antiemetic, for use as a complete therapeutic substitute for an IV antiemetic at the time of chemotherapy treatment, not to exceed a 48-hour dosage regimen
Medicare Statute 4557

⊘ Q0179 Ondansetron HCl, 8 mg, oral, FDA-approved prescription antiemetic, for use as a complete therapeutic substitute for an IV antiemetic at the time of chemotherapy treatment, not to exceed a 48-hour dosage regimen
Medicare Statute 4557

⊘ Q0180 Dolasetron mesylate, 100 mg, oral, FDA-approved prescription antiemetic, for use as a complete therapeutic substitute for an IV antiemetic at the time of chemotherapy treatment, not to exceed a 24-hour dosage regimen
Medicare Statute 4557

⊘ Q0181 Unspecified oral dosage form, FDA-approved prescription antiemetic, for use as a complete therapeutic substitute for a IV antiemetic at the time of chemotherapy treatment, not to exceed a 48-hour dosage regimen
Medicare Statute 4557

▶✳ Q0182 Dermal and epidermal, tissue of non-human origin, with or without other bioengineered or processed elements, without metabolically active elements, per square centimeter

✳ Q0183 Dermal tissue, of human origin, with and without other bioengineered or processed elements, but without metabolically active elements, per square centimeter

Q0184 Deleted 12/31/02

Q0185 Deleted 01/01/02, Cross Reference J7340

⊘ Q0187 Factor VIIa (coagulation factor, recombinant) per 1.2 mg
MCM 2049

⊘ Q1001 New technology intraocular lens category 1 as defined in Federal Register notice, Vol 65, dated May 3, 2000

⊘ Q1002 New technology intraocular lens category 2 as defined in Federal Register notice, Vol 65, dated May 3, 2000

⊘ Q1003 New technology intraocular lens category 3 as defined in Federal Register notice

⊘ Q1004 New technology intraocular lens category 4 as defined in Federal Register notice

⊘ Q1005 New technology intraocular lens category 5 as defined in Federal Register notice

◆ Q2001 Oral, cabergoline, 0.5 mg
MCM 2049.5

⊘ Q2002 Injection, Elliott's B solution, per milliliter
MCM 2049, Medicare Statute 1861S2B

⊘ Q2003 Injection, aprotinin, 10,000 KIU
MCM 2049, Medicare Statute 1861S2B

⊘ Q2004 Irrigation solution for treatment of bladder calculi, for example renacidin, per 500 ml
MCM 2049, Medicare Statute 1861S2B

⊘ Q2005 Injection, corticorelin ovine triflutate, per dose
MCM 2049, Medicare Statute 1861S2B

⊘ Q2006 Injection, digoxin immune fab (ovine), per vial
MCM 2049, Medicare Statute 1861S2B

⊘ Q2007 Injection, ethanolamine oleate, 100 mg
MCM 2049, Medicare Statute 1861S2B

⊘ Q2008 Injection, fomepizole, 15 mg
MCM 2049, Medicare Statute 1861S2B

⊘ Q2009 Injection, fosphenytoin, 50 mg
MCM 2049, Medicare Statute 1861S2B

Q2010 Deleted 12/31/03

⊘ Q2011 Injection, hemin, per 1 mg
MCM 2049, Medicare Statute 1861S2B

⊘ Q2012 Injection, pegademase bovine, 25 IU
MCM 2049, Medicare Statute 1861S2B

⊘ Q2013 Injection, pentastarch, 10% solution, per 100 cc
MCM 2049, Medicare Statute 1861S2B

⊘ Q2014 Injection, sermorelin acetate, 0.5 mg
Medicare Statute 1861S2B MCM 2049

Q2015 Deleted 01/01/02

Q2016 Deleted 01/01/02

⊘ Q2017 Injection, teniposide, 50 mg
MCM 2049, Medicare Statute 1861S2B

⊘ Q2018 Injection, urofollitropin, 75 IU
MCM 2049, Medicare Statute 1861S2B

⊘ Q2019 Injection, basiliximab, 20 mg
MCM 2049, Medicare Statute 1861S2B

⊘ Q2020 Injection, histrelin acetate, 10 mg
MCM 2049, Medicare Statute 1861S2B

⊘ Q2021 Injection, lepirudin, 50 mg
MCM 2049, Medicare Statute 1861S2B

⊘ Q2022 Von Willebrand factor complex, human, per IU
MCM 2049.5, CIM 35-30

⊘ Q3000 Supply of radiopharmaceutical diagnostic imaging agent, rubidium Rb-82, per dose

⊘ Q3001 Radioelements for brachytherapy, any type, each
MCM 15022

⊘ Q3002 Supply of radiopharmaceutical diagnostic imaging agent, gallium Ga-67, per mCi
MCM 15022

⊘ Q3003 Supply of radiopharmaceutical diagnostic imaging agent, technetium Tc99m bicisate, per unit dose
MCM 15022

⊘ Q3004 Supply of radiopharmaceutical diagnostic imaging agent, xenon Xe-133, per 10 mCi
MCM 15022

✪ Q3005   Supply of radiopharmaceutical diagnostic imaging agent, technetium Tc99m mertiatide, per mCi
MCM 15022

✪ Q3006   Supply of radiopharmaceutical diagnostic imaging agent, technetium Tc99m gluceptate, per 5 mCi
MCM 15022

✪ Q3007   Supply of radiopharmaceutical diagnostic imaging agent, sodium phosphate P32, per mCi
MCM 15022

✪ Q3008   Supply of radiopharmaceutical diagnostic imaging agent, indium In-111 pentetreotide, per 3 mCi
MCM 15022

✪ Q3009   Supply of radiopharmaceutical diagnostic imaging agent, technetium Tc99m oxidronate, per millicurie
MCM 15022

✪ Q3010   Supply of radiopharmaceutical diagnostic imaging agent, technetium Tc99m–labeled red blood cells, per millicurie
MCM 15022

✪ Q3011   Supply of radiopharmaceutical diagnostic imaging agent, chromic phosphate P32 suspension, per millicurie
MCM 15022

✪ Q3012   Supply of oral radiopharmaceutical diagnostic imaging agent, cyanocobalamin cobalt Co57, per 0.5 mCi
MCM 15022

Q3013   Deleted 01/01/02, Cross Reference J3395

✳ Q3014   Telehealth originating site facility fee

Q3017   Deleted 03/31/02

✳ Q3019   ALS vehicle used, emergency transport, no ALS level services furnished.

✳ Q3020   ALS vehicle used, non-emergency transport, no ALS level service furnished

◆ Q3021   Injection, hepatitis B vaccine, pediatric or adolescent, per dose

◆ Q3022   Injection, hepatitis B vaccine, adult, per dose

◆ Q3023   Injection, hepatitis B vaccine, immunosuppressed patients (including renal dialysis patients), per dose

✪ Q3025   Injection, interferon beta-1a, 11 mcg for intramuscular use
MCM 2049

◆ Q3026   Injection, interferon beta-1a, 11 mcg for subcutaneous use

Q3030   Deleted 12/31/02, Cross Reference J7317

▶✪ Q3031   Collagen skin test
CIM 65-9

✳ Q4001   Casting supplies, body cast adult, with or without head, plaster

✳ Q4002   Cast supplies, body cast adult, with or without head, fiberglass

✳ Q4003   Cast supplies, shoulder cast, adult (11 years +), plaster

✳ Q4004   Cast supplies, shoulder cast, adult (11 years +), fiberglass

✳ Q4005   Cast supplies, long arm cast, adult (11 years +), plaster

✳ Q4006   Cast supplies, long arm cast, adult (11 years +), fiberglass

✳ Q4007   Cast supplies, long arm cast, pediatric (0-10 years), plaster

✳ Q4008   Cast supplies, long arm cast, pediatric (0-10 years), fiberglass

✳ Q4009   Cast supplies, short arm cast, adult (11 years +), plaster

✳ Q4010   Cast supplies, short arm cast, adult (11 years +), fiberglass

✳ Q4011   Cast supplies, short arm cast, pediatric (0-10 years), plaster

✳ Q4012   Cast supplies, short arm cast, pediatric (0-10 years), fiberglass

✳ Q4013   Cast supplies, gauntlet cast (includes lower forearm and hand), adult (11 years +), plaster

✳ Q4014   Cast supplies, gauntlet cast (includes lower forearm and hand), adult (11 years +), fiberglass

✳ Q4015   Cast supplies, gauntlet cast (includes lower forearm and hand), pediatric (0-10 years), plaster

✳ Q4016   Cast supplies, gauntlet cast (includes lower forearm and hand), pediatric (0-10 years), fiberglass

✳ Q4017   Cast supplies, long arm splint, adult (11 years +), plaster

✳ Q4018   Cast supplies, long arm splint, adult (11 years +), fiberglass

✳ Q4019   Cast supplies, long arm splint, pediatric (0-10 years), plaster

✳ Q4020   Cast supplies, long arm splint, pediatric (0-10 years), fiberglass

✳ Q4021   Cast supplies, short arm splint, adult (11 years +), plaster

✳ Q4022   Cast supplies, short arm splint, adult (11 years +), fiberglass

✳ Q4023   Cast supplies, short arm splint, pediatric (0-10 years), plaster

✳ Q4024   Cast supplies, short arm splint, pediatric (0-10 years), fiberglass

✳ Q4025   Cast supplies, hip spica (one or both legs), adult (11 years +), plaster

✳ Q4026   Cast supplies, hip spica (one or both legs), adult (11 years +), fiberglass

✳ Q4027   Cast supplies, hip spica (one or both legs), pediatric (0-10 years), plaster

✳ Q4028   Cast supplies, hip spica (one or both legs), pediatric (0-10 years), fiberglass

✳ Q4029   Cast supplies, long leg cast, adult (11 years +), plaster

✳ Q4030   Cast supplies, long leg cast, adult (11 years +), fiberglass

* Q4031 Cast supplies, long leg cast, pediatric (0-10 years), plaster
* Q4032 Cast supplies, long leg cast, pediatric (0-10 years), fiberglass
* Q4033 Cast supplies, long leg cylinder cast, adult (11 years +), plaster
* Q4034 Cast supplies, long leg cylinder cast, adult (11 years +), fiberglass
* Q4035 Cast supplies, long leg cylinder cast, pediatric (0-10 years), plaster
* Q4036 Cast supplies, long leg cylinder cast, pediatric (0-10 years), fiberglass
* Q4037 Cast supplies, short leg cast, adult (11 years +), plaster
* Q4038 Cast supplies, short leg cast, adult (11 years +), fiberglass
* Q4039 Cast supplies, short leg cast, pediatric (0-10 years), plaster
* Q4040 Cast supplies, short leg cast, pediatric (0-10 years), fiberglass
* Q4041 Cast supplies, long leg splint, adult (11 years +), plaster
* Q4042 Cast supplies, long leg splint, adult (11 years +), fiberglass
* Q4043 Cast supplies, long leg splint, pediatric (0-10 years), plaster
* Q4044 Cast supplies, long leg splint, pediatric (0-10 years), fiberglass
* Q4045 Cast supplies, short leg splint, adult (11 years +), plaster
* Q4046 Cast supplies, short leg splint, adult (11 years +), fiberglass
* Q4047 Cast supplies, short leg splint, pediatric (0-10 years), plaster
* Q4048 Cast supplies, short leg splint, pediatric (0-10 years), fiberglass
* Q4049 Finger splint, static
* Q4050 Cast supplies, for unlisted types and materials of casts
* Q4051 Splint supplies, miscellaneous (includes thermoplastics, strapping, fasteners, padding and other supplies)
  Q4052 Deleted 12/31/03, Cross Reference J2353
  Q4053 Deleted 12/31/03, Cross Reference J2505
▶⊙ Q4054 Injection, darbepoetin alfa, 1 mcg (for ESRD on dialysis) MCM 4273.1
▶⊙ Q4055 Injection, epoetin alfa, 1000 units (for ESRD on dialysis) MCM 4273.1
▶* Q4075 Injection, acyclovir, 5 mg
▶* Q4076 Injection, dopamine HCl, 40 mg
▶* Q4077 Injection, treprostinil, 1 mg
  Q4078 Deleted 12/31/03, Cross Reference A9526

Injection Codes for Epoetin Alfa

Q9920-Q9940 Deleted 12/31/03

DOMESTIC RADIOLOGY SERVICES (R0000-R5999)
Transportation/Setup of Portable X-Ray Equipment

⊙ R0070 Transportation of portable x-ray equipment and personnel to home or nursing home, per trip to facility or location, one patient seen
MCM 2070.4, MCM 5244B
⊙ R0075 Transportation of portable x-ray equipment and personnel to home or nursing home, per trip to facility or location, more than one patient seen, per patient
MCM 2070.4, MCM 5244B
⊙ R0076 Transportation of portable ECG to facility or location, per patient
MCM 2070.1, MCM 2070.4, CIM 50-15

TEMPORARY NATIONAL CODES (S0009-S9999)

  S0009 Deleted 12/31/03
◆ S0012 Butorphanol tartrate, nasal spray, 25 mg
◆ S0014 Tacrine HCl, 10 mg
◆ S0016 Injection, amikacin sulfate, 500 mg
◆ S0017 Injection, aminocaproic acid, 5 gm
◆ S0020 Injection, bupivacaine HCl, 30 ml
◆ S0021 Injection, cefoperazone sodium, 1 gm
◆ S0023 Injection, cimetidine HCl, 300 mg
  S0024 Deleted 01/01/02
◆ S0028 Injection, famotidine, 20 mg
  S0029 Deleted 01/01/02, Cross Reference J1450
◆ S0030 Injection, metronidazole, 500 mg
◆ S0032 Injection, nafcillin sodium, 2 gm
◆ S0034 Injection, ofloxacin, 400 mg
◆ S0039 Injection, sulfamethoxazole and trimethoprim, 10 ml
◆ S0040 Injection, ticarcillin disodium and clavulanate potassium, 3.1 gm
◆ S0071 Injection, acyclovir sodium, 50 mg
◆ S0072 Injection, amikacin sulfate, 100 mg
◆ S0073 Injection, aztreonam, 500 mg
◆ S0074 Injection, cefotetan disodium, 500 mg
◆ S0077 Injection, clindamycin phosphate, 300 mg
◆ S0078 Injection, fosphenytoin sodium, 750 mg
  S0079 Deleted 12/31/03
◆ S0080 Injection, pentamidine isethionate, 300 mg

◆ S0081   Injection, piperacillin sodium, 500 mg

S0085   Deleted 12/31/02, Cross Reference J1590

S0086   Deleted 01/01/02, Cross Reference J3395

S0087   Deleted 12/31/02, Cross Reference J9010

◆ S0088   Imatinib, 100 mg

◆ S0090   Sildenafil citrate, 25 mg

◆ S0091   Granisetron hydrochloride, 1 mg (for circumstances falling under the Medicare statute, use Q0166)

◆ S0092   Injection, hydromorphone hydrochloride, 250 mg (loading dose for infusion pump)

◆ S0093   Injection, morphine sulfate, 500 mg (loading dose for infusion pump)

S0096   Deleted 01/01/02

►◆ S0104   Zidovudine, oral, 100 mg

◆ S0106   Bupropion HCl sustained release tablet, 150 mg, per bottle of 60 tablets

►◆ S0107   Injection, omalizumab, 25 mg

◆ S0108   Mercaptopurine, oral, 50 mg

S0112   Deleted 12/31/02, Cross Reference J0880

◆ S0114   Injection, treprostinil sodium, 0.5 mg

►◆ S0115   Bortezomib, 3.5 mg

◆ S0122   Injection, menotropins, 75 IU

S0124   Deleted 12/31/03

◆ S0126   Injection, follitropin alfa, 75 IU

◆ S0128   Injection, follitropin beta, 75 IU

S0130   Deleted 12/31/03

◆ S0132   Injection, ganirelix acetate, 250 mcg

S0135   Deleted 12/31/03

►◆ S0136   Clozapine, 25 mg

►◆ S0137   Didanosine (DDI), 25 mg

►◆ S0138   Finasteride, 5 mg

►◆ S0139   Minoxidil, 10 mg

►◆ S0140   Saquinavir, 200 mg

►◆ S0141   Zalcitabine (DDC), 0.375 mg

◆ S0155   Sterile dilatant for epoprostenol, 50 ml

◆ S0156   Exemestane, 25 mg

◆ S0157   Becaplermin gel 0.01%, 0.5 gm

►◆ S0158   Injection, laronidase, 0.58 mg

►◆ S0159   Injection, agalsidase beta, 35 mg

►◆ S0160   Dextroamphetamine sulfate, 5 mg

►◆ S0161   Calcitrol, 0.25 mcg

►◆ S0162   Injection, efalizumab, 125 mg

►◆ S0163   Injection, risperidone, long acting, 12.5 mg

►◆ S0164   Injection, pantoprazole sodium, 40 mg

►◆ S0165   Injection, abarelix, 100 mg

◆ S0170   Anastrozole, oral, 1 mg

◆ S0171   Injection, bumetanide, 0.5 mg

◆ S0172   Chlorambucil, oral, 2 mg

◆ S0173   Dexamethasone, oral, 4 mg

◆ S0174   Dolasetron mesylate, oral 50 mg (for circumstances falling under the Medicare statute, use Q0180)

◆ S0175   Flutamide, oral, 125 mg

◆ S0176   Hydroxyurea, oral, 500 mg

◆ S0177   Levamisole HCl, oral, 50 mg

◆ S0178   Lomustine, oral, 10 mg

◆ S0179   Megestrol acetate, oral, 20 mg

◆ S0181   Ondansetron HCl, oral, 4 mg (for circumstances falling under the Medicare statute, use Q0179)

◆ S0182   Procarbazine HCl, oral, 50 mg

◆ S0183   Prochlorperazine maleate, oral, 5 mg (for circumstances falling under the Medicare statute, use Q0164-Q0165)

◆ S0187   Tamoxifen citrate, oral, 10 mg

◆ S0189   Testosterone pellet, 75 mg

◆ S0190   Mifepristone, oral, 200 mg

◆ S0191   Misoprostol, oral 200 mcg

S0193   Deleted 12/31/03

►◆ S0194   Dialysis/stress vitamin supplement, oral, 100 capsules

◆ S0195   Pneumococcal conjugate vaccine, polyvalent, intramuscular, for children from five years to nine years of age who have not previously received the vaccine

⇒◆ S0199   Medically induced abortion by oral ingestion of medication including all associated services and supplies (e.g., patient counseling, office visits, confirmation of pregnancy by HCG, ultrasound to confirm duration of pregnancy, ultrasound to confirm completion of abortion), except drugs

►◆ S0201   Partial hospitalization services, less than 24 hours, per diem

S0206   Deleted 12/31/02, Cross Reference modifier SU

►◆ S0207   Paramedic intercept, non-hospital based ALS service (non-voluntary), non-transport

◆ S0208   Paramedic intercept, hospital-based ALS service (non-voluntary), non-transport

◆ S0209   Wheelchair van, mileage, per mile

◆ S0215   Non-emergency transportation; mileage per mile

◆ S0220   Medical conference by a physician with interdisciplinary team of health professionals or representatives of community agencies to coordinate activities of patient care (patient is present); approximately 30 minutes

◆ S0221   Medical conference by a physician with interdisciplinary team of health professionals or representatives of community agencies to coordinate activities of patient care (patient is present); approximately 60 minutes

◆ S0250   Comprehensive geriatric assessment and treatment planning performed by assessment team

◆ S0255   Hospice referral visit (advising patient and family of care options) performed by nurse, social worker, or other designated staff

◆ S0260   History and physical (outpatient or office) related to surgical procedure (list separately in addition to code for appropriate evaluation and management service)

◆ S0302   Completed EPSDT service (list in addition to code for appropriate evaluation and management service)

◆ S0310   Hospitalist services (list separately in addition to code for appropriate evaluation and management service)

▶◆ S0315   Disease management program; initial assessment and initiation of the program

▶◆ S0316   Follow-up/assessment

▶◆ S0317   Disease management program; per diem

▶◆ S0320   Telephone calls by a registered nurse to a disease management program member for monitoring purposes; per month

◆ S0340   Lifestyle modification program for management of coronary artery disease, including all supportive services; first quarter/stage

◆ S0341   Lifestyle modification program for management of coronary artery disease, including all supportive services; second or third quarter/stage

◆ S0342   Lifestyle modification program for management of coronary artery disease, including all supportive services; fourth quarter/stage

◆ S0390   Routine foot care; removal and/or trimming of corns, calluses and/or nails and preventive maintenance in specific medical conditions (e.g., diabetes), per visit

◆ S0395   Impression casting of a foot performed by a practitioner other than the manufacturer of the orthotic

◆ S0400   Global fee for extracorporeal shock wave lithotripsy treatment of kidney stone(s)

◆ S0500   Disposable contact lens, per lens

◆ S0504   Single vision prescription lens (safety, athletic, or sunglass), per lens

◆ S0506   Bifocal vision prescription lens (safety, athletic, or sunglass), per lens

◆ S0508   Trifocal vision prescription lens (safety, athletic, or sunglass), per lens

◆ S0510   Non-prescription lens (safety, athletic, or sunglass), per lens

◆ S0512   Daily wear specialty contact lens, per lens

◆ S0514   Color contact lens, per lens

◆ S0516   Safety eyeglass frames

◆ S0518   Sunglasses frames

◆ S0580   Polycarbonate lens (list this code in addition to the basic code for the lens)

◆ S0581   Nonstandard lens (list this code in addition to the basic code for the lens)

◆ S0590   Integral lens service, miscellaneous services reported separately

◆ S0592   Comprehensive contact lens evaluation

◆ S0601   Screening proctoscopy

◆ S0605   Digital rectal examination, annual

◆ S0610   Annual gynecological examination, new patient

◆ S0612   Annual gynecological examination, established patient

▶◆ S0618   Audiometry for hearing aid evaluation to determine the level and degree of hearing loss

◆ S0620   Routine ophthalmological examination including refraction; new patient

◆ S0621   Routine ophthalmological examination including refraction; established patient

◆ S0622   Physical exam for college, new or established patient (list separately) in addition to appropriate evaluation and management code)

◆ S0630   Removal of sutures; by a physician other than the physician who originally closed the wound

◆ S0800   Laser in situ keratomileusis (lasik)

◆ S0810   Photorefractive keratectomy (PRK)

◆ S0812   Phototherapeutic keratectomy (PTK)

◆ S0820   Computerized corneal topography, unilateral

S0830   Deleted 4/01/04

◆ S1001   Deluxe item, patient aware (list in addition to code for basic item)

◆ S1002   Customized item (list in addition to code for basic item)

◆ S1015   IV tubing extension set

◆ S1016   Non-polyvinyl chloride (PVC) IV administration set, for use with drugs that are not stable in PVC (e.g., paclitaxel)

◆ S1025   Inhaled nitric oxide for the treatment of hypoxic respiratory failure in the neonate; per diem

◆ S1030   Continuous noninvasive glucose monitoring device, purchase (for physician interpretation of data, use CPT code

◆ S1031   Continuous noninvasive glucose monitoring device, rental, including sensor, sensor replacement, and download to monitor (for physician interpretation of data, use CPT code

▶◆ S1040   Cranial remolding orthosis, rigid, with soft interface material, custom fabricated, includes fitting and adjustment(s)

S2052   Deleted 01/01/02

◆ S2053   Transplantation of small intestine and liver allografts

◆ S2054   Transplantation of multivisceral organs

◆ S2055   Harvesting of donor multivisceral organs, with preparation and maintenance of allografts; from cadaver donor

◆ S2060   Lobar lung transplantation

◆ S2061   Donor lobectomy (lung) for transplantation, living donor

◆ S2065   Simultaneous pancreas kidney transplantation

▶ ◆ S2070   Cystourethroscopy, with ureteroscopy and/or pyeloscopy; with endoscopic laser treatment of ureteral calculi (includes ureteral catheterization)

◆ S2080   Laser-assisted uvulopalatoplasty (LAUP)

▶ ◆ S2082   Laparoscopy, surgical; gastric restrictive procedure, adjustable gastric band includes placement of subcutaneous port)

▶ ◆ S2083   Adjustment of gastric band diameter via subcutaneous port by injection or aspiration of saline

▶ ◆ S2085   Laparoscopy, gastric restrictive procedure, with gastric bypass for morbid obesity, with short limb (less than 100 cm) roux-en-y gastroenterostomy

▶ ◆ S2090   Ablation, open, one or more renal tumor(s); cryosurgical

▶ ◆ S2091   Ablation, percutaneous, one or more renal tumor(s); cryosurgical

▶ ◆ S2095   Transcatheter occlusion or embolization for tumor destruction, percutaneous, any method, using yttrium-90 microspheres

◆ S2102   Islet cell tissue transplant from pancreas allogeneic

◆ S2103   Adrenal tissue transplant to brain

◆ S2107   Adoptive immunotherapy i.e. development of specific anti-tumor reactivity (e.g. tumor-infiltrating lymphocyte therapy) per course of treatment

◆ S2112   Arthroscopy, knee, surgical for harvesting of cartilage (chondrocyte cells)

▶ ◆ S2113   Arthroscopy, knee, surgical for implantation of cultured analogous chondrocytes

◆ S2115   Osteotomy, periacetabular, with internal fixation

◆ S2120   Low-density lipoprotein (LDL) apheresis using heparin-induced extracorporeal LDL precipitation

◆ S2130   Endoluminal radiofrequency ablation of refluxing saphenous vein

▶ ◆ S2131   Endovascular laser ablation of long or short saphenous vein, with or without proximal ligation or division

▶ ◆ S2135   Neurolysis, by injection, of metatarsal neuroma/interdigital neuritis, any interspace of the foot

◆ S2140   Cord blood harvesting for transplantation, allogeneic

◆ S2142   Cord blood–derived stem cell transplantation, allogeneic

⇒ ◆ S2150   Bone marrow or blood-derived stem cells (peripheral or umbilical), allogeneic or autologous, harvesting, transplantation, and related complications; including: pheresis and cell preparation/storage; marrow ablative therapy; drugs; supplies; hospitalization with outpatient follow-up; medical/surgical, diagnostic, emergency, and rehabilitative services; and the number of days of pre- and post-transplant care in the global definition

▶ ◆ S2152   Solid organ(s), complete or segmental, single organ or combination of organs; deceased or living donor(s), procurement, transplantation, and related complications; including: drugs; supplies; hospitalization with outpatient follow-up; medical/surgical, diagnostic, emergency, and rehabilitative services; and the number of days of pre- and post-transplant care in the global definition

S2180   Deleted 12/31/02, Cross Reference 38242*

◆ S2202   Echosclerotherapy

◆ S2205   Minimally invasive direct coronary artery bypass surgery involving mini-thoracotomy or mini-sternotomy surgery, performed under direct vision; using arterial graft(s), single coronary arterial graft

◆ S2206   Minimally invasive direct coronary artery bypass surgery involving mini-thoracotomy or mini-sternotomy surgery, performed under direct vision; using arterial graft(s), two coronary arterial grafts

◆ S2207   Minimally invasive direct coronary artery bypass surgery involving mini-thoracotomy or mini-sternotomy surgery, performed under direct vision; using venous graft only, single coronary venous graft

◆ S2208   Minimally invasive direct coronary artery bypass surgery involving mini-thoracotomy or mini-sternotomy surgery, performed under direct vision; using single arterial and venous graft(s), single venous graft

◆ S2209   Minimally invasive direct coronary artery bypass surgery involving mini-thoracotomy or mini-sternotomy surgery, performed under direct vision; using two arterial grafts and single venous graft

◆ S2211   Transcatheter placement of intravascular stent(s), carotid artery, percutaneous, unilateral (if performed bilaterally, use −50 modifier)

▶ ◆ S2213   Implantation of gastric electrical stimulation device

S2220 Deleted 01/01/02

▶◆ S2225 Myringotomy, laser-assisted

▶◆ S2230 Implantation of magnetic component of semi-implantable hearing device on ossicles in middle ear

▶◆ S2235 Implantation of auditory brain stem implant

◆ S2250 Uterine artery embolization for uterine fibroids

▶◆ S2255 Hysteroscopy, surgical; with occlusion of oviducts bilaterally by micro-inserts for permanent sterilzation

◆ S2260 Induced abortion, 17-24 weeks, any surgical method

▶◆ S2262 Abortion for maternal indications, 25 weeks or greater

▶◆ S2265 Abortion for fetal indications, 25-28 weeks

▶◆ S2266 Abortion for fetal indication, 29-31 weeks

▶◆ S2267 Abortion for fetal indication, 32 weeks or greater

◆ S2300 Arthroscopy, shoulder, surgical; with thermally induced capsulorrhaphy

◆ S2340 Chemodenervation of abductor muscle(s) of vocal cord

◆ S2341 Chemodenervation of adductor muscle(s) of vocal cord

◆ S2342 Nasal endoscopy for post-operative debridement following functional endoscopic sinus surgery, nasal and/or sinus cavity(s), unilateral or bilateral

◆ S2350 Diskectomy, anterior, with decompression of spinal cord and/or nerve root(s) including osteophytectomy; lumbar, single interspace

◆ S2351 Diskectomy, anterior, with decompression of spinal cord and/or nerve root(s) including osteophytectomy; lumbar, each additional interspace (list separately in addition to code for primary procedure)

◆ S2360 Percutaneous vertebroplasty, one vertebral body, unilateral or bilateral injection; cervical

◆ S2361 Each additional cervical vertebral body (list separately in addition to code for primary procedure)

▶◆ S2362 Kyphoplasty, one vertebral body, unilateral or bilateral injection

▶◆ S2363 Kyphoplasty, one vertebral body, unilateral or bilateral injection; each additional vertebral body (list separately in addition to code for primary procedure)

◆ S2370 Intradiscal electrothermal therapy, single interspace

◆ S2371 Each additional interspace (list separately in addition to code for primary procedure)

◆ S2400 Repair, congenital diaphragmatic hernia in the fetus using temporary tracheal occlusion, procedure performed in utero

◆ S2401 Repair, urinary tract obstruction in the fetus, procedure performed in utero

◆ S2402 Repair, congenital cystic adenomatoid malformation in the fetus, procedure performed in utero

◆ S2403 Repair, extralobar pulmonary sequestration in the fetus, procedure performed in utero

◆ S2404 Repair, myelomeningocele in the fetus, procedure performed in utero

◆ S2405 Repair of sacrococcygeal teratoma in the fetus, procedure performed in utero

◆ S2409 Repair, congenital malformation of fetus, procedure performed in utero, not otherwise classified

◆ S2411 Fetoscopic laser therapy for treatment of twin-to-twin transfusion syndrome (TTTS)

▶◆ S3000 Diabetic indicator; retinal eye exam, dilated, bilateral

◆ S3600 Stat laboratory request (situations other than S3601)

◆ S3601 Emergency stat laboratory charge for patient who is homebound or residing in a nursing facility

◎ S3620 Newborn metabolic screening panel, includes test kit, postage, and the laboratory tests specified by the sate for inclusion in this panel (e.g., galactose, hemoglobin; electrophoresis; hydroxyprogesterone; 17-D; phenylalanine (PKU); and thyroxine, total)

▶◆ S3625 Maternal serum triple marker screen including alpha-fetoprotein (AFP), estriol, and human chorionic gonadotropin (hCG)

◆ S3630 Eosinophil count, blood, direct

◆ S3645 Human immunodeficiency virus-1 (HIV-1) antibody testing of oral mucosal transudate

◆ S3650 Saliva test, hormone level; during menopause

◆ S3652 Saliva test, hormone level; to assess preterm labor risk

▶◆ S3655 Antisperm antibodies test (immunobead)

◆ S3701 Immunoassay for nuclear matrix protein 22 (NMP-22), quantitative

◆ S3708 Gastrointestinal fat absorption study

◆ S3818 Complete gene sequence analysis; BRCA1 gene

◆ S3819 Complete gene sequence analysis; BRCA2 gene

▶◆ S3820 Complete BRAL1 and BRCA2 gene sequence analysis for susceptibility to breast and ovarian cancer

▶◆ S3822 Single mutation analysis (in individual with a known BRCA1 or BRCA2 mutation in the family) for susceptibility to breast and ovarian cancer

▶◆ S3823 Three-mutation BRCA1 and BRCA2 analysis for susceptibility to breast and ovarian cancer in Ashkenazi individuals

▶◆ S3828 Complete gene sequence analysis; MLH1 gene

▶◆ S3829 Complete gene sequence analysis; MLH2 gene

◆ S3830 Complete MLH and MLH gene sequence analysis for hereditary nonpolyposis colorectal cancer (HNPCC) genetic testing

◆ S3831 Single-mutation analysis (in individual with a known MLH and MLH mutation in the family) for hereditary non-polyposis colorectal cancer (HNPCC) genetic testing

▶◆ S3833 Complete APC gene sequence analysis for susceptibility to familial adenomatous polyposis (FAP) and attenuated FAP

▶◆ S3834 Single-mutation analysis (in individual with a known APC mutation in the family) for susceptibility to familial adenomatous polyposis (FAP) and attenuated FAP

◆ S3835 Complete gene sequence analysis for cystic fibrosis genetic testing

◆ S3837 Complete gene sequence analysis for hemochromatosis genetic testing

▶◆ S3840 DNA analysis for germline mutations of the ret proto-oncogene for susceptibility to multiple endocrine neoplasia type 2

▶◆ S3841 Genetic testing for retinoblastoma

▶◆ S3842 Genetic testing for von Hippel-Lindau disease

▶◆ S3843 DNA analysis of the F5 gene for susceptibility to Factor V leiden thrombophilia

▶◆ S3844 DNA analysis of the connexin 26 gene (GJB2) for susceptibility to congenital, profound deafness

▶◆ S3845 Genetic testing for alpha-thalassemia

▶◆ S3846 Genetic testing for hemoglobin E beta-thalassemia

▶◆ S3847 Genetic testing for Tay-Sachs disease

▶◆ S3848 Genetic testing for Gaucher disease

▶◆ S3849 Genetic testing for Niemann-Pick disease

▶◆ S3850 Genetic testing for sickle cell anemia

▶◆ S3851 Genetic testing for Canavan disease

▶◆ S3852 DNA analysis for APOE epilson 4 allele for susceptibility to Alzheimer's disease

▶◆ S3853 Genetic testing for myotonic muscular dystrophy

▶◆ S3890 DNA analysis, fecal, for colorectal cancer screening

◆ S3900 Surface electromyography (EMG)

◆ S3902 Ballistrocardiogram

◆ S3904 Masters two step

S3906 Deleted 01/01/02

◆ S4005 Interim labor facility global (labor occurring but not resulting in delivery)

◆ S4011 In vitro fertilization (IVF); including but not limited to identification and incubation of mature oocytes, fertilization with sperm, incubation of embryo(s), and subsequent visualization for determination of development

◆ S4013 Complete cycle, gamete intrafallopian transfer (GIFT), case rate

◆ S4014 Complete cycle, zygote intrafallopian transfer (ZIFT), case rate

◆ S4015 Complete in vitro fertilization cycle, not otherwise specified, case rate

◆ S4016 Frozen in vitro fertilization cycle, case rate

◆ S4017 Incomplete cycle, treatment canceled prior to stimulation, case rate

◆ S4018 Frozen embryo transfer procedure cancelled before transfer, case rate

◆ S4020 In vitro fertilization procedure cancelled before aspiration, case rate

◆ S4021 In vitro fertilization procedure cancelled after aspiration, case rate

◆ S4022 Assisted oocyte fertilization, case rate

◆ S4023 Donor egg cycle, incomplete, case rate

◆ S4025 Donor services for in vitro fertilization (sperm or embryo), case rate

◆ S4026 Procurement of donor sperm from sperm bank

◆ S4027 Storage of previously frozen embryos

◆ S4028 Microsurgical epididymal sperm aspiration (MESA)

◆ S4030 Sperm procurement and cryopreservation services; initial visit

◆ S4031 Sperm procurement and cryopreservation services; subsequent visit

◆ S4035 Stimulated intrauterine insemination (IUI), case rate

◆ S4036 Intravaginal culture (IVC), case rate

◆ S4037 Cryopreserved embryo transfer, case rate

◆ S4040 Monitoring and storage of cryopreserved embryos, per 30 days

◆ S4981 Insertion of levonorgestrel-releasing intrauterine system

◆ S4989 Contraceptive intrauterine device (IUD) (e.g. Progestasert), including implants and supplies

◆ S4990 Nicotine patches, legend

◆ S4991 Nicotine patches, non-legend

◆ S4993 Contraceptive pills for birth control

◆ S4995 Smoking cessation gum

◆ S5000 Prescription drug, generic

◆ S5001 Prescription drug, brand name

S5002   Deleted 01/01/02
S5003   Deleted 01/01/02
◆ S5010   5% dextrose and 45% normal saline, 1000 ml
◆ S5011   5% dextrose in lactated Ringer's, 1000 ml
◆ S5012   5% dextrose with potassium chloride, 1000 ml
◆ S5013   5% dextrose/45% normal saline with potassium chloride and magnesium sulfate, 1000 ml
◆ S5014   5% dextrose/45% normal saline with potassium chloride and magnesium sulfate, 1500 ml
S5016   Deleted 01/01/02
S5017   Deleted 01/01/02
S5018   Deleted 01/01/02
S5019   Deleted 01/01/02
S5020   Deleted 01/01/02
S5021   Deleted 01/01/02
S5022   Deleted 01/01/02
S5025   Deleted 01/01/02
◆ S5035   Home infusion therapy, routine service of infusion device (e.g., pump maintenance)
◆ S5036   Home infusion therapy, repair of infusion device (e.g., pump repair)
▶◆ S5100   Day care services, adult; per 15 minutes
▶◆ S5101   Day care services, adult; per half day
▶◆ S5102   Day care services, adult; per diem
▶◆ S5105   Day care services, center-based; services not included in program fee, per diem
▶◆ S5108   Home care training to home care client, per 15 minutes
▶◆ S5109   Home care training to home care client, per session
▶◆ S5110   Home care training, family; per 15 minutes
▶◆ S5111   Home care training, family; per session
▶◆ S5115   Home care training, non-family; per 15 minutes
▶◆ S5116   Home care training, non-family; per session
▶◆ S5120   Chore services; per 15 minutes
▶◆ S5121   Chore services; per diem
▶◆ S5125   Attendant care services; per 15 minutes
▶◆ S5126   Attendant care services; per diem
▶◆ S5130   Homemaker service, NOS; per 15 minutes
▶◆ S5131   Homemaker service, NOS; per diem
▶◆ S5135   Companion care, adult (e.g., IADL/ADL); per 15 minutes
▶◆ S5136   Companion care, adult (e.g., IADL/ADL); per diem
▶◆ S5140   Foster care, adult; per diem
▶◆ S5141   Foster care, adult; per month
▶◆ S5145   Foster care, therapeutic, child; per diem
▶◆ S5146   Foster care, therapeutic, child; per month
▶◆ S5150   Unskilled respite care, not hospice; per 15 minutes

▶◆ S5151   Unskilled respite care, not hospice; per diem
▶◆ S5160   Emergency response system; installation and testing
▶◆ S5161   Emergency response system; service fee, per month (excludes installation and testing)
▶◆ S5162   Emergency response system; purchase only
▶◆ S5165   Home modifications; per service
▶◆ S5170   Home delivered meals, including preparation; per meal
▶◆ S5175   Laundry service, external, professional; per order
▶◆ S5180   Home health respiratory therapy, initial evaluation
▶◆ S5181   Home health respiratory therapy, NOS, per diem
▶◆ S5185   Medication reminder service, non-face-to-face; per month
▶◆ S5190   Wellness assessment, performed by non-physician
▶◆ S5199   Personal care item, NOS, each
◆ S5497   Home infusion therapy, catheter care/maintenance, not otherwise classified; includes administration services, professional pharmacy services, care coordination, and all necessary supplies and equipment (drugs and nursing visits coded separately), per diem
◆ S5498   Home infusion therapy, catheter care/maintenance, simple (single lumen), includes administrative services, professional pharmacy services, care coordination and all necessary supplies and equipment, (drugs and nursing visits coded separately), per diem
◆ S5501   Home infusion therapy, catheter care/maintenance, complex (more than one lumen), includes administrative services, professional pharmacy services, care coordination, and all necessary supplies and equipment (drugs and nursing visits coded separately), per diem
◆ S5502   Home infusion therapy, catheter care/maintenance, implanted access device, includes administrative services, professional pharmacy services, care coordination and all necessary supplies and equipment, (drugs and nursing visits coded separately), per diem (use this code for interim maintenance of vascular access not currently in use)
S5503   Deleted 01/01/02
◆ S5517   Home infusion therapy, all supplies necessary for restoration of catheter patency or declotting
◆ S5518   Home infusion therapy, all supplies necessary for catheter repair

◆ S5520 Home infusion therapy, all supplies (including catheter) necessary for a peripherally inserted central venous catheter (PICC) line insertion

◆ S5521 Home infusion therapy, all supplies (including catheter) necessary for a midline catheter insertion

◆ S5522 Home infusion therapy, insertion of PICC, nursing services only (no supplies or catheter included)

◆ S5523 Home infusion therapy, insertion of midline central venous catheter, nursing services only (no supplies or catheter included)

▶◆ S5550 Insulin, rapid onset, 5 units

▶◆ S5551 Insulin, most rapid onset (Lispro or Aspart); 5 units

▶◆ S5552 Insulin, intermediate acting (NPH or Lente); 5 units

▶◆ S5553 Insulin, long acting; 5 units

▶◆ S5560 Insulin delivery device, reusable pen; 1.5 ml size

▶◆ S5561 Insulin delivery device, reusable pen; 3 ml size

▶◆ S5565 Insulin cartridge for use in insulin delivery device other than pump; 150 units

▶◆ S5566 Insulin cartridge for use in insulin delivery device other than pump; 300 units

▶◆ S5570 Insulin delivery device, disposable pen (including insulin); 1.5 ml size

▶◆ S5571 Insulin delivery device, disposable pen (including insulin); 3 ml size

S8001 Deleted 01/01/02

S8002 Deleted 12/31/02, Cross Reference A9522

S8003 Deleted 12/31/02, Cross Reference A9523

▶◆ S8004 Radioimmunopharmaceutical localization of targeted cells; whole body

◆ S8030 Scleral application of tantalum ring(s) for localization of lesions for proton beam therapy

◆ S8035 Magnetic source imaging

◆ S8037 Magnetic resonance cholangiopancreatography (MRCP)

◆ S8040 Topographic brain mapping

◆ S8042 Magnetic resonance imaging (MRI), low-field

◆ S8049 Intraoperative radiation therapy (single administration)

◆ S8055 Ultrasound guidance for multifetal pregnancy reduction(s), technical component (only to be used when the physician doing the reduction procedure does not perform the ultrasound, guidance is included in the CPT code for multifetal pregnancy reduction-59866*)

▶◆ S8075 Computer analysis of full-field digital mammogram and further physician review for interpretation, mammography (list separately in addition to code for primary procedure)

◆ S8080 Scintimammography (radioimmunoscintigraphy of the breast), unilateral, including supply of radiopharmaceutical

◆ S8085 Fluorine-18 fluorodeoxyglucose (F-18 FDG) imaging using dual-head coincidence detection system (non-dedicated postiron emissition test [PET] scan)

◆ S8092 Electron beam computed tomography (also known as ultrafast CT, cine CT)

◆ S8095 Wig (for medically or congenitally induced hair loss)

◆ S8096 Portable peak flow meter

◆ S8097 Asthma kit (including but not limited to portable peak expiratory flow meter, instructional video, brochure, and/or spacer)

◆ S8100 Holding chamber or spacer for use with an inhaler or nebulizer; without mask

◆ S8101 Holding chamber or spacer for use with an inhaler or nebulizer; with mask

S8105 Deleted 12/31/02

◆ S8110 Peak expiratory flow rate (physician services)

▶◆ S8120 Oxygen contents, gaseous, 1 unit equals 1 cubic foot

▶◆ S8121 Oxygen contents, liquid, 1 unit equals 1 pound

S8180 Deleted 12/31/03

S8181 Deleted 12/31/03

◆ S8182 Humidifier, heated, used with ventilator, non-servo-controlled

◆ S8183 Humidifier, heated, used with ventilator, dual servo-controlled with temperature monitoring

◆ S8185 Flutter device

◆ S8186 Swivel adaptor

◆ S8189 Tracheostomy supply, not otherwise classified

◆ S8190 Electronic spirometer (or micro spirometer)

S8200 Deleted 12/31/02, Cross Reference E0483

S8205 Deleted 12/31/02, Cross Reference E0483

◆ S8210 Mucus trap

◆ S8260 Oral orthotic for treatment of sleep apnea, includes fitting, fabrication, and materials

◆ S8262 Mandibular orthopedic repositioning device, each

◆ S8265 Haberman feeder for cleft lip/palate

S8401 Deleted 12/31/02, Cross Reference A4529, A4530

S8402 Deleted 01/01/02

S8403 Deleted 12/31/02

*CPT only © 2003. *Current Procedural Terminology, 2004, Professional Edition,* American Medical Association. All Rights Reserved.

1256   ☼ **Special coverage instructions**   ◆ **Not covered by or valid for Medicare**   ✳ **Carrier discretion**   ◀▶ **New**   ◀▥▥▶ **Revised**

S8404   Deleted 12/31/02, Cross Reference A4531, A4532

S8405   Deleted 12/31/02, Cross Reference A4535

◆ S8415   Supplies for home delivery of infant

◆ S8420   Gradient pressure aid (sleeve and glove combination), custom made

◆ S8421   Gradient pressure aid (sleeve and glove combination), ready made

◆ S8422   Gradient pressure aid (sleeve), custom made, medium weight

◆ S8423   Gradient pressure aid (sleeve), custom made, heavy weight

◆ S8424   Gradient pressure aid (sleeve), ready made

◆ S8425   Gradient pressure aid (glove), custom made, medium weight

◆ S8426   Gradient pressure aid (glove), custom made, heavy weight

◆ S8427   Gradient pressure aid (glove), ready made

◆ S8428   Gradient pressure aid (gauntlet), ready made

◆ S8429   Gradient pressure exterior wrap

◆ S8430   Padding for compression bandage, roll

◆ S8431   Compression bandage, roll

S8433   Deleted 12/31/02, Cross Reference A4280

◆ S8450   Splint, prefabricated, digit (specify digit by use of modifier)

◆ S8451   Splint, prefabricated, wrist or ankle

◆ S8452   Splint, prefabricated, elbow

▶◆ S8460   Camisole, post-mastectomy

◆ S8490   Insulin syringes (100 syringes, any size)

S8945   Deleted 12/31/03

▶◆ S8948   Application of a modality (requiring constant provider attendance) to one or more areas; low-level laser; each 15 minutes

◆ S8950   Complex lymphedema therapy, each 15 minutes

▶◆ S8990   Physical or manipulative therapy performed for maintenance rather than restoration

◆ S8999   Resuscitation bag (for use by patient on artificial respiration during power failure or other catastrophic event)

◆ S9001   Home uterine monitor with or without associated nursing services

◆ S9007   Ultrafiltration monitor

◆ S9015   Automated electroencephalogram (EEG) monitoring

◆ S9022   Digital subtraction angiography (use in addition to CPT code for the procedure for further identification)

S9023   Deleted 01/01/02

◆ S9024   Paranasal sinus ultrasound

◆ S9025   Omnicardiogram/cardiointegram

◆ S9034   Extracorporeal shockwave lithotripsy for gall stones (if performed with ERCP, use 43265)

S9035   Deleted 01/01/02

◆ S9055   Procuren or other growth factor preparation to promote wound healing

◆ S9056   Coma stimulation per diem

◆ S9061   Home administration of aerosolized drug therapy (e.g., pentamidine); administrative services, professional pharmacy services, care coordination, all necessary supplies and equipment (drugs and nursing visits coded separately), per diem

◆ S9075   Smoking cessation treatment

◆ S9083   Global fee urgent care centers

S9085   Deleted 01/01/02

◆ S9088   Services provided in an urgent care center (list in addition to code for service)

◆ S9090   Vertebral axial decompression, per session

◆ S9092   Canolith repositioning, per visit

◆ S9098   Home visit, phototherapy services (e.g. Bili-Lite), including equipment rental, nursing services, blood draw, supplies, and other services, per diem

◆ S9109   Congestive heart failure telemonitoring, equipment rental, including telescale, computer system and software, telephone connections, and maintenance, per month

◆ S9117   Back school, per visit

◆ S9122   Home health aide or certified nurse assistant, providing care in the home; per hour

⇒◆ S9123   Nursing care, in the home; by registered nurse, per hour (use for general nursing care only, not to be used when CPT codes 99500-99602* can be used)

◆ S9124   Nursing care, in the home; by licensed practical nurse, per hour

◆ S9125   Respite care, in the home, per diem

◆ S9126   Hospice care, in the home, per diem

◆ S9127   Social work visit, in the home, per diem

◆ S9128   Speech therapy, in the home, per diem

◆ S9129   Occupational therapy, in the home, per diem

◆ S9131   Physical therapy; in the home, per diem

◆ S9140   Diabetic management program, follow-up visit to non-physician provider

◆ S9141   Diabetic management program, follow-up visit to physcian provider

◆ S9145   Insulin pump initiation, instruction in initial use of pump (pump not included)

▶◆ S9150   Evaluation by ocularist

S9200   Deleted 01/01/02

◆ S9208　Home management of preterm labor, including administrative services, professional pharmacy services, care coordination, and all necessary supplies or equipment (drugs and nursing visits coded separately), per diem (do not use this code with any home infusion per diem code)

◆ S9209　Home management of preterm premature rupture of membranes (PPROM), including administrative services, professional pharmacy services, care coordination, and all necessary supplies or equipment (drugs and nursing visits coded separately), per diem (do not use this code with any home infusion per diem code)

S9210　Deleted 01/01/02

◆ S9211　Home management of gestational hypertension, includes administrative services, professional pharmacy services, care coordination and all necessary supplies and equipment (drugs and nursing visits coded separately); per diem (do not use this code with any home infusion per diem code)

◆ S9212　Home management of postpartum hypertension, includes administrative services, professional pharmacy services, care coordination, and all necessary supplies and equipment (drugs and nursing visits coded separately), per diem (do not use this code with any home infusion per diem code)

◆ S9213　Home management of preeclampsia, includes administrative services, professional pharmacy services, care coordination, and all necessary supplies and equipment (drugs and nursing services coded separately); per diem (do not use this code with any home infusion per diem code)

◆ S9214　Home management of gestational diabetes, includes administrative services, professional pharmacy services, care coordination, and all necessary supplies and equipment (drugs and nursing visits coded separately); per diem (do not use this code with any home infusion per diem code)

S9216　Deleted 12/31/02, Cross Reference S9211

S9217　Deleted 12/31/02, Cross Reference S9212

S9218　Deleted 12/31/02, Cross Reference S9213

S9220　Deleted 01/01/02
S9225　Deleted 01/01/02
S9230　Deleted 01/01/02
S9300　Deleted 01/01/02
S9308　Deleted 01/01/02

S9310　Deleted 01/01/02

◆ S9325　Home infusion therapy, pain management infusion; administrative services, professional pharmacy services, care coordination, and all necessary supplies and equipment, (drugs and nursing visits coded separately), per diem (do not use this code with S9326, S9327 or S9328)

◆ S9326　Home infusion therapy, continuous (twenty-four hours or more) pain management infusion; administrative services, professional pharmacy services, care coordination and all necessary supplies and equipment (drugs and nursing visits coded separately), per diem

◆ S9327　Home infusion therapy, intermittent (less than twenty-four hours) pain management infusion; administrative services, professional pharmacy services, care coordination, and all necessary supplies and equipment (drugs and nursing visits coded separately), per diem

◆ S9328　Home infusion therapy, implanted pump pain management infusion; administrative services, professional pharmacy services, care coordination, and all necessary supplies and equipment (drugs and nursing visits coded separately), per diem

◆ S9329　Home infusion therapy, chemotherapy infusion; administrative services, professional pharmacy services, care coordination, and all necessary supplies and equipment (drugs and nursing visits coded separately), per diem (do not use this code with S9330 or S9331)

◆ S9330　Home infusion therapy, continuous (twenty-four hours or more) chemotherapy infusion; administrative services, professional pharmacy services, care coordination, and all necessary supplies and equipment (drugs and nursing visits coded separately), per diem

◆ S9331　Home infusion therapy, intermittent (less than twenty-four hours) chemotherapy infusion; administrative services, professional pharmacy services, care coordination, and all necessary supplies and equipment (drugs and nursing visits coded separately), per diem

▶◆ S9335　Home therapy, hemodialysis; administrative services, professional pharmacy services, care coordination, and all necessary supplies and equipment (drugs and nursing services coded separately), per diem

◆ S9336 Home infusion therapy, continuous anticoagulant infusion therapy (e.g. heparin), administrative services, professional pharmacy services, care coordination and all necessary supplies and equipment (drugs and nursing visits coded separately), per diem

◆ S9338 Home infusion therapy, immunotherapy therapy; (e.g., intravenous immunoglobulin, interferon); administrative services, professional pharmacy services, care coordination, and all necessary supplies and equipment (drug and nursing visits coded separately), per diem

◆ S9339 Home therapy; peritoneal dialysis, administrative services, professional pharmacy services, care coordination and all necessary supplies and equipment (drugs and nursing visits coded separately), per diem

◆ S9340 Home therapy; enteral nutrition; administrative services, professional pharmacy services, care coordination, and all necessary supplies and equipment (enteral formula and nursing visits coded separately), per diem

◆ S9341 Home therapy; enteral nutrition via gravity; administrative services, professional pharmacy services, care coordination, and all necessary supplies and equipment (enteral formula and nursing visits coded separately), per diem

◆ S9342 Home therapy; enteral nutrition via pump; administrative services, professional pharmacy services, care coordination, and all necessary supplies and equipment (enteral formula and nursing visits coded separately), per diem

◆ S9343 Home therapy; enteral nutrition via bolus; administrative services, professional pharmacy services, care coordination, and all necessary supplies and equipment (enteral formula and nursing visits coded separately), per diem

◆ S9345 Home infusion therapy, anti-hemophilic agent infusion therapy (e.g. Factor VIII); administrative services, professional pharmacy services, care coordination, and all necessary supplies and equipment (drugs and nursing visits coded separately), per diem

◆ S9346 Home infusion therapy, alpha-1-proteinase inhibitor (e.g., Prolastin); administrative services, professional pharmacy services, care coordination, and all necessary supplies and equipment (drugs and nursing visits coded separately), per diem

◆ S9347 Home infusion therapy, uninterrupted, long-term, controlled rate IV or subcutaneous infusion therapy (e.g. Epoprostenol); administrative services, professional pharmacy services, care coordination, and all necessary supplies and equipment (drugs and nursing visits coded separately), per diem

◆ S9348 Home infusion therapy, sympathomimetic/inotropic agent infusion therapy (e.g., Dobutamine); administrative services, professional pharmacy services, care coordination, all necessary supplies and equipment (drugs and nursing visits coded separately), per diem

◆ S9349 Home infusion therapy, tocolytic infusion therapy; administrative services, professional pharmacy services, care coordination, and all necessary supplies and equipment (drugs and nursing visits coded separately), per diem

◆ S9351 Home infusion therapy, continuous antiemetic infusion therapy; administrative services, professional pharmacy services, care coordination, all necessary supplies and equipment (drugs and nursing visits coded separately), per diem

◆ S9353 Home infusion therapy, continuous insulin infusion therapy; administrative services, professional pharmacy services, care coordination, and all necessary supplies and equipment (drugs and nursing visits coded separately), per diem

◆ S9355 Home infusion therapy, chelation therapy; administrative services, professional pharmacy services, care coordination, and all necessary supplies and equipment (drugs and nursing visits coded separately), per diem

◆ S9357 Home infusion therapy, enzyme replacement IV therapy; (e.g. Imiglucerase); administrative services, professional pharmacy services, care coordination, and all necessary supplies and equipment (drugs and nursing visits coded separately), per diem

◆ S9359 Home infusion therapy, anti-tumor necrosis factor IV therapy; (e.g. Infliximab); administrative services, professional pharmacy services, care coordination, and all necessary supplies and equipment (drugs and nursing visits coded separately), per diem

◆ S9361 Home infusion therapy, diuretic IV therapy; administrative services, professional pharmacy services, care coordination, and all necessary supplies and equipment (drugs and nursing visits coded separately), per diem

◆ S9363 Home infusion therapy, anti-spasmotic IV therapy; administrative services, professional pharmacy services, care coordination, and all necessary supplies and equipment (drugs and nursing visits coded separately), per diem

◆ S9364 Home infusion therapy, total parenteral nutrition (TPN); administrative services, professional pharmacy services, care coordination, and all necessary supplies and equipment including standard TPN formula (lipids, specialty amino acid formulas, drugs other than in standard formula and nursing visits coded separately) per diem (do not use with home infusion codes S9365-S9368 using daily volume scales)

◆ S9365 Home infusion therapy, total parenteral nutrition (TPN); one liter per day, administrative services, professional pharmacy services, care coordination, and all necessary supplies and equipment including standard TPN formula (lipids, specialty amino acid formulas, drugs other than in standard formula and nursing visits coded separately), per diem

◆ S9366 Home infusion therapy, total parenteral nutrition (TPN); more than one liter but no more than two liters per day, administrative services, professional pharmacy services, care coordination, and all necessary supplies and equipment including standard TPN formula; (lipids, specialty amino acid formulas, drugs other than in standard formula and nursing visits coded separately), per diem

◆ S9367 Home infusion therapy, total parenteral nutrition (TPN); more than two liters but no more than three liters per day, administrative services, professional pharmacy services, care coordination, and all necessary supplies and equipment including standard TPN formula; (lipids, specialty amino acid formulas, drugs other than in standard formula and nursing visits coded separately), per diem

◆ S9368 Home infusion therapy, total parenteral nutrition (TPN); more than three liters per day, administrative services, professional pharmacy services, care coordination, and all necessary supplies and equipment (includes standard TPN formula; (lipids, specialty amino acid formulas, drugs other than in standard formula and nursing visits coded separately), per diem

◆ S9370 Home therapy, intermittent antiemetic injection therapy; administrative services, professional pharmacy services, care coordination, and all necessary supplies and equipment (drugs and nursing visits coded separately), per diem

◆ S9372 Home therapy; intermittent anti-coagulant injection therapy (e.g. heparin); administrative services, professional pharmacy services, care coordination, and all necessary supplies and equipment (drugs and nursing visits coded separately), per diem (do not use this code for flushing of infusion devices with heparin to maintain patency)

◆ S9373 Home infusion therapy, hydration therapy; administrative services, professional pharmacy services, care coordination, and all necessary supplies and equipment (drugs and nursing visits coded separately), per diem (do not use with hydration therapy codes S9374-S9377 using daily volume scales)

◆ S9374 Home infusion therapy, hydration therapy; one liter per day, administrative services, professional pharmacy services, care coordination, and all necessary supplies and equipment (drugs and nursing visits coded separately), per diem

◆ S9375 Home infusion therapy, hydration therapy; more than one liter but no more than two liters per day, administrative services, professional pharmacy services, care coordination, and all necessary supplies and equipment (drugs and nursing visits coded separately), per diem

◆ S9376 Home infusion therapy, hydration therapy; more than two liters but no more than three liters per day, administrative services, professional pharmacy services, care coordination, and all necessary supplies and equipment (drugs and nursing visits coded separately), per diem

◆ S9377 Home infusion therapy, hydration therapy; more than three liters per day, administrative services, professional pharmacy services, care coordination, and all necessary supplies (drugs and nursing visits coded separately), per diem

◆ S9379 Home infusion therapy, infusion therapy, not otherwise classified; administrative services, professional pharmacy services, care coordination, and all necessary supplies and equipment (drugs and nursing visits coded separately), per diem

◆ S9381 Delivery or service to high risk areas requiring escort or extra protection, per visit

S9395 Deleted 01/01/02

◆ S9401 Anti-coagulation clinic, inclusive of all services except laboratory tests, per session

S9420 Deleted 01/01/02
S9423 Deleted 01/01/02
S9425 Deleted 01/01/02

◆ S9430 Pharmacy compounding and dispensing services

▶◆ S9434 Modified solid food supplements for inborn errors of metabolism

◆ S9435 Medical foods for inborn errors of metabolism

◆ S9436 Childbirth preparation/Lamaze classes, non-physician provider, per session

◆ S9437 Childbirth refresher classes, non-physician provider, per session

◆ S9438 Cesarean birth classes, non-physician provider, per session

◆ S9439 Vaginal birth after cesarean (VBAC) classes, non-physician provider, per session

◆ S9441 Asthma education, non-physician provider, per session

◆ S9442 Birthing classes, non-physician provider, per session

◆ S9443 Lactation classes, non-physician provider, per session

◆ S9444 Parenting classes, non-physician provider, per session

◆ S9445 Patient education, not otherwise classified, non-physician provider, individual, per session

◆ S9446 Patient education, not otherwise classified, non-physician provider, group, per session

◆ S9447 Infant safety (including cardiopulmonary resuscitation [CPR]) classes, non-physician provider, per session

◆ S9449 Weight management classes, non-physician provider, per session

◆ S9451 Exercise classes, non-physician provider, per session

◆ S9452 Nutrition classes, non-physician provider, per session

◆ S9453 Smoking cessation classes, non-physician provider, per session

◆ S9454 Stress management classes, non-physician provider, per session

◆ S9455 Diabetic management program, group session

◆ S9460 Diabetic management program, nurse visit

◆ S9465 Diabetic management program, dietitian visit

◆ S9470 Nutritional counseling, dietitian visit

◆ S9472 Cardiac rehabilitation program, non-physician provider, per diem

◆ S9473 Pulmonary rehabilitation program, non-physician provider, per diem

◆ S9474 Enterostomal therapy by a registered nurse certified in enterostomal therapy, per diem

◆ S9475 Ambulatory setting substance abuse treatment or detoxification services, per diem

▶◆ S9476 Vestibular rehabilitation program, non-physician provider, per diem

◆ S9480 Intensive outpatient psychiatric services, per diem

▶◆ S9484 Crisis intervention mental health services, per hour

◆ S9485 Crisis intervention mental health services, per diem

▶◆ S9490 Home infusion therapy, corticosteroid infusion; administrative services, professional pharmacy services, care coordination, and all necessary supplies and equipment (drugs and nursing visits coded separately), per diem

◆ S9494 Home infusion therapy, antibiotic, antiviral, or anti-fungal therapy; administrative services, professional pharmacy services, care coordination, and all necessary supplies and equipment (drug and nursing visits coded separately, per diem), (do not use with home infusion codes for hourly dosing schedules S9497-S9504)

◆ S9497 Home infusion therapy, antibiotic, antiviral, or anti-fungal therapy; once every 3 hours; administrative services, professional pharmacy services, care coordination, and all necessary supplies and equipment (drugs and nursing visits coded separately), per diem

◆ S9500 Home infusion therapy, antibiotic, antiviral, or anti-fungal therapy; once every 24 hours; administrative services, professional pharmacy services, care coordination, and all necessary supplies and equipment (drugs and nursing visits coded separately), per diem

◆ S9501 Home infusion therapy, antibiotic, antiviral, or anti-fungal therapy; once every 12 hours; administrative services, professional pharmacy services, care coordination, and all necessary supplies and equipment (drugs and nursing visits coded separately), per diem

◆ S9502 Home infusion therapy, antibiotic, antiviral, or anti-fungal therapy; once every 8 hours, administrative services, professional pharmacy services, care coordination, and all necessary supplies and equipment (drugs and nursing visits coded separately), per diem

◆ **S9503** Home infusion therapy, antibiotic, antiviral, or anti-fungal; once every 6 hours; administrative services, professional pharmacy services, care coordination, and all necessary supplies and equipment (drugs and nursing visits coded separately), per diem

◆ **S9504** Home infusion therapy, antibiotic, antiviral, or anti-fungal; once every 4 hours; administrative services, professional pharmacy services, care coordination, and all necessary supplies and equipment (drugs and nursing visits coded separately), per diem

S9524 Deleted 03/31/03
S9526 Deleted 01/01/02
S9527 Deleted 01/01/02
S9528 Deleted 01/01/02

◆ **S9529** Routine venipuncture for collection of specimen(s), single home bound, nursing home, or skilled nursing facility patient

S9533 Deleted 01/01/02
S9535 Deleted 01/01/02

◆ **S9537** Home therapy; hematopoietic hormone injection therapy (e.g. erythropoietin, G-CSF, GM-CSF); administrative services, professional pharmacy services, care coordination, and all necessary supplies and equipment (drugs and nursing visits coded separately), per diem

◆ **S9538** Home transfusion of blood product(s); administrative services, professional pharmacy services, care coordination and all necessary supplies and equipment (blood products, drugs, and nursing visits coded separately), per diem

S9539 Deleted 01/01/02

◆ **S9542** Home injectable therapy; not otherwise classified, including administrative services, professional pharmacy services, care coordination, and all necessary supplies and equipment (drugs and nursing visits coded separately), per diem

S9543 Deleted 04/01/02
S9545 Deleted 01/01/02
S9546 Deleted 09/30/03
S9550 Deleted 01/01/02
S9555 Deleted 01/01/02

◆ **S9558** Home infusion therapy; growth hormone, including administrative services, professional pharmacy services, care coordination, and all necessary supplies and equipment (drugs and nursing visits coded separately), per diem

◆ **S9559** Home infusion therapy; interferon, including administrative services, professional pharmacy services, care coordination, and all necessary supplies and equipment (drugs and nursing visits coded separately), per diem

◆ **S9560** Home injectable therapy; hormonal therapy (e.g.; Leuprolide, Goserelin), including administrative services, professional pharmacy services, care coordination, and all necessary supplies and equipment (drugs and nursing visits coded separately), per diem

◆ **S9562** Home injectable therapy, palivizumab, including administrative services, professional pharmacy services, care coordination, and all necessary supplies and equipment (drugs and nursing visits coded separately), per diem

◆ **S9590** Home therapy, irrigation therapy (e.g. sterile irrigation of an organ or anatomical cavity); including administrative services, professional pharmacy services, care coordination, and all necessary supplies and equipment (drugs and nursing visits coded separately), per diem

S9800 Deleted 12/31/02, Cross Reference S9802, S9803
S9802 Deleted 06/30/03
S9803 Deleted 06/30/03
S9806 Deleted 12/31/03

◆ **S9810** Home therapy; professional pharmacy services for provision of infusion, specialty drug administration, and/or disease state management, not otherwise classified, per hour (do not use this code with any per diem code)

▶◆ **S9900** Services by authorized Christian Science Practitioner for the process of healing, per diem; not to be used for rest or study; excludes in-patient services

◆ **S9970** Health club membership, annual
◆ **S9975** Transplant related lodging, meals and transportation, per diem
▶◆ **S9976** Lodging, per diem, not otherwise specified
▶◆ **S9977** Meals, per diem, not otherwise specified
◆ **S9981** Medical records copying fee, administrative
◆ **S9982** Medical records copying fee, per page
◆ **S9986** Not medically necessary service (patient is aware that service not medically necessary)
▶◆ **S9988** Services provided as part of phase I clinical trial

⊘ **Special coverage instructions** ◆ **Not covered by or valid for Medicare** ✳ **Carrier discretion** ◀▶ **New** ◀▦▦▶ **Revised**

◆ S9989 Services provided outside of the United States of America (list in addition to code[s] for services[s])

◆ S9990 Services provided as part of a phase II clinical trial

◆ S9991 Services provided as part of a phase III clinical trial

◆ S9992 Transportation costs to and from trial location and local transportation costs (e.g., fares for taxicab or bus) for clinical trial participant and one caregiver/companion

◆ S9994 Lodging costs (e.g., hotel charges) for clinical trial participant and one caregiver/companion

◆ S9996 Meals for clinical trial participant and one caregiver/companion

◆ S9999 Sales tax

NATIONAL T CODES FOR STATE MEDICAID AGENCIES (T1000-T9999)

Not Valid For Medicare

◆ T1000 Private duty/independent nursing service(s), licensed, up to 15 minutes

◆ T1001 Nursing assessment/evaluation

◆ T1002 RN services, up to 15 minutes

◆ T1003 Licensed practical nurse/licensed nurse (LPN/LVN) services, up to 15 minutes

◆ T1004 Services of a qualified nursing aide, up to 15 minutes

◆ T1005 Respite care services, up to 15 minutes

◆ T1006 Alcohol and/or substance abuse services, family/couple counseling

◆ T1007 Alcohol and/or substance abuse services, treatment plan development and/or modification

T1008 Deleted 03/31/03

◆ T1009 Child sitting services for children of the individual receiving alcohol and/or substance abuse services

◆ T1010 Meals for individuals receiving alcohol and/or substance abuse services (when meals not included in the program)

T1011 Deleted 03/31/03

◆ T1012 Alcohol and/or substance abuse services, skills development

◆ T1013 Sign language or oral interpreter services, per 15 minutes

◆ T1014 TEL health transmission, per minute, professional services bill separately

◆ T1015 Clinic visit/encounter, all-inclusive

◆ T1016 Case Management, each 15 minutes

◆ T1017 Targeted Case Management, each 15 minutes

◆ T1018 School-based IEP services, bundled

◆ T1019 Personal care services, per 15 minutes, not for an in-patient or resident of a hospital, nursing facility, ICF/MR or IMD, part of the individualized plan of treatment (code may not be used to identify services provided by home health aide or certified nurse assistant)

◆ T1020 Personal care services, per diem, not for an inpatient or resident of a hospital, nursing facility, ICF/MR or IMD, part of the individualized plan of treatment (code may not be used to identify services provided by home health aide or certified nurse assistant)

◆ T1021 Home health aide or certified nurse assistant, per visit

◆ T1022 Contracted home health agency services, all services provided under contract, per day

◆ T1023 Screening to determine the appropriateness of consideration of an individual for participation in a specified program, project or treatment protocol, per encounter

◆ T1024 Evaluation and treatment by an integrated, specialty team contracted to provide coordinated care to multiple or severely handicapped children, per encounter

◆ T1025 Intensive, extended multidisciplinary services provided in a clinic setting to children with complex medical, physical, mental and psychosocial impairments, per diem

◆ T1026 Intensive, extended multidisciplinary services provided in a clinic setting to children with complex medical, physical, medical and psychosocial impairments, per hour

◆ T1027 Family training and counseling for child development, per 15 minutes

◆ T1028 Assessment of home, physical and family environment, to determine suitability to meet patient's medical needs

◆ T1029 Comprehensive environmental lead investigation, not including laboratory analysis, per dwelling

◆ T1030 Nursing care, in the home, by registered nurse, per diem

◆ T1031 Nursing care, in the home, by licensed practical nurse, per diem

◆ T1500 Diaper/incontinent pant, reusable/washable, any size, each

◆ T1502 Administration of oral, intramuscular and/or subcutaneous medication by health care agency/professional, per visit

◆ T1999 Miscellaneous therapeutic items and supplies, retail purchases, not otherwise classified; identify product in "remarks"

◆ T2001   Non-emergency transportation; patient attendant/escort
◆ T2002   Non-emergency transportation; per diem
◆ T2003   Non-emergency transportation; encounter/trip
◆ T2004   Non-emergency transport; commercial carrier, multi-pass
◆ T2005   Non-emergency transportation: non-ambulatory stretcher van
◆ T2006   Ambulance response and treatment, no transport
◆ T2007   Transportation waiting time, air ambulance and non-emergency vehicle, one-half (1/2) hour increments
▶◆ T2010   Preadmission screening and resident review (PASRR) level I identification screening, per screen
▶◆ T2011   Preadmission screening and resident review (PASRR) level II evaluation, per evaluation
▶◆ T2012   Habilitation, educational; waiver, per diem
▶◆ T2013   Habilitation, educational, waiver; per hour
▶◆ T2014   Habilitation, prevocational, waiver; per diem
▶◆ T2015   Habilitation, prevocational, waiver; per hour
▶◆ T2016   Habilitation, residential, waiver; per diem
▶◆ T2017   Habilitation, residential, waiver; 15 minutes
▶◆ T2018   Habilitation, supported employment, waiver; per diem
▶◆ T2019   Habilitation, supported employment, waiver; per 15 minutes
▶◆ T2020   Day habilitation, waiver; per diem
▶◆ T2021   Day habilitation, waiver; per 15 minutes
▶◆ T2022   Case management, per month
▶◆ T2023   Targeted case management; per month
▶◆ T2024   Service assessment/plan of care development, waiver
▶◆ T2025   Waiver services; not otherwise specified (NOS)
▶◆ T2026   Specialized childcare, waiver; per diem
▶◆ T2027   Specialized childcare, waiver; per 15 minutes
▶◆ T2028   Specialized supply, not otherwise specified, waiver
▶◆ T2029   Specialized medical equipment, not otherwise specified, waiver
▶◆ T2030   Assisted living, waiver; per month
▶◆ T2031   Assisted living; waiver, per diem
▶◆ T2032   Residential care, not otherwise specified (NOS), waiver; per month
▶◆ T2033   Residential care, not otherwise specified (NOS), waiver; per diem
▶◆ T2034   Crisis intervention, waiver; per diem

▶◆ T2035   Utility services to support medical equipment and assistive technology/devices, waiver
▶◆ T2036   Therapeutic camping, overnight, waiver; each session
▶◆ T2037   Therapeutic camping, day, waiver; each session
▶◆ T2038   Community transition, waiver; per service
▶◆ T2039   Vehicle modifications, waiver; per service
▶◆ T2040   Financial management, self-directed, waiver; per 15 minutes
▶◆ T2041   Supports brokerage, self-directed, waiver; per 15 minutes
▶◆ T2042   Hospice routine home care; per diem
▶◆ T2043   Hospice continuous home care; per hour
▶◆ T2044   Hospice inpatient respite care; per diem
▶◆ T2045   Hospice general inpatient care; per diem
▶◆ T2046   Hospice long term care, room and board only; per diem
▶◆ T2048   Behavioral health; long-term care residential (non-acute care in a residential treatment program where stay is typically longer than 30 days), with room and board, per diem
▶◆ T2101   Human breast milk processing, storage and distribution only
▶◆ T5001   Positioning seat for persons with special orthopedic needs, for use in vehicles
▶◆ T5999   Supply, not otherwise specified

VISION SERVICES (V0000-V2999)

Frames

⊘ V2020   Frames, purchases
          MCM 2130
◆ V2025   Deluxe frame
          MCM 3045.4

Spectacle Lenses

NOTE: If a CPT procedure code for supply of spectacles or a permanent prosthesis is reported, recode with the specific lens type listed below. For aphakic temporary spectacle correction, see CPT.*

Single Vision, Glass or Plastic

✳ V2100   Sphere, single vision, plano to plus or minus 4.00, per lens

---

* V2101   Sphere, single vision, plus or minus 4.12 to plus or minus 7.00d, per lens
* V2102   Sphere, single vision, plus or minus 7.12 to plus or minus 20.00d, per lens
* V2103   Spherocylinder, single vision, plano to plus or minus 4.00d sphere, 0.12 to 2.00d cylinder, per lens
* V2104   Spherocylinder, single vision, plano to plus or minus 4.00d sphere, 2.12 to 4.00d cylinder, per lens
* V2105   Spherocylinder, single vision, plano to plus or minus 4.00d sphere, 4.25 to 6.00d cylinder, per lens
* V2106   Spherocylinder, single vision, plano to plus or minus 4.00d sphere, over 6.00d cylinder, per lens
* V2107   Spherocylinder, single vision, plus or minus 4.25 to plus or minus 7.00 sphere, 0.12 to 2.00d cylinder, per lens
* V2108   Spherocylinder, single vision, plus or minus 4.25d to plus or minus 7.00d sphere, 2.12 to 4.00d cylinder, per lens
* V2109   Spherocylinder, single vision, plus or minus 4.25 to plus or minus 7.00d sphere, 4.25 to 6.00d cylinder, per lens
* V2110   Sperocylinder, single vision, plus or minus 4.25 to 7.00d sphere, over 6.00d cylinder, per lens
* V2111   Spherocylinder, single vision, plus or minus 7.25 to plus or minus 12.00d sphere, 0.25 to 2.25d cylinder, per lens
* V2112   Spherocylinder, single vision, plus or minus 7.25 to plus or minus 12.00d sphere, 2.25d to 4.00d cylinder, per lens
* V2113   Spherocylinder, single vision, plus or minus 7.25 to plus or minus 12.00d sphere, 4.25 to 6.00d cylinder, per lens
* V2114   Spherocylinder, single vision, sphere over plus or minus 12.00d, per lens
* V2115   Lenticular (myodisc), per lens, single vision
   V2116   Deleted 12/31/03
   V2117   Deleted 12/31/03
* V2118   Aniseikonic lens, single vision
▶ ⊙ V2121   Lenticular lens, per lens, single MCM 2130B
* V2199   Not otherwise classified, single vision lens

Bifocal, Glass or Plastic

* V2200   Sphere, bifocal, plano to plus or minus 4.00d, per lens
* V2201   Sphere, bifocal, plus or minus 4.12 to plus or minus 7.00d, per lens
* V2202   Sphere, bifocal, plus or minus 7.12 to plus or minus 20.00d, per lens
* V2203   Spherocylinder, bifocal, plano to plus or minus 4.00d sphere, 0.12 to 2.00d cylinder, per lens

* V2204   Spherocylinder, bifocal, plano to plus or minus 4.00d sphere, 2.12 to 4.00d cylinder, per lens
* V2205   Spherocylinder, bifocal, plano to plus or minus 4.00d sphere, 4.25 to 6.00d cylinder, per lens
* V2206   Spherocylinder, bifocal, plano to plus or minus 4.00d sphere, over 6.00d cylinder, per lens
* V2207   Spherocylinder, bifocal, plus or minus 4.25 to plus or minus 7.00d sphere, 0.12 to 2.00d cylinder, per lens
* V2208   Spherocylinder, bifocal, plus or minus 4.25 to plus or minus 7.00d sphere, 2.12 to 4.00d cylinder, per lens
* V2209   Spherocylinder, bifocal, plus or minus 4.25 to plus or minus 7.00d sphere, 4.25 to 6.00d cylinder, per lens
* V2210   Spherocylinder, bifocal, plus or minus 4.25 to plus or minus 7.00d sphere, over 6.00d cylinder, per lens
* V2211   Spherocylinder, bifocal, plus or minus 7.25 to plus or minus 12.00d sphere, 0.25 to 2.25d cylinder, per lens
* V2212   Spherocylinder, bifocal, plus or minus 7.25 to plus or minus 12.00d sphere, 2.25 to 4.00d cylinder, per lens
* V2213   Spherocylinder, bifocal, plus or minus 7.25 to plus or minus 12.00d sphere, 4.25 to 6.00d cylinder, per lens
* V2214   Spherocylinder, bifocal, sphere over plus or minus 12.00d, per lens
* V2215   Lenticular (myodisc), per lens, bifocal
   V2216   Deleted 12/31/03
   V2217   Deleted 12/31/03
* V2218   Aniseikonic, per lens, bifocal
* V2219   Bifocal seg width over 28 mm
* V2220   Bifocal add over 3.25d
▶ ⊙ V2221   Lenticular lens, per lens, bifocal MCM 2130B
* V2299   Specialty bifocal (by report)

Trifocal, Glass or Plastic

* V2300   Sphere, trifocal, plano to plus or minus 4.00d, per lens
* V2301   Sphere, trifocal, plus or minus 4.12 to plus or minus 7.00d per lens
* V2302   Sphere, trifocal, plus or minus 7.12 to plus or minus 20.00, per lens
* V2303   Spherocylinder, trifocal, plano to plus or minus 4.00d sphere, 0.12 to 2.00d cylinder, per lens
* V2304   Spherocylinder, trifocal, plano to plus or minus 4.00d sphere, 2.25 to 4.00d cylinder, per lens
* V2305   Spherocylinder, trifocal, plano to plus or minus 4.00d sphere, 4.25 to 6.00 cylinder, per lens

* V2306 Spherocylinder, trifocal, plano to plus or minus 4.00d sphere, over 6.00d cylinder, per lens
* V2307 Spherocylinder, trifocal, plus or minus 4.25 to plus or minus 7.00d sphere, 0.12 to 2.00d cylinder, per lens
* V2308 Spherocylinder, trifocal, plus or minus 4.25 to plus or minus 7.00d sphere, 2.12 to 4.00d cylinder, per lens
* V2309 Spherocylinder, trifocal, plus or minus 4.25 to plus or minus 7.00d sphere, 4.25 to 6.00d cylinder, per lens
* V2310 Spherocylinder, trifocal, plus or minus 4.25 to plus or minus 7.00d sphere, over 6.00d cylinder, per lens
* V2311 Spherocylinder, trifocal, plus or minus 7.25 to plus or minus 12.00d sphere, 0.25 to 2.25d cylinder, per lens
* V2312 Spherocylinder, trifocal, plus or minus 7.25 to plus or minus 12.00d sphere, 2.25 to 4.00d cylinder, per lens
* V2313 Spherocylinder, trifocal, plus or minus 7.25 to plus or minus 12.00d sphere, 4.25 to 6.00d cylinder, per lens
* V2314 Spherocylinder, trifocal, sphere over plus or minus 12.00d, per lens
* V2315 Lenticular (myodisc), per lens, trifocal
  V2316 Deleted 12/31/03
  V2317 Deleted 12/31/03
* V2318 Aniseikonic lens, trifocal
* V2319 Trifocal seg width over 28 mm
* V2320 Trifocal add over 3.25d
▶ ◉ V2321 Lenticular lens, per lens, trifocal
  MCM 2130B
* V2399 Specialty trifocal (by report)

Variable Asphericity

* V2410 Variable asphericity lens, single vision, full field, glass or plastic, per lens
* V2430 Variable asphericity lens, bifocal, full field, glass or plastic, per lens
* V2499 Variable sphericity lens, other type

Contact Lenses

If a CPT procedure code for supply of contact lens is reported, recode with specific lens type listed below (per lens).

* V2500 Contact lens, PMMA, spherical, per lens
* V2501 Contact lens, PMMA, toric or prism ballast, per lens
* V2502 Contact lens PMMA, bifocal, per lens
* V2503 Contact lens PMMA, color vision deficiency, per lens

* V2510 Contact lens, gas permeable, spherical, per lens
* V2511 Contact lens, gas permeable, toric, prism ballast, per lens
* V2512 Contact lens, gas permeable, bifocal, per lens
* V2513 Contact lens, gas permeable, extended wear, per lens
◉ V2520 Contact lens, hydrophilic, spherical, per lens
  CIM 45-7, CIM 65-1
◉ V2521 Contact lens, hydrophilic, toric, or prism ballast, per lens
  CIM 45-7, CIM 65-1
◉ V2522 Contact lens, hydrophilic, bifocal, per lens
  CIM 45-7, CIM 65-1
◉ V2523 Contact lens, hydrophilic, extended wear, per lens
  CIM 45-7, CIM 65-1
* V2530 Contact lens, scleral, gas impermeable, per lens (for modification, see contact lens, 92325*)
◉ V2531 Contact lens, scleral, gas permeable, per lens (for contact lens modification, see 92325*)
  CIM 65-3
* V2599 Contact lens, other type

Low Vision Aids

If a CPT procedure code for supply of low vision aid is reported, recode with specific systems listed below.

* V2600 Hand-held low vision aids and other nonspectacle mounted aids
* V2610 Single lens spectacle mounted low vision aids
* V2615 Telescopic and other compound lens system, including distance vision telescopic, near vision telescopes and compound microscopic lens system

Prosthetic Eye

◉ V2623 Prosthetic eye, plastic, custom
  MCM 2133
* V2624 Polishing/resurfacing of ocular prosthesis
* V2625 Enlargement of ocular prosthesis
* V2626 Reduction of ocular prosthesis
◉ V2627 Scleral cover shell
  CIM 65-3
* V2628 Fabrication and fitting of ocular conformer
* V2629 Prosthetic eye, other type

Intraocular Lenses

○ V2630 Anterior chamber intraocular lens
MCM 2130

○ V2631 Iris supported intraocular lens
MCM 2130

○ V2632 Posterior chamber intraocular lens
MCM 2130

Miscellaneous

* V2700 Balance lens, per lens
* V2710 Slab off prism, glass or plastic, per lens
* V2715 Prism, per lens
* V2718 Press-on lens, Fresnel prism, per lens
* V2730 Special base curve, glass or plastic, per lens

V2740-V2743 Deleted 12/31/03

○ V2744 Tint, photochromatic, per lens
MCM 2130B

▶○ V2745 Addition to lens, tint, any color, solid, gradient or equal, excludes photochromatic, any lens material, per lens
MCM 2130B

○ V2750 Anti-reflective coating, per lens
MCM 2130B

○ V2755 U-V lens, per lens
MCM 2130B

▶◆ V2756 Eye glass case

* V2760 Scratch resistant coating, per lens

▶○ V2761 Mirror coating, any type, solid, gradient or equal, any lens material, per lens
MCM 2130B

▶○ V2762 Polarization, any lens material, per lens
MCM 2130B

* V2770 Occluder lens, per lens
* V2780 Oversize lens, per lens
* V2781 Progressive lens, per lens

▶○ V2782 Lens, index 1.54 to 1.65 plastic or 1.60 to 1.79 glass, excludes polycarbonate, per lens
MCM 2130B

▶○ V2783 Lens, index greater than or equal to 1.66 plastic or greater than or equal to 1.80 glass, excludes polycarbonate, per lens
MCM 2130B

▶○ V2784 Lens, polycarbonate or equal, any index, per lens
MCM 2130B

* V2785 Processing, preserving and transporting corneal tissue

▶○ V2786 Specialty occupational multifocal lens, per lens
MCM 2130B

* V2790 Amniotic membrane for surgical reconstruction, per procedure

▶* V2797 Vision supply, accessory and/or service component of another HCPCS vision code

* V2799 Vision service, miscellaneous

HEARING SERVICES (V5000-V5299)

NOTE: These codes are for non-physician services.

◆ V5008 Hearing screening
MCM 2320

◆ V5010 Assessment for hearing aid
Medicare Statute 1862A7

◆ V5011 Fitting/orientation/checking of hearing aid
Medicare Statute 1862A7

◆ V5014 Repair/modification of a hearing aid
Medicare Statute 1862A7

◆ V5020 Conformity evaluation
Medicare Statute 1862A7

◆ V5030 Hearing aid, monaural, body worn, air conduction
Medicare Statute 1862A7

◆ V5040 Hearing aid, monaural, body worn, bone conduction
Medicare Statute 1862A7

◆ V5050 Hearing aid, monaural, in the ear
Medicare Statute 1862A7

◆ V5060 Hearing aid, monaural, behind the ear
Medicare Statute 1862A7

◆ V5070 Glasses, air conduction
Medicare Statute 1862A7

◆ V5080 Glasses, bone conduction
Medicare Statute 1862A7

◆ V5090 Dispensing fee, unspecified hearing aid
Medicare Statute 1862A7

◆ V5095 Semi-implantable middle ear hearing prosthesis
Medicare Statute 1862a7

◆ V5100 Hearing aid, bilateral, body worn
Medicare Statute 1862A7

◆ V5110 Dispensing fee, bilateral
Medicare Statute 1862A7

◆ V5120 Binaural, body
Medicare Statute 1862A7

◆ V5130 Binaural, in the ear
Medicare Statute 1862A7

◆ V5140 Binaural, behind the ear
Medicare Statute 1862A7

◆ V5150 Binaural, glasses
Medicare Statute 1862A7

◆ V5160 Dispensing fee, binaural
Medicare Statute 1862A7

◆ V5170 Hearing aid, CROS, in the ear
Medicare Statute 1862A7

◆ V5180 Hearing aid, CROS, behind the ear
Medicare Statute 1862A7

◆ V5190 Hearing aid, CROS, glasses
Medicare Statute 1862A7

◆ V5200 Dispensing fee, CROS
Medicare Statute 1862A7

◆ V5210 Hearing aid, BICROS, in the ear
Medicare Statute 1862A7

◆ V5220 Hearing aid, BICROS, behind the ear
Medicare Statute 1862A7

◆ V5230 Hearing aid, BICROS, glasses
Medicare Statute 1862A7

◆ V5240 Dispensing fee, BICROS
Medicare Statute 1862A7

◆ V5241 Dispensing fee, monaural hearing aid, any type
Medicare Statute 1862A7

◆ V5242 Hearing aid, analog, monaural, completely in the ear canal (CIC)
Medicare Statute 1862A7

◆ V5243 Hearing aid, analog, monaural, in the canal (ITC)
Medicare Statute 1862A9

◆ V5244 Hearing aid, digitally programmable analog, monaural, CIC
Medicare Statute 1862A7

◆ V5245 Hearing aid, digitally programmable, analog, monaural, ITC
Medicare Statute 1862A7

◆ V5246 Hearing aid, digitally programmable analog, monaural, in the ear (ITE)
Medicare Statute 1862A7

◆ V5247 Hearing aid, digitally programmable analog, monaural, behind the ear (BTE)
Medicare Statute 1862A7

◆ V5248 Hearing aid, analog, binaural, CIC
Medicare Statute 1862A7

◆ V5249 Hearing aid, analog, binaural, ITC
Medicare Statute 1862A7

◆ V5250 Hearing aid, digitally programmable analog, binaural, CIC
Medicare Statute 1862A7

◆ V5251 Hearing aid, digitally programmable analog, binaural, ITC
Medicare Statute 1862A7

◆ V5252 Hearing aid, digitally programmable, binaural, ITE
Medicare Statute 1862A7

◆ V5253 Hearing aid, digitally programmable, binaural, BTE
Medicare Statute 1862A7

◆ V5254 Hearing aid, digital, monaural, CIC
Medicare Statute 1862A7

◆ V5255 Hearing aid, digital, monaural, ITC
Medicare Statute 1862A7

◆ V5256 Hearing aid, digital, monaural, ITE
Medicare Statute 1862A7

◆ V5257 Hearing aid, digital, monaural, BTE
Medicare Statute 1862A7

◆ V5258 Hearing aid, digital, binaural, CIC
Medicare Statute 1862A7

◆ V5259 Hearing aid, digital, binaural, ITC
Medicare Statute 1862A7

◆ V5260 Hearing aid, digital, binaural, ITE
Medicare Statute 1862A7

◆ V5261 Hearing aid, digital, binaural, BTE
Medicare Statute 1862A7

◆ V5262 Hearing aid, disposable, any type, monaural
Medicare Statute 1862A7

◆ V5263 Hearing aid, disposable, any type, binaural
Medicare Statute 1862A7

◆ V5264 Ear mold/insert, not disposable, any type
Medicare Statute 1862A7

◆ V5265 Ear mold/insert, disposable, any type
Medicare Statute 1862A7

◆ V5266 Battery for use in hearing device
Medicare Statute 1862A7

◆ V5267 Hearing aid supplies/accessories
Medicare Statute 1862A7

◆ V5268 Assistive listening device, telephone amplifier, any type
Medicare Statute 1862A7

◆ V5269 Assistive listening device, alerting, any type
Medicare Statute 1862A7

◆ V5270 Assistive listening device, television amplifier, any type
Medicare Statute 1862A7

◆ V5271 Assistive listening device, television caption decoder
Medicare Statute 1862A7

◆ V5272 Assistive listening device, TDD
Medicare Statute 1862A7

◆ V5273 Assistive listening device, for use with cochlear implant
Medicare Statute 1862A7

◆ V5274 Assistive listening device, not otherwise specified
Medicare Statute 1862A7

◆ V5275 Ear impression, each
Medicare Statute 1862A7

◆ V5298 Hearing aid, not otherwise classified
Medicare Statute 1862a7

☉ V5299 Hearing service, miscellaneous
MCM 2320

Speech-Language Pathology Services

NOTE: These codes are for non-physician services.

◆ V5336 Repair/modification of augmentative communicative system or device (excludes adaptive hearing aid)
Medicare Statute 1862A7

➠◆ V5362 Speech screening
MCM 2320

➠◆ V5363 Language screening
MCM 2320

➠◆ V5364 Dysphagia screening
MCM 2320

2004 TABLE OF DRUGS

IA—Intra-arterial administration
IV—Intravenous administration
IM—Intramuscular administration
IT—Intrathecal
SC—Subcutaneous administration
INH—Administration by inhaled solution
VAR—Various routes of administration
OTH—Other routes of administration
ORAL—Administered orally

Intravenous administration includes all methods, such as gravity infusion, injections, and timed pushes. The "VAR" posting denotes various routes of administration and is used for drugs that are commonly administered into joints, cavities, tissues, or topical applications, in addition to other parenteral administrations. Listings posted with "OTH" indicate other administration methods, such as suppositories or catheter injections.

A

Abbokinase, *see* Urokinase
Abbokinase, Open Cath, *see* Urokinase

Abciximab	10 mg	IV	J0130

Abelcet, *see* Amphotericin B lipid complex
ABLC, *see* Amphotericin B

Acetazolamide sodium	up to 500 mg	IM, IV	J1120
Acetylcysteine, unit dose form	per gram	INH	J7608

Achromycin, *see* Tetracycline
ACTH, *see* Corticotropin
Acthar, *see* Corticotropin
Actimmune, *see* Interferon gamma 1-B
Activase, *see* Alteplase recombinant

Acyclovir	5 mg		Q4075

Adenocard, *see* Adenosine
Adenoscan, *see* Adenosine

Adenosine	6 mg	IV	J0150
Adenosine	30 mg	IV	J0152

Adrenalin Chloride, *see* Adrenalin, epinephrine

Adrenalin, epinephrine	up to 1 ml ampule	SC, IM	J0170

Adriamycin PFS, *see* Doxorubicin HCl
Adriamycin RDF, *see* Doxorubicin HCl
Adrucil, *see* Fluorouracil
Aggrastat, *see* Tirofiban hydrochloride
A-hydroCort, *see* Hydrocortisone sodium phosphate
Akineton, *see* Biperiden

Alatrofloxacin mesylate, injection 100 mg		IV	J0200
Albuterol	up to 5 mg	INH	J7621
Albuterol, concentrated form	per mg	INH	J7618
Albuterol, unit dose form	per mg	INH	J7619
Aldesleukin	per single use vial	IM, IV	J9015

Aldomet, *see* Methyldopate HCl

Alefacept	0.5 mg		J0215
Alemtuzumab	10 mg		J9010

Alferon N, *see* Interferon alfa-n3

Alglucerase	per 10 units	IV	J0205

Alkaban-AQ, *see* Vinblastine sulfate
Alkeran, *see* Melphalan, oral

Alpha-1-proteinase inhibitor (human)	per 10 mg	IV	J0256
Alprostadil, injection	1.25 mcg	OTH injection	J0270 J0275
Alprostadil, urethral suppository		OTH	
Alteplase recombinant	per 1 mg	IV	J2997

Alupent, *see* Metaproterenol sulfate or Metaproterenol, compounded
Amcort, *see* Triamcinolone diacetate
A-Methapred, *see* Methylprednisolone sodium succinate
Amgen, *see* Interferon alpha-con-1

Amifostine	500 mg	IV	J0207
Aminolevalinic acid HCl	unit dose (354 mg)	OTH	J7308
Aminophylline/Aminophyllin	up to 250 mg	IV	J0280
Amiodarone HCl	30 mg	IV	J0282
Amitriptyline HCl	up to 20 mg	IM	J1320
Amobarbital	up to 125 mg	IM, IV	J0300

Amphocin, *see* Amphotericin B

Amphotericin B	50 mg	IV	J0285
Amphotericin B lipid complex	10 mg	IV	J0287 J0289
Ampicillin sodium	up to 500 mg	IM, IV	J0290
Ampicillin sodium/sulbactam sodium	per 1.5 gm	IM, IV	J0295

Amygdalin, *see* Laetrile, Amygdalin, vitamin B-17
Amytal, *see* Amobarbital
Anabolin LA 100, *see* Nandrolone decanoate
Ancef, *see* Cefazolin sodium
Andrest 90-4, *see* Testosterone enanthate and estradiol valerate
Andro-Cyp, *see* Testosterone cypionate
Andro-Cyp 200, *see* Testosterone cypionate
Andro L.A. 200, *see* Testosterone enanthate
Andro-Estro 90-4, *see* Testosterone enanthate and estradiol valerate
Andro/Fem, *see* Testosterone cypionate and estradiol cypionate
Androgyn L.A., *see* Testosterone enanthate and estradiol valerate
Androlone-50, *see* Nandrolone phenpropionate
Androlone-D 100, *see* Nandrolone decanoate
Andronaq-50, *see* Testosterone suspension
Andronaq-LA, *see* Testosterone cypionate
Andronate-200, *see* Testosterone cypionate

Andronate-100, *see* Testosterone cypionate			
Andropository 100, *see* Testosterone enanthate			
Andryl 200, *see* Testosterone enanthate			
Anectine, *see* Succinylcholine chloride			
Anergan 25, *see* Promethazine HCl			
Anergan 50, *see* Promethazine HCl			
Anistreplase	30 units	IV	J0350
Anti-Inhibitor	per IU	IV	J7198
Antispas, *see* Dicyclomine HCl			
Antithrombin III (human)	per IU	IV	J7197
Anzemet, *see* Dolasetron mesylate injection			
A.P.L., *see* Chorionic gonadotropin			
Apresoline, *see* Hydralazine HCl			
Aprotinin	10,000 KIU		Q2003
AquaMEPHYTON, *see* Vitamin K			
Aralen, *see* Chloroquine HCl			
Aramine, *see* Metaraminol			
Aranesp, *see* Darbepoietin Alfa			
Arbutamine	1 mg	IV	J0395
Aredia, *see* Pamidronate disodium			
Arfonad, *see* Trimethaphan camsylate			
Aristocort Forte, *see* Triamcinolone diacetate			
Aristocort Intralesional, *see* Triamcinolone diacetate			
Aristospan Intra-Articular, *see* Triamcinolone hexacetonide			
Aristospan Intralesional, *see* Triamcinolone hexacetonide			
Arrestin, *see* Trimethobenzamide HCl			
Arsenic trioxide	1 mg	IV	J9017
Asparaginase	10,000 units	IV, IM	J9020
Astramorph PF, *see* Morphine sulfate			
Atgam, *see* Lymphocyte immune globulin			
Ativan, *see* Lorazepam			
Atropine, concentrated form	per mg	INH	J7635
Atropine, unit dose form	per mg	INH	J7636
Atropine sulfate	up to 0.3 mg	IV, IM, SC	J0460
Atrovent, *see* Ipratropium bromide			
Aurothioglucose	up to 50 mg	IM	J2910
Autologous cultured chondrocytes implant			J7330
Autoplex T, *see* Hemophilia clotting factors			
Avonex, *see* Interferon beta-1a			
Azathioprine	50 mg	ORAL	J7500
Azathioprine, parenteral	100 mg	IV	J7501
Azithromycin, dihydrate	1 gm	ORAL	Q0144
Azithromycin, injection	500 mg	IV	J0456

B

Baclofen	10 mg	IT	J0475
Baclofen for intrathecal trial	50 mcg	OTH	J0476
Bactocill, *see* Oxacillin sodium			
BAL in oil, *see* Dimercaprol			
Banflex, *see* Orphenadrine citrate			
Basiliximab	20 mg		Q2019
BCG (Bacillus Calmette and Guérin), live	per vial instillation	IV	J9031
Beclomethasone inhalation solution, unit dose form	per mg	INH	J7622
Bena-D 10, *see* Diphenhydramine HCl			
Bena-D 50, *see* Diphenhydramine HCl			
Benadryl, *see* Diphenhydramine HCl			
Benahist 10, *see* Diphenhydramine HCl			
Benahist 50, *see* Diphenhydramine HCl			
Ben-Allergin-50, *see* Diphenhydramine HCl			
Benefix, *see* Factor IX, recombinant			
Benoject-10, *see* Diphenhydramine HCl			
Benoject-50, *see* Diphenhydramine HCl			
Bentyl, *see* Dicyclomine			
Benztropine mesylate	per 1 mg	IM, IV	J0515
Berubigen, *see* Vitamin B-12, cyanocobalamin			
Betalin 12, *see* Vitamin B-12, cyanocobalamin			
Betameth, *see* Betamethasone sodium phosphate			
Betamethasone acetate & betamethasone sodium phosphate	3 mg of ea	IM	J0702
Betamethasone inhalation solution, unit dose form	per mg	INH	J7624
Betamethasone sodium phosphate	4 mg	IM, IV	J0704
Betaseron, *see* Interferon beta-1b			
Bethanechol chloride	up to 5 mg	SC	J0520
Bicillin L-A, *see* Penicillin G benzathine			
Bicillin C-R 900/300, *see* Penicillin G procaine and penicillin G benzathine			
Bicillin C-R, *see* Penicillin G benzathine and penicillin G procaine			
BiCNU, *see* Carmustine			
Biperiden lactate	per 5 mg	IM, IV	J0190
Bitolterol mesylate, concentrated form	per mg	INH	J7628
Bitolterol mesylate, unit dose form	per mg	INH	J7629
Bivalirudin	1 mg		J0583
Blenoxane, *see* Bleomycin sulfate			
Bleomycin sulfate	15 units	IM, IV, SC	J9040
Botulinum toxin type A	per unit	IM	J0585
Botulinum toxin type B	per 100 units	IM	J0587
Brethine, *see* Terbutaline sulfate or Terbutaline, compounded			
Bricanyl Subcutaneous, *see* Terbutaline sulfate			
Brompheniramine maleate	per 10 mg	IM, SC, IV	J0945
Bronkephrine, *see* Ethylnorepinephrine HCl			

Bronkosol, *see* Isoetharine HCl			
Budesonide inhalation solution, concentrated form	0.25 mg	INH	J7633
Budesonide inhalation solution, unit dose form	0.25 mg	INH	J7626
Buprenorphine Hydrochloride	0.1 mg		J0592
Busulfan	2 mg	ORAL	J8510
Butorphanol tartrate	2 mg		J0595
C			
Cabergoline	0.5 mg	ORAL	Q2001
Cafcit, *see* Caffeine citrate			
Caffeine citrate	5 mg	IV	J0706
Caine-1, *see* Lidocaine HCl			
Caine-2, *see* Lidocaine HCl			
Calcijex, *see* Calcitriol			
Calcimar, *see* Calcitonin-salmon			
Calcitonin-salmon	up to 400 units	SC, IM	J0630
Calcitriol	0.1 mcg	IM	J0636
Calcium Disodium Versenate, *see* Edetate calcium disodium			
Calcium gluconate	per 10 ml	IV	J0610
Calcium glycerophosphate & calcium lactate	per 10 ml	IM, SC	J0620
Calphosan, *see* Calcium glycerophosphate & calcium lactate			
Camptosar, *see* Irinotecan			
Capecitabine	150 mg	ORAL	J8520
	500 mg	ORAL	J8521
Carbocaine with Neo-Cobefrin, *see* Mepivacaine			
Carbocaine, *see* Mepivacaine			
Carboplatin	50 mg	IV	J9045
Carmustine	100 mg	IV	J9050
Carnitor, *see* Levocarnitine			
Carticel, *see* Autologous cultured chondrocytes			
Caspofungin Acetate	5 mg	IV	J0637
Cefadyl, *see* Cephapirin sodium			
Cefazolin sodium	up to 500 mg	IV, IM	J0690
Cefepime hydrochloride	500 mg	IV	J0692
Cefizox, *see* Ceftizoxime sodium			
Cefotaxime sodium	per 1 g	IV, IM	J0698
Cefoxitin sodium	1 g	IV, IM	J0694
Ceftazidime	per 500 mg	IM, IV	J0713
Ceftizoxime sodium	per 500 mg	IV, IM	J0715
Ceftriaxone sodium	per 250 mg	IV, IM	J0696
Cefuroxime sodium, sterile	per 750 mg	IM, IV	J0697
Celestone Phosphate, *see* Betamethasone sodium phosphate			
Celestone Soluspan, *see* Betamethasone acetate and betamethasone sodium phosphate			
CellCept, *see* Mycophenolate mofetil			
Cel-U-Jec, *see* Betamethasone sodium phosphate			
Cenacort Forte, *see* Triamcinolone diacetate			
Cenacort A-40, *see* Triamcinolone acetonide			
Cephalothin sodium	up to 1 g	IM, IV	J1890
Cephapirin sodium	up to 1 g	IV, IM	J0710
Ceredase, *see* Alglucerase			
Cerezyme, *see* Imiglucerase			

Cerubidine, *see* Daunorubicin HCl			
Chealamide, *see* Endrate ethylenediamine-tetra-/ acetic acid			
Chloramphenicol sodium succinate	up to 1 g	IV	J0720
Chlordiazepoxide HCl	up to 100 mg	IM, IV	J1990
Chloromycetin Sodium Succinate, *see* Chloramphenicol sodium succinate			
Chloroprocaine HCl	per 30 ml	VAR	J2400
Chlorpromazine HCl, oral	10 mg	ORAL	Q0171
	25 mg	ORAL	Q0172
Chloroquine HCl	up to 250 mg	IM	J0390
Chlorothiazide sodium	per 500 mg	IV	J1205
Chlorpromazine HCl	10 mg	ORAL	Q0171
	25 mg	ORAL	Q0172
	up to 50 mg	IM, IV	J3230
Chorex-5, *see* Chorionic gonadotropin			
Chorex-10, *see* Chorionic gonadotropin			
Chorignon, *see* Chorionic gonadotropin			
Chorionic gonadotropin	per 1,000 USP units	IM	J0725
Choron-10, *see* Chorionic gonadotropin			
Cidofovir	375 mg	IV	J0740
Cilastatin sodium, imipenem	per 250 mg	IV, IM	J0743
Cipro IV, *see* Ciprofloxacin			
Ciprofloxacin	200 mg	IV	J0706
Cisplatin, powder or solution	per 10 mg	IV	J9060
Cisplatin	50 mg	IV	J9062
Cladribine	per mg	IV	J9065
Claforan, *see* Cefotaxime sodium			
Clonidine HCl	1 mg	epidural	J0735
Cobex, *see* Vitamin B-12, cyanocobalamin			
Codeine phosphate	per 30 mg	IM, IV, SC	J0745
Codimal-A, *see* Brompheniramine maleate			
Cogentin, *see* Benztropine mesylate			
Colchicine	per 1 mg	IV	J0760
Colistimethate sodium	up to 150 mg	IM, IV	J0770
Coly-Mycin M, *see* Colistimethate sodium			
Compa-Z, *see* Prochlorperazine			
Compazine, *see* Prochlorperazine			
Cophene-B, *see* Brompheniramine maleate			
Copper contraceptive, intrauterine	—	OTH	J7300
Cordarone, *see* Amiodarone HCl			
Corgonject-5, *see* Chorionic gonadotropin			
Corticorelin ovine triflutate	per dose		Q2005
Corticotropin	up to 40 units	IV, IM, SC	J0800
Cortrosyn, *see* Cosyntropin			
Cosmegen, *see* Dactinomycin			
Cosyntropin	per 0.25 mg	IM, IV	J0835
Cotranzine, *see* Prochlorperazine			
Cromolyn sodium, unit dose form	per 10 mg	INH	J7631
Crysticillin 300 A.S., *see* Penicillin G procaine			

Crysticillin 600 A.S., *see* Penicillin G procaine			
Cyclophosphamide	100 mg	IV	J9070
	200 mg	IV	J9080
	500 mg	IV	J9090
	1 g	IV	J9091
	2 g	IV	J9092
Cyclophosphamide, lyophilized	100 mg	IV	J9070
	200 mg	IV	J9080
	500 mg	IV	J9090
	1 g	OV	J9091
	2g	IV	J9092
Cyclophosphamide, oral	25 mg	ORAL	J8530
Cyclosporine, oral	25 mg	ORAL	J7515
	100 mg	ORAL	J7502
Cyclosporine, parenteral	250 mg	IV	J7516
Cytarabine	100 mg	SC, IV	J9100
	500 mg	SC, IV	J9110
Cytarabine liposome	10 mg		J9098
Cytomegalovirus immune globulin intravenous (human)	per vial	IV	J0850
Cytosar-U, *see* Cytarabine			
Cytovene, *see* Ganciclovir sodium			
Cytoxan, *see* Cyclophosphamide; cyclophosphamide, lyophilized; and cyclophosphamide, oral			

D

D-5-W, infusion	1000 cc	IV	J7070
Dacarbazine	100 mg	IV	J9130
	200 mg	IV	J9140
Daclizumab	25 mg	IV	J7513
Dactinomycin	0.5 mg	IV	J9120
Dalalone, *see* Dexamethasone sodium phosphate			
Dalalone L.A., *see* Dexamethasone acetate			
Dalteparin sodium	per 2500 IU	SC	J1645
Darbepoetin Alfa	1 mcg		Q4054
	5 mcg		J0880
	1000 units		Q0137
Daunorubicin citrate, liposomal formulation	10 mg	IV	J9151
Daunorubicin HCl	10 mg	IV	J9150
DaunoXome, (*see* Daunorubicin citrate)			
DDAVP, *see* Desmopressin acetate			
Decadron Phosphate, *see* Dexamethasone sodium phosphate			
Decadron, *see* Dexamethasone sodium phosphate			
Decadron-LA, *see* Dexamethasone acetate			
Deca-Durabolin, *see* Nandrolone decanoate			
Decaject, *see* Dexamethasone sodium phosphate			
Decaject-L.A., *see* Dexamethasone acetate			
Decolone-50, *see* Nandrolone decanoate			
Decolone-100, *see* Nandrolone decanoate			
De-Comberol, *see* Testosterone cypionate and estradiol cypionate			
Deferoxamine mesylate	500 mg	IM, SC, IV	J0895
Dehist, *see* Brompheniramine maleate			

Deladumone, *see* Testosterone enanthate and estradiol valerate			
Deladumone OB, *see* Testosterone enanthate and estradiol valerate			
Delatest, *see* Testosterone enanthate			
Delatestadiol, *see* Testosterone enanthate and estradiol valerate			
Delatestryl, *see* Testosterone enanthate			
Delta-Cortef, *see* Prednisolone, oral			
Delestrogen, *see* Estradiol valerate			
Demadex, *see* Torsemide			
Demerol HCl, *see* Meperidine HCl			
Denileukin diftitox	300 mcg		J9160
DepAndro 100, *see* Testosterone cypionate			
DepAndro 200, *see* Testosterone cypionate			
DepAndrogyn, *see* Testosterone cypionate and estradiol cypionate			
DepGynogen, *see* Depo-estradiol cypionate			
DepMedalone 40, *see* Methylprednisolone acetate			
DepMedalone 80, *see* Methylprednisolone acetate			
Depo-estradiol cypionate	up to 5 mg	IM	J1000
Depogen, *see* Depo-estradiol cypionate			
Depoject, *see* Methylprednisolone acetate			
Depo-Medrol, *see* Methylprednisolone acetate			
Depopred-40, *see* Methylprednisolone acetate			
Depopred-80, *see* Methylprednisolone acetate			
Depo-Provera, *see* Medroxyprogesterone acetate			
Depotest, *see* Testosterone cypionate			
Depo-Testadiol, *see* Testosterone cypionate and estradiol cypionate			
Depotestogen, *see* Testosterone cypionate and estradiol cypionate			
Depo-Testosterone, *see* Testosterone cypionate			
Desferal Mesylate, *see* Deferoxamine mesylate			
Desmopressin acetate	1 mcg	IV, SC	J2597
Dexacen LA-8, *see* Dexamethasone acetate			
Dexacen-4, *see* Dexamethasone sodium phosphate			
Dexamethasone, concentrated form	per mg	INH	J7637
Dexamethasone, unit form	per mg	INH	J7638
Dexamethasone acetate	1 mg	IM	J1094
Dexamethasone sodium phosphate	1 mg	IM, IV, OTH	J1100
Dexasone, *see* Dexamethasone sodium phosphate			
Dexasone L.A., *see* Dexamethasone acetate			

Dexferrum, *see* Iron dextran			
Dexone, *see* Dexamethasone sodium phosphate			
Dexone LA, *see* Dexamethasone acetate			
Dexrazoxane HCl	250 mg	IV	J1190
Dextran 40	500 ml	IV	J7100
Dextran 75	500 ml	IV	J7110
Dextrose 5%/normal saline solution	500 ml = 1 unit	IV	J7042
Dextrose/water (5%)	500 ml = 1 unit	IV	J7060
D.H.E. 45, *see* Dihydroergotamine			
Diamox, *see* Acetazolamide sodium			
Diazepam	up to 5 mg	IM, IV	J3360
Diazoxide	up to 300 mg	IV	J1730
Dibent, *see* Dicyclomine HCl			
Dicyclomine HCl	up to 20 mg	IM	J0500
Didronel, *see* Etidronate disodium			
Diethylstilbestrol diphosphate	250 mg	IV	J9165
Diflucan, see Fluconazole			
Digoxin	up to 0.5 mg	IM, IV	J1160
Digoxin immune Fab (ovine)	per vial		Q2006
Dihydrex, *see* Diphenhydramine HCl			
Dihydroergotamine mesylate	per 1 mg	IM, IV	J1110
Dilantin, *see* Phenytoin sodium			
Dilaudid, *see* Hydromorphone HCl			
Dilocaine, *see* Lidocaine HCl			
Dilomine, *see* Dicyclomine HCl			
Dilor, *see* Dyphylline			
Dimenhydrinate	up to 50 mg	IM, IV	J1240
Dimercaprol	per 100 mg	IM	J0470
Dimethyl sulfoxide, *see* DMSO, Dimethyl sulfoxide			
Dinate, *see* Dimenhydrinate			
Dioval, *see* Estradiol valerate			
Dioval 40, *see* Estradiol valerate			
Dioval XX, *see* Estradiol valerate			
Diphenacen-50, *see* Diphenhydramine HCl			
Diphenhydramine HCl, injection	up to 50 mg	IV, IM	J1200
Diphenhydramine HCl, oral	50 mg	ORAL	Q0163
Dipyridamole	per 10 mg	IV	J1245
Disotate, *see* Endrate ethylenediamine-tetra-acetic acid			
Di-Spaz, *see* Dicyclomine HCl			
Ditate-DS, *see* Testosterone enanthate and estradiol valerate			
Diuril Sodium, *see* Chlorothiazide sodium			
D-Med 80, *see* Methylprednisolone acetate			
DMSO, Dimethyl sulfoxide	50%, 50 ml	OTH	J1212
Dobutamine HCl	per 250 mg	IV	J1250
Dobutrex, *see* Dobutamine HCl			
Docetaxel	20 mg	IV	J9170
Dolasetron mesylate, injection	10 mg	IV	J1260
Dolasetron mesylate, tablets	100 mg	ORAL	Q0180
Dolophine HCl, *see* Methadone HCl			
Dommanate, *see* Dimenhydrinate			
Dopamine HCl	40 mg		Q4076
Dornase alpha, unit dose form	per mg	INH	J7639
Doxercalciferol	1 mcg	IV	J1270
Doxil, *see* Doxorubicin HCl, lipid			
Doxorubicin HCl	10 mg	IV	J9000
Doxorubicin HCl, all lipid	10 mg	IV	J9001
Dramamine, *see* Dimenhydrinate			
Dramanate, *see* Dimenhydrinate			
Dramilin, *see* Dimenhydrinate			
Dramocen, *see* Dimenhydrinate			
Dramoject, *see* Dimenhydrinate			
Dronabinol, oral	2.5 mg	ORAL	Q0167
Dronabinol, oral	5 mg	ORAL	Q0168
Droperidol	up to 5 mg	IM, IV	J1790
Drug administered through a metered dose inhaler		INH	J3535
Droperidol and fentanyl citrate	up to 2 ml ampule	IM, IV	J1810
DTIC-Dome, *see* Dacarbazine			
Dua-Gen L.A., *see* Testosterone enanthate and estradiol valerate cypionate			
Duoval P.A., *see* Testosterone enanthate and estradiol valerate			
Durabolin, *see* Nandrolone phenpropionate			
Duraclon, *see* Clonidine HCl			
Dura-Estrin, *see* Depo-estradiol cypionate			
Duracillin A.S., *see* Penicillin G procaine			
Duragen-10, *see* Estradiol valerate			
Duragen-20, *see* Estradiol valerate			
Duragen-40, *see* Estradiol valerate			
Duralone-40, *see* Methylprednisolone acetate			
Duralone-80, *see* Methylprednisolone acetate			
Duralutin, *see* Hydroxyprogesterone caproate			
Duramorph, *see* Morphine sulfate			
Duratest-100, *see* Testosterone cypionate			
Duratest-200, *see* Testosterone cypionate			
Duratestrin, *see* Testosterone cypionate and estradiol cypionate			
Durathate-200, *see* Testosterone enanthate			
Dymenate, *see* Dimenhydrinate			
Dyphylline	up to 500 mg	IM	J1180
E			
Edetate calcium disodium	up to 1000 mg	IV, SC, IM	J0600
Edetate disodium	per 150 mg	IV	J3520

Elavil, *see* Amitriptyline HCl			
Ellence, *see* Epirubicin HCl			
Elliott's B solution	per ml	OTH	Q2002
Elspar, *see* Asparaginase			
Emete-Con, *see* Benzquinamide			
Eminase, *see* Anistreplase			
Enbrel, *see* Etanercept			
Endrate ethylenediamine-tetra-acetic acid, *see* Edetate disodium			
Enovil, *see* Amitriptyline HCl			
Enoxaparin sodium	10 mg	SC	J1650
Epinephrine, adrenalin	up to 1 ml ampule	SC, IM	J0170
Epirubicin hydrochloride	2 mg		J9178
Epoetin alfa	1000 units		Q4055
Epoprostenol	0.5 mg	IV	J1325
Eptifibatide, injection	5 mg	IM, IV	J1327
Ergonovine maleate	up to 0.2 mg	IM, IV	J1330
Ertapenem sodium	500 mg		J1335
Erythromycin lactobionate	500 mg	IV	J1364
Estra-D, *see* Depo-estradiol cypionate			
Estra-L 20, *see* Estradiol valerate			
Estra-L 40, *see* Estradiol valerate			
Estra-Testrin, *see* Testosterone enanthate and estradiol valerate			
Estradiol Cypionate, *see* Depo-estradiol cypionate			
Estradiol L.A., *see* Estradiol valerate			
Estradiol L.A. 20, *see* Estradiol valerate			
Estradiol L.A. 40, *see* Estradiol valerate			
Estradiol valerate	up to 10 mg	IM	J1380
	up to 20 mg	IM	J1390
	up to 40 mg	IM	J0970
Estro-Cyp, *see* Depo-estradiol cypionate			
Estrogen, conjugated	per 25 mg	IV, IM	J1410
Estroject L.A., *see* Depo-estradiol cypionate			
Estrone	per 1 mg	IM	J1435
Estrone 5, *see* Estrone			
Estrone Aqueous, *see* Estrone			
Estronol, *see* Estrone			
Estronol-L.A., *see* Depo-estradiol cypionate			
Etanercept, injection	25 mg	IM, IV	J1438
Ethanolamine	100 mg		Q2007
Ethyol, *see* Amifostine			
Etidronate disodium	per 300 mg	IV	J1436
Etopophos, *see* Etoposide			
Etoposide	10 mg	IV	J9181
	100 mg	IV	J9182
Etoposide, oral	50 mg	ORAL	J8560
Everone, *see* Testosterone enanthate			
F			
Factor VIIa (coagulation factor, recombinant)	per mg	IV	Q0187
Factor VIII (anti-hemophilic factor, human)	per IU	IV	J7190
Factor VIII (anti-hemophilic factor, porcine)	per IU	IV	J7191
Factor VIII, (anti-hemophilic factor, recombinant)	per IU	IV	J7192
Factor IX (anti-hemophilic factor, purified, non-recombinant)	per IU	IV	Q0160
Factor IX (anti-hemophilic factor, recombinant)	per IU	IV	Q0161
Factor IX, complex	per IU	IV	J7194
Factors, other hemophilia clotting	per IU	IV	J7196
Factrel, *see* Gonadorelin HCl			
Feiba VH Immuno, *see* Factors, other hemophilia clotting			
Fentanyl citrate	0.1 mg	IM, IV	J3010
Ferrlecit, *see* Sodium ferric-gluconate complex in sucrose injection			
Filgrastim (G-CSF)	300 mcg	SC, IV	J1440
	480 mcg	SC, IV	J1441
Flexoject, *see* Orphenadrine citrate			
Flexon, *see* Orphenadrine citrate			
Flolan, *see* Epoprostenol			
Floxuridine	500 mg	IV	J9200
Fluconazole	200 mg	IV	J1450
Fludara, *see* Fludarabine phosphate			
Fludarabine phosphate	50 mg	IV	J9185
Flunisolide inhalation solution, unit dose form	per mg	INH	J7641
Fluorouracil	500 mg	IV	J9190
Folex, *see* Methotrexate sodium			
Folex PFS, *see* Methotrexate sodium			
Follutein, *see* Chorionic gonadotropin			
Fomepizole	1.5 mg		Q2008
Fomivirsen sodium	1.65 mg	Intraocular	J1452
Fondaparinux sodium	0.5 mg		J1652
Fortaz, *see* Ceftazidime			
Foscarnet sodium	per 1,000 mg	IV	J1455
Foscavir, *see* Foscarnet sodium			
Fosphenytoin	50 mg		Q2009
FUDR, *see* Floxuridine			
Fulvestrant	25 mg		J9395
Fungizone Intravenous, *see* Amphotericin B			
Furomide M.D., *see* Furosemide			
Furosemide	up to 20 mg	IM, IV	J1940
G			
Gamastan, *see* Gamma globulin and Immune globulin			
Gamma globulin	1 cc	IM	J1460
	2 cc	IM	J1470
	3 cc	IM	J1480
	4 cc	IM	J1490
	5 cc	IM	J1500
	6 cc	IM	J1510
	7 cc	IM	J1520
	8 cc	IM	J1530
	9 cc	IM	J1540
	10 cc	IM	J1550
	over 10 cc	IM	J1560
Gammar, *see* Gamma globulin and immune globulin			
Gammar-IV, *see* Immune globulin intravenous (human)			
Gamulin RH, *see* Rho(D) immune globulin			
Ganciclovir, implant	4.5 mg	OTH	J7310

Ganciclovir sodium	500 mg	IV	J1570
Garamycin, gentamicin	up to 80 mg	IM, IV	J1580
Gatifloxacin	10 mg	IV	J1590
Gemcitabine HCl	200 mg	IV	J9201
Gemtuzumab ozogamicin	5 mg	IV	J9300
Gemzar, *see* Gemcitabine HCl			
Gentamicin Sulfate, *see* Garamycin, gentamicin			
Gentran, *see* Dextran 40			
Gentran 75, *see* Dextran 75			
Gesterol 50, *see* Progesterone			
Glatiramer acetate	20 mg		J1595
Glucagon HCl	per 1 mg	SC, IM, IV	J1610
Glukor, *see* Chorionic gonadotropin			
Glycopyrrolate, concentrated form	per 1 mg	INH	J7642
Glycopyrrolate, unit dose form	per 1 mg	INH	J7643
Gold sodium thiomalate	up to 50 mg	IM	J1600
Gonadorelin HCl	per 100 mcg	SC, IV	J1620
Gonic, *see* Chorionic gonadotropin			
Goserelin acetate implant	per 3.6 mg	SC	J9202
Granisetron HCl, injection	100 mcg	IV	J1626
Granisetron HCl, oral	1 mg	ORAL	Q0166
Gynogen L.A. "A10," *see* Estradiol valerate			
Gynogen L.A. "A20," *see* Estradiol valerate			
Gynogen L.A. "A40," *see* Estradiol valerate			
H			
Haldol, *see* Haloperidol			
Haloperidol	up to 5 mg	IM, IV	J1630
Haloperidol decanoate	per 50 mg	IM	J1631
Hectorol, *see* Doxercalciferol			
Hemin	per 1 mg		Q2011
Hemofil M, *see* Factor VIII			
Hemophilia clotting factors (e.g., anti-inhibitors)	per IU	IV	J7198
Hemophilia clotting factors, NOC	per IU	IV	J7199
Hepatitis B vaccine			Q3021-Q3023
Hep-Lock, *see* Heparin sodium (heparin lock flush)			
Heparin sodium	1,000 units	IV, SC	J1644
Heparin sodium (heparin lock flush)	10 units	IV	J1642
Herceptin, *see* Trastuzumab			
Hexadrol Phosphate, *see* Dexamethasone sodium phosphate			
Histaject, *see* Brompheniramine maleate			
Histerone 50, *see* Testosterone suspension			
Histerone 100, *see* Testosterone suspension			
Histrelin acetate	10 mg		Q2020
Hyalgan, *see* Sodium hyaluronate			
Hyaluronidase	up to 150 units	SC, IV	J3470
Hyate:C, *see* Factor VIII (anti-hemophilic factor, porcine)			
Hybolin Improved, *see* Nandrolone phenpropionate			
Hybolin Decanoate, *see* Nandrolone decanoate			
Hycamtin, *see* Topotecan			

Hydralazine HCl	up to 20 mg	IV, IM	J0360
Hydrate, *see* Dimenhydrinate			
Hydrochlorides of opium alkaloids	up to 20 mg	IM, SC	J2480
Hydrocortisone acetate	up to 25 mg	IV, IM, SC	J1700
Hydrocortisone sodium phosphate	up to 50 mg	IV, IM, SC	J1710
Hydrocortisone succinate sodium	up to 100 mg	IV, IM, SC	J1720
Hydrocortone Acetate, *see* Hydrocortisone acetate			
Hydrocortone Phosphate, *see* Hydrocortisone sodium phosphate			
Hydromorphone HCl	up to 4 mg	SC, IM, IV	J1170
Hydroxyzine HCl	up to 25 mg	IM	J3410
Hydroxyzine pamoate	25 mg	ORAL	Q0177
	50 mg	ORAL	Q0178
Hylan G-F 20	16 mg	OTH	J7320
Hyoscyamine sulfate	up to 0.25 mg	SC, IM, IV	J1980
Hyperstat IV, *see* Diazoxide			
Hyper-Tet, *see* Tetanus immune globulin, human			
HypRho-D, *see* Rho(D) immune globulin			
Hyrexin-50, *see* Diphenhydramine HCl			
Hyzine-50, *see* Hydroxyzine HCl			
I			
Ibutilide fumarate	1 mg	IV	J1742
Idamycin, *see* Idarubicin HCl			
Idarubicin HCl	5 mg	IV	J9211
Ifex, *see* Ifosfamide			
Ifosfamide	per 1 g	IV	J9208
Ilotycin, *see* Erythromycin gluceptate			
Imferon, *see* Iron dextran			
Imiglucerase	per unit	IV	J1785
Imitrex, *see* Sumatriptan succinate			
Immune globulin	per 500 mg	IV	J1561
Immune globulin, anti-thymocyte globulin	25 mg	IV	J7504
Immune globulin intravenous	1 gm	IV	J1563
	10 mg	IV	J1564
Immunosuppressive drug, not otherwise classified			J7599
Imuran, *see* Azathioprine			
Inapsine, *see* Droperidol			
Inderal, *see* Propranolol HCl			
Infed, *see* Iron dextran-			
Infergen, *see* Interferon alfa-1			
Infliximab, injection	10 mg	IM, IV	J1745
Innohep, *see* Tinzarparin			
Innovar, *see* Droperidol with fentanyl citrate			
Insulin	5 units	SC	J1815
	50 units	SC	J1817
Insulin lispro	up to 50 units	SC	K0548
Intal, *see* Cromolyn sodium or Cromolyn sodium, compounded			
Integrilin, injection, *see* Eptifibatide			
Interferon alphacon-1, recombinant	1 mcg	SC	J9212

Interferon alfa-2a, recombinant	3 million units	SC, IM	J9213
Interferon alfa-2b, recombinant	1 million units	SC, IM	J9214
Interferon alfa-n3 (human leukocyte derived)	250,000 IU	IM	J9215
Interferon beta-1a	33 mcg	IM	J1825
	11 mcg	IM	Q3025
	11 mcg	SC	Q3026
Interferon beta-1b	0.25 mg	SC	J1830
Interferon gamma-1b	3 million units	SC	J9216
Intrauterine copper contraceptive, *see* Copper contraceptive, intrauterine			
Ipratropium bromide, unit dose form	per mg	INH	J7644
Irinotecan	20 mg	IV	J9206
Iron dextran	50 mg	IV, IM	J1750
Iron sucrose	1 mg	IV	J1756
Irrigation solution for Tx of bladder calculi	per 50 ml	OTH	Q2004
Isocaine HCl, *see* Mepivacaine			
Isoetharine HCl, concentrated form	per mg	INH	J7648
Isoetharine HCl, unit dose form	per mg	INH	J7649
Isoproterenol HCl, concentrated form	per mg	INH	J7658
Isoproterenol HCl, unit dose form	per mg	INH	J7659
Isuprel, *see* Isoproterenol HCl			
Itraconazole	50 mg	IV	J1835

J

Jenamicin, *see* Garamycin, gentamicin			

K

Kabikinase, *see* Streptokinase			
Kaleinate, *see* Calcium gluconate			
Kanamycin sulfate	up to 75 mg	IM, IV	J1850
Kanamycin sulfate	up to 500 mg	IM, IV	J1840
Kantrex, *see* Kanamycin sulfate			
Keflin, *see* Cephalothin sodium			
Kefurox, *see* Cufuroxime sodium			
Kefzol, *see* Cefazolin sodium			
Kenaject-40, *see* Triamcinolone acetonide			
Kenalog-10, *see* Triamcinolone acetonide			
Kenalog-40, *see* Triamcinolone acetonide			
Kestrone 5, *see* Estrone			
Ketorolac tromethamine	per 15 mg	IM, IV	J1885
Key-Pred 25, *see* Prednisolone acetate			
Key-Pred 50, *see* Prednisolone acetate			
Key-Pred-SP, *see* Prednisolone sodium phosphate			
K-Flex, *see* Orphenadrine citrate			
Klebcil, *see* Kanamycin sulfate			
Konate-HP, *see* Factor VIII			
Kogenate, *see* Factor VIII			
Konakion, *see* Vitamin K, phytonadione, etc.			

Konyne 80, *see* Factor IX, complex			
Kutapressin	up to 2 ml	SC, IM	J1910
Kytril, *see* Granisetron HCl			

L

L.A.E. 20, *see* Estradiol valerate			
Laetrile, Amygdalin, vitamin B-17			J3570
Lanoxin, *see* Digoxin			
Largon, *see* Propiomazine HCl			
Lasix, *see* Furosemide			
L-Caine, *see* Lidocaine HCl			
Lepirudin	50 mg		Q2021
Leucovorin calcium	per 50 mg	IM, IV	J0640
Leukine, *see* Sargramostim (GM-CSF)			
Leuprolide acetate (for depot suspension)	3.75 mg	IM	J1950
	7.5 mg	IM	J9217
Leuprolide acetate	per 1 mg	IM	J9218
Leuprolide acetate implant	65 mg		J9219
Leustatin, *see* Cladribine			
Levalbuterol HCl, concentrated form	0.5 mg	INH	J7618
Levalbuterol HC1, unit form	0.5 mg	INH	J7619
Levaquin I.U., *see* Levofloxacin			
Levocarnitine	per 1 gm	IV	J1955
Levo-Dromoran, *see* Levorphanol tartrate			
Levofloxacin	250 mg	IV	J1956
Levonorgestrel releasing intrauterine contraceptive	52 mg	OTH	J7302
Levorphanol tartrate	up to 2 mg	SC, IV	J1960
Levsin, *see* Hyoscyamine sulfate			
Levulan Kerastick, *see* Aminolevulinic acid HC1			
Librium, *see* Chlordiazepoxide HCl			
Lidocaine HCl	10 mg	IV	J2001
Lidoject-1, *see* Lidocaine HCl			
Lidoject-2, *see* Lidocaine HCl			
Lincocin, *see* Lincomycin HCl			
Lincomycin HCl	up to 300 mg	IV	J2010
Linezolid	200 mg	IV	J2020
Liquaemin Sodium, *see* Heparin sodium			
Lioresal, *see* Baclofen			
LMD (10%), *see* Dextran 40			
Lovenox, *see* Enoxaparin sodium			
Lorazepam	2 mg	IM, IV	J2060
Lufyllin, *see* Dyphylline			
Luminal Sodium, *see* Phenobarbital sodium			
Lunelle, *see* Medroxyprogesterone acetate/estradiol cypionate			
Lupron, *see* Leuprolide acetate			
Lymphocyte immune globulin			
anti-thymocyte globulin, equine	250 mg	IV	J7504
anti-thymocyte, globulin, rabbit	25 mg	IV	J7511
Lyophilized, *see* Cyclophosphamide, lyophilized			

M

Magnesium sulfate	500 mg		J3475

Mannitol	25% in 50 ml	IV	J2150
Marmine, *see* Dimenhydrinate			
Maxipime, *see* Cefepime hydrochloride			
Mechlorethamine HCl (nitrogen mustard), HN2	10 mg	IV	J9230
Medralone 40, *see* Methylprednisolone acetate			
Medralone 80, *see* Methylprednisolone acetate			
Medrol, *see* Methylprednisolone			
Medroxyprogesterone acetate	50 mg	IM	J1051
	150 mg	IM	J1055
Medroxyprogesterone acetate/estradiol cypionate	5 mg/25 mg	IV	J1056
Mefoxin, *see* Cefoxitin sodium			
Melphalan HCl	50 mg	IV	J9245
Melphalan, oral	2 mg	ORAL	J8600
Menoject LA, *see* Testosterone cypionate and estradiol cypionate			
Mepergan Injection, *see* Meperidine and promethazine HCl			
Meperidine HCl	per 100 mg	IM, IV, SC	J2175
Meperidine and promethazine HCl	up to 50 mg	IM, IV	J2180
Mepivacaine HCL	per 10 ml	VAR	J0670
Meropenem	100 mg		J2185
Mesna	200 mg	IV	J9209
Mesnex, *see* Mesna			
Metaprel, *see* Metaproterenol sulfate			
Metaproterenol sulfate, concentrated form	per 10 mg	INH	J7668
Metaproterenol sulfate, unit dose form	per 10 mg	INH	J7669
Metaraminol bitartrate	per 10 mg	IV, IM, SC	J0380
Metastron, *see* Strontium-89 chloride			
Methadone HCl	up to 10 mg	IM, SC	J1230
Methergine, *see* Methylergonovine maleate			
Methocarbamol	up to 10 ml	IV, IM	J2800
Methotrexate, oral	2.5 mg	ORAL	J8610
Methotrexate sodium	5 mg	IV, IM, IT, IA	J9250
	50 mg	IV, IM, IT, IA	J9260
Methotrexate LPF, *see* Methotrexate sodium			
Methylergonovine maleate	up to 0.2 mg	IM, IV	J2210
Methyldopate HCl	up to 250 mg	IV	J0210
Methylergonovine maleate	up to 0.2 mg		J2210
Methylprednisolone, oral	per 4 mg	ORAL	J7509
Methylprednisolone acetate	20 mg	IM	J1020
	40 mg	IM	J1030
	80 mg	IM	J1040
Methylprednisolone sodium succinate	up to 40 mg	IM, IV	J2920
	up to 125 mg	IM, IV	J2930
Metoclopramide HCl	up to 10 mg	IV	J2765
Miacalcin, *see* Calcitonin-salmon			
Midazolam HCl	per 1 mg	IM, IV	J2250
Milrinone lactate	per 5 mg	IV	J2260
Mirena, *see* Levonorgestrel releasing intrauterine contraceptive			
Mithracin, *see* Plicamycin			
Mitomycin	5 mg	IV	J9280
	20 mg	IV	J9290
	40 mg	IV	J9291
Mitoxantrone HCl	per 5 mg	IV	J9293
Monocid, *see* Cefonicid sodium			
Monoclate-P, *see* Factor VIII			
Monoclonal antibodies, parenteral	5 mg	IV	J7505
Mononine, *see* Factor IX, purified, non-recombinant			
Morphine sulfate	up to 10 mg	IM, IV, SC	J2270
	100 mg	IM, IV, SC	J2271
Morphine sulfate, preservative-free	per 10 mg	IM, IV, SC	J2275
Moxifloxacin	100 mg		J2280
M-Prednisol-40, *see* Methylprednisolone acetate			
M-Prednisol-80, *see* Methylprednisolone acetate			
Mucomyst, *see* Acetylcysteine or Acetylcysteine, compounded			
Mucosol, *see* Acetylcysteine			
Muromonab-CD3	5 mg	IV	J7505
Muse, *see* Alprostadil			
Mustargen, *see* Mechlorethamine HCl			
Mustargen, *see* Mechlorethamine HCl			
Mutamycin, *see* Mitomycin			
Mycophenolate mofetil	250 mg	ORAL	J7517
Myleran, *see* Busulfan			
Mylotarg, *see* Gemtuzumab ozogamicin			
Myobloc, *see* Botulinum toxin type B			
Myochrysine, *see* Gold sodium thiomalate			
Myolin, *see* Orphenadrine citrate			
N			
Nalbuphine HCl	per 10 mg	IM, IV, SC	J2300
Naloxone HCl	per 1 mg	IM, IV, SC	J2310
Nandrobolic L.A., *see* Nandrolone decanoate			
Nandrolone decanoate	up to 50 mg	IM	J2320
	up to 100 mg	IM	J2321
	up to 200 mg	IM	J2322
Narcan, *see* Naloxone HCl			
Naropin, *see* Ropivacaine HCl			
Nasahist B, *see* Brompheniramine maleate			
Nasal vaccine inhalation		INH	J3530
Navane, *see* Thiothixene			
Navelbine, *see* Vinorelbine tartrate			
ND Stat, *see* Brompheniramine maleate			
Nebcin, *see* Tobramycin sulfate			
NebuPent, *see* Pentamidine isethionate			
Nembutal Sodium Solution, *see* Pentobarbital sodium			
Neocyten, *see* Orphenadrine citrate			
Neo-Durabolic, *see* Nandrolone decanoate			
Neoquess, *see* Dicyclomine HCl			
Neosar, *see* Cyclophosphamide			
Neostigmine methylsulfate	up to 0.5 mg	IM, IV, SC	J2710

Neo-Synephrine, *see* Phenylephrine HCl

Nervocaine 1%, *see* Lidocaine HCl

Nervocaine 2%, *see* Lidocaine HCl

Nesacaine, *see* Chloroprocaine HCl

Nesacaine-MPF, *see* Chloroprocaine HCl

Nesiritide	0.5 mg		J2324

Neumega, *see* Oprelvekin

Neupogen, *see* Filgrastim (G-CSF)

Neutrexin, *see* Trimetrexate glucuronate

Nipent, *see* Pentostatin

Nordryl, *see* Diphenhydramine HCl

Norflex, *see* Orphenadrine citrate

Norzine, *see* Thiethylperazine maleate

Not otherwise classified drugs			J3490
Not otherwise classified drugs	other than INH, administered thru DME		J7799
Not otherwise classified drugs	INH, administered thru DME		J7699
Not otherwise classified drugs, anti-neoplastic	—		J9999
Not otherwise classified drugs, chemotherapeutic		ORAL	J8999
Not otherwise classified drugs, immunosuppressive	—		J7599
Not otherwise classified drugs, nonchemotherapeutic		ORAL	J8499

Novantrone, *see* Mitoxantrone HCl

Novo Seven, *see* Factor VIIa

NPH, *see* Insulin

Nubain, *see* Nalbuphine HCl

Nulicaine, *see* Lidocaine HCl

Numorphan, *see* Oxymorphone HCl

Numorphan H.P., *see* Oxymorphone HCl

O

Octreotide Acetate, injection	1 mg	IM	J2352
	25 mcg	IV, SQ	J2354

Oculinum, *see* Botulinum toxin type A

Odansetron HCl	1 mg	IV	J2405

O-Flex, *see* Orphenadrine citrate

Omnipen-N, *see* Ampicillin

Oncaspar, *see* Pegaspargase

Oncovin, *see* Vincristine sulfate

Ondansetron HCl, oral	8 mg	ORAL	Q0179
Oprelvekin	5 mg	SC	J2355

Oraminic II, *see* Brompheniramine maleate

Ormazine, *see* Chlorpromazine HCl

Orphenadrine citrate	up to 60 mg	IV, IM	J2360

Orphenate, *see* Orphenadrine citrate

Or-Tyl, *see* Dicyclomine

Oxacillin sodium	up to 250 mg	IM, IV	J2700
Oxaliplatin	0.5 mg		J9263
Oxymorphone HCl	up to 1 mg	IV, SC, IM	J2410
Oxytetracycline HCl	up to 50 mg	IM	J2460
Oxytocin	up to 10 units	IV, IM	J2590

P

Paclitaxel	30 mg	IV	J9265
Pamidronate disodium	per 30 mg	IV	J2430
Papaverine HCl	up to 60 mg	IV, IM	J2440

Paragard T 380 A, *see* Copper contraceptive, intrauterine

Paraplatin, *see* Carboplatin

Paricalcitol, injection	1 mcg	IV, IM	J2501
Pegademase bovine	25 IU		Q2012
Pegaspargase	per single dose vial	IM, IV	J9266
Pegfilgrastim	6 mg		J2505
Penicillin G benzathine	up to 600,000 units	IM	J0560
	up to 1,200,000 units	IM	J0570
	up to 2,400,000 units	IM	J0580
Penicillin G benzathine and penicillin G procaine	up to 600,000 units	IM	J0530
	up to 1,200,000 units	IM	J0540
	up to 2,400,000 units	IM	J0550
Penicillin G potassium	up to 600,000 units	IM, IV	J2540
Penicillin G procaine, aqueous	up to 600,000 units	IM, IV	J2510
Pentamidine isethionate	per 300 mg	INH	J2545
Pentastarch, 10%	per 100 ml		Q2013
Pentazocine HCl	up to 30 mg	IM, SC, IV	J3070
Pentobarbital sodium	per 50 mg	IM, IV, OTH	J2515
Pentostatin	per 10 mg	IV	J9268

Permapen, *see* Penicillin G benzathine

Perphenazine, injection	up to 5 mg	IM, IV	J3310
Perphenazine, tablets	4 mg	ORAL	Q0175
	8 mg	ORAL	Q0176

Persantine IV, *see* Dipyridamole

Pfizerpen, *see* Penicillin G potassium

Pfizerpen A.S., *see* Penicillin G procaine

Phenazine 25, *see* Promethazine HCl

Phenazine 50, *see* Promethazine HCl

Phenergan, *see* Promethazine HCl

Phenobarbital sodium	up to 120 mg	IM, IV	J2560
Phentolamine mesylate	up to 5 mg	IM, IV	J2760
Phenylephrine HCl	up to 1 ml	SC, IM, IV	J2370
Phenytoin sodium	per 50 mg	IM, IV	J1165

Photofrin, *see* Porfimer sodium

Phytonadione (Vitamin K)	per 1 mg	IM, SC, IV	J3430
Piperacillin/Tazobactam Sodium, injection	1.125 g	IV	J2543

Pitocin, *see* Oxytocin

Plantinol AQ, *see* Cisplatin

Plas + SD, *see* Plasma, pooled multiple donor			
Plasma, cryoprecipitate reduced	each unit		P9044
Plasma, pooled multiple donor, frozen, each unit		IV	P9023
Platinol, *see* Cisplatin			
Plicamycin	2,500 mcg	IV	J9270
Polocaine, *see* Mepivacaine			
Polycillin-N, *see* Ampicillin			
Porfimer Sodium	75 mg	IV	J9600
Potassium chloride	per 2 mEq	IV	J3480
Pralidoxime chloride	up to 1 g	IV, IM, SC	J2730
Predalone-50, *see* Prednisolone acetate			
Predcor-25, *see* Prednisolone acetate			
Predcor-50, *see* Prednisolone acetate			
Predicort-50, *see* Prednisolone acetate			
Prednisone	per 5 mg	ORAL	J7506
Prednisolone, oral	5 mg	ORAL	J7510
Prednisolone acetate	up to 1 ml	IM	J2650
Predoject-50, *see* Prednisolone acetate			
Pregnyl, *see* Chorionic gonadotropin			
Premarin Intravenous, *see* Estrogen, conjugated			
Prescription, chemotherapeutic, not otherwise specified		ORAL	J8999
Prescription, nonchemotherapeutic, not otherwise specified		ORAL	J8499
Primacor, *see* Milrinone lactate			
Primaxin I.M., *see* Cilastatin sodium, imipenem			
Primaxin I.V., *see* Cilastatin sodium, imipenem			
Priscoline HCl, *see* Tolazoline HCl			
Pro-Depo, *see* Hydroxyprogesterone Caproate			
Procainamide HCl	up to 1 g	IM, IV	J2690
Prochlorperazine	up to 10 mg	IM, IV	J0780
Prochlorperazine maleate, oral	5 mg	ORAL	Q0164
	10 mg	ORAL	Q0165
Profasi HP, *see* Chorionic gonadotropin			
Profilnine Heat-Treated, *see* Factor IX			
Progestaject, *see* Progesterone			
Progesterone	per 50 mg		J2675
Prograf, *see* Tacrolimus, oral or parenteral			
Prokine, *see* Sargramostim (GM-CSF)			
Prolastin, *see* Alpha 1-proteinase inhibitor (human)			
Proleukin, *see* Aldesleukin			
Prolixin Decanoate, *see* Fluphenazine decanoate			
Promazine HCl	up to 25 mg	IM	J2950
Promethazine HCl, injection	up to 50 mg	IM, IV	J2550
Promethazine HCl, oral	12.5 mg	ORAL	Q0169
	25 mg	ORAL	Q0170
Pronestyl, *see* Procainamide HCl			
Proplex T, *see* Factor IX			
Proplex SX-T, *see* Factor IX			
Propranolol HCl	up to 1 mg	IV	J1800

Prorex-25, *see* Promethazine HCl			
Prorex-50, *see* Promethazine HCl			
Prostaphlin, *see* Procainamide HCl			
Prostigmin, *see* Neostigmine methylsulfate			
Protamine sulfate	per 10 mg	IV	J2720
Protirelin	per 250 mcg	IV	J2725
Prothazine, *see* Promethazine HCl			
Protopam Chloride, *see* Pralidoxime chloride			
Proventil, *see* Albuterol sulfate, compounded			
Prozine-50, *see* Promazine HCl			
Pulmicort Respules, *see* Budesonide			
Pyridoxine HCl	100 mg		J3415
Q			
Quelicin, *see* Succinylcholine chloride			
Quinupristin/dalfopristin	500 mg (150/350)	IV	J2770
R			
Ranitidine HCl, injection	25 mg	IV, IM	J2780
Rapamune, *see* Sirolimus			
Rasburicase	0.5 mg		J2783
Recombinate, *see* Factor VIII			
Redisol, *see* Vitamin B-12 cyanocobalamin			
Regitine, *see* Phentolamine mesylate			
Reglan, *see* Metoclopramide HCl			
Regular, *see* Insulin			
Relefact TRH, *see* Protirelin			
Remicade, *see* Infliximab, injection			
Reo Pro, *see* Abciximab			
Rep-Pred 40, *see* Methylprednisolone acetate			
Rep-Pred 80, *see* Methylprednisolone acetate			
RespiGam, *see* Respiratory Syncytial Virus			
Respiratory Syncytial Virus Immune-globulin	50 mg	IV	J1565
Retavase, *see* Reteplase			
Reteplase	18.8 mg	IV	J2993
Retrovir, *see* Zidovudine			
Rheomacrodex, *see* Dextran 40			
Rhesonativ, *see* Rho(D) immune globulin, human			
Rheumatrex Dose Pack, *see* Methotrexate, oral			
Rho(D) immune globulin, human	1 dose package, 300 mcg	IM	J2790
	1 dose package, 50 mcg	IM	J2798
Rho(D)immune globulin (human), solvent detergent	100 IU	IV	J2792
RhoGAM, *see* Rho(D) immune globulin, human			
Ringer's lactate infusion	up to 1,000 cc	IV	J7120

Rituxan, *see* Rituximab

Rituximab	100 mg	IV	J9310

Robaxin, *see* Methocarbamol

Rocephin, *see* Ceftriaxone sodium

Roferon-A, *see* Interferon alfa-2A, recombinant

Ropivacaine HCl	1 mg		J2795

Rubex, *see* Doxorubicin HCl

Rubramin PC, *see* Vitamin B-12 cyanocobalamin

S

Saline solution	5% dextrose, 500 ml	IV	J7042
	infusion, 250 cc	IV	J7050
	infusion, 1,000 cc	IV	J7030
Saline solution, sterile	500 ml = 1 unit	IV, OTH	J7040
	up to 5 cc	IV, OTH	J7051

Sandimmune, *see* Cyclosporine

Sandoglobulin, *see* Immune globulin intravenous (human)

Sandostatin Lar Depot, *see* Octreotide

Sargramostim (GM-CSF)	50 mcg	IV	J2820
Secobarbital sodium	up to 250 mg	IM, IV	J2860

Seconal, *see* Secobarbital sodium

Selestoject, *see* Betamethasone sodium phosphate

Sermorelin acetate	0.5 mg		Q2014
Sinusol-B, *see* Brompheniramine maleate	per 2 ml	IV	J2912
Sirolimus	1 mg	ORAL	J7520
Sodium chloride, 0.9%	per 2 ml		J2912
Sodium ferricgluconate in sucrose	12.5 mg		J2916
Sodium hyaluronate	5 mg	OTH	J7316

Solganal, *see* Aurothioglucose

Solu-Cortef, *see* Hydrocortisone sodium phosphate			J1710

Solu-Medrol, *see* Methylprednisolone sodium succinate

Solurex, *see* Dexamethasone sodium phosphate

Solurex LA, *see* Dexamethasone acetate

Somatrem	1 mg		J2940
Somatropin	1 mg		J2941

Sparine, *see* Promazine HCl

Spasmoject, *see* Dicyclomine HCl

Spectinomycin HCl	up to 2 g	IM	J3320

Sporanox, *see* Itraconazole

Staphcillin, *see* Methicillin sodium

Stilphostrol, *see* Diethylstilbestrol diphosphate

Streptase, *see* Streptokinase

Streptokinase	per 250,000 IU	IV	J2995

Streptomycin Sulfate, *see* Streptomycin

Streptomycin	up to 1 g	IM	J3000
Streptozocin	1 gm	IV	J9320
Strontium-89 chloride	per 10 ml	IV	J3005

Sublimaze, *see* Fentanyl citrate

Succinylcholine chloride	up to 20 mg	IV, IM	J0330
Sumatriptan succinate	6 mg	SC	J3030

Supartz *see* Sodium hyaluronate

Surostrin, *see* Succinycholine chloride

Sus-Phrine, *see* Adrenalin, epinephrine

Synercid, *see* Quinupristin/dalfopristin

Synkavite, *see* Vitamin K, phytonadione, etc.

Syntocinon, *see* Oxytocin

Synvisc, *see* Hylan G-F 20

Sytobex, *see* Vitamin B-12 cyanocobalamin

T

Tacrolimus, oral	per 1 mg	ORAL	J7507
Tacrolimus, parenteral	5 mg		J7515

Talwin, *see* Pentazocine HCl

Taractan, *see* Chlorprothixene

Taxol, *see* Paclitaxel

Taxotere, *see* Docetaxel

Tazidime, *see* Ceftazidime

Technetium TC Sestamibi	per dose		A9500

TEEV, *see* Testosterone enanthate and estradiol valerate

Temozolomide	5 mg	ORAL	J8700
Tenecteplase	50 mg		J3100
Teniposide	50 mg		Q2017

Tequin, *see* Gatifloxacin

Terbutaline sulfate	up to 1 mg	SC, IV	J3105
Terbutaline sulfate, concentrated form	per 1 mg	INH	J7680
Terbutaline sulfate, unit dose form	per 1 mg	INH	J7681

Terramycin IM, *see* Oxytetracycline HCl

Testa-C, *see* Testosterone cypionate

Testadiate, *see* Testosterone enanthate and estradiol valerate

Testadiate-Depo, *see* Testosterone cypionate

Testaject-LA, *see* Testosterone cypionate

Testaqua, *see* Testosterone suspension

Test-Estro Cypionates, *see* Testosterone cypionate and estradiol cypionate

Test-Estro-C, *see* Testosterone cypionate and estradiol cypionate

Testex, *see* Testosterone propionate

Testoject-50, *see* Testosterone suspension

Testoject-LA, *see* Testosterone cypionate

Testone LA 200, *see* Testosterone enanthate

Testone LA 100, *see* Testosterone enanthate

Testosterone Aqueous, *see* Testosterone suspension

Testosterone enanthate and estradiol valerate	up to 1 cc	IM	J0900
Testosterone enanthate	up to 100 mg	IM	J3120
	up to 200 mg	IM	J3130

Testosterone cypionate	up to 100 mg	IM	J1070
	1 cc, 200 mg	IM	J1080
Testosterone cypionate and estradiol cypionate	up to 1 ml	IM	J1060
Testosterone propionate	up to 100 mg	IM	J3150
Testosterone suspension	up to 50 mg	IM	J3140
Testradiol 90/4, see Testosterone enanthate and estradiol valerate			
Testrin PA, see Testosterone enanthate			
Tetanus immune globulin, human	up to 250 units	IM	J1670
Tetracycline	up to 250 mg	IM, IV	J0120
Thallous Chloride TL 201	per MCI		A9505
Theelin Aqueous, see Estrone			
Theophylline	per 40 mg	IV	J2810
TheraCys, see BCG live			
Thiamine HCl	100 mg		J3411
Thiethylperazine maleate, injection	up to 10 mg	IM	J3280
Thiethylperazine maleate, oral	10 mg	ORAL	Q0174
Thiotepa	15 mg	IV	J9340
Thorazine, see Chlorpromazine HCl			
Thymoglobulin, see Immune globulin, anti-thymocyte			
Thypinone, see Protirelin			
Thyrogen, see Thyrotropin Alfa			
Thyrotropin Alpha, injection	0.9 mg	IM, SC	J3240
Tice BCG, see BCG live			
Ticon, see Trimethobenzamide HCl			
Tigan, see Trimethobenzamide HCl			
Tiject-20, see Trimethobenzamide HCl			
Tinzarparin	1000 IU	SC	J1655
Tirofiban hydrochloride, injection	12.5 mg	IM, IV	J3245
TNKase, see, Tenecteplase			
Tobi, see Tobramycin, inhalation solution			
Tobramycin, inhalation solution	300 mg	INH	J7682
Tobramycin sulfate	up to 80 mg	IM, IV	J3260
Tofranil, see Imipramine HCl			
Tolazoline HCl	up to 25 mg	IV	J2670
Topotecan	4 mg	IV	J9350
Toradol, see Ketorolac tromethamine			
Torecan, see Thiethylperazine maleate			
Tornalate, see Bitolterol mesylate			
Torsemide	10 mg/ml	IV	J3265
Totacillin-N, see Ampicillin			
Trastuzumab	10 mg	ORAL	J9355
Treprostinil	1 mg		Q4077
Tri-Kort, see Triamcinolone acetonide			
Triam-A, see Triamcinolone acetonide			
Triamcinolone, concentrated form	per 1 mg	INH	J7683
Triamcinolone, unit dose	per 1 mg	INH	J7684
Triamcinolone acetonide	per 10 mg	IM	J3301
Triamcinolone diacetate	per 5 mg	IM	J3302
Triamcinolone hexacetonide	per 5 mg	VAR	J3303

Triflupromazine HCl	up to 20 mg	IM, IV	J3400
Trilafon, see Perphenazine			
Trilog, see Triamcinolone acetonide			
Trilone, see Triamcinolone diacetate			
Trimethobenzamide HCl, injection	up to 200 mg	IM	J3250
Trimethobenzamide HCl, oral	250 mg	ORAL	Q0173
Trimetrexate glucuronate	per 25 mg	IV	J3305
Triptorelin Pamoate	3.75 mg		J3315
Trisenox, see Arsenic trioxide			
Trobicin, see Spectinomycin HCl			
Trovan, see Alatrofloxacin mesylate			
U			
Ultrazine-10, see Prochlorperazine			
Unasyn, see Ampicillin sodium/sulbactam sodium			
Unclassified drugs (see also Not otherwise classified)			J3490
Unspecified oral antiemetic			Q0181
Urea	up to 40 gm	IV	J3350
Ureaphil, see Urea			
Urecholine, see Bethanechol chloride			
Urofollitropin	75 IU		Q2018
Urokinase	5,000 IU vial	IV	J3364
	250,000 IU vial	IV	J3365
V			
V-Gan 25, see Promethazine HCl			
V-Gan 50, see Promethazine HCl			
Valergen 10, see Estradiol valerate			
Valergen 20, see Estradiol valerate			
Valergen 40, see Estradiol valerate			
Valertest No. 1, see Testosterone enanthate and estradiol valerate			
Valertest No. 2, see Testosterone enanthate and estradiol valerate			
Valium, see Diazepam			
Valrubicin, intravesical	200 mg	OTH	J9357
Valstar, see Valrubicin			
Vancocin, see Vancomycin HCl			
Vancoled, see Vancomycin HCl			
Vancomycin HCl	up to 500 mg	IV, IM	J3370
Vasoxyl, see Methoxamine HCl			
Velban, see Vinblastine sulfate			
Velsar, see Vinblastine sulfate			
Venofer, see Iron sucrose			
Ventolin, see Albuterol sulfate			
VePesid, see Etoposide and Etoposide, oral			
Versed, see Midazolam HCl			
Verteporfin	15 mg	IV	J3395

Vesprin, *see* Triflupromazine HCl

Viadur, *see* Leuprolide acetate implant

Vinblastine sulfate	1 mg	IV	J9360

Vincasar PFS, *see* Vincristine sulfate

Vincristine sulfate	1 mg	IV	J9370
	2 mg	IV	J9375
	5 mg	IV	J9380
Vinorelbine tartrate	per 10 mg	IV	J9390

Vistaject-25, *see* Hydroxyzine HCl

Vistaril, *see* Hydroxyzine HCl

Vistide, *see* Cidofovir

Visudyne, *see* Verteporfin

Vitamin K, phytonadione, menadione, menadiol sodium diphosphate	per 1 mg	IM, SC, IV	J3430
Vitamin B-12 cyanocobalamin	up to 1,000 mcg	IM, SC	J3420
Von Willebrand factor complex, human	per IU	IV	Q2022
Voriconazole	10 mg		J3465

W

Wehamine, *see* Dimenhydrinate

Wehdryl, *see* Diphenhydramine HCl

Wellcovorin, *see* Leucovorin calcium

Win Rho SD, *see* Rho(D)immune globulin (human), solvent detergent

Wyamine Sulfate, *see* Mephentermine sulfate

Wycillin, *see* Penicillin G procaine

Wydase, *see* Hyaluronidase

X

Xeloda, *see* Capecitabine

Xopenex, *see* Albuterol

Xylocaine HCl, *see* Lidocaine HCl

Z

Zanosar, *see* Streptozocin

Zantac, *see* Ranitidine HCl-Zemplar, *see* Paricalcitol

Zenapax, *see* Daclizumab

Zetran, *see* Diazepam

Zidovudine	10 mg	IV	J3485

Zinacef, *see* Cefuroxime sodium

Ziprasidone Mesylate	10 mg		J3486

Zithromax, *see* Azithromycin dihydrate

Zithromax I.V., *see* Azithromycin, injection

Zofran, *see* Ondansetron HCl

Zoladex, *see* Goserelin acetate implant

Zoledronic Acid			J3487

Zolicef, *see* Cefazolin sodium

Zosyn, *see* Piperacillin

A

Abciximab, J0130
Abdomen
  dressing holder/binder, A4462
  pad, low profile, L1270
  supports, pendulous, L0920, L0930
Abduction control, each, L2624
Abduction rotation bar, foot, L3140–
  L3170
Absorption dressing, A6251–A6256
Access system, A4301
Accessories
  ambulation devices, E0153–E0159
  artificial kidney and machine (*see also* ESRD), E1510–E1699
  beds, E0271–E0280, E0300–E0326
  wheelchairs, E0950–E1030, E1050–
    E1298, E2300–E2399, K0001–
    K0109
Acetazolamide sodium, J1120
Acetylcysteine, inhalation solution,
  J7608
Acyclovir, Q4075
Adenosine, J0150, J0152
Adhesive, A4364
  disc or foam pad, A5126
  remover, A4365, A4455
  support, breast prosthesis, A4280
  tape, A4454, A6265
Administrative, Miscellaneous and In-
  vestigational, A9000–A9999
Adrenalin, J0170
Aerosol
  compressor, E0571, E0572
  compressor filter, K0178–K0179
  mask, K0180
AFO, E1815, E1830, L1900–L1990, L4392,
  L4396
Aggrastat, J3245
A-hydroCort, J1710
Air ambulance (*see also* Ambulance),
  A0030, A0040
Air bubble detector, dialysis, E1530
Air fluidized bed, E0194
Air pressure pad/mattress, E0176, E0186,
  E0197
Air travel and nonemergency transpor-
  tation, A0140
Alarm, pressure, dialysis, E1540

Alatrofloxacin mesylate, J0200
Albumin, human, P9041, P9042
Albuterol, all formulations, inhalation
  solution, concentrated, J7618
Albuterol, all formulations, inhalation
  solution, unit dose, J7619
Albuterol, all formulations, inhalation
  solution, J7621
Alcohol, A4244
Alcohol wipes, A4245
Aldesleukin (IL2), J9015
Alefacept, J0215
Alemtuzumab, J9010
Alert device, A9280
Alginate dressing, A6196–A6199
Alglucerase, J0205
Alpha-1-proteinase inhibitor, human,
  J0256
Alprostadil
  injection, J0270
  urethral suppository, J0275
Alteplase recombinant, J2997
Alternating pressure mattress/pad,
  A4640, E0180, E0181, E0277
Ambulance, A0021–A0999
  air, A0430, A0431, A0435, A0436
  disposable supplies, A0382–A0398
  oxygen, A0422
Ambulation device, E0100–E0159
Aminophylline, J0280
Amiodarone HCl, J0282
Amitriptyline HCl, J1320
Ammonia N-13, A9526
Ammonia test paper, A4774
Amniotic membrane, V2790
Amobarbital, J0300
Amphotericin B, J0285
Amphotericin B Lipid Complex, J0287–
  J0289
Ampicillin sodium, J0290
Ampicillin sodium/sulbactam sodium,
  J0295
Amputee
  adapter, wheelchair, E0959
  prosthesis, L5000–L7510, L7520, L7900,
    L8400–L8465
  stump sock, L8470–L8490
  wheelchair, E1170–E1190, E1200,
    K0100
Amygdalin, J3570

Anesthesia
  dialysis, A4735
Anistreplase, J0350
Ankle splint, recumbent, K0126–K0130
Ankle-foot orthosis (AFO), L1900–
  L1990, L2106–L2116, L4392, L4396
Anterior-posterior-lateral orthosis,
  L0520, L0550–L0565, L0700, L0710
Anterior-posterior-lateral-rotary ortho-
  sis, L0340–L0440
Anterior-posterior orthosis, L0320,
  L0330, L0530
Antiemetic, oral, Q0163–Q0181
Anti-hemophilic factor (Factor VIII),
  J7190–J7192
Anti-inhibitors, per I.U., J7198
Anti-neoplastic drug, NOC, J9999
Antithrombin III, J7197
Apnea monitor, E0608
Appliance
  cleaner, A5131
  pneumatic, E0655–E0673
Aprotinin, Q2003
Aqueous
  shunt, L8612
  sterile, J7051
Arbutamine HCl, J0395
Arch support, L3040–L3100
  intralesional, J3302
Arm, wheelchair, E0973
Arsenic trioxide, J9017
Artificial
  kidney machines and accessories (*see
    also* Dialysis), E1510–E1699
  larynx, L8500
Asparaginase, J9020
Assessment
  audiologic, V5008–V5020
  cardiac output, M0302
  speech, V5362–V5364
Astramorph, J2275
Atropine, inhalation solution, concen-
  trated, J7635
Atropine, inhalation solution, unit dose,
  J7636
Atropine sulfate, J0460
Audiologic assessment, V5008–V5020
Aurothioglucose, J2910
Azathioprine, J7500, J7501
Azithromycin injection, J0456

B

Back supports, L0500–L0960
Baclofen, J0475, J0476
Bacterial sensitivity study, P7001
Bag
  drainage, A4357
  irrigation supply, A4398
  urinary, A5112, A4358
Bandage, A4441–A4456
Basiliximab, Q2019
Bathtub
  chair, E0240
  stool or bench, E0245, E0247–E0248
  transfer rail, E0246
  wall rail, E0241, E0242
Battery, K0082–K0087, L7360, L7364–
    L7368
  charger, E1066, K0088, K0089, L7362,
    L7366
  replacement for blood glucose moni-
    tor, A4254
  replacement for TENS, A4630
  ventilator, A4611–A4613
  wheelchair, A4631
BCG live, intravesical, J9031
Beclomethasone inhalation solution,
    J7622
Bed
  air fluidized, E0194
  cradle, any type, E0280
  drainage bag, bottle, A4357, A5102
  hospital, E0250–E0270, E0298–E0301
  pan, E0275, E0276
  rail, E0305, E0310
  safety enclosure frame/canopy, E0316
Below knee suspension sleeve, L5674,
    L5675
Belt
  extremity, E0945
  ostomy, A4367
  pelvic, E0944
  safety, K0031
  wheelchair, E0978, E0979
Bench, bathtub (see also **Bathtub**),
    E0245
Benefix, *see* Factor IX, Q0161

Benesch boot, L3212–L3214
Benztropine, J0515
Betadine, A4246, A4247
Betameth, J0704
Betamethasone inhalation solution,
    J7624
Betamethasone acetate and betametha-
    sone sodium phosphate, J0702
Betamethasone sodium phosphate, J0704
Bethanechol chloride, J0520
Bicarbonate dialysate, A4705
Bifocal, glass or plastic, V2200–V2299
Bilirubin (phototherapy) light, E0202
Binder, A4465
Biofeedback device, E0746
Bioimpedance, electrical, cardiac output,
    M0302
Biperiden lactate, J0190
Bitolterol mesylate, inhalation solution,
    concentrated, J7628
Bitolterol mesylate, inhalation solution,
    unit dose, J7629
Bivalirudin, J0583
Bladder calculi irrigation solution,
    Q2004
Bladder capacity test, ultrasound, G0050
Bleomycin sulfate, J9040
Blood
  Congo red, P2029
  fresh frozen plasma, P9017
  glucose monitor, E0607, E2100, E2101
  glucose test, A4253
  granulocytes, pheresis, P9050
  leak detector, dialysis, E1560
  leukocyte poor, P9016
  mucoprotein, P2038
  platelets, P9019
  platelets, irradiated, P9032
  platelets, leukocytes reduced, P9031
  platelets, leukocytes reduced, irradi-
    ated, P9033
  platelets, pheresis, P9034
  platelets, pheresis, irradiated, P9036
  platelets, pheresis, leukocytes reduced,
    P9035
  platelets, pheresis, leukocytes reduced,
    irradiated, P9037

  pressure monitor, A4660, A4663,
    A4670
  pump, dialysis, E1620
  red blood cells, deglycerolized, P9039
  red blood cells, irradiated, P9038
  red blood cells, leukocytes reduced,
    P9016
  red blood cells, leukocytes reduced, ir-
    radiated, P9040
  red blood cells, washed, P9022
  strips, A4253
  supply, P9010–P9022
  testing supplies, A4770
  tubing, A4750, A4755
Blood collection devices accessory,
    A4257, E0620
Body jacket
  lumbar-sacral orthosis (spinal), L0500–
    L0565, L0600, L0610
  scoliosis, L1300, L1310
Body sock, L0984
Bond or cement, ostomy skin, A4364
Bone mineral density study, G0062,
    G0063
Boot
  pelvic, E0944
  surgical, ambulatory, L3260
Botulinum toxin type A, J0585
Botulinum toxin type B, J0587
Brachytherapy radioelements, Q3001
Brachytherapy source, A9670
Breast prosthesis, L8000–L8035, L8600
Breast prosthesis, adhesive skin sup-
    port, A4280
Breast pump
  accessories, A4281-4286
  electric, any type, E0603
  heavy duty, hospital grade, E0604
  manual, any type, E0602
Breathing circuit, A4618
Brompheniramine maleate, J0945
Budesonide inhalation solution, J7626,
    J7633
Buprenorphine hydrochloride, J0592
Bus, nonemergency transportation,
    A0110
Butorphanol tartrate, J0595

C

Cradle, bed, E0280
Crib, E0300
Cromolyn sodium, inhalation solution, unit dose, J7631
Crutches, E0110–E0118
  accessories, A4635–A4637, K0102
Cryoprecipitate, each unit, P9012
CTLSO, L1000–L1120, L0700, L0710
Cuirass, E0457
Culture sensitivity study, P7001
Cushion, wheelchair, E0962–E0965, E0977
Cyanocobalamin Cobalt CO57, Q3012
Cycler dialysis machine, E1594
Cyclophosphamide, J9070–J9092
Cyclophosphamide, lyophilized, J9093–J9097
Cyclophosphamide, oral, J8530
Cyclosporine, J7502, J7515, J7516
Cylinder tank carrier, K0104
Cytarabine, J9110
Cytarabine liposome, J9098
Cytomegalovirus immune globulin (human), J0850

D

Dacarbazine, J9130, J9140
Daclizumab, J7513
Dactinomycin, J9120
Dalalone, J1100
Dalteparin sodium, J1645
Darbepoetin Alfa, J0880, Q0137, Q4054
Daunorubicin citrate, J9151
Daunorubicin HCl, J9150
DaunoXome, see Daunorubicin Citrate
Decubitus care equipment, E0176–E0199
Deferoxamine mesylate, J0895
Defibrillator, external, E0617, K0606
  battery, K0607
  electrode, K0609
  garment, K0608
Deionizer, water purification system, E1615
Delivery/set-up/dispensing, A9901
Denileukin diftitox, J9160
Depo-estradiol cypionate, J1000
Desmopressin acetate, J2597
Detector, blood leak, dialysis, E1560
Device, water collection (for nebulizer), K0177
Dexamethasone acetate, J1094
Dexamethasone, inhalation solution, concentrated, J7637
Dexamethasone, inhalation solution, unit dose, J7638

Dexamethasone sodium phosphate, J1100
Dextran, J7100
Dextrose
  saline (normal), J7042
  water, J7060, J7070
Dextrostick, A4772
Diagnostic
  radiology services, R0070–R5999
Dialysate concentrate additives, A4765
Dialysate solution, A4700, A4705, A4728
Dialysate testing solution, A4760
Dialysis
  air bubble detector, E1530
  bath conductivity, meter, E1550
  chemicals/antiseptics solution, A4674
  continuous ambulatory peritoneal dialysis (CAPD) supply kit, A4900
  continuous cycling peritoneal dialysis (CCPD) supply kit, A4901
  disposable cycler set, A4671
  equipment, E1510–E1702
  extension line, A4672–A4673
  filter, A4680
  fluid barrier, E1575
  forceps, A4910
  kit, A4820, A4914
  measuring cylinder, A4921
  pressure alarm, E1540
  shunt, A4740
  supplies, A4650–A4927
  thermometer, A4910
  tourniquet, A4910
  unipuncture control system, E1580
  venous pressure clamp, A4918
Dialyzer, A4690
  holder, A4919
Diaper, T1500, T1501
Diaper, adult incontinence garment, A4360
Diazepam, J3360
Diazoxide, J1730
Dicyclomine HCl, J0500
Diethylstilbestrol diphosphate, J9165
Digoxin, J1160
Digoxin immune fab (ovine), Q2006
Dihydroergotamine mesylate, J1110
Dimenhydrinate, J1240
Dimercaprol, J0470
Dimethyl sulfoxide (DMSO), J1212
Diphenhydramine HCl, J1200
Dipyridamole, J1245
Disarticulation
  lower extremities, prosthesis, L5000–L5999
  upper extremities, prosthesis, L6000–L6692
Disposable supplies, ambulance, A0382, A0384, A0392–A0398

Distilled water (for nebulizer), K0182
DMSO, J1212
Dobutamine HCl, J1250
Docetaxel, J9170
Dolasetron mesylate, J1260
Dome and mouthpiece (for nebulizer), A7016
Dopamine HCl, Q4076
Dornase alpha, inhalation solution, unit dose form, J7639
Doxercalciferol, J1270
Doxil, J9001
Doxorubicin HCl, J9000, J9001
Drainage
  bag, A4347, A4357, A4358
  board, postural, E0606
  bottle, A5102
Dressing (see also Bandage), A6020–A6406
  alginate, A6196–A6199
  collagen, A6020–A6024
  composite, A6200–A6205
  contact layer, A6206–A6208
  foam, A6209–A6215
  gauze, A6216–A6230, A6402–A6406
  holder/binder, A4462
  hydrocolloid, A6234–A6241
  hydrogel, A6242–A6248
  specialty absorptive, A6251–A6256
  tape, A4454, A6265
  transparent film, A6257–A6259
  tubular, K0620
Droperidol, J1790
  and fentanyl citrate, J1810
Dropper, A4649
Drugs (see also Table of Drugs)
  administered through a metered dose inhaler, J3535
  chemotherapy, J8500–J9999
  dispensing fee for DME drugs, E0590
  disposable delivery system, 5 ml or less per hour, A4306
  disposable delivery system, 50 ml or greater per hour, A4305
  immunosuppressive, J7500–J7599
  infusion supplies, A4230–A4232, A4221, A4222
  inhalation solutions, J7608–J7699
  not otherwise classified, J3490, J7599, J7699, J7799, J8499, J8999, J9999
  prescription, oral, J8499, J8999
Dry pressure pad/mattress, E0179, E0184, E0199
Durable medical equipment (DME), E0100–E1830, K Codes
Duraclon, see Clonidine
Dyphylline, J1180

E

Ear mold, V5264
Echocardiography injectable contrast material, A9700
Edetate calcium disodium, J0600
Edetate disodium, J3520
Eggcrate dry pressure pad/mattress, E0179, E0184, E0199
Elastic
 bandage, A4460
 gauze, A6263, A6405
Elbow
 disarticulation, endoskeletal, L6450
 orthosis (EO), E1800, L3700–L3740, L3760
 protector, E0191
Electrical work, dialysis equipment, A4870
Electrocardiogram strips,
 monitoring, G0004–G0007
 physician interpretation, G0016
 tracing, G0015
 transmission, G0015, G0016
Electrodes, per pair A4556
Elevating leg rest, K0195
Elliott's b solution, Q2002
EMG, E0746
Eminase, J0350
Endarterectomy, chemical, M0300
Endoscope sheath, A4270
Endoskeletal system, addition, L5858, L5925
Enoxaparin sodium, J1650
Enteral
 feeding supply kit (syringe) (pump) (gravity), B4034–B4036
 formulae, B4150–B4156
 nutrition infusion pump (with alarm) (without), B9000, B9002
Epinephrine, J0170
Epirubicin HCl, J9178
Epoetin alpha, for non-ESRD use, Q0136, Q4055
Epoprostenol, J1325
Ergonovine maleate, J1330
Ertapenem sodium, J1335
Erythromycin lactobionate, J1364
ESRD (End Stage Renal Disease; *see also* Dialysis)
 machines and accessories, E1500–E1699
 plumbing, A4870
 supplies, A4651–A4929
Estrogen conjugated, J1410
Estrone (5, Aqueous), J1435
Ethanolamine oleate, Q2007
Etidronate disodium, J1436
Etoposide, J9181, J9182
Etoposide, oral, J8560
Exercise equipment, A9300
External
 ambulatory infusion pump, E0781, E0784
 power, battery components, L7360–L7499
 power, elbow, L7160–L7191
 urinary supplies, A4356–A4359

Extremity belt/harness, E0945
Eye
 case, V2756
 lens (contact) (spectacle), V2100–V2615
 pad, A4610–A4612
 prosthetic, V2623, V2629
 service (miscellaneous), V2700–V2799

F

Faceplate, ostomy, A4361, K0428
Face tent, oxygen, A4619
Factor VIII, anti-hemophilic factor, J7190–J7192
Factor IX, J7193, J7194, J7195
Family Planning Education, H1010
Fecal leukocyte examination, G0026
Fentanyl citrate, J3010
Fentanyl citrate and droperidol, J1810
Fern test, Q0114
Filgrastim (G-CSF), J1440, J1441
Filler, wound
 alginate dressing, A6199
 foam dressing, A6215
 hydrocolloid dressing, A6240, A6241
 hydrogel dressing, A6248
 not elsewhere classified, A6261, A6262
Film, transparent (for dressing), A6257–A6259
Filter
 aerosol compressor, A7014
 CPAP device, K0188, K0189
 dialysis carbon, A4680
 ostomy, A4368
 tracheostoma, A4481
 ultrasonic generator, A7014
Fistula cannulation set, A4730
Flowmeter, E0440, E0555, E0580
Floxuridine, J9200
Fluconazole, injection, J1450
Fludarabine phosphate, J9185
Fluid barrier, dialysis, E1575
Flunisolide inhalation solution, J7641
Fluorouracil, J9190
Foam dressing, A6209–A6215
Foam pad adhesive, A5126
Folding walker, E0135, E0143
Foley catheter, A4312–A4316, A4338–A4346
Fomepizole, Q2008
Fomivirsen sodium intraocular, J1452
Fondaparinux sodium, J1652
Footdrop splint, L4398
Footplate, E0175, E0970, L3031
Footwear, orthopedic, L3201–L3265
Forceps, dialysis, A4910
Forearm crutches, E0110, E0111
Foscarnet sodium, J1455
Fosphenytoin, Q2009
Fracture
 bedpan, E0276
 frame, E0920, E0930, E0946–E0948
 orthosis, L2102–L2136, L3980–L3986
 orthotic additions, L2180–L2192, L3995

Fragmin, *see* Dalteparin sodium
Frames (spectacles), V2020, V2025
Fulvestrant, J9395
Furosemide, J1940

G

Gadolinium, A4647
Gallium Ga 67, Q3002
Gamma globulin, J1460–J1561
Ganciclovir, implant, J7310
Ganciclovir sodium, J1570
Garamycin, J1580
Gas system
 compressed, E0424, E0425
 gaseous, E0430, E0431, E0441, E0443
 liquid, E0434–E0440, E0442, E0444
Gastrostomy/jejunostomy tubing, B4084
Gastrostomy tube, B4085
Gatifloxacin, J1590
Gauze (*see also* Bandage)
 elastic, A6263, A6405
 impregnated, A6222–A6230, A6231–A6233, A6266
 nonelastic, A6264, A6406
 nonimpregnated, A6216–A6221, A6402–A6404
Gel
 conductive, A4558
 pressure pad, E0178, E0185, E0196
Gemcitabine HCl, J9201
Gemtuzumab ozogamicin, J9300
Generator
 implantable neurostimulator, E0751
 ultrasonic with nebulizer, E0574
Gentamicin (Sulfate), J1580
Glasses
 air conduction, V5070
 binaural, V5120–V5150
 bone conduction, V5080
 frames, V2020, V2025
 hearing aid, V5230
Glatiramer acetate, Q2010
Gloves, A4927
Glucagon HCl, J1610
Glucose monitor with integrated lancing/blood sample collection, E2101
Glucose monitor with integrated voice synthesizer, E2100
Glucose test strips, A4253, A4772
Gluteal pad, L2650
Glycopyrrolate, inhalation solution concentrated, J7642
Glycopyrrolate, inhalation solution, unit dose, J7643
Gold sodium thiomalate, J1600
Gomco drain bottle, A4912
Gonadorelin HCl, J1620
Goserelin acetate implant (*see also* Implant), J9202
Grab bar, trapeze, E0910, E0940
Grade-aid, wheelchair, E0974
Granisetron HCl, J1626
Gravity traction device, E0941
Gravlee jet washer, A4470

H

Hair analysis (excluding arsenic), P2031
Hallus-Valgus dynamic splint, L3100
Hallux prosthetic implant, L8642
Haloperidol, J1630
    decanoate, J1631
Halo procedures, L0810–L0860
Halter, cervical head, E0942
Hand finger orthosis, prefabricated,
    L3923
Hand restoration, L6900–L6915
    partial prosthesis, L6000–L6020
    orthosis (WHFO), E1805, E1825,
        L3800–L3805, L3900–L3954
    rims, wheelchair, E0967
Handgrip (cane, crutch, walker), A4636
Harness, E0942, E0944, E0945
Harvard pressure clamp, dialysis, A4920
Headgear (for positive airway pressure
    device), K0185
Hearing devices, V5000–V5299, L8614
Heat
    application, E0200–E0239
    infrared heating pad system, A4639,
        E0221
    lamp, E0200, E0205
    pad, E0210, E0215, E0237, E0238,
        E0249
Heater (nebulizer), E1372
Heel
    elevator, air, E0370
    protector, E0191
    shoe, L3430–L3485
    stabilizer, L3170
Helicopter, ambulance (see also Ambu-
    lance)
Helmet, cervical, L0100, L0110
Helmet, head, E0701
Hemin, Q2011
Hemi-wheelchair, E1083–E1086
Hemipelvectomy prosthesis, L5280,
    L5340
Hemodialysis
    kit, A4820
    machine, E1590
Hemodialyzer, portable, E1635
Hemofil M, J7190
Hemoglobin, Q0116
Hemophilia clotting factor, J7190–J7198
Hemophilia clotting factor, NOC, J7199
Hemostats, A4850
Hemostix, A4773
Heparin infusion pump, dialysis, E1520
Heparin lock flush, J1642
Heparin sodium, A4800, J1644
Hepatitis B vaccine, Q3021–Q3023
Hep-Lock (U/P), J1642
Hexalite, A4590
Hip
    disarticulation prosthesis, L5250,
        L5270, L5330
    orthosis (HO), L1600–L1690
Hip-knee-ankle-foot orthosis (HKAFO),
    L2040–L2090
Histrelin acetate, Q2020
HKAFO, L2040–L2090
Home Health Agency Services, T0221
Hot water bottle, E0220
Humidifier, A7046, E0550–E0562
Hyaluronate, sodium, J7316
Hyaluronidase, J3470
Hydralazine HCl, J0360
Hydraulic patient lift, E0630

Hydrocollator, E0225, E0239
Hydrocolloid dressing, A6234–A6241
Hydrocortisone
    acetate, J1700
    sodium phosphate, J1710
    sodium succinate, J1720
Hydrogel dressing, A6242–A6248,
    A6231–A6233
Hydromorphone, J1170
Hydroxyzine HCl, J3410
Hylan G-F 20, J7320
Hyoscyamine Sulfate, J1980
Hyperbaric oxygen chamber, topical, A4575
Hypertonic saline solution, J7130

I

Ibutilide Fumarate, J1742
Ice
    cap, E0230
    collar, E0230
Idarubicin HCl, J9211
Ifosfamide, J9208
Imiglucerase, J1785
Immune globulin intravenous, J1563–
    J1564
Immunosuppressive drug, not other-
    wise classified, J7599
Implant
    access system, A4301
    aqueous shunt, L8612
    breast, L8600
    cochlear, L8614, L8619
    collagen, urinary tract, L8603
    contraceptive, A4260
    ganciclovir, J7310
    hallux, L8642
    indium III-in Pentetreotide, Q3008
    infusion pump, programmable, E0783,
        E0786
    joint, L8630, L8641, L8658
    lacrimal duct, A4262, A4263
    metacarpophalangeal joint, L8630
    metatarsal joint, L8641
    neurostimulator electrodes, E0752
    neurostimulator pulse generator, E0756
    neurostimulator radiofrequency re-
        ceiver, E0757
    not otherwise specified, L8699
    ocular, L8610
    ossicular, L8613
    osteogenesis stimulator, E0749
    percutaneous access system, A4301
    replacement implantable intraspinal
        catheter, E0785
    synthetic, urinary, L8606
    urinary tract, L8603, L8606
    vascular graft, L8670
Impregnated gauze dressing, A6222–
    A6230, K0535–K0537
Incontinence
    appliances and supplies, A4310–A4355,
        A4356–A4360, A5071–A5075,
        A5102–A5114, K0280, K0281
    products, A4521–A4538
    treatment system, E0740
Indium in 111 carpromab pendetide,
    A9507
Indwelling catheter insertion, G0002
Infliximab injection, J1745
Infusion
    pump, ambulatory, with administra-
        tive equipment, E0781

pump, heparin, dialysis, E1520
pump, implantable, E0782, E0783
pump, implantable, refill kit, A4220
pump, insulin, E0784
pump, mechanical, reusable, E0779, E0780
pump, uninterrupted infusion of Epi-
    prostenol, K0455
supplies, A4221, A4222, A4230–A4232
therapy, other than chemotherapeutic
    drugs, Q0081
Inhalation solution (see also drug name),
    J7608–J7699
Injections (see also drug name), J0120–J7320
    contrast material, during MRI, A4643
    supplies for self-administered, A4211
Insertion, indwelling catheter, G0002
Insertion tray, A4310–A4316
Insulin, J1815, J1817
Insulin lispro, K0548
Interferon
    Alpha, J9212–J9215
    Beta-1a, J1825, Q3025–Q3026
    Beta-1b, J1830
    Gamma, J9216
Intermittent
    assist device with continuous positive
        airway pressure device, E0470–
        E0472
    peritoneal dialysis system, E1592
    positive pressure breathing (IPPB) ma-
        chine, E0500
Interphalangeal joint, prosthetic im-
    plant, L8658, L8659
Interscapular thoracic prosthesis
    endoskeletal, L6570
    upper limb, L6350–L6370
Intraconazole, J1835
Intraocular lenses, V2630–V2632
Intrapulmonary percussive ventilation
    system, E0481
Intrauterine copper contraceptive,
    J7300
Iobenguane sulfate I-131, A9508
Iodine swabs/wipes, A4247
IPD
    supply kit, A4905
    system, E1592
IPPB machine, E0500
Ipratropium bromide, inhalation solu-
    tion, unit dose, J7644
Irinotecan, J9206
Iron Dextran, J1750
Iron sucrose, J1756
Irrigation/evacuation system, bowel
    control unit, E0350
    disposable supplies for, E0352
Irrigation solution for bladder calculi,
    Q2004
Irrigation supplies, A4320–A4323,
    A4355, A4397–A4400
Isoetharine HCL, inhalation solution,
    concentrated, J7648
Isoetharine HCL, inhalation solution,
    unit dose, J7649
Isolates, B4150, B4152
Isoproterenol HCL, inhalation solution,
    concentrated, J7658
Isoproterenol HCL, inhalation solution,
    unit dose, J7659
IV pole, each, E0776, K0105

J

Jacket
body (LSO) (spinal), L0500–L0565
scoliosis, L1300, L1310
Jenamicin, J1580
Joint supportive device/garment, A4464

K

Kanamycin sulfate, J1840, J1850
Kartop patient lift, toilet or bathroom
(*see also* Lift), E0625
Ketorolac thomethamine, J1885
Kidney
ESRD supply, A4650–A4927
system, E1510
wearable artificial, E1632
Kits
continuous ambulatory peritoneal dialysis (CAPD), A4900
continuous cycling peritoneal dialysis (CCPD), A4901
dialysis, A4910
enteral feeding supply (syringe) (pump) (gravity), B4034–B4036
fistula cannulation (set), A4730
intermittent peritoneal dialysis (IPD) supply, A4905
parenteral nutrition, B4220–B4224
surgical dressing (tray), A4550
tracheostomy, A4625
Knee
disarticulation, prosthesis, L5150, L5160
joint, miniature, L5826

orthosis (KO), E1810, L1800–L1885
Knee-ankle-foot orthosis (KAFO), L2000–L2039, L2126–L2136
addition, high strength, lightweight material, L2755
Kutapressin, J1910
Kyphosis pad, L1020, L1025

L

Laboratory tests
chemistry, P2028–P2038
microbiology, P7001
miscellaneous, P9010–P9615, Q0111–Q0115
toxicology, P3000–P3001, Q0091
Lacrimal duct implant
permanent, A4263
temporary, A4262
Lactated Ringer's infusion, J7120
Laetrile, J3570
Lancet, A4258, A4259
Larynx, artificial, L8500
Laser blood collection device and accessory, E0620, A4257
Lead investigation, T1029
Lead wires, per pair, A4557
Leg
bag, A4358, A5105, A5112
extensions for walker, E0158
rest, elevating, K0195
rest, wheelchair, E0990
strap, replacement, A5113–A5114
Legg Perthes orthosis, L1700–L1755
Lens
aniseikonic, V2118, V2318

contact, V2500–V2599
eye, V2100–V2615, V2700–V2799
intraocular, V2630–V2632
low vision, V2600–V2615
progressive, V2781
Lepirudin, Q2021
Leucovorin calcium, J0640
Leukocyte examination, fecal, G0026
Leukocyte poor blood, each unit, P9016
Leuprolide acetate, J1950, J9217, J9218, J9219
Levocarnitine, J1955
Levofloxacin, J1956
Levonorgestrel, (contraceptive), implants and supplies, A4260
Levorphanol tartrate, J1960
Lidocaine HCl, J2001
Lift
patient (includes seat lift), E0621–E0635
shoe, L3300–L3334
Lincomycin HCl, J2010
Linezolid, J2020
Liquid barrier, ostomy, A4363
Lodging, recipient, escort nonemergency transport, A0180, A0200
Lorazepam, J2060
LSO, L0500–L0565
Lubricant, A4402, A4332
Lumbar flexion, L0540
Lumbar-sacral orthosis (LSO), L0500–L0565
Lymphocyte immune globulin, J7504, J7511

M

Magnesium sulphate, J3475
Maintenance contract, ESRD, A4890
Manipulation of spine, chiropractic, A2000
Mannitol, J2150
Mask
  aerosol, K0180
  oxygen, A4620, A4621
Mastectomy
  bra, L8000
  form, L8020
  prosthesis, L8030, L8600
  sleeve, L8010
Mattress
  air pressure, E0186
  alternating pressure, E0277
  dry pressure, E0184
  gel pressure, E0196
  hospital bed, E0271, E0272
  non-powered, pressure reducing, E0373
  overlay, E0371–E0372
  powered, pressure reducing, E0277
  water pressure, E0187
Measuring cylinder, dialysis, A4921
Mechlorethamine HCl, J9230
Medical and surgical supplies, A4206–A8999
Medroxyprogesterone acetate, J1051, J1055
Medroxyprogesterone acetate/estradiol cypionate, J1056
Melphalan HCl, J9245
Melphalan, oral, J8600
Meperidine, J2175
Meperidine and promethazine, J2180
Mepivacaine HCl, J0670
Meropenem, J2185
Mesna, J9209
Metabolically active tissue, Q0184
Metabolically active D/E tissue, Q0185
Metacarpophalangeal joint, prosthetic implant, L8630, L8631
Metaproterenol sulfate, inhalation solution, concentrated, J7668
Metaproterenol sulfate, inhalation solution, unit dose, J7669
Metaraminol bitartrate, J0380
Metatarsal joint, prosthetic implant, L8641
Meter, bath conductivity, dialysis, E1550
Methadone HCl, J1230
Methocarbamol, J2800
Methotrexate, oral, J8610
Methotrexate sodium, J9250, J9260
Methyldopate HCl, J0210
Methylergonovine maleate, J2210
Methylprednisolone
  acetate, J1020–J1040
  oral, J7509
  sodium succinate, J2920, J2930
Metoclopramide HCl, J2765

Microbiology test, P7001
Midazolam HCl, J2250
Mileage, ambulance, A0380, A0390
Mini-bus, nonemergency transportation, A0120
Milrinone lactate, J2260
Mitomycin, J9280–J9291
Mitoxantrone HCl, J9293
Modalities, with office visit, M0005–M0008
Moisture exchanger for use with invasive mechanical ventilation, A4483
Moisturizer, skin, A6250
Monitor
  apnea, E0608
  blood glucose, E0607, E0609
  blood pressure, A4670
  pacemaker, E0610, E0615
Monitoring and recording, EKG, G0004–G0007
Monoclonal antibodies, J7505
Mononine, Q0160
Morphine sulfate, J2270, J2271
  sterile, preservative-free, J2275
Mouthpiece (for respiratory equipment), A4617
  and dome (for nebulizer), K0181
Moxifloxacin, J2280
MRI contrast material, A4643
Mucoprotein, blood, P2038
Multiaxial ankle, L5986
Multidisciplinary services, H2000–H2001, T1023–T1028
Multiple post collar, cervical, L0180–L0200
Multi-Podus type AFO, L4396
Muromonab-CD3, J7505
Mycophenolate mofetil, J7517

N

Nalbuphine HCl, J2300
Naloxone HCl, J2310
Nandrolone
  decanoate, J2320–J2322
Narrowing device, wheelchair, E0969
Nasal application device, K0183
Nasal pillows/seals (for nasal application device), K0184
Nasal vaccine inhalation, J3530
Nasogastric tubing, B4081, B4082
Nebulizer, E0570–E0585
  aerosol compressor, E0571
  aerosol mask, A7015
  corrugated tubing, disposable, A7010
  corrugated tubing, non-disposable, A7011
  distilled water, K0182
  drug dispensing fee, E0590
  filter, disposable, A7013
  filter, non-disposable, A7014

heater, E1372
  large volume, disposable, prefilled, A7008
  large volume, disposable, unfilled, A7007
  not used with oxygen, durable, glass, A7017
  pneumatic, administration set, A7003, A7005, A7006
  pneumatic, nonfiltered, A7004
  portable, E0570
  small volume, A7003–A7005
  ultrasonic, E0575
  ultrasonic, dome and mouthpiece, A7016
  ultrasonic, reservoir bottle, non-disposable, A7009
  water collection device, large volume nebulizer, A7012
Needle, A4215
  dialysis, A4655
  non-coring, A4212
  with syringe, A4206–A4209
Negative pressure wound therapy pump, E2402
  accessories, A6550–A6551
Neonatal transport, ambulance, base rate, A0225
Neostigmine methylsulfate, J2710
Nerve stimulator with batteries, E0765
Nesiritide injection, J2324
Neuromuscular stimulator, E0745
Neurostimulator
  electrodes, E0753
  programmer, E0754
  pulse generator, E0756
  receiver, E0757
  transmitter, E0758
Nonchemotherapy drug, oral, NOS, J8499
Noncovered services, A9270
Nonelastic gauze, A6264, A6406
Nonemergency transportation, A0080–A0210
Nonimpregnated gauze dressing, A6216–A6221, A6402–A6404
Nonmetabolic active tissue, Q0183
Nonprescription drug, A9150
Not otherwise classified drug, J3490, J7599, J7699, J7799, J8499, J8999, J9999, Q0181
NPH, J1820
NTIOL category 1, Q1001
NTIOL category 2, Q1002
NTIOL category 3, Q1003
NTIOL category 4, Q1004
NTIOL category 5, Q1005
Nursing care, T1030–T1031
Nutrition
  enteral infusion pump, B9000, B9002
  parenteral infusion pump, B9004, B9006
  parenteral solution, B4164–B5200

O

Occipital/mandibular support, cervical, L0160
Octreotide acetate, J2353, J2354
Ocular prosthetic implant, L8610
Ondansetron HCl, J2405
One arm, drive attachment, K0101
Oprelvekin, J2355
O & P supply/accessory/service, L9900
Oropharyngeal suction catheter, A4628
Orphenadrine, J2360
Orthopedic shoes
    arch support, L3040–L3100
    footwear, L3201–L3265
    insert, L3000–L3030
    lift, L3300–L3334
    miscellaneous additions, L3500–L3595
    positioning device, L3140–L3170
    transfer, L3600–L3649
    wedge, L3340–L3420
Orthotic additions
    carbon graphite lamination, L2755
    fracture, L2180–L2192, L3995
    halo, L0860
    lower extremity, L2200–L2999, L4320
    ratchet lock, L2430
    scoliosis, L1010–L1120, L1210–L1290
    shoe, L3300–L3595, L3649
    spinal, L0970–L0984
    upper extremity joint, L3956
    upper limb, L3810–L3890, L3970–L3974, L3995
Orthotic devices
    ankle-foot (AFO; see also Orthopedic shoes), E1815, E1816, E1830, L1900–L1990, L2102–L2116, L3160
    anterior-posterior, L0320, L0330, L0530
    anterior-posterior-lateral, L0520, L0550–L0565, L0700, L0710
    anterior-posterior-lateral-rotary, L0340–L0440

cervical, L0100–L0200
cervical-thoracic-lumbar-sacral (CTLSO), L0700, L0710
elbow (EO), E1800, E1801, L3700–L3740
fracture, L2102–L2136, L3980–L3986
halo, L0810–L0830
hand (WHFO), E1805, E1825, L3800, L3805, L3807, L3900–L3954
hand, finger, prefabricated, L3923
hip (HO), L1600–L1690
hip-knee-ankle-foot (HKAFO), L2040–L2090
interface material, E1820
knee (KO), E1810, E1811, L1800–L1885
knee-ankle-foot (KAFO; see also Orthopedic shoes), L2000–L2038, L2122–L2136
Legg Perthes, L1700–L1755
lumbar flexion, L0540
lumbar-sacral (LSO), L0500–L0565
multiple post collar, L0180–L0200
not otherwise specified, L0999, L1499, L2999, L3999, L5999, L7499, L8039, L8239
pneumatic splint, L4350–L4380
pronation/supination, E1818
repair or replacement, L4000–L4210
replace soft interface material, L4390–L4394
sacroiliac, L0600–L0620
scoliosis, L1000, L1499
shoe, see Orthopedic shoes
shoulder (SO), L1840, L3650–L3677
shoulder-elbow-wrist-hand (SEWHO), L3960–L3969
side bar disconnect, L2768
spinal, cervical, L0100–L0200
spinal, DME, K0112–K0116
thoracic, L0210

thoracic-hip-knee-ankle (THKO), L1500–L1520
thoracic-lumbar-sacral (TLSO), L0300–L0440
toe, E1830
torso supports, L0900–L0960
wrist-hand-finger (WHFO), E1805, E1806, E1825, L3800, L3805, L3900–L3954
Ossicular prosthetic implant, L8613
Osteogenesis stimulator, E0747–E0749, E0760
Ostomy
    accessories, A5093
    belt, A4396
    pouches, A4416–A4434
    skin barrier, A4401–A4449
    supplies, A4361–A4421, A5051–A5149
Oxacillin sodium, J2700
Oxaliplatin, J9263
Oximeter devices, E0454, A4609
Oxygen
    ambulance, A0422
    catheter, transtracheal, A7018
    chamber, hyperbaric, topical, A4575
    concentrator, E1390–E1391
    mask, A4620, A4621
    medication supplies, A4611–A4627
    rack/stand, E1355
    regulator, E1353
    respiratory equipment/supplies, A4611–A4627, E0424–E0480
    supplies and equipment, E0425–E0444, E0455
    tent, E0455
    tubing, A4616
    water vapor enriching system, E1405, E1406
Oxymorphone HCl, J2410
Oxytetracycline HCl, J2460
Oxytocin, J2590

P

Pacemaker monitor, E0610, E0615
Paclitaxel, J9265
Pad
  gel pressure, E0178, E0185, E0196
  heat, E0210, E0215, E0217, E0238, E0249
  orthotic device interface, E1820
  sheepskin, E0188, E0189
  water circulating cold with pump, E0218
  water circulating heat with pump, E0217
  water circulating heat unit, E0249
  wheelchair, low pressure and positioning, E0192
Pail, for use with commode chair, E0167
Palate, prosthetic implant, L8618
Pamidronate disodium, J2430
Pan, for use with commode chair, E0167
Papanicolaou (Pap) screening smear, P3000, P3001, Q0091
Papaverine HCl, J2440
Paraffin, A4265
Paraffin bath unit, E0235
Paramagnetic contrast material, (Gadolinium), A4647
Paramedic intercept, rural, Q0186
Parenteral nutrition
  administration kit, B4224
  pump, B9004, B9006
  solution, B4164–B5200
  supply kit, B4220, B4222
Paricalcitol, J2501
Parking fee, nonemergency transport, A0170
Paste, conductive, A4558
Patella, prosthetic implant, L8640
Pathology and laboratory tests, miscellaneous, P9010–P9615
Patient support system, E0636
PEFR, peak expiratory flow rate meter, A4614
Pegademase bovine, Q2012
Pegaspargase, J9266
Pegfilgrastim, J2505
Pelvic belt/harness/boot, E0944
Penicillin
  G benzathine/G benzathine and penicillin G procaine, J0530–J0580
  G potassium, J2540
  G procaine, aqueous, J2510
Pentamidine isethionate, J2545
Pentastarch, 10% solution, Q2013
Pentazocine HCl, J3070
Pentobarbital sodium, J2515
Pentostatin, J9268
Percussor, E0480
Percutaneous access system, A4301
Peroneal strap, L0980
Peroxide, A4244
Perphenazine, J3310
Personal care services, T1019–T1021
Personal comfort item, A9190
Pessary, A4561, A4562
PET myocardial perfusion imaging, G0030–G0047

Phenobarbital sodium, J2560
Phentolamine mesylate, J2760
Phenylephrine HCl, J2370
Phenytoin sodium, J1165
Phisohex solution, A4246
Photofrin, see Porfimer sodium
Phototherapy light, E0202
Phytonadione, J3430
Pillow, cervical, E0943
Pinworm examination, Q0113
Plasma
  multiple donor, pooled, frozen, P9023
  protein fraction, P9018
  single donor, fresh frozen, P9017
Plastazote, L3002, L3252, L3253, L3265, L5654–L5658
Platelet
  concentrate, each unit, P9019
  rich plasma, each unit, P9020
Platform attachment
  forearm crutch, E0153
  walker, E0154
Plicamycin, J9270
Plumbing, for home ESRD equipment, A4870
Pneumatic
  appliance, E0655–E0673, L4350–L4380
  compressor, E0650–E0652
  splint, L4350–L4380
  tire, wheelchair, E0953
Pneumatic nebulizer
  administration set, small volume, filtered, A7006
  administration set, small volume, non-filtered, A7003
  administration set, small volume, non-filtered, non-disposable, A7005
  small volume, disposable, A7004
Porfimer, J9600
Portable
  equipment transfer, R0070–R0076
  hemodialyzer system, E1635
  nebulizer, E1375
  x-ray equipment, Q0092
Positioning seat, T5001
Positive airway pressure device, accessories, A7030–A7039, E0561–E0562
Positive expiratory pressure device, E0484
Post-coital examination, Q0115
Post-voiding residual, ultrasound, G0050
Postural drainage board, E0606
Potassium chloride, J3480
Potassium hydroxide (KOH) preparation, Q0112
Pouch
  fecal collection, A4330
  ostomy, A4375–A4378, A5051–A5054, A5061–A5065
  urinary, A4379–A4383, A5071–A5075
Pralidoxime chloride, J2730
Prednisolone
  acetate, J2650
  oral, J7506, J7510
Prednisone, J7506
Preparation kits, dialysis, A4914

Preparatory prosthesis, L5510–L5595
  chemotherapy, J8999
  nonchemotherapy, J8499
Pressure
  alarm, dialysis, E1540
  pad, A4640, E0176–E0199
  ventilator, E0454
Procainamide HCl, J2690
Prochlorperazine, J0780
Prolotherapy, M0076
Promazine HCl, J2950
Promethazine HCl, J2550
Promethazine and meperidine, J2180
Propranolol HCl, J1800
Prosthesis
  artificial larynx battery/accessory, L8505
  breast, L8000–L8035, L8600
  eye, L8610, L8611, V2623–V2629
  fitting, L5400–L5460, L6380–L6388
  foot/ankle one piece system, L5979
  hand, L6000–L6020, L6025
  implants, L8600–L8690
  larynx, L8500
  lower extremity, L5700–L5999, L8640–L8642
  mandible, L8617
  maxilla, L8616
  maxillofacial, provided by a non-physician, L8040–L8048
  miscellaneous service, L8499
  ocular, V2623–V2629
  repair of, L7520, L8049
  socks (shrinker, sheath, stump sock), L8400–L8485
  taxes, orthotic/prosthetic/other, L9999
  tracheo-esophageal, L8507-L8509
  upper extremity, L6000–L6999
  vacuum erection system, L7900
  voice amplifier, E1904
Prosthetic additions
  lower extremity, L5610–L5999
  upper extremity, L6600–L7274
Protamine sulfate, J2720
Protectant, skin, A6250
Protector, heel or elbow, E0191
Protirelin, J2725
Pulse generator, E2120
Pump
  alternating pressure pad, E0182
  ambulatory infusion, E0781
  ambulatory insulin, E0784
  blood, dialysis, E1620
  breast, E0602-E0604
  enteral infusion, B9000, B9002
  external infusion, E0779
  heparin infusion, E1520
  implantable infusion, E0782, E0783
  implantable infusion, refill kit, A4220
  infusion, supplies, A4230, A4232, K0110–K0111
  negative pressure wound therapy, K0538
  parenteral infusion, B9004, B9006
  suction, portable, E0600
  suction, supplies, K0190–K0192
  water circulating pad, E0236
Purification system, A4880, E1610, E1615
Pyridoxine HCl, J3415

Q

Quad cane, E0105
Quinupristin/dalfopristin, J2770

R

Rack/stand, oxygen, E1355
Radial head, prosthetic implant, L8620
Radioelements for brachytherapy, Q3001
Radiofrequency transmitter, E0758, E0759
Radiology service, R0070–R0076
Radiopharmaceutical diagnostic imaging agent, A4641, A4642, A9500, A9507, A9512–A9532, Q3002–Q3004
Radiopharmaceutical, therapeutic, A9600, A9605
Rail
   bathtub, E0241, E0242, E0246
   bed, E0305, E0310
   toilet, E0243
Rasburicase, J2783
Reciprocating peritoneal dialysis system, E1630
Red blood cells, P9021, P9022
Reduction pneumoplasty, G0061

Regular insulin, J1820
Regulator, oxygen, E1353
Repair
   contract, ESRD, A4890
   durable medical equipment, E1340
   maxillofacial prosthesis, L8049
   orthosis, L4000–L4130
   prosthetic, L7500, L7510, K0285
Replacement
   battery, A4254, A4630, A4631
   components, ESRD machine, E1640
   pad (alternating pressure), A4640
   tanks, dialysis, A4880
   tip for cane, crutches, walker, A4637
   underarm pad for crutches, A4635
Reservoir bottle (for ultrasonic nebulizer), K0174
RespiGam, see Respiratory syncytial virus immune globulin
Respiratory
   Heated humidifier used with PAP, K0531

Invasive assist with backup, K0534
Noninvasive assist with backup, K0533
Noninvasive assist without backup, K0532
Respiratory syncytial virus immune globulin, J1565
Restraint, any type, E0710
Reteplase, J2993
Rho(D) immune globulin, human, J2788, J2790, J2792
Rib belt, thoracic, A4572, L0210, L0220
Ringer's lactate infusion, J7120
Ring, ostomy, A4404
Rituximab, J9310
Robin-Aids, L6000, L6010, L6020, L6855, L6860
Rocking bed, E0462
Rollabout chair, E1031
Ropivacaine Hcl, J2795
Rubidium Rb-82, Q3000

S

T

Tables, bed, E0274, E0315
Tacrolimus, oral, J7507
Tacrolimus, parenteral, J7515
Tape, A4454, A6265, K0265
Taxi, nonemergency transportation, A0100
Technetium Tc 99m Bicisate, Q3003
Technetium TC 99m Depreotide, A9511
Technetium Tc 99m Disofenin, A9510
Technetium Tc 99m Gluceptate, Q3006
Technetium Tc 99m–labeled red blood cells, Q3010
Technetium Tc 99m Oxidronate, Q3009
Technetium Tc 99M Sestamibi, A9500
TEEV, J0900
Telehealth, Q3014
Telehealth transmission, T1014
Temozolomide, oral, J8700
Tenecteplase, J3100
Teniposide, Q2017
TENS, A4595, E0720–E0749
Tent, oxygen, E0455
Terbutaline sulfate, J3105
Terbutaline sulfate, inhalation solution, concentrated, J7680
Terbutaline sulfate, inhalation solution, unit dose, J7681
Terminal devices, L6700–L6895
Testosterone
  aqueous, J3140
  cypionate and estradiol cypionate, J1060
  enanthate, J3120, J3130
  enanthate and estradiol valerate, J0900
  propionate, J3150
  suspension, J3140
Tetanus immune globulin, human, J1670
Tetracycline, J0120
Thallous chloride TL 201, A9505
Theophylline, J2810
Therapeutic lightbox, A4634, E0203
Therapy
  activity, Q0082
  occupational, H5300
  physical (evaluation/treatment), Q0086
Thermometer, A4931–A4932
Thermometer, dialysis, A4910
Thiamine HCl, J3411
Thiethylperazine maleate, J3280
Thiotepa, J9340
Thoracic-hip-knee-ankle (THKAO), L1500–L1520
Thoracic-lumbar-sacral orthosis (TLSO)
  scoliosis, L1200–L1290
  spinal, K0618–K0619, L0300–L0440
Thoracic orthosis, L0210
Thymol turbidity, blood, P2033
Thyrotropin, Alfa, J3240
Tinzarparin, sodium, J1655
Tip (cane, crutch, walker) replacement, A4637
Tire, wheelchair, E0996, E0999, E1000

Tissue-based surgical dressings, Q0183–Q0185
Tissue of human origin, J7340, J7342, J7350
TLSO, L0300–L0440, L1200–L1290
Tobramycin, inhalation solution, unit dose, J7682
Tobramycin sulfate, J3260
Toilet accessories, E0167–E0179, E0243, E0244, E0625
Tolazoline HCl, J2670
Toll, nonemergency transport, A0170
Tool kit, dialysis, A4910
Topical hyperbaric oxygen chamber, A4575
Topotecan, J9350
Torsemide, J3265
Torso support, L0900–L0960
Tourniquet, dialysis, A4910
Tracheostoma heat moisture exchange system, A7501–A7509
Tracheostomy
  care kit, A4629
  filter, A4481
  speaking valve, L8501
  supplies, A4632, A4629, A7523–A7524
  tube, A7520–A7522
Tracheotomy mask or collar, A7525–A7526
Traction device, ambulatory, E0830
Traction equipment, E0840–E0948
Transcutaneous electrical nerve stimulator (TENS), E0720–E0749
Transducer protector, dialysis, E1575
Transfer board or device, E0972
Transfer (shoe orthosis), L3600–L3640
Transfer system with seat, E1035
Transparent film (for dressing), A6257–A6259
Transportation
  ambulance, A0021–A0999, Q3019–Q3020
  corneal tissue, V2785
  EKG (portable), R0076
  handicapped, A0130
  nonemergency, A0080–A0210, T2001–T2005
  service, including ambulance, A0021–A0999, T2006
  taxi, nonemergency, A0100
  toll, nonemergency, A0170
  volunteer, nonemergency, A0080, A0090
  x-ray (portable), R0070, R0075
Transtracheal oxygen catheter, A7018
Trapeze bar, E0910, E0940
Trapezium, prosthetic implant, L8625
Tray
  insertion, A4310–A4316
  irrigation, A4320
  surgical (see also kits), A4550
  wheelchair, E0950
Triamcinolone, J3301–J3303
  acetonide, J3301
  diacetate, J3302
  hexacetonide, J3303

inhalation solution, concentrated, J7683
inhalation solution, unit dose, J7684
Triflupromazine HCl, J3400
Trifocal, glass or plastic, V2300–V2399
Trimethobenzamide HCl, J3250
Trimetrexate glucuronate, J3305
Triptorelin pamoate, J3315
Truss, L8300–L8330
Tube/Tubing
  anchoring device, A5200
  blood, A4750, A4755
  corrugated, for nebulizer, K0175, K0176
  CPAP device, K0187
  drainage extension, A4331
  gastrostomy, B4084, B4085, B4086
  irrigation, A4355
  laryngectomy, A4622
  nasogastric, B4081, B4082
  oxygen, A4616
  serum clotting time, A4771
  stomach, B4083
  suction pump, each, A7002
  tire, K0064, K0068, K0078, K0091, K0093, K0095, K0097
  tracheostomy, A4622
  urinary drainage, K0280

U

Ultrasonic nebulizer, E0575
Ultrasonic nebulizer reservoir bottle, K0174
Ultrasound bladder capacity test, G0050
Ultrasound bone mineral study, G0133
Ultraviolet cabinet, E0690
Ultraviolet light therapy system, A4633, E0691–E0694
Unclassified drug, J3490
Unipuncture control system, dialysis, E1580
Upper extremity addition, locking elbow, L6693
Upper extremity fracture orthosis, L3980–L3999
Upper limb prosthesis, L6000–L7499
Urea, J3350
Ureterostomy supplies, A4454–A4590
Urethral suppository, Alprostadil, J0275
Urinal, E0325, E0326
Urinary
  catheter, A4338-A4346, A4351-A4353, K0410, K0411
  collection and retention (supplies), A4310–A4359, K0407, K0408, K0410, K0411
  tract implant, collagen, L8603
  tract implant, synthetic, L8606
Urine
  sensitivity study, P7001
  tests, A4250
Urofollitropin, Q2018
Urokinase, J3364, J3365
U-V lens, V2755

V

Vabra aspirator, A4480
Vaccination, administration
  hepatitis B, G0010
  influenza virus, G0008
  pneumococcal, G0009
Vancomycin HCl, J3370
Vaporizer, E0605
Vascular
  catheter (appliances and supplies),
    A4300–A4306
  graft material, synthetic, L8670
Vasoxyl, J3390
Venipuncture, routine specimen collection, G0001
Venous pressure clamp, dialysis, A4918
Ventilator
  battery, A4611–A4613
  moisture exchanger, disposable,
    A4483
  negative pressure, E0460
  volume, stationary or portable, E0450,
    E0461
Verteporfin, J3395
Vest, safety, wheelchair, E0980
Vinblastine sulfate, J9360
Vincristine sulfate, J9370–J9380
Vinorelbine tartrate, J9390
Vision service, V2020–V2799
Vitamin B-12 cyanocobalamin, J3420
Vitamin K, J3430
Voice amplifier, L8510
Voice prosthesis, L8511–L8514
Voriconazole, J3465

W

Waiver, T2012–T2050
Walker, E0130–E0149
  accessories, A4636, A4637
  attachments, E0153–E0159

Walking splint, L4386
Water
  collection device (for nebulizer),
    K0177
  distilled (for nebulizer), A7018
  pressure pad/mattress, E0177, E0187,
    E0198
  purification system (ESRD), E1610,
    E1615
  softening system (ESRD), E1625
  sterile, A4712, A4714, A4319
  tanks (dialysis), A4880
Wedges, shoe, L3340–L3420
Wet mount, Q0111
Wheel attachment, rigid pickup walker,
  E0155
Wheelchair, E0950–E1298, K0001–
  K0108
  accessories, E0192, E0950–E1030,
    E1065–E1069, E2300–E2399
  amputee, E1170–E1200
  back, fully reclining, manual, E1226
  battery, A4631
  bearings, K0452
  component or accessory, not otherwise
    specified, K0108
  motorized, E1210–E1213
  narrowing device, E0969
  power add-on, E0983–E0984
  shock absorber, E1015–E1018
  specially sized, E1220, E1230
  stump support system, K0551
  tire, E0996, E0999, E1000
  transfer board or device, E0972
  tray, K0107
  van, nonemergency, A0130
  youth, E1091
WHFO with inflatable air chamber,
  L3807
WHO, wrist extension, L3914
Whirlpool equipment, E1300–E1310
Wipes, A4245, A4247

Wound cleanser, A6260
Wound cover
  alginate dressing, A6196–A6198
  collagen dressing, A6020–A6024
  foam dressing, A6209–A6214
  hydrocolloid dressing, A6234–A6239
  hydrogel dressing, A6242–A6247
  non-contact wound warming cover,
    and accessory, E0231, E0232
  specialty absorptive dressing, A6251–
    A6256
Wound filler
  alginate dressing, A6199
  collagen based, A6010
  foam dressing, A6215
  hydrocolloid dressing, A6240, A6241
  hydrogel dressing, A6248
  not elsewhere classified, A6261, A6262
Wound pouch, A6154
Wrist
  disarticulation prosthesis, L6050, L6055
  hand/finger orthosis (WHFO), E1805,
    E1825, L3800–L3954

X

Xenon Xe 133, Q3004
X-ray equipment, portable, Q0092,
  R0070, R0075
Xylocaine HCl, J2000

Z

Zidovudine, J3485
Ziprasidone mesylate, J3486
Zoledronic acid, J3487

APPENDIX A

MEDICARE CARRIERS MANUAL (MCM), SELECT

CENTERS FOR MEDICARE AND MEDICAID SERVICES (CMS) INTERNET-ONLY MANUALS (IOM)

The CMS manuals are currently undergoing a major transformation as the paper-based manuals are being phased out and the new internet-only manuals (IOM) are implemented. During the transition, users are to check both sets of manuals to insure the use of current policies and procedures. The internet-only manuals will be the official copy of the manuals and will be maintained in the CMS central office.

Effective October 1, 2003, the CMS will no longer issue program memoranda (PMs) containing new policies and procedure as this information will be contained in the IOM.

The paper-based Coverage Issue Manual (CIM) is to be replaced by the internet-only National Coverage Determinations Manual (NCD). The NCD is organized by categories such as supplies and medical procedures. The manual will contain Chapter 1, which outlines the CMS determinations regarding coverage, and Chapter 2, which contains the HCPCS codes that correlate to each of the CMS determinations. CPT categories are also used in Chapter 2 of the manual. The CMS Coverage Web page http://www.cms.hhs.gov/medcov contains information about pending National Coverage Determinations and also provides access to a database of National Coverage Determinations, National Coverage Analyses, and Local Medical review Policies.

The paper-based Medicare Carriers Manual (MCM) will be replaced by the internet-only manual, publications 100. The CMS Manual System will include the following functional areas:

Pub 100	Introduction
Pub 100-01	Medicare General Information, Eligibility, and Entitlement
Pub 100-02	**Medicare Benefit Policy**
Pub 100-03	**Medicare National Coverage Determinations**
Pub 100-04	**Medicare Claims Processing**
Pub 100-05	**Medicare Secondary Payer**
Pub 100-06	Medicare Financial Management
Pub 100-07	Medicare State Operations
Pub 100-08	Medicare Program Integrity
Pub 100-09	**Medicare Contractor Beneficiary and Provider Communications**
Pub 100-10	Medicare Quality Improvement Organization
Pub 100-11	Reserved
Pub 100-12	State Medicaid
Pub 100-13	Medicate State Children's Health Insurance Program
Pub 100-14	Medicare End Stage Renal Disease Network Organization
Pub 100-15	**Medicare State Buy-In**
Pub 100-16	Medicare Managed Care
Pub 100-17	Medicare Business Partners Systems Security
Pub 100-18	Medicare Business Partners Security Oversight
Pub 100-19	Demonstrations
Pub 100-20	**One-Time Notification**

The publications in bold in the above list are the publications that are included in the initial release.

At this time, many sections of the internet-only manuals were not available, so this edition of this text references both the paper based and internet only manuals of CIM and MCM. The CMS web site contains the latest develops on the IOM at www.cms.gov/manuals/ .

To assist in the transformation, the CMS has provided crosswalks indication the location of the paper-based material and the new location of the material in the internet-based manual. Following is a crosswalk for the CIM to NCD.

MEDICARE NATIONAL COVERAGE DETERMINATIONS (NCD) MANUAL

Crosswalk CIM to NCD Sections—The column on the far right (column 3) is in CIM sequence. Column 1 shows the NDC Manual section. Note that the sections in the NCD are in CPT category sequence and not in Medicare benefit category sequence.

NCD Section	Title	CIM Section
310.1	Routine Costs in Clinical Trails	CIM 30-1
10.8.1	Stem Cell Transplantation	CIM 35.30.1
100.7	Colonic Irrigation	CIM 35-1
20.29	Hyperbaric Oxygen Therapy	CIM 35-10
80.2	Photodynamic Therapy	CIM 35-100
250.4	Treatment of Actinic Keratosis	CIM 35-101
160.25	Multiple Electroconvulsive Therapy (MECT)	CIM 35-103
260.5	Intestinal and Multivisceral Transplantation	CIM 35-104
230.3	Sterilization	CIM 35-11
140.4	Plastic Surgery to Correct "Moon Face"	CIM 35-12
150.7	Prolotherapy; Joint Sclerotherapy, and Ligamentous Injections with Sclerosing Agents	CIM 35-13
70.1	Consultations With a Beneficiary's Family and Associates	CIM 35-14
240.7	Postural Drainage Procedures and Pulmonary Exercises	CIM 35-15
80.11	Vitrectomy	CIM 35-16
160.1	Induced Lesions of Nerve Tracts	CIM 35-17
30.4	Electrosleep Therapy	CIM 35-18
30.6	Intravenous Histamine Therapy	CIM 35-19
150.1	Manipulation	CIM 35-2
160.2	Treatment of Motor Function Disorders with Electric Nerve Stimulation	CIM 35-20
10.3	Inpatient Hospital Pain Rehabilitation Programs	CIM 35-21
10.4	Outpatient Hospital Pain Rehabilitation Programs	CIM 35-21.1
130.1	Inpatient Hospital Stays for the Treatment of Alcoholism	CIM 35-22
130.2	Outpatient Hospital Services for Treatment of Alcoholism	CIM 35-22
130.6	Treatment of Drug Abuse (Chemical Dependency)	CIM 35-22.2
130.5	Treatment of Alcoholism and Drug Abuse in a Freestanding Clinic	CIM 35-22.3
130.3	Chemical Aversion Therapy for Treatment of Alcoholism	CIM 35-23
130.4	Electrical Aversion Therapy for Treatment of Alcoholism	CIM 35-23.1
230.4	Diagnosis and Treatment of Impotence	CIM 35-24
20.10	Cardiac Rehabilitation Programs	CIM 35-25
40.5	Treatment of Obesity	CIM 35-26
30.1	Biofeedback Therapy	CIM 35-27
30.1.1	Biofeedback Therapy For The Treatment Of Urinary Incontinence	CIM 35-27.1
50.5	Oxygen Treatment of Inner Ear/Carbon Therapy	CIM 35-29
240.3	Heat Treatment, Including the Use of Diathermy and Ultra-Sound for Pulmonary Conditions	CIM 35-3
110.8	Blood Platelet Transfusions	CIM 35-30
270.4	Treatment Of Decubitus Ulcers	CIM 35-31
100.8	Intestinal By-Pass Surgery	CIM 35-33
230.2	Uroflowmetric Evaluations	CIM 35-33
20.23	Fabric Wrapping of Abdominal Aneurysms	CIM 35-34
20.28	Therapeutic Embolization	CIM 35-35

NCD Section	Title	CIM Section
20. 01	Vertebral Artery Surgery	CIM 35-37
20. 2	Extracranial-Intracranial (EC-IC) Arterial Bypass Surgery	CIM 35-37
110.15	Ultrafiltration, Hemoperfusion and Hemofiltration	CIM 35-38
80.6	Intraocular Photography	CIM 35-39
50.8	Ultrasonic Surgery	CIM 35-4
100.1	Gastric Bypass Surgery for Obesity	CIM 35-40
150.5	Diathermy Treatment	CIM 35-41
130.7	Withdrawal Treatments for Narcotic Addictions	CIM 35-42
10.1	Use Of Visual Tests Prior To And General Anesthesia During Cataract Surgery	CIM 35-44
20.25	Cardiac Catheterization Performed in Other Than a Hospital Setting	CIM 35-45
160.3	Assessing Patients Suitability for Electrical Nerve Stimulation	CIM 35-46
160.7.1	Assessing Patients Suitability for Electrical Nerve Stimulation Therapy	CIM 35-46
140.2	Breast Reconstruction Following Mastectomy	CIM 35-47
150.2	Osteogenic Stimulator	CIM 35-48
160.11	Osteogenic Stimulation	CIM 35-48
110.1	Hyperthermia for Treatment of Cancer	CIM 35-49
30.8	Cellular Therapy	CIM 35-5
50.7	Cochleostomy with Neurovascular Transplant for Meniere's Disease	CIM 35-50
130.8	Hemodialysis for Treatment of Schizophrenia	CIM 35-51
140.5	Laser Procedures	CIM 35-52
260.1	Adult Liver Transplantation	CIM 35-53
260.2	Pediatric Liver Transplantation	CIM 35-53.1
80.7	Refractive Keratoplasty	CIM 35-54
240.6	Transvenous (Catheter) Pulmonary Embolectomy	CIM 35-55
150.8	Fluidized Therapy Dry Heat for Certain Musculoskeletal Disorders	CIM 35-56
160.8	Electroencephalographic Monitoring During Surgical Procedures Involving the Cerebral Vasculature	CIM 35-57
160.9	Electroencephalographic (EEG) Monitoring During Open-Heart Surgery	CIM 35-57.1
20.3	Thoracic Duct Drainage (TDD) In Renal Transplants	CIM 35-58
100.2	Endoscopy	CIM 35-59
30.2	Thermogenic Therapy	CIM 35-6
110.14	Apheresis (Therapeutic Pheresis)	CIM 35-60
140.3	Transsexual Surgery	CIM 35-61
160.14	Invasive Intracranial Pressure Monitoring	CIM 35-62
50.6	Tinnitus Masking	CIM 35-63
20.21	Chelation Therapy for Treatment of Atherosclerosis	CIM 35-64
100.6	Gastric Freezing	CIM 35-65
250.1	Treatment of Psoriasis	CIM 35-66
170.2	Melodic Intonation Therapy	CIM 35-67
100.9	Implantation of Anti-Gastroesophageal Reflux Device	CIM 35-69
20.18	Carotid Body Resection/Carotid Body Denervation	CIM 35-7
40.3	Closed-Loop Blood Glucose Control Device (CBGCD)	CIM 35-70
110.16	Nonselective (Random) Transfusions and Living Related Donor Specific Transfusions (DST) in Kidney Transplantation	CIM 35-71
160.15	Electrotherapy for Treatment of Facial Nerve Palsy (Bell's Palsy)	CIM 35-72
100.10	Injection Sclerotherapy for Esophageal Variceal Bleeding	CIM 35-73

NCD Section	Title	CIM Section
20.20	External Counterpulsation (ECP) for Severe Angina	CIM 35-74
20.11	Intraoperative Ventricular Mapping	CIM 35-75
150.4	Neuromuscular Electrical Stimulator (NMES) in the Treatment of Disuse Atrophy	CIM 35-77
160.12	Neuromuscular Electrical Stimulation (NMES) in the Treatment of Disuse Atrophy	CIM 35-77
20.12	Diagnostic Endocardial Electrical Stimulation (Pacing)	CIM 35-78
10.6	Anesthesia in Cardiac Pacemaker Surgery	CIM 35-79
20.8.3	Anesthesia in Cardiac Pacemaker Surgery	CIM 35-79
30.3	Acupuncture	CIM 35-8
230.1	Treatment of Kidney Stones	CIM 35-81
260.3	Pancreas Transplants	CIM 35-82
100.3	24-Hour Ambulatory Esophegeal pH Monitoring	CIM 35-83
160.4	Steroetactic Cingulotomy as a Means of Psychosurgery	CIM 35-84
20.4	Implantation of Automatic Defibrillators	CIM 35-85
100.11	Gastric Balloon for Treatment of Obesity	CIM 35-86
260.9	Heart Transplants	CIM 35-87
110.4	Extracorporeal Photopheresis	CIM 35-88
170.3	Speech Pathology Services for the Treatment of Dysphagia	CIM 35-89
80.10	Phaco-Emulsification Procedure (Cataract Extraction)	CIM 35-9
20.5	Extracorporeal Immunoadsorption (ECI) Using Protein A Columns	CIM 35-90
100.13	Laproscopic Cholecystectomy	CIM 35-91
30.5	Transcendental Meditation	CIM 35-92
240.1	Lung Volume Reduction Surgery (Reduction Pneumoplasty)	CIM 35-93
20.6	Transmyocardial Revascularization (TMR)	CIM 35-94
20.26	Partial Ventriculectomy	CIM 35-95
230.9	Cryosurgery of Prostate	CIM 35-96
160.16	Vertebral Axial Decompression (VAX-D)	CIM 35-97
270.1	Electrostimulation in the Treatment of Wounds	CIM 35-98
140.1	Abortion	CIM 35-99
160.17	L-Dopa	CIM 45-1
30.7	Laetrile and Related Substances	CIM 45-10
10.5	Autogenous Epidural Blood Graft	CIM 45-11
270.5	Porcine Skin and Gradient Pressure Dressings	CIM 45-12
70.3	Physician's Office Within an Institution—Coverage of Services and Supplies Incident to a Physician's Services	CIM 45-15
110.2	Certain Drugs Distributed by the National Cancer Institute	CIM 45-16
160.20	Transfer Factor For Treatment of Multiple Sclerosis	CIM 45-17
110.5	Granulocyte Transfusions	CIM 45-18
10.2	Transcutaneous Electrical Nerve Stimulation (TENS) for Acute Post-Operative Pain	CIM 45-19
20.22	Ethylenediamine-Tetra-Acetic (EDTA) Chelation Therapy for Treatment of Atherosclerosis	CIM 45-20
110.6	Scalp Hypothermia During Chemotherapy to Prevent Hair Loss	CIM 45-21
260.7	Lymphocyte Immune Globulin, Anti-Thymocyte Globulin (Equine)	CIM 45-22
230.12	Dimethyl Sulfoxide (DMSO)	CIM 45-23

NCD Section	Title	CIM Section
110.3	Anti-Inhibitor Coagulant Complex (AICC)	CIM 45-24
160.13	Supplies Used in the Delivery of Transcutaneous Electrical Nerve Stimulation (TENS) and Neuromuscular Electrical Stimulation (NMES)	CIM 45-25
270.3	Platelet-Derived Wound Healing Formula	CIM 45-26
110.7	Blood Transfusions	CIM 45-27
110.9	Antigens Prepared for Sublingual Administration	CIM 45-28
110.10	Intravenous Iron Therapy	CIM 45-29
40.4	Insulin Syringe	CIM 45-3
80.3	Photosensitive Drugs	CIM 45-30
250.3	Intravenous Immune Globulin For The Treatment Of Autoimmune Mucutaneous Blistering Diseases	CIM 45-31
230.19	Levocarnitine for Use in the Treatment of Carnitine Deficiency in ESRD Patients	CIM 45-32
150.6	Vitamin B12 Injections to Strengthen Tendons; Ligaments; etc; of the Foot	CIM 45-4
80.1	Hydrophilic Contact Lens for Corneal Bandage	CIM 45-7
70.2.1	Services Provided for the Diagnosis and Treatment of Diabetic Sensory Neuropathy with Loss of Protective Sensation (aka Diabetic Peripheral Neuropathy)	CIM 50.8.1
20.8.1	Cardiac Pacemaker Evaluation Services	CIM 50-1
20.8.1.1	Transtelephonic Monitoring of Cardiac Pacemakers	CIM 50-1
230.6	Vabra Aspirator	CIM 50-10
220.1	Computerized Tomography	CIM 50-12
220.2	Magnetic Resonance Imaging	CIM 50-13
220.3	Magnetic Resonance Angiography	CIM 50-14
20.15	Electrocardiographic Services	CIM 50-15
250.2	Hemorheograph	CIM 50-16
190.4	Electron Microscope	CIM 50-18
70.4	Pronouncement of Death	CIM 50-19
110.13	Cytotoxic Food Tests	CIM 50-2
190.2	Diagnostic Pap Smears	CIM 50-20
230.11	Diagnostic Pap Smears	CIM 50-20
210.2	Screening Pap Smears and Pelvic Examinations for Early Detection of Cervical or Vaginal Cancer	CIM 50-20.1
220.4	Mammograms	CIM 50-21
110.12	Challenge Ingestion Food Testing	CIM 50-22
190.1	Histocompatibility Testing	CIM 50-23
190.6	Hair Analysis	CIM 50-24
100.4	Esophageal Manometry	CIM 50-25
260.6	Dental Examination Prior to Kidney Transplantation	CIM 50-26
220.7	Xenon Scan	CIM 50-27
70.5	Hospital and Skilled Nursing Facility Admission Diagnostic Procedures	CIM 50-28
190.3	Cytogenetic Studies	CIM 50-29
20.13	HIS Bundle Study	CIM 50-3
220.8	Nuclear Radiology Procedure	CIM 50-30
160.10	Evoked Response Tests	CIM 50-31
20.7	Percutaneous Transluminal Angioplasty (PTA)	CIM 50-32
300.1	Obsolete or Unreliable Diagnostic Tests	CIM 50-34
190.5	Sweat Test	CIM 50-35
220.6	Positron Emission Tomography (PET) Scans	CIM 50-36
20.17	Noninvasive Tests of Carotid Function	CIM 50-37
80.8	Endothelial Cell Photography	CIM 50-38
160.21	Telephone Transmission of EEGs	CIM 50-39
160.22	Ambulatory EEG Monitoring	CIM 50-39.1
230.5	Gravlee Jet Washer	CIM 50-4

NCD Section	Title	CIM Section
160.5	Sterotaxic Depth Electrode Implantation	CIM 50-40
190.7	Human Tumor Stem Cell Drug Sensitivity Assays	CIM 50-41
20.19	Ambulatory Blood Pressure Monitoring	CIM 50-42
220.9	Digital Subtraction Angiography	CIM 50-43
150.3	Bone (Mineral) Density Studies	CIM 50-44
190.8	Lymphocyte Mitogen Response Assays	CIM 50-45
30.9	Transillumination Light Scanning or Diaphanography	CIM 50-46
20.27	Cardiointegram (CIG) as an Alternative to Stress Test or Thallium Stress Test	CIM 50-47
220.10	Portable Hand-Held X-Ray Instrument	CIM 50-48
80.9	Computer Enhanced Perimetry	CIM 50-49
220.11	Thermography	CIM 50-5
20.24	Displacement Cardiography	CIM 50-50
100.5	Diagnostic Breath Analyses	CIM 50-51
190.9	Serologic Testing for Acquired Immunodeficiency Syndrome (AIDS)	CIM 50-52
110.11	Food Allergy Testing and Treatment	CIM 50-53
20.16	Cardiac Output Monitoring By Electrical Bioimpedance	CIM 50-54
210.1	Prostate Cancer Screening Tests	CIM 50-55
190.11	Home Prothrombin Time INR Monitoring for Anticoagulation Management	CIM 50-56
160.23	Current Perception Threshold/Sensory Nerve Conduction Threshold Test (sNCT)	CIM 50-57.1
220.12	Single Photon Emission Computed Tomograph (SPECT)	CIM 50-58
220.13	Percutaneous Image-Guided Breast Biopsy	CIM 50-59
20.14	Plethysmography	CIM 50-6
220.5	Ultrasound Diagnostic Procedures	CIM 50-7
70.2	Consultation Services Rendered By a Podiatrist in a Skilled Nursing Facility	CIM 50-8
100.12	Gastrophotography	CIM 50-9
230.7	Water Purification and Softening Systems Used in Conjunction with Home Dialysis	CIM 55-1
230.13	Peridex CAPD Filter Set	CIM 55-2
230.14	Ultrafiltration Monitor	CIM 55-3
40.2	Home Blood Glucose Monitors	CIM 60-11 and CIM 60-14
280.14	Infusion Pumps	CIM 60-14
280.5	Safety Roller	CIM 60-15
280.6	Pneumatic Compression Devices	CIM 60-16
240.4	Continuous Positive Airway Pressure (CPAP)	CIM 60-17
280.7	Hospital Beds	CIM 60-18
280.8	Air-Fluidized Bed	CIM 60-19
280.13	Transcutaneous Electrical Nerve Stimulators (TENS)	CIM 60-20
240.5	Intrapulmonary Percussive Ventilator (IPV)	CIM 60-21
160.18	Vagus Nerve Stimulation for Treatment of Seizures	CIM 60-22
50.1	Speech Generating Devices	CIM 60-23
230.8	Non-Implantable Pelvic Flood Electrical Stimulator	CIM 60-24
270.2	Noncontact Normothermic Wound Therapy (NNWT)	CIM 60-25
280.2	White Cane for Use by a Blind Person	CIM 60-3
240.2	Home Use of Oxygen	CIM 60-4
280.9	Power Operated Vehicles That May Be Used as Wheelchairs	CIM 60-5
280.3	Specially Sized Wheelchairs	CIM 60-6
20.8.2	Self-Contained Pacemaker Monitors	CIM 60-7
280.4	Seat Lift	CIM 60-8
280.1	Durable Medical Equipment Reference List	CIM 60-9

NCD Section	Title	CIM Section
80.5	Scleral Shell	CIM 65.3
80.4	Hydrophilic Contact Lenses	CIM 65-1
180.2	Enteral and Parenteral Nutritional Therapy	CIM 65-10
230.16	Bladder Stimulators (Pacemakers)	CIM 65-11
160.19	Phrenic Nerve Stimulator	CIM 65-13
50.3	Cochlear Implantation	CIM 65-14
20.9	Artificial Hearts and Related Devices	CIM 65-16
50.4	Tracheostomy Speaking Valve	CIM 65-165
230.17	Urinary Drainage Bags	CIM 65-17
230.18	Sacral Nerve Stimulation for Urinary Incontinence	CIM 65-18
160.24	Deep Brain Stimulation for Essential Tremor and Parkinson's Disease	CIM 65-19
230.15	Electrical Continence Aid	CIM 65-2
160.6	Carotid Sinus Nerve Stimulator	CIM 65-4
50.2	Electronic Speech Aids	CIM 65-5
20.8	Cardiac Pacemakers	CIM 65-6
80.12	Intraocular Lenses (IOLs)	CIM 65-7
160.7	Electrical Nerve Stimulators	CIM 65-8
230.10	Incontinence Control Devices	CIM 65-9
280.11	Corset Used as Hernia Support	CIM 70-1
280.12	Sykes Hernia Control	CIM 70-2
280.10	Prosthetic Shoe	CIM 70-3
170.1	Institutional and Home Care Patient Education Programs	CIM 80-1
40.1	Diabetes Outpatient Self-Management Training	CIM 80-2
180.1	Medical Nutrition Therapy	CIM 80-3
290.1	Home Health Visits to a Blind Diabetic	CIM 90-1
290.2	Home Health Nurses' Visits to Patients Requiring Heparin Injections	CIM 90-2

The crosswalk for the Medicare Carriers Manual (MCM) is too extensive to display in this text, but can be accessed at www.cms.hhs.gov/manuals/ .

2005 WHEN PART B EXPENSES ARE INCURRED (100-2, 15, §20)

2005.1 Physicians' Expense for Surgery, Childbirth, and Treatment for Infertility (100-2, 15, §20.1)

A. Surgery and Childbirth.—Skilled medical management is appropriate throughout the events of pregnancy, beginning with diagnosis, continuing through delivery, and ending after the necessary postnatal care. Similarly, in the event of termination of pregnancy, regardless of whether terminated spontaneously or for therapeutic reasons (i.e., where the life of the mother would be endangered if the fetus were brought to term), the need for skilled medical management and/or medical services is equally important as in those cases carried to full term. After the infant is delivered and is a separate individual, items and services furnished to the infant are not covered on the basis of the mother's eligibility.

Most surgeons and obstetricians bill patients an all-inclusive package charge intended to cover all services associated with the surgical procedure or delivery of the child. All expenses for surgical and obstetrical care, including preoperative/prenatal examinations and tests and postoperative/postnatal services are considered incurred on the date of surgery or delivery, as appropriate. This policy applies whether the physician bills on a package charge basis, or itemizes his/her bill separately for these items.

Occasionally, a physician's bill may include charges for additional services not directly related to the surgical procedure or the delivery. Such charges are considered incurred on the date the additional services are furnished.

The above policy applies only where the charges are imposed by one physician or by a clinic on behalf of a group of physicians. Where charges are imposed by more than one physician for surgical or obstetrical services, all preoperative/prenatal and postoperative/postnatal services performed by the physician who per-

formed the surgery or delivery are considered incurred on the date of the surgery or delivery. Expenses for services rendered by other physicians are considered incurred on the date they were performed.

B. Treatment for Infertility.—Reasonable and necessary services associated with treatment for infertility are covered under Medicare. Infertility is a condition sufficiently at variance with the usual state of health to make it appropriate for a person who normally is expected to be fertile to seek medical consultation and treatment. Coordinate with PROs to see that utilization guidelines are established for this treatment if inappropriate utilization or abuse is suspected.

2049 DRUGS AND BIOLOGICALS (100-2, 15, §50, 17, §10)

Generally, drugs and biologicals are covered only if all of the following requirements are met:

- They meet the definition of drugs or biologicals (see section 50.1);
- They are of the type that cannot be self-administered (see section 50.2);
- They meet all the general requirements for coverage of items as incident to a physician's services (see sections 50.1 and 50.3);
- They are reasonable and necessary for the diagnosis or treatment of the illness or injury for which they are administered according to accepted standards of medical practice (see section 50.4);
- They are not excluded as immunizations (see section 50.4.4.2); and
- They have not been determined by the FDA to be less than effective. (See section 50.4.4)

Medicare Part B does generally not cover drugs that can be self-administered, such as those in pill form, or are used for self-injection. However, the statute provides for the coverage of some self-administered drugs. Examples of self-administered drugs that are covered include blood-clotting factors, drugs used in immunosuppressive therapy, erythropoietin for dialysis patients, osteoporosis drugs for certain homebound patients, and certain oral cancer drugs. (See §110.3 for coverage of drugs, which are necessary to the effective use of Durable Medical Equipment (DME) or prosthetic devices.)

2049.1 Definition of Drug or Biological. (100-2, 15, §50.1)—
Drugs and biologicals must be determined to meet the statutory definition. Under the statute section 1861(+)(1), payment may be made for a drug or biological only where it is included, or approved for inclusion, in the latest official edition of the United States Pharmacopoeia-National Formulary (USP-NF), the United States Pharmacopoeia Drug Information (USPDI), or the American Dental Association (ADA) Guide to Dental Therapeutics, except for those drugs and biologicals unfavorably evaluated in the ADA Guide to Dental Therapeutics. Combination drugs are also included in the definition of drugs if the combination itself or all of the therapeutic ingredients of the combination are included, or approved for inclusion, in any of the above drug compendia.

Drugs and biologicals are considered approved for inclusion in a compendium if approved under the established procedure by the professional organization responsible for revision of the compendium.

2049.2 Determining Self-Administration of Drug or Biological. (100-2, 15, §50.2)—The Medicare program provides limited benefits for outpatient prescription drugs. The program covers drugs that are furnished "incident to" a physician's service provided that the drugs are not usually self-administered by the patients who take them. Section 112 of the Benefits, Improvements & Protection Act of 2000 (BIPA) amended sections 1861(s)(2)(A) and 1861(s)(2)(B) of the Act to redefine this exclusion. The prior statutory language referred to those drugs "which cannot be self-administered." Implementation of the BIPA provision requires interpretation of the phrase "not usually self-administered by the patient".

A. Policy—Fiscal intermediaries and carriers are instructed to follow the instructions below when applying the exclusion for drugs that are usually self-administered by the patient. Each individual contractor must make its own individual determination on each drug. Contractors must continue to apply the policy that not only the drug is medically reasonable and necessary for any individual claim, but also that the route of administration is medically reasonable and necessary. That is, if a drug is available in both oral and injectable forms, the injectable form of the drug must be medically reasonable and necessary as compared to using the oral form.

For certain injectable drugs, it will be apparent due to the nature of the condition(s) for which they are administered or the usual course of treatment for those conditions, they are, or are not, usually self-administered. For example, an injectable drug used to treat migraine headaches is usually self-administered. On the other hand, an injectable drug, administered at the same time as chemotherapy, used to treat anemia secondary to chemotherapy is not usually self-administered.

B. Administered—The term "administered" refers only to the physical process by which the drug enters the patient's body. It does not refer to whether the process is supervised by a medical professional (for example, to observe proper technique or side-effects of the drug). Only injectable (including intravenous) drugs are eligible for inclusion under the "incident to" benefit. Other routes of administration including, but not limited to, oral drugs, suppositories, topical medications are all considered to be usually self-administered by the patient.

C. Usually—For the purposes of applying this exclusion, the term "usually" means more than 50 percent of the time for all Medicare beneficiaries who use the drug. Therefore, if a drug is self-administered by more than 50 percent of Medicare beneficiaries, the drug is excluded from coverage and the contractor may not make any Medicare payment for it. In arriving at a single determination as to whether a drug is usually self-administered, contractors should make a separate determination for each indication for a drug as to whether that drug is usually self-administered.

After determining whether a drug is usually self-administered for each indication, contractors should determine the relative contribution of each indication to total use of the drug (i.e., weighted average) in order to make an overall determination as to whether the drug is usually self-administered. For example, if a drug has three indications, is not self-administered for the first indication, but is self administered for the second and third indications, and the first indication makes up 40 percent of total usage, the second indication makes up 30 percent of total usage, and the third indication makes up 30 percent of total usage, then the drug would be considered usually self-administered.

Reliable statistical information on the extent of self-administration by the patient may not always be available. Consequently, CMS offers the following guidance for each contractor's consideration in making this determination in the absence of such data:

1. Absent evidence to the contrary, presume that drugs delivered intravenously are not usually self-administered by the patient.

2. Absent evidence to the contrary, presume that drugs delivered by intramuscular injection are not usually self-administered by the patient. (Avonex, for example, is delivered by intramuscular injection, not usually self-administered by the patient.) The contractor may consider the depth and nature of the particular intramuscular injection in applying this presumption. In applying this presumption, contractors should examine the use of the particular drug and consider the following factors:

3. Absent evidence to the contrary, presume that drugs delivered by subcutaneous injection are self-administered by the patient. However, contractors should examine the use of the particular drug and consider the following factors:

A. Acute Condition—Is the condition for which the drug is used an acute condition? If so, it is less likely that a patient would self-administer the drug. If the condition were longer term, it would be more likely that the patient would self-administer the drug.

B. Frequency of Administration—How often is the injection given? For example, if the drug is administered once per month, it is less likely to be self-administered by the patient. However, if it is administered once or more per week, it is likely that the drug is self-administered by the patient.

In some instances, carriers may have provided payment for one or perhaps several doses of a drug that would otherwise not be paid for because the drug is usually self-administered. Carriers may have exercised this discretion for limited coverage, for example, during a brief time when the patient is being trained under the supervision of a physician in the proper technique for self-administration. Medicare will no longer pay for such doses. In addition, contractors may no longer pay for any drug when it is administered on an outpatient emergency basis, if the drug is excluded because it is usually self-administered by the patient.

D. Definition of Acute Condition—For the purposes of determining whether a drug is usually self-administered, an acute condition means a condition that begins over a short time period, is likely to be of short duration and/or the expected course of treatment is for a short, finite interval. A course of treatment consisting of scheduled injections lasting less than two weeks, regardless of frequency or route of administration, is considered acute. Evidence to support this may include Food and Drug administration (FDA) approval language, package inserts, drug compendia, and other information.

E. By the Patient—The term "by the patient" means Medicare beneficiaries as a collective whole. The carrier includes only the patients themselves and not other individuals (that is, spouses, friends, or other care-givers are not considered the patient). The determination is based on whether the drug is self-administered by the patient a majority of the time that the drug is used on an outpatient basis by Medicare beneficiaries for medically necessary indications. The carrier ignores all instances when the drug is administered on an inpatient basis.

The carrier makes this determination on a drug-by-drug basis, not on a beneficiary-by-beneficiary basis. In evaluating whether beneficiaries as a collective whole self-administer, individual beneficiaries who do not have the capacity to self-administer any drug due to a condition other than the condition for which they are taking the drug in question are not considered. For example, an individual afflicted with paraplegia or advanced dementia would not have the capacity to self-administer any injectable drug, so such individuals would not be included in the population upon which the determination for self-administration by the patient was based. Note that some individuals afflicted with a less severe stage of an otherwise debilitating condition would be included in the population upon which the determination for "self-administered by the patient" was based; for example, an early onset of dementia.

F. Evidentiary Criteria—Contractors are only required to consider the following types of evidence: peer reviewed medical literature, standards of medical practice, evidence-based practice guidelines, FDA approved label, and package inserts. Contractors may also consider other evidence submitted by interested individuals or groups subject to their judgment.

Contractors should also use these evidentiary criteria when reviewing requests for making a determination as to whether a drug is usually self-administered, and requests for reconsideration of a pending or published determination.

Please note that prior to the August 1, 2002, one of the principal factors used to determine whether a drug was subject to the self-administered exclusion was whether the FDA label contained instructions for self-administration. However, CMS notes that under the new standard, the fact that the FDA label includes instructions for self-administration is not, by itself, a determining factor that a drug is subject to this exclusion.

G. Provider Notice of Noncovered Drugs—Contractors must describe on their Web site the process they will use to determine whether a drug is usually self-administered and thus does not meet the "incident to" benefit category. Contractors must publish a list of the injectable drugs that are subject to the self-administered exclusion on their Web site, including the data and rationale that led to the determination. Contractors will report the workload associated with developing new coverage statements in CAFM 21208.

Contractors must provide notice 45 days prior to the date that these drugs will not be covered. During the 45-day time period, contractors will maintain existing medical review and payment procedures. After the 45-day notice, contractors may deny payment for the drugs subject to the notice.

Contractors must not develop local medical review policies (LMRPs) for this purpose because further elaboration to describe drugs that do not meet the 'incident to' and the 'not usually self-administered' provisions of the statute are unnecessary. Current LMRPs based solely on these provisions must be withdrawn. LMRPs that address the self-administered exclusion and other information may be reissued absent the self-administered drug exclusion material. Contractors will report this workload in CAFM 21206. However, contractors may continue to use and write LMRPs to describe reasonable and necessary uses of drugs that are not usually self-administered.

H. Conferences Between Contractors—Contractors' Medical Directors may meet and discuss whether a drug is usually self-administered without reaching a formal consensus. Each contractor uses its discretion as to whether or not it will participate in such discussions. Each contractor must make its own individual determinations, except that fiscal intermediaries may, at their discretion, follow the determinations of the local carrier with respect to the self-administered exclusion.

I. Beneficiary Appeals—If a beneficiary's claim for a particular drug is denied because the drug is subject to the "self-administered drug" exclusion, the beneficiary may appeal the denial. Because it is a "benefit category" denial and not a denial based on medical necessity, an Advance Beneficiary Notice (ABN) is not required. A "benefit category" denial (i.e., a denial based on the fact that there is no benefit category under which the drug may be covered) does not trigger the financial liability protection provisions of Limitation On Liability (under §1879 of the Act). Therefore, physicians or providers may charge the beneficiary for an excluded drug.

J. Provider and Physician Appeals—A physician accepting assignment may appeal a denial under the provisions found in Chapter 29 of the Medicare Claims Processing Manual.

K. Reasonable and Necessary—Carriers and fiscal intermediaries will make the determination of reasonable and necessary with respect to the medical appropriateness of a drug to treat the patient's condition. Contractors will continue to make the determination of whether the intravenous or injection form of a drug is appropriate as opposed to the oral form. Contractors will also continue to make the determination as to whether a physician's office visit was reasonable and necessary. However, contractors should not make a determination of whether it was reasonable and necessary for the patient to choose to have his or her drug administered in the physician's office or outpatient hospital setting. That is, while a physician's office visit may not be reasonable and necessary in a specific situation, in such a case an injection service would be payable.

L. Reporting Requirements—Each carrier and intermediary must report to CMS, every September 1 and March 1, its complete list of injectable drugs that the contractor has determined are excluded when furnished incident to a physician's service on the basis that the drug is usually self-administered. The CMS anticipates that contractors will review injectable drugs on a rolling basis and publish their list of excluded drugs as it is developed. For example, contractors should not wait to publish this list until every drug has been reviewed. Contractors must send their exclusion list to the following e-mail address: drugdata@cms.hhs.gov a template that CMS will provide separately, consisting of the following data elements in order:

1. Carrier Name
2. State
3. Carrier ID#
4. HCPCS
5. Descriptor
6. Effective Date of Exclusion
7. End Date of Exclusion
8. Comments

Any exclusion list not provided in the CMS mandated format will be returned for correction.

To view the presently mandated CMS format for this report, open the file located at: *http://cms.hhs.gov/manuals/pm_trans/AB02_139a.zip*

2049.3 Incident-to Requirements. (100.2, 15, §50.3, 100-4, 8-§60.3)—In order to meet all the general requirements for coverage under the incident-to provision, an FDA approved drug or biological must:

- Be of a form that is not usually self-administered;
- Must be furnished by a physician; and
- Must be administered by the physician, or by auxiliary personnel employed by the physician and under the physician's personal supervision.

The charge, if any, for the drug or biological must be included in the physician's bill, and the cost of the drug or biological must represent an expense to the physician. Drugs and biologicals furnished by other health professionals may also meet these requirements. (See §§170, 180, 190 and 200 for specific instructions.)

Whole blood is a biological, which cannot be self-administered and is covered when furnsihed incident to a physician's services. Payment may also be made for blood fractions if all coverage requirements are satisfied and the blood deductible has been met.

2049.4 Approved use of Drug. (100-2, 15, §50.4-50.4.4.1, 100-4, 18, §10.2)—Use of the drug or biological must be safe and effective and otherwise reasonable and necessary. (See section the Medicare Benefit Policy Manual, Chapter 16, "General Exclusions from Coverage," §20.) Drugs or biologicals approved for marketing by the Food and Drug Administration (FDA) are considered safe and effective for purposes of this requirement when used for indications specified on the labeling. Therefore you may pay for the use of an FDA approved drug or biological, if:

- It was injected on or after the date of the FDA's approval;
- It is reasonable and necessary for the individual patient; and
- All other applicable coverage requirements are met.

The Carrier, DMERC, or intermediary will deny coverage for drugs and biologicals that have not received final marketing approval by the FDA unless you receive instructions from HCFA to the contrary. For specific guidelines on coverage of Group C cancer drugs, see the Medicare National Coverage Determinations Manual.

If there is reason to question whether the FDA has approved a drug or biological for marketing, obtain satisfactory evidence of FDA approval. Acceptable evidence includes:

- A copy of the FDA's letter to the drug's manufacturer approving the new drug application (NDA)
- Listing of the drug or biological in the FDA's Approved Drug Products or FDA Drug and Device Product Approvals
- A copy of the manufacturer's package insert, approved by the FDA as part of the labeling of the drug, containing its recommended uses and dosage, as well as possible adverse reactions and recommended precautions in using it
- Information from the FDA's Web site

When necessary, the RO may be able to help in obtaining information.

(50.4.2 Unlabeled Use of Drug) An unlabeled use of a drug is a use that is not included as an indication on the drug's label as approved by the FDA. FDA-approved drugs used for indications other than what is indicated on the official label may be covered under Medicare if the carrier determines the use to be medically accepted, taking into consideration the major drug compendia, authoritative medical literature, and/or accepted standards of medical practice. In the case of drugs used in an anti-cancer chemotherapeutic regimen, unlabeled uses are covered for a medically accepted indication as defined in section 50.5.

(50.4.3 Examples of Not Reasonable and Necessary) Determinations as to whether medication is reasonable and necessary for an individual patient should be made on the same basis as all other such determinations (i.e., with the advice of medical consultants and with reference to accepted standards of medical practice and the medical circumstances of the individual case). The following guidelines identify three categories with specific examples of situations in which medications would not be reasonable and necessary according to accepted standards of medical practice.

1. Not for Particular Illness.—Medications given for a purpose other than the treatment of a particular condition, illness, or injury are not covered (except for certain immunizations). Exclude the charge for medications, e.g., vitamins, given simply for the general good and welfare of the patient and not as accepted therapy for a particular illness.

2. Injection Method Not Indicated.—Medication given by injection (parenterally) is not covered if standard medical practice indicates that the administration of the medication by mouth (orally) is effective and is an accepted or preferred method of administration. For example, the accepted standards of medical practice for the treatment of certain diseases is to initiate therapy with parenteral penicillin and to complete therapy with oral penicillin. Exclude the entire charge for penicillin injections given after the initiation of therapy if oral penicillin is indicated unless there are special medical circumstances that justify additional injections.

3. Excessive Medications.— Medications administered for treatment of a disease that exceed the frequency or duration of injections indicated by accepted standards of medical practice are not covered. For example, the accepted standard of medical practice in the maintenance treatment of pernicious anemia is one vitamin B-12 injection per month. Exclude the entire charge for injections given in excess of this frequency unless there are special medical circumstances that justify additional injections.

Supplement the guidelines as necessary with guidelines concerning appropriate use of specific injections in other situations. Use the guidelines to screen out questionable cases for special review, further development, or denial when the injection billed for would not be reasonable and necessary. Coordinate any type of drug treatment review with the PRO.

If a medication is determined not to be reasonable and necessary for diagnosis or treatment of an illness or injury according to these guidelines, exclude the entire charge (i.e., for both the drug and its administration). Also exclude from payment any charges for other services (such as office visits) that were primarily for the purpose of administering a noncovered injection (i.e., an injection that is not reasonable and necessary for the diagnosis or treatment of an illness or injury).

(50.4.4.1) A. Antigens.—Payment may be made for a reasonable supply of antigens that have been prepared for a particular patient if: (1) the antigens are prepared by a physician who is a doctor of medicine or osteopathy, and (2) the physician who prepared the antigens has examined the patient and has determined a plan of treatment and a dosage regimen.

Antigens must be administered in accordance with the plan of treatment and by a doctor of medicine or osteopathy or by a properly instructed person (who could be the patient) under the supervision of the doctor. The associations of allergists that CMS consulted advised that a reasonable supply of antigens is considered to be not more than a 12-week supply of antigens that has been prepared for a particular patient at any one time. The purpose of the reasonable supply limitation is to assure that the antigens retain their potency and effectiveness over the period in which they are to be administered to the patient. (See sections 20.2 and 50.2.)

(50.4.4.2) B. Immunizations.—Vaccinations or inoculations are excluded as immunizations unless they are directly related to the treatment of an injury or direct exposure to a disease or condition, such as antirabies treatment, tetanus antitoxin or booster vaccine, botulin antitoxin, antivenin sera, or immune globulin. In the absence of injury or direct exposure, preventive immunization (vaccination or inoculation) against such diseases as smallpox, polio, diphtheria, etc., is not covered. However, pneumococcal, hepatitis B, and influenza virus vaccines are exceptions to this rule. (See items A, B and C below.) In cases where a vaccination or inoculation is excluded from coverage, deny the entire charge.

A. Pneumococcal Pneumonia Vaccinations.— Effective for services furnished on or after May 1, 1981, the Medicare Part B program covers pneumococcal pneumonia vaccine and its administration when furnished in compliance with any applicable State law by any provider of services or any entity or individual with a supplier number. This includes revaccination of patients at highest risk of pneumococcal infection. Typically, these vaccines are administered once in a lifetime except for persons at highest risk. Effective July 1, 2000, Medicare does not require for coverage purposes that the vaccine must be ordered by a doctor of medicine or osteopathy. Therefore, the beneficiary may receive the vaccine upon request without a physician's order and without physician supervision.

An initial vaccine may be administered only to persons at high risk (see below) of pneumococcal disease. Revaccination may be administered only to persons at highest risk of serious pneumococcal infection and those likely to have a rapid decline in pneumococcal antibody levels, provided that at least 5 years have passed since receipt of a previous dose of pneumococcal vaccine.

Persons at high risk for whom an initial vaccine may be administered include all people age 65 and older; immunocompetent adults who are at increased risk of pneumococcal disease or its complications because of chronic illness (e.g., cardiovascular disease, pulmonary disease, diabetes mellitus, alcoholism, cirrhosis, or cerebrospinal fluid leaks); and individuals with compromised immune systems (e.g., splenic dysfunction or anatomic asplenia, Hodgkin's disease, lymphoma, multiple myeloma, chronic renal failure, HIV infection, nephrotic syndrome, sickle cell disease, or organ transplantation).

Persons at highest risk and those most likely to have rapid declines in antibody levels are those for whom revaccination may be appropriate. This group includes persons with functional or anatomic asplenia (e.g., sickle cell disease, splenectomy), HIV infection, leukemia, lymphoma, Hodgkin's disease, multiple myeloma, generalized malignancy, chronic renal failure, nephrotic syndrome, or other conditions associated with immunosuppression such as organ or bone marrow transplantation, and those receiving immunosuppressive chemotherapy. Routine revaccination of people age 65 or older who are not at highest risk is not appropriate.

Those administering the vaccine should not require the patient to present an immunization record prior to administering the pneumococcal vaccine, nor should they feel compelled to review the patient's complete medical record if it is not available. Instead, provided that the patient is competent, it is acceptable for them to rely on the patient's verbal history to determine prior vaccination status. If the patient is uncertain about his/her vaccination history in the past 5 years, the vaccine should be given. However, if the patient is certain he/she was vaccinated in the last 5 years, the vaccine should not be given. If the patient is certain that the vaccine was given and that more than 5 years have passed since receipt of the previous dose, revaccination is not appropriate unless the patient is at highest risk.

B. Hepatitis B Vaccine.—With the enactment of P.L. 98-369, coverage under Part B was extended to hepatitis B vaccine and its administration, furnished to a Medicare beneficiary who is at high or intermediate risk of contracting hepatitis B. This coverage is effective for services furnished on or after September 1, 1984. High-risk groups currently identified include (see exception below):

- End stage renal disease (ESRD) patients;
- Hemophiliacs who receive Factor VIII or IX concentrates;
- Clients of institutions for the mentally retarded;
- Persons who live in the same household as a hepatitis B virus (HBV) carrier;
- Homosexual men; and
- Illicit injectable drug abusers.

Intermediate risk groups currently identified include:

- Staff in institutions for the mentally retarded; and
- Workers in health care professions who have frequent contact with blood or blood-derived body fluids during routine work.

EXCEPTION: Persons in the above-listed groups would not be considered at high or intermediate risk of contracting hepatitis B, however, if there is laboratory evidence positive for antibodies to hepatitis B. (ESRD patients are routinely tested for hepatitis B antibodies as part of their continuing monitoring and therapy.)

For Medicare program purposes, the vaccine may be administered upon the order of a doctor of medicine or osteopathy by home health agencies, skilled nursing facilities, ESRD facilities, hospital outpatient departments, persons recognized under the incident to physicians' services provision of law, and doctors of medicine and osteopathy.

A charge separate from the ESRD composite rate will be recognized and paid for administration of the vaccine to ESRD patients.

C. Influenza Virus Vaccine.—Effective for services furnished on or after May 1, 1993, the Medicare Part B program covers influenza virus vaccine and its administration when furnished in compliance with any applicable State law by any provider of services or any entity or individual with a supplier number. Typically, these vaccines are administered once a year in the fall or winter. Medicare does not require for coverage purposes that the vaccine must be ordered by a doctor of medicine or osteopathy. Therefore the beneficiary may receive the vaccine upon request without a physician's order and without physician supervision.

(50.4.5) C. Unlabeled Use For Anti-Cancer Drugs.—Effective January 1, 1994, unlabeled uses of FDA-approved drugs and biologicals used in an anti-cancer chemotherapeutic regimen for a medically accepted indication are evaluated under the conditions described in this paragraph. A regimen is a combination of anti-cancer agents that has been clinically recognized for the treatment of a specific type of cancer. An example of a drug regimen is: Cyclophosphamide + vincristine + prednisone (CVP) for non-Hodgkin's lymphoma.

In addition to listing the combination of drugs for a type of cancer, there may be a different regimen or combinations that are used at different times in the history of the cancer (induction, prophylaxis of CNS involvement, post remission, and relapsed or refractory disease). A protocol may specify the combination of drugs, doses, and schedules for administration of the drugs. For purposes of this provision, a cancer treatment regimen includes drugs used to treat toxicities or side effects of the cancer treatment regimen when the drug is administered incident to a chemotherapy treatment. Contractors must not deny coverage based solely on the absence of FDA-approved labeling for the use, if the use is supported by one of the following and the use is not listed as "not indicated" in any of the three compendia. (See note at the end of this subsection.)

A. American Hospital Formulary Service Drug Information.—Drug monographs are arranged in alphabetical order within therapeutic classifications. Within the text of the monograph, information concerning indications is provided, including both labeled and unlabeled uses. Unlabeled uses are identified with daggers. The text must be analyzed to make a determination whether a particular use is supported.

B. American Medical Association Drug Evaluations.—Drug evaluations are organized into sections and chapters that are based on therapeutic classifications. The evaluation of a drug provides information concerning indications, including both labeled and unlabeled uses. Unlabeled uses are not specifically identified as such. The text must be analyzed to make a determination whether a particular use is supported. In making these determinations, also refer to the AMA Drug Evaluations Subscription, Volume III, section 17 (Oncolytic Drugs), chapter 1 (Principles of Cancer Chemotherapy), tables 1 and 2.

Table 1, Specific Agents Used in Cancer Chemotherapy, lists the anti-neoplastic agents that are currently available for use in various cancers. The indications presented in this table for a particular anti-cancer drug include labeled and unlabeled uses (although they are not identified as such). Any indication appearing in this table is considered to be a medically accepted use.

Table 2, Clinical Responses to Chemotherapy, lists some of the currently preferred regimens for various cancers. The table headings include (1) type of cancer, (2) drugs or regimens currently preferred, (3) alternative or secondary drugs or regimens, and (4) other drugs or regimens with reported activity.

A regimen appearing under the preferred or alternative/secondary headings is considered to be a medically accepted use.

A regimen appearing under the heading "Other Drugs or Regimens with Reported Activity" is considered to be for a medically accepted use provided:

- The preferred and alternative/secondary drugs or regimens are contraindicated; or
- A preferred and/or alternative/secondary drug or regimen was used but was not tolerated or was ineffective; or
- There was tumor progression or recurrence after an initial response.

C. United States Pharmacopoeia Drug Information (USPDI).—Monographs are arranged in alphabetical order by generic or family name. Indications for use appear as accepted, unaccepted, or insufficient data. An indication is considered to be a medically accepted use only if the indication is listed as accepted. Unlabeled uses are identified with brackets. A separate indications index lists all indications included in USPDI along with the medically accepted drugs used in treatment or diagnosis.

D. A Use Supported by Clinical Research that Appears in Peer Reviewed Medical Literature.—This applies only when an unlabeled use does not appear in any of the compendia or is listed as insufficient data or investigational. If an unlabeled use of a drug meets these criteria, contact the compendia to see if a report regarding this use is forthcoming. If a report is forthcoming, use this information as a basis for your decision making. The compendium process for making decisions concerning unlabeled uses is very thorough and continuously updated. Peer-reviewed medical literature includes scientific, medical, and pharmaceutical publications in which original manuscripts are published, only after having been critically reviewed for scientific accuracy, validity, and reliability by unbiased independent experts. This does not include in-house publications of pharmaceutical manufacturing companies or abstracts (including meeting abstracts).

In determining whether there is supportive clinical evidence for a particular use of a drug, your medical staff (in consultation with local medical specialty groups) must evaluate the quality of the evidence in published, peer-reviewed medical literature. When evaluating this literature, consider (among other things) the following:

- The prevalence and life history of the disease when evaluating the adequacy of the number of subjects and the response rate. While a 20% response rate may be adequate for highly prevalent disease states, a lower rate may be adequate for rare diseases or highly unresponsive conditions.
- The effect on the patient's well-being and other responses to therapy that indicate effectiveness, e.g., a significant increase in survival rate or life expectancy or an objective and significant decrease in the size of the tumor or a reduction in symptoms

related to the tumor. Stabilization is not considered a response to therapy.
• The appropriateness of the study design. Consider:

1. Whether the experimental design in light of the drugs and conditions under investigation is appropriate to address the investigative question. (For example, in some clinical studies, it may be unnecessary or not feasible to use randomization, double blind trials, placebos, or crossover.);

2. That nonrandomized clinical trials with a significant number of subjects may be a basis for supportive clinical evidence for determining accepted uses of drugs; and

3. That case reports are generally considered uncontrolled and anecdotal information and do not provide adequate supportive clinical evidence for determining accepted uses of drugs.

The Carrier will use peer reviewed medical literature appearing in the following publications:

• American Journal of Medicine;
• Annals of Internal Medicine;
• The Journal of the American Medical Association;
• Journal of Clinical Oncology;
• Blood;
• Journal of the National Cancer Institute;
• The New England Journal of Medicine;
• British Journal of Cancer;
• British Journal of Hematology;
• British Medical Journal;
• Cancer;
• Drugs;
• European Journal of Cancer (formerly the European Journal of Cancer and Clinical Oncology);
• Lancet; or
• Leukemia.

The Carrier is not required to maintain copies of these publications. If a claim raises a question about the use of a drug for a purpose not included in the FDA-approved labeling or the compendia, ask the physician to submit copies of relevant supporting literature.

Unlabeled uses may also be considered medically accepted if determined by you to be medically accepted generally as safe and effective for the particular use.

NOTE: If a use is identified as not indicated by CMS or the FDA, or if a use is specifically identified as not indicated in one or more of the three compendia mentioned, or if you determine based on peer-reviewed medical literature that a particular use of a drug is not safe and effective, the off-label usage is not supported and therefore the drug is not covered.

(50.4.6) 5. Less Than Effective Drug.—This is a drug that has been determined by the Food and Drug Administration (FDA) to lack substantial evidence of effectiveness for all labeled indications. Also, a drug that has been the subject of a Notice of an Opportunity for a Hearing (NOOH) published in the Federal Register before being withdrawn from the market, and for which the Secretary has not determined there is a compelling justification for its medical need, is considered less than effective. This includes any other drug product that is identical, similar, or related. Payment may not be made for a less than effective drug.

Because the FDA has not yet completed its identification of drug products that are still on the market, existing FDA efficacy decisions must be applied to all similar products once they are identified.

(50.4.7) 6. Denial of Medicare Payment for Compounded Drugs Produced in Violation of Federal Food, Drug, and Cosmetic Act.—The Food and Drug Administration (FDA) has found that, from time to time, firms established as retail pharmacies engage in mass production of compounded drugs, beyond the normal scope of pharmaceutical practice, in violation of the Federal Food, Drug, and Cosmetic Act (FFDCA). By compounding drugs on a large scale, a company may be operating as a drug manufacturer within the meaning of the FFDCA, without complying with requirements of that law. Such companies may be manufacturing drugs that are subject to the new drug application (NDA) requirements of the FFDCA, but for which FDA has not approved an NDA or which are misbranded or adulterated. If the manufacturing and processing procedures used by these facilities have not been approved by the FDA, the FDA has no assurance that the drugs these companies are producing are safe and effective. The safety and effectiveness issues pertain to such factors as chemical stability, purity, strength, bioequivalency, and biovailability.

Section 1862(a)(1)(A) of the Act requires that drugs must be reasonable and necessary in order to be covered under Medicare. This means, in the case of drugs, they must have been approved for marketing by the FDA. Section 50.4.1 instructs carriers to deny coverage for drugs that have not received final marketing approval by the FDA, unless instructed otherwise by CMS. Section 2300.1 instructs carriers to deny coverage of services related to the use of noncovered drugs as well. Hence, if DME or a prosthetic device is used to administer a noncovered drug, coverage is denied for both the nonapproved drug and the DME or prosthetic device.

In those cases in which the FDA has determined that a company is producing compounded drugs in violation of the FFDCA, Medicare does not pay for the drugs because they do not meet the FDA approval requirements of the Medicare program. In addition, Medicare does not pay for the DME or prosthetic device used to administer such a drug if the FDA determines that a required NDA has not been approved or that the drug is misbranded or adulterated.

The CMS will notify you when the FDA has determined that compounded drugs are being produced in violation of the FFDCA. Do not stop Medicare payment for such a drug unless you are notified that it is appropriate to do so through a subsequent instruction. In addition, if you or ROs become aware that other companies are possibly operating in violation of the FFDCA, notify:

Centers for Medicare and Medicaid Services
7500 Security Blvd.
Baltimore, MD 21244-1850

2049.5 Self-Administered Drugs and Biologicals. (100.2, 15, §50, 100-4, 8-§60.3)—Medicare Part B does not cover drugs that are self-administered unless the statute provides for such coverage. This statute explicitly provides coverage for blood clotting factors, drugs used in immunosuppressive therapy, erythropoietin for dialysis patients, certain oral anti-cancer drugs, and oral anti-nausea drugs when used in certain situations.

(50.5.1) A. Immunosuppressive Drugs.—Until January 1, 1995, immunosuppressive drugs are covered under Part B for a period of 1 year following discharge from a hospital for a Medicare-covered organ transplant. The CMS interpreted the 1-year period after the date of the transplant procedure to mean 365 days from the day on which an inpatient is discharged from the hospital. Beneficiaries are eligible to receive additional Part B coverage within 18 months after the discharge date for drugs furnished in 1995; within 24 months for drugs furnished in 1996; within 30 months for drugs furnished in 1997; and within 36 months for drugs furnished after 1997.

For immunosuppressive drugs furnished on or after December 21, 2000, this time limit for coverage is eliminated.

Covered drugs include those immunosuppressive drugs that have been specifically labeled as such and approved for marketing by the FDA. (This is an exception to the standing drug policy which permits coverage of FDA approved drugs for **nonlabeled** uses, where such uses are found to be reasonable and necessary in an individual case.)

Covered drugs also include those prescription drugs, such as prednisone, that are used in conjunction with immunosuppressive drugs as part of a therapeutic regimen reflected in FDA-approved labeling for immunosuppressive drugs. Therefore, antibiotics, hypertensives, and other drugs that are not directly related to rejection are not covered.

The FDA has identified and approved for marketing the following specifically labeled immunosuppressive drugs. They are:

- Sandimmune (cyclosporine), Sandoz Pharmaceutical;
- Imuran (azathioprine), Burroughs Wellcome;
- Atgam (antithymocyte globulin), Upjohn;
- Orthoclone OKT3 (Muromonab-CD3), Ortho Pharmaceutical;
- Prograf (tacrolimus), Fujisawa USA, Inc;
- Celicept (mycophenolate mefetil, Roche Laboratories;
- Daclizumab (Zenapax);
- Cyclophosphamide (Cytoxan);
- Prednisone; and
- Prednosolone.

The CMS expects contractors to keep informed of FDA additions to the list of immunosuppressive drugs.

(50.5.2) B. Erythropoietin (EPO).— The statute provides that EPO is covered for the treatment of anemia for patients with chronic renal failure who are on dialysis. Coverage is available regardless of whether the drug is administered by the patient or the patient's caregiver. EPO is a biologically engineered protein that stimulates the bone marrow to make new red blood cells.

NOTE: Non-ESRD patients who are receiving EPO to treat anemia induced by other conditions such as chemotherapy or the drug zidovudine (commonly called AZT) must meet the coverage requirements in section 50.

EPO is covered for the treatment of anemia for patients with chronic renal failure who are on dialysis when:

- It is administered in the renal dialysis facility; or
- It is self-administered in the home by any dialysis patient (or patient caregiver) who is determined competent to use the drug and meets the other conditions detailed below.

NOTE: Payment may not be made for EPO under the incident to provision when EPO is administered in the renal dialysis facility. (See section 5202.4.)

Also, in the office setting, reimbursement will be made for the administration charge only for non-ESRD patients receiving EPO.

(50.5.2.1 Requirements for Medicare Coverage for EPO) Medicare covers EPO and items related to its administration for dialysis patients who use EPO in the home when the following conditions are met.

A. Patient Care Plan.—A dialysis patient who uses EPO in the home must have a current care plan (a copy of which must be maintained by the designated back-up facility for Method II patients) for monitoring home use of EPO that includes the following:

1. Review of diet and fluid intake for aberrations as indicated by hyperkalemia and elevated blood pressure secondary to volume overload;

2. Review of medications to ensure adequate provision of supplemental iron;

3. Ongoing evaluations of hematocrit and iron stores;

4. Reevaluation of the dialysis prescription taking into account the patient's increased appetite and red blood cell volume;

5. Method for physician and facility (including back-up facility for Method II patients) follow-up on blood tests and a mechanism (such as a patient log) for keeping the physician informed of the results;

6. Training of the patient to identify the signs and symptoms of hypotension and hypertension; and

7. The decrease or discontinuance of EPO if hypertension is uncontrollable.

B. Patient Selection.—The dialysis facility, or the physician responsible for all dialysis-related services furnished to the patient, must make a comprehensive assessment that includes the following:

1. Pre-selection monitoring. The patient's hematocrit (or hemoglobin), serum iron, transferrin saturation, serum ferritin, and blood pressure must be measured.

2. Conditions the patient must meet. The assessment must find that the patient meets the following conditions:

(a) Is a dialysis patient;

(b) Has a hematocrit (or comparable hemoglobin level) that is as follows:

• For a patient who is initiating EPO treatment, no higher than 30 percent unless there is medical documentation showing the need for EPO despite a hematocrit (or comparable hemoglobin level) higher than 30 percent. Patients with severe angina, severe pulmonary distress, or severe hypotension may require EPO to prevent adverse symptoms even if they have higher hematocrit or hemoglobin levels.

• For a patient who has been receiving EPO from the facility or the physician, between 30 and 36 percent; and

(c) Is under the care of:

• A physician who is responsible for all dialysis-related services and who prescribes the EPO and follows the drug labeling instructions when monitoring the EPO home therapy; and

• A renal dialysis facility that establishes the plan of care and monitors the progress of the home EPO therapy.

3. The assessment must find that the patient or a caregiver meets the following conditions:

• Is trained by the facility to inject EPO and is capable of carrying out the procedure;

• Is capable of reading and understanding the drug labeling; and

• Is trained in, and capable of observing, aseptic techniques.

4. Care and storage of drug. The assessment must find that EPO can be stored in the patient's residence under refrigeration and that the patient is aware of the potential hazard of a child's having access to the drug and syringes.

C. Responsibilities of Physician or Dialysis Facility.—The patient's physician or dialysis facility must:

• Develop a protocol that follows the drug label instructions;

• Make the protocol available to the patient to ensure safe and effective home use of EPO;

• Through the amounts prescribed, ensure that the drug on hand at any time does not exceed a 2-month supply; and

• Maintain adequate records to allow quality assurance for review by the network and State survey agencies. For Method II patients, current records must be provided to and maintained by the designated back-up facility.

• The dialysis facility must submit claims for EPO, if the facility provides it.

See the Medicare Claims Processing Manual, Chapter 11, "End Stage Renal Disease," for instructions for billing and processing claims for EPO under Method 1 and Method 2. Note that hematocrit readings are required on claims. It is expected that the ESRD facility or hospital outpatient department will maintain the following information in each patient's medical record to permit the review of the medical necessity of EPO.

1. Diagnostic coding;
2. Most recent creatinine prior to initiation of EPO therapy;
3. Date of most recent creatinine prior to initiation of EPO therapy;
4. Most recent hematocrit (HCT) prior to initiation of EPO therapy;
5. Date of most recent hematocrit (HCT) prior to initiation of EPO therapy;
6. Dosage in units/kg;

7. Weight in kgs; and
8. Number of units administered.

(50.5.3) C. *Oral Anti-Cancer Drugs.*—Effective January 1, 1994, Medicare Part B coverage is extended to include oral anti-cancer drugs that are prescribed as anti-cancer chemotherapeutic agents providing they have the same active ingredients and are used for the same indications as anti-cancer chemotherapeutic agents that would be covered if they were not self-administered and they were furnished incident to a physician's service as drugs and biologicals.

For an oral anti-cancer drug to be covered under Part B, it must;

- Be prescribed by a physician or other practitioner licensed under State law to prescribe such drugs as anti-cancer chemotherapeutic agents;
- Be a drug or biological that has been approved by the Food and Drug Administration (FDA);
- Have the same active ingredients as a non-self-administrable anti-cancer chemotherapeutic drug or biological that is covered when furnished incident to a physician's service. The oral anti-cancer drug and the non-self-administrable drug must have the same chemical/generic name as indicated by the FDA's "Approved Drug Products" (Orange Book), "Physician's Desk Reference" (PDR), or an authoritative drug compendium;
- Be used for the same indications, including unlabeled uses, as the non-self-administrable version of the drug; and
- Be reasonable and necessary for the individual patient.

(50.5.4) D. *Oral Anti-Nausea Drugs.*—Effective January 1, 1998, Medicare also covers self-administered anti-emetics which are necessary for the administration and absorption of the anti-neoplastic chemotherapeutic agents when a high likelihood of vomiting exists. The anti-emetic drug is covered as a necessary means for administration of the antineoplastic chemotherapeutic agents. Oral drugs prescribed for use with the primary drug, which enhance the anti-neoplastic effect of the primary drug or permit the patient to tolerate the primary anti-neoplastic drug in higher doses for longer periods are not covered. Self-administered anti-emetics to reduce the side effects of nausea and vomiting brought on by the primary drug are not included beyond the administration necessary to achieve drug absorption.

Section 1861(s)(2) of the Act extends coverage to oral anti-emetic drugs that are used as full replacement for intravenous dosage forms of a cancer regimen under the following conditions:

- Coverage is provided only for oral drugs approved by the Food and Drug Administration (FDA) for use as anti-emetics;
- The oral anti-emetics must either be administered by the treating physician or in accordance with a written order from the physician as part of a cancer chemotherapy regimen;
- Oral anti-emetics drugs administered with a particular chemotherapy treatment must be initiated within 2 hours of the administration of the chemotherapeutic agent and may be continued for a period not to exceed 48 hours from that time; and
- The oral anti-emetic drugs provided must be used as a full therapeutic replacement for the intravenous anti-emetic drugs that would have otherwise been administered at the time of the chemotherapy treatment.

Only drugs pursuant to a physician's order at the time of the chemotherapy treatment qualify for this benefit. The dispensed number of dosage units may not exceed a loading dose administered within 2 hours of that treatment, plus a supply of additional dosage units not to exceed 48 hours of therapy.

Oral drugs that are not approved by the FDA for use as anti-emetics and that are used by treating physicians adjunctively in a manner incidental to cancer chemotherapy are not covered by this benefit and are not reimbursable within the scope of this benefit.

It is recognized that a limited number of patients will fail on oral anti-emetic drugs. Intravenous anti-emetics may be covered (subject to the rules of medical necessity) when furnished to patients who fail on oral anti-emetic therapy.

More than one oral anti emetic drug may be prescribed and may be covered for concurrent use if needed to fully replace the intravenous drugs that otherwise would be given.

(50.5.5) E. Hemophilia Clotting Factors.—Section 1861(s)(2)(I) of the Act provides Medicare coverage of blood clotting factors for hemophilia patients competent to use such factors to control bleeding without medical supervision, and items related to the administration of such factors. Hemophilia, a blood disorder characterized by prolonged coagulation time, is caused by deficiency of a factor in plasma necessary for blood to clot. (The discovery in 1964 of a cryoprecipitate rich in antihemophilic factor activity facilitated management of acute bleeding episodes.) For purposes of Medicare Part B coverage, hemophilia encompasses the following conditions:

- Factor VIII deficiency (classic hemophilia);
- Factor IX deficiency (also termed plasma thromboplastin component (PTC) or Christmas factor deficiency); and
- Von Willebrand's disease.

Claims for blood clotting factors for hemophilia patients with these diagnoses may be covered if the patient is competent to use such factors without medical supervision.

The amount of clotting factors determined to be necessary to have on hand and thus covered under this provision is based on the historical utilization pattern or profile developed by the carrier for each patient. It is expected that the treating source (e.g., a family physician or comprehensive hemophilia diagnostic and treatment center) has such information. From this data, the contractor is able to make reasonable projections concerning the quantity of clotting factors anticipated to be needed by the patient over a specific period of time. Unanticipated occurrences involving extraordinary events, such as automobile accidents of inpatient hospital stays, will change this base line data and should be appropriately considered. In addition, changes in a patient's medical needs over a period of time require adjustments in the profile. (See section 5245 for payment policies.)

2070 DIAGNOSTIC X-RAY, DIAGNOSTIC LABORATORY, AND OTHER DIAGNOSTIC TESTS (100-2, 15, §80, 100-4, 16-§2070)

2070.1 Independent Laboratories. (100-1, 5, §90.2, 100-2, 15, §80.1, 100-4, 16-§10, 10.1, 110.4)—Section 1833 and 1861 of the Act provides for payment of clinical laboratory services under Medicare Part B. Clinical laboratory services involve the biological, microbiological, serological, chemical, immunohematological, hematological, biophysical, cytological, pathological, or other examination of materials derived from the human body for the diagnosis, prevention, or treatment of a disease or assessment of a medical condition. Laboratory services must meet all applicable requirements of the Clinical Laboratory Improvement Amendments of 1988 (CLIA), as set forth at 42 CFR part 493. Section 1862(a)(1)(A) of the Act provides that Medicare payment may not be made for services that are not reasonable and necessary. Clinical laboratory services must be ordered and used promptly by the physician who is treating the beneficiary as described in 42CFR410.32(a), or by a qualified nonphysician practitioner, as described in 42CFR410.32(a)(3).

See the Medicare Claims Processing Manual Chapter 16 for related claims processing instructions.

80.1.1 Certification Changes B3-2070.1.E—Each page of the lists of approved specialties also includes a column "Certification Changed" in which the following codes are used:

"C" indicates a change in the laboratory's approved certification since the preceding listing.

"A" discloses an accretion.

"TERM"—Laboratory not approved for payment after the indicated date which follows the code. The reason for termination also is given in the following codes:

1. Involuntary termination—no longer meets requirements

2. Voluntary withdrawal

3. Laboratory closed, merged with other interests, or organizational change

4. Ownership change with new ownership participating under different name

5. Ownership change with new owner not participating

6. Change in ownership—new provider number assigned

7. Involuntary termination—failure to abide by agreement

8. Former "emergency" hospital now fully participating

80.1.2 Carrier Contacts With Independent Clinical Laboratories
B3-2070.1.F—An important role of the carrier is as a communicant of necessary information to independent clinical laboratories. Experience has shown that the failure to inform laboratories of Medicare regulations and claims processing procedures may have an adverse effect on prosecution of laboratories suspected of fraudulent activities with respect to tests performed by, or billed on behalf of, independent laboratories. United States Attorneys often have to prosecute under a handicap or may simply refuse to prosecute cases where there is no evidence that a laboratory has been specifically informed of Medicare regulations and claims processing procedures.

Carriers must follow the Provider Education and Training (PET) guidelines to assure that laboratories are aware of Medicare regulations and the carrier's policy when any changes are made in coverage policy or claims processing procedures. The PET guidelines require carriers to use various methods of communication (such as print, Internet, face-to-face instruction). Newsletters/bulletins that contain program and billing information must be produced at least quarterly and posted on the carrier Web site where duplicate copies may be obtained.

Some items which should be communicated to laboratories and responsibilities that laboratories are required to perform are:

- The requirements to have the same fee schedule for Medicare and private patients;
- To specify whether the tests are manual or automated;
- To document fully the medical necessity for pickup of specimens from a skilled nursing facility or a beneficiary's home, and
- In cases when a laboratory service is referred from one independent laboratory to another independent laboratory, to identify the laboratory actually performing the test.

Additionally, when carrier professional relations representatives make personal contacts with particular laboratories, the representative should prepare and retain reports of contact indicating dates, persons present, and issues discussed. Finally, carriers should inform independent laboratories that the Medicare National Coverage Determinations Manual as well as other guidelines contained in the manual for determining medical necessity are on the Web site. Carriers should also publish local guidelines on its Web site; the carrier should not duplicate national instructions here. Timely paper or electronic communications concerning the Internet publications to independent laboratories new to the carrier's service area are essential.

80.1.3 Independent Laboratory Service to a Patient in the Patient's Home or an Institution B3-2070.1.G—Where it is medically necessary for an independent laboratory to visit a patient to obtain a specimen, the service would be covered in the following circumstances:

1. Patient Confined to Home—If a patient is confined to the home or other place of residence used as his or her home (see §60.4.1 for the definition of a "homebound patient"), medical necessity would exist (e.g., where a laboratory technician draws a blood specimen). However, where the specimen is a type which would require only the services of a messenger and would not require the skills of a laboratory technician, e.g., urine or sputum, a specimen pickup service would not be considered medically necessary.

2. Place of Residence is an Institution—Medical necessity could also exist where the patient's place of residence is an institution, including a skilled nursing facility that does not perform venipunctures. This would apply even though the institution meets the basic definition of a skilled nursing facility and would not ordinarily be considered a beneficiary's home. (This policy is intended for independent laboratories only and does not expand the range of coverage of services to homebound patients under the incident to provision.) A trip by an independent laboratory technician to a facility (other than a hospital) for the purpose of performing a venipuncture is considered medically necessary only if:

a. The patient was confined to the facility; and

b. The facility did not have on duty personnel qualified to perform this service.

When facility personnel actually obtained and prepared the specimens for the independent laboratory to pick them up, the laboratory provides this pickup service as a service to the facility in the same manner as it does for physicians.

2130 PROSTHETIC DEVICES (100-2, 15, §120)

Prosthetic devices, other than dental devices and renal dialysis machines, are covered CORF services. Prosthetic devices are defined as devices that replace all or part of an internal body or external body member (including contiguous tissue), or that replace all or part of the function of a permanently inoperative or malfunctioning internal body organ or external body member.

Coverage of a prosthetic device includes all services necessary for forumulating its design, material, and component selection; measurement, fittings, static and dynamic alignments; and instructing the patient in its use. Such coverage is included as an integral part of the fabrication of the device.

Orthotic devices are those orthopedic appliances or apparatus used to support, align, prevent, or correct deformities, or to improve the function of moveable parts of the body. As with prosthetic devices, the coverage of an orthosis includes its design, materials, measurements, fabrications, testing, fitting, or training in the use of the orthosis.

2133 LEG, ARM, BACK, AND NECK BRACES, TRUSSES, AND ARTIFICIAL LEGS, ARMS, AND EYES (100-2, 15, §130)

These appliances are covered under Part B when furnished incident to physicians' services or on a physician's order. A brace includes rigid and semi-rigid devices that are used for the purpose of supporting a weak or deformed body member or restricting or eliminating motion in a diseased or injured part of the body. Elastic stockings, garter belts, and similar devices do not come within the scope of the definition of a brace. Back braces include, but are not limited to, special corsets, e.g., sacroiliac, sacrolumbar, dorsolumbar corsets and belts. A terminal device (e.g., hand or hook) is covered under this provision whether an artificial limb is required by the patient. (See section 2323.) Stump stockings and harnesses (including replacements) are also covered when these appliances are essential to the effective use of the artificial limb.

Adjustments to an artificial limb or other appliance required by wear or by a change in the patient's condition are covered when ordered by a physician.

Adjustments, repairs and replacements are covered even when the item had been in use before the user enrolled in Part B of the program so long as the device continues to be medically required.

2150 CLINICAL PSYCHOLOGIST SERVICES (100.2, 15, §160, 100-4, 12-§160, 170, 170.1)

(160) A. Clinical Psychologist Defined.—To qualify as a CP, a practitioner must meet the following requirements:

- Hold a doctoral degree in psychology;
- Be licensed or certified, on the basis of the doctoral degree in

psychology, by the State in which he or she practices, at the independent practice level of psychology to furnish diagnostic, assessment, preventive, and therapeutic services directly to individuals.

B. Qualified Clinical Psychologist Services Defined.—Effective July 1, 1990, the diagnostic and therapeutic services of CPs and services and supplies furnished incident to such services are covered as the services furnished by a physician or as incident to physician's services are covered. However, the CP must be legally authorized to perform the services under applicable licensure laws of the State in which they are furnished.

C. Types of Clinical Psychologist Services That May Be Covered.—CPs may provide the following services:

• Diagnostic and therapeutic services that the CP is legally authorized to perform in accordance with State law and/or regulation. Pay all qualified CPs based on the fee schedule for their diagnostic and therapeutic services. Also, pay those practitioners who do not meet the requirements for a CP on the basis of the physician fee schedule for the provision of diagnostic services under §80.2.
• Services and supplies furnished incident to a CP's services are covered if the requirements that apply to services incident to a physician's services, as described in §60 are met. These services must be:

1. Mental health services that are commonly furnished in CPs' offices;

2. An integral, although incidental, part of professional services performed by the CP;

3. Performed under the direct personal supervision of the CP, i.e., the CP must be physically present and immediately available; and

4. Furnished without charge or included in the CP's bill.

Any person involved in performing the service must be an employee of the CP (or an employee of the legal entity that employs the supervising CP) under the common law control test of the Act, as set forth in 20 CFR 404.1007 and §RS 2101.020 of the Retirement and Survivors Insurance part of the Social Security Program Operations Manual System.

Be familiar with appropriate State laws and/or regulations governing a CP's scope of practice. The development of lists of appropriate services may prove useful.

D. Noncovered Services.—The services of CPs are not covered if they are otherwise excluded from Medicare coverage even though a clinical psychologist is authorized by State law to perform them. For example, §1862(a)(1)(A) of the Act excludes from coverage services that are not "reasonable and necessary for the diagnosis or treatment of an illness or injury or to improve the functioning of a malformed body member." Therefore, even though the services are authorized by State law, the services of a CP that are determined to be not reasonable and necessary are not covered. Additionally, any therapeutic services that are billed by CPs under CPT psychotherapy codes that include medical evaluation and management services are not covered.

E. Requirement for Consultation.—When applying for a Medicare provider number, a CP must submit to the carrier a signed Medicare provider/supplier enrollment form that indicates an agreement to the effect that, contingent upon the patient's consent, he or she will attempt to consult with the patient's attending or primary care physician in accordance with accepted professional ethical norms, taking into consideration patient confidentiality.

If the patient assents to the consultation, the CP must attempt to consult with the patient's physician within a reasonable time after receiving the consent. If the CP's attempts to consult directly with the physician are not successful, the CP must notify the physician within a reasonable time that he or she is furnishing services to the patient. Additionally, the CP must document, in the patient's medical record, the date the patient consented or declined consent to consultations, the date of consultation, or, if attempts to

consult did not succeed, that date and manner of notification to the physician.

The only exception to the consultation requirement for CPs is in cases where the patient's primary care or attending physician refers the patient to the CP. Also, neither a CP nor a primary care or attending physician may bill Medicare or the patient for this required consultation.

See H.R. Conf. Rep. No. 386, 101st Cong., 1st Sess. 789 (1989).

F. Payment Methodology Limitation.—All covered therapeutic services furnished by qualified CPs are subject to the outpatient mental health services limitation in Pub 100-1, Medicare General Information, Eligibility, and Entitlement Manual, Chapter 3, "Deductibles, Coinsurance Amounts, and Payment Limitations," §30, (i.e., only 62½ percent of expenses for these services are considered incurred expenses for Medicare purposes). The limitation does not apply to diagnostic services.

G. Assignment Requirement.—Make all claims for covered services rendered by CPs on an assignment basis.

2152 CLINICAL SOCIAL WORKER SERVICES (100-2, 15, §170, 100-4, 12-§150)

See the Medicare Claims Processing Manual Chapter 12, Physician/Nonphysician Practitioners, §150, "Clinical Social Worker Services," for payment requirements.

A. Clinical Social Worker Defined.—Section 1861(hh) of the Act defines a "clinical social worker" as an individual who:

• Possesses a master's or doctor's degree in social work;
• Has performed at least 2 years of supervised clinical social work; and either:
• Is licensed or certified as a clinical social worker by the State in which the services are performed; or
• In the case of an individual in a State that does not provide for licensure or certification, has completed at least 2 years or 3,000 hours of post master's degree supervised clinical social work practice under the supervision of a master's level social worker in an appropriate setting such as a hospital, SNF, or clinic.

B. Clinical Social Worker Services Defined.—Section 1861(hh)(2) of the Act defines "clinical social worker services" as those services that the CSW is legally authorized to perform under State law (or the State regulatory mechanism provided by State law) of the State in which such services are performed for the diagnosis and treatment of mental illnesses. Services furnished to an inpatient of a hospital or an inpatient of an SNF that the SNF is required to provide as a requirement for participation are not included. The services that are covered are those that are otherwise covered if furnished by a physician or as incident to a physician's professional service.

C. Covered Services.—Coverage is limited to the services a CSW is legally authorized to perform in accordance with State law (or State regulatory mechanism established by State law). The services of a CSW may be covered under Part B if they are:

• The type of services that are otherwise covered if furnished by a physician, or as incident to a physician's service. (See section 30 for a description of physicians' services and §70 of Pub 100-1, the Medicare General Information, Eligibility, and Entitlement Manual, Chapter 5, for the definition of a physician.);
• Performed by a person who meets the definition of a CSW (see subsection A.); and
• Not otherwise excluded from coverage.

Carriers should become familiar with the State law or regulatory mechanism governing a CSW's scope of practice in your service area.

D. Noncovered Services.—Services of a CSW are not covered when furnished to inpatients of a hospital or to inpatients of a SNF if the services furnished in the SNF are those that the SNF is required to furnish as a condition of participation in Medicare. In addition, CSW services are not covered if they are otherwise excluded from Medicare coverage even though a CSW is authorized by State law to perform them. For example, the Medicare law excludes from coverage services that are not "reasonable and necessary for the diagnosis or treatment of an illness or injury or to improve the functioning of a malformed body member."

E. Outpatient Mental Health Services Limitation.—All covered therapeutic services furnished by qualified CSWs are subject to the outpatient psychiatric services limitation in section Pub 100-1, Medicare General Information, Eligibility, and Entitlement Manual, Chapter 3, "Deductibles, Coinsurance Amounts, and Payment Limitations," §30, (i.e., only 62.5 percent of expenses for these services are considered incurred expenses for Medicare purposes). The limitation does not apply to diagnostic services.

F. Assignment Requirement.—Assignment is required.

2210 PAYABLE PHYSICAL THERAPY (PT) (100-2, 15, §230)

A. General.—To be covered PT services, the services must relate directly and specifically to an active written treatment regimen established by the physician after any needed consultation with the qualified physical therapist and must be reasonable and necessary to the treatment of the individual's illness or injury. Effective July 18, 1984, a plan of treatment for OPT services may be established by either the physician or the qualified physical therapist providing such services. Services related to activities for the general good and welfare of patients, e.g., general exercises to promote overall fitness and flexibility and activities to provide diversion or general motivation, do not constitute PT services for Medicare purposes.

Services furnished beneficiaries must constitute PT where entitlement to benefits is at issue. Since the OPT benefit under Part B provides coverage only of PT services, payment can be made only for those services that constitute PT.

There is a limit for the amount of therapy expenses that is recognized as payable for some years. See the Medicare Claims Processing Manual, Chapter 5, §10.2, for a complete description of this financial limitation.

B. Reasonable and Necessary.—To be considered reasonable and necessary, the following conditions must be met:

- The services must be considered under accepted standards of medical practice to be a specific and effective treatment for the patient's condition.
- The services must be of such a level of complexity and sophistication or the condition of the patient must be such that the services required can be safely and effectively performed only by a qualified physical therapist or under his supervision. Services that do not require the performance or supervision of a physical therapist are not considered reasonable or necessary PT services, even if they are performed or supervised by a physical therapist. (When you determine the services furnished were of a type that could have been safely and effectively performed only by a qualified physical therapist or under his/her supervision, presume that such services were properly supervised. However, this assumption is rebuttable, and, if in the course of processing claims you find that PT services are not being furnished under proper supervision, deny the claim and bring this matter to the attention of the Division of Survey and Certification of the RO.)
- The development, implementation, management, and evaluation of a patient care plan constitute skilled physical therapy services when, because of the beneficiary's condition, those activities require the skills of a physical therapist to meet the beneficiary's needs, promote recovery, and ensure medical safety. Where the skills of a physical therapist are needed to manage and periodically reevaluate the appropriateness of a maintenance program because of an identified danger to the patient, those reasonable and necessary management and evaluation services could be covered, even if the skills of a therapist are not needed to carry out the activities performed as part of the maintenance program.
- While a beneficiary's particular medical condition is a valid factor in deciding if skilled physical therapy services are needed, a beneficiary's diagnosis or prognosis should never be the sole factor in deciding that a service is or is not skilled. The key issue is whether the skills of a physical therapist are needed

to treat the illness or injury, or whether the services can be carried out by nonskilled personnel.
- A service that ordinarily would be performed by nonskilled personnel could be considered a skilled physical therapy service in cases in which there is clear documentation that, because of special medical complications, a skilled physical therapist is required to perform or supervise the service. However, the importance of a particular service to a beneficiary or the frequency with which it must be performed does not, by itself, make a nonskilled service into a skilled service.
- There must be an expectation that the patient's condition will improve significantly in a reasonable (and generally predictable) period of time, or the services must be necessary for the establishment of a safe and effective maintenance program required in connection with a specific disease state.
- The amount, frequency, and duration of the services must be reasonable.

NOTE: Claims for PT services denied because they are not considered reasonable and necessary are excluded by section 1862(a)(1) of the Act and are thus subject to consideration under the waiver of liability provision in section 1879 of the Act.

2210.3 Application of Guidelines. (100-2, 15, §230.3)—The following discussion illustrates the application of the above guidelines to some of the more common physical therapy modalities and procedures utilized in the treatment of patients:

1. Hot Pack, Hydrocollator, Infra-Red Treatments, Paraffin Baths and Whirlpool Baths.—Heat treatments of this type and whirlpool baths do not ordinarily require the skills of a qualified physical therapist. However, in a particular case the skills, knowledge, and judgment of a qualified physical therapist might be required in such treatments or baths, e.g., where the patient's condition is complicated by circulatory deficiency, areas of desensitization, open wounds, or other complications. Also, if such treatments are given prior to but as an integral part of a skilled physical therapy procedure, they would be considered part of the physical therapy service.

2. Gait Training.—Gait evaluation and training furnished a patient whose ability to walk has been impaired by neurological, muscular, or skeletal abnormality require the skills of a qualified physical therapist. However, if gait evaluation and training cannot reasonably be expected to improve significantly the patient's ability to walk, such services would not be considered reasonable and necessary. Repetitive exercises to improve gait or maintain strength and endurance, and assistive walking, such as provided in support for feeble or unstable patients, are appropriately provided by supportive personnel, e.g., aides or nursing personnel and do not require the skills of a qualified physical therapist.

3. Ultrasound, Shortwave, and Microwave Diathermy Treatments.—These modalities must always be performed by or under the supervision of a qualified physical therapist, and, therefore, such treatments constitute physical therapy.

4. Range of Motion Tests.—Only the qualified physical therapist may perform range of motion tests and, therefore, such tests would constitute physical therapy.

5. Therapeutic Exercises.—Therapeutic exercises that must be performed by or under the supervision of a qualified physical therapist due either to the type of exercise employed or to the condition of the patient would constitute physical therapy. Range of motion exercises require the skills of a qualified physical therapist only when they are part of the active treatment of a specific disease that has resulted in a loss or restriction of mobility (as evidenced by physical therapy notes showing the degree of motion lost and the degree to be restored) and such exercises, either because of their nature or the condition of the patient, may only be performed safely and effectively by or under the supervision of a qualified physical therapist. Generally, range of motion exercises that are not related to the restoration of a specific loss of function but rather are related to the maintenance of function (see section 2210.2) do not require the skills of a qualified physical therapist.

2303 SERVICES NOT REASONABLE AND NECESSARY (100-2, 16, §20)

Items and services that are not reasonable and necessary for the diagnosis or treatment of illness or injury, or to improve the functioning of a malformed body member; e.g., payment *cannot* be made for the rental of a special hospital bed to be used by the patient in his home unless it was a reasonable and necessary part of the patient's treatment. See also section 80.

A health care item or service for the purpose of causing, or assisting to cause, the death of any individual (assisted suicide) is not covered. This prohibition does not apply to the provision of an item or service for the purpose of alleviating pain or discomfort, even if such use may increase the risk of death, so long as the item or service is not furnished for the specific purpose of causing death.

2323 FOOT CARE (100-2, 16, §100, 290)

A. Treatment of Subluxation of Foot.—Subluxations of the foot are defined as partial dislocations or displacements of joint surfaces, tendons ligaments, or muscles of the foot. Surgical or non-surgical treatments undertaken for the sole purpose of correcting a subluxated structure in the foot as an isolated entity are not covered.

However, medical or surgical treatment of subluxation of the ankle joint (talo-crural joint) is covered. In addition, reasonable and necessary medical or surgical services, diagnosis, or treatment for medical conditions that have resulted from or are associated with partial displacement of structures is covered. For example, if a patient has osteoarthritis that has resulted in a partial displacement of joints in the foot, and the primary treatment is for the osteoarthritis, coverage is provided.

B. Exclusion of Coverage.—The following foot care services are generally excluded from coverage under both Part A and Part B. Exceptions to this general exclusion for limited treatment of routine foot care services are described in subsections A.2 and B. (See section 4120 for procedural instructions in applying foot care exclusions.)

1. Treatment of Flat Foot.—The term "flat foot" is defined as a condition in which one or more arches of the foot have flattened out. Services or devices directed toward the care or correction of such conditions, including the prescription of supportive devices, are not covered.

2. Routine Foot Care.—Except as provided in subsection B, routine foot care is excluded from coverage. Services that normally are considered routine and not covered by Medicare include the following:

- The cutting or removal of corns and calluses;
- The trimming, cutting, clipping, or debriding of nails; and
- Other hygienic and preventive maintenance care, such as cleaning and soaking the feet, the use of skin creams to maintain skin tone of either ambulatory or bedfast patients, and any other service performed in the absence of localized illness, injury, or symptoms involving the foot.

3. Supportive Devices for Feet.—Orthopedic shoes and other supportive devices for the feet generally are not covered. However, this exclusion does not apply to such a shoe if it is an integral part of a leg brace, and its expense is included as part of the cost of the brace. Also, this exclusion does not apply to therapeutic shoes furnished to diabetics.

C. Exceptions to Routine Foot Care Exclusion

1. Necessary and Integral Part of Otherwise Covered Services.—In certain circumstances, services ordinarily considered to be routine may be covered if they are performed as a necessary and integral part of otherwise covered services, such as diagnosis and treatment of ulcers, wounds, or infections.

2. Treatment of Warts on Foot.—The treatment of warts (including plantar warts) on the foot is covered to the same extent as services provided for the treatment of warts located elsewhere on the body.

3. Presence of Systemic Condition.—The presence of a systemic condition such as metabolic, neurologic, or peripheral vascular disease may require scrupulous foot care by a professional that in the absence of such condition(s) would be considered routine (and, therefore, excluded from coverage). Accordingly, foot care that would otherwise be considered routine may be covered when systemic condition(s) result in severe circulatory embarrassment or areas of diminished sensation in the individual's legs or feet. (See subsection A.

In these instances, certain foot care procedures that otherwise are considered routine (e.g., cutting or removing corns and calluses, or trimming, cutting, clipping, or debriding nails) may pose a hazard when performed by a nonprofessional person on patients with such systemic conditions. (See §290.G for procedural instructions.)

4. Mycotic Nails.—In the absence of a systemic condition, treatment of mycotic nails may be covered.

The treatment of mycotic nails for an ambulatory patient is covered only when the physician attending the patient's mycotic condition documents that (1) there is clinical evidence of mycosis of the toenail, and (2) the patient has marked limitation of ambulation, pain, or secondary infection resulting from the thickening and dystrophy of the infected toenail plate.

The treatment of mycotic nails for a nonambulatory patient is covered only when the physician attending the patient's mycotic condition documents that (1) there is clinical evidence of mycosis of the toenail, and (2) the patient suffers from pain or secondary infection resulting from the thickening and dystrophy of the infected toenail plate.

For the purpose of these requirements, documentation means any written information that is required by the carrier in order for services to be covered. Thus, the information submitted with claims must be substantiated by information found in the patient's medical record. Any information, including that contained in a form letter, used for documentation purposes is subject to carrier verification in order to ensure that the information adequately justifies coverage of the treatment of mycotic nails.

D. Systemic Conditions That Might Justify Coverage.—Although not intended as a comprehensive list, the following metabolic, neurologic, and peripheral vascular diseases (with synonyms in parentheses) most commonly represent the underlying conditions that might justify coverage for routine foot care.

- Diabetes mellitus*
- Arteriosclerosis obliterans (A.S.O., arteriosclerosis of the extremities, occlusive peripheral arteriosclerosis)
- Buerger's disease (thromboangiitis obliterans)
- Chronic thrombophlebitis*
- Peripheral neuropathies involving the feet—
  - Associated with malnutrition and vitamin deficiency*
    - Malnutrition (general, pellagra)
    - Alcoholism
    - Malabsorption (celiac disease, tropical sprue)
    - Pernicious anemia
  - Associated with carcinoma*
  - Associated with diabetes mellitus*
  - Associated with drugs and toxins*
  - Associated with multiple sclerosis*
  - Associated with uremia (chronic renal disease)*
  - Associated with traumatic injury
  - Associated with leprosy or neurosyphilis
  - Associated with hereditary disorders
    - Hereditary sensory radicular neuropathy
    - Angiokeratoma corporis diffusum (Fabry's)
    - Amyloid neuropathy

When the patient's condition is one of those designated by an asterisk (*), routine procedures are covered only if the patient is under the active care of a doctor of medicine or osteopathy who documents the condition.

E. Supportive Devices for Feet.—Orthopedic shoes and other supportive devices for the feet generally are not covered. However, this exclusion does not apply to such a shoe if it is an integral part of a leg brace, and its expense is included as part of the cost of the brace. Also, this exclusion does not apply to therapeutic shoes furnished to diabetics.

F. Presumption of Coverage.—In evaluating whether the routine services can be reimbursed, a presumption of coverage may be made where the evidence available discloses certain physical and/or clinical findings consistent with the diagnosis and indicative of severe peripheral involvement. For purposes of applying this presumption the following findings are pertinent:

Class A Findings

• Nontraumatic amputation of foot or integral skeletal portion thereof.

Class B Findings

• Absent posterior tibial pulse;
• Advanced trophic changes as: hair growth (decrease or absence) nail changes (thickening) pigmentary changes (discoloration) skin texture (thin, shiny) skin color (rubor or redness) (Three required); and
• Absent dorsalis pedis pulse.

Class C Findings

• Claudication;
• Temperature changes (e.g., cold feet);
• Edema;
• Paresthesias (abnormal spontaneous sensations in the feet); and
• Burning.

The presumption of coverage may be applied when the physician rendering the routine foot care has identified:

1. A Class A finding;
2. Two of the Class B findings; or
3. One Class B and two Class C findings.

Cases evidencing findings falling short of these alternatives may involve podiatric treatment that may constitute covered care and should be reviewed by the intermediary's medical staff and developed as necessary.

For purposes of applying the coverage presumption where the routine services have been rendered by a podiatrist, the contractor may deem the active care requirement met if the claim or other evidence available discloses that the patient has seen an M.D. or D.O. for treatment and/or evaluation of the complicating disease process during the 6-month period prior to the rendition of the routine-type services. The intermediary may also accept the podiatrist's statement that the diagnosing and treating M.D. or D.O. also concurs with the podiatrist's findings as to the severity of the peripheral involvement indicated.

Services ordinarily considered routine might also be covered if they are performed as a necessary and integral part of otherwise covered services, such as diagnosis and treatment of diabetic ulcers, wounds, and infections.

G. Application of Foot Care Exclusions to Physician's Services.—The exclusion of foot care is determined by the nature of the service. Thus, payment for an excluded service should be denied whether performed by a podiatrist, osteopath, or a doctor of medicine, and without regard to the difficulty or complexity of the procedure.

When an itemized bill shows both covered services and noncovered services not integrally related to the covered service, the portion of charges attributable to the noncovered services should be denied. (For example, if an itemized bill shows surgery for an ingrown toenail and also removal of calluses not necessary for the performance of toe surgery, any additional charge attributable to removal of the calluses should be denied.)

In reviewing claims involving foot care, the carrier should be alert to the following exceptional situations:

1. Payment may be made for incidental noncovered services performed as a necessary and integral part of, and secondary to, a covered procedure. For example, if trimming of toenails is required for application of a cast to a fractured foot, the carrier need not allocate and deny a portion of the charge for the trimming of the nails. However, a separately itemized charge for such excluded service should be disallowed. When the primary procedure is covered the administration of anesthesia necessary for the performance of such procedure is also covered.

2. Payment may be made for **initial** diagnostic services performed in connection with a specific symptom or complaint if it seems likely that its treatment would be covered even though the resulting diagnosis may be one requiring only noncovered care.

The name of the M.D. or D.O. who diagnosed the complicating condition must be submitted with the claim. In those cases, where active care is required, the approximate date the beneficiary was last seen by such physician must also be indicated.

NOTE: Section 939 of P.L. 96-499 removed "warts" from the routine foot care exclusion effective July 1, 1981.

Relatively few claims for routine-type care are anticipated considering the severity of conditions contemplated as the basis for this exception. Claims for this type of foot care should not be paid in the absence of convincing evidence that nonprofessional performance of the service would have been hazardous for the beneficiary because of an underlying systemic disease. The mere statement of a diagnosis such as those mentioned in §D above does not of itself indicate the severity of the condition. Where development is indicated to verify diagnosis and/or severity the carrier should follow existing claims processing practices which may include review of carrier's history and medical consultation as well as physician contacts.

The rules in §290.F concerning presumption of coverage also apply.

Codes and policies for routine foot care and supportive devices for the feet are not exclusively for the use of podiatrists. These codes must be used to report foot care services regardless of the specialty of the physician who furnishes the services. Carriers must instruct physicians to use the most appropriate code available when billing for routine foot care.

2455 MEDICAL INSURANCE BLOOD DEDUCTIBLE (100-1, 3-§20.5.2)

A. General.—Program payment under Part B may not be made for the first three units of whole blood, or packed red cells, received by a beneficiary in a calendar year. For purpose of the blood deductible, a unit of whole blood means a pint of whole blood. The term "whole blood" means human blood from which none of the liquid or cellular components has been removed. Where packed red cells are furnished, a unit of packed red cells is considered equivalent to a pint of whole blood. After the three unit deductible has been satisfied, payment may be made for all blood charges, subject to the normal coverage and reasonable charge criteria.

NOTE: Blood is a biological and can be covered under Part B only when furnished incident to a physician's services. (See sections 2050.1ff. for a more complete explanation of services rendered "incident to a physician's services.")

B. Application of the Blood Deductible.—The blood deductible applies only to whole blood or packed red cells. Other components of blood such as platelets, fibrinogen, plasma, gamma globulin, and serum albumin are not subject to the blood deductible. These components of blood are covered biologicals.

The blood deductible involves only the charges for the blood (or packed red cells). Charges for the administration of blood or packed cells are not subject to the blood deductible. Accordingly, although payment may not be made for the first three pints of blood and/or units of packed red cells furnished to a beneficiary in a calendar year, payment may be made (subject to the cash deductible) for the administration charges for all covered pints or units including the first three furnished in a calendar year.

The blood deductible applies only to the first three pints and/or units furnished in a calendar year, even though more than one physician or clinic furnished blood. Furthermore, to count toward the deductible, the blood must be covered with respect to all applicable criteria (i.e., it must be medically necessary, it must be furnished incident to a physician's services, etc.). (See section 2050.5.)

C. Physician or Supplier Right to Charge for Deductible Blood.—A physician or other supplier who accepts assignment may bill a beneficiary the reasonable charge for unreplaced deductible blood (i.e., any of the first three units in a calendar year) but may not charge for blood that has been replaced.

Once a physician or supplier accepts a replacement unit of whole blood or packed red cells from a beneficiary or another individual acting on his behalf, the beneficiary may not be charged for the blood.

When a supplier accepts blood donated in advance, in anticipation of need by a specific beneficiary, whether the beneficiary's own blood, that is, an autologous donation, or blood furnished by another individual or blood assurance group, such donations are considered replacement for units subsequently furnished the beneficiary.

D. Distinction Between Blood Charges and Blood Administration Charges.—Since the blood deductible applies only to charges for blood and does not apply to charges for blood administration, these two charges must be considered separately. Where a bill for unreplaced blood shows only a single blood charge, break down the charge between blood and blood administration in accordance with the supplier's customary charges for these items. If the supplier does not customarily bill separately for blood and for blood administration, the portion of the single charge that is considered to be a charge for blood is determined by reference to the established reasonable charge in the locality as it applies to blood. The remainder of the charge is considered a blood administration charge.

E. Relationship to Other Deductibles.—Part B payment for all blood administration charges and for blood charges after the beneficiary has received three pints and/or units in a calendar year is subject to the annual cash deductible and coinsurance provisions. Expenses incurred in meeting the Part B blood deductible do not count as incurred expenses under Part B for purposes of meeting the cash deductible or for purposes of payment.

There is also a Part A blood deductible applicable to the first three pints of whole blood or equivalent units of packed red cells received by a beneficiary in a benefit period. The Part A and Part B blood deductibles are applied separately.

F. Example of Application of the Part B Blood Deductible.—In 1991, a beneficiary received three pints of blood from a physician for which the total charge is $100 per pint. (The physician does not specify how much of the charge is for blood, and how much is for blood administration.) The physician accepted assignment and submitted a claim for Part B payment.

Determine that the beneficiary has not met any part of the Part B blood deductible and has met only $40 of the cash deductible. You determine that the physician's customary charge for blood administration is $50 per unit and that it is reasonable. Consequently, charges for blood administration are $50 per unit or a total of $150 for the three units furnished, and charges for blood are $50 per unit or a total of $150 for the three units furnished. The beneficiary replaces one pint of blood. Since the beneficiary had not met any of the Part B blood deductible, none of the $150 in blood charges are payable, nor may any of such charges be applied to satisfy the annual cash deductible ($100). Of the $150 in blood administration charges, $60 is applied to satisfy the beneficiary's unmet cash deductible, and a payment of $72 is made on the remaining $90 in charges ($90 x 80%). Since the physician accepted assignment and since the beneficiary replaced one pint of blood, the physician may charge the beneficiary the reasonable charge only for the two remaining deductible pints.

2470 OUTPATIENT MENTAL HEALTH TREATMENT LIMITATION (100.1, 3, §30-30.3, 100.4, 12-§210)

Regardless of the actual expenses a beneficiary incurs for treatment of mental, psychoneurotic, and personality disorders while the beneficiary is not an inpatient of a hospital at the time such expenses are incurred, the amount of those expenses that may be recognized for Part B deductible and payment purposes is limited to 62.5 percent of the Medicare allowed amount for those services. This limitation is called the outpatient mental health treatment limitation. Expenses for diagnostic services (e.g., psychiatric testing and evaluation to diagnose the patient's illness) are not subject to this limitation. This limitation applies only to therapeutic services and to services performed to evaluate the progress of a course of treatment for a diagnosed condition.

3045 FILING THE REQUEST - ASSIGNMENTS (100.4, 1-§30.3)

3045.4 Effect of Assignment Upon Purchase of Cataract Glasses from Participating Physician or Supplier. (100.4, 1-§30.3.5)—A pair of cataract glasses is composed of two distinct products: a professional product (the prescribed lenses) and a retail commercial product (the frames). The frames serve not only as a holder of lenses but also as an article of personal apparel. As such, they are usually selected on the basis of personal taste and style. Although Medicare will pay only for standard frames, most patients want deluxe frames. Participating physicians and suppliers cannot profitably furnish such deluxe frames unless they can make an extra (non-covered) charge for the frames even though they accept assignment.

Therefore a participating physician or supplier (whether an ophthalmologist, optometrist, or optician) who accepts assignment on cataract glasses with deluxe frames may charge the Medicare patient the difference between his usual charge to private pay patients for glasses with standard frames and his usual charge to such patients for glasses with deluxe frames, in addition to the applicable deductible and coinsurance on glasses with standard frames, if all of the following requirements are met:

A. The participating physician or supplier has standard frames available, offers them for sale to the patient, and explains to the patient the price and other differences between standard and deluxe frames.

B. The participating physician or supplier obtains from the patient (or his representative) and keeps on file the following signed and dated statement:

Name of Patient   Medicare Claim Number

Having been informed that an extra charge is being made by the physician or supplier for deluxe frames, that this extra charge is not covered by Medicare, and that standard frames are available for purchase from the physician or supplier at no extra charge, I have chosen to purchase deluxe frames.

_____

Signature   Date

C. The participating physician or supplier itemizes on his claim his actual charge for the lenses, his actual charge for the standard frames, and his actual extra charge for the deluxe frames (charge differential).

Once the assigned claim for deluxe frames has been processed, the carrier will follow the ABN instructions as described in section 60.

3045.7 Mandatory Assignment and Other Requirements for Home Dialysis Supplies and Equipment Paid Under Method II On Claims Submitted to Carriers. (100.4, 1-§30.3.8, 100.4, 8-§90.2, 90.3, 90.3.1, 90.3.3, 20-§30.8, 140.3)—DMERCs pay only on an assignment basis for home dialysis supplies and equipment furnished a beneficiary who has selected Method II.

Refer to Chapter 8 and Chapter 20 for more information.

A. General.—Effective for services furnished on or after February 1, 1990, pay only on an assignment basis for home dialysis supplies and equipment furnished a beneficiary who has selected

Method II. There is also a monthly payment limitation: $1974.45 for continuous cycling peritoneal dialysis (CCPD) and $1490.85 for all other methods of dialysis. (Note, however, that beneficiaries are permitted to have on hand one month's emergency reserve supplies.) This payment may be made to only one supplier per beneficiary. (See sections 4270-4271.)

B. Billing Instructions.—Claims for these supplies must be completed as follows:

- You may allow suppliers to bill for more than one month's supplies at a time. However, the date of service field must identify the month for which the supplies are purchased, so that you can apply the monthly payment limit. This may be accomplished by using a separate line for each month's supplies or by using inclusive service dates and the units field.

Example: In July 1990, a supplier bills for 2 CCPD supply kits. The first kit was supplied for the patient's use in June, and the second for use in July.

If the supplier lists both kits on the same line, that item must include the following information:

- Date of service: From: 060190 To 073190
- Procedure Code: A4900
- Units: 2

If the supplier lists each month's supplies on a separate line, the inclusive dates of service for each month are the first to the last date of each month (e.g., 060190 to 063090).

- Modifier "QR" must be used to designate the one month's emergency reserve supplies. This allows you to identify situations in which the payment limit for a given month may be exceeded if an emergency reserve is billed for in addition to regular monthly supplies. It also allows you to ensure that emergency supplies are not purchased more frequently than required.
- HCPCS code A4901 identifies CCPD supplies.

3060 CLAIMS, FILING, JURISDICTION AND DEVELOPMENT PROCEDURES (100-4, 1-§§10.1.7, 30.2)

3060.6 Payment Under Reciprocal Billing Arrangements.—(100-4, 30.2.10) The patient's regular physician may submit the claim, and (if assignment is accepted) receive the Part B payment, for covered visit services (including emergency visits and related services) that the regular physician arranges to be provided by a substitute physician on an occasional reciprocal basis, if:

- The regular physician is unavailable to provide the visit services;
- The Medicare patient has arranged or seeks to receive the visit services from the regular physician;
- The substitute physician does not provide the visit services to Medicare patients over a continuous period of longer than 60 days; and
- The regular physician identifies the services as substitute physician services meeting the requirements of this section by entering in item 24d of Form CMS-1500 HCPCS Q5 modifier (service furnished by a substitute physician under a reciprocal billing arrangement) after the procedure code. When Form CMS-1500 is next revised, provision will be made to identify the substitute physician by entering his/her unique physician identification number (UPIN) on the form and cross-referring the entry to the appropriate service line item(s) by number(s). Until further notice, the regular physician must keep in file a record of each service provided by the substitute physician, associated with the substitute physician's UPIN, and make this record available to you upon request.

If the only substitution services a physician performs in connection with an operation are postoperative services furnished during the period covered by the global fee, these services need not be identified on the claim as substitution services.

A physician may have reciprocal arrangements with more than one physician. The arrangements need not be in writing.

The term "covered visit service" includes not only those services ordinarily characterized as a covered physician visit, but also any other covered items and services furnished by the substitute physician or by others as incident to his/her services.

"Incident to" services furnished by staff of a substitute physician or regular physician are covered if furnished under the supervision of each.

A "continuous period of covered visit services" begins with the first day on which the substitute physician provides covered visit services to Medicare Part B patients of the regular physician, and it ends with the last day on which the substitute physician provides these services to these patients before the regular physician returns to work. This period continues without interruption on days on which no covered visit services are provided to patients on behalf of the regular physician or are furnished by some other substitute physician on behalf of the regular physician. A new period of covered visit services can begin after the regular physician has returned to work.

Example: The regular physician goes on vacation on June 30, 1992, and returns to work on September 4, 1992. A substitute physician provides services to Medicare Part B patients of the regular physician on July 2, 1992, and at various times thereafter, including August 30th and September 2, 1992. The continuous period of covered visit services begins on July 2nd and runs through September 2nd, a period of 63 days. Since the September 2nd services are furnished after the expiration of 60 days of the period, the regular physician is not entitled to bill and receive direct payment for them. The substitute physician must bill for these services in his/her own name. The regular physician may, however, bill and receive payment for the services that the substitute physician provides on his/her behalf in the period July 2nd through August 30th.

The requirements for the submission of claims under reciprocal billing arrangements are the same for assigned and unassigned claims.

A. Physician Medical Group Claims Under Reciprocal Billing Arrangements.—The requirements of this section generally do not apply to the substitution arrangements among physicians in the same medical group where claims are submitted in the name of the group. On claims submitted by the group, the group physician who actually performed the service must be identified in the manner described in §30.2.13 with one exception. When a group member provides services on behalf of another group member who is the designated attending physician for a hospice patient, the Q5 modifier may be used **by the designated attending physician** to bill for services related to a hospice patient's terminal illness that were performed by another group member.

For a medical group to submit assigned and unassigned claims for the covered visit services of a substitute physician who is **not** a member of the group and for an independent physician to submit assigned and unassigned claims for the substitution services of a physician who **is** a member of a medical group, the following requirements must be met:

- The regular physician is unavailable to provide the visit services;
- The Medicare patient has arranged or seeks to receive the visit services from the regular physician; and
- The substitute physician does not provide the visit services to Medicare patients over a continuous period of longer than 60 days.

Substitute billing services are billed for each entity as follows:

- The medical group must enter in item 24d of Form CMS-1500 the HCPCS code modifier Q5 after the procedure code.
- The independent physician must enter in item 24 of Form CMS-1500 HCPCS code modifier Q5 after he procedure code.
- The designated attending physician for a hospice patient (receiving services related to a terminal illness) bills the Q5 modifier in item 24 of Form CMS-1500 when another group member covers for the attending physician.

- A record of each service provided by the substitute physician must be kept on file and associated with the substitute physician's UPIN. The record must be made available to the carrier upon request.
- In addition, the medical group physician for whom the substitution services are furnished must be identified by his/her provider identification number (PIN) in block 24k of the appropriate line item.

Physicians who are members of a group but who bill in their own names are treated as independent physicians for purposes of applying the requirements of this section.

Carriers should inform physicians of the compliance requirements when billing for services of a substitute physician. The physician notification should state that, in entering the Q5 modifier, the regular physician (or the medical group, where applicable) is certifying that the services are covered visit services furnished by the substitute physician identified in a record of the regular physician which is available for inspection, and are services for which the regular physician (or group) is entitled to submit the claim. Carriers should include in the notice that penalty for false certifications may be civil or criminal penalties for fraud. The physician's right to receive payment or to submit claims or accept any assignments may be revoked. The revocation procedures are set forth in §40.

If a line item includes the code Q5 certification, carriers assume that the claim meets the requirements of this section in the absence of evidence to the contrary. Carriers need not track the 60-day period or validate the billing arrangement on a prepayment basis, absent postpayment findings that indicate that the certifications by a particular physician may not be valid.

When carriers make Part B payment under this section, they determine the payment amount as though the regular physician provided the services. The identification of the substitute physician is primarily for purposes of providing an audit trail to verify that the services were furnished, not for purposes of the payment or the limiting charge. Also, notices of noncoverage are to be given in the name of the regular physician.

3060.7 Payment Under Locum Tenens Arrangements (100.4, 1-§30.2.11)

A. Background.—It is a longstanding and widespread practice for physicians to retain substitute physicians to take over their professional practices when the regular physicians are absent for reasons such as illness, pregnancy, vacation, or continuing medical education, and for the regular physician to bill and receive payment for the substitute physician's services as though he/she performed them himself/herself. The substitute physician generally has no practice of his/her own and moves from area to area as needed. The regular physician generally pays the substitute physician a fixed amount per diem, with the substitute physician having the status of an independent contractor rather than of an employee. These substitute physicians are generally called "locum tenens" physicians.

Section 125(b) of the Social Security Act Amendments of 1994 makes this procedure available on a permanent basis. Thus, beginning January 1, 1995, a regular physician may bill for the services of "locum tenens" physicians. A regular physician is the physician who is normally scheduled to see a patient. Thus, a regular physician may include physician specialists (such as a cardiologist, oncologist, urologist, etc.).

B. Payment Procedure.—A patient's regular physician may submit the claim, and (if assignment is accepted) receive the Part B payment, for covered visit services (including emergency visits and related services) of a locum tenens physician who is not an employee of the regular physician and whose services for patients of the regular physician are not restricted to the regular physician's offices, if:

- The regular physician is unavailable to provide the visit services;
- The Medicare beneficiary has arranged or seeks to receive the visit services from the regular physician;

- The regular physician pays the locum tenens for his/her services on a per diem or similar fee-for-time basis;
- The substitute physician does not provide the visit services to Medicare patients over a continuous period of longer than 60 days; and
- The regular physician identifies the services as substitute physician services meeting the requirements of this section by entering HCPCS Q6 modifier (service furnished by a locum tenens physician) after the procedure code. When Form CMS-1500 is next revised, provision will be made to identify the substitute physician by entering his/her unique physician identification number (UPIN).

If the only substitution services a physician performs in connection with an operation are postoperative services furnished during the period covered by the global fee, these services need not be identified on the claim as substitution services.

The requirements for the submission of claims under reciprocal billing arrangements are the same for assigned and unassigned claims.

C. Medical Group Claims Under Locum Tenens Arrangements.—For a medical group to submit assigned and unassigned claims for the services a locum tenens physician provides for patients of the regular physician who is a member of the group, the requirements of subsection B must be met. For purposes of these requirements, per diem or similar fee-for-time compensation that the group pays the locum tenens physician is considered paid by the regular physician. Also, a physician who has left the group and for whom the group has engaged a locum tenens physician as a temporary replacement may still be considered a member of the group until a permanent replacement is obtained. The group must enter in item 24d of Form CMS-1500 the HCPCS Q6 modifier after the procedure code. Until further notice, the group must keep in file a record of each service provided by the substitute physician, associated with the substitute physician's UPIN, and make this record available to you upon request. In addition, the medical group physician for whom the substitution services are furnished must be identified by his/her provider identification number (PIN) on block 24k of the appropriate line item.

Physicians who are members of a group but who bill in their own names are generally treated as independent physicians for purposes of applying the requirements of subsection A for payment for locum tenens physician services. Compensation paid by the group to the locum tenens physician is considered paid by the regular physician for purposes of those requirements. The term "regular physician" includes a physician who has left the group and for whom the group has hired the locum tenens physician as a replacement.

3312 EVIDENCE OF MEDICAL NECESSITY FOR DURABLE MEDICAL EQUIPMENT (100-8—[Program Integrity Manual])

Section 3312 has been moved to Chapter 8 of the Program Integrity Manual.

3350.3 Claims Coding Requirements. (100-4, 12-§90.3)—Physicians must indicate that their services were provided in an incentive-eligible rural or urban HPSA by using one of the following modifiers:

- QB—physician providing a service in a rural HPSA; or
- QU—physician providing a service in an urban HPSA.

3350.4 Payment. (100-4, 12-§90.4.4)—The incentive payment is 10 percent of the amount actually paid, not the approved amount. Pay the incentive payment for services identified on either assigned or unassigned claims.

Do not include the incentive payment with each claim payment. Establish a quarterly schedule for issuing incentive payments. These payments are taxable and must be reported to the IRS.

Prepare a list to accompany each payment. Include a line item for each assigned claim represented in the incentive check and a "summary" item showing the number of unassigned claims represented. The sum of the line items and the "summary" items should equal the amount of the check.

3350.5 Services Eligible for HPSA Bonus Payments (100-4, 12-§90.4.5)

A. Information in the Professional Component/Technical Component (PC/TC) Indicator Field of the Medicare Physician Fee Schedule Database.—Use the information in the Professional Component/Technical Component (PC/TC) indicator field of the Medicare Physician Fee Schedule Database to identify professional services eligible for HPSA bonus payments. The following are the rules to apply in determining whether to pay the bonus on services furnished within a geographic HPSA and billed with a QB or QU modifier, as appropriate.

PC/TC Indicator	HPSA Payment Policy
0	Pay the HPSA bonus.
1	Globally billed. Only the professional component of this service qualifies for the HPSA bonus payment. The HPSA bonus cannot be paid on the technical component of globally billed services.

ACTION: Return the service as unprocessable. Instruct the provider to re-bill the service as two components with separate charges for the professional component (billed with the "26" and "HPSA" modifiers) and the technical component (billed with the "TC" modifier but not the "HPSA" modifier). (See §3350.6(A).)

1	Professional Component (modifier 26). Pay the bonus.
1	Technical Component (modifier TC). Do not pay the bonus. (See §3350.6(B).)
2	Professional Component only. Pay the bonus.
3	Technical Component only. Do not pay the bonus. (See §3350.6(B).)
4	Global test only. Only the professional component of this service qualifies for the HPSA bonus payment.

ACTION: Return the service as unprocessable. Instruct the provider to re-bill the service as separate professional and technical component procedure codes. The HPSA modifier should only be used with the professional component code. (See §3350.6(A).)

5	Incident to codes. Do not pay the bonus. (See §3350.6(B).)
6	Laboratory physician interpretation codes. Pay the bonus.
7	Physical therapy service. Do not pay the bonus. (See §3350.6(B).)
8	Physician interpretation codes. Pay the bonus.
9	Concept of PC/TC does not apply. Do not pay the bonus. (See §3350.6(B).)

NOTE: Codes that have a status of "X" on the Medicare Physician Fee Schedule Database (MFSDB) have been assigned PC/TC indicator 9 and are not considered physician services for MFSDB payment purposes. Therefore, the HPSA bonus payment will not be paid for these codes.

B. Anesthesia Codes (CPT Codes 00100 through 01999*) that Do Not Appear on the MFSDB.—Anesthesia codes (CPT codes 00100 through 01999*) do not appear on the MFSDB. However, when a medically necessary anesthesia service is furnished within a HPSA area by a physician, a HPSA bonus is payable.

To claim a HPSA payment for anesthesia, physician's bill codes 00100 through 01999 with modifiers QY, QK, AD, AA, or GC to signify that the anesthesia service was performed by a physician, and also include one of the HPSA modifiers (QB or QU).

4105 DURABLE MEDICAL EQUIPMENT, PROSTHETIC, AND ORTHOTIC SUPPLIES (100.4, 20-§100.2.3)

Sections 4105–4105.7 have been deleted and moved to the Program Integrity Manual (PIM).

4107 DURABLE MEDICAL EQUIPMENT BILLING AND PAYMENT CONSIDERATIONS UNDER THE FEE SCHEDULE (100.4, 20-§§20 and 20.4)

(20) Section 1834 of the Act requires the use of fee schedules under Medicare Part B for reimbursement of durable medical equipment (DME) and for prosthetic and orthotic devices, beginning January 1, 1989. Payment is limited to the lower of the actual charge for the equipment or the fee established.

Beginning with fee schedule year 1991, CMS calculates the updates for the fee schedules and national limitation amounts and provides the contractors with the revised payment amounts. The CMS calculates most fee schedule amounts and provides them to the carriers, DMERCs, FIs and RHHIs. However, for some services CMS asks carriers to calculate local fee amounts and to provide them to CMS to include in calculation of national amounts. These vary from update to update, and CMS issues special related instructions to carriers when appropriate.

Parenteral and enteral nutrition services paid on and after January 1, 2002 are paid on a fee schedule. This fee schedule also is furnished by CMS. Prior to 2002, payment amounts for PEN were determined under reasonable charge rules, including the application of the lowest charge level (LCL) restrictions.

The CMS furnishes fee schedule updates (DMEPOS, PEN, etc.) at least 30 days prior to the scheduled implementation. FIs use the fee schedules to pay for covered items, within their claims processing jurisdictions, supplied by hospitals, home health agencies, and other providers. FIs consult with DMERCs and where appropriate with carriers on filling gaps in fee schedules.

The CMS furnishes the fee amounts annually, or as updated if special updates should occur during the year, to carriers and FIs, including DMERCs and RHHIs, and to other interested parties (including the Statistical Analysis DMERC (SADMERC), Railroad Retirement Board (RRB), Indian Health Service, and United Mine Workers).

(20.4) The fee schedule file provided by CMS contains HCPCS codes and related prices subject to the DMEPOS fee schedules, including application of any update factors and any changes to the national limited payment amounts. The file does not contain fees for drugs that are necessary for the effective use of DME. It also does not include fees for items for which fee schedule amounts are not established. See Chapter 23 for a description of pricing for these. The CMS releases via program issuance, the gap-filled amounts and the annual update factors for the various DMEPOS payment classes:

- IN = Inexpensive/routinely purchased . . . DME;
- FS = Frequency Service . . . DME;
- CR = Capped Rental . . . DME;
- OX = Oxygen and Oxygen Equipment . . . OXY;
- OS = Ostomy, Tracheostomy and Urologicals . . . P/O;
- S/D = Surgical Dressings . . . S/D;
- P/O = Prosthetics and Orthotics . . . P/O;
- SU = Supplies . . . DME; and
- TE = TENS . . . DME,

RHHIs need to retrieve data from all of the above categories. Regular FIs need to retrieve data only from categories P/O, S/D and SU. FIs need to retrieve the SU category in order to be able to price supplies on Part B SNF claims.

4107.1 General Billing and Claims Processing. (100.4, 20-§100)—

Benefit policies are set forth in the Medicare Benefit Policy Manual, Chapter 15, §§110-130.

Program integrity policies for DMEPOS are set forth in the Medicare Program Integrity Manual, Chapter 5.

---

*CPT only © 2003. *Current Procedural Terminology, 2004, Professional Edition*, American Medical Association. All Rights Reserved.

See Chapter 21 for applicable MSN messages.

See Chapter 22 for Remittance Advice coding.

4107.2 Rent/Purchase Decisions. (100-4, 20-§30.5)—For services provided on or after October 1, 1988, discontinue making rent/purchase decisions on rental claims. For purchase claims with dates of service before January 1, 1989, continue to make rent/purchase decisions. Discontinue making rent/purchase decisions for purchase claims with dates of service on or after January 1, 1989. Do not pay for oxygen delivery systems, items requiring frequent and substantial servicing or capped rental items that were purchased on or after June 1, 1989.

4107.3 Comparability and Inherent Reasonableness Limitations. (100-4, 20-§30.5)—For services provided on or after January 1, 1989, do not apply the comparable circumstances provision. Also, for services provided between January 1, 1989 and December 31, 1990, do not apply the special payment limitation provisions.

4107.4 15-Month Ceiling on Capped Rental Items. (100-4, 20-§30.5)—Ensure that your system accurately computes the 15 month period for capped rental items.

4107.5 Transcutaneous Electrical Nerve Stimulator (TENS). (100-4, 20-§30.1.2)—To permit an attending physician time to determine whether purchase of a TENS unit is medically appropriate, ensure that your system allows no more than 10 percent of the fee schedule purchase amount for up to 2 months of rental prior to purchase. Do not apply the rentals toward the purchase allowance.

4107.6 Written Order Prior to Delivery. (100-3, 1-§256)—Ensure that your system will pay for the equipment listed below only when the supplier has a written order in hand prior to delivery. Otherwise, do not pay for that item even if a written order is subsequently furnished. However, you can pay for a similar item if it is subsequently provided by an unrelated supplier that has a written order in hand prior to delivery. The HCPCS codes for the equipment requiring a written order are:

- E0180
- E0181
- E0182
- E0183
- E0184
- E0185
- E0188
- E0189
- E0190
- E0192
- E0195
- E0620
- E0720
- E0730
- E1230

4107.7 Special Requirements for Oxygen Claims. (100-4, 20-§130.6)—There are a number of billing considerations for oxygen claims.

A. Monthly Billing.—Fee schedule payments for stationary oxygen system rentals are all inclusive and represent a monthly allowance per beneficiary. Accordingly, a supplier must bill on a monthly basis for stationary oxygen equipment and contents furnished during a rental month.

A portable equipment add-on is also payable when portable oxygen is prescribed and you determine it to be medically necessary in accordance with Medicare coverage requirements. The portable add-on must be claimed in order to be paid.

Claims may be submitted when expenses are incurred for initial rentals of oxygen systems, or no sooner than the monthly anniversary date in the case of an established oxygen patient. In the latter situation, suppliers must indicate the monthly volume of oxygen contents delivered, rounded in accordance with subsection D3.

Where the beneficiary has purchased a stationary system (other than a concentrator and/or a portable delivery system), oxygen contents must be billed and paid on a monthly basis, except for unassigned oxygen contents claims submitted by a beneficiary. For beneficiary filed claims, allow, on a claim-by-claim basis, the

submitted charge until the applicable monthly fee for oxygen contents has been met.

B. Reduced Number of HCPCS Codes.—The number of HCPCS codes for billing of oxygen claims have been reduced.

C. Use of Payment Modifiers.—The monthly payment amount for stationary oxygen is subject to adjustment depending on the amount of oxygen prescribed (liters per minute (LPM)), and whether or not portable oxygen is also prescribed. To make proper payment adjustments, supplier claims must indicate the appropriate HCPCS modifier described below, if applicable. On unassigned claims, suppliers should indicate this information on the itemized bill.

If the prescribed amount of oxygen is less than 1 LPM, the modifier is "QE". Reduce the monthly payment amount for stationary oxygen by 50 percent.

If the prescribed amount of oxygen is greater than 4 LPM, the modifier is "QG". Increase the monthly payment amount for stationary oxygen by 50 percent. Conduct prepayment medical review of these claims.

If the prescribed amount of oxygen exceeds 4 LPM and portable oxygen is prescribed, the modifier is "QF". Increase the monthly payment for stationary oxygen by the higher of 50 percent of the monthly stationary oxygen payment amount, or the fee schedule amount for the portable oxygen add-on. Conduct a prepayment medical review of these claims.

D. Units Required.—Excluding concentrators, suppliers must furnish units of oxygen contents in Item 24F of their CMS-1500 claims, or the itemized bill furnished to the beneficiary for unassigned claims.

1. Initial Oxygen Claims.—When submitting an initial claim for rental of a gaseous or liquid oxygen delivery system, units of oxygen contents furnished for the first month need not be indicated. Base your payment upon the lower of the actual charge for the initial rental month or the monthly payment amount.

2. Subsequent Oxygen Claims.—For dates of service subsequent to the initial rental month, suppliers should indicate actual content usage for the month billed or, if billed prospectively, the actual content usage during the previous rental month, rounded in accordance with subsection D3. Base your payment determination on the lower of the actual charge submitted or the monthly payment amount.

For applying these instructions, treat claims submitted under recertifications of continuing and uninterrupted need for oxygen therapy as subsequent claims if a change in suppliers is not involved.

If a change in suppliers has occurred, apply the initial rule in subsection D.1 above for specifying oxygen contents delivered for the initial rental month by the new supplier.

Develop subsequent rental claims for gaseous or liquid oxygen delivery systems that do not include "unit" information.

3. Rounding of Oxygen Contents.—For stationary gas system rentals, suppliers should indicate, in item 24F of the CMS-1500, oxygen contents in unit multiples of 50 cubic feet, rounded to the nearest increment of 50. For example, if 73 cubic feet of oxygen was delivered during the rental month, the item 24F unit entry "01" indicates the nearest 50 cubic foot increment. For stationary liquid systems, units of contents should be specified in multiples of 10 pounds of liquid contents delivered, rounded to the nearest 10 pound increment. For example, if 63 pounds of liquid oxygen were delivered during the applicable rental month billed, the unit entry "06" is made in Item 24F. For units of portable contents only (i.e., no stationary gas or liquid system used), round to the nearest five cubic feet or one liquid pound, respectively.

Periodically audit supplier records to verify that gaseous and liquid content usage is reported correctly.

E. Conserving Device Modifier.—Suppliers must indicate if an oxygen conserving device is being used with an oxygen delivery system by using HCPCS modifier "QH".

4107.8 EOMB Messages. (100.4, 20-§100, 130.2, 130.3, 130.4, 130.5)—The following EOMB messages are suggested:

A. General

- "This is the maximum approved amount for this item." (Use when payment is reduced for a line item.)

B. Inexpensive/Frequently Purchased Equipment

- "The total approved amount for this item is whether this item is purchased or rented." (Use in first month.)
- "This is your next to last rental payment."
- "This is your last rental payment."
- "This item has been rented up to the Medicare payment limit."
- "The approved amount has been reduced by the previously approved rental amounts."

4120 FOOT CARE (100-2, 16, §100)

NOTE: See §4281 for the relationship between foot care and the coverage and billing of the diagnosis and treatment of peripheral neuropathy with loss of protective sensation (LOPS) in people with diabetes.

4120.1 Application of Foot Care Exclusions to Physicians' Services. (100-2, 16, §100)—The exclusion of foot care is determined by the nature of the service. Thus, reimbursement for an excluded service should be denied whether performed by a podiatrist, osteopath, or a doctor of medicine, and without regard to the difficulty or complexity of the procedure.

When an itemized bill shows both covered services and noncovered services not integrally related to the covered service, the portion of charges attributable to the noncovered services should be denied. (For example, if an itemized bill shows surgery for an ingrown toenail and also removal of calluses not necessary for the performance of toe surgery, any additional charge attributable to removal of the calluses should be denied.)

In reviewing claims involving foot care, the carrier should be alert to the following exceptional situations:

1. Payment may be made for incidental noncovered services performed as a necessary and integral part of, and secondary to, a covered procedure. For example, if trimming of toenails is required for application of a cast to a fractured foot, the carrier need not allocate and deny a portion of the charge for the trimming of the nails. However, a separately itemized charge for such excluded service should be disallowed. When the primary procedure is covered the administration of anesthesia necessary for the performance of such procedure is also covered.

2. Payment may be made for initial diagnostic services performed in connection with a specific symptom or complaint if it seems likely that its treatment would be covered even though the resulting diagnosis may be one requiring only noncovered care.

3. Payment may be made for routine-type foot care such as cutting or removal of corns, calluses, or nails when the patient has a systemic disease of sufficient severity that unskilled performance of such procedure would be hazardous.

a. Claims for such routine services would show in item 7D of the SSA-1490 the complicating systemic disease. Where these services were rendered by a podiatrist this item should also include the name of the MD or DO who diagnosed the complicating condition. In those cases where active care is required, the approximate date the beneficiary was last seen by such physician must also be indicated.

NOTE: Section 939 of P.L. 96-499 removed "warts" from the routine foot care exclusion effective July 1, 1981.

b. Relatively few claims for routine-type care are anticipated considering the severity of conditions contemplated as the basis for this exception. Claims for this type of foot care should not be paid in the absence of convincing evidence that nonprofessional performance of the service would have been hazardous for the beneficiary because of an underlying systemic disease. The mere statement of a diagnosis such as those mentioned in section 2323C does not of itself indicate the severity of the condition.

Where development is indicated to verify diagnosis and/or severity the carrier should follow existing claims processing practices that may include review of carrier's history and medical consultation as well as physician contacts.

c. A presumption of coverage may be made by the carrier where the claim or other evidence available discloses certain physical and/or clinical findings consistent with the diagnosis and indicative of severe peripheral involvement. For purposes of applying this presumption, the following findings are pertinent:

- Class A Findings
  —Nontraumatic amputation of foot or integral skeletal portion thereof
- Class B Findings
  —Absent posterior tibial pulse
  —Advanced trophic changes as (three required): hair growth (decrease or absence); nail changes (thickening); pigmentary changes (discoloration); skin texture (thin, shiny); skin color (rubor or redness)
  —Absent dorsalis pedis pulse
- Class C Findings
  —Claudication
  —Temperature changes (e.g., cold feet)
  —Edema
  —Paresthesia (abnormal spontaneous sensations in the feet)
  —Burning

The presumption of coverage may be applied when the physician rendering the routine foot care has identified: (1) a Class A finding; (2) two of the Class B findings; or (3) one Class B and two Class C findings. Case evidencing findings falling short of these alternatives may involve podiatric treatment that may constitute covered care and should be reviewed by the carrier's medical staff and developed as necessary.

For purposes of applying the coverage presumption where the routine services have been rendered by a podiatrist, the carrier may deem the active care requirement met if the claim or other evidence available discloses that the patient has seen an MD or DO for treatment and/or evaluation of the complicating disease process during the 6-month period prior to the rendition of the routine-type service or had come under such care shortly after the services were furnished usually as a result of a referral.

4120.2 Application of the "Reasonable and Necessary" Limitation to Foot Care Services. (100.2, 16, §100.1)—In evaluating claims for foot care services, in addition to determining whether any of the other statutory limitations apply, carriers should assure that payment is made only for services that are "reasonable and necessary" for diagnosis or treatment of an illness or injury or to improve the functioning of a malformed body member. Determinations as to whether a foot care service is reasonable and necessary should be made on the same basis as all other such determinations—that is, with the advice of medical consultants and with reference to accepted standards of medical practice and the circumstances of the individual case. With appropriate professional consultation, guidelines should be established concerning the scope, frequency, and duration of services that would constitute reasonable and necessary utilization of services for various foot conditions; these guidelines should be used to screen out for denial, claims in which the services billed would clearly not be reasonable and necessary and to screen out questionable cases for special review or further development.

For example, infections of the feet and toenails that cause pain or deformity of sufficient degree to markedly limit ambulation may require a variety of medical services such as physical examination, and laboratory tests for the purpose of diagnosing the existence and type of infectious condition (and differentiating it from other types of dermatoses), prescription of a regimen of treatment, periodic examinations throughout the course of treatment to evaluate the status of the lesion and watch for complicating factors, and active treatment by one or a combination of the following modalities:

(1) Surgical excision (avulsion) of the affected nail(s);
(2) Mechanical debridement of the lesion;
(3) Topical treatment; or
(4) Systemic treatment.

With the appropriate advice from physicians who treat foot infections (e.g., dermatologists, podiatrists and surgeons), guidelines should be developed concerning accepted standards of medical practice with respect to appropriate utilization of the above types of services for different types of infectious conditions, taking into account such factors as the indications for various modalities of treatment, the required duration of different courses of therapy, and the required frequency of follow-up evaluation examinations. For example, when a physician prescribes a topical medication for an infection, patients are usually expected to perform most of the treatment by themselves at home (or if residing in nursing homes or skilled nursing facilities, etc., the staff of the facility is expected to perform most of the treatment), with perhaps occasional follow-up visits to (or by) the physician for evaluation of the status of the lesion. As part of the initial diagnostic and follow-up evaluation visits, the physician may cleanse the lesion and apply medication and these services would, of course, be covered where they are an accepted integral component of such visits; however, if the patient regularly comes to the physician to receive the care that he is expected to perform himself at home and there are no special medical circumstances relating to the infection warranting such special care, this would represent excessive utilization of physicians' services and should be excluded.

Carriers' utilization guidelines should enable them to identify where a course of therapy involves more frequent follow-up visits than are the accepted standards of physician care for that modality of therapy and to deny payment for such excessive visits unless there is documentation of special medical circumstances relating to the infection justifying the extra visits. For instance, in the case of claims for patients whose initial course of treatment includes a medically necessary visit to the physician for mechanical debridement of a mycotic lesion of the toenail, carriers must use a 60-day claims processing screen for identifying excessive follow-up services for the patient (i.e., the presumption would be that only one follow-up visit is covered every 60 days following the end of the initial treatment period unless medical documentation is submitted that supports more frequent visits). Similarly, utilization guidelines should identify when visits extend beyond the period of follow-up evaluation that is the accepted standard for a particular course of treatment for an infection and to deny payment for visits beyond the period unless development reveals complications in the infectious condition necessitating more prolonged treatment.

4173 POSITRON EMISSION TOMOGRAPHY (PET) SCANS BACKGROUND (100.4, 13-§60)

4173.1 Conditions for Medicare Coverage of Pet Scans for Noninvasive Imaging of the Perfusion of the Heart (100-4, 13-§60)

4173.2 Conditions of Coverage of PET Scans for Characterization of Solitary Pulmonary Nodules (SPNs) and PET Scans Using FDG to Initially Stage Lung Cancer (100-4, 13-§60.2)

4173.3 Conditions of Coverage of PET Scans for Recurrence of Colorectal Cancer, Staging and Characterization of Lymphoma, and Recurrence of Melanoma (100-4, 13-§60.2)

4173.4 Billing Requirements for PET Scans (100-4, 13-§60.2)

4173.5 HCPCS and Modifiers for PET Scans (100-4, 13-§60.2)

4173.6 Claims Processing Instructions for PET Scan Claims. (100.4, 13-§60)—Positron emission tomography (PET) is a noninvasive imaging procedure that assesses perfusion and the level of metabolic activity in various organ systems of the human body. A positron camera (tomograph) is used to produce cross-sectional tomographic images by detecting radioactivity from a radioactive tracer substance (radiopharmaceutical) that is administered intravenously into the patient.

For dates of service on and after March 14, 1995, Medicare covers one use of PET scans, i.e., imaging of the perfusion of the heart using Rubidium 82 (Rb 82), provided that the following conditions are met:

- The PET is done at a PET imaging center with a PET scanner that has been approved by the FDA;
- The PET scan is a rest alone or rest with pharmacologic stress PET scan, used for noninvasive imaging of the perfusion of the heart for the diagnosis and management of patients with known or suspected coronary artery disease, using Rb 82; and
- Either the PET scan is used in place of, but not in addition to, a single photon emission computed tomography (SPECT) or the PET scan is used following a SPECT that was found inconclusive.

(HCPCS Codes G0030 -G0047, G0210-G0234, G0252-G0254, 78454)—For procedures furnished on or after March 14, 1995, carriers pay for PET procedure of the heart under the limited coverage policy above and set forth in the Medicare National Coverage Determinations Manual.

The Medicare National Coverage Determinations Manual contains additional coverage instructions to indicate the conditions under which a PET scan is performed. FIs process claims for the technical component with HCPCS codes under Revenue Code 0404 (Positron Emission Tomography).

HCPCS	Definition
G0030	PET myocardial perfusion imaging, (following previous PET, G0030-G0047); single study, rest or stress (exercise and/or pharmacologic)
G0031	PET myocardial perfusion imaging, (following previous PET, G0030-G0047); multiple studies, rest or stress (exercise and/or pharmacologic)
G0032	PET myocardial perfusion imaging, (following rest SPECT, 78464); single study, rest or stress (exercise and/or pharmacologic)
G0033	PET myocardial perfusion imaging, (following rest SPECT, 78464); multiple studies, rest or stress (exercise and/or pharmacologic)
G0034	PET myocardial perfusion imaging, (following stress SPECT, 78465); single study, rest or stress (exercise and/or pharmacologic)
G0035	PET myocardial perfusion imaging, (following stress SPECT, 78465); multiple studies, rest or stress (exercise and/or pharmacologic)
G0036	PET myocardial perfusion imaging, (following coronary angiography, 93510-93529); single study, rest or stress (exercise and/or pharmacologic)
G0037	PET myocardial perfusion imaging, (following coronary angiography, 93510-93529); multiple studies, rest or stress (exercise and/or pharmacologic)
G0038	PET myocardial perfusion imaging, (following stress planar myocardial perfusion, 78460; single study, rest or stress (exercise and/or pharmacologic)
G0039	PET myocardial perfusion imaging, (following stress planar myocardial perfusion, 78460; multiple studies, rest or stress (exercise and/or pharmacologic)
G0040	PET myocardial perfusion imaging, (following stress echocardiogram, 93350); single study, rest or stress (exercise and/or pharmacologic)
G0041	PET myocardial perfusion imaging, (following stress echocardiogram, 93350); multiple studies, rest or stress (exercise and/or pharmacologic)
G0042	PET myocardial perfusion imaging, (following stress nuclear ventriculogram, 78481 or 78483); single study, rest or stress (exercise and/or pharmacologic)
G0043	PET myocardial perfusion imaging, (following stress nuclear ventriculogram 78481 or 78483); multiple studies, rest or stress (exercise and/or pharmacologic)
G0044	PET myocardial perfusion imaging, (following rest ECG, 93000); single study, rest or stress (exercise and/or pharmacologic)
G0045	PET myocardial perfusion imaging, (following rest ECG, 93000); multiple studies, rest or stress (exercise and/or pharmacologic)

HCPCS	Definition
G0046	PET myocardial perfusion imaging, (following stress ECG, 93015); single study, rest or stress (exercise and/or pharmacologic)
G0047	PET myocardial perfusion imaging, (following stress ECG, 93015); multiple studies, rest or stress (exercise and/or pharmacologic)

Effective July 1, 1999, Medicare expanded coverage of PET scans to include the evaluation of recurrent colorectal cancer in patients with rising levels of carinoembryonic antigen (CEA), for the staging of lymphoma (both Hodgkins and non-Hodgkins) when the PET scan substitutes for a gallium scan or lymphangiogram, and for the staging of recurrent melanoma prior to surgery, provided certain conditions are met. All three indications are covered only when using the radiopharmaceutical FDA (2-[flourine-18]-fluoro-2-deoxy-D-glucose), and are further predicated on the legal availability of FDG for use in such scans.

HCPCS codes for PET scans when performed on or after July 1, 1999, are listed below.

HCPCS	Definition
G0163	Code deleted effective 6-30-2001. Position Emission tomography (PET), whole body, for recurrence of colorectal metastatic cancer
G0215	Code effective 1-1-2002. PET imaging whole body, full and partial ring PET scanners only, restaging colorectal cancer (replaces code G0163)
G0164	Code deleted effective 6-30-01. Position emission Tomography (PET), whole body, for staging and characterization of lymphoma.
G0221	Code effective 1-1-2002. Positron Emission Tomography (PET), imaging whole body, initial staging; lymphoma (replaces code G0164).
G0222	Code effective 1-1-2002. PET imaging whole body; restaging; lymphoma (replaces G0164)
G0165	Code deleted effective 6-30-01. Position Emission Tomography (PET), whole body, for recurrence of melanoma or melanoma metastatic cancer
G0218	Code effective 1-1-2002. PET imaging whole body, restaging; melanoma (replaces code G0165)

FIs pay these codes based on the technical component of the fee schedule when billed by SNFs. They are reported to FIs with revenue code 0404 (Positron Emission Tomography).

60.1 Expanded Coverage of PET Scans for Claims With Dates of Service on or After July 1, 2002 (Rev. 1, 10-01-03) AB-02-115.— Effective for claims received on or after July 1, 2001, CMS will no longer require the designation of the four PET Scan modifiers (N, E, P, S) and that no paper documentation needs to be submitted up front with PET scan claims. Documentation requirements such as physician referral and medical necessity determination are to be maintained by the provider as part of the beneficiary's medical record. This information must be made available to the carrier or FI upon request of additional documentation to determine appropriate payment of an individual claim.

See the Medicare National Coverage Determinations Manual for specific coverage criteria for PET Scans. Coverage is expanded for PET scans to include the following effective July 1, 2001:

• Scans performed with dedicated full-ring scanners will be covered. Gamma camera systems with at least a 1 inch thick crystal are eligible for coverage in addition to those already approved by CMS (FDA approved);
• The provider must maintain on file the doctor's referral and documentation that the procedure involved:

  a. Only FDA approved drugs and devices and,

  b. Did not involve investigational drugs, or procedures using investigational drugs, as determined by the FDA;

• The ordering physician is responsible for certifying the medical necessity of the study according to the conditions. The physician must have documentation in the beneficiary's medical

record to support the referral supplied to the PET scan provider;

The following is a brief summary of the expanded coverage.

• PET is covered for diagnosis, initial staging and restaging of non-small cell lung cancer (NSCLC).
• Usage of PET for colorectal cancer has been expanded to include diagnosis, staging, and restaging.
• Usage of PET for the initial staging, and restaging of both Hodgkin's and non-Hodgkin's disease.
• Usage of PET for the diagnosis, initial staging, and restaging of melanoma. **(PET Scans are NOT covered for the evaluation of regional nodes.)**
• Medicare covers PET for the diagnosis, initial staging, and restaging of esophageal cancer.
• Usage of PET for Head and Neck Cancers. **(PET scans for head and neck cancer is NOT covered for central nervous system or thyroid cancers.)**
• Usage of PET following an inconclusive single photon emission computed tomography (SPECT) only for myocardial viability. In the event that a patient has received a SPECT and the physician finds the results to be inconclusive, only then may a PET scan be ordered utilizing the proper documentation.
• Usage of PET for pre-surgical evaluation for patients with refractory seizures.

  A. Limitations.—For staging and restaging: PET is covered in either/or both of the following circumstances:

• The stage of the cancer remains in doubt after completion of a standard diagnostic workup, including conventional imaging (computed tomography, magnetic resonance imaging, or ultrasound); and/or
• The clinical management of the patient would differ depending on the stage of the cancer identified. PET will be covered for restaging after the completion of treatment for the purpose of detecting residual disease, for detecting suspected recurrence, or to determine the extent of a known recurrence. Use of PET would also be considered reasonable and necessary if it could potentially replace one or more conventional imaging studies when it is expected that conventional study information is insufficient for the clinical management of the patient.

PET is not covered for other diagnostic uses, and is not covered for screening (testing of patients without specific symptoms). Use of PET to monitor tumor response during the planned course of therapy (i.e. when no change in therapy is being contemplated) is not covered

  B. Frequency.—In the absence of national frequency limitations, for all indications covered on and after July 1, 2001, contractors can, if necessary, develop frequency limitations on any or all covered PET scan services.

  C. HCPCS for PET Scans.—G0210 through G0230 are new HCPCS codes effective for claims with dates of service on and after July 1, 2001. Note that G0211 replaces G0126. HCPCS G0215 replaces G0163. HCPCS G0218 replaces code G0165. HCPCS G0221 and G0222 replace G0164. HCPCS G0219 is for noncovered indications.

  D. Carrier Claims.—Claims for PET scan services must be billed on the Form-CMS 1500 or the electronic equivalent with the appropriate HCPCS and diagnosis codes to the carrier. **Effective for claims received on or after July 1, 2001, PET modifiers will be discontinued and are no longer a claims processing requirement for PET scan claims.** Therefore, July 1, 2001, and after the MSN messages regarding the use of PET modifiers can be discontinued. The type of service (TOS) for the new PET scan procedure codes is TOS 4, Diagnostic Radiology.

  E. FI Claims.—Claims for PET scan procedures must be billed to the FI on Form CMS-1450 (UB-92) or the electronic equivalent with the appropriate diagnosis, HCPCS "G" codes to indicate the conditions under which a PET scan was done. These codes represent the technical component costs associated with these procedures when furnished to hospital and SNF outpatients. They are paid under the Outpatient Prospective Payment System to hospitals and under the Medicare Physician Fee schedule when billed by a SNF. Institutional providers bill these codes under Revenue Code 0404 (PET scan).

60.2 Expanded Coverage of PET Scans for Claims with Dates of Service on or After October 1, 2002 (Rev. 1, 10-01-03) AB-02-065.—Effective for dates of service on or after October 1, 2002, Medicare will cover FDG PET as an adjunct to other imaging modalities for staging and restaging for locoregional, recurrence or metastasis. Monitoring treatment of a locally advanced breast cancer tumor and metastatic breast cancer when a change in therapy is contemplated is also covered as an adjunct to other imaging modalities. The baseline PET study for monitoring should be done under the code for staging or restaging.

Effective for dates of service on or after October 1, 2002, Medicare continues to have a national non-coverage determination for initial diagnosis of breast cancer and initial staging of axillary lymph nodes. Medicare coverage now includes PET as an adjunct to standard imaging modalities for staging patients with distant metastasis or restaging patients with locoregional recurrence or metastasis; as an adjunct to standard imaging modalities for monitoring for women with locally advanced and metastatic breast cancer when a change in therapy is contemplated.

In the absence of national frequency limitations, contractors can, if necessary, develop reasonable frequency limitations for breast cancer.

A. HCPCS Codes for Breast Cancer PET Scans Performed on or After October 1, 2002.—G0252 through G0254 are applicable codes for billing breast cancer PET scans performed on or after October 1, 2002.

B. HCPCS Codes for Myocardial Viability PET Scans Performed on or After October 1, 2002.—G0230, 78459 are applicable for myocardial viability PET scans performed on or after October 1, 2002.

NOTE: The National Coverage Determinations Manual contains a description of coverage. FDG Positron Emission Tomography is a minimally invasive diagnostic procedure using positron camera [tomograph] to measure the decay of radioisotopes such as FDG. The CMS determined that the benefit category for the requested indications fell under §1861(s)(3) of the Act diagnostic service.)

C. Billing and Payment Requirements.—FI claims for PET scan procedures must be billed on Form CMS-1450 (UB-92) or the electronic equivalent with the appropriate diagnosis HCPCS "G" codes to indicate the conditions under which a PET scan was done. These codes represent the technical component costs associated with these procedures when furnished to hospital outpatients, and are paid under the Outpatient Prospective Payment System. Providers bill these codes under Revenue Code 0404 (PET scan). Applicable bill types include: 12X, 13X, 21X, 22X, 23X, and 85X.

Payment pricing information for HCPCS codes are effective October 2002, in the Medicare Physician Fee Schedule.

60.2.1 Coverage for Myocardial Viability AB-02-065.—FDG PET is covered for the determination of myocardial viability following an inconclusive single photon computed tomography test (SPECT) from July 1, 2001, through September 30, 2002. Only full ring scanners are covered as the scanning medium for this service from July 1, 2001, through December 31, 2001. However, as of January 1, 2002, full and partial ring scanners are covered for myocardial viability following an inconclusive SPECT.

Beginning October 1, 2002, Medicare will cover FDG PET for the determination of myocardial viability as a primary or initial diagnostic study prior to revascularization, and will continue to cover FDG PET when used as a follow-up to an inconclusive SPECT. However, if a patient received a FDG PET study with inconclusive results, a follow-up SPECT is not covered. FDA full and partial ring PET scanners are covered.

In the event that a patient receives a SPECT with inconclusive

results, a PET scan may be performed and covered by Medicare. However, a SPECT is not covered following a FDG PET with inconclusive results. See the Medicare National Coverage Determinations Manual for specific frequency limitations for Myocardial Viability following an inconclusive SPECT.

In the absence of national frequency limitations, contractors can, if necessary develop reasonable frequency limitations for myocardial viability.

Documentation that these conditions are met should be maintained by the referring physician as part of the beneficiary's medical record.

60.3 FI Post-Payment Review (Rev. 1, 10-01-03).—As with any claim, but particularly in view of the limitations on this coverage, Medicare may decide to conduct post-payment reviews to determine that the use of PET scans is consistent with coverage instructions. SNFs must keep patient record information on file for each Medicare patient for whom a PET scan claim is made. These medical records will be used in any post-payment reviews and must include the information necessary to substantiate the need for the PET scan. These records must include standard information (e.g., age, sex, and height) along with sufficient patient histories to allow determination that the steps required in the coverage instructions were followed. Such information must include, but is not limited to, the date, place and results of previous diagnostic tests (e.g., cytopathology and surgical pathology reports, CT), as well as the results and reports of the PET scan(s) performed at the center. If available, such records should include the prognosis derived from the PET scan, together with information regarding the physician or institution to which the patient proceeded following the scan for treatment or evaluation. The ordering physician is responsible for forwarding appropriate clinical data to the PET scan facility.

60.4 Use of Gamma Cameras and Full Ring and Partial Ring PET Scanners for PET Scans (Rev. 1, 10-01-03) AB-01-168.—See the Medicare National Coverage Determinations Manual concerning 2-[F-18] Fluoro-D-Glucose (FDG) PET scanners and details about coverage.

On July 1, 2001, HCPCS codes G0210–G0230 were added to allow billing for all currently covered indications for FDG PET. Although the codes do not indicate the type of PET scanner, these codes should be used until January 1, 2002, by providers to bill for services in a manner consistent with the coverage policy. Effective January 1, 2002, these codes have new descriptors to properly reflect the type of PET scanner used. Also effective January 1, 2002, there are four new G codes for covered conditions that may be billed if a gamma camera is used for the PET scan. As of January 1, 2002, providers should bill using the revised HCPCS codes G0120–G0234. Payment is based on the Medicare Fee Schedule.

4182 PROSTATE CANCER SCREENING TESTS AND PROCEDURES (100-4, 18-§50)

4182.1 Coverage Summary. (100-4, 18-§50)

4182.2 Requirements for Submitting Claims. (100-4, 18-§50.3)

4182.3 HCPCS Codes and Payment Requirements. (100-4, 18-§50.2, 50.3)

4182.4 Calculating the Frequency. (100-4, 18-§50.6)

4182.5 CWF Edits. (100-4, 18-§50.6)

4182.6 Correct Coding Requirements. (100-4, 18-§50.3.1)

4182.7 Diagnosis Coding Requirements. (100-4, 18-§50.5)

4182.8 Denial Messages. (100.4, 18-§50.7, 50.8)

50 PROSTATE CANCER SCREENING TESTS AND PROCEDURES (Rev. 1, 10-01-03) B3-4182, A3-3616

Sections 1861(s)(2)(P) and 1861(oo) of the Act (as added by §4103

HCPCS Code; Type of Service (TOS)	Description	Payment	
		Requirements	Methodology/Fee Schedule
G0102; TOS = 1	Prostate cancer screening; digital rectal examination	1. Performed on a male Medicare beneficiary over 50 years of age (i.e., for services starting at least one day after the beneficiary attained age 50). 2. Performed by one of the following, who is authorized under State law to perform the examination, is fully knowledgeable about the beneficiary, and is responsible for explaining the results of the examination to the beneficiary: a. Doctor of medicine or osteopathy b. Qualified physician assistant c. Qualified nurse practitioner d. Qualified clinical nurse specialist e. Qualified certified nurse midwife 3. Performed at a frequency no greater than once every 12 months (See §4182.4).	1. Refer to the physician's fee schedule. 2. Apply deductible and coinsurance. 3. Claims from physicians for these examinations where assignment was not taken are subject to the Medicare limiting charge. (See §7555). 4. Correct Coding Initiative requirements apply. See §4182.6
G0103; TOS = 5	Prostate cancer screening; PSA test	1. Performed on a male Medicare beneficiary over 50 years of age (i.e., for services starting at least one day after the beneficiary attained age 50) 2. Ordered by one of the following, who is authorized under State law to perform the examination, is fully knowledgeable about the beneficiary, and is responsible for explaining the results of the examination to the beneficiary: a. Physician (doctor of medicine or osteopathy) b. Qualified physician assistant c. Qualified nurse practitioner d. Qualified clinical nurse specialist e. Qualified certified nurse midwife 3. Performed at a frequency no greater than once every 12 months. (See §4182.4.)	1. Refer to the clinical laboratory fee schedule; payment for this test is the same as for code "84153*, PSA; total." 2. Do not apply deductible and coinsurance.

*CPT only © 2003. *Current Procedural Terminology, 2004, Professional Edition,* American Medical Association. All Rights Reserved.

of the Balanced Budget Act of 1997), provide for Medicare Part B coverage of certain prostate cancer screening tests subject to certain coverage, frequency, and payment limitations. Effective for services furnished on or after January 1, 2000, Medicare Part B covers prostate cancer screening tests/procedures for the early detection of prostate cancer. Coverage of prostate cancer screening tests includes the following procedures furnished to an individual for the early detection of prostate cancer:

• Screening digital rectal examination, and
• Screening prostate specific antigen (PSA) blood test.

Each test may be paid at a frequency of once every 12 months for men who have attained age 50 (i.e., starting at least one day after they have attained age 50), if at least 11 months have passed following the month in which the last Medicare-covered screening digital rectal examination was performed (for digital rectal exams) or PSA test was performed (for PSA tests).

50.1 Definitions (Rev. 1, 10-01-03). A3-3616.A.1 and 2

A. Screening Digital Rectal Examination.—Screening digital rectal examination means a clinical examination of an individual's prostate for nodules or other abnormalities of the prostate. This screening must be performed by a doctor of medicine or osteopathy (as defined in §186l(r)(1) of the Act), or by a physician assistant, nurse practitioner, clinical nurse specialist, or by a certified nurse mid-wife (as defined in §1861(aa) and §1861(gg) of the Act),

who is authorized under State law to perform the examination, fully knowledgeable about the beneficiary, and would be responsible for explaining the results of the examination to the beneficiary.

B. Screening Prostate Specific Antigen (PSA) Tests.—Screening prostate specific antigen (PSA) is a test that measures the level of prostate specific antigen in an individual's blood. This screening must be ordered by the beneficiary's physician or by the beneficiary's physician assistant, nurse practitioner, clinical nurse specialist, or certified nurse midwife (the term "physician" is defined in §1861(r)(1) of the Act to mean a doctor of medicine or osteopathy and the terms "physician assistant, nurse practitioner, clinical nurse specialist, or certified nurse midwife" are defined in §1861(aa) and §1861(gg) of the Act) who is fully knowledgeable about the beneficiary, and who would be responsible for explaining the results of the test to the beneficiary.

50.2 Deductible and Coinsurance (Rev. 1, 10-01-03). B3-4182.3—
The screening PSA test is a lab test to which neither deductible nor coinsurance apply.

Both deductible (if unmet) and coinsurance are applicable to screening rectal examinations.

50.3 Payment Method—FIs and Carriers (Rev. 1, 10-01-03). B3-4182.3, A3-3616.C—Screening PSA tests (G0103) are paid under the clinical diagnostic lab fee schedule.

Screening rectal examinations (G0102) are paid under the MPFS except for the following bill types identified (FI only). Bill types not identified are paid under the MPFS.

- 12X = Outpatient Prospective Payment System
- 13X = Outpatient Prospective Payment System
- 14X = Outpatient Prospective Payment System
- 71X = Included in All Inclusive Rate
- 73X = Included in All Inclusive Rate
- 85X = Cost (Payment should be consistent with amounts paid for code 84153 or code 86316.)

RHCs and FQHCs should include the charges on the claims for future inclusion in encounter rate calculations.

50.3.1 Correct Coding Requirements for Carrier Claims (Rev. 1, 10-01-03). B3-4182.6—Billing and payment for a Digital Rectal Exam (DRE) (G0102) is bundled into the payment for a covered E/M service (CPT codes 99201–99456 and 99499)* when the two services are furnished to a patient on the same day. If the DRE is the only service or is provided as part of an otherwise noncovered service, HCPCS code G0102 would be payable separately if all other coverage requirements are met.

50.4 HCPCS, Revenue, and Type of Service Codes (Rev. 1, 10-01-03).—The appropriate bill types for billing the FI on Form CMS-1450 or its electronic equivalent are 12X, 13X, 14X, 22X, 23X, 71X, 73X, 75X, and 85X.

HCPCS code G0102—for prostate cancer screening digital rectal examination.

- Carrier TOS is 1
- FI revenue code is 0770

HCPCS code G0103—for prostate cancer screening PSA tests

- Carrier TOS is 5
- FI revenue code is 030X

50.5 Diagnosis Coding (Rev. 1, 10-01-03). B3-4182.7—Prostate cancer screening digital rectal examinations and screening Prostate Specific Antigen (PSA) blood tests must be billed using screening ("V") code V76.44 (Special Screening for Malignant Neoplasms, Prostate).

50.6 Calculating Frequency (Rev. 1, 10-01-03). A3-3616.D and E, B3-4182.4, B3-4182.5—Calculating Frequency—To determine the 11-month period, the count starts beginning with the month after the month in which a previous test/procedure was performed.

Example: The beneficiary received a screening prostate specific antigen test in January 2002. Start counts beginning February 2002. The beneficiary is eligible to receive another screening prostate specific antigen test in January 2003 (the month after 11 months have passed).

Common Working File (CWF) Edits

Beginning October 1, 2000, the following CWF edits were implemented for dates of service January 1, 2000, and later, for prostate cancer screening tests and procedures for the following:

- Age;
- Frequency;
- Sex; and
- Valid HCPCS code.

50.7 MSN Messages (Rev. 1, 10-01-03). B3-4182.8.B, A3-3616.F—If a claim for screening prostate specific antigen test or a screening digital rectal examination is being denied because of the age of the beneficiary, FIs use MSN message 18.13:

This service is not covered for patients under 50 years of age.

The Spanish version of this MSN message should read:

Este servicio no está cubierto hasta después de que el beneficiario cumpla 50 años.

Carriers use MSN Message 18.19:

This service is not covered until after the patient's 50th birthday.

The Spanish version of this MSN message should read:

Este servicio no está cubierto hasta después de que el beneficiario cumpla 50 años.

If the claim for screening prostate specific antigen test or screening digital rectal examination is being denied because the time period between the same test or procedure has not passed, FIs and carriers use MSN message 18.14:

Service is being denied because it has not been 12 months since your last test/procedure) of this kind.

The Spanish version of this MSN message should read:

Este servicio está siendo denegado ya que no han transcurrido (12, 24, 48) meses desde el último (examen/procedimiento) de esta clase.

50.8 Remittance Advice Notices (Rev. 1, 10-01-03). B3-4182.8, A3-3616.G—If the claim for a screening prostate antigen test or screening digital rectal examination is being denied because the patient is less than 50 years of age, ANSI X12N 835.

- Claim adjustment reason code 6 "the procedure/revenue code is inconsistent with the patient's age," at the line level; and
- Remark code M140 "Service is not covered until after the patient's 50th birthday, i.e., no coverage prior to the day after the 50th birthday."

If the claim for a screening prostate specific antigen test or screening digital rectal examination is being denied because the time period between the test/procedure has not passed, contractors use ANSI X12N 835 claim adjustment reason code 119 "Benefit maximum for this time period has been reached" at the line level.

If the claim for a screening prostate antigen test or screening digital rectal examination is being denied due to the absence of diagnosis code V76.44 on the claim, use ANSI X12N 835 claim adjustment reason code 47, "This (these) diagnosis(es) is (are) not covered, missing, or invalid."

4270. ESRD BILL PROCESSING PROCEDURES (100.4, 8-§70, 80, 90, 90.1, 90.3, 2, 130)

4270.1 Home Dialysis Supplies and Equipment. (100.4, 8-§60.4.4, 90.1, 90.2, 90.2.2)

60.4.4 Home Patients (Rev. 1, 10-01-03). B3-4270.1—Medicare covers EPO, including items related to its administration for dialysis patients who use EPO in the home, when requirements for a patient care plan and patient selection as described in the Medicare Benefit Policy Manual, Chapter 11, are met.

When EPO is prescribed for a home patient, it may be either administered in a facility, e.g., the one shown on the Form CMS-382 (home patient selection form) or furnished by a facility or Method II supplier for self-administration to a home patient determined to be competent to administer this drug. For EPO furnished for self-administration to Method I and Method II home patients determined to be competent, the facility bills its FI and the Method II supplier bills its DMERC. No additional payment is made for training a prospective self-administering patient or retraining an existing home patient to self-administer EPO.

In accordance with the Code of Federal Regulations (CFR), Method II patients who self-administer erythropoeitin (EPO) may obtain EPO only from either their Method II supplier, or a Medicare certified ESRD facility. (See 42 CFR 414.335.)

In this case, the DMERC makes payment at the same rate that applies to facilities. Program payment may not be made for EPO furnished by a physician to a patient for self-administration.

90.1 DMERC Denials for Beneficiary Submitted Claims Under

---

*CPT only © 2003. *Current Procedural Terminology, 2004, Professional Edition,* American Medical Association. All Rights Reserved.

Method II (Rev. 1, 10-01-03). A3-3170.6, A3-3644.3, A3-3644.3.A—E, HO-238.2.C, HO-238.3, HO-238.3.A, B3-2231.3.A and B, B3-2231, B3-4270.1, PRM-1-2709.2.A—Under Method II, beneficiaries may not submit any claims and cannot receive payment for any benefits for home dialysis equipment and supplies. DMERCs must deny unassigned and beneficiary submitted claims with the following MSN messages.

MSN # 16.6: "This item or service cannot be paid unless the provider accepts assignment."

Spanish: "Este articulo o servicio no se pagará a menos de que el proveedor acepte asignación."

MSN # 16.7: "Your provider must complete and submit your claim."

Spanish: "Su proveedor debe completar y someter su reclamación."

MSN # 16.36: "If you have already paid it, you are entitled to a refund from this provider."

Spanish: "Si usted ya lo ha pagado, tiene derecho a un reebolso de su proveedor."

0.2 Requirements for Payment by the DMERC (Rev. 1, 10-01-03). B3-4270.1, B3-3045.7—DMERCS may make payment to home dialysis suppliers only if all of the following conditions are met:

- The beneficiary has elected Method II and to receive home dialysis equipment and supplies from an independent supplier. (Method II);
- The supplier is not a Medicare approved dialysis facility;
- The supplier accepts assignment for all Method II equipment and supplies;
- The supplier agrees to be the beneficiary's sole supplier for all home dialysis equipment and supplies;
- The supplier agrees to bill on a monthly basis for the quantity of supplies appropriate for that period. (However, there is one exception to this rule. Beneficiaries are permitted to have one month's supplies in reserve in case of emergency.);
- The supplier maintains a written certification in its files that it has a written agreement with a Medicare approved dialysis facility under which the facility will furnish all necessary support, backup, and emergency dialysis services, for each beneficiary the supplier services. (For Medicare beneficiaries who are also entitled to military or veterans benefits, a military or Veteran's Administration (VA) hospital satisfies this requirement.) As of July 1, 2002, suppliers are required to use a modifier (Specific required documentation on file) on any claim for services requiring such a backup agreement. See §90.4 for more information. The supplier may not provide supplies or services to the beneficiary, or submit a claim to the DMERC, until they have a valid written support service facility agreement for that beneficiary. The dialysis facility must be a reasonable distance from the beneficiary's home in order to furnish these services. Determine a reasonable distance by considering such variables as terrain, whether the patient's home is located in a rural or urban area, and the usual distances traveled and time in transit by patients in the area in obtaining health care services;
- In cases where a supplier cannot establish an agreement with a support service facility that is within a reasonable distance from the patient's home, the supplier must establish a written agreement with a support service facility outside of the geographic area of the patient's home. However, in this situation, the support service facility must establish a written agreement with a dialysis facility within the beneficiary's geographic region to provide any required in-facility dialysis treatments. In this situation, the support service facility will be responsible for providing all other necessary services for the patient, and must provide for the coordination of the patient's care and monitor the patient through frequent visits to the patient's home. The signed agreement with the Method II supplier must stipulate how the support services facility will provide each of the required support services. The written agreement must include documentation to support the arrangement with the local facility for any needed in-facility services;

- The supplier reports to the backup facility within 30 days all items and services that it furnishes to the patient so that the facility can record this information in the patient's medical record; and
- The supplies and equipment are reasonable and necessary for that patient.

90.2.2 DMERC (Rev. 1, 10-01-03) **Letter Explaining Requirements to Method II Supplier. B3-4270.1 updated with transmittal B3-1729 (11-01)**—DMERCs must explain the Medicare requirements to every Method II supplier they service. Below is a sample letter to use.

Dear Method II Supplier:

Our records show that you supply home dialysis equipment and/or supplies to Medicare home dialysis beneficiaries who have chosen payment Method II. Effective February 1, 1990, there is a limit on the amount that a dialysis supplier may be paid under Method II.

The payment limit for Method II benefits for all forms of dialysis except continuous cycling peritoneal dialysis (CCPD) cannot exceed the median composite rate for hospital-based dialysis facilities. This rate is $1,974.45 for continuous cycling peritoneal dialysis (CCPD) and $1,490.85 for all other methods of dialysis. These limits are subject to the usual Medicare Part B deductible and coinsurance amounts.

There are additional requirements for Method II benefits. Each Method II beneficiary that did not choose Method II before February 1, 1990 must certify in writing that he/she deals with a single supplier for all home dialysis equipment and supplies. Beneficiaries who chose Method II before February 1, 1990, are presumed to meet this requirement and need not submit this certification. If a beneficiary chooses Method II on or after February1, 1990, the beneficiary (or the dialysis facility or the supplier on the beneficiary's behalf) must write the following in Block 8 of the Form CMS-382:

"I certify that I have only one Method II supplier."

As a Method II home dialysis supplier, in order to be paid Medicare benefits, the supplier must:

- Be the beneficiary's sole supplier for all home dialysis equipment and supplies needed by the beneficiary;
- Accept assignment of Medicare benefits for home dialysis equipment and supplies. If the supplier does not accept assignment, inform your Medicare beneficiaries that the supplier does not accept assignment and that, therefore, Medicare CANNOT pay for his/her home dialysis equipment or supplies;
- Maintain written certifications that there is a written agreement with a Medicare approved dialysis facility under which the facility will furnish all necessary support, backup, and emergency dialysis services for each beneficiary you serve. Support services include, but are not limited to, maintaining the patient's medical record and providing information required by the ESRD network. For each Medicare beneficiaries, there must be an agreement with a dialysis facility that is a reasonable distance from the beneficiary's home. The CMS determines a reasonable distance by considering such variables as terrain, whether the beneficiary's home is in an urban or rural area, and the usual distances traveled and time in transit by patients in the area when obtaining health services. In cases where an agreement with a support service facility cannot be established that is within a reasonable distance from the patient's home, a written agreement with a support service facility outside of the geographic area of the patient's home must be established. In this situation, the support service facility must establish a written arrangement with a dialysis facility within the beneficiary's geographic region to provide any required in-facility dialysis treatments. In this situation, the support service facility will be responsible for providing all other necessary services for the beneficiary and must provide for the coordination of the patient's care and monitor the patient through frequent visits to the patient's home. The signed agreement with the Method II supplier must stipulate how the support services facility will provide each of the required support services. The written agreement must include documentation to support the arrange-

ment with the local facility for any needed in-facility services. Suppliers may not provide services or submit a claim to Medicare before this agreement is obtained. They need not identify individual beneficiaries.

- Report to the support service dialysis facility within 30 days all items and services that are furnished to the patient so that this information can be recorded by the facility in the medical record; and

- Agree to generally bill once a month and for only one month's quantity of supplies at a time. In the event that a beneficiary becomes a hospital inpatient for at least three days (not counting the day of admission or discharge), suppliers must prorate the following month's supply bills to account for supplies the beneficiary did not use while an inpatient.

130 PHYSICIANS AND SUPPLIER (NONFACILITY) BILLING FOR ESRD SERVICES—GENERAL (Rev. 1, 10-01-03) B3-4270 updated with Transmittal 1729

Payment for renal-related physicians' services to ESRD patients is made in either of the following ways:

- Under the Monthly Capitation Payment (MCP) (see §140 below for an explanation of the MCP); or
- Using the daily codes for ESRD services (CPT codes 90922-90925)* with units that represent the number of days services were furnished.
- Under the Initial method (IM)

The carrier receives bills (Form CMS--1500 or electronic equivalent) from physicians for services furnished ESRD beneficiaries. DMERCs receive bills for equipment and supplies for Method II beneficiaries. Intermediaries receive bills from ESRD facilities. Lab bills from CLIA certified independent dialysis facilities were billed to the carrier before September 1, 1997, and to the FI beginning on that date. Other certified labs continue to bill the carrier.

4270.2 Bill Review of Laboratory Services. (100-4, 8-§60.1, 90, 16-§40.6, 16-§60.1.3)

60.1 Lab Services (Rev. 1, 10-01-03). A3-3644.1, PRM-1-2711.1, B3-4270.2, RDF-322, A3-3167.3—See the Medicare Benefit Policy Manual, Chapter 11, for a description of lab services included in the composite rate.

Independent laboratories and independent dialysis facilities with the appropriate clinical laboratory certification in accordance with CLIA may be paid for ESRD clinical laboratory tests that are separately billable. The laboratories and independent dialysis facilities are paid for separately billable clinical laboratory tests according to the Medicare laboratory fee schedule for independent laboratories. Independent dialysis facilities billing for separately billable laboratory tests that they perform must submit claims to the FI. Independent laboratories must bill the carrier.

Hospital-based laboratories providing separately billable laboratory service to hospital dialysis patients of the hospital's dialysis facility bill separately and are paid in accordance with the outpatient lab provisions. However, where the hospital lab does tests for an independent dialysis facility or for another hospital's facility, the non-patient billing provisions apply.

Clinical laboratory tests can be performed individually or in predetermined groups on automated profile equipment. Automated profiles and application of the "50 percent rule" can be found in Chapter 16 of this manual.

A specimen collection fee determined by CMS (as of this writing, up to $3.00) will be allowed for ESRD Method II billing only in the following circumstances:

- Drawing a blood sample through venipuncture (i.e., inserting into a vein a needle with a syringe or vacutainer to draw the specimen).
- Collecting a urine sample by catheterization.

Laboratory tests for Hemodialysis, Intermittent Peritoneal Dialysis (IPD), Continuous Cycling Peritoneal Dialysis (CCPD), and Hemofiltration (as specifically listed below) are usually performed for dialysis patients and are routinely covered at the frequency specified in the absence of indications to the contrary, i.e., no documentation of medical necessity is required other than knowledge of the patient's status as an ESRD beneficiary. When any of these tests is performed at a frequency greater than that specified, the additional tests are separately billable and are covered only if they are medically justified by accompanying documentation. A diagnosis of ESRD alone is not sufficient medical evidence to warrant coverage of the additional tests. The nature of the illness or injury (diagnosis, complaint, or symptom) requiring the performance of the test(s) must be present on the claim. Such information must be furnished using the ICD-9-CM coding system.

Per Treatment

All hematocrit, hemoglobin, and clotting time tests furnished incident to dialysis treatments

Weekly

Prothrombin time for patients on anticoagulant therapy
Serum Creatinine

Weekly or Thirteen Per Quarter

BUN
Monthly

Serum Calcium	Serum Bicarbonate	Alkaline Phosphatase
Serum Potassium	Serum Phosphorous	AST, SGOT
Serum Chloride	Total Protein	LDH
CBC	Serum Albumin	

Automated Battery of Tests.—If an automated battery of tests, such as the SMA-12, is performed and contains most of the tests listed in one of the weekly or monthly categories, it is not necessary to **separately** identify any tests in the battery that are not listed.

Guidelines for Separately Billable Tests for Hemodialysis, IPD, CCPD, and Hemofiltration

Serum Aluminum—one every 3 months
Serum Ferritin—one every 3 months

90 METHOD II BILLING (Rev. 1, 10-01-03) A3-3644.A, RO-2-3440.C, B3-4270, B3-4271, B3-4270.1, B3-4270.2, B3-34271, PRM-1-2740, A3-3644.3

Physicians and independent laboratories, must submit claims (Form CMS-1500 or electronic equivalent) to their local carrier for services furnished to end stage renal disease (ESRD) beneficiaries. Suppliers of Method II dialysis equipment and supplies will submit their claims (Form CMS-1500 or electronic equivalent) to the appropriate Durable Medical Equipment Regional Carriers (DMERCs). All ESRD facilities must submit their claims to their appropriate FI.

The amount of Medicare payment under Method II for home dialysis equipment and supplies may NOT exceed $1974.45 for continuous cycling peritoneal dialysis (CCPD) and $1490.85 for all other methods of dialysis.

All laboratory tests furnished to home dialysis patients who have selected payment Method II (see §70.1 above), are billed to and paid by the carrier at the fee schedule, if the tests are performed by an independent laboratory for an independent dialysis facility patient.

If the beneficiary elects to deal directly with a supplier and make arrangements for securing the necessary supplies and equipment to dialyze at home, and chooses Method II, he/she deals directly with a supplier of home dialysis equipment and supplies (this supplier is not a dialysis facility). A supplier other than a facility bills the DMERC. There can be only one supplier per beneficiary, and the supplier must accept assignment. The beneficiary is responsible for any unmet Part B deductible and the 20 percent coinsurance.

---

*CPT only © 2003. *Current Procedural Terminology, 2004, Professional Edition*, American Medical Association. All Rights Reserved.

Only a supplier that is not a dialysis facility may submit a claim to a DMERC for home dialysis supplies and equipment. Suppliers will submit these claims on Form CMS-1500, or electronic equivalent. Under Method II, beneficiaries may not submit any claims and cannot receive payment for any benefits for home dialysis equipment and supplies.

The supplier must have a written agreement with a Medicare approved dialysis facility that will provide all necessary support, backup, and emergency dialysis services. The dialysis facility will not receive a regular per treatment payment for a patient who chooses Method II.

However, if the facility provides any support services, backup, and emergency dialysis services to a beneficiary who selects this option, the facility is reimbursed for the items or services it furnishes. Hospital-based facilities are paid the reasonable cost of support services, subject to the lesser of cost or charges provisions of §1833(a)(2)(A) of the Act. Independent facilities are paid on a reasonable charge basis for any home dialysis support services they furnish.

A. Description of Support Services.—Support services specifically applicable to home patients include but are not limited to:

• Surveillance of the patient's home adaptation, including provisions for visits to the home in accordance with a written plan prepared and periodically reviewed by a team that includes the patient's physician and other professionals familiar with the patient's condition;
• Furnishing dialysis-related emergency services;
• Consultation for the patient with a qualified social worker and a qualified dietician;
• Maintaining a record-keeping system which assures continuity of care;
• Maintaining and submitting all required documentation to the ESRD network;
• Assuring that the water supply is of the appropriate quality;
• Assuring that the appropriate supplies are ordered on an ongoing basis;
• Arranging for the provision of all ESRD laboratory tests;
• Testing and appropriate treatment of water used in dialysis;
• Monitoring the functioning of dialysis equipment;
• All other necessary dialysis services as required under the ESRD conditions for coverage;
• Watching the patient perform CAPD and assuring that it is done correctly, and reviewing with the patient any aspects of the technique he/she may have forgotten, or informing the patient of modification in apparatus or technique;
• Documenting whether the patient has or has not had peritonitis that requires physician intervention or hospitalization, (unless there is evidence of peritonitis, a culture for peritonitis is not necessary);
• Inspection of the catheter site; and
• Since home dialysis support services include maintaining a medical record for each home dialysis patient, the Method II supplier must report to the support service dialysis facility within 30 days all items and services that it furnished to the patient so that the facility can record this information in the patient's medical record.

The services must be furnished in accordance with the written plan required for home dialysis patients. See the Medicare Benefit Policy Manual, Chapter 15, for coverage of telehealth services, and this manual, Chapter 12 for billing telehealth.

Each of the support services may be paid routinely at a frequency of once per month. Any support services furnished in excess of this frequency must be documented for being reasonable and necessary. For example, the patient may contract peritonitis and require an unscheduled connecting tube change.

B. Reasonableness Determinations.—Support services (which include the laboratory services included under the composite rate for in-facility patients) are paid on a reasonable charge basis to independent facilities and a reasonable cost basis to hospital-based facilities, subject to the Method II payment cap (refer to §140). A reasonable cost/charge determination must be made for

each individual support service furnished to home patients. With respect to the connecting tube change, facilities may bill Medicare for the personnel services required to change the connecting tube, but must look to the Method II supplier for payment for the connecting tube itself.

The payment cap is not a payment rate that is paid automatically each month. Accordingly, in no case may the FI routinely pay any monthly amount for support services without a claim that shows the services actually furnished.

40.6 Billing for End Stage Renal Disease (ESRD) Related Laboratory Tests (Rev. 1, 10-01-03). PM AB-98-7, PRM 1 2711, B3-4270.2—Hemodialysis, Intermittent Peritoneal Dialysis (IPD), and Continuous Cycling Peritoneal Dialysis (CCPD) Tests

With some exceptions, laboratory tests for hemodialysis, intermittent peritoneal dialysis (IPD), and continuous cycling peritoneal dialysis (CCPD) are included in the ESRD composite rate.

For a particular date of service to a beneficiary, if 50 percent or more of the covered laboratory tests are noncomposite rate tests Medicare allows separate payment beyond that included in the composite rate

For a description of what laboratory tests and other tests are included in the composite rate and under what conditions such tests may qualify for additional payment in addition to the composite rate, see the Medicare Benefit Policy Manual Chapter 11, "End Stage Renal Disease (ESRD)," and Chapter 8 of this manual.

Clinical diagnostic laboratory tests included under the composite rate payment are paid through the composite rate paid by the FI.

40.6.1 Automated Multi-Channel Chemistry (AMCC) Tests for ESRD Beneficiaries—FIs (Rev. 1, 10-01-03). A-03-033—Medicare will apply the following rules to Automated Multi-Channel Chemistry (AMCC) tests for ESRD beneficiaries:

• Payment is at the lowest rate for services performed by the same provider, for the same beneficiary, for the same date of service.
• The facility must identify, for a particular date of service, the AMCC tests ordered that are included in the composite rate and those that are not included. See Chapter 8 for the composite rate tests for Hemodialysis, Intermittent Peritoneal Dialysis (IPD), Continuous Cycling Peritoneal Dialysis (CCPD), Hemofiltration, and Continuous Ambulatory Peritoneal Dialysis (CAPD).
• If 50 percent or more of the covered tests are included under the composite rate payment, then all submitted tests are included within the composite payment. In this case, no separate payment in addition to the composite rate is made for any of the separately billable tests.
• If less than 50 percent of the covered tests are composite rate tests, all AMCC tests submitted for that Date of Service (DOS) for that beneficiary are separately payable.
• A noncomposite rate test is defined as any test separately payable outside of the composite rate or beyond the normal frequency covered under the composite rate that is reasonable and necessary.

(See §100.6 for details regarding pricing modifiers.)

The FI shared system must calculate the number of AMCC tests provided for any given date of service. The FI sums all AMCC tests with a CD modifier and divides the sum of all tests with a CD, CE, and CF modifier for the same beneficiary and provider for any given date of service

If the result of the calculation for a date of service is 50 percent or greater, the FI does not pay for the tests.

If the result of the calculation for a date of service is less than 50 percent, the FI pays for all of the tests.

All tests for a date of service must be billed on the monthly ESRD bill. Providers must send in an adjustment if they identify additional tests that have not been billed.

The organ and disease oriented panels (80049, 80051, 80054, and 80058) are subject to the 50 percent rule. Laboratory tests that are not covered under the composite rate and that are furnished to CAPD end stage renal disease (ESRD) patients dialyzing at home are billed in the same way as any other test furnished home patients.

Business Requirements for ESRD Reimbursement of AMCC Tests:

Requirement Number	Requirements	Responsibility
1.1	The FI shared system must RTP a claim for AMCC tests when a claim for that date of service has already been submitted.	Shared system
1.2	Based upon the presence of the CD, CE and CF payment modifiers, identify the AMCC tests ordered that are included and not included in the composite rate payment	Shared system
1.3	Based upon the determination of requirement 1.2, if 50 percent or more of the covered tests are included under the composite rate, no separate payment is made.	Shared system
1.4	Based upon the determination of requirement 1.2, if less than 50 percent are covered tests included under the composite rate, all AMCC tests for that date of service are payable.	Shared system
1.5	Reject line items that contain a procedure (identified in exhibit 1 and 2) with a modifier CE and a modifier 91 and no line item on the claim with modifier CE and no modifier 91.	Shared system
1.6	Reject line items that contain a procedure (identified in exhibits 1 and 2) with a modifier CF and a modifier 91 and no line item on the claim with modifier CF and no modifier 91.	Shared system
1.7	FI must return any claims for additional tests for any date of service within the billing period when the provider has already submitted a claim. Instruct the provider to adjust the first claim.	FI or Shared system
1.8	Do not apply the 50/50 rule to line items for one of the chemistries in exhibits 1 or 2 that contain modifiers CE or CF and modifier 91 on the line item.	Shared system

Examples of the Application of the 50/50 Rule

The following examples are to illustrate how claims should be paid. The percentages in the action section represent the number of composite rate tests over the total tests. If this percentage is 50 percent or greater, no payment should be made for the claim.

Example 1:

Provider Name: Jones Hospital

DOS 2/1/02

Claim/Services 82040* Mod 1
82310 Mod 1
82374 Mod 1
82435 Mod 1
82947 Mod 3
84295 Mod 3

82040 Mod 1 (Returned as duplicate)
84075 Mod 2
82310 Mod 2
84155 Mod 2

ACTION: 9 services total, 2 non-composite rate tests, 3 composite rate tests beyond the frequency, 4 composite rate tests; 4/9 = 44.4% <50% pay at ATP 09

Example 2:

Provider Name: Bon Secours Renal Facility

DOS 2/15/02

Claim/Services 82040* Mod 2 and Mod 91
84450 Mod 2
82310 Mod 2
82247 Mod 3
82465 No modifier present
82565 Mod 3
84550 Mod 3
82042 Mod 1
84075 Mod 2
82435 Mod 2
82550 Mod 3
82947 Mod 3
82977 Mod 3

ACTION: 11 services total, 6 non-composite rate tests, 4 composite rate tests beyond the frequency, 1 composite rate test; 1/11 = .09.4% <50% pay at ATP 11

Example 3:

Provider Name: Sinai Hospital Renal Facility

Bene 1: DOS 4/02/02

Claim/Services 82565* Mod 1
83615 Mod 1
82247 Mod 3
82248 Mod 3
82040 Mod 1
82450 Mod 1
82565 Mod 2
84550 Mod 3
82248 Mod 3 (Duplicate)

ACTION: 8 services total, 4 composite rate tests; 4/8 = 50%, therefore no payment is made

Example 4:

Provider Name: Dr. Andrew Ross

Bene 1: DOS 6/01/02

Claim/Services 84460* Mod 3
82247 Mod
82248 Mod 3
82040 Mod 1
84075 Mod 1
84450 Mod 1

ACTION: 6 services total, 3 non-composite rate tests and 3 composite rate tests; 3/6 = 50%, therefore no payment. An overpayment should be recovered for the ATP 03 payment amount.

40.6.2 Claims Processing for Separately Billable Tests for ESRD Beneficiaries (Rev. 1, 10-01-03).—Clinical laboratory tests can be performed individually or in predetermined groups on automated profile equipment. If a test profile is performed see §40.6.1. If a clinical laboratory test is performed individually, see §40.6.2.1 or §40.6.2.2 depending upon whether the patient is treated in a hospital-based or independent dialysis facility

40.6.2.1 Separately Billable ESRD Laboratory Tests Furnished by Hospital-Based Facilities (Rev. 1, 10-01-03).—Hospital-based facilities are reimbursed for the separately billable ESRD laboratory tests furnished to their outpatients following the same rules that apply to all other Medicare covered outpatient laboratory services furnished by a hospital.

40.6.2.2 Separately Billable ESRD Laboratory Tests Furnished to

Patients of Independent Dialysis Facilities—FIs.—In accord with Medicare program rules, the FI pays the laboratory that provided the service for all separately billable ESRD clinical laboratory services furnished to patients of independent dialysis. Independent dialysis facilities with appropriate clinical laboratory certification may bill their FI for any separately billable clinical laboratory tests they perform. The FI pays both laboratories and independent dialysis facilities for separately billable clinical laboratory tests according to the Medicare clinical laboratory fee schedule.

60.1.3 Specimen Drawing for Dialysis Patients (Rev. 1, 10-01-03). A3 3644.1, PR 2711.1, B3-4270.2, PUB-29 322—See the Medicare Benefit Policy Manual, Chapter 11, for a description of laboratory services included in the composite rate.

Independent laboratories and independent dialysis facilities with the appropriate clinical laboratory certification in accordance with CLIA may be paid for ESRD clinical laboratory tests that are separately billable. The laboratories and independent dialysis facilities are paid for separately billable clinical laboratory tests according to the Medicare laboratory fee schedule for independent laboratories. Independent dialysis facilities billing for separately billable laboratory tests that they perform must submit claims to the FI. Independent laboratories must bill the carrier.

Hospital-based laboratories providing laboratory service to hospital dialysis patients of the hospital's dialysis facility are paid in accordance with the outpatient laboratory provisions. However, where the hospital laboratory does tests for an independent dialysis facility or for another hospital's facility, the nonpatient billing provisions apply (see §20.1).

Clinical laboratory tests can be performed individually or in predetermined groups on automated profile equipment. A specimen collection fee determined by CMS (as of this writing, up to $3.00) will be allowed only in the following circumstances:

- Drawing a blood sample through venipuncture (i.e., inserting into a vein a needle with a syringe or vacutainer to draw the specimen).
- Collecting a urine sample by catheterization.

Special rules apply when such services are furnished to dialysis patients. The specimen collection fee is not separately payable for y patients dialyzed in the facility or for patients dialyzed at home under reimbursement Method I. Payment for this service is included under the ESRD composite rate, regardless of whether the laboratory test itself is included in the composite rate or is separately billable.

Fees for taking specimens from home dialysis patients, who have elected reimbursement Method II may be paid separately, provided all other criteria for payment are met. Also, fees for taking specimens in the hospital setting, but outside of the dialysis unit, for use in performing laboratory tests not included in the ESRD composite rate may be paid separately.

4273 CLAIMS FOR PAYMENT FOR EPOETIN ALFA (EPO) (100-4, 8-§60.4)

4273.1 Completion of Initial Claim for EPO. (100-4, 8-§60.4.2, 60.4.2.1)

60.4 Erythropoietin (EPO) (Rev. 1, 10-01-03). A3-3644.D.1–D.3, PRM-1-2710.3.A–D, RDF-207.5.A–C, B3-2049.5.B, B3-2049.3.B.1, PM AB 97-2, PM AB-00-76, PM A-01-106, RDF-319—Coverage rules for EPO are explained in the Medicare Benefit Policy Manual, Chapter 11.

Intermediaries pay for EPO to independent ESRD facilities (facilities that are not classified as hospital based) as an add-on amount to the composite rate. No additional payment is made to administer EPO, whether in a facility or a home.

If the beneficiary obtains EPO from a supplier for self-administration, the supplier bills the DMERC and the DMERC pays at the rate shown in §60.4.3

Where EPO is administered in a hospital outpatient department for home dialysis or for patients with chronic renal failure (but not yet on dialysis), payment for EPO is paid under hospital outpatient PPS rules.

Program payment may not be made to a physician for EPO for self-administration. Where EPO is payable as "incident to services" the regular carrier processes the claim.

EPO Payment Methodology

Type of provider	Composite Add on Payment	OPPS	DMERC FEE	No separate payment
In-facility freestanding ESRD facility	X			
In-facility provider based ESRD facility	X			
Hospital OP not on dialysis		X		
Self-administer Home Method I	X			
Self administer Home Method II			X	
Incident to physician in facility or for self-administration*				X

* Medicare pays for a drug if self-administered by a dialysis patient and would still pay the facility if the doctor administered it incident to in a facility.

The Dialysis Outcomes Quality Initiative recommends a threshold hematocrit value range of 33 to 36 percent. National policy requires FIs and carriers to identify practitioners with an atypical number of patients with hematocrit levels above a 90-day rolling average of 37.5 percent for routine medical; review activities, such as provider education or pre-payment reviews. That is, medical documentation is not required for a single value over 36 percent. However, FIs and carriers must make a determination upon post payment review if the treating physician argues it is medically necessary to have a target hematocrit that is greater than 36 percent (which would then exceed the rolling average of 37.5 percent). These hematocrit requirements apply only to EPO furnished as an ESRD benefit under §1881(b) of the Social Security Act (the Act). EPO furnished incident to a physician's service is not included in this policy. Carriers have discretion for local policy for EPO furnished as "incident to service."

60.4.1 EPO Facility Billing Requirements Using UB-92/Form CMS-1450 (Rev. 1, 10-01-03). A3-3644, PRM-1-2710.3—Revenue codes 0634 and 0635 are used to report EPO. Code 0634 reports the number of administrations under 10,000 units and 0635 reports the number of administrations of 10,000 or more.

The number of units of EPO administered during the billing period is reported with value code 68.

The hematocrit reading taken prior to the last administration of EPO during the billing period must also be reported on the UB-92/Form CMS-1450 with value code 49.

The hemoglobin reading taken during the billing period must be reported on the UB-92/Form CMS-1450 with value code 48.

Either the hematocrit or the hemoglobin reading is required. The FI must retain the hematocrit (hct) or hemoglobin (hgb) reading in format accessible to the claims process for use to average readings for a 90-day period on future claims.

The statutory payment allowance for EPO is the only allowance for the drug and its administration when used for ESRD patients. Payment for medical supplies needed for the administration of EPO, whether in the home or in a facility, is included in the Medicare payment rate for EPO.

4450 PARENTERAL AND ENTERAL NUTRITION (PEN) (100-4, 20-§100.2.2, 100.2.2.3)

100.2 Certificates of Medical Necessity (CMN) (Rev. 1, 10-01-03). B3-3312—For certain items or services billed to the DME Regional Carrier (DMERC), the supplier must receive a signed Certificate of Medical Necessity (CMN) from the treating physician. CMNs are not required for the same items when billed by HHAs to RHHIs. Instead, the items must be included in the physician's signed orders on the home health plan of care. See the Medicare Program Integrity Manual, Chapter 6.

The FI will inform other providers (see §01 for definition pf provider) of documentation requirements.

Contractors may ask for supporting documentation beyond a CMN.

Refer to the local DMERC Web site described in §10 for downloadable copies of CMN forms.

See the Medicare Program Integrity Manual, Chapter 5, for specific Medicare policies and instructions on the following topics:

- Requirements for supplier retention of original CMNs
- CMN formats, paper and electronic
- List of currently approved CMNs and items requiring CMNs
- Supplier requirements for submitting CMNs
- Requirements for CMNs to also serve as a physician's order
- Civil monetary penalties for violation of CMN requirements
- Supplier requirements for completing portions of CMNs
- Physician requirements for completing portions of CMNs

100.2.1. Completion of Certificate of Medical Necessity Forms (Rev. 1, 10-01-03).

1. SECTION A:—(This may be completed by supplier.)

a. Certification Type/Date—If this is an initial certification for this patient, the date (MM/DD/YY) is indicated in the space marked "INITIAL". If this is a revised certification (to be completed when the physician changes the order, based on the patient's changing clinical needs), the initial date is indicated in the space marked "INITIAL", **and** the revision date is indicated in the space marked "REVISED". If this is a recertification, the initial date is indicated in the space marked "INITIAL", **and** the recertification date is indicated in the space marked "RECERTIFICATION". Whether a REVISED or RECERTIFIED CMN is submitted, the INITIAL date as well as the REVISED or RECERTIFICATION date is always furnished.

b. Patient Information—This indicates the patient's name, permanent legal address, telephone number, and his/her health insurance claim number (HICN) as it appears on his/her Medicare card and on the claim form.

c. Supplier Information—This indicates the name of the company (supplier name), address, telephone number, and the Medicare supplier number assigned by the National Supplier Clearinghouse (NSC).

d. Place of Service—This indicates the place in which the item is being used, i.e., patient's home is 12, skilled nursing facility (SNF) is 31, or end stage renal disease (ESRD) facility is 65. See chapter 23 for place of service codes.

e. Facility Name—This indicates the name and complete address of the facility, if the place of service is a facility.

f. HCPCS Codes—This is a list of all HCPCS procedure codes for items ordered that require a CMN. Procedure codes that do not require certification are not listed on the CMN.

g. Patient Date of Birth (DOB), Height, Weight, and Sex—This indicates patient's DOB (MM/DD/YY), height in inches, weight in pounds, and sex (male or female).

h. Physician Name and Address—This indicates the treating physician's name and complete mailing address.

i. UPIN—This indicates the treating physician's unique physician identification number (UPIN).

j. Physician's Telephone Number—This indicates the telephone number where the treating physician can be contacted (preferably where records would be accessible pertaining to this patient) if additional information is needed.

2. SECTION B:—(This may not be completed by the supplier. While this section may be completed by a non-physician clinician, or a physician employee, it must be reviewed by the treating physician. Contractors publish this requirement about section B in their bulletins at least annually.)

a. Estimated Length of Need—This indicates the estimated

length of need (the length of time (in months) the physician expects the patient to require use of the ordered item). If the treating physician expects that the patient will require the item for the duration of his/her life, 99 is entered. For recertification and revision CMNs, the cumulative length of need (the total length of time in months from the initial date of need) is entered.

b. Diagnosis Codes—Listed in the first space is the ICD-9 code that represents the primary reason for ordering this item. Additional ICD-9 codes that would further describe the medical need for the item (up to 3 codes) are also listed. A given CMN may have more than one item billed, and for each item, the primary reason for ordering may be different. For example, a CMN is submitted for a manual wheelchair (K0001) and elevating leg rests (K0195). The primary reason for K0001 is stroke, and the primary reason for K0195 is edema.

c. Question Section—This section is used to gather clinical information regarding the patient's condition, the need for the DME, and supplies.

d. Name of Person Answering Section B Questions—If a clinical professional other than the treating physician (e.g., home health nurse, physical therapist, dietician, or a physician employee) answers the questions in section B, he/she must **print** his/her name, give his/her professional title, and the name of his/her employer, where indicated. If the **treating physician** answered the questions, this space may be left blank.

3. SECTION C:—(This is completed by the supplier.)

a. Narrative Description of Equipment and Cost—The supplier indicates (1) a narrative description of the item(s) ordered, as well as all options, accessories, supplies, and drugs; (2) the supplier's charge for each item, option, accessory, supply, and drug; and (3) the Medicare fee schedule allowance for each item, option, accessory, supply, or drug, if applicable.

4. SECTION D:—(This is completed by the treating physician.)

a. Physician Attestation—The treating physician's signature certifies the CMN that he/she is reviewing includes sections A, B, C, and D, the answers in section B are correct, and the self-identifying information in section A is correct.

b. Physician Signature and Date—After completion and/or review **by the treating physician** of sections A, B, and C, the treating physician must sign and date the CMN in section D, verifying the attestation appearing in this section. The treating physician's signature also certifies the items ordered are medically necessary for this patient. Signature and date stamps are not acceptable.

Certifications and recertifications may not be altered by "whiting out" or "pasting over" and entering new data. Such claims are denied and suppliers that show a pattern of altering CMNs are identified for educational contact and/or audit.

Also suppliers who have questionable utilization or billing practices or who are under sanction are considered for audit.

100.2.2 Evidence of Medical Necessity for Parenteral and Enteral Nutrition (PEN) Therapy (Rev. 1, 10-01-03). B3-3324, B3-4450

—PEN coverage is determined by information provided by the treating physician and the PEN supplier. A completed certification of medical necessity (CMN) must accompany and support initial claims for PEN to establish whether coverage criteria are met and to ensure that the PEN therapy provided is consistent with the attending or ordering physician's prescription. Contractors ensure that the CMN contains pertinent information from the treating physician. Uniform specific medical data facilitate the review and promote consistency in coverage determinations and timelier claims processing.

The medical and prescription information on a PEN CMN can be most appropriately completed by the treating physician or from information in the patient's records by an employee of the physician for the physician's review and signature. Although PEN suppliers sometimes may assist in providing the PEN services, they cannot complete the CMN since they do not have the same access to patient information needed to properly enter medical or prescription information. Contractors use appropriate professional relations issuances, training sessions, and meetings to ensure that all persons and PEN suppliers are aware of this limitation of their role.

When properly completed, the PEN CMN includes the elements of a prescription as well as other data needed to determine whether Medicare coverage is possible. This practice will facilitate prompt delivery of PEN services and timely submittal of the related claim.

100.2.2.1 Scheduling and Documenting Certifications and Recertifications of Medical Necessity for PEN (Rev. 1, 10-01-03).—A certification for PEN therapy must accompany the initial claim submitted. The initial certification is valid for six months. Contractors establish the schedule on a case-by-case basis for recertifying the need for PEN therapy. A change in prescription for a beneficiary past the initial certification period does not restart the certification process.

A period of medical necessity ends when PEN services are not medically required for 2 consecutive months. The entire certification process, if required, begins after 2 consecutive months have elapsed.

A revised certification or a change in prescription may impact on the payment levels of PEN services. A revised certification is appropriate when there is a change:

- In the treating physician's orders in the category of nutrients and/or calories prescribed;
- By more than one liter in the daily volume of parenteral solutions;
- From home-mix to pre-mix or pre-mix to home-mix parenteral solutions;
- From enteral to parenteral or parenteral to enteral therapy; or
- In the method of infusion (e.g., from gravity-fed to pump-fed).

100.2.2.2 Completion of the Elements of PEN CMN (Rev. 1, 10-01-03).—The patient's name, address, and HICN and the nature of the certification (i.e., initial, renewed, or revised) must be entered on all certifications by the supplier, physician, or physician's designated employees. The supplier identifying information is required on all PEN certifications.

All medical and prescription information must be completed from the patient's records by the attending/ordering physician, or an employee of the physician authorized to act on the physician's behalf, and reviewed and signed by the physician.

1. Place of Service.—The CMN must identify the site where the patient is receiving PEN services. A patient may receive services at home, in a nursing home setting (e.g., skilled nursing facility), or another site that must be indicated by the supplier/physician.

2. Patient's General Condition.—The attending physician must complete information about the patient's age, height, and weight. The general condition of the patient also includes an estimated duration of therapy (i.e., in months, years, or for life), the ambulatory status, and whether the patient is conscious. The physician should also indicate food allergies/sensitivities, other medical treatments, therapies, and/or medical conditions that may affect the patient's nutritional needs.

3. Patient's Clinical Assessment.—The attending physician must indicate all the diagnoses related to the PEN therapy and describe the patient's functional impairment of the digestive tract that precludes the enteral patient from swallowing and the parenteral patient from absorbing nutrients. The physician must certify that PEN therapy meets the requirement that a patient is not able to maintain weight and strength due to pathology or nonfunction of the ingestion system and that the enteral therapy serves as the source of nutrition for the patient who has a functioning digestive tract, but whose disability prevents ingestion of sufficient nutrients to the alimentary tract for metabolism. Nutritional supplements for patients capable of ingesting normally, even if required to maintain weight and strength, cannot be covered under the prosthetic device benefit. The physician must have a basis for certifying or recertifying the need for PEN services. The physician is expected to see the patient within 30 days prior to certifying or

recertifying PEN services. However, if the physician did not see the patient, he/she must explain why and describe what other monitoring methods were used to evaluate the patient's PEN needs.

4. Patient's Nutritional Prescription.—Subsequent to an examination of the patient and/or a review of the patient's medical information, the attending physician must complete the patient's nutritional requirements (prescription) to certify the PEN therapy provided.

For the parenteral patient, the CMN must contain the following information:

- The infusion frequency per week,
- The route of administration,
- A reason for the use of pre-mixed parenteral formulas,
- An explanation for the use of special formulas such as hepatic, renal, or stress
- formulas, and
- The amino acid/dextrose formula components of the parenteral solution mix.

Amino acids serve as a source of protein. Adult parenteral nutrition patients generally need 1 to 1.5 grams of protein per day for each kilogram (2.2 pounds) of body weight. Dextrose concentrations less than 10 percent must be explained by the physician. The physician must document the reason for using more than 12 units (@ 500ml per unit) of lipids per month.

Parenteral nutrition may be either "self-mixed" (i.e., the patient is taught to prepare the nutrient solution aseptically) or "premixed" (i.e., the nutrient solution is prepared by trained professionals employed or contracted by the PEN supplier). The attending physician must provide information to justify the reason for "pre-mixed" parenteral nutrient solutions.

Renal dialysis patients sometimes undergo parenteral therapy to replace fluids and nutrients lost during dialysis. Patients are usually infused less than daily and parenteral feeding is often supplemental and, therefore, not covered as a PEN benefit. The renal dialysis patient must meet all the requirements for PEN coverage. The attending physician must document that the patient, despite the need for renal dialysis, suffers from a permanently impaired functional impairment that precludes swallowing or absorption of nutrients.

For the enteral patient, the attending physician must include the following information on the CMN:

- The name of the nutrient product or nutrient category,
- The number of calories per day (100 calories = 1 unit),
- The frequency per day,
- The method of administration (i.e., syringe, gravity, or pump),
- The route of administration (i.e., nasogastric tube, gastrostomy tube, jejunostomy tube, percutaneous enteral gastrostomy tube, or naso-intestinal tube), and
- The reason for the use of a pump.

Categories of enteral nutrition are based on the composition and source of ingredients in each enteral nutrient product. Category IB of enteral nutrients contains products that are natural intact protein/protein isolates commonly known as blenderized nutrients. Additional documentation is required to justify the necessity of Category IB nutrients. The attending physician must provide sufficient information to indicate that the patient:

- Has an intolerance to nutritionally equivalent (semi-synthetic) products;
- Had a severe allergic reaction to a nutritionally equivalent (semi-synthetic) product; or
- Was changed to a blenderized nutrient to alleviate adverse symptoms expected to be of permanent duration with continued use of semi-synthetic products.

Enteral nutrient categories III through VI require additional medical justification for coverage. These categories represent formulas for special needs or use.

- Category III (code B4153): hydrolyzed protein/amino acids. These products contain a high nitrogen availability as a result of chemical treatment to reduce high molecular protein compounds into smaller molecules and amino acids that are easier to digest.

- Category IV (code B4154): defined formulas for special metabolic needs and conditions such as abnormal glucose tolerance, renal disease, liver disease, HIV, respiratory insufficiency, and malnutrition.
- Category V (code B4155): modular components (proteins, carbohydrates, fats).
- Category VI (code B4156): standardized nutrients. These products contain low residue ingredients.

If the patient exhibits a problem with any particular formula in Nutrient Category I (HCPCS B4150) or II (HCPCS B4152), the physician must document the unfavorable events that resulted in prescribing a higher category formula.

Generally, daily enteral intake of 750 to 2,000 calories is considered sufficient to maintain body weight. Patients with medical complications may require an intake outside the range. The attending physician must document the reason for prescribing less than 750 calories per day or more than 2000 calories per day.

Enteral nutrition may be administered by syringe, gravity, or pump. The attending physician must specify the reason that necessitates the use of an enteral feeding pump. Some enteral patients may experience complications associated with syringe or gravity method of administration. Contractors provide coverage for enteral pumps if the medical necessity is documented by the attending physician on the CMN. Examples of circumstances that indicate the need for a pump include, but are not limited to:

- Aspiration or Dumping Syndrome;
- Severe diarrhea remedied by regulated feeding;
- Insulin-dependent diabetics who require a flow rate of less than 100cc's per hour for proper regulation of nutrients;
- Patients with congestive heart failure who require a pump to prevent circulatory overload; or
- Patients with a jejunostomy tube for feeding.

The DMERC reviews the claims to ensure that the equipment for which payment is claimed is consistent with that prescribed (e.g., expect a claim for an I.V. pole, if a pump is used).

5. Attending Physician's Signature and Identification.—A handwritten, original signature and date must be on each certification. The form must be dated to show reasonable association to the dates of active PEN therapy. The full name, address, telephone number (including area code), and Unique Physician Identification Number (UPIN) allows the contractor to determine if the prescriber is authorized to order Medicare services and facilitate claims development.

6. PEN Supplier's Identification.—The PEN supplier's name, address, telephone number, and PEN identification number must be on each certification. This information allows the contractor to determine if the supplier is authorized to provide PEN supplies and facilitate claims development.

100.2.2.3 DMERC Review of Initial PEN Certifications (Rev. 1, 10-01-03). B3-4450—In reviewing the claim and the supporting data on the CMN, the DMERC compares certain items, especially pertinent dates of treatment. For example, the start date of PEN coverage cannot precede the date of physician certification. The estimated duration of therapy must be contained on the CMN. This information is used to verify that the test of permanence is met. Once coverage is established, the estimated length of need at the start of PEN services will determine the recertification schedule.

The information shown on the certification must support the need for PEN supplies as billed. A diagnosis must show a functional impairment that precludes the enteral patient from swallowing and the parenteral patient from absorbing nutrients.

Initial assigned claims with the following conditions are denied without development:

- Inappropriate or missing diagnosis or functional impairment;
- Estimated duration of therapy is less than 90 consecutive days;
- Duration of therapy is not listed;

- Supplies have not been provided;
- Supplies were provided prior to onset date of therapy; and
- Stamped physician's signature.

Unassigned claims are developed for missing or incomplete information.

A. Revised Certifications/Change in Prescription.—A revised certification is required when:

- There is a change in the attending physician's orders in the category of nutrients and/or calories prescribed;
- There is a change by more than one liter in the daily volume of parenteral solutions;
- There is a change from home-mix to pre-mix or pre-mix to home-mix parenteral solutions;
- There is a change from enteral to parenteral or parenteral to enteral therapy; or
- There is a change in the method of infusion (e.g., from gravity-fed to pump-fed).

PEN payments are not adjusted unless a revised or renewed certification documents the necessity for the change. Payment levels for the most current certification or recertification may not be changed unless a prescription change is documented by a new recertification.

The DMERC may adjust the recertification schedule as needed.

5102.3 Transition to Fee Schedule-Relationship to Prior Rules. (100-4, 20-§40.1)

40.1 General (Rev. 1, 10-01-03). B3-5102.2.G, B3-5102.3—Contractors pay for maintenance and servicing of purchased equipment in the following classes:

- inexpensive or frequently purchased,
- customized items, other prosthetic and orthotic devices, and
- capped rental items purchased in accordance with §30.5.2 or §30.5.3.

They do not pay for maintenance and servicing of purchased items that require frequent and substantial servicing, or oxygen equipment. (Maintenance and servicing may be paid for purchased items in these two classes if they were purchased prior to June 1, 1989). Reasonable and necessary charges include only those made for parts and labor that are not otherwise covered under a manufacturer's or supplier's warranty. Contractors pay on a lump-sum, as needed basis based on their individual consideration for each item. Payment may not be made for maintenance and servicing of rented equipment other than maintenance and servicing for PEN pumps (under the conditions of §40.3) or the maintenance and servicing fee established for capped rental items in §40.2.

Servicing of equipment that a beneficiary is purchasing or already owns is covered when necessary to make the equipment serviceable. The service charge may include the use of "loaner" equipment where this is required. If the expense for servicing exceeds the estimated expense of purchasing or renting another item of equipment for the remaining period of medical need, no payment can be made for the amount of the excess. Contractors investigate and deny cases suggesting malicious damage, culpable neglect or wrongful disposition of equipment as discussed in BPM Chapter 15 where they determine that it is unreasonable to make program payment under the circumstances. Such cases are referred to the program integrity specialist in the RO.

5112 PAYMENT TO PSYCHOLOGISTS (100-4, 12-§160.1)

160.1 Payment (Rev. 1, 10-01-03)—Diagnostic testing services are not subject to the outpatient mental health limitation. Refer to §210, below, for a discussion of the outpatient mental health limitation.

The diagnostic testing services performed by a psychologist (who is not a clinical psychologist) practicing independently of an institution, agency, or physician's office are covered as other diagnostic tests if a physician orders such testing. Medicare covers this type of testing as an outpatient service if furnished by any psychologist who is licensed or certified to practice psychology in the State or jurisdiction where he or she is furnishing services or, if the jurisdiction does not issue licenses, if provided by any practicing psychologist. (It is CMS' understanding that all States, the District of Columbia, and Puerto Rico license psychologists, but that some trust territories do not. Examples of psychologists, other than clinical psychologists, whose services are covered under this provision include, but are not limited to, educational psychologists and counseling psychologists.)

To determine whether the diagnostic psychological testing services of a particular independent psychologist are covered under Part B in States which have statutory licensure or certification, carriers must secure from the appropriate State agency a current listing of psychologists holding the required credentials. In States or territories which lack statutory licensing and certification, carriers must check individual qualifications as claims are submitted. Possible reference sources are the national directory of membership of the American Psychological Association, which provides data about the educational background of individuals and indicates which members are board-certified, and records and directories of the State or territorial psychological association. If qualification is dependent on a doctoral degree from a currently accredited program, carriers must verify the date of accreditation of the school involved, since such accreditation is not retroactive. If the reference sources listed above do not provide enough information (e.g., the psychologist is not a member of the association), carriers must contact the psychologist personally for the required information. Carriers may wish to maintain a continuing list of psychologists whose qualifications have been verified.

Medicare excludes expenses for diagnostic testing from the payment limitation on treatment for mental/psychoneurotic/personality disorders.

Carriers must identify the independent psychologist's choice whether or not to accept assignment when performing psychological tests.

Carriers must accept an independent psychologist claim only if the psychologist reports the name/UPIN of the physician who ordered a test.

Carriers pay nonparticipating independent psychologists at 95 percent of the physician fee schedule allowed amount. Carriers pay participating independent psychologists at 100 percent of the physician fee schedule allowed amount.

Independent psychologists are identified on the provider file by specialty code 62 and provider type 35.

5113 PAYMENT TO CLINICAL SOCIAL WORKERS (100-4, 12-§150)

150 CLINICAL SOCIAL WORKER (CSW) SERVICES (Rev. 1, 10-01-03) B3-2152, B3-17000

See Medicare Benefit Policy Manual, Chapter 15, for coverage requirements.

Assignment of benefits is required.

Payment is at 75 percent of the physician fee schedule.

CSWs are identified on the provider file by specialty code 80 and provider type 56.

Medicare applies the outpatient mental health limitation to all covered therapeutic services furnished by qualified CSWs. Refer to §210, below, for a discussion of the outpatient mental health limitation. The modifier "AJ" must be applied on CSN services.

5114 PAYMENT FOR DIAGNOSTIC LABORATORY SERVICES (100.4, 16-§10, 10.2, 50.5.1, 90.1, 90.1.1, 90.2, 100-4, 23-§40)

10.2 General Explanation of Payment (Rev. 1, 10-01-03). B3-5114, HO-437, A3-3628, B3-5114.1, AB-03-076—Outpatient laboratory services can be paid in different ways:

• Physician Fee Schedule;
• Reasonable costs (Critical Access Hospitals (CAH) only);

NOTE: When the CAH bills a 14X bill type as a reference laboratory, the CAH is paid under the laboratory fee schedule.

• Laboratory Fee Schedule;
• Outpatient Prospective Payment System, (OPPS) except for most hospitals in the state of Maryland that are subject to waiver; or
• Reasonable Charge

Annually, CMS distributes a list of codes and indicates the payment method. Carriers and FIs pay as directed by this list. Neither deductible nor coinsurance applies to HCPCS codes paid under the laboratory fee schedule; further, deductible and coinsurance do not apply to HCPCS laboratory codes paid via reasonable cost to CAHs. The majority of outpatient laboratory services are paid under the laboratory fee schedule or the OPPS.

Carriers and FIs are responsible for applying the correct fee schedule for payment of clinical laboratory tests. FIs must determine which hospitals meet the criteria for payment at the 62 percent fee schedule. Only sole community hospitals with qualified hospital laboratories are eligible for payment under the 62 percent fee schedule. Generally, payment for diagnostic laboratory tests that are not subject to the clinical laboratory fee schedule is made in accordance with the reasonable charge or physician fee schedule methodologies (or reasonable costs for CAHs).

For Clinical Diagnostic Laboratory services denied due to frequency edits contractors must use standard health care adjustment reason code 151—"Payment adjusted because the payer deems the information submitted does not support this many services."

50.5.1 Referral Laboratory Services (Rev. 1, 10-01-03). B3-3102, B3-5114—The referring independent laboratory may obtain Medicare reimbursement for medically necessary covered tests if no more than 30 percent of the total annual clinical laboratory tests requested for the referring laboratory are performed by another laboratory.

If the specimen is drawn or received by an independent laboratory approved under the Medicare program and the laboratory performs a covered test but refers the specimen to another laboratory in a different carrier jurisdiction for additional tests, the carrier servicing the referring laboratory retains jurisdiction for services performed by the other laboratory only if it has, in house, the appropriate certification information as well as appropriate fee schedule allowance(s) of the performing laboratory. If the carrier with jurisdiction of the referring laboratory does not have this information, in house, the claims for services performed by other laboratories must be transferred to the carrier servicing the laboratory that performed the service. This rule applies whether or not the referring and reference laboratories are owned and controlled by the same entity or the reference laboratory deals only with other laboratories and not with patients and third party payers. In such cases, the referring independent laboratory must identify the performing laboratory on its bills.

NOTE: In no case should jurisdiction be determined by the location of a nonapproved pickup station.

If the approved independent laboratory that draws or receives the specimen does not perform covered services, but refers the specimen to another independent laboratory in a different carrier jurisdiction, the rules cited above apply.

90.1 Laboratory Tests Utilizing Automated Equipment (Rev. 1, 10-01-03). B3-5114, HO-437, A3-3628—Clinical laboratory tests are covered under Medicare if they are reasonable and necessary for the diagnosis or treatment of an illness or injury. Because of the numerous technological advances and innovations in the clinical laboratory field and the increased availability of automated testing equipment, no distinction is generally made in determining payment for individual tests because of either (1) the sites where the service is performed, or (2) the method of the testing process used, whether manual or automated. Whether the test is actually performed manually or with automated equipment, the services are considered similar and the payment is the same.

However, where groups of tests that are billed individually may be done as a panel or profile, a determination must be made about whether payment should be made at the individual rate or at the panel or profile rate.

90.1.1 Automated Test Listing (Rev. 1, 10-01-03). B3-5114, HO-

437, A3-3628, PMs AB-97-5, AB-97-7, AB-97-17—Profiles are specific groupings of blood chemistries that enable physicians to more accurately diagnose their patients' medical problems. While the component tests in automated profiles may vary somewhat from one laboratory to another, or from one physician's office or clinic to another, in order to develop appropriate payment amounts, contractors group together those profile tests that can be performed at the same time on the same equipment. The carrier or FI must group together the individual tests in the profile when billed separately and consider the price of the related automated profile test. Payment cannot exceed the lower of the profile price or the totals of the prices of all the individual tests. (This rule is applicable also if the tests are done manually.) The profile HCPCS code and each individual test is priced at the lower of the billed charge or the fee amount; and payment is made at the lower of the profile/panel price or the total of the prices for all covered components.

Payment is made only for those tests in an automated profile that meet Medicare coverage rules. Where only some of the tests in a profile of tests are covered, payment cannot exceed the amount that would have been paid if only the covered tests had been ordered. For example, the use of the 12-channel serum chemistry test to determine the blood sugar level in a proven case of diabetes is unreasonable because the results of a blood sugar test performed separately provide the essential information. Normally, the payment allowance for a blood sugar test is lower than the payment allowance for the automated profile of tests. In no event, however, may payment for the covered tests exceed the payment allowance for the profile.

However, the carrier prices and pays the 1-22 automated multi-channel chemistry tests tested in §90.2 at the lowest possible amount in accordance with §90.3.

90.2 Organ or Disease Oriented Panels (Rev. 1, 10-01-03). B3-5114, HO-437, A3-3628—Organ or disease panels must be paid at the lower of the billed charge, the fee amount for the panel, or the sum of the fee amounts for all components. When panels contain one or more automated tests, the carrier determines the correct price for the panel by comparing the price for the automated profile laboratory tests with the sum of the fee amounts for individual tests. Payment for the total panel may not exceed the sum total of the fee amounts for individual covered tests. All Medicare coverage rules apply.

The carrier shared system must calculate the correct payment amount. The CMS furnishes fee prices for each code but the carrier system must compare individual codes billed with codes and prices for related individual tests. (With each HCPCS update, HCPCS codes are reviewed and the system is updated). Once the codes are identified, carriers publish panel codes to providers.

The only acceptable Medicare definition for the component tests included in the CPT codes for organ or disease oriented panels is the American Medical Association (AMA) definition of component tests. The CMS will not pay for the panel code unless all of the tests in the definition are performed. If the laboratory has a custom panel that includes other tests, in addition to those in the defined CPT or HCPCS panels, the additional tests, whether on the list of automated tests or not, are billed separately in addition to the CPT or HCPCS panel code.

NOTE: If a laboratory chooses, it can bill each of the component tests of these panels individually, but payment will be based upon the above rules.

TABLE OF CHEMISTRY PANELS

Chemistry	CPT Code*	Hepatic Function Panel 80076	Basic Metabolic 80048	Comprehensive Metabolic 80053	Renal Function Panel 80069	Lipid* Panel 80061	Electrolyte Panel 80051
Albumin	82040	X		X	X		
Alkaline phosphatase	84075	X		X			
ALT (SGPT)	84460	X		X			
AST (SGOT)	84450	X		X			
Bilirubin, total	82247	X		X			
Bilirubin, direct	82248	X					
Calcium	82310		X	X	X		
Chloride	82435		X	X	X		X
Cholesterol	82465					X	
CK, CPK	82550						
CO2 (bicarbonate)	82374		X	X	X		X
Creatinine	82565		X	X	X		
GGT	82977						
Glucose	82947		X	X	X		
LDH	83615						
Phosphorus	84100				X		
Potassium	84132		X	X	X		X
Protein, total	84155	X		X			
Sodium	84295		X	X	X		X
Triglycerides	84478					X	
Urea nitrogen (BUN)	84520		X	X	X		
Uric Acid	84550						

*CPT only © 2003. *Current Procedural Terminology, 2004, Professional Edition,* American Medical Association. All Rights Reserved.

100.4 Not Otherwise Classified Clinical Laboratory Tests (Rev. 1, 10-01-03).—The following codes for unlisted or not otherwise classified (NOC) clinical laboratory tests are not subject to the NLA:

81099	*87999
84999	88299
85999	89399
86999	

NOC codes shall suspend for review and the carrier shall determine a price for them.

40 CLINICAL DIAGNOSTIC LABORATORY FEE SCHEDULE (Rev. 1, 10-01-03). B3-5114, B3-5114.1, A3-3628, AB-01-162, AB-02-163

The Medicare Claims Processing Manual, Chapter 16, "Laboratory Services From Independent Labs, Physicians, and Providers," provides background and additional information for payment of laboratory services.

Clinical diagnostic laboratory tests—whether performed in a physician's office, by an independent laboratory, or by a hospital laboratory for its outpatients—are paid based on fee schedules. This section sets out rules for use of these schedules.

The fee schedule amounts are adjusted annually to reflect changes in the Consumer Price Index (CPI) for all Urban Consumers (U.S. city average), or as otherwise specified by legislation. Adjustments are applied and amounts are determined by CMS and published for contractor use and also on CMS Web site. Contractors are notified when and where updates are published.

For a cervical or vaginal smear test (pap smear), payment is the lesser of the local fee or the national limitation amount, but not less than the national minimum payment amount. However, in no case may payment for these tests exceed actual charges. The Part B deductible and coinsurance do not apply.

Regardless of whether a diagnostic laboratory test is performed in a physician's office, by an independent laboratory, or by a hospital laboratory for its outpatients or nonpatients, it is considered a laboratory service. When a hospital laboratory performs diagnostic laboratory tests for nonhospital patients, the laboratory is functioning as an independent laboratory.

National minimum limitation amounts are established each year for cervical or vaginal smear clinical laboratory tests. These payment amounts are published each year in Program Memoranda issued by CMS. The affected CPT laboratory test codes for the national minimum payment amount are also identified in the annual Program Memorandum.*

National maximum limitation amounts may also be established for certain services and are also published each year in Program Memoranda issued by CMS.

Carriers and Intermediaries pay the lowest of the applicable current fee schedule, the actual charge, or the NLA. This applies to all clinical diagnostic laboratory tests except:

- Laboratory tests furnished to a hospital inpatient whose stay is covered under Part A;
- Laboratory tests performed by a Skilled Nursing Facility (SNF) for its own SNF inpatients and reimbursed under Part A or Part B and any laboratory tests furnished under arrangements to an SNF inpatient with Part A coverage. (The only covered source for laboratory services furnished under Part A is the SNF itself or a hospital with which the facility has a transfer agreement in effect.);
- Laboratory tests furnished by hospital-based or independent ESRD dialysis facilities that are included under the ESRD composite rate payment;
- Laboratory tests furnished by hospitals in States or areas which have been granted demonstration waivers of Medicare reimbursement principles for outpatient services. The State of Maryland has been granted such demonstration waivers;
- Laboratory tests furnished to inpatients of a hospital with a waiver under §602(k) of the 1983 Amendments to the Act. This section of the Act provides that an outside supplier may bill under Part B

for laboratory and other nonphysician services furnished to inpatients that are otherwise paid only though the hospital;
- Laboratory tests furnished to patients of rural health clinics (RHCs) under an all inclusive rate;
- Laboratory tests provided by a participating health maintenance organization (HMO) or health care prepayment plan (HCPP) to an enrolled member of the plan; and
- Laboratory tests furnished by a hospice.

40.1 Access to Clinical Diagnostic Lab Fee Schedule Files (Rev. 1, 10-01-03). AB-01-162—The annual laboratory fee schedule data file should be retrieved electronically through CMS' mainframe telecommunications system, formerly referred to as the National Data Mover.

For each test code, if the contractor's system retains only the pricing amount, they should load the data from the field named "60% Pricing Amt." For each test code, if the contractor's system has been developed to retain the local fee and the NLA, they may load the data from the fields named "60% Local Fee Amt" and "60% Natl Limit Amt" to use to determine payment. For clinical laboratory test codes for cervical or vaginal smear tests (listed in Chapter 16, "Laboratory Services from Independent Labs, Physicians, and Providers," §80.3) load the data from the field named "60% Pricing Amt" to reflect the lower of the local fee or the NLA, but not less than the national minimum payment amount. The fields named "62% Local Fee Amt," "62% Natl Limit Amt," and "62% Pricing Amt" should be used by intermediaries for payment of clinical laboratory tests performed by a sole community hospital's qualified laboratory.

The 3-month grace period for deleted codes is defined in the above in §20.4 and begins January 1.

Internet access to annual laboratory fee schedule data is available at the following CMS Web address: http://www.cms.hhs.gov/clia/clsites.asp or http://www.cms.hhs.gov/paymentsystems/. It is available in multiple formats: Excel, text, and comma delimited.

40.2 Carrier Record Layout for Clinical Laboratory Fee Schedule (Rev. 1, 10-01-03). PM AB-01-162, AB-02-163—The instructions for each annual update contain the actual data set name for that year. The Data Set Name is included with each annual update instructions.

Data Element Name	Picture	Location	Comment
HCPCS Code	X(05)	1–5	
Carrier Number	X(05)	6–10	
Locality	X(02)	11–12	00 = Denotes Single Carrier State
			01 = North Dakota
			02 = South Dakota
			20 = Puerto Rico
			40 = New Hampshire
			50 = Vermont
60% Local Fee	9(05)V99	13–19	
62% Local Fee	9(05)V99	20–26	
60% Natl Limit Amt	9(05)V99	27–33	
62% Natl Limit Amt	9(05)V99	34–40	
60% Pricing Amt	9(05)V99	41–47	
62% Pricing Amt	9(05)V99	48–54	
Gap-Fill Indicator	X(01)	55–55	0 = No Gap-fill Required
			1 = Carrier Gap-fill
			2 = Special Instructions Apply
Modifier	X(02)	56–57	Where modifier is shown, QW denotes a CLIA waive test.
Filler	X(03)	58–60	

40.3 Intermediary and Regional Home Health Intermediary (RHHI) Record Layout for Clinical Laboratory Fee Schedule (Rev. 1, 10-01-03). PM AB-01-162, A-01-104, AB-02-163—The instructions for each annual update contain the actual file name for

---

*CPT only © 2003. *Current Procedural Terminology, 2004, Professional Edition,* American Medical Association. All Rights Reserved.

that year. The Data Set Name is included with each annual update instructions.

Record Length = 60
Record Format = FB
Block Size = 6000
Character Code = EDBCIC
Sort Sequence = Carrier, Locality, HCPCS Code

Header Record

Data Element Name	Picture	Location	Comment
Label	X(03)	1–3	Value = Lab
Filler	X(07)	4–10	
Filler	X(08)	11–15	
Filler	X(04)	16–22	
Date Fee Update	X(08)	23–30	YYYYMMDD
Filler	X(22)	31–52	
Date File Created	X(08)	53–60	YYYYMMDD

Data Record

Data Element Name	Picture	Location	Comment
HCPCS	X(05)	1–5	
Filler	X(04)	6–9	
60% Pricing Amt	9(05)V99	10–16	
62% Pricing Amt	9(05)V99	17–23	
Filler	X(07)	24–30	
Carrier Number	X(05)	31–35	
Locality	X(02)	36–37	00 = Denotes Single State Carrier
			01 = North Dakota
			02 = South Dakota
			20 = Puerto Rico
			40 = New Hampshire
			50 = Vermont
Filler	X(23)	38–60	

40.4 Gap-Filled Fees Submitted to CMS by Carriers (Rev. 1, 10-01-03). AB-01-162, AB-02-163—In accordance with §531(b) of the Benefits Improvement and Protection Act of 2000 (BIPA), CMS solicits public comments on determining payment amounts for new laboratory tests. The CMS hosts an annual public meeting to allow parties the opportunity to provide input to the payment determination process. The CMS employs one of two approaches to establishing payment amounts for new laboratory test codes, crosswalking and gap-filling. After considering public input regarding the new test codes, CMS determines which approach is most appropriate for each new test code.

If the new test is comparable to an existing test, the new test is "crosswalked" to the existing test, and it is assigned the local fee for the existing test and the corresponding NLA. The new test code and payment amounts are included in the updated laboratory fee schedule annually.

If CMS determines that the laboratory fee schedule includes no sufficiently comparable test to permit crosswalking, CMS instructs carriers to "gap-fill" the payment amount for the new test code. Gap-filling is an empirical process of determining a payment amount in a locality using available information sources. Usually the period during which gap-filled payment amounts are instructed is the year following the introduction of a new code. During this period, carriers establish and use these payment amounts; they may be revised in the course of the year. Also during this period, carriers must report the gap-fill amounts to their ROs which are then forwarded to CMS CO. The CMS considers the gap-fill amounts and uses them to establish the fees for the new test code in the next update of the laboratory fee schedule.

In determining gap-fill amounts, the sources of information carriers should examine, if available, include: charges for the test and routine discounts to charges; resources required to perform the test; payment amounts determined by other payers; and charges, payment amounts, and resources required for other tests that may be comparable or otherwise relevant. Carriers may consider

other sources of information as appropriate, including clinical studies and information provided by clinicians practicing in the area, manufacturers, or other interested parties. To assist each carrier in establishing a gap-fill amount, carriers' Medical Directors may meet and share information regarding the new test, though without reaching a formal consensus.

Establishing payment amounts for new laboratory tests is inherently difficult, precisely because these tests are new and as a result the types and extent of information available about them may be limited. Because the circumstances of different tests may vary significantly, specifying in detail a method of using the various information sources outlined above does not appear appropriate at this time. However, CMS designates a new test code for gap-filling in instances where no test code seems sufficiently similar to make a crosswalk approach appropriate. Accordingly, carriers should not determine a gap-fill amount by crosswalking to the payment amount for another test code.

After determining a gap-fill amount, a carrier may consider if a least costly alternative to a new test exists. If a carrier determines a least costly alternative test exists, the carrier may adopt the payment amount of the least costly alternative test as the gap-fill amount for the new test code. The least costly alternative amount will be considered the local fee, and CMS will use this payment amount in establishing the NLA. However in this case, the carrier must report two payment amounts, the gap-fill amount prior to determination of a least costly alternative and the payment amount that the carrier has determined to be the least costly alternative.

Carriers should also communicate the gap-fill amounts to corresponding intermediaries. Carriers can seek assistance from RO staff to facilitate communication of the gap-fill amounts to intermediaries. The list of codes which carriers are required to gap-fill each year are communicated in the annual instructions.

Carriers provide their RO with gap-fill fees according to the date communicated by CMS (usually May), to be used by CMS-Central for the development of subsequent or later laboratory fee schedules. Carriers submit the gap-fill fees in a right-justified format. These gap-fill data should be transmitted in an ASCII file with the following file specifications to MStevenson@cms.hhs.gov with a copy to Agreenberg@cms.hhs.gov to assist with coordinated collection of the gap-fill fees.

Data Set Name: CLXXXXX.TXT*   (ASCII File)
(*Denotes carrier 5 - digit number)

Gap-filled Fees Record Layout

Data Element Name	Picture	Location	Comment
Year	X(4)	1–4	Set to Year (e.g., 2003)
HCPCS Code	X(5)	5–9	
Modifier	X(2)	10–11	
Carrier Number	X(5)	12–16	
Locality	X(2)	17–18	00 = Denotes Single State Carrier
			01 = North Dakota
			02 = South Dakota
			20 = Puerto Rico
			40 = New Hampshire
			50 = Vermont
Gap-fill Amount	9(5)V99	19–25	Prior to any determination of a least costly alternative
Least Costly Alternative Amount	9(5)V99	26–32	
Least Costly Alternative Code	X(5)	33–37	

40.4.1 Carriers Forward HCPCS Gap Fill Amounts to Fiscal Intermediaries (Rev. 1, 10-01-03). CMS Memo 9-13-02 HCPCS Gap-fillR3.doc—Any carrier that establishes a HCPCS gap fill payment rate for its own use, or at the request of an FI, must forward the information to the contacts at all FIs/RHHIs with providers in the carrier service area.

Carriers that establish HCPCS gap-fill payment rates for their own needs should forward the information to FI/RHHIs as soon as practicable. FIs are to contact the appropriate carrier to request a gap fill payment rate with 5 working days of the suspension of claims containing HCPCS codes(s) for which payment rate is needed and has not been forwarded. Carriers must provide the payment rate to the requesting FI/RHHI (and all other FI/RHHIs with providers in that common jurisdiction) within 10 working days of receipt of the request.

Requests for policy clarification in carrier establishing the HCPCS gap fill payment rates or FI/RHHI procedures for the use thereof should be directed to the respective Regional Office HCPCS business function experts (BFE). Examples of the need for FI consultation with the BRE are coverage questions and receipt of unresolved significant inconsistencies in fee amounts from different carriers for the same HCPCS. The FI should consult the carriers with disparate fees before contacting the BFE.

An intermediary experiencing delay in replies or nonresponses from a carrier should alert it respective Consortium Contractor Management Staff (CCMS) Contract Manager (CM). The CM will coordinate with his/her counterpart assigned to the carrier to achieve more timely action by the carrier.

It is the FI's responsibility to ascertain the amount or consult with the carrier, CCMS-CM, or BFE timely. Intermediary requests to apply CC 15 to claims which are paid untimely solely because of a delay in ascertaining a HCPCS gap fill amount from the carrier should be addressed to the respective CM. The CM will contact the HCPCS BFE for a decision. Requests for application of CC 15 to claims for which the FI did not request the gap fill payment rate within 5 working days of the claim suspension and/or did not seek timely advice from the RO BFE concerning application of gap fill amount will not be honored. Additionally, if the carrier replied at least five days before the expiration of the payment floor, CC 15 requests will **not** be honored.

5114.1 Payment for Outpatient Clinical Diagnostic Laboratory Tests Using Fee Schedules and for Specimen Collection. (100-4, 16-§10.2, 20, 20.1, 30.1, 30.2, 30.3, 40.1, 40.4, 40.7, 50.1, 60, 60.1, 60.1.1, 60.2, 80.4, 100, 110, 23-§40)

10.2 General Explanation of Payment (Rev. 1, 10-01-03). B3-5114, HO-437, A3-3628, B3-5114.1, AB-03-076—Outpatient laboratory services can be paid in different ways:

- Physician Fee Schedule;
- Reasonable costs (Critical Access Hospitals (CAH) only);

NOTE: When the CAH bills a 14X bill type as a reference laboratory, the CAH is paid under the laboratory fee schedule.

- Laboratory Fee Schedule;
- Outpatient Prospective Payment System, (OPPS) except for most hospitals in the state of Maryland that are subject to waiver; or
- Reasonable Charge

Annually, CMS distributes a list of codes and indicates the payment method. Carriers and FIs pay as directed by this list. Neither deductible nor coinsurance applies to HCPCS codes paid under the laboratory fee schedule; further, deductible and coinsurance do not apply to HCPCS laboratory codes paid via reasonable cost to CAHs. The majority of outpatient laboratory services are paid under the laboratory fee schedule or the OPPS.

Carriers and FIs are responsible for applying the correct fee schedule for payment of clinical laboratory tests. FIs must determine which hospitals meet the criteria for payment at the 62 percent fee schedule. Only sole community hospitals with qualified hospital laboratories are eligible for payment under the 62 percent fee schedule. Generally, payment for diagnostic laboratory tests that are not subject to the clinical laboratory fee schedule is made in accordance with the reasonable charge or physician fee schedule methodologies (or reasonable costs for CAHs).

For Clinical Diagnostic Laboratory services denied due to frequency edits contractors must use standard health care adjustment reason code 151—"Payment adjusted because the payer deems the information submitted does not support this many services."

20 CALCULATION OF PAYMENT RATES—CLINICAL LABORATORY TEST FEE SCHEDULES (Rev. 1, 10-01-03) HO-437, A3-3628, PM AB-98-7, B3-5114.1

Under Part B, for services rendered on or after July 1, 1984, clinical laboratory tests performed in a physician's office, by an independent laboratory, or by a hospital laboratory for its outpatients are reimbursed on the basis of fee schedules. Current exceptions to this rule are CAH laboratory services as described in §10, and services provided by hospitals in the State of Maryland.

Medicare pays the lesser of:

- Actual charges;
- The fee schedule amount for the State or a local geographic area; or
- A national limitation amount (NLA) for the HCPCS code as provided by §1834(h) of the Act.

Annually, CMS furnishes to carriers and FIs the proper amount to pay for each HCPCS code for each local geographic area. This includes a calculation of whether a national limitation amount or the local fee schedule amount is to be used.

This information is available to the public on the CMS Web site in public use files.

20.1 Initial Development of Laboratory Fee Schedules (Rev. 1, 10-01-03). HO-437, A3-3628, B3-5114.1.C—Initially, each carrier established the fee schedules on a carrier-wide basis (not to exceed a statewide basis). If a carrier's area includes more than one State, the carrier established a separate fee schedule for each State. The carrier determined the fee schedule amount based on prevailing charges for laboratory billings by physicians and independent laboratories billing the carrier. Carriers set the fees at 60 percent of prevailing charges. FIs used the same fee schedules to pay outpatient hospital laboratory services. They set the fee at 62 percent of carrier prevailing charges. Subsequently, except for sole community hospitals, which continue to be paid at the 62 percent rate, FIs changed payments to hospital laboratories to the "60 percent fee schedule."

In 1994, CMS took over the annual update and distribution of clinical laboratory fee schedules. The CMS updates the fee schedule amounts annually to reflect changes in the Consumer Price Index (CPI) for all Urban Consumers (U.S. city average), or as otherwise specified by legislation.

Effective for hospital outpatient tests furnished by a hospital on or after April 1, 1988, to receive the 62 percent fee the hospital must be a sole community hospital. Otherwise, the fee is the "60 percent fee schedule." If a hospital is uncertain whether it meets the qualifications of a sole community hospital it can seek assistance from the FI or the RO.

For tests to hospital nonpatients, the fee is 60 percent of the carrier prevailing charge. If a hospital laboratory acts as an independent laboratory, i.e., performs tests for persons who are nonhospital patients; or if the hospital laboratory is not a qualified hospital laboratory, the services are reimbursed using the 60 percent fee schedule or the adjusted fee schedule, as appropriate.

See §10.1 for the definition of a hospital outpatient.

30.1 Mandatory Assignment for Laboratory Tests (Rev. 1, 10-01-03). B3-5114.1—Unless a laboratory, physician, or medical group accepts assignment, the carrier makes no Part B payment for laboratory tests paid on the laboratory fee schedule. Laboratories, physicians, or medical groups that have entered into a participation agreement must accept assignment. Sanctions of double the violation charges, civil money penalties (up to $2,000 per violation), and/or exclusion from the program for a period of up to five years may be imposed on physicians and laboratories, with the exception of rural health clinic laboratories, that knowingly, willfully, and repeatedly bill patients on an unassigned basis. However, sole community physicians and physicians who are the sole source of an essential specialty in a community are not excluded from the program. Whenever a carrier is notified of a sanction action for this reason, the carrier does not pay for any laboratory services unless the services were furnished within 15 days after the date on the exclusion or suspension notice to the practitioner, and:

- It is the first claim filed for services rendered to that beneficiary after the date on the notice of suspension or exclusion; or
- It is filed with respect to services furnished within 15 days of the date on the first notice of denial of claims to the beneficiary. (Fifteen days are allowed for the notice to reach the beneficiary.)

Carriers refer questions on payment procedures to the Sanctions Coordinator in the RO.

Carriers process laboratory claims inadvertently submitted as unassigned as if they were assigned. (See §50.)

For purposes of this section, the term assignment includes assignment in the strict sense of the term as well as the procedure under which payment is made, after the death of the beneficiary, to the person or entity that furnished the service, on the basis of that person's or entity's agreement to accept the Medicare payment as the full charge or fee for the service.

30.2 Deductible and Coinsurance Application for Laboratory Tests (Rev. 1, 10-01-03). B3-2462, B3-5114.1, A3-3215, HHA-160— Neither the annual cash deductible nor the 20 percent coinsurance apply to:

- Clinical laboratory tests performed by a physician, laboratory, or other entity paid on an assigned basis;
- Specimen collection fees; or
- Travel allowance related to laboratory tests (e.g., collecting specimen).

Codes on the physician fee schedule are generally subject to the Part B deductible and coinsurance, although exceptions may be noted for a given code in the MPFS or through formal Medicare instructions such as temporary instructions and requirements for specific services noted in this manual.

Any laboratory code paid at reasonable charge is subject to the Part B deductible and coinsurance, unless otherwise specified in the description of coverage and payment rules.

Neither deductible nor coinsurance is applied to payment for codes on the laboratory fee schedule that are made to CAHs.

30.3 Method of Payment for Clinical Laboratory Tests—Place of Service Variation (Rev. 1, 10-01-03). HO-437, A3-3628, B3-5114.1, PM A-01-31— The following apply in determining the amount of Part B payment for clinical laboratory tests, including those furnished under method II for ESRD beneficiaries:

Independent laboratory or a physician or medical group— Payment to an independent laboratory or a physician or medical group is the lesser of the actual charge, the fee schedule amount or the national limitation amount. Part B deductible and coinsurance do not apply.

Reference laboratory— For tests performed by a reference laboratory, the payment is the lesser of the actual charge by the billing laboratory, the fee schedule amount, or the national limitation amount. (See §50.5 for carrier jurisdiction details.) Part B deductible and coinsurance do not apply.

Outpatient or a nonpatient of the hospital— Payment to a hospital for tests furnished for an outpatient or a nonpatient of the hospital is the lesser of the actual charge, the 60 percent fee schedule amount, or the 60 percent NLA. Part B deductible and coinsurance do not apply.

Inpatient without Part A— Payment to a hospital for tests performed for an inpatient without Part A coverage is made on a reasonable cost basis and is subject to Part B deductible and coinsurance. Payment to a SNF inpatient without Part A coverage is made under the laboratory fee schedule.

Inpatient or SNF patient with Part A— Payment to a hospital for laboratory tests furnished to an inpatient whose stay is covered under Part A, is included in the PPS rate for PPS facilities or is made on a reasonable cost basis for non-PPS hospitals. Payment for lab services for beneficiaries in a Part A stay in a SNF, other than a swing bed in a CAH are included in the SNF PPS rate. For

such services provided in a swing bed CAH, payment is made on a reasonable cost basis.

Sole community hospital— Payment to a sole community hospital for tests furnished for an outpatient of that hospital, is the least of the actual charge, the 62 percent fee schedule amount, or the 62 percent NLA. The Part B deductible and coinsurance do not apply.

Waived Hospitals— Payment to a hospital which has been granted a waiver of Medicare payment principles for outpatient services is subject to Part B deductible and coinsurance unless otherwise waived as part of an approved waiver. Specifically, laboratory fee schedules do not apply to laboratory tests furnished by hospitals in States or areas that have been granted demonstration waivers of Medicare reimbursement principles for outpatient services. The State of Maryland has been granted such demonstration waivers. This also may apply to hospitals in States granted approval for alternative payment methods for paying for hospital outpatient services under §1886(c) of the Act.

Critical Access Hospital— For a CAH being reimbursed under the "Standard Method" of reimbursement (See Chapter 4), payment for clinical laboratory services furnished as an outpatient service is made on a reasonable cost basis. Critical Access Hospitals choosing the "Standard Method" are paid under the fee schedule for services when they function as a reference laboratory (bill type 14X).

CAHs choosing the "Optional Method" of reimbursement (see Chapter 4) are reimbursed at reasonable cost for non-professional clinical laboratory services and at 115 percent of the fee schedule for professional clinical laboratory services.

Beneficiaries are not liable for any coinsurance, deductible, co-payment, or other cost sharing amount with respect to CAH clinical laboratory services.

Dialysis facility— Payment to a hospital-based or independent dialysis facility for laboratory tests included under the ESRD composite rate payment and performed for a patient of that facility, is included in the facility's composite rate payment for these tests and is subject to the Part B deductible and coinsurance. Laboratory tests that are not included under the ESRD composite rate payment; and are performed by an independent laboratory or a provider-based laboratory for dialysis patients of independent dialysis facilities or provider based facilities; are paid in addition to the composite rate payment and are subject to the fee schedule limits. This also applies to all laboratory tests furnished to home dialysis patients who have selected Payment Method II. These limits are 60 percent for all tests unless performed by a qualified hospital laboratory in a sole community hospital; in which case the 62 percent rate applies. The laboratory performing the tests must bill.

Rural health clinic— Payment to a rural health clinic (RHC) for laboratory tests performed for a patient of that clinic is not included in the all-inclusive rate and may be billed separately by the laboratory (including a laboratory that is part of a hospital that hosts a hospital based RHC). Payment for the laboratory service is not subject to Part B deductible and coinsurance. (See §40.4 for details on RHC billing.)

Enrolled in Managed Care— Payment to a participating health maintenance organization (HMO) or health care prepayment plan (HCPP) for laboratory tests provided to a Medicare beneficiary who is an enrolled member is included in the monthly capitation amount.

Nonenrolled Managed Care— Payment to a participating HMO or HCPP for laboratory tests performed for a patient who is not a member is the lesser of the actual charge, or the fee schedule, or the NLA. The Part B deductible and coinsurance do not apply.

Hospice— Payment to a hospice for laboratory tests performed by the hospice is included in the hospice rate.

40.1 Laboratories Billing for Referred Tests (Rev. 1, 10-01-03). B3-5114.1.E— Section 1833(h) (5) of the Act provides that a referring laboratory may bill for tests for Medicare beneficiaries performed on or after May 1, 1990, by a reference laboratory only if the referring laboratory meets certain exceptions. In the case of a test performed at the request of a laboratory by another laboratory, payment may be made to the referring laboratory but only if one of the following three exceptions is met:

- The referring laboratory is located in, or is part of, a rural hospital;
- One of the following relationships exists between the referring laboratory and the entity performing the tests:
  - The referring laboratory is wholly owned by the entity performing such test;
  - the referring laboratory wholly owns the entity performing such test; or
  - both the referring laboratory and the entity performing such test are wholly-owned by a third entity (collectively, a related referring laboratory); or
- Not more than 30 percent of the clinical laboratory tests for which a nonrelated referring laboratory receives requests for testing during the year in which the test are performed by another laboratory.

In the case of a clinical laboratory test provided under an arrangement (as defined in §1861(w)(1)) made by a hospital, CAH or SNF, payment is made to the hospital or SNF.

Examples of 30 Percent Exception:

1. A laboratory receives requests for 200 tests, performs 139 tests, and refers 61 tests to a nonrelated laboratory.

All tests referred to a non-related laboratory are counted. Thus, 30.5 percent (61/200) of the tests are considered tests referred to a non-related laboratory and, since this exceeds the 30 percent standard, the referring laboratory may not bill for any Medicare beneficiary laboratory tests referred to a non-related laboratory.

2. A laboratory receives requests for 200 tests, performs 139 tests and refers 15 to a related laboratory and 46 to a nonrelated laboratory. Only 23 percent of the tests were referred to nonrelated laboratories. Since this is less than 30 percent, the referring laboratory may bill for all tests.

NOTE: This provision of §6111(b) of OBRA of 1989 has no effect on hospitals that are paid under §1833(h)(5)(A)(iii).

NOTE: Laboratory services provided to a SNF inpatient under Part A are billed by the SNF, not the laboratory, due to consolidated billing for SNFs.

40.7 Billing for Noncovered Clinical Laboratory Tests (Rev. 1, 10-01-03). B3-5114.1—Ordinarily, neither a physician nor a laboratory bills the Medicare Program for noncovered tests. However, if the beneficiary (or his/her representative) contends that a clinical laboratory test which a physician or laboratory believes is noncovered may be covered, the physician or laboratory must file a claim that includes the test to effectuate the beneficiary's right to a Medicare determination. The physician or laboratory annotates the claim that he/she believes that the test is noncovered and is submitting it at the beneficiary's insistence. Before furnishing a beneficiary a test which the physician or laboratory believes is excluded from coverage as not reasonable and necessary (rather than excluded from coverage as part of a routine physical checkup), the physician or laboratory must obtain a signed Advanced Beneficiary Notice (ABN) from the beneficiary (or representative) that the physician or laboratory has informed him/her of the noncoverage of the test and that there will be a charge for the test. This protects the physician or laboratory against possible liability for the test under the limitation of liability provision.

See Chapter 30, regarding Advance Beneficiary Notices (ABN) and demand bills.

50.1 Referring Laboratories (Rev. 1, 10-01-03). B3-5114.1—Effective with services rendered on or after January 1, 1991, carriers deny bills from a referring laboratory for tests performed by a reference laboratory unless the carrier is informed in writing by the referring laboratory that the referring laboratory meets one of the exception criteria in §40.1.

If it is later found that a referring laboratory does not, in fact, meet an exception criterion, the carrier should recoup payment for the referred tests improperly billed. If, after carrier notification, the referring laboratory persists in not identifying the laboratory to which the test(s) were referred, the carrier advises the RO. The RO takes whatever action is necessary to correct the problem.

60 SPECIMEN COLLECTION FEE AND TRAVEL ALLOWANCE (Rev. 1, 10-01-03) B3-5114.1

60.1 Specimen Collection Fee (Rev. 1, 10-01-03). B3-5114.1, A3-3628—In addition to the amounts provided under the fee schedules, the Secretary shall provide for and establish a nominal fee to cover the appropriate costs of collecting the sample on which a clinical laboratory test was performed and for which payment is made with respect to samples collected in the same encounter.

A specimen collection fee is allowed in circumstances such as drawing a blood sample through venipuncture (i.e., inserting into a vein a needle with syringe or vacutainer to draw the specimen) or collecting a urine sample by catheterization. A specimen collection fee is not allowed for blood samples where the cost of collecting the specimen is minimal (such as a throat culture or a routine capillary puncture for clotting or bleeding time). This fee will not be paid to anyone who has not extracted the specimen. Only one collection fee is allowed for each type of specimen for each patient encounter, regardless of the number of specimens drawn. When a series of specimens is required to complete a single test (e.g., glucose tolerance test), the series is treated as a single encounter.

60.1.1 Physician Specimen Drawing (Rev. 1, 10-01-03). HO-437, A3-3628, B3-5114.1—Medicare allows a specimen collection fee for physicians only when (1) it is the accepted and prevailing practice among physicians in the locality to make separate charges for drawing or collecting a specimen, and (2) it is the customary practice of the physician performing such services to bill separate charges for drawing or collecting the specimen.

60.2 Travel Allowance (Rev. 1, 10-01-03). HO-437, A3-3628.F, B3-5114.1K; PM-AB-99-49—In addition to a specimen collection fee allowed under §60.1, Medicare, under Part B, covers a specimen collection fee and travel allowance for a laboratory technician to draw a specimen from either a nursing home patient or homebound patient under §1833(h)(3) of the Act and payment is made based on the clinical laboratory fee schedule. The travel allowance is intended to cover the estimated travel costs of collecting a specimen and to reflect the technician's salary and travel costs.

The additional allowance can be made only where a specimen collection fee is also payable, i.e., no travel allowance is made where the technician merely performs a messenger service to pick up a specimen drawn by a physician or nursing home personnel. The travel allowance may not be paid to a physician unless the trip to the home, or to the nursing home was solely for the purpose of drawing a specimen. Otherwise travel costs are considered to be associated with the other purposes of the trip.

The travel allowance is not distributed by CMS. Instead, the carrier must calculate the travel allowance for each claim using the following rules for the particular Code. The following HCPCS codes are used for travel allowances:

Per Mile Travel Allowance (P9603)

- The minimum "per mile travel allowance" is 75 cents. The per mile travel allowance is to be used in situations where the average trip to patients' homes is longer than 20 miles round trip, and is to be pro-rated in situations where specimens are drawn or picked up from non-Medicare patients in the same trip.—one way, in connection with medically necessary laboratory specimen collection drawn from homebound or nursing home bound patient; prorated miles actually traveled (carrier allowance on per mile basis); or
- The per mile allowance was computed using the Federal mileage rate plus an additional 44 cents a mile to cover the technician's time and travel costs. Contractors have the option of

establishing a higher per mile rate in excess of the minimum (75 cents a mile in cy 2000) if local conditions warrant it. The minimum mileage rate will be reviewed and updated in conjunction with the clinical lab fee schedule as needed. At no time will the laboratory be allowed to bill for more miles than are reasonable or for miles not actually traveled by the laboratory technician.

Example 1: In CY 2000, a laboratory technician travels 60 miles round trip from a lab in a city to a remote rural location, and back to the lab to draw a single Medicare patient's blood. The total reimbursement would be $45.00 (60 miles x .75 cents a mile), plus the specimen collection fee of $3.00.

Example 2: In CY 2000, a laboratory technician travels 40 miles from the lab to a Medicare patient's home to draw blood, and then travels an additional 10 miles to a non-Medicare patient's home and then travels 30 miles to return to the lab. The total miles traveled would be 80 miles. The claim submitted would be for one half of the miles traveled or $30.00 (40 $\times$ .75), plus specimen collection fee of $3.00.

Flat Rate (P9604)

The CMS will pay a minimum of $7.50 one way flat rate travel allowance. The flat rate travel allowance is to be used in areas where average trips are less than 20 miles round trip. The flat rate travel fee is to be pro-rated for more than one blood drawn at the same address, and for stops at the homes of Medicare and non-Medicare patients. The laboratory does the pro-ration when the claim is submitted based on the number of patients seen on that trip. The specimen collection fee will be paid for each patient encounter.

This rate is based on an assumption that a trip is an average of 15 minutes and up to 10 miles one way. It uses the Federal mileage rate and a laboratory technician's time of $17.66 an hour, including overhead. Contractors have the option of establishing a flat rate in excess of the minimum of $7.50, if local conditions warrant it. The minimum national flat rate will be reviewed and updated in conjunction with the clinical laboratory fee schedule, as necessitated by adjustments in the Federal travel allowance and salaries.

The claimant identifies round trip travel by use of the LR modifier

Example 3: A laboratory technician travels from the laboratory to a single Medicare patient's home and returns to the laboratory without making any other stops. The flat rate would be calculated as follows: 2 $\times$ $7.50 for a total trip reimbursement of $15.00, plus the specimen collection fee.

Example 4: A laboratory technician travels from the laboratory to the homes of five patients to draw blood, four of the patients are Medicare patients and one is not. An additional flat rate would be charged to cover the 5 stops and the return trip to the lab (6 $\times$ $7.50 = $45.00). Each of the claims submitted would be for $9.00 ($45.00/5 = $9.00). Since one of the patients is non-Medicare, four claims would be submitted for $9.00 each, plus the specimen collection fee for each.

Example 5: A laboratory technician travels from a laboratory to a nursing home and draws blood from 5 patients and returns to the laboratory. Four of the patients are on Medicare and one is not. The $7.50 flat rate is multiplied by two to cover the return trip to the laboratory (2 $\times$ $7.50 = $15.00) and then divided by five (1/5 of $15.00 = $3.00). Since one of the patients is non-Medicare, four claims would be submitted for $3.00 each, plus the specimen collection fee.

If a carrier determines that it results in equitable payment, the carrier may extend the former payment allowances for additional travel (such as to a distant rural nursing home) to all circumstances where travel is required. This might be appropriate, for example, if the carrier's former payment allowance was on a per mile basis. Otherwise, it should establish an appropriate allowance and inform the suppliers in its service area. If a carrier decides to establish a new allowance, one method is to consider developing a travel allowance consisting of:

• The current Federal mileage allowance for operating personal automobiles, plus a personnel allowance per mile to cover personnel costs based upon an estimate of average hourly wages and average driving speed.

Carriers must prorate travel allowance amounts claimed by suppliers by the number of patients (including Medicare and non-Medicare patients) from whom specimens were drawn on a given trip.

The carrier may determine that payment in addition to the routine travel allowance determined under this section is appropriate if:

• the patient from whom the specimen must be collected is in a nursing home or is homebound; and
• the clinical laboratory tests are needed on an emergency basis outside the general business hours of the laboratory making the collection.

80.4 Oximetry (Rev. 1, 10-01-03). B3-5114.1—Certain blood gas levels are determined either by invasive means through use of a blood specimen for a clinical laboratory test or by noninvasive means through ear or pulse oximetry, which is not considered a clinical laboratory test. CPT code 82792 is used for invasive oximetry. HCPCS code M0592 is used for ear and pulse oximetry. Code M0592 is not subject to fee schedules.

100 CPT CODES SUBJECT TO AND NOT SUBJECT TO THE CLINICAL LABORATORY FEE SCHEDULE (Rev. 1, 10-01-03) HO-437, A3-3628, B3-5114.1

For fee schedule purposes, clinical laboratory services include most laboratory tests listed in codes 80048-89399 of CPT-1996. The CMS issues an update to the laboratory fee schedule each year, with information about whether prices have been determined by CMS or whether the individual carrier must determine the allowable charge.

Codes not included are not paid under the laboratory fee schedule but may be paid under the MPFS if covered for Medicare.

110 COORDINATION BETWEEN CARRIERS AND OTHER ENTITIES (Rev. 1, 10-01-03) B3-5114.1

110.1 Coordination Between Carriers and FIs/RRB (Rev. 1, 10-01-03).—The carrier furnishes copies of fees that are locally established under the fee schedules (price code = 22) to Medicare FIs and to the appropriate RRB carrier. The carrier must provide updates at least 30 days prior to the carrier's scheduled implementation of the update. The FIs add these fees to system fee schedule tables to use in paying for hospital laboratory tests performed for both outpatients of the hospital and persons who are not patients of the hospital. The RRB contractor uses the fee schedules in paying for outpatient clinical laboratory tests.

FIs and the RRB may consult with carriers on filling gaps in fee schedules for tests where the carrier may not have established an amount. If an FI or the RRB carrier has bills for payment on laboratory tests for which the carrier has not furnished amounts, it consults with the area carrier. If necessary the area carrier consults with other nearby carriers.

110.2 Coordination With Medicaid (Rev. 1, 10-01-03).—Carriers furnish copies of the fee schedules and the annual update (including NLAs where applicable) to State agencies (SAs). Carriers provide updates to SAs at least 30 days prior to the scheduled implementation. To obtain Federal matching funds for clinical laboratory services, State Medicaid agencies may not pay more than Medicare pays for the services and specimen collections.

Since the fee schedule provisions were implemented on a carrier wide basis, a State may have more than one carrier servicing Medicare beneficiaries residing in the State. A Medicaid agency for such a State may, if it deems necessary, use the fee schedules of either one or both of the carriers to meet the Federal fund-matching requirement. State Medicaid agencies may consult with ROs concerning the fee schedule, the NLAs, and specimen collection provisions.

110.3 Coordination With FIs and Providers (Rev. 1, 10-01-03). HO-437, A3-3628—There may be procedures hospitals bill for outpatients that are not included in the fee schedule. Where gaps occur, hospitals should work out procedures with the FI so that the hospital can secure the missing information promptly. Price Codes established by the carrier to fill gaps are valid until replaced by the earlier of permanent codes or the next annual update.

110.4 Carrier Contacts With Independent Clinical Laboratories (Rev. 1, 10-01-03). B3-2070.1.F—An important role of the carrier is as a communicant of necessary information to independent clinical laboratories. Failure to inform independent laboratories of Medicare regulations and claims processing procedures may have an adverse effect on prosecution of laboratories suspected of fraudulent activities with respect to tests performed by, or billed on behalf of, independent laboratories. United States Attorneys often must prosecute under a handicap or may refuse to prosecute cases where there is no evidence that a laboratory has been specifically informed of Medicare regulations and claims processing procedures.

To assure that laboratories are aware of Medicare regulations and carrier's policy, notification must be sent to independent laboratories when any changes are made in coverage policy or claims processing procedures. Additionally, to completely document efforts to fully inform independent laboratories of Medicare policy and the laboratory's responsibilities, previously issued newsletters should be periodically re-issued to remind laboratories of existing requirements.

Some items which should be discussed are the requirements to have the same charges for Medicare and private patients, to document fully the medical necessity for collection of specimens from a skilled nursing facility or a beneficiary's home, and, in cases when a laboratory service is referred from one independent laboratory to another independent laboratory, to identify the laboratory actually performing the test.

Additionally, when carrier professional relations representatives make personal contacts with particular laboratories, they should prepare and retain reports of contact indicating dates, persons present, and issues discussed.

40 CLINICAL DIAGNOSTIC LABORATORY FEE SCHEDULE (Rev. 1, 10-01-03) B3-5114, B3-5114.1, A3-3628, AB-01-162, AB-02-163

The Medicare Claims Processing Manual, Chapter 16, "Laboratory Services From Independent Labs, Physicians, and Providers," provides background and additional information for payment of laboratory services.

Clinical diagnostic laboratory tests—whether performed in a physician's office, by an independent laboratory, or by a hospital laboratory for its outpatients—are paid based on fee schedules. This section sets out rules for use of these schedules.

The fee schedule amounts are adjusted annually to reflect changes in the Consumer Price Index (CPI) for all Urban Consumers (U.S. city average), or as otherwise specified by legislation. Adjustments are applied and amounts are determined by CMS and published for contractor use and also on CMS Web site. Contractors are notified when and where updates are published.

For a cervical or vaginal smear test (pap smear), payment is the lesser of the local fee or the national limitation amount, but not less than the national minimum payment amount. However, in no case may payment for these tests exceed actual charges. The Part B deductible and coinsurance do not apply.

Regardless of whether a diagnostic laboratory test is performed in a physician's office, by an independent laboratory, or by a hospital laboratory for its outpatients or nonpatients, it is considered a laboratory service. When a hospital laboratory performs diagnostic laboratory tests for nonhospital patients, the laboratory is functioning as an independent laboratory.

National minimum limitation amounts are established each year

for cervical or vaginal smear clinical laboratory tests. These payment amounts are published each year in Program Memoranda issued by CMS. The affected CPT laboratory test codes for the national minimum payment amount are also identified in the annual Program Memorandum.

National maximum limitation amounts may also be established for certain services and are also published each year in Program Memoranda issued by CMS.

Carriers and Intermediaries pay the lowest of the applicable current fee schedule, the actual charge, or the NLA. This applies to all clinical diagnostic laboratory tests except:

- Laboratory tests furnished to a hospital inpatient whose stay is covered under Part A;
- Laboratory tests performed by a Skilled Nursing Facility (SNF) for its own SNF inpatients and reimbursed under Part A or Part B and any laboratory tests furnished under arrangements to an SNF inpatient with Part A coverage. (The only covered source for laboratory services furnished under Part A is the SNF itself or a hospital with which the facility has a transfer agreement in effect.);
- Laboratory tests furnished by hospital-based or independent ESRD dialysis facilities that are included under the ESRD composite rate payment;
- Laboratory tests furnished by hospitals in States or areas which have been granted demonstration waivers of Medicare reimbursement principles for outpatient services. The State of Maryland has been granted such demonstration waivers;
- Laboratory tests furnished to inpatients of a hospital with a waiver under §602(k) of the 1983 Amendments to the Act. This section of the Act provides that an outside supplier may bill under Part B for laboratory and other nonphysician services furnished to inpatients that are otherwise paid only though the hospital;
- Laboratory tests furnished to patients of rural health clinics (RHCs) under an all inclusive rate;
- Laboratory tests provided by a participating health maintenance organization (HMO) or health care prepayment plan (HCPP) to an enrolled member of the plan; and
- Laboratory tests furnished by a hospice.

40.1 Access to Clinical Diagnostic Lab Fee Schedule Files (Rev. 1, 10-01-03). AB-01-162—The annual laboratory fee schedule data file should be retrieved electronically through CMS' mainframe telecommunications system, formerly referred to as the National Data Mover.

For each test code, if the contractor's system retains only the pricing amount, they should load the data from the field named "60% Pricing Amt." For each test code, if the contractor's system has been developed to retain the local fee and the NLA, they may load the data from the fields named "60% Local Fee Amt" and "60% Natl Limit Amt" to use to determine payment. For clinical laboratory test codes for cervical or vaginal smear tests (listed in Chapter 16, "Laboratory Services from Independent Labs, Physicians, and Providers," §80.3) load the data from the field named "60% Pricing Amt" to reflect the lower of the local fee or the NLA, but not less than the national minimum payment amount. The fields named "62% Local Fee Amt," "62% Natl Limit Amt," and "62% Pricing Amt" should be used by intermediaries for payment of clinical laboratory tests performed by a sole community hospital's qualified laboratory.

The 3-month grace period for deleted codes is defined in the above in §20.4 and begins January 1.

Internet access to annual laboratory fee schedule data is available at the following CMS Web address: http://www.cms.hhs.gov/clia/clsites.asp or http://www.cms.hhs.gov/paymentsystems/. It is available in multiple formats: Excel, text, and comma delimited.

40.2 Carrier Record Layout for Clinical Laboratory Fee Schedule (Rev. 1, 10-01-03). PM AB-01-162, AB-02-163—The instructions for each annual update contain the actual data set name for that year. The Data Set Name is included with each annual update instructions.

Data Element Name	Picture	Location	Comment
HCPCS Code	X(05)	1–5	
Carrier Number	X(05)	6–10	
Locality	X(02)	11–12	00 = Denotes Single Carrier State
			01 = North Dakota
			02 = South Dakota
			20 = Puerto Rico
			40 = New Hampshire
			50 = Vermont
60% Local Fee	9(05)V99	13–19	
62% Local Fee	9(05)V99	20–26	
60% Natl Limit Amt	9(05)V99	27–33	
62% Natl Limit Amt	9(05)V99	34–40	
60% Pricing Amt	9(05)V99	41–47	
62% Pricing Amt	9(05)V99	48–54	
Gap-Fill Indicator	X(01)	55–55	0 = No Gap-fill Required
			1 = Carrier Gap-fill
			2 = Special Instructions Apply
Modifier	X(02)	56–57	Where modifier is shown, QW denotes a CLIA waive test.
Filler	X(03)	58–60	

40.3 Intermediary and Regional Home Health Intermediary (RHHI) Record Layout for Clinical Laboratory Fee Schedule (Rev. 1, 10-01-03). PM AB-01-162, A-01-104, AB-02-163—The instructions for each annual update contain the actual file name for that year. The Data Set Name is included with each annual update instructions.

Record Length = 60
Record Format = FB
Block Size = 6000
Character Code = EDBCIC
Sort Sequence = Carrier, Locality, HCPCS Code

Header Record

Data Element Name	Picture	Location	Comment
Label	X(03)	1–3	Value = Lab
Filler	X(07)	4–10	
Filler	X(08)	11–15	
Filler	X(04)	16–22	
Date Fee Update	X(08)	23–30	YYYYMMDD
Filler	X(22)	31–52	
Date File Created	X(08)	53–60	YYYYMMDD

Data Record

Data Element Name	Picture	Location	Comment
HCPCS	X(05)	1–5	
Filler	X(04)	6–9	
60% Pricing Amt	9(05)V99	10–16	
62% Pricing Amt	9(05)V99	17–23	
Filler	X(07)	24–30	
Carrier Number	X(05)	31–35	
Locality	X(02)	36–37	00 = Denotes Single State Carrier
			01 = North Dakota
			02 = South Dakota
			20 = Puerto Rico
			40 = New Hampshire
			50 = Vermont
Filler	X(23)	38–60	

40.4 Gap-Filled Fees Submitted to CMS by Carriers (Rev. 1, 10-01-03). AB-01-162, AB-02-163—In accordance with §531(b) of the Benefits Improvement and Protection Act of 2000 (BIPA), CMS

solicits public comments on determining payment amounts for new laboratory tests. The CMS hosts an annual public meeting to allow parties the opportunity to provide input to the payment determination process. The CMS employs one of two approaches to establishing payment amounts for new laboratory test codes, crosswalking and gap-filling. After considering public input regarding the new test codes, CMS determines which approach is most appropriate for each new test code.

If the new test is comparable to an existing test, the new test is "crosswalked" to the existing test, and it is assigned the local fee for the existing test and the corresponding NLA. The new test code and payment amounts are included in the updated laboratory fee schedule annually.

If CMS determines that the laboratory fee schedule includes no sufficiently comparable test to permit crosswalking, CMS instructs carriers to "gap-fill" the payment amount for the new test code. Gap-filling is an empirical process of determining a payment amount in a locality using available information sources. Usually the period during which gap-filled payment amounts are instructed is the year following the introduction of a new code. During this period, carriers establish and use these payment amounts; they may be revised in the course of the year. Also during this period, carriers must report the gap-fill amounts to their ROs which are then forwarded to CMS CO. The CMS considers the gap-fill amounts and uses them to establish the fees for the new test code in the next update of the laboratory fee schedule.

In determining gap-fill amounts, the sources of information carriers should examine, if available, include: charges for the test and routine discounts to charges; resources required to perform the test; payment amounts determined by other payers; and charges, payment amounts, and resources required for other tests that may be comparable or otherwise relevant. Carriers may consider other sources of information as appropriate, including clinical studies and information provided by clinicians practicing in the area, manufacturers, or other interested parties. To assist each carrier in establishing a gap-fill amount, carriers' Medical Directors may meet and share information regarding the new test, though without reaching a formal consensus.

Establishing payment amounts for new laboratory tests is inherently difficult, precisely because these tests are new and as a result the types and extent of information available about them may be limited. Because the circumstances of different tests may vary significantly, specifying in detail a method of using the various information sources outlined above does not appear appropriate at this time. However, CMS designates a new test code for gap-filling in instances where no test code seems sufficiently similar to make a crosswalk approach appropriate. Accordingly, carriers should not determine a gap-fill amount by crosswalking to the payment amount for another test code.

After determining a gap-fill amount, a carrier may consider if a least costly alternative to a new test exists. If a carrier determines a least costly alternative test exists, the carrier may adopt the payment amount of the least costly alternative test as the gap-fill amount for the new test code. The least costly alternative amount will be considered the local fee, and CMS will use this payment amount in establishing the NLA. However in this case, the carrier must report two payment amounts, the gap-fill amount prior to determination of a least costly alternative and the payment amount that the carrier has determined to be the least costly alternative.

Carriers should also communicate the gap-fill amounts to corresponding intermediaries. Carriers can seek assistance from RO staff to facilitate communication of the gap-fill amounts to intermediaries. The list of codes which carriers are required to gap-fill each year are communicated in the annual instructions.

Carriers provide their RO with gap-fill fees according to the date communicated by CMS (usually May), to be used by CMS-Central for the development of subsequent or later laboratory fee schedules. Carriers submit the gap-fill fees in a right-justified format. These gap-fill data should be transmitted in an ASCII file with the following file specifications to MStevenson@cms.hhs.gov with a copy to Agreenberg@cms.hhs.gov to assist with coordinated collection of the gap-fill fees.

Data Set Name: CLXXXXX.TXT*   (ASCII File)
(*Denotes carrier 5 - digit number)

Gap-filled Fees Record Layout

Data Element Name	Picture	Location	Comment
Year	X(4)	1–4	Set to Year (e.g., 2003)
HCPCS Code	X(5)	5–9	
Modifier	X(2)	10–11	
Carrier Number	X(5)	12–16	
Locality	X(2)	17–18	00 = Denotes Single State Carrier
			01 = North Dakota
			02 = South Dakota
			20 = Puerto Rico
			40 = New Hampshire
			50 = Vermont
Gap-fill Amount	9(5)V99	19–25	Prior to any determination of a least costly alternative
Least Costly Alternative Amount	9(5)V99	26–32	
Least Costly Alternative Code	X(5)	33–37	

40.4.1 Carriers Forward HCPCS Gap Fill Amounts to Fiscal Intermediaries (Rev. 1, 10-01-03). CMS Memo 9-13-02 HCPCS Gap-fillR3.doc—Any carrier that establishes a HCPCS gap fill payment rate for its own use, or at the request of an FI, must forward the information to the contacts at all FIs/RHHIs with providers in the carrier service area.

Carriers that establish HCPCS gap-fill payment rates for their own needs should forward the information to FI/RHHIs as soon as practicable. FIs are to contact the appropriate carrier to request a gap fill payment rate with 5 working days of the suspension of claims containing HCPCS codes(s) for which payment rate is needed and has not been forwarded. Carriers must provide the payment rate to the requesting FI/RHHI (and all other FI/RHHIs with providers in that common jurisdiction) within 10 working days of receipt of the request.

Requests for policy clarification in carrier establishing the HCPCS gap fill payment rates or FI/RHHI procedures for the use thereof should be directed to the respective Regional Office HCPCS business function experts (BFE). Examples of the need for FI consultation with the BRE are coverage questions and receipt of unresolved significant inconsistencies in fee amounts from different carriers for the same HCPCS. The FI should consult the carriers with disparate fees before contacting the BFE.

An intermediary experiencing delay in replies or nonresponses from a carrier should alert it respective Consortium Contractor Management Staff (CCMS) Contract Manager (CM). The CM will coordinate with his/her counterpart assigned to the carrier to achieve more timely action by the carrier.

It is the FI's responsibility to ascertain the amount or consult with the carrier, CCMS-CM, or BFE timely. Intermediary requests to apply CC 15 to claims which are paid untimely solely because of a delay in ascertaining a HCPCS gap fill amount from the carrier should be addressed to the respective CM. The CM will contact the HCPCS BFE for a decision. Requests for application of CC 15 to claims for which the FI did not request the gap fill payment rate within 5 working days of the claim suspension and/or did not seek timely advice from the RO BFE concerning application of gap fill amount will not be honored. Additionally, if the carrier replied at least five days before the expiration of the payment floor, CC 15 requests will **not** be honored.

15030 SUPPLIES

Make a separate payment for supplies furnished in connection with a procedure only when one of the two following conditions exists:

A. HCPCS codes A4500, A4200, and A4263 are billed in conjunction with the appropriate procedure in the Medical Physician Fee Schedule Data Base (place of service is physician's office); or

B. The supply is a pharmaceutical or radiopharmaceutical diagnostic imaging agent (including codes A4641 through A4647); pharmacologic stressing agent (code J1245); or therapeutic radionuclide (CPT code 79900*). The procedures performed are:

- Diagnostic radiologic procedures (including diagnostic nuclear medicine) requiring pharmaceutical or radiopharmaceutical contrast media and/or pharmocological stressing agent,
- Other diagnostic tests requiring a pharmacological stressing agent,
- Clinical brachytherapy procedures (other than remote afterloading high intensity brachytherapy procedures (CPT codes 77781 through 77784*), for which the expendable source is included in the TC RVUs), or Therapeutic nuclear medicine procedures.

APPENDIX B

COVERAGE ISSUES MANUAL (CIM), SELECT

30-1 ROUTINE COSTS IN CLINICAL TRIALS (310.1)

Effective for items and services furnished on or after September 19, 2000, Medicare covers the routine costs of qualifying clinical trials, as such costs are defined below, as well as reasonable and necessary items and services used to diagnose and treat complications arising from participation in all clinical trials. All other Medicare rules apply.

Routine costs of a clinical trial include all items and services that are otherwise generally available to Medicare beneficiaries (i.e., there exists a benefit category, it is not statutorily excluded, and there is not a national noncoverage decision) that are provided in either the experimental or the control arms of a clinical trial **except**:

- The investigational item or service, itself;
- Items and services provided solely to satisfy data collection and analysis needs and that are not used in the direct clinical management of the patient (e.g., monthly CT scans for a condition usually requiring only a single scan); and
- Items and services customarily provided by the research sponsors free of charge for any enrollee in the trial.

Routine costs in clinical trials include:

- Items or services that are typically provided absent a clinical trial (e.g., conventional care);
- Items or services required solely for the provision of the investigational item or service (e.g., administration of a noncovered chemotherapeutic agent), the clinically appropriate monitoring of the effects of the item or service, or the prevention of complications; and
- Items or services needed for reasonable and necessary care arising from the provision of an investigational item or service—in particular, for the diagnosis or treatment of complications.

This policy does not withdraw Medicare coverage for items and services that may be covered according to local medical review policies or the regulations on category B investigational device exemptions (IDE) found in 42 CFR 405.201-405.215, 411.15, and 411.406. For information about LMRPs, refer to www.lmrp.net, a searchable database of Medicare contractors' local policies.

For noncovered items and services, including items and services for which Medicare payment is statutorily prohibited, Medicare only covers the treatment of complications arising from the delivery of the noncovered item or service and unrelated reasonable and necessary care. (Refer to MCM §§2300.1 and MIM 3101.) However, if the item or service is not covered by virtue of a national noncoverage policy in the Coverage Issues Manual and is the focus of a qualifying clinical trial, the routine costs of the clinical trial (as defined above) will be covered by Medicare but the noncovered item or service, itself, will not.

A. Requirements for Medicare Coverage of Routine Costs.— Any clinical trial receiving Medicare coverage of routine costs must meet the following three requirements:

1. The subject or purpose of the trial must be the evaluation of an item or service that falls within a Medicare benefit category (e.g., physicians' service, durable medical equipment, diagnostic test) and is not statutorily excluded from coverage (e.g., cosmetic surgery, hearing aids).

2. The trial must not be designed exclusively to test toxicity or disease pathophysiology. It must have therapeutic intent.

3. Trials of therapeutic interventions must enroll patients with diagnosed disease rather than healthy volunteers. Trials of diagnostic interventions may enroll healthy patients in order to have a proper control group.

The three requirements above are insufficient by themselves to qualify a clinical trial for Medicare coverage of routine costs. Clinical trials also should have the following desirable character-istics; however, some trials, as described below, are presumed to meet these characteristics and are automatically qualified to receive Medicare coverage:

1. The principal purpose of the trial is to test whether the intervention potentially improves the participants' health outcomes;

2. The trial is well-supported by available scientific and medical information or it is intended to clarify or establish the health outcomes of interventions already in common clinical use;

3. The trial does not unjustifiably duplicate existing studies;

4. The trial design is appropriate to answer the research question being asked in the trial;

5. The trial is sponsored by a credible organization or individual capable of executing the proposed trial successfully;

6. The trial is in compliance with Federal regulations relating to the protection of human subjects; and

7. All aspects of the trial are conducted according to the appropriate standards of scientific integrity.

B. Qualification Process for Clinical Trials.—Using the authority found in §1142 of the Act (cross-referenced in §1862(a)(1)(E) of the Act), the Agency for Healthcare Research and Quality (AHRQ) will convene a multi-agency Federal panel (the "panel") composed of representatives of the Department of Health and Human Services research agencies (National Institutes of Health (NIH), Centers for Disease Control and Prevention (CDC), the Food and Drug Administration (FDA), AHRQ, and the Office of Human Research Protection), and the research arms of the Department of Defense (DOD) and the Department of Veterans Affairs (VA) to develop qualifying criteria that will indicate a strong probability that a trial exhibits the desirable characteristics listed above. These criteria will be easily verifiable, and where possible, dichotomous. Trials that meet these qualifying criteria will receive Medicare coverage of their associated routine costs. This panel is not reviewing or approving individual trials. The multi-agency panel will meet periodically to review and evaluate the program and recommend any necessary refinements to CMS.

Clinical trials that meet the qualifying criteria will receive Medicare coverage of routine costs after the trial's lead principal investigator certifies that the trial meets the criteria. This process will require the principal investigator to enroll the trial in a Medicare clinical trials registry, currently under development.

Some clinical trials are automatically qualified to receive Medicare coverage of their routine costs because they have been deemed by AHRQ, in consultation with the other agencies represented on the multi-agency panel to be highly likely to have the above-listed seven desirable characteristics of clinical trials. The principal investigators of these automatically qualified trials do not need to certify that the trials meet the qualifying criteria, but must enroll the trials in the Medicare clinical trials registry for administrative purposes, once the registry is established.

Effective September 19, 2000, clinical trials that are deemed to be automatically qualified are:

1. Trials funded by NIH, CDC, AHRQ, CMS, DOD, and VA;

2. Trials supported by centers or cooperative groups that are funded by the NIH, CDC, AHRQ, CMS, DOD and VA;

3. Trials conducted under an investigational new drug application (IND) reviewed by the FDA; and

4. Drug trials that are exempt from having an IND under 21 CFR 312.2(b)(1) will be deemed automatically qualified until the qualifying criteria are developed and the certification process is in place. At that time the principal investigators of these trials must certify that the trials meet the qualifying criteria in order to main-

tain Medicare coverage of routine costs. This certification process will only affect the future status of the trial and will not be used to retroactively change the earlier deemed status.

Medicare will cover the routine costs of qualifying trials that either have been deemed to be automatically qualified or have certified that they meet the qualifying criteria unless CMS's Chief Clinical Officer subsequently finds that a clinical trial does not meet the qualifying criteria or jeopardizes the safety or welfare of Medicare beneficiaries.

Should CMS find that a trial's principal investigator misrepresented that the trial met the necessary qualifying criteria in order to gain Medicare coverage of routine costs, Medicare coverage of the routine costs would be denied under §1862(a)(1)(E) of the Act. In the case of such a denial, the Medicare beneficiaries enrolled in the trial would not be held liable (i.e., would be held harmless from collection) for the costs consistent with the provisions of §§1879, 1842(l), or 1834(j)(4) of the Act, as applicable. Where appropriate, the billing providers would be held liable for the costs and fraud investigations of the billing providers and the trial's principal investigator may be pursued.

Medicare regulations require Medicare+Choice (M+C) organizations to follow CMS's national coverage decisions. This NCD raises special issues that require some modification of most M+C organizations' rules governing provision of items and services in and out of network. The items and services covered under this NCD are inextricably linked to the clinical trials with which they are associated and cannot be covered outside of the context of those clinical trials. M+C organizations therefore must cover these services regardless of whether they are available through in-network providers. M+C organizations may have reporting requirements when enrollees participate in clinical trials, in order to track and coordinate their members' care, but cannot require prior authorization or approval.

35-3 HEAT TREATMENT, INCLUDING THE USE OF DIATHERMY AND ULTRASOUND FOR PULMONARY CONDITIONS—NOT COVERED (240.3)

There is no physiological rationale or valid scientific documentation of effectiveness of diathermy or ultrasound heat treatments for asthma, bronchitis, or any other pulmonary condition, and for such purpose this treatment cannot be considered reasonable and necessary within the meaning of section 1862(a)(1) of the law.

Cross-refer: §150.5.

35-5 CELLULAR THERAPY—NOT COVERED (30.8)

Cellular therapy involves the practice of injecting humans with foreign proteins like the placenta or lungs of unborn lambs. Cellular therapy is without scientific or statistical evidence to document its therapeutic efficacy and, in fact, is considered a potentially dangerous practice. Accordingly, cellular therapy is not considered reasonable and necessary within the meaning of section 1862(a)(1) of the law.

35-10 HYPERBARIC OXYGEN THERAPY (20.29)

For purposes of coverage under Medicare, hyperbaric oxygen (HBO) therapy is a modality in which the entire body is exposed to oxygen under increased atmospheric pressure.

A. Covered Conditions.—Program reimbursement for HBO therapy will be limited to that which is administered in a chamber (including the one man unit) and is limited to the following conditions:

1. Acute carbon monoxide intoxication.
2. Decompression illness.
3. Gas embolism.
4. Gas gangrene.
5. Acute traumatic peripheral ischemia. HBO therapy is a valuable adjunctive treatment to be used in combination with accepted standard therapeutic measures when loss of function, limb, or life is threatened.

6. Crush injuries and suturing of severed limbs. As in the previous conditions, HBO therapy would be an adjunctive treatment when loss of function, limb, or life is threatened.
7. Progressive necrotizing infections (necrotizing fasciitis, Meleney ulcer).
8. Acute peripheral arterial insufficiency.
9. Preparation and preservation of compromised skin grafts (not for primary management of wounds), (ICD-9-CM diagnosis 996.52, excludes artifical skin grafts).
10. Chronic refractory osteomyelitis, unresponsive to conventional medical and surgical management.
11. Osteoradionecrosis as an adjunct to conventional treatment.
12. Soft tissue radionecrosis as an adjunct to conventional treatment.
13. Cyanide poisoning.

The following use of HBO is covered for services rendered on or after 2/22/84.

14. Actinomycosis, only as an adjunct to conventional therapy when the disease process is refractory to antibiotics and surgical treatment.
15. Diabetic wounds of the lower extremities in patients who meet the following three criteria:

    a. Patient has type I or type II diabetes and has a lower extremity wound that is due to diabetes;

    b. Patient has a wound classified as Wagner grade III or higher; and

    c. Patient has failed an adequate course of standard wound therapy.

The use of HBO therapy is covered as adjunctive therapy only after there are no measurable signs of healing for at least 30 days of treatment with standard wound therapy and must be used in addition to standard wound care. Standard wound care in patients with diabetic wounds includes: assessment of a patient's vascular status and correction of any vascular problems in the affected limb if possible, optimization of nutritional status, optimization of glucose control, debridement by any means to remove devitalized tissue, maintenance of a clean, moist bed of granulation tissue with appropriate moist dressings, appropriate off-loading, and necessary treatment to resolve any infection that might be present. Failure to respond to standard wound care occurs when there are not measurable signs of healing for at least 30 consecutive days. Wounds must be evaluated at least every 30 days during administration of HBO therapy. Continued treatment with HBO therapy is not covered if measurable signs of healing have not been demonstrated within any 30-day period of treatment.

B. Noncovered Conditions.—All other indications not specified under section 35-10 (A) are not covered under the Medicare program. No program payment may be made for any conditions other than those listed in section 35-10 (A).

No program payment may be made for HBO in the treatment of the following conditions:

1. Cutaneous, decubitus, and stasis ulcers.
2. Chronic peripheral vascular insufficiency.
3. Anaerobic septicemia and infection other than clostridial.
4. Skin burns (thermal).
5. Senility.
6. Myocardial infarction.
7. Cardiogenic shock.
8. Sickle cell anemia.
9. Acute thermal and chemical pulmonary damage, i.e., smoke inhalation with pulmonary insufficiency.

10. Acute or chronic cerebral vascular insufficiency.

11. Hepatic necrosis.

12. Aerobic septicemia.

13. Nonvascular causes of chronic brain syndrome (Pick's disease, Alzheimer's disease, Korsakoff's disease).

14. Tetanus.

15. Systemic aerobic infection.

16. Organ transplantation.

17. Organ storage.

18. Pulmonary emphysema.

19. Exceptional blood loss anemia.

20. Multiple Sclerosis.

21. Arthritic Diseases.

22. Acute cerebral edema.

C. Topical Application of Oxygen.—This method of administering oxygen does not meet the definition of HBO therapy as stated above. Also, its clinical efficacy has not been established. Therefore, no Medicare reimbursement may be made for the topical application of oxygen. (Cross refer: section 35-31.)

35-13 PROLOTHERAPY, JOINT SCLEROTHERAPY, AND LIGAMENTOUS INJECTIONS WITH SCLEROSING AGENTS—NOT COVERED (150.7)

The medical effectiveness of the above therapies has not been verified by scientifically controlled studies. Accordingly, reimbursement for these modalities should be denied on the ground that they are not reasonable and necessary as required by section 1862(a)(1) of the law.

35-20 TREATMENT OF MOTOR FUNCTION DISORDERS WITH ELECTRIC NERVE STIMULATION—NOT COVERED (160.2)

While electric nerve stimulation has been employed to control chronic intractable pain for some time, its use in the treatment of motor function disorders, such as multiple sclerosis, is a recent innovation, and the medical effectiveness of such therapy has not been verified by scientifically controlled studies. Therefore, where electric nerve stimulation is employed to treat motor function disorders, no reimbursement may be made for the stimulator or for the services related to its implantation since this treatment cannot be considered reasonable and necessary.

NOTE: For Medicare coverage of deep brain stimulation for essential tremor and Parkinson's disease, see §65-19.

NOTE: Medicare coverage of deep brain stimulation by implantation of a stimulator device is not prohibited. Therefore, coverage of deep brain stimulation provided by an implanted deep brain stimulator is at the carrier's discretion.

35-27 BIOFEEDBACK THERAPY (30.1)

Biofeedback therapy provides visual, auditory or other evidence of the status of certain body functions so that a person can exert voluntary control over the functions, and thereby alleviate an abnormal bodily condition. Biofeedback therapy often uses electrical devices to transform bodily signals indicative of such functions as heart rate, blood pressure, skin temperature, salivation, peripheral vasomotor activity, and gross muscle tone into a tone or light, the loudness or brightness of which shows the extent of activity in the function being measured.

Biofeedback therapy differs from electromyography, which is a diagnostic procedure used to record and study the electrical properties of skeletal muscle. An electromyography device may be used to provide feedback with certain types of biofeedback.

Biofeedback therapy is covered under Medicare only when it is reasonable and necessary for the individual patient for muscle reeducation of specific muscle groups or for treating pathological muscle abnormalities of spasticity, incapacitating muscle spasm,

or weakness, and more conventional treatments (heat, cold, massage, exercise, support) have not been successful. This therapy is not covered for treatment of ordinary muscle tension states or for psychosomatic conditions.

(See CMS-Pub. 14-3, sections 2200ff., 2215, and 4161; CMS-Pub. 13-3, section 3133.3, 3148, and 3149; CMS-Pub. 10, section 242 and 242.5 for special physical therapy requirements. See also sections 35-20 and 65-8.)

35-27.1 BIOFEEDBACK THERAPY FOR THE TREATMENT OF URINARY INCONTINENCE (30.1.1)

Biofeedback therapy for the treatment of urinary incontinence (Effective for services performed on or after July 1, 2001.) This policy applies to biofeedback therapy rendered by a practitioner in an office or other facility setting.

Biofeedback is covered for the treatment of stress and/or urge incontinence in cognitively intact patients who have failed a documented trial of pelvic muscle exercise (PME) training. Biofeedback is not a treatment, per se, but a tool to help patients learn how to perform PME. Biofeedback-assisted PME incorporates the use of an electronic or mechanical device to relay visual and/or auditory evidence of pelvic floor muscle tone, in order to improve awareness of pelvic floor musculature and to assist patients in the performance of PME.

A failed trial of PME training is defined as no clinically significant improvement in urinary incontinence after completing 4 weeks of an ordered plan of pelvic muscle exercises to increase periurethral muscle strength.

Contractors may decide whether or not to cover biofeedback as an initial treatment modality.

Home use of biofeedback therapy is not covered.

35-31 TREATMENT OF DECUBITUS ULCERS (270.4)

An accepted procedure for healing decubitus ulcers is to remove dead tissue from the lesions and to keep them clean to promote the growth of new tissue. This may be accomplished by hydrotherapy (whirlpool) treatments. Hydrotherapy (whirlpool) treatment for decubitus ulcers is a covered service under Medicare for patients when treatment is reasonable and necessary. Some other methods of treating decubitus ulcers, the safety and effectiveness of which have not been established, are not covered under the Medicare program. Some examples of these types of treatments are: ultraviolet light, low intensity direct current, topical application of oxygen, and topical dressings with Balsam of Peru in castor oil.

35-34 FABRIC WRAPPING OF ABDOMINAL ANEURYSMS— NOT COVERED (20.23)

Fabric wrapping of abdominal aneurysms is not a covered Medicare procedure. This is a treatment for abdominal aneurysms which involves wrapping aneurysms with cellophane or fascia lata. This procedure has not been shown to prevent eventual rupture. In extremely rare instances, external wall reinforcement may be indicated when the current accepted treatment (excision of the aneurysm and reconstruction with synthetic materials) is not a viable alternative, but external wall reinforcement is not fabric wrapping. Accordingly, fabric wrapping of abdominal aneurysms is not considered reasonable and necessary within the meaning of section 1862(a)(1) of the Act.

35-41 DIATHERMY TREATMENT (150.5)

High-energy pulsed-wave diathermy machines have been found to produce some degree of therapeutic benefit for essentially the same conditions and to the same extent as standard diathermy. Accordingly, when the contractor's medical staff has determined that the pulsed-wave diathermy apparatus used is one which is considered therapeutically effective, the treatments are considered a covered service, but only for those conditions for which standard diathermy is medically indicated and only when rendered by a physician or incident to a physician's professional services.

Further, when the charge for covered pulsed-wave diathermy treatment is substantially in excess of that which is reasonable for standard diathermy, payment is based on the reasonable charge for standard diathermy (CPT-4 code 97024,* ICD-9-CM code 93.34).

Cross-refer: §35-3.

35-46 ASSESSING PATIENT'S SUITABILITY FOR ELECTRICAL NERVE STIMULATION THERAPY (160.3)

Electrical nerve stimulation is an accepted modality for assessing a patient's suitability for ongoing treatment with a transcutaneous or an implanted nerve stimulator. Accordingly, program payment may be made for the following techniques when used to determine the potential therapeutic usefulness of an electrical nerve stimulator:

A. Transcutaneous Electrical Nerve Stimulation (TENS).—This technique involves attachment of a transcutaneous nerve stimulator to the surface of the skin over the peripheral nerve to be stimulated. It is used by the patient on a trial basis and its effectiveness in modulating pain is monitored by the physician, or physical therapist. Generally, the physician or physical therapist is able to determine whether the patient is likely to derive a significant therapeutic benefit from continuous use of a transcutaneous stimulator within a trial period of 1 month; in a few cases this determination may take longer to make. Document the medical necessity for such services which are furnished beyond the first month. (See section 45-25 for an explanation of coverage of medically necessary supplies for the effective use of TENS.)

If TENS significantly alleviates pain, it may be considered as primary treatment; if it produces no relief or greater discomfort than the original pain, electrical nerve stimulation therapy is ruled out. However, where TENS produces incomplete relief, further evaluation with percutaneous electrical nerve stimulation may be considered to determine whether an implanted peripheral nerve stimulator would provide significant relief from pain. (See section 35-46B.)

Usually, the physician or physical therapist providing the services will furnish the equipment necessary for assessment. Where the physician or physical therapist advises the patient to rent the TENS from a supplier during the trial period rather than supplying it himself/herself, program payment may be made for rental of the TENS as well as for the services of the physician or physical therapist who is evaluating its use. However, the combined program payment which is made for the physician's or physical therapist's services and the rental of the stimulator from a supplier should not exceed the amount which would be payable for the total service, including the stimulator, furnished by the physician or physical therapist alone.

B. Percutaneous Electrical Nerve Stimulation (PENS).—This diagnostic procedure which involves stimulation of peripheral nerves by a needle electrode inserted through the skin is performed only in a physician's office, clinic, or hospital outpatient department. Therefore, it is covered only when performed by a physician or incident to physician's service. If pain is effectively controlled by percutaneous stimulation, implantation of electrodes is warranted.

As in the case of TENS (described in subsection A), generally the physician should be able to determine whether the patient is likely to derive a significant therapeutic benefit from continuing use of an implanted nerve stimulator within a trial period of 1 month. In a few cases, this determination may take longer to make. The medical necessity for such diagnostic services which are furnished beyond the first month must be documented.

NOTE: Electrical nerve stimulators do not prevent pain but only alleviate pain as it occurs. A patient can be taught how to employ the stimulator, and once this is done, can use it safely and effectively without direct physician supervi-

sion. Consequently, it is inappropriate for a patient to visit his physician, physical therapist or an outpatient clinic on a continuing basis for treatment of pain with electrical nerve stimulation. Once it is determined that electrical nerve stimulation should be continued as therapy and the patient has been trained to use the stimulator, it is expected that a stimulator will be implanted or the patient will employ the TENS on a continual basis in his home. Electrical nerve stimulation treatments furnished by a physician in his office, by a physical therapist or outpatient clinic are excluded from coverage by section 1862(a)(1) of the law. (See section 65-8 for an explanation of coverage of the therapeutic use of implanted peripheral nerve stimulators under the prosthetic devices benefit. See section 60-20 for an explanation of coverage of the therapeutic use of TENS under the durable medical equipment benefit.)

35-47 BREAST RECONSTRUCTION FOLLOWING MASTECTOMY (140.2)

During recent years there has been a considerable change in the treatment of diseases of the breast such as fibrocystic disease, and cancer. While extirpation of the disease remains of primary importance, the quality of life following initial treatment is increasingly recognized as of great concern. The increased use of breast reconstruction procedures is due to several factors:

- A change in epidemiology of breast cancer, including an apparent increase in incidence;
- Improved surgical skills and techniques;
- The continuing development of better prostheses; and
- Increasing awareness by physicians of the importance of post-surgical psychological adjustment.

Reconstruction of the affected and the contralateral unaffected breast following a medically necessary mastectomy is considered a relatively safe and effective noncosmetic procedure. Accordingly, program payment may be made for breast reconstruction surgery following removal of a breast for any medical reason.

Program payment may not be made for breast reconstruction for cosmetic reasons. (Cosmetic surgery is excluded from coverage under section 1862(a)(10) of the Social Security Act.)

35-48 OSTEOGENIC STIMULATION (150.2)

Electrical stimulation to augment bone repair can be attained either invasively or noninvasively. Invasive devices provide electrical stimulation directly at the fracture site either through percutaneously placed cathodes or by implantation of a coiled cathode wire into the fracture site. The power pack for the latter device is implanted into soft tissue near the fracture site and subcutaneously connected to the cathode, creating a self-contained system with no external components. The power supply for the former device is externally placed and the leads connected to the inserted cathodes. With the noninvasive device, opposing pads, wired to an external power supply, are placed over the cast. An electromagnetic field is created between the pads at the fracture site.

1. Noninvasive Stimulator.—The noninvasive stimulator device is covered only for the following indications:

- Nonunion of long bone fractures;
- Failed fusion, where a minimum of 9 months has elapsed since the last surgery;
- Congenital pseudarthroses; and
- As an adjunct to spinal fusion surgery for patients at high risk of pseudarthrosis due to previously failed spinal fusion at the same site or for those undergoing multiple level fusion. A multiple level fusion involves 3 or more vertebrae (e.g., L3-L5, L4-S1, etc).

2. Invasive (Implantable) Stimulator.—The invasive stimulator device is covered only for the following indications:

- Nonunion of long bone fractures;
- As an adjunct to spinal fusion surgery for patients at high risk of pseudarthrosis due to previously failed spinal fusion at the

same site or for those undergoing muliple level fusion. A multiple level fusion involves 3 or more vertebrae (e.g., L3-L5, L4-S1, etc).

Effective for services performed on or after September 15, 1980, nonunion of long bone fractures, for both noninvasive and invasive devices, is considered to exist only after six or more months have elapsed without healing of the fracture.

Effective for services performed on or after April 1, 2000, nonunion of long bone fractures, for both noninvasive and invasive devices, is considered to exist only when serial radiographs have confirmed that fracture healing has ceased for three or more months prior to starting treatment with the electrical osteogenic stimulator. Serial radiographs must include a minimum of two sets of radiographs, each including multiple views of the fracture site, separated by a minimum of 90 days.

B. Ultrasonic Osteogenic Stimulators.—An ultrasonic osteogenic stimulator is a non-invasive device that emits low intensity, pulsed ultrasound. The ultrasound signal is applied to the skin surface at the fracture location via ultrasound conductive gel in order to stimulate fracture healing.

Effective for services performed on or after January 1, 2001, ultrasonic osteogenic stimulators are covered as medically reasonable and necessary for the treatment of non-union fractures. In demonstrating nonunion of fractures, we would expect:

1. A minimum of two sets of radiographs obtained prior to starting treatment with the osteogenic stimulator, separated by a minimum of 90 days. Each radiograph must include multiple views of the fracture site accompanied with a written interpretation by a physician stating that there has been no clinically significant evidence of fracture healing between the two sets of radiographs.

2. Indications that the patient failed at least one surgical intervention for the treatment of the fracture.

Non-unions of the skull, vertebrae, and those that are tumor-related are excluded from coverage. The ultrasonic osteogenic stimulator may not be used concurrently with other non-invasive osteogenic devices. The national non-coverage policy related to ultrasonic osteogenic stimulators for fresh fractures and delayed unions remains in place. This policy relates only to non-union as defined above.

35-61 TRANSSEXUAL SURGERY (140.3)

Transsexual surgery, also known as sex reassignment surgery or intersex surgery, is the culmination of a series of procedures designed to change the anatomy of transsexuals to conform to their gender identity. Transsexuals are persons with an overwhelming desire to change anatomic sex because of their fixed conviction that they are members of the opposite sex. For the male-to-female, transsexual surgery entails castration, penectomy and vulva-vaginal construction. Surgery for the female-to-male transsexual consists of bilateral mammectomy, hysterectomy and salpingo-oophorectomy, which may be followed by phalloplasty and the insertion of testicular prostheses.

Transsexual surgery for sex reassignment of transsexuals is controversial. Because of the lack of well-controlled, long-term studies of the safety and effectiveness of the surgical procedures and attendant therapies for transsexualism, the treatment is considered experimental. Moreover, there is a high rate of serious complications for these surgical procedures. For these reasons, transsexual surgery is not covered.

35-64 CHELATION THERAPY FOR TREATMENT OF ATHEROSCLEROSIS (20.21)

Chelation therapy is the application of chelation techniques for the therapeutic or preventive effects of removing unwanted metal ions from the body. The application of chelation therapy using ethylenediamine-tetra-acetic acid (EDTA) for the treatment and prevention of atherosclerosis is controversial. There is no widely accepted rationale to explain the beneficial effects attributed to

this therapy. Its safety is questioned and its clinical effectiveness has never been established by well designed, controlled clinical trials. It is not widely accepted and practiced by American physicians. EDTA chelation therapy for atherosclerosis is considered experimental. For these reasons, EDTA chelation therapy for the treatment or prevention of atherosclerosis is not covered.

Some practitioners refer to this therapy as chemoendarterectomy and may also show a diagnosis other than atherosclerosis, such as arteriosclerosis or calcinosis. Claims employing such variant terms should also be denied under this section.

Cross-refer: section 45-20

35-65 GASTRIC FREEZING (100.6)

Gastric freezing for chronic peptic ulcer disease is a non-surgical treatment which was popular about 20 years ago but now is seldom done. It has been abandoned due to a high complication rate, only temporary improvement experienced by patients, and lack of effectiveness when tested by double-blind, controlled clinical trials. Since the procedure is now considered obsolete, it is not covered.

35-74 EXTERNAL COUNTERPULSATION (ECP) FOR SEVERE ANGINA—COVERED (20.20)

External counterpulsation (ECP), commonly referred to as enhanced external counterpulsation, is a non-invasive outpatient treatment for coronary artery disease refractory to medical and/or surgical therapy. Although ECP devices are cleared by the Food and Drug Administration (FDA) for use in treating a variety of cardiac conditions, including stable or unstable angina pectoris, acute myocardial infarction, and cardiogenic shock. The use of this device to treat cardiac conditions other than stable angina pectoris is not covered, since only that use has developed sufficient evidence to demonstrate its medical effectiveness. Non Coverage of hydraulic versions of these types of devices remains in force.

Coverage is provided for the use of ECP for patients who have been diagnosed with disabling angina (Class III or Class IV, Canadian Cardiovascular Society Classification or equivalent classification) who, in the opinion of a cardiologist or cardiothoracic surgeon, are not readily amenable to surgical intervention, such as PTCA or cardiac bypass because: (1) their condition is inoperable, or at high risk of operative complications or post-operative failure; (2) their coronary anatomy is not readily amenable to such procedures; or (3) they have co-morbid states which create excessive risk.

A full course of therapy usually consists of 35 one-hour treatments which may be offered once or twice daily, usually 5 days per week. The patient is placed on a treatment table where the lower trunk and lower extremities are wrapped in a series of three compressive air cuffs which inflate and deflate in synchronization with the patient's cardiac cycle.

During diastole the three sets of air cuffs are inflated sequentially (distal to proximal) compressing the vascular beds within the muscles of the calves, lower thighs, and upper thighs. This action results in an increase in diastolic pressure, generation of retrograde arterial blood flow, and an increase in venous return. The cuffs are deflated simultaneously just prior to systole, which produces a rapid drop in vascular impedance, a decrease in ventricular workload, and an increase in cardiac output.

The augmented diastolic pressure and retrograde aortic flow appear to improve myocardial perfusion, while systolic unloading appears to reduce cardiac workload and oxygen requirements. The increased venous return coupled with enhanced systolic flow appears to increase cardiac output. As a result of this treatment, most patients experience increased time until onset of ischemia, increased exercise tolerance, and a reduction in the number and severity of anginal episodes. Evidence was presented that this effect lasted well beyond the immediate post-treatment phase, with patients symptom-free for several months to two years.

This procedure must be done under direct supervision of a physician.

35-77 NEUROMUSCULAR ELECTRICAL STIMULATION (NMES) (150.4)

Neuromuscular electrical stimulation (NMES) involves the use of a device which transmits an electrical impulse to activate muscle groups by way of electrodes. There are two broad categories of NMES. One type of device stimulates the muscle when the patient is in a resting state to treat muscle atrophy. The second type is used to enhance functional activity of neurologically impaired patients.

Treatment of Muscle Atrophy

Coverage of NMES to treat muscle atrophy is limited to the treatment of patients with disuse atrophy where the nerve supply to the muscle is intact, including brain, spinal cord and peripheral nerves and other nonneurological reasons for disuse atrophy. Examples include casting or splinting of a limb, contracture due to scarring of soft tissue as in burn lesions, and hip replacement surgery (until orthotic training begins). (See CIM 45-25 for an explanation of coverage of medically necessary supplies for the effective use of NMES).

Use for Walking in Patients with Spinal Cord Injury (SCI)

The type of NMES that is used to enhance the ability to walk of SCI patients is commonly referred to as functional electrical stimulation (FES). These devices are surface units that use electrical impulses to activate paralyzed or weak muscles in precise sequence. Coverage for the use of NMES/FES is limited to SCI patients, for walking, who have completed a training program, which consists of at least 32 physical therapy sessions with the device over a period of 3 months. The trial period of physical therapy will enable the physician treating the patient for his or her spinal cord injury to properly evaluate the person's ability to use these devices frequently and for the long term. Physical therapy sessions are only covered in the inpatient hospital, outpatient hospital, comprehensive outpatient rehabilitation facilities, and outpatient rehabilitation facilities. The physical therapy necessary to perform this training must be directly performed by the physical therapist as part of a one-on-one training program; this service cannot be done unattended.

The goal of physical therapy must be to train SCI pateints on the use of NMES/FES devices to achieve walking, not to reverse or retard muscle atrophy.

Coverage for NMES/FES for walking will be limited to SCI patients with all of the following characteristics:

1. Persons with intact lower motor units (L1 and below) (both muscle and peripheral nerve);

2. Persons with muscle and joint stability for weight bearing at upper and lower extremities that can demonstrate balance and control to maintain an upright support posture independently;

3. Persons that demonstrate brisk muscle contraction to NMES and have sensory perception of electrical stimulation sufficient for muscle contraction;

4. Persons that possess high motivation, commitment and cognitive ability to use such devices for walking;

5. Persons that can transfer independently and can demonstrate independent standing tolerance for at least 3 minutes;

6. Persons that can demonstrate hand and finger function to manipulate controls;

7. Persons with at least 6-month post recovery spinal cord injury and restorative surgery;

8. Persons without hip and knee degenerative disease and no history of long bone fracture secondary to osteoporosis; and

9. Persons who have demonstrated a willingness to use the device long-term.

NMES/FES for walking will not be covered in SCI patients with any of the following:

1. Persons with cardiac pacemakers;

2. Severe scoliosis or severe osteoporosis;

3. Skin disease or cancer at area of stimulation;

4. Irreversible contracture; or

5. Autonomic dysreflexia.

The only settings where therapists with the sufficient skills to provide these services are employed, are inpatient hospitals, outpatient hospitals, comprehensive outpatient rehabilitation facilities and outpatient rehabilitation facilities. The physical therapy necessary to perform this training must be part of a one-on-one training program.

Additional therapy after the purchase of the DME would be limited by our general policies on coverage of skilled physical therapy.

All other uses of NMES remain non-covered.

(Also reference Medicare Carriers Manual, Part 3, Claims-§2210 and Medicare Intermediary Manual, Part 3, Claims-§3653—See—Maintenance Program 271.1)

35-90 EXTRACORPOREAL IMMUNOADSORPTION (ECI) USING PROTEIN A COLUMNS (20.5)

Extracorporeal immunoadsorption (ECI), using protein A columns, has been developed for the purpose of selectively removing circulating immune complexes (CIC) and immunoglobulins (IgG) from patients in whom these substances are associated with their diseases. The technique involves pumping the patient's anticoagulated venous blood through a cell separator from which 1 to 3 liters of plasma are collected and perfused over adsorbent columns, after which the plasma rejoins the separated, unprocessed cells and is retransfused to the patient.

For claims with dates of service on or after January 1, 2001, Medicare covers the use of Protein A columns for the treatment of ITP. In addition, Medicare will cover Protein A columns for the treatment of rheumatoid arthritis (RA) under the following conditions:

1. Patient has severe RA. Patient disease is active, having > 5 swollen joints, > 20 tender joints, and morning stiffness > 60 minutes.

2. Patient has failed an adequate course of a minimum of 3 Disease Modifying Anti-Rheumatic Drugs (DMARDs). Failure does not include intolerance.

Other uses of these columns are currently considered to be investigational and, therefore, not reasonable and necessary under the Medicare law. (See '1862(a)(1)(A) of the Act.)

35-93 LUNG VOLUME REDUCTION SURGERY (REDUCTION PNEUMOPLASTY, ALSO CALLED LUNG SHAVING OR LUNG CONTOURING) UNILATERAL OR BILATERAL BY OPEN OR THORACOSCOPIC APPROACH FOR TREATMENT OF EMPHYSEMA OR CHRONIC OBSTRUCTIVE PULMONARY DISEASE—NOT GENERALLY COVERED (240.1)

Lung volume reduction surgery (LVRS) or reduction pneumoplasty, also referred to as lung shaving or lung contouring, is performed on patients with severe emphysema in order to allow the remainin compressed lung to expand, and thus, improve respiratory function.

Covered Indications

Medicare-covered LVRS approaches are limited to bilateral excision of a damaged lung with stapling performed via median sternotomy or video-assisted thoracoscopic surgery.

1. National Emphysema Treatment Trial (NETT) participants (effective for services performed on or after August 11, 1997):

Medicare provides coverage to those beneficiaries who are participating in the NETT trial for all services integral to the study and for which the Medicare statute does not prohibit coverage.

2. Medicare will only consider LVRS reasonable and necessary when all of the following requirements are met (effective for services performed on or after January 1, 2004):

a. The patient satisfies all the criteria outlined below:

Assessment	Criteria
History and physical examination	Consistent with emphysema BMI, ≤31.1 kg/m² (men) or ≤32.3 kg/m² (women) Stable with ≤20 mg prednisone (or equivalent) qd
Radiographic	High Resolution Computer Tomography (HRCT) scan evidence of bilateral emphysema
Pulmonary function (pre-rehabilitation)	Forced expiratory volume in one second (FEV₁) ≤ 45% predicted (≥15% predicted if age ≥70 years) Total hung capacity (TLC) ≥ 100% predicted post-bronchodilator Residual volume (RV) ≥ 150% predicted post-bronchodilator
Arterial blood gas level (pre-rehabilitation)	PCO₂, ≤60 mm Hg (PCO₂, ≤55 mm Hg if 1-mile above sea level) PO₂, ≥45 mm Hg on room air (PO₂, ≥30 mm Hg if 1-mile above sea level)
Cardiac assessment	Approval for surgery by cardiologist if any of the following are present: Unstable angina; left-ventricular ejection fraction (LVEF) cannot be estimated from the echocardiogram; LVEF <45%; dobutamine-radionuclide cardiac scan indicates coronary artery disease or ventricular dysfunction; arrhythmia (>5 premature ventricular contractions per minute; cardiac rhythm other than sinus; premature ventricular contractions on EKG at rest)
Surgical assessment	Approval for surgery by pulmonary physician, thoracic surgeon, and anesthesiologist post-rehabilitation
Exercise	Post-rehabilitation 6-min walk of ≥140 m; able to complete 3 min unloaded pedaling in exercise tolerance test (pre- and post-rehabilitation)
Consent	Signed consents for screening and rehabilitation
Smoking	Plasma continine level ≤13.7 ng/mL (or arterial carboxyhemoglobin ≤2.5% if using nicotine products) Nonsmoking for 4 months prior to initial interview and throughout evaluation for surgery
Preoperative diagnostic and therapeutic program adherence	Must complete assessment for and program of preoperative services in preparation for surgery

b. In addition, the patient must have:

• Severe upper lobe predominant emphysema (as defined by radiologist assessment of upper lobe predominance on CT scan), or

• Severe non-upper lobe emphysema with low exercise capacity.

Patients with low evercise capacity are those whose maximal exercise capacity is at or below 25 watts for women and 40 watts (w) for men after completion of the preoperative therapeutic program in preparation for LVRS. Exercise capacity is measured by incremantal, maximal, symptom-limited exercise with a cycle ergometer utilizing 5 or 10 watt/minute ramp on 30% oxygen after 3 minutes of unloaded pedaling.

c. The surgery must be performed at facilities that were identified by the National Heart, Lung, and Blood Institute to meet the thresholds for participation in the NETT, and at sites

that have been approved by Medicare as lung transplant facilities. These facilities are listed on our Web site at *www.cms.hhs.gov/coverage/lvrsfacility.pdf*. The CMS is currently working to develop accreditation standards for facilities to perform LVRS and when implemented, will consider LVRS to be reasonable and necessary only at accredited facilities.

d. The surgery must be preceded and followed by a program of diagnostic and therapeutic services consistent with those provided in the NETT and designed to maximize the patient's potential to successfully undergo and recovery from surgery. The program must include a 6- to 10-week series of at least 16, and no more than 20, preoperative sessions, each lasting a minimum of 2 hours. It must also include at least 6, and no more than 10, postoperative sessions, each lasting a minimum of 2 hours, within 8 to 9 weeks of the LVRS. This program must be consistent with the care plan developed by the treating physician following performance of a comprehensive evaluation of the patient's medical, psychosocial and nutritional needs, be consistent with the preoperative and postoperative services provided in the NETT, and arranged, monitored, and performed under the coordination of the facility where the surgery takes place.

Noncovered Indications

1. LVRS is not covered in any of the following clinical circumstances:

a. Patient characteristics carry a high risk for perioperative morbidity and/or mortality;

b. The disease is unsuitable for LVRS;

c. Medical conditions or other circumstances make it likely that the patient will be unable to complete the preoperative and postoperative pulmonary diagnostic and therapeutic program required for surgery;

d. The patient presents with FEV₁ ≤ 20% of predicted value, and either homogeneous distribution of emphysema on CT scan, or carbon monoxide diffusing capacity of ≤20% of predicted value (high-risk group identified October 2001 by the NETT); or

e. The patient satisfies the criteria outlined above in section 2(a), and has severe, non-upper lobe emphysema with high exercise capacity. High exercise capacity is defined as a maximal workload at the completion of the preoperative diagnostic and therapeutic program that is above 25 w for women and 40 w for men (under the measurement conditions for cycle ergometry specified above).

2. All other indications for LVRS not otherwise specified remain noncovered.

(This NCD last reviewed October 2003.)

35-96 CRYOSURGERY OF PROSTATE (Effective for services performed on or after July 1, 1999) (230.9)

Cryosurgery of the prostate gland, also known as cryosurgical ablation of the prostate (CSAP), destroys prostate tissue by applying extremely cold temperatures in order to reduce the size of the prostate gland. It is safe and effective, as well as medically necessary and appropriate, as primary treatment for patients with clinically localized prostate cancer, Stages T1–T3.

Cryosurgery of the prostate as a salvage therapy is not covered for any services performed prior to June 30, 2001.

35-103 MULTIPLE ELECTROCONVULSIVE THERAPY (MECT) (Effective for services provided on or after April 1, 2003) (160.25)

The clinical effectiveness of the multiple-seizure electroconvulsive therapy has not been verified by scientifically controlled studies. In addition, studies have demonstrated an increased risk of adverse effects with multiple seizures. Accordingly, MECT cannot be considered reasonable and necessary and is not covered by the Medicare program.

45-4 VITAMIN B12 INJECTIONS TO STRENGTHEN TENDONS, LIGAMENTS, ETC., OF THE FOOT—NOT COVERED (150.6)

Vitamin B12 injections to strengthen tendons, ligaments, etc., of the foot are not covered under Medicare because (1) there is no evidence that vitamin B12 injections are effective for the purpose of strengthening weakened tendons and ligaments, and (2) this is nonsurgical treatment under the subluxation exclusion. Accordingly, vitamin B12 injections are not considered reasonable and necessary within the meaning of section 1862(a)(1) of the Act.

See Intermediary Manual sections 3101.3 and 3158, and Carriers Manual, sections 2050.5 and 2323.

45-7 HYDROPHILIC CONTACT LENS FOR CORNEAL BANDAGE (80.1)

Some hydrophilic contact lenses are used as moist corneal bandages for the treatment of acute or chronic corneal pathology, such as bullous keratopathy, dry eyes, corneal ulcers and erosion, keratitis, corneal edema, descemetocele, corneal ectasis, Mooren's ulcer, anterior corneal dystrophy, neurotrophic keratoconjunctivitis, and for other therapeutic reasons.

Payment may be made under section 1861(s)(2) of the Act for a hydrophilic contact lens approved by the Food and Drug Administration (FDA) and used as a supply incident to a physician's service. Payment for the lens is included in the payment for the physician's service to which the lens is incident. Contractors are authorized to accept an FDA letter of approval or other FDA published material as evidence of FDA approval. (See §80.4 for coverage of a hydrophilic contact lens as a prosthetic device.) See the Medicare Benefit Policy Manual, Chapter 15, "Covered Medical and Other Health Services," and the Medicare Benefit Policy Manual, Chapter 6, "Hospital Services Covered Under Part B," §20.4

45-10 LAETRILE AND RELATED SUBSTANCES—NOT COVERED (30.7)

Laetrile (and the other drugs called by the various terms mentioned below) have been used primarily in the treatment or control of cancer. Although the terms "Laetrile," "laetrile," "amygdalin," "Sarcarcinase," "vitamin B-17," and "nitriloside" have been used interchangeably, the chemical identity of the substances to which these terms refer has varied.

The FDA has determined that neither Laetrile nor any other drug called by the various terms mentioned above, nor any other product which might be characterized as a "nitriloside" is generally recognized (by experts qualified by scientific training and experience to evaluate the safety and effectiveness of drugs) to be safe and effective for any therapeutic use. Therefore, use of this drug cannot be considered to be reasonable and necessary within the meaning of section 1862(a)(1) of the Act and program payment may not be made for its use or any services furnished in connection with its administration.

A hospital stay only for the purpose of having laetrile (or any other drug called by the terms mentioned above) administered is not covered. Also, program payment may not be made for laetrile (or other drug noted above) when it is used during the course of an otherwise covered hospital stay, since the FDA has found such drugs to not be safe and effective for any therapeutic purpose.

45-15 PHYSICIAN'S OFFICE WITHIN AN INSTITUTION— COVERAGE OF SERVICES AND SUPPLIES INCIDENT TO A PHYSICIAN'S SERVICES (70.3)

When a physician establishes an office within a nursing home or other institution, coverage of services and supplies furnished in the office must be determined in accordance with the "incident to a physician's professional service" provision (see the Medicare Benefit Policy Manual, Chapter 6, "Hospital Services Covered Under Part B," §20.4.1 or the Medicare Benefit Policy Manual, Chapter 15, "Covered Medical and Other Health Services," §60.1) as in any physician's office. A physician's office within an institution must be confined to a separately identified part of the facility that is used solely as the physician's office and cannot be construed to

extend throughout the entire institution. Thus, services performed outside the "office" area would be subject to the coverage rules applicable to services furnished outside the office setting.

In order to accurately apply the criteria in the Medicare Benefit Policy Manual, Chapters 6, §20.4.1, or Chapter 15, "Covered Medical and Other Health Services," §60.1, the contractor gives consideration to the physical proximity of the institution and physician's office. When his office is located within a facility, a physician may not be reimbursed for services, supplies, and use of equipment which fall outside the scope of services "commonly furnished" in physician's offices generally, even though such services may be furnished in his institutional office. Additionally, make a distinction between the physician's office practice and the institution, especially when the physician is administrator or owner of the facility. Thus, for their services to be covered under the criteria in the Medicare Benefit Policy Manual, Chapter 6, §20.4.1, or the Medicare Benefit Policy Manual, Chapter 15, "Covered Medical and Other Health Services," §60.1, the auxiliary medical personnel must be members of the office staff rather than of the institution's staff, and the cost of supplies must represent an expense to the physician's office practice. Finally, services performed by the employees of the physician outside the "office" area must be **directly** supervised by the physician; his presence in the facility as a whole would not suffice to meet this requirement. (In **any** setting, of course, supervision of auxiliary personnel in and of itself is not considered a "physician's professional service" to which the services of the auxiliary personnel could be an incidental part, i.e., in addition to supervision, the physician must perform or have performed a personal professional service to the patient to which the services of the auxiliary personnel could be considered an incidental part.) Denials for failure to meet any of these requirements would be based on §1861(s)(2)(A) of the Act.

Establishment of an office within an institution would not modify rules otherwise applicable for determining coverage of the physician's personal professional services within the institution. However, in view of the opportunity afforded to a physician who maintains such an office for rendering services to a sizable number of patients in a short period of time or for performing frequent services for the same patient, claims for physicians' services rendered under such circumstances would require careful evaluation by the carrier to assure that payment is made only for services that are reasonable and necessary.

Cross-refer: The Medicare Benefit Policy Manual, Chapter 15, "Covered Medical and Other Health Services." The Medicare Benefit Policy Manual, Chapter 6, "Hospital Services Covered Under Part B," §20.4.1.

45-16 CERTAIN DRUGS DISTRIBUTED BY THE NATIONAL CANCER INSTITUTE (110.2)

Under its Cancer Therapy Evaluation, the Division of Cancer Treatment of the National Cancer Institute (NCI), in cooperation with the Food and Drug Administration, approves and distributes certain drugs for use in treating terminally ill cancer patients. One group of these drugs, designated as Group C drugs, unlike other drugs distributed by the NCI, are not limited to use in clinical trials for the purpose of testing their efficacy. Drugs are classified as Group C drugs only if there is sufficient evidence demonstrating their efficacy within a tumor type and that they can be safely administered.

A physician is eligible to receive Group C drugs from the Divison of Cancer Treatment only if the following requirements are met:

- A physician must be registered with the NCI as an investigator by having completed an FD-Form 1573;
- A written request for the drug, indicating the disease to be treated, must be submitted to the NCI;
- The use of the drug must be limited to indications outlined in the NCI's guidelines; and
- All adverse reactions must be reported to the Investigational Drug Branch of the Division of Cancer Treatment.

In view of these NCI controls on distribution and use of Group C drugs, intermediaries may assume, in the absence of evidence to the contrary, that a Group C drug and the related hospital stay are covered if all other applicable coverage requirements are satisfied.

If there is reason to question coverage in a particular case, the matter should be resolved with the assistance of the local PSRO, or if there is none, the assistance of your medical consultants.

Information regarding those drugs which are classified as Group C drugs may be obtained from:

Office of the Chief, Investigational Drug Branch
Division of Cancer Treatment, CTEP, Landow Building
Room 4C09, National Cancer Institute
Bethesda, Maryland 20205

45-20 ETHYLENEDIAMINE-TETRA-ACETIC (EDTA) CHELATION THERAPY FOR TREATMENT OF ATHEROSCLEROSIS (20.22)

The use of EDTA as a chelating agent to treat atherosclerosis, arteriosclerosis, calcinosis, or similar generalized condition not listed by the FDA as an approved use is not covered. Any such use of EDTA is considered experimental.

See section 35-64 for an explanation of this conclusion.

45-22 LYMPHOCYTE IMMUNE GLOBULIN, ANTI-THYMOCYTE GLOBULIN (EQUINE) (260.7)

The lymphocyte immune globulin preparations are biologic drugs not previously approved or licensed for use in the management of renal allograft rejection. A number of other lymphocyte immune globulin products of equine, lapine, and murine origin are currently under investigation for their potential usefulness in controlling allograft rejections in human transplantation. These biologic drugs are viewed as adjunctive to traditional immunosuppressive products such as steroids and anti-metabolic drugs. At present, lymphocyte immune globulin preparations are not recommended to replace conventional immunosuppressive drugs, but to supplement them and to be used as alternatives to elevated or accelerated dosing with conventional immunosuppressive agents.

The FDA has approved one lymphocyte immune globulin preparation for marketing, lymphocyte immune globulin, anti-thymocyte globulin (equine). This drug is indicated for the management of allograft rejection episodes in renal transplantation. It is covered under Medicare when used for this purpose. Other forms of lymphocyte globulin preparation which the FDA approves for this indication in the future may be covered under Medicare.

45-23 DIMETHYL SULFOXIDE (DMSO) (230.12)

DMSO is an industrial solvent produced as a chemical byproduct of paper production from wood pulp. The Food and Drug Administration has determined that the only purpose for which DMSO is safe and effective for humans is in the treatment of the bladder condition, interstitial cystitis. Therefore, the use of DMSO for all other indications is not considered to be reasonable and necessary. Payment may be made for its use only when reasonable and necessary for a patient in the treatment of interstitial cystitis.

45-24 ANTI-INHIBITOR COAGULANT COMPLEX (AICC) (110.3)

Anti-inhibitor coagulant complex, AICC, is a drug used to treat hemophilia in patients with factor VIII inhibitor antibodies. AICC has been shown to be safe and effective and has Medicare coverage when furnished to patients with hemophilia A and inhibitor antibodies to factor VIII who have major bleeding episodes and who fail to respond to other, less expensive therapies.

45-25 SUPPLIES USED IN THE DELIVERY OF TRANSCUTANEOUS ELECTRICAL NERVE STIMULATION (TENS) AND NEUROMUSCULAR ELECTRICAL STIMULATION (NMES) (160.13)

Transcutaneous Electrical Nerve Stimulation (TENS) and/or Neuromuscular Electrical Stimulation (NMES) can ordinarily be deliv-

ered to patients through the use of conventional electrodes, adhesive tapes and lead wires. There may be times, however, where it might be medically necessary for certain patients receiving TENS or NMES treatment to use, as an alternative to conventional electrodes, adhesive tapes and lead wires, a form-fitting conductive garment (i.e., a garment with conductive fibers which are separated from the patients' skin by layers of fabric).

A form-fitting conductive garment (and medically necessary related supplies) may be covered under the program only when:

　　1. It has received permission or approval for marketing by the Food and Drug Administration;

　　2. It has been prescribed by a physician for use in delivering covered TENS or NMES treatment; and

　　3. One of the medical indications outlined below is met:

• The patient cannot manage without the conductive garment because there is such a large area or so many sites to be stimulated and the stimulation would have to be delivered so frequently that it is not feasible to use conventional electrodes, adhesive tapes and lead wires;
• The patient cannot manage without the conductive garment for the treatment of chronic intractable pain because the areas or sites to be stimulated are inaccessible with the use of conventional electrodes, adhesive tapes and lead wires;
• The patient has a documented medical condition such as skin problems that preclude the application of conventional electrodes, adhesive tapes and lead wires;
• The patient requires electrical stimulation beneath a cast either to treat disuse atrophy, where the nerve supply to the muscle is intact, or to treat chronic intractable pain; or
• The patient has a medical need for rehabilitation strengthening (pursuant to a written plan of rehabilitation) following an injury where the nerve supply to the muscle is intact.

A conductive garment is not covered for use with a TENS device during the trial period specified in section 35-46 unless:

　　4. The patient has a documented skin problem prior to the start of the trial period; and

　　5. The carrier's medical consultants are satisfied that use of such an item is medically necessary for the patient.

(See conditions for coverage of the use of TENS in the diagnosis and treatment of chronic intractable pain in sections 35-46 and 60-20 and the use of NMES in the treatment of disuse atrophy in section 35-77.)

45-30 PHOTOSENSITIVE DRUGS (80.3)

Verteporfin

Verteporfin, a benzoporphyrin derivative, is an intravenous lipophilic photosensitive drug with an absorption peak of 690 nm. This drug was first approved by the Food and Drug Administration (FDA) on April 12, 2000, and subsequently, approved for inclusion in the United States Pharmacopoeia on July 18, 2000, meeting Medicare's definition of a drug when used in conjunction with ocular photodynamic therapy (see §80.2, "Photodynamic Therapy") when furnished intravenously incident to a physician's service. For patients with age-related macular degeneration, Verteporfin is only covered with a diagnosis of neovascular age-related macular degeneration (ICD-9-CM 362.52) with predominately classic subfoveal choroidal neovascular (CNV) lesions (where the area of classic CNV occupies ≥50 percent of the area of the entire lesion) at the initial visit as determined by a fluorescein angiogram (CPT code 92235*). Subsequent follow-up visits will require a fluorescein angiogram prior to treatment. OPT with verteporfin is covered for the above indication and will remain noncovered for all other indications related to AMD (see §80.2). OPT with Verteporfin for use in non-AMD conditions is elgible for coverage through individual contractor discretion.

---

*CPT only © 2003. *Current Procedural Terminology, 2004 Professional Edition*, American Medical Association. All Rights Reserved.

50 DIAGNOSTIC SERVICES (20.8.1)

50-1 Cardiac Pacemaker Evaluation Services—Medicare covers a variety of services for the post-implant follow-up and evaluation of implanted cardiac pacemakers. The following guidelines are designed to assist contractors in identifying and processing claims for such services.

NOTE: These new guidelines are limited to lithium battery-powered pacemakers, because mercury-zinc battery-powered pacemakers are no longer being manufactured and virtually all have been replaced by lithium units. Contractors still receiving claims for monitoring such units should continue to apply the guidelines published in 1980 to those units until they are replaced.

There are two general types of pacemakers in current use—single-chamber pacemakers, which sense and pace the ventricles of the heart, and dual-chamber pacemakers which sense and pace both the atria and the ventricles. These differences require different monitoring patterns over the expected life of the units involved. One fact of which contractors should be aware is that many dual-chamber units may be programmed to pace only the ventricles; this may be done either at the time the pacemaker is implanted or at some time afterward. In such cases, a dual-chamber unit, when programmed or reprogrammed for ventricular pacing, should be treated as a single-chamber pacemaker in applying screening guidelines.

The decision as to how often any patient's pacemaker should be monitored is the responsibility of the patient's physician who is best able to take into account the condition and circumstances of the individual patient. These may vary over time, requiring modifications of the frequency with which the patient should be monitored. In cases where monitoring is done by some entity other than the patient's physician, such as a commercial monitoring service or hospital outpatient department, the physician's prescription for monitoring is required and should be periodically renewed (at least annually) to assure that the frequency of monitoring is proper for the patient. Where a patient is monitored both during clinic visits and transtelephonically, the contractor should be sure to include frequency data on both types of monitoring in evaluating the reasonableness of the frequency of monitoring services received by the patient.

Since there are over 200 pacemaker models in service at any given point, and a variety of patient conditions that give rise to the need for pacemakers, the question of the appropriate frequency of monitorings is a complex one. Nevertheless, it is possible to develop guidelines within which the vast majority of pacemaker monitorings will fall and contractors should do this, using their own data and experience, as well as the frequency guidelines which follow, in order to limit extensive claims development to those cases requiring special attention.

Guidelines for Transtelephonic Monitoring of Cardiac Pacemakers

A. General.—Transtelephonic monitoring of pacemakers is coming into increasingly widespread use, with the services being furnished by commercial suppliers, hospital outpatient departments and physicians' offices.

Telephone monitoring of cardiac pacemakers as described below is medically efficacious in identifying early signs of possible pacemaker failure, thus reducing the number of sudden pacemaker failures requiring emergency replacement. All systems which monitor the pacemaker rate (bpm) in both the free-running and/or magnetic mode are effective in detecting subclinical pacemaker failure due to battery depletion. More sophisticated systems are also capable of detecting internal electronic problems within the pulse generator itself and other potential problems. In the case of dual chamber pacemakers in particular, such monitoring may detect failure of synchronization of the atria and ventricles, and the need for adjustment and reprogramming of the device.

NOTE: The transmitting device furnished to the patient is simply one component of the diagnostic system, and is not covered as durable medical equipment. Those engaged in trans-telephonic pacemaker monitoring should reflect the costs of the transmitters in setting their charges for monitoring.

B. Definition of Transtelephonic Monitoring.—In order for transtelephonic monitoring services to be covered, the services must consist of the following elements:

1. A minimum 30-second readable strip of the pacemaker in the free-running mode;

2. Unless contraindicated, a minimum 30-second readable strip of the pacemaker in the magnetic mode; and

3. A minimum 30 seconds of readable ECG strip.

C. Frequency Guidelines for Transtelephonic Monitoring.—The guidelines below constitute a system which contractors should use, in conjunction with their knowledge of local medical practices, to screen claims for transtelephonic monitoring prior to payment. It is important to note that they are not recommendations with respect to a minimum frequency for such monitorings, but rather a maximum frequency (within which payment may be made without further claims development). As with previous guidelines, more frequent monitorings may be covered in cases where contractors are satisfied that such monitorings are medically necessary; e.g., based on the condition of the patient, or with respect to pacemakers exhibiting unexpected defects or premature failure. Contractors should seek written justification for more frequent monitorings from the patient's physician and/or any monitoring service involved.

These guidelines are divided into two broad categories—Guideline I, which will apply to the majority of pacemakers now in use, and Guideline II, which will apply only to pacemaker systems (pacemaker and leads) for which sufficient long-term clinical information exists to assure that they meet the standards of the Inter-Society Commission for Heart Disease Resources (ICHD) for longevity and end-of-life decay. (The ICHD standards are: (1) 90 percent cumulative survival at 5 years following implant; and (2) an end-of-life decay of less than a 50 percent drop of output voltage and less than 20 percent deviation of magnet rate, or a drop of 5 beats per minute or less, over a period of 3 months or more.) Contractors should consult with their medical advisers and other appropriate individuals and organizations (such as the North American Society of Pacing and Electrophysiology, which publishes product reliability information) should questions arise over whether a pacemaker system meets the ICHD standards.

The two groups of guidelines are then further broken down into two general categories—single chamber and dual-chamber pacemakers. Contractors should be aware that the frequency with which a patient is monitored may be changed from time to time for a number of reasons, such as a change in the patient's overall condition, a reprogramming of the patient's pacemaker, the development of better information on the pacemaker's longevity or failure mode, etc. Consequently, changes in the proper set of guidelines may be required. Contractors should inform physicians and monitoring services to alert contractors to any changes in the patient's monitoring prescription that might necessitate changes in the screening guidelines applied to that patient. (Of particular importance is the reprogramming of a dual-chamber pacemaker to a single-chamber mode of operation. Such reprogramming would shift the patient from the appropriate dual-chamber guideline to the appropriate single-chamber guideline.)

Guideline I

1. Single-chamber pacemakers:
   1st month—every 2 weeks.
   2nd through 36th month—every 8 weeks.
   37th month to failure—every 4 weeks.

2. Dual-chamber pacemaker:
   1st month—every 2 weeks.
   2nd through 6th month—every 4 weeks.
   7th through 36th month—every 8 weeks.
   37th month to failure—every 4 weeks.

Guideline II

1. Single-chamber pacemakers:
   1st month—every 2 weeks.
   2nd through 48th month—every 12 weeks.
   49th through 72nd month—every 8 weeks.
   Thereafter—every 4 weeks.

2. Dual-chamber pacemaker:
   1st month—every 2 weeks.
   2nd through 30th month—every 12 weeks.
   31st through 48th month—every 8 weeks.
   Thereafter—every 4 weeks.

D. Pacemaker Clinic Services

1. General—Pacemaker monitoring is also covered when done by pacemaker clinics. Clinic visits may be done in conjunction with transtelephonic monitoring or as a separate service; however, the services rendered by a pacemaker clinic are more extensive than those currently possible by telephone. They include, for example, physical examination of patients and reprogramming of pacemakers. Thus, the use of one of these types of monitoring does not preclude concurrent use of the other.

2. Frequency Guidelines—As with transtelephonic pacemaker monitoring, the frequency of clinic visits is the decision of the patient's physician, taking into account, among other things, the medical condition of the patient. However, contractors can develop monitoring guidelines that will prove useful in screening claims. The following are recommendations for monitoring guidelines on lithium-battery pacemakers:

a. For single-chamber pacemakers—twice in the first 6 months following implant, then once every 12 months.

b. For dual-chamber pacemakers—twice in the first 6 months, then once every 6 months.

50-15 ELECTROCARDIOGRAPHIC SERVICES (20.15)

Reimbursement may be made under Part B for electrocardiographic (EKG) services rendered by a physician or incident to his/her services or by an approved laboratory or an approved supplier of portable X-ray services. Since there is no coverage for EKG services of any type rendered on a screening basis or as part of a routine examination, the claim must indicate the signs and symptoms or other clinical reason necessitating the services.

A separate charge by an attending or consulting physician for EKG interpretation is allowed only when it is the normal practice to make such charge in addition to the regular office visit charge. No payment is made for EKG interpretations by individuals other than physicians.

On a claim involving EKG services furnished by a laboratory or a portable X-ray supplier, identify the physician ordering the service and, when the charge includes both the taking of the tracing and its interpretation, include the identity of the physician making the interpretation. No separate bill for the services of a physician is paid unless it is clear that he/she was the patient's attending physician or was acting as a consulting physician. The taking of an EKG in an emergency, i.e., when the patient is or may be experiencing what is commonly referred to as a heart attack, is covered as a laboratory service or a diagnostic service by a portable X-ray supplier only when the evidence shows that a physician was in attendance at the time the service was performed or immediately thereafter.

Where EKG services are rendered in the patient's home and the laboratory's or portable X-ray supplier's charge is higher than that imposed for the same service when performed in the laboratory or portable X-ray supplier's office, the medical need for home service should be documented. In the absence of such justification, reimbursement for the service if otherwise medically necessary should be based on the reasonable charge applicable when performed in the laboratory or X-ray supplier's office.

The documentation required in the various situations mentioned above must be furnished not only when the laboratory or porta-

ble X-ray supplier bills the patient or carrier for its service, but also when such a facility bills the attending physician who, in turn, bills the patient or carrier for the EKG services. (In addition to the evidence required to document the claim, the laboratory or portable X-ray supplier must maintain in its records the referring physician's written order and the identity of the employee taking the tracing.)

Long-term EKG monitoring, also referred to as long-term EKG recording, Holter recording, or dynamic electrocardiography, is a diagnostic procedure which provides a continuous record of the electrocardiographic activity of a patient's heart while he is engaged in his daily activities.

The basic components of the long-term EKG monitoring systems are a sensing element, the design of which may provide either for the recording of electrocardiographic information on magnetic tape or for detecting significant variations in rate or rhythm as they occur, and a component for either graphically recording the electrocardiographic data or for visual or computer assisted analysis of the information recorded on magnetic tape. The long-term EKG permits the examination in the ambulant or potentially ambulant patient of as many as 70,000 heartbeats in a 12-hour recording while the standard EKG which is obtained in the recumbent position, yields information on only 50 to 60 cardiac cycles and provides only a limited data base on which diagnostic judgments may be made.

Many patients with cardiac arrhythmias are unaware of the presence of an irregularity in heart rhythm. Due to the transient nature of many arrhythmias and the short intervals in which the rhythm of the heart is observed by conventional standard EKG techniques, the offending arrhythmias can go undetected. With the extended examination provided by the long-term EKG, the physician is able not only to detect but also to classify various types of rhythm disturbances and waveform abnormalities and note the frequency of their occurrence. The knowledge of the reaction of the heart to daily activities with respect to rhythm, rate, conduction disturbances, and ischemic changes are of great assistance in directing proper therapy and rehabilitation.

This modality is valuable in both inpatient and outpatient diagnosis and therapy. Long-term monitoring of ambulant or potentially ambulant inpatients provides significant potential for reducing the length of stay for post-coronary infarct patients in the intensive care setting and may result in earlier discharge from the hospital with greater assurance of safety to the patients. The indications for the use of this technique, noted below, are similar for both inpatients and outpatients.

The long-term EKG has proven effective in detecting transient episodes of cardiac dysrhythmia and in permitting the correlation of these episodes with cardiovascular symptomatology. It is also useful for patients who have symptoms of obscure etiology suggestive of cardiac arrhythmia. Examples of such symptoms include palpitations, chest pain, dizziness, light-headedness, near syncope, syncope, transient ischemic episodes, dyspnea, and shortness of breath.

This technique would also be appropriate at the time of institution of any arrhythmic drug therapy and may be performed during the course of therapy to evaluate response. It is also appropriate for evaluating a change of dosage and may be indicated shortly before and after the discontinuation of anti-arrhythemic medication. The therapeutic response to a drug whose duration of action and peak of effectiveness is defined in hours cannot be properly assessed by examining 30 to 40 cycles on a standard EKG rhythm strip. The knowledge that all patients placed on anti-arrhythmic medication do not respond to therapy and the known toxicity of anti-arrhythmic agents clearly indicate that proper assessment should be made on an individual basis to determine whether medication should be continued and at what dosage level.

The long-term EKG is also valuable in the assessment of patients with coronary artery disease. It enables the documentation of etiology of such symptoms as chest pain and shortness of breath. Since the standard EKG is often normal during the intervals between the episodes of precordial pain, it is essential to obtain EKG information while the symptoms are occurring. The long-term EKG has enabled the correlation of chest symptoms with the objective evidence of ST-segment abnormalities. It is appropriate for patients who are recovering from an acute mycardial infarction or coronary insufficiency before and after discharge from the hospital, since it is impossible to predict which of these patients is subject to ventricular arrhythmias on the basis of the presence or absence of rhythm disturbances during the period of initial coronary care. The long-term EKG enables the physician to identify patients who are at a higher risk of dying suddenly in the period following an acute myocardial infarction. It may also be reasonable and necessary where the high-risk patient with known cardiovascular disease advances to a substantially higher level of activity which might trigger increased or new types of arrhythmias necessitating treatment. Such a high-risk case would be one in which there is documentation that acute phase arrhythmias have not totally disappeared during the period of convalesence.

In view of recent developments in cardiac pacemaker monitoring techniques (see CIA 50-1), the use of the long-term EKG for routine assessment of pacemaker function can no longer be justified. Its use for the patient with an internal pacemaker would be covered only when he has symptoms suggestive of arrhythmia not revealed by the standard EKG or rhythm strip.

These guidelines are intended as a general outline of the circumstances under which the use of this diagnostic procedure would be warranted. Each patient receiving a long-term EKG should be evaluated completely, prior to performance of this diagnostic study. A complete history and physical examination should be obtained and the indications for use of the long-term EKG should be reviewed by the referring physician.

The performance of a long-term EKG does not necessarily require the prior performance of a standard EKG. Nor does the demonstration of a normal standard EKG preclude the need for a long-term EKG. Finally, the demonstration of an abnormal standard EKG does not obviate the need for a long-term EKG if there is suspicion that the dysrhythmia is transient in nature.

A period of recording of up to 24 hours would normally be adequate to detect most transient arrhythmias and provide essential diagnostic information. The medical necessity for longer periods of monitoring must be documented.

Medical documentation for adjudicating claims for the use of the long-term EKG should be similar to other EKG services, X-ray services, and laboratory procedures. Generally, a statement of the diagnostic impression of the referring physician with an indication of the patient's relevant signs and symptoms should be sufficient for purposes of making a determination regarding the reasonableness and medical necessity for the use of this procedure. However, the intermediaries or carriers should require whatever additional documentation their medical consultants deem necessary to properly adjudicate the individual claim where the information submitted is not adequate.

It should be noted that the recording device furnished to the patient is simply one component of the diagnostic system and a separate charge for it will not be recognized under the durable medical equipment benefit.

Patient-Activated EKG Recorders, distributed under a variety of brand names, permit the patient to record an EKG upon manifestation of symptoms, or in response to a physician's order (e.g., immediately following strong exertion). Most such devices also permit the patient to simultaneously voice-record in order to describe symptoms and/or activity. In addition, some of these devices permit transtelephonic transmission of the recording to a physician's office, clinic, hospital, etc., having a decoder/recorder for review and analysis, thus eliminating the need to physically transport the tape. Some of these devices also permit a "time sampling" mode of operation. However, the "time sampling" mode is not covered—only the patient-activated mode of operation, when used for the indications described below, is covered at this time.

Services in connection with patient-activated EKG recorders are covered when used as an alternative to the long-term EKG monitoring (described above) for similar indications—detecting and characterizing symptomatic arrhythmias, regulation of anti-arrhythmic drug therapy, etc. Like long-term EKG monitoring, use of these devices is covered for evaluating patients with symptoms of obscure etiology suggestive of cardiac arrhythmia such as palpitations, chest pain, dizziness, lightheadedness, near syncope, syncope, transient ischemic episodes, dyspnea and shortness of breath.

As with long-term EKG monitors, patient-activated EKG recorders may be useful for both inpatient and outpatient diagnosis and therapy. While useful for assessing some post-coronary infarct patients in the hospital setting, these devices should not, however, be covered for outpatient monitoring of recently discharged post-infarct patients.

Computer Analyzed Electrocardiograms.—Computer interpretation of EKGs is recognized as a valid and effective technique which will improve the quality and availability of cardiology services. Reimbursement may be made for such computer service when furnished in the setting and under the circumstances required for coverage of other electrocardiographic services. Where either a laboratory's or a portable x-ray supplier's charge for EKG services includes the physician review and certification of the printout as well as the computer interpretation, the certifying physician must be identified on the CMS-1490 before the entire charge can be considered a reimbursable charge. Where the laboratory's (or portable x-ray supplier's) reviewing physician is not identified, the carrier should conclude that no professional component is involved and make its charge determination accordingly. If the supplying laboratory (or portable x-ray supplier when supplied by such a facility) does not include professional review and certification of the hard copy, a charge by the patient's physician may be recognized for the service. In any case the charge for the physician component should be substantially less than that for physician interpretation of the conventional EKG tracing in view of markedly reduced demand on the physician's time where computer interpretation is involved. Considering the unit cost reduction expected of this innovation, the total charge for the complete EKG service (taking of tracing and interpretation) when computer interpretation is employed should never exceed that considered reasonable for the service when physician interpretation is involved.

Transtelephonic Electrocardiographic Transmissions (Formerly Referred to as EKG Telephone Reporter Systems).—Effective for services furnished on and after March 1, 1980, coverage is extended to include the use of transtelephonic electrocardiographic (EKG) transmissions as a diagnostic service for the indications described below, when performed with equipment meeting the standards described below, subject to the limitations and conditions specified below. Coverage is further limited to the amounts payable with respect to the physician's service in interpreting the results of such transmissions, including charges for rental of the equipment. The device used by the beneficiary is part of a total diagnostic system and is not considered durable medical equipment.

1. Covered Uses.—The use of transtelephonic EKGs is covered for the following uses:

a. To detect, characterize, and document symptomatic transient arrhythmias;

b. To overcome problems in regulating antiarrhythmic drug dosage;

c. To carry out early posthospital monitoring of patients discharged after myocardial infarction; (only if 24-hour coverage is provided, see 4. below).

Since cardiology is a rapidly changing field, some uses other than those specified above may be covered if, in the judgment of the contractor's medical consultants, such a use was justifiable in the particular case. The enumerated uses above represent uses for which a firm coverage determination has been made, and for which contractors may make payment without extensive claims development or review.

2. Specifications for Devices.—The devices used by the patient are highly portable (usually pocket-sized) and detect and convert the normal EKG signal so that it can be transmitted via ordinary telephone apparatus to a receiving station. At the receiving end, the signal is decoded and transcribed into a conventional EKG. There are numerous devices available which transmit EKG readings in this fashion. For purposes of Medicare coverage, however, the transmitting devices must meet at least the following criteria:

a. They must be capable of transmitting EKG Leads, I, II, or III;

b. These lead transmissions must be sufficiently comparable to readings obtained by a conventional EKG to permit proper interpretation of abnormal cardiac rhythms.

3. Potential for Abuse—Need for Screening Guidelines.—While the use of these devices may often compare favorably with more costly alternatives, this is the case only where the information they contribute is actively utilized by a knowledgeable practitioner as part of overall medical management of the patient. Consequently, it is vital that contractors be aware of the potential for abuse of these devices, and adopt necessary screening and physician education policies to detect and halt potentially abusive situations. For example, use of these devices to diagnose and treat suspected arrhythmias as a routine substitute for more conventional methods of diagnosis, such as a careful history, physical examination, and standard EKG and rhythm strip would not be appropriate. Moreover, contractors should require written justification for use of such devices in excess of 30 consecutive days in cases involving detection of transient arrhythmias.

Contractors may find it useful to review claims for these devices with a view toward detecting patterns of practice which may be useful in developing schedules which may be adopted for screening such claims in the future.

4. Twenty-Four Hour Coverage.—No payment may be made for the use of these devices to carry out early posthospital monitoring of patients discharged after myocardial infarction unless provision is made for 24 hour coverage in the manner described below.

Twenty-four hour coverage means that there must be, at the monitoring site (or sites) an experienced EKG technician receiving calls; tape recording devices do not meet this requirement. Further, such technicians should have immediate access to a physician, and have been instructed in when and how to contact available facilities to assist the patient in case of emergencies.

Cross-refer: CMS-Pub. 13-3, sections 3101.5, 3110, 3112.3, CMS-Pub. 14-3, sections 2070, 2255, 2050.1

50-17 LABORATORY TESTS—CRD PATIENTS

A. Laboratory tests are essential to monitor the progress of CRD patients. The following list and frequencies of tests constitute the level and types of routine laboratory tests that are covered. Bills for other types of tests are considered non-routine. Routine tests at greater frequencies must include medical justification. Non-routine tests generally are justified by the diagnosis. The routinely covered regimen includes the following tests:

Per Dialysis
All hematocrit or hemoglobin and clotting time tests furnished incident to dialysis treatments.
Per Week
Prothrombin time for patients on anticoagulant therapy
Serum creatinine
Per Week or Thirteen Per Quarter
BUN
Monthly

CBC	Serum calcium
Serum potassium	Serum chloride
Serum bicarbonate	Serum phosphorous
Total protein	Serum albumin
Alkaline phosphatase	AST, SGOT
LDH	

Guidelines for tests other than those routinely performed include:
Serum aluminum—one every 3 months
Serum ferritin—one every 3 months

The following tests for hepatitis B are covered when patients first enter a dialysis facility: hepatitis B surface antigen (HBsAg) and Anti-HBs. Coverage of future testing in these patients depends on their serologic status and on whether they have been successfully immunized against hepatitis B virus. The following table summarizes the frequency of serologic surveillance for hepatitis B. Tests furnished according to this table do not require additional documentation and are paid separately because payment for maintenance dialysis treatments does not take them into account.

Vaccination and Serologic Status	Frequency of Screening	
	HBsAg Patients	Anti-HBs Patients
UNVACCINATED		
Susceptible	Monthly	Semiannually
HBsAg carrier	Annually	None
Anti-HBs-positive*	None	Annually
VACCINATED		
Anti-HBs-positive*	None	Annually
Low level or no anti-HBs	Monthly	Semiannually

*At least 10 sample ration units by radioimmunoassay or positive by enzyme immunoassay.

Patients who are in the process of receiving hepatitis B vaccines, but have not received the complete series, should continue to be routinely screened as susceptible. Between one and six months after the third dose, all vaccines should be tested for anti-HBs to confirm their response to the vaccine. Patients who have a level of anti-HBs of at least 10 sample ratio units (SRUs) by radioimmunoassay (RIA) or who are positive by enzyme immunoassay (EIA) are considered adequate responders to vaccine and need be tested only for anti-HBs annually to verify their immune status. If anti-HBs drops below 10 SRUs by RIA or is negative by EIA, a booster dose of hepatitis B vaccine should be given.

B. Laboratory tests are subject to the normal coverage requirements. If the laboratory services are performed by a free-standing facility, be sure it meets the conditions of coverage for independent laboratories.

50-20 DIAGNOSTIC PAP SMEARS (190.2)

A diagnostic Pap smear and related medically necessary services are covered under Medicare Part B when ordered by a physician under one of the following conditions:

• Previous cancer of the cervix, uterus, or vagina that has been or is presently being treated;
• Previous abnormal Pap smear;
• Any abnormal findings of the vagina, cervix, uterus, ovaries, or adnexa;
• Any significant complaint by the patient referrable to the female reproductive system; or
• Any signs or symptoms that might in the physician's judgment reasonably be related to a gynecologic disorder.

In respect to the last bullet, the contractor's medical staff must determine whether in a particular case a previous malignancy at another site is an indication for a diagnostic Pap smear or whether the test must be considered a screening Pap smear as described in section 50-20.1. Use the following CPT codes for indicating diagnostic Pap smears:

• 88150* Cytopathology, smears, cervical or vaginal (e.g., Papanicolaou), up to three smears; screening by technician under physician supervision; *or*
• 88151* Cytopathology, smears, cervical or vaginal (e.g., Papanicolaou), up to three smears; requiring interpretation by physician.

50-20.1 Screening PAP Smears and Pelvic Examinations for Early Detection of Cervical or Vaginal Cancer (210.2)

A screening Pap smear and related medically necessary services provided to a woman for the early detection of cervical cancer (including collection of the sample of cells and a physician's interpretation of the test results) and pelvic examination (including clinical breast examination) are covered under Medicare Part B when ordered by a physician (or authorized practitioner) under one of the following conditions:

- She has not had such a test during the preceding 3 years or is a woman of childbearing age (section 1861(nn) of the Act).
- There is evidence (on the basis of her medical history or other findings) that she is at high risk of developing cervical cancer and her physician (or authorized practitioner) recommends that she have the test performed more frequently than every 3 years.

High risk factors for cervical and vaginal cancer are:

- Early onset of sexual activity (under 16 years of age)
- Multiple sexual partners (five or more in a lifetime)
- History of sexually transmitted disease (including HIV infection)
- Fewer than three negative or any Pap smears within the previous 7 years; and
- DES (diethylstilbestrol)-exposed daughters of women who took DES during pregnancy.

NOTE: Claims for Pap smears must indicate the beneficiary's low or high risk status by including the appropriate ICD-9-CM on the line item (Item 24E of the CMS-1500).

- V76.2, special screening for malignant neoplasms of the cervix, **indicates low risk**; and
- V15.89, other specified personal history presenting hazards to health, **indicates high risk.**

If Pap smear or pelvic exam claims do not point to one of these diagnosis codes, the claim will reject in the Common Working File. Claims can contain up to four diagnosis codes, but the one pointed to on the line item must be either V76.2 or V15.89.

Definitions:

A woman as described in section 1861(nn) of the Act is a woman who is of childbearing age and has had a Pap smear test during any of the preceding 3 years that indicated the presence of cervical or vaginal cancer or other abnormality, or is at high risk of developing cervical or vaginal cancer.

A woman of childbearing age is one who is premenopausal and has been determined by a physician or other qualified practitioner to be of childbearing age, based upon the medical history or other findings.

"Other qualified practitioner," as defined in 42 CFR 410.56(a) includes a certified nurse midwife (as defined in section 1861(gg) of the Act), or a physician assistant, nurse practitioner, or clinical nurse specialist (as defined in section 1861(aa) of the Act) who is authorized under State law to perform the examination.

Screening Pelvic Examination:

Section 4102 of the Balanced Budget Act of 1997 provides for coverage of screening pelvic examinations (including a clinical breast examination) for all female beneficiaries, subject to certain frequency and other limitations. A screening pelvic examination (including a clinical breast examination) should include at least seven of the following eleven elements:

- Inspection and palpation of breasts for masses or lumps, tenderness, symmetry, or nipple discharge.
- Digital rectal examination including sphincter tone, presence of hemorrhoids, and rectal masses. Pelvic examination (with or without specimen collection for smears and cultures) including:
- External genitalia (e.g., general appearance, hair distribution, or lesions).
- Urethral meatus (e.g., size, location, lesions, or prolapse).
- Urethra (e.g., masses, tenderness, or scarring).
- Bladder (e.g., fullness, masses, or tenderness).

- Vagina (e.g., general appearance, estrogen effect, discharge lesions, pelvic support, cystocele, or rectocele).
- Cervix (e.g., general appearance, lesions, or discharge).
- Uterus (e.g., size, contour, position, mobility, tenderness, consistency, descent, or support).
- Adnexa/parametria (e.g., masses, tenderness, organomegaly, or nodularity).
- Anus and perineum.

This description is from Documentation Guidelines for Evaluation and Management Services, published in May 1997 and was developed by Medicaid Services Centers for Medicare & the American Medical Association.

50-24 HAIR ANALYSIS—NOT COVERED (190.6)

Hair analysis to detect mineral traces as an aid in diagnosing human disease is not a covered service under Medicare.

The correlation of hair analysis to the chemical state of the whole body is not possible at this time, and therefore this diagnostic procedure cannot be considered to be reasonable and necessary under section 1862(a)(1) of the law.

50-36 POSITRON EMISSION TOMOGRAPHY (PET) SCANS (220.6)

I. General Description

Positron emission tomography (PET) is a noninvasive diagnostic imaging procedure that assesses the level of metabolic activity and perfusion in various organ systems of the [human] body. A positron camera (tomograph) is used to produce cross-sectional tomographic images, which are obtained from positron emitting radioactive tracer substances (radiopharmaceuticals) such as 2-[F-18] Fluoro-D-Glucose (FDG), that are administered intravenously to the patient.

The following indications may be covered for PET under certain circumstances. Details of Medicare PET coverage are discussed later in this section. Unless otherwise indicated, the clinical conditions below are covered when PET utilizes FDG as a tracer.

NOTE: All other uses of PET scans not listed in this manual are NOT covered.

Clinical Condition	Effective Date	Coverage
Solitary Pulmonary Nodules (SPNs)	January 1, 1998	Characterization
Lung Cancer (Non Small Cell)	January 1, 1998	Initial staging
Lung Cancer (Non Small Cell)	July 1, 2001	Diagnosis, staging and restaging
Esophageal Cancer	July 1, 2001	Diagnosis, staging and restaging
Colorectal Cancer	July 1, 1999	Determining location of tumors if rising CEA level suggests recurrence
Colorectal Cancer	July 1, 2001	Diagnosis, staging and restaging
Lymphoma	July 1, 1999	Staging and restaging only when used as an alternative to Gallium scan
Lymphoma	July 1, 2001	Diagnosis, staging and restaging
Melanoma	July 1, 1999	Evaluating recurrence prior to surgery as an alternative to a Gallium scan
Melanoma	July 1, 2001	Diagnosis, staging and restaging; Non-covered for evaluating regional nodes

Clinical Condition	Effective Date	Coverage
Breast Cancer	October 1, 2002	As an adjunct to standard imaging modalities for staging patients with distant metastasis or restaging patients with locoregional recurrence or metastasis; as an adjunct to standard imaging modalities for monitoring tumor response to treatment for women with locally advanced and metastatic breast cancer when a change in therapy is anticipated.
Head and Neck Cancers (excluding CNS and thyroid)	July 1, 2001	Diagnosis, staging and restaging
Myocardial Viability	July 1, 2001 to September 30, 2002	Covered only following inconclusive SPECT
Myocardial Viability	October 1, 2002	Primary or initial diagnosis, or following an inconclusive SPECT prior to revascularization. SPECT may not be used following an inconclusive PET scan.

Refractory Seizures	July 1, 2001	Covered for pre-surgical evaluation only
Perfusion of the heart using Rubidium 82* tracer	March 14, 1995	Covered for noninvasive imaging of the perfusion of the heart

* Not FDG-PET.

II. General Conditions of Coverage

A. Allowable FDG PET Systems

1. Definitions: For purposes of this section,

a. "Any FDA approved" means all systems approved or cleared for marketing by the FDA to image radionuclides in the body.

b. "FDA approved" means that the system indicated has been approved for cleared for marketing by the FDA to image radionuclides in the body.

c. "Certain coincidence sytems" refers to the systems that have all the following features:

- crystal at least 5/8-inch thick
- techniques to minimize or correct for scatter and/or randoms, and
- digital detectors and iterative reconstruction.

Scans performed with gamma camera PET systems with crystals thinner than 5/8-inch will not be covered by Medicare. In addition, scans performed with systems with crystals greater than or equal to 5/8-inch in thickness, but that do not meet the other listed design characteristics are not covered by Medicare.

2. Allowable PET systems by covered clinical indication:

	Allowable Type of FDG PET System		
Covered Clinical Condition	Prior to July 1, 2001	July 1, 2001 through December 31, 2001	On or after January 1, 2002
Characterization of single pulmonary nodules	Effective 1/1/1998, any FDA approved	Any FDA approved	FDA approved: Full ring Partial ring Certain coincidence systems
Initial staging of lung cancer (non small cell)	Effective 1/1/1998, any FDA approved	Any FDA approved	FDA approved: Full ring Partial ring Certain coincidence systems
Evaluating recurrence of melanoma prior to surgery as an alternative to a gallium scan	Effective 7/1/1999, any FDA approved	Any FDA approved	FDA approved: Full ring Partial ring Certain coincidence systems
Diagnosis, staging, and restaging of colorectal cancer	Not covered by Medicare	Full ring	FDA approved: Full ring Partial ring
Diagnosis, staging, and restaging of esophageal cancer	Not covered by Medicare	Full ring	FDA approved: Full ring Partial ring
Diagnosis, staging, and restaging of head and neck cancers (excluding CNS and thyroid)	Not covered by Medicare	Full ring	FDA approved: Full ring Partial ring
Diagnosis, staging, and restaging of lung cancer (non small cell)	Not covered by Medicare	Full ring	FDA approved: Full ring Partial ring
Diagnosis, staging, and restaging of lymphoma	Not covered by Medicare	Full ring	FDA approved: Full ring Partial ring
Diagnosis, staging, and restaging of melanoma (noncovered for evaluating regional nodes)	Not covered by Medicare	Full ring	FDA approved: Full ring Partial ring

	Allowable Type of FDG PET System		
Covered Clinical Condition	Prior to July 1, 2001	July 1, 2001 through December 31, 2001	On or after January 1, 2002
Determination of myocardial viability only following an inconclusive SPECT	Not covered by Medicare	Full ring	FDA approved: Full ring Partial ring
Presurgical evaluation of refractory seizures	Not covered by Medicare	Full ring	FDA approved: Full ring Partial ring
Breast Cancer	Not covered	Not covered	Effective October 1, 2002, Full and partial ring
Myocardial Viability Primary or initial diagnosis prior to revascularization	Not covered	Not covered	Effective October 1, 2002, Full and partial ring

B. Regardless of any other terms or conditions, all uses of FDG PET scans, in order to be covered by the Medicare program, must meet the following general conditions as of July 1, 2001:

1. PET scans are covered for those indications otherwise listed in this document. For indications covered beginning July 1, 2001, scans performed with dedicated full-ring scanners will be covered. In the decision memorandum of December 15, 2000, CMS had indicated that gamma camera systems with at least a 1 inch thick crystal would be eligible for coverage. However, coverage of PET using camera-based systems is now under further review as a separate national coverage determination. A final decision on what systems other than dedicated PET will be eligible for coverage, if any, will be announced prior to July 1, 2001. For those indications covered prior to July 1, 2001, all PET scanners approved or cleared for marketing by the FDA remain covered.

2. The provider of the PET scan should maintain on file the doctor's referral and documentation that the procedure involved only FDA approved drugs and devices, as is normal business practice.

3. The ordering physician is responsible for documenting the medical necessity of the study and that it meets the conditions specified in the instructions. The physician should have documentation in the beneficiary's medical record to support the referral to the PET scan provider.

4. Medicare coverage is predicated upon the use of PET scans with FDG for the purpose of development of appropriate treatment plans for patients. CMS will evaluate both the data produced by claims for these services, and data obtained from other sources, to determine whether, and to what extent, this coverage policy may need additional modification in order to assure that the services covered are medically effective for the treatment of Medicare beneficiaries.

III. Covered Indications for PET Scans and Limitations/Requirements for Usage

For all uses of PET relating to malignancies the following conditions apply:

1. Diagnosis: PET is covered only in clinical situations in which the PET results may assist in avoiding an invasive diagnostic procedure, or in which the PET results may assist in determining the optimal anatomical location to perform an invasive diagnostic procedure. In general, for most solid tumors, a tissue diagnosis is made prior to the performance of PET scanning. PET scans following a tissue diagnosis are performed for the purpose of staging, not diagnosis. Therefore, the use of PET in the diagnosis of lymphoma, esophageal, and colorectal cancers as well as in melanoma should be rare.

PET is not covered for other diagnostic uses, and is not covered for screening (testing of patients without specific signs and symptoms of disease).

2. Staging and or Restaging: PET is covered in clinical situations in which 1) (a) the stage of the cancer remains in doubt after completion of a standard diagnostic workup, including conventional imaging (computed tomography, magnetic resonance imaging, or ultrasound) or (b) the use of PET would also be considered reasonable and necessary if it could potentially replace one or more conventional imaging studies when it is expected that conventional study information is insufficient for the clinical management of the patient and 2) clinical management of the patient would differ depending on the stage of the cancer identified. PET will be covered for restaging after the completion of treatment for the purpose of detecting residual disease, for detecting suspected recurrence or to determine the extent of a known recurrence. Use of PET would also be considered reasonable and necessary if it could potentially replace one or more conventional imaging studies when it is expected that conventional study information is insufficient for the clinical management of the patient.

3. Monitoring: Use of PET to monitor tumor response during the planned course of therapy (i.e. when no change in therapy is being contemplated) is not covered, except for breast cancer. Restaging only occurs after a course of treatment is completed, and this is covered, subject to the conditions above.

NOTE: In the absence of national frequency limitations, contractors may, if necessary, develop frequency requirements on any or all of the indications covered on and after July 1, 2001.

IV. Coverage of PET for Perfusion of the Heart Using Rubidium 82

Effective for services performed on or after March 14, 1995, PET scans performed at rest or with pharmacological stress used for noninvasive imaging of the perfusion of the heart for the diagnosis and management of patients with known or suspected coronary artery disease using the FDA-approved radiopharmaceutical Rubidium 82 (Rb 82) are covered, provided the requirements below are met.

Requirements:

• The PET scan, whether at rest alone, or rest with stress, is performed in place of, but not in addition to, a single photon emission computed tomography (SPECT); or
• The PET scan, whether at rest alone or rest with stress, is used following a SPECT that was found to be inconclusive. In these cases, the PET scan must have been considered necessary in order to determine what medical or surgical intervention is required to treat the patient. (For purposes of this requirement, an inconclusive test is a test(s) whose results are equivocal, technically uninterpretable, or discordant with a patient's other clinical data and must be documented in the beneficiary's file.)
• For any PET scan for which Medicare payment is claimed for dates of services prior to July 1, 2001, the claimant must submit additional specified information on the claim form (including

proper codes and/or modifiers), to indicate the results of the PET scan. The claimant must also include information on whether the PET scan was done after an inconclusive noninvasive cardiac test. The information submitted with respect to the previous noninvasive cardiac test must specify the type of test done prior to the PET scan and whether it was inconclusive or unsatisfactory. These explanations are in the form of special G codes used for billing PET scans using Rb 82. Beginning July 1, 2001 claims should be submitted with the appropriate codes.

V. Coverage of FDG PET for Lung Cancer

The coverage for FDG PET for lung cancer, effective January 1, 1998, has been expanded. Beginning July 1, 2001 usage of FDG PET for lung cancer has been expanded to include diagnosis, staging, and restaging (see section III) of the disease.

A. Effective for services performed on or after January 1, 1998, Medicare covers regional FDG PET chest scans, on any FDA approved scanner, for the characterization of single pulmonary nodules (SPNs). The primary purpose of such characterization should be to determine the likelihood of malignancy in order to plan future management and treatment for the patient.

Beginning July 1, 2001, documentation should be maintained in the beneficiary's medical file at the referring physician's office to support the medical necessity of the procedure, as is normal business practice.

Requirements:

• There must be evidence of primary tumor. Claims for regional PET chest scans for characterizing SPNs should include evidence of the initial detection of a primary lung tumor, usually by computed tomography (CT). This should include, but is not restricted to, a report on the results of such CT or other detection method, indicating an indeterminate or possibly malignant lesion, not exceeding four centimeters (cm) in diameter.
• PET scan claims must include the results of concurrent thoracic CT (as noted above), which is necessary for anatomic information, in order to ensure that the PET scan is properly coordinated with other diagnostic modalities.
• In cases of serial evaluation of SPNs using both CT and regional PET chest scanning, such PET scans will not be covered if repeated within 90 days following a negative PET scan.

NOTE: A tissue sampling procedure (TSP) is not routinely covered in the case of a negative PET scan for characterization of SPNs, since the patient is presumed not to have a malignant lesion, based upon the PET scan results. When there has been a negative PET, the provider must submit additional information with the claim to support the necessity of a TSP, for review by the Medicare contractor.

B. Effective for services performed from January 1, 1998 through June 30, 2001, Medicare approved coverage of FDG PET for initial staging of non-small-cell lung carcinoma (NSCLC).

Limitations: This service is covered only when the primary cancerous lung tumor has been pathologically confirmed; claims for PET must include a statement or other evidence of the detection of such primary lung tumor. The evidence should include, but is not restricted to, a surgical pathology report, which documents the presence of an NSCLC. Whole body PET scan results and results of concurrent computed tomography (CT) and follow-up lymph node biopsy must be properly coordinated with other diagnostic modalities. Claims must include both:

• The results of concurrent thoracic CT, necessary for anatomic information, and
• The results of any lymph node biopsy performed to finalize whether the patient will be a surgical candidate. The ordering physician is responsible for providing this biopsy result to the PET facility.

NOTE: Where the patient is considered a surgical candidate, (given the presumed absence of metastatic NSCLC unless medical review supports a determination of medical necessity of a biopsy) a lymph node biopsy will not be covered in the case of a negative CT and negative PET. A

lymph node biopsy will be covered in all other cases, i.e., positive CT + positive PET; negative CT + positive PET; positive CT + negative PET.

C. Beginning July 1, 2001, Medicare covers FDG PET for diagnosis, staging, and restaging of NSCLC. Documentation should be maintained in the beneficiary's medical file to support the medical necessity of the procedure, as is normal business practice.

Requirements: PET is covered in either/or both of the following circumstances:

• Diagnosis—PET is covered only in clinical situations in which the PET results may assist in avoiding an invasive diagnostic procedure, or in which the PET results may assist in determining the optimal anatomical location to perform an invasive diagnostic procedure. In general, for most solid tumors, a tissue diagnosis is made prior to the performance of PET scanning. PET scans following a tissue diagnosis are performed for the purpose of staging, not diagnosis. Therefore, the use of PET in the diagnosis of lymphoma, esophageal, and colorectal cancers as well as in melanoma should be rare.
• Staging and/or Restaging—PET is covered in clinical situations in which 1) (a) the stage of the cancer remains in doubt after completion of a standard diagnostic workup, including conventional imaging (computed tomography, magnetic resonance imaging, or ultrasound) or (b) the use of PET would also be considered reasonable and necessary if it could potentially replace one or more conventional imaging studies when it is expected that conventional study information is insufficient for the clinical management of the patient and 2) clinical management of the patient would differ depending on the stage of the cancer identified. PET will be covered for restaging after the completion of treatment for the purpose of detecting residual disease, for detecting suspected recurrence or to determine the extent of a known recurrence. Use of PET would also be considered reasonable and necessary if it could potentially replace one or more conventional imaging studies when it is expected that conventional study information is insufficient for the clinical management of the patient.

Documentation should be maintained in the beneficiary's medical record at the referring physician's office to support the medical necessity of the procedure, as is normal business practice.

VI. Coverage of FDG PET for Esophageal Cancer

A. Beginning July 1, 2001, Medicare covers FDG PET for the diagnosis, staging, and restaging of esophageal cancer. Medical evidence is present to support the use of FDG PET in pre-surgical staging of esophageal cancer.

Requirements: PET is covered in either/or both of the following circumstances:

• Diagnosis - PET is covered only in clinical situations in which the PET results may assist in avoiding an invasive diagnostic procedure, or in which the PET results may assist in determining the optimal anatomical location to perform an invasive diagnostic procedure. In general, for most solid tumors, a tissue diagnosis is made prior to the performance of PET scanning. PET scans following a tissue diagnosis are performed for the purpose of staging, not diagnosis. Therefore, the use of PET in the diagnosis of lymphoma, esophageal and colorectal cancers as well as in melanoma should be rare.
• Staging and/or Restaging - PET is covered in clinical situations in which 1) (a) the stage of the cancer remains in doubt after completion of a standard diagnostic workup, including conventional imaging (computed tomography, magnetic resonance imaging, or ultrasound) or (b) the use of PET would also be considered reasonable and necessary if it could potentially replace one or more conventional imaging studies when it is expected that conventional study information is insufficient for the clinical management of the patient, and 2) clinical management of the patient would differ depending on the stage of the cancer identified. PET will be covered for restaging after the completion of treatment for the purpose of detecting residual disease, for detecting suspected recurrence, or to determine the extent of a known recurrence. Use of PET would also be consid-

ered reasonable and necessary if it could potentially replace one or more conventional imaging studies when it is expected that conventional study information is insufficient for the clinical management of the patient.

Documentation should be maintained in the beneficiary's medical record at the referring physician's office to support the medical necessity of the procedure, as is normal business practice.

VII. Coverage of FDG PET for Colorectal Cancer

Medicare coverage of FDG PET for colorectal cancer where there is a rising level of carcinoembryonic antigen (CEA) was effective July 1, 1999 through June 30, 2001. Beginning July 1, 2001, usage of FDG PET for colorectal cancer has been expanded to include diagnosis, staging, and restaging of the disease(see part III).

A. Effective July 1, 1999, Medicare covers FDG PET for patients with recurrent colorectal carcinomas, which are suggested by rising levels of the biochemical tumor marker CEA.

1. Frequency Limitations: Whole body PET scans for assessment of recurrence of colorectal cancer cannot be ordered more frequently than once every 12 months unless medical necessity documentation supports a separate re-elevation of CEA within this period.

2. Limitations: Because this service is covered only in those cases in which there has been a recurrence of colorectal tumor, claims for PET should include a statement or other evidence of previous colorectal tumor, through June 30, 2001.

B. Beginning July 1, 2001, Medicare coverage has been expanded for colorectal carcinomas for diagnosis, staging and restaging. New medical evidence supports the use of FDG PET as a useful tool in determining the presence of hepatic/extrahepatic metastases in the primary staging of colorectal carcinoma, prior to selecting a treatment regimen. Use of FDG PET is also supported in evaluating recurrent colorectal cancer beyond the limited presentation of a rising CEA level where the patient presents clinical signs or symptoms of recurrence.

Requirements: PET is covered in either/both of the following circumstances:

• Diagnosis - PET is covered only in clinical situations in which the PET results may assist in avoiding an invasive diagnostic procedure, or in which the PET results may assist in determining the optimal anatomical location to perform an invasive diagnostic procedure. In general, for most solid tumors, a tissue diagnosis is made prior to the performance of PET scanning. PET scans following a tissue diagnosis are performed for the purpose of staging, not diagnosis. Therefore, the use of PET in the diagnosis of lymphoma, esophageal, and colorectal cancers as well as in melanoma should be rare.

• Staging and/or Restaging - PET is covered in clinical situations in which 1) (a) the stage of the cancer remains in doubt after completion of a standard diagnostic workup, including conventional imaging (computed tomography, magnetic resonance imaging, or ultrasound) or (b) the use of PET would also be considered reasonable and necessary if it could potentially replace one or more conventional imaging studies when it is expected that conventional study information is insufficient for the clinical management of the patient, and 2) clinical management of the patient would differ depending on the stage of the cancer identified. PET will be covered for restaging after the completion of treatment for the purpose of detecting residual disease, for detecting suspected recurrence, or to determine the extent of a known recurrence. Use of PET would also be considered reasonable and necessary if it could potentially replace one or more conventional imaging studies when it is expected that conventional study information is insufficient for the clinical management of the patient.

Documentation that these conditions are met should be maintained by the referring physician in the beneficiary's medical record, as is normal business practice.

VIII. Coverage of FDG PET for Lymphoma

Medicare coverage of FDG PET to stage and re-stage lymphoma

as alternative to a Gallium scan, was effective July 1, 1999. Beginning July 1, 2001 usage of FDG PET for lymphoma has been expanded to include diagnosis, staging and restaging (see section III) of the disease.

A. Effective July 1, 1999, FDG PET is covered for the staging and restaging of lymphoma.

Requirements:

• FDG PET is covered only for staging or follow-up restaging of lymphoma. Claims must include a statement or other evidence of previous diagnosis of lymphoma when used as an alternative to a Gallium scan.

• To ensure that the PET scan is properly coordinated with other diagnostic modalities, claims must include the results of concurrent computed tomography (CT) and/or other diagnostic modalities when they are necessary for additional anatomic information.

• In order to ensure that the PET scan is covered only as an alternative to a Gallium scan, no PET scan may be covered in cases where it is done within 50 days of a Gallium scan done by the same facility where the patient has remained during the 50-day period. Gallium scans done by another facility less than 50 days prior to the PET scan will not be counted against this screen. The purpose of this screen is to assure that PET scans are covered only when done as an alternative to a Gallium scan within the same facility. We are aware that, in order to assure proper patient care, the treating physician may conclude that previously performed Gallium scans are either inconclusive or not sufficiently reliable.

Frequency Limitation for Restaging: PET scans will be allowed for restaging no sooner than 50 days following the last staging PET scan or Gallium scan, unless sufficient evidence is presented to convince the Medicare contractor that the restaging at an earlier date is medically necessary. Since PET scans for restaging are generally done following cycles of chemotherapy, and since such cycles usually take at least 8 weeks, we believe this screen will adequately prevent medically unnecessary scans while allowing some adjustments for unusual cases. In all cases, the determination of the medical necessity for a PET scan for re-staging lymphoma is the responsibility of the local Medicare contractor.

Beginning July 1, 2001, documentation should be maintained in the beneficiary's medical record at the referring physician's office to support the medical necessity of the procedure, as is normal business practice.

B. Effective for services performed on or after July 1, 2001, the Medicare program has broadened coverage of FDG PET for the diagnosis, staging and restaging of lymphoma.

Requirements: PET is covered in either/both of the following circumstances:

• Diagnosis - PET is covered only in clinical situations in which the PET results may assist in avoiding an invasive diagnostic procedure, or in which the PET results may assist in determining the optimal anatomical location to perform an invasive diagnostic procedure. In general, for most solid tumors, a tissue diagnosis is made prior to the performance of PET scanning. PET scans following a tissue diagnosis are performed for the purpose of staging, not diagnosis. Therefore, the use of PET in the diagnosis of lymphoma, esophageal, and colorectal cancers as well as in melanoma should be rare.

• Staging and/or Restaging - PET is covered in clinical situations in which 1) (a) the stage of the cancer remains in doubt after completion of a standard diagnostic workup, including conventional imaging (computed tomography, magnetic resonance imaging, or ultrasound) or (b) the use of PET would also be considered reasonable and necessary if it could potentially replace one or more conventional imaging studies when it is expected that conventional study information is insufficient for the clinical management of the patient, and 2) clinical management of the patient would differ depending on the stage of the cancer identified. PET will be covered for restaging after the completion of treatment for the purpose of detecting residual disease, for detecting suspected recurrence, or to determine the extent of a known recurrence. Use of PET would also be considered reasonable and necessary if it could potentially replace one or more conventional imaging studies when it is expected that conventional study information is insufficient for the clinical management of the patient.

Documentation that these conditions are met should be maintained by the referring physician in the beneficiary's medical record, as is normal business practice.

IX. Coverage of FDG PET for Melanoma

Medicare covered the evaluation of recurrent melanoma prior to surgery when used as an alternative to a Gallium scan, effective July 1, 1999. For services furnished on or after July 1, 2001 FDG PET is covered for the diagnosis, staging, and restaging of malignant melanoma (see part III). FDG PET is not covered for the use of evaluating regional nodes in melanoma patients.

A. Effective for services furnished July 1, 1999 through June 30, 2001, in the case of patients with recurrent melanoma prior to surgery, FDG PET (when used as an alternative to a Gallium scan) is covered for tumor evaluation.

Frequency Limitations: Whole body PET scans cannot be ordered more frequently than once every 12 months, unless medical necessity documentation, maintained in the beneficiaries medical record, supports the specific need for anatomic localization of possible recurrent tumor within this period.

Limitations: The FDG PET scan is covered only as an alternative to a Gallium scan. PET scans can not be covered in cases where it is done within 50 days of a Gallium scan done by the same PET facility where the patient has remained under the care of the same facility during the 50-day period. Gallium scans done by another facility less than 50 days prior to the PET scan will not be counted against this screen. The purpose of this screen is to assure that PET scans are covered only when done as an alternative to a Gallium scan within the same facility. We are aware that, in order to assure proper patient care, the treating physician may conclude that previously performed Gallium scans are either inconclusive or not sufficiently reliable to make the determination covered by this provision. Therefore, we will apply this 50-day rule only to PET scans done by the same facility that performed the Gallium scan.

Beginning July 1, 2001, documentation should be maintained in the beneficiary's medical file at the referring physician's office to support the medical necessity of the procedure, as is normal business practice.

B. Effective for services performed on or after July 1, 2001 FDG PET scan coverage for the diagnosis, staging and restaging of melanoma (not the evaluation regional nodes) has been broadened.

Limitations: PET scans are not covered for the evaluation of regional nodes.

Requirements: PET is covered in either/both of the following circumstances:

• Diagnosis—PET is covered only in clinical situations in which the PET results may assist in avoiding an invasive diagnostic procedure, or in which the PET results may assist in determining the optimal anatomical location to perform an invasive diagnostic procedure. In general, for most solid tumors, a tissue diagnosis is made prior to the performance of PET scanning. PET scans following a tissue diagnosis are performed for the purpose of staging, not diagnosis. Therefore, the use of PET in the diagnosis of lymphoma, esophageal, and colorectal cancers as well as in melanoma should be rare.

• Staging and/or Restaging—PET is covered in clinical situations in which 1) (a) the stage of the cancer remains in doubt after completion of a standard diagnostic workup, including conventional imaging (computed tomography, magnetic resonance imaging, or ultrasound) or (b) the use of PET would also be considered reasonable and necessary if it could potentially replace one or more conventional imaging studies when it is expected that conventional study information is insufficient for the clinical management of the patient, and 2) clinical manage-

ment of the patient would differ depending on the stage of the cancer identified. PET will be covered for restaging after the completion of treatment for the purpose of detecting residual disease, for detecting suspected recurrence, or to determine the extent of a known recurrence. Use of PET would also be considered reasonable and necessary if it could potentially replace one or more conventional imaging studies when it is expected that conventional study information is insufficient for the clinical management of the patient.

Documentation that these conditions are met should be maintained by the referring physician in the beneficiary's medical file, as is normal business practice.

X. Coverage of FDG PET for Head and Neck Cancers (Cancers of the central nervous system (CNS) and thyroid are not covered)

Effective for services performed on or after July 1, 2001, Medicare will provide coverage for cancer of the head and neck, excluding the central nervous system (CNS) and thyroid. The head and neck cancers encompass a diverse set of malignancies of which the majority is squamous cell carcinomas. Patients may present with metastases to cervical lymph nodes but conventional forms of diagnostic imaging fail to identify the primary tumor. Patients that present with cancer of the head and neck are left with two options either to have a neck dissection or to have radiation of both sides of the neck with random biopsies. PET scanning attempts to reveal the site of primary tumor to prevent the adverse effects of random biopsies or unneeded radiation.

Limitations: PET scans for head and neck cancers are not covered for CNS or thyroid cancers.

Requirements: PET is covered in either/or both of the following circumstances:

• Diagnosis—PET is covered only in clinical situations in which the PET results may assist in avoiding an invasive diagnostic procedure, or in which the PET results may assist in determining the optimal anatomical location to perform an invasive diagnostic procedure. In general, for most solid tumors, a tissue diagnosis is made prior to the performance of PET scanning. PET scans following a tissue diagnosis are performed for the purpose of staging, not diagnosis. Therefore, the use of PET in the diagnosis of lymphoma, esophageal, and colorectal cancers as well as in melanoma should be rare.

• Staging and/or Restaging—PET is covered in clinical situations in which 1) (a) the stage of the cancer remains in doubt after completion of a standard diagnostic workup, including conventional imaging (computed tomography, magnetic resonance imaging, or ultrasound) or (b) the use of PET would also be considered reasonable and necessary if it could potentially replace one or more conventional imaging studies when it is expected that conventional study information is insufficient for the clinical management of the patient, and 2) clinical management of the patient would differ depending on the stage of the cancer identified. PET will be covered for restaging after the completion of treatment for the purpose of detecting residual disease, for detecting suspected recurrence, or to determine the extent of a known recurrence. Use of PET would also be considered reasonable and necessary if it could potentially replace one or more conventional imaging studies when it is expected that conventional study information is insufficient for the clinical management of the patient.

Documentation that these conditions are met should be maintained by the referring physician in the beneficiary's medical record, as is normal business practice.

XI. Coverage of FDG PET for Myocardial Viability

The identification of patients with partial loss of heart muscle movement or hibernating myocardium is important in selecting candidates with compromised ventricular function to determine appropriateness for revascularization. Diagnostic tests such as FDG PET distinguish between dysfunctional but viable myocardial tissue and scar tissue in order to affect management decisions in patients with ischemic cardiomyopathy and left ventricular dysfunction.

FDG PET is covered for the determination of myocardial viability following an inconclusive SPECT from July 1, 2001 through September 30, 2002. Only fully ring PET scanners are covered from July 1, 2001 through December 31, 2001. However, as of January 1, 2002, full and partial ring scanners are covered.

Beginning October 1, 2002, Medicare covers FDG PET for the determination of myocardial viability as a primary or initial diagnostic study prior to revascularization, or following an inconclusive SPECT. Studies performed by full and partial ring scanners are covered.

Limitations: In the event that a patient has received a single photon computed tomography test (SPECT) with inconclusive results, a PET scan may be covered. However, if a patient received a FDG PET study with inconclusive results, a follow up SPECT is not covererd.

Documentation that these conditions are met should be maintained by the referring physician in the beneficiary's medical record, as is normal business practice.

(See §50-58 of the CIM for SPECT coverage.)

XII. Coverage of FDG-PET for Refractory Seizures

Beginning July 1, 2001, Medicare will cover FDG-PET for pre-surgical evaluation for the purpose of localization of a focus of refractory seizure activity.

Limitations: Covered only for pre-surgical evaluation.

Documentation that these conditions are met should be maintained by the referring physician in the beneficiary's medical record, as is normal business practice.

XIII. Breast Cancer

Beginning October 1, 2002, Medicare covers FDG PET as an adjunct to other imaging modalities for staging patients with distant metastasis, or restaging patients with locoregional recurrence or metastasis. Monitoring treatment of a breast cancer tumor when a change in therapy is contemplated is also covered as an adjunct to other imaging modalities.

Limitations: Effective October 1, 2002, Medicare continues to have a national non-coverage determination for initial diagnosis of breast cancer and staging of axillary lymph nodes. Medicare coverage for staging patients with distant metastasis or restaging patients with locoregional recurrence or metastasis; and for monitoring tumor response to treatment for women with locally advanced and metastatic breast cancer when a change in therapy is anticipated, is only covered as an adjunct to other imaging modalities.

Documentation that these conditions are met should be maintained by the referring physician in the beneficiary's medical record, as is normal business practice.

50-44 BONE (MINERAL) DENSITY STUDIES (150.3)

Bone (mineral) density studies are used to evaluate diseases of bone and/or the responses of bone diseases to treatment. The studies assess bone mass or density associated with such diseases as osteoporosis, osteomalacia, and renal osteodystrophy. Various single or combined methods of measurement may be required to: (a) diagnose bone disease, (b) monitor the course of bone changes with disease progression, or (c) monitor the course of bone changes with therapy. Bone density is usually studied by using photodensitometry, single or dual photon absorptiometry, or bone biopsy. The following bone (mineral) density studies are covered under Medicare:

A. Single Photon Absorptiometry.—A non-invasive radiological technique that measures absorption of a monochromatic photon beam by bone material. The device is placed directly on the patient, uses a low dose of radionuclide, and measures the mass absorption efficiency of the energy used. It provides a quantitative measurement of the bone mineral of cortical and trabecular bone, and is used in assessing an individual's treatment response at appropriate intervals.

Single photon absorptiometry is covered under Medicare when used in assessing changes in bone density of patients with osteodystrophy or osteoporosis when performed on the same individual at intervals of 6 to 12 months.

B. Bone Biopsy.—A physiologic test which is a surgical, invasive procedure. A small sample of bone (usually from the ilium) is removed, generally by a biopsy needle. The biopsy sample is then examined histologically, and provides a qualitative measurement of the bone mineral of trabecular bone. This procedure is used in ascertaining a differential diagnosis of bone disorders and is used primarily to differentiate osteomalacia from osteoporosis.

Bone biopsy is covered under Medicare when used for the qualitative evaluation of bone no more than four times per patient, unless there is special justification given. When used more than four times on a patient, bone biopsy leaves a defect in the pelvis and may produce some patient discomfort.

C. Photodensitometry (Radiographic Absorptiometry).—A noninvasive radiological procedure that attempts to assess bone mass by measuring the optical density of extremity radiographs with a photodensitometer, usually with a reference to a standard density wedge placed on the film at the time of exposure. This procedure provides a quantitative measurement of the bone mineral of cortical bone, and is used for monitoring gross bone change.

The following bone (mineral) density study is not covered under Medicare: dual photon absorptiometry. A noninvasive radiological technique that measures absorption of a dichromatic beam by bone material. This procedure is not covered under Medicare because it is still considered to be in the investigational stage.

50-50 DISPLACEMENT CARDIOGRAPHY (20.24)

Displacement cardiography, including cardiokymography and photokymography, is a noninvasive diagnostic test used in evaluating coronary artery disease.

A. Cardiokymography.—(Effective for Services Rendered on or after October 12, 1988).—Cardiokymography is a covered service only when it is used as an adjunct to electrocardiographic stress testing in evaluating coronary artery disease and only when the following clinical indications are present:

• For male patients, atypical angina pectoris or nonischemic chest pain; or
• For female patients, angina, either typical or atypical.

B. Photokymography.—not covered. Photokymography remains excluded from coverage.

50-54 CARDIAC OUTPUT MONITORING BY ELECTRICAL BIOIMPEDANCE—NOT COVERED (Effective for services performed on or after July 1, 1999) (20.16)

Cardiac monitoring using electrical bioimpedance, a form of plethysmography, is covered, effective for services furnished on or after July 1, 1999, for the uses and conditions described below. Contractors should be aware that this technology is in the process of being proven for additional uses. Therefore, the uses below represent the current situation. Contractors may cover additional uses when they believe there is sufficient evidence of the medical effectiveness of such uses.

These devices utilize electrical bioimpedance to noninvasively produce hemodynamic measurements of cardiac output, specifically, stroke volume, contractility, systemic vascular resistance, and thoracic fluid content. These devices are covered for the following uses:

1. Noninvasive diagnosis or monitoring of hemodynamics in patients with suspected or known cardiovascular disease;

2. Differentiation of cardiogenic from pulmonary causes of acute dyspnea;

3. Optimization of atrioventricular interval for patient with A/V sequential cardiac pacemakers;

4. Patients with need of determination for intravenous inotropic therapy;

5. Post heart transplant myocardial biopsy patients; and,

6. Patients with a need for fluid management.

Not covered at this time are the use of such devices for any monitoring of patients with proven or suspected disease involving severe regurgitation of the aorta, or for patients with minute ventilation (MV) sensor function pacemakers, since the device may adversely affect the functioning of that type of pacemaker. Also, these devices do not render accurate measurements in cardiac bypass patients while on a cardiopulmonary bypass machine, but do provide accurate measurements prior to and post bypass pump.

Covered uses of cardiac output monitoring by electrical bioimpedance should be billed using HCPCS code M0302.

50-55 PROSTATE CANCER SCREENING TESTS—COVERED
(210.1)

A. General—Section 4103 of the Balanced Budget Act of 1997 provides for coverage of certain prostate cancer screening tests subject to certain coverage, frequency, and payment limitations. Medicare will cover prostate cancer screening tests/procedures for the early detection of prostate cancer.

Coverage of prostate cancer screening tests includes the following procedures furnished to an individual for the early detection of prostate cancer:

• Screening digital rectal examination; and
• Screening prostate specific antigen blood test.

B. Screening Digital Rectal Examinations—Screening digital rectal examinations (HCPCS code G0102) are covered at a frequency of once every 12 months for men who have attained age 50 (at least 11 months have passed following the month in which the last Medicare-covered screening digital rectal examination was performed). Screening digital rectal examination means a clinical examination of an individual's prostate for nodules or other abnormalities of the prostate. This screening must be performed by a doctor of medicine or osteopathy (as defined in section 1861(r)(1) of the Act), or by a physician assistant, nurse practitioner, clinical nurse specialist, or certified nurse midwife (as defined in section 1861(aa) and section 1861(gg) of the Act) who is authorized under State law to perform the examination, fully knowledgeable about the beneficiary's medical condition, and would be responsible for using the results of any examination performed in the overall management of the beneficiary's specific medical problem.

C. Screening Prostate Specific Antigen Tests.—Screening prostate specific antigen tests (code G0103) are covered at a frequency of once every 12 months for men who have attained age 50 (at least 11 months have passed following the month in which the last Medicare-covered screening prostate specific antigen test was performed). Screening prostate specific antigen tests (PSA) means a test to detect the marker for adenocarcinoma of prostate. PSA is a reliable immunocytochemical marker for primary and metastatic adenocarcinoma of prostate. This screening must be ordered by the beneficiary's physician or by the beneficiary's physician assistant, nurse practitioner, clinical nurse specialist, or certified nurse midwife (the term "attending physician" is defined in section 1861(r)(1) of the Act to mean a doctor of medicine or osteopathy and the terms "physician assistant, nurse practitioner, clinical nurse specialist, or certified nurse midwife" are defined in section 1861(aa) and section 1861(gg) of the Act) who is fully knowledgeable about the beneficiary's medical condition, and who would be responsible for using the results of any examination (test) performed in the overall management of the beneficiary's specific medical problem.

55 DIALYSIS EQUIPMENT

55-1 WATER PURIFICATION AND SOFTENING SYSTEMS USED IN CONJUNCTION WITH HOME DIALYSIS
(230.7)

A. Water Purification Systems.—Water used for home dialysis

should be chemically free of heavy trace metals and/or organic contaminants which could be hazardous to the patient. It should also be as free of bacteria as possible but need not be biologically sterile. Since the characteristics of natural water supplies in most areas of the country are such that some type of water purification system is needed, such a system used in conjunction with a home dialysis (either peritoneal or hemodialysis) unit is covered under Medicare.

There are two types of water purification systems which will satisfy these requirements:

• Deionization—The removal of organic substances, mineral salts of magnesium and calcium (causing hardness), compounds of fluoride and chloride from tap water using the process of filtration and ion exchange; or

• Reverse Osmosis—The process used to remove impurities from tap water utilizing pressure to force water through a porous membrane.

Use of both a deionization unit and reverse osmosis unit in series, theoretically to provide the advantages of both systems, has been determined medically unnecessary since either system can provide water which is both chemically and bacteriologically pure enough for acceptable use in home dialysis. In addition, spare deionization tanks are not covered since they are essentially a precautionary supply rather than a current requirement for treatment of the patient.

Activated carbon filters used as a component of water purification systems to remove unsafe concentrations of chlorine and chloramines are covered when prescribed by a physician.

B. Water Softening System.—Except as indicated below, a water softening system used in conjunction with home dialysis is excluded from coverage under Medicare as not being reasonable and necessary within the meaning of section 1862(a)(1) of the law. Such a system, in conjunction with a home dialysis unit, does not adequately remove the hazardous heavy metal contaminants (such as arsenic) which may be present in trace amounts.

A water softening system may be covered when used to pretreat water to be purified by a reverse osmosis (RO) unit for home dialysis where:

• The manufacturer of the RO unit has set standards for the quality of water entering the RO (e.g., the water to be purified by the RO must be of a certain quality if the unit is to perform as intended);
• The patient's water is demonstrated to be of a lesser quality than required; and
• The softener is used only to soften water entering the RO unit, and thus, used only for dialysis. (The softener need not actually be built into the RO unit, but must be an integral part of the dialysis system.)

C. Developing Need When a Water Softening System Is Replaced with a Water Purification Unit in an Existing Home Dialysis System.—The medical necessity of water purification units must be carefully developed when they replace water softening systems in existing home dialysis systems. A purification system may be ordered under these circumstances for a number of reasons. For example, changes in the medical community's opinions regarding the quality of water necessary for safe dialysis may lead the physician to decide the quality of water previously used should be improved, or the water quality itself may have deteriorated. Patients may have dialyzed using only an existing water softener previous to Medicare ESRD coverage because of inability to pay for a purification system. On the other hand, in some cases, the installation of a purification system is not medically necessary. Thus, when such a case comes to your attention, ask the physician to furnish the reason for the changes. Supporting documentation, such as the supplier's recommendations or water analysis, may be required. All such cases should be reviewed by your medical consultants.

Cross-refer: Intermediary Manual, sections 3113, 3643 (item 1c); Carriers Manual, sections 2100, 2100.2 2130, 2105 (item 1c); Hospital Manual, section 235.

55-2 PERIDEX CAPD FILTER SET—NOT COVERED (230.13)

The Peridex Filter Set is used by home continuous ambulatory peritoneal dialysis (CAPD) patients. The Peridex Filter Set is designed to provide sterile filtration during infusion of the dialysis solution in a beneficiary's peritoneal cavity; included in the filter set is a bacterial filter designed to block peritonitis-causing organisms and thus reduce the incidence of peritonitis.

Based upon advice of our medical consultants, we have determined that the Peridex CAPD Filter Set cannot be covered at this time by Medicare because it has not yet been shown to be safe and effective in preventing peritonitis.

55-3 ULTRAFILTRATION MONITOR (Effective for services performed on and after July 11, 1983.) (230.14)

The Ultrafiltration Monitor is designed to reduce the clinical risks of overfiltration and underfiltration during hemodialysis. Overfiltration is the removal of too much fluid from body tissues and underfiltration is removal of too little fluid.

Covered: Ultrafiltration and ultrafiltration monitoring as a component of hemodialysis has an established and critical role in maintaining the well-being of ESRD patients and is a covered service. The Ultrafiltration Monitor is covered under the Medicare program when it is used to calculate fluid rates for those recipients who present difficult fluid management problems. Determine the medical necessity of this device on a case-by-case basis.

Not Covered: Ultrafiltration, independent of conventional dialysis, is considered experimental, and technology exclusively designed for this purpose is not covered under Medicare.

60 DURABLE MEDICAL EQUIPMENT

60-3 WHITE CANE FOR USE BY A BLIND PERSON—NOT COVERED (280.2)

A white cane for use by a blind person is more an identifying and self-help device rather than an item which makes a meaningful contribution in the treatment of an illness or injury.

60-4 HOME USE OF OXYGEN (240.2)

A. General.—Medicare coverage of home oxygen and oxygen equipment under the durable medical equipment (DME) benefit (see 1861(s)(6) of the Act) is considered reasonable and necessary only for patients with significant hypoxemia who meet the medical documentation, laboratory evidence, and health conditions specified in subsections B, C, and D. This section also includes special coverage criteria for portable oxygen systems. Finally, a statement on the absence of coverage of the professional services of a respiratory therapist under the DME benefit is included in subsection F.

B. Medical Documentation.—Initial claims for oxygen services must include a completed Form CMS-484 (Certificate of Medical Necessity: Oxygen) to establish whether coverage criteria are met and to ensure that the oxygen services provided are consistent with the physician's prescription or other medical documentation. The treating physician's prescription or other medical documentation must indicate that the other forms of treatment (e.g., medical and physical therapy directed at secretions, bronchospasm and infection) have been tried, have not been sufficiently successful, and oxygen therapy is still required. While there is no substitute for oxygen therapy, each patient must receive optimum therapy before long-term home oxygen therapy is ordered. Use Form CMS-484 for recertifications. (See the Medicare Program Integrity Manual, Chapter 5, for completion of Form CMS-484.)

The medical and prescription information in section B of Form CMS-484 can be completed only by the treating physician, the physician's employee, or another clinician (e.g., nurse, respiratory therapist, etc.) as long as that person is not the DME supplier. Although hospital discharge coordinators and medical social workers may assist in arranging for physician-prescribed home oxygen, they do not have the authority to prescribe the services. Suppliers may not enter this information. While this section may

be completed by a nonphysician clinician or a physician employee, it must be reviewed and the form CMS-484 signed by the attending physician.

A physician's certification of medical necessity for oxygen equipment must include the results of specific testing before coverage can be determined.

Claims for oxygen must also be supported by medical documentation in the patient's record. Separate documentation is used with electronic billing. This documentation may be in the form of a prescription written by the patient's attending physician who has recently examined the patient (normally within a month of the start of therapy) and must specify:

- A diagnosis of the disease requiring home use of oxygen;
- The oxygen flow rate; and
- An estimate of the frequency, duration of use (e.g., 2 liters per minute, 10 minutes per hour, 12 hours per day), and duration of need (e.g., 6 months or lifetime).

NOTE: A prescription for "Oxygen PRN" or "Oxygen as needed" does not meet this last requirement. Neither provides any basis for determining if the amount of oxygen is reasonable and necessary for the patient.

A member of the carrier's medical staff should review all claims with oxygen flow rates of more than 4 liters per minute before payment can be made.

The attending physician specifies the type of oxygen delivery system to be used (i.e., gas, liquid, or concentrator) by signing the completed form CMS-484. In addition the supplier or physician may use the space in section C for written confirmation of additional details of the physician's order. The additional order information contained in section C may include the means of oxygen delivery (mask, nasal, cannula, etc.), the specifics of varying flow rates, and/or the noncontinuous use of oxygen as appropriate. The physician confirms this order information with his or her signature in section D.

New medical documentation written by the patient's attending physician must be submitted to the carrier in support of revised oxygen requirements when there has been a change in the patient's condition and need for oxygen therapy.

Carriers are required to conduct periodic, continuing medical necessity reviews on patients whose conditions warrant these reviews and on patients with indefinite or extended periods of necessity as described in the Medicare Program Integrity Manual, Chapter 5, "Items and Services Having Special DMERC Review Considerations." When indicated, carriers may also request documentation of the results of a repeat arterial blood gas or oximetry study.

NOTE: Section 4152 of OBRA 1990 requires earlier recertification and retesting of oxygen patients who begin coverage with an arterial blood gas result at or above a partial pressure of 55 or an arterial oxygen saturation percentage at or above 89. (See the Medicare Claims Processing Manual, Chapter 20, "Durable Medical Equipment, Prosthetics and Orthotics, and Supplies (DMEPOS)," §100.2.3, for certifications and retesting schedules.)

C. Laboratory Evidence.—Initial claims for oxygen therapy must also include the results of a blood gas study that has been ordered and evaluated by the attending physician. This is usually in the form of a measurement of the partial pressure of oxygen (PO2) in arterial blood. A measurement of arterial oxygen saturation obtained by ear or pulse oximetry, however, is also acceptable when ordered and evaluated by the attending physician and performed under his or her supervision or when performed by a qualified provider or supplier of laboratory services. When the arterial blood gas and the oximetry studies are both used to document the need for home oxygen therapy and the results are conflicting, the arterial blood gas study is the preferred source of documenting medical need. A DME supplier is not considered a qualified provider or supplier of laboratory services for purposes of these guidelines. This prohibition does not extend to the results of a blood gas test conducted by a hospital certified to do such tests. The conditions under which the laboratory tests are performed must be specified in writing and submitted with the initial claim, i.e., at rest, during exercise, or during sleep.

The preferred sources of laboratory evidence are existing physician and/or hospital records that reflect the patient's medical condition. Since it is expected that virtually all patients who qualify for home oxygen coverage for the first time under these guidelines have recently been discharged from a hospital where they submitted to arterial blood gas tests, the carrier needs to request that such test results be submitted in support of their initial claims for home oxygen. If more than one arterial blood gas test is performed during the patient's hospital stay, the test result obtained closest to, but no earlier than 2 days prior to, the hospital discharge date is required as evidence of the need for home oxygen therapy.

For those patients whose initial oxygen prescription did not originate during a hospital stay, blood gas studies should be done while the patient is in the chronic stable state, i.e., not during a period of an acute illness or an exacerbation of their underlying disease.

Carriers may accept an attending physician's statement of recent hospital test results for a particular patient, when appropriate, in lieu of copies of actual hospital records.

A repeat arterial blood gas study is appropriate when evidence indicates that an oxygen recipient has undergone a major change in their condition relevant to home use of oxygen. If the carrier has reason to believe that there has been a major change in the patient's physical condition, it may ask for documentation of the results of another blood gas or oximetry study.

D. Health Conditions.—Coverage is available for patients with significant hypoxemia in the chronic stable state i.e., not during a period of acute illness or an exacerbation of their underlying disease, if: (1) The attending physician has determined that the patient has a health condition outlined in subsection D1, (2) The patient meets the blood gas evidence requirements specified in subsection D3, and (3) The patient has appropriately tried other alternative treatment measures without complete success. (See subsection B.)

1. Conditions for Which Oxygen Therapy May Be Covered:

• A severe lung disease, such as chronic obstructive pulmonary disease, diffuse interstitial lung disease, cystic fibrosis bronchiectasis; widespread pulmonary neoplasm; or
• Hypoxia-related symptoms or findings that might be expected to improve with oxygen therapy. Examples of these symptoms and findings are pulmonary hypertension, recurring congestive heart failure due to chronic cor pulmonale, erythrocytosis, impairment of the cognitive process, nocturnal restlessness, and morning headache.

2. Conditions for Which Oxygen Therapy Is Not Covered:

• Angina pectoris in the absence of hypoxemia. This condition is generally not the result of a low oxygen level in the blood, and there are other preferred treatments;
• Breathlessness without cor pulmonale or evidence of hypoxemia. Although intermittent oxygen use is sometimes prescribed to relieve this condition, it is potentially harmful and psychologically addicting;
• Severe peripheral vascular disease resulting in clinically evident desaturation in one or more extremities. There is no evidence that increased PO_2 improves the oxygenation of tissues with impaired circulation; or
• Terminal illnesses that do not affect the lungs.

3. Covered Blood Gas Values.—If the patient has a condition specified in subsection D1, the carrier must review the medical documentation and laboratory evidence that has been submitted for a particular patient (see subsections B and C) and determine if coverage is available under one of the three group categories outlined below.

a. Group I.—Except as modified in subsection D, coverage is provided for patients with significant hypoxemia evidenced by any of the following:

(1) An arterial PO_2 at or below 55 mm Hg, or an arterial oxygen saturation at or below 88 percent, taken at rest, breathing room air.

(2) An arterial PO_2 at or below 55 mm Hg, or an arterial oxygen saturation at or below 88 percent, taken during sleep for a patient who demonstrates an arterial PO_2 at or above 56 mm Hg, or an arterial oxygen saturation at or above 89 percent, while awake; or a greater than normal fall in oxygen level during sleep (a decrease in arterial PO_2 more than 10 mm Hg, or decrease in arterial oxygen saturation more than 5 percent) associated with symptoms or signs reasonably attributable to hypoxemia (e.g., impairment of cognitive processes and nocturnal restlessness or insomnia). In either of these cases, coverage is provided only for use of oxygen during sleep, and then only one type of unit will be covered. Portable oxygen, therefore, would not be covered in this situation.

(3) An arterial PO_2 at or below 55 mm Hg or an arterial oxygen saturation at or below 88 percent, taken during exercise for a patient who demonstrates an arterial PO_2 at or above 56 mm Hg, or an arterial oxygen saturation at or above 89 percent, during the day while at rest. In this case, supplemental oxygen is provided for during exercise if there is evidence the use of oxygen improves the hypoxemia that was demonstrated during exercise when the patient was breathing room air.

b. Group II.—Except as modified in subsection D, coverage is available for patients whose arterial PO_2 is 56 to 59 mm Hg or whose arterial blood oxygen saturation is 89 percent, if there is evidence of:

(1) Dependent edema suggesting congestive heart failure;

(2) Pulmonary hypertension or cor pulmonale, determined by measurement of pulmonary artery pressure, gated blood pool scan, echocardiogram, or "P" pulmonale on EKG (P wave greater than 3 mm in standard leads II, III, or AVF); or

(3) Erythrocythemia with a hematocrit greater than 56 percent.

c. Group III.—Except as modified in subsection D, carriers must apply a rebuttable presumption that a home program of oxygen use is not medically necessary for patients with arterial PO_2 levels at or above 60 mm Hg, or arterial blood oxygen saturation at or above 90 percent. In order for claims in this category to be reimbursed, the carrier's reviewing physician needs to review any documentation submitted in rebuttal of this presumption and grant specific approval of the claims. The CMS expects few claims to be approved for coverage in this category.

d. Variable Factors That May Affect Blood Gas Values.—In reviewing the arterial PO_2 levels and the arterial oxygen saturation percentages specified in subsections D3A, B and C, the carrier's medical staff must take into account variations in oxygen measurements that may result from such factors as the patient's age, the altitude level, or the patient's decreased oxygen carrying capacity.

E. Portable Oxygen Systems.—A patient meeting the requirements specified below may qualify for coverage of a portable oxygen system either (1) by itself or (2) to use in addition to a stationary oxygen system. Portable oxygen is not covered when it is provided only as a backup to a stationary oxygen system. A portable oxygen system is covered for a particular patient if:

• The claim meets the requirements specified in subsections A-D, as appropriate; and
• The medical documentation indicates that the patient is mobile in the home and would benefit from the use of a portable oxygen system in the home. Portable oxygen systems are not covered for patients who qualify for oxygen solely based on blood gas studies obtained during sleep.

F. Respiratory Therapists.—Respiratory therapists' services are not covered under the provisions for coverage of oxygen services under the Part B durable medical equipment benefit as outlined above. This benefit provides for coverage of home use of oxygen and oxygen equipment, but does not include a professional component in the delivery of such services.

(See §280.1, and the Medicare Benefit Policy Manual, Chapter 15, "Covered Medical and Other Health Services," §110)

60-5 POWER-OPERATED VEHICLES THAT MAY BE USED AS WHEELCHAIRS (280.9)

Power-operated vehicles that may be appropriately used as wheelchairs are covered under the durable medical equipment provision.

These vehicles have been appropriately used in the home setting for vocational rehabilitation and to improve the ability of chronically disabled persons to cope with normal domestic, vocational and social activities. They may be covered if a wheelchair is medically necessary and the patient is unable to operate a wheelchair manually.

A specialist in physical medicine, orthopedic surgery, neurology, or rheumatology must provide an evaluation of the patient's medical and physical condition and a prescription for the vehicle to assure that the patient requires the vehicle and is capable of using it safely. When an intermediary determines that such a specialist is not reasonably accessible, e.g., more than 1 day's round trip from the beneficiary's home, or the patient's condition precludes such travel, a prescription from the beneficiary's physician is acceptable.

The intermediary's medical staff reviews all claims for a power-operated vehicle, including the specialists' or other physicians' prescriptions and evaluations of the patient's medical and physical conditions, to insure that all coverage requirements are met. (See section 60-9 and Intermediary Manual, Part 3, section 3629.)

60-6 SPECIALLY SIZED WHEELCHAIRS (280.3)

Payment may be made for a specially sized wheelchair even though it is more expensive than a standard wheelchair. For example, a narrow wheelchair may be required because of the narrow doorways of a patient's home or because of a patient's slender build. Such difference in the size of the wheelchair from the standard model is not considered a deluxe feature.

A physician's certification or prescription that a special size is needed is not required where you can determine from the information in file or other sources that a specially sized wheelchair (rather than a standard one) is needed to accommodate the wheelchair to the place of use or the physical size of the patient.

To determine the reasonable charge in these cases, use the criteria set out in Carriers Manual, sections 5022, 5022.1, 5200, and 5205, as necessary.

Cross-refer: Intermediary Manual, sections 3113.2C, 3642.1, 3643 (item 3); Carriers Manual, sections 2100.2c, 2105, 4105.2, 5107; Hospital Manual, sections 235.2c, 420.1 (item 13).

60-7 SELF-CONTAINED PACEMAKER MONITORS (20.8.2)

Self-contained pacemaker monitors are accepted devices for monitoring cardiac pacemakers. Accordingly, program payment may be made for the rental or purchase of either of the following pacemaker monitors when it is prescribed by a physician for a patient with a cardiac pacemaker:

A. Digital Electronic Pacemaker Monitor.—This device provides the patient with an instantaneous digital readout of his pacemaker pulse rate. Use of this device does not involve professional services until there has been a change of five pulses (or more) per minute above or below the initial rate of the pacemaker; when such change occurs, the patient contacts his physician.

B. Audible/Visible Signal Pacemaker Monitor.—This device produces an audible and visible signal which indicates the pacemaker rate. Use of this device does not involve professional services until a change occurs in these signals; at such time, the patient contacts his physician.

NOTE: The design of the self-contained pacemaker monitor makes it possible for the patient to monitor his pacemaker periodically and minimizes the need for regular visits to the outpatient department of the provider.

Therefore, documentation of the medical necessity for pacemaker evaluation in the outpatient department of the provider should be obtained where such evaluation is employed in addition to the self-contained pacemaker monitor used by the patient in his home.

Cross-refer: section 50-1

60-8 SEAT LIFT (280.4)

Reimbursement may be made for the rental or purchase of a medically necessary seat lift when prescribed by a physician for a patient with severe arthritis of the hip or knee and patients with muscular dystrophy or other neuromuscular diseases when it has been determined the patient can benefit therapeutically from use of the device. In establishing medical necessity for the seat lift, the evidence must show that the item is included in the physician's course of treatment, that it is likely to effect improvement, or arrest or retard deterioration in the patient's condition, and that the severity of the condition is such that the alternative would be chair or bed confinement.

Coverage of seat lifts is limited to those types which operate smoothly, can be controlled by the patient, and effectively assist a patient in standing up and sitting down without other assistance. Excluded from coverage is the type of lift which operates by a spring release mechanism with a sudden, catapult-like motion and jolts the patient from a seated to a standing position. Limit the payment for units which incorporate a recliner feature along with the seat lift to the amount payable for a seat lift without this feature.

Cross-refer: Carriers Manual, section 5107

60-9 DURABLE MEDICAL EQUIPMENT REFERENCE LIST (280.1)

The durable medical equipment (DME) list which follows is designed to facilitate your processing of DME claims. This section is designed to be used as a quick reference tool for determining the coverage status of certain pieces of DME and especially for those items which are commonly referred to by both brand and generic names. The information contained herein is applicable (where appropriate) to all DME coverage determinations discussed in the DME portion of this manual. The list is organized into two columns. The first column lists alphabetically various generic categories of equipment on which national coverage decisions have been made by CMS; and the second column notes the coverage status of each equipment category.

In the case of equipment categories that have been determined by CMS to be covered under the DME benefit, the list outlines the conditions of coverage that must be met if payment is to be allowed for the rental or purchase of the DME by a particular patient, or cross-refers to another section of the manual where the applicable coverage criteria are described in more detail. With respect to equipment categories that cannot be covered as DME, the list includes a brief explanation of why the equipment is not covered. This DME list will be updated periodically to reflect any additional national coverage decisions that CMS may make with regard to other categories of equipment.

When you receive a claim for an item of equipment which does not appear to fall logically into any of the generic categories listed, you have the authority and responsibility for deciding whether those items are covered under the DME benefit. These decisions must be made by each contractor based on the advice of its medical consultants, taking into account:

• The general DME coverage instructions in the Carriers Manual, section 2100ff and Intermediary Manual, section 3113ff (see below for brief summary);

• Whether the item has been approved for marketing by the Food and Drug Administration (FDA) (see Carriers Manual, section

2303.1 and Intermediary Manual, section 3151.1) and is otherwise generally considered to be safe and effective for the purpose intended; and
• Whether the item is reasonable and necessary for the individual patient.

As provided in the Carriers Manual, section 2100.1, and Intermediary Manual, section 3113.1, the term DME is defined as equipment which:

• Can withstand repeated use; i.e., could normally be rented, and used by successive patients;
• Is primarily and customarily used to serve a medical purpose;
• Generally is not useful to a person in the absence of illness or injury; and
• Is appropriate for use in a patient's home.

Durable Medical Equipment Reference List

Air Cleaners—deny—environmental control equipment; not primarily medical in nature (section 1861(n) of the Act)

Air Conditioners—deny—environmental control equipment; not primarily medical in nature (section 1861(n) of the Act)

Air-Fluidized Bed—(*See* section 60-19.)

Alternating Pressure Pads—covered if patient has, or is highly susceptible to, and matresses and decubitus ulcers and patient's physician has Lambs Wool Pads specified that he will be supervising its use in connection with his course of treatment.

Audible/Visible Signal—(*See* Self-Contained Pacemaker Monitor.) Pacemaker Monitor

Augmentative Communication Device—(*See* speech Generating Devices. Section 60-23.)

Bathtub Lifts—deny—convenience item; not primarily medical in nature (section 1861(n) of the Act)

Bathtub Seats—deny—comfort or convenience item; hygienic equipment; not primarily medical in nature (section 1861(n) of the Act)

Bead Bed—(*See* section 60-19.)

Bed Baths (home type)—deny—hygienic equipment; not primarily medical in nature (section 1861(n) of the Act)

Bed Lifter (bed elevator)—deny—not primarily medical in nature (section 1861(n) of the Act).

Bedboards—deny—not primarily medical in nature (section 1861(n) of the Act)

Bed Pans (autoclavable hospital type)—covered if patient is bed confined

Bed Side Rails—(*See* Hospital Beds, section 60-18.)

Beds—Lounge (power or manual)—deny—not a hospital bed; comfort or convenience item; not primarily medical in nature (section 1861(n) of the Act)

Beds—Oscillating—deny—institutional equipment; inappropriate for home use

Bidet Toilet Seat—(*See* Toilet Seats.)

Blood Glucose Analyzer—deny—unsuitable for home use (*See* section 60-11.)

Blood Glucose Monitor—covered if patient meets certain conditions (*See* section 60-11.)

Braille Teaching Texts—deny—educational equipment; not primarily medical in nature (section 1861(n) of the Act)

Canes—covered if patient's condition impairs ambulation (*See* section 1861(m).)

Carafes—deny—convenience item; not primarily medical in nature (section 1861(n) of the Act)

Catheters—deny—nonreusable disposable supply (section l861(n) of the Act)

Commodes—covered if patient is confined to bed or room

NOTE: The term "room confined" means that the patient's condition is such that leaving the room is medically contraindicated. The accessibility of bathroom facilities generally would not be a factor in this determination. However, confinement of a patient to his home in a case where there are no toilet facilities in the home may be equated to room confinement. Moreover, payment may also be made if a patient's medical condition confines him to a floor of his home and there is no bathroom located on that floor (*See* Hospital Beds in section 60-18 for definition of "bed confinement".)

Communicator—deny—convenience item; not primarily medical in nature (See section 60-23. Speech Generating Devices)

Continuous Passive Motion—Continuous Passive Motion (CPM) devices are covered for patients who have received a total knee replacement. To qualify for coverage, use of the device must commence within two days following surgery. In addition, coverage is limited to that portion of the three week period following surgery during which the device is used in the patient's home.

There is insufficient evidence to justify coverage of these devices for longer periods of time or for other applications.

Continuous Positive Airway Pressure (CPAP)—(*See* section 60-17.)

Crutches—covered if patient's condition impairs ambulation

Cushion Lift Power Seat—(*See* Seat Lifts.)

Dehumidifiers (room or central heating system type)—deny—environmental control equipment; not primarily medical in nature (section 1861(n) of the Act)

Diathermy Machines (standard wave types)—deny—inappropriate for home use (*See* section 35-41.)

Digital Electronic Pacemaker Monitor—(*See* Self-Contained Pacemaker Monitor.)

Disposable Sheets and Bags—deny—nonreusable disposable supplies (section 1861(n) of the Act)

Elastic Stockings—deny—nonreusable supply; not rental-type items (section 1861(n) of the Act)

Electric Air Cleaners—deny—(*See* Air Cleaners.) (section 1861(n) of the Act)

Electric Hospital Beds—(*See* Hospital Beds section 60-18.)

Electrical Stimulation for Wounds—deny—inappropriate for home use

Electrostatic Machines—deny—(*See* Air Cleaners and Air Conditioners.) (section 1861(n) of the Act)

Elevators—deny—convenience item; not primarily medical in nature (section 1861(n) of the Act)

Emesis Basins—deny—convenience item; not primarily medical in nature (section 1861(n) of the Act)

Esophageal Dilator—deny—physician instrument; inappropriate for patient use

Exercise Equipment—deny—not primarily medical in nature (section 1861(n) of the Act)

Fabric Supports—deny—nonreusable supplies; not rental-type item (section 1861(n) of the Act)

Face Masks (oxygen)—covered if oxygen is covered (*See* section 60-4.)

Face Masks (surgical)—deny—nonreusable disposable items (section 1861(n) of the Act)

Flowmeter—(*See* Medical Oxygen Regulators)

Fluidic Breathing Assister—(*See* IPPB Machines.)

Fomentation Device—(*See* Heating Pads.)

Gel Flotation Pads and Mattresses—(*See* Alternating Pressure Pads.)

Grab Bars—deny—self-help device; not primarily medical in nature (section 1861(n) of the Act)

Heat and Massage Foam Cushion Pad—deny—not primarily medical in nature; personal comfort item (section 1861(n) and 1862(a)(6) of the Act)

Heating and Cooling Plants—deny—environmental control equipment; not primarily medical in nature (section 1861(n) of the Act)

Heating Pads—covered if the contractor's medical staff determines patient's medical condition is one for which the application of heat in the form of a heating pad is therapeutically effective.

Heat Lamps—covered if the contractor's medical staff determines patient's medical condition is one for which the application of heat in the form of a heat lamp is therapeutically effective.

Hospital Beds—(See section 60-18.)

Hot Packs—(See Heating Pads.)

Humidifiers (oxygen)—(See Oxygen Humidifiers.)

Humidifiers (room or central heating system types)—deny—environmental control equipment; not medical in nature (section 1861(n) of the Act)

Hydraulic Lift—(See Patient Lifts.)

Incontinent Pads—deny—non-reusable supply; hygienic item (section 1861(n) of the Act.)

Infusion Pumps—For external and implantable pumps, see section 60-14. If the pump is used with an enteral or parenteral malnutritional therapy system, see section 65-10 to 65.10.2 0.2 for special coverage rules.

Injectors (hypodermic jet devices for injection of insulin)—deny—noncovered self-administered drug supply; pressure powered devices (section 1861(s)(2)(A) of the Act)

IPPB Machines—covered if patient's ability to breathe is severely impaired

Iron Lungs—(See Ventilators.)

Irrigating Kit—deny—nonreusable supply; hygienic equipment (section 1861(n) of the Act)

Lambs Wool Pads—covered under same conditions as alternating pressure pads and mattresses

Leotards—deny—(See Pressure Leotards.) (section 1861(n) of the Act)

Lymphedema Pumps (segmental and non-segmental therapy types)—covered (See section 60-16.)

Massage Devices—deny—personal comfort items; not primarily medical in nature (section 1861(n) and 1862(a)(6) of the Act)

Mattress—covered only where hospital bed is medically necessary (Separate charge for replacement mattress should not be allowed where a hospital bed with mattress is rented.) (See section 60-18.)

Medical Oxygen Regulators—covered if patient's ability to breathe is severely impaired (See section 60-4.)

Mobile Geriatric Chair—(See Rolling Chairs.)

Motorized Wheelchairs—(See Wheelchairs (power operated).)

Muscle Stimulators—Covered for certain conditions (See section 35-77.)

Nebulizers—covered if patient's ability to breathe is severely impaired

Oscillating Beds—deny—institutional equipment—inappropriate for home use

Overbed Tables—deny—convenience item; not primarily medical in nature (section 1861(n) of the Act)

Oxygen—covered if the oxygen has been prescribed for use in connection with medically necessary durable medical equipment (See section 60-4.)

Oxygen Humidifiers—covered if a medical humidifier has been prescribed for use in connection with medically necessary durable medical equipment for purposes of moisturizing oxygen (See section 60-4.)

Oxygen Regulators (Medical)—(See Medical Oxygen Regulators.)

Oxygen Tents—(See section 60-4.)

Paraffin Bath Units (Portable)—(See Paraffin Bath Units [Portable].)

Paraffin Bath Units (Standard)—deny—institutional equipment; inappropriate for home use

Parallel Bars—deny—support exercise equipment; primarily for institutional use; in the home setting other devices (e.g., a walker) satisfy the patient's need

Patient Lifts—covered if contractor's medical staff determines patient's condition is such that periodic movement is necessary to effect improvement or to arrest or retard deterioration in his condition.

Percussors—covered for mobilizing respiratory tract secretions in patients with chronic obstructive lung disease, chronic bronchitis, or emphysema, when patient or operator of powered percussor has received appropriate training by a physician or therapist, and no one competent to administer manual therapy is available.

Portable Oxygen Systems:

    1. Regulated (adjustable—covered under conditions specified in flow rate) section 60-4. Refer all claims to medical staff for this determination.

    2. Preset (flow rate—deny—emergency, first-aid, or not adjustable) precautionary equipment; essentially not therapeutic in nature.

Portable Paraffin Bath Units—covered when the patient has undergone a successful trial period of paraffin therapy ordered by a physician and the patient's condition is expected to be relieved by long term use of this modality.

Portable Room Heaters—deny—environmental control equipment; not primarily medical in nature (section 1861(n) of the Act)

Portable Whirlpool Pumps—deny—not primarily medical in nature; personal comfort items (section 1861(n) and 1862(a)(6) of the Act)

Postural Drainage Boards—covered if patient has a chronic pulmonary condition

Preset Portable Oxygen Units—deny—emergency, first-aid, or precautionary equipment; essentially not therapeutic in nature

Pressure Leotards—deny—nonreusable supply, not rental-type item (section 1861(n) of the Act)

Pulse Tachometer—deny—not reasonable or necessary for monitoring pulse of homebound patient with or without a cardiac pacemaker

Quad-Canes—(See Walkers.)

Raised Toilet Seats—deny—convenience item; hygienic equipment; not primarily medical in nature (section 1861(n) of the Act)

Reflectance Colorimeters—(See Blood Glucose Analyzer.)

Respirators—(See Ventilators.)

Rolling Chairs—covered if the contractor's medical staff determines that the patient's condition is such that there is a medical need for this item and it has been prescribed by the patient's physician in lieu of a wheelchair. Coverage is limited to those roll about chairs having casters of at least 5 inches in diameter and specifically designed to meet the needs of ill, injured, or otherwise impaired individuals. Coverage is denied for the wide range of chairs with smaller casters as are found in general use in homes, offices, and institutions for many purposes not related to the care or treatment of ill or injured persons. This type is not primarily medical in nature. (section 1861(n) of the Act)

Safety Roller—(*See* section 60-15.)

Sauna Baths—deny—not primarily medical in nature; personal comfort items (section 1861(n) and (1862(a)(6) of the Act)

Seat Lift—covered under the conditions specified in section 60-8. Refer all to medical staff for this determination.

Self-Contained Pacemaker—covered when prescribed by a physician. Monitor for a patient with a cardiac pacemaker (*See* section 50-1C and 60-7.)

Sitz Bath—covered if the contractor's medical staff determines patient has an infection or injury of the perineal area and the item has been prescribed by the patient's physician as a part of his planned regimen of treatment in the patient's home.

Spare Tanks of Oxygen—deny—convenience or precautionary supply

Speech Teaching Machine—deny—education equipment; not primarily medical in nature (section 1861(n) of the Act)

Stairway Elevators—deny—(*See* Elevators.) (section l861(n) of the Act)

Standing Table—deny—convenience item; not primarily medical in nature (section 1861(n) of the Act)

Steam Packs—these packs are covered under the same condition as a heating pad (*See* Heating Pads.)

Suction Machine—covered if the contractor's medical staff determines that the machine specified in the claim is medically required and appropriate for home use without technical or professional supervision.

Support Hose—deny (*See* Fabric Supports.) (section 1861(n) of the Act)

Surgical Leggings—deny—nonreusable supply; not rental-type item (section 1861(n) of the Act)

Telephone Alert Systems—deny—these are emergency communications systems and do not serve a diagnostic or therapeutic purpose

Telephone Arms—deny—convenience item; not medical in nature (section 1861(n) of the Act)

Toilet Seats—deny—not medical equipment (section 1861(n) of the Act)

Traction Equipment—covered if patient has orthopedic impairment requiring traction equipment which prevents ambulation during the period of use. (Consider covering devices usable during ambulation; e.g., cervical traction collar, under the brace provision.)

Trapeze Bars—covered if patient is bed confined and the patient needs a trapeze bar to sit up because of respiratory condition, to change body position for other medical reasons, or to get in and out of bed.

Treadmill Exerciser—deny—exercise equipment; not primarily medical in nature (section 1861(n) of the Act)

Ultraviolet Cabinet—covered for selected patients with generalized intractable psoriasis. Using appropriate consultation, the contractor should determine whether medical and other factors justify treatment at home rather than at alternative sites, e.g., outpatient department of a hospital.

Urinals (autoclavable hospital type)—covered if patient is bed confined

Vaporizers—covered if patient has a respiratory illness

Ventilators—covered for treatment of neuromuscular diseases, thoracic restrictive diseases, and chronic respiratory failure consequent to chronic obstructive pulmonary disease. Includes both positive and negative pressure types.

Walkers—covered if patient's condition impairs ambulation (*See* also section 60-15.)

Water and Pressure Pads and Mattresses—(*See* Alternating Pressure Pads and Mattresses.)

Wheelchairs—covered if patient's condition is such that without the use of a wheelchair he would otherwise be bed or chair confined. An individual may qualify for a wheelchair and still be considered bed confined.

Wheelchairs (power operated) and wheelchairs with other special features—covered if patient's condition is such that a wheelchair is medically necessary and the patient is unable to operate the wheelchair manually. Any claim involving a power wheelchair or a wheelchair with other special features should be referred for medical consultation since payment for the special features is limited to those which are medically required because of the patient's condition. (See section 60-5 for power operated and section 60-6 for specially sized wheelchairs.)

NOTE: A power-operated vehicle that may appropriately be used as a wheelchair can be covered. (*See* section 60-5 for coverage details.)

Whirlpool Bath Equipment—covered if patient is homebound and has a (standard) condition for which the whirlpool bath can be expected to provide substantial therapeutic benefit justifying its cost. Where patient is not homebound but has such a condition, payment is restricted to the cost of providing the services elsewhere; e.g., an outpatient department of a participating hospital, if that alternative is less costly. In all cases, refer claim to medical staff for a determination.

Whirlpool Pumps—deny—(*See* Portable Whirlpool Pumps.) (section 1861(n) of the Act)

White Cane—deny—(*See* section 60-3.)

60-11 HOME BLOOD GLUCOSE MONITORS (230.16)

There are several different types of blood glucose monitors which use reflectance meters to determine blood glucose levels. Medicare coverage of these devices varies, both with respect to the type of device and the medical condition of the patient for whom the device is prescribed.

Reflectance colorimeter devices used for measuring blood glucose levels in clinical settings are not covered as durable medical equipment for use in the home because their need for frequent professional recalibration makes them unsuitable for home use. However, some types of blood glucose monitors which use a reflectance meter specifically designed for home use by diabetic patients may be covered as durable medical equipment, subject to the conditions and limitations described below.

Blood glucose monitors are meter devices which read color changes produced on specially treated reagent strips by glucose concentrations in the patient's blood. The patient, using a disposable sterile lancet, draws a drop of blood, places it on a reagent strip and, following instructions which may vary with the device used, inserts it into the device to obtain a reading. Lancets, reagent strips, and other supplies necessary for the proper functioning of the device are also covered for patients for whom the device is indicated. Home blood glucose monitors enable certain patients to better control their blood glucose levels by frequently checking and appropriately contacting their attending physician for advice and treatment. Studies indicate that the patient's ability to carefully follow proper procedures is critical to obtaining satisfactory results with these devices. In addition, the cost of the devices, with their supplies, limits economical use to patients who must make frequent checks of their blood glucose levels. Accordingly, coverage of home blood glucose monitors is limited to patients meeting the following conditions:

- The patient must be an insulin-treated diabetic;
- The patient's physician states that the patient is capable of being trained to use the particular device prescribed in an appropriate manner. In some cases, the patient may not be able to perform this function, but a responsible individual can be trained to use the equipment and monitor the patient to assure that the intended effect is achieved. This is permissible if the record is properly documented by the patient's physician; and
- The device is designed for home rather than clinical use.

There is also a blood glucose monitoring system designed especially for use by those with visual impairments. The monitors used in such systems are identical in terms of reliability and sensitivity to the standard blood glucose monitors described above. They differ by having such features as voice synthesizers, automatic timers, and specially designed arrangements of supplies and materials to enable the visually impaired to use the equipment without assistance.

These special blood glucose monitoring systems are covered under Medicare if the following conditions are met:

- The patient and device meet the four conditions listed above for coverage of standard home blood glucose monitors; and
- The patient's physician certifies that he or she has a visual impairment severe enough to require use of this special monitoring system.

The additional features and equipment of these special systems justify a higher reimbursement amount than allowed for standard blood glucose monitors. Separately identify claims for such devices and establish a separate reimbursement amount for them. For those carriers using HCPCS, the procedure code and definition is: EO609—Blood Glucose Monitor—with special features (e.g., voice synthesizers, automatic timer).

60-14 INFUSION PUMPS (280.14)

The following indications for treatment using infusion pumps are covered under medicare:

A. External Infusion Pumps.—

1. Iron Poisoning (Effective for Services Performed On or After 9/26/84).—When used in the administration of deferoxamine for the treatment of acute iron poisoning and iron overload, only external infusion pumps are covered.

2. Thromboembolic Disease (Effective for Services Performed On or After 9/26/84).—When used in the administration of heparin for the treatment of thromboembolic disease and/or pulmonary embolism, only external infusion pumps used in an institutional setting are covered.

3. Chemotherapy for Liver Cancer (Effective for Services Performed On or After 1/29/85).—The external chemotherapy infusion pump is covered when used in the treatment of primary hepatocellular carcinoma or colorectal cancer where this disease is unresectable or where the patient refuses surgical excision of the tumor.

4. Morphine for Intractable Cancer Pain (Effective for Services Performed On or After 4/22/85).—Morphine infusion via an external infusion pump is covered when used in the treatment of intractable pain caused by cancer (in either an inpatient or outpatient setting, including a hospice).

5. Continuous Subcutaneous Insulin Infusion Pumps (CSII) (Effective for Services Performed On or After 4/1/2000).—An external infusion pump and related drugs/supplies are covered as medically necessary in the home setting in the following situation: Treatment of diabetes.

In order to be covered, patients must meet criterion A or B:

(A) The patient has completed a comprehensive diabetes education program and has been on a program of multiple daily injections of insulin (i.e., at least 3 injections per day), with frequent self-adjustments of insulin dose, for at least 6 months prior to initiation of the insulin pump and has documented frequency of glucose self-testing an average of at least four times per day during the 2 months prior to initiation of the insulin pump, and meets one or more of the following criteria while on the multiple daily injection regimen:

(1) Glycosylated hemoglobin level (HbAlc) > 7.0%

(2) History of recurring hypoglycemia

(3) Wide fluctuations in blood glucose before mealtime

(4) Dawn phenomenon, with fasting blood sugars frequently exceeding 200 mg/dl

(5) History of severe glycemic excursions

(B) The patient with diabetes has been on a pump prior to enrollment in Medicare and has documented frequency of glucose self-testing an average of at least four times per day during the month prior to Medicare enrollment. Diabetes needs to be documented by a fasting C-peptide level that is less than or equal to 110 percent of the lower limit of normal of the laboratory's measurement method. (Effective for Services Performed on or after January 1, 2002)

Continued coverage of the insulin pump would require that the patient has been seen and evaluated by the treating physician at least every 3 months. The pump must be ordered by and follow-up care of the patient must be managed by a physician who manages multiple patients with CSII and who works closely with a team including nurses, diabetes educators, and dietitians who are knowledgeable in the use of CSII.

Subcutaneous insulin infusion pumps will continue to be denied as not medically necessary and reasonable for all Type II diabetics, including insulin-requiring Type II diabetics.

6. Other uses of external infusion pumps are covered if the contractor's medical staff verifies the appropriateness of the therapy and of the prescribed pump for the individual patient.

NOTE: Payment may also be made for drugs necessary for the effective use of an external infusion pump as long as the drug being used with the pump is itself reasonable and necessary for the patient's treatment.

B. Implantable Infusion Pumps.—

1. Chemotherapy for Liver Cancer (Effective for Services Performed On or After 9/26/84).—The implantable infusion pump is covered for intra-arterial infusion of 5-FUdR for the treatment of liver cancer for patients with primary hepatocellular carcinoma or Duke's Class D colorectal cancer, in whom the metastases are limited to the liver, and where (1) the disease is unresectable or (2) where the patient refuses surgical excision of the tumor.

2. Anti-Spasmodic Drugs for Severe Spasticity.—An implantable infusion pump is covered when used to administer anti-spasmodic drugs intrathecally (e.g., baclofen) to treat chronic intractable spasticity in patients who have proven unresponsive to less invasive medical therapy as determined by the following criteria:

- As indicated by at least a 6-week trial, the patient cannot be maintained on noninvasive methods of spasm control, such as oral anti-spasmodic drugs, either because these methods fail to control adequately the spasticity or produce intolerable side effects, and
- Prior to pump implantation, the patient must have responded favorably to a trial intrathecal dose of the anti-spasmodic drug.

3. Opioid Drugs for Treatment of Chronic Intractable Pain.—An implantable infusion pump is covered when used to administer opioid drugs (e.g., morphine) intrathecally or epidurally for treatment of severe chronic intractable pain of malignant or non-malignant origin in patients who have a life expectancy of at least 3 months and who have proven unresponsive to less invasive medical therapy as determined by the following criteria:

- The patient's history must indicate that he/she would not respond adequately to noninvasive methods of pain control, such as systemic opioids (including attempts to eliminate physical and behavioral abnormalities which may cause an exaggerated reaction to pain); and
- A preliminary trial of intraspinal opioid drug administration must be undertaken with a temporary intrathecal/epidural catheter to substantiate adequately acceptable pain relief and degree of side effects (including effects on the activities of daily living) and patient acceptance.

4. Coverage of Other Uses of Implanted Infusion Pumps.—Determinations may be made on coverage of other uses of implanted infusion pumps if the contractor's medical staff verifies that:

- The drug is reasonable and necessary for the treatment of the individual patient;

- It is medically necessary that the drug be administered by an implanted infusion pump; and
- The FDA approved labeling for the pump must specify that the drug being administered and the purpose for which it is administered is an indicated use for the pump.

5. Implantation of Infusion Pump Is Contraindicated.—The implantation of an infusion pump is contraindicated in the following patients:

- Patients with a known allergy or hypersensitivity to the drug being used (e.g., oral baclofen, morphine, etc.);
- Patients who have an infection;
- Patients whose body size is insufficient to support the weight and bulk of the device; and
- Patients with other implanted programmable devices since crosstalk between devices may inadvertently change the prescription.

NOTE: Payment may also be made for drugs necessary for the effective use of an implantable infusion pump as long as the drug being used with the pump is itself reasonable and necessary for the patient's treatment.

The following indications for treatment using infusion pumps are not covered under Medicare:

A. External Infusion Pumps.—

1. Vancomycin (Effective for Services Beginning On or After September 1, 1996).—Medicare coverage of vancomycin as a durable medical equipment infusion pump benefit is not covered. There is insufficient evidence to support the necessity of using an external infusion pump, instead of a disposable elastomeric pump or the gravity drip method, to administer vancomycin in a safe and appropriate manner.

B. Implantable Infusion Pump.—

1. Thromboembolic Disease (Effective for Services Performed On or After 9/26/84).—According to the Public Health Service, there is insufficient published clinical data to support the safety and effectiveness of the heparin implantable pump. Therefore, the use of an implantable infusion pump for infusion of heparin in the treatment of recurrent thromboembolic disease is not covered.

2. Diabetes—Implanted infusion pumps for the infusion of insulin to treat diabetes is not covered. The data do not demonstrate that the pump provides effective administration of insulin.

60-15 SAFETY ROLLER (280.5)

"Safety roller" is the generic name applied to devices for patients who cannot use standard wheeled walkers. They may be appropriate, and therefore covered, for some patients who are obese, have severe neurological disorders, or restricted use of one hand, which makes it impossible to use a wheeled walker that does not have the sophisticated braking system found on safety rollers.

In order to assure that payment is not made for a safety roller when a less expensive standard wheeled walker would satisfy the patient's medical needs, carriers refer safety roller claims to their medical consultants. The medical consultant determines whether some or all of the features provided in a safety roller are necessary, and therefore covered and reimbursable. If it is determined that the patient could use a standard wheeled walker, the charge for the safety roller is reduced to the charge of a standard wheeled walker.

Some obese patients who could use a standard wheeled walker if their weight did not exceed the walker's strength and stability limits can have it reinforced and its wheel base expanded. Such modifications are routine mechanical adjustments and justify a moderate surcharge. In these cases the carrier reduces the charge for the safety roller to the charge for the standard wheeled walker plus the surcharge for modifications.

In the case of patients with medical documentation showing severe neurological disorders or restricted use of one hand which makes it impossible for them to use a wheeled walker that does not have a sophisticated braking system, a reasonable charge for the safety roller may be determined without relating it to the

reasonable charge for a standard wheeled walker. (Such reasonable charge should be developed in accordance with the instructions in Medicare Carriers Manual, sections 5010 and 5205.)

Cross Refer: Carriers Manual, sections 2100ff., section 60-9.

60-16 PNEUMATIC COMPRESSION DEVICES (280.6)

Lymphedema

Lymphedema is the swelling of subcutaneous tissues due to the accumulation of excessive lymph fluid. The accumulation of lymph fluid results from an impairment to the normal clearing function of the lymphatic system and/or from an excessive production of lymph. Lymphedema is divided into two broad classes according to etiology. Primary lymphedema is a relatively uncommon, chronic condition which may be due to such causes as Milroy's Disease or congenital anomalies. Secondary lymphedema, which is much more common, results from the destruction of or damage to formerly functioning lymphatic channels, such as surgical removal of lymph nodes or post radiation fibrosis, among other causes.

Pneumatic compression devices are covered in the home setting for the treatment of lymphedema if the patient has undergone a four-week trial of conservative therapy and the treating physician determines that there has been no significant improvement or if significant symptoms remain after the trial. The trial of conservative therapy must include use of an appropriate compression bandage system or compression garment, exercise, and elevation of the limb. The garment may be prefabricated or custom-fabricated but must provide adequate graduated compression.

Chronic Venous Insufficiency With Venous Statis Ulcers

Chronic venous insufficiency (CVI) of the lower extremities is a condition caused by abnormalities of the venous wall and valves, leading to obstruction or reflux of blood flow in the veins. Sings of CVI include hyperpigmentation, statis dermatitis, chronic edema, and venous ulcers.

Pneumatic compression devices are covered in the home setting for the treatment of CVI of the lower extremities only if the patient has one or more venous statis ulcer(s) which have failed to heal after a 6 month trial of conservative therapy directed by the treating physician. The trial of conservative therapy must include a compression bandage system or compression garment, appropriate dressings for the wound, exercise, and elevation of the limb.

General Coverage Criteria

Pneumatic compression devices are covered only when prescribed by a physician and when they are used with appropriate physician oversight, i.e., physician evaluation of the patient's condition to determine medical necessity of the device, assuring suitable instruction in the operation of the machine, a treatment plan defining the pressure to be used and the frequency and duration of use, and ongoing monitoring of use and response to treatment.

The determination by the physician of the medical necessity of a pneumatic compression device must include (1) the patient's diagnosis and prognosis; (2) symptoms and objective findings, including measurements which establish the severity of the condition; (3) the reason the device is required, including the treatments which have been tried and failed, and (4) the clinical response to an initial treatment with the device. The clinical response includes the change in pre-treatment measurements, ability to tolerate the treatment session and parameters, and ability of the patient (or caregiver) to apply the device for continued use in the home.

The only time that a segmented, calibrated gradient pneumatic compression device (HCPCs code E0652) would be covered is when the individual has unique characteristics that prevent them from receiving satisfactory pneumatic compression treatment using a nonsegmented device in conjunction with a segmented appliance or a segmented compression device without manual control of pressure in each chamber.

Cross Refer: §60-9.

60-17 CONTINUOUS POSITIVE AIRWAY PRESSURE (CPAP) (240.4)

CPAP is a noninvasive technique for providing low levels of air pressure from a flow generator, via a nose mask, through the nares. The purpose is to prevent the collapse of the oropharyngeal walls and the obstruction of airflow during sleep, which occurs in obstructive sleep apnea (OSA). The diagnosis of OSA requires documentation of at least 30 episodes of apnea, each lasting a minimum of 10 seconds, during 6 to 7 hours of recorded sleep. The use of CPAP is covered under Medicare when used in adult patients with moderate or severe OSA for whom surgery is a likely alternative to CPAP.

Initial claims must be supported by medical documentation (separate documentation where electronic billing is used), such as a prescription written by the patient's attending physician, that specifies:

• a diagnosis of moderate or severe obstructive sleep apnea, and
• surgery is a likely alternative.

The claim must also certify that the documentation supporting a diagnosis of OSA (described above) is available.

The use of CPAP devices are covered under Medicare when ordered and prescribed by the licensed treating physician to be used in adult patients with OSA if either of the following criteria using the Apnea-Hypopnea Index (AHI) are met:

AHI ≥ 15 events per hour, or

AHI ≥ 5 and ≤ 14 events per hour with documented symptoms of excessive daytime sleepiness, impaired cognition, mood disorders or insomnia, or documented hypertension, ischemic heart disease or history of stroke.

The AHI is equal to the average number of episodes of apnea and hypopnea per hour and must be based on a minimum of 2 hours of sleep recorded by polysomnography using actual recorded hours or sleep (i.e., the AHI may not be extrapolated or projected).

Apnea is defined as a cessation of airflow for at least 10 seconds. Hypopnea is defined as an abnormal respiratory event lasting at least 10 seconds with at least 30% reduction in thoracoabdominal movement or airflow as compared to baseline, and with at least a 4% oxygen desaturation.

The polysomnography must be performed in a facility-based sleep study laboratory, and not in the home or in a mobile facility.

Initial claims for CPAP devices must be supported by information contained in the medical record indicating that the patient meets Medicare's stated coverage criteria.

Cross Refer: section 280.1.

60-18 HOSPITAL BEDS (280.7)

A. General Requirements for Coverage of Hospital Beds.—A physician's prescription, and such additional documentation as the contractors' medical staffs may consider necessary, including medical records and physicians' reports, must establish the medical necessity for a hospital bed due to one of the following reasons:

• The patient's condition requires positioning of the body; e.g., to alleviate pain, promote good body alignment, prevent contractures, avoid respiratory infections, in ways not feasible in an ordinary bed; or
• The patient's condition requires special attachments that cannot be fixed and used on an ordinary bed.

B. Physician's Prescription.—The physician's prescription, which must accompany the initial claim, and supplementing documentation when required, must establish that a hospital bed is medically necessary. If the stated reason for the need for a hospital bed is the patient's condition requires positioning, the prescription or other documentation must describe the medical con-

dition, e.g., cardiac disease, chronic obstructive pulmonary disease, quadriplegia or paraplegia, and also the severity and frequency of the symptoms of the condition, that necessitates a hospital bed for positioning.

If the stated reason for requiring a hospital bed is the patient's condition requires special attachments, the prescription must describe the patient's condition and specify the attachments that require a hospital bed.

C. Variable Height Feature.—In well documented cases, the contractors' medical staffs may determine that a variable height feature of a hospital bed, approved for coverage under subsection A above, is medically necessary and, therefore, covered, for one of the following conditions:

• Severe arthritis and other injuries to lower extremities; e.g., fractured hip. The condition requires the variable height feature to assist the patient to ambulate by enabling the patient to place his or her feet on the floor while sitting on the edge of the bed;
• Severe cardiac conditions. For those cardiac patients who are able to leave bed, but who must avoid the strain of "jumping" up or down;
• Spinal cord injuries, including quadriplegic and paraplegic patients, multiple limb amputee and stroke patients. For those patients who are able to transfer from bed to a wheelchair, with or without help; or
• Other severely debilitating diseases and conditions, if the variable height feature is required to assist the patient to ambulate.

D. Electric Powered Hospital Bed Adjustments.—Electric powered adjustments to lower and raise head and foot may be covered when the contractor's medical staff determines that the patient's condition requires frequent change in body position and/or there may be an immediate need for a change in body position (i.e., no delay can be tolerated) and the patient can operate the controls and cause the adjustments. Exceptions may be made to this last requirement in cases of spinal cord injury and brain damaged patients.

E. Side Rails.—If the patient's condition requires bed side rails, they can be covered when an integral part of, or an accessory to, a hospital bed.

Cross refer: Carriers Manual, section 5015.4

60-19 AIR-FLUIDIZED BED (280.8)

An air-fluidized bed uses warm air under pressure to set small ceramic beads in motion which simulate the movement of fluid. When the patient is placed in the bed, his body weight is evenly distributed over a large surface area which creates a sensation of "floating." Medicare payment for home use of the air-fluidized bed for treatment of pressure sores can be made if such use is reasonable and necessary for the individual patient.

A decision that use of an air-fluidized bed is reasonable and necessary requires that:

• The patient has a stage 3 (full thickness tissue loss) or stage 4 (deep tissue destruction) pressure sore;
• The patient is bedridden or chair bound as a result of severely limited mobility;
• In the absence of an air-fluidized bed, the patient would require institutionalization;
• The air-fluidized bed is ordered in writing by the patient's attending physician based upon a comprehensive assessment and evaluation of the patient after completion of a course of conservative treatment designed to optimize conditions that promote wound healing. This course of treatment must have been at least one month in duration without progression toward wound healing. This month of prerequisite conservative treatment may include some period in an institution as long as there is documentation available to verify that the necessary conservative treatment has been rendered.
• Use of wet-to-dry dressings for wound debridement, begun during the period of conservative treatment and which continue beyond 30 days, will not preclude coverage of air-fluidized bed. Should additional debridement again become necessary, while a

pant is using an air-fluidized bed (after the first 30-day
cose of conservative treatment) that will not cause the air-
fluized bed to become non-covered. In all instances documen-
tain verifying the continued need for the bed must be avail-
al.
- Cservative treatment must include:
  - Frequent repositioning of the patient with particular atten-
    tion to relief of pressure over bony prominences (usually
    every 2 hours);
  - Use of a specialized support surface (Group II) designed to
    reduce pressure and shear forces on healing ulcers and to
    prevent new ulcer formation;
  - Necessary treatment to resolve any wound infection;
  - Optimization of nutrition status to promote wound healing;
  - Debridement by any means (including wet to dry
    dressings-which does not require an occlusive covering) to
    remove devitalized tissue from the wound bed;
  - Maintenance of a clean, moist bed of granulation tissue with
    appropriate moist dressings protected by an occlusive cover-
    ing, while the wound heals.

A trained adult caregiver is available to assist the patient with
activities of daily living, fluid balance, dry skin care, repositioning, recognition and management of altered mental status, dietary needs, prescribed treatments, and management and support of the air-fluidized bed system and its problems such as
leakage;
- A physician directs the home treatment regimen, and reevalu-
  ates and recertifies the need for the air-fluidized bed on a
  monthly basis; and
- All other alternative equipment has been considered and ruled
  out.

Home use of the air-fluidized bed is not covered under any of the
following circumstances:

- The patient has coexisting pulmonary disease (the lack of firm
  back support makes coughing ineffective and dry air inhalation
  thickens pulmonary secretions);
- The patient requires treatment with wet soaks or moist wound
  dressings that are not protected with an impervious covering
  such as plastic wrap or other occlusive material;
- The caregiver is unwilling or unable to provide the type of care
  required by the patient on an air-fluidized bed;
- Structural support is inadequate to support the weight of the
  air-fluidized bed system (it generally weighs 1600 pounds or
  more);
- Electrical system is insufficient for the anticipated increase in
  energy consumption; or
- Other known contraindications exist.

Coverage of an air-fluidized bed is limited to the equipment
itself. Payment for this covered item may only be made if the
written order from the attending physician is furnished to the
supplier prior to the delivery of the equipment. Payment is not
included for the caregiver or for architectural adjustments such as
electrical or structural improvement.

Cross refer: Carriers Manual, section 5102.2

60-23 SPEECH GENERATING DEVICES (50.1)

Effective January 1, 2001, augmentative and alternative communication devices or communicators, which are hereafter referred to
as "speech generating devices" are now considered to fall within
the DME benefit category established by §1861(n) of the Act.
They may be covered if the contractor's medical staff determines
that the patient suffers from a severe speech impairment and that
the medical condition warrants the use of a device based on the
following definitions.

Definition of Speech Generating Devices.—Speech generating
devices are defined as speech aids that provide an individual
who has a severe speech impairment with the ability to meet his
functional speaking needs. Speech generating are characterized
by:

- Being a dedicated speech device, used solely by the individual
  who has a severe speech impairment;

- May have digitized speech output, using pre-recorded messages, less than or equal to 8 minutes recording time;
- May have digitized speech output, using pre-recorded
  messages, greater than 8 minutes recording time;
- May have synthesized speech output, which requires message
  formulation by spelling and device access by physical contact
  with the device-direct selection techniques;
- May have synthesized speech output, which permits multiple
  methods of message formulation and multiple methods of device access; or
- May be software that allows a laptop computer, desktop computer or personal digital assistant (PDA) to function as a speech
  generating device.
- Devices that would not meet the definition of speech generating
  devices and therefore, do not fall within the scope of §1861(n)
  of the Act are characterized by:
- Devices that are not dedicated speech devices, but are devices
  that are capable of running software for purposes other than for
  speech generation, e.g., devices that can also run a word processing package, an accounting program, or perform other non-
  medical function.
- Laptop computers, desktop computers, or PDAs, which may be
  programmed to perform the same function as a speech generating device, are non-covered since they are not primarily medical
  in nature and do not meet the definition of DME. For this
  reason, they cannot be considered speech generating devices for
  Amedicare coverage purposes.
- A devices that is useful to someone without severe speech impairment is not considered a speech generating devices for
  Medicare coverage purposes.

60-24 NON-IMPLANTABLE PELVIC FLOOR ELECTRICAL STIMULATOR (230.8)

Non-implantable pelvic floor electrical stimulators provide neuromuscular electrical stimulation through the pelvic floor with the
intent of strengthening and exercising pelvic floor musculature.
Stimulation is generally delivered by vaginal or anal probes connected to an external pulse generator.

The methods of pelvic floor electrical stimulation vary in location,
stimulus frequency (Hz), stimulus intensity or amplitude (mA),
pulse duration (duty cycle), treatments per day, number of treatment days per week, length of time for each treatment session,
overall time period for device use and between clinic and home
settings. In general, the stimulus frequency and other parameters
are chosen based on the patient's clinical diagnosis.

Pelvic floor electrical stimulation with a non-implantable stimulator is covered for the treatment of stress and/or urge urinary
incontinence in cognitively intact patients who have failed a documented trial of pelvic muscle exercise (PME) training.

A failed trial of PME training is defined as no clinically significant improvement in urinary continence after completing 4 weeks
of an ordered plan of pelvic muscle exercises designed to increase
periurethral muscle strength.

65 PROSTHETIC DEVICES

65-1 HYDROPHILIC CONTACT LENSES (80.4)

Hydrophilic contact lenses are eyeglasses within the meaning of
the exclusion in section 1862(a)(7) of the law and are not covered
when used in the treatment of nondiseased eyes with spherical
ametrophia, refractive astigmatism, and/or corneal astigmatism.
Payment may be made under the prosthetic device benefit, however, for hydrophilic contact lenses when prescribed for an
aphakic patient.

Contractors are authorized to accept an FDA letter of approval or
other FDA published material as evidence of FDA approval.

(See §80.1 for coverage of a hydrophilic lens as a corneal bandage.)

Cross-refer: The Medicare Benefit Policy Manual, Chapter 15,
"Covered Medical and Other Health Services," §100 and §120
The Medicare Benefit Policy Manual, Chapter 16, "General Exclu-
sions from Coverage," §20 and §90.

65-3 SCLERAL SHELL (80.5)

Scleral shell (or shield) is a catch-all term for different types of hard scleral contact lenses.

A scleral shell fits over the entire exposed surface of the eye as opposed to a corneal contact lens which covers only the central non-white area encompassing the pupil and iris. Where an eye has been rendered sightless and shrunken by inflammatory disease, a scleral shell may, among other things, obviate the need for surgical enucleation and prosthetic implant and act to support the surrounding orbital tissue.

In such a case, the device serves essentially as an artificial eye. In this situation, payment may be made for a scleral shell under section 1861(s)(8) of the Act.

Scleral shells are occasionally used in combination with artificial tears in the treatment of "dry eye" of diverse etiology. Tears ordinarily dry at a rapid rate, and are continually replaced by the lacrimal gland. When the lacrimal gland fails, the half-life of artificial tears may be greatly prolonged by the use of the scleral contact lens as a protective barrier against the drying action of the atmosphere. Thus, the difficult and sometimes hazardous process of frequent instillation of artificial tears may be avoided. The lens acts in this instance to substitute, in part, for the functioning of the diseased lacrimal gland and would be covered as a prosthetic device in the rare case when it is used in the treatment of "dry eye."

Cross-refer: The Medicare Benefit Policy Manual, Chapter 15, "Covered Medical and Other Health Services," §120 and §130. The Medicare Benefit Policy Manual, Chapter 1, "Inpatient Hospital Services," §40 and §120.1.

65-5 ELECTRONIC SPEECH AIDS (50.2)

Electronic speech aids are covered under Part B as prosthetic devices when the patient has had a laryngectomy or his larynx is permanently inoperative. There are two types of speech aids. One operates by placing a vibrating head against the throat; the other amplifies sound waves through a tube which is inserted into the user's mouth. A patient who has had radical neck surgery and/or extensive radiation to the anterior part of the neck would generally be able to use only the "oral tube" model or one of the more sensitive and more expensive "throat contact" devices.

Cross-refer: The Medicare Benefit Policy Manual, Chapter 15, "Covered Medical and Other Health Services," §120.

65-7 INTRAOCULAR LENSES (IOLs) (80.12)

An intraocular lens, or pseudophakos, is an artificial lens which may be implanted to replace the natural lens after cataract surgery. Intraocular lens implantation services, as well as the lens itself, may be covered if reasonable and necessary for the individual. Implantation services may include hospital, surgical, and other medical services, including pre-implantation ultrasound (A-scan) eye measurement of one or both eyes.

Cross-refer: The Medicare Benefit Policy Manual, Chapter 6, "Hospital Services Covered Under Part B," §10. The Medicare Benefit Policy Manual, Chapter 15, "Covered Medical and Other Health Services," §120. The Medicare Benefit Policy Manual, Chapter 16, "General Exclusions from Coverage," §20 and §90.

8 ELECTRICAL NERVE STIMULATORS (160.7)

general classifications of electrical nerve stimulators are employed to treat chronic intractable pain: peripheral nerve stimula- and central nervous system stimulators.

Implanted Peripheral Nerve Stimulators.—Payment may be under the prosthetic device benefit for implanted peripheral stimulators. Use of this stimulator involves implantation of des around a selected peripheral nerve. The stimulating le is connected by an insulated lead to a receiver unit s implanted under the skin at a depth not greater than 1/ Stimulation is induced by a generator connected to an unit which is attached to the skin surface over the re-

ceiver unit. Implantation of electrodes requires surgery and usually necessitates an operating room.

NOTE: Peripheral nerve stimulators may also be employe to assess a patient's suitability for continued treatment th an electric nerve stimulator. As explained in section 3 6, such use of the stimulator is covered as part of the al diagnostic service furnished to the beneficiary rather tn as a prosthesis.

B. Central Nervous System Stimulators (Dorsal Column d Depth Brain Stimulators).—The implantation of central nerve system stimulators may be covered as therapies for the relief chronic intractable pain, subject to the following conditions:

1. Types of Implantations.—There are two types of implant tions covered by this instruction:

    a. Dorsal Column (Spinal Cord) Neurostimulation.—Th surgical implantation of neurostimulator electrodes within th dura mater (endodural) or the percutaneous insertion of elec trodes in the epidural space is covered.

    b. Depth Brain Neurostimulation.—The stereotactic im plantation of electrodes in the deep brain (e.g., thalamus and periaqueductal gray matter) is covered.

2. Conditions for Coverage.—No payment may be made for the implantation of dorsal column or depth brain stimulators or services and supplies related to such implantation, unless all of the conditions listed below have been met:

    a. The implantation of the stimulator is used only as a late resort (if not a last resort) for patients with chronic intractable pain;

    b. With respect to item a, other treatment modalities (pharmacological, surgical, physical, or psychological therapies) have been tried and did not prove satisfactory, or are judged to be unsuitable or contraindicated for the given patient;

    c. Patients have undergone careful screening, evaluation and diagnosis by a multidisciplinary team prior to implantation. (Such screening must include psychological, as well as physical evaluation);

    d. All the facilities, equipment, and professional and support personnel required for the proper diagnosis, treatment training, and followup of the patient (including that required to satisfy item c must be available; and

    e. Demonstration of pain relief with a temporarily implanted electrode precedes permanent implantation.

Contractors may find it helpful to work with PROs to obtain the information needed to apply these conditions to claims.

See Intermediary Manual, section 3110.4 and section 35-20 and 35-27.

65-9 INCONTINENCE CONTROL DEVICES (230.10)

A. Mechanical/Hydraulic Incontinence Control Devices.—Mechanical/hydraulic incontinence control devices are accepted as safe and effective in the management of urinary incontinence in patients with permanent anatomic and neurologic dysfunctions of the bladder. This class of devices achieves control of urination by compression of the urethra. The materials used and the success rate may vary somewhat from device to device. Such a device is covered when its use is reasonable and necessary for the individual patient.

B. Collagen Implant.—A collagen implant, which is injected into the submucosal tissues of the urethra and/or the bladder neck and into tissues adjacent to the urethra, is a prosthetic device used in the treatment of stress urinary incontinence resulting from intrinsic sphincter deficiency (ISD). ISD is a cause of stress urinary incontinence in which the urethral sphincter is unable to contract and generate sufficient resistance in the bladder, especially during stress maneuvers.

Prior to collagen implant therapy, a skin test for collagen sensitivity must be administered and evaluated over a 4 week period.

In male patients, the evaluation must include a complete history and physical examination and a simple cystometrogram to determine that the bladder fills and stores properly. The patient then is asked to stand upright with a full bladder and to cough or otherwise exert abdominal pressure on his bladder. If the patient leaks, the diagnosis of ISD is established.

In female patients, the evaluation must include a complete history and physical examination (including a pelvic exam) and a simple cystometrogram to rule out abnormalities of bladder compliance and abnormalities of urethral support. Following that determination, an abdominal leak point pressure (ALLP) test is performed. Leak point pressure, stated in cm H2O, is defined as the intra-abdominal pressure at which leakage occurs from the bladder (around a catheter) when the bladder has been filled with a minimum of 150 cc fluid. If the patient has an ALLP of less than 100 cm H2O, the diagnosis of ISD is established.

To use a collagen implant, physicians must have urology training in the use of a cystoscope and must complete a collagen implant training program.

Coverage of a collagen implant, and the procedure to inject it, is limited to the following types of patients with stress urinary incontinence due to ISD:

- Male or female patients with congenital sphincter weakness secondary to conditions such as myelomeningocele or epispadias;
- Male or female patients with acquired sphincter weakness secondary to spinal cord lesions;
- Male patients following trauma, including prostatectomy and/or radiation; and
- Female patients without urethral hypermobility and with abdominal leak point pressures of 100 cm H2O or less.

Patients whose incontinence does not improve with 5 injection procedures (5 separate treatment sessions) are considered treatment failures, and no further treatment of urinary incontinence by collagen implant is covered. Patients who have a reoccurrence of incontinence following successful treatment with collagen implants in the past (e.g., 6 to 12 months previously) may benefit from additional treatment sessions. Coverage of additional sessions may be allowed but must be supported by medical justifica-

See Intermediary Manual, §3110.4.

C. Non-Implantable Pelvic Floor Electrical Stimulator.—(See section 60-24)

65-10 ENTERAL AND PARENTERAL NUTRITIONAL THERAPY COVERED AS PROSTHETIC DEVICE (180.2)

There are patients who, because of chronic illness or trauma, cannot be sustained through oral feeding. These people must rely on either enteral or parenteral nutritional therapy, depending upon the particular nature of their medical condition.

Coverage of nutritional therapy as a Part B benefit is provided under the prosthetic device benefit provision, which requires that the patient must have a permanently inoperative internal body organ or function thereof. Therefore, enteral and parenteral nutritional therapy are not covered under Part B in situations involving temporary impairments. Coverage of such therapy, however, does not require a medical judgment that the impairment giving rise to the therapy will persist throughout the patient's remaining years. If the medical record, including the judgment of the attending physician, indicates that the impairment will be of long and indefinite duration, the test of permanence is considered met.

If the coverage requirements for enteral or parenteral nutritional therapy are met under the prosthetic device benefit provision, related supplies, equipment and nutrients are also covered under the conditions in the following paragraphs and the Medicare Benefit Policy Manual, Chapter 15, "Covered Medical and Other Health Services," §120.

65-10.1 Parenteral Nutrition Therapy.—Daily parenteral nutrition is considered reasonable and necessary for a patient with severe pathology of the alimentary tract which does not allow absorption of sufficient nutrients to maintain weight and strength commensurate with the patient's general condition.

Since the alimentary tract of such a patient does not function adequately, an indwelling catheter is placed percutaneously in the subclavian vein and then advanced into the superior vena cava where intravenous infusion of nutrients is given for part of the day. The catheter is then plugged by the patient until the next infusion. Following a period of hospitalization, which is required to initiate parenteral nutrition and to train the patient in catheter care, solution preparation, and infusion technique, the parenteral nutrition can be provided safely and effectively in the patient's home by nonprofessional persons who have undergone special training. However, such persons cannot be paid for their services, nor is payment available for any services furnished by nonphysician professionals except as services furnished incident to a physician's service.

For parenteral nutrition therapy to be covered under Part B, the claim must contain a physician's written order or prescription and sufficient medical documentation to permit an independent conclusion that the requirements of the prosthetic device benefit are met and that parenteral nutrition therapy is medically necessary. An example of a condition that typically qualifies for coverage is a massive small bowel resection resulting in severe nutritional deficiency in spite of adequate oral intake. However, coverage of parenteral nutrition therapy for this and any other condition must be approved on an individual, case-by-case basis initially and at periodic intervals of no more than 3 months by the carrier's medical consultant or specially trained staff, relying on such medical and other documentation as the carrier may require. If the claim involves an infusion pump, sufficient evidence must be provided to support a determination of medical necessity for the pump. Program payment for the pump is based on the reasonable charge for the simplest model that meets the medical needs of the patient as established by medical documentation.

Nutrient solutions for parenteral therapy are routinely covered. However, Medicare pays for no more than one month's supply of nutrients at any one time. Payment for the nutrients is based on the reasonable charge for the solution components unless the medical record, including a signed statement from the attending physician, establishes that the beneficiary, due to his/her physical or mental state, is unable to safely or effectively mix the solution and there is no family member or other person who can do so. Payment will be on the basis of the reasonable charge for more expensive pre-mixed solutions only under the latter circumstances.

65-10.2 Enteral Nutrition Therapy.—Enteral nutrition is considered reasonable and necessary for a patient with a functioning gastrointestinal tract who, due to pathology to or nonfunction of the structures that normally permit food to reach the digestive tract, cannot maintain weight and strength commensurate with his or her general condition. Enteral therapy may be given by nasogastric, jejunostomy, or gastrostomy tubes and can be provided safely and effectively in the home by nonprofessional persons who have undergone special training. However, such persons cannot be paid for their services, nor is payment available for any services furnished by nonphysician professionals except as services furnished incident to a physician's service.

Typical examples of conditions that qualify for coverage are head and neck cancer with reconstructive surgery and central nervous system disease leading to interference with the neuromuscular mechanisms of ingestion of such severity that the beneficiary can not be maintained with oral feeding. However, claims for Part coverage of enteral nutrition therapy for these and any oth conditions must be approved on an individual, case-by-case bas Each claim must contain a physician's written order or prescrip tion and sufficient medical documentation (e.g., hospital reco clinical findings from the attending physician) to permit an i pendent conclusion that the patient's condition meets the requ ments of the prosthetic device benefit and that enteral nut therapy is medically necessary. Allowed claims are to b viewed at periodic intervals of no more than 3 months b contractor's medical consultant or specially trained staff, and additional medical documentation considered necessary is to be obtained as part of this review.

Medicare pays for no more than one month's supply of enteral nutrients at any one time.

If the claim involves a pump, it must be supported by sufficient medical documentation to establish that the pump is medically necessary, i.e., gravity feeding is not satisfactory due to aspiration, diarrhea, dumping syndrome. Program payment for the pump is based on the reasonable charge for the simplest model that meets the medical needs of the patient as established by medical documentation.

65-10.3 Nutritional Supplementation—Some patients require supplementation of their daily protein and caloric intake. Nutritional supplements are often given as a medicine between meals to boost protein-caloric intake or the mainstay of a daily nutritional plan. Nutritional supplementation is not covered under Medicare Part B.

65-11 BLADDER STIMULATORS (PACEMAKERS)—NOT COVERED (230.16)

There are a number of devices available to induce emptying of the urinary bladder by using electrical current which forces the muscles of the bladder to contract. These devices (commonly known as bladder stimulators or pacemakers) are characterized by the implantation of electrodes in the wall of the bladder, the rectal cones, or the spinal cord. While these treatments may effectively empty the bladder, the issue of safety involving the initiation of infection, erosion, placement, and material selection has not been resolved. Further, some facilities previously using electronic emptying have stopped using this method due to the pain experienced by the patient.

The use of spinal cord electrical stimulators, rectal electrical stimulators, and bladder wall stimulators is not considered reasonable and necessary. Therefore, no program payment may be made for these devices or for their implantation.

65-14 COCHLEAR IMPLANTATION (50.3)

A cochlear implant device is an electronic instrument, part of which is implanted surgically to stimulate auditory nerve fibers, and part of which is worn or carried by the individual to capture, analyze, and code sound. Cochlear implant devices are available in single channel and multi-channel models. The purpose of implanting the device is to provide an awareness and identification of sounds and to facilitate communication for persons who are profoundly hearing impaired.

Medicare coverage is provided only for those patients who meet all of the following selection guidelines.

A. General.—

• Diagnosis of bilateral severe-to-profound sensorineural hearing impairment with limited benefit from appropriate hearing (or vibrotactile) aids;

Cognitive ability to use auditory clues and a willingness to undergo an extended program of rehabilitation;

eedom from middle ear infection, an accessible cochlear lu-
n that is structurally suited to implantation, and freedom
m lesions in the auditory nerve and acoustic areas of the
ral nervous system;

ontraindications to surgery; and

evice must be used in accordance with the FDA-approved
ng.

ults.—Cochlear implants may be covered for adults (over
for prelinguistically, perilinguistically, and postlinguisti-
fened adults. Postlinguistically deafened adults must
ate test scores of 30 percent or less on sentence recogni-
from tape recorded tests in the patient's best listening

C. Children.—Cochlear implants may be covered for prelinguistically and postlinguistically deafened children aged 2 through 17. Bilateral profound sensorineural deafness must be demonstrated by the inability to improve on age appropriate closed-set word identification tasks with amplification.

65-16 TRACHEOSTOMY SPEAKING VALVE (20.9)

A trachea tube has been determined to satisfy the definition of a prosthetic device, and the tracheostomy speaking valve is an add-on to the trachea tube which may be considered a medically necessary accessory that enhances the function of the tube. In other words, it makes the system a better prosthesis. As such, a tracheostomy speaking valve is covered as an element of the trachea tube which makes the tube more effective.

65-18 SACRAL NERVE STIMULATION FOR URINARY INCONTINENCE (230.18)

Effective January 1, 2002, sacral nerve stimulation is covered for the treatment of urinary urge incontinence, urgency-frequency syndrome, and urinary retention. Sacral nerve stimulation involves both a temporary test stimulation to determine if an implantable stimulator would be effective and a permanent implantation in appropriate candidates. Both the test and the permanent implantation are covered.

The following limitations for coverage apply to all three indications:

(1) Patient must be refractory to conventional therapy (documented behavioral, pharmacologic and/or surgical corrective therapy) and be an appropriate surgical candidate such that implantation with anesthesia can occur.

(2) Patients with stress incontinence, urinary obstruction, and specific neurologic diseases (e.g., diabetes with peripheral nerve involvement) which are associated with secondary manifestation of the above three indications are excluded.

(3) Patient must have had a successful test stimulation in order to support subsequent implantation. Before a patient is eligible for permanent implantation, he/she must demonstrate a 50% greater improvement through test stimulation. Improveme
measured through voiding diaries.

(4) Patient must be able to demonstrate adequate ability to record voiding diary data such that clinical results of the implant procedure can be properly evaluated.

70 BRACES—TRUSSES—ARTIFICIAL LIMBS AND EYES

70-1 CORSET USED AS HERNIA SUPPORT (280.11)

A hernia support (whether in the form of a corset or truss) which meets the definition of a brace is covered under Part B under section 1861(s)(9) of the Act.

See Intermediary Manual, section 3110.5; Medicare Carriers Manual, section 2133; and Hospital Manual, section 228.5.

70-2 SYKES HERNIA CONTROL (280.12)

Based on professional advice, it has been determined that the Sykes hernia control (a spring-type, U-shaped, strapless truss) is not functionally more beneficial than a conventional truss. Make program reimbursement for this device only when an ordinary truss would be covered. (Like all trusses, it is only of benefit when dealing with a reducible hernia.) Thus, when a charge for this item is substantially in excess of that which would be reasonable for a conventional truss used for the same condition, base reimbursement on the reasonable charges for the conventional truss.

See Intermediary Manual, section 3110.5; Medicare Carriers Manual, section 2133; and Hospital Manual, section 228.5.